Plumb's™

Veterinary Drug Handbook

10TH Edition

James A. Budde, PharmD, DICVP
Dawn M. McCluskey, DVM

Distributed by
John Wiley & Sons, Inc

PUBLISHED BY:
Educational Concepts, LLC, dba VetMedux
Tulsa, OK

WORLDWIDE PRINT DISTRIBUTION BY:
Wiley-Blackwell
111 River Street
Hoboken, NJ 07030
877-762-2974
www.wiley.com/wiley-blackwell
Wiley-Blackwell is an imprint of John Wiley & Sons, formed
by the merger of Wiley's global scientific, technical, and medical business
with Blackwell Publishing.

ISBN: 9781394172207
x 2023 1

SKY10064824_011524

To Donald Plumb,
for his vision and determination to create, nurture,
and grow *Plumb's® Veterinary Drug Handbook* into the most respected
and valued veterinary drug information resource.

~

To the veterinarians, veterinary healthcare staff, students, and pharmacists
who rely on this resource as they care for animals large and small.

~

James A. Budde and Dawn M. McCluskey,
on behalf of the entire Plumb's® Team

Editor Emeritus

Donald C. Plumb, PharmD, FSVHP (Honorary)

THE PLUMB'S® TEAM & VETMEDUX

Editors: Veterinary Medicine

Dawn M. McCluskey, DVM
Veterinary Officer, Pharmacy

Jordy L. Waller, DVM
Assistant Veterinary Officer, Pharmacy

Editors: Veterinary Pharmacy

James A. Budde, PharmD, DICVP
Senior Pharmacy Officer

Chloe A. Ciarrocchi, PharmD, DICVP
Assistant Pharmacy Officer

Editorial

Samantha Farley, MPS
Managing Editor

Katy Drawhorn
Associate Editor

Lindsay Roberts
Projects Editor

Carol Watkins
Editorial Assistant

Publishing Operations

Elizabeth Green
Founder & CEO

Amy Mohl, DVM
Chief Medical Officer

Michelle Munkres, MA
Executive Editor

Mistretta Design Group, LLC
Design

Consultants and Contributors

Consulting Editors

Todd M. Archer, DVM, MS, DACVIM
College of Veterinary Medicine, Mississippi State University
Mississippi State, MS

Michele Barletta, DVM, MS, PhD, DACVAA
College of Veterinary Medicine, University of Georgia
Athens, GA

Ashley M. Bell, PharmD, FSVHP
College of Veterinary Medicine, North Carolina State University
Raleigh, NC

Elaine Blythe, RPh, PharmD
School of Veterinary Medicine, St. Matthew's University
Grand Cayman Island, BWI

Alison Clode, DVM, DACVO
Ophthalmology Section Editor
Port City Veterinary Referral Hospital, InTown Veterinary Group
Portsmouth, NH

Megan Flanigan, PharmD, FSVHP
College of Veterinary Medicine, The Ohio State University
Columbus, OH

Shannon E. Grady, PharmD, FSVHP
College of Veterinary Medicine, The Ohio State University
Columbus, OH

Tamara Grubb, DVM, PhD, DACVAA
Veterinary Clinical Sciences, Washington State University
Pullman, WA

Sandra N. Koch, DVM, MS, DACVD
Dermatology and Otic Sections Editor
College of Veterinary Medicine, University of Minnesota
St. Paul, MN

Brian A. Scansen, DVM, MS, DACVIM (Cardiology), FVIR
College of Veterinary Medicine and Biomedical Sciences, Colorado State University
Fort Collins, CO

Erica Earnhardt Wassack, PharmD, DICVP, FSVHP, FACVP
College of Veterinary Medicine, Mississippi State University
Mississippi State, MS

Contributors & Reviewers

Derek Adrian, DVM, PhD
Graduate Research Assistant, North Carolina State University Comparative Biomedical Sciences (Pharmacology)*
Raleigh, NC
*Affiliation at the time of contribution

Michael D. Apley, DVM, PhD, DACVCP
College of Veterinary Medicine, Kansas State University
Manhattan, KS

Lora R. Ballweber, DVM, MS, DACVM, DEVPC
College of Veterinary Medicine and Biomedical Sciences, Colorado State University
Fort Collins, CO

Heidi Banse, DVM, PhD, DACVIM
School of Veterinary Medicine, Louisiana State University
Baton Rouge, LA

Darren Berger, DVM, DACVD
College of Veterinary Medicine, Iowa State University
Ames, IA

Alex Bianco, DVM, MS, DACVIM (LAIM)
College of Veterinary Medicine, University of Minnesota
St. Paul, MN

Alex Blutinger, VMD, DACVECC
Veterinary Emergency Group
New York, NY

Benjamin Brainard, VMD, DACVAA, DACVECC
College of Veterinary Medicine, University of Georgia
Athens, GA

Andrew Bugbee, DVM, DACVIM (SAIM)
College of Veterinary Medicine, University of Georgia
Athens, GA

Theresa Burns, DVM, MS, PhD, DACVIM (LAIM)
College of Veterinary Medicine, The Ohio State University
Columbus, OH

Jennifer Buur, DVM, PhD, DACVCP
College of Veterinary Medicine, Western University of Health Sciences
Pomona, CA

Julie Byron, DVM, MS, DACVIM (SAIM)
College of Veterinary Medicine, The Ohio State University
Columbus, OH

Renee Carter, DVM, DACVO
School of Veterinary Medicine, Louisiana State University
Baton Rouge, LA

Amanda Cavanagh, DVM, DACVECC
College of Veterinary Medicine and Biomedical Sciences, Colorado State University
Fort Collins, CO

Marjorie L. Chandler, DVM, MS, MANZCVSc, DACVN, DACVIM, DECVIM-CA, MRCVS
Vets Now Referrals
Glasgow, Scotland

Peter S. Chapman, BVetMed (Hons), DECVIM-CA, DACVIM, MRCVS
Veterinary Specialty and Emergency Center
Levittown, PA

Bruce Christensen, DVM, MS, DACT
Kokopelli Assisted Reproductive Services
Elk Grove, CA

Martha G. Cline, DVM, DACVIM (Nutrition)
Red Bank Veterinary Hospital
Tinton Falls, NJ

Leah A. Cohn, DVM, PhD, DACVIM
Veterinary Health Center, University of Missouri
Columbia, MO

Audrey K. Cook, BVMS, MSc VetEd, DACVIM, DECVIM, DABVP (Feline)
College of Veterinary Medicine, Texas A&M University
College Station, TX

Johnny R. Cross, DVM, DACVIM (Neurology)
VCA Advanced Veterinary Care
Fishers, IN

Gigi Davidson, RPh, DICVP, FSVHP (Honorary), FACVP
VetPharm Consulting and College of Veterinary Medicine, North Carolina State University
Raleigh, NC

Elizabeth Davis, DVM, PhD, DACVIM (LAIM)
College of Veterinary Medicine, Kansas State University
Manhattan, KS

Jennifer L. Davis, DVM, PhD, DACVIM, DACVCP
Virginia-Maryland College of Veterinary Medicine
Blacksburg, VA

Patricia Dowling, DVM, MSc, DACVIM (LAIM), DACVCP
Western College of Veterinary Medicine, University of Saskatchewan
Saskatoon, SK, Canada

Sue Duran, RPh, MS, PhD, DICVP, FSVHP
College of Veterinary Medicine, Auburn University
Auburn, AL

Lisa Ebner, DVM, MS, DACVAA, CVA
College of Veterinary Medicine, Lincoln Memorial University
Harrogate, TN

Marion Ehrich, MS, PhD, DABT, ATS
Virginia-Maryland College of Veterinary Medicine
Blacksburg, VA

Lauren Eichstadt-Forsythe, PharmD, DICVP, FSVHP
College of Veterinary Medicine, University of Illinois
Urbana, IL

Steve Ensley, DVM, MS, PhD
College of Veterinary Medicine, Kansas State University
Manhattan, KS

Timothy Fan, DVM, PhD, DACVIM (SAIM), DACVIM (Oncology)
College of Veterinary Medicine, University of Illinois
Urbana, IL

Claire Fellman, DVM, PhD, DACVIM (SAIM), DACVCP
Cummings School of Veterinary Medicine, Tufts University
North Grafton, MA

Hathaway Fiocchi, DVM, DACVIM (SAIM)
Mobile Veterinary Specialists
Boston, MA

Berit Fischer, DVM, DACVAA, CCRP, CVA
Crown Veterinary Specialists and Associates
Lebanon, NJ

Lauralei L. Fisher-Cronkhite, PharmD, DICVP, FSVHP
College of Veterinary Medicine, Oregon State University
Corvallis, OR

Alex Gallagher, DVM, MS, DACVIM (SAIM)
Columbia Veterinary Emergency Trauma and Specialty
Columbia, SC

José García-López, VMD, BS, DACVS, DACVSMR
New Bolton Center, University of Pennsylvania
Kennett Square, PA

Laura D. Garrett, DVM, DACVIM (Oncology)
College of Veterinary Medicine, University of Illinois
Urbana, IL

Jessica Gaskins Garten, RPh, PharmD, DICVP, FSVHP
College of Veterinary Medicine, University of Florida
Gainesville, FL

Ronette Gehring, BVSc, MMedVet (Pharm), MRCVS, DACVCP, DECVPT
Faculty of Veterinary Medicine, Utrecht University
Utrecht, Netherlands

Alexandria Gochenauer, PharmD, FSVHP
College of Veterinary Medicine, University of Illinois
Urbana, IL

Shannon Grady, PharmD, DICVP, FSVHP
College of Veterinary Medicine, The Ohio State University
Columbus, OH

Lynelle Graham, DVM, MS, DACVAA
College of Veterinary Medicine, North Carolina State University
Durham, NC

Sarah Gray, DVM, DACVECC
Horizon Veterinary Specialists
Ventura, CA

Margaret Gruen, DVM, MVPH, PhD, DACVB
College of Veterinary Medicine, North Carolina State University
Raleigh, NC

Wilson E. Gwin, RPh, DICVP, FSVHP
College of Veterinary Medicine, Purdue University
West Lafayette, IN

Devon Hague, DVM, DACVIM (Neurology)
College of Veterinary Medicine, University of Illinois
Urbana, IL

Tiffany Hall, DVM, DACVIM, DACVECC
Equine Medical Center of Ocala
Ocala, FL

Karyn Harrell, DVM, DACVIM
College of Veterinary Medicine, North Carolina State University
Raleigh, NC

Eleanor C. Hawkins, DVM, DACVIM
College of Veterinary Medicine, North Carolina State University
Raleigh, NC

Trina Hazzah, DVM, DACVIM (Oncology), CVCH
Green Nile, Inc.
Los Angeles, CA

Rikki Horne, PharmD, FSVHP
College of Veterinary Medicine, The Ohio State University
Columbus, OH

Maria Angeles Jimenez Lozano, DVM, CertVA, DECVAA, MRCVS
North Downs Specialist Referrals
Bletchingley, Surrey, United Kingdom

Rebecca Johnson, DVM, MS, PhD, DACVAA
School of Veterinary Medicine, University of Wisconsin
Madison, WI

Ray Kaplan, DVM, PhD, DEVPC, DACVM (Parasitology)
College of Veterinary Medicine, University of Georgia
Athens, GA

Shawn Kearns, DVM, DACVIM
Angell Animal Medical Center
Boston, MA

Nina Kieves, DVM, DACVS, DACVSMR, CCRT
College of Veterinary Medicine, The Ohio State University
Columbus, OH

Heather K. Knych, DVM, MS, PhD, DACVCP
School of Veterinary Medicine, University of California, Davis
Davis, CA

Kendan W. Kuo, DVM, MS, DACVECC
College of Veterinary Medicine, Auburn University
Auburn, AL

Mary A. Labato, DVM, DACVIM
Cummings School of Veterinary Medicine, Tufts University
North Grafton, MA

Jeffrey Lakritz, DVM, PhD, DACVIM (LAIM), DACVCP
College of Veterinary Medicine, The Ohio State University
Columbus, OH

Daniel K. Langlois, DVM, DACVIM
College of Veterinary Medicine, Michigan State University
East Lansing, MI

Jean-Pierre Lavoie, DMV, DACVIM (LAIM)
Faculty of Veterinary Medicine, Université de Montréal
Saint-Hyacinthe, Quebec, Canada

Yuri A. Lawrence, DVM, PhD, MS, MA, DACVIM (SAIM)
Lawrence Mobile Internal Medicine Consulting Services
Austin, TX

Elizabeth Layne, DVM, DACVD
Montana Veterinary Dermatology
Bozeman, MT

Stacey Leach, DVM, DACVIM (Cardiology)
Veterinary Health Center, University of Missouri
Columbia, MO

Amandine T. Lejeune, DVM, DACVIM (Oncology)
School of Veterinary Medicine, University of California, Davis
Davis, CA

Cynthia Leveille-Webster, DVM, DACVIM
Cummings School of Veterinary Medicine, Tufts University
New Grafton, MA

Heather Lindell-Tally, PharmD, BSPh, RPh, DICVP, FSVHP
Atlanta Vet, Inc. and University of Georgia
Athens, GA

Mark Lowrie, MA, VetMB, MVM, DECVN, MRCVS
Dovecote Veterinary Hospital
Castle Donington, Derby, United Kingdom

Shane Lyon, DVM, MS, DACVIM (SAIM)
College of Veterinary Medicine, Kansas State University
Manhattan, KS

Sophie Mainguy-Seers, DMV, DES, DACVIM (LAIM)
Faculty of Veterinary Medicine, Université de Montréal
Saint-Hyacinthe, Quebec, Canada

Khursheed Mama, DVM, DACVAA
College of Veterinary Medicine and Biomedical Sciences, Colorado State University
Fort Collins, CO

Tara Marmulak, PharmD, DICVP, FSVHP
College of Veterinary Medicine and Biomedical Sciences, Colorado State University
Fort Collins, CO

Lara Maxwell, DVM, PhD, DACVCP
College of Veterinary Medicine, Oklahoma State University
Stillwater, OK

Elisa Mazzaferro, DVM, MS, PhD, DACVECC
Cornell University Veterinary Specialists
Stamford, CT

Tamara McArdle, DVM, DABVP
Albuquerque Cat Clinic
Albuquerque, NM

Katrina L. Mealey, DVM, PhD, DACVIM, DACVCP
College of Veterinary Medicine, Washington State University
Pullman, WA

Emma G. Meyer, PharmD, FSVHP, DICVP
Costco Pharmacy
Apex, NC

Gillian Miner, PharmD
School of Veterinary Medicine, University of Wisconsin-Madison
Madison, WI

Andrew Moorhead, DVM, MS, PhD, DACVM (Parasitology)
College of Veterinary Medicine, University of Georgia
Athens, GA

Carolyn O'Brien, BVSc, MVetClinStud, PhD, FANZCVS
Melbourne Cat Vets
Fitzroy, Victoria, Australia

Adesola Odunayo, DVM, MS, DACVECC
College of Veterinary Medicine, University of Florida
Gainesville, FL

William Oldenhoff, DVM, DACVD
Access Specialty Animal Hospitals
Woodland Hills, CA

Thierry Olivry, DrVet, PhD, DACVD, DECVD
College of Veterinary Medicine, North Carolina State University*
Raleigh, NC
*Affiliation at the time of contribution

Garret Pachtinger, VMD, DACVECC
Veterinary Emergency Group

Carly Patterson, DVM, DACVIM (SAIM)
College of Veterinary Medicine, Texas A&M University
College Station, TX

Kursten Pierce, DVM, DACVIM (Cardiology)
College of Veterinary Medicine, North Carolina State University
Raleigh, NC

Amy Pike, DVM, DACVB, IAABC-CABC
Animal Behavior Wellness Center
Fairfax, VA

Robert Poppenga, DVM, PhD, DABVT
School of Veterinary Medicine, University of California, Davis
Davis, CA

Nicola Pusterla, DVM, PhD, DACVIM (LAIM), DAVDC-Equine
School of Veterinary Medicine, University of California, Davis
Davis, CA

Bruno H. Pypendop, DrMedVet, DrVetSci, DACVAA
School of Veterinary Medicine, University of California, Davis
Davis, CA

Jane Quandt, DVM, MS, DACVAA, DACVECC
College of Veterinary Medicine, University of Georgia
Athens, GA

Rebecca L. Quinn, DVM, DACVIM
Cape Cod Veterinary Specialists
Buzzards Bay, MA

Lisa Radosta, DVM, DACVB
Florida Veterinary Behavior Service
West Palm Beach, FL

Katherine Raines, PharmD, FSVHP
College of Veterinary Medicine, Mississippi State University
Mississippi State, MS

Jennifer M. Reinhart, DVM, MS, PhD, DACVIM (SAIM), DACVCP
College of Veterinary Medicine, University of Illinois
Urbana, IL

Elizabeth Rozanski, DVM, DACVIM, DACVECC
Cummings School of Veterinary Medicine, Tufts University
New Grafton, MA

Erin E. Runcan, DVM, DACT
College of Veterinary Medicine, The Ohio State University
Columbus, OH

Kirk Ryan, DVM, DACVIM
School of Veterinary Medicine, Louisiana State University
Baton Rouge, LA

Thomas Schermerhorn, VMD, DACVIM
College of Veterinary Medicine, Kansas State University
Manhattan, KS

Kai-Biu Shiu, BVMS, MRCVS, DACVIM (Oncology)
VCA Veterinary Emergency Service and Veterinary Specialty Center
Madison, WI

Andrew Simpson, DVM, MS, DACVD
VCA Aurora Animal Hospital
Aurora, IL

Margaret M. Sleeper, VMD, DACVIM (Cardiology)
College of Veterinary Medicine, University of Florida
Gainesville, FL

Lesley Smith, DVM, DACVAA
School of Veterinary Medicine, University of Wisconsin-Madison
Madison, WI

Emily Sorah, PharmD, DICVP, FSVHP, FACVP
College of Veterinary Medicine, North Carolina State University
Raleigh, NC

Laura Staats, PharmD, DICVP
School of Veterinary Medicine, University of Wisconsin-Madison
Madison, WI

Bryden Stanley, BVMS, MVETSC, MACVSC, DACVS
College of Veterinary Medicine, Michigan State University
East Lansing, MI

Jörg Steiner, MedVet, DrMedVet, PhD, DACVIM, DECVIM-CA, AGAF
College of Veterinary Medicine, Texas A&M University
College Station, TX

Jason W. Stull, VMD, MPVM, PhD, DACVPM
College of Veterinary Medicine, The Ohio State University
Columbus, OH

Karen Sueda, DVM, DACVB
VCA West Los Angeles Animal Hospital
Los Angeles, CA

Douglas H. Thamm, VMD, DACVIM (Oncology)
College of Veterinary Medicine and Biomedical Sciences, Colorado State University
Fort Collins, CO

Cory Theberge, PhD
Clear Eyes Partners
Brunswick, ME

Justin D. Thomason, DVM, DACVIM (Cardiology)
College of Veterinary Medicine, Kansas State University
Manhattan, KS

Lauren Trepanier, DVM, PhD, DACVIM (SAIM), DACVCP
School of Veterinary Medicine, University of Wisconsin
Madison, WI

Mark Troxel, DVM, DACVIM (Neurology)
Massachusetts Veterinary Referral Hospital
Woburn, MA

Heather D. S. Walden, MS, PhD
College of Veterinary Medicine, University of Florida
Gainesville, FL

Ashlee Watts, DVM, PhD, DACVS
Veterinary Medical Teaching Hospital, Texas A&M University
College Station, TX

J. Scott Weese, DVM, DVSc, DACVIM
Ontario Veterinary College, University of Guelph
Guelph, Ontario, Canada

Lois Wetmore, DVM, MS, ScD, DACVAA
Cummings School of Veterinary Medicine, Tufts University
North Grafton, MA

Shelby Williams, PharmD, DICVP, FSVHP
School of Veterinary Medicine, University of Wisconsin
Madison, WI

Tina Wismer, DVM, DABVT, DABT
ASPCA Animal Poison Control Center
Champaign, IL

Bonnie D. Wright, DVM, DACVAA
Mistral Vet
Fort Collins, CO

Aurora Zoff, DVM (Hons), CertAVP(VA), DACVAA, MRCVS
North Downs Specialist Referrals
Bletchingley, Surrey, United Kingdom

In Appreciation

LET'S CONSIDER just what Donald Plumb started back in 1991. From its utilitarian roots as the University of Minnesota Veterinary Pharmacy Formulary, that spiral-bound "orange virus" was elevated into the first edition of *Plumb's® Veterinary Drug Handbook*. With a distribution center located in his basement and staffed by his wife, Shirley Werlein Plumb, veterinary medicine finally had a drug information resource.

The subsequent editions of *Plumb's® Veterinary Drug Handbook* expanded not only the book's content, but also its reach. The handbook has been printed in multiple languages and has been sold to veterinarians around the world. With his same entrepreneurial spirit, Dr. Plumb forayed into digital publication as a way to provide easy access to the information found in the handbook. In 2014, with vision inspired by VetMedux CEO and founder, Elizabeth Green, Dr. Plumb was able to bring the handbook onto a modern web platform and mobile app.

By 2018, Dr. Plumb was pleased with the roadmap that the Brief Media (now VetMedux) team had designed for the handbook, and he entrusted his life's work to our care. The Plumb's® team is honored to carry on this legacy through close collaboration with veterinary specialists, veterinary pharmacists, and our audience—without whom the content of Plumb's® would not be possible.

In this 10th edition of *Plumb's® Veterinary Drug Handbook*, we on the Plumb's® team, on behalf of veterinarians and their patients across the globe, offer our most profound gratitude to Dr. Plumb for his vision and commitment to the safety of animals under veterinary care.

Just look at what he started.

Preface

FROM ITS UTILITARIAN INCEPTION as a formulary for the University of Minnesota Veterinary Teaching Hospital, to the subsequent 9 editions of *Plumb's® Veterinary Drug Handbook*, Donald Plumb created a widely respected and profoundly impactful veterinary drug reference. Today, a new Plumb's® team is answering the call to transform content to meet the emerging informational needs of a fast-paced clinical setting, as well as to serve the need for up-to-date information not limited by the confines of a printed book. Alongside the digital innovations in how veterinary drug information is delivered at **plumbs.com**, the 10th edition of *Plumb's® Veterinary Drug Handbook* continues the mission to serve as a single-volume reference to assist veterinarians when making critical therapy decisions about their patients as well as provide trusted counsel to pharmacists serving pet owners.

This 10th edition presents trusted drug information in the consistent, easy-to-use (and understand) Plumb's® format readers far and wide have become accustomed to in their daily clinical practice. From the ***Prescriber Highlights*** that capture the most important elements for at-a-glance comprehension to the ***Dosage Forms*** section and everything in between, Plumb's® provides pertinent information needed when prescribing drugs to veterinary patients. The sequence of the monograph sections provides fine details about what conditions the drug is used for (***Uses/Indications***), the drug's mechanism of action (***Pharmacology/Actions***), ***Pharmacokinetics***, and what concerns the prescriber should be aware of before prescribing a drug to a patient (eg, ***Contraindications/Precautions/Warnings, Adverse Effects, Reproductive/Nursing Safety, Overdose/Acute Toxicity, Drug Interactions***); ***Monitoring*** of drug therapy and information related to drug characteristics (eg, ***Chemistry/Synonyms, Storage/Stability, Compounding/Compatibility Considerations***) may also influence treatment. The ***References*** section has been significantly expanded and is available digitally; readers may explore specific details from the cited literature by accessing each drug's references at **wiley.com/go/budde/plumb**.

Plumb's® is committed to antimicrobial stewardship and has included globally accepted designations for each antibiotic monograph to alert the prescriber to the critically important choice to be made when using this class of drugs.

All of these important details factor into the decisions of whether and how to use a particular drug for a particular patient; dosages should be chosen only based on the totality of information, and response to therapy should be monitored accordingly.

This edition also includes rigorous peer review and infusion of relevant clinical details to further support a veterinarian's critical decisions when treating patients. Every effort has been made to continue presenting information in a manner that will help to minimize misunderstandings and reduce the risk for a medication error.

The reference that was once compiled by one person has now been expanded to include the efforts of a team of board-certified veterinary specialists and veterinary pharmacists. The Plumb's® team recognizes that information changes so rapidly that it is impossible for one person to keep up and have all the answers; as a result, we have assembled a team of experts to scour the primary and secondary literature and revise the monograph content to incorporate updates from these sources. Woven throughout this entire process are the tireless and never-ending efforts of the editors, who ensure that the content herein is clear and concise.

Each monograph, including the ***Ophthalmic*** and ***Topical Dermatologic and Otic Agents***, in this edition has been updated and 36 new monographs have been added (see ***Table***). These new monographs include therapeutic entities recently introduced into the veterinary marketplace, or are human drugs that either have been increasingly incorporated into veterinary practice, or were determined (often via feedback submitted from readers via plumbs.com) to be useful additions to this reference. Converse to the additions of new content, some content has been removed, either because the drug is no longer marketed, more effective or safer alternatives are now available, available information supporting the drug's use is lacking, or because the drug is no longer considered to have a place in therapy.

As with the first edition of *Plumb's® Veterinary Drug Handbook*, it may still be helpful to describe what this book is *not*. It is not intended to be a pharmacology textbook, nor medical chemistry tome, nor compounding manual. It is not merely a compilation of pharmacokinetic data, recitation of drug interactions, or simple repetition of product labels. Instead, *Plumb's® Veterinary Drug Handbook* captures the best of all of these—and more.

With information ever-changing, the Plumb's® team recognizes the need for regularly updated resources to be delivered at the speed of clinical practice. Digital advancements to Plumb's® content—including drug monograph updates, medication guides, and the profession's first and only veterinary-specific drug interaction checker—are available to those who purchase a subscription at **plumbs.com**.

Our vision in this 10th edition is to guide the most critical decisions in veterinary medicine. We hope this edition of *Plumb's® Veterinary Drug Handbook* helps busy veterinary practitioners provide the best possible care for their patients.

NEW CONTENT

Cannabidiol
Cefquinome
Cholestyramine
Ciclesonide
Crofelemer
Dextromethorphan
Dipyrone
Eprinomectin/Praziquantel
Exenatide
Fenofibrate
Frunevetmab
Honey, Topical
Imidacloprid, Systemic
Insulins

- General information
- Aspart
- Detemir
- Glargine
- Lente
- Lispro
- NPH
- Protamine Zinc
- Regular

Linezolid
Lidocaine Ophthalmic
Lotilaner
Medetomidine/Vatinoxan
Polymyxin B
Reserpine
Rifaximin
Ropinirole
Selamectin/Sarolaner
Spironolactone/Benazepril
Tigilanol Tiglate
Valacyclovir
Verdinexor
Vinorelbine

Antimicrobials in Human and Veterinary Medicine: A Global Classification**
Veterinarian's Guide to Writing Prescriptions**

CONTENT REMOVED*

Acetohydroxamic Acid
Acitretin
Aminopentamide
Aztreonam
Baclofen
Benzonatate
Boldenone
Bumetanide
Busulfan
Butaphosan/Cyanocobalamin
Candesartan
Captopril
Carbamazepine
Chlordiazepoxide ± Clidinium
Chlorpropamide
Chromium
Danazol
Dexpanthenol
Dihydrotachysterol
Disopyramide
Echothiophate Iodide Ophthalmic
Emedastine Ophthalmic
Ethyl Lactate
Etidronate
Flavoxate
Glimepiride
Glutamine
Indoxacarb ± Permethrin, Topical
Iodixanol
Ipodate
Isosorbide
Lithium
Mercaptopurine
Methohexital
Methyltestosterone
Metipranolol Ophthalmic
Mibolerone
Nandrolone
Naproxen
Neomycin Ophthalmic
Pancuronium
Paregoric
Pentazocine
Phenytoin
Polysulfated Glycosaminoglycan, Ophthalmic
Primidone
Protamine
Schirmer Tear Test Ophthalmic
Silymarin
Sodium Polystyrene Sulfonate
Thioguanine
Thiotepa
Triclosan, Topical
Trypan Blue
Valproic Acid
Vanadium
Vardenafil
Zafirlukast

Abbreviations Used in Prescription Writing**
Canine & Feline Animal Blood Products**
Importation of Unapproved Drugs into the USA**

---

* The content of these monographs remains available in archived status at Plumb's® Veterinary Drugs (plumbs.com); however, the content has not been updated and may be incomplete or inaccurate.

** Appendix item

Notes and Cautions

How to Use This Book

The information found in this reference is meant to be an aggregate of drug information that is relevant and important to clinical settings. The core focus of the content is to help veterinary and pharmacy professionals make safe, informed prescribing decisions when treating the animals in their care. The content is not meant to be an exhaustive text of related pharmacology or case management information; readers are encouraged to consult other resources and experts for these purposes. Pharmacologic and clinical case management concepts are not discussed.

Although this reference is used globally, it presents information in the context of US regulations. It is the responsibility of the reader to understand relevant local regulations related to, but not limited by, the use, storage, and withdrawal times for specific drugs in specific species.

Great care has been taken to carefully organize the content in this reference so that readers can readily find the information they need. Although the most commonly accessed information is in the ***Dosages*** section, it is important for readers to turn their attention to other sections of the monograph (eg, ***Contraindications/Precautions/Warnings, Drug Interactions***) to understand the complete drug profile.

The ***Client Information*** section is now presented with language from the perspective of the prescriber speaking to the client. This presentation allows the information to be readily copied into client handouts. The bullet points are not exhaustive and are intended to convey the most important information to the client. A complete set of thorough Veterinary Medication Guides with client-friendly language can be accessed with a subscription to plumbs.com.

Dosages and Extra-Label Drug Use

The drug dosages listed for the various species in this reference come from a variety of sources, and there has been a concerted effort to ensure all dosages are referenced to their primary source and to indicate where dosages only have anecdotal support. Although a sincere effort has been made to ensure that the dosages and information included in this book are accurate and reflect the original source's information, errors can occur; it is recommended that the reader refer to the original reference or the approved labeling information of the product for additional information and verification of all dosages. Please note that the ***References*** section from each monograph is available digitally; specific details from the cited literature can be found by accessing each drug's references at **wiley.com/go/budde/plumb**.

Information in the ***Dosages*** section is organized by species so that prescribers can quickly access the dosage they need. Each monograph lists the applicable species in the same order for a consistent format; when relevant, label dosages of a particular species are always presented first. Any dosage listing that deviates from the US label is clearly delineated as extra-label. Please note that the presentation of drug information is centered on US-labeled products; foreign labels that differ from US labels are considered extra-label in this US-based reference. Extra-label dosages are not necessarily endorsed by the manufacturer, the Food and Drug Administration (FDA), or the Plumb's® authors. Veterinarians are responsible, per the Animal Medical Drug Use Clarification Act (AMDUCA), for the appropriate use of medications. For further information, see ***Extra-Label Drug Use*** in the ***Appendix*** section.

Drug Interactions

Drug interaction identification and evaluation is an art and is slowly emerging in veterinary medicine; relatively little specific information is known on this subject for the variety of species treated. Although drug interactions can be clinically significant and potentially life-threatening in veterinary patients, most of the interactions listed in the drug monographs are derived from human medicine (which is only slightly more informed than veterinary medicine on this topic) and are often included primarily to serve as cautions to the prescriber to be alert for unforeseen outcomes or to enhance monitoring associated with the drug therapy. Additionally, it is likely there are many other clinically significant interactions between drugs that are not listed; prescribers are reminded that the risk for adverse drug interactions increases with the number of different medications given to an individual patient. For situations when a patient is receiving multiple medications, consultation with a veterinary pharmacist or veterinary clinical pharmacologist is highly encouraged.

Abbreviations

To minimize medication errors, abbreviations such as SID, BID, or q8h are not used. In the ***Dosage Forms*** section, the terms Rx or OTC are noted in parentheses after a listed dosage form. If Rx, the drug is considered to be a prescription or legend product and requires a prescription. OTC denotes that the item is available "over-the-counter" and does not legally require a prescription for purchase. Note, however, that use of "human" OTC medications in veterinary species is considered extra-label drug use and, per AMDUCA, must be undertaken only under the supervision of a veterinarian.

Trade and Proprietary Names

Trade names or proprietary names are both italicized and capitalized and then followed by the registered trademark symbol (eg, *Amoxi-Tabs*®). This notation may not accurately represent the drug's official registered copyright, trademark, or licensed status (eg, ™). For clarity, the registered trademark symbol (®) and italics have not been used in the index. Where listed, trade names are typically the innovator product(s), particularly those names listed at the top of each monograph. Additional names, including chemical and foreign trade names, can be found in the ***Chemistry/Synonyms*** section. Newly branded, generic products are continually released and ever-changing, and the listing in this reference may not be complete.

Errors

If an error is found or suspected, please contact our team at **plumbs.com/about/contact-us/** so the concern can be appropriately addressed. Errors that have been found in this edition and previous editions can be found at **plumbs.com/handbook-errata-10th-edition/**.

DISCLAIMER

CONTENTS

SYSTEMIC MONOGRAPHS

Acarbose

(ay-***kar***-bose) *Precose®, Glucobay®*

Antidiabetic Agent, Alpha Glucosidase Inhibitor

Prescriber Highlights

- ► Antihyperglycemic agent that reduces the rate and amount of glucose absorbed from the gut after a meal; may be useful in dogs and cats with mild hyperglycemia; unlikely to be effective when used as the sole therapy for management of diabetes mellitus
- ► Contraindications include a known hypersensitivity to the drug, diabetic ketoacidosis, inflammatory bowel disease, colonic ulceration, partial intestinal obstruction or predisposition to obstruction, or chronic intestinal disease with marked disorders of digestion or absorption, as well as in patients that are underweight or in cases in which excessive GI gas formation would be detrimental.
- ► Adverse effects can limit the drug's usefulness and include dose-dependent loose stools, diarrhea, and flatulence.
- ► Give with meals (preferably right before feeding); this drug is not as effective if feeding ad libitum.

Uses/Indications

Acarbose may be useful in reducing blood glucose concentrations in cases of mild to moderate hyperglycemia (250-350 mg/dL range) in dogs and cats with non-insulin-dependent diabetes mellitus and as adjunctive treatment for insulin-dependent diabetes mellitus. Acarbose may be useful in dogs or cats when insulin activity peaks too soon.[1]

In healthy cats, acarbose resulted in a 5% to 7.5% reduction in postprandial glucose area under the curve (AUC) and a 35% to 45% reduction in postprandial insulin AUC as compared to no treatment.[2] In diabetic cats, acarbose apparently is most effective in cats that refuse to eat a low carbohydrate diet and consume their food within a short time after acarbose is given. Acarbose given in conjunction with a high carbohydrate diet has an effect similar to feeding an ultra-low carbohydrate diet.[3] Acarbose is usually not effective in animals with reduced appetites (eg, cats with advanced chronic kidney disease). Acarbose may be considered in dogs when glycemic control is poor and the cause is not determined.[4] Acarbose is unlikely to give adequate glucose control when used alone; dietary therapy and other antihyperglycemic agents (eg, insulin) are typically recommended instead.

Pharmacology/Actions

Acarbose competitively inhibits pancreatic alpha-amylase and alpha-glucosidases found in the small intestine. This inhibition delays the digestion of complex carbohydrates and disaccharides to glucose and other monosaccharides, which causes glucose to be absorbed in lesser amounts lower in the GI tract. This reduced absorption decreases blood glucose and insulin requirements during the postprandial hyperglycemic phase. Acarbose has no effect on lactase nor does it enhance insulin secretion.

Pharmacokinetics

In dogs, ≈4% of an oral dose is absorbed; in humans, only ≈2% of an oral dose is absorbed from the gut and then excreted by the kidneys. Practically all of the remaining drug in the gut is metabolized by intestinal bacterial flora. Patients with severe renal dysfunction attain serum levels ≈5 times those of normal patients.

Contraindications/Precautions/Warnings

Acarbose is contraindicated in patients with known hypersensitivity to the drug, diabetic ketoacidosis, inflammatory bowel disease, colonic ulceration, partial intestinal obstruction or predisposition to obstruction, and chronic intestinal disease with marked disorders of digestion or absorption, as well as when excessive GI gas formation would be detrimental. Acarbose is contraindicated in patients with low body weight (may also apply to patients with normal body weight), as the drug may have deleterious effects on nutrition status. Use caution in patients with renal dysfunction or severe liver disease.

Adverse Effects

Adverse effects reported in cats include flatulence, soft stools, and diarrhea. In dogs, adverse effects include soft or watery stools, diarrhea, and weight loss.[4] These adverse effects are more likely at higher doses and may outweigh treatment benefits.[5]

Although acarbose alone does not cause hypoglycemia, it may contribute to it by reducing the rate and amount of glucose absorbed when the patient is receiving other hypoglycemic agents (eg, insulin, oral hypoglycemic drugs).

Dose-related increases in hepatic transaminases have been reported rarely in humans.

Reproductive/Nursing Safety

Studies in laboratory animals have demonstrated no evidence of fetal harm or impaired fertility. Weigh any potential risks versus benefits in pregnant animals.

It is not known if acarbose is excreted in maternal milk. Acarbose is likely safe to use during nursing because it is minimally absorbed.

Overdose/Acute Toxicity

Acute overdoses are likely to only cause diarrhea and flatulence; no treatment should be necessary. If acute hypoglycemia occurs secondary to other hypoglycemic agents, parenteral glucose should be administered. Use glucose (eg, dextrose) instead of sucrose when treating orally, as the absorption of oral glucose is not inhibited by acarbose.

For patients that have experienced or are suspected to have experienced an overdose, it is strongly encouraged that a 24-hour poison consultation center that specializes in providing information specific for veterinary patients be consulted. For general information related to overdose and toxin exposures, as well as contact information for poison control centers, refer to ***Appendix***.

Drug Interactions

The following drug interactions have either been reported or are theoretical in humans or animals receiving acarbose and may be of significance in veterinary patients. Unless otherwise noted, use together is not necessarily contraindicated, but weigh the potential risks and perform additional monitoring when appropriate.

- **Charcoal, Activated**: Intestinal adsorbents may reduce the efficacy of acarbose.
- **Digoxin**: Acarbose may reduce digoxin blood concentrations.
- **Hyperglycemic Agents** (eg, **calcium channel blockers, corticosteroids, estrogens, phenothiazines, thiazides, thyroid hormones**): May reduce or negate the effects of acarbose
- **Hypoglycemic agents** (eg, **insulin, sulfonylureas**): May increase the risk for hypoglycemia
- **Pancreatin, Pancrelipase,** or **Amylase**: Exogenous enzyme formulations may reduce the efficacy of acarbose.

Laboratory Considerations

- Increased serum aminotransferase (ALT) and bilirubin levels have been noted in some humans taking high dosages for a long period.

Dosages

DOGS:

Adjunctive treatment for diabetes mellitus (extra-label): Initially, 12.5 – 25 mg/dog (NOT mg/kg) PO with each meal (usually twice daily). Give only at time of feeding (right before). If response is inadequate after 2 weeks, the dosage may be titrated up to 50 mg/dog (NOT mg/kg) PO twice daily. For dogs weighing greater than 10 to 25 kg (22 to 55.1 lb), a further increase up to 100 mg/dog (NOT mg/kg) twice daily may be considered if response has been inadequate.

CATS:

Adjunctive treatment for diabetes mellitus (extra-label): 12.5 mg/cat (NOT mg/kg) PO twice daily with a meal.[2,3,6,7] One study found acarbose to be ineffective in healthy cats fed a low carbohydrate diet.[6]

Monitoring

- Serum glucose
- Adverse effects (eg, diarrhea, flatulence)
- Liver enzymes

Client Information

- For best results, give this drug right before feeding your animal. Tablets may be split or crushed and mixed with food just prior to administration.
- Diarrhea and/or gas are the most likely side effects.
- Acarbose does not cause low blood sugar; however, it may contribute to it if the animal is getting other drugs that lower blood sugar (including insulin). Call your veterinarian immediately if you see signs of low blood sugar (eg, seizures [ie, convulsions], collapse, rear leg weakness or paralysis, muscle twitching, unsteadiness, tiredness, depression).
- It may take up to 2 weeks for the drug to work.

Chemistry/Synonyms

Acarbose, a complex oligosaccharide antihyperglycemic agent, occurs as a white to off-white powder, is soluble in water, and has a pK_a of 5.1.

Acarbose may also be known as Bay-g-5421, *Asucrose®*, *Glicobase®*, *Glucobay®*, *Glucor®*, *Glumida®*, *Prandase®*, or *Precose®*.

Storage/Stability

Do not store tablets above 25°C (77°F), and protect them from moisture.

Compatibility/Compounding Considerations

Tablets may be split or crushed and mixed with food just prior to administration.

Dosage Forms/Regulatory Status

VETERINARY-LABELED PRODUCTS: NONE

HUMAN-LABELED PRODUCTS:

Acarbose Oral Tablets: 25 mg, 50 mg, and 100 mg; *Precose®*, generic; (Rx)

References

For the complete list of references, see **wiley.com/go/budde/plumb**

Acepromazine

Acetylpromazine

(***ase***-pro-ma-zeen) *PromAce®*

Phenothiazine Sedative/Tranquilizer

Prescriber Highlights

- ▶ Used as a sedative/tranquilizer, or in balanced anesthetic or analgesic protocols; also used as adjunctive treatment of urethral obstruction in male cats and laminitis in horses
- ▶ Clinical dosages are significantly lower than those listed on the United States-approved label.
- ▶ Time to onset (15 minutes, up to 30 minutes for full effect) and duration of action (3 to 4 hours, up to 6 to 8 hours in some animals) are relatively long as compared with other sedatives such as the alpha-2 agonists.
- ▶ Does not have a reversal agent
- ▶ Provides no analgesic effects but can be combined with analgesics (eg, opioids) to enhance sedation and increase duration of analgesia (ie, neuroleptanalgesia). Use a low dose of acepromazine when combining with other sedatives or anesthetic drugs.
- ▶ Acepromazine has minimal to no impact on respiratory function but may cause significant hypotension and hypothermia; it should be avoided or dose-reduced in debilitated animals, especially those with predicted or pre-existing hypotension or hepatic insufficiency; and used with caution in patients with moderate to severe cardiac disease that cannot tolerate reduced blood pressures.
- ▶ Dogs with the multidrug sensitivity gene *(MDR1) mutation (also known as ABCB1*-1delta) are overly sensitive to effects and require dose reduction or avoidance.
- ▶ Use with caution as a sole sedative in aggressive dogs as dogs may be prone to startling and occasional dogs experience worsening of aggression and CNS stimulation.
- ▶ May cause penile prolapse in horses, but associated permanent penile dysfunction is very rare.

Uses/Indications

Acepromazine is FDA-approved for use in dogs, cats, and horses. Labeled indications for dogs and cats include as an aid in controlling intractable animals and alleviating itching as a result of skin irritation, as an antiemetic to control vomiting associated with motion sickness, and as a preanesthetic agent.[1]

Acepromazine has a wide safety margin and is one of the most commonly used sedatives/tranquilizers in small animal species, with less frequent use in large animal species. The injectable formulation is used primarily as a preanesthetic agent or for procedural sedation. Sedation with acepromazine is mainly indicated for use in healthy patients or patients with mild systemic disease. Because acepromazine has minimal effects on respiratory function, it can be a useful tranquilizer/sedative in small animal species with upper airway obstruction (eg, laryngeal paralysis). The long duration of action can be advantageous in some situations (eg, can promote smoother recovery from anesthesia in excited/anxious animals) but can be problematic in others (eg, can delay discharge in same-day sedation/anesthesia procedures).

Acepromazine has been used as one part of a multimodal protocol to resolve urethral obstruction in male cats without the need for urethral catheterization[2]; this protocol may be beneficial in situations where client financial constraints limit treatment and would otherwise result in euthanasia.

Acepromazine has no analgesic effects; however, when combined with opioid analgesics, acepromazine can enhance sedation and prolong the opioid analgesic effect (neuroleptanalgesia). Acepromazine also has antihistamine and antiemetic effects; however, it is not commonly used for these indications due to availability of more specific and effective treatment options.

The oral form of acepromazine is most commonly used to decrease an animal's response to stress or fear-inducing stimuli like loud noises (eg, fireworks, thunder) or travel. Whether acepromazine causes anxiolysis or only sedation in these situations is unknown and controversial. Specific drugs that cause fewer adverse effects are available for behavioral modification associated with anxiety in dogs and cats.

In horses, acepromazine is labeled for use as an aid in controlling fractious animals and in conjunction with local anesthesia for various procedures and treatments.[1] It is also commonly used in horses at low doses (0.005 – 0.04 mg/kg) as a preanesthetic agent for mild sedation and for its potential antiarrhythmic effects.[3] Acepromazine has also been administered to horses with laminitis to improve blood flow to the distal limb.[4–6]

Although not FDA-approved, acepromazine is used as a tranquilizer in other species such as cattle, sheep, goats, swine, and rabbits. Acepromazine has been shown to reduce the incidence of halothane-induced malignant hyperthermia in susceptible pigs.[7]

Pharmacology/Actions

Acepromazine is a phenothiazine neuroleptic agent. Although the exact mechanisms of action are not fully understood, phenothiazines block postsynaptic dopamine receptors in the CNS and may inhibit the release of dopamine and increase its turnover rate. They are thought to depress portions of the reticular activating system that assist in the control of body temperature, basal metabolic rate, emesis, vasomotor tone, hormonal balance, and alertness. In addition, phenothiazines have varying degrees of anticholinergic, antihistaminic, antispasmodic, and alpha-adrenergic blocking effects.

The primary desired effect for the use of acepromazine in veterinary medicine is tranquilization/sedation. Additional desirable pharmacologic actions of acepromazine include its use as a muscle relaxant, antiemetic, antiarrhythmic (blockade of myocardial alpha-1 receptors), and antispasmodic. Examples of muscle relaxant/antispasmodic effects include relief of clinical signs in a mare with urethral spasms[8] and reduction of urethral pressure in cats anesthetized with halothane.[9]

Vasodilation secondary to alpha-1 receptor blockade can contribute to hypotension with potential reflex tachycardia; however, mild vasodilation can be beneficial in some dogs and cats with cardiac disease in which systemic vasodilation or a decrease in afterload is desired, as in moderate to severe mitral regurgitation. In this case, acepromazine 0.005 – 0.01 mg/kg is adequate. A combination of acepromazine and an opioid is commonly used for sedation of patients for cardiac imaging because of the limited to no impact on cardiac function. In one study, acepromazine 0.02 mg/kg combined with butorphanol 0.2 mg/kg administered IM to dogs provided adequate sedation for echocardiography with only mild changes on measured variables.[10] In dogs, premedication with acepromazine caused a moderate decrease in blood pressure without significantly altering glomerular filtration rate or renal blood flow.[11]

Acepromazine may decrease respiratory rate, but studies have demonstrated that little or no effect occurs with regard to blood gas status, pH, and/or oxyhemoglobin saturation.[12–15]

A dose-dependent decrease in hematocrit can be seen within 30 minutes after administration to dogs and horses. Hematocrit values in horses may decrease ≈20% of predose values; this change is due to increased splenic sequestration of red blood cells, which has been demonstrated in dogs.[13,16–18] Although the red blood cells return to circulation, this effect may not occur until after recovery from anesthesia and could exacerbate decreased oxygen delivery during anesthesia of anemic patients. Acepromazine may transiently reduce platelet count and aggregation; however, platelet function and hemostasis are not altered.[19,20]

Although acepromazine use was historically avoided in epileptic animals and in those that were susceptible to seizures (eg, postmyelography), recent research has disproved this effect and shown that acepromazine may have some anticonvulsant activity. In a study, acepromazine did not significantly alter EEG in healthy dogs.[21] In other studies, acepromazine caused no seizures, even in high-risk dogs, and actually decreased seizures in some actively convulsing dogs.[22–24]

Acepromazine can delay gastric emptying, reduce lower esophageal tone, and slow GI motility in dogs, cats, horses, cattle, and likely other species.[25–28] This effect is not likely to have a clinical impact in most animals but could influence GI motility studies[25] and potentially increase the risk for gastric reflux.

Other pharmacologic actions are discussed in the ***Adverse Effects*** section.

Pharmacokinetics

In dogs that receive acepromazine 1.3 – 1.5 mg/kg, oral bioavailability is ≈20% and elimination half-lives are ≈7.1 hours (IV) and 16 hours (PO).[29]

In horses, acepromazine 0.3 mg/kg IV has a fairly high volume of distribution (6.6 L/kg) and is more than 99% protein bound.[17] The onset of action is fairly slow, requiring up to 15 minutes following IV administration, with peak effects seen in 30 to 60 minutes. Elimination half-life is ≈3 hours. In one study, horses appeared sedated (based on chin-to-ground measurement) within 5 minutes of IV administration as compared with 15 minutes for oral and sublingual administration (0.09 mg/kg for all routes); sedation lasted 2 hours.[30] Elimination half-lives after oral, sublingual, and IV administration were 8.6 hours, 6.7 hours, and 5.2 hours, respectively.

Acepromazine is metabolized in the liver with both conjugated and unconjugated metabolites eliminated in the urine.[1,31] Metabolites may be found in equine plasma up to 24 hours and urine up to 144 hours after IV administration.[32]

Contraindications/Precautions/Warnings

Acepromazine potentiates the toxicity of organophosphates (including those found in flea collars) and procaine hydrochloride, and it is contraindicated in patients that are receiving or exposed to those agents.[1] There are no other absolute contraindications.

In the United States, the parenteral formulation is only available as a 10 mg/mL concentration. Dilution of the drug or use of very small syringes (eg, tuberculin syringes, U-100 insulin syringes) is important for safe administration to small animal patients. For instance, at a dose of 0.03 mg/kg, a 10-kg (22-lb) dog would receive 0.03 mL of 10 mg/mL acepromazine.

In all species, the tranquilization effects of acepromazine can be overridden by patient arousal, so it cannot always be relied on when used alone as a restraining agent. The effects of acepromazine may be individually variable and breed dependent. Animals will require lower doses of general anesthetics after receiving acepromazine. This is a dose-dependent effect that is true for all species and all inhalant anesthetics in current clinical use.

Acepromazine has no analgesic effects; animals should be treated with appropriate analgesics to control pain. Sedation of painful patients without provision of analgesia can result in the inability to identify pain behaviors with a subsequent negative impact on animal health and welfare.

Acepromazine does not have a reversal agent and requires hepatic metabolism for termination of effect; thus, it should either not be used or should be used cautiously at the low end of the dose range in animals with moderate hepatic dysfunction (eg, some geriatric and pediatric patients) and avoided if the disease/dysfunction is severe.[1,33]

Because of its potential hypotensive effects, acepromazine should either not be used or be used cautiously at the low end of the dose range in patients with mild cardiac disease that may not tolerate drops in blood pressure or in those with decreased sympathetic nervous system response to hypotension (eg, general debilitation, obtundation, neonates, some pediatric and geriatric patients) and avoided in patients with significant cardiac disease, hypovolemia, dehydration, hypotension, or shock.[1,33]

Acepromazine may decrease platelet aggregation and should be avoided or used with caution in patients with coagulopathies or thrombocytopenia.[19,20] Use acepromazine with caution in anemic animals, as splenic red blood cells will exacerbate signs associated with the anemic condition.[34] Acepromazine-mediated splenic engorgement (see ***Pharmacology/Actions***) can make performing a splenectomy difficult; consider other premedication agents for this surgery.

In all species, IV injections should be administered slowly,[1] which is recommended for most sedatives/anesthetic agents to avoid sudden profound sedation or paradoxical excitement. Acepromazine should not be administered intra-arterially, as it may cause severe CNS excitement/depression, seizures, and death.

Acepromazine's vasodilatory effects may be deleterious in compromised horses (eg, acute colic, cantharidin toxicosis, dehydration/hypovolemia, hypotension/shock). In a study of healthy horses, IV infusion of norepinephrine at 1 µg/kg/minute reversed the hypotensive effects of 0.1 mg/kg acepromazine IV.[35]

Breed-specific concerns include dogs with *MDR1* gene mutation (also known as *ABCB1*-1delta), which may develop a more pronounced sedation that persists longer than expected.[36] The drug is best completely avoided in *MDR1*-mutant dogs because there is no reversal, but if no other option is available, the dose should be reduced by 25% in dogs that are heterozygous and by 30% to 50% in dogs that are homozygous for the *MDR1* gene mutation (mutant/mutant).[36,37] Spontaneous fainting or syncope due to sinoatrial block caused by excessive vagal tone has been observed in some dogs, particularly boxers and other brachycephalic breeds; a low acepromazine dose should be used with or without atropine in these patients.[38] **NOTE:** This issue has only been reported in boxers (and *not* other brachycephalic breeds) and may be present in a familial line, as it is rarely reported, especially outside the UK. When there is a history of this type of syncope, or if it is suspected because of excessive sinus arrhythmia, it may be advantageous to control the dysrhythmia with atropine administered just before the acepromazine.[38]

Acepromazine should be used very cautiously as a restraining agent in aggressive dogs, as it may make the animal more prone to startle and react to noises or other sensory inputs and can potentially make them more aggressive; it is best used in combination with other restraining agents in these situations. In some geriatric patients, very low doses have been associated with prolonged effects of the drug, likely due to slowed hepatic metabolism. Anecdotally, giant breeds appear to be sensitive to the drug, whereas terrier breeds appear to be somewhat resistant to its effects; however, this is most likely based on use of body weight instead of body surface area for dose calculation.[34]

Adverse Effects

The potential for acepromazine-mediated hypotension and possible reflex tachycardia should be considered during treatment planning. This effect is mediated by central mechanisms and through the alpha-adrenergic antagonistic action of the drug. Secondary tachycardia may accompany the hypotension.[1] Cardiovascular collapse (secondary to bradycardia and hypotension) can occur after rapid IV injection[1] and has been reported in dogs following IM administration of supraclinical doses (1 mg/kg).[39] Atropine may be used to treat this effect.[38] Splenic sequestration of red blood cells may cause transient decreases in PCV. See ***Pharmacology/Actions***.

Occasionally, an animal may develop the contradictory clinical signs of aggressiveness and generalized CNS stimulation after receiving acepromazine. For orally administered acepromazine tablets, mild respiratory distress (ie, reverse sneeze) has been reported and does not have an effect on the desired action of the drug.

Acepromazine causes prolapse of the nictitating membrane and has been shown to decrease tear production in cats[40] and rabbits.[41]

In horses, acepromazine may cause protrusion of the penis; this effect is dose-related and may last for 2 or more hours.[17] Permanent penile dysfunction in horses and ponies is possible, but a retrospective study found the risk to be extremely low (less than or equal to 1 in 10,000).[42] The main contributor to permanent penile dysfunction is prolonged protrusion and subsequent penile edema followed by inability to retract the penis and worsening edema. If using acepromazine in male horses, ensure penile retraction occurs within 1 hour of protrusion.

Acepromazine inhibits the voltage-gated K+ channel (Kv11.1), which may induce repolarization disorders and lead to drug–drug interactions that prolong the QT interval[43]; however, this seems to have no clinical impact.

IM administration may cause transient pain at the injection site, which is possibly related to the injection itself rather than the drug. SC administration may be less painful than IM while providing similar sedation.[44]

In addition to the legal aspects (ie, extra-label; not FDA-approved) of using acepromazine in cattle, the drug may cause regurgitation of ruminal contents when sedation is followed by general anesthesia.

Reproductive/Nursing Safety

Acepromazine injection is listed as contraindicated in pregnant animals on at least one international drug label[38]; however, acepromazine has been used safely in late-term pregnant cattle[45] and ferrets.[46] Use of the drug in cesarean sections in dogs and cats is not recommended because of the prolonged duration of recovery and potential for hypotension. Excretion of the drug in milk has not been evaluated; however, acepromazine has been used in mares to promote lactation (secondary to increased prolactin production) and facilitate adoption of orphan foals. In one case report, acepromazine (30 mg IM every 8 hours for 48 hours) administered to a thoroughbred mare increased milk production, calmed the mare, and promoted bonding with an orphan foal while having no impact on the mare's concurrent pregnancy.[47]

Because safety has not been established in animals, this drug should only be used when the maternal benefits outweigh the potential risks to offspring.

Overdose/Acute Toxicity

LD_{50} in mice is 59 mg/kg after IV administration, 130 mg/kg after SC administration, and 200 mg/kg after oral administration.[48] A toxicity study in dogs reported no adverse effects in dogs receiving 20 – 40 mg/kg over 6 weeks[1]; however, anecdotally, adverse effects have been reported in dogs receiving single doses between 20 and 42 mg/kg. Dogs have survived oral doses up to 220 mg/kg, but overdoses can cause severe hypotension, CNS depression, pulmonary edema, and/or hyperemia of the internal organs.[1] Acepromazine overdose can also cause extrapyramidal effects (eg, tremor, catalepsy, rigidity, excitement, sweating, seizures) via dopamine blockade.[49]

Because of the relatively low toxicity of acepromazine, most overdoses can be handled by monitoring the animal and treating clinical signs as they occur; massive oral overdoses should be treated by gastric decontamination if possible. Hypotension should be treated initially with IV fluids; alpha-adrenergic pressor agents (eg, norepinephrine, phenylephrine; *not* epinephrine) can be considered if IV fluid therapy does not maintain adequate blood pressure. **NOTE:** Epinephrine is contraindicated for treatment of acute hypotension produced by phenothiazine-derivative tranquilizers since further depression of blood pressure can occur.[1,33] This phenomenon is known as epinephrine reversal and could occur when epinephrine is administered after an alpha-adrenergic antagonist (eg, acepromazine). In these situations, the peripheral beta-adrenergic effects of epinephrine will predominate, resulting in relaxation of the vascular smooth musculature and hypotension.

Seizures may be controlled with benzodiazepines. Doxapram has been suggested as an antagonist to the CNS depressant effects of acepromazine, and one study in dogs found that doxapram 1.25 mg/kg IV significantly reduced sedation scores and did not induce panting.[50] See ***Doxapram***.

For patients that have experienced or are suspected to have experienced an overdose, consultation with a 24-hour poison consultation center specializing in providing veterinary-specific information is recommended. For general information related to overdose and toxin exposures, as well as contact information for poison control centers, refer to ***Appendix***.

Drug Interactions

The following drug interactions have either been reported or are theoretical in humans or animals receiving acepromazine or other phenothiazines and may be of significance in veterinary patients. Unless otherwise noted, use together is not necessarily contraindicated, but the potential risks should be weighed, and additional monitoring performed when appropriate.

- **Alpha-2 Agonists** (eg, **dexmedetomidine, xylazine**): Additive risk for CNS depression when used with acepromazine
- **Anesthetic Agents** (eg, **alfaxalone, isoflurane, ketamine**): Additive CNS depression is possible.
- **Antipyretics** (eg, **acetaminophen, dipyrone, NSAIDs**): Possible increased risk for hypothermia with concurrent use
- **Antacids, Aluminum-, Calcium- or Magnesium-Containing:** Concomitant use of acepromazine or other phenothiazines with antacids may cause reduced GI absorption of oral phenothiazines; administration should be separated by at least 2 hours to minimize this effect (with acepromazine being administered before the antacid).[51]
- **Anticholinergic Agents** (eg, **atropine, glycopyrrolate, hyoscyamine**): Increased risk of anticholinergic effects (eg, dry mucous membranes, constipation, urinary retention)
- **Antidiarrheal Mixtures** (eg, **bismuth subsalicylate, kaolin/pectin**): Concomitant use of acepromazine or other phenothiazines with antidiarrheal mixtures may reduce GI absorption of oral phenothiazines; administration should be separated by at least 2 hours to minimize this effect (with acepromazine being administered before the antidiarrheal mixture).[51]
- **Barbiturates** (eg, **pentobarbital, phenobarbital**): Causes additive CNS depression when used with acepromazine. Although this effect is desirable when the 2 drugs/drug classes are used for anesthesia or euthanasia, it may not be desirable if the barbiturates are being used for seizure control in conscious patients.
- **Benzodiazepines** (eg, **diazepam, midazolam**): Additive risk for CNS depression when used with acepromazine
- **Cannabidiol:** Additive risk for CNS depression
- **Cimetidine:** Cimetidine may increase chlorpromazine concentrations; no information for structurally related acepromazine, but combination could lead to excessive sedation and hypotension. Avoid combination if possible.
- **Cisapride:** Concurrent use with acepromazine and other phenothiazines may increase risk for QT interval prolongation, cardiac arrhythmias, torsade de pointes, and death. Acepromazine may reduce prokinetic effect of cisapride. Concurrent use of cisapride with acepromazine or other phenothiazines should be avoided.
- **Dopaminergic Agonists** (eg, **bromocriptine, cabergoline, pergolide**): Concurrent use may reduce the efficacy of both drugs and should be avoided
- **Emetics** (eg, **apomorphine, ropinirole**): Acepromazine may reduce the effectiveness of emetics as well as increased risk for sedation and hypotension.
- **Epinephrine:** Contraindicated in the treatment of acute hypotension produced by acepromazine or other phenothiazines, as further depression of blood pressure can occur (also referred to as epinephrine reversal)
- **Fluoxetine:** May increase chlorpromazine concentration in humans due to inhibition of CYP2D6; the relevance of this interaction for acepromazine use in veterinary species is uncertain
- **Hypotensive Agents** (eg, **amlodipine, benazepril, enalapril, telmisartan**): Concurrent use of acepromazine with hypotensive agents may increase risk for hypotension; monitor blood pressure.
- **Methocarbamol:** Concurrent use may cause additive CNS depression.
- **Metoclopramide:** Concurrent use may increase risk for extrapyramidal adverse effects (eg, tremor, catalepsy, rigidity, excitement, sweating, seizures). Acepromazine may reduce prokinetic effect of metoclopramide.
- **Opioids** (eg, **buprenorphine, fentanyl, morphine**): May enhance the hypotensive effects of the phenothiazines; dosage of acepromazine may need to be reduced when used with an opioid
- **Organophosphate Agents:** Acepromazine should not be given within one month of treatment with or accidental exposure to these agents as organophosphate toxicity may be potentiated.
- **QT Prolonging Agents** (eg, **cisapride, domperidone, erythromycin, sotalol**): Concurrent use may increase risk for QT prolongation and should be avoided.
- **Procaine:** Although not clinically documented, procaine activity may be enhanced by phenothiazines and some resources state that concurrent use with acepromazine is contraindicated.[1,33]
- **Propranolol:** Increased blood concentrations of both propranolol and acepromazine may result if administered concurrently.
- **Quinidine:** Concurrent use with acepromazine or other phenothiazines may cause additive cardiac depression.
- **Sucralfate:** May reduce GI absorption of oral phenothiazines

Laboratory Considerations

- Acepromazine does not alter the results of **glucose tolerance testing** in dogs.[52]
- Because acepromazine has antihistamine effects, it can decrease the wheal-and-flare response to antigens during **intradermal skin testing**. In dogs and cats, it has been suggested that antihistamines be discontinued at least 2 weeks before testing.[53]

Dosages

NOTES:

1. Acepromazine does not provide analgesia; addition of an analgesic agent is required when pain relief is needed.
2. Administer IV doses slowly; allow at least 15 minutes for onset of action.[1]

DOGS & CATS:

NOTE: The label dosage for dogs and cats is considered by most clinicians to be 10 to 100 times (or more) greater than is necessary for most indications. The labeled indications are provided below, but the use of lower, extra-label dosages is strongly recommended.

Dogs: **As an aid in tranquilization, controlling intractable ani-**

mals, and alleviating itching as a result of skin irritation; as an antiemetic to control vomiting associated with motion sickness; and as a preanesthetic agent (label dosage; FDA-approved): 0.55 – 2.2 mg/kg PO (dose may be repeated as required), or 0.55 – 1.1 mg/kg IV, IM, or SC[1,33]

Cats: **As an aid in controlling intractable animals and alleviating itching as a result of skin irritation, as an antiemetic to control vomiting associated with motion sickness, and as a preanesthetic agent** (label dosage; FDA approved): 1.1 – 2.2 mg/kg IV, IM, or SC[1]

Sedation, tranquilization, premedication, or restraint (extra-label):

1. Injectable: 0.01 – 0.1 mg/kg IV (slowly), IM, or SC generally as a single dose but could be repeated if initial dose is ineffective or after sedative effects have dissipated and continued sedation is desired. Maximum sedation in most patients likely occurs at 0.05 mg/kg.[34] Numerous anesthesia references recommend that total dose should not exceed more than 3 mg (total dose/dog; NOT mg/kg)[54,55]; however, some references recommend a maximum dose of 4 mg (total dose/dog; NOT mg/kg).[38,56] This is especially true in large breed dogs[55] who appear more "sensitive" to higher dosages of acepromazine, which is actually due to dosing on a mg/kg basis rather than on a body surface area basis.[34]
   a. Anesthetic premedication: 0.02 – 0.05 mg/kg IM, SC, or slow IV. Lower doses (ie, 0.02 – 0.03 mg/kg) are sufficient for most patients, especially when the drug is combined with an opioid. The lower end of the dosing range should be used for IV administration. Following acepromazine administration, anesthetic induction agent doses can often be reduced by ≈30%.
   b. Tranquilization/sedation: 0.03 – 0.125 mg/kg IM, SC, or slow IV.[38] Dosages in the preanesthetic range are often sufficient, especially when combined with an opioid. The lower end of the dosing range should be used for IV administration. Lower doses should be used for tranquilization and higher doses used for sedation. Typically administered as a single dose but could be repeated if initial dose was ineffective or after sedative effects have dissipated and continued sedation is desired; long-term use is not recommended.
2. Oral: Anecdotal dose recommendations vary widely but generally these are similar to the labeled dose range of 0.55 – 2.2 mg/kg PO, although some clinicians think that doses at the higher end of this range are too high. If oral doses require repeating, they are usually given every 6 to 12 hours. Acepromazine also may be given in combination with an anxiolytic medication (eg, gabapentin, trazodone).
3. Transmucosal (TM)
   a. Sedation for cats (anecdotal): Using injectable formulations, 0.05 – 0.1 mg/kg combined with buprenorphine 0.03 mg/kg and administered TM 30 to 90 minutes prior to appointment
   b. Sedation for dogs: Acepromazine 0.025 – 0.05 mg/kg OTM should be administered 30 minutes before the scheduled appointment given in combination with an anxiolytic medication (eg, gabapentin, trazodone), as in the "Chill Protocol" in which the animal receives gabapentin ≈12 hours prior to leaving the home for the veterinary hospital and melatonin and gabapentin PO ≈ 2 hours prior.[57]

Adjunctive treatment of urethral obstruction in male cats (extra-label): 0.25 mg/cat (NOT mg/kg) IM OR 2.5 mg/cat (NOT mg/kg) PO every 8 hours in combination with medetomidine 0.1 mg IM every 24 hours and buprenorphine 0.075 mg PO every 8 hours.[2] Acepromazine is not recommended in obtunded cats as profound hypotension and hypoventilation could occur. See *Contraindications/Precautions/Warnings*.

HORSES:

As an aid in controlling fractious animals and in conjunction with local anesthesia for various procedures and treatments (label dosage; FDA-approved): 0.044 – 0.088 mg/kg (2 – 4 mg/100 lb [45 kg] body weight) IV (slowly), IM, or SC[1]

Sedation, tranquilization, premedication (extra-label): When used alone, acepromazine is usually dosed similarly to the label: 0.02 – 0.1 mg/kg IM, IV, or SC. When used in combination with drugs such as butorphanol as a premedication or to increase blood flow in the treatment of laminitis, recommended doses are usually on the low end of this range. Repeat doses should be limited and ideally not given more frequently than every 36 hours.

Anesthetic premedication, to facilitate restraint, or for sedation during travel (extra-label): Preanesthetic: 0.02 – 0.05 mg/kg IM or slow IV; sedation/restraint: 0.05 – 0.1 mg/kg IM or slow IV. Administer up to 15 minutes prior to the desired effect and await clinical signs of tranquilization before travel or subsequent administration of anesthetic. The low end of the dose range is generally adequate. For tranquilization, adjust dose to maintain desired effect for the duration of travel or procedure.[58,59] These doses can also be used to sedate mares during extended separation from their foals.

Sedation in donkeys: 0.1 mg/kg IV produced sedation ≈10 minutes after administration, which lasted ≈80 minutes.[60,61] In general, horse doses are appropriate for donkeys, but the higher end of the dose range may be necessary to adequately sedate mules.
Laminitis (extra-label): 0.04 – 0.066 mg/kg IM, IV, or SC[5,6,62]

CATTLE:

All dosages are extra-label.
a) **Sedation**: 0.01 – 0.02 mg/kg IV or 0.03 – 0.1 mg/kg IM[63]
b) **Mild sedation or tranquilization**: 0.02 – 0.05 mg/kg IV, 0.02 – 0.1 mg/kg IM[64]
c) **Sedative 1 hour before local anesthesia**: 0.1 mg/kg IM[64]

SHEEP & GOATS:

Sedation (extra-label): 0.05 – 0.1 mg/kg IM.[65] Sedation in sheep was equivalent when acepromazine 0.03 mg/kg IM was administered either with morphine 0.3 mg/kg IM or buprenorphine 0.02 mg/kg IM.[66] The low end of the dose is generally adequate.

SWINE:

NOTE: When used as a single agent in swine, the effects of acepromazine are inconsistent and may be inadequate.

Sedation (extra-label):
a) 0.1 – 0.2 mg/kg IV, IM,[67] or SC[68]
b) 0.03 – 0.1 mg/kg IM[65,69]

Brief periods of immobilization (extra-label): Acepromazine 0.5 mg/kg in combination with ketamine 15 mg/kg IM.[67] Atropine 0.044 mg/kg IM will reduce salivation and bronchial secretions.[70]

FERRETS:

All dosages are extra-label.
a) **Tranquilization:** 0.25 – 0.75 mg/kg IM or SC[46] ; the lower to mid-range of the dosage is generally adequate.
b) **Premedication:** 0.1 – 0.25 mg/kg IM or SC; may cause hypotension/hypothermia[71]

RABBITS, RODENTS, & SMALL MAMMALS:

All dosages are extra-label.
a) **Rabbits: Sedative/tranquilization**: 0.75 – 1 mg/kg IM. Effect should begin 10 minutes after administration and last for 1 to 2 hours.[63,72]

b) **Rabbits: Premedication:** 0.2 – 1 mg/kg SC, IM[73,74]
c) **Mice, rats, hamsters, guinea pigs, chinchillas:** 0.5 – 1.5 mg/kg IM, SC; 0.5 – 2.5 mg/kg PO. Can be used IP in some species. Use in gerbils is not recommended by some clinicians.[75]

Monitoring

- Cardiac rate and rhythm, blood pressure (critical), end-tidal carbon dioxide ($ETCO_2$), and pulse oximetry (recommended)
- PCV and total protein, especially in borderline anemic patients and patients with current or expected blood loss
- Degree of sedation/tranquilization
- Male horses should be checked to make sure the penis retracts and is not injured.
- Body temperature (especially if ambient temperature is very hot or cold)

Client Information

- This medicine will have the best effect when it is given by mouth 45 to 60 minutes before the procedure or travel. Sedative or tranquilizing effects (sleepiness) and side effects may last up to 24 hours. Your veterinarian may recommend a trial dose a few days before travel to see how your animal reacts to the medicine.
- Animals sedated with this medicine may startle easily in response to sounds or other sudden stimuli. Use caution when approaching your animal as this effect can occasionally make them more aggressive. If this occurs, isolate your animal in a safe environment and contact your veterinarian.
- Keep treated animal in a quiet environment at a comfortable temperature.
- This medicine may cause a harmless pinkish to reddish-brown discoloration of your animal's urine. This change is not to be worried about.
- Do not give additional medicines to tranquilize or sedate your animal unless instructed to do so by your veterinarian.

Chemistry/Synonyms

Acepromazine maleate (formerly acetylpromazine maleate) is a phenothiazine derivative that occurs as an odorless, bitter-tasting, yellow powder. One gram is soluble in 27 mL of water, 13 mL of alcohol, or 3 mL of chloroform. The injection is a clear, pale yellow to yellow solution.

Acepromazine maleate may also be known as ACE, *Aceproject®*, *Aceprotabs®*, acetylpromazine maleate, *Acevet®*, ACP, *Atravet®*, *Notensil®*, *PromAce®*, and *Plegicil®*.

Storage/Stability

Store tablets and injection protected from light at 20°C to 25°C (68°F-77°F), with excursions permitted between 15°C and 30°C (59°F-86°F). Tablets should be stored in tight containers. There is no limit to the number of vial punctures throughout the full expiry period.[1]

Compatibility/Compounding Considerations

Compatibility is dependent on factors such as pH, concentration, temperature, and diluent used; specialized references or a hospital pharmacist should be consulted for more specific information.

A study evaluating the stability, sterility, pH, particulate formation, and efficacy of compounded ketamine, acepromazine, and xylazine (KAX) in laboratory rodents supported the finding that the drugs are stable and efficacious for at least 180 days after mixing if stored at room temperature in the dark.[76] When injectable acepromazine is mixed with ketamine and xylazine and diluted with 0.9% saline, drug potency dropped below 90% between 1 and 2 months when stored in syringes at room temperature but retained more than 90% potency for 3 months when stored in syringes under refrigeration.[77] **NOTE:** Admixtures with ketamine or other controlled substances must be stored according to DEA requirements.

Combinations of acepromazine mixed with atropine, buprenorphine, chloral hydrate, meperidine, and oxymorphone have been commonly used, but studies documenting their compatibility and stability were not located. Both glycopyrrolate and diazepam have been reported to be physically **incompatible** with phenothiazines; however, glycopyrrolate has been demonstrated to be **compatible** with promazine HCl for injection.

Dosage Forms/Regulatory Status

VETERINARY-LABELED PRODUCTS:

The Association of Racing Commissioners International (ARCI) has designated this drug as a class 3 substance. Use of this drug may not be allowed in certain animal competitions. Check rules and regulations before entering in a competition while this medication is being administered. Contact local racing authorities for further guidance. See ***Appendix*** for more information.

Acepromazine Maleate for Injection: 10 mg/mL for injection in 50 mL vials; *PromAce®*, generic; (Rx). FDA-approved forms available for use in dogs, cats, and horses not intended for food. Requires dilution or small syringes for safe and accurate dosing in small animals.

Acepromazine Maleate Tablets: 10 mg and 25 mg in bottles of 100 and 500 tablets; *PromAce®*, generic; (Rx)

In other countries, acepromazine is formulated in oral gels and powders and in varying strengths of injectable solutions (eg, 2 mg/mL, 25 mg/mL).

When used in an extra-label manner in food animals, it is recommended to contact Food Animal Residue Avoidance Databank (FARAD; see ***Appendix***) for further guidance.

HUMAN-LABELED PRODUCTS: NONE

References

For the complete list of references, see **wiley.com/go/budde/plumb**

Acetaminophen

APAP, Paracetamol

(ah-seet-a-***min***-a-fen) *Tylenol®*

Analgesic, Antipyretic

Prescriber Highlights

- **Contraindicated in cats and ferrets at any dosage**
- At recommended dosages, not overly toxic to dogs, rodents, or rabbits. Dogs are more susceptible than humans to red blood cell toxicity, so dose carefully.
- Often used in combined dosage forms with codeine, tramadol, or hydrocodone

Uses/Indications

Acetaminophen is used as an oral analgesic or antipyretic in dogs, horses, and small mammals. It may be particularly beneficial for the treatment of chronic pain conditions in dogs for which other analgesics (eg, NSAIDS, opioids) should not be used. In a clinical trial, acetaminophen was as effective as meloxicam and carprofen for postsurgical analgesia in bitches undergoing elective ovariohysterectomy.[1] For moderate pain, acetaminophen may be used in combination products containing codeine, hydrocodone, or tramadol. See the ***Codeine***, ***Tramadol***, and ***Hydrocodone Combinations*** monographs for more information on the use of acetaminophen combination preparations.

Acetaminophen has also been used for research purposes to measure gastric emptying in a variety of large animal species.[2-5]

Pharmacology/Actions

Acetaminophen's exact mechanisms of action are not completely understood. It produces analgesia and antipyresis via inhibition of cyclooxygenase and peroxidase sites on prostaglandin H_2 synthetase.[6] In addition, serotonergic activity may contribute to the drug's analgesic effect.[7] Unlike aspirin, acetaminophen does not possess significant anti-inflammatory activity or inhibit platelet function when given at clinically recommended dosages.

Pharmacokinetics

In dogs, acetaminophen oral bioavailability is 45%. Peak concentrations occur 20 to 50 minutes after oral dosing. Protein binding is ≈25%, and volume of distribution is 0.9 L/kg. Clearance is 1.5 to 2 L/kg/hour. Elimination half-life is ≈1 to 4 hours and appears to vary by breed.[8-13] Maximum plasma concentration, time at maximum concentration, and bioavailability are not affected by feeding in dogs.[14] In a study of hospitalized dogs receiving acetaminophen orally or rectally, rectal absorption was only 30% that of oral administration, and the drug did not reach concentrations associated with efficacy.[12]

In horses, peak concentration is reached ≈60 to 80 minutes after oral administration. Bioavailability is 91%. Volume of distribution is 0.82 to 2.7 L/kg and protein binding is 49%. Clearance is ≈0.25 L/kg/hour and elimination half-life is ≈2 to 4 hours.[11,15-17]

Acetaminophen was found to be stable in rumen fluid from cattle[18] and goats.[5] Oral bioavailability in cattle was 70%, peak concentration was reached after 1.4 hours, and elimination half-life was 2.4 hours.[18] In goats, oral bioavailability (16%) appeared to be limited, not by ruminal activity, but by first-pass metabolism.[5] Volume of distribution was 1.4 L/kg, and clearance was 53 mL/kg/minute.[19]

Similar bioavailability (42% to 75%) and half-lives (0.6 to 1.2 hours) were observed in a multi-species study that included pigs, turkeys, and chickens.[11]

Contraindications/Precautions/Warnings

Acetaminophen is contraindicated in cats at any dosage. Severe methemoglobinemia, hematuria, and icterus can be seen. Cats are deficient in glucuronyl transferases and are therefore unable to sufficiently glucuronidate acetaminophen; this leads to formation of active toxic metabolites (eg, free oxygen radicals) that cause oxidative injury and results in methemoglobinemia and formation of Heinz bodies in red blood cells. Acetaminophen should not be used in ferrets,[20] as in vitro studies indicate they may be as sensitive to acetaminophen as cats. At this time, acetaminophen should also not be used in sugar gliders or hedgehogs, as its safety has not been determined.

Dogs do not metabolize acetaminophen as well as humans do and its use must be judicious. Although dogs are not as sensitive as cats to acetaminophen, they may still be susceptible to methemoglobinemia when acetaminophen is prescribed at high dosages. Anecdotally, some dogs may be idiosyncratically sensitive to acetaminophen and some dogs may develop hepatotoxicity if acetaminophen is used chronically at therapeutic doses.[21]

Adverse Effects

At suggested dosages in dogs, there is potential for adverse renal, hepatic, GI, and hematologic effects. Higher dosages (3 times recommended) can cause keratoconjunctivitis sicca. In horses given acetaminophen for 14 days, increased total bilirubin and reduced sorbitol dehydrogenase activity were noted, and evidence of mild portal inflammation was noted on liver biopsies.[15]

Reproductive/Nursing Safety

Acetaminophen crosses the placenta.[22] Absolute reproductive safety has not been established; however, acetaminophen is considered relatively safe for occasional use in pregnancy.[23-25] In laboratory animals given acetaminophen at doses 0.85 to 1.2 times the maximum human dose (MHD, 4 g/day), reduced fetal weight and skeletal ossification, and focal renal and hepatic necrosis were observed.[26] Abnormal sperm and reduced testicular weight were noted in animals given 1.2 times MHD.[26]

Acetaminophen is excreted in milk in low concentrations with reported milk:plasma ratios of 0.91 to 1.42 at 1 and 12 hours, respectively; it is considered acceptable to administer to pregnant women.[27] In nursing human infants, no adverse effects have been reported.

Because safety has not been established in animals, this drug should only be used when the maternal benefits outweigh the potential risks to offspring.

Overdose/Acute Toxicity

Cats are highly susceptible to methemoglobinemia development because of their inability to glucuronidate acetaminophen, and there is no dose for cats that is considered safe. In the first few hours following ingestion, cats may present with swelling of the face and limbs. Doses of 40 mg/kg can cause methemoglobinemia, although some cats have been reported to develop it at 10 mg/kg. Because cats can develop methemoglobinemia rapidly after ingestion of acetaminophen, do not delay N-acetylcysteine treatment, and preferably give the first dose IV. See ***N-Acetylcysteine***. Clinical signs associated with methemoglobinemia include respiratory distress, cyanosis, depression, hypothermia, weakness, edema, and death. Hepatotoxicity occurs at higher doses; most cats are presented with methemoglobinemia signs before signs of hepatotoxicity develop.[28]

In dogs, hepatotoxicity generally occurs at doses greater than 75 – 100 mg/kg,[29,30] and clinical signs (eg, icterus, vomiting, anorexia, abdominal pain; coagulopathy, hypoglycemia, hepatic encephalopathy in severe cases) usually develop within 24 to 48 hours after ingestion. Many authors advise intervention with doses greater than 50 mg/kg. Methemoglobinemia generally occurs with doses greater than 200 mg/kg with clinical signs similar to those seen in cats. Signs typically develop 1 to 4 hours postexposure and persist for 12 to 48 hours. If the patient is left untreated, death can occur between 18 to 36 hours postexposure. Keratoconjunctivitis sicca can be seen with doses greater than 30 mg/kg, with clinical signs first seen 48 to 72 hours after exposure.[28]

For overdoses in dogs or cats, standard GI decontamination techniques with supportive care should be administered when applicable. Further treatment with N-acetylcysteine, *S*-adenosyl-methionine (SAMe), oxygen, and blood transfusions may be warranted.[29,31-34]

For patients that have experienced or are suspected to have experienced an overdose, consultation with a 24-hour poison consultation center specializing in providing veterinary-specific information is recommended. For general information related to overdose and toxin exposures, as well as contact information for poison control centers, refer to ***Appendix***.

Drug Interactions

The following drug interactions with acetaminophen have either been reported or are theoretical in humans or animals and may be of significance in veterinary patients. Unless otherwise noted, use together is not necessarily contraindicated, but weigh the potential risks and perform additional monitoring when appropriate.

- **Anesthetics, Local** (eg, **bupivacaine, lidocaine, mepivacaine, ropivacaine**): Concurrent use may increase the risk for methemoglobinemia.
- **Barbiturates** (eg, **phenobarbital, primidone**): Increased conversion of acetaminophen to hepatotoxic metabolites; potentially increased risk for hepatotoxicity
- **Cholestyramine:** May reduce oral acetaminophen absorption; administer separately
- **Chloramphenicol:** Increased acetaminophen concentration noted in humans; veterinary significance is unclear.
- **Dipyrone:** Combined used may increase risk for hepatocellular injury.

- **Doxorubicin**: May deplete hepatic glutathione, leading to increased hepatic toxicity
- **Fenbendazole**: May increase the risk for hepatotoxicity (study done in mice)[35]
- **Isoniazid**: Increased conversion of acetaminophen to hepatotoxic metabolites with possible increased risk for hepatotoxicity
- **Leflunomide**: May increase the risk for hepatotoxicity
- **Metoclopramide:** May increase acetaminophen absorption
- **Metyrapone**: May reduce acetaminophen conjugation, potentially increasing formation of toxic acetaminophen metabolites
- **Penicillin G Benzathine and/or Procaine**: Concurrent use of the benzathine and/or procaine penicillin G salts may increase risk for methemoglobinemia.
- **Phenothiazines** (eg, **acepromazine**): Possible increased risk for hypothermia
- **Probenecid**: May increase acetaminophen concentration and alter its metabolism, potentially increasing formation of toxic acetaminophen metabolites
- **Propylene Glycol**: Foods containing propylene glycol (often found in wet cat foods) may increase the severity of acetaminophen-induced methemoglobinemia or Heinz body formation.
- **Rifampin**: May increase the risk for hepatotoxicity
- **Verdinexor**: Increases of serum concentration of either drug are possible due to competitive inhibition of glutathione S-transferase. Avoid combination if possible or monitor closely for adverse effects of each drug if combination cannot be avoided.
- **Warfarin**: Although acetaminophen is relatively safe to use, large doses may potentiate anticoagulant effects.

Laboratory Considerations

- False positive results may occur for urinary **5-hydroxyindoleacetic acid** (serotonin metabolite).

Dosages

NOTE: For dosages of acetaminophen combination products (with codeine or hydrocodone), refer to the individual *Codeine* and *Hydrocodone Combinations* monographs, respectively.

DOGS:

Analgesic or antipyretic (extra-label): 10 – 15 mg/kg PO or rectally every 8 hours; if using long-term (ie, more than 5 days), consider giving every 12 hours at the lower end of dosing range.

HORSES:

Analgesic or antipyretic (extra-label): 20 mg/kg PO once as single dose, or given twice daily[36,37]

RABBITS/RODENTS/SMALL MAMMALS:

Analgesic (extra-label): Using Children's *Tylenol*®, 1 – 2 mg acetaminophen/mL of drinking water. Effective for controlling mild to moderate pain[38–41]

Monitoring

- When used at recommended doses for pain control in otherwise healthy patients, little monitoring should be necessary. However, with chronic therapy, baseline and periodic liver, renal, and hematologic monitoring may be warranted, particularly when clinical signs occur.

Client Information

- Must **NEVER** be used in **cats**. Do **NOT** use in ferrets.
- Watch for side effects and contact your veterinarian if you see any of the following: dog stops eating, whites of the eyes become yellowish, continued vomiting or diarrhea, or blood seen in vomit or stool.
- Do **NOT** give more than your veterinarian prescribes. Unless your veterinarian instructs, do **NOT** give with other pain or fever medicine.
- Keep out of reach of children.

Chemistry/Synonyms

A synthetic nonopioid analgesic, acetaminophen (also known as paracetamol) occurs as a crystalline white powder with a slightly bitter taste. It is soluble in boiling water and freely soluble in alcohol. Acetaminophen is known in the UK as paracetamol.

Acetaminophen may also be known as paracetamol, *N*-acetyl-*p*-aminophenol, MAPAP or APAP; many trade names are available, *Tylenol*® is one common name.

Storage/Stability

Acetaminophen products should be stored at temperatures less than 40°C (104°F). Do not freeze the oral solution or suspension.

Compatibility/Compounding Considerations

Nonextended-release tablets may be split or crushed and mixed with food immediately prior to administration.

Dosage Forms/Regulatory Status

VETERINARY-LABELED PRODUCTS: NONE

The Association of Racing Commissioners International (ARCI) has designated this drug as a class 4 substance. See *Appendix* for more information. Use of this drug may not be allowed in certain animal competitions. Check rules and regulations before entering in a competition while this medication is being administered. Contact local racing authorities for further guidance.

HUMAN-LABELED PRODUCTS:

There are many different trade names and products of acetaminophen available commercially. The most commonly known trade name is *Tylenol*®. Acetaminophen is available in 160 mg, 325 mg, and 500 mg tablets, capsules, or caplets; 80 mg chewable tablets; 650 mg extended-release tablets; 32 mg/mL oral liquids, and 60 mg, 80 mg, 120 mg, 125 mg, 250 mg, 325 mg, and 650 mg rectal suppositories. Combinations with other analgesics (aspirin, codeine phosphate, hydrocodone, tramadol, or oxycodone) or antihistamines (diphenhydramine) are also available.

References

For the complete list of references, see **wiley.com/go/budde/plumb**

Acetazolamide
Acetazolamide Sodium

(a-set-a-***zole***-a-mide) *Diamox*®

Carbonic Anhydrase Inhibitor Diuretic; Antiglaucoma Agent

Prescriber Highlights

- ► May be used to treat metabolic alkalosis or glaucoma in small animals and hyperkalemic periodic paralysis (HYPP) in horses
- ► Contraindicated in patients with significant hepatic, renal, pulmonary, or adrenocortical insufficiency, hyponatremia, hypokalemia, hyperchloremic acidosis, or electrolyte imbalance
- ► Give oral doses with food if GI upset occurs.
- ► Electrolytes and acid–base status should be monitored with chronic or high-dose therapy.
- ► Monitor with tonometry if using for glaucoma.

Uses/Indications

Acetazolamide has been used principally in veterinary medicine for its diuretic action and its effects on aqueous humor production in the treatment of metabolic alkalosis and glaucoma, respectively. This drug may be useful as an adjunctive treatment for increased CSF pressures associated with syringomyelia in dogs[1]; however, acetazolamide was ineffective in reducing clinical signs or the ventricle:brain ratio in dogs with idiopathic communicating hydrocephalus.[2]

In horses, acetazolamide is used as a preventive and/or treatment for HYPP.

In humans, the drug has been used as adjunctive therapy for treatment of epilepsy and acute high-altitude sickness.

Pharmacology/Actions

Carbonic anhydrase inhibitors (CAIs) act via a noncompetitive, reversible inhibition of the enzyme carbonic anhydrase. Inhibition reduces the formation of hydrogen and bicarbonate ions from carbonic acid, which reduces the availability of these ions for active transport into body secretions.

Within the eye, the pharmacologic effect of CAIs is decreased formation of aqueous humor, which reduces intraocular pressure (IOP). Within the kidney, the pharmacologic effect of CAIs is increased renal tubular secretion of sodium and potassium and, to a greater extent, bicarbonate, leading to increased urine alkalinity and volume. Acetazolamide has some anticonvulsant activity, which is independent of its diuretic effects. This mechanism is not fully understood but may be caused by an effect on carbonic anhydrase in the brain or induction of metabolic acidosis.

In a study comparing the effects of acetazolamide and methazolamide in anesthetized cats, methazolamide did not reduce the hypoxic ventilatory response, but acetazolamide did. The study authors believe this response was not a result of carbonic anhydrase inhibition but instead was caused by acetazolamide's effects on carotid bodies or type I cells.[3]

Pharmacokinetics

One report states that in small animal species given acetazolamide 22 mg/kg (2 to 5 times the standard dosage), the onset of action for reduction of IOP is 30 minutes, maximal effects occur after 2 to 4 hours, and duration of action is ≈4 to 6 hours.[4]

In horses, IV administration of acetazolamide results in a high mean clearance rate (4.5 mL/kg/min) and a short mean residence time (1.71 hours). Immediate-release formulations show a low oral bioavailability (25%) with maximum concentrations of 1.9 µg/mL.[5]

In humans, the drug is well absorbed after oral administration, with peak concentrations occurring within 1 to 3 hours. The drug is distributed throughout the body, and the highest concentrations are found in the kidneys, plasma, and erythrocytes. Within 24 hours of oral tablet administration, an average of 90% of the drug is excreted unchanged into the urine by tubular secretion and passive reabsorption processes.

Contraindications/Precautions/Warnings

Carbonic anhydrase inhibitors (CAIs) are contraindicated in patients hypersensitive to them and in patients with significant hepatic disease (may precipitate hepatic coma), renal or adrenocortical insufficiency, hyponatremia, hypokalemia, hyperchloremic acidosis, or other electrolyte imbalances. This class of drugs should not be used in patients with severe pulmonary obstruction that are unable to increase alveolar ventilation.

Acetazolamide should be used with caution in patients with severe respiratory acidosis or in those with pre-existing hematologic abnormalities. Chronic, high-dose administration may lead to decreased exercise capacity, hypercapnia, and respiratory acidosis in healthy horses during exercise.[6]

Although acetazolamide is a sulfonamide, cross-reactivity with antibacterial sulfonamides or furosemide does not appear to occur.[7] Do not confuse acetaZOLAMIDE with acetoHEXAMIDE or acetaMINOPHEN.

Adverse Effects

Potential adverse effects include GI disturbances (eg, nausea, vomiting, diarrhea, anorexia), CNS effects (eg, sedation, depression, weakness, excitement, paresthesias), hematologic effects (eg, bone marrow depression), renal effects (eg, crystalluria, dysuria, renal colic, polyuria), hypokalemia, hyperchloremia, hyperglycemia, hyponatremia, hyperuricemia, hepatic insufficiency, dermatologic effects (eg, rash), and hypersensitivity reactions, which includes Stevens-Johnson syndrome and toxic epidermal necrolysis. Acidosis occurred after IV administration of high-dose acetazolamide in dogs, and 3 dogs displayed mild tremors that resolved within 1 hour after administration.[8]

At the dosages used for HYPP in horses, adverse effects are reportedly uncommon.[9]

Reproductive/Nursing Safety

Acetazolamide crosses the placenta in unknown quantities. Acetazolamide has caused limb defects in laboratory animals and reduced fetal weight and incisor development in rats.[10] No effects on fertility were noted in rats. Fetal toxicity has been noted when the drug has been used in pregnant humans.

Acetazolamide is excreted in milk. Because safety has not been established in animals, this drug should only be used when the maternal benefits outweigh the potential risks to offspring. If unavoidable, use milk replacer instead of allowing offspring to nurse.

Overdose/Acute Toxicity

Information regarding overdose with this drug is not available. Monitor serum electrolytes, venous blood gases (including pH), hydration status, and CNS status during an acute overdose; treat clinical signs and provide supportive treatment. Acetazolamide is dialyzable.

For patients that have experienced or are suspected to have experienced an overdose, consultation with a 24-hour poison consultation center specializing in providing veterinary-specific information is recommended. For general information related to overdose and toxin exposures, as well as contact information for poison control centers, refer to *Appendix*.

Drug Interactions

The following drug interactions have either been reported or are theoretical in humans or animals receiving acetazolamide and may be of significance in veterinary patients. Unless otherwise noted, use together is not necessarily contraindicated, but weigh the potential risks and perform additional monitoring when appropriate.

- **Cyclosporine**: Acetazolamide may increase concentrations.
- **Digoxin**: As acetazolamide may cause hypokalemia, there is an increased risk for digoxin toxicity.
- **Drugs Affecting Potassium** (eg, **amphotericin B, corticosteroids** [eg, **dexamethasone, prednis(ol)one**], **corticotropin, or other diuretics**): Concomitant use may exacerbate potassium depletion.
- **Folic Acid Antagonists** (eg, **pyrimethamine, sulfadiazine, sulfadimethoxine, trimethoprim**): May augment folic acid antagonism
- **Insulin**: Rarely, CAIs interfere with the hypoglycemic effects of insulin.
- **Methenamine Compounds**: Acetazolamide may negate methenamine effects in the urine.
- **Methotrexate:** May augment folic acid antagonism
- **Phenobarbital**: Acetazolamide-induced alkaline urine may increase urinary excretion and compromise efficacy.
- **Primidone**: May reduce primidone absorption and serum concentration
- **Procainamide**: Acetazolamide-induced alkaline urine may decrease urinary excretion of procainamide; procainamide toxicity is possible.
- **Quinidine**: Acetazolamide-induced alkaline urine may decrease urinary excretion of quinidine; quinidine toxicity is possible.

- **Salicylates** (eg, **aspirin, bismuth subsalicylate**): Increased risk for acetazolamide accumulation and toxicity; increased risk for metabolic acidosis
- **Sodium Bicarbonate**: Increased risk for development of renal calculi
- **Tricyclic Antidepressants (TCAs**; eg, **amitriptyline, clomipramine**): Acetazolamide-induced alkaline urine may decrease TCA urinary excretion.

Laboratory Considerations

- CAIs alkalinize the urine, which can cause false positive results for **urine protein** when using bromphenol blue reagent (*Albustix®, Albutest®, Labstix®*), sulfosalicylic acid (*Bumintest®, Exton's® Test Reagent*), nitric acid ring test, or heat and acetic acid test methods.
- Carbonic anhydrase inhibitors may **decrease iodine uptake** via the thyroid gland in hyperthyroid or euthyroid patients and, therefore, lower thyroid hormone concentrations.
- May interfere with HPLC determination of **theophylline** concentrations.

Dosages

DOGS:

Adjunctive therapy for treatment of glaucoma or metabolic alkalosis (extra-label): 4 – 10 mg/kg PO every 8 to 12 hours or IV once

Paroxysmal dyskinesias (extra-label): From a case report, 4 mg/kg PO every 8 hours[11]

CATS:

Adjunctive therapy for treatment of glaucoma (extra-label): 6 – 8 mg/kg PO every 8 to 12 hours

HORSES:

Prevention or adjunctive therapy for treatment of hyperkalemic periodic paralysis (HYPP) episodes (extra-label): 2.2 – 4.4 mg/kg PO twice daily[9,12]

Monitoring

- Intraocular pressure (tonometry) if used for glaucoma
- Venous blood gases if used for treatment of metabolic alkalosis
- Serum electrolytes
- Baseline and periodic CBC with differential and serum chemistry profile if using chronically
- Other adverse effects (eg, vomiting diarrhea, sedation, weakness)

Client Information

- The most common side effect of this drug is stomach upset; giving with food may help reduce this effect.
- Contact your veterinarian immediately if unusual panting or rapid breathing, weakness, staggering, behavior changes, tremors, or seizures (ie, convulsions) are seen.
- Horses must have access to **fresh** water and food while taking this medication.
- Animals will need ongoing laboratory tests while taking this medicine. Do not miss these important follow-up visits.

Chemistry/Synonyms

Acetazolamide, a CAI, occurs as a white to faintly yellowish-white, odorless, crystalline powder with pK_as of 7.4 and 9.1. It is slightly soluble in water and sparingly soluble in hot water (90°C-100°C [194°F-212°F]) and alcohol. Acetazolamide sodium occurs as a white lyophilized solid and is freely soluble in water. The injection has a pH of 9.2 after reconstitution with sterile water for injection.

Acetazolamide may also be known as acetazolam, acetazolamidum, or sodium acetazolamide; *Diamox®* is one of many trade names that are available.

Storage/Stability

Acetazolamide tablets or unreconstituted powder for injection should be stored at room temperature of 20°C to 25°C (68°F-77°F) in a tightly closed container.

After reconstitution, the injection is stable for 3 days when refrigerated or 12 hours at room temperature and should be used within 12 hours.

Compatibility/Compounding Considerations

Acetazolamide sodium for injection is reportedly physically **compatible** with all commonly used IV solutions and cimetidine HCl for injection. Compatibility is dependent on factors such as pH, concentration, temperature, and diluent used; specialized references or a hospital pharmacist should be consulted for more specific information.

Directions for reconstitution of injection: Reconstitute 500 mg vial with at least 5 mL of sterile water for injection; use within 12 hours after reconstitution. For IV use only due to alkaline pH.

Compounded preparation stability: Acetazolamide oral suspension stability when compounded from commercially available tablets has been published.[13] Triturating 12 250 mg tablets with 60 mL of *Ora-Plus®* and qs ad to 120 mL with *Ora-Sweet®* (or *Ora-Sweet® SF*) yields a 25 mg/mL suspension that retains greater than 90% potency for 60 days stored at both 5°C (41°F) and 25°C (77°F). The optimal stability of acetazolamide aqueous liquids is within a pH range of 3 to 5; stability decreases at pH values greater than 9. Compounded preparations of acetazolamide should be protected from light.

Dosage Forms/Regulatory Status

VETERINARY-LABELED PRODUCTS: NONE

The Association of Racing Commissioners International (ARCI) has designated this drug as a class 4 substance. See ***Appendix*** for more information. Use of this drug may not be allowed in certain animal competitions. Check rules and regulations before entering in a competition while this medication is being administered. Contact local racing authorities for further guidance.

HUMAN-LABELED PRODUCTS:

Acetazolamide Oral Tablets: 125 mg, 250 mg; generic; (Rx)

Acetazolamide Extended-Release Oral Capsules: 500 mg; generic; (Rx)

Acetazolamide Sodium Injection (Lyophilized Powder for Solution): 500 mg; generic; (Rx)

References

For the complete list of references, see **wiley.com/go/budde/plumb**

Acetic Acid

Vinegar

(ah-***see***-tick ***ass***-id)

GI Acidifier

Prescriber Highlights

- ► Used primarily for treatment of nonprotein nitrogen-induced ammonia toxicosis (eg, secondary to urea poisoning) in ruminants or enterolith prevention in horses
- ► Do not use concentrated acetic acid; use only vinegar (3%-5% acetic acid).
- ► Contraindicated if lactic acidosis (eg, grain overload, rumen acidosis) is possible
- ► Administered via stomach tube

Uses/Indications

Acetic acid is used for its acidifying qualities in ruminants to treat nonprotein nitrogen-induced (eg, urea poisoning) ammonia toxicosis. It is also used as a potential adjunctive treatment to prevent enterolith formation in horses by reducing colonic pH.

Pharmacology/Actions

Acetic acid in the rumen lowers pH by shifting ammonia (NH_3) to ammonium ions (NH_4^+) to reduce ammonia absorption; it may also slow the hydrolysis of urea.

Pharmacokinetics

No information is noted.

Contraindications/Precautions/Warnings

Acetic acid should not be administered to ruminants until lactic acidosis (eg, grain overload, rumen acidosis) is ruled out.

Do **NOT** use concentrated forms of acetic acid; use only vinegar (3%-5% acetic acid).

Adverse Effects

Because of the unpleasant taste and potential for causing mucous membrane irritation, it is generally recommended to administer acetic acid via stomach tube.

Overdose/Acute Toxicity

When acetic acid is used for appropriate indications, there is little likelihood of serious toxicity occurring after minor overdoses. Because of its potential corrosiveness, the greatest concern is when a concentrated form of acetic acid is mistakenly used.

Drug Interactions

There are no documented drug interactions with oral acetic acid. Because of its acidic qualities, acetic acid could theoretically affect the pharmacokinetics of several drugs, which may have clinical significance in veterinary species. Unless otherwise noted, use together is not necessarily contraindicated, but the potential risks should be weighed and additional monitoring performed when appropriate.

- **Aspirin**: Acidified urine can decrease the excretion of salicylates.
- **Azole Antifungals** (eg, **itraconazole, ketoconazole**): Acetic acid may increase absorption of azole antifungal agents.
- **Iron**: Acetic acid may increase iron absorption.
- **Phenobarbital**: Acidified urine can decrease the excretion of phenobarbital.
- **Quinidine**: Acidified urine can decrease the excretion of quinidine.

Dosages

CATTLE/RUMINANTS:

Urea poisoning/nonprotein nitrogen-induced ammonia toxicosis (extra-label): Using 5% acetic acid (ie, vinegar), infuse 4 – 10 L (for cattle) or 250 mL – 1 L (sheep/goats) into the rumen.[1] Follow with cold water (up to 30 L in cattle; 2 – 8 L in sheep/goats) to reduce rumen temperature and reduce formation of urea. Repeat treatment as required if clinical signs reoccur.

HORSES:

Adjunctive treatment for enterolith prevention (extra-label): Using 5% acetic acid (ie, vinegar), add 250 mL/450 kg (250 mL/990 lb) body weight to food once daily.

Chemistry/Synonyms

Glacial acetic acid is $C_2H_4O_2$. Acetic acid has a distinctive odor and a sharp acid taste. It is miscible with water, alcohol, or glycerin. Much confusion can occur with the percentages of $C_2H_4O_2$ contained in various acetic acid solutions. Acetic Acid USP is defined as having a concentration of 36% to 37% $C_2H_4O_2$. Diluted Acetic Acid NF contains 5.7% to 6.3% w/v of $C_2H_4O_2$. Solutions containing ≈3% to 5% w/v of $C_2H_4O_2$ are commonly known as vinegar. Be certain of the concentration of the product you are using and your dilutions.

Acetic acid may also be known as E260, eisessig (glacial acetic acid), essigsäure, etanoico, or ethanoic acid.

Storage/Stability

Acetic acid solutions should be stored in airtight containers.

Compatibility/Compounding Considerations

If diluting more concentrated forms of acetic acid to concentrations equivalent to vinegar (3% to 5%), use safety precautions to protect eyes and skin. It is strongly recommended to have someone check your calculations to prevent potentially serious consequences.

Dosage Forms/Regulatory Status

VETERINARY-LABELED PRODUCTS: NONE

HUMAN-LABELED PRODUCTS: NONE

No systemic products are commercially available. Acetic acid (in various concentrations) may be purchased from chemical supply houses. Distilled white vinegar is available in gallon sizes from grocery stores or mass merchandisers.

References

For the complete list of references, see **wiley.com/go/budde/plumb**

Acetylcysteine

N-Acetylcysteine

NAC, ACC

(assah-teel-***sis***-tay-een) *Mucomyst®*

Antidote; Mucolytic

Prescriber Highlights

- ► Used primarily as a treatment for acetaminophen toxicity or other hepatotoxic conditions in which glutathione synthesis is inhibited or oxidative stress occurs
- ► When using as an antidote, if possible, give first dose IV; oral doses should be given on an empty stomach and via gastric tube.
- ► Has also been used as an inhaled solution for its mucolytic effect and, anecdotally, orally for treating degenerative myelopathy
- ► Administration via nebulization has caused hypersensitivity and bronchospasm.
- ► Dilute prior to IV administration; use a 0.2 micron in-line filter if administering inhalation solution IV

Uses/Indications

Acetylcysteine (*N*-acetylcysteine, NAC) is used in veterinary medicine as both a mucolytic agent in the pulmonary tree and as a treatment for acetaminophen, xylitol, or phenol toxicity in small animals. It potentially could be useful in the adjunctive treatment of sulfonamide hypersensitivity, sago palm hepatotoxicity, mushroom hepatotoxicity, doxorubicin-induced hepatotoxicity, cadmium toxicity, or phenazopyridine toxicity.[1-4] Acetylcysteine may also be used topically in the eye to halt the melting effect of collagenases and proteinases on the cornea (see ***Acetylcysteine Ophthalmic***).

Acetylcysteine has been used anecdotally with aminocaproic acid to treat degenerative myelopathy in dogs, but efficacy data are lacking.

In horses with strangles (ie, *Streptococcus equi* subsp *equi* infection), acetylcysteine instilled into the guttural pouch has been used to help break up chondroids and avoid the need for surgical removal.[5] Acetylcysteine enemas have been used in neonatal foals to break up meconium refractory to repeated enemas. In mares in estrus, intrauterine acetylcysteine instillation could potentially be useful as an adjunctive treatment of endometritis, as acetylcysteine appears to have anti-inflammatory effects on equine endometrial cells and improves pregnancy rates.[6,7]

Pharmacology/Actions

When administered into the pulmonary tree, acetylcysteine reduces the viscosity of both purulent and nonpurulent secretions and expedites the removal of these secretions via coughing, suction, or postural drainage. The free sulfhydryl group on the drug is believed to reduce disulfide linkages in mucoproteins; this effect is most pronounced at a pH from 7 to 9. The drug has no effect on living tissue or fibrin.

In the management of toxicity, acetylcysteine acts as a thiol donor, stimulating glutathione synthesis, and is a free radical scavenger. It also improves hepatic blood flow through increased production of nitric oxide. In acetaminophen hepatotoxicity, glutathione stores are maintained allowing elimination via nontoxic metabolites.

When administered to sick dogs ($n = 30$) during the first 48 hours of hospitalization, acetylcysteine stabilized erythrocyte glutathione concentrations, but when compared with the placebo group, illness severity scores and survival rates were unchanged.[8]

Pharmacokinetics

When given orally, some acetylcysteine is absorbed from the GI tract. Oral bioavailability in healthy cats has been reported as ≈20%.[9] When administered via nebulization or intratracheally into the pulmonary tract, most of the drug is involved in the sulfhydryl-disulfide reaction and the remainder is absorbed. Absorbed drug is converted (deacetylated) into cysteine in the liver and then further metabolized. Elimination half-life in cats is ≈0.8 hours (IV) and ≈1.3 hours (PO). The authors postulated that oral doses of 100 mg/kg may be effective in cats when treating chronic diseases, but additional studies are required to confirm safety and efficacy.[9]

Contraindications/Precautions/Warnings

Acetylcysteine is contraindicated (for pulmonary indications) in animals hypersensitive to it. Use as an antidote has no contraindications.

Acetylcysteine administration via inhalation (nebulization) may cause bronchospasm, and this drug should be used very cautiously, if at all, in animals with bronchospastic conditions (eg, asthma, bronchitis).

Oral or IV administration requires dilution to a 5% (50 mg/mL) solution. Although acetylcysteine is not labeled for injection, this route is used anecdotally; a 0.2 micron in-line filter must be used when giving IV. The taste and smell of the solution is unpleasant (sulfurous), and taste-masking agents (eg, colas, juices) have been used in humans. Because oral dosing of these drugs may be difficult in animals, gastric tubes may be necessary.

Adverse Effects

When given orally for acetaminophen toxicity, acetylcysteine can cause GI effects (eg, nausea, vomiting) and rarely, urticaria.

IV administration appears to be well-tolerated in veterinary patients. IV boluses in humans have caused changes in blood pressure (ie, hyper- or hypotension), GI effects, erythema and flushing 30 to 60 minutes after infusion, and hypersensitivity reactions (eg, in humans, rash, hypotension, wheezing).

Adverse effects reported when acetylcysteine is administered into the pulmonary tract include hypersensitivity, stomatitis, chest tightness, bronchoconstriction, and bronchial or tracheal irritation. A sticky residue may be noted on the face following nebulization with a mask. A study in cats with experimentally induced asthma demonstrated that endotracheal nebulization with acetylcysteine increased airway resistance and caused other adverse effects in some cats, including increased airway secretions, cough, and unilateral strabismus.[10]

Reproductive/Nursing Safety

Acetylcysteine crosses the placenta. Reproduction studies in rabbits and rats have not demonstrated any evidence of teratogenic or embryotoxic effects when used in doses up to 3 times normal. Studies in laboratory animals have not demonstrated impaired fertility.

It is unknown whether acetylcysteine enters milk. Because safety has not been established, this drug should only be used when the maternal benefits outweigh the potential fetal risks.

Overdose/Acute Toxicity

The LD_{50} of acetylcysteine in dogs is 1 g/kg (PO) and 700 mg/kg (IV). It is believed that acetylcysteine is quite safe (with the exception of the adverse effects listed above) in most overdose situations.

For patients that have experienced or are suspected to have experienced an overdose, consultation with a 24-hour poison consultation center specializing in providing veterinary-specific information is recommended. For general information related to overdose and toxin exposures, as well as contact information for poison control centers, refer to *Appendix*.

Drug Interactions

- ACTIVATED CHARCOAL: The use of activated charcoal as a gut adsorbent of acetaminophen is controversial, as charcoal may also adsorb orally-administered acetylcysteine.
- NITROGLYCERIN: May enhance hypotension when given IV concomitantly with acetylcysteine

Dosages

DOGS/CATS:

Maintain or restore glutathione levels for the adjunctive treatment of hepatotoxicity associated with oxidative damage (extra-label): Initial dose 140 – 180 mg/kg IV (dilute to 5% and give via slow IV using a 0.2 micron filter over 15 to 20 minutes) or 280 mg/kg PO (via gastric tube), followed by 70 mg/kg PO or IV every 6 hours for a minimum of 7 treatments.[2,11-13] Large overdoses may require up to 17 doses. IV administration is preferred in serious intoxications or in animals with uncontrolled vomiting.

Canine degenerative myelopathy (extra-label): 25 mg/kg PO every 8 hours for 2 weeks, then every 8 hours every other day. The 20% solution should be diluted to 5% with chicken broth or suitable diluent. Used in conjunction with aminocaproic acid at a dosage of 500 mg per dog (NOT mg/kg) PO every 8 hours indefinitely. Adjunctive treatments may include prednisone (0.25 – 0.5 mg/kg PO daily for 10 days, then every other day), Vitamin C (1000 mg PO every 12 hours), and Vitamin E (1000 units PO every 12 hours). **NOTE:** No treatment has been shown to be effective in published trials.[14]

Adjunctive treatment of hepatic lipidosis (extra-label): Identify underlying cause of anorexia and provide a protein replete feline diet, give acetylcysteine at 140 mg/kg IV over 20 minutes, then 70 mg/kg IV every 12 hours; dilute 10% acetylcysteine with saline 1:4 and administer IV using a 0.2 micron filter.[15] See also *Carnitine*.

HORSES:

To help break up chondroids in the guttural pouch (extra-label): Instill 20% solution.[5]

In neonatal foals to break up meconium refractory to repeated enemas (extra-label): 8 g in 20 g sodium bicarbonate in 200 mL water (pH of 7.6), give as enema as needed to effect[16] or with foal in lateral recumbency, insert a 30 Fr Foley catheter with a 30-cc bulb for a retention enema. Using gravity flow, slowly infuse 100 – 200 mL of 4% acetylcysteine solution and retain for 30 to 45 minutes. IV fluids and pain medication should be considered. Monitor for possible bladder distention.[17]

Monitoring

- When used for inhalational therapy (ie, nebulization), monitor for bronchoconstriction (eg, coughing, wheezing, dyspnea)

- When used for applicable toxicities, monitoring will depend on inciting cause. Some examples include:
  - CBC with methemoglobin value when applicable (eg, acetaminophen toxicity)
  - Serum chemistry profile with electrolytes
  - Hydration status

Client Information

- This agent should be used only in a clinically supervised setting.

Chemistry/Synonyms

The *N*-acetyl derivative of *L*-cysteine, acetylcysteine occurs as a white, crystalline powder with a slight acetic odor. It is freely soluble in water or alcohol.

Acetylcysteine may also be known as *N*-acetylcysteine or *N*-acetyl-*L*-cysteine, NAC, 5052 acetylcysteinum, NSC-111180, *Acetadote®*, *Mucomyst®*, *Cetylev®*, or *ACC®*.

Storage/Stability

When unopened, vials of acetylcysteine should be stored at room temperature, 15°C to 30°C (59°F-86°F). The product labeled for IV use states that it should be used within 24 hours of first use, and that unused portions should be discarded. However, when stored at room temperature (under fluorescent lighting) or under refrigeration, 20% injection repackaged in 3 mL oral syringes (600 mg/3 mL; for oral use) is physically and chemically stable for 6 months.[18] Unopened vials of acetylcysteine solution for inhalation should be stored at 20°C to 25°C (68°F-77°F) with excursions permitted to 15°C to 30°C (59°F-86°F). Opened vials should be kept refrigerated and used within 96 hours.

The color of acetylcysteine solutions may turn from essentially colorless to a slight pink or purple once the vial is opened or the stopper is punctured, but color change does not affect quality or concentration.

Compatibility/Compounding Considerations

Acetylcysteine injection (20%) is hyperosmolar and must be diluted before IV administration. It is **compatible** with dextrose 5% (D5W), sodium chloride 0.45% injection (half-normal saline), and water for injection. Acetylcysteine is **incompatible** with oxidizing agents; solutions can become discolored and liberate hydrogen sulfide when exposed to rubber, copper, and iron, and during autoclaving. It does not react to aluminum, stainless steel, glass, or plastic. If the solution becomes light purple in color, potency is not appreciably affected, but it is best to use nonreactive materials when giving the drug via nebulization. Acetylcysteine solutions are **incompatible** with amphotericin B, ampicillin sodium, erythromycin lactobionate, tetracycline, oxytetracycline, iodized oil, hydrogen peroxide, and trypsin.

In veterinary medicine, acetylcysteine 20% is usually diluted with a compatible solution (see above) to a concentration of 5% (final concentration of 50 mg/mL). This concentration can be obtained by adding 1 part injection (20%) to 3 parts of diluent.

One study reports anacetylcysteine 1.25% solution (12.5 mg/mL) that was created using 0.05 mL of acetylcysteine 20% solution and 0.75 mL of Ciprodex® (ciprofloxacin 0.3% and dexamethasone 0.1%). This study found the solution to be stable for 15 days when refrigerated at 4°C (39°F).[19]

Dosage Forms/Regulatory Status

VETERINARY-LABELED PRODUCTS: NONE

HUMAN-LABELED PRODUCTS:

Acetylcysteine Injection: 20% (200 mg/mL) in 30 mL single-dose vials, preservative free; *Acetadote®*, generic; (Rx). Contains EDTA

Acetylcysteine Oral Capsules: 500 mg and 600 mg; (Rx and OTC). May be labeled as a nutritional product

Acetylcysteine Inhalation or Oral Solution: 10% and 20% (as sodium) in 4 mL, 10 mL, and 30 mL vials; generic; (Rx) **NOTE**: If using this product for dilution and then intravenous dosing, it is preferable to use a 0.2 micron in-line filter. Contains EDTA

References

For the complete list of references, see **wiley.com/go/budde/plumb**

Acyclovir

Acycloguanosine, ACV

(ay-***sye***-kloe-vir) *Zovirax®*

Antiviral, Nucleoside

Prescriber Highlights

- ▶ Used primarily in birds for *psittacid alphaherpesvirus*-1 (PsHV-1; Pacheco's Disease)
- ▶ May be nephrotoxic when given rapidly IV and cause tissue necrosis in birds when given IM
- ▶ Do not use in cats because of the risk for myelosuppression and significant renal and hepatic toxicity.
- ▶ Oral use may cause GI distress.
- ▶ Adjust dosage in patients with renal insufficiency.

Uses/Indications

Acyclovir may be useful in the treatment of herpes infections in a variety of avian species. Specifically, this drug may be effective in the treatment of *psittacid alphaherpesvirus*-1 (PsHV-1; formerly known as Pacheco's Disease) when administered early in the course of disease (ie, before clinical signs occur).

In horses, acyclovir was investigated as a treatment for equine herpesvirus type 5 (EHV-5)[1,2] and equine herpesvirus type 1 (EHV-1) myeloencephalopathy,[3] but clinical efficacy was not proven. Bioavailability of oral acyclovir is poor,[4,5] but IV acyclovir may be an option in neonatal foals. Valacyclovir has better bioavailability and has demonstrated clinical efficacy.[6-8]

Despite mild efficacy against feline herpesvirus type 1 (FHV-1), acyclovir should not be used in cats due to a high potential for toxicity and low bioavailability. Other, less toxic, antiviral agents in the same class (eg, famciclovir) can be considered for this indication.

Acyclovir has been used as adjunctive treatment for canine herpesvirus in puppies.[9] Acyclovir may be of benefit in the prophylactic treatment of canine parvovirus in dogs.[10]

Pharmacology/Actions

Acyclovir is a purine (guanine) analogue with antiviral activity against a variety of viruses, including herpes simplex (types I and II), cytomegalovirus, Epstein–Barr, and varicella-zoster. It is preferentially converted by viral thymidine kinase into the active triphosphate form, which is incorporated into viral DNA where it inhibits viral DNA replication.

Pharmacokinetics

After a single IV or IM acyclovir dose in Quaker parakeets, elimination half-life was ≈40 minutes, and IM bioavailability was 90%.[11]

Bioavailability in horses after oral administration is low (ie, less than 4%).[4-6] Oral doses of up to 20 mg/kg may not yield sufficient concentrations to treat equine herpes virus, but some accumulation may occur with prolonged oral administration. Elimination half-lives in dogs[12] and cats[13] is ≈3 hours. In horses, the elimination half-life is ≈2 hours for total plasma concentration of acyclovir and ≈12 hours for unbound (free) plasma concentration of acyclovir.[6]

In dogs, acyclovir bioavailability varies according to the dose. At doses of 20 mg/kg and below, bioavailability is ≈80% but declines to ≈50% at 50 mg/kg. Sustained-release tablets (not commercially available in the United States) have better bioavailability than standard tablets.[12]

In humans, acyclovir is poorly absorbed after oral administration (ie, ≈20%), and absorption is not significantly affected by the presence of food. Acyclovir is widely distributed throughout body tissues and fluids, including the brain, semen, and CSF. It has low protein binding and crosses the placenta. Acyclovir is primarily metabolized in the liver and has a half-life of ≈3 hours in humans.

Contraindications/Precautions/Warnings

Acyclovir is contraindicated in patients hypersensitive to it or related antiviral drugs. Use with caution in patients with dehydration, pre-existing renal or hepatic impairment, hypoxia, neurologic deficits, or electrolyte abnormalities. Dosage reduction is recommended in humans with significant renal impairment.

Acyclovir for injection has a pH of ≈11 and should be administered by slow IV infusion (1 hour for humans) after dilution to a drug concentration less than or equal to 7 mg/mL.

Do not use in cats because of the risk for myelosuppression, hepatic necrosis, and renal tubular necrosis.[14]

Adverse Effects

With parenteral therapy, potential adverse effects include thrombophlebitis, acute renal failure, and encephalopathic changes (rare). IV administration of acyclovir over 15 minutes in a horse resulted in tremors, sweating, and colic.[5]

GI disturbances may occur with either oral or parenteral therapy.

Reproductive/Nursing Safety

Acyclovir crosses the placenta, but rodent studies have not demonstrated any teratogenic effects.[15]

Acyclovir crosses into maternal milk, but associated adverse effects have not been noted.

Because safety has not been established in animals, this drug should only be used when the maternal benefits outweigh the potential risks to offspring.

Overdose/Acute Toxicity

Acute oral overdose is unlikely to cause significant toxicity. GI signs (eg, vomiting, diarrhea) and lethargy predominate with overdoses less than 150 mg/kg. Acute kidney injury is possible with higher dosages; consider GI decontamination with acyclovir overdoses of 150 mg/kg or higher.[16] Crystalluria and increased renal values occurred with acyclovir 188.7 mg/kg in a dog.

Acyclovir is removed by hemodialysis but not by peritoneal dialysis. Precipitation of the drug in renal tubules and acute renal failure have been noted in humans.

For patients that have experienced or are suspected to have experienced an overdose, consultation with a 24-hour poison consultation center specializing in providing veterinary-specific information is recommended. For general information related to overdose and toxin exposures, as well as contact information for poison control centers, refer to ***Appendix.***

Drug Interactions

The following drug interactions with acyclovir have either been reported or are theoretical in humans or animals and may be of significance in veterinary patients. Unless otherwise noted, use together is not necessarily contraindicated, but weigh the potential risks and perform additional monitoring when appropriate.

- **Aminophylline/Theophylline**: Concurrent use may increase theophylline concentrations. Monitor theophylline concentrations.
- **Meperidine**: Concurrent use may increase concentrations of meperidine and normeperidine, increasing the risk for lethargy, agitation, and seizures. Avoid combination
- **Mycophenolate:** Concurrent oral administration may increase concentrations of both acyclovir and mycophenolate. Greatest risk may be in patients with impaired renal function. Use this combination cautiously. Monitor mycophenolate concentrations and signs of toxicity from both medications.
- **Nephrotoxic Medications** (eg, **aminoglycosides** [eg, **amikacin, gentamicin**], **amphotericin B, cyclosporine**): Concurrent administration of IV acyclovir with nephrotoxic medications may increase the potential for nephrotoxicity. Amphotericin B may potentiate the antiviral effects of acyclovir, but it also increases the chances for development of nephrotoxicity.
- **Probenecid**: Concurrent use may increase acyclovir exposure by inhibiting renal clearance.
- **Zidovudine**: Concurrent use with zidovudine may cause additional CNS depression.

Dosages

BIRDS:

Treatment and prophylaxis of *psittacid alphaherpesvirus*-1 (PsHV-1, Pacheco's Disease; extra-label):

Treatment: 80 mg/kg PO (oral gavage) or IM (once; can cause tissue necrosis) every 8 hours for 7 to 14 days

Prophylaxis: After an initial dose of 25 mg/kg IM, acyclovir may be added to drinking water at 1 mg/mL or to food at 400 mg/quart of seed for at least 7 days.

Herpesvirus:

1. 80 mg/kg PO (oral gavage) every 8 hours[17]
2. 240 mg/kg applied to feed[17]
3. Quaker parakeets: 80 mg/kg PO every 8 hours for 7 days[11,18]
4. Raptors: 330 mg/kg PO every 12 hours[19,20]

HORSES:

Equine herpes infections (extra-label): 10 mg/kg IV (over 1 hour) every 12 hours[4,5,21]

DOGS:

Adjunctive treatment of neonatal canine herpesvirus infection (extra-label): 10 mg/kg PO every 6 hours for 5 days[9]

Prophylaxis for canine parvovirus (CPV) infections in puppies (extra-label): In a small, experimentally induced CPV-2 infection study, acyclovir 20 mg/kg IV every 8 hours for 5 days prevented clinical signs and virus replication.[10]

Monitoring

- Renal function tests (BUN, serum creatinine) with prolonged or IV therapy

Client Information

- Side effects are usually limited to gastrointestinal problems (eg, diarrhea, vomiting, lack of appetite).
- For birds, acyclovir is usually given in water or mixed with seed or peanut butter.
- Your animal will need ongoing laboratory tests while taking this medication. Do not miss these important follow-up visits.

Chemistry/Synonyms

Acyclovir, an antiviral agent, occurs as a white, crystalline powder; 1.3 mg is soluble in 1 mL of water. Acyclovir sodium has a solubility greater than 100 mg/mL in water; however, at a pH of 7.4 at 37°C (98.6°F), it is practically all unionized with a solubility of only 2.5 mg/mL in water. Each gram of acyclovir sodium contains 4.2 mEq of sodium.

Acyclovir may be known as ACV, aciclovirum, acycloguanosine, acyclovir, BW-248U, *Acic®*, *Aciclobene®*, *Aciclotyrol®*, *Acivir®*, *Acyrax®*, *Cicloviral®*, *Geavir®*, *Herpotern®*, *Isavir®*, *Nycovir®*, *Supraviran®*, *Viclovir®*, *Virherpes®*, *Viroxy®*, *Xorox®*, or *Zovirax®*.

Storage/Stability

Acyclovir capsules and tablets should be stored in tight, light-resistant containers at room temperature (15°C-25°C [59°F-77°F]). Acyclovir suspension and sodium sterile powder should be stored at room temperature (20°C-25°C [68°F-77°F]); do not refrigerate. Reconstituted solution should be used within 12 hours. Unused portions of acyclovir injection should be discarded.

Compatibility/Compounding Considerations

When reconstituting acyclovir sodium, do not use bacteriostatic water with parabens, as precipitation may occur. The manufacturer does not recommend using bacteriostatic water for injection with benzyl alcohol because of the potential toxicity in neonates. After further dilution to a concentration less than or equal to 7 mg/mL with a standard electrolyte or dextrose solution, the resulting solution is stable at 25°C (77°F) for 24 hours.

Acyclovir is reportedly **incompatible** with biologic or colloidal products (eg, blood products or protein-containing solutions), dopamine, dobutamine, foscarnet, meperidine, and morphine. Many other drugs have been shown to be **compatible** in specific situations. Compatibility is dependent on factors such as pH, concentration, temperature, and diluent used; consult specialized references or a hospital pharmacist for more specific information.

Dosage Forms/Regulatory Status

VETERINARY-LABELED PRODUCTS: NONE

HUMAN-LABELED PRODUCTS:

Acyclovir Oral Tablets: 400 mg and 800 mg; *Zovirax®*,generic; (Rx)

Acyclovir Oral Capsules: 200 mg; *Zovirax®*, generic; (Rx)

Acyclovir Oral Suspension: 40 mg/mL in 473 mL bottles; *Zovirax®*, generic; (Rx)

Acyclovir Injection (for IV infusion only): 50 mg/mL (as sodium) in 10 mL vials or as 500 mg lyophilized powder for reconstitution; generic; (Rx)

Acyclovir Buccal Tablets: 50 mg; *Sitavig®*; (Rx). Tablet remains in contact with oral mucosa for ≈14 hours; veterinary use is doubtful.

Topical 5% creams and ointments are also available.

References

For the complete list of references, see **wiley.com/go/budde/plumb**

Afoxolaner

(ah-***fox***-ah-lan-er) *NexGard®*

Isoxazoline Ectoparasiticide

Prescriber Highlights

- Chewable oral tablet for use in dogs and puppies 8 weeks of age and older and weighing at least 1.8 kg (4 lb)
- Labeled for monthly treatment and prevention of flea infestations and for monthly treatment and control of American dog tick, black-legged tick, lone star tick, and brown dog tick infestations
- Indicated for the prevention of *Borrelia burgdorferi* infections as a direct result of killing *Ixodes scapularis* vector ticks before disease transmission occurs
- Used for extra-label treatment of generalized demodicosis and *Sarcoptes scabiei* var *canis*
- Appears to be well-tolerated when administered at the label dosage
- FDA has warned that drugs in the isoxazoline class have the potential to cause neurologic adverse effects (eg, muscle tremors, ataxia, seizures) in dogs and cats.

Uses/Indications

Afoxolaner chewable tablets are approved by the FDA for monthly treatment and prevention of flea infestations (*Ctenocephalides felis*) and for the monthly treatment and control of American dog tick (*Dermacentor variabilis*, also called wood tick), black-legged tick (*Ixodes scapularis*, also called deer tick), lone star tick (*Amblyomma americanum*), and brown dog tick (*Rhipicephalus sanguineus*) infestations in dogs and puppies 8 weeks of age and older with a body weight of 1.8 kg (4 lb) or greater. The drug is also indicated for the prevention of *Borrelia burgdorferi* infections via killing *Ixodes scapularis* vector ticks before disease transmission occurs.

Afoxolaner has demonstrated efficacy in dogs for the treatment of generalized demodicosis,[1-3] sarcoptic mange,[4,5] cutaneous myiasis,[6] bedbugs,[7] and ear mite (*Otodectes cynotis*) infestations,[8,9] as well as against sand fly (*Phlebotomus perniciosus;* vector for canine leishmaniosis) and dog flea (*Ctenocephalides canis*) infestations.[10-13] Afoxolaner has also been shown to be effective in the treatment of other tick infestations (eg, *Dermacentor reticulatus, Haemaphysalis longicornis, Ixodes hexagonus, Ixodes holocyclus, Ixodes ricinus*) in dogs.[12,13]

Afoxolaner's effectiveness with flea control has been shown to be effective in preventing infestations by *Dipylidium caninum* (flea tapeworm).[13] Under experimental conditions, an afoxolaner and milbemycin combination product (not available in the US) also effectively reduced flea exposure and thus reduced infections by *Dipylidium caninum* in dogs.[14] Monthly administration of the combination product was 100% effective against canine thelaziosis (*Thelazia callipaeda*) in a European field study.[15]

Afoxolaner was successfully used to treat otodectic mange in naturally infested cats, eradicating mites within 48 hours of treatment and maintaining efficacy for 65 days.[16] The drug controlled flea populations in cats under experimental conditions.[17]

Afoxolaner has demonstrated efficacy against *Sarcoptes scabiei* in pigs[18,19] and *Goniodes Pavonis* in peacocks and pheasants.[20]

Pharmacology/Actions

Afoxolaner is in the isoxazoline family of insecticides and acaracides. In the parasite CNS, isoxazolines block pre- and postsynaptic transfer of chloride ions across cell membranes by inhibiting gamma-aminobutyric acid (GABA)-mediated ligand-gated chloride channels. Prolonged neuronal hyperexcitation results in paralysis and death of susceptible insects and ticks. The difference between GABA receptor sensitivities of insects/acarines as compared with mammals is believed to be the reason for differential toxicity. Insects and acarines must feed on dogs to ingest afoxolaner. Onset of action against fleas is within 4 hours of administration, with 99% effectiveness at 8 hours (ie, before fleas can lay eggs). Against ticks, the onset of action is within 48 hours, and may be as fast as 8 to 12 hours after infestation for some tick species.[21,22] Afoxolaner kills adult fleas and ticks only after they have bitten and fed.

Pharmacokinetics

In dogs, afoxolaner is reported to be rapidly absorbed, with a bioavailability of ≈75% and peak concentrations occurring between 2 to 6 hours. Food does not impair absorption. Protein binding is very high (more than 99%). Elimination is via biliary excretion of free afoxolaner and renal excretion of hepatically biotransformed metabolites. Terminal elimination half-life is ≈15 days.

Contraindications/Precautions/Warnings

There are no contraindications when afoxolaner is used as directed on the product label. The drug is labeled for use in puppies 8 weeks of age and older and weighing more than 1.8 kg (4 lb). Use with caution in dogs with a history of seizures or epilepsy. Drugs in the isoxazoline class have the potential to cause neurologic adverse effects, including muscle tremors, ataxia, and seizures.[23] These effects have been noted in patients with and without a history of neurologic disorders.

Adverse Effects

In preapproval field studies (415 dogs given monthly afoxolaner doses for 3 consecutive months), serious adverse effects were not noted, although 2 dogs with a history of seizures had a seizure during the study (causation could not be determined). The most prevalent adverse effect noted was vomiting (4.1%). Other adverse effects reported (more than 1%) included dry flaky skin (3.1%), diarrhea (3.1%), lethargy (1.7%), and anorexia (1.2%). Neurologic (hyperactivity, panting, ataxia, muscle tremors, seizures),[23] dermal (erythema, dermatitis), and hypersensitivity (hives, swelling) reactions have been reported.

Reproductive/Nursing Safety

Although studies in laboratory animals have not demonstrated teratogenic effects or any adverse effect on male or female reproductive capacity,[12] the US product label states that safe use in breeding, pregnant, or lactating dogs has not been evaluated.[24]

Because safety has not been established in animals, this drug should only be used when the maternal benefits outweigh the potential risks to offspring.

Overdose/Acute Toxicity

No information was located for acute toxicity in dogs. Oral doses up to 1000 mg/kg in rats and 2000 mg/kg in mice were not lethal. Dogs receiving doses of 5 times the maximum label dose for 3 treatments every 28 days, followed by 3 treatments every 14 days (for a total of 6 treatments), did not show clinically relevant effects related to treatment on physical examination, body weight, food consumption, clinical pathology (hematology, clinical chemistries, or coagulation tests), gross pathology, histopathology, or organ weights.[24] Vomiting occurred throughout the study, with a similar incidence in the treated and control groups.

For patients that have experienced or are suspected of having experienced an overdose, consultation with a 24-hour poison consultation center specializing in providing veterinary-specific information is recommended. For general information related to overdose and toxin exposures, as well as contact information for poison control centers, refer to *Appendix*.

Drug Interactions

None have been reported. In a field study, afoxolaner was safely used concurrently with vaccines, anthelmintics, antibiotics (including topicals), steroids, NSAIDS, anesthetics, and antihistamines.[24]

Laboratory Considerations

None were noted.

Dosages

DOGS:

Treatment and prevention of flea infestations *(Ctenocephalides felis)*, and the treatment and control of black-legged tick *(Ixodes scapularis)*, American dog tick *(Dermacentor variabilis)*, lone star tick *(Amblyomma americanum)*, and brown dog tick *(Rhipicephalus sanguineus)* infestations, and for the prevention of *Borrelia burgdorferi* infections in dogs and puppies 8 weeks of age and older, with a body weight of 1.8 kg (4 lb) or greater, for 1 month (label dosage; FDA-approved): Minimum dosage is 2.5 mg/kg (1.14 mg/lb) PO once per month.[24] The package insert has a dosing table for the various tablet sizes:

Body weight	Tablet size (mg)	Number of tablets
1.8 kg to 4.5 kg (4 lb to 10 lb)	11.3	1
4.6 kg to 10.9 kg (10.1 lb to 24 lb)	28.3	1
11 kg to 27.3 kg (24.1 lb to 60 lb)	68	1
27.4 kg to 55 kg (60.1 lb to 121 lb)	136	1
Greater than 54.6 kg (121 lb)	Administer the appropriate combination of chewable tablets.	

Generalized demodicosis (extra-label):

a) At least 2.5 mg/kg orally on days 0, 14, 28, and 56[1]
b) 2.7 – 7 mg/kg PO once per month until 2 negative skin scrapings are obtained 1 month apart[12]

***Sarcoptes scabiei var canis* infestations** (extra-label): At least 2.5 mg/kg orally on days 0 and 28[4,12,13]

***Otodectes synotis* infection** (extra-label): 2.5 mg/kg PO once,[13] or once monthly for 2 months[9]

CATS:

Ear mite (*Otodectes cynotis*) infestation (extra-label): 2.5 mg/kg PO as a single dose[16]

Cat flea (*Ctenocephalides felis*) infestation (extra-label): Under experimental conditions, 2.5 mg/kg PO as a single dose[16]

PIGS:

Sarcoptes scabiei var suis (extra-label): 2.5 mg/kg PO as a single dose[18,19,25]

BIRDS:

Bird louse (*Goniodes pavonis*) (extra-label): 2.5 mg/kg PO as a single dose [20,26]

Monitoring

- Clinical efficacy
- Adverse effects

Client Information

- Afoxolaner can be administered with or without food.
- Be sure your animal consumes the complete dose. Watch your animal for a few minutes after giving the medication to be sure it doesn't spit out any part of the dose.
- If your animal vomits within 2 hours of receiving the medication, give another full dose. If a dose is missed, give it when you remember and start a new monthly dosing schedule.
- Treatment may start at any time of the year. In areas where fleas and ticks are common year-round, monthly treatment should continue for the entire year.
- To minimize the likelihood of flea and tick reinfestation, treat all animals within a household with an approved flea and tick control product.
- Afoxolaner kills adult fleas and ticks only after they have bitten your animal but before the fleas or ticks can lay eggs or transmit disease. Existing flea eggs will hatch and must feed in order to be killed.
- Keep this medicine out of the reach of other animals and children. Keep the tablets in the original packaging until you are ready to give the medicine to your animal.
- Contact your veterinarian if you see any side effects, including neurologic problems, such as tremors, difficulty walking, or seizures.

Chemistry/Synonyms

Afoxolaner has a molecular weight of 625.87 g/mol and has the chemical composition 1-Naphthalenecarboxamide, 4-[5-[3-chloro-5-(trifluoromethyl)-phenyl]-4,5-dihydro-5-(trifluoromethyl)-3-isoxazolyl]-N-[2-oxo-2-[(2,2,2 trifluoroethyl)amino]ethyl. Afoxolaner is lipophilic, hydrophobic, and non-ionizable. Its ATCvet code is QP-53BX04. It is also known as *NexGard*®, and *NexGard*® *Spectra* (afoxolaner and milbemycin).

Storage/Stability

Store chewable tablets at or below 30°C (86°F) with excursions permitted up to 40°C (104°F).

Compatibility/Compounding Considerations

No specific information was noted.

Dosage Forms/Regulatory Status

VETERINARY-LABELED PRODUCTS:

Afoxolaner Chewable (beef-flavored) Tablets: 11.3 mg, 28.3 mg, 68 mg, and 136 mg; *NexGard*®; (Rx). Available in color-coded packages of 1, 3, or 6 chewables. FDA-approved (NADA 141-406) for use in dogs.

HUMAN-LABELED PRODUCTS: NONE

References

For the complete list of references, see **wiley.com/go/budde/plumb**

Aglepristone

(a-gle-***pris***-tone) Alizin®, Alizine®

Progesterone Receptor Antagonist

Prescriber Highlights

- ► Injectable progesterone receptor antagonist used for pregnancy termination in many species; may also be of benefit to induce parturition in dogs, for medical treatment of pyometra complex in dogs or cats, and for mammary fibroadenomatous hyperplasia in cats
- ► Not currently available in the US; marketed for use in dogs in several other countries
- ► Adverse effects include anorexia, localized injection site inflammation, excitation, depression, injection-related pain, diarrhea, hematological/biochemical changes, and uterine infections.
- ► This medication should not be handled or administered by pregnant women.

Uses/Indications

Aglepristone is labeled (in the UK and elsewhere) for pregnancy termination in bitches up to 45 days after mating. In early pregnancy, aglepristone is nearly 100% effective at preventing implantation.[1] In midterm pregnancy, aglepristone terminates pregnancy in ≈95% of cases.[2]

In dogs, aglepristone, in combination with oxytocin, may also prove useful to induce parturition[3,4] or in treating pyometra complex[5-8] (often in combination with a prostaglandin F analogue such as cloprostenol). Additional potential clinical uses in dogs include treatment of insulin-resistant diabetes mellitus (for which ovariectomy/ovariohysterectomy is not an option),[9] acromegaly,[10] benign vaginal tumors,[11,12] and progesterone receptor-positive mammary carcinomas.[13]

In cats, aglepristone may be of benefit for pregnancy termination, but reports on its efficacy as a single agent range from only 50% to 87%.[14-18] In separate studies, the addition of misoprostol,[6] cabergoline,[7] or cloprostenol[8] each increased the abortion rate to 100%. Aglepristone may also be useful for treating mammary hyperplasia[19,20] or pyometra[21] in cats.

Aglepristone may be useful for parturition induction in ewes.[22,23]

In rabbits, aglepristone injected on days 6 and 7 after mating prevented implantation in 100% of does (n = 13).[24] Subsequent fertility was unaffected, with 5 of 5 does becoming pregnant.

Pharmacology/Actions

Aglepristone is a synthetic steroid that competitively antagonizes progesterone at the P4 progesterone receptor. In dogs, it has an affinity for uterine progesterone receptors ≈3 times that of endogenous progesterone.[25] In queens, affinity is ≈9 times greater than the endogenous hormone.[26] As progesterone is necessary for maintaining pregnancy, aglepristone terminates pregnancy or induces parturition. Pregnancy termination (resorption or abortion) occurs within 4 to 7 days of administration.[25,27]

When aglepristone is used for treating pyometra in dogs, it can cause opening of the cervix and resumption of myometrial contractility.

Aglepristone does not appreciably affect circulating plasma concentrations of progesterone, cortisol, prostaglandins, or oxytocin. Plasma concentrations of prolactin are increased within 12 hours when aglepristone is used in dogs during midpregnancy; this effect is likely the cause of mammary gland congestion often seen in these dogs. Aglepristone has been shown to have inhibitory effects on progesterone receptor-positive canine mammary carcinoma cells.[28] Endogenous progesterone secretion during diestrus or pregnancy, or administration of exogenous progesterone derivatives for contraception, can stimulate hypersecretion of mammary growth hormone (GH), which can secondarily lead to insulin resistance. Progesterone-induced acromegaly is the most common form of acromegaly in dogs and usually appears after prolonged administration of progestogens, or during the luteal phase in older intact females.

Aglepristone also binds to glucocorticoid receptors with affinity similar to dexamethasone but without glucocorticoid activity[25]; it can prevent endogenous or exogenously administered glucocorticoids from binding and acting at these sites.

Pharmacokinetics

In dogs, after injecting 2 doses of aglepristone 10 mg/kg SC 24 hours apart, peak serum concentrations occur ≈2.5 days later and mean residence time is ≈6 days.[25] Excretion of the drug occurs slowly, with 80% of the dose excreted over 24 days. The majority (90%) of the drug is excreted via the feces.

Contraindications/Precautions/Warnings

Aglepristone is contraindicated in animals with documented hypersensitivity to it and during pregnancy, unless it is used for pregnancy termination or inducing parturition.[25] Do not use aglepristone in animals in poor health, with diabetes, or with impaired hepatic or renal function. Because of its antagonistic effects on glucocorticoid receptors, the drug should not be used in animals with hypoadrenocorticism or a genetic predisposition to hypoadrenocorticism. Use with caution in animals with chronic obstructive-airway disease, or with cardiovascular disease, particularly bacterial endocarditis. Medical management of pyometra (eg, aglepristone) is contraindicated in bitches with severe or life-threatening conditions (eg, hepatorenal failure, suspected peritonitis).[8,26]

This medication should not be handled or administered by pregnant women.

Adverse Effects

Aglepristone is in an oil-alcohol base and localized pain and inflammatory reactions (ie, edema, skin thickening, ulceration, localized lymph node enlargement) have been noted at the injection site.[25] Size and intensity of injection reactions have been correlated with injection volume. Resolution of pain generally occurs shortly after injection; other injection site reactions usually resolve within 2 to 4 weeks. The manufacturer recommends light massage of the injection site after administration. Larger dogs should not receive more than

5 mL at any one SC injection site; severe local reactions can be avoided if the drug is administered into the scruff of the neck.[25]

Systemic adverse effects reported from field trials include anorexia (25%), localized injection site inflammation (23%), excitation (23%), depression (21%), injection-related pain (17%), diarrhea (13%), uterine infections (3.4%), and vomiting (2%).[25] Tachycardia has also been reported in cats treated with aglepristone for fibroadenomatous hyperplasia.[19] Transient and reversible changes in hematologic (neutrophilia, neutropenia, thrombocytosis, hematocrit variation, lymphocytosis, lymphopenia) or biochemical (elevated BUN, creatinine, chloride, potassium, sodium, liver enzymes [ALT, ALP, AST]) laboratory parameters were seen in 4.5% of dogs treated.[25]

When aglepristone is used for pregnancy termination, a brown mucoid vaginal discharge can be seen ≈24 hours before fetal expulsion. This discharge can persist for an additional 3 to 5 days. If the drug is used in bitches after the 20th day of gestation, abortion may be accompanied with other signs associated with parturition (eg, inappetence, restlessness, mammary congestion, lactation). Bitches may return to estrus in as little as 45 days after pregnancy termination.[25]

Reproductive/Nursing Safety

Unless used for pregnancy termination or at term to induce parturition, aglepristone is contraindicated during pregnancy.

One study using aglepristone to induce parturition (day 58 post mating) demonstrated no significant differences in weight gain between those puppies in the treatment group as compared with those in the control group, suggesting that aglepristone did not have an effect on milk production of treated bitches.[4]

Overdose/Acute Toxicity

When aglepristone was administered at 3 times the recommended dose (30 mg/kg), bitches demonstrated no untoward systemic effects.[25] Localized reactions were noted at the injection site, presumably due to the larger volumes injected.

For patients that have experienced or are suspected to have experienced an overdose, consultation with a 24-hour poison consultation center specializing in providing veterinary-specific information is recommended. For general information related to overdose and toxin exposures, as well as contact information for poison control centers, refer to ***Appendix***.

Drug Interactions

The following drug interactions have either been reported or are theoretical in humans or animals receiving aglepristone and may be of significance in veterinary patients. Unless otherwise noted, use together is not necessarily contraindicated, but weigh the potential risks and perform additional monitoring when appropriate.

- **Progestins** (**natural** or **synthetic**): Could theoretically reduce the efficacy of each other
- **Glucocorticoids** (eg, **prednis(ol)one**): Aglepristone could reduce the efficacy of glucocorticoid treatment.[25]
- **Ketoconazole, Itraconazole, Erythromycin**: May interact with aglepristone presumably via inhibiting CYP3A and/or P-glycoprotein[25]

Laboratory Considerations

None are noted.

Dosages

WARNING: Because accidental injection of this product can induce abortion, it should not be administered or handled by pregnant women.

DOGS:

Termination of pregnancy up to day 45 after mating (extra-label): 10 mg/kg SC; repeat one time, 24 hours after the first injection.[25] Administer into the scruff of the neck; a light massage of the injection site is recommended after administration. A maximum of 5 mL should be injected at any one site. In case of partial abortion or no abortion, repeat treatment may be recommended 10 days after the initial dose, between days 30 and 45 after mating.

Induction of parturition (extra-label): At day 60 (NOT before day 58), post-estimated luteinizing hormone (LH) surge, 15 mg/kg SC and another dose 24 hours later.[3,29] **NOTE:** This treatment may not be safe for all breeds and should only be done in conjunction with other modalities (eg, fetal ultrasound, drop in progesterone levels) to ensure adequate fetal maturation. Use standard protocols to assist with birth (including oxytocin to assist in pup expulsion if necessary) or to intervene if parturition does not proceed.

Adjunctive therapy for pyometra (extra-label): **NOTE:** Additional therapies (eg, IV fluids, antibiotics) may be necessary based on clinical presentation.

a. 10 mg/kg SC on days 1 and 2, and then every 7th and 8th day (eg, days 7 and 8, days 14 and 15) until the end of treatment (ie, return to clinically healthy status).[30] A median of 4 doses (range 2 to 5 doses) were given. Antimicrobial therapy was administered concurrently.
b. 10 mg/kg SC once daily on days 1, 2, and 8 in combination with cloprostenol 1 µg/kg SC on days 3 to 7.[5] If pyometra was not resolved, additional aglepristone doses were administered on days 14 and 28.[5,31]

Insulin-resistant diabetes mellitus in intact bitches for which ovariectomy/ovariohysterectomy is not an option (extra-label): In addition to PZI insulin, aglepristone 10 mg/kg SC at days 1, 2, 9, and 17 during the luteal phase improved glycemic control in diabetic bitches with diestrus-induced insulin resistance ($n = 8$).[9] The effects of the treatment were significant from day 12, with reductions in the dose of insulin needed to control glycemia.

Progesterone-induced acromegaly (extra-label): Aglepristone 10 mg/kg SC at days 1, 8, 15, and 22 resulted in a reduction in mean plasma concentrations of GH and IGF-1 in affected beagle bitches ($n = 5$).[10] Once the source of progesterone has been eliminated (eg, ovariectomy, withdrawal of exogenous progestogens), the prognosis is good. Long-term efficacy and safety data are lacking.

Benign vaginal tumors (extra-label): 10 mg/kg SC on days 1 (day of diagnosis), 2, 8, 15, 28, and 35 (based on a case report of a vaginal fibroma in which tumor size was noticeably reduced on day 45)[11]

Progesterone receptor-positive mammary carcinomas (extra-label): 20 mg/kg SC on days 1 and 8. On day 15, reduced proliferation was observed in progesterone receptor-positive tumors.[13]

CATS:

Termination of pregnancy up to day 45 (extra-label)**:** 10 mg/kg SC every 24 hours for 2 doses [14-18,32] One study used 15 mg/kg SC every 24 hours for 2 doses. [17] The addition of cabergoline,[16] cloprostenol,[18] or misoprostol[15] may increase efficacy.

Pyometra (extra-label): 10 mg/kg SC on days 1, 2, 7, and 14 (if not cured) with concurrent antibiotic therapy

Mammary fibroadenomatous hyperplasia (extra-label)**:**

a) 10 – 15 mg/kg SC on days 1, 2, and 7.[19,20,33] Weekly treatment should be made until resolution of signs and may be required for several weeks. Cats that have been treated with a long-acting progestin (eg, medroxyprogesterone acetate) may require longer durations of treatment to prevent relapse.
b) 20 mg/kg SC every 7 days also has been used[19]

SHEEP:

Parturition induction, pregnancy toxemia (extra-label): 5 – 10 mg/kg SC once daily for 2 consecutive days[22,23]

RABBITS:

Prevention of fetal implantation (extra-label): 10 mg/kg SC twice 24 hours apart on days 6 and 7 after mating[24]

Monitoring

- Clinical efficacy
- For pregnancy termination: Ultrasonography 10 days after treatment and at least 30 days after mating[25]
- For induction of parturition:
  - Ultrasonography to verify fetal viability (eg, fetal intestinal peristalsis, kidney corticomedullary distinction)
  - Serum progesterone concentration: A decrease in endogenous progesterone concentration may indicate the appropriate time to administer aglepristone. **NOTE:** Progesterone concentrations are not intended to monitor efficacy of aglepristone.
- For pyometra: CBC and chemistry panel, culture and susceptibility, ultrasonography
- For insulin-resistant diabetes mellitus: serial blood glucose
- Adverse effects (see ***Adverse Effects***)

Client Information

- Only veterinary professionals should handle and administer this product.
- This medication should not be handled or administered by pregnant women.
- It is essential that your dog be evaluated by your veterinarian 7 to 10 days after treatment to ensure it has been effective.
- When using this drug for pregnancy termination in bitches, it should be understood that it might only be 95% effective in terminating pregnancy when used between days 26 and 45.
- When aglepristone is used to terminate a pregnancy, a brown mucoid vaginal discharge can be seen ≈24 hours before fetal expulsion.
- Bitches may exhibit the following after treatment: inflammation at the injection site, lack of appetite, excitement, restlessness or depression, or diarrhea.
- Contact your veterinarian if your bitch exhibits a purulent or hemorrhagic discharge after treatment or if vaginal discharge persists 3 weeks after treatment.
- When this drug is used to treat pyometra, there is risk for treatment failure (10% treatment failure in cats and 19% recurrence after 2 years[5] in dogs), and ovariohysterectomy may be required.[8,30,32]

Chemistry/Synonyms

Aglepristone is a synthetic steroid. The manufactured injectable dosage form is in a clear, yellow, oily, nonaqueous vehicle that contains arachis oil and ethanol. No additional antimicrobial agent is added to the injection.

Aglepristone may also be known as *Alizin*®, *Alizine*®, RU-534, or RU-46534.

Storage/Stability

Aglepristone injection should be stored below 25°C (77°F) and protected from light. The manufacturer recommends using the product within 28 days of withdrawing the first dose.

Compatibility/Compounding Considerations

Although no incompatibilities have been reported, because of aglepristone's oil/alcohol vehicle formulation, it should not be mixed with any other medication.

Dosage Forms/Regulatory Status

VETERINARY-LABELED PRODUCTS:

NOTE: Not presently available or approved for use in the US. In other countries: Aglepristone Injection: 30 mg/mL in 5 mL, 10 mL, and 30 mL vials; *Alizin*® or *Alizine*®; (Rx)

HUMAN-LABELED PRODUCTS: NONE

References

For the complete list of references, see **wiley.com/go/budde/plumb**

Albendazole

(al-***ben***-da-zole) *Albenza*®, *Valbazen*®

Antiparasitic

Prescriber Highlights

- ▶ Broad-spectrum anthelmintic with activity against a variety of nematodes, trematodes, cestodes, and protozoa
- ▶ FDA-approved for cattle and sheep as well as nonlactating goats
- ▶ Contraindicated with hepatic failure, during the first trimester of pregnancy, and in lactating does and female dairy cattle of breeding age
- ▶ Usually well-tolerated when used at label dosage in indicated animal species
- ▶ Due to significant toxicity, extra-label use in dogs, cats, crias, pigeons, or doves is not recommended.

Uses/Indications

Albendazole is FDA-approved in cattle and sheep for the removal and control of adult liver flukes, heads and segments of tapeworms, adult and fourth-stage larvae of lung worms, stomach worms, and intestinal worms. Albendazole is FDA-approved for the treatment of adult *Fasciola hepatica* in nonlactating goats.

Albendazole has been used (extra-label) for the treatment of *Encephalitozoon cuniculi* in rabbits.[1,2]

Albendazole is also used (extra-label) in small mammals (eg, dogs and cats) and swine for endoparasite control. However, because of the availability of safer alternatives and concerns about bone marrow toxicity,[3,4] it is not recommended for use in dogs or cats.

Pharmacology/Actions

Benzimidazole antiparasitic agents have a broad spectrum of activity against a variety of pathogenic internal parasites. In susceptible parasites, their mechanism of action disrupts intracellular microtubular transport systems by binding tubulin, preventing tubulin polymerization, and inhibiting microtubule formation. Benzimidazoles are also believed to act at higher concentrations to disrupt metabolic pathways within the helminth, and inhibit metabolic enzymes, including malate dehydrogenase and fumarate reductase.

In cattle, albendazole activity and efficacy have been demonstrated against adult and fourth-stage larvae of *Ostertagia ostertagi, Haemonchus* spp, *Trichostrongylus* spp, *Nematodius* spp, *Cooperia* spp, *Bunostomum phlebotomum, Oesphagostomum* spp, adult *Fasciola hepatica, Dictacaulus vivaparus*, and *Moniezia* spp.[5] Activity against other parasites species and/or life cycle stages is probable.

In sheep, albendazole activity and efficacy have been demonstrated against adult and fourth-stage larvae of *Ostertagia circumcincta, Marshallagia marshalli, Haemonchus contortus, Trichostrongylus* spp, *Nematodius* spp, *Cooperia* spp, *Oesphagostomum* spp, *Chabertia ovina*, adult and larval *Dictacaulus filaria*, adult *Fasciola hepatica, Fascioides magna, Moniezia expansa*, and *Thysanosoma actinoides*.[5] Activity against other parasites species and/or life cycle stages is probable.

Pharmacokinetics

Albendazole pharmacokinetics were studied in cattle, sheep, and goats.[6] The drug was undetectable in the plasma of all three species after oral administration due to rapid metabolism to albendazole sulfone (inactive) and albendazole sulfoxide (active; also known as ricobendazole). Peak albendazole sulfoxide concentration was reached after 11 hours in cattle, and ≈24 hours in sheep and goats. AUC_{last} was highest in goats (30 µg/hour/mL) compared to sheep

(23 µg/hour/mL) or cattle (14 µg/hour/mL), but AUC_{last}/dose was greatest in sheep (42 µg/hour/mL/mg, versus 17 and 10 µg/hour/mL/mg in goats and cattle, respectively).

Calves that were fasted 24 to 48 hours prior to receiving intraruminal albendazole had significantly higher peak albendazole sulfone concentration, area under the curve (AUC), and mean residence time (MRT) compared to fed calves,[7,8] whereas fasting periods of 6 to 12 hours increased AUC and MRT.[8] Albendazole sulfoxide peak concentration and AUC were higher in sheep that were fasted or had reduced feed rations compared to sheep that were fed normal rations.[9] However, in goats albendazole sulfoxide AUC and half-life were higher and longer when albendazole was administered with food.[10]

In humans, albendazole is widely distributed throughout the body. It is extensively metabolized in the liver.

Contraindications/Precautions/Warnings

The drug is not FDA-approved for use in lactating dairy cattle. The manufacturer recommends not administering to female cattle during the first 45 days of pregnancy or for 45 days after removal of bulls. In sheep or goats, it should not be administered to ewes or does during the first 30 days of pregnancy or for 30 days after removal of rams or bucks. Because a withdrawal time in milk has not been established, the drug is not to be used in lactating does or in female dairy cattle of breeding age.

Accurate estimates of animal weight result in the most effective use of the drug.

Pigeons and doves may be susceptible to albendazole toxicity (intestinal crypt epithelial necrosis and bone marrow hypoplasia).[11] Albendazole toxicosis also has been noted in rabbits, many of whom received higher dosages than are recommended[12]; use with caution.

Adverse Effects

Albendazole is tolerated without significant adverse effects when dosed in cattle, goats, or sheep at recommended dosages.

Dogs may develop anorexia. Cats may exhibit adverse effects of mild lethargy, depression, anorexia, and resistance to receiving albendazole when it is used to treat *Paragonimus kellicotti* infections. Albendazole has been implicated in causing neutropenia and aplastic anemia in dogs and cats.[3,4] In cases where fenbendazole is efficacious, it is preferred.

Reproductive/Nursing Safety

Albendazole has been associated with teratogenic and embryotoxic effects in rats and rabbits at doses less than those used clinically,[4] and dose-related teratogenic effects in sheep when given early in pregnancy.[13] The manufacturer recommends not administering to female cattle during the first 45 days of pregnancy or for 45 days after removal of bulls.[5] In sheep and goats, it should not be administered to ewes or does during the first 30 days of pregnancy or for 30 days after removal of rams or bucks.

Albendazole is excreted in milk.[14] Safety during nursing has not been established.

Because safety has not been established in animals, this drug should only be used when the maternal benefits outweigh the potential risks to offspring.

Overdose/Acute Toxicity

Doses of 300 mg/kg (30 times recommended) and 75 mg/kg (10 times recommended) have caused death in cattle[4] and sheep,[13] respectively. Doses of 45 mg/kg (4.5 times recommended) did not cause any adverse effects in cattle. Albendazole 19 – 100 mg/kg/day caused severe diarrhea, neutropenia, and multiple organ failure in crias, and lethargy, fever, diarrhea, and neutropenia in adult alpacas.[15] Cats receiving 100 mg/kg/day for 14 to 21 days showed signs of weight loss, neutropenia, and mental dullness.

For patients that have experienced or are suspected to have experienced an overdose, it is strongly encouraged to consult with a 24-hour poison consultation center that specializes in providing information specific for veterinary patients. For general information related to overdose and toxin exposures, as well as contact information for poison control centers, refer to ***Appendix***.

Drug Interactions

The following drug interactions with albendazole have either been reported or are theoretical in humans or animals and may be of significance in veterinary patients. Unless otherwise noted, use together is not necessarily contraindicated, but weigh the potential risks and perform additional monitoring when appropriate.

- **CIMETIDINE**: May increase albendazole concentrations in bile and cystic fluid
- **DEXAMETHASONE**: May increase albendazole serum concentrations
- **IVERMECTIN**: Albendazole sulfoxide (active metabolite) AUC was decreased, and ivermectin AUC was increased in lambs that received albendazole coadministered with ivermectin.[16,17]
- **PRAZIQUANTEL**: May increase albendazole serum concentrations
- **THEOPHYLLINE DERIVATIVES** (eg, **aminophylline, theophylline**): May decrease theophylline concentrations

Laboratory Considerations

None are noted.

Dosages

CATTLE:

Removal and control of liver flukes, tapeworms, adult and fourth-stage larvae of stomach worms (including fourth-stage inhibited larvae of *Ostertagia ostertagi*), intestinal worms, and lungworms (label dosage; FDA-approved): 10 mg/kg PO (4 mL/45.3 kg [100 lb] of body weight) as a single dose.[5] Re-treat as necessary. **NOTE**: Not approved for use in female dairy cattle of breeding age.

SHEEP:

Removal and control of liver flukes, tapeworms, adult and fourth-stage larvae of stomach worms (including fourth-stage inhibited larvae of *Ostertagia ostertagi*), intestinal worms, and lungworms (label dosage; FDA-approved): 7.5 mg/kg PO (3 mL/45.3 kg [100 lb] of body weight) as a single dose.[5] Re-treat as necessary.

GOATS:

Treatment of adult liver flukes in nonlactating goats (label dosage; FDA-approved): 10 mg/kg PO (4 mL/45.3 kg [100 lb] of body weight) as a single dose.[5] Re-treat as necessary.

CAMELIDS:

Susceptible GI helminths (extra-label): 15 mg/kg PO as a single dose[18]

RABBITS/RODENTS/SMALL MAMMALS:

a) **Rabbits**: ***E cuniculi*-induced phacoclastic uveitis** (extra-label): 30 mg/kg PO once daily for 30 days, then 15 mg/kg PO once daily for 30 days[19]
b) **Rabbits**: ***E cuniculi*** (extra-label): 20 mg/kg PO once daily for 10 days[20]
c) **Chinchillas**: ***Giardia* spp** (extra-label): 50 – 100 mg/kg PO once daily for 3 days[21]

Monitoring

- Efficacy (eg, pre- and post-fecal flotation or fecal egg count reduction test [FECRT])
- Adverse effects, particularly if used in non-FDA-approved species or at dosages higher than recommended
- Consider monitoring CBC and liver enzymes (every 4 to 6 weeks) if treating long-term (more than 1 month)

Client Information

- Shake well before administering.
- This medicine can be given with or without food. If your animal vomits or acts sick after receiving the drug on an empty stomach, try giving the next dose with food. If vomiting continues, contact your veterinarian.
- Contact your veterinarian if your animal develops vomiting, diarrhea, or yellowing of the eyes, skin, or gums (ie, jaundice).

Chemistry/Synonyms

A benzimidazole anthelmintic structurally related to mebendazole, albendazole has a molecular weight of 265. It is insoluble in water and soluble in alcohol.

Albendazole may also be known as albendazolum, SKF-62979, *Valbazen*®, or *Albenza*®. Many other trade names are available. Albendazole sulfoxide is also known as ricobendazole.

Storage/Stability

Albendazole suspension should be stored at room temperature 20°C to 25°C (68°F-77°F). Protect from freezing. Shake well before use. Albendazole tablets should be stored at 20°C to 30°C (68°F-86°F).

Compatibility/Compounding Considerations

No specific information noted

Dosage Forms/ Regulatory Status

VETERINARY-LABELED PRODUCTS:

Albendazole Suspension: 113.6 mg/mL (11.36%) in 500 mL, 1 L, 5 L; *Valbazen® Suspension*; (OTC). FDA-approved for use in cattle (see ***Contraindications/Precautions/Warnings)***, goats, and sheep (do not administer to does or ewes during the first 30 days of pregnancy or for 30 days after removal of bucks or rams). Slaughter withdrawal time for cattle is 27 days at labeled doses.[5] Slaughter withdrawal time for goats and sheep is 7 days at labeled dose. Because milk withdrawal time has not been established, do not use in lactating does or in female dairy cattle of breeding age.

HUMAN-LABELED PRODUCTS:

Albendazole Oral Tablets: 200 mg; *Albenza*®, generic; (Rx)

References

For the complete list of references, see **wiley.com/go/budde/plumb**

Albumin, Human

Albumin, Canine

(al-***byoo***-min)

Natural Protein Colloid

Prescriber Highlights

- ► Used to increase intravascular oncotic pressure and organ perfusion and decrease edema secondary to crystalloid fluid replacement, particularly in critically ill animals with reversible diseases or conditions when hypoalbuminemia is present
- ► Contraindications include in patients that have demonstrated hypersensitivity to albumin products.
- ► Significant adverse effects are possible, especially immune-mediated reactions when using albumin products in a species other than which it was derived (xeno-albumin products).
- ► Lyophilized canine albumin products are available commercially in the United States, but limited safety and efficacy data are available. Local or regional availability may vary.

Uses/Indications

Human serum albumin (HSA) and canine serum albumin (CSA) may be useful as colloid fluid replacement therapy in critically ill small animal species. Albumin therapy may be considered in patients that are severely hypoalbuminemic (albumin less than 2.0 g/dL), severely edematous, have systemic inflammatory response syndrome or sepsis, or have increased vascular permeability. Human albumin is typically used in small animal species due to availability; however, using albumin products in species other than which they are derived (xeno-albumin) can pose considerable risks. There is limited information available on the use of human albumin in cats.

The administration of 10% human albumin may be useful in dogs with reversible disease that are clinically affected by marked hypoalbuminemia (serum albumin less than 1.5 g/dL) and low colloid osmotic pressure (COP; less than 14 mm Hg). Dogs with surgical diseases and septic peritonitis should be especially considered because of the role of albumin in wound healing; however, given the risk for complications and uncertain positive outcomes, it should be used with extreme caution in critically ill dogs.[1]

One review of human albumin use in small animal species suggests the use of 25% human albumin in patients with refractory hypotension; refractory hypotension associated with gastric dilation-volvulus; patients that are severely hypoalbuminemic (albumin less than 1.5 g/dL or less than 1.8 g/dL) and dehydrated/hypovolemic with ongoing losses (eg, peritonitis, pleural effusion); septic patients that are hypoalbuminemic (combined with FFP); patients with protein-losing enteropathy before surgical biopsy; and markedly hypoalbuminemic patients that continue to vomit (likely attributable to bowel edema).[2]

Another review on fluid therapy in emergent small animal species recommended that the use of HSA be reserved for critically ill patients with a life-threateningly low albumin (eg, septic peritonitis) and that it should not be routinely used for patients with a low COP, as safer synthetic colloids (eg, hydroxyethyl starch) can be used. In dogs, CSA appears to be a safer option than HSA, but outcomes such as hospitalization time and survival time compared to untreated dogs with similar conditions are unknown. Comparative, prospective studies are needed.[3]

Pharmacology/Actions

Albumin provides 75% to 80% of the oncotic pressure of plasma. When albumin is given therapeutically, it increases intravascular oncotic pressure and can cause mobilization of fluids from the interstitial into the intravascular space.

Albumin (for its species) also has other actions, including binding and transport of drugs, ions, hormones, lipids, and metals (including iron); maintenance of endothelial integrity and permeability control; wound healing; antioxidant properties; free radical scavenging; metabolic and acid–base functions; decreasing platelet aggregation; and augmenting antithrombin and serving as a thiol-group. It is unknown what effect, if any, xeno-albumin has on these actions.

Pharmacokinetics

Endogenous circulating albumin represents 30% to 40% of total body albumin. Elimination of exogenously administered canine albumin is estimated to be between 20 to 24 days with a half-life of 10 to 12 days. The kinetics of human albumin in dogs or cats is not well described.

Contraindications/Precautions/Warnings

A history of hypersensitivity to human or canine albumin is a specific contraindication for use. Because of the risk for hypersensitivity, repeat administration of xeno-albumin is relatively contraindicated[4]; in otherwise healthy animals that are only volume depleted, its use should be avoided. In one study, no dog was eligible to receive additional human albumin 7 days following initial administration due to its antigenicity.[1]

Dogs with a pre-existing condition resulting in volume overload should be monitored carefully during administration of hyperosmolar products such as canine albumin. Dogs with anemia or extreme dehydration should not receive canine albumin unless concurrent red blood cell products or appropriate fluid therapy is first administered.[5]

Adverse Effects

The incidence of adverse effects reported in retrospective studies in dogs and cats with human albumin vary widely, but these effects can be serious. Immediate (type I hypersensitivity; anaphylaxis) and delayed (type III hypersensitivity; serum sickness) hypersensitivity reactions are possible when using human albumin in dogs and cats[6]; these effects can be serious, and deaths have occurred. Immediate adverse effects reported include facial edema, vomiting, urticaria, hyperthermia, and shock. Should facial edema occur, diphenhydramine should be given at 1 – 2 mg/kg IM and repeated every 8 hours as required.[2] Delayed adverse effects can include lethargy, lameness, edema, cutaneous lesions/vasculitis, vomiting, inappetence, renal failure, and coagulopathies.

Although no hypersensitivity reactions were observed during 28-day follow-up periods in prospective trials with clinically ill dogs and cats, these finding contrast with previous research.[7,8] A retrospective study evaluating 25% albumin (human) in critically ill dogs and cats found that it could be safely administered and increased albumin levels and systemic blood pressure[9]; however, another retrospective study[1] evaluating human serum albumin (HSA) in 73 critically ill dogs found that although albumin increased serum albumin, total protein, and colloid osmotic pressure (COP), 23% of treated dogs developed at least 1 adverse effect that could potentially have been caused by albumin. The authors caution that given the risks for complications and uncertain positive influence, thoughtful consideration and extreme care must be taken when deciding whether to administer HSA transfusions to critically ill dogs; these concerns should be discussed with clients, and frequent monitoring should always be used.

An Italian retrospective study evaluating 5% HSA in 418 dogs and 170 cats with critical illnesses, severe hypersensitivity reactions such as anaphylaxis, angioedema, or urticaria were not noted in any patient record.[10] In no case was it necessary to discontinue or interrupt the albumin infusion due to adverse effects. Diarrhea, hyperthermia, or tremors were noted in 43% of dogs and 36% of cats treated. A combination of these adverse reactions was seen in 32% of dogs and 34% of cats. Adverse reactions that developed 1 day or more after treatment were noted in 28% of dogs and 11% of cats. Reactions beyond day 3 were not recorded. Perivascular inflammation at catheter sites following albumin administration were seen in 17% of dogs and 34% of cats. This study did not measure changes in total protein, colloid oncotic pressure, or albumin.

The incidence of adverse effects in dogs associated with HSA appears to be higher in healthy dogs than in critically ill dogs, possibly due to the blunted immune response that can be seen in critically ill patients. In a study of 6 healthy dogs given 2 mL/kg of 25% HSA during a 1-hour period, an immediate hypersensitivity reaction (eg, vomiting, facial edema) was seen in 1 dog; delayed adverse reactions were seen 5 to 13 days after albumin was administered in all 6 dogs (including lethargy, lameness, peripheral edema, ecchymoses, vomiting, and anorexia). Delayed complications in 2 of these dogs resulted in death due to renal failure and coagulopathy and were suspected to have occurred because of serum sickness secondary to type III hypersensitivity reactions. Another dog had shock and sepsis secondary to a multidrug-resistant *Escherichia coli* infection.[11] In another study in 9 healthy dogs that were given 1 or 2 infusions of HSA (25% at an initial infusion rate of 0.5 mL/kg/hour that was increased incrementally to a maximum of 4 mL/kg/hour), adverse effects were seen after the first or second infusion in 3 dogs. Anaphylactoid reactions were observed in 1 of 9 dogs during the first infusion and in the 2 dogs that were administered a second infusion. Two dogs developed severe edema and urticaria 6 or 7 days after the initial infusion. All dogs developed anti-HSA antibodies.[4]

The adverse effect profile for canine serum albumin (CSA) use in dogs is not well described. One study of 14 dogs with septic peritonitis demonstrated minimal adverse effects (1 dog developed tachypnea) that could have been attributable to albumin administration.[12] Safety studies in healthy normovolemic beagles where canine albumin was administered once weekly for 4 weeks did not show any evidence of adverse effects or antibody formation.

Although the risk appears low, transmission of infectious agents from albumin products is possible. Rash, nausea, vomiting, tachycardia, and hypotension have been reported in humans, but hypersensitivity reactions are very rare.

Reproductive/Nursing Safety

Albumin products are unlikely to pose much risk to the fetus, particularly when used appropriately. Albumin excretion into maternal milk is not known, but it is unlikely to be harmful.

Because safety has not been established in animals, this drug should only be used when the maternal benefits outweigh the potential risks to offspring.

Overdose/Acute Toxicity

To avoid the effects of hyperalbuminemia/hyperproteinemia, albumin levels should be monitored. During treatment with albumin, it is thought that serum albumin should not exceed 2.5 g/dL. Some clinicians use a more conservative upper limit of 2 g/dL.

For patients that have experienced or are suspected to have experienced an overdose, consultation with a 24-hour poison consultation center specializing in providing veterinary-specific information is recommended. For general information related to overdose and toxin exposures, as well as contact information for poison control centers, refer to *Appendix*.

Drug Interactions

Although the administration of exogenous albumin could bind drugs that are highly bound to plasma proteins and affect the amount of free drug circulating, clinical significance is unlikely.

Laboratory Considerations

- Exogenous administration of albumin may temporarily decrease serum concentrations of calcium.

Dosages

DOGS:

Using human albumin (extra-label):

a) In nonemergent situations, give a test dose of 0.25 mL/kg/hour over 15 minutes while monitoring heart rate, respiratory rate, and temperature (baseline before transfusion and at end of test dose). Discontinue infusion if facial swelling or other signs of anaphylaxis develop. The range for a CRI after a bolus administration is 0.1 – 1.7 mL/kg/hour (0.025 – 0.425 g/kg) over 4 to 72 hours. Suggested maximum volume for slow IV push to treat hypotension is 4 mL/kg (1 g/kg), with a reported average volume of 2 mL/kg (0.5 g/kg). Suggested maximum volume when administered continuously over 72 hours is 25 mL/kg (6.25 g/kg); the reported average of overall volume administered is 5 mL/kg (1.25 g/kg). Infusions are empirically selected to meet low normal values. Shorter infusion times are most commonly used for refractory hypotension.[2]

b) One protocol suggested to calculate albumin deficit (g) is 10 × (serum albumin desired – serum albumin of patient) × body weight (kg) × 0.3. Alternatively, 0.5 – 1.25 g/kg has been suggested. Calculated dose of human albumin is aseptically diluted to a 10% solution with 0.9% sodium chloride and administered over a 12-hour period with a transfusion filter.[1]

c) 2 mL/kg of 25% human serum albumin (HSA) IV over 2 hours, followed by 0.1 – 0.2 mL/kg/hour IV for 10 hours (total dose of 2 g/kg). Alternatively, calculate the albumin deficit and replace it over 6 to 12 hours: albumin deficit = 10 × (desired albumin – patient albumin) × body weight in kg × 0.3.[13]

Using canine albumin: Reconstitute lyophilized powder with 0.9% sodium chloride, *Normosol R*®, or 5% dextrose to desired concentration according to product label.

a) **Hypovolemic shock**: Using a 16% solution, give 1 mL/minute up to a total of 2.5 – 5 g/kg (15.6 – 31.2 mL/kg).

b) **Hypoalbuminemia**:

i. Using a 5% solution, administer up to 2 g/kg/day based on clinical condition.[5]

ii. Using a 5% solution, give 800 mg/kg IV over 6 hours. **NOTE**: Study was done in hypoalbuminemic dogs following surgical source control for septic peritonitis.[12]

CATS:

Using 5% (NOT 25%) human albumin: 2 mL/kg/hour IV over 5 to 10 hours to a maximum of 10 – 20 mL/kg/day. Infusion was repeated on subsequent days if serum albumin concentration was less than 2 g/dL.[8] All cats showed clinical improvement, and 50% of cats attained serum albumin concentration above 2 g/dL.

Monitoring

- Pre- and post-treatment serum albumin; 2 – 2.5 g/dL is a common target for serum albumin concentrations.
- Pre- and post-treatment colloid osmotic pressure (COP), if possible; a target COP of 14 – 20 mm Hg has been suggested.[1]
- Baseline and periodic body temperature, respiratory rate, blood pressure, and heart rate
- Adverse effects
- Signs of volume overload (eg, increased respiratory rate, increased central venous pressure)
- Monitor for delayed reactions, which can occur weeks after administration.

Client Information

- This medicine must be given in an inpatient setting.
- Clients should understand and accept the risks, costs, and monitoring associated with the use of albumin.

Chemistry/Synonyms

Human serum albumin (HSA) is a highly soluble, globular protein with a molecular weight of 66,500. The 5% solution has a colloid osmotic pressure (COP) similar to that of normal plasma. Amino acid homology of HSA and canine serum albumin (CSA) is ≈79%, but the CSA molecule is 2 kDalton larger and has a different relative charge and isoelectric point.

HSA may also be known as Alb, albumine, HSA, or albuminum. "Salt-poor" albumin is a misnomer, but still occasionally used as a designation for 25% albumin. There are a variety of trade name products.

Storage/Stability

- 5% solution: Human serum albumin (HSA) 5% solution is stable for 3 years, providing storage temperature does not exceed 30°C (86°F). Protect this product from freezing.
- 25% and 20% solutions: Store this product at room temperature not exceeding 30°C (86°F). Do not freeze it. Do not use this product after expiration date.

Do not use solutions if they appear turbid or if sediment is noted. Solutions should not be used if more than 4 hours have passed since the container was entered, as they contain no preservatives. Do not use solutions that have been frozen.

The lyophilized canine serum albumin (CSA) product should be stored at 4°C to 6°C (39.2°F-42.7°F; refrigerated) until use.[5] Product is stable for 15 months as labeled. After rehydration, it should be used within 24 hours.

Compatibility/Compounding Considerations

Human serum albumin (HSA) may be administered either in conjunction with or combined with other parenteral products such as whole blood, plasma, saline, glucose, or sodium lactate. It is reportedly **compatible at Y-site** with usual carbohydrate or electrolyte solutions, diltiazem, or midazolam. The canine serum albumin (CSA) product label warns **not** to add supplementary medication or mix with other medicinal products including whole blood or plasma, but that it can be given in conjunction with saline.

Do not mix albumin with protein hydrolysates, amino acid solutions, or solutions containing alcohol.

When preparing HSA for administration, use only 16-gauge needles or dispensing pins with 20 mL vial sizes and larger. Needles or dispensing pins should only be inserted within the stopper area delineated by the raised ring. The stopper should be penetrated perpendicular to the plane of the stopper within the ring.

CSA 5 gram lyophilized should be rehydrated with 0.9% sterile saline (sodium chloride 0.9%) or *Normosol* R® as the diluent. Dextrose 5% may also be used. Adding 30 mL of sterile saline will yield a 16% (166 mg/mL) solution and 100 mL will yield a 5% (50 mg/mL) solution.

DO NOT use sterile water to rehydrate the product. After addition of the diluent, gently swirl the solution intermittently to avoid foaming until all the powder is rehydrated. Once diluent is added, the vial may be warmed in 37°C (98.6°F) water bath to speed rehydration. Do not aggressively agitate the bottle, as foaming may occur. Rehydration may take 15 to 30 minutes with gentle swirling. CSA may be administered in conjunction with or combined with whole blood, packed red blood cells, plasma, saline, or dextrose.

Dosage Forms/Regulatory Status

VETERINARY-LABELED PRODUCTS:

Albumin, Canine, lyophilized 5 g, without preservatives or plasma byproducts; (Animal Blood Resources International). Labeled for IV use in dogs by or on the order of licensed veterinarian. **NOTE**: This is not an FDA-approved product.

HUMAN-LABELED PRODUCTS:

Albumin, Human: 5%, 20%, 25%, in various sizes; *Albuked*®, *Albuminar*®, *AlbuRX*®, *Albutein*®, *Flexbumin*®, *Kedbumin*®, *Plasbumin*®, generic; (Rx). FDA-approved

References

For the complete list of references, see **wiley.com/go/budde/plumb**

Albuterol

Salbutamol

(al-***byoo***-ter-ole) *Proventil*®, *Ventolin*®

Beta-Adrenergic Agonist

Prescriber Highlights

- ► Used primarily as a bronchodilator; available in oral and inhaled dosage forms
- ► Can be used to improve hypoxemia in horses under general anesthesia
- ► Use with caution in patients with cardiac dysrhythmias or dysfunction, seizure disorders, hypertension, or hyperthyroidism
- ► May be teratogenic at high doses and delay labor

Uses/Indications

Albuterol is used principally in cats[1,2] and horses[3] for its effects on bronchial smooth muscle to alleviate acute bronchospasm. True bronchoconstriction is rare in dogs, but albuterol may be a useful treatment in these cases. The inhalation aerosol formulation has been used to improve hypoxemia in anesthetized horses[4]; however, in normal horses, albuterol does not appear to improve physiologic response to exercise.[5,6]

Administration of inhaled albuterol can be facilitated using masks combined with aerosol chambers. In horses, the device used does not appear to significantly impact drug delivery or response.[7] Under laboratory conditions, lack of adherence to the "best practice" inhaler technique (ie, angle device is held against the face, elapsed time, or shaking the inhaler between doses) did not change the amount of albuterol delivery.[8]

Pharmacology/Actions

Albuterol is a sympathomimetic drug that preferentially stimulates beta-2-adrenergic receptors found primarily in vascular smooth muscle (including bronchial, GI, and uterine tissues) to cause relaxation of bronchial smooth muscle, reduced airway resistance, vasodilation, and tocolysis, as well as to inhibit the release of bronchoconstrictive mediators from mast cells. At recommended doses, albuterol spares the beta-1 receptor found primarily in the heart, thus lowering the likelihood of cardiac adverse effects. Albuterol's specificity is not as precise at higher doses, and some beta-1 activity may occur, resulting in tachycardia and increased myocardial contractility. Beta-adrenergic agonists promote a shift of potassium from the serum into the cell, perhaps via stimulation of Na^+-K^+-ATPase, which may cause a temporary decrease in serum potassium concentration.

In horses, albuterol (racemic) produces bronchodilation for ≈30 to 60 minutes.[3,9] The bronchodilatory effects of the R-form (levalbuterol) are comparable to the racemic form but last twice as long (120 minutes).[9] In cats, inflammatory markers in bronchoalveolar lavage (BAL) fluid were lower after levalbuterol use (twice daily for 2 weeks) as compared with racemic albuterol.[10]

Pharmacokinetics

The specific pharmacokinetics of this agent have not been thoroughly studied in domestic animals.

In general, albuterol is absorbed rapidly and well after oral administration in humans. After nebulization, less than 20% of a dose is systemically absorbed. Effects occur within 5 minutes after oral inhalation and 30 minutes after oral administration (eg, tablets). Albuterol does not cross the blood-brain barrier but does cross the placenta. Duration of effect generally persists for 3 to 6 hours after nebulization and up to 12 hours after oral administration (depending on dosage form [eg, tablets, syrup]). The drug is extensively metabolized in the liver, principally to the inactive metabolite, albuterol 4'-O-sulfate. After oral administration, the serum half-life in humans has been reported to be 2.7 to 5 hours.

Contraindications/Precautions/Warnings

Albuterol is contraindicated in patients that are hypersensitive to it or to other sympathomimetics. It should be used with caution in patients with diabetes, glaucoma, hyperthyroidism, hypertension, hypokalemia, seizure disorders, or cardiac disease (especially if concurrent arrhythmias are present).

Do not confuse albuterol with atenolol, or salbutamol with salmeterol.

Adverse Effects

Most adverse effects are dose-related and are consistent with other sympathomimetic agents, including increased heart rate, tremors, CNS excitement (ie, nervousness), and dizziness. These effects are generally transient and mild and usually do not require discontinuation of therapy. Transient hypokalemia has been reported in humans receiving beta-adrenergic agents; potassium supplementation is rarely required. In humans, hyperglycemia, cardiac arrhythmia, paradoxical bronchospasm, immediate hypersensitivity reactions, and pulmonary edema have also been reported.[11]

In cats, the S-form of albuterol may potentially increase airway inflammation. As "regular" albuterol is the racemic form (R,S-albuterol), it may also increase airway inflammation, and its use in cats should likely be limited only to acute rescue treatment and not long-term treatment.[10] In addition, some cats do not like the hissing sound during the actuation of the metered-dose inhaler or the taste of the drug/vehicle.

Mild tachycardia, premature ventricular complexes, increases and decreases in blood pressure, and profound sweating have been reported when aerosol albuterol has been administered via the breathing system to horses under general anesthesia for improvement of partial pressure of oxygen in arterial blood.[4,12] Hypokalemia has also been noted.[13,14] When high doses of beta-agonists are administered to horses via nebulization, adverse effects can include twitching, sweating, and excitement.

Reproductive/Nursing Safety

Albuterol crosses the placenta and is teratogenic (cleft palate) in rodents at doses lower than that used clinically in humans. This drug should only be used during pregnancy (particularly the oral dosage forms) when the potential benefits outweigh the risks. Use during the late stages of pregnancy may inhibit uterine contractions, and it may delay pre-term labor after oral administration. Fetal hyperglycemia and tachycardia may occur.

It is not known whether albuterol is excreted in milk. Use it with caution in nursing patients.

Overdose/Acute Toxicity

The oral LD_{50} of albuterol in mice and rats is reported to be greater than 2 g/kg.[15] Significant toxicity can occur in small animals after an oral overdose, or in dogs that bite into the metered-dose inhalers. Clinical signs of significant overdose after systemic administration (including when dogs bite into an aerosol canister) can include arrhythmias (eg, tachycardia, extrasystole), hypertension, lethargy, fever, vomiting, panting/tachypnea, polyuria/polydipsia, mydriasis, hypokalemia, hyperlactatemia, hyperglycemia, tremors, and CNS stimulation.[16-19] A retrospective study of 501 dogs with acute exposure to albuterol (most commonly due to biting/piercing an inhaler) noted the following: signs were rapid in onset (within 1 to 3 hours); the most common clinical signs included tachycardia (≈81%), tachypnea (≈33%), depression (21%), and vomiting (≈19%); and hypokalemia was reported in ≈21%, and arrhythmias occurred in 3.4% of dogs.[20] Overall, 6% of dogs remained subclinical while 94% developed clinical signs, with 2 dogs (0.4%) dying. In a dog that received ≈4 times the recommended dose for 2 years, sinus tachycardia, marked QT interval prolongation, P waves partially merged with previous prominent T waves, and mild ST-segment depression were reported. Other findings included severe hypokalemia, metabolic acidosis, and hyperlactatemia.[17] One case report describes acute nontraumatic rhabdomyolysis in a greyhound after albuterol toxicosis.[21]

If an animal has recently ingested tablets and the animal does not have significant cardiac or CNS effects, the situation should be handled like other overdoses (ie, GI decontamination procedures). For inhalation exposure (eg, when a dog bites into an aerosol canister), decontamination is generally not effective. If cardiac arrhythmias require treatment, a beta-blocking agent (eg, propranolol[16] or esmolol[22]) can be used, and in one study ≈40% of dogs required a beta-blocker.[20] Diazepam can be used for tremors. Potassium supplementation may be required (16% in one study[20]), but be alert for rebound hyperkalemia.[18]

For patients that have experienced or are suspected of having experienced an overdose, it is strongly encouraged to consult with a 24hour poison consultation center that specializes in providing information specific for veterinary patients. For general information related to overdose and toxin exposures, as well as contact information for poison control centers, refer to the ***Appendix***.

Drug Interactions

The following drug interactions have either been reported or are theoretical in humans or animals receiving albuterol (primarily when albuterol is given orally, not via inhalation) and may be of significance in veterinary patients. Unless otherwise noted, use together is not necessarily contraindicated, but weigh the potential risks and perform additional monitoring when appropriate.

- **Beta-Adrenergic Blocking Agents** (eg, **atenolol, propranolol**): May antagonize the actions of albuterol
- **Digoxin**: Albuterol may increase the risk for cardiac arrhythmias.
- **Diuretics**: Hypokalemia caused by diuretics may be acutely exacerbated by albuterol use.
- **Inhaled Anesthetics** (eg, **isoflurane**): Albuterol may predispose patients to ventricular arrhythmias, particularly those with preexisting cardiac disease—use cautiously.
- **Monoamine Oxidase Inhibitors** (MAOIs; eg, **amitraz, linezolid, selegiline**): May potentiate the vascular effects of albuterol
- **Succinylcholine**: Concurrent use may result in enhanced neuromuscular blockade.
- **Sympathomimetic Amines, Other** (eg, **phenylpropanolamine**): Use with albuterol may increase the risk for developing adverse cardiovascular effects.
- **Theophylline**: May result in decreased theophylline concentrations. The combination may result in additive CNS stimulation and increased risk for hypokalemia and cardiac arrhythmias; sudden death has occurred in laboratory animals.
- **Tricyclic antidepressants** (eg, **amitriptyline, clomipramine**): May potentiate the vascular effects of albuterol

Dosages

DOGS:

Bronchodilator for bronchoconstriction (extra-label): 0.02 – 0.05 mg/kg (20 – 50 µg/kg) PO every 8 to 12 hours.[23] Start at the low end of the dosing range and assess for efficacy and adverse effects. Increase dose and/or frequency if the response is not adequate and adverse effects are acceptable.

CATS:

Bronchodilator for intermittent, short-term treatment of feline asthma (extra-label): 1 puff (90 µg) may be repeated up to 3 times every 5 to 15 minutes.[1,24] Use with an appropriate spacer and mask (eg, *Aerokat*®). **Albuterol** should not be used on a long-term basis (see ***Adverse Effects***); the continued need for this drug may indicate a lack of control of underlying inflammation. Inhaled corticosteroids (eg, fluticasone) are recommended for long-term use to control inflammation. **NOTE**: Cats with status asthmaticus may respond faster with injectable terbutaline. See ***Terbutaline***.

Bronchoconstriction associated with bronchoscopy, bronchoalveolar lavage (BAL), or endotracheal wash (extra-label): Using an albuterol plus ipratropium combination MDI, 2 puffs (albuterol 200 µg and ipratropium 40 µg) administered prior to sedation through a spacing chamber[2]

HORSES:

Bronchodilator for acute (rescue) treatment of severe equine asthma (SEA) (extra-label):

a. **Using a handheld device** (eg, ***AeroHippus***®, ***Equine Haler***®): 2 to 3 puffs (180 – 270 µg total dose; NOT µg/kg) initially; may repeat up to 3 times every 5 to 15 minutes. In addition to environmental management, consider using inhaled corticosteroids (eg, fluticasone 5 minutes after albuterol), as tolerance to albuterol alone can develop rapidly.
b. 3 to 6 puffs (360 – 720 µg total dose; NOT µg/kg) every 3 hours[3]

Hypoxemia under general anesthesia (extra-label): Use a canister adaptor between the Y-piece of the anesthesia machine breathing system and the endotracheal tube of the patient. Administer a total of 2 µg/kg just before the inhalation phase of the respiratory cycle.[4,25]

Recovery of BAL fluid (extra-label): 1 puff (1 µg/kg) as a single dose administered via *EquiHaler*® before sedation and 30 minutes before BAL[26]

CATTLE:

Respiratory distress syndrome in premature calves (extra-label): 25 µg/kg via nebulization every 6 hours; may also be nebulized in combination with fluticasone 15 µg/kg every 12 hours, furosemide 1 mg/kg nebulized every 12 hours, or both[27]

Monitoring

- Improvement of clinical signs
- Arterial blood gases (as indicated)
- Heart rate and rhythm (ECG if warranted)
- Thoracic auscultation
- Baseline and periodic serum potassium

Client Information

- Contact your veterinarian if your animal's condition deteriorates or the animal becomes acutely ill.
- If using the aerosol form, shake product canister well before using, then attach the canister to the spacer/mask. The device must be primed by depressing the canister prior to first use or if it has been unused for prolonged periods. Be certain how to appropriately administer the product to maximize effectiveness.
- Do not puncture or use near an open flame. Do not allow exposure to temperatures greater than 48.9°C (120°F), as the canister could explode if kept in the heat. Keep out of reach of children and animals.
- When using inhaled albuterol with an appropriate spacer/facemask (eg, *Aerokat*®) in cats, the following tips have been recommended:
  a. Allow the cat to get used to and investigate the device (eg, leave the device by food bowl) over several days.
  b. Reward (eg, via praise, food, catnip, stroking) fearless approaches to the device, and start placing the device near the cat's face.
  c. Practice placing the mask over the cat's face without anything in the chamber.
  d. Preload the chamber with a puff of albuterol (in addition to the dose required).
  e. Make sure the mask is placed snugly over the muzzle for 4 to 6 breaths.

Chemistry/Synonyms

Albuterol sulfate, a synthetic sympathomimetic amine, occurs as a white crystalline powder. It is soluble in water and slightly soluble in alcohol. Albuterol sulfate inhalation solution is a clear colorless to light yellow solution. One milligram of albuterol is equivalent to 1.2 mg of albuterol sulfate.

Albuterol sulfate may also be known as salbutamol hemisulphate, salbutamol sulphate, or salbutamoli sulfas; many trade names are available.

Storage/Stability

Store oral albuterol products between 2°C and 30°C (36°F-86°F) in well-closed containers. Store inhaled metered-dose aerosols at room temperature (eg, 15°C-25°C [59°F-77°F]), as temperatures above or below may impair device performance; do not allow exposure to temperatures above 48.9°C (120°F) or the canister may explode. Solutions for nebulization may be stored in the refrigerator or at room temperature of 2°C to 25°C (36°F-77°F). Discard solutions if they become colored. Protect all albuterol products from light.

Compatibility/Compounding Considerations

Albuterol solution for nebulization may be mixed with other medications formulated for nebulization.

Dosage Forms/Regulatory Status

VETERINARY-LABELED PRODUCTS: NONE

The Association of Racing Commissioners International (ARCI) has designated this drug as a class 3 substance. Use of this drug may not be allowed in certain animal competitions. Check rules and regulations before entering a competition while this medication is being administered. Contact local racing authorities for further guidance. See ***Appendix*** for more information.

HUMAN-LABELED PRODUCTS:

Albuterol Oral Tablets: 2 mg and 4 mg; generic; (Rx)

Albuterol Extended-Release Oral Tablets: 4 mg and 8 mg; generic; (Rx)

Albuterol Oral Syrup: 2 mg (as sulfate)/5 mL in 473 mL; generic; (Rx)

Albuterol Aerosol for Inhalation: Each actualization (puff) delivers 90 µg. Now labeled as 108 µg albuterol sulfate in 6.7 g, 8 g, 8.5 g, and 18 g. Some canisters have 60 actuations, and some have 200 actuations; *Proventil HFA®*, *Ventolin HFA®*, *ProAir HFA®*;(Rx)

Albuterol Solution for Inhalation (Nebulization): 0.083% (2.5 mg/3 mL) in 3 mL UD vials; 0.021% (0.63 mg/3 mL), and 0.042% (1.25 mg/3 mL) preservative-free in 3 mL UD vials; 0.5% (5 mg/mL) in 0.5 mL ampules and 20 mL with dropper (must be diluted); generic; (Rx)

Albuterol and Ipratropium Solution for Inhalation: 14.7 g aerosol metered-dose inhaler containing 20 µg ipratropium bromide (an inhaled anticholinergic) and 100 µg albuterol sulfate per puff; *Combivent® Respimat*, generic; (Rx); and 3 mL unit dose solution for inhalation (neb) containing 0.5 mg ipratropium bromide and 3 mg albuterol; *DuoNeb®*, generic; (Rx)

Also available: Albuterol dry-powder inhalers (requires deep inhalation to activate)

References

For the complete list of references, see **wiley.com/go/budde/plumb**

Alendronate

(a-***len***-droe-nate) *Fosamax®*

Bone Resorption Inhibitor

Prescriber Highlights

- ► Oral bisphosphonate that reduces osteoclastic bone resorption. Potentially useful for refractory hypercalcemia, bone pain, osteosarcoma, and feline tooth resorption
- ► There is little experience using this drug in animals; adverse effect profile and dosages may significantly change with more experience and clinical research.
- ► Potentially can cause esophageal erosions; risks are not clear for dogs or cats.
- ► Accurate dosing may be difficult; bioavailability is adversely affected by the presence of food in the stomach.

Uses/Indications

Use of alendronate in small animal species has been limited, but this drug has been used in treating idiopathic hypercalcemia in cats,[1-3] and reducing feline tooth resorption.[4] It can also be used in dogs for reducing pain associated with bone tumors and as an osteosarcoma treatment adjuvant.[5]

Pharmacology/Actions

Alendronate, like other bisphosphonates, binds to bone hydroxyapatite, inhibits osteoclast function and thereby reduces bone resorption. Secondary actions that may contribute to therapeutic usefulness in osteogenic neoplasms include promoting apoptosis and inhibiting osteoclastogenesis, angiogenesis, and cancer cell proliferation.[6]

Pharmacokinetics

Specific pharmacokinetic values are limited for dogs and unavailable for cats. Oral bioavailability in all species studied is less than 2%. In humans, alendronate sodium has very low oral bioavailability (less than 1%), and the presence of food in the stomach can reduce bioavailability further to negligible amounts. In women, taking the medication with coffee or orange juice reduced bioavailability by 60% when as compared with plain water.

Absorbed drug is rapidly distributed to bone or excreted in the urine. The drug is reportedly not highly plasma protein-bound in dogs, but it is in rats.[7] Alendronate appears to accumulate on subgingival tooth surfaces and bordering alveolar bone.[4] Plasma concentrations are virtually undetectable after therapeutic dosing.[7]

Alendronate is not metabolized, and drug taken up by bone is eliminated very slowly. It is estimated that the terminal elimination half-life is ≈1000 days in dogs and ≈10 years in humans; however, once incorporated into bone, alendronate is no longer active.

Contraindications/Precautions/Warnings

Alendronate is contraindicated in patients hypersensitive to it. Bisphosphonates may cause upper GI adverse reactions (eg, esophagitis, esophageal ulcers), and alendronate is contraindicated in human patients with esophageal abnormalities (eg, strictures, achalasia) that cause delayed esophageal emptying and those who cannot stand or sit upright for 30 minutes after administration. The drug is not recommended for use in human patients with severe renal dysfunction (CrCl less than 35 mL/minute). Hypocalcemia must be corrected prior to alendronate use. Calcium and vitamin D should be supplemented if dietary intake is inadequate.

Bisphosphonate use in humans has been associated with osteonecrosis of the jaw; one case has been reported in a cat.[8] Risk factors in humans include poor oral hygiene, invasive dental procedures (extractions, implants), cancer diagnosis, concurrent medication therapy (chemotherapy, corticosteroid use), and comorbidities (anemia, infection, coagulopathy).

Alendronate use in small animals should be considered investigational at this point. Limited research and experience, dosing questions, risks for esophageal irritation or ulcers, and medication expense all are potential hindrances to its therapeutic usefulness.

Adverse Effects

There is little information on the specific adverse effect profile of alendronate in dogs or cats. In humans, alendronate can cause upper GI irritation and erosions. See ***Contraindications/Precautions/Warnings.*** GI upset, vomiting, and inappetence have been anecdotally reported in dogs receiving the drug. It has been suggested that after administration, walking or playing with the dog for 30 minutes may reduce the incidence of esophageal problems. In cats, buttering the lips after administration to induce salivation and reduce esophageal transit time has been suggested.

Other potential adverse effects of concern include atypical fractures and musculoskeletal pain.

Reproductive/Nursing Safety

Alendronate at dosages of 2 mg/kg in rats caused decreased post-implantation survival rates and at 1 mg/kg caused decreased weight gain in healthy pups.[9] Higher dosages (10 mg/kg) caused incomplete fetal ossification of several bone types. Hypocalcemia in the dam resulted in protracted parturition. No adverse fetal effects were noted in pregnant rabbits given alendronate during periods of organogenesis.

Although it is unknown whether alendronate enters maternal milk, it would be unexpected that measurable quantities would be found in milk or that it would be absorbed in clinically significant amounts in nursing offspring.

Because safety has not been established in animals, this drug should only be used when the maternal benefits outweigh the potential risks to offspring.

Overdose/Acute Toxicity

No lethality was observed in dogs receiving doses up to 200 mg/kg.[9] Lethality in mice and rats was seen at dosages starting at 966 mg/kg and 552 mg/kg, respectively. Observed adverse effects associated with overdoses included hypocalcemia, hypophosphatemia, and upper GI reactions.

A recently ingested overdose should be treated with orally administered antacids or milk to bind the drug and reduce absorption. Do not induce vomiting. Monitor serum calcium and phosphorus, and treat the patient supportively.

For patients that have experienced or are suspected to have experienced an overdose, it is strongly encouraged to consult with a 24-hour poison consultation center that specialize in providing information specific for veterinary patients. For general information related to overdose and toxin exposures, as well as contact information for poison control centers, refer to *Appendix*.

Drug Interactions

The following drug interactions with alendronate have either been reported or are theoretical in humans or animals and may be of significance in veterinary patients. Unless otherwise noted, use together is not necessarily contraindicated, but weigh the potential risks and perform additional monitoring when appropriate.

- **AMINOGLYCOSIDES** (eg, **amikacin, gentamicin**): Concurrent use may increase the risk of hypocalcemia and nephrotoxicity. Use combination cautiously and monitor for signs of hypocalcemia.
- **ASPIRIN**: Theoretically increased risk for GI toxicity and renal impairment; however, data are lacking.
- **CALCIUM, ALUMINUM,** and **MAGNESIUM,** or **OTHER POLYVALENT CATION-CONTAINING ORAL PRODUCTS**: Likely to significantly decrease oral bioavailability of alendronate. Patients should receive nothing by mouth other than water for 2 hours before and 30 minutes after oral administration of alendronate.
- **DIURETICS, LOOP** (eg, **furosemide**): Concurrent use may increase risk for hypocalcemia. Monitor calcium levels and renal function.
- **ESTROGENS** (eg, **diethylstilbestrol, estradiol**): Concurrent use may increase effects on bone density.
- **H_2 RECEPTOR ANTAGONISTS** (eg, **famotidine, ranitidine**): Concurrent use may increase levels of both drugs.
- **NSAIDs** (eg, **carprofen, meloxicam, robenacoxib**): Theoretically increased risk for GI toxicity and renal impairment; however, data are lacking. Use together cautiously and monitor renal function and signs of gastrointestinal toxicity.
- **PROTON PUMP INHIBITORS** (eg, **omeprazole, pantoprazole**): Concurrent use may decrease effects of alendronate. Avoid combination.

Laboratory Considerations

- Alendronate may interfere with technitium-99m-diphosphonate bone scans.

Dosages

DOGS:

Refractory hypercalcemia or to reduce pain associated with bone tumors (extra-label): **NOTE**: There is little experience using this drug in dogs. Reported dosages include 10 mg/dog (NOT mg/kg) PO once daily on an empty stomach[5] or 2 mg/kg PO once daily on an empty stomach.[10]

CATS:

Idiopathic hypercalcemia (extra-label): Initially 5 – 10 mg/cat (NOT mg/kg) PO once weekly; most cats started treatment at 10 mg/cat (NOT mg/kg) weekly.[3] Following administration, give 6 mL tap water PO by syringe, then butter the nasal planum to increase salivation. By the end of the 6-month period, 1 cat was receiving 15 mg (total dose; NOT mg/kg) and 4 cats 20 mg (total dose; NOT mg/kg) per week. Alendronate was well-tolerated and decreased ionized Ca in most cats for the 6-month period of observation.

Tooth resorption (extra-label): 9 mg/kg PO twice per week slowed or arrested the progression of tooth resorption.[4]

Monitoring

- Serum ionized calcium (iCa). Usually repeated monthly; adjust alendronate dose to maintain iCa in the target range.
- GI adverse effects. **NOTE**: Depending on diagnosis (eg, hypercalcemia, adjunctive treatment of osteogenic sarcomas, or feline resorptive lesions), other monitoring of serum electrolytes (eg, total calcium, phosphorus, potassium, sodium) or disease-associated signs may be required.

Client Information

- Do not break, split, or crush tablets unless your veterinarian has instructed you to do so.
- Must be given with water on an empty stomach. Food can prevent the drug from being absorbed and make it ineffective; do not offer food for at least 30 minutes after a dose is given. Offer your animal water after dosing to reduce the chances of throat or esophagus problems.
- If your animal vomits or acts sick after receiving the drug, try walking, exercising, or playing with your animal after dosing; encouraging it to drink water; or spreading butter on the lips (to stimulate salivation).
- Alendronate has not been used in many animals. Possible side effects include vomiting, lack of appetite, throat or esophagus ulcers or sores, or bone pain. Contact your veterinarian if you see

any other side effects of concern while your animal is taking this medicine.

- This medication can be given for various lengths of time. Be sure you understand how long your veterinarian wants you to continue giving this medication. Prescription refills may be necessary before the therapy will be complete. Before stopping this medication, talk to your veterinarian, as there may be important reasons to continue its use.
- Your veterinarian will need to monitor your animal closely while receiving this medicine. Do not miss these important follow-up visits.

Chemistry/Synonyms

Alendronate sodium is a synthetic analogue of pyrophosphonate with the chemical name (4-amino-1-hydroxy-1-phosphono-butyl) phosphonic acid. One mg is soluble in 1 L of water.

Alendronate may also be known as alendronic acid, acide alendronique, acido alendronico, acidum alendronicum, *Adronat*®, *Alendros*®, *Arendal*®, *Onclast*®, or *Fosamax*®.

Storage/Stability

Alendronate tablets should be stored in tightly closed containers at room temperature 20°C to 25°C (68°F-77°F); excursions permitted to 15°C to 30°C (59°F-86°F). The oral solution should be stored at room temperature; do not freeze.

Compatibility/Compounding Considerations

No specific information noted

Dosage Forms/Regulatory Status

VETERINARY-LABELED PRODUCTS: NONE

HUMAN-LABELED PRODUCTS:

Alendronate Oral Tablets: 5, 10, 35, 40, and 70 mg (also effervescent tablet); *Fosamax*®, generic; (Rx). A 70 mg tablet combined with vitamin D3 (*Fosamax® Plus D*, 70 µg or 140 µg) is also available.

Alendronate Oral Solution: 70 mg (as base) in 75 mL; raspberry flavor; *Fosamax*®, generic; (Rx)

References

For the complete list of references, see **wiley.com/go/budde/plumb**

Alfaxalone

(al-***fax***-ah-lone) *Alfaxan*®

Intravenous Anesthetic

Prescriber Highlights

- ► Injectable (IV) anesthetic agent labeled for dogs and cats and indexed for use in multiple minor species; used extra-label in many species
- ► Used extra-label IM for sedation/premedication/light anesthesia in cats, small dogs, and a variety of small mammals, and other species. IM administration can be limited to animals of a smaller body size because of the large injectate volume required in larger animals.
- ► Provides no analgesia
- ► Respiratory depression/apnea can occur, particularly if administered rapidly IV.
- ► When used as a sole agent, opisthotonos, muscle tremors, hyperreactivity, and excitement can occur. To facilitate smoother patient recovery, a lower alfaxalone dose can be used in conjunction with premedication drugs.
- ► DEA Schedule IV (C-IV) controlled substance

Uses/Indications

Alfaxalone is FDA approved for use in cats and dogs for induction and maintenance of anesthesia, and for induction of anesthesia followed by maintenance with an inhalant anesthetic.

Alfaxalone has been used, with mixed results, for light anesthesia in the assessment of laryngeal motion in dogs. One study in premedicated dogs (methadone 0.2 mg/kg IM and acepromazine 0.01 mg/kg IM) concluded that alfaxalone (0.5 – 2 mg/kg IV) was comparable to propofol (1 – 4 mg/kg IV) for assessing laryngeal motion in non-brachycephalic versus brachycephalic dogs[1]; however, another study showed that thiopentone 7.5 mg/kg IV (not currently available in the United States) or propofol 3 mg/kg IV may be superior for assessing laryngeal motion as compared with alfaxalone 1.5 mg/kg IV.[2] The addition of doxapram 2.5 mg/kg IV to the protocol improved assessment of laryngeal motion.[3]

Alfaxalone has also been administered alone as a deep IM injection (extra-label in the United States) to cats to provide dose-dependent light to heavy sedation but it may cause tremors, ataxia, and opisthotonos-like posture.[4] The level of sedation from alfaxalone alone is generally not adequate for fractious cats. IM administration is limited to patients with a small body size (domestic cat-sized and smaller) because a larger body size will require an inappropriately large volume of injectate.

In cats, alfaxalone combined with midazolam or butorphanol and administered IM has been used to facilitate echocardiography. Compared to dexmedetomidine, alfaxalone has less of an impact on echocardiographic parameters.[5,6]

Because of its fast onset, which facilitates titration of low doses administered IV 'to effect', alfaxalone may be considered for use in high-risk patients[7]; however, dose-dependent cardiorespiratory depression, similar to that caused by propofol, can occur so alfaxalone doses should be kept as low as possible in these patients. It is also useful in sighthounds.[7,8]

Although not approved for use in horses, alfaxalone may be useful as an injectable induction agent or part of a total IV anesthesia (TIVA) protocol for short-term field anesthesia procedures.[9-13] Alfaxalone may also be useful in combination with medetomidine and butorphanol for procedures lasting up to 60 minutes[14]; however, due to the large volumes required, it is not commonly used in this species.

Alfaxan® Mulitdose IDX is an FDA-index product indicated for a variety of routes of administration including IV, IM, and intraperitoneal in captive, nonfood-producing reptiles, amphibians, ornamental fish, birds, nonhuman primates, rodents, mustelids, marsupials, and ungulates.[15] Alfaxalone has also been used extra-label in a variety of species including small mammals, rabbits, sheep, alpacas, goats, pigs, deer, fish, primates, amphibians, and reptiles.[16-32] The absorption of alfaxalone from IM and intraperitoneal injection sites facilitates use in these species, especially when IV access is a challenge.

Pharmacology/Actions

Alfaxalone is a neuroactive steroid molecule with properties of a general anesthetic. The primary mechanism for the anesthetic action of alfaxalone is the modulation of neuronal cell membrane chloride ion transport, which is induced by binding alfaxalone to gamma-aminobutyric acid (GABA) cell surface receptors. Alfaxalone has no analgesic properties.

In dogs, recumbency typically occurs 60 seconds after the start of IV injection, and intubation can be performed within 1 to 2 minutes. In dogs not given a preanesthetic agent, the duration of anesthesia from a single induction dose of alfaxalone is ≈5 to 10 minutes; duration may be longer in dogs given preanesthetic agents. In cats, effects of anesthesia are typically observed within 60 seconds after the start of injection, and intubation can be performed within 1 to 2 minutes. In cats not given a preanesthetic agent, the duration of anesthesia after being given a single induction dose of alfaxalone ranges between 15 to 30 minutes; duration may be longer in cats given preanesthetic agents. However, in field trials, the duration was shorter in premedicated dogs and cats, likely due to a lower alfaxalone dose needed for induction.[33]

In preapproval field studies, patient recovery times (ie, extubation to head lift) following administration of alfaxalone averaged 22 minutes in dogs and 15 minutes in cats that did not receive a preanesthetic agent, and 15 minutes in dogs and 17 minutes in cats that did receive a preanesthetic agent. At labeled doses, dogs and cats are expected to recover to sternal recumbency in 60 to 80 minutes.[33]

Propofol 10 mg/kg compared to alfaxalone 5 mg/kg administered IV to unpremedicated cats caused rapid loss of consciousness without apnea or clinically relevant changes in physiologic parameters.[34] Transient hypoxemia was more profound with propofol whereas more adverse events (ataxia, muscle tremors) in recovery occurred with alfaxalone.[34]

Pharmacokinetics

In dogs, the volume of distribution after a single injection of alfaxalone at 2 mg/kg is ≈2.5 L/kg, clearance is ≈54 mL/kg/minute, and elimination terminal half-life is ≈27 minutes.[35] A study done in greyhounds showed similar results when dogs were not premedicated; however, greyhounds premedicated with acepromazine and morphine had substantially longer (ie, 5 times) anesthetic durations, elimination half-life was ≈19% longer, and clearance was ≈24% lower than dogs not premedicated.[8]

In cats, the volume of distribution of alfaxalone is ≈2 L/kg. Clearance is dosage dependent with doses of 5 mg/kg (clinical dose) averaging 25.1 mL/kg/minute and doses of 25 mg/kg (supraclinical dose) averaging 14.8 mL/kg/minute. The elimination half-lives at these doses are 45.2 and 76.6 minutes, respectively. Alfaxalone has nonlinear pharmacokinetics in cats, but there is no clinically relevant accumulation with administration of multiple doses.[36]

Cat and dog hepatocyte (in vitro) studies have shown that alfaxalone undergoes phase I (cytochrome P450-dependent) and phase II (conjugation-dependent) metabolism in both species. Cats and dogs form the same 5 phase I metabolites. Phase II metabolites in cats are alfaxalone sulfate and alfaxalone glucuronide, with only alfaxalone glucuronide found in dogs. Alfaxalone metabolites are likely to be eliminated from dogs and cats by hepatic/fecal and renal routes, which is similar to other species studied.[37]

In adult horses given IV premedication that consisted of acepromazine, xylazine, and guaifenesin, alfaxalone's plasma elimination half-life was ≈33 minutes, volume of distribution was 1.6 L/kg, and plasma clearance was 33 mL/kg/minute.[38] In neonatal foals given a premedication of butorphanol, alfaxalone's plasma elimination half-life was ≈23 minutes, volume of distribution was 0.6 L/kg, and plasma clearance was 20 mL/kg/minute.[39]

Contraindications/Precautions/Warnings

Alfaxalone is contraindicated in patients with a known hypersensitivity to alfaxalone or its components or when general anesthesia and/or sedation are contraindicated. This drug should not be used with other IV general anesthetic agents (eg, propofol).[40,41] Because postinduction apnea can occur, alfaxalone should only be used if the patient can be continuously monitored and if appropriate oxygen supplementation, maintenance of the patient's airway, and artificial ventilation can be immediately provided.

Appropriate pain control should be administered because alfaxalone does not provide analgesia.

For induction, administer IV over ≈60 seconds, to effect, until clinical signs show the onset of anesthesia, titrating administration against the response of the patient. **This drug must be given slowly IV (see *Dosages*); rapid IV administration or overdose can cause cardiorespiratory depression or apnea.** Apnea can occur following induction or after the administration of maintenance boluses. The use of preanesthetic agents may reduce the alfaxalone induction dose. The choice and amount of phenothiazine, alpha$_2$-adrenergic receptor agonist, benzodiazepine, or opioid will influence the response of the patient to an induction dose of alfaxalone.[33]

Patients should be in an appropriate facility and under sufficient supervision during the postanesthetic recovery period. Animals in recovery should not be handled or disturbed, as psychomotor excitement can occur; premedication with a benzodiazepine may increase this likelihood.[33]

Caution is advised in patients with significant hepatic dysfunction, as they may require lower doses or increased dose intervals to maintain anesthesia.[42] Caution is also advised for senior, critically ill, or debilitated animals.

IM use of the preservative-free formulation in cats is approved in some countries.[41] The multidose formulation that contains preservatives is approved for IV-only administration in all countries; however, it has been used IM (extra-label) in dogs and cats. IM administration is limited to patients with small body size (domestic cat-sized and smaller) because a larger body size will require an inappropriately large volume of injectate. Alfaxalone used IM in dogs produces dose-dependent neurologic depression; lateral recumbency; and decreases in respiratory rate, rectal temperature, and blood pressure. Transient hypoxemia and muscular tremors can occur, but recovery may be satisfactory, especially if appropriate premedications are administered.[43] Similar to dogs, alfaxalone used IM in cats causes dose-dependent sedation and lateral recumbency. Ataxia, muscular tremors, and opisthotonus-like posture can be observed after IM and IV administration.[4,44]

The US label states that safe use of alfaxalone in cats younger than 4 weeks and dogs younger than 10 weeks has not been evaluated. A study in kittens (n = 34; ≈6 to 11 weeks) concluded that alfaxalone is a suitable anesthetic induction agent for premedicated kittens younger than 12 weeks and anesthetic maintenance with supplemental doses of alfaxalone may be a suitable alternative in kittens when inhalant maintenance is not feasible.[45] A similar study in puppies (n = 25; ≈6-11 weeks) concluded that alfaxalone is a suitable induction agent for premedicated puppies younger than 12 weeks that require anesthesia for surgical or diagnostic procedures; however, 2 of the puppies had excited recoveries and 1 puppy had an unacceptable anesthetic maintenance period characterized by prolonged apnea.[46]

Adverse Effects

Alfaxalone is relatively safe for a general anesthetic agent; with respiratory depression and apnea being the biggest concerns. These adverse effects can be exacerbated depending on the administration rate and premedication agents used. Respiratory depression following induction is more common when alfaxalone is administered rapidly IV.[47]

In field studies, 40% of dogs and 16% of cats experienced postinduction apnea (defined as cessation of breathing for 30 seconds or more), with a mean duration of 100 seconds in dogs and 60 seconds in cats.[33] The drug should be given slowly IV and the patient should be closely monitored. Slow administration (≈0.5 mg/kg per minute, which equals 0.05 mL/kg/minute of the 10 mg/mL product) caused apnea in 25% of dogs premedicated with dexmedetomidine and methadone. Administration at 2 mg/kg/minute caused apnea in 100% of dogs with the same premedications.[47] Slow administration also resulted in a lower induction dose needed to achieve endotracheal intubation. Once the patient is sufficiently anesthetized, alfaxalone administration should be discontinued, and an endotracheal tube placed. It is advisable to provide supplemental oxygen and monitor oxygen saturation (SpO_2). Cardiac arrhythmias may occur but are thought to occur primarily due to hypoxemia/hypercapnia; oxygen therapy is recommended as the primary treatment, followed by specific therapy for the arrhythmia(s), if required.

The cardiodepressant effects of alfaxalone, along with the vasodilatory effects of inhalant anesthetics, can cause hypotension.

Transient hypertension can also be noted, possibly due to increased sympathetic activity. Minimal cardiac effects have been found in dogs when alfaxalone is used in combination with butorphanol and midazolam.[48] In dogs, the heart rate is preserved or increased when alfaxalone is used in combination with fentanyl.[49] Alfaxalone given IM with dexmedetomidine caused a mild decrease in heart rate and oxygen saturation in cats.[50] Tachycardia, hypertension, and hypoxemia were observed in calves anesthetized with alfaxalone.[51] The cardiac index in horses reached 68% of baseline value after alfaxalone induction and was maintained between 74% to 90% during TIVA[52]; however, another study did not detect differences in cardiovascular function between TIVA using either propofol or alfaxalone with medetomidine/gauifenesin.[53]

As with most anesthetics, hypothermia during and after anesthesia is likely; providing external heat sources and monitoring the patient's core body temperature are recommended.

Induction of general anesthesia with alfaxalone can increase intraocular pressure (IOP) in dogs. Administering premedication drugs (ie, acepromazine/butorphanol, dexmedetomidine/hydromorphone) did not counteract the effect of alfaxalone on IOP.[54] In another study, the increase in IOP was only transient up to 2 minutes after induction and was followed by a decrease in IOP. Alfaxalone also caused a decrease in tear production.[55]

Excitement (eg, disorientation, nervousness, violent movements), vocalization, paddling, trembling, and myoclonus have been reported in dogs and cats during recovery.[56-58] In dogs premedicated with morphine and acepromazine, administration of midazolam before alfaxalone reduced excitement as compared with administration of midazolam after alfaxalone.[59] Sedative drugs used in combination with alfaxalone can improve recovery[60] and, especially in cats, recovery should ideally be in a quiet room. Paddling and muscle tremors occurred during recovery in 6 out of 8 horses following administration of alfaxalone TIVA.[52]

One case of anaphylaxis to alfaxalone has been described in a dog.[61]

Reproductive/Nursing Safety

Safe use of alfaxalone has not been established in animals that are pregnant or lactating; however, alfaxalone is used routinely for cesarean sections in dogs and cats. A study that compared the survival time of puppies born to bitches that were given a constant rate infusion (CRI) of alfaxalone, as compared with bitches given isoflurane after induction with alfaxalone, found that although bitches given a CRI of alfaxalone had longer recovery times and their puppies had lower Apgar scores, no difference was found in the survival rate of puppies in both groups.[62] Studies in pregnant mice, rats, and rabbits have not demonstrated deleterious effects on gestation of the treated animals or on the reproductive performance of their offspring. The effects of alfaxalone on fertility have not been evaluated.

Because safety has not been established in animals, this drug should only be used when the maternal benefits outweigh the potential risks to offspring.

Overdose/Acute Toxicity

Hypoventilation, apnea, and hypotension are the most likely consequences of overdoses up to 5 times the induction dose (20 mg/kg IV in dogs and 50 mg/kg IV in cats).[33] Marked cardiorespiratory depression and prolonged apnea and hypoxia occurred in cats receiving 50 mg/kg[33,63] and in a cat that received an alfaxalone CRI at 10 times the recommended rate due to a calculation error.[64] Cardiac arrhythmias are possible. Extended monitoring with appropriate cardiopulmonary support may be required.

For patients that have experienced or are suspected to have experienced an overdose, consultation with a 24-hour poison consultation center specializing in providing veterinary-specific information is recommended. For general information related to overdose and toxin exposures, as well as contact information for poison control centers, refer to ***Appendix***.

Drug Interactions

The US label states that alfaxalone may be used (**NOTE:** *therapeutic* compatibility, not *pharmaceutical* compatibility) with benzodiazepines, opioids, $alpha_2$ agonists, and phenothiazines, as commonly used in surgical practice. The Australia/New Zealand label states that alfaxalone has been safely used in combination with the following premedications: acepromazine, atropine, methadone, butorphanol, diazepam, and xylazine. Concomitant use of alfaxalone with other CNS depressants is expected to potentiate the depressant effects of either drug, and appropriate dose adjustments should be made.

The following drug interactions have either been reported or are theoretical in humans or animals receiving alfaxalone and may be of significance in veterinary patients. Unless otherwise noted, use together is not necessarily contraindicated, but the potential risks must be weighted and additional monitoring performed when appropriate.

- **Propofol, Thiopental:** The UK label states that alfaxalone **should not** be used with **other intravenous anesthetics.**

Laboratory Considerations

None noted

Dosages

NOTES:

1. Alfaxalone is used in many different combinations with other agents. The following are representative, but not necessarily inclusive; it is suggested to refer to a recent veterinary anesthesia reference for more information.[65,66]
2. Do not confuse CRI dosages listed as mg or mL per kg/*HOUR* with those listed as mg or mL per kg/*minute*.
3. Product label information should be referred to for more specific information. The distinction between the label and extra-label use and dosages (US, UK) for this drug should be noted, as approved label information varies between countries.

DOGS:

Induction of general anesthesia (label dosage; FDA-approved): 1.5 – 4.5 mg/kg IV in dogs with no preanesthetic agents given.[33] In dogs that received a preanesthetic drug, alfaxalone induction doses were reduced by 23% to 50%, depending on the combination of preanesthetic drugs given. Average IV alfaxalone induction doses ranged from 1.1 mg/kg in dogs that received an $alpha_2$-adrenergic agonist to 1.7 mg/kg in dogs that received benzodiazepine/opioid/acepromazine. Use of a preanesthetic drug appeared to decrease the occurrence of apnea following alfaxalone induction. The dose-sparing effect of alfaxalone depends on the potency, dose, and time of administration of the preanesthetic drugs used prior to induction. To avoid anesthetic overdose, titrate the administration of alfaxalone against the response of the patient. Additional doses of alfaxalone, similar to those used for anesthetic maintenance (1.2 – 2.2 mg/kg IV), may be administered to facilitate intubation in the patient.[33]

Maintenance of anesthesia (label dosage; FDA-approved): Following induction of anesthesia with alfaxalone and intubation, anesthesia may be maintained using intermittent IV boluses or an inhalant anesthetic agent.[33] A maintenance bolus of 1.2 – 1.4 mg/kg provides an additional 6 to 8 minutes of anesthesia in preanesthetized dogs. A dose of 1.5 – 2.2 mg/kg IV provides an additional 6 to 8 minutes of anesthesia in nonpreanesthetized dogs. Clinical responses may vary and are determined by the dose, rate of administration, and frequency of maintenance injections. Administration of additional low doses, similar to maintenance doses, may be required to facilitate the transition to inhalant maintenance anesthesia.[33]

Induction of general anesthesia (extra-label):
Without premedication, 3 mg/kg IV; with premedication, 2 mg/kg IV[41,42]

a) Following premedication with either medetomidine 4 µg/kg (0.004 mg/kg) IM or butorphanol 0.1 mg/kg IM, the average alfaxalone induction dose was 1.2 mg/kg IV. When medetomidine 4 µg/kg (0.004 mg/kg) is combined with butorphanol 0.1 mg/kg IM for premedication, the average alfaxalone induction dose was 0.8 mg/kg IV.[67]
b) Following premedication with methadone 0.2 mg/kg IM, the average alfaxalone dose required to permit endotracheal intubation was ≈1.7 mg/kg IV. When methadone 0.2 mg/kg is combined with dexmedetomidine 3 µg/kg (0.003 mg/kg) IM, the average alfaxalone induction dose was ≈1.4 mg/kg IV (a 16% reduction of the alfaxalone dose).[68]

Maintenance of anesthesia (extra-label):

a) Following induction, the dog should be intubated, and anesthesia maintained with alfaxalone or an inhalation anesthetic agent. Maintenance doses of alfaxalone may be given as supplemental boluses or as an IV CRI. If alfaxalone is being used for anesthetic maintenance for procedures that last more than 5 to 10 minutes, a butterfly needle or catheter can be securely placed in the vein, and small amounts of alfaxalone can be subsequently injected to maintain the required level and duration of anesthesia. Alfaxalone has been used safely and effectively in dogs for procedures that last up to 1 hour. In most cases, the average duration of recovery when alfaxalone is given for anesthetic maintenance is often longer than when an inhalant gas is used as a maintenance agent.[33,42] Following are dosages suggested for maintenance of anesthesia, based on data taken from controlled laboratory and field studies and that represent the average amount of drug required to provide maintenance anesthesia for dogs; however, the actual dose should be based on the response of the individual patient[42]:

Bolus dose for each 10 minutes of maintenance	Unpremedicated dogs	Premedicated dogs
mg/kg	1.3 – 1.5	1 – 1.2
mL/kg (using 10 mg/mL concentration)	0.13 – 0.15	0.1 – 0.12

IV CRI dose	Unpremedicated dogs	Premedicated dogs
mg/kg/HOUR	8 – 9	6 – 7
mg/kg/minute	0.13 – 0.15	0.1 – 0.12
mL/kg/minute (using 10 mg/mL concentration)	0.013 – 0.015	0.01 – 0.012

b) After administration of premedications and induction drugs, general anesthesia can be maintained with dosages of 0.16 – 0.2 mg/kg/minute IV CRI.[69] This range should be considered as a starting point and should be modified according to the patient's response.

Sedation for short procedures - intramuscular (extra-label): Alfaxalone 0.5 or 1 mg/kg combined with dexmedetomidine 3 µg/kg (0.003 mg/kg) and methadone 0.3 mg/kg and administered IM provided recumbency and sedation that was deeper and had a longer duration than dexmedetomidine and methadone at these doses without alfaxalone, but without differences between the two alfaxalone doses.[70] Decreases for all physiologic variables (eg, heart and respiratory rate, body temperature), except for noninvasive blood pressure, occurred and oxygen supplementation was provided due to the low SpO_2. Recoveries were deemed 'acceptable.'

Heavy sedation/light anesthesia - intramuscular (extra-label): Alfaxalone 1 – 2.5 mg/kg combined with medetomidine 0.005 mg/kg and butorphanol 0.3 mg/kg and administered IM provided anesthetic depth appropriate for intubation with clinically acceptable physiologic parameters.[71] Increasing the alfaxalone to 5 mg/kg IM caused extreme hypoxemia in some dogs; however, when only medetomidine OR butorphanol (at the same doses) were combined with alfaxalone at 2.5 – 5 mg/kg IM, extreme hypoxemia did not occur.

CATS:

Induction of general anesthesia (label dosage; FDA-approved): 2.2 – 9.7 mg/kg IV in cats with no preanesthetic agents given. In cats that received a preanesthetic drug, alfaxalone induction doses were reduced by 10% to 43%, depending on the combination of preanesthetic drugs given. Average induction doses ranged from 2.3 mg/kg IV in cats that received benzodiazepine/opioid/phenothiazine to 3.6 mg/kg IV in cats that received benzodiazepine/phenothiazine or an alpha$_2$-adrenergic agonist with or without a phenothiazine. The dose-sparing effect of alfaxalone depends on the potency, dose, and time of administration of the preanesthetic drugs used prior to induction. To avoid anesthetic overdose, titrate the administration of alfaxalone against the response of the patient. Additional doses of alfaxalone, similar to those used for anesthetic maintenance (1.1 – 1.5 mg/kg IV), may be administered to facilitate intubation of the patient.[33]

Maintenance of anesthesia (label dosage; FDA-approved): Following induction of anesthesia with alfaxalone and intubation, anesthesia may be maintained using intermittent IV boluses or an inhalant anesthetic agent. A maintenance bolus of 1.1 – 1.3 mg/kg provides an additional 7 to 8 minutes of anesthesia in preanesthetized cats. A dose of 1.4 – 1.5 mg/kg provides an additional 3 to 5 minutes of anesthesia in nonpreanesthetized cats. Clinical responses may vary and are determined by the dose, rate of administration, and frequency of maintenance injections. Administration of additional low doses, similar to maintenance doses, may be required to facilitate the transition to inhalant maintenance anesthesia.[33]

Induction (extra-label):

1. With or without premedication, 5 mg/kg IV[41,42]
2. Administration of a 'priming dose' of alfaxalone 0.25 mg/kg IV over 60 seconds to cats sedated with dexmedetomidine and methadone IM followed by alfaxalone induction administered at 0.5 mg/kg/minute IV CRI resulted in a ≈30% lower overall alfaxalone dosage required for orotracheal intubation.[72]

Maintenance of anesthesia (extra-label):

1. Following induction, the cat should be intubated, and anesthesia maintained with alfaxalone or an inhalation anesthetic agent. Maintenance doses of alfaxalone may be given as supplemental boluses or as an IV CRI. If alfaxalone is being used for anesthetic maintenance for procedures that last more than 5 to 10 minutes, a butterfly needle or catheter can be placed in the vein, and small amounts of alfaxalone can be subsequently injected to maintain the required level and duration of anesthesia. Alfaxalone has been used safely and effectively in cats for procedures that last up to 1 hour. In most cases,

the average duration of recovery when alfaxalone is given for anesthetic maintenance is often longer than when an inhalant gas is used as a maintenance agent.[42] Following are dosages suggested for maintenance of anesthesia, based on data taken from controlled laboratory and field studies and that represent the average amount of drug required to provide maintenance anesthesia for cats; however, the actual dose should be based on the response of the individual patient[42]:

Bolus dose for each 10 minutes of maintenance	Unpremedicated cats	Premedicated cats
mg/kg	1.6 – 1.8	1.1 – 1.3
mL/kg (using 10 mg/mL concentration)	0.16 – 0.18	0.11 – 0.13

IV CRI dose	Unpremedicated cats	Premedicated cats
mg/kg/HOUR	10 – 11	7 – 8
mg/kg/minute	0.16 – 0.18	0.11 – 0.13
mL/kg/minute (using 10 mg/mL concentration)	0.016 – 0.018	0.011 – 0.013

2. After administration of premedications and induction drugs, general anesthesia can be maintained with alfaxalone 0.16 – 0.2 mg/kg/minute.[73] This range should be considered as a starting point and should be modified according to the patient's response.
3. Two studies were conducted in cats undergoing ovariohysterectomy. In the first study, alfaxalone was given at 1.7 mg/kg IV at induction with medetomidine 20 µg/kg (0.02 mg/kg) IM and morphine 0.3 mg/kg IM followed by alfaxalone at 0.18 mg/kg/minute for maintenance.[74] In the second study, alfaxalone was given at 0.2 mg/kg IV every 20 seconds to effect with butorphanol 0.2 mg/kg IM and either acepromazine 0.1 mg/kg IM or medetomidine 20 µg/kg (0.02 mg/kg) IM followed by alfaxalone at 10 mg/kg/HOUR for maintenance.[75] A 3-step infusion regimen produced alfaxalone concentrations closer to the target concentration than a single infusion rate.[76]

Sedation for short procedures - subcutaneous (extra-label): In a study in hyperthyroid cats, alfaxalone 3 mg/kg and butorphanol 0.2 mg/kg were drawn up in the same syringe and administered as a single SC injection in the region dorsal to the right hip; maximum sedation occurred 45 minutes after the injection was given. Blood pressure, heart rate, and respiration rate were all significantly decreased. Blood pressure monitoring is recommended. Further studies are required to determine whether these sedative, respiratory, and cardiovascular effects are similar in euthyroid cats.[77]

Sedation for short procedures - intramuscular (extra-label): Alfaxalone 3 mg/kg, dexmedetomidine 10 µg/kg (0.01 mg/kg), and butorphanol 0.2 mg/kg were drawn up in the same syringe and administered IM in the lumbar muscle prior to castration. Respiration rate decreased significantly but SpO_2 remained within normal limits during the procedure. The rectal temperature also decreased significantly.[78] Another study using alfaxalone 1 mg/kg IM, dexmedetomidine 5 µg/kg (0.005 mg/kg) IM, and butorphanol 0.2 mg/kg IM reported a sedation time of 90 minutes with excellent recovery quality and acceptable cardiovascular stability.[79] Alfaxalone 1.5 mg/kg combined with hydromorphone 0.1 mg/kg and midazolam 0.2 mg/kg administered IM provided more profound sedation and easier IV catheterization than alfaxalone and hydromorphone without midazolam.[80]

Sedation for blood donation - intramuscular (extra-label): Alfaxalone 2 – 3 mg/kg combined with butorphanol 0.2 – 0.4 mg/kg and given IM for healthy cats undergoing blood donation[81,82]

Sedation for echocardiography - intramuscular (extra-label): Alfaxalone 2 mg/kg combined with methadone 0.3 mg/kg +/- ketamine 1 mg/kg administered IM to cats provided sedation with no clinically meaningful effects on echocardiographic variables.[83] Sedation with alfaxalone in combination with methadone was mild whereas the addition of ketamine provided adequate sedation for diagnostic procedures.

Heavy sedation/light anesthesia - intramuscular (extra-label): 5 – 10 mg/kg IM. Variability in response may be minimized by giving a deep IM injection in the quadriceps muscle mass.[41] Most practitioners deem this unacceptable because of the large volume of drug injected IM, which may cause discomfort to the cat.

EQUINE:

Induction of general anesthesia (extra-label):

a. Premedication with medetomidine 6 µg/kg (0.006 mg/kg) and midazolam 0.02 mg/kg followed by alfaxalone 1 mg/kg IV bolus over 10 seconds resulted in sternal recumbency 49 seconds (median) after injection, and recovery (ie, time to first attempt to stand) 44 minutes after administration.[84] In a subsequent study, horses were given alfaxalone 1 or 2 mg/kg IV following IV administration of the same premedications.[85] Recovery occurred in 50 minutes after alfaxalone 1 mg/kg and in 90 minutes after 2 mg/kg. Hypoxemia occurred with both doses but was more profound following 2 mg/kg.
b. In donkeys sedated with xylazine 2 mg/kg IM followed by alfaxalone 1 mg/kg IV and midazolam 0.05 mg/kg IV, times to lateral recumbency, first movement, and standing were 29 seconds, 27 minutes, and 58 minutes, respectively. Although an alfaxalone and midazolam combination was deemed acceptable, donkeys given midazolam and ketamine recovered more quickly and with better quality.[86]

Constant rate infusion (extra-label): In a study, horses were premedicated with medetomidine 5 µg/kg (0.005 mg/kg) in combination with midazolam 20 µg/kg (0.02 mg/kg) IV. Anesthesia was induced with rapid injection of 5% guaifenesin 100 mg/kg IV with alfaxalone 1 mg/kg IV. Anesthesia was maintained with sevoflurane and alfaxalone 0.5 mg/kg/HOUR IV CRI in combination with medetomidine 3 µg/kg/HOUR (0.003 mg/kg/HOUR) IV CRI; sevoflurane requirements were reduced by ≈25%, but 20% of horses given alfaxalone experienced an excitatory response during recovery.[13]

Total IV anesthesia (extra-label):

a. After IV premedication with acepromazine 0.03 mg/kg and xylazine 1 mg/kg and induction with IV guaifenesin 35 mg/kg and alfaxalone 1 mg/kg, alfaxalone IV infusion was started at 5 mg/kg/HOUR; median TIVA infusion rate was 3.1 mg/kg/HOUR. TIVA was maintained for 180 minutes. Six of the 8 horses exhibited muscle tremors and paddling following cessation of the infusion but all horses stood without incident on the first or second attempt with a good to excellent recovery.[52]
b. After premedication with medetomidine 5 µg/kg (0.005 mg/kg) IV and butorphanol 0.02 mg/kg IV, anesthesia was induced with guaifenesin 10 mg/kg IV followed by alfaxalone 1 mg/kg IV; anesthesia was maintained with

guaifenesin 80 mg/kg/*HOUR* IV CRI, medetomidine 3 µg/kg/*HOUR* (0.003 mg/kg/*HOUR*) IV CRI, and alfaxalone 1.5 mg/kg/*HOUR* IV CRI. Mild cardiorespiratory depression occurred, and supplemental oxygen was provided to prevent hypoxemia. Recovery was good to excellent.[53]

CATTLE:

Sedation (extra-label): Alfaxalone 1.2 mg/kg IV given to calves premedicated with xylazine 0.1 mg/kg IM produced smooth induction and facilitated endotracheal intubation.[51]

GOATS:

Induction of general anesthesia (extra-label): Induction of anesthesia with alfaxalone 2 mg/kg IV in combination with lidocaine 1 – 4 mg/kg IV was followed by alfaxalone 6.7 mg/kg/*HOUR* IV CRI and lidocaine 6 mg/kg/*HOUR* IV CRI.[32] In a separate study, xylazine premedication (0.05 mg/kg IV) decreased the alfaxalone induction dose from 4 mg/kg IV to 2.3 mg/kg IV, provided antinociception, and supported stable cardiovascular parameters; however, SpO_2 was decreased for 20 minutes, and supplemental oxygen was needed.[87]

RABBITS:

Deep sedation (extra-label):

a) Alfaxalone 2.5 mg/kg IM in adult healthy rabbits[88]
b) Deeper sedation occurred with alfaxalone 5 mg/kg in combination with dexmedetomidine 100 µg/kg (0.1 mg/kg) either IV or IM than with alfaxalone alone at the same dose/route.[89] As with other species, dose-dependent respiratory depression is common and supplemental oxygen is recommended.

Induction of general anesthesia (extra-label): In adult healthy rabbits, alfaxalone 6 mg/kg IM in combination with butorphanol 0.3 mg/kg and dexmedetomidine 200 µg/kg (0.2 mg/kg) IM produced recumbency and sedation with a more consistent and prolonged (57 ± 3 minutes) loss of toe-pinch response than alfaxalone alone or combined with midazolam or with either butorphanol or dexmedetomidine alone.[90]

FERRETS:

Induction of general anesthesia (extra-label): **NOTE**: Alfaxalone is NOT recommended to be used as a single agent or in combination with tramadol in ferrets.[91] Death may result if alfaxalone is used at doses greater than or equal to 10 – 20 mg/kg IV.[91]

a) Satisfactory anesthesia is provided when alfaxalone is administered at 2.5 mg/kg IV in combination with medetomidine 20 µg/kg (0.02 mg/kg) IM and lasts ≈60 minutes.[91]
b) Alfaxalone 2.5 or 5 mg/kg combined with butorphanol 0.2 mg/kg administered IM in the epaxial muscles of young healthy ferrets resulted in dose-dependent sedation with only minor cardiorespiratory depression.[92] Because of the large volume, the 5 mg/kg alfaxalone dose was divided and half injected into both left and right epaxial muscles.

Monitoring

- Level of anesthesia/CNS effects
- Ventilatory status (eg, respiratory rate/depth/pattern, mucous membrane color, SpO_2, $ETCO_2$)
- Cardiovascular status (eg, cardiac rate/rhythm, blood pressure)
- Body temperature
- Intraocular pressure as indicated in susceptible animals

Chemistry/Synonyms

Alfaxalone is 3-alpha-hydroxy-5-alpha-pregnane-11,20-dione and has a molecular weight of 332.5. Alfaxalone is a white to creamy white powder and is practically insoluble in water or mineral spirits, soluble in alcohol, and freely soluble in chloroform.

The commercial injectable formulations occur as clear, colorless sterile solutions. Alfaxalone is a water-soluble formulation that contains 2-hydroxypropyl-beta-cyclodextrin (HPCD) as the solubilizing agent. Another product containing alfaxalone, *Saffan®*, was marketed in the 1970s as an IV anesthetic agent for cats, but it contained a polyethoxylated castor oil as the solubilizing agent, which caused significant histamine release via mast cell degranulation. *Saffan®* was subsequently removed from the market.

Alfaxalone may also be known as alfaksaloni, alfaxalon, alfaxalona, alfaxalonum, alphaxalone, or GR-2/234. A common trade name is *Alfaxan®*.

Storage/Stability

Alfaxalone solutions for injection should be stored at a controlled room temperature of 20°C to 25°C (68°F-77°F) with excursions permitted between 15°C to 30°C (59°F-86°F). The Australia and New Zealand labels state *…contains no preservatives. Solution should be removed from the vial using aseptic technique. Contents of broached vials should preferably be used within 24 hours, but may be stored if necessary, at 4°C* [49.2°F] *for up to 7 days provided contamination is avoided. Do not use broached vials if the solution is not clear, colorless and free from particulate matter.*[41]

Alfaxalone multidose vials contain preservatives, including ethanol, benzethonium chloride, chlorocresol, and should be used within 28 days of when the vial is first punctured. Discard unused drug after 28 days. *Alfaxan® Multidose IDX*, which contains the same preservatives, is approved for 56 days of use after first vial puncture. A preservative-free formulation remains available in some countries.

As a controlled substance, alfaxalone must be stored in an area that is substantially constructed and securely locked in accordance with DEA regulations. Follow applicable local, state, and federal rules regarding disposal of unused or wasted controlled drugs.

Compatibility/Compounding Considerations

Compatibility is dependent on factors such as pH, concentration, temperature, and diluent used; consult specialized references or a hospital pharmacist for more specific information.

The US product label states that it should not be mixed with other therapeutic agents prior to administration.[33] When the alfaxalone formulation containing preservatives is mixed with some drugs, including butorphanol, in the same syringe, anecdotal reports describe a cloudy nature to the injectate.

Dosage Forms/Regulatory Status

VETERINARY-LABELED PRODUCTS:

Alfaxalone Injection: 10 mg/mL in 10 and 20 mL multidose vials; *Alfaxan® Multidose*; (Rx). FDA approved for use in cats and dogs; NADA #141-342. (Rx; C-IV).

Alfaxalone Injection: 10 mg/mL in 10 mL multidose vials; *Alfaxan® Multidose IDX*; (Rx). FDA indexed (MIF 900-031) for a use in a variety of non-food-producing minor species including reptiles, amphibians, ornamental fish, birds, non-human primates, rodents, mustelids, marsupials, and minor species ungulates. (Rx; C-IV)

HUMAN-LABELED PRODUCTS: NONE

References

For the complete list of references, see **wiley.com/go/budde/plumb**

Alfentanil

(al-***fen***-ta-nil) *Alfenta*®

Opioid Agonist

Prescriber Highlights

- ▶ Injectable, potent opioid that may be useful for adjunctive anesthesia and analgesia in dogs and cats
- ▶ Use with caution in patients with head injury, pulmonary disease or impaired respiration, or impaired hepatic or renal function.
- ▶ Limited veterinary experience and published data available to draw conclusions on adverse effects in veterinary species; bradycardia has been observed in dogs; cats and horses may experience CNS excitation.
- ▶ Overdoses are associated with CNS and respiratory depression; naloxone may be used to reverse opioid effects.
- ▶ Dose may need adjustment in geriatric patients and those with hepatic disease; obese patients should have dose calculated based on lean body weight.
- ▶ DEA Schedule II (C-II) controlled substance

Uses/Indications

An opioid analgesic, alfentanil may be a useful alternative to fentanyl for anesthesia, analgesia, or sedation in dogs and cats.

Pharmacology/Actions

Alfentanil is a potent mu opioid agonist with the typical opioid sedative, analgesic, and anesthetic properties. When comparing analgesic potencies after IM injection, alfentanil 0.4 – 0.8 mg is equivalent to fentanyl 0.1 – 0.2 mg and morphine ≈10 mg.

In dogs, the use of alfentanil decreased the required dose of propofol target-controlled infusion to maintain the animal under general anesthesia, but did not provide any cardiovascular benefits and increased the incidence of hypoxemia compared to propofol alone.[1] In cats, plasma alfentanil concentrations of 500 ng/mL decreased the isoflurane MAC by 16% to 35%.[2,3] No significant reduction in halothane MAC was observed with alfentanil use in horses.[4]

Pharmacokinetics

In dogs, the drug's steady state volume of distribution is ≈0.6 L/kg, clearance is ≈19 to 30 mL/kg/minute, and the terminal half-life is ≈20 to 60 minutes.[5,6] In cats, alfentanil's elimination half-life is ≈2 to 3 hours, volume of distribution (steady state) is ≈0.9 L/kg, and clearance is 12 mL/minute/kg.[7,8]

In humans, onset of anesthetic action occurs within 2 minutes after IV dosing and within 5 minutes of IM injection. Peak effects occur ≈15 minutes after IM injection. Alfentanil has a volume of distribution of 0.4 to 1 L/kg.[9] Approximately 90% of the drug is bound to plasma proteins. Alfentanil is primarily metabolized in the liver to inactive metabolites that are excreted by the kidneys into the urine; only ≈1% of the drug is excreted unchanged into the urine. Total body clearance in humans ranges from 1.6 to 17.6 mL/minute/kg. Clearance is decreased by ≈50% in patients with alcoholic cirrhosis or in those that are obese. Clearance is reduced by ≈30% in geriatric patients. Elimination half-life in humans is ≈100 minutes.[9] Veterinary significance of this human data is unclear.

Contraindications/Precautions/Warnings

Alfentanil is contraindicated in patients hypersensitive to opioids. In humans, initial dose reduction may be required in geriatric or debilitated patients, particularly those with diminished cardiopulmonary function; the dose for obese patients is calculated based on lean body weight.[9] Use with caution in patients with head injury, with pulmonary disease or impaired respiration, and with impaired hepatic or renal function.

Because of alfentanil's potency and potential for significant adverse effects, it should only be used in situations in which sufficient monitoring and patient support capabilities (eg, intubation, ventilation) are available.

Opioid analgesics are contraindicated in patients stung by scorpions (eg, *Centruroides* spp) as they may potentiate venom effects.[10]

Do not confuse alfentanil with fentanyl, remifentanil, or sufentanil. Because of the potency of alfentanil, the use of a tuberculin syringe to measure doses less than 1 mL, in addition to a double-check system for dose calculation and measurement, is recommended.

Adverse Effects

Limited information is available regarding alfentanil's adverse effect profile in veterinary patients, and adverse effects are expected to be dose-related and consistent with other opioid agonists. Although tachycardia and increased blood pressure have been observed in cats,[11] bradycardia has been reported in dogs.[5,12] Bradycardia is usually responsive to anticholinergic agents; however, one study in dogs found that concurrent atropine improved heart rate but increased the risk of hypotension.[13] Clinicians should consider administration of atropine prior to or together with alfentanil.

In conscious cats, mydriasis and excitement after an IV bolus has been noted[7]; healthy cats anesthetized with alfentanil-propofol combination had a significant decrease in blood pressure as compared to cats anesthetized with remifentanil-propofol.[14] Respiratory depression has been recorded in cats[11] and horses.[15] Increased blood pressure[4] and locomotor activity[16-18] has been observed after IV administration to horses.

In humans, common adverse effects include nausea, vomiting, bradycardia or tachycardia, hyper- or hypotension, apnea, and postoperative respiratory depression. Dose-related skeletal muscle rigidity can also occur, and neuromuscular blockers are routinely used when the patient is under general anesthesia and mechanically ventilated to counteract this effect. Alfentanil has rarely been associated with asystole, hypercarbia, and hypersensitivity reactions. Significance of these findings remains unclear in veterinary patients.

Reproductive/Nursing Safety

Placental transfer of alfentanil has been reported in humans.[9] When alfentanil is administered systemically to women directly before parturition, infants may show behavioral alterations (hypotonia, depression) associated with opioids. High alfentanil doses given to laboratory animals for 10 to 30 days have been associated with embryotoxicity, which may be due to direct effects of the drug caused by prolonged administration. Teratogenicity was not observed in rats or rabbits.[9]

Alfentanil is excreted into human breast milk; caution is advised when administering alfentanil to nursing women.[9]

Because safety has not been established in animals, this drug should only be used when the maternal benefits outweigh the potential risks to offspring.

Overdose/Acute Toxicity

Alfentanil LD_{50} in dogs is 60 – 88 mg/kg IV.[9] Severe overdoses may cause circulatory collapse, pulmonary edema, seizures, cardiac arrest, and death. Less severe overdoses may cause CNS and respiratory depression, coma, hypotension, muscle flaccidity, and miosis. Doses of 30 micrograms/kg IV have caused agitation, incoordination, and excitement in dogs.[19]

Treatment is a combination of supportive therapy, as necessary, and the administration of an opioid antagonist (eg, ***Naloxone***). Although alfentanil has a relatively rapid half-life, multiple doses of naloxone may be necessary.

For patients that have experienced or are suspected to have experienced an overdose, consultation with a 24-hour poison consultation center specializing in providing veterinary-specific information

is recommended. For general information related to overdose and toxin exposures, as well as contact information for poison control centers, refer to *Appendix*.

Drug Interactions

The following drug interactions with alfentanil have either been reported or are theoretical in humans or animals and may be of significance in veterinary patients. Unless otherwise noted, use together is not necessarily contraindicated, but weigh the potential risks and perform additional monitoring when appropriate.

- ANTICHOLINERGIC AGENTS (eg, **acepromazine, amitriptyline, atropine, clomipramine, glycopyrrolate**): Concurrent use may increase risk for urinary retention, constipation, and CNS and respiratory depression.
- BETHANECHOL: Concurrent use may antagonize the beneficial effects of bethanechol on GI motility. Avoid combination.
- BRADYCARDIA-CAUSING AGENTS (eg, **amiodarone, anesthetic agents, beta-adrenergic antagonists** [eg, **atenolol, propranolol**], **digoxin**): May produce bradycardia or hypotension if used concurrently with alfentanil
- CNS DEPRESSANTS (eg, **anesthetic agents, barbiturates** [eg, **phenobarbital**], **benzodiazepines** [eg, **diazepam, midazolam**], **cannabidiol**): Concurrent use may increase the risk for CNS and/or respiratory depression. Monitor and adjust doses accordingly.
- DESMOPRESSIN: Concurrent use may increase concentrations of desmopressin and increase risk for water intoxication and/or hyponatremia, which can progress to seizures, coma, respiratory arrest, and death. Monitor electrolytes and renal function.
- DIURETICS (eg, **furosemide**): Opioids may decrease therapeutic effects of diuretics.
- DOMPERIDONE: Concurrent use may antagonize the GI effects of domperidone.
- DRUGS THAT INDUCE HEPATIC ISOENZYMES (eg, **griseofulvin, mitotane, phenobarbital**): Concurrent use may decrease concentration of alfentanil. Monitor clinical response and adjust dosages accordingly.
- DRUGS THAT INHIBIT HEPATIC ISOENZYMES (eg, **cimetidine, diltiazem, erythromycin, fluconazole, itraconazole, ketoconazole**): May increase the half-life and decrease the clearance of alfentanil leading to prolonged effects and an increased risk for respiratory depression. Monitor for adverse effects, and consider adjusting doses accordingly.
- HIGHLY PROTEIN-BOUND DRUGS (eg, **amiodarone, furosemide, NSAIDs** [eg, **carprofen, meloxicam**]): Because alfentanil is highly bound to plasma proteins (greater than 90%), it could theoretically displace other highly bound drugs, causing a transient increase in serum concentrations of each drug. These interactions are unlikely to be of clinical concern because increased free drug concentrations will equilibrate through increased clearance. Monitor for adverse effects of each drug when using this combination.
- HYPOTENSIVE AGENTS (eg, **amlodipine, enalapril, telmisartan**): Concurrent use may increase risk for bradycardia, hypotension, and orthostasis. Use combination with caution; monitor blood pressure and heart rate.
- IFOSFAMIDE: Concurrent use may increase risk for neurotoxicity including somnolence, confusion, hallucinations, blurred vision, urinary incontinence, seizures, and coma. Use cautiously and monitor.
- IOHEXOL: Concurrent use of opioids with intrathecal iohexol may increase risk for seizures. Opioids should be withheld for 48 hours before and 24 hours after intrathecal administration of iohexol.
- LOPERAMIDE: Concurrent use may increase risk for constipation.
- MONOAMINE OXIDASE INHIBITORS (MAOIs; eg, **amitraz, selegiline**): Concurrent use may increase risk for anxiety, confusion, hypotension, respiratory depression, cyanosis, and coma. MAOIs should be withheld for 14 days prior to administration of opioids. Avoid combination.
- NEUROMUSCULAR BLOCKING AGENTS (eg, **atracurium, pancuronium**): Concurrent use may increase risk for tachycardia, bradycardia, and/or hypotension. Use combination with caution; monitor heart rate and blood pressure.
- PROKINETIC AGENTS (eg, **cisapride, erythromycin, metoclopramide**): Concurrent use may antagonize the prokinetic effects.

Laboratory Considerations

- Opioids may increase biliary tract pressure, resulting in increased plasma **amylase** and **lipase** values up to 24 hours following their administration.

Dosages

NOTE: In obese patients, calculate doses based on lean body weight.

DOGS:

Anesthetic premedication (extra-label): Alfentanil 5 – 10 μg/kg IV[20,21]

Analgesia (extra-label):

a. Loading dose of alfentanil 0.5 – 1 μg/kg IV followed by alfentanil 0.5 – 1 μg/kg/minute IV CRI[22]
b. Intraoperative analgesia in patients with intracranial disease: 0.2 μg/kg/minute IV[23]

Anesthetic agent (extra-label):

a) Induction dose following premedication (choose one)
   i. Alfentanil 2.1 – 10 μg/kg in combination with propofol 2 mg/kg and administered IV [13,24] OR
   ii. Alfentanil 1 – 40 μg/kg IV in combination with midazolam[19]
b) Maintenance dose (choose one)
   i. Less than or equal to alfentanil 1 μg/kg/min IV CRI with concurrent propofol 0.4 mg/kg/min IV CRI (using 2 separate fluid pumps)[25] OR
   ii. Alfentanil 4 – 5 micrograms/kg/min IV CRI with concurrent midazolam 0.005 mg/kg/min IV CRI (using 2 separate fluid pumps)[19]
c) Adjunct to anesthesia: Alfentanil 2 – 5 μg/kg IV every 20 minutes[20,26]

CATS:

Analgesic adjunct to anesthesia (extra-label): Loading dose of alfentanil 5 – 10 μg/kg IV followed by alfentanil 0.8 – 1 μg/kg per minute IV CRI.[14,27] In both studies, anesthesia was induced with propofol and maintenance with alfentanil-propofol combination began 20 minutes after induction.

Monitoring

- Anesthetic and/or analgesic efficacy
- Cardiac and respiratory rate; blood pressure
- Pulse oximetry or other methods to measure blood oxygenation when used for anesthesia

Client Information

- Alfentanil is a potent opioid that should only be used under the guidance of licensed veterinarians in a setting where adequate patient monitoring is available.

Chemistry/Synonyms

A phenylpiperidine opioid anesthetic-analgesic related to fentanyl, alfentanil HCl occurs as a white to off-white powder. It is freely soluble in alcohol, water, chloroform, or methanol. The commercially available injection has a pH of 4 to 6 and contains sodium chloride for isotonicity. Alfentanil is more lipid soluble than morphine, but less so than fentanyl.

Alfentanil may also be known as alfentanyl, *Alfenta®*, *Alfast®*, *Fanaxal®*, *Fentalim®*, *Limifen®*, or *Rapifen®*.

Storage/Stability

Alfentanil injection should be stored protected from light at controlled room temperature (20°C-25°C; 68°F-77°F).

Alfentanil is a DEA schedule II controlled substance that should be stored in an area that is substantially constructed and securely locked. Follow applicable local, state, and federal rules regarding disposal of unused or wasted controlled drugs.

Compatibility/Compounding Considerations

In concentrations up to 80 µg/mL, alfentanil injection has been shown to be **compatible** with sodium chloride 0.9%, dextrose 5%, dextrose 5% in sodium chloride 0.9%, and lactated Ringer's solution.[9]

Compatibility is dependent on factors such as pH, concentration, temperature, and diluent used; specialized references or a hospital pharmacist should be consulted for more specific information.

Dosage Forms/Regulatory Status

VETERINARY-LABELED PRODUCTS: NONE.

The Association of Racing Commissioners International (ARCI) has designated this drug as a class 1 substance. See the ***Appendix*** for more information. Use of this drug may not be allowed in certain animal competitions. Check rules and regulations before entering in a competition while this medication is being administered. Contact local racing authorities for further guidance.

HUMAN-LABELED PRODUCTS:

Alfentanil HCl for injection: 500 µg (as base)/mL in 2 mL, 5 mL, 10 mL, and 20 mL ampules; preservative-free; *Alfenta®*, generic; (Rx, C-II)

References

For the complete list of references, see **wiley.com/go/budde/plumb**

Allopurinol

(al-oh-***pyoor***-i-nol) *Zyloprim®*

Xanthine Oxidase Inhibitor; Purine Analogue

Prescriber Highlights

- ▶ Used to reduce uric acid in dogs, cats, reptiles, and birds; adjunctive treatment for leishmaniasis in dogs and cats
- ▶ Use with caution in patients with renal or hepatic dysfunction.
- ▶ Contraindicated in red-tailed hawks and should be used with caution, if at all, in other raptors
- ▶ A low purine diet is recommended with long-term treatment.
- ▶ Most common adverse effects are GI-related, but hypersensitivity reactions, increased liver enzymes, or renal events (eg, mineralization, uroliths) can occur.
- ▶ Many potential drug interactions

Uses/Indications

The primary veterinary uses for allopurinol are for the treatment and prevention of recurrent uric acid and hyperuricosuric calcium oxalate uroliths in dogs, particularly Dalmatians. It has also been used to treat gout in pet birds and reptiles.[1]

Allopurinol has been used as an alternative treatment for canine and feline leishmaniasis. Although it appears to have moderate clinical efficacy, treatment duration is several months and does not result in a full cure.[2]

There are also minimal data to support its use to treat trypanosomiasis infections.[3]

Pharmacology/Actions

Allopurinol and its metabolite, oxypurinol, inhibit the enzyme xanthine oxidase, which is responsible for the conversion of oxypurines (eg, hypoxanthine, xanthine) to uric acid. Allopurinol does not increase the renal excretion of uric acid, nor does it possess any anti-inflammatory or analgesic activity.

Allopurinol inhibits *Leishmania* spp activity by limiting available purines in the host that are required for protozoal survival. Allopurinol is taken up by the protozoa and metabolized into a toxic compound (4-amino-pyrazole-pyrimidine), which incorporates into the parasite's RNA, causing death.[4,5]

Allopurinol, by inhibiting xanthine oxidase, can inhibit the formation of superoxide anion radicals and provide protection against hemorrhagic shock and myocardial ischemia in laboratory conditions. However, the clinical use of the drug in cardiovascular diseases requires further study.[6]

Pharmacokinetics

In dogs, oral bioavailability was similar to that in humans (≈90%) with a serum half-life of ≈2 and 4 hours for allopurinol and oxypurinol, respectively. Food does not appear to alter absorption. Absorption is non-linear with oral and intravenous administration and therefore high doses are not recommended.[7] In Dalmatians, absorption rates were variable between subjects, with peak levels occurring within 1 to 3 hours after oral dosing. Elimination half-life is ≈2.7 hours.[8] The drug exhibits good systemic absorption, but CNS penetration is limited.

In horses, oral bioavailability of allopurinol is ≈15% and the drug is rapidly converted to oxypurinol.[9] Elimination half-life is ≈5 to 6 minutes for allopurinol and ≈1.1 hours for oxypurinol.

Neither allopurinol nor oxypurinol are bound to plasma proteins, but both drugs are excreted into milk.

Contraindications/Precautions/Warnings

Allopurinol is contraindicated in patients with previous hypersensitivity reactions and should be used with caution in patients with hepatic or renal dysfunction. Dosage reductions and increased monitoring are warranted in these cases.

Allopurinol does not appear to be effective in dissolving urate uroliths in dogs with portovascular anomalies.[10,11]

This drug is not recommended for use in red-tailed hawks. Dosages of 50 mg/kg PO once daily caused clinical signs of vomiting and hyperuricemia with renal dysfunction. Dosages of 25 mg/kg PO once daily were safe but not effective in reducing plasma uric acid.[12] Use with caution in other raptors.

Adverse Effects

Adverse effects in dogs are uncommon with allopurinol when fed low purine diets. Xanthine coatings have formed around ammonium urate uroliths in dogs consuming purines. Xanthinuria has been noted in dogs receiving allopurinol for the treatment of leishmaniasis.[13,14] Renal mineralization and urolithiasis were also noted in 6% of dogs.[14] Prolonged allopurinol at doses greater than 30 mg/kg/day may result in xanthine urolithiasis.[10] Consider a low purine diet if allopurinol is required for chronic therapy.[15] Adverse GI effects may include nausea, vomiting, anorexia, or diarrhea.

In humans, the most common adverse effects include rash, diarrhea, nausea, acute gout attacks, and ALT/AST elevations. Other less common adverse effects include bone marrow suppression, severe dermatologic reactions, hepatitis, and vasculitis. Humans with renal dysfunction are at risk for further decreases in renal function and other severe adverse effects unless dosages are reduced.

Reproductive/Nursing Safety

Although the safe use of allopurinol during pregnancy has not been established, dosages up to 20 times normal in rats and rabbits have not demonstrated decreases in fertility or evidence of fetal harm. Intraperitoneal administration to pregnant mice was associated with increased fetal death and malformations.

Allopurinol and oxypurinol are excreted into milk; use caution when allopurinol is administered to a nursing dam.

Overdose/Acute Toxicity

One source lists the allopurinol oral LD_{50} in mice as 78 mg/kg,[16-18] whereas other sources list 500 – 700 mg/kg. Clinical signs associated with overdose can include vomiting (seen in dogs at doses of more than 44 mg/kg) and trembling. There is no known antidote for allopurinol, but it is dialyzable.

For patients that have experienced or are suspected to have experienced an overdose, it is strongly encouraged to consult with a 24-hour poison consultation center that specialize in providing information specific for veterinary patients. For general information related to overdose and toxin exposures, as well as contact information for poison control centers, refer to ***Appendix***.

Drug Interactions

The following drug interactions with allopurinol have either been reported or are theoretical in humans or animals and may be of significance in veterinary patients. Unless otherwise noted, use together is not necessarily contraindicated, but weigh the potential risks and perform additional monitoring when appropriate.

- **Aluminum Hydroxide**: May decrease absorption of allopurinol
- **Angiotensin-Converting Enzyme Inhibitors** (ACEIs; eg, **benazepril, enalapril**). In humans, this combination may increase risk for hypersensitivity reactions to allopurinol. The veterinary significance of this interaction is unknown.
- **Aminopenicillins** (eg, **amoxicillin, ampicillin**): In humans, this combination may increase risk for hypersensitivity reactions to allopurinol. The veterinary significance of this interaction is unknown.
- **Azathioprine** or **Mercaptopurine**: Allopurinol may increase the serum concentration of mercaptopurine (azathioprine's active metabolite) and promote formation of active thioguanine nucleotides. Consider therapy modification or reduce the dose of immunosuppressive agent by 25% to 33% initially.
- **Cyclophosphamide**: Increased risk for bone marrow suppression
- **Cyclosporine**: Increased cyclosporine concentration may occur.
- **Diuretics** (eg, **chlorothiazide, furosemide, hydrochlorothiazide**): May increase serum concentration of allopurinol
- **Theophylline/Aminophylline**: Allopurinol may decrease metabolism, thereby increasing their serum levels.
- **Uricosuric Agents** (eg, **probenecid, sulfinpyrazone**): May increase the renal excretion of oxypurinol and thereby reduce xanthine oxidase inhibition; in treatment of hyperuricemia, the additive effects on blood uric acid may be beneficial.
- **Urinary Acidifiers** (eg, **ammonium chloride, methionine**): May reduce the solubility of uric acid in the urine and induce urolithiasis

Dosages

DOGS:

Dissolution of urate uroliths (extra-label): 15 mg/kg PO every 12 hours for up to 4 weeks.[11] Use in conjunction with low-purine, alkalinizing, diuretic diets.

Prevention of urate uroliths (extra-label): 5 – 7 mg/kg PO every 12 to 24 hours.[11] **NOTE:** Prolonged high doses of allopurinol may result in xanthine uroliths; use in conjunction with increased water intake and low-purine, alkalinizing, diuretic diets to reduce recurrences and lessen need to use intermittent higher dose dissolution protocols.

Leishmaniasis (extra-label): Improved efficacy when used in combination with an antimonial drug

a) Allopurinol 10 – 15 mg/kg PO twice daily for 6 to 12 months plus meglumine antimoniate (N-methylglucamine antimoniate) 75 – 100 mg/kg SC once daily for 1 to 2 months.[19]

b) Alternatively, allopurinol 10 – 15 mg/kg PO twice daily for 6 to 12 months plus miltefosine 2 mg/kg PO once daily for 4 weeks[20,21]

c) As monotherapy, dosages range from 5 – 20 mg/kg PO every 12 hours for 2 to 24 months.[4] **NOTE:** Initiate allopurinol at 5 mg/kg PO twice daily in dogs with renal dysfunction.

CATS:

Leishmaniasis (extra-label): 10 – 20 mg/kg PO every 12 or 24 hours long-term[22]

BIRDS:

Gout (extra-label):

a) Highly variable dosages (300 – 830 mg/L) for drinking water administration have been reported.[23]

b) **In budgies and cockatiels**: Crush one 100 mg tablet into 10 mL of water. Add 20 drops of this solution to 30 mL (1 oz) of drinking water.[24]

c) **In parakeets**: As above for budgies and cockatiels or give 1 drop 4 times daily.[25]

REPTILES:

Gout in lizards or iguanas (extra-label): 20 – 25 mg/kg PO once daily.[1] Reported dosages in reptiles range from 10 to 50 mg/kg.[23]

Monitoring

- Hydration status
- Baseline and periodic CBC and serum chemistry profile
- Baseline and periodic urinalysis (including pH) to check if urine pH is greater than or equal to 7
- Periodic urinary tract imaging (eg, ultrasound) to monitor for recurrence of calculi
- In dogs with leishmaniasis, monitor clinical response, reduction in UPPC,[26-28] saliva IgG2 and IgA antibodies,[29] and normalization of acute-phase proteins (eg, C-reactive protein, haptoglobin, ferritin, paraoxanase).[30]

Laboratory Considerations

- None

Client Information

- May be given with food if vomiting occurs
- Always provide access to fresh clean water while your animal is taking this medicine.
- When this drug is used long-term in dogs, low-purine diets are recommended.
- Contact your veterinarian immediately if you observe a rash, unusual tiredness, or yellowing of the whites of the eyes.
- If using in drinking water for birds or reptiles, make a fresh solution every day.

Chemistry/Synonyms

A xanthine oxidase inhibitor, allopurinol occurs as a tasteless, fluffy white to off-white powder with a slight odor. Its melting point is more than 350°C (662°F) and it has a pK_a of 9.4. Oxypurinol, its active metabolite, has a pK_a of 7.7. Allopurinol is very slightly soluble in water and alcohol and insoluble in diethyl ether.

Allopurinol may also be known as allopurinolum, BW-56-158, HPP, or NSC-1390; many trade names are available.

Storage/Stability

Allopurinol tablets should be stored between 20°C to 25°C (68°F to 77°F) in tightly closed containers and protected from light.[31]

Compatibility/Compounding Considerations

Compounded preparation stability: An extemporaneous suspension for oral use can be prepared from the commercially available tablets. Triturate eight 300 mg tablets of allopurinol with 60 mL of *Ora-Plus*® and qs ad to 120 mL with *Ora-Sweet*® (or *Ora-Sweet*® *SF*). This formulation yields a 20 mg/mL suspension that retains more than 95% potency for at least 60 days stored at both 5°C (41°F) and 25°C (77°F). Compounded preparations of allopurinol should be protected from light.[32]

Dosage Forms/Regulatory Status

VETERINARY-LABELED PRODUCTS: NONE

The FEI (International Federation for Equestrian Sports) lists this drug as a "prohibited substance - banned."[33]

HUMAN-LABELED PRODUCTS:

Allopurinol Oral Tablets: 100 and 300 mg; *Zyloprim*® generic; (Rx)

References

For the complete list of references, see **wiley.com/go/budde/plumb**

Alprazolam

(al-***prah***-zoe-lam) *Xanax*®

Benzodiazepine

Prescriber Highlights

- Oral benzodiazepine that may be useful for adjunctive behavioral treatment in dogs and cats
- Contraindicated in aggressive animals (controversial) and animals with benzodiazepine hypersensitivity
- Use with caution in patients with hepatic or renal disease
- Adverse effects include sedation, unintended negative behavior changes, and paradoxical responses. Physical dependence is a possibility. May impede training or performance of working animals
- Many drug interactions are possible.
- DEA Schedule IV (C-IV) controlled substance

Uses/Indications

Alprazolam may be useful for adjunctive therapy in anxious and/or aggressive dogs or in dogs that demonstrate panic reactions and for managing anxiety while a long-term drug (eg, selective serotonin reuptake inhibitor [SSRI], other serotonin-enhancing drug) reaches therapeutic concentrations.[1,2] When alprazolam is used to treat anxiety related to a triggering event (eg, storm, fireworks), it is most effective when administered 30 to 60 minutes prior to the event. Alprazolam may be useful in cats for adjunctive treatment of anxiety disorders and inappropriate elimination, and, unlike oral diazepam, alprazolam has not been implicated in causing liver failure in cats. A case report described the successful use of alprazolam to facilitate bonding in a mare that was aggressive when her foal attempted to nurse.[3]

At low doses, alprazolam may have less of an effect on motor function than diazepam.

Pharmacology/Actions

Alprazolam exhibits similar pharmacologic actions as other benzodiazepines; subcortical levels (primarily limbic, thalamic, and hypothalamic) of the CNS are depressed, which produces anxiolytic, sedative, skeletal muscle relaxant, and anticonvulsant effects. The exact mechanism of action is unknown, but postulated mechanisms include antagonism of serotonin, increased release of and/or facilitation of gamma-aminobutyric acid (GABA) activity, and diminished release or turnover of acetylcholine in the CNS.

Benzodiazepine-specific receptors have been located in the mammalian brain, kidney, liver, lungs, and heart. In all species studied, receptors are lacking in the white matter.

Pharmacokinetics

The pharmacokinetics of alprazolam have not been described for dogs or cats.

In adult horses, alprazolam was detected in serum 30 minutes after administration of a single oral dose (0.04 mg/kg), and peak plasma levels occurred in a median of 3 hours. Elimination half-life was ≈16 hours.[4]

In humans, alprazolam is well absorbed with peak plasma concentrations occurring in 1 to 2 hours. Alprazolam is widely distributed throughout the body and readily crosses the blood-brain barrier; it is 80% bound to plasma proteins. It is metabolized in the liver primarily by cytochrome P450 3A4 (CYP3A4) to at least 2 metabolites, including alpha-hydroxy-alprazolam, which is pharmacologically active.[5] Elimination half-lives range from 6 to 27 hours; half-life is extended in cases of hepatic disfunction and obesity. Alprazolam is primarily excreted in the urine as unchanged drug and metabolites.

Contraindications/Precautions/Warnings

Alprazolam is contraindicated in patients with known hypersensitivity to the drug. Some clinicians also believe that benzodiazepines are contraindicated in aggressive dogs, as anxiety may restrain the animal from aggressive tendencies; however, this remains controversial.[6] Some clinicians recommend administering alprazolam for the first time at the clinic with the owner present to monitor for adverse effects (eg, excessive sedation) or for a paradoxical reaction (ie, worsening of clinical signs [eg, CNS excitement, including increased excitability, aggression, and anxiety]) to the drug. If unacceptable sedation occurs, the dosage can be lowered. If a paradoxical response occurs, alprazolam may not be an acceptable treatment for that animal; however, it has been suggested that higher dosages may alleviate the paradoxical reaction.[6] Caution is advised in debilitated or geriatric patients and patients with hepatic or renal disease or narrow-angle glaucoma. Benzodiazepines may impair the abilities of working animals.

Chronic use of alprazolam may induce physical dependence,[7] and if the drug is to be discontinued, the dosage must be gradually decreased (tapered) over several weeks.

Alprazolam, like other benzodiazepines, has the potential for drug abuse and drug diversion in humans; caution is advised when prescribing this drug.

Adverse Effects

Benzodiazepines can cause sedation, increased appetite, and transient ataxia. Animals may rarely exhibit a paradoxical response following administration. See ***Contraindications/Precautions/Warnings***.

There have been sporadic reports of cats developing idiosyncratic hepatic failure after receiving oral, but not injectable, diazepam (not dose-dependent) for several days.[8] See ***Diazepam*** for more information related to hepatic changes that may occur. Although this adverse effect has not been reported for alprazolam, oral benzodiazepines should be used with caution in cats. See ***Monitoring***.

Benzodiazepines have an amnestic effect which may impede the ability of the animal to learn and may delay training.[5,6]

Reproductive/Nursing Safety

Diazepam and other benzodiazepines have been implicated in causing congenital abnormalities in humans when they are administered during the first trimester of pregnancy. Infants born to mothers that received large doses of benzodiazepines shortly before delivery have been reported to suffer from apnea, impaired metabolic response to cold stress, difficulty in feeding, hyperbilirubinemia, and hypotonia.[5] Withdrawal symptoms have occurred in infants whose mothers took benzodiazepines chronically during pregnancy. The veterinary significance of these effects is unclear, but the use of these agents during the first trimester of pregnancy should only occur when the benefits clearly outweigh the risks associated with their use.

Alprazolam enters human breast milk. Case reports have noted drowsiness, depression, and withdrawal symptoms in infants exposed to alprazolam while breastfeeding.[5] In humans, alprazolam is not recommended while breastfeeding.[9]

Because safety of alprazolam has not been established in animals, this drug should only be used when the maternal benefits outweigh the potential risks to offspring.

Overdose/Acute Toxicity

Overdoses of alprazolam are generally limited to CNS signs. CNS depression can be seen, and the severity is generally dose-dependent. Hypotension, respiratory depression, and cardiac arrest have been reported in humans but apparently are rare. The acute LD_{50} in rats for alprazolam is greater than 330 mg/kg.[10] Life-threatening signs in small animals are rare. Some animals may be presented with a paradoxical-type reaction (eg, disorientation, vocalization, agitation). At times, those signs may be followed by CNS depression.

Common clinical signs seen in dogs with alprazolam overdose include ataxia, hyperactivity/agitation, lethargy/sedation, and vomiting; in cats, the common clinical signs include ataxia, vocalization, agitation, polyphagia, and lethargy.

Massive overdoses can lead to CNS and respiratory depression or hypotension. Gastric decontamination can be considered. The decision to give activated charcoal should be weighed carefully, as, in some cases, there is a risk for aspiration pneumonia in an obtunded patient, which may outweigh the benefit. Use of analeptic agents (eg, caffeine, doxapram) is generally not recommended. Flumazenil can be used to reverse respiratory depression or severe CNS depression. The half-life of flumazenil is short, and the animal may require multiple doses of the drug. See *Flumazenil*.

For patients that have experienced or are suspected to have experienced an overdose, consultation with a 24-hour poison consultation center specializing in providing veterinary-specific information is recommended. For general information related to overdose and toxin exposures, as well as contact information for poison control centers, refer to *Appendix*.

Drug Interactions

The following drug interactions with alprazolam have either been reported or are theoretical in humans or animals and may be of significance in veterinary patients. Unless otherwise noted, use together is not necessarily contraindicated, but the potential risk must be weighed and additional monitoring performed when appropriate.

- **Amiodarone**: Concurrent use may increase bioavailability and pharmacologic effects of benzodiazepines. Sedation levels should be monitored, and benzodiazepine doses adjusted accordingly.
- **Antacids, Aluminum-, Calcium- and Magnesium-Containing**: May slow the rate but not the extent of oral absorption; administering antacids 2 hours apart from alprazolam may help avoid this potential interaction
- **Antihypertensive Agents** (eg, **amlodipine, enalapril, telmisartan**): May increase risk for hypotension and orthostasis. Blood pressure monitoring is needed.
- **Azole Antifungals** (eg, **fluconazole, itraconazole, ketoconazole**): Metabolism of alprazolam may be decreased, and excessive sedation may occur. This combination is contraindicated in humans.
- **Carbonic Anhydrase Inhibitors (CAIs)** (eg, **acetazolamide, methazolamide**): Benzodiazepines may interfere with the beneficial effects of CAIs by inhibiting respiratory responses to hypoxia; combination should be avoided.
- **CNS Depressant Agents** (eg, **anesthetic agents, antihistamines** (first generation), **barbiturates, cannabidiol, narcotics**): Combination may increase the risk for CNS and/or respiratory depression. Sedation levels should be monitored and doses adjusted accordingly.
- **Digoxin**: Serum digoxin concentrations may be increased; monitor serum digoxin concentrations and for clinical signs associated with digoxin toxicity (eg, arrhythmias, vomiting, diarrhea, inappetence).
- **Fluoxetine, Fluvoxamine**: Metabolism of alprazolam may be decreased and cause excessive sedation.
- **Hepatic Enzyme Inducers** (eg, **dexamethasone, mitotane**): Concurrent use may decrease benzodiazepine concentrations. Clinical response should be monitored and doses adjusted accordingly.
- **Hepatic Enzyme Inhibitors** (eg, **cimetidine, diltiazem, grapefruit juice, isoniazid**): Metabolism of alprazolam may be decreased and cause excessive sedation.
- **Ifosfamide:** Concurrent use may increase the risk for ifosfamide-induced neurotoxic effects. Careful monitoring of the level of sedation is recommended, and both drugs should be discontinued if signs of encephalopathy occur.
- **Macrolide Antibiotics** (eg, **clarithromycin, erythromycin**): Metabolism of alprazolam may be decreased, and excessive sedation may occur.
- **Macrocyclic Lactones** (eg, **ivermectin, milbemycin oxime**): Benzodiazepine effects may be potentiated by concurrent macrocyclic lactone use.
- **Maropitant:** Concurrent benzodiazepine administration with the human drug aprepitant may increase benzodiazepine exposure via inhibition of CYP3A4. Interaction may apply to maropitant.
- **Non-Depolarizing Neuromuscular Blockers** (eg, **atracurium, pancuronium**): Concurrent use may potentiate, attenuate, or have no effect. Respiratory status should be monitored.
- **Opioids** (eg, **buprenorphine, hydromorphone, tramadol**): May increase the risk for cardiorespiratory and CNS depression
- **Phenobarbital:** Concurrent use of phenobarbital and benzodiazepines may increase the risk for respiratory depression.
- **Propofol:** May increase the risk for cardiorespiratory depression
- **Rifampin:** May induce hepatic microsomal enzymes and decrease the pharmacologic effects of benzodiazepines
- **Theophylline/Aminophylline:** Concurrent use may decrease the levels and effectiveness of benzodiazepines. Withdrawing theophylline from a stable patient may increase the risk for benzodiazepine toxicity. Sedation levels should be monitored and doses adjusted accordingly.
- **Tricyclic Antidepressants** (eg, **amitriptyline, clomipramine, imipramine**): Alprazolam may increase concentrations of these drugs; clinical significance is not known, and clomipramine and alprazolam have been used together anecdotally to manage phobias (eg, thunderstorm phobia). However, concurrent use may increase the risk for CNS and/or respiratory depression. Anticholinergic effects may be additive.
- **Yohimbine:** Limited data indicate that yohimbine may decrease therapeutic effects of anxiolytic drugs.

Laboratory Considerations

- Benzodiazepines may decrease the thyroidal uptake of I^{123} or I^{131}.

Dosages

DOGS:

Adjunctive treatment of canine anxiety disorders or phobias (extra-label): 0.02 – 0.1 mg/kg (usually 0.02 – 0.05 mg/kg initially) PO every 6 to 12 hours as needed. If used for acute phobias (eg, fireworks, thunderstorms), the drug should be given 30 to 60 minutes before the expected trigger.

CATS:

Adjunctive treatment of feline anxiety disorders, phobias, or house soiling/marking (extra-label): 0.125 – 0.25 mg/cat (NOT mg/kg) PO every 8 to 24 hours. If used for phobias, the drug should be given 30 to 60 minutes before the expected trigger.

Adjunctive treatment of highly aroused felines before transport to a veterinary visit (extra-label): 0.5 – 1 mg/cat (NOT mg/kg) 1 hour prior to leaving for veterinary visit[11]

HORSES:

Facilitating mare-foal bonding (extra-label): One case study reported 0.035 mg/kg PO every 8 to 12 hours for facilitating healthy mare–foal bonding and behavior in an aggressive mare.[3]

Monitoring

- Efficacy
- Adverse effects
- Monitoring hepatic enzymes should be considered, particularly with chronic therapy.

Client Information

- Alprazolam is often used to help treat or prevent fears and anxiety in dogs and cats.
- When alprazolam is used for thunderstorm phobias or other triggers (eg, separation anxiety) that upset your animal, try to give your animal the drug about 30 to 60 minutes before the triggering event.
- This medicine may be given with or without food. If your animal vomits or acts sick after receiving the drug on an empty stomach, try giving the next dose with food or a small treat. If vomiting continues, contact your veterinarian.
- Contact your veterinarian immediately if you see yellowing of the whites of the eyes of your animal or if your animal's gums have a yellowish tint.
- Sleepiness is the most common side effect, but sometimes the drug can change behavior or work in the opposite way (ie, cause hyperactive behavior) from what is expected.
- This drug may increase appetite, especially in cats.
- Alprazolam is classified as a schedule IV (C-IV) controlled drug by the federal Drug Enforcement Agency (DEA). Use of this medication in animals or humans other than those for whom it is prescribed is illegal.

Chemistry/Synonyms

Alprazolam is a benzodiazepine. It occurs as a white to off-white crystalline powder and is soluble in alcohol and insoluble in water.

Alprazolam may also be known as D65 MT, U 31889, or alprazolamum; many trade names are available internationally.

Storage/Stability

Alprazolam tablets should be stored at room temperature in tight, light-resistant containers. The orally disintegrating tablets should be stored at room temperature and protected from moisture. The oral solution should be stored at room temperature, protected from light, and discarded 90 days after opening. Alprazolam is a DEA Schedule IV (C-IV) controlled substance that should be stored in an area that is substantially constructed and securely locked. Follow applicable local, state, and federal rules regarding disposal of unused or wasted controlled drugs.

Compatibility/Compounding Considerations

Compounded preparation stability: An alprazolam oral suspension compounded from commercially available tablets has been published.[12] Triturating sixty (60) alprazolam 2 mg tablets with 60 mL of *Ora-Plus*® and *qs ad* to 120 mL with *Ora-Sweet*® (or *Ora-Sweet*® SF) yields a 1 mg/mL oral suspension that retains more than 90% potency for 60 days when stored at 5°C (41°F) and 25°C (77°F). Compounded preparations of alprazolam should be protected from light.

Dosage Forms/Regulatory Status

VETERINARY-LABELED PRODUCTS: NONE

The Association of Racing Commissioners International (ARCI) has designated this drug as a class 2 substance. Use of this drug may not be allowed in certain animal competitions. Check rules and regulations before entering in a competition while this medication is being administered. Contact local racing authorities for further guidance. See ***Appendix*** for more information.

HUMAN-LABELED PRODUCTS:

Alprazolam Oral Tablets: 0.25 mg, 0.5 mg, 1 mg, and 2 mg; *Xanax*®, generic; (Rx; C-IV)

Alprazolam Extended-release Oral Tablets: 0.5 mg, 1 mg, 2 mg, and 3 mg; *Xanax XR*®, generic; (Rx; C-IV)

Alprazolam Orally Disintegrating Tablets: 0.25 mg, 0.5 mg, 1 mg, and 2 mg; *Niravam*®, generic; (Rx; C-IV)

Alprazolam Oral Solution: 1 mg/mL in 30 mL; *Alprazolam Intensol*®; (Rx; C-IV)

References

For the complete list of references, see **wiley.com/go/budde/plumb**

Altrenogest

(al-***tre***-noe-jest) *Regu-Mate*®, *Matrix*®

Oral Progestin

Prescriber Highlights

- ► Used in mares to suppress estrus or maintain pregnancy in those that are progestin deficient
- ► Used in swine to synchronize estrus
- ► Contraindicated in mares or gilts with previous or current uterine inflammation
- ► May be used in dogs for luteal deficiency or to prevent premature delivery
- ► Readily absorbed by the skin; wear protective gloves (not latex) when handling
- ► The National Institute for Occupational Safety and Health (NIOSH) classifies progestins as hazardous drugs; use appropriate precautions when handling.

Uses/Indications

Altrenogest is FDA-approved for use in mares to suppress estrus and allow a more predictable occurrence of estrus following withdrawal of the drug.[1] It is used clinically to establish normal estrous cycles at the end of the transitional period from anestrus to the normal breeding season, to facilitate management of prolonged estrus conditions, or to facilitate scheduled breeding; it also helps maintain high-risk pregnancies (eg, placentitis, history of early embryonic loss, embryo transfer recipients). Mares with considerable follicular activity (mares with 1 or more follicles that are 20 mm or greater in size) are more likely to respond to altrenogest than are mares with inactive ovaries and small follicles.[1] Mares that have been in estrus for 10 days or more and have active ovaries are also considered excellent candidates for progestin treatment.

Altrenogest has been demonstrated to maintain pregnancy in ovariectomized mares and may be of benefit in mares that abort due to subtherapeutic progestin levels.[2]

Some altrenogest products are FDA-approved for synchronization of estrus in sexually mature gilts that have had at least 1 estrous cycle.[3] It has been shown that feeding altrenogest to sows that are nursing small litters during late lactation improves fertility and increases ovulation rate and subsequent litter size.[4]

Altrenogest has been used extra-label in dogs for luteal insufficiency and as a treatment to prevent premature delivery.

Pharmacology/Actions

Endogenous progestins are primarily produced by the corpus luteum; they transform proliferative endometrium to secretory endometrium, enhance myometrial hypertrophy, and inhibit spontaneous uterine contraction. Altrenogest acts via negative feedback to decrease plasma concentrations of endogenous gonadotrophin hormones (LH and FSH). Low gonadotrophin concentrations cause regression of large follicles and do not allow the growth of small follicles, resulting in an absence of estrus and ovulation during treatment. When treatment is discontinued, plasma LH concentration increases to stimulate follicular growth and maturation.

In normally cycling mares, altrenogest is effective for minimizing the necessity for estrus detection, for the synchronization of estrus, and for permitting scheduled breeding. Estrus typically occurs 2 to 5 days after treatment is completed and most mares ovulate between 8 to 15 days after withdrawal.

Progestins have some degree of estrogenic, anabolic, and androgenic activity.

Pharmacokinetics

After oral dosing of altrenogest 0.044 mg/kg PO (recommended dose) in horses, the time to peak concentration has been reported to range from 15 minutes to 4 hours.[5] Elimination half-life has been reported to be between 2.5 and 8.5 hours.[6] Altrenogest appears to be primarily eliminated in the urine. Peak urine concentrations occur 3 to 6 hours after oral dosing. Urine concentrations were detectable up to 12 days postadministration. Altrenogest 150 mg IM produced peak serum concentrations between 9 and 24 hours postdose.[7] The elimination half-life was ≈15 hours and plasma concentrations remained above 0.5 ng/mL for 148 hours after dosing.

Altrenogest has been shown to be rapidly absorbed after rectal administration to horses; however, rectal administration results in decreased bioavailability and shorter half-life and time at therapeutic concentration than oral dosing.[6]

In gilts that were given altrenogest 20 mg/kg PO once daily for 18 days, peak plasma concentrations were achieved after ≈2 to 3 hours.[8] Half-life on days 1 and 18 was ≈7 and 10 hours, respectively. There was no significant accumulation of drug seen after 18 days.

Contraindications/Precautions/Warnings

Altrenogest is contraindicated in stallions and geldings[9] and mares that have a history of uterine inflammation (ie, acute, subacute, or chronic endometritis).[1,9] Natural or synthetic gestagen therapy may exacerbate existing low-grade or "smoldering" uterine inflammation into a fulminating uterine infection[1]; therefore, the use of progestational agents in mares with chronic uterine infections should be avoided, as the agents may enhance the infection process. When altrenogest is used to maintain pregnancy, luteal insufficiency should be documented, and infectious causes of pregnancy loss should be ruled out prior to altrenogest therapy; altrenogest therapy should be discontinued within 24 hours of the mare's due date,[10] and 2 to 7 days prior to the bitch's anticipated whelping date.[11] Avoid administering altrenogest to pregnant bitches during the first trimester.[12]

Pregnant mares with GI disease may not absorb oral altrenogest adequately and injectable progesterone is preferred.[13]

In swine, underdosing can lead to the formation of cystic follicles.[3]

WARNING FOR THOSE HANDLING THIS DRUG[1]:

Individuals who should not handle this product include:

1. Women
   a. Who are or suspect they are pregnant
   b. With known or suspected carcinoma of the breast
   c. With known or suspected estrogen-dependent neoplasia
   d. With undiagnosed vaginal bleeding
2. Anyone with
   a. Thrombophlebitis or thromboembolic disorders or with a history of these events
   b. Cerebral-vascular or coronary artery disease
   c. A benign or malignant tumor that developed during the use of oral contraceptives or other estrogen-containing products
   d. Liver dysfunction/disease

Altrenogest is readily absorbed by the skin and can penetrate porous (eg, latex, rubber) gloves; absorption can be increased from areas covered by these occlusive materials. It is recommended to wear impermeable (eg, nitrile, vinyl) gloves for dermal protection.

If skin exposure occurs, wash the skin immediately with soap and water. If eye exposure occurs, flush the eyes immediately with water for 15 minutes and seek medical attention. If swallowed, seek medical attention and do NOT induce vomiting, as vomiting should be supervised by a physician because of potential pulmonary damage via aspiration of oil base.

Altrenogest should not enter water courses as this may be dangerous for fish and other aquatic organisms.[14]

The National Institute for Occupational Safety and Health (NIOSH) classifies progestins as hazardous drugs; personal protective equipment (PPE) should be used accordingly to minimize the risk for exposure.

Adverse Effects

Adverse effects of altrenogest appear to be minimal when used at labeled dosages.[15]

Progestogens may induce cystic endometrial hyperplasia and pyometra in bitches.[16]

Reproductive/Nursing Safety

Altrenogest administration to rats during the embryogenic stage of pregnancy caused masculinization of female genitalia when it was given at high doses (manyfold greater than the recommended equine dose).

Because safety has not been established in animals, this drug should only be used when the maternal benefits outweigh the potential risks to offspring.

Overdose/Acute Toxicity

The LD_{50} of altrenogest is 176 mg/kg in rats and 233 mg/kg in mice.[17] Dogs tolerated an oral dose up to 400 mg/kg.[17] No information was located regarding the effects of an accidental acute overdose in horses or other species.

For patients that have experienced or are suspected to have experienced an overdose, consultation with a 24-hour poison consultation center specializing in providing veterinary-specific information is recommended. For general information related to overdose and toxin exposures, as well as contact information for poison control centers, refer to *Appendix*.

Drug Interactions

The following drug interactions with altrenogest have either been reported or are theoretical in humans or animals and may be of significance in veterinary patients. Unless otherwise noted, use together is not necessarily contraindicated, but weigh the potential risks and perform additional monitoring when appropriate.

- **Dinoprost:** Altrenogest may reduce the effects of dinoprost.
- **Heparins** (eg, **enoxaparin, heparin**): Concurrent use of progestins may decrease anticoagulant effects of heparin or low-molecular weight heparins.
- **Hypoglycemic Agents** (eg, **glipizide, insulins**): Altrenogest may reduce blood glucose-lowering effects.
- **Rifampin:** Concurrent use may decrease progestin activity, due to microsomal enzyme induction with resultant increase in progestin metabolism. The clinical significance of this potential interaction is unknown.
- **Phenobarbital:** Concurrent use may decrease progestin activity due to microsomal enzyme induction with resultant increase in progestin metabolism.

Laboratory Considerations

- Unlike exogenously administered progesterone, altrenogest does not interfere or cross-react with progesterone assays.

Dosages

DOGS:

Luteal insufficiency (extra-label): 0.05 – 0.1 mg/kg PO once daily[11,12,18,19]

HORSES:

Suppression of estrus for synchronization (label dosage; FDA-approved): Administer 1 mL/49.9 kg (110 lb) body weight (0.044 mg/kg) PO once daily for 15 consecutive days. May administer altrenogest directly on the animal's tongue using a dose syringe or on the usual grain ration[1]

Suppression of estrus in normally cycling mares (extra-label): 0.3 mg/kg IM every 5 to 7 days[9]

Long-term suppression of estrus (extra-label): 0.044 mg/kg PO daily[20]

Prevention of abortion/pregnancy loss (extra-label): 0.088 mg/kg PO once daily[21]

Maintain pregnancy in mares with deficient progesterone levels (extra-label): 0.044 mg/kg PO once daily. Three options for treatment:

a) Treat until day 60 of pregnancy or greater AND measurement of endogenous progesterone level of greater than 4 ng/mL;
b) Treat until day 120 of pregnancy; or
c) Treat until end of pregnancy[22]

Maintain pregnancy in mares with deficient progesterone levels and at risk of early embryonic death or abortion (extra-label): 0.3 mg/kg IM on the fifth day after ovulation; repeat every 5 days until day 120 of gestation[9]

Maintain pregnancy in mares with placentitis: 22 – 44 mg/mare (NOT mg/kg) PO daily[23]

Rectal administration for the above indications when oral administration is not possible (extra-label): 0.088 mg/kg rectally every 4 to 8 hours.[6] From a pharmacokinetic study; the clinical efficacy of this dosage has not been studied.

SWINE:

Synchronization of estrus in sexually mature gilts that have had at least 1 estrous cycle (label dosage; FDA-approved): Administer 6.8 mL (15 mg)/gilt (NOT mg/kg) once daily for 14 consecutive days.[3] Apply as a top-dressing on a portion of gilt's daily feed allowance. Estrus should occur 4 to 9 days after completing treatment. To synchronize estrus in a group of gilts, treat all gilts daily for the same 14-day period.

Synchronization of estrus in sexually mature gilts that have had at least 1 estrous cycle (extra-label): 15 mg/gilt (NOT mg/kg) once daily for 18 consecutive days[24]

Monitoring

- Monitor pregnancy via ultrasonography and progesterone concentration[12]

Client Information

MANUFACTURER WARNING FOR THOSE HANDLING THIS DRUG:

Individuals who should not handle this product include:

1. Women
   a. Who are or suspect they are pregnant
   b. With known or suspected carcinoma of the breast
   c. With known or suspected estrogen-dependent neoplasia
   d. With undiagnosed vaginal bleeding
2. Anyone with
   a. Thrombophlebitis or thromboembolic disorders or with a history of these events
   b. Cerebral-vascular or coronary artery disease
   c. A benign or malignant tumor which developed during the use of oral contraceptives or other estrogen-containing products
   d. Liver dysfunction/disease

- Additionally, the FDA has issued a warning that exposure to these products may cause reproductive system disorders or other adverse effects. Although both men and women can be affected, the FDA cautions that teenage girls may be at highest risk.
- Individuals handling altrenogest products should wear impermeable (eg, nitrile or vinyl; NOT latex) protective gloves.
- The outside of the medicine containers and syringes should be kept clean of medicine residue, and any medicine that is spilled should be cleaned and decontaminated according to package insert instructions.
- Altrenogest can be absorbed after skin contact. Absorption can be increased if the medicine is covered by occlusive materials (eg, under latex gloves). If this medicine comes into contact with skin, wash off immediately with soap and water. If the eyes are exposed, flush the eyes with water for 15 minutes and get medical attention. If the product is swallowed, do not induce vomiting and contact a physician or poison control center.
- This medication is prohibited from use in an extra-label manner to enhance food and/or fiber production in animals.
- Altrenogest should not enter water courses as this may be dangerous for fish and other aquatic organisms.
- This medication is considered to be a hazardous drug as defined by the National Institute for Occupational Safety and Health (NIOSH). Talk with your veterinarian or pharmacist about the use of personal protective equipment when handling this medicine.

Chemistry/Synonyms

An orally administered synthetic progestational agent, altrenogest has a chemical name of 17 alpha-allyl-17-beta-hydroxyestra-4,9,11-trien-3-one.

Altrenogest may also be known as allyl trenbolone, A-35957, A-41300, RH-2267, or RU-2267, *Regu-Mate®*, *Altren®*, *Altresyn®*, *ChronoMate®*, *Matrix®*, or *Virbagest®*.

Storage/Stability

Altrenogest oral solution should be stored at or below 25°C (77° F); do not expose to temperatures exceeding 50°C (122°F). Altrenogest is extremely sensitive to light; dispense in light-resistant containers.

Compatibility/Compounding Considerations

No specific information is noted.

Dosage Forms/Regulatory Status

VETERINARY-LABELED PRODUCTS:

Altrenogest 0.22% (2.2 mg/mL) in oil solution in 150 mL and 1000 mL bottles; *Regu-Mate*®, generic (Rx). FDA-approved for use in horses that are not intended for food. This medication is banned in racing animals in some countries.

Altrenogest 0.22% (2.2 mg/mL) in 1000 mL bottles; *Matrix*®, generic; (OTC). FDA-approved for use in sexually mature gilts that have had at least 1 estrous cycle. Gilts must not be slaughtered for human consumption for 21 days after the last treatment. The FDA prohibits the extra-label use of this medication, including to enhance food and/or fiber production in animals.

HUMAN-LABELED PRODUCTS: NONE

References

For the complete list of references, see **wiley.com/go/budde/plumb**

Aluminum Hydroxide

(ah-***loo***-min-um hye-***droks***-ide) *Amphojel*®

Oral Antacid/Phosphate Binder

Prescriber Highlights

- Used to treat hyperphosphatemia in small animals and sometimes as an antacid for gastric ulcers
- Chronic use may lead to electrolyte abnormalities; possible aluminum toxicity.
- Many potential drug interactions
- Bulk dried powder available from several sources

Uses/Indications

Orally administered aluminum hydroxide is used to reduce hyperphosphatemia in patients with chronic kidney disease when dietary phosphorus restriction fails to maintain serum phosphorus concentrations in the normal range. Occasionally, it has been used as an oral antacid in veterinary patients, although its short duration of action for this purpose may make its use less practical.

Pharmacology/Actions

Aluminum salts reduce the amount of phosphorus absorbed from the intestine by physically binding to dietary phosphorus to form insoluble aluminum phosphate, which is then excreted in the feces. When used as an antacid, the hydroxyl ion interacts with hydrogen ions in the stomach to increase gastric/abomasal pH.

Contraindications/Precautions/Warnings

Aluminum-containing antacids may inhibit gastric emptying; use cautiously in patients with gastric outlet obstruction. Also, use with caution in patients prone to developing constipation. Aluminum may accumulate in patients with renal failure.

Adverse Effects

In small animals, the most likely adverse effect of aluminum hydroxide is constipation. Hypophosphatemia can develop if the patient is receiving a low phosphate diet and chronically receives aluminum antacids.

Potentially, aluminum toxicity could occur with prolonged use. Although previously believed unlikely to occur in small animals, at least 2 dogs with renal failure have developed aluminum toxicity after receiving aluminum-containing phosphate binders.[1] Osteomalacia related to hypophosphatemia or aluminum accumulation is also possible with chronic use. Aluminum-containing and calcium-containing phosphate binders may be used in combination to reduce the dose of each and reduce the risk for aluminum toxicity or hypercalcemia.

Reproductive/Nursing Safety

Use during pregnancy and lactation has not been studied; however, it is considered generally safe since oral absorption of this drug is poor.

Because safety has not been established in animals, this drug should only be used when the maternal benefits outweigh the potential risks to offspring.

Overdosage/Acute Toxicity

Acute toxicity is unlikely with an oral overdose. If necessary, GI effects (eg, constipation) and electrolyte imbalances that may occur with acute or chronic overdose should be treated based on clinical presentation.

For patients that have experienced or are suspected to have experienced an overdose, it is strongly encouraged to consult with one of the 24-hour poison consultation centers that specialize in providing information specific for veterinary patients. For general information related to overdose and toxin exposures, as well as contact information for poison control centers, refer to *Appendix*.

Drug Interactions

The following drug interactions with aluminum hydroxide have either been reported or are theoretical in humans or animals and may be of significance in veterinary patients. Unless otherwise noted, use together is not necessarily contraindicated, but weigh the potential risks and perform additional monitoring when appropriate.

- **DIAZEPAM**: Concurrent aluminum may increase diazepam absorption.
- **QUINIDINE:** Increased gastric pH caused by aluminum hydroxide can potentially **increase** the absorption of basic drugs such as **quinidine;** separate from aluminum hydroxide by at least 2 hours.
- **VITAMIN D ANALOGUES** (eg, **calcitriol, ergocalciferol**): May increase aluminum absorption. Avoid combination.

Aluminum hydroxide can **decrease** the amount absorbed (orally) or the pharmacologic effect of the drugs listed below; separate oral doses of aluminum hydroxide and these drugs by at least 2 hours to help reduce the potential for this interaction.

- **ALLOPURINOL**
- **ASPIRIN**
- **AZOLE ANTIFUNGALS** (eg, **itraconazole, ketoconazole**)
- **CEFPODOXIME**
- **CORTICOSTEROIDS** (eg, **dexamethasone, prednis(ol)one**)
- **DIGOXIN**
- **ETHAMBUTOL**
- **FEXOFENADINE**
- **FLUOROQUINOLONES** (eg, **enrofloxacin, marbofloxacin**)
- **GABAPENTIN**
- **H_2 ANTAGONISTS** (eg, **famotidine, ranitidine**)
- **IRON SALTS** (eg, **ferrous sulfate**)
- **ISONIAZID** (INH)
- **MYCOPHENOLATE**
- **PENICILLAMINE**
- **PHENOTHIAZINES** (eg, **acepromazine, chlorpromazine**)
- **PHENYTOIN**
- **SOTALOL**
- **TETRACYCLINES** (eg, **doxycycline, minocycline**)
- **THYROID HORMONES**

Doses

NOTE: All dosages are extra-label.

DOGS/CATS:

Hyperphosphatemia secondary to chronic kidney disease (extra-label): 30 – 100 mg/kg per day as adjunct to reduced dietary phosphorus.[2-4] Aluminum hydroxide gel powder (USP) is preferred, as it can be mixed with food and is tasteless. Dose is divided and mixed with *each* meal. Start at low end of dosage range and adjust upward every 4 to 6 weeks until desired serum phosphorus is attained (see *Monitoring*). If a reduced-phosphorus diet and higher dosages of aluminum hydroxide do not adequately control serum phosphorus, consider adding a lanthanum- or calcium-based (eg, calcium acetate, calcium carbonate) phosphate binder to reduce the chances for aluminum toxicity.

RABBITS/RODENTS/SMALL MAMMALS:

Hyperphosphatemia in chinchillas (extra-label): Aluminum hydroxide gel: 1 mL/animal (NOT mL/kg) PO as needed

Hyperphosphatemia in Guinea pigs (extra-label): 0.5 – 1 mL per animal (NOT mL/kg) PO as needed[5]

REPTILES:

Hyperphosphatemia (extra-label): 100 mg/kg PO every 12 to 24 hours[6]

CATTLE:

Antacid (extra-label): 15 – 60 mg/kg PO every 8 – 24 hours.[7] Efficacy in adult cattle is questionable since the drug becomes diluted in the rumen and may not provide therapeutic benefit in the abomasum.

Abomasal ulcers in calves using a combination of aluminum hydroxide and magnesium hydroxide (extra-label): 25 mL (each mL contains aluminum hydroxide 0.1 g/mL and magnesium hydroxide 0.09 g/mL) PO every 8 hours.[8] **NOTE:** this study was done in healthy calves; based on the results from this study, this dose is expected to be beneficial for ill calves with abomasal ulcers.

HORSES:

Adjunctive gastroduodenal ulcer therapy in foals (extra-label): Aluminum/magnesium hydroxide suspension: 15 mL (total dose) 4 times a day[9]

Monitoring

- After beginning therapy, check serum phosphorus (after a 12-hour fast) every 4 to 6 weeks until target phosphorous levels are attained. Once phosphorous levels are stable, check phosphorous levels at the time of renal chemistry rechecks (eg, every 12 weeks). For chronic kidney disease (CKD), the International Renal Interest Society (IRIS) recommends a target phosphorous range for dogs and cats at each stage:
  - Stage 2 CKD target phosphorous levels: greater than 2.7 and less than 4.6 mg/dL (0.9 – less than 1.5 mmol/L)
  - Stage 3 CKD target phosphorous levels: greater than 2.7 and less than 5.0 mg/dL (0.9 – less than 1.6 mmol/L)
  - Stage 4 CKD target phosphorous levels: greater than 2.7 and less than 6.0 mg/dL (0.9 – less than 1.9 mmol/L)
- To monitor for aluminum toxicity, watch for development of neuromuscular effects, progressive decreases in mean cell volume (MCV), and microcytosis.

Client Information

- Oral aluminum hydroxide products are available without prescription (OTC) but should be used under the supervision of your veterinarian.
- Bulk powder or compounded capsules are easier to administer than liquids or suspensions. Shake the suspension thoroughly prior to administration.
- Must be given either just before feeding or mixed in food to be effective.
- Can cause constipation or decreased appetite
- Report to your veterinarian any unusual signs, such as weakness, difficulty walking, or stumbling.

Chemistry/Synonyms

Dried Aluminum Hydroxide Gel (CAS Registry: 21645-51-2) occurs as a white, odorless, tasteless, amorphous powder. It is insoluble in water or alcohol. The USP 36 standard allows varying amounts of basic aluminum carbonate and bicarbonate, but it must contain no less than 76.5% of $Al(OH)_3$.

Aluminum hydroxide may also be known as aluminium hydroxide.

Storage/Stability

Store powder forms in airtight containers. Liquid formulations should not be allowed to freeze.

Compatibility/Compounding Considerations

Because aluminum hydroxide powder USP can vary in the concentration of aluminum hydroxide (must be 76.5% or greater) and powders can vary in density, volume measurements can only approximate actual weight. However, ¼ teaspoonful (1.25 mL) of the dried USP powder has been reported to contain ≈300 mg of aluminum hydroxide.

Dosage Forms/Regulatory Status

VETERINARY-LABELED PRODUCTS: NONE

HUMAN-LABELED PRODUCTS:

Aluminum Hydroxide Concentrated Gel Suspension/Liquid (**NOTE:** These products are usually flavored (mint) and not well accepted by dogs or cats): 320 mg/5 mL in 473 mL; UD 15 mL and 30 mL; generic; (OTC)

Aluminum Hydroxide Gel, Dried Powder, USP; bulk powder is available from a variety of sources including many compounding pharmacies. See: http://goo.gl/1lYJk for additional source information.

NOTE: There are also many products available that have aluminum hydroxide and a magnesium or calcium salt (eg, *Maalox®*) that are used as antacids. All oral aluminum and magnesium hydroxide preparations are OTC.

References

For the complete list of references, see **wiley.com/go/budde/plumb**

Amantadine

(a-***man***-ta-deen) *Symmetrel®*

Antiviral; NMDA Antagonist

Prescriber Highlights

- Limited published efficacy or safety data, although clinical experience suggests it is useful in adjunctive treatment for chronic pain in small animal species
- Historically dosed every 24 hours; however, based on pharmacokinetic data, the same dose given every 12 hours may be more effective
- Dogs may exhibit agitation and GI effects, especially early in treatment.
- Large interpatient variations of pharmacokinetics in horses limit its therapeutic usefulness.
- Overdoses are potentially very serious; it may need to be compounded to accurately dose small animals.
- Extra-label use is prohibited by the FDA in chickens, turkeys, and ducks.

Uses/Indications

Although amantadine may have efficacy and clinical usefulness against some veterinary viral diseases, presently the greatest interest for its use in small animal species is in the adjunctive treatment of neuropathic[1] or chronic pain,[2] often in those in which opioids do not provide adequate analgesia or who are intolerant of higher opioid doses. It is generally considered ineffective when used alone[3]; use in combination with an NSAID, opioid, or gabapentin/pregabalin is typical.[1,4] Several weeks may be required to break a pain cycle.[5,6] It has been suggested for use as an early intervention in the treatment of pain associated with osteosarcomas.[7]

Amantadine has also been investigated for treatment of equine-2 influenza virus in a horse[8]; however, because of expense, interpatient variability in oral absorption and other pharmacokinetic parameters, and the potential for causing seizures after IV dosing, it is not commonly used for treatment.

In humans, amantadine is used for parkinsonian syndrome and drug-induced extrapyramidal effects; its use for the treatment and prophylaxis of influenza A is no longer recommended.[9] As in veterinary medicine, the effect of amantadine on NMDA receptors in humans is of active interest, particularly its use as a coanalgesic with opioids and in the reduction of opioid tolerance development.

Pharmacology/Actions

Like ketamine, dextromethorphan, and memantine, amantadine inhibits the NMDA receptor by stabilizing it in the closed state.[10] Within the CNS, chronic pain can be maintained or exacerbated when glutamate or aspartate bind to this receptor. It is believed that this receptor is particularly important in allodynia (ie, sensation of pain resulting from a normally non-noxious stimulus). Amantadine is expected to produce analgesic effects when pain or CNS sensitization is already present. Although there is limited evidence that amantadine alone provides analgesia,[2] it is thought that it may help alleviate chronic pain when used in combination with other analgesics (eg, opioids, NSAIDs).[3]

Amantadine's antiviral activity is limited to strains of influenza A. Although its complete mechanism of action is unknown, it inhibits viral replication by interfering with influenza A virus M2 protein, preventing release of viral RNA into the host cell, and possibly inhibiting viral replication. Influenza A variants have demonstrated resistance to amantadine's antiviral action, and it is currently not recommended for the treatment or prophylaxis of influenza A.[9]

Amantadine's antiparkinsonian activity is not well understood, but it apparently increases dopamine concentrations in the brain. The drug appears to have potentiating effects on dopaminergic neurotransmission in the CNS, is an NMDA antagonist, and has anticholinergic activity.

Pharmacokinetics

In dogs, oral bioavailability of amantadine is reportedly very high.[11] A study in nonfasted greyhounds showed an oral dose of 2.8 mg/kg was well tolerated, and maximum concentration, time to maximum concentration, and terminal half-life were 271 ng/mL, 1 to 4 hours, and 4.9 hours respectively. This study also suggested that the "every 24-hour dose interval" should be re-evaluated.[12] The drug is renally eliminated.[11]

In cats, bioavailability was very high after oral administration, and peak levels occurred ≈2 hours after dosing. After IV administration, the steady-state volume of distribution was ≈4.3 L/kg and clearance (mean) was 8.2 mL/minute/kg.[13] Elimination half-life was 5.5 to 6 hours.

In horses, amantadine had a very wide interpatient variability of absorption after oral dosing (10 – 20 mg/kg); bioavailability ranged from 40% to 60% and was not affected by feed.[8] The elimination half-life in horses was ≈3.5 hours, and the steady-state volume of distribution was ≈5 L/kg.

In Amazon parrots, the time to maximum concentration was ≈3 to 4 hours, and half-life was 21 to 23 hours.[14]

In humans, amantadine was well absorbed after oral administration with peak plasma concentrations occurring ≈3 hours after dosing.[15] Volume of distribution was 3 to 8 L/kg, and protein binding was ≈67%. Amantadine is primarily eliminated via renal mechanisms. Oral clearance was ≈0.28 L/hour/kg and half-life was ≈16 hours. Clearance is reduced in patients with renal impairment, and half-life may double.

Contraindications/Precautions/Warnings

In humans, amantadine is contraindicated in patients with known hypersensitivity to it[15] or to rimantadine, and in those with end-stage renal disease. It should be used with caution in patients with hepatic disease, renal disease (dosage adjustment may be required), congestive heart failure, active psychoses, eczematoid dermatitis, seizure disorders, or untreated angle-closure glaucoma. The drug is no longer recommended for the treatment or prevention of influenza A in humans due to high levels of amantadine resistance among circulating influenza strains.[9] In 2006, the FDA banned the use of amantadine and other influenza antivirals in chickens, turkeys, and ducks.

The human liquid dosage form has an unpleasant taste.

Do not confuse AMANTadine with RIMantadine, AMIOdarone, or RANITidine.

Adverse Effects

Experience with amantadine in domestic animals is limited, and its adverse effect profile is not well described. It has been reported that dogs given amantadine occasionally develop agitation, flatulence, loose stools, or diarrhea, particularly early in treatment. Experience in cats is limited, and an adverse effect profile has yet to be fully elucidated, but some clinicians report that GI effects are more likely than in dogs.

Reproductive/Nursing Safety

In rats, amantadine 50 – 100 mg/kg/day PO (ie, ≈1.5 to 3 times the maximum recommended human dose) throughout pregnancy was embryotoxic and caused fetal malformations and reduced fetal weight.[15] Fertility was slightly impaired in rats that were given 32 mg/kg/day.

Amantadine is excreted into maternal milk; its use is not recommended in nursing women.[16] Veterinary significance is unclear.

Because safety has not been established, this drug should only be used when the maternal benefits outweigh the potential risks to offspring.

Overdose/Acute Toxicity

The oral LD_{50} in mice and rats is 700 to 800 mg/kg and 25 to 50 mg/kg in humans.[17] The toxic amantadine dose reported for cats is 30 mg/kg[18]; behavioral effects may be noted at 15 mg/kg in dogs and cats.

Clinical signs associated with overdose in dogs include tremors, anxiety, ataxia, hypersalivation, and/or vomiting.

In humans, overdoses as low as 1 gram (total dose) have been associated with fatalities. Cardiac dysfunction (eg, arrhythmias, hypertension, tachycardia), pulmonary edema, CNS toxicity (eg, tremors, seizures, psychosis, agitation, coma), hyperthermia, renal dysfunction, and respiratory distress syndrome have all been documented. There is no known specific antidote for amantadine overdose. Treatment should consist of GI decontamination when appropriate, intensive monitoring (including ECG), and supportive therapy. Hydration and urinary acidification, with or without diuresis, may increase renal amantadine excretion. The drug is poorly removed by hemodialysis. Physostigmine has been suggested for cautious use in treating CNS effects.

For patients that have experienced or are suspected to have experienced an overdose, consultation with a 24-hour poison consultation center specializing in providing veterinary-specific information is recommended. For general information related to overdose and

toxin exposures, as well as contact information for poison control centers, refer to *Appendix*.

Drug Interactions

The following drug interactions with amantadine have either been reported or are theoretical in humans or animals and may be of significance in veterinary patients. Unless otherwise noted, use together is not necessarily contraindicated, but weigh the potential risks and perform additional monitoring when appropriate.

- Anticholinergic Drugs (eg, **atropine, glycopyrrolate, oxybutynin**): Amantadine may enhance anticholinergic effects.
- Antihistamines (eg, **diphenhydramine, hydroxyzine**): Amantadine may enhance anticholinergic effects.
- Carbonic Anhydrase Inhibitors (eg, **acetazolamide**): May increase amantadine concentration
- CNS Stimulants (eg, **caffeine, methylphenidate**, **selegiline**): Concomitant use with amantadine may increase the drug's CNS stimulatory effects.
- Glucagon: Amantadine's anticholinergic effects may increase GI adverse effects of glucagon.
- Phenothiazines (eg, **acepromazine**): Amantadine may enhance anticholinergic effects.
- Quinidine, Quinine: Renal clearance of amantadine may be reduced.
- QT Prolonging Drugs (eg, **amiodarone, cisapride, procainamide, sotalol**): May increase the risk for arrhythmias
- Sulfa-/Trimethoprim: May decrease the excretion of amantadine, yielding higher blood concentrations of amantadine
- Tramadol: Concomitant use with amantadine may increase the risk for seizures because tramadol at high doses has caused seizures in humans[19] and amantadine can lower the seizure threshold[15]; however, an increased risk for seizures with this drug combination appears unlikely in a clinical setting at recommended dosages. Monitor for sedation or other neurologic adverse effects if using this combination.
- Triamterene: May decrease the excretion of amantadine, yielding higher blood concentrations of amantadine
- Tricyclic Antidepressants (eg, **amitriptyline, clomipramine**): May enhance the anticholinergic effects of amantadine
- Urinary Acidifiers (eg, **methionine, ammonium chloride, ascorbic acid**): May increase the excretion of amantadine
- Urinary Alkalinizers (eg, **sodium bicarbonate, potassium citrate**): May decrease the excretion of amantadine

Laboratory Considerations

- No laboratory interactions identified

Dosages

DOGS/CATS:

Adjunctive analgesia, including neuropathic pain and to prevent "wind-up" pain (extra-label): 3 – 5 mg/kg PO once daily.[1,4] Anecdotally, it is suggested to start at the lower end of the dosing range and increase slowly, if needed. Pharmacokinetic studies suggest administration every 12 hours may be needed.[3,12,13]

Monitoring

- Adverse effects (ie, GI effects, anxiety, restlessness, dry mouth)
- Efficacy

Client Information

- Give this medicine as directed by your veterinarian. The benefits of this medicine may take a week or more to be seen.
- Gastrointestinal effects (eg, loose stools, gas, diarrhea) or some agitation may occur, particularly early in treatment. Contact your veterinarian if these become serious or persist.
- Overdoses with this medication can be serious. Be sure to keep this medicine out of reach of other pets and children.

Chemistry/Synonyms

An adamantane class antiviral agent with NMDA antagonist properties, amantadine HCl occurs as a white to off-white, bitter crystalline powder that is freely soluble in water and soluble in alcohol. Commercial dosage forms contain amantadine HCl, and strength is expressed and calculated as amantadine base. 1.24 mg amantadine HCl contains 1 mg amantadine.

Amantadine HCl may also be known as adamantanamine HCl, *Endantadine®*, *GOCOVRI®*, *Osmolex®*, and *Symmetrel®*.

Storage/Stability

Tablets, capsules, and the oral solution should be stored in tight, light-resistant containers at room temperature 20°C to 25°C (68°F-77°F), with excursions permitted to 15°C to 30°C (59°F-86°F). Avoid freezing the liquid.

Compatibility/Compounding Considerations

No specific information is noted.

Dosage Forms/Regulatory Status

VETERINARY-LABELED PRODUCTS: NONE

The International Federation for Equestrian Sports lists this drug as a "prohibited substance – controlled medication."[20] Use of this drug may not be allowed in certain animal competitions. Check rules and regulations before entering in a competition while this medication is being administered. Contact local racing authorities for further guidance.

HUMAN-LABELED PRODUCTS:

Amantadine HCl Oral Tablets and Capsules: 100 mg; generic; (Rx)

Amantadine HCl Oral Solution/Syrup: 50 mg/5mL (10 mg/mL) in 480 mL; generic; (Rx). **NOTE:** It is reported that the oral liquid has a bad taste and may not be accepted by veterinary patients.

Amantadine HCl extended-release oral tablets and capsules (*Osmolex® ER, GOCOVRI®*) are available. They are not directly equivalent to immediate-release amantadine capsules and have not been studied in veterinary patients.

In 2006, the FDA banned the extra-label use of amantadine and other influenza antivirals in chickens, turkeys, and ducks.

References

For the complete list of references, see **wiley.com/go/budde/plumb**

Amikacin, Systemic

(am-i-***kay***-sin) *Amikin®, Amiglyde-V®*

Aminoglycoside Antibiotic

Prescriber Highlights

- ► Parenteral aminoglycoside antibiotic that has good activity against a variety of bacteria, predominantly gram-negative aerobic bacilli and staphylococci; ineffective against anaerobic bacteria
- ► Adverse effects include nephrotoxicity, ototoxicity, and neuromuscular blockade.
- ► Cats may be more sensitive to toxic effects.
- ► Risk factors for toxicity include pre-existing renal disease, age (both neonatal and geriatric), fever, sepsis, and dehydration.

Uses/Indications

Although parenteral use of amikacin is only FDA approved in dogs, it is often used in most species for treatment of serious gram-negative and staphylococcal infections when the adverse effects of other aminoglycosides are a concern. Because aminoglycosides have an inherent toxicity and should be administered parenterally, use should be limited to treatment of serious infections with either a documented lack of susceptibility to other, less toxic antibiotics or in cases in which the clinical situation dictates immediate treatment of a presumed gram-negative infection before culture and susceptibility results are reported.

It is widely accepted that aminoglycosides should be given once a day in most patients (mammals). This dosing regimen yields higher peak concentrations with resultant greater bacterial kill. Because aminoglycosides exhibit a postantibiotic effect, surviving susceptible bacteria generally do not replicate as rapidly, even when antibiotic concentrations are below the MIC. Periods in which antibiotic concentrations are low may also decrease the "adaptive resistance" (ie, bacteria take up less drug in the presence of continuous exposure) that can occur.

Amikacin is also FDA-approved for intrauterine infusion in mares and is used via intraarticular injection (extra-label) in foals to treat gram-negative septic arthritis. In horses with septic arthritis, intravenous regional limb perfusion (IVRLP) using amikacin is actively being researched.[1-3]

Amikacin is also used topically for treatment of otitis externa in dogs—often in combination with EDTA-Triz[4]—and may be impregnated in materials (eg, PMMA beads, gels) for local treatment of infections, particularly implant-associated surgical site infections.

The World Health Organization (WHO) has designated amikacin as a Critically Important, High Priority antimicrobial for human medicine.[5]

Pharmacology/Actions

Similar to other aminoglycoside antibiotics, amikacin acts on susceptible bacteria by irreversibly binding to the 30S ribosomal subunit, thereby, inhibiting protein synthesis.[6] Amikacin is considered a bactericidal, concentration-dependent antibiotic.

Amikacin's spectrum of activity includes coverage against many aerobic gram-negative and some aerobic gram-positive bacteria, including *Escherichia coli* and most species of *Klebsiella* spp, *Proteus* spp, *Pseudomonas* spp, *Salmonella* spp, *Enterobacter* spp, *Serratia* spp, *Shigella* spp, *Mycoplasma* spp, and *Staphylococcus* spp. Several strains of *Pseudomonas aeruginosa*, *Proteus* spp, and *Serratia* spp that are resistant to gentamicin will be killed by amikacin. Amikacin is ineffective against anaerobic bacteria, viruses, fungi, and protozoa.

In an in vitro study with canine *E coli* isolates, amikacin demonstrated additive or synergistic antimicrobial activity when given in combination with ceftazidime and amoxicillin/clavulanate but not in combination with enrofloxacin or marbofloxacin.[7]

Antimicrobial activity of aminoglycosides is enhanced in an alkaline environment but inhibited by the presence of pus or organic debris.

Pharmacokinetics

Amikacin, like the other aminoglycosides, is not appreciably absorbed after oral, dermal, or intrauterine administration or urinary bladder irrigations but is absorbed when used in irrigations during surgical procedures or in regional limb perfusion. Systemic absorption of amikacin from impregnated beads is not described; plasma amikacin concentration was undetectable 24 hours after SC placement of an amikacin-impregnated dextrose cross-linked gel[8] but is minimal for gentamicin in PMMA beads on dogs[9] and in calcium sulfate beads in goats.[10] With IM administration in dogs and cats, peak concentrations occur after 30 to 60 minutes. SC injection results in slightly delayed peak concentrations and more variability than after IM injection. Bioavailability from extravascular injection (IM or SC) is greater than 90%.

After absorption, aminoglycosides are distributed primarily in the extracellular fluid and are found in ascitic, pleural, pericardial, peritoneal, synovial, and abscess fluids; high levels are found in sputum, bronchial secretions, and bile. Aminoglycosides are minimally protein bound (ie, less than 20%) to plasma proteins.[11] Aminoglycosides do not readily cross the blood-brain barrier and do not penetrate ocular tissue. CSF concentrations are unpredictable and range from 0% to 50% of those found in the serum. Therapeutic concentrations are found in bone, heart, gallbladder, and lung tissues after parenteral administration. Prostate concentrations have not been adequately assessed in animals, but amikacin has been shown to be effective for the treatment of chronic bacterial prostatitis in humans when fluoroquinolones cannot be used.[12] A maximum distal interphalangeal joint synovial fluid concentration of 600 µg/mL was reached 15 minutes after intravenous regional limb perfusion (IVRLP) in healthy adult horses; however, significant interpatient variability was noted. A maximum serum amikacin concentration of 19 µg/mL was reached 25 minutes after IVRLP.[13] Aminoglycosides tend to accumulate in certain tissues (eg, inner ear, kidneys), contributing to the toxicity seen in those tissues. Volumes of distribution have been reported to be 0.15 to 0.3 L/kg in adult cats and dogs, and 0.26 to 0.58 L/kg in horses. Volumes of distribution may be significantly larger in neonates and juvenile animals due to their higher extracellular fluid fractions. Aminoglycosides cross the placenta; fetal concentrations range from 15% to 50% of those found in maternal serum.

Elimination of aminoglycosides after parenteral administration occurs almost entirely by glomerular filtration. The approximate elimination half-life for amikacin has been reported to be 5 hours in foals, 1.14 to 2.3 hours in adult horses, 2.2 to 2.7 hours in calves, 1 hour in cows, 1.5 hours in sheep, and 0.5 to 2 hours in dogs and cats. Patients with decreased renal function can have a significantly prolonged half-life. In humans with normal renal function, elimination rates can be highly variable with aminoglycoside antibiotics.

Contraindications/Precautions/Warnings

Aminoglycosides are contraindicated in animals that are hypersensitive to them. Often, these drugs are the only effective agents in treating severe gram-negative or multidrug resistant staphylococcal infections; thus, there are no absolute contraindications to their use. However, these drugs should be used with extreme caution in animals with pre-existing renal disease; concomitant monitoring and dosage interval adjustments should be used as needed. Other risk factors for the development of toxicity include patient age (neonatal and geriatric patients), fever, sepsis, and dehydration.

Aminoglycosides can cause irreversible ototoxicity, so they should be used with caution, especially in working and guide dogs, and should be avoided when treating otitis if an intact tympanic membrane cannot be confirmed. Amikacin is considered less ototoxic than gentamicin or streptomycin.[14]

Aminoglycosides should be used with caution in animals with neuromuscular disorders (eg, myasthenia gravis) because of the drug's neuromuscular blocking activity.

Sight hounds may require reduced dosages of aminoglycosides, as they have significantly lower volumes of distribution.

Aminoglycosides are eliminated primarily through renal mechanisms and should be used cautiously in neonatal or geriatric animals; consider periodic therapeutic drug monitoring and serum chemistry profiles with dosage adjustments as needed.

Adverse Effects

Aminoglycosides can be nephrotoxic and ototoxic. The nephrotoxic (ie, tubular necrosis) mechanisms are not completely understood but are probably related to interference with phospholipid metabolism in the lysosomes of proximal renal tubular cells, resulting in leakage of proteolytic enzymes into the cytoplasm. The risk for nephrotoxicity increases with prolonged therapy and is predominantly associated with accumulation of amikacin within tubular cells, which is more likely to occur with repeated lower doses as compared with higher doses with prolonged (ie, every 24 hour) dosing intervals. Nephrotoxicity is usually manifested by nonoliguric renal failure, with increases in serum BUN and creatinine and decreases in urine specific gravity and creatinine clearance. Proteinuria and abnormal urine sediment (eg, casts, renal tubular cells, glycosuria) may be seen. Nephrotoxicity is usually reversible after the drug is discontinued. Although amikacin is less nephrotoxic than other aminoglycosides, the incidence of nephrotoxicity is poorly described, and caution and monitoring are required.

Ototoxicity (ie, eighth cranial nerve toxicity) can manifest through hearing loss and/or vestibular clinical signs (eg, nystagmus, head tilt) and may be irreversible. Vestibular clinical signs are more frequent with use of streptomycin, gentamicin, or tobramycin. Hearing loss is more frequent with use of amikacin or neomycin.[15] However, hearing loss or vestibular clinical signs can occur with use of any of these drugs. Cats are apparently more sensitive to the vestibular effects of aminoglycosides.[16]

Aminoglycosides can also cause neuromuscular blockade, facial edema, pain and inflammation at the injection site, peripheral neuropathy, and hypersensitivity reactions. Rarely, GI clinical signs and hematologic and hepatic effects have been reported.

An in vitro study found that amikacin caused rapid, dose-dependent cytotoxicity in equine joint cells[17]; additional in vivo studies are required to confirm these findings.

Reproductive/Nursing Safety

Aminoglycosides can cross the placenta and although rare, may cause eighth cranial nerve toxicity or nephrotoxicity in fetuses. Nephrotoxicity has occurred in fetal rats. Because the drug should only be used in serious infections, the benefits of therapy may exceed the potential risks. There is no evidence that amikacin impairs fertility; amikacin does not appear to affect sperm quality,[18] however, the preservative in the intrauterine infusion may impair sperm viability.[19]

Aminoglycosides are excreted in milk. Although it is possible that amikacin ingested with milk could alter the GI microbiota and cause diarrhea, low levels of amikacin in milk are unlikely to be of significant concern.

Overdose/Acute Toxicity

Two treatments have been recommended in case of inadvertent overdose:

1) Hemodialysis, which is effective in reducing serum drug concentrations but is not a viable option for most veterinary patients.
2) Peritoneal dialysis, which also reduces serum drug concentrations but is much less effective. Amikacin is less affected by this approach than are tobramycin or gentamicin, and it is assumed that reduction in serum concentrations will also be minimized.

For patients that have experienced or are suspected to have experienced an overdose, consultation with a 24-hour poison consultation center specializing in providing veterinary-specific information is recommended. For general information related to overdose and toxin exposures, as well as contact information for poison control centers, refer to *Appendix.*

Drug Interactions

The following drug interactions have either been reported or are theoretical in humans or animals receiving amikacin and may be of significance in veterinary patients. Unless otherwise noted, use together is not necessarily contraindicated, but weigh the potential risks and perform additional monitoring when appropriate.

- Anesthetics, General (eg **isoflurane, ketamine, propofol**): Concomitant use with general anesthetics could potentiate neuromuscular blockade.
- Cephalosporins: Concurrent use of aminoglycosides with cephalosporins is somewhat controversial. Potentially, cephalosporins could cause additive nephrotoxicity when used with aminoglycosides, but this interaction has only been well-documented with cephaloridine and cephalothin (both of which are no longer marketed). The potential synergistic effect[7] may outweigh these unlikely risks; however, concurrent use of third- or fourth-generation cephalosporins with amikacin, results in abundant and typically unnecessary duplication of the gram-negative spectrum.
- Diuretics, Loop (eg, **furosemide, torsemide**): Concurrent use with loop diuretics may increase the nephrotoxic or ototoxic potential of aminoglycosides.
- Diuretics, Osmotic (eg, **mannitol**): Concurrent use with osmotic diuretics may increase the nephrotoxic or ototoxic potential of the aminoglycosides.
- Magnesium, Systemic (eg, **magnesium sulfate**): Concomitant use could increase the risk for neuromuscular blockade.
- Nephrotoxic drugs, Other (eg, **amphotericin B, cisplatin, polymyxin B, vancomycin**): Potential for increased risk for nephrotoxicity
- Neuromuscular Blocking Agents (eg, **atracurium, pancuronium**): Concomitant use with neuromuscular blocking agents could potentiate neuromuscular blockade.
- NSAIDs (eg, **carprofen, firocoxib, flunixin, meloxicam, phenylbutazone, robenacoxib**): Increased risk of nephrotoxicity
- Penicillins: May have synergistic effects against some bacteria[7]; some potential for physical inactivation of aminoglycosides in vitro (do not mix together) and in vivo (patients in renal failure)

Laboratory Considerations

- **Amikacin serum concentrations** may be falsely decreased if the patient is also receiving **beta-lactam antibiotics** and the serum is stored prior to analysis. It is recommended that if the assay is delayed, samples be frozen and, if possible, drawn at times when the beta-lactam antibiotic is at a trough.

Dosages

DOGS:

Susceptible infections and empirical therapy (extra-label): 15 – 30 mg/kg IV, IM, SC once daily. Septic patients may be started at 20 – 30 mg/kg IV once daily. **NOTE**: Dosage should be adjusted based on kidney function and serum amikacin concentrations when possible. When renal function is significantly decreased (eg, IRIS stage II or III) and less nephrotoxic drugs cannot be used, the dose amount remains the same but the dosing interval should be increased. See *Monitoring.*

CATS:

Susceptible infections and empirical therapy (extra-label): 10 – 15 mg/kg IV, IM, SC once daily. Septic patients may be started at 20 mg/kg IV once daily. **NOTE**: Dosage should be adjusted based on renal function and serum levels when possible. When renal function is significantly decreased (eg, IRIS stage II or III) and less nephrotoxic drugs cannot be used, the dose amount remains the same but the dosing interval should be increased. See *Monitoring.*

HORSES:

Uterine infections (endometritis, metritis, pyometra) caused by susceptible organisms (label dosage; FDA approved): 2 g mixed with 200 mL sterile normal saline (0.9% sodium chloride for injection) and aseptically infused into the uterus daily for 3 consecutive days[19]

Susceptible infections and empirical therapy (extra-label):

Adults: 10 mg/kg IV or IM once daily

Neonatal foals: 20 – 25 mg/kg IV or IM once daily. It is strongly recommended to individualize the dose based on therapeutic drug monitoring.

Treatment of septic joints (extra-label): Intra-articular administration: 125 – 250 mg/horse (NOT mg/kg) IA once daily[20]

Intravenous regional limb perfusion (IVRLP) administration in standing adult horses (extra-label):

a) 2 g (diluted to 30 – 60 mL with sterile saline) via cephalic vein, with 10 to 20 minute tourniquet time.[13,21,22] The addition of penicillin G sodium at 10 million units has resulted in variable retention time in the synovium.[23,24]

b) 1 g (diluted to 30 – 120 mL with sterile saline), with 30 minute tourniquet time reached therapeutic concentration in the thoracic limb distal phalangeal joint but not in the radiocarpal joint.[25]

NOTE: Despite the procedure's name (ie, IVRLP), amikacin is absorbed systemically and potentially reaches therapeutic concentrations.[13]

NEW WORLD CAMELIDS:

Susceptible infections and empirical therapy: 18 mg/kg IV or IM every 24 hours (once daily)[26]

BIRDS:

Susceptible infections:

a) 15 mg/kg IM or SC every 12 hours[27]

b) **Gram-negative infections resistant to gentamicin**: Dilute commercial solution and administer 15 – 20 mg/kg (0.015 – 0.02 mg/g) IM once or twice daily.[28]

c) **Intravenous regional limb perfusion (IVRLP) administration in chickens:** From a case report: Using the medial metatarsal vein, 5.3 mg/kg IV with flunixin 1.3 mg/kg were infused, with 15 minute tourniquet time.[29]

d) **Mycobacterial infections in psittacines**: 15 mg/kg twice daily (route not specified, assume IM)[30]

REPTILES:

Gram-negative respiratory disease: 3.5 mg/kg IM, SC, or via lung catheter every 3 to 10 days for 30 days[31]

Snakes:

a) 5 mg/kg IM (forebody) loading dose, then 2.5 mg/kg IM every 72 hours for 7 to 9 treatments. Commonly used in respiratory infections. Use a lower dose for *Python curtus*.[32]

b) **Gopher snakes**: In a study, 5 mg/kg IM loading dose, then 2.5 mg/kg IM every 72 hours. House snakes were at the high end of their preferred optimum ambient temperature.[33]

TURTLES/TORTOISES:

a) **Bacterial shell diseases**: 10 mg/kg (route not specified; assume IM) daily in water turtles and every other day in land turtles and tortoises for 7 to 10 days. Used commonly with a beta-lactam antibiotic. It is recommended to begin therapy with 20 mL/kg fluid injection. Maintain hydration and monitor uric acid levels when possible.[34]

b) **Gopher tortoises**: 5 mg/kg IM every 48 hours at 30°C (86°F)[35]

c) **Crocodilians**: 2.25 mg/kg IM every 72 to 96 hours[36]

FERRETS:

Susceptible infections (extra-label):

a) 8 – 16 mg/kg IM or IV once daily[37]

b) 8 – 16 mg/kg/day SC, IM, IV divided every 8 to 24 hours[38]

RABBITS/RODENTS/SMALL MAMMALS:

Rabbits (extra-label):

a) 8 – 16 mg/kg SC, IM, or IV daily dose (may be divided and given every 8-24 hours). Increased efficacy and decreased toxicity are possible if given once daily. If given IV, dilute product into 4 mL/kg of saline and administer over 20 minutes.[39]

b) 5 – 10 mg/kg SC, IM, or IV divided every 8 to 24 hours

Guinea pigs (extra-label): 10 – 15 mg/kg SC, IM, or IV divided every 8 to 24 hours

Chinchillas (extra-label):

a) 10 – 15 mg/kg SC, IM, or IV divided every 8 to 24 hours

b) 2 – 5 mg/kg SC, IM every 8 to 12 hours[40]

Hamsters, rats, mice (extra-label): 10 mg/kg SC or IM every 12 hours (twice daily)

Prairie dogs (extra-label): 5 mg/kg SC or IM every 12 hours (twice daily)[38]

FISH:

Susceptible infections: 5 mg/kg IM loading dose, then 2.5 mg/kg every 72 hours for 5 treatments[41]

Monitoring

- Efficacy (eg, culture, clinical signs, WBC count, and clinical signs associated with infection).

  Therapeutic drug monitoring would be ideal but is rarely available. When available, collect plasma samples 30 minutes after administration and immediately before the next dose to measure peak and trough concentrations, respectively. Target concentrations in veterinary patients have not been well-established. In humans, peak levels of 20 – 25 µg/mL (25 – 40 µg/mL for sepsis) have been recommended, whereas in foals, a target peak of 40 µg/mL has been stated.[42] In humans, trough levels of less than 8 µg/mL are recommended.
- Adverse effect monitoring is essential. Baseline serum renal chemistry testing (eg, creatinine) and urinalysis (including specific gravity and sediment evaluation) are recommended and should be repeated every 3 to 5 days during therapy. **NOTE:** A decrease in urine specific gravity is often the initial sign of impending nephrotoxicity; casts in the urine can be transient and a lack of casts does not rule out renal toxicity.
- Gross monitoring of vestibular or auditory toxicity is recommended.

Client Information

- You may give subcutaneous injections at home if you have received appropriate training, but routine monitoring of therapy for efficacy and toxicity by a veterinarian is still required.
- Permanent hearing loss and severe damage to the kidneys can occur with use of this medicine. Contact your veterinarian immediately if your animal develops a head tilt, hearing loss (ie, not responding to noise), loss of balance, poor appetite, low energy level, and/or vomiting.
- While taking this medicine, your animal will need to be closely monitored by your veterinarian. Do not miss these important follow-up visits.
- Use in food producing animals is controversial. Be sure to talk with your veterinarian about the long withdrawal periods associated with this medicine.

Chemistry/Synonyms

Amikacin, a semisynthetic aminoglycoside derived from kanamycin, occurs as a white, crystalline powder that is sparingly soluble in water. The sulfate salt is formed during the manufacturing process. 1.3 g of amikacin sulfate is equivalent to 1 g of amikacin. Amikacin may also be expressed in terms of units. 50,600 units are equal to 50.9 mg of base. The commercial injection is a clear to straw-colored solution, and the pH is adjusted to 3.5 to 5.5 with sulfuric acid.

Amikacin sulfate may also be known as amikacin sulphate, amikacini sulfas, or BB-K8; many trade names are available.

Storage/Stability

Amikacin sulfate for injection should be stored at room temperature (20°C-25°C [68°F to 77°F]); freezing or temperatures above 40°C (104°F) should be avoided. Solutions may become very pale yellow with time, but this does not indicate a loss of potency.

Amikacin is stable for at least 2 years at room temperature. Autoclaving commercially available solutions at 15 pounds of pressure at 120°C (248°F) for 60 minutes did not result in any loss of potency. Gamma sterilization of amikacin-impregnated plaster of Paris (calcium sulfate) or polymethylmethacrylate beads did not alter antimicrobial efficacy.[43]

Compatibility/Compounding Considerations

When given IV, amikacin should be diluted into suitable IV diluent (eg, normal saline, D5W, LRS) and administered over at least 30 minutes. Amikacin diluted to 0.25 – 5 mg/mL is stable for 24 hours at room temperature, 60 days when refrigerated (4°C [39.2°F]), and 30 days when frozen (-15°C [5°F]). Discard solution if particulates or discoloration are present.[19]

Amikacin sulfate is reportedly **compatible** and stable in all commonly used IV solutions and with the following drugs: ascorbic acid injection, bleomycin sulfate, calcium chloride/gluconate, cefoxitin sodium, chloramphenicol sodium succinate, chlorpheniramine maleate, cimetidine HCl, clindamycin phosphate, dimenhydrinate, diphenhydramine HCl, epinephrine HCl, hyaluronidase, hydrocortisone sodium phosphate/succinate, lincomycin HCl, metronidazole (with or without sodium bicarbonate), norepinephrine bitartrate, pentobarbital sodium, phenobarbital sodium, phytonadione, prochlorperazine edisylate, promethazine HCl, sodium bicarbonate, succinylcholine chloride, vancomycin HCl, and verapamil HCl.

The following drugs or solutions are reportedly **incompatible** or only **compatible in specific situations** with amikacin: amphotericin B, ampicillin sodium, cefazolin sodium, chlorothiazide sodium, dexamethasone sodium phosphate, erythromycin gluceptate, heparin sodium, oxytetracycline HCl, penicillin G potassium, phenytoin sodium, potassium chloride (in dextran 6% in sodium chloride 0.9%; stable with potassium chloride in "standard" solutions), vitamin B complex with C, and warfarin sodium. Compatibility is dependent on factors such as pH, concentration, temperature, and diluent used; consult specialized references or a hospital pharmacist for more specific information.

In vitro inactivation of aminoglycoside antibiotics by beta-lactam antibiotics is well-documented. Although amikacin is less susceptible to this effect, it is usually recommended to avoid mixing these compounds together in the same syringe or IV bag unless administration occurs promptly. See also ***Drug Interactions*** and ***Laboratory Considerations***.

Dosage Forms/Regulatory Status

VETERINARY-LABELED PRODUCTS:

Amikacin Sulfate Injection: 50 mg (of amikacin base) per mL in 50 mL vials; (Rx). FDA approved for use in dogs. Although this drug is still listed in the FDA's Green Book of approved animal drugs, it may not be commercially available.

Amikacin Sulfate Intrauterine Solution: 250 mg (of amikacin base) per mL in 48 mL vials; (Rx). FDA approved for use in horses not intended for food.

Warning: Amikacin is not FDA approved for use in cattle or other food-producing animals in the United States. Drug residues may persist for long periods, particularly in renal tissue. For guidance with determining use and withdrawal times, contact FARAD (see ***Appendix*** for contact information).

HUMAN-LABELED PRODUCTS:

Amikacin Injection: 50 mg/mL and 250 mg/mL in 2 mL and 4 mL; generic; (Rx)

References

For the complete list of references, see **wiley.com/go/budde/plumb**

Aminocaproic Acid

(a-***mee***-noe-ka-***proe***-ik ***as***-id)

Epsilon Aminocaproic Acid (EAC), *Amicar®*

Hemostatic

Prescriber Highlights

- May be useful for treating hypofibrinolysis in dogs and horses and postoperative bleeding in greyhounds; efficacy for the treatment of degenerative myelopathies in dogs is questionable
- Contraindicated in disseminated intravascular coagulation (DIC)
- Infrequently causes GI distress
- Rapid IV administration may cause hypotension and bradycardia

Uses/Indications

Aminocaproic acid is potentially useful for the treatment of hyperfibrinolysis and as a prophylaxis for postoperative bleeding, especially in greyhounds or other sighthounds.[1,2] In dogs, 20 – 100 mg/kg PO inhibited fibrinolysis in an in vitro model of hyperfibrinolysis.[3] A retrospective study did not show a correlation between administration of aminocaproic acid and the packed cell volume (PCV) prior to transfusion or packed red blood cell transfusion dose in dogs with different bleeding disorders, including neoplastic disease.[4] Aminocaproic acid has also been used to help stabilize clots and slow bleeding in horses with guttural pouch hemorrhage.[5] A study in horses found that aminocaproic acid was not effective in preventing or reducing the severity of exercise-induced pulmonary hemorrhage (EIPH).[6]

Aminocaproic acid has been used as a treatment for degenerative myelopathy (seen primarily in German shepherds), but no controlled studies documenting its efficacy have been noted. In one study evaluating aminocaproic acid given concurrently with acetylcysteine and vitamins B, C, and E, no improvement was noted and all dogs in the study had a worsening of neurological signs over time.[7]

There is some interest in evaluating aminocaproic acid for the adjunctive treatment of immune-mediated thrombocytopenia in dogs, but the drug's efficacy and safety for this purpose has yet to be investigated. In humans, the drug is primarily used for treatment of hyperfibrinolysis-induced hemorrhage.

Pharmacology/Actions

Aminocaproic acid inhibits fibrinolysis via its inhibitory effects on plasminogen activator substances and some antiplasmin activity. Much higher plasma concentrations (511.7 µg/mL) are required in dogs than in humans (122 µg/mL) to completely inhibit fibrinolysis.[8] In horses, a plasma concentration of 5.8 µg/mL is sufficient to inhibit fibrinolysis.[9]

Aminocaproic acid is thought to affect degenerative myelopathy via its antiprotease activity, thereby reducing the activation of inflammatory enzymes that damage myelin.

Pharmacokinetics

Pharmacokinetic data have been studied in dogs. After oral administration of an injectable aminocaproic acid solution at 20, 50, and 100 mg/kg maximum concentration was ≈30, 69, and 166 µg/mL (respectively), time until maximum concentration was 63, 42, and 54 minutes (respectively), terminal half-life was 70, 69, and 77 minutes (respectively), volume of distribution/bioavailability was 594, 589, and 575 mL), and total body clearance/bioavailability was 6.1, 6, and 5.2 mL/minute (respectively). The pharmacokinetic data of an oral formulation (tablet) administered at 100 mg/kg were similar to the injectable formulation given orally at the same dose.[3]

In a study in which aminocaproic acid 70 mg/kg IV was given to horses over 20 minutes, the drug was distributed rapidly, and plasma levels remained above the proposed therapeutic concentration of 130 μg/mL for 1 hour after the end of the infusion.[10] Elimination half-life was 2.3 hours. The authors proposed that a 15 mg/kg/hour IV CRI after the original infusion would maintain more prolonged therapeutic levels.

In humans, the drug is rapidly and completely absorbed after oral administration. The drug is well distributed in both intravascular and extravascular compartments and penetrates cells, including RBCs. Aminocaproic acid does not bind to plasma proteins. Terminal half-life is ≈2 hours in humans, and the drug is primarily renally excreted as unchanged drug. Clearance is markedly reduced in patients with severe renal impairment.

Contraindications/Precautions/Warnings

Aminocaproic acid is contraindicated in patients with active intravascular clotting, especially those with disseminated intravascular coagulation (DIC), which can result in fatal thrombus formation. Do not administer in the absence of laboratory confirmation of hyperfibrinolysis (eg, thromboelastography). In patients with upper urinary tract bleeding, glomerular capillary thrombosis or clots in the renal pelvis and ureters can form. In patients with pre-existing cardiac, renal, or hepatic disease, this drug should only be used when the benefits outweigh the risks; dosage reduction may be needed in patients with renal impairment.

The product label states that rapid IV injection of undiluted aminocaproic acid is not recommended in humans.[11]

Subendocardial hemorrhage and fatty degeneration of the myocardium have been reported in dogs.

Do not confuse the brand names *Amicar®* with amikacin or *Omacor®* (omega-3-acid ethyl esters).

Adverse Effects

Aminocaproic acid appears to be well tolerated. Approximately 1% of dogs treated with oral aminocaproic acid show clinical signs of GI irritation. This drug can potentially cause hyperkalemia, particularly in renally impaired patients.

In humans, myositis and skeletal muscle weakness with muscle fiber necrosis has occurred rarely; if this occurs, the potential for cardiac muscle damage should also be considered. Rapid IV administration can cause hypotension or bradycardia.

Reproductive/Nursing Safety

Impaired fertility has been noted when aminocaproic acid was administered to rats of either sex. Animal studies for the safe use of aminocaproic acid during pregnancy have not been conducted.[12]

It is unknown if aminocaproic acid is excreted in milk. Because safety has not been established in animals, this drug should only be used when the maternal benefits outweigh the potential risks to offspring.

Overdose/Acute Toxicity

There is very limited information on overdoses with aminocaproic acid. The IV lethal dose in dogs is reportedly 2.3 g/kg.[12] At lower IV overdoses, tonic-clonic seizures were noted in some dogs.[11] There is no known antidote, but the drug is dialyzable.

For patients that have experienced or are suspected to have experienced an overdose, it is strongly encouraged that a 24-hour poison consultation center that specializes in providing information specific for veterinary patients be consulted. For general information related to overdose and toxin exposures, as well as contact information for poison control centers, refer to *Appendix*.

Drug Interactions

- There are no reported drug interactions of clinical significance.
- Blood Products: Concurrent administration with factor IX complex concentrates or anti-inhibitor coagulant may increase the risk for thrombosis.

Laboratory Considerations

- **Serum potassium** may be elevated by aminocaproic acid, especially in patients with pre-existing chronic kidney disease.

Dosages

NOTE: Aminocaproic acid solution for injection administered orally to dogs produced a similar pharmacologic effect as aminocaproic acid tablets.[3]

DOGS:

Antifibrinolytic to reduce delayed-onset bleeding after surgery in greyhounds (extra-label): 500 mg/dog (≈15.6-17.5 mg/kg) PO every 8 hours for 5 days beginning the night of surgery.[1,2] Data suggest canine dosing extrapolated from human data may result in suboptimal plasma concentrations after in vitro thromboelastograph (TEG) analysis revealed canine plasma was hypercoagulable as compared with human plasma.[8]

Bleeding secondary to hyperfibrinolysis (extra-label): From a case report, 33 mg/kg IV every 6 hours.[13] Modified TEG analysis showed normalization of the fibrinolytic response after discontinuation of the drug.

Pericardial effusion secondary to right atrial mass (extra-label): 50 mg/kg PO 3 or 4 times daily. Compounded formulation did not significantly delay recurrence of pericardial effusion or improve survival.[14]

Active bleeding (extra-label): Average dose was ≈17.5 mg/kg IV in dogs presented with active bleeding caused by neoplastic disease, postsurgical bleeding, or bleeding from other causes.[4] **NOTE:** Dogs may require higher dosages of aminocaproic acid as compared with humans,[8] and an in vitro model found that a single dose of 100 mg/kg PO inhibited fibrinolysis more effectively than did 20 mg/kg PO.[3]

Adjunctive treatment of degenerative myelopathy (extra-label): Aminocaproic acid 500 mg/dog (NOT mg/kg) PO every 8 hours indefinitely. Other treatments included acetylcysteine 25 mg/kg PO 3 times daily, prednisolone 1 mg/kg PO daily for 15 days then every other day for 30 days, vitamin C 500 mg PO every 12 hours, and vitamin E 2000 IU PO every 24 hours. From a retrospective study of 12 dogs,[7] disease progressed in all the dogs, and the authors questioned the benefit of treatment.

HORSES:

Antifibrinolytic for guttural pouch hemorrhage (extra-label): 40 mg/kg IV bolus, followed by 10 – 20 mg/kg every 6 hours.[15] Data suggest current equine dosing regimens may be higher than necessary after in vitro analysis revealed that the aminocaproic acid plasma concentration needed to inhibit fibrinolysis in horses was $^{1}/_{20}$ of the concentration needed in human plasma.[9]

Monitoring

- Thromboelastography (TEG)
- Signs of bleeding
- Creatine kinase in patients receiving long-term therapy; discontinue the drug if elevations occur

Client Information

- Your veterinarian will need to do regular blood tests to monitor how well your animal is tolerating this medicine. Do not miss these important follow-up visits.
- Use of this drug for treatment of degenerative myelopathy is considered investigational—meaning there is not a large amount of evidence that this treatment is helpful for this condition. Contact your veterinarian if you have any concerns about your animal while it is receiving this medication.

Chemistry/Synonyms

Aminocaproic acid, an inhibitor of fibrinolysis, is a synthetic monamino carboxylic acid occurring as a fine, white crystalline powder. It is slightly soluble in alcohol, freely soluble in water, and has pK_as of 4.43 and 10.75. The injectable product is pH adjusted to ≈6.8.

Aminocaproic acid may also be known as acidum aminocaproicum, CL-10304 CY-116, EACA, epsilon aminocaproic acid, 6-aminohexanoic acid, JD-177, NSC-26154, *Acepramin®*, *Amicar®*, *Caprac-id®*, *Capramol®*, *Caproamin®*, *Caprolisin®*, *Epsicaprom®*, *Hemocaprol®*, *Hemocid®*, *Hexalense®*, or *Ipsilon®*.

Storage/Stability

Products should be stored at controlled room temperature (20°C-25°C [68°F-77°F]). Avoid freezing liquid preparations. Dilutions in normal saline or dextrose 5% in water at concentrations of 10 and 100 mg/mL had 98% potency that was retained for 7 days at 4°C (39.2°F) and 23°C (73.4°F).[16] Discoloration will occur if aldehydes or aldehydic sugars are present. Dilution with dextrose 5% in water produced discoloration but had no effect on potency.[16]

Compatibility/Compounding Considerations

Compatible with sodium chloride 0.9%, dextrose 5% in water, and lactated Ringer's injection for dilution

Dosage Forms/Regulatory Status

VETERINARY-LABELED PRODUCTS: NONE

The ARCI (Association of Racing Commissioners International) has designated this drug as a class 4 substance. See ***Appendix*** for more information. The FEI (International Federation for Equestrian Sports) lists this drug as a *prohibited substance - controlled medication*. Use of this drug may not be allowed in certain animal competitions. Check rules and regulations before entering in a competition while this medication is being administered. Contact local racing authorities for further guidance.

HUMAN-LABELED PRODUCTS:

Aminocaproic Acid; Oral Tablets: 500 mg and 1000 mg; *Amicar®*; (Rx)

Aminocaproic Acid Oral Syrup: 250 mg/mL in 237 mL; *Amicar®*; (Rx)

Aminocaproic Acid Injection: 250 mg/mL in 20 mL vials; generic; (Rx)

References

For the complete list of references, see **wiley.com/go/budde/plumb**

Aminophylline

(am-in-***off***-i-lin)

Phosphodiesterase Inhibitor Bronchodilator

Prescriber Highlights

- ▶ Parenteral form of theophylline
- ▶ Bronchodilator drug with mild diuretic activity
- ▶ Used as an adjunct therapy for chronic cough caused by tracheitis and bronchitis associated with airway collapse; may also be used to relieve cough in patients with respiratory disease that complicates management of congestive heart failure
- ▶ Narrow therapeutic index in humans, but dogs appear to be less susceptible to toxic effects at higher plasma concentrations.
- ▶ Many potential drug interactions. Fluoroquinolones (eg, enrofloxacin) can increase theophylline concentrations substantially.

Uses/Indications

Aminophylline is the parenteral form for administering theophylline. Theophyllines (ie, aminophylline, theophylline) are used primarily for their bronchodilatory effects, especially in animals with cough. Aminophylline also may be used to manage sick sinus syndrome and other bradyarrhythmias.[1]

Theophylline could potentially be of benefit in dogs with pulmonary arterial hypertension if the underlying cause is chronic obstructive pulmonary disease (COPD).[2]

Although theophyllines are still used, especially in animals with cough, they must be used cautiously because of their adverse effects and toxicity.

Pharmacology/Actions

Aminophylline competitively inhibits phosphodiesterase (PDE) III (and PDE IV to a lesser extent), thereby increasing amounts of cyclic AMP (cAMP) that then increase the release of endogenous epinephrine. The increased concentrations of cAMP may also inhibit the release of histamine and the slow-reacting substance of anaphylaxis (SRS-A). The myocardial and neuromuscular transmission effects of aminophylline may be a result of translocating intracellular ionized calcium. Adenosine antagonism may contribute to CNS stimulant effects.

Methylxanthines have anti-inflammatory effects, increase mucociliary clearance, enhance corticosteroid activity, and support respiratory muscles.[3,4] Aminophylline directly relaxes smooth muscles in the bronchi and pulmonary vasculature; smooth muscle relaxant effects also occur in the uterus, as well as the biliary and GI tracts. In addition, aminophylline may induce diuresis, vasodilate arterioles and veins, increase gastric acid secretion, and inhibit mast cell release. Aminophylline has weak chronotropic and inotropic action, improves diaphragm contractility, stimulates the CNS, and can cause respiratory stimulation (centrally mediated).

Pharmacokinetics

Theophylline is distributed throughout the extracellular fluids and body tissues. It crosses the placenta and is distributed into milk (70% of serum concentrations). In dogs, at therapeutic serum concentrations, only ≈7% to 14% is bound to plasma proteins. After IV administration of aminophylline to greyhounds, mean theophylline Vdss was 0.72 L/kg.[5] The volume of distribution in cats is reported to be 0.46 L/kg,[6] and in horses, 0.85 to 1.6 L/kg.[7-9] Because of the low volumes of distribution and theophylline's low lipid solubility, obese patients should be dosed on a lean body weight basis.

In ruminating calves, oral bioavailability is 93%, volume of distribution is 0.8 L/kg, and elimination half-life is 6.4 hours.[10] In adult camels, protein binding is ≈33%, volume of distribution is ≈0.8 L/kg, and elimination half-life is ≈11 hours.[11] Oral bioavailability in goats and camels is 90%.[12] In goats, volume of distribution is 1.4 L/kg and elimination half-life is ≈2 hours.[12]

Because of the low volume of distribution and theophylline's low lipid solubility, obese patients should be dosed on a lean body weight basis.

Theophylline is metabolized primarily in the liver (in humans) to 3-methylxanthine, which has weak bronchodilator activity. Renal clearance contributes only ≈10% to the overall plasma clearance of theophylline. In humans, wide interpatient variations in serum half-lives and resultant serum concentrations occur. It could be expected that similar variability exists in veterinary patients, particularly those with concurrent illnesses. The reported elimination half-lives (mean values) in various species are ≈9 hours in dogs,[5] ≈7.8 hours in cats,[6] ≈11 hours in pigs, and ≈12 to 17 hours in horses.[8,9] Note that the pharmacokinetics of long-acting theophylline products vary with the modified (ie, extended) release mechanism, and duration of effect may vary between 8 and 24 hours in humans.

Contraindications/Precautions/Warnings

Aminophylline is contraindicated in patients that are hypersensitive to xanthines (including aminophylline, theobromine, caffeine). Use in dogs with a history of epileptiform seizures is contraindicated.[13]

Aminophylline should be administered with caution in patients with severe cardiac disease, seizure disorders, gastric ulcers, hyperthyroidism, renal or hepatic disease, severe hypoxia, or severe hypertension. Aminophylline clearance is decreased ≈50% in patients with hepatic disease or CHF, and a 50% decrease in dosage has been suggested for patients in hepatic failure.[14] Clearance is decreased to a lesser extent by hypothyroidism, fever, and sepsis. Because it may cause or worsen pre-existing arrhythmias, patients with cardiac tachyarrhythmias should receive aminophylline only with caution and enhanced monitoring. Neonatal and geriatric patients may have decreased clearances of aminophylline and be more sensitive to its toxic effects.

In humans, exposure to secondhand smoke may increase aminophylline clearance; whether the same occurs in animals is unknown.

Aminophylline causes intense local pain when administered IM and is rarely used or recommended for administration via this route.

Adverse Effects

Aminophylline can produce CNS stimulation and GI irritation after administration by any route. Most adverse effects are related to the serum concentration of the drug and may be indicative of toxic blood concentrations; dogs appear to tolerate concentrations that may be toxic to humans.

Tachycardia was noted in dogs with a plasma theophylline concentration greater than 30 µg/mL.[15] Undiluted or rapid infusions of aminophylline can cause cardiac arrhythmias, hypotension, tremors, and acute respiratory failure. Under experimental conditions, 10 mg/kg aminophylline by rapid IV administration failed to elicit arrhythmias in healthy dogs.[16]

Tachycardia and excitement have been noted in horses.[17] Transient CNS excitement (eg, tremors) and GI disturbances (eg, vomiting, anorexia) may occur when starting therapy but generally are mild and resolve spontaneously.

Dogs and cats can exhibit clinical signs of nausea and vomiting, insomnia, increased gastric acid secretion, diarrhea, polyphagia, polydipsia, and polyuria. Adverse effects in horses generally are dose-related and may include nervousness, excitability (with auditory, tactile, or visual stimulation), tremors, diaphoresis, tachycardia, and ataxia. Seizures or cardiac arrhythmias may occur in cases of overdose.

Reproductive/Nursing Safety

Aminophylline has been shown to reduce uterine contractions; it crosses the placenta but has not been shown to be teratogenic in mice or rats.

Theophylline is distributed into milk (70% of serum concentrations). Use with caution in nursing patients.

Because safety has not been established in animals, this drug should only be used when the maternal benefits outweigh the potential risks to offspring.

Overdose/Acute Toxicity

In humans, clinical signs of toxicity (see *Adverse Effects*) are usually associated with serum drug concentrations greater than 20 µg/mL and become more severe as the serum concentration exceeds that value. Tachycardia, arrhythmia, and CNS effects (eg, seizures, hyperthermia) are considered the most life-threatening aspects of toxicity. Hypokalemia and acid-base disturbances also may occur. Dogs and cats appear to tolerate serum concentrations greater than 20 µg/mL. The ASPCA Animal Poison Control Center (APCC) reported 86 single-agent exposures to theophylline from 2009 to 2013. Of the 75 dogs exposed, 27 had clinical signs, with tachycardia (48%) reported most commonly.

Treatment of theophylline toxicity is supportive. GI decontamination with activated charcoal, which blocks theophylline absorption, can be considered[18,19] and is more effective in reducing theophylline exposure than inducing emesis. Patients with seizures should have an adequate airway maintained and be treated with an IV benzodiazepine (eg, diazepam, midazolam). Patients should be continuously monitored for cardiac arrhythmias and tachycardia. Fluid and electrolytes should be monitored and corrected as necessary.

Hyperthermia may be treated with phenothiazines[20] and tachycardia treated with propranolol if either condition is considered life-threatening. Theophylline is removed by hemodialysis, which may be an option in cases in which activated charcoal cannot be administered.

For patients that have experienced or are suspected to have experienced an overdose, it is strongly encouraged to consult with a 24-hour poison consultation center that specializes in providing information specific for veterinary patients. For general information related to overdose and toxin exposures, as well as contact information for poison control centers, refer to *Appendix*.

Drug Interactions

The following drug interactions with aminophylline or theophylline have either been reported or are theoretical in humans or animals and may be of significance in veterinary patients. Unless otherwise noted, use together is not necessarily contraindicated, but weigh the potential risks and perform additional monitoring when appropriate.

- KETAMINE: Theophylline with ketamine can cause an increased incidence of seizures and cardiac arrhythmias.
- SYMPATHOMIMETICS (eg, **beta agonists** [eg, **albuterol**], **ephedrine, isoproterenol, phenylpropanolamine**): Toxic synergism (eg, CNS stimulation, arrhythmias) can occur if theophylline is used concurrently with sympathomimetics (especially ephedrine) or possibly isoproterenol. Concurrent use with beta sympathomimetics is contraindicated according to the UK product label.[13]

The following drugs can *increase* or *decrease* theophylline concentrations:

- ISONIAZID
- LOOP DIURETICS (eg, **furosemide**)

The following drugs can *decrease* theophylline concentrations:

- ALBENDAZOLE
- BARBITURATES (eg, **phenobarbital**): Can induce CYP enzymes and increase theophylline metabolism in dogs (not cats)
- CHARCOAL, ACTIVATED
- HERBAL AGENTS (eg, **fenugreek, garden cress**)[21]
- KETOCONAZOLE

- **Rifampin**
- **Sympathomimetics** (eg, **beta agonists** [eg, **albuterol**], **ephedrine, isoproterenol, phenylpropanolamine**)

The following drugs can *increase* theophylline concentrations:

- Allopurinol
- **Beta-Blockers, Non-Selective** (eg, **propranolol**)
- **Calcium Channel Blockers** (eg, **diltiazem, verapamil**)
- **Chloramphenicol:** Consider decreasing the dose of theophylline by 30% to 50% or extending the dosing interval.
- **Cimetidine**
- **Corticosteroids** (eg, **dexamethasone, prednis(ol)one**)
- **Estrogen**
- **Fluconazole**
- **Fluoroquinolones** (eg, **enrofloxacin, ciprofloxacin**): If adding either, consider reducing the dose of theophylline by 30% or extending the dosing interval. Monitor for toxicity/efficacy. **Marbofloxacin** decreases clearance of theophylline in dogs but not with clinical significance. In animals with renal impairment, marbofloxacin may interfere with theophylline metabolism in a clinically relevant manner.[22]
- **Interferon Alfa**
- **Macrolides** (eg, **clarithromycin, erythromycin**)
- **Methotrexate**
- **Mexiletine**
- **Selective Serotonin Reuptake Inhibitors** (SSRIs; eg, **fluoxetine**)
- **Thiabendazole**
- **Thyroid Hormones** (in hypothyroid patients)

Theophylline may *decrease* the effects of the following drugs:

- **Benzodiazepines** (eg, **diazepam, midazolam**)
- **Lithium**
- **Pancuronium**
- **Propofol**[23]

Laboratory Considerations

- Theophylline can cause falsely elevated values of **serum uric acid** if measured by the Bittner or colorimetric methods. Values are not affected if using the uricase method.
- Immunoassays are specific for theophylline. If using a spectrophotometric method of assay, theophylline serum concentrations can be falsely elevated by **furosemide, phenylbutazone, probenecid, theobromine, caffeine, sulfathiazole, chocolate**, or **acetaminophen**. **Cefazolin** may interfere with HPLC assays. The Schack and Wexler method of determining theophylline concentrations may be affected by large doses of **thiamine**.

Dosages

NOTES:

1. Theophyllines have a relatively low therapeutic index; determine doses carefully. Calculate doses based on lean body weight.
2. Dosage conversions between aminophylline and theophylline can be performed using the information found in the *Chemistry* section.

DOGS/CATS:

Bronchodilator (extra-label): 3 – 11 mg/kg IV or IM every 6 to 12 hours. Dogs may require the higher end of the dosage range and may be dosed every 6 to 8 hours. For cats, the low end of the dosing range is used and given every 12 hours. If effective, switch to oral therapy (theophylline) as soon as possible. When giving IV, do not push. Preferably administer over at least several minutes or as an infusion.

HORSES:

Adjunctive treatment of severe equine asthma (SEA; formerly known as recurrent airway obstruction [RAO]); (extra-label): 5 – 14 mg/kg IV every 8 to 12 hours.[17,24] IV infusion should be in ≈1 liter of IV fluids given over 20 to 60 minutes. Rarely recommended because of narrow therapeutic index. Consider monitoring serum aminophylline concentrations.

CATTLE

Bronchoconstriction secondary to smoke inhalation (extra-label): 6 – 10 mg/kg IV or PO three times daily[25]

Monitoring

- Therapeutic efficacy
- Clinical signs of toxicity: tachycardia, vomiting, diarrhea, seizures
- Consider measuring serum theophylline concentrations for patients not responding to therapy or that have clinical signs of toxicity. The therapeutic serum concentrations of theophylline in humans are generally described to be ≈10 µg/mL. In small animals, serum concentrations can be monitored by measuring the trough concentration; the concentration should be greater than 8 – 10 µg/mL. **NOTE**: Some clinicians recommend not exceeding 15 µg/mL in horses.[17]

Client Information

- Injectable aminophylline should only be used in an inpatient setting or under the direct supervision of a veterinarian.

Chemistry/Synonyms

Aminophylline occurs as bitter-tasting, white or slightly yellow granules or powder, with a slight ammoniacal odor and a pK_a of 5.

Aminophylline is soluble in water and insoluble in alcohol. One mg of aminophylline (hydrous) contains ≈0.79 mg of theophylline (anhydrous). Conversely, 1 mg of theophylline (anhydrous) is equivalent to 1.27 mg aminophylline (hydrous).

Aminophylline also may be known as aminofilina, aminophyllinum, euphyllinum, metaphyllin, theophyllaminum, theophylline and ethylenediamine, theophylline ethylenediamine compound, or theophyllinum ethylenediaminum; many trade names are available.

Storage/Stability

Aminophylline for injection should be stored in single-use containers in which carbon dioxide has been removed. It should be stored at 20°C to 25°C (68°F-77°F) and protected from freezing and light. Upon exposure to air (carbon dioxide), aminophylline will absorb carbon dioxide, lose ethylenediamine, and liberate free theophylline that can precipitate out of solution. Do not inject aminophylline solutions that contain either precipitate or visible crystals.

Compatibility/Compounding Considerations

Compatibility is dependent on factors such as pH, concentration, temperature, and diluent used; consult specialized references or a hospital pharmacist for more specific information.

Aminophylline for injection is reportedly **compatible** when mixed with commonly used IV solutions, but it may be **incompatible** with 10% fructose or invert sugar solutions. Aminophylline is reportedly **compatible** when mixed with the following drugs: calcium gluconate, chloramphenicol sodium succinate, dexamethasone sodium phosphate, dopamine HCl, erythromycin lactobionate, heparin sodium, hydrocortisone sodium succinate, lidocaine HCl, metronidazole with sodium bicarbonate, phenobarbital sodium, potassium chloride, sodium bicarbonate, sodium iodide, terbutaline sulfate, and verapamil HCl.

Aminophylline is reportedly **incompatible** (or data conflict) with the following drugs: amikacin sulfate, ascorbic acid injection, bleomycin sulfate, clindamycin phosphate, corticotropin, dimenhydrinate, dobutamine HCl, doxorubicin HCl, epinephrine HCl, erythromycin gluceptate, hydralazine HCl, hydroxyzine HCl, insulin (regular), isoproterenol HCl, meperidine HCl, methadone HCl, methylprednisolone sodium succinate, morphine sulfate, norepinephrine bitartrate, oxytetracycline, penicillin G potassium, pentazocine lactate, procaine HCl, prochlorperazine, promazine HCl, promethazine HCl, vancomycin HCl, and vitamin B complex with C.

Dosage Forms/Regulatory Status

VETERINARY-LABELED PRODUCTS: NONE

The Association of Racing Commissioners International (ARCI) has designated this drug as a class 3 substance. See ***Appendix*** for more information.

HUMAN-LABELED PRODUCTS:

Aminophylline Injection: 25 mg/mL (equivalent to 19.7 mg/mL of theophylline) in 10 mL and 20 mL vials; generic; (Rx)

Oral aminophylline tablets have been discontinued for the US market. See the ***Theophylline*** monograph for information on using oral products.

References

For the complete list of references, see **wiley.com/go/budde/plumb**

Amiodarone

(a-mee-oh-***da***-rone) *Cordarone®, Nexterone®, Pacerone®*

Antiarrhythmic Class III

Prescriber Highlights

- Antiarrhythmic agent used in dogs for arrhythmias associated with systolic dysfunction or for cardioversion from atrial fibrillation to sinus rhythm; very limited experience warrants cautious use. May take several days to weeks to have an effect
- When combined with itraconazole, is an effective treatment for *Trypanosoma cruzi* infection (Chagas disease).
- May be useful in horses for cardioversion from atrial fibrillation, supraventricular tachycardia, or ventricular tachycardia to sinus rhythm
- Contraindications include cardiogenic shock, or bradyarrhythmias (eg, second- and third-degree heart block, sinus node dysfunction) and iodine hypersensitivity. Use caution in patients with thyroid dysfunction; can exacerbate or cause hypo- or hyperthyroidism
- Adverse effects in dogs include GI disturbances (eg, nausea, vomiting, anorexia). Corneal deposits, neutropenia, pulmonary fibrosis, thrombocytopenia, bradycardia, hepatotoxicity, and positive Coombs tests have been reported. IV formulations containing polysorbate 80 (*Tween® 80*) can cause serious histaminergic effects in dogs.
- Limited use in horses precludes a full adverse effect profile; pelvic limb weakness, diarrhea and increased bilirubin have been reported when used IV for cardioversion.
- Many potential drug interactions

Uses/Indications

Because of its potential toxicity and limited experience with use in canine and equine patients, amiodarone is generally used only when other less toxic or commonly used drugs are ineffective. Amiodarone may be useful in dogs and horses for cardioversion from atrial fibrillation to sinus rhythm and in dogs for arrhythmias in which the benefit outweighs the risk (eg, refractory arrhythmia associated with systolic dysfunction).

Amiodarone combined with itraconazole reduced mortality and clinical signs of *Trypanosoma cruzi* infection (Chagas disease) in dogs.[1]

Successful use of a constant rate infusion of amiodarone for cardioversion of supraventricular tachycardia has been reported in a horse.[2] It was unsuccessful in cardioverting a llama with lone atrial fibrillation.[3]

Pharmacology/Actions

Amiodarone's mechanism of action is not fully understood; it acts primarily as a potassium channel blocker that possesses unique pharmacology from other antiarrhythmic agents. It can be best classified as a class III antiarrhythmic agent that also blocks sodium and calcium channels and beta-adrenergic receptors. Major properties include prolongation of myocardial cell action-potential duration and refractory period.

The trypanocidal effects of amiodarone in *T cruzi* appear to be mediated by disruption of calcium homeostasis, sterol production, and blockade of the protease cruzipain.[1]

Pharmacokinetics

Amiodarone may be administered parenterally or orally. It is widely distributed throughout the body and can accumulate and persist in adipose tissue. Amiodarone concentrations in myocardial cells[4] and adipose tissue[5] are significantly higher than in plasma. Amiodarone is metabolized by the liver into desethylamiodarone, which is active. After oral administration of a single dose in healthy dogs, amiodarone's plasma half-life averaged 7.5 hours, but repeated dosing increased its half-life to 3.2 days.[5]

In horses, amiodarone has a low oral bioavailability (6% to 34%) and peak concentrations of amiodarone and desethylamiodarone occur ≈7 to 8 hours after an oral dose. After IV administration, amiodarone is rapidly distributed with a high apparent volume of distribution of 31 L/kg. In horses, amiodarone is highly bound to plasma proteins (96%). Clearance was 0.35 L/kg/hour and median elimination half-lives for amiodarone and desethylamiodarone after IV administration were ≈51 and 75 hours, respectively compared to 24 and 59 hours, respectively, after oral administration.[6]

In humans, oral absorption is slow and variable, with bioavailabilities ranging from 22% to 86%. Elimination half-lives for amiodarone and desethylamiodarone range from 2.5 to 10 days after a single dose but average 53 days and 60 days, respectively, with chronic dosing.

Contraindications/Precautions/Warnings

Amiodarone is considered contraindicated in patients that are hypersensitive to it or iodine, or that have cardiogenic shock, severe sinus node dysfunction with severe sinus bradycardia, second- and third-degree atrioventricular block, or bradycardial syncope. Amiodarone should be used with caution in patients with thyroid dysfunction.

One report has shown Doberman pinschers with ventricular arrhythmias to be at higher risk for toxicity, particularly hepatic and GI toxicity, from amiodarone. This report concludes that amiodarone should be used cautiously in Doberman pinschers with preclinical left ventricular systolic dysfunction prior to receiving other antiarrhythmic agents.[7]

Amiodarone inhibits peripheral conversion of thyroxine T4 to triiodothyronine T3, and in humans may cause hypothyroidism (more common); rarely, amiodarone can also lead to iodine-induced hyperthyroidism or a destructive thyroiditis in humans.[8]

Adverse Effects

GI effects (eg, anorexia, vomiting) are the most likely adverse effects in canine patients.[1] Hepatopathy (eg, bilirubinemia, increased hepatic enzymes) has been reported in dogs on amiodarone.[1,9] Because hepatic effects can occur before clinical signs are noted, routine serial evaluation of liver enzymes and bilirubin is recommended; laboratory abnormalities may require 6 to 8 weeks to resolve. Amiodarone dosage should be reduced, or the drug discontinued if hepatopathy develops.[10] Other adverse effects reported in dogs include bradycardia, neutropenia, thrombocytopenia, keratopathy,[11,12] regenerative anemia, and a positive Coombs test.[13] Corneal deposits may be seen in dogs treated with amiodarone, but this affect apparently occurs less frequently in dogs than in humans.

A case series of 5 dogs administered IV amiodarone reported pruritus, erythema, subcutaneous edema, hives, agitation, tachypnea, and hypotension.[14] The authors postulated that the solvent polysorbate 80 found in the IV solutions could be the cause of these effects. A newer IV formulation, *Nexterone®*, does not contain polysorbate 80 or benzyl alcohol. One study of 17 dogs receiving *Nexterone®* showed no adverse effects after a 2 mg/kg bolus followed by a 0.8 mg/kg/hour infusion.[15] Under experimental conditions, decreased myocardial contractility was noted at 12.5 – 15 mg/kg IV.[16]

Horses treated with IV amiodarone for 36 hours or longer developed short-term hind limb weakness and diarrhea.[17,18]

In human patients, adverse effects are very common while on amiodarone therapy (eg, nausea and vomiting). The effects that most commonly cause discontinuation of the drug include pulmonary infiltrates or pulmonary fibrosis (sometimes fatal), liver enzyme elevations, congestive heart failure, bradycardia, paroxysmal ventricular tachycardia, peripheral neuropathy, and thyroid dysfunction (hypo- or hyperthyroidism). Some individuals develop a bluish tint to their skin. Optic neuropathy or neuritis has been reported.

Reproductive/Nursing Safety

In laboratory animals, amiodarone has been embryotoxic and fetotoxic at doses 3 times the maximum recommended human dose, and congenital bony malformations and thyroid abnormalities have been detected in offspring. Use during pregnancy only when the potential benefits outweigh the risks of the drug. Amiodarone may reduce male and female fertility.

Amiodarone is excreted in milk, and adverse effects in nursing infants have been reported. Use during nursing is not recommended.

Overdose/Acute Toxicity

Clinical overdose experience is limited; adverse effects include hypotension, bradycardia, cardiogenic shock, AV block, and hepatotoxicity. Treatment is supportive. Bradycardia may be managed with beta agonists (eg, isoproterenol) or a pacemaker; hypotension may be managed with positive inotropic agents or vasopressors. Neither amiodarone nor its active metabolite is dialyzable.

For patients that have experienced or are suspected to have experienced an overdose, it is strongly encouraged to consult with a 24-hour poison consultation center that specialize in providing information specific for veterinary patients. For general information related to overdose and toxin exposures, as well as contact information for poison control centers, refer to ***Appendix***.

Drug Interactions

Several potentially significant interactions can occur with amiodarone. The following is a partial list of interactions that have either been reported or are theoretical in humans or animals and may be of significance in veterinary patients. Unless otherwise noted, use together is not necessarily contraindicated, but weigh the potential risks and perform additional monitoring when appropriate.

Amiodarone may significantly **increase** the serum levels and/or pharmacologic or toxic effects of:

- **BETA-ADRENERGIC ANTAGONISTS** (eg, **atenolol, metoprolol, propranolol**)
- **CALCIUM-CHANNEL BLOCKERS** (CCBs; eg, **amlodipine, diltiazem**): Possible potentiation of bradycardia, AV block or sinus arrest
- **DIGOXIN:** May increase digoxin concentration and risk for bradycardia
- **CYCLOPHOSPHAMIDE**
- **CYCLOSPORINE:** May also increase creatinine
- **DEXTROMETHORPHAN**
- **LIDOCAINE (SYSTEMIC)**
- **METHOTREXATE** (with prolonged amiodarone administration)
- **PROCAINAMIDE**
- **QUINIDINE**
- **WARFARIN**

Amiodarone may **prolong the QT interval**, which may be additive and lead to cardiac arrhythmias when administered with the following drugs:

- **ANTIARRHYTHMICS** (eg, **disopyramide, procainamide, quinidine, sotalol**)
- **AZOLE ANTIFUNGALS** (eg, **itraconazole, ketoconazole**)
- **CISAPRIDE**
- **FLUOROQUINOLONE ANTIBIOTICS** (some, such as **moxifloxacin**, possibly **pradofloxacin**, but NOT **enrofloxacin, marbofloxacin**)
- **MACROLIDE ANTIBIOTICS** (eg, **azithromycin, erythromycin**)
- **OPIOIDS** (ie, **buprenorphine, methadone**)
- **SEROTONIN HT_3 ANTAGONISTS** (eg, **granisetron, ondansetron**)

Other amiodarone drug interactions:

- **ANESTHETICS, GENERAL** (eg, **isoflurane, propofol**): Increased risks for hypotension or arrhythmias
- **CHOLESTYRAMINE:** May decrease amiodarone concentration
- **CIMETIDINE**: Increased amiodarone levels
- **OPIOIDS** (eg, **fentanyl, morphine**): Possible hypotension, bradycardia
- **RIFAMPIN**: Decreased amiodarone levels
- **THEOPHYLLINE**: Amiodarone may reduce theophylline metabolism

Laboratory Considerations

- Although most human patients remain euthyroid while receiving amiodarone, it may cause an increase in **serum T_4** and **serum reverse T_3** concentrations, and a reduction in **serum T_3** concentrations.
- Amiodarone may cause a **positive Coombs** test result.[13]

Dosages

NOTE: Some human references state that because of the potential for drug interactions with previous drug therapies, the life-threatening nature of the arrhythmias being treated, and the unpredictability of response to amiodarone, the drug should initially be given (loaded) over several days in an inpatient setting where adequate monitoring can occur.

DOGS:

Atrial fibrillation or ventricular arrhythmias (extra-label): Dosages for oral amiodarone are not well established, and there is significant variation in recommendations. At present, no well-controlled, prospective studies evaluating dosage regimens in clinically ill dogs could be located.

1. 5 – 7.5 mg/kg per day PO[19]; a retrospective study concluded that amiodarone might be a safe and effective alternative drug for the treatment of arrhythmias with myocardial dysfunction that are not controlled with commonly used antiarrhythmic drugs.
2. Due to its unique pharmacokinetics, an initial loading dosage of 8 – 10 mg/kg PO twice daily for 1 week then reduce to 5 – 10 mg/kg PO once daily thereafter. [20,21]

Ventricular tachycardia, supraventricular tachycardia, or atrial flutter refractory to other antiarrhythmic therapy (extra-label): Using polysorbate 80-free formulation (ie, *Nexterone®*, 2 mg/kg IV over 10 minutes followed by 0.8 mg/kg/hour IV CRI for 6 hours and then 0.5 mg/kg/hour thereafter).[15] A dedicated central venous catheter and an in-line filter are recommended for IV administration.[22] In the study, for patients in cardiopulmonary arrest, doses ranged from 3 – 12 mg/kg IV with a CRI of 0.05 – 18 mg/kg/hour.

T cruzi **infection** (extra-label): Amiodarone loading dose: 15 mg/kg PO every 12 hours for 7 days, followed by 15 mg/kg PO every 24 hours for 14 days. Maintenance dose: 7.5 mg/kg PO every 24 hours. Itraconazole 10 mg/kg PO (rounded down to the nearest 100 mg increment dose) every 24 hours (**NOTE:** Itraconazole 100 mg PO every 48 hours was administered to dogs with low body weight) was concurrently initiated on the first day of amiodarone therapy. [1] Treatment continued for 12 months. A minority of dogs (15%) initiated amiodarone at the maintenance dose (ie, the loading dose was omitted). Amiodarone dose was reduced by half if adverse effects occurred.

HORSES:

Atrial fibrillation, supraventricular tachycardia, or ventricular tachycardia (extra-label): 5 mg/kg/hour IV CRI for 1 hour, followed by 0.83 mg/kg/hour IV CRI for 23 hours and then 1.9 mg/kg/hour IV CRI for the following 30 hours.[17,23] Infusion was discontinued when conversion occurred or when any adverse effects were noted. Four of 6 horses converted from atrial fibrillation as well as 1 horse from supraventricular tachycardia and 1 from ventricular tachycardia. One horse with supraventricular tachycardia also was given amiodarone at 5 mg/kg PO every 24 hours with strict stall rest for 2 weeks.[2]

Monitoring

- Intermittent or continuous ECG
- Adverse effects (eg, inappetence, vomiting, diarrhea)
- The human therapeutic serum amiodarone concentrations of 1 – 2.5 µg/mL are believed to apply to dogs as well. One study in horses[18] suggests adverse effects may be more common when amiodarone concentration exceeds 2.5 µg/mL, although a dose relationship was not noted in another study.[23]
- Baseline and periodic CBC, liver panel, thyroid function tests, blood pressure, and thoracic radiographs as indicated. One reference recommends that liver enzymes be monitored monthly during therapy; if liver enzymes become abnormal, it is recommended the dosage be reduced or the drug be discontinued.[10]
- *T cruzi*: PCR and/or serology to assess therapeutic effectiveness

Client Information

- This drug has not been used often in dogs, and therefore not all side effects are known. The most commonly reported side effects seen in dogs are vomiting and lack of appetite. Consult your veterinarian if there are any unexpected effects.
- Amiodarone may interact with other medications. Make sure your veterinarian is aware of all medications and supplements your animal is receiving.
- Your veterinarian will need to monitor your animal while on this medication. Do not miss these important follow-up visits.

Chemistry/Synonyms

An iodinated benzofuran, amiodarone is unique structurally and pharmacologically from other antiarrhythmic agents. Amiodarone occurs as a white to cream colored lipophilic powder having a pK_a of ≈6.6. Amiodarone 200 mg tablets each contain ≈75 mg of iodine. Generic forms of the injectable solution contain polysorbate 80 and benzyl alcohol. *Nexterone*® pre-filled IV bags contain dextrose 42.1 mg/mL but do not contain benzyl alcohol or polysorbate 80.

Amiodarone HCl may also be known as amiodaroni hydrochloridum, L-3428, 51087N, or SKF-33134-A; *Cordarone*®, *Nexterone*® and *Pacerone*® are among many trade names available.

Storage/Stability

Tablets should be stored in airtight containers, at room temperature 20°C to 25°C (68°F-77°F) and protected from light.

Injection should be stored at room temperature and protected from light, freezing, or excessive heat. While administering, light protection is not necessary.

Compatibility/Compounding Considerations

Compatibility is dependent on factors such as pH, concentration, temperature, and diluent used; specialized references or a hospital pharmacist should be consulted for more specific information.

IV preparations should be diluted with 5% dextrose in water (D5W). Amiodarone is reportedly **compatible** with dobutamine, lidocaine, potassium chloride, procainamide, propafenone, and verapamil. Variable compatibility is reported with furosemide and quinidine gluconate. Do not admix supplemental medications with *Nexterone*®.

Compounded preparation stability: Amiodarone oral suspension compounded from commercially available tablets has been published.[24] Triturating 1 tablet of amiodarone 200 mg with 20 mL of *Ora-Plus*® and quantity sufficient to make to 40 mL with *Ora-Sweet*® (or *Ora-Sweet®SF*) yields a 5 mg/mL oral suspension that retains more than 90% potency for 91 days stored at 5°C. Compounded preparations of amiodarone should be protected from light. Amiodarone suspensions may be stored at room temperature during short periods (eg, travel).

Dosage Forms/Regulatory Status

VETERINARY-LABELED PRODUCTS: NONE

The Association of Racing Commissioners International (ARCI) has designated this drug as a class 4 substance. See ***Appendix*** for more information.

HUMAN-LABELED PRODUCTS:

Amiodarone Oral Tablets: 100 mg, 200 mg, and 400 mg; generic; (Rx)

Amiodarone Injection Solution: 50 mg/mL in 3 mL and 9 mL single-dose vials, and 18 mL single-dose vials or multi-dose vials; 3 mL prefilled syringes; generic; (Rx)

Amiodarone Injection Solution: 150 mg/100 mL and 360 mg/200 mL prefilled IV bags (contains 42.1 mg/mL dextrose as diluent); *Nexterone*®; (Rx)

References

For the complete list of references, see **wiley.com/go/budde/plumb**

Amitriptyline

(a-mih-***trip***-ti-leen) *Elavil*®

Tricyclic Antidepressant; Antipruritic; Neuropathic Pain Modifier

Prescriber Highlights

- ► Tricyclic antidepressant used primarily for behavior disorders, neuropathic pain, and pruritus in small animals
- ► May reduce seizure thresholds in epileptic animals
- ► The most likely adverse effects include sedation and anticholinergic effects; there is risk for serotonin syndrome when amitriptyline is used concurrently with serotonergic drugs.
- ► May take a few weeks to see clinical effects; taper medication when discontinuing
- ► Many possible drug interactions
- ► Overdose can be serious.
- ► Use may decrease total triiodothyronine (tT3), total thyroxine (tT4), and free T4 (fT4) concentrations in dogs and cats; baseline thyroid testing should be performed prior to initiating therapy.

Uses/Indications

Amitriptyline is a tricyclic antidepressant (TCA) that has been used for the treatment of behavior conditions (eg, separation anxiety, generalized anxiety) and pruritus[1] in dogs, as well as to treat excessive grooming, spraying, pica, and anxiety in cats. Clomipramine is an FDA-approved TCA for use in dogs and is therefore often chosen over amitriptyline in cases where a TCA is needed for the treatment of behavior-modifying indications. A retrospective study also suggests clomipramine is more effective than amitriptyline.[2] One study demonstrated that amitriptyline was not effective in the treatment of aggressive dogs that were concomitantly undergoing behavior modification; however, the dose may have been inadequate.[3]

Amitriptyline may be useful for adjunctive treatment of chronic neuropathic pain in dogs[4] and cats. Although studies have questioned the drug's use for adjunctive treatment of lower urinary tract disease in cats,[5,6] amitriptyline appears to still be anecdotally used for analgesic and/or urethral antispasmodic effects.

Amitriptyline appears effective in reducing feather plucking in birds.[7,8]

Pharmacology/Actions

Amitriptyline (and its active metabolite, nortriptyline) is a tricyclic antidepressant (TCA) with a complicated pharmacologic profile that includes blockage of serotonin and norepinephrine reuptake pumps (thereby increasing neurotransmitter concentrations), sedation, and central and peripheral anticholinergic activity. Other pharmacologic effects include alpha-1 adrenergic antagonism, stabilizing mast cells via H1 receptor antagonism, and antagonism of glutamate receptors and sodium channels. TCAs act similar to phenothiazines in altering avoidance behaviors in animals.

Amitriptyline potentiated the minimum alveolar concentration (MAC)-sparing effects of remifentanil in rats.[9]

Pharmacokinetics

Amitriptyline is rapidly absorbed from both the GI tract and parenteral injection sites, but transdermal (PLO gel-based) absorption in cats is poor.[10] Absolute bioavailability is low, with one study noting only 6% bioavailability after a single oral dose (4 mg/kg) was administered to greyhounds.[11] Absorption appears to be increased when amitriptyline is administered with food.[12] Low oral bioavailability in dogs may reflect both incomplete absorption and first-pass metabolism to inactive metabolites. Further investigation is necessary.[11]

Peak concentrations occur 1 to 2 hours after oral administration in dogs[11-13] and cats[10] and within 2 to 12 hours in other species. Amitriptyline is highly bound to plasma proteins and enters the CNS. The drug is metabolized in the liver to several metabolites, including nortriptyline, which is active. In a study of 12 crossbreed dogs, the elimination half-life of amitriptyline and nortriptyline was 4.5 hours and 12.3 hours, respectively.[13] In greyhounds, the mean terminal half-life was 4 to 10 hours, and the terminal half-life of nortriptyline was 6.2 to 9.6 hours.[11] Because tricyclic antidepressants (TCAs) are metabolized through glucuronidation, cats may be more sensitive to TCAs than dogs.[14]

Amitriptyline has been administered intrathecally and epidurally in sheep; the concentration-time profiles were highly variable, with a bioavailability of 55% and 1.3%, respectively.[15]

One study in birds saw significantly varied absorption and elimination constants. Elimination half-life varied from 1.6 to 91.2 hours.[16]

Contraindications/Precautions/Warnings

Amitriptyline is contraindicated in patients that are hypersensitive to it or other tricyclic antidepressants (TCAs). Concomitant use with monoamine oxidase inhibitors is contraindicated in humans. Use amitriptyline with extreme caution in animals with seizure disorders, as tricyclic agents may reduce seizure thresholds. In cats, at standard doses, epileptiform pathology was noted on EEG, and sustained discharges and generalized seizures occurred at higher (20 – 25 mg/kg IV) doses.[17] Use amitriptyline with caution in animals with thyroid disorders, urinary retention, hepatic disorders, renal disorders, KCS, glaucoma, cardiac rhythm disorders, diabetes, or adrenal tumors. Although amitriptyline may prolong the QTc interval in humans, ECG abnormalities did not occur in healthy dogs with behavioral conditions treated with standard doses of amitriptyline.[18,19]

Because data are lacking about the impact of amitriptyline on the QT interval in animals, this drug should be used with caution in patients that have pre-existing cardiac disease.

Amitriptyline should not be given on an as-needed basis; it needs to be given continuously and may require several weeks to see a positive response. If discontinuing amitriptyline, the dose should be slowly tapered over 2 to 3 weeks to minimize the risks for signs of withdrawal.

Adverse Effects

The most predominant adverse effects seen with tricyclic antidepressants (TCAs) are related to sedation and anticholinergic (eg, constipation, urinary retention) properties. Occasionally, dogs exhibit hyperexcitability and, rarely, develop seizures; however, adverse effects can affect various systems, including cardiac (eg, dysrhythmias), hematologic (eg, bone marrow suppression), GI (eg, vomiting, diarrhea), and endocrine (eg, hyperglycemia, hyponatremia). After oral administration, vomiting may be more likely in fasted dogs.[12]

Adverse effects seen in cats include sedation, hypersalivation, urinary retention, anorexia, thrombocytopenia, neutropenia, unkempt hair coat, vomiting/nausea, ataxia, disorientation, and cardiac conductivity disturbances.[5,20]

Reduced reverse triiodothyronine (rT3), total thyroxine (tT4), and free T4 (fT4) concentrations may occur in dogs and cats.[21,22]

Dystonia and akathisia were described in a macaw that was given a single dose of amitriptyline.[23]

Reproductive/Nursing Safety

In humans, amitriptyline crosses the placenta, and isolated reports of limb reduction abnormalities in fetuses have been noted. Amitriptyline enters maternal milk in levels similar to or greater than those found in maternal serum. In humans, amitriptyline is considered a drug for which the effect on nursing infants is unknown but may be of concern.[24]

Because safety has not been established in animals, this drug should only be used when the maternal benefits outweigh potential risks.

Overdose/Acute Toxicity

Overdose with tricyclic antidepressants (TCAs) can cause life-threatening conditions (eg, arrhythmias, cardiorespiratory collapse). Under experimental conditions, dogs receiving amitriptyline by IV infusion developed cardiotoxicity after an average cumulative dose of 36 mg/kg, and convulsions occurred in 42% of dogs.[25] Other common clinical signs in dogs and cats include lethargy, ataxia, and vomiting. IV fat emulsion therapy (*Intralipid®*) is thought to trap amitriptyline in plasma during overdose and lower brain concentration; however, severe hypotension occurred in 10% of pigs,[26] and amitriptyline mortality rates were not affected in rats.[27]

For patients that have experienced or are suspected to have experienced an overdose, consultation with a 24-hour poison consultation center specializing in providing veterinary-specific information is recommended. For general information related to overdose and toxin exposures, as well as contact information for poison control centers, refer to ***Appendix***.

Drug Interactions

In humans, amitriptyline is a substrate of CYP3A4, 2C9, and 2D6. The following drug interactions with amitriptyline either have been reported or are theoretical in humans or animals and may be of significance in veterinary patients. Unless otherwise noted, use together is not necessarily contraindicated, but weigh the potential risks and perform additional monitoring when appropriate.

- ACETAZOLAMIDE/DICHLORPHENAMIDE: Concurrent use may increase amitriptyline concentrations by alkalinizing urine.
- ALPHA-2 ADRENERGIC AGONISTS (eg, **clonidine**, **detomidine**, **dexmedetomidine**, **medetomidine**): Concurrent use may increase the risk for CNS and respiratory depression, hypertension, and bradycardia. Tricyclic antidepressants (TCAs) may interfere with the antihypertensive effects of alpha-2 agonists. Use cautiously in combination.
- AMANTADINE: Concurrent use may increase the risk for urinary retention, constipation, ileus, hyperthermia, heat stroke, anticholinergic intoxication syndrome, and QT interval prolongation. Use cautiously in combination.
- AMMONIUM CHLORIDE: Concurrent use may decrease tricyclic antidepressant concentrations by acidifying urine.
- ANESTHETIC AGENTS (eg, **isoflurane**, **ketamine**): Concurrent use may increase the risk for hypotension, CNS depression, QT interval prolongation, torsade de pointes, and death.
- ANTHRACYCLINES (eg, **doxorubicin**): Concurrent use may cause additive effects on the QT interval.
- ANTICHOLINERGIC AGENTS (eg, **atropine**, **doxepin**, **glycopyrrolate**, **meclizine**, **oxybutynin**): Concurrent use may increase the risk for constipation, ileus, urinary retention, CNS depression, and anticholinergic intoxication syndrome.
- ANTIHISTAMINES (eg, **cetirizine**, **chlorpheniramine**, **diphenhydramine**, **hydroxyzine**): Concurrent use may increase the risk for constipation, ileus, urinary retention, CNS depression, and anticholinergic intoxication syndrome.
- ANTIHYPERTENSIVE AGENTS: Concurrent use may result in additive hypotension and orthostasis.
- APOMORPHINE: Concurrent use may increase the risk for QT interval prolongation, torsade de pointes, and death.
- AZOLE ANTIFUNGALS (eg, **itraconazole**, **ketoconazole**): Concurrent use increases the risk for CNS toxicity, constipation, ileus, urinary retention, and QT interval prolongation.
- BARBITURATES (eg, **thiopental**): Concurrent use may cause additive respiratory depression. Amitriptyline concentrations may decrease.
- BENZODIAZEPINES (eg, **diazepam**, **midazolam**): Concurrent use may increase the risk for CNS and/or respiratory depression. Anticholinergic effects may be additive.
- BETA-2 ADRENERGIC AGONISTS (eg, **albuterol**, **clenbuterol**): Concurrent use may increase the risk for arrhythmias, hypertension, hyperpyrexia, flattening of the T-wave, and QT interval prolongation. Use cautiously in combination.
- BETHANECHOL: Amitriptyline may antagonize the cholinergic effects of bethanechol. Avoid combination.
- BROMOCRIPTINE: Amitriptyline may enhance the CNS depression and respiratory depression effects of bromocriptine. Concurrent use may increase the risk for serotonin syndrome.
- BUSPIRONE: Concurrent use may increase the risk for CNS depression and serotonin syndrome. Avoid combination.
- CANNABIDIOL: Concurrent use may increase the risk for CNS depression.
- CARBAMAZEPINE: Concurrent use may decrease concentrations of amitriptyline by induction of CYP450 enzymes, and carbamazepine concentrations may be increased by an undetermined mechanism. Amitriptyline may decrease anticonvulsant effects of carbamazepine.
- CIMETIDINE: May inhibit amitriptyline hepatic metabolism and increase the risk for toxicity
- CYPROHEPTADINE: Concurrent use may decrease efficacy of amitriptyline by decreasing serotonin concentrations, may increase the risk for CNS depression, and anticholinergic effects may be additive.
- DESMOPRESSIN: Concurrent use may increase the risk for water intoxication and/or hyponatremia, which can progress to seizure, coma, respiratory depression, and death. Electrolytes and renal function should be monitored.
- DIAZOXIDE: Concurrent use may increase the risk for hypotension and orthostasis, with greatest risk during initial treatment or dose escalation.
- DILTIAZEM: May increase amitriptyline concentrations
- DOBUTAMINE/DOPAMINE: Concurrent use may increase the risk for hypertension, tremors, and cardiac dysrhythmias. Avoid concurrent use except in emergency cases.
- DOMPERIDONE: Concurrent use may increase the risk for QT interval prolongation, cardiac arrhythmias, torsade de pointes, and death. Efficacy of domperidone may be decreased. Avoid combination.
- ERYTHROMYCIN: Concurrent use may increase the risk for QT interval prolongation and cardiac arrhythmias.
- ESTROGENS: May decrease effect and increase toxicity of amitriptyline; mechanism and clinical significance are not established.
- FLUCONAZOLE: Concurrent use may increase the risk for QT interval prolongation.
- FLUMAZENIL: Flumazenil use in animals suspected of TCA overdose may increase the risk for seizures and arrhythmias.[25]
- FLUOROQUINOLONES (eg, **ciprofloxacin**, **enrofloxacin**): Concurrent use may increase the risk for QT interval prolongation, torsade de pointes, and death.
- HYDROXYCHLOROQUINE: Concurrent use may increase the risk for QT interval prolongation.
- IFOSFAMIDE: Concurrent use may increase neurotoxicity of ifosfamide.
- IOHEXOL: Concurrent use may increase the risk for seizures associated with intrathecal administration of iohexol.
- LEUPROLIDE: Concurrent use may increase the risk for QT interval prolongation, torsade de pointes, and death.
- LEVETIRACETAM: Concurrent use may increase the risk for CNS and respiratory depression.
- LITHIUM: Concurrent use may increase the risk for neurotoxicity, including serotonin syndrome.
- MACROLIDES (eg, **azithromycin**, **clarithromycin**): Concurrent use may increase the risk for QT interval prolongation, torsade de pointes, and death.
- METHYLPHENIDATE: Concurrent use may increase concentrations of amitriptyline and increase the risk for hypertension, cardiac effects, and CNS stimulation, including increased risk for serotonin syndrome.
- METOCLOPRAMIDE: Amitriptyline may reduce the prokinetic effect of metoclopramide. Combination may also result in additive sedation or CNS depression.
- METRONIDAZOLE: Concurrent use may increase the risk for QT interval prolongation, cardiac arrhythmias, and torsade de pointes.
- MIRTAZAPINE: Concurrent use may increase the risk for constipation, urinary retention, CNS depression, and serotonin syndrome.

- **Mitotane**: Mitotane may induce CYP3A4 and reduce amitriptyline exposure and effectiveness.
- **Monoamine Oxidase Inhibitors** (eg, **amitraz**, **furazolidone**, **linezolid**, **methylene blue**, **procarbazine**, **selegiline**): There is a potential risk for life-threatening serotonin syndrome. Concurrent use is contraindicated. A 14-day washout period between the 2 drugs should be observed.
- **Muscle Relaxants** (eg, **baclofen**, **dantrolene**, **methocarbamol**): Concurrent use may increase the risk for CNS and respiratory depression. Loss of muscle tone and memory has been reported with baclofen use in humans.
- **Nitroglycerin**: Concurrent use may increase the risk for hypotension and orthostasis. Amitriptyline may reduce topical nitroglycerin absorption.
- **Nitroprusside**: Concurrent use may increase the risk for hypotension and orthostasis.
- **Nonsteroidal Anti-Inflammatory Drugs** (NSAIDS; eg, **carprofen**, **meloxicam**, **robenacoxib**): Concurrent use may increase the risk for bleeding. Use cautiously, especially in animals with other risk factors
- **Octreotide**: Concurrent use may increase the risk for serotonin syndrome, QT interval prolongation, and torsade de pointes. Avoid combination.
- **Opioids** (eg, **buprenorphine**, **butorphanol**, **fentanyl**, **methadone, morphine**): Concurrent use may increase the risk for constipation, urinary retention, CNS depression, respiratory depression, and serotonin syndrome.
- **Pergolide**: Concurrent use may increase the risk for CNS depression.
- **Phenothiazines** (eg, **acepromazine**, **chlorpromazine**): Concurrent use may increase concentrations of either drug, increasing the risk for CNS depression, hypotension, prolongation of the QT interval, constipation, ileus, urinary retention, and anticholinergic intoxication syndrome.
- **Phenoxybenzamine:** Concurrent use may increase the risk for hypotension and orthostasis.
- **Physostigmine:** Amitriptyline may negate the clinical effects of physostigmine
- **Potassium Chloride**: Concurrent use of oral, solid dosage forms of potassium chloride may increase the risk for upper GI injury. Combination is contraindicated.
- **Pregabalin**: Concurrent use may increase the risk for CNS depression.
- **Primidone/Phenobarbital:** Concurrent use may antagonize the anticonvulsant effects of primidone. Primidone may decrease amitriptyline concentration by inducing hepatic metabolism. CNS and respiratory depressant effects may be additive.
- **QT Prolonging Agents** (eg, **cisapride**, **procainamide**, **quinidine**, **sotalol**): Concurrent use may increase the risk for QT interval prolongation, cardiac arrhythmias, torsade de pointes, and death. May potentiate anticholinergic effects of some agents (eg, **quinidine**). Avoid concurrent use.
- **Rifampin**: Concurrent use may decrease amitriptyline concentrations by inducing hepatic metabolism.
- **Selective Serotonin Reuptake Inhibitors** (SSRIs; eg, **fluoxetine**, **paroxetine**, **sertraline**): Concurrent use may increase amitriptyline concentrations and increase the risk for serotonin syndrome. NOTE: SSRIs and TCAs (eg, **amitriptyline**) are often used together in veterinary behavior medicine, but enhanced monitoring for adverse effects is suggested.
- **Serotonin Receptor Antagonists** (eg, **dolasetron**, **ondansetron**): Concurrent use may increase the risk for serotonin syndrome, QT interval prolongation, and torsade de pointes.
- **Sulfamethoxazole/Trimethoprim:** Concurrent use may increase the risk for QT interval prolongation, torsade de pointes, and death.
- **Sulfonylureas** (eg, **glimepiride**, **glipizide**, **glyburide**): Concurrent use may increase hypoglycemia effects by an undetermined mechanism.
- **Sympathomimetic Agents** (eg, **phenylpropanolamine**): Concurrent use may increase the risk for hypertension, arrhythmias, tachycardia, and fever.
- **Tamsulosin:** Concurrent use may increase the risk for hypotension and orthostasis.
- **Terbinafine**: Concurrent use may increase amitriptyline concentrations. Interaction may persist for weeks following discontinuation of terbinafine. Avoid combination.
- **Thyroid Agents** (eg, **levothyroxine**): Concurrent use may potentiate effects of both drugs and may increase the risk for tachycardia, hypothyroidism, and thyrotoxicosis.
- **Tramadol**: Increased risk for serotonin syndrome; veterinary clinical significance is not known, but one source states that TCAs should not be administered concurrently with tramadol.[27,28]
- **Trazodone**: Concurrent use may increase the risk for constipation, ileus, urinary retention, CNS depression, serotonin syndrome, and anticholinergic intoxication syndrome. Avoid combination.
- **Vasopressors** (eg, **ephedrine**, **epinephrine**, **norepinephrine**, **vasopressin**): Concurrent use may increase the risk for hypertension, tremors, QT prolongation, cardiac dysrhythmias, and death. Avoid concurrent use except in emergency cases.
- **Warfarin**: Concurrent use may increase or decrease anticoagulant effects of warfarin.
- **Yohimbine**: Concurrent use may enhance the pressor effects of yohimbine by inhibiting reuptake of norepinephrine. Avoid combination.
- **Zonisamide**: Concurrent use may increase the risk for CNS depression and drowsiness

Laboratory Considerations

- **Metyrapone:** The response to metyrapone may be decreased by amitriptyline.
- **Blood glucose:** Tricyclics may alter (ie, increase or decrease) blood glucose levels.

Dosages

NOTE: Several weeks of therapy may be needed to see maximal effects. If discontinuing, taper the drug off slowly over 2 to 3 weeks, although more rapid taper can be undertaken when significant TCA toxicity is present.

DOGS:

Adjunctive treatment (with behavior modification and anxiolytics if required) of anxiety disorders (extra-label): Initially, 1 – 2 mg/kg PO every 12 hours for 2 to 4 weeks. May gradually increase dose by 1 mg/kg as tolerated to a maximum of 4 mg/kg PO twice daily

Adjunctive treatment of pruritus (after other more conventional therapies have failed) (extra-label): 1 – 2.2 mg/kg PO every 12 hours; ≈33% of dogs responded[1,29]

Adjunctive treatment of chronic (especially neuropathic) pain (extra-label): 1 – 2 mg/kg PO every 12 hours.[4] Doses up to 3 – 4 mg/kg PO every 12 hours may be tried.[25] If discontinuing, taper the drug slowly over 2 to 3 weeks.

CATS:

Clinical signs related to idiopathic cystitis (extra-label): 2.5 – 12.5 mg/cat (NOT mg/kg) PO once daily at night or

0.5 – 1 mg/kg PO once daily at night.[20,30] Neither 5 mg/cat[5] (NOT mg/kg) nor 10 mg/cat[6] (NOT mg/kg) once daily for 7 days reduced short-term lower urinary tract disease signs (eg, hematuria, pollakiuria).

Adjunctive treatment of behavior disorders amenable to tricyclics (anxiety, fear, adjunct in self-harm behaviors) (extra-label): 0.5 – 1.5 mg/kg PO every 24 hours.[31] Start at the lower end of the dosing range and gradually increase as tolerated. If discontinuing, gradually taper off the dosage.

Adjunctive treatment of pruritus (after other more conventional therapies have failed) (extra-label): 2.5 – 12.5 mg/cat (NOT mg/kg) PO once daily or 2.5 – 7.5 mg/cat (NOT mg/kg) twice daily.[32] To minimize adverse effects, start at the low end of the dosing range (2.5 mg/cat [NOT mg/kg] once daily) and gradually increase as tolerated. The drug may need to be compounded to give an accurate dose and to improve palatability (fish or cod liver oil).

Adjunctive treatment of chronic pain, including neuropathic (extra-label): 2.5 – 12.5 mg/cat (NOT mg/kg) PO once daily or 1 – 4 mg/kg PO every 12 to 24 hours[33]

BIRDS:

Adjunctive treatment of feather plucking (extra-label): 1 – 2 mg/kg PO every 12 to 24 hours.[7] Anecdotal reports indicate some usefulness. Barring adverse effects, a more prolonged course of therapy may be necessary to determine efficacy.[34] A pharmacokinetic study suggested doses up to 9 mg/kg may be necessary, although adverse effects are possible in some birds.[16]

Monitoring

- Clinical efficacy
- Adverse effects
- Baseline CBC, serum chemistry profile, urinalysis, and baseline thyroid testing[21,35] (eg, tT4, thyroid panel) prior to therapy, 1 month after initial therapy, and yearly thereafter
- Baseline ECG is recommended prior to therapy. Tricyclics can widen QRS complexes, prolong PR intervals, and invert or flatten T-waves on ECG; significance in animals is not fully understood.

Client Information

- This medication should be given with food.
- It can take several days to weeks to determine if the drug is effective.
- Consult your veterinarian before discontinuing this medication; do not stop suddenly.
- The most common side effects are drowsiness (sleepiness), dry mouth, and constipation; be sure your animal has access to water.
- Contact your veterinarian immediately if you see serious (rare) side effects like abnormal bleeding, fever, seizures, and/or very fast or irregular heart rate.
- Overdoses can be very serious; keep this medicine out of reach of animals and children.
- Tell your veterinarian if your animal has worn a flea and tick collar containing amitraz in the past 2 weeks.

Chemistry/Synonyms

Amitriptyline HCl, a tricyclic dibenzocycloheptene-derivative antidepressant, occurs as a white or practically white, odorless or practically odorless crystalline powder that is freely soluble in water or alcohol. It has a bitter, burning taste and a pK_a of 9.4.

Pharmaceutical dosage forms contain amitriptyline hydrochloride and express potency as amitriptyline base.

Amitriptyline may also be known as amitriptylini hydrochloridum; many trade names are available.

Storage/Stability

Amitriptyline tablets should be stored at room temperature.

Compatibility/Compounding Considerations

No specific information is noted. Transdermal (PLO-gel based) absorption is poor in cats.[10]

Dosage Forms/Regulatory Status

VETERINARY-LABELED PRODUCTS: NONE

The Association of Racing Commissioners International (ARCI) has designated this drug as a class 2 substance. Use of this drug may not be allowed in certain animal competitions. Check rules and regulations before entering in a competition while this medication is being administered. Contact local racing authorities for further guidance. See the *Appendix* for more information.

HUMAN-LABELED PRODUCTS:

Amitriptyline HCl Tablets: 10 mg, 25 mg, 50 mg, 75 mg, 100 mg, and 150 mg; generic; (Rx)

References

For the complete list of references, see **wiley.com/go/budde/plumb**

Amlodipine

(am-**loe**-**di**-peen) *Norvasc®, Amodip®*

Calcium-Channel Blocker

Prescriber Highlights

- ► Dihydropyridine calcium-channel blocker often used for treatment of systemic arterial hypertension
- ► Caution should be used in patients with heart disease and hepatic dysfunction
- ► Potential to cause anorexia and hypotension in cats, especially early in therapy
- ► Gingival hyperplasia has been reported as a long-term adverse effect in dogs; may occur rarely in cats.

Uses/Indications

Oral amlodipine is used to treat systemic hypertension in dogs and cats and is considered the drug of choice for managing hypertension.[1-3] Hypertension in small animals is typically secondary to other diseases (eg, acute or chronic kidney disease, hyperthyroidism, hyperadrenocorticism) and is most often seen in middle-aged or geriatric cats and dogs.

Systemic activation of the renin-angiotensin-aldosterone system (RAAS) does not appear to be a major contributor of hypertension in cats with chronic kidney disease.[1] Cats are often presented with acute clinical signs (eg, blindness, seizures, collapse, disorientation, paresis/paralysis). Dogs and cats are considered hypertensive if repeated systolic blood pressure measurements exceed 160 mm Hg or if a single elevated blood pressure measurement is present in the setting of target organ damage (eg, eyes, heart, brain, kidneys). Antihypertensive therapy may improve ophthalmic lesions and restore vision in a minority of patients with blindness secondary to hypertension.[4] Amlodipine has been shown to significantly increase plasma renin activity in cats that are azotemic and hypertensive, which is a similar response to that seen in human studies.[5] Target systolic blood pressure values of less than 140 to 150 mm Hg[1,2] are recommended to minimize target organ damage from hypertension. Amlodipine has not been shown to reduce mortality in hypertensive cats.[2,5,6] In one study evaluating hypertensive cats treated with amlodipine 0.125 – 0.5 mg/kg for 28 days, the mean decrease in systolic blood pressure was 28 mm Hg,[7] but even larger blood pressure reduction (49 mm Hg) has been reported.[6]

In dogs, amlodipine therapy is typically initiated after a RAAS inhibitor (eg, ACE-inhibitor, angiotensin-receptor blocker) because of the high prevalence of chronic kidney disease in hypertensive dogs.[2] In one study of hypertensive dogs, secondary to acute kidney injury, amlodipine therapy at a median dose of 0.38 mg/kg/day was associated with a decrease in systolic blood pressure of 24 mm Hg and correction of severe systemic hypertension in 10 of 11 dogs within 24 hours.[8] In a retrospective review of dogs with severe hypertension, dogs treated with amlodipine for 1 week had a reduction in blood pressure of 18 mm Hg, as compared with 29 mm Hg when treated with telmisartan and 46 mm Hg when treated with a combination of amlodipine and telmisartan.[9] In a small case series (n = 5 dogs), dogs with an average pretreatment systolic arterial blood pressure (SBP) of 215 mm Hg had their SBP reduced to 180 mm Hg when treated with a combination of amlodipine and benazepril, but SBP was reduced to 142 mm Hg when treatment was changed to amlodipine and telmisartan.[10]

Pharmacology/Actions

Amlodipine is a dihydropyridine L-type calcium-channel blocker, which inhibits voltage-gated calcium channels in cardiac and vascular smooth muscle. Amlodipine has a higher affinity for L-type calcium channels and some affinity for T-type calcium channels. In the kidney, L-type calcium channels are found primarily in afferent (prerenal) arterioles. Amlodipine has a greater effect on vascular smooth muscle, where it acts as a peripheral arteriolar vasodilator and reduces afterload. Amlodipine slightly depresses impulse formation (automaticity) and conduction velocity in cardiac muscle. Amlodipine has mild diuretic activity after an initial dose in dogs.[11,12] Amlodipine has been shown to activate the RAAS when used alone in healthy dogs at higher dosages (0.57 mg/kg twice daily).[13] Use of amlodipine with an ACE inhibitor partially blocks this effect.[13,14]

In client-owned cats with systemic hypertension treated with amlodipine as the sole antihypertensive agent (in combination with a phosphate-restricted diet if azotemic), a significant decline in UPC (urine protein:creatinine) was found in cats treated with amlodipine.[15]

Pharmacokinetics

In cats, amlodipine volume of distribution is ≈10 L/kg. In vitro protein binding in cat plasma is 97%. In healthy cats, plasma concentrations approach steady-state by 2 weeks at 0.125 mg/kg/day. Total plasma clearance is estimated to be 2.3 mL/minute/kg. Amlodipine is extensively metabolized by the liver, and elimination half-life is 53 hours.[16] In cats, effects on systemic blood pressure are usually seen within 4 hours of administration and may persist for an additional ≈30 hours.[17]

In dogs, amlodipine bioavailability is 88% after oral administration, with peak concentration occurring at 4 to 6 hours. Amlodipine is widely distributed (volume of distribution, 25 L/kg) and extensively metabolized. Reported elimination half-life ranges from 7 to 30 hours.[18,19]

In humans, amlodipine's bioavailability does not appear to be altered by the presence of food in the gut. The drug is slowly but almost completely absorbed after oral administration and is reported to be absorbed after rectal administration. In humans, peak plasma concentrations occur between 6 and 9 hours after administration and effects on blood pressure are correspondingly delayed. Amlodipine has high plasma protein-binding characteristics (≈93%). However, drug interactions associated with potential displacement from these sites have not been elucidated. Amlodipine is slowly but extensively metabolized to inactive compounds in the liver. Terminal plasma half-life is ≈35 hours in healthy humans but is prolonged in the elderly and in those patients with hypertension or hepatic dysfunction.

Contraindications/Precautions/Warnings

Amlodipine is contraindicated in patients hypersensitive to it, in shock, with documented hypotension, with severe aortic stenosis (due to an inability to increase stroke volume in response to peripheral vasodilation), or with severe hepatic failure. It should also be used cautiously in patients that are at risk for developing hypotension or patients with hepatic disease. Amlodipine use for pulmonary hypertension in dogs is not recommended, as systemic hypotension can occur without substantive improvements in pulmonary arterial pressures.[20]

There is concern that using amlodipine alone for treating hypertension with renal disease may expose glomeruli to higher pressures secondary to efferent arteriolar constriction, which is caused by localized increases in renin-angiotensin-aldosterone (RAAS) activity, allowing progressive damage to glomeruli. It is postulated that using an ACE inhibitor with amlodipine may help prevent this occurrence.[21] The concurrent use of ACE inhibitors with amlodipine in animals with chronic kidney disease and hypertension is routine, though evidence supporting this approach is lacking. Notably, treatment of hypertension in cats with amlodipine as a sole antihypertensive agent appeared to limit proteinuria, which led to improved survival.[15]

Adverse Effects

In a placebo-controlled study in hypertensive cats, the adverse effect profile for amlodipine-treated cats (eg, emesis, inappetence, diarrhea, lethargy, dehydration) was similar to placebo.[7] Hypotension and bradycardia are possible; however, because of amlodipine's relatively slow onset of action, these effects are usually absent in cats. Cats may infrequently develop azotemia, hypokalemia, reflex tachycardia, and weight loss. Gingival hyperplasia is also possible but occurs only rarely.[16]

Dogs may also experience inappetence, lethargy, and hypotension. Reversible gingival hyperplasia has been reported when amlodipine has been administered long term in dogs; incidence in the retrospective study was 8.5%.[22] Diffuse peripheral edema has been reported in dogs and this may or may not respond to medical treatment and discontinuation of amlodipine.[23]

Headache and peripheral edema are common side effects in humans taking amlodipine.

Reproductive/Nursing Safety

The UK-approved feline tablet product label states *the safety of amlodipine has not been established during pregnancy or lactation in cats.* Although no evidence of impaired fertility was noted in rats given 8 times the maximum human daily dose, amlodipine has been shown to be fetotoxic (ie, intrauterine death rates increased five-fold) in laboratory animals (eg, rats, rabbits) at very high doses.[24] No evidence of teratogenicity or mutagenicity was observed in laboratory animal studies. Amlodipine can prolong labor in rats.

Amlodipine enters maternal milk in small amounts.

Because safety has not been established in animals, this drug should only be used when the maternal benefits outweigh the potential risks to offspring.

Overdose/Acute Toxicity

Limited experience with other calcium-channel blockers in humans has shown that an overdose of amlodipine may result in profound hypotension and reflex tachycardia.[24] From 2009 to 2013, 578 dogs and 140 cats with single agent exposures to amlodipine were reported to the ASPCA Animal Poison Control Center; 19% of dogs and 22% of cats showed clinical signs (see ***Table***).

	DOGS	CATS
Total number reported	578	140
Number showing clinical signs	108 (19%)	31 (22%)
Hypotension	32%	23%
Tachycardia	39%	23%
Hypertension	13%	23%
Lethargy	26%	13%
Vomiting	18%	not reported

Other possible clinical signs in dogs are respiratory problems (including pulmonary edema), bradycardia, depression, hyperglycemia, and cardiac arrhythmias.[12] Rare clinical signs include azotemia, hypokalemia, hyponatremia, hyperkalemia, acidosis, tremors/fasciculations, and seizures.

The following treatments are recommended for patients with different levels of toxicosis:

- For massive overdoses, treat early with gut decontamination, crystalloid fluids, IV calcium, and supportive treatment.
- For subclinical patients exposed within 2 hours, gut decontamination strategies (eg, induction of emesis, gastric lavage, activated charcoal administration) should be considered.
- For stable, clinical patients, gastric lavage or activated charcoal should be considered; induction of emesis is contraindicated.
- For unstable, clinical patients, first stabilize the patient before gut decontamination strategies are attempted.

Intravenous fluid therapy, IV calcium, vasopressors, and atropine are considered first-line therapies, as is high-dose insulin euglycemic therapy, for patients showing clinical signs associated with an amlodipine overdose.[12] Additional interventions may include beta-agonists, IV lipid emulsion therapy,[25] glucagon, and/or a temporary pacemaker.[12] Close monitoring of the cardiovascular system (eg, blood pressure, ECG), respiratory system (eg, rate and character), nervous system (eg, mental status), electrolytes, and blood chemistry should be implemented 12 to 24 hours or longer following exposure.[12]

For patients that have experienced or are suspected to have experienced an overdose, consultation with a 24-hour poison consultation center specializing in providing veterinary-specific information is recommended. For general information related to overdose and toxin exposures, as well as contact information for poison control centers, refer to *Appendix*.

Drug Interactions

The following drug interactions have either been reported or are theoretical in humans or animals receiving amlodipine and may be of significance in veterinary patients. Unless otherwise noted, use together is not necessarily contraindicated, but the potential risks must be weighed, and additional monitoring performed when appropriate.

- **Beta-Adrenergic Receptor Antagonists** (eg, **atenolol, propranolol**): Concurrent use may reduce blood pressure, heart rate and contractility, particularly in animals with ventricular dysfunction.[16]
- **Calcium Channel Blockers, Other** (eg, **diltiazem**): Concurrent use may reduce blood pressure, heart rate and contractility, particularly in animals with ventricular dysfunction.[16]
- **Clopidogrel**: Amlodipine may decrease the antithrombotic effect of clopidogrel.
- **Cyclosporine**: Amlodipine may increase cyclosporine concentrations.
- **CYP3A4 Strong Inhibitors** (eg, **ketoconazole, itraconazole**): Amlodipine concentrations may be increased.
- **CYP3A4 Inducers** (eg, **rifampin**): Amlodipine concentrations may be decreased.
- **Tacrolimus:** Amlodipine may increase tacrolimus concentrations.
- **Hypotensive Agents** (eg, **enalapril, telmisartan**): Although antihypertensive combinations are commonly used to manage hypertension, they may have additive blood pressure lowering effects when used with amlodipine.

Laboratory Considerations

- No specific concerns noted.

Dosages

DOGS:

Adjunctive treatment of systemic hypertension and as an afterload reducer for refractory heart failure (extra-label): 0.1 – 0.25 mg/kg PO every 24 hours[2,26]; should begin at the low end of the dose range. In dogs, amlodipine is generally added after ACE-inhibitor (eg, benazepril) therapy has been initiated.

Hypertensive Emergency (extra-label): 0.2 - 0.4 mg/kg PO every 24 hours.[2] Doses of up to 0.6 mg/kg PO every 24 hours may used, but close monitoring is warranted.

CATS:

Systemic hypertension (extra-label):

a) 0.625 – 1.25 mg/cat (ie, ¼ – ½ of a 2.5 mg tablet/cat; NOT mg/kg) PO once daily. Therapy should be initiated with a lower dose (0.625 mg/cat [NOT mg/kg]) and blood pressure rechecked in 1 to 3 weeks; the dose can be doubled[1,7] (up to 2.5 mg/cat [NOT mg/kg] PO once daily maximum) if owner compliance is confirmed and blood pressure remains elevated (see ***Monitoring***). It has been suggested that higher doses (1.25 mg/cat [NOT mg/kg]) can be beneficial if systolic blood pressure is greater than 200 mm Hg and potassium plasma concentrations are low.[27] In cats with proteinuria, an ACE inhibitor (eg, benazepril) can be added.[1,2]

b) 0.125 – 0.25 mg/kg PO daily.[16] After 14 days of treatment, the dose may be doubled or increased up to 0.5 mg/kg once daily if adequate clinical response has not been achieved (eg, systolic blood pressure remaining over 150 mm Hg or a decrease of less than 15% from the pretreatment measurement).

Hypertensive Emergency (extra-label): 0.2 - 0.4 mg/kg PO every 24 hours.[2] Dosage up to 0.6 mg/kg PO every 24 hours may used, but close monitoring is warranted.

BIRDS:

Systemic hypertension (extra-label): Initially, 0.4 mg/kg PO every 24 hours[28]; increased dose or frequency may be needed.

Monitoring

- Blood pressure. A general guideline for treating hypertension is to maintain systolic blood pressure below 160 mm Hg, with a long-term goal of maintaining a systolic blood pressure less than 150 mm Hg to minimize the risk for target organ damage.[1] In cats without evidence of target organ damage, blood pressure should be reassessed every 1 to 3 weeks, with evaluation of clinical signs for target organ damage, until an adequate response is seen.[1] If the response is inadequate, dose increases are typically made at intervals of 7 days or more.[1] In cats with evidence of target organ damage at the time of diagnosis or cats with systolic blood pressure greater than 200 mm Hg, it is recommended to closely monitor the cat for the first 24 to 72 hours after initiation of therapy.[1] Dose adjustments can be made sooner than 7 days if systolic blood pressure remains above 200 mm Hg or if there is ongoing target organ damage.[1] If the response to amlodipine is inadequate, or if there is additional disease present (eg, persistent proteinuria), treatment with a secondary antihypertensive agent (eg, telmisartan or an ACE inhibitor) may be warranted in addition to amlodipine.[1] Once systolic blood pressure is controlled, patient reevaluation (including blood pressure and clinical signs of target organ damage) should occur at least every 3 months.[1] Although the preceding approach applies to cats, a comparable approach is considered for most dogs with systemic hypertension.[2]
- Fundic examination to monitor for retinal hemorrhage or retinal detachment
- Echocardiogram and/or thoracic radiographs to assess for target organ damage (ie, ventricular remodeling and/or cardiac enlargement caused by hypertension)

- Serum renal chemistry profile (BUN, creatinine), SDMA, and urine protein:creatinine should be monitored every 3 to 4 months in dogs and cats receiving amlodipine or more frequently if clinically indicated. As chronic kidney disease is a common condition underlying hypertension, monitoring renal function and proteinuria during antihypertensive therapy is appropriate. Serum potassium concentrations should also be evaluated periodically, again related to potential presence of chronic kidney disease.

Client Information

- Amlodipine may be given with or without food.
- Do not skip doses, as this may result in poor blood pressure control and organ damage.
- Side effects are not common but can include reduced appetite and low energy level, especially early in treatment. Overgrowth of the gums can occur, which is more common in dogs than cats.
- Amlodipine is typically a long-term medication and will require frequent follow-up veterinary visits. Once blood pressure is normalized and patients are feeling well, most cats and dogs are evaluated by their veterinarian every 3 to 4 months. Do not miss these important follow-up visits.

Chemistry/Synonyms

Amlodipine besylate, a dihydropyridine calcium channel-blocking agent, is a white crystalline powder that is slightly soluble in water and sparingly soluble in alcohol.

Amlodipine besylate may also appear as amlodipini besilas, UK-48340-26, or UK-48340-11 (amlodipine maleate); many trade names are available.

Storage/Stability

Store amlodipine tablets at 20°C to 25°C (68°F-77°F); excursions permitted to 15°C to 30°C (59°F-86°F) in tight, light-resistant containers. When splitting the UK-approved veterinary chewable tablets, the remaining portion should be returned to the blister packaging and discarded after 24 hours.[16]

Compatibility/Compounding Considerations

Compounded preparation stability: Amlodipine oral suspension compounded from commercially available tablets has been published.[29] Triturating six (6) amlodipine 5 mg tablets with 15 mL of *Ora-Plus*® and *qs ad* to 30 mL with *Ora-Sweet*® yields a 1 mg/mL oral suspension that retains more than 90% potency for 91 days stored at 5°C (41°F) and 25°C (77°F). Compounded preparations of amlodipine should be protected from light.

Amlodipine compounded into a topical PLO-based gel failed to control blood pressure in hypertensive cats.[30]

Dosage Forms/Regulatory Status

VETERINARY-LABELED PRODUCTS:

Amlodipine Chewable Tablets: 1.25 mg; *Amodip*® (available in the United Kingdom; not available in the United States); POM-V. Indicated for treatment of systemic hypertension in cats.

The Association of Racing Commissioners International (ARCI) has designated this drug as a class 4 substance. See the ***Appendix*** for more information. Use of this drug may not be allowed in certain animal competitions. Check rules and regulations before entering in a competition while this medication is being administered. Contact local racing authorities for further guidance.

HUMAN-LABELED PRODUCTS:

Amlodipine Oral Tablets: 2.5 mg, 5 mg, and 10 mg; *Norvasc*®, generic; (Rx)

Fixed-dose combination products with benazepril (*Lotrel*®) and atorvastatin (*Caduet*®) are available.

References

For the complete list of references, see **wiley.com/go/budde/plumb**

Ammonium Chloride

(ah-***moe***-nee-um)

Urinary-Acidifying Agent

Prescriber Highlights

- May be used for urinary acidification to treat and prevent struvite urolithiasis, to enhance renal excretion of some toxins (eg, strychnine), and to enhance the efficacy of certain antimicrobials when treating UTIs
- May also be used for ammonia tolerance testing in patients with normal baseline ammonia levels and without clinical signs of hepatic encephalopathy
- Contraindicated in patients with hepatic failure or uremia
- GI upset (nausea, vomiting, diarrhea) is the primary adverse effect of oral dosage forms.
- Urinary acidification may increase the risk for oxalate urolithiasis; metabolic acidosis can occur.
- Unpalatable; addition of sugar (not molasses) may improve palatability to goats and sheep.

Uses/Indications

Ammonium chloride can be used as an urinary-acidifying agent to help prevent and dissolve uroliths that form in alkaline urine (eg, struvite), to enhance renal excretion of some toxins (eg, strontium, strychnine) or drugs (eg, quinidine), or to enhance the efficacy of certain antimicrobials (eg, chlortetracycline, methenamine mandelate, nitrofurantoin, oxytetracycline, penicillin G, or tetracycline) when treating UTIs.

Feeding of acidifying commercial feline diets can successfully minimize struvite urolith formation,[1] and ammonium chloride can be considered for cats for whom these diets are not or cannot be fed.

Ammonium chloride is recommended to help prevent uroliths in small ruminants, but dietary changes can significantly affect the drug's efficacy for this purpose. When ammonium chloride is used continually, renal compensatory mechanisms may negate ammonium chloride's urinary pH-lowering effects, so pulse therapy may be more effective for these species.[2]

Ammonium chloride may also be used for ammonia tolerance testing in dogs and cats to test liver function.[3-5] See ***Contraindications/Precautions/Warnings.***

Pharmacology/Actions

The acidification properties of ammonium chloride are caused by its dissociation into chloride and ammonium ions in vivo. The ammonium cation is converted by the liver to urea with the release of a hydrogen ion. This ion combines with bicarbonate to form water and carbon dioxide. In the extracellular fluid, chloride ions combine with fixed bases and decrease the alkaline reserves in the body. The net effects are decreased serum bicarbonate levels and a decrease in blood and urine pH.

Excess chloride ions delivered to the kidney are not completely reabsorbed by the tubules and are excreted with cations (principally sodium) and water. This diuretic effect is usually compensated for in the kidneys after a few days of therapy.

Pharmacokinetics

No information was located on the pharmacokinetics of this agent in veterinary species. In humans, ammonium chloride is rapidly absorbed from the GI tract. The liver converts ammonium ions to urea, which is excreted in the urine.

Contraindications/Precautions/Warnings

Ammonium chloride is contraindicated in patients with severe hepatic disease or if the baseline ammonia measurement is elevated prior to ammonia tolerance testing, as ammonia may accumulate and cause toxicity (ie, hepatic encephalopathy).[6] In general, ammonium chloride should not be administered to uremic patients because it can intensify any existing metabolic acidosis in these patients. Additionally, ammonium chloride should not be used in patients with severe renal insufficiency that have metabolic alkalosis secondary to vomiting; sodium depletion can occur. In these cases, sodium chloride repletion, with or without ammonium chloride administration, should be performed to correct both sodium and chloride deficits.

Ammonium chloride is contraindicated in patients with urate or oxalate calculi or respiratory acidosis with high total CO_2 and buffer base. Ammonium chloride alone cannot correct hypochloremia with secondary metabolic alkalosis due to intracellular potassium chloride depletion; potassium chloride must be administered to these patients.

Use ammonium chloride with caution in patients with pulmonary insufficiency or cardiac edema.

A high roughage/concentrate ratio diet can decrease the urine pH, thus lowering the effect of ammonium chloride in horses.[7]

Adverse Effects

Development of metabolic acidosis (sometimes severe) can occur during or after treatment with ammonium chloride. Gastric irritation, nausea, and vomiting may be associated with oral dosing of the drug. Urinary acidification is associated with an increased risk for calcium oxalate urolith formation.

Reproductive/Nursing Safety

Ammonium chloride does not appear to cross the placenta, but large doses may result in metabolic acidosis in the dam and offspring. In humans, the drug is considered compatible for use during pregnancy and is likely compatible during lactation.[8] Because safety has not been established in animals, this drug should only be used when the maternal benefits outweigh the potential risks to offspring.

Overdose/Acute Toxicity

Clinical signs of overdose may include nausea, vomiting, excessive thirst, hyperventilation, bradycardias or other arrhythmias, and progressive CNS depression. Profound metabolic acidosis and hypokalemia may be noted on laboratory results.

Treatment should consist of correcting the metabolic acidosis by administering sodium bicarbonate or sodium acetate IV. Hypokalemia should be treated using a suitable potassium product; frequent acid-base and electrolyte monitoring should be performed until the patient is stable.

For patients that have experienced or are suspected to have experienced an overdose, consultation with a 24-hour poison consultation center specializing in providing veterinary-specific information is recommended. For general information related to overdose and toxin exposures, as well as contact information for poison control centers, refer to *Appendix*.

Drug Interactions

The following drug interactions have either been reported or are theoretical in humans or animals receiving ammonium chloride and may be of significance in veterinary patients. Unless otherwise noted, use together is not necessarily contraindicated, but weigh the potential risks and perform additional monitoring when appropriate.

- **Aluminum Hydroxide:** Avoid frequent use with ammonium chloride as urine acidification could be negated.
- **Aminoglycosides** (eg, **gentamicin**): Aminoglycoside antibiotics are more effective in an alkaline medium; urine acidification may diminish the effectiveness of these drugs in treating bacterial UTIs.
- **Aspirin:** Increased risk for salicylate toxicity as acidic urine can decrease the urinary excretion of salicylate.
- **Carbonic Anhydrase Inhibitors** (CAIs; eg, **acetazolamide, dichlorphenamide, methazolamide**): Concurrent use with ammonium chloride may increase risk for hyperchloremia and metabolic acidosis.
- **Erythromycin:** Erythromycin is more effective in an alkaline medium; urine acidification may diminish the effectiveness of this drug in treating bacterial UTIs.
- **Methadone:** Ammonium chloride may decrease methadone efficacy.
- **Quinidine:** Urine acidification caused by ammonium chloride may increase renal excretion of quinidine.

Dosages

DOGS:

Urine acidification (extra-label):

a. 20 mg/kg PO every 8 hours[9]
b. **Adjunctive toxicosis management:** 100 mg/kg PO every 12 hours[10]

Ammonia tolerance testing (extra-label): Patient must be fasted 12 hours prior to ammonia tolerance testing. Prior to beginning this test, measure a baseline ammonia level. **NOTE**: Special handling is required for accurate analysis of ammonia in blood samples. If the ammonia level is elevated, the patient has already failed the test; do not proceed with the administration of ammonium chloride, as this can result in profound hepatic encephalopathy. To complete the test, 2 options are available:

a. Administer 2 mL/kg of a 5% solution of ammonium chloride deep in the rectum. Measure serum ammonia concentrations at 20 minutes and 40 minutes post ammonium chloride administration.[4,5]
b. Oral challenge can be performed by administering ammonium chloride 100 mg/kg (maximum dose = 3 g) PO either in solution (dissolved in 20 to 50 mL warm water) or in gelatin capsules. Measure serum ammonia concentration at 30 minutes post ammonium chloride administration.

CATS:

Urine acidification (extra-label): 20 mg/kg PO every 12 hours[9,11]

Ammonia tolerance testing (extra-label): Patient must be fasted prior to ammonia tolerance testing. Prior to beginning this test, measure a baseline ammonia level. **NOTE**: Special handling is required for accurate analysis of ammonia in blood samples. If the ammonia level is elevated, the patient has already failed the test; do not proceed with the administration of ammonium chloride, as this can make the patient profoundly hepatic encephalopathy. To complete the test, 2 options are available:

a. Administer 2 mL/kg of a 5% solution of ammonium chloride deep in the rectum. Measure serum ammonia concentrations at 20 minutes and 40 minutes post ammonium chloride administration.
b. Oral challenge can be performed by administering with ammonium chloride 100 mg/kg (maximum dose = 3 grams) PO either in solution (dissolved in 20 to 50 mL warm water) or in gelatin capsules. Measure serum ammonia concentration at 30 minutes post ammonium chloride administration.

HORSES:

Urine acidification (extra-label): 100 mg/kg PO twice daily.[12] Ammonium salts are unpalatable and will have to be dosed via stomach tube or dosing syringe.

Urinary acidifier to enhance renal excretion of strychnine (extra-label): 132 mg/kg PO[13]

SHEEP/GOATS:

Urolithiasis prevention (extra-label):

a. 200 – 300 mg/kg PO twice daily for 3 days and then off for 4 days; continue 7-day recurring cycles. Start dose at 200 mg/kg, and increase dose until urine pH is less than 6.5.[2]
b. 450 mg/kg (2.25% of dry matter intake) PO daily maintained urine pH less than 6.5 in a study of goats.[14] Animals were fed orchard grass diet.
c. Of the daily dry matter, 0.5% to 1% will acidify urine but can be unpalatable. Table sugar (not molasses) may improve palatability.[15,16]

Monitoring

When using ammonium chloride as part of ammonia tolerance testing, be sure to record a baseline serum ammonia concentration prior to administration. If baseline ammonia is elevated, ammonia tolerance testing should not be done. See ***Contraindications/Precautions/Warnings.***

- Urine pH of less than or equal to 6.5 is the recommended goal of therapy
- Blood pH if there are clinical signs of toxicity or evidence of acid-base disturbance
- Clinical signs associated with ammonia toxicity (eg, hepatic encephalopathy)

When used to acidify the urine for the treatment of toxicosis[10]:

- Urine pH: baseline then hourly until treatment is complete
- Serum sodium and potassium: baseline then every 1 to 2 hours until treatment is complete
- Blood pressure: baseline then periodic as needed for patient's condition

Client Information

- Contact your veterinarian if your animal exhibits signs of nausea (may appear as excessive drooling, poor appetite), vomiting, excessive thirst, hyperventilation, progressive lethargy, or weakness.
- For this medication to work, give it exactly as your veterinarian has prescribed.
- Granules have a bitter taste. Mixing the medicine with food or giving the medicine with a dosing syringe may be helpful patients.
- While your animal is taking this medication, it is important to return to your veterinarian for all recommended examinations. Do not miss these important follow-up visits.

Chemistry/Synonyms

An acid-forming salt, ammonium chloride occurs as colorless crystals or as a fine or coarse white crystalline powder. It is somewhat hygroscopic and has a cool, saline taste. When dissolved in water, the temperature of the solution is decreased. One gram is soluble in ≈3 mL of water at room temperature and 1.4 mL at 100°C (212°F). One gram is soluble in ≈100 mL of alcohol.

One gram of ammonium chloride contains 18.7 mEq of ammonium and chloride ions. The commercially available concentrate for injection (26.75%) contains 5 mEq of each ion per mL and contains disodium edetate as a stabilizing agent. The pH of the concentrate for injection is ≈5.

Ammonium chloride may also be known as muriate of ammonia and sal ammoniac.

Storage/Stability

Ammonium chloride powder should be stored at room temperature, protected from moisture and light and with adequate ventilation.[17]

Compatibility/Compounding Considerations

Ammonium chloride should not be titrated with strong oxidizing agents (eg, potassium chlorate) as explosive compounds may result.

Compatibility is dependent on factors such as pH, concentration, temperature, and diluent used; specialized references or a hospital pharmacist should be consulted for more specific information.

Dose Forms/Regulatory Status

VETERINARY-LABELED PRODUCTS:

NOTE: The following may not be FDA-approved products, as they are marketed for veterinary use but not located in the FDA Green Book.

Ammonium Chloride Solution: 20% (200 mg/mL) solution in 60 mL bottles; *Fus-Sol*® (OTC). Also contains dl-Methionine and unspecified B vitamins.

Ammonium Chloride Solution: 2% (20 mg/mL) in 1 L, 2.5 L, and 20 L bottles; generic; (OTC). (Also contains potassium iodide 2%)

When used in large animals, feed-grade ammonium chloride powder can be obtained from feed mills (OTC).

HUMAN-LABELED PRODUCTS: NONE

References

For the complete list of references, see **wiley.com/go/budde/plumb**

Amoxicillin

(a-mox-i-***sill***-in) *Amoxi-Tabs*®, *Amoxi-Drops*®, *Bimox*®

Aminopenicillin

Prescriber Highlights

- ▶ Bactericidal aminopenicillin with the same spectrum as ampicillin; ineffective against bacteria that produce beta-lactamase
- ▶ Most common adverse effects are GI-related, but hypersensitivity and other adverse effects can occur (rare).

Uses/Indications

Amoxicillin is FDA-approved for oral use in dogs and cats to treat infections caused by many gram-positive and gram-negative bacteria (see ***Pharmacology/Actions***) and for intra-mammary infusion for the treatment of bovine mastitis in lactating cows. The drug also has been used in an extra-label fashion to treat a wide range of bacterial infections in other species. Amoxicillin is an effective first choice for bacterial cystitis, streptococcal infections, and other infections caused by non-beta-lactamase–producing bacteria. It is commonly used in treatment protocols for *Helicobacter* spp gastric infections in a variety of species. Amoxicillin/clavulanate is often used in small animals because of its enhanced efficacy against many beta-lactamase–producing bacteria. Amoxicillin may also be combined with an antibiotic that has greater gram-negative activity (eg, fluoroquinolones) for broad-spectrum empirical coverage.

The World Health Organization has designated amoxicillin as a Critically Important, High Priority antimicrobial for human medicine.[1] The Office International des Epizooties (OIE) has designated amoxicillin as a Veterinary Critically Important Antimicrobial (VCIA) Agent in avian, bovine, caprine, equine, ovine, and swine species.[2]

Pharmacology/Actions

Amoxicillin is a time-dependent, bactericidal agent that acts by inhibiting cell wall synthesis. Amoxicillin generally shares the same spectrum of activity and uses as ampicillin, although there may be slight differences in activity against certain organisms. Higher serum concentrations may be attained with amoxicillin as compared with ampicillin because amoxicillin is better absorbed orally (in nonruminants). Separate serum and urinary clinical breakpoints are available; ampicillin sensitivity is used to predict amoxicillin activity.

Penicillins are bactericidal against susceptible bacteria and act by inhibiting mucopeptide synthesis in the cell wall, which results in a defective barrier and an osmotically unstable spheroplast. The exact mechanism for this effect has not been definitively determined, but beta-lactam antibiotics have been shown to bind to several enzymes (eg, carboxypeptidases, transpeptidases, endopeptidases) in the bacterial cytoplasmic membrane involved with cell wall synthesis. Beta-lactam antibiotics have different affinities for these enzymes (ie, penicillin-binding proteins), which may help explain the difference in drug activity spectrums not explained by the influence of beta-lactam-ases. Like other beta-lactam antibiotics, penicillins are generally considered more effective against actively growing bacteria.

Aminopenicillins (ie, broad-spectrum or ampicillin penicillins) have increased activity against many strains of gram-negative aerobes not covered by natural penicillins or penicillinase-resistant penicillins, including some strains of *Escherichia coli, Klebsiella* spp, and *Haemophilus* spp. Like the natural penicillins, aminopenicillins are susceptible to inactivation by beta-lactamase–producing bacteria (eg, many *Staphylococcus* spp, *E coli*). Although not as active as natural penicillins, aminopenicillins have activity against many anaerobic bacteria, including clostridial organisms. Organisms that are generally not susceptible include *Pseudomonas aeruginosa, Serratia* spp, indole-positive *Proteus* spp (*Proteus mirabilis* is susceptible), *Enterobacter* spp, *Citrobacter* spp, and *Acinetobacter* spp. Aminopenicillins are ineffective against methicillin-resistant staphylococci and are inactive against mycobacteria, *Mycoplasma* spp, *Rickettsia* spp, fungi, protozoa, and viruses.

Potassium clavulanate, sulbactam, and tazobactam are beta-lactamase inhibitors that, when combined with penicillins, can extend the spectrum of those penicillins. These combinations are often effective against many beta-lactamase–producing strains of otherwise resistant *E coli, Pasteurella* spp, *Staphylococcus* spp, *Klebsiella* spp, and *Proteus* spp.

Pharmacokinetics

Amoxicillin trihydrate is stable in the presence of gastric acid. After oral administration, amoxicillin bioavailability is highly variable between species. Food will decrease the rate but not the extent of oral absorption and many clinicians suggest giving the drug with food, particularly if there is concomitant GI distress. In dogs, amoxicillin bioavailability was 64% to 77% following oral administration.[3] In cats, one study found the bioavailability to be ≈77%.[4] Amoxicillin serum concentrations will generally be 1.5 to 3 times greater than those of ampicillin after equivalent oral doses. In dogs following oral administration, maximum plasma concentrations of 11 to 21 µg/mL were reached after ≈1.38 to 2 hours.[3,5] In cats following a 10 mg/kg oral dose, maximum plasma concentrations of 5.89 µg/mL were reached in 1.69 hours.[4]

In sheep and goats, peak concentrations occurred ≈4.2 hours after IM administration.[6]

After absorption, the volume of distribution for amoxicillin is ≈0.28 to 0.71 L/kg in dogs[33] and 0.86 L/kg in cats.[4] The drug is widely distributed to most body tissues and fluids. When meninges are inflamed, amoxicillin will cross into the CSF in concentrations ranging from 10% to 60% of those found in serum. Very low concentrations of the drug are found in the aqueous humor; low concentrations are found in tears, sweat, and saliva. Protein binding in dogs is ≈13%.

Amoxicillin is eliminated primarily unchanged via renal mechanisms, principally by tubular secretion; however, some of the drug is metabolized by hydrolysis to penicilloic acids (inactive) and then excreted in the urine. Elimination half-lives of amoxicillin have been reported to be 0.91 to 1.52 hours in dogs[7,8] and ≈1.25 hours in cats.[4] Clearance in cats is reportedly 0.45 L/hour/kg.[4] In cats with azotemic chronic kidney disease given amoxicillin-clavulanic acid, amoxicillin concentration was significantly lower in the urine and somewhat higher in serum when compared to cats without kidney disease.[9]

After IM administration, the elimination half-life is 4.7 hours in sheep and 6.9 hours in goats.[6]

Milk yield had no effect on amoxicillin pharmacokinetic parameters after intramammary administration in dairy cows.[10]

Contraindications/Precautions/Warnings

Penicillins are contraindicated in patients with a history of hypersensitivity to them. Penicillins should be used cautiously in patients with a documented hypersensitivity to other beta-lactam antibiotics (eg, cephalosporins, cephamycins, carbapenems), as there may be cross-reactivity.

Systemic antibiotics should not be administered orally to patients with septicemia, shock, or other grave illnesses, as absorption of the medication from the GI tract may be significantly delayed or diminished. Parenteral—preferably IV—routes should be used for these cases.

Oral beta-lactam antibiotics and macrolides should not be administered to rabbits, guinea pigs, chinchillas, hamsters, or other small mammals, as severe enteritis and clostridial enterotoxemia may occur.

Adverse Effects

Adverse effects caused by penicillins are not typically serious and have a relatively low frequency of occurrence.

Hypersensitivity reactions unrelated to dose can occur with these agents and can manifest as rashes (including severe cutaneous reactions), fever, eosinophilia, neutropenia, agranulocytosis, thrombocytopenia, leukopenia, anemia, lymphadenopathy, or anaphylaxis.

When penicillins are given orally, they may cause GI effects (eg, anorexia, vomiting, diarrhea). Because penicillins may alter gut flora, antibiotic-associated diarrhea can occur and can allow for the proliferation of resistant bacteria in the colon (ie, superinfections). Healthy dogs that are given oral amoxicillin have had their gut flora altered with a shift in balance toward gram-negative bacteria that included resistant species of Enterobacteriaceae.[11]

Neurotoxicity (eg, ataxia in dogs) has been associated with high doses or prolonged use of penicillins. Although the penicillins are not considered hepatotoxic, elevated liver enzymes have been reported with their use. Other effects reported in dogs include tachypnea, dyspnea, edema, and tachycardia.

Reproductive/Nursing Safety

Penicillins have been shown to cross the placenta; safe use during pregnancy has not been firmly established, but it is not believed to be teratogenic. Milk levels of amoxicillin are considered low. Amoxicillin concentration in milk is roughly half that found in plasma in lactating cows.[12]

Because safety has not been established in animals, this drug should only be used when the maternal benefits outweigh the potential risks to offspring.

Overdosage/Acute Toxicity

Acute oral penicillin overdoses are unlikely to cause significant problems other than GI distress, but other effects are possible (see *Adverse Effects*). In humans, very high dosages (≈300 mg/kg) of parenteral penicillins, especially in patients with renal disease, have induced CNS effects.

For patients that have experienced or are suspected to have experienced an overdose, consultation with a 24-hour poison consultation center specializing in providing veterinary-specific information is recommended. For general information related to overdose and toxin exposures, as well as contact information for poison control centers, refer to ***Appendix***.

Drug Interactions

The following drug interactions with amoxicillin have either been reported or are theoretical in humans or animals and may be of significance in veterinary patients. Unless otherwise noted, use together is not necessarily contraindicated, but the potential risks must be weighed and additional monitoring performed when appropriate.

- **Aminoglycosides** (eg, **amikacin**, **gentamicin**): Beta-lactam antibiotics can inactivate aminoglycosides in vitro (and in vivo in patients with chronic kidney disease).
- **Bacteriostatic Antimicrobials** (eg, **chloramphenicol**, **erythromycin**, other **macrolides**, **sulfonamides**, **tetracyclines**): Because there is evidence of in vitro antagonism between beta-lactam antibiotics and bacteriostatic antibiotics, use together has not generally been recommended in the past, but the clinical significance of this is unclear.
- **Methotrexate (MTX)**: Amoxicillin may decrease the renal excretion of MTX, causing increased MTX concentrations and potential MTX toxic effects.
- **Mycophenolate**: May decrease mycophenolate concentrations by decreasing concentrations of mycophenolate's active metabolite
- **Probenecid**: Competitively blocks the tubular secretion of most penicillins, thereby increasing serum concentrations and serum half-lives
- **Warfarin**: Concurrent use may increase risk for bleeding.

Laboratory Considerations

- Amoxicillin may cause false positive **urine glucose determinations** when using cupric sulfate solution (Benedict's Solution, *Clinitest*®). Tests utilizing glucose oxidase (*Tes-Tape*®, *Clinistix*®) are not affected by amoxicillin.
- As penicillins and other beta-lactams can inactivate **aminoglycosides** in vitro (and in vivo in patients in renal failure), serum concentrations of aminoglycosides may be falsely decreased if the patient is also receiving beta-lactam antibiotics, particularly when the serum is stored prior to analysis. It is recommended that if the assay is delayed, samples be frozen and, if possible, drawn at times when the beta-lactam antibiotic is at a trough.

Dosages

NOTE: The following FDA-approved label indications and dosages are not accepted by most clinicians today as being consistently efficacious.

DOGS:

Respiratory tract infections (tonsillitis, tracheobronchitis), genitourinary tract infections (cystitis), GI tract infections (bacterial gastroenteritis), and soft tissue infections (abscesses, lacerations, and wounds) due to *Staphylococcus aureus*, *Streptococcus* spp, Escherichia *coli*, and *Proteus mirabilis*. Bacterial dermatitis due to *Staphylococcus aureus*, *Streptococcus* spp, and *Proteus mirabilis* (label dosage; FDA-approved): 11 mg/kg PO twice daily for 5 to 7 days or 48 hours after all clinical signs have subsided. If no improvement is seen in 5 days, review diagnosis and change therapy.[13]

Systemic infections (extra-label): 11 – 22 mg/kg PO every 8 hours; duration of treatment should be dictated by indication and clinical response.

Sporadic bacterial cystitis (extra-label): 11 – 15 mg/kg PO every 8 to 12 hours. Duration of treatment requires more study but recent recommendations for sporadic bacterial cystitis are 3 to 5 days of treatment.[14]

Recurrent (2 or more episodes of clinical bacterial cystitis per 6 months or 3 per 12 months) bacterial cystitis (extra-label): 11 – 15 mg/kg PO every 8 to 12 hours for 3 to 5 days, as for sporadic bacterial cystitis. Longer courses (1 to 2 weeks) may be considered for persistent or relapsing infections.[14]

Borreliosis (Lyme disease) (extra-label): 20 mg/kg PO 3 times daily for 30 days[15]

***Helicobacter* spp gastritis infections using triple therapy** (extra-label):

a) Amoxicillin 11 mg/kg PO every 8 hours in combination with metronidazole 15.4 mg/kg every 8 hours and bismuth subsalicylate suspension (original *Pepto-Bismol*®) 0.22 mL/kg (3.85 mg/kg) PO every 4 to 6 hours for 3 weeks[16]
b) Amoxicillin 15 mg/kg every 12 hours in combination with metronidazole 10 mg/kg PO every 12 hours and bismuth subsalicylate 262 mg tablets given based on body weight (less than 5 kg (11 lb) = 0.25 tablet; 5 to 9.9 kg (11 to 21.8 lb) = 0.5 tablet; 10 to 24.9 kg (22 to 54.8 lb) = 1 tablet; greater than 25 kg = 2 tablets) every 12 hours for 2 weeks[17]
c) Amoxicillin 22 mg/kg PO every 12 hours in combination with metronidazole 11 – 15 mg/kg PO every 12 hours and bismuth subsalicylate suspension 0.22 mL/kg (3.85 mg/kg) PO every 6 to 8 hours for 3 weeks[18]

CATS:

Upper respiratory tract infections due to *Staphylococcus aureus*, *Streptococcus* spp, and *E coli*. Genitourinary tract infections (cystitis) due to *Staphylococcus aureus*, *Streptococcus* spp, *E coli*, and *Proteus mirabilis*. GI tract infections due to *E coli*. Skin and soft tissue infections (abscesses, lacerations, and wounds) due to *Staphylococcus aureus*, *Streptococcus* spp, *E coli*, and *Pasteurella multocida* (label dosage; FDA-approved): 50 mg/cat (NOT mg/kg) or 11 – 22 mg/kg once daily for 5 to 7 days or 48 hours after all clinical signs have subsided. If no improvement is seen in 5 days, review diagnosis and change therapy[13]

Systemic infections (extra-label): 11 – 22 mg/kg PO every 8 hours; duration of treatment should be dictated by indication and clinical response.

Sporadic bacterial cystitis (extra-label): 11 – 15 mg/kg PO every 8 to 12 hours for 3 to 5 days[14]

Recurrent (2 or more episodes of clinical bacterial cystitis per 6 months or 3 per 12 months) bacterial cystitis (extra-label): 11 – 15 mg/kg PO every 8 to 12 hours for 3 to 5 days, as for sporadic bacterial cystitis.[14] Longer courses (1 to 2 weeks) may be considered for persistent or relapsing infections.

***Helicobacter* spp gastritis infections using triple therapy** (extra-label): Amoxicillin 11 – 22 mg/kg PO every 8 hours in combination with metronidazole 11 – 15.4 mg/kg PO every 8 - 12 hours and bismuth subsalicylate suspension (original Pepto-Bismol®) 0.22 mL/kg (3.85 mg/kg) PO every 4 to 8 hours and for 3 weeks[16,18]

***Helicobacter* spp gastritis infections using quadruple therapy** (extra-label): Amoxicillin 10 – 20 mg/kg PO 3 times daily in combination with metronidazole 10 mg/kg PO twice daily and bismuth subsalicylate (262 mg tablets; *Pepto-Bismol*®) ¼ tablet/cat (total dose) PO twice daily, ± H2 blocker (eg, famotidine) or omeprazole for 2 weeks[19]

CATTLE:

Mastitis in lactating cows (label dosage; FDA approved): 62.5 mg (contents of one syringe) intramammary infusion in each affected quarter every 12 hours for a total of 3 doses.[20] Before administration, milk udder completely, thoroughly wash and then dry udder and teat, and next clean and disinfect teat with alcohol swabs (provided with product). After completing the infusion, withdraw the syringe, and massage medication up into the milk cistern.

BIRDS:

Susceptible infections (extra-label):

a) 125 mg/kg PO every 12 hours. Mix oral solution to double strength to a final concentration of 125 mg/mL[21]
b) 100 mg/kg IM, SC, PO every 8 hours[22]

FERRETS:

Helicobacter **spp gastritis infections using triple therapy** (extra-label):

a) Amoxicillin 20 mg/kg PO every 12 hours, with metronidazole 20 mg/kg PO every 12 hours and bismuth subsalicylate 17.5 mg/kg PO every 8 hours for 21 days. Sucralfate 25 mg/kg PO every 8 hours and famotidine 0.5 mg/kg PO every 24 hours may also be used. Fluids and assisted feeding should be continued while the primary cause of disease is investigated.[23]
b) Amoxicillin 10 mg/kg, metronidazole 20 mg/kg, and bismuth subsalicylate 17.5 mg/kg, all given PO 3 times daily for 3 to 4 weeks[24]
c) Amoxicillin 30 mg/kg, metronidazole 20 mg/kg, and bismuth subsalicylate 17.5 mg/kg, all given PO 3 times daily for 3 to 4 weeks[25]

RABBITS/RODENTS/SMALL MAMMALS:

See *Contraindications/Precautions/Warnings.*

Hedgehogs (extra-label): 15 mg/kg IM, SC, or PO every 12 hours[26]

REPTILES:

Susceptible infections for all species (extra-label): 22 mg/kg PO every 12 to 24 hours; not useful unless used in combination with aminoglycosides.[27]

Monitoring

- Efficacy: resolution of clinical signs
- Culture and susceptibility as indicated for clinical condition being treated
- Urine culture may be considered after 5 to 7 days when treating bacterial cystitis for longer periods of time.[14] It is important to note that positive cultures taken at this time should prompt questioning the owner about compliance and further investigation as to why the infection has not been eliminated (eg, underlying pathology [eg, cystic calculi, neoplasia]); a positive culture at this time should not simply prompt a change in antibiotic choice. A negative culture during this time frame does not necessarily guarantee resolution of the infection.

Client Information

- It is preferred that the oral suspension be refrigerated but this is not absolutely necessary. Any unused oral suspension should be discarded after 14 days.
- This medicine can be given with or without food, but gastrointestinal side effects (eg, poor appetite, nausea, vomiting) might be prevented if this medicine is given with food.
- The most common side effects are diarrhea, vomiting, and loss of appetite.
- It is important to give this medication exactly as prescribed and to complete the full course of treatment, even if your animal seems better. Missing doses or stopping treatment early may result in treatment failure.
- Amoxicillin should not be given to rabbits, guinea pigs, chinchillas, hamsters, rodents, or other "pocket pets", as life-threatening diarrhea may occur.

Chemistry/Synonyms

Commercially available dosage forms contain amoxicillin trihydrate, which occurs as a practically odorless, white, crystalline powder that is sparingly soluble in water. Amoxicillin differs structurally from ampicillin only by having an additional hydroxyl group on the phenyl ring.

Amoxicillin may also be known as amoxycillin, p-hydroxyampicillin, or BRL 2333; many trade names are available.

Storage/Stability

Amoxicillin capsules, tablets, and powder for oral suspension should be stored at room temperature (15°C-30°C [59°F-86°F]) in tight containers. After reconstitution, the oral suspension can be stored at room temperature or refrigerated (refrigeration preferred); any unused product should be discarded after 14 days. Intramammary syringes should be stored at or below 24°C (75°F).

Compatibility/Compounding Considerations

No specific information is noted.

Dosage Forms/Regulatory Status

VETERINARY-LABELED PRODUCTS:

Amoxicillin Oral Tablets: 50 mg, 100 mg, 150 mg, 200 mg, and 400 mg; *Amoxi-Tabs®*, *Bimox®*; generic; (Rx). FDA-approved for use in dogs and cats.

Amoxicillin Powder for Oral Suspension: 50 mg/mL (after reconstitution) in 15 mL or 30 mL bottles; *Amoxi-Drops®*, *Bimox®*, generic; (Rx). FDA-approved for use in dogs and cats.

Amoxicillin Intramammary Infusion: 62.5 mg in 10 mL syringes; *Amoxi-Mast®*; (Rx). FDA-approved to treat subclinical infectious mastitis in lactating cows. NADA 55-100. (Rx). Withdrawal times: milk— 60 hours after last treatment; slaughter—12 days

HUMAN-LABELED PRODUCTS:

Amoxicillin Oral Tablets (chewable): 125 mg, 200 mg, 250 mg, and 400 mg; *Amoxil®*, generic; (Rx)

Amoxicillin Oral Tablets: 500 mg and 875 mg; *Amoxil®*, generic; (Rx)

Amoxicillin Oral Capsules: 250 mg and 500 mg; *Amoxil®*, generic; (Rx)

Amoxicillin Powder for Oral Suspension: 125 mg/5 mL (25 mg/mL) in 80 mL, 100 mL, and 150 mL; 200 mg/5 mL (40 mg/mL) in 50 mL, 75 mL, and 100 mL; 250 mg/5 mL (50 mg/mL) in 80 mL, 100 mL, and 150 mL; 400 mg/5 mL (80 mg/mL) in 50 mL, 75 mL, and 100 mL; *Amoxil®*, *Trimox®*, generic; (Rx)

Amoxicillin Oral Extended-Release Tablets: 775 mg in 30s and UD 10s; *Moxatag®*; (Rx)

References

For the complete list of references, see **wiley.com/go/budde/plumb**

Amoxicillin/Clavulanate

Amoxicillin/Clavulanic Acid

(a-mox-i-***sill***-in clav-yue-***lan***-ate) *Clavamox®, Augmentin®*

Potentiated Aminopenicillin

Prescriber Highlights

- Bactericidal aminopenicillin with beta-lactamase inhibitor that expands its spectrum, increasing susceptibility of bacteria that are resistant to amoxicillin via beta-lactamase production.
- Most common adverse effects are GI-related; hypersensitivity and other adverse effects may occur but are rare.
- As compared with veterinary-labeled products, human-labeled products contain different ratios of amoxicillin:clavulanate and product strengths are expressed in terms of amoxicillin (only), whereas veterinary products are expressed as the sum of both compounds.

Uses/Indications

Amoxicillin/clavulanate potassium tablets and oral suspension products are used in dogs and cats for the treatment of urinary tract, skin (eg, wounds, pyoderma), canine periodontal disease, and soft tissue (eg, abscesses) infections caused by susceptible organisms, particularly gram-positive bacteria and anaerobes. It is also indicated for respiratory tract infections, although it is ineffective against *Mycoplasma* spp, and resistance to *Bordetella* spp is an increasing problem in some regions.

The World Health Organization has designated amoxicillin/clavulanate as a Critically Important antimicrobial for human medicine.[1] The Office International des Epizooties (OIE) has designated amoxicillin/clavulanate as a Veterinary Critically Important Antimicrobial (VCIA) Agent in avian, bovine, caprine, equine, ovine, and swine species.[2]

Pharmacology/Actions

Amoxicillin is a time-dependent, bactericidal agent that acts by inhibiting cell wall synthesis. Amoxicillin generally shares the same spectrum of activity and uses as ampicillin but is better absorbed orally (in nonruminants) and attains higher serum levels. Separate serum and urinary clinical breakpoints are available.

Penicillins are bactericidal against susceptible bacteria and act by inhibiting mucopeptide synthesis in the cell wall, which results in a defective barrier and an osmotically unstable spheroplast. The exact mechanism for this effect has not been definitively determined, but beta-lactam antibiotics have been shown to bind to several enzymes (eg, carboxypeptidases, transpeptidases, endopeptidases) within the bacterial cytoplasmic membrane that are involved with cell wall synthesis. The different affinities that various beta-lactam antibiotics have for these enzymes (also known as penicillin-binding proteins [PBPs]) help explain the differences in the drugs' spectrums of activity that are not explained by the influence of beta-lactamases. Like other beta-lactam antibiotics, penicillins are generally considered to be more effective against actively growing bacteria.

Aminopenicillins (ie, broad-spectrum or ampicillin penicillins) have increased activity against many strains of gram-negative aerobes not covered by either the natural penicillins or penicillinase-resistant penicillins, including some strains of *Escherichia coli*, *Klebsiella* spp, and *Haemophilus* spp. Like the natural penicillins, aminopenicillins are susceptible to inactivation by beta-lactamase–producing bacteria (eg, *Staphylococcus* spp, *E coli*). Although not as active as natural penicillins, aminopenicillins have activity against many anaerobic bacteria, including clostridial organisms. Organisms that are generally not susceptible include *Pseudomonas aeruginosa*, *Serratia* spp, indole-positive *Proteus* spp (*Proteus mirabilis* is susceptible), *Enterobacter* spp, *Citrobacter* spp, and *Acinetobacter* spp. Aminopenicillins are ineffective against methicillin-resistant staphylococci and are inactive against mycobacteria, *Mycoplasma* spp, *Rickettsia* spp, fungi, protozoa, and viruses.

Clavulanic acid has only weak antibacterial activity when used alone and is only available in fixed-dose oral combinations with amoxicillin. Clavulanic acid acts by competitively and irreversibly binding to beta-lactamases (including types II, III, IV, and V) and penicillinases produced by staphylococci. Staphylococci that are resistant to penicillinase-resistant penicillins (eg, oxacillin) are considered resistant to amoxicillin/potassium clavulanate, despite susceptibility testing that may indicate otherwise. Amoxicillin with potassium clavulanate is usually ineffective against type I cephalosporinases. Members of the family Enterobacteriaceae, particularly *Pseudomonas aeruginosa*, often produce these plasmid-mediated cephalosporinases. When clavulanic acid is combined with amoxicillin, there is little, if any, synergistic activity against organisms already susceptible to amoxicillin, but amoxicillin-resistant strains (due to beta-lactamase inactivation) may be covered.

When Kirby-Bauer susceptibility testing is performed, the *Augmentin*® disk (human-product trade name) is often used. Because the amoxicillin:clavulanic acid ratio of 2:1 in the susceptibility tests may not correspond to in vivo drug levels, susceptibility testing may not always accurately predict efficacy for this combination. A urinary tract-specific breakpoint in dogs and cats for amoxicillin/clavulanate is reported as less than 8/4 µg/mL because of the greater drug levels that are achieved in urine. This breakpoint should only be used for cystitis—not pyelonephritis, for which serum breakpoints should be applied.

Pharmacokinetics

Amoxicillin trihydrate is stable in the presence of gastric acid. After oral administration, amoxicillin bioavailability is highly variable between species. Food will decrease the rate but not the extent of oral absorption, and many clinicians suggest giving the drug with food, particularly if there is concomitant GI distress. In dogs, amoxicillin bioavailability was 64% to 77% following oral administration.[3] In cats, one study found the bioavailability to be ≈77%.[4] Amoxicillin serum levels will generally be 1.5 to 3 times greater than those of ampicillin after equivalent oral doses. In dogs following oral administration, maximum plasma concentrations of 11 to 21 µg/mL were reached after ≈1.38 to 2 hours.[3,5] In cats following a 10 mg/kg oral dose, maximum plasma concentrations of 5.89 µg/mL were reached in 1.69 hours.[4]

After absorption, the volume of distribution for amoxicillin is ≈0.28 to 0.71 L/kg in dogs[3] and 0.86 L/kg in cats.[4] The drug is widely distributed to most body tissues and fluids. When meninges are inflamed, amoxicillin will cross into the CSF in concentrations ranging from 10% to 60% of those found in serum. Very low levels of the drug are found in the aqueous humor, and low levels are found in tears, sweat, and saliva. Protein binding in dogs is ≈13%.

Amoxicillin is eliminated primarily unchanged via renal mechanisms, principally by tubular secretion; however, some of the drug is metabolized by hydrolysis to penicilloic acids (inactive) and then excreted in the urine. Elimination half-lives of amoxicillin have been reported to be 0.91 to 1.52 hours in dogs[6] and ≈1.25 hours in cats.[4] Clearance in cats is reportedly 0.45 L/hour/kg.

There is no evidence to suggest that the addition of clavulanic acid significantly alters amoxicillin pharmacokinetics.[6] As a time-dependent antimicrobial, duration of time above the MIC is critical, so frequent dosing is necessary.

Clavulanate potassium is stable in the presence of gastric acid and is readily absorbed. In dogs following oral administration, maximum plasma concentrations of 2.06 to 2.3 µg/mL were reached after 0.95 to 1.05 hours.[5] In cats following oral administration, bioavailability of clavulanic acid was ≈98%, with maximum plasma concentrations of 1.41 µg/mL reached in 1.03 hours.[4]

Clavulanic acid has an apparent volume of distribution of 0.32 L/kg in dogs and 0.93 L/kg in cats.[4] It is distributed (with amoxicillin) into the lungs, pleural fluid, and peritoneal fluid. Low concentrations of both drugs are found in the saliva, sputum, and CSF (uninflamed meninges). Higher concentrations in the CSF are expected when meninges are inflamed,[7] but it is questionable whether therapeutic concentrations are attainable. Clavulanic acid is 13% bound to proteins in dog serum.

Clavulanic acid is apparently extensively metabolized in dogs and rats, primarily to 1-amino-4-hydroxybutan-2-one. It is unknown whether this compound possesses any beta-lactamase–inhibiting activity. The drug is also excreted unchanged in the urine via glomerular filtration. In dogs, 34% to 52% of a dose is excreted in the urine as unchanged drug and metabolites, 25% to 27% is eliminated in the feces, and 17% into respired air. Urine levels of active drug are considered high but may be only ≈20% of those of amoxicillin. In cats with azotemic chronic kidney disease given amoxicillin\clavulanic acid, amoxicillin concentration was significantly lower in the urine and somewhat higher in serum when compared to cats without kidney disease.[8]

Elimination half-lives of clavulanic acid are reported to be 0.71 to 0.83 hours in dogs[5] and 0.71 hours in cats.[4] Clearance in cats is reportedly 0.92 L/hour/kg.[4]

Contraindications/Precautions/Warnings

Penicillins are contraindicated in patients with a history of hypersensitivity to them. Penicillins should be used cautiously in patients with documented hypersensitivity to other beta-lactam antibiotics (eg, cephalosporins, cefamycins, carbapenems) as there may be cross-reactivity.

Systemic antibiotics should not be administered orally in patients with septicemia, shock, or other grave illnesses, as absorption of the medication from the GI tract may be significantly delayed or diminished. Parental routes should be used for these cases.

Oral beta-lactam antibiotics and macrolides should not be administered to rabbits, guinea pigs, chinchillas, or hamsters, as serious enteritis and clostridial enterotoxemia may occur.

Adverse Effects

Adverse effects with the penicillins are usually not serious and have a relatively low frequency of occurrence.

Hypersensitivity reactions unrelated to dose can occur with these agents and can manifest as rashes (including severe cutaneous reactions), fever, eosinophilia, neutropenia, agranulocytosis, thrombocytopenia, leukopenia, anemia, lymphadenopathy, or anaphylaxis.

When penicillins are given orally, they may cause GI effects (eg, anorexia, vomiting, diarrhea). Because the penicillins may alter GI microbiota, antibiotic-associated diarrhea can occur and can allow for the proliferation of resistant bacteria in the colon (ie, superinfections). Probiotic use reduced GI abnormalities and diarrhea in laboratory cats that received amoxicillin/clavulanate.[9]

Cats diagnosed with chronic kidney disease (CKD) that were azotemic were more likely to experience multiple adverse effects when compared to CKD cats without azotemia.[8]

Neurotoxicity (eg, ataxia in dogs) has been associated with high doses or prolonged use of penicillins. Although the penicillins are not considered hepatotoxic, elevated liver enzymes have been reported with their use. Other effects reported in dogs include tachypnea, dyspnea, edema, and tachycardia.

Reproductive/Nursing Safety

Penicillins have been shown to cross the placenta. Safe use during pregnancy has not been firmly established, but it is not believed to be teratogenic.

Amoxicillin and clavulanic acid are found in milk in low concentrations. Because safety has not been established in animals, this drug should only be used when the maternal benefits outweigh the potential risks to offspring.

Overdosage/Acute Toxicity

Acute oral penicillin overdoses are unlikely to cause significant problems other than GI distress, but other effects are possible (see *Adverse Effects*). In humans, very high doses of parenteral penicillins, especially in patients with renal disease, have induced CNS effects.

For patients that have experienced or are suspected to have experienced an overdose, consultation with a 24-hour poison consultation center specializing in providing veterinary-specific information is recommended. For general information related to overdose and toxin exposures, as well as contact information for poison control centers, refer to ***Appendix***.

Drug Interactions

The following drug interactions with amoxicillin/clavulanate have either been reported or are theoretical in humans or animals and may be of significance in veterinary patients. Unless otherwise noted, use together is not necessarily contraindicated, but the potential risks should be weighed and additional monitoring should be performed when appropriate.

- **Aminoglycosides** (eg, **gentamicin**): beta-lactams can inactivate aminoglycosides in vitro (and in vivo in patients with chronic kidney disease).
- **Bacteriostatic Antimicrobials** (eg, **chloramphenicol, erythromycin, minocycline** and other **macrolides, tetracyclines, sulfonamides**): Because there is evidence of in vitro antagonism between beta-lactam antibiotics and bacteriostatic antibiotics, use together generally has not been recommended in the past; however, the clinical significance of this is unclear.
- **Leflunomide**: Prior, concurrent, or subsequent use of amoxicillin/clavulanate with leflunomide without observing washout may increase the risk for hepatotoxicity.
- **Methotrexate (MTX)**: Amoxicillin may decrease the renal excretion of MTX, causing increased MTX concentrations and potential MTX toxic effects.
- **Mycophenolate**: May decrease concentrations of mycophenolate by decreasing concentrations of mycophenolate's active metabolite
- **Probenecid**: Competitively blocks the tubular secretion of most penicillins, thereby increasing serum concentrations and serum half-lives
- **Warfarin**: Concurrent use of amoxicillin/clavulanate may increase the risk for warfarin-induced bleeding.

Laboratory Considerations

- Amoxicillin may cause false positive **urine glucose determinations** when cupric sulfate solution (Benedict's Solution, *Clinitest®*) is used. Tests using glucose oxidase (*Tes-Tape®, Clinistix®*) are not affected by amoxicillin.
- Because penicillins and other beta-lactam antibiotics can inactivate **aminoglycosides** in vitro (and in vivo in patients in renal failure), serum concentrations of aminoglycosides may be falsely decreased if the patient is also receiving beta-lactam antibiotics, particularly when the serum is stored prior to analysis. It is recommended that if there is a delay in running the assay, samples should be frozen and, if possible, drawn at times when the beta-lactam antibiotic is at a trough.

Dosages

NOTE: All dosages listed are for combined quantities of both drugs (unless otherwise noted).

DOGS:

<u>Skin and soft tissue infections</u> such as wounds, abscesses, cellulitis, superficial and deep pyoderma due to susceptible strains of the following organisms: beta-lactamase–producing *Staphylococcus aureus*, non-beta-lactamase–producing *Staphylococcus aureus*, *Staphylococcus* spp, *Streptococcus* spp, and *Escherichia coli*. <u>Periodontal infections</u> due to susceptible strains of both aerobic and anaerobic bacteria (label dosage; FDA-approved): 13.75 mg/kg PO twice daily.[10] Skin and soft tissue infections such as abscesses, cellulitis, wounds, superficial/juvenile pyoderma, and periodontal infections should be treated for 5 to 7 days or for 48 hours after all signs have subsided. If no response is seen after 5 days of treatment, therapy should be discontinued and the case reevaluated. Deep pyoderma may require treatment for 21 days; the maximum duration of treatment should not exceed 30 days.

Sporadic bacterial cystitis (extra-label): 12.5 – 25 mg/kg PO every 8 to 12 hours for 3 to 5 days is an acceptable option but is not recommended as empirical therapy (ie, without or before culture and susceptibility testing); amoxicillin (without clavulanic acid) achieves high concentrations in the urine and is preferred for empirical therapy.[11]

Pyoderma (extra-label):

a) **Superficial pyoderma:** 12.5 – 25 mg/kg PO twice daily[12] for 21 to 28 days up to a maximum of 90 days[13]; fair evidence available to support moderate to high efficacy[13]

b) **Deep pyoderma:** 12.5 – 25 mg/kg PO twice daily for at least 28 days, up to a maximum of 90 days[13]; good level of evidence for high efficacy[13]

Endocarditis (chronic therapy) secondary to a susceptible strain of *Staphylococcus* spp (extra-label): 20 mg/kg PO 3 times daily for 6 to 8 weeks[14]

Canine infectious respiratory disease complex when a bacterial component is involved (extra-label): 11 mg/kg PO every 12 hours (twice daily) as a first-line treatment option for bacterial upper respiratory tract infection not suspected to be caused by *Mycoplasma* spp[15]

CATS:

<u>Skin and soft tissue infections</u> such as wounds, abscesses, and cellulitis/dermatitis due to susceptible strains of the following organisms: beta-lactamase–producing *Staphylococcus aureus*, nonbeta-lactamase–producing *Staphylococcus aureus*, *Staphylococcus* spp, *Streptococcus* spp, *E coli*, *Pasteurella multocida*, and *Pasteurella* spp. <u>UTIs</u> due to susceptible strains of *E coli*. (label dosage; FDA-approved): 62.5 mg/cat (NOT mg/kg) PO twice daily.[10] Skin and soft tissue infections such as abscesses and cellulitis/dermatitis should be treated for 5 to 7 days or 48 hours after all signs have subsided, not to exceed 30 days. If no response is seen after 3 days of treatment, therapy should be discontinued and the case re-evaluated. UTIs may require treatment for 10 to 14 days or longer. The maximum duration of treatment should not exceed 30 days. Therapy may be initiated prior to obtaining results from bacteriological and susceptibility studies. A culture should be obtained prior to treatment to determine susceptibility of the organisms to this drug. Following determination of susceptibility results and clinical response to medication, therapy may be reevaluated.

Sporadic bacterial cystitis (extra-label): 12.5 – 25 mg/kg PO every 8 to 12 hours for 3 to 5 days is an acceptable option but is not recommended as empirical therapy (ie, without or before culture and susceptibility testing); amoxicillin (without clavulanic acid) achieves high concentrations in the urine and is preferred for empirical therapy.[11]

Upper respiratory tract disease (URTD) with a bacterial component (extra-label): 12.5 mg/kg PO every 12 hours[15,16]

BIRDS:

Susceptible infections (extra-label): 50 – 100 mg/kg PO every 6 to 8 hours[17]

FERRETS:

Susceptible infections (extra-label): 10 – 20 mg/kg PO every 8 to 12 hours[18,19]

Monitoring

- Efficacy: resolution of clinical signs
- Culture and susceptibility as indicated for clinical condition being treated.
- Urine culture may be considered after 5 to 7 days when treating bacterial cystitis for longer periods of time.[11] It is important to note that positive cultures taken at this time should prompt questioning the owner about compliance and further investigation as to why the infection has not been eliminated (eg, underlying pathology [eg, cystic calculi, neoplasia]); a positive culture at this time should not simply prompt a change in antibiotic choice. A negative culture during this time frame does not necessarily guarantee resolution of the infection.

Client Information

- The oral suspension should preferably be refrigerated; any unused oral suspension should be discarded after 10 days.
- This medicine can be given with or without food, but gastrointestinal side effects might be prevented if this medicine is given with food.
- The most common side effects are diarrhea, vomiting, and loss of appetite
- It is important to give this medication exactly as prescribed and to complete the full course of therapy, even if your animal seems better. Missing doses or stopping treatment early may result in treatment failure.
- Do NOT give this drug to rabbits, guinea pigs, chinchillas, hamsters, rodents, or other "pocket pets," as life-threatening diarrhea may occur.

Chemistry/Synonyms

Commercially available dosage forms contain amoxicillin trihydrate, which occurs as a practically odorless, white, crystalline powder that is sparingly soluble in water. Amoxicillin differs structurally from ampicillin only by having an additional hydroxyl group on the phenyl ring.

Clavulanate potassium is a beta-lactamase inhibitor; it occurs as an off-white crystalline powder, has a pK_a of 2.7 (as the acid), and is very soluble in water and slightly soluble in alcohol at room temperatures. Although available in commercially available preparations as the potassium salt, potency is expressed in terms of clavulanic acid.

Amoxicillin may also be known as amoxycillin, p-hydroxyampicillin, or BRL 2333; many trade names are available. Clavulanate potassium may also be known as clavulanic acid, BRL-14151K, or kalii clavulanas.

Storage/Stability

Clavulanate products should be stored at temperatures below 25°C (77°F), and some tablet formulations specify storage at 20°C to 25°C (68°F-77°F). Potassium clavulanate is very susceptible to moisture and should be protected from excessive humidity.

After reconstitution, oral suspensions are stable for 10 days when refrigerated. Unused portions should be discarded after that time. At room temperature, suspensions labeled for human use are reportedly stable for 48 hours. The veterinary oral suspension requires refrigeration and is reconstituted by adding 14 mL of water and shaking vigorously.

Compatibility/Compounding Considerations

No specific information is noted.

Dosage Forms/Regulatory Status

VETERINARY-LABELED PRODUCTS:

Oral Tablets and Chewable Tablets (4:1 amoxicillin:clavulanic acid ratio):

62.5 mg: Amoxicillin 50 mg/12.5 mg clavulanic acid (as the potassium salt); 125 mg: Amoxicillin 100 mg/25 mg clavulanic acid (as the potassium salt); 250 mg: Amoxicillin 200 mg/50 mg clavulanic acid (as the potassium salt); 375 mg: Amoxicillin 300 mg/75 mg clavulanic acid (as the potassium salt); *Clavamox® Tablets*, *Clavamox® Chewable*, generic; (Rx). FDA-approved for use in dogs and cats.

Powder for Oral Suspension:

Amoxicillin 50 mg/12.5 mg clavulanic acid (as the potassium salt) per mL in 15 mL dropper bottles; *Clavamox® Drops*, generic; (Rx). FDA-approved for use in dogs and cats.

HUMAN-LABELED PRODUCTS:

NOTE: Human-labeled amoxicillin/clavulanate products have varying ratios of amoxicillin:clavulanate ranging from 2:1 to 7:1. Additionally, human products are generally expressed in potency only as the amoxicillin component (eg, *Augmentin® 875* contains 875 mg of amoxicillin and 125 mg of clavulanic acid), whereas the veterinary products are expressed as the total of both drugs.

Amoxicillin (as trihydrate)/Clavulanic Acid (as potassium salt) Tablets: Amoxicillin 250 mg/125 mg clavulanic acid; Amoxicillin 500 mg/125 mg clavulanic acid; Amoxicillin 875 mg/125 mg clavulanic acid; *Augmentin®*, generic (Rx)

Chewable Tablets: Amoxicillin 125 mg/31.25 mg clavulanic acid; Amoxicillin 200 mg/28.5 mg clavulanic acid; 250 mg/62.5 mg clavulanic acid and 400 mg/57 mg clavulanic acid; *Augmentin®*, generic; (Rx)

Powder for Oral Suspension—Amoxicillin/Clavulanic Acid (as potassium salt) after reconstitution: Amoxicillin 125 mg/31.25 mg clavulanic acid per 5 mL in 75 mL, 100 mL, and 150 mL; Amoxicillin 200 mg/28.5 mg clavulanic acid per 5 mL in 50 mL, 75 mL, and 100 mL; Amoxicillin 250 mg/62.5 mg clavulanic acid per 5 mL in 75 mL, 100 mL, and 150 mL; Amoxicillin 400 mg/57 mg clavulanic acid per 5 mL in 50 mL, 75 mL, and 100 mL; 600 mg/42.9 mg clavulanic acid per 5 mL in 75 mL, 100 mL, 125 mL, and 200 mL; *Augmentin®*and *Augmentin ES-600®*, *Amoclan®*, generic; (Rx)

Amoxicillin 1000 mg/62.5 mg clavulanic acid oral extended-release tablet; *Augmentin XR®*, generic; (Rx)

References

For the complete list of references, see **wiley.com/go/budde/plumb**

Amphotericin B

(am-foe-***ter***-i-sin ***bee***) *Abelcet®,AmBisome®, Fungizone®*

Antifungal

Prescriber Highlights

- Systemic antifungal used for serious mycotic infections
- Must be parenterally administered (IV or SC infusion) for systemic infections
- Three different forms available on US market: conventional, formulated with sodium deoxycholate (generic); lipid complex (*Abelcet®*); and liposomal (*AmBisome®*). Each form has different reconstitution instructions, dilution, stability, storage, and dosage recommendations; thus, they are not interchangeable.
- Nephrotoxicity is the biggest concern, particularly with the deoxycholate form; newer products (lipid complex and liposomal) are less nephrotoxic and penetrate into tissues better but are more expensive.
- Renal function monitoring is essential.
- Many potential drug interactions

Uses/Indications

Amphotericin B has activity against most systemic fungal pathogens in numerous animal species, but because the potential exists for severe toxicity, its use should generally be limited to severe, life-threatening infections, progressive disease unresponsive to other antifungals, or in cases in which antifungal susceptibility warrants its use.

The liposomal form of amphotericin B can also be used to treat leishmaniasis and, although this form can be clinically effective, relapses inevitably occur. Additionally, concerns about the development of amphotericin B-resistant *Leishmania* strains in human leishmaniasis has prompted the World Health Organization (WHO) to discourage the use of amphotericin B in the treatment of dogs with leishmaniasis.[1,2]

Pharmacology/Actions

Amphotericin B is generally fungistatic, but it can be fungicidal against some organisms depending on drug concentration. This drug acts by binding to sterols (primarily ergosterol) in the fungal cell membrane and altering the permeability of the membrane, allowing intracellular potassium and other cellular constituents to leak out. Because bacteria and rickettsial organisms do not contain sterols, amphotericin B has no activity against them. Mammalian cell membranes also contain sterols (primarily cholesterol) and the drug's toxicity may be a result of a similar mechanism of action, although amphotericin B binds less strongly to cholesterol than ergosterol.

Amphotericin B has in vitro activity against a variety of fungal organisms, including *Blastomyces* spp, *Aspergillus* spp, *Paracoccidioides* spp, *Coccidioides* spp, *Histoplasma* spp, *Cryptococcus* spp, *Mucor* spp, and *Sporothrix* spp. Although absolute resistance to amphotericin B is rare, some strains of *Aspergillus* spp and *Sporothrix* spp have high minimum inhibitory concentration (MIC) values. Additionally, amphotericin B has in vivo activity against some protozoa species, including *Leishmania* spp and *Naegleria* spp. *Leishmania* spp have ergostane-based sterols in their cell membranes, which may explain amphotericin B's efficacy for treating this organism.

Pharmacokinetics

In humans, amphotericin B is poorly absorbed from the GI tract and must be administered parenterally to achieve sufficient concentrations to treat systemic fungal infections. After IV injection, the drug reportedly penetrates well into most tissues except for the pancreas, muscle, bone, aqueous humor, or pleural, pericardial, synovial, and peritoneal fluids. The drug enters the pleural cavity and joints when inflamed. CSF concentrations are ≈3% of those found in the serum. Approximately 90% to 95% of amphotericin in the vascular compartment is bound to serum proteins.[3] The newer lipid forms of amphotericin B have higher penetration into the lungs, liver, and spleen than the conventional form. The lipid complex formulation reaches higher peak plasma concentrations and has a larger volume of distribution (131 L/kg) as compared with conventional formulations (5 L/kg).[4]

The metabolic pathways of amphotericin B are not known, but amphotericin B exhibits biphasic elimination. In humans, an initial serum half-life of ≈24 hours and a longer terminal half-life of ≈15 days have been described for the conventional formulation.[3] Seven weeks after treatment has stopped, amphotericin B can still be detected in the urine. Approximately 2% to 5% of the drug is recovered in the urine in unchanged (biologically active) form.

Contraindications/Precautions/Warnings

Amphotericin B is contraindicated in patients that are hypersensitive to it.[3] Only use amphotericin B to treat severe, life-threatening infections, progressive disease unresponsive to other antifungals, or in cases in which it is indicated by antifungal susceptibility results.

Because of the serious nature of the diseases treated with systemic amphotericin B, it is not absolutely contraindicated in patients with renal disease, but it should be used cautiously with adequate monitoring and only when safer options (eg, fluconazole, itraconazole) have failed.

Do not confuse amphotericin B formulations. Each amphotericin B formulation (ie, deoxycholate [conventional], lipid complex, or liposomal) has different reconstitution instructions, dilution, stability, storage, and dosage recommendations; thus, they are not interchangeable. Because of the toxicity of this drug, dose calculations and solution preparation procedures should be double-checked.

Adverse Effects

Amphotericin B is known for its nephrotoxic effects; most mammalian patients will show some degree of renal toxicity after receiving the drug. The proposed mechanism of nephrotoxicity is via renal vasoconstriction, with a subsequent reduction in glomerular filtration rate. The drug may directly act as a toxin to renal epithelial cells. Renal damage may be more common, irreversible, and more severe in patients that receive higher doses or have pre-existing renal disease. Renal tubular acidosis, nephrogenic diabetes insipidus, hypokalemia, and hypomagnesemia can be associated with amphotericin B nephrotoxicity. Usually, renal function will return to normal after treatment is halted but may require several months to do so. As compared with dogs, cats may be more sensitive to nephrotoxic effects. Newer forms of amphotericin B (lipid complex and liposomal) are more hydrophobic than the deoxycholate form and significantly reduce the nephrotoxic qualities of the drug in humans.[3-6] Because higher doses may then be used, these forms may also have enhanced effectiveness. A study in dogs showed that amphotericin B lipid complex was 8 to 10 times less nephrotoxic than the conventional form.[7] However, newer forms may be associated with more infusion related-reactions such as phlebitis.

Several dosing regimens have been used in an attempt to reduce nephrotoxicity in dogs and cats treated with amphotericin B deoxycholate (conventional amphotericin B), including pretreatment with sodium[8] and/or mannitol,[6] but mannitol is not commonly used in veterinary medicine for this purpose. A tubuloglomerular feedback mechanism that induces vasoconstriction and decreased GFR has been postulated for amphotericin B toxicity, and increasing sodium load at the glomerulus may help prevent that feedback. Slow IV infusion with large volumes of fluid may also decrease nephrotoxicity.[9] A diluted SC infusion technique (see ***Dosages***) that may mimic slow IV infusion has been employed in dogs and cats to potentially reduce nephrotoxic potential and allow outpatient administration.[10] None of these techniques have been proven in animals to be superior over another.

Other adverse effects that have been reported with amphotericin B use in mammals include lethargy, restlessness, anorexia, vomiting, hypokalemia, distal renal tubular acidosis, hypomagnesemia, phlebitis, tachycardia, tachypnea, cardiac arrhythmia, bronchospasm, hypotension, nonregenerative anemia, fever (may be reduced by pretreatment with NSAIDs or a low dosage of steroids), polyuria, and collapse.[3] Sterile abscesses have been reported in dogs (20 kg [44.1 lb]) that were administered amphotericin B as a SC injection at concentrations of 25 mg/L (NOT mg/mL); however, these abscesses did not occur when the amphotericin B concentration was less than or equal to 20 mg/L (NOT mg/mL).[10] Calcinosis cutis has been reported in dogs that were treated with amphotericin B.[11,12] Cats with cryptococcosis (CNS involvement) may have increased neurologic signs within the first 3 days of treatment; this is possibly due to an inflammatory response to dying organisms.

In horses receiving amphotericin B via IV regional limb perfusion, adverse effects included limb edema and pain on palpation (42%) and inflammation at injection site (33%); adverse effects resolved within 14 days.[13]

In birds, nephrotoxicity does not appear to occur with amphotericin B use (possibly because of the drug's shorter half-life in birds[14]); however, it may cause myelosuppression.[15]

Amphotericin B has been documented to increase creatine kinase concentrations in humans.[16]

Reproductive/Nursing Safety

The safety of amphotericin B during pregnancy has not been established; however, in humans, amphotericin B has been shown to cross the placenta and enter fetal circulation. No reports of teratogenicity have been associated with any amphotericin formulation used at clinically relevant dosages and the drug is considered to be compatible with pregnancy in humans.[3,4,17,18]

It is unknown if amphotericin B crosses into breast milk. Although oral amphotericin B is poorly bioavailable, the risk to nursing offspring remains unknown.

Because safety has not been established in animals, this drug should only be used when the maternal benefits outweigh the potential risks to offspring.

Overdose/Acute Toxicity

No case reports were located regarding acute IV overdose of amphotericin B. The reported LD_{50} following IV administration is 6 mg/kg (nephrotoxicity) in dogs and 5 mg/kg (neurotoxicity) in rabbits.[19] Beagles receiving amphotericin B liposomal 8 – 16 mg/kg IV once daily for up to 30 days lost 25% or more of their body weight, beginning on the third day of treatment.[20] If an accidental overdose is administered, giving fluids and mannitol may minimize renal toxicity.[19]

For patients that have experienced or are suspected to have experienced an overdose, consultation with a 24-hour poison consultation center specializing in providing veterinary-specific information is recommended. For general information related to overdose and toxin exposures, as well as contact information for poison control centers, refer to ***Appendix.***

Drug Interactions

The following drug interactions have either been reported or are theoretical in humans or animals receiving amphotericin B and may be of significance in veterinary patients. Unless otherwise noted, use together is not necessarily contraindicated, but weigh the potential risks and perform additional monitoring when appropriate.

- **CORTICOSTEROIDS** (eg, **dexamethasone, prednis(ol)one**): May exacerbate the potassium-losing effects of amphotericin B
- **DIGOXIN**: Amphotericin B-induced hypokalemia may exacerbate digoxin toxicity.
- **FLUCYTOSINE**: In vitro synergy between amphotericin B and flucytosine may occur against strains of *Cryptococcus* spp and *Candida* spp, but increased flucytosine toxicity may also occur.
- **HIGHLY PROTEIN BOUND DRUGS** (eg, azole antifungals, furosemide, NSAIDs): Because amphotericin B is highly bound to plasma proteins (90%-95%), it could theoretically displace other highly bound drugs, causing a transient increase in serum levels of each drug. These interactions are unlikely to be of clinical concern because increased free drug levels will equilibrate through increased clearance. Monitor for adverse effects of each drug when using this combination.
- **NEPHROTOXIC DRUGS** (eg, **aminoglycosides, cisplatin, cyclosporine**): Because the renal effects of other nephrotoxic drugs may be additive with amphotericin B, avoid the concurrent or sequential use of these agents if possible.
- **POTASSIUM-DEPLETING DRUGS** (eg, **thiazide** or **loop diuretics**): May increase risk for hypokalemia
- **NEUROMUSCULAR BLOCKERS** (eg, **atracurium, tubocurarine**): Amphotericin B-induced hypokalemia may enhance neuromuscular blockade.
- **ZIDOVUDINE** (AZT): Potential for increased myelotoxicity or nephrotoxicity

Laboratory Interactions

- Amphotericin B liposomal may cause false elevations in **serum phosphate** when using the PHOSm assay[3]

Dosages

NOTE: Because of the potential toxicity, expense (drug, associated administration costs, and laboratory tests), and the necessity for parenteral administration, amphotericin B treatment in animals is generally reserved for treating serious systemic fungal infections. See ***Uses/Indications***. Dosage recommendations (initial dosages, frequency of administration, and cumulative doses) can vary widely depending on the disease/organism treated, formulation used, species, and route of administration. The cumulative dose is the total amount of amphotericin B administered to the patient over the entire treatment period. Solid evidence supporting any specific dose is lacking.

DOGS:

Serious susceptible systemic fungal infections (extra-label):

Deoxycholate formulations (conventional amphotericin B)

a) Initially, 0.5 mg/kg IV every other day; practically, 3 times per week (eg, Monday, Wednesday, and Friday). The calculated drug dose should be diluted in dextrose 5% (1:50) and administered slowly IV over 4 to 6 hours; the slow IV route is more commonly recommended for dogs. Cumulative dose recommendations vary and are dependent on patient response and drug toxicity; most recommendations range from 9 – 12 mg/kg. Patients must be kept well hydrated before and during treatment, but care must be taken to avoid fluid overload.

b) Initially, 0.5 – 0.75 mg/kg SC 1 to 3 times per week.[10,21] The calculated drug dose should initially be diluted to a concentration of 5 mg/mL and then the patient's calculated dose is further diluted into 350 to 500 mL of sodium chloride 0.45%/dextrose 2.5% and injected SC between the scapulae. Alternatively, the SC fluid (without amphotericin B) can be injected first and then the amphotericin B dose can then be injected into the SC fluid "lump." Cumulative dose recommendations vary and are dependent on patient response and drug toxicity; most recommendations range from 8 – 26 mg/kg. [5,10,21-23] See ***Contraindications/Precautions/Warnings*** about SC administration.

Lipid formulations (**NOTE:** Most clinicians recommend using these formulations in animals with preexisting renal disease or that have developed renal toxicity with the deoxycholate form.)

a) Amphotericin B lipid complex (ABLC; *Abelcet®*): 1 – 3.3 mg/kg IV over 2 hours. Cumulative dose recommendations vary and depend on patient response and drug toxicity; recommended cumulative doses range from 8 – 12 mg/kg[24,25] to 24 – 30 mg/kg. One protocol published for use of ABLC treatment of blastomycosis in dogs follows[5,24]: Calculate the patient's ABLC dosage (1 mg/kg) and dilute the appropriate volume of reconstituted ABLC to a concentration of 1 mg/mL in dextrose 5%. For 30 minutes before ABLC administration, begin an LRS IV infusion at 2.5 times the maintenance rate. Immediately before ABLC administration, discontinue LRS, and flush the IV fluid line with dextrose 5%. Infuse the ABLC dose in dextrose 5% over 2 hours. Once the ABLC infusion is complete, flush the IV fluid line with dextrose 5% again and restart LRS at 2.5 times the maintenance rate and continue for 120 minutes after ABLC treatment.

b) Liposomal formulation (*Ambisome®*): 3.3 mg/kg IV once daily for 3 days (10 mg/kg cumulative dose); or 3 mg/kg IV once daily for either 4 doses (days 1, 2, 3, and 10) or 5 doses (days 1, 2, 3, 4, and 10 [cumulative dose: 12 – 15 mg/kg])[26]

CATS:

Serious susceptible systemic fungal infections (extra-label):

Deoxycholate formulations (conventional amphotericin B)

a) Initially, 0.25 mg/kg IV every other day[27]; practically, 3 times per week (eg, Monday, Wednesday, and Friday). The calculated drug dose should be diluted in dextrose 5% (1:50) and administered slowly IV over 4 to 6 hours. Cumulative dose recommendations vary and depend on patient response and drug toxicity; most recommendations range from 6 – 9 mg/kg, but recommendations as low as 4 mg/kg to as high as 16 mg/kg have been noted.[27] Patients must be kept well hydrated before and during treatment, but care must be taken to avoid fluid overload.

b) Initially, 0.5 mg/kg SC 1 to 3 times per week.[10,21] The calculated drug dose should initially be diluted to a concentration of 5 mg/mL and then patient's dose is further diluted into 350 mL of sodium chloride 0.45%/dextrose 2.5% and injected SC between the scapulae. Alternatively, the SC fluid (without amphotericin B) can be injected first, and the amphotericin B dose can then be injected into the SC fluid "lump." Cumulative dose recommendations vary and are dependent on patient response and drug toxicity; most recommendations range from 16 – 20 mg/kg.[10,21,22,28]

Lipid formulations: 1 – 3.3 mg/kg IV over 1 to 2 hours. Cumulative dose recommendations vary and are dependent on patient response and drug toxicity; most recommendations are in the 12 mg/kg range. See the above dosage protocol for dogs [5,29]

HORSES:

NOTE: Using amphotericin B systemically in adult equids can be inordinately expensive, and there is little consensus on dosage regimens.

Serious susceptible systemic fungal infections (extra-label): Using deoxycholate (conventional), initial dose 0.3 mg/kg IV (in 1 L of dextrose 5%) over at least 1 hour; increase dose by 0.1 – 0.15 mg/kg per day on each of the next 2 days. Withhold treatment for 1 to 3 days, then administer 0.5 – 0.6 mg/kg IV every 2 to 3 days (practically, 3 times per week). Treatment has continued for up to one month, or until a cumulative dosage of 6.75 mg/kg has been reached. Oral sodium chloride has been suggested to reduce nephrotoxicity. If toxicity occurs, a dose may be skipped, dosage may be reduced, or dosage interval may be lengthened.[30,31]

Limb pythiosis using IV regional limb perfusion (IRLP; extra-label): After surgical excision of granulation tissue and thermocautery, a catheter is placed in a superficial vein of the affected limb next to the lesion, and a tourniquet is placed above the injection site. Dilute amphotericin B 50 mg (formulation not specified) with 50 mL LRS and administer over 5 minutes. Remove IV catheter 10 minutes post-administration, and apply firm manual pressure over the injection site. Release the tourniquet 45 minutes after administration and bandage the debrided area. Administer a second treatment of amphotericin B if kunkers and/or dark red or black exuberant granulation tissue (necrotic areas) are still observed 14 days after surgery.[13]

Fungal endometritis: 200 – 250 mg/horse (NOT mg/kg) by intrauterine infusion. (NOTE: Amphotericin B formulation was not specified but is assumed to be the conventional/deoxycholate form.) Little science is available for recommending dosages, volume infused, frequency, or diluents. Most intrauterine treatments are commonly performed every day or every other day for 3 to 7 days.[32]

LLAMAS:

Serious susceptible systemic fungal infections (extra-label; from a single case report): Llama with coccidioidomycosis received a test dose of amphotericin 1 mg/llama (NOT mg/kg), then 0.3 mg/kg IV over 4 hours, followed by 3 L of LRS with 1.5 mL of B-complex and 20 mEq of KCl added. Subsequent doses were increased by 10 mg and given every 48 hours until reaching 1 mg/kg every 48 hours IV for 6 weeks. (NOTE: Amphotericin B formulation was not specified but is assumed to be the conventional/deoxycholate form.) The animal tolerated therapy well, but treatment was ultimately unsuccessful.[33]

BIRDS:

Susceptible systemic fungal infections (extra-label):

a) Amphotericin B (conventional) 1.5 mg/kg IV every 12 hours for 3 to 5 days or intratracheally at 1 mg/kg every 12 hours, or 0.3 – 1 mg/mL nebulized for 15 minutes 2 to 4 times daily[34]
b) **Raptors and psittacines with aspergillosis**: Deoxycholate formulation (conventional amphotericin B) 1.5 mg/kg IV every 8 hours for 3 days with flucytosine or follow with flucytosine. May also use intratracheally at 1 mg/kg diluted in sterile water every 8 to 24 hours for 3 days in conjunction with flucytosine or nebulized (1 mg/mL of saline) for 15 minutes every 12 hours. May cause bone marrow suppression[15]
c) **Macrorhabdiasis (*Microrhabdus ornithogaster*)**: Amphotericin B (conventional) 100 – 150 mg/kg PO every 12 hours for 30 days; treatment can be stressful, and failures are common especially with shorter durations of treatment.[35]

RABBITS:

Serious susceptible systemic fungal infections (extra-label): Amphotericin B (conventional) 1 mg/kg/day IV[36]

REPTILES (MOST SPECIES):

Susceptible fungal respiratory infections (extra-label): Anecdotally, amphotericin B (conventional) 1 mg/kg diluted in saline and given intratracheally every 24 hours for 14 to 28 treatments[37]

Monitoring

Also see *Adverse Effects*

- Baseline and periodic (eg, weekly, before each dose) CBC, chemistry panel including electrolytes, and urinalysis during treatment based on clinical presentation and progression of disease
- Several different recommendations have been made regarding stopping treatment when a certain BUN is reached. Most clinicians recommend stopping amphotericin B treatment—at least temporarily—if BUN reaches 30 to 40 mg/dL, if serum creatinine reaches more than 3 mg/dL, or if other clinical signs of systemic toxicity develop (eg, serious depression, vomiting).

Client Information

- Amphotericin B is used to treat serious infections in animals.
- Because the drug requires special handling and frequent bloodwork, it is administered in the veterinarian's clinic.
- Your veterinarian will need to monitor your animal while being treated with this medicine. Do not miss these important follow-up visits.

Chemistry/Synonyms

A polyene macrolide antifungal agent produced by *Streptomyces nodosus*, amphotericin B occurs as a yellow to orange, odorless, or practically odorless powder. It is insoluble in water and anhydrous alcohol. Amphotericin B is amphoteric and can form salts in acidic or basic media. These salts are more water-soluble but possess less antifungal activity than the parent compound. Each mg of amphotericin B must contain not less than 750 µg of anhydrous drug. Amphotericin A may be found as a contaminant in concentrations not exceeding 5%. The commercially available powder for injection contains sodium deoxycholate as a solubilizing agent.

Amphotericin B is available in several formulations. Amphotericin B deoxycholate may also be known as amphotericin generic, AMB, conventional amphotericin B, or *Fungizone®*. Amphotericin B lipid complex may also be known as ABLC or *Abelcet®*. Amphotericin B liposome may also be known as liposomal amphotericin B, lip-AmB, ABL, L-AMB, or *Ambisome®*.

Storage/Stability

The following information is for the conventional (deoxycholate; generic) and lipid complex (ABLC; *Abelcet®*) forms of amphotericin B. If using the liposomal form (*AmBisome®*), refer to the package insert for detailed information.

Vials of amphotericin B deoxycholate powder for injection (conventional; generic) should be stored in the refrigerator (2°C-8°C [36°F-46°F]) and protected from light and moisture. Reconstitution of the powder must be done with sterile water for injection (no preservatives—see directions for preparation in ***Dosage Forms/Regulatory Status***).

After reconstitution of conventional amphotericin B, if protected from light, the solution is stable for 24 hours at room temperature and for 1 week if kept refrigerated. After diluting with dextrose 5% (must have pH more than 4.3) for IV use, the manufacturer recommends continuing to protect the solution from light during administration. Additional studies, however, have shown that potency remains largely unaffected if the solution is exposed to light for 8 to 24 hours.

One reference states that for avian use, the conventional amphotericin B can be diluted with sterile water, divided into 10 mL aliquots using aseptic technique, and stored at -20°C (-4°F) for ≈1 month.[38] However, published data documenting the stability of the drug for this practice have not been located.

Amphotericin B lipid complex vials should be refrigerated at 2°C to 8°C (36°F-46°F) and protected from light and freezing. The manufacturer recommends keeping the vials in their original cartons until use. When diluted in dextrose 5% for administration, the manufacturer states that it can be stored for 48 hours when refrigerated and then an additional 6 hours at room temperature. However, other sources have stated that at a concentration of 1 mg/mL in dextrose 5%, it is stable for 10 days when refrigerated.

Amphotericin B liposomal vials should be stored at temperatures up to 25°C (77°F). Once reconstituted, the concentrated product may be stored for up to 24 hours at 2°C to 8°C (36°F-46°F); do not freeze. Administration should begin within 6 hours after the concentrated product is further diluted with dextrose 5%. Discard unused portions.

Compatibility/Compounding Considerations

Compatibility is dependent on factors such as pH, concentration, temperature, and diluent used; specialized references or a hospital pharmacist should be consulted for more specific information.

Amphotericin B deoxycholate (conventional; generic) is **compatible** with the following solutions and drugs: dextrose 5%, dextrose 5% in sodium chloride 0.2%, heparin sodium, heparin sodium with hydrocortisone sodium phosphate, hydrocortisone sodium phosphate/succinate, and sodium bicarbonate.

Amphotericin B (conventional; generic) is **incompatible** with the following solutions and drugs: sodium chloride 0.9%, lactated Ringer's, D5-sodium chloride 0.9%, D5-lactated Ringer's, amino acids 4.25%-dextrose 25%, amikacin, calcium chloride/gluconate, chlorpromazine HCl, cimetidine HCl, diphenhydramine HCl, dopamine HCl, edetate calcium disodium (CaEDTA), gentamicin sulfate, oxytetracycline HCl, penicillin G potassium/sodium, polymyxin B sulfate, potassium chloride, prochlorperazine mesylate, tetracycline

HCl, and verapamil HCl.[17]

Directions for reconstitution/administration: Using strict aseptic technique and a 20 gauge or larger needle, rapidly inject 10 mL of sterile water for injection (without a bacteriostatic agent) directly into the lyophilized cake; immediately shake well until solution is clear.[17] A 5 mg/mL colloidal solution results. Further dilute (1:50) for administration to a concentration of 0.1 mg/mL with D5W (pH more than 4.2). An in-line filter may be used during administration but must have a pore diameter more than 1 µm.

Amphotericin B lipid complex is **compatible** with dextrose 5%, but it is **incompatible** with sodium chloride 0.9% or other electrolyte solutions.[4]

Directions for dilution/administration: The suspension must be diluted in dextrose 5% for administration.[4] Shake the vial gently so that no sediment remains on the vial bottom. Withdraw the dose using a syringe and needle. Attach the 5 µm filter needle that is supplied with the vial, and add the drug suspension into a bag of D5W. One filter needle may be used for up to 4 vials of drug. The final concentration is usually 1 mg/mL, although 2 mg/mL may be used in cases that require a smaller infusion volume. The bag is shaken just prior to infusion; it should not be used if foreign matter is present. If delivery proceeds over more than 2 hours, the bag should be shaken every 2 hours. Use a separate infusion line or flush an existing line with D5W prior to administration.

Amphotericin B liposomal is **compatible** with D5W, but it is **incompatible** with sodium chloride 0.9%.[3]

Directions for reconstitution/administration: Reconstitute the lyophilized material by adding 12 mL sterile water for injection and shake immediately and vigorously for at least 30 seconds; continue shaking until completely dispersed.[3] Withdraw the required amount of amphotericin B liposomal from the vial into a sterile syringe, attach the provided 5 micron filter needle to the syringe, and add the drug suspension to a sufficient volume of dextrose to achieve a final amphotericin B concentration between 1 – 2 mg/mL, although lower concentration (0.2 – 0.5 mg/mL) may be used to provide an appropriate fluid volume for administration. Use a separate infusion line or flush an existing line with D5W prior to administration. An in-line filter may be used during administration but must have a pore diameter more than 1 µm. Administer amphotericin B liposomal IV infusion over a period of ≈120 minutes, although infusion time may be reduced to ≈60 minutes in patients in whom the treatment is well tolerated.

Dosage Forms/Regulatory Status

VETERINARY-LABELED PRODUCTS: NONE

HUMAN-LABELED PRODUCTS:

Amphotericin B (conventional; deoxycholate) Powder for Injection: 50 mg in vials; generic; (Rx)

Amphotericin B Lipid-complex Suspension Injection: 100 mg/20 mL (as lipid complex) in vials with 5 µm filter needles: *Abelcet®*; (Rx)

Amphotericin B Liposome for Injection: 50 mg in single-dose vials with 5 µm filter; *AmBisome®*; (Rx)

References

For the complete list of references, see **wiley.com/go/budde/plumb**

Ampicillin

Ampicillin Sodium

Ampicillin Trihydrate

(am-pi-***sill***-in) *Princillin®, Omnipen®, Polyflex®*

Aminopenicillin

Prescriber Highlights

- Bactericidal aminopenicillin with same spectrum as amoxicillin (ineffective against bacteria that produce beta-lactamase)
- Poor oral absorption in dogs and cats limits use to parenteral routes; amoxicillin is preferred for oral administration
- Ampicillin trihydrate (*Polyflex®*) must **not** be given IV.
- Adverse effects are infrequent; GI-related effects are most common, but hypersensitivity and other adverse effects occur rarely.

Uses/Indications

In dogs and cats, ampicillin is not well absorbed after oral administration, and its oral use has largely been supplanted by amoxicillin. Ampicillin is used commonly in parenteral dosage forms in all species when an aminopenicillin is indicated. At high doses, ampicillin is still an effective drug for treating penicillin-susceptible enterococci, particularly *Enterococcus faecium*, streptococci, staphylococci, and Enterobacterales. It is often used in combination with a drug with better gram-negative activity (eg, fluoroquinolone, aminoglycoside) when broad-spectrum empirical coverage is needed. It is highly effective against streptococci. The use of ampicillin for staphylococci and Enterobacteriaceae is limited by an increasing prevalence of beta-lactamase–producing strains. Ampicillin can be used as an alternate treatment for leptospirosis when oral doxycycline is not tolerated.[1-3] An aminoglycoside (eg, gentamicin) is often added to treat serious *Enterococcus* spp infections caused by penicillin-sensitive organisms for synergistic activity. Ampicillin is sometimes used for perioperative prophylaxis, but the lack of efficacy against beta-lactamase–producing bacteria limits its efficacy.

The World Health Organization has designated ampicillin as a Critically Important, High Priority antimicrobial for human medicine.[4] The Office International des Epizooties (OIE) has designated ampicillin as Veterinary Critically Important Antimicrobial (VCIA) Agents in avian, bovine, caprine, equine, ovine, and swine species.[5]

Pharmacology/Actions

Like other penicillins, ampicillin is a time-dependent, bactericidal agent that acts by inhibiting cell wall synthesis. Ampicillin and the other aminopenicillins have increased activity against many strains of gram-negative aerobes not covered by either the natural penicillins or penicillinase-resistant penicillins, including some strains of *Escherichia coli, Klebsiella* spp, and *Haemophilus* spp. Like the natural penicillins, aminopenicillilns are susceptible to inactivation by beta-lactamase–producing bacteria (eg, staphylococci, Enterobacterales).

Although they are not as active as the natural penicillins, aminopenicillins do have activity against many anaerobic bacteria, including clostridial organisms. Organisms that are generally not susceptible include *Pseudomonas aeruginosa, Serratia* spp, indole-positive *Proteus* (*Proteus mirabilis* is susceptible), *Enterobacter* spp, *Citrobacter* spp, and *Acinetobacter* spp. The aminopenicillins also are inactive against rickettsial organisms, mycobacteria, fungi, *Mycoplasma* spp, and viruses.

To reduce the inactivation of penicillins by beta-lactamases, potassium clavulanate and sulbactam have been developed to inactivate these enzymes and extend the spectrum of those penicillins. See ***Ampicillin/Sulbactam*** or ***Amoxicillin/Clavulanate***.

Pharmacokinetics

Ampicillin anhydrous and trihydrate are relatively stable in the presence of gastric acid. After oral administration, ampicillin is absorbed ≈30% to 55% in humans (taken on an empty stomach) and monogastric animals. Because amoxicillin oral absorption is ≈75% to 92%, ampicillin is not recommended for oral administration in animals. Food will decrease the rate and extent of oral absorption.

When ampicillin is administered parenterally (ie, IM, SC), the trihydrate salt will achieve serum concentrations of approximately one-half those of a comparable dose of the sodium salt. The trihydrate parenteral dosage form should not be used in cases in which higher MICs are required for treating systemic infections.

After absorption, the volume of distribution for ampicillin is ≈0.3 L/kg in humans and dogs, 0.167 L/kg in cats, and 0.16 to 0.5 L/kg in cattle. The drug is widely distributed to many tissues, including the liver, lungs, prostate (humans), muscle, bile, and ascitic, pleural, and synovial fluids. Ampicillin will cross into the CSF only when meninges are inflamed, reaching concentrations of 10% to 60% those found in serum. Low concentrations of the drug are found in the aqueous humor, tears, sweat, and saliva. Although ampicillin crosses the placenta, it is thought to be relatively safe to use during pregnancy. Ampicillin is ≈20% bound to plasma proteins, primarily albumin.

Ampicillin is eliminated primarily through renal mechanisms, principally by tubular secretion, resulting in high concentrations of active drug in the urine. Some of the drug is metabolized by hydrolysis to penicilloic acids (inactive) then excreted in the urine. Elimination half-lives of ampicillin have been reported as 45 to 80 minutes in dogs and cats and 60 minutes in swine.

Contraindications/Precautions/Warnings

Penicillins are contraindicated in patients with a history of hypersensitivity to them. Because there may be cross-reactivity, penicillins should be used cautiously in patients with documented hypersensitivity to other beta-lactam antibiotics (eg, cephalosporins, cefamycins, carbapenems).

The trihydrate form (*Polyflex*®) must not be given IV, as there is a high risk for anaphylaxis and sudden death. Ampicillin sodium for injection is the only form of ampicillin that may be administered IV.

Ampicillin sodium should be used with caution in azotemic dogs; increased plasma drug concentrations, AUC, and increased elimination half-life have been documented in one study.[6] Dosage adjustment (ie, reduced dosing frequency) may be needed.

In humans, ampicillin has been shown to lower seizure threshold and should be used with caution with any drug that also lowers seizure threshold[7]; significance in veterinary patients is not known.

Penicillins, cephalosporins, and macrolides should not be administered to rabbits, guinea pigs, chinchillas, or hamsters, as serious enteritis and clostridial enterotoxemia may occur.

Adverse Effects

Adverse effects with penicillins are usually not serious and have a relatively low frequency of occurrence.

Hypersensitivity reactions unrelated to dose can occur with these agents and manifest as rashes, fever, eosinophilia, neutropenia, agranulocytosis, thrombocytopenia, leukopenia, anemia, lymphadenopathy, or anaphylaxis.

When given orally, penicillins may cause GI effects (eg, anorexia, vomiting, diarrhea). Because penicillins may also alter the gut microbiota, antibiotic-associated diarrhea can occur and allow the proliferation of resistant bacteria in the colon (ie, superinfections).

Neurotoxicity (eg, ataxia in dogs) has been associated with very high doses or prolonged use. Although penicillins are not considered hepatotoxic, elevated liver enzymes have been reported. Other effects reported in dogs include tachypnea, dyspnea, edema, and tachycardia.

Reproductive/Nursing Safety

Penicillins have been shown to cross the placenta; although safe use during pregnancy has not been firmly established, there has not been any documented teratogenic problem associated with these drugs.

Milk concentrations of ampicillin are considered low. In lactating dairy cattle, the milk:plasma ratio is about 0.3.

Because safety has not been established in animals, this drug should only be used when the maternal benefits outweigh the potential risks to offspring.

Overdose/Acute Toxicity

Acute oral penicillin overdoses are unlikely to cause significant problems other than GI distress, but other effects are possible (see ***Adverse Effects***). In humans, high doses of parenteral penicillins, particularly in patients with renal disease, have induced CNS effects.

For patients that have experienced or are suspected to have experienced an overdose, consultation with a 24-hour poison control center specializing in providing veterinary-specific information is recommended. For general information related to overdose and toxin exposures, as well as contact information for poison control centers, refer to ***Appendix***.

Drug Interactions

The following drug interactions with ampicillin either have been reported or are theoretical in humans or animals and may be of significance in veterinary patients. Unless otherwise noted, use together is not necessarily contraindicated, but the potential risks should be weighed and additional monitoring should be performed when appropriate.

- **ALLOPURINOL**: In humans, concurrent use has been implicated in increased occurrences of skin rashes; veterinary significance of this interaction is unknown.
- **AMINOGLYCOSIDES** (eg, **amikacin**, **gentamicin**): Beta-lactam antibiotics can inactivate aminoglycosides in vitro (and in vivo in patients with chronic kidney disease).
- **ATENOLOL**: Concurrent oral use may decrease atenolol bioavailability.
- **BACTERIOSTATIC ANTIMICROBIALS** (eg, **chloramphenicol, erythromycin,** and **other macrolides, tetracyclines, sulfonamides**): Because there is evidence of in vitro antagonism between beta-lactam antibiotics and bacteriostatic antibiotics, use together has generally not been recommended, but actual clinical importance is not clear and is currently in doubt.
- **DICHLORPHENAMIDE:** Concurrent use may increase hypokalemia risk.
- **METHOTREXATE (MTX)**: Ampicillin may decrease the renal excretion of MTX, causing increased levels and potential toxic effects.
- **MYCOPHENOLATE**: Concurrent use may reduce levels or effects of mycophenolate.
- **PROBENECID**: Competitively blocks the tubular secretion of most penicillins, thereby increasing serum levels and serum half-lives
- **PROTON PUMP INHIBITORS (PPIs**; eg, **omeprazole**, **pantoprazole**): May reduce absorption of oral ampicillin
- **WARFARIN**: Concurrent use may decrease vitamin K production and increase risk for bleeding.

Laboratory Considerations

- Ampicillin may cause false-positive **urine glucose determinations** with the use of cupric sulfate solution (Benedict's Solution, *Clinitest*®). Tests using glucose oxidase (*Tes-Tape*®, *Clinistix*®) are not affected by ampicillin.
- Because penicillins and other beta-lactams can inactivate **aminoglycosides** in vitro (and in vivo in patients in renal failure), serum concentrations of aminoglycosides may be falsely decreased if the

patient is also receiving beta-lactam antibiotics, particularly when the serum is stored prior to analysis. It is recommended that samples should be drawn at times when the beta-lactam antibiotic is at a trough level and, if the assay cannot be run right away, samples should be frozen immediately.

Dosages

DOGS/CATS:

Ampicillin *trihydrate* (*Polyflex*®) injection (label dosage; FDA-approved): **NOTE**: Although the following indications and dosages are on the FDA-approved label, the label dosages are not accepted by most clinicians today as being consistently efficacious because of the listed low doses and dosing interval.

Indications: Respiratory Tract Infections: Upper respiratory infections, tonsillitis and bronchopneumonia due to hemolytic streptococci, *Staphylococcus aureus, Escherichia coli, Proteus mirabilis,* and *Pasteurella* spp. Urinary Tract Infections due to *Proteus mirabilis, E coli, Staphylococcus* spp, hemolytic streptococci, and *Enterococcus* spp. GI Infections due to *Enterococcus* spp, *Staphylococcus* spp, and *E coli*. Skin, Soft Tissue, and Postsurgical Infections: Abscesses, pustular dermatitis, cellulitis and infections of the anal gland due to *E coli, Proteus mirabilis,* hemolytic streptococci, *Staphylococcus* spp, and *Pasteurella* spp. **Dosage**: 6.6 mg/kg SC or IM twice daily.[8] The dosage will vary according to the animal being treated, the severity of the infection, and the animal's response. Treatment for 3 days is usually adequate, but treatment should be continued for 48 to 72 hours after the animal has become afebrile or there is resolution of clinical signs associated with infection.

Adjunctive antibiotic therapy for sepsis (empiric therapy) or susceptible systemic infections (extra-label): Ampicillin *sodium* 20 – 40 mg/kg IV every 6 to 8 hours; usually used in combination with an antibiotic that enhances coverage for gram-negative organisms (eg, aminoglycoside, fluoroquinolone). Enterococci infections may require much higher ampicillin dosages (40 – 100 mg/kg).

Leptospirosis in dogs (extra-label): Ampicillin *sodium* 20 mg/kg IV every 6 hours if vomiting or other adverse reactions, or the need for parenteral treatment preclude doxycycline administration.[9]

Acute treatment in dogs of endocarditis secondary to a susceptible strain of *Streptococcus canis* (extra-label): Ampicillin *sodium* 20 – 40 mg/kg IV every 6 to 8 hours[10]

HORSES:

Ampicillin *sodium* injection (label dosage; FDA-approved): **NOTE**: Although the following indications and dosages are on the FDA-approved label, the label dosages are not accepted by most today as being consistently efficacious.

Indications: Respiratory Tract Infections: Bacterial infections caused by susceptible strains of *Staphylococcus* species, *Streptococcus* spp, *E coli,* and *Proteus mirabilis.* Skin and soft tissue infections: Bacterial infections caused by susceptible strains of *Staphylococcus* spp, *E coli,* and *Proteus mirabilis.* **Dosage**: 6.6 mg/kg IV or IM twice daily.[11] Treatment should be continued 48 hours after all clinical signs of infection have subsided.

Susceptible infections (extra-label): Ampicillin *sodium* 20 mg/kg IV or IM every 6 to 8 hours

Streptococcal lower airway infections (extra-label): Ampicillin *sodium* 15 mg/kg IV every 12 hours from a pharmacokinetic study. Ampicillin concentrations in pulmonary epithelial lining fluid (PELF) are above minimum inhibitory concentration (MIC) values for at least 12 hours. Treatment of other bacterial pathogens requires susceptibility testing and possibly more frequent dosing, depending on MIC.[12]

Foals (extra-label): Ampicillin *sodium* 15 – 30 mg/kg IV or IM every 6 to 8 hours[11]

CATTLE

Ampicillin *trihydrate* (*Polyflex*®) injection (label dosage; FDA-approved):

Indications: Respiratory Tract Infections: Bacterial pneumonia (shipping fever, calf pneumonia and bovine pneumonia) caused by *Aerobacter* spp, *Klebsiella* spp, *Staphylococcus* spp, *Streptococcus* spp, *Pasteurella multocida*, and *E coli* susceptible to ampicillin trihydrate. **Dosage**: 4.4 – 11 mg/kg once daily IM.[8] Do not treat for more than 7 days. Treatment for 3 days is usually adequate, but treatment should be continued for 48 to 72 hours after the animal has become afebrile or there is resolution of clinical signs associated with infection. One study looked at the effects of dosing twice daily and concluded that there was no significant effect of dosing interval on achieving therapeutic concentrations in the milk, lochial fluid, and endometrial tissue.[13]

Respiratory infections: (extra-label): Ampicillin *trihydrate* (*Polyflex*®) 22 mg/kg SC every 12 hours[14]

Surgical prophylaxis (extra-label): Ampicillin *sodium* 5 g IV as a single dose administered ≈15 minutes prior to the first incision[15]

FERRETS:

Susceptible infections (extra-label): 5 – 10 mg/kg IM, SC, or IV twice daily[16]

RODENTS/SMALL MAMMALS:

a) **Rabbits, Guinea pigs, Chinchillas, Hamsters** (extra-label): Not recommended as it can cause a fatal enterocolitis[17]
b) **Gerbils, Mice, Rats** (extra-label): 20 – 100 mg/kg PO, SC, or IM every 8 to 12 hours[18]
c) **Hedgehogs** (extra-label): 10 mg/kg IM or PO once daily[19]

REPTILES:

Respiratory tract infections (extra-label): 50 mg/kg SC or IM every 12 hours[20]

Monitoring

- Because penicillins usually have minimal toxicity associated with their use, monitoring for efficacy is usually all that is required unless toxic signs develop. Serum levels and therapeutic drug monitoring are not routinely done with these agents.

Client Information

- Antibiotic given by injection under the skin or into the muscle. Do not administer into the vein. Be sure you understand how to safely give this medicine to your animal.
- Your animal's signs of infections should improve within 2 or 3 days of starting treatment. Contact your veterinarian if your animal appears to not be responding to treatment.
- Follow recommended drug residue withholding times if you are administering to an animal that will be used for human food.

Chemistry/Synonyms

As semisynthetic aminopenicillins, ampicillin anhydrous and trihydrate occur as practically odorless, white, crystalline powders that are slightly soluble in water. At usual temperatures (less than 42°C [107.6°F]), ampicillin anhydrous is more soluble in water than the trihydrate (13 mg/mL vs 6 mg/mL at 20°C [68°F]). Ampicillin anhydrous or trihydrate oral suspensions have a pH of 5 to 7.5 after reconstitution with water. After reconstitution, ampicillin trihydrate for injection is pale white to yellow in color.

Ampicillin sodium occurs as an odorless or practically odorless, white to off-white, crystalline hygroscopic powder. It is very soluble in water or other aqueous solutions. After reconstitution, ampicillin sodium has a pH of 8 to 10 at a concentration of 10 mg/mL. Commercially available ampicillin sodium for injection has ≈3 mEq of sodium per gram of ampicillin.

Potency of the ampicillin salts is expressed in terms of ampicillin anhydrous.

Ampicillin may also be known as aminobenzylpenicillin, ampicillinum, ampicillinum anhydricum, anhydrous ampicillin, AY-6108, BRL-1341, NSC-528986, or P-50; many trade names are available.

Storage/Stability

Ampicillin trihydrate (*Polyflex®*) powder for injection should be stored at or below 25°C (77°F), with excursions permitted up to 30°C (86°F). After reconstitution, it is stable for 3 months when refrigerated.

Ampicillin anhydrous or trihydrate capsules and powder for oral suspension should be stored at room temperature (15°C-30°C [59°F-86°F]). After reconstitution, the oral suspension is stable for 14 days if refrigerated (2°C-8°C [36°F-46°F]) or 7 days when kept at room temperature.

Ampicillin sodium powder for injection should be stored at room temperature (15°C-30°C [59°F-86°F]). The drug is relatively unstable after reconstitution and should be used within 1 hour of reconstitution. As the concentration of the drug in solution increases, the stability of the drug decreases. Dextrose may also speed the destruction of the drug by acting as a catalyst in the hydrolysis of ampicillin.

Although most sources recommend using solutions of ampicillin sodium immediately, studies have demonstrated that refrigeration at 4°C (39.2°F) increases stability of reconstituted solutions. In sterile water for injection, ampicillin sodium solutions are stable at 30 mg/mL for up to 48 hours and at 20 mg/mL or less for up to 72 hours. In 0.9% sodium chloride, ampicillin sodium solutions are stable at 30 mg/mL for up to 24 hours and at 20 mg/mL or less for up to 48 hours.

Compatibility/Compounding Considerations

Compatibility is dependent on factors such as pH, concentration, temperature, and diluent used; specialized references or a hospital pharmacist should be consulted for more specific information.

Ampicillin sodium is reportedly **Y-site compatible** with the following solutions and additives: aminocaproic acid, asparaginase, azithromycin, carboplatin, cisplatin, clarithromycin, cytarabine, dexmedetomidine hydrochloride, dexrazoxane, doxapram hydrochloride, doxorubicin hydrochloride (liposomal), fat emulsions, gemcitabine hydrochloride, heparin sodium, levofloxacin, mannitol, methadone hydrochloride, metronidazole, pantoprazole sodium, *Plasma-Lyte A*, potassium chloride, propofol, vinblastine sulfate, vincristine sulfate, voriconazole, and zoledronic acid.

Ampicillin sodium injection has ***variable or uncertain Y-site compatibility*** with amikacin sulfate, ascorbic acid (vitamin C), atracurium besylate, atropine sulfate, butorphanol tartrate, calcium chloride, calcium gluconate, cefazolin sodium, cefotaxime, cefotetan disodium, ceftazidime, ceftriaxone sodium, cefuroxime, chloramphenicol sodium succinate, clindamycin phosphate, cyclophosphamide, cyclosporine, dexamethasone sodium succinate, digoxin, diltiazem hydrochloride, dopamine hydrochloride, edetate calcium disodium, epinephrine hydrochloride, epinephrine sulfate, erythromycin lactobionate, esmolol hydrochloride, famotidine, fentanyl citrate, furosemide, gentamicin sulfate, glycopyrrolate, heparin sodium, hydralazine hydrochloride, hydrocortisone sodium succinate, hydromorphone hydrochloride, insulin (regular), lactated Ringer's solution, lidocaine hydrochloride, magnesium sulfate, mechlorethamine hydrochloride, metoclopramide hydrochloride, morphine sulfate, multiple vitamins injection, naloxone hydrochloride, nitroglycerin, nitroprusside, norepinephrine bitartrate, oxytocin, penicillin G potassium, penicillin G sodium, pentobarbital sodium, phenobarbital sodium, phytonadione (vitamin K_1), polymyxin B sulfate, potassium chloride, procainamide, propranolol hydrochloride, ranitidine hydrochloride, sodium bicarbonate, succinylcholine chloride, theophylline, thiamine hydrochloride (vitamin B_1), tobramycin sulfate, and vasopressin.

Ampicillin sodium is reportedly **incompatible** with the following additives: aminophylline, amiodarone hydrochloride, amphotericin B cholesteryl sulfate complex, amphotericin B conventional colloidal, amphotericin B lipid complex, amphotericin B liposome, buprenorphine hydrochloride, chlorpromazine hydrochloride, diazepam, diphenhydramine hydrochloride, dobutamine hydrochloride, doxorubicin hydrochloride, doxycycline hyclate, fluconazole, ketamine hydrochloride, lorazepam, midazolam hydrochloride, mitoxantrone hydrochloride, mycophenolate mofetil hydrochloride, ondansetron hydrochloride, phenytoin sodium, prochlorperazine edisylate, prochlorperazine mesylate, protamine sulfate, tranexamic acid, trimethoprim-sulfamethoxazole, and vinorelbine tartrate.

Dosage Forms/Regulatory Status

VETERINARY-LABELED PRODUCTS:

Ampicillin Trihydrate Injection Powder for Suspension: 25 g (of ampicillin) vials; *Polyflex®*; (Rx). NADA 055-030. FDA-approved for use in dogs, cats, and cattle. Withdrawal times at labeled doses (cattle, do not treat for more than 7 days): Milk = 48 hours (4 milkings); Slaughter = 6 days (144 hours).

Ampicillin Sodium Powder for Injection: 1 g and 3 g vials; generic; (Rx). NADA # 200-335. FDA-approved for use in horses not intended for meat production.

The following products are listed in the FDA Green Book, but marketing status is uncertain.

Ampicillin Trihydrate Soluble Powder: 88.2 mg (of ampicillin) per gram of powder; *Princillin®*; (Rx). FDA-approved for use in swine. Withdrawal times at labeled doses: Slaughter = 24 hours.

Ampicillin Trihydrate Capsules: 125 mg, 250 mg, and 500 mg (of ampicillin) capsules; *Princillin®*; (Rx). FDA-approved for use in dogs and cats.

Ampicillin Trihydrate Tablets: 50 mg and 100 mg (of ampicillin) tablets; *Ampi-Tab®* (Rx). FDA-approved for use in dogs.

Ampicillin Anhydrous Capsules: 125 mg and 250 mg (of ampicillin) capsules; *Omnipen®*; (Rx). FDA-approved for use in dogs and cats.

HUMAN-LABELED PRODUCTS:

Ampicillin Sodium Powder for Injection: 125 mg, 250 mg, 500 mg, 1 g, 2 g, and 10 g in vials; generic; (Rx)

Ampicillin Oral Capsules (as trihydrate): 250 mg and 500 mg; generic; (Rx)

Ampicillin (as trihydrate) Powder for Oral Suspension: 125 mg/5 mL (25 mg/mL) and 250 mg/5 mL (50 mg/mL) when reconstituted; generic; (Rx)

References

For the complete list of references, see **wiley.com/go/budde/plumb**

Ampicillin/Sulbactam

(am-pi-***sill***-in; sul-***bak***-tam) *Unasyn®*

Potentiated Aminopenicillin

Prescriber Highlights

- ▶ Parenteral potentiated aminopenicillin that may be used to treat infections for which amoxicillin/clavulanate would be appropriate, but an injectable antibiotic is required
- ▶ May be used for surgical prophylaxis
- ▶ Hypersensitivity reactions possible; contraindicated in patients with documented severe hypersensitivity to penicillins
- ▶ Usually administered SC, IM, or IV every 6 to 8 hours

Uses/Indications

The addition of sulbactam to ampicillin broadens ampicillin's spectrum through inhibition of some beta-lactamases.

Ampicillin/sulbactam may be indicated when parenteral therapy is required for the treatment of aerobic or anaerobic gram-positive and gram-negative infections. In dogs and cats, ampicillin/sulbactam may be considered when oral amoxicillin/clavulanate is not viable (eg, patient NPO, in cases of critical illness [eg, sepsis, pneumonia, other severe infections]), or for surgical prophylaxis. For broad spectrum uses, ampicillin/sulbactam is often combined with another drug such as a fluoroquinolone or aminoglycoside to provide enhanced gram-negative coverage.

The World Health Organization (WHO) has designated ampicillin/sulbactam as a Critically Important, High Priority antimicrobial in human medicine.[1] The Office International des Epizooties (OIE) has designated ampicillin/sulbactam as Veterinary Critically Important Antimicrobial (VCIA) Agents in avian, bovine, and swine species.[2]

Pharmacology/Actions

Ampicillin is a time-dependent bactericidal agent that acts via inhibition of cell wall synthesis. Penicillins are bactericidal against susceptible bacteria and act by inhibition of mucopeptide synthesis in the cell wall, which results in a defective barrier and an osmotically unstable spheroplast. The exact mechanism for this effect has not been definitively determined, but beta-lactam antibiotics have been shown to bind to several enzymes in the bacterial cytoplasmic membrane that are involved with cell wall synthesis (eg, carboxypeptidases, transpeptidases, endopeptidases). Various beta-lactam antibiotics have different affinities for these enzymes (ie, penicillin-binding proteins), which helps explain the differences in spectrums of activity not explained by the influence of beta-lactamases. Like other beta-lactam antibiotics, penicillins are generally considered to be more effective against actively growing bacteria.

Sulbactam has some intrinsic antibacterial activity against some bacteria (eg, *Neisseria* spp, *Moraxella* spp, *Bacteroides* spp); however, for most bacteria, sulbactam alone does not achieve levels sufficient to act as an antibacterial agent. Sulbactam binding to certain penicillin-binding proteins may explain its activity and, when used in combination with ampicillin, synergistic effects may result. On an mg-for-mg basis, clavulanic acid is a more potent beta-lactamase inhibitor than sulbactam, but sulbactam offers reduced likelihood of inducing chromosomal beta-lactamases, greater tissue penetration, and stability.

When sulbactam is combined with ampicillin, ampicillin's spectrum of activity is extended to bacteria (eg, *Escherichia coli*, *Pasteurella* spp, *Staphylococcus* spp, *Klebsiella* spp, *Proteus* spp) that produce beta-lactamases of Richmond-Sykes types II through VI that would otherwise render ampicillin ineffective. Sulbactam binds to beta-lactamases, thereby protecting the beta-lactam ring of ampicillin from hydrolysis. The efficacy of sulbactam involves how well it binds the specific beta-lactamase and the relative levels of sulbactam and beta-lactamase. In cases in which there is a high bacterial bioburden or bacteria are producing large amounts of beta-lactamase, efficacy may be limited. Other aerobic bacteria that may be susceptible to ampicillin/sulbactam include *Streptococcus* spp, *Listeria monocytogenes*, *Bacillus anthracis*, *Salmonella* spp, *Pasteurella* spp, and *Acinetobacter* spp. Anaerobic bacterial infections caused by *Clostridium* spp, *Bacteroides* spp, *Fusobacterium* spp, *Peptostreptococcus* spp, and *Propionibacterium* spp may also be susceptible to ampicillin/sulbactam.[3-5] Similar to amoxicillin/clavulanic acid, ampicillin/sulbactam can be used in the treatment of bacterial respiratory tract infections, although ampicillin/sulbactam is ineffective against *Mycoplasma* spp and resistance in *Bordetella* spp is an increasing problem in some regions. In general, ampicillin/sulbactam is excellent for beta-lactamase–producing gram-positive aerobic and anaerobic bacteria, but less effective for beta-lactamase–producing gram-negative bacteria.

Methicillin-resistant staphylococci are resistant to ampicillin/sulbactam. Ampicillin/sulbactam is usually ineffective against AmpC (type I) cephalosporinases, and efficacy against extended-spectrum beta-lactamase–producing bacteria is variable and often unpredictable. There is little—if any—synergistic activity against organisms already susceptible to ampicillin.

Pharmacokinetics

See ***Ampicillin*** for pharmacokinetic information.

Because sulbactam sodium is not appreciably absorbed from the GI tract, this medication must be given parenterally. A covalently linked double ester form of ampicillin/sulbactam (ie, sultamicillin) is orally absorbed, but this combination is not commercially available in the US. When sulbactam is administered parenterally (ie, IV, IM), its pharmacokinetic profile closely mirrors that of ampicillin's pharmacokinetic profile in most species studied. In a study of calves, plasma concentrations of sulbactam during the elimination phase were consistently higher than those of ampicillin, leading the study authors to propose using a higher ratio (greater than 2:1 ampicillin/sulbactam) if the combination is used in calves.[6]

A regional IV limb perfusion (RIVLP; 45-minute duration) with ampicillin/sulbactam (1.5 g; ratio, 2:1; total volume, 4 mL) administered in the dorsal common digital vein of the right rear limb of healthy, adult nonlactating cattle resulted in peak ampicillin serum concentrations of ≈5 mg/mL in the perfused limb and 2 mg/mL in the synovial fluid of the metatarsophalangeal joint 1 hour after RIVLP. Ampicillin concentration in synovial fluid remained above 8 µg/mL for 19 hours. Maximum systemic ampicillin concentration was 2.5 µg/mL 5.4 hours after RIVLP. Sulbactam pharmacokinetics followed trends similar to ampicillin.[7]

Contraindications/Precautions/Warnings

Penicillins are contraindicated in patients with a history of severe hypersensitivity (anaphylaxis) to them. Because cross-reactivity can occur, penicillins should be used cautiously in patients documented as being hypersensitive to other beta-lactam antibiotics (eg, cephalosporins, cephamycins, carbapenems).

Ampicillin/sulbactam is contraindicated in humans with a history of ampicillin/sulbactam-associated cholestatic jaundice or hepatic dysfunction; veterinary significance is unknown. In humans, ampicillin has been shown to lower seizure threshold and should be used with caution with any drug that also lowers seizure threshold[8]; significance in veterinary patients is not known.

Increased plasma ampicillin drug concentrations, AUC, and increased elimination half-life have been documented in azotemic dogs.[9] Dosage adjustment (ie, reduced dosing frequency) may be needed.

Penicillins, cephalosporins, and macrolides should not be administered to rabbits, guinea pigs, chinchillas, or hamsters, as serious enteritis and clostridial enterotoxemia may occur.

Adverse Effects

IM injections may be painful, as pH of the solution is high. IV injections may cause thrombophlebitis and phlebitis. Although hypersensitivity reactions to penicillins occur infrequently in animals, they can be severe (anaphylaxis), particularly after IV administration.

Hepatotoxicity (ie, cholestatic hepatitis, cholestasis) has been reported in some humans receiving ampicillin/sulbactam. Toxicity is usually reversible with discontinuation of therapy, but deaths have been reported. Veterinary significance is unknown.

High doses or increased CNS penetration of penicillins have been associated with neurotoxicity (eg, ataxia in dogs).[10] Although penicillins are not considered to be hepatotoxic, elevated liver enzymes have been reported in some dogs. Other effects reported in dogs include tachypnea, dyspnea, edema, and tachycardia. GI disturbances are possible, and *Clostridium difficile*-associated diarrhea (CDAD) has been reported in humans.

Reproductive/Nursing Safety

Both ampicillin and sulbactam have been shown to cross the placenta. Ampicillin/sulbactam should be used only when the potential benefits outweigh the risks.

Both ampicillin and sulbactam are distributed into human breast milk in low concentrations but are considered to be compatible with breastfeeding. Nursing offspring should be monitored for GI disturbances.

Overdose/Acute Toxicity

Neurologic effects (eg, ataxia) have rarely been reported, and risk increases with higher doses or conditions that can lead to increased CNS penetration (eg, meningitis); should these signs develop, the risks for continued use should be weighed with those associated with dose reduction or use of a different antibiotic. In humans, particularly those with renal disease, high doses of parenteral penicillins have induced CNS effects.

For patients that have experienced or are suspected to have experienced an overdose, consultation with a 24-hour poison control center specializing in providing veterinary-specific information is recommended. For general information related to overdose and toxin exposures, as well as contact information for poison control centers, refer to ***Appendix***.

Drug Interactions

The following drug interactions with ampicillin/sulbactam either have been reported or are theoretical in humans or animals and may be of significance in veterinary patients. Unless otherwise noted, use together is not necessarily contraindicated, but the potential risks should be weighed and additional monitoring performed when appropriate.

- **Allopurinol**: In humans, concurrent use has been implicated in increased occurrences of skin rashes; veterinary significance of this interaction is unknown.
- **Aminoglycosides** (eg, **amikacin, gentamicin**): Beta-lactam antibiotics can inactivate aminoglycosides in vitro (and in vivo in patients with chronic kidney disease).
- **Bacteriostatic Antimicrobials** (eg, **chloramphenicol, erythromycin and other macrolides, tetracyclines, sulfonamides**): Because there has been evidence of in vitro antagonism between beta-lactam antibiotics and bacteriostatic antibiotics, use together generally has not been recommended, but actual clinical importance is not clear and is currently in doubt.
- **Dichlorphenamide:** Concurrent use may increase risk for hypokalemia.
- **Methotrexate (MTX)**: Ampicillin may decrease the renal excretion of MTX, causing increased MTX concentrations and potential toxic effects.
- **Mycophenolate**: Concurrent use may reduce concentrations or effects of mycophenolate.
- **Probenecid**: Can reduce the renal tubular secretion of both ampicillin and sulbactam, thereby maintaining higher systemic concentrations for a longer period. This potentially beneficial interaction requires further investigation before dosing recommendations can be made for veterinary patients.
- **Warfarin:** Concurrent use may decrease vitamin K production and increase risk for bleeding.

Laboratory Considerations

- Ampicillin may cause false-positive **urine glucose determinations** when using cupric sulfate solution (Benedict's solution, *Clinitest*®). Tests using glucose oxidase (*Test-Tape*®, *Clinistix*®) are not affected by ampicillin.
- Because penicillins and other beta-lactams can inactivate **aminoglycosides** in vitro and in vivo in patients in renal failure or when penicillins are used in larger doses, serum concentrations of aminoglycosides may be falsely decreased, particularly when the serum is stored prior to analysis. It is recommended that samples should be drawn at times when the beta-lactam antibiotic is at a trough level, and if the assay cannot be run right away, samples should be frozen immediately.

Dosages

DOGS/CATS:

NOTE: Dosages are listed for combined amounts of ampicillin/sulbactam.

Empiric antibiotic therapy in critically ill animals (extra-label): 22 – 30 mg/kg IV every 6 to 8 hours; used in combination with a parenteral drug with gram-negative activity (eg, aminoglycoside, fluoroquinolone)

Infections susceptible to amoxicillin/clavulanate in patients unable to receive oral doses (extra-label): 22 mg/kg SC, IV, or IM every 8 hours

Surgical prophylaxis (extra-label): 22 mg/kg IV ≈1 hour prior to incision; redosing can be performed intraoperatively every 2 hours if needed based on duration of surgery.

Monitoring

- Because penicillins usually have minimal toxicity associated with their use, monitoring for efficacy is usually all that is required unless toxic signs develop.
- Periodic liver panel (eg, liver enzymes, bilirubin) in patients with pre-existing hepatic dysfunction
- Serum concentrations and therapeutic drug monitoring are not routinely performed.

Client Information

- Because of the dosing intervals required, this drug is best administered to inpatients only.

Chemistry/Synonyms

Commercial drug formulations contain sodium salts of both ampicillin and sulbactam in a 2:1 ratio (eg, ampicillin, 250 mg; sulbactam, 125 mg). Ampicillin sodium/sulbactam sodium for injection occurs as a white to off-white powder that is freely soluble in water or other aqueous solutions. The reconstituted solution is yellow to pale yellow and has a pH of 8 to 10.

Ampicillin/sulbactam may also be known as *Ampibactan*®, *Bacimex*®, *Begalin-P*®, *Bethacil*®, *Comabactan*®, *Galotam*®, *Loricin*®, *Sulam*®, *Sulperazon*®, *Synergistin*®, *Unacid*®, *Unacim*®, *Unasyn*®, or *Unasyna*®.

Storage/Stability

Ampicillin/sulbactam powder should be stored at temperatures at or below 30°C (86°F).

Compatibility/Compounding Considerations

Compatibility is dependent on factors such as pH, concentration, temperature, and diluent used; specialized references or a hospital pharmacist should be consulted for more specific information.

Diluents for reconstituting the powder for IV use reported to be **compatible** with ampicillin/sulbactam include sterile water for injection and 0.9% sodium chloride. If the powder is reconstituted to a concentration of 30 mg/mL (combined concentration), the resultant solution is stable for 72 hours at 4°C (39.2°F) or 8 hours at room temperature. After reconstitution and before administration, the solution can either be given slowly IV over 5 to 20 minutes or be further diluted into a 50- or 100-mL bag of 0.9% sodium chloride and administered IV over 15 to 30 minutes.

When ampicillin/sulbactam is reconstituted for IM use, sterile water for injection or 0.5% or 2% lidocaine HCl for injection may be used as a diluent; 3.2 mL of diluent should be added to the 1.5 g vial and 6.4 mL of diluent to the 3 g vial. After reconstitution, the solution should be administered within 1 hour.

Ampicillin/sulbactam injection is **compatible** with vancomycin when mixed at concentrations of 50/25 mg/mL of ampicillin/sulbactam and 20 mg/mL or less of vancomycin. Ampicillin/sulbactam is **Y-site compatible** with aminocaproic acid, asparaginase, azithromycin, carboplatin, cisplatin, cytarabine, dexmedetomidine hydrochloride, doxorubicin hydrochloride (liposomal), fat emulsions, gemcitabine hydrochloride, hydromorphone hydrochloride, methadone hydrochloride, metronidazole, pamidronate disodium, pantoprazole sodium, sodium acetate, vinblastine sulfate, vincristine sulfate, voriconazole, and zoledronic acid.

Ampicillin/sulbactam injection has ***variable or uncertain Y-site compatibility*** with amikacin sulfate, aminophylline, ascorbic acid (vitamin C), atracurium besylate, atropine sulfate, buprenorphine hydrochloride, butorphanol tartrate, calcium chloride, calcium gluconate, cefazolin sodium, cefotetan disodium, cefotaxime, ceftazidime, ceftriaxone sodium, cefuroxime, chloramphenicol sodium succinate, clindamycin phosphate, cyclosporine, dexamethasone sodium succinate, dextrose 5% in water, digoxin, diltiazem hydrochloride, diphenhydramine hydrochloride, dopamine hydrochloride, epinephrine hydrochloride, erythromycin lactobionate, esmolol hydrochloride, famotidine, fentanyl citrate, fluconazole, furosemide, gentamicin sulfate, glycopyrrolate, heparin sodium, insulin (regular), lactated Ringer's solution (LRS), lidocaine hydrochloride, magnesium sulfate, mannitol, metoclopramide, morphine sulfate, multiple vitamins injections, naloxone hydrochloride, nitroglycerin, nitroprusside sodium, norepinephrine bitartrate, oxytocin, penicillin G potassium, penicillin G sodium, pentobarbital sodium, phenobarbital sodium, polymyxin B sulfate, potassium chloride, procainamide hydrochloride, ranitidine hydrochloride, sodium bicarbonate, thiamine hydrochloride (vitamin B_1), and vasopressin.

Administration of ampicillin diluted in LRS has been shown to decrease ampicillin concentrations by ≈30%; therefore, coadministration with LRS (ie, through the same fluid line) should be performed with caution.[11]

Ampicillin/sulbactam is **Y-site incompatible** with amiodarone hydrochloride, amphotericin B conventional, amphotericin B liposomal, ciprofloxacin, diazepam, dobutamine hydrochloride, doxorubicin hydrochloride, doxycycline hyclate, hydralazine hydrochloride, hydrocortisone sodium succinate, hydroxyzine hydrochloride, lorazepam, mechlorethamine hydrochloride, methylprednisolone sodium succinate, midazolam hydrochloride, mitoxantrone hydrochloride, mycophenolate mofetil hydrochloride, ondansetron hydrochloride, phenytoin sodium, quinidine gluconate, trimethoprim/sulfamethoxazole, tranexamic acid, and vinorelbine tartrate.

Dosage Forms/Regulatory Status

VETERINARY-LABELED PRODUCTS: NONE

HUMAN-LABELED PRODUCTS:

Ampicillin Sodium/Sulbactam Sodium Powder (injection): 1.5 g (ampicillin sodium 1 g; sulbactam sodium 0.5 g) and 3 g (ampicillin sodium 2 g; sulbactam sodium 1 g) in vials; 15 g (ampicillin sodium 10 g; sulbactam sodium 5 g) in bulk; *Unasyn®*, generic; (Rx)

References

For the complete list of references, see **wiley.com/go/budde/plumb**

Amprolium

(am-proe-***lee***-um) *AmproMed®, Corid®*

Anticoccidial

Prescriber Highlights

- Thiamine analogue coccidiostat
- Prolonged high doses may cause thiamine deficiency; length of treatment usually does not exceed 14 days
- Occasionally may cause GI or neurologic effects
- May be unpalatable

Uses/Indications

Amprolium is FDA-approved for the treatment and prevention of *Eimeria bovis* and *Eimeria zurnii* in calves, and for the treatment of coccidiosis in poultry.

Although there are no FDA-approved products in the US for dogs, swine, sheep, or goats, amprolium has also been used in these species for the control of coccidiosis.

Pharmacology/Actions

By mimicking the structure of thiamine, amprolium competitively inhibits thiamine utilization by the parasite preferentially; amprolium has this same effect in the host but to a far less extent.[1]

Amprolium is a coccidiostat. It has good activity against *Eimeria tenella* and *Eimeria acervulina* in poultry and can be used as a therapeutic agent against these organisms. Amprolium only has marginal activity or weak activity against *Eimeria maxima, Eimeria mivati, Eimeria necatrix*, and *Eimeria brunetti*; it is often used in combination with other agents (eg, ethopabate) to improve control against these organisms.

Amprolium acts primarily upon the first-generation trophozoites and schizonts in enterocytes, preventing differentiation of the merozoites; it also suppresses the sexual stages and sporulation of the oocysts.

Pharmacokinetics

Chickens receiving amprolium 20 mg/kg PO demonstrated the following pharmacokinetic values: maximum blood concentrations at 4 hours; volume of distribution, 0.5 L/kg; clearance, 1.98 mL/kg/min.[2]

Contraindications/Precautions/Warnings

Amprolium is not recommended to be used for more than 12 days in puppies.

The undiluted liquid is reportedly unpalatable. Excessive dietary thiamine can reduce or reverse the anticoccidial activity of the drug.

Adverse Effects

In dogs, neurologic disturbances (eg, "stargazing", opisthotonos, central blindness, circling, ataxia), depression, anorexia, and diarrhea have been reported but are rare and likely dose related. See *Overdose/Acute Toxicity* for treatment recommendations.

High dosages or long-term use of amprolium may induce neurologic signs because of thiamine deficiency (eg, polioencephalomalacia [PEM], cerebrocortical necrosis). Parenteral thiamine (vitamin B1) can be used for treatment.

Overdose/Acute Toxicity

Amprolium has induced polioencephalomalacia (PEM) in sheep when administered at 880 mg/kg (16 times the normal dose) for 3 to 6 weeks[3] and at 1000 mg/kg for 3 to 5 weeks. Erythrocyte production has also been shown to cease in lambs receiving these high dosages.

Overdoses of amprolium can produce neurologic signs (eg, "stargazing", opisthotonos, central blindness, circling, ataxia). Treatment should consist of stopping amprolium therapy and administering parenteral thiamine. See *Thiamine* for more information.

For patients that have experienced or are suspected to have experienced an overdose, consultation with a 24-hour poison consultation center specializing in providing veterinary-specific information is recommended. For general information related to overdose and toxin exposures, as well as contact information for poison control centers, refer to *Appendix*.

Drug Interactions

The following drug interactions have either been reported or are theoretic in animals receiving amprolium and may be of significance in veterinary patients:

- **Thiamine**: Exogenously administered thiamine in high doses may reverse or reduce the efficacy of amprolium.

Dosages

DOGS:

Coccidiosis (extra-label):

a. **Using the 20% powder***[4]: a) Small dogs less than 10 kg [22 lb] anticipated adult weight): 60 – 100 mg/dog (NOT mg/kg) placed in a gelatin capsule and given PO once daily for 7 to 12 days. Large pups (greater than 10 kg [22 lb] anticipated adult weight): 110 – 200 mg/dog (NOT mg/kg) placed in a gelatin capsule and given PO once daily for 7 to 12 days. b) In food, for pups or bitches: 250 – 300 mg/dog (NOT mg/kg) using the 20% powder on food once daily for 7 to 12 days. ***NOTE**: Using the 20% powder, a 100 mg dose will equate to 500 mg powder; a 200 mg dose = 1 g powder; a 250 - 300 mg dose = 1.25 g - 1.5 g powder.
b. **In water**: a) 30 mL of the 9.6% solution in 3.8 liters (1 gallon) of water (no other water provided) for 7 to 10 days[4] OR b) 1.5 tablespoonsful (22.5 mL) of the 9.6% solution in 3.8 liters (1 gallon) of water to be used as the sole drinking water source; treatment not to exceed 10 days.[5] Monitor water consumption both for treatment and hydration assurance. Rarely, some dogs may not drink the amprolium water because of its bitter taste. In situations where dogs are cohabitants, it is necessary to place enough treated water for all to have access.
c. **Combination therapy**: Amprolium 150 mg/kg in combination with sulfadimethoxine 25 mg/kg PO every 24 hours for 14 days[6]

CATS:

Coccidiosis (extra-label):

1. **Using the 20% powder:** 60 – 100 mg/cat (NOT mg/kg) PO once daily for 7 days[6]
2. **In water:** 1.5 teaspoonful (7.5 mL) of the 9.6% solution in 3.8 liters (1 gallon) of water per day for 10 days[5]
3. **Combination therapy:** Amprolium 150 mg/kg in combination with sulfadimethoxine 25 mg/kg PO every 24 hours for 14 days[7]

CATTLE:

As an aid in the treatment and prevention of coccidiosis caused by *Eimeria bovis* and *Eimeria zuernii* in calves (label dosage; FDA-approved)): See product labels for additional information.

1. 5-day *treatment* protocol: 10 mg/kg daily PO for 5 days
2. 21-day *prevention* protocol: 5 mg/kg daily PO for 21 days. Can be administered either as an oral drench or mixed into the sole source of fresh drinking water. [8,9]

SHEEP/GOATS:

Coccidiosis (extra-label):

1. **Lambs**: 55 mg/kg daily PO for 19 days[10]
2. **Goat kids**: 50 mg/kg daily PO for 5 days will effectively reduce the fecal shedding of *Eimeria* spp oocysts without inducing neurologic disease.[11]

CAMELIDS (NEW-WORLD):

Eimeria macusaniensis (extra-label): Using a 1.5% solution, 10 mg/kg PO once daily for 10 to 15 days; supplement with thiamine 10 mg/kg SC every 5 days during treatment.[12]

SWINE:

Coccidiosis treatment (extra-label): 25 – 65 mg/kg PO once or twice daily for 3 to 4 days[10]

AVIAN:

1. **Treatment of coccidiosis in growing chickens, turkeys, and laying hens** (label dosage; FDA-approved): Administer 0.012% solution in the sole source of drinking water for 3 to 5 days, then as 0.006% solution for an additional 1 to 2 weeks.[13] Severe outbreaks may require higher initial dosages; see product labels for additional information.
2. **Coccidiosis in pet birds** (extra-label):
   a. 15 – 30 mg/kg/day PO for 1 to 5 days; repeat 5 days later[14]
   b. **In water:** Using the 9.6% solution, 1 – 2.5 mL per liter of water for 5 days or longer.[14,15] Cages should be steam cleaned to prevent reinfection. Supplement diet with B vitamins. Toucans and mynahs are resistant to some strains.

FERRETS:

Coccidiosis (extra-label): 19 mg/kg once daily[16]

RABBITS/RODENTS/SMALL MAMMALS:

Coccidiosis (extra-label):

1. **Rabbits**: Using 9.6% solution, 1 mL/7 kg (15 lb) (≈0.15 mL/kg) PO once daily for 5 days. Diluted in drinking water: 0.5 mL of 9.6% solution/500 mL for 10 days[17]
2. **Gerbils, Mice, Rats, Hamsters**: 10 – 20 mg/kg divided and given SC or IM every 8 to 24 hours
3. **Chinchillas**: 10 – 15 mg/kg per day divided and given SC, IM, or IV every 8 to 24 hours[18]

Monitoring

- Clinical efficacy
- Hydration, body weight
- If using in high dosages (extra-label), watch for neurologic signs (eg, "stargazing," opisthotonos, central blindness, circling, ataxia).

Chemistry/Synonyms

Amprolium hydrochloride, a structural analogue of thiamine (vitamin B_1), occurs as a white or almost white, odorless or nearly odorless powder. One gram is soluble in 2 mL of water and is slightly soluble in alcohol.

Amprolium may also be known as amprocidi, *Amprol®*, *Ampromed®*, *Corid®*, *Coxoid®*, or *Coxiprol®*.

Storage/Stability

Unless otherwise instructed by the manufacturer, store amprolium products at room temperature 15°C to 30°C (59°F-86°F).

Compatibility/Compounding Considerations

No specific information is noted.

Dosage Forms/Regulatory Status

VETERINARY-LABELED PRODUCTS:

Amprolium Oral Solution: 9.6% (96 mg/mL) in 473 mL and 1 gallon bottles; *Corid®*, generic; (OTC). FDA-approved for use in calves (not veal calves). Slaughter withdrawal (when used as labeled) = 24 hours. A withdrawal period has not been established for preruminating calves.

Amprolium Oral Solution: 9.6% (96 mg/mL) in 473 mL and 1 gallon bottles; *Amprol®*, generic; (OTC). FDA-approved for use in growing chickens, turkeys, and laying hens. Withdrawal information is not included on the FDA label.

Amprolium Soluble Powder: 20% (200 mg/g) in 283.5 g pouches *Corid®*; (OTC). FDA-approved for use in calves (not veal calves). NADA #033-165. Slaughter withdrawal (when used as labeled) = 24 hours. A withdrawal period has not been established for preruminating calves.

Amprolium Soluble Powder: 20% (200 mg/g) in 283.5 g pouches *Amprol® 128*; generic; (OTC). FDA-approved for use in growing chickens, turkeys, and laying hens; withdrawal information is not included on the FDA label.

There are also available medicated feeds (amprolium alone) and combination products (medicated feeds, feed additives) containing amprolium with other therapeutic agents. These products may be labeled for use in calves, chickens, and/or turkeys.

HUMAN-LABELED PRODUCTS: NONE

References

For the complete list of references, see **wiley.com/go/budde/plumb**

Antivenom, *Latrodectus mactans*

Antivenom, Black Widow Spider

(an-tie-**ven**-nin lah-tro-dec-tus mack-tans) *Antivenom, Antidote*

Antivenin and antivenom are synonymous terms and are used interchangeably throughout the monograph to avoid confusion between the currently preferred term (antivenom) and the term used on the product label (antivenin). NOTE: Veterinary poison control centers can offer current, detailed treatment recommendations (consultation fees may apply). See ***Important Contact Information***.

Prescriber Highlights

- Neutralizes the venom of black widow spiders. Early antivenom administration (within 4 to 6 hours of envenomation) is associated with greater efficacy, but later administration can still be effective.
- May cause hypersensitivity reactions (acute and delayed)
- Product may be difficult for veterinarians to obtain in a timely manner in emergent situations; consider keeping this product on hand in areas where envenomation occurs more commonly.
- It is recommended to contact a veterinary poison control center for current treatment recommendations and assistance in locating and acquiring antivenom.

Uses/Indications

Black widow spider antivenom is used to treat envenomation by *Latrodectus mactans* (black widow spider). Cats, horses, and camels are considered to be extremely sensitive to the alpha-latrotoxin in the spider venom, whereas dogs are considered more resistant.[1,2] Clinical signs associated with envenomation occur within 8 hours of the spider bite and are primarily neuromuscular (eg, severe pain, seizures, muscle spasms [especially in the chest wall, abdomen, and other large muscle mass areas], which may progress to flaccid paralysis in cats) and cardiovascular (eg, hypertension, tachycardia, cardiovascular collapse); secondary respiratory compromise may result from muscular rigidity and lead to death if not treated. Within 24 hours, affected animals may lose up to 20% of their body weight. Cats may also develop hypersalivation and GI signs (eg, vomiting, diarrhea[3]); death is very common in this species.[1]

Pharmacology/Actions

Antivenoms act by binding to venom toxins and thereby neutralizing venom-induced effects in patients via passive immunization of immunoglobulins obtained from horses that are hyperimmunized with the venom of *Latrodectus mactans*.

The use of antivenom early in the course of therapy is emphasized. Improvement in clinical signs may occur as early as 30 minutes after administration,[1,2] and complete recovery may be seen within 6 to 8 hours.[2]

Pharmacokinetics

No pharmacokinetic information was located.

Contraindications/Precautions/Warnings

Because there is a risk for anaphylaxis secondary to the equine immunoglobulins contained in this product, many clinicians recommend performing sensitivity testing before administration; however, antivenom sensitivity testing is frequently unreliable, with false positive and negative results.[4] Delayed serum sickness may occur several days to a couple weeks following antivenom administration. Antivenom dilution with and administration in IV fluids should be undertaken with extreme caution because of the risk of hypertension resulting from envenomation.

Adverse Effects

Anaphylaxis secondary to the product's equine serum origin may occur; the incidence is rare in humans (less than 0.6%).[1] Although rare, there is the possibility of life-threatening hypersensitivity reactions; appropriate resuscitative drugs (eg, epinephrine) and equipment should be readily available. The FDA-approved product contains a small vial of normal equine serum to perform intradermal hypersensitivity testing. Alternatively, a 1:10 dilution of the antivenom administered intracutaneously at a dose of 0.02 – 0.03 mL has been suggested as a test for hypersensitivity. Wheal formation and erythema indicate a positive reaction and are generally seen within 30 minutes of administration. A negative response does not ensure that anaphylaxis will be avoided during treatment; slow IV administration is usually sufficient to identify animals that will react to the product. A pretreatment dose of diphenhydramine is often recommended before administering antivenom, primarily to sedate the patient and, theoretically, to reduce any possible allergic reactions to the antivenom.

Epinephrine (0.01 mg/kg IM and repeated at 15- to 20-minute intervals until the patient is stable) has been recommended if early signs of anaphylaxis occur (clinical signs vary by species and include vomiting/diarrhea [dogs], dyspnea [cats/ruminants], nausea, pruritus, pyrexia, and hyperemia of the inner pinnae). Stopping the infusion, administering histamine H_1- and H_2-receptor antagonists (eg, diphenhydramine and famotidine, respectively), and restarting the infusion 5 minutes later at a slower rate may allow the dose to be administered without further problems.[5] In severe envenomation, patients exhibiting allergic reactions to antivenom can still receive it; administration of antivenom as a slow IV infusion with concomitant diphenhydramine (and possibly epinephrine) has been suggested.

Muscle cramps have also been reported in humans following antivenom administration.

Reproductive/Nursing Safety

The safe use of black widow spider antivenom during pregnancy or lactation has not been established; however, it has been used successfully in human pregnancies.[6-8]

Because safety has not been established in animals, this drug should only be used when the maternal benefits outweigh the potential risks to offspring.

Drug Interactions

The following drug interactions with black widow spider antivenom have either been reported or are theoretical in humans or animals and may be of significance in veterinary patients. Unless otherwise noted, use together is not necessarily contraindicated, but the veterinarian must weigh the potential risks and perform additional monitoring when appropriate.

- Beta-Adrenergic Receptor Antagonists (eg, **atenolol, propranolol**): May mask the early signs associated with anaphylaxis
- Opioids (eg, **morphine**): Opioid-induced histamine release may obscure clinical signs associated with anaphylaxis.
- Respiratory Depressants (eg, **alpha-2 agonists, barbiturates, benzodiazepines**): Concomitant use of respiratory depressant drugs may exacerbate the respiratory depression caused by envenomation.

Dosages

DOGS/CATS:

Black widow spider envenomation (extra-label):

a) After reconstituting the antivenom, add the contents of 1 vial to 100 mL of 0.9% sodium chloride and administer IV over 30 minutes. Pretreatment with diphenhydramine 2 – 4 mg/kg SC may help calm the patient and may protect against allergic reactions from the antivenom. If signs of an allergic reaction occur (eg, pyrexia, dyspnea, vomiting/diarrhea, pruritus), discontinue the infusion, and give a second dose of diphenhydramine. If allergic reactions abate, may restart infusion at a slower rate; if they recur, stop the infusion, and seek consultation. See *Adverse Effects*. Use care with the administration of IV fluids, as envenomation can cause significant hypertension. Benzodiazepines (eg, diazepam, midazolam) or methocarbamol may alleviate muscle cramping.[3,9]

b) Dissolve contents of one vial of antivenom and add to 100 – 200 mL of warm 0.9% sodium chloride and infuse IV over 2 to 6 hours. Administer diphenhydramine 0.5 – 1 mg/kg SC prior to infusion.[10]

Monitoring

- Signs associated with an allergic response to the antivenom (eg, anaphylaxis, anaphylactic-like reactions, serum sickness); hyperemia of the inner ear pinnae may be a good marker.[1]
- Respiratory and cardiac rate
- Blood pressure
- Serum chemistry (in particular, blood glucose, which is commonly elevated with envenomations); creatine kinase
- CBC
- Urine output; urinalysis

Client Information

- Clients must be made aware of the potential for anaphylaxis, as well as the expenses associated with treatment, monitoring (including for delayed serum sickness), and hospitalization.
- Some animals may experience an allergic reaction ("serum sickness") to antivenom products 1 to 2 weeks after administration. Inform your veterinarian if your animal develops a fever, rash, or appears to have muscle or joint pain (eg, stiffness, limited ability to move around).

Chemistry/Synonyms

This product is concentrated serum immunoglobulins obtained from horses immunized with the venom of the black widow spider. It is provided as a refined, lyophilized product. When this product is reconstituted as directed, the color of the antivenom ranges from light (straw) to very dark (iced tea); however, the color has no effect on potency.

Storage/Stability

Store the product in the refrigerator 2°C to 8°C (36°F-46°F). Do not freeze. Discard unused portion.

Compatibility/Compounding Considerations

Reconstitute the lyophilized product by adding 2.5 mL of sterile water for injection; shake the vial to completely dissolve the contents. Inspect the dissolved product to make sure no particulate is evident. For IV use, further dilute the solution in 10 to 100 mL of normal saline injection.

Dosage Forms/Regulatory Status

VETERINARY-LABELED PRODUCTS: NONE

HUMAN-LABELED PRODUCTS:

Antivenin (*Latrodectus mactans*) Powder for Injection: greater than or equal to 6000 antivenin units/vial in single-use vials. Only 2 vials may be ordered at a time. (Rx). FDA-approved. Product comes packaged with a 1 mL vial of normal horse serum that may be used for sensitivity testing.

References

For the complete list of references, see **wiley.com/go/budde/plumb**

Antivenom, Crotalidae

(an-tie-**ven**-in cro-**tal**-ih-day)

Antivenin®, RattlerAntivenin®, VenomVet®

Antivenom, Antidote

Antivenin and antivenom are synonymous terms and are used interchangeably throughout the monograph to avoid confusion between the currently preferred term (antivenom) and the term used on the product label (antivenin). NOTE: Veterinary poison control centers can offer current, detailed treatment recommendations (consultation fees may apply). See ***Important Contact Information.***

Prescriber Highlights

- Neutralizes the venom of Crotalidae snakes. Early antivenom administration (within 4 to 6 hours of envenomation) is associated with greater efficacy, but later administration can still be effective.
- May cause hypersensitivity reactions (acute and delayed)
- Product may be difficult for veterinarians to obtain in a timely manner in emergent situations; consider keeping this product on hand in areas where envenomation occurs more commonly.
- Treatment with antivenom requires economic consideration, as product costs range from hundreds to thousands of dollars.
- It is recommended to contact a veterinary poison control center for current treatment recommendations and assistance in locating and acquiring antivenom.

Uses/Indications

Three equine-derived veterinary antivenom products are available and indicated for the treatment of envenomation from native North American Crotalidae snakes (ie, venomous pit viper snakes including rattlesnakes, copperheads, and cottonmouths/water moccasins) in dogs and horses. They also may be effective for envenomation from several Central and South American snake species (fer-de-lance, lancehead, Central and South American rattlesnake), or in other species (eg, habu, mamushi [Japanese moccasin]).[1]

An ovine-derived F(ab) product is indicated for North American Crotalidae snake envenomation in humans, and has been used successfully in dogs.[2] An equine-derived $F(ab')_2$ is approved for human use, but efficacy data in animals are lacking.

Many factors contribute to the potential for venom toxicity (eg, patient age, body weight, and general health; location of bite site[s]; number of bites; age, species, and size of snake). Antivenom treatment, along with crystalloid fluid therapy and analgesia, is considered the mainstay treatment for moderate to severe pit viper envenomation.[3] Early administration (within 4 to 6 hours) is ideal, but antivenom treatment administered up to 24 hours after a snakebite can still be effective.[3]

There are no studies comparing efficacy or safety of the various antivenom products, and antivenom use in animals can be dictated by local availability in veterinary clinics and affordability.

Pharmacology/Actions

Antivenoms are venom toxin-specific antibodies that bind venom toxins and thereby neutralize venom-induced toxic effects. Antivenom use is a passive immunization process that uses toxin-specific immunoglobulins or antibody fragments, such as F(ab) and $F(ab')_2$, obtained from horses or sheep hyperimmunized with snake venom(s) or specific venom components. Antivenom can be very effective in halting and reversing venom-related coagulation abnormalities or neurotoxicity (depending on the specific antivenom given and time to treatment).

Pharmacokinetics

Specific product-related information was not located. Because of their variable molecular mass differences, the 3 antibody types that compose individual antivenom types have different individual pharmacokinetics. IgG antibodies have a low volume of distribution, the longest half-life, and are eliminated via extrarenal mechanisms. F(ab) fragments reach the extravascular compartments easily, are catabolized by the kidney, and have a rapid clearance via the kidneys. $F(ab')_2$ fragments exhibit an intermediate pharmacokinetic profile between IgG and F(ab).[4] For example, it has been reported that the $F(ab')_2$ antibody fragment antivenom (*Antivipmyn®*) is cleared from the body faster than IgG (ACP, or *Polyvet-ICP®*) but slower than the F(ab) antibody fragment (*CroFab®*).[3]

Contraindications/Precautions/Warnings

Equine- or ovine-derived antivenoms should be used cautiously or not at all in animals with known sensitivities to equine or ovine proteins. Although rare, there is the possibility of life-threatening hypersensitivity reactions; appropriate resuscitative drugs (eg, epinephrine) and equipment should be readily available. Administer the antivenom IV slowly and monitor closely for the first 10 minutes of the infusion to observe for signs of hypersensitivity reactions. Use antihistamines, tranquilizers, sedatives, and analgesics with care as they may mask important clinical signs.[1] In particular, opioid-induced histamine release may obscure clinical signs associated with anaphylaxis.

Historically, diluted antivenom given intradermally (typically 1:10 dilution) was suggested as a test for hypersensitivity. This practice is no longer commonly recommended secondary to false negative and false positive results occurring.[5]

Adverse Effects

Three of the veterinary-labeled antivenom products (and the human-labeled product, *Anavip®*) are derived from equine proteins, and the risk for anaphylactic-like reactions in small animal species should be considered when administration is determined to be necessary.[5] Type I hypersensitivity was noted in dogs receiving an equine-derived polyvalent product, including both whole IgG[6-8] and $F(ab')_2$.[9] This same concern should be considered if using the ovine-derived F(ab) antivenom (*CroFab®*), although the risk for adverse effects, including anaphylaxis, may be lower.[2,5]

Epinephrine (0.01 mg/kg IM and repeated at 15- to 20-minute intervals until the patient is stable) has been recommended if early signs of anaphylaxis occur (clinical signs vary by species and include vomiting/diarrhea [dogs], dyspnea [cats/ruminants], nausea, pruritus, pyrexia, and hyperemia of the inner pinnae).[3] Stopping the infusion, administering histamine H_1- and H_2-receptor antagonists (eg, diphenhydramine and famotidine, respectively), and restarting the infusion 5 minutes later at a slower rate may allow the dose to be administered without further problems.[3,10] In severe envenomation, patients exhibiting allergic reactions to antivenom can still receive it; administration of antivenom as a slow IV infusion with concomitant diphenhydramine (and possibly epinephrine) has been suggested.[10]

In a case series, type I hypersensitivity was reported in 26 of 115 cats receiving antivenom and was more likely to occur when infusion time was completed in less than 1 hour.[11] Premedication with diphenhydramine ± corticosteroids did not significantly alter the occurrence of type I hypersensitivity reactions.

Antivenom-associated serum sickness has been reported in dogs after treatment using Antivenin (Crotalidae) Polyvalent (ACP),[6,7,12] and a retrospective study of 218 dogs reported signs of delayed hypersensitivity/serum sickness in 2 of the 218 dogs.[13] Although it is believed that the fractionated antibody products would have less antigenic potential than full IgG preparations, hypersensitivity reactions are still possible especially when an increased number of vials are required. Other potential adverse effects from antivenom administration include hypocalcemia, urticaria, GI effects (eg, vomiting, diarrhea), changes in heart rate and rhythm (eg, tachycardia, bradycardia), changes in blood pressure, and agitation/trembling.

Reproductive/Nursing Safety

There are no data available regarding Antivenin (Crotalidae) Polyvalent (ACP) use in pregnant or lactating bitches, queens, or mares. Potential benefits may warrant use of antivenom in pregnancy despite potential risks. *Crofab®* has been successfully used in humans during the third trimester of pregnancy.[14] Product has been used in late gestation with subsequent healthy litters.[15]

Safety during nursing has not been established but it would unlikely pose much risk. Because safety has not been established in animals, this drug should only be used when the maternal benefits outweigh the potential risks to offspring.

Drug Interactions

The following drug interactions with antivenin have either been reported or are theoretical in humans or animals and may be of significance in veterinary patients. Unless otherwise noted, use together is not necessarily contraindicated, but weigh the potential risks and perform additional monitoring when appropriate.

- **Analgesics/Sedatives** (eg, **acepromazine, dexmedetomidine, fentanyl):** Although analgesia, reducing excessive movement, and **administration of** other supportive treatments are important parts of treating envenomation; drugs that can mask the clinical signs associated with the venom (eg, analgesics and sedatives) should initially be used with caution.
- **Antihistamines, H_1 Receptor Antagonists** (eg, **diphenhydramine**): Antihistamines may mask clinical signs of envenomation[1]; however, diphenhydramine is routinely used by many clinicians to treat snakebite in dogs.[3,8] Additionally, antihistamines are indicated for the management of antivenom hypersensitivity reactions.[3]
- **Beta-Adrenergic Receptor Antagonists** (eg, **atenolol, propranolol**): May mask the early signs associated with anaphylaxis
- **Opioids** (eg, **morphine**): Opioid-induced histamine release may obscure clinical signs associated with anaphylaxis.

Laboratory Considerations

- None noted

Dosages

NOTES:

1. Early administration of antivenom increases effectiveness.
2. The treatment of pit viper snakebite involves significant supportive treatment and monitoring beyond administration of antivenom. It is highly recommended to refer to specialized references[3,10] and consult with an animal poison control center for guidance beyond what is listed in this monograph. See *Important Contact Information.*
3. The number of vials for each patient will depend on the bite size, relative amount of venom injected, the body mass of the patient (smaller patients may require higher doses as venom amount/kg body weight is higher), duration of time after the bite, snakebite severity score, coagulation times, and clinician judgment.[10]

DOGS:

Antivenin® — **Crotalidae (North and South American Snakebite) polyvalent antiserum of equine origin**

a) **Label dosage; USDA-licensed**: Administer 1 to 5 rehydrated vials of antivenom (ie, 10 – 50 mL) IV. Additional doses may be given every 2 hours as required. If unable to give IV, may administer IM as close to bite as practical.[1]

b) **Extra-label:** Average dose required is 1 to 2 vials of antivenom (ie, 10 – 20 mL), although multiple vials may be necessary. Initially, give 1 vial by adding it to 100 – 250 mL of crystalloid fluids (eg, sodium chloride 0.9%) and administering IV slowly over 3 to 5 minutes; monitor patient for clinical signs related to an allergic reaction. See *Adverse Effects.* If no adverse effects are observed, increase the infusion rate and administer the remaining volume IV slowly over 30 minutes. In smaller patients, adjust infusion volume to prevent fluid overload.[10] Repeat antivenom treatment as clinically indicated, particularly if clotting defects persist.

RattlerAntivenin® — **North American Crotalidae polyvalent antivenom of equine origin** (label dosage; USDA-licensed): Administer using a filtered IV set. Typically, 1 or 2 doses of antivenom (ie, 50 – **100 mL**) are adequate regardless of body size (small or large canine). Product can be administered prior to, concomitantly, or following other IV fluids. Administer antivenom IV slowly during the initial 10 minutes; monitor patient for clinical signs related to an allergic reaction. See *Adverse Effects.* If no adverse effects occur, administer the remaining volume IV slowly to effect over 20 to 60 minutes. If adverse effects develop, stop infusion for 5 to 10 minutes, and reinitiate at a slower infusion rate. If adverse effects persist, discontinue administration.[15]

VenomVet® —**North American Pit Viper polyvalent Crotalidae F(ab')$_2$ antivenom of equine origin** (label dosage; USDA-licensed): Dilute each vial of antivenom with 100 – 150 mL crystalloid fluid (eg, sodium chloride 0.9%). Administer IV slowly during the initial 10 minutes; monitor patient for clinical signs related to an allergic reaction. See *Adverse Effects.* Do not inject product at the site of snakebite or perifocal area. Full dose should be delivered IV slowly over 30 to 60 minutes. Treatment may be discontinued once clinical signs of envenomation resolve.[16]

Crotalidae polyvalent immune F(ab) antivenom of ovine origin (extra-label): Administer contents of a single vial either as a single dose, or by giving ½ of the vial contents initially and the remaining portion administered 6 hours later (keep product refrigerated in between dosing).[2] To administer, dilute antivenom vial contents with sodium chloride 0.9% 250 mL. Administer the first 25 – 50 mL IV slowly during the first 10 minutes; monitor patient for clinical signs related to an allergic reaction. See *Adverse Effects.* If no adverse effects occur, administer the remaining volume IV slowly to effect over 45 to 60 minutes. Critical patients may need to have undiluted antivenom administered via IV push over 5 to 10 minutes.[17]

CATS:

Antivenin® — **Crotalidae (North and South American Snakebite) polyvalent antiserum of equine origin** (extra-label): Average dose required for cats is 1 to 2 vials of antivenom (ie, 10 – 20 mL), although multiple vials may be necessary. Initially, give 1 vial by adding it to 100 – 250 mL of crystalloid fluids (eg, sodium chloride 0.9%) and administering 1 to 2 mL IV slowly over 3 to 5 minutes; monitor patient for clinical signs related to an allergic reaction. See *Adverse Effects.* If no adverse effects are observed, increase the infusion rate and administer the remaining volume IV slowly over 30 minutes to 2 hours).[10,11] Adjust infusion volume to prevent fluid overload. A multicenter retrospective study in cats suggested no mortality benefit of antivenom administration (1 vial, 10 mL), but did not report on other envenomation sequelae (eg, hemostasis, neurologic status, or cardiovascular conduction abnormalities).

HORSES:

RattlerAntivenin® — **North American Crotalidae polyvalent antivenom of equine origin** (label dosage; USDA-approved): Administer using a filtered IV set. Typically, 1 or 2 doses of antivenom (ie, 50 – 100 mL) are adequate regardless of body size, administered within 24 hours of envenomation. Product can be administered prior to, concurrently, or following other fluids. Administer IV slowly to effect over 20 to 60 minutes. Administer slowly during the initial 10 minutes; monitor for signs of hypersensitivity and anaphylaxis (eg, angioedema, hypotension, respiratory distress, urticaria). If these clinical signs develop, stop administration for 5 to 10 minutes, and reinitiate as a slower infusion rate. If adverse effects persist, discontinue administration.[15]

Antivenin® — **North and South American Crotalidae polyvalent antiserum of equine origin** (extra-label): Administer 1 to 2 vials diluted in 250 – 500 mL saline or lactated Ringer's slowly IV.[1] **NOTE:** Use of this product is only recommended in horses exhibiting systemic effects from envenomation. Administer antihistamines as needed.

Monitoring

- Signs associated with an allergic response to the antivenom (eg, urticaria, facial swelling, dyspnea, anaphylaxis, anaphylactic-like reactions, serum sickness)
- CBC with platelets; coagulation parameters (eg, PT, aPTT, ACT), thromboelastography, and fibrinogen
- Serum chemistry profile; hydration status
- ECG

Client Information

- Clients must be made aware of the potential for anaphylaxis as well as the financial expenses associated with treatment, monitoring, and hospitalization.
- Some animals may experience an allergic reaction ("serum sickness") to antivenom products 1 to 2 weeks after administration. Inform your veterinarian if your animal develops a fever, rash, or appears to have muscle or joint pain (eg, stiffness, limited ability to move around).

Chemistry/Synonyms

Available veterinary (and human) antivenom products are concentrated serum immunoglobulins (either whole IgG, or the venom-binding portion as either F(ab) or F(ab')$_2$ fragments) obtained from horses or sheep immunized with the venoms of several species of Crotalidae ("pit viper") snakes. Commercially available products are provided as refined, lyophilized products with diluent, presolubilized injectable solution, or plasma preparation.

Antivenin and antivenom are interchangeable terms.

Antivenin (Crotalidae) Polyvalent may also be known as ACP. Crotalidae Polyvalent Immune F(ab) (Ovine) may also be known as OPCA.

Storage/Stability

Antivenin (Crotalidae) Polyvalent (equine origin) North and South American Snakebite Antiserum; *Antivenin*®: Do not store above 37°C (98°F); avoid freezing and excessive heat. After reconstitution, the vial should be used immediately.

Antivenin Crotalidae Polyvalent (equine origin) North American Crotalidae Antivenom; *Rattler Antivenin*®: Product should be kept frozen below -5°C (23°F) until use. May be thawed in warm (not hot) water over 2 to 5 minutes (not to exceed 10 minutes). May be kept at room temperature 15°C to 27°C (60°F to 80°F) for up to 6 hours. May warm to body temperature immediately before administration.

Antivenin Polyvalent Crotalidae F(ab')$_2$ (equine origin) Injectable Solution North American Pit Viper Antivenin; *VenomVet*®: Refrigerate at 2°C to 8°C (36°F-46°F).

Crotalidae Polyvalent Immune F(ab) (ovine origin), human product, should be stored in the refrigerator at 2°C to 8°C (36°F-46°F) and used within 4 hours of reconstitution. Do not freeze. Storage at -20°C to 25°C (-4°F-77°F) is permitted for no longer than 7 days.

The Crotalidae Immune (F(ab')$_2$ (equine origin), human product, should be stored at a room temperature of 25°C (77°F), with brief temperature excursions up to 40°C (104°F) permitted; do not freeze. Use within 6 hours of reconstitution.

Compatibility/Compounding Considerations

Antivenin (Crotalidae) Polyvalent (ACP; equine origin) North and South American Snakebite Antiserum; *Antivenin*®: Reconstitute each vial with the diluent provided; gently swirl the vial (may require several minutes; do not shake) to prevent excessive foaming. Warming the vial to body temperature may speed up reconstitution. Once reconstituted, the vial contents are often added to a crystalloid IV solution (D_5W, normal saline often recommended) for infusion.

Antivenin Crotalidae Polyvalent (equine origin) North American Crotalidae Antivenom; *RattlerAntivenin*®: Product does not require reconstitution or dilution (do not mix with other fluids); however, other fluids can be administered concurrently. Administer using a filtered IV set.

Antivenin Polyvalent Crotalidae F(ab')$_2$ (equine origin) Injectable Solution North American Pit Viper Antivenin; *VenomVet*®: Product does not require reconstitution, but does require dilution to 100 to 150 mL in crystalloid fluid.

Crotalidae Polyvalent Immune Fab (ovine origin), human product: Each product vial requires reconstitution with 18 mL of 0.9% sodium chloride for injection and dissolution via manual inversion; do not shake. Further dilution of reconstituted product in 0.9% saline (250 mL total volume) is required.

The Crotalidae Immune F(ab')$_2$ (equine origin), human product: Each product vial requires reconstitution 10 mL 0.9% sodium chloride for injection. Further dilution of reconstituted product in 0.9% saline (250 mL total volume) is required.

Dosage Forms/Regulatory Status

VETERINARY-LABELED PRODUCTS:

Antivenin Crotalidae Polyvalent (equine origin) North and South American Snakebite Antiserum: Product is single-dose vial lyophilized IgG provided with a single 10 mL vial of diluent. *Antivenin*®; (Rx). USDA permit #124; labeled for use in dogs.

Antivenin Crotalidae Polyvalent (equine origin) North American Crotalidae Antivenom: 50 mL mini-IV bags of frozen, whole IgG antivenom. *RattlerAntivenin*®, Antidote 3 *RattlerAntivenin*®; (Rx). USDA veterinary license #614; labeled for use in dogs 8 weeks of age and older, and horses of any age.

Antivenin Polyvalent Crotalidae F(ab')$_2$ (equine origin) Injectable Solution North American Pit Viper Antivenin: Product box contains 1 liquid nonpyrogenic 10 mL sterile vial of antibody fragment preparation (antibodies in which the Fc fragments have been enzymatically removed, reducing the potential for allergic reactions). *VenomVet*™; (Rx). USDA veterinary license #444A; labeled for use in dogs 6 months of age and older.

Because product may be difficult for veterinarians to obtain in a timely manner during emergent situations, consider keeping this product on hand in regions where envenomation occurs more commonly.

HUMAN-LABELED PRODUCTS:

Antivenin Crotalidae Polyvalent Immune Fab (ovine origin) Powder for Injection (lyophilized): 1 g total protein per single-use vial; *CroFab*®; (Rx) FDA approved. **NOTE:** The cost of this product may prohibit its use in veterinary patients.

Crotalidae Immune F(ab')$_2$ (equine origin) Lyophilized Powder for Solution for Injection: 120 mg total protein per single-use vial; *Anavip*®; (Rx) FDA approved. **NOTE:** The cost of this product may prohibit its use in veterinary patients.

References

For the complete list of references, see **wiley.com/go/budde/plumb**

Antivenom, North American Coral Snake

(an-tie-***ven***-nin)

Antivenom; Antidote

Antivenin and antivenom are synonymous terms and used interchangeably throughout the monograph to avoid confusion between the currently preferred term (antivenom) and the term used on the product label (antivenin). ***NOTE:*** Veterinary poison control centers can offer current, detailed treatment recommendations (consultation fees may apply). See ***Important Contact Information.***

Prescriber Highlights

- ► Neutralizes the venom of Eastern and Texas coral snakes. Early antivenom administration (within 4 to 6 hours of envenomation) is associated with greater efficacy, but later administration can still be effective.
- ► May cause hypersensitivity reactions (acute and delayed)
- ► Patients may require mechanical ventilation despite antivenom therapy.
- ► Product may be difficult for veterinarians to obtain in a timely manner in emergent situations; consider keeping this product on hand in areas where envenomation occurs more commonly.
- ► Treatment with antivenom requires economic consideration, as product costs range from hundreds to thousands of dollars.
- ► It is recommended to contact a veterinary poison control center for current treatment recommendations and assistance in locating and acquiring antivenom.

Uses/Indications

This antivenom is indicated for the treatment of envenomation from North American coral snakes of the genus *Micrurus*. It is specific for the Eastern coral snake (*Micrurus fulvius fulvius*) and will provide cross-neutralization with the Texas coral snake (*Micrurus fulvius tenere*). Coral snake envenomation is relatively uncommon in the US and, of the bites that occur to humans, ≈60% do not result in clinically significant envenomation.[1]

Pharmacology/Actions

Coral snake venom primarily causes neurotoxicity (flaccid paralysis) and clinical signs may be delayed for hours. Intravascular hemolysis associated with anemia and hemoglobinuria has been reported in dogs.[1] Coral snake antivenom acts via venom toxin-specific antibodies that bind venom toxins, thereby neutralizing venom-induced toxic effects.

Toxin-specific immunoglobulins are obtained from horses that have been hyperimmunized with Eastern coral snake venom. Each vial of antivenom will neutralize ≈2 mg of *Micrurus fulvius fulvius* venom.

Pharmacokinetics

The pharmacokinetics of coral snake antivenom have not been described in veterinary species.

Contraindications/Precautions/Warnings

Coral snake antivenom should not be administered prophylactically to subclinical animals for which a bite is questionable. It should be administered with caution in animals with a confirmed history of hypersensitivity to equine serum and in animals with a history of asthma or other allergic tendencies.[2] Although rare, there is the possibility of life-threatening hypersensitivity reactions; appropriate resuscitative drugs (eg, epinephrine) and equipment should be readily available. Professional veterinary judgment is required to determine if the potential benefit of antivenom administration outweighs the risk. Performing sensitivity testing before antivenom administration may be considered, but this practice is questionable due to false negative and false positive results occurring[1] and most clinicians recommend particularly close observation during the initial IV infusion of 1 – 2 mL of diluted antivenom solution over 3 to 5 minutes.[3] Coral snake antivenom will not neutralize *Micruroides euryxanthus* (Sonoran or Arizona coral snake) venom.

Use antihistamines, tranquilizers, sedatives, and analgesics with care as they may mask important clinical signs and augment the respiratory depressant effects of the venom. Additionally, opioid-induced histamine release may obscure clinical signs associated with anaphylaxis.

Adverse Effects

The most significant adverse effects are associated with hypersensitivity reactions. Anaphylaxis (or anaphylactic-like reactions) secondary to the equine serum proteins in this product may occur, but the incidence is low. Serum sickness (fever, rash, arthralgia, myalgia) may also occur days following antivenom administration.

Epinephrine (0.01 mg/kg IM and repeated at 15- to 20-minute intervals until the patient is stable) has been recommended if early signs of anaphylaxis occur (clinical signs vary by species and include vomiting/diarrhea [dogs], dyspnea [cats/ruminants], nausea, pruritus, pyrexia, and hyperemia of the inner pinnae). Stopping the infusion, administering histamine H_1- and H_2-receptor antagonists (eg, diphenhydramine and famotidine, respectively), and restarting the infusion 5 minutes later at a slower rate may allow the dose to be administered without further problems.[1,4] In severe envenomation, patients exhibiting allergic reactions to antivenom can still receive it; administration of antivenom as a slow IV infusion with concomitant diphenhydramine (and possibly epinephrine) has been suggested.

Reproductive/Nursing Safety

Snake antivenoms have been successfully administered in humans during pregnancy, and typically what is beneficial for the mother's health is also beneficial for the fetus[5]; it is likely that this also applies to veterinary species.

Safety during nursing has not been established for snake antivenoms but it would unlikely pose much risk. Because safety has not been established in animals, this drug should only be used when the maternal benefits outweigh the potential risks to offspring.

Drug Interactions

The following drug interactions with antivenom have either been reported or are theoretical in humans or animals and may be of significance in veterinary patients. Unless otherwise noted, use of these together is not necessarily contraindicated, but the potential risks must be weighed, and additional monitoring performed as needed.

- **Beta-Adrenergic Receptor Antagonists**: May mask the early signs associated with anaphylaxis
- **CNS and/or Respiratory Depressants** (eg, **alpha-2 agonists, barbiturates, benzodiazepines**): Although analgesia, reducing excessive movement, and administration of other supportive therapy are important parts of treating envenomation, drugs that can mask the clinical signs, or potentially worsen CNS and respiratory depression associated with the coral snake envenomation (eg, analgesics, sedatives) should initially be used with caution.
- **Opioids** (eg, **morphine**): Concurrent use of opioids is considered contraindicated in coral snake envenomation as it may augment the respiratory depressant effects of the venom. Clinical signs caused by opioid-induced histamine release may also obscure the diagnosis of anaphylaxis to the antivenom.

Laboratory Considerations

None noted

Dosages

NOTES:

1. Early administration of antivenom increases effectiveness.
2. Treatment for coral snake envenomation may require significant supportive treatment and monitoring beyond administration of antivenom. It is highly recommended to refer to specialized references[6] and consult with an animal poison control center for guidance beyond what is listed in this monograph. See ***Important Contact Information***.
3. The dose required is based on the relative amount of venom injected and the body mass of the patient.[1] Smaller patients may require higher doses (as venom amount/kg body weight is higher).

DOGS/CATS:

Eastern and Texas coral snake envenomation (extra-label): Average dose required for a dog or cat is 1 to 2 vials of antivenom. Dilute each vial into 100 – 250 mL of crystalloid fluids (eg, sodium chloride 0.9%).[1,2] Initial infusion should be 1 – 2 mL IV slowly over 3 to 5 minutes; observe patient for clinical signs related to an allergic reaction. See ***Adverse Effects***. If no adverse effects are observed, the remaining dose can be administered at a rate that is comfortable for the patient based on body weight and general condition. Administer additional vials as indicated by the progression of the condition.[1]

HORSES:

Eastern and Texas coral snake envenomation (extra-label): Administer 1 to 2 vials slowly IV diluted in 250 – 500 mL sodium chloride 0.9% or lactated Ringer's.[7]

Monitoring

- Animals suspected of having a coral snake envenomation should be hospitalized with close observation for 24 to 48 hours postbite.
- Signs associated with an allergic reaction to the antivenom (eg, urticaria, facial swelling, dyspnea, anaphylaxis, anaphylactic-like reactions, serum sickness)
- Respiratory rate and character, pulse oximetry; mechanical ventilation may be necessary.
- Neurologic assessment: muscle weakness, paralysis, convulsions

Client Information

- Clients must be made aware of the potential for anaphylaxis as well as the economic costs associated with antivenom treatment, patient monitoring, and hospitalization.
- Some animals may experience an allergic reaction ("serum sickness") to antivenom products 1 to 2 weeks after administration. Inform your veterinarian if your animal develops a fever, rash, or appears to have muscle or joint pain (eg, stiffness, limited ability to move around).

Chemistry/Synonyms

Antivenom is composed of serum immunoglobulins obtained from horses that have been hyperimmunized with coral snake venom. The antivenom is provided as a refined lyophilized product with a suitable diluent. Antivenin and antivenom are interchangeable terms.

North American coral snake antivenom may also be known as NACSA or *Antivenin*®.

Storage/Stability

Unreconstituted product vials should be stored at 2°C to 8°C (36°F-46°F). Avoid freezing and excessive heat. After reconstitution, vials of antivenom that have been further diluted should be used within 4 hours.

Compatibility/Compounding Considerations

Reconstitute each vial of antivenom with 10 mL of the supplied diluent (sterile water for injection), aiming the diluent stream at the center of the lyophilized pellet. Gentle swirling may be used to hasten dissolution of the lyophilized powder; do not shake. Complete reconstitution may require 30 minutes or longer. Once vials have been reconstituted with the provided diluent, further dilution with normal saline for injection is required. Stability of the antivenom when diluted in other fluids (eg, LRS), and compatibility with other drugs, is unknown.

Dosage Forms/Regulatory Status

VETERINARY-LABELED PRODUCTS: NONE

HUMAN-LABELED PRODUCTS:

North American Coral Snake Antivenin (Equine) Lyophilized for Solution for IV Injection provided as single-use vials with 1 vial of diluent (10 mL water for injection). FDA-approved biologic; (Rx). Product can be obtained through the human-labeled pharmaceutical supply chain.

References

For the complete list of references, see **wiley.com/go/budde/plumb**

Apomorphine

(a-poe-*mor*-feen) *Apokyn*®, *Emedog*®

Emetic

Prescriber Highlights

- ► Rapid-acting, centrally mediated emetic used in dogs; rarely used in cats because it is often ineffective
- ► Contraindicated in certain species that are unable to vomit (eg, rodents, rabbits) and when vomiting may be deleterious (eg, impending coma, seizures, aspiration, ingestion of a corrosive substance)
- ► Can cause protracted vomiting; naloxone should reverse CNS effects or cardiorespiratory depression but not vomiting or cardiovascular effects. Recovery is usually within a few hours.
- ► The National Institute for Occupational Safety and Health (NIOSH) classifies apomorphine as a hazardous drug; use appropriate precautions when handling.

Uses/Indications

Apomorphine is used primarily as an emetic in dogs; it induces vomiting in 90% to 100% of dogs.[1,2] In a retrospective study of foreign body ingestion, apomorphine-induced vomiting successfully removed the object in ≈75% of dogs.[3] Apomorphine is rarely used in cats; and if emesis is indicated, an alpha 2 adrenergic agonist (eg, dexmedetomidine) is generally preferred.[4]

Pharmacology/Actions

Apomorphine stimulates dopamine receptors in the chemoreceptor trigger zone, which induces vomiting. This drug can cause both CNS depression and stimulation, but it tends to cause stimulatory effects. At high doses, medullary centers can be affected with resultant respiratory depression. In humans, apomorphine has an affinity for alpha-adrenergic receptors.

Pharmacokinetics

Apomorphine is slowly absorbed after oral administration and has unpredictable efficacy when it is given by this route; therefore, it is usually administered parenterally or via the subconjunctival sac. After SC injection, the drug is rapidly and almost completely absorbed, with effective concentrations reached in 10 minutes and peak concentrations reached in 25 minutes.[5] When apomorphine is administered intranasally, the mean time to reach the maximum plasma concentrations (T_{max}), the mean C_{max}, and the mean half-life ($t_{1/2}$) were 19.17 minutes, 36.14 ng/mL, and 29.85 minutes, respectively.[6] Median time to cause emesis may occur as soon as 1 minute (range, 1-5 minutes) after IV administration[2,7] and ≈13.5 minutes (range, 3-32 minutes) after SC injection; IM administration appears to have the slowest onset.[5] Duration of emesis for each route is ≈30 to 45 minutes.[1,5]

Apomorphine is primarily conjugated in the liver and then excreted in the urine. Its elimination half-life in dogs is 30 to 64 minutes. In humans, higher peak concentration (25%) and overall drug exposure (10%) may occur in patients that have hepatic impairment.

Contraindications/Precautions/Warnings

Emetics can be an important aspect in the treatment of orally ingested toxins, but they must be used judiciously. Most emetics cause emesis when administered within 2 hours of foreign material or toxin ingestion[8]; however, induction of emesis should be performed as soon as possible, especially for cases of toxin ingestion. Emetics should not be used in rodents or rabbits because these patients are either unable to vomit or do not have stomach walls strong enough to tolerate emesis. Emetics are also contraindicated in patients that are hypoxic, have evidence of cardiovascular shock or respiratory distress, are actively having seizures, and/or lack normal pharyngeal reflexes (ie, laryngeal paralysis). The risks and benefits of administering an emetic should also be considered for animals with a recurrent history of aspiration pneumonia, seizures, coma, severe CNS depression or deteriorating CNS function, or extreme physical weakness. Emetics should also be withheld in patients that have previously vomited repeatedly. Because of the risk for additional esophageal or gastric injury with emesis, emetics are contraindicated in patients that have ingested a sharp object, strong acids, alkalis, or other caustic agents. Because of the risk for aspiration, emetics are usually contraindicated after petroleum distillate ingestion but may be employed when the risk for toxicity of the compound is greater than the risk for aspiration. Use of emetics after ingestion of strychnine or other CNS stimulants may precipitate seizures.

Emetics generally do not remove more than 80% of the material in the stomach (usually 40% to 60%),[9] and successful induction of emesis does not signal the end of appropriate monitoring or therapy. In addition to the contraindications outlined above, apomorphine should not be used in patients with oral opioid or other CNS depressant (eg, barbiturates) toxicity or in patients hypersensitive to morphine. Patients with hepatic impairment may have prolonged drug effects.

If vomiting does not occur in the expected time after apomorphine administration, repeated doses are unlikely to induce emesis and may cause clinical signs of toxicity.

The use of apomorphine in cats is controversial, as it is thought to be much less effective than alpha-2 agonists and, possibly, less safe.

In humans, IV crystallization leading to thrombus formation and pulmonary embolism has occurred following administration of apomorphine IV and use by the IV route is not advised.[10] These adverse effects have not been reported in animals and the IV route is commonly used for toxicity cases due to rapid onset of emesis.

The National Institute for Occupational Safety and Health (NIOSH) classifies apomorphine as a hazardous drug; personal protective equipment (PPE) should be used accordingly to minimize the risk for exposure.

Adverse Effects

Protracted nausea and vomiting are the main adverse effects seen with typical apomorphine doses. The severity of emesis and CNS depression is increased in dogs with the multidrug sensitivity gene (*MDR1)* mutation (also known as *ABCB1-1*delta); use apomorphine with caution in these dogs.[11] Sedation (44%) and tachycardia (16%) were reported in a study and were more likely to occur when apomorphine was given in the subconjunctival sac.[2] Other adverse effects after ophthalmic administration include lethargy, hypersalivation, persistent nausea, and eye redness/irritation. Hypotension and CNS or respiratory depression are usually associated with overdoses. Protracted vomiting after ophthalmic administration may be averted by washing the conjunctival sac with sterile saline or ophthalmic rinsing solution. Anecdotal reports of corneal ulcers have been noted after conjunctival administration.

In humans, hypotension, syncope, prolongation of the QT interval, and sudden episodes of sleepiness have been reported.[10] In contrast, low dose of apomorphine (0.01 mg/kg IV) exerted positive chronotropic and inotropic effects in dogs without affecting any electrophysiological variables.[12] When 0.1 mg/kg IV was administered, no hemodynamic effects were noted, and only an increase in the effective refractory period was reported.

Reproductive/Nursing Safety

The reproductive safety of this drug has not been established; weigh the risks versus the potential benefits before use. Teratogenicity (eg, fetal malformation, death) has been noted in laboratory animals. There were no changes in reproductive parameters in male dogs treated daily (0.01 – 0.4 mg/kg/day) for 6 months.[13]

Apomorphine is excreted into maternal milk.[14] Monitor nursing puppies for adverse effects; consider a milk replacer.

Because safety has not been established in animals, this drug should only be used when the maternal benefits outweigh the potential risks to offspring.

Overdose/Acute Toxicity

Excessive doses of apomorphine may result in respiratory and/or cardiac depression, CNS stimulation (eg, excitement, seizures), depression, or protracted vomiting. Naloxone may reverse CNS and respiratory effects but does not reverse apomorphine-induced cardiovascular effects or necessarily stop the vomiting.[15] Naloxone increases and prolongs the emetic effect of apomorphine by blockading mu receptors.[5]

Recovery generally occurs in 2 to 3 hours. Atropine has been suggested to treat severe bradycardia. Protracted hypersalivation or vomiting can be treated with maropitant or metoclopramide.[16]

In experimental studies, high doses of apomorphine (after 0.1 mg/kg SC) caused decreased motor activity, behavior changes (eg, anxiety, pacing, limb flicking), hyperesthesia, hallucinations, and hypersalivation in cats (after 0.5 or 2 mg/kg SC).[17]

For patients that have experienced or are suspected to have experienced an overdose, it is strongly encouraged to consult with a 24-hour poison control center that specializes in providing information specific for veterinary patients. For general information related to overdose and toxin exposures, as well as contact information for poison control centers, refer to the ***Appendix***.

Drug Interactions

The following drug interactions with apomorphine either have been reported or are theoretical in humans or animals and may be of significance in veterinary patients. Unless otherwise noted, use together is not necessarily contraindicated, but weigh the potential risks and perform additional monitoring when appropriate.

- **ANTIDOPAMINERGIC DRUGS** (eg, **metoclopramide, phenothiazines**): May negate the emetic effects of apomorphine
- **ANTIHISTAMINES, SEDATING** (eg, **chlorpheniramine, diphenhydramine**): Added sedative effects may occur.
- **BARBITURATES** (eg, **phenobarbital**): Additive CNS or respiratory depression and hypotension may occur.
- **CNS DEPRESSANT DRUGS** (eg, **alpha-2 adrenergic agonists** [eg, **dexmedetomidine**], **benzodiazepines** [eg, **alprazolam, diazepam, midazolam**], **gabapentin, propofol**): Additive CNS or respiratory depression may occur.
- **HYPOTENSIVE AGENTS** (eg, **amlodipine, enalapril, furosemide, hydralazine, prazosin**): May have additive hypotensive effects
- **MAROPITANT:** Negates the emetic effects of apomorphine[18]
- **MECLIZINE:** May negate the emetic effects of apomorphine. Additive sedative effects may occur.
- **NALOXONE:** Emetic effect may be prolonged.[5] Naloxone can reverse the respiratory depressant effects (but not the emetic or cardiovascular effects) of apomorphine.
- **NITROGLYCERIN:** May increase the risk for hypotension
- **NITROPRUSSIDE:** May increase the risk for hypotension
- **ONDANSETRON:** May negate the emetic effects of apomorphine. A human patient that received ondansetron and apomorphine developed severe hypotension.[10] In humans, use together is contraindicated.
- **OPIOIDS** (eg, **hydromorphone, morphine**): Additive CNS or respiratory depression may occur; use together cautiously.
- **PENTOXIFYLLINE:** May increase the risk for hypotension
- **QT PROLONGING DRUGS** (eg, **amiodarone, cisapride, clomipramine, quinidine, sotalol**): May increase the risk for QT prolongation

- **Serotonin Antagonists** (eg, **mirtazapine, trazodone**): May negate the emetic effects of apomorphine. A human patient that received ondansetron and apomorphine developed severe hypotension.[10] In humans, use together is contraindicated.
- **Sildenafil:** May increase the risk for hypotension

Dosages

DOGS:

Induction of emesis (extra-label):

a. 0.01 – 0.04 mg/kg IV, SC, or IM.[1,2,7,14,19-21] **NOTE**: Induction of emesis is fastest with IV administration followed by SC; IM route has the longest lag time until emesis occurs.

b. 0.25 mg/kg PO (one 6.5 mg tablet per 26 kg)[16]

c. Subconjunctival route: Place a 6.25 mg tablet (whole or crushed; not available in the US) under the conjunctiva.[16] Alternatively, a crushed tablet (typically 6.25 mg) can be dissolved in a saline solution (0.9% sodium chloride) instilled in the conjunctival sac. **NOTE**: Solutions must be prepared fresh to be effective. Remove the tablet and rinse with water or saline solution after emesis (resulting in a dose to effect).[1,22]

FERRETS:

Induction of emesis (extra-label):

a) 0.04 mg/kg IV, IM, or SC[23-25]

b) 0.25 mg/kg subconjunctivally[26]

Monitoring

- CNS, respiratory, and cardiac systems should be monitored.
- Vomitus should be quantified, examined for contents, and saved for possible later analysis.

Client Information

- This medicine should only be given by your veterinarian.
- This medication is considered to be a hazardous drug as defined by the National Institute for Occupational Safety and Health (NIOSH). Talk with your veterinarian or pharmacist about the use of personal protective equipment when handling this medicine.

Chemistry/Synonyms

Apomorphine is a centrally acting emetic that occurs as a white powder or minute, white or grayish-white crystals, and is sparingly soluble in water or alcohol.

Apomorphine HCl may also be known as apomorphini hydrochloridum, *APO-go*®, *APO-go Pen*®, *Apofin*®, *Apokinon*®, *Apokyn*®, *Apometic*®, *Apomine*®, *Britaject*®, *Emedog*®, *Ixense*®, *Taluvian*®, or *Uprima*®.

Storage/Stability

Apomorphine soluble tablets should be stored in tight containers at room temperature (15°C-30°C [59°F-86°F]) and protected from moisture and light.

Apomorphine gradually darkens in color when exposed to light and air. Discolored (ie, green to turquoise) tablets and solutions should be discarded. Apomorphine solutions are more stable in acidic versus alkaline solutions. An apomorphine 0.3% solution has a pH of ≈3 to 4.

Compatibility/Compounding Considerations

Solutions of apomorphine can be made by solubilizing tablets in at least 1 to 2 mL of either sterile water for injection or 0.9% sodium chloride for injection. After being sterilized by filtration, the solution is stable for 2 days if protected from light and air and stored in the refrigerator. Do not use solutions that are discolored or form a precipitate after filtering.

Compounded preparation stability: Apomorphine injectable solution compounded from the active pharmaceutical ingredient (API) has been published.[27] Dissolving 10 mg apomorphine with 0.1% sodium metabisulfite in sterile water to a final volume of 10 mL and filtering through a 0.22 µm sterilizing filter yields a 2.5 mg/mL sterile solution that retains potency for 2 months stored at 25°C (77°F). Compounded preparations of apomorphine should be protected from light. Solutions of apomorphine should not be autoclaved, as autoclaving results in the development of a green color.

Dosage Forms/Regulatory Status

VETERINARY-LABELED PRODUCTS:

Apomorphine HCl Injection: 1 mg/mL in 1 mL ampules; *Emedog*®; available in the United Kingdom; (POM-V)

Apomorphine HCl Tablet: 6.5 mg; available in Australia/New Zealand; (Rx)

Pharmaceutical dosage forms of apomorphine can be difficult to obtain and compounding pharmacies may be required to obtain the drug.

HUMAN-LABELED PRODUCTS:

Apomorphine HCl Injection: 10 mg/mL in 3 mL cartridges; *Apokyn*®; (Rx)

References

For the complete list of references, see **wiley.com/go/budde/plumb**

Apramycin

(a-pra-***mye***-sin) *Apralan*®

Aminoglycoside

Prescriber Highlights

- Orally administered antibiotic for bacterial enteritis in pigs, calves, and poultry
- Apramycin is no longer available in the US, but products labeled for use in pigs, calves, and poultry remain available in some countries.
- Contraindicated in animals hypersensitive to apramycin, animals with renal disease, calves with a functional rumen, and cats.
- May be partially absorbed in neonates

Uses/Indications

Apramycin is no longer commercially available in the US, but it is used in some countries for the treatment of bacterial enteritis (eg, colibacillosis, salmonellosis) in pigs, calves, and poultry.

The World Health Organization (WHO) has designated aminoglycosides as a Critically Important, High Priority antimicrobial in human medicine.[1] The Office International des Epizooties (OIE) has designated apramycin as a Veterinary Critically Important Antimicrobial (VCIA) in avian, bovine, lagomorph, ovine, and swine species.[2]

Pharmacology/Actions

Apramycin is an aminoglycoside-aminocyclitol that is bactericidal against many gram-negative bacteria (eg, *Escherichia coli*, *Pseudomonas* spp, *Salmonella* spp, *Klebsiella* spp, *Proteus* spp, *Pasteurella* spp, *Treponema hyodysenteriae*, *Bordetella bronchiseptica*), *Staphylococcus* spp, and *Mycoplasma* spp. It prevents protein synthesis by susceptible bacteria by binding to the 30S ribosomal subunit.

There are public health concerns about the widespread use of apramycin in pigs, as apramycin resistance in *E coli* caused by the *aac(3)-IV* gene also confers resistance toward other aminoglycosides (eg, gentamicin, tobramycin); treated animals may become a reservoir for transfer of resistant genes or bacteria to humans.[3,4]

Pharmacokinetics

After oral administration, apramycin is partially absorbed, particularly in neonates. Absorption decreases substantially with the age of the animal. The absorbed drug is eliminated unchanged via the kidneys.

Apramycin is absorbed when administered orally to neonatal swine at single dosage levels of 10, 30, and 100 mg/kg, with peak blood concentrations observed at 1 to 4 hours postadministration; detectable serum apramycin concentrations persist for 12 to 24 hours. Considerable variation in postadministration blood concentrations is observed; however, the concentration detected is generally commensurate with the dose.

After IV administration to goats, apramycin has a volume of distribution (steady-state) of 0.26 L/kg, clearance of 2.8 mL/minute/kg, and an elimination half-life of 1.3 hours.[5]

Contraindications/Precautions/Warnings

Do not use in known cases of apramycin hypersensitivity. The drug has a wide margin of safety when used orally. Apramycin is contraindicated in cats, in calves with a functional rumen and in patients with kidney disorders.[6]

Because apramycin is delivered in feed or drinking water, animals that are not eating or drinking should receive alternative (parenteral) antimicrobial therapy.

Adverse Effects

When used as labeled, the manufacturer does not list any adverse reactions. Fecal softness has been observed in 1- to 3-day-old piglets. Although not documented, as with other aminoglycosides, ototoxicity and nephrotoxicity could occur if significant amounts of apramycin are systemically absorbed.

Reproductive/Nursing Safety

Apramycin is safe to use in breeding swine.[7] Fetal toxicity has been observed in rabbits given apramycin between days 6 and 18 of pregnancy.[6]

Because safety has not been established in other animals, this drug should only be used when the maternal benefits outweigh the potential risks to offspring.

Overdose/Acute Toxicity

No mortality was observed following oral doses of 1250 mg/kg in pigs, 520 mg/kg in dogs, or 5200 mg/kg in mice.[7]

For patients that have experienced or are suspected to have experienced an overdose, consultation with a 24-hour poison consultation center specializing in providing veterinary-specific information is recommended. For general information related to overdose and toxin exposures, as well as contact information for poison control centers, refer to *Appendix*.

Drug Interactions

The following drug interactions have either been reported or are theoretical in humans or animals receiving oral neomycin and may apply to apramycin and be of significance in veterinary patients. Unless otherwise noted, use together is not necessarily contraindicated, but weigh the potential risks and perform additional monitoring when appropriate.

- CEPHALOSPORINS (eg, **ceftiofur, cephalexin**): Concurrent use may enhance the nephrotoxic effect of neomycin.
- CYCLOSPORINE: Neomycin may increase the nephrotoxic potential of cyclosporine.
- DIGOXIN: Oral neomycin with orally administered digoxin may result in decreased absorption of digoxin. Separating the doses of the 2 medications may not alleviate this effect. Some human patients (less than 10%) metabolize digoxin in the GI tract, and neomycin may increase serum digoxin levels in these patients. It is recommended that therapeutic drug monitoring be performed if oral neomycin is added or withdrawn from the drug regimen of a patient stabilized on a digitalis glycoside.
- MANNITOL: Concurrent use should be avoided, as it may enhance the nephrotoxic effect of neomycin.
- METHOTREXATE: Absorption may be reduced by oral neomycin but is increased by oral kanamycin (found in *Amforal®*).
- NEUROMUSCULAR-BLOCKING AGENTS (eg, **atracurium, pancuronium**): Concomitant use with neuromuscular blocking agents could potentiate neuromuscular blockade.[6]
- OTOTOXIC, NEPHROTOXIC DRUGS: Although only minimal amounts of neomycin are absorbed after oral or rectal administration, concurrent use of other ototoxic or nephrotoxic drugs with neomycin should be done with caution. Topical use for the treatment of otitis should be avoided if an intact tympanic membrane has not been confirmed.
- PENICILLIN V POTASSIUM (**oral**): Oral neomycin should not be given concurrently with oral penicillin V Potassium, as malabsorption of the penicillin may occur.
- VANCOMYCIN: May enhance the nephrotoxic effect of neomycin
- VITAMIN K ANTAGONISTS (eg, **warfarin**): Oral neomycin may decrease the amount of vitamin K absorbed from the gut; this may have ramifications for patients receiving oral anticoagulants.

Laboratory Considerations

None have been noted.

Dosages

NOTE: All dosages are expressed as mg/kg apramycin sulfate.

CATTLE:

Treatment of colibacillosis or salmonellosis in calves (extra-label): 72 mg/kg PO once daily for 5 consecutive days, administered in drinking water (as sole source of water), milk, or milk replacer.[6]

SWINE:

Bacterial enteritis in weaned piglets caused by *Escherichia coli* (extra-label): 22.5 mg/kg PO once daily for 7 consecutive days, administered in drinking water (as sole source of water)[6]

POULTRY:

Treatment of *Escherichia coli* septicemia in young chickens (extra-label): 144 mg/kg PO once daily for 5 consecutive days, administered in drinking water (as sole source of water)[6]

RABBITS:

Treatment and metaphylaxis of bacterial enteritis caused by *Escherichia coli* (extra-label): 36 mg/kg PO once daily for 5 consecutive days, administered in drinking water (as sole source of water)[6]

Monitoring

- Clinical efficacy

Chemistry/Synonyms

Apramycin is an aminocyclitol antibiotic produced from *Streptomyces tenebrarius*; it is a light to medium brown powder that is soluble in water. Aminocyclitols are closely related to the aminoglycosides.

Apramycin may also be known as nebramycin factor 2, nebramcyin II, apramycine, apramicina, AIDS166733, *Apralan®*, *Actavis®*, or *Abylan®*.

Storage/Stability

Store apramycin powder in a cool dry place, in tightly closed containers, protected from moisture. Store at temperatures less than 25°C (77°F). If exposed to rust (eg, a rusty waterer), the drug can be inactivated. Opened product should be used within 28 days.[6,7]

- Discard any medicated water not consumed within 24 hours and milk replacer within 6 hours.

- Prepare solutions in milk and reconstituted milk replacer immediately before use. Discard any medicated milk or milk replacer not consumed within 1 hour. Milk replacer should not exceed 40°C (104°F) when mixing in apramycin powder.

Compatibility/Compounding Considerations

Do not mix with other medications.[6]

Dosage Forms/Regulatory Status

VETERINARY-LABELED PRODUCTS:

None in the US. A swine product, Apramycin Sulfate Soluble Powder 37.5 g and 48 g (base) bottle; *Apralan*®; (OTC), was formerly marketed in the US and is still available in several countries.

In the UK: Apramycin Soluble Powder: 1 g sachets and 50 g (apramycin activity) in 220 mL; *Apralan Soluble Powder*®; (POM-V). Refer to local regulations for withdrawal times.

HUMAN-LABELED PRODUCTS: NONE

References

For the complete list of references, see **wiley.com/go/budde/plumb**

Ascorbic Acid

Vitamin C

(a-***skor***-bik ***ass***-id)

Vitamin, Antioxidant

Prescriber Highlights

- Used to prevent and treat scurvy in guinea pigs
- Antioxidant sometimes used in dogs and cats to treat ingestion of certain toxicants (eg, acetaminophen)
- At recommended dosages, there are minimal adverse effects; may exacerbate liver injury in copper toxicosis
- May alter laboratory results (eg, urine dipstick, fecal occult blood, serum bilirubin)

Uses/Indications

Ascorbic acid (vitamin C) is used to prevent and treat scurvy in guinea pigs.

Ascorbic acid is sometimes recommended as an antioxidant as part of treatment for ingestion of toxicants that can cause methemoglobinemia (eg, acetaminophen, phenazopyridine, monomethylhydrazine-containing mushrooms) or hepatotoxicity.

In small animal species, ascorbic acid can be a urinary acidifier, but its efficacy is questionable, and it is rarely used for this purpose. Previously, ascorbic acid was used to treat copper-induced hepatopathy in dogs but has fallen into disfavor (see ***Contraindications/Precautions/Warnings***). Supplementation to dogs that are experiencing a stressful situation (eg, intensive care) does not appear warranted.[1]

Pharmacology/Actions

Exogenously supplied ascorbic acid is a dietary requirement in some exotic species (eg, rainbow trout, coho salmon), guinea pigs, and primates. Domestic species synthesize ascorbic acid in vivo to meet their nutritional needs. Ascorbic acid is used in tissue repair and collagen formation; it is also important for maintaining blood vessel integrity and immune function. Some oxidation-reduction reactions and substrate metabolism (iron, folic acid, norepinephrine, histamine, phenylalanine, tyrosine, some drug enzyme systems) include ascorbic acid. Iron absorption and storage require ascorbic acid. Protein, lipid, and carnitine synthesis may require ascorbic acid. As an antioxidant for the adjunctive treatment of toxins that cause methemoglobinemia and/or hepatotoxicity, ascorbic acid serves as a reducing agent that neutralizes reactive oxygen compounds (eg, hydrogen peroxide), and it can increase conversion of methemoglobin to oxyhemoglobin, and act as a substrate for the antioxidant enzyme ascorbate peroxidase.

Pharmacokinetics

Human data suggest ascorbic acid is generally well absorbed in the jejunum after oral administration. Absorption is an active process and saturated at high doses. Only IV administration of vitamin C produces high plasma and urine concentrations.[2] Ascorbic acid is widely distributed with ≈25% bound to plasma proteins. Biotransformation of ascorbic acid occurs in the liver. When the body is saturated with ascorbic acid and blood concentrations exceed the renal threshold, the drug is readily excreted unchanged in the urine.

In guinea pigs, most ascorbic acid is eliminated in the urine.[3] Some ascorbic acid is metabolized to carbon dioxide, with peak elimination occurring 30 minutes after oral administration.[4]

Contraindications/Precautions/Warnings

High-dose ascorbic acid should be used cautiously in patients with diabetes mellitus because of laboratory interactions (see ***Laboratory Considerations***), and in patients that are susceptible to calcium oxalate, cystine, or urate urolithiasis.

In patients with copper-associated chronic hepatitis, ascorbic acid may increase copper's oxidative damage to the liver and should be avoided.[5]

Some dosage forms may contain benzyl alcohol as a preservative. In human newborns, benzyl alcohol and derivatives can potentially displace bilirubin from protein-binding sites, and caution for use in human neonates is advised. It is unclear if benzyl alcohol has the same effect in guinea pigs; formulations containing benzyl alcohol should not be administered to cats.

Adverse Effects

At usual doses, ascorbic acid has minimal adverse effects. Occasionally, GI disturbances have occurred in humans. Higher doses may increase urate, oxalate, or cystine urolithiasis, particularly in susceptible patients.

Reproductive/Nursing Safety

The reproductive safety of ascorbic acid has not been studied, but ascorbic acid is generally considered safe at moderate dosages during pregnancy and lactation.

Overdose/Acute Toxicity

Large doses may result in diarrhea (due to an osmotic effect and increased peristalsis) and potentially urolithiasis. Single doses of 0.5 g/kg in dogs; 1 g/kg in cats; 2 g/kg in rabbits; and 5 g/kg in guinea pigs, rats, and mice were well tolerated.[6] Treatment should consist of monitoring and hydration.

Drug Interactions

The following drug interactions with ascorbic acid (high dosages) have either been reported or are theoretical in humans or animals and may be of significance in veterinary patients. Unless otherwise noted, use together is not necessarily contraindicated, but weigh the potential risks and perform additional monitoring when appropriate.

- **Aluminum Hydroxide**: Increased absorption of aluminum hydroxide may occur with coadministration with ascorbic acid; administration should be separated by at least 2 hours to minimize effects.
- **Aminoglycosides** (eg, **gentamicin**) These drugs are more effective in an alkaline medium; urine acidification may diminish these drugs' effectiveness in treating bacterial urinary tract infections.
- **Copper**: Add ascorbic acid to total parenteral nutrition last to minimize drug degradation from copper.
- **Cyclosporine**: Concentrations of cyclosporine may be decreased with concomitant ascorbic acid administration.

- **Deferoxamine**: Ascorbic acid may be synergistic with deferoxamine in removing iron and may cause cardiac muscle dysfunction. Use with caution, particularly in patients with pre-existing cardiac disease.
- **Erythromycin**: This antibiotic is more effective in an alkaline medium; urine acidification may diminish the antimicrobial's effectiveness in treating bacterial urinary tract infections.
- **Estrogens** (eg, **estradiol, estriol**): Ascorbic acid may increase estrogen concentration.
- **Iron Salts**: Presence of ascorbic acid may enhance the oral absorption of iron salts.
- **Quinidine**: Urine acidification may increase renal excretion.

Laboratory Considerations

- **Urine dipstick tests**: Large amounts of vitamin C can cause false increases in urine test results measured by copper reduction methods, and false decreases in results measured by glucose oxidase methods; significant interference with other urine dipstick test results (eg, blood) may also occur.[7]
- **Stool occult blood**: False-negative results may occur if vitamin C is administered within 48 to 72 hours of an amine-dependent test.
- **Bilirubin, serum**: Vitamin C may decrease concentrations.
- **Aspartate aminotransferase (AST)**: Vitamin C may increase concentrations.
- **Creatinine**: Vitamin C can cause a false increase in serum and urine creatinine concentrations.

Dosages

DOGS/CATS:

Antioxidant for adjunctive treatment of toxin-induced (eg, **acetaminophen, phenazopyridine) methemoglobinemia** (extra-label): 30 – 33 mg/kg PO every 6 hours. Efficacy is questionable,[8] particularly because high plasma concentrations of ascorbic acid are probably not achieved after oral dosing.

HORSES:

Adjunctive treatment of erythrocyte oxidative injury (eg, red maple toxicity; extra-label):

1. 10 – 20 g/horse (NOT g/kg) PO once daily[9]
2. 30 – 50 mg/kg IV twice daily diluted in 5 – 10 L of crystalloid fluids[10]

Urinary acidifier (extra-label): 1 – 2 g/kg PO daily[11]

As adjunctive therapy for perinatal asphyxia syndrome in foals (extra-label): 100 mg/kg per day IV[12]

CATTLE:

Vitamin C-responsive dermatitis in calves (extra-label): 3 g/calf (NOT g/kg) SC once or twice[13]

RABBITS:

Stool softener (extra-label): 100 mg/kg PO every 12 hours[14]; may reduce cecal absorption of clostridial endotoxins

GUINEA PIGS:

Prevention of scurvy (extra-label): **NOTE:** Daily ascorbic acid requirement is 15 – 30 mg/kg/day[15,16] (daily requirements for adult, nonbreeding guinea pigs is 10 mg/kg/day, whereas breeding/growing animals require 30 mg/kg/day; pregnant females may require 30-45 mg/kg/day[17]).

1. 10 – 30 mg/kg/day PO, SC, or IM[18]
2. Add ascorbic acid 200 mg to 1 L of dechlorinated water and add to drinking water bottle; water must be changed daily to ensure adequate ascorbic acid concentrations. Use this route of administration with caution as the water supplementation may cause the guinea pig to not drink as well.[15]

Treatment of scurvy (extra-label): 100 mg/kg/day PO or SC during deficient states, pregnancy, stress, and illness.[19]

Monitoring

Monitoring depends on the underlying clinical condition being treated.

Client Information

- Vitamin C is most commonly used in guinea pigs to prevent scurvy (vitamin C deficiency).
- If mixing vitamin C in water, use dechlorinated water and change solution daily. Administering via syringe is preferable to placing in drinking water.

Chemistry/Synonyms

Ascorbic acid occurs as a white to slightly yellow crystal or powder. Although freely soluble in water, ascorbic acid is sparingly soluble in alcohol. The parenteral solution has a pH of 5.5 to 7.

Ascorbic acid may also be known as acidum ascorbicum, L-ascorbic acid, cevitamic acid, E300, or vitamin C; many trade names are available.

Storage/Stability

Protect from air and light. Ascorbic acid will slowly darken with light exposure; slight discoloration does not affect potency. Over time ascorbic acid will decompose with the production of CO_2. Open ampules carefully. To reduce potentially excessive pressure within ampules, store refrigerated and open while cold. Pressure release may be required prior to medication withdrawal.

Compatibility/Compounding Considerations

Compatibility is dependent on factors such as pH, concentration, temperature, and diluent used; consult specialized references or a hospital pharmacist for more specific information.

Ascorbic acid for injection is **compatible** with most commonly used IV solutions (eg, lactated Ringer's solution), but is **incompatible** with many drugs when mixed in syringes or IV bags.

Dosage Forms/Regulatory Status

VETERINARY-LABELED PRODUCTS:

Parenteral Injection: 250 mg/mL (as sodium ascorbate) in 100 mL and 250 mL vials; generic; (Rx or OTC depending on labeling)

Ascorbic Acid Powder: Concentrations vary; (OTC)

HUMAN-LABELED PRODUCTS:

Vitamin C or Ascorbic Acid Oral Tablets and Capsules: 100 mg, 250 mg, 500 mg, 1000 mg, and 1500 mg; generic; (OTC)

Ascorbic Acid Oral Extended-release Tablets: 500 mg, 1000 mg, and 1500 mg; generic; (OTC)

Ascorbic Acid Oral Crystals or Powder: Concentrations vary; (OTC)

Ascorbic Acid Oral Liquid/Solution: 100 mg/mL in 50 mL and 500 mg/5 mL; *Cecon®*, generic; (OTC)

Ascorbic Acid Injection: 500 mg/mL in 50 mL vials; *Ascor L 500®* (0.025% EDTA, preservative-free), generic; (Rx)

References

For the complete list of references, see **wiley.com/go/budde/plumb**

Asparaginase

(a-***spar***-a-gin-ase)

Antineoplastic

Prescriber Highlights

- Antineoplastic agent used in some protocols for treatment of lymphomas and leukemias in dogs and cats
- Adverse effects include hypersensitivity reactions (eg, vomiting, diarrhea, urticaria, pruritus, dyspnea, restlessness, hypotension, collapse) and effects on protein synthesis (eg, GI effects, hemorrhagic pancreatitis, hepatotoxicity, coagulation disorders).
- Bone marrow suppression is rare. Asparaginase does not cause significant GI mucosal toxicity.
- Teratogenic in laboratory animals
- Should be given IM or SC; not IV, as IV administration may increase the risk for anaphylaxis
- *Escherichia coli*-derived asparaginase is not therapeutically equivalent to asparaginase *Erwinia chrysanthemi* (*Erwinaze*®).
- Availability of commercial, *E coli*-derived asparaginase may be limited, and doses may need to be obtained from a compounding pharmacy.

Uses/Indications

Asparaginase has been used in combination with other agents in the treatment of lymphoid malignancies, most commonly high-grade lymphoma. The drug is thought to be most useful for inducing disease remission (in combinatorial regimens), rescue protocols, and treatment of fragile patients presented with severe comorbidities that preclude the safe use of traditional cytotoxic agents. Asparaginase may also be beneficial in the treatment of leukemias, particularly acute lymphocytic leukemia (ALL).

Asparaginase as part of an initial treatment canine lymphoma protocol is optional, as results of a retrospective study[1] in dogs showed no statistical difference in dogs treated with or without asparaginase (as part of a standard CHOP protocol) in regards to response rate, remission or survival rate, remission or survival duration, or prevalence of toxicity and treatment delay. Asparaginase is still commonly used at the beginning of the feline CHOP protocol because it has a favorable adverse effect profile and potent anticancer activities.

Pharmacology/Actions

Some malignant cells are unable to synthesize asparagine and are dependent on exogenous asparagine for DNA and protein synthesis. Asparaginase catalyzes asparagine into ammonia and aspartic acid. The antineoplastic activity of asparaginase is greatest during the postmitotic (G_1) cell phase. Although normal cells can synthesize asparagine intracellularly, some normal cells with a high rate of protein synthesis require exogenous asparagine and may be adversely affected by asparaginase.

Resistance to asparaginase can develop rapidly, but cross-resistance between asparaginase and other antineoplastic agents is not apparent.

Asparaginase possesses antiviral activity, but its toxicity prevents it from being clinically useful for this indication.

Pharmacokinetics

Asparaginase is not absorbed from the GI tract and must be given either SC or IM. After IM injection, serum concentrations of asparaginase are ≈½ of those after IV injection. Because of its high molecular weight, asparaginase does not diffuse readily out of the capillaries, and ≈80% of the drug remains within the intravascular space.

Asparaginase administered IM to cats significantly reduces asparagine concentrations within 2 days, but the effect is lost within 7 days.[2]

Contraindications/Precautions/Warnings

Asparaginase is contraindicated in patients that have exhibited anaphylaxis to the drug or have existing or a history of pancreatitis, thrombosis, or hemorrhagic events. Asparaginase should be used with caution in patients with pre-existing hepatic, renal, hematologic, GI, and CNS dysfunction or when high protein synthesis is required for tissue repair.

Monitor the patient for 1 hour after administration for signs of hypersensitivity reactions; epinephrine, diphenhydramine; corticosteroids should be readily available. Prior asparaginase use can increase the risk for immunologic hypersensitivity.

No specific precautions are required for handling asparaginase, but it is considered a contact irritant, and contact with eyes, skin, and the upper respiratory tract should be avoided.

Adverse Effects

Asparaginase adverse effects are classified in 2 main categories: hypersensitivity reactions and effects on protein synthesis. Clinical signs of hypersensitivity reactions include vomiting, diarrhea, urticaria, pruritus, dyspnea, restlessness, hypotension, and collapse. The likelihood of hypersensitivity reactions increases with subsequent doses because of the antigenicity of asparaginase. Following the first treatment cycle, many oncologists now recommend administering antihistamines (eg, diphenhydramine at 2 mg/kg) in dogs prior to administration of subsequent doses. If a hypersensitivity reaction occurs, diphenhydramine (0.2 – 0.5 mg/kg slow IV), dexamethasone sodium phosphate (1 – 2 mg/kg IV), IV fluids, and, if severe, epinephrine (0.1 – 0.3 mg IV [total dose]) have been suggested.[3] Hypersensitivity reaction in cats is considered unlikely.[4]

The effects of asparaginase on protein synthesis can result in hemorrhagic pancreatitis or other GI disturbances, hepatotoxicity, and coagulation defects. Large doses may be associated with hyperglycemia secondary to altered insulin synthesis. Subclinical hyperammonemia[5] and a case report of acute hyperammonemia in a dog have been reported.[6]

Reproductive/Nursing Safety

For sexually intact patients, verify pregnancy status prior to administration. Asparaginase is teratogenic in laboratory animals. At doses below those used clinically, asparaginase caused pulmonary, renal, and skeletal malformations. Therapeutic doses resulted in exencephaly and skeletal anomalies.

It is unknown if the drug is excreted in milk. Use with caution, if at all, in nursing patients.

Because safety has not been established in animals, this drug should only be used when the maternal benefits outweigh the potential risks to offspring.

Overdose/Acute Toxicity

Limited information was located regarding overdoses with this agent. Toxicity secondary to the protein-synthesis–altering effects of asparaginase would be expected. In dogs, it has been reported that the maximally tolerated dose of asparaginase is 10,000 units/kg and the LD_{50} is 50,000 units/kg. Supportive treatment is recommended in the event of overdose.

For patients that have experienced or are suspected to have experienced an overdose, consultation with a 24-hour poison consultation center specializing in providing veterinary-specific information is recommended. For general information related to overdose and toxin exposures, as well as contact information for poison control centers, refer to ***Appendix.***

Drug Interactions

The following drug interactions with asparaginase have either been reported or are theoretical in humans or animals and may be of significance in veterinary patients. Unless otherwise noted, use together is not necessarily contraindicated, but weigh the potential risks and perform additional monitoring when appropriate.

- **Anticoagulants** (eg, **clopidogrel, heparin, rivaroxaban, warfarin**): Increased risk for bleeding
- **Aspirin and Other Salicylates** (eg, **bismuth subsalicylate**): Increased risk for bleeding
- **Corticosteroids** (eg, **dexamethasone, predniso(lo)ne**): Use with asparaginase may increase the risk for hyperglycemia; in humans, asparaginase is usually administered after the corticosteroid. Asparaginase may increase dexamethasone concentration.
- **Cytarabine**: Asparaginase may reduce cytarabine effectiveness against tumor cells until serum asparagine concentrations return to normal.
- **Immunosuppressants** (eg, **cyclosporine, mycophenolate**): Excessive immune suppression may increase the risk for infection or lymphoproliferation.
- **Methotrexate**: Asparaginase may reduce methotrexate effectiveness against tumor cells until serum asparagine concentrations return to normal.
- **NSAIDs** (eg, **carprofen, meloxicam, robenacoxib**): Increased risk for bleeding
- **Vaccines, Modified Live Virus**: Use with caution during chemotherapy protocols.
- **Vincristine**: In humans, increased toxicity (neuropathy and erythropoiesis disruption) may occur when asparaginase is given IV concurrently with or before vincristine. Myelosuppression reportedly occurs in a minority of dogs treated with asparaginase (IM or SC) and vincristine (IV); some veterinary oncologists separate administration by a few days to a week, but others do not feel this is necessary.

Laboratory Considerations

- **Serum ammonia and urea nitrogen**: Concentrations may be increased by the action of the drug.
- **Thyroxine-binding globulin (TBG)**: Asparaginase may cause rapid (within 2 days) and profound decreases in circulating TBG, which may alter interpretation of thyroid function studies; values may return to normal after ≈4 weeks.
- **Serum hepatic chemistry abnormalities**: Hyperbilirubinemia and elevated transaminases have been reported in humans.

Dosages

NOTE: Because of the potential toxicity of this drug to patients, veterinary staff, and pet owners and because chemotherapy indications, treatment protocols, monitoring, and safety guidelines often change, the following dosages should be used only as a general guide. Consultation with a veterinary oncologist and referral to current veterinary oncology references[7-11] are strongly recommended.

DOGS:

Lymphoreticular malignancies (eg, **lymphoma, leukemia**) (extra-label): 400 units/kg or 10,000 units/m^2 (NOT units/kg) IM or SC, with a maximum dose of 10,000 units per patient. **NOTE**: Many oncologists recommend pretreatment with an antihistamine such as diphenhydramine 2 mg/kg IM or SC.

Transmissible venereal tumor (TVT; extra-label): Asparaginase 200 units/kg or 5000 units/m^2 (NOT units/kg) SC in week 1, vincristine 0.025 mg/kg IV in week 2. The 2-week cycle was repeated until the tumor was undetectable; total duration ranged from 2 to 5 weeks. Complete response was reported in 12 out of 13 dogs.[12]

CATS:

Lymphoreticular malignancies (eg, **lymphoma, leukemia**): (extra-label): 400 units/kg or 10,000 units/m^2 (NOT units/kg) IM or SC, with a maximum dose of 10,000 units per patient

Monitoring

- Baseline and periodic CBC, serum chemistry profile (including amylase and lipase), and coagulation profile
- Bone marrow evaluation as necessary based on initial diagnosis

Client Information

- This drug can cause severe toxicity, including drug-related death.
- Contact your veterinarian if your animal shows signs of itching, difficulty breathing, very low energy levels, vomiting, poor appetite, severe diarrhea, abnormal bleeding (including bloody diarrhea), bruising, and/or yellowing of the eyes, skin, or gums (ie, jaundice).
- While taking this medicine, your animal will need to be closely monitored by your veterinarian. Do not miss these important follow-up visits.
- Exposure to other animals (eg, from dog parks, animal competitions) can put your animal at serious risk for infection during chemotherapy treatment. Talk with your veterinarian about when it will be safe to return to these activities.

Chemistry/Synonyms

Asparaginase is an enzyme derived from *Escherichia coli* and occurs as a white or almost white, slightly hygroscopic powder that is soluble in water. Asparaginase in this form is not commercially available. The only commercially available product in the United States is *Erwinaze*® (asparaginase *Erwinia chrysanthemi*), a lyophilized powder that is not therapeutically equivalent to *E coli*-derived asparaginase. Activity of asparaginase is expressed in terms of International Units (I.U.) or units.

Asparaginase may also be known as A-ase, ASN-ase, colo-aspase, L-asparaginase, L-asparagine amidohydrolase, MK-965 NSC-109229, Re-82-TAD-15, *Crasnitin*®, *Crasnitine*®, *Elspar*®, *Erwinase*®, *Kidrolase*®, *L-Asp*®, *Laspar*®, *Leucogen*®, *Leunase*®, *Paronal*®, or *Serasa*®.

Storage/Stability

Asparaginase powder for injection should be at 2°C to 8°C (36°F-46°F) unless labeling states otherwise. Reconstituted *Kidrolase*® may be stored refrigerated for more than 72 hours. Asparaginase prepared by compounding pharmacies should be stored in accordance with instructions on the product label.

Solutions should be used only if clear; turbid solutions should be discarded. Upon standing, gelatinous fibers may be noted in the solution occasionally. These may be removed with a 5-micron filter without loss of potency.[3] Some loss of potency may occur if a 0.2-micron filter is used. The solution may be gently mixed or swirled while reconstituting, but vigorous shaking or inversion of the vial should be avoided. Recommended IV diluents include D_5W or sodium chloride 0.9%.

Compatibility/Compounding Considerations

Compatible with sodium chloride 0.9% and dextrose 5% in water for dilution

Dosage Forms/Regulatory Status

VETERINARY-LABELED PRODUCTS: NONE

HUMAN-LABELED PRODUCTS:

No commercial products with *E coli*-derived asparaginase are available. *Elspar*® (asparaginase powder for injection) has been discontinued in the United States. Compounding pharmacies or FDA-registered outsourcing facilities may be able to compound asparaginase using bulk chemical, which has been shown to have a similar safety profile.[13] *Kidrolase*® is an equivalent Canadian product available in 10,000 unit vials.

Asparaginase *Erwinia chrysanthemi* Powder for Injection, lyophilized: 10,000 units in 3 mL vials (preservative-free); *Erwinaze*®;

(Rx). **NOTE:** *E coli*-derived asparaginase is not considered therapeutically equivalent to asparaginase *Erwinia chrysanthemi* because of differences in enzyme characteristics.

References

For the complete list of references, see **wiley.com/go/budde/plumb**

Aspirin

(***ass***-pir-in) *ASA, Acetylsalicylic Acid*

Antiplatelet agent; Nonsteroidal Anti-Inflammatory Drug (NSAID)

Prescriber Highlights

- NSAID historically used for analgesic, anti-inflammatory, and antiplatelet effects in various species. Use in dogs and cats has been superseded by safer and/or more effective alternatives.
- Contraindicated in patients hypersensitive to aspirin or that have active GI bleeding; relatively contraindicated in patients with bleeding disorders, GI disease, asthma, concurrent glucocorticoid or other NSAID use, or renal insufficiency
- Aspirin has a long half-life in cats (ie, ≈30 hours; dose carefully); dogs are relatively sensitive to GI adverse effects (eg, ulcerations, vomiting, diarrhea).
- Avoid use in pregnant animals.
- Many drug and laboratory interactions

Uses/Indications

Aspirin is an NSAID used for its analgesic, antipyretic, and antiplatelet effects.

When treatment with cyclosporine is required, aspirin therapy may be advisable to offset cyclosporine-induced thromboxane synthesis.[1] Although aspirin appears to be effective as an antiplatelet agent, clopidogrel appears to be a safer and more effective antiplatelet drug in cats and dogs.[2,3]

Experimental studies in healthy horses failed to demonstrate reliable antiplatelet effects.[4,5]

Pharmacology/Actions

Aspirin inhibits cyclooxygenase (COX-1, prostaglandin synthetase), thereby reducing prostaglandin and thromboxane (TXA2) synthesis. These effects are thought to be how aspirin produces analgesia and reduces fever, platelet aggregation, and inflammation. Most cells synthesize new COX; however, platelets are not able to synthesize new COX, resulting in an irreversible inhibition of platelet aggregation. A study in dogs investigated platelet function effects of various aspirin doses and showed that doses less than 1 mg/kg/day or at 10 mg/kg/day did not have a statistically significant effect on platelet aggregation. Doses of 12 mg/kg/day inhibited platelet function and aggregation.[6] Variability in canine platelet response to aspirin appears to be due both to interindividual patient sensitivity to aspirin and differences in pharmacokinetics.[7] Aspirin appears to have minimal effect on platelet aggregation in cattle[8] and horses.[9]

Aspirin may decrease the clinical signs of experimentally induced anaphylaxis in calves and ponies.

Although aspirin does not directly inhibit COX-2, aspirin along with lipoxygenase (LOX), can modify COX-2 to produce the aspirin-triggered lipoxin (ATL) compound, which may have gastric mucosal protective actions.[10-12] This effect may explain why aspirin tends to have reduced gastric damaging effects when used over time.

Pharmacokinetics

Aspirin is rapidly absorbed from the stomach and proximal small intestine in monogastric animals. The rate of absorption is dependent on stomach content, gastric emptying times, tablet disintegration rates, and gastric pH. In cattle, oral doses of 50 mg/kg did not achieve therapeutic concentrations.[13]

During absorption, aspirin is partially hydrolyzed to salicylic acid, which is distributed widely throughout the body. The highest concentrations of salicylate are found in the liver, heart, lungs, renal cortex, and plasma. Aspirin's plasma protein binding is variable depending on species as well as serum salicylate and albumin concentrations. Lower salicylate concentrations are 90% protein bound, and higher salicylate concentrations are 70% protein bound.

Salicylate is metabolized in the liver primarily by conjugation with glycine and glucuronic acid via glucuronyl transferase. Cats are deficient in this enzymatic pathway, resulting in prolonged half-lives of 27 to 45 hours; this may cause drug accumulation. Minor metabolites formed include gentisic acid; 2,3-dihydroxybenzoic acid; and 2,3,5-trihydroxybenzoic acid. Gentisic acid appears as the only active metabolite, but low concentrations have an insignificant therapeutic role. Metabolism is determined by first-order and dose-dependent kinetics, depending on the metabolic pathway. Serum half-life is ≈8 hours in dogs, ≈38 hours in cats, and an average of 1.5 hours in humans. In general, steady-state serum concentrations increase to levels (proportionally) higher than expected with dose increases. These effects have not been well studied in domestic animals.

Kidneys rapidly excrete salicylate and its metabolites via filtration and renal tubular secretion. Significant tubular reabsorption occurs and is pH dependent. Raising urine pH to 5 to 8 can significantly increase salicylate excretion. Salicylate and metabolites may be removed using peritoneal dialysis or more rapidly by using hemodialysis.

Contraindications/Precautions/Warnings

Aspirin is contraindicated in patients that have demonstrated previous hypersensitivity reactions to aspirin or other salicylates or have GI erosions and ulcerations. Concurrent corticosteroid use may significantly increase the risk for GI pathology (eg, mucosal hemorrhages, erosions, ulcerations)[14]; presumably, concurrent NSAIDs have a similar risk. Relative contraindications include patients with hemorrhagic disorders, asthma, or renal insufficiency.

Aspirin should be used cautiously in cats due to their inability to rapidly metabolize and excrete salicylates. Neonatal animals are at risk for toxicity if given adult doses of aspirin.

High protein binding to plasma albumin indicates that patients with hypoalbuminemia may require lower aspirin dosages to prevent clinical signs of toxicity. Aspirin should be used cautiously in patients with severe hepatic failure or diminished renal function.

Aspirin therapy should be discontinued 1 week prior to surgical procedures because of its effects on platelet aggregation. In animals at high risk for thrombotic complications, some studies have advocated that aspirin should be discontinued 48 hours prior to surgical procedures.[15] Desmopressin acetate has been shown to reverse aspirin-induced platelet dysfunction in 3 dogs that required emergent surgery.[16]

Adverse Effects

The most common adverse effect of aspirin at therapeutic doses is GI irritation (eg, nausea, anorexia, vomiting, diarrhea). Varying degrees of occult GI blood loss may occur[14]; severe blood loss can cause anemia and panhypoproteinemia. In dogs, plain uncoated aspirin may irritate the gastric mucosa more than buffered aspirin or enteric-coated tablets. Hypersensitivity reactions in dogs are rarely reported. See *Overdose/Acute Toxicity*.

Reproductive/Nursing Safety

Salicylate crosses the placenta, and fetal levels may exceed those found in the mother. High-dose aspirin (ie, 400 mg/kg/day) was fetotoxic and teratogenic when administered to pregnant beagles.[17] Salicylates are possible teratogens and have been shown to delay parturition; their use should be avoided during pregnancy, particularly during the later stages.[18]

Aspirin is excreted in human breast milk; veterinary significance is uncertain. Use with caution in nursing animals.

Overdose/Acute Toxicity

Clinical signs of mild toxicity (ie, less than 50 mg/kg) in dogs and cats include depression, anorexia, vomiting (may contain fresh blood or look like coffee grounds [ie, digested blood]), and diarrhea. Ingestions of greater than 100 mg/kg (in dogs) and 80 mg/kg (in cats) may cause hyperthermia tachypnea (ie, hyperventilation secondary to an initial respiratory alkalosis), increased respiratory rate, muscular weakness, pulmonary and cerebral edema, hypernatremia, hypokalemia, ataxia, and seizures; coma and eventual death are possible if left untreated.

There were 1939 single agent exposures to aspirin reported to the ASPCA Animal Poison Control Center (APCC) from 2009 to 2013. Of the 1749 dogs exposed, 712 had clinical signs; common signs included vomiting (75%), lethargy (21%), panting (9%), hyperthermia (8%), and bloody vomiting (7%). Of the 177 cats exposed, 54 had clinical signs; common signs included vomiting (56%), anorexia (22%), lethargy (13%), and bloody vomiting (6%).

Acute overdose treatment initially consists of gastric decontamination (if ingestion occurred within 12 hours), activated charcoal with an oral cathartic, IV fluid therapy, and gastroprotectants (eg, misoprostol); serial laboratory monitoring (eg, venous blood gas, electrolytes) may also be necessary. Balanced isotonic crystalloid IV solutions (eg, lactated Ringer's, *Normosol-R*, Plasmalyte-A) are preferred to treat dehydration and acid–base disturbances; additional treatment for metabolic acidosis may be required. Animals with severe metabolic derangements may require peritoneal dialysis, continuous renal replacement therapy (CRRT), or hemodialysis.

For patients that have experienced or are suspected to have experienced an overdose, it is strongly encouraged that a 24-hour poison consultation center that specializes in providing information specific for veterinary patients be consulted. For general information related to overdose and toxin exposures, as well as contact information for poison control centers, refer to *Appendix*.

Drug Interactions

The following drug interactions have either been reported or are theoretical in humans or animals receiving aspirin and may be of significance in veterinary patients. Unless otherwise noted, use together is not necessarily contraindicated, but weigh the potential risks and perform additional monitoring when appropriate.

- Ace inhibitors (eg, **benazepril, enalapril**): The effects of ACE inhibitors may be decreased with concomitant aspirin use; nephrotoxic effects of ACE inhibitors may be increased with concomitant aspirin use.
- Alendronate: Increased risk for upper GI adverse effects when used concurrently with aspirin
- Aminoglycosides (eg, **amikacin, gentamicin**): Some clinicians feel aspirin should not be given concomitantly with aminoglycoside antibiotics because of an increased likelihood for developing nephrotoxicity; however, the clinical significance of this interaction is unclear. Weigh the risks versus benefits when contemplating therapy.
- Anticoagulants, Oral (eg, **rivaroxaban, warfarin**): Concomitant aspirin use may increase the risk for bleeding.
- Calcium Channel Blockers, Nondihydropyridine (eg, **diltiazem**): The antiplatelet effects of aspirin may be increased with concurrent use, increasing the risk for bleeding.
- Carbonic Anhydrase Inhibitors (eg, **acetazolamide, dichlorphenamide**): High dose aspirin therapy used concurrently with dichlorphenamide is considered contraindicated, as metabolic acidosis may result.[19] Use caution with other carbonic anhydrase inhibitors.
- Clopidogrel: Concomitant aspirin use may increase the risk for bleeding.
- Corticosteroids (eg, **dexamethasone, prednis(ol)one**): Corticosteroids may increase the clearance of salicylates, decrease salicylate serum levels, and increase the risk for GI bleeding. One study in dogs showed no significant difference in gastric mucosal injury when ultra-low–dose aspirin (0.5 mg/kg/day) was added to prednisone therapy[20]; however, the addition of aspirin increased the incidence of mild self-limiting diarrhea.
- Digoxin: In dogs, aspirin demonstrates increased plasma levels of digoxin by decreasing digoxin clearance.
- Furosemide: Furosemide may compete with renal excretion of aspirin and delay aspirin excretion. Accumulated aspirin may cause clinical signs of toxicity in animals receiving high aspirin doses. Furosemide diuretic effect may be diminished.
- Glucosamine: Concomitant aspirin use may increase the risk for bleeding.
- Heparin: Concomitant aspirin use may increase the risk for bleeding.
- Hyaluronidase: The therapeutic benefits of hyaluronidase may be decreased; higher hyaluronidase doses may be required.
- Insulin: Hypoglycemic effects may be potentiated by aspirin.
- Methotrexate: Aspirin may displace methotrexate from plasma proteins and reduce renal tubular methotrexate excretion, increasing the risk for methotrexate toxicity.
- NSAIDs (eg, **carprofen, deracoxib, meloxicam**): Increased chance for developing GI ulceration exists when used concomitantly. Animals receiving aspirin therapy that will be replaced with a COX-2 NSAID should have a washout period of 3 to 10 days from when aspirin is discontinued and the NSAID is started.[21] In cats, it is recommended that a washout period of ≈7 to 10 days be used when aspirin therapy is switched to another NSAID.[22]
- Omega-3 Fatty Acids: May augment antiplatelet effects and the risk for bleeding[23]
- Pentosan Polysulfate Sodium: May increase the risk for bleeding
- Phenobarbital: Hepatic enzyme induction by phenobarbital may increase aspirin metabolism.
- Probenecid: At usual doses, aspirin may antagonize the uricosuric effects of probenecid.
- Selective Serotonin Reuptake Inhibitors (SSRIs; eg, **fluoxetine, paroxetine, sertraline**): The antiplatelet effects of aspirin may be increased with concurrent use, increasing the risk for bleeding.
- Spironolactone: Aspirin may inhibit the diuretic activity of spironolactone.
- Sulfonylureas (eg, **glipizide, glyburide**): Hypoglycemic effects may be potentiated by aspirin.
- Tetracycline: Antacids in buffered aspirin may chelate tetracycline products if given simultaneously; separate doses by at least 1 hour.
- Tiludronate: Serum concentrations of tiludronate may be decreased with concurrent aspirin therapy.
- Urinary Acidifying Drugs (eg, **ammonium chloride, ascorbic acid, methionine**): Urine acidifiers can decrease renal excretion of salicylates.
- Urinary Alkalinizing Drugs: (eg, **acetazolamide, sodium bicarbonate**): Urine alkalinizers significantly increase the renal excretion of salicylates.
- Valproic Acid, Divalproex: Serum concentrations of valproate products may be increased with concurrent aspirin therapy.
- Vitamin E: The antiplatelet effects of aspirin may be increased with concurrent use, increasing the risk for bleeding.

Laboratory Considerations

- At high doses, aspirin may cause false-positive results for **urinary glucose** if using the cupric sulfate method (eg, *Clinitest*®, Benedict's solution) or false-negative results if using the glucose oxidase method (eg, *Clinistix*®, *Tes-Tape*®).
- **Urinary ketones** measured by the ferric chloride method (ie, Gerhardt's method) may be affected if salicylates are in the urine (reddish-color produced during reaction). Salicylates may interfere with fluorescent methods used to determine urine **5-hydroxyindoleacetic acid (5-HIAA)**. Falsely elevated **vanillylmandelic acid (VMA)** may be seen with most methods if salicylates are in the urine. Falsely lowered **VMA** levels may be seen if using the Pisano method.
- Urinary excretion of **xylose** may be decreased if aspirin is given concurrently.
- Falsely elevated **serum uric acid** values may be measured if using colorimetric methods.
- Aspirin can decrease serum concentrations of **total T4** (ie, **thyroxine**).

Dosages

NOTE: There are no FDA-approved products or dosages for veterinary patients; all dosages listed here are extra-label.

DOGS:

Decrease platelet aggregation; antithrombotic: 2 – 10 mg/kg PO once daily. The ideal aspirin dosage, if any, for prevention of thromboembolism in dogs is unknown due to conflicting data and study limitations.[24-26]

Immune-mediated hemolytic anemia (IMHA): 1 – 2 mg/kg PO every 24 hours in combination with clopidogrel.[27]

Analgesic/antipyretic/anti-inflammatory: Anecdotal dosages range from 10 – 20 mg/kg PO of buffered aspirin every 12 hours to 20 – 30 mg/kg PO every 8 to 12 hours. NSAIDs that are FDA approved for dogs are preferred over aspirin because they have significantly fewer GI effects.

CATS:

Analgesic/antipyretic/anti-inflammatory: 10 mg/kg PO every 2 to 3 days (anecdotal); practically, ½ to one 81 mg tablet (ie, baby aspirin) on Monday, Wednesday, and Friday weekly.

Antithrombotic: High dose: 10 mg/kg PO every 2 to 3 days. Low dose: 5 mg per cat (NOT mg/kg) PO every third day. Clopidogrel appears superior to aspirin as an antiplatelet agent.[28,29]

HORSES:

Antiplatelet adjunctive treatment of laminitis: 5 – 10 mg/kg PO every 24 to 48 hours or 20 mg/kg PO every 4 to 5 days[30]

CATTLE:

Analgesic: 100 mg/kg PO every 12 hours[31,32]

FERRETS:

Analgesic: 10 – 20 mg/kg PO once daily[33]

RABBITS/RODENTS/SMALL MAMMALS:

Rabbits: 5 – 20 mg/kg PO once daily for low-grade analgesia[34]

Mice, Rats, Gerbils, Hamsters: 100 – 150 mg/kg PO every 4 hours

Guinea pigs: 87 mg/kg PO[35]

Monitoring

- Analgesic and/or antipyretic effects
- Adverse effects such as inappetence, lethargy, vomiting, and/or diarrhea
- Platelet function (ie, buccal mucosal bleeding time [BMBT]), including platelet aggregometry or platelet activation[2,26,28,36,37]
- Packed cell volume (PCV) and fecal occult blood (eg, guaiac) tests if indicated

Client Information

- Contact your veterinarian if your animal shows any signs of a decreased or lack of appetite, vomiting, diarrhea, and/or excessive bleeding or bruising.
- Black, tarry feces are a sign of serious internal bleeding and should be reported to your veterinarian immediately.

Chemistry/Synonyms

Aspirin is the salicylate ester of acetic acid. The compound occurs as a white crystalline powder or tabular or needle-like crystals. Aspirin is a weak acid with a pK_a of 3.5; it is slightly soluble in water and freely soluble in alcohol. Each gram of aspirin contains ≈760 mg of salicylate.

Aspirin may also be known as ASA, acetylsal acid, acetylsalicylic acid, acidum acetylsalicylicum, polopiryna, or salicylic acid acetate; many trade names are available.

Storage/Stability

Aspirin tablets should be stored in tight, moisture-resistant containers. Do not use products past the expiration date or if a strong vinegar-like odor is emitting from the bottle.

Aspirin is stable in dry air but readily hydrolyzes to acetate and salicylate when exposed to water or moist air; it then exudes a strong vinegar-like odor. The addition of heat speeds the hydrolysis rate. In aqueous solutions, aspirin is most stable at a pH of 2 to 3 and least stable at a pH less than 2 or greater than 8. In cases in which an aqueous solution is needed as a dosage form, the commercial aspirin-containing product *Alka-Seltzer*® remains stable for 10 hours at room temperature after dissolving in water, and 90 hours when refrigerated.[38]

Compatibility/Compounding Considerations

Compounded preparation stability: Aspirin is hydrolyzed by water to degradative byproducts, acetic acid and salicylic acid.

Although pharmacists compound aspirin suspensions in fixed oils, the long-term stability of these preparations is unknown.

Dosage Forms/Regulatory Status

VETERINARY-LABELED PRODUCTS:

NOTE: There are no known products that are FDA approved for use in animals. Aspirin predates formal FDA-approval regulations for its use in animals. There are no meat or milk withdrawal times listed for food-producing animals. In the interest of public health of salicylate-sensitive humans, contact the Food Animal Residue Avoidance Databank (FARAD) for further guidance with determining use and withdrawal times. See ***Appendix***.

Aspirin Tablets (Enteric-Coated): 81 mg; (OTC). Labeled for use in dogs

Aspirin Tablets (Buffered, Microencapsulated, Chewable for dogs): 60 mg, 120 mg, 150 mg, 300 mg, and 450 mg; *Canine Aspirin Chewable Tablets for Small & Medium* (150 mg) or *Large Dogs*® (450 mg); (OTC). Labeled for use in dogs

Aspirin Tablets 60 grains (3.9 g): Aspirin 60 Grains (OTC, Rx); Rx is labeled for use in horses, foals, cattle, calves, sheep, and swine; not for use in horses intended for food or in lactating dairy animals

Aspirin Boluses 240 grains (15.6 g): Aspirin 240 Grains Boluses, Aspirin Bolus (various); (OTC). Labeled for use in horses, foals, cattle, and calves; not for use in lactating animals

Aspirin Boluses 480 grains (31.2 g): Aspirin 480 Grains Boluses (various); (OTC). Labeled for use in mature horses and cattle

Aspirin Powder: 1 lb (various); (OTC); Aspirin Powder Molasses-Flavored 50% acetylsalicylic acid in base; Aspirin USP 204 g/lb (apple flavored); Acetylsalicylic acid; (OTC). Labeled for use in horses, foals, cattle, calves, sheep, swine, and poultry

Aspirin Granules: 2.5 gram per 39 mL scoop (apple and molasses flavor); *Arthri-Eze Aspirin Granules®*; (OTC). Labeled for use in horses

Aspirin Liquid Concentrate (equivalent to 12% aspirin) for Dilution in Drinking Water in 32 oz bottles; (OTC). Labeled for addition to drinking water for swine, poultry, beef cattle, and dairy cattle

The Association of Racing Commissioners International (ARCI) has designated this drug as a class 4 substance. See *Appendix*.

HUMAN-LABELED PRODUCTS:

Aspirin, Tablets; chewable: 81 mg (1.25 grains); many trade names, generic; (OTC)

Aspirin, Tablets; plain uncoated: 325 mg (5 grains), and 500 mg (7.8 grains); many trade names, generic; (OTC)

Aspirin, Tablets; enteric coated: 81 mg, 325 mg, 500 mg, and 650 mg (10 grains); many trade names, generic; (OTC)

Aspirin, Tablets; extended-controlled release: 81 mg, 650 mg; many trade names, generic; (OTC)

Aspirin, Tablets; buffered uncoated: 324 mg (5 grains) and 325 mg (5 grains), with aluminum and/or magnesium salts; many trade names, generic; (OTC)

Aspirin, Tablets; buffered coated: 325 mg and 500 mg; many trade names, generic; (OTC)

Rectal suppositories, chewing gum, and effervescent oral dosage forms are commercially available for humans.

References

For the complete list of references, see **wiley.com/go/budde/plumb**

Atenolol

(a-***ten***-oh-lol) *Tenormin®*

Beta-Adrenergic Blocker

Prescriber Highlights

- Relatively specific beta-1-blocker used primarily for ventricular hypertrophy and tachyarrhythmias in small animals
- Minimal beta-2-blocking activity at recommended doses; comparatively safe for use in animals with asthma
- Contraindicated in patients with bradycardic arrhythmias or that are hypersensitive to it
- Negative inotrope, so caution is advised in patients with CHF, chronic kidney disease, and sinus node dysfunction
- Higher dosages may mask clinical signs of hyperthyroidism or hypoglycemia; may cause hyper- or hypoglycemia—use with caution in fragile diabetics.
- Usually well-tolerated, but primary adverse effects are lethargy, hypotension, or diarrhea
- If discontinuing therapy, gradual withdrawal is recommended.

Uses/Indications

Atenolol may be useful in the treatment of supraventricular tachyarrhythmias, premature ventricular complexes (PVCs, VPCs), and systemic arterial hypertension. It has also been used to reduce clinical signs of thyrotoxicosis in cats. A study evaluating atenolol as monotherapy for treating systemic hypertension in cats with hyperthyroidism found that most cats had a decrease in heart rate, but blood pressure was not controlled (defined as less than 160 mmHg) in 70% of cases, and additional drug therapy (eg, amlodipine or ACE inhibitor) was required.[1]

Although atenolol has been used in cats with subclinical hypertrophic cardiomyopathy, its utility is unproven. Atenolol given to cats with subclinical HCM had decreased heart rate, murmur grade, and LVOT obstruction, and to a lesser degree, frequency of ventricular ectopy.[2] However, it is still unclear if occurrence of sudden cardiac death or long-term outcome is influenced by atenolol administration.[2] A study (prospective, observational, open-label, clinical cohort) found no significant difference in mortality between subclinical cats treated or not treated with atenolol.[3]

Atenolol is often prescribed for semilunar (ie, aortic, pulmonary) valve stenosis; however, a retrospective study of dogs with subvalvular aortic stenosis failed to identify increased survival in those receiving atenolol as compared with those receiving no treatment.[4] In dogs, atenolol has also been used in combination with mexiletine to control arrhythmias associated with arrhythmogenic right ventricular cardiomyopathy (also known as boxer cardiomyopathy).[5]

Atenolol is relatively safe to use in animals with bronchospastic disease (eg, asthma).

Pharmacology/Actions

Atenolol is a relatively specific beta-1-blocker. At higher dosages, this specificity may be lost and beta-2-blockade can occur. Atenolol does not possess intrinsic sympathomimetic activity like pindolol, nor does it possess membrane-stabilizing activity like pindolol or propranolol. Cardiovascular effects secondary to atenolol's negative inotropic and chronotropic actions include decreased sinus heart rate, slowed AV conduction, diminished cardiac output at rest and during exercise, decreased myocardial oxygen demand, reduced blood pressure, and inhibition of isoproterenol-induced tachycardia.[6]

Pharmacokinetics

In humans, only ≈50% to 60% of an oral dose is absorbed, but it is absorbed rapidly. In cats, atenolol is reported to have a bioavailability of ≈90%.[6] The drug has very low protein binding characteristics (5% to 15%) and is distributed well into most tissues. Atenolol has low lipid solubility and, unlike propranolol, only small amounts of atenolol are distributed into the CNS. Atenolol is minimally biotransformed in the liver; 40% to 50% is excreted unchanged in the urine and the bulk of the remainder is excreted in the feces unchanged as unabsorbed drug. Reported half-lives are 3.2 hours in dogs, 3.7 hours in cats,[6] and 6 to 7 hours in humans.[7] Duration of the beta blockade effect lasts for ≈12 hours in cats[6] and between 6 to 12 hours in dogs.[8] A study investigating the ability of atenolol to attenuate the heart rate response to isoproterenol in healthy dogs supported a dosing interval of less than 24 hours.[8]

Contraindications/Precautions/Warnings

Atenolol is contraindicated in patients hypersensitive to it and in patients with overt or decompensated heart failure, cardiogenic shock, greater than first-degree heart block, or sinus bradycardia. Atenolol may cause increased morbidity in cats with left-sided CHF caused by hypertrophic cardiomyopathy.[9]

Atenolol should be used cautiously in patients with significant renal insufficiency; dosage reduction is suggested in cats with reduced renal function.[10]

At high dosages, atenolol can mask the clinical signs associated with hypoglycemia. It can also cause hypoglycemia or hyperglycemia and, therefore, should be used cautiously in labile diabetic patients. In humans, atenolol use should be avoided in patients with untreated pheochromocytoma, and this is most likely applicable for veterinary patients as well.

Atenolol can mask the clinical signs (eg, tachycardia, hypertension) associated with thyrotoxicosis.

Genetic variants in the canine adrenoreceptor-1 (*ADRB1*) gene have been identified in dogs, and dogs with the polymorphism had lower heart rates both at baseline and while receiving atenolol than unaffected dogs.[11]

Exacerbation of signs has been reported following abrupt cessation of beta-blockers in humans. It is recommended to withdraw therapy gradually when patients have been receiving this drug chronically.

Adverse Effects

Adverse effects most commonly occur in geriatric animals or those that have acute decompensating heart disease. Adverse effects that are considered to be clinically relevant include bradycardia, inappetence, lethargy and depression, impaired AV conduction, CHF or worsening of heart failure, hypotension, hypoglycemia, and bronchoconstriction (less so with beta-1-specific drugs [eg, atenolol]). Syncope and diarrhea have also been reported in dogs with beta-blockers. Lethargy and hypotension may be noted within 1 hour of administration.

In a case report, atenolol therapy was suggested to have exacerbated keratoconjunctivitis sicca in a dog.[12]

Reproductive/Nursing Safety

Atenolol crosses the placenta, and maternal and fetal serum concentrations are similar. Use during pregnancy does not appear to cause fetal structural anomalies in laboratory animals, but embryotoxicity and fetotoxicity have been noted in animals given 50 mg/kg/day. Fetal growth restriction has been observed in humans and animals, and in humans is correlated with length of atenolol use. Atenolol use during the antenatal period may result in beta blockade (eg, hypoglycemia, bradycardia) in newborns.[13]

Atenolol is excreted into, and accumulates in, human breast milk, reaching concentrations significantly greater than in human plasma. Due to the possibility of beta blockade in nursing animals, consider use of milk replacer.[13]

Overdose/Acute Toxicity

In dogs, clinical signs associated with overdose include bradycardia or tachycardia, lethargy, vomiting, and hypotension. Clinical signs in cats include hypo- or hypertension, bradycardia or tachycardia, lethargy, and vomiting.

Humans have apparently survived doses up to 5 g.[7] Clinical signs in humans are extensions of the drug's pharmacologic effects (eg, hypotension, bradycardia, bronchospasm, cardiac failure, hypoglycemia, hyperkalemia).

If overdose is from a recent oral ingestion, GI decontamination, including charcoal administration, may be considered. Monitor ECG, blood glucose, potassium, and blood pressure. For adverse cardiovascular effects, treatment is based on clinical signs. Use fluids and pressor agents (ie, dopamine or norepinephrine) to treat hypotension. Bradycardia may be treated with atropine. If atropine fails, isoproterenol given cautiously has been recommended. Insulin and dextrose may be needed for treatment of hyperkalemia and hypoglycemia. Use of a temporary artificial pacemaker may be necessary. Cardiac failure can be treated with pimobendan, diuretics, and oxygen. Glucagon may increase heart rate and blood pressure and reduce the cardiodepressant effects of atenolol.

For patients that have experienced or are suspected to have experienced an overdose, it is strongly encouraged to consult with a 24-hour poison consultation center that specializes in providing information specific for veterinary patients. For general information related to overdose and toxin exposures, as well as contact information for poison control centers, refer to *Appendix*.

Drug Interactions

The following drug interactions have either been reported or are theoretical in humans or animals receiving atenolol and may be of significance in veterinary patients. Unless otherwise noted, use together is not necessarily contraindicated, but weigh the potential risks and perform additional monitoring when appropriate.

- ALPHA-1 ADRENERGIC ANTAGONISTS (eg, **prazosin, tamsulosin**): Increased risk for hypotension
- AMIODARONE: Increased risk for bradycardia, hypotension, and cardiac arrest
- AMPICILLIN: May decrease atenolol bioavailability
- ANESTHETICS (**myocardial depressant agents**; eg, **halothane**): Additive myocardial depression may occur with the concurrent use of atenolol and myocardial depressant anesthetic agents. Reduction in dose or avoidance the day of anesthesia has been advised.
- ANTACIDS, ALUMINUM-, CALCIUM-, OR MAGNESIUM-CONTAINING: Can reduce oral absorption of atenolol; separate oral doses by 2 hours if possible.
- ANTIDIABETIC AGENTS (eg, **acarbose, chlorpropamide, insulin, sulfonylureas** [eg, **glipizide, glyburide**]): Beta-blockers can alter blood glucose levels and/or mask signs of hypoglycemia.
- BETA-2 ADRENERGIC AGONISTS (eg, **albuterol, terbutaline**): At higher doses, atenolol may impair bronchodilation.
- BETHANECHOL: Concurrent administration may increase the risk for adverse effects of bethanechol, including cardiac conduction abnormalities and bronchoconstriction.
- BROMOCRIPTINE: Atenolol may enhance the vasoconstriction of ergot alkaloids causing hypertension and peripheral ischemia.
- BUPIVACAINE: May increase bupivacaine concentration
- BUSPIRONE: Concurrent use may increase the risk for hypotension and orthostasis.
- DIAZEPAM: Concurrent use may increase the risk for hypotension and orthostasis.
- DIAZOXIDE: Concurrent use may increase the risk for hypotension and orthostasis.
- DIPHENHYDRAMINE: Concurrent use may increase the risk for hypotension and orthostasis.
- DOXEPIN: Concurrent use may increase the risk for hypotension and orthostasis.
- CABERGOLINE: Concurrent use may enhance vasoconstriction effects of cabergoline.
- CALCIUM-CHANNEL BLOCKERS (eg, **amlodipine, diltiazem, verapamil**): Concurrent use may increase the risk for hypotension and bradycardia.
- CLONIDINE: Atenolol may exacerbate rebound hypertension after clonidine therapy is stopped. Risk for AV block may be increased.
- CORTICOSTEROIDS (eg, **dexamethasone, prednis(ol)one**): May interfere with the effects of atenolol by causing sodium and fluid retention
- DIGOXIN: Potential for increased bradycardia and/or digitalis toxicity. If used together, digoxin levels, heart rate, and blood pressure should be closely monitored.
- DISOPYRAMIDE: Increased adverse effects (eg, severe bradycardia, asystole, heart failure) of disopyramide may occur. If possible, avoid combination, or monitor closely if both must be used.
- DIURETICS, LOOP (eg, **furosemide**): Concurrent use may increase the risk for hyperglycemia and hypertriglyceridemia.
- DOBUTAMINE: Concurrent use may lead to increased peripheral resistance, increasing the risk for hypertension.
- DOLASETRON: Concurrent use may lead to PR and/or QRS interval prolongation, increasing the risk for bradycardia and heart block.
- DOPAMINE: Concurrent use may lead to increased peripheral resistance, increasing the risk for hypertension.
- GLUCAGON: Atenolol may inhibit the hyperglycemic effects of glucagon.

- **Hypotensive Agents** (eg, **enalapril, hydralazine, nitroprusside, sildenafil, telmisartan**): Concurrent use may increase the risk for hypotension.
- **Lidocaine:** May increase lidocaine concentration
- **Methimazole/Carbimazole:** Ability to alter the pharmacokinetics of atenolol
- **NSAIDs** (eg, **carprofen, meloxicam, robenacoxib**): Potential for reduced hypotensive effects
- **Opioid, Partial Agonists** (eg, buprenorphine, butorphanol): Concurrent use may increase the risk for hypotension and orthostasis.
- **Phenothiazines** (eg, **acepromazine, chlorpromazine**): May exhibit enhanced hypotensive effects
- **Reserpine:** Potential for additive effects (eg, hypotension, bradycardia)
- **Sympathomimetics** (eg, **albuterol, beta-effects of epinephrine, clenbuterol, metaproterenol, phenylpropanolamine, terbutaline**): May have their actions blocked by atenolol and may, in turn, reduce the efficacy of atenolol
- **Warfarin:** Mild prolongation of prothrombin time is possible.
- **Yohimbine:** May reduce atenolol efficacy

Dosages

DOGS:

Beta-blockade indications (eg, **tachyarrhythmias, obstructive heart disease)** (extra-label): 0.25 – 1.5 mg/kg PO every 12 hours.[14,15] Practically 6.25 mg (1/4 of a 25 mg tablet) to 50 mg per dog twice daily. Dosage is often started on the low end and titrated upward with atrial fibrillation or left ventricular systolic dysfunction; the high end of the dosing range is used for subvalvular aortic stenosis or pulmonary valve stenosis.

Arrhythmogenic right ventricular cardiomyopathy (also known as boxer cardiomyopathy) (extra-label): Atenolol 0.3 – 0.6 mg/kg PO every 12 hours in combination with mexiletine 5 – 8 mg/kg PO every 8 hours[5]

CATS:

Beta-blockade indications (eg, hypertrophic cardiomyopathy, tachycardia due to hyperthyroidism, hypertension [usually in combination with other drugs]; extra-label):

a. Initially, 6.25 mg/cat (NOT mg/kg) (ie, ¼ of a 25 mg tablet) PO every 12 hours. Dosage may be titrated upward (eg, 12.5 mg in the morning and 6.25 mg in the evening)[3,16,17]
b. **Tachycardia due to hyperthyroidism** 1 – 2 mg/kg PO every 12 hours[1]
c. **Dosage adjustment based on IRIS CKD staging**[10]:
   IRIS stage II: 0.19 mg/kg PO every 12 to 24 hours
   IRIS stage III: 0.125 mg/kg PO every 12 to 24 hours
   IRIS stage IV: 0.06 mg/kg PO every 24 hours

FERRETS:

Left ventricular hypertrophy (extra-label):

a) 6.25 mg/ferret (NOT mg/kg) PO once daily[18]
b) 3.125 – 6.25 mg/ferret (NOT mg/kg) PO once daily[19,20] (⅛ to ¼ of a 25 mg tablet)

Monitoring

- Heart rate, pulse quality
- ECG
- Blood pressure
- Cardiac function (ie, echocardiography)
- Baseline and periodic renal panel with electrolytes
- Adverse effects

Client Information

- To be effective, the animal must receive all doses as prescribed.
- Notify your veterinarian if your animal becomes lethargic or exercise intolerant, develops shortness of breath or a cough, or develops a change in behavior or attitude.
- Do not stop therapy without first discussing with your veterinarian.
- While on this medication, your animal will need to be monitored periodically with blood tests and special heart testing. Do not miss these important follow-up visits.

Chemistry/Synonyms

Atenolol, a beta-1-adrenergic blocking agent, occurs as a white, crystalline powder. At 37°C (98.6°F), 26.5 mg is soluble in 1 mL of water. The pH of the commercially available injection is adjusted to 5.5 to 6.5.

Atenolol may also be known as atenololum or ICI-66082; many trade names are available.

Storage/Stability

Tablets should be stored at room temperature of 20°C to 25°C (68°F-77°F) and protected from heat, light, and moisture.

Compatibility/Compounding Considerations

Atenolol tablets may be crushed or split/cut into quarters or halves for appropriate dosing.

Compounded preparation/stability:

1) Atenolol oral suspensions should be compounded with sugar-free vehicles. Atenolol oral suspension compounded from either active pharmaceutical ingredients (API) or commercially available tablets has been published.[21] Triturating an appropriate amount of API or tablets with equal volumes of *Ora-Plus®* and *Ora-Sweet® SF* yields a 2 mg/mL oral suspension that retains more than 90% potency for 90 days stored at both 5°C (41°F) and 25°C (77°F). This investigation also reveals that the presence of sugars (*Ora-Sweet®* and simple syrup) reduces the potency of compounded atenolol suspensions to less than 90% in 7 to 14 days after compounding. Atenolol preparations are most stable at pH 4. Atenolol should be stored protected from light, as exposure to ultraviolet light results in drug decomposition at all pH ranges.
2) Atenolol suspension (flavored) 25 mg/mL. In a study, 150 mL batches were prepared by adding atenolol powder (3.75 g), PEG 4500 (51 g), processed beef and pork flavor powder (15 g), sodium saccharin (1.8 g), and 50 mL of distilled water then vigorously shaken.[22] Distilled water was added to volume (150 mL), shaken again, and stored in the refrigerator. Stability is still to be established, but pharmacokinetics in cats were comparable to tablets.

Dosage Forms/Regulatory Status

VETERINARY-LABELED PRODUCTS: NONE

The Association of Racing Commissioners International (ARCI) has designated this drug as a class 3 substance. See *Appendix* for more information. Use of this drug may not be allowed in certain animal competitions. Check rules and regulations before entering in a competition while this medication is being administered. Contact local racing authorities for further guidance.

HUMAN-LABELED PRODUCTS:

Atenolol Oral Tablets: 25 mg, 50 mg, and 100 mg; *Tenormin®*, generic; (Rx). Atenolol oral solution (5 mg/mL) may be available in some countries.

References

For the complete list of references, see **wiley.com/go/budde/plumb**

Atipamezole

(at-i-***pam***-a-zole) *Antisedan®, Revertidine®*

Alpha-2-Adrenergic Antagonist

Prescriber Highlights

- ▶ Reversal agent for alpha-2-adrenergic agonists (eg, dexmedetomidine, medetomidine, xylazine)
- ▶ Effects of atipamezole may subside before nontoxic concentrations of the offending agent are reached; repeat dosing may be necessary
- ▶ May reverse effects rapidly, including analgesia; animals should be observed and protected from self-harm or causing harm to others. When appropriate, alternative analgesia (non- alpha-2-adrenergic agonists) is recommended prior to atipamezole administration.
- ▶ Adverse effects may include vomiting, diarrhea, hypersalivation, tremors, or excitation.
- ▶ No safety data are available for use of this drug in pregnant or lactating animals.

Uses/Indications

Atipamezole is labeled for use in dogs as a reversal agent for dexmedetomidine and medetomidine. It is also used for reversal of other alpha-2-adrenergic agonists (eg, amitraz, detomidine, xylazine) in a wide range of species.

Pharmacology/Actions

Atipamezole competitively inhibits alpha-2-adrenergic receptors, thereby acting as a reversal agent for alpha-2-adrenergic agonists (eg, dexmedetomidine, medetomidine). Atipamezole reduces sedation, decreases blood pressure, increases heart and respiratory rates, and reduces the analgesic effects of alpha-2-adrenergic agonists. Atipamezole antagonizes the diuretic action of xylazine in dogs[1] and decreases medetomidine-induced tear production in cats 15 minutes after administration.[2] Atipamezole does not completely reverse the sedative and bradycardic effects in horses when administered 1 hour after sublingual detomidine gel.[3]

Pharmacokinetics

In dogs, peak plasma concentration occurs within ≈10 minutes after IM administration. Atipamezole is metabolized in the liver to compounds that are eliminated in the urine. Average plasma elimination half-life is ≈2 to 3 hours.

In horses, atipamezole has an average clearance and elimination half-life of 25 mL/kg/min and 53 minutes, respectively, after sublingual administration of detomidine gel.[3]

Contraindications/Precautions/Warnings

Atipamezole is contraindicated in patients hypersensitive to it.

Because reversal can occur rapidly, care should be exercised, as animals emerging from sedation and analgesia may exhibit apprehensive or aggressive behaviors. After reversal, animals should be protected from falling. Additional analgesia with a non-alpha-2-adrenergic agonist (eg, opioids) should be considered, especially after painful procedures.

When used as a reversal agent or as an antidote for alpha-2-agonist toxicity, effects of atipamezole may subside before nontoxic concentrations of the offending agent are reached; repeat dosing may be necessary.

Adverse Effects

Potential adverse effects include occasional vomiting, diarrhea, hypersalivation, tremors, and brief excitation or apprehensiveness. Transient fluctuations in blood pressure (ie, hypotension followed by hypertension) and increased respiratory rate may occur. Severe arterial hypotension has been noted in cats.[4]

In reptiles, IV administration reportedly can cause profound hypotension.[5,6]

Reproductive/Nursing Safety

The manufacturer states that atipamezole is not recommended in pregnant or lactating animals or in animals intended for breeding due to lack of data establishing safety in these animals.[7]

Because safety has not been established in animals, atipamezole should only be used when the maternal benefits outweigh the potential risks to offspring.

Overdose/Acute Toxicity

Dogs receiving up to 10 times the labeled dosage exhibited panting, excitement, trembling, vomiting, soft or liquid feces, vasodilation of sclera, and some muscle injury at the IM injection site. Increased serum ALT and creatine kinase activity may occur. Specific overdose therapy is generally not necessary.

Drug Interactions

The following drug interactions have either been reported or are theoretical in humans or animals receiving atipamezole and may be of significance in veterinary patients. Unless otherwise noted, use together is not necessarily contraindicated, but weigh the potential risks and perform additional monitoring when appropriate.

- ALPHA-2-ADRENERGIC AGONISTS (eg, **amitraz, brimonidine, clonidine, detomidine, xylazine**). Atipamezole reduces the effects (toxic or therapeutic) of these agents by competing for alpha-2-adrenergic receptors. **NOTE**: This action is an expected outcome when atipamezole is used as a reversal agent.
- ALPHA-1-ADRENERGIC ANTAGONISTS (eg, **prazosin**): Atipamezole is a relatively specific alpha-2 blocker, but it can also partially block alpha-1 receptors, especially at high dosages, and reduce the effects of prazosin.

Dosages

DOGS:

Reversal of dexmedetomidine or medetomidine (label dosage; FDA-approved): 3750 μg/m² (NOT μg/kg) IM to reverse IV dexmedetomidine or medetomidine, and 5000 μg/m² (NOT μg/kg) IM to reverse IM dexmedetomidine or medetomidine. The product label provides dose tables in μg/kg and mL based on body weight.[7]

Reversal of dexmedetomidine or medetomidine (extra-label): 100 μg/kg IV or IO (intraosseous) as part of CPR to reverse alpha-2 agonists. Dosage is based on dexmedetomidine 10 μg/kg. If a higher dose of dexmedetomidine was administered, increase this dose accordingly.[8]

Reversal of oral transmucosal alpha-2-adrenergic agonists (extra-label):

1. Under experimental conditions, atipamezole 100 μg/kg IM administered 150 minutes after administration of detomidine buccal gel reversed detomidine effects in ≈6 to 9 minutes.[9]
2. From case reports in 2 dogs, atipamezole doses of 0.16 mg/kg IM or 0.04 mg/kg IM successfully reversed the effects of transmucosally-administered dexmedetomidine injection solution.[10]

Amitraz toxicity (extra-label): 50 μg/kg IM; dose may need to be repeated every 4 to 6 hours, as the half-life of amitraz is longer than atipamezole in dogs.[11]

CATS:

Reversal of medetomidine, when used alone or in combination with other sedatives or analgesics (extra-label): Administer a volume of atipamezole IM equal to the administered volume of medetomidine.[12]

Reversal of dexmedetomidine or medetomidine (extra-label): 100 µg/kg IV or IO as part of CPR to reverse alpha-2 agonists. Dosage is based on a 10 µg/kg dexmedetomidine dosage. If a higher dose of dexmedetomidine was administered, increase this dose accordingly.[8] For example, atipamezole 125 µg/kg IM was used in cats receiving dexmedetomidine 25 µg/kg as part of a multimodal analgesic protocol,[13] and 200 µg/kg IM followed 80 µg/kg medetomidine administration.[14]

Reversal of dexmedetomidine constant rate infusion (extra-label): 15 – 30 µg/kg IM, given upon discontinuation of dexmedetomidine CRI.[15]

Reversal of xylazine when used as an emetic (extra-label): 25 – 50 µg/kg IM or IV (slowly)[16]

HORSES:

Reversal of alpha-2-adrenergic agonist (eg, amitraz, xylazine) toxicity (extra-label): 0.1 mg/kg IV has been suggested.[17]

Reversal of dexmedetomidine-containing total IV anesthesia in foals (extra-label): 50 µg/kg IM if recovery was prolonged without return of swallow reflex, with 30 minutes of sternal recumbency within 60 minutes[18]

CATTLE:

NOTE: As a rule of thumb, if induction included ketamine or tiletamine/zolazepam, do not reverse alpha-2-adrenergic agonist sooner than 30 minutes, ideally 60 minutes, after induction. This timeframe will allow enough ketamine or tiletamine to be metabolized.

Reversal of alpha-2-adrenergic agonists (eg, detomidine, xylazine; extra-label):

1. 0.02 – 0.1 mg/kg IV to effect[19]
2. 0.02 – 0.06 mg/kg IV; average dose 0.03 mg/kg.[20] Cattle were immobilized with detomidine and tiletamine-zolazepam; average atipamezole administration was ≈20 minutes after anesthetic combination, and time to standing was ≈13 minutes after atipamezole administration.

Reversal of medetomidine sedation in cattle (adults and calves; extra-label): 0.1 mg/kg IV[21] or 0.2 mg/kg IV[22]

Reversal of xylazine immobilization or sedation in bovine calves (extra-label):

1. 0.03 mg/kg IV.[21,23] Lateral recumbency occurred ≈10 minutes after atipamezole administration.[23]
2. IM atipamezole dose at ¼ the xylazine dose; IV atipamezole 1/5 or 1/8- times the xylazine doses[24]

Reversal of detomidine epidural in bovine calves (extra-label): 0.05 mg/kg IV[25]

SHEEP/GOATS:

NOTE: As a rule of thumb, if induction included ketamine or tiletamine/zolazepam, do not reverse alpha-2-adrenergic agonist sooner than 30 minutes, ideally 60 minutes, after induction. This timeframe will allow enough ketamine or tiletamine to be metabolized.

Reversal of alpha-2-adrenergic agonists (eg, **detomidine, xylazine**; extra-label):

1. 0.02 – 0.1 mg/kg IV to effect[19]
2. 0.1 – 0.2 mg/kg IM or slow IV[26,27]

Reversal of medetomidine in sheep and goats: 0.2 mg/kg IV[22,28,30]

CAMELIDS:

NOTE: As a rule of thumb, if induction included ketamine or tiletamine/zolazepam, do not reverse alpha-2-adrenergic agonist sooner than 30 minutes, ideally 60 minutes, after induction. This timeframe will allow enough ketamine or tiletamine to be metabolized.

Reversal of alpha-2-adrenergic agonists (eg, **detomidine, xylazine**; extra-label):

1. 0.02 – 0.1 mg/kg IV to effect[19]
2. 0.1 – 0.2 mg/kg IM or slow IV[26,27]

Reversal of medetomidine in llamas: 0.125 mg/kg IV[31]

BIRDS:

Reversal agent for alpha-2-adrenergic agonists (eg, xylazine, dexmedetomidine; extra-label):

1. 0.5 mg/kg IM[32]
2. 250 µg/kg intranasally has been reported in pigeons. Antagonism of adverse cardiorespiratory and sedative effects, but not complete recovery, was observed within 10 minutes of atipamezole administration.[33]

RABBITS/RODENTS/SMALL MAMMALS:

Rabbits: reversal of medetomidine (extra-label): 0.5 mg/kg IM or SC; 0.25 mg/kg IV.[34] Alternatively, 0.75 mg/kg IV or IM[35]

Mice, Rats, Chinchillas, Gerbils, Hamsters, Guinea pigs: reversal of xylazine or medetomidine (extra-label): 0.1 – 1 mg/kg IM, IP, IV, or SC[36,37]

REPTILES:

NOTE: Reversal in reptiles may take longer (up to 1 hour) than in other species. Do **NOT** give IV as profound hypotension can occur.[5]

Reversal agent for alpha-2-adrenergic agonists (extra-label):

1. **Ball pythons** (extra label): 0.5 mg/kg SC[38]
2. **American alligators** (extra label): Adults 0.7 mg/kg IM, juveniles 1.2 mg/kg IM; administer in either masseter (jaw), or in triceps muscle in the front leg opposite that used to administer medetomidine.[39]
3. **Leopard geckos** (extra label): 1 mg/kg SC[40]
4. **Western Santa Cruz tortoises** (extra label): 0.5 mg/kg IM[41]
5. **Chinese box turtles** (extra label): 0.5 mg/kg IM administered in the right pectoralis major[42]

Monitoring

- Level of sedation and analgesia
- Heart rate and blood pressure
- Body temperature

Client Information

- Atipamezole should be administered by veterinary professionals only.
- Vomiting, diarrhea, hypersalivation, excitation, and tremors may occasionally be seen.
- If side effects are severe or persist after leaving the veterinary hospital, contact your veterinarian.

Chemistry/Synonyms

Atipamezole is an imidazole alpha-2-adrenergic antagonist. The injection is a clear, colorless solution.

Atipamezole HCl may also be known as MPV-1248 or *Antisedan®*, *Revertidine®*.

Storage/Stability

Atipamezole HCl injection should be stored at room temperature of 15°C to 30°C (59°F-86°F) and protected from light. Use within 90 days of first vial puncture.

Compatibility/Compounding Considerations

No specific information noted

Dosage Forms/Regulatory Status

VETERINARY-LABELED PRODUCTS:

Atipamezole HCl for Injection: 5 mg/mL in 10 mL multidose vials; *Antisedan®*, *Revertidine®*; (Rx). FDA-approved for use in dogs.

HUMAN-LABELED PRODUCTS: NONE

References

For the complete list of references, see **wiley.com/go/budde/plumb**

Atovaquone

(ah-*toe*-va-kwone) *Mepron®*

Oral Antiprotozoal Agent

Prescriber Highlights

- Atovaquone in combination with azithromycin appears effective in treating dogs with *Babesia gibsoni* infections and in cats for treating cytauxzoonosis. Alone, atovaquone is a second-line agent (after potentiated sulfonamides) for pneumocystosis in dogs.
- Limited use thus far; appears well tolerated by dogs and cats

Uses/Indications

Atovaquone, as a single agent, may be of benefit for treating pneumocystosis in dogs, but it is considered second-line therapy after potentiated sulfonamides.

Atovaquone in combination with azithromycin appears effective in treating dogs with *Babesia gibsoni* (Asian genotype) infections, particularly in dogs not immunosuppressed or splenectomized. A prospective, unmasked study in dogs comparing atovaquone in combination with azithromycin (AA) with a protocol using clindamycin, diminazene, and imidocarb (CDI) found that CDI had higher recovery and lower relapse rates, albeit longer therapy duration and slower reduction in parasite numbers than AA. The authors concluded that CDI was effective for initial therapy and when the M121I gene in *B gibsoni* had mutated.[1] Atovaquone with proguanil (combination product *Malarone®*), alone or in combination with doxycycline, also has demonstrated efficacy in dogs with *Babesia gibsoni* (Asian genotype) infections.[2] Dogs infected with *Babesia conradae* were PCR negative for infection after receiving atovaquone in combination with azithromycin[3,4]; this combination was also effective for treating dogs with piroplasmosis caused by *B vulpes* (also known as *B microti*-like piroplasm and *Theileria annae*).[5]

Atovaquone in combination with azithromycin is recommended for treatment of *Cytauxzoon felis* infections in cats.[6,7]

Pharmacology/Actions

Atovaquone's antiprotozoal mechanism of action is not completely understood. It is believed that the hydroxynaphthoquinones, like atovaquone, target protozoal cytochrome b (cytb) which selectively inhibits protozoan mitochondrial electron transport and causes inhibition of *de novo* pyrimidine synthesis. Unlike mammalian cells, certain protozoa cannot salvage preformed pyrimidines. Mutations in the *Babesia gibsoni* cytochrome b gene (M121I, M128I, or M128V) confer atovaquone resistance by affecting the drug's site of action.[1,8,9] Atovaquone treatment for *B gibsoni* in dogs may reduce recurrent parasite susceptibility to the drug.[10,11]

Cytauxzoon felis genotype *cytb1* may predict response to treatment with azithromycin and atovaquone combination[12]; however, resistance to atovaquone may occur during treatment.[13]

Atovaquone is not effective against viral, fungal, or bacterial infections.

Pharmacokinetics

Pharmacokinetic data for dogs or cats were not located. In humans after oral administration, bioavailability ranges from 23% to 47%. The presence of food, particularly high in fat, can increase bioavailability significantly (2+ fold over fasted administration). The drug is highly bound to human plasma proteins (99.9%) and concentrations in the CSF are approximately 1% of those found in plasma.

Elimination half-life in people is about 70 hours presumably due to enterohepatic recycling. There may be limited hepatic metabolism, but the bulk of absorbed drug is eventually eliminated unchanged in the feces.

Contraindications/Precautions/Warnings

No absolute contraindications for using atovaquone in dogs or cats have been documented. Animals with malabsorption syndromes or that cannot take the drug with food should have alternate therapies considered.

The drug is contraindicated in human patients that develop or have a prior history of hypersensitivity reactions to the drug.[14]

Adverse Effects

Atovaquone use in dogs and cats has been limited and the adverse effect profile is not well known. One study[15] using atovaquone in combination with azithromycin for treating *Babesia gibsoni* infections in 10 dogs reported that no adverse effects were noted. The combination product containing atovaquone and proguanil (*Malarone®*) may cause vomiting in dogs.[2]

In humans treated with atovaquone, rashes (up to 39% of treated patients) and gastrointestinal effects (nausea, vomiting, diarrhea) are the most frequently reported adverse effects.[14] Rashes or diarrhea may necessitate discontinuation of therapy. Other adverse effects reported in humans include hypersensitivity reactions, increased liver enzymes, CNS effects (headache, dizziness, insomnia), hyperglycemia, hyponatremia, fever, neutropenia, and anemia.

Reproductive/Nursing Safety

Studies in pregnant rats with atovaquone plasma concentrations approximately 2 to 3 times those found in humans receiving therapeutic dosages revealed no increase in teratogenicity.[14] Similar studies in rabbits showed increased maternal and fetal toxicity (decreased fetal growth and increased early fetal resorption).[14]

Little information is available on the safety of this drug during lactation. In rats, milk levels were approximately ⅓ those found in maternal plasma.[14] It is unlikely atovaquone in milk poses much risk to nursing animals.

Because safety has not been established in animals, this drug should only be used when the maternal benefits outweigh the potential risks to offspring.

Overdose/Acute Toxicity

Limited information is available for any species. Minimum toxic doses have not been established; laboratory animals have tolerated doses up to 31.5 grams. The current recommendation for treating overdoses is supportive, based on clinical signs.

For patients that have experienced or are suspected to have experienced an overdose, consultation with a 24-hour poison consultation center specializing in providing veterinary-specific information is recommended. For general information related to overdose and toxin exposures, as well as contact information for poison control centers, refer to ***Appendix***.

Drug Interactions

The following drug interactions with atovaquone either have been reported or are theoretical in humans or animals and may be of significance in veterinary patients. Unless otherwise noted, use together is not necessarily contraindicated, but weigh the potential risks and perform additional monitoring when appropriate.

- **Highly Protein-Bound Drugs** (eg, **azole antifungals, furosemide, NSAIDs**): Because atovaquone is highly bound to plasma proteins (99.9%), it could theoretically displace other highly bound drugs, causing a transient increase in serum levels of each drug. These interactions are unlikely to be of clinical concern because increased free drug concentrations will equilibrate through increased clearance. Monitor for adverse effects of each drug when using this combination.

- **Metoclopramide**: Can decrease atovaquone plasma concentrations; use together only when no other options are available[14]
- **Rifampin**: Can decrease atovaquone plasma concentrations; concomitant use with atovaquone is not recommended[14]
- **Tetracycline**: Can decrease atovaquone plasma concentrations[14]

Laboratory Considerations

- None

Doses

DOGS:

Babesia gibsoni **(Asian genotype),** ***B conradae*****, or** ***B microti-like*** **(also known as** ***Theileria annae*** **or** ***B vulpes*****) infections** (extra-label): Atovaquone 13.3 mg/kg PO every 8 hours with a fatty meal in combination with azithromycin 10 mg/kg PO every 24 hours for 10 days. Reserve immunosuppressive therapy for cases that do not respond within 3 to 5 days.[1,8,15-18] Single-agent treatment with atovaquone 30 mg/kg PO twice daily for 7 days cleared parasites within 2 days, but parasites re-appeared on blood smears 33 days after the last treatment.[10]

Babesia gibsoni **(Asian genotype) infections** (extra-label): Using atovaquone with proguanil (combination tablet, *Malarone*®), atovaquone 17 – 25 mg/kg PO and proguanil 7 – 10 mg/kg PO every 12 hours with a fatty meal for 10 days with or without doxycycline 5 mg/kg PO every 12 hours for 30 days[2]

Pneumocystosis (extra-label): 15 mg/kg PO every 24 hours for 3 weeks[19]

CATS:

Cytauxzoonosis| ***Cytauxzoon felis*** (extra-label): Atovaquone 15 mg/kg PO every 8 hours in combination with azithromycin 10 mg/kg PO once daily (every 24 hours) for 10 days. All cases were also treated with IV fluids and most received heparin.[6,7] Consider placing a feeding tube to reduce the stress of administering these oral medications and ensure food intake to maximize antimicrobial absorption.

Monitoring

- Monitoring for therapy for *Babesia gibsoni* in dogs should include surveillance for potential adverse effects and signs for clinical efficacy.
- Baseline and periodic CBCs

Client Information

- Store medication at room temperature and away from bright light.
- Before using, shake bottle gently. This medicine may come as a thick suspension that can make measurement difficult. After drawing the medicine into the syringe, allow the medicine to settle into the syringe to remove air bubbles and ensure the full amount has been measured.
- To increase absorption from the gastrointestinal tract, give with food high in fat (eg, ice cream, tuna oil, butter, meat fat).
- If your veterinarian has placed a feeding tube in your animal to help with feeding and medication delivery, be sure you understand how to care for it.
- Side effects in dogs and cats for this medication are not well known. Report any significant effects such as rash, or severe or persistent vomiting or diarrhea, to your veterinarian.

Chemistry/Synonyms

Atovaquone is a synthetic, hydroxy-1,4-naphthoquinone antiprotozoal agent. It occurs as a yellow powder that is highly lipid soluble, insoluble in water and slightly soluble in alcohol.

Atovaquone may also be known as BW-556C, Atovacuona, Atovakvon, Atovakvoni, Atovaquonnum, *Malanil*®, *Mepron*®, or *Wellvone*®.

Storage/Stability

The commercially available oral suspension should be stored in a tight container at room temperature (15°C-25°C [59°F-77°F]) in tight containers and protected from bright light; do not freeze.

Compatibility/Compounding Considerations

In one study, 39 of 42 dogs in a shelter facility responded to treatment with compounded atovaquone capsules.[17]

Dosage Forms/Regulatory Status

VETERINARY-LABELED PRODUCTS: NONE.

HUMAN-LABELED PRODUCTS:

Atovaquone Oral Suspension: 150 mg/mL (750 mg/5mL) in 210 mL bottles and in 5 mL and 10 mL unit-dose containers; citrus flavor; *Mepron*®; (Rx)

A combination tablet product containing atovaquone and proguanil HCl is available that has labeled indications (human) for malaria prophylaxis and treatment. It is available in two formulations, atovaquone 62.5 mg with proguanil 25 mg (*Malarone Pediatric*®) and atovaquone 250 mg with proguanil 100 mg (*Malarone*®).

References

For the complete list of references, see **wiley.com/go/budde/plumb**

Atracurium

(a-tra-***cure***-ee-um) *Tracrium*®

Nondepolarizing Neuromuscular Blocker

Prescriber Highlights

- Nondepolarizing neuromuscular blocking agent with minimal cardiovascular effects. It is valuable in patients under general anesthesia for which complete muscle relaxation is desired.
- Intraurethral administration of atracurium may assist patients with upper motor neuron urinary bladder signs and assist with urethral plug removal in male cats.
- Should not be given as a sole agent. It does *not* provide analgesia or sedation. Administer after general anesthesia has been induced.
- Reversal agents should be readily available when atracurium is used; effects can be reversed with cholinesterase inhibitors (eg, neostigmine, pyridostigmine).
- Administration of atracurium requires familiarization with ventilatory support and the monitoring required for safe use and to minimize risk for overdose.
- Store neuromuscular blockers segregated from other medications and with prominent warnings to mitigate the risk of inadvertent use

Uses/Indications

Atracurium is indicated as an adjunct to inhalant or IV general anesthesia to produce complete muscle relaxation during surgical procedures or mechanical ventilation and to facilitate endotracheal intubation. Atracurium is also used to aid in central bulbus positioning during ophthalmic surgery.

Intraurethral administration of atracurium in male cats with urethral plugs has been shown to increase the proportion (64% vs. 15% control) of obstruction removal.[1] Intraurethral administration also assisted with manual urinary bladder expression in dogs and cats with urine retention secondary to upper motor neuron signs (eg, T3-L3 myelopathy).[2]

Atracurium can be used safely in patients with significant renal or hepatic insufficiency.[3]

Pharmacology/Actions

Atracurium is a nondepolarizing neuromuscular blocking agent; it does not provide any analgesia or sedation.[4] It competitively binds cholinergic receptor sites on the motor end-plate to antagonize acetylcholine, and results in paralysis of striated muscles. Atracurium is considered ¼ to ⅓ as potent as pancuronium.

Neuromuscular blockade (NMB) can be variably potentiated when used with different general anesthetic agents. A study in dogs demonstrated that, when compared with propofol, sevoflurane prolonged atracurium-induced NMB by about 15 minutes.[5]

At recommended doses, atracurium exhibits minimal cardiovascular effects, unlike most nondepolarizing neuromuscular blockers, and will not counteract bradycardia or vagal stimulation induced by other agents. At doses in excess of those used clinically, atracurium can stimulate histamine release. In humans receiving atracurium, less than 1% exhibit clinically significant adverse reactions or histamine release.

Pharmacokinetics

Atracurium has low liposolubility, limiting its ability to cross biological membranes.[6] In humans, maximal neuromuscular blockade generally occurs within 3 to 5 minutes after IV administration.[4] The duration of maximal blockade increases as the dose increases. In conjunction with balanced anesthesia, the duration of blockade generally persists for 20 to 35 minutes.

Systemic alkalosis may diminish the degree and duration of blockade; acidosis may potentiate it. Recovery times do not appreciably change after giving maintenance doses, so predictable neuromuscular blocking effects can be attained when the drug is administered at regular intervals. However, resistance may develop with chronic use.

Atracurium is metabolized by ester hydrolysis and Hofmann elimination that occur independent of renal or hepatic function. Physiologic pH and temperature can affect the elimination of atracurium. Increased body temperature can enhance drug elimination. Ester hydrolysis is enhanced by decreases in pH, while Hofmann elimination is reduced by decreases in pH.

Contraindications/Precautions/Warnings

Atracurium should not be given as a sole agent; it does *not* provide analgesia or sedation.[4] Atracurium should only be administered once general anesthesia has been induced and when endotracheal and ventilatory support and anticholinesterase reversal agents are readily available.[4]

Atracurium is contraindicated in patients that are hypersensitive to it and should be used cautiously in patients with a history of hypersensitivity to other neuromuscular blocking agents due to the risk of cross-sensitivity.[4] Neuromuscular blocking agents must be used with extreme caution in patients suffering from conditions that may potentiate neuromuscular blockade, such as electrolyte abnormalities and myasthenia gravis (MG). Atracurium has been used safely in dogs with MG at 16 to 20% of the recommended dose with close monitoring of neuromuscular transmission throughout the procedure.[7]

Caution is advised in patients where significant histamine release would be hazardous (eg, severe cardiovascular disease, asthma). In anesthetized dogs, partial neuromuscular blockade with atracurium decreases spontaneous ventilation and impairs the response to hypercarbia.[8] Atracurium has also been administered to dogs with centronuclear myopathy without significant adverse effects; however, these dogs required a longer recovery time.[9]

Recurarization has occurred due to residual atracurium in IV ports and fluid lines.[10,11]

Inadvertent administration of neuromuscular blocking agents to patients for which they were not intended may cause significant harm, including death. Neuromuscular blocking agents should be sequestered from other medications, and with access limited to those familiar with their use.[12] Prominent placement of warning labels (eg, "paralyzing agent- causes respiratory arrest," "causes respiratory paralysis; patient must be ventilated") on storage containers is highly recommended.

Adverse Effects

Clinically significant adverse effects are rare (less than 1%) in humans receiving recommended doses of atracurium and are usually secondary to histamine release.[4] They can include allergic reactions, inadequate or prolonged neuromuscular blockade, hypotension (usually manifesting in patients with pre-existing cardiovascular disease), vasodilation, bradycardia, tachycardia, dyspnea, bronchospasm, laryngospasm, rash, urticaria, or a reaction at the injection site. The risk of histamine release can be reduced by decreasing the initial dose or administration over 1 to 2 minutes.

An atracurium metabolite, laudanosine, is a CNS stimulant that may induce seizures.[4] The risk of seizures appears quite low in most patients, but may be increased with prolonged atracurium use or possibly in patients with hepatic impairment (laudanosine is hepatically cleared). In a case series, 3 pediatric dogs that had received atracurium CRI experienced new-onset seizures in the initial 24 hours following extubation.[13]

Infusion of anatracurium 0.5 mg/mL solution into the urinary bladder via sterile catheter appears to deliver sufficient atracurium to cross the urethral mucosa to induce at least partial paralysis of the urethral muscles without causing systemic adverse effects.[2]

Reproductive/Nursing Safety

Atracurium has demonstrated teratogenicity in rabbits at clinically relevant doses.[4] It is unknown if atracurium is excreted in human milk.

Because safety has not been established in animals, this drug should only be used when the maternal benefits outweigh the potential risks to offspring.

Overdose/Acute Toxicity

The IV LD_{50} in non-ventilated male mice, female mice, and rats was 1.9, 2.01, and 1.31 mg/kg, respectively.[4] Deaths occurred within 2 minutes due to respiratory paralysis.

Monitoring muscle twitch responses to peripheral nerve stimulation can minimize overdose risk.[4] Overdose signs can include histamine release (see ***Adverse Effects***), prolonged duration of muscle blockade, and cardiovascular effects (primarily hypotension); death may occur due to respiratory failure. Significant cardiovascular adverse effects in dogs have been reported with inadvertent overdoses.[14]

In addition to maintaining the patient's airway and providing appropriate cardiovascular support (eg, IV fluid administration, vasopressors), reversal of blockade may be accomplished by administering an anticholinesterase agent (eg, neostigmine 0.02 – 0.04 mg/kg IV) in conjunction with an anticholinergic (eg, atropine, glycopyrrolate).[15-18] Reversal is typically complete within 8 to 10 minutes. Because the duration of action of atracurium may be longer than the reversal agent, careful observation and monitoring are required, and re-administration of the reversal agent may be necessary.

For patients that have experienced or are suspected to have experienced an overdose, consultation with a 24-hour poison consultation center specializing in providing veterinary-specific information is recommended. For general information related to overdose and toxin exposures, as well as contact information for poison control centers, refer to ***Appendix***.

Drug Interactions

The following drug interactions with atracurium have either been reported or are theoretical in humans or animals and may be of significance in veterinary patients. Unless otherwise noted, use together is not necessarily contraindicated, but weigh the potential risks and perform additional monitoring when appropriate.

- **Acetylcholinesterase Inhibitors** (eg, **neostigmine, pyridostigmine**): Antagonizes effect of neuromuscular blocking actions of atracurium. This effect can be used advantageously to reverse neuromuscular blockade.

- **Corticosteroids (eg, dexamethasone, prednis(ol)one)**: May enhance unwanted neuromuscular effects of corticosteroids (eg, muscle weakness). Consider therapy modification.
- **Other Muscle Relaxant Drugs** (eg, **alpha-2 agonists [eg, dexmedetomidine, xylazine], diazepam, methocarbamol**): May cause a synergistic or antagonistic effect
- **Phenobarbital:** Concomitant administration may decrease the effects and duration of neuromuscular blockade.
- **Succinylcholine:** May speed the onset of action and enhance the neuromuscular blocking actions of atracurium. Do not give atracurium until succinylcholine effects have diminished.

The following drugs may enhance and/or prolong the neuromuscular blocking activity of atracurium:

- **Aminoglycosides** (eg, **amikacin, gentamicin**[19,20])
- **Amphotericin B**
- **Anesthetics, Inhalant** (eg, **isoflurane,**[21] **sevoflurane**[5])
- **Antiarrhythmic Agents** (eg, **procainamide, quinidine**)
- **Beta Adrenergic Receptor Antagonists** (eg, **atenolol, propranolol**)
- **Calcium Channel Blockers** (eg, **amlodipine, diltiazem**)
- **Cyclosporine** (systemic)
- **Diuretics** (eg, **furosemide, hydrochlorothiazide**)
- **Lincosamide Antibiotics** (eg, **clindamycin**)
- **Lithium:** Competes with sodium and decreases acetylcholine release
- **Magnesium Salts** (parenteral route only)
- **Polymyxin B**
- **Tetracyclines** (eg, **doxycycline, minocycline**)
- **Vancomycin**

Dosages

NOTE: Administration of atracurium requires familiarization with the monitoring required for safe use and to minimize risk for overdose; mechanical ventilation and cardiovascular monitoring are required when administering atracurium.

DOGS:

Muscle relaxation during surgical procedures or endotracheal intubation (extra-label): 0.1 – 0.25 mg/kg IV initially; subsequent doses 0.1 mg/kg IV. Do not dose more frequently than every 20 to 30 minutes in critical patients unless a peripheral nerve stimulator is applied or voluntary movement is observed. Positive pressure ventilation, preferably mechanical, is required.[15,18,22-25]

Induction of respiratory muscle paralysis during mechanical ventilation: Loading dose: 0.2 – 0.5 mg/kg IV, then 5 minutes later, 3 – 9 µg/kg/min IV CRI.[26] Use dextrose 5% or sodium chloride 0.9% for diluent; do not mix with other drugs. Respiratory and cardiovascular monitoring should be provided.

Central positioning of bulbus for ophthalmic surgery: One treatment of 0.2 mg/kg IV under general anesthesia.[27,28] Subsequent doses of atracurium 0.1 mg/kg IV if needed during prolonged surgery. **NOTE:** No obvious mydriatic effect was found.

Urinary retention post-spinal cord lesion: Infuse 2 – 4 mL of atracurium 0.5 mg/mL solution into the urinary bladder via sterile placement of a urinary catheter. The volume administered is 2 mL for dogs weighing less than 10 kg (22 lb), 3 mL for dogs weighing 10 to 20 kg (22 to 44 lb), and 4 mL for dogs weighing over 20 kg (44 lb). The catheter is left in place for 5 minutes following the infusion. The urethral infusion is made using 0.2 mL of 10 mg/mL atracurium diluted in 3.8 mL of 0.9% saline to obtain a final volume of 4 mL with a concentration of 0.5 mg/mL of atracurium.[2]

CATS:

Adjunctive muscle relaxation during IV anesthesia and analgesia (extra-label)**:** 0.1 – 0.25 mg/kg IV initially; subsequent doses 0.1 mg/kg IV. Do not dose more frequently than every 20 to 30 minutes in critical patients unless a peripheral nerve stimulator is applied or voluntary movement is observed. Positive pressure ventilation, preferably mechanical, is required.[23,25,29]

Induction of respiratory muscle paralysis during mechanical ventilation: Loading dose: 0.2 – 0.5 mg/kg IV, then 5 minutes later, 3 – 9 µg/kg/min IV CRI.[26,30] Use dextrose 5% or sodium chloride 0.9% for diluent; do not mix with other drugs. Respiratory and cardiovascular monitoring should be provided.

Removal of urethral plugs in male cats and urinary retention post spinal cord lesion (extra-label): 0.2 mL of 10 mg/mL injection diluted in 3.8 mL of normal saline; final concentration 0.5 mg/mL. Instill 2 mL of this diluted solution via a urinary catheter with steady, gentle pressure over 5 minutes while the urethra is pressed with two fingers to prevent leakage. Retrograde flushing with saline is performed for a maximum of 20 seconds. If the obstruction is not removed with the first attempt, repeat the procedure.[1,2]

RABBITS/RODENTS/SMALL MAMMALS:

Muscle relaxation for periophthalmic surgery in rabbits (extra-label): 0.1 mg/kg IV[31]

HORSES:

Muscle relaxation during surgical procedures (extra-label): 0.07 – 0.2 mg/kg IV.[32-35] Subsequent doses of 0.04 mg/kg IV have been used.[33] Another source reported repeat doses of 10 – 30 mg per horse (NOT mg/kg).[34]

Central positioning of bulbus for ophthalmic surgery (extra-label): 0.1 mg/kg IV under general anesthesia. Relaxation occurred after ≈9 minutes and lasted ≈25-30 minutes.[36,37]

LLAMAS:

Muscle relaxation during surgical procedures (extra-label): 0.15 mg/kg IV; subsequent doses 0.08 mg/kg IV[38]

Central positioning of bulbus for ophthalmic surgery (extra-label): 0.2 mg/kg IV under general anesthesia[39]

SHEEP:

Muscle relaxation during surgical procedures in lambs (extra-label): 0.5 mg/kg IV; subsequent doses 0.17 mg/kg IV[21,40]

Monitoring

- Level of neuromuscular blockade. It is strongly recommended to be familiar with techniques required to monitor the level of neuromuscular blockade (eg, acceleromyography, train of four twitch ratio) when using atracurium.[35] Visual or tactile assessments of the level of blockade are inaccurate and unreliable. Correct placement of electrodes is essential to minimize direct muscle stimulation and prevent misinterpretation of the degree of the blockade and minimize risk for overdose.
- Assess ventilation (eg, arterial blood gas, $ETCO_2$)
- Heart rate and rhythm
- Blood pressure

Labaratory Considerations

- None noted.

Client Information

- Only professionals familiar with the use of atrucurium should use this drug.

Chemistry/Synonyms

Atracurium is a synthetic, nondepolarizing neuromuscular blocking agent. It is a bisquaternary, non-choline diester structurally similar to metocurine and tubocurarine. It occurs as white to pale yellow powder with a pH of 3.25 to 3.65; 50 mg is soluble in 1 mL of water, 200 mg is soluble in 1 mL of alcohol, and 35 mg is soluble in 1 mL of normal saline.

Atracurium besylate may also be known as 33A74, atracurium besilate, BW-33A, *Abbottracurium®*, *Atracur®*, *Faulcurium®*, *Ifacur®*, *Laurak®*, *Mycurium®*, *Relatrac®*, *Sitrac®*, *Trablok®*, *Tracrium®*, or *Tracur®*.

Storage/Stability

The commercially available injection occurs as a clear, colorless solution. Store intact atracurium vials between 2°C to 8°C (36°F to 46°F) and protect against freezing. According to the US prescribing information, once removed from refrigeration to room temperature (25°C [77°F]), use within 14 days is recommended.[4] At room temperature, ≈5% potency loss occurs each month; when refrigerated, a 6% potency loss occurs over a year's time. Dilutions of 0.2 mg/mL or 0.5 mg/mL in sodium chloride 0.9%, dextrose 5% in water, or dextrose 5% in sodium chloride 0.9% are stable for up to 24 hours at room temperature or under refrigeration.[4]

Compatibility/Compounding Considerations

Compatibility is dependent on factors, such as pH, concentration, temperature, and diluent used; specialized references or a hospital pharmacist should be consulted for more specific information.

Compatible with sodium chloride 0.9%, dextrose 5% in water, and dextrose 5% in sodium chloride 0.9% for dilution. **Compatible** in a syringe with alfentanil, fentanyl, midazolam, and sufentanil.

Y-site administration is **incompatible** with propofol, diazepam, and thiopental. Atracurium should not be mixed in the same IV bag or syringe or given through the same needle as alkaline drugs (eg, barbiturates) or solutions (eg, sodium bicarbonate) as precipitation may occur.

Dosage Forms/Regulatory Status

VETERINARY-LABELED PRODUCTS: NONE.

The Association of Racing Commissioners International (ARCI) has designated this drug as a class 2 substance. The use of this drug may not be allowed in some animal competitions. Check rules and regulations before entering a competition while this medication is being administered. Contact local racing authorities for further guidance.

The International Federation for Equestrian Sports (FEI) lists this drug as a prohibited substance - banned.

HUMAN-LABELED PRODUCTS:

Atracurium Besylate Injection: 10 mg/mL in 5 mL single-use and 10 mL multi-use vials; *Tracrium®*, generic; (Rx)

References

For the complete list of references, see **wiley.com/go/budde/plumb**

Atropine

(*a*-troe-peen)

Anticholinergic, Antidote

See also ***Atropine Ophthalmic***

Prescriber Highlights

- Prototype antimuscarinic agent used for a variety of indications (eg, treatment or prevention of bradycardia, anesthetic premedication, antidote for cholinergic agents and toxins)
- Contraindicated when anticholinergic effects would be detrimental (eg, narrow-angle glaucoma, tachycardia, ileus, urinary obstruction, hypertrophic or restrictive cardiomyopathy, isoxazole mushroom toxicity)
- Adverse effects are dose-related and anticholinergic in nature (ie, dry respiratory and gastrointestinal [including oral] secretions, initial bradycardia (occasionally) then tachycardia, slowed GI motility, urine retention, and mydriasis/cycloplegia).
- Many drug interactions

Uses/Indications

The principal veterinary indications for systemic atropine include:

- As a preanesthetic to prevent, or during anesthesia to treat, vagally-mediated bradycardia. Treatment of bradyarrhythmias as they occur is recommended/preferred over indiscriminate use of atropine to prevent arrhythmias because atropine-mediated adverse effects (eg, tachycardia) can be detrimental in some patients (eg, patients with cardiac disease). Anticholinergics are more commonly needed for procedures that increase vagal tone (eg, ophthalmologic procedures and procedures that result in traction of the viscera).
- As a preanesthetic agent to prevent or reduce secretions of the oral/respiratory tract. This use has significantly declined as modern inhalants are unlikely to cause hypersecretion.
- Treatment of sinus bradycardia, sinoatrial arrest, and incomplete atrioventricular (AV) block
- During cardiopulmonary resuscitation
- To differentiate vagally-mediated bradycardia from other causes
- As an antidote for overdoses of cholinergic agents (eg, physostigmine) or to mitigate adverse effects from therapeutic use (eg, prior to an edrophonium test for diagnosing myasthenia gravis, pretreatment for imidocarb diproprionate[1]
- As an antidote for organophosphate, carbamate, muscarinic mushroom, or blue-green algae intoxication
- To reduce secretions that are a result of hypersialosis
- Adjunctive treatment of bronchoconstrictive disease, although atropine use results in greater systemic adverse effects than does N-butylscopolammonium bromide (butylscopolamine)[2]
- In conjunction with anticholinesterases (edrophonium, neostigmine) administered for reversal of drugs used for nondepolarizing neuromuscular blockade (eg, curare derivatives)

Pharmacology/Actions

Atropine, like other antimuscarinic agents, competitively inhibits acetylcholine or other cholinergic stimulants at postganglionic parasympathetic neuroeffector sites. Pharmacologic effects are dose related. Salivation, bronchial secretions, and sweating (not in horses or other species under adrenergic rather than cholinergic control of sweating) are inhibited at low doses. At moderate systemic doses, atropine dilates and inhibits accommodation of the pupil,[3] increases intraocular pressure,[4,5] and increases heart rate (and myocardial oxygen consumption), although heart rate may decrease initially. High doses decrease GI and urinary tract motility, and very high doses inhibit gastric secretion. High doses may also block nicotinic receptors at the autonomic ganglia and at the neuromuscular junction.

In a retrospective study, a positive response to atropine predicted successful medical treatment in dogs with sick sinus syndrome.[6] This is also true for most other vagally-mediated bradyarrhythmias.

Pharmacokinetics

Atropine sulfate is well absorbed after oral administration, IM injection, inhalation, or endotracheal administration.[7] After IV administration, peak effects in heart rates occur within 3 to 4 minutes. The pharmacokinetic profile after intraosseous administration to healthy pigs was comparable to the IV route.[8]

Atropine is well distributed throughout the body and crosses into the CNS and placenta.

Atropine is metabolized in the liver and excreted into the urine. Approximately 30% to 50% of a dose is excreted unchanged into the urine. The plasma half-life in humans has been reported to be between 2 and 3 hours.

As compared with glycopyrrolate, atropine has a faster onset, shorter duration of action, and causes more profound tachycardia. See ***Glycopyrrolate.***

In healthy horses administered topical atropine sulfate 1% ophthalmic solution in 1 eye every 6 hours the first day, then every 12 hours for 4 days, atropine was not detected in serum, and no objective evidence of ileus was noted.[9] A small but significant increase in heart rate was noted in healthy dogs receiving 3 doses of atropine 1% ophthalmic solution in each eye every 6 hours.[10] Gut sounds were reduced by ≈50% in healthy sheep given atropine eye drops.[11]

Contraindications/Precautions/Warnings

Atropine is contraindicated in those hypersensitive to it or other anticholinergic drugs and in those with narrow-angle glaucoma,[4] posterior synechiae, tachycardia secondary to thyrotoxicosis or cardiac insufficiency, myocardial ischemia, hypertrophic or restrictive cardiomyopathy, unstable cardiac status during acute hemorrhage, asthma, and urine retention caused by bladder outlet obstruction (eg, prostatic hyperplasia). Atropine is also contraindicated in the treatment of poisoning with isoxazole mushrooms (eg, *Amanita muscaria, A pantherine, Tricholoma muscarium*) that contain muscimol and/or ibotenic acid.[12] Atropine's pharmacologic actions are similar to ibotenic acid and may worsen clinical signs of isoxazole mushroom poisoning.

Alpha-2 agonist-mediated bradycardia is primarily a reflex secondary to alpha-2-mediated vasoconstriction with a resultant increase in blood pressure. Administration of anticholinergic agents in dogs or cats at the same time or after alpha-2 agonists leads to adverse cardiovascular effects (secondary tachycardia, prolonged hypertension, and cardiac arrhythmias).[13-15] The routine use of anticholinergics simultaneously with, or after, dexmedetomidine in dogs or cats is neither recommended nor necessary because blood pressure is generally normal to high. During anesthesia, if both the heart rate AND the blood pressure are low, an anticholinergic drug (atropine or glycopyrrolate) can be used as part of blood pressure support.[16] Another treatment option is reversal of the alpha-2 agonist (see ***Atipamezole***).

Antimuscarinic agents should be used with extreme caution in animals with known or suspected GI infections and inflammatory diseases (eg, severe ulcerative colitis), ileus, obstructive GI disease (eg, pyloric stenosis, foreign body obstruction), and GI toxin exposure. Atropine or other antimuscarinic agents can decrease GI motility and prolong retention of the causative agent(s) or toxin(s), resulting in prolonged clinical signs. Antimuscarinic agents must also be used with extreme caution in animals with autonomic neuropathy (eg, myasthenia gravis [unless used to reverse adverse muscarinic effects secondary to therapy]).

Antimuscarinic agents should be used with caution in animals with hepatic or renal disease, hyperthyroidism, hypertension, CHF, tachyarrhythmia, or esophageal reflux and in geriatric or pediatric animals. Antimuscarinic agents may also reduce the epinephrine dose at which epinephrine promotes arrhythmias.

Systemic atropine should be used cautiously, or not at all, in horses, as it may decrease gut motility and induce colic in susceptible animals. Use of atropine in ruminants may result in inappetence and rumen stasis that can persist for several days.

Atropine may aggravate some signs seen with amitraz toxicity, leading to hypertension and further inhibition of peristalsis. It is not recommended for treating bradycardia secondary to dexmedetomidine. See ***Drug Interactions***.

Atropine is reportedly not effective in treating bradycardia in puppies younger than 14 days of age or kittens younger than 11 days of age.[17] Anticholinergic induced tachycardia can exacerbate myocardial oxygen deficits and cause myocardial damage.[18]

Some rabbit populations have endogenous atropinesterase that breaks down atropine, rendering it ineffective; glycopyrrolate is often the anticholinergic of choice in this species. See ***Glycopyrrolate.***[19]

Atropine impairs sweat gland function in species with cholinergic control of sweating, and hyperthermia may develop in susceptible animals that receive the drug in warm ambient temperatures.

Adverse Effects

Adverse effects are exacerbations of the drug's pharmacologic effects and are generally dose related. At standard doses, effects tend to be mild in relatively healthy animals. The more severe effects typically occur with high or toxic doses. GI effects can include dry mouth (ie, xerostomia), increased viscosity of secretions, dysphagia, constipation, and vomiting. Respiratory secretions may become viscous and more difficult to clear from the airway. Genitourinary effects may include urinary retention. CNS effects may include stimulation, drowsiness, ataxia, seizures, and respiratory depression. Sedation and/or agitation can occur after atropine administration to conscious patients and could (rarely) impact anesthetic recovery. Ophthalmic effects include mydriasis, cycloplegia, photophobia, and an increase in intraocular pressure. Cardiovascular effects include sinus tachycardia (usually transient), increased myocardial oxygen consumption, bradycardia (initially, or at very low doses), hypertension, hypotension, tachyarrhythmia (eg, premature ventricular complexes [PVCs], ventricular tachycardia), and circulatory failure. The latter effects are generally related to excessively high dosages.

Reproductive/Nursing Safety

Atropine use in pregnancy may cause fetal tachycardia. In humans, atropine rapidly crosses the placenta,[20] but human data suggest there is low risk for use during pregnancy.

Atropine may be excreted into the breast milk; however, no human adverse events have been reported, and limited human data suggest it is probably compatible with lactation in humans.[20]

Because safety has not been established in animals, this drug should only be used when the maternal benefits outweigh the potential risks to offspring.

Overdose/Acute Toxicity

For signs of atropine toxicity see ***Adverse Effects*** above. CNS depression occurs with larger doses, and medullary depression is the most common cause of overdose-related death.

GI decontamination with activated charcoal and saline cathartics may be warranted if there has been a recent oral ingestion. Treatment consists of supportive care measures (eg, maintaining hydration, providing respiratory support, managing arrhythmia). Do not use phenothiazines, as they may contribute to anticholinergic effects. Standard treatments for shock may be necessary. Atropine is not removed by dialysis.

The use of physostigmine is controversial and should probably be reserved for animals that exhibit extreme agitation and are at risk for injuring themselves or others, or for cases in which supraventricular tachycardia or sinus tachycardia are severe or life-threatening.

For patients that have experienced or are suspected to have experienced an overdose, it is strongly encouraged that a 24-hour poison consultation center that specializes in providing information specific for veterinary patients be consulted. For general information related to overdose and toxin exposures, as well as contact information for poison control centers, refer to *Appendix*.

Drug Interactions

The following drug interactions with atropine have either been reported or are theoretical in humans or animals and may be of significance in veterinary patients. Unless otherwise noted, use together is not necessarily contraindicated, but weigh the potential risks and perform additional monitoring when appropriate.

- **Acetylcholinesterase Inhibitors** (eg, **edrophonium, neostigmine**): May reduce atropine effects. Atropine may intentionally be administered immediately prior AChI to prevent peripheral muscarinic effects.
- **Alpha-2 Agonists** (eg, **dexmedetomidine, medetomidine, xylazine**): Use of atropine with alpha-2 agonists may significantly increase arterial blood pressure, heart rate, and the incidence of arrhythmia.[21,22] Clinical use of atropine or glycopyrrolate to prevent or treat bradycardia caused by alpha-2 agonists is controversial and use together is discouraged; this may be particularly important when using higher doses of the alpha-2 agonist. See *Contraindications/Precautions/ Warnings*.
- **Amitraz**: Atropine may aggravate some signs seen with amitraz toxicity, leading to hypertension and further inhibition of peristalsis.
- **Cholinergic Agents** (eg, **bethanechol, pilocarpine**): Concurrent use of cholinergic agonists and antagonists should be avoided.
- **Corticosteroids** (eg, **prednis(ol)one**): Long-term use may increase intraocular pressure.
- **Domperidone**: Atropine may reduce domperidone efficacy.
- **Epinephrine**: May reduce dose at which epinephrine promotes arrhythmias
- **Ketoconazole**: Increased gastric pH may decrease GI absorption; administer oral atropine 2 hours after ketoconazole.
- **Latanoprost**: Atropine counteracted the miotic effect of latanoprost without altering intraocular pressure (IOP) in healthy dogs.[23]
- **Loperamide**: Concurrent use may further reduce GI motility and increase risk of ileus and constipation.
- **Metoclopramide**: Atropine and its derivatives may antagonize the actions of metoclopramide.
- **Monoamine Oxidase (MAO) Inhibitors** (eg, **linezolid, selegiline**): Concurrent use with atropine may increase risk for hypertensive crisis.
- **Potassium Salts (oral)**: Reduced GI motility may increase risk for GI irritation from solid oral dosage forms of potassium.
- **Promotility Agents** (eg, **cisapride, erythromycin, metoclopramide**): Atropine may antagonize effects on GI peristalsis.

The following drugs may enhance the activity or toxicity of atropine and its derivatives:

- **Amantadine**
- **Anticholinergic Agents (other)** (eg, **glycopyrrolate, hyoscyamine, oxybutynin**)
- **Antihistamines** (eg, **diphenhydramine, hydroxyzine**)
- **Opioids** (eg, **fentanyl, hydromorphone, methadone, morphine**)
- **Phenothiazines** (eg, **acepromazine, chlorpromazine**)
- **Procainamide**
- **Primidone**
- **Skeletal Muscle Relaxants** (eg, **cyclobenzaprine, dantrolene, dicyclomine, methocarbamol**)
- **Tricyclic antidepressants** (eg, **amitriptyline, doxepin, clomipramine**)

Laboratory Considerations

None noted

Dosages

NOTE: FDA approval has not been required for atropine products in animals. All dosages should be considered extra-label.

DOGS/CATS:

Preanesthetic adjuvant: Generally, 0.02 – 0.04 mg/kg IM or IV. Consider smaller doses (0.01 mg/kg) in geriatric or debilitated animals. The veterinary label lists 0.06 mg/kg IV, IM, or SC, but this is not currently recommended.

During cardiopulmonary cerebral resuscitation (CPCR) efforts to block vagal tone and treat/eliminate bradyarrhythmias: Atropine at 0.04 mg/kg IV or intraosseous (IO) is most likely to be useful (although not strongly supported in the literature) in dogs and cats with asystole or pulseless electrical activity (PEA) associated with high vagal tone. Due to a lack of any clear detrimental effects, routine use of atropine during CPR can be considered (0.04 mg/kg IV or IO; may repeat every other BLS [basic life support] cycle, which are 2 minutes in duration). Intratracheal administration (preferably past the level of the carina) at 0.15 – 0.2 mg/kg (diluted 1:10 in saline or water) can be considered when IV or IO access is not possible.[24]

Atropine response test (ART):

- **Rishniw Preference**: 1) Record ECG at baseline; 2) administer atropine at 0.04 mg/kg IV; 3) wait 15 minutes; and 4) record ECG for at least 2 minutes (use slow paper speed). If the response is incomplete, repeat steps 2 through 4. Persistent sinus tachycardia at greater than 140 bpm is expected in most dogs with vagally-mediated bradycardia.
- **Kittleson Preference**: 1) Record ECG at baseline; 2) administer atropine at 0.04 mg/kg SC; 3) wait 30 minutes; and 4) record ECG for at least 2 minutes (use slow paper speed). Persistent sinus tachycardia at greater than 140 bpm is expected in most dogs with vagally-mediated bradycardia.[25]

Organophosphate (OP) and carbamate toxicity:

a) If poisoning or overdose is suspected: Obtain baseline heart rate; give test dose of atropine at 0.02 mg/kg IV. If heart rate increases and pupils dilate, organophosphate toxicity is not likely. Look for other causes of signs, as it generally requires 10 times (0.2 mg/kg) the test dose to resolve muscarinic signs of OP/carbamate poisoning. Muscarinic signs (eg, SLUDDE [salivation, lacrimation, urination, defecation, dyspnea, emesis], miosis, bradycardia) can be treated with atropine at 0.2 mg/kg (administer ¼ of the dose IV, remainder IM or SC). Repeat as required. Atropine will not reverse nicotinic (eg, muscular weakness) or CNS (eg, seizures) effects.[26] See *Overdose/Acute Toxicity*.

b) Atropine 0.025 – 0.2 mg/kg IV repeated until clinical signs of poisoning are relieved. Several sequential injections may be required, depending on the severity of the poisoning. In severe cases, give ¼ of the dose IM or by slow IV injection and the remainder SC; in less severe cases, give the whole dose SC. The frequency of the dose administered should be such that the recurrence of moderate or severe signs of poisoning are treated, typically at 3- to 4-hour intervals. Atropine is only effective several minutes after administration and maximum effect may be delayed 5 to 10 minutes after injection.[27]

Muscarinic mushroom toxicity: Initially, atropine at 0.04 mg/kg (administer ¼ of the dose IV, remainder IM or SC). Dose can be titrated up and repeated if needed to control severe signs; avoid overtreating. Muscarinic signs (eg, SLUDDE [salivation, lacrimation, urination, defecation, dyspnea, emesis], miosis, bradycardia) usually resolve in 30 minutes. Give supportive care (eg, IV fluids) as needed.[28] **WARNING:** Atropine is contraindicated in the management of poisoning with isoxazole mushrooms (eg, *Amanita muscaria, A pantherine, Tricholoma muscarium*) that contain muscimol and/or ibotenic acid.[12]

FERRETS:

Premedication and treatment of vagally-mediated bradycardia: 0.04 – 0.05 mg/kg IV, SC, or IM[29] or intratracheally for CPR

RABBITS/RODENTS/SMALL MAMMALS:

Premedication and treatment of vagally-mediated bradycardia in rodents (rats, mice, guinea pigs): 0.04 – 0.05 mg/kg IM, SC, IP

Premedication and treatment of vagally-mediated bradycardia in rabbits: 0.05 – 0.25 mg/kg IM, SC. Atropine is ineffective in ≈50% of rabbits due to the presence of atropinase, so glycopyrrolate is preferred.

Organophosphate and carbamate toxicity: 10 mg/kg SC every 20 minutes[30]

CATTLE:

Organophosphate and carbamate toxicity: 0.5 – 1 mg/kg; give ¼ of the dose IV and the remainder SC or IM; repeat and titrate dose as required.

HORSES

Vagal-induced bradyarrhythmia: **NOTE**: This use is uncommon because bradycardia and bradyarrhythmias, like second-degree AV block (Mobitz Type 1) are normal in horses.

a) 0.01 – 0.02 mg/kg IV[31]
b) 0.03 – 0.06 mg/kg SC[27]

Bronchodilator: 0.1 – 0.15 mg/kg IV[32] (practically, 5 – 7 mg IV per horse [450 kg; 990 lb] [NOT mg/kg]) can serve as a rescue medication in cases of severe airway obstruction; however, it is not commonly used because it has a short duration of action (0.5 to 2 hours), and adverse effects (eg, ileus, CNS toxicity, tachycardia, increased mucus secretion, impaired mucociliary clearance) limit its use to a single rescue dose.[33] ***Butylscopolamine*** appears better tolerated and equally effective.[2]

Organophosphate and carbamate toxicity:

a) 0.2 mg/kg (administer ¼ of the dose IV, remainder IM or SC); repeat every 1.5 to 6 hours as necessary to control clinical signs associated with toxicity. Mydriasis and absence of salivation can be used as therapy endpoints. Do not overuse, as ileus is a concern.
b) 0.025 – 0.2 mg/kg repeated until clinical signs of poisoning are relieved. In severe cases, give ¼ of the dose IM or by slow IV injection and the remainder SC; in less severe cases, give the whole dose SC. The frequency of the dose administered should be such that the recurrence of moderate or severe signs of poisoning are treated, typically at 3- to 4-hour intervals. Atropine is only effective several minutes after administration and maximum effect may be delayed 5 to 10 minutes after injection.

SWINE:

Organophosphate and carbamate toxicity:

a) 0.2 mg/kg (administer ¼ of the dose IV, remainder IM or SC); repeat every 1.5 to 6 hours as necessary to control clinical signs associated with toxicity. Mydriasis and absence of salivation can be used as therapy endpoints.
b) 0.025 – 0.2 mg/kg repeated until clinical signs of poisoning are relieved. In severe cases, give ¼ of the dose IM or by slow IV injection and the remainder SC; in less severe cases, give the whole dose SC. The frequency of the dose administered should be such that the recurrence of moderate or severe signs of poisoning are treated, typically at 3- to 4-hour intervals. Atropine is only effective several minutes after administration and maximum effect may be delayed 5 to 10 minutes after injection.

Adjunctive preanesthetic agent: 0.02 – 0.04 mg/kg IV or IM[34,35]

SHEEP/GOATS:

Organophosphate and carbamate toxicity: 0.6 – 1 mg/kg (administer ¼ – ⅓ of the dose IV, remainder SC). Given every 4 to 5 hours as needed, but should be slowed down or stopped to avoid GI stasis and bloat.[36,37]

NEW WORLD CAMELIDS:

Organophosphate and carbamate toxicity: 0.2 – 0.4 mg/kg (administer ½ dose IV, ½ dose SC)

BIRDS:

Organophosphate and carbamate toxicity:

a) 0.2 mg/kg IM every 3 to 4 hours as needed. Use with pralidoxime (except in raptors) at 10 – 20 mg/kg IM every 8 to 12 hours as needed. Do not use pralidoxime to treat carbamate poisoning. To assist in diagnosing organophosphate poisoning (in conjunction with history and clinical signs) in birds presenting with bradycardia, atropine at 0.02 mg/kg IV may be given. If bradycardia does not reverse, organophosphate toxicity should be considered.[38]
b) **Raptors**: 0.5 mg/kg; (administer ¼ of the dose IV, remainder IM). Repeat 3 or 4 times per day if bradycardia persists.[39]

Preanesthetic agent: 0.04 – 0.1 mg/kg IM or SC once[40]

During cardiopulmonary cerebral resuscitation (CPCR) efforts for adjunctive treatment of bradycardia: 0.2 mg/kg IV with ventilation and epinephrine (0.1 mg/kg diluted in saline and into the trachea)[41]

REPTILES:

Organophosphate and carbamate toxicity in most species: 0.1 – 0.2 mg/kg SC or IM as needed[42]

Ptyalism in tortoises: 0.05 mg/kg SC or IM once daily[42]

Monitoring

Dependent on dose and indication:

- Heart rate and rhythm
- Blood pressure
- GI motility (via auscultation) in horses and potentially in ruminants
- Urination, defecation capability
- Hydration; dry mouth and secretions (eg, respiratory)

Client Information

- Injections of atropine should only be performed by veterinary staff and in the clinic where adequate monitoring is available.
- Be sure your animal has free access to plenty of fresh, clean water when receiving this medicine. Encourage drinking if dry mouth is a problem.
- Animals treated with atropine may have dilated pupils and experience difficulty urinating or passing feces (constipation) for a short period of time afterward. Contact your veterinarian if these problems continue, or if your animal appears weak, has low energy or is unable to urinate and defecate normally.

Chemistry/Synonyms

Atropine sulfate, the prototype tertiary amine antimuscarinic agent, is derived from naturally occurring atropine. Commercial dosage forms contain atropine sulfate, which has greater solubility than atropine. Atropine is a racemic mixture of D-hyoscyamine and

L-hyoscyamine. The L-form of the drug is active; the D-form has practically no antimuscarinic activity. Atropine sulfate occurs as colorless and odorless crystals or white, crystalline powder. One gram of atropine sulfate is soluble in 0.5 mL of water, 5 mL of alcohol, or 2.5 mL of glycerin. Aqueous solutions are practically neutral or only slightly acidic. Commercially available injections may have the pH adjusted to 3 to 6.5.

Atropine may also be known as DL-hyoscyamine. Atropine sulfate may also be known as atrop. sulph., atropine sulphate, or atropini sulfas; many trade names are available.

Storage/Stability

Atropine sulfate for injection should be stored at room temperature between 15°C and 30°C (59°F-86°F).

Compatibility/Compounding Considerations

Compatibility is dependent on factors such as pH, concentration, temperature, and diluent used; consult specialized references or a veterinary hospital pharmacist for more specific information.

Atropine sulfate for injection is reportedly **compatible** with the following agents: butorphanol, chlorpromazine, cimetidine (not with pentobarbital), dimenhydrinate, diphenhydramine, dobutamine, fentanyl, glycopyrrolate, hydromorphone, meperidine, morphine, nalbuphine, pentazocine, pentobarbital (for 5 minutes, not 24 hours), perphenazine, prochlorperazine, promazine, promethazine (also with meperidine), and scopolamine.

Atropine sulfate is reported physically **incompatible** with methohexital (forms a haze after 15 minutes) and norepinephrine.

Dosage Forms/Regulatory Status

VETERINARY-LABELED PRODUCTS:

Atropine Sulfate for Injection: 0.54 mg/mL (1/120 grain) in 100 mL vials; (Rx)

Atropine Sulfate for Injection: 15 mg/mL (organophosphate treatment), 100 mL vial; (Rx)

Atropine is labeled for use in dogs, cats, horses, cattle, sheep, and swine in the United States, but FDA approval has not been required. No withdrawal times are mandated when used in food animals in the United States, but the Food Animal Residue Avoidance Databank (FARAD) recommends a 28-day meat and 6-day milk withdrawal time when used in food animals at doses up to 0.2 mg/kg.[43] For guidance in determining use and associated withdrawal times, contact FARAD (see ***Important Contact Information*** in ***Appendix***).

The Association of Racing Commissioners International (ARCI) has designated this drug as a class 3 substance. See ***Appendix*** for more information.

HUMAN-LABELED PRODUCTS:

Atropine Sulfate for Injection:
0.05 mg/mL in 5 mL syringes; (Rx)

0.1 mg/mL in 5 mL and 10 mL syringes; (Rx)

0.3 mg/mL in 1 mL and 30 mL vials; (Rx)

0.4 mg/mL in 1 mL amps and 1 mL, 20 mL, and 30 mL vials; (Rx)

0.5 mg/mL in 1 mL and 30 mL vials and 5 mL syringes; (Rx)

0.6 mg/mL in 1 mL amps; (Rx)

0.8 mg/mL in 0.5 mL and 1 mL amps and 0.5 mL syringes; (Rx)

1 mg/mL in 1 mL amps and vials and 10 mL syringes; (Rx)

0.5 mg, 1 mg, and 2 mg prefilled auto-injectors; *AtroPen*®; (Rx)

Historically, atropine tablets (0.4 or 0.6 mg; Rx) have been available.

References

For the complete list of references, see **wiley.com/go/budde/plumb**

Auranofin

(au-***rane***-oh-fin) *Ridaura*®

Oral Gold Immunosuppressive

Prescriber Highlights

- ► May be used for pemphigus complex and idiopathic polyarthritis in dogs or cats, and possibly as adjunctive treatment for osteosarcoma in dogs
- ► Requires intensive monitoring
- ► Contraindications include systemic lupus erythematosus (as it exacerbates the condition) and hypersensitivity to gold products.
- ► Renal, hepatic, and GI toxicity possible; dose-dependent immune-mediated thrombocytopenia, hemolytic anemia, or leukopenia have been observed
- ► Expensive; doses may need to be compounded

Uses/Indications

Auranofin treats idiopathic polyarthritis and pemphigus complex in dogs and cats. It is also anecdotally reported to be useful for eosinophilic granuloma complex, plasma cell pododermatitis, and stomatitis in cats. Clinicians report that auranofin may be less toxic but also less efficacious than injectable gold (aurothioglucose; no longer marketed). Limited information is published on the safety and efficacy in dogs and cats; therefore, auranofin should be reserved for cases that are unresponsive to or do not tolerate more conventional immunomodulatory therapy, such as glucocorticoids and azathioprine.

Auranofin is also being studied for its potential anticancer effects.[1-3] In dogs with osteosarcoma, a significant increase in overall survival was observed when auranofin was added to standard-of-care treatment (ie, amputation and carboplatin), specifically in male dogs.[1]

Pharmacology/Actions

Auranofin is an orally available gold salt. Gold has anti-inflammatory, antirheumatic, immunomodulating, and antimicrobial effects. The exact mechanisms for these actions are not well understood. Gold is taken up by macrophages, which inhibits phagocytosis and may inhibit lysosomal enzyme activity. Gold inhibits the release of histamine and decreases prostaglandin production. Auranofin suppresses helper T cells without affecting suppressor T-cell populations. It also has in vitro inhibitory effect on DNA, RNA, and protein synthesis.

The antineoplastic effects of auranofin are thought to be due to inhibition of thioredoxin reductase (TrxR2) and reactive oxygen-induced apoptosis.[1-3] Inhibition of TrxR2 is thought to be the mechanism by which auranofin decreases lung metastases of osteosarcoma.[3,4]

Auranofin is also being studied for its potential antimicrobial effects,[5-12] including broad and potent in vitro and in vivo antifungal activity, which suggests that auranofin might be a promising novel antifungal, mainly considering its ability to cross the blood–brain barrier.[13] More research is needed to determine the clinical utility of these effects.

Pharmacokinetics

Auranofin is rapidly metabolized, and pharmacokinetic data are based on gold concentrations rather than auranofin drug concentrations.

In dogs, gold from orally administered auranofin was 15% to 38% absorbed, and the half-life of gold was 19.5 days; excretion occurred primarily via the feces.[14]

In humans, auranofin is absorbed when given by mouth (20% to 25% of the gold), primarily in the small and large intestines.[15] Auranofin is moderately plasma protein bound. Auranofin crosses the placenta and is distributed into maternal milk. Tissues with the highest concentrations of gold are kidneys, spleen, lungs, adrenal glands, and liver. Accumulation of gold does not appear to occur. About 15% of an administered dose (60% of the absorbed dose) is excreted by the kidneys, the remainder in the feces.

Contraindications/Precautions/Warnings

Gold salts are contraindicated in systemic lupus erythematosus due to potential disease exacerbation, and in patients with a history of adverse reactions to gold products. Do not use in animals with suppressed bone marrow or animals receiving other bone marrow suppressive agents, such as azathioprine or cyclophosphamide. Only administer auranofin to animals when other less expensive and less toxic therapies are ineffective. Ensure all parties are aware of the potential pitfalls of auranofin therapy and are willing to accept the associated risks and expenses.

Adverse Effects

Dogs may exhibit dose-dependent immune-mediated thrombocytopenia,[16] hemolytic anemia, or leukopenia. If an immune response occurs, it is recommended to discontinue auranofin and administer steroids. Auranofin has a high incidence of dose-dependent GI disturbances, particularly diarrhea in dogs.[17,18] This generally resolves with dose reduction or discontinuation of the drug. Renal toxicity may manifest as proteinuria. Hepatotoxicity may occur. Renal and hepatic toxicities are less likely than either the GI or hematologic effects (eg, thrombocytopenia, anemia, leukopenia). Dermatoses (including toxic epidermal necrolysis) and corneal and oral ulcers have been associated with auranofin therapy.

Reproductive/Nursing Safety

Auranofin has been demonstrated to be teratogenic and maternotoxic in rabbits[15]; it should not be used during pregnancy unless the owner accepts the potential risks for use.

Following auranofin administration, gold is excreted in the milk of rodents. Trace amounts appear in the serum and red blood cells of nursing offspring. Gold may cause adverse effects in nursing offspring; switching to milk replacer is recommended if auranofin is continued. Gold is slowly excreted; persistence in milk will occur even after drug discontinuation.

Overdose/Acute Toxicity

Limited data are available. The minimum lethal oral dose in rats is 30 mg/kg. Recommend employing gastric-emptying protocols after acute overdoses when applicable. Chelating agents (eg, penicillamine, dimercaprol) for severe toxicities are controversial. One human patient overdosed over 10 days and developed various neurologic sequelae, but eventually (after 3 months) recovered completely after drug discontinuation and chelation therapy.

For patients that have experienced or are suspected of having experienced an overdose, consultation with a 24-hour poison consultation center specializing in providing veterinary-specific information is recommended. For general information related to overdose and toxin exposures, as well as contact information for poison control centers, refer to *Appendix*.

Drug Interactions

The following drug interactions with auranofin have either been reported or are theoretical in humans or animals and may be of significance in veterinary patients. Unless otherwise noted, use together is not necessarily contraindicated, but weigh the potential risks and perform additional monitoring when appropriate.

- Antimalarial Drugs (eg, **primaquine, quinacrine**): Use with gold salts is not recommended due to the increased potential for hematologic or renal toxicity.
- Immunosuppressive Agents (eg, **azathioprine, high-dose corticosteroids, leflunomide, pyrimethamine**): Auranofin's safety when used with these agents has not been established; use with caution.
- Myelosuppressive Agents (eg, **chlorambucil, chloramphenicol, cyclophosphamide**): Concurrent use may increase the risk for myelosuppression.
- Penicillamine: Use with gold salts is not recommended due to the increased potential for hematologic or renal toxicity.
- Theophylline, Aminophylline: Decreased theophylline concentration may occur

Laboratory Considerations

- In humans, response to **tuberculin skin tests** may be enhanced; veterinary significance is unclear.

Dosages

DOGS:

Immune-mediated skin diseases in patients unresponsive to or that cannot tolerate conventional therapy (eg, glucocorticoids or azathioprine) (extra-label): 0.05 – 0.2 mg/kg PO every 12 hours (up to 9 mg/day total dose per dog); often in conjunction with glucocorticoids. Allow a 4-week "washout" before starting therapy after azathioprine discontinuation. A lag phase of 6 to 12 weeks can occur before seeing a response. If remission is achieved, pulse therapy of 1 – 2 mg/kg PO every other week for one month and then once monthly can be attempted. If remission is maintained for 6 months, one can attempt discontinuation.

Adjunct therapy for osteosarcoma in addition to standard first-line therapy (eg, surgery and carboplatin) (extra-label): 6 mg/dog (NOT mg/kg) PO every 3 days for dogs weighing less than 15 kg (33 lb), 9 mg/dog (NOT mg/kg) PO every 3 days for dogs weighing more than 15 kg (33 lb)[1]

CATS:

Immune-mediated skin diseases (eg, feline pemphigus, eosinophilic granuloma complex, plasma cell pododermatitis, and stomatitis) (extra-label): 0.2 – 0.3 mg/kg PO every 12 hours; must be reformulated for accurate dosing[19]

Monitoring

The following should be performed prior to therapy, then monthly for 2 to 3 months, then every other month:

- Hepatic and renal function tests
- Urinalysis
- CBC, with platelet counts; **NOTE**: eosinophilia may denote impending reaction.

Client Information

- May require several months before seeing a positive response.
- Requires commitment to the twice-daily dosing schedule
- Discuss therapy costs and potential side effects before initiating therapy.
- While your animal is taking this medication, it is important to return to your veterinarian for laboratory work. Do not miss these important follow-up visits.

Chemistry/Synonyms

Auranofin is an orally administered gold compound that occurs as a white, odorless, crystalline powder. It is slightly soluble in water and soluble in alcohol. Auranofin contains 29% gold.

Auranofin may also be known as SKF-39162, SKF-D-39162, *Crisinor®, Crisofin®, Goldar®, Ridaura®,* or *Ridauran®.*

Storage/Stability

Store capsules in tight, light-resistant containers at 15C° to 30°C (59°F-86°F).

Compatibility/Compounding Considerations

No specific information was noted.

Dosage Forms/Regulatory Status

VETERINARY-LABELED PRODUCTS: NONE

HUMAN-LABELED PRODUCTS:

Auranofin Capsules: 3 mg; *Ridaura*®; (Rx)

References

For the complete list of references, see **wiley.com/go/budde/plumb**

Azathioprine

(ay-za-***thye***-oh-preen) *Imuran*®, *Azasan*®

Immunosuppressant

Prescriber Highlights

- Purine-antagonist, immunosuppressive agent used in dogs for a variety of autoimmune diseases
- Not generally used in cats, as they are highly sensitive to myelosuppression
- May take several weeks for immunosuppression to occur; doses are given daily the first 2 weeks
- Often used in combination with corticosteroids to reduce doses and frequency of each drug
- Myelosuppression is the principal adverse effect; GI effects include GI distress, anorexia, pancreatitis, hepatotoxicity. Use with caution in patients with hepatic disease.
- Known mutagen and teratogen
- The National Institute for Occupational Safety and Health (NIOSH) classifies azathioprine as a hazardous drug; use appropriate precautions when handling.

Uses/Indications

In dogs, azathioprine is used primarily as an immunosuppressive agent in the treatment of immune-mediated diseases, but no large, controlled, prospective studies documenting its efficacy were located. In patients with immune-mediated hemolytic anemia, azathioprine is often recommended at the start of treatment in combination with other drugs. Azathioprine is often used in combination with corticosteroids (eg, prednis(ol)one) for synergy and to reduce the incidence of adverse effects of each drug by allowing dosage reductions and, eventually, every other day dosing of each drug.

When used in combination with cyclosporine, azathioprine has been used to prevent rejection of MHC-matched renal allografts in dogs.

Pharmacology/Actions

Azathioprine antagonizes purine metabolism by causing breaks in DNA and RNA secondary to incorporation into nucleic acids and termination of the replication process. Cellular metabolism may become disrupted by the drug's ability to inhibit coenzyme formation. Evidence suggests azathioprine interferes with CD28 costimulation of T lymphocytes by converting the costimulatory signal from CD28 to trigger apoptosis.[1]

Azathioprine has greater activity on delayed hypersensitivity and cellular immunity than on humoral antibody responses. Clinical response to azathioprine may not be observed for up to 5 weeks.

Pharmacokinetics

Azathioprine is poorly absorbed from the GI tract. It is rapidly metabolized to 6-mercaptopurine (6-MP), which is then taken up by lymphocytes and erythrocytes. The remaining drug in the plasma is further metabolized in the liver and GI tract and excreted by the kidneys. Only minimal amounts of either azathioprine or mercaptopurine are excreted unchanged. Half-life is variable and estimated to be 2 hours. Azathioprine and mercaptopurine are 30% protein bound.

Cats have low activity of thiopurine methyltransferase (TPMT) (ie, one of the routes used to metabolize azathioprine). Approximately 11% of humans have low TPMT activity; these patients have a greater incidence of bone marrow suppression but also greater azathioprine efficacy. Dogs have variable TPMT activity similar to that seen in humans. This may explain why some canine breeds respond better to and/or develop more myelotoxicity than others. TPMT activity is lower in giant schnauzers and much higher in Alaskan malamutes than in other breeds. However, one study in dogs did not show significant correlation between TPMT activity in RBCs and drug toxicity.[2]

Contraindications/Precautions/Warnings

Azathioprine is contraindicated in patients with previous hypersensitivity reactions and should be used cautiously in patients with hepatic or renal dysfunction. Because azathioprine suppresses the immune system, animals may be at an increased risk for infections or neoplastic illnesses with long-term use.

Use of azathioprine in cats is rarely recommended, as they are more susceptible to azathioprine's myelosuppressive effects because of TPMT deficiencies.

In humans, chronic immunosuppression with azathioprine has been shown to increase the risk for malignancy (eg, lymphoma, skin cancer) and serious infection.

Prescription/order errors have occurred when azithromycin and azathioprine have been confused. The use of "tall man" letters (ie, writing part of the drug's name in upper case) on prescriptions/orders may reduce the risk for errors: aZITHROmycin; azaTHIOprine.

The National Institute for Occupational Safety and Health (NIOSH) classifies azathioprine as a hazardous drug; personal protective equipment (PPE) should be used accordingly to minimize the risk for exposure.

Adverse Effects

The principal adverse effects associated with azathioprine in dogs are GI effects (eg, vomiting, anorexia, diarrhea), bone marrow suppression, pancreatitis, and hepatotoxicity.[4] In dogs, there is a reported 8% incidence of myelosuppression, manifested primarily as leukopenia, but poorly regenerative anemia and thrombocytopenia have also been seen.[5,6] Myelosuppression typically occurs after several months of treatment.[5] Hepatotoxicity has also been described, and a retrospective study of 34 dogs reported a 15% incidence of subclinical increases in ALT and ALP activities occurring within the first several weeks of treatment, with only 1 dog showing signs related to hepatotoxicity (ie, anorexia, diarrhea).[5] However, marked myelosuppression and/or hepatotoxicity appear to be idiosyncratic (not dose dependent); these effects may be reversible if caught early enough and with drug withdrawal.[7]

In dogs recovering from immune-mediated hemolytic anemia, taper the drug dose slowly over several months and monitor for early signs of relapse. Rapid withdrawal can lead to a relapse of disease.

Reproductive/Nursing Safety

Azathioprine crosses the placenta and is mutagenic and teratogenic (eg, skeletal malformation, visceral anomalies) in laboratory animals at clinical doses. This drug has caused fetal harm during human pregnancies. Avoid use during pregnancy whenever possible. Decreased spermatogenesis and reduced sperm viability have been demonstrated in mice.[8]

The azathioprine metabolite 6-MP is distributed into maternal milk; a milk replacer should be used while the dam is receiving azathioprine.[8]

Because safety has not been established in animals, this drug should only be used when the maternal benefits outweigh the potential risks to offspring.

Overdose/Acute Toxicity

The oral LD_{50} for single doses of azathioprine in mice and rats are 2500 mg/kg and 400 mg/kg, respectively.[9]

There were 122 single agent exposures to azathioprine reported to the ASPCA Animal Poison Control Center (APCC) from 2009 to 2013. Common clinical signs observed following an overdose include vomiting and anorexia; increased liver enzyme activity and thrombocytopenia may also occur. Supportive treatment and GI decontamination protocols are recommended in the event of an overdose. The drug is partially dialyzable (≈45% removed) because of moderate protein binding.

For patients that have experienced or are suspected to have experienced an overdose, it is strongly encouraged that a 24-hour poison consultation center that specializes in providing information specific for veterinary patients be consulted. For general information related to overdose and toxin exposures, as well as contact information for poison control centers, refer to ***Appendix***.

Drug Interactions

The following drug interactions have either been reported or are theoretical in humans or animals receiving azathioprine and may be of significance in veterinary patients. Unless otherwise noted, use together is not necessarily contraindicated, but weigh the potential risks and perform additional monitoring when appropriate.

- ACE Inhibitors (eg, **benazepril, enalapril**): Increased potential for hematologic toxicity
- Allopurinol: The hepatic metabolism of azathioprine may be decreased by concomitant administration of allopurinol; in humans, the azathioprine dose should be reduced to ¼ or ⅓ of the usual dose if both drugs will be used together.
- Aminosalicylates (eg, **mesalamine, olsalazine, sulfasalazine**): Increased risk for azathioprine toxicity
- Myelosuppressive Agents, Other (eg, **cyclophosphamide, leflunomide, sulfa-/trimethoprim**): Increased potential for hepatic and hematologic toxicities
- NonDepolarizing Muscle Relaxants (eg, **pancuronium, tubocurarine**): The neuromuscular blocking activity of these drugs may be inhibited or reversed by azathioprine.
- Purine Antagonists (eg, **mercaptopurine, mycophenolate, thioguanine**): Increased risk for toxicity due to similar mechanism of action
- Vaccines (live and inactivated): May diminish vaccine efficacy and enhance adverse effects of vaccines
- Warfarin: Potential for reduced anticoagulant effect

Laboratory Considerations

- None

Doses

DOGS:

Immunosuppressive agent (all dosages listed below are extra-label; no prospective studies supporting any dosage protocol were noted): Many anecdotal protocols for use of azathioprine exist. General recommendations are to initially give 2 mg/kg PO every 24 hours for 1 to 4 weeks, then reduce the dosage to 0.5 – 2 mg/kg PO every other day. After treatment has started, a lag period of at least 1 week, and often as long as 3 to 5 weeks, is required before significant clinical immunosuppressive effect can be observed. Some treatment protocols include concurrent glucocorticoid administration. During the maintenance phase of treatment (ie, every other day administration), glucocorticoids are often given on days azathioprine is not given. Sample dosage protocols follow:

a) **Inflammatory bowel disease**: Initially, 2 mg/kg PO every 24 hours for 2 weeks, then tapered to 2 mg/kg PO every other day for 2 to 4 weeks, then 1 mg/kg PO every other day. It may take 2 to 6 weeks before beneficial effects are seen.[10]

b) **Immune-mediated hemolytic anemia (IMHA) and or immune-mediated thrombocytopenia (IMT)**: In conjunction with immunosuppressive doses of glucocorticoids (eg, prednis(ol)one), give azathioprine 2 mg/kg or 50 mg/m^2 PO every 24 hours for 2 to 3 weeks, then reduce azathioprine to every other day.[7,11,12]

c) **Adjunctive therapy for myasthenia gravis in nonresponsive patients**: 2 mg/kg PO every 24 hours for 2 weeks, then every 48 hours.[13] CBC should be repeated every week for the first month and then monthly thereafter. Azathioprine should be discontinued if WBC counts fall below 4,000 cells/μL or neutrophil counts are less than 1,000 cells/μL. Reevaluate serum AChR antibody concentrations every 4 to 6 weeks. Taper azathioprine to every other day when clinical remission occurs and serum AChR antibody concentrations are normalized.[14]

d) **Perianal fistulas (anal furunculosis)**: Initially, 2 mg/kg PO every 24 hours until there is a reduction in the size, number, or inflammation of the fistula, total WBC count is less than 5000 cells/μL, neutrophil count is less than 3500 cells/μL, or platelet count is less than 160,000 cells/μL. Then, reduce azathioprine to 2 mg/kg PO every other day for 12 weeks, unless myelosuppression develops. After 12 weeks, reduce dose to 1 mg/kg PO every other day for 12 months. In addition, give prednisone 2 mg/kg PO every 24 hours for the first 2 weeks of therapy, then 1 mg/kg PO every 24 hours for 2 weeks, and then discontinue. In a study in which all dogs were placed on a limited antigen diet, no correlation with efficacy and lymphocyte blastogenesis effect was seen.[15] The complete or partial remission rate was 64% of treated dogs, which is less than systemic cyclosporine or topical tacrolimus treatment.

e) **Reduce inflammation associated with chronic hepatitis**: Initially, 2.2 mg/kg PO every 24 hours in combination with corticosteroids. After 1 to 2 weeks, decrease dose to every other day.[16]

f) **Adjunctive therapy for with immune-mediated glomerular disease**: 2 mg/kg PO every 24 hours for 1 to 2 weeks, then 1 – 2 mg/kg PO every other day[17]

g) **Immune-mediated polyarthritis**: 2 mg/kg PO every 24 hours for 2 weeks, then tapered to a maintenance dosage of 0.5 mg/kg every other day[18]

h) **Meningoencephalomyelitis of undetermined etiology (MUE) in dogs**: In conjunction with corticosteroid therapy, azathioprine is initially started at 2 mg/kg PO every 24 hours for 2 weeks, then decreased to every other day.[19]

FERRETS:

Immunosuppressive agent for inflammatory bowel disease (extra-label; no prospective studies supporting any dosage protocol were noted): Treatment includes prednisone 1 mg/kg PO every 12 to 24 hours, azathioprine 0.9 mg/kg PO every 24 to 72 hours, and dietary management.[20]

HORSES:

Immunosuppressive agent (extra-label; no prospective studies supporting any dosage protocol were noted): 3 mg/kg PO every 24 hours. Although clinical experiences are still limited, azathioprine appears to be a relatively safe immunosuppressive treatment in horses.[21]

Monitoring

- Closely monitor CBC (including platelets) and serum chemistry profile (including liver enzymes [eg, ALT, ALP]). Baseline and periodic testing every 2 weeks for the first 2 months, then every 1 to 2 months during the course of therapy is recommended.[7]
  a. Some clinicians recommend reducing the dose by 25% if

the WBC count is between 5,000 to 7,000 cells/µL. If the WBC count is less than 5,000 cells/µL (or neutrophil count <1000 cells/µL), treatment should be discontinued until leukopenia resolves.

b. Hepatotoxicity is defined as a greater than 2-fold increase in ALT activity as compared to pretreatment values. In one study, 15% of dogs treated with azathioprine for clinical disease developed hepatotoxicity, requiring an azathioprine dosage adjustment in all affected dogs.[16]

- Serum cPLI analysis for possible pancreatitis, if indicated
- Signs of infection
- Efficacy

Client Information

- This drug can cause severe toxicity, including drug-related tumors or death; routine testing to detect toxic effects is necessary. Do not miss these important follow-up appointments.
- May be given with food to minimize gastrointestinal side effects
- May take up to 6 weeks to see positive effects
- Pregnant women should avoid handling this drug; caregivers should wash their hands or wear disposable gloves when handling this drug.
- Do not stop the drug unless your veterinarian tells you to do so.
- Watch for fever, reduced activity, bruising, bleeding, vomiting, lack of appetite, yellowing of whites of eyes, gums, skin).
- The medication is considered to be a hazardous drug as defined by the National Institute for Occupational Safety and Health (NIOSH). Talk with your veterinarian or pharmacist about the use of personal protective equipment when handling this medicine.

Chemistry/Synonyms

Azathioprine, which is related structurally to adenine, guanine, and hypoxanthine, is a purine-antagonist antimetabolite that is used primarily for its immunosuppressive properties. Azathioprine occurs as an odorless, pale-yellow powder that is insoluble in water and slightly soluble in alcohol. Azathioprine sodium powder for injection occurs as a bright-yellow, amorphous mass. After reconstitution with sterile water for injection to a concentration of 10 mg/mL, azathioprine has a pH of ≈9.6.

Azathioprine/azathioprine sodium may also be known as azathioprinum, BW-57322, or NSC-39084; many trade names are available.

Storage/Stability

Azathioprine tablets should be stored between 20°C to 25°C (68°F-77°F) in well-closed containers and protected from light.[7]

The sodium powder for injection should be stored at room temperature and protected from light. The powder is reportedly stable at neutral or acidic pH but will hydrolyze to mercaptopurine in alkaline solutions. This conversion is enhanced upon warming or in the presence of sulfhydryl-containing compounds (eg, cysteine). After reconstitution, the injection should be used within 24 hours, as no preservative is present.

Compatibility/Compounding Considerations

Compatible with sodium chloride 0.45% or 0.9% and dextrose 5% in water for dilution

Compounded preparation stability: Azathioprine oral suspension has been compounded from commercially available tablets.[22] Triturating 120 azathioprine 50 mg tablets with 60 mL of *Ora-Plus®* and qs ad to 120 mL with *Ora-Sweet®* (or *Ora-Sweet® SF*) yields a 50 mg/mL suspension that retains greater than 90% potency for 60 days stored at both 5°C (41°F) and 25°C (77°F). The stability of azathioprine aqueous liquids decreases in the presence of alkaline pH. Optimal stability is reported to be between 5.5 to 6.5. Compounded preparations of azathioprine should be protected from light.

Dosage Forms/Regulatory Status

VETERINARY-LABELED PRODUCTS: NONE

The International Federation for Equestrian Sports (FEI) lists this drug as a *prohibited substance - banned.* Use of this drug may not be allowed in certain animal competitions. Check rules and regulations before entering in a competition while this medication is being administered. Contact local racing authorities for further guidance.

HUMAN-LABELED PRODUCTS:

Azathioprine Tablets: 50 mg, 75 mg, and 100 mg; *Azasan®*, *Imuran®*, generic (50 mg only); (Rx)

Azathioprine Sodium Injection: 100 mg (as sodium)/vial in 20 mL vials; generic; (Rx)

References

For the complete list of references, see **wiley.com/go/budde/plumb**

Azithromycin

(ay-zith-roe-***my***-sin) Zithromax®

Macrolide Antibiotic

Prescriber Highlights

- ▶ Oral and parenteral macrolide antibiotic useful for treating a variety of bacterial, rickettsial, and protozoal infections
- ▶ Long tissue half-lives in dogs and cats
- ▶ Contraindications include hypersensitivity to macrolides.
- ▶ Use with caution in patients with hepatic dysfunction and in adult horses
- ▶ Adverse effects include potential GI effects (eg, anorexia, vomiting, diarrhea), but this drug has fewer adverse effects as compared with erythromycin.

Uses/Indications

Azithromycin is used to treat a variety of bacterial, rickettsial, and protozoal infections. Azithromycin has some anti-inflammatory and immunomodulatory effects[1,2]; however, the clinical relevance of these effects in veterinary species is unknown. Azithromycin has GI promotility properties in humans, and it has been used anecdotally as a prokinetic in dogs and cats.[3]

Azithromycin has been used to treat canine papillomatosis[4,5]; however, its effectiveness for this indication is unclear as the lesions may have regressed without treatment.

Azithromycin is anecdotally used in cats with recurrent and refractory rhinosinusitis; however, this drug is best reserved for select cases (ie, when chlamydiosis is not likely and other antimicrobial agents [eg, doxycycline, amoxicillin] are not viable options).[6]

Azithromycin has potential in the treatment of *Rhodococcus equi* infections in foals. Azithromycin combined with doxycycline was as effective as an azithromycin/rifampin combination for the treatment of *Rhodococcus equi.*[7] Although azithromycin's pharmacokinetics support oral dosing in adult horses, concerns for potential antimicrobial-associated enterocolitis indicate necessary caution when using this antibiotic in adult horses.[8]

The World Health Organization (WHO) has designated azithromycin as a Critically Important, Highest Priority antimicrobial for human medicine.[9]

Pharmacology/Actions

Azithromycin inhibits protein synthesis by penetrating bacterial cell walls and binding the 50S ribosomal subunits in susceptible bacteria. Azithromycin is a bacteriostatic antibiotic. Azithromycin can accumulate and persist in macrophages, neutrophils, and pulmonary epithelial lining fluid.

Azithromycin has a relatively broad antibacterial spectrum with excellent in vitro activity against most gram-positive bacteria, and greater gram-negative activity (including *Salmonella* spp, *Bordetella* spp, *Pasteurella* spp, and *Haemophilus influenzae*) than most other macrolides. Activity against *Campylobacter* spp, *Brucella* spp, *Bartonella* spp, and *Borrelia* spp is variable. It has good activity against *Mycoplasma* spp and *Chlamydia* spp; however, it is important to note that treatment regimens for *Mycoplasma haemofelis*[10] and *Chlamydophila felis*[11] in cats may result in clinical resolution, but azithromycin is ineffective in eradicating these infections, and thus treatment for these infections with azithromycin is not recommended. Azithromycin also has activity against *Mycobacterium* spp, but it is not recommended for *Mycobacterium avium* complex.

Azithromycin's antiprotozoal effect against *Babesia* spp and *Toxoplasma* spp is through inhibition of apicoplast (ie, DNA-containing organelles) protein translation, which results in protozoal progeny death.[12]

Azithromycin has been used to treat cryptosporidiosis in various species, but there is limited understanding of its potential efficacy for this use. In immunocompromised humans,[13] azithromycin has been shown to improve clinical symptoms related to infection but does not have an effect on *Cryptosporidium* spp shedding. It is unclear if azithromycin may have a similar result when it is used in animals. A positive effect on clinical signs and oocyst shedding has been identified in calves.[14] Azithromycin combined with toltrazuril was more effective than either agent alone in promoting rapid clinical recovery in calves with cryptosporidiosis.[15]

Azithromycin combined with atovaquone appears to be effective in the treatment of dogs with *Babesia gibsoni* infections[12,16,17] as well as piroplasmosis caused by *Babesia microti*-like piroplasm[18] and theileriosis.[19] Azithromycin (used alone or in combination with minocycline) demonstrated efficacy against *Pythium insidiosum* in an experimental rabbit model.[20]

Pharmacokinetics

In comparison to erythromycin, azithromycin has better absorption characteristics, longer tissue half-lives, and higher concentrations in tissues and WBCs. Concentrations of azithromycin are high in bronchial secretions and pulmonary epithelial lining fluid; it has excellent ocular penetration.

In dogs, azithromycin has 97% oral bioavailability. Peak serum concentration occurred ≈2 hours after oral administration. Tissue concentrations do not mirror serum concentrations after multiple doses. Serum half-life was ≈50 hours, and tissue half-lives in dogs may be up to 90 hours. Skin concentrations are 3.5 to 12 times higher than serum concentrations.[21] Azithromycin exhibits concentrations in canine external ear canals.[22] More than 50% of an oral dose is excreted unchanged in bile.[23]

In cats, azithromycin has 58% oral bioavailability and peak concentration is reached after 0.85 hours. Tissue half-lives in cats are less than in dogs and range from 13 hours in adipose tissue to 72 hours in cardiac muscle. Cats excrete ≈66% of a dose unchanged in bile.[23]

In foals, azithromycin is variably absorbed after oral administration, with a mean systemic bioavailability ranging from 40% to 60%. The effect of food on absorption is unclear. Azithromycin has a very high volume of distribution (11.6 to 18.6 L/kg). Elimination half-life is ≈20 to 26 hours. The drug concentrates in bronchoalveolar cells and pulmonary epithelial fluid. Elimination half-life in polymorphonuclear leukocytes is ≈2 days.[24-26] In adult horses, intragastric administration (tablets suspended in 500 mL of water) resulted in an average oral bioavailability of 45%, with peak levels occurring ≈1 hour after administration. Plasma elimination half-life after IV dosing was ≈18 hours. Plasma concentrations after a single intragastric dose remained above MIC_{90} for 6 to 12 hours for beta-hemolytic streptococci, *Pasteurella* spp, and *Staphylococcus* spp. For these bacteria, intracellular concentrations of azithromycin in alveolar macrophages were above MIC_{90} for at least 48 hours and in neutrophils for at least 120 hours after a dose.[8]

In goats, azithromycin has an elimination half-life of 32.5 hours (IV) and 45 hours (IM), an apparent volume of distribution (steady-state) of 34.5 L/kg, and a clearance of 0.85 L/kg/hour.[27]

In sheep, azithromycin has an average elimination half-life of 48 hours (IV) and 61 hours (IM), an apparent volume of distribution (steady-state) of 34.5 L/kg, and a clearance of 0.52 L/kg/hour.[28]

In rabbits, azithromycin has an elimination half-life of 24.1 hours (IV) and 25.1 hours (IM). IM injection has a high bioavailability but causes some degree of muscle damage at the injection site.[29]

Contraindications/Precautions/Warnings

Azithromycin is contraindicated in animals that are hypersensitive to any macrolide antibiotic. There have been anecdotal reports of fatal colitis in adult horses, and the drug should be used with extreme caution, if at all, in these patients.

Caution should be used when using azithromycin in patients with impaired hepatic function because this drug is primarily eliminated via liver metabolism.

Prolonged QT intervals can occur with use of azithromycin, which increases the risk for cardiac arrhythmias, including torsades de pointes. Caution should be used when combining azithromycin with other medications (eg, azole antifungals, cisapride, dolasetron, moxifloxacin, erythromycin, ondansetron) that may prolong QT intervals especially in animals with underlying heart disease. (See *Drug Interactions*)

Exacerbation of symptoms related to myasthenia gravis or a new onset of syndromes have been reported in human patients taking azithromycin.[30] The clinical significance in veterinary patients is unknown.

Prescription order errors for azithromycin and azathioprine have occurred. Use of tall man letters (eg, aZITHROmycin, azaTHIOprine) may reduce the risk for errors.

Adverse Effects

Azithromycin can cause vomiting, reduced appetite, and diarrhea in small animals. As compared with erythromycin, azithromycin has significantly fewer GI adverse effects. Local reactions have occurred in patients receiving IV azithromycin.

In a small preliminary study of horses administered azithromycin 10 mg/kg PO once daily for 5 days, no life-threatening adverse effects were observed[8]; however, anecdotally, azithromycin use in adult horses has resulted in fatal colitis. Anhidrosis has been noted in foals but appears to be less significant than with erythromycin.[31] Some self-limiting GI adverse effects (eg, decreased appetite, change in fecal consistency) were observed, which raises concerns for potential serious antimicrobial-associated enterocolitis.[7]

Reproductive/Nursing Safety

Safe use of azithromycin during pregnancy has not been fully established; therefore, it should only be used when it is clearly necessary. Humans excrete low amounts of azithromycin in breast milk. The clinical significance in veterinary patients is unknown.

Because safety has not been established in animals, this drug should only be used when the maternal benefits outweigh the potential risks to offspring.

Overdose/Acute Toxicity

Acute oral overdoses are unlikely to cause significant morbidity other than vomiting, diarrhea, and GI cramping.

For patients that have experienced or are suspected to have experienced an overdose, consultation with a 24-hour poison consultation center specializing in providing veterinary-specific information is recommended. For general information related to overdose and

toxin exposures, as well as contact information for poison control centers, refer to *Appendix*.

Drug Interactions

The following drug interactions with azithromycin either have been reported or are theoretical in humans or animals and may be of significance in veterinary patients. Unless otherwise noted, use together is not necessarily contraindicated, but the potential risks must be weighed and additional monitoring performed when appropriate.

- **Amiodarone**: Increased risk for QT prolongation when combined with azithromycin
- **Antacids, Oral** (eg, **magnesium-** and **aluminum-containing**): May reduce the rate of absorption of azithromycin; administration is suggested to be separated by 2 hours.
- **Azole Antifungals** (eg, **ketoconazole, voriconazole**): Azithromycin may prolong QT intervals. This effect may be increased when it is combined with other agents that also prolong QT intervals and/or alter azithromycin metabolism.
- **Cisapride**: No data exist on azithromycin, but other macrolides (eg, **clarithromycin**) are contraindicated with cisapride due to risk for QT prolongation; caution is advised.
- **Cyclosporine**: Azithromycin may increase cyclosporine blood levels; careful monitoring is necessary.
- **Digoxin**: Increased risk for digoxin toxicity when used concurrently
- **Estriol**: Azithromycin may decrease estriol's therapeutic effect.
- **Leflunomide**: Azithromycin may increase risk for hepatotoxicity.
- **Methotrexate**: Azithromycin may increase methotrexate levels and risk for hepatotoxicity.
- **Ondansetron**: Increased risk for QT prolongation when combined with azithromycin
- **P-Glycoprotein Substrates** (eg, **colchicine, doxorubicin, morphine, vincristine**): Azithromycin inhibits p-glycoprotein transport mechanisms and may increase serum concentrations of certain substrates mediated by this transport system.
- **Procainamide**: Increased risk for QT prolongation when combined with azithromycin
- **Quinidine**: Increased risk for QT prolongation when combined with azithromycin
- **Quinolones** (eg, **ciprofloxacin, enrofloxacin**): Increased risk for QT prolongation when combined with azithromycin
- **Sotalol**: Increased risk for QT prolongation when combined with azithromycin
- **Tacrolimus**: Azithromycin may increase tacrolimus blood levels; careful monitoring is necessary.
- **Theophylline**: Azithromycin may reduce theophylline metabolism and increase risk for toxicity.
- **Warfarin**: Increased risk for bleeding; careful monitoring is necessary.

Dosages

DOGS:

Susceptible infections (extra-label): There is significant variability in anecdotal dosing recommendations. Most recommendations are 5 – 10 mg/kg PO once daily for 3 to 7 days. Because of the drug's pharmacokinetics, after a few days of once-a-day dosing, some clinicians recommend every-other-day dosing, or giving higher doses (eg, 10 – 15 mg/kg) twice per week; these dosing regimens may be effective for longer-term treatment of some infections. 10 mg/kg PO every 24 hours for 3 days, weekly, has been recommended for skin infections,[21] although clinical data are lacking and azithromycin is not a recommended drug in recent superficial bacterial folliculitis guidelines.[32]

a) ***Babesia gibsoni*** **or** ***Babesia microti*** (extra-label): azithromycin 10 mg/kg PO every 24 hours in combination with atovaquone 13.3 mg/kg PO every 8 hours with a fatty meal for 10 days. Reserve immunosuppressive therapy for cases not rapidly responding (3 to 5 days) to antiprotozoal therapy.[16,18,33]

b) **Theileriosis** (extra-label): Azithromycin 10 mg/kg PO every 24 hours in combination with atovaquone 13.3 mg/kg PO every 8 hours with a fatty meal for 10 days[19]

c) **Cryptosporidiosis** (extra-label): 5 – 10 mg/kg PO twice daily for 5 to 7 days

GI promotility (extra-label): 2 mg/kg IV, PO every 8 hours[3]

Reducing gingival hyperplasia caused by cyclosporine (extra-label): 10 mg/kg PO once daily for 4 to 6 weeks[34,35]

Papillomatosis (extra-label): 10 mg/kg PO every 24 hours for 10 days[4]

CATS:

Susceptible infections (extra-label): There is significant variability in dosing recommendations. Most clinicians recommend 5 – 10 mg/kg PO every 24 hours for 3 to 7 days. Some infections require longer treatment durations (see below). Based on the drug's pharmacokinetics, after a few days of once-daily dosing, some clinicians recommend every-48-hour dosing or giving higher doses (eg, 10 – 15 mg/kg) twice weekly; these dosing regimens may be effective for longer-term treatment. Sample indications and treatment recommendations follow:

a) **Upper respiratory infections** (extra-label): 5 – 10 mg/kg PO every 24 hours for 5 days, then every 72 hours (ie, every third day) long-term. After an initial positive response to azithromycin, therapy should be continued for 6 to 8 weeks without changing the antibiotic.

b) **Bartonellosis** (extra-label): 10 mg/kg PO every 24 hours for 21 days. Response to therapy is rapid; most cats with anterior uveitis will show significant improvement in less than one week. Recurrence after 21 days of treatment with good flea control is low. Treatment failure in *Bartonella*-positive cats indicates a polymicrobial disease syndrome.[36]

c) **Cryptosporidiosis** (extra-label): 10 mg/kg PO every 24 hours; optimal duration of therapy is unknown but is usually several weeks.[37] This treatment may be helpful for cats that are intolerant or nonresponsive to tylosin.

d) **Cytauxzoonosis** (extra-label): 10 mg/kg PO every 24 hours in combination with atovaquone 15 mg/kg PO every 8 hours for 10 days.[38,39] All cases were also treated with IV fluids and most received heparin.[38,39] Consider placing a feeding tube to reduce the stress of administering these oral medications, and ensure food intake to maximize antimicrobial absorption

e) **Toxoplasmosis** (extra-label): 10 mg/kg PO every 24 hours for a minimum of 4 weeks

GI promotility (extra-label): 2 mg/kg IV, PO every 8 hours[3]

HORSES:

Rhodococcus equi **in foals** (extra-label): 10 mg/kg PO every 24 hours in combination with rifampin 5 mg/kg PO every 12 hours.[40,41] Based on the drug's pharmacokinetics (persistence in bronchoalveolar cells and pulmonary epithelial lining fluid) after 5 days of once-daily treatment, consideration should be given for every-48-hours dosing in foals responding to treatment.[41] **NOTE**: Combination therapy with azithromycin/rifampin was shown to be inferior to clarithromycin/rifampin.[40]

CATTLE:

Cryptosporidiosis in calves (extra-label): 20 mg/kg PO once daily for 6 days in combination with toltrazuril 20 mg/kg PO every other day for 3 treatments.[15] Alternatively, azithromycin 1500 mg/calf (NOT mg/kg) PO once daily for 7 days[14]

RABBITS:

Staphylococcal osteomyelitis (extra-label): 50 mg/kg PO every 24 hours in combination with rifampin 40 mg/kg PO every 12 hours[42]

Jaw abscesses (extra-label): 15 – 30 mg/kg PO every 24 hours. Systemic antibiotic treatment is continued for 2 to 4 weeks postoperatively. Owners need to be advised to discontinue treatment if anorexia or diarrhea occurs.[43]

GUINEA PIGS:

Pneumonia (extra-label)**:** 15 – 30 mg/kg PO every 24 hours. Owners need to be advised to discontinue treatment if their animal develops soft stools.[44]

BIRDS:

Chlamydiosis (study done in experimentally infected cockatiels) (extra-label): 40 mg/kg PO every 48 hours for 21 days was used to treat experimentally infected cockatiels; this treatment was effective as a 21- or 45-day treatment with doxycycline. Dosed via metallic feeding tube into crop using commercially available human oral suspension.[45]

Monitoring

- Clinical efficacy
- Adverse effects (eg, vomiting, diarrhea, inappetence)

Client Information

- Give this medicine as directed by your veterinarian.
- Oral suspension should be shaken well before each use. Store the suspension at room temperature (do not refrigerate). It is preferable to give suspension when the animal has an empty stomach.
- Any unused oral suspension should be discarded after 10 days.
- Contact your veterinarian if your animal develops persistent or severe diarrhea or vomiting, or if your animal's condition worsens after the start of therapy.

Chemistry/Synonyms

Semisynthetic azalide macrolide antibiotics azithromycin dihydrate and azithromycin monohydrate occur as white crystalline powder. In 1 mL of water at neutral pH and 37°C (98.6°F), 39 mg are soluble. Although commercial preparations are available as dihydrates and monohydrates, potency is noted as the anhydrous form.

Azithromycin may also be known as azithromycinum, acitromicina, CP-62993, or XZ-450; many trade names are available.

Storage/Stability

Commercially available tablets should be stored at room temperature less than 30°C (86°F). Oral suspension products for reconstitution should be stored at room temperatures between 5°C to 30°C (41°F-86°F) before reconstitution. After reconstitution, the multiple-dose product may be stored at room temperatures between 5°C to 30°C (41°F-86°F) for up to 10 days, then discarded. The single-dose packets should be given immediately after reconstitution.

Intact injectable product should be stored at room temperature below 30°C (86°F). After reconstitution with sterile water for injection, solutions containing 100 mg/mL will be stable for 24 hours if stored below 30°C (86°F). Further diluted solution of 2 mg/mL or less will remain physically and chemically stable for 24 hours at room temperature and up to 7 days if refrigerated at 5°C (41°F).

Compatibility/Compounding Considerations

Compatibility is dependent on factors such as pH, concentration, temperature, and diluent used; specialized references or a hospital pharmacist can be consulted for more specific information.

500-mg vials can be reconstituted with 4.8 mL of sterile water for injection using a nonautomated 5-mL syringe (vials are supplied under vacuum). 1 mL will contain 100 mg of azithromycin.

Azithromycin injection must be further diluted in a compatible IV solution and administered by IV infusion over 1 to 3 hours. It is physically and chemically **compatible** with: 0.45% and 0.9% sodium chloride, 5% Dextrose, lactated Ringer's solution (LRS), 5% Dextrose with 0.225% or 0.45% sodium chloride, *Normosol-M* and 5% Dextrose, *Normosol R* and 5% Dextrose, and LRS and 5% Dextrose. When azithromycin injection is diluted into 250 to 500 mL of a compatible solution, it remains physically and chemically stable for 24 hours at room temperature and up to 7 days if refrigerated at 5°C (41°F).

Azithromycin is **Y-site compatible** with ampicillin, ampicillin/sulbactam, buprenorphine, butorphanol, calcium salts, doxycycline, hydromorphone, magnesium sulfate, mannitol, metronidazole, ondansetron, pantoprazole, ranitidine, sodium bicarbonate, and vasopressin. Azithromycin is **incompatible** or has **variable compatibility** with midazolam, amikacin, famotidine, furosemide, gentamicin, morphine, and potassium chloride (KCl).

Dosage Forms/Regulatory Status

VETERINARY-LABELED PRODUCTS: NONE

Preparations compounded for dogs and cats may be available from compounding pharmacies.

HUMAN-LABELED PRODUCTS:

Azithromycin Oral Tablets: 250 mg, 500 mg, and 600 mg (as dihydrate); *Zithromax*®, generic; (Rx)

Azithromycin Powder for Oral Suspension (banana-cherry and cherry flavors): After reconstitution: 100 mg/5 mL (20 mg/mL) in 15 mL bottles; 200 mg/5 mL (40 mg/mL) in 15 mL, 22.5 mL, and 30 mL bottles (as monohydrate); 1 gram per packet in single-dose packets (as dihydrate); *Zithromax*®, generic; (Rx); 2 grams; *Zmax*®, brand (Rx)

Azithromycin Powder for Injection (lyophilized): 500 mg in 10 mL vials (as dihydrate); *Zithromax*®, generic; (Rx)

References

For the complete list of references, see **wiley.com/go/budde/plumb**

Benazepril

(ben-***a***-za-pril) *Lotensin*®

Angiotensin Converting Enzyme (ACE) Inhibitor

See also ***Spironolactone/Benazepril***

Prescriber Highlights

- Used to treat heart failure, hypertension, chronic kidney disease (CKD), and proteinuria in dogs and cats
- Not recommended for use in patients with acute kidney injury. Should be used with caution in volume-depleted patients, and in patients with increased serum creatinine, hyponatremia, coronary or cerebrovascular insufficiency, collagen vascular disease (eg, systemic lupus erythematosus [SLE]), and hematologic disorders
- Adverse effects are uncommon. GI disturbances are the most likely adverse effect, but hypotension, renal dysfunction, and hyperkalemia are possible.
- Avoid use during pregnancy

Uses/Indications

Benazepril may be useful as a vasodilator in the treatment of congestive heart failure (CHF). Reasonable evidence exists to support the theory that angiotensin converting enzyme (ACE) inhibitors increase survival (as compared with placebo) in dogs with dilated cardiomyopathy and mitral valve disease,[1,2] although pimobendan monotherapy appears to be superior to benazepril alone.[3–5] Benazepril/spironolactone was also superior to benazepril in dogs with CHF and receiving furosemide in a blinded, multi-center clinical trial.[6] Amlodipine was superior to benazepril in lowering left atrial pressure in a small study of dogs with experimentally induced mitral valve regurgitation.[7] In dogs with Stage C heart disease (myxomatous mitral valve disease and mitral regurgitation resulting in CHF) and Stage D heart disease (myxomatous mitral valve disease and mitral regurgitation resulting in CHF refractory to standard treatment), a consensus recommendation from the ACVIM is to use an ACE inhibitor such as benazepril as part of multimodal therapy.[8]

Use of benazepril in dogs with heart disease prior to CHF (eg, dogs with Stage B2 myxomatous mitral valve disease indicating mitral regurgitation and cardiac remodeling resulting in cardiomegaly but without clinical signs) remains controversial.[8,9,9–11] Although one retrospective study suggested a benefit of benazepril in subclinical dogs with myxomatous mitral valve disease,[9] a prospective placebo-controlled study failed to show the benefit of benazepril/spironolactone in subclinical disease with cardiac remodeling (Stage B2). In a retrospective study of Doberman pinschers with subclinical dilated cardiomyopathy, benazepril appeared to delay the progression to overt disease compared to dogs receiving no ACE inhibitor.[12] The benefit, or lack of benefit, of ACE inhibitors in dogs with heart disease may relate to dose, with a retrospective study suggesting a twice daily dosing of ACE inhibitors was predictive of 2-year survival.[13]

In cats with heart disease, including subclinical cats and those with CHF, no benefit of benazepril therapy was observed in a prospective, randomized, blinded clinical trial of 151 cats.[14] In horses, a short-term (28 day) study of benazepril showed improved echocardiographic changes for horses with left-sided valvular regurgitation compared to placebo.[15]

Benazepril may also be used in the treatment of systemic hypertension.[16] One study of dogs with hyperadrenocorticism found that benazepril controlled high blood pressure in 18 of 31 hypertensive dogs, with the other 13 dogs requiring additional medication (ie, amlodipine) for control.[17]

ACE inhibitors may also be used in the adjunctive treatment of chronic kidney disease (CKD)[18,19] and for treatment of protein-losing glomerulonephropathies. Studies demonstrate that benazepril reduces urine protein:creatinine (UP:C) ratios over the progression of canine[18] and feline[20] CKD. Benazepril has been shown to increase survival in cats with CKD associated with a UP:C ratio greater than or equal to 0.8.[21] In one comparative feline study, telmisartan and benazepril each reduced UP:C as compared with baseline, but only the reduction by telmisartan reached statistical significance.[22] Benazepril is cleared via both renal and hepatic routes in contrast to enalapril (primarily renal), potentially allowing it to be more safely administered in patients with decreased renal function. Benazepril may also be an effective treatment for idiopathic renal hematuria in dogs.[23]

Outside of the United States (eg, United Kingdom, Australia), benazepril is indicated for reducing protein loss associated with chronic kidney disease in dogs and cats and for the treatment of heart failure in dogs. In the United States, a combination product (*Cardalis*®) in a fixed dose with spironolactone is approved with concurrent diuretic therapy for the management of clinical signs of mild, moderate, or severe CHF in dogs.

Pharmacology/Actions

Benazepril is a prodrug and has little pharmacologic activity of its own. After being hydrolyzed in the liver to benazeprilat, the drug inhibits the conversion of angiotensin-I to angiotensin-II by inhibiting angiotensin-converting enzyme (ACE). Angiotensin-II is a vasoconstrictor that stimulates production of aldosterone in the adrenal cortex. By blocking angiotensin-II formation, ACE inhibitors generally reduce blood pressure in hypertensive patients and vascular resistance in patients with CHF. Decreased angiotensin-II and aldosterone also reduce sodium/water retention and can limit cardiac fibrosis and remodeling.[24,25] Aldosterone breakthrough (ie, insufficient suppression of aldosterone secretion) has been documented with ACE-I use in healthy dogs.[26,27]

When administered to dogs with heart failure at low doses (0.1 mg/kg every 12 hours), benazepril improved clinical signs but did not significantly affect blood pressure.[28]

ACE inhibitors' proteinuric-reducing effects are most likely a result of reduced intraglomerular hypertension from a vasodilating effect on efferent glomerular arterioles. Reduction in glomerular hypertension may be accompanied by an increase in serum creatinine concentration.

In cats with CKD, benazepril has been shown to reduce systemic arterial pressure and glomerular capillary pressure while increasing renal plasma flow and preserving glomerular filtration rate (GFR). It may also help improve appetite. There is no evidence that ACE inhibitors reduce pathologic cardiac hypertrophy in cats.

Benazepril (0.5 mg/kg PO once daily) effectively inhibited ACE in healthy adult horses[29] and, at higher doses (1 – 4 mg/kg PO as a single dose), attenuated response to angiotensin-I.[30] Benazepril use increased cardiac output in horses with left-sided valvular regurgitation, and echocardiographic assessments suggested a reduced afterload.[15]

Like enalapril and lisinopril, but not captopril, benazepril does not contain a sulfhydryl group. ACE inhibitors containing sulfhydryl groups (eg, captopril) may have a greater tendency to cause immune-mediated reactions.

Pharmacokinetics

After oral administration in healthy dogs, benazepril is rapidly absorbed and converted into the active metabolite benazeprilat, with peak concentrations of benazeprilat occurring ≈75 minutes after administration. Protein binding is ≈85%. Unlike enalaprilat, which is ≈95% cleared in dogs via renal mechanisms, benazeprilat is cleared via both renal (45%) and hepatic (55%) routes. Benazeprilat terminal half-life is ≈19 hours.[31]

In cats, peak benazeprilat concentrations are reached 2 hours after administration. Inhibition of ACE is long-lasting (half-life, 16 to 23 hours) due to high affinity of benazeprilat to ACE; however, free benazeprilat is eliminated relatively quickly (half-life, 2.4 hours). Only 15% of benazeprilat is eliminated via renal excretion in cats, with 85% excreted via biliary routes. Because benazeprilat exhibits nonlinear binding to ACE in cats, doses over 0.25 mg/kg PO produced only small incremental increases in peak effect or duration of ACE inhibition.[32]

In humans, ≈37% of the dose is absorbed after oral administration, and food apparently does not affect the extent of absorption. Approximately 95% of the parent drug and active metabolite are bound to serum proteins. Benazepril and benazeprilat are primarily eliminated via the kidneys, and mild-to-moderate renal dysfunction apparently does not significantly alter elimination, as biliary clearance may compensate somewhat for reductions in renal clearances. Hepatic dysfunction or age does not appreciably alter benazeprilat concentrations.

Contraindications/Precautions/Warnings

Benazepril is contraindicated in patients that have demonstrated hypersensitivity to ACE inhibitors.

ACE inhibitors should be used with caution in patients with hyponatremia or sodium depletion, hypotension, hypovolemia, coronary or cerebrovascular insufficiency, or preexisting hematologic abnormalities,[21] or a collagen vascular disease (eg, systemic lupus erythematosus [SLE]). Patients with severe CHF or that recently received aggressive diuretic therapy should be monitored very closely for progressive azotemia following initiation of therapy.

Because ACE inhibitors may decrease GFR and worsen azotemia, they are generally avoided in critically ill patients with acute kidney injury.

Benazepril can potentially be confused with *Benadryl®* on written prescriptions and written or verbal orders. Use tall man letters to distinguish (ie, benAZEPril, benADRYl).

Adverse Effects

Benazepril's adverse effect profile in dogs is not well described. Adverse effects of other ACE inhibitors in dogs usually center around GI distress (eg, anorexia, vomiting, diarrhea); fatigue, lethargy, ataxia, and incoordination have also been observed. Potentially, hypotension, renal dysfunction, and hyperkalemia could occur. Plasma creatinine concentration may increase at the start of therapy in patients with CKD or dehydration.

In one study evaluating cats with CKD and nonazotemic cats with cardiac disease and comparing pretreatment and posttreatment values, with all cats receiving a mean dosage of benazepril 0.79 mg/kg orally once daily, no cats experienced systemic hypotension, and only 1 cat (out of 24) with CKD experienced hyperkalemia during days 31 through 60; no cats in the nonazotemic group experienced hyperkalemia.[15]

Reproductive/Nursing Safety

Benazepril crosses the placenta.[33] ACE inhibitor use in rodents has resulted in decreased fetal weights and increased fetal and maternal death rates. In rats, use of ACE inhibitors at label dosages during the second and third trimesters is associated with fetal malformation, and fetal and neonatal morbidity and mortality. In humans, benazepril is to be discontinued as soon as pregnancy is detected. In some countries where benazepril is approved for veterinary use, it is contraindicated to use during pregnancy or lactation.[31]

Benazepril is distributed into human breastmilk in very small amounts and is not expected to cause adverse effects in a nursing infant.[33,34]

Because safety has not been established in animals, this drug should only be used when the maternal benefits outweigh the potential risks to offspring.

Overdose/Acute Toxicity

In healthy cats given mild overdoses (2 mg/kg PO once daily for 52 weeks), only increased food consumption and weight gain were noted.[21] Reduced red blood cell (RBC) counts occurred in healthy cats given 10 mg/kg/day and healthy dogs receiving 150 mg/kg/day for 12 months.[21] A 200-fold overdose was tolerated in dogs without incident.[21] In overdose situations, the primary concern is hypotension. Supportive treatment is recommended, including volume expansion with appropriate IV fluid therapy if hypotension is documented and cardiac function will tolerate volume expansion. Because of the drug's long duration of action, prolonged monitoring and treatment may be required. Recent massive overdoses should be managed using standard decontamination protocols as appropriate.

There were 298 single agent exposures to benazepril reported to the ASPCA Animal Poison Control Center (APCC) between 2009 and 2013. Of the 256 dogs exposed, 30 showed clinical signs (ie, vomiting [33%], lethargy [27%], tachycardia [27%], hypotension [17%]).

For patients that have experienced or are suspected to have experienced an overdose, consultation with a 24-hour poison consultation center specializing in providing veterinary-specific information is recommended. For general information related to overdose and toxin exposures, as well as contact information for poison control centers, refer to ***Appendix***.

Drug Interactions

The following drug interactions have either been reported or are theoretical in humans or animals receiving benazepril and may be of significance in veterinary patients. Unless otherwise noted, use together is not necessarily contraindicated, but the potential risks should be weighed and additional monitoring performed when appropriate.

- **ALLOPURINOL:** Concurrent use may cause severe hypersensitivity reactions, neutropenia, agranulocytosis, or serious infections.
- **ALPHA-2 ADRENERGIC AGONISTS** (eg, **dexmedetomidine**): Concurrent use may result in additive effects on blood pressure and heart rate.
- **ANTIDIABETIC AGENTS** (eg, **insulin, oral agents**): Possible increased risk for hypoglycemia; enhanced monitoring is recommended
- **ANTIHISTAMINES** (eg, **diphenhydramine**): Concurrent use may result in additive hypotension.
- **ANTIHYPERTENSIVE AGENTS** (eg, **amlodipine**): Concurrent use may result in hypotension or hypovolemia. Concurrent use of multiple antihypertensive agents may be required to control hypertension in some animals.
- **APOMORPHINE:** Concurrent use may potentiate the hypotensive effects of benazepril.
- **ANGIOTENSIN RECEPTOR ANTAGONISTS (ARBS)** (eg, **candesartan, telmisartan**): Concurrent use may increase the risk for adverse effects such as hypotension, syncope, hyperkalemia, changes in renal function, or acute renal insufficiency.
- **ASPIRIN**: Aspirin may potentially negate the decrease in systemic vascular resistance induced by ACE inhibitors; however, one study in dogs using low-dose aspirin showed that the hemodynamic effects of enalaprilat (active metabolite of enalapril, a related drug) were not affected.
- **AZATHIOPRINE**: Concurrent use may result in an increased risk for neutropenia or leukopenia.
- **BARBITURATES**: Concurrent use may enhance the hypotensive effects of benazepril.
- **BENZODIAZEPINES** (eg, **alprazolam, diazepam, midazolam**): Concurrent use may lead to low blood pressure.
- **BUSPIRONE:** Concurrent use may increase risk for hypotension.
- **CABERGOLINE:** Concurrent use may lead to additive hypotension.
- **CORTICOSTEROIDS** (eg, **dexamethasone, prednis(ol)one**): May decrease antihypertensive effects by causing fluid and sodium retention
- **CYCLOSPORINE:** Concurrent administration may increase the risk for hyperkalemia or precipitate acute renal failure.
- **DALTEPARIN/ENOXAPARIN:** Concurrent use may increase risk for hyperkalemia.
- **DIAZOXIDE:** Concurrent use may lead to hypotension and orthostasis.
- **DIURETICS** (eg, **furosemide, hydrochlorothiazide**): Potential for increased hypotensive effects. May be used concurrently for management of heart failure.
- **DIURETICS, POTASSIUM-SPARING** (eg, **spironolactone, triamterene**): Concurrent use may increase hyperkalemic effects. Enhanced monitoring of serum potassium concentration is recommended.
- **FENOLDOPAM:** Concurrent administration may theoretically increase the risk for severe hypotension.
- **FURAZOLIDONE:** Concurrent use may increase risk for hypotension.

- **Glycerin:** Concurrent use may increase risk for hypovolemia and hypotension.
- **Heparin:** Concurrent use may increase the risk for hyperkalemia.
- **Interferon Alfa:** Concurrent use may increase risk for granulocytopenia.
- **Iodinated Contrast Agents** (eg, **iohexol**): Concurrent use may increase risk for nephrotoxicity.
- **Iron:** Benazepril may increase severity and risk for systemic adverse effects associated with parenteral administration of iron.
- **Lanthanum:** In theory, lanthanum may bind with drugs in the GI tract and interfere with absorption. Lanthanum should be given 2 hours before or after benazepril.
- **Lithium:** Increased serum lithium concentrations possible; increased monitoring is required
- **Methotrexate:** Concurrent use may potentiate risk for liver injury.
- **Mirtazapine:** Concurrent administration may result in additive hypotension and orthostasis.
- **Muscle Relaxants** (eg, **methocarbamol**): Concurrent use may have additive blood pressure lowering effects.
- **Naltrexone:** Concurrent administration may increase risk for hepatotoxicity.
- **Nitroglycerin:** Benazepril may enhance the vasodilatory and hypotensive effects.
- **Non-Steroidal Anti-Inflammatory Drugs (NSAIDs,** eg, **carprofen, meloxicam, robenacoxib):** Potentially could increase the risk for nephrotoxicity and/or reduce efficacy of the ACE inhibitor in animals with cardiac or renal disease; monitoring is advised[35,36]
- **Opioids** (eg, **hydrocodone, morphine**)**:** Concurrent use may result in additive hypotension and orthostasis.
- **Pentoxifylline:** Concurrent use may increase risk for hypotension.
- **Pergolide:** Concurrent use may increase risk for severe hypotensive episodes.
- **Phenothiazines** (eg, **acepromazine**): Concurrent administration may cause orthostatic hypotension and syncope associated with vasodilation.
- **Polyethylene Glycol 3350:** Concurrent use may increase risk for fluid and electrolyte imbalances leading to renal impairment, cardiac arrhythmias, or seizures.
- **Potassium Supplements:** Increased risk for hyperkalemia
- **Prazosin:** Concurrent use can cause additive hypotension.
- **Pregabalin:** Concurrent use may increase risk for angioedema.
- **Procarbazine:** Concurrent use can cause additive hypotension and orthostasis.
- **QT Prolonging Agents** (eg, **amiodarone, cisapride, fluoroquinolones, ondansetron**): Concurrent use may increase risk for QTc prolongation and arrhythmias.
- **Selegiline:** Concurrent use can cause additive hypotension and orthostasis.
- **Sildenafil:** Concurrent use may potentiate the blood pressure lowering effects of benazepril and cause orthostasis and hypotension.
- **Sulfamethoxazole/Trimethoprim:** Concurrent use may increase the risk for hyperkalemia.
- **Thioguanine:** Concurrent use may potentiate risk for liver injury.
- **Trazodone:** Concurrent use may result in additive hypotension and orthostasis.
- **Tricyclic Antidepressants** (eg, **amitriptyline, clomipramine**): Concurrent use may result in additive hypotension and orthostasis.

Laboratory Considerations

- When **iodohippurate sodium I^{123}/I^{134}** or **Technetium Tc^{99} pentetate renal imaging** is used in patients with renal artery stenosis, ACE inhibitors may cause a reversible decrease in localization and excretion of these agents in the affected kidney that may lead to confusion in test interpretation.

Dosages

DOGS:

Adjunctive treatment of heart failure (extra-label):

a. Initially, 0.25 – 0.5 mg/kg PO once daily. Dosage may be increased up to 0.5 – 1 mg/kg PO once daily[31] **NOTE:** ACE inhibitor dosing remains somewhat controversial with one retrospective study in dogs suggesting twice daily dosing of ACE inhibitors were predictive of 2-year survival.[13]

b. 0.5 mg/kg PO every 12 hours for chronic Stage C heart failure. Use in addition to furosemide (typically 2 mg/kg PO twice daily, up to 8 mg/kg total dose per day), pimobendan (0.25 – 0.3 mg/kg PO every 12 hours), and spironolactone (2 mg/kg PO every 12 to 24 hours).[8]

Adjunctive treatment of proteinuria (extra-label): Begin with 0.5 mg/kg PO every 24 hours. Many dogs will need dosage increases to minimize proteinuria (see ***Monitoring***). Dose can be gradually increased by 0.5 mg/kg per day to a maximum of 2 mg/kg PO per day. Total daily doses can be divided and given every 12 hours.[37] Combination therapy with telmisartan may result in better results than benazepril alone.[38]

Control of systemic hypertension (extra-label): 0.5 mg/kg PO every 12 to 24 hours initially; may increase incrementally up to 2 mg/kg PO twice daily[16]

CATS:

Adjunctive treatment of hypertrophic heart failure (extra-label): Although evidence of efficacy is lacking, some recommend 0.25 – 0.5 mg/kg PO every 12 to 24 hours.

Adjunctive treatment of hypertension (extra-label): Benazepril 0.5 mg/kg PO every 12 hours in cats that do not have blood pressure controlled with amlodipine alone or in those with concurrent proteinuria. Amlodipine or telmisartan are considered first-line agents.[16]

Reduction of proteinuria associated with CKD (extra-label): Most recommend 0.5 – 1 mg/kg PO once daily.[31] Some anecdotal dosage recommendations state that some cats may require the drug every 12 hours but that higher dosages may worsen preexisting azotemia; caution is advised.

HORSES:

Adjunctive treatment of valvular heart disease (extra-label): May have benefit at 1 mg/kg PO every 12 hours in horses with mitral and aortic valve regurgitation.[15]

Monitoring

- Clinical signs of CHF
- Serum electrolytes, creatinine, BUN, and UP:C ratio (if abnormal at baseline) 3 to 14 days after initiation of therapy; recommendation is for dogs with Stage C heart failure[8] but likely applies for other indications as well. **NOTE:** Plasma creatinine concentration may increase at the start of therapy in patients with CKD.
- Blood pressure (if treating hypertension or if clinical signs associated with hypotension arise)

Client Information

- This medicine may be given with or without food. It is usually well tolerated but vomiting and diarrhea can occur. Give with food if vomiting or lack of appetite becomes a problem.

- If your animal develops a rash or signs of infection occur (eg, fever), contact your veterinarian immediately.
- It is important to give benazepril to your animal as directed by your veterinarian. Do not stop or change the dose without your veterinarian's guidance.
- Your animal will need to have regular blood pressure and laboratory tests performed while receiving benazepril. Do not miss these important follow-up visits.

Chemistry/Synonyms

Commercial dosage forms contain benazepril HCl. Benazepril HCl occurs as a white to off-white crystalline powder that is soluble in water and ethanol. Benazepril does not contain a sulfhydryl group in its structure.

Benazepril may also be known as CGS-14824A (benazepril or benazepril hydrochloride). Many trade names are available; veterinary trade names include *Apex® Benazemav®*, *Benefortin®*, *Bexepril®*, *Nelio®*, *Prilben®, and Vetace®.*

Storage/Stability

Benazepril tablets (and combination products) should be stored at temperatures less than 30°C (86°F) and protected from moisture. They should be dispensed in airtight containers. Unused half tablets of chewable veterinary formulations (approved outside the United States) should be returned to the original blister space inside the original carton and used within 1 to 2 days.

Compatibility/Compounding Considerations

No specific information noted

Dosage Forms/Regulatory Status

VETERINARY-LABELED PRODUCTS:

Available in a fixed-dose combination product with spironolactone (*Cardalis®*): 20/2.5 mg spironolactone/benazepril, 40/5 mg, and 80/10 mg

None in the United States. Outside the United States (eg, Australia, Canada, EU, UK): Benazepril Tablets: 2.5 mg, 5 mg, and 20 mg; *Fortekor®* is one example; (POM-V/Rx). Labeled for use in cats to reduce proteinuria associated with chronic kidney disease and to treat heart failure in dogs. Also available as tablets combined with pimobendan or spironolactone.

The Association of Racing Commissioners International (ARCI) has designated this drug as a class 3 substance. Use of this drug may not be allowed in certain animal competitions. Check rules and regulations before entering in a competition while this medication is being administered. Contact local racing authorities for further guidance. See the ***Appendix*** for more information.

HUMAN-LABELED PRODUCTS:

Benazepril HCl Oral Tablets: 5 mg, 10 mg, 20 mg, and 40 mg; *Lotensin®*, generic; (Rx)

Also available in fixed-dose combination products containing amlodipine (*Lotrel®*) or hydrochlorothiazide (*Lotensin HCT®*)

References

For the complete list of references, see **wiley.com/go/budde/plumb**

Betamethasone (Systemic)

(bet-ta-**meth**-a-sone) *Celestone®*

Glucocorticoid

NOTE: For topical or otic use, see ***Betamethasone, Topical*** and ***Corticosteroid/Antimicrobial Preparations***

Prescriber Highlights

- ► Long-acting injectable glucocorticoid; 25 to 40 times more potent than hydrocortisone; no mineralocorticoid activity
- ► Primary use is intra-articular administration in horses; may be used to improve pulmonary condition in preterm puppies.
- ► Relatively safe when used intra-articularly; some systemic absorption occurs, although systemic adverse effects are uncommon.
- ► Teratogenic; may cause preterm labor if administered early in third trimester

Uses/Indications

In veterinary medicine, betamethasone for systemic or intra-articular effects is usually administered as an injection combining betamethasone sodium phosphate (prompt effect) and betamethasone acetate (sustained effect). It can be used when an injectable glucocorticoid that has both rapid- and long-acting effects is desired.

In dogs, prenatal maternal administration of betamethasone improves preterm neonatal pulmonary conditions (ie, improved gas exchange capacity) but not surfactant production, as occurs in humans.[1,2]

In horses, intra-articular injection of betamethasone sodium phosphate/acetate can be useful for treating pain and inflamed joints; pain relief can last up to 4 weeks after injection.[3]

Comparing IV or PO glucocorticoid potency, betamethasone 0.75 mg is approximately equivalent to dexamethasone 0.75 mg, prednisone 5 mg, methylprednisolone 4 mg, or hydrocortisone 20 mg (intra-articular or IM may be different).

Pharmacology

Betamethasone is a long-acting glucocorticoid with a biologic half-life of over 300 hours. Glucocorticoids have effects on almost every cell type and system in mammals.

Cardiovascular system: Glucocorticoids can reduce capillary permeability and enhance vasoconstriction. A clinically insignificant positive inotropic effect can occur after glucocorticoid administration. This drug's vasoconstrictive properties and increased blood volume can result in increased blood pressure.

Cells: Glucocorticoids can inhibit fibroblast proliferation, macrophage response to migration inhibiting factor, sensitization of lymphocytes, and the cellular response to mediators of inflammation; they can also stabilize lysosomal membranes.

CNS/autonomic nervous system: Glucocorticoids can lower the seizure threshold, alter mood and behavior, diminish response to pyrogens, stimulate appetite, and maintain alpha rhythm. Glucocorticoids are necessary for normal adrenergic receptor sensitivity.

Endocrine system: When an animal is not stressed, glucocorticoids suppress the release of corticotropin (adrenocorticotropic hormone [ACTH]) from the anterior pituitary, which reduces or prevents the release of endogenous corticosteroids. Stress factors (eg, renal disease, liver disease, diabetes) may occasionally nullify the suppressing aspects of exogenously administered steroids. The release of thyroid-stimulating hormone (TSH), follicle-stimulating hormone (FSH), prolactin, and luteinizing hormone may be reduced when glucocorticoids are administered at pharmacologic doses. Conversion of thyroxine (T4) to triiodothyronine (T3) may be reduced by glucocorticoids, and plasma levels of parathyroid hormone may be increased. Glucocorticoids may inhibit osteoblast function. Vasopressin (antidiuretic hormone [ADH]) activity is reduced at the renal tubules and diuresis may occur. Glucocorticoids inhibit insulin binding to insulin receptors and the postreceptor effects of insulin.

Fluid and electrolyte balance: Glucocorticoids can increase renal potassium and calcium excretion, sodium and chloride reabsorption, and extracellular fluid volume. Hypokalemia and/or hypocalcemia rarely occur. Diuresis may develop following glucocorticoid administration.

GI tract and hepatic system: Glucocorticoids increase the secretion of gastric acid, pepsin, and trypsin. They alter the structure of mucin and decrease mucosal cell proliferation. Iron salts and calcium absorption are decreased, whereas fat absorption is increased. Hepatic changes can include increased fat and glycogen deposits in hepatocytes and increased serum levels of ALT and gamma-glutamyl transpeptidase (GGT). Significant increases can be seen in serum ALP. Glucocorticoids can cause minor increases in bromosulfophthalein (BSP) retention time.

Hematopoietic system: Glucocorticoids can increase the number of circulating platelets, neutrophils, and RBCs, but platelet aggregation is inhibited. Decreased amounts of lymphocytes (peripheral), monocytes, and eosinophils are seen because glucocorticoids can sequester these cells into the lungs and spleen and can prompt decreased release from bone marrow; removal of old RBCs becomes diminished. Glucocorticoids can cause involution of lymphoid tissue.

Immune system (also see **Cells and Hematopoietic system**): Glucocorticoids can decrease circulating levels of T-lymphocytes; inhibit lymphokines; inhibit neutrophil, macrophage, and monocyte migration; reduce production of interferon; and inhibit phagocytosis, chemotaxis, antigen processing, and intracellular killing. Specific acquired immunity is affected less than nonspecific immune responses. Glucocorticoids can also antagonize the complement cascade and mask the clinical signs of infection. Mast cells are decreased in number and histamine synthesis is suppressed. Many of these effects only occur at high doses and species have different responses.

Metabolic effects: Glucocorticoids stimulate gluconeogenesis. Lipogenesis is enhanced in certain areas of the body (eg, abdomen), and adipose tissue can be redistributed away from the extremities to the trunk. Fatty acids are mobilized from tissues and their oxidation is increased. Plasma levels of triglycerides, cholesterol, and glycerol are increased. Protein is mobilized from most areas of the body (not the liver).

Musculoskeletal: Glucocorticoids may cause muscular weakness, atrophy, and osteoporosis. Bone growth can be inhibited via growth hormone and somatomedin inhibition, increased calcium excretion, and inhibition of vitamin D activation. Resorption of bone can be enhanced. Fibrocartilage growth is also inhibited.

Ophthalmic: Prolonged corticosteroid use (both systemic or topically to the eye) can cause increased intraocular pressure and glaucoma, cataracts, and exophthalmos.

Skin: Thinning of dermal tissue and skin atrophy can be seen with glucocorticoid therapy. Hair follicles can become distended, and alopecia may occur.

Pharmacokinetics

Betamethasone is absorbed into systemic circulation after intra-articular administration to horses.[4] After administration of a 9 mg (total) dose in one joint, peak plasma concentration is reached within 4.5 to 8 hours, and terminal elimination half-life is 4 to 8 hours. After two 15 mg doses administered concurrently in 2 joints, peak plasma and urine concentrations occurred at 0.8 hours and 7.1 hours, respectively, and plasma half-life was 9.2 hours.[5]

Contraindications/Precautions/Warnings

Betamethasone is contraindicated in patients that are hypersensitive to it or any of its excipients. Intra-articular glucocorticoids are contraindicated in the presence of septic arthritis.[4] Because betamethasone injected into joints is absorbed systemically, it should not be used in the face of acute infections.[4]

Systemic use of glucocorticoids is generally considered contraindicated in systemic fungal infections (unless used for replacement therapy in patients with hypoadrenocorticism) and when administered IM in patients with idiopathic thrombocytopenia. Use of sustained-release injectable glucocorticoids is contraindicated for chronic corticosteroid therapy of systemic diseases.

Regardless of the route of administration, betamethasone should be used with caution in patients who have or have history of congestive heart failure (CHF); pre-existing cardiac disease; chronic kidney disease; diabetes mellitus; pre-existing GI disease or history of GI ulcers; or in horses with pituitary pars intermedia dysfunction (PPID) or are at high risk of developing laminitis (eg, history of laminitis, obesity).

Animals that have received chronic, systemic glucocorticoids should be tapered off the drug slowly to allow endogenous adrenocorticotrophic hormone (ACTH) and endogenous corticosteroid to return to function. If the animal undergoes a stressful event (eg, surgery, trauma, illness) during the tapering process or until normal adrenal and pituitary function resume, additional glucocorticoids should be administered.

Do not administer betamethasone suspension for injection by the IV route.

Adverse Effects

Adverse effects are generally associated with long-term systemic administration of this class of drugs, especially if the drugs are administered at high doses or not on an alternate-day regimen. Effects generally manifest as clinical signs of hyperadrenocorticism (eg, polydipsia [PD], polyphagia [PP], polyuria [PU]). When administered to young, growing animals, glucocorticoids can delay growth. See ***Pharmacology***.

In dogs, PD, PP, and PU may all be seen with short-term "burst" therapy as well as with alternate-day maintenance therapy on days when the drug is administered. Adverse effects in dogs associated with long-term use can include dull, dry hair coat; weight gain; panting; poor wound healing; vomiting; diarrhea; elevated liver enzymes; pancreatitis; GI ulceration; hyperlipidemia; activation or worsening of diabetes mellitus; muscle wasting; and behavior changes (eg, depression, lethargy, aggression). Discontinuation of the drug may be necessary; changing to an alternate glucocorticoid (eg, prednis(ol)-one) may also alleviate the problem. With the exceptions of PD, PP, and PU, adverse effects associated with anti-inflammatory dosages are relatively uncommon. Adverse effects associated with immunosuppressive dosages (eg, GI ulceration, infection, poor wound healing) are more common and potentially more severe (eg, pulmonary thromboembolism), especially with long-term use.

Cats generally require higher doses of betamethasone than dogs for clinical effect but tend to develop fewer adverse effects. Occasionally, PD, PP, PU with weight gain, GI ulceration, vomiting, diarrhea, or depression can be seen; however, the development of PU/PD/PP may indicate the development of diabetes mellitus, and diabetes mellitus should be ruled out if these signs develop. Long-term, high-dose therapy can lead to the similar effects seen in dogs.

When used systemically in horses, betamethasone, like other glucocorticoids, may potentially increase the risk for laminitis. Injection site reactions are the most common adverse effect in horses receiving the drug by the intra-articular route. Although systemic absorption of corticosteroids is possible after intra-articular administration, when administered by that route to adult horses, betamethasone sodium phosphate/acetate does not appear to have deleterious effects.[6] However, there is a slight risk for infection (septic arthritis) and postcorticosteroid reactive synovitis after intra-articular injection. In one report, 2 horses developed hyperglycemia after receiving intra-articular betamethasone.[7]

Reproductive/Nursing Safety

Betamethasone has been demonstrated to cause decreased sperm output and semen volume and increased percentages of abnormal sperm in dogs. Corticosteroids have been shown to be teratogenic (eg, reduced fetal growth, cleft palate, deformed forelegs, phocomelia, and anasarca). In developing sheep, betamethasone reduced CNS myelination[8] and affected testicular development in male fetuses.[9] The first stage of parturition may be induced when corticosteroids, including betamethasone,[2] are administered in the third trimester of pregnancy. Betamethasone injection (0.5 mg on day 55) has been shown in pregnant dogs to induce premature labor. No long-term negative clinical effects in preterm puppies (delivered by C-section on day 58) were detected, and glucocorticoid treatment appeared to enhance vital organ maturation.[10]

Corticosteroids appear in milk and could suppress growth, interfere with endogenous corticosteroid production, or cause other unwanted effects in the nursing offspring. Use with caution in nursing dams.

Overdose/Acute Toxicity

Acute overdoses of glucocorticoids rarely cause serious problems. Clinical signs associated with an overdose reflect the adverse effect profile. Should clinical signs occur, use supportive treatment (eg, fluid therapy, GI protection) as needed.

For patients that have experienced or are suspected to have experienced an overdose, consultation with a 24-hour poison consultation center specializing in providing veterinary-specific information is recommended. For general information related to overdose and toxin exposures, as well as contact information for poison control centers, refer to ***Appendix.***

Drug Interactions

Drug interactions are considered unlikely with intra-articular betamethasone administration. The following drug interactions have either been reported or are theoretical in humans or animals receiving betamethasone *systemically* and may be of significance in veterinary patients. Unless otherwise noted, use together is not necessarily contraindicated, but weigh the potential risks and perform additional monitoring when appropriate.

- AMPHOTERICIN B: May cause hypokalemia when administered concomitantly with glucocorticoids
- ANTICHOLINESTERASE AGENTS (eg, **neostigmine, pyridostigmine**): In patients with myasthenia gravis, concomitant glucocorticoid and anticholinesterase agent administration may lead to profound muscle weakness; if possible, discontinue anticholinesterase medication at least 24 hours prior to corticosteroid administration.
- AZOLE ANTIFUNGALS (eg, **itraconazole, ketoconazole**): Glucocorticoid clearance may be reduced, and the AUC increased.
- CHOLESTYRAMINE: May increase glucocorticoid clearance
- CYCLOPHOSPHAMIDE: Glucocorticoids may inhibit the hepatic metabolism of cyclophosphamide; dosage adjustments may be required.
- CYCLOSPORINE: Concomitant administration of glucocorticoids and cyclosporine may increase the blood levels of each drug by mutually inhibiting hepatic metabolism; clinical significance is not clear.
- DIGOXIN: When glucocorticoids are used concurrently with digitalis glycosides, the risk for digitalis toxicity may be increased should hypokalemia develop; diligent monitoring of potassium and digitalis glycoside levels is recommended.
- DIURETICS, POTASSIUM-DEPLETING (eg, **furosemide, thiazides**): May cause hypokalemia when administered concomitantly with glucocorticoids
- ESTROGENS (eg, **DES, estriol**): May decrease glucocorticoid clearance
- INSULIN: Requirements may increase in patients receiving glucocorticoids.
- ISONIAZID: Serum levels may be decreased by glucocorticoid
- MITOTANE: May alter the metabolism of glucocorticoids; higher-than-usual doses of glucocorticoids may be necessary to treat mitotane-induced adrenal insufficiency.
- NONSTEROIDAL ANTI-INFLAMMATORY DRUGS (**NSAIDs;** eg, **flunixin, phenylbutazone**): May result in increased risk for GI ulceration or bleeding
- PHENOBARBITAL: May result in decreased betamethasone efficacy
- RIFAMPIN: May increase the metabolism of glucocorticoids
- SALICYLATES (eg, **aspirin, bismuth subsalicylate**): Glucocorticoids may reduce salicylate blood levels and may increase the risk for GI ulceration.
- THEOPHYLLINE: Alterations of pharmacologic effects of either drug can occur.
- VACCINES, MODIFIED-LIVE: Patients receiving corticosteroids at immunosuppressive dosages should generally not receive live attenuated-virus vaccines as virus replication may be augmented; diminished immune response may occur after vaccine, toxoid, or bacterin administration in patients receiving glucocorticoids.

Laboratory Considerations

The following laboratory interactions have either been reported or are theoretical in humans or animals receiving betamethasone *systemically* and may be of significance in veterinary patients receiving betamethasone locally:

- Glucocorticoids may increase **serum cholesterol** and **urine glucose** levels.
- Glucocorticoids may decrease **serum potassium.**
- Glucocorticoids can suppress the release of thyroid-stimulating hormone (TSH) and reduce T_3 and T_4 values; thyroid gland atrophy has been reported after chronic glucocorticoid administration.
- Uptake of **I^{131}** by the thyroid may be decreased by glucocorticoids.
- Reactions to **skin tests** may be suppressed by glucocorticoids.
- False-negative results of the **nitroblue tetrazolium test** for systemic bacterial infections may be induced by glucocorticoids.
- Betamethasone does not cross-react with the cortisol assay.

Dosages

DOGS:

Control of pruritus (label dosage; FDA-approved): 0.25 – 0.5 mL/9 kg (20 lb; NOT mL/kg [lb]) body weight IM.[11] Dose chosen is dependent on severity of condition. May repeat when necessary. Relief averages 3 weeks in duration. Do not exceed more than 4 injections. **NOTE**: Product is no longer marketed in the US.

Pulmonary maturation in preterm puppies (extra-label): 0.5 mg/kg IM administered to the bitch at 55 to 57 days postovulation[1,2,12]

HORSES:

Control of pain and inflammation associated with osteoarthritis (label dosage; FDA-approved): 9 mg/joint (NOT mg/kg) by intra-articular injection in up to 2 joints[4]

Intra-articular administration (extra-label): Most dosage recommendations range from 3 – 18 mg/joint (NOT mg/kg) intra-articularly. Repeat doses should be limited to the minimum required to achieve soundness.

Monitoring

Monitoring of glucocorticoid therapy is dependent on its reason for use, dosage, agent used, dosage schedule (daily versus alternate day therapy), route of administration, duration of therapy, and the animal's age and condition. The following list may not be appropriate or complete for all animals; use clinical assessment and judgment should adverse effects be noted:

- Body weight, appetite, GI signs (eg, anorexia, vomiting, diarrhea)
- Signs of edema
- Serum electrolytes
- Total plasma protein, albumin
- Blood glucose
- Growth and development in young animals
- Adrenocorticotrophic hormone (ACTH) stimulation test, if concerned about iatrogenic hyperadrenocorticism

Client Information

- Carefully follow the instructions for how to give this medicine to your animal. Do not suddenly stop giving this medicine without talking to your veterinarian.
- Do not give other medications (including over-the-counter [OTC] medication) or nonsteroidal anti-inflammatory (NSAID) medications while your pet is on this medication without talking to your veterinarian first.
- There are many potential side effects that can be seen with these drugs, including increased or decreased appetite, vomiting, abnormal stool, and increased thirst and urination. Contact your veterinarian if these effects become severe or worsen.
- While your animal is taking this medication, it is important to return to your veterinarian for periodic examinations and blood work. Do not miss these important follow-up visits.

Chemistry/Synonyms

A synthetic glucocorticoid, betamethasone has been manufactured as the base and as the dipropionate, acetate, and sodium phosphate salts. The base is used for oral dosage forms. The sodium phosphate and acetate salts are used in injectable preparations. The dipropionate salt is used in topical formulations.

Betamethasone occurs as an odorless, white to practically white crystalline powder. It is insoluble in water and practically insoluble in alcohol. The acetate salt occurs as a white or creamy-white odorless powder. It is practically insoluble in water and soluble in alcohol. The sodium phosphate salt occurs as an odorless, white to practically white hygroscopic powder. It is freely soluble in water and slightly soluble in alcohol.

Betamethasone may also be known as flubenisolone, *BetaVet*®, or *Celestone*®.

Storage/Stability

The combination injectable product should be stored between 20°C to 25°C (68°F-77°F) and protected from light. Shake well before using.

Compatibility/Compounding Considerations

Compatibility is dependent on factors such as pH, concentration, temperature, and diluent used; specialized references or a hospital pharmacist should be consulted for more specific information.

If coadministration with a local anesthetic is desired, lidocaine 1% or 2% (without parabens or phenol) mixed with betamethasone sodium phosphate/acetate injection has been suggested.[13] The lidocaine should be drawn into the syringe after the dose of betamethasone is drawn up. Do not add lidocaine to the vial of betamethasone.

Dosage Forms/Regulatory Status

VETERINARY-LABELED PRODUCTS:

The Association of Racing Commissioners International (ARCI) has designated betamethasone as a class 4 substance. Use of this drug may not be allowed in certain animal competitions. Check rules and regulations before entering in a competition while this medication is being administered. Contact local racing authorities for further guidance. See ***Appendix*** for more information.

Betamethasone Injectable suspension: 6 mg/mL as 3.15 mg betamethasone sodium phosphate and 2.85 mg betamethasone acetate in 5 mL single-dose vials; *BetaVet*®; (Rx). FDA-approved for use in horses. Not for use in horses intended for human consumption

Intra-articular injection: Betamethasone acetate 12 mg/mL (equivalent to 10.8 mg betamethasone) and 3.9 mg/mL betamethasone disodium phosphate (equivalent to 3 mg of betamethasone); *Betavet Soluspan Suspension*®; (Rx). FDA-approved for use in horses. This product is listed in the FDA Green Book is no longer marketed.

Betamethasone valerate is also found in several otic and topical products either as a single agent or in combination with gentamicin.

HUMAN-LABELED PRODUCTS:

Betamethasone Injection: betamethasone (as sodium phosphate) 3 mg/mL and betamethasone acetate 3 mg/mL suspension in 5 mL multi-dose vials; *Celestone Soluspan*®, generic; (Rx)

Various topical formulations are also available.

References

For the complete list of references, see **wiley.com/go/budde/plumb**

Bethanechol

(beh-***than***-e-kole) *Urecholine*®

Cholinergic

Prescriber Highlights

- Cholinergic agent used primarily to increase urinary bladder contractility; bethanechol can also be used as a prokinetic agent and for treatment of clinical signs associated with dysautonomia. May be useful for adjunctive treatment of equine gastric ulcer syndrome (EGUS)
- Principal contraindications are GI or urinary tract obstructions or when the integrity of the urinary bladder wall is of concern.
- Adverse effects are related to cholinergic effects and include salivation, lacrimation, urination, defecation, GI distress, emesis, and miosis (ie, SLUDGE-M).
- Cholinergic crisis is possible when injecting bethanechol IV or IM; atropine should be readily available.

Uses/Indications

Bethanechol can be used to stimulate urinary bladder contractions in small animal species. This drug appears to be most effective in the treatment of acute and partial detrusor atony secondary to acute urinary bladder overdistension and partial neurogenic lesions and when given in combination with other agents (eg, alpha-adrenergic antagonists, benzodiazepines) to reduce urethral resistance. A pilot study in healthy beagles showed no changes in urethral or urinary bladder function after bethanechol treatment was given for 15 days.[1] Bethanechol can be used as an esophageal prokinetic. This drug can also be used as a general GI prokinetic agent, but other agents (eg, metoclopramide, cisapride) are better tolerated.

Bethanechol has been shown to increase abomasum and duodenum contractility in both healthy dairy cattle and cattle with left displacement of the abomasum (LDA)[2]; however, bethanechol did not alter the abomasal emptying rate in calves.[3]

In horses, bethanechol has been suggested as an adjunctive prokinetic agent for treatment of equine gastric ulcer syndrome (EGUS) and in cases with adynamic ileus and gastroduodenal reflux.[4-6]

Pharmacology/Actions

Bethanechol directly stimulates cholinergic receptors. Its effects are principally muscarinic and has negligible nicotinic activity at recommended dosages. This drug is more resistant to hydrolysis than acetylcholine by cholinesterase and, therefore, has an increased duration of activity.

Pharmacologic effects include increased esophageal peristalsis and lower esophageal sphincter tone, increased tone and peristaltic activity of the stomach and intestines, increased gastric and pancreatic secretions, increased tone of the detrusor muscle of the urinary bladder, and decreased bladder capacity. High parenteral dosages can result in adverse effects related to cholinergic effects on other systems (eg, increased bronchial secretions and constriction, miosis, lacrimation, salivation). When administered SC or PO, bethanechol's effects are predominantly seen in the GI and urinary tracts. A ceiling effect (ie, decreased response despite higher dosages) can be seen secondary to receptor desensitization and calcium depletion.

Pharmacokinetics

No information was located on the pharmacokinetics of this agent in veterinary species. In humans, bethanechol is poorly absorbed from the GI tract, and the onset of action is usually within 30 to 90 minutes after oral administration. After SC administration, effects begin within 5 to 15 minutes and usually peak within 30 minutes. The duration of action after oral administration may last up to 6 hours after large doses and 2 hours after SC administration. SC administration yields a more enhanced effect on urinary tract stimulation than oral administration.

Bethanechol does not enter the CNS when administered at recommended doses; other distribution aspects of the drug are not known. The metabolic and excretory fate of bethanechol has not been described.

Contraindications/Precautions/Warnings

Bethanechol is contraindicated in animals with a known hypersensitivity to the drug. Additional contraindications to bethanechol therapy include urinary outflow obstruction, when the integrity of the urinary bladder wall is of concern (eg, after recent bladder surgery), hyperthyroidism, peptic ulcer disease or when other inflammatory GI lesions are present, recent GI surgery with resection and anastomosis, GI obstruction or peritonitis, hypersensitivity to the drug, epilepsy, bronchoconstrictive disease (eg, asthma), hypotension, severe bradycardia or vagotonia, and vasomotor instability. Bethanechol should only be used in conjunction with another agent that will sufficiently reduce outflow resistance (eg, diazepam, dantrolene [striated muscle], phenoxybenzamine [smooth muscle]) when urinary outflow resistance is increased due to enhanced urethral tone (not mechanical obstruction).

Retrograde urinary reflux to the kidney may occur if bethanechol fails to relax the urethral sphincter.

Adverse Effects

When administered orally to small animal species, adverse effects are usually mild; vomiting, diarrhea, salivation, and anorexia are the effects most likely to occur. Cardiovascular effects (eg, tachycardia, arrhythmias, hypotension) and respiratory effects (eg, asthma, dyspnea) are typically only seen after overdose or with high doses given SC. Bethanechol may stimulate pancreatic stimulation of amylase and lipase, and serum bilirubin and AST may be increased due to retention caused by contraction of the sphincter of Oddi.

In horses, salivation, lacrimation, and abdominal pain (colic) are potential adverse effects.

IV or IM use is not recommended; however, the IV route may be necessary in an emergency situation. Severe cholinergic reactions are likely if the drug is given IV. **If injecting the drug (IV or IM), it is recommended that atropine be immediately available.**

Reproductive/Nursing Safety

No data were located regarding bethanechol use in pregnant animals. It is unknown if bethanechol is distributed into milk.

Because safety has not been established in animals, this drug should only be used when the maternal benefits outweigh the potential risks to offspring.

Overdose/Acute Toxicity

Clinical signs of overdose are cholinergic in nature. Muscarinic effects (eg, salivation, urination, defecation) are usually seen with PO or SC administration. If given IM or IV, a cholinergic crisis can occur; circulatory collapse, bloody diarrhea, shock, and cardiac arrest are possible.

Treatment for bethanechol toxicity is atropine (see ***Atropine***). Epinephrine may also be used to treat clinical signs of bronchospasm (see ***Epinephrine***).

For patients that have experienced or are suspected to have experienced an overdose, consultation with a 24-hour poison consultation center specializing in providing veterinary-specific information is recommended. For general information related to overdose and toxin exposures, as well as contact information for poison control centers, refer to ***Appendix***.

Drug Interactions

The following drug interactions have either been reported or are theoretical in humans or animals receiving bethanechol and may be of significance in veterinary patients. Unless otherwise noted, use together is not necessarily contraindicated, but weigh the potential risks and perform additional monitoring when appropriate.

- **Anticholinergic Drugs** (eg, **atropine, glycopyrrolate, propantheline**): Can antagonize bethanechol's effects
- **Beta Adrenergic Antagonists**: May increase the risk for arrhythmias and bronchospasm
- **Cholinergic Drugs** (eg, **neostigmine, physostigmine, pyridostigmine**): Because of additional cholinergic effects, bethanechol should generally not be used concomitantly with other cholinergic drugs.
- **Ganglionic Blocking Drugs** (eg, **mecamylamine, trimethaphan**): Can produce severe GI and hypotensive effects
- **Quinidine, Procainamide**: Can antagonize the effects of bethanechol

Laboratory Considerations

- None noted

Dosages

NOTE: The injectable product is no longer commercially available in the United States.

DOGS:

Increase urinary bladder contractility caused by detrusor muscle atony or treatment for clinical signs related to dysautonomia (extra-label): 2.5 mg – 25 mg/dog (NOT mg/kg) PO 3 times daily. Some dogs may respond to twice-daily administration.

GI prokinetic (extra-label): 5 – 15 mg/dog (NOT mg/kg) PO every 8 hours. May give up to 25 mg/dog (NOT mg/kg) every 8 hours. Improvement in esophageal motility in dogs with megaesophagus is possible.[7,8]

CATS:

Increase urinary bladder contractility caused by detrusor muscle atony or treatment for clinical signs related to dysautono-

mia (extra-label): 1.25 mg (¼ of a 5 mg tablet) – 7.5 mg/cat (NOT mg/kg) PO 3 times daily. Some cats may respond to twice daily dosing.

HORSES:

Increase urinary bladder contractility caused by detrusor muscle atony (extra-label): 0.025 – 0.075 mg/kg SC every 8 hours for 2 to 3 doses, then 0.25 – 0.75 mg/kg PO 2 to 4 times daily. If no response after 5 days, discontinue therapy. **NOTE:** The PO dose is 10 times that of the SC dose.

Adjunctive treatment for equine gastric ulcer syndrome (EGUS) (extra-label): 0.025 – 0.03 mg/kg SC every 4 to 8 hours until no reflux, then 0.3 – 0.4 mg/kg PO 3 to 4 times daily[9-11]

CATTLE:

Adjunctive treatment for cecal dilation/dislocation (CDD); (extra-label): 0.07 mg/kg SC 3 times daily for 2 days, if clinical signs are mild, defecation is present, and rectal examination does not reveal torsion or retroflexion. If these criteria are not met or no improvement is seen within 24 hours of medical therapy, surgical therapy is recommended. **NOTE:** Compounded preparations are required, as no products are commercially available.[12]

Monitoring

- Clinical efficacy
- Urination frequency, urine volume, and urinary bladder palpation
- Adverse effects including signs of colic

Client Information

- This drug is prescribed to help animals urinate more easily. In horses, it may be used to treat gastric ulcer syndrome.
- It is recommended that food be given with this medicine to reduce nausea and/or vomiting.
- In dogs and cats, side effects include vomiting, diarrhea, lack of appetite, and increased drooling. Contact your veterinarian if any of these signs are severe, worsen, or continue to be a problem.
- In horses, side effects include watery eyes, drooling, and signs of colic. Contact your veterinarian if any of these signs are severe, worsen, or continue to be a problem.

Chemistry/Synonyms

Bethanechol, a synthetic cholinergic ester that is structurally and pharmacologically related to acetylcholine, occurs as a slightly hygroscopic white or colorless crystalline powder with a slight, amine-like or fishy odor. It exhibits polymorphism, with one form melting at 211°C (411°F) and the other form at 219°C (426°F). The drug is freely soluble in water and alcohol.

Bethanechol chloride may also be known as carbamylmethylcholine chloride, *Duvoid*®, *Miotonachol*®, *Muscaran*®, *Myo Hermes*®, *Myocholine*®, *Myotonine*®, *Ucholine*®, *Urecholine*®, *Urocarb*®, or *Urotonine*®.

Storage/Stability

Bethanechol tablets should be stored in air-tight, light-resistant containers at room temperature 20°C to 25°C (68°F-77°F).

Compatibility/Compounding Considerations

No specific information has been noted.

Information on bethanechol oral suspension compounded from commercially available tablets has been published.[13] Triturating 12 bethanechol 50 mg tablets with 60 mL of *Ora-Plus*® and qs ad to 120 mL with *Ora-Sweet*® (or *Ora-Sweet® SF*) yields a 5 mg/mL oral suspension that retains more than 90% potency for 60 days stored at both 5°C (41°F) and 25°C (77°F). Compounded preparations of bethanechol should be protected from light.

Dosage Forms/Regulatory Status

VETERINARY-LABELED PRODUCTS: NONE

The Association of Racing Commissioners International (ARCI) has designated this drug as a class 4 substance. See the ***Appendix*** for more information. Use of this drug may not be allowed in certain animal competitions. Check rules and regulations before entering in a competition while this medication is being administered. Contact local racing authorities for further guidance.

HUMAN-LABELED PRODUCTS:

Bethanechol Chloride Oral Tablets: 5 mg, 10 mg, 25 mg, and 50 mg; *Urecholine*®, generic; (Rx)

An injectable product was formerly commercially available; a compounding pharmacy may be able to prepare a bethanechol injectable form.

References

For the complete list of references, see **wiley.com/go/budde/plumb**

Bisacodyl

(bis-a-***koe***-dill) *Dulcolax*®

Laxative

Prescriber Highlights

- ▶ Stimulant laxative used short-term in dogs and cats
- ▶ Contraindicated in patients with GI obstruction
- ▶ Adverse effects include GI cramping and diarrhea
- ▶ Do not administer with milk products or liquid antacids; tablets should not be crushed or split.

Uses/Indications

Bisacodyl oral and rectal products are used as stimulant laxatives in dogs and cats. Efficacy is improved when patients are adequately hydrated prior to administration.

In preparation of dogs for colonoscopy, bisacodyl in combination with sodium phosphate +/- warm water enema produced a colon-cleansing effect which appeared to be less effective than that achieved with a polyethylene glycol (PEG)-electrolyte solution.[1]

Pharmacology/Actions

A stimulant laxative, bisacodyl is thought to produce catharsis by increasing peristalsis via direct stimulation on the intramural nerve plexuses of intestinal smooth muscle. Bisacodyl has been shown to increase fluid and ion accumulation in the colon thereby enhancing catharsis.

Pharmacokinetics

Bisacodyl is minimally absorbed after either oral or rectal administration. Intestinal or bacterial enzymes convert it to an active desacetyl metabolite, which is excreted in the feces. Onset of action is generally 6 to 10 hours after oral administration and 15 minutes to 1 hour after rectal administration.

Contraindications/Precautions/Warnings

Bisacodyl is contraindicated in patients that are hypersensitive to it. Stimulant laxatives are contraindicated in animals with GI obstruction (not constipation), undiagnosed rectal bleeding, or when the animal is at risk for intestinal perforation. Use with caution in patients with infiltrative bowel disease, acute GI conditions, or dehydration. Review specific product labels carefully as some may contain other active ingredients (eg, docusate).

Bisacodyl should only be used short-term, as long-term use can damage myenteric neurons.

Adverse Effects

Bisacodyl has relatively few adverse effects when used occasionally; abdominal discomfort (cramping), nausea, or diarrhea may be noted after use.

Reproductive/Nursing Safety

Because there is minimal bisacodyl absorption following administration, the risk to the fetus or the nursing offspring is expected to be limited.

Because safety has not been established in animals, this drug should only be used when the maternal benefits outweigh the potential risks to offspring.

Overdose/Acute Toxicity

The reported LD_{50} in a dog after oral administration is 15 g/kg.[2] Overdoses may result in severe cramping, diarrhea, vomiting and, potentially, fluid and electrolyte imbalances. Animals should be monitored and given replacement parenteral fluids and electrolytes as necessary.

For patients that have experienced or are suspected to have experienced an overdose, consultation with a 24-hour poison control center specializing in providing veterinary-specific information is recommended. For general information related to overdose and toxin exposures, as well as contact information for poison control centers, refer to ***Appendix.***

Drug Interactions

The following drug interactions either have been reported or are theoretical in humans or animals receiving bisacodyl and may be of significance in veterinary patients. Unless otherwise noted, use together is not necessarily contraindicated, but weigh the potential risks and perform additional monitoring when appropriate.

- **Antacids, Aluminum-, Calcium- or Magnesium-Containing/ Milk**: Do not give antacids or milk within an hour of bisacodyl tablets as it may cause premature disintegration of the enteric coating resulting in a diminished therapeutic effect.
- **Oral Medications**: Stimulant laxatives may potentially decrease GI transit time thereby affecting absorption of other oral medications. Separate doses by 2 hours if possible.

Dosages

DOGS/CATS:

Cathartic (extra-label): Anecdotally, one 5 mg tablet/cat or small dog (NOT tablet/kg) PO once daily; one to three 5 mg tablets (5 – 15 mg)/dog (NOT tablets/kg) PO once daily for medium to large dogs. Do not break or crush tablets.

Client Information

- This medicine is a stimulant laxative used in dogs and cats.
- Do not crush, split, or allow your animal to chew tablets.
- Diarrhea, stomach pain, and cramping can occur.
- Do not give milk (dairy) products or liquid antacids within one hour of giving the oral tablets as it can dissolve the protective coating on the tablets.
- If you are giving other oral medicines to your animal, try to give them two hours apart from the bisacodyl oral dose. Bisacodyl can prevent other medicines from being absorbed properly.
- Bisacodyl should only be used on an occasional basis; long-term, regular use can cause harm to the intestinal tract.

Chemistry/Synonyms

A diphenylmethane laxative, bisacodyl occurs as white to off-white crystalline powder. It is practically insoluble in water and sparingly soluble in alcohol.

Bisacodyl may also be known as bisacodylum; many trade names are available.

Storage/Stability

Bisacodyl suppositories, enemas, and enteric-coated tablets should be stored at temperatures less than 25°C (77°F) and protected from humidity.

Compatibility/Compounding Considerations

Do not crush tablets. The 10 mg suppositories can be cut lengthwise to deliver a 5 mg rectal dose.

Dosage Forms/Regulatory Status

VETERINARY-LABELED PRODUCTS: NONE

HUMAN-LABELED PRODUCTS:

Bisacodyl Enteric-coated Oral Tablets: 5 mg; *Dulcolax®*, generic; (OTC). **NOTE**: Some *Dulcolax®* products may contain other active ingredients (eg, docusate); check product label carefully.

Bisacodyl Rectal Suppositories: 10 mg: *Dulcolax®*, generic; (OTC)

Bisacodyl Rectal Enema: 10 mg/30 mL; (OTC)

References

For the complete list of references, see **wiley.com/go/budde/plumb**

Bismuth Subsalicylate

BSS

(***biz***-mith sub-sa-***liss***-ih-layt) *Pepto-Bismol®*

Antidiarrheal; Gastroprotectant

Prescriber Highlights

- ► Used to treat diarrhea and as a component of triple/quadruple therapy for treating *Helicobacter* GI infections
- ► High doses may cause salicylism; use with caution in cats.
- ► Constipation/impaction may occur.
- ► May change feces color to gray-black or greenish-black
- ► Bismuth is radiopaque and may interfere with GI radiographic testing.
- ► Refrigeration may improve palatability.
- ► Possible teratogen

Uses/Indications

In veterinary medicine, bismuth subsalicylate products are used to treat diarrhea, as a gastroprotectant, and as a component of triple or quadruple therapy for treating *Helicobacter* GI infections.

In humans, bismuth subsalicylate is used to treat other GI symptoms (indigestion, cramps, gas pains) and in the treatment and prophylaxis of traveler's diarrhea.

Pharmacology/Actions

Bismuth subsalicylate is thought to possess gastroprotectant, anti-endotoxic, and weak antimicrobial properties in the GI tract. It is believed that the parent compound is cleaved in the small intestine into bismuth carbonate and salicylate. The protectant, anti-endotoxic, and weak antimicrobial properties are thought to be derived from the bismuth. The salicylate component has antiprostaglandin activity that may contribute to its effectiveness and reduce clinical signs associated with secretory diarrheas.

Pharmacokinetics

No pharmacokinetic information specific to veterinary medicine has been located. In humans, the amount of bismuth absorbed is negligible, whereas the salicylate component is rapidly and completely absorbed. Salicylates are highly bound to plasma proteins and are metabolized in the liver to salicylic acid. Salicylic acid, conjugated salicylate metabolites, and any absorbed bismuth are all excreted renally.

Bismuth subsalicylate did not alter gastric pH in healthy adult horses.[1]

Contraindications/Precautions/Warnings

Salicylate absorption may occur. Do not use in patients hypersensitive to aspirin or other salicylates. Use of this product in patients with preexisting bleeding disorders or GI ulcers may exacerbate underlying conditions. Because of the potential for adverse effects caused by the salicylate component, this drug should be used cautiously, if at all, in cats. Antidiarrheal products are not a substitute for adequate fluid and electrolyte therapy when required.

Adverse Effects

Bismuth subsalicylate may change stool color to a gray-black or greenish-black; do not confuse with melena. One case report of a rhesus macaque suggests that chronic use may cause renal pigmentation.[2]

In human infants and debilitated individuals, use of this product may cause fecal impaction.

Reproductive/Nursing Safety

Salicylates are possible teratogens and have been shown to delay parturition; in humans, their use should be avoided during pregnancy, particularly during later stages.[3] Use with caution in pregnant animals.

Salicylates are excreted into human breast milk, and salicylate toxicity is possible.[3] Use with caution in nursing dams.

Overdose/Acute Toxicity

Bismuth subsalicylate liquid/suspension contains ≈8.7 mg/mL salicylate. Two tablespoons (30 mL) are approximately equivalent to one 325 mg aspirin tablet. Products containing bismuth may cause neurotoxicity at high doses. Common clinical signs in dogs include diarrhea, lethargy, vomiting, ataxia, weakness, and panting. Common clinical signs in cats include diarrhea, lethargy, and inappetence. See ***Aspirin*** for more information.

For patients that have experienced or are suspected to have experienced an overdose, consultation with a 24-hour poison consultation center specializing in providing veterinary-specific information is recommended. For general information related to overdose and toxin exposures, as well as contact information for poison control centers, refer to ***Appendix***.

Drug Interactions

The following drug interactions have either been reported or are theoretical in humans or animals receiving bismuth subsalicylate and may be of significance in veterinary patients. Unless otherwise noted, use together is not necessarily contraindicated, but weigh the potential risks and perform additional monitoring when appropriate.

- **Aspirin**: Because bismuth subsalicylate contains salicylate, concomitant administration with aspirin may increase salicylate serum concentrations and increase risk for adverse effects (eg, GI ulceration).
- **Angiotensin Converting Enzyme Inhibitors** (**ACEIs**; eg, **benazepril, enalapril**): Salicylates may enhance the nephrotoxic effects and reduce the effectiveness of ACE inhibitors. Monitor appropriately.
- **Anticoagulants** (eg, **heparin, rivaroxaban, warfarin**): May increase bleeding risk
- **Clopidogrel**: May have additive antiplatelet effects
- **Corticosteroids** (eg, **dexamethasone, prednis(ol)one**): Corticosteroids may increase the clearance of salicylates, decrease salicylate serum concentrations, and increase GI bleeding risk.
- **Loop Diuretics** (eg, **furosemide**): Salicylates may decrease the diuretic effect of loop diuretics. The serum concentration of salicylates may be increased by loop diuretics.
- **Methotrexate**: Aspirin may displace methotrexate from plasma proteins, increasing the risk for methotrexate toxicity.
- **NSAIDs** (eg, **carprofen, meloxicam, robenacoxib**): Concomitant administration with NSAIDs may increase the risk of bleeding.
- **Tetracycline Antibiotics** (eg, **doxycycline**): Products containing bismuth can decrease the absorption of orally administered tetracycline products. If both agents are to be used, separate drugs by at least 2 hours and administer tetracycline first. If necessary, tetracyclines may be given 6 hours after bismuth administration.

Laboratory Considerations

- At high doses, salicylates may cause false-positive results for **urinary glucose** if using the cupric sulfate method (*Clinitest®*, Benedict's solution) and false-negative results if using the glucose oxidase method (*Clinistix®* or *Tes-Tape®*).
- **Urinary ketones** measured by the ferric chloride method (Gerhardt) may be affected if salicylates are in the urine (reddish color produced).
- Salicylates in the urine may interfere with **5-HIAA** determinations by the fluorometric method.
- Falsely elevated **vanillylmandelic acid (VMA)** may be seen with most methods used if salicylates are in the urine. Falsely lowered VMA concentrations may be seen if using the Pisano method.
- Urinary excretion of **xylose** may be decreased if salicylates are given concurrently.
- Falsely elevated **serum uric acid** concentrations may be measured if using colorimetric methods.
- As bismuth is radiopaque, it may interfere with GI tract radiologic examinations.

Dosages

NOTE: Liquid doses below refer to suspensions of bismuth subsalicylate that are 17.5 mg/mL (1.75%) (eg, veterinary suspensions, original *Pepto-Bismol®* liquid) unless otherwise specified. Several over-the-counter products list dosages for dogs, cats, horses, cattle, and swine; however, none of the products or labeling are FDA-approved.

DOGS:

Acute diarrhea or as a GI "coating agent" (extra-label): Liquid: 0.25 – 2 mL/kg (4.4 – 35 mg/kg) PO 3 to 4 times per day

***Helicobacter* gastritis infections using triple therapy** (extra-label):

a) Bismuth subsalicylate suspension (original *Pepto-Bismol®*) 0.22 mL/kg (3.85 mg/kg) PO every 4 to 6 hours in combination with metronidazole 15.4 mg/kg and amoxicillin 11 mg/kg PO every 8 hours for 3 weeks[4]

b) Bismuth subsalicylate 262 mg tablets given based on body weight (less than 5 kg (11 lb) = 0.25 tablet; 5 to 9.9 kg (11 to 21.8 lb)= 0.5 tablet; 10 to 24.9 kg (22 to 54.8 lb) = 1 tablet; greater than 25 kg = 2 tablets) every 12 hours in combination with metronidazole 10 mg/kg PO every 12 hours and amoxicillin 15 mg/kg every 12 hours for 2 weeks[5]

c) Bismuth subsalicylate suspension 0.22 mL/kg (3.85 mg/kg) PO every 6 to 8 hours in combination with metronidazole 11 – 15 mg/kg PO every 12 hours and amoxicillin 22 mg/kg PO every 12 hours for 3 weeks[6]

CATS:

Diarrhea (extra-label): 0.5 – 1 mL/kg (8.8 – 17.5 mg/kg) PO every 12 hours. Use cautiously in cats; recommend not treating for more than 3 days[7]

***Helicobacter* gastritis infections using triple therapy** (extra-label): Bismuth subsalicylate suspension (original *Pepto-Bismol®*) 0.22 mL/kg (3.85 mg/kg) PO every 4 to 8 hours in combination with metronidazole 11 – 15.4 mg/kg PO every 8 to 12 hours and amoxicillin 11 – 22 mg/kg PO every 8 hours for 3 weeks[4,6]

***Helicobacter* gastritis infections using quadruple therapy** (extra-label): Bismuth subsalicylate (262 mg tablets; *Pepto-Bismol®*) ¼ tablet/cat (total dose) PO twice daily, ± H_2 blocker (eg, famotidine) or omeprazole in combination with metronidazole

10 mg/kg PO twice daily and amoxicillin 10 – 20 mg/kg PO 3 times daily for 2 weeks[8]

HORSES:

Diarrhea in foals (extra-label):

a) 60 – 120 mL/foal (NOT mL/kg) PO 2 to 4 times per day. **NOTE:** This dose equates to 21 – 42 mg/kg for a 50-kg foal (46.2-92.4 mg/lb for a 110-lb foal).

b) 2 – 5 mL/kg (35 – 87.5 mg/kg) PO divided into 2 to 4 doses[9]

CATTLE:

Diarrhea in cattle (labeled dose, not FDA-approved): 180 – 300 mL/calf (NOT mL/ kg) PO every 2 to 3 hours

Diarrhea in calves (labeled dose, not FDA-approved): 90 – 120 mL/calf (NOT mL/kg) PO every 2 to 3 hours

Diarrhea in calves (extra-label): 60 – 90 mL/calf (NOT mL/kg) PO 2 to 4 times per day

SWINE:

Diarrhea in baby pigs (extra-label): 2 – 5 mL/piglet (35 – 87.5 mg; total dose, NOT mg/kg) PO 2 to 4 times a day for 2 days

FERRETS:

***Helicobacter* gastritis infections using triple therapy** (extra-label):

a) Bismuth subsalicylate 7.5 mg/kg PO in combination with metronidazole 20 mg/kg PO and amoxicillin 30 mg/kg PO every 8 hours for 21-28 days[10]

b) Bismuth subsalicylate 17.5 mg/kg PO every 8 hours in combination with metronidazole 20 mg/kg PO every 12 hours and amoxicillin 20 mg/kg PO every 12 hours for 21 days. Used with gastroprotectants (famotidine and sucralfate)[11]

Monitoring

- Clinical efficacy
- Fluid and electrolyte status in severe diarrhea

Client Information

- Use with caution in cats, as they may be sensitive to the salicylate (aspirin-like compound).
- May cause constipation
- Do not give other drugs to your animal within 2 hours of this drug unless directed by your veterinarian.
- Shake the suspension well; store in the refrigerator to improve palatability. Do not mix with milk.
- May cause stool to change color to a gray-black or greenish-black. This may not indicate a problem. Contact your veterinarian if your animal tires easily or if the stool becomes tarry and black.
- May cause tongue discoloration

Chemistry/Synonyms

Bismuth subsalicylate occurs as a white or nearly white tasteless, odorless powder and contains ≈50% bismuth. It is insoluble in water, glycerin, and alcohol.

Bismuth subsalicylate may also be known as BSS, basic bismuth salicylate, bismuth oxysalicylate, bismuth salicylate, bismuthi subsalicylas, *Bismu-kote*®, *Bismukote*®, *Bismupaste*®, *Bismatrol*®, *Bismed*®, *Bismusal*®, *Bismylate*®, *Bisval*®, *Corrective*®, *Equi-Phar*®, *Gastrocote*®, *Jatrox*®, *Kalbeten*®, *Katulcin-R*®, *Oral-Pro Biz-Cote*®, *PalaBIS*®, *Peptic Relief*®, *Pink Biscoat*®, *Pink Bismuth Rose*®, or *Ulcolind Wismut*®; many other human trade names are available.

Storage/Stability

Bismuth subsalicylate should be stored protected from light. Unless otherwise labeled, store at room temperature (15 °C-30° C [59°F-86° F]); do not freeze.

Compatibility/Compounding Considerations

Bismuth subsalicylate is **incompatible** with mineral acids and iron salts. When exposed to alkali bicarbonates, bismuth subsalicylate decomposes with effervescence.

Compatibility is dependent on factors such as pH, concentration, temperature, and diluent used; specialized references or a hospital pharmacist should be consulted for more specific information.

Dosage Forms/Regulatory Status

VETERINARY-LABELED PRODUCTS:

NOTE: Veterinary labeling does not imply that the product is FDA-approved.

Bismuth Subsalicylate Paste: 5% (50 mg/mL); 10% (100 mg/mL); (OTC). Depending on product, labeled for use in small, medium, and large dogs; 20% (200 mg/mL); (OTC). Labeled for use in horses

Bismuth Subsalicylate Oral Suspension: 1.75% (17.5 mg/mL; 262 mg/15 mL). Many trade names available, generic; (OTC). Available in gallons. Labeled for use in cattle, horses, calves, foals, dogs, and cats. Each mL contains ≈8.7 mg salicylate.

Bismuth Subsalicylate Tablets (each tablet contains 262 mg of bismuth subsalicylate): Labeled for use in dogs; (OTC). One tablet contains ≈102 mg salicylate.

HUMAN-LABELED PRODUCTS:

Bismuth Subsalicylate (BSS) Liquid/Suspension: 87 mg/5 mL; 130 mg/15 mL; 262 mg/15 mL; 524 mg/15 mL; 525 mg/15 mL; in 120 mL, 236 mL, 237 mL, 240 mL, 355 mL, 360 mL, and 480 mL; many trade names including *Pepto-Bismol*®, *Kaopectate*®, *Pink Bismuth*; (OTC). **NOTE**: Regular strength (262 mg BSS/15 mL) contains 8.7 mg/mL salicylate; Extra-Strength (525 mg BSS/15 mL) contains 15.7 mg/mL of salicylate.

Bismuth Subsalicylate Tablets and Caplets: 262 mg (regular and chewable); Many trade names including *Pepto-Bismol*®, *Kaopectate*®; (OTC). One tablet contains ≈102 mg of salicylate.

References

For the complete list of references, see **wiley.com/go/budde/plumb**

Bleomycin

(blee-oh-***mye***-sin) *Blenoxane*®

Antineoplastic

Prescriber Highlights

- ► Antibiotic antineoplastic agent infrequently used for a variety of neoplasms in dogs and cats; intralesional administration may have promise.
- ► Two main toxicity types: acute (fever, anorexia, vomiting, and allergic reactions) and delayed (dermatologic effects, stomatitis, pneumonitis, and pulmonary fibrosis)
- ► Do not exceed total dosage recommendations.
- ► Clinical monitoring for adverse toxicity required when used systemically
- ► The National Institute for Occupational Safety and Health (NIOSH) classifies bleomycin as a hazardous drug; use appropriate precautions when handling.

Uses/Indications

Bleomycin has been used in treatment of lymphomas, oral squamous cell carcinomas, teratomas, and nonfunctional thyroid tumors in both dogs and cats, although more recent evidence suggests extremely limited single-agent activity in canine lymphoma.[1] Bleomycin may be promising for intralesional treatment for localized tumors with or without concomitant electropermeabilization.[2,3] Intralesional bleomycin has been successfully used to treat dogs with acanthomatous ameloblastoma.[4,5]

Pharmacology/Actions

Bleomycin is an antibiotic that has activity against a variety of gram-negative and gram-positive bacteria and some fungi; however, its cytotoxicity to eukaryote cells prevents it from being clinically useful as an antimicrobial drug.

Bleomycin has both a DNA binding site and a site that binds to the ferrous form of iron. By serving as an electron acceptor from the ferrous ion to an oxygen atom in the DNA strand, bleomycin cleaves DNA and causes cellular apoptosis.

Resistance to bleomycin can result from reduced cellular uptake of the drug, reduced ability to damage DNA, increased rates of DNA repair by the cell and drug inactivation by the enzyme bleomycin hydrolase.

Pharmacokinetics

Pharmacokinetic information in veterinary species was not located. In humans, bleomycin is not appreciably absorbed from the GI tract and must be administered parenterally.[6] It is mainly distributed to the lungs, kidneys, skin, lymphatics, and peritoneum. Following IM or SC administration in humans, bleomycin reaches peak concentration within 30 to 60 minutes. In humans with normal renal function, terminal half-life is 2 to 4 hours. In humans, 60% to 70% of a dose is excreted as active drug in the urine.

Contraindications/Precautions/Warnings

Because bleomycin is a cytotoxic agent with a low therapeutic index, it should only be used in clinical facilities able to actively monitor and handle potential complications. Bleomycin is contraindicated in patients with previous hypersensitivity reactions and should be used cautiously in patients with preexisting pulmonary disease or adverse pulmonary effects from prior therapy. Dosage reduction may be necessary for patients with significant renal impairment. Bleomycin can be teratogenic; it should only be used in pregnant animals when the owners accept the associated risks.

A total cumulative bleomycin dose of 125 – 200 mg/m² should not be exceeded in order to reduce the risk of pulmonary toxicity.

The National Institute for Occupational Safety and Health (NIOSH) classifies bleomycin as a hazardous drug; personal protective equipment (PPE) should be used accordingly to minimize the risk for exposure.[7]

Adverse Effects

Toxicity falls into two broad categories: acute and delayed. Acute toxicities include fever, anorexia, mild vomiting, and allergic reactions including anaphylaxis. Delayed toxic effects include dermatologic effects (eg, erythema, hyperpigmentation, rash, and tenderness of the skin), stomatitis, pneumonitis, and pulmonary fibrosis. The latter 2 delayed toxic effects have been associated with drug-induced fatalities. Initial signs associated with pulmonary toxicity include pulmonary interstitial edema with alveolar hyaline membrane formation and hyperplasia of type II alveolar macrophages. Pulmonary toxicity is potentially reversible if cessation of treatment occurs prior to irreversible damage and appropriate supportive care instituted. Unlike many other antineoplastic agents, bleomycin does not usually cause myelotoxicity, but thrombocytopenia, leukopenia, and slight decreases in hemoglobin levels are possible. Renal toxicity and hepatotoxicity are also possible. When administered to dogs at 0.5 units/kg, adverse effects were infrequent and mostly GI related.[1]

To reduce the likelihood of pulmonary toxicity and other adverse effects, a total cumulative dose of 125 – 200 mg/m² should not be exceeded.

Reproductive/Nursing Safety

It is not known if bleomycin enters milk; it is not recommended to nurse while receiving the medication.

Because safety has not been established in animals, this drug should only be used when the maternal benefits outweigh the potential risks to offspring.

Overdose/Acute Toxicity

The intravenous LD_{50} in mice is 53 mg/kg.[8] Due to the potential for serious toxicity associated with this agent, dosage calculations should be checked thoroughly to avoid overdosing. There is no known antidote.

Drug Interactions

The following drug interactions have either been reported or are theoretical in humans or animals receiving bleomycin and may be of significance in veterinary patients. Unless otherwise noted, use together is not necessarily contraindicated, but weigh the potential risks and perform additional monitoring when appropriate.

- **ANESTHETICS, GENERAL:** Use of general anesthetics in patients treated previously with bleomycin should be done with caution. Bleomycin sensitizes lung tissue to oxygen (even to concentrations of inspired oxygen considered to be safe) and rapid deterioration of pulmonary function with postoperative pulmonary fibrosis can occur.
- **PRIOR OR CONCOMITANT CHEMOTHERAPY, RADIATION THERAPY, OR IMMUNOSUPPRESSANTS:** Can lead to increased hematologic, mucosal, and pulmonary toxicities
- **GRANULOCYTE COLONY-STIMULATING FACTORS** (eg, **filgrastim**): Can increase risk for pulmonary toxicity
- **NEPHROTOXIC AGENTS** (eg, **aminoglycosides, amphotericin B, cisplatin, iohexol**): Can increase risk for nephrotoxicity
- **VACCINES (LIVE AND INACTIVATED):** Bleomycin may diminish vaccine efficacy and enhance adverse effects of vaccines.

Laboratory Considerations

None

Dosages

NOTE: Because of the potential toxicity of this drug to patients, veterinary personnel, and clients, and because chemotherapy indications, treatment protocols, monitoring, and safety guidelines change often, the following dosages should only be used as a general guide. Consultation with a veterinary oncologist and referral to current veterinary oncology references[9,10-13] are strongly recommended.

SMALL ANIMALS:

Antineoplastic agent (extra-label): 10 mg/m² (NOT mg/kg) OR 0.3 – 0.5 mg/kg (**NOTE:** 1 unit = 1 mg), IV, SC, or intralesionally. Some protocols use the drug once daily for a few days and then reduce to once weekly; some give the drug once weekly initially.[4,14] To reduce the likelihood of pulmonary toxicity, a total cumulative dose of 125 – 200 mg/m² should not be exceeded. Bleomycin has also been administered in combination with electrochemotherapy.[3,15]

Monitoring

- Efficacy
- Pulmonary toxicity: Obtain thoracic radiographs (baseline and on a regular basis—in humans they are recommended every 1 to 2 weeks); lung auscultation (dyspnea and fine rales may be early signs of toxicity); other initial signs associated with pulmonary toxicity include pulmonary interstitial edema with alveolar hyaline membrane formation and hyperplasia of type II alveolar macrophages.
- Baseline and periodic CBC and serum chemistry profiles (to monitor for potential renal, hepatic, and hematologic toxicities.
- Total dose accumulation (not to exceed a total cumulative dose of 125 – 200 mg/m²)

Client Information

- Bleomycin is a chemotherapy medicine. This medicine can be hazardous to other animals and people that come in contact with it. On the day your animal receives this medicine and then for a few days afterward, all bodily waste (urine, feces, litter), blood, or vomit should only be handled while wearing disposable gloves. Seal the waste in a plastic bag and then place both the bag and gloves in with the regular trash.

- Bleomycin can have serious side effects, including lung damage that could result in death. Be sure to immediately report to your veterinarian any changes to your animal's breathing pattern or quality (eg, shortness of breath, wheezing).
- This medication is considered to be a hazardous drug as defined by the National Institute for Occupational Safety and Health (NIOSH). Talk with your veterinarian or pharmacist about the use of personal protective equipment when handling this medicine.

Chemistry/Synonyms

An antibiotic antineoplastic agent, bleomycin sulfate is obtained from *Streptomyces verticullis*. It occurs as a cream colored, lyophilized powder that is soluble in water and slightly soluble in alcohol. After reconstitution, the pH of the solution ranges from 4.5 to 6. Bleomycin is assayed microbiologically. One unit of bleomycin is equivalent to 1 mg of the reference Bleomycin A_2 standard.

Bleomycin sulfate may also be known as bleomycin sulphate, bleomycini sulfas, *Bileco®*, *Blanoxan®*, *Blenamax®*, *Blenoxane®*, *Bleo®*, *Bleo-S®*, *Bleo-cell®*, *Bleocin®*, *Bleolem®*, *Blio®*, *Blocamicina®*, *Bonar®*, *Oil Bleo®*, or *Tecnomicina®*.

Storage/Stability

Store unopened vials at 2°C to 8°C (36°F-46°F). After reconstituting with sterile saline, sterile water, or bacteriostatic water, the resulting solution is stable for 24 hours.

Compatibility/Compounding Considerations

Compatibility is dependent upon factors such as pH, concentration, temperature, and diluent used; consult specialized references or a hospital pharmacist for more specific information.

Compatible with sodium chloride 0.9% for dilution. Dilution or reconstitution in dextrose 5% in water demonstrated a loss of potency. Bleomycin sulfate is reported to be **incompatible** for Y-site administration with the following drugs: amphotericin B, dantrolene, diazepam, phenytoin, and tigecycline.

Dosage Forms/Regulatory Status

VETERINARY-LABELED PRODUCTS: NONE

HUMAN-LABELED PRODUCTS:

Bleomycin Sulfate lyophilized powder for injection: 15 units and 30 units per vial; *Blenoxane®*, generic; (Rx)

References

For the complete list of references, see **wiley.com/go/budde/plumb**

Bromides

Potassium Bromide

Sodium Bromide

(***broe***-mide) *KBroVet®-CA1*

Anticonvulsant

Prescriber Highlights

- ► Primary or adjunctive therapy for seizure disorders in dogs; rarely used in cats, as it can cause eosinophilic bronchitis
- ► Very long half-life; must give loading dose to achieve therapeutic bromide concentrations faster.
- ► Most prevalent adverse effect in dogs is sedation, especially when the drug is used with phenobarbital. Polyphagia with resultant weight gain is also commonly noted, particularly in the first few months of therapy. Polydipsia and polyuria can also be seen.
- ► Monotherapy with bromide may require higher serum bromide concentration, and risk for toxicity is significantly increased.
- ► Do not feed salty snacks or make abrupt dietary changes; keep chloride in diet stable.
- ► Toxic effects include profound sedation to stupor, ataxia, tremors, hindlimb paresis, or other CNS manifestations.
- ► Dosages for sodium bromide are not the same as potassium bromide; check dosages carefully.

Uses/Indications

Bromide is used as both primary and adjunctive therapy to control seizures in dogs. Historically, bromide was only recommended for use as monotherapy in patients with phenobarbital hepatotoxicity. Potassium bromide is conditionally approved by the FDA for control of seizures due to idiopathic epilepsy.[1] Bromides also are used by some as a primary treatment or as add-on therapy in dogs with inadequate seizure control receiving phenobarbital alone. A study comparing phenobarbital with bromide as a first-choice antiepileptic drug for treatment of epilepsy in dogs found that although both were reasonable choices, phenobarbital was more effective (seizure eradication in 85% of phenobarbital treated and 52% of bromide treated) and better tolerated during the first 6 months of treatment.[2] Potassium bromide or phenobarbital have been demonstrated to be efficacious as add-on therapy for improved seizure control in dogs with idiopathic epilepsy refractory to imepitoin alone, with a response rate of 79% and 69%, respectively.[3]

The high incidence of adverse pulmonary effects precludes routine bromide use in cats.[4,5]

Pharmacology/Actions

Bromide's anti-seizure activity is thought to be the result of its generalized depressant effects on neuronal excitability and activity. Bromide ions compete with chloride transport across cell membranes resulting in membrane hyperpolarization, thereby raising seizure threshold and limiting the spread of epileptic discharges.

Pharmacokinetics

Bromides are well-absorbed after oral administration, primarily in the small intestine. Oral bioavailability in dogs averages 46%,[6] but there can be wide interpatient variability. The presence of food does not appear to affect absorption. Bromides are also well-absorbed after solutions are administered rectally in dogs (bioavailability, 60%-100%). Bromide is distributed in the extracellular fluid and mimics the volume of distribution of chloride (0.2 – 0.4 L/kg).[6,7] It is not bound to plasma proteins and readily enters the CSF (in dogs, ≈80% of serum concentration).[7] Bromide is predominantly excreted unchanged via renal mechanisms. The half-life in dogs has been reported to be ≈15 days,[7] and steady-state serum concentrations are reached after ≈4 months.[7] Alterations in serum chloride levels[8] or diminished renal function can significantly affect bromide elimination rates.

In sheep, when sodium bromide is given IV, the half-life is ≈16 days, and when potassium bromide is given orally, the half-life is ≈14 to 15 days. The oral bioavailability of potassium bromide in sheep is ≈92%.[9]

Contraindications/Precautions/Warnings

Older animals and those with comorbidities may be prone to intolerance (see ***Adverse Effects***) at serum drug concentrations that are tolerated by younger, healthier dogs. Because bromides are primarily renally eliminated, patients with renal dysfunction may require dosage adjustments to minimize risk for bromide toxicity. Potentially, large loading doses of potassium bromide could affect serum potassium concentrations. Use with caution in dogs with an underlying condition that may predispose to electrolyte imbalances[1] (eg, unregulated hypoadrenocorticism or diabetes mellitus).

Potassium bromide must **never** be administered IV due to risk of cardiotoxicity from potassium; use sodium bromide if IV regimen is required.

Because bromides have been associated with serious adverse pulmonary effects in cats,[4,5] they should be used with extreme caution. Some state that the drug should not be used in cats.[1]

Adverse Effects

A systematic review and meta-analysis of adverse effects of antiepileptic drugs in dogs showed strong evidence for potassium bromide safety profile as monotherapy and weak as an adjunctive therapy.[10] Although no statistical significance was found, there was a trend for imepitoin, levetiracetam, and phenobarbital to have a safer profile than bromide. The most common type I adverse effects (dose-dependent and predictable) were ataxia followed by sedation, polyuria, polydipsia, polyphagia, paraparesis, hyperactivity, vomiting, and increased serum ALP and ALT activity. Less commonly, constipation or diarrhea, anorexia, aggression, tetraparesis, skin conditions (eg, panniculitis[11]), euthyroid sick syndrome, anisocoria, and chronic clinical hepatopathy/toxicity, as well as increased serum chloride, bile acids, and AST activity. Type II adverse effects (idiosyncratic dose-independent and unpredictable) were pancreatitis (most common adverse effect reported), followed by panniculitis, generalized appendicular repetitive myoclonus, neuromyopathy with generalized lower motor signs, and hyperchloremia with a negative anion gap.[10]

Ataxia and sedation are common and typically transient (lasting up to 3 weeks); conversely, some dogs show signs of irritability and restlessness. Bromide use reduced trainability in epileptic dogs.[12] GI effects, particularly during oral loading doses, may be reduced or avoided by giving with food or dividing the dose. If the patient cannot tolerate the GI effects (eg, vomiting) of potassium bromide and divided doses with food do not alleviate the problem, switching to sodium bromide may be considered. Potentially, large loading doses of potassium bromide could affect serum potassium concentrations.

In cats, pulmonary adverse effects (eg, cough, dyspnea, eosinophilic bronchitis) have been associated with bromide therapy,[4,5] and its use is rarely recommended. Peribronchial infiltrates may be seen on radiographs and dyspnea may be serious or fatal. Signs appear to be reversible in most cats once bromides are discontinued. Other adverse effects in cats include polydipsia, sedation, and weight gain.

Reproductive/Nursing Safety

Reproductive safety has not been evaluated in veterinary patients. Human infants have suffered bromide intoxication and growth delays after maternal ingestion of bromides during pregnancy. Bromide intoxication has also been reported in human infants breastfeeding from mothers taking bromides.

Because safety has not been established in animals, this drug should only be used when the maternal benefits outweigh the potential risks to offspring.

Overdose/Acute Toxicity

Toxicity is more likely with chronic overdoses, but acute overdoses are possible. Toxicity is generally associated with higher serum bromide concentrations (greater than 2.5 mg/mL), but some dogs can show toxic signs at lower concentrations. Neurotoxic effects are most common and present as profound sedation to stupor or coma, ataxia, tremors, mydriasis, or other CNS manifestations (eg, upper and lower motor neuron signs with tetraparesis/paraparesis, megaesophagus). Hypersalivation, vomiting, and diarrhea are common. In addition, animals that have developed bromism (acute or chronic) may develop signs of muscle pain, conscious proprioceptive deficits, anisocoria, hyporeflexia, and other neurologic deficits.

Standard GI decontamination should be employed after a known acute overdose. Death after an acute oral ingestion is apparently rare as vomiting generally occurs spontaneously. Administration of parenteral 0.9% sodium chloride or oral sodium chloride with parenteral glucose and diuretics (eg, furosemide) may be helpful in reducing bromide loads in either acutely or chronically intoxicated individuals.

For patients that have experienced or are suspected to have experienced an overdose, it is strongly encouraged to consult with a 24-hour poison consultation center that specialize in providing information specific for veterinary patients. For general information related to overdose and toxin exposures, as well as contact information for poison control centers, refer to ***Appendix.***

Drug Interactions

The following drug interactions have either been reported or are theoretical in humans or animals receiving bromides and may be of significance in veterinary patients. Unless otherwise noted, use together is not necessarily contraindicated, but weigh the potential risks and perform additional monitoring when appropriate.

- **Anticonvulsants, Other** (eg, **levetiracetam, phenobarbital, zonisamide**): May increase risk for CNS depression
- **Antihistamines** (eg, **cetirizine**, **diphenhydramine**): May increase risk for CNS depression
- **Benzodiazepines** (eg, **alprazolam, diazepam, midazolam**): May increase risk for CNS depression
- **CNS Sedating Drugs, Miscellaneous** (eg, **acepromazine, methocarbamol, trazodone**): Because bromides can cause CNS depression, other CNS sedating drugs may cause additive sedation.
- **Diuretics** (eg, **furosemide, thiazides**): May enhance the excretion of bromides thereby affecting seizure control and dosage requirements
- **IV Fluids Containing Sodium:** Can reduce serum bromide concentrations. Lactated Ringer's and normal saline reduced serum bromide concentration by 14%.[13]
- **Low/High Salt (Sodium Chloride) Diets**: Bromide toxicity can occur if chloride ion ingestion is markedly reduced. Patients on low-salt diets may be at risk. Conversely, additional sodium chloride in the diet (including prescription diets high in chloride) could reduce serum bromide concentrations, affecting seizure control. Keep chloride content of diet relatively constant while bromides are being administered. If chloride content must be altered, monitor serum bromide concentrations more frequently.[14]
- **Opioids** (eg, **buprenorphine, hydrocodone, morphine, tramadol**): May increase risk for CNS depression. Tramadol appears

to lower seizure threshold in humans[15]; veterinary significance is uncertain.

- **Tricyclic Antidepressants** (eg, **amitriptyline, clomipramine**): May increase risk for CNS depression

Laboratory Considerations

- **Gold chloride assay for serum bromide.** This assay is considered reliable for serum bromide concentrations below 4 mg/mL, but at concentrations above 4 mg/mL, results can become nonlinear and may not be accurate.
- **Chloride, serum**. See ***Drug Interactions*** regarding chloride. Bromide interferes with serum chloride determinations, yielding falsely high results.
- **Hypertriglyceridemia, lipemia.** May interfere with colorimetric assays for serum bromide and give falsely elevated bromide values. A 12-hour fast prior to drawing levels has been recommended.[16]
- Potassium bromide does not affect **canine thyroid function test** results.[17,18]

Dosages

DOGS:

NOTE: Unless otherwise noted, the following dosages are for potassium bromide. If substituting sodium bromide, reduce dosage by 15%.

Controls of seizures associated with idiopathic epilepsy (Label dosage; FDA-conditionally approved): 25 – 68 mg/kg PO once daily; adjust based on clinical response.[1,19] The median dosage in the efficacy trial was 37 mg/kg/day PO.

Epilepsy *loading* dosage (extra-label): Because of the long serum elimination half-life (weeks) in dogs (it may take up to 4 to 5 months for blood levels to reach steady-state concentrations), many dosing recommendations include an initial oral loading dose regimen to reduce the time required to attain therapeutic concentrations. In dogs that are unable to eat, the dose can be divided and given rectally every 4 hours.

1. Potassium bromide 450 mg/kg PO divided into 14 doses, given every 12 hours for 7 days (ie, 32 mg/kg PO every 12 hours for 7 days)[20]
2. Potassium bromide 600 mg/kg PO loading dose given in 5 to 10 equally divided doses over 17 to 48 hours in addition to the 30 mg/kg/day PO maintenance dose. 84% of dogs had bromide concentrations within the therapeutic range within 24 hours of completion of this protocol, 13% had concentrations below the therapeutic range, and 3% had a concentration above the therapeutic range.[21]
3. Sodium bromide 3% in sterile water can potentially be administered IV as an infusion over at least 8 hours, but this must be done with caution, as there is little clinical experience giving the drug IV and there are no commercially available IV preparations available; an in-line IV filter is required. Sodium bromide dosage is 15% less than the potassium bromide dosage. **NOTE:** Potassium bromide must **NOT** be administered IV; IV regimen is for sodium bromide only.

Epilepsy *maintenance* dosage (extra-label): 30 – 40 mg/kg PO once daily or divided into 2 daily doses.[20-22] Some state that if using bromide as an add-on drug in dogs already on phenobarbital, a lower initial dosage of 15 – 30 mg/kg PO once daily should be used. Adjust dosages based on clinical efficacy, adverse effects, and serum bromide concentrations (see ***Monitoring***). Dosage increases should generally be in less than 5 mg/kg increments, particularly when prescribing at the higher end of the dosing range. A retrospective study found that dosage increases of 5 mg/kg increased the risk for toxicity (bromism) by almost 5-fold.[23]

Monitoring

- Efficacy/toxicity. One review of the safety of potassium bromide in dogs states that clinical signs may be a better indication of the appropriateness of treatment than is monitoring serum bromide concentration alone.[24]
- Serum bromide concentrations. In dogs, therapeutic bromide concentrations are generally agreed to be 1 to 3 mg/mL (100 to 300 mg/dL; 1000-3000 mg/L; 12.5-37.5 mmol/L). Concentrations in the lower range may be effective for dogs also receiving phenobarbital therapy and the higher range for dogs on bromide alone. Measure serum bromide concentration once steady state is achieved (ie, 3 to 4 months after initiating therapy or dose changes).[25] Thereafter, monitor bromide concentrations every 6 to 12 months or sooner if seizure control lessens (ie, patient has more than 3 seizures prior to next scheduled examination) or if signs of bromide toxicity occur.[22] Once steady state is reached, the time of day (hours postdose) for sampling for bromide measurement is not critical (ie, sample may be obtained regardless of when the last dose was administered)[22,25]; however, a 12-hour fast prior to blood draw is desirable to reduce interference from triglycerides.[16]

Client Information

- This medicine may be given with or without food.
- The dose may either be sprinkled on the dog's food (assuming the food is consumed entirely) or squirted in the side of the mouth. If mixed with food, elevate the food bowl.
- Dose measurements of bromide solutions should be done with an oral dosing syringe or other accurate measuring device.
- Dogs that cannot tolerate the gastrointestinal effects (eg, vomiting, poor appetite) of potassium bromide with single daily doses may better tolerate doses divided through the day and given with food.
- Do not give salty snacks or salty food or change your dog's diet without talking with your veterinarian first.
- Most common side effect is drowsiness (usually improves in a few weeks). Some dogs will consume more water or food than usual.
- Watch for serious side effects that may indicate that the dosage is too high, including behavior changes, difficulty walking, stumbling, incoordination, severe vomiting, difficulty swallowing.

Chemistry

Potassium bromide occurs as a white, odorless, cubical crystal or crystalline powder. One gram will dissolve in 1.5 mL of water. Potassium bromide contains 67.2% bromide. Each gram contains 8.4 mEq (mMol) of potassium and bromide.

Sodium bromide occurs as a white, odorless cubical crystal or granular powder. One gram will dissolve in 1.2 mL of water. Sodium bromide contains 77.7% bromide.

Because of the different molecular weights of sodium and potassium, with respect to actual bromide content, sodium bromide solutions of 250 mg/mL contain ≈20% more bromide than potassium bromide 250 mg/mL solution. This is generally not clinically significant *unless* changing from one salt to another in a given patient.

Storage/Stability

Unless otherwise labelled, store in tight containers at room temperature 15°C to 30°C (59°F-86°F). Compounded solutions may be stored for up to 1 year in clear or brown glass or plastic containers at room temperature. Refrigerating the solution may help reduce the chance for microbial growth but may cause crystals or precipitants to form. Should precipitation occur, warming the solution should resolubilize the bromide.

Compatibility/Compounding Considerations

Bromides can precipitate out alkaloids in solution. Mixing with strong oxidizing agents can liberate bromine. Metal salts can precipitate solutions containing bromides. Sodium bromide is hygroscopic; potassium bromide is not.

To compound a solution with a concentration of 250 mg/mL, 25 g of potassium bromide is weighed; a sufficient amount of distilled water is added to a final volume of 100 mL; potassium bromide dissolves easily in water, sodium bromide may take longer to dissolve. Flavoring agents are not usually necessary for patient acceptance. USP grade (preferred) or reagent grade (specify American Chemical Society [ACS] grade) powder/crystals may be obtained from various chemical supply houses to compound an acceptable oral product.

Dosage Forms/Regulatory Status

VETERINARY-LABELED PRODUCTS:

Potassium Bromide Chewable Tablets: 250 mg and 500 mg in 60- or 180- count bottles; *KBroVet®-CA1; (Rx).* Contains liver flavor. A potassium bromide 250 mg/mL oral solution using the same trade name is also commercially available but is not included in the conditional approval under NADA #141-544.

References

For the complete list of references, see **wiley.com/go/budde/plumb**

Bromocriptine

(broe-moe-***krip***-teen) *Cycloset®, Parlodel®*

Dopamine Agonist/Prolactin Inhibitor

Prescriber Highlights

- ▶ Synthetic ergot derivative historically used in dogs for estrus induction or treatment of pseudocyesis; in horses for pituitary pars intermedia dysfunction (PPID) or inappropriate lactation; in cats for acromegaly or mammary hyperplasia
- ▶ Cabergoline (another synthetic ergot derivative) is generally preferred for use in small animal species, due to its safety profile and low incidence of adverse effects as compared with bromocriptine.
- ▶ Pergolide is generally preferred (over bromocriptine) for the treatment of PPID in horses.
- ▶ Many adverse effects possible; GI (emesis), CNS depression, and hypotension are most common.
- ▶ Interferes with lactation

Uses/Indications

Bromocriptine has historically been used treat acromegaly in cats; inappropriate lactation[1] and pituitary pars intermedia dysfunction (PPID) in horses; and for pregnancy termination, pyometra, and pseudopregnancy in dogs; however, other dopamine agonists (eg, cabergoline for dogs and cats, pergolide for horses) have largely replaced bromocriptine due to their greater efficacy and safety as well as a more favorable adverse effect profile.

In humans, bromocriptine is used to treat hyperprolactinemia, Parkinson disease, and type 2 diabetes mellitus.

Pharmacology/Actions

Bromocriptine is an ergot alkaloid-derived dopamine (D_2) receptor agonist that exhibits multiple pharmacologic actions.[2] It inhibits prolactin release from the anterior pituitary, thereby reducing serum prolactin. The mechanism for this action is by a direct effect on the pituitary and/or stimulating postsynaptic dopamine receptors in the hypothalamus to cause the release of prolactin-inhibitory factor. Bromocriptine also activates dopaminergic receptors in the neostriatum of the brain and lowers growth hormone concentrations in patients with acromegaly. In humans with type 2 diabetes mellitus, it has been shown to counteract insulin resistance and subsequently reduce hepatic glucose output, serum triglycerides, and free fatty acids.

Pharmacokinetics

The pharmacokinetics of bromocriptine have not been reported in domestic animals. In humans, due to a high first-pass effect, only ≈7% of a bromocriptine dose reaches the systemic circulation.[3] Distribution characteristics are not well-described, but in humans, it is highly bound (90%-96%) to serum albumin. In humans, bromocriptine is metabolized by the liver primarily by CYP3A4 to inactive and nontoxic metabolites; it has a half-life of ≈5 to 6 hours.[2,3] Elimination occurs predominantly by the fecal route.

Contraindications/Precautions/Warnings

Bromocriptine is generally contraindicated in patients that are hypersensitive to ergot derivatives (eg, cabergoline)[3] or during pregnancy unless termination of pregnancy is desired. Patients that are intolerant of cabergoline may not tolerate bromocriptine.

In humans, bromocriptine is contraindicated in lactating or postpartum patients, and in patients that have uncontrolled hypertension as additive hypertension could occur.[3] Use with caution in patients with hypertension that are already being treated with antihypertensive medications as syncope may result. Bromocriptine should also be used with caution in patients with hepatic disease as the metabolism of the drug may be reduced.[3]

Adverse Effects

Bromocriptine may cause a plethora of adverse effects that are usually dose-related and minimized with dosage reduction. Common adverse effects include nausea, vomiting sedation, fatigue, and hypotension (particularly with the first dose, but it may persist). In dogs, bromocriptine is more likely to cause emesis as compared with cabergoline. Reducing the dose and administering with food may help minimize adverse GI effects. Cats may develop psychoactive effects with long-term administration.[4] Hypoglycemia has been documented in humans receiving bromocriptine[3]; incidence in veterinary species is unknown.

Reproductive/Nursing Safety

Because bromocriptine is an ergot alkaloid, toxicities associated with some of the naturally occurring ergot alkaloid toxins (eg, fescue toxicity) may occur and result in abortion, prolonged gestation with dystocia, and/or thickened or retained placenta in pregnant mares. Reduced implantation and embryolethality has been documented in laboratory species receiving high doses of bromocriptine.[3]

In humans, bromocriptine use during lactation is contraindicated because bromocriptine inhibits lactation.[3] The same effect is expected to occur in lactating veterinary patients and administration of bromocriptine to lactating animals is not recommended..

Overdose/Acute Toxicity

Overdoses may cause vomiting, severe nausea, lethargy, hypothermia, tachycardia, and profound hypotension. Standard GI decontamination techniques (eg, emesis induction, activated charcoal) should be employed when applicable; however, emesis often occurs spontaneously from the overdose, and induction of emesis may not be necessary. Cardiovascular monitoring (eg, blood pressure, heart rate) and supportive care should be provided based on clinical presentation.

For patients that have experienced or are suspected to have experienced an overdose, consultation with a 24-hour poison consultation center specializing in providing veterinary-specific information is recommended. For general information related to overdose and toxin exposures, as well as contact information for poison control centers, refer to ***Appendix.***

Drug Interactions

The following drug interactions have either been reported or are theoretical in humans or animals receiving bromocriptine and may be of significance in veterinary patients. Unless otherwise noted, use

together is not necessarily contraindicated, but weigh the potential risks and perform additional monitoring when appropriate.

- **Amitriptyline**: May increase prolactin concentrations; bromocriptine dose may need to be increased
- **Azole Antifungals** (eg, **itraconazole, ketoconazole**): May increase bromocriptine concentrations
- **Butyrophenones** (eg, **azaperone, haloperidol**): May increase prolactin concentrations, and bromocriptine doses may need to be increased
- **Cyclosporine**: May increase cyclosporine concentrations
- **Erythromycin, Clarithromycin**: May increase bromocriptine concentrations
- **Estrogens** (eg, **estradiol, estriol**): May interfere with the intended effects of bromocriptine
- **Ergot Alkaloids, Other** (eg, **cabergoline, metergoline, pergolide**): Concomitant use of bromocriptine with other ergot alkaloids is not recommended. In humans receiving this combination, nausea, vomiting, lethargy, severe hypertension, and myocardial infarction has occurred[2,3]; a similar effect is expected in veterinary patients.
- **Ethanol**: Use of bromocriptine with alcohol may cause a disulfiram-type reaction (eg, nausea, vomiting).
- **Hypotensive Medications** (eg, **amlodipine, enalapril, opioids**): May cause additive hypotension if used with bromocriptine
- **Metoclopramide**: May cause prolactin release in dogs, thereby negating the effects of bromocriptine for treating pseudopregnancy
- **Monoamine Oxidase Inhibitors (MAOIs**; eg, **amitraz, linezolid, selegiline**): Avoid the use of bromocriptine with these compounds.
- **Octreotide**: May increase bromocriptine concentrations
- **Phenothiazines** (eg, **acepromazine, chlorpromazine**): May increase prolactin concentrations; bromocriptine dose may need to be increased
- **Progestins**: May interfere with the intended effects of bromocriptine
- **Reserpine**: May increase prolactin concentrations; bromocriptine dose may need to be increased
- **Sympathomimetics** (eg, **phenylpropanolamine**): Enhanced bromocriptine effects have been reported in humans (rare), including ventricular tachycardia and cardiac dysfunction.[2]

Laboratory Considerations

- None

Dosages

DOGS:

Pseudocyesis (pseudopregnancy) | suppression of lactation (extra-label): 10 µg/kg PO every 8 to 12 hours for 7 to 10 days[5]

Adjunctive treatment of pyometra (extra-label): 25 µg/kg PO 3 times daily in combination with prostaglandin[6]

Estrus induction (extra-label): 20 – 50 µg/kg PO twice daily.[7] NOTE: Not often recommended for this indication

Pregnancy termination (extra-label): 15 – 30 µg/kg PO every 12 hours in conjunction with a prostaglandin (eg, cloprostenol).[8] NOTE: Not often recommended for this indication

CATS:

NOTE: Bromocriptine may need to be compounded for use in cats.

Adjunctive treatment of acromegaly (extra-label): Initial dose of 200 µg/cat (NOT µg/kg) PO once daily. May have some effect, especially in reducing insulin requirements[9]

Adjunctive treatment of mammary fibroadenomatous hyperplasia (extra-label): 250 µg/cat (NOT µg/kg) PO.[10] **NOTE**: Not often recommended for this indication.

HORSES:

Pituitary pars intermedia dysfunction (PPID; extra-label):

a) 30 – 90 µg/kg twice daily PO or SC, but its use is limited[11]

b) 5000 µg/horse (NOT µg/kg) IM every 12 hours for 6 weeks.[12] See **Compatibility/Compounding Considerations.**

Inappropriate lactation (extra-label): 40 µg/kg PO twice daily for 10 days. Dosage based on a case report and administered in conjunction with local hydrotherapy (20 minutes twice daily); milking restricted to times when the mare was in extreme discomfort[1]

Monitoring

- Monitoring for efficacy is dependent on the reason for use.
- Adverse effects (eg, lethargy, hyporexia, vomiting)
- Blood pressure
- Serum progesterone

Client Information

- In horses, this drug is usually injected into the muscle (IM) or under the skin (SC) twice a day. If your veterinarian has instructed you to give this medication by shot in the muscle or under the skin, be sure you understand the proper places and technique to give it.
- Vomiting, fatigue, and low blood pressure are possible. For dogs and cats, giving this medicine with food may help to decrease vomiting.
- Long-term use of this medicine in cats may cause behavior changes (eg, head and body shaking, flicking of legs). Contact your veterinarian if you have any concerns.

Chemistry/Synonyms

Bromocriptine mesylate—a dopamine agonist and prolactin inhibitor—is a semisynthetic ergot alkaloid derivative. It occurs as a yellowish-white powder and is slightly soluble in water and sparingly soluble in alcohol.

Bromocriptine mesylate may also be known as bromocryptine, brom-ergocryptine, 2-bromergocryptine, bromocriptine methanesulphonate, bromocriptini mesilas, 2-bromo-alpha-ergocryptine mesylate, 2-bromoergocryptine monomethanesulfonate, or CB-154 (bromocriptine); many trade names are available.

Storage/Stability

Protect tablets and capsules from light and store them in tight containers at 20°C to 25°C (68°F-77°F).

Compatibility/Compounding Considerations

A case report described the preparation of an injectable formulation for IM use: bromocriptine mesylate 70 mg was added to 7 mL of a solution of 80% normal saline and 20% absolute alcohol (v/v). Final concentration is 1% (10 mg/mL).[12]

Dosage Forms/Regulatory Status

VETERINARY-LABELED PRODUCTS: NONE

The Association of Racing Commissioners International (ARCI) has designated this drug as a class 2 substance. Use of this drug may not be allowed in certain animal competitions. Check rules and regulations before entering a competition while this medication is being administered. Contact local racing authorities for further guidance. See the ***Appendix*** for more information.

HUMAN-LABELED PRODUCTS:

Bromocriptine Mesylate Oral Capsules: 5 mg; *Parlodel®*, generic; (Rx)

Bromocriptine Mesylate Oral Tablets: 0.8 and 2.5 mg; *Cycloset®*, *Parlodel®*, generic; (Rx)

References

For the complete list of references, see **wiley.com/go/budde/plumb**

Budesonide

(bue-***des***-oh-nide) *Entocort EC®, Uceris®*
Glucocorticoid

Prescriber Highlights

- ▶ Orally administered, locally active glucocorticoid that may be useful in treating chronic inflammatory enteropathies in small animal species
- ▶ Has been proposed for treating patients that are intolerant of systemic steroids; evidence of fewer adverse effects as compared with other oral glucocorticoids is lacking, and HPA axis suppression has been documented.
- ▶ Inhalation therapy may be useful in cats with asthma or horses with severe equine asthma, but currently available inhaled dosage forms may preclude use.
- ▶ Drug interactions with CYP3A inhibitors and antacids have been reported.
- ▶ Embryocidal and teratogenic in rats and rabbits
- ▶ Expense may be an issue, but generic forms are available; may need to be compounded to smaller dosage strengths.

Uses/Indications

Most veterinary interest is in budesonide's potential oral use to treat inflammatory intestinal diseases in small animal species that are intolerant of systemic corticosteroids. In studies of dogs with chronic inflammatory enteropathies (previously termed inflammatory bowel disease [IBD]), modest clinical and/or histopathologic response was noted with commercial budesonide capsules, whereas all dogs receiving placebo had worsening of disease.[1,2] One study demonstrated that budesonide powder (not commercial capsules) and prednisone were equally efficacious at inducing remission in dogs with inflammatory bowel disease, but no difference in adverse effects was noted.[3] Anecdotally, budesonide may be effective for some cats with chronic inflammatory enteropathies.[4]

Inhalational dosage forms are available for treating asthma or allergic rhinitis in humans. Inhaled budesonide has improved clinical signs in cats with asthma and chronic bronchitis[5] and significantly improved pulmonary function in horses with severe equine asthma (SEA; formerly known as recurrent airway obstruction [RAO]).[6] However, in the US, the mode of inhalation of commercially available products is not compatible with the space chambers used in veterinary medicine, which may preclude usage.

Pharmacology/Actions

Budesonide is a potent glucocorticoid (15 times more potent than prednisolone) with high topical activity. It has weak mineralocorticoid activity. By delaying drug dissolution until reaching the duodenum, the commercial enteric-coated formulations control release of the drug so it can exert its topical anti-inflammatory activity in the intestines. Although the drug is absorbed from the gut into the portal circulation, it has a high first-pass metabolism effect through the liver that reduces systemic blood concentrations and resultant glucocorticoid effects of the drug. However, suppression of the HPA axis has been demonstrated in dogs,[7-10] cats,[5] and horses.[6]

Pharmacokinetics

Budesonide's pharmacokinetics have been reported in healthy dogs. With oral administration of a controlled-release formulation, the drug has a bioavailability of 10% to 20%. When dosed at 10 µg/kg, half-life is ≈2 hours and clearance 2.2 L/hour/kg. At 100 µg/kg, half-life is mildly prolonged to 2 to 3 hours. In dogs with inflammatory bowel disease, budesonide (as the commercial oral product) is apparently rapidly absorbed with peak concentrations occurring at 1 hour post dosing.[2]

Upon oral administration of the commercially available product in humans, budesonide is nearly completely absorbed from the gut, but time to achieve peak concentrations are widely variable (30 to 600 minutes). The presence of food in the gut may delay absorption but does not impact the amount of drug absorbed. Because of a high first-pass effect, only ≈10% of a dose is systemically bioavailable in healthy adults. In patients with Crohn's disease, oral bioavailability may be twice that initially, but with further dosing, reduces to amounts similar to healthy subjects. Budesonide's mean volume of distribution in humans ranges from 2.2 to 3.9 L/kg. The drug is completely metabolized, and metabolites are excreted in the feces and urine. Budesonide's terminal half-life is ≈4 hours.

After nebulization, budesonide is detectable in the plasma and urine of horses for up to 96 hours and 120 hours, respectively.[11]

Contraindications/Precautions/Warnings

Budesonide is contraindicated in patients hypersensitive to it. Because budesonide can cause systemic corticosteroid effects, it should be used with caution in any patient in which glucocorticoid therapy may be problematic, including those with GI ulcers, active infections, diabetes mellitus, or cataracts. Risk for systemic effects may be increased in patients with hepatic impairment; dosage reduction may be required.

Because budesonide suppresses the HPA axis, exogenous steroid administration should be considered for animals undergoing stressful procedures, such as surgery.

Adverse Effects

In humans, budesonide causes few glucocorticoid adverse effects when it is used for courses of therapy no longer than 8 weeks in duration. However, budesonide has been shown to cause significant HPA axis suppression in dogs when using commercial formulations,[8-10] and when using compounded budesonide powder.[7] One study failed to show a decreased incidence of adverse systemic effects compared to prednisone.[3] A tendency towards less severe adverse effects was observed with budesonide, but this finding was not statistically significant. Increases in liver enzyme activity were seen in this study but were not noted in other studies. Of note, as budesonide is a potent glucocorticoid that is locally active in the GI tract, local adverse effects, such as GI erosion, ulceration, and even perforation are possible when budesonide is overdosed.

Inhaled budesonide reduced cortisol concentration in horses,[6] and resulted in HPA axis suppression in cats.[5]

Reproductive/Nursing Safety

Budesonide had no effect on fertility in rats at SC doses up to 80 µg/kg. As with other corticosteroids, budesonide has been demonstrated to be embryocidal and teratogenic in rats and rabbits. Because safety has not been established in animal species, this drug should only be used when the maternal benefits outweigh the potential fetal risks.

Specific data on budesonide concentrations in maternal milk are not available and the manufacturer warns against use by nursing women; however, because of the drug's high first-pass effect, the amounts are unlikely to be of clinical significance to nursing animal offspring.

Overdose/Acute Toxicity

Budesonide doses of 200 mg/kg were lethal in mice. Overdoses of glucocorticoids used alone are unlikely to cause harmful effects, but GI signs that are sometimes severe can be seen in dogs. If clinical signs occur, use supportive treatment if required. Chronic use of glucocorticoids can lead to serious adverse effects. Refer to ***Adverse Effects*** for more information.

For patients that have experienced or are suspected to have experienced an overdose, it is strongly encouraged to consult with a 24-hour poison consultation center that specializes in providing information specific for veterinary patients. For general information related to overdose and toxin exposures, as well as contact information for poison control centers, refer to ***Appendix***.

Drug Interactions

The following drug interactions have either been reported or are theoretical in humans or animals receiving budesonide and may be of significance in veterinary patients. Unless otherwise noted, combined use is not necessarily contraindicated, but the potential risks should be carefully weighed and additional monitoring should be performed when appropriate.

- **Aspirin:** Increased risk for GI erosion, ulceration, or perforation
- **Nonsteroidal Anti-Inflammatory Drugs (NSAIDs; eg, carprofen, meloxicam, robenacoxib)**: Increased risk for GI erosion, ulceration, or perforation
- **Oral Antacids**: Because the dissolution of the drug's coating is pH dependent, separate the administration of oral antacids from budesonide by at least 2 hours. Other drugs that potentially would increase gastric pH (eg, famotidine, omeprazole) do not significantly impact the oral pharmacokinetics of the drug.[12]

Because the hepatic enzyme CYP3A extensively metabolizes budesonide, drugs that inhibit this isoenzyme can significantly increase the amount of drug that enters the systemic circulation.

- **Azole Antifungals** (eg, **fluconazole, itraconazole, ketoconazole):** Concomitant ketoconazole is known to increase budesonide area under the curve (AUC) by 8-fold.[12]
- **Cimetidine**[12]
- **Cyclosporine**
- **Diltiazem**
- **Erythromycin**
- **Grapefruit Juice Powder**

Laboratory Considerations

- **Intradermal skin testing (IDST)** for allergens: Inhaled budesonide (for 1 month) eliminated skin reactivity in 3/6 cats tested. A 2-week withdrawal period is suggested if performing IDST but may not be necessary if using serum IgE testing for allergies.[13]

Dosages

DOGS

Adjunctive treatment of chronic inflammatory enteropathies (extra-label)**:** Initial dosage recommendations vary, but practically: body weight 3 to 7 kg: 1 mg (must be compounded), 7.1 to 15 kg: 2 mg (must be compounded), 15.1 to 30 kg: 3 mg (commercially available), greater than 30 kg: 5 mg (must be compounded) PO once daily[3] OR 3 mg/m^2 (NOT mg/kg) PO once daily.[7] Once adequately controlled, gradual reductions in dosage amounts or frequency (every other day) are desirable.

CATS:

Adjunctive treatment of chronic inflammatory enteropathies (extra-label): Most cats tolerate oral glucocorticoids, but in those that cannot and especially in diabetic cats, budesonide can be considered: 3 mg/m^2 (NOT mg/kg) PO once daily[14,15] or 0.5 – 0.75 mg/cat (NOT mg/kg) PO once daily.[4] **NOTE**: These dosages require reformulation to provide the appropriate dose.

HORSES

Adjunctive treatment of severe equine asthma (**SEA**; extra-label): 1.8 mg total dose (NOT mg/kg) twice daily. The drug was delivered as 8 actuations via Respimat® inhalation device and using an equine-specific nostril adapter.[6]

Monitoring

- Efficacy (improved clinical signs)
- Adverse effects, including possible HPA axis suppression

Client Information

- Do not crush capsules or allow animals to chew them. Do not open capsules unless your veterinarian has instructed you to do so.
- Once your animal has been taking this drug for a while, don't stop giving it unless instructed to do so by your veterinarian. Serious withdrawal effects can occur if the medication is stopped suddenly.
- In dogs, stomach or intestinal ulcers, perforation, or bleeding can occur. If your animal stops eating or has a low energy level or you notice a high fever, black tarry stools, or bloody vomit (may look like coffee grounds), contact your veterinarian immediately.
- Side effects (eg, increased panting, appetite, thirst, and need to urinate) are possible, especially when the medication is used long-term, but are less likely to occur than with other medications in this class. Other side effects could include lethargy, muscle weakness, changes in skin and hair/coat, weight gain, and/or pot belly. Contact your veterinarian if these side effects occur.

Chemistry/Synonyms

Budesonide, a nonhalogenated glucocorticoid, occurs as a white to off-white odorless, tasteless powder. It is practically insoluble in water, freely soluble in chloroform, and sparingly soluble in alcohol. The commercially available capsules contain a granulized micronized form of the drug that is enteric coated to protect it from dissolution in gastric juice but that dissolves at pH greater than 5.5. In humans, this pH usually corresponds with the drug reaching the duodenum. After dissolution of the outer coating, budesonide is released from an inner core in a time-dependent manner. The commercially available tablet contains an outer coating that dissolves at or above pH 7.0, followed by a controlled release of budesonide from the inner tablet core.

Budesonide may also be known as S 1320, *Entocord*®, *Entocort EC*®, *Uceris*®, Pulmicort®, and *Rhinocort*®.

Storage/Stability

Budesonide oral capsules should be stored in tight containers at room temperature (20°C-25°C [68°F-77°F]), protected from light and moisture. Exposures to temperatures as low as 15°C (59°F) and as high as 30°C (86°F) are permitted.

Compatibility/Compounding Considerations

If reformulating into smaller capsules, do not alter (damage) the micronized enteric-coated sugar spheres inside the capsules.

Dosage Forms/Regulatory Status

VETERINARY-LABELED PRODUCTS: NONE

The Association of Racing Commissioners International (ARCI) has designated this drug as a class 4 substance. See ***Appendix*** for more information. Use of this drug may not be allowed in certain animal competitions. Check rules and regulations before entering in a competition while this medication is being administered. Contact local racing authorities for further guidance.

HUMAN-LABELED PRODUCTS:

Budesonide Extended-Release Capsules: 3 mg and 9 mg (micronized); *Entocort EC*®, *Uceris*®, generic; (Rx)

Budesonide Extended-Release Tablets: 6 mg and 9 mg; *Uceris*®; (Rx)

Budesonide capsules intended for human use may need to be compounded into dosage strengths suitable for dogs and cats, but the enteric-coated sugar spheres found inside the capsule should not be altered or damaged.

Budesonide Inhalation Suspension (for nebulization): 0.25 mg and 0.5 mg in 2 mL ampules; generic; (Rx). The budesonide oral inhaler is a breath-actuated device that is not amenable for typical veterinary use.

References

For the complete list of references, see **wiley.com/go/budde/plumb**

Bupivacaine

(byoo-***piv***-a-kane) *Sensorcaine®, Marcaine®*

Local Anesthetic

*For information regarding liposomal bupivacaine extended-release formulation, please refer to **Bupivacaine Liposome**.*

Prescriber Highlights

- ▶ Local anesthetic with slower onset (20 to 30 minutes) and longer duration of action (3 to 5 hours) than others in its class
- ▶ Do not convert dosing from any other formulations of bupivacaine to bupivacaine liposome injection suspension or vice versa.
- ▶ Unintended systemic administration or absorption can lead to severe cardiac and CNS adverse effects, including death.
- ▶ Adverse effects are unlikely when the correct administration technique is used. Clinicians should be knowledgeable in the diagnosis and management of local anesthetic toxicity, and resources for treating acute emergencies must be readily available.
- ▶ Patients susceptible to malignant hyperthermia should receive intensified monitoring.

Uses/Indications

Bupivacaine is used in most species to produce local or regional analgesia and anesthesia for surgery and diagnostic or therapeutic procedures. It is also used for caudal and lumbar epidural anesthesia. Local analgesia can have a MAC-sparing effect on inhalant anesthesia, and leads to better postoperative recovery following orthopedic surgery in dogs.[1,2] The duration of analgesia can be extended when bupivacaine is combined with dexmedetomidine for femoral and sciatic nerve blocks in dogs.[3]

Epidural bupivacaine results in reduced intraoperative opioid use[4] and may have a MAC-sparing effect.[5] To provide a longer duration of epidural analgesia, bupivacaine can be combined with buprenorphine.[3]

Additional local anesthetic administration techniques for bupivacaine include intrathecal administration[6] or intraperitoneal spraying[7-10] for incision closure.

Some clinicians prefer a combination of lidocaine (faster onset) and bupivacaine (longer duration) but studies in a variety of species suggest the onset of effect is similar to that of either lidocaine or bupivacaine alone[11-14] and the duration of analgesia is shorter than bupivacaine alone (but longer than lidocaine alone).[11,13,15-18] To achieve a faster onset but longer duration nerve block, use only lidocaine prior to the procedure and repeat the block at the end of the procedure using only bupivacaine.

An extensive description of most common local blocks and epidural/spinal injection in small animals can be found in other reference texts.[19-22]

Pharmacology/Actions

Local anesthetics block sodium ion channels on the nerve cell membrane, thereby altering electrical excitability, depolarization, and action potential propagation. They block the generation and conduction of impulses in motor, sensory, and autonomic nerve fibers around the site of application. Nerve fiber diameter, conduction velocity, and myelination determine loss of nerve function. Clinically, the progressive loss of nerve function occurs in the following order: pain, temperature, touch, proprioception, and skeletal muscle tone. Anesthetic effect is lost in reverse order.

Bupivacaine produces analgesia typically within 20 to 30 minutes after local administration and persists for 3 to 5 hours. Compared to lidocaine, bupivacaine has a slower onset and longer duration of action.

Pharmacokinetics

Local anesthetics are absorbed from their site of administration into the systemic circulation. Systemic absorption increases when administration is repeated in the head and neck region and/or injected into highly vascularized sites.

In dogs, peak plasma concentrations occurred 11 minutes after intra-articular administration and elimination half-life was 1 hour.[23] After epidural use, plasma levels peaked after 5 minutes, and half-life was 3 hours.[24] Intermittent wound infusion of bupivacaine 0.25% solution (2 mg/kg) via wound catheter in dogs resulted in a measurable bupivacaine concentration of 0.25 to 0.35 µg/mL, which is below the known toxic concentration (ie, 2.5 µg/mL).[25]

In cats, peak plasma concentrations have been noted 17 to 30 minutes after administration, with an elimination half-life of 4.8 hours.[26,27]

In humans, peak levels occur ≈15 to 30 minutes after administration. Systemically absorbed drug distributes into all tissues, including the CNS. Protein binding is ≈95%, which may limit but not prevent it from crossing the placenta and being excreted in milk. It is hepatically metabolized and is excreted in the urine, principally as metabolites. Elimination half-life in humans is ≈2.5 hours in adults, and ≈8 hours in neonates.

Epinephrine may be added to bupivacaine formulations at a very low concentration (5 µg/mL) to cause vasoconstriction at the site of administration, thereby reducing the rate of systemic absorption. Commercial bupivacaine products containing epinephrine are available. Epinephrine prolongs the duration of action at the site of administration, as well as minimizing systemic bupivacaine toxicity.

Contraindications/Precautions/Warnings

Bupivacaine is contraindicated in patients with a known hypersensitivity to it or to another amide-type local anesthetic, and for obstetrical paracervical block anesthesia. Epidural use is contraindicated in patients with severe CNS disease. Use with caution in patients with hepatic disease or impaired cardiovascular function. Bupivacaine is more cardiotoxic than other local anesthetic agents and should never be administered IV. When used for IV regional anesthesia (Bier Block) in humans, bupivacaine has been linked to cardiac arrest and death; veterinary significance is unclear.

Epidural injections should be administered incrementally, with aspiration prior to injection. Local anesthetics with preservatives should not be used for epidural or caudal anesthesia.

Bupivacaine products that contain epinephrine should be used with caution, if at all, in patients with cardiovascular disease or hyperthyroidism, or for anesthesia of the digits, ears, nose, or penis. Avoid bupivacaine/epinephrine when nerve integrity or collateral circulation is compromised as it causes intense vasoconstriction and diminished blood flow; ischemic injury could result.

Hyperbaric bupivacaine (bupivacaine solutions with dextrose) produces a different pharmacological effect and is not interchangeable with bupivacaine solution formulated in sterile water. Hyperbaric bupivacaine should not be used for peripheral nerve blocks.

Adverse Effects

Local anesthetics are generally well tolerated when administered correctly. Adverse effects are related to high plasma concentrations, which may result from the dosage or bupivacaine concentration used, rapid absorption from the injection site, and unintentional intravascular or subarachnoid injection.

Cardiovascular adverse effects include hypotension, bradycardia, AV block, and decreased cardiac output. Either CNS excitation (restlessness, tremors) or depression (drowsiness, loss of consciousness) may occur. Nausea and vomiting are also noted. See ***Overdose/Acute Toxicity.*** Chondrolysis has occurred in humans receiving intra-articular injections, but was considered unlikely to occur in dogs.[28] Intra-articular use in horses induced an anabolic effect in one small study.[29]

Reproductive/Nursing Safety

Bupivacaine crosses the placenta, and the fetal to maternal ratio is ≈0.2 to 0.4. Developmental toxicity was noted in rats and rabbits receiving bupivacaine 40 mg/kg SC and 22 mg/kg SC, respectively, and decreased pup survival was noted in rats. Because safety has not been established in animal species, this drug should only be used when the maternal benefits outweigh the potential fetal risks. An example of when it may be used is a line block of the linea alba prior to cesarean section. Bupivacaine will decrease inhalant anesthesia requirements and thus decrease cardiovascular and respiratory depression effects to the neonates.

Bupivacaine is excreted in human milk in small amounts; significance in veterinary medicine is not known. Use with caution in lactating dams.

Overdose/Acute Toxicity

Toxic blood levels are most likely to occur after unintended intravascular administration. To avoid this, ALWAYS aspirate before injecting the local anesthetic. Toxic effects may occur rapidly and simultaneously. Cardiac conduction and excitability are depressed and may lead to AV block, ventricular arrhythmias, and cardiac arrest; arrhythmias may be refractory to treatment. In addition, myocardial contractility is depressed and peripheral vasodilation occurs, leading to decreased cardiac output and arterial blood pressure. Central nervous system stimulation (restlessness, tremors, and shivering progressing to seizures) may be followed by CNS depression, coma, and respiratory arrest. The mean convulsive dose in cats was 3.8 mg/kg IV and the mean cardiotoxic dose was 18.4 mg/kg IV.[30] In dogs, mean convulsive dose was 4.1 mg/kg IV[31] and the mean cardiotoxic dose was ≈20 mg/kg IV.[32] The LD_{50} in mice is 6 – 8 mg/kg IV.

If signs of overdose are present, management must begin with delivery of oxygen via a patent airway as successful oxygen delivery may prevent convulsions caused by toxicity. Benzodiazepines and barbiturates can be used for seizure management but may cause further CNS depression. Cardiovascular support should be provided and may include IV fluids and vasopressor drugs (eg, dobutamine, norepinephrine). Prolonged resuscitative efforts may be required. Lipid emulsion 20% 1.5 mL/kg IV over 30 minutes can be beneficial.[33,34] See ***Fat Emulsion, Intravenous.***

For patients that have experienced or are suspected to have experienced an overdose, it is strongly encouraged to consult with a 24-hour poison consultation center that specialize in providing information specific for veterinary patients. For general information related to overdose and toxin exposures, as well as contact information for poison control centers, refer to ***Appendix.***

Drug Interactions

The following drug interactions have either been reported or are theoretical in humans or animals receiving bupivacaine and may be of significance in veterinary patients. Unless otherwise noted, use together is not necessarily contraindicated, but weigh the potential risks and perform additional monitoring when appropriate.

- **Angiotensin-Converting Enzyme Inhibitors** (ACEIs; eg, **benazepril, enalapril**): Increased risk for bradycardia and hypotension
- **Beta-Adrenergic Antagonists:** (eg, **atenolol, esmolol, propranolol, sotalol**): May increase serum bupivacaine concentrations by reducing bupivacaine clearance

Severe, prolonged hypertension may result when using bupivacaine/epinephrine combination products with the following:

- **Ergot Alkaloids**
- **Monoamine Oxidase Inhibitors** (MAOIs; eg, **amitraz, linezolid, selegiline**)
- **Tricyclic Antidepressants** (TCAs ; eg, **amitriptyline, clomipramine**
- **Vasopressors** (eg, **dobutamine, norepinephrine**)

Laboratory Interactions

- None noted

Dosages

NOTES:

1. Bupivacaine product concentration, administration volume, site of administration, administration technique (eg, gentle needle insertion, aspiration prior to injection), and underlying patient condition(s) are important interrelated factors that determine bupivacaine's safe and effective use.
2. All dosages are extra-label.

DOGS:

Local anesthesia (tissue infiltration):

1. Using 0.25% or 0.5% bupivacaine solution, 1 – 2 mg/kg[1]
2. Using 0.5% bupivacaine solution, 0.5 mg/kg combined with dexmedetomidine 0.1 µg/kg[3]
3. Using 0.5% bupivacaine solution, mix with equal volume of 2% lidocaine solution to speed onset of effect[15]

Intraperitoneal administration ovariohysterectomy: 3 mg/kg intraperitoneal to linea alba prior to closure.[8,10] 4.4 mg/kg using 0.25% bupivacaine also appears to be effective.[35,36]

Retrobulbar injection: 0.5 mg/kg using 0.5% bupivacaine solution.[37]

NOTE: Peribulbar injection may produce more reliable analgesia.[38]

Epidural:

1. Using 0.5% bupivacaine solution, 1.25 mg/kg[18]
2. Using 0.5% bupivacaine solution, 1 mg/kg combined with morphine 1% preservative-free solution, 0.1 mg/kg[39-41]
3. Using 0.5% bupivacaine solution, 1 mg/kg combined with buprenorphine 4 µg/kg[3]
4. Using 0.5% bupivacaine solution, 1 mg/kg combined with dexmedetomidine 0.05 % solution, 4 µg/kg.[41] Using 0.5% bupivacaine solution, 2 mg/kg combined with dexmedetomidine 7 µg/kg.[42] Note: These doses may increase risk for cranial spread of the local anesthetic, which can impair respiration by blocking intercostal nerves.
5. Using 0.5% bupivacaine solution, 1 – 2 mg/kg; greater efficacy with the higher dosage.[43] If using 0.25% bupivacaine solution, 0.6 mL/kg appears to be the optimal volume for epidural use.[44]

CATS:

Local anesthesia (tissue infiltration): 1.1 mg/kg using 0.5% bupivacaine solution.[45] Most experts consider 1 mg/kg the appropriate dose for cats, but one study safely used 2 mg/kg using 0.5% bupivacaine solution to infiltrate a surgical wound site.[46]

Intraperitoneal administration during ovariohysterectomy (OVH):

1. Using 0.25% bupivacaine solution, 2 mg/kg divided into 3 equal volumes and instilled in the right and left ovarian pedicles, and caudal uterus immediately before OVH using a 3 mL syringe attached to a 22 G IV catheter. Surgery proceeded ≈2 minutes later. [7] Similar results were obtained using bupivacaine 0.25% with epinephrine 2 µg/kg.[47]

2. Using 0.5% bupivacaine solution, 2 mg/kg divided equally into the right and left ovarian suspensory ligaments, uterine body just caudal to bifurcation, and to the subcutaneous tissue between the closed abdominal muscle fascia and subcuticular layers[48]

Retrobulbar injection: 0.7 – 1 mg/kg using 0.5% bupivacaine solution[26,49]

Epidural: Using 0.5% bupivacaine solution, 1.5 – 2.5 mg/kg lumbosacral epidural.[17] Bupivacaine 0.22 mg/kg caudal epidural using 0.5% solution. The addition of preservative-free morphine (0.1 mg/kg) to the epidural modestly (12%) reduced propofol requirements without significantly changing rescue analgesia.[5]

HORSES:

Continuous peripheral nerve block: In an experimental setting using a bupivacaine 0.125% solution, a 3 mL bolus infused through a nerve block catheter, followed by 2 mL/hour infusion over 6 days, suppressed mechanical hoof withdrawal response.[50]

Caudal epidural for perineal analgesia: 0.04 mg/kg bupivacaine using 0.25% solution, or 0.02 mg/kg bupivacaine combined with morphine 0.1 mg/kg <u>OR</u> ketamine 0.5 mg/kg injected into the epidural space. All 3 treatments were effective; bupivacaine plus morphine produced a longer duration of analgesia (5.25 hours vs 3.5 to 4 hours with the other drug combinations).[51]

CATTLE:

Caudal epidural: 0.05 – 0.06 mg/kg using 0.5% bupivacaine solution; analgesia improved with the higher dose.[14]

SHEEP & GOATS:

Local anesthesia (tissue infiltration):

1. 1.25 – 2 mg/kg using 0.5% bupivacaine solution[52-54]
2. 0.2 mL/kg (NOT mg/kg) using 0.5% bupivacaine solution[55]

Perineural administration in forelimbs: 2 mL/animal (NOT mL/kg) using 0.5% bupivacaine solution. A combination block using equal volumes of lidocaine and bupivacaine had similar onset of analgesia but shorter duration than bupivacaine alone.[11]

Lumbar epidural:

1. Bupivacaine 0.5 mg/kg injected into the epidural space[56]
2. In sheep, bupivacaine 0.5 mg/kg injected into the epidural space produced analgesia and fewer cardiovascular or respiratory adverse effects than bupivacaine 0.25 mg/kg combined with either fentanyl 2 µg/kg or methadone 0.3 mg/kg.[57]
3. In goats, using 0.5% bupivacaine solution 0.8 – 1.2 mg/kg combined with methadone 0.22 mg/kg and administered via thoracolumbar epidural resulted in longer duration of analgesia than bupivacaine alone.[58]

SMALL MAMMALS (RABBITS, GUINEA PIGS, CHINCHILLAS, RODENTS):

Local anesthesia (tissue infiltration): 1 mg/kg[59]

Epidural: 1.5 mg/kg using 0.5% bupivacaine into the coccygeal spinal canal of rabbits provided hind limb, perineal, and tail analgesia. Subarachnoid bupivacaine distribution was not observed, but inadvertent vascular entry may occur.[60]

REPTILES, AMPHIBIANS:

Local anesthesia (tissue infiltration): using 0.25% or 0.5% bupivacaine solution, 1 – 2 mg/kg; dilute up to 1:1 to expand volume if needed (diluent not provided, assume sterile water for injection or normal saline—Plumb).[61]

Spinal anesthesia: using 0.5% bupivacaine solution, 1 mg/kg intrathecally at the level of the coccygeal vertebrae of tortoises and turtles; provides regional analgesia for ≈2 hours[62]

Monitoring

- Adequacy of analgesia and anesthesia
- Cardiovascular and respiratory function as well as state of consciousness after each injection

Client Information

- This medication causes temporary loss of feeling. The area where it was injected may not have usual function for several hours.
- This drug should only be used by or on the order of a licensed veterinarian familiar with its use and in a setting where adequate patient monitoring can be performed.

Chemistry/Synonyms

Bupivacaine hydrochloride is an aminoacyl local anesthetic related to mepivacaine and lidocaine, with an amide linkage between the aromatic nucleus and the piperidine group. It occurs as a white crystalline powder that is freely soluble in ethanol and soluble in water. It has a pK_a of 8.1. Solutions are clear and colorless, with a pH 4 to 6.5. Solutions that contain epinephrine have a pH 3.5 to 5.5.

Bupivacaine hydrochloride is also known as AH-2250, LAC-43, Win-11318, bupivakaiinihydrokloridi, *Longocain*®, *Sensorcaine*®, and *Marcaine*®.

Storage/Stability

Bupivacaine HCl should be stored at room temperature, 20°C to 25°C (68°F-77°F). Solutions that contain epinephrine should be protected from light. Bupivacaine stored under field conditions for equine use was found to maintain pH and potency without microbial contamination in a variety of storage conditions and with repeated vial use over 12 months.[63]

Compatibility/Compounding Considerations

Compatibility is dependent upon factors such as pH, concentration, temperature, and diluent used; consult specialized references or a hospital pharmacist for more specific information.

Bupivacaine HCl is **compatible** with D5W and 0.9% sodium chloride solutions and the following drugs (partial list): ampicillin sodium, buprenorphine, epinephrine, fentanyl citrate, hydromorphone, ketamine, lidocaine, morphine sulfate, and penicillin G sodium/potassium. Bupivacaine HCl is reported to be **variably compatible** with sodium bicarbonate, and to be **incompatible** with mepivacaine.

Bupivacaine combinations with epinephrine are commercially available. When preparing this combination in the clinic, the recommended final concentration of epinephrine is 5 µg/mL. To reach this concentration, add 0.1 mg (0.1 mL) of epinephrine (1 mg/mL) to 20 mL of local anesthetic.

Dose Forms/Regulatory Status

VETERINARY-LABELED PRODUCTS: NONE.

The Association of Racing Commissioners International (ARCI) has designated this drug as a class 2 substance. See the ***Appendix*** for more information. Use of this drug may not be allowed in certain animal competitions. Check rules and regulations before entering in a competition while this medication is being administered. Contact local racing authorities for further guidance.

HUMAN-LABELED PRODUCTS:

Bupivacaine HCl Solution: 0.25% (2.5 mg/mL) in 10 mL and 30 mL single-dose vials, and 50 mL multidose vials; 0.5% (5 mg/mL) in 10 mL and 30 mL single-dose vials or ampules, and 50 mL multidose vials; 0.75% (7.5 mg/mL) in 10 mL, 20 mL, and 30 mL single-dose vials; *Sensorcaine*®-MPF, *Marcaine*®, generic; (Rx)

Bupivacaine HCl Solution with Epinephrine: bupivacaine 0.25% (2.5 mg/mL) with epinephrine 5 µg/mL (1:200,000) in 10 mL and 30 mL single-dose vials and 50 mL multidose vials; bupivacaine 0.5% (5 mg/mL) with epinephrine 5 µg/mL (1:200,000) in 10 mL and 30 mL single-dose vials and 50 mL multidose vials; bupivacaine 0.75% (7.5 mg/mL) with epinephrine 5 µg/mL (1:200,000) in 30 mL single-dose vials; *Sensorcaine®*-MPF with epinephrine, *Marcaine®* with epinephrine, generic; (Rx)

Bupivacaine solutions with dextrose (hyperbaric bupivacaine) are not interchangeable with bupivacaine solution formulated in sterile water and should not be used for peripheral nerve blocks.

References

For the complete list of references, see **wiley.com/go/budde/plumb**

Bupivacaine Liposome

(byoo-***piv***-ah-kane ***lye***-poh-zoam) *Nocita®*

Local Anesthetic

For information regarding immediate-release bupivacaine, please refer to ***Bupivacaine***

Prescriber Highlights

- FDA-approved injectable suspension for postoperative analgesia following cranial cruciate ligament surgery (dogs) and onychectomy (cats)
- Do not convert dosing from any other formulations of bupivacaine to bupivacaine liposome injection suspension or vice versa.
- May be diluted with a less than or equal volume of 0.9% NaCl or lactated Ringer's solution to obtain a volume sufficient to cover the surgical site. Do NOT dilute with water or other hypotonic solutions.
- Potentially effective for 72 hours postsurgery
- Adverse effects are unlikely when the correct administration technique is used. Clinicians should be knowledgeable in the diagnosis and management of local anesthetic toxicity, and resources for treating acute emergencies must be readily available.
- When used as labeled, very low incidence of adverse effects

Uses/Indications

Bupivacaine liposome injectable suspension is FDA-approved for use in dogs to infiltrate the tissue layers of the surgical site at the time of incision closure (only) to provide local postoperative analgesia for cranial cruciate ligament (CCL) surgery. It is also FDA-approved for use in cats as a peripheral nerve block to provide regional analgesia following onychectomy.

A study has shown that approximately twice as many patients (both dogs and cats) receiving bupivacaine liposome were deemed to have adequate pain control (assessed using established pain scales) compared to those receiving treatment control at all assessed time points up to 72 hours postsurgery.[1] In a pilot field study, 14 of 24 dogs receiving bupivacaine liposome just prior to closure following CCL surgery were considered treatment success (based on established pain scales) at 24 hours compared to 4 of 22 receiving a placebo during the same time period; at 72 hours postsurgery, 9 of 24 dogs were considered treatment success compared to 2 of 22 dogs receiving a placebo.[2]

Although the veterinary-labeled product states that safe use with surgical procedures other than CCL surgery has not been evaluated, the companion product labeled for use in humans (*Exparel®*) is indicated for administration into sites that meet criteria based on size of the surgical site, volume of drug required, and patient factors (eg, to produce postsurgical analgesia).[3]

Pharmacology/Actions

Bupivacaine is an amide local anesthetic. Local anesthetics block the generation and conduction of impulses through all nerve fibers (sensory, motor, and autonomic). These local anesthetics prevent conduction of nerve impulses by decreasing permeability of the nerve cell membrane to sodium ions. This blocking of the sodium channels results in a decreased depolarization rate of the nerve membrane, thus increasing the threshold for electrical excitability and preventing propagation of the action potential.[4]

The liposome form encapsulates the drug, and bupivacaine exerts its effects only after leaving the lipid vesicle. Liposomal bupivacaine releases bupivacaine slowly at the injection site and provides a longer duration of anesthetic action than the standard bupivacaine solution.

Pharmacokinetics

In order to assess systemic uptake of bupivacaine from the liposome encapsulated bupivacaine preparation, bupivacaine liposome 9 mg/kg SC was administered to dogs and cats.[1] Dogs had a median time to maximum serum concentration (T_{max}) of 30 minutes and an elimination half-life of 36.2 hours. Cats had a T_{max} of 10 hours and bupivacaine was measurable for up to 120 hours postinjection.

Intra-articular administration of bupivacaine liposome injectable suspension to horses resulted in sustained bupivacaine concentration in the joint for up to 96 hours.[5] See ***Contraindications/Precautions/Warnings.***

In humans, peak drug concentrations occur 30 minutes to 2 hours after infiltration. The drug is 95% protein bound. Hepatic metabolism is extensive to the metabolite pipecoloxylidide. Bupivacaine AUC is increased 50% in patients with hepatic dysfunction. Bupivacaine is renally eliminated, predominantly as metabolites.[6]

Contraindications/Precautions/Warnings

Do not administer by IV or intra-arterial injection, as adverse cardiovascular (eg, arrhythmias, hypotension, hypertension) or neurologic (eg, tremors, seizures) effects can occur. Although local anesthetic agents have been used intra-articularly, administration by this route is contraindicated due to risk for chondrolysis.[1] Although the veterinary label of bupivacaine liposome does not mention epidural or intrathecal administration, the human label does not recommend use by these routes.

Because they are not bioequivalent, do not convert dosages from any other formulations of bupivacaine to bupivacaine liposome injection suspension and vice versa.

Safe use has not been evaluated in dogs or cats younger than 5 months of age, with cardiac disease, or with hepatic or renal impairment.[1] Because bupivacaine is metabolized by the liver and excreted by the kidneys, use with caution in patients with impaired renal or hepatic function.[6]

Bupivacaine liposome is not indicated for preincisional or preprocedural locoregional anesthetic techniques that require deep and complete sensory block in the area of administration as its ability to achieve effective anesthesia has not been studied.

Wear gloves when handling to prevent accidental exposure.[1]

Bupivacaine is contraindicated for obstetrical paracervical block anesthesia in human patients. Fetal bradycardia and death have been reported.[6]

Adverse Effects

Bupivacaine must exit the liposomes to exert its pharmacologic effect. In a safety study,[7] liposomal bupivacaine demonstrated a favorable safety profile after intravascular administration compared to standard bupivacaine solution.

In preapproval field studies, the following adverse effects were reported in treated dogs (incidence more than 1%): discharge from incision site (3.3%), incisional inflammation (2.4%), vomiting (2.4%), isosthenuria ± proteinuria (1.6%), and increased ALP (1.6%). The placebo treated cohort did not report any of these effects.[1]

In preapproval field studies in cats undergoing onychectomy, the following adverse effects were reported in treated cats (incidence more than 1%): body temperature equal to or more than 39.4°C (103 °F) (6.7%), surgical site infection (3.3%), chewing/licking surgical site (2.5%), and diarrhea (1.7%).[1]

Adverse effects reported to occur in human patients (incidence more than 10%) include nausea, constipation, and vomiting.[3]

Reproductive/Nursing Safety

The label states that safe use of bupivacaine liposome has not been evaluated in dogs or cats that are intended for breeding or are pregnant or lactating. Bupivacaine, once released from the liposome, can cross the placenta and some animal reproduction studies have demonstrated adverse effects at high dosages. Bupivacaine used for epidural, caudal, or pudendal block anesthesia for human patients during labor and delivery can cause varying degrees of maternal, fetal, and neonatal toxicity.[6] Use with caution in pregnant dogs and cats.

Bupivacaine and its metabolite (pipecoloxylidide) can cross into maternal milk in low concentrations. There does not appear to be information documenting any effects on milk production or harm to nursing offspring; bupivacaine liposome is likely safe to use in nursing mothers.

Overdose/Acute Toxicity

In safety studies, dogs receiving 1.5 to 5 times the labeled dose SC twice weekly all survived the 4-week study. No clinically relevant treatment-related effects on clinical observations, physical examination, body weight, ECG, hematology, serum chemistry, urinalysis, coagulation, or organ weights were detected. When used as labeled, acute toxicity is unlikely unless administered intravascularly. Intravascular administration may result in cardiovascular (eg, dysrhythmias, blood pressure fluctuation) and neurologic (eg, tremors, ataxia, seizures) adverse effects, although one study found that bupivacaine liposome 4.5 mg/kg IV had a favorable safety profile compared to bupivacaine HCl 0.75 mg/kg IV.[7]

In cats receiving up to 3 times the labeled dose (31.8 mg/kg) every 9 days for 3 doses as a right femoral nerve block (suprainguinal approach), 1 cat developed a suppurative, open necrotic wound in the right stifle after the second injection and was euthanized. Right limb impairment occurred in 23 of 24 cats and lasted between 1 to 5 days. Histopathology findings at the injection site included inflammation, mineralization, and myofiber degeneration and necrosis. No clinically relevant treatment-related effects on ECG, hematology, serum chemistry, urinalysis, coagulation, or organ weights were detected.

Management of bupivacaine overdose must begin with delivery of oxygen via a patent airway. Benzodiazepines and barbiturates can be used for seizure management but may cause further CNS depression. Cardiovascular support should be provided and may include IV fluids and vasopressor drugs. Prolonged resuscitative efforts may be required. Lipid emulsion 20% 1.5 mL/kg IV over 30 minutes can be beneficial.[8,9]

For patients that have experienced or are suspected to have experienced an overdose, it is strongly encouraged to consult with a 24-hour poison consultation center that specialize in providing information specific for veterinary patients. For general information related to overdose and toxin exposures, as well as contact information for poison control centers, refer to ***Appendix.***

Drug Interactions

The following drug interactions have either been reported or are theoretical in humans or animals receiving bupivacaine liposome and may be of significance in veterinary patients. Unless otherwise noted, use together is not necessarily contraindicated, but weigh the potential risks and perform additional monitoring when appropriate.

- **ANTISEPTICS, TOPICAL** (eg, **chlorhexidine, povidone iodine**): Do not allow contact with topical antiseptics; wait for these agents to dry before administering drug.[1]
- **BUPIVACAINE, INJECTABLE, AND OTHER AMIDE LOCAL ANESTHETICS** (eg, **lidocaine, mepivacaine**): Use with bupivacaine liposome may increase toxic effects. The veterinary label warns, *Do not administer concurrently with bupivacaine HCl, lidocaine, or other amide local anesthetics. A safe interval from time of bupivacaine HCl, lidocaine, or other amide local anesthetic administration to time of Nocita® administration has not been determined.*[1] However, the human bupivacaine liposome label states that other formulations of bupivacaine should not be administered within 96 hours following administration of bupivacaine liposome[3]; the label also states that liposomal bupivacaine may be administered 20 minutes or more after local administration of lidocaine.
- **HYALURONIDASE**: May increase local anesthetic toxicity or increase adverse effects

Laboratory Considerations

- None noted

Dosages

NOTES:

1. Do not shake vial. Invert the vial multiple times to re-suspend the particles immediately before withdrawal of the product from the vial.[1]
2. Prior to injection, aspirate to check for negative pressure at the injection site to prevent inadvertent intravascular administration.
3. See ***Compatibility/Compounding Considerations*** prior to diluting or combining bupivacaine liposome with any other drugs.

DOGS:

Single-dose infiltration into the surgical site to provide local postoperative analgesia for cranial cruciate ligament surgery (label dose; FDA-approved): 5.3 mg/kg (0.4 mL/kg) is administered by infiltration injection into the tissue layers at the time of incisional closure. Wear gloves when handling. Administer with a 25-gauge or larger bore needle.

Inject slowly into the tissues using an infiltration injection technique. Do not allow contact with topical antiseptics (eg, povidone iodine, chlorhexidine); wait for these agents to dry before instilling drug. To obtain adequate coverage, infiltrate all of the tissues in each surgical closure layer. Aspirate frequently to prevent intravascular administration. May be administered undiluted or diluted with up to an equal volume (1:1 by volume) of normal (0.9%) sterile saline or lactated Ringer's solution to obtain a volume sufficient to cover the surgical site. Do not dilute with water or other hypotonic solutions. Analgesic effects may persist up to 72 hours.[1]

CATS:

Peripheral nerve block to provide regional postoperative analgesia following onychectomy (label dose; FDA-approved): 5.3 mg/kg (0.4 mL/kg) per forelimb (ie, 10.6 mg/kg per cat) as a 4-point nerve block prior to forelimb onychectomy. Aspirate prior to injecting to prevent intravascular administration. See table below and refer to the product label for administration instructions. Wear gloves when handling. Administer with a 25-gauge or larger bore needle. Do NOT dilute prior to use as nerve block in cats. Analgesic effects may persist up to 72 hours.[1]

Site of 4-point nerve block	% of total forelimb volume	Dose volume (mL/kg)	Instructions
Superficial branch of the radial nerve	35%	0.14	At the center of the limb, on the dorsal aspect at the level of the antebrachiocarpal joint, insert the needle subcutaneously with the bevel up. Advance the needle subcutaneously and inject adjacent to the confluence of the accessory cephalic and cephalic veins.
Dorsal branch of the ulnar nerve	20%	0.08	Palpate a groove between the accessory carpal bone (in the base of the carpal pad) and the styloid process of the ulna. Distal to this groove, insert the needle subcutaneously with the bevel up and advance the needle proximally. Inject once the tip reaches the midpoint of the groove.
Median nerve and superficial branch of the palmar branch of the ulnar nerve	40%	0.16	Insert the needle subcutaneously with the bevel up lateral to the distal tip of the accessory carpal pad and advance the needle medially ⅔ the width of the limb, until the tip is located near the base of the first digit. Inject ⅔ of the volume at this point and the remaining volume while withdrawing the needle. Gently massage for 5 seconds.
Deep branch of the palmar branch of the ulnar nerve	5%	0.02	Orient the needle perpendicular to the long axis of the limb at the level of the accessory carpal bone. Insert the needle subcutaneously and advance the needle laterally until it contacts the medial aspect of the accessory carpal bone. Redirect the needle dorsally by rotating the needle 90°, advance it along the medial side of the accessory carpal bone 2 to 3 mm until it penetrates the flexor retinaculum, and inject.

Incisional block following ovariohysterectomy (extra-label): 5.4 mg/kg diluted to 5 mL with 0.9% NaCl into a syringe with a 22-gauge, 1-inch needle; after linea alba closure 2.5 mL was injected under the rectus sheath in a continuous line on both sides of the incision. After closure of the subcutaneous layer the remaining 2.5 mL was slowly injected at least 5 mm away from the incision such that a continuous line of anesthetic extended around the entire incision. Pain scores remained low for up to 68 hours after surgery, and reduced the need for postoperative robenacoxib use.[10]

Monitoring

- Adequate postsurgical analgesia is indicative of efficacy.
- If there was a significant chance that intravascular administration occurred, monitor for possible toxicity (eg, arrhythmias, changes in blood pressure, CNS excitation).

Client Information

- If your animal is discharged before 72 hours, monitor them for signs associated with pain and infection (eg, discharge, swelling). Be sure to contact your veterinarian if you are concerned about an infection. If an infection occurs, the anesthetic used to control the pain will not work well and it will cause your animal to be more painful.

Chemistry/Synonyms

Bupivacaine is an amide-type local anesthetic structurally related to lidocaine and mepivacaine. Chemically it is 1-butyl-*N*-(2,6-dimethylphenyl)-2-piperidinecarboxamide with a molecular weight of 288.4.

Bupivacaine liposome injectable suspension is a sterile, nonpyrogenic, and preservative-free white to off-white aqueous suspension of multivesicular lipid-based particles containing bupivacaine. Each mL contains 13.3 mg bupivacaine. Inactive ingredients and their nominal concentrations are cholesterol, 4.7 mg/mL; 1,2-dipalmitoyl-sn-glycero-3-phospho-rac-(1-glycerol) (DPPG), 0.9 mg/mL; tricaprylin, 2.0 mg/mL; and 1,2-dierucoylphosphatidylcholine (DEPC), 8.2 mg/mL.

Storage/Stability

Unopened vials should be stored refrigerated between 2°C and 8°C (36°F-46°F). Do not freeze. Unopened bottles may be held at a controlled room temperature of 20°C to 25°C (68°F-77°F) for up to 30 days.

Do not puncture the vial multiple times. Once the vial stopper has been punctured with a sterile needle, draw out the dose into a sterile syringe. Each syringe should be prepared for single patient use only. Discard the vial after all doses are withdrawn. Following withdrawal from the vial into a syringe, *Nocita*® may be stored at a controlled room temperature between 20°C and 25°C (68°F-77°F) for up to 4 hours. After 4 hours, the syringe must be discarded.[1] A study evaluating use of bupivacaine liposome injectable suspension single-dose vials in a multidose fashion (repeated vial entry over 5 days when stored both under refrigeration as well as at room temperature) found no bacterial growth, and free bupivacaine concentration remained stable for 4 days.[11]

According to the human label, bupivacaine liposome should not be administered if the stopper is bulging or if the vial is suspected of having been frozen or exposed to high temperatures.[6]

Compatibility/Compounding Considerations

Compatibility is dependent on factors such as pH, concentration, temperature, and diluent used; specialized references or a hospital pharmacist should be consulted for more specific information.

May be administered to dogs undiluted or diluted with up to an equal volume (1:1 by volume) of normal (0.9%) sterile saline or lactated Ringer's solution to obtain a volume sufficient to cover the surgical site. Do not dilute with water or other hypotonic solutions; this will result in disruption of the liposomal particles. Mixing with non-bupivacaine-based local anesthetics, including lidocaine (infiltrated or topical), may cause an immediate release of bupivacaine from the liposomes.[12] The product label states "do not dilute [bupivacaine liposome] prior to use as a nerve block in cats".[1]

The human label product includes similar diluent recommendations but with larger volumes, reflecting the common practice of combining bupivacaine HCL with bupivacaine liposome. This practice does not appear to be needed in veterinary medicine and no studies have been done to assess any possible advantage of such practice. When bupivacaine HCl and bupivacaine liposome are both used in the same patient, it is important to remember that the toxic effects of these products are additive; these drugs should be co-administered with caution, and the patient should be monitored for neurologic and cardiovascular effects related to toxicity.[6]

Dosage Forms/Regulatory Status

VETERINARY-LABELED PRODUCTS:

Bupivacaine Liposome Injectable Suspension 1.3% (13.3 mg/mL) in 10 mL and 20 mL single-use vials; *Nocita*®; (Rx). Approved for use in dogs and cats; NADA #141-461

HUMAN-LABELED PRODUCTS:

Bupivacaine Liposome Injectable Suspension 1.3% (13.3 mg/mL) in 10 mL and 20 mL single-use vials; *Exparel*®; (Rx)[6]

References

For the complete list of references, see **wiley.com/go/budde/plumb**

Buprenorphine

(byoo-pre-***nor***-feen) *Buprenex*®, *Simbadol*®, *Zorbium*®

Opioid Partial Agonist

Prescriber Highlights

- ▶ Partial mu-opioid agonist used primarily as an injectable and buccal (ie, oral transmucosal [OTM]) analgesic, especially in cats
- ▶ Often used as a component of short-term immobilization and anesthetic drug combinations
- ▶ Buccal/OTM administration is well tolerated and can be effective, but bioavailability is low by this route, as is standard (0.3 mg/mL) buprenorphine administered SC.
- ▶ Longer onset of action and longer duration of action as compared with most other opioids
- ▶ Rarely, may cause respiratory depression
- ▶ Because of tight buprenorphine receptor binding, standard doses of naloxone may not completely reverse drug effects.
- ▶ DEA Schedule III (C-III) controlled substance

Uses/Indications

Buprenorphine is most often used as an analgesic for mild to moderate pain or in preanesthetic drug combinations in small animals. In most species, buprenorphine provides less analgesia than pure mu-opioid agonists (eg, morphine, hydromorphone) and it is less sedating than most other opioids (particularly butorphanol). For acute pain control, buprenorphine may have the disadvantage of a longer onset of action than other opioids.

In dogs, an isoflurane MAC-sparing effect occurs at IV dosages of 0.01 mg/kg, 0.05 mg/kg, and 0.1 mg/kg[1] but methadone (0.3 mg/kg) provided more effective presurgical analgesia than buprenorphine (0.02 mg/kg) in dogs sedated with acepromazine and medetomidine prior to undergoing ovariohysterectomy (OHE).[2] Use of the feline-labeled *Simbadol*® (0.02 mg/kg IM) prior to surgery in dogs (pretreated with acepromazine and carprofen and undergoing ovariohysterectomy) provided similar postoperative analgesia as standard buprenorphine (0.02 mg/kg IM) but more dogs in the standard buprenorphine group (3/12) required postoperative rescue analgesia (vs 0/12 for *Simbadol*®).[3] Oral transmucosal (OTM) administration can provide effective analgesia (0.02 and 0.12 mg/kg were studied)[4] but bioavailability is low and variable with this route.[5] When used epidurally in combination with bupivacaine for stifle arthroplasty, buprenorphine produced sufficient analgesia for up to 24 hours.[6] Buprenorphine/bupivacaine combination for infraorbital nerve block had an isoflurane-sparing effect and extended the duration of analgesia to 48 to 96 hours.[7]

In cats, one product (*Simbadol*®) is a high-concentration (1.8 mg/mL), long-duration (72 hour) form of buprenorphine that is FDA-approved for SC administration for the control of postoperative pain associated with surgical procedures. A transdermal buprenorphine solution is FDA-approved for the control of postoperative pain. It is applied by veterinary staff in the clinic or hospital 1 to 2 hours prior to surgical procedures and provides analgesia for 4 days.[8]

In one study, when combined with medetomidine (0.002 mg/kg), standard concentration buprenorphine (0.3 mg/mL; 0.002 mg/kg) given IM provided equivalent analgesia to that provided by butorphanol (0.4 mg/kg) or methadone (0.5 mg/kg).[9] Combined with dexmedetomidine (0.001 mg/kg), butorphanol (0.4 mg/kg) provided better sedation and less vomiting than buprenorphine (0.02 mg/kg) when administered IM to cats.[10] With standard buprenorphine, buccal/OTM administration can be a practical, effective method for controlling postoperative pain. However, IV or IM administration of buprenorphine provides better postoperative (OHE) analgesia as compared with SC or buccal/OTM administration, and the cats receiving buprenorphine by the OTM route experienced a high prevalence of treatment failure.[11] Multidose injectable formulations may be less palatable to cats when given by the OTM route than the preservative-free formulation.[12] Combining opioids such as buprenorphine with short-term NSAIDs for postoperative pain control provides better analgesia than buprenorphine alone.[13]

In the UK and Australia, there are licensed buprenorphine products that are labeled for postoperative analgesia in dogs, cats, and horses and potentiation of the sedative effects of centrally acting agents in dogs and horses.

Pharmacology/Actions

Buprenorphine has partial agonist activity at the mu receptor and is a kappa-receptor antagonist. Buprenorphine is considered 30 times more potent than morphine and exhibits many of the same actions as the pure opioid agonists. It produces a dose-related analgesia; however, at higher doses, analgesic effects may plateau. Buprenorphine has a high affinity for, and slow dissociation from, mu receptors in the CNS, which may explain its relatively long duration of action. In dogs, sedative effects are generally seen after 15 minutes, but analgesia may not develop fully until 30 minutes postadministration. Analgesia is unlikely to persist for 12 hours unless pain is mild. A 6- to 8-hour duration of analgesic effect is often reported but analgesia may be as short as 4 hours, with high variability between cats.[13] Multimodal analgesia with frequent pain assessment is recommended. The high-concentration, long duration buprenorphine product lasts 72 hours when given SC to cats.

The cardiovascular effects of buprenorphine may cause a decrease in both blood pressure and cardiac rate. Rarely, human patients may exhibit increases in blood pressure and cardiac rate. Respiratory depression is a possibility and decreased respiratory rates have been noted in horses treated with buprenorphine. GI effects appear to be minimal in cats treated with buprenorphine.

Pharmacokinetics

In cats, buprenorphine is rapidly and completely absorbed when given IM.[14] Peak concentrations after SC injection can vary widely; blood concentrations are low and do not appear to correlate with analgesic effect. Buprenorphine has a volume of distribution at steady-state (VD_{ss}) of ≈3 to 8 L/kg and a clearance of ≈8 to 20 mL/kg per minute. Elimination half-life is ≈6 to 7 hours. When administered by the buccal/OTM route, bioavailability is low and highly variable (≈20% to 30%).[13,15] The human transdermal patch buprenorphine (*Transtec*®; UK) applied to cats has demonstrated widely variable blood concentrations and, without a loading dose, does not appear to provide adequate analgesia. Individual variability in response to buprenorphine administration by all administration routes, especially SC and OTM, has been reported. Some cats may not receive sufficient analgesia from buprenorphine.[13]

In dogs, oral bioavailability is very low (5%), but buprenorphine administered via the buccal/OTM route is ≈35% to 50% absorbed.[5] Elimination half-life ranges from 4 to 9 hours,[16] and wide interpatient variability exists. In a small pilot study, application of topical buprenorphine patches showed that plasma concentrations increased during the first 36 hours, then remained between 0.7 and 1 ng/mL during the study period.[17] In greyhounds, when buprenorphine was administered IV, the volume of distribution, plasma clearance, and terminal half-life were 3.54 L/kg, 10.3 mL/minute/kg, and 3.96 hours, respectively.[18] A pharmacokinetic study in 6 mongrel dogs resulted in a volume of distribution, plasma clearance, and terminal half-life of 4.68 L/kg, 23.3 mL/minute/kg, and 3.97 hours,[19] respectively, when buprenorphine was administered IV, and a terminal half-life of 12.74 hours when the extended-release injection was administered SC.[20]

In horses, the onset of action is ≈15 minutes after IV dosing. Buprenorphine is variably absorbed after IM administration and bioavailability is ≈50% to 80%.[21] Volume of distribution is ≈2.5 to 3 L/kg.[22,23] The peak effect occurs within 30 to 45 minutes and the duration of action may last up to 8 hours. Elimination half-life after an IV or IM dose is ≈3.5 to 6 hours.[22,23] Because acepromazine exhibits a similar onset and duration of action, many equine clinicians favor using acepromazine in combination with buprenorphine. One study found plasma buprenorphine concentrations between 0.34 and 2.45 ng/mL after IV administration of 10 µg/kg.[24] In foals younger than 21 days of age, buprenorphine 0.01 – 0.02 mg/kg IV had a VD_{ss} of 6.5 L/kg; clearance was 56 mL/kg/minute, and elimination half-life was ≈2 hours.[25] The same dosage administered sublingually was only 25% bioavailable, and plasma concentration reached the presumed therapeutic concentration briefly in only one foal; however, physiologic changes did occur, indicating absorption of the drug. The therapeutic concentration could be lower in foals than in other species.

Elimination half-life was 1 to 2.7 hours after IV and SC administration in alpacas, and SC bioavailability was 64%.[26]

The distribution of the drug has not been well studied. Data from work done in rats reflect that buprenorphine concentrates in the liver but is also found in the brain, GI tract, and placenta. It is highly bound (96%) to plasma proteins (not albumin).

In most species, buprenorphine is metabolized in the intestinal wall and liver[27,28] by N-dealkylation likely via CYP3A4 (forming norbuprenorphine, which is active). Buprenorphine and norbuprenorphine also undergo glucuronidation; metabolites are then eliminated by biliary excretion into the feces (≈70%) and urinary excretion (≈27%).

Contraindications/Precautions/Warnings

The drug is contraindicated in patients with a known hypersensitivity to it or other opioids.

Because of the potential for decreased clearance with subsequent exaggerated/prolonged effects, all opioids should be used with caution in patients that have hypothyroidism, impaired hepatic function, or adrenocortical insufficiency (Addison's disease), and in pediatric, geriatric, or severely debilitated patients.

Rarely, patients may develop respiratory depression from buprenorphine; therefore, it should be used cautiously in patients with compromised pulmonary function. Like other opioids, buprenorphine must be used with caution in patients with head trauma, increased CSF pressure, or other CNS dysfunction (eg, coma), as any degree of respiratory depression could result in excessive partial pressure of arterial carbon dioxide with a subsequent increase in intracranial pressure.

Patients with severe hepatic dysfunction may eliminate the drug more slowly than normal patients. Buprenorphine may increase bile duct pressure and should be used cautiously in patients with biliary tract disease[29]; however, this appears to not have any clinical impact. As with all opioids, buprenorphine should also be used with caution in horses that show signs of diminished GI tract motility.

Opioid analgesics are contraindicated in patients stung by scorpions (eg, *Centruroides* spp), as these drugs may potentiate venom effects.[30]

Mild sedation can occur in both dogs and cats, making buprenorphine an important component of a preanesthetic protocol; however, excitement can occur in horses and, less commonly, in cats, as is true of other opioids. Mild postoperative hyperthermia can occur in cats.[28]

Because buprenorphine can cause excitement in horses, when it is used as a preoperative analgesic, an IV sedative should be administered prior to, or in conjunction with, the buprenorphine injection.[22,23]

The standard formulation of buprenorphine by the SC route is not recommended due to poor absorption. Buprenorphine should not be administered via the intrathecal or peridural routes.

The transdermal solution requires ≈30 minutes to dry, and once dried the risk for human buprenorphine exposure following contact of the administration site is limited. Clinic staff should use personal protective equipment (impermeable gloves, eye protection, laboratory coat) when preparing or administering any of the concentrated buprenorphine products.[8]

Adverse Effects

Although rare, respiratory depression appears to be the major adverse effect. Other adverse effects (eg, sedation, nausea, vomiting, bradycardia, excitement [primarily cats and horses]) may be noted but generally occur less frequently as compared with other opioids.

In dogs, as with other opioids, salivation, bradycardia, hypothermia, agitation, dehydration, and miosis have been reported. Tachycardia, vomiting, and high blood pressure rarely occur. Injection site reactions and skin lesions have been noted with the non-FDA-approved extended-release injectable formulation and are most likely due to a reaction to the vehicle.[31] SC administration of high-concentration buprenorphine to dogs resulted in varying degrees of sedation, reduced appetite, panting, whining, and hyperptyalism.[20]

In cats, as with other opioids, mydriasis and behavioral effects (eg, excessive purring, pacing, rubbing, hiding) can be seen. Vomiting, salivation, anorexia, and hyperthermia occur rarely; however, hyperthermia was observed in ≈28% of cats on the day after surgery; constipation and mydriasis also were noted.[32] Vomiting occurred in 55% of cats receiving buprenorphine/dexmedetomidine combination with only 5% vomiting in cats receiving dexmedetomidine/butorphanol.[10] In a study, high doses of standard buprenorphine (0.24, 0.72, and 1.2 mg/kg/day SC) for 9 consecutive days were well tolerated in young cats. Adverse effects included hyperactivity, tachycardia, difficulty in handling, disorientation, agitation, and mydriasis.[33]

In horses, buprenorphine may cause ataxia, excitement, and diminished gut sounds, but colic has not been a major concern. All horses ($n = 4$) developed constipation after receiving a single SC or IM dose of an experimental sustained-release buprenorphine formulation.[34] Administration with a sedative (eg, acepromazine, detomidine) may help decrease excitement and cardiac and respiratory rates.

In rabbits, SC buprenorphine reduced food and water intake, GI transit, and fecal output.[35,36]

The primary adverse effect seen in humans is sedation, with an incidence of ≈66%.[29] Buprenorphine may cause urine retention or difficulty voiding, particularly with high IV doses or epidural administration.

Reproductive/Nursing Safety

Safe use of veterinary buprenorphine formulations in breeding, pregnant, or lactating animals has not been established. The drug crosses the placenta. Although no controlled studies have been performed in domestic animals or humans, the drug has exhibited no evidence of teratogenicity or causing impaired fertility in laboratory animals. Early fetal death and postimplantation loss have been noted in rats.[27] The *Vetergesic*® 0.3 mg/mL solution for injection for dogs and cats label (Canada) states that the drug is contraindicated preoperatively for cesarean section due to concerns for respiratory depression in offspring.[27]

In rats, maternal milk buprenorphine concentration equaled or exceeded that of plasma[27]; however, maternal milk buprenorphine concentrations are low in humans[37] and no adverse effects were seen in 4-week-old infants nursing from buprenorphine-treated women.[38] There are no data for commonly encountered veterinary species.

Because safety has not been established in animals, this drug should only be used when the maternal benefits outweigh the potential risks to offspring.

Overdose/Acute Toxicity

The intraperitoneal LD_{50} of buprenorphine has been reported to be 243 mg/kg in rats. The ratio of lethal dose to effective dose is at least 1000:1 in rodents. Because of the apparent high index of safety, life-threatening acute overdoses should be rare in veterinary medicine, but most overdoses will cause clinical signs. Common findings in dogs (in decreasing frequency) include vocalization, ataxia, hypersalivation, hypothermia, and lethargy.

Treatment with naloxone and doxapram has been suggested for cases of acute overdoses causing respiratory or cardiac effects.[27] Secondary to buprenorphine's high affinity for the mu-opioid receptor, high doses and/or repeated doses of naloxone may be required to treat respiratory depression. See ***Naloxone***.

For patients that have experienced or are suspected to have experienced an overdose, consultation with a 24 hour poison consultation center specializing in providing veterinary-specific information is recommended. For general information related to overdose and toxin exposures, as well as contact information for poison control centers, refer to ***Appendix***.

Drug Interactions

The following drug interactions have either been reported or are theoretical in humans or animals receiving buprenorphine and may be of significance in veterinary patients. Unless otherwise noted, use together is not necessarily contraindicated, but the potential risks should be weighed, and additional monitoring performed when appropriate. **NOTE**: Drug interactions may be positive rather than adverse (eg potentiation of local anesthetic effects when combined with buprenorphine).

- ANESTHETICS, LOCAL (eg, **mepivacaine, bupivacaine**): When buprenorphine and the local anesthetic agent are combined in the same syringe and injected perineurally, the anesthetic action may be potentiated.
- ANTICONVULSANTS (eg, **phenobarbital, phenytoin**): May decrease plasma buprenorphine concentrations
- BENZODIAZEPINES (eg, **diazepam, midazolam**): Case reports of humans developing respiratory/cardiovascular/CNS depression; use combination with caution
- CNS DEPRESSANT AGENTS (eg, **anesthetic agents, antihistamines, barbiturates, benzodiazepines, phenothiazines, tranquilizers**): May cause increased CNS or cardiorespiratory depression when used with buprenorphine
- DESMOPRESSIN: The concurrent use of desmopressin and opioids may increase the risk for hyponatremia.
- ERYTHROMYCIN: Can increase plasma buprenorphine concentrations
- HALOTHANE: Reduced hepatic blood flow during anesthesia can increase buprenorphine effects.
- KETOCONAZOLE, ITRACONAZOLE, FLUCONAZOLE: Can increase plasma buprenorphine concentrations
- METOCLOPRAMIDE: Concurrent use of metoclopramide and buprenorphine may increase the risk for CNS depression.
- MONOAMINE OXIDASE INHIBITORS (MAOIs; eg, **selegiline, amitraz**): Possible additive effects or increased CNS depression; combination is not recommended in humans due to additional risk for serotonin syndrome[29]
- NALOXONE: Will reduce analgesia but is less effective at reversing buprenorphine effects as compared with other opioids
- OPIOIDS (PURE MU-AGONISTS) (eg, **fentanyl, hydromorphone**): Buprenorphine may potentially antagonize some analgesic effects but may also reverse some of the sedative and respiratory depressant effects of pure agonists.
- PANCURONIUM: If used with buprenorphine, may cause increased conjunctival changes
- PHENOBARBITAL: Concurrent use of phenobarbital and buprenorphine may result in increased risk for CNS depression and/or decreased plasma concentrations of buprenorphine.
- QT PROLONGING AGENTS (eg, **cisapride, quinidine, sotalol**): Concurrent use can increase the risk for life-threatening arrhythmias in humans; significance in veterinary patients is unknown.
- RIFAMPIN: Potentially decreased plasma buprenorphine concentrations
- SEROTONERGIC AGENTS (eg, **clomipramine, fluoxetine, mirtazapine, trazodone**): Concurrent use may increase the risk for serotonin syndrome.[29]
- TRAMADOL: May increase the risk for serotonin syndrome and respiratory depression[29]

Laboratory Considerations

None noted

Dosages

DOGS:

Analgesia (all extra-label):

a) **General use:** 5 – 30 µg/kg (0.005 – 0.03 mg/kg) IV or IM every 4 to 6 hours; consider extended dosing interval to 8 to 12 hours for treating mild pain. **NOTE**: SC administration of buprenorphine does not provide clinical analgesia due to erratic drug absorption.[39]

b) **Constant rate infusion (CRI):** Following an IV loading dose of 5 – 10 µg/kg (0.005 – 0.01 mg/kg), 2 – 4 µg/kg/hour IV CRI has been suggested. Acceptable analgesia was described in a pharmacokinetic study evaluating a loading dose of 15 µg/kg (0.015 mg/kg) IV administered after recovery from anesthesia, followed by 2.5 µg/kg/hour IV CRI for 6 hours.[40]

c) **Postoperative analgesia**: 10 – 20 µg/kg (0.01 – 0.02 mg/kg) IV or IM.[41,42] For further pain relief, repeat if necessary with 10 µg/kg (0.01 mg/kg) after 3 to 4 hours or 20 µg/kg (0.02 mg/kg) every 5 to 6 hours; exact timing is based on expected duration of the dose administered, degree of pain, and results of pain assessment.

d) **Postoperative analgesia using the feline-labeled buprenorphine product (*Simbadol®*)**: In dogs undergoing ovariohysterectomy, buprenorphine 20 µg/kg (0.02 mg/kg) IV, IM in combination with acepromazine 0.02 mg/kg IM as a premedication followed by carprofen 4.4 mg/kg SC administered after induction of anesthesia provided immediate postoperative analgesia (duration not determined).[39]

e) **Buccal (oral transmucosal; OTM) for postsurgical analgesia**: Based on study results, the authors concluded that 120 µg/kg (0.12 mg/kg) buccally before OHE was an effective analgesic with minimal intraoperative and postoperative adverse effects.[43] Under experimental conditions, 30 µg/kg (0.03 mg/kg) provided antinociceptive effects.[44]

Premedication before surgery or as an anesthetic adjunct (extra-label): **NOTE:** Many potential combinations have been suggested; the following are examples and are not inclusive. For additional information, refer to anesthesia-specific references.

a) In one study, buprenorphine 20 µg/kg (0.02 mg/kg) was

combined in the same syringe with either acepromazine 0.03 mg/kg or dexmedetomidine (dosed by body surface area at 250 μg/m^2) and injected IM prior to induction of anesthesia. IV catheters were placed 30 to 45 minutes after premedication, and general anesthesia was induced with propofol or alfaxalone. Meloxicam 0.2 mg/kg IV was given after induction and before surgery started. General anesthesia was maintained with isoflurane. Both combinations (buprenorphine with either acepromazine or dexmedetomidine) resulted in suitable anesthesia and analgesia for dogs undergoing elective procedures; some animals required additional analgesia within 4 hours of the premedication. Postsurgical analgesic differences were not clinically significant.[45]

b) In another study, the efficacy and cardiorespiratory effects of a combination of dexmedetomidine 15 μg/kg, ketamine 3 mg/kg, and either buprenorphine 40 μg/kg, butorphanol 0.2 mg/kg, or hydromorphone 0.05 mg/kg as a single IM injection (with or without reversal by atipamezole) in dogs undergoing castration was tested. Supplemental isoflurane was used when anesthesia was considered inadequate during surgery. The authors concluded that the most suitable analgesic with this drug combination was buprenorphine and that the use of atipamezole after surgery shortened recovery times.[46]

CATS:

Analgesia:

a) **Control of postoperative pain associated with surgical procedures** (label dosage; FDA-approved):
   i. Using the high-concentration SC injection (*Simbadol*®): 0.24 mg/kg SC once daily for up to 3 days.[28] Administer the first dose ≈1 hour prior to surgery. Do not dispense for administration at home by the pet owner due to the risks associated with the high concentration of *Simbadol*® (1.8 mg/mL) compared with other buprenorphine products.
   ii. Using the transdermal solution (*Zorbium*®): The label dosage provides a dosage range of 2.7 – 6.7 mg/kg, and the duration of analgesia is 4 days.[8] Apply to healthy and non-injured skin at the dorsal cervical region; part hair prior to application. Administer in the veterinary clinic or hospital 1 to 2 hours prior to surgical procedure.
   - For cats weighing 1.2 to 3 kg (2.6 to 6.6 lb): 0.4 mL (8 mg)
   - For cats weighing greater than 3 kg (6.6 lb) and up to 7.5 kg (16.5 lb): 1 mL (20 mg)

b) **General use and postoperative analgesia** (extra-label): 10 – 30 μg/kg (0.01 – 0.03 mg/kg) standard buprenorphine IM, IV, or buccal/OTM every 4 to 8 hours. Dosages at the high end of the dosing range may be required for more severe pain. **NOTE**: If using buccal/OTM, suggest using upper end of dosing range or higher (up to 0.05 mg/kg). Use of high-concentration buprenorphine (*Simbadol*®) 0.12 – 0.24 mg/kg buccal/OTM provided analgesia under experimental conditions with a duration of 8 to 12 hours (not 24 hours as provided by SC administration).[47]

c) **Constant rate infusion** (extra-label): Although not reported in cats, anecdotally the use as an infusion is the same as that used in dogs.

Premedication before surgery or as an anesthetic adjunct (extra-label): **NOTE:** Many potential combinations have been suggested; the following are examples and are not inclusive. For additional information, refer to anesthesia-specific references.

a) 0.01 – 0.03 mg/kg buprenorphine IM either 30 minutes prior to or combined with medetomidine 0.1 mg/kg (or dexmedetomidine 0.05 – 0.08 mg/kg) and ketamine 10 mg/kg and given IM for a brief, light plane of anesthesia. Inhalant may be needed for longer-term anesthesia or moderate-severe pain-level procedures.[48] Atipamezole can be used to reverse the alpha-2 agonist, if desired.

b) In one study, buprenorphine at 20 μg/kg (0.02 mg/kg) was combined in the same syringe with either acepromazine 0.03 mg/kg or dexmedetomidine (dosed by body surface area at 250 μg/m^2) and injected IM. IV catheters were placed 30 to 45 minutes after premedication and general anesthesia induction was done using propofol or alfaxalone. Meloxicam was given IV (0.3 mg/kg) after induction before surgery started. General anesthesia was maintained with isoflurane. Both combinations (buprenorphine with either acepromazine or dexmedetomidine) resulted in suitable anesthesia and analgesia for cats undergoing elective procedures; some animals required additional analgesia within 4 hours of the premedication. Cats given dexmedetomidine were more sedated than when acepromazine was used. Analgesic effect differences postsurgery were not clinically significant.[45]

c) In a study assessing analgesia after OHE, one of the protocols used was: 10 minutes prior to surgery, ketamine 60 mg/m^2 (≈3 mg/kg), midazolam 3 mg/m^2 (≈0.2 mg/kg), medetomidine 600 μg/m^2 (≈30 μg/kg), and buprenorphine 180 μg/m^2 (≈9 μg/kg) were combined and given as a single IM injection in the quadriceps muscles. In addition, either carprofen (4 mg/kg) or meloxicam (0.3 mg/kg) was given SC. All protocols in the study provided adequate analgesia.[49]

HORSES:

Neuroleptanalgesia (all extra-label):

a) 4 – 10 μg/kg (0.004 – 0.01 mg/kg) IV; usually given with a sedative such as acepromazine and/or detomidine.[50-52] IM administration could also be used, but bioavailability may be reduced, and onset of action delayed.

b) **Analgesia**: 10 μg/kg (0.01 mg/kg) IV, given 5 minutes after administration of an IV sedative.[41] A single dose may be repeated if necessary, after no less than 1 to 2 hours. A case report noted 6 μg/kg (0.006 mg/kg) sublingually every 12 hours provided analgesia to a 5-month-old filly with a C1 fracture.[53]

c) **To potentiate sedation**: 5 μg/kg (0.005 mg/kg) IV given 5 minutes after administration of an IV sedative.[41] The dose may be repeated after 10 minutes if necessary.

SHEEP:

Sedation (extra-label): 0.02 mg/kg combined with acepromazine 0.03 mg/kg and given IM provided similar sedation as morphine/acepromazine.[54]

SWINE:

Analgesic (extra-label): 0.04 mg/kg IM once effectively reduced lameness[55] and alleviated castration-related pain behaviors[56] in piglets.

FERRETS:

Analgesic (extra-label): 0.01 – 0.05 mg/kg SC or IM 2 to 3 times daily.[57] Anecdotally can use as a preanesthetic/anesthetic adjunct combined with an alpha-2 agonist and ketamine at the same dosages listed for cats.

RABBITS/GUINEA PIGS:

Analgesic (all extra-label):

a) **Rabbits**:
   1. 0.05 mg/kg SC, IM, or IV every 4 to 12 hours; 0.5 mg/kg rectally every 12 hours[58]
   2. One study in rabbits found that a compounded buprenorphine extended release (ER) formulation was at least as

effective as commercially available buprenorphine for postoperative analgesia. The ER formulation was prepared using FDA-approved buprenorphine powder and a proprietary polymer matrix. The product was administered at 0.12 mg/kg SC as a single injection and compared with commercially available buprenorphine at 0.02 mg/kg SC every 12 hours.[59]

b) **Guinea pigs**: 0.05 mg/kg SC or IV every 4 to 12 hours [60]

Premedication or anesthetic adjunct in rabbits (all extra-label):

a) **Compromised patients**: 0.05 – 0.1 mg/kg SC[61]

b) Buprenorphine 0.03 – 0.05 mg/kg IM or SC either 30 minutes before or combined with medetomidine 0.25 mg/kg (or dexmedetomidine 0.125 mg/kg) and ketamine 15 mg/kg IM or SC for a brief, light plane of anesthesia. Inhalant may be needed for longer-term anesthesia or moderate-severe pain-level procedures.[62] Atipamezole can be used to reverse the alpha-2 agonist, if desired.

c) **Healthy animals before uncomplicated elective procedures**: buprenorphine 0.02 – 0.06 mg/kg combined with midazolam (0.25 – 0.5 mg/kg) and given IM within 20 minutes of procedure; used with a local or line incisional block using lidocaine and bupivacaine [63]

MICE/RATS:

Analgesic:

a) **Mice:**

i. **Postprocedural pain control** (label dosage, FDA-indexed):

- Using extended-release buprenorphine suspension: 3.25 mg/kg SC as a single injection.[64] If needed, a single repeat dose may be administered 72 hours after the initial dose.
- Using extended-release buprenorphine solution: 1 – 1.5 mg/kg SC[65]

ii. **Using standard buprenorphine** (extra-label): 0.05 – 0.1 mg/kg SC every 12 hours[60]

b) **Rats:**

i. **Postprocedural pain control using extended-release buprenorphine product** (label dosage, FDA-indexed): 0.65 mg/kg SC as a single injection.[64] If needed, a single repeat dose may be administered 72 hours after the initial dose.

ii. **Using standard buprenorphine** (extra-label): 0.01 – 0.05 mg/kg SC or IV every 8 to 12 hours or 0.1 – 0.25 mg/kg PO every 8 to 12 hours[60]

Monitoring

- Analgesic efficacy (pain scores)
- Respiratory effects (respiratory rate, $ETCO_2$, SpO_2)
- Cardiac effects (heart rate, ECG, blood pressure)
- Body temperature (in cats, due to potential development of hyperthermia)

Client Information

- Buprenorphine is an opioid analgesic often used for short-term pain relief. It is given either by injection or buccally (ie, oral transmucosally [OTM]; squirted into the side of the mouth).
- When giving buccally/OTM to cats, gently squirt or drip just under the tongue or in the cheek pouch for the best effect. The doses are very small for this potent drug, so be sure you are giving the exact amount your veterinarian has prescribed.
- Sedation is the most common side effect.
- Buprenorphine is classified as a schedule III (C-III) controlled drug by the federal Drug Enforcement Agency (DEA) and requires a new written prescription for refills. Use of this medication in animals or humans other than those for whom they are prescribed is illegal.

Chemistry/Synonyms

Buprenorphine is a thebaine derivative and a synthetic partial-opioid agonist. It occurs as a white crystalline powder with a solubility of 17 mg/mL in water and 42 mg/mL in alcohol. The commercially available injectable product (*Buprenex*®) has a pH of 3.5 to 5 and is a sterile solution of the drug dissolved in D_5W. Terms of potency are expressed in terms of buprenorphine. The commercial human product contains 0.324 mg/mL of buprenorphine HCl, which is equivalent to 0.3 mg/mL of buprenorphine. Autoclaving may considerably decrease drug potency.

Buprenorphine HCl may also be known as buprenorphini hydrochloridum, CL-112302, NIH-8805, UM-952; trade names include *Animalgesics*®, BupaqB, *Buprenex*®, *Buprenodale*®, *EthiqaXR*®, *Simbadol*®, Suboxone®, *Subutex*®, and *Temgesic*®, and *Vetergesic*®.

Storage/Stability

Buprenorphine Injection 1.8 mg/mL (*Simbadol*®) should be stored at temperatures up to 25°C (77°F) and protected from light and excessive heat (greater than 40°C [104°F]). The vial has a 56-day in-use shelf-life.

Buprenorphine transdermal solution should be stored at temperatures up to 25°C (77°F) and protected from light.

As a controlled substance, buprenorphine must be stored in an area that is substantially constructed and securely locked in accordance with DEA regulations. Follow applicable local, state, and federal rules regarding disposal of unused or wasted controlled drugs.

Store buprenorphine extended-release injectable suspension vials (*Ethiqa XR*®) at temperatures between 15°C and 25°C (59°F-77°F) or refrigerated. Do not freeze. Discard 28 days after broaching. Wear gloves when handling. Allow drug to reach room temperature before administration.

Store buprenorphine extended-release injectable solution (*BupreLab-Rat*®) between 15° and 30°C (59°-86°F). Discard 28 days after broaching.

Buprenorphine 0.3 mg/mL injection should be stored at 20°C to 25°C (68°F-77°F) and protected from prolonged exposure to light. Temperatures above 40°C (104°F) or below freezing should be avoided.

Compatibility/Compounding Considerations

Compatibility is dependent on factors such as pH, concentration, temperature, and diluent used; specialized references or a hospital pharmacist should be consulted for more specific information.

Buprenorphine is reported to be **compatible** with the following IV solutions and drugs: acepromazine, atropine, diphenhydramine, D5W, D5W with normal saline, glycopyrrolate, haloperidol, hydroxyzine, lactated Ringer's solution, normal saline, scopolamine, and xylazine. Although no published data could be located to support stability for these combinations, buprenorphine injection has also been mixed in syringes with detomidine, dexmedetomidine, ketamine, medetomidine, and midazolam.

Buprenorphine is reportedly **incompatible** with diazepam and lorazepam.

An in vitro study demonstrated that a 3 mg/mL buprenorphine solution compounded for buccal/OTM use was stable for at least 90 days when stored at room temperature or refrigerated.[66] A buccal/OTM buprenorphine suspension was prepared by dissolving a 2 mg sublingual tablet in 0.6 mL deionized water and adding to 6 mL simple syrup (final concentration, 0.3 mg/mL). The product had a pH of 3.9 and was stable for 21 days at room temperature or refrigerated. A pharmacokinetic study using this formulation showed that peak concentration and AUC were ≈45% and ≈50% lower, respectively, with the compounded product as compared with the commercial injection (0.3 mg/mL).[67]

Buprenorphine injection (0.3 mg/mL) diluted 1:10 with bacteriostatic saline experienced less than 10% drug loss when stored in glass vials for 180 days either refrigerated or at room temperature. Storage in plastic syringes for 180 days resulted in more than 80% loss at room temperature and 28% loss refrigerated.[68]

Dosage Forms/Regulatory Status

VETERINARY-LABELED PRODUCTS:

The Association of Racing Commissioners International (ARCI) has designated this drug as a class 2 substance. Use of this drug may not be allowed in certain animal competitions. Check rules and regulations before entering in a competition while this medication is being administered. Contact local racing authorities for further guidance. See ***Appendix*** for more information.

Buprenorphine Injection 1.8 mg/mL in 10 mL multidose vials; *Simbadol*®; (Rx; DEA C-III). FDA-approved (NADA #141-434) for use in cats

Buprenorphine Transdermal Solution: 20 mg/mL in 0.4 mL or 1 mL applicator tubes; *Zorbium*®; (Rx; DEA C-III). FDA-approved (NADA #141-547) for use in cats

Buprenorphine Extended-Release Injectable Suspension: 1.3 mg/mL (buprenorphine hydrochloride, equivalent to 1.2 mg/mL buprenorphine) as a lipid-encapsulated formulation in 1.6 and 3 mL multidose vials; *EthiqaXR*®; (Rx; C-III). Not FDA-approved; legally marketed as an FDA-indexed product under MIF 900-014. Extra-label use is prohibited.

Buprenorphine Extended-Release Injectable Solution: 1 mg/mL in 5 mL multidose vials; *BupreLab-Rat*; Rx; C-III). Not FDA-approved; legally marketed as an FDA-indexed product under MIF 900-006. Extra-label use is prohibited.

A compounded sustained-release formulation by ZooPharm has been used in several domestic and wildlife species, such as dogs,[69] cats,[70] rabbits,[59] Göttingen minipigs,[71] sheep,[72,73] elephant seals,[74] and macaques.[75]

HUMAN-LABELED PRODUCTS:

Buprenorphine HCl for Injection: 0.324 mg/mL (equivalent to 0.3 mg/mL buprenorphine); 1 mL amps, vials, and syringes; *Buprenex*, generic; (Rx, C-III)

Buprenorphine HCl Sublingual Tablets: 2 mg and 8 mg (as base); generic; (Rx, DEA C-III)

References

For the complete list of references, see **wiley.com/go/budde/plumb**

Buspirone

(byoo-***spye***-rone) *BuSpar*®

Anxiolytic

Prescriber Highlights

- Nonbenzodiazepine anxiolytic agent used in dogs and cats.
- May take a week or more to be effective; not appropriate for acute treatment of situational anxieties
- Use with caution in patients with severe hepatic or renal disease.
- Adverse effects are relatively uncommon; cats may exhibit behavior changes.
- Many potential drug interactions

Uses/Indications

Buspirone may be effective in treating certain behavior disorders in dogs and cats, principally those that are phobia-related and those associated with social interactions. Buspirone may also be useful for urine spraying,[1] fear-related behavior,[2] or psychogenic alopecia[3] in cats. Approximately 50% of cats show a decrease in urine marking when buspirone is given, and the drug may be more effective in multi-cat households than in single-cat households.[1]

Although no comparative studies have been performed, other drugs (eg, fluoxetine, clomipramine) are likely more effective.

Pharmacology/Actions

Buspirone is an anxioselective agent. Thus, unlike benzodiazepines, buspirone does not possess any anticonvulsant or muscle relaxant activity and little sedative or psychomotor impairment activity. Buspirone does not have significant affinity for benzodiazepine receptors and does not affect GABA binding. It appears to act as a partial agonist at serotonin (5-HT_{1A}) receptors and as an agonist/antagonist of dopamine (D2) receptors in the CNS. In neurons, buspirone slows neuronal serotonin depletion.

Pharmacokinetics

In a limited study done in 6 cats,[4] oral administration of buspirone gave peak concentrations in ≈1.4 hours, but oral bioavailability appeared to be significantly lower than in humans. Transdermal administration of buspirone (PLO-base) did not yield detectable concentrations (ELISA method). However, a study comparing the effects of oral versus transdermal buspirone on urine marking indicated a significant reduction in urine marking frequency for both groups and there was no difference in efficacy between the two groups. This study administered the medication for 35 days and included 17 cats in each group.[5]

In humans, buspirone is rapidly and completely absorbed but a high first-pass effect limits systemic bioavailability to ≈5%. Binding to plasma proteins is very high (95%). In rats, the highest tissue concentrations are found in the lungs, kidneys, and fat. Lower concentrations are found in the brain, heart, skeletal muscle, plasma, and liver. The elimination half-life (in humans) is ≈2 to 4 hours. Buspirone is hepatically metabolized to several metabolites (including the active 1-PP). These metabolites are primarily excreted in the urine.

Contraindications/Precautions/Warnings

Buspirone is contraindicated in patients hypersensitive to it. Clearance of buspirone may be reduced in animals with either significant renal or hepatic disease, therefore increasing the risk for adverse effects. Because buspirone may blunt disinhibitory neural processes, it should be used with caution in aggressive animals. Sedation is possible, although less than with other anxiolytic drugs; use this drug with caution in working or service dogs, as their level of alertness may be affected.

Because buspirone often takes a week or more for effect, it should not be used as the sole therapy for situational anxieties.

Do not confuse BusPIRone and BuPROPion.

Adverse Effects

Buspirone is generally well-tolerated; adverse effects are usually minimal. Bradycardia, GI disturbances (eg, inappetence, vomiting), and stereotypic behaviors (eg, excessive grooming, pacing) are possible. Cats may demonstrate increased affection, which may be the desired effect. In multi-cat households, cats that have previously been extremely timid in the face of repeated aggression from other cats may, after receiving buspirone, become less anxious and more assertive.

In humans, the most likely adverse effect profile seen with buspirone includes dizziness, headache, nausea, anorexia, and restlessness; other neurologic effects (including sedation) may be noted. Rarely, tachycardias and other cardiovascular clinical signs may be present.

Reproductive/Nursing Safety

Although the drug has not been proven safe during pregnancy, doses up to 30 times the labeled human dose in rabbits and rats demonstrated no teratogenic effects.[6] Because safety has not been established in animals, this drug should only be used when the maternal benefits outweigh the potential fetal risks.

Buspirone and its metabolites have been detected in the milk of lactating rats; avoid use during nursing if possible.

Overdose/Acute Toxicity

Limited information is available. Hypertension, increased total peripheral resistance, and increased urinary volume and electrolyte loss occurred in dogs given 0.3 – 3 mg/kg IV.[7] The oral LD_{50} in dogs is 586 mg/kg.[8] Oral overdoses may produce vomiting, dizziness, drowsiness, miosis, and gastric distention. Standard overdose protocols should be followed after ingestion has been determined.

For patients that have experienced or are suspected to have experienced an overdose, it is strongly encouraged to consult with a 24-hour poison consultation center that specialize in providing information specific for veterinary patients. For general information related to overdose and toxin exposures, as well as contact information for poison control centers, refer to ***Appendix.***

Drug Interactions

The following drug interactions have either been reported or are theoretical in humans or animals receiving buspirone and may be of significance in veterinary patients. Unless otherwise noted, use together is not necessarily contraindicated, but weigh the potential risks and perform additional monitoring when appropriate.

- **Alpha-2-Adrenergic Agonists** (eg, **dexmedetomidine, xylazine**): May increase risk for CNS and respiratory depression
- **Alpha-2-Adrenergic Antagonists** (eg, **phenoxybenzamine, prazosin, tamsulosin**): May increase risk for hypotension and orthostasis
- **Anesthetic Agents** (eg, **isoflurane, ketamine, propofol**): May increase risk for CNS and respiratory depression
- **Angiotensin Converting Enzyme Inhibitors** (ACEIs; eg, **enalapril**): May increase risk for hypotension and orthostasis
- **Angiotensin Receptors Blockers** (eg, **telmisartan**): May increase risk for hypotension and orthostasis
- **Antihistamines** (eg, **cetirizine, chlorpheniramine**): May increase risk for CNS and respiratory depression
- **Apomorphine:** May increase risk for CNS depression, somnolence, and dizziness
- **Azole Antifungals** (eg, **fluconazole, ketoconazole**): May slow metabolism of buspirone, thus potentially significantly increasing buspirone concentrations
- **Barbiturates** (eg, **methohexital, phenobarbital**): May increase risk for CNS and respiratory depression
- **Benzodiazepines** (eg, **alprazolam, midazolam**): May increase risk for CNS depression
- **Bromocriptine:** May increase risk for CNS and respiratory depression and serotonin syndrome
- **Calcium Channel Blockers** (**amlodipine, diltiazem, verapamil**): May increase risk for hypotension and orthostasis. Diltiazem and verapamil may increase buspirone plasma concentrations and adverse effects.
- **Carbamazepine:** May result in decreased buspirone concentrations
- **Cimetidine:** May increase buspirone concentrations
- **Clarithromycin/Erythromycin:** May slow metabolism of buspirone, thus potentially significantly increasing buspirone concentrations
- **Danazol:** May slow metabolism of buspirone, thus potentially significantly increasing buspirone concentrations
- **Diazoxide:** May increase risk for hypotension and orthostasis
- **Digoxin:** Buspirone may displace digoxin from protein binding sites. Clinical significance is uncertain.
- **Diuretics** (eg, **bumetanide, furosemide**): May increase risk for hypotension and orthostasis
- **Felbamate:** May increase risk for CNS depression
- **Fenoldopam:** May increase risk for hypotension and orthostasis
- **Flavoxate:** May increase risk for CNS and respiratory depression
- **Gabapentin:** May increase risk for CNS depression
- **Grapefruit Juice (powder):** May cause increased buspirone plasma concentrations and adverse effects
- **Glucocorticoids** (eg, **dexamethasone, prednis(ol)one**): May increase metabolism of buspirone
- **Ifosfamide:** May increase neurotoxic effects of ifosfamide
- **Levetiracetam:** May increase risk for CNS and respiratory depression
- **Lithium:** May increase risk for serotonin syndrome and CNS and respiratory depression
- **Magnesium Sulfate:** Concurrent use of high doses of magnesium sulfate may increase risk for CNS and respiratory depression.
- **Methylene Blue:** May increase risk for serotonin syndrome
- **Metoclopramide:** May increase risk for CNS and respiratory depression and neuroleptic malignant syndrome
- **Minocycline IV:** May increase CNS depression due to magnesium content of the IV formulation
- **Mirtazapine:** May increase risk for serotonin syndrome
- **Mitotane:** May decrease buspirone concentrations
- **Monoamine Oxidase Inhibitors** (MAOIs; eg, **amitraz, linezolid, selegiline**): Concurrent buspirone use, or use within 14 days of discontinuing MAOI, is contraindicated because dangerous hypertension and serotonin syndrome may occur.
- **Muscle Relaxants** (eg, **baclofen, methocarbamol**): May increase risk for CNS and respiratory depression
- **Opioids** (eg, **fentanyl, morphine**): May increase risk for severe respiratory depression, coma, and death
- **Phenothiazines** (eg, **acepromazine, chlorpromazine**): May increase risk for CNS and respiratory depression
- **Pergolide:** May increase risk for CNS and respiratory depression
- **Phenylbutazone:** May increase rate of buspirone metabolism
- **Pregabalin:** May increase risk for CNS and respiratory depression
- **Procarbazine:** May inhibit metabolism of buspirone, increasing risk for serotonin syndrome and dangerous hypertension
- **Rifampin:** May cause decreased buspirone plasma concentrations
- **Serotonin Antagonists** (eg, **dolasetron, ondansetron**): May increase risk for serotonin syndrome
- **Selective Serotonin Reuptake Inhibitors** (SSRIs; eg, **fluoxetine, paroxetine**): May increase risk for serotonin syndrome. SSRIs may decrease metabolism of buspirone. Concurrent use may increase psychiatric signs. Dosage reductions may be necessary to minimize adverse effects.
- **Tramadol:** May increase risk for serotonin syndrome and CNS and respiratory depression
- **Trazodone:** Use with buspirone may cause increased ALT and increased risk for serotonin syndrome.
- **Tricyclic Antidepressants** (TCAs; eg, **amitriptyline, clomipramine**): May increase the risk for serotonin syndrome. Dosage reductions may be necessary to minimize adverse effects.

- **Valproic Acid/Divalproex:** May increase risk for CNS and respiratory depression
- **Vasodilators** (eg, **hydralazine**, **nitroglycerin**, **nitroprusside**): May increase risk for hypotension and orthostasis
- **Zonisamide**: May increase risk for CNS and respiratory depression

Dosages

DOGS:

Adjunctive treatment of low-grade anxieties and fears (extra-label): Most recommendations fall into a range of 0.5 – 1 mg/kg PO every 8 to 12 hours, but anecdotal recommendations as high as 2 mg/kg have been noted. Some recommendations have maximum dosage limits of 10 – 15 mg/dog (NOT mg/kg) PO every 8 to 12 hours.

CATS:

Adjunctive treatment of low-grade anxieties and fears, urine spraying, and overgrooming (extra-label): 0.5 – 1 mg/kg PO every 12 hours. Practically, using 5 mg tablets: 2.5 – 7.5 mg/cat (NOT mg/kg) PO every 12 hours[9]

Monitoring

- Efficacy
- Adverse effects

Client Information

- May be given either with food or on an empty stomach. If animal vomits or acts sick after receiving it on an empty stomach, give with food or small treat to see if this helps.
- May take a few weeks for the full benefits of this medication to be noticeable. Best used in conjunction with behavioral therapy.
- This medication has many potential drug interactions. Be sure your veterinarian is aware of all medicines you give your animal, including vitamins, supplements, and herbal therapies.
- If your animal has worn a flea or tick collar in the past two weeks, let your veterinarian know. Do not start new flea/tick products without discussing with your veterinarian first.
- Buspirone is usually well-tolerated by dogs and cats. Cats may show increased friendliness during buspirone treatment.

Chemistry/Synonyms

An arylpiperazine derivative azapirone anxiolytic agent, buspirone HCl differs structurally from the benzodiazepines. It occurs as a white crystalline powder with solubility at 25°C (77°F) of 865 mg/mL in water and ≈20 mg/mL in alcohol.

Buspirone HCl may also be known as MJ-9022; many trade names are available. A common trade name is *BuSpar®*.

Storage/Stability

Buspirone HCl tablets should be stored in air-tight, light-resistant containers at room temperature 20°C to 25°C (68°F-77°F).

Compatibility/Compounding Considerations

No specific information noted

Dose Forms/Regulatory Status

VETERINARY-LABELED PRODUCTS: NONE

The Association of Racing Commissioners International (ARCI) has designated buspirone as a class 2 substance. See ***Appendix*** for more information. Use of this drug may not be allowed in certain animal competitions. Check rules and regulations before entering in a competition while this medication is being administered. Contact local racing authorities for further guidance.

HUMAN-LABELED PRODUCTS:

Buspirone HCl Oral Tablets: 5 mg (4.6 mg as base), 7.5 mg (6.85 mg as base), 10 mg (9.1 mg as base), 15 mg (13.7 mg as base), and 30 mg (27.4 mg as base); generic; (Rx). 5 and 10 mg tablets have a bisecting score, whereas 15 and 30 mg tablets are trisected (allows splitting into ⅓ tablet).

References

For the complete list of references, see **wiley.com/go/budde/plumb**

Butorphanol

(byoo-***tor***-fa-nol) *Stadol®, Torbutrol®, Torbugesic®*

Antitussive, Opioid Partial Agonist

Prescriber Highlights

- ► Opioid agonist/antagonist used in a variety of species as an analgesic, premedication, or antitussive; effects are reversible with naloxone.
- ► Moderately effective analgesic for horses; however, more effective options are available for moderate to severe pain in small animal species
- ► Primarily used as a sedative in small animal species as analgesia is mild and of short duration. Provides mild to moderate sedation in ruminants
- ► Contraindicated or should be used with caution in patients with liver disease, hypothyroidism, renal insufficiency, Addison's disease, head trauma, increased intracranial pressure, or other CNS dysfunction (eg, coma) and in geriatric or severely debilitated patients; however, butorphanol has a wide safety margin and effects are reversible, thus it is commonly used in patients with most of these conditions.
- ► Dose should be reduced in dogs with *MDR1 (ABCB-1)* mutation.
- ► Potential adverse effects include ataxia and sedation. Anorexia or diarrhea (rare) may occur in dogs and cats. In horses, reduced intestinal sounds secondary to slowed GI motility; CNS excitement is possible.
- ► DEA Schedule IV (C-IV) controlled substance

Uses/Indications

Butorphanol is FDA-approved for use in dogs to relieve chronic nonproductive cough associated with tracheobronchitis, tracheitis, tonsillitis, laryngitis, and pharyngitis originating from inflammatory conditions of the upper respiratory tract.[1] In cats, butorphanol is labeled for the relief of pain caused by major or minor trauma or pain associated with surgical procedures.[2] It is also used in both dogs and cats as an adjunctive preanesthetic medication or analgesic. As compared with other opioid analgesics, butorphanol is not very effective for treating pain in small animal species as it is less potent and has a short duration of action, necessitating frequent administration. Due to its kappa effects, butorphanol can be an effective reversal agent for the CNS and respiratory depressant effects of mu-opioid agonists (eg, morphine, hydromorphone) without completely reversing the analgesic effects. Because of the short duration (≈50 minutes in dogs[3] and 90 minutes in cats[4]) and mild analgesia but effective sedation, butorphanol is more commonly used as a sedative than an analgesic. Combining butorphanol with an alpha-2 agonist enhances both analgesia and sedation in dogs and cats.

Butorphanol is FDA-approved for use in adult horses and yearlings for relief of pain associated with colic.[5] In horses, combining butorphanol with an alpha-2 agonist (eg, detomidine, xylazine) appears to enhance analgesia and sedation. Buprenorphine provided better postoperative analgesia than butorphanol in horses undergoing elective surgery[6]; however, buprenorphine may be more likely to cause increased locomotor activity and excitement than butorphanol.[7]

Butorphanol has also been used as an analgesic and/or sedative in cattle, camelids, small ruminants, small mammals, and several wildlife species. Butorphanol use in reptiles is somewhat controversial, and most studies show it has minimal analgesic or anesthetic-sparing activity in many of these species. The same is true for birds.

Pharmacology/Actions

Butorphanol is considered to be, on a weight basis, 4 to 7 times more potent an analgesic (ie, agonist) than morphine, 15 to 30 times more potent than pentazocine, and 30 to 50 times more potent than meperidine; however, a ceiling effect is reached at higher doses, where analgesia is no longer enhanced and may be reduced. Its agonist activity is thought to occur primarily at the kappa- and sigma-opioid receptors as well as in the analgesic receptors in the limbic system (subcortical and spinal levels). Its use as an analgesic in small animals has been less useful as compared with other opioids, primarily because of its short duration of action and ability to alleviate only mild to moderate pain.

The antagonist potency of butorphanol at mu-opioid receptors is considered to be ≈30 times that of pentazocine and 1/40 that of naloxone and will antagonize the effect of true opioid agonists (eg, morphine, meperidine, oxymorphone).

In addition to its analgesic qualities, butorphanol has significant antitussive activity. The drug has 15 to 20 times the oral antitussive activity of codeine or dextromethorphan in dogs. In dogs, butorphanol has been shown to elevate the CNS respiratory center threshold to CO_2, but, unlike pure mu-opioid agonists, it does not depress respiratory center sensitivity. Butorphanol, unlike morphine, apparently does not cause histamine release in dogs. CNS depression may occur in dogs receiving butorphanol, whereas CNS excitation has been noted (usually at high dosages) in horses and dogs.

As with other opioid agonists, butorphanol can cause a decrease in heart rate secondary to increased parasympathetic tone and mild decreases in arterial blood pressure. However, increased heart rates have been noted in horses after IV injection.[8]

The risk for physical dependence appears minimal in veterinary patients.

Pharmacokinetics

In general, butorphanol is absorbed completely in the gut when administered orally, but, because of a high first-pass effect, only ≈1/6 of the administered dose reaches systemic circulation. The drug is completely absorbed following IM administration.

Butorphanol is well-distributed, with the highest concentrations (of the parent compound and metabolites) found in the liver, kidneys, and intestine. Concentrations in the lungs, endocrine tissues, spleen, heart, adipose tissue, and blood cells are also higher than those found in plasma. In humans, ≈80% of the drug is bound to plasma proteins.

Butorphanol is metabolized in the liver, primarily by hydroxylation. Other methods of metabolism include N-dealkylation and conjugation. The metabolites of butorphanol do not exhibit any analgesic activity. These metabolites, and the parent compound, are mainly excreted into the urine (only 5% is excreted unchanged), but 11% to 14% of a dose is excreted into the bile and eliminated with the feces. Terminal half-lives reported in various species include the following: cats, ≈5 to 6 hours (IM/OTM); dogs, 2.6 hours (IM/SC); dairy cattle, 82 minutes[9] and goats, 1.87 hours (IV) and 2.75 hours (IM).

In adult horses, the onset of action after IV administration is ≈3 minutes, with peak analgesic effect at 15 to 30 minutes. The duration of action in horses may be up to 4 hours after a single dose. After a single 0.1 mg/kg IV dose, volume of distribution is ≈1.4 L/kg, clearance is ≈12 mL/minute/kg, and elimination half-life is 6 hours.[8] After SC administration, bioavailability is ≈87% and half-life is ≈5.3 hours.[10] Another study suggested that the half-life in conscious horses is ≈44 minutes with a clearance of 21 mL/kg/minute after a single 0.1 – 0.13 mg/kg IV dose.[11]

Bioavailability after IM injections in adult horses is relatively low (≈37%).[12] In neonatal foals, IM bioavailability is ≈67%, and peak concentrations occurred ≈6 minutes after administration. Terminal half-life was ≈2 hours after IV administration.[13]

In ferrets given a single dose of 0.3 mg/kg SC, peak concentration was reached after 13.3 minutes, and elimination half-life was 91 minutes.[14]

In parrots, butorphanol compounded at 8.3 mg/mL in a sterile 25% poloxamer 407 gel and administered at 12.5 mg/kg SC reached a peak concentration at 1.3 hours and provided analgesia for 4 to 8 hours; however, further studies are required to support clinical use.[15]

Contraindications/Precautions/Warnings

Butorphanol is contraindicated in patients with known hypersensitivity to it. All opioids should potentially be used with caution in patients with hypothyroidism, severe renal insufficiency, adrenocortical insufficiency (Addison's), or obstructive respiratory disease and in geriatric or severely debilitated patients.

Like other opioids, butorphanol must be used with caution in patients with head trauma, increased intracranial pressure, or other CNS dysfunction (eg, coma). It should be used cautiously with other sedatives or analgesics.

Dogs with MDR1 mutations may develop a more pronounced sedation that persists longer than normal. The Washington State University Veterinary Clinical Pharmacology Lab (http://vcpl.vetmed.wsu.edu) recommends reducing the dosage by 25% in dogs heterozygous for the *MDR1* gene (also known as *ABCB1* gene) mutation and by 30% to 50% in dogs homozygous (mutant/mutant) for the mutation. However, clinically there seems to be a minimal impact and butorphanol effects are reversible so avoidance of butorphanol in these patients is not generally necessary.

Manufacturers state that butorphanol should not be used in animals with a history of liver disease or with severe hepatic or renal dysfunction, and, because of its effects on suppressing cough, "it should not be used in conditions of the lower respiratory tract associated with copious mucous production." The drug should be used cautiously in dogs with heartworm disease, as safety for butorphanol has not been established in these patients.

In turtles and tortoises, butorphanol may not be an effective analgesic and may cause respiratory depression.[16]

Opioid analgesics are contraindicated in patients stung by scorpions (eg, *Centruroides* spp) as they may potentiate venom effects.[17]

Because butorphanol injection is available in different concentrations (see ***Dosage Forms/Regulatory Status***), careful attention should be paid to which concentration is being used when drawing up dosages. Doses should not be ordered in mLs.

Butorphanol is commonly administered with other medications in the same syringe. Due to the negative pressure in the vial, it may become contaminated with other medications. Although one study showed the contamination to be below clinically important levels in 10 mL vials,[18] 50 mL vials may reach significant levels. Caution should be used in critically ill patients when drawing from a previously used vial if the practice of drawing up multiple medications in the same syringe is employed.

Adverse Effects

Adverse effects reported in dogs and cats include sedation, excitement, respiratory depression, ataxia, mydriasis, disorientation, hypersalivation, anorexia, vomiting, or diarrhea (rarely). Sedation with butorphanol and dexmedetomidine can decrease tear production and may require treatment with a tear substitute.[65] Antitussive effect may result in mucus accumulation in the respiratory tract. Although adverse cardiovascular effects are uncommon, bradycardia may occur and can be treated with anticholinergic agents (eg, atropine, glycopyrrolate). Adverse effects are generally less severe than those seen with pure agonists.

Adverse effects in horses may include transient bradycardia, ataxia, and sedation, but restlessness, shivering, and excitement have also been noted. Although reported to have minimal effects on the GI tract, butorphanol has the potential to decrease intestinal motility, and ileus is possible. Horses may exhibit increased heart rates and CNS excitement (eg, tossing and jerking of head, increased ambulation, augmented avoidance response to auditory stimuli), particularly with rapid IV administration of high doses (0.2 mg/kg). Very high doses IV (1 – 2 mg/kg) may lead to the development of nystagmus, salivation, seizures, hyperthermia, and decreased GI motility. It has been suggested that when used for analgesia in horses, butorphanol administered as a continuous rate IV infusion can minimize adverse effects and maximize analgesia as compared with bolus dosing but GI transit time may be delayed.[19] When administered to horses recovering from abdominal surgery for colic, butorphanol CRI slowed GI motility but did not cause signs of colic and resulted in decreased pain-related behavioral scores compared to horses receiving only NSAIDs.[20] However, butorphanol may delay GI transit without affecting somatic nociception as measured by thermal threshold response when it is administered to healthy, nonpainful horses as a CRI in combination with lidocaine, ketamine, or lidocaine/ketamine.[21] Both the presence of pain and the duration of infusion (24 vs 96 hours, respectively) could explain the difference in outcomes.

Reproductive/Nursing Safety

Butorphanol crosses the placenta and neonatal plasma concentrations are approximately equivalent to maternal concentrations. Although no controlled studies have been performed in domestic animals or humans, in laboratory animals the drug has exhibited no evidence of teratogenicity or of causing impaired fertility but has increased the rate of stillbirth and postimplantation losses.[22] Butorphanol is not recommend for use in pregnant bitches or queens or breeding males (feline, equine).[1,2,5]

In humans, butorphanol can be distributed into milk,[23] but not in amounts that would cause concern in nursing offspring.

Because safety has not been established in animals, this drug should only be used when the maternal benefits outweigh the potential risks to offspring.

Overdose/Acute Toxicity

Acute life-threatening overdoses with butorphanol are unlikely. The LD_{50} in dogs is reportedly 50 mg/kg.[1] However, because butorphanol injection is available in different dosage strengths (0.5 mg/mL, 2 mg/mL, and 10 mg/mL) for veterinary use, inadvertent overdoses could occur in small animals. It has been suggested that animals exhibiting clinical signs of overdose (eg, CNS effects, cardiovascular changes (including, profound bradycardia, respiratory depression) be treated immediately with IV naloxone. Additional supportive measures (eg, fluids, O_2, vasopressor agents, mechanical ventilation) may be required. Should seizures occur and persist, diazepam may be used for control.

For patients that have experienced or are suspected of having experienced an overdose, consultation with a 24-hour poison consultation center specializing in providing veterinary-specific information is recommended. For general information related to overdose and toxin exposures, as well as contact information for poison control centers, refer to *Appendix*.

Drug Interactions

The following drug interactions have either been reported or are theoretical in humans or animals receiving butorphanol and may be of significance in veterinary patients. Unless otherwise noted, use together is not necessarily contraindicated, but the potential risks should be weighed and additional monitoring performed when appropriate.

- Alpha-2 Receptor Agonists (eg, **dexmedetomidine, xylazine**): Concurrent use may increase risk for bradycardia
- Angiotensin Converting Enzyme Inhibitors (eg, **benazepril, enalapril**): Concurrent use may increase risk for hypotension and orthostasis.
- Anticholinergics (eg, **atropine, glycopyrrolate**): Concurrent use may increase risk for CNS depression, urinary retention, constipation, and ileus.
- Antidiarrheals: Concurrent use can lead to severe constipation and ileus.
- Apomorphine: Concurrent use may increase risk for CNS depression.
- Beta-adrenergic Receptor Antagonists (eg, **atenolol, carvedilol**): Concurrent use may increase risk for hypotension and orthostasis.
- Bromocriptine: Concurrent use may increase CNS depression and respiratory depression.
- Calcium-Channel Blockers (eg, **amlodipine, diltiazem**): Concurrent use may increase risk for hypotension and orthostasis.
- Cannabidiol: Concurrent use may enhance the CNS depressant effect of opioids.
- Clopidogrel: Concurrent use of clopidogrel and opioid agonists may result in reduced efficacy of clopidogrel.
- CNS Depressants (eg, **anesthetic agents, antihistamines, anticonvulsants, benzodiazepines, phenothiazines, barbiturates, muscle relaxants, tranquilizers, opioids**): May cause increased CNS or respiratory depression when used with butorphanol; dosage may need to be decreased
- CYP 3A Inhibitors (eg, **cimetidine, erythromycin, itraconazole**): May decrease metabolism of butorphanol, increasing risk for respiratory depression and apnea
- Desmopressin: Concurrent use may increase concentrations and pharmacologic activity of desmopressin, increasing risk for hyponatremia and water intoxication.
- Diuretics (eg, **furosemide, hydrochlorothiazide**): Concurrent use may increase risk for hypotension and orthostasis.
- Fenoldopam: Concurrent use may increase risk for hypotension and orthostasis.
- Hydromorphone: In cats, butorphanol administered 30 minutes after hydromorphone reduced the duration of hydromorphone antinociception.[24]
- Ifosfamide: Concurrent use may increase risk for neurotoxic effects of ifosfamide, including sleepiness, confusion, hallucinations, extrapyramidal clinical signs, seizures, psychotic behavior, and coma.
- Inhalant Anesthetics (eg, **isoflurane, sevoflurane**): Opioids may decrease MAC anesthetic requirements.
- Iohexol: Concurrent use of intrathecal iohexol may increase risk for seizures. Butorphanol should be withheld 48 hours before and 24 hours after intrathecal iohexol if possible.
- Metoclopramide: The prokinetic effects of metoclopramide may be decreased and risk for CNS depression may be increased.
- Minocycline: Minocycline may enhance the CNS depressant effects of opioids.
- Monoamine Oxidase Inhibitors (MAOIs; eg, **furazolidone, methylene blue, selegiline, procarbazine**): Concurrent use may increase risk for anxiety, confusion, respiratory depression, hypotension, cyanosis, and coma by an unknown mechanism. A 14-day washout should be observed between discontinuation of furazolidone and initiation of butorphanol.
- Opioids (eg, **fentanyl, hydrocodone, morphine**): Butorphanol may potentially antagonize some analgesic effects and will also reverse some of the sedative and respiratory depressant effects of pure agonists. Withdrawal effects may occur in patients receiving

chronic opioid therapy.

- **Pancuronium:** If used with butorphanol, may cause increased conjunctival changes
- **Phenoxybenzamine:** Concurrent use may result in additive hypotension and orthostasis.
- **Polyethylene Glycol:** Concurrent use may increase risk for seizures associated with the use of bowel cleansing preparations.
- **Selective Serotonin Reuptake Inhibitors** (eg, **fluoxetine, sertraline**): Concurrent use may increase risk for CNS or respiratory depression and serotonin syndrome.
- **Tamsulosin:** Concurrent use may increase risk for hypotension and orthostasis.
- **Theophylline:** Could decrease metabolism of butorphanol
- **Tramadol:** Concurrent use may increase risk for seizures, CNS depression, and respiratory depression.
- **Tricyclic Antidepressants** (eg, **amitriptyline, clomipramine**): Concurrent use may increase risk for CNS and respiratory depression, constipation, and urinary retention.
- **Vasodilators** (eg, **hydralazine, nitroglycerin, nitroprusside**): Concurrent use may result in additive hypotension and orthostasis.

Laboratory Considerations

None noted

Dosages

NOTE: Potency of veterinary-labeled products is expressed as butorphanol base, whereas the human product strength is labeled as the tartrate salt; these formulations are not equal. All dosages are expressed in mg/kg of the base activity. As a rough conversion, 1.5 mg butorphanol tartrate will provide 1 mg butorphanol base.

DOGS:

Antitussive (label dosage; FDA-approved):

a) *Injection*: 0.055 mg/kg SC every 6 to 12 hours; may be increased to 0.11 mg/kg SC every 6 to 12 hours.[25] Treatment should not normally be required for longer than 7 days.

b) *Oral*: 0.55 mg/kg PO every 6 to 12 hours; may increase dose to 1.1 mg/kg PO every 6 to 12 hours.[1,25] Treatment should not normally be required for longer than 7 days.[26]

Analgesic (extra-label):

a) 0.2 – 0.4 mg/kg IV, IM, SC is the most common range chosen, but 0.1 – 0.5 mg/kg IV, IM, SC can also be used. Butorphanol provides only mild to moderate analgesia (potentially better visceral than somatic analgesia but this is controversial); duration of sedative action is 2 to 4 hours, but analgesic action may be less than 1 hour.[3,27]

b) **Constant rate infusion (CRI):** 0.2 mg/kg IV as a loading dose followed by 0.1 – 0.24 mg/kg/hour IV CRI. Dosages as high as 0.4 mg/kg/hour can be used but may cause sedation.

c) **Epidural analgesic**: 0.25 mg/kg diluted with preservative-free saline or local anesthetic (to a total volume of 0.2 mL/kg with a maximum of 6 mL) injected into the lumbosacral epidural space. Onset of action is less than 30 minutes and duration is 2 to 4 hours. This method of delivery has predominantly supraspinal effects.[28]

In combination as an anesthetic or sedative adjunct (extra-label): **NOTE:** There are many potential combinations that have been suggested; the following are examples and are not inclusive. For additional information, refer to other anesthesia-specific references.[29,30]

a) **In combination with acepromazine for dogs undergoing OHE or gastroduodenoscopy**: butorphanol 0.3 – 0.4 mg/kg with acepromazine 0.02 mg/kg IV[31] or in the same syringe and given IM[31-33]

b) **In combination with dexmedetomidine:** butorphanol 0.4 mg/kg IM has been combined with dexmedetomidine at 5 – 10 µg/kg IM for echocardiography. This combination results in sedation, but with decreased heart rate, cardiac output, and the development of valvular regurgitation. Caution should be used when giving this drug combination to dogs with cardiovascular disease.[34] Butorphanol 0.15 mg/kg with dexmedetomidine 0.01 mg/kg IM produced superior antinociceptive effects under experimental conditions.[35]

c) **In combination with dexmedetomidine and ketamine ('doggie magic') to provide anesthesia and pain management:** see ***Dexmedetomidine*** or ***Ketamine***

d) **In combination with medetomidine**: butorphanol 0.4 mg/kg IM can be combined with medetomidine 2.5 µg/kg IM to provide moderate to deep sedation for 20 to 30 minutes; there will be a decrease in heart rate.[36]

e) **In combination with medetomidine and alfaxalone IM:** butorphanol 0.25 – 0.3 mg/kg in combination with medetomidine 2.5 – 5 µg/kg, and (preservative-free) alfaxalone 1 – 2.5 mg/kg IM provided anesthetic effect without severe cardiorespiratory depression[37,38]; however, substantial cardiorespiratory depression was noted when butorphanol 0.1 mg/kg has been combined with medetomidine 10 µg/kg and (preservative-free) alfaxalone 1.5 mg/kg IM to induce anesthesia/analgesia.[39]

f) **In combination with medetomidine and midazolam:**

i. **Dogs requiring light to moderate sedation for short procedures (eg, nail trims, radiographs):** butorphanol 0.2 mg/kg with medetomidine 0.001 – 0.01 mg/kg ± midazolam 0.05 – 0.2 mg/kg; combined and administered IM

ii. **Dogs requiring more sedation**: butorphanol 0.2 mg/kg with medetomidine 0.01 – 0.02 mg/kg and midazolam 0.05 – 0.2 mg/kg; combined and administered IM. Consider adding tiletamine/zolazepam or ketamine at 1 – 2 mg/kg if insufficient sedation from above drug combination. For painful procedures, consider adding buprenorphine at 0.02 – 0.04 mg/kg or substituting butorphanol or buprenorphine with either morphine 0.5 – 1 mg/kg or hydromorphone 0.1 – 0.2 mg/kg.[40]

g) **In combination with midazolam:** butorphanol 0.2 mg/kg IV followed by midazolam 0.1 mg/kg IV was deemed a good option for contrast-enhanced ultrasonography of the duodenum.[41]

h) **In combination with midazolam and alfaxalone IV:** butorphanol 0.2 mg/kg IV followed by midazolam 0.2 mg/kg IV, then administration of alfaxalone 2 mg/kg IV over 1 minute, provides excellent quality of induction and good to excellent recovery with minimal cardiopulmonary effects in healthy dogs. Time from induction to extubation was ≈29 minutes and to standing was ≈36 minutes.[42]

Reversal agent for the sedative and respiratory depressant effects of mu-agonist opioids (extra-label): 0.05 – 0.1 mg/kg IV; the benefit of using butorphanol over naloxone is that butorphanol does not completely reverse analgesic effects.[43]

CATS:

Analgesic:

a) **Relief of pain caused by major or minor trauma, or pain associated with surgical procedures** (label dosage; FDA-approved): 0.4 mg/kg SC. The dose may be repeated up to 4 times daily for up to 2 days.[44]

b) **Relief of pain** (extra-label): 0.1 – 0.5 mg/kg IV, IM, or SC; provides only mild to moderate analgesia (potentially better visceral than somatic analgesia but this is controversial). Duration of sedative action is 2 to 4 hours, but analgesic action may be 1 to 2 hours or less.[4,45]

c) **Postoperative CRI** (usually in combination with ketamine; extra-label) for mild to moderate pain: Loading dose of butorphanol 0.1 – 0.2 mg/kg IV, followed by butorphanol 0.1 – 0.2 mg/kg/hour IV CRI. Ketamine may be added for complementary analgesia with a loading dose of 0.1 mg/kg IV followed by ketamine 0.4 mg/kg/hour IV CRI. Opioid and ketamine IV CRI combinations may allow dose reductions for both drugs.[46]
d) **Epidural analgesic** (extra-label): 0.25 mg/kg, diluted with preservative-free saline or local anesthetic (to a total volume of 0.2 mL/kg) and injected into the lumbosacral epidural space. Onset of action is less than 30 minutes with a duration of 2 to 4 hours. This drug delivery combination has predominantly supraspinal effects.[28]

Prevention of dexmedetomidine-induced emesis (extra-label): butorphanol 0.1 – 0.2 mg/kg IM when given concurrently with dexmedetomidine[47]

In combination as an anesthetic or sedative adjunct (extra-label): **NOTE:** There are many potential combinations that have been suggested; the following are examples and are not inclusive. For additional information, refer to other anesthesia-specific references.[29,30]

a) **In combination with ketamine, midazolam, and medetomidine:** In the study assessing analgesia after OHE,[48] one of the protocols used was: Ten minutes prior to surgery, ketamine 60 mg/m^2 (≈3 mg/kg), midazolam 3 mg/m^2 (≈0.2 mg/kg), medetomidine 600 µg/m^2 (≈30 µg/kg), and butorphanol 6 mg/m^2 (≈0.3 mg/kg) were combined and given as a single IM injection in the quadriceps muscles. Additionally, either carprofen (4 mg/kg) or meloxicam (0.3 mg/kg) were given SC. All protocols in the study provided adequate analgesia.
b) **In combination with dexmedetomidine:** Butorphanol 0.4 mg/kg in combination with dexmedetomidine 10 µg/kg IM provided adequate sedation and was superior to dexmedetomidine/buprenorphine combination.[47,49]
c) **In combination with midazolam and ketamine OR dexmedetomidine:** From a small (n = 6) healthy cat crossover study, butorphanol 0.4 mg/kg in combination with midazolam 0.4 mg/kg and ketamine 3 mg/kg IM provided acceptable sedation and minimal cardiovascular changes.[50] Substituting dexmedetomidine 5 µg/kg for ketamine produced excellent sedation and recovery but caused more cardiovascular depression and hematologic changes.
d) **In combination with alfaxalone:**
   i. **SC dosing for sedation during short procedures:** In a study in hyperthyroid cats,[51] butorphanol 0.2 mg/kg in combination with (preservative-free) alfaxalone 3 mg/kg drawn up in the same syringe and administered as a single SC injection in the region dorsal to the right hip. Maximum sedation occurred 45 minutes postadministration. Blood pressure, heart rate, and respiratory rate were all significantly decreased. Monitoring blood pressure is recommended. Further studies are required to determine whether the sedative, respiratory, and cardiovascular effects are similar in euthyroid cats.
   ii. **IM dosing:**
      - Rapid, deep, short duration sedation can be achieved with butorphanol 0.2 mg/kg and (preservative-free) alfaxalone 2 mg/kg IM; recumbency attained within 36 ± 4.4 minutes. Cats had smooth recovery with no adverse effects.[52]
      - Another study combined butorphanol 0.4 mg/kg IM with (preservative-free) alfaxalone 2 – 3 mg/kg IM to achieve sedation in cats sufficient to undergo phlebotomy; median recumbency time was 53 minutes, and no adverse effects were noted.[66]
      - Butorphanol 0.4 mg/kg and (preservative-free) alfaxalone 2 – 3 mg/kg IM provided sufficient restraint for blood donation.[53]
      - In cats undergoing diagnostic imaging or noninvasive procedures, butorphanol 0.2 mg/kg IM with (preservative-free) alfaxalone 5 mg/kg IM yielded better sedation than a lower alfaxalone dose (2 mg/kg IM).[54]
      - Butorphanol 0.3 mg/kg with alfaxalone 3 mg/kg combined and injected IM; injection into the supraspinatus muscle produced faster and superior sedation as compared to injection into the quadriceps muscle.[55]
e) **In combination with dexmedetomidine and alfaxalone OR ketamine for anesthetic induction:**
   i. Butorphanol 0.3 mg/kg, dexmedetomidine 25 µg/kg, and alfaxalone 2 mg/kg combined and given IM[56]
   ii. Butorphanol 0.2 mg/kg and dexmedetomidine 10 µg/kg combined with *either* (preservative-free) alfaxalone 3 mg/kg OR ketamine 5 mg/kg IM produced acceptable anesthesia for short procedures.[57]
   iii. A study evaluated efficacy and cardiorespiratory effects of a combination of butorphanol 0.2 mg/kg combined with dexmedetomidine 25 µg/kg and ketamine 3 mg/kg as a single IM injection (with or without reversal by atipamezole) in cats undergoing castration. Cats also received meloxicam 0.2 mg/kg SC immediately prior to the conclusion of surgery.
   iv. **Short-term restraint:** butorphanol 0.3 mg/kg with dexmedetomidine 5 µg/kg +/- ketamine 3 mg/kg mixed in the same syringe and administered IM. Duration of sedation is longer when ketamine is added.[58]
   v. **'Kitty magic' to provide anesthesia and pain management:** see ***Dexmedetomidine*** or ***Ketamine***
f) **In combination with medetomidine and alfaxalone as injectable anesthesia:** butorphanol 0.2 mg/kg, medetomidine 20 µg/kg, and (preservative-free) alfaxalone 5 mg/kg mixed in the same syringe and administered IM. Analgesia lasted ≈1 hour and recovery took 2 hours.[59]

Reversal agent for sedative and respiratory depressant effects of mu-opioid receptor agonists (eg, fentanyl, hydromorphone, morphine; extra-label): 0.05 – 0.1 mg/kg IV. The benefit of using butorphanol over naloxone is that butorphanol does not completely reverse analgesic effects[43]; however, one study showed that butorphanol administration decreased the duration of hydromorphone analgesic effects in cats.[24]

HORSES (EQUIDS):

Analgesic:

a) **Relief of pain associated with colic in adult horses and yearlings** (label dosage; FDA-approved): 0.1 mg/kg IV every 3 to 4 hours; duration of therapy not to exceed 48 hours[5]
b) **SC administration** (extra-label): 0.1 mg/kg SC. This route of administration provided less marked physiologic and behavioral effects as compared with the same dose given IV.[10]
c) **Constant rate infusion** (CRI; extra-label): There is evidence that giving butorphanol via a CRI may provide better analgesia and reduce the potential for adverse effects.[19]
   i. **Postceliotomy:** Butorphanol 13 µg/kg/hour IV CRI and

continued for 24 hours; therapy was combined with flunixin 1.1 mg/kg IV every 12 hours; administration started at the end of celiotomy.[20] Although horses treated with this combination had delayed passage of feces following surgery, no horses experienced colic, pain scores were significantly decreased, less weight was lost, and recovery scores were improved. Treated horses were discharged 3 days sooner, on average, than those treated with flunixin alone.[20]

ii. **Sedation**: Sedation with butorphanol 17.8 µg/kg in combination with xylazine 1 mg/kg IV followed by butorphanol 23.7 µg/kg/hour IV CRI may be useful.[60] Horses sedated with the same protocol and receiving butorphanol/xylazine infusions had more ataxia and instances of falling and occasionally inadequate sedation.

iii. **Standing procedures**: butorphanol (loading dose, 18 µg/kg IV; CRI, 25 µg/kg/hour) combined with romifidine (loading dose, 80 µg/kg IV; CRI, 29 µg/kg/hour) for standing dentistry and ophthalmologic procedures.[61]

iv. Butorphanol 0.02 mg/kg combined with dexmedetomidine 3.5 µg/kg and given as an initial IV bolus followed by butorphanol 0.024 mg/kg/hour with dexmedetomidine 3.5 µg/kg/hour IV CRI provided clinically sufficient sedation for 30 minutes.[62]

d) **Foals** (extra-label): Most recommend dosages of ≈0.1 mg/kg IV or IM. One study in pony foals (both neonatal and older) found that 0.1 mg/kg IV, but not 0.05 mg/kg IV, significantly raised the thermal nociceptive threshold[63]; however, a pharmacokinetic study in neonatal foals found that dosages of 0.05 mg/kg IV significantly changed behaviors (increased nursing, sedation).[63] Because elimination half-life in foals is longer than in adults, repeat doses may be considered every 4 to 6 hours, when needed.

Sedative and analgesic in combination with other agents (extra-label): Several protocols have been described using butorphanol in conjunction with an alpha-2 receptor agonist (eg, xylazine, romifidine, detomidine); often, butorphanol is used at a lower dose than labeled (eg, 0.02 – 0.05 mg/kg).

a) Premedicate with xylazine 1 mg/kg IV OR 2 mg/kg IM 5 to 10 minutes (longer for IM route) before induction of anesthesia with ketamine 2 mg/kg IV. Horse must be adequately sedated (head to knees) before giving the ketamine, as ketamine alone can cause muscle rigidity. If adequate sedation does not occur, either: 1) Re-dose xylazine using up to half the original dose. 2) Add butorphanol 0.02 – 0.04 mg/kg IV. Butorphanol can be given with the original xylazine premedication if the horse is suspected to be difficult to tranquilize (eg, high-strung thoroughbreds) or added before the ketamine induction. This drug combination improves induction quality, increases analgesia, and increases recumbency time by ≈5 to 10 minutes. 3) Give diazepam 0.03 mg/kg IV. Mix the diazepam with the ketamine. This combination will improve induction quality when sedation is marginal, improve muscle relaxation during anesthesia, and prolong anesthesia by ≈5 to 10 minutes. 4) Guaifenesin 5% solution administered IV to effect can also be added to increase sedation and muscle relaxation.[64]

b) Butorphanol 0.05 – 0.1 mg/kg in combination with romifidine 0.05 – 0.1 mg/kg IV.[65] Sedation onset and duration were ≈5 minutes and ≈60 minutes, respectively. Analgesia lasted ≈30 minutes.[66]

c) Butorphanol 0.02 mg/kg IV in combination with detomidine 8 µg/kg IV[67]

Intravenous anesthetic protocol (extra-label):

a) **Procedures in standing horses**: butorphanol 0.018 mg/kg and romifidine 0.08 mg/kg IV bolus followed by butorphanol 0.025 mg/kg/hour and romifidine 0.029 mg/kg/hour[61]

b) **Standing laparoscopic ovariectomy:** Butorphanol 0.01 mg/kg IV and medetomidine 5 µg/kg IV bolus; to maintain sedation, bolus doses of butorphanol 0.004 mg/kg IV and medetomidine 1 µg/kg IV were repeated every 15 minutes.[68]

Analgesia and sedation of donkeys (extra label): One study recommended a combination of butorphanol 0.05 mg/kg and *either* detomidine 0.04 mg/kg OR romifidine 0.08 mg/kg IV.[69] These combinations provided safe and effective sedation with complete analgesia in standing donkeys. Another study recommended xylazine 0.5 mg/kg and butorphanol 0.04 mg/kg IV.[70]

CATTLE:

Analgesic (extra-label): When used alone in cattle, butorphanol has been recommended anecdotally at 0.02 – 0.04 mg/kg IV or SC every 4 hours.

Analgesia, sedation/restraint in calves (extra-label): Butorphanol 0.1 mg/kg with xylazine 0.1 mg/kg provided reliable recumbent restraint in healthy Holstein-Friesian calves[71]

Analgesia, sedation/restraint, and disassociation from a noxious procedure in combination as "ketamine stun" (extra-label):

a) **IV administration:** Butorphanol 0.01 – 0.025 mg/kg with xylazine 0.02 – 0.05 mg/kg and ketamine 0.05 – 0.5 mg/kg IV; doses at upper end of these ranges should produce recumbency, while lower doses are expected to produce standing restraint; duration of effect is ≈15 minutes.[72]

b) **IM/SC administration:** Butorphanol 0.02 – 0.1 mg/kg with xylazine 0.02 – 0.05 mg/kg and ketamine 0.04 – 0.1 mg/kg IM or SC; doses at upper end of these ranges should produce recumbency for ≈ 45 minutes, whereas lower doses are expected to produce standing restraint for 60 to 90 minutes. SC administration provides slightly longer duration of effect than IM.[72]

CRI in calves: in isoflurane-anesthetized calves, butorphanol 0.1 mg/kg IV followed by 20 µg/kg/minute IV CRI. Hemodynamic variables were unaffected, and recovery was uneventful.[73]

GOATS:

Premedication (extra-label): A combination of midazolam 0.3 mg/kg and butorphanol 0.1 mg/kg IM has been used to decrease the amount of IV alfaxalone needed for induction of general anesthesia.[74] Cardiorespiratory parameters were within clinically accepted limits.

CAMELIDS:

Analgesic and sedative (extra-label): Most butorphanol dosage recommendations fall between 0.05 – 0.1 mg/kg IM or IV every 4 to 6 hours. Several dose protocols have been suggested for combining butorphanol with other sedative and/or anesthetic agents:

a) As an anesthetic: Butorphanol 0.07 – 0.1 mg/kg with ketamine 0.2 – 0.3 mg/kg and xylazine 0.2 – 0.3 mg/kg combined and given IV OR butorphanol 0.05 – 0.1 mg/kg with ketamine 0.2 – 0.5 mg/kg and xylazine 0.2 – 0.5 mg/kg combined and given IM[75]

b) Procedural pain relief (eg, castrations) when recumbency (up to 30 minutes) is desired: *Alpacas*: Butorphanol 0.046 mg/kg with xylazine 0.46 mg/kg and ketamine 4.6 mg/kg combined and given IM. *Llamas*: Butorphanol 0.037 mg/kg with xylazine 0.37 mg/kg and ketamine 3.7 mg/kg combined and given IM. May administer 50% of original dose of ketamine and xylazine during anesthesia to prolong effect up to 15 minutes. If doing castrations on 3 or more animals sequentially, it is acceptable to make up a bottle of the drug mixture: Add butorphanol 10 mg (1 mL) and xylazine 100 mg (1 mL) to ketamine 1 g (10 mL vial). This mixture is dosed at 1 mL/18 kg (40 lb) for alpacas and 1 mL per 22 kg (50 lb) for llamas. Handle quietly and allow plenty of time before starting procedure. Expect 20 minutes of surgical time; patient should stand 45 minutes to 1 hour after injection.[75]

c) **Alpacas**: Ketamine 4 mg/kg with xylazine 0.4 mg/kg and butorphanol 0.04 mg/kg combined and given IM resulted in ≈30 minutes of anesthesia time for castrations. Additional anesthesia (⅓ the induction dose) was given at the discretion of the anesthetist.[76]

BIRDS:

Analgesic (extra-label):

a) Butorphanol 1 – 4 mg/kg IM has been suggested in birds, but dose frequencies range from every 2 to 24 hours. Limited pharmacokinetic studies in birds suggest that frequent dosing may be necessary in birds, raising issues of the practicality of using this drug.[77]

b) Butorphanol 2 mg/kg IM every 2 hours was used in broiler chickens undergoing terminal surgical procedures.[78]

Anesthesia/sedation in psittacid species (extra-label):

a) Butorphanol 1 mg/kg IM with midazolam 0.5 mg/kg IM in the pectoral muscle provided good anesthetic premedication prior to isoflurane. The combination improved induction quality and reduced induction time and isoflurane concentration required for anesthetic maintenance without adverse effects on cardiorespiratory parameters.[79]

b) In cockatiels, butorphanol 3 mg/kg combined with midazolam 3 mg/kg and given intranasally provided rapid, deep sedation with no adverse effects.[67]

FERRETS:

Analgesic (extra-label): Because butorphanol appears to have shorter duration of action, buprenorphine is more commonly recommended for use as an analgesic in ferrets, but a butorphanol CRI of 0.1 – 0.2 mg/kg can be useful. Recommended analgesic dosages generally range from 0.1 – 0.4 mg/kg IM, IV, or SC every 2 to 6 hours.

Anesthetic adjunct (extra-label):

a) Butorphanol 0.1 mg/kg, ketamine 5 mg/kg, medetomidine 80 µg/kg. Combine in one syringe and give IM. May need to supplement with isoflurane 0.5% to 1.5% for abdominal surgery[80]

b) Butorphanol 0.2 mg/kg with xylazine 2 mg/kg IM[32]

c) Butorphanol 0.2 mg/kg with tiletamine/zolazepam 1.5 mg/kg and xylazine 1.5 mg/kg IM; may reverse xylazine with yohimbine 0.05 mg/kg IM

RABBITS/RODENTS/SMALL MAMMALS:

Analgesic (extra-label):

a) **Rabbits**: Butorphanol dosage recommendations generally range from 0.1 – 0.5 mg/kg SC, IM, or IV every 2 to 4 hours. An IV CRI dosage of 0.1 – 0.2 mg/kg/hour has also been recommended.[81]

b) **Rabbits:** Intranasal dexmedetomidine 0.1 mg/kg with midazolam 2 mg/kg and butorphanol 0.4 mg/kg produces profound sedation and analgesia lasting 45 minutes, with moderate sedation lasting another 25 minutes. Residual central nervous system impairment lasted up to 100 minutes. Because blood pressure and respiratory rates decrease with this drug combination, oxygen supplementation and careful monitoring are required. Use cautiously in compromised rabbits.[82]

c) **Rodents and Guinea pigs**: 1 – 2 mg/kg SC every 4 hours

d) **Chinchillas**:

i. Butorphanol 0.2 – 2 mg/kg SC every 2 to 4 hours[83]

ii. Butorphanol 0.5 mg/kg with (preservative-free) alfaxalone 5 mg/kg IM resulted in rapid anesthesia but of inconsistent depth and quality.[84]

Monitoring

- Analgesic and/or antitussive efficacy
- Respiratory rate and depth
- Appetite and bowel function
- CNS effects
- Heart rate

Client Information

- Be sure to tell your veterinarian if you notice any significant changes in your animal's behavior, appetite, bowel or urinary habits.
- This medicine is a controlled substance. Keep it in a secure location out of reach of children and animals.
- Butorphanol is classified as a schedule IV controlled drug by the federal Drug Enforcement Agency (DEA). Use of this medication in animals or humans other than those for whom it is prescribed is illegal.

Chemistry/Synonyms

Butorphanol tartrate is a synthetic narcotic agonist-antagonist and a morphinan derivative related structurally to morphine but that exhibits pharmacologic actions similar to other partial agonists (eg, pentazocine, nalbuphine). The compound occurs as a white crystalline powder that is sparingly soluble in water and insoluble in alcohol. It has a bitter taste and a pK_a of 8.6. The commercial injection has a pH of 3 to 5.5. One mg of butorphanol tartrate is equivalent to 0.68 mg of butorphanol base.

Butorphanol tartrate may also be known as levo-BC-2627 (butorphanol), *Alvegesic*®, *Butador*®, *Butomidor*®, *Butordyne*®, *Butorgesic*®, *Dolorex*®, *Equanol*®, *Stadol*®, *Torbutrol*®, *Torbugesic*®, *Torphadine*®, and *Verstadol*®.

Storage/Stability

The injectable product should be stored out of bright light and at controlled room temperature (20°C-25°C [68°F-77°F]), with excursions between 15°C to 30°C (59°F-86°F). The US label states to use contents within 4 months of first puncture. UK/AU/Canadian labels state to discard vial 28 days after first use.

Butorphanol is a controlled substance that should be stored in an area that is substantially constructed and securely locked. Follow applicable local, state, and federal rules regarding disposal of unused or wasted controlled drugs.

Compatibility/Compounding Considerations

Label information from butorphanol products approved in other countries state that butorphanol should not be mixed with any other drug in the same syringe. The injectable butorphanol product is reported to be **compatible** with the following drugs when mixed in the same syringe: acepromazine, atropine, chlorpromazine, diphenhydramine, fentanyl, hydroxyzine, meperidine, metoclopramide, midazolam, morphine, pentazocine, perphenazine, prochlorperazine, promethazine, scopolamine, and xylazine. Although studies confirming compatibility were not located, butorphanol is reportedly also compatible with preservative-free alfaxalone, detomidine, dexmedetomidine, ketamine, and medetomidine.

Butorphanol is reportedly **incompatible** with the following agents: alfaxalone from multi-dose vials (preservatives may form precipitate), dimenhydrinate, and pentobarbital sodium. It is unlikely to be compatible with diazepam.

Butorphanol has been compounded in a 8.3 mg/mL gel using a sterile 25% poloxamer 407 gel. Administration of this product in parrots at 12.5 mg/kg SC reached a peak concentration at 1.3 hours, and provided analgesia for 4 to 8 hours, but further studies are required to support clinical use.[15]

Dosage Forms/Regulatory Status

NOTE: Butorphanol is a class IV controlled substance. The veterinary product (*Torbutrol*®, *Torbugesic*®) strengths are listed as base activity, whereas the human product strength is labeled as the tartrate salt; these formulations are not equal.

VETERINARY-LABELED PRODUCTS:

Butorphanol Tartrate Injection: 2 mg/mL (activity as base) in 10 mL vials. *Torbugesic®-SA*, generic; (Rx, C-IV). FDA-approved for use in cats. NADA #141-047

Butorphanol Tartrate Injection: 10 mg/mL (activity as base) in 10 mL and 50 mL vials; *Torbugesic®*, *Dolorex®*, *Butorphic®*, generic; (Rx, C-IV). FDA-approved for use in horses not intended for food

Butorphanol Tartrate Tablets: 1 mg, 5 mg, and 10 mg (activity as base) tablets; bottles of 100; *Torbutrol®*; (Rx, C-IV). FDA-approved for use in dogs. NADA #103-390. **NOTE: Although this product is still listed in FDA's Green Book of approved animal drugs, it may no longer be commercially available in the United States.**

The Association of Racing Commissioners International (ARCI) has designated this drug as a class 3 substance. Use of this drug may not be allowed in certain animal competitions. Check rules and regulations before entering in a competition while this medication is being administered. Contact local racing authorities for further guidance. See ***Appendix*** for more information.

Food Animal Residue Avoidance Databank (FARAD) recommends a 5-day meat withdrawal and 3-day milk withdrawal with butorphanol use.[85]

HUMAN-LABELED PRODUCTS:

Butorphanol Tartrate Injection: 1 mg/mL (as tartrate salt; equivalent to 0.68 mg base) in 1 mL vials; 2 mg/mL (as tartrate salt) in 1 mL and 2 mL vials; generic; (Rx, C-IV)

Butorphanol Nasal Spray: 10 mg/mL in 2.5 mL metered dose; generic; (Rx, C-IV)

References

For the complete list of references, see **wiley.com/go/budde/plumb**

Butylscopolamine

N-Butylscopolammonium Bromide (NBB) Hyoscine Butylbromide, Butylscopolamine Bromide

(***byoo***-tel-skoe-***pahl***-ah-***meen***) *Buscopan®*

Quaternary Ammonium Antispasmodic and Anticholinergic

Prescriber Highlights

- Injectable anticholinergic used in horses
- Labeled for treating colic associated with spasmodic colic, flatulent colic, and simple impactions. May be an alternative to atropine or glycopyrrolate for treating bradycardia or acute episodes of severe equine asthma (SEA)
- Shorter-acting than atropine; only labeled for a single dose IV. Extra-label IM dosing has a longer duration of action.
- Not for use in patients with ileus or when decreased GI motility may be harmful
- Adverse effects include transient tachycardia, pupil dilation, decreased secretions, and dry mucous membranes.

Uses/Indications

N-butylscopolammonium bromide (NBB) injection is indicated (per the label) for control of abdominal pain (colic) associated with spasmodic colic, flatulent colic, and simple impactions in horses. As compared with butorphanol, NBB provided superior analgesia for ponies in a balloon model of abdominal pain.[1] It may also be of benefit in horses in combination with oxytocin to treat esophageal obstruction (choke) and as an aid to performing rectal examinations,[2] including colonoscopy. It can be considered an alternative to atropine as a positive chronotropic agent in horses[3] and has demonstrated bronchodilatory effects in horses with severe equine asthma (SEA),[4,5] although it does not improve yield during bronchoalveolar lavage.[6] NBB may be used to facilitate ophthalmic examination.[7]

Pharmacology/Actions

N-butylscopolammonium reduces GI peristalsis and rectal pressure via its anticholinergic actions by competitively inhibiting muscarinic receptors on smooth muscle. It has some bronchodilatory and chronotropic effects in horses. The bronchodilatory effects are observed within 10 minutes of IV administration, and dissipate within 1 hour.[4] NBB has shorter duration of action than atropine. It appears to have brief (15 to 20 minutes) visceral colorectal distention antinociceptive effects in horses.[8]

Pharmacokinetics

Limited information is available for horses. After an IV dose, the drug is eliminated within 48 hours in urine and feces equally. Estimated elimination half-life is ≈6 hours.

Contraindications/Precautions/Warnings

N-butylscopolammonium is labeled as contraindicated in horses with impaction colic associated with ileus or those with glaucoma.

NBB might be useful for equine ileal impactions by reducing intestinal spasm, but further studies are needed to confirm these effects and impaction is still listed as a contraindication.[9]

Because NBB can increase heart rate, use with caution in horses with systemic cardiovascular compromise.[10]

Adverse Effects

Adverse effects include transient tachycardia and hypertension, and a period of ≈20 to 30 minutes of decreased borborygmal sounds after IV dosing. Transient pupil dilation can be noted. Other effects include decreased secretions and dry mucous membranes.

Because this drug can cause increases in heart rate, heart rate cannot be used as a valid pain indicator for 30 minutes after injection.

When used for labeled indications, a lack of response may indicate a more serious problem that may require surgery or more aggressive care.[11]

Reproductive/Nursing Safety

Because no data are available to document safety, the manufacturer does not recommend use in nursing foals or pregnant or lactating mares.

Overdose/Acute Toxicity

Doses up to 10 times (3 mg/kg) the recommended amount were administered to horses as part of preapproval studies.[12] Clinical effects noted included dilated pupils (returned to normal in 4 to 24 hours), tachycardia (returned to normal within 2 hours) and dry mucous membranes (returned to normal in 1 to 2 hours). Gut motility was inhibited but returned to baseline within 4 hours and normal feces were seen within 6 hours. Two of the 4 horses treated at 10 times the recommended dose developed mild signs of colic that resolved without further treatment.

For patients that have experienced or are suspected to have experienced an overdose, it is strongly encouraged to consult with a 24-hour poison consultation center that specialize in providing information specific for veterinary patients. For general information related to overdose and toxin exposures, as well as contact information for poison control centers, refer to ***Appendix***.

Drug Interactions

The following drug interactions have either been reported or are theoretical in animals receiving N-butylscopolammonium bromide and may be of significance in veterinary patients. Unless otherwise noted, use together is not necessarily contraindicated, but weigh the potential risks and perform additional monitoring when appropriate.

- **Anticholinergic Agents** (eg, **atropine, glycopyrrolate**): May cause additive anticholinergic effects
- **Metoclopramide** (and other drugs that have cholinergic-like actions on the GI tract): These drugs and NBB may counteract one another's actions on GI smooth muscle.
- **Xylazine**: In healthy horses, NBB with xylazine can cause significant hypertension and cardiac tachyarrhythmias; may falsely influence surgical decision-making and prognosis in horses with colic.[10]

Laboratory Considerations
- No specific concerns noted

Dosages
HORSES:

Control of abdominal pain (colic) associated with spasmodic colic, flatulent colic, simple impactions (label dosage; FDA-approved): 0.3 mg/kg (30 mg or 1.5 mL per 100 kg (220 lb) of body weight) slowly IV, one time[12]

Control of abdominal pain (colic) associated with spasmodic colic, flatulent colic, simple impactions (extra-label): 0.3 mg/kg IM[13]

Esophageal obstruction (extra-label): NBB 0.3 mg/kg IV with oxytocin 0.11 – 0.22 units/kg IV once. Oxytocin should be avoided in mares, or dose significantly reduced; do NOT use in pregnant mares.[14]

Monitoring
- Heart rate (**NOTE:** Heart rate cannot be used as indicator for pain for the first 30 minutes after administration.)
- GI motility via gut sounds and feces output

Client Information
- Because an accurate patient assessment must be performed prior to the use of this medication and it requires IV administration and subsequent monitoring, this drug should only be administered by your veterinarian.

Chemistry/Synonyms
N-butylscopolammonium bromide, a derivative of scopolamine, is a synthetic, quaternary ammonium antispasmodic-anticholinergic agent. It occurs as a white crystalline substance that is soluble in water.

N-butylscopolammonium bromide may also be known as butylscopolamine bromide, hyoscine butylbromide, hyoscine N-butylbromide, scopolamini butylbromidum, hyoscini butylbromidum, *Buscopan®*, or *Buscapina®*.

Storage/Stability
The commercially available injection should be stored at or below 25°C (77°F) with excursions permitted up to 30°C (86°F).

Compatibility/Compounding Considerations
No specific information noted

Dosage Forms/Regulatory Status
VETERINARY-LABELED PRODUCTS:

N-butylscopolammonium bromide injection: 20 mg/mL in 50 mL multidose vials; *Buscopan®*; (Rx). NADA #141-228. FDA-approved for use in horses. Do not use in horses intended for human consumption

HUMAN-LABELED PRODUCTS:

None in the United States. There are several products with the trade name *Buscopan®* or *Buscapina®* available in many countries. Refer to actual product labels as ingredients and concentrations may vary.

References
For the complete list of references, see **wiley.com/go/budde/plumb**

Cabergoline

(ka-***ber***-goe-leen) *Dostinex®, Galastop®*

Dopamine Agonist/Prolactin Inhibitor

Prescriber Highlights
- ► Synthetic ergot derivative used for reducing prolactin levels in bitches and queens for medical treatment of pyometra, inducing and synchronizing estrus, inducing abortion, treating pseudopregnancy, mastitis, and pre-surgery for mammary tumors.
- ► Appears to be well tolerated in dogs and cats; vomiting has been reported, but adverse effects are much less than with bromocriptine.
- ► May need to be compounded for accurate dosing in cats and small dogs
- ► The National Institute for Occupational Safety and Health (NIOSH) classifies cabergoline as a hazardous drug; use appropriate precautions when handling.

Uses/Indications
For dogs and cats, cabergoline may be useful for medical treatment of pyometra, inducing and synchronizing estrus, treatment of primary or secondary anestrus, mastitis, pseudopregnancy, as a treatment prior to mammary tumor surgery, and for pregnancy termination in the second half of pregnancy. Cabergoline has also been used for post-spay aggression and anxiety in dogs and cats particularly when the surgery is performed during the luteal phase.

Cabergoline has been used in psittacines (primarily cockatiels) for adjunctive treatment of reproductive-related disorders, particularly persistent egg laying.[1-3]

Pharmacology/Actions
Cabergoline is an ergot alkaloid-derived dopamine (D_2) receptor agonist that exhibits multiple pharmacologic actions. It has a high affinity for dopamine$_2$ (D_2) receptors and a long duration of action. It exerts a direct inhibitory effect on the secretion of prolactin from the anterior pituitary gland. Its effect in inducing estrus is presumably due to its dopamine agonist effects on GnRH secretion rather than its effects on prolactin. When compared to bromocriptine, cabergoline has greater D_2 receptor specificity, longer duration of action, and less tendency to cause vomiting.

Pharmacokinetics
The pharmacokinetics of cabergoline have not been reported for dosages commonly used in dogs or cats. In humans, the drug is absorbed after oral dosing but its absolute bioavailability is not known.[4] Food does not appear to significantly alter absorption. The drug is extensively distributed throughout the body and is moderately bound to plasma proteins (40%). Cabergoline is extensively metabolized in the liver via hydrolysis. Half-life is estimated to be around 60 hours. Duration of pharmacologic action may persist for 48 hours or more. Elimination occurs by fecal (≈60%) and renal (≈22%) routes. Renal dysfunction does not appear to significantly alter elimination characteristics of the drug, but in severe hepatic insufficiency C_{max} and AUC are substantially increased.[4]

Contraindications/Precautions/Warnings
Cabergoline is contraindicated in patients that are hypersensitive to ergot derivatives (eg, bromocriptine)[4] or during pregnancy unless termination of pregnancy is desired. Patients that do not tolerate bromocriptine may not tolerate cabergoline.

In humans, bromocriptine is contraindicated in patients that have uncontrolled hypertension as additive hypertension could occur[4]; use with caution in those with hypertension that are already being treated with antihypertensive medications as syncope may result.[5,6]

It should be used with caution in patients with hepatic disease as the metabolism of the drug may be reduced.[6]

When using to induce estrus, it is recommended to wait at least 4 months after the prior cycle to allow the uterus to recover.

The National Institute for Occupational Safety and Health (NIOSH) classifies cabergoline as a hazardous drug; personal protective equipment (PPE) should be used accordingly to minimize the risk for exposure. Pregnant or nursing women, or women trying to become pregnant should avoid handling the medication due to reproductive risks.

Adverse Effects

Cabergoline is usually well tolerated by animal patients; it may cause lethargy and decreased appetite. Vomiting has been reported (most commonly after first few doses) but may be alleviated by reducing the dose and/or administering with food.[6,7] Dogs receiving cabergoline for more than 14 days may exhibit changes in coat color or texture[8]; this effect is likely reversible with drug withdrawal.

Human patients have reported postural hypotension, dizziness, headache, nausea, and vomiting while receiving cabergoline.[4]

Reproductive/Nursing Safety

This drug can cause spontaneous abortion in pregnant dogs or cats because prolactin is luteotrophic in these species.

Because cabergoline suppresses prolactin, it should not be used in nursing dams. A study in rats detected significant levels of cabergoline and its metabolites in maternal milk.[4]

Because safety has not been established in animals, this drug should only be used when the maternal benefits outweigh the potential risks to offspring.

Overdose/Acute Toxicity

Overdose information is not available for dogs or cats and remains limited for humans. It is postulated that cabergoline overdoses in people could cause hypotension, nasal congestion, syncope, or hallucinations.

Standard GI decontamination techniques (eg, emesis induction, activated charcoal) should be employed when applicable; however, emesis may occur spontaneously from the overdose and induction of emesis may not be necessary. Cardiovascular monitoring (eg, blood pressure, heart rate) and supportive care should be provided based on clinical presentation.

For patients that have experienced or are suspected to have experienced an overdose, consultation with a 24-hour poison control center specializing in providing veterinary-specific information is recommended. For general information related to overdose and toxin exposures, as well as contact information for poison control centers, refer to ***Appendix***.

Drug Interactions

The following drug interactions either have been reported or are theoretical in humans or animals receiving cabergoline and may be of significance in veterinary patients. Unless otherwise noted, use together is not necessarily contraindicated, but weigh the potential risks and perform additional monitoring when appropriate.

- **Butyrophenones** (eg, **azaperone, haloperidol**): Use of cabergoline with dopamine (D_2) antagonists may reduce the efficacy of both drugs and should be avoided.
- **Hypotensive Drugs** (eg, **amlodipine, enalapril, telmisartan**): Because cabergoline may have hypotensive effects, concomitant use with other hypotensive drugs may cause additive hypotension. Avoid concomitant use.
- **Macrolide Antibiotics** (eg, **clarithromycin**): Cabergoline concentration may be elevated.
- **Metoclopramide**: Use with cabergoline may reduce the efficacy of both drugs and use together should be avoided.
- **Phenothiazines** (eg, **acepromazine, chlorpromazine**): Use of cabergoline with dopamine (D_2) antagonists may reduce the efficacy of both drugs and should be avoided.
- **Reserpine**: May increase prolactin concentrations, and cabergoline doses may need to be increased

Laboratory Considerations

- None

Dosages

Because of the dosage differences in animals versus human patients and the strength of the commercially available product in the US, a compounding pharmacist must usually reformulate this medication (especially in cats and small dogs).

DOGS:

Estrus induction (extra-label):

a) Most commonly recommended: cabergoline 5 µg/kg PO once daily until 2 to 8 days after onset of proestrus or 14 to 42 days of treatment.[9] Proestrus occurs within 6 to 30 days.

b) 0.6 µg/kg PO once daily.[10] Continue treatment until day 2 after the onset of the first signs of proestrus, or until day 42 without signs of proestrus; 81% (22 of 27) of dogs treated at this low dose showed proestrus between days 4 and 48.

Pseudocyesis (pseudopregnancy) |suppression of lactation (extra-label):

a) 5 µg/kg PO once daily for 4 to 6 consecutive days depending on the severity of the clinical condition.[7] If signs do not resolve after a course of treatment, or if they recur, treatment may be repeated.

b) **Adjunctive treatment of pyometra** (extra-label): cabergoline 5 µg/kg PO in combination with cloprostenol 1 µg/kg SC once a day for 7 days with oral antibiotic therapy and supportive hydration. If no response, continue cloprostenol (without cabergoline) and any supportive treatment required for another 7 days.[12-14] See ***Monitoring***.

Abortifacient (extra-label):

a) Between gestation days 35 and 45: cabergoline 5 µg/kg PO once daily for 7 days in food and cloprostenol 1 µg/kg SC (after a tenfold dilution with physiologic saline) on days 1 and 3 given at least 8 hours after food. If pregnancy not terminated by day 8, continue cabergoline (at same dose) until day 12.[15] See ***Monitoring***.

b) Between gestation days 22 and 23: cabergoline 10 µg/kg PO once daily for 10 days[16]

Presurgical treatment mammary tumors (extra-label): 5 µg/kg PO 5 to 7 days prior to surgery aids in the detection of the tumors, decreases postsurgical reactions, and promotes recovery.[17]

CATS:

Abortifacient (extra-label):

a) At 30 days postcoitus, cabergoline 5 µg/kg PO once daily in combination with cloprostenol 5 µg/kg SC every 48 hours for 7 to 13 days was used to induce abortion.[18]

b) Cabergoline 15 µg/kg PO once daily with or without alfaprostol 10 µg/kg SC every other day was effective at terminating pregnancy when treatments were started on days 25 to 42 of pregnancy.[19]

Pseudocyesis (pseudopregnancy) | suppression of lactation (extra-label): 5 µg/kg PO once daily[6,20]

Presurgical treatment mammary tumors (extra-label): 5 µg/kg PO 5 to 7 days prior to surgery aids in the detection of the tumors, decreases postsurgical reactions, and promotes recovery.[17]

BIRDS:

Persistent egg laying in psittacines (extra-label):

a) Initially 10 – 20 µg/kg PO daily[1]; higher dosages were also used. Treatment is done in combination with removal of males and altered light cycle. Further work needed to determine the dose rate.[2]

b) 10 – 50 µg/kg PO every 12 to 24 hours[3]

Monitoring

- Monitoring for efficacy is dependent on the reason for use.
- Adverse effects (eg, lethargy, hyporexia, vomiting)
- Serum progesterone concentrations can be measured to assess response to cabergoline and client's adherence to therapy

Client Information

- Give this medicine with food to help prevent vomiting.
- Usually well tolerated by dogs and cats
- Because this drug has a higher risk for causing birth defects and affecting pregnancy or nursing, pregnant or nursing women should be very careful not to accidentally take it. Wear disposable gloves when giving doses or handling the drug, and avoid inhaling any dust from split or crushed tablets.
- This medication is considered to be a hazardous drug as defined by the National Institute for Occupational Safety and Health (NIOSH). Talk with your veterinarian or pharmacist about the use of personal protective equipment when handling this medicine.

Chemistry/Synonyms

Cabergoline, a synthetic, ergot-derivative, dopamine agonist similar to bromocriptine, occurs as a white powder that is insoluble in water and soluble in ethanol or chloroform. The commercially available tablets also contain the inactive ingredients leucine and lactose.

Cabergoline may also be known as FCE-21336, cabergolina, *Cabaser*®, *Actualene*®, *Sostilar*®, *Dostinex*®, *Finilac*®, *Galastop*®, or *Kelactin*®.

Storage/Stability

The commercially available tablets should be stored at controlled room temperature (20°C-25°C [68°F-77°F]).

The veterinary oral solution (available in EU and UK) should be stored below 25°C and protected from light. Do not refrigerate. Once opened, it should be used within 28 days.

Compatibility/Compounding Considerations

It has been reported that cabergoline is unstable or degrades in aqueous suspensions and if compounded into a liquid that will not be used immediately, should be compounded into a lipid-based product. Aqueous preparations should be used immediately and the remainder discarded. In one report a 10 µg/mL solution was prepared by dissolving one 0.5 mg [500 µg] commercial tablets in 50 mL of warm distilled water; the dose was administered within 15 minutes of preparation and the remaining solution was discarded.[21]

Dosage Forms/Regulatory Status

VETERINARY-LABELED PRODUCTS: NONE IN THE UNITED STATES

Cabergoline is available in Europe as a 50 µg/mL oral solution. An injectable product, *Galastop*® Injectable, is available in some countries.

HUMAN-LABELED PRODUCTS:

Cabergoline Oral Tablets: 0.5 mg (500 µg); generic; (Rx)

References

For the complete list of references, see **wiley.com/go/budde/plumb**

Caffeine

(***kaf***-een) *Cafcit*®

CNS Stimulant

Prescriber Highlights

- ► May be useful for respiratory acidosis in foals and as an adjunctive treatment for pneumonia in dogs
- ► Use with caution in patients with cardiovascular or seizure disorders, or a history of GI bleeding
- ► Adverse effects include increased locomotor activity, GI effects, increased heart rate, and glucose dysregulation.
- ► Use with caution in patients with cardiac, hepatic, or renal disease, or those at risk for GI bleeding
- ► Tolerance may develop; physical withdrawal symptoms may occur if stopped abruptly.

Uses/Indications

Caffeine may be used in foals with hypercapnia and respiratory acidosis,[1,2] although it appears to be less effective than doxapram. While there is support for a beneficial effect on equine exercise performance,[3] other evidence suggests caffeine has no effect.[4] In dogs, caffeine has been used anecdotally as adjunctive treatment with pneumonia.

In humans, caffeine is used to treat episodes of prolonged apnea in premature infants.

Pharmacology/Actions

Caffeine is a methylxanthine, like theophylline and theobromine; however, it has weaker respiratory, cardiac, and diuretic effects and more potent CNS effects. Caffeine antagonizes phosphodiesterase (via nonselective inhibition, which results in accumulation of cyclic AMP and GMP and increased transmission through these pathways) and adenosine A1 and A2 receptors to cause stimulation of the respiratory center via vagal and vasomotor pathways. This respiratory center stimulation may result in increased tidal volume and diaphragm contractility. Caffeine may also stimulate release of catecholamines, and beta-1 and beta-2-adrenergic effects may cause tachycardia and hypertension, but at high doses, hypotension and reduced peripheral vascular resistance may result. Caffeine can constrict cerebral blood vessels. Increased renal blood flow, combined with reduced proximal tubular sodium reabsorption, produces a mild diuresis. The drug also increases intraocular pressure, skeletal muscle contraction, and parietal cell acid release in the stomach.

Tolerance to caffeine's stimulating effects may occur rapidly.

Pharmacokinetics

In dogs, peak concentrations are reached 1.6 hours after oral administration; elimination half-life is ≈3.2 hours.[5]

In horses, caffeine is variably absorbed after oral administration, with bioavailability between 39% to 100%.[6,7] CNS penetration lags behind blood concentrations.[8] It has an elimination half-life between 10 to 21 hours after IV administration[6,7,9] that may be shortened by exercise.[10] Theophylline is one of many metabolites formed after caffeine administration in horses.[8]

In camelids, elimination half-life was 11 hours in male alpacas and 16 hours in female llamas.[11]

In humans, caffeine is readily absorbed, and peak concentration occurs within 30 to 120 minutes after oral administration. Food does not alter absorption. It is widely distributed, and CNS concentrations approximate plasma concentrations. Protein binding is ≈35%. In adults, caffeine is almost completely metabolized in the liver, including by CYP1A2; metabolites are excreted in the urine. Hepatic metabolism in neonates is immature and results in most of the drug being excreted unchanged in the urine; hepatic metabolism similar to adults is reached by ≈9 months of age. Elimination half-lives are 3 to 7 hours in adults, but 3 to 4 days in neonates.

Contraindications/Precautions/Warnings

Caffeine is contraindicated in patients hypersensitive to it or any of its components. Use caffeine with caution in patients with cardiovascular or seizure disorders, or a history of GI bleeding. Lower dosages may be required for patients with hepatic or renal disease. Cases of necrotizing enterocolitis occurred in human infants during FDA approval studies, although a causal relationship with caffeine has not been fully established.[12]

Adverse Effects

Excessive CNS stimulation may cause tremors, irritability, and decreased sleep. Increased locomotor activity in horses correlates with blood and CNS caffeine concentrations.[8] Caffeine may increase heart rate and blood pressure and disrupt blood glucose regulation. Nausea, vomiting, and inappetence may also occur. Physical withdrawal signs (eg, restlessness, irritability) may occur if drug administration is stopped abruptly.

Reproductive/Nursing Safety

Caffeine crosses the placenta. Reduced reproductive performance and embryotoxicity occurred in male rats receiving 50 mg/kg SC daily for 4 days.[12] Low rates of cleft palate occurred in pregnant mice implanted with sustained release caffeine pellets.

Caffeine is found in human breast milk at ≈50% to 75% of plasma concentrations. Moderate intake by breastfeeding women is generally considered safe, although poor sleep may be noted in nursing infants.[13]

Because safety has not been established in animals, this drug should only be used when the maternal benefits outweigh the potential risks to offspring.

Overdose/Acute Toxicity

Hypokalemia, hyperglycemia, tachycardia, hypertension (possibly followed by hypotension), metabolic acidosis, fever, hypertonia, rhabdomyolysis, and seizures may occur with caffeine overdose.[14] Serious toxicity in humans is associated with serum caffeine concentration greater than 50 micrograms/mL.[12] In human pediatric patients, toxicity may be seen at 35 mg/kg PO; an estimated oral lethal dose in adults is 150 – 200 mg/kg. Caffeine toxicosis has occurred in horses after ingestion of coffee husks used for bedding.[15]

Treatment is mainly supportive based on clinical presentation.[12] GI decontamination with activated charcoal should be considered. Blood pressure, ECG, electrolytes, and acid-base status should be monitored. Treat seizures with benzodiazepines (eg, diazepam, midazolam). Caffeine is dialyzable.

For patients that have experienced or are suspected to have experienced an overdose, consultation with a 24-hour poison control center specializing in providing veterinary-specific information is recommended. For general information related to overdose and toxin exposures, as well as contact information for poison control centers, refer to ***Appendix***.

Drug Interactions

In humans, caffeine is metabolized by CYP1A2. The following drug interactions either have been reported or are theoretical in humans or animals receiving caffeine and may be of significance in veterinary patients. Unless otherwise noted, use together is not necessarily contraindicated, but weigh the potential risks and perform additional monitoring when appropriate.

- **BETA-ADRENERGIC RECEPTOR AGONISTS** (eg, **albuterol, dobutamine, epinephrine**): Inotropic effects may be enhanced.
- **CIMETIDINE**: May reduce caffeine metabolism by 50% to 70%
- **ESTROGENS**: May reduce caffeine metabolism
- **CIPROFLOXACIN, ENROFLOXACIN**: May reduce caffeine metabolism
- **MEXILETINE**: May reduce caffeine metabolism by 30% to 50%
- **PHENOBARBITAL**: May increase caffeine metabolism
- **PHENYLPROPANOLAMINE**: May increase plasma caffeine concentrations. Combination increases blood pressure to greater extent than either drug alone.
- **TERBINAFINE**: May reduce caffeine metabolism
- **THEOPHYLLINE**: May have additive adverse effects. Premature human neonates metabolize theophylline to caffeine; horses metabolize caffeine to theophylline.[8]

Laboratory Interactions

- Falsely elevated **serum urate** when measured by the Bittner method
- Increases in urine levels of **catecholamines, vanillylmandelic** acid and **5-hydroxyindoleacetic acid** may occur.

Dosages

NOTE: Dosages are expressed in terms of caffeine base. See ***Chemistry/Synonyms***.

DOGS:

Adjunctive treatment of pneumonia (extra-label):

a) 5 – 10 mg/kg IV every 6 to 8 hours diluted and administered slowly over at least 30 minutes[16]
b) 10 mg/kg PO was used in a single-dose pharmacokinetic study.[5]

HORSES:

Respiratory acidosis and apnea in foals (extra-label): Loading dose: 7.5 – 12 mg/kg PO; maintenance dosage: 2.5 – 5 mg/kg PO every 12 to 24 hours[1,2,17,18]

Improving exercise performance in adult horses (extra-label): 5 mg/kg IV improved short-duration, intense exercise performance in Arabians.[3] A separate study using 2.5 mg/kg IV did not have an effect on any performance variable in physically fit thoroughbreds.[4] See ***Dosage Forms/Regulatory Status***.

Monitoring

- Respiratory character and rate, heart rate and rhythm, blood pressure
- Thoracic radiographs, pulse oximetry, and arterial blood gas as indicated by clinical condition

Client Information

- Caffeine is only administered by veterinary professionals; it may cause increased alertness and disrupt your animal's normal sleep pattern.
- Vomiting, diarrhea, and decreased appetite are possible side effects.

Chemistry/Synonyms

Caffeine is a methylxanthine. Caffeine citrate occurs as a bitter white powder that is freely soluble in water and soluble in alcohol. Caffeine citrate is ≈50% anhydrous caffeine. That is, each 1 mL of 20 mg/mL caffeine citrate solution and injection provides 10 mg caffeine base.

Caffeine citrate is also known as citrated caffeine, *Cafcit®*, and *Peyona®*.

Storage/Stability

Caffeine citrate should be stored at room temperature 20°C to 25°C (68°F-77°F). Caffeine citrate oral solutions and injections do not contain preservatives, and unused portions should be discarded.

Compatibility/Compounding Considerations

Compatibility is dependent on factors such as pH, concentration, temperature, and diluent used; specialized references or a hospital pharmacist should be consulted for more specific information.

Caffeine citrate for injection is reportedly **compatible** with dextrose-containing solutions, as well as the following drugs (partial list): calcium gluconate, dexamethasone sodium phosphate, diphenhydramine, dobutamine HCl, dopamine HCl, doxapram, fentanyl citrate, heparin, ketamine HCl, lidocaine HCl, morphine sulfate, and potassium chloride. The drug is reportedly **incompatible** with furosemide and pantoprazole.

Dosage Forms/Regulatory Status

VETERINARY-LABELED PRODUCTS: NONE

The Association of Racing Commissioners International (ARCI) has designated this drug as a class 2 substance. Use of this drug may not be allowed in certain animal competitions. Check rules and regulations before entering in a competition while this medication is being administered. Contact local racing authorities for further guidance.

HUMAN-LABELED PRODUCTS:

Caffeine Citrate for Injection: 20 mg/mL in 3 mL vials; *Cafcit®*, generic; (Rx)

Caffeine Citrate Oral Solution: 20 mg/mL in 3 mL vials; generic; (Rx)

References

For the complete list of references, see **wiley.com/go/budde/plumb**

Calcitonin

(kal-si-***toe***-nin) *Miacalcin®, Calcimar®*

Osteoclast-Inhibiting Hormone

Prescriber Highlights

- Hormone used primarily to control hypercalcemia in dogs and reptiles. Very short duration of action in dogs and can be expensive
- Hypersensitivity possible. May cause GI effects
- Young animals may be extremely sensitive to effects.
- Do not confuse with calcitriol.

Uses/Indications

In small animals and reptiles, calcitonin has been used as adjunctive therapy to control hypercalcemia. It may be of use in the adjunctive treatment of pain that originates from bone. Calcitonin's use in veterinary medicine has been limited by expense, availability, and development of resistance to its effects after several days of treatment.

Pharmacology/Actions

Calcitonin has a multitude of physiologic effects. It principally acts on bone, inhibiting osteoclastic bone resorption. By reducing tubular reabsorption of calcium, phosphate, sodium, magnesium, potassium, and chloride, it promotes their renal excretion. Calcitonin also increases jejunal secretion of water, sodium, potassium, and chloride (not calcium).

Pharmacokinetics

Calcitonin is destroyed in the gut after oral administration and therefore must be administered parenterally. In humans, the onset of effect after IV administration of calcitonin salmon is immediate. After IM or SC administration, onset occurs within 15 minutes, with maximal effects occurring in ≈4 hours. Duration of action is 6 to 12 hours after IM or SC injection. The drug is believed to be rapidly metabolized by the kidneys and in blood and peripheral tissues.

Contraindications/Precautions/Warnings

Calcitonin is contraindicated in animals hypersensitive to it. Patients with a history of hypersensitivity to other related proteins may be at risk. Young animals are reportedly up to 100 times more sensitive to calcitonin than are older animals (adults).[1,2] Hypocalcemia must be corrected prior to use whenever calcitonin is being used for an indication other than hypercalcemia.

Do not confuse calcitriol with calcitonin. Consider writing orders and prescriptions using tall man lettering; calciTONIN and calciTRIOL.

Adverse Effects

There is not a well-documented adverse effect profile for calcitonin in domestic animals; however, anorexia and vomiting have been reported in dogs. Overmedicating with this drug can lead to hypocalcemia. The following effects are documented in humans and potentially could be seen in animals: diarrhea, anorexia, vomiting, swelling and pain at injection site, and redness and peripheral paresthesias. Rarely, allergic reactions may occur. Tachyphylaxis (resistance to drug therapy with time) may occur in some treated dogs.

Reproductive/Nursing Safety

There is little information on the reproductive safety of calcitonin; however, it does not cross the placenta. Very high doses have resulted in decreased birth weight in rabbits, presumably due to the drug's metabolic effects.

Calcitonin has been shown to inhibit lactation in rats. Safe use during nursing has not been established.

Because safety has not been established in animals, this drug should only be used when the maternal benefits outweigh the potential risks to offspring.

Overdose/Acute Toxicity

Very limited data are available. Nausea and vomiting have been reported after accidental overdose injections. Chronic overdosing can lead to hypocalcemia.

For patients that have experienced or are suspected to have experienced an overdose, consultation with a 24-hour poison consultation center specializing in providing veterinary-specific information is recommended. For general information related to overdose and toxin exposures, as well as contact information for poison control centers, refer to ***Appendix.***

Drug Interactions

The following drug interactions have either been reported or are theoretical in humans or animals receiving calcitonin and may be of significance in veterinary patients. Unless otherwise noted, use together is not necessarily contraindicated, but weigh the potential risks and perform additional monitoring when appropriate.

- **Calcium-Containing Products**: May interfere with the efficacy of calcitonin
- **Lithium**: Concurrent use may result in decreased lithium concentrations and loss of lithium efficacy.
- **Pamidronate:** Although pamidronate and calcitonin are used together in human medicine, studies do not show any benefit when these drugs are used together in dogs.[3]
- **Vitamin D Analogues** (eg, **calcitriol, cholecalciferol**): May interfere with the efficacy of calcitonin

Dosages

DOGS:

Vitamin D toxicity, hypercalcemia (extra-label): Calcitonin treatment is not routinely recommended due to expense, frequency of dosing, and limited efficacy. In a recent review of management of hypercalcemia associated with cholecalciferol and vitamin D analogues,[4] the authors stated that the following protocol using calcitonin could be used but, due to inconsistent results, some patients becoming refractory to treatment, and the potential for greater soft tissue mineralization, they prefer substituting pamidronate for calcitonin: 1) Normal saline; twice maintenance; forced diuresis; maintain diuresis until calcium levels have dropped; 2) Furosemide 2.5 – 4.5 mg/kg PO 3 to 4 times a day or 0.5 mg/kg/hour via continuous IV infusion; 3) Either dexamethasone 1 mg/kg SC or IV divided 4 times daily, or prednisone 2 – 3 mg/kg PO twice daily;

4) Calcitonin 4 – 6 units/kg SC 2 to 3 times a day

REPTILES:

Hypercalcemia in green iguanas: 1.5 units/kg SC every 8 hours in combination with fluid therapy for several weeks if necessary[5]

Nutritional secondary hyperparathyroidism (NSHP):

1) If reptile is not hypocalcemic: 50 units/kg IM once weekly for 2 to 3 doses[6]
2) Correct husbandry problems and correct hypocalcemia with calcium and vitamin D. Once calcium level is normal and the animal is on oral calcium supplementation (usually about 7 days after starting therapy), give calcitonin at 50 units/kg IM weekly for 2 to 3 doses. Supportive care can be tapered once the animal becomes stable.[7]

Monitoring

- Serum-ionized (if possible) calcium. Directly measured serum-ionized calcium is a better indicator of calcium status than is total calcium but requires specific collection techniques and analyzers. Refer to your laboratory's guidelines or your analyzer's instructions.
- Phosphorus, BUN, and creatinine
- Hydration status
- Urine sediment for cast formation

Chemistry/Synonyms

Calcitonin is a 32-amino acid polypeptide with a molecular weight of ≈3600. Calcitonin is available commercially as either calcitonin human or calcitonin salmon, both of which are synthetically prepared. The potency of calcitonin salmon is typically expressed in international units (IU) but is expressed as units in this reference. Calcitonin salmon is ≈50 times more potent than calcitonin human on a per-weight basis.

Calcitonin salmon may also be known as calcitonin-salmon, calcitoninum salmonis, salmon calcitonin, SCT-1, or *Calcimar*®; many other trade names are available internationally.

Storage/Stability

Calcitonin salmon for injection should be stored in the refrigerator (2°C-8°C [36°F-46°F]).

Compatibility/Compounding Considerations

No specific information noted

Dosage Forms/Regulatory Status

VETERINARY-LABELED PRODUCTS: NONE

HUMAN-LABELED PRODUCTS:

Calcitonin Salmon for Injection: 200 units/mL in 2 mL vials; *Miacalcin*®; (Rx)

References

For the complete list of references, see **wiley.com/go/budde/plumb**

Calcitriol

(kal-si-***trye***-ole) *Rocaltrol*®, *Calcijex*®, *Active Vitamin* D_3

Vitamin D Analogue

Prescriber Highlights

- ▶ Vitamin D analogue that is used in dogs and cats for treatment of hypocalcemia and chronic kidney disease (CKD)
- ▶ Contraindications include hypercalcemia, hyperphosphatemia. Use cautiously in patients with malabsorption syndromes, calcium oxalate uroliths
- ▶ Adverse effects including hypercalcemia, hypercalciuria, and hyperphosphatemia are the greatest concern.
- ▶ Administer on an empty stomach to minimize promotion of calcium absorption and risk for hypercalcemia
- ▶ Do not confuse with calcitonin

Uses/Indications

Calcitriol is combined with oral calcium therapy for the long-term treatment of hypocalcemia associated with hypoparathyroidism. It has been shown to confer a survival benefit in dogs with CKD,[1] but there is only weak evidence to support calcitriol use in cats.[2] The decision remains unclear on how soon in the course of CKD calcitriol should be employed; it can reportedly improve cats' appetite and general wellbeing. Calcitriol may be a useful adjunctive drug for treating certain neoplasias (eg, mast cell tumors) as it may potentiate some chemotherapy agents.[3] It may also be of benefit in treating some types of refractory dermatopathies (eg, primary idiopathic seborrhea).[4]

Pharmacology/Actions

Calcitriol is a vitamin D analogue. Vitamin D is considered a hormone that, in conjunction with parathormone (PTH) and calcitonin, regulates calcium homeostasis in the body. Active analogues (or metabolites) of vitamin D enhance calcium absorption from the GI tract, promote reabsorption of calcium by the renal tubules, and increase the rate of accretion and resorption of minerals in bone. Unlike other forms of vitamin D, calcitriol does not require renal activation for it to be effective.

Pharmacokinetics

If fat absorption is normal, vitamin D analogues are readily absorbed from the GI tract (small intestine). Bile is required for adequate absorption and patients with steatorrhea or hepatic or biliary disease will have diminished absorption. Calcitriol has an onset of action of 1 to 4 days and a duration of action of less than 2 weeks.[5,6]

Contraindications/Precautions/Warnings

Calcitriol is contraindicated in patients with hypercalcemia, vitamin D toxicity, or abnormal sensitivity to the effects of vitamin D. Withhold treatment if hypercalcemia develops; resume treatment with a lower dosage only after calcium normalizes.[7] It should be used with extreme caution in patients with hyperphosphatemia (many clinicians believe hyperphosphatemia or a combined calcium-phosphorous product of more than 70 is a contraindication to the use of vitamin D analogues). Using calcitriol in patients with hyperphosphatemia can increase risks for tissue mineralization with additional renal tissue damage and dysfunction. Generally, calcium and phosphorus levels should be in the low normal range before beginning treatment, and adequate hydration maintained during therapy.[7]

As calcitriol can promote hypercalciuria, it should be used with caution in animals susceptible to calcium oxalate uroliths.

Monitoring of serum calcium levels is mandatory while using this drug.

Calcitriol absorption may be impaired in patients with malabsorption syndromes, resulting in reduced or unpredictable efficacy.

Do not confuse calcitriol with calcitonin. Consider writing orders and prescriptions using tall man letters: calciTONIN and calciTRIOL.

Adverse Effects

Although hypercalcemia is a known adverse effect, calcitriol administered in low dosages to dogs with CKD infrequently causes hypercalcemia, unless it is used with a calcium-containing phosphorus binder, particularly calcium carbonate. Signs of hypercalcemia include polydipsia, polyuria, and anorexia. Hyperphosphatemia may also occur with calcitriol therapy and patients' serum phosphate levels should be normalized before therapy is begun. Tissue calcification has been demonstrated in dogs with marginally elevated calcitriol concentration after chronic (up to 26 weeks) administration.[7]

Reproductive/Nursing Safety

Calcitriol has proven to be teratogenic in rabbits, but not in rats, when given at doses several times higher than those used therapeutically.[7] Reduced fetal weight, skeletal abnormalities, hypercalcemia in the offspring, and reduced pup survival have been observed. Because safety has not been established in animal species, this drug should only be used when the maternal benefits outweigh the potential fetal risks.

Calcitriol is passed into human breast milk. Safe use during lactation has not been established.

Overdose/Acute Toxicity

Overdose can cause hypercalcemia, hypercalciuria, and hyperphosphatemia. Intake of excessive calcium and phosphate may also cause the same effect. Clinical signs may include vomiting, diarrhea, anorexia, and lethargy; azotemia may occur. Hypercalcemia may require several days to up to 1 week to resolve. Acute ingestions should be managed using established protocols for removal or prevention of the drug being absorbed from the GI tract. Orally administered cholestyramine or mineral oil may reduce absorption and enhance fecal elimination.

Hypercalcemia secondary to chronic dosing of the drug should be treated by temporarily discontinuing calcitriol (not dose reduction) and exogenous calcium therapy. If the hypercalcemia is severe, a bisphosphonate (eg, pamidronate), furosemide, calcium-free IV fluids (eg, normal saline), urine acidification, and corticosteroids may be employed.

For patients that have experienced or are suspected to have experienced an overdose, it is strongly encouraged to consult with a 24-hour poison consultation center that specializes in providing information specific for veterinary patients. For general information related to overdose and toxin exposures, as well as contact information for poison control centers, refer to ***Appendix.***

Drug Interactions

The following drug interactions have either been reported or are theoretical in humans or animals receiving calcitriol and may be of significance in veterinary patients. Unless otherwise noted, use together is not necessarily contraindicated, but weigh the potential risks and perform additional monitoring when appropriate.

- **Aluminum-containing Phosphorus Binding Agents** (eg, **aluminum hydroxide**): Calcitriol may increase aluminum absorption.
- **Barbiturates** (eg, **phenobarbital, primidone**): May induce hepatic enzyme systems and increase the metabolism of vitamin D analogues thus decreasing their activity
- **Calcium Channel Blockers** (eg, **amlodipine, diltiazem, verapamil**): Calcitriol-induced hypercalcemia may antagonize the effects of calcium channel blocking agents.
- **Calcium-containing Phosphorus Binding Agents** (eg, **calcium acetate, calcium carbonate**): Use with calcitriol may induce hypercalcemia.
- **Cholestyramine:** May reduce calcitriol absorption; separate administration by several hours.
- **Corticosteroids** (eg, **dexamethasone, prednis(ol)one**): Can nullify the effects of vitamin D analogues
- **Digoxin**: Hypercalcemia increases the risk for digoxin toxicity.
- **Magnesium-Containing Products** (eg, **magnesium hydroxide**): Concurrent use may result in hypermagnesemia.
- **Sevelamer**: May reduce calcitriol absorption; separate administration by several hours.
- **Sucralfate**: Calcitriol may increase aluminum absorption.
- **Thiazide Diuretics** (eg, **chlorothiazide, hydrochlorothiazide**): May cause hypercalcemia when given in conjunction with vitamin D analogues

Laboratory Considerations

- **Serum cholesterol** levels may be falsely elevated by vitamin D analogues when using the Zlatkis-Zak reaction for determination.

Dosages

DOGS:

Cases of secondary hyperparathyroidism and slow progression of chronic kidney disease (CKD) (extra-label):

1. Recommended initial dosage: 1.5 – 3.5 ng/kg PO once daily, preferably in the evening on an empty stomach, to minimize calcium absorption and risk for hypercalcemia. Strong evidence supports use of calcitriol in dogs with IRIS CKD Stages 3 and 4.[8] Do not exceed calcitriol dosages of 5 ng/kg per day. If hypercalcemia develops, try giving double the daily dose every other day to reduce GI calcium absorption. Lifelong treatment is required.[9]
2. 2 – 2.5 ng/kg/day PO given on an empty stomach; maximum of 5 ng/kg/day. If hypercalcemia occurs, administer twice the daily dose every other day (eg, 2 ng/kg PO per day becomes 4 ng/kg every other day).[10]

Long-term maintenance of hypocalcemia-associated hypoparathyroidism (extra-label):

1. 30 – 60 ng/kg/day PO on an empty stomach. Combine with oral calcium to reduce vitamin D dose requirements.[11]
2. Initially, 20 – 30 ng/kg/day PO divided in two daily doses for 2 to 4 days.[6] Maintenance dosage 5 – 15 ng/kg/day

Primary idiopathic seborrhea (extra-label): 10 ng/kg PO once daily. Give on an empty stomach[4]

CATS:

Secondary hyperparathyroidism associated with CKD (extra-label):

1. 1.5 – 3.5 ng/kg PO daily given separately from meals[12]
2. 2.5 – 3.5 ng/kg PO once daily[13]

Long-term maintenance of hypocalcemia associated with hypoparathyroidism (extra-label):

1. 30 – 60 ng/kg/day PO. Maximal effect is in 1 to 4 days. Combine with oral calcium to reduce vitamin D dose requirements. Adjust dose by monitoring serum calcium.[11]
2. Initial dose 20 – 30 ng/kg/day PO for 2 to 4 days then decrease to 10 – 20 ng/kg/day PO for long-term management. Maximal effect is in 1 to 4 days. Oral calcium supplementation should also be provided initially but can usually be tapered and discontinued within a week of starting calcitriol. [14]
3. Initially, 20 – 30 ng/kg/day PO divided in 2 daily doses for 2 to 4 days.[6] Maintenance dosage 5 – 15 ng/kg/day

Monitoring

- Monitoring preventive dose: Assess serum calcium on days 7 and 14 after starting calcitriol and then every 6 months. Serum creatinine should be measured every 1 to 3 months. If hypercalcemia occurs, stop calcitriol for 1 week to determine if the drug is causing the hypercalcemia or if it is due to another cause (eg, too little calcitriol).

- Serum calcium: baseline and at 1 week after starting calcitriol therapy, then every 2 to 4 weeks thereafter. **NOTE**: Directly measured serum ionized calcium (ie, biologically active fraction) is a better indicator of calcium status than total calcium and requires specific collection techniques and analyzers. Refer to your laboratory's or analyzer's instructions. It is recommended to consult a veterinary endocrinology reference for a more thorough discussion of calcium measurement and monitoring.
- Serum phosphorous, magnesium, and creatinine. Baseline and at 1 week after starting calcitriol therapy, then every 2 to 4 weeks thereafter.
- Serum calcium (total) x phosphate product should remain below 70.[5,15]
- Baseline and periodic serum PTH levels: Monitor as above and determine PTH levels at 4 to 6 weeks after starting calcitriol. If PTH remains elevated, increase calcitriol dose by 1 – 2 ng/kg/day, but do not exceed 6.6 ng/kg/day unless also monitoring ionized calcium. If higher daily doses are required (5 – 7 ng/kg/day), a pulsed-dosing strategy may be considered; this is usually ≈20 ng/kg given twice weekly PO at bedtime on an empty stomach.[16]
- Clinical efficacy (eg, improved appetite, activity level, slowed progression of disease)

Client Information

- Best given on an empty stomach; some recommend giving at night.
- Watch for signs of high blood calcium (eg, greater thirst and urination, reduced or lack of appetite) and low blood calcium (eg, muscle tremors, twitching, stiffness, weakness, stiff gait, unsteadiness, behavioral changes, seizures, facial itching). If any of these signs are seen, contact your veterinarian immediately.
- Do not give calcium supplements or antacids (eg, *Tums*®) without your veterinarian's approval.

Chemistry/Synonyms

Calcitriol, a vitamin D analogue, is synthesized for pharmaceutical use. It is a white crystalline compound and is insoluble in water.

Calcitriol may also be known as calcitrolo, calcitriolum, 1,25-dihydroxycholecalciferol, 1-α,25 dihydrocholecalciferol, 1α, 25-Dihydroxyvitamin D_3, or 1,25-DHCC, 1,25-dihidroxyvitamin D_3, Ro 21-5535, U 49562, or *Rocaltrol*®.

Storage/Stability

Protect from light. Store oral calcitriol products in air-tight, light-resistant containers at room temperature 15°C to 30°C (59°F-86°F). The injection should be stored at 20°C to 25°C (68°F-77°F). It does not contain preservatives; any remaining drug should be discarded after opening ampule.

Compatibility/Compounding Considerations

No specific information noted

Dosage Forms/Regulatory Status

VETERINARY-LABELED PRODUCTS: NONE

HUMAN-LABELED PRODUCTS:

Note: Most doses are expressed in nanograms/kg (ng/kg); to convert µg to ng: 1 µg = 1000 ng, 0.25 µg = 250 ng. Reformulation by a compounding pharmacy may be required to assure accurate dosing, especially in smaller patients.

Calcitriol Oral Capsules: 0.25 and 0.5 µg; *Rocaltrol*®, generic; (Rx)

Calcitriol Oral Solution: 1 µg/mL in 15 mL bottles; *Rocaltrol*®, generic; (Rx)

Calcitriol Injection: 1 µg/mL and 2 µg/mL in 1 mL single-dose amps and vials; generic; (Rx)

Topical calcitriol is also available.

References

For the complete list of references, see **wiley.com/go/budde/plumb**

Calcium Acetate

(***kal***-see-um ***ass***-ah-tate) *Calphron*®

Oral Phosphate Binder

Prescriber Highlights

- Oral calcium salt used as a phosphorus binding agent in treating hyperphosphatemia associated with chronic kidney disease
- Must monitor serum phosphorus and calcium; hypercalcemia is possible but less likely from calcium acetate when compared to other calcium salts (eg, calcium carbonate)

Uses/Indications

Calcium acetate is administered orally to treat hyperphosphatemia in patients with chronic kidney disease. Secondary to its phosphorus binding efficiency and lower concentration of elemental calcium, calcium acetate is considered the most effective of the calcium-based phosphorus-binding agents and has the lowest potential for causing hypercalcemia.

Pharmacology/Actions

When calcium acetate is given with meals, it binds to dietary phosphorus and forms calcium phosphate, an insoluble compound that is eliminated in the feces. Calcium acetate is soluble over a wide pH range and therefore, available for binding phosphorus in the stomach and proximal small intestine. Calcium acetate binds ≈50% more phosphorous than calcium carbonate. Calcium acetate is less likely to cause hypercalcemia than calcium carbonate. Unlike calcium citrate, calcium acetate does not promote aluminum absorption.

Pharmacokinetics

No information was located on the pharmacokinetics of calcium acetate in dogs and cats. In humans, ≈30% is absorbed when given with food.

Contraindications/Precautions/Warnings

This agent should not be used when hypercalcemia is present. Because hypercalcemia can result from administering oral calcium products to animals with chronic kidney disease, adequate monitoring of serum ionized calcium and phosphorus is required.

Use calcium-containing phosphate binders with caution in patients with a serum calcium x phosphorus product greater than 60.

Calcium acetate decreases systemic absorption of dietary phosphorous; patients who are not eating will not benefit from this treatment to lower serum phosphorous levels.

Using calcium-based phosphate binders and calcitriol together is controversial. Some authors state that the combination is contraindicated, whereas others state that intensified monitoring for hypercalcemia is required.

Adverse Effects

Hypercalcemia and extraosseous (soft tissue) calcification are the primary concerns associated with calcium acetate, especially when using high doses long-term. Adequate monitoring is required.

In humans, GI intolerance (nausea) has been reported.

Reproductive/Nursing Safety

No reproductive safety studies were located, and the human label states that it is not known whether the drug causes fetal harm. However, it would be surprising if calcium acetate caused teratogenic effects.

It would be expected that calcium acetate would be safe to administer during lactation.

Overdose/Acute Toxicity

Acute overdoses could potentially cause hypercalcemia. Patients should be monitored, and their clinical signs treated. If the dose was massive and recent, consider using standard protocols to empty the GI tract.

For patients that have experienced or are suspected to have experienced an overdose, consultation with a 24-hour poison consultation center specializing in providing veterinary-specific information is recommended. For general information related to overdose and toxin exposures, as well as contact information for poison control centers, refer to ***Appendix***.

Drug Interactions

The following drug interactions have either been reported or are theoretical in humans or animals receiving calcium acetate and may be of significance in veterinary patients. Unless otherwise noted, use together is not necessarily contraindicated, but weigh the potential risks and perform additional monitoring when appropriate.

- ASPIRIN: Concurrent use may result in decreased salicylate effectiveness.
- ATENOLOL: Concurrent use may result in reduced atenolol efficacy.
- BISPHOSPHONATES, ORAL (eg, **alendronate**): Concurrent oral administration may reduce bisphosphonate absorption. If combination is required, separate doses by at least 2 hours if possible.
- CALCIUM CHANNEL BLOCKERS (eg, **amlodipine**, **diltiazem, verapamil**): Concurrent use may reduce the therapeutic effects of calcium channel blockers.
- CEFPODOXIME: Concurrent use may result in decreased cefpodoxime efficacy.
- CEFTRIAXONE: Concurrent use may result in formation of ceftriaxone-calcium precipitates. This combination is contraindicated in human neonates.
- DIGOXIN: Calcium acetate is not recommended for use in human patients that are on digoxin therapy, as hypercalcemia may cause serious arrhythmias.
- FLUOROQUINOLONES (eg, **enrofloxacin, marbofloxacin**): Oral calcium-containing products can reduce absorption of fluoroquinolones. If combination is required, separate doses by at least 2 hours.
- IRON: Concurrent use may result in decreased iron effectiveness.
- KETOCONAZOLE: Concurrent use may result in decreased ketoconazole exposure.
- LEVOTHYROXINE: Oral calcium products may reduce levothyroxine absorption if given at the same time. Separate doses by at least 2 hours if possible.
- PENICILLAMINE: Oral calcium-containing products can reduce penicillamine absorption.
- PHOSPHATES, ORAL: Concurrent use may result in decreased phosphate absorption.
- SUCRALFATE: Concurrent use may result in decreased sucralfate efficacy.
- TETRACYCLINES (eg, **doxycycline, minocycline**): Oral calcium-containing products can reduce absorption of tetracyclines. If combination is required, separate doses by at least 2 hours.
- THIAZIDE DIURETICS (eg, **chlorothiazide/hydrochlorothiazide**): Concurrent use may increase risk of hypercalcemia.
- TRIENTENE: Oral calcium-containing products can reduce trientene absorption.
- VITAMIN D ANALOGUES (eg, **calcitriol, cholecalciferol, ergocalciferol**): Concurrent use may increase risk of hypercalcemia.

Laboratory Considerations

- **Hemolyzed blood samples** or **hyperlipidemia:** Can cause falsely elevated total calcium reports
- **Heparin**: Sodium or lithium heparin may bind small amounts of ionized calcium. Heparinized samples are acceptable provided that careful attention is paid to the concentration of heparin in the final sample.
- **Hyperbilirubinemia:** Can cause falsely low total calcium reports
- **Oxalate, citrate, ethylenediaminetetraacetic acid (EDTA):** These anticoagulants in blood sample collection tubes can bind calcium and cause falsely low total calcium reports.

Dosages

DOGS/CATS:

Hyperphosphatemia associated with chronic kidney disease, in conjunction with a low-phosphorus diet (extra-label): 60 – 90 mg/kg/day PO divided and given with food, mixed with food, or just prior to each meal. Therapy usually begins at the lower end of the recommended dose range and is adjusted upward as needed every 4 to 6 weeks until the therapeutic target is reached. Monitor ionized calcium; hypercalcemia is possible. Decrease dose if serum calcium exceeds normal limits.[1-3]

Hyperphosphatemia associated with chronic kidney disease, in conjunction with a low-phosphorus diet (extra-label): Initially, 30 – 60 mg/kg/day PO in divided doses and mixed with food at each meal. Adjust dose to achieve target phosphorus concentration.[4,5]

Monitoring

- Serum phosphorus (after a 12-hour fast) and ionized calcium: monitor values at 4- to 6-week intervals initially, then once stable, recheck every 3 months.[4,5] Some clinicians recommend more frequent intervals (eg, every 10 to 14 days) initially, particularly in patients at higher risk for hypercalcemia. **NOTE:** Directly measured serum ionized calcium is a better indicator of calcium status than total calcium, but requires specific collection techniques and/or analyzers.[6]

Client Information

- Give this medicine with meals; either just before feeding or mixed into food. Your veterinarian may prescribe additional doses to be administered between meals.
- Contact your veterinarian if your animal develops increased thirst and urinations, vomiting, decreased appetite, or low energy level while receiving this medicine.
- While your animal is taking this medicine, your veterinarian will need to perform periodic blood tests to know how well the medicine is working. Do not miss these important follow-up visits.

Chemistry/Synonyms

Calcium acetate is a white, odorless, hygroscopic powder that is freely soluble in water and slightly soluble in alcohol. Each gram contains ≈254 mg of elemental calcium.

Calcium acetate may also be known as calcii acetas, acetato de calcio, kalcio acetates, kalciumacetat, or kalciumasetaatti, *Calphron®*, *PhosLo®*.

Storage/Stability

The commercially available tablets, capsules, and gelcaps should be stored at room temperature (25°C [77°F]); excursions are permitted to 15°C to 30°C (59°F-86°F).

Compatibility/Compounding Considerations

No specific information noted

Dosage Forms/Regulatory Status

VETERINARY-LABELED PRODUCTS: NONE

HUMAN-LABELED PRODUCTS:

Calcium Acetate Oral Tablets: 667 mg (169 mg elemental calcium); *Calphron®*, generic; (Rx)

Calcium Acetate Oral Capsules and Gelcaps: 667 mg (169 mg elemental calcium); generic; (Rx)

Calcium Acetate Oral Solution: 667 mg/5 mL (169 mg elemental calcium); *Phoslyra®*; (Rx)

References

For the complete list of references, see **wiley.com/go/budde/plumb**

Calcium, IV (-Borogluconate, -Chloride, -Gluconate)

(kal-***see***-um)

Essential Cation

Prescriber Highlights

- Used IV to treat or prevent severe hypocalcemia, and effects of acute hyperkalemia and hypermagnesemia; SC administration is somewhat controversial.
- Contraindications include ventricular fibrillation or hypercalcemia.
- Determine dosages carefully as calculations can be confusing.
- Must be given slowly IV to avoid adverse effects
- Must monitor therapy carefully; frequency of monitoring depends on condition and response to therapy
- Many potential drug interactions as well as drug and fluid incompatibilities

Uses/Indications

Parenteral calcium is used to treat confirmed hypocalcemia, calcium channel blocker toxicity, hypermagnesemia, and/or hyperkalemia. Parenteral calcium salts include calcium gluconate, calcium borogluconate, and calcium chloride. Calcium gluconate is generally preferred as it is less irritating to vascular tissues.

Routine administration of IV calcium during CPR is not recommended as administration does not improve the odds of survival. However, it may be considered in cases with moderate to severe hypocalcemia and hyperkalemia.[1]

Pharmacology/Actions

Calcium is an essential element that is required for many functions, including nervous and musculoskeletal system function, cell membrane and capillary permeability, and activation of enzymatic reactions.

Pharmacokinetics

After administration, ionized calcium enters the extracellular fluid and is rapidly incorporated into skeletal tissue. Calcium administration does not necessarily stimulate new bone formation. Approximately 99% of total body calcium is stored in bone. Of circulating calcium, ≈50% is bound to serum proteins or complexed with anions and ≈50% is found in the ionized form. Total serum calcium is dependent on serum protein concentrations. Total serum calcium changes by ≈0.8 mg/dL for every 1.09 g/dL change in serum albumin. Calcium crosses the placenta and is distributed into milk.

Calcium is eliminated primarily (≈80%) in the feces, consisting of both unabsorbed calcium and calcium excreted into the bile and pancreatic fluids. Only small amounts of calcium are excreted in the urine as most cationic calcium is filtered by the glomeruli and reabsorbed by the tubules and ascending loop of Henle. Vitamin D, parathyroid hormone, and thiazide diuretics decrease the amount of calcium excreted by the kidneys. Loop diuretics (eg, furosemide), calcitonin, and somatotropin increase calcium renal excretion.

Contraindications/Precautions/Warnings

Calcium is contraindicated in patients with ventricular fibrillation or hypercalcemia. Parenteral calcium should not be administered to patients with serum calcium levels above normal. Calcium should be used cautiously in patients receiving digitalis glycosides (eg, digoxin) or those with cardiac or renal disease. Due to its acidifying nature, calcium chloride should be used with caution in patients with respiratory failure, respiratory acidosis, or renal disease.

Hypocalcemia may not resolve in some animals until they receive magnesium supplementation.[2,3]

Rapid IV injection of calcium can cause hypotension, cardiac arrhythmias (eg, bradycardia, ST segment elevation, or QT interval shortening), and cardiac arrest. Dilution prior to administration may help promote a safer injection rate, and thus reduce risks associated with rapid injection.

Administration of calcium salts by SC or IM routes has been associated with severe injection site reactions, including tissue necrosis, and is not recommended.[3]

Parenteral treatment using calcium should be considered "High Alert" with dosages double-checked by another person.

Adverse Effects

Hypercalcemia can be associated with calcium therapy, particularly in patients with cardiac or renal disease; animals should be adequately monitored. Calcium chloride may be more irritating to vascular tissue than other parenteral salts and is more likely to cause hypotension. Rapid IV injection of calcium can cause hypotension, cardiac arrhythmias, and cardiac arrest. Calcinosis cutis has been observed in animals receiving diluted 10% calcium gluconate SC; this effect is more prevalent in small dogs or cats and those with concurrent hypophosphatemia.

Venous irritation may occur after IV administration. If calcium salts are accidentally infused perivascularly, stop the infusion. Treatment then may include infiltrating the affected area with normal saline SC, corticosteroids administered SC locally, applying heat to and elevating the area, and infiltrating the affected area with a local anesthetic and hyaluronidase.

Reproductive/Nursing Safety

Although parenteral calcium products have not been proven safe for use during pregnancy, they are often used before, during, and after parturition in cows, ewes, bitches, and queens to treat parturient paresis secondary to hypocalcemia.

In humans, calcium crosses the placenta and is excreted in milk. Calcium salts are considered compatible with pregnancy and lactation.[4]

Overdose/Acute Toxicity

Hypercalcemia can occur with parenteral therapy, oral therapy in combination with vitamin D, or increased parathyroid hormone levels. Treat hypercalcemia by withholding calcium therapy and other calcium elevating drugs (eg, vitamin D analogues). Mild hypercalcemia will usually resolve without further intervention when renal function is adequate. Moderate to marked hypercalcemia should be treated with IV fluid diuresis using normal saline and administering a loop diuretic (eg, furosemide) to increase sodium and calcium excretion. Potassium and magnesium must be monitored and replaced as necessary. ECG should also be monitored during treatment. Corticosteroids (and in humans, calcitonin and hemodialysis) have also been employed in treating hypercalcemia.

Horses with functional kidneys can eliminate large amounts of calcium; hypercalcemia from excessive calcium administration is rare, especially if the horse is receiving fluid therapy.

For patients that have experienced or are suspected to have experienced an overdose, consultation with a 24-hour poison consultation center specializing in providing veterinary-specific information is recommended. For general information related to overdose and toxin exposures, as well as contact information for poison control centers, refer to ***Appendix.***

Drug Interactions

The following drug interactions have either been reported or are theoretical in humans or animals receiving calcium and may be of significance in veterinary patients. Unless otherwise noted, use together is not necessarily contraindicated, but weigh the potential risks and perform additional monitoring when appropriate.

- **Bisphosphonates** (eg, **alendronate, pamidronate, zoledronic acid):** Bisphosphonate use may result in hypocalcemia.
- **Calcitonin:** Calcium administration may interfere with the calcium-lowering effects of calcitonin.
- **Calcium Channel Blockers** (eg, **amlodipine, diltiazem, verapamil**): IV calcium may antagonize the effects of calcium channel blocking agents.
- **Digoxin**: Patients on digoxin therapy are more susceptible to developing arrhythmias if receiving IV calcium (especially if given rapidly); use with caution.
- **Dobutamine**: Calcium salts may decrease the therapeutic effects of dobutamine.
- **Loop Diuretics** (eg, **furosemide**): Loop diuretics promote calcium excretion.[5]
- **Magnesium Sulfate**: Parenteral calcium can neutralize the effects of hypermagnesemia or magnesium toxicity secondary to parenteral magnesium sulfate.
- **Neuromuscular Blockers** (eg, **atracurium, pancuronium, vecuronium**): Parenteral calcium may reverse the effects of nondepolarizing neuromuscular blocking agents.
- **Potassium Supplements**: Patients receiving both parenteral calcium and potassium supplementation may have an increased chance of developing cardiac arrhythmias—use cautiously.
- **Thiazide Diuretics** (eg, **chlorothiazide, hydrochlorothiazide**): May cause hypercalcemia and metabolic alkalosis when used in conjunction with large doses of calcium
- **Vitamin D Analogues** (eg, **calcitriol, ergocalciferol**): Concurrent use may increase risk for hypercalcemia. Monitor calcium and phosphate and watch for signs of hypercalcemia.

Laboratory Considerations

- **Hemolyzed blood samples** or **hyperlipidemia:** Can cause falsely elevated total calcium reports
- **Heparinized blood collection tubes**: Sodium or lithium heparin may bind small amounts of ionized calcium. Heparinized samples are acceptable provided that careful attention is paid to the concentration of heparin in the final sample
- **Hyperbilirubinemia:** Can cause falsely lower total calcium levels
- **Oxalate, citrate, ethylenediaminetetraacetic acid (EDTA) blood collection tubes**: These anticoagulants in blood sample collection tubes can bind calcium and cause falsely low total calcium reports.

Dosages

NOTES:

1. **WARNING**: Dosing parenteral calcium can be confusing and potentially dangerous. Depending on the reference, dosages can be listed by mL/kg, mEq/kg, mmol/kg, or mg/kg. These may be for the calcium salt being used OR for elemental calcium. Calcium chloride 10% (100 mg/mL) injection contains ≈3 times more **elemental calcium** per mL than calcium gluconate 10% (100 mg/mL). See ***Contraindications/Precautions/Warnings.***
2. Patient response (ie, improvement of clinical signs) determines the final dose of calcium. Patients must be continually monitored during the infusion. See ***Monitoring.*** Stop infusion immediately if a pronounced change in rate or rhythm is detected.
3. Rapid IV injection of calcium can cause hypotension, cardiac arrhythmias (eg, bradycardia, ST segment elevation, or QT interval shortening), and cardiac arrest. Dilution prior to administration may help promote a safer injection rate, thus reducing risks associated with rapid injection.

Calcium source	Elemental calcium (mg/mL)
Calcium gluconate 10% injection	9.3
Calcium chloride 10% injection	27.3

DOGS/CATS:

Treatment of clinical signs associated with hypocalcemia (ie, tetany, seizures; extra-label): 5 – 15 mg/kg of <u>elemental</u> calcium IV *slowly* over 10 to 30 minutes. This dosage corresponds to*:

a. **Calcium <u>gluconate</u> 10% injection:** 0.54 – 1.61 mL/kg (NOT mg/kg)
b. **Calcium <u>chloride</u> 10% injection:** 0.18 – 0.55 mL/kg (NOT mg/kg)

***NOTE:** If using other concentrations or other salts (eg, calcium borogluconate), the <u>actual volume to inject will vary</u> depending on the concentration of the solution and which salt is being used.

Short-term maintenance after tetany has been corrected using a constant rate infusion (CRI; extra-label)**:** 2.5 – 3.5 mg/kg/hour of <u>elemental</u> calcium IV CRI. Dilute in compatible IV solution (eg, lactated Ringer's, 0.9% sodium chloride; see ***Compatibility/Compatibility Considerations*** for more information). The goal of treatment is to maintain calcium within the normal range, and to wean off parenteral calcium as soon as oral calcium and vitamin D take effect and serum calcium concentration remains stable. Parenteral calcium is preferably given by constant rate infusion (**calcium <u>gluconate</u>** or **calcium <u>chloride</u>**) or subcutaneous administration (**calcium <u>gluconate</u>** only).

Hyperkalemic cardiotoxicity (extra-label): elemental calcium 4.65 – 9.3 mg/kg (0.5 – 1 mL/kg calcium <u>gluconate</u> 10%) IV *slowly* over 10 to 20 minutes. Rapidly corrects arrhythmias but effects are very short (10 to 15 minutes). **NOTE:** IV calcium treatment can antagonize the cardiotoxic effects of potassium but does not reduce potassium concentrations. IV dextrose (0.5 – 1 g/kg body weight with or without regular insulin) can be administered to lower serum K+ concentrations.[6]

Adjunctive therapy for nonobstructive dystocia (extra-label): In most cases, calcium is given *before* oxytocin to improve contraction strength. See ***Oxytocin*** for further information.

a. Elemental calcium 9 mg/kg IV *slowly* infusion (≈ 1 mL/kg calcium gluconate 10%); dogs 20 kg or greater received a total dose of 180 mg elemental calcium (total dose, NOT mg/kg; ≈ 20 mL calcium gluconate 10%)[7]
b. Elemental calcium median dose 3.8 mg/kg (0.41 mL/kg calcium gluconate 10%) IV *slowly*[8]
c. Elemental calcium ≈2 mg/kg (0.2 mL/kg calcium gluconate 10% solution) IV *slowly*[9]

HORSES:

Hypocalcemia (extra-label):

a) **Mild hypocalcemia**: add 50 mL of 23% **calcium borogluconate** per 5 L of lactated Ringer's solution (LRS); administer IV at twice maintenance rate; this is sufficient to restore normocalcemia. Horses with functional kidneys can eliminate large amounts of calcium; hypercalcemia from excessive calcium administration is rare, especially when the horse is receiving fluid therapy.

b) **Severe hypocalcemia**: add 100 – 150 mL of 23% **calcium borogluconate** per 5 L of LRS. In animals with chronic or refractory hypocalcemia, PO supplementation with **calcium carbonate** (limestone) 100 – 300 g/horse/day (NOT g/kg) or dicalcium phosphate 100 – 200 g/horse/day (NOT g/kg) should be considered. Adding vitamin D treatment is questionable and some horses may develop toxicity from hypervitaminosis D; however, low doses of vitamin D might benefit horses with decreased calcium absorption and reabsorption.

c) **Calcium gluconate injection**: 150 – 250 mg/kg IV *slowly* to effect (intraperitoneal route may also be used)[10]

d) **Lactation tetany**: 250 mL per 450 kg (992 lb) body weight of a standard commercially available solution that also contains magnesium and phosphorous IV *slowly* while auscultating heart. If no improvement of clinical signs after 10 minutes, repeat dosing. Intensity in heart sounds should be noted, with only an infrequent extrasystole.[11]

e) **During general anesthesia for colic surgery**: If serum ionized calcium is less than 1.1 mmol/L (2.2 mEq/L or 4.4 mg/dL), administer **calcium gluconate** 10 mg/kg IV *slowly* over 30 to 60 minutes.[12]

CATTLE:

Hypocalcemia (labeled dosage; not FDA approved): 250 – 500 mL IV *slowly*. Some product labels also state that the intraperitoneal route may be used. **NOTE:** There are no known products that are FDA-approved for use in animals. Calcium predates formal FDA approval regulations for its use in animals.

Hypocalcemia (extra-label): **Calcium gluconate** injection: 150 – 250 mg/kg IV *slowly* to effect (intraperitoneal route may also be used)[10]

SHEEP/GOATS:

Hypocalcemia (extra-label):

a) **Calcium borogluconate** 23% is ≈50 – 75 mL/45 kg (100 lb) body weight (NOT mL/kg) IV *slowly*. Slow IV infusion of calcium should show immediate clinical response. May also be given SC.

b) **Sheep**: **Calcium gluconate** 150 – 250 mg/kg IV *slowly* to effect (intraperitoneal route may also be used)[10]

SWINE:

Hypocalcemia (extra-label): **Calcium gluconate** 150 – 250 mg/kg IV *slowly* to effect (intraperitoneal route may also be used)[10]

BIRDS:

Hypocalcemic tetany (extra-label): **Calcium gluconate** 50 – 100 mg/kg IV *slowly* to effect; may be diluted and given IM if a vein cannot be located[13]

Egg-bound birds (extra-label): Initially, **calcium gluconate** 1% solution 0.01 – 0.02 mL/g IM. Provide moist heat (26°C to 29°C [80°F-85°F]) and allow 24 hours for bird to pass egg.[14] **NOTE**: calcium gluconate 1% must be compounded; dilute the 10% solution with a compatible solution.

REPTILES:

Egg binding in combination with oxytocin (extra-label): **Calcium glubionate**: 10 – 50 mg/kg IM and oxytocin 1 – 10 units/kg IM as needed until calcium levels back to normal or egg binding is resolved. Use care when giving multiple injections. Calcium with oxytocin is not as effective in lizards as in other species.[15]

Monitoring

- During IV administration, monitor temperature, pulse, respiratory rate, and continuous monitoring of heart rate and rhythm with an ECG. If bradycardia, shortened QT interval, or ST segment elevation occurs, temporarily stop the calcium infusion.
- Serum ionized calcium every 4 to 6 hours; more frequent monitoring may be required based on response to therapy. Directly measured serum ionized calcium is a better indicator of calcium status than total calcium but requires specific collection techniques and analyzers.[3,16]
- Serum magnesium, phosphorous, and potassium when indicated. Calcium x phosphorus product should be less than 60
- Serum PTH (parathyroid hormone) if indicated
- Renal chemistry panel initially and as needed during therapy

Chemistry

Several different salts of calcium are available in various formulations. Calcium gluceptate and calcium chloride are freely soluble in water; calcium lactate is soluble in water; calcium gluconate and calcium glycerophosphate are sparingly soluble in water, and calcium phosphate and carbonate are insoluble in water. Calcium gluconate for injection has a pH of 6.0 to 8.2 and calcium chloride for injection has a pH of 5.5 to 7.5.

To determine approximate elemental calcium content *per gram* of various calcium salts:

Calcium borogluconate: 90 mg (4.6 mEq; 2.3 mmol)
Calcium chloride: 273 mg (13.6 mEq; 6.8 mmol)
Calcium glubionate: 66 mg (3.29 mEq; 1.64 mmol)
Calcium gluceptate: 82 mg (4.08 mEq; 2.04 mmol)
Calcium gluconate: 93 mg (4.65 mEq; 2.32 mmol)

Storage/Stability

Calcium gluconate, calcium borogluconate, and calcium chloride injectable formulations should be stored at room temperature 20°C to 25°C (68°F-77°F) and protected from freezing.

Compatibility/Compounding Considerations

Compatibility is dependent on factors such as pH, concentration, temperature, and diluent used; specialized references or a hospital pharmacist should be consulted for more specific information.

Calcium chloride for injection is reportedly **compatible** with the following IV solutions and drugs: amikacin sulfate, ascorbic acid, chloramphenicol sodium succinate, dopamine HCl, hydrocortisone sodium succinate, isoproterenol HCl, lidocaine HCl, norepinephrine bitartrate, penicillin G potassium/sodium, pentobarbital sodium, phenobarbital sodium, sodium bicarbonate, verapamil HCl, and vitamin B complex with C.

Calcium chloride for injection **compatibility information conflicts** or is dependent on diluent or concentration factors with the following drugs or solutions: fat emulsion 10%, dobutamine HCl, oxytetracycline HCl, and tetracycline HCl. Compatibility is dependent upon factors such as pH, concentration, temperature, and diluent used.

Calcium chloride for injection is reportedly **incompatible** with the following solutions or drugs: amphotericin B and chlorpheniramine maleate.

Calcium gluconate for injection is reportedly **compatible** with the following IV solutions and drugs: sodium chloride 0.9% for injection, lactated Ringer's injection, dextrose 5% to 20%, dextrose-lactated Ringer's injection, dextrose-saline combinations, amikacin sulfate, aminophylline, ascorbic acid injection, chloramphenicol sodium succinate, corticotropin, dimenhydrinate, erythromycin gluceptate, heparin sodium, hydrocortisone sodium succinate, lidocaine HCl, norepinephrine bitartrate, penicillin G potassium/sodium, phenobarbital sodium, potassium chloride, tobramycin sulfate, vancomycin HCl, verapamil, and vitamin B complex with C.

Calcium gluconate compatibility information conflicts or is dependent on diluent or concentration factors with the following drugs or solutions: phosphate salts, oxytetracycline HCl, and prochlorperazine edisylate. Compatibility is dependent upon factors such as pH, concentration, temperature, and diluent used.

Calcium gluconate is reportedly **incompatible** with the following solutions or drugs: IV fat emulsion, amphotericin B, ceftriaxone, dobutamine HCl, methylprednisolone sodium succinate, metoclopramide, or fluids containing bicarbonate, or phosphate.

Dosage Forms/Regulatory Status

VETERINARY-LABELED PRODUCTS:

NOTE: Not necessarily a complete list. Veterinary-labeled products may not be FDA-approved, as they do not appear in the Green Book.

Calcium Gluconate 23% (mg/mL; equivalent to 20.7 mg [1.07 mEq] elemental calcium per mL), in 500 mL bottles; generic; (OTC). Some formulations may contain boric acid (ie, calcium borogluconate). Labeled for use in cattle. No withdrawal times are required.

Products are also available that include calcium, phosphorus, potassium, magnesium and/or dextrose; refer to the individual product's labeling for specific dosage information. Trade names for these products include *Norcalciphos®*, and *Cal-Dextro® Special, #2, C,* and *K*; (Rx).

Oral Products: No products containing only calcium (as a salt) are available commercially with veterinary labeling. There are several products (eg, *Pet-Cal®* and *Osteoform® Improved*) that contain calcium with phosphorous and vitamin D (plus other ingredients in some preparations).

HUMAN-APPROVED PRODUCTS: (NOT A COMPLETE LIST)

Calcium Gluconate Injection 10% (100 mg/mL; equivalent to 9.3 mg [0.465 mEq] elemental calcium per mL), preservative-free in 10 mL and 50 mL single-dose vials and 100 mL pharmacy bulk vials; generic; (Rx)

Calcium Chloride Injection 10% (100 mg/mL; equivalent to 27.3 mg [1.36 mEq] elemental calcium per mL) in 10 mL vials, and syringes; generic; (Rx)

References

For the complete list of references, see **wiley.com/go/budde/plumb**

Calcium, Oral (-Carbonate, -Gluconate, -Lactate)

(***kal***-see-um)

Oral Phosphate Binder and Antacid (Calcium Carbonate); Calcium Supplement (Calcium Carbonate and Calcium Gluconate)

Prescriber Highlights

- Calcium carbonate is used as a phosphorus binding agent for treating hyperphosphatemia associated with chronic kidney disease and as a calcium supplement in animals with chronic hypocalcemia. It could also be used as an oral antacid but is rarely recommended for this purpose in small animals.
- Calcium gluconate and calcium lactate are alternative oral calcium supplements.
- Serum phosphorus and calcium concentrations must be monitored during therapy.

See also ***Calcium Acetate***

Uses/Indications

Calcium carbonate can be used for oral administration to treat hyperphosphatemia in patients with chronic kidney disease and as a calcium supplement in animals with chronic hypocalcemia. Unlike calcium citrate, calcium carbonate does not promote aluminum absorption. Calcium carbonate could also be used as an oral antacid but is rarely recommended for this purpose in small animals.

Calcium gluconate and calcium lactate are alternatives to calcium carbonate as an oral calcium supplement.

Pharmacology/Actions

When calcium carbonate is given with meals, it binds to dietary phosphorus and forms calcium phosphate, an insoluble compound that is eliminated in the feces. Calcium carbonate is more likely than calcium acetate to cause hypercalcemia because calcium carbonate binds ≈50% as much phosphorous as calcium acetate, making it less effective as a phosphorus binding agent and resulting in higher concentrations of elemental calcium.

Pharmacokinetics

No information was located on the pharmacokinetics of calcium carbonate, calcium gluconate, or calcium lactate in dogs and cats. In humans, calcium carbonate is converted to calcium chloride by gastric acid. Oral calcium absorption is influenced by a variety of factors, including intestinal pH, vitamin D status, and the administered dose. Approximately ≈80% calcium is eliminated in the feces, and ≈20% is renally eliminated.

Contraindications/Precautions/Warnings

Calcium salts should not be used when hypercalcemia is present. Because hypercalcemia can result from administering oral calcium products to animals with kidney disease, monitoring of serum ionized calcium and phosphorus concentrations is required. Because oral calcium reduces dietary phosphorus absorption, treatment will be ineffective in animals that are not eating.

Use calcium-containing phosphate binders with caution in patients with serum calcium-phosphorus product concentrations greater than or equal to 60.

Using calcium-based phosphate binders and calcitriol together is controversial. Some authors state that the combination is contraindicated, whereas others state that intensified monitoring for hypercalcemia is required.

Adverse Effects

Hypercalcemia and extraosseous (soft tissue) calcification are the primary concerns associated with calcium carbonate, especially when using high dosages long-term; adequate monitoring is required.

In humans, nausea and constipation have been reported while taking this drug.

Reproductive/Nursing Safety

In humans, calcium crosses the placenta and is excreted in milk; calcium salts are considered compatible with pregnancy and lactation.[1]

Overdose/Acute Toxicity

Potentially, acute overdoses could cause hypercalcemia in susceptible animals. Patients should be monitored and treated based on clinical signs. If overdose was massive and recent, consider using standard protocols to empty the gut.

Drug Interactions

The following drug interactions have either been reported or are theoretical in humans or animals receiving oral calcium-containing products and may be of significance in veterinary patients. Unless otherwise noted, use together is not necessarily contraindicated, but weigh the potential risks and perform additional monitoring when appropriate.

- **Aspirin**: Concurrent use may result in decreased salicylate effectiveness.
- **Azole Antifungals** (eg, **itraconazole**, **ketoconazole,** but *not* **fluconazole**)**:** Concurrent use may result in decreased antifungal exposure.
- **Bisphosphonates, Oral** (eg, **alendronate**). Concurrent oral administration may reduce bisphosphonate absorption.
- **Calcitriol**: If administered with calcium carbonate, may lead to hypercalcemia; if calcitriol is used concomitantly, intensified monitoring for hypercalcemia is mandatory.
- **Cefpodoxime**: Concurrent use may result in decreased cefpodoxime effectiveness.
- **Corticosteroids** (eg, **dexamethasone, prednis(ol)one**): Calcium may reduce corticosteroid bioavailability.
- **Digoxin**: Calcium carbonate is not recommended for use in human patients that are on digoxin therapy as hypercalcemia may cause serious arrhythmias.
- **Fluoroquinolones** (eg, **enrofloxacin**): Oral calcium-containing products can reduce absorption of fluoroquinolones; if both calcium carbonate and a fluoroquinolone are required, separate doses by at least 2 hours.
- **H_2 Receptor Antagonists** (eg, **famotidine, ranitidine**): Reducing stomach acid may lower the phosphorous binding capacity of calcium carbonate.
- **Levothyroxine**: Oral calcium products may reduce levothyroxine absorption if given at the same time. Separate doses by at least 2 hours if possible.
- **Loop Diuretics** (eg, **furosemide**): Loop diuretics promote calcium excretion.[2]
- **Mycophenolate**: Oral calcium-containing products can reduce absorption of mycophenolate.
- **Oral Phosphates**: Concurrent use may result in decreased phosphate absorption.
- **Propranolol**: Concurrent use may result in decreased propranolol bioavailability.
- **Proton Pump Inhibitors** (eg, **omeprazole**): Reducing stomach acid may lower the phosphorous binding capacity of calcium carbonate. Omeprazole reduces dietary calcium digestibility[3]; the effect, if any, on calcium supplementation is unclear.
- **Quinidine**: Oral calcium-containing products can decrease quinidine excretion.
- **Rifampin:** Oral calcium-containing products can reduce absorption of rifampin; if both calcium carbonate and rifampin are required, separate doses by at least 2 hours.
- **Sotalol**: Oral calcium-containing products can reduce sotalol absorption.
- **Sucralfate**: Concurrent use may result in decreased sucralfate efficacy.
- **Tetracyclines** (eg, **doxycycline, minocycline**): Oral calcium-containing products can reduce absorption of tetracyclines; if both calcium carbonate and a tetracycline are required, separate doses by at least 2 hours.
- **Thiazide Diuretics** (eg, **chlorothiazide/hydrochlorothiazide**): Concurrent use may increase risk of hypercalcemia.
- **Verapamil**: Concurrent use may result in reversal of hypotensive effects.

Laboratory Considerations

When using to treat hypocalcemia:

- **Hemolyzed blood samples** or **hyperlipidemia:** Can cause falsely elevate total calcium concentrations
- **Heparinized blood collection tubes**: Sodium or lithium heparin may bind small amounts of ionized calcium. Heparinized samples are acceptable provided that careful attention is paid to the concentration of heparin in the final sample.
- **Hyperbilirubinemia:** Can cause falsely lower total calcium concentrations
- **Oxalate, citrate, ethylenediaminetetraacetic acid (EDTA) blood collection tubes**: These anticoagulants in blood sample collection tubes can bind calcium and cause falsely low total calcium concentrations.

Dosages

DOGS/CATS:

Hyperphosphatemia associated with chronic kidney disease using a low-phosphorus diet (extra-label): Calcium carbonate 30 – 60 mg/kg PO per day *divided* and given with food or just prior to each meal.[4,5] Doses up to 90 – 150 mg/kg/day PO may be needed.[6] Therapy usually begins at the lower end of the recommended dose range and is adjusted upward as needed every 4 to 6 weeks until the serum phosphorus target is reached. Decrease dose if serum calcium exceeds normal limits. See ***Chemistry/Synonyms***.

Calcium supplement for chronic hypocalcemia: Dogs (total dose/dog, NOT mg/kg): ≈1250 mg (toy breeds) – 10 g (giant breeds) of calcium carbonate PO per day. This dosage is equivalent to 0.5 – 4 g/dog (NOT mg/kg) of elemental calcium PO per day. Cats: 1250 mg – 2.5 g/cat (NOT mg/kg) (0.5 – 1 g/cat of elemental calcium) PO per day. See ***Chemistry/Synonyms***.

Monitoring

The IRIS guidelines suggest monitoring serum phosphorus and calcium concentrations every 4 to 6 weeks initially, then, once stable, at 12-week intervals.[4,5] However, some recommend more frequent intervals (ie, initially every 10 to 14 days), particularly in patients at higher risk for hypercalcemia.

- Serum phosphorus (after a 12-hour fast): 2.7 – 4.6 mg/dL is the goal for Stage 2 patients and is ideal for all stages. More realistic goals for Stage 3 and 4 patients are less than 5 mg/dL and less than 6 mg/dL, respectively.
- Serum ionized (if possible) calcium: Directly measured serum ionized calcium is a better indicator of calcium status than total calcium but requires specific collection techniques and analyzers.[7] The IRIS guidelines suggest a goal for total calcium of less than 12 mg/dL in cats.
- Calcium x phosphorus product less than 60

Client Information

- Give medication with meals, either just before the animal eats or mixed into its food.

- Your veterinarian may prescribe additional doses to be administered between meals if additional calcium is required; give only with meals unless your veterinarian instructs you to do otherwise.
- Use of this medication requires ongoing laboratory monitoring.

Chemistry/Synonyms

Calcium carbonate occurs as a fine, white, odorless, microcrystalline powder. It is practically insoluble in water, but water solubility is increased by presence of carbon dioxide or ammonium salts. Calcium carbonate dissolves with effervescence in hydrochloric acid. It is insoluble in alcohol. Calcium carbonate may also be known as calcii carbonas, E170, or precipitate chalk. A common oral dosage form trade name is *Tums*®. One gram of calcium carbonate contains 400 mg of elemental calcium (40%).

Calcium gluconate is a white or almost-white, crystalline or granular powder. It is sparingly soluble in water and freely soluble in boiling water. One gram of calcium gluconate contains 90 mg of elemental calcium (9%).

Calcium lactate is a white or almost-white, crystalline or granular powder. It is soluble in water (freely soluble in boiling water) and slightly soluble in alcohol. It may also be known as calcii lactas. One gram of calcium lactate contains 130 mg of elemental calcium (13%).

When using oral calcium supplements, adjust the dose to give an equivalent amount of elemental calcium as provided by the chosen calcium salt. For example, 1 g of calcium gluconate contains 90 mg of elemental calcium, 1 g of calcium lactate contains 130 mg of elemental calcium, and 1 g of calcium carbonate contains 400 mg of elemental calcium.

Storage/Stability

The commercially available tablets, capsules, and gel caps should be stored at room temperature (25°C [77°F]); excursions are permitted at 15°C to 30°C (59°F-86°F).

Compatibility/Compounding Considerations

No specific information was noted.

Dosage Forms/Regulatory Status

VETERINARY-LABELED PRODUCTS: NONE.

An oral nutritional supplement (*Epakitin*®) (not FDA-approved) contains calcium carbonate 10% (100 mg/g) and chitosan (8%).

HUMAN-LABELED PRODUCTS:

Calcium Carbonate: Many oral products are available, and all are OTC. Dosage forms include chewable and regular tablets in strengths ranging from 420 mg (168 mg calcium) to 1250 mg (500 mg calcium; common sizes are 500 mg [200 mg calcium] and 750 mg [300 mg calcium]), oral powders (1000 mg/packet [400 mg calcium]), suspensions (1250 mg/5 mL), and capsules (600 mg [240 mg calcium]); generic.

Calcium Gluconate: Generally available as 500 mg (45 mg calcium), 650 mg (58.5 mg calcium), and 1 g (90 mg calcium) oral tablets; all are OTC.

Calcium Lactate Tablets: 325 mg (42.3 mg calcium) and 650 mg (84.5 mg calcium); generic; OTC

References

For the complete list of references, see **wiley.com/go/budde/plumb**

Cannabidiol (CBD)

(can-na-bi-***dye***-ole) *Epidiolex*®

Cannabinoid

NOTE: The information presented in this monograph is for products containing only cannabidiol (CBD); extrapolation of this information to "full-spectrum" products will not accurately predict safety or efficacy.

Prescriber Highlights

- ► The use of cannabidiol (CBD) in animals has not been approved by the FDA. State and local laws vary, and practitioners should consult independent legal counsel to determine their compliance obligations with respect to the veterinary use of CBD.
- ► Naturally occurring cannabinoid that has been used to treat canine osteoarthritis and epilepsy
- ► In veterinary species, efficacy for specific conditions and optimal dosages are under investigation.
- ► Contraindications include hypersensitivity to CBD.
- ► Use with caution in patients with hepatic impairment; dosage reduction may be needed
- ► Withdraw gradually when discontinuing its use as an anticonvulsant.
- ► CBD appears to be well tolerated at dosages that have been studied; hypersalivation, diarrhea, emesis, increased liver enzymes, lethargy, and ataxia have been noted.
- ► Products that also contain tetrahydrocannabinol (THC) appear more likely to cause adverse effects; choose products carefully, as formulations may contain varying amounts of CBD as well as other cannabinoids (eg, THC) or impurities.

Uses/Indications

Cannabidiol (CBD) use in veterinary medicine is an area of active investigation. CBD has shown benefit as an analgesic for canine osteoarthritis[1-3] and has reduced seizure frequency in dogs with epilepsy.[4] CBD controlled pruritic behavior in dogs with atopic dermatitis.[5] One study found no difference between CBD and placebo for relieving clinical signs associated with osteoarthritis in dogs.[6] Low-dose CBD (1.4 mg/kg daily PO) lacked efficacy as an anxiolytic in dogs with noise phobia.[7]

Although most studies have focused on CBD, the products used in many studies contained varying amounts of other cannabinoids. The impact of these other cannabinoids on the safety and efficacy of CBD products remains unclear. See ***Chemistry/Synonyms*** for further information.

Pharmacology/Actions

Cannabidiol (CBD) is a lipophilic, nonintoxicating cannabinoid that can bind to CB_2 cannabinoid receptors, which are primarily found in the periphery (ie, immune system) and have little to no psychotropic effects. Activation of these receptors is thought to prevent inflammatory cytokine release.[8,9] CBD also interacts with many (over 65) noncannabinoid receptors,[10] including the serotonin 1A receptor (5-$HT1_A$), which may help alleviate anxiety, insomnia, pain, and nausea; it also acts on the vanilloid receptor (TRPV1), which assists in perception of pain, inflammation, and body temperature.[11,12] The anticonvulsant effect of CBD in humans is not thought to be due to a direct effect on cannabinoid receptors.[13]

In contrast, tetrahydrocannabinol (THC) is a cannabinoid primarily targeting CB_1 receptors, which modulate calcium and potassium ion influx and appear to inhibit excitatory and inhibitory neurotransmitter release.[14] The CB_1 receptor is found primarily in the CNS and is involved in cognitive function, emotion, movement, and hunger. THC is considered intoxicating and is responsible for the "high" associated with marijuana use in humans.[8,15]

Alterations in the canine metabolome were observed after 3 weeks of cannabidiol administration to healthy dogs; the physiologic relevance of this finding warrants further investigation.[16]

Pharmacokinetics

Assessment of cannabidiol (CBD) pharmacokinetics is complicated by the lack of standardized CBD formulations.

Absorption of CBD after oral administration appears to be limited by an extensive first-pass effect.[14,17] In dogs, bioavailability after transdermal application to the pinna was ≈9% relative to oral administration.[18] CBD is widely distributed into tissues and is highly lipophilic.[8,19] Elimination half-life of CBD is ≈1 to 4 hours following single doses,[1,20,21] but is ≈14 to 25 hours following 28 days of CBD administration.[22] When CBD was administered IV, half-life varied between 7 and 9 hours.[23,24]

In cats that were given a single dose of a CBD fish oil formulation, peak concentration of 43 ng/mL occurred 1 to 4 hours after administration; AUC was 164 ng/hour/mL and half-life was 1.7 hours.[21]

In horses, orally administered CBD (in oil) was readily absorbed, with peak concentration occurring ≈3 to 5 hours after dosing.[25,26] Peak concentration following pelleted CBD occurred at ≈2.5 hours.[27] Terminal half-life ranged from 8.5 to 15 hours following single or repeated (4 to 6 weeks) administration.[25-27]

In humans, peak CBD concentration is reached ≈2 to 2.5 hours after administration.[13] Administration with food increases absorption, leading to a 4- to 5-fold increase of C_{max} and a 3- to 4-fold increase in AUC. The drug is widely distributed, and protein binding exceeds 94%. CBD is extensively metabolized, primarily in the liver but also in the GI tract, by CYP2C19, CYP3A4, UGT1A7, UGT1A9, and UGT2B7. At least one metabolite (7-OH-CBD) is active. Half-life is ≈60 hours, and elimination occurs via the feces.

Contraindications/Precautions/Warnings

Cannabidiol (CBD) is contraindicated in patients that are hypersensitive to it or to other components of the formulation. Use CBD with caution in patients with hepatic dysfunction; dosage reduction is recommended in humans with hepatic impairment, and it is assumed that this applies to veterinary patients.

When it is used to control seizures, CBD should be discontinued gradually, as rapid withdrawal can increase the risk for seizures.[13]

Adverse Effects

When cannabidiol (CBD) is administered at 4 mg/kg/day PO (the dosage most commonly used in studies), it appears to be well tolerated. Occasional GI effects[6,28] (eg, hypersalivation, diarrhea, emesis) and lethargy may occur, but CBD is without apparent effect on voluntary daily activity in dogs.[22,29] Decreased body weight was noted in one study of healthy dogs, despite food intake being considered adequate.[22] Higher dosages and/or products that also contain tetrahydrocannabinol (THC) appear more likely to cause adverse CNS effects (eg, hyperesthesia, static ataxia) in dogs.[22,30] A case of Stevens-Johnson syndrome has been documented in one dog after receiving a CBD-containing product.[31] Increases (2 times the upper limit of normal) in ALP were noted in healthy dogs and were not associated with adverse effects, and in one study increases in ALP were more common at higher dosage (12 mg/kg/day) as compared with lower dosages (1 – 4 mg/kg/day).[28]

Cats experienced low rates of lethargy and ataxia following administration of CBD-infused oil; emesis and hypersalivation also occurred, but these effects appeared to be due to the medium-chain triglyceride oil in the formulation.[32] One cat was reported to have an increased ALT (3 times the upper limit of normal).[21]

Horses receiving CBD for up to one week showed no adverse GI or behavioral effects, or changes in activity (step count).[25,27] In one study in 12 horses receiving CBD for 6 weeks,[26] 10 horses gained weight (average 18.5 kg), and elevated liver enzymes were noted in 8 horses. Additionally, all horses experienced mild decreases in total calcium, although ionized calcium remained within the reference range. Hypocalcemia and elevated liver enzymes normalized within 10 days of discontinuing CBD.

Reproductive/Nursing Safety

Administration of cannabidiol (CBD) 150 – 250 mg/kg/day to pregnant rats increased embryofetal mortality, decreased growth, delayed sexual maturation, and caused small testes and reduced fertility in male offspring.[13] Administration of CBD to rabbits caused decreased birth weights, and reproductive system changes.

CBD is excreted in human maternal milk following maternal medical or recreational use of cannabis products,[33] and in mouse milk following intraperitoneal injections of CBD.[34] It is unknown if CBD is excreted in maternal milk following oral administration.[13]

Because safety has not been established in animals, this drug should only be used when the maternal benefits outweigh the potential risks to offspring.

Overdose/Acute Toxicity

Cannabidiol (CBD) products may contain more or less CBD than is stated on the product label.[35] They also may contain varying amounts of tetrahydrocannabinol (THC), which may increase the risk for adverse effects or toxicity. Although the ASCPA has not seen an increase in calls from states that have legalized recreational marijuana, animal clinics in Colorado have reported significant increases in marijuana exposures.[19,36] Because recreational use of marijuana remains illegal in many states, clients may be reluctant to discuss possible exposures to marijuana or treatment with cannabis products, including CBD. For that reason, some clients may need reassurance when taking a history.

Clinical signs of a CBD overdose can include hypersalivation, emesis, lethargy, diarrhea, and ataxia.

Treatment of a significant cannabinoid overdose may consist of GI decontamination (inducing emesis, activated charcoal) for recent ingestion or if a significant amount remains in the stomach, and supportive treatment (eg, IV fluids, antiemetics). Additionally, butorphanol may be used for agitation and a benzodiazepine (eg, diazepam, midazolam) may be administered to control seizures as indicated. IV lipid emulsion may be useful.[8] Anecdotally, most overdoses of cannabinoids do not require intervention; placing the animal in a dark, quiet room can minimize stimulations while the animal is intoxicated.

For patients that have experienced or are suspected to have experienced an overdose, it is strongly encouraged to consult with one of the 24-hour poison control centers that specialize in providing information specific for veterinary patients. For general information related to overdose and toxin exposures, as well as contact information for poison control centers, refer to ***Appendix.***

Drug Interactions

In humans, cannabidiol (CBD) is a substrate of CYP3A4 and CYP2C19; therefore, it may affect concentrations of drugs metabolized by CYP2C19 and CYP1A2. The following drug interactions either have been reported or are theoretical in humans or animals receiving CBD and may be of significance in veterinary patients. Unless otherwise noted, use together is not necessarily contraindicated, but weigh the potential risks and perform additional monitoring when appropriate.

- **Amiodarone:** Concurrent use may lead to increased CBD concentration.[13,37,38]
- **Azole Antifungals** (eg, **fluconazole**, **itraconazole, ketoconazole**, **voriconazole**): Increased CBD concentration is possible; there is possible additive hepatotoxicity risk.[13,37,38]

- **Benzodiazepines**: Concurrent use with CBD may lead to increased concentrations of certain benzodiazepines (eg, **alprazolam, diazepam**; not midazolam).[11,13] Concurrent use may increase risk for sedation and respiratory depression.
- **Central Nervous System (CNS) Depressants** (eg, **acepromazine, gabapentin, pregabalin, tramadol, trazodone**): Concurrent use with other CNS depressants increases risk for sedation.[13,38]
- **Chloramphenicol:** Concurrent use may lead to increased CBD concentration.[13,37,38]
- **Cimetidine:** Concurrent use may lead to increased CBD concentration.[13,37,38]
- **Clopidogrel**: CBD may decrease formation of clopidogrel active metabolite. Clopidogrel may increase CBD concentration.[13,37,38]
- **Dexamethasone:** Concurrent use may lead to decreased CBD concentration.[13,38,39]
- **Diltiazem:** Concurrent use may lead to increased CBD concentration.[13,37,38]
- **Fenofibrate**: Increased fenofibrate concentration may occur when used concurrently with CBD.
- **Fluoxetine:** Concurrent use may lead to increased CBD concentration and risk for serotonin syndrome.[13,37,38]
- **Glipizide**: CBD may decrease glipizide metabolism, increasing hypoglycemic effect.
- **Hepatotoxic Drugs** (eg, **lomustine, prednis(ol)one, sex-steroid hormones** [eg, **estrogens, progestins**]): Concurrent use with valproate and clobazam increased serum liver transaminases.[13] It is suggested to use CBD cautiously with other hepatotoxic drugs.
- **Lidocaine**: Increased lidocaine concentration is possible with concurrent use.
- **Loperamide**: Increased loperamide concentration is possible with concurrent use.
- **Nonsteroidal Anti-Inflammatory Drugs (NSAIDs)** (eg, **carprofen, meloxicam**): Concurrent use with CBD oil for 4 weeks resulted in no apparent adverse effects or significant laboratory value changes in dogs.[1]
- **Opioids** (eg, **fentanyl, methadone, morphine, tramadol**): Increased risk for CNS depression
- **Phenobarbital:** A pharmacokinetic interaction was not observed in healthy dogs, but possible additive risk for CNS depression or hepatotoxicity.[40]
- **Propofol:** CBD use may increase propofol concentration.
- **Proton Pump Inhibitors** (eg, **omeprazole, pantoprazole**): Concurrent use may lead to increased CBD concentration.[13,37,38]
- **Rifampin:** May decrease CBD concentration[13,38,39]
- **Sildenafil**: CBD may increase sildenafil concentrations.
- **Theophylline/Aminophylline:** CBD may increase theophylline concentration.
- **Tricyclic Antidepressants (TCAs**; eg, **amitriptyline, clomipramine**): Concurrent use increased risk for cardiovascular effects (hypotension, tachycardia).[38]
- **Warfarin**: CBD may prolong prothrombin times and increase the risk for bleeding.

Laboratory Considerations

- Cannabidiol may cause a false-positive on **cannabis screening** tests, particularly if the product administered was a full- or mislabeled broad-spectrum product.

Dosages

NOTES:

1. Effective cannabidiol (CBD) dosages remain under investigation and are yet to be fully determined. The dosages listed below represent recommendations from peer-reviewed studies using products that contain <u>only</u> CBD and do not accurately reflect dosage recommended for full-spectrum products. Some clinicians recommend starting with lower dosages and slowly escalating to the dosages presented below.
2. In humans, dosage reductions of 50% and 80% are recommended for patients with moderate and severe hepatic impairment, respectively.[13] Until veterinary-specific information becomes available, it is suggested to reduce initial dosages in veterinary patients with hepatic impairment.
3. Be sure to fully understand and comply with local, state, or provincial regulations related to CBD. See ***Dosage Forms/Regulatory Status***.

DOGS:

Osteoarthritis (extra-label): 2 mg/kg PO, OTM every 12 hours[2]

Epilepsy (extra-label): 2.5 mg/kg PO every 12 hours in addition to current therapy. The authors hypothesize that a higher dosage may be more effective.[4]

Monitoring

- Clinical efficacy
- Liver enzymes (ALP, ALT) and bilirubin at baseline; at 1, 3, and 6 months after initiating therapy and then as clinically indicated during ongoing therapy[13]
- Adverse effects (eg, vomiting, salivation, sedation, ataxia)

Client Information

- Although there is limited information available, it appears cannabidiol (CBD) is well tolerated by dogs and cats.
- Giving CBD with food will increase the amount of medicine that is absorbed, but CBD can be given with or without food. It is important to give CBD the same way each time.
- If your animal vomits or acts sick after receiving the drug on an empty stomach, try giving the next dose with food or a small treat. If vomiting continues, contact your veterinarian.
- Information regarding the use of CBD in animals is continually emerging and other side effects may be discovered. Contact your veterinarian if you notice any unexplained side effects or abnormal behaviors in your animal.
- Do not give your animal a CBD product without first discussing it with your veterinarian. Some products contain ingredients other than CBD that could be harmful to your animal.

Chemistry/Synonyms

Cannabidiol (CBD) is a cannabinoid derived from the *Cannabis sativa L* plant that occurs as a white to pale yellow crystalline solid that is soluble in oils and organic solvents and is insoluble in water. The FDA-approved product (*Epidiolex*®) contains sesame seed oil and 7.9% (w/v) dehydrated alcohol.[13]

Cannabidiol may also be known as CBD or *Epidiolex*®.

Cannabis sativa L contains more than 100 cannabinoids, of which CBD and tetrahydrocannabinol (THC) are the most well-known but others may exert a pharmacologic effect. Hemp is distinguished from marijuana by THC concentration: Although hemp and marijuana can both be from the *Cannabis sativa L* plant, **hemp** contains not more than 0.3% THC (dry weight), whereas **marijuana** contains more than 0.3% THC.[41] That is, hemp and marijuana are varieties or cultivars of the same plant but differ in THC concentration. CBD may only be legally produced from hemp grown under the restrictions established by the 2018 Farm Bill.[41]

Storage/Stability

The product FDA-approved for human use (*Epidiolex*®) should be stored upright at 20°C to 25°C (68°F-77°F), with permitted excursions between 15°C to 30°C (59°F-86°F); keep the cap tightly closed.[13] Do not freeze. Use product within 12 weeks of opening. Unless otherwise instructed by the manufacturer, store other cannabidiol (CBD) products at room temperature in tightly closed containers.

Compatibility/Compounding Considerations

Many compounded formulations are available. It is recommended to request a certificate of analysis that demonstrates product potency and purity. A 3-fold difference in cannabidiol (CBD) concentration was discovered between batches of commercially supplied CBD in oil.[26]

Dosage Forms/Regulatory Status

Other than the product FDA-approved for human use (*Epidiolex®*), cannabidiol (CBD) products are compounded, and as such, product quality (eg, potency, purity, stability) is not overseen or enforced by the FDA. Considerations for selecting a product include:

1. Choose a product made from hemp, not marijuana. Legally, CBD oil products must be derived from hemp and must contain less than 0.3% tetrahydrocannabinol (THC). Because hemp contains minimal amounts of THC, using a product derived from hemp will limit the amount of THC present. Legally grown hemp is no longer a controlled substance under federal law, but it may be a controlled substance in individual states. See ***Chemistry/Synonyms*** for further information.
2. Request a certificate of analysis (COA). Reputable companies will provide a COA of their products stating CBD, THC, or other cannabinoid content. Some companies will also confirm the absence of other harmful toxins (eg, pesticides, microbes, residual solvents, heavy metals).
3. Using CBD in animals has not been approved by the FDA. State and local laws vary, and practitioners should consult independent legal counsel to determine their compliance obligations with respect to the veterinary use of CBD.

VETERINARY-LABELED PRODUCTS: NONE

The Association of Racing Commissioners International (ARCI) has designated CBD as a class 2 substance. Use of this drug may not be allowed in certain animal competitions. Check rules and regulations before entering in a competition while this medication is being administered. Contact local racing authorities for further guidance. See ***Appendix*** for more information.

HUMAN-LABELED PRODUCTS:

Cannabidiol Solution: 100 mg/mL in 60 mL or 100 mL bottles; *Epidiolex®*; (Rx)

References

For the complete list of references, see **wiley.com/go/budde/plumb**

Capromorelin

(***kap***-roe-moe-***rel***-in) *Elura®, Entyce®*

Appetite Stimulant

Prescriber Highlights

- FDA-approved to stimulate appetite in dogs, and for management of weight loss in cats with chronic kidney disease
- Ghrelin-receptor agonist that stimulates growth hormone release and causes the feeling of hunger
- Contraindications include hypersensitivity and acromegaly (hypersomatotropism) in cats.
- Use with caution in dogs and cats with hepatic dysfunction, in dogs with renal insufficiency, and in cats with cardiac disease or severe dehydration. Hyperglycemia has occurred in healthy cats given labeled doses of capromorelin; use in diabetic patients has not been evaluated and may not be appropriate.
- Adverse effects include vomiting, hypersalivation, hiding behavior (cats), diarrhea, and polydipsia; some cats have developed hypotension and bradycardia after administration.

Uses/Indications

Capromorelin is labeled for the stimulation of appetite in dogs and for the management of weight loss in cats with chronic kidney disease (CKD).

In preapproval studies, dogs given capromorelin for 4 to 7 days had an ≈60% increase in food consumption and ≈6% weight gain as compared with the baseline.[1] In a clinical field study, 68.6% of dogs receiving capromorelin experienced increased appetite based on owner observation as compared with 44.6% of dogs that received the vehicle control. In the same study, 76% of dogs receiving capromorelin gained weight (1.8% increase) as compared with 44.6% of dogs that received the control (0.1% increase).[2] A post-approval study demonstrated that healthy beagles treated with capromorelin had an average 60% increase in food consumption compared to an 11% decrease in placebo-treated dogs.[3]

In cats with CKD, field studies demonstrated a 3.3% increase in body weight after 2 weeks of treatment, and 5.2% increase after 8 weeks.[4] In healthy laboratory cats receiving capromorelin, food consumption increased by 25% to 45% and body weight increased by 4% to 6.6% as compared with an 11% food consumption increase and 1% decrease in body weight in cats receiving a placebo.[5,6] In a safety study, cats given capromorelin 6 mg/kg PO once daily for 91 days had a nonsignificant increase in food consumption but significant weight gain.[6] Further studies are warranted to establish efficacy.

Pharmacology/Actions

Capromorelin is a ghrelin-receptor agonist that stimulates growth hormone (GH) release and causes release of insulin-like growth factor 1 (IGF1). Serum GH and cortisol increased in healthy dogs given capromorelin for 7 days, and levels returned to baseline 8 hours after administration; the magnitude of GH and cortisol elevations were diminished by days 4 and 7 as compared with day 1. Increased IGF1 levels were sustained throughout the 7-day study period.[7] Sustained elevation of IGF1 was also noted in cats.[8]

Ghrelin appears to regulate cardiac, gastric, and pancreatic function and may result in anxiety. In mice, exogenous ghrelin accelerates gastric emptying and intestinal transit.[9] At the spinal cord level, capromorelin stimulates bladder emptying in mice[10] and colonic motility in rats.[11,12]

In addition to stimulating appetite and the effects described above in rats, ghrelin and ghrelin-receptor agonists have been shown to stimulate bone formation, increase muscle mass, and have anti-inflammatory and immunomodulatory effects.[13]

Pharmacokinetics

In dogs, ≈44% of an oral dose is absorbed[14] and peak levels are reached within 1 hour. Protein binding is ≈50%. Hepatic metabolism is primarily via cytochrome P450 3A4 isozyme (CYP3A4) and CYP3A5. Elimination half-life is ≈1.2 hours. Capromorelin (primarily as metabolites) is excreted in urine (≈37%) and feces (≈62%) within 72 hours of oral administration. Capromorelin does not accumulate with repeated administration.[1,15]

In fasted healthy cats, capromorelin peak concentration is reached within 0.25 to 1 hour after administration.[4] Giving with food delays time to peak concentration (0.5 to 4 hours) and reduces capromorelin peak concentration by ≈50% and exposure (AUC) by ≈40% compared to fasted cats.[4] Half-life in fasted cats is 1.1 hours.

Contraindications/Precautions/Warnings

Capromorelin is contraindicated in patients hypersensitive to it or its components. Avoid use in cats with acromegaly (hypersomatotropism). Caution should be used in dogs and cats with hepatic dysfunction, in dogs with renal insufficiency, and in cats with cardiac disease or severe dehydration. Although the manufacturer recommends using capromorelin with caution in dogs with renal insufficiency, cats with CKD enrolled in a pilot study gained weight and tolerated the drug.[16] Blood glucose may increase for several hours after administration to cats[4,17]; capromorelin use in diabetic or prediabetic cats has not been evaluated and may not be appropriate.

Drug interactions are possible in dogs concurrently treated with CYP3A4 and CYP3A5 inducers and inhibitors, but specific interactions have not been reported to date. See ***Drug Interactions***.

Adverse Effects

Adverse effects reported in dogs during clinical trials included diarrhea, vomiting, polydipsia, hypersalivation, flatulence, nausea, abdominal discomfort, increased gut sounds, and lethargy.[15] Elevated BUN and phosphorus have also been noted.

In cats with CKD (median age 15 years and 67% with Stage 2 CKD) receiving capromorelin 2 mg/kg/day, reported adverse effects included vomiting, hypersalivation, inappetence, hiding behavior, lethargy, anemia, dehydration, progression of CKD stage, diarrhea, upper respiratory infection, UTI, and hyperglycemia. Emesis, increased salivation, lip smacking, and head shaking reportedly occurred immediately after administration and resolved within a few minutes.[4,6,17] Clinical signs of bradycardia and hypotension may occur after administration, reaching peak effect after 1 hour, and resolving within 4 hours[4]; anecdotally, in some instances, hypotension may be profound enough to require fluid resuscitation. Hypotension appears to decrease in magnitude with repeated dosing. In healthy cats, insulin secretion and glycemic control decreased during the first several days of treatment; significance in diabetic patients has not been ascertained.[17]

Reproductive/Nursing Safety

The manufacturer recommends capromorelin not be used in breeding, pregnant, or lactating bitches or queens, as safety studies have not been performed for these animals.[4,15]

Overdose/Acute Toxicity

In safety studies in dogs, capromorelin (7 mg/kg/day and 40 mg/kg/day) was associated with increased salivation, red and swollen paws, increased liver weight, and hepatocellular vacuolation. In dogs receiving capromorelin at 17.5 times the label dose for up to 12 months, the drug was generally well tolerated and resulted in statistically insignificant decreased RBC count, hemoglobin, and hematocrit as compared with a placebo. Dose-related increased cholesterol and alkaline phosphatase were also noted.[7] Increased PR interval was noted on the ECG in dogs receiving either 7 mg/kg/day or 40 mg/kg/day; however, no evidence of cardiac toxicity was noted on physical examination or cardiac histopathology.[1]

Cats receiving capromorelin (6 mg/kg/day PO) for 91 days tolerated treatment well with no significant alterations in clinical pathology.[8] One cat receiving capromorelin 10.5 mg/kg/day as part of a safety study developed hyperglycemia and was euthanized after the onset of diabetic ketoacidosis.[4] Cats receiving capromorelin (up to 60 mg/kg/day PO) for 14 days experienced a greater frequency of emesis, hypersalivation, and lethargy as compared with the control group.[6]

For patients that have experienced or are suspected to have experienced an overdose, consultation with a 24-hour poison consultation center specializing in providing veterinary-specific information is recommended. For general information related to overdose and toxin exposures, as well as contact information for poison control centers, refer to ***Appendix***.

Drug Interactions

No drug interactions with capromorelin have been reported. Capromorelin is metabolized by CYP3A4 and CYP3A5 in dogs. In feline field studies, capromorelin was used concurrently with parenteral fluids, methimazole, amlodipine, antibiotics, laxatives, antiparasitics, and antiemetics.[18] The following drug interactions are theoretical in animals receiving capromorelin and may be of significance in veterinary patients. Unless otherwise noted, use together is not necessarily contraindicated, but the potential risks must be weighed, and additional monitoring performed when appropriate.

- **CYP3A4 Inhibitors** (eg, **amiodarone, cimetidine, diltiazem, erythromycin, itraconazole, ketoconazole**): May reduce capromorelin metabolism in dogs
- **CYP3A4 Inducers** (eg, **phenobarbital**, **rifampin**): May increase capromorelin metabolism in dogs

Laboratory Interactions

- None noted

Dosages

DOGS:

Appetite stimulation (label dosage; FDA-approved): 3 mg/kg PO once daily. **NOTE**: The effectiveness of capromorelin solution has not been evaluated beyond 4 days of treatment.[15]

CATS:

Management of weight loss in cats with chronic kidney disease (label dosage; FDA-approved): 2 mg/kg PO once daily 30 minutes before routine feeding.[4] Readminister the dose if the cat receives only a partial dose, or if the cat vomits within 15 minutes of administration.

Appetite stimulation (extra-label): 1 – 3 mg/kg PO once daily for up to 21 days[5]

Monitoring

- Food and fluid intake
- Body weight
- Adverse effects (eg, vomiting, diarrhea, inappetence, lethargy)
- Additional monitoring as applicable to address underlying condition(s)

Client Information

- Gently shake the bottle prior to withdrawing the appropriate amount of solution using the provided syringe (dog product only). Rinse syringe between treatment doses.
- Store medication out of reach of other pets and children.
- Drooling, vomiting, and head shaking may occur shortly after administration.
- Common side effects in dogs include vomiting and frequent urination. In cats, vomiting, hypersalivation, lack of appetite, hiding behavior, and lethargy have been noted.

- When giving this medicine to cats:
  a) Administer the dose 30 minutes prior to feeding.
  b) Only readminister if a partial dose is received, or if your cat vomits within 15 minutes.

Chemistry/Synonyms
Capromorelin is a growth hormone secretagogue-receptor agonist. The commercial oral solutions contain capromorelin tartrate. No solubility data was located.

Capromorelin is also known as AT-002, RQ-5, CP-424391, *Entyce*®, and *Elura*®.

Storage/Stability
Capromorelin should be stored at or below 30°C (86°F) and kept out of reach of children and pets.

Compatibility/Compounding Considerations
None noted

Dosage Forms/Regulatory Status
VETERINARY-LABELED PRODUCTS:

Capromorelin Flavored Solution: 30 mg/mL in 10 mL, 15 mL, and 30 mL bottles; *Entyce*®; (Rx). FDA-approved for use in dogs. NADA #141-457

Capromorelin Flavored Solution: 20 mg/mL in 15 mL bottles; *Elura*®; (Rx). FDA-approved for use in cats. NADA #141-536

HUMAN-LABELED PRODUCTS: NONE

References
For the complete list of references, see **wiley.com/go/budde/plumb**

Carbimazole
(kar-***bi***-ma-zole) *Vidalta*®

Antithyroid

Prescriber Highlights
- ► Prodrug of methimazole; used for treatment of feline hyperthyroidism
- ► Contraindications include hypersensitivity to carbimazole or methimazole and in cats with abnormal red or white blood cell counts, thrombocytopenia, coagulopathies, severe liver disease, diabetes mellitus, or with signs of autoimmune disease. Use with caution in cats with existing renal or hepatic disease.
- ► Most adverse effects occur within the first 3 months of treatment; vomiting, hyporexia, and lethargy are the most frequent. Eosinophilia, leukopenia, and lymphocytosis are usually transient. Rare but serious effects include self-induced excoriations, bleeding, hepatopathy, thrombocytopenia, agranulocytosis, immune-mediated hemolytic anemia, immune-mediated thrombocytopenia, and acquired myasthenia gravis.
- ► Dosing requirements may change with time.
- ► Typically administered PO; give with food. Do not crush or split tablets.
- ► The National Institute for Occupational Safety and Health (NIOSH) classifies methimazole (the active carbimazole metabolite) as a hazardous drug; use appropriate precautions when handling.

Uses/Indications
Carbimazole (a prodrug of methimazole) and methimazole are considered by most clinicians to be the agents of choice for treatment of feline hyperthyroidism and hyperthyroidism-associated clinical signs in cats.[1]

Pharmacology/Actions
Carbimazole is converted almost entirely to methimazole in vivo. Methimazole inhibits thyroid peroxidase and interferes with iodine incorporation into tyrosyl residues of thyroglobulin, thereby inhibiting thyroid hormone synthesis. It also inhibits iodinated tyrosyl residues from coupling to form iodothyronine. Methimazole has no effect on the release or activity of thyroid hormones already formed or in general circulation.

Pharmacokinetics
Carbimazole is rapidly absorbed from the GI tract and rapidly and nearly totally converted to methimazole.[1] Administering carbimazole with food increases bioavailability. Because of differences in molecular weight (carbimazole 5 mg vs methimazole 3 mg), to attain an equivalent serum concentration, the dose of carbimazole for oral administration must be ≈2 times that of methimazole.[2]

In cats, the volume of distribution of methimazole is variable (0.12 – 0.84 L/kg). Methimazole apparently concentrates in thyroid tissue and biologic effects persist beyond measurable blood concentrations. After oral dosing, plasma elimination half-life ranges from 2.3 to 10.2 hours. There is usually a 1- to 3-week lag time between starting the drug and significant reductions in serum T_4. Timed-release formulations of carbimazole can extend methimazole (active metabolite) half-life and allow once-daily dosing. Carbimazole may be amenable for use transdermally with twice-daily dosing in cats to control hyperthyroidism.

In dogs, methimazole has a serum half-life of 8 to 9 hours.

Contraindications/Precautions/Warnings
Carbimazole is contraindicated in patients that are hypersensitive to it or methimazole. It should not be used in patients with concurrent systemic diseases (eg, severe primary liver disease, diabetes mellitus[1]) or with hematologic abnormalities (eg, anemia, neutropenia, lymphopenia, thrombocytopenia), coagulopathies, or autoimmune disease.[1,3] Use with caution in cats with preexisting hepatic disease.

Because carbimazole is a prodrug and is converted into methimazole, cats that have had prior severe reactions to methimazole should not receive carbimazole.[1]

Treatment of hyperthyroid cats with methimazole can unmask underlying renal disease because lowering thyroid hormone levels decreases glomerular filtration rates.[4] As such, a cat's renal parameters should be monitored closely during treatment (see ***Monitoring***).[5] In a study, a significant reduction in serum creatinine was noted after restoration of euthyroidism in cats with iatrogenic hypothyroidism caused by methimazole or carbimazole.[6]

The prevalence of moderate to severe thyroid disease (eg, large thyroid tumors, multifocal disease, intrathoracic thyroid masses) increased with the duration of hyperthyroidism, despite ongoing methimazole use; the authors speculated that this finding may indicate a progressive nature of feline hyperthyroidism that is not stopped by maintaining euthyroidism with methimazole.[7]

The National Institute for Occupational Safety and Health (NIOSH) classifies methimazole (the active carbimazole metabolite) as a hazardous drug representing an occupational hazard to healthcare workers; wash hands after handling and use personal protective equipment (PPE) accordingly to minimize the risk for exposure.[8]

Consider writing part of the drug's name in uppercase letters (tall man designations) on prescriptions/orders to reduce the risk for errors. Do not confuse carbiMAZOLe with carbamazEPINE or CARBOplatin. Additionally, do not write prescriptions for this drug using the abbreviation SID. Many nonveterinary pharmacists are unfamiliar with this abbreviation and could interpret it as another abbreviation (eg, QID).

Adverse Effects
Most adverse effects associated with carbimazole or methimazole use in cats occur within the first 3 months of therapy.[9] In cats receiving carbimazole, vomiting, anorexia, and lethargy occur most frequent-

ly[1,10] (≈10%), are often transient, and can typically be managed with a dosage reduction.[11] Eosinophilia, leukopenia, and/or lymphocytosis may be noted in ≈5% of cats[12]; these hematologic effects are usually also transient and generally do not require drug withdrawal unless the blood dyscrasia is persistent or severe.[1]

Methimazole and carbimazole may also rarely cause self-induced excoriations and hepatopathy, and potentially trigger immune-mediated hemolytic anemia and immune-mediated thrombocytopenia in cats[1,9,13-15]; these more serious effects generally require withdrawal of the drug. In one study, increased antinuclear antibodies (ANA) were noted in ≈22% of all cats receiving methimazole, and in ≈50% of cats receiving methimazole for greater than 6 months, but none of the cats had signs of a lupus-like syndrome.[9] The occurrence of ANA is dose dependent,[16] and although elevated ANA have historically been viewed as an indication for dose reduction, this may not be necessary in the absence of clinical signs or other indications of autoimmune disease.[9] Rarely, cats treated with methimazole or carbimazole have developed acquired myasthenia gravis that requires drug withdrawal.[17,18] One case report indicated that a cat developed hypersensitivity vasculitis after receiving carbimazole.[19]

Potentially, treatment with methimazole or carbimazole could unmask underlying renal dysfunction in some cats.[20] The hyperthyroid state may increase GFR and, by treating the hyperthyroidism, this effect is abolished.

Reproductive/Nursing Safety

Carbimazole has been associated with teratogenic and embryotoxic effects in rats.[1] Do not use carbimazole in pregnant animals as it may also affect offspring thyroid development or function.

Methimazole enters milk and reaches concentrations higher than those found in maternal serum.[1] If treatment with carbimazole is necessary for nursing queens, switch to milk replacer for nursing animals.

Overdose/Acute Toxicity

Acute toxicity that may be seen with overdoses includes those effects listed in ***Adverse Effects***. Agranulocytosis, thrombocytopenia, autoimmune hemolytic anemia, GI bleeding (potentially with hematemesis), hepatitis, and nephritis are perhaps the most serious effects that may be seen.[1] Coat and skin abnormalities (erythema, alopecia) can also occur. Treatment of overdose/toxicity consists of following standard protocols for handling an oral ingestion (eg, empty stomach, administer charcoal if not contraindicated) and to treat supportively and based on clinical signs.

For patients that have experienced or are suspected to have experienced an overdose, consultation with a 24-hour poison consultation center specializing in providing veterinary-specific information is recommended. For general information related to overdose and toxin exposures, as well as contact information for poison control centers, refer to ***Appendix***.

Drug Interactions

The following drug interactions have either been reported or are theoretical in humans or animals receiving carbimazole or methimazole and may be of significance in veterinary patients. Unless otherwise noted, use together is not necessarily contraindicated, but veterinarians should weigh the potential risks and perform additional monitoring when appropriate.

- **ANTICOAGULANTS** (eg, **heparin, rivaroxaban**): Methimazole may potentiate anticoagulant activity.
- **BENZIMIDAZOLE ANTIPARASITICS** (eg, **albendazole, fenbendazole, thiabendazole**): Concurrent use with methimazole can reduce hepatic oxidation of benzimidazoles and increase blood levels of the parent drug or its metabolites.[1,16,21-23]
- **BETA-ADRENERGIC ANTAGONISTS** (eg, **atenolol, propranolol**): Beta-blocker dose may need to be decreased once the patient becomes euthyroid.[16]
- **CHLORAMPHENICOL:** Combination with carbimazole may increase the risk for myelosuppression
- **DIGOXIN**: Correction to euthyroidism reduces digoxin clearance,[16] resulting in increased digoxin exposure and risk for toxicity. A reduction in the digoxin dose may be needed when the patient becomes euthyroid.
- **DIPYRONE:** Combination with carbimazole may increase the risk for myelosuppression.
- **IODINE 131:** There was no difference in response to radioiodine based on when methimazole was discontinued relative to I^{131} administration.[24]
- **PHENOBARBITAL**: Concurrent use of phenobarbital may reduce the clinical effectiveness of carbimazole.
- **PREDNIS(OL)ONE:** A reduction in predniso(lo)ne dose may be needed when the patient becomes euthyroid.
- **THEOPHYLLINE**: Theophylline dose may need to be reduced once the patient becomes euthyroid.[16]
- **WARFARIN**: In humans with hyperthyroidism, the metabolism of vitamin K clotting factors is increased, resulting in increased sensitivity to oral anticoagulants.[25] By reducing the effects of hyperthyroidism, methimazole may decrease clotting factor metabolism, thus reducing the effects of warfarin. However, patients that are euthyroid on methimazole and receiving warfarin may develop hypoprothrombinemia if methimazole is stopped and they become thyrotoxic again. Methimazole also has antivitamin K activity, so anticoagulants may be potentiated by methimazole.[16] Recommendation: If methimazole and warfarin are used together, increased monitoring of anticoagulant effect is warranted.

Laboratory Considerations

- Methimazole and carbimazole may affect **serum fructosamine** levels in diabetic cats. Increased serum fructosamine after 6 weeks of treatment has been reported. It has been recommended that serum fructosamine not be used to initially diagnose or assess the adequacy of diabetic control in cats with concurrent hyperthyroidism until hyperthyroidism is controlled for at least 6 weeks.[26]
- **TECHNETIUM-99M PERTECHNETATE:** Carbimazole administration should be discontinued at least 2 weeks prior to thyroid scintigraphy, as it may interfere with accurate detection of ectopic thyroid tissue.[12,27,28]

Dosages

CATS:

Hyperthyroidism:

a) **Immediate-release tablets** (extra-label): Most dosage recommendations are initially 5 mg/cat (NOT mg/kg) PO every 8 to 12 hours.[10,12,15] Once a euthyroid state is established, the dosage amount or frequency is slowly decreased to the lowest effective dose. Most cats will require 2.5 – 5 mg/cat (NOT mg/kg) PO every 12 hours, but some cats can be controlled on once-daily dosing.[12,29]

b) **Sustained-release tablets** (extra-label): 15 mg/cat (NOT mg/kg) PO once daily at the same time each day.[1,30] 10 mg/cat (NOT mg/kg) PO once daily can be considered for cats with moderate hyperthyroidism (TT_4 between 50 and 100 nmol/L; 3.9 – 7.8 µg/dL). Adjust dosage within a range of 10 – 25 mg/cat/day (NOT mg/kg) in 5 mg increments depending on clinical signs and TT_4 (**NOTE**: Tablets cannot be split, so combinations of 10 mg and 15 mg tablets must be used). If cat requires doses less than 10 mg/day, use alternate-day dosing (eg, 10 – 15 mg/cat [NOT mg/kg] every other day), or consider different treatment.

Monitoring

During the first 3 months of therapy (baseline and after every 3 and 6 weeks of treatment or dosage change)[5,16]:

- Physical examination to include body weight, body condition score, heart rate, and fundic examination
- Blood pressure
- CBC (including platelet count)
- Serum chemistry profile
- Serum TT_4: Blood samples can be collected at any time (ie, do not need to be collected at a prescribed time after methimazole treatment).
- Serum fT_4: Note that this assay is not indicated as a sole monitoring parameter for hyperthyroidism.
- Serum TSH: May be useful to evaluate for iatrogenic hypothyroidism
- **NOTE:** Cats receiving higher dosages should be monitored more frequently.

After stabilization (at least 3 months of therapy)[16]:

- Body weight
- Blood pressure
- TT_4 at 3- to 6-month intervals
- Other diagnostic tests as indicated by adverse effects

Client Information

- Give this medicine with food. Do not crush or split tablets.
- For this medication to work, give it exactly as your veterinarian prescribed.
- This medicine will decrease excessive thyroid hormones but does not cure the condition. It may take several weeks before your cat shows improvement.
- While your cat is taking this medicine, your cat will require close monitoring with regular examinations by your veterinarian as well as blood tests. Do not miss these important follow-up visits.
- Treatment is long term, often for the remainder of your cat's life.
- Most side effects (including vomiting, decreased appetite, or low energy level occur in the first 3 months of therapy. If any of these side effects are seen, stop giving this medicine to your cat and contact your veterinarian before restarting this medicine.
- Serious side effects are rare. If your cat develops yellow skin, eyes, or gums (*jaundice*) or becomes intensely itchy, discontinue this medicine and contact your veterinarian immediately.
- Wash your hands with soap and water after handling the medicine (even if gloves are worn) or used litter.
- Pregnant women or women who may become pregnant, nursing mothers, or people with low thyroid hormones should avoid handling carbimazole. If this is not possible, wear disposable gloves while handling this medication and cat litter or bodily fluids (ie, feces, blood, saliva) of treated animals. Do not reuse gloves. Once used, the gloves should be thrown away in the trash.
- This medication is considered to be a hazardous drug as defined by the National Institute for Occupational Safety and Health (NIOSH). Talk with your veterinarian or pharmacist about the use of personal protective equipment when handling this medicine.

Chemistry/Synonyms

A thioimidazole-derivative antithyroid drug, carbimazole occurs as a white to creamy white powder with a characteristic odor. It is slightly soluble in water and soluble in alcohol.

Carbimazole may also be known as carbimazolum, *Basolest®*, *Camazol®*, *Carbimazole®*, *Carbazole®*, *Carbistad®*, *Cazole®*, *Neo Tomizol®*, *NeoMercazole®*, *Neo-Thyreostat®*, *Thyrostat®*, *Tyrazol®*, *Vidalta®*, or *Neo-morphazole®*.

Storage/Stability

Unless otherwise labeled, carbimazole tablets should be stored at room temperature (not above 77°F [25°C]) in tightly closed containers and protected from light.[1] Do not remove desiccants from manufacturer's bottle.

Compatibility/Compounding Considerations

No specific information was noted. Do not crush or break the prolonged-release tablets.[1]

Dosage Forms/Regulatory Status

VETERINARY-LABELED PRODUCTS: NONE IN THE UNITED STATES

In some countries: Carbimazole Oral Prolonged-Release Tablets: 10 mg and 15 mg; *Vidalta®*; (POM-V)

HUMAN-LABELED PRODUCTS:

There are no FDA-approved products in the United States; elsewhere it may be available as:

Carbimazole Oral Tablets: 5 mg, 10 mg, 15 mg, and 20 mg. Many trade names available outside the US; (POM)

References

For the complete list of references, see **wiley.com/go/budde/plumb**

Carboplatin

(***kar***-boe-pla-tin) *Paraplatin®*

Antineoplastic

Prescriber Highlights

- ▶ Platinum antineoplastic agent used for a variety of carcinomas and sarcomas. In general, less nephrotoxic and fewer GI adverse effects as compared to cisplatin.
- ▶ Unlike cisplatin, carboplatin may be used safely in cats.
- ▶ Contraindicated in patients with a history of hypersensitivity to carboplatin or other platinum agents, and with severe bone marrow depression. Use with caution in patients with hepatic or renal disease, or active infection.
- ▶ Primary adverse effects include bone marrow suppression (dose-limiting toxicity) and GI upset. Neutrophil nadir in dogs typically occurs around day 14 or 21 after administration.
- ▶ Embryotoxic, teratogenic
- ▶ The National Institute for Occupational Safety and Health (NIOSH) classifies carboplatin as a hazardous drug; use appropriate precautions when handling.

Uses/Indications

Carboplatin is a broad-spectrum antineoplastic agent used to treat a variety of neoplastic diseases, including carcinoma (squamous cell carcinoma, ovarian carcinoma, pulmonary carcinoma, nasal carcinoma, anal sac apocrine gland adenocarcinoma,[1] colonic adenocarcinoma, urinary tract carcinoma,[2] hepatocellular carcinoma, and thyroid adenocarcinoma), melanoma,[3] and sarcoma (osteosarcoma[4]).

Unlike cisplatin, systemic carboplatin appears to be safe and well-tolerated in cats.[5,6]

Intracavitary carboplatin may be used to treat carcinomatosis and other malignant effusions.[7] Interventional radiology techniques can be used to facilitate intra-arterial carboplatin administration for the treatment of lower urinary tract carcinoma.[8] Carboplatin may be considered for intralesional use in conditions such as equine sarcoids[9] and to treat adenocarcinoma in birds.[10,11] Carboplatin beads and poloxamer gel have also been used locally. They have been well tolerated in different species (equines, canines, and felines), though efficacy has not been thoroughly established.[12-14]

Carboplatin is a radiation sensitizing agent.[15] Small studies have shown the tolerability of carboplatin in combination with other chemotherapy agents, such as toceranib[16] or 5-fluorouracil[1716,17]; however, further studies are needed to determine the efficacy of these combinations.

Pharmacology/Actions

Carboplatin is an antineoplastic agent. Its chemical reactivity is nonspecific, but the primary cytotoxic effect is thought to be due to intra- and interstrand DNA cross-linking that causes single- and double-stranded DNA breakage, impairs DNA replication, RNA transcription, and protein synthesis, leading to cell death and inhibition of tumor growth.[18]

Acquired resistance to carboplatin has been reported and is thought to be due to several mechanisms.[19]

Pharmacokinetics

After IV administration, carboplatin is well distributed throughout the body and is not protein-bound.[18] The highest concentrations are found in the liver, kidney, skin, and neoplastic tissue. The metabolism and elimination of carboplatin are complex. After degradation into platinum and platinum-complexed compounds, they become highly protein-bound and are slowly eliminated by the kidneys. In dogs, almost ½ of the dose is excreted unchanged in the urine within 24 hours. After 72 hours, ≈70% of the platinum administered is secreted in the urine.

Contraindications/Precautions/Warnings

Carboplatin is contraindicated in patients hypersensitive to it or other platinum-containing compounds (eg, cisplatin). It is also contraindicated in patients with severe bone marrow suppression or significant bleeding. Bone marrow suppression is the dose-limiting toxicity of carboplatin.[18] Bone marrow suppression is dose-dependent, and blood counts should be monitored frequently during treatment. Patients with severe carboplatin-induced myelosuppression should be allowed to recover their blood cell counts before additional therapy.

Caution is advised in patients with active infections and preexisting renal or hepatic disease. The elimination of carboplatin is impaired in cats with renal insufficiency, which increases the risk for myelosuppression.

Do not confuse CARBOplatin with CISplatin. Consider using tall man lettering when writing orders or prescriptions. Carboplatin is considered a high alert medication (medication that requires special safeguards to reduce the risk for errors). Consider instituting practices such as redundant drug dosage and volume checking and special alert labels.[20]

Aluminum can react with carboplatin, causing precipitates and loss of potency. Thus, for the preparation or administration of carboplatin, needles or administration sets containing aluminum parts should NOT be used.[18]

The National Institute for Occupational Safety and Health (NIOSH) classifies carboplatin as a hazardous drug; personal protective equipment (PPE) should be used accordingly to minimize the risk for exposure.[21]

Adverse Effects

The dose-limiting toxicity of carboplatin in dogs and cats is bone marrow suppression, particularly neutropenia or thrombocytopenia. Bone marrow suppression is dose-dependent, and neutrophil and platelet nadirs most commonly occur on day 14 or day 21 after treatment.[5,22] Bone marrow suppression can also lead to secondary complications, such as infection and bleeding. In dogs, lithium carbonate did not prevent carboplatin-induced thrombocytopenia.[23]

In dogs, myelosuppression associated with carboplatin is related to patient body weight.[24] Dogs weighing less than 15 kg (33 lb) appear to be at a higher risk of developing myelosuppression after treatment with carboplatin. One study found that dogs weighing less than 10 kg (22 lb) were 3.5 times more likely to develop severe (grade 3 or 4) neutropenia and 2.5 times more likely to develop severe (grade 3 or 4) thrombocytopenia than dogs 10 kg (22 lb) or greater. Dogs weighing less than 15 kg (33 lb) were 3 times more likely to develop severe (grade 3 or 4) neutropenia than dogs weighing 15 kg (33 lb) or more.

Other than myelosuppression, most adverse effects in dogs and cats are GI-related and include vomiting, diarrhea, and inappetence.

GI effects usually occur 2 to 5 days after a dose. In general, carboplatin is associated with fewer adverse effects in dogs compared to cisplatin with reduced nephrotoxicity and vomiting.

One case of a dog developing a cutaneous delayed hypersensitivity reaction has been reported.[25] In humans, sterile hemorrhagic cystitis (SHC) is a rare adverse effect. One case of a dog developing SHC has been reported in the veterinary literature.[26] Although carboplatin is classified as an irritant rather than a vesicant, necrosis associated with extravasation and suspected cases of extravasation have been reported in dogs.

Hepatotoxicity (increased serum bilirubin and liver enzymes) is observed in about 15% of humans treated with carboplatin. Other potential adverse effects include nephrotoxicity, neuropathies, and ototoxicity. These adverse effects occur less frequently with carboplatin therapy than with cisplatin therapy. Anaphylactoid reactions have been reported rarely in humans who have received platinum-containing compounds (eg, cisplatin). Some dogs receiving chemotherapy will have minor hair coat changes (eg, shagginess, loss of luster). Breeds with continuously growing hair coats (eg, poodles, terriers, Afghan hounds, or old English sheepdogs) are more likely to experience significant alopecia.

Reproductive/Nursing Safety

For sexually intact patients, verify pregnancy status before administration. Carboplatin is fetotoxic and embryotoxic in rats. The risks of its use during pregnancy should be weighed with its potential benefits.

It is unknown whether carboplatin enters maternal milk. In humans, it is recommended to discontinue nursing if the mother is receiving the drug.

Overdose/Acute Toxicity

The intravenous LD_{50} in dogs and mice is 31.2 mg/kg and 89.36 mg/kg, respectively. Anticipated complications of overdose would be secondary to bone marrow suppression and hepatic toxicity.[18] If overdose is suspected, patients should be monitored for neurotoxicity, ototoxicity, hepatotoxicity, and nephrotoxicity. Treatment is supportive as there is no known antidote.

For patients that have experienced or are suspected of having experienced an overdose, consultation with a 24-hour poison consultation center specializing in providing veterinary-specific information is recommended. For general information on overdose and toxin exposures, as well as contact information for poison control centers, refer to ***Appendix.***

Drug Interactions

The following drug interactions have either been reported or are theoretical in humans or animals receiving carboplatin and may be of significance in veterinary patients. Unless otherwise noted, use together is not necessarily contraindicated, but veterinarians should weigh the potential risks and perform additional monitoring when appropriate.

- **AMINOGLYCOSIDES** (eg, **gentamicin**): Potential for increased risk of nephrotoxicity and ototoxicity
- **MYELOSUPPRESSIVE AGENTS** (eg, **antineoplastics, immunosuppressants, iron chelators**): Concurrent use with other bone marrow depressant medication may result in additive myelosuppression; avoid combination when possible.
- **NEPHROTOXIC AGENTS** (eg, **aminoglycosides**): Renal effects of nephrotoxic compounds may be potentiated by carboplatin.
- **RADIATION THERAPY**: Potential for increased hematologic toxicity
- **TIGILANOL TIGLATE:** The tigilanol tiglate administration proto-

col does not permit concurrent use of other antineoplastic drugs. Avoid combination.

- VACCINES (live and inactivated): Myelosuppressive drugs may diminish vaccine efficacy and enhance adverse effects of vaccines.

Laboratory Considerations

- None noted

Dosages

NOTES:

1. Because of the potential toxicity of this drug to patients, veterinary personnel, and clients, and because chemotherapy indications, treatment protocols, monitoring, and safety guidelines often change, the following dosages should be used only as a general guide. Consultation with a veterinary oncologist and referral to current veterinary oncology references[27-31] are strongly recommended.
2. Dosages are commonly listed as mg/m². Do not confuse with mg/kg dosages. See ***Appendix*** for a conversion table.
3. Do not confuse CISplatin and CARBOplatin dosages; CISplatin dosages are much lower.

The following is a usual dosage range for carboplatin and should be used only as a general guide (dosage may need adjustment in patients with reduced renal function or bone marrow suppression):

DOGS:

- **Chemotherapeutic agent** (extra-label): 250 – 300 mg/m² IV every 3 weeks. For dogs weighing 15 kg or less, consider lower doses, such as 240 mg/m² (or 10 mg/kg), due to increased risk of toxicity at typical starting doses.[24] Consider lower doses if using in combination with toceranib (*Palladia®*); one study found the maximum tolerated dose of carboplatin to be 200 mg/m² with this combination.[16]

CATS:

- **Chemotherapeutic agent** (extra-label): 240 – 260 mg/m² IV every 3 weeks.[5] Lower carboplatin doses of 180 – 200 mg/m² have also been reported.[5,6]

Monitoring

- Baseline CBC, serum chemistry profile, and urinalysis
- Frequency of hematologic monitoring depends on the protocol employed. Consultation with a veterinary oncologist is recommended.
- CBC 1, 2, and 3 weeks after the first treatment.
  a) If absolute neutrophil count is less than 1000/µL or platelet count is less than 50,000/µL at weeks 1 or 2, then reduce the next dosage by 10% to 20%. Be sure to recheck the CBC before the following treatment.
  b) If absolute neutrophil count is less than 2000/µL or platelet count is less than 75,000/µL the day of treatment, then delay scheduled treatment until blood cell counts have recovered, then either reduce dose by 10% to 20% or change to an every 4-week dosing interval).
  c) For subsequent treatments, a CBC is needed just before each treatment if the patient is stable and the dosage remains unchanged.
  - Chemistry panel every 3 months initially, then every 6 months once stable
  - Tumor measurement and radiography at least monthly (eg, every 4 to 6 weeks)

Client Information

- Carboplatin is a chemotherapy (cancer) drug. The drug and its byproducts can be hazardous to people and other animals that come in contact with it. The drug and its metabolites will stay in your pet's system for a few days after treatment. Therefore, on the day of and for a few days after treatment, wear disposable gloves to handle all bodily waste (urine, feces), blood, or vomit.
- If possible, keep treated dogs in a separate area of the yard, and use a separate litter box for cats. Clean up all pet waste right away whenever possible. Double bag waste, seal, and throw away in the regular trash. Completely change litter and disinfect litter box a few days after the dose was given.
- If any accidents occur in the house (vomit, urine, feces), absorb as much as possible with paper towels, double bag, and discard in the trash, then clean the area with a diluted bleach solution.
- Carboplatin may be toxic to the gastrointestinal tract and cause vomiting and gastrointestinal upset. Carboplatin may also cause changes in blood cell counts, which may cause an increased risk of bleeding, bruising, infection, lethargy, bloody diarrhea, and shortness of breath. Contact your veterinarian immediately if you notice these signs or if you have any other concerns.
- This medication is considered to be a hazardous drug as defined by the National Institute for Occupational Safety and Health (NIOSH). Talk with your veterinarian or pharmacist about the use of personal protective equipment when handling this medicine.

Chemistry/Synonyms

Carboplatin, like cisplatin, is a platinum-containing antineoplastic agent. It is supplied as a clear, odorless aqueous solution with a pH of 5 to 7. It has a solubility of 14 mg/mL in water and insoluble in ethanol, acetone, and dimethylacetamide.

Carboplatin may also be known as cis-Diammine-1,1-cyclobutanedicarboxylato-platinum; carboplatinum; CBDCA; JM-8; or NSC-241240. Many trade names are available.

Storage/Stability

Protect the solution for injection from light and store at 25°C (77°F); excursions permitted from 15°C to 30°C (59°F-86°F). Multidose vials maintain microbial, chemical, and physical stability for up to 14 days following multiple needle entries.[32] After dilution, the manufacturer recommends discarding unused portions after 8 hours.[33] However, other sources suggest discarding after 24 hours.[34]

Compatibility/Compounding Considerations

Compatibility is dependent upon factors such as pH, concentration, temperature, and diluent used. Consult specialized references or a hospital pharmacist for more specific information.

The commercially available solution can be infused directly (usually over 15 minutes) or further diluted to as low as 0.5 mg/mL. Carboplatin is **compatible** with 5% dextrose in water, 5% dextrose in sodium chloride (0.2%, 0.45%, or 0.9%), and normal saline for dilution. Carboplatin is **incompatible** for Y-site administration with amphotericin B, chlorpromazine, diazepam, lansoprazole, leucovorin calcium, phenytoin, procainamide, and thiopental. It is **compatible** for admixture with cisplatin, etoposide, floxuridine, ifosfamide, and paclitaxel.

Because aluminum can displace platinum from carboplatin, the solution should not be prepared, stored, or administered where aluminum-containing items can come into contact with the solution. Should carboplatin come into contact with aluminum, a black precipitate will form, and the product should not be used.

Carboplatin prepared in a proprietary liquid polymer delivery system steadily released platinum over the 28-day investigation period. The clinical efficacy of the compounded formulation was not assessed, but thrombocytopenia and neutropenia were noted.[35]

Intralesional carboplatin in poloxamer gel was reported in one case as an adjunct to surgery and systemic carboplatin therapy. Carboplatin 10 mg/mL injection was mixed with an equal volume of poloxamer 407 gel in a sterile environment ≈15 minutes before use. While efficacy was unclear, no adverse wound healing or myelosuppressive effects were observed as a result of the intralesional dose.[14]

Multiple studies have looked at carboplatin impregnated calcium sulfate hemihydrate beads with variable results. Overall, CSH appears to be an effective carrier for carboplatin in vitro, and beads appear well-tolerated in vivo. However, caution is required regarding its use due to variability in compounded formulations and hazards associated with compounding.[12,36,37]

Dosage Forms/Regulatory Status

VETERINARY-LABELED PRODUCTS: NONE

HUMAN-LABELED PRODUCTS:

Carboplatin Injection: 10 mg/mL in 5 mL, 15 mL, 45 mL, 60 mL, and 100 mL multi-dose vials; generic; (Rx)

References

For the complete list of references, see **wiley.com/go/budde/plumb**

Carnitine

Levocarnitine

(***kar***-ni-teen) *Carnitor*®

Nutrient

Prescriber Highlights

- ► Nutrient required for normal fat utilization and energy metabolism
- ► May be useful as adjunctive therapy in dogs for cysteine or urate urolithiasis and cardiomyopathies (eg, dilated cardiomyopathy, doxorubicin induced); in cats, as adjunctive therapy for feline hepatic lipidosis
- ► Use only L (levo-) forms.
- ► Preferably give with meals

Uses/Indications

Levocarnitine may be useful as adjunctive therapy for dogs with cysteine or urate urolithiasis and dilated cardiomyopathy (DCM); however, only ≈5% with dilated cardiomyopathy respond to supplementation. It may also protect against doxorubicin-induced cardiomyopathy. It may also be beneficial in the adjunctive treatment of valproic acid toxicity.

In cats, levocarnitine has been recommended as a useful adjunctive therapy in feline hepatic lipidosis by facilitating hepatic lipid metabolism, but its use for this indication is somewhat controversial.

Pharmacology/Actions

Levocarnitine is an endogenous substance; it is required for normal fat utilization and energy metabolism in mammalian species. It serves to facilitate entry of long-chain fatty acids into cellular mitochondria, where they can be used during oxidation for energy production. Cardiac and skeletal muscle are significant sites for levocarnitine storage and activity.

Severe chronic deficiency is generally a result of an inborn genetic defect where levocarnitine utilization is impaired and not the result of dietary insufficiency. Effects seen in levocarnitine deficiency may include hypoglycemia, progressive myasthenia, hepatomegaly, DCM, hepatic coma, neurologic disturbances, encephalopathy, hypotonia, and lethargy.

D-carnitine lacks biologic activity, and competitively inhibits levocarnitine (L-carnitine) function.

Pharmacokinetics

In humans, levocarnitine is rapidly absorbed via the GI tract via passive and active mechanisms with a bioavailability of about 15%.[1,2] Half-life is ≈17 hours. Exogenously administered levocarnitine is eliminated primarily in the urine.

Contraindications/Precautions/Warnings

There are no known contraindications to levocarnitine use.

Products not specifically labeled as "levocarnitine" may contain D-carnitine, and should be avoided (see ***Pharmacology/Actions***).

In humans with severely compromised renal function, chronic administration of large doses of oral levocarnitine may result in accumulation or potentially toxic metabolites; the significance of this finding for veterinary patients is uncertain.[1]

Do not confuse levoCARNitine with levetiracetam.

Adverse Effects

Adverse effect profile is minimal. GI upset (eg, nausea, vomiting, diarrhea) is the most likely effect that may be noted and is usually associated with high doses.[3] Human patients have reported increased body odor while taking supplemental carnitine.

Reproductive/Nursing Safety

Studies done in rats and rabbits have demonstrated no teratogenic effects. It is generally believed that levocarnitine is safe for use in pregnancy though documented safety during pregnancy has not been established. Levocarnitine is distributed in milk.

Because safety has not been established in animals, this drug should only be used when the maternal benefits outweigh the potential risks to offspring.

Overdose/Acute Toxicity

Levocarnitine is a relatively safe drug; the LD_{50} in rats is 5.4 g/kg IV and in mice is 19.2 g/kg PO. In humans, there are no reports of toxicity following overdose, although diarrhea may occur with large doses.[1]

For patients that have experienced or are suspected to have experienced an overdose, consultation with a 24-hour poison consultation center specializing in providing veterinary-specific information is recommended. For general information related to overdose and toxin exposures, as well as contact information for poison control centers, refer to ***Appendix***.

Drug Interactions

The following drug interactions either have been reported or are theoretical in humans or animals receiving levocarnitine and may be of significance in veterinary patients. Unless otherwise noted, use together is not necessarily contraindicated, but weigh the potential risks and perform additional monitoring when appropriate.

- **VALPROIC ACID:** Patients receiving valproic acid may require higher dosages of levocarnitine.

Dosages

DOGS:

Myocardial carnitine deficiency associated with dilated cardiomyopathy (extra-label):

a) 100 – 200 mg/kg PO every 8 to 12 hours[3]; response to treatment may require 2 to 4 months

b) Adjunctive treatment of American cocker spaniels with dilated cardiomyopathy: carnitine 1 g with taurine 500 mg PO 2 to 3 times daily[4,5]

Systemic carnitine deficiency (extra-label): 50 – 100 mg/kg PO every 8 hours[3,6,7]

CATS:

Adjunctive therapy for severe hepatic lipidosis (extra-label): 250 – 500 mg/cat (NOT mg/kg) PO per day[8-10]

Monitoring

- Depends on indication for use; examples include:
    a) DCM: resting respiratory rate, echocardiographic measurements to monitor myocardial function, body weight
    b) Hepatic lipidosis: baseline and periodic serum liver chemistry panels, appetite, body weight
- Adverse effects (eg, diarrhea)
- Baseline and periodic plasma carnitine concentrations

Client Information

- This medicine usually causes no side effects but vomiting or diarrhea can occur with larger doses. Giving this medicine with food may help with these side effects.
- If using a powder form of this medicine, mix it into your animal's food as directed by your veterinarian.
- Do NOT use any carnitine product that contains D-carnitine; use only L-carnitine.
- Most dogs that respond to carnitine therapy for dilated cardiomyopathy will require other medication to control their condition.

Chemistry/Synonyms

Levocarnitine (the L-isomer of carnitine) is an amino acid derivative, synthesized in vivo from methionine and lysine. It occurs as a white hygroscopic crystalline powder that is soluble in water and insoluble in acetone.

Carnitine may also be known as vitamin B_T, L-carnitine, or levocarnitinum; many trade names are available.

Storage/Stability

Levocarnitine formulations should be stored at room temperature 20°C to 25°C (68°F-77°F).

Compatibility/Compounding Considerations

No specific information noted

Dosage Forms/Regulatory Status

VETERINARY-LABELED PRODUCTS: NONE

HUMAN-LABELED PRODUCTS:

Levocarnitine Oral Tablets: 330 mg and 500 mg; *Carnitor*®, generic; (Rx and OTC)

Levocarnitine or L-Carnitine Oral Capsules: 250 mg, 300 mg, and 400 mg; generic; (OTC)

Levocarnitine Oral Solution: 100 mg/mL in 118 mL; *Carnitor*®, generic; (Rx – regular and sugar free [saccharin] available)

NOTE: L-carnitine may also be available in bulk powder form or other capsule strengths from local health food stores. Check labels to ensure products do not contain D-Carnitine (see ***Pharmacology/Actions***).

References

For the complete list of references, see **wiley.com/go/budde/plumb**

Carprofen

(kar-***pro***-fen) *Rimadyl*®, *Carprieve*®, *Carprovet*®, *Norocarp*®, *Novox*®, *quellin*®, *Rovera*®, *Vetprofen*®

Nonsteroidal Anti-inflammatory Drug (NSAID)

Prescriber Highlights

- ▶ NSAID used in a variety of domestic animal species
- ▶ Contraindications include use in dogs with bleeding disorders (eg, Von Willebrand disease) or dogs with a history of serious reactions to it or other propionic-class NSAIDs.
- ▶ Caution advised in geriatric patients or those with preexisting chronic diseases (eg, inflammatory bowel disease, renal or hepatic insufficiency) or taking certain medications (eg, corticosteroids, nephrotoxic agents)
- ▶ Mild GI effects (eg, vomiting, diarrhea, constipation, inappetence) and/or lethargy are the most common adverse effects, but incidence is low (less than 2%).
- ▶ Rare cause of idiosyncratic hepatic failure; liver enzymes should be monitored

Uses/Indications

Carprofen is labeled for the pain and inflammation associated with osteoarthritis and for control of postoperative pain associated with soft tissue and orthopedic surgeries in dogs.[1] An evaluation of the scientific literature concluded that there is evidence to support the clinical benefit of longer-term (more than 28 days) NSAID use with a low risk for serious adverse effects in dogs with chronic osteoarthritis,[2] although others note that most studies of NSAIDs were conducted in nongeriatric, healthy dogs.[3] Carprofen injection prior to surgery has a sevoflurane minimum alveolar concentration (MAC)-sparing effect.[4] Carprofen has demonstrated a survival benefit in dogs with prostatic carcinoma.[5]

Carprofen may also be of benefit in other species. Outside the United States, carprofen is registered for use in horses, cattle, and cats. Little data exist to support safe use of carprofen beyond short-term administration in cats, and adverse GI effects (eg, vomiting) have been reported in cats given more than a single dose.

Pharmacology/Actions

Like other NSAIDs, carprofen can exhibit analgesic, anti-inflammatory, and antipyretic activity, most likely through inhibition of cyclooxygenase, phospholipase A_2, and prostaglandin synthesis. However, its relatively weak inhibition of prostaglandin synthesis suggests that other mechanisms may also be responsible for carprofen's pharmacologic effects.[6] Carprofen appears to be more sparing of COX-1 in vitro and, in dogs, appears to have fewer COX-1 effects (eg, GI ulceration, platelet inhibition, renal damage) as compared with older non-COX–2 specific agents. The specificity of carprofen's COX-2 effects appears to be species-, dose-, and tissue-dependent. Carprofen use in horses and cats does not appear to be as COX-2 specific as it is when used in dogs.

Pharmacokinetics

When administered orally to dogs, carprofen is rapidly absorbed and has over 90% bioavailability. Peak serum concentrations occur 1 to 3 hours after oral administration. Subcutaneous administration delays the rate of absorption but results in comparable total drug absorption within 12 hours. The drug is highly bound to plasma proteins (99%) and has a low volume of distribution (0.12 to 0.22 L/kg). Carprofen is extensively metabolized in the liver, primarily via glucuronidation and oxidative processes. Approximately 70% to 80% of a dose is eliminated in feces and 10% to 20% is eliminated in urine. Some enterohepatic recycling of the drug occurs.

In dogs, the elimination half-life of carprofen is ≈8 hours, with the S form having a longer half-life than the R form.[1]

In cats, the average half-life of carprofen is 20 hours; however, there is a high degree of interpatient variability (9 to 49 hours). Half-life is not necessarily a good predictor of duration of effect, as the drug's high affinity for tissue proteins may act as a reservoir for the drug in inflamed tissues. However, one study showed that although the terminal half-life was longer in interstitial fluid than in plasma, there was no difference between unbound drug concentrations in inflamed versus control interstitial fluid.[7]

In horses, bioavailability following oral administration is 75% to 100%. Plasma protein binding is high (99%). Following intramuscular injection, half-life ranges from 23 to 43 hours.[8]

In adult cattle, the half-life is ≈30 to 65 hours.[9,10] In calves younger than 10 weeks, the half-life is ≈43 hours.[11]

Contraindications/Precautions/Warnings

In healthy dogs, carprofen has minor effects on bleeding times and platelet aggregation but remains contraindicated in dogs with bleeding disorders (eg, Von Willebrand disease, thrombocytopenia) due to increased risk for impaired hemostasis. Carprofen is also contraindicated in animals with prior serious reactions to it or other propionic-class anti-inflammatory agents (eg, ketoprofen, naproxen, ibuprofen). It should be used with caution in geriatric animals or those with preexisting conditions and diseases (eg, GI ulceration, dehydration, hypoproteinemia, cardiovascular disease, inflammatory bowel disease, renal or hepatic insufficiency). Using parenteral fluids during general anesthesia should be considered to decrease the risk for NSAID-induced perioperative renal injury. Carprofen use inhibited bone healing in healthy dogs that received the drug for 120 days following tibial osteotomy.[12]

The manufacturer states that the safe use of carprofen in dogs younger than 6 weeks has not been established.

Adverse Effects

Adverse effects are uncommon with carprofen use in dogs; mild GI effects (eg, vomiting, diarrhea, constipation, inappetence) and/or lethargy are most common, but incidence is low (less than 2%). Subclinical GI erosions have been demonstrated in dogs receiving carprofen chronically.[13,14] Development of hepatocellular damage and/or renal disease is a rare but serious possibility. Preexisting renal insufficiency, dehydration, and sodium depletion can increase the risk for renal toxicity. Other reported adverse effects include neurologic (eg, ataxia, paresis, paralysis, seizures, vestibular signs, disorientation), behavior (eg, sedation, lethargy, hyperactivity, restlessness, aggression), hematologic (eg, immune-mediated hemolytic anemia and thrombocytopenia, blood-loss anemia, epistaxis), dermatologic (eg, pruritus, alopecia, moist dermatitis, panniculitis, vasculitis, ventral ecchymosis), hypersensitivity (eg, facial swelling, hives, erythema), and serious GI effects (eg, ulceration, pancreatitis). Swelling and warmth at injection sites may be noted.

The reported incidence of hepatopathy is ≈0.05% or less in dogs. Geriatric dogs or dogs with chronic diseases (eg, inflammatory bowel disease, renal or hepatic insufficiency) may be at greater risk for development of hepatotoxicity while receiving this drug, but the effect may be idiosyncratic and unpredictable. Labrador retrievers have been associated with ≈25% of the initially reported cases of hepatic syndrome; however, Labrador retrievers are most commonly treated with this drug, and it is not believed that this breed has a greater chance to develop this hepatic syndrome. Pretreatment patient evaluation, as well as discussion with the owner regarding the potential risks versus benefits of therapy, is advised before therapy is initiated. There are rare case reports of neutrophilic dermatosis (ie, Sweet's syndrome).[15,16]

Carprofen has been used in cats, but, because cats have limited ability to glucuronidate, there is a greater potential for drug accumulation with resultant adverse effects. In particular, cats appear to be more susceptible for development of renal adverse effects from NSAIDs. Prolonged administration of carprofen in cats has also caused adverse GI effects. Development of hepatotoxicity does not appear to be a significant concern with NSAID use in cats, possibly because cats do not form significant amounts of glucuronidated metabolites.

Reproductive/Nursing Safety

The manufacturer states that safe use of carprofen in pregnant dogs, dogs used for breeding purposes, or lactating bitches has not been established. Carprofen (up to 20 mg/kg) has been given to pregnant rats during days 7 to 15 of gestation. Although no teratogenic effects were noted in pups, the drug did delay parturition, and there was an increased number of dead pups at birth.

Carprofen given 1 hour after parturition to first-lactation cows increased milk yield during the 305-day lactation period, increased pregnancy rates, and reduced calving interval and somatic counts.[17]

Because safety has not been established in animals, this drug should only be used when the maternal benefits outweigh the potential risks to offspring.

Overdose/Acute Toxicity

In toxicologic studies on dogs, repeated administration of up to 10 times the recommended dose resulted in few adverse effects. Some dogs exhibited hypoalbuminemia, melena, or slight increases in ALT. However, postmarketing surveillance suggests there may have been significant interpatient variability in response to acute or chronic overdoses. According to the ASPCA Animal Poison Control Center (APCC) database, vomiting has been reported after administration of a dose as low as 5.3 mg/kg in dogs and 3.9 mg/kg in cats. Based on reports to the APCC from 2009 to 2013, clinical signs in dogs or cats may include vomiting, lethargy, diarrhea, anorexia, elevated liver enzymes, and azotemia. The APCC level of concern for renal damage is 50 mg/kg in dogs and 8 mg/kg in cats.

This drug is an NSAID, and an overdose can lead to GI and renal effects. Decontamination with emetics and/or activated charcoal is appropriate. For toxic doses in which GI effects are expected, the use of GI protectants is warranted. If renal effects are also expected, fluid diuresis is warranted. Therapeutic plasma exchange may be beneficial.[18] IV lipid emulsion therapy was successfully used to manage caprofen toxicity in a cat.[19]

For patients that have experienced or are suspected to have experienced an overdose, consultation with a 24-hour poison consultation center specializing in providing veterinary-specific information is recommended. For general information related to overdose and toxin exposures, as well as contact information for poison control centers, refer to ***Appendix***.

Drug Interactions

NOTE: Although the manufacturer does not list any specific drug interactions in the package insert, it cautions against concomitant carprofen use with other ulcerogenic drugs (eg, **corticosteroids**, other **NSAIDs**) unless the animal is closely monitored for adverse effects. Although a multiday washout period may be appropriate when switching from one NSAID to another, there does not appear to be any credible evidence to support this (except with ***Aspirin***).

The following drug interactions have either been reported or are theoretical in humans or animals receiving NSAIDS, including carprofen, and may be of significance in veterinary patients. Unless otherwise noted, use together is not necessarily contraindicated, but the potential risks must be weighed and additional monitoring performed when appropriate.

- **Anticoagulants** (eg, **coumarin** or **indanedione derivatives, heparin,** or **thrombolytic agents**): NSAID-induced inhibition of platelet aggregation and GI ulceration may be hazardous in animals receiving anticoagulant or thrombolytic therapy.

- **ACE Inhibitors** (eg, **benazepril, enalapril**): ACE inhibitors act through the effects of vasodilatory prostaglandins on renal function, so NSAIDs may decrease their effectiveness; however, one study in dogs receiving tepoxalin (an NSAID) did not show any adverse effects. It is unknown what effects, if any, occur if other NSAIDs and ACE inhibitors are used together in dogs.
- **Aspirin** or **Other NSAIDS**: Concurrent administration with carprofen may increase the risk for toxicity (eg, GI ulceration). Animals receiving aspirin therapy that will be replaced with a COX-2 NSAID should undergo a washout period of 3 to 10 days between stopping aspirin and starting the NSAID.[20]
- **Corticosteroids**: Concomitant administration with NSAIDs may increase the risk for GI adverse effects.
- **Cyclosporine** or **Other Nephrotoxic Medications**: The risk for drug-induced nephrotoxicity may be increased when NSAIDs and other nephrotoxic medications are coadministered, in part because NSAIDs can increase the plasma concentrations of nephrotoxic drugs through inhibition of renal prostaglandin.
- **Dacarbazine; Dactinomycin**: Concurrent use with NSAIDs may increase risk for bleeding.
- **Desmopressin**: Concurrent use may increase risk for water intoxication and/or hyponatremia. Electrolytes and renal function should be monitored.
- **Digoxin**: Carprofen may increase serum concentrations of digoxin; caution is advised in patients with severe cardiac failure.
- **Dinoprost**: NSAIDs may inhibit prostaglandin synthesis.
- **Highly Protein Bound Drugs** (eg, **phenytoin, valproic acid, oral anticoagulants, other anti-inflammatory agents, salicylates, sulfonamides, sulfonylurea antidiabetic agents**): Because carprofen is highly bound to plasma proteins (99%), it could potentially displace other highly bound drugs; increased serum concentrations may occur. Although these interactions are typically not a clinical concern, caution is advised when these drugs are used together. Cefovecin does not significantly affect the pharmacokinetics of the active S(+) enantiomer of carprofen.[21]
- **Insulin** or **Oral Antidiabetic Agents**: The hypoglycemic effects of insulin and antidiabetic agents may be increased by NSAIDs because prostaglandins contribute to regulation of glucose metabolism.
- **Loop Diuretics** (eg, **furosemide**): Carprofen may reduce the diuretic, saluretic, and antihypertensive effects by inhibiting prostaglandin synthesis. Concurrent use of NSAIDs and diuretics may increase the risk for renal insufficiency secondary to decreased renal blood flow. In dogs, glomerular filtration rate has been shown to decrease after 8 days of concurrent use.[22]
- **Methotrexate**: NSAIDs may cause increased and prolonged methotrexate plasma concentrations due to decreased protein binding and/or renal excretion. Serious toxicity has occurred when NSAIDs have been used concomitantly with methotrexate; extreme caution is advised when these drugs are used together, especially during high-dose methotrexate infusion therapy.
- **Nonsteroidal Anti-Inflammatory Drugs (NSAIDs), Other**: Concomitant administration with other NSAIDs should be avoided.
- **Selective Serotonin Reuptake Inhibitors** (SSRIs; eg, **fluoxetine**): Concurrent use of this drug class may increase antiplatelet effects of NSAIDs.
- **Tricyclic Antidepressants** (eg, **clomipramine**): Concurrent use of this drug class may increase antiplatelet effects of NSAIDs.

Laboratory Considerations

- In dogs, carprofen may slightly lower **Free T_4, Total T_4,** and **TSH** concentrations.
- Increases in liver enzyme values, including **ALP, ALT, lactate dehydrogenase (LDH), and other transaminases**, may be detected. Concurrent administration of phenobarbital, rifampin, or other hepatic enzyme-inducing agents may also elevate liver enzymes and interfere with interpretation of these tests.
- Prolonged bleeding times
- Decreased **hematocrit** or **hemoglobin** due to GI bleeding, microbleeding, and/or hemodilution caused by fluid retention
- **Leukocyte and platelet count** may be decreased.
- Serum **potassium** concentrations may be increased.
- NSAIDs may decrease renal function, which will be reflected in renal function tests (eg, increased serum **creatinine** coupled with consistently lowered **urine specific gravity**).

Dosages

DOGS:

Anti-inflammatory and analgesic (label dose): 4.4 mg/kg PO once daily, or divided and given as 2.2 mg/kg PO twice daily. Dose should be rounded down to the nearest half-caplet increment. For postoperative pain, carprofen should be administered at 4.4 mg/kg SC ≈2 hours before the procedure.[1]

CATS:

Anti-inflammatory and analgesic:

Warning: Extreme caution is advised, particularly with continued administration. All dosages listed are extra-label in the United States.

a) 4 mg/kg SC or IV once for treatment of postoperative pain; best given preoperatively at the time of induction of anesthesia[23]
b) 12.5 mg/cat (adult) (NOT mg/kg) PO or SC once weekly[24]

HORSES: (NOTE: ARCI UCGFS CLASS 4 DRUG)

Anti-inflammatory and analgesic (extra-label): 0.7 mg/kg IV once; dose may be repeated every 24 hours up to a total of 5 days.[25]

CATTLE:

Reduce pyrexia or clinical signs in acute infectious respiratory disease and acute mastitis (extra-label in United States): 1.4 mg/kg IV or SC once[26]

SHEEP:

Anti-inflammatory and analgesic agent (extra-label): 8 mg/kg PO once daily (every 24 hours)[27]

FERRETS:

Anti-inflammatory and analgesic (extra-label): 1 – 4 mg/kg SC every 12 to 24 hours; 4 mg/kg PO once daily (every 24 hours)

RABBITS/RODENTS/SMALL MAMMALS:

Anti-inflammatory and analgesic (all are extra-label):

a) **Rabbits**: 2 – 4 mg/kg PO every 12 to 24 hours; 4 mg/kg SC[28]
b) **Rats/mice**: 5 mg/kg SC every 12 to 24 hours[29]
c) **Guinea pigs/chinchillas**: 4 mg/kg SC every 12 to 24 hours[29]

BIRDS:

Anti-inflammatory and analgesic (all are extra-label):

a) 2 mg/kg PO every 8 to 24 hours[30]
b) 1 mg/kg SC; single-dose study demonstrated increased walking ability in lame chickens.[31]
c) 1 – 4 mg/kg IM, IV, PO[32]

REPTILES:

Anti-inflammatory (extra-label): 1 – 4 mg/kg IV, IM, SC, PO every 24 to 72 hours[32]

Monitoring

- Baseline parameters should be established before therapy is started, especially in geriatric dogs, in dogs with chronic diseases, or when prolonged treatment is likely. Physical examination, CBC, serum chemistry profile (including liver and renal parameters), and urinalysis should be evaluated. Liver enzymes should be reassessed 2 to 4 weeks after starting carprofen therapy and at 3- to 6-month intervals. Carprofen should be discontinued if problems arise.
- Clinical efficacy
- Signs of potential adverse effects include: inappetence, diarrhea, vomiting, melena, polyuria, polydipsia, anemia, jaundice, lethargy, behavior changes, ataxia, and seizures.
- Chronic therapy: Clinicians should consider repeating CBC, urinalysis, and serum chemistry profiles as needed.

Client Information

- Read and understand the client information sheet provided with this medication; contact your veterinarian with any questions or concerns.
- May be given with or without food, but food may reduce the chances for stomach problems.
- Most dogs tolerate carprofen well, but rarely some dogs can develop ulcers or serious kidney and liver problems. Watch for changes in bowel movements, behavior or activity level (ie, more or less active than normal), and/or drinking (ie, frequency, amount consumed) or urination (ie, frequency, color, or smell) habits; signs of decreased appetite, vomiting, muscle weakness (eg, stumbling, clumsiness), seizures (ie, convulsions) or aggression; and yellowing of gums, skin, or whites of the eyes (jaundice).
- Store flavored, chewable tablets out of reach of animals and children to avoid accidental ingestion.
- Periodic laboratory tests are recommended to check liver and kidney function. Do not miss these important follow-up visits.

Chemistry/Synonyms

Carprofen, a propionic acid derivative nonsteroidal anti-inflammatory agent, occurs as a white crystalline compound. It is practically insoluble in water and freely soluble in ethanol at room temperature. Carprofen has an S(+) enantiomer and R(-) enantiomer. The commercial product contains a racemic mixture of both. The S(+) enantiomer has greater anti-inflammatory potency than the R(-) form.

Carprofen may also be known as C-5720, Ro-20-5720/000, *Rimadyl*®, *Carprovet*®, *Vetprofen*®, *Zinecarp*®, *Canidryl*®, *Novox*®, *Aventicarp*®, *Rycarfa*®, *Rimifin*®, *Carpox*®, *Prolet*®, *Tergive*®, *Carprodyl*®, or *Norocarp*®.

Storage/Stability

Store the commercially available caplets or chewable tablets at room temperature (15°C-30°C [59°F-86°F]).

Store the commercially available injection (in the United States) in the refrigerator (2°C-8°C [36°F-46°F]). Once broached, store the injection at temperatures up to 25°C (77°F) for 28 days.

Compatibility/Compounding Considerations

Compounded preparation stability: Carprofen oral suspension compounded from commercially available tablets has been published.[33] In adaptation of that work, triturating 1 carprofen 100 mg tablet with 10 mL of *Ora-Plus*® and *qs* ad to 20 mL with *Ora-Sweet*® will yield a 5 mg/mL suspension that retains 90% potency for 21 days stored at both 5°C (41°F) and 25°C (77°F). Compounded preparations of carprofen should be protected from light.

A 1:10 dilution of carprofen injection with sterile water maintained potency for over 28 days when stored at room temperature or refrigerated; no bacterial contamination or endotoxin was detected.[34]

Dosage Forms/Regulatory Status

VETERINARY-LABELED PRODUCTS:

Carprofen Scored Caplets: 25 mg, 75 mg, and 100 mg; *Rimadyl*® *Caplets*, *Novox*®, *Carprieve*®, *Rovera*®, *Norocarp*®, generic; (Rx). FDA-approved for use in dogs

Carprofen Flavored Tablets: 25 mg, 75 mg, and 100 mg: *Carprovet*®, *Truprofen*®, *Vetprofen*® (Rx). FDA-approved for use in dogs

Carprofen Chewable Tablets: 25 mg, 75 mg, and 100 mg; *quellin*® (soft chewable; scored), *Rimadyl*®, *Carprieve*®, *Novox*®, *Truprofen*®, generic; (Rx). FDA-approved for use in dogs

Carprofen Sterile Injectable Solution: 50 mg/mL in 20 mL multidose vials; *Rimadyl*®; generic; (Rx). FDA-approved for use in dogs

Outside the United States, carprofen injection is labeled for use in dogs, cats, cattle (slaughter withdrawal, 21 days; milk withdrawal, 0 hours), and in horses not intended for human consumption.

The Association of Racing Commissioners International (ARCI) has designated this drug as a class 4 substance. See ***Appendix*** for more information. Use of this drug may not be allowed in certain animal competitions. Check rules and regulations before entering in a competition while this medication is being administered. Contact local racing authorities for further guidance.

HUMAN-LABELED PRODUCTS: NONE

References

For the complete list of references, see **wiley.com/go/budde/plumb**

Carvedilol

(kar-***ve***-dil-ole) *Coreg*®

Alpha- and Beta-Adrenergic Antagonist

Prescriber Highlights

- ► Nonselective beta-adrenergic blocker with selective alpha1-adrenergic blocking activity that could be useful as adjunctive treatment of congestive heart failure in dogs
- ► Negative inotrope, which may prohibit its use in patients with CHF, as it could cause worsening of their condition
- ► Additional adverse effects that may demonstrate intolerance include lassitude, inappetence, and hypotension.

Uses/Indications

Carvedilol may be useful as adjunctive therapy in the treatment of congestive heart failure (specifically, dilated cardiomyopathy) in dogs. One study[1] performed in a small number of dogs with dilated cardiomyopathy showed that carvedilol dosed at 0.3 mg/kg PO every 12 hours for 3 months did not produce any significant improvements in neurohormonal activation, heart size, or owner-perceived quality of life. The authors stated that dosages greater than 0.3 mg/kg every 12 hours are likely to be required to effect changes in ventricular remodeling and function.

In a retrospective study, 38 dogs (33 were Cavalier King Charles spaniels) with stage B2 (left-sided heart enlargement without CHF) chronic valvular heart disease were treated with carvedilol. The average initial dosages of 0.31 mg/kg PO twice daily and average uptitration target dosages of 1.11 mg/kg PO twice daily were well tolerated.[2] The median survival was 48.5 months. Additional prospective studies to assess efficacy are warranted.

In a study in dogs, carvedilol attenuated the development of systolic dysfunction of pacing-induced dilated cardiomyopathy and inhibited cardiac apoptosis and fibrosis in the heart; however, there was an enlargement of the left ventricle and atrium.[3]

In one study, when carvedilol was combined with conventional therapy (benazepril, digoxin, ±furosemide, ±spironolactone, ±hydrochlorothiazide) for acquired chronic mitral valve disease in dogs, it improved the quality of life and the heart disease stage classification.[4] It has also been shown that carvedilol can suppress atrial fibrillation inducibility and oxidative stress of the atrial tissue[5] and autonomic nerve activity and paroxysmal atrial tachycardia.[6]

Pharmacology/Actions

Carvedilol is a nonselective, beta-adrenergic blocker with selective alpha$_1$-adrenergic blocking activity. Although beta-blockers have negative inotropic effects, long-term dosing in humans with dilated cardiomyopathy can be beneficial in reducing morbidity and mortality. Patients in heart failure chronically activate their sympathetic nervous system, thereby leading to tachycardia, activation of the renin-angiotensin-aldosterone system, down-regulation of beta-receptors, induction of myocyte necrosis and myocyte energy substrate, and calcium ion handling. By administering beta-blockers, these negative effects may be reversed or diminished. As carvedilol also inhibits alpha$_1$-adrenergic activity, it can cause vasodilation and reduce afterload. Carvedilol has free radical scavenging and antidysrhythmic effects that could be beneficial in patients with heart failure.

Pharmacokinetics

In dogs, a pilot study[7] showed the bioavailability of carvedilol after oral dosing (standard tablets) averaged about 23% in the 4 dogs studied; however, in 3 of the 4 dogs, the bioavailability ranged from 3% to 10%. The volume of distribution averaged about 1.4 L/kg; the elimination half-life was about 100 minutes. At least 15 different metabolites of carvedilol have been identified after dosing in dogs. The most predominant metabolisms in dogs are hydroxylation of the carbazolyl ring and glucuronidation of the parent compound. No pharmacokinetic data were located for the extended-release oral capsules (*Coreg CR*®) in dogs.

In cats, oral carvedilol has a relatively low mean bioavailability (15.7%) with a wide interpatient variation. Peak concentrations occur about one-hour post oral dose. The elimination half-life is about 4.5 hours.[8]

In humans, carvedilol is rapidly and extensively absorbed, but due to a high first-pass effect, its bioavailability is about 30%. The drug is extensively bound to plasma proteins (98%). It is extensively metabolized, and the R(+) enantiomer is metabolized 2 to 3 times greater than the S(-) form during the first pass. Both the R(+) and S(-) enantiomers have equal potency as nonspecific beta- or alpha-adrenergic blockers. CYP2D6 and CYP2C9 are the P450 isoenzymes most responsible for hepatic metabolism. Some of these metabolites have pharmacologic activity. Metabolites are primarily excreted via the bile and feces. The elimination half-life of carvedilol in humans is about 8 to 9 hours.

Contraindications/Precautions/Warnings

In humans, carvedilol is contraindicated in patients with decompensated heart failure, bronchial asthma, second- or third- degree AV block, sick sinus syndrome (unless artificially paced), severe bradycardia, cardiogenic shock, and hypersensitivity to the drug. Dogs with similar conditions should not receive the drug. Patients with hepatic insufficiency should receive the drug with caution.

Too rapid dose up-titration can cause cardiac decompensation.[9] Do not discontinue carvedilol abruptly; in humans, tapering over 1 to 2 weeks is recommended.

Adverse Effects

Veterinary experience with carvedilol is sparse, and an accurate portrayal of adverse effects in dogs has yet to be elucidated. Too rapid dose escalation can cause decompensation in patients with heart failure; cautious dosage titration is mandatory. Dogs that do not tolerate the medication may show signs of inappetence, lassitude, or hypotension.

In humans, carvedilol use has resulted in hypotension, bradycardia, bronchospasm, hyperglycemia and on rare occasions, caused mild hepatocellular injury.[9]

Reproductive/Nursing Safety

In rats and rabbits, carvedilol increased postimplantation loss.[9]

It is unknown if carvedilol enters maternal milk in dogs, but it does enter milk in rats.[9] Use it with caution in nursing patients.

Because safety has not been established in animals, this drug should only be used when the maternal benefits outweigh the potential risks to offspring.

Overdose/Acute Toxicity

The acute oral LD_{50} in healthy rats and mice is greater than 8 g/kg.[10] Clinical signs associated with large overdoses of carvedilol include severe hypotension, cardiac insufficiency, bradycardia, cardiogenic shock, and death due to cardiac arrest. Gut-emptying protocols should be considered if ingestion was recent. In humans, bradycardia is treated with atropine. Cardiovascular function is supported with glucagon and sympathomimetics (eg, dobutamine, epinephrine).

Clinical signs associated with an overdose in dogs include lethargy, bradycardia, hypotension, hypertension, and tachycardia; in cats, lethargy and vomiting are the most common clinical signs.

For patients that have experienced or are suspected to have experienced an overdose, consultation with a 24-hour poison consultation center specializing in providing veterinary-specific information is recommended. For general information related to overdose and toxin exposures, as well as contact information for poison control centers, refer to ***Appendix.***

Drug Interactions

The following drug interactions have either been reported or are theoretical in humans or animals receiving carvedilol and may be of significance in veterinary patients. Unless otherwise noted, use together is not necessarily contraindicated, but weigh the potential risks and perform additional monitoring when appropriate.

- **Antidiabetic Agents, Oral** (eg, **glipizide, metformin**): Carvedilol may enhance the blood-glucose-lowering effects of antidiabetic agents.
- **Amiodarone**: Concurrent use may result in bradycardia, hypotension, sinus arrest, and AV block.
- **Beta-Adrenergic Receptor Antagonists** (eg, **atenolol, propranolol**): Use with carvedilol may cause additive effects
- **Calcium Channel Blockers** (eg, **amlodipine, diltiazem, verapamil**): Increased risk for hypotension and bradycardia; may precipitate heart failure in patients with pre-existing cardiac conditions
- **Cimetidine**: May decrease metabolism and increase the AUC of carvedilol
- **Clonidine**: Carvedilol may potentiate the cardiovascular effects of clonidine.
- **Cyclosporine**: Carvedilol may increase cyclosporine concentrations.
- **Digoxin**: Carvedilol can increase (in humans) digoxin plasma concentrations by ≈15% and increase the risk for complete heart block.[9]
- **Dobutamine**: Concurrent use may lead to decreased dobutamine efficacy.
- **Doxorubicin**: Concurrent use may result in increased doxorubicin exposure.
- **Epinephrine**: Concurrent use may result in hypertension, bradycardia, and resistance to epinephrine in anaphylaxis.
- **Fluoxetine, Paroxetine:** May increase R(+) carvedilol concentrations and increase alpha$_1$ blocking effects (vasodilation)

- **Hypotensive Agents** (eg, **enalapril, telmisartan**): Concurrent use may increase the risk for hypotension.
- **Insulin**: Carvedilol may enhance the blood-glucose-lowering effects of insulin or other antidiabetic agents.
- **Methimazole**: Concurrent use may alter the metabolism of carvedilol.
- **Nonsteroidal Anti-inflammatory Drugs (NSAIDs**; eg, **carprofen, meloxicam, robenacoxib**): Concurrent use may lead to decreased antihypertensive effects of carvedilol.
- **Opioids** (eg, **fentanyl, hydrmorphone, methadone**): Increased risk for hypotension and bradycardia. Concurrent use with morphine may lead to increased morphine exposure.
- **Quinidine**: May increase R(+)carvedilol concentrations and increase alpha$_1$ blocking effects that lead to vasodilation.
- **Rifampin**: Can decrease carvedilol plasma concentrations by as much as 70%.[9]
- **Reserpine**: May increase risk for bradycardia and hypotension
- **Vincristine**: Concurrent use may lead to increased vincristine plasma concentrations.
- **Yohimbine**: Concurrent use may lead to decreased carvedilol efficacy.

Laboratory Considerations

- No specific laboratory interactions or considerations were noted.

Dosages

DOGS:

Adjunctive treatment of stage B myxomatous mitral valve disease (extra-label):

a) From a retrospective study: Carvedilol at an initial dose of 0.31 mg/kg (mean) PO twice daily and a target dose of 1.11 mg/kg (mean) PO twice daily is safe and well tolerated in dogs with stage B1 and early stage B2 when an uptitration protocol is used that involves a 50% to 100% increase in dose every 7 to 14 days until the target dose is reached.[11]

b) Initial dose 0.15 – 0.2 mg/kg PO twice daily for 1 week. After evaluating blood pressure and heart rate, the dose can be increased to 0.3 mg/kg PO twice daily.[4,12]

Adjunctive treatment of pseudoephedrine toxicosis (extra-label): From a case report, 0.5 mg/kg PO twice daily[13]

Monitoring

- Adverse effects (eg, lethargy, inappetence, collapse)
- Blood pressure, heart rate
- Resting respiratory rate
- ECG and cardiac function (ie, echocardiography)
- Plasma drug concentrations may be useful.

Client Information

- This medication is best given with food.
- When starting this medicine for your animal, your veterinarian may begin with a low dose and gradually increase the dose over time. It is critical to be aware of the changing doses and not administer more at one time than your veterinarian prescribes. Do not stop the medication without talking with your veterinarian first.
- If the initial doses are too high, it may cause your animal's condition to worsen and show signs of loss of appetite, depression, lack of energy, or weakness. If any of these clinical signs occur, call your veterinarian immediately.
- Do NOT store compounded liquids of carvedilol in the refrigerator.

Chemistry/Synonyms

Carvedilol, a nonselective beta-adrenergic blocker with selective alpha$_1$-adrenergic blocking activity, occurs as a white to off-white crystalline powder that is practically insoluble in water, dilute acids, and gastric or intestinal fluids. It is sparingly soluble in ethanol. The compound exhibits polymorphism and contains both R(+) and S(-) enantiomers. It is a basic lipophilic compound.

Carvedilol may also be known as BM-14190, carvedilolum, *Cardilol®*, *Cardiol®*, *Carloc®*, *Carvil®*, *Carvipress®*, *Coreg®*, *Coritensil®*, *Coropres®*, *Dilatrend®*, *Dilbloc®*, *Dimitone®*, *Divelol®*, *Eucardic®*, *Hybridil®*, *Kredex®*, or *Querto®*.

Storage/Stability

Store carvedilol tablets and extended-release capsules below 30°C (86°F), protected from moisture. Dispense them in tight, light-resistant containers.

Compatibility/Compounding Considerations

Compounded preparation stability: Carvedilol oral suspension compounded from commercially available tablets has been published[14] ; however, HPLC analysis of drug samples in this study gave inconsistent and variable results, indicating a loss of potency at refrigerated temperatures compared with room temperature. Results of this study do not necessarily confirm that carvedilol is stable when prepared as an oral liquid.

Another published[15] compounded oral suspension with documented 90-day stability to accurately dose dogs is to powder 25 mg tablets and add enough de-ionized water to make a paste, allowing the tablet coating to dissolve. Then, suspend the paste in a commercially available simple syrup to a concentration of either 2 mg/mL or 10 mg/mL. Store the medication in amber bottles at temperatures not exceeding 25°C (77°F) and protect from light for up to 90 days. Shake well before administering.

Dosage Forms/Regulatory Status

VETERINARY-LABELED PRODUCTS: NONE

The Association of Racing Commissioners International (ARCI) has designated this drug as a class 3 substance. Use of this drug may not be allowed in certain animal competitions. Check rules and regulations before entering in a competition while this medication is being administered. Contact local racing authorities for further guidance. See the ***Appendix*** for more information.

HUMAN-LABELED PRODUCTS:

Carvedilol Oral Tablets: 3.125 mg, 6.25 mg, 12.5 mg, and 25 mg; *Coreg®*, generic; (Rx)

Carvedilol extended-release oral capsules are available; however, no information about use in veterinary species was located for this dosage form.

References

For the complete list of references, see **wiley.com/go/budde/plumb**

Caspofungin

(kas-poe-***fun***-jin) *Cancidas®*

Parenteral Antifungal

Prescriber Highlights

- Parenteral antifungal that has potential for treating invasive aspergillosis or disseminated candidal infections in companion animals
- Very limited clinical experience in veterinary medicine
- Must be given slow IV

Uses/Indications

Caspofungin has potential for treating invasive aspergillosis or disseminated candidal infections in companion animals, although limited information on its use in dogs or cats is available.

Pharmacology/Actions

Caspofungin is an echinocandin antifungal agent. These drugs inhibit beta-glucan synthase, thereby blocking the synthesis of beta-(1,3)-D-glucan, a component found in cell walls of filamentous fungi. Beta-(1,3)-D-glucan is not present in mammalian cells.

Caspofungin has activity against *Aspergillus* spp and *Candida* spp and is effective in treating pneumonia caused by *Pneumocystis carinii*. Because it contains very little beta-glucan synthase, *Cryptococcus neoformans* infections are not effectively treated with caspofungin.[1]

An in vitro study found that caspofungin had significant, but only minimal to moderate inhibition of *Pythium insidiosum* and a *Lagenidium* spp.[2]

Pharmacokinetics

In cats given caspofungin 1 mg/kg IV infused over 1 hour, peak concentration was 14.8 µg/mL after the first dose and 19.8 µg/mL at steady state; trough concentration was ≈5 µg/mL. Clearance was 18 mL/kg/minute, and elimination half-life was 14.5 hours.[3]

In humans, the drug is not appreciably absorbed from the gut and must be administered IV. Protein binding (primarily to albumin) is high (97%), and the drug is distributed to tissues over a 36- to 48-hour period. Caspofungin is slowly metabolized via hydrolysis and N-acetylation. It also spontaneously degrades chemically. Caspofungin exhibits polyphasic elimination, but little is excreted or biotransformed during the first 30 hours postadministration. Elimination half-life for the primary phase is about 10 hours; the secondary phase between 40 and 50 hours. Excretion, consisting mostly as metabolites, is via the feces and urine. Only small amounts (1% to 2%) are excreted unchanged into the urine.[4]

Contraindications/Precautions/Warnings

No specific information is available for veterinary patients. Caspofungin is contraindicated in human patients that are hypersensitive to it. Elevated liver enzyme tests, hepatic necrosis, and hepatic failure have been observed in humans; dosage adjustment is recommended in humans with moderate hepatic impairment. No information is available for use in patients with significant hepatic impairment; avoid use.

Adverse Effects

An adverse effect profile for animals has not been determined. Diarrhea and transient fever have been observed in healthy cats given caspofungin.[3]

In humans, caspofungin is generally well tolerated. Nausea and diarrhea have been noted. Histamine-mediated signs have occurred (eg, rash, facial swelling, pruritus) and anaphylaxis has been reported. IV site reactions (eg, pain, redness, phlebitis) and elevated liver enzymes have also been reported.[4]

Reproductive/Nursing Safety

Fertility and reproductive performance were not affected by the IV administration of caspofungin to rats at doses up to 5 mg/kg.[4] Studies in pregnant rats and rabbits demonstrated changes in fetal ossification and increased fetal resorption. The drug should be avoided during the first trimester of pregnancy unless the benefits associated with treating outweigh the risks.

Caspofungin is distributed into milk in rats.[4] Although no data are available, because the drug is not appreciably absorbed from the gut, it would be expected that caspofungin would be safe to administer during lactation.

Because safety has not been established in animals, this drug should only be used when the maternal benefits outweigh the potential risks to offspring.

Overdose/Acute Toxicity

Limited information is available. Doses of 210 mg (about 3 times) in humans were well tolerated.[4] Some monkeys receiving 5 – 8 mg/kg (≈4 to 6 times the recommended dose) over 5 weeks developed sites of microscopic subcapsular necrosis on their livers.

For patients that have experienced or are suspected of having experienced an overdose, consultation with a 24-hour poison consultation center specializing in providing veterinary-specific information is recommended. For general information related to overdose and toxin exposures, as well as contact information for poison control centers, refer to ***Appendix***.

Drug Interactions

The following drug interactions have either been reported or are theoretical in humans or animals receiving caspofungin and may be of significance in veterinary patients. Unless otherwise noted, use together is not necessarily contraindicated, but veterinarians should weigh the potential risks and perform additional monitoring when appropriate.

- **CYCLOSPORINE**: Increased caspofungin plasma concentrations and increased risk for elevated liver enzymes
- **DEXAMETHASONE**: Reduced caspofungin plasma concentrations
- **RIFAMPIN**: Reduced caspofungin plasma concentrations

Laboratory Considerations

- None noted

Dosages

DOGS:

Treatment of *Aspergillus deflectus* (extra-label): From a case report in a dog that had disease progression despite treatment with other antifungals (eg, voriconazole, amphotericin B lipid complex), caspofungin 1 mg/kg IV over 1 hour every 24 hours[5]; the drug was diluted in 250 mL 0.9% sodium chloride. Rapid clinical improvement and resolution of lymphadenomegaly was noted after 6 weeks of treatment, at which time caspofungin was administered 3 times weekly for 2 months, then on 3 consecutive days every 3 weeks for 4 months, then discontinued. One month later, small numbers of *A deflectus* (sensitive to caspofungin) were noted in urine culture. Twice-weekly caspofungin treatment was administered for 2 weeks, and urine culture again was negative. Treatment was continued on 3 consecutive days every 3 weeks. One year later, the dog showed clinical signs of disease recurrence, and enlarged mesenteric lymph nodes revealed fungal hyphae with marked necrosis.

CATS:

- **Sino-orbital aspergillosis** (extra-label):
  - a) 1 mg/kg IV once daily for 14 to 22 days.[6,7] The calculated dose was administered in 20 mL 0.9% sodium chloride and infused over 1 hour.[7]
  - b) From a pharmacokinetic study, 1 mg/kg IV loading dose followed by 0.75 mg/kg IV every 24 hours yielded the optimal ratio of peak caspofungin concentration to minimum effective concentration (C_{max}:MEC).[3] This dosage was effectively used in 2 cats with sino-orbital aspergillosis; treatment continued for 2 to 3 weeks.[8] Alternatively, 1 mg/kg IV loading dose followed by 1 mg/kg IV every 72 hours yielded a similar C_{max}:MEC.

Monitoring

- Clinical efficacy
- Baseline and periodic CBC, serum electrolytes, liver enzymes, bilirubin
- Clinical signs associated with infusion reactions (eg, pyrexia, blood pressure changes, tachycardia)

Client Information

- This medication is appropriate for inpatient use only.

- Clients should understand the investigational nature and the associated expense of using this drug in veterinary patients.

Chemistry/Synonyms

Caspofungin acetate is a semisynthetic echinocandin compound produced from a fermentation product of *Glarea lozoyensis*. It occurs as a white to off-white powder that is freely soluble in water and slightly soluble in ethanol. The commercially available lyophilized powder for injection also contains acetic acid, sodium hydroxide, mannitol, and sucrose.

Caspofungin may also be known as caspofungina, caspofungine, caspofungini, kaspofungiinia, kaspofungina, L-743873, MK-0991, or *Cancidas*®.

Storage/Stability

The commercially available product should be stored refrigerated 2° to 8°C (36°F-46°F). Refer to the package insert for very specific directions on preparing the solution for IV use. Reconstituted solutions must be further diluted within 1 hour. Caspofungin diluted in saline or lactated Ringer's may be stored for 24 hours at room temperature below 25°C (below 77°F), or 48 hours if refrigerated. Unused portions should be discarded.

Do not use this product if the solution is cloudy or has precipitated.

Compatibility/Compounding Considerations

Compatibility is dependent on factors such as pH, concentration, temperature, and diluent used; specialized references or a hospital pharmacist should be consulted for more specific information.

Caspofungin must be infused slowly diluted in lactated Ringer's or sodium chloride containing solutions. It is not stable in dextrose-containing IV solutions. Do not mix or infuse caspofungin with any other medications.[4]

Dosage Forms/Regulatory Status

VETERINARY-LABELED PRODUCTS: NONE

HUMAN-LABELED PRODUCTS:

Caspofungin Acetate Lyophilized Powder for Injection: 50 mg and 70 mg in single-use vials; *Cancidas*®; (Rx)

References

For the complete list of references, see **wiley.com/go/budde/plumb**

Cefaclor

(**sef**-a-klor) *Ceclor*®

Oral Second-Generation Cephalosporin

Prescriber Highlights

- More active against some gram-negative bacteria than first-generation cephalosporins (eg, cephalexin, cefadroxil)
- It is potentially useful when an oral cephalosporin is desired to treat bacterial infections that are susceptible to cefaclor but resistant to first-generation cephalosporins.
- Limited clinical experience in veterinary medicine
- Contraindications include hypersensitivity to cefaclor or other cephalosporins.
- The most likely adverse effects in small animal species are GI related.

Uses/Indications

Cefaclor may be useful in uncommon situations when an oral cephalosporin is desired to treat infections that are susceptible to cefaclor but resistant to first-generation cephalosporins, such as cephalexin or cefadroxil. However, little information is available on the clinical use of cefaclor in small animals.

The World Health Organization (WHO) has designated cefaclor as a Highly Important antimicrobial for human medicine.[1]

Pharmacology/Actions

Cefaclor, like other cephalosporins, is bactericidal and acts via inhibiting cell wall synthesis. Its spectrum of activity is similar to that of cephalexin, but it has a broader spectrum to include activity against gram-negative bacteria, including strains of *Escherichia coli*, *Klebsiella pneumoniae*, and *Proteus mirabilis* (but not most other *Proteus*). It is ineffective against enterococci, *Enterobacter*, most *Pseudomonas* spp, methicillin-resistant staphylococci, and extended-spectrum beta-lactamase (ESBL)–producing gram-negative bacteria.

Pharmacokinetics

Limited information is available on the pharmacokinetics of cefaclor in dogs, and no information is currently available for cats. In dogs, about 75% of an oral dose is absorbed, but an apparent first-pass effect reduces bioavailability to about 60%.[2] Cefaclor is distributed to many tissues, but concentrations are lower in interstitial fluid than those found in serum. High concentrations are excreted into the urine unchanged. Bile concentrations are higher than those found in serum. Dogs appear to metabolize a greater percentage of cefaclor than do rats, mice, or humans. The elimination half-life is ≈2 hours in dogs.[3] Pharmacokinetic information for the extended-release oral tablets in dogs was not located.

In humans, cefaclor is well absorbed after oral administration; food delays, but does not appreciably alter, the amount of cefaclor absorbed when immediate-release capsules are used. The bioavailability of extended-release tablets is decreased by 23% when taken on an empty stomach and the maximum concentration is decreased by 67% and should therefore be given with food. The drug is widely distributed, crosses the placenta, and enters breast milk.[4] Up to 85% of a dose is excreted unchanged into the urine; elimination half-life is less than 1 hour in patients with normal renal function.

Contraindications/Precautions/Warnings

Cefaclor is contraindicated in humans that are hypersensitive to it and other cephalosporins. Cefaclor must be cautiously used in patients with an allergy to penicillin.[5] Use with caution in patients with severe renal impairment.[6]

Cefaclor can be easily confused with other cephalosporins. Consider writing orders and prescriptions using tall man lettering: CefaCLOR.

Adverse Effects

As use of cefaclor in animals has been limited, a comprehensive adverse effect profile has not been determined. In humans, cefaclor is generally well-tolerated but commonly can cause GI effects (eg, nausea, diarrhea). Hypersensitivity reactions including anaphylaxis are possible; cefaclor appears to cause a higher incidence of serum-sickness-like reactions than other cephalosporins, particularly in children who have received multiple courses of treatment. In humans, it is estimated that up to 15% of patients who are hypersensitive to penicillins will also be hypersensitive to cephalosporins.[5]

Rare adverse effects reported include erythema multiforme, rash, increases in liver function tests, and transient increases in BUN and serum creatinine. High doses or prolonged use of cephalosporins have been associated with neurotoxicity, neutropenia, agranulocytosis, thrombocytopenia, hepatitis, interstitial nephritis, and tubular necrosis.

Reproductive/Nursing Safety

Cefaclor cross the placenta. Studies performed in pregnant mice and rats (doses up to 12 times the human dose) and ferrets (doses up to 3 times the human dose) demonstrated no overt fetal harm.[6]

Cefaclor enters maternal milk in low concentrations, and alteration to gut microbiome is possible in the nursing offspring with resultant diarrhea. Cefaclor is considered compatible with breastfeeding in humans.[4]

Because safety has not been established in animals, this drug should only be used when the maternal benefits outweigh the potential risks to offspring.

Overdose/Acute Toxicity

Cefaclor appears quite safe in dogs. Acute oral cephalosporin overdoses are unlikely to cause significant problems other than GI distress, but other, more serious effects are possible. See ***Adverse Effects***. Dogs given daily PO doses of 200 mg/kg/day (10 times the normal dosage) for 30 days developed soft stools and occasional emesis.[7] Two dogs in this study group developed transient moderate decreases in hemoglobin. One dog in another study group that was given 400 mg/kg/day (20 times the normal dosage) for 1 year developed a reversible thrombocytopenia.

For patients that have experienced or are suspected to have experienced an overdose, consultation with a 24-hour poison consultation center specializing in providing veterinary-specific information is recommended. For general information related to overdose and toxin exposures, as well as contact information for poison control centers, refer to ***Appendix.***

Drug Interactions

The following drug interactions have either been reported or are theoretical in humans or animals receiving cefaclor and may be of significance in veterinary patients. Unless otherwise noted, use together is not necessarily contraindicated, but weigh the potential risks and perform additional monitoring when appropriate.

- **Aminoglycosides**: The nephrotoxic effects of aminoglycosides may be enhanced by second-generation cephalosporins.
- **Antacids (aluminum-, calcium-** or **magnesium- containing)**: Reduces the extent of absorption of extended-release cefaclor tablets in humans; separate doses by at least 2 hours
- **Probenecid**: Reduces renal excretion of cefaclor
- **Warfarin**: Rare reports of increased anticoagulant effects when used concomitantly with cefaclor

Laboratory Considerations

- Cefaclor may cause false-positive **urine glucose determinations** when using the copper reduction method (Benedict's solution, Fehling's solution, *Clinitest*®); tests utilizing glucose oxidase (*Tes-Tape*®, *Clinistix*®) are not affected.
- When using the Jaffe reaction to measure **serum or urine creatinine**, cefaclor given in high doses may result in falsely elevated values.
- In humans, particularly with azotemia, cephalosporins have caused a false-positive direct **Coombs test**.
- Cefaclor may also result in falsely elevated **17-ketosteroid** values in urine.

Dosages

DOGS/CATS:

Susceptible infections (extra-label): 7 – 20 mg/kg PO every 8 hours

Monitoring

- Clinical efficacy
- Patients with renal insufficiency should have periodic renal function monitored.

Client Information

- This medicine works best when given without food. If your animal vomits or develops a lack of appetite while receiving the medicine, it can be administered with food.
- The most common side effects are diarrhea, vomiting, and loss of appetite.
- Be sure to give the medication to your animal as long as your veterinarian has prescribed, even if your animal seems better.
- Cephalosporin antibiotics have an odor that resembles cat urine.

Chemistry/Synonyms

Cefaclor occurs as a white to off-white powder that is slightly soluble in water.

Cefaclor may also be known as cefaclorum, cefaklor, cefkloras, kefakloori, or compound 99638. There are many internationally registered trade names.

Storage/Stability

Store cefaclor capsules, tablets, and powder for suspension in tight containers at room temperature (15°C-30°C [59°F-86°F]). After reconstituting, store the oral suspension in a tight container in the refrigerator. Discard it after 14 days.

Compatibility/Compounding Considerations

No specific information was noted.

Dosage Forms/Regulatory Status

VETERINARY-LABELED PRODUCTS: NONE

HUMAN-LABELED PRODUCTS:

Cefaclor Oral Capsules: 250 mg and 500 mg; generic; (Rx)

Cefaclor Extended-Release Oral Tablets: 500 mg; generic; (Rx)

Cefaclor Powder for Oral Suspension: 125 mg/5 mL (25 mg/mL), 187 mg/5 mL (37.4 mg/mL), 250 mg/5 mL (50 mg/mL), and 375 mg/5 mL (75 mg/mL), generic; (Rx)

References

For the complete list of references, see **wiley.com/go/budde/plumb**

Cefadroxil

(sef-a-***drox***-ill) *Duricef*®

First-Generation Cephalosporin

Prescriber Highlights

- ► Oral antibiotic indicated in dogs and cats for bacterial cystitis or skin/soft tissue infections
- ► Usually well-tolerated; adverse GI effects (eg, anorexia, vomiting, diarrhea) may occur
- ► May be administered with or without food; however, administering the drug with food may help prevent GI upset.
- ► Severe renal impairment may require dose adjustment.

Uses/Indications

Cefadroxil is FDA-approved for use in dogs for genitourinary tract infections (cystitis) caused by susceptible strains of *Escherichia coli, Proteus mirabilis,* and *Staphylococcus aureus* and skin and soft tissue infections including cellulitis, pyoderma, dermatitis, wound infections, and abscesses caused by susceptible strains of *S aureus.* In cats, cefadroxil is labeled for treatment of genitourinary tract infections (cystitis) caused by susceptible strains of *Escherichia coli, Proteus mirabilis,* and *Staphylococcus aureus;* and skin and soft tissue infections including abscesses, wound infections, cellulitis, and dermatitis caused by susceptible strains of *Pasteurella multocida, S aureus, Staphylococcus epidermidis, and Streptococcus* spp.

This antibiotic is used primarily for its activity against staphylococci, particularly for pyoderma.[1,2] Because of high urine concentrations, cefadroxil can be an effective drug for treatment of bacterial cystitis caused by most gram-negative pathogens.

The World Health Organization (WHO) has designated first-generation cephalosporins as Highly Important antimicrobials for human medicine.[3] The Office International des Epizooties (OIE) has designated first-generation cephalosporins as Veterinary Highly Important Antimicrobial (VHIA) agents in veterinary medicine.[4]

Pharmacology/Actions

Cephalosporins are considered time dependent and bactericidal against susceptible bacteria, and they act by inhibiting mucopeptide synthesis in the cell wall, which results in a defective barrier and an osmotically unstable spheroplast. The exact mechanism for this effect has not been definitively determined, but beta-lactam antibiotics have been shown to bind to several enzymes (eg, carboxypeptidases, transpeptidases, endopeptidases) in the bacterial cytoplasmic membrane that are involved in cell wall synthesis. The different affinities that various beta-lactam antibiotics have for these enzymes (also known as penicillin-binding proteins [PBPs]) help explain the differences in spectrums of activity of these drugs that are not explained by the influence of beta-lactamases. Like other beta-lactam antibiotics, cephalosporins are generally considered to be more effective against actively growing bacteria. For bactericidal activity, cephalosporin levels should exceed bacterial MIC for ≈40% of the dose interval for staphylococcal infections and ≈60% of the dose interval for streptococcal infections.[5]

Although there may be differences in MICs for individual first-generation cephalosporins, their spectrums of activity are similar. First-generation cephalosporins generally possess excellent coverage against most gram-positive pathogens (with the exception of enterococci). They have variable to poor coverage against most gram-negative pathogens. These drugs are active in vitro against streptococci, staphylococci, *Proteus mirabilis,* and some strains of *Escherichia coli, Klebsiella* spp, *Actinobacillus* spp, and *Pasteurella* spp. Methicillin-resistant staphylococci are resistant to this class of antibiotics. In vitro susceptibility is generally predictive of the potential for in vivo efficacy. Cefadroxil is inactive against *Enterococcus* spp, *Pseudomonas* spp, *Rickettsia* spp, mycobacteria, *Mycoplasma* spp, fungi, and viruses.

Pharmacokinetics

Cefadroxil is reportedly well-absorbed after oral administration to dogs regardless of feeding state.[6] After an oral dose of 22 mg/kg, peak serum concentrations of ≈18.6 µg/mL occur within 1 to 2 hours of dosing. Only ≈20% of the drug is bound to canine plasma proteins. The drug is excreted into the animal's urine and has a half-life of ≈2 hours. Over 50% of a dose can be recovered unchanged in the urine within 24 hours of dosing.

In cats, the serum half-life has been reported as ≈3 hours.

Oral absorption of cefadroxil suspension in adult horses was characterized as poor and erratic. In a study done in foals, oral bioavailability ranged from 36% to 99.8% (mean, 58.2%); mean elimination half-life was 3.75 hours after oral dosing.[7,8] Oral absorption becomes more rapid as foals age, but bioavailability decreases significantly.

Contraindications/Precautions/Warnings

Cephalosporins are contraindicated in patients with a history of hypersensitivity to them. Because there may be cross-reactivity, cephalosporins should be used cautiously in patients that have a documented hypersensitivity to other beta-lactam antibiotics (eg, penicillins, cefamycins, carbapenems).

Cefadroxil should be used with caution in patients with significant renal impairment; dose adjustment may be required. However, this guidance is likely only necessary for patients with severe renal disease, and there is no guidance for optimal dose and frequency changes in animals with renal disease. In humans with significant renal dysfunction, dosing frequency is decreased.[9]

In general, oral antibiotics such as cefadroxil should not be used for patients with septicemia, shock, or other grave illnesses, as absorption of the medication from the GI tract may be significantly delayed or diminished.

Cefadroxil can be easily confused with other cephalosporins. Consider writing orders and prescriptions using tall man lettering: cefaDROXil.

Some formulations of cefadroxil may contain sodium benzoate or benzoic acid.

Adverse Effects

Adverse effects with cephalosporins are usually mild and have a relatively low frequency of occurrence. When cephalosporins are given orally, they may cause GI effects (eg, anorexia, vomiting, diarrhea). Administering the drug with a small meal may help alleviate these effects. Because cephalosporins may alter GI microbiota, antibiotic-associated diarrhea can occur and allow the proliferation of resistant bacteria in the colon (superinfections).

Hypersensitivity reactions unrelated to dose can occur with these agents and can manifest as rashes, fever, eosinophilia, lymphadenopathy, or anaphylaxis. The use of cephalosporins in patients that are documented to be hypersensitive to penicillin-class antibiotics is controversial. In humans, it is estimated that up to 15% of patients that are hypersensitive to penicillins will also be hypersensitive to cephalosporins.[10] The incidence of cross-reactivity in veterinary patients is unknown.

Although cephalosporins (particularly cephalothin) have the potential for causing nephrotoxicity, at clinically used doses in patients with normal renal function, the risks for the occurrence of this adverse effect appear minimal.

High doses or prolonged use of cephalosporins have been associated with neurotoxicity, neutropenia, agranulocytosis, thrombocytopenia, hepatitis, positive Coombs test, interstitial nephritis, and tubular necrosis. Except for tubular necrosis and neurotoxicity, these effects have an immunologic component.

Reproductive/Nursing Safety

Cephalosporins cross the placenta. Cefadroxil did not demonstrate teratogenicity in laboratory animals,[9] and cefadroxil is considered compatible with human pregnancy.[11]

Cefadroxil is excreted into human breast milk in clinically insignificant amounts[12] and the drug is considered compatible with nursing.[11]

Because safety has not been established in animals, this drug should only be used when the maternal benefits outweigh the potential risks to offspring.

Overdose/Acute Toxicity

Acute oral cephalosporin overdoses are unlikely to cause significant problems other than GI distress, but other, more serious effects are possible. See ***Adverse Effects***.

For patients that have experienced or are suspected to have experienced an overdose, consultation with a 24-hour poison consultation center specializing in providing veterinary-specific information is recommended. For general information related to overdose and toxin exposures, as well as contact information for poison control centers, refer to ***Appendix.***

Drug Interactions

The following drug interactions either have been reported or are theoretical in humans or animals receiving cefadroxil and may be of significance in veterinary patients. Unless otherwise noted, use together is not necessarily contraindicated, but weigh the potential risks and perform additional monitoring when appropriate.

- **Nephrotoxic Drugs**: Concurrent use of parenteral aminoglycosides or other nephrotoxic drugs (eg, amphotericin B) with cephalosporins is somewhat controversial. Cephalosporins could potentially cause additive nephrotoxicity when used with these drugs, but this interaction has only been well-documented with cephaloridine (no longer marketed). Caution is advised when using these drug combinations.

- **Probenecid**: Competitively blocks the tubular secretion of most cephalosporins, thereby increasing serum levels and serum half-lives
- **Vitamin K Antagonists:** Cephalosporins may enhance the anticoagulant effects of vitamin K antagonists (eg, warfarin).

Laboratory Considerations

- Cephalosporins may cause false-positive **urine glucose determinations** when a cupric sulfate solution (Benedict's solution, *Clinitest*®, Fehling's solution) is used. Tests using glucose oxidase (*Tes-Tape*®, *Clinistix*®) are not affected by cephalosporins.
- When the Jaffe reaction is used to measure **serum or urine creatinine**, high-dose cefadroxil may cause falsely elevated values.
- In humans, particularly in those with azotemia, cephalosporins may cause a false-positive direct **Coombs test.**
- Cephalosporins may also cause falsely elevated **17-ketosteroid** values in urine.
- Cephalosporins may falsely decrease serum **albumin** measurements.
- **Cefazolin-surrogate susceptibility** is not a good predictor of cefadroxil susceptibility.[13,14]

Dosages

DOGS:

Susceptible genitourinary or skin/soft tissue infections (label dosage; FDA-approved): **NOTE**: The label specifies treatment duration times for various infections, but these duration times are outdated and and may no longer apply.

- **Skin/soft tissue infections caused by susceptible strains of *Staphylococcus aureus*:** 22 mg/kg PO twice daily (ie, every 12 hours) for a minimum of 3 days[15,16]; continue treatment for at least 48 hours after the dog becomes afebrile or clinical signs resolve. If no improvement is seen after 3 days of treatment, discontinue therapy and re-evaluate the case. Do not treat for more than 30 days.
- **Genitourinary infections (cystitis) caused by susceptible strains of *Escherichia coli, Proteus mirabilis, and S aureus*:** 22 mg/kg PO twice daily (ie, every 12 hours) for a minimum of 7 days[15,16]; continue treatment for at least 48 hours after the dog becomes afebrile or clinical signs resolve. If no improvement is seen after 3 days of treatment, discontinue therapy and re-evaluate the case. Do not treat for more than 30 days.

Superficial pyoderma (extra-label): 22 – 35 mg/kg PO twice daily (ie, every 12 hours) for 28 to 42 days[1,17]

Deep pyoderma (extra-label): Either 20 mg/kg PO twice daily (ie, every 12 hours) or 40 mg/kg PO once daily (ie, every 24 hours) for 21 days[1]

Bacterial cystitis (extra-label): 12 – 25 mg/kg PO every 12 hours for 3 to 5 days.[18] **NOTE**: Chronic urethrocystitis or pyelonephritis are best initially treated with a veterinary-labeled fluoroquinolone or cefpodoxime, pending culture and susceptibility results.[18]

CATS:

Susceptible infections (label dosage; FDA-approved): **NOTE**: The label specifies treatment frequency and duration times for various infections, but these duration times are outdated and may no longer apply.

- **Skin/soft tissue infections caused by susceptible strains of *S aureus*:** 22 mg/kg PO twice daily (ie, every 12 hours) for a minimum of 3 days[15,16]; continue treatment for at least 48 hours after the cat becomes afebrile or clinical signs resolve. If no improvement is seen after 3 days of treatment, discontinue therapy and re-evaluate the case. Do not treat for more than 30 days.
- **Skin/soft tissue infections caused by susceptible strains of *Pasteurella multocida, S aureus, Staphylococcus epidermidis,* and *Streptococcus* spp:** 22 mg/kg PO once daily (ie, every 24 hours)[15,16]; continue treatment for at least 48 hours after the cat becomes afebrile or clinical signs resolve. If no improvement is seen after 3 days of treatment, discontinue therapy and re-evaluate the case. Do not treat for more than 21 days.
- **Genitourinary infections (cystitis) caused by susceptible strains of *E coli, P mirabilis, and S aureus*:** 22 mg/kg PO twice daily (ie, every 12 hours) for a minimum of 7 days[15,16]; continue treatment for at least 48 hours after the cat becomes afebrile or clinical signs resolve. If no improvement is seen after 3 days of treatment, discontinue therapy and re-evaluate the case. Do not treat for more than 30 days.

FERRETS:

Susceptible infections (extra-label): 15 – 20 mg/kg PO twice daily[19]

Monitoring

- Culture and susceptibility testing as indicated by clinical condition
- Because cephalosporins usually have minimal toxicity associated with their use, monitoring for efficacy is often all that is required.
- Patients with diminished renal function may require intensified monitoring of renal parameters (eg, BUN, creatinine, urinalysis).

Client Information

- This medicine can be given with or without food, but GI side effects (eg, loss of appetite, vomiting, diarrhea) might be prevented if given with food. If your animal vomits or acts sick after receiving this medication on an empty stomach, try administering the next dose with food or a small treat. If vomiting continues, contact your veterinarian.
- The most common side effects are vomiting, diarrhea, and loss of appetite.
- Be sure to give this antibiotic to your pet as long as your veterinarian has prescribed, even if your animal seems better.
- This antibiotic has an odor that resembles cat urine.

Chemistry/Synonyms

A semisynthetic cephalosporin antibiotic, cefadroxil occurs as a white to yellowish-white, crystalline powder that is soluble in water and slightly soluble in alcohol. The commercially available product is available as the monohydrate.

Cefadroxil may also be known as BL-S578, cefadroxilum, cephadroxil, or MJF-11567-3; many trade names are available.

Storage/Stability

Cefadroxil tablets, capsules, and powder for oral suspension should be stored at room temperature (20°C-25°C [68°F-77°F]) with temperature excursions (15°C-30°C [59°F-86°F]) permitted in tight containers. After reconstitution, the oral suspension is stable for 14 days when kept refrigerated (4°C[39°F]).[15]

Compatibility/Compounding Considerations

No specific information is noted.

Dosage Forms/Regulatory Status

VETERINARY-LABELED PRODUCTS:

Cefadroxil Oral Tablets: 50 mg, 100 mg, 200 mg, and 1000 mg tablets; *Cefa-tabs*®; (Rx). FDA-approved for use in dogs and cats. NADA #119-688. Product is not marketed but remains listed in the FDA Green Book.

Cefadroxil Powder for Oral Suspension: 50 mg/mL in 15 mL and 50 mL bottles; *Cefa-Drops*®; (Rx). FDA-approved for use in dogs and cats. NADA #140-684. Product is not marketed but remains listed in the FDA Green Book.

HUMAN-LABELED PRODUCTS:

Cefadroxil Oral Tablets: 1 g; generic; (Rx)

Cefadroxil Oral Capsules: 500 mg; generic; (Rx)

Cefadroxil Powder for Oral Suspension: 250 mg/5 mL (50 mg/mL) and 500 mg/5 mL (100 mg/mL) in 50 mL, 75 mL (500 mg/5 mL only), and 100 mL; generic; (Rx)

References

For the complete list of references, see **wiley.com/go/budde/plumb**

Cefazolin

(sef-*a*-zoe-lin) *Ancef®, Kefzol®, Zolicef®*

First-Generation Cephalosporin

Prescriber Highlights

- First-generation parenteral cephalosporin; often used for surgical prophylaxis for gram-positive coverage
- May cause hypersensitivity reactions
- Can cause pain on IM injection; give IV slowly over 3 to 5 minutes (or more, as needed).

Uses/Indications

Cefazolin is used in several animal species when an injectable first-generation cephalosporin is indicated. Cefazolin is used for surgical prophylaxis, particularly for orthopedic surgery and other procedures in which *Staphylococcus* spp is the most common cause of surgical site infections.

Because cefazolin is a time-dependent antibiotic, where time above minimal inhibitory concentration (MIC) is the critical factor, constant rate IV infusion protocols may be used to maintain serum and tissue concentrations above MIC.

The World Health Organization (WHO) has designated cefazolin as a Highly Important antimicrobial for human medicine.[1] The Office International des Epizooties (OIE) has designated cefazolin as a Veterinary Highly Important Antimicrobial (VHIA) Agent in bovine, caprine, and ovine species.[2]

Pharmacology/Actions

Cephalosporins are considered time dependent and bactericidal against susceptible bacteria, and they act by inhibiting mucopeptide synthesis in the cell wall, which results in a defective barrier and an osmotically unstable spheroplast. The exact mechanism for this effect has not been definitively determined, but beta-lactam antibiotics have been shown to bind to several enzymes (eg, carboxypeptidases, transpeptidases, endopeptidases) in the bacterial cytoplasmic membrane that are involved in cell wall synthesis. The different affinities that various beta-lactam antibiotics have for these enzymes (also known as penicillin-binding proteins [PBPs]) help explain the differences in spectrums of activity of these drugs that are not explained by the influence of beta-lactamases. Like other beta-lactam antibiotics, cephalosporins are generally considered to be more effective against actively growing bacteria.

Cefazolin is a first-generation cephalosporin that exhibits activity against most gram-positive pathogens (excluding enterococci) and variable to poor coverage against most gram-negative pathogens. Cephalosporins are active in vitro against streptococci, staphylococci, *Proteus mirabilis,* and some strains of *Escherichia coli, Klebsiella* spp, *Actinobacillus* spp, and *Pasteurella* spp. With the exception of *Bacteroides fragilis*, most anaerobes are susceptible to first-generation cephalosporins. Bacterial resistance is of increasing concern, particularly with methicillin-resistant staphylococci and extended spectrum beta-lactamase (ESBL) producing Enterobacterales. Cefazolin is inactive against *Enterococcus* spp, *Pseudomonas* spp, *Rickettsia* spp, mycobacteria, *Mycoplasma* spp, fungi, and viruses.

Although the spectrum of activity among first-generation cephalosporins are similar, there may be differences in their individual MICs. Plasma concentrations of less than or equal to 2 µg/mL are believed to be effective for most bacteria not inherently resistant to the drug or those that have acquired resistance. For bactericidal activity, cephalosporin levels should exceed bacterial MIC for at least 40% of the dose interval for staphylococcal infections and ≈60% of the dose interval for streptococcal infections.[3]

Pharmacokinetics

Cefazolin is not appreciably absorbed after oral administration and must be given parenterally to achieve therapeutic serum concentrations; it is excreted unchanged by the kidneys into the urine. Elimination half-life may be significantly prolonged in patients with severely diminished renal function.

In dogs, peak concentrations occur ≈30 to 90 minutes after IM administration. The apparent volume of distribution at steady state (Vd_{ss}) is 700 mL/kg, and total body clearance is 10.4 mL/kg/minute. Elimination half-life is ≈45 to 70 minutes.[4,5] In one study of dogs undergoing gonadectomy and receiving 25 mg/kg IV, cefazolin Vd_{ss} and clearance were 400 mL/kg and 150 mL/kg/hour; half-life was 3 hours.[6] Approximately 64% of clearance can be attributed to renal tubular secretion. Cefazolin is ≈16% to 28% bound to plasma proteins in dogs. Penetration into pancreatic tissue is poor. Cefazolin concentration in interstitial fluid remained above 4 µg/mL for 4 hours after a single dose of 22 mg/kg IV was administered to beagles and for 5 hours after 22 mg/kg IV and 22 mg/kg IM (combined, 44 mg/kg) were administered to beagles.[4] Administration of 22 mg/kg IV every 2 hours during surgery was predicted to maintain serum cefazolin concentrations at least 10 times MIC for 3 to 4 hours; 8 mg/kg IV every hour during surgery was also suggested as an option.[5] A concentration of cefazolin (ie, 4 µg/mL) in the surgical wound was maintained for longer than 12 hours by administering cefazolin (20 mg/kg IV) at the beginning of surgery and repeating administration via SC injection 6 hours later.[7]

In cats given a single dose of cefazolin 20 mg/kg IV, peak plasma concentration (initial peak plasma concentration [$Cp_{(0)}$]) was 134.8 µg/mL, Vd_{ss} was 290 mL/kg, and elimination half-life was 1.2 hours. Eighty-four percent of the dose was eliminated within 6 hours after administration. Tissue:plasma concentration ratios ranged from 0.18 to 0.58, and plasma concentration remained above 2 µg/mL for up to 4 hours in all cats.[8]

In horses, the apparent Vd_{ss} is 190 mL/kg; total body clearance is 5.51 mL/kg/minute with a serum elimination half-life of 38 minutes when given IV and 84 minutes after IM injection (gluteal muscles). Bioavailability after IM administration is ≈80%. Cefazolin is about 4% to 8% bound to equine plasma proteins.[9] Probenecid administration is expected to alter the kinetics of cefazolin because of the significant tubular secretion of cefazolin. One study performed in horses[10] did not show any effect from probenecid, but the authors concluded that the dosage of probenecid used in the study may have been subtherapeutic in this species.

In calves, the volume of distribution is 165 mL/kg, with a terminal elimination half-life of 49 to 99 minutes after IM administration.[11]

Contraindications/Precautions/Warnings

Cephalosporins are contraindicated in patients with a history of hypersensitivity to them. Because there may be cross-reactivity, cephalosporins should be used cautiously in patients with a documented hypersensitivity to other beta-lactam antibiotics (eg, penicillins, cefamycins, carbapenems). Cephalosporin use in small mammals (eg, hamsters, guinea pigs) may cause antibiotic-induced enterocolitis; a 25% mortality rate was reported in guinea pigs that received 100 mg IM every 6 hours for 5 days.

Cefazolin should be used with caution in patients with significant renal impairment; dose adjustment may be required. However, this guidance is likely only necessary for patients with severe renal disease, and there is no guidance for optimal dose and frequency changes in animals with renal disease. In humans with significant renal dysfunction, dosing frequency is decreased.[12]

Cefazolin can be easily confused with other cephalosporins. Consider writing orders and prescriptions using tall man lettering (ie, ceFAZolin).

Adverse Effects

Adverse effects with cephalosporins are usually mild and have a relatively low frequency of occurrence.

Hypersensitivity reactions unrelated to dosage can occur with these agents and can manifest as a rash, fever, eosinophilia, lymphadenopathy, or anaphylaxis. Use of cephalosporins in patients documented to be hypersensitive to penicillin-class antibiotics is controversial. In humans, it is estimated that up to 15% of patients that are hypersensitive to penicillins will also be hypersensitive to cephalosporins.[13] The incidence of cross-reactivity in veterinary patients is unknown.

Cephalosporins can cause pain at the injection site with IM administration, although this effect occurs less with cefazolin than with other related agents. Sterile abscesses or other severe local tissue reactions are possible but are much less common. Thrombophlebitis is also possible after IV administration of this drug class.

Although cephalosporins (particularly cephalothin) have the potential for causing nephrotoxicity at clinically used doses in patients with normal renal function, risks for the occurrence of this adverse effect appear minimal.

High doses or prolonged use have been rarely associated with neurotoxicity, neutropenia, agranulocytosis, thrombocytopenia, hepatitis, positive Coombs test, interstitial nephritis, and tubular necrosis. These effects, with the exception of tubular necrosis and neurotoxicity, have an immunologic component. Cefazolin may be more likely than other cephalosporins to cause seizures at very high doses. A case of status epilepticus was reported after cefazolin was mistakenly injected into the subarachnoid space of a dog undergoing lumbar myelography[14]; the dog in this case had no previous history of seizures.

Reproductive/Nursing Safety

Cephalosporins have been shown to cross the placenta and, although safety during pregnancy has not been firmly established, there are no documented teratogenic problems associated with these drugs. Cefazolin should only be used when the potential benefits outweigh the risks. In humans, cefazolin is compatible with pregnancy.[15] The pharmacokinetics of cefazolin are changed in pregnant women, resulting in a shorter half-life, a smaller area under the curve (AUC), and an increased clearance and volume of distribution.

Cefazolin is compatible with breastfeeding in humans, although it is distributed into milk and could potentially alter the neonatal gut flora. Cefazolin should be used with caution in nursing dams.

Overdose/Acute Toxicity

Cefazolin LD_{50} in rats and mice is greater than 2000 mg/kg.[16] Cephalosporin overdoses are unlikely to cause significant problems, but other effects are possible (see ***Adverse Effects***). Very high doses given rapidly IV can cause seizures.

For patients that have experienced or are suspected to have experienced an overdose, consultation with a 24-hour poison control center specializing in providing veterinary-specific information is recommended. For general information related to overdose and toxin exposures, as well as contact information for poison control centers, refer to ***Appendix***.

Drug Interactions

The following drug interactions with cefazolin either have been reported or are theoretical in humans or animals and may be of significance in veterinary patients. Unless otherwise noted, use together is not necessarily contraindicated, but the potential risks must be weighed and additional monitoring performed when appropriate.

- **Aminoglycosides and Other Nephrotoxic Drugs**: Concurrent use of parenteral aminoglycosides or other nephrotoxic drugs (eg, **amphotericin B, furosemide**) with cephalosporins is somewhat controversial. Cephalosporins could potentially cause additive nephrotoxicity when used with these drugs, but this interaction has only been well-documented with cephaloridine (no longer marketed). Caution is advised when using these drug combinations.
- **Probenecid**: Competitively blocks the tubular secretion of most cephalosporins, thereby increasing serum levels and serum half-lives
- **Vitamin K Antagonists** (eg, **warfarin**): Cephalosporins may enhance the anticoagulant effects of vitamin K antagonists.

Laboratory Considerations

- Cephalosporins may cause false-positive **urine glucose determinations** when used with cupric sulfate solution (eg, Benedict's solution, Fehling's solution, *Clinitest®*). Tests using glucose oxidase (eg, *Tes-Tape®, Clinistix®*) are not affected by cephalosporins.
- When the Jaffe reaction is used to measure **serum or urine creatinine**, high-dose cefazolin may cause falsely elevated values.
- Cephalosporins may also cause falsely elevated **17-ketosteroid** values in urine.
- In humans, particularly those with azotemia, cephalosporins have caused a false-positive direct **Coombs test**.
- Cephalosporins may falsely decrease serum **albumin** measurements.
- Prothrombin time may be increased.

Dosages

NOTES:

1. If injecting IM, the drug must be injected into a large muscle mass.
2. IV injections should be given slowly (ie, over 3 to 5 minutes).

DOGS/CATS:

Surgical prophylaxis (extra-label): 20 – 22 mg/kg IV slowly 30 to 60 minutes prior to incision and repeated every 90 to 120 minutes until wound closure

Susceptible infections (extra-label):

a) 15 – 35 mg/kg IV (slowly), IM (large muscle), or SC every 6 to 8 hours. A typical dosage is 20 mg/kg every 8 hours.

b) **CRI**: Loading dose of 1.3 mg/kg IV slowly, then 1.2 mg/kg/hour IV[17]

c) **Empirical dosage adjustment for renal insufficiency in cats**: 20 mg/kg every 12 hours IV (slow), IM (large muscle), or SC if CrCL is greater than or equal to 0.15 mL/kg/minute (roughly a serum creatinine up to 5.5 mg/dL); decrease frequency to every 24 hours if CrCL is less than 0.15 mL/kg/minute (roughly a serum creatinine of 8.5 mg/dL or more).[18] **NOTE:** These recommendations have been extrapolated from human data.

HORSES:

Susceptible infections (extra-label): 25 mg/kg IV slowly or IM every 6 to 8 hours

REPTILES:

Susceptible infections in chelonians (extra-label): 22 mg/kg IM once daily (every 24 hours)[19]

Monitoring

- Culture and susceptibility testing as indicated by clinical condition
- Because cephalosporins usually have minimal toxicity associated with their use, monitoring for efficacy is often all that is required.
- For patients with diminished renal function, consider intensified monitoring of renal parameters (eg, BUN, creatinine, urinalysis).

Chemistry/Synonyms

Commercial cefazolin dosage forms contain cefazolin sodium. Cefazolin sodium, an injectable, semisynthetic cephalosporin antibiotic, occurs as a practically odorless (or with faint odor), white to off-white, crystalline powder or lyophilized solid. It is freely soluble in water and very slightly soluble in alcohol. Each gram of the injection contains 2 mEq of sodium. After reconstitution, the solution for injection has a pH of 4.5 to 6 and a light-yellow to yellow color.

Cefazolin sodium may also be known as 46083, cefazolinum natricum, cephazolin sodium, or SKF-41558; many trade names are available.

Storage/Stability

Cefazolin sodium powder for injection and solutions for injection should be protected from light. The powder for injection should be stored at room temperature (20°C-25°C [68°F-77°F]) but may be exposed to 15°C to 30°C (59°F-86°F) temperatures; temperatures above 40°C (104°F) should be avoided. The frozen solution for injection should be stored at temperatures no higher than -20°C (-4°F). Once thawed (at room temperature or under refrigeration), the solution will be stable for 48 hours at room temperature or 30 days if refrigerated. The solution should not be refrozen.

After reconstitution, the solution will be stable for 24 hours if kept at room temperature or for 10 days if refrigerated (5°C [41°F]). If, after reconstitution, the solution is immediately frozen in the original container, the preparation will be stable for at least 12 weeks when stored at -20°C (-4°F).

Darkening of cefazolin powder or solution may occur but does not affect potency.

Compatibility/Compounding Considerations

Compatibility is dependent on factors such as pH, concentration, temperature, concomitant drugs, and diluent used; clinicians should consult specialized references or a hospital pharmacist for more specific information.

The following solutions are reportedly **compatible** with cefazolin: amino acids 4.25%/dextrose 25%, D_5W in Ringer's, D_5W in lactated Ringer's, D_5W in sodium chloride 0.2% to 0.9%, D_5W, $D_{10}W$, Ringer's injection, lactated Ringer's injection, and normal saline. The following drugs are reportedly **Y-site compatible** with cefazolin: amiodarone in normal saline (incompatible in dextrose), atracurium, calcium gluconate, famotidine, cyclophosphamide, dexmedetomidine, diltiazem, doxorubicin liposome, heparin, hetastarch, regular insulin, lidocaine, magnesium sulfate, midazolam, metronidazole, morphine, propofol, ranitidine, vancomycin (concentration-dependent), vecuronium, verapamil, and vitamin B-complex.

The following drugs or solutions are reportedly **incompatible** or only compatible in specific situations with cefazolin: amikacin, ascorbic acid injection, bleomycin, calcium chloride/gluconate, cimetidine, cisapride, erythromycin gluceptate, lidocaine, oxytetracycline, pentobarbital, polymyxin B, tetracycline, and vitamin B-complex with C injection.

Cefazolin beads prepared by addition to polymethyl methacrylate (PMMA) reduced bead compression strength but not bending strength.[20] Neither the heat of polymerization nor steam sterilization affected cefazolin activity in PMMA beads. Under experimental conditions, antibacterial effect was maintained for 9 days[21] and 30 days,[22] but a combination of cefazolin and amikacin did not maintain the antibacterial effect.[22] Approximately 35% of the total amount of cefazolin incorporated into PMMA beads was eluted over 15 days as compared with 95% of cefazolin in calcium sulfate (ie, plaster of Paris) beads. Freshly prepared cefazolin beads in calcium sulfate eluted more drug than stored beads, but storage conditions (eg, exposure to light, room temperature, refrigeration) over 6 months had little effect on drug elution.[23]

Dosage Forms/Regulatory Status

VETERINARY-LABELED PRODUCTS: NONE

HUMAN-LABELED PRODUCTS:

Cefazolin Sodium Powder for Injection: 500 mg, 1 g, 2 g, 10 g, and 20 g, in vials and piggyback vials; 100 g and 300 g in flex containers; generic; (Rx)

Cefazolin Sodium for Injection (Iso-osmotic IV infusion): 1 g in 4% dextrose and 2 g in 3% dextrose, 50 mL plastic containers, or duplex bags; generic; (Rx)

References

For the complete list of references, see **wiley.com/go/budde/plumb**

Cefepime

(***sef***-eh-pim) *Maxipime®*

Fourth-Generation Cephalosporin

Prescriber Highlights

- ► Injectable fourth-generation cephalosporin that is more active against some gram-negative and gram-positive bacteria than third-generation cephalosporins
- ► Potentially useful for treating neonatal foals and dogs with serious infections, where more commonly used antimicrobials are not options
- ► Limited clinical experience with this drug in veterinary medicine
- ► Adverse GI effects (eg, diarrhea) are possible. Injection site reactions have occurred following IM injections in dogs.

Uses/Indications

Cefepime is a semi-synthetic fourth-generation cephalosporin with enhanced activity against many gram-negative and gram-positive pathogens. It may be useful in treating severe infections in dogs or foals, particularly when aminoglycosides, fluoroquinolones, or other more commonly used beta-lactam drugs are ineffective or contraindicated. As with other fourth-generation cephalosporins, the use of this critically important human drug in veterinary patients should be limited to patients with culture and susceptibility testing results that indicate its use is necessary.

The World Health Organization (WHO) has designated cefepime as a Critically Important, Highest Priority antimicrobial for human medicine.[1]

Pharmacology/Actions

Cefepime, like other cephalosporins, is usually bactericidal and acts by inhibiting cell wall synthesis. It is classified as a fourth- generation cephalosporin, implying it has increased gram-negative activity (particularly against *Pseudomonas* spp) and better activity against many gram-positive bacteria than would be seen with the third-generation agents. Cefepime has activity against many gram-positive aerobes, including staphylococci, streptococci, and Enterobacteriaceae (eg, *Escherichia coli, Enterobacter* spp). Cefepime has good activity against many gram-negative bacteria and has better activity (than other cephalosporins) against many Enterobacteriaceae, including *Enterobacter* spp, *E coli*, *Proteus* spp, and *Klebsiella* spp. It is considered an antipseudomonal cephalosporin, with activity against *Pseudomonas* spp being similar to, or slightly less than, that of ceftazidime (a third-generation cephalosporin). It has limited activity against extended-spectrum beta-lactamase (ESBL) producing bacteria.

Cefepime also has activity against certain atypical organisms like *Mycobacterium avium-intracellulare* complex but is not a suitable antibiotic for monotherapy.

Some anaerobes are susceptible to cefepime; however, *Bacteroides* spp is typically resistant.

Cefepime does not readily induce beta-lactamases and is highly resistant to hydrolysis by them. Cefepime is ineffective against enterococci, *Listeria monocytogenes,* and methicillin-resistant staphylococci.

Pharmacokinetics

Cefepime is not absorbed from the GI tract and must be administered parenterally. In dogs, cefepime's volume of distribution at steady state is ≈0.14 L/kg, elimination half-life is about 1.1 hours, and clearance is about 0.13 L/kg/hour.[2]

In neonatal foals, cefepime's volume of distribution at steady state is ≈0.18 L/kg, elimination half-life is about 1.65 hours, and clearance is about 0.08 L/kg/hour.[2]

In calves, the volume of distribution at steady state is ≈0.21 L/kg, elimination half-life is about 2.38 hours, and clearance is about 1.1 mL/minute/kg. Cefepime has a bioavailability of 95.7% following IM administration in this species.[3]

In ewes, the volume of distribution at steady state is ≈0.32 L/kg, and the elimination half-life is about 1.76 hours. Clearance is 2.37 mL/minute/kg. Cefepime has a bioavailability of 86.8% after IM administration.[4]

In humans, the volume of distribution is about 18 L in adults; 20% of the drug is bound to plasma proteins.[5] The elimination half-life is about 2 hours. Approximately 85% of a dose is excreted unchanged into the urine; less than 1% is metabolized.

Contraindications/Precautions/Warnings

No specific information is available regarding contraindications in veterinary patients. Cefepime is contraindicated in human patients that are hypersensitive to it or other cephalosporins. Dosage adjustment is recommended in humans with severe renal impairment.

Cefepime can be easily confused with other cephalosporins. Consider writing orders and prescriptions using tall man lettering: cefePIME.

Adverse Effects

As use of cefepime in animals has been very limited, a comprehensive adverse effect profile has not been determined.

There are some reports of dogs or foals having loose stools or diarrhea after receiving cefepime.[2] IM injections may be painful (may be alleviated by combining with lidocaine 1% as diluent). Lameness and injection site edema were observed in dogs receiving IM cefepime.[6]

Human patients generally tolerate cefepime well. Injection site inflammation and rashes occur in ≈1% of treated patients.[5] GI effects (eg, dyspepsia, diarrhea) occur in less than 1% of treated patients. Hypersensitivity reactions, including anaphylaxis, are possible. In humans, it is estimated that up to 15% of patients who are hypersensitive to penicillins will also be hypersensitive to cephalosporins.[7] Rarely, patients with renal dysfunction who have received cefepime without any dosage adjustments will develop neurologic effects (see ***Overdose/Acute Toxicity*** section).

Reproductive/Nursing Safety

Studies performed in pregnant mice, rats, and rabbits demonstrated no overt fetal harm.[5]

Cefepime enters maternal milk in low concentrations, and alteration to gut microbiome is possible in the nursing offspring with resultant diarrhea. It is considered compatible with breastfeeding in pregnant women.[8]

Because safety has not been established in animals, this drug should only be used when the maternal benefits outweigh the potential risks to offspring.

Overdose/Acute Toxicity

No specific information was located regarding acute toxicity in veterinary patients. Acute oral cephalosporin overdoses are unlikely to cause significant problems other than GI distress, but other, more serious effects are possible. See ***Adverse Effects***.

Humans with impaired renal function receiving inadvertent overdoses have developed encephalopathy, seizures, and neuromuscular excitability.

For patients that have experienced or are suspected to have experienced an overdose, consultation with a 24-hour poison consultation center specializing in providing veterinary-specific information is recommended. For general information related to overdose and toxin exposures, as well as contact information for poison control centers, refer to ***Appendix.***

Drug Interactions

The following drug interactions have either been reported or are theoretical in humans or animals receiving cefepime and may be of significance in veterinary patients. Unless otherwise noted, use together is not necessarily contraindicated, but weigh the potential risks and perform additional monitoring when appropriate.

- **AMINOGLYCOSIDES**: Potential for increased risk for nephrotoxicity; monitor renal function
- **PROBENECID**: Probenecid may increase the serum concentration of cephalosporins.
- **VITAMIN K ANTAGONISTS** (eg, **warfarin**): Cephalosporins may increase the concentration of vitamin K antagonists.

Laboratory Considerations

- Cefepime may cause false-positive **urine glucose determinations** when using the copper reduction method (Benedict's solution, Fehling's solution, *Clinitest®*); tests utilizing glucose oxidase (*Tes-Tape®*, *Clinistix®*) are not affected by cephalosporins.
- In humans, particularly with azotemia, cephalosporins have caused a false-positive direct **Coombs test.**

Dosages

DOGS/CATS:

Susceptible infections (extra-label): Based on pharmacokinetic studies, 40 mg/kg IV over 30 minutes every 6 hours has been recommended for dogs.[2] Anecdotal sources state that it can be given to dogs and cats at 50 mg/kg IM or IV every 8 hours or as a CRI using 1.4 mg/kg IV as a loading dose, followed by 1.1 mg/kg/hour IV CRI.

HORSES:

Susceptible gram-negative infections in foals: 11 mg/kg IV over 30 minutes every 8 hours.[2,9] Its use has been limited primarily to neonates for whom aminoglycoside cannot be used.

Monitoring

- Clinical efficacy
- Patients with renal insufficiency should have periodic renal function monitored.

Client Information

- This medicine should only be given by veterinary professionals.

Chemistry/Synonyms

Cefepime HCl occurs as a white to off-white, non-hygroscopic powder that is freely soluble in water.

Cefepime may also be known as BMY-28142, cefepimi, or cefepima; internationally registered trade names include *Axepime®*, *Biopime®*, *Cefepen®*, *Ceficad®*, *Cemax®*, *Cepim®*, *Cepimix®*, *Forpar®*, *Maxcef®*, *Maxipime®*, and *Maxil®*.

Storage/Stability

Store the powder for injection and *Duplex®* containers between 20°C and 25°C (68°F-77°F), with excursions to 15°C to 30°C (59°F-86°F) allowed by some manufacturers. Protect the powder from light. Some manufacturers store the powder between 2°C and 25°C (46°F-77°F). Refer to package insert for further information.

Generally, the solution is stable for up 24 hours at room temperature and up to 7 days if kept refrigerated.

Store *GALAXY®* containers at or below -20°C (-4°F). Once thawed, the solution is stable for 7 days under refrigeration or 24 hours at room temperature.

Compatibility/Compounding Considerations

It is possible to reconstitute and administer cefepime with several diluents, including normal saline and D_5W. Drugs that may be admixed with cefepime include amikacin (but not gentamicin or tobramycin), ampicillin up to 40 mg/mL, and clindamycin. These admixtures have varying times at which they remain stable. Compatibility is dependent on factors such as pH, concentration, temperature, and diluent used; specialized references or a hospital pharmacist should be consulted for more specific information.

Dosage Forms/Regulatory Status

VETERINARY-LABELED PRODUCTS: NONE

HUMAN-LABELED PRODUCTS:

Cefepime Powder for Injection: 500 mg, 1 g, and 2 g in 15 mL and 20 mL vials, ADD-Vantage vials, and 100 mL piggyback bottles; *Maxipime®*, generic; (Rx)

Cefepime Injection Solution: 1 g/50 mL, and 2 g/50 mL single-dose *DUPLEX®* containers with 5% dextrose; generic; (Rx)

References

For the complete list of references, see **wiley.com/go/budde/plumb**

Cefixime

(sef-***ix***-eem) *Suprax®*

Third-Generation Cephalosporin

Prescriber Highlights

- Oral third-generation cephalosporin that may be useful in dogs and cats, but that has a limited spectrum compared to most other third-generation cephalosporins
- Contraindications include hypersensitivity to cefixime or other cephalosporins.
- May need to adjust dose if the patient has renal disease
- Adverse effects primarily include GI distress, but hypersensitivity reactions are possible.

Uses/Indications

Cefixime is a third-generation cephalosporin with broad-spectrum antibacterial properties. Uses for cefixime are limited in veterinary medicine, in large part because of the availability of other approved third-generation cephalosporins. Its use should be reserved for those times when infections are caused by susceptible gram-negative organisms where oral treatment is indicated or when FDA-approved fluoroquinolones are either contraindicated or ineffective. Given the enhanced antibacterial spectrum and similarity in the adverse effects compared to other third-generation cephalosporins (eg, cefpodoxime), there would rarely be an indication for this antibiotic in veterinary patients.

The World Health Organization (WHO) has designated cefixime as a Critically Important, Highest Priority antimicrobial for human medicine.[1]

Pharmacology/Actions

Like other cephalosporins, cefixime inhibits bacterial cell wall synthesis. It is considered bactericidal. Cefixime's primary spectrum of activity is against gram-negative bacteria in the family Enterobacteriaceae, including *Escherichia* spp, *Proteus* spp, and *Klebsiella* spp. It is resistant to penicillinases but is inactivated by extended-spectrum beta-lactamases (EBSLs). Unlike veterinary third-generation cephalosporins, it has limited activity against gram-positive bacteria. Against streptococci, it is efficacious but has a limited effect. Cefixime is not efficacious against *Bordetella* spp, *Campylobacter* spp, *Enterobacter* spp, *Proteus* spp, *Pseudomonas aeruginosa,* and *Enterococcus* spp; it has limited efficacy against anaerobes. Because of the difference in the spectrum of cefixime compared to commonly tested third-generation cephalosporins (eg, ceftiofur, cefpodoxime, cefovecin), specific testing for cefixime susceptibility is required.

Pharmacokinetics

Cefixime is relatively rapidly absorbed after oral administration. Bioavailability in the dog is about 50%. Food may impede the rate, but not the extent, of absorption. The suspension may have a higher bioavailability than tablets. The drug is highly bound to plasma proteins in the dog (about 90%).[2] It is unknown if the drug penetrates into the CSF.

Elimination of cefixime is by both renal and nonrenal means, but serum half-lives are prolonged in patients with decreased renal function. In dogs, the elimination half-life is about 7 hours.[2]

Contraindications/Precautions/Warnings

Cefixime is contraindicated in patients hypersensitive to it or other cephalosporins. Because cefixime is excreted by the kidneys, dosages and/or dosing frequency may need to be adjusted in patients with significantly diminished renal function. Use with caution in patients with seizure disorders and patients allergic to penicillins.

Cefixime can be easily confused with other cephalosporins. Consider writing orders and prescriptions using tall man lettering: cefIXIME.

Adverse Effects

Cefixime use in animals has been limited, and a comprehensive adverse effect profile has not been determined. Adverse effects in dogs may include GI distress (eg, vomiting) and hypersensitivity reactions (eg, urticaria and pruritus, possibly fever).

In humans, it is estimated that up to 15% of patients who are hypersensitive to penicillins will also be hypersensitive to cephalosporins.[3]

Reproductive/Nursing Safety

Cefixime is has not been shown to be teratogenic but should only be used during pregnancy when indicated.[4] In humans, cefixime is considered compatible with pregnancy.[5] Cefixime is considered compatible with breastfeeding in humans.[5]

Because safety has not been established in animals, this drug should only be used when the maternal benefits outweigh the potential risks to offspring.

Overdose/Acute Toxicity

Cephalosporin overdoses are unlikely to cause significant problems, but other effects are possible. See ***Adverse Effects***.

Drug Interactions

The following drug interactions have either been reported or are theoretical in humans or animals receiving cefixime and may be of significance in veterinary patients. Unless otherwise noted, use together is not necessarily contraindicated, but weigh the potential risks and perform additional monitoring when appropriate.

- **Probenecid**: Competitively blocks the tubular secretion of most cephalosporins, thereby increasing serum levels and serum half-lives.
- **Salicylates** (eg, **aspirin**): May displace cefixime from plasma protein binding sites; the clinical significance is unclear.
- **Vitamin K Antagonists** (eg, **warfarin**): Cephalosporins may enhance the anticoagulant effects of vitamin K antagonists.

Laboratory Considerations

- Cefixime may cause false-positive **urine glucose determinations** when using cupric sulfate solution (Fehling's solution, Benedict's solution, *Clinitest*®). Tests utilizing glucose oxidase (*Tes-Tape*®, *Clinistix*®) are not affected.
- If using the nitroprusside test for determining **urinary ketones**, cefixime may cause false-positive results.
- May cause a false-positive direct **Coombs test**.
- When using the Jaffe reaction to measure serum or urine creatinine, cefixime in high doses may cause falsely elevated values.

Dosages

DOGS/CATS:

Susceptible infections (extra-label): Dosage recommendations range from 5 mg/kg PO once or twice daily for UTIs, to 10 – 12.5 mg/kg PO twice daily for systemic infections. As other third-generation cephalosporins (eg, cefpodoxime) have a superior antibacterial spectrum, there would rarely be an indication for this antibiotic in veterinary patients.

Monitoring

- Efficacy
- Adverse effects

Client Information

- This medicine works best when given without food. If your animal vomits or develops a lack of appetite while receiving the medicine, try administering with food.
- The most common side effects are diarrhea, vomiting, and loss of appetite.
- Be sure to give the medication to your animal as long as your veterinarian has prescribed, even if your animal seems better.
- Cephalosporin antibiotics have an odor that resembles cat urine.

Chemistry/Synonyms

Cefixime is an oral third-generation semisynthetic cephalosporin antibiotic. It is available commercially as the trihydrate. Cefixime occurs as a white to slightly yellowish-white crystalline powder with a characteristic odor and a pK_a of 3.73. Solubility in water is pH-dependent. At a pH of 3.2, 0.5 mg/mL is soluble and 18 mg/mL at pH 4.2. The oral suspension is strawberry flavored and, after reconstitution, has a pH of 2.5 to 4.2.

Cefixime may also be known as cefiximum, CL-284635, FK-027, FR-17027, and *Suprax*®; many internationally registered trade names are available.

Storage/Stability

Cefixime powder for suspension should be stored at room temperature (20°C-25°C [68°F-77°F]) in tight containers. The reconstituted oral suspension may be stored in the refrigerator or at room temperature and should be discarded after 14 days.

Compatibility/Compounding Considerations

No specific information noted.

Dosage Forms/Regulatory Status

VETERINARY-LABELED PRODUCTS: NONE

HUMAN-LABELED PRODUCTS:

Cefixime Oral Capsules: 400 mg; *Suprax*®; (Rx)

Cefixime Oral Chewable Tablets: 100 mg and 200 mg; *Suprax*®; (Rx)

Cefixime Powder for Oral Suspension: 100 mg/5 mL (20 mg/mL) in 50 mL, 75 mL, 100 mL; 200 mg/5 mL (40 mg/mL) in 25 mL, 37.5 mL, 50 mL, 75 mL, and 100 mL; 500 mg/5 mL (100 mg/mL) in 10 mL and 20 mL; *Suprax*®; 100 mg/5 mL (20 mg/mL) in 50 mL; 200 mg/5 mL (40 mg/mL) in 50 mL and 75 mL; generic; (Rx)

References

For the complete list of references, see **wiley.com/go/budde/plumb**

Cefotaxime

(sef-oh-***taks***-eem) *Claforan*®

Third-Generation Cephalosporin

Prescriber Highlights

- Third-generation cephalosporin for parenteral use
- May cause hypersensitivity reactions, granulocytopenia, or diarrhea
- Causes pain on IM injection; give IV over at least 3 to 5 minutes
- Extra-label use in food-producing animals is prohibited by the FDA.

Uses/Indications

In the United States, there are no cefotaxime products FDA-approved for veterinary species, but it has been used clinically in several species when an injectable third-generation cephalosporin may be indicated. Uses include treatment of susceptible bone, joint, and CNS infections, surgical prophylaxis, and as empiric therapy for bacterial sepsis.

The World Health Organization has designated cefotaxime as a Critically Important, Highest Priority antimicrobial for human medicine.[1] The Office International des Epizooties (OIE) has designated third-generation cephalosporins as Veterinary Critically Important Antimicrobial (VHIA) agents in veterinary medicine.[2]

Pharmacology/Actions

Cefotaxime is a third-generation injectable cephalosporin agent and, like other cephalosporins, it inhibits bacteria cell wall synthesis. It is bactericidal and time-dependent. Cefotaxime has a relatively wide spectrum of activity against both gram-positive and gram-negative bacteria. Although less active against *Staphylococcus* spp. than the first-generation agents, it still has significant activity against those and other gram-positive cocci, except *Enterococcus* spp. Cefotaxime, like the other third-generation agents, has extended coverage of gram-negative aerobes particularly in the Enterobacterales, including *Klebsiella* spp, *E coli*, and *Salmonella* spp. Many anaerobes are also susceptible to cefotaxime including strains of *Bacteroides fragilis*, *Clostridium* spp, *Fusobacterium* spp, *Peptococcus* spp, and *Peptostreptococcus* spp. Cefotaxime is as effective as penicillins for treating leptospirosis in humans. Like most other third-generation cephalosporins, cefotaxime is ineffective against *Serratia* spp, *Proteus vulgaris*, *Acinetobacter* spp, *Citrobacter* spp, and *Enterobacter* spp ("SPACE" organisms), as well as *Pseudomonas aeruginosa*, methicillin-resistant staphylococci, and extended spectrum beta-lactamase (ESBL)-producing Enterobacterales.

Because third-generation cephalosporins exhibit specific activities against bacteria, a 30 µg cefotaxime disk should be used when performing Kirby-Bauer disk susceptibility tests for this antibiotic.

Pharmacokinetics

Cefotaxime is not appreciably absorbed after oral administration and must be given parenterally to attain therapeutic serum concentrations. After administration, the drug is widely distributed in body tissues including bone, prostatic fluid (human), aqueous humor, bile, and ascitic and pleural fluids. Cefotaxime crosses the placenta and activity in amniotic fluid either equals or exceeds that in maternal serum. Cefotaxime distributes into milk in low concentrations. In humans, ≈13% to 40% of the drug is bound to plasma proteins.

Unlike the first-generation cephalosporins (and most second-generation agents), cefotaxime will enter the CSF in therapeutic concentrations (at high dosages) when the patient's meninges are inflamed.

Cefotaxime is partially metabolized by the liver to desacetylcefotaxime which exhibits some antibacterial activity. Desacetylcefotaxime is partially degraded to inactive metabolites by the liver. Cefotaxime and its metabolites are primarily excreted in the urine. Because tubular secretion is involved in the renal excretion of the drug, in several species probenecid has been demonstrated to prolong the serum half-life of cefotaxime.

Pharmacokinetic parameters in certain veterinary species follow: In dogs, the apparent volume of distribution at steady state is 480 mL/kg, and total body clearance is 10.5 mL/minute/kg after IV injection. Serum elimination half-lives of 45 minutes when given IV, 50 minutes after IM injection, and 103 minutes after SC injection have been noted. Bioavailability is about 87% after IM injection and ≈100% after SC injection.[3]

In cats, total body clearance is ≈3 mL/minute/kg after IV injection and the serum elimination half-life is about 1 hour. Bioavailability is about 93% to 98% after IM injection.

In foals, several pharmacokinetic studies have been performed with reported values for volume of distribution ranging from 0.29 L/kg to 4.2 L/kg. Half-life is around 1 hour, and clearance is ≈0.32 L/kg/hour.

Contraindications/Precautions/Warnings

Cephalosporins are contraindicated in patients with a history of hypersensitivity to them. Because there may be cross-reactivity, use cephalosporins cautiously in patients that have a documented hypersensitivity to other beta-lactam antibiotics (eg, penicillins, cefamycins, carbapenems).

Patients with significant renal impairment may need dosage adjustments.

In humans, rapid administration (less than 1 minute) via central line may cause potentially life-threatening arrhythmias.[4]

Cefotaxime can be easily confused with other cephalosporins. Consider writing orders and prescriptions using tall man letters: cefoTAXime.

Adverse Effects

Adverse effects with the cephalosporins are usually mild and have a relatively low frequency of occurrence. In humans, the most common adverse effects are pain and inflammation at the injection site, rash, diarrhea, nausea, and vomiting.[5]

Hypersensitivity reactions, unrelated to dosage, can occur with these agents and can manifest as rashes, fever, eosinophilia, lymphadenopathy, or anaphylaxis. The use of cephalosporins in patients documented to be hypersensitive to penicillin-class antibiotics is controversial. In humans, it is estimated that up to 15% of patients hypersensitive to penicillins will also be hypersensitive to cephalosporins.[6] The incidence of cross-reactivity in veterinary patients is unknown.

Cephalosporins can cause pain at the injection site when administered intramuscularly. Sterile abscesses or other severe local tissue reactions are also possible but much less common. Thrombophlebitis is also possible after IV administration of these drugs.

Because the cephalosporins may also alter gut flora, antibiotic-associated diarrhea can occur and allow the proliferation of resistant bacteria in the colon (superinfections).

High doses or very prolonged use has been associated with neurotoxicity, neutropenia, agranulocytosis, thrombocytopenia, hepatitis, positive Coombs test, interstitial nephritis, and tubular necrosis.[7] Except for tubular necrosis and neurotoxicity, these effects have an immunologic component.

Reproductive/Nursing Safety

Cephalosporins have been shown to cross the placenta. No evidence of embryotoxicity or fetotoxicity was observed in pregnant laboratory animals given cefotaxime at doses similar to those used clinically in humans.[4]

Cefotaxime is excreted in milk in small quantities.[4] Alteration of the intestinal biome in the offspring with resultant diarrhea is theoretically possible when using this antibiotic; however, in humans, cefotaxime is considered compatible with breast feeding.[8]

Because safety has not been established in animals, this drug should only be used when the maternal benefits outweigh the potential risks to offspring.

Overdose/Acute Toxicity

Cephalosporin overdoses are unlikely to cause significant problems, but other effects are possible (see ***Adverse Effects*** section).

For patients that have experienced or are suspected to have experienced an overdose, consultation with a 24-hour poison control center specializing in providing veterinary-specific information is recommended. For general information related to overdose and toxin exposures, as well as contact information for poison control centers, refer to ***Appendix.***

Drug Interactions

The following drug interactions either have been reported or are theoretical in humans or animals receiving cefotaxime and may be of significance in veterinary patients. Unless otherwise noted, use together is not necessarily contraindicated, but weigh the potential risks and perform additional monitoring when appropriate.

- **Aminoglycosides** (eg, **gentamicin**): Potential for increased risk of nephrotoxicity—monitor renal function; however, aminoglycosides and cephalosporins may have synergistic or additive actions against some gram-negative bacteria (Enterobacteriaceae).
- **Nephrotoxic Drugs** (eg, **amphotericin B, furosemide**): Concurrent use with cephalosporins could potentially cause additive nephrotoxicity, although this is somewhat controversial. Use together cautiously and monitor renal function closely.
- **Probenecid**: Competitively blocks the tubular secretion of most cephalosporins, thereby increasing serum levels and serum half-lives.
- **Vitamin K Antagonists**: Cephalosporins may enhance the anticoagulant effects of vitamin K antagonists (eg, warfarin).

Laboratory Considerations

- In humans, particularly with azotemia, cephalosporins have caused a false-positive direct **Coombs test**.
- Cephalosporins may cause falsely elevated **17-ketosteroid** values in urine.
- Cefotaxime like most other cephalosporins, may cause a **false-positive urine glucose determination** when using the cupric sulfate solution test (eg, *Clinitest*®, Benedict's solution or Fehling's solution).

Dosages

DOGS/CATS:

Susceptible infections (extra-label):

a) *Intermittent infusion*: Dosage recommendations vary widely, ranging from 20 – 80 mg/kg IV, SC, or IM every 6 to 12 hours. A common anecdotal dosage is 40 – 50 mg/kg IV, SC, or IM every 8 hours. Alternatively, 20 – 40 mg/kg IV, IM, SC every 6 to 12 hours has also been suggested. Use the higher end of the dosing range when treating meningitis.

b) *Continuous-rate infusion*: initial IV load of 3.2 mg/kg IV followed by 5 mg/kg/hour IV CRI

HORSES:

Susceptible infections (extra-label):

a) **Neonatal foals**: 40 mg/kg IV every 6 hours.[9-11] Alternatively, based on a pharmacokinetic study, foals were given a 40 mg/kg IV bolus followed by a CRI 120 mg/kg/day (5 mg/kg/hour) IV the first day. On subsequent days foals were given a CRI 160 mg/kg/day (6.66 mg/kg/hour) IV.[12]

b) **Foals**: As regional perfusion for adjunctive treatment of septic arthritis: 1 g cefotaxime in 20 mL of saline. Tourniquet above and below joint. Inject antibiotic solution and leave tourniquet in place for 20 minutes.[13]

BIRDS:

Susceptible infections (extra-label):

a) 50 – 100 mg/kg IM or IV every 8 to 12 hours[14]

b) **Ratites** (young birds): 25 mg/kg IM 3 times daily[15]

c) **Bacterial infections, including bacterial hepatitis**: 75 – 100 mg/kg IM or IV every 4 to 8 hours[16,17]

REPTILES:

Susceptible infections (extra-label):

a) 20 – 40 mg/kg IM once daily for 7 to 14 days[18]

b) Chelonians: 20 – 40 mg/kg IM once daily (every 24 hours)[19]

c) Nebulized antibiotic therapy: 100 mg/animal (NOT mg/kg) twice daily[20]

Monitoring

- Efficacy: culture and susceptibility as indicated by underlying condition being treated
- Patients with diminished renal function may require intensified renal monitoring.

Chemistry/Synonyms

A semisynthetic, third-generation aminothiazolyl cephalosporin, cefotaxime sodium occurs as an odorless, white to off-white crystalline powder with a pK_a of 3.4. It is sparingly soluble in water and slightly soluble in alcohol. Potency of cefotaxime sodium is expressed in terms of cefotaxime. One gram of cefotaxime (sodium) contains 2.2 mEq of sodium.

Cefotaxime sodium may also be known as cefotaximum natricum, CTX, HR-756, RU-24756 and *Claforan*®; many other trade names are available internationally.

Storage/Stability

Cefotaxime sodium sterile powder for injection should be stored at 20°C to 25°C (68°F-77°F) and protected from light. Depending on storage conditions, the powder or solutions may darken which may indicate a loss in potency. Cefotaxime is not stable in solutions with pH is greater than 7.5 (sodium bicarbonate). The reconstituted solution is stable for 12 to 24 hours below 22°C (71.6°F) (concentration dependent), 7 to 10 days when stored below 5°C (41°F) in original container and 13 weeks when frozen.

Compatibility/Compounding Considerations

Compatibility is dependent upon factors such as pH, concentration, temperature, and diluent used; consult specialized references or a hospital pharmacist for more specific information. All commonly used IV fluids and the following drugs are reportedly **compatible** with cefotaxime: clindamycin, metronidazole, and verapamil.

Do not mix cefotaxime with aminoglycosides.

Dosage Forms/Regulatory Status

VETERINARY-LABELED PRODUCTS: NONE

HUMAN-LABELED PRODUCTS:

Cefotaxime Sodium Powder for Injection: 500 mg, 1 g, 2 g, and 10 g in vials, bottles, infusion bottles and *ADD-Vantage* system vials; *Claforan*®, generic; (Rx)

References

For the complete list of references, see **wiley.com/go/budde/plumb**

Cefotetan

(***sef***-oh-tee-tan) *Cefotan*®

Second-Generation Cephalosporin (cephamycin)

Prescriber Highlights

- Second-generation parenteral cephalosporin (cephamycin) similar to cefoxitin, with more activity against gram-negative bacteria than first- and other second-generation cephalosporins
- Pharmacokinetic profile of cefotetan is better (and it may be more effective against *Escherichia coli* in dogs) than cefoxitin, although cefotetan is rarely used in animals and clinical data are lacking.
- Contraindications include hypersensitivity to cefotetan or cephalosporins.
- Adverse effects are unlikely; however, cefotetan could increase risk for bruising or bleeding.
- If severe renal dysfunction occurs with cefotetan, may need to increase time between doses.

Uses/Indications

Cefotetan is similar to second-generation cephalosporins, with relatively broad-spectrum activity against gram-positive and gram-negative bacteria. It may be a reasonable choice for treating serious infections caused by susceptible bacteria, including *Escherichia coli* or anaerobes. It appears to be well tolerated in small animals and may be given less frequently than cefoxitin. Although extended spectrum beta-lactamase (ESBL)-producing bacteria are often susceptible to cefotetan in vitro, evidence of clinical efficacy is lacking and cephamycins are not recommended.

The World Health Organization (WHO) has designated cefotetan as a Highly Important antimicrobial for human medicine.[1]

Pharmacology/Actions

Cefotetan, like cefoxitin, is a cephamycin antimicrobial and classified with second-generation cephalosporins. It has most of the same properties of second-generation cephalosporins except it is not affected by extended spectrum beta-lactamases (ESBLs) in vitro. It is usually bactericidal and acts by inhibiting mucopeptide synthesis in the bacterial cell wall.

As with second-generation cephalosporins, cefotetan has activity against gram-positive and gram-negative bacteria, with enhanced gram-negative activity compared with first-generation cephalosporins. Cefotetan's in vitro activity against aerobes include *Escherichia coli, Proteus* spp, *Klebsiella* spp, *Salmonella* spp, *Staphylococcus* spp, and *Streptococcus* spp. It also has efficacy against most anaerobes, including *Actinomyces* spp, *Clostridium* spp, *Propionibacterium* spp, and many strains of *Bacteroides* spp. Cefotetan is generally ineffective against *Pseudomonas aeruginosa* and enterococci, as well as methicillin-resistant staphylococci. Because in vitro susceptibility to cefotetan is rarely tested, cefoxitin susceptibility is used for clinical decision making.

Pharmacokinetics

Cefotetan is not appreciably absorbed after oral administration and must be given parenterally to achieve therapeutic serum concentrations. The drug is well distributed into most tissues, but it only has limited penetration into the CSF. Cefotetan is primarily excreted unchanged by the kidneys into the urine via both glomerular filtration (primarily) and tubular secretion. Elimination half-lives may be significantly prolonged in patients with severely diminished renal function.

Contraindications/Precautions/Warnings

Cephamycins are contraindicated in patients that have a history of hypersensitivity to them. Because there may be cross-reactivity, use cephamycins cautiously in patients that are documented to be hypersensitive to other beta-lactam antibiotics (eg, penicillins, cephalosporins, or carbapenems). Cefotetan may prolong prothrombin time and increase the risk for bruising or bleeding.

Cefotetan can be easily confused with other cephalosporins. Consider writing orders and prescriptions using tall man lettering: cefoTEtan.

Adverse Effects

There is little information on the adverse effect profile of this medication in veterinary species, but it appears to be well tolerated. In humans, less than 5% of patients report adverse effects.[2] Because cefotetan contains an N-methylthiotetrazole side chain (like cefoperazone), it may have a greater tendency to cause hematologic effects (eg, hypoprothrombinemia) or disulfiram-like reactions (eg, vomiting) than other parenteral cephalosporins.

Hypersensitivity reactions unrelated to dose can occur with these agents and can manifest as rashes, fever, eosinophilia, lymphadenopathy, or full-blown anaphylaxis. The use of cephalosporins in patients that are documented to be hypersensitive to penicillin-class antibiotics is controversial. In humans, it is estimated that up to 15% of patients who are hypersensitive to penicillins will also be hypersensitive to cephalosporins.[3] The incidence of cross-reactivity in veterinary patients is unknown.

Cephalosporins can cause pain at the injection site when they are administered IM. Sterile abscesses or other severe local tissue reactions are also possible but are less common. Thrombophlebitis is also possible after IV administration of these drugs.

Even when they are administered parenterally, cephalosporins may alter the gut microbiome, resulting in antibiotic-associated diarrhea or the proliferation of resistant bacteria in the colon (superinfections).

Although cephalosporins (particularly cephalothin) have the potential for causing nephrotoxicity at clinically used doses in patients with normal renal function, the risks for the occurrence of this adverse effect appear minimal. High doses or very prolonged use has been associated with neurotoxicity, neutropenia, agranulocytosis, thrombocytopenia, hepatitis, positive Coombs test, interstitial nephritis, and tubular necrosis. Except for tubular necrosis and neurotoxicity, these effects have an immunologic component.

Reproductive/Nursing Safety

Cefotetan did not demonstrate impaired fertility or harm to the fetus when administered to laboratory animals.[2,4] In humans, cefotetan is considered compatible with pregnancy.

Cefotetan enters maternal milk in low concentrations, and alteration to gut microbiome is possible in the nursing offspring with resultant diarrhea. Cefotetan is considered compatible with breastfeeding in humans.[5]

Because safety has not been established in animals, this drug should only be used when the maternal benefits outweigh the potential risks to offspring.

Overdose/Acute Toxicity

Cephalosporin overdoses are unlikely to cause significant problems. In mice, the LD_{50} is 5 to 6.4 grams/kg IV, and in rats it is 6.8 to 8.5 grams/kg IV.[4] Cefotetan is unlikely to cause adverse effects, unless it is massively or chronically overdosed; seizures are possible. Treat these overdoses supportively.

For patients that have experienced or are suspected to have experienced an overdose, consultation with a 24-hour poison control center specializing in providing veterinary-specific information is recommended. For general information related to overdose and toxin exposures, as well as contact information for poison control centers, refer to the ***Appendix***.

Drug Interactions

The following drug interactions either have been reported or are theoretical in humans or animals receiving cefotetan and may be of significance in veterinary patients. Unless otherwise noted, use together is not necessarily contraindicated, but weigh the potential risks and perform additional monitoring when appropriate.

- **ALCOHOL** (eg, **ethylene glycol**): A disulfiram reaction is possible.
- **AMINOGLYCOSIDES/NEPHROTOXIC DRUGS**: The concurrent use of parenteral aminoglycosides or other nephrotoxic drugs (eg, **amphotericin B**) with cephalosporins is somewhat controversial. Potentially, cephalosporins could cause additive nephrotoxicity when used with these drugs, but this interaction has only been well documented with cephaloridine (no longer marketed). In vitro studies have demonstrated that cephalosporins can have synergistic or additive activity against certain bacteria when used with aminoglycosides, but they should not be mixed together (administer separately).
- **PROBENECID**: May increase the serum concentration of cephalosporins
- **VITAMIN K ANTAGONISTS** (eg, **warfarin**): Cephalosporins may enhance the anticoagulant effects of vitamin K antagonists.

Laboratory Considerations

- Cefotetan may cause false-positive **urine glucose determinations** when using cupric sulfate solution (Benedict's solution, *Clinitest®*, Fehling's solution). Tests utilizing glucose oxidase (*Tes-Tape®*, *Clinistix®*) are not affected.
- When using the Jaffe reaction to measure **serum or urine creatinine**, cefotetan in high doses may cause falsely elevated values.
- In humans, particularly with azotemia, cephalosporins have caused a false-positive direct **Coombs test**.
- Cephalosporins may also cause falsely elevated **17-ketosteroid** values in urine.

Dosages

DOGS/CATS:

Susceptible infections (extra-label):

a) 30 mg/kg IV every 8 hours or 30 mg/kg SC every 12 hours[6]

b) Empirical dosage adjustment for renal insufficiency: If creatinine clearance (CrCl) is 0.15 to 0.4 mL/kg/minute (in cats, roughly a serum creatinine between 4.9 – 5.5 mg/dL [433 – 486 µmol/L]) consider dosing once daily (every 24 hours); if CrCl is less than 0.15 mL/kg/minute (in cats, roughly a serum creatinine of 8.5 mg/dL [751 µmol/L]), consider dosing every 48 hours.[7]

Surgical (GI surgery) prophylaxis (extra-label): 30 mg/kg IV 30 to 60 minutes prior to incision. Intraoperative re-dosing should not be required because of the long half-life of the drug.

Monitoring

- Because cephalosporins usually have minimal toxicity associated with their use, monitoring for efficacy is usually all that is required.
- Patients with diminished renal function may require intensified renal monitoring and decreased dosage frequency. Serum levels and therapeutic drug monitoring are not routinely done with these agents.

Chemistry/Synonyms

A semisynthetic cephamycin similar to cefoxitin, cefotetan disodium occurs as a white to pale yellow, lyophilized powder. It is very soluble in water and alcohol. The injection contains ≈3.5 mEq of sodium per gram of cefotetan and after reconstitution has a pH of 4 to 6.5.

Cefotetan Disodium may also be known as ICI-156834, YM-09330, *Apacef*, *Apatef*, *Cefotan*®, *Ceftenon*®, *Cepan*®, *Darvilen*®, or *Yamatetan*®.

Storage/Stability

The sterile powder for injection should be stored at 20°C to 25°C (68°F-77°F) and protected from light. A darkening of the powder with time does not indicate lessened potency. After reconstituting with sterile water for injection, the resultant solution is stable for 24 hours at 25°C (77°F), 96 hours at 5°C (21°F), and 7 days at -20°C (-4°F).

Dosage Forms/Regulatory Status

VETERINARY-LABELED PRODUCTS: NONE

HUMAN-LABELED PRODUCTS:

Cefotetan Disodium Powder for Solution: 1 g, 2 g, and 10 g in 10 mL and 20 mL vials, and 1 g and 2 g premixed bags (with dextrose); generic; (Rx)

References

For the complete list of references, see **wiley.com/go/budde/plumb**

Cefovecin

(sef-oh-**vee**-sin) *Convenia*®

Third-generation Cephalosporin

Prescriber Highlights

- Long-acting injectable cephalosporin labeled in the United States for treatment of skin infections in dogs and cats. Labeled in the United Kingdom, European Union, and Australia as adjunctive treatment for periodontal disease and UTIs.
- Primary benefit is for patients with owners that have difficulty adhering to an oral dosing regimen or when oral antibiotics are not tolerated or absorbed.
- Cefovecin use should be carefully considered as third-generation cephalosporins are critically important for human medicine.
- Usually well tolerated
- Effectiveness against systemic (non-UTI) *Escherichia* coli or other Enterobacterales (eg *Enterobacter* spp) infections is limited because of high protein binding and the inability to reach adequate drug concentrations for an adequate period of time.

Uses/Indications

In the United States, cefovecin is FDA-approved to treat canine skin infections (secondary superficial pyoderma, abscesses, wounds) caused by susceptible strains of *Staphylococcus intermedius* and *Streptococcus canis* (group G) and feline skin infections (wounds, abscesses) caused by susceptible strains of *Pasteurella multocida*.[1] A review of antibiotic efficacy for the treatment of superficial and deep pyoderma in dogs found a good level of evidence for high efficacy when treating superficial pyoderma and a fair level of evidence for moderate to high efficacy when treating deep pyoderma.[2] Cefovecin's long half-life in dogs and cats allows for a single dose or extended dosing intervals (determined by organism susceptibility and minimum inhibitory concentration [MIC]) for treatment of a variety of other infections.

In other countries, cefovecin is labeled for use in dogs to treat skin and soft tissue infections caused by *S pseudintermedius*, beta-hemolytic streptococci, *Escherichia coli*, and/or *P multocida*[3-5]; for treatment of UTI associated with *E coli* and/or *Proteus* spp,[3,4] and/or *S intermedius*[1] [1]; and as an adjunctive treatment for mechanical or surgical periodontal therapy for severe infections of the gingival and periodontal tissues associated with *Porphyromonas* spp and *Prevotella* spp.[3-5] In cats, cefovecin is also labeled for treatment of skin infections caused by *P multocida*, *Fusobacterium* spp, *Bacteroides* spp, *Prevotella oralis*, beta-hemolytic streptococci, and/or *S pseudintermedius*, and treatment of UTIs associated with *E coli*.[3,4] The Working Group of the International Society for Companion Animal Infectious Diseases recommended that cefovecin be used for treating UTIs in dogs and cats *only* when oral treatment is problematic.[6]

A study evaluating treatment of upper respiratory tract infections in cats found that single-dose cefovecin appeared to be less effective than oral amoxicillin/clavulanic acid and oral doxycycline.[7] It has been shown that 2 doses of cefovecin, given 14 days apart, appears to be as effective as 4 weeks of therapy with amoxicillin or doxycycline for the treatment of canine Lyme borreliosis.[8,9]

Cefovecin, in combination with diligent supportive therapies (eg, SC fluid therapy, antiemetics) and monitoring, may be a considered for outpatient treatment of canine parvoviral enteritis when hospitalization is not an option.[10]

The World Health Organization (WHO) has designated cefovecin as a Critically Important, Highest Priority antimicrobial for human medicine.[11] The World Organisation for Animal Health (OIE) classifies third-generation cephalosporins as a Veterinary Critically Important Antimicrobial Agent (VCIA).[12]

Pharmacology/Actions

Cefovecin is a third-generation cephalosporin antibiotic, but it is not as active against gram-negative organisms as other antibiotics of this class (eg, cefotaxime, ceftazidime). Cefovecin's mechanism of action in susceptible bacteria, like other beta-lactams, is to bind to and disrupt the actions of bacterial penicillin-binding proteins (ie, transpeptidase and carboxypeptidase), thereby interfering with bacterial cell wall synthesis and resulting in bactericidal activity.[1]

Cefovecin is not active against *Pseudomonas* spp, methicillin-resistant staphylococci, enterococci, or *Bordetella bronchiseptica*.[3] Extrapolation of results of other third-generation cephalosporins should be avoided because of the reduced activity of cefovecin against gram-negative organisms (eg, susceptibility to cefotaxime does not necessarily indicate susceptibility to cefovecin). Cefovecin's effectiveness against systemic (non-UTI) *Escherichia coli* or other Enterobacterales (eg, *Enterobacter* spp) is limited because the drug's extensive protein binding result in the inability to reach adequate free drug concentrations for an adequate period of time for these organisms.[12]

Cefovecin rapidly cleared spirochetes and reduced antibodies in dogs with experimentally induced Lyme borreliosis.[8]

Pharmacokinetics

Cefovecin is completely absorbed after SC injection in dogs and cats. Peak concentrations occur ≈6 hours after administration in dogs and ≈2 hours after administration in cats. Cefovecin is highly bound to plasma proteins (dogs, 98.5%; cats, 99.8%) that slowly dissociate and give cefovecin a long elimination half-life. Because cefovecin exhibits nonlinear kinetics in dogs and cats, an increased dose does not proportionally increase the plasma concentration. The following additional pharmacokinetic values are listed on the product label:

Pharmacokinetic value	Canine	Feline
Terminal plasma elimination half-life	133 ± 16 hours (5.5 days)	166 ± 18 hours (6.9 days)
Maximum total plasma concentration	121 ± 51 µg/mL	141 ± 12 µg/mL
Volume of distribution (steady-state)	0.122 ± 0.011 L/kg	0.090 ± 0.010 L/kg
Total body clearance	0.76 ± 0.13 mL/hour/kg	0.35 ± 0.40 mL/hour/kg

Elimination of cefovecin is primarily via renal mechanisms; the majority is excreted unchanged in urine, but a small amount is excreted unchanged in bile. Cefovecin may persist in the body for up to 65 days and be excreted in urine at therapeutic concentrations for 14 days in dogs and 21 days in cats.

Several small pharmacokinetic studies have been done in other species. In alpacas, after IV injection, the elimination half-life of cefovecin was ≈10.28 hours, volume of distribution was 85.76 mL/kg, and clearance was 7.07 mL/hour/kg. After SC injection, the elimination half-life was ≈16.87 hours. This study found that cefovecin had lower levels of protein binding in this species (≈79%) than in dogs and cats.[13] One study in healthy horses showed that intra-articular injection of cefovecin in the radiocarpal joint was well tolerated and after a single dose of 240 mg, the maximum plasma concentration of 5.54 µg/mL was achieved at ≈4 hours.[14] The concentration remained above 1 µg/mL in the joint for 28 hours after administration, although therapeutic use is still unclear. Many other studies are available that report the pharmacokinetics of a variety of animal species (eg, sea otters,[15] copper rockfish,[16] Patagonian sea lions,[17] cheetahs,[18] lions,[19] koalas,[20] tigers,[21] mice[22]); an exhaustive listing of this information is beyond the scope of this reference.

Cefovecin's usefulness appears to be limited for certain species. Shorter half-lives and a larger volume of distribution (possibly due to lower protein binding) in birds and reptiles[23] may indicate that cefovecin offers no advantage over current treatments for these species.[24] A short elimination half-life was also found in rhesus monkeys (≈6.6 hours), and cefovecin did not reach a sufficient concentration over the MIC of bacteria found in infected skin wounds.[25]

Hypoproteinemia may alter cefovecin pharmacokinetics; however, there are no studies that support or refute this.

Contraindications/Precautions/Warnings

Cephalosporins are contraindicated in patients with a history of hypersensitivity to them. Because there may be cross-reactivity, cephalosporins should be used cautiously in patients with a documented hypersensitivity to other beta-lactam antibiotics (eg, penicillins, cefamycins, carbapenems). Anaphylaxis has been reported with the use of cefovecin.[1]

Safe use in dogs or cats younger than 4 months, with long-term use, or with IV or IM administration has not been established[1]; in other countries, there is a warning against use in dogs or cats younger than 8 weeks.[3,4] Cefovecin should be used with caution in patients with significant renal impairment; dose adjustment may be required. However, this guidance is likely only necessary for patients with severe renal disease. There is no guidance for optimal dose and frequency changes in animals with renal disease.

Cephalosporin use in small mammals (eg, guinea pigs, rabbits) is not recommended, as it may cause antibiotic-induced enterocolitis.[3,4]

Humans with beta-lactam allergies should exercise caution while handling this product.

Cefovecin can be easily confused with other cephalosporins. Consider writing orders and prescriptions using tall man lettering: cefoVECin.

Adverse Effects

Cefovecin appears to be well tolerated in dogs and cats. Emesis, diarrhea, anorexia, and injection site reactions are possible. Premarketing (in United States) studies in dogs and cats found no significant increase in adverse effect types or rates when compared with control; however, treated animals did have some changes in laboratory values. Several dogs had mild to moderate increases in liver enzymes (eg, ALT, gamma-glutamyl transferase [GGT]).[26] In 147 treated cats, 4 had mild increases in ALT concentrations, 24 had increases in BUN, and 6 had moderately elevated serum creatinine values.[26]

In the FDA's Cumulative Veterinary Adverse Drug Experience Reports (through April 2013), the most common adverse effects listed in decreasing order of frequency are:

- Dogs: depression/lethargy, anorexia, vomiting
- Cats: anorexia, depression/lethargy, vomiting

Hypersensitivity reactions, anaphylaxis, and death associated with cefovecin are possible and have been reported. The manufacturer also states, *Occasionally, cephalosporins and NSAIDs have been associated with myelotoxicity, thereby creating a toxic neutropenia.* Other hematologic reactions seen with cephalosporins include neutropenia, anemia, hypoprothrombinemia, thrombocytopenia, prolonged prothrombin time (PT) and partial thromboplastin time (PTT), platelet dysfunction, and transient increases in serum aminotransferases (eg, ALT, AST).

In healthy dogs, beta-lactam resistance in fecal *E coli* and the bla(CMY-2) gene were increased after cefovecin treatment as compared with dogs that received a placebo.[27]

Because cefovecin can persist in the body for up to 65 days, adverse effects that require prolonged treatment may occur.

Reproductive/Nursing Safety

The manufacturer states that safe use in breeding or lactating animals has not been determined. Product labeling in the European Union states, *treated animals should not be used for breeding for 12 weeks after the last administration.*[3] However, cephalosporins are generally considered safe for use during pregnancy and lactation and veterinarians and owners can weigh any risks of using the drug versus potential benefits to the dam and offspring.

Overdose/Acute Toxicity

Acute overdoses should be relatively safe. Dogs receiving cefovecin SC up to 180 mg/kg (22.5 times the label dose) showed injection site irritation, vocalization, edema, vomiting, and diarrhea. Edema resolved within 8 to 24 hours.[1] Cats given the same dose (22.5 times the label dose) showed the same signs but had lower mean WBC counts 10 days after treatment as compared with controls, and one cat had a small amount of bilirubinuria on day 10.

For patients that have experienced or are suspected to have experienced an overdose, consultation with a 24-hour poison consultation center specializing in providing veterinary-specific information is recommended. For general information related to overdose and toxin exposures, as well as contact information for poison control centers, refer to ***Appendix***.

Drug Interactions

Because cefovecin is highly bound to plasma proteins, it could theoretically displace other highly bound drugs causing a transient increase in serum concentrations of each drug. These interactions are unlikely to be of clinical concern because increased free drug levels will equilibrate through increased clearance. Monitor for adverse effects of each drug when using together. In experimental, in vitro systems, cefovecin has been shown to increase free concentrations of **carprofen, furosemide, doxycycline,** and **ketoconazole**. Other highly protein-bound drugs that could theoretically compete with cefovecin for binding and cause adverse effects include **maropitant, other NSAIDs, propofol, anticonvulsants, cardiac medication, and behavior medication.**[1] However, actual clinical significance has not been established and a recent report concluded that a clinically significant drug interaction is unlikely from the concurrent administration of **carprofen** and cefovecin in dogs.[28]

Laboratory Considerations

- Cephalosporins may cause false positive **urine glucose determinations** when the copper reduction method (Benedict's solution, Fehling's solution, *Clinitest*®) is used; tests using glucose oxidase (*Tes-Tape*®, *Clinistix*®) are not affected by cephalosporins.
- When the Jaffe reaction is used to measure **serum or urine cre-**

atinine, cephalosporins (not ceftazidime or cefotaxime) given in high dosages may cause falsely elevated values.

- Cephalosporins may cause falsely lowered **albumin** levels when certain tests are used to measure albumin.
- In humans, particularly those with azotemia, cephalosporins have caused a false positive direct **Coombs test**.
- Cephalosporins may also cause falsely elevated **17-ketosteroid** values in urine.

Dosages

DOGS:

Skin infections due to susceptible strains of *Staphylococcus intermedius* or *Streptococcus canis* (group G) (label dosage; FDA-approved): 8 mg/kg SC once.[1] A second injection (same dosage/route) may be administered if response to therapy is not complete after 7 days for *S intermedius* infections and after 14 days for *S canis* (group G) infections. Maximum treatment should not exceed 2 injections.

Susceptible skin and soft tissue infections (extra-label): 8 mg/kg SC once. If required, treatment may be repeated at 14-day intervals, up to 3 additional times.[3,4]

UTIs and severe infections of the gingival and periodontal tissues (extra-label; for indicated organisms, see ***Uses/Indications***): 8 mg/kg SC once [3,4]

Lyme disease (extra-label): 8 mg/kg SC, with a second dose repeated after 14 days was effective in eliminating spirochetes and reducing *Borrelia burgdorferi* antibodies in experimentally induced Lyme borreliosis.[8]

CATS:

Skin infections (eg, wounds, abscesses) caused by susceptible strains of *Pasteurella multocida* (label dosage; FDA-approved): 8 mg/kg SC as a single, one-time SC injection.[1] Therapeutic concentrations are maintained for ≈7 days for *P multocida* infections.

Susceptible skin and soft tissue infections (extra-label): 8 mg/kg SC once. If required, a second treatment may be repeated 14 days after the first injection.[3,4]

UTI and severe infections of the gingival and periodontal tissues (extra-label): 8 mg/kg SC once[3,4,6]

Monitoring

- Culture and susceptibility testing as indicated by clinical condition. Because cefovecin has prolonged excretion, optimal timing of the sampling for posttreatment urine culture is unclear; however, testing 3 weeks after the last dose may be reasonable.[6]
- Because cephalosporins usually have minimal toxicity associated with their use, monitoring for efficacy is often all that is required.
- Patients with diminished renal function may require intensified monitoring of renal parameters (eg, BUN, creatinine, urinalysis).

Client Information

- This medicine must be injected; it does not work when given by mouth.
- Medication is well tolerated in dogs and cats, but vomiting, diarrhea, or lack of appetite can occur.
- Antibiotic effect is long-lasting after a single injection in dogs and cats, and side effects can occur up to 2 months after an injection.
- If giving this medicine to your animal at home, be sure you understand how to do the injections.
- Store this medicine in the refrigerator, protected from light. Discard any unused medicine after 56 days.

Chemistry/Synonyms

Cefovecin sodium is a third-generation cephalosporin antibacterial agent with a molecular weight of 475.5. Each mL of reconstituted lyophilized powder contains cefovecin sodium equivalent to 80 mg of cefovecin; methylparaben (1.8 mg) and propylparaben (0.2 mg) are added as preservatives, and sodium citrate dihydrate (5.8 mg) and citric acid monohydrate (0.1 mg), sodium hydroxide, or hydrochloric acid are added to adjust pH.

Cefovecin sodium may also be known as UK-287074-02, cefovecina sodica, céfovécine sodique, or natrii cefovecinum. A trade name is *Convenia*®.

Storage/Stability

Store the powder and the reconstituted product protected from light in the original carton and refrigerate at 2°C to 8°C (36°F-46°F); do not freeze. Use the entire contents of the vial within 56 days of reconstitution. Cefovecin is light-sensitive. Although the color of the solution may vary from clear to amber at reconstitution and may darken over time, if the solution is stored as recommended, color does not adversely affect potency.

Compatibility/Compounding Considerations

To deliver the appropriate dose, the vial should be aseptically reconstituted with 10 mL of sterile water for injection. The vial should be shaken then allowed to sit until all material is visually dissolved. The resulting solution contains cefovecin sodium equivalent to 80 mg/mL of cefovecin.

Dosage Forms/Regulatory Status

VETERINARY-LABELED PRODUCTS:

Cefovecin Sodium (lyophilized) 800 mg (of cefovecin) per 10 mL multidose vial (80 mg/mL when reconstituted); *Convenia*®; (Rx). FDA-approved as labeled for use in dogs and cats. NADA #141-285. 320 mg/4 mL vials may be available in other countries.

HUMAN-LABELED PRODUCTS: NONE

References

For the complete list of references, see **wiley.com/go/budde/plumb**

Cefoxitin

(se-***fox***-i-tin) *Mefoxin*®

Second-Generation Cephalosporin (Cephamycin)

Prescriber Highlights

- ▶ Parenteral antimicrobial effective against most gram-positive cocci and gram-negative rods, and against some anaerobes
- ▶ Potentially causes hypersensitivity reactions, thrombocytopenia, and diarrhea
- ▶ Causes pain on IM injection; IV injections should be given over 3 to 5 minutes (or longer)
- ▶ Dosage reductions may be needed for patients with renal insufficiency.

Uses/Indications

Cefoxitin has been used clinically in several species when an injectable second-generation cephalosporin is indicated; however, no cefoxitin products are FDA-approved for veterinary species in the United States. Cefoxitin has been used in treatment protocols for dogs with parvoviral enteritis.[1]

Pharmacology/Actions

Cefoxitin is a cephamycin, not a true cephalosporin; however, it is usually classified as a second-generation antibacterial agent. Cefoxitin has activity against most gram-positive cocci, but activity is less on a per weight basis than with first-generation cephalosporin agents. Cefoxitin has better activity against *Escherichia coli, Klebsiella* spp, *Campylobacter* spp, *Proteus* spp, and other gram-negative bacteria compared to first-generation cephalosporin agents. Extended spectrum beta-lactamase (ESBL) producing gram-negative bacteria are typically susceptible to cefoxitin in vitro but in vivo response is unpredictable.

Bacterial resistance to cefoxitin is a growing concern. Methicillin-resistant staphylococci and AmpC producing gram-negative bacteria are resistant to cefoxitin. Cefoxitin resistance is commonly used as an in vitro marker for methicillin resistance in *Staphylococcus aureus*. Activity against enterococci and *Pseudomonas* spp is poor.

The World Health Organization has designated cefoxitin as a Highly Important antimicrobial for human medicine.[2]

Pharmacokinetics

In dogs ($n = 4$) after 30 mg/kg doses (IV, SC), plasma cefoxitin concentrations remained greater than MIC_{90} (*Escherichia coli*) for 4 to 6 hours after an IV dose and ≈8 hours after SC administration.[3]

In cats after 30 mg/kg doses, peak concentrations are similar when given IV or IM, and IM bioavailability is ≈90%. Apparent volume of distribution is 0.32 L/kg, clearance is 0.14 L/hour/kg, and elimination half-life is ≈1.5 hours. No significant accumulation occurs when dosed at 30 mg/kg every 8 or 12 hours, and time of MIC (estimated for cefoxitin) is similar after IV or IM administration: 75% every 8 hours or 50% every 12 hours.[4]

In horses, the apparent volume of distribution at steady state is 120 mL/kg, total body clearance is 4.32 mL/min/kg, and serum elimination half life is 49 minutes. Bioavailability after IM injection was 77%.[5]

In calves, the volume of distribution is 318 mL/kg, and terminal elimination half-life is 67 minutes after IV dosing and 81 minutes after IM administration. Cefoxitin is ≈50% bound to calf plasma proteins. Probenecid (40 mg/kg) has been demonstrated to significantly prolong elimination half-lives.[6]

In humans, cefoxitin is not appreciably absorbed after oral administration and must be given parenterally to achieve therapeutic serum concentrations. Cefoxitin is distributed into pleural and joint fluids.[7] The drug is primarily excreted unchanged by the kidneys into the urine via both tubular secretion and glomerular filtration, and high urinary concentrations are reached. Approximately 2% of a dose is metabolized to descarbamylcefoxitin, which is inactive. Elimination half-life is ≈1 hour but may be significantly prolonged in patients with markedly diminished renal function.

Contraindications/Precautions/Warnings

Cephalosporins are contraindicated in patients with a history of hypersensitivity to them. Because cross-reactivity may occur, use cephalosporins cautiously in patients with documented hypersensitivity to other beta-lactam antibiotics (eg, penicillins, cephamycins, carbapenems).

Patients with renal insufficiency may need dosage adjustments.

Cephalosporins in small mammals such as Syrian hamsters and guinea pigs may cause antibiotic-induced enterocolitis.

Cefoxitin can be easily confused with other cephalosporins. Writing part of the drug's name in uppercase on prescriptions/orders may reduce the risk of errors: CefOXitin. Do not confuse cefoxitin with *Cytoxan®* (cyclophosphamide).

Adverse Effects

Adverse effects with cephalosporins are usually not serious and have a relatively low frequency of occurrence.

Hypersensitivity reactions, unrelated to dosage, can occur with cephalosporins and can manifest as rashes, fever, eosinophilia, lymphadenopathy, or anaphylaxis. The use of cephalosporins in patients documented to be hypersensitive to penicillin-class antibiotics is controversial. In humans, ≈1% to 15% of patients hypersensitive to penicillins will also be hypersensitive to cephalosporins. The incidence of cross-reactivity in veterinary patients is unknown.

Cephalosporins can cause pain at the injection site when administered IM. Sterile abscesses or other severe local tissue reactions are also possible but are less common. Thrombophlebitis is possible after IV administration of cephalosporins.

Even when administered parenterally, cephalosporins may alter gut microbiota, causing antibiotic-associated diarrhea or proliferation of resistant bacteria in the colon (superinfections).

Although cephalosporins (particularly cephalothin) have the potential for causing nephrotoxicity at clinical dosages in patients with normal renal function, risks for the occurrence of this adverse effect appear minimal. High doses or prolonged use in humans has been associated with neurotoxicity (eg, seizures), neutropenia, agranulocytosis, thrombocytopenia, hepatitis, positive Coombs test, interstitial nephritis, and tubular necrosis. Except for tubular necrosis and neurotoxicity, these effects have an immunologic etiology.

Reproductive/Nursing Safety

Cephalosporins have been shown to cross the placenta. No teratogenic or fetal toxic effects were observed in studies performed in mice and rats. In humans, cefoxitin is considered compatible with pregnancy.[8]

Cefoxitin can be distributed into human milk in low concentrations. It is unlikely to pose significant risk to nursing offspring but may cause alterations in bowel flora. In humans, cefoxitin is considered compatible with breastfeeding.[8]

Overdose/Acute Toxicity

Cephalosporin overdoses are unlikely to cause significant adverse effects. The IV LD_{50} in mice is 8 g/kg.[7]

For patients that have experienced or are suspected to have experienced an overdose, it is strongly encouraged to consult with a 24-hour poison consultation center that specializes in providing information specific for veterinary patients. For general information related to overdose and toxin exposures, as well as contact information for poison control centers, refer to ***Appendix.***

Drug Interactions

The following drug interactions have either been reported or are theoretical in humans or animals receiving cefoxitin and may be of significance in veterinary patients. Unless otherwise noted, use together is not necessarily contraindicated, but weigh the potential risks and perform additional monitoring when appropriate.

- **AMINOGLYCOSIDES**: The concurrent use of parenteral aminoglycosides with cephalosporins is somewhat controversial. Potentially, cephalosporins could cause additive nephrotoxicity when used with these drugs, but this interaction has only been well documented with cephaloridine (no longer marketed). In vitro studies have demonstrated that cephalosporins can have synergistic or additive activity against certain bacteria when used with aminoglycosides, but they should be administered separately.
- **NEPHROTOXIC DRUGS** (eg, **amphotericin B, furosemide, iohexol**): Concurrent use with cefoxitin could cause additive nephrotoxicity.
- **PROBENECID**: Probenecid approximately doubled cefoxitin half-life and mean residence time in calves.[6]
- **VITAMIN K ANTAGONISTS** (eg, **warfarin**): Cephalosporins may enhance the anticoagulant effects of vitamin K antagonists.

Laboratory Considerations

- **Methicillin-resistant staphylococci**: Although cefoxitin resistance is widely used as an indicator of methicillin resistance in *S aureus*, it is a less effective indicator for *Staphylococcus pseudintermedius*. Cefoxitin resistance in *S pseudintermedius* indicates methicillin resistance; however, false negative results can occur.[9]
- Except for cefotaxime, cephalosporins may cause false-positive **urine glucose determinations** when using cupric sulfate solution (Benedict's solution, Fehling's solution, *Clinitest®*). Tests

utilizing glucose oxidase (*Tes-Tape®, Clinistix®*) are not affected by cephalosporins.

- When using the Jaffe reaction to measure **serum or urine creatinine**, cephalosporins (except ceftazidime and cefotaxime) in high dosages may cause falsely elevated values.
- In humans, particularly with azotemia, cephalosporins have caused a false-positive direct **Coombs test**.
- Cephalosporins may cause falsely elevated **17-ketosteroid** values in urine.

Dosages

DOGS/CATS:

Susceptible infections (extra-label): 30 mg/kg IV or IM every 6 to 8 hours[10,11]

Surgical (GI and orthopedic) prophylaxis (extra-label): 20 – 30 mg/kg IV, IM 30 to 60 minutes prior to incision. May repeat 1 time in 2 to 4 hours

HORSES:

Susceptible infections (extra-label): Foals: 20 mg/kg IV every 4 to 6 hours[12]

Monitoring

- Because cephalosporins are usually associated with minimal toxicity, monitoring for efficacy is typically all that is required.
- Patients with diminished renal function may require intensified renal monitoring.

Chemistry/Synonyms

Cefoxitin sodium, a cephamycin, is a semisynthetic antibiotic that is derived from cephamycin C produced by *Streptomyces lactamdurans*. It occurs as a white to off-white, somewhat hygroscopic powder or granules with a faint but characteristic odor. It is very soluble in water and only slightly soluble in alcohol. Each gram of cefoxitin sodium contains 2.3 mEq of sodium.

Cefoxitin may also be known as MK-306, L-620-388, cefoxitinum, cefoxitina, cefoxitine, *Mefoxin®*, *Mefoxitin®*, *Cefociclin®*, or *Cefoxin®*.

Storage/Stability

Cefoxitin sodium powder for injection should be stored between 2°C and 25°C (36°F-77°F) and should not be exposed to temperatures greater than 50°C (122°F). Once the 1 g and 2 g vials are reconstituted with sterile water for injection, 0.9% sodium chloride or 5% dextrose to 100 mg/mL, the solution is stable for 6 hours at room temperature and for 7 days if refrigerated below 5°C (41°F), while the bulk pharmacy 10 g vials are stable for 4 hours after initial entry. The solution may be diluted further to 50 to 1000 mL, which provides an additional 18 hours of stability at room temperature or an additional 48 hours under refrigeration.

Inactivated dual chamber bags of cefoxitin with dextrose should be stored at 20°C to 25°C (68°F-77°F) with excursions permitted to 15°C to 30°C (59°F-86°F). Do not freeze. Once activated, use the contents within 12 hours if stored at room temperature or within 7 days if stored under refrigeration.

The powder or reconstituted solution may darken but this does not affect the potency of the product.

Compatibility/Compounding Considerations

Compatibility is dependent on factors such as pH, concentration, temperature, and diluent used; consult specialized references or a hospital pharmacist for more specific information.

All commonly used IV fluids and the following drugs are reportedly **compatible** with cefoxitin: amikacin sulfate, cimetidine HCl, gentamicin sulfate, kanamycin sulfate, mannitol, metronidazole, multivitamin infusion concentrate, sodium bicarbonate, tobramycin sulfate, and vitamin B complex with vitamin C.

Dosage Forms/Regulatory Status

VETERINARY-LABELED PRODUCTS: NONE

HUMAN-LABELED PRODUCTS:

Cefoxitin Sodium Powder for Injection: 1 g, 2 g, and 10 g in vials; generic; (Rx)

Cefoxitin Sodium Injection Solution (with dextrose): 1 g and 2 g in 50 mL dual chamber bags; generic; (Rx)

References

For the complete list of references, see **wiley.com/go/budde/plumb**

Cefpodoxime

(sef-poe-***docks***-eem) *Simplicef®, Vantin®*

Third-Generation Cephalosporin

Prescriber Highlights

- ► Oral third-generation cephalosporin that may be useful in dogs and cats
- ► Contraindications: Known hypersensitivity to cephalosporins and beta-lactam antibiotics
- ► Adverse effects are primarily GI-related; hypersensitivity is possible.

Uses/Indications

In dogs, cefpodoxime is labeled for the treatment of skin infections caused by susceptible strains of *Staphylococcus pseudintermedius, Staphylococcus aureus, Streptococcus canis, Escherichia coli, Proteus mirabilis*, and *Pasteurella multocida*. Although not currently FDA approved for use in cats, cefpodoxime may be useful in this species. Cefpodoxime can be used to treat UTIs in dogs and cats.[1]

The World Health Organization (WHO) has designated cefpodoxime as a Critically Important (Highest Priority) antimicrobial in human medicine.[2]

Pharmacology/Actions

Like other cephalosporins, cefpodoxime binds penicillin-binding proteins, inhibiting bacterial cell wall synthesis and resulting in bacterial cell lysis. It is considered a time-dependent bactericidal antibiotic that is relatively resistant to bacterial beta lactamases.

Cefpodoxime is characterized as a third-generation cephalosporin. Although cefpodoxime has activity against many gram-negative bacteria in the Enterobacteriaceae family, including many *Escherichia* spp, *Proteus* spp, and *Klebsiella* spp, MICs with cefpodoxime are often significantly higher than with other third-generation drugs (eg, cefotaxime, ceftazidime). Against wild-type *Escherichia coli*, cefpodoxime has a MIC that is 8 times greater than cefotaxime's and 4 times greater than ceftazidime's.[3] Cefpodoxime has good activity against methicillin-susceptible staphylococci and many streptococci. Cefpodoxime has no activity against fungi, viruses, or parasites.

Cefpodoxime is not effective against the "SPACE" organisms (ie, *Serratia* spp, *Pseudomonas* spp, *Acinetobacter* spp, *Citrobacter* spp, *Enterobacter* spp), *Enterococcus* spp, anaerobes, or methicillin-resistant staphylococci. An ongoing concern is the development of resistance to third-generation cephalosporins by *E coli* and other gram-negative bacteria, mainly through the production of extended-spectrum beta-lactamases (ESBLs).

Due to potential differences between cefpodoxime and other third-generation cephalosporins, cefpodoxime-specific disks or dilutions should be used to determine susceptibility rather than susceptibility being inferred from other third-generation cephalosporins.

Pharmacokinetics

Cefpodoxime proxetil is not active as an antibiotic. Cefpodoxime is active after the proxetil ester is cleaved in vivo, which occurs rapidly and almost completely in the intestine. After administration of single oral doses of 5 or 10 mg/kg in dogs, bioavailability is ≈63%, the volume of distribution is 150 mL/kg, peak concentration is ≈16 µg/mL, and time to peak concentration is 2.2 hours. The concentration of a free drug in the skin and SC fluid is 1.7 µg/mL and 3 µg/mL, respectively.[4] The elimination half-life is 4.7 to 5.7 hours.[4–6] High levels of the drug are found in urine, and ≈70% to 95% is excreted unchanged.[4] ≈83% of the drug is bound to plasma proteins.[5] Oral bioavailability between the oral suspension and tablets is equivalent.[6]

In neonatal foals (7 to 14 days old), an oral suspension dose of 10 mg/kg can produce peak levels in ≈1.7 hours and a maximum serum concentration of ≈0.8 µg/mL. The elimination half-life is ≈7 hours. In a study, levels in synovial and peritoneal fluids were similar to those found in the serum, but no drug was detected in CSF.[7] Half-life in 3- to 4-month-old foals and adult horses is 6.2 hours and 3.8 hours, respectively.[7]

In humans, cefpodoxime proxetil is ≈40% to 50% absorbed from the GI tract.[8] Food does not alter the rate but may increase the extent of absorption. Cefpodoxime penetrates most tissue well; it is unknown if it penetrates into CSF. ≈20% to 30% of the drug is bound to plasma or serum proteins. It is eliminated in both the urine and feces. Serum half-life is 2 to 3 hours but may be prolonged in patients with impaired renal function; hepatic dysfunction does not alter elimination half-life.[8]

Contraindications/Precautions/Warnings

Cefpodoxime is contraindicated in patients hypersensitive to it or to other beta-lactam antibiotics (eg, penicillins, other cephalosporins).

Because cefpodoxime is excreted by the kidneys, doses and/or dose frequency may need to be adjusted in patients with significantly diminished renal function. However, there is limited guidance regarding when and how to reduce doses. In humans, cefpodoxime should be used with caution in patients with seizure disorders; this warning is not listed on the veterinary label. It is not known whether this concern applies to veterinary patients receiving cefpodoxime at the label dosage.

Cefpodoxime can be easily confused with other cephalosporins. Consider writing orders and prescriptions using tall man lettering: cefPODOXime.

Adverse Effects

The most likely adverse effects in dogs include inappetence, diarrhea, vomiting, and lethargy. Hypersensitivity and pemphigus-like drug reactions are rare but possible.

Rarely, blood dyscrasias may be seen following high doses of cephalosporins.

Reproductive/Nursing Safety

Cefpodoxime has not been shown to be teratogenic, but it should be used during pregnancy only when clearly indicated. The safety of cefpodoxime proxetil in dogs used for breeding, pregnant dogs, or lactating bitches has not been demonstrated.[9] In humans, cefpodoxime is considered compatible with pregnancy.[10]

In humans, cefpodoxime enters maternal milk in concentrations up to 16% of that of maternal serum levels.[8] Alteration of the gut microbiota with resultant diarrhea is theoretically possible.[8] Cefpodoxime should be used cautiously in nursing patients.

Because safety has not been established in animals, this drug should only be used when the maternal benefits outweigh the potential risks to offspring.

Overdose/Acute Toxicity

Cephalosporin overdoses are unlikely to cause significant problems, but other effects are possible. See ***Adverse Effects***.

For patients that have experienced or are suspected of having experienced an overdose, consultation with a 24-hour poison consultation center specializing in providing veterinary-specific information is recommended. For general information related to overdose and toxin exposures, as well as contact information for poison control centers, refer to ***Appendix***.

Drug Interactions

The following drug interactions have either been reported or are theoretical in humans or animals receiving cefpodoxime and may be of significance in veterinary patients. Unless otherwise noted, use together is not necessarily contraindicated, but weigh the potential risks and perform additional monitoring when appropriate.

- **Aminoglycosides and Other Nephrotoxic Drugs**: The concurrent use of parenteral aminoglycosides or other nephrotoxic drugs (eg, **amphotericin B**) with cephalosporins is somewhat controversial. Cephalosporins can cause additive nephrotoxicity when used with these drugs, but this interaction has only been well documented with cephaloridine, which is no longer marketed. *In vitro* studies have demonstrated that cephalosporins can have synergistic or additive activity against certain bacteria when used with aminoglycosides.
- **Antacids** (eg, **aluminum hydroxide**, **magnesium hydroxide**): Drugs that can increase stomach pH may decrease the peak levels and extent of absorption of cefpodoxime.
- **Histamine$_2$ (H_2) Receptor Antagonists** (eg, **famotidine**): H_2 antagonists may decrease peak levels and extent of absorption of cefpodoxime. Oral doses should be separated by at least 2 hours.
- **Probenecid**: Competitively blocks the tubular secretion of most cephalosporins, thereby increasing serum levels and serum half-lives
- **Proton-Pump Inhibitors** (**PPIs**; eg, **omeprazole**, **pantoprazole**): Concurrent use with cefpodoxime may reduce serum cefpodoxime concentrations.
- **Vitamin K Antagonists** (eg, **warfarin**): Cephalosporins may enhance the anticoagulant effects of vitamin K antagonists (eg, warfarin).

Laboratory Considerations

- Cefpodoxime may cause false-positive **urine glucose determinations** when using cupric sulfate solution (Benedict's solution, *Clinitest®*, Fehling's solution). Tests using glucose oxidase (*Tes-Tape®*, *Clinistix®*) are not affected by cephalosporins.
- Cefpodoxime may cause false-positive results when the nitroprusside test is used for determining **urinary ketones**.
- Cephalosporins (except ceftazidime and cefotaxime) in high doses may cause falsely elevated values when the Jaffe reaction is used to measure **serum or urine creatinine**.
- In humans, particularly humans with azotemia, cephalosporins have caused a false-positive direct **Coombs test** result.

Dosages

DOGS:

NOTE: Whether this drug should be used as a first- or second-tier drug is of debate, as the broader gram-negative coverage provided by this drug as compared with other antimicrobials commonly used to treat pyoderma is rarely necessary.[11] Supporting antimicrobial stewardship, narrow-spectrum cephalosporins, such as cephalexin, should always be considered prior to considering broad-spectrum cephalosporins, such as cefpodoxime.

Susceptible skin infections (wounds and abscesses) (label dosage; FDA approved): 5 – 10 mg/kg PO once daily for 5 to 7 days or 2 to 3 days beyond the cessation of clinical signs, up to a maximum of 28 days.[9] Treatment of acute infections should not be continued for more than 3 to 4 days if no response to therapy is seen. May be given with or without food.

Deep pyoderma (extra-label): 5 - 10 mg/kg PO once daily until 1 to 2 weeks after clinical resolution. Extended treatment duration (eg, 8 to 12 weeks) may be required. Higher doses may be needed for bacteria with MICs greater than 0.5 µg/mL.[4]

Bacterial cystitis (extra-label): 5 – 10 mg/kg PO every 24 hours.[1] Urinary excretion data supports cefpodoxime proxetil effectiveness in the treatment of UTIs in dogs, although not as a first-line option.[4]

CATS:

Susceptible skin and soft tissue infections (extra-label): 5 mg/kg PO every 12 hours or 10 mg/kg PO once daily until complete clinical resolution (extrapolated from human dose)[12]

HORSES:

Foals (neonates) with bacterial infections (extra-label): From a pharmacokinetic study, 10 mg/kg PO every 6 to 12 hours.[7] Additional studies are required to confirm clinical efficacy and safety. Safety in adult horses has not been established, and cefpodoxime should be avoided in horses beyond the neonatal period due to the risk for severe colitis seen with other oral beta-lactam antimicrobials.

Monitoring

- Clinical efficacy
- Adverse effects

Client Information

- Can be given with or without food, but GI side effects might be prevented if the medication is given with food.
- Most common side effects are diarrhea, vomiting, and loss of appetite.
- Be sure to give as long as your veterinarian has prescribed, even if your animal seems better.
- Cephalosporin antibiotics have an odor that resembles cat urine, but this is normal.

Chemistry/Synonyms

Cefpodoxime proxetil, an oral semisynthetic aminothiazolyl third-generation cephalosporin, is a prodrug that is hydrolyzed *in vivo* to cefpodoxime. The esterified form (proxetil) enhances lipid solubility and oral absorption. Potency is expressed in mg of cefpodoxime.

Cefpodoxime proxetil may also be known as CS-807; R-3763, U-76252, U-76253, *Banan*®, *Biocef*®, *Cefodox*®, *Cepodem*®, *Garia*®, *Instana*®, *Kelbium*®, *Orelox*®, *Otreon*®, *Podomexef*®, *Simplicef*®, or *Vantin*®.

Storage/Stability

Store tablets and unreconstituted powder between 20°C and 25°C (68°F and 77°F) in well-closed containers. After reconstitution, store the oral suspension in the refrigerator between 2°C and 8°C (36°F and 46°F) and discard after 14 days.

Dosage Forms/Regulatory Status

VETERINARY-LABELED PRODUCTS:

Cefpodoxime Proxetil Tablets: 100 mg and 200 mg; *Simplicef*®, Cefpoderm®, generic; (Rx). FDA approved for use in dogs. NADA #141-232

HUMAN-LABELED PRODUCTS:

Cefpodoxime Proxetil Oral Tablets: 100 mg and 200 mg; *Vantin*®, generic; (Rx)

Cefpodoxime Proxetil Granules for Suspension, Oral: 50 mg/5 mL (10 mg/mL) and 100 mg/5 mL (20 mg/mL) in 50 mL, 75 mL, and 100 mL bottles; *Vantin*®, generic; (Rx)

References

For the complete list of references, see **wiley.com/go/budde/plumb**

Cefquinome

(sef-***kwi***-nohm) *Cobactan*®, *Ceffect*®

Fourth-Generation Cephalosporin

Prescriber Highlights

- Antibacterial agent used in horses, cattle, and pigs
- Appears safe when used according to the label
- Not an approved drug in the United States; extra-label use of cephalosporins in major food-producing animals is prohibited by the FDA.

Uses/Indications

Cefquinome is approved in some countries for the treatment of susceptible gram-positive and gram-negative infections in cattle, pigs, and horses.

The following table lists the veterinary species with indications for cefquinome use.

Species	Indication(s)
Horses	Respiratory diseases caused by *Streptococcus equi* subsp *zooepidemicus*
Foals	Severe bacterial infections that carry a high risk for *Escherichia coli* septicemia
Cattle*	Respiratory disease caused by *Pasteurella multocida*, *Mannheimia haemolytica*, or *Histophilus somni* Digital dermatitis, infectious bulbar necrosis, and acute interdigital necrobacillosis (ie, foot rot) Acute *E coli* mastitis with signs of systemic involvement
Dry dairy cattle*	Subclinical mastitis at the time of drying off and for the prevention of new bacterial infections caused by *Staphylococcus aureus*, *S dysgalactiae*, *S uberis*, *S agalactiae*, and coagulase-negative staphylococci
Lactating dairy cattle*	Clinical mastitis caused by susceptible bacteria (including *S aureus*, *S uberis*, *S dysgalactiae*, and *E coli*)
Calves*	*E coli* septicemia
Pigs*	Bacterial infections of the lungs and respiratory tract caused by *P multocida*, *Haemophilus parasuis*, *Actinobacillus pleuropneumoniae*, *S suis*, and other cefquinome-sensitive organisms Mastitis, metritis, agalactia (MMA) syndrome caused by *E coli*, *Staphylococcus* spp, *Streptococcus* spp, and other cefquinome-sensitive organisms
Piglets*	Reduction of mortality in cases of meningitis caused by *S suis* Arthritis caused by *Streptococcus* spp, *E coli*, and other cefquinome-sensitive organisms Epidermitis (eg, mild or moderate lesions) caused by *S hyicus*

*In the United States, cefquinome use in food-producing animals is considered extra-label and is therefore prohibited by the FDA.

The World Health Organization (WHO) has designated fourth-generation cephalosporins such as cefquinome as Critically Important, Highest Priority antimicrobials for human medicine.[1] The Office International des Epizooties (OIE) has designated cefquinome as a Veterinary Critically Important Antimicrobial (VCIA) Agent in bovine, caprine, equine, lagomorph, ovine, and swine species.[2]

Pharmacology/Actions

Cefquinome is a fourth-generation cephalosporin with time-dependent bactericidal activity. Like other cephalosporins, this drug interferes with bacterial cell wall synthesis, which causes the cell to become more susceptible to lysis and results in cell death. Cefquinome is not an antiviral, antifungal, or antiparasitic drug.

Cefquinome penetrates the outer membrane of gram-negative bacteria more readily than other cephalosporins. This drug is not hydrolyzed by plasmid-mediated or AmpC-type cephalosporinases but may be hydrolyzed by some extended-spectrum beta-lactamases (ESBLs). To minimize selection of resistant bacteria strains carrying ESBLs, cefquinome use should be reserved for clinical conditions that have responded poorly to first-line treatment and, whenever possible, cefquinome use should be based on susceptibility testing. Cefquinome is ineffective against methicillin-resistant staphylococci.

Cefquinome has excellent gram-negative activity and retains good activity against gram-positive bacteria. In vitro, cefquinome has antibiotic activity against gram-positive and gram-negative bacteria (including *Staphylococcus* spp, *Streptococcus dysgalactiae, S agalactiae, S uberis, S equi* subsp *zooepidemicus, Clostridium* spp, *Corynebacterium pyogenes, Erysipelothrix rhusiopathiae, Actinobacillus* spp, *Bacteroides* spp, *Bacillus* spp, *Citrobacter* spp, *E coli, A pleuropneumoniae, Fusobacterium* spp, *Haemophilus* spp, *Klebsiella* spp, *Mannheimia haemolytica, Pasteurella* spp, *Prevotella* spp, *Proteus* spp, *Salmonella* spp, and *Serratia marcescens*).

In Europe, ≈98% of bacterial isolates in cattle and pigs were susceptible to cefquinome, with a minimum inhibitory concentration (MIC) ranging from less than 0.004 µg/mL to 2 µg/mL and a resistance breakpoint of 4 µg/mL.[3]

Pharmacokinetics

In adult horses given cefquinome at 1 mg/kg IM, the drug is completely absorbed, and peak concentration (2.5 µg/mL) occurs 1 hour after administration. Protein binding is minimal. The time above MIC for *Streptococcus equi* subsp *zooepidemicus* is ≈12 hours, and the elimination half-life is 2 hours. In foals, bioavailability is 87% after IM administration. Peak concentration (1.8 µg/mL) occurs within 1 hour of administration, and the elimination half-life is 1.4 hours.[4]

In cattle given cefquinome at 1 mg/kg IM or SC, a peak serum concentration of 2 µg/mL is reached within 90 to 120 minutes. Protein binding is minimal. This drug is excreted unchanged in urine, and the elimination half-life is 2.5 hours.[3] The average cefquinome concentration in milk is 19 µg/mL 12 hours after intramammary administration and ≈2.5 µg/mL after the animal is milked a second time following the last infusion.[5]

In sheep, cefquinome has been shown to accumulate after repeated SC doses given every 24 hours. One study showed statistically significant increases in AUC and maximum concentration between Day 1 and Day 5.[6]

In goats, peak concentration of cefquinome is 2.37 µg/mL and terminal elimination half-life is 4.85 hours. Elimination is prolonged when coadministered with ketoprofen in goats.[7]

In pigs or piglets, a peak serum concentration of 5 µg/mL is reached within 15 to 60 minutes after administration of 2 mg/kg IM. Protein binding is poor, and 12 hours after administration, the drug is able to penetrate into CSF fluid at a concentration similar to plasma. Elimination half-life is ≈9 hours.[3]

Cefquinome is not absorbed after oral administration.

Contraindications/Precautions/Warnings

Cephalosporins are contraindicated in patients with a history of hypersensitivity to them. Because there may be cross-reactivity, caution is advised in patients that have a documented hypersensitivity to other beta-lactam antibiotics (eg, penicillins, cefamycins, carbapenems). Isolated cases of hypersensitivity reactions have been noted in cattle.

In the United States, cefquinome use in food-producing animals is considered extra-label and is therefore prohibited by the FDA.

Cefquinome is renally excreted. Dosage modification may be necessary in patients with reduced or impaired renal function.

It is important not to confuse cefQUINome with other cephalosporins.

Adverse Effects

When used according to label instructions, cefquinome appears to be well tolerated. Local tissue reactions at the injection site have been noted to last 15 to 28 days after administration.[3,4]

Reproductive/Nursing Safety

Cephalosporins cross the placenta. Reproductive toxicity studies in laboratory animals did not show teratogenic or fetotoxic effects. No information is available regarding reproductive toxicity in horses, cattle, or swine. Intramammary suspensions have demonstrated no evidence of reproductive toxicity in cattle.

Safe use of cefquinome, including intramammary infusions, in nursing animals has not been established.

Because safety has not been established in animals, this drug should only be used when the maternal benefits outweigh the potential risks to offspring.

Overdose/Acute Toxicity

Dosages up to 20 mg/kg/day IV in cattle and 10 mg/kg/day in pigs and piglets have been well tolerated.[3,4]

For patients that have experienced or are suspected to have experienced an overdose, consultation with a 24-hour poison consultation center specializing in providing veterinary-specific information is recommended. For general information related to overdose and toxin exposures, as well as contact information for poison control centers, refer to ***Appendix***.

Drug Interactions

The following drug interactions with cefquinome have either been reported or are theoretical in animals or humans receiving similar cephalosporins and may be of significance in veterinary patients. Unless otherwise noted, use together is not necessarily contraindicated, but the potential risks should be weighed and additional monitoring performed when appropriate:

- AMINOGLYCOSIDES: Concurrent use may increase the risk for nephrotoxicity.
- CHLORAMPHENICOL: Concurrent use with some cephalosporins may reduce antibacterial effectiveness; interaction may apply to cefquinome. Combination should be avoided.
- PROBENECID: Concurrent use can increase cephalosporin exposure; interaction may apply to cefquinome.

Laboratory Considerations

No specific laboratory interactions or considerations were noted for cefquinome. The following class effects are known regarding cephalosporins:

- Except for cefotaxime, cephalosporins may cause false positive **urine glucose determinations** when using cupric sulfate solution (eg, Benedict's solution, *Clinitest*®). Tests using glucose oxidase (eg, *Tes-Tape*®, *Clinistix*®) are not affected by cephalosporins.
- When the Jaffe reaction is used to measure serum or urine creatinine, cephalosporins (not ceftazidime or cefotaxime) given in high dosages may cause falsely elevated values.

- In humans, particularly those with azotemia, cephalosporins have caused a false positive direct **Coombs test**.
- Cephalosporins may also cause falsely elevated **17-ketosteroid** values in urine.

Dosages

HORSES:

Respiratory disease caused by *Streptococcus equi* subsp *zooepidemicus* (extra-label): 1 mg/kg IV or IM once daily for 5 to 10 consecutive days. Treatment should be stopped 2 days after clinical signs cease. Diagnosis should be re-evaluated if no response to treatment is seen in 3 to 4 days.[1,4]

In foals, severe bacterial infections with a high risk for septicemia caused by *Escherichia coli* (extra-label): 1 mg/kg IV or IM twice daily for 6 to 14 consecutive days. It is recommended to begin treatment with IV doses for 3 days followed with IM injections. Treatment should be stopped 3 days after clinical signs cease. Diagnosis should be re-evaluated if no response to treatment is seen in 3 to 4 days.[4]

NOTE: The following dosages are approved in some countries outside the United States; however, because cefquinome is not FDA-approved, all use is considered extra-label in the United States. FDA prohibition of extra-label use of cephalosporins in major food animal species effectively bans cefquinome use in food-producing animals in the United States.

CATTLE:

Susceptible infections (extra-label use prohibited in United States): 1 mg/kg IM once daily for 2 to 5 consecutive days depending on indication and age. The cervical neck region is the preferred injection site, and subsequent injection sites should be rotated.[3]

SWINE:

Susceptible infections (extra-label use prohibited in United States): 2 mg/kg IM once daily for 2 to 5 consecutive days depending on indication and age. The cervical neck region is the preferred injection site, and subsequent injection sites should be rotated.[3]

Monitoring

- Clinical efficacy
- Adverse effects
- Culture and susceptibility as appropriate

Client Information

- Handle this medicine with caution if you have an allergy to penicillin or cephalosporin antibiotics.
- Clean and disinfect teat and orifice prior to intramammary infusion.
- Follow all withdrawal instructions for production animals.
- In the United States, the FDA prohibits the extra-label use of cephalosporins in food-producing animals.

Chemistry/Synonyms

Cefquinome is structurally related to other beta-lactam antibiotics. Commercial dosage forms contain cefquinome sulfate; 1.19 mg cefquinome sulfate contains 1 mg cefquinome. Cefquinome sulfate occurs as a powder or crystal that can be white, faint/pale yellow, beige, or brown. Cefquinome 2.5% suspension for injection contains ethyl oleate and is light brown. The 7.5% suspension for injection has a white to off-white color. Cefquinome intramammary suspensions contain a paraffin vehicle.

Cefquinome may also be known as *Cobactan*®, *Ceffect*®, *Cefimam*®, or *Cephaguard*®.

Storage/Stability

Store cefquinome products protected from light at a controlled room temperature of 25°C (77°F). Cefquinome 45 mg/mL solution should be refrigerated (2°C-8°C [36°F-46°F]) after reconstitution. Manufacturers of cefquinome for injection state the following discard intervals:

- 25 mg/mL solution: 28 days after first use or 25 vial punctures; store vial in original carton
- 45 mg/mL solution: 10 days after reconstitution (refrigerated) or after 20 punctures of vial stopper
- 75 mg/mL suspension: 28 days after first use

Compatibility/Compounding Considerations

A study tested the stability of cefquinome sulfate after it was diluted to 5 mg/mL and stored in polyvinyl chloride mini bags at 6°C (42.8°F; refrigerated), 22°C (71.6°F; room temperature), and -20°C (-4°F; frozen). Refrigerated cefquinome solutions were stable over the 6 day study interval when diluted with sterile water, 0.9% sodium chloride, 0.9% sodium chloride with glucose, lactated Ringer's solution, and multielectrolytic isotonic fluid and were less stable when stored at room temperature. Frozen solutions were stable for the 30-day study interval.[8]

Dosage Forms/Regulatory Status

VETERINARY-LABELED PRODUCTS:

NOTE: In the United States, cefquinome use in food producing animals is considered extra-label and, therefore, is prohibited by the FDA.

Cefquinome Suspension for Injection: 25 mg/mL in 50 mL and 100 mL vials; *Cobactan*®, *Ceffect*®; (POM-V). Available in Europe, United Kingdom, and New Zealand. Withholding periods vary by product and country of origin; it is important to read and follow the label instructions.

Cefquinome Solution for Injection: 45 mg/mL in 30 mL and 100 mL powder vial bundled with solvent vial; *Cobactan*®; (POM-V). Available in Europe and United Kingdom. Not to be used in horses producing milk for human consumption. Withholding periods vary by product and country of origin; it is important to read and follow label instructions.

Cefquinome Suspension for Injection: 75 mg/mL in 50 mL, 100 mL, and 250 mL vials; *Cobactan*®; (POM-V). Available in Europe and United Kingdom. Not to be used in dairy cows producing milk for human consumption or within 2 months prior to first calving in heifers intended to produce milk for human consumption. Withholding periods vary by product and country of origin; it is important to read and follow label instructions.

Cefquinome Intramammary Infusion for Lactating Cows: 75 mg cefquinome in 8 g tubes in cartons of 3, 15, 20, or 24 syringes; *Cephaguard*® Milking Cow, *Cefimam*® LC, *Cobactan*® LC; (POM-V). For the treatment of clinical mastitis in lactating cows. Withholding periods vary by product and country of origin; it is important to read and follow label instructions.

Cefquinome Intramammary Infusion for Dry Cows: 150 mg in 3 g tubes in cartons of 20, 24, or 60 syringes or buckets of 120 syringes. *Cefimam*® DC, *Cephaguard*® DC; (POM-V). For the treatment of subclinical mastitis at drying off and prevention of new bacterial infections in dairy cows during the dry period; not for treatment of mastitis. If there is erroneous use during lactation, milk will need to be discarded for 35 days. Withholding periods vary by product and country of origin; it is important to read and follow label instructions.

HUMAN-LABELED PRODUCTS: NONE

References

For the complete list of references, see **wiley.com/go/budde/plumb**

Ceftazidime

(sef-*taz*-i-deem) *Ceptaz®, Fortaz®, Tazicef®*

Third-Generation Cephalosporin

Prescriber Highlights

- Parenteral antibacterial primarily used for serious systemic *Pseudomonas* spp infections in dogs and cats as well as for broad-spectrum antimicrobial coverage in reptiles
- Constant rate IV infusion or frequent parenteral administration may be necessary in dogs and cats with serious systemic *Pseudomonas* spp infections.
- Use with caution in patients with renal insufficiency; dosing interval may need to be increased.
- May cause hypersensitivity reactions, granulocytopenia, thrombocytopenia, diarrhea, and mild azotemia
- May cause pain on IM injection; SC injection may be less painful.

Uses/Indications

Ceftazidime is a third-generation cephalosporin with antipseudomonal properties. It is effective against *Pseudomonas* spp, Enterobacteriaceae, and other gram-negative bacteria. Ceftazidime is usually reserved for use in patients with severe infections that cannot be treated with licensed veterinary alternatives and when other antimicrobial agents such as aminoglycosides are not indicated because of their potential toxicity. Ceftazidime is of particular interest in treating gram-negative infections in reptiles because of its long half-life in many species.

The World Health Organization has designated ceftazidime as a Critically Important (Highest Priority) antimicrobial for human medicine.[1]

Pharmacology/Actions

Ceftazidime is a third-generation injectable cephalosporin. It is bactericidal and acts via its inhibition of enzymes responsible for bacterial cell wall synthesis. The third-generation cephalosporins retain much of the gram-positive activity of the first- and second-generation agents but have expanded gram-negative activity. As with the second-generation agents, enough variability exists with individual bacterial sensitivities that susceptibility testing is necessary for most bacteria. Unlike most other third-generation cephalosporins, ceftazidime is considered an anti-pseudomonal cephalosporin, but resistance can be present. Ceftazidime is ineffective against extended-spectrum beta-lactamase (ESBL)–producing bacteria and methicillin-resistant staphylococci, as well as enterococci.

Because susceptibility of various bacteria to the third-generation cephalosporin antibiotics is unique to a given agent, ceftazidime-specific disks or dilutions must be used to determine susceptibility. Resistance of *Pseudomonas* spp to other third-generation cephalosporins does not necessarily indicate resistance to ceftazidime because of the poor anti-pseudomonal activity of most other cephalosporins.

Pharmacokinetics

Ceftazidime is not appreciably absorbed after oral administration. In dogs after SC injection, the terminal half-life of ceftazidime was 0.8 hours; a 30 mg/kg dose resulted in drug concentrations greater than the serum breakpoint for *Pseudomonas aeruginosa* for 4.3 hours. When ceftazidime was administered as a 4.1 mg/kg/hour CRI (after a loading dose of 4.4 mg/kg), mean serum concentration was greater than 165 µg/mL.[2] Another study in dogs reported average terminal elimination half-lives between 1 and 2 hours after IV, IM, or SC dosing.[3]

In cats, ceftazidime is ≈83% bioavailable after IM administration. It has an apparent volume of distribution of 0.18 L/kg and a clearance of 0.19 L/kg/hr. Elimination half-life is ≈0.8 hours (IV) to 1 hour (IM).[4]

In neonatal foals, bioavailability was 90% after IM administration, and median half-life was 2 hours.[5] Synovial ceftazidime concentrations declined rapidly following regional limb perfusion in horses.[6] Clinical use by this route is not recommended because concentration exceeded MIC for only 2 to 6 hours.

Ceftazidime is widely distributed throughout the body, including into bone and CSF, and is primarily excreted unchanged by the kidneys via glomerular filtration. As renal tubular excretion does not play a major role in the drug's excretion, probenecid does not affect elimination kinetics.

Two studies have examined the pharmacokinetics of ceftazidime in lactating animals. One study compared ceftazidime pharmacokinetics between nonlactating and lactating Creole goats. A dose of 10 mg/kg was given IV or IM. The elimination half-life when ceftazidime was given IV was ≈2.3 hours in nonlactating goats and 1.6 hours in lactating goats. The volume of distribution was 200 mL/kg in nonlactating goats and 238 mL/kg in lactating goats. Bioavailability after IM injection was excellent at 96% to 113%. Half-life was similar to half-life after IV injection. The maximum serum concentration was 67.5 µg/mL in lactating goats and 31.9 µg/mL in nonlactating goats. Penetration into the milk was 18% after IV dosing and 14% after IM dosing. No ceftazidime was detected in the milk after 96 hours.[7] A similar study was performed in lactating dromedary camels. The camels were given a 10 mg/kg dose either IV or IM. The half-life was ≈2.85 hours after IV administration and 3.2 hours after IM administration. Bioavailability after IM administration was 93%. The maximum mean serum concentration was 32.43 µg/mL. The volume of distribution was 0.21 L/kg. Penetration into the milk was ≈10.8% for IV dosing and 12.8% for IM dosing.[8] Both sets of authors concluded that systemic ceftazidime may be a useful treatment for mastitis but further clinical studies are needed.

Contraindications/Precautions/Warnings

Ceftazidime is contraindicated in patients that have had allergic reactions to cephalosporins in the past. Because cross-reactivity may occur, use cephalosporins cautiously in patients that have a documented hypersensitivity to other beta-lactam antibiotics (eg, penicillins, cephamycins, carbapenems).

Ceftazidime is primarily excreted via the kidneys and may accumulate in patients with markedly impaired renal function; use with caution and adjust dose as required. The risk of neurologic toxicity (eg, seizures, myoclonus, encephalopathy) is increased in patients with renal impairment.

Ceftazidime can be easily confused with other cephalosporins. Consider writing part of the drug's name in uppercase letters (tall-man designations) on prescriptions/orders to reduce the risk of errors, for example, cefTAZidime.

Adverse Effects

Because veterinary use of ceftazidime has been limited, a full adverse effect profile has not been determined for veterinary patients. GI effects have been reported in dogs that have received the drug SC. When given IM, pain may be noted at the injection site; in animals, pain on injection could also occur after SC administration.

Hypersensitivity reactions, hemolytic anemia, and GI signs have been reported in humans and may not apply to veterinary patients.

Pseudomembranous colitis (*Clostridium difficile*) may occur in patients receiving this antibiotic. Increased serum liver enzyme (eg, ALT, AST, LDH, GGT) activity have been described in 1% to 8% of human patients given ceftazidime[9]; significance in veterinary medicine is unknown.

Reproductive/Nursing Safety

Cephalosporins have been shown to cross the placenta. No teratogenic effects were demonstrated in studies in pregnant mice and rats given up to 40 times labeled doses of ceftazidime.[9] In humans, ceftazidime is considered compatible with pregnancy.[10]

Because of the drug's low oral absorbability, it is unlikely to be harmful to nursing offspring, but alterations to GI microbiota of nursing animals could occur. In humans, ceftazidime is considered compatible with breastfeeding.[10]

Because safety has not been established in animals, this drug should only be used when the maternal benefits outweigh the potential risks to offspring.

Overdose/Acute Toxicity

An acute overdose in patients with normal renal function is unlikely to be of great concern; but in humans with renal insufficiency, overdose of ceftazidime has caused seizures, encephalopathy, coma, neuromuscular excitability, asterixis, and myoclonia.[9] Treatment of signs associated with overdose is primarily based on clinical signs and is supportive. Hemodialysis could be used to enhance elimination. Ceftazidime is cleared significantly during continuous renal replacement therapies (CRRTs).

For patients that have experienced or are suspected to have experienced an overdose, consultation with a 24-hour poison consultation center specializing in providing veterinary-specific information is recommended. For general information related to overdose and toxin exposures, as well as contact information for poison control centers, refer to ***Appendix***.

Drug Interactions

The following drug interactions have either been reported or are theoretical in humans or animals receiving ceftazidime and may be of significance in veterinary patients. Unless otherwise noted, use together is not necessarily contraindicated, but weigh the potential risks and perform additional monitoring when appropriate.

- **Aminoglycosides** (eg, **amikacin, gentamicin**): The concurrent use of parenteral aminoglycosides with cephalosporins is somewhat controversial. Potentially, cephalosporins could cause additive nephrotoxicity when used with these drugs, but this interaction has only been well documented with cephaloridine (no longer marketed). In vitro studies have demonstrated that cephalosporins can have synergistic or additive activity against certain bacteria when used with aminoglycosides,[11] but they should be administered separately.
- **Nephrotoxic Drugs** (eg, **amphotericin B, furosemide, iohexol**): Concurrent use with ceftazidime may cause additive nephrotoxicity.
- **Chloramphenicol**: May be antagonistic to ceftazidime's effects on gram-negative bacilli; concurrent use is not recommended.
- **Vitamin K Antagonists** (eg, **warfarin**): Cephalosporins may enhance the anticoagulant effect of vitamin K antagonists.

Laboratory Considerations

- Except for cefotaxime, cephalosporins may cause false-positive **urine glucose determinations** when using cupric sulfate solution (Benedict's solution, Fehling's solution, *Clinitest*®). Tests utilizing glucose oxidase (*Tes-Tape*®, *Clinistix*®) are not affected by cephalosporins.
- In humans, particularly with azotemia, cephalosporins have caused a false-positive direct **Coombs test**.
- Cephalosporins may also cause falsely elevated **17-ketosteroid** values in urine.
- **Prothrombin time** may be prolonged.
- When using **Kirby-Bauer disk diffusion** procedures for testing susceptibility, a specific 30 µg ceftazidime disk should be used. An inhibition zone of 18 mm or greater indicates the organism is susceptible, 15 to 17 mm is intermediate, and 14 mm or less is resistant. When using a dilution susceptibility procedure, an organism with a MIC of 8 µg/mL or less is considered susceptible, 16 µg/mL is intermediate, and 32 µg/mL or greater is resistant. With either susceptibility method, infections caused by organisms with intermediate susceptibility may be effectively treated if the infection is limited to tissues in which the drug concentrates, or when a higher-than-normal dose is used.

Dosages

DOGS:

Susceptible *Pseudomonas aeruginosa* infections (extra-label):

1. **Based on a pharmacokinetics/pharmacodynamics (PK/PD) study:** 30 mg/kg IV, IM, SC every 4 hours or given as a continuous IV infusion (CRI) with a loading dose of 4.4 mg/kg and a CRI infusion rate of 4.1 mg/kg/hr. The authors recommended that these regimens be tested in clinical trials of dogs with *P aeruginosa* infections and that ceftazidime should be reserved for those dogs with *P aeruginosa* isolates that are resistant to or develop adverse effects to aminoglycosides and fluoroquinolones.[2]
2. **Based on a PK/PD study:** The authors concluded that ceftazidime administered at 20 mg/kg IV or 25 mg/kg IM, SC every 8 hours should be a useful alternative to aminoglycosides and fluoroquinolones for the empirical treatment of most *P aeruginosa* infections in dogs. However, higher doses may be needed and clinical trials must be conducted to verify these recommendations.[3]

CATS:

Susceptible infections (extra-label): Based on a PK/PD study: 30 mg/kg IM every 8 hours should be effective, but for *Pseudomonas* spp infections, ceftazidime would either need to be dosed much more frequently (every 2 to 4 hours) or as a CRI similar to the dose suggested for dogs (loading dose of 4.4 mg/kg and a CRI infusion rate of 4.1 mg/kg/hour).[4]

HORSES:

Susceptible infections in neonatal foals (extra-label): 25 mg/kg IV or IM every 8 hours. Based on a single-dose pharmacokinetic study in healthy neonatal foals[5]

REPTILES:

Susceptible infections (extra-label): 20 mg/kg IM or SC every 72 hours (every 3 days)[12]

Bacterial infections in snakes, particularly for Enterobacteriaceae or *P aeruginosa* infections (extra-label): 20 mg/kg IM every 72 hours at 30°C (86°F)[13,14]

Chelonians (extra-label): 50 mg/kg IM once daily (every 24 hours)[15]

Wild turtles (extra-label): 20 mg/kg IM as a single dose is predicted to maintain ceftazidime concentration above MIC of most wild-type bacteria.[16]

Monitoring

- Culture and susceptibility as indicated
- Baseline and periodic serum renal and hepatic chemistry panel (eg, BUN, creatinine, ALT, ALP), urinalysis
- For patients with renal insufficiency, monitor for neurotoxicity (eg, seizures, myoclonus)
- Because veterinary use of ceftazidime has been limited, a full adverse effect profile has not been determined for veterinary patients. Pet owners should be encouraged to be in communication about any adverse effects that could be caused by the drug.

Client Information

- Ceftazidime must be injected under the skin (subcutaneously); it is not effective when given by mouth.
- Closely follow storage requirements and discard dates.
- This medicine may cause GI side effects; however, because this

drug is not used commonly in animals, other side effects could occur that are not known. Be sure to contact your veterinarian if you have any concerns about how your animal is responding to this medicine.

- Be sure your animal has access to plenty of fresh water while receiving this medicine.
- Discard used needles and syringes in a puncture-resistant ("sharps") container immediately after use, making sure you do not attempt to disconnect the needle from the syringe or recap the needle. Do not reuse needles or syringes. Your veterinarian or pharmacist will help you obtain these containers as well as disposing them when full, or therapy is complete.

Chemistry/Synonyms

A semisynthetic, third-generation cephalosporin antibiotic, ceftazidime occurs as a white to cream-colored crystalline powder that is slightly soluble in water (5 mg/mL) and insoluble in alcohol, chloroform, and ether. The pH of a 0.5% solution in water is between 3 and 4.

Ceftazidime may also be known as ceftazidimum, GR-20263, LY-139381, *Fortaz*®, *Ceptaz*®, *Tazicef*®, and *Tazidime*®; many trade names are used internationally.

Storage/Stability

Commercially available powders for injection should be stored at 20°C to 25°C (68°F-77°F) and protected from light.

Commercial products contain sodium carbonate (*Fortaz*®, *Tazicef*®), which releases carbon dioxide (effervesces) when reconstituted. Vials are under negative pressure; do not allow pressure to normalize before adding diluent.

Once reconstituted, the solution retains potency for 12 hours at room temperature and 3 days when refrigerated. Some manufacturers state that the solution is stable for 24 hours at room temperature and 7 days when refrigerated. Consult the package insert for further information.

Activated Duplex containers must be used within 12 hours if at room temperature or 3 days if refrigerated.

Once thawed, the premixed frozen solution is stable for 8 hours at room temperature or 3 days under refrigeration. Do not refreeze.

Ceftazidime reconstituted with sterile water to 100 mg/mL and frozen at -20°C (-4°F) in glass vials or plastic syringes retained greater than 90% potency for 91 days; once thawed, the solution may be stored at room temperature for 24 hours or refrigerated for 7 days.[17,18]

Compatibility/Compounding Considerations

Compatibility is dependent upon factors such as pH, concentration, temperature, and diluent used; consult specialized references or a hospital pharmacist for more specific information.

Ceftazidime is **compatible** with the following diluents when being prepared for IM (or SC) injection: sterile or bacteriostatic water for injection, 0.5% or 1% lidocaine. Once reconstituted, ceftazidime is **compatible** with several IV fluids including D5W, 0.9% and 0.45% sodium chloride, Ringer's injection, and lactated Ringer's injection.

Do not use sodium bicarbonate solution for a diluent. Ceftazidime is **compatible** with additives of clindamycin, fluconazole, heparin, and potassium chloride. Ceftazidime is **incompatible** with gentamicin, pantoprazole, ranitidine, and vancomycin.

Dosage Forms/Regulatory Status

VETERINARY-LABELED PRODUCTS: NONE

HUMAN-LABELED PRODUCTS:

Ceftazidime Powder for Injection: 500 mg, 1 g, 2 g, and 6 g in 20 mL and 100 mL vials, infusion packs, *ADD-Vantage* vials and piggyback vials; *Fortaz*®, *Tazicef*®, generic; (Rx)

References

For the complete list of references, see **wiley.com/go/budde/plumb**

Ceftiofur Crystalline Free Acid

(sef-***tee***-oh-fur) *Excede*®

Third-Generation Cephalosporin

Prescriber Highlights

- ► Veterinary-only third-generation cephalosporin labeled for use in horses, cattle, and swine
- ► Oil-based suspension maintains concentrations of ceftiofur and metabolites above MIC for more than 96 hours after a single IM or SC injection.
- ► Administered IM in swine and horses. Administered SC at the posterior aspect of ear in cattle. **Inadvertent intra-arterial injection is likely to result in sudden death.**
- ► Potentially causes hypersensitivity reactions, granulocytopenia, thrombocytopenia, or diarrhea
- ► Shake well prior to use.

Uses/Indications

In horses, ceftiofur CFA is FDA-approved for the treatment of lower respiratory tract infections caused by susceptible strains of *Streptococcus equi* ssp *zooepidemicus*.

In beef and dairy cattle, ceftiofur crystalline free acid (CCFA) is FDA approved for the treatment of bovine respiratory diseases (BRD, shipping fever, pneumonia) associated with *Mannheimia haemolytica, Pasteurella multocida,* and *Histophilus somni* and for the treatment of foot rot (interdigital necrobacillosis) associated with *Fusobacterium necrophorum* and *Porphyromonas levii.*[1] In beef and nonlactating dairy cattle, CCFA is indicated for the control of respiratory disease in animals at high risk for developing BRD associated with *M haemolytica*, *P multocida*, and *H somni*. Additionally, this antibiotic is indicated for the treatment of acute metritis in lactating dairy cattle (0 to 10 days postpartum) associated with bacterial organisms susceptible to ceftiofur.

In swine, ceftiofur CFA is FDA-approved for the treatment and control of swine respiratory disease (SRD) associated with *Actinobacillus pleuropneumoniae, P multocida, Haemophilus parasuis,* and *Streptococcus suis.*

The World Health Organization has designated third-generation cephalosporins as Critically Important (Highest Priority) antimicrobials for human medicine.[2] The Office International des Epizooties (OIE) has designated ceftiofur as a Veterinary Critically Important Antimicrobial (VCIA) Agent in avian, bovine, caprine, equine, lagomorph, ovine, and swine species.[3]

Pharmacology/Actions

Ceftiofur is a time-dependent, bactericidal, third-generation cephalosporin antibiotic active against a variety of gram-positive and gram-negative bacteria and anaerobes. Like other cephalosporins, it inhibits bacteria cell wall synthesis. Ceftiofur is not active against *Pseudomonas* spp or enterococci. Acquired resistance is increasingly common, particularly in staphylococci (methicillin-resistant staphylococci) and Enterobacteriaceae (extended spectrum beta-lactamase (ESBL) or extended spectrum cephalosporinase producers).

Ceftiofur is rapidly cleaved into furoic acid and desfuroylceftiofur (active). Desfuroylceftiofur inhibits cell wall synthesis (at stage 3) of susceptible multiplying bacteria and exhibits a spectrum of activity similar to that of cefotaxime, also a third-generation cephalosporin. Parent ceftiofur and the primary metabolite are equally potent and assays to measure microbial sensitivity (plasma and tissue levels) are based on ceftiofur equivalents (CE). The protein binding activity of ceftiofur creates a reservoir effect to maintain active levels at the site of infection.

In cattle, ceftiofur has a broad range of in vitro activity against a variety of pathogens, including *Pasteurella* spp, *Streptococcus* spp,

Staphylococcus spp, *Salmonella* spp, and *E coli*. In dairy cattle with metritis treated with systemic ceftiofur, the effects on postpartum inflammation and fever significantly improved the cure rate, milk yield, and rectal temperature in cows with fever and vaginal discharge or dystocia.[4]

In swine, CCFA at a single IM dose of 5 mg/kg (2.27 mg/lb) provides concentrations of ceftiofur and desfuroylceftiofur-related metabolites in plasma that are multiples above the MIC_{90} for an extended period of time for the SRD label pathogens *Actinobacillus pleuropneumoniae, Pasteurella multocida, Haemophilus parasuis,* and *Streptococcus suis.*

Pharmacokinetics

CCFA is formulated in a caprylic-capric triglyceride acid/cottonseed oil base that allows slow and sustained release from the site of injection to provide prolonged therapeutic concentrations with a single injection.[5,6]

In horses, CCFA at 6.6 mg/kg IM is relatively slowly absorbed and eliminated. After the first dose, the time to peak serum level is ≈22 hours and after a second dose 96 hours after the first, time to peak serum drug levels was ≈16 hours.[7] When given at this dosage, the drug and its active metabolites stay above the determined therapeutic concentration (0.2 µg/mL) for susceptible strains of *Streptococcus equi* subsp *zooepidemicus* for 10 days.

In cattle, SC administration of CCFA—in the middle third of the posterior aspect of the ear of beef and nonlactating dairy cattle or in the posterior aspect of the ear where it attaches to the head of beef, nonlactating dairy, and lactating dairy cattle—provides therapeutic concentrations of ceftiofur and desfuroylceftiofur-related metabolites in plasma above the MIC_{90} for BRD pathogens (*Pasteurella multocida, Mannheimia haemolytica,* and *Histophilus somni*) for generally not less than 150 hours after single administration. Pharmacokinetic studies indicate that base of ear (BOE) administration in dairy cattle is therapeutically equivalent to middle of ear (MOE) administration in beef cattle, with blood levels at therapeutic threshold within 2 hours of administration at both sites using labeled doses.

CCFA 6.6 mg/kg SC in neonatal calves to treat diarrhea (extra-label) provided plasma concentrations above the therapeutic target of 2 µg/mL for at least 3 days following a single dose.[5]

In swine, therapeutic plasma levels for the parent compound and primary metabolite, desfuroylceftiofur, are reached within 1 hour of administration.[8] Plasma levels remained above the MIC for nearly 100% of target SRD pathogens for an average of 8 days.

Approximate half-lives of ceftiofur/desfuroylceftiofur after administration of 6.6 mg/kg SC in a variety of species include alpacas, 45 hours[9]; goats, 37 to 49 hours[10-12]; and elephants, 84 hours.[13] In elephants, a dose of 6.6 mg/kg SC provided adequate plasma concentrations for 7 to 10 days.

In sheep, adequate therapeutic serum concentrations of CCFA for treatment of disease caused by *M haemolytica* and *P multocida* were achieved following SC administration in the right cervical region with a single dose of 6.6 mg/kg. The dosing interval for CCFA in sheep is suggested to be 48 to 72 hours. Adverse systemic reactions were not observed.[14]

A single dose of CCFA (30 mg/kg) administered IM or SC to bearded dragons yielded plasma concentrations of ceftiofur and its metabolites more than 1 µg/mL for more than 288 hours.[6] The author reports the SC route was preferred over the IM route because of less variability in plasma concentrations and greater ease of administration. The author's analysis suggests that a single dose of 30 mg/kg SC may be used to treat infections susceptible to ceftiofur in bearded dragons.

In red-tailed hawks, study results suggest that CCFA could be administered IM in the pectoral region at 10 or 20 mg/kg to treat infections with ceftiofur-susceptible bacteria.[15] Administration resulted in little to no inflammation at the injection site.

Contraindications/Precautions/Warnings

Cephalosporins are contraindicated in patients with a history of hypersensitivity to them. Hypersensitivity reactions unrelated to dosage can occur with cephalosporin antibiotics and manifest as rashes, fever, eosinophilia, lymphadenopathy, or anaphylaxis. The use of cephalosporins in patients documented to be hypersensitive to penicillin class antibiotics is controversial. In humans, it is estimated that 1% to 15% of patients hypersensitive to penicillins will also be hypersensitive to cephalosporins. The incidence of cross-reactivity in veterinary patients is unknown; however, because there may be cross-reactivity, use cephalosporins cautiously in patients that are documented hypersensitive to other beta-lactam antibiotics (eg, penicillins, cephamycins, carbapenems).

In horses, the manufacturer warns that if acute diarrhea is observed after dosing, additional doses should not be administered and appropriate therapy for diarrhea should be initiated.[7] Ceftiofur use has not been evaluated in horses less than 4 months of age and in breeding, pregnant, or lactating horses. The long-term effects on injection sites have not been evaluated in this species. Additionally, the manufacturer warns that due to the extended exposure in horses, based on the drug's pharmacokinetic properties, adverse reactions may require prolonged monitoring and care, as ≈17 days are needed to eliminate 97% of the dose from the body.

Administer to cattle by the SC route only. Inadvertent intra-arterial injection is likely to result in sudden death.

Ceftiofur can be easily confused with other cephalosporins. Consider writing orders and prescriptions using tall man letters: cefTIOfur. Do not confuse the three distinct formulations for this drug (HCl, sodium, and CFA).

Adverse Effects

Adverse effects with the cephalosporins are usually not serious and have a relatively low frequency of occurrence, but cephalosporins can cause allergic reactions in sensitized patients. Topical exposures to such antimicrobials, including ceftiofur, may elicit mild to severe allergic reactions in some patients. Repeated or prolonged exposure may lead to sensitization.

In horses, CCFA may cause firmness, swelling, sensitivity, and/or edema at the injection site and diarrhea, soft or loose stools, ataxia, muscle tremors, and allergic reactions.[7] When used in an extra-label manner (long-term weekly SC injections), significantly greater swelling occurred at the injection site compared to that observed after single IM administration.[16] Clinical signs consistent with foot pain were noted in healthy horses undergoing a pharmacokinetic study, but causal relationship with ceftiofur was not definitively determined.[7]

Following SC injection in the middle third of the posterior aspect of the ear of cattle, thickening and swelling (characterized by aseptic cellular infiltrate) of the ear may occur.[1] As with other parenteral injections, localized postinjection bacterial infections may result in abscess formation. Attention to hygienic procedures can minimize occurrence. Following SC injections at the posterior aspect of the ear where it attaches to the head (base of the ear), areas of discoloration and signs of inflammation may persist for at least 13 days, potentially resulting in trim loss of edible tissue at slaughter. Injection of volumes greater than 20 mL in the middle third of the ear may result in open draining lesions in a small percentage of cattle.

Reproductive/Nursing Safety

The manufacturer states that the effects of ceftiofur on bovine reproductive performance, pregnancy, and lactation have not been determined,[1] and the safety of ceftiofur has not been demonstrated for pregnant swine or swine intended for breeding.[8] Ceftiofur use has not been evaluated in breeding, pregnant, or lactating horses.[7] However, cephalosporins as a class are relatively safe for use during pregnancy, and teratogenic or embryotoxic effects would not be anticipated.

Target animal safety studies report administration of a single dose of ceftiofur CFA at the base of the ear in high-producing dairy cattle did not adversely affect milk production compared to untreated controls. Ceftiofur in maternal milk would be unlikely pose significant risk to offspring.

Overdose/Acute Toxicity

Cephalosporin overdoses are unlikely to cause significant problems other than injection site reactions or GI distress, but other effects are possible (see ***Adverse Effects***). Use of this drug in excess of labeled dosages or via unapproved routes of administration may cause violative residues; contact FARAD (see ***Appendix***) for assistance in determining appropriate withdrawal times in these circumstances.

Equine safety data: Dosages up to 20 mg/kg IM every 4 days for 6 doses given to healthy horses resulted in injection-site reactions (eg, edema, firmness) but no treatment-related GI findings.[7]

Cattle safety data: Results from a 5-day tolerance study in feeder calves indicated that ceftiofur sodium was well-tolerated at 55 mg ceftiofur equivalents/kg (25 times the highest recommended dose) for 5 consecutive days. Ceftiofur administered IM had no adverse systemic effects.[1]

Swine safety data: Results from a 5-day tolerance study in normal feeder pigs indicated that ceftiofur sodium was well-tolerated when administered at 125 mg ceftiofur equivalents/kg (more than 25 times the highest recommended daily dosage) for 5 consecutive days. Ceftiofur administered IM to pigs produced no overt adverse signs of toxicity.[8]

For patients that have experienced or are suspected to have experienced an overdose, consultation with a 24-hour poison consultation center specializing in providing veterinary-specific information is recommended. For general information related to overdose and toxin exposures, as well as contact information for poison control centers, refer to ***Appendix.***

Drug Interactions

The following drug interactions have either been reported or are theoretical in humans or animals receiving ceftiofur and may be of significance in veterinary patients. Unless otherwise noted, use together is not necessarily contraindicated, but weigh the potential risks and perform additional monitoring when appropriate.

- **Aminoglycosides** (eg, **amikacin, gentamicin**): The concurrent use of parenteral aminoglycosides with cephalosporins is somewhat controversial. Potentially, cephalosporins could cause additive nephrotoxicity when used with these drugs, but this interaction has only been well-documented with cephaloridine (no longer marketed). In vitro studies have demonstrated that cephalosporins can have synergistic or additive activity against certain bacteria when used with aminoglycosides,[17] but the drugs should be administered at separate times.
- **Nephrotoxic Drugs** (eg, **amphotericin B, furosemide, iohexol**): Concurrent use with ceftiofur may cause additive nephrotoxicity.
- **Probenecid**: Competitively blocks the tubular secretion of most cephalosporins, thereby increasing serum levels and serum half-lives.

Laboratory Considerations

NOTE: Considerations listed below are for cefotaxime, which is structurally similar to ceftiofur; these considerations may apply to ceftiofur.

- Except for cefotaxime, cephalosporins may cause false-positive **urine glucose determinations** when using cupric sulfate solution (Benedict's solution, *Clinitest®*). Tests using glucose oxidase (*Tes-Tape®*, *Clinistix®*) are not affected by cephalosporins.
- When using the Jaffe reaction to measure **serum or urine creatinine**, cephalosporins (not ceftazidime or cefotaxime) at high dosages may cause falsely elevated values.
- In humans, particularly with azotemia, cephalosporins have caused a false-positive direct **Coombs test.**[18]
- Cephalosporins may also cause falsely elevated **17-ketosteroid** values in urine.

Dosages

HORSES:

Equine strangles *(Streptococcus equi* subsp ***zooepidemicus)*** (label dosage; FDA-approved): 6.6 mg/kg IM; repeat in 4 days. A maximum of 20 mL per injection site may be administered.

Susceptible bacterial infection in neonatal foals (extra-label): 13.2 mg/kg SC every 48 hours. **NOTE**: Dosage is based on a pharmacokinetic study in healthy foals.[19]

CATTLE:

Treatment of Bovine Respiratory Disease (BRD) and bovine foot rot (label dosage for beef, nonlactating dairy, and lactating dairy cattle; FDA-approved): 6.6 mg/kg (3 mg/lb) as a single injection SC in the posterior aspect of the ear base where it attaches to the head (1.5 mL sterile suspension per 45.3 kg [100 lb] BW).[1] In beef and nonlactating dairy cattle, it may also be administered as a single SC injection in the middle third of the posterior aspect of the ear at the same dosage. Most animals will respond to treatment within 3 to 5 days. If no improvement is observed, the diagnosis should be re-evaluated.

Control of BRD (label dosage for beef and nonlactating dairy cattle only at high risk of developing BRD; FDA-approved): 6.6 mg/kg (3 mg/lb) as a single injection SC in the middle third of the posterior aspect of the ear OR in the posterior aspect of the ear base where it attaches to the head (1.5 mL sterile suspension per 45.3 kg [100 lb] BW).[1]

Acute metritis in lactating dairy cattle (labeled dosage; FDA-approved): 6.6 mg/kg (3 mg/lb) as a single injection SC in the posterior aspect of the ear base where it attaches to the head (1.5 mL sterile suspension per 45.3 kg [100 lb] BW).[1] Repeat this dose in the opposite ear ≈72 hours following the initial dose.

GOATS:

Susceptible bacterial infection (extra-label): 6.6 mg/kg SC once. **NOTE**: dosage based on a pharmacokinetic study in healthy female goats.[11]

SWINE:

Swine Respiratory Disease (label dosage; FDA-approved): Administer by IM injection in the postauricular region of the neck as a single dosage of 5 mg/kg (1 mL sterile suspension per 20 kg [44 lb] BW).[8] No more than 2 mL should be injected in a single injection site. Pigs heavier than 40 kg (88 lb) will require more than one injection. Most animals will respond to treatment within 3 to 5 days. If no improvement is observed, the diagnosis should be re-evaluated.

RABBITS:

Susceptible bacterial infection (extra-label): 40 mg/kg SC every 24 to 72 hours. **NOTE:** Dosage is based on a single-dose pharmacokinetic study in healthy New Zealand White rabbits.[20]

Monitoring

Because cephalosporins usually have minimal toxicity associated with their use, monitoring for efficacy is usually all that is required.

Patients with diminished renal function may require intensified renal monitoring. Therapeutic drug monitoring is not typically done.

Client Information

- Be sure you know how to administer this medication safely. **Injection of this form of ceftiofur into a blood vessel can result in sudden death of the animal.**
- This drug must be injected as a shot; it does not work when given by mouth. In cattle, it is injected under the skin (SC) in the ear; in swine, it is given into the muscle in the neck, behind the ear; in horses, it is given into the muscle (IM).
- Antibiotic effect is long-lasting after a single injection under the skin in cattle, pigs, and horses.
- Follow recommended withholding times when using in an animal that will be used for human food.
- Persons with a known hypersensitivity to penicillin or cephalosporins should handle this drug carefully to avoid accidental exposure.

Chemistry/Synonyms

CCFA contains 200 mg/mL of ceftiofur in a caprylic/capric triglyceride and cottonseed oil base. It has a molecular weight of 523.58.

CCFA may also be known as CM-31916, ceftiofuri, or *Excede*®.

Storage/Stability

CCFA cattle and swine products should be stored at a controlled room temperature 20°C to 25°C (68°F-77°F). Shake well before using. Contents should be used within 12 weeks after the first dose is removed.

Compatibility/Compounding Considerations

No specific information noted

Dosage Forms/Regulatory Status

VETERINARY-LABELED PRODUCTS:

Ceftiofur Crystalline Free Acid equivalent to 200 mg/mL ceftiofur in 100 mL and 250 mL vials; *Excede*® Sterile Suspension. FDA-approved for use in horses, beef, lactating and nonlactating cattle. Following labeled use as either a single-dose or 2-dose regimen, no milk discard period is required, but a 13-day pre-slaughter withdrawal period is required after the last treatment. Do not use in calves to be processed for veal, or in horses intended for human consumption. A withdrawal period has not been established for this product in preruminating calves. Use of doses in excess of 6.6 mg/kg or administration by unapproved routes (SC injection in the neck or IM injection) may cause violative residues.

Ceftiofur Crystalline Free Acid equivalent to 100 mg/mL ceftiofur in 100 mL vials; *Excede® for Swine*; (Rx). Following labeled use as a single treatment, a 14-day preslaughter withdrawal period is required. Doses in excess of label directions or administration by an unapproved route may result in illegal residues in edible tissues.

In 2012, the FDA prohibited extra-label use of cephalosporin in major food animal species (see ***Extra-Label Drug Use***).

HUMAN-LABELED PRODUCTS: NONE

References

For the complete list of references, see **wiley.com/go/budde/plumb**

Ceftiofur HCl

(sef-***tee***-oh-fur) *Excenel® RTU EZ, Cefenil® RTU, Spectramast®*

Third-Generation Cephalosporin

Prescriber Highlights

- ► A veterinary-only third-generation cephalosporin approved as an intramammary infusion for dairy cattle and as an injection (given daily) for swine and cattle
- ► Withdrawal times in cattle vary based on product formulations.
- ► Potentially causes hypersensitivity reactions, granulocytopenia, thrombocytopenia, or diarrhea
- ► IM injection route can cause pain in small animal species.

Uses/Indications

In cattle, ceftiofur HCl is FDA-approved for the treatment of the following bacterial diseases: Bovine respiratory diseases (eg, BRD, shipping fever, pneumonia) associated with *Mannheimia haemolytica, Pasteurella multocida,* and *Histophilus somni*; acute bovine interdigital necrobacillosis (foot rot, pododermatitis) associated with *Fusobacterium necrophorum* and *Bacteroides melaninogenicus*; and acute metritis (0 to 14 days postpartum) associated with bacterial organisms susceptible to ceftiofur.

The intramammary syringe for dry dairy cattle (*Spectramast DC*®) is FDA-approved for the treatment of subclinical mastitis in dairy cattle (at the time of dry off) associated with *Staphylococcus aureus, Streptococcus dysgalactiae,* and *Streptococcus uberis*. The intramammary syringe for lactating dairy cattle (*Spectramast LC*®) is labeled for the treatment of clinical mastitis in lactating dairy cattle associated with coagulase-negative staphylococci, *Streptococcus dysgalactiae,* and *Escherichia coli* and the treatment of diagnosed subclinical mastitis associated with coagulase-negative staphylococci and *Streptococcus dysgalactiae*.

In swine, ceftiofur HCl injection is FDA-approved for the treatment and control of swine bacterial respiratory disease associated with *Actinobacillus (Haemophilus) pleuropneumoniae, Pasteurella multocida, Salmonella choleraesuis,* and *Streptococcus suis*.

The World Health Organization has designated third-generation cephalosporins as Critically Important (Highest Priority) antimicrobials for humans.[1] The Office International des Epizooties (OIE) has designated ceftiofur as a Veterinary Critically Important Antimicrobial (VCIA) Agent in avian, bovine, caprine, equine, lagomorph, ovine, and swine species.[2]

Pharmacology/Actions

Ceftiofur is a third-generation, time-dependent, bactericidal cephalosporin antibiotic that is active against a variety of gram-positive and gram-negative bacteria and that, like other cephalosporins, inhibits bacteria cell wall synthesis.

Ceftiofur is rapidly cleaved into furoic acid and desfuroylceftiofur (active). Desfuroylceftiofur inhibits cell-wall synthesis (at stage 3) of susceptible multiplying bacteria and exhibits a spectrum of activity similar to that of cefotaxime (a third-generation cephalosporin). Parent ceftiofur and the primary metabolite are equally potent and assays to measure microbial sensitivity (plasma and tissue levels) are based on ceftiofur equivalents (CE). The protein-binding activity of ceftiofur creates a reservoir effect to maintain active levels at the site of infection.

In cattle, ceftiofur has a broad range of in vitro activity against a variety of pathogens, including *Pasteurella* spp, *Streptococcus* spp, *Staphylococcus* spp, *Salmonella* spp, and *Escherichia coli*.

In swine, ceftiofur HCl has activity against the pathogens *Actinobacillus pleuropneumoniae, Pasteurella multocida, Haemophilus parasuis,* and *Streptococcus suis* for an extended period of time.

Ceftiofur is ineffective against methicillin-resistant staphylococci, extended-spectrum beta-lactamase–producing gram-negative bacteria, and enterococci.

Pharmacokinetics

In cattle and swine, ceftiofur is rapidly metabolized to desfuroylceftiofur, the primary and active metabolite. In cattle, the peak total ceftiofur concentration (ceftiofur + desfuroylceftiofur) of ≈9.2 µg/mL is reached ≈1.7 hours and 2.25 hour after IM and SC administration, respectively, and elimination half-life is 29 to 33 hours.[3] Total ceftiofur plasma concentration remained above 0.2 µg/mL for ≈41 hours after administration of a single SC or IM dose of 5 mg/kg (**NOTE:** This exceeds the FDA-approved dose).[3]

The elimination kinetics of ceftiofur HCl in milk when used in an extra-label manner to treat coliform mastitis has been studied. Milk samples were tested after two 300 mg doses (6 mL) administered 12 hours apart into the affected mammary quarters. The samples tested at less than the tolerance level for this drug set by FDA by 7 hours after the last intramammary administration. However, the authors noted considerable variability in the time required for samples from individual cows and mammary gland quarters to consistently have drug residues less than the tolerance level and reported that elimination rates of the drug may be related to milk production. Therefore, cows producing smaller volumes of milk may have prolonged withdrawal times.[4]

In lactating dairy cattle, active ceftiofur concentrations were measured after the administration of 1 mg/kg SC in healthy dairy cattle within 24 hours of calving. Drug concentrations were found to exceed MIC in uterine tissues and lochial fluid for common pathogens.[5]

In swine given 5 mg/kg IM, the peak total ceftiofur concentration (ceftiofur + desfuroylceftiofur) of 19.7 µg/mL is reached after ≈1.5 hours, elimination half-life is 20 hours, and total ceftiofur plasma concentration remained above 0.2 µg/mL for 82.5 hours.[3] A study measuring tissue distribution following IM injection of varying doses to swine revealed the highest concentration was detected in the kidneys, followed by the lungs, liver, and muscle tissues.[6]

Contraindications/Precautions/Warnings

Cephalosporins are contraindicated in patients with a history of hypersensitivity to them. Hypersensitivity reactions unrelated to dosage can occur with cephalosporin antibiotics and manifest as rashes, fever, eosinophilia, lymphadenopathy, or anaphylaxis. Use of cephalosporins in patients documented to be hypersensitive to penicillin-class antibiotics is controversial. In humans, it is estimated that 1% to 15% of patients hypersensitive to penicillins will also be hypersensitive to cephalosporins. The incidence of cross-reactivity in veterinary patients is unknown; however, because there may be cross-reactivity, use cephalosporins cautiously in patients that are documented hypersensitive to other beta-lactam antibiotics (eg, penicillins, cephamycins, carbapenems).

In cattle, after IM or SC administration, areas of discoloration at the site may result in trim loss of edible tissues at slaughter. Discard milk obtained during treatment with intramammary (LC) product.

In swine, areas of discoloration associated with the injection site may result in trim-out of edible tissues at slaughter.

The injectable product should not be given in a vein or artery.

Ceftiofur can be easily confused with other cephalosporins. Consider writing orders and prescriptions using tall man letters: cefTIOfur. Do not confuse the 3 distinct formulations for this drug (HCl, sodium, and crystalline free acid [CFA]). Branded drug names may not be consistent internationally (eg, in Canada, *Excenel®* contains ceftiofur sodium, whereas in the US, *Excenel® RTU EZ* contains ceftiofur HCl).

Adverse Effects

Adverse effects with the cephalosporins are usually not serious and have a relatively low frequency of occurrence, but cephalosporins can cause allergic reactions in sensitized individuals. Topical exposures to such antimicrobials, including ceftiofur, may elicit mild to severe allergic reactions in some individuals. Repeated or prolonged exposure may lead to sensitization.

Injection-site reactions (eg, swelling, erythema, firmness) occur in ≈59% in cattle following SC administration but appear to be uncommon (less than 0.4%) with IM administration.[3]

Reproductive/Nursing Safety

The manufacturer states that the effects of ceftiofur on bovine reproductive performance, pregnancy, and lactation have not been determined, and the safety of ceftiofur has not been demonstrated for pregnant swine or swine intended for breeding. However, cephalosporins as a class are relatively safe for use during pregnancy, and teratogenic or embryotoxic effects would not be anticipated.

Ceftiofur in maternal milk would be unlikely pose significant risk to offspring.

Overdose/Acute Toxicity

Cephalosporin overdoses are unlikely to cause significant problems other than GI distress, but other effects are possible (see ***Adverse Effects*** section). Use of this drug in excess of labeled dosages or by unapproved routes of administration may cause violative residues. Contact FARAD (see ***Appendix***) for assistance in determining appropriate withdrawal times in circumstances where the drug has been used at higher-than-labeled dosages.

Cattle safety data: Results from a 5-day tolerance study in feeder calves indicated that ceftiofur sodium (proven to be equivalent to ceftiofur HCl) was well tolerated at 55 mg ceftiofur equivalents/kg (25 times the highest recommended dose) for 5 consecutive days. Ceftiofur administered IM had no adverse systemic effects.[7]

Swine safety data: Results from a 5-day tolerance study in normal feeder pigs indicated that ceftiofur sodium (proven to be equivalent to ceftiofur HCl) was well-tolerated when administered at 125 mg ceftiofur equivalents/kg (more than 25 times the highest recommended daily dosage) for 5 consecutive days. Ceftiofur administered IM to pigs produced no overt adverse signs of toxicity.[7]

For patients that have experienced or are suspected to have experienced an overdose, consultation with a 24-hour poison consultation center specializing in providing veterinary-specific information is recommended. For general information related to overdose and toxin exposures, as well as contact information for poison control centers, refer to ***Appendix***.

Drug Interactions

The following drug interactions have either been reported or are theoretical in humans or animals receiving ceftiofur and may be of significance in veterinary patients. Unless otherwise noted, use together is not necessarily contraindicated, but weigh the potential risks and perform additional monitoring when appropriate.

- **Aminoglycosides** (eg, **amikacin, gentamicin**): Concurrent use of parenteral aminoglycosides with cephalosporins is somewhat controversial. Potentially, cephalosporins could cause additive nephrotoxicity when used with these drugs, but this interaction has only been well-documented with cephaloridine (no longer marketed). In vitro studies have demonstrated that cephalosporins can have synergistic or additive activity against certain bacteria when used with aminoglycosides,[8] but the drugs should be administered at separate times.
- **Nephrotoxic Drugs** (eg, **amphotericin B, furosemide, iohexol**): Concurrent use with ceftiofur may cause additive nephrotoxicity.
- **Probenecid**: Competitively blocks the tubular secretion of most cephalosporins thereby increasing serum levels and serum half-lives.

Laboratory Considerations

NOTE: Considerations listed below are for cefotaxime, which is structurally similar to ceftiofur; these considerations may apply to ceftiofur.

- Except for cefotaxime, cephalosporins may cause false-positive **urine glucose determinations** when cupric sulfate solution (Benedict's solution, *Clinitest*®) is used. Tests using glucose oxidase (*Tes-Tape*®, *Clinistix*®) are not affected by cephalosporins.
- When the Jaffe reaction is used to measure **serum or urine creatinine**, cephalosporins (not ceftazidime or cefotaxime) at high dosages may cause falsely elevated values.
- In humans, particularly those with azotemia, cephalosporins have caused a false-positive direct **Coombs test**.[9]
- Cephalosporins may also cause falsely elevated **17-ketosteroid** values in urine.

Dosages

CATTLE:

Bovine respiratory disease (BRD) and acute bovine interdigital necrobacillosis (label dosage; FDA-approved): 1.1 – 2.2 mg/kg IM or SC (1 – 2 mL sterile suspension per 45kg [100 lb]) daily for a total of 3 consecutive days.[3,10] Additional treatments may be administered on days 4 and 5 for animals that do not show a satisfactory response. For BRD only. Based on an assessment of the severity of disease, pathogen susceptibility and clinical response, can administer 2.2 mg/kg IM or SC every other day on days 1 and 3 (48-hour interval). Do not inject more than 15 mL per injection site.

Acute postpartum metritis (label dosage; FDA-approved): 2.2 mg/kg IM or SC (2 mL sterile suspension per 45 kg [100 lb]) daily for 5 consecutive days.[3,10] Do not inject more than 15 mL per injection site.

Subclinical mastitis in dairy cattle at time of dry off associated with *Staphylococcal aureus, Streptococcus dysgalactiae,* or *Streptococcus uberis* (label dosage; FDA-approved): Infuse one syringe of *Spectramast*® *DC* into each affected quarter at the time of dry off.[12]

Clinical or diagnosed subclinical mastitis in lactating dairy cattle associated with coagulase-negative staphylococci *Streptococcus dysgalactiae* or *Escherichia coli* (label dosage; FDA-approved): Infuse one syringe of *Spectramast*® *LC* into each affected quarter.[13] Repeat this treatment in 24 hours. For extended duration therapy, once daily treatment may be repeated for up to 8 consecutive days.

Neonatal salmonellosis (extra-label): Ceftiofur HCl 5 mg/kg IM once daily for 5 days[11]

SWINE:

Swine bacterial respiratory infections (label dosage; FDA-approved): 3 – 5 mg/kg IM (1 mL of sterile suspension per 10 to 16.7 kg [22 to 37 lb] body weight) every 24 hours for a total of 3 consecutive days[3,10]

Monitoring

Because minimal toxicity is associated with use of cephalosporins, monitoring for efficacy is usually all that is required. Patients with diminished renal function may require intensified renal monitoring. Therapeutic drug monitoring is not typically done.

Client Information

For the injectable product:

- Be sure you know how to administer this medication safely.
- This drug must be given as a shot under the skin or into the muscle only; do not give in a vein or artery. It does not work when given by mouth.
- Do not give more than 15 mL at one site.
- May cause discoloration of the skin at the injection site
- Follow recommended drug residue withholding times if you are administering to an animal that will be used for human food.

For the intramammary product:

- Wash teats thoroughly with warm water mixed with a suitable antiseptic and dry thoroughly.
- Milk udder out completely.
- Wipe end of affected teat with provided alcohol pad; use a separate pad for each teat.
- Insert tip of syringe into teat canal and push plunger to dispense entire contents.
- Massage quarter to distribute suspension into the milk cistern.
- Follow recommended drug residue withholding times.

Chemistry/Synonyms

Ceftiofur HCl is a semisynthetic third-generation cephalosporin. Ceftiofur HCl is a weak acid, acid-stable, and water soluble with a molecular weight of 560. The RTU injectable sterile suspension is a ready-to-use formulation that contains ceftiofur hydrochloride equivalent to 50 mg ceftiofur, 5.73 mg aluminum monostearate, 1.03 mg sorbitan monooleate, and medium chain triglycerides. The RTU EZ injectable sterile suspension is a ready-to-use formulation that contains ceftiofur hydrochloride equivalent to 50 mg ceftiofur, 2.50 mg polyoxyethylene sorbitan monooleate (polysorbate 80), 6.5 mg water for injection in a caprylic/capric triglyceride (*Miglyol* 812) suspension. Both *Spectramast*® products are sterile, oil-based suspensions of ceftiofur HCl.

Ceftiofur HCl may also be known as U-64279A, ceftiofuri hydrochloridium, *Cefenil*® *RTU, Excenel*® *RTU*, or *Excenel*® *RTU EZ*.

Storage/Stability

The ready-to-use injectable product should be stored at room temperature (either 20°C to 25°C (68°F-77°F) or less than 30°C (86°F), depending on the product used; consult product label). Shake well before using; protect from freezing. Contents should be used within 42 days after first dose is removed.

The intramammary syringes should be stored at controlled room temperature 20°C to 25°C (68°F-77°F). Protect from light. Store plastets in carton until used.

Compatibility/Compounding Considerations

No specific information noted

Dosage Forms/Regulatory Status

VETERINARY-LABELED PRODUCTS:

Ceftiofur HCl Sterile Suspension for injection, 50 mg/mL in 100 mL and 250 mL vials; *Cefenil*® RTU; (Rx). FDA-approved for use in cattle and swine. Slaughter withdrawal = 3 days in cattle; 4 days in swine. There is no required milk discard time.

Ceftiofur HCl Sterile Suspension for injection, 50 mg/mL in 100 mL and 250 mL vials; *Excenel*® RTU EZ; (Rx). FDA-approved for use in cattle (not veal calves) and swine. Slaughter withdrawal = 4 days in cattle (withdrawal period not determined in pre-ruminating calves); 4 days in swine if injected volume is less than/equal to 5 mL, and 6 days if volume is greater than 5 mL but less than or equal to 15 mL. There is no required milk discard time.

Ceftiofur HCl Sterile Suspension for Intramammary Infusion in Dry Cows 500 mg ceftiofur equivalents (as the HCl) per 10 mL syringe (plastets) in packages of 12 or 144 syringes with 70% isopropyl alcohol pads; *Spectramast*® *DC*; (Rx). Slaughter withdrawal for cattle = 16 days (no slaughter withdrawal required for neonatal calves born from treated cows)

Ceftiofur HCl Sterile Suspension for Intramammary Infusion in

Lactating Cows 125 mg ceftiofur equivalents (as the HCl) per 10 mL syringe (plastets) in packages of 12 or 144 syringes with 70% isopropyl alcohol pads; *Spectramast® LC*; (Rx). Cattle slaughter withdrawal = 2 days; milk discard = 72 hours

In 2012, the FDA prohibited extra-label use of cephalosporin in major food animal species. (See ***Extra-Label Drug Use***)

HUMAN-LABELED PRODUCTS: NONE

References

For the complete list of references, see **wiley.com/go/budde/plumb**

Ceftiofur Sodium

(sef-***tee***-oh-fur) *Naxcel®, Ceftiflex®*

Third-Generation Cephalosporin

Prescriber Highlights

- ► A veterinary-only third-generation cephalosporin approved for use in dogs, horses, cattle, sheep/goats, swine, and poultry. Also used in an extra-label manner in a variety of other species
- ► Potentially causes hypersensitivity reactions, granulocytopenia, thrombocytopenia, or diarrhea
- ► Causes pain on IM injection in small animals

Uses/Indications

In dogs, ceftiofur is labeled for treatment of canine UTIs associated with *Escherichia coli* and *Proteus mirabilis*.

In horses, ceftiofur is labeled for treatment of respiratory infections associated with *Streptococcus equi* subsp *zooepidemicus*.

In cattle, ceftiofur sodium is FDA-approved for treatment of bovine respiratory disease (BRD; eg, shipping fever, pneumonia) associated with *Mannheimia haemolytica*, *Pasteurella multocida*, and *Histophilus somni*. It is also indicated for treatment of acute bovine interdigital necrobacillosis (eg, foot rot, pododermatitis) associated with *Fusobacterium necrophorum* and *Bacteroides melaninogenicus*.

In swine, ceftiofur is labeled for treatment and control of swine bacterial respiratory disease (eg, swine bacterial pneumonia) associated with *Actinobacillus (Haemophilus) pleuropneumoniae*, *Pasteurella multocida*, *Salmonella choleraesuis*, and *Streptococcus suis*.

In sheep and goats, ceftiofur is labeled for treatment of sheep/caprine respiratory disease (eg, sheep/goat pneumonia) associated with *Mannheimia haemolytica* and *Pasteurella multocida*.

In day-old chicks and poults, ceftiofur is labeled for control of early mortality associated with *Escherichia coli* organisms susceptible to ceftiofur.

Ceftiofur has also been used in an extra-label manner in a variety of veterinary species (see ***Dosages***) to treat infections susceptible to a third-generation cephalosporin.

The World Health Organization (WHO) has designated third-generation cephalosporins as Critically Important, Highest Priority antimicrobials for human medicine.[1] The Office International des Epizooties (OIE) has designated ceftiofur as a Veterinary Critically Important Antimicrobial (VCIA) Agent in avian, bovine, caprine, equine, lagomorph, ovine, and swine species.[2]

Pharmacology/Actions

Ceftiofur is a third-generation cephalosporin and a time-dependent bactericidal antibiotic active against a variety of gram-positive and gram-negative bacteria; like other cephalosporins, it inhibits bacteria cell wall synthesis.

Ceftiofur is rapidly cleaved into furoic acid and desfuroylceftiofur (active). Desfuroylceftiofur inhibits cell wall synthesis (at stage 3) of susceptible multiplying bacteria and exhibits a spectrum of activity similar to that of cefotaxime (ie, a third-generation cephalosporin). Parent ceftiofur and the primary metabolite are equally potent and assays to measure microbial sensitivity (plasma and tissue levels) are based on ceftiofur equivalents (CE). Ceftiofur has a broad range of in vitro activity against a variety of pathogens, including *Pasteurella* spp, *Streptococcus* spp, *Staphylococcus* spp, *Salmonella* spp, and *Escherichia coli*. It is ineffective against methicillin-resistant staphylococci, extended spectrum beta-lactamase-producing gram-negative bacteria, and enterococci.

Pharmacokinetics

In cattle, ceftiofur sodium and HCl have practically equivalent pharmacokinetic parameters. The following pharmacokinetic values for cattle are for the active metabolite desfuroylceftiofur. The volume of distribution in cattle is ≈0.3 L/kg. Peak concentrations are ≈7 µg/mL after IM injection of *Naxcel®*, but areas under the curve and elimination half-lives (≈8-12 hours) for both forms of the drug are practically equal. Peak concentrations occur 30 to 45 minutes after IM dosing. Pharmacokinetic parameters of ceftiofur sodium are similar for either SC or IM injection in cattle.

In dairy goats given ceftiofur 1.1 mg/kg or 2.2 mg/kg IV or IM, 100% bioavailability was demonstrated via the IM route. After 5 daily IM doses of the drug, serum concentrations were found to be dose proportional.[3] Lactating does eliminate the drug more rapidly as compared with nonlactating does.[4]

Ceftiofur sodium given IM to beef cattle, dairy cattle, swine, and sheep is absorbed quickly and metabolized rapidly to desfuroylceftiofur (DFC), which can be further converted to desfuroylceftiofur cysteine disulfide (DCCD), condensed to a dimer, or bound to proteins or other macromolecules. New determinative and confirmatory methods by liquid chromatography-mass spectrometry (LC-MS) have been developed and validated for DCCD in bovine kidney, liver, and muscle to modernize the drug residue monitoring approach.[5]

In horses, 2 g of ceftiofur was administered via regional IV perfusion or systemic IV to determine radiocarpal joint synovial fluid and plasma concentrations.[6] Mean synovial fluid concentrations were higher for the regional IV perfusion than systemic IV administration. The study concluded that regional IV perfusion induced significantly higher intra-articular antibiotic concentrations in the radiocarpal joint as compared with systemic IV administration. In addition, synovial fluid drug concentrations remained above the MIC for common pathogens longer than 24 hours.[6] A separate study evaluating regional IV perfusion found plasma concentration above common bacterial MIC 12 hours after administration and SC tissue concentration above MIC for 24 hours.[7]

In foals, administration of ceftiofur sodium 2.2 mg/kg once daily for 5 days (5 total doses) via nebulization was well-tolerated, and desfuroylceftiofur acetamide concentrations in plasma and pulmonary epithelial lining fluid remained above the MIC required to inhibit the growth of 90% of *Streptococcus equi* subsp *zooepidemicus* for ≈24 hours after administration, suggesting further investigation for treatment of bacterial infections of the lower respiratory tract in horses.[8] Terminal half-life in pregnant pony mares was ≈3 to 4 hours after IM administration.[9]

In dogs, ceftiofur sodium only attains effective concentrations in urine.[10]

Contraindications/Precautions/Warnings

Cephalosporins are contraindicated in patients with a history of hypersensitivity to them. Hypersensitivity reactions unrelated to dosage can occur with cephalosporin antibiotics and manifest as rashes, fever, eosinophilia, lymphadenopathy, or anaphylaxis. The use of cephalosporins in patients documented to be hypersensitive to penicillin class antibiotics is controversial. In humans, it is estimated that 1% to 15% of patients hypersensitive to penicillins will also be hypersensitive to cephalosporins. The incidence of cross-reactivity in veterinary patients is unknown; however, because there may be cross-reactivity, use cephalosporins cautiously in patients that are documented to be hypersensitive to other beta-lactam antibiotics (eg, penicillins, cephamycins, carbapenems).

Ceftiofur can be easily confused with other cephalosporins. Consider writing orders and prescriptions using tall man letters: cefTIOfur. Do not confuse the 3 distinct formulations for this drug (HCl, sodium, and crystalline free acid [CFA]). Branded drugs names may not be consistent internationally (eg, in Canada, *Excenel®* contains ceftiofur sodium; in the US *Excenel® RTU EZ* contains ceftiofur HCl).

Adverse Effects

Adverse effects with cephalosporins are usually not serious and have a relatively low frequency of occurrence, but cephalosporins can cause allergic reactions in sensitized patients. Topical exposures to such antimicrobials, including ceftiofur, may elicit mild to severe allergic reactions in some patients. Repeated or prolonged exposure may lead to sensitization.

Following SC administration of ceftiofur sodium in the neck, small areas of discoloration at the site may persist beyond 5 days, potentially resulting in trim loss of edible tissue at slaughter. Localized postinjection bacterial infections may result in abscess formation in cattle; attention to hygienic procedures can minimize their occurrence.

Reproductive/Nursing Safety

The manufacturer states that the effects of ceftiofur on bovine reproductive performance, pregnancy, and lactation have not been determined, and the safety of ceftiofur has not been demonstrated in pregnant swine or swine intended for breeding. However, cephalosporins as a class are relatively safe for use during pregnancy, and teratogenic or embryotoxic effects would not be anticipated.

Most cephalosporins are excreted in milk in small quantities. The active ceftiofur metabolite was present in colostrum of pony mares at 3% to 33% of maternal serum values.[9] Modification/alteration of GI microbiota with resultant diarrhea in the nursing patient is theoretically possible. When given as labeled, there are no milk withdrawal times necessary for ceftiofur products in dairy cattle.

Overdose/Acute Toxicity

Cephalosporin overdoses are unlikely to cause significant problems other than GI distress, but other effects are possible (see ***Adverse Effects***). Use of this drug in excess of labeled dosages or via unapproved routes of administration may cause violative residues; contact FARAD (see ***Appendix***) for assistance in determining appropriate withdrawal times in these circumstances.

No toxicity was noted during safety studies in cattle, swine, sheep, and goats given up to 25 times the highest labeled dosage for each species, in chicks given up to 100 mg/kg SC, and in poults given up to 400 mg/kg SC. Colitis and diarrhea occurred in horses receiving 22 – 55 mg/kg/day IV. Thrombocytopenia and anemia were noted in dogs given 2.2 – 11 mg/kg/day SC for 42 days.[4]

Swine safety data: results from a 5-day tolerance study in normal feeder pigs indicated ceftiofur sodium was well-tolerated when administered at 125 mg ceftiofur equivalents/kg (more than 25 times the highest recommended daily dosage) for 5 consecutive days. Ceftiofur administered IM to pigs produced no overt adverse signs of toxicity.[4]

Cattle safety data: results from a 5-day tolerance study in feeder calves indicated ceftiofur sodium was well-tolerated when administered at 55 mg ceftiofur equivalents/kg (25 times the highest recommended dose) for 5 consecutive days. Ceftiofur administered IM had no adverse systemic effects.[4]

For patients that have experienced or are suspected to have experienced an overdose, consultation with a 24-hour poison consultation center specializing in providing veterinary-specific information is recommended. For general information related to overdose and toxin exposures, as well as contact information for poison control centers, refer to ***Appendix***.

Drug Interactions

The following drug interactions have either been reported or are theoretical in humans or animals receiving ceftiofur and may be of significance in veterinary patients. Unless otherwise noted, use together is not necessarily contraindicated, but weigh the potential risks and perform additional monitoring when appropriate.

- **AMINOGLYCOSIDES** (eg, **amikacin, gentamicin**): Concurrent use of parenteral aminoglycosides with cephalosporins is somewhat controversial. Potentially, cephalosporins could cause additive nephrotoxicity when used with these drugs, but this interaction has only been well-documented with cephaloridine (no longer marketed). In vitro studies have demonstrated that cephalosporins can have synergistic or additive activity against certain bacteria when used with aminoglycosides,[11] but the drugs should be administered at separate times.
- **NEPHROTOXIC DRUGS** (eg, **amphotericin B, furosemide, iohexol**): Concurrent use with ceftiofur may cause additive nephrotoxicity.
- **PROBENECID**: Competitively blocks the tubular secretion of most cephalosporins, thereby increasing serum levels and serum half-lives

Laboratory Considerations

NOTE: Considerations listed below are for cefotaxime, which is structurally similar to ceftiofur; these considerations may apply to ceftiofur.

- Except for cefotaxime, cephalosporins may cause false-positive **urine glucose determinations** when using cupric sulfate solution (Benedict's solution, *Clinitest®*). Tests using glucose oxidase (*Tes-Tape®, Clinistix®*) are not affected by cephalosporins.
- When using the Jaffe reaction to measure **serum** or **urine creatinine**, cephalosporins (not ceftazidime or cefotaxime) at high dosages may cause falsely elevated values.
- In humans, particularly those with azotemia, cephalosporins have caused a false-positive direct **Coombs test**.[12]
- Cephalosporins may also cause falsely elevated **17-ketosteroid** values in urine.

Dosages

DOGS:

UTIs associated with *Escherichia coli* and *Proteus mirabilis* (label dosage; FDA-approved): 2.2 mg/kg SC every 24 hours for 5 to 14 days (0.1 mL reconstituted sterile solution per 2.2 kg [5 lb] body weight)[4]

Susceptible Infections (extra-label):

a) **UTI**: 2 mg/kg SC every 12 to 24 hours[13]
b) **Neonatal septicemia**: 2.5 mg/kg SC every 12 hours for no longer than 5 days; presumptive therapy with vitamin K_1 (0.01 – 1 mg/neonate [NOT mg/kg] SC) may be used in puppies younger than 48 hours.[14,15]
c) 5 mg/kg IV or SC every 12 hours is predicted to treat susceptible bacteria with MIC less than or equal to 4 µg/mL; based on a single-dose pharmacokinetic study[16]

CATS:

Susceptible Infections (extra-label):

a) **UTI**: 2 mg/kg SC every 12 to 24 hours[13]
b) **Neonatal septicemia**: 2.5 mg/kg SC every 12 hours for no longer than 5 days; presumptive therapy with vitamin K_1 (0.01 – 1 mg/neonate [NOT mg/kg] SC) may be used in kittens younger than 48 hours.[14,15]

c) 5 mg/kg IV or SC every 12 hours is predicted to treat susceptible bacteria with MIC less than or equal to 4 µg/mL; based on a single-dose pharmacokinetic study[17]

HORSES:

Respiratory infections associated with *Streptococcus equi* subsp *zooepidemicus* (label dosage; FDA-approved): 2.2 – 4.4 mg/kg IM (2 – 4 mL reconstituted sterile solution per 45 kg [100 lb] body weight) daily; continue for 48 hours after clinical signs have disappeared.[4] A maximum of 10 mL may be administered per injection site. Do not exceed 10 days of treatment.

Susceptible Infections in adults (extra-label): 2.5 – 3.2 mg/kg IV loading dose, followed by 200 – 285.12 µg/kg/hour (3.33 to 4.75 µg/kg/minute) IV CRI[18,19]

Susceptible Infections in foals (extra-label):

a) Based on a pharmacokinetic study, a bolus loading dose of 1.26 mg/kg IV followed immediately by 2.86 µg/kg/minute IV CRI. Daily dose is ≈5.4 mg/kg. This dosage could presumably be used to treat bacteria with an MIC of less than or equal to 4 µg/mL. Once clinical condition improves, dosing can be switched from CRI daily to IM every 12 hours.[20]
b) 2.2 – 5 mg/kg IM every 12 hours[21]

CATTLE:

Bovine respiratory disease (BRD) and acute bovine interdigital necrobacillosis (label dosage; FDA-approved): 1.1 – 2.2 mg/kg IM or SC (1 – 2 mL reconstituted sterile solution per 45 kg [100 lb] body weight) daily for a total of 3 consecutive days.[22] Additional treatments may be given on days 4 and 5 for animals that do not show a satisfactory response (ie, not recovered) after the initial 3 treatments.

SHEEP/GOATS:

Respiratory disease associated with *Mannheimia haemolytica* and *Pasteurella multocida* (label dosage; FDA-approved): 1.1 – 2.2 mg/kg IM (1 – 2 mL reconstituted sterile solution per 45 kg [100 lb] body weight) daily for a total of 3 consecutive days.[4] Additional treatments may be given on days 4 and 5 for animals that do not show a satisfactory response (ie, not recovered) after the initial 3 treatments. When used in lactating does, the high end of the dosage is recommended.

SWINE:

Swine bacterial respiratory infections associated with *Actinobacillus (Haemophilus) pleuropneumoniae, P multocida, Salmonella choleraesuis* and *Streptococcus suis* (label dosage; FDA-approved): 3 – 5 mg/kg IM (1 mL of reconstituted sterile solution per 10 to 16.7 kg [22 to 37 lb] body weight) daily for a total of 3 consecutive days[4]

BIRDS:

Control of early mortality associated with *E coli* (label dosage; FDA-approved):

a) **Day-old turkey poults**: 0.17 – 0.5 mg/poult (NOT mg/kg) SC in the neck region.[4] 1 mL of the 50 mg/mL reconstituted solution will treat ≈100- to 294-day-old poults.
b) **Day-old chicks**: 0.08 – 0.2 mg/chick (NOT mg/kg) SC in the neck region.[4] 1 mL of the 50 mg/mL reconstituted solution will treat ≈250- to 625-day-old chicks. A sterile, 26-gauge needle and syringe or properly cleaned automatic injection machine should be used.

REPTILES:

Susceptible Infections (extra-label):

a) **Chelonians**: 4 mg/kg IM once daily for 2 weeks. Commonly used in respiratory infections[23]
b) For microbes susceptible at more than 2 µg/mL, 5 mg/kg, IM or SC, every 24 hours[24]; based on a pharmacokinetic study in green iguanas
c) **Bacterial pneumonia**: 2.2 mg/kg IM every 24 to 48 hours; keep patient at upper end of ideal temperature range[25]

Monitoring

Because cephalosporins usually have minimal toxicity associated with their use, monitoring for efficacy is usually all that is required. Patients with diminished renal function may require intensified renal monitoring. Therapeutic drug monitoring is not typically done.

Client Information

- This drug must be injected; it does not work when given by mouth.
- Pain is possible when this drug is injected in the muscle. If given at home to small animals, it is usually given via injection under the skin (ie, subcutaneously).
- Observe recommended withholding times if injecting an animal that will be used for human food.

Chemistry/Synonyms

Ceftiofur sodium is a semisynthetic third-generation cephalosporin that is a weak acid, acid-stable, and water-soluble.

Ceftiofur sodium may also be known as CM 31-916, U 64279E, ceftiofen sodium, *Excenel*® (not *Excenel® RTU*), *Naxcel*®, *Ceftiflex*®, or *Accent*®.

Storage/Stability

Concentrated ceftiofur sodium powder for reconstitution should be stored at room temperature (20°C-25°C [68°F-77°F]). Protect from light. Color of the cake may vary from off-white to tan, but this does not affect potency.[4]

After reconstitution with bacteriostatic water or sterile water for injection, the solution is stable for up to 7 days when refrigerated at 2°C to 8°C (36°F-46°F) and for 12 hours at room temperature (20°C-25°C [68°F-77°F]).

There is a one-time salvage procedure for the reconstituted product. At the end of day 7 refrigeration or 12-hour room temperature storage following reconstitution, any remaining reconstituted product may be frozen for up to 8 weeks without loss in potency or other chemical properties. To use this salvaged product at any time during the 8-week storage period, hold the vial under warm running water, gently swirling the container to accelerate thawing, or allow the frozen material to thaw at room temperature. Rapid freezing or thawing may result in vial breakage. Any product not used immediately upon thawing should be discarded.[4]

Compatibility/Compounding Considerations

No specific information is noted.

Dosage Forms/Regulatory Status

VETERINARY-LABELED PRODUCTS:

Ceftiofur Sodium Powder for Injection: 50 mg ceftiofur/mL when reconstituted in 1 g and 4 g vials; *Naxcel*®[4]; *Excenel*® (in Canada), *Ceftiflex*®, generic; (Rx). FDA-approved for various indications in cattle, swine, sheep, goats, horses, dogs, and day-old chicks or turkey poults. Withdrawal times: Cattle: 4-day slaughter withdrawal time is required. No milk discard time is required. Swine: A 4-day slaughter withdrawal time is required. Sheep/Goats: No slaughter withdrawal time or milk discard time is required. Not to be used in horses intended for human consumption.

- In 2012, the FDA prohibited cephalosporin extra-label drug use in major food animal species. (See ***Extra-Label Drug Use***)

HUMAN-LABELED PRODUCTS: NONE

References

For the complete list of references, see **wiley.com/go/budde/plumb**

Ceftriaxone

(sef-try-**ax**-ohn) *Rocephin®*
Third-Generation Cephalosporin

Prescriber Highlights

- ▶ Injectable antibiotic used to treat serious bacterial infections
- ▶ Achieves therapeutic concentrations in CNS; long half-life
- ▶ Adverse effects include hypersensitivity reactions and injection site reactions (eg, skin tightness, induration).
- ▶ Administer ceftriaxone IV over 30 minutes (or longer). Pain on IM injection is reduced when reconstituted with lidocaine.
- ▶ **In the United States, extra-label drug use of cephalosporins is restricted in food-producing animals.**

Uses/Indications

Ceftriaxone is used to treat serious infections (particularly against susceptible Enterobacteriaceae) that are not susceptible to other agents or when aminoglycosides are not indicated because of their potential toxicity. Its long half-life, good CNS penetration, and activity against *Borrelia burgdorferi* have also made ceftriaxone a potential choice for treating Lyme borreliosis and other infections in animals. Although ceftriaxone has been reported for the treatment of uncomplicated lower UTI,[1] its use is not recommended for this purpose.[2] In dogs, ceftriaxone's lower protein binding and shorter half-life (when compared with humans) give it no advantage over the other parenteral third-generation cephalosporins. In horses, intraperitoneal ceftriaxone successfully treated cases of septic peritonitis.[3]

The World Health Organization (WHO) classifies third-generation cephalosporins as Critically Important, Highest Priority antimicrobials for human medicine.[4] The Office International des Epizooties (OIE) has designated third-generation cephalosporins as Veterinary Critically Important Antimicrobial (VCIA) agents in avian, bovine, ovine, and swine species.[5]

Pharmacology/Actions

Ceftriaxone is a third-generation injectable cephalosporin agent that is bactericidal and displays time-dependent killing. Third-generation cephalosporins retain the gram-positive activity of the first- and second-generation agents, but have much expanded gram-negative activity. This class of antibiotics is often chosen for their excellent gram-negative coverage and significantly less toxic potential (as compared with the aminoglycosides). As with the second-generation cephalosporins, enough variability exists with individual bacterial sensitivities that susceptibility testing is necessary.

Ceftriaxone is ineffective against methicillin-resistant staphylococci, enterococci, extended-spectrum beta-lactamase (ESBL)-producing Enterobacterales, and AmpC-producing Enterobacterales. It generally has excellent activity against gram-negative bacteria; however, it is not a good choice for *Serratia* spp, *Pseudomonas* spp, some *Proteus* spp, *Citrobacter* spp, and *Enterobacter* spp ("SPICE" organisms).

Pharmacokinetics

In humans, ceftriaxone is not absorbed after oral administration and must be given parenterally. It is widely distributed throughout the body and highly bound (95%-98%) to plasma proteins. Ceftriaxone crosses into the CNS; CSF concentrations are higher when meninges are inflamed. Ceftriaxone is excreted by both renal and biliary mechanisms; elimination half-lives are ≈6 to 11 hours.

In dogs, ceftriaxone bioavailability after IM or SC administration was equal after IV administration, but peak concentrations occur much faster after IM (≈30 minutes) than SC (80 minutes) administration.[6] Peak concentrations are higher with IM administration than with SC, but total area under the curve is similar for both routes. Elimination half-life is longer after SC administration (1.73 hours) than after either IM (1.17 hours) or IV administration (0.88 hours). The authors of the study concluded that once or twice daily IM or SC injections of 50 mg/kg should be adequate to treat most susceptible infections in dogs.

In a study of cats, ceftriaxone was well-absorbed when administered IM and SC.[7] Elimination half-life averaged between 1.5 and 2 hours. Protein binding was not determined.

One study compared healthy cows with endometritic cows.[8] After a single ceftriaxone IV dose, elimination half-life was about 1 hour in healthy cows, clearance was 0.3 L/kg/hour, and volume of distribution was 0.5 L/kg. In endometritic cows, elimination half-life was slightly longer at 1.56 hours, clearance was 0.56 L/kg/hour, and volume of distribution was 1.55 L/kg.

Contraindications/Precautions/Warnings

Cephalosporins are contraindicated in patients with a history of hypersensitivity to them. Because there may be cross-reactivity, cephalosporins should be used cautiously in patients that have a documented hypersensitivity to other beta-lactam antibiotics (eg, penicillins, cefamycins, carbapenems).

Human patients that have significant renal insufficiency with concomitant hepatic impairment may need dosage adjustments[9]; the relevance of this finding for veterinary patients is unclear.

Ceftriaxone can be easily confused with other cephalosporins. Consider writing orders and prescriptions using tall man lettering: cefTRIAXone.

Adverse Effects

Because use of ceftriaxone is limited in veterinary patients, an accurate adverse effect profile has not been determined. Pain at the injection site has been reported.[6,7] In dogs, very high dosages (100 mg/kg per day) of ceftriaxone have caused sludge in the bile.

One case report describes 2 horses that were experimentally infected with *Borrelia burgdorferi* and experienced anaphylactoid reactions (ie, nonimmunologic anaphylaxis) after receiving ceftriaxone treatment.[10] Each horse was supposed to receive 25 mg/kg IV, but both infusions were stopped early because of the reaction. Both horses had previously received penicillin without any problems. It is unclear whether the reactions were due to the drug itself, caused by a reaction between the drug and the infection, or due to massive die-off of the bacteria.

The following adverse effects have been reported in humans and may or may not apply to veterinary patients: hematologic effects, including eosinophilia (6%), thrombocytosis (5%), leukopenia (2%), and, more rarely, anemia, neutropenia, lymphopenia, and thrombocytopenia.[9] Approximately 2% to 4% of humans get diarrhea. Hypersensitivity reactions (usually a rash) have been noted. Increased serum concentrations of liver enzymes, BUN, creatinine, and urine casts have been described in ≈1% to 3% of patients.

Reproductive/Nursing Safety

Cephalosporins cross the placenta. Teratogenic effects were not demonstrated in studies in pregnant mice and rats that received up to 20 times the label doses of ceftriaxone.[9] Ceftriaxone is considered compatible with human pregnancy.[11]

Ceftriaxone enters maternal milk in low concentrations.[12] Ceftriaxone is considered compatible with breastfeeding in humans.[11]

Because safety has not been established in animals, this drug should only be used when the maternal benefits outweigh the potential risks to offspring.

Overdose/Acute Toxicity

All beagles receiving ceftriaxone 300 mg/kg/day IV developed soft or mucoid feces and diarrhea; emesis was common.[13] As limited information is available, overdoses should be monitored and treated supportively based on clinical signs.

For patients that have experienced or are suspected to have experienced an overdose, consultation with a 24-hour poison consultation center specializing in providing veterinary-specific information is recommended. For general information related to overdose and toxin exposures, as well as contact information for poison control centers, refer to ***Appendix.***

Drug Interactions

The following drug interactions either have been reported or are theoretical in humans or animals receiving ceftriaxone and may be of significance in veterinary patients. Unless otherwise noted, use together is not necessarily contraindicated, but weigh the potential risks and perform additional monitoring when appropriate.

- **Aminoglycosides and other Nephrotoxic Drugs** (eg, **amphotericin B**): Concurrent use of parenteral aminoglycosides or other nephrotoxic drugs with cephalosporins is somewhat controversial. Cephalosporins could cause additive nephrotoxicity when used with these drugs, but this interaction has only been well-documented with cephaloridine (no longer marketed). In vitro studies have demonstrated that cephalosporins can have synergistic or additive activity against certain bacteria when used with aminoglycosides.
- **Calcium Salts, Intravenous (IV)**: Concomitant use with calcium-containing solutions has caused fatal calcium/ceftriaxone precipitates in lungs and kidneys of neonatal humans. Do not mix with calcium or administer calcium-containing solutions (eg, lactated Ringers, Hartmann's solution) or products within 48 hours of ceftriaxone administration. There have been no reported interactions between oral calcium products and ceftriaxone.

Laboratory Considerations

- Because bacterial sensitivity to third-generation cephalosporin antibiotics is unique, when Kirby-Bauer disk diffusion procedures are employed for testing susceptibility, a specific ceftriaxone 30 µg disk should be used. A cephalosporin-class disk containing cephalothin should not be used to test for ceftriaxone susceptibility.
- Except for cefotaxime, cephalosporins may cause false-positive **urine glucose determinations** when cupric sulfate solution (Benedict's solution, Fehling's solution, *Clinitest*®) is used. Tests that use glucose oxidase (*Tes-Tape*®, *Clinistix*®) are not affected by cephalosporins.
- Ceftriaxone in high concentrations (50 µg/mL or greater) may cause falsely elevated **serum creatinine** levels when manual methods of testing are used. Automated methods do not appear to be affected.

Dosages

NOTE: In humans, it is recommended that IV infusions be administered over 30 minutes (60 minutes in neonates) at concentrations between 10 – 40 mg/mL.[9]

DOGS:

Susceptible infections (extra-label): 50 mg/kg IM or SC once or twice daily,[6] based on a pharmacokinetic study

Borreliosis | Lyme disease | *Borrelia burgdorferi* infection (extra-label): 25 mg/kg IV or SC once daily for 14 to 30 days[14]

Infective endocarditis caused by *Streptococcus canis* (extra-label): 20 mg/kg IV twice daily for 2 weeks, followed by long-term treatment with oral antibiotics[15]

CATS:

Susceptible infections (extra-label): 25 mg/kg IM or SC every 12 hours[7], based on a pharmacokinetic study

Borreliosis | Lyme disease | *Borrelia burgdorferi* infection (extra-label): 25 mg/kg IV or SC once daily for 14 to 30 days[14]

HORSES:

Susceptible infections (extra-label): 25 – 50 mg/kg every 12 hours IV or IM[16]

Adjuvant treatment for septic peritonitis (extra-label): 25 mg/kg diluted in 250 mL of warmed 0.9% sodium chloride and administered intraperitoneally once daily until resolution of clinical signs and laboratory parameters.[3] Used in combination with parenteral antimicrobial therapy (eg, gentamicin) and supportive treatment. The study authors recommend reserving intraperitoneal ceftriaxone for aggressive cases or cases that have failed to respond to routine antibiotics.

Monitoring

- Culture and susceptibility testing as indicated by clinical condition
- Because cephalosporins usually have minimal toxicity associated with their use, monitoring for efficacy is usually all that is required.
- With long-term administration, consider periodic monitoring of CBC, chemistry panel, and urinalysis.

Client Information

- This drug must be injected; it does not work when given by mouth.
- This drug causes pain when administered in the muscle. If the drug is given at home to small animals, it usually is administered by injecting under the skin (subcutaneously).

Chemistry/Synonyms

A third-generation cephalosporin, ceftriaxone sodium occurs as a white to yellowish-orange crystalline powder. It is soluble in water (400 mg/mL at 25°C [77°F)). Potencies of commercial products are expressed in terms of ceftriaxone. One gram of ceftriaxone sodium contains 3.6 mEq of sodium.

Ceftriaxone sodium may also be known as ceftriaxonum natricum, Ro-13-9904, or Ro-13-9904/000; many trade names are available.

Storage/Stability

The sterile powder for reconstitution should be stored between 20°C to 25°C (68°F-77°F) and protected from light.

After reconstituting with sterile water, 0.9% sodium chloride, or D_5W, ceftriaxone solutions (at concentrations of up to 100 mg/mL) are stable for 2 days at room temperature and for 10 days when refrigerated. Solutions of 250 mg/mL are stable for 24 hours at room temperature and 3 days when refrigerated. At concentrations of 10 – 40 mg/mL, solutions frozen at -20°C (-4°F) are stable for 26 weeks. Reconstituted solutions do not need to be protected from normal light; solution color may darken over time.

Solutions reconstituted with 1% lidocaine to a concentration of 100 – 350 mg/mL are stable for 24 hours at room temperature and 3 days when refrigerated.

Compatibility/Compounding Considerations

When ceftriaxone is used IM in humans, it may be reconstituted with lidocaine 1% (10 mg/mL, without epinephrine) to reduce pain on administration.

Compatibility is dependent on factors such as pH, concentration, temperature, and diluent used; specialized references or a hospital pharmacist should be consulted for more specific information.

Ceftriaxone is **compatible** with dextrose 5% and sodium chloride 0.9%. The manufacturer does not recommend admixing any other anti-infective drugs with ceftriaxone sodium, but amikacin and metronidazole are reported to be **compatible**.

Do not mix with calcium or calcium-containing solutions (eg, lactated Ringer's) or administer simultaneously **(Y-site)** with calcium or calcium-containing products (see ***Drug Interactions***) as a precipitate may form.

Regulatory Status

VETERINARY-LABELED PRODUCTS: NONE

NOTE: Extra-label use of cephalosporins in food-producing animals is restricted. Contact the Food Animal Residue Avoidance Databank (FARAD) for guidance in determining withdrawal periods.

HUMAN-LABELED PRODUCTS:

Ceftriaxone Injection Powder for Solution: 250 mg, 500 mg, 1 g, 2 g, 10 g, and 100 g (as base) in vials, single-use duplex containers, and in bulk; generic; (Rx). *Rocephin*® has been discontinued in the United States.

References

For the complete list of references, see **wiley.com/go/budde/plumb**

Cefuroxime

Cefuroxime Axetil

Cefuroxime Sodium

(sef-yoor-***oks***-eem) *Ceftin*®, *Zinacef*®

Second-Generation Cephalosporin

Prescriber Highlights

- Oral and parenterally administered second-generation cephalosporin that is more active against some gram-negative bacteria than first-generation (eg, cephalexin, cefazolin) cephalosporins
- Potentially useful in small animals when a cephalosporin is desired but there is resistance to first-generation cephalosporins, or when slightly enhanced gram-negative coverage is desired for surgical prophylaxis
- Limited clinical experience in veterinary medicine
- Adverse effects most commonly seen in small animal species are GI-related

Uses/Indications

Cefuroxime is a semi-synthetic second-generation cephalosporin with enhanced activity against some gram-negative pathogens when compared with the first-generation agents. Cefuroxime is available in both oral and parenteral dosage forms. It may be useful in small animal species when a cephalosporin is desired to treat bacterial infections that are resistant to first-generation cephalosporins, when slightly enhanced gram-negative coverage is desired for surgical prophylaxis, or for the treatment of bacterial meningitis or other CNS infections in which inflamed meninges will allow cefuroxime to penetrate into the CNS. Little information is available regarding the clinical use of cefuroxime in small animal species.

The World Health Organization (WHO) has designated cefuroxime as a Highly Important antimicrobial for human medicine.[1] The Office International des Epizooties (OIE) has designated cefuroxime as a Veterinary Highly Important Antimicrobial (VHIA) Agent in bovine species.[2]

Pharmacology/Actions

Cefuroxime, like other cephalosporins, is a time-dependent bactericidal antibiotic and acts by inhibiting cell wall synthesis. Its spectrum of activity is similar to that of cephalexin, but it is more active against gram-negative bacteria, including strains of *Escherichia coli*, *Klebsiella pneumoniae*, *Salmonella* spp, and *Enterobacter* spp. It is not effective against methicillin-resistant *Staphylococcus* spp, *Pseudomonas* spp, *Serratia* spp, or *Enterococcus* spp and it has little activity against *Bacteroides fragilis*. It is also ineffective against extended-spectrum beta-lactamase (ESBL)–producing bacteria.

Pharmacokinetics

In dogs, cefuroxime is rapidly distributed after IV injection. The volume of distribution is about 0.49 L/kg. The elimination half-life is ≈1.12 hours. When cefuroxime is given at 20 mg/kg IM, the elimination half-life is 1.13 hours, bioavailability is ≈80%, and peak plasma concentration is 23 µg/mL. When given at the same dose SC, the elimination half-life is 1.04 hours, bioavailability is ≈77%, and peak plasma concentration is 15.4 µg/mL. Clearance is 0.34 L/kg/hour for both routes. The authors concluded that cefuroxime given at 20 mg/kg IM or IV every 11 hours, or SC every 12 hours, would be effective for bacteria with an MIC less than or equal to 1 µg/mL, but the interval would need to be shortened to every 8 hours (IM or SC) for bacteria with an MIC less than or equal to 4 µg/mL; however, further pharmacokinetic and pharmacodynamic studies as well as clinical trials are needed.[3]

In goats, after 40 mg/kg is administered, IM bioavailability is high and protein binding is low. Volume of distribution is about 0.46 L/kg. Elimination half-life is about 2.1 hours (IM).

In humans, cefuroxime axetil is well absorbed after oral administration and is rapidly hydrolyzed in the intestinal mucosa and circulation to the parent compound.[4] Bioavailability ranges on average from 37% (fasted) to 52% (with food). Peak serum concentrations occur in about 2 to 3 hours after oral dosing. When the sodium salt is administered IM, peak concentrations occur within 15 minutes to 1 hour. Cefuroxime is widely distributed after absorption, including to the bone, aqueous humor, and joint fluid.[4,5] Therapeutic levels can be attained in the CSF if meninges are inflamed. Binding to human plasma proteins ranges from 35 to 50%. Cefuroxime is primarily excreted unchanged in the urine; elimination half-life in patients with normal renal function is between 1 to 2 hours.

Contraindications/Precautions/Warnings

No specific information is available for veterinary patients. In humans, cefuroxime is contraindicated in patients that are hypersensitive to it or other cephalosporins. Dosage adjustment is recommended in humans with severe renal impairment.

Cefuroxime can be easily confused with other cephalosporins. Consider writing orders and prescriptions using tall man lettering: cefUROXime.

Adverse Effects

As use of cefuroxime in animals has been limited, a comprehensive adverse effect profile has not been determined. A 6-month toxicity study of oral cefuroxime axetil given at dosages ranging from 100 mg/kg/day to 1600 mg/kg/day in beagles demonstrated little adversity associated with cefuroxime.[6] At the highest dosing levels (≈80 times the recommended dose), some vomiting and slight suppression of body weight gain were noted. Minor reductions in neutrophils and red blood cells and prolonged prothrombin times were also seen.

When cefuroxime is used clinically in dogs, GI effects (eg, inappetence, vomiting, diarrhea) would be the most likely expected adverse effects, but incidence rates are not known.

The use of cephalosporins in patients documented to be hypersensitive to penicillin-class antibiotics is controversial. In humans, it is estimated that up to 15% of patients that are hypersensitive to penicillins will also be hypersensitive to cephalosporins[7].

Cefuroxime is generally well-tolerated in humans. Injection site inflammation can occur when cefuroxime is used IV. GI effects (eg, nausea, diarrhea) may occur, but are not frequently reported. Eosinophilia and hypersensitivity reactions (including anaphylaxis) are possible. Neurologic effects (eg, hearing loss, seizures), pseudomembranous colitis, serious dermatologic reactions (eg, toxic epidermal necrolysis [TEN], Stevens-Johnson syndrome), hematologic effects (eg, pancytopenia, thrombocytopenia), and interstitial nephritis have been reported rarely.

Reproductive/Nursing Safety

Studies performed in pregnant mice at dosages of up to 6400 mg/kg and rabbits at 400 mg/kg demonstrated no adverse fetal effects. In humans, cefuroxime is considered compatible with pregnancy.[8]

Cefuroxime enters maternal milk in low concentrations. Although cefuroxime is likely safe for nursing offspring, the potential for adverse effects cannot be ruled out, particularly alterations to gut flora with resultant diarrhea. In humans, cefuroxime is considered compatible with breast feeding.[8]

Because safety has not been established in animals, this drug should only be used when the maternal benefits outweigh the potential risks to offspring.

Overdose/Acute Toxicity

Beagles receiving daily dosages of up to 1600 mg/kg/day orally tolerated cefuroxime well (see ***Adverse Effects***).[6]

Cerebral irritation with seizures has been reported with large overdoses in humans. Plasma concentrations of cefuroxime can be reduced with hemodialysis or peritoneal dialysis.

For patients that have experienced or are suspected to have experienced an overdose, consultation with a 24-hour poison consultation center specializing in providing veterinary-specific information is recommended. For general information related to overdose and toxin exposures, as well as contact information for poison control centers, refer to ***Appendix.***

Drug Interactions

The following drug interactions either have been reported or are theoretical in humans or animals receiving cefuroxime and may be of significance in veterinary patients. Unless otherwise noted, use together is not necessarily contraindicated, but weigh the potential risks and perform additional monitoring when appropriate.

- **Aminoglycosides** (eg, **gentamicin**): Potential for increased risk of nephrotoxicity—monitor renal function; however, aminoglycosides and cephalosporins may have synergistic or additive actions against some gram-negative bacteria (Enterobacteriaceae).
- **Antacids, Aluminum-, Calcium-, or Magnesium-Containing**: Antacids may decrease serum levels of oral cefuroxime. Separate doses by 1 to 2 hours.
- **H_2-Receptor Antagonists** (eg, **famotidine, ranitidine**): H_2 antagonists may significantly decrease the absorption of cefuroxime. Concurrent use is not recommended.
- **Nephrotoxic Drugs** (eg, **amphotericin B, furosemide**): Concurrent use with cephalosporins could potentially cause additive nephrotoxicity, although this is somewhat controversial. Use together cautiously and monitor renal function closely.
- **Probenecid**: Reduced renal excretion of cefuroxime.
- **Proton Pump Inhibitors** (eg, **omeprazole, pantoprazole**): Cefuroxime absorption may be significantly decreased. Concurrent use is not recommended.
- **Sodium Bicarbonate**: Cefuroxime absorption may be decreased. Separate doses by 1 to 2 hours.
- **Vitamin K Antagonists**: Cephalosporins may enhance the anticoagulant effects of vitamin K antagonists (eg, warfarin).

Laboratory Considerations

- Cefuroxime may cause false-positive **urine glucose determinations** when using the copper reduction method (Benedict's solution, Fehling's solution, *Clinitest®*); tests utilizing glucose oxidase (*Tes-Tape®*, *Clinistix®*) are not affected by cephalosporins.
- In humans, particularly with azotemia, cephalosporins have caused a false-positive direct **Coombs test.**

Dosages

DOGS/CATS:

Susceptible infections (extra-label):

a) Oral: Anecdotally, 10 – 15 mg/kg IV every 8 to 12 hours
b) Parenteral: From a small PK study, 20 mg/kg SC every 12 hours for bacteria with MIC less than or equal to 1 µg/mL OR 20 mg/kg IM or SC every 8 hours for bacteria with MIC less than or equal to 4 µg/mL[3]

Surgical prophylaxis (extra-label): 20 – 50 mg/kg IV slowly (over at least 3 to 5 minutes) ≈30 minutes prior to surgery (often given at induction) and every 1.5 to 3 hours during surgery

GOATS:

Susceptible infections for organisms with MIC less than or equal to 1 µg/mL (extra-label): 40 mg/kg IM every 12 hours based on a pharmacokinetic study[9]

Monitoring

- Because cephalosporins usually have minimal toxicity associated with their use, monitoring for efficacy is usually all that is required.
- Patients with diminished renal function may require intensified renal monitoring.
- Therapeutic drug monitoring is not routinely done with these agents.

Client Information

- Give this medicine with food.
- Do not crush tablets. This medicine has a bitter taste. Contact your veterinarian if you have trouble medicating your animal.
- The most common side effects are diarrhea, vomiting, and loss of appetite. Contact your veterinarian if your animal develops severe vomiting/diarrhea or rash/itching.
- Be sure to give this medicine to your animal as long as your veterinarian has prescribed, even if your animal seems better.
- Cephalosporin antibiotics have an odor that resembles cat urine, but this is normal.

Chemistry/Synonyms

Cefuroxime axetil occurs as a white or almost white powder that is insoluble in water and slightly soluble in dehydrated alcohol.

Cefuroxime sodium occurs as a white or almost white hygroscopic powder that is freely soluble in water.

Cefuroxime may also be known as CCI-15641, cefuroxim, cefuroxima, cefuroximum, cefuroksiimi, or cefuroksimas; many internationally registered trade names are available.

Storage/Stability

Cefuroxime axetil tablets should be stored in tight containers at room temperature (15°C-30°C [59°F-86°F]); protect from excessive moisture.

The powder for suspension should be stored at 2°C to 30°C [36°F-86°F]. Once reconstituted, it should be kept refrigerated (2°C to 8°C [36°F-46°F]) and any unused suspension should be discarded after 10 days.

The powder for injection should be stored at room temperature (15°C-30°C [59°F-86°F]) and protected from light. The powder may darken, but this does not indicate any loss of potency. When the powder is reconstituted with sterile water to a concentration of 90 mg/mL, the resulting solution is stable for 24 hours at room temperature; 48 hours, if refrigerated. The 7.5 g pharmacy bulk container is stable for 7 days when reconstituted to 95 mg/mL and kept under refrigeration. Any of these containers may be further diluted into a compatible IV solution such as 5% dextrose, 0.9% sodium chloride, or Ringer's, and the resulting solution is stable for 24 hours at room temperature or up to 7 days if refrigerated. The powder for injection may be reconstituted at up to 90 mg/mL and then immediately frozen in a Viaflex mini-bag containing 50 to 100 mL of 0.9% sodium chloride or 5% dextrose. This solution is stable for up to 6 months when it is stored at -20°C (-4°F). Thaw at room temperature and do not refreeze. Thawed solutions are stable for 24 hours at room temperature or 7 days under refrigeration.

Compatibility/Compounding Considerations

Compatibility is dependent upon factors such as pH, concentration, temperature, and diluent used; consult specialized references or a hospital pharmacist for more specific information.

Cefuroxime is **compatible** with dextrose 5 and 10%, Ringer's injection, lactated Ringer's, and sodium chloride 0.9%. Drugs that are reportedly **compatible** when mixed with cefuroxime for IV use include clindamycin, furosemide, and metronidazole. Drugs that may be given at a Y-site with a cefuroxime infusion running include morphine, hydromorphone, and propofol. Cefuroxime is **incompatible** with aminoglycosides, ciprofloxacin, and ranitidine.

Dosage Forms/Regulatory Status

VETERINARY-LABELED PRODUCTS: NONE

HUMAN-LABELED PRODUCTS:

Cefuroxime Axetil Oral Tablets (film coated): 125 mg, 250 mg, and 500 mg; *Ceftin®*, generic; (Rx)

Cefuroxime Axetil Oral Suspension: 25 mg/mL and 50 mg/mL (125 mg/5 mL and 250 mg/5 mL; as base) when reconstituted in 50 mL and 100 mL; generic; (Rx)

Cefuroxime Sodium for Injection: 750 mg, 1.5 g, 7.5 g, and 225 g (as sodium); *Zinacef®*, generic; (Rx)

References

For the complete list of references, see **wiley.com/go/budde/plumb**

Cephalexin

(sef-a-***lex***-in) *Rilexine®, Keflex®*

First-Generation Cephalosporin

Prescriber Highlights

- First-generation oral cephalosporin. Some countries may have an injectable form.
- May be administered with food (especially if GI upset occurs)
- Most likely adverse effects are GI in nature; hypersensitivity reactions are possible

Uses/Indications

Cephalexin is labeled for the treatment of secondary superficial bacterial pyoderma in dogs caused by susceptible strains of *Staphylococcus pseudintermedius*. Cephalexin is also often used extra-label for other bacterial skin infections such as deep pyoderma. Cephalexin has also been used clinically in cats, ferrets, reptiles, and birds, particularly for susceptible staphylococcal infections. Cephalexin is considered a first-tier drug for the treatment of bacterial skin infections.[1,2]

Cephalexin may not be effective in patients with history of lack of response to other cephalosporins, multiple antibiotic use, and multidrug resistance. Before using cephalexin in these cases, antimicrobial culture and susceptibility testing is recommended. Additionally, topical antimicrobial therapy using antibacterial agents and biocides with proven anti-staphylococcal efficacy should be considered prior to systemic antibiotics, including cephalexin, for any surface or superficial pyoderma and wound infections, particularly those that are mild or associated with localized lesions or due to methicillin-resistant infections, to help reduce antibiotic pressure and antimicrobial resistance.[3]

The World Health Organization (WHO) has designated cephalexin as a Highly Important antimicrobial for human medicine.[4] The Office International des Epizooties (OIE) has designated cephalexin as a Veterinary Highly Important Antimicrobial (VHIA) Agent in bovine, caprine, equine, ovine, and swine species.[5]

Pharmacology/Actions

Cephalexin is a first-generation cephalosporin that exhibits activity against bacteria usually covered by this class. First-generation cephalosporins generally possess excellent coverage against most gram-positive pathogens (excluding enterococci); they are active in vitro against streptococci and staphylococci. Because first-generation cephalosporins have variable coverage against most gram-negative pathogens, their usefulness for these bacteria is mainly for treatment of lower UTIs because of the high drug concentrations achieved in urine. With the exception of *Bacteroides fragilis*, most anaerobes are susceptible to the first-generation agents. Resistance is of increasing concern, particularly with methicillin-resistant staphylococci and extended-spectrum beta-lactamase (ESBL) producing Enterobacteriaceae.

Cephalexin is inactive against *Enterococcus* spp, *Pseudomonas* spp, *Rickettsia* spp, mycobacteria, *Mycoplasma* spp, fungi, and viruses.

Cephalosporins are considered time-dependent and bactericidal against susceptible bacteria, and they act by inhibiting mucopeptide synthesis in the cell wall, which results in a defective barrier and an osmotically unstable spheroplast. The exact mechanism for this effect has not been definitively determined, but beta-lactam antibiotics have been shown to bind to several enzymes (eg, carboxypeptidases, transpeptidases, endopeptidases) in the bacterial cytoplasmic membrane that are involved in cell wall synthesis. The different affinities that various beta-lactam antibiotics have for these enzymes (also known as penicillin-binding proteins [PBPs]) help explain the differences in spectrums of activity of these drugs that are not explained by the influence of beta-lactamases. Like other beta-lactam antibiotics, cephalosporins are generally considered to be more effective against actively growing bacteria. For bactericidal activity, cephalosporin levels should exceed bacterial MIC for at least 40% of the dose interval for staphylococcal infections and ≈60% of the dose interval for streptococcal infections.[6]

Pharmacokinetics

In a study in dogs and cats, peak serum concentrations reached 18.6 µg/mL ≈1.8 hours after a mean oral dose of 12.7 mg/kg in dogs and reached 18.7 µg/mL ≈2.6 hours after an oral dose of 22.9 mg/kg in cats.[7] Elimination half-lives ranged from 1 to 2 hours in both species. Bioavailability after oral administration is ≈90% in dogs and ≈60% in cats.[8,9] A different study found that protein binding of cephalexin in dogs is low (21%) and elimination half-life in interstitial fluid (protein unbound) is ≈3.2 hours, as compared with 4.7 hours in total plasma.[10] The FDA-approved tablets that were administered at 22 mg/kg orally to fasted dogs yielded peak concentrations of 21.7 µg/mL 1.4 hours after administration; when the tablets were given with food, a lower peak concentration (17 µg/mL) was reached more quickly (1.2 hours). Elimination half-lives were 7.3 hours fasted and 8.8 hours given with food. The drug is renally eliminated.

There may be temporal differences in pharmacokinetics depending on the time of day the drug is administered. Six beagles given cephalexin orally at 10:00 and 22:00 had significantly lower peak concentrations (77%) after the 22:00 dose as compared with the 10:00 dose. In addition, the elimination half-life was ≈50% longer with the evening dose as compared with the morning dose. Clinical significance is not clear, as times above an MIC of 0.5 µg/mL were not different.[11]

In horses, oral cephalexin has low bioavailability (≈5%) and a short plasma half-life (≈2 hours), and at dosages of 30 mg/kg PO every 8 hours, plasma and interstitial concentrations were achieved to only treat gram-positive bacteria with MIC less than 0.5 μg/mL.[12]

An oil-based suspension of the sodium salt is available in several countries for IM or SC injection in animals. In calves, the sodium salt had 74% bioavailability after IM injection and a serum half-life of ≈90 minutes. When 7.5 mg/kg was injected either SC or IM in adult cattle, the 20% suspension had longer durations of time above MIC_{90} for common gram-positive pathogens when injected SC as compared with IM (11 to 14 hours vs 8 to 9 hours).[13] In the United States, extra-label use of cephalosporins in food animals is prohibited by the FDA.

After oral administration in humans, cephalexin is rapidly and completely absorbed, although absorption can be delayed. Food apparently has little impact on absorption.

Contraindications/Precautions/Warnings

Cephalexin is contraindicated in patients with a history of hypersensitivity to it and other cephalosporins. Because there may be cross-reactivity, cephalexin should be used cautiously in patients that are documented hypersensitive to other beta-lactam antibiotics (eg, penicillins, cephamycins, carbapenems). Use of cephalosporins in patients that are documented to be hypersensitive to penicillin-class antibiotics is controversial. In humans, it is estimated that 1% to 15% of patients hypersensitive to penicillins will also be hypersensitive to cephalosporins.[14] The incidence of cross-reactivity in veterinary patients is unknown.

Oral systemic antibiotics should not be administered in patients with septicemia, shock, or other grave illnesses, as absorption of the medication from the GI tract may be significantly delayed or diminished. Parenteral routes (preferably IV) should be used for these cases. Although cephalexin has been used in some small mammal species, products licensed in the United Kingdom state: *Do not use in rabbits, guinea pigs, hamsters and gerbils, and other small rodents*; potentially serious enterocolitis can result. Similar risks are likely in horses.

In humans, it is recommended to use cephalosporins with caution in those with significantly impaired renal function. Although the relevance of this finding in veterinary patients is unclear, a dosage reduction (eg, prolonged dosing interval) may be considered in patients with marked renal impairment.

Cephalexin can be easily confused with other cephalosporins. Writing orders and prescriptions using tall man letters may help: cephaLEXin.

Adverse Effects

Adverse effects associated with cephalexin are usually not serious and have a relatively low frequency of occurrence.

When given orally, cephalexin may cause GI effects (eg, salivation, vomiting, diarrhea, anorexia). Administration with a small meal may help alleviate these effects. Because cephalexin may also alter the gut microbiome, antibiotic-associated diarrhea or proliferation of resistant bacteria in the colon can occur.

Cephalexin has reportedly caused lethargy, pruritus, salivation, tachypnea, and excitability in dogs, and emesis and fever in cats. Rarely, cephalexin has been implicated in causing serious skin reactions (eg, erythema multiforme, toxic epidermal necrolysis, cutaneous vasculitis, and pemphigus foliaceus) in small animals. Hypersensitivity reactions unrelated to dosage can occur with these agents and can manifest as a rash, fever, eosinophilia, lymphadenopathy, interstitial nephritis, or anaphylaxis. Although apparently uncommon, the true incidence of these effects is not known.

Nephrotoxicity can occur (rare) during therapy with cephalexin, but patients that have renal dysfunction, are receiving other nephrotoxic drugs, or are geriatric may be more susceptible.

High doses or very prolonged use has been associated with neurotoxicity, neutropenia, agranulocytosis, thrombocytopenia, hepatitis, positive Coombs test, interstitial nephritis, and tubular necrosis. Longer prothrombin times have also been noted. Except for tubular necrosis and neurotoxicity, these effects have an immunologic component.

Reproductive/Nursing Safety

Cephalosporins have been shown to cross the placenta and safe use during pregnancy has not been firmly established.[6] There have been no documented teratogenic problems associated with these drugs.

Small amounts of cephalexin may be distributed into maternal milk; it could potentially affect gut flora in neonates. It should be used with caution in nursing patients.

Because safety has not been established in animals, this drug should only be used when the maternal benefits outweigh the potential risks to offspring.

Overdose/Acute Toxicity

Acute oral cephalosporin overdoses are unlikely to cause significant problems other than GI distress (eg, salivation, vomiting, diarrhea), but other effects are possible. See ***Adverse Effects***. Dogs receiving 110 mg/kg every 8 hours developed sporadic GI effects (eg, salivation, vomiting, diarrhea); increased ALT and decreased total protein were also noted but not considered clinically relevant. The drug is removed by dialysis.

For patients that have experienced or are suspected to have experienced an overdose, consultation with a 24-hour poison control center specializing in providing veterinary-specific information is recommended. For general information related to overdose and toxin exposures, as well as contact information for poison control centers, refer to ***Appendix***.

Drug Interactions

The following drug interactions have either been reported or are theoretical in humans or animals receiving cephalexin and may be of significance in veterinary patients. Unless otherwise noted, use together is not necessarily contraindicated, but the potential risks should be weighed, and additional monitoring performed when appropriate.

- **AMINOGLYCOSIDES AND OTHER NEPHROTOXIC DRUGS:** Concurrent use of parenteral aminoglycosides or other nephrotoxic drugs (eg, amphotericin B, furosemide) with cephalosporins is somewhat controversial. Cephalosporins could cause additive nephrotoxicity when used with these drugs, but this interaction has only been well documented with cephaloridine (no longer marketed). In vitro studies have demonstrated that cephalosporins can have synergistic or additive activity against certain bacteria when used with aminoglycosides.
- **CHOLESTYRAMINE:** Cephalexin absorption may be reduced.
- **ESTROGENS** (eg, **estriol**)**:** Cephalexin disruption of GI flora may alter enterohepatic recirculation, which may decrease estrogen effectiveness.
- **METFORMIN:** Metformin levels may be increased.
- **METOCLOPRAMIDE:** Metoclopramide given IV may increase cephalexin peak concentration and AUC when given prior to oral cephalexin.[15]
- **OMEPRAZOLE:** Omeprazole may reduce peak cephalexin concentration and AUC and may delay oral absorption in adult dogs; however, time above MIC was not altered.[16]
- **PROBENECID**: May competitively block the tubular secretion of most cephalosporins, thereby increasing serum levels and serum half-lives
- **WARFARIN**: May increase risk for bleeding
- **ZINC (ORAL)**: Cephalexin absorption may be reduced.

Laboratory Considerations

- Most laboratories use cephalothin as the class representative for testing veterinary isolates for susceptibility to other first-generation cephalosporins, including cephalexin. One study established cephalexin breakpoints of less than or equal to 2 µg/mL (susceptible), 4 µg/mL (intermediate), and more than or equal to 8 µg/mL (resistant) for isolates obtained from dogs, particularly for *Staphylococcus pseudintermedius* isolates, and recommended that cephalothin should not be used for susceptibility testing of cephalexin for veterinary bacterial pathogens, and canine-specific breakpoints should be used for testing susceptibility.[17]

- Cephalexin may cause false positive **urine glucose determinations** when cupric sulfate solution (Benedict's solution, *Clinitest*®) is used. Tests using glucose oxidase (*Tes-Tape*®, *Clinistix*®) are not affected.
- When the Jaffe reaction is used to measure **serum creatinine or urine creatinine**, cephalexin in high dosages may cause falsely elevated values.
- Cephalexin may cause falsely elevated **urine 17-ketosteroid** values.
- In humans, particularly those with azotemia, cephalexin has caused a false positive direct and indirect **Coombs test** result.
- **Prothrombin time** may be increased.
- False elevation of **urine protein** may occur.
- Cephalexin may falsely decrease **albumin** measurements.

Dosages

DOGS:

Susceptible skin infections (label dosage; FDA-approved): 22 mg/kg PO twice daily for 28 days. Appropriate culture and susceptibility tests should be performed before treatment, and antimicrobial therapy should be adjusted accordingly.

Susceptible skin infections (extra-label):

a) 15 – 30 mg/kg PO every 12 hours is often recommended.[1] Some believe that the higher end of the dosage range may be more effective. Good evidence to support treatment duration is lacking, but continuing treatment for 7 days (superficial pyoderma) or 14 days (deep pyoderma) after clinical signs have resolved is commonly recommended.

b) 25 mg/kg PO every 12 hours for up to 3 weeks.[18] Treatment should be reassessed if no improvement is seen after 14 days.

c) 15 – 30 mg/kg PO twice daily.[19] Treat for at least 15 days in cases of superficial infectious dermatitis and at least 28 days in cases of deep infectious dermatitis.

Susceptible UTIs (extra-label):

a) 12 – 25 mg/kg PO every 12 hours[20]

b) 15 – 30 mg/kg PO twice daily for 14 days[19,21]

c) 20 mg/kg PO every 12 hours for 10 days is recommended for sporadic bacterial cystitis[20]

CATS:

Susceptible skin infections (extra-label):

a) 22 – 30 mg/kg PO every 12 hours is often recommended. Good evidence to support treatment duration is lacking, but continuing treatment for 7 days (superficial pyoderma) or 14 days (deep pyoderma) after clinical signs have resolved is commonly recommended.

b) 15 mg/kg PO twice daily for 5 days for wounds and abscesses and 14 days at least in case of pyoderma.[8] The treatment must be continued for 10 days once the lesions have disappeared.

Susceptible UTIs (extra-label):

a) 12 – 25 mg/kg PO every 12 hours[20]

b) 15 mg/kg PO twice daily for 10 to 14 days for lower UTIs due to *E coli* and *Proteus mirabilis*[8,21]

c) 20 mg/kg PO every 12 hours for 10 days is recommended for sporadic bacterial cystitis.[20]

RODENTS & SMALL MAMMALS:

Susceptible infections in guinea pigs (extra-label): 50 mg/kg IM every 24 hours[22] **NOTE**: Use with caution in small mammals. See ***Contraindications/Precautions/Warnings***.

FERRETS:

Susceptible infections (extra-label): 15 – 25 mg/kg PO every 8 to 12 hours[23]

REPTILES:

Susceptible infections (extra-label): 20 – 40 mg/kg PO every 12 to 24 hours[24]

BIRDS:

Susceptible infections (extra-label):

a) 35 – 50 mg/kg PO every 6 hours (using suspension)[25]

b) 40 – 100 mg/kg PO every 6 hours[26]

Monitoring

- Because cephalosporins usually have minimal toxicity associated with their use, monitoring for efficacy is usually all that is required.
- Culture and susceptibility when indicated (eg, clinical condition does not improve, recurring infection, intracellular bacterial rods seen on cytology, history of multi-drug resistant infection)
- Therapeutic drug monitoring is not routinely done with these agents.

Client Information

- This medicine can be given with or without food, but gastrointestinal side effects might be prevented if given with food.
- Most common side effects are diarrhea, vomiting, and loss of appetite. Contact your veterinarian if your animal develops severe vomiting/diarrhea or rash/itching.
- Be sure to give this drug for as long as your veterinarian has prescribed, even if your animal seems better.
- Cephalosporin antibiotics have an odor that resembles cat urine, but this is normal.

Chemistry/Synonyms

Cephalexin is a semisynthetic oral cephalosporin. As the monohydrate, cephalexin occurs as a bitter-tasting, white to off-white crystalline powder. It is slightly soluble in water and practically insoluble in alcohol.

Cephalexin may also be known as cefalexin, 66873, or cefalexinum; many trade names are available.

Storage/Stability

Cephalexin tablets, chewable tablets, capsules, and powder for oral suspension should be stored at room temperature (15°C-30°C; 59°F-86°F) in tight containers. After reconstitution, the oral suspension is stable for 2 weeks when refrigerated.

Compatibility/Compounding Considerations

No specific information noted

Dosage Forms/Regulatory Status

VETERINARY-LABELED PRODUCTS:

Cephalexin Chewable Tablets (scored): 75 mg, 150 mg, 300 mg, and 600 mg; *Rilexine*®; (Rx). Approved for use in dogs. NADA #141-326.

In the UK and other countries, there are other oral dosage forms licensed for dogs and cats. Trade names include *Cefaceptin®*, *Ceporex®*, *Cephaforte®*, *Cephorum®*, *Cefaseptin®*, *Kefvet®*, and *Therios®*. Sodium cephalexin 180 mg/mL suspension for injection (*Ceporex®*) also is available in the United Kingdom for use in dogs, cats, and cattle.

HUMAN-LABELED PRODUCTS:

Cephalexin Oral Capsules: 250 mg, 333 mg, 500 mg, and 750 mg; generic; (Rx)

Cephalexin Oral Tablets: 250 mg and 500 mg; generic; (Rx)

Cephalexin Powder for Oral Suspension: 125 mg/5 mL (25 mg/mL) and 250 mg/5 mL (50 mg/mL) after reconstitution in 100 mL and 200 mL; *Keflex®*, generic; (Rx)

References

For the complete list of references, see **wiley.com/go/budde/plumb**

Cephapirin
Cephapirin Benzathine
Cephapirin Sodium

(sef-a-***pye***-rin) *ToDAY®, ToMORROW®*

First-Generation Cephalosporin

Prescriber Highlights

- ▶ First-generation intramammary cephalosporin; also used via intrauterine infusions for endometritis
- ▶ Drug has potential to cause hypersensitivity reactions
- ▶ Available as both dry and lactating cow treatments; follow withdrawal times.

Uses/Indications

An intramammary cephapirin sodium product is FDA-approved in the United States for treatment of mastitis in lactating dairy cows, and cephapirin benzathine is FDA-approved in dry cows. In the United States, there are no longer parenterally administered cephapirin products available. An intrauterine suspension is available in some countries.

The lay literature is replete with reports on the extra-label use of the mastitis products to treat thrush or topical wounds in equids; however, this practice is not supported by peer-reviewed scientific literature and the use of antibacterial agents in the absence of a veterinarian's supervision is strongly discouraged.

The World Health Organization (WHO) has designated first-generation cephalosporins as Highly Important antimicrobials for human medicine.[1] The Office International des Epizooties (OIE) has designated cephapirin as a Veterinary Highly Important Antimicrobial (VHIA) Agent in bovine species.[2]

Pharmacology/Actions

Cephapirin is a first-generation cephalosporin that exhibits activity against bacteria usually covered by this class. Although there may be differences in minimum inhibitory concentration (MIC) for individual first-generation cephalosporins, their spectrums of activity are similar. They generally possess excellent coverage against most gram-positive pathogens (excluding enterococci) and variable coverage against most gram-negative pathogens. These drugs are very active in vitro against streptococci and staphylococci. With the exception of *Bacteroides fragilis*, most anaerobes are very susceptible to the first-generation agents. Resistance is of increasing concern, particularly with methicillin-resistant staphylococci and extended-spectrum beta-lactamase (ESBL)-producing Enterobacteriaceae.

Cephalexin is inactive against *Enterococcus* spp, *Rickettsia* spp, mycobacteria, *Mycoplasma* spp, fungi, and viruses.

Cephalosporins are considered time-dependent and bactericidal against susceptible bacteria, and they act by inhibiting mucopeptide synthesis in the cell wall, which results in a defective barrier and an osmotically unstable spheroplast. The exact mechanism for this effect has not been definitively determined, but beta-lactam antibiotics have been shown to bind to several enzymes (eg, carboxypeptidases, transpeptidases, and endopeptidases) in the bacterial cytoplasmic membrane that are involved in cell wall synthesis. The different affinities that various beta-lactam antibiotics have for these enzymes (also known as penicillin-binding proteins [PBPs]) help explain the differences in spectrums of activity of these drugs that are not explained by the influence of beta-lactamases. Like other beta-lactam antibiotics, cephalosporins are generally considered to be more effective against actively growing bacteria. For bactericidal activity, cephalosporin levels should exceed bacterial MIC for ≈40% of the dose interval for staphylococcal infections and ≈60% of the dose interval for streptococcal infections.

Pharmacokinetics

In cattle, when cephapirin is administered systemically, the apparent volume of distribution has been reported as 0.335 to 0.399 L/kg, total body clearance is 12.66 mL/minute/kg, and serum elimination half-life is ≈64 to 70 minutes.

When cephapirin sodium was administered to healthy (no mastitis) dairy cattle via intramammary infusion, it was rapidly metabolized to the active metabolite desacetylcephapirin in milk.[3] Time above MIC_{90} for common mastitis pathogens and time to reach FDA tolerance concentrations was similar whether the cow was milked 2 or 3 times daily. Additionally, giving the second dose 16 hours later (rather than 12 hours as labeled) to cows that were milked 3 times daily caused no significant effect on withdrawal times or times above MIC. Cows with low daily milk production (less than 25 kg) appeared to absorb more cephapirin systemically and had longer mean residence times than those with high milk production. The authors caution that extended withdrawal times would be prudent in cows with very low milk production and that more studies are required to determine the pharmacokinetics in animals with mastitis.

Contraindications/Precautions/Warnings

Cephalosporins are contraindicated in patients with a history of hypersensitivity to them. Because there may be cross-reactivity, use cephalosporins cautiously in patients that are documented to be hypersensitive to other beta-lactam antibiotics (eg, penicillins, cefamycins, or carbapenems).

Adverse Effects

Adverse effects from cephalosporins are usually not serious and have a relatively low frequency of occurrence.

Potentially, hypersensitivity reactions could occur with intramammary infusion. Hypersensitivity reactions unrelated to dosage can occur with these agents and can manifest as rashes, fever, eosinophilia, lymphadenopathy, or anaphylaxis. The use of cephalosporins in patients documented to be hypersensitive to penicillin-class antibiotics is controversial. In humans, it is estimated that up to 15% of patients that are hypersensitive to penicillins will also be hypersensitive to cephalosporins.[4] The incidence of cross-reactivity in veterinary patients is unknown.

Reproductive/Nursing Safety

Cephalosporins have been shown to cross the placenta and safe use during pregnancy has not been firmly established, but neither have there been any documented teratogenic problems associated with these drugs.

Because safety has not been established in animals, this drug should only be used when the maternal benefits outweigh the potential risks to offspring.

Overdose/Acute Toxicity

No clinical effects would be expected but if used at doses or rates higher than labeled, withdrawal times may be prolonged.

For patients that have experienced or are suspected to have experienced an overdose, consultation with a 24-hour poison consultation center specializing in providing veterinary-specific information is recommended. For general information related to overdose and toxin exposures, as well as contact information for poison control centers, refer to ***Appendix***.

Drug Interactions

There are no significant concerns when cephapirin is used via the intramammary or intrauterine routes.

Laboratory Considerations

- No significant concerns when cephapirin is used via the intramammary route or intrauterine routes
- A cephalothin disk is usually used to determine bacterial susceptibility to this antibiotic when using the Kirby-Bauer method.

Dosages

CATTLE:

Mastitis in cows caused by susceptible strains of *Streptococcus agalactiae* and *Staphylococcus aureus* including strains resistant to penicillin (label dosage; FDA-approved):

a) **Lactating cow** (cephapirin *sodium*): Just prior to administration, completely milk out the udder, clean and dry teat area, then disinfect teat tip with an alcohol wipe and allow to dry.[L] Insert tip of syringe into teat canal; push plunger to instill entire contents of one syringe (10 mL; cephapirin 200 mg) into each infected quarter; repeat once only, 12 hours after initial dose. Massage quarter gently and do not milk out for 12 hours.

b) **Dry cow** (cephapirin *benzathine*): Perform treatment at the time of drying off and no later than 30 days prior to calving.[6] Just prior to administration, completely milk out all four quarters, then wash the udder and teats with warm water and a suitable dairy antiseptic; allow to dry. Disinfect the teat tip with an alcohol wipe, using a separate swab for each teat; allow to dry. Insert tip of syringe into teat canal; push plunger to instill entire contents of one syringe (10 mL; cephapirin 300 mg) into each infected quarter. Massage quarter gently.

Subacute and chronic endometritis (at least 14 days after parturition) caused by cephapirin-sensitive bacteria (extra-label): Using the intrauterine suspension, instill syringe contents (cephapirin 500 mg) through the cervix into the lumen of the uterus; depending on response may re-treat in 7 to 14 days if clinical signs persist. May be used one day after insemination. If pyometra is present, pretreatment with a prostaglandin is recommended to cause luteolysis and expel debris from the uterus.[7]

Monitoring

- Because cephalosporins usually have minimal toxicity associated with their use, monitoring for efficacy is usually all that is required.

Client Information

- Follow all label information and milk and slaughter withdrawal times.

Chemistry/Synonyms

A semisynthetic cephalosporin antibiotic, cephapirin sodium occurs as a white to off-white crystalline powder with a faint odor. It is very soluble in water and slightly soluble in alcohol. Each gram of the injection contains 2.36 mEq of sodium. After reconstitution, the solution for injection has a pH of 6.5 to 8.5.

Cephapirin sodium may also be known as BL-P-1322, cefapirin, cefapyrin, cefapirinum natricum, *Metricure*®, *ToDAY*®, or *ToMORROW*®.

Storage/Stability

Cephapirin intramammary syringes should be stored at controlled room temperature (15°C-30°C [59°F-86°F]); avoid excessive heat. Do not freeze.

Compatibility/Compounding Considerations

No specific information is noted.

Dosage Forms/Regulatory Status

VETERINARY-LABELED PRODUCTS:

Cephapirin Sodium Mastitis Tube: cephapirin 200 mg/10 mL tube; *ToDAY*®; (OTC). FDA-approved for use in lactating dairy cattle. Milk withdrawal = 96 hours; slaughter withdrawal = 4 days

Cephapirin Benzathine Mastitis Tube: cephapirin 300 mg/10 mL tube; *ToMORROW*®; (OTC). FDA-approved for use in dry dairy cattle. Milk withdrawal = 72 hours after calving and must not be administered within 30 days of calving; slaughter withdrawal = 42 days.

Cephapirin is excluded from the 2012 FDA/CVM ban on ELDU of cephalosporins in food-producing animals. There are multiple reports from the lay literature on the extra-label use of the mastitis products to treat thrush or topical wounds in equids.

In many countries, including Canada, Australia, and the UK, cephapirin benzathine 500 mg intrauterine infusion syringes are available for treating endometritis in dairy or beef cattle. *Metricure*®; (Rx). Milk and meat withdrawal times may vary with each country; refer to each specific label, but commonly, milk withdrawal = 0 hours and meat withdrawal = 48 hours.

HUMAN-LABELED PRODUCTS: NONE

References

For the complete list of references, see **wiley.com/go/budde/plumb**

Cetirizine

(se-***tih***-ra-zeen) *Zyrtec*®

Antihistamine, Second Generation

Prescriber Highlights

- ► Oral, relatively nonsedating antihistamine
- ► No significant anticholinergic or serotonergic effects
- ► Recommended dosages for dogs and cats vary widely
- ► Can potentially cause vomiting, hypersalivation, or somnolence in small animals

Uses/Indications

Cetirizine is an H_1 receptor blocking antihistamine agent that may be useful for the adjunctive treatment of histamine-mediated pruritic and allergic conditions, including respiratory allergies (eg, nasal and ocular discharge, sneezing), urticaria, and insect bite hypersensitivity in dogs and cats. Although antihistamines are commonly used to treat canine atopic dermatitis, cetirizine does not appear effective for the treatment of chronic and acute flares of canine atopic dermatitis.[1-3] Guidelines for atopic dermatitis treatment in dogs state that antihistamines have modest efficacy; cetirizine should be given continuously (ie, daily) as preventive therapy before an acute flare.[3,4] Moreover, one randomized double-blinded crossover study showed that cetirizine was effective in preventing cutaneous allergic reactions in healthy dogs.[5]

An open clinical trial administering cetirizine in cats with allergic skin disease showed pruritus reduction in 41% of cats.[6] A separate randomized double-blind placebo-controlled crossover study investigated cetirizine at 1 mg/kg/day PO for 14 days for the control of pruritus in cats with feline atopic skin syndrome. The study showed there were no statistically significant differences between cetirizine and placebo regarding clinical and pruritus scores.[7]

Cetirizine may also have a role in treating allergic conditions, including dermatographism[8] and seasonal headshaking[9] in horses. However, one controlled study showed no apparent benefit from a 3-week trial treating insect bite hypersensitivity in horses.[10] Cetirizine appears to reduce the risk for recurrence of eosinophilic keratitis in horses.[11]

Pharmacology/Actions

Cetirizine hydrochloride, a metabolite of hydroxyzine, is a nonsedating antihistamine (ie, it does not cross the blood-brain barrier as compared with first-generation drugs) that selectively inhibits peripheral H_1 receptors. Cetirizine inhibited histamine and anticanine immunoglobulin E (IgE)-mediated skin reactions (wheals) in dogs.[2,12] Cetirizine administered for 6 days at 2 mg/kg/day PO to healthy dogs was effective in preventing immediate- and late-phase cutaneous allergic reactions.[5] It also appears to decrease histamine release from basophils in some species; in cats, cetirizine or cyproheptadine do not reduce eosinophilic airway inflammation (experimentally produced).[13] Cetirizine does not possess significant anticholinergic or antiserotonergic effects. Tolerance to its antihistamine effects is thought not to occur.

Pharmacokinetics

In dogs, peak concentration occurred 4 to 7 hours after oral administration,[2] and elimination half-life was ≈10 hours.[2,12]

In a study of cats receiving an oral dose of 5 mg/cat (NOT mg/kg), protein binding was 88%, volume of distribution was 0.24 L/kg, and clearance was ≈0.3 mL/kg/minute.[14] The terminal elimination half-life was ≈10 hours. The mean plasma concentrations remained above 0.72 µg/mL (a concentration reported to be effective for humans) for 24 hours after administration.

In horses, peak concentration occurred 0.7 hours after oral administration.[15] The terminal elimination half-life was reported to be between 3.5 and 6 hours, with trough plasma concentrations of ≈16 to 18 ng/mL after 0.2 mg/kg PO, and ≈45 ng/mL after 0.4 mg/kg PO.[15-17] Another study showed a longer terminal half-life for cetirizine of 7.13 hours in exercised Thoroughbred horses.[18] Drug accumulation does not appear to occur in horses.[16]

After oral administration to humans, cetirizine peak concentrations occur in ≈1 hour. Food can delay but not affect the extent of absorption. Cetirizine is 93% bound to human plasma proteins, and brain concentrations are ≈10% of those found in plasma. Approximately 80% of the drug is excreted in the urine, primarily as unchanged drug. Terminal elimination half-life is ≈8 hours; antihistaminic effect generally persists for 24 hours after administration. Elimination half-life is ≈12 hours in geriatric adults. Its elimination was shown to be slowed in individuals with liver disease.[19]

Contraindications/Precautions/Warnings

No specific information is available for veterinary patients. In humans, cetirizine is contraindicated in those that are hypersensitive to it or hydroxyzine. Avoidance or dose adjustment is recommended in geriatric humans or in humans with severe renal or hepatic impairment.

The combination product containing pseudoephedrine (eg, *Zyrtec-D®*) is not appropriate for use in dogs or cats. Commercially available liquid formulations may contain propylene glycol, which is toxic to cats; orally disintegrating tablets may contain xylitol, which is toxic to dogs.

Adverse Effects

Cetirizine appears to be well tolerated in dogs and cats. Vomiting or hypersalivation after administration may occur in some dogs.[1] Drowsiness has been reported in small dogs given higher doses.

A pharmacokinetic/pharmacodynamic study performed in a small number of horses yielded no visible adverse effects.

In humans, the primary adverse effects reported have been drowsiness (13%) and dry mouth (5%). Hypersensitivity reactions, increased liver enzymes, hepatitis, and cholestasis have been rarely reported. Additionally, pruritus after discontinuation of cetirizine has been reported in humans.[20]

Reproductive/Nursing Safety

Cetirizine did not impair fertility or reproductive performance in mice or rats. In pregnant mice, rats, and rabbits, doses ≈40 times, 180 times, and 220 times the human dose (respectively)—when compared on an mg/m^2 basis—caused no teratogenic effects. Results from a retrospective study in humans suggested that exposure to cetirizine was not associated with adverse pregnancy outcomes in the fetuses above background rates.[21] One prospective study determined that cetirizine does not appear to be associated with increased teratogenic risk.[22]

In beagles, ≈3% of a dose was excreted into milk. Cetirizine enters human breastmilk, and one study estimated the relative infant dose to be ≈1.8% at 24 hours.[23] In humans, international guidelines recommend cetirizine as an acceptable choice if an antihistamine is required during breastfeeding. Small infrequent doses of cetirizine are likely tolerated during breastfeeding; however, larger doses or long-term use may cause drowsiness and other adverse effects in the infant or reduce milk production, mainly when combined with a sympathomimetic, such as pseudoephedrine, or before lactation is settled.[24]

Because safety has not been established, this drug should only be used when the maternal benefits outweigh the potential fetal risks.

Overdose/Acute Toxicity

Limited information is available. Reported minimum lethal oral doses for mice and rats are 237 mg/kg (95 times the human adult dose on an mg/m^2 basis) and 562 mg/kg (460 times the human adult dose on an mg/m^2 basis), respectively. In cases of overdose, cetirizine may cross into the CNS and cause neurologic signs (eg, hyperactivity, lethargy); it may also cause vomiting, panting, mydriasis, and tachycardia. Cetirizine does not appreciably prolong the QT interval on ECG at high serum levels.

Overdoses of cetirizine products that also contain pseudoephedrine (eg, *Zyrtec-D®*) may be serious.

For patients that have experienced or are suspected of having experienced an overdose, it is strongly encouraged that a 24-hour poison consultation center that specializes in providing veterinary-specific information be consulted. For general information related to overdose and toxin exposures, as well as contact information for poison control centers, refer to ***Appendix***.

Drug Interactions

The following drug interactions have either been reported or are theoretical in humans or animals receiving cetirizine and may be of significance in veterinary patients. Unless otherwise noted, use together is not necessarily contraindicated, but weigh the potential risks and perform additional monitoring when appropriate.

- **CNS DEPRESSANTS** (eg, **acepromazine, benzodiazepines, opioids**): Additive CNS depression or sedation is possible.
- **IVERMECTIN**: The use of ivermectin 12 hours prior to cetirizine significantly increased cetirizine exposure (area under the curve [AUC]) by 60% and elimination half-life by 18% in horses. Administration of ivermectin 90 minutes prior to cetirizine did not produce the same effect. Clinical significance is unknown.[15]
- **P-GLYCOPROTEIN SUBSTRATES** (eg, **cyclosporine, digoxin, vincristine**): Cetirizine has been shown to be a p-glycoprotein inhibitor (however, not a metabolite of the CYP450 system)[25]; therefore, avoidance or care should be taken with coadministration of cetirizine with p-glycoprotein substrate drugs.[26]

Laboratory Considerations

- **Intradermal allergy testing (IDT)**: Suppression of IDT results may persist for 1 to 2 weeks after discontinuation of cetirizine; it is recommended that treatment be discontinued at least 2 weeks prior to testing.[27]

Dosages

DOGS:

Pruritus associated with atopic dermatitis (extra-label): 1 – 4 mg/kg PO once daily with or without food.[2,12,27] Cetirizine should be given continuously (ie, daily) as preventive therapy before an acute flare.[3,4] Reduced efficacy was noted in one study[1] at lower dosages (1 mg/kg PO every 24 hours), as well as in dogs with acute[28] or chronic[3] atopic dermatitis.

CATS:

Adjunctive treatment of pruritus (extra-label):

a) Based on an open trial: 5 mg/cat (NOT mg/kg) PO once daily; 41% of cats had pruritus reduced.[29]

b) Anecdotal: 0.5 – 1 mg/kg or 2.5 – 5 mg/cat (NOT mg/kg) PO every 12 to 24 hours

HORSES:

Antihistamine (extra-label): 0.2 – 0.4 mg/kg PO every 12 hours[9,16]; a subsequent study did not support this dose as being efficacious.[10]

Eosinophilic keratitis (extra-label): 0.4 mg/kg PO twice daily[11]

Monitoring

- Clinical efficacy (trial periods to determine an individual antihistamine's efficacy are usually 1 to 2 weeks long)
- Adverse effects (eg, vomiting, somnolence)

Client Information

- Use antihistamines on a regular ongoing basis in animals that respond well. Antihistamines work better when used before an animal has been exposed to an allergen.
- Cetirizine may cause less drowsiness or sleepiness than other antihistamines, but this effect is still possible.
- **Only use products that contain cetirizine as a single active ingredient.** Any other ingredients (eg, pain relievers, decongestants) found in human-label combination products can be toxic to animals.
- Cetirizine may be given with or without food. If your animal vomits or acts sick after receiving the drug on an empty stomach, try giving the next dose with food or a small treat. If vomiting continues, contact your veterinarian.

Chemistry/Synonyms

Cetirizine is a piperazine derivative that occurs as a white to almost white crystalline powder that is freely soluble in water. A 5% solution has a pH of 1.2 to 1.8. Commercial formulations contain cetirizine HCl.

Cetirizine may also be known as UCB-P071, P-071, cetirizina, cetirizini, cetirizin, ceterizino, or *Zyrtec*®; many internationally registered trade names are available.

Storage/Stability

Store cetirizine tablets and syrup at room temperature 20°C to 25°C (68°F-77°F).

Compatibility/Compounding Considerations

No specific information has been noted.

Dosage Forms/Regulatory Status

VETERINARY-LABELED PRODUCTS: NONE

The Association of Racing Commissioners International (ARCI) has designated this drug as a class 4 substance. Use of this drug may not be allowed in certain animal competitions. Check rules and regulations before entering in a competition while this medication is being administered. Contact local racing authorities for further guidance. See ***Appendix*** for more information.

HUMAN-LABELED PRODUCTS:

Cetirizine HCl Oral Tablets (film-coated): 5 mg and 10 mg; *Zyrtec*®, generic; (OTC)

Cetirizine HCl Chewable Tablets: 5 mg and 10 mg; *Zyrtec*®; (OTC). Available in fruit flavors.

Cetirizine HCl Oral Syrup or Solution: 1 mg/mL in 118 mL and 473 mL; *Zyrtec*®, generic; (OTC). Available in bubble gum or fruit flavors. May contain propylene glycol

Cetirizine 10 mg is also available in liquid gel caps and orally disintegrating tablet formulations. Combination products are available but are not appropriate for use in small animals. Disintegrating tablets may contain xylitol.

References

For the complete list of references, see **wiley.com/go/budde/plumb**

Charcoal, Activated

(***char***-kole) *ToxiBan*®, *Actidose*®

Oral Adsorbent

Prescriber Highlights

- ▶ Orally administered adsorbent for ingested toxins and drug overdoses; consider consulting with an animal poison control center before use
- ▶ Some formulations contain a cathartic (eg, sorbitol). Use caution when administering with cathartics; monitor closely for dehydration and electrolyte disturbances (eg, hypernatremia, hyperkalemia).
- ▶ Contraindications include administration to animals with a reduced gag reflex or at risk for aspiration pneumonia (eg, megaesophagus, CNS depression), decreased peristalsis, hypernatremia, or hyperosmolar states (eg, diabetic ketoacidosis).
- ▶ Not effective for treatment of inorganic molecules (eg, iron), mineral acid or alkali ingestion
- ▶ Adverse effects include emesis with rapid administration, dehydration, hypernatremia, constipation, or diarrhea.
- ▶ Charcoal stains clothing and animal fur.

Uses/Indications

Activated charcoal is administered orally to prevent or reduce systemic absorption of certain drugs or toxins in the GI tract. To enhance elimination of the charcoal-toxin moiety, an osmotic cathartic (eg, sorbitol; combinations are commercially available) is often given with activated charcoal. In humans, the benefit of adding a cathartic remains unproven. There is little need to administer a cathartic if significant diarrhea is already present. One study suggested single-dose activated charcoal alone was equally as effective as activated charcoal with sorbitol (as a cathartic) in reducing the serum concentration of carprofen following overdose in dogs.[1]

In humans, a single dose of activated charcoal is recommended when a potentially toxic amount of a substance (known to be adsorbed by charcoal) has been ingested in the past hour[2]; this same recommendation appears to also apply to veterinary patients.[1]

Pharmacology/Actions

Activated charcoal has a large surface area and adsorbs many chemicals and drugs via ion–ion, hydrogen bonding, dipole, and Van der Waals forces in the upper GI tract, thereby preventing or reducing their absorption. Efficiency of adsorption increases with the molecular size of the toxin, and poorly water-soluble organic substances are better adsorbed than small, polar, water-soluble organic compounds.

Although activated charcoal also adsorbs various nutrients and enzymes from the gut, there are generally no significant impacts on nutritional needs when used for acute poisonings.

Activated charcoal slurries are most effective in adsorbing most toxins.[3] Charcoal is most effective if given within 1 hour of toxin ingestion and is generally not recommended over 4 hours postingestion unless the exposure involves a drug that is enterohepatically recirculated.[1,2]

Pharmacokinetics

Activated charcoal is not absorbed or metabolized in the gut. Activated charcoal slurries can slow GI transit times; thus, an osmotic cathartic (eg, sorbitol) is often given concurrently to enhance expulsion of the toxin-charcoal moiety. See ***Contraindications/Precautions/Warnings***.

An in vitro study demonstrated that the presence of dog food can reduce the adsorptive capacity of activated charcoal, but the authors concluded the reduction was clinically insignificant.[4]

Contraindications/Precautions/Warnings

Activated charcoal should not be used for mineral acids, salt toxicosis (including paintballs and homemade play dough), hydrocarbons, or caustic alkalis, as it is either ineffective or dangerous (eg, risk for bowel perforation) with these substances. Although activated charcoal is not contraindicated with ethanol, methanol, ethylene glycol, xylitol, caustic alkalis, nitrates, sodium chloride/chlorate, petroleum distillates, mineral acids, heavy metals (eg, lithium), or iron salts, it is ineffective in adsorbing these products and may obscure GI lesions during endoscopy. Administration of activated charcoal (after orogastric lavage) for acute cyanide ingestion may be helpful if administered within 1 hour; however, it is not a replacement for use of cyanide antidotes.[5,6]

Animals with a decreased gag reflex or that are otherwise at risk for aspiration pneumonia (eg, megaesophagus, CNS depression) should not be given activated charcoal without adequate airway protection (ie, endotracheal intubation). Administration of activated charcoal via a nasogastric tube may be appropriate in these situations; however, if clinical signs related to the toxicity are already present, the benefit of activated charcoal treatment may not outweigh the risk for potential complications (eg, aspiration pneumonia) related to its administration. Other potential contraindications to charcoal therapy include a history of decreased peristalsis, recent GI surgery, GI obstruction or ileus, GI perforation, hypernatremia and other hyperosmolar states (eg, acute kidney injury, diabetic ketoacidosis), or imminent GI surgery or endoscopy. The ability of activated charcoal to adsorb toxicants (and therefore, its efficacy) decreases significantly 1 to 2 hours after toxicant ingestion[2]; however, delayed or repeated activated charcoal administration may be effective for agents that are enterohepatically recirculated (eg, caffeine, cannabinoids, phenobarbital, theobromine, theophylline, bromethalin, pyrethrins, marijuana, NSAIDs, organophosphate insecticides, ivermectin, digoxin, antidepressants).[2,7]

If multiple doses of activated charcoal are administered, it has been recommended that only the first dose contain the cathartic to prevent diarrhea, dehydration, and potentially hypernatremia.[8,9] Check the product label to ensure the appropriate product is being used at the appropriate time, as some commercial products contain a combination of activated charcoal and a cathartic in a premixed solution. Contraindications to cathartic use include absent bowel sounds, recent abdominal trauma, recent bowel surgery, intestinal obstruction, intestinal perforation, ingestion of a corrosive substance, volume depletion, hypotension, and electrolyte imbalance.

Although over-the-counter tablets are available to control flatulence and bloating, they are not as effective.[3]

Separate administration of any other orally administered therapeutic agents by at least 2 to 4 hours, as activated charcoal will adsorb the drug while in the GI tract. Administer any needed drugs parenterally when possible.

Endoscopic examination may be difficult after activated charcoal administration.[10] Feces will appear black when it is eliminated, making detection of melena challenging.

Adverse Effects

Rapid GI administration of charcoal can induce emesis. If aspiration occurs after activated charcoal is administered, acute pneumonitis and aspiration pneumonia[10] may result and lead to chronic pneumonitis. Charcoal can cause either constipation or diarrhea; in one study, diarrhea was more likely in dogs receiving repeated charcoal doses.[1] Prolonged constipation may cause release of the toxin from the activated charcoal; monitor stool production. Products containing sorbitol may cause loose stools, vomiting, and abdominal cramping. In humans, most activated charcoal complications are due to aspiration or inadvertent administration in the lungs; this likely also applies to veterinary patients.

Dehydration and hypernatremia may occur after administration of activated charcoal (with sorbitol[11] or without[12]), presumably due to an osmotic effect pulling water into the GI tract. Low sodium fluids (eg, dextrose 5%, 0.45% NaCl/dextrose 2.5%) and warm water enemas can be administered to alleviate the hypernatremic effect.[12] Increased osmolality and serum lactate has also been observed following activated charcoal administration.[13]

Charcoal powder stains, and dry powder is a respiratory irritant that tends to aerosolize across wide areas.

Reproductive/Nursing Safety

Charcoal is unlikely to cause embryo- or fetotoxicity or toxicity to nursing offspring, as it is not absorbed into the systemic circulation. Maternal benefits of activated charcoal treatment are likely to outweigh any potential risks to offspring.

Overdose/Acute Toxicity

The most likely effect from administering too much activated charcoal is induction of emesis with risk for aspiration. Activated charcoal that contains a cathartic (eg, sorbitol) can cause electrolyte abnormalities and dehydration. See ***Adverse Effects*** for more information.

For patients that have experienced or are suspected to have experienced an overdose, consultation with a 24-hour poison consultation center specializing in providing veterinary-specific information is recommended. For general information related to overdose and toxin exposures, as well as contact information for poison control centers, refer to ***Appendix***.

Drug Interactions

The following drug interactions have either been reported or are theoretical in humans or animals receiving charcoal and may be of significance in veterinary patients. Unless otherwise noted, use together is not necessarily contraindicated, but weigh the potential risks and perform additional monitoring when appropriate.

- ACEPROMAZINE: Risk for GI obstruction may be increased by drugs that slow GI motility.
- ANTICHOLINERGIC AGENTS (eg, **atropine, glycopyrrolate, hyoscyamine, meclizine, oxybutynin**): Risk for GI obstruction may be increased by drugs that slow GI motility.
- ANTIDIARRHEAL AGENTS (eg, **diphenoxylate, loperamide**): Risk for GI obstruction may be increased by drugs that slow GI motility.
- ANTIHISTAMINE H_1-RECEPTOR ANTAGONISTS (eg, **diphenhydramine, hydroxyzine**): Risk for GI obstruction may be increased by drugs that slow GI motility.
- DAIRY PRODUCTS: May reduce the adsorptive capacity of activated charcoal

- **Mineral Oil**: May reduce the adsorptive capacity of activated charcoal
- **Opioids** (eg, **butorphanol, hydrocodone, morphine, tramadol**): Risk for GI obstruction may be increased by drugs that slow GI motility.
- **Orally Administered Drugs**: Separate administration of any other orally administered therapeutic agents by at least 3 hours, as the charcoal will adsorb the drug while in the GI tract. Administer any needed drugs parenterally when possible.
- **Polyethylene Glycol ± Electrolyte Solutions** (eg, *Miralax®*, *GoLytely®*): May reduce the adsorptive capacity of activated charcoal
- **Tricyclic Antidepressants** (TCA; eg, **amitriptyline, clomipramine, doxepin**): Risk for GI obstruction may be increased by drugs that slow GI motility.

Laboratory Considerations

- A false-positive **ethylene glycol test** may result from products that contain sorbitol or polyethylene glycol.

Dosages

NOTE: Depending on the toxin exposure, recommendations for using activated charcoal can vary. It is highly recommended to contact an animal poison control center for specific guidance on using activated charcoal in veterinary patients.

DOGS & CATS:

Adjunctive treatment for toxin ingestion (extra-label): 1 – 2 g/kg PO but doses up to 5 g/kg have been described. Charcoal with sorbitol is commonly employed (only with the first dose) to reduce GI transit time. For drugs and toxins that undergo enterohepatic recirculation (eg, caffeine, phenobarbital, theobromine, theophylline, bromethalin, pyrethrins, marijuana, NSAIDs, organophosphate insecticides, ivermectin, digoxin, antidepressants), multiple subsequent doses of activated charcoal WITHOUT sorbitol at 1 – 2 g/kg PO every 4 to 8 hours for 24 to 48 hours is recommended. Dogs and cats with no clinical signs may freely consume the charcoal suspension if administered via syringe. A small amount of food may be added to the solution to enhance palatability.[4] In animals exhibiting clinical signs, administration of activated charcoal suspensions may be done via a nasogastric tube, as it may be better accepted, easier to place (especially in cats), and offer a greater margin of safety; always ensure adequate airway protection.[7,8,14,15]

HORSES:

Adjunctive treatment for toxin ingestion (extra-label):

a) 1 – 2 g/kg PO as a slurry through a stomach tube, with or without a cathartic[16]
b) Up to 750 g/horse (NOT g/kg) PO.[17] Make a slurry by mixing with up to 4 L (depending on animal's size) of warm water, and administer via stomach tube. Leave in stomach for 20 to 30 minutes then give a cathartic to hasten removal of toxicants.

RUMINANTS:

Plant intoxication (extra-label): 1 – 5 g/kg PO.[18] Multidose activated charcoal is beneficial for a number of plant intoxications, including oleander. Administration of a cathartic mixed in the activated charcoal slurry helps to hasten elimination of contents from the GI tract. Commonly used cathartics include sodium sulfate (ie, Glauber's salts), magnesium sulfate (ie, Epsom salt), and sorbitol. Sodium or magnesium sulfate can be administered at 250 – 500 mg/kg PO mixed in the activated charcoal slurry. Sorbitol (70%) can be administered at 3 mL/kg PO and also mixed in the activated charcoal slurry.

General treatment for toxicosis (extra-label): 1 – 3 g/kg PO every 8 – 12 hours[19]

FERRETS:

Adjunctive treatment for toxin ingestion (extra-label): 1 – 3 g/kg PO, usually via syringe or gastric tube. Repeat doses may be indicated if the drug or toxin undergoes enterohepatic recirculation.[20]

Monitoring

- Monitoring for efficacy of charcoal is usually dependent on the toxin/drug's mechanism of action, extent of toxicity, and patient's clinical signs.
- When activated charcoal is given with a cathartic, repeated serum sodium measurements (eg, every 8 to 12 hours) are recommended to address potential hypernatremia before clinical signs (eg, tremors, ataxia, seizures) occur. Serum sodium increases can be seen 6 to 10 hours after cathartic administration.[11]
- Hydration status
- Stool production: prolonged constipation can cause the toxin to be released from activated charcoal.

Client Information

- Activated charcoal should be used under the guidance of a licensed veterinarian. Monitor your animal for at least 4 hours after the drug is given to watch for weakness, unsteadiness, tremors, or convulsions. Contact your veterinarian immediately if these signs occur.
- Charcoal can permanently stain clothing and fur.
- It is expected that your animal's feces will be black when the charcoal is passed.

Chemistry/Synonyms

Activated charcoal occurs as a fine, black, odorless, tasteless powder that is insoluble in water or alcohol. Commercially available activated charcoal products may differ in their adsorptive properties, but 1 g must adsorb 100 mg of strychnine sulfate in 50 mL of water to meet USP standards.

Activated charcoal may also be known as AC, active carbon, activated carbon, carbo activatus, adsorbent charcoal, decolorizing carbon, or medicinal charcoal. There are many trade names available. Activated charcoal with sorbitol may be known as ACS.

Storage/Stability

Store activated charcoal in well-closed glass or metal containers or in the manufacturer's supplied container.

Compatibility/Compounding Considerations

No specific information is noted.

Dosage Forms/Regulatory Status

NOTE: Carefully read label to determine if the product also contains a cathartic; avoid multiple administrations of cathartic-containing combinations.

VETERINARY-LABELED PRODUCTS:

The following products are labeled for veterinary use, but there are no oral activated charcoal products listed as FDA-approved on the FDA's Green Book website.

Activated charcoal 47.5%, kaolin 10%, sorbitol 20% granules (free flowing and wettable) in 453.6 g (1 lb) bottles and 5 kg (11.02 lb) pails; *ToxiBan® Granules*; (OTC). Labeled for use in both large and small animal species

Activated charcoal 10.4%, kaolin 6.25% suspension in 240 mL bottles; *ToxiBan® Suspension*; (OTC). Labeled for use in both large and small animal species

Activated charcoal 10%, kaolin 6.25%, sorbitol 10% suspension in 240 mL bottles; *ToxiBan® Suspension* with *Sorbitol*; (OTC). Labeled for use in small animal species

Activated charcoal 10%, attapulgite 20%, sodium chloride 35 mg/mL, potassium chloride 35 mg/mL gel/paste in 80 mL and 300 mL; *D-Tox-Besc®, Activated Charcoal Gel with Electrolytes®*; (OTC). Labeled for use in small and large animal species

Activated hardwood charcoal and thermally activated attapulgite clay (concentrations not labeled) in an aqueous gel suspension in 8 fl oz bottle, 60 mL tube, and 300 mL tube with easy dose syringe; *UAA® (Universal Animal Antidote) Gel*; (OTC). Labeled for use in dogs and cats and for grain overload in ruminants

HUMAN-LABELED PRODUCTS:

Activated charcoal oral powder: 15 g, 30 g, 40 g, 120 g, 240 g, and UD 30 g; generic; (OTC)

Activated charcoal oral liquid/suspension with sorbitol: 25 g in 120 mL and 50 g in 240 mL; *Actidose® with Sorbitol*, generic; (OTC)

Activated charcoal liquid/suspension without sorbitol: 208 mg/mL to 12.5 g in 60 mL, 15 g in 72 mL, 25 g in 120 mL, and 50 g in 240 mL; *Actidose-Aqua®*, generic; (OTC)

Activated charcoal oral granules: 25 g; *EZ Char®*; (OTC)

References

For the complete list of references, see **wiley.com/go/budde/plumb**

Chlorambucil

(klor-***am***-byoo-sil) *Leukeran®*

Antineoplastic, Immunosuppressant

Prescriber Highlights

- Nitrogen mustard derivative antineoplastic and immunosuppressant in dogs, cats, and horses
- Caution: Pre-existing bone marrow depression or infection
- Adverse effects: Primarily myelosuppression and GI toxicity
- Known teratogen; National Institute for Occupational Safety and Health (NIOSH) hazardous drug; use appropriate precautions when handling.

Uses/Indications

Chlorambucil may be useful as part of multidrug protocols in a variety of neoplastic diseases, including lymphocytic leukemia, T-cell lymphoma,[1] GI lymphoma,[2,3] multiple myeloma, lymphangiosarcoma,[4] mast cell tumor,[5] cutaneous plasmacytosis, polycythemia vera, macroglobulinemia, and ovarian adenocarcinoma. Chlorambucil may also be used as a solo metronomic agent for some neoplasias (eg, hemangiosarcoma, transitional cell carcinoma).[6,7] It may also be useful as adjunctive therapy for some immune-mediated conditions (eg, inflammatory bowel disease, nonerosive arthritis, immune-mediated hemolytic anemia, immune-mediated skin disease).[8,9]

Pharmacology/Actions

Chlorambucil is an aromatic nitrogen mustard derivative and an alkylating antineoplastic agent. Its chemical reactivity is nonspecific, but the primary cytotoxic effect is due to alkylation of cancer cell DNA strands resulting in cross-linking and cellular apoptosis. Immunosuppressive effects may not be noted until 2 to 4 weeks after starting the drug.

Acquired resistance to chlorambucil has been reported and is thought to be caused by several mechanisms.[10]

Pharmacokinetics

Chlorambucil is rapidly and completely absorbed after oral administration, reaching C_{max} in ≈1 hour. It is highly bound to plasma proteins. Although it is unknown if chlorambucil crosses the blood–brain barrier, neurologic adverse effects have been reported. Chlorambucil is extensively metabolized in the liver primarily to the active metabolite phenylacetic acid mustard. Phenylacetic acid mustard is further metabolized to other metabolites that are excreted in the urine. Terminal half-life is 1.5 hours in humans.

Contraindications/Precautions/Warnings

Chlorambucil is contraindicated in patients with a history of hypersensitivity to it or other alkylating agents. It should be used with caution in patients with pre-existing bone marrow depression, patients susceptible to bone marrow depression (including patients receiving long-standing maximum-tolerated dose chemotherapy), or patients that have an active systemic infection. Because chlorambucil is hepatically metabolized, use with caution in patients with hepatic impairment.

Because chlorambucil is a chemotherapy agent with potential to cause teratogenic effects, proper and safe handling methods are recommended to reduce personal and occupational exposure.[11] The National Institute for Occupational Safety and Health (NIOSH) classifies chlorambucil as a hazardous drug.[12]

Adverse Effects

The most common major adverse effect associated with chlorambucil therapy is myelosuppression (eg, anemia, leukopenia, thrombocytopenia). Myelosuppression may occur gradually, with nadirs occurring within 7 to 14 days of the start of therapy. Recovery generally takes from 7 to 14 days. Severe bone marrow depression, an uncommon adverse effect occurring more often with prolonged (months to years) therapy, can result in pancytopenia that may require months to years for recovery. GI toxicity (eg, vomiting, diarrhea) is more common with higher (20 mg in humans) pulse doses. Hepatotoxicity was noted in 23% of dogs in one study.[5] Alopecia and delayed regrowth of shaven hair have been reported in dogs; breeds with a continuously growing hair coat (eg, poodles, terriers, Afghan hounds, old English sheepdogs) are more likely to experience significant hair loss. Lower-dose metronomic therapy (4 mg/m^2 [NOT mg/kg] once daily) in dogs is associated with a lower incidence of adverse effects. One study that evaluated several metronomic dose schedules found that dogs receiving 6 mg/m^2 (NOT mg/kg) once daily and 8 mg/m^2 (NOT mg/kg) once daily were at higher risk for adverse effects (GI and hematologic) as compared with dogs that received 4 mg/m^2 (NOT mg/kg) once daily. In addition, higher dosages of metronomic chlorambucil did not improve tumor response.[13]

One case report of neurotoxicity (eg, facial twitching, myoclonus, agitation, seizures) in a cat has been reported.[14] In addition, acquired Fanconi syndrome has been reported in 4 cats receiving chlorambucil and corticosteroids. Partial or complete resolution of Fanconi syndrome was seen in 3 of 4 cats within 3 months of discontinuing chlorambucil therapy.[15] In another report, chlorambucil was suspected of causing seizures in a dog.[16]

In humans, skin reactions that may progress to erythema multiforme or toxic epidermal necrolysis have been reported rarely. Bronchopulmonary dysplasia with pulmonary fibrosis, neurotoxicity, uric acid nephropathy, and hepatotoxicity have also been reported. Secondary malignancies may occur.

Reproductive/Nursing Safety

Chlorambucil has been documented to cause teratogenic effects in laboratory animals. Use during pregnancy only when the benefits to the dam outweigh the potential risks. In humans, chlorambucil has caused prolonged or permanent azoospermia in men, amenorrhea in women, and both reversible and irreversible infertility, particularly when given during pre-puberty and puberty.

It is unknown whether chlorambucil enters maternal milk. In humans, it is recommended to discontinue nursing if the mother is receiving the drug.

Because safety has not been established in animals, this drug should only be used when the maternal benefits outweigh the potential risks to offspring.

Overdose/Acute Toxicity

The oral LD_{50} of chlorambucil in rats and mice is 76 mg/kg and 80 mg/kg, respectively. Experiences with acute overdoses in humans have been limited, but doses of up to 5 mg/kg resulted in neurologic (seizures) toxicity and pancytopenia (nadirs at 1 to 6 weeks postingestion). All patients recovered without long-term sequelae. Supportive treatment and gut emptying protocols are recommended following an overdose but beware of rapidly changing neurologic status if inducing vomiting. CBC should be monitored for several weeks following an overdose, and blood component therapy may be necessary. Chlorambucil is not dialyzable.

For patients that have experienced or are suspected to have experienced an overdose, consultation with a 24-hour poison center specializing in providing veterinary-specific information is recommended. For general information related to overdose and toxin exposures, as well as contact information for poison control centers, refer to ***Appendix***.

Drug Interactions

The following drug interactions have either been reported or are theoretical in humans or animals receiving chlorambucil and may be of significance in veterinary patients. Unless otherwise noted, use together is not necessarily contraindicated, but weigh the potential risks and perform additional monitoring when appropriate.

- **Myelosuppressive Agents** (eg, **antineoplastics, immunosuppressants, iron chelators**): Concurrent use with other bone marrow depressant medications may result in additive myelosuppression; avoid combination when possible.
- **Vaccines** (live and inactivated): Chlorambucil may diminish vaccine efficacy and enhance adverse effects of vaccines.

Laboratory Considerations

- Chlorambucil may raise **serum uric acid** concentrations. Drugs such as allopurinol may be required to control hyperuricemia in some patients.

Dosages

NOTE: Because of the potential toxicity of this drug to patients, veterinary personnel, and clients, and because chemotherapy indications, treatment protocols, monitoring, and safety guidelines often change, the following dosages should be used only as a general guide. Consultation with a veterinary oncologist and referral to current veterinary oncology references[17-21] are strongly recommended.

WARNINGS:

1. Chlorambucil dosages are commonly based on surface area (mg/m²). Do not confuse with citations that list dosages in mg/kg. Commercial tablet size (2 mg) may make precise dosing difficult without compounding.
2. **Tablets should not be crushed, split, or formulated into a liquid**, unless adequate environmental, personal, and occupational exposure can be safeguarded.

DOGS:

Immunosuppressive agent (extra-label): Commonly dosed at 1.95 – 4.5 mg/m² (NOT mg/kg) once daily. Dosages are generally rounded to the nearest 2 mg. Following remission, chlorambucil has been dosed every other day for maintenance.[8] Use lowest dosage that will control condition. Often used in conjunction with prednisolone

Inflammatory colorectal polyps (extra-label): Consider in dogs with inflammatory colorectal polyps that do not respond well to traditional therapies (based on a retrospective study of 6 dachshunds): average chlorambucil initial dose: 2 mg/m² (NOT mg/kg) PO once daily used in combination with ***EITHER*** prednisolone 0.47 mg/kg PO once daily ***OR*** firocoxib 6.2 mg/kg PO daily (average). A positive response was seen in 5 of 6 dogs.[22]

Antineoplastic agent (metronomic) (all are extra-label):

a) **Chronic lymphocytic leukemia:** 3 – 6 mg/m² (NOT mg/kg) PO every day for 1 to 2 weeks, then decrease to 3 – 6 mg/m² (NOT mg/kg) PO every other day as determined by routine hematologic screening and cancer response.[23] Concurrently with chlorambucil, prednis(ol)one can be used at a dosage of 1 mg/kg PO every day for 1 to 2 weeks, then 0.5 mg/kg PO every other day thereafter.
b) **Mast cell tumor**: 4 – 6 mg/m² (NOT mg/kg) PO every 48 hours for 8 weeks. Chlorambucil treatment followed 3 or 4 sessions of lomustine 60 – 90 mg/m² (NOT mg/kg) every 21 days.[5]
c) **Lymphoma and other lymphoreticular neoplasia OR as a substitute for cyclophosphamide in the COP or CHOP protocol if sterile hemorrhagic cystitis occurs**: 1.4 mg/kg PO once on the same schedule as cyclophosphamide, in substitute of cyclophosphamide[23]
d) **Metronomic chemotherapeutic agent (eg, hemangiosarcoma, transitional cell carcinoma)** (extra-label): 4 mg/m² (NOT mg/kg) PO once daily. For dogs weighing more than 8 kg (17.6 lb), the dose is rounded to the nearest 2 mg; for dogs weighing less than or equal to 8 kg (17.6 lb), the dose is compounded to 4 mg/m² (NOT mg/kg).[6,7]

CATS:

Immunosuppressive agent (extra-label): Chlorambucil is generally considered a second-line immunosuppressant (after glucocorticoids) in cats and often used in conjunction with prednisolone. Anecdotal chlorambucil dosing recommendations vary and the commercial tablet size (2 mg) may make precise dosing difficult without compounding. For immune-mediated conditions, chlorambucil is commonly dosed initially at 0.1 – 0.2 mg/kg (≈1.5 – 4 mg/m² PO once daily). If using the entire 2 mg tablet, chlorambucil is dosed in a practical manner every 48 hours for cats weighing more than 4 kg (8.8 lb) and every 72 hours for cats weighing less than 4 kg (8.8 lb). Once remission occurs, the dose is reduced or the dosing interval (often every 3 to 4 days) is extended to an interval that still controls the condition.

Low-grade GI lymphoma; chronic lymphocytic leukemia (extra-label): Several protocols using chlorambucil with prednisolone have had a relatively high degree of efficacy, including:

a) Chlorambucil 15 mg/m² (NOT mg/kg) PO once daily for 4 days repeated every 3 weeks, and prednisolone initially at 3 mg/kg PO once daily[24]
b) Chlorambucil 20 mg/m² (NOT mg/kg) (rounded to nearest 2 mg) PO once every 2 weeks and prednisolone 2 mg/kg PO once daily[25]
c) Chlorambucil 2 mg/cat (NOT mg/m² or mg/kg) PO every 2 to 3 days (48-72 hours) and prednisolone 5 – 10 mg PO every 12 to 24 hours[26]

HORSES:

Adjunctive therapy in treating lymphoma using the LAP protocol (extra-label): Cytarabine 200 – 300 mg/m² (NOT mg/kg) SC or IM once every 1 to 2 weeks; chlorambucil 20 mg/m² (NOT mg/kg) PO every 2 weeks (alternating with cytarabine) and prednisone 1.1 – 2.2 mg/kg PO every other day. If this protocol is ineffective (no response seen in 2-4 weeks), add vincristine at 0.5 mg/m² (NOT mg/kg) IV once weekly.[27]

FERRETS:

Adjunctive therapy in treating lymphoma (extra-label): As part of a multiagent protocol, 2 mg total dose (NOT mg/kg) PO in weeks 11 and 20 of a 20-week protocol

Monitoring

- Efficacy
- Baseline CBC, serum chemistry profile, urinalysis
- Frequency of hematologic monitoring depends on protocol employed. Consultation with a veterinary oncologist is recommended. Recommendation for patients receiving continuous dosing without breaks is CBC 1 month after starting treatment, then CBC/serum chemistry profile every 2 to 3 months thereafter or earlier if patient is presented for unexpected changes in behaviors (eg, weight loss, fever, reduced activity, and/or appetite). For patients receiving bolus dosing with hiatus between treatment, CBC is recommended 1 week after each treatment. If neutrophils are less than 2500/µL or platelets less than 75,000/µL, stop chlorambucil until patient has recovered, and reduce dose by 10% to 20% or increase dosing interval. Other references recommend CBCs at 0, 1, 2, 4, 8, and 12 weeks and then every 3 to 6 months[28] or, in cats, CBCs at 2 to 3 weeks after starting therapy and every 3 to 6 months thereafter.[29]
- For sexually intact patients, verify pregnancy status prior to administration.

Client Information

- Bone marrow depression can occur. The greatest effects on bone marrow usually occur within a few weeks after treatment. Your veterinarian will do blood tests to watch for bone marrow depression, but if you see bleeding, bruising, or fever (indicating an infection), or if your animal tires easily, contact your veterinarian right away.
- Chlorambucil may be toxic to the gastrointestinal tract and cause vomiting and gastrointestinal upset. Chlorambucil may cause changes in blood cell counts, which may cause increased risk for bleeding, bruising, infection, lethargy, bloody diarrhea, and shortness of breath. Contact your veterinarian immediately if you notice these or any other atypical signs. Contact your veterinarian immediately if you notice abnormal bleeding, bruising, depression, infection, shortness of breath, or bloody diarrhea.
- It is important to follow your veterinarian's orders in administering this medication as prescribed to help minimize the risk for side effects.
- Routine bloodwork is recommended to monitor for changes in blood cell counts and liver and kidney laboratory values while the animal is on this medication. Do not miss these important follow-up visits.
- Handle this drug with caution. Wear gloves when administering medication or cleaning up your animal's waste. Those who are pregnant, attempting to conceive, or nursing should not administer the drug or clean up the animal's waste.
- Hair loss and delayed regrowth of shaven hair have been reported in dogs; breeds with a continuously growing hair coat (eg, poodles, terriers, Afghan hounds, old English sheepdogs) are more likely to experience significant hair loss.
- This medication is considered to be a hazardous drug as defined by the National Institute for Occupational Safety and Health (NIOSH). Talk with your veterinarian or pharmacist about the use of personal protective equipment when handling this medicine.

Chemistry/Synonyms

Chlorambucil is a nitrogen mustard derivative antineoplastic agent. It occurs as an off-white, slightly granular powder. It is soluble in diethyl ether or acetone but is considered insoluble in water with a pK_a of 5.75.

Chlorambucil may also be known as CB-1348, NSC-3088, WR-139013, chlorambucilum, chloraminophene, chlorbutinum, *Chloraminophene*®, *Leukeran*®, or *Linfolysin*®.

Storage/Stability

Chlorambucil tablets should be stored in light-resistant, well-closed containers under refrigeration (2°C -8°C [36°F-46°F]). Tablets can be stored at a maximum of 30°C (86°F) for up to 1 week.

Compatibility/Compounding Considerations

Compounding chlorambucil should only be undertaken in facilities where adequate environmental and personnel exposure can be safeguarded.

Compounded preparation stability: For chlorambucil 2 mg/mL oral suspension, crush 60 2 mg oral tablets completely and suspend in 30 mL of methylcellulose 1%. Dilute with a sufficient amount of syrup for a final total volume of 60 mL. A 2 mg/mL oral suspension retains 90% potency for 7 days at 5°C (41°F).

Suspensions of chlorambucil stored at room temperature rapidly decompose with losses greater than 15% in 1 day. Chlorambucil is rapidly hydrolyzed independently of pH, but minimal hydrolysis occurs at pH 2. Refrigeration slows hydrolysis.

Compounded chlorambucil capsules demonstrated variable potency (71% to 104% of labeled strength), and stability and potency should be considered when prescribing compounded oral chemotherapy.[30]

Dosage Forms/Regulatory Status

VETERINARY-LABELED PRODUCTS: NONE

HUMAN-LABELED PRODUCTS:

Chlorambucil Oral Tablets (film-coated): 2 mg; *Leukeran*®; (Rx)

References

For the complete list of references, see **wiley.com/go/budde/plumb**

Chloramphenicol

(klor-am-***fen***-i-kole) *Chloromycetin*®, *Victeon*®

Antibacterial

Prescriber Highlights

- ► Broad-spectrum antibiotic with good tissue penetration, including in the eye, CNS, and prostate
- ► Use in food animals is prohibited by the FDA.
- ► Use should be avoided or pursued with extreme caution in animals with preexisting hematologic disorders or hepatic failure as well as in animals that are pregnant, or that are neonates. Doses may need to be reduced in animals with hepatic or renal insufficiency.
- ► Lower dosages are used in cats, for which there is a greater risk for complications, particularly with long-term use (ie, longer than 14 days).
- ► GI adverse effects are possible; there is also the potential for myelosuppression, especially with high-dose, long-term treatment.
- ► National Institute for Occupational Safety and Health (NIOSH) Hazardous Drug; use appropriate precautions when handling

Uses/Indications

Because of potential adverse effects in animals and human exposure concerns, chloramphenicol should only be used when other antimicrobial agents are not viable options. Chloramphenicol is used in small animal species and horses for the treatment of a variety of bacterial infections, particularly those caused by streptococci, staphylococci, and anaerobes. In dogs, chloramphenicol is indicated for the treatment of bacterial pneumonia, canine respiratory disease complex, as well as ocular infections, otitis media, and UTIs caused by susceptible bacteria. This antibiotic is also potentially useful for the treatment of methicillin-resistant staphylococcal infections and bacterial prostatitis caused by susceptible bacteria. In cats, it is used for the treatment of haemobartonellosis, chlamydiosis, ocular infections, and UTIs. Chloramphenicol appears relatively safe to use in hindgut-fermenting species (eg, rabbits, guinea pigs, horses).

The World Health Organization (WHO) has designated chloramphenicol as a Highly Important antimicrobial for human medicine.[1]

Pharmacology/Actions

Chloramphenicol usually acts as a time-dependent, bacteriostatic antibiotic, but it can be bactericidal at higher concentrations or against some susceptible organisms. Chloramphenicol acts by binding to the 50S ribosomal subunit of susceptible bacteria, thereby preventing bacterial protein synthesis. Erythromycin, clindamycin, lincomycin, and tylosin also bind to the same bacterial ribosomal subunit, but unlike these other antibiotics, chloramphenicol appears to also have an affinity for mitochondrial ribosomes of rapidly proliferating mammalian cells (eg, bone marrow) that may result in reversible bone marrow suppression.

Chloramphenicol has a wide spectrum of activity against many aerobic and anaerobic gram-positive and gram-negative organisms. Gram-positive aerobic organisms that are generally susceptible to chloramphenicol include many streptococci and staphylococci. Some strains of methicillin-resistant staphylococci are susceptible. Chloramphenicol is also effective against some gram-negative aerobes, including *Neisseria* spp, *Brucella* spp, *Salmonella* spp, *Proteus* spp, *Shigella* spp, and *Haemophilus* spp. Many anaerobic bacteria (eg, *Clostridium* spp, *Bacteroides* spp [including *B fragilis*], *Fusobacterium* spp, *Veillonella* spp) are susceptible to chloramphenicol. Chloramphenicol also has activity against *Nocardia* spp, *Chlamydia* spp, *Mycoplasma* spp, and *Rickettsia* spp. This antibiotic is ineffective for the treatment of viral, fungal, or parasitic infections

Antimicrobial resistance appears to be mediated by enzymatic acetylation and inactivation by chloramphenicol acetyltransferases, efflux pumps, or altered ribosomal binding sites.[2-4]

At present, the Clinical and Laboratory Standards Institute (CLSI) has established a susceptibility breakpoint for most human bacterial pathogens at an MIC target of 8 µg/mL. Some studies show that equine plasma concentrations did not reach the recommended MIC target.[5-7]

Pharmacokinetics

Chloramphenicol is rapidly absorbed after oral administration; peak serum concentrations occur ≈30 minutes after administration. The compounded oral suspension produces significantly lower peak serum concentrations when administered to horses[5] and fasted cats. The palmitate and sodium succinate salts are hydrolyzed to the base in the GI tract and liver.

Chloramphenicol is widely distributed throughout the body, and although the highest concentrations are found in the liver and kidney, the drug attains therapeutic concentrations for some pathogens in most tissues and fluids, including the aqueous and vitreous humor and synovial fluid. CSF concentrations may be up to 50% of those in the serum when meninges are uninflamed and higher when meninges are inflamed. There may be a 4- to 6-hour lag time before CSF peak concentrations occur. Chloramphenicol concentrations in the prostate are ≈50% of those in the serum. Because only a small amount of the drug is excreted unchanged in the urine in dogs, chloramphenicol is not a good option for treatment of lower UTIs. The volume of distribution of chloramphenicol has been reported as 1.6 – 1.8 L/kg in dogs, 2.4 L/kg in cats, and 1.41 L/kg in horses. Chloramphenicol is ≈30% to 60% bound to plasma proteins. A recent study in horses indicated that plasma chloramphenicol concentrations after oral administration of chloramphenicol base (50 mg/kg) were lower than previously reported, resulting in a recommendation to evaluate the MIC of the causative bacterium before using this drug.[7]

The elimination half-life has been reported as 1.1 to 5 hours (average, ≈2.4 hours) in dogs, less than 1 hour in foals and ponies, and 4 to 8 hours in cats. The elimination half-life in birds is highly variable across species, ranging from 26 minutes in pigeons to nearly 5 hours in bald eagles and peafowl.[8]

In most species, chloramphenicol undergoes hepatic metabolism primarily via glucuronidative mechanisms. Parent drug (≈10%) and metabolites (≈90%) are predominantly renally eliminated (ie, only ≈5% to 15% of the drug is excreted unchanged in the urine). Cats have less ability to glucuronidate drugs, so ≈25% of a dose is excreted unchanged in the urine.

Contraindications/Precautions/Warnings

The FDA prohibits use of chloramphenicol in food animals.

Chloramphenicol is contraindicated in those hypersensitive to it. Because of the potential for hematopoietic toxicity, chloramphenicol should be used with extreme caution, if at all, in animals with preexisting hematologic abnormalities, especially preexisting anemia. Chloramphenicol should be used with caution in animals with impaired hepatic or renal function, as drug accumulation can occur; dosage adjustments may be needed in these patients. Chloramphenicol should only be used in animals in hepatic failure when no other effective antibiotics are available and then only with prolonged treatment intervals. Consideration should be given to monitoring WBC and RBC counts in animals in which long-term use (greater than 14 days) is anticipated. See also ***Reproductive/Nursing Safety***.

Use with caution in cats. Dosages for dogs and cats are significantly different.

Chloramphenicol should be used with caution in neonatal animals, particularly in young kittens. In human neonates, circulatory collapse (ie, Gray syndrome) has occurred with chloramphenicol use.[9] This syndrome is probably caused by toxic drug accumulation secondary to an inability to conjugate the drug or excrete the conjugate effectively.

The National Institute for Occupational Safety and Health (NIOSH) classifies chloramphenicol as a hazardous drug; personal protective equipment (PPE) should be used accordingly to minimize the risk for exposure.[10]

Do not confuse chloramphenicol with chlorambucil, chlorpheniramine, or chlorpromazine.

Adverse Effects

Although chloramphenicol toxicity in humans has been greatly discussed in the literature, it is generally considered to have a low order of toxicity in adult companion animals when administered appropriately. A retrospective review found that in 51 dogs treated with chloramphenicol at recommended doses (≈50 mg/kg) for methicillin-resistant *Staphylococcus pseudintermedius* (MRSP) pyoderma, 53% developed adverse effects that included GI signs (47%), lethargy (14%), shaking (8%), and increased liver enzymes (6%).[11] Anemia, panting, and aggression were reported in individual dogs. GI signs and rear limb weakness were noted in another retrospective review.[12] Peripheral neuropathy (ie, rear limb weakness) anecdotally appears to be more common in large-breed dogs, which may be more likely due to ease of recognition of this clinical sign versus a truly increased incidence. As there is no evidence that peripheral neuropathy is dose-related, treatment of large-breed dogs at the lower end of the dose range should be weighed against consequences of treatment failure.

Development of aplastic anemia (reported in humans) does not appear to be a significant problem for veterinary patients[9]; however, a dose-related bone marrow suppression (reversible) has been seen in all species, primarily with long-term therapy. Early signs of bone marrow toxicity can include vacuolation of many of the early cells of the myeloid and erythroid series, as well as lymphocytopenia and neutropenia. Thrombocytopenia associated with chloramphenicol use in cats has been reported.

Other possible adverse effects include anorexia, vomiting, diarrhea, and depression. Chloramphenicol in guinea pigs can have a negative effect on the cardiovascular system, as seen by ECG changes (eg, shortened P waves, P-R interval, QRS complex).[13]

Cats tend to be more sensitive to developing adverse effects to chloramphenicol than dogs, but this is likely because the drug's half-life is longer in cats due to poor glucuronidation capacity. Cats given higher-than-label feline dosages for prolonged periods (eg, 50 mg/kg every 12 hours for 2 to 3 weeks) may experience a high incidence of adverse effects, including bone marrow hypoplasia, and should be closely monitored.

Reproductive/Nursing Safety

Chloramphenicol should not be administered to dogs maintained for breeding purposes, as significant disorders in gonad morphology and function have been noted under experimental conditions.[14] Chloramphenicol readily crosses the placenta to achieve concentrations at 75% of maternal blood. The drug may decrease protein synthesis in the fetus, particularly in the bone marrow. It should be given with extreme caution during pregnancy and only when the maternal benefits of therapy clearly outweigh the risks to the fetus.

Because chloramphenicol is found in milk in humans at 50% of serum concentrations, the drug should be given with extreme caution to nursing animals, particularly within the first week of giving birth. Use of an alternative antimicrobial is recommended during nursing.[15]

Overdose/Acute Toxicity

Dosages of 200 mg/kg/day for up to 4 months were tolerated by dogs,[14] but cats show toxicity at 60 mg/kg daily within 14 days.[16]

Because of the potential for serious bone marrow toxicity, large overdoses of oral chloramphenicol should be handled by GI decontamination using standard protocols followed by supportive care based on clinical presentation. For more information on chloramphenicol toxicity, see ***Adverse Effects***.

For patients that have experienced or are suspected to have experienced an overdose, consultation with a 24-hour poison consultation center specializing in providing veterinary-specific information is recommended. For general information related to overdose and toxin exposures, as well as contact information for poison control centers, refer to ***Appendix***.

Drug Interactions

Chloramphenicol is a cytochrome P450 CYP2B11 inhibitor in dogs and may possibly inhibit other CYP isoenzymes in dogs and other species. The following drug interactions have either been reported or are theoretical in humans or animals receiving chloramphenicol and may be of significance in veterinary patients. (**NOTE**: Cats may be particularly susceptible to chloramphenicol's effects on the hepatic metabolism of other drugs.)

- **ACETAMINOPHEN:** Concurrent use of chloramphenicol and acetaminophen resulted in increased serum concentrations of chloramphenicol in one human study, but subsequent studies have contradicted that result. There are no veterinary data for this interaction.
- **AMINOGLYCOSIDES** (eg, **amikacin, gentamicin, streptomycin**): May cause antibacterial antagonism; clinical significance, if any, is not clear
- **ANTI-ANEMIA DRUGS** (eg, **epoetin, folic acid, iron, vitamin B_{12}**): Chloramphenicol may delay hematopoietic response.
- **ASPIRIN AND OTHER SALICYLATES** (eg, **bismuth subsalicylate**): Chloramphenicol may delay hepatic metabolism of the salicylate and therefore potentiate toxicity.
- **BETA-LACTAM ANTIBIOTICS** (eg, **cephalosporins, penicillins**): May cause antibacterial antagonism; clinical significance, if any, is not clear
- **CIMETIDINE:** May reduce the metabolism of chloramphenicol, increasing the risk for toxicity
- **CYCLOPHOSPHAMIDE:** Chloramphenicol may reduce formation of the active cyclophosphamide metabolite and reduce cyclophosphamide efficacy. Additive myelosuppression may occur.
- **CYCLOSPORINE:** May increase the risk for cyclosporine toxicity
- **DIPYRONE:** May increase the risk for myelosuppression
- **GLIPIZIDE:** Chloramphenicol may decrease sulfonylurea metabolism and increase the risk for hypoglycemia.
- **KETAMINE:** Chloramphenicol may prolong effects. Chloramphenicol did not prolong anesthesia in dogs receiving xylazine/ketamine in a study.[17]
- **LEVAMISOLE:** Fatalities have been reported after concomitant levamisole and chloramphenicol administration; avoid using these agents together.
- **LIDOCAINE**: Chloramphenicol may delay hepatic metabolism.
- **METHADONE**: Chloramphenicol inhibits hepatic metabolism and increases methadone effects.[18]
- **MIDAZOLAM**: Chloramphenicol may prolong effects.
- **MYELOSUPPRESSIVE DRUGS** (eg, **azathioprine, interferons, methimazole, toceranib**): May cause additive bone marrow depression
- **OPIOIDS:** Chloramphenicol can significantly inhibit metabolism and prolong opioid effects.
- **PENTOBARBITAL**: Chloramphenicol has been demonstrated to prolong the duration of pentobarbital anesthesia by 120% in dogs and 260% in cats,[19,20] but there was no prolonged duration in guinea pigs.[21]
- **PHENOBARBITAL/PRIMIDONE**: Chloramphenicol may inhibit phenobarbital metabolism, and phenobarbital may decrease chloramphenicol concentrations. Interaction does not apply to chloramphenicol ophthalmic ointment.[22,23]
- **PROPOFOL**: Chloramphenicol may prolong anesthesia.
- **RIFAMPIN**: May decrease serum chloramphenicol concentrations
- **VORICONAZOLE**: Chloramphenicol may increase voriconazole concentration.

Laboratory Considerations

- False positive **glucosuria** (glycosuria) has been reported, but the incidence is unknown.

Dosages

NOTE: Because of potential adverse effects in animals and human exposure concerns, chloramphenicol should only be used when other antimicrobial agents are not viable options.

DOGS:

Susceptible GI, pulmonary, and urinary bacterial infections (label dosage; FDA-approved): 55 mg/kg PO every 6 hours[14]

Susceptible infections (extra-label):

a) 25 – 50 mg/kg PO every 6 to 8 hours, continuing for 3 to 5 days after the animal has become free of clinical signs or afebrile[24]
b) 40 – 50 mg/kg PO, IV, SC, IM every 8 hours.[25,26] Dosages up to 60 mg/kg PO every 8 hours may be necessary for some infections. IV doses should be administered over at least 1 minute.

CATS:

Susceptible infections (extra-label): 12.5 – 20 mg/kg every 12 hours PO, IV, IM, or SC.[25] Practically, it is often administered at

50 mg/cat (NOT mg/kg) PO every 12 hours.

HORSES:

NOTE: All are extra-label.

Susceptible infections:

a) **Adult horses**:45 – 60 mg/kg PO every 8 hours; 45 – 60 mg/kg IM, SC, or IV every 6 to 8 hours[27]
b) **Foals**: 20 mg/kg PO or IV every 4 hours[28]
c) **Foals**: Chloramphenicol sodium succinate: 25 – 50 mg/kg IV every 4 to 8 hours; chloramphenicol base or palmitate: 40 – 50 mg/kg PO every 6 to 8 hours[29]
d) **Regional limb perfusion**: 2000 mg diluted to 100 mL perfusion volume with sterile saline.[30]

BIRDS:

Susceptible infections (extra-label):

a) Chloramphenicol sodium succinate: 80 mg/kg IM 2 to 3 times daily, 50 mg/kg IV 3 to 4 times daily
b) Chloramphenicol sodium succinate: 50 mg/kg IM or IV every 8 hours[31]

FERRETS:

Susceptible infections (extra-label): 50 mg/kg PO, SC, IV every 12 hours

RABBITS/RODENTS/SMALL MAMMALS:

a) **Rabbits** (extra-label): 30 – 50 mg/kg PO, SC, IM, IV every 8 to 24 hours[32]
b) **Hedgehogs** (extra-label): 50 mg/kg PO every 12 hours; 30 – 50 mg/kg SC, IM, IV, or intraosseous (IO) every 12 hours[33]
c) **Chinchillas** (extra-label): 30 – 50 mg/kg PO, SC, IM every 12 hours
d) **Gerbils, guinea pigs, hamsters, mice, rats** (extra-label): 20 – 50 mg/kg (succinate salt) SC every 6 to 12 hours[34]
e) **Pneumonia in guinea pigs** (extra-label): 30 – 50 mg/kg PO every 12 hours[35]

REPTILES:

Susceptible infections (extra-label):

a) For most species using the sodium succinate salt: 20 – 50 mg/kg IM or SC for up to 3 weeks. Chloramphenicol is often a good initial choice until susceptibility results are available.[36]
b) 30 – 50 mg/kg/day IV or IM for 7 to 14 days[37]

Monitoring

- Baseline and periodic (eg, every 1 to 2 weeks) CBC during treatment
- Clinical efficacy
- Culture and susceptibility testing is recommended prior to treatment, as this drug should typically be reserved for treatment of infections in which more commonly used drugs are not appropriate.
- Adverse effects (eg, GI adverse effects, hindlimb weakness)

Client Information

- Wear gloves when handling this medicine and avoid contact with the drug, especially around your mouth, nose, or eyes. Avoid crushing pills.
- For this medication to work, give it exactly as your veterinarian has prescribed. Missing a dose can cause the medicine to not work properly for your animal.
- This medicine is best given with food as it has an extremely bitter taste that can make administration of the tablets difficult.
- The most common side effects are stomach upset, vomiting, and diarrhea. Cats may be more likely to experience serious side effects.
- This medicine is banned for use in animals to be used for food, including egg-laying chickens and dairy animals.
- This medication is considered to be a hazardous drug as defined by the National Institute for Occupational Safety and Health (NIOSH). Talk with your veterinarian or pharmacist about the use of personal protective equipment when handling this medicine.

Chemistry/Synonyms

Chloramphenicol, originally isolated from *Streptomyces venezuelae*, is now produced synthetically. It occurs as fine, white to grayish, yellow-white, elongated plates or needle-like crystals with a pK_a of 5.5. It is soluble in alcohol and propylene glycol, and ≈2.5 mg are soluble in 1 mL of water at 25°C (77°F).

Chloramphenicol sodium succinate occurs as a white to light yellow powder. It is freely soluble in both water and alcohol.

Chloramphenicol may also be known as chloramphenicolum, chloranfenicol, cloranfenicol, kloramfenikol, or laevomycetinum; *Chloromycetin®* and *Viceton®* are common trade names.

Storage/Stability

Chloramphenicol tablets should be stored in tight containers at or below 25°C (77°F) and in a dry place. The sodium succinate powder for injection should be stored between 20°C and 25°C (68°F-77°F). After reconstituting the sodium succinate injection with sterile water, the solution is stable for 30 days at room temperature or 6 months if frozen. The solution should be discarded if it becomes cloudy.

Compatibility/Compounding Considerations

Compatibility is dependent on factors such as pH, concentration, temperature, and diluent used; consult specialized references or a hospital pharmacist for more specific information.

Reconstitute each chloramphenicol sodium succinate 1g vial with 10 mL sterile water for injection or 5% dextrose solution.

The following drugs and solutions are reportedly **compatible** with chloramphenicol sodium succinate injection: all commonly used IV fluids, amikacin sulfate, aminophylline, amphotericin B lipid complex, ampicillin sodium (in syringe for 1 hour), atropine, buprenorphine, calcium chloride/gluconate, cefazolin, cyclosporine, dexamethasone sodium phosphate, ephedrine, fentanyl, furosemide, heparin, hydrocortisone sodium succinate, hydromorphone, lidocaine, magnesium sulfate, mannitol, methylprednisolone sodium succinate, metoclopramide, metronidazole, morphine, naloxone, norepinephrine, oxytocin, penicillin G potassium/sodium, pentobarbital, phenobarbital, phenylephrine, piperacillin/tazobactam, plasma protein fraction, potassium chloride, ranitidine, sodium bicarbonate, tobramycin, vasopressin, verapamil, and vitamin B-complex with vitamin C.

The following drugs and solutions are reportedly **incompatible** (or compatibility data conflicts) with chloramphenicol sodium succinate injection: amiodarone, ascorbic acid, ceftazidime, chlorpromazine, diazepam, diltiazem, diphenhydramine, dobutamine, dopamine, famotidine, fluconazole, gentamicin, glycopyrrolate, hydroxyzine, midazolam, ondansetron, oxytetracycline, pantoprazole, sulfa-/trimethoprim, and vancomycin.

FDA-approved chloramphenicol tablets dissolved in water with *Karo®* syrup added just prior to administration to horses demonstrated greater bioavailability, higher peak concentration, and area under the curve (AUC) as compared with compounded chloramphenicol paste and suspension.[5] The study also noted that tablets required ≈5.5 hours to dissolve.

Dosage Forms/Regulatory Status

VETERINARY-LABELED PRODUCTS:

Chloramphenicol Oral Tablets: 250 mg, 500 mg, and 1 g; *Viceton®*; (Rx). FDA-approved for use in dogs. NADA #055-059

Chloramphenicol is prohibited by the FDA for use in food animals.

HUMAN-LABELED PRODUCTS:

Chloramphenicol Powder for Injection: 1 gram vials (100 mg/mL as sodium succinate when reconstituted); generic; (Rx). **NOTE**: this product is no longer commercially available.

References

For the complete list of references, see **wiley.com/go/budde/plumb**

Chlorothiazide

(klor-oh-***thye***-a-zide) *Diuril®*

Thiazide Diuretic

Prescriber Highlights

- Thiazide diuretic used for nephrogenic diabetes insipidus
- Contraindications include hypersensitivity to the drug; pregnancy is a relative contraindication.
- Use with extreme caution or avoid in cases of severe renal disease, pre-existing electrolyte and/or water balance abnormalities, impaired hepatic function, hyperuricemia, calcium oxalate urolithiasis, systemic lupus erythematosus (SLE), or diabetes mellitus.
- Adverse effects include hypokalemia, hypochloremic alkalosis, other electrolyte imbalances, hyperuricemia, and GI effects.
- Many drug–drug and laboratory test interactions

Uses/Indications

Thiazides are used for the treatment of systemic hypertension, ascites, hypermagnesemia, and nephrogenic diabetes insipidus (DI); they are also used as adjunctive therapy in patients with central DI.[1-3]

In veterinary medicine, furosemide has largely supplanted the use of thiazides as a general diuretic. If a thiazide diuretic is necessary, hydrochlorothiazide is preferred for use in dogs and cats. Chlorothiazide is also FDA-approved for use in dairy cattle for the treatment of postparturient udder edema,[4] but the veterinary-labeled product is no longer marketed in the United States.

Pharmacology/Actions

Thiazide diuretics act by interfering with the transport of sodium ions across the renal tubular epithelium, possibly by altering the metabolism of tubular cells. The principal site of action is at the cortical diluting segment of the nephron (between the proximal and distal convoluted tubules), which results in enhanced excretion of sodium, chloride, and water. Thiazides also increase the excretion of potassium, magnesium, phosphate, iodide, and bromide and decrease the glomerular filtration rate (GFR). Plasma renin and resulting aldosterone levels are increased, which contributes to the hypokalemic effects of the thiazides. Bicarbonate excretion is increased, but effects on urine pH are usually minimal. Thiazides usually initially have a hypercalciuric effect, but with continued therapy, calcium excretion is significantly decreased. Thiazides can cause or exacerbate hyperglycemia in diabetic patients or induce diabetes mellitus in prediabetic patients.

In nephrogenic diabetes insipidus, the administration of a thiazide diuretic can result in a paradoxical decrease in urine output. The proposed mechanism for this effect is related to sodium reduction. Thiazide diuretics reduce the reabsorption of sodium and chloride in the distal tubule of the nephron. This initially results in sodium loss and extracellular volume contraction, which results in increased reabsorption of sodium and water in the proximal tubule. Less filtrate is presented to the distal nephron and collecting duct and is subsequently excreted as urine.

The antihypertensive effects of thiazides are well-known, and these agents are used extensively in human medicine for treating essential hypertension. The exact mechanism of this effect has not been established.

Pharmacokinetics

The pharmacokinetics of thiazides have not been studied in domestic animals. In humans, chlorothiazide is only 10% to 21% absorbed after oral administration. The onset of diuretic activity occurs in 1 to 2 hours and peaks at about 4 hours. The serum half-life is ≈1 to 2 hours, and the duration of activity is 6 to 12 hours. Chlorothiazide is not metabolized and is eliminated almost entirely as unchanged drug via the urine. Like all thiazides, the antihypertensive effects of chlorothiazide can be delayed by several days.

Contraindications/Precautions/Warnings

Thiazides are contraindicated in patients that are anuric or hypersensitive to any one of these agents. Although many sources state that thiazides are contraindicated in patients that are hypersensitive to sulfonamides, clear evidence for cross-reactivity has not been established in humans or animals.

Thiazides should be used with extreme caution, if at all, in patients with severe renal disease or with preexisting electrolyte or water balance abnormalities, impaired hepatic function (may precipitate hepatic coma), hyperuricemia, systemic lupus erythematosus (SLE), or diabetes mellitus. Patients with conditions that may lead to electrolyte or water balance abnormalities (eg, vomiting, diarrhea) should be monitored carefully. The use of chlorothiazide is not recommended in patients with calcium oxalate urolithiasis, as it has been demonstrated to increase renal calcium excretion, particularly at higher doses[5]; if a thiazide diuretic is required in these patients, hydrochlorothiazide should be used instead.

Adverse Effects

Hypokalemia is one of the most common adverse effects associated with thiazides but rarely causes clinical signs or progresses further; however, monitoring of serum potassium is recommended with chronic therapy.

Hypochloremic metabolic alkalosis (with hypokalemia) may develop, especially if there are other causes of potassium and chloride loss (eg, vomiting, diarrhea, potassium-losing nephropathies) or if the patient has cirrhotic liver disease. Dilutional hyponatremia and hypomagnesemia may also occur. Hyperparathyroid-like effects of hypercalcemia and hypophosphatemia have been reported in humans but have not led to effects, such as nephrolithiasis, bone resorption, or peptic ulceration.

Hyperuricemia can occur but it is usually subclinical.

Other possible adverse effects include vomiting, diarrhea, pancreatitis, hypersensitivity, dermatologic reactions, polyuria, hematologic toxicity, hyperglycemia, hyperlipidemias, and orthostatic hypotension.

Reproductive/Nursing Safety

Thiazides cross the placenta and are contraindicated in pregnant patients that are otherwise healthy and have only mild edema, as newborn human infants have developed thrombocytopenia when their mother received thiazides. Chlorothiazide did not impair fertility in rats that were given doses up to 60 mg/kg/day.

Chlorothiazide enters maternal milk and can reduce milk volume and suppress lactation. Because of the risk for idiosyncratic or hypersensitivity reactions, it is recommended that these drugs not be used in lactating female patients or nursing mothers. In general, either discontinuation of the drug or nursing is recommended in humans.

Overdose/Toxicity

Acute overdose may cause dehydration and electrolyte problems (eg, hyponatremia, hypokalemia), CNS effects (lethargy, coma, seizures), and GI effects (eg, hypermotility, GI distress). Transient increases in BUN have also been reported.

Treatment consists of GI decontamination after recent oral ingestion using standard protocols. Avoid giving concomitant cathartics, as they may exacerbate the fluid and electrolyte imbalances that may ensue. Monitor and treat electrolyte and water balance abnormalities supportively. Monitor respiratory, CNS, and cardiovascular status; treat clinical signs supportively.

For patients that have experienced or are suspected to have experienced an overdose, consultation with a 24-hour poison consultation center specializing in providing veterinary-specific information is recommended. For general information related to overdose and toxin exposures, as well as contact information for poison control centers, refer to ***Appendix.***

Drug Interactions

The following drug interactions have either been reported or are theoretical in humans or animals receiving chlorothiazide and may be of significance in veterinary patients. Unless otherwise noted, use together is not necessarily contraindicated, but weigh the potential risks and perform additional monitoring when appropriate.

- **Amphotericin B**: Use with thiazides can lead to increased risk for severe hypokalemia.
- **Bromides:** May enhance bromide excretion and reduce seizure control
- **Calcium Salts** (eg, **calcium carbonate, calcium acetate**): Hypercalcemia may be exacerbated if thiazides are concurrently administered with vitamin D or calcium salts.
- **Corticosteroids** (eg, **dexamethasone, prednis(ol)one corticotropin**):Use with thiazides can lead to increased risk for severe hypokalemia.
- **Diazoxide**: Increased risk for hyperglycemia, hyperuricemia, and hypotension may occur.
- **Digoxin**: Thiazide-induced hypokalemia, hypomagnesemia, and/or hypercalcemia may increase the likelihood of digitalis toxicity.
- **Furosemide**: May have additive diuretic and hypokalemic effect
- **Hypoglycemic Agents** (eg, **acarbose, glipizide, insulin, metformin**): Thiazides may cause or exacerbate hyperglycemia in diabetic patients; increase in doses of hypoglycemic agents may be required.
- **Hypotensive Agents** (eg, **amlodipine, enalapril, telmisartan**): May have additive hypotensive effect
- **Lithium**: Thiazides can increase serum lithium concentrations.
- **Methenamine**: Thiazides can alkalinize urine and reduce methenamine effectiveness.
- **Nonsteroidal Anti-inflammatory Drugs** (**NSAIDs**; eg, **carprofen, meloxicam, robenacoxib**): Thiazides may increase risk for renal toxicity, and NSAIDs may reduce diuretic actions of thiazides.
- **Nondepolarizing Neuromuscular Blocking Agents** (eg, **atracurium, rocuronium, vecuronium**: Nondepolarizing neuromuscular-blocking agents' response or duration may be increased in patients receiving thiazide diuretics.
- **Probenecid**: Blocks thiazide-induced uric acid retention (used to therapeutic advantage)
- **Quinidine**: Half-life may be prolonged by thiazides (thiazides can alkalinize the urine).
- **Vitamin D** (eg, **cholecalciferol, ergocalciferol**): Hypercalcemia may be exacerbated if thiazides are concurrently administered with vitamin D or its analogues.

Laboratory Considerations

- **Amylase**: Thiazides can increase serum amylase values in subclinical patients and those in the developmental stages of acute pancreatitis (humans).
- **Cortisol**: Thiazides can decrease the renal excretion of cortisol.
- **Estrogen, Urinary**: Thiazides may falsely decrease total urinary estrogen when a spectrophotometric assay is used.
- **Hydroxycorticosteroids:** Thiazides may decrease urinary corticosteroid values by interfering in vitro with the absorbance in the modified Glenn-Nelson technique for urinary 17-hydroxycorticosteroids.
- **Parathyroid-Function Tests**: Thiazides may elevate serum calcium; discontinuing thiazides prior to testing is recommended.
- **Phenolsulfonphthalein (PSP)**: Thiazides can compete for secretion at proximal renal tubules.
- **Pheochromocytoma:** Thiazides may cause false-negative results with **histamine, phentolamine,** or **tyramine** tests.
- **Protein-Bound Iodine**: Thiazides may decrease values.
- **Triiodothyronine Resin Uptake Test**: Thiazides may slightly reduce uptake.

Dosages

DOGS/CATS:

Congestive heart failure (CHF) (label dosage; FDA-approved): 11 – 22 mg/kg PO 2 or 3 times daily. Severe conditions may require higher doses.[4]

Some dogs may have an adequate response to intermittent doses (eg, administered for 3 to 5 days per week).[4] **NOTE:** Most clinicians recommend furosemide as a general diuretic for CHF.

Diuresis or treatment for nephrogenic diabetes insipidus (extra-label): 20 – 40 mg/kg PO every 12 hours[6]

Monitoring

- Baseline and periodic serum electrolytes, BUN, creatinine, glucose
- Hydration status
- Blood pressure, if indicated
- CBC, if indicated

Client Information

- When beginning this medicine, your animal may urinate more frequently than normal.
- This medicine may be given with or without food. Provide your animal with access to fresh water at all times and encourage normal food intake.
- Because this drug can change electrolytes (salts) in the blood, your veterinarian will want to do more frequent testing.
- Contact your veterinarian immediately if you notice weakness, collapse, head tilt, lack of urination, or a racing heartbeat.

Chemistry/Synonyms

Chlorothiazide is a thiazide diuretic and occurs as a white to practically white odorless crystalline powder that has a slightly bitter taste. It is very slightly soluble in water and slightly soluble in alcohol.

Chlorothiazide may also be known as chlorothiazidum, clorotiazida, *Azide*®, *Diuril*®, or *Saluric*®.

Storage/Stability

Store the oral suspension at room temperature (15°C to 30°C [59° to 86°F]) and protected from freezing.[7]

Compatibility/Compounding Considerations

None

Dosage Forms/Regulatory Status

VETERINARY-LABELED PRODUCTS: NONE

The Association of Racing Commissioners International (ARCI) has designated this drug as a class 4 substance. See the ***Appendix*** for more information.

HUMAN-LABELED PRODUCTS:

Chlorothiazide Oral Suspension: 50 mg/mL in 237 mL; *Diuril*®; (Rx)

Chlorothiazide Sodium Powder for Injection (lyophilized): 500 mg (0.25 g mannitol) in 20 mL vials; *Diuril*®; (Rx)

References

For the complete list of references, see **wiley.com/go/budde/plumb**

Chlorpheniramine

(klor-fen-***ir***-a-meen) *Chlor-Trimeton*®

Antihistamine, First Generation

Prescriber Highlights

- Used principally for antihistaminic and antipruritic properties; used as adjunctive agent for atopic dermatitis
- Contraindications include known hypersensitivity to the drug.
- Use with caution in patients with narrow-angle glaucoma, hypertension, GI or urinary obstruction, hyperthyroidism, and cardiovascular disease.
- Adverse effects include sedation, anticholinergic effects, and GI effects.
- Chlorpheniramine may be found OTC in combination with other drugs that may be toxic to animals (eg, acetaminophen, pseudoephedrine).

Uses/Indications

Chlorpheniramine is a first-generation antihistamine that may be useful in dogs and cats for the adjunctive treatment of histamine-mediated pruritic and allergic conditions (eg, urticaria, insect-bite hypersensitivity). Guidelines for atopic dermatitis treatment in dogs state there is no conclusive evidence regarding the efficacy of oral first-generation antihistamines in the treatment of chronic and acute flares of canine atopic dermatitis, with only highly variable therapeutic efficacy reported anecdotally; chlorpheniramine should be given continuously (ie, daily) as preventive therapy before an acute flare.[1,2]

The response to chlorpheniramine, as with other antihistamines in dogs and cats, is individualized and not predictable. One patient may respond to one formulation but not another. Chlorpheniramine, when combined with hydroxyzine, has potentially shown better results in reducing clinical signs of canine atopic dermatitis in ≈1 of 3 treated dogs,[3] and pruritus improved by more than 25% in 10 of 17 dogs.[4] In pruritic cats, chlorpheniramine has been shown to have an antipruritic effect when combined with oral omega-3 and -6 fatty acid supplements.[5]

First-generation antihistamines may also be used as adjunctive therapy for mast cell tumors and to prevent local histamine release during surgical excision of mast cell tumors.

Pharmacology/Actions

H_1-receptor antagonist antihistamines competitively inhibit histamine H_1 receptors; they do not inactivate or prevent the release of histamine but can prevent histamine's action on the cell. In addition to its antihistaminic effects, chlorpheniramine also has varying degrees of anticholinergic, sedative, tranquilizing, antispasmodic, local anesthetic, mild bronchodilator, and antiemetic activities.

Pharmacokinetics

Pharmacokinetic information for chlorpheniramine in small animals is limited. In dogs, chlorpheniramine has an oral bioavailability of 10% to 40% that is considered dose-dependent with extensive drug distribution to the extravascular tissues.[6] The mean distribution half-life was reported to be 12.5 minutes with an elimination half-life of ≈1.7 hours.

In healthy thoroughbred horses, administration of 0.5 mg/kg IV plasma drug disposition was very rapid, with the mean terminal half-life and total body clearance calculated as 2.7 hours and 0.7 L/hour/kg, respectively. The observed maximal inhibition of wheal formation at 0.5 hours after administration of 0.1 and 0.5 mg/kg IV were 37.8% and 60.6%, respectively. Administration of d-chlorpheniramine at 0.5 mg/kg PO resulted in a bioavailability of 38%, with a peak plasma concentration at 1 hour and a maximal inhibition of wheal formation of 39% at 2 hours, suggesting that a larger dose rate and more frequent intervals may be needed to maintain therapeutic concentrations in horses.[7]

In humans, chlorpheniramine is well absorbed after oral administration, but bioavailability is 25% to 60% due to first-pass metabolism. The apparent steady-state volume of distribution is 2 to 12 L/kg, and 33% to 70% is bound to plasma proteins. Chlorpheniramine is metabolized in the liver and practically all the drug (as metabolites and unchanged drug) is excreted in the urine. In human patients with normal renal and hepatic function, the terminal serum half-life of the drug ranges from 13.2 to 43 hours. Half-life is increased with renal dysfunction; children have a decreased half-life.

Contraindications/Precautions/Warnings

Chlorpheniramine is contraindicated in patients that are hypersensitive to it or other antihistamines in its class. Because of its anticholinergic activity, chlorpheniramine should be used with caution in animals with narrow-angle glaucoma, prostatic hypertrophy, pyloroduodenal or bladder neck obstruction, and pulmonary diseases with minimal mucosal secretions. In addition, the drug should be used cautiously in animals with hyperthyroidism, cardiovascular disease, hypertension, or renal dysfunction. Palatability of this drug is also an issue in cats.

Do not confuse chlorPHENiramine with clomiPRAMINE or chlorpromAZINE.

Adverse Effects

The most common adverse effects are CNS depression (eg, lethargy, sedation)[8] and GI effects (eg, constipation, diarrhea, vomiting, anorexia). The sedative effects of antihistamines may adversely affect the performance of working dogs. With continued administration the sedative effects of antihistamines may diminish over time. Anticholinergic effects (eg, dry mouth, urine and fecal retention) are possible. Chlorpheniramine may cause paradoxical excitement in cats.

Reproductive/Nursing Safety

Laboratory animals given 50 to 85 times the human dose (based on weight) experienced no reproductive impairment or fetal harm. The drug is considered compatible with pregnancy.

Chlorpheniramine is excreted into milk; use with caution in dams and nursing neonates.

Because safety has not been established in animals, this drug should only be used when the maternal benefits outweigh the potential risks to offspring.

Overdose/Acute Toxicity

Overdose of first-generation antihistamines may cause CNS stimulation (eg, hyperexcitability, seizures) or depression (eg, lethargy, coma), anticholinergic effects, respiratory depression, and/or death. A 9-month-old dachshund that ingested 25 mg/kg showed signs of ataxia, tremors, bradycardia, coma, and cardiac arrest and died within 11 hours of ingestion.[9] Another source states not to use dosages greater than 1.1 mg/kg/day in dogs, as sudden death has occurred.[10]

Treatment consists of GI decontamination (if ingestion was oral) using standard protocols. Induce emesis if the patient is alert and CNS status is stable. A saline cathartic and/or activated charcoal may be given after emesis or gastric lavage. Treatment should be performed using supportive therapy based on clinical signs.

For patients that have experienced or are suspected to have expe-

rienced an overdose, consultation with a 24-hour poison consultation center specializing in providing veterinary-specific information is recommended. For general information related to overdose and toxin exposures, as well as contact information for poison control centers, refer to ***Appendix***.

Drug Interactions

The following drug interactions have either been reported or are theoretical in humans or animals receiving chlorpheniramine and may be of significance in veterinary patients. Unless otherwise noted, use together is not necessarily contraindicated, but weigh the potential risks and perform additional monitoring when appropriate.

- **Acetylcholinesterase Inhibitors** (eg, **neostigmine, pyridostigmine**): Chlorpheniramine may reduce effects of acetylcholinesterase inhibitors.
- **Anticholinergic Agents** (eg, **atropine, glycopyrrolate, oxybutynin**): Additive anticholinergic effects may occur when chlorpheniramine is used concomitantly with other anticholinergic agents.
- **Anticoagulants** (eg, **heparin, warfarin**): May partially counteract the anticoagulation effects of heparin or warfarin
- **CNS Depressant Drugs, Other** (eg, **acepromazine, ketamine, methocarbamol, mirtazapine, phenobarbital, trazodone**): Additive CNS depression may be seen if combining chlorpheniramine with other CNS depressant medications.
- **Monoamine Oxidase Inhibitors** (MAOIs; eg, **amitraz, amitriptyline, selegiline**): May prolong and exacerbate anticholinergic effects
- **Opioids** (eg, **buprenorphine, fentanyl, hydromorphone, methadone, morphine, tramadol**): Additive CNS depression and anticholinergic effects may occur.
- **Potassium Supplements, Oral**: The risk of focal upper GI injury caused by solid oral dosage forms of potassium salts may be increased by agents that reduce GI transit.
- **Prokinetics** (eg, **cisapride, metoclopramide**): Chlorpheniramine may reduce the effects of prokinetic agents.
- **Tricyclic Antidepressants** (eg, **amitriptyline, clomipramine**): Additive CNS depression and anticholinergic effects may occur.

Laboratory Considerations

- **Intradermal allergy testing (IDT)**: Although antihistamines may suppress IDT results, it is recommended that chlorpheniramine be discontinued a minimum of 2 days, but optimally 7 days prior to testing.[11]

Dosages

DOGS:

Adjunctive treatment and prevention of histamine-related pruritic conditions or as a mild sedative (extra-label): Most recommendations range from 0.2 – 0.5 (maximum) mg/kg PO every 8 to 12 hours. Using commercially available oral tablets, this is usually rounded off to the nearest 2 mg, with doses ranging from 2 – 8 mg/dog (NOT mg/kg) 2 to 3 times per day.

CATS:

Adjunctive treatment and prevention of histamine-related pruritic conditions or as a mild sedative (extra-label): Most recommended dosages are 1 – 4 mg/cat (NOT mg/kg) PO 2 to 3 times per day. Commonly administered at 2 mg/cat (NOT mg/kg) twice daily.[5,12] Some cats may be controlled with once-daily administration.

HORSES:

Adjunctive treatment and prevention of histamine-related pruritic conditions such as insect-bite hypersensitivity (extra-label): 0.25 mg/kg PO every 12 hours[13] **NOTE**: A pharmacokinetic study found a single dose of 0.5 mg/kg PO to be less efficacious than other antihistamines.[7]

BIRDS:

Adjunctive treatment (prevention) of histamine-related pruritic conditions or as a mild sedative (extra-label): One 4 mg tablet in one cup (240 mL; 8 oz) of bottled water to be used as drinking water; changed daily[14]

FERRETS:

Adjunctive treatment (prevention) of histamine-related pruritic conditions or as a mild sedative (extra-label): 1 – 2 mg/kg PO 2 to 3 times per day[15]

Monitoring

- Clinical efficacy; trial periods to determine an antihistamine's efficacy are usually 1 to 2 weeks in duration
- Adverse effects

Client Information

- This medicine may be difficult to give to cats, as it has a bitter taste. Acceptance by cats may be improved by dipping the split tablet into tuna juice, butter, or petrolatum, or by placing split tablets into empty gelatin capsules.
- Antihistamines should be used on a regular ongoing basis in animals that respond well to the medicine. Antihistamines work better when used before an animal has been exposed to an allergen.
- Drowsiness/sleepiness can occur with this medication, but this effect will usually lessen with time. Cats sometimes become excited after receiving the drug.
- Dry mouth, decreased gastrointestinal activity (including constipation), and urine retention (less frequent urinations) are possible.
- Use caution with over the counter (OTC) formulations, as other potentially toxic drugs (eg, acetaminophen, pseudoephedrine) may be combined in the product. Be sure to select a product that only contains chlorpheniramine.
- If using a sustained-release product, do not split or crush the tablets. If using a long-acting capsule, you may empty the contents of the capsule over food, but do not allow the beads to dissolve before the animal eats the food.

Chemistry/Synonyms

Chlorpheniramine maleate, a propylamine (alkylamine) antihistaminic agent, occurs as an odorless white crystalline powder with a melting point between 130°C and 135°C (266°F-275°F) and a pK_a of 9.2. One gram is soluble in ≈4 mL of water or 10 mL of alcohol.

Chlorpheniramine maleate may also be known as chlorphenamini maleas, chlorprophenypyridamine, or CAS No 113-92-8; many trade names are available; a commonly known brand is *Chlor-Trimeton®*.

Storage/Stability

All chlorpheniramine products should be stored at room temperature (15°C-30°C [59°F-86°F]) and protected from light. Avoid freezing the oral solution.

Compatibility/Compounding Considerations

Timed-release forms of the drug should not be crushed or allowed to dissolve in liquids.

Dosage Forms/Regulatory Status

VETERINARY-LABELED PRODUCTS: NONE

The Association of Racing Commissioners International (ARCI) has designated this drug as a class 4 substance. Use of this drug may not be allowed in certain animal competitions. Check rules and regulations before entering in a competition while this medication is being administered. Contact local racing authorities for further guidance. See ***Appendix*** for more information.

HUMAN-LABELED PRODUCTS:

Chlorpheniramine Maleate Oral Tablets: 4 mg tablets; (OTC)

Chlorpheniramine Maleate Extended-Release Tablets: 12 mg; (OTC)

Chlorpheniramine Maleate Oral Syrup: 2 mg/5 mL in 118 mL; (OTC)

Chlorpheniramine Maleate Oral Drops: 2 mg/mL in 60 mL; (OTC)

Many combination products are available that combine chlorpheniramine with decongestants, analgesics, and/or antitussives, but these generally should not be used in animals due to the potential for unpredictable adverse effects.

References

For the complete list of references, see **wiley.com/go/budde/plumb**

Chlorpromazine

(klor-***proe***-ma-zeen) *Thorazine*

Phenothiazine Sedative/Antiemetic

Prescriber Highlights

- Prototype phenothiazine used primarily as an antiemetic; may be particularly useful in treating motion sickness in cats
- Provides no analgesic effects
- Contraindications include hypersensitivity and use in horses; relative contraindications include use in hypovolemic animals, or animals with tetanus or strychinine intoxication.
- Use should be avoided or dose-reduced in debilitated animals, especially those with predicted or pre-existing hypotension or hepatic insufficiency; and use with caution in patients with moderate to severe cardiac disease that cannot tolerate reduced blood pressures
- Adverse effects may include significant hypotension, cardiac rate abnormalities, or hypo- or hyperthermia; extrapyramidal effects may occur in cats that are given high doses
- Inject diluted solution IV slowly
- Dogs with the multidrug sensitivity gene (MDR1) mutation (also known as *ABCB1*-1delta) may be overly sensitive to effects and require dose reduction.

Uses/Indications

Clinical use of chlorpromazine has diminished, but it is still occasionally used for its antiemetic and tranquilizing/sedating effects in small animals. Although it was previously the principal phenothiazine used in veterinary medicine, chlorpromazine has been largely supplanted by acepromazine.

Chlorpromazine (or acepromazine) can be useful in patients exhibiting severe anxiety, tachycardia, or hypertension secondary to a toxin or overdose of amphetamine-like attention-deficit disorder (ADD)/attention-deficit/hyperactivity disorder (ADHD) medications, selective serotonin reuptake inhibitors (SSRIs), antidepressants (or other agents that can cause serotonin syndrome), or the paradoxical CNS stimulation that can be seen with overdoses of human sleep aids (eg, eszopiclone, zolpidem).[1] As an antiemetic, chlorpromazine use is limited to normotensive or hypertensive patients, as it causes hypotension. It will inhibit apomorphine-induced emesis in dogs but not in cats. Chlorpromazine will also inhibit the emetic effects of morphine in dogs. It does not inhibit emesis caused by copper sulfate or digitalis glycosides.

Pharmacology/Actions

Chlorpromazine has similar pharmacologic effects as acepromazine but is less potent and has a longer duration of action. For further information, refer to ***Acepromazine***.

Pharmacokinetics

Chlorpromazine is absorbed rapidly after oral administration but undergoes extensive first-pass metabolism in the liver. The drug is also well-absorbed after IM injection, but the onset of action is slower than after IV administration.

Chlorpromazine is distributed throughout the body, and brain concentrations are higher than those in plasma. Approximately 95% of chlorpromazine in plasma is bound to plasma proteins (primarily albumin).

The drug is extensively metabolized, principally in the liver and kidneys, but little specific information is available regarding its excretion in dogs and cats.

Contraindications/Precautions/Warnings

Chlorpromazine is contraindicated in patients that are hypersensitive to it. Use chlorpromazine cautiously and in smaller doses in animals with hepatic dysfunction, cardiac disease, or general debilitation. Because of its hypotensive effects, phenothiazines are relatively contraindicated in patients with hypovolemia or shock and in those with tetanus or strychnine intoxication due to effects on the extrapyramidal system. Because of adverse CNS effects (eg, ataxia, panic reaction), this drug is not recommended for use in horses.

Chlorpromazine has no analgesic effects; animals should be treated with appropriate analgesics to control pain. Animals may require lower doses of general anesthetics when receiving phenothiazines in their premedications.

Phenothiazines should be used cautiously as restraining agents in aggressive dogs; they may make the animal more prone to startle and react to noises or other sensory inputs.

IV injections must be diluted with saline to concentrations of no more than 1 mg/mL and administered slowly. Chlorpromazine causes severe muscle discomfort and swelling when injected IM in rabbits; therefore, chloropromazine should only be administered IV in this species.

Breed-specific concerns include dogs with *MDR1* gene mutation (also known as *ABCB1*-1delta), which may develop a more pronounced sedation that persists longer than expected.[2] The drug is best completely avoided in *MDR1*-mutant dogs because there is no reversal, but if no other option is available, the dose should be reduced by 25% in dogs that are heterozygous and by 30% to 50% in dogs that are homozygous for the *MDR1* gene mutation (mutant/mutant).

Consider writing part of the drug's name in uppercase letters (ie, tall man designations) on prescriptions/orders to reduce the risk for errors. Do not confuse chlorproMAZINE with chlordiazePOXIDE, clomiPRAMINE, prochlorperazine, or promethazine.

Adverse Effects

In addition to the possible effects listed in the ***Acepromazine*** monograph (eg, hypotension, contradictory effects such as CNS stimulation and bradycardia), chlorpromazine may cause extrapyramidal signs (eg, tremors, shivering, rigidity, loss of the righting reflexes) in cats when used at high doses; lethargy, diarrhea, and loss of anal sphincter tone may also be seen.

Horses may develop ataxia, paradoxical excitation, and unpredictable behavior (eg, thrashing). These ataxic periods may cycle with periods of sedation. Because of these adverse effects, chlorpromazine is rarely used in equine medicine.

Reproductive/Nursing Safety

Embryotoxicity and increased neonatal mortality have been demonstrated in rodents. Chlorpromazine is excreted into maternal milk, and safety to nursing offspring cannot be assured.[3]

Because safety has not been established in animals, this drug should only be used when the maternal benefits outweigh the potential risks to offspring.

Overdose/Acute Toxicity

Most small overdoses cause only somnolence; larger overdoses can cause serious effects including coma, agitation, seizures, arrhythmias, hypotension, tachycardia, and extrapyramidal effects (eg, tremors, shivering, rigidity, loss of the righting reflexes).

Most overdoses can be handled by monitoring the patient and providing supportive care based on presenting signs; oral overdoses should be treated by GI decontamination if possible. IV lipid emulsion therapy may also be helpful.[4] Seizures may be controlled with barbiturates or diazepam. Hypotension should be treated initially with IV fluids; alpha-adrenergic pressor agents (eg, norepinephrine, phenylephrine; *not* epinephrine) can be considered if IV fluid therapy does not maintain adequate blood pressure. NOTE: The FDA label states *Epinephrine is contraindicated for treatment of acute hypotension produced by phenothiazine-derivative tranquilizers since further depression of blood pressure can occur.*[5,6] This phenomenon, known as epinephrine reversal, can occur when epinephrine is administered after an alpha-adrenergic antagonist (eg, chlorpromazine). In these situations, the peripheral beta-adrenergic effects of epinephrine will predominate, resulting in relaxation of the vascular smooth musculature and hypotension.

For patients that have experienced or are suspected to have experienced an overdose, consultation with a 24-hour poison control center specializing in providing veterinary-specific information is recommended. For general information related to overdose and toxin exposures, as well as contact information for poison control centers, refer to ***Appendix.***

Drug Interactions

The following drug interactions have either been reported or are theoretical in humans or animals receiving chlorpromazine or other phenothiazines and may be of significance in veterinary patients. Unless otherwise noted, use together is not necessarily contraindicated, but weigh the potential risks and perform additional monitoring when appropriate.

- **ANTIPYRETICS** (eg, **acetaminophen, dipyrone, NSAIDs**): Possible increased risk for hypothermia with concurrent use
- **ANTACIDS, ALUMINUM-, CALCIUM- OR MAGNESIUM-CONTAINING:** May cause reduced GI absorption of oral phenothiazines
- **ANTIDIARRHEAL MIXTURES** (eg, **kaolin/pectin, bismuth subsalicylate mixtures**): May cause reduced GI absorption of oral phenothiazines
- **BROMOCRIPTINE:** Phenothiazines may antagonize effects of bromocriptine and increase risk for dizziness, hypotension, and drowsiness.
- **BUSPIRONE:** Concurrent use may increase the risk for neuroleptic malignant syndrome and serotonin syndrome.
- **CABERGOLINE:** Concurrent use may decrease the efficacy of both medications. Increased risk for serotonin syndrome and neuroleptic malignant syndrome may occur.
- **CALCIUM CHANNEL BLOCKERS** (eg, **amlodipine, diltiazem, verapamil**): Concurrent use may increase risk for hypotension and orthostasis. Monitor blood pressure, especially at initiation of therapy or with parenteral administrations of phenothiazines. Slow-dose titration is advisable.
- **CNS DEPRESSANT AGENTS** (eg, **barbiturates, cannabidiol, anesthetics**): May cause additive CNS depression if used with phenothiazines
- **DESMOPRESSIN:** Concurrent use may increase risk for water intoxication and/or hyponatremia. Electrolytes and renal function should be monitored.
- **DIAZOXIDE:** Concurrent use may increase risk for hypotension and orthostasis. Phenothiazines may increase the risk for hyperglycemic effects from diazoxide.
- **DOXORUBICIN:** Chlorpromazine may increase levels of doxorubicin.
- **EMETICS** (eg, **apomorphine, ropinirole**): May reduce the effectiveness of emetics as well as increase risk for sedation and hypotension
- **EPINEPHRINE/NOREPINEPHRINE:** Phenothiazines block alpha-adrenergic receptors, and concomitant epinephrine can lead to unopposed beta activity, causing vasodilation and increased cardiac rate.
- **LAXATIVES** (eg, **bisacodyl**): Overuse of laxatives may cause electrolyte loss, increasing the risk for cardiovascular adverse effects with chlorpromazine.
- **LOOP DIURETICS** (eg, **bumetanide, furosemide**): Concurrent use may cause hypomagnesemia and hypokalemia, increasing the risk for cardiac arrhythmias.
- **METOCLOPRAMIDE:** Concurrent use with metoclopramide may increase risk for extrapyramidal adverse effects (eg, tremor, catalepsy, rigidity, excitement, sweating, seizures).
- **OPIOIDS** (eg, **buprenorphine, fentanyl, morphine**): May enhance the hypotensive effects of the phenothiazines; dosages of chlorpromazine may need to be reduced when used with an opioid.
- **ORGANOPHOSPHATE AGENTS:** Phenothiazines should not be given within one month of these antiparasitic agents, as their effects may be potentiated.
- **PHYSOSTIGMINE:** Toxicity may be enhanced by chlorpromazine.
- **PROPRANOLOL:** Increased blood concentrations of both drugs may result if propranolol is administered with phenothiazines.
- **QT PROLONGING AGENTS** (eg, **cisapride, domperidone, erythromycin** and **sotalol**): Concurrent use may increase risk for QTc prolongation and should be avoided.
- **QUINIDINE:** May cause additive cardiac depression
- **SUCRALFATE:** May reduce GI absorption of oral phenothiazines
- **TRICYCLIC ANTIDEPRESSANTS** (eg, **amitriptyline, clomipramine, doxepin**): Concurrent use may increase levels of either agent and may increase risk for serotonin syndrome, QT interval prolongation, and anticholinergic intoxication.

Dosages

DOGS/CATS:

Antiemetic or sedative (extra-label): Most recommendations range from 0.2 – 0.5 mg/kg IM or SC every 6 to 8 hours. IV dosage recommendations can vary widely (0.05 – 0.5 mg/kg [dogs] or 0.025 – 0.5 mg/kg [cats] IV every 6 to 8 hours). It is advised when giving the drug IV to start at the lower end of the dosage range and increase dosage as necessary (to effect) while monitoring blood pressure.

CATTLE:

Premedication for cattle undergoing standing procedures (extra-label): 0.2 – 1 mg/kg IM (may cause regurgitation if animal undergoes general anesthesia)[7]

SHEEP/GOATS:

a) **Sedative or premedicant in sheep and goats** (extra-label): 0.55 – 4.4 mg/kg IV or 2.2 – 6.6 mg/kg IM[8]
b) **Goats** (extra-label): 2 – 3.5 mg/kg IV every 5 to 6 hours[9]

SWINE:

Premedication (extra-label): 1 mg/kg IM[7]

Restraint (extra-label): 1.1 mg/kg IM (effects peak in 45 to 60 minutes); prior to barbiturate anesthesia: 2 – 4 mg/kg IM[9]

Monitoring

- Cardiac rate and rhythm and blood pressure (critical); end-tidal carbon dioxide ($ETCO_2$) and pulse oximetry (recommended)
- PCV and total protein, especially in borderline anemic patients and patients with current or expected blood loss
- Degree of sedation/tranquilization
- Body temperature (especially if ambient temperature is very hot or cold)

Client Information

- Causes sedation (sleepiness)
- Sedative or tranquilizing effects (sleepiness) and side effects may last up to 24 hours.
- Keep treated animal in a quiet environment at a comfortable temperature. Avoid getting this medication on hands or clothing; a skin rash (contact dermatitis) may develop.
- This medicine may cause a harmless pinkish to reddish-brown discoloration of your animal's urine. This change is not to be worried about.

Chemistry/Synonyms

Chlorpromazine is a propylamino-phenothiazine derivative and is the prototypic phenothiazine agent. It occurs as a white to slightly creamy white, odorless, bitter-tasting crystalline powder. One g is soluble in 1 mL of water and 1.5 mL of alcohol. The commercially available injection is a solution of chlorpromazine HCl in sterile water at a pH of 3 to 5.

Chlorpromazine HCl may also be known as aminazine or chlorpromazini hydrochloridum; many trade names are available.

Storage/Stability

Protect from light and store at room temperature 15°C to 30°C (59°F-86°F); avoid freezing. Do not store in plastic syringes or IV bags for prolonged periods as the drug may adsorb to plastic.

Chlorpromazine will darken with prolonged exposure to light; do not use solutions that are darkly colored or those in which precipitates have formed. A slight yellowish color will not affect potency or efficacy.

Compatibility/Compounding Considerations

Compatibility is dependent upon factors such as pH, concentration, temperature, and diluent used; consult specialized references or a hospital pharmacist for more specific information.

The following products have been reported to be **compatible** when mixed with chlorpromazine HCl injection: all commonly used IV electrolyte solutions, ascorbic acid, atropine sulfate, butorphanol tartrate, diphenhydramine, fentanyl citrate, glycopyrrolate, heparin sodium, hydromorphone HCl, hydroxyzine HCl, lidocaine HCl, meperidine, metoclopramide, metaraminol bitartrate, morphine sulfate, pentazocine lactate, promazine HCl, promethazine, scopolamine HBr, and tetracycline HCl.

Alkaline solutions will cause the drug to oxidize. The following products have been reported as being **incompatible** when mixed with chlorpromazine: aminophylline, amphotericin B, chloramphenicol sodium succinate, chlorothiazide sodium, dimenhydrinate, methohexital sodium, penicillin G potassium, pentobarbital sodium, phenobarbital sodium, and thiopental sodium.

Dosage Forms/Regulatory Status

VETERINARY-LABELED PRODUCTS: NONE

The Association of Racing Commissioners International (ARCI) has designated this drug as a class 1 substance. Use of this drug may not be allowed in certain animal competitions. Check rules and regulations before entering in a competition while this medication is being administered. Contact local racing authorities for further guidance.

HUMAN-LABELED PRODUCTS:

Chlorpromazine Injection: 25 mg/mL in 1 mL and 2 mL amps; generic; (Rx)

References

For the complete list of references, see **wiley.com/go/budde/plumb**

Chlortetracycline

(klor-te-tra-***sye***-kleen) *Aureomycin®*

Tetracycline Antibiotic

Prescriber Highlights

- Tetracycline antibiotic used primarily in water or feed treatments or topically for ophthalmic use
- Many bacteria are now resistant; may still be useful to treat *Mycoplasma* spp, *Rickettsia* spp, spirochetes, and *Chlamydia* spp
- Contraindications include hypersensitivity to the drug. Use chlortetracycline with extreme caution during pregnancy
- Use with caution in patients with liver or renal insufficiency
- Adverse effects include GI distress, staining of developing teeth and bones, superinfections, and photosensitivity.

Uses/Indications

There are a variety of FDA-approved chlortetracycline products for use in food animals. This antibiotic may also be useful in treating susceptible infections in cats, birds, and small mammals (excluding guinea pigs).

The World Health Organization (WHO) has designated tetracyclines as Highly Important antimicrobials for human medicine.[1] The Office International des Epizooties (OIE) has designated chlortetracycline as a Veterinary Critically Important Antimicrobial (VCIA) Agent in avian, bovine, caprine, equine, lagomorph, ovine, and swine species.[2]

Pharmacology/Actions

Tetracyclines generally act as bacteriostatic antibiotics inhibiting protein synthesis by reversibly binding to 30S ribosomal subunits of susceptible organisms, thereby preventing protein transcription. Tetracyclines are also believed to alter cytoplasmic membrane permeability in susceptible organisms. In high concentrations, tetracyclines can inhibit protein synthesis in mammalian cells.

As a class, the tetracyclines have activity against most *Mycoplasma* spp, spirochetes (including *Borrelia burgdorferi*), *Chlamydia* spp, and *Rickettsia* spp. The tetracyclines have activity against some gram-positive bacteria, including strains of staphylococci and streptococci, but resistance of these organisms is increasing. Additional gram-positive bacteria that are usually susceptible to tetracyclines include *Actinomyces* spp, *Bacillus anthracis*, *Clostridium perfringens*, *Clostridium tetani*, and *Listeria monocytogenes*. Tetracyclines usually have in vitro and in vivo activity against the following gram-negative bacteria: *Bordetella* spp, *Brucella* spp, *Bartonella* spp, *Haemophilus* spp, *Pasteurella multocida*, *Shigella* spp, and *Yersinia pestis*. Many or most strains of *Escherichia coli*, *Klebsiella* spp, *Bacteroides* spp, *Enterobacter* spp, *Proteus* spp, and *Pseudomonas aeruginosa* are resistant to the tetracyclines.

Oxytetracycline, chlortetracycline, and tetracycline share nearly identical spectrums of activity and patterns of cross-resistance, and a tetracycline susceptibility disk is often used for in vitro testing for chlortetracycline susceptibility.

Pharmacokinetics

Refer to ***Oxytetracycline*** for general information on the pharmacokinetics of tetracyclines.

Contraindications/Precautions/Warnings

Chlortetracycline is contraindicated in patients that are hypersensitive to it or other tetracyclines. Because tetracyclines can delay fetal skeletal development and discolor deciduous teeth, they should only be used in the last half of pregnancy when the benefits outweigh the fetal risks. Oxytetracycline, chlortetracycline, and tetracycline are considered more likely to cause these abnormalities than doxycycline or minocycline.

In patients with renal insufficiency or hepatic impairment, chlortetracycline must be used cautiously. Lower than normal dosages are recommended, in addition to enhanced monitoring of renal and hepatic function. Avoid concurrent administration of other nephrotoxic or hepatotoxic drugs.

Because it may cause clostridial enterotoxemia in guinea pigs, chlortetracycline should not be used in this species.

Adverse Effects

Chlortetracycline given to young animals can cause discoloration of bones and teeth to a yellow, brown, or gray color. High dosages or chronic administration may delay bone growth and healing.

In humans, tetracyclines at high levels can exert a catabolic effect that can cause an increase in BUN and/or hepatotoxicity, particularly in patients with preexisting renal dysfunction.[3] As renal function deteriorates secondary to drug accumulation, this effect may be exacerbated.

In ruminants, high oral doses can cause ruminal microflora depression and ruminoreticular stasis.

In small animals, tetracyclines can cause nausea, vomiting, anorexia, and diarrhea. Cats do not tolerate oral tetracycline or oxytetracycline very well; signs of colic, fever, hair loss, and depression may be seen. There are reports that long-term tetracycline use may cause urolith formation in dogs.[4]

Horses that are under stress (eg, from surgery, anesthesia, trauma) may exhibit severe diarrhea after receiving tetracyclines (especially with oral administration).

Tetracycline therapy (especially long term) may result in overgrowth (superinfections) of nonsusceptible bacteria or fungi.

Tetracyclines have been associated with photosensitivity reactions and, rarely, hepatotoxicity or blood dyscrasias.

Reproductive/Nursing Safety

Tetracyclines cross the placenta; they are embryotoxic when used early in pregnancy and can retard fetal skeletal growth and permanently discolor teeth.

Tetracyclines are excreted in milk, but because much of the drug will be bound to calcium in milk, it is unlikely to be of significant risk to nursing animals.

Because safety has not been established in animals, this drug should only be used when the maternal benefits outweigh the potential risks to offspring.

Overdose/Acute Toxicity

Tetracyclines are generally well tolerated after acute overdoses. Dogs given more than 400 mg/kg/day orally or 100 mg/kg/day IM of oxytetracycline did not demonstrate any toxicity. Oral overdoses would most likely be associated with GI disturbances (vomiting, anorexia, and/or diarrhea). Should the patient develop severe emesis or diarrhea, fluids and electrolytes should be monitored and replaced if necessary. Chronic overdoses may lead to drug accumulation and nephrotoxicity.

High oral doses given to ruminants can cause ruminal microflora depression and ruminoreticular stasis. Rapid IV injection of undiluted propylene-glycol-based products can cause intravascular hemolysis with resultant hemoglobinuria.

Rapid IV injection of tetracyclines has induced transient collapse and cardiac arrhythmias in several species, presumably due to chelation with intravascular calcium ions. Overdose quantities of drug could exacerbate this effect if given too rapidly IV. If the drug must be given rapidly IV (less than 5 minutes), some clinicians recommend pretreating the animal with IV calcium gluconate.

For patients that have experienced or are suspected to have experienced an overdose, consultation with a 24-hour poison consultation center specializing in providing veterinary-specific information is recommended. For general information related to overdose and toxin exposures, as well as contact information for poison control centers, refer to ***Appendix.***

Drug Interactions

The following drug interactions have either been reported or are theoretical in humans or animals receiving chlortetracycline and may be of significance in veterinary patients. Unless otherwise noted, use together is not necessarily contraindicated, but weigh the potential risks and perform additional monitoring when appropriate.

- **Beta-Lactam or Aminoglycoside Antibiotics**: Bacteriostatic drugs, like the tetracyclines, may interfere with bactericidal activity of the penicillins, cephalosporins, and aminoglycosides; however, there is some controversy regarding the actual clinical significance of this interaction.
- **Cholestyramine:** May decrease absorption of tetracyclines
- **Digoxin**: Tetracyclines may increase the bioavailability of digoxin in a small percentage of patients (human) and lead to digoxin toxicity. These effects may persist for months after discontinuation of the tetracycline.
- **Divalent or Trivalent Cations** (eg, **oral antacids, saline cathartics** or other **orally-administered products containing aluminum (eg, sucralfate), bismuth, calcium, iron, magnesium, or zinc cations**): When orally administered, tetracyclines can chelate divalent or trivalent cations that can decrease the absorption of the tetracycline or the other drug if it contains these cations; it is recommended that all oral tetracyclines be given at least 1 to 2 hours before or after the cation-containing products.
- **Lanthanum:** May decrease absorption of tetracyclines
- **Retinoid Acids** (eg, **acitretin, vitamin A**): May increase the potential for the occurrence of intracranial hypertension. Combination is contraindicated.
- **Warfarin**: Tetracyclines may depress plasma prothrombin activity, and anticoagulant dosage adjustment may be needed.

Laboratory Considerations

- Tetracyclines (excluding minocycline) may cause falsely elevated values of **urine catecholamines** when using fluorometric methods of determination.
- Tetracyclines can reportedly cause false positive **urine glucose** results if using the cupric sulfate method of determination (Benedict's reagent, *Clinitest*®), but this may be the result of ascorbic acid that is found in some parenteral formulations of tetracyclines. Tetracyclines have also reportedly caused false negative results in determining urine glucose when using the glucose oxidase method (*Clinistix*®, *Tes-Tape*®).

Dosages

CATS:

Prevent recurrence of *Mycoplasma* spp or chlamydial conjunctivitis in large catteries where topical therapy is impractical (extra-label): Soluble chlortetracycline powder in food at a dose of 50 mg/cat (NOT mg/kg) daily for 1 month[5]

BIRDS:

All dosages are extra-label. Refer to product labels for FDA-approved dosing rates in poultry and withdrawal times.

a) **Chlamydiosis**: In small birds, add chlortetracycline to food in a concentration of 0.05%; larger psittacines require 1% chlortetracycline.[6]

b) **Pigeons**: 50 mg/kg PO every 6 to 8 hours; or 1000 – 1500 mg/gallon drinking water; in warm weather, mix fresh every 12 hours. Best used in combination with tylosin for ornithosis complex; calcium inhibits absorption; therefore, grit and layer pellets should be withheld during treatment.[7]

RABBITS/RODENTS/SMALL MAMMALS:

All dosages are extra-label.

a) **Rabbits**: 50 mg/kg PO every 12 to 24 hours[8]
b) **Chinchillas**: 50 mg/kg PO every 12 hours[9]
c) **Hamsters**: 20 mg/kg IM or SC every 12 hours[10]
d) **Mice**: 25 mg/kg SC or IM every 12 hours[10]
e) **Rats**: 6 – 10 mg/kg SC or IM every 12 hours[10]

Monitoring

- Adverse effects
- Clinical efficacy
- Long-term use or in susceptible patients: baseline and periodic renal, hepatic, hematologic evaluations

Client Information

- Avoid giving this drug orally within 1 to 2 hours of feeding milk or other dairy products.
- When this medicine is given orally, it should be administered on an empty stomach 1 to 2 hours before or after consumption of food, milk, other dairy products, and minerals such as calcium or iron. If your animal vomits or acts sick after receiving the medicine on an empty stomach, give it with a small amount of food to see if this helps. If vomiting continues, contact your veterinarian.
- Chlortetracycline may permanently stain teeth and interfere with developing bones in young animals.
- If used in food animals, follow label dosages and withdrawal times.

Chemistry/Synonyms

Chlortetracycline is a tetracycline antibiotic that occurs as yellow odorless crystals. It is slightly soluble in water.

Chlortetracycline may also be known as clortetraciclina, A-377, NRRL-2209, or SF-66; *Aureomycin®* is a common trade name.

Storage/Stability

Chlortetracycline should be stored in tight containers and protected from light.

Compatibility/Compounding Considerations

No specific information is noted.

Dosage Forms/Regulatory Status

VETERINARY-LABELED PRODUCTS:

There are several feed additive/water mix preparations available containing chlortetracycline. The Type A Medicated Feed Article products require a VFD. There are also combination products containing chlortetracycline and sulfamethazine (*Aureomycin Sulmet®*, *Aureo S 700®*); chlortetracycline, sulfamethazine, and penicillin G (*Aureomix 500®*, *Pennclor SP 250®, and 500®*); and chlortetracycline, sulfathiazole, and penicillin G (*Aureozol 500®*); (Rx)

HUMAN-LABELED PRODUCTS: NONE

References

For the complete list of references, see **wiley.com/go/budde/plumb**

Cholestyramine

(**ko**-less-**tər**-a-meen) *Questran®, Prevalite®*

Bile-Acid Sequestrant

Prescriber Highlights

- ► May bind drugs that undergo enterohepatic recirculation in dogs and cats and thus may be helpful in the treatment of toxicoses associated with those drugs
- ► Avoid using formulations with xylitol for veterinary patients.
- ► Adverse effects can include constipation, bloating, and decreased appetite.
- ► Not commonly used in veterinary patients

Uses/Indications

Cholestyramine may be used to treat toxicoses of enterohepatically recirculated agents[1] (eg, cholecalciferol,[2,3] amiodarone, digoxin, NSAIDs,[4] vincristine).[5] In a case report of a dog with cyanotoxin (blue-green algae, microcystin) exposure, clinical improvement was noted within 48 hours of cholestyramine administration.[6] Cholestyramine may also be beneficial in patients with diarrhea caused by bile acid malabsorption.[7-9] In addition, cholestyramine reduces cholesterol in dogs.[10]

In small mammals, cholestyramine has been used to manage enterotoxemia caused by penicillin in guinea pigs[11] and clindamycin in rabbits.[12] Cholestyramine also increased survival rate in a rabbit model of brodifacoum poisoning.[13]

In humans, cholestyramine is used as an adjunct to lifestyle changes to reduce total cholesterol and low-density lipoprotein (LDL) concentrations. The drug also reduces pruritus in patients with partial cholestasis, partial biliary obstruction, and/or biliary cirrhosis.[14] Other uses include management of diarrhea, including *Clostridium difficile* enterocolitis, and non-life–threatening cases of cardiac glycoside (eg, digoxin) toxicosis.

Pharmacology/Actions

Cholestyramine is a nonabsorbable resin that binds to anionic bile acids in the small intestines in exchange for cholestyramine's chloride ions to form an insoluble complex that prevents enterohepatic recirculation of bile acids and thus reduces serum bile acid concentrations.[14]

In humans, the resulting excretion of bile acids stimulates the liver to convert cholesterol to bile acids, which leads to decreased serum cholesterol and plasma LDL concentrations. Chloestyramine's maximal effect on bile acid and cholesterol concentrations can be seen after ≈3 weeks of therapy.

Cholestyramine was also shown to bind microcystin-LR in experimental rat models of blue-green algae hepatotoxicity.[15]

Pharmacokinetics

Cholestyramine is not systemically available, as it is not absorbed after oral administration. The insoluble complex formed by cholestyramine and bile acids is excreted in the feces.

Contraindications/Precautions/Warnings

Cholestyramine should not be used in patients that are hypersensitive to it or with GI or complete biliary obstruction or biliary cirrhosis. Cholestyramine may increase triglyceride concentrations and is contraindicated in humans with triglyceride concentrations greater than 300 mg/dL. The drug should be used with caution in patients with renal insufficiency, volume depletion, mild hypertriglyceridemia, and cholelithiasis.[14] Adequate patient hydration status should be ensured prior to initiating therapy. Prolonged use can result in hyperchloremic acidosis. Patients receiving cholestyramine long term may benefit from folic acid and fat-soluble vitamin supplementation (eg, vitamin K).

Adverse Effects

Veterinary use is limited, and little is known regarding the adverse effects of cholestyramine in veterinary patients. In a study of healthy beagles, a 14-day course of cholestyramine was well tolerated but increased fecal output and decreased nutrient digestibility were observed.[16]

Constipation is the most common adverse effect in humans and may lead to fecal impaction. Other adverse effects include bloating, flatulence, steatorrhea, nausea, and anorexia. Impaired absorption of fat-soluble vitamins associated with long-term cholestyramine use may lead to bleeding disorders and osteoporosis.[14] Increased triglyceride concentrations may occur. Cholestyramine is poorly tolerated in humans due to the GI adverse effects, which leads to discontinuation of therapy in ≈70% of patients.[17,18]

Hyperchloremic metabolic acidosis may occur due to liberation of large quantities of chloride anions; this risk appears to be greater with high cholestyramine doses or long-term use, or when the drug is used in patients with low body weights. Altered absorption and/or excretion of other electrolytes (eg, calcium, nitrogen, phosphorus) is also possible.

Reproductive/Nursing Safety

Reproductive safety in veterinary patients is not known.

Because cholestyramine is not absorbed, it does not cross the placenta or enter into breast milk; however, cholestyramine impairs fat-soluble vitamin absorption for the dam, which may have consequences for the offspring (eg, reduced vitamin concentration in milk). Therefore, cholestyramine should be used with caution in pregnant or nursing patients; vitamin supplementation and/or a milk replacer should be considered.

Because safety of cholestyramine has not been established in animals, it should only be used when the maternal benefits outweigh the potential risks to offspring.

Overdose/Acute Toxicity

Because cholestyramine is not absorbed, there is little to no risk for systemic toxicity. Adverse GI effects, including risk for GI obstruction, are the primary concern. Continued GI motility should be ensured, and electrolytes and serum chemistry profiles should be monitored.

For patients that have experienced or are suspected to have experienced an overdose, consultation with a 24-hour poison consultation center specializing in providing veterinary-specific information is recommended. For general information related to overdose and toxin exposures, as well as contact information for poison control centers, refer to ***Appendix.***

Drug Interactions

Cholestyramine can bind to and decrease the absorption of many orally administered medications. Acidic drugs and drugs that undergo enterohepatic recirculation are particularly susceptible. Other oral drugs should be administered at least 1 hour before or 4 to 6 hours or longer after administering cholestyramine. The following drug interactions include those drugs/drug classes in which absorption has either been reported or is theoretical in humans or animals receiving cholestyramine and may be of significance in veterinary patients; unless otherwise noted, use together is not necessarily contraindicated, but the potential risks should be weighed and additional monitoring performed when appropriate:

- **ACETAMINOPHEN**
- **AMIODARONE**
- **DIGOXIN**
- **ESTROGENS** (eg, **estriol**)
- **GLUCOCORTICOIDS** (eg, **dexamethasone, hydrocortisone, prednis(ol)one**)
- **FISH OIL SUPPLEMENTS**
- **FOLIC ACID**
- **GEMFIBROZIL**
- **GLIPIZIDE**
- **IRON SALTS**
- **ISOTRETINOIN**
- **LEFLUNOMIDE:** Separating administration times will not prevent an interaction.
- **LEVOTHYROXINE**
- **LOOP DIURETICS** (eg, **furosemide, torsemide**)
- **METHOTREXATE**
- **METRONIDAZOLE**
- **MYCOPHENOLATE**
- **NONSTEROIDAL ANTI-INFLAMMATORY DRUGS** (NSAIDs; eg, **carprofen, meloxicam, piroxicam**)
- **PHENOBARBITAL**
- **PHOSPHATE SUPPLEMENTS (ORAL)**
- **PROGESTERONE**
- **PROPRANOLOL**
- **SPIRONOLACTONE:** Concurrent use may increase risk for hyperkalemic metabolic acidosis.
- **TESTOSTERONE**
- **TETRACYCLINES** (eg, **doxycycline, minocycline**)
- **THIAZIDE DIURETICS** (eg, **hydrochlorothiazide**)
- **URSODIOL**
- **VANCOMYCIN (ORAL):** Combination is contraindicated.
- **VITAMIN A**
- **VITAMIN D** (eg, **calcitriol, cholecalciferol**)
- **VITAMIN E**
- **VITAMIN K:** Concomitant cholestyramine may bind to vitamin K and worsen underlying coagulopathy.
- **WARFARIN:** Combination may increase or decrease anticoagulant effect of warfarin.

Laboratory Considerations

- None have been noted.

Dosages

DOGS:

Vincristine overdose (extra-label): 100 mg/kg PO every 12 hours for 5 days; concurrent treatments included activated charcoal 13 mL/kg once, sorbitol 3 mL/kg PO for 3 days (frequency not specified), folinic acid 3 mg/m² PO every 24 hours for 3 days, antibiotics (NOTE: Antibiotic coverage should be appropriate for leukopenic patients), and filgrastim 5 µg/kg SC every 24 hours for 5 days.[5]

Reduction of NSAID exposure (extra-label): 2.5 g/dog (NOT g/kg) diluted in 20 mL of water PO (gavage), followed by 20 mL of water as a rinse administered 3 times daily.[4]

Bile acid diarrhea (extra-label): 2 – 3 g/dog (NOT g/kg) PO twice daily. From a case report of 2 dogs refractory to management of diarrhea, including dietary trials, probiotics, cyclosporine therapy, fecal transplantation, and metronidazole.[19]

Cholecalciferol toxicosis: 0.3 – 1 g/kg, dissolved in liquid and administered orally every 8 hours for 4 days; administer in between activated charcoal doses.[3]

CATS:

Reduction of NSAID exposure (extra-label): From experimental studies, cholestyramine 1 g/cat (NOT mg/kg) PO administered immediately prior to flunixin injection has been shown to significantly reduce volume of distribution and mean residence time.[20]

RABBITS/GUINEA PIGS:

Antibiotic-induced enterotoxaemia (extra-label): 2 g/animal (NOT g/kg) cholestyramine diluted in 20 mL of water and administered orally once daily for 21 days.[12,21] Dose may be divided over 24 hours.

Monitoring

- Clinical efficacy
- Adverse effects
- Prothrombin time with long-term use

Client Information

- The most common side effects are constipation, bloating, abdominal discomfort, flatulence, and loss of appetite.
- Always mix cholestyramine powder with water or other fluids or into high-moisture content foods (eg, applesauce). Do not give dry powder, as intestinal irritation or obstruction may result.
- Give medicine with a meal
- Other drugs should be given at least 1 hour before or at least 4 to 6 hours after giving cholestyramine.

Chemistry/Synonyms

Cholestyramine is the chloride salt of a basic polymeric anion exchange resin. It is hydrophilic but insoluble in water and alcohol. The drug occurs as a white to off-white fine powder, although the appearance of manufactured dose forms varies based on the presence and amounts of inactive ingredients (eg, sweeteners, dyes).

Cholestyramine may also be known as colestyramine, *Cholebar*®, *Olestyr*®, *Prevalite*®, or *Questran*®.

Storage/Stability

Store cholestyramine powder at a controlled room temperature between 20°C and 25°C (68°F-77°F). Excursions are permitted between 15°C and 30°C (59°F-86°F). Protect from moisture until time of use.

Compatibility/Compounding Considerations

Cholestyramine has been applied topically as a 5% to 15% compounded ointment or paste for perianal skin irritation due to fecal exposure[22,23] or following hemorrhoidectomy[24] or ileostomy.[25]

Dosage Forms/Regulatory Status

VETERINARY-LABELED PRODUCTS: NONE

HUMAN-LABELED PRODUCTS:

Cholestyramine Powder for Suspension: Formulations vary: 4 g cholestyramine in 210 g, 231 g, or 378 g containers or canisters measured with provided scoop to deliver 5 to 9 g total powder weight, or in individual packets, pouches, or sachets containing 5.5 to 9 g total powder weight; *Questran*®, generic; (Rx). Scoops in bulk containers may not be interchanged between products.

Cholestyramine Light Powder for Suspension: 4 g cholestyramine measured with provided scoop to deliver 5.5 g or 5.7 g total powder weight in 202, 210 g, 231 g, or 339 g containers or canisters or in individual pouches or sachets containing 5.5 g or 5.7 g total powder weight; *Questran® Light, Prevalite*®, generic. (Rx). Contains aspartame. Scoops may not be interchanged between products.

References

For the complete list of references, see **wiley.com/go/budde/plumb**

Chorionic Gonadotropin

hCG, HCG

(kor-ee-***on***-ic goe-***nad***-oh-troe-pin) *Chorulon*®

Reproductive Hormone

Prescriber Highlights

- Human glycoprotein hormone that mimics luteinizing hormone; used for a variety of theriogenology conditions in many species
- *For parenteral use only*
- Contraindications include androgen-responsive neoplasias and hypersensitivity to the drug.
- Adverse effects are rare and include anaphylactic reaction.
- The National Institute of Occupational Safety and Health (NIOSH) classifies chorionic gonadotropin as a hazardous drug; use appropriate precautions when handling.

Uses/Indications

The veterinary FDA-approved human chorionic gonadotropin (hCG) product is used parenterally in cows for the treatment of nymphomania (frequent or constant heat) caused by cystic ovaries and as an aid to improve spawning function in male and female brood finfish.[1] It has been used for other purposes in several species; refer to the ***Dosages*** section for more information.

Pharmacology/Actions

Chorionic gonadotropin (CG) mimics the effects of luteinizing hormone (LH). In males, CG stimulates the differentiation of testicular interstitial (Leydig) cells and produces androgens. Hormonal treatment of cryptorchidism with human chorionic gonadotropin (hCG) is controversial in humans and domestic animals.

In females, hCG is primarily used in an extra-label fashion as an ovulation-inducing agent. In bitches, administration of hCG induces estrogen secretion during anestrus and can, therefore, be used to identify spayed bitches with ovarian remnants.[2]

Pharmacokinetics

Human chorionic gonadotropin (hCG) is destroyed in the GI tract after oral administration, so it must be given parenterally. After IM injection, peak plasma concentrations occur in about 6 hours.

hCG is distributed primarily to the ovaries in females and to the testes in males, but some hCG may also be distributed to the proximal tubules in the renal cortex.

hCG is eliminated from the blood in a biphasic manner. The initial elimination half-life in humans is about 11 hours and the terminal half-life is ≈23 hours.

Contraindications/Precautions/Warnings

In humans, chorionic gonadotropin (hCG) is contraindicated in patients with prostatic carcinoma or other androgen-dependent neoplasias, precocious puberty, or those with a previous hypersensitivity reaction to hCG. No labeled contraindications for veterinary patients were noted, but these human contraindications should be used as guidelines.

Antibody production to hCG has been reported after repetitive use; however, despite this effect, pharmacological activity (induction of ovulation) is expected to remain unaltered.

The National Institute for Occupational Safety and Health (NIOSH) classifies hCG as a hazardous drug; personal protective equipment (PPE) should be used accordingly to minimize the risk for exposure.

Adverse Effects

Repeated doses of chorionic gonadotropin (hCG) may cause abortion in mares prior to the 35th day of pregnancy, possibly because of increased estrogen levels.[3] Potentially, hypersensitivity reactions are possible with this agent. Anaphylactic reactions are rare, and several practitioners have anecdotally reported mares showing transient hives and respiratory distress immediately following hCG administration. Problems associated with using *PG 600*® in dogs for estrus induction include unpredictability of response, potential for allergic reactions, and premature luteal failure.[4]

In humans, hCG has caused pain at the injection site, gynecomastia, headache, depression, irritability, restlessness, and edema.

Reproductive/Nursing Safety

In humans, chorionic gonadotropin (hCG) and its metabolites have been found in maternal milk.[5] There are no similar studies with animals reported following administration of hCG.

Because safety has not been established in animals, this drug should only be used when the maternal benefits outweigh the potential risks to offspring.

Overdose/Acute Toxicity

No overdose cases have been reported with chorionic gonadotropin.

Drug Interactions

No interactions have apparently been reported with chorionic gonadotropin.

Laboratory Considerations

None

Dosages

NOTE: Unless otherwise noted, dosages refer to the use of chorionic gonadotropin (hCG) (*Chorulon*®).

DOGS:

hCG challenge test to determine if testicular tissue remains in neutered male dogs (extra-label): 44 µg/kg hCG IM and take a 4-hour post sample. **NOTE:** Contact your laboratory for specific recommendations for testing. Various protocols exist including taking a sample for resting testosterone level.

hCG challenge test to identify the presence of ovarian tissue in presumably spayed bitches or those suspected to have ovarian remnants (extra-label): 200 – 500 units/dog (NOT units/kg) IV and take a blood sample before and 90 minutes after the treatment. Submit plasma samples for determination of estradiol concentrations. Highly variable response; results may be inconclusive.

Produce luteinization of a follicular cyst (extra-label): 500 – 1000 units/dog (NOT units/kg) IM; repeat in 48 hours or once daily for 3 days

Improve semen quality in male dogs with oligospermia (extra-label): 500 – 1000 units/dog (NOT units/kg) IM.[6] Semen quality expected to improve transiently between 2 to 4 weeks after treatment.

CATS:

hCG challenge test to determine if testicular tissue remains in neutered male cats (extra-label): Various protocols exist including: Take baseline serum testosterone sample, administer 250 units/cat (NOT units/kg) IM; take second sample 4 hours later. **NOTE:** Contact your laboratory for specific recommendations for testing.

hCG challenge test to identify the presence of ovarian tissue in presumably spayed queens or those suspected to have ovarian remnants (extra-label): 500 units/cat (NOT unit/kg) IM between 1 and 3 days following the onset of estrus behavior and take a blood sample before hCG administration and 7 days later. Submit plasma samples for determination of progesterone concentrations.[7]

Infertility, reduced libido, cryptorchidism in male cats (extra-label): 50 – 100 units/cat (NOT unit/kg) IM; repeat if necessary[8]

Induction of ovulation in female cats (extra-label): 100 – 500 units/cat (NOT unit/kg) IM on day 1 or days 1 and 2 of estrus. Alternatively, 250 units/cat (NOT unit/kg) IM on days 2 and 3 of estrus, coupled with mating 3 times per day at 3-hour intervals for the first 3 days of estrus[9]

HORSES:

Induction of ovulation (extra-label in the United States): 1500 – 3000 units/horse (NOT units/kg) IV to mares in estrus with more than 30 to 35 mm follicle. Ovulation is expected to occur within 48 hours from administration.[10]

hCG challenge test to determine if testicular tissue remains in a gelding (extra-label): Take baseline serum testosterone sample, administer 10,000 units IV; take samples 30 minutes, 1 hour, and 24 hours later.[11,12] **NOTE:** Contact your laboratory for specific recommendations for testing as various protocols exist.

Induction of testicular descent in cryptorchids (less than 2 years of age): 2500 units/horse (NOT units/kg) IM twice weekly for 4 weeks.[13] Four of eight horses responded to therapy.

CATTLE:

Treatment of ovarian cysts (label dosage): The reconstituted contents of one vial (10,000 units; 10 mL) should be administered as a single deep IM injection. Dose may be repeated in 14 days if the animal's behavior or rectal examination of the ovaries indicates the necessity for retreatment.[1]

Induction of ovulation (extra-label): 1500 or 2000 units/cow (NOT units/kg) IM will induce ovulation in cows subjected to estrus synchronization protocols.

SHEEP:

Induction of estrus (extra-label in the United States): 400 – 800 units eCG (*Pregnecol*®, not available in the United States) IM or SC in the anterior half of the neck. (Adapted from product label; *Pregnecol*®)

GOATS:

Induction of estrus (extra-label in the United States): 200 – 600 units eCG (*Pregnecol*®, not available in the United States) IM or SC in the anterior half of the neck. (Adapted from product label; *Pregnecol*®)

SWINE:

Induction of fertile estrus (heat) in healthy prepuberal (non-cycling) gilts over 5 ½ months of age and weighing at least 85 kg (187 lb) or in healthy sows at weaning that are experiencing delayed return to estrus (labeled dosage): One dose (5 mL) of reconstituted *PG 600*® injected into the gilt or sow's neck behind the ear. Prepuberal gilts should be injected when they are selected for addition to the breeding herd. Sows should be injected at weaning during periods of delayed return to estrus. (Adapted from product label; *PG 600*®)

BIRDS:

Reduce feather plucking (especially in female birds); (extra-label): 500 – 1000 units/kg IM; dosage is empirical.[14] If no response in 3 days, repeat. If no response after second injection, unlikely to be of benefit at any dose. If reduces feather plucking, will need to repeat after 4 to 6 weeks. Major drawback is that with repeated usage, time between treatments is reduced.

FISH:

Improve spawning function in male and female brood finfish (labeled dosage): Administer IM just ventral to the dorsal fin for 1 to 3 injections.[1] See product label for weight-based dosing based on species of fish.

Chemistry/Synonyms

A gonad-stimulating polypeptide secreted by the human placenta, chorionic gonadotropin (hCG) is obtained from the urine of pregnant women. It occurs as a white or practically white amorphous lyophilized powder. It is soluble in water and practically insoluble in alcohol. One international unit (called units in this reference) of hCG is equal to 1 USP unit. There are at least 1500 USP units per mg.

This drug may also be known as human chorionic gonadotropin, HCG, hCG, LH 500, CG, chorionic gonadotrophin, dynatropin, gonadotropine chorionique, gonadotrophinum chorionicum, choriogonadotrophin, chorionogonadotropin, pregnancy-urine hormone, PU, equine chorionic gonadotropin, eCG, pregnant mare serum gonadotropin, or PMSG; there are many trade names internationally.

Storage/Stability

Store *Chorulon®* powder for injection at room temperature (15°C-30°C [59°F-86°F]) and protected from light. Store *PG 600®* in the refrigerator (2°C-8°C [36°F-46°F]). After reconstitution, the resultant solution is stable for 30 to 90 days (depending on the product) when stored at 2°C to 15°C (36°F-59°F). The labels for *Chorulon®* and *PG 600®* state to use the vial immediately after reconstituting with the supplied diluent.[1,15] Alternatively, freezing of unused hCG in aliquots can be used to maximize the use of the veterinary preparation that typically contains 10,000 units.[10]

Compatibility/Compounding Considerations

No specific information is noted.

Dosage Forms/Regulatory Status

VETERINARY-LABELED PRODUCTS:

Chorionic Gonadotropin (hCG) Injection: 10,000 units per 10 mL double vial packs containing 10,000 USP units per vial with bacteriostatic water for injection; single dose 10 mL vials of freeze-dried powder and five 10 mL vials of sterile diluent; *Chorulon®*; (Rx). FDA-approved for use in cows and finfish. In fish intended for human consumption, the total dose administered (all injections combined) should not exceed 25,000 units (25 mL) per fish. No withdrawal time is required when used as labeled.

Chorionic Gonadotropin freeze-dried powder: Single dose 5 mL vials when reconstituted contains pregnant mare serum gonadotropin (equine chorionic gonadotrophin, eCG, PMSG) 400 units and human chorionic gonadotropin (hCG) 200 units; five dose 25 mL vials that when reconstituted contain pregnant mare serum gonadotropin (PMSG) 2000 units and human chorionic gonadotropin (hCG) 1000 units; *PG 600®*; (OTC). FDA-approved for use in swine (prepubertal gilts and sows at weaning); no meat withdrawal time is required when used as labeled.

HUMAN-LABELED PRODUCTS:

Chorionic Gonadotropin (Human) Powder for Injection: 5000 units/vial with 10 mL diluent (to make 500 units/mL); 10,000 units/vial with 10 mL diluent (to make 1000 units/mL); 20,000 units/vial with 10 mL diluent (to make 2000 units/mL) in 10 mL vials; *Novarel®*, *Pregnyl®*, generic; (Rx)

References

For the complete list of references, see **wiley.com/go/budde/plumb**

Ciclesonide

(sye-***kles***-oh-nide) *Aservo® EquiHaler®*

Glucocorticoid, Inhaled

Prescriber Highlights

- Indicated for management of clinical signs associated with severe equine asthma. May be combined with other asthma treatment modalities
- Clinical improvement may be delayed by several days.
- Ciclesonide is not a bronchodilator and should not be used for management of acute bronchospasm.
- Use with caution in patients with active respiratory infection, chronic nephritis, congestive heart failure, equine pituitary pars intermedia dysfunction (PPID), and when there is higher risk for, or a history of, laminitis.
- Common adverse effects include nasal discharge and cough during or after administration; leukocytosis, nasal irritation, and sneezing may also occur but are uncommon.
- Drug is delivered via intranasal inhalation into the horse's left nostril; the inhaler device should have a snug fit into the nostril to ensure delivery of a complete dose.
- Unlike traditional human inhaler devices, ciclesonide does not require shaking prior to administration, and the device contents are neither pressurized nor contain aerosol propellants.
- Be sure to explain proper use of the inhalation device; dispense this drug with the manufacturer's user manual.

Uses/Indications

Ciclesonide is indicated for the management of clinical signs associated with severe equine asthma. It may be used in addition to other treatment strategies (eg, bronchodilators, environmental management).[1] Under experimental conditions, ciclesonide treatment was comparable with oral dexamethasone in reducing measures of experimentally induced airway obstruction in asthmatic horses, but ciclesonide did not reduce serum cortisol.[2] Roughly 85% to 92% of horses accepted the drug's inhaler device.[3] In a study, improvement in clinical score and owner-perceived quality of life were observed in horses that received ciclesonide.[4]

In some regions (eg, UK,[5] EU[6], ciclesonide is approved for summer pasture-associated severe equine asthma.

Pharmacology/Actions

Ciclesonide, a glucocorticoid with potent anti-inflammatory activity, is a prodrug converted into des-ciclesonide by esterases in the respiratory tract.[7] Des-ciclesonide has an affinity 12 times that of dexamethasone for human glucocorticoid receptors, and 120 times greater than the parent drug. Des-ciclesonide demonstrates inhibitory activities against a variety of cell types (eg, mast cells, eosinophils, basophils, lymphocytes, macrophages, neutrophils) as well as against pro-inflammatory mediators (eg, histamine, eicosanoids, leukotrienes, cytokines) involved in the pathophysiology of asthma. Cortisol suppression was not observed at the labeled dosage in the equine species.[5] For a more thorough discussion of glucocorticoid effects, refer to the ***Glucocorticoid*** monograph.

Pharmacokinetics

Ciclesonide is a prodrug rapidly de-esterified to the active component des-ciclesonide, which is detectable within 5 minutes of administration. Des-ciclesonide plasma concentration peaks 30 minutes after administration, and increasing doses result in greater-than-proportional increases in peak concentration. Absolute systemic bioavailability of ciclesonide is 5% to 17%, and apparent systemic bioavailability of des-ciclesonide is 34% to 59%. Peak des-ciclesonide concentration is higher and more variable in lightweight horses (defined as body weight of 121.5 to 260.5 kg [266 to 574 lb]) compared with average weight horses. Drug accumulation is minimal with the labeled dosage. Ciclesonide volume of distribution is ≈26 L/kg in horses, and protein binding of des-ciclesonide in other species has been found to be ≈98% with less than 1% of the unbound drug found in the systemic circulation.[5,6] Enterohepatic recirculation may occur.[6] Half-life is 2 to 5 hours for ciclesonide and 3 to 6 hours for des-ciclesonide. The drug and metabolite are excreted primarily via the feces.[1,5,6]

Contraindications/Precautions/Warnings

Ciclesonide is contraindicated in patients that are hypersensitive to it.

Clinical improvement is expected to be delayed by several days after initiating therapy.[5] Ciclesonide is not a bronchodilator, and should not be used for management of acute bronchospasm.

Corticosteroids may worsen existing bacterial, viral, or fungal infections, and active respiratory infection should be ruled out prior to ciclesonide use; use with caution, if at all, in patients with active respiratory infection. The drug should be used with caution in horses with chronic nephritis, congestive heart failure, equine pituitary pars intermedia dysfunction (PPID), or in horses at higher risk for, or with a history of, laminitis.

Ensure that the device fits snugly in the patient's *left* nostril, as an incomplete dose may be delivered with a poor fit.

When transferring from systemic steroid therapy to inhaled glucocorticoids, systemic therapy may need to be slowly weaned to avoid acute adrenal insufficiency, and additional glucocorticoid therapy may be required during periods of acute stress, severe asthma attacks occurring during the withdrawal stage, or after transfer to inhaled steroids.

Adverse Effects

Common adverse effects reported[1] with ciclesonide nasal inhalation include cough during or after inhalation and nasal discharge; however, the incidence of these effects (≈17% and ≈10%, respectively) was similar to that reported for placebo inhalation. Adverse effects that might be attributable to ciclesonide include leukocytosis or neutrophilia (6.1%), nasal irritation (eg, soreness, redness, scabs) or bleeding (3% to 6%), sneezing (3%), increased sorbitol dehydrogenase (≈1.5%), and hives (0.6%).[1] The inhalation solution contains ethanol, which could cause ocular irritation if a dose inadvertently comes in contact with the horse's eyes.

According to the United States product label, laminitis developed in 3 horses, 2 of which had a history or prior evidence of laminitis.[1] In a large, placebo-controlled study of severe equine asthma, reported adverse events were minimal, and laminitis was not reported in any horses in the ciclesonide treatment arm ($n = 110$).[4]

Reproductive/Nursing Safety

Safe use of ciclesonide in pregnant mares has not been established. Ciclesonide was not found to be teratogenic in rats, but doses as low as 5 µg/kg/day SC administered to pregnant rabbits caused decreased body weight and fetal loss, reduced fetal weight, cleft palate, and skeletal abnormalities.[8] Corticosteroids that are administered during the last trimester may induce premature parturition leading to dystocia and fetal death, and therefore ciclesonide should only be used if the benefit to the mare outweighs the potential harm.

Safe use in lactating mares has not been established.

Ciclesonide should only be used in pregnant or lactating mares if the maternal benefit justifies the potential risk to offspring.

Overdosage/Acute Toxicity

Clinical signs in horses receiving up to 3 times the labeled dosage included mucoid and seromucoid nasal discharge, and weight loss (mean estimated weight loss of 24 kg [52.9 lb]).[1,6] Facial asymmetry was observed in 2 horses, one of which resolved during treatment. Cortisol was suppressed in 2 lightweight horses receiving 3 times the label dose. No other pathological changes were identified.

The oral LD_{50} in rats is over 2,000 mg/kg. Inhaled doses up to 5.3 mg/kg/day administered to rats for 2 weeks resulted in reduced food intake and body weight, and reduced organ weights in the spleen, thymus, and adrenal gland. Inhaled doses up to 1.8 mg/kg/day administered to dogs for 4 weeks resulted in reduced body weight and dose-dependent decrease in cortisol concentration as well as adrenal gland atrophy.[6] A reduced cortisol response to ACTH stimulation also was noted.

For patients that have experienced or are suspected to have experienced an overdose, it is strongly encouraged to consult with one of the 24-hour poison consultation centers that specialize in providing information specific for veterinary patients. For general information related to overdose and toxin exposures, as well as contact information for poison control centers, refer to ***Appendix.***

Drug Interactions

Coadministration of ciclesonide with clenbuterol was tolerated in a small number of horses.[9] The following drug interactions have either been reported or are theoretical in humans or animals receiving ciclesonide and may be of significance in veterinary patients. Unless otherwise noted, use together is not necessarily contraindicated, but weigh the potential risks and perform additional monitoring when appropriate.

- ASPIRIN: May increase risk for GI or renal toxicity
- BETA-BLOCKERS (eg, **atenolol, propranolol**): May exacerbate asthma signs
- CORTICOSTEROIDS (eg, **fludrocortisone, prednis(ol)one**): Concurrent use of inhaled ciclesonide with corticosteroids may increase the risk for GI or renal toxicity.
- KETOCONAZOLE: Concomitant use of ciclesonide with ketoconazole increased des-ciclesonide plasma concentration.[8]
- NONSTEROIDAL ANTI-INFLAMMATORY DRUGS (NSAIDs; eg, **phenylbutazone, firocoxib**): Combined use of ciclesonide with NSAIDs may increase the risk for GI or renal toxicity.
- PROTEIN-BOUND DRUGS (eg, **oral anticoagulants, other anti-inflammatory agents, salicylates, sulfonamides, sulfonylurea antidiabetic agents, valproic acid**): Because ciclesonide is highly bound to plasma proteins (≈98%), it could theoretically displace other highly bound drugs, causing a transient increase in serum levels of each drug. These interactions are unlikely to be of clinical concern because increased free drug levels will equilibrate through increased clearance. Monitor for adverse effects of each drug when using this combination.

Laboratory Considerations

- **Intradermal allergy testing (IDT)**: The effects of inhaled ciclesonide on intradermal allergy testing results are unknown. Systemic glucocorticoids suppress IDT results in horses[10] and inhaled budesonide suppresses IDT results in cats.[11]

Dosages

HORSES:

Severe equine asthma (label dosage; FDA-approved): Initially, 8 actuations (2744 µg ciclesonide)/horse twice daily for 5 days, followed by 12 actuations (4116 µg ciclesonide)/horse once daily for 5 days. **NOTE:** Dosage is independent of body weight. Total treatment duration is 10 days.[1]

Monitoring

- Clinical efficacy
- Adverse effects
- Because this is a new drug with a novel drug delivery system, suspected adverse effects should be reported to the manufacturer.

Client Information

- Dispense the drug with the manufacturer-supplied user manual, which contains very detailed instructions for use of the inhalation device.
- Be sure you understand how to properly activate the device, and how to administer doses. Shaking of the device is not required. Administer doses in a well-ventilated area.
- Ensure the inhaler device fits snugly into the left nostril prior to administering doses. An insecure fit may incompletely deliver doses.
- The device's breath indicator should be seen to curve inward with each inhalation and outward with exhalation. Reposition the device for a more secure fit in the nostril if these movements are not seen. Deliver a dose ("puff") at the *beginning* of an inhalation.
- The device is made to be used with only the left hand (ie, one-handed), while the right hand holds or controls the horse.
- The fill indicator displays the approximate percentage of doses available in the device. The device mechanism will continue to work even if no drug remains in the chamber. Discard after completion of a 10-day treatment course, even if the fill indicator reads above 0%.
- Discuss other equine asthma treatment options (eg, soaking hay, use of airway dilating medication) with your veterinarian.
- Contact your veterinarian if your horse's condition does not improve or worsens.
- Discharging the device will release the medicine into the air and could result in human exposure. It may be appropriate to wear an aerosol-filtering mask during administration. Ask your veterinarian or pharmacist for guidance.
- Not for use in humans. Pregnant women should not administer this product.

Chemistry/Synonyms

Ciclesonide is a nonhalogenated glucocorticoid that occurs as a white to yellow-white powder.[8] It is practically insoluble in water and freely soluble in ethanol. The commercial solution is a clear, colorless to yellow solution that also contains ethanol 0.84% but does not contain propellants.

Ciclesonide may also be known as *Aservo® EquiHaler®* for equine use, or *Alvesco®, Omnaris®, or Zetonna®* for human use.

Storage/Stability

Ciclesonide inhaler is a nonpressurized device. Store at 15°C to 30°C (59°F-86°F); excursions permitted up to 40°C (104°F).[1] Protect from freezing. Use within 12 days of activation. Discard after a 10-day treatment course has finished, even if the fill indicator reads above 0%.[1]

Compatibility/Compounding Considerations

None noted

Dosage Forms/Regulatory Status

VETERINARY-LABELED PRODUCTS:

The Association of Racing Commissioners International (ARCI) has designated other inhaled glucocorticoids (eg, budesonide, fluticasone) as class 4 substances. Use of this drug may not be allowed in certain animal competitions. Check rules and regulations before entering in a competition while this medication is being administered. Contact local racing authorities for further guidance. See ***Appendix*** for more information.

Ciclesonide Inhalation Spray: 343 µg/actuation in a 140-dose prefilled, nonpressurized nasal inhalation device containing ciclesonide 30 mg/mL; *Aservo® EquiHaler®*;(Rx). NADA #141-533. Each device contains enough doses for a 10-day treatment course. **NOTE**: Although human-labeled products containing ciclesonide are available, they are not intended to be used with this device. Do not use in horses intended for human consumption.

HUMAN-LABELED PRODUCTS:

Ciclesonide Metered Aerosol: 80 and 160 µg/actuation in pressurized metered dose inhalers containing 60 actuations; *Alvesco®*;(Rx)

Ciclesonide Metered Nasal Aerosol Solution: 37 µg/actuation; *Zetonna®*; (Rx)

Ciclesonide Metered Nasal Suspension: 50 37 µg/actuation; *Omnaris®*; (Rx)

References

For the complete list of references, see **wiley.com/go/budde/plumb**

Cimetidine

(sye-***met***-i-deen) *Tagamet®*

Histamine H_2 Receptor Antagonist

Prescriber Highlights

- Prototype H_2-receptor antagonist primarily used to reduce GI acid production. Newer H_2-antagonists (eg, ranitidine, famotidine) and other antacid agents (eg, omeprazole) are preferred due to greater efficacy, longer duration of activity, and/or fewer drug interactions.
- Use with caution in geriatric patients or those with hepatic or renal insufficiency
- Many drug interactions are possible.

Uses/Indications

Cimetidine use in veterinary and human medicine has been supplanted by newer agents that are more effective, need less frequent dosing, and do not have as many drug-interaction concerns. Cimetidine has also been used in the past as an adjunctive treatment for acetaminophen toxicity in cats; however, cimetidine may increase the risk of methemoglobinemia[1,2] in cats and some consider its use contraindicated.[2] Of note, adjunctive cimetidine use in the management of acetaminophen overdose was not effective in humans[3] and is not recommended.[4]

Historically, cimetidine has been used in veterinary medicine for the treatment and/or prophylaxis of gastric, abomasal, and duodenal ulcers; uremic gastritis; stress-related or drug-induced erosive gastritis; esophagitis; duodenal gastric reflux; and esophageal reflux. It has also been employed to treat hypersecretory conditions associated with gastrinomas and systemic mastocytosis. Cimetidine has also been used investigationally as an immunomodulating agent in dogs.

Cimetidine has been used for the treatment of melanomas in horses,[5] but efficacy is unproven.[6]

Pharmacology/Actions

At the H_2 receptors of the parietal cells, cimetidine competitively inhibits histamine, thereby reducing gastric acid output both during basal conditions and when stimulated by food, pentagastrin, histamine, or insulin. Gastric emptying time, pancreatic or biliary secretion, and lower esophageal pressures are not altered by cimetidine. By decreasing the amount of gastric acid secretions, cimetidine also decreases pepsin secretion.

Cimetidine has an apparent immunomodulating effect, as it has been demonstrated to reverse suppressor T-cell–mediated immune suppression. It also possesses weak anti-androgenic activity.

Pharmacokinetics

In dogs, the oral bioavailability of cimetidine is reported to be ≈75% to 95%; food can significantly reduce oral bioavailability. Serum half-life is 1.3 to 1.6 hours and volume of distribution is 1.2 L/kg.[7]

In horses, after oral administration, bioavailability is only ≈30%; after IV administration the steady-state volume of distribution is 1.1 L/kg, median plasma clearance is 0.44 L/kg/hour, and half-life is ≈2.2 hours.[8] Separately, a half-life of 7 hours was reported after oral administration.[9]

In humans, cimetidine is rapidly and well absorbed after oral administration, but a small amount is metabolized in the liver before entering the systemic circulation (first-pass effect). The oral bioavailability is 70% to 80%. Food may delay absorption and slightly decrease the amount absorbed, but when given with food, peak concentrations occur when the stomach is not protected by the buffering capabilities of the ingesta. Cimetidine is well distributed in body tissues and only 15% to 20% is bound to plasma proteins. Cimetidine is metabolized in the liver and excreted unchanged by the kidneys. More of the drug is excreted by the kidneys when administered parenterally (75%) than when given orally (48%). The average serum half-life of 2 hours can be prolonged in elderly patients and patients with renal or hepatic disease.

Contraindications/Precautions/Warnings

Cimetidine is contraindicated in patients with known hypersensitivity to the drug.

Cimetidine should be used cautiously in geriatric patients and patients with significantly impaired hepatic or renal function. In humans meeting these criteria, increased risk of CNS effects (confusion) may occur; dosage reductions may be necessary. Acid-suppressing therapy has been associated with increased risk of pneumonia in humans.[10]

Cimetidine inhibits CYP450 microsomal enzymes and may alter the metabolism of other drugs (see ***Drug Interactions*** below).

Adverse Effects

Adverse effects appear to be quite rare in animals at the dosages generally used. Potential adverse effects (documented in humans) include mental confusion, headache (upon discontinuation of the drug), increased liver transaminase activity (ie, increased ALT, AST), pancreatitis, and gynecomastia. Rarely, myalgia, arthralgia, and agranulocytosis may develop; if given rapidly IV, transient cardiac arrhythmias may be seen. Pain at the injection site may occur after IM administration.

Reproductive/Nursing Safety

Cimetidine crosses the placenta. No fetal harm was observed in laboratory animals given up to 40 times the normal human cimetidine dose.[11] In humans it is considered compatible with pregnancy.[12] High doses in humans have been associated with impotence[11]; relevance for veterinary patients is unknown.

Cimetidine is distributed into milk; although safety during nursing is not assured, it is usually considered compatible with nursing in humans.[12]

Overdose/Acute Toxicity

Clinical experience with cimetidine overdose is limited. In laboratory animals, toxic doses have been associated with tachycardia and respiratory failure.[11] The oral LD_{50} in mice is 2550 mg/kg.[13] If these signs occur, consider respiratory support and treatment with beta-adrenergic antagonists (eg, atenolol, propranolol). Peritoneal dialysis does not appreciably enhance the removal of cimetidine from the body.

For patients that have experienced or are suspected to have experienced an overdose, consultation with a 24-hour poison center specializing in providing veterinary-specific information is recommended. For general information related to overdose and toxin exposures, as well as contact information for poison control centers, refer to ***Appendix***.

Drug Interactions

The following drug interactions have either been reported or are theoretical in humans or animals receiving cimetidine and may be of significance in veterinary patients. Unless otherwise noted, use together is not necessarily contraindicated, but weigh the potential risks and perform additional monitoring when appropriate.

- **Antacids** (eg, **aluminum- and/or magnesium-containing agents**): May decrease the absorption of cimetidine; stagger doses (separate by 2 hours if possible).
- **Cefpodoxime, Cefuroxime:** Concurrent use may decrease antibacterial efficacy.
- **Clopidogrel:** Concurrent use may result in decreased clopidogrel efficacy because of lack of metabolism to its active form. However, the clinical effects of this are unclear.[14]
- **Iron Preparations, Oral** (eg, **ferrous sulfate**): Cimetidine may decrease iron absorption.
- **Itraconazole, Ketoconazole:** Cimetidine may decrease the absorption of these drugs; give these medications at least 2 hours before cimetidine.
- **Myelosuppressive Drugs**: Cimetidine may exacerbate leukopenias when used with myelosuppressive agents.
- **Tolazoline**: Concurrent use may result in decreased tolazoline efficacy.

Cimetidine may inhibit the hepatic microsomal enzyme system and thereby reduce the metabolism, prolong serum half-lives, and increase the serum concentrations of several drugs. It may also reduce the hepatic blood flow and reduce the amount of hepatic extraction of drugs that have a high first-pass effect, resulting in increased risk of adverse effects and toxicity. Affected drugs include:

- **Benzodiazepines** (eg, **alprazolam, diazepam, midazolam**)
- **Beta-Blockers** (eg, **atenolol, carvedilol, propranolol**)
- **Calcium Channel Blockers** (eg, **diltiazem, verapamil,** *not* **amlodipine**)
- **Carbamazepine**
- **Chloramphenicol**
- **Cisapride**
- **Cyclosporine** (no overall effect was found in dogs,[15] but interaction may apply to other species)
- **Domperidone**
- **Doxepin**
- **Epirubicin** (avoid combination)
- **Fluorouracil**
- **Glipizide/Glyburide**
- **Lidocaine**
- **Loratadine**
- **Metformin**
- **Metronidazole**
- **Mirtazapine**
- **Opioids** (eg, **alfentanil, fentanyl, hydrocodone**)
- **Pentoxifylline**
- **Praziquantel**
- **Procainamide**
- **Quinidine**
- **Sildenafil**
- **Selective Serotonin Reuptake Inhibitors** (SSRIs; eg, **fluoxetine, sertraline**)
- **Tamsulosin**
- **Theophylline**
- **Terbinafine**
- **Tramadol:** Cimetidine increases tramadol bioavailability.[16]
- **Triamterene**
- **Tricyclic Antidepressants** (TCAs; eg, **amitriptyline, clomipramine**)
- **Warfarin**

Laboratory Considerations

- **Creatinine**: Cimetidine may cause small increases in plasma creatinine concentrations early in therapy; these increases are generally mild, nonprogressive, and have disappeared when therapy is discontinued.
- **Gastric Acid Secretion Tests**: H_2-receptor antagonists may antagonize the effects of histamine and pentagastrin in the evaluation of gastric acid secretion; it is recommended that H_2-receptor antagonists be discontinued at least 24 hours before performing this test.
- **Intradermal allergy testing (IDT):** H_2-receptor antagonists may inhibit histamine responses[17]; based on half-life in dogs, consider discontinuing cimetidine at least 24 hours before performing this test in this species

Dosages

DOGS/CATS:

Esophagitis, gastritis, ulcer disease (extra-label): 5 – 10 mg/kg PO every 6 to 8 hours

HORSES:

Gastroprotectant, reduce stomach acid (extra-label): 300 – 600 mg per foal (NOT mg/kg) PO 3 to 4 times daily

Melanomas, adjunctive treatment (extra-label): 1.6 – 7.5 mg/kg PO once to twice daily.[6,18] Efficacy is questionable at these dosages, and 1 author[18] speculates that higher doses may be needed.

FERRETS:

Stress-induced GI ulcers (extra-label): 5 – 10 mg/kg PO 3 times daily[19]

RABBITS/RODENTS/SMALL MAMMALS:

Rabbits: GI ulceration (extra-label): 5 – 10 mg/kg PO every 8 to 12 hours[20]

Mice, rats, gerbils, hamsters, guinea pigs, chinchillas (extra-label): 5 – 10 mg/kg PO every 6 to 12 hours[21]

Monitoring

- Clinical efficacy (dependent on reason for use); monitored by decrease in clinical signs, endoscopic examination, intragastric pH, blood in feces
- Adverse effects if noted
- If drug interactions are possible, adverse or toxic effects of other drug therapy

Client Information

- Used to reduce stomach acid and to treat or prevent stomach ulcers
- Doses often need to be given 2 to 4 times per day; signs may recur if dosages are missed.
- Cimetidine interacts with many other medications. Do not give your animal new medicines without your veterinarian's approval.
- Cimetidine is available OTC (over the counter; without a prescription), but only give it to your animal if your veterinarian recommends it.

Chemistry/Synonyms

An H_2-receptor antagonist, cimetidine HCl occurs as a white to off-white crystalline powder. It has what is described as an "unpleasant" odor and a pK_a of 6.8. Cimetidine is sparingly soluble in water and soluble in alcohol.

Cimetidine HCl occurs as a white crystalline powder and is very soluble in water and soluble in alcohol. It has a pK_a of 7.11, and the commercial injection has a pH of 3.8 to 6.0.

Cimetidine may also be known as cimetidinum or SKF-92334; many trade names are available.

Storage/Stability

Cimetidine products should be stored protected from light in airtight containers and kept at room temperature, 20°C to 25°C (68°F-77°F).

Compatibility/Compounding Considerations

Compatibility is dependent on factors such as pH, concentration, temperature, and diluent used; specialized references or a hospital pharmacist should be consulted for more specific information.

Compounded preparation stability: Cimetidine oral suspension has been compounded from commercially available tablets.[22] Triturating twenty-four (24) cimetidine 300 mg tablets with 10 mL of glycerin and a sufficient quantity (up to 120 mL) of simple syrup yields a 60 mg/mL oral suspension that retains greater than 90% potency for 17 days stored at 4°C (39°F). Apply "shake well" and "refrigerate" labels to the compounded product.

Dosage Forms/Regulatory Status

VETERINARY-LABELED PRODUCTS: NONE.

The Association of Racing Commissioners International (ARCI) has designated this drug as a class 5 substance. See ***Appendix*** for more information. Use of this drug may not be allowed in certain animal competitions. Check rules and regulations before entering in a competition while this medication is being administered. Contact local racing authorities for further guidance.

HUMAN-LABELED PRODUCTS:

Cimetidine Oral Tablets: 200 mg, 300 mg, 400 mg, and 800 mg; *Tagamet®*, generic; (Rx, OTC)

Cimetidine HCl Oral Solution: 300 mg (as HCl)/5 mL in 240 mL, 480 mL, and UD 5 mL; generic; (Rx)

A parenteral solution was formerly available in the US but has been withdrawn.

References

For the complete list of references, see **wiley.com/go/budde/plumb**

Ciprofloxacin

(sip-roe-***flox***-a-sin) *Cipro®*

Fluoroquinolone Antibiotic

Prescriber Highlights

- ▶ Human-label fluoroquinolone antibiotic; in dogs and cats, oral bioavailability can be very low and unpredictable.
- ▶ Injectable products are formulated for IV administration only.
- ▶ Contraindicated in animals with a history of hypersensitivity to it or other fluoroquinolones
- ▶ When possible, avoid use in young, growing animals because of the potential negative impact on cartilage development.
- ▶ Caution is advised in patients with hepatic or renal insufficiency or dehydration.
- ▶ Adverse effects include GI distress, CNS stimulation, crystalluria, or hypersensitivity.
- ▶ Many potential drug interactions
- ▶ FDA prohibits extra-label use in food animals.

Uses/Indications

Ciprofloxacin is a broad-spectrum antibiotic with good gram-negative coverage. Because of its similar spectrum of activity, ciprofloxacin could be used as an alternative to enrofloxacin when an IV product is desired. It is important to note that ciprofloxacin and enrofloxacin cannot be considered equivalent because of pharmacokinetic differences (see ***Pharmacokinetics***). Because of ciprofloxacin's poor and variable bioavailability, there is little justification for its use in place of fluoroquinolones approved for veterinary use. Further, it has been suggested that human breakpoints for susceptibility should not be applied to isolates from dogs (and presumably cats) because of ciprofloxacin's poor bioavailability and because a much lower breakpoint should be used.[1]

The World Health Organization (WHO) has designated ciprofloxacin as a Critically Important, Highest Priority antimicrobial in human medicine.[2]

Pharmacology/Actions

Ciprofloxacin is a bactericidal and concentration-dependent antibiotic, with susceptible bacteria cell death occurring within 20 to 30 minutes of exposure. Ciprofloxacin has demonstrated a significant postantibiotic effect in both gram-negative and gram-positive bacteria and is active in both the stationary and growth phases of bacterial replication. Its mechanism of action is not thoroughly understood, but it is believed to act by inhibiting bacterial DNA-gyrase (a type II topoisomerase), thereby preventing DNA supercoiling and DNA synthesis.

Enrofloxacin and ciprofloxacin have similar spectrums of activity. Both agents have good activity against many gram-negative bacilli and cocci, including most species and strains of *Pseudomonas aeruginosa*, *Klebsiella* spp, *Escherichia coli*, *Enterobacter* spp, *Campylobacter* spp, *Shigella* spp, *Salmonella* spp, *Aeromonas* spp, *Haemophilus* spp, *Proteus* spp, *Yersinia* spp, *Serratia* spp, and *Vibrio* spp. Other organisms that are generally susceptible include *Brucella* spp, *Chlamydia trachomatis*, staphylococci (including penicillinase-producing and some methicillin-resistant strains), *Mycoplasma* spp, and *Mycobacterium* spp (except *Mycobacterium avium* subsp *paratuberculosis*, the etiologic agent for Johne's disease). However, acquired resistance is increasingly common in some important pathogens (eg, *Pseudomonas* spp, *Staphylococcus* spp, enterobacteriales [ie, *Escherichia coli*]). Ciprofloxacin has weak activity against streptococci and enterococci and is not recommended in the treatment of these infections; it is ineffective against anaerobes.

It is recommended that human breakpoints for susceptibility should not be applied to isolates from dogs because of ciprofloxacin's poor bioavailability and because a much lower breakpoint should be used. Even with a lower breakpoint, high doses are required. A dosage of 25 mg/kg PO once daily was estimated to have only an 18% chance of attaining a target AUC/MIC of 100 for bacteria with an MIC of 0.25 µg/mL.[1]

Development of resistance to this class of antibiotics is a concern with many bacteria, particularly *E coli*, staphylococci, and *P aeruginosa*. In a study of pigs receiving ciprofloxacin orally, *E coli* MIC increased 16-fold after only 3 days of treatment but decreased after the drug was stopped.[3] Temporary ciprofloxacin exposure to canine *E coli* isolates increased expression of drug efflux pumps, which are mechanisms for drug resistance.[4]

Pharmacokinetics

Ciprofloxacin is the active metabolite of enrofloxacin. Approximately 10% to 40% of circulating enrofloxacin is metabolized to ciprofloxacin in most species. Approximately 15% to 50% of both ciprofloxacin and enrofloxacin are eliminated unchanged in the urine by tubular secretion and glomerular filtration. Enrofloxacin and ciprofloxacin are metabolized to various metabolites that are less active than the parent compounds. These metabolites are eliminated in the urine and feces. Because of the dual means of elimination (ie, renal and hepatic), patients with severely impaired renal function may have slightly prolonged half-lives and higher serum concentrations but may not require dosage adjustment.

In dogs, ciprofloxacin's bioavailability is variable and significantly less than enrofloxacin, likely due to incomplete dissolution of tablets formulated for human use. In one study, after oral tablets (250 mg/dog [NOT mg/kg]) were administered to beagles, bioavailability ranged from 32% to 80% (mean, 58%). Administration of a 10 mg/mL solution given via stomach tube resulted in more uniform and consistent bioavailability (71%).[5] Improved absorption with an oral solution was confirmed in another study.[6] In dogs given a target dose of 25 mg/kg PO, the AUC was 13.6 to 22.5 µg/hour/mL.[1,5,7] Volume of distribution in the same study was 10.7 L/kg and peak plasma concentration was 1.9 µg/mL.[1] Elimination half-life has been reported to be 2.9 to 3.7 hours for IV administration[5,6] and 2.5 to 4.35 hours for PO administration.[1,5]

Oral bioavailability in cats can be very low. A study found that the oral bioavailability average in cats was ≈33%. After IV dosing, volume of distribution (steady-state) was ≈3.9 L/kg; clearance was ≈0.64 L/hour/kg; and elimination half-life averaged ≈4.5 hours.[8]

In a study in healthy mares, oral bioavailability was 10.5%.[9] Studies of the oral bioavailability in ponies have shown that ciprofloxacin is poorly absorbed (2% to 12%),[10] whereas enrofloxacin in foals is apparently well absorbed.[11] Terminal half-life in horses after PO and IV administration was 3.6 hours and 5.8 hours, respectively.[9] Minimal systemic absorption and exposure occurred after intrauterine ciprofloxacin administration to mares in estrus.[12] Following a single intrauterine infusion, resultant intrauterine lumen ciprofloxacin concentration was 148 µg/mL (± 33 µg/mL) and 91 µg/mL (± 51 µg/mL) 24 hours after infusion into healthy mares. Mean intrauterine concentrations 12 hours postinfusion were 10 to 40 times the MIC_{90} for *Klebsiella pneumoniae, Pseudomonas aeruginosa,* and *S equi* subsp *zooepidemicus*; at 24 hours postinfusion the intrauterine concentration was 1.2 to 5 times MIC_{90}. For *Escherichia coli*, ciprofloxacin concentration was 2000 times greater than MIC_{90} at both 12 and 24 hours postinfusion.[12]

In humans, the oral bioavailability of ciprofloxacin has been reported to be between 50% to 85%. The volume of distribution in adults is ≈2 L/kg to 3.5 L/kg, and it is ≈20% to 40% bound to serum proteins. High tissue concentrations are found in the kidneys, gallbladder, liver, and lungs.

Contraindications/Precautions/Warnings

There are potential concerns for cartilage damage in growing animals, although the incidence and highest risk periods are poorly defined. Bubble-like changes in articular cartilage have been noted when the drug was given at 2 to 5 times the recommended doses for 30 days, although clinical signs have only been reported at 5 times the recommended dose.[13] The need for fluoroquinolones must be balanced with the potential risk in dogs younger than 8 months of age. To avoid cartilage damage, treatment for large- and giant-breed dogs may need to wait until 12 to 18 months of age, respectively. Quinolones are also contraindicated in patients hypersensitive to them.

Because ciprofloxacin has occasionally been reported to cause crystalluria, animals should not be allowed to become dehydrated during therapy. In humans, ciprofloxacin has been associated with CNS stimulation and should be used with caution in patients with seizure disorders.[14] Patients with severe renal or hepatic impairment may require dosage adjustments to prevent drug accumulation. Fluoroquinolones increase risk for QTc interval prolongation in humans and should be used with caution in veterinary patients with cardiac disease. In humans, fluoroquinolones may exacerbate muscle weakness in patients with myasthenia gravis.[14]

No reports of retinal toxicity secondary to ciprofloxacin in cats have been located. Although retinal toxicity appears to be less likely than with a high dose of enrofloxacin (ciprofloxacin is less lipophilic than enrofloxacin), use of an alternative fluoroquinolone can be considered.

Adverse Effects

Potential adverse effects include cartilage abnormalities in young, growing animals (see ***Contraindications/Precautions/Warnings***); GI distress (eg, vomiting, anorexia, esophagitis, diarrhea); crystalluria/urolithiasis (dogs); CNS stimulation; and hypersensitivity reactions (dogs).

In a pharmacokinetic study in healthy mares,[9] IV ciprofloxacin caused agitation, excitement, and muscle fasciculation, and all horses experienced diarrhea. After oral administration, diarrhea, colitis, laminitis, and endotoxemia occurred, necessitating humane euthanasia in 3 of the 8 (≈39%) horses.[9] In mares receiving an intrauterine ciprofloxacin infusion, 3 of 10 horses had cytological evidence of intrauterine inflammation.[12]

In humans, systemic fluoroquinolones, including ciprofloxacin, have been associated with disabling and potentially irreversible serious adverse effects, including tendonitis and tendon rupture, peripheral neuropathy, and CNS effects (eg, convulsions, increased intracranial pressure, lowered seizure threshold). In humans, fluoroquinolones may also alter cardiac conduction and cause prolongation of the QTc interval, especially in those with a history of QTc interval prolongation, electrolyte disorders, and cardiac disease.

Reproductive/Nursing Safety

Ciprofloxacin crosses the placenta. Studies in laboratory animals have not demonstrated adverse fetal outcomes; however, because of ciprofloxacin's adverse effects on cartilage, it should be used cautiously in pregnant animals.

Ciprofloxacin is distributed into milk. In lactating cows given a CRI of ciprofloxacin (prohibited in the United States) for 7 days, ≈6% of the ciprofloxacin dose was transferred to milk, and ciprofloxacin concentration in milk was 45 times higher than in plasma. Milk from the cows was fed to calves, but oral absorption was negligible, and the drug did not accumulate in the calf.[15] No adverse effects have been reported in nursing human infants of mothers receiving ciprofloxacin.

Because safety has not been fully established in animals, this drug should only be used when the maternal benefits outweigh the potential risks to offspring.

Overdose/Acute Toxicity

Little specific information in veterinary patients is available. See ***Enrofloxacin*** for more information.

For patients that have experienced or are suspected to have experienced an overdose, consultation with a 24-hour poison consultation center specializing in providing veterinary-specific information is recommended. For general information related to overdose and toxin exposures, as well as contact information for poison control centers, refer to ***Appendix***.

Drug Interactions

In hepatic microsomes from healthy beagles, select fluoroquinolones (ie, ofloxacin, orbifloxacin, ciprofloxacin, enrofloxacin, norfloxacin) were shown to inhibit CYP1A activity, with ciprofloxacin the most likely to have clinically relevant drug interactions.[16] The following drug interactions have either been reported or are theoretical in humans or animals receiving ciprofloxacin and may be of significance in veterinary patients. Unless otherwise noted, use together is not necessarily contraindicated, but the potential risks should be weighed and additional monitoring performed when appropriate.

- ALUMINUM-, CALCIUM-, AND MAGNESIUM-CONTAINING ORAL PRODUCTS: May bind to fluoroquinolones and prevent absorption; doses of these products should be separated from ciprofloxacin by at least 2 hours
- ANTIBIOTICS, OTHER (eg, **aminoglycosides, extended spectrum penicillins, third-generation cephalosporins**): Synergism may occur against some bacteria (particularly *Pseudomonas aeruginosa*), but this is unpredictable. Although enrofloxacin and ciprofloxacin have minimal activity against anaerobes, in vitro synergy has been reported when used with clindamycin against strains of *Peptostreptococcus* spp, *Lactobacillus* spp, and *Bacteroides fragilis*.
- BLOOD GLUCOSE LOWERING AGENTS (eg, **insulin, sulfonylureas** [eg, **glipizide, glyburide**]): Fluoroquinolones may enhance hypoglycemic effect of blood glucose lowering agents.
- CORTICOSTEROIDS (eg, **dexamethasone, prednis[ol]one**): Concomitant use with fluoroquinolones may increase the risk for tendonitis and tendon rupture.
- CYCLOSPORINE (**systemic**): Fluoroquinolones may exacerbate nephrotoxicity and reduce the metabolism of cyclosporine.
- DOXORUBICIN: Ciprofloxacin may increase doxorubicin exposure in humans. Combination may also increase the risk for QT prolongation.
- DRUGS THAT PROLONG QT INTERVAL (eg, **azithromycin, chlorpromazine, cisapride, fluconazole, fluoxetine, ketoconazole, methadone, ondansetron, quinidine, sotalol**): Combinations with ciprofloxacin may increase the risk for QTc prolongation; concurrent use of cisapride and ciprofloxacin is contraindicated in humans.
- FENTANYL: Ciprofloxacin may increase fentanyl effects.
- FLUNIXIN: Enrofloxacin increases the AUC and prolongs the elimination half-life of flunixin in dogs, which could increase flunixin toxicity. Flunixin decreases the C_{max} of enrofloxacin in dogs, which could decrease antibiotic efficacy. Interaction may apply to ciprofloxacin.
- IRON, ZINC (**oral**): Concomitant administration may decrease fluoroquinolone absorption; doses should be separated by at least 2 hours.
- LANTHANUM: Concomitant administration decreases ciprofloxacin absorption by 50% in humans; use of an alternate phosphate binder is recommended.
- LEVOTHYROXINE: Ciprofloxacin may decrease levothyroxine efficacy.
- MAGNESIUM (**parenteral**): May bind to fluoroquinolones and prevent absorption; doses of these products being administered by the same route as ciprofloxacin should be separated by at least 2 hours
- METHOTREXATE (MTX): Concomitant administration may increase MTX concentrations and increase the risk for toxicity.
- MYCOPHENOLATE: Ciprofloxacin may decrease mycophenolic acid exposure.
- NITROFURANTOIN: May antagonize the antimicrobial activity of fluoroquinolones; concomitant use is not recommended
- PROBENECID: Blocks renal tubular secretion of ciprofloxacin and may increase ciprofloxacin serum concentrations and elimination half-life. Monitor for increased ciprofloxacin adverse effects (eg, nausea, diarrhea).
- SEVELAMER: Concomitant administration decreases ciprofloxacin absorption by 50% in humans; administer ciprofloxacin at least 2 hours before or 6 hours after sevelamer.
- SILDENAFIL: Concomitant use with ciprofloxacin may increase sildenafil serum concentrations and adverse effects.[13]
- SUCRALFATE: Concomitant oral administration may inhibit GI absorption of ciprofloxacin; doses of these drugs should be separated by at least 2 hours.[7,13]
- THEOPHYLLINE DERIVATIVES (eg, **aminophylline, theophylline**): Enrofloxacin reduces theophylline metabolism in dogs, increasing theophylline serum concentration by 30% to 50%[17]; interaction likely applies to ciprofloxacin.
- WARFARIN: Concomitant use may increase anticoagulant effects of warfarin.

Laboratory Considerations

- In some humans, fluoroquinolones have caused increases in **liver**

enzymes, **BUN**, and **creatinine** and decreases in **hematocrit**. The clinical relevance of these mild changes in veterinary patients is unknown.

Dosages

NOTES:

1) Considering improved bioavailability of other approved fluoroquinolones after oral administration, ciprofloxacin is best reserved for use when an IV fluoroquinolone is indicated and a fluoroquinolone approved for veterinary use is not available.
2) Ciprofloxacin IV should be administered slowly to reduce the risk for vein irritation. In humans, IV ciprofloxacin is given as a diluted solution (0.5 – 2 mg/mL) by slow IV infusion over 60 minutes into a large vein.

DOGS:

Susceptible infections (extra-label): 25 mg/kg PO or 20 mg/kg IV slowly once daily. **NOTE**: Because of the drug's variable oral bioavailability in dogs, a dosage of 25 mg/kg PO once daily may not achieve adequate drug exposure for bacteria with an MIC greater than 0.06 µg/mL, despite the human breakpoint (1 µg/mL) often used by laboratories.[1,7]

Bacterial pyoderma (extra-label): 30 mg/kg PO once daily[18]

UTI (extra-label): 30 mg/kg PO once daily[19]

CATS:

Susceptible infections (extra-label): 20 – 25 mg/kg PO or IV slowly once daily

UTI (extra-label): 30 mg/kg PO once daily[19]

HORSES:

Endometritis (extra-label): 600 mg/horse (NOT mg/kg) via intrauterine infusion. **NOTE:** Dosage based on a pharmacokinetic study in healthy mares.[12]

BIRDS:

NOTE: Higher doses administered once daily are considered more clinically appropriate than lower, twice-daily dosages.

Susceptible gram-negative infections (extra-label):

a) 20 – 40 mg/kg PO twice daily using ciprofloxacin 500 mg tablets. Crushed tablets mix into the suspension well but must be shaken before administering.[20]
b) 20 mg/kg PO every 12 hours[21]
c) 10 – 15 mg/kg PO every 12 hours[22]

FERRETS:

NOTE: Higher doses administered once daily are considered more clinically appropriate than lower, twice-daily dosages.

Susceptible infections (extra-label):

a) 10 – 30 mg/kg PO every 24 hours[23]
b) 5 – 15 mg/kg PO twice daily[24]

RABBITS/RODENTS/SMALL MAMMALS:

NOTE: Higher doses administered once daily are considered more clinically appropriate than lower, twice-daily dosages.

a) **Rabbits** (extra-label): 5 – 20 mg/kg PO every 12 to 24 hours[24]
b) **Pasteurellosis in rabbits** (extra-label):
   i. 15 – 20 mg/kg PO twice daily for a minimum of 14 days in mild cases and up to several months in chronic infections[25]
   ii. 20 mg/kg IV, PO once daily based on a pharmacokinetic study.[26]
c) **Chinchillas, gerbils, guinea pigs, hamsters, mice, rats** (extra-label): 5 – 20 mg/kg PO every 12 to 24 hours[24]

Monitoring

- Clinical efficacy
- Adverse effects

Client Information

- This medicine should be given without food and on an empty stomach. However, it may be given with a small amount of food or treat if your animal experiences an upset stomach (eg, salivating, refusing to eat, vomiting). Contact your veterinarian if upset stomach persists.
- Do not give this medicine at the same time as other drugs or vitamins that contain calcium, iron, or aluminum, as these can reduce the amount that gets absorbed.
- Ciprofloxacin may cause joint abnormalities if used in young, pregnant, or nursing animals.
- The most common side effects are vomiting, nausea, and diarrhea.

Chemistry/Synonyms

Ciprofloxacin HCl, a fluoroquinolone antibiotic, occurs as a faintly yellowish to yellow crystalline powder. It is slightly soluble in water. Ciprofloxacin is related structurally to the veterinary FDA-approved drug enrofloxacin (enrofloxacin has an additional ethyl group on the piperazinyl ring).

Ciprofloxacin may also be known as ciprofloxacine, ciprofloxacinum, ciprofloxacino, Bay-q-3939, or *Cipro®*.

Storage/Stability

Unless otherwise directed by the manufacturer, ciprofloxacin tablets should be stored in airtight containers at temperatures less than 30°C (86°F). Protect this product from strong UV light. The injection should be stored at 5°C to 25°C (41°F-77°F) and protected from light and freezing.

Compatibility/Compounding Considerations

Compatibility is dependent on factors such as pH, concentration, temperature, and diluent used. Specialized references or a hospital pharmacist should be consulted for more specific information.

Ciprofloxacin should be diluted to a concentration of 1 to 2 mg/mL in 5% dextrose, 0.9% sodium chloride, or lactated Ringer's solution (LRS) prior to IV administration. Diluted solutions in 5% dextrose, 0.9% sodium chloride, or LRS from 0.5 to 2 mg/mL are stable for up to 14 days at room temperature or in the refrigerator.

The manufacturer recommends administering IV ciprofloxacin alone and temporarily discontinuing other solutions or drugs while ciprofloxacin is being administered; however, other sources state that ciprofloxacin injection is reportedly **compatible** with the following IV solutions and drugs: 5% dextrose, 5% dextrose with 0.22% or 0.45% sodium chloride, Ringer's solution, lactated Ringer's solution (LRS), 0.9% sodium chloride; **Y-site compatible with** amikacin sulfate, amiodarone, aztreonam, calcium gluconate, ceftazidime, cimetidine, clarithromycin, cyclophosphamide, cyclosporine, cytarabine, dexmedetomidine, diltiazem, diphenhydramine, dobutamine, dopamine, fluconazole, gentamicin, hydromorphone, lidocaine, metoclopramide, metronidazole, midazolam, mycophenolate mofetil hydrochloride, ondansetron, oxytocin, potassium chloride (KCl), ranitidine, tobramycin, vancomycin, voriconazole, and vitamin B complex.

Ciprofloxacin injection is reportedly **incompatible** with aminocaproic acid, aminophylline, amphotericin B, ampicillin/sulbactam, azithromycin, cefepime, cefuroxime, clindamycin, dexamethasone sodium phosphate, furosemide, heparin sodium, magnesium sulfate, meropenem, methylprednisolone sodium succinate, pantoprazole, piperacillin/tazobactam, potassium phosphate, propofol, sodium bicarbonate, and sodium phosphate.

The pH of the IV solution in vials ranges from 3.3 to 3.9, and pH of the IV solution in PVC bags ranges from 3.5 to 4.6.

Dosage Forms/Regulatory Status

VETERINARY-LABELED PRODUCTS: NONE

HUMAN-LABELED PRODUCTS:

Ciprofloxacin Oral Tablets: 100 mg, 250 mg, 500 mg, 750 mg, and 1000 mg; *Cipro®*, generic; (Rx)

Ciprofloxacin Extended-Release Oral Tablets: 500 mg and 1000 mg; *Cipro XR®*, generic; (Rx)

Ciprofloxacin Solution for Injection: 200 mg and 400 mg in 100 mL and 200 mL, respectively, in 5% dextrose flexible containers (0.2%); *Cipro® I.V.*, generic; (Rx)

In the United States, the FDA has banned extra-label use of ciprofloxacin (and other fluoroquinolones) in food animals.

References

For the complete list of references, see **wiley.com/go/budde/plumb**

Cisapride

(***sis***-a-pride)

Promotility Agent

Prescriber Highlights

- Oral GI prokinetic agent used in several species for GI stasis, gastroesophageal reflux, and constipation/megacolon (cats)
- Not commercially available; must be obtained from a compounding pharmacy
- Contraindications include hypersensitivity to the drug and use for patients in which increased GI motility could be harmful (eg, GI perforation, obstruction, hemorrhage).
- Unlike in humans, cisapride-induced arrhythmias have not been reported in veterinary patients.
- Adverse effects appear to be minimal in veterinary patients; vomiting, diarrhea, and abdominal discomfort can occur.
- Many drug interactions are possible.

Uses/Indications

Proposed uses for cisapride in small animal species include treatment of gastroesophageal reflux, reflux esophagitis, and primary gastric motility disorders. It may be used for the prevention of reflux and aspiration pneumonia in dogs during surgery.[1-3] Cisapride has been found to be useful in the treatment of constipation and megacolon in cats. Cisapride has also been proposed to enhance detrusor contractility in dogs with micturition disorders,[4] but it is not commonly used for this purpose. Cisapride has limited efficacy in conditions of esophageal dysmotility.

Pharmacology/Actions

Cisapride is a 5-HT_4-receptor agonist that enhances the release of acetylcholine at the myenteric plexus without stimulating nicotinic or muscarinic receptors or inhibiting acetylcholinesterase activity. Cisapride is also a 5-HT_1- and 5-HT_3-receptor antagonist of the enteric cholinergic neurons; it is a direct 5-HT_2-alpha-receptor agonist on colonic smooth muscle. The drug stimulates smooth muscle contraction (thus increasing lower esophageal peristalsis and sphincter pressure), [1,5] increases gastric contractions,[6] accelerates gastric emptying,[7] and promotes small[8,9] and large[10] intestinal motility. Cisapride blocks dopaminergic receptors to a lesser extent than metoclopramide and does not increase gastric acid secretion. Cisapride stimulates distal esophageal smooth muscle and is considered ineffective for distal esophageal dysmotility in dogs due to the striated muscle of that species' distal esophagus. In horses, cisapride attenuated the gastric hypomotility effects of endotoxin under experimental conditions[7], and it increased GI motility and rate of passage in horses with chronic grass sickness.[11] Cisapride may be preferred to promote colonic activity over metoclopramide, as it does not cause collapse when it is given IV. Cisapride did not increase gastric or intestinal contractility in the bovine abomasal antrum or proximal duodenal smooth muscle preparations.[12]

Pharmacokinetics

In dogs, the oral bioavailability of cisapride has been reported as ≈53%.[13] It is widely distributed into tissues and has a high volume of distribution. Plasma protein binding is 95%. Cisapride is hepatically metabolized to mostly inactive compounds, with ≈25% of an oral dose eliminated in the urine and ≈70% in the feces, and ≈23% of the dose is excreted unchanged in the feces.[14] Half-life in dogs is reported as ≈4 to 10 hours[13]; a study evaluating lower esophageal pressure in dogs after cisapride administration (0.5 mg/kg PO) found that effects were absent after 7 hours.[15]

In cats, the oral bioavailability is variable but averages 30%, and the elimination half-life is ≈5 to 6 hours.[16]

In horses, the oral bioavailability is ≈50%, the volume of distribution is 1.5 L/kg, and clearance is ≈0.5 L/hour/kg.[17] The elimination half-life is ≈2 hours.[17,18] The drug is not appreciably absorbed after rectal administration.[18,19]

In humans, cisapride is rapidly absorbed after oral administration. Bioavailability is 35% to 40%, indicating substantial first-pass metabolism. The drug is ≈98% bound to plasma proteins and well distributed throughout the body. Cisapride is extensively metabolized in the liver, primarily by CYP3A4.[20] The elimination half-life is ≈6 to 12 hours.[21]

Contraindications/Precautions/Warnings

Cisapride is contraindicated in patients in which increased GI motility could be harmful (eg, perforation, obstruction, GI hemorrhage) or in patients that are hypersensitive to the drug. Use it with caution in patients with significant hepatic impairment and in patients with mechanical obstruction, GI perforation, or GI hemorrhage. Correct hypokalemia and hypomagnesemia prior to use; use cisapride with caution in patients that may experience precipitous decreases in plasma potassium (eg, potassium-wasting diuretics, insulin).

In humans, cisapride therapy has resulted in QTc prolongation leading to fatal arrhythmias (eg, torsade de pointes, ventricular tachycardia, ventricular fibrillation) and is contraindicated in patients with QTc prolongation or other conditions (eg, AV block, cardiomyopathy) that predispose to or potentiate QTc prolongation, including drugs that inhibit CYP3A. Significance in veterinary species is unclear; cisapride-induced arrhythmias have not been reported in veterinary patients.

Adverse Effects

Cisapride appears to be safe in small animal species at recommended dosages. Occasionally, vomiting, diarrhea, and abdominal discomfort may be noted. Although no reports have been noted in dogs or cats, prolonged QT intervals or other cardiac arrhythmias are possible.

In humans, the primary adverse effects are GI related with diarrhea and abdominal pain most commonly reported, but the drug was removed from the market due to concerns with QT-interval prolongation.[22]

Reproductive/Nursing Safety

Cisapride at high dosages (greater than 40 mg/kg/day) caused fertility impairment in female rats.[23] At doses 12 to 100 times the maximum recommended dose, cisapride caused embryotoxicity and fetotoxicity in rabbits and rats. Its use during pregnancy should occur only when the benefits outweigh the risks.

Cisapride is excreted in maternal milk; use it with caution in nursing mothers.

Overdose/Acute Toxicity

LD_{50} doses in various laboratory animal species range from 160 to 4000 mg/kg. The reported oral lethal dose in dogs is 640 mg/kg.[24] In one reported human overdose of 540 mg, the patient developed GI distress and pollakiuria. The most common adverse effects seen in dogs and cats are diarrhea, lethargy, ataxia, hypersalivation, muscle fasciculations, agitation, abnormal behavior, hyperthermia, ataxia and incoordination, and possibly seizures (dogs).[24]

Significant overdoses should be handled using standard gastric decontamination protocols when appropriate; supportive therapy should be initiated when required. Activated charcoal is effective in binding unabsorbed cisapride.

For patients that have experienced or are suspected of having experienced an overdose, consultation with a 24-hour poison consultation center specializing in providing veterinary-specific information is recommended. For general information related to overdose and toxin exposures, as well as contact information for poison control centers, refer to ***Appendix***.

Drug Interactions

In humans, cisapride is a substrate of CYP3A4. The following drug interactions have either been reported or are theoretical in humans or animals receiving cisapride and may be of significance in veterinary patients. Unless otherwise noted, use together is not necessarily contraindicated, but weigh the potential risks and perform additional monitoring when appropriate.

- **Anticholinergic Agents** (eg, **atropine**): Use of anticholinergic agents may diminish the effects of cisapride.
- **Benzodiazepines**: Cisapride may enhance the sedative effects of alcohol or benzodiazepines.
- **Cyclosporine**: Cisapride may increase the risk for cyclosporine toxicity.
- **Diuretics, Potassium Wasting** (eg, **furosemide**): Hypokalemia may increase the risk for cardiac arrhythmias.
- **Highly Protein Bound Drugs** (eg, **nonsteroidal anti-inflammatory agents [NSAIDs], oral anticoagulants, salicylates, sulfonamides, sulfonylurea antidiabetic agents, valproic acid**): Because cisapride is highly bound to plasma proteins, it could theoretically displace other highly bound drugs, causing a transient increase in serum concentrations of each drug. These interactions are unlikely to be of clinical concern because increased free drug concentrations will equilibrate through increased clearance. Monitor for adverse effects of each drug when using this combination.
- **Insulin**: Insulin-induced decrease in plasma potassium concentration may increase the risk for cardiac arrhythmias.
- **Opioids** (eg, **fentanyl, morphine**): May diminish the effects of cisapride
- **Oral Drugs With A Narrow Therapeutic Index** (eg, **digoxin, warfarin**): Closer monitoring of serum drug concentrations may be needed when adding or discontinuing cisapride, as cisapride can decrease GI transit times and potentially affect the absorption of other oral drugs.
- **Warfarin**: Cisapride may enhance anticoagulant effects; additional monitoring and anticoagulant dosage adjustments may be required.

As cisapride is metabolized via CYP450 (3A4 in humans), the following medications/foods that can inhibit this enzyme may lead to increased cisapride concentrations and an increased risk for cisapride cardiotoxicity:

- **Amiodarone**
- **Azole Antifungals** (eg, **fluconazole, itraconazole, ketoconazole**)
- **Chloramphenicol**
- **Cimetidine**
- **Fluvoxamine**
- **Grapefruit Juice/Powder**
- **Macrolide Antibiotics** (**except azithromycin**): **NOTE:** Erythromycin did not alter cisapride pharmacodynamics in one study in dogs.
- **Ondansetron**

The following drugs may increase QTc interval, and use with cisapride may increase this risk:

- **Amiodarone**
- **Domperidone**
- **Fluoroquinolones** (eg, **ciprofloxacin, moxifloxacin**)
- **Macrolide Antibiotics** (including **azithromycin**): Dose-related QT prolongation occurred in dogs receiving an erythromycin and cisapride combination, but arrhythmias were not observed.[25]
- **Methadone**
- **Phenothiazines** (eg, **promethazine**, possibly **acepromazine**)
- **Procainamide**
- **Quinidine**
- **Sotalol**
- **Tricyclic Antidepressants** (eg, **amitriptyline, clomipramine, doxepin**)

Dosages

DOGS:

Promotility agent (extra-label): Initially, 0.1 – 0.5 mg/kg PO every 8 to 12 hours; some gastroenterologists recommend administering 30 minutes before feeding. Some sources state that dosages (gradually increased) up to 1 mg/kg PO every 8 hours may be required (if tolerated).[26]

Reduce gastroesophageal reflux and aspiration pneumonia in anesthetized dogs: Cisapride 1 mg/kg IV combined with esomeprazole (1 mg/kg IV) 11.5 hours prior to anesthesia.[2] Alternately, cisapride 1 mg/kg IV infusion (diluted in 100 or 150 mL 0.9% sodium chloride) beginning 90 minutes prior to anesthesia induction. Half of the admixed volume is delivered over the first 60 minutes, and if vital parameters (eg, TPR) are acceptable, the remaining volume is administered over 30 minutes.[3] (**NOTE:** Finding a compounding pharmacy to prepare cisapride for injection can be difficult.)

CATS:

Promotility agent (extra-label):

a) Initially, 2.5 mg/cat (NOT mg/kg) PO twice daily, preferably 15 to 30 minutes before food. Dosages may be titrated upwards, if tolerated, to as high as 7.5 mg/cat (NOT mg/kg) PO 3 times daily in large cats. Cats with hepatic insufficiency may need dosage interval extensions.[27-29]
b) 1 mg/kg PO every 8 hours, or 1.5 mg/kg PO every 12 hours based on a study in 7 healthy cats[16]
c) 2.5 mg/cat (NOT mg/kg) PO every 8 hours in cats less than 5 kg (11 lb); 5 mg/cat (NOT mg/kg) PO every 8 hours in cats greater than 5 kg (11 lb)[26]

HORSES:

Promotility agent in foals with periparturient asphyxia (extra-label): 10 mg/horse (NOT mg/kg) PO every 6 to 8 hours. Adequate time for healing of damaged bowel before using prokinetic agents is essential.[30]

Chronic grass sickness (extra-label): 0.1 mg/kg IM 3 times daily for 7 days, or 0.8 mg/kg PO 3 times daily for 7 days[11]

Promotility agent in adult horses: In a study of 7 clinically healthy male horses, cisapride was administered at a dose of 0.22 mg/kg PO every 8 hours for 2 days.[31] GI transit time, bowel movements per day, and stool weight were significantly improved with cisapride as compared with the control phase (no drug).

RABBITS/RODENTS/SMALL MAMMALS:

Promotility agent (extra-label):

a) **Mice, rats, gerbils, hamsters, guinea pigs, chinchillas**: 0.1 – 0.5 mg/kg PO every 12 hours[32]

b) **Rabbits for GI stasis**: 0.5 mg/kg PO every 6 to 12 hours. With IV or SC fluids, depending on the amount of dehydration, feeding a high-fiber slurry, with or without metoclopramide (0.2 – 1 mg/kg PO, SC every 6 to 8 hours). Begin after first stools were produced or no intestinal obstruction appreciated. It may be synergistic if used with ranitidine (0.5 mg/kg IV every 24 hours).[33,34]

c) **Ileus if GI tract not obstructed in guinea pigs, chinchillas**: 0.5 mg/kg every 8 to 12 hours (*Route not specified; assume PO*)[35]

Monitoring

- Efficacy
- Adverse effects
- ECG in patients with underlying cardiac disease (eg, arrhythmias) or concurrently receiving other potentially pro-arrhythmic drugs

Client Information

- Side effects are not common, but vomiting, diarrhea, and abdominal discomfort can occur.
- This medicine may be given with or without food.
- Give this medicine as directed by your veterinarian.
- Other medications can interact with cisapride, so be sure to tell your veterinarian and pharmacist what medications (including vitamins, supplements, or herbal therapies) you give your animal, including the amount and time you give each.

Chemistry/Synonyms

Cisapride is a substituted piperidinyl benzamide and is structurally but not pharmacologically related to procainamide and metoclopramide. It is available commercially as a monohydrate, but the potency is expressed in terms of the anhydrate.

Cisapride may also be known as cisapridum or R-51619; many trade names are registered.

Storage/Stability

Unless otherwise instructed by the manufacturer, store cisapride tablets in tight, light-resistant containers at room temperature.

Compatibility/Compounding Considerations

Compounded preparation stability: Cisapride oral suspension compounded from commercially available tablets has been published.[36] Triturating twelve (12) cisapride 10 mg tablets with 60 mL of *Ora-Plus*® and add *Ora-Sweet*® *qs ad* to 120 mL, with pH finally adjusted to 7 with sodium bicarbonate. This yields a 1 mg/mL oral suspension that retains greater than 90% potency for 60 days stored at both 5°C (41°F) and 25°C (77°F). Although cisapride tablets are no longer commercially available, the active pharmaceutical ingredient powder (medicinal grade) may be used to compound suitable oral suspensions of cisapride. Compounded preparations of cisapride should be protected from light. A cisapride 1 mg/mL suspension formulated in a 1:1 combination of simple syrup and methylcellulose 1% was found to be stable for 28 days at room temperature and for 91 days when refrigerated.[37] **NOTE:** Medicinal-grade cisapride should be purchased from FDA-approved pharmacies and must be of USP quality. The USP has an approved monograph with stability information.

Compatibility is dependent on factors such as pH, concentration, temperature, and diluent used; specialized references or a hospital pharmacist should be consulted for more specific information. Anecdotally, compounded cisapride injection is incompatible when mixed in the same syringe as cefazolin injection.

Dosage Forms/Regulatory Status

VETERINARY-LABELED PRODUCTS: NONE

HUMAN-LABELED PRODUCTS: NONE

Because of adverse effects in humans, cisapride has been removed from the US market. It may be available from compounding pharmacies.

References

For the complete list of references, see **wiley.com/go/budde/plumb**

Cisplatin

(***sis***-pla-tin) *Platinol*®

Antineoplastic

Prescriber Highlights

- ► Platinum antineoplastic agent used for a variety of carcinomas and sarcomas
- ► **Systemic use is contraindicated in cats.**
- ► Contraindicated in patients with preexisting significant renal impairment or myelosuppression
- ► Drug-related deaths possible
- ► The most common adverse effects include vomiting (pretreat with antiemetic), nephrotoxicity (use forced saline diuresis), ototoxicity, and myelosuppression. Many other adverse effects are possible.
- ► Must be given as slow IV infusion; rapid administration (less than 5 minutes) may increase toxicity
- ► The National Institute for Occupational Safety and Health (NIOSH) classifies cisplatin as a hazardous drug; use appropriate precautions when handling; it is teratogenic, fetotoxic, and may cause azoospermia.

Uses/Indications

The systemic use of cisplatin is presently limited to treatment of dogs with a variety of neoplastic diseases including squamous cell carcinoma, transitional cell carcinoma, ovarian carcinoma, osteosarcoma, nasal carcinoma, and thyroid adenocarcinoma. There is some evidence that efficacy for transitional cell carcinoma can be enhanced with concurrent NSAIDs.[1]

Cisplatin may also be useful for the palliative control of neoplastic pulmonary effusions after intracavitary administration.[2,3]

Intralesional injections of compounded cisplatin suspension in oil or as cisplatin-impregnated beads have been used for intralesional treatment of skin tumors (sarcoids) in horses. Cisplatin also shows some promise as an electrochemotherapy agent for treating incompletely excised mast cell tumors or sarcomas[4] in dogs,[5] sarcoids in horses,[6] incompletely excised injection site sarcomas in cats,[7] (ie, injected into tumor margins, *not* systemically administered), and potentially fibromas in birds.[8]

Cisplatin has also been used successfully as a topical treatment for equine hoof cankers.[9]

Various studies have investigated the use of liposomal cisplatin and cisplatin in hyaluronan nanoparticle carriers; however, current data do not support the use of these formulations.[10–13]

Pharmacology/Actions

Cisplatin is an antineoplastic agent. Its chemical reactivity is nonspecific, but the primary cytotoxic effect is thought to be due to intra- and interstrand DNA cross-linking that causes single- and double-stranded DNA breakage, impairs DNA replication, RNA transcription and protein synthesis, leading to cell death and inhibition of tumor growth.

Acquired resistance to cisplatin has been reported and is thought to be due to several mechanisms.[14]

Pharmacokinetics

After administration, the drug concentrates in the liver, lungs, ovaries, uterus, and kidneys. Cisplatin is highly protein bound (90%) and is renally excreted.

In dogs, cisplatin exhibits a biphasic elimination profile. The initial plasma half-life is short (≈20 to 50 minutes), but the terminal phase is much longer (≈60 to 80 hours). Approximately 80% of a dose can be recovered as free platinum in the urine within 48 hours of cisplatin dosing in dogs.[15]

Contraindications/Precautions/Warnings

Systemic cisplatin use is contraindicated in cats because of severe dose-related primary pulmonary toxicities (dyspnea, hydrothorax, pulmonary edema, mediastinal edema, and death). Death can occur within 2 to 4 days of administration. Cats given intralesional chemotherapy have also developed sarcomas at the injection site.[16] Cisplatin is also contraindicated in patients with significant preexisting renal impairment, myelosuppression, or a history of hypersensitivity to it or other platinum-containing compounds (eg, carboplatin).

Cisplatin-induced nephrotoxicity is dose-related. Ensure adequate hydration before, during, and after administration and monitor renal values. Because of the diuresis required prior to and after dosing, cisplatin should be used with caution in patients with congestive heart failure. Cumulative renal toxicity, ototoxicity, and neurotoxicity have been reported in humans. Ocular toxicity has also been reported in humans with standard doses. Cisplatin should **not** be administered IM or SC due to the risk for tissue irritation.

Cisplatin is classified as a highly emetogenic chemotherapeutic agent; patients should be premedicated with antiemetics.[17]

Owners must understand the importance of immediately reporting any signs associated with toxicity (eg, abnormal bleeding, bruising, abnormal urination, depression, infection, shortness of breath).

Do not confuse CISplatin with CARBOplatin. Consider using tall man lettering when writing orders or prescriptions. Cisplatin is considered a high alert medication (medication that requires special safeguards to reduce the risk for errors). Consider instituting practices such as redundant drug dosage and volume checking and special alert labels.[18]

Aluminum can react with cisplatin, causing precipitates and loss of potency. Thus, for the preparation or administration of cisplatin, needles or administration sets containing aluminum parts should NOT be used.[17]

The National Institute for Occupational Safety and Health (NIOSH) classifies cisplatin as a hazardous drug; personal protective equipment (PPE) should be used accordingly to minimize the risk for exposure.[19]

Adverse Effects

In dogs, the most frequent adverse effect seen after cisplatin treatment is vomiting, usually occurring within 6 hours after dosing and can persist for 1 to 6 hours. Maropitant, ondansetron, dolasetron, metoclopramide, and butorphanol have all been used successfully as antiemetics when given prior to cisplatin administration.

Nephrotoxicity is the dose-limiting toxicity in humans. Nephrotoxicity is cumulative and dose related. Diuresis and adequate hydration can significantly reduce the incidence and severity of nephrotoxicity in the majority of dogs. Methimazole 40 mg/kg IV has been demonstrated in experimental models to protect against cisplatin-induced nephrotoxicity in dogs.[20,21] Other agents being investigated to reduce cisplatin-induced nephrotoxicity include edaravone[22] and vitamin E/cod liver oil[23]; however, further research is required for these agents.

Ototoxicity (high-frequency permanent hearing loss and tinnitus) has been reported, but incidence in dogs is not known. Coadministration of antioxidants (eg, vitamins A and E, glutathione) has been proposed to help protect against cisplatin-induced ototoxicity. The use of these supplements is somewhat controversial, as theoretically they could also reduce cisplatin's antitumor efficacy.[24] In humans, ototoxicity is cumulative.

Other adverse effects include myelosupppression (thrombocytopenia, granulocytopenia), anorexia, diarrhea (including hemorrhagic diarrhea), seizures, peripheral neuropathies, electrolyte abnormalities (eg, hypokalemia, hypomagnesemia), hyperuricemia, increased liver enzymes, anaphylactic reactions, and death. Some dogs receiving chemotherapy will have minor hair coat changes (eg, shagginess, loss of luster). Breeds with continuously growing hair coats (eg, poodles, terriers, Afghan hounds, or old English sheepdogs) are more likely to experience significant alopecia.

Reproductive/Nursing Safety

For sexually intact patients, verify pregnancy status prior to administration. Cisplatin's safe use in pregnancy has not been established. It is teratogenic and embryotoxic in mice.[25] In human males, the drug may cause azoospermia and impaired spermatogenesis.

Cisplatin is excreted in milk. In humans, it is recommended to discontinue nursing if the mother is receiving this drug.

Overdose/Acute Toxicity

The minimum lethal dose in dogs is reportedly 2.5 mg/kg (≈80 mg/m^2). At this dose, a dog exhibited hematological changes and nephrotoxicity. The IV LD_{50} in mice is 11 mg/kg. In humans, overdoses may result in kidney failure, liver failure, deafness, ocular toxicity, severe myelosuppression, nausea/vomiting, neuritis, and death.[17] Treatment is supportive as there is no known antidote.

For patients that have experienced or are suspected to have experienced an overdose, consultation with a 24-hour poison consultation center specializing in providing veterinary-specific information is recommended. For general information related to overdose and toxin exposures, as well as contact information for poison control centers, refer to ***Appendix***.

Drug Interactions

The following drug interactions have either been reported or are theoretical in humans or animals receiving cisplatin and may be of significance in veterinary patients. Unless otherwise noted, use together is not necessarily contraindicated, but weigh the potential risks and perform additional monitoring when appropriate.

- **Aminoglycosides** (eg, **gentamicin**): Potential for increased risk for nephrotoxicity and ototoxicity; if possible, delay aminoglycoside administration by at least 2 weeks after cisplatin.
- **Amphotericin B**: Potential for increased nephrotoxicity
- **Carboplatin**: Human patients previously treated with carboplatin have an increased risk for developing neurotoxicity or ototoxicity after receiving cisplatin.
- **Furosemide** (and other **loop diuretics**): Potential for increased nephrotoxicity and ototoxicity
- **Iohexol**: Potential for increased nephrotoxicity
- **Myelosuppressive Agents** (eg, **antineoplastics, immunosuppressants, iron chelators**): Concurrent use with other bone marrow depressant medication may result in additive myelosuppression; avoid combination when possible.
- **Nonsteroidal Anti-inflammatory Drugs (NSAIDs**; eg, **carprofen, flunixin, meloxicam**): Potential for increased nephrotoxicity
- **Polymyxin B:** Potential for increased nephrotoxicity and ototoxicity
- **QT Prolonging Agents** (eg, **acepromazine, amiodarone, cisapride, quinidine, sotalol**): Potential increased risk for QT interval prolongation, cardiac arrhythmias, and torsade de pointes
- **Tigilanol Tiglate:** The tigilanol tiglate administration protocol does not permit concurrent use of other antineoplastic drugs. Avoid combination.

- **Vaccines** (live and inactivated): Myelosuppressive drugs may diminish vaccine efficacy and enhance adverse effects of vaccines.
- **Verdinexor:** Concurrent use may increase serum concentration of either drug due to competitive inhibition of glutathione S-transferase. Avoid combination if possible or monitor closely for adverse effects of each drug if combination cannot be avoided.

Laboratory Considerations

- None noted

Dosages

NOTES:

1. Because of the potential toxicity of this drug to patients, veterinary personnel, and clients, and because chemotherapy indications, treatment protocols, and monitoring and safety guidelines often change, the following dosages should only be used as a general guide. Consultation with a veterinary oncologist and referral to current veterinary oncology references[26-30] are strongly recommended.
2. Dosages are commonly listed as mg/m^2. Do not confuse with mg/kg doses. See ***Appendix*** for conversion table.
3. Do not confuse CISplatin and CARBOplatin dosages; CARBOplatin doses are much higher.

DOGS:

Potentially susceptible carcinomas and sarcomas (extra-label): The following is a usual dosage range for cisplatin and should only be used as a general guide: Dogs: 50 – 60 mg/m^2 (NOT mg/kg) IV over 20 minutes to several hours every 3 to 5 weeks.[31-33] Dogs must undergo saline diuresis before <u>and</u> after cisplatin therapy to reduce the potential for nephrotoxicity.

Intracavitary administration for palliative control of neoplastic pulmonary effusions (extra-label): Administer 0.9% sodium chloride 10 mL/kg/hour IV for 4 hours prior to treating. Then, administer cisplatin 50 mg/m^2 (NOT mg/kg) diluted in 0.9% sodium chloride to a total volume of 250 mL/m^2).[2,3] Warm diluted cisplatin solution to body temperature. Place a 16 gauge over-the-needle catheter into the pleural space using sterile technique. Remove as much pleural fluid as possible and then slowly infuse diluted cisplatin solution through same catheter. Once infusion is completed, remove catheter. May repeat administration every 3 to 4 weeks as needed to control effusion. On resolution, discontinue therapy after the fourth treatment. Restart if neoplastic effusion recurs.

HORSES:

Intralesional injection of skin tumors (extra-label): Following hazardous drug protocols, add cisplatin powder 10 mg to 1 mL of water and 2 mL of medical-grade sesame oil. Resultant solution contains cisplatin 3.3 mg/mL. Inject cisplatin solution at 1 mg/cm^3 of tumor bed intralesionally with a small gauge needle (22 to 25 gauge) attached to an extension set with luer-lock connections. Inject in multiple planes no more than 0.6 to 1 cm apart. Because the volume of tumor is difficult to measure, the rule of thumb is to discontinue injection when fluid extrudes from the skin surface. Because recurrence at the periphery of the treated area is the primary cause of treatment failure, injection into 1 to 2 cm of normal tissue surrounding the tumor has been recommended. Intralesional injection is generally repeated at 2-week intervals for 4 total treatments.[6,34]

Monitoring

- Baseline CBC, serum electrolytes, serum renal and liver chemistry profiles, and urinalysis
- Repeat tests before each dose and as needed if signs of toxicity develop.
  a) Delay scheduled treatments if absolute neutrophil count is less than 2000/µL, platelet count is less than 100,000/µL, serum creatinine is elevated above normal reference range for the patient, or if electrolyte or acid-base imbalance is present.
- Tumor measurement and radiography at least monthly (eg, every 4 to 6 weeks)[1]
  a) Dogs demonstrating complete or partial remission, or stable disease should continue to receive additional cisplatin therapy.
  b) Dogs that have progressive disease should have cisplatin therapy stopped and receive alternate therapies, if warranted.
- Regular neurologic examinations as indicated by clinical presentation.

Client Information

- Care should be taken to avoid contact with the administration site.
- Cisplatin is a chemotherapy (anticancer) drug. The drug and its byproducts can be hazardous to humans and other animals that come in contact with it. The drug and its metabolites will stay in your pet's system for a few days after treatment. Therefore, on the day of and for a few days after treatment, all bodily waste (urine, feces, soiled litter), blood, or vomit should only be handled while wearing disposable gloves.
- If possible, keep treated dog in a separate area of the yard. Clean up all pet waste right away whenever possible. Double bag waste, seal, and throw away in the regular trash.
- If any accidents occur in the house (vomit, urine, feces), absorb as much as possible with paper towels, double bag, and discard in the trash, then clean area with a diluted bleach solution.
- The most common side effects are vomiting and kidney toxicity.
- Bone marrow suppression can occur. The greatest effects on bone marrow usually occur within a few weeks after treatment. Your veterinarian will do blood tests to watch for this, but if you see bleeding, bruising, fever (indicating an infection), or if your animal becomes tired easily or develops shortness of breath, contact your veterinarian immediately.
- Contact your veterinarian immediately if your pet has any signs associated with toxicity (eg, abnormal bleeding, bruising, urination, depression, infection, shortness of breath).
- This medication is considered to be a hazardous drug as defined by the National Institute for Occupational Safety and Health (NIOSH). Talk with your veterinarian or pharmacist about the use of personal protective equipment when handling this medicine.

Chemistry/Synonyms

An inorganic platinum-containing antineoplastic, cisplatin occurs as white powder. It is soluble in water or saline. The drug is also available commercially as a solution for injection that is odorless and clear. Cisplatin injection (premixed solution) has a pH of 3.7 to 6.

Cisplatin may also be known as cis-Platinum II, cis-DDPCDDP, cis-diamminedichloroplatinum, cisplatina, cisplatinum, cis-platinum, DDP, NSC-119875, Peyrone's salt, or platinum diamminodichloride; many trade names are available.

Storage/Stability

The injection should be protected from light and stored at 20°C to 25°C (68°F-77°F); do not refrigerate, as a precipitate may form. During infusion, the injection should be protected from direct bright sunlight, but does not need to be protected from normal room incandescent or fluorescent lights. The manufacturer recommends that diluted solutions be administered within 24 hours as the solution contains no preservatives. Following initial entry, vials are stable at room temperature for 7 days under fluorescent light and 28 days protected from light.

Compatibility/Compounding Considerations

Compatibility is dependent on factors such as pH, concentration, temperature, and diluent used; consult specialized references or a hospital pharmacist for more specific information.

Cisplatin is **compatible** with 5% dextrose in sodium chloride (0.2%, 0.45%, or 0.9%) and sodium chloride (0.225%, 0.3%, 0.45%, or 0.9%) for dilution. It is also **compatible** in syringes with bleomycin sulfate, cyclophosphamide, fluorouracil, furosemide, heparin sodium, leucovorin calcium, methotrexate, metoclopramide, vinblastine sulfate, and vincristine sulfate.

Cisplatin is **incompatible** with amphotericin B, cefepime, diazepam, regular insulin, lansoprazole, pantoprazole, piperacillin-tazobactam, and 2 in 1 TPN mixtures for y-site administration.

Because aluminum can displace platinum from cisplatin, the solution should not be prepared, stored, or administered where aluminum-containing items can come into contact with the solution. If cisplatin comes into contact with aluminum, a black precipitate will form and the product should not be used.

Dosage Forms/Regulatory Status

VETERINARY-LABELED PRODUCTS: NONE

HUMAN-LABELED PRODUCTS:

Cisplatin Injection: 1 mg/mL in 50 mL, 100 mL, and 200 mL multi-dose vials; *Platinol AQ*®, generic; (Rx)

Cisplatin lyophilized powder for injection: 10 and 50 mg in vials; *Platinol*®; (Rx)

Cisplatin powder or compounded formulations appropriate for intralesional injection may be available from compounding pharmacies.

References

For the complete list of references, see **wiley.com/go/budde/plumb**

Citrate, Potassium

(*si*-trate) *Urocit-K*®

Alkalinizing Agent

Prescriber Highlights

- Orally administered precursor to bicarbonate; used to treat hypokalemia and for urinary alkalization and treatment of chronic metabolic acidosis; may be useful in prevention of calcium oxalate urolith formation
- Contraindications include severe myocardial damage, acute or chronic kidney failure, active UTI with any type of urolithiasis, hyperkalemia, conditions that predispose to hyperkalemia (ie, hypoadrenocorticism, diabetic ketoacidosis, acute dehydration) and GI ulcers. Potassium citrate tablets are contraindicated in patients with delayed gastric emptying, esophageal disease, or intestinal obstruction.
- Most prevalent adverse effect is GI distress, but hyperkalemia, fluid retention, and metabolic alkalosis can also occur. Severe GI adverse effects (eg, GI perforation and ulceration) may also occur especially with the solid forms of potassium citrate.
- Adequate serum electrolyte and urine pH monitoring is mandatory.

Uses/Indications

Potassium citrate (*Urocit-K*®) has been used to increase urine pH to make conditions less favorable for the formation of calcium oxalate and uric acid uroliths. Compounds containing potassium (eg, potassium citrate) can also be used for treatment of hypokalemia. As a bicarbonate precursor, potassium citrate may help inhibit the increased activity of osteoclasts and improve bone health in patients with metabolic acidosis.

The optimal dosage and overall efficacy of potassium citrate supplementation on the reduction of calcium oxalate uroliths in veterinary patients have not been fully elucidated.[1] A single study evaluating its use in normal dogs found no difference in relative supersaturation (RSS) of calcium oxalate and failed to demonstrate a significant increase in urinary citrate between control and study groups, although a subset of miniature schnauzers experienced a significant decrease in calcium oxalate RSS and increased urinary citrate excretion. A difference in urinary pH was detected between groups, with the study group having a higher urinary pH for a longer part of the day than the control group.[2]

Potassium citrate may be beneficial for treatment of hypokalemia in patients with Fanconi syndrome but cannot replace sodium bicarbonate in correcting metabolic acidosis. It should be noted that this treatment (ie, Gonto protocol) has not been evaluated in a clinical study but is used extensively in the management of Fanconi syndrome.[3,4]

Alkalization of urine can help restore pH to inhibit new calcium nephrolith formation in humans with distal renal tubular acidosis.

Pharmacology/Actions

Citrate salts are oxidized in the liver to form bicarbonate, thereby acting as systemic and urinary alkalinizing agents. Specifically, metabolism of absorbed citrate produces an alkaline load, increasing urinary pH, and raises urinary citrate by affecting citrate clearance.[5] The citric acid component of multicomponent products is converted only to carbon dioxide and water and has only a temporary effect on systemic acid–base status. Citrate also forms a complex with calcium to decrease urinary concentrations of calcium oxalate. The urinary alkalinizing effects of the citrate increase the solubility of uric acid.

Pharmacokinetics

Absorption and oxidation are nearly complete after oral administration; less than 5% of a citrate dose is excreted unchanged.[6]

Contraindications/Precautions/Warnings

Contraindications for products containing potassium citrate include aluminum toxicity, severe myocardial damage, severe renal impairment, hyperkalemia, acute kidney injury (with azotemia or oliguria), and calcium or struvite uroliths associated with an active UTI. Additional contraindications for potassium citrate include conditions that predispose to hyperkalemia (eg, adrenal insufficiency, acute dehydration, advanced kidney disease, uncontrolled diabetes mellitus). Potassium citrate *tablets* are particularly contraindicated in patients with GI ulceration or with conditions that increase the risk of GI mucosal damage due to prolonged contact with the tablet (eg, delayed gastric emptying conditions, esophageal compression, or intestinal obstruction).

Potassium citrate should be used with caution in patients with impaired potassium excretion (eg, heart failure, chronic renal failure), or in patients with hepatic impairment as they may have decreased ability to metabolize citrate to bicarbonate.

Adverse Effects

The primary adverse effects noted with potassium citrate products are GI in nature (eg, nausea, vomiting, diarrhea). Potassium citrate products have the potential to cause hyperkalemia, especially in animals predisposed to developing hyperkalemia (eg, adrenal insufficiency, acute dehydration, advanced kidney disease, uncontrolled diabetes mellitus). Because patients with hyperkalemia may present subclinically until cardiovascular collapse or muscle paralysis occurs, periodic electrolyte monitoring is recommended when prescribing potassium citrate. See ***Monitoring***.

Oral liquids containing potassium citrate can have a bitter taste, making patient acceptance difficult.

Solid forms of potassium citrate may cause esophageal, gastric or intestinal ulcers, obstructions, or perforations; this risk may be increased in patients with pre-existing GI disease.

Reproductive/Nursing Safety

As long as dosages do not result in hypernatremia, hyperkalemia, or metabolic alkalosis of the dam, potassium citrate products should not cause fetal harm.

No specific data are available on the safety of citrates during nursing, but no documented adverse effects have been reported.

In humans, potassium citrate is most likely compatible during pregnancy and nursing.[7]

Because safety has not been established in animals, this drug should only be used when the maternal benefits outweigh the potential risks to offspring.

Overdose/Acute Toxicity

Signs related to overdose and acute toxicity are generally related to GI distress (eg, diarrhea, nausea, vomiting) and ulceration, metabolic alkalosis, or hyperkalemia. Treatment is based on clinical signs with IV fluids and/or other supportive care (eg, GI mucosal protectants) as needed. Hyperkalemia, hypernatremia, and metabolic alkalosis should be treated if warranted.

For patients that have experienced or are suspected to have experienced an overdose, consultation with a 24-hour poison consultation center specializing in providing veterinary-specific information is recommended. For general information related to overdose and toxin exposures, as well as contact information for poison control centers, refer to ***Appendix***.

Drug Interactions

The following drug interactions have either been reported or are theoretical in humans or animals receiving citrates and may be of significance in veterinary patients. Unless otherwise noted, use together is not necessarily contraindicated, but weigh the potential risks and perform additional monitoring when appropriate.

- **Aluminum-Containing Phosphate Binders:** Increased risk for aluminum toxicity and systemic alkalosis, particularly in patients with advanced kidney disease
- **Antacids**: Citrate alkalinizers used with antacids (particularly those containing bicarbonate or aluminum salts) may cause systemic alkalosis and aluminum toxicity (aluminum antacids only), particularly in animals with advanced kidney disease. Sodium citrate combined with sodium bicarbonate may cause hypernatremia and, in animals with pre-existing uric acid stones, the development of calcium stones.
- **Anticholinergic Agents** (eg, **aminopentamide, atropine, oxybutynin, tricyclic antidepressants**): Anticholinergic drugs may reduce GI motility and therefore prolong GI transit time, which increases the risk for GI erosions or ulceration from potassium citrate tablets.
- **Antidiarrheal Agents** (eg, **diphenoxylate, loperamide**): Prolonged GI transit time may increase the risk for GI erosions or ulceration from extended-release potassium citrate formulations.
- **Aspirin**: Alkalinized urine can increase the excretion of salicylates.
- **Digoxin**: Hyperkalemia increases the risk for digoxin-induced cardiac toxicity.
- **Fluoroquinolones**: The solubility of ciprofloxacin and enrofloxacin is decreased in an alkaline environment. Patients with alkaline urine should be monitored for signs of crystalluria.
- **Lithium**: Alkalinized urine can decrease excretion of lithium.
- **Methenamine**: Concurrent use with methenamine is not recommended, as it requires an acidic urine for efficacy.
- **Opioids** (eg, **butorphanol, morphine, tramadol**): May prolong GI transit time, increasing the risk for GI erosions or ulceration from extended-release potassium citrate formulations
- **Phenobarbital**: Alkalinized urine can increase excretion of phenobarbital.[8]
- **Quinidine**: Alkalinized urine can decrease excretion of quinidine.
- **Sympathomimetic Agents** (eg, **amphetamines, ephedrine, pseudoephedrine**): Alkalinized urine can decrease excretion of these drugs and therefore increase the risk for adverse effects.
- **Tetracyclines**: Alkalinized urine can decrease excretion of tetracyclines.

With potassium citrate products, the following agents may lead to increases in serum potassium concentrations (including severe hyperkalemia), particularly in patients with advanced kidney disease:

- **ACE Inhibitors** (eg, **benazepril, enalapril, lisinopril**)
- **Angiotensin Receptors Blockers** (ARBs; eg, **telmisartan**)
- **Heparin**
- **Nonsteroidal Anti-inflammatory Drugs** (NSAIDs; eg, **carprofen, meloxicam**)
- **Potassium-Containing Drugs and Foods**
- **Potassium-Sparing Diuretics** (eg, **spironolactone; triamterene**)

Dosages

NOTE: No prospective studies supporting any dosage protocol were noted.

DOGS:

Adjunctive therapy to inhibit calcium oxalate formation (extra-label): Potassium citrate 50 – 75 mg/kg PO every 12 hours.[2] If urine pH is already greater than 7.5, do not use potassium citrate. Usually used with dietary therapy; some recommend concurrent use of hydrochlorothiazide.

Adjunctive therapy of chronic kidney disease as a potassium supplement and alkalinizing agent (extra-label): Potassium citrate 40 – 60 mg/kg (0.4 – 0.6 mEq/kg) PO every 8 to 12 hours[9]

Fanconi syndrome, as part of the Gonto protocol (extra-label): Dosing based on serum potassium concentrations[4]:

- K+= 1.5 to 2.0 mEq/L: give 15 mEq (1620 mg potassium citrate) PO every 12 hours
- K+= 2.1 to 2.75 mEq/L, give 10 mEq (1080 mg potassium citrate) PO every 12 hours
- K+= 2.76 to 3.75 mEq/L, give 5 mEq (540 mg potassium citrate) PO every 12 hours

CATS:

Adjunctive therapy to inhibit calcium oxalate formation (extra-label): Initial potassium citrate dosage recommendations range from 50 – 75 mg/kg PO every 12 hours. Efficacy is not well-established in cats.

Adjunctive therapy of hypokalemia associated with chronic kidney disease (extra-label): Below are suggested starting dosages. Dose should be adjusted based on serial measurements of serum potassium during treatment.

a) 40 – 60 mg/kg PO daily divided into 2 to 3 doses[9,10]
b) From a retrospective study, 0.04 – 1.34 mEq/kg OR 0.25 – 2.8 mEq/cat (NOT mEq/kg) PO daily[11]
c) 1 – 4 mEq/cat (NOT mEq/kg) PO every 12 hours[12]

Adjunctive therapy of metabolic acidosis associated with chronic kidney disease (extra-label): Start with 40 – 60 mg/kg PO every 8 to 12 hours when renal diet is insufficient to maintain appropriate acid-base status with CKD; may also be used in conjunction with oral sodium bicarbonate.[9] Dose adjustments should be based on serial measurements of acid-base status once therapy has started.

Monitoring

Depending on patient's condition, product chosen, and reason for use:

- Serum potassium, sodium, bicarbonate, and chloride:
  - *Dogs:* Monitor serum potassium and bicarbonate concentrations every 7 to 14 days to establish the final maintenance dosage when used as potassium supplement and urinary alkalinizer. Target serum bicarbonate concentration should be between 18 to 24 mmol/L.[13]
  - *Cats:* Monitor serum potassium and bicarbonate concentrations every 7 to 14 days to establish the final maintenance dosage. Target serum bicarbonate concentration should be between 15 to 24 mmol/L.[14]
- Venous blood gas
- Urinalysis with urine pH
- Serum BUN, creatinine

Client Information

- This medication can be used to prevent the formation of calcium oxalate bladder and kidney stones. In animals with chronic kidney disease, it can be used to increase blood potassium concentrations and prevent acids from accumulating in the body.
- Usually given with or mixed into food. Provide free access to water after each dose.
- Use of this medication requires periodic laboratory monitoring to ensure patient safety and adequate treatment.

Chemistry/Synonyms

Potassium citrate occurs as odorless transparent crystals or a white granular powder with a cooling, saline taste. It is freely soluble in water. There is ≈1 mEq of potassium in every 108 mg of potassium citrate.

Potassium citrate may also be known as citrate of potash or citric acid tripotassium salt monohydrate. Sodium citrate and citric acid solutions may also be known as Shohl's solution.

Storage/Stability

Store potassium citrate products in tight containers at room temperature of 20°C to 25°C (68°F-77°F) unless otherwise recommended by the manufacturer.

Compatibility/Compounding Considerations

No specific information noted

Dosage Forms/Regulatory Status

VETERINARY-LABELED PRODUCTS:

Potassium Citrate Tablets: 675 mg (6.25 mEq of potassium); *CitraVet®* (also contains liver flavoring), generic; (OTC). Labeled for dogs and cats, but does not appear to be an FDA-approved product

Potassium Citrate and Fatty Acids Granules: Each 5 g (1 scoop) contains potassium citrate 300 mg (≈2.8 mEq of potassium) and total fatty acids 423 mg; also contains several amino acids—quantities not labeled; *Nutrived® Potassium Citrate Granules for Cats and Dogs*; (OTC). Does not appear to be an FDA-approved product

Potassium Citrate and Cranberry Extract Chewable Tablets: Potassium citrate 680 mg (6.25 mEq of potassium) and cranberry extract 113.3 mg; generic; (OTC). Does not appear to be an FDA-approved product

Potassium Citrate, Cranberry Extract, and Fatty Acids Granules: Each 5 g (1 scoop) contains potassium citrate 300 mg (≈2.8 mEq of potassium), cranberry extract 50 mg, and total fatty acids 423 mg; generic; (OTC). Does not appear to be an FDA-approved product

HUMAN-LABELED PRODUCTS:

Potassium Citrate Extended-Release Oral Tablets: 5 mEq (540 mg), 10 mEq (1080 mg), and 15 mEq (1620 mg); *Urocit-K®*, generic; (Rx)

Potassium Citrate/Sodium Citrate Combinations:

Tablets: Potassium citrate 50 mg and sodium citrate 950 mg; *Citrolith®*; (Rx)

Syrup: Potassium citrate 550 mg, sodium citrate 500 mg, and citric acid 334 mg/5 mL (1 mEq of potassium, 1 mEq of sodium per mL; equivalent to 2 mEq of bicarbonate) in 120 mL and 480 mL; *Polycitra®*; (Rx)

Solution: Potassium citrate 550 mg, sodium citrate 500 mg, and citric acid 334 mg /5 mL (1 mEq of potassium, 1 mEq of sodium per mL; equivalent to 2 mEq of bicarbonate) in 120 mL and 480 mL; *Polycitra-LC®*; (Rx)

Potassium citrate 1100 mg and citric acid 334 mg/5 mL (2 mEq of potassium/mL; equivalent to 2 mEq of bicarbonate) in 120 mL and 480 mL; *Polycitra-K®*; (Rx)

Crystals for reconstitution: potassium citrate 3300 mg and citric acid 1002 mg per UD packet (equivalent to 30 mEq of bicarbonate) in single-dose packets; *Polycitra-K®*; (Rx)

Potassium Citrate, Sodium Citrate/Citric Acid Solutions:

Potassium citrate monohydrate 550 mg, sodium citrate dihydrate 500 mg, and citric acid monohydrate 334 mg per 5 mL (1 mEq of potassium and 1 mEq of sodium per mL; equivalent to 2 mEq of bicarbonate) in 60-oz bottles; *Cytra-LC®*; (Rx)

Potassium citrate monohydrate 1100 mg and citric acid monohydrate 334 mg per 5 mL (2 mEq of potassium per mL; equivalent to 2 mEq of bicarbonate) in 473 mL; *Cytra-K®*; (Rx)

Potassium citrate monohydrate 3300 mg and citric acid monohydrate 1002 mg (30 mEq of potassium; equivalent to 30 mEq of bicarbonate) in unit-dose packets; *Citra-K Crystals*; (Rx)

References

For the complete list of references, see **wiley.com/go/budde/plumb**

Clarithromycin

(klar-***ith***-ro-my-sin) *Biaxin®*

Macrolide Antibiotic

Prescriber Highlights

- ▶ Macrolide antibiotic that may be useful for treating atypical mycobacterial infections or *Helicobacter* spp infections in dogs, cats, and ferrets and *Rhodococcus equi* infections in foals.
- ▶ Use with caution in hindgut fermenters (eg, adult horses, rabbits).
- ▶ Appears to be well tolerated by domestic animals, but common adverse effects include GI upset.
- ▶ Many potential drug interactions

Uses/Indications

In small animal medicine, clarithromycin is primarily of interest in treating atypical mycobacterial and *Helicobacter* spp infections in cats and ferrets. However, one study used quadruple therapy (amoxicillin, clarithromycin, metronidazole, and a proton pump inhibitor) and demonstrated this drug combination did not eradicate *Helicobacter pylori* in 4/13 treated cats and might only cause transient suppression.[1] A 21-day treatment course is recommended for eliminating *Helicobacter* spp infections in dogs.[2] In equine medicine, clarithromycin may be used to treat *Rhodococcus equi* infections in foals, but drug interactions with rifampin and development of resistance[3] raise questions for its usefulness.

The World Health Organization has designated clarithromycin

as a Critically Important, Highest Priority antimicrobial for human medicine.[4]

Pharmacology/Actions

Similar to other macrolide antibiotics, clarithromycin penetrates susceptible bacterial cell walls and binds to the 50S ribosomal subunit, inhibiting protein synthesis. The macrolide class of antibiotics is usually bacteriostatic but may be bactericidal at high concentrations in susceptible organisms. Clarithromycin's spectrum of activity is similar to that of erythromycin, but it also has activity against several bacteria that are not easily treated with other antibiotics (eg, mycobacteria). The activity against gram-positive aerobic cocci is also similar to that of erythromycin. Clarithromycin is typically not effective against methicillin-resistant staphylococci. It is also ineffective against *Pseudomonas,* Enterobacterales (eg, *Escherichia coli*), and enterococci. Clarithromycin has activity against *Rhodococcus equi.* It has activity against gram-negative aerobic bacteria, including *Haemophilus influenzae, Pasteurella multocida, Legionella pneumophila, Bordetella pertussis,* and *Campylobacter* spp. Clarithromycin has inhibitory activity against a variety of mycobacteria, including *Mycobacterium avium complex* and *Mycobacterium leprae,* and good activity against *Mycoplasma pneumoniae* and *Ureaplasma urealyticum.* Other organisms where clarithromycin may have therapeutic usefulness include *Nocardia* spp, *Toxoplasma gondii, H pylori, Borrelia burgdorferi, Bartonella* spp, and *Cryptosporidium parvum.*

Clarithromycin also has immunomodulatory effects via impacts on cell-mediated immunity, but the clinical implications are not clear. It has been suggested that clarithromycin can have effects against biofilm production by staphylococci. One study showed no impact on *Staphylococcus pseudintermedius.*

Pharmacokinetics

In dogs, clarithromycin bioavailability ranges from 60% to 83%. Higher values are obtained when given to fasted animals.[5] Elimination half-life following oral administration is ≈4.6 to 5.9 hours.

In foals, clarithromycin is apparently well absorbed (≈50% to 60%) after intragastric administration, with peak serum concentrations occurring about 1.6 hours after dosing. The elimination half-life is about 5.4 hours.[6] However, when it is used with chronic rifampin treatment, oral bioavailability can be reduced by 90%.[7]

Clarithromycin is well distributed throughout the body, reaching therapeutic concentrations in body fluids and most tissues, including the eye and prostate.

Contraindications/Precautions/Warnings

Clarithromycin is contraindicated in human patients who are hypersensitive to it or other macrolide antibiotics (eg, erythromycin, azithromycin).

Use clarithromycin cautiously in hindgut fermenters (eg, adult horses, rabbits, guinea pigs), as these species appear to be at increased risk for developing diarrhea and enteritis.

Adverse Effects

Clarithromycin is relatively well tolerated in dogs, cats, ferrets, and foals. Like all orally administered antibiotics, GI disturbances (eg, inappetence, vomiting, diarrhea) are possible. The incidence of diarrhea in foals may be higher than with other macrolides. Pinnal or generalized erythema may be associated with this drug when used in cats. Orange staining of skin is possible. Clarithromycin may cause anhidrosis in foals but to a lesser degree than erythromycin.[8]

Adverse effects in humans include GI adverse effects (primarily nausea, vomiting, abdominal pain, abnormal taste, diarrhea)[9] that, when compared with erythromycin, are milder and occur less frequently. Approximately 4% of treated humans develop transient, mildly elevated BUN levels. Rarely, prolonged QT interval, hepatotoxicity, thrombocytopenia, or hypersensitivity reactions have been reported. Pseudomembranous colitis secondary to *Clostridium difficile* has been reported after clarithromycin use.[9,10]

Reproductive/Nursing Safety

Teratogenic studies in rats and rabbits failed to document any teratogenic effects in some studies; however, at high dosages (yielding plasma concentrations 2 to 17 times those achieved in humans with the maximum recommended dosages) in pregnant rats, rabbits, and monkeys, some teratogenic effects (cleft palate, cardiovascular abnormalities, fetal growth retardation) were noted.[9]

Clarithromycin is excreted into the milk of lactating animals, and concentrations may be higher in milk than in the dam's plasma, but this is unlikely to be of clinical significance.

Because safety has not been established in animals, this drug should only be used when the maternal benefits outweigh the potential risks to offspring.

Overdose/Acute Toxicity

Generally, overdoses of clarithromycin are usually not serious with only GI effects seen. A dog that ingested clarithromycin 5 g/kg developed nausea, vomiting, and hemorrhage.[11,12] Patients ingesting large overdoses may be given activated charcoal with a cathartic to remove any unabsorbed drug. Forced diuresis, peritoneal dialysis, or hemodialysis do not appear to be effective in removing clarithromycin from the body.

For patients that have experienced or are suspected of having experienced an overdose, consultation with a 24-hour poison center specializing in providing veterinary-specific information is recommended. For general information related to overdose and toxin exposures, as well as poison control centers' contact information, refer to ***Appendix.***

Drug Interactions

The following drug interactions have either been reported or are theoretical in humans or animals receiving clarithromycin and may be of significance in veterinary patients. Unless otherwise noted, use together is not necessarily contraindicated, but weigh the potential risks and perform additional monitoring when appropriate.

- **ANTICOAGULANTS** (eg, **rivaroxaban, warfarin**): Clarithromycin may potentiate the effects of oral anticoagulant drugs.
- **COLCHICINE**: Increased risk for colchicine toxicity. In humans with normal renal or hepatic function a reduced colchicine dose is recommended, but concurrent use is contraindicated with renal or hepatic impairment.
- **CYCLOSPORINE**: Clarithromycin can significantly increase oral bioavailability of cyclosporine in cats and dogs and reduce dosage requirements by 30% to 35%.[13,14]
- **DIGOXIN**: Clarithromycin may increase the serum concentrations of digoxin.
- **LEFLUNOMIDE**: Increased risk for hepatotoxicity
- **QT INTERVAL PROLONGATION DRUGS** (eg, **amiodarone, cisapride, procainamide, sotalol**): Combinations with clarithromycin may increase the risk for QT prolongation. Concurrent cisapride and clarithromycin are contraindicated in humans.
- **RIFAMPIN**: Can significantly decrease the oral bioavailability of clarithromycin in foals and can negate its efficacy.[7,15]
- **ZIDOVUDINE**: Clarithromycin may decrease serum concentrations of zidovudine.

Like erythromycin, clarithromycin can inhibit the metabolism of other drugs that use the CYP3A subfamily of the cytochrome P450 enzyme system, thereby increasing exposure to those agents. Depending on the therapeutic index of the drug(s) involved, therapeutic drug monitoring and/or dosage reduction may be required if the medications must be used together. These drugs include:

- **AZOLE ANTIFUNGALS** (eg, **itraconazole, ketoconazole**): May increase concentration of each other, and also increase risk for QT interval prolongation

- **Benzodiazepines** (eg, **alprazolam, diazepam, midazolam**)
- **Bromocriptine, Cabergoline**
- **Buspirone**
- **Calcium Channel Blockers** (**amlodipine, diltiazem**)
- **Cannabidiol**
- **Chemotherapeutic Agents** (**doxorubicin, vinblastine, vincristine**): Clarithromycin may increase the serum concentration of chemotherapy drugs.
- **Corticosteroids** (eg, **dexamethasone, methylprednisolone, triamcinolone**)
- **Disopyramide** (also risk for QT interval prolongation)
- **Ketamine**
- **Mitotane** (also may decrease clarithromycin concentration)
- **Opioid Analgesics** (eg, **fentanyl, hydrocodone, methadone, morphine**)
- **Quinidine** (also risk for QT interval prolongation)
- **Sildenafil**
- **Tacrolimus** (**systemic**)
- **Theophylline/Aminophylline**

Laboratory Considerations

- None noted

Dosages

DOGS:

Susceptible infections (extra-label): 5 – 10 mg/kg PO twice daily

Severe or refractory cases of canine leproid granuloma syndrome (extra-label): Clarithromycin 15 – 25 mg/kg total daily dose PO divided every 8 to 12 hours combined with rifampin 10 – 15 mg/kg PO once daily. Treatment is usually continued for 4 to 8 weeks until lesions are substantially reduced in size and ideally have resolved completely.[16]

CATS:

Susceptible infections (extra-label): 7.5 mg/kg PO every 12 hours

Feline leprosy syndrome and other opportunist mycobacteria (extra-label):

NOTE: Combination therapy using two or more antibiotics has been recommended and appears more efficacious than single antibiotic therapy. Prolonged treatment courses are often needed (2 to 14 months) and should be continued for at least 2 months beyond the resolution of the lesions. Several treatment protocols have been suggested (see below). No evidence was located that clearly supports one over the other.

a) Clarithromycin 7.5 – 15 mg/kg PO twice daily in combination with pradofloxacin 3 mg/kg PO once daily and <u>either</u> rifampin 10 – 15 mg/kg PO once daily OR clofazimine 4 – 10 mg/kg PO once daily (alternatively, clofazimine can be given at 25 – 50 mg/cat (NOT mg/kg) PO every 24 to 48 hours)[17]
b) Clarithromycin 62.5 mg/cat (NOT mg/kg) PO every 12 hours combined with doxycycline 5 mg/kg PO every 12 hours, or enrofloxacin (or marbofloxacin) 5 mg/kg PO once daily, or clofazimine 8 – 12 mg/kg PO once daily, and/or rifampin 10 – 15 mg/kg PO once daily[18]

Nocardia **(*N nova*) infections** (extra-label): Combination therapy with amoxicillin 20 mg/kg PO twice daily with clarithromycin 62.5 – 125 mg/cat (NOT mg/kg) PO twice daily and/or doxycycline 5 mg/kg or higher PO twice daily[19]

H pylori **infections** (extra-label):

a) Using quadruple therapy: Amoxicillin 20 mg/kg PO twice daily, metronidazole 20 mg/kg PO twice daily, clarithromycin 7.5 mg/kg PO twice daily, and omeprazole 0.7 mg/kg every 8 hours for 14 days. Treatment did not eradicate the organism in 4 of 13 cats in the study.[1]
b) Using triple therapy (anecdotal): Amoxicillin 20 mg/kg PO twice daily, clarithromycin 7.5 mg/kg PO twice daily, and metronidazole 10 mg/kg PO twice daily for 14 to 21 days. Further studies are required before clear guidelines can be made. The author recommends a 21-day treatment only for patients with clinical signs associated with infection and that have biopsy-confirmed *Helicobacter* spp infection and gastritis.[20]

HORSES:

Rhodococcus equi **infection in foals** (extra-label): 7.5 mg/kg PO twice daily in combination with rifampin based on a retrospective study[21]

Lawsonia intracellularis **(equine proliferative enteropathy [EPE]) infections in foals** (extra-label): Chloramphenicol 50 mg/kg PO every 6 to 8 hours and oxytetracycline 10 mg/kg IV once daily (every 24 hours), followed by doxycycline 10 mg/kg PO every 12 hours or clarithromycin 7.5 mg/kg PO every 12 hours. Treatment length is determined by clinical response, but 3 weeks minimum is recommended.[22]

FERRETS:

Helicobacter mustelae **infections** (extra-label):

a) Clarithromycin 12.5 mg/kg PO every 12 hours in combination with ranitidine bismuth citrate (**NOTE:** Not currently available in the US but may be available from compounding pharmacies) 24 mg/kg PO every 12 hours for 14 days. Same dosing regimen but given every 8 hours is also published.[23]
b) Clarithromycin 12.5 – 50 mg/kg every 8 to 24 hours with omeprazole at 0.7 mg/kg PO once daily[24]
c) Clarithromycin 12.5 mg/kg PO every 12 hours, along with metronidazole 20 mg/kg PO every 8 hours[25]

Monitoring

- Clinical efficacy
- Adverse effects

Client Information

- This medicine can be given with or without food. Give with food if stomach upset or vomiting occurs.
- May cause stomach and intestinal pain and cramping when given by mouth
- Cats may experience reddening of the skin (especially the ears) while taking this medicine.
- Do not give this medicine to rabbits, gerbils, guinea pigs, hamsters, or adult horses/ponies.
- Many possible drug interactions. Tell your veterinarian and pharmacist what other medications you are giving your animal.
- If using the oral suspension, keep it at room temperature and discard it after 14 days. Do not refrigerate.

Chemistry/Synonyms

Clarithromycin is a semi-synthetic macrolide antibiotic related to erythromycin. It differs from erythromycin by the methylation of position 6 in the lactone ring. Clarithromycin occurs as a white to off-white crystalline powder. It is practically insoluble in water, slightly soluble in ethanol, and soluble in acetone. It is slightly soluble in a phosphate buffer at a pH of 2 to 5.

Clarithromycin may also be known as 6-*O*-methylerythromycin, TE-031, and A-56268. *Biaxin®* is a common trade name.

Storage/Stability

Store tablets in well-closed containers at controlled room temperature (20°C to 25°C [68°F-77°F]) with excursions permitted to 15°C to 30°C (59°F-86°F). Store the granules for reconstitution into an oral suspension in well-closed containers at 15°C to 30°C (59°F to 86°F). After reconstitution, store the oral suspension at room temperature (do not refrigerate) and discard any unused drug after 14 days.

Compatibility/Compounding Considerations

No specific information was noted.

Dosage Forms/Regulatory Status

VETERINARY-LABELED PRODUCTS: NONE

HUMAN-LABELED PRODUCTS:

Clarithromycin Regular and Film-Coated Oral Tablets: 250 mg and 500 mg; Extended-release Tablets: 500 mg and 1000 mg; *Biaxin®* & *Biaxin XL®*, generic; (Rx).

Clarithromycin Granules for Oral Suspension: 125 mg/5 (25 mg/mL) mL and 250 mg/5 mL (50 mg/mL) in 50 mL and 100 mL; *Biaxin®*, generic; (Rx).

A pre-packaged combination containing lansoprazole, amoxicillin, and clarithromycin for *H pylori* in humans is marketed as *Prevpak®*; (Rx).

References

For the complete list of references, see **wiley.com/go/budde/plumb**

Clemastine

(***klem***-as-teen) *Dayhist®*

First-Generation Antihistamine

Prescriber Highlights

- Oral antihistamine with greater anticholinergic activity and fewer sedative effects as compared with other first-generation antihistamines
- Poor pharmacokinetic profile for oral administration in dogs and horses
- Use with caution in patients with prostatic hypertrophy, bladder neck obstruction, severe cardiac failure, angle-closure glaucoma, or pyloroduodenal obstruction.
- Most likely adverse effects in dogs are sedation, paradoxic hyperactivity, and anticholinergic effects (eg, dryness of mucous membranes); in cats, diarrhea

Uses/Indications

Clemastine may be used for relief of clinical signs of histamine$_1$-related allergic conditions. One uncontrolled study investigating the efficacy of clemastine in dogs with atopic dermatitis reported that 29.1% showed good to excellent response[1] however, a retrospective study in dogs with canine atopic dermatitis observed that clemastine had a lower positive response rate compared with other H$_1$-receptor antihistamines.[2] Guidelines for atopic dermatitis treatment in dogs state that antihistamines have modest efficacy; they should be given continuously (ie, daily) as preventative therapy before an acute flare.[3,4] In allergic cats, one open clinical trial showed that pruritus improved in 50% of the cats when clemastine was administered at 0.68 mg/cat (NOT mg/kg) PO twice daily, as compared with 0.34 mg/cat (NOT mg/kg) PO twice daily for 14 days.[5]

Pharmacology/Actions

Like other H$_1$-receptor antihistamines, clemastine acts by competing with histamine for H$_1$-receptor sites on effector cells. They do not block histamine release but can antagonize its effects. Clemastine has greater anticholinergic activity with fewer sedative effects as compared with other first-generation antihistamines.

Pharmacokinetics

In dogs, oral bioavailability is very low (3%). Clemastine has a high volume of distribution (13.4 L/kg; 98% protein bound) and clearance (2.1 L/hr/kg). After IV administration, clemastine completely inhibited wheal formation for 7 hours; elimination half-life was ≈4 hours. Oral administration of 0.5 mg/kg only yielded minor inhibition of wheal formation. The authors of the study concluded that most oral dosage regimens in the literature are likely to give too low a systemic exposure of the drug to allow effective therapy.[6]

In horses, clemastine has poor oral bioavailability (3%-4%), a volume of distribution at steady-state of 3.8 L/kg, a clearance (TBC) of 0.79 L/hour/kg, and a terminal half-life of ≈5.4 hours. The duration of effect after IV administration was ≈5 hours. The authors concluded that the drug is not appropriate for oral administration in horses and must be dosed at least 3 to 4 times a day IV to maintain therapeutic plasma concentrations.[7]

In humans, clemastine has a variable bioavailability (20% to 70%); its distribution is not well characterized, but it does distribute into milk. Metabolic fate has not been clearly determined, but clemastine appears to be extensively metabolized, with metabolites eliminated in the urine. In humans, its duration of action is ≈12 hours.

Contraindications/Precautions/Warnings

Clemastine is contraindicated in patients hypersensitive to it. It should be used with caution in patients with prostatic hypertrophy, bladder neck obstruction, severe cardiac failure, angle-closure glaucoma, or pyloroduodenal obstruction.

Adverse Effects

The most likely adverse effects seen in dogs receiving clemastine are sedation, paradoxical hyperactivity, and anticholinergic effects (eg, dryness of mucous membranes). Urinary incontinence, dysuria, and stranguria with profound depression was reported in 3/102 dogs treated with clemastine, necessitating discontinuation of treatment in one study.[1] In cats, diarrhea has been noted most commonly; one cat reportedly developed a fixed drug reaction while on this medication.

Reproductive/Nursing Safety

Clemastine has been tested in pregnant lab animals in dosages up to 312 times the label dosage without evidence of harm to fetuses. However, because safety has not been established in other species, its use during pregnancy should be weighed carefully.

Clemastine enters maternal milk and may potentially cause adverse effects in offspring. Use with caution, especially with newborns. Because safety has not been established in animals, this drug should only be used when the maternal benefits outweigh the potential risks to offspring.

Overdose/Acute Toxicity

There are no specific antidotes available. Significant overdoses should be handled using standard gut emptying protocols, when appropriate, and supportive therapy should be initiated. The adverse effects seen with overdoses are an extension of the drug's side effects; principally CNS depression (although CNS stimulation may be seen), anticholinergic effects (eg, severe drying of mucous membranes, tachycardia, urinary retention, hyperthermia), and possibly hypotension. Physostigmine may be considered to treat serious CNS anticholinergic effects and diazepam employed to treat seizures, if necessary.

For patients that have experienced or are suspected to have experienced an overdose, consultation with a 24-hour poison consultation center specializing in providing veterinary-specific information is recommended. For general information related to overdose and toxin exposures, as well as contact information for poison control centers, refer to ***Appendix***.

Drug Interactions

The following drug interactions either have been reported or are theoretical in humans or animals receiving clemastine and may be of significance in veterinary patients. Unless otherwise noted, use together is not necessarily contraindicated, but weigh the potential risks and perform additional monitoring when appropriate.

- **Anticholinergic Agents** (eg, **atropine, glycopyrrolate**): Additive anticholinergic effects (eg, dry eyes, urinary retention, constipation) possible
- **CNS Depressant Medications** (eg, **anesthetics, benzodiazepines, opioids**): Additive CNS depression may be seen if combining clemastine with other CNS depressant medications.
- **Monoamine Oxidase Inhibitors** (**MAOIs**; eg, **furazolidone, amitraz, linezolid, selegiline**): May intensify the anticholinergic effects of clemastine

Laboratory Considerations

Intradermal allergy testing (IDT): IV clemastine can completely inhibit wheal formation in dogs for 7 hours.[8] A 7-day withdrawal prior to IDT is considered optimal; a 2-day withdrawal should be considered the minimum.[9]

Dosages

DOGS:

Antihistamine: Usual dosages are ≈0.05 – 0.1 mg/kg PO every 12 hours[1]; however, 0.5 mg/kg (10 times most published doses) PO in dogs only inhibited histamine-induced wheal formation to a slight degree.[8] Anecdotally, higher dosages, such as 1 mg/kg PO every 12 hours, may be needed to achieve beneficial antipruritic response. Other antihistamines with better bioavailability in dogs may be considered.

CATS:

Antihistamine (extra-label): 0.34 – 0.68 mg/cat (NOT mg/kg) PO twice daily. **NOTE:** Clemastine 0.68 mg/cat (NOT mg/kg) twice daily appears to be more efficacious based on one open label clinical trial.[5]

Monitoring

- Efficacy
- Adverse effects

Client Information

- Antihistamines are used on a regular, ongoing basis in animals that respond to them. They work better if used before exposure to an allergen and prior to allergy flare.
- Drowsiness (sleepiness) can occur with this medication but usually this lessens with time.
- Use caution with over-the-counter formulations as other potentially toxic drugs may be combined in the products. Be sure to only use products that contain clemastine as a single ingredient.
- Cats can develop diarrhea.

Chemistry/Synonyms

Also known as meclastine fumarate or mecloprodin fumarate, clemastine fumarate is an ethanolamine antihistamine. It occurs as an odorless faintly yellow crystalline powder. It is very slightly soluble in water and sparingly soluble in alcohol.

Clemastine fumarate may also be known by the following synonyms and internationally registered trade names: clemastini fumaras or HS-592; a common trade name is *Dayhist*®. *Tavist*®is no longer commercially available.

Storage/Stability

Oral tablets and solution should be stored in tight, light resistant containers at room temperature.

Compatibility/Compounding Considerations

No specific information noted

Dosage Forms/Regulatory Status

VETERINARY-LABELED PRODUCTS: NONE

The Association of Racing Commissioners International (ARCI) has designated this drug as a class 3 substance. Use of this drug may not be allowed in certain animal competitions. Check rules and regulations before entering in a competition while this medication is being administered. Contact local racing authorities for further guidance. See the ***Appendix*** for more information.

HUMAN-LABELED PRODUCTS:

Clemastine Fumarate Oral Tablets: 1.34 mg as fumarate (equivalent to 1 mg clemastine), 2.68 mg (equivalent to 2 mg clemastine); *Dayhist®Allergy*, generic; (OTC)

Clemastine Fumarate Oral Syrup: 0.67 mg/5 mL (equivalent to 0.5 mg clemastine) in 120 mL bottles; generic; (OTC)

References

For the complete list of references, see **wiley.com/go/budde/plumb**

Clenbuterol

(klen-***byoo***-ter-ol) *Ventipulmin*®

Beta-2-Adrenergic Agonist

Prescriber Highlights

- Beta-2-adrenergic agonist used in horses as a short-term bronchodilator for the management of airway obstruction and as a uterine relaxant for dystocia
- Extra-label use in food animals is prohibited in the United States.
- In pregnant animals, clenbuterol antagonizes the effects of dinoprost (prostaglandin F2 alpha) and oxytocin and can diminish normal uterine contractility.
- Acute adverse effects include tachycardia, muscle tremors, sweating, restlessness, and urticaria.
- Long-term administration may cause tachyphylaxis and deleterious effects on endocrine, immune, and reproductive functions.

Uses/Indications

Clenbuterol is FDA-approved for use in horses as a bronchodilator in the management of airway obstruction (eg, severe equine asthma [SEA], formerly known as recurrent airway obstruction [RAO]).[1] Clenbuterol has been shown to increase tracheal mucociliary clearance rate, which may be useful in horses to prevent pneumonia that can develop from long-distance travel.[2] It has been used both parenterally and orally as a uterine relaxant in the adjunctive treatment of dystocia.

Clenbuterol has been used as a repartitioning agent in food-producing animals, but its use for this purpose is banned in the United States, as relay toxicity has been documented in humans.[3] It is rarely used in small animal species.

Pharmacology/Actions

Like other beta-2 agonists, clenbuterol is believed to act by stimulating production of cyclic adenosine monophosphate (cAMP) through the activation of adenyl cyclase. Beta-2 agonists produce more smooth muscle relaxation activity (ie, bronchial, vascular, uterine smooth muscle) than beta-1 cardiac effects (positive inotropy, lusitropy, chronotropy). Clenbuterol appears to have secondary modes of action in horses, as it can inhibit the release of proinflammatory cytokines (eg, interleukin 1 beta and tumor necrosis factor alpha) from macrophages, increase mucociliary clearance, and reduce mucus production.[2,4]

Tachyphylaxis has been observed with an increase in tracheal mucociliary clearance rate (TMCR) after 12 days of administration[5] and histamine-induced airway reactivity after 21 days of administration.[6] Long-term use (greater than 21 days) of clenbuterol has been theorized to desensitize sweat glands in horses, as these glands also contain beta-2 adrenergic receptors. Studies that have tested this theory were not well powered and did not show a desensitization of sweat glands.[6] High-dose clenbuterol (3.2 µg/kg PO twice daily) downregulates genes encoding beta-2-adrenergic receptors.[7] Clenbuterol reduces the number and responsiveness of beta-2 receptors, but concurrent dexamethasone can prevent this effect.[8]

Clenbuterol has anabolic activity in humans and cattle. In horses, it can increase muscle mass,[9] but any performance increases are offset by a negative ergonomic effect. The drug attenuates skeletal muscle changes (eg, heave lines) in horses with severe equine asthma (SEA).[10] Clenbuterol has also been shown to decrease body fat percentage in adult horses.[11]

When clenbuterol was administered IV to healthy horses, aerobic capacity was not improved, insulin levels were increased, and treadmill velocities for defined heart rates were reduced as compared with the control group.[12] Clenbuterol administration does not appear to confer additional benefit to furosemide in healthy horses with exercise-induced pulmonary hemorrhage (EIPH).[13]

Clenbuterol administration at the low end of the labeled dosage (0.8 µg/kg [route of administration unknown] every 12 hours) for 14 days improved cardiac function in horses with SEA.[14] Long-term administration of clenbuterol in horses can cause decreased aerobic performance, which may be due to effects on thermoregulation. Clenbuterol can induce cardiac hypertrophy and infiltration of collagen in cardiac muscle and can suppress cortisol response to exercise. Long-term clenbuterol administration in combination with exercise training can diminish immune function by reducing numbers of monocytes and CD8+ T cells.[15] Anti-inflammatory effects have been demonstrated in horses experimentally challenged with endotoxin.[16,17]

In pregnant mares, clenbuterol can inhibit uterine tone and contractility,[18] but these effects are not considered detrimental. In non-pregnant mares, clenbuterol's effects on uterine contractility may potentially increase risks for mating-induced endometritis. Some studies have shown that clenbuterol can impair reproductive function in stallions.[19]

Pharmacokinetics

In horses, peak plasma concentrations occur ≈2 hours after oral administration, and oral bioavailability is ≈84%.[20] After multiple oral doses, the drug's volume of distribution is ≈1.6 L/kg[20] and the highest concentrations of the drug are found in the liver, lungs, and left ventricle.[21] The manufacturer states that the duration of effect varies from 6 to 8 hours. In a study, average clearance was 94 mL/kg/hour, and half-life was ≈10 to 13 hours after a single dose[20], although another study noted a half-life of ≈46 hours after oral administration of 3.2 µg/kg twice daily.[22] Seventy percent to ninety percent of a dose is excreted by the kidneys. Urinary concentrations of clenbuterol are ≈100 times greater than those found in plasma and can persist at quantifiable levels for 288 hours (12 days) in urine after the last oral dose.[20]

Contraindications/Precautions/Warnings

Clenbuterol is contraindicated in animals that are hypersensitive to it and in horses that are suspected of having cardiovascular impairment. Extra-label use in food animals is prohibited in the United States.

Pregnant women are advised to avoid risk for exposure to clenbuterol.[23]

In human athletes, clenbuterol has been touted as an alternative to anabolic steroids for muscle development and body fat reduction; however, its use for this purpose is prohibited.[24] Those prescribing this medication should be alert for scams to divert clenbuterol for this purpose.

Adverse Effects

Muscle tremors, sweating, restlessness, urticaria, tachycardia, and ataxia may be noted, particularly early in the course of therapy. Creatine kinase elevations have been noted in some horses.

A few studies performed in rats[25] and dogs[26] have shown that clenbuterol causes skeletal and cardiac muscle apoptosis. Studies in horses have not shown this adverse effect.[27] A recent case study in a human documented rhabdomyolysis subsequent to clenbuterol use for muscle-building effects.[28]

One study in adult horses found that a dosage of 0.8 µg/kg PO twice daily for 21 days resulted in significant decreases in body fat with no loss in body weight.[11] Adverse effects such as muscle tremors, tachycardia, and electrolyte abnormalities have been observed in humans after ingestion of animals that have been treated with clenbuterol.

Reproductive/Nursing Safety

Clenbuterol's safety in breeding stallions and brood mares has not been established. Clenbuterol should not be used in pregnant mares near full-term, as it antagonizes the effects of prostaglandin F2 alpha and oxytocin and can diminish normal uterine contractility. Clenbuterol reportedly induces abortion in pregnant animals. Clenbuterol crosses the placenta and is detectable in milk. In countries where clenbuterol is approved for human use, the label states to avoid use during breastfeeding.

Overdose/Acute Toxicity

Clinical signs associated with overdose/acute toxicity are similar its adverse effects.

In a report of 3 horses with clenbuterol toxicosis due to incorrectly compounded clenbuterol products, horses received oral dosages between 10 – 100 µg/kg. Sinus tachycardia, muscle tremors, hyperhidrosis, colic, hyperglycemia, hyperbilirubinemia, azotemia, and elevated liver enzymes and creatine kinase activity were noted.[29] Elevated temperature and agitation/excitation occurred in 2 of the 3 horses. Cardiomyopathy, skeletal and cardiac muscle necrosis, laminitis, and/or rhabdomyolysis led to euthanasia in 2 of the horses.[29]

Depending on dose and species, GI decontamination may be appropriate. Supportive therapy may include fluid and electrolyte management, insulin, and administration of parenteral beta-blockers (eg, propranolol) to control heart rate and rhythm and elevated blood pressure. Benzodiazepines can be used to manage agitation or seizures.

For patients that have experienced or are suspected to have experienced an overdose, consultation with a 24-hour poison consultation center specializing in providing veterinary-specific information is recommended. For general information related to overdose and toxin exposures, as well as contact information for poison control centers, refer to ***Appendix***.

Drug Interactions

The following drug interactions have either been reported or are theoretical in humans or animals receiving clenbuterol and may be of significance in veterinary patients. Unless otherwise noted, use together is not necessarily contraindicated, but the potential risks should be weighed and additional monitoring performed when appropriate.

- **Anesthetics, Inhalant** (eg, **isoflurane**): Use of clenbuterol with inhalation anesthetics may predispose patients to arrhythmias. In a study, transient hypotension was noted in dogs receiving clenbuterol IV at the time of surgery.[30]
- **Beta Blockers** (eg, **propranolol, sotalol**): May antagonize clenbuterol's effects
- **Digoxin**: Use with digitalis glycosides may increase the risk for cardiac arrhythmias.

- **Dinoprost**: Clenbuterol may antagonize the effects of dinoprost (prostaglandin F2 alpha).[23]
- **Oxytocin**: Clenbuterol may antagonize the effects of oxytocin.[23,31]
- **Sympathomimetic Amines, Other** (eg, **albuterol, phenylpropanolamine**): Concomitant administration with other sympathomimetic amines may enhance the adverse effects of clenbuterol.
- **Theophylline/Aminophylline:** May enhance the adverse effects (eg, tachycardia, CNS stimulation) of clenbuterol
- **Tricyclic antidepressants** (eg, **amitriptyline, clomipramine**): May potentiate the vascular effects of clenbuterol
- **Xylazine**: Clenbuterol may antagonize the uterine contractility effects of xylazine[32]; this effect likely applies to other alpha-2 agonists.

Dosages

HORSES:

Management of airway obstruction (label dosage; FDA-approved): Initially, 0.8 µg/kg PO twice daily for 3 days; if no improvement, dose can be increased to 1.6 µg/kg twice daily for 3 days; if no improvement, dose can be increased to 2.4 µg/kg twice daily for 3 days; if no improvement, dose can be increased to 3.2 µg/kg twice daily for 3 days; if no improvement, therapy should be discontinued. Recommended duration of therapy is 30 days, then it should be withdrawn and therapy should be reevaluated. If signs return, the above stepwise dosage schedule can be reinitiated.[1] **NOTE:** One study of horses with SEA noted increased airway reactivity and reduced bronchodilatory effects after 21 days of administration of clenbuterol. Use clenbuterol no longer than is needed for clinical benefit.[6]

Adjunctive treatment for dystocia emergencies (extra-label): 300 µg/500 kg (1102 lb) mare IV slowly (**NOTE:** Parenteral formulation not available commercially in the United States). The drug's fast onset of action when given IV allows the veterinarian to decide quickly if uterine relaxation will correct the problem. Clenbuterol is particularly useful when repelling the equine fetus to allow manipulation of the head and limbs. May be used in combination with sedatives, analgesics, and tranquilizers. Xylazine or detomidine may inhibit the uterine relaxant effects of clenbuterol.[33]

CATTLE:

Uterine relaxant in cattle (extra-label): 300 µg/cow (NOT µg/kg) slow IV once. May be used during embryo transfer or during the final stages of pregnancy, including labor. **NOTE**: IV formulation not available in the United States. Extra-label use of clenbuterol in food-producing animals is prohibited by the FDA.[23]

Monitoring

- Clinical efficacy
- Adverse effects

Client Information

- This medicine is usually used in horses with asthma or airway obstruction to relax muscles and improve breathing.
- Clenbuterol may be used to treat difficult delivery (*dystocia*) emergencies in mares.
- This medicine can be used to prevent labor and thus, it should be used with caution in pregnant animals.
- Seek immediate medical attention if accidental ingestion occurs in humans.
- Extra-label use in food animals in the United States is illegal. Use may also be prohibited in show or racing horses. Check rules and regulations before entering your animal in a competition while this medication is being administered.

Chemistry/Synonyms

Clenbuterol HCl is a substituted phenylaminoethanol beta-2-adrenergic agonist. It is very slightly soluble in water and has a molecular weight of 313.65. The commercial syrup is a colorless solution.

Clenbuterol HCl may also be known as NAB-365, clebuterolum, *Bronchopulmin®*, *Dilaterol®*, *Planipart®*, *Respipulmin®*, *Spiropent®*, or *Ventipulmin®*.

Storage/Stability

The commercially available syrup should be stored at or below 25°C (77°F); avoid freezing. The manufacturer warns to replace the safety cap on the bottle when not in use.

Clenbuterol injection should be stored below 25°C (77°F) and discarded 28 days after first use.

Compatibility/Compounding Considerations

No specific information is noted.

Dosage Forms/Regulatory Status

VETERINARY-LABELED PRODUCTS:

Clenbuterol HCl Oral Syrup: 72.5 µg/mL in 100 mL and 330 mL bottles; *Ventipulmin® Syrup*; (Rx). NADA #140-973. Do not use in horses intended for human consumption.

Clenbuterol HCl for Injection: 0.03 mg/mL (30 µg/mL) in 10 mL vials; *Planipart®* (POM-V, CD [Sch 4 pt 2])

Extra-label clenbuterol use in food animals is prohibited by federal United States law.

Association of Racing Commissioners International (ARCI) Uniform Classification Guidelines for Foreign Substances (UCGFS) Class 3 Drug. Use of this drug may not be allowed in certain animal competitions. Check rules and regulations before entering in a competition while this medication is being administered. Contact local racing authorities for further guidance. See ***Appendix*** for more information.

HUMAN-LABELED PRODUCTS: NONE

References

For the complete list of references, see **wiley.com/go/budde/plumb**

Clindamycin

(klin-da-***mye***-sin) *Antirobe®, Cleocin®*

Lincosamide Antibiotic

Prescriber Highlights

- ▶ Used for broad-spectrum coverage against many anaerobes, gram-positive aerobic cocci, and *Toxoplasma* spp
- ▶ Contraindicated in hindgut fermenters (eg, horses, rodents, ruminants, lagomorphs) and patients that are hypersensitive to lincosamides
- ▶ Use with caution in patients with liver or renal dysfunction; dose reduction should be considered if the dysfunction is severe.
- ▶ Potential adverse effects include gastroenteritis, and esophageal injuries if dry pilled.

Uses/Indications

Labeled indications for clindamycin include treatment of skin infections (eg, wounds, abscesses), dental infections, and osteomyelitis (in dogs) caused by coagulase-positive staphylococci (ie, *Staphylococcus aureus*, *Staphylococcus intermedius*), *Streptococcus* spp (in cats), *Bacteroides fragilis*, *Prevotella melaninogenicus*, *Fusobacterium necrophorum*, and *Clostridium perfringens*.[1]

Clindamycin is also used for a variety of protozoal infections, including toxoplasmosis, but high doses may be required to achieve adequate CNS concentrations.

The World Health Organization (WHO) has designated clindamycin as a Highly Important antimicrobial for human medicine.[2] The Office International des Epizooties (OIE) has designated lincosamides as Veterinary Highly Important Antimicrobial (VHIA) Agents in veterinary species.[3]

Pharmacology/Actions

Lincosamide antibiotics may act as bacteriostatic or bactericidal agents, depending on the concentration of the drug at the infection site and the susceptibility of the organism. Lincosamides act by binding to the 50S ribosomal subunit of susceptible bacteria, thereby inhibiting peptide bond formation and protein synthesis of the bacterial cell wall. The lincosamides—lincomycin and clindamycin—share mechanisms of action and have similar spectrums of activity, although lincomycin is usually less active against susceptible organisms. Complete cross-resistance occurs between the 2 drugs, and at least partial cross-resistance occurs between lincosamides and erythromycin.

Most aerobic gram-positive cocci are susceptible to lincosamides. Clindamycin has excellent activity against staphylococci and streptococci. Other organisms that are generally susceptible include *Corynebacterium diphtheriae*, *Nocardia asteroides*, *Erysipelothrix* spp, and *Mycoplasma* spp. Enterococci are inherently resistant. Acquired resistance is a potential problem, particularly among staphylococci. Inducible resistance to clindamycin is common in methicillin-resistant *Staphylococcus aureus* (MRSA) and occurs less commonly in other methicillin-resistant staphylococci.[4-6] Methicillin-resistant staphylococci, particularly methicillin-resistant *Staphylococcus pseudintermedius*, are usually resistant to clindamycin. This resistance cannot be detected with routine testing and can lead to treatment failure. Testing for inducible clindamycin resistance is important in any *Staphylococcus* spp that have been reported as erythromycin-resistant or in cases in which erythromycin susceptibility has not been reported; erythromycin-susceptible staphylococci will not be inducibly resistant.[5,6] Streptococcal resistance is rare.

Most anaerobic bacteria are susceptible to lincosamides. There is a low prevalence of resistance in the *Bacteroides fragilis* group.

Clindamycin has activity against a variety of protozoal organisms, but it may be more suppressive than curative in the treatment of *Toxoplasma gondii* infections. Clindamycin can have a delayed onset of action (1 to 3 days), and drug concentrations may not be high enough to achieve complete efficacy. Clindamycin is not effective against the extracellular tachyzoites associated with these protozoal infections.

Pharmacokinetics

In dogs, oral bioavailability is ≈73%, and the elimination half-life is reportedly 5 hours after oral administration and 10 to 13 hours after SC administration. The volume of distribution is ≈0.9 L/kg. Half-life may be longer with higher dosages. One study in dogs found a mean half-life of ≈4 hours after administration of 5.5 mg/kg PO every 12 hours as compared with 7 to 10 hours after administration of 11 mg/kg PO every 24 hours; overall drug exposure (area under the curve $[AUC]_{0\text{-}24}$/MIC) was higher with the higher, once-daily dose.[7]

In cats, clindamycin half-life after a dose of 11 mg/kg is ≈16 hours (capsules) and 8 hours (liquid). The volume of distribution is ≈1.6 L/kg to 3 L/kg. The highest concentrations are found in the lungs, liver, spleen, jejunum, and colon.

In humans, the drug is rapidly absorbed from the gut, and ≈90% of the total dose is absorbed. Food decreases the rate of absorption but not the extent. Peak serum concentrations are attained ≈45 to 60 minutes after oral administration. After IM administration, peak concentrations are attained ≈1 to 3 hours postinjection.

Clindamycin is distributed in most tissue and fluids. Therapeutic concentrations are achieved in bone, synovial fluid, bile, pleural fluid, peritoneal fluid, skin, and myocardial tissue. Clindamycin also penetrates well into abscesses, scar tissue, and WBCs. CNS concentrations may only reach 40% of those found in serum if meninges are inflamed and use for this indication in humans is not recommended. Clindamycin does not penetrate the eye at concentrations required to treat infections. Clindamycin is ≈93% bound to plasma proteins. The drug crosses the placenta and can be distributed in milk at concentrations equal to those in plasma.

Clindamycin palmitate and clindamycin phosphate are inactive, and hydrolysis in vivo to free (active) clindamycin usually occurs rapidly. Clindamycin is partially metabolized in the liver to both active and inactive metabolites. The unchanged drug and metabolites are excreted in the urine, feces, and bile; however, active drug concentrations in urine are poor (low). Halflives can be prolonged in patients with severe renal or hepatic dysfunction.

Contraindications/Precautions/Warnings

Clindamycin should never be administered undiluted as a bolus.[8] A calculated dose should be administered by IV intermittent infusion over at least 10 to 60 minutes (see ***Dosages***).

Although there have been case reports of parenteral administration of lincosamides to horses, cattle, and sheep, lincosamides are contraindicated in hind-gut fermenters, such as horses, ruminants, rabbits, hamsters, chinchillas, and guinea pigs, as serious GI effects, including death, can occur. Clindamycin is also contraindicated in patients with known hypersensitivity to it or lincomycin.

Clindamycin has been implicated in causing esophagitis and, potentially, esophageal strictures in small animal species.[9] Dry pilling should be avoided when administering this drug.

Patients with severe renal and/or hepatic disease should receive the drug with caution; the manufacturer suggests monitoring serum clindamycin levels in dogs or cats receiving high-dose therapy.[1]

In humans, it has been suggested to use the drug with caution in patients with atopy or a history of GI disease, particularly colitis; the significance of this suggestion for veterinary patients is not known.

Clindamycin use is becoming more scrutinized and restricted in humans due to the risk for severe *Clostridium difficile* infection and *Clostridium difficile*–associated diarrhea (CDAD). Clindamycin in 5% dextrose injection therapy has been associated with severe colitis, which may end up fatal. Though of lesser concern in dogs and cats, it may need to be monitored.

Adverse Effects

Reported adverse effects after oral administration in dogs and cats include gastroenteritis (eg, emesis, loose stool, infrequently bloody diarrhea [dogs]). In a study of healthy cats, administration of a symbiotic (prebiotic and probiotic mixture) 1 hour after administration of oral clindamycin reduced antibiotic-associated GI signs.[10] In rabbits, cholestyramine reduced enterotoxemia caused by IV clindamycin administration.[11]

There have been case reports of esophageal injuries (eg, esophagitis, strictures) in cats when solid dose forms were administered without food or a water bolus. Cats may occasionally show signs of hypersalivation or lip-smacking after oral administration. IM injections reportedly cause pain at the injection site.

In humans, eye pain and contact dermatitis have been reported.

Reproductive/Nursing Safety

Clindamycin crosses the placenta, and cord blood concentrations are ≈46% of those found in maternal serum. Safe use in dogs and cats during pregnancy has not been established, but the drug has not been implicated in causing teratogenic effects.

Clindamycin is distributed in milk; nursing puppies or kittens of mothers receiving the drug may develop diarrhea; however, in humans, the American Academy of Pediatrics considers clindamycin compatible with breastfeeding.

Because safety has not been established in animals, this drug should only be used when the maternal benefits outweigh the potential risks to offspring.

Overdose/Acute Toxicity

There is little information available regarding overdoses of this drug. In dogs, oral dosages of up to 300 mg/kg/day for up to 1 year did not result in toxicity. Dogs receiving 600 mg/kg/day for 6 months developed anorexia, vomiting, and weight loss; erosive gastritis and focal gallbladder necrosis were found on necropsy. Cats that received 110 mg/kg/day for 15 days or 55 mg/kg/day for 42 days displayed little evidence of toxicity.[1] Hyporexia, vomiting, and/or diarrhea occurred in healthy research cats that received oral clindamycin ≈35 mg/kg/day.[12]

For patients that have experienced or are suspected of having experienced an overdose, consultation with a 24-hour poison consultation center specializing in providing veterinary-specific information is recommended. For general information related to overdose and toxin exposures, as well as contact information for poison control centers, refer to ***Appendix***.

Drug Interactions

The following drug interactions have either been reported or are theoretical in humans or animals receiving clindamycin and may be of significance in veterinary patients. Unless otherwise noted, use together is not necessarily contraindicated, but weigh the potential risks and perform additional monitoring when appropriate.

- **Aminoglycosides:** Clindamycin has been reported to antagonize the bactericidal activity of aminoglycosides in vitro.
- **CYP3A Inducers** (eg, **phenobarbital, rifampin**): In humans, clindamycin is a substrate of CYP3A isoenzymes, and inducers of this isoenzyme may reduce plasma clindamycin concentration and decrease antimicrobial effectiveness.[13] Veterinary significance is uncertain.
- **CYP3A Inhibitors** (eg, **clarithromycin**, **ketoconazole**): In humans, clindamycin is a substrate of CYP3A isoenzymes and inhibitors of this isoenzyme may increase plasma clindamycin concentration and risk for adverse effects. Veterinary significance is uncertain.
- **Cyclosporine**: Clindamycin has been reported to reduce levels in humans, but this apparently does not occur in dogs.
- **Erythromycin**: In vitro antagonism when used with clindamycin; concomitant use should likely be avoided.
- **Neuromuscular Blocking Agents** (eg, **atracurium, pancuronium**): Clindamycin possesses intrinsic neuromuscular blocking activity and should be used cautiously with other neuromuscular blocking agents.

Laboratory Considerations

- **Slight increases in serum liver enzymes** (AST, ALT, ALP) can occur. Apparently, no clinical significance has been associated with these increases.

Dosages

NOTE: Clindamycin should never be administered IV as an undiluted bolus. The calculated dose should be administered by IV intermittent infusion over at least 10 to 60 minutes at a maximum rate of 30 mg/minute (do not exceed 1200 mg/hour). The final concentration for administration should not exceed 18 mg/mL.

DOGS:

Skin infections (eg, wounds, abscesses) and dental infections (label dosage; FDA-approved): 5.5 – 33 mg/kg PO every 12 hours for a maximum of 28 days.[1] If no response after 3 to 4 days, the drug should be discontinued.

Osteomyelitis (label dosage; FDA-approved): 11 – 33 mg/kg PO every 12 hours for a minimum of 28 days[1]

Pyoderma, superficial (extra-label): 5.5 – 10 mg/kg PO every 12 hours.[14] Fair level of evidence for moderate to high efficacy.[15] Pharmacokinetic studies have suggested 11 mg/kg PO every 24 hours to be at least equal, if not more effective, than 5.5 mg/kg PO every 12 hours.[7,16]

Pyoderma, deep (extra-label): 11 mg/kg PO every 12 to 24 hours for at least 1 week beyond clinical resolution

Systemic infections (eg, sepsis); (extra-label): 10 mg/kg slow IV infusion every 12 hours.[17,18] **NOTE:** Broad-spectrum coverage requires an additional antibiotic (eg, aminoglycoside, fluoroquinolone) for protection against gramnegative organisms.

Surgical prophylaxis for gram-positive aerobes and anaerobic coverage prior to dental procedure (extra-label): 11 – 22 mg/kg PO every 12 to 24 hours for 5 days prior to dental cleaning[19]; however, there is no evidence that this practice minimizes the risk for bacterial translocation from the oral cavity during a dentistry procedure.[20]

Surgical prophylaxis for gram-positive aerobes and anaerobic coverage when beta-lactam antibiotics are contraindicated (extra-label):

a) 5 – 11 mg/kg PO 60 minutes preoperatively[21]
b) 10 mg/kg slow IV infusion to be completed 30 minutes before incision[21]

Susceptible protozoal infections (extra-label):

a) ***Babesia gibsonii:***
   i. Begin therapy with diminazene aceturate 2 mg/kg SC every 48 hours for 3 doses. Once complete, begin (day 8 of a treatment regimen) clindamycin 25 mg/kg PO twice daily for 21 days. This treatment regimen was shown to reduce infection relapse rates.[22]
   ii. In cases of atovaquone resistance, clindamycin 30 mg/kg PO every 12 hours with diminazene aceturate 3.5 mg/kg IM once on the first day of treatment and imidocarb dipropionate 6 mg/kg SC once on the day after diminazene administration; the average duration of treatment was 6 weeks.[23]
   iii. Alternative after atovaquone and azithromycin failed to eliminate infection on PCR test: Clindamycin 25 mg/kg PO twice daily in combination with metronidazole 15 mg/kg PO twice daily and doxycycline 5 mg/kg PO once daily for 30 to 90 days[24]
b) ***Hepatozoon canis***: Clindamycin 10 mg/kg PO every 8 hours in combination with sulfadiazine/trimethoprim 15 mg/kg PO every 12 hours and pyrimethamine 0.25 mg/kg PO every 24 hours (or ponazuril 10 mg/kg PO every 12 hours) for 14 days.[25]
c) **Other protozoal (eg, *Neospora* spp,[26] *Toxoplasma* spp) infections**: Most recommendations for adjunctive treatment are clindamycin 12.5 mg/kg PO every 12 hours for at least 2 weeks or longer. Additional drugs are often used (eg, sulfadiazine/trimethoprim, pyrimethamine).

CATS:

Skin infections (eg, deep wounds, abscesses) and dental infections (label dosage; FDA-approved): 11 – 33 mg/kg PO every 24 hours.[1] In cases of acute infections, therapy should not continue for more than 3 to 4 days if no clinical response is seen. The maximum labeled treatment period is 14 days.

Systemic infections (eg, sepsis); (extra-label): 10 mg/kg slow IV infusion every 12 hours.[17,18] Up to 33 mg/kg PO every 12 hours may be considered in refractory infections that are still susceptible to clindamycin. **NOTE:** Broad-spectrum coverage requires an additional antibiotic (eg, aminoglycoside, fluoroquinolone) for protection against gram-negative organisms.

Surgical prophylaxis for gram-positive aerobes and anaerobic coverage when beta-lactam antibiotics are contraindicated (extra-label):

a) 11 mg/kg PO 60 minutes preoperatively[21]

b) 10 mg/kg slow IV infusion to be completed 30 minutes before incision[27]

Toxoplasmosis (extra-label): 10 – 12 mg/kg slow IV infusion every 12 hours until able to tolerate oral administration for a total of 4 weeks.[28] Patients with uveitis should receive topical, oral, or parenteral glucocorticoids to reduce the risk for secondary glaucoma and lens luxations.[29]

BIRDS:

Susceptible infections (extra-label):

a) 25 mg/kg PO every 8 hours[30]

b) For mild spore-forming enteric bacterial infections: 50 mg/kg PO every 12 hours for 5 to 10 days[31]

FERRETS:

Susceptible infections (extra-label): 5 – 10 mg/kg PO every 12 hours[32]

REPTILES:

Susceptible anaerobic infections (extra-label):

a) 5 mg/kg PO every 24 hours[33]

b) Respiratory infections (eg, anaerobes, mycoplasma): 5 mg/kg PO every 24 hours for 14 days[34]

Monitoring

- Clinical efficacy
- Culture and susceptibility testing as warranted by clinical presentation
- Adverse effects, particularly vomiting and severe diarrhea
- Periodic CBC and liver and kidney chemistry profiles if therapy persists for more than 30 days[13]

Client Information

- This medicine is an antibiotic that is used to treat infections of skin, wounds, and bone, but is also useful in the treatment of toxoplasmosis.
- Give this medicine as directed by your veterinarian.
- Do not give this medicine to horses, cattle, sheep, goats, deer, rabbits, mice, rats, hamsters, or guinea pigs, as it may cause fatal diarrhea.
- This medicine may be given with or without food. Do not dry pill, as doing so may cause throat burns. Give a small amount of food or water (slightly over a teaspoonful) after pilling.
- This medicine has a very bitter taste and may require disguising in food to get the animal to take it.
- Be sure to let your veterinarian know if your animal has any severe, prolonged, or bloody vomiting or diarrhea.

Chemistry/Synonyms

Clindamycin, a semisynthetic derivative of lincomycin, is available as hydrochloride hydrate, phosphate ester, and palmitate hydrochloride. The potency of all 3 salts is expressed as milligrams of clindamycin. The hydrochloride occurs as a white to practically white crystalline powder. The phosphate occurs as a white to off-white hygroscopic crystalline powder. The palmitate HCl occurs as a white to off-white amorphous powder. All may have a faint characteristic odor and are freely soluble in water. With the phosphate, ≈400 mg is soluble in 1 mL of water. Clindamycin has a pK_a of 7.45. The commercially available injection has a pH of ≈6 (range, 5.5 to 7).

Clindamycin HCl may also be known as chlorodeoxylincomycin hydrochloride, (7S)-chloro-7-deoxy-lincomycin hydrochloride, clindamycini hydrochloridum, U-28508, or U-25179E; many trade names are available.

Storage/Stability

Clindamycin capsules and the palmitate powder for oral solution should be stored at controlled room temperature 20°C to 25°C (68°F to 77°F). After reconstitution, do not refrigerate the palmitate oral solution (human product), as thickening may occur. It is stable for 2 weeks at room temperature. The veterinary oral solution should be stored at room temperature and has an extended shelf life.

Store clindamycin phosphate injection at controlled room temperature. If refrigerated or frozen, crystals may form, which resolubilize on warming.

Compatibility/Compounding Considerations

Compatibility is dependent on factors, such as pH, concentration, temperature, and diluent used; specialized references or a hospital pharmacist should be consulted for more specific information.

Clindamycin for injection is reportedly **compatible** for at least 24 hours in the following IV infusion solutions: dextrose 5%, dextrose 10%, dextrose combinations with Ringer's solution, lactated Ringer's, and sodium chloride, sodium chloride 0.9%, Normosol R, Ringer's solution, and lactated Ringer's solution.

Clindamycin for injection is reportedly **compatible** with the following drugs: amikacin sulfate, amphotericin B (cholesteryl, lipid complex, and liposomal), aztreonam, buprenorphine, butorphanol, calcium salts, cefazolin sodium, cefoperazone sodium, cefotaxime sodium, ceftazidime sodium, cefuroxime sodium, dobutamine, doxycycline, famotidine, furosemide, gentamicin sulfate, heparin sodium, hydrocortisone sodium succinate, ketamine, lidocaine, methylprednisolone sodium succinate, magnesium sulfate, metoclopramide HCl, metronidazole, morphine sulfate, ondansetron, penicillin G potassium/sodium, piperacillin/tazobactam sodium, potassium chloride, sodium bicarbonate, tobramycin HCl (not in syringes), verapamil HCl, and vitamin-B complex with C.

Drugs that are reportedly **incompatible** with clindamycin include aminophylline, amphotericin B (conventional colloid), ampicillin sodium, ciprofloxacin, diazepam, midazolam, quinidine gluconate, ranitidine HCl, pantoprazole, trimethoprim/sulfamethoxazole, and ceftriaxone sodium.

In a study, clindamycin impregnated in calcium hemihydrate beads failed to elute in a concentration above the MIC for common infecting bacteria.[35]

Dosage Forms/Regulatory Status

VETERINARY-LABELED PRODUCTS:

Clindamycin HCl Oral Capsules: 25 mg, 75 mg, and 150 mg; *Antirobe®*; (Rx). NADA #120-161. FDA-approved for use in dogs

Clindamycin HCl Oral Tablets: 25 mg, 75 mg, and 150 mg; *Clintabs®*; (Rx). NADA #200-316. FDA-approved for use in dogs

Clindamycin HCl Oral Solution: 25 mg/mL in 30 mL bottles; *Antirobe® Aquadrops, Clinsol®*, generic; (Rx). NADA #135-940. FDA-approved for use in dogs and cats

HUMAN-LABELED PRODUCTS:

Clindamycin HCl Oral Capsules: 75 mg, 150 mg, and 300 mg; *Cleocin®*, generic; (Rx)

Clindamycin Palmitate HCl Granules for Oral Solution: 75 mg/5 mL in 100 mL; *Cleocin® Pediatric*, generic; (Rx)

Clindamycin Phosphate Solution Concentrate for Injection: 150 mg/mL in 2 mL, 4 mL, and 6 mL single-dose vials and 2 mL, 4 mL, and 6 mL *ADD-Vantage®* delivery vials; 150 mg, 300 mg, 600 mg, and 900 mg in 50 mL or 60 mL with 5% dextrose flexible bags; *Cleocin®*, generic; (Rx)

Also available in topical and vaginal preparations

References

For the complete list of references, see **wiley.com/go/budde/plumb**

Clodronate

Clodronic Acid

(kloe-***dron***-ayte) *OSPHOS®*

Bisphosphonate

Prescriber Highlights

- Bisphosphonate approved for clinical signs associated with navicular syndrome in horses
- Contraindications include patients with known hypersensitive to it or those with impaired renal function or a history of renal disease.
- Do not administer concurrently with NSAIDs (eg, phenylbutazone).
- Adverse effects include abdominal pain (colic), discomfort, and agitation.
- Given IM; dose is divided into 3 equal injections. Single-use vial; discard unused drug.
- May be re-administered every 3 to 6 months if initially effective

Uses/Indications

In horses, clodronate is indicated for the control of clinical signs associated with navicular syndrome.[1] Based on a pre-approval study, 75% of treated horses were deemed a treatment success, defined as an improvement in lameness grade in the primarily affected limb by at least 1 AAEP grade and no worsening of lameness grade in the other forelimb on Day 56 after treatment. Clinical improvement was most evident at 2 months posttreatment; approximately 65% of horses that responded to initial treatment maintained their level of improvement through the 6-month evaluation.

A human-labeled (E.U.) IV form was used in a study to determine the effects of clodronate (4 mg/kg in 150 mL 0.9% NaCl IV infusion 24 hours post vitamin D_3 administration; administration rate not reported) on vitamin D_3-induced hypercalcemia in dogs. The authors concluded that clodronate may be useful within the first 24 hours to treat vitamin D_3-induced hypercalcemia in dogs, but that further studies are necessary to define toxicity and appropriate dosing.[2]

Liposome-encapsulated clodronate (LCP) is preferentially phagocytosed by osteoclasts, macrophages, and dendritic cells, which then undergo apoptosis. Therefore, LCP may be clinically useful for treating certain autoimmune diseases. Research is ongoing to evaluate LCP for the management of immune-mediated hemolytic anemia and malignant histiocytosis in dogs.[3]

Pharmacology/Actions

Clodronate is a bisphosphonate that inhibits bone resorption by binding to calcium phosphate crystals thereby inhibiting their formation and dissolution, and by directly inhibiting osteoclast cell function. Clodronate's mechanism of action for treating navicular disease is not well understood.

Pharmacokinetics

After IM injection in horses, clodronate disodium is rapidly absorbed and cleared from the plasma. Plasma half-life of the parent compound is relatively fast (≈2 to 3 hours). Like other bisphosphonates, a percentage of bioavailable clodronate is taken up by bone and then slowly excreted over a sustained period of time (months to years). The actual residence time in equine bone has not been established.

Contraindications/Precautions/Warnings

Clodronate is contraindicated in animals with a known hypersensitivity to clodronate or clodronic acid, in horses with impaired renal function or with a history of renal disease, or in pregnant or lactating mares.[1] See ***Reproductive/Nursing Safety***. Do not administer concurrently with NSAIDs (eg, phenylbutazone). See ***Drug Interactions***.

Use with caution in horses younger than 4 years of age as the drug has not been evaluated in this age group.[1] Since bisphosphonates can affect bone, they may affect bone growth in young, growing horses.

As a class, bisphosphonates are renally excreted and may be associated with GI and renal toxicity. Use clodronate with caution in patients receiving other potentially nephrotoxic drugs (eg, aminoglycosides).[1] Animals should be well-hydrated prior to and after clodronate administration.

Use with caution in horses with conditions affecting mineral or electrolyte homeostasis (eg, hyperkalemic periodic paralysis, hypocalcemia) as bisphosphonates can affect plasma concentrations of electrolytes (eg, calcium, magnesium, and potassium) immediately posttreatment, with effects lasting up to several hours.[1]

Adverse Effects

In pre-approval field studies, the following adverse reactions in horses were reported: Within 2 hours of injection: discomfort, agitation, pawing, or signs of colic (reported together; incidence rate 9%); lip licking (5.4%); yawning (4.5%); head shaking (2.7%); and injection site swelling (1.8%). One horse (of 111) developed colic that required treatment and another, hives, and pruritus. Other reported adverse effects (partial listing) include renal failure, polydipsia, polyuria, anorexia, lethargy, hypercalcemia, hyperkalemia, hyperactivity, recumbency, and injection site reactions.[1]

Reduced bone turnover and remodeling may lead to increased bone fragility, especially when given at high doses or with long-term use.[1]

Reproductive/Nursing Safety

Bisphosphonates have been shown to cause fetal developmental abnormalities in laboratory animals and uptake into fetal bone may be greater than into maternal bone creating a possible risk for fetal skeletal or other abnormalities.[1]

Although oral bioavailability is likely very low, bisphosphonates may be excreted in milk and absorbed by nursing animals.

Because safety has not been established in animals, this drug should only be used when the maternal benefits outweigh the potential risks to offspring.

Overdose/Acute Toxicity

Five of 6 horses given single doses of 5 times the labeled dosage (9 mg/kg) IM divided evenly into 5 separate injection sites showed changes in attitude (eg, agitation, nervousness, pawing, circling, and tail twitching) within 6 minutes of the dose. Four of 6 also showed excessive yawning, flehmen, tongue rolling, head shaking, and head bobbing. All horses developed mild to moderate muscle fasciculations between 2 and 30 minutes posttreatment. By 30 minutes posttreatment, 4 of 6 also developed signs of discomfort and possible abdominal pain including full body stretching, repetitive lying down and rising, and kicking at the abdomen. At approximately 1 hour posttreatment, 1 horse exhibited agitation and clinical signs of colic requiring medical therapy. This horse responded to medical therapy and was clinically normal at 7 hours posttreatment. Three of 6 developed temporary gait abnormalities that included mild to moderate hypermetria, spasticity, or mild ataxia. Four of 6 developed mildly elevated BUN concentrations by 48 hours posttreatment and one had a creatinine concentration slightly above the reference range (2.0 mg/dL; reference range 0.9-1.9 mg/dL) for 12 hours posttreatment.

For patients that have experienced or are suspected to have experienced an overdose, consultation with a 24-hour poison control center specializing in providing veterinary-specific information is recommended. For general information related to overdose and toxin exposures, as well as contact information for poison control centers, refer to ***Appendix***.

Drug Interactions

The following drug interactions either have been reported or are theoretical in humans or animals receiving clodronate and may be of significance in veterinary patients. Unless otherwise noted, use together is not necessarily contraindicated, but weigh the potential risks and perform additional monitoring when appropriate.

- **Aminoglycosides** (eg, **amikacin, gentamicin**): Potential for additive effects in lowering serum calcium concentrations and increasing risk for nephrotoxicity and should not be given for 72 hours after receiving clodronate.[1,4]
- **Digoxin**: May increase digoxin concentrations; use together with caution.
- **Furosemide (or other loop diuretics)**: Increased risk of hypocalcemia; use together with caution.
- **Nonsteroidal Anti-Inflammatory Drugs** (NSAIDs; eg, **flunixin, phenylbutazone**): Concurrent use may increase the risk for renal insufficiency or failure.[1,4]
- **Tetracyclines** (eg, **oxytetracycline**): As tetracyclines can reduce serum calcium concentrations, they should not be given for 72 hours after administration of clodronate[4]

Laboratory Considerations

- No specific information noted

Dosages

HORSES:

Control of clinical signs associated with navicular syndrome (label dosage; FDA-approved): 1.8 mg/kg IM (up to a maximum dose of 900 mg/ horse; NOT mg/kg).[1] Divide the total volume equally and administer into three separate injection sites. If no response to initial therapy, re-evaluate patient. In horses that initially respond but do not maintain clinical improvement for 6 months, it may be re-administered at 3- to 6-month intervals based on recurrence of clinical signs. In horses that respond initially and maintain clinical improvement for 6 months, re-administer after clinical signs recur. **NOTE:** Anecdotal reports suggest that administering the dose over a 2-day period (eg, half dose on day one and second half of dose on day two) reduces postinjection reactions and nephrotoxicity.

Control of clinical signs associated with navicular syndrome (extra-label): 1.53 mg/kg IM (up to a maximum dose of 765 mg/horse; NOT mg/kg).[4] Divide the total volume equally and administer into 3 separate injection sites.

Monitoring

- Efficacy
- Serum renal chemistry panel to include creatinine, calcium, phosphorous, magnesium, potassium at baseline and prior to each treatment
- Hydration status before and after each treatment
- Water intake and urine output for 3 to 5 days posttreatment
- Baseline and periodic urinalysis
- Adverse effects (eg, signs of colic, agitation, and/or abnormal behavior)

Client Information

- Watch your horse for at least two hours after treatment for agitation, signs of colic, and other abnormal behavior, such as head shaking and lip licking. If your horse seems uncomfortable, nervous, or experiences cramping, hand-walk your horse for 15 minutes. Contact your veterinarian if signs don't resolve or if your horse displays other abnormal signs.
- Be sure your horse has access to plenty of clean, fresh water at all times before and for 3 to 5 days after treatment. Make sure your horse is drinking and urinating adequately. Contact your veterinarian if you notice any changes to your horse's drinking, appetite, or urinations.
- Do not administer other medications to your horse in the days before and after treatment without first discussing with your veterinarian.

Chemistry/Synonyms

Clodronate disodium, a non-amino, chloro-containing bisphosphonate, occurs as a white or almost white, crystalline powder. It is freely soluble in water, practically insoluble in alcohol, and slightly soluble in methyl alcohol. A 5% solution in water has a pH of 3 to 4.5. Sodium hydroxide is used in the equine product to adjust pH. Clodronic acid is also used to describe the active entity in some research or products. 60 mg of clodronate disodium is equivalent to 51 mg of clodronic acid.

Clodronate disodium may also be known as 177501, BM-06.011, ZK-00091106, clodronate sodium, sodium clodronate, dichloromethane diphosphonate, or dichloromethylene diphosphonate disodium.

Storage/Stability

Store at controlled room temperature 25°C (77°F) with excursions between 15°C to 30°C (59°F-86°F) permitted. Discard unused vial contents; single use vial and does not contain a preservative.

Compatibility/Compounding Considerations

Do not mix the IM injection with other medications or solutions.

Dosage Forms/Regulatory Status

VETERINARY-LABELED PRODUCTS:

Clodronate Disodium Injection 60 mg/mL, 15 mL/single-use vial; *OSPHOS*®; (Rx). FDA-approved (NADA #141-427) for use in horses not intended for human consumption

Association of Racing Commissioners International (ARCI) Uniform Classification Guidelines for Foreign Substances (UCGFS) Class 3 Drug. Use of this drug may not be allowed in certain animal competitions. Check rules and regulations before entering in a competition while this medication is being administered. Contact local racing authorities for further guidance. See ***Appendix*** for more information.

HUMAN-LABELED PRODUCTS:

None in the United States; both injectable and oral products may be available elsewhere.

References

For the complete list of references, see **wiley.com/go/budde/plumb**

Clofazimine

(kloe-***fa***-zi-meen) *Lamprene®*
Antimycobacterial Antibiotic

Prescriber Highlights

- ► Antimycobacterial antibiotic that may be used as part of multi-drug therapy for leprosy-like or *Mycobacterium avium*-related diseases in small animals.
- ► Use in humans has been restricted to minimize the emergence of resistant strains and preserve its efficacy in patients with leprosy. May be difficult for veterinarians to obtain
- ► Clinical experience and documentation supporting its use in veterinary patients are very limited.
- ► Clofazimine stains skin, eyes, bodily fluids, and excreta. It has dose-limiting GI adverse effects.
- ► Availability may be a concern.

Uses/Indications

In small animals, clofazimine is sometimes used as part of multi-drug therapy against non-tuberculous *Mycobacterium* infection, primarily leprosy-like or *M avium* complex (MAC)-related disease states.

In humans, clofazimine is used primarily as part of a multi-drug regimen in the treatment of all forms of leprosy (with rifampin and dapsone) or the treatment of MAC (with at least two of the following agents: clarithromycin or azithromycin, rifampin or rifabutin, and ethambutol).

The World Health Organization (WHO) has designated clofazimine as a Highly Important antimicrobial for human medicine.[1]

Pharmacology/Actions

Clofazimine binds to mycobacterial DNA and inhibits growth. It is considered to be slowly bactericidal against susceptible organisms. Clofazimine has activity against a variety of mycobacteria, including *Mycobacterium leprae, Mycobacterium tuberculosis, M avium* complex (MAC), *Mycobacterium bovis*, and *Mycobacterium chelonae*. Clofazimine is ineffective against most other bacteria, fungi, and protozoa. Resistance is thought to occur only rarely; cross-resistance with dapsone or rifampin apparently does not happen. Clofazimine may have some activity against *Leishmania* spp. Clofazimine has anti-inflammatory and immunosuppressive effects, but the mechanisms of action for these effects are not understood. Clofazimine is a red dye that may discolor tissue, skin, and bodily fluids (see ***Adverse Effects***).

Pharmacokinetics

Clofazimine's pharmacokinetics have apparently not been determined in domestic animals. In humans, the microcrystalline form of the drug is variably absorbed after oral administration. Bioavailability ranges from 45% to 70%. Food enhances absorption, but increasing the dosage decreases the percentage absorbed. Clofazimine is highly lipid-soluble and is distributed primarily to lipid tissue and the reticuloendothelial system. Throughout the body, macrophages take up clofazimine. The drug crosses the placenta and is distributed into milk but does not apparently cross into the CNS or CSF. Clofazimine is retained in the body for an extended time; its elimination half-life from tissues is at least 70 days long. Bile excretion may be responsible for most of the drug's excretion, but excretion in sputum, sebum, and sweat may also contribute.

Contraindications/Precautions/Warnings

It is suggested that clofazimine be used with caution in patients with pre-existing GI conditions, such as diarrhea or abdominal pain.

Adverse Effects

There is very limited clinical experience with this medication in domestic animals, and its adverse effect profile is not well documented. Apparently, the skin, eye, and excretion discoloration (described below) also occur in animals. GI effects have been reported. A dog receiving clofazimine and rifampin to treat canine leproid granuloma developed hepatotoxicity. There is a report of one cat treated with clofazimine developing a photosensitization reaction.[2]

In humans, clofazimine is usually well-tolerated, particularly at dosages of 100 mg/day or less. The most troubling adverse effect in many human patients is the dose-related discoloration (pink to brownish-black) of skin, eyes, and body fluids, which occurs in most patients. This discoloration can persist for months to years after clofazimine has been discontinued. GI effects (pain, nausea, vomiting, diarrhea) occur frequently and are dose related. Other adverse effects (CNS, increased liver enzymes, etc.) are reported in less than 1% of patients receiving the drug.

Reproductive/Nursing Safety

In rats, clofazimine impaired fertility, reducing implantation rates and the number of offspring. Large doses (12 to 25 times) demonstrated no teratogenic effects in rats or rabbits, but some effects were noted in mice. The World Health Organization (WHO) states that the drug is safe for use during pregnancy when used as part of one of their treatment protocols for leprosy.

Clofazimine enters maternal milk, and skin discoloration of nursing offspring can occur.

Because safety has not been established in animals, this drug should only be used when the maternal benefits outweigh the potential risks to offspring.

Overdose/Acute Toxicity

Limited data are available; the LD_{50} for rabbits is 3.3 g/kg and is greater than 5 g/kg in mice, rats, and guinea pigs. Treatment, if required, would include gut emptying and supportive care. Contact an animal poison control center for additional guidance.

For patients that have experienced or are suspected to have experienced an overdose, consultation with a 24-hour poison consultation center specializing in providing veterinary-specific information is recommended. For general information related to overdose and toxin exposures, as well as poison control centers' contact information, refer to ***Appendix.***

Drug Interactions

The following drug interactions have either been reported or are theoretical in humans or animals receiving clofazimine and may be of significance in veterinary patients. Unless otherwise noted, use together is not necessarily contraindicated, but weigh the potential risks and perform additional monitoring when appropriate.

- ANTACIDS: May reduce clofazimine concentrations
- DAPSONE: There is weak evidence that suggests dapsone may reduce the anti-inflammatory effects of clofazimine; the clinical significance is unclear.
- ISONIAZID: May reduce the clofazimine levels in the skin and increase the amounts in plasma and urine; the clinical significance is unclear.
- QT PROLONGING AGENTS (eg, **amiodarone, cisapride, quinidine, sotalol**): May increase risk of QT interval prolongation and serious cardiac arrhythmias

Laboratory Considerations

- None noted

Dosages

DOGS:

M avium-intracellulare **complex infections, some other non-tuberculous mycobacterial infections (especially rapidly growing** ***Mycobacterium*****), and canine leproid granuloma syndrome** (extra-label): 4 – 8 mg/kg PO once a day for 4 weeks, usually as part of a multi-drug protocol[3]

CATS:

***M avium-intracellulare* complex infections, feline leprosy, other non-tuberculous mycobacterial infections, or feline leprosy** (extra-label): 4 – 10 mg/kg (or 25 – 50 mg/cat [NOT mg/kg]) PO every 24 to 48 hours for 4 weeks, usually as part of a multi-drug protocol

BIRDS:

Avian mycobacteriosis (extra-label): Treatment protocols include: **1**) rifampin 45 mg/kg, ethambutol 30 mg/kg, and clofazimine 6 mg/kg PO once daily; or **2**) ethambutol 20 mg/kg every 12 hours, cycloserine 5 mg/kg every 12 hours, enrofloxacin 15 mg/kg every 12 hours, and clofazimine 1.5 mg/kg PO once daily; (recommended regime for raptors). Regular monitoring of fecal samples is needed; antifungal medication may be required. Surgery for discrete nodules may be curative.[4]

Monitoring

- Efficacy against mycobacterial disease
- Adverse effects (primarily GI, but consider monitoring hepatic function in dogs)

Client Information

- Unless otherwise instructed, give this medication with food.
- This medication may cause your animal's skin to turn color (usually pink, but from red to orange to brown). It may also cause discoloring of tears, urine, feces, and other body fluids to a brownish-black color. This discoloration may persist for many months after therapy is concluded.

Chemistry/Synonyms

Clofazimine is a phenazine dye antimycobacterial agent. It occurs as an odorless or nearly odorless, reddish-brown powder that is highly insoluble in water. In room temperature alcohol, clofazimine's solubility is 1 mg/mL.

Clofazimine may also be known as B-663, G-30320, NSC-141046, Chlofazimine, *Clofozine®*, *Hansepran®*, *Lamcoin®*, *Lamprene®*, or *Lampren®*.

Storage/Stability

Clofazimine oral capsules should be stored in tight containers, protected from moisture at temperatures less than 30°C (86°F).

Compatibility/Compounding Considerations

The commercially available capsules are a micronized form of the drug in a wax matrix base; it may be difficult to obtain an accurate dosage for small animals. It is suggested to contact a compounding pharmacist for advice.

A topical clofazimine formulation, which successfully treated a dog with leproid granuloma, was prepared by incorporating the contents of 40 capsules' contents (crushed inside a plastic bag) into 100 g petroleum ointment. No potency or stability testing was performed on the resulting ointment, but it was found effective when used for a 2-month treatment course.[5]

Dosage Forms/Regulatory Status

VETERINARY-LABELED PRODUCTS: NONE

HUMAN-LABELED PRODUCTS: NONE

In November 2004, clofazimine (*Lamprene®*) became available in the US only on a limited basis. It may be obtained for treating human leprosy cases by contacting the National Hansen's Disease Program (NHDP) of the US Department of Health and Human Services, Health Resources and Services Administration. The NHDP may make clofazimine available for other uses in rare circumstances; contact 800-642-2477 or email HRSANHDPCLINIC@hrsa.gov. Its status for use in veterinary patients is uncertain at the time of writing (2021); approach the FDA Center for Veterinary Medicine (see appendix) for more information.

References

For the complete list of references, see **wiley.com/go/budde/plumb**

Clomipramine

(kloe-***mi***-pra-meen) *Clomicalm®, Anafranil®*

Tricyclic Antidepressant

Prescriber Highlights

- ▶ FDA-approved for use in conjunction with behavior modification in dogs with separation anxiety that may manifest as inappropriate barking, destructive behavior, and/or inappropriate elimination
- ▶ May be used extra-label in cats for urine spraying and in birds for treatment of feather-picking
- ▶ Use is contraindicated in male breeding dogs and in animals with a history of seizures.
- ▶ Caution is advised in animals with liver disease, cardiac arrhythmia, increased intraocular pressure, pre-existing liver disease, reduced GI motility, or urinary retention disorders.
- ▶ Common adverse effects include urine and fecal retention, sedation, vomiting, diarrhea, anticholinergic effects (eg, dry mouth, tachycardia); cats may be more sensitive than dogs.
- ▶ Use may decrease total triiodothyronine (tT3), total thyroxine (tT4), and free T4 (fT4) concentrations in dogs and cats; baseline thyroid testing should be performed prior to therapy.

Uses/Indications

Clomipramine is a tricyclic antidepressant (TCA) labeled for use in dogs as part of a comprehensive behavioral management program to treat separation anxiety. When used in conjunction with behavior training for separation anxiety, both the time to improvement and the final result were improved as compared with behavioral training alone.[1] Clomipramine may also be used in an extra-label manner for compulsive disorder and noise phobias.[2,3] Clomipramine appeared to be more effective than amitriptyline, but equivalent to fluoxetine and dog-appeasing pheromone, in controlling compulsive behavior in dogs.[4–6] In beagles, short-term use had a modest effect on reducing fear and anxiety related to ground transport.[7] **NOTE:** This drug was not effective in reducing canine aggression toward human family members.[8]

Clomipramine may also be useful in cats, particularly for urine spraying.[9–12] Clomipramine was as effective as fluoxetine in reducing urine marking in one study in cats.[10] The usefulness of clomipramine in cats with psychogenic alopecia is unclear, with efficacy demonstrated in a case series[13] but no benefit observed in a prospective, double-blinded, study.[14]

Clomipramine has been used to treat feather-picking in birds.[15]

Pharmacology/Actions

Although the exact mechanism of action of TCAs is not fully understood, it is believed that their most significant effects result from preventing neurotransmitter reuptake at the neuronal membrane. Clomipramine is predominantly an inhibitor of serotonin (5-HT) reuptake, but it also has effects on norepinephrine and possibly other neurotransmitters. Desmethylclomipramine, clomipramine's active metabolite, primarily inhibits noradrenergic uptake and may be responsible for the majority of the drug's adverse effects (in humans). Clomipramine also binds to histamine-1 (H_1) receptors and antagonizes alpha-1 adrenergic and muscarinic acetylcholine receptors.

Pharmacokinetics

In dogs, an extensive first-pass effect limits clomipramine oral bioavailability (17%). Peak concentration is reached ≈1.5 to 2 hours after a single oral dose and ≈3 to 4 hours with repeated oral administration. The presence of food increases clomipramine bioavailability, peak concentration, and area under the curve by ≈20% to 25%. Clomipramine accumulates with repeated oral administration. Volume of distribution is 3.8 L/kg. Clomipramine is rapidly converted in the liver to its active metabolite (ie, desmethylclomipramine). Both the parent drug and the active metabolite are highly bound to plasma proteins (96%). The elimination half-life of clomipramine is ≈6 to 7 hours and of desmethylclomipramine is ≈2 hours. The parent and metabolite are further metabolized by glucuronidation.[1,16-18]

Cats appear to metabolize clomipramine more slowly than dogs,[19] and wide interpatient variability in pharmacokinetic parameters have been shown after single oral doses. Male cats may metabolize clomipramine more slowly than female cats.[19,20] In a limited (6 subject) pharmacokinetic study, oral bioavailability averaged 90%, time to peak concentration was ≈6 hours, and elimination half-life was 12.3 hours.[21]

In humans, the drug is well absorbed from the GI tract, but a substantial first-pass effect reduces its systemic bioavailability to ≈50%. The presence of food in the gut does not significantly alter absorption of the drug. Clomipramine is highly lipophilic and widely distributed throughout the body, with an apparent volume of distribution of 17 L/kg. Both clomipramine and its active metabolite (ie, desmethylclomipramine) cross the blood–brain barrier, and significant concentrations are found in the brain. Clomipramine is metabolized principally in the liver to several metabolites, including desmethylclomipramine, which is active. Approximately ⅔ of these metabolites are eliminated in the urine and the rest in the feces. After a single dose, the elimination half-life of clomipramine averages 32 hours and desmethylclomipramine averages 69 hours, but there is wide interpatient variation.

Contraindications/Precautions/Warnings

Clomipramine is contraindicated in those hypersensitive to it or other TCAs. Concomitant use (or use within 14 days before or after treatment) with monoamine oxidase inhibitors (eg, selegiline or amitraz [including collars]) is contraindicated. Use of clomipramine is also contraindicated in dogs with a history of seizures or concomitantly with drugs that lower the seizure threshold. Epileptiform pathology and sustained generalized discharges occurred in cats given clomipramine.[22] Safety in dogs less than 6 months of age has not been studied.[1]

TCAs should be used cautiously in animals with hyperthyroidism or in those that are receiving thyroid supplementation, as there may be an increased risk for cardiac rhythm abnormalities. Clomipramine impairs synthesis of thyroxine (T4); concentrations of tT3, tT4, and free T4 may be reduced by 16% to 35% in dogs and cats.[23,24]

Because of its anticholinergic effects, use clomipramine with caution in animals with decreased GI motility, urinary retention, cardiovascular disease (especially cardiac rhythm disturbances), narrow angle glaucoma, or increased intraocular pressure.[1,25] Caution should also be used in animals with pre-existing hepatic disease.

If discontinuing clomipramine, the manufacturer recommends tapering the medication to minimize the risk for signs of withdrawal.[1] Clomipramine should be discontinued for as long as clinically feasible prior to elective surgery using general anesthetic agents.

Do not confuse clomiPRAMINE with chlorproMAZINE.

Adverse Effects

The primary adverse effects reported in dogs are anorexia, emesis, diarrhea, dry mouth, elevation of liver enzymes, and sedation/lethargy/depression. Significant ECG abnormalities were not identified in small studies in dogs[26,27] or cats.[23] One case of a dog developing pancreatitis after receiving clomipramine has been published.[28]

Cats have been reported to be more susceptible than dogs to developing adverse effects, including anticholinergic effects (eg, dry mouth, mydriasis, urine retention, constipation), sedation, and diarrhea; this may be the result of slower elimination of the active (desmethyl) metabolite in cats.

Adverse effects reported in birds include ataxia, drowsiness, and regurgitation.

Although therapeutic effects may take several weeks to be seen, adverse effects can occur early in the course of treatment.

Reproductive/Nursing Safety

Clomipramine crosses the placenta. Embryotoxic and fetotoxic effects were noted in mice and rats given clomipramine at dosages up to 20 times the usual maximum human dosage. Data in other domestic species appear to be lacking. The manufacturer warns not to use in breeding male dogs, as studies of high-dose toxicity (12.5 times the maximum label-recommended dose) demonstrated testicular hypoplasia. Long-term administration (8 weeks) in mice resulted in decreased sperm count and motility; these effects were reversed after discontinuing clomipramine.[29]

Clomipramine has been detected in human milk. Use clomipramine with caution in nursing animals or consider using a milk replacer.

Because safety has not been established in animals, this drug should only be used when the maternal benefits outweigh the potential risks to offspring.

Overdose/Acute Toxicity

Clomipramine has a narrow margin of safety; significant clinical signs (eg, ataxia, mydriasis, tremors) can be seen at or slightly above therapeutic range (2 – 3 mg/kg, APCC database). Dogs receiving 20 mg/kg experienced bradycardia and sporadic SA and AV block.[30] Overdoses of tricyclic antidepressants can be life-threatening (ie, arrhythmias, seizures, cardiorespiratory collapse). In dogs, lethal doses are ≈50 – 100 mg/kg/day PO.

Clinical signs seen in dogs with a clomipramine overdose include lethargy/sedation, tachycardia, vomiting, vocalization, and ataxia; common signs seen in cats include mydriasis, lethargy, tachycardia, ataxia, vocalization, and agitation.

Clomipramine oral overdoses should be treated with standard decontamination measures if appropriate for the animal; IV lipid emulsion therapy may be beneficial.

For patients that have experienced or are suspected to have experienced an overdose, consultation with a 24-hour poison consultation center specializing in providing veterinary-specific information is recommended. For general information related to overdose and toxin exposures, as well as contact information for poison control centers, refer to ***Appendix.***

Drug Interactions

The following drug interactions have either been reported or are theoretical in humans or animals receiving clomipramine and may be of significance in veterinary patients. Unless otherwise noted, use together is not necessarily contraindicated, but weigh the potential risks and perform additional monitoring when appropriate.

- ALPHA-2-ADRENERGIC AGONISTS (eg, **dexmedetomidine, xylazine**): Increased risk for CNS and respiratory depression and bradycardia. Use cautiously in combination.
- AMLODIPINE: Increased risk for hypotension
- ANESTHETIC AGENTS (eg, **alfaxalone, isoflurane, ketamine, propofol**): Discontinue clomipramine as long as clinically feasible prior to elective surgery with general anesthetic agents.[1,31]
- ANGIOTENSIN CONVERTING ENZYME INHIBITORS (ACEIs; eg, **benazepril, enalapril**): Increased risk for hypotension
- ANGIOTENSIN RECEPTOR BLOCKERS (ARBs; eg, **telmisartan**): Increased risk for hypotension
- ANTICHOLINERGIC AGENTS (eg, **atropine, glycopyrrolate, oxy-**

butynin): Because of the additive anticholinergic effects, use cautiously with clomipramine.

- ANTIHISTAMINES (eg, **cetirizine, chlorpheniramine, diphenhydramine, hydroxyzine**): Concurrent use may increase risk for CNS depression and additive anticholinergic effects. Avoid combination or monitor for sedation, tachycardia, ileus, mydriasis, or constipation.
- AZOLE ANTIFUNGALS (eg, **itraconazole, ketoconazole**): Concurrent use may increase the risk for QT-interval prolongation.
- BARBITURATES (eg, **pentobarbital, phenobarbital**): May result in decreased clomipramine efficacy or additive adverse effects.[31] Monitor clomipramine efficacy.
- BUSPIRONE: Increased risk for CNS depression and serotonin syndrome
- CIMETIDINE: May inhibit tricyclic antidepressant metabolism and increase the risk for toxicosis
- CNS DEPRESSANTS (eg, **cannabidiol, diazepam, methocarbamol, pregabalin**): Because of the additive CNS effects, use cautiously with clomipramine.
- CYPROHEPTADINE: May antagonize the serotonergic effects of tricyclic antidepressants
- DEXTROMETHORPHAN: Increased risk for serotonin syndrome
- FLUMAZENIL: Flumazenil use in animals suspected of TCA overdose may increase the risk for seizures and arrhythmias.[32]
- FLUOROQUINOLONES (eg, **enrofloxacin, marbofloxacin, pradofloxacin**): Concurrent use may increase the risk for QT-interval prolongation.
- LEVOTHYROXINE: Concurrent use may increase therapeutic and toxic effects of both levothyroxine and clomipramine.
- METOCLOPRAMIDE: Concurrent use may increase the risk for extrapyramidal reactions or neuroleptic malignant syndrome; combination is contraindicated in humans. No data available for veterinary patients. Avoid combination or use conservative doses and monitor carefully.
- MIRTAZAPINE: Increased risk for constipation, urinary retention, CNS depression, and serotonin syndrome
- MONOAMINE OXIDASE INHIBITORS (eg, **amitraz, furazolidone, linezolid, methylene blue, procarbazine, selegiline**): Concomitant use (within 14 days) with monoamine oxidase inhibitors is contraindicated (serotonin syndrome).
- OPIOIDS (eg, **buprenorphine, butorphanol, fentanyl, meperidine, methadone, morphine**): Concurrent use may result in additive CNS and respiratory depression; rarely, serotonin syndrome has been reported in humans. Monitor closely for adverse effects.
- PENTAZOCINE: Increased risk for serotonin syndrome
- QT PROLONGING AGENTS (eg, **amiodarone, cisapride, procainamide, quinidine, sotalol**): Increased risk for QT-interval prolongation and tricyclic adverse effects
- SELECTIVE SEROTONIN REUPTAKE INHIBITOR (SSRIs; eg, **fluoxetine, paroxetine, sertraline**): Concurrent use may increase the risk for serotonin syndrome. In dogs, if switching from treatment with clomipramine to an SSRI, a 3- to 4-day washout period has been recommended.[33]
- SEROTONIN RECEPTOR ANTAGONISTS (eg, **dolasetron, ondansetron**): Concurrent use may increase the risk for serotonin syndrome.
- SYMPATHOMIMETIC AGENTS (eg, **albuterol, ephedrine, phenylpropanolamine**): Use in combination with sympathomimetic agents may increase the risk for cardiac effects (eg, arrhythmias, hyperpyrexia, hypertension).
- TRAMADOL: In humans, concurrent use may increase the risk for serotonin syndrome and seizures; veterinary clinical significance is not known, but one source states that tricyclic antidepressants (eg, amitriptyline, clomipramine), should not be administered concurrently with tramadol.[34]
- TRAZODONE: Concurrent use may cause additive CNS depression and may increase the risk for serotonin syndrome in humans.
- TRICYCLIC ANTIDEPRESSANTS (TCAs; eg, **amitriptyline, doxepin, imipramine**): Concurrent use of two tricyclic antidepressants should be avoided due to increased risk for serotonin syndrome, anticholinergic adverse effects, and cardiac arrhythmias.
- YOHIMBINE: Concurrent use may increase the risk for hypertension.

Laboratory Considerations

- **Metapyrone stimulation test**: The response to metapyrone may be decreased by clomipramine.
- **Blood glucose**: TCAs may alter (ie, increase or decrease) blood glucose concentrations.

Dosages

NOTE: Dosages are generally started at the low end and increased gradually (ie, every 2 weeks) until efficacy is noted or limited by adverse effects. Up to 8 weeks of treatment are required to determine efficacy. Discontinuation of the drug should be done gradually, preferably over several weeks.

DOGS:

Separation anxiety (label dosage; FDA-approved): 2 – 4 mg/kg PO once daily or divided twice daily in conjunction with a comprehensive behavior management program.[1]

Adjunctive treatment of behavioral conditions (extra-label): 1 – 2 mg/kg PO twice daily initially and eventually up to 3 mg/kg PO once to twice daily[35]; up to 4 mg/kg PO twice daily was well tolerated in one study.[3] Dosages are generally started at the low end and increased gradually (ie, every 2 weeks) until efficacy is noted or limited by adverse effects. Up to 8 weeks of treatment are required to determine efficacy.[4] When used for treatment of situational anxiety/phobias, it is recommended by many clinicians that this drug should be used in conjunction with a benzodiazepine (eg, alprazolam) as necessary.[2] When behavioral modification treatment efficacy is established, doses may be reduced in many animals.

CATS:

Adjunctive treatment of behavioral conditions (extra-label): 0.25 – 1 mg/kg PO once daily,[9-11,36] in combination with behavior modification therapy. Practically, 2.5 – 5 mg/cat (NOT mg/kg) PO once daily

BIRDS:

Adjunctive treatment of feather-picking (extra-label): From a study in cockatoos, 3 mg/kg PO every 12 hours.[15] Reported dosages range from 0.5 – 9 mg/kg PO every 12 to 24 hours.[37]

Monitoring

- Clinical efficacy
- Adverse effects
- Baseline CBC, serum chemistry profile, urinalysis, and baseline thyroid testing[23,24] (eg, tT4, thyroid panel) prior to therapy, 1 month after initial therapy, and yearly, thereafter.
- Baseline ECG is recommended prior to therapy. TCAs can widen QRS complexes, prolong PR intervals, and invert or flatten T-waves on ECG; significance in animals is not fully understood.

Client Information

- This medicine works best when used with behavior therapy.
- It may take several weeks to determine if this medicine is working.
- This medicine may be given with or without food; giving with

food may reduce the risk for vomiting.

- The most common side effects are drowsiness/sleepiness, dry mouth, and constipation; be sure your animal has access to fresh, clean water.
- Rare side effects that can be serious include abnormal bleeding, fever, seizures, or very fast or irregular heartbeat. Contact your veterinarian immediately if you see any of these signs.
- An overdose can be very serious. Be sure to keep this medicine out of reach of animals and children.
- Tell your veterinarian if your animal has worn a flea or tick collar in the past 2 weeks. Do not use a new flea and tick collar on your animal without talking to your veterinarian first.
- Do not suddenly stop giving this medicine to your animal. If you want to stop giving the medication before the prescription is completed, first contact your veterinarian. There may be an important reason to continue its use. Clomipramine must be tapered off slowly or your animal may suffer uncomfortable withdrawal signs including vomiting, anxiety, and shaking.

Chemistry/Synonyms

Clomipramine HCl, a dibenzazepine-derivative tricyclic antidepressant, occurs as a white to off-white crystalline powder and is freely soluble in water.

Clomipramine HCl may also be known as chlorimipramine hydrochloride, clomipramini hydrochloridum, G-34586, monochlorimipramine hydrochloride, *Anafranil®*, *Clofranil®*, *Clomav®*, *Clomicalm®*, *Clopram®*, *Clopress®*, *Equinorm®*, *Hydiphen®*, *Maronil®*, *Novo-Clopamine®*, *Placil®*, *Tranquax®*, or *Zoiral®*.

Storage/Stability

The commercially available veterinary tablets should be stored in a dry place at a controlled room temperature (15°C-30°C [59°F-86°F]) in the original closed container. The (human label) capsules should be stored at 20°C-25°C (68°F-77°F) in tight containers and protected from moisture.

Compatibility/Compounding Considerations

No specific information noted

Dosage Forms/Regulatory Status

VETERINARY-LABELED PRODUCTS:

Clomipramine HCl Oral Tablets: 5 mg, 20 mg, 40 mg, and 80 mg; *Clomicalm®*; generic; (Rx). FDA approved for use in dogs. NADA #141-120

The Association of Racing Commissioners International (ARCI) has designated this drug as a class 2 substance. See the ***Appendix*** for more information. Use of this drug may not be allowed in certain animal competitions. Check rules and regulations before entering in a competition while this medication is being administered. Contact local racing authorities for further guidance.

HUMAN-LABELED PRODUCTS:

Clomipramine Oral Capsules: 25 mg, 50 mg, and 75 mg; *Anafranil®*; generic; (Rx)

References

For the complete list of references, see **wiley.com/go/budde/plumb**

Clonazepam

(kloe-***na***-ze-pam) *Klonopin®*

Benzodiazepine

Prescriber Highlights

- ► Benzodiazepine anticonvulsant used primarily as adjunctive therapy for short-term treatment of epilepsy in dogs and for long-term adjunctive treatment of epilepsy in cats; may also be used as an anxiolytic, particularly when a longer-acting benzodiazepine is desired
- ► Contraindicated in patients with hypersensitivity to benzodiazepines, narrow angle glaucoma, or significant liver disease. May exacerbate myasthenia gravis
- ► If using for treatment of seizures, discontinue use gradually.
- ► Sedation and ataxia are the most prevalent adverse effects. Cats may experience hepatic necrosis, but it is believed this is less likely to occur than with diazepam.
- ► Dogs may develop a tolerance to efficacy over a few weeks.
- ► Schedule-IV controlled substance in the United States
- ► The National Institute for Occupational Safety and Health (NIOSH) classifies clonazepam as a hazardous drug; use appropriate precautions when handling.

Uses/Indications

Clonazepam is used primarily as a short-term adjunctive anticonvulsant for the treatment of epilepsy in dogs. It has been considered for long-term adjunctive therapy in dogs not controlled with more standard therapies, but, like diazepam, tolerance tends to develop within a few weeks of treatment. Clonazepam can also be used as an anxiolytic agent or as a muscle relaxant.

Clonazepam has been used as an anxiolytic and in the treatment of epilepsy in cats. The availability of oral dispersible tablets (ODT) in strengths from 0.125 mg may make dosing in cats easier than with other dosage forms.

Pharmacology/Actions

Clonazepam and other benzodiazepines depress CNS subcortical levels (primarily limbic, thalamic, and hypothalamic), thereby producing anxiolytic, sedative, skeletal muscle relaxation, and anticonvulsant effects. The exact mechanism of action is unknown, but postulated mechanisms include antagonism of serotonin, increased release of and/or facilitation of gamma-aminobutyric acid (GABA) activity, and diminished release or turnover of acetylcholine in the CNS. Benzodiazepine-specific receptors have been located in the mammalian brain, kidney, liver, lung, and heart. In all species studied, receptors are lacking in the white matter.

Pharmacokinetics

In dogs, clonazepam's oral bioavailability is variable (ie, 20%-60%), but absorption is rapid. Protein binding is ≈82%, and the drug rapidly crosses into the CNS. Clonazepam exhibits saturation kinetics in dogs, as elimination rates are dose-dependent.

In humans, the drug is well absorbed from the GI tract, crosses the blood–brain barrier and placenta, and is metabolized in the liver to several metabolites that are excreted in the urine. Peak serum levels occur ≈3 hours after oral administration. Half-life ranges from 19 to 40 hours.

Contraindications/Precautions/Warnings

Clonazepam is contraindicated in patients that are hypersensitive to it or other benzodiazepines or have significant liver dysfunction or acute narrow angle glaucoma. Benzodiazepines have been reported to exacerbate myasthenia gravis. Use with caution in patients with renal or hepatic impairment. Clonazepam should be used cautiously in aggressive patients.

Clonazepam orally dispersible tablets (ODT) that contain xylitol (unknown quantity) should be used with caution in dogs.

Tolerance (usually noted after several weeks) to the anticonvulsant effects has been reported in dogs. Dosage adjustment may restore efficacy.

In patients chronically treated with clonazepam at high doses for seizure control, the drug should be tapered off, as status epilepticus may be precipitated; vomiting and diarrhea may also occur during the withdrawal period.

Do not confuse clonazepam with clonidine or other benzodiazepines (eg, clorazepate, lorazepam). Consider writing orders and prescriptions using tall man letters (eg, clonazePAM).

The National Institute for Occupational Safety and Health (NIOSH) classifies clonazepam as a hazardous drug; personal protective equipment (PPE) should be used accordingly to minimize the risk for exposure.[1]

Adverse Effects

There is limited information on the adverse effect profile of this drug in domestic animals. Sedation (or excitement) and ataxia may occur.[2] The effect, if any, of clonazepam on working dogs is unknown.

In cats, clonazepam may cause sedation and ataxia. Acute hepatic necrosis has been documented from oral administration of diazepam in cats[3]; other benzodiazepines (eg, clonazepam) may cause similar adverse effects.

Clonazepam has been reported to cause various adverse effects in humans. Some of the more significant effects include hypotonia, ataxia, sedation, increased salivation, hypersecretion in upper respiratory passages, GI effects (eg, vomiting, constipation, diarrhea), transient elevations of liver enzymes, and hematologic effects (eg, anemia, leukopenia, thrombocytopenia).

Reproductive/Nursing Safety

Clonazepam crosses the placenta. Teratogenic effects (eg, cleft palate, fused sternebrae, limb defects) have been seen in rabbits and rats receiving clinical doses.[4] Neonates may experience signs of withdrawal if the dam has received clonazepam during the later stages of pregnancy.

Clonazepam is excreted into maternal milk. Use with caution in nursing dams.

Overdose/Acute Toxicity

Overdoses commonly cause sedation, depression, and ataxia. Some animals have paradoxical signs (eg, hyperactivity, disorientation, vocalization). Emesis is generally not indicated. With mild to moderate overdoses, animals can often be monitored at home, as long as the animal is rousable and does not show paradoxical signs; animals should be confined and stimulation kept to a minimum. Paradoxical excitation can be treated with a mild sedative (eg diphenhydramine).

Common clinical signs seen in dogs with a clonazepam overdose include ataxia, sedation, agitation, and vomiting; common signs seen in cats include ataxia, sedation, and agitation.

Massive overdoses can lead to CNS and respiratory depression or hypotension. Gastric decontamination can be considered. Use of analeptic agents (eg, caffeine, doxapram) is generally not recommended. Flumazenil can be used to reverse respiratory depression or severe CNS depression. The half-life of flumazenil is short and the animal may require multiple doses of the drug. Flumazenil may precipitate seizures in epileptic patients or patients chronically receiving clonazepam antiseizure therapy.

For patients that have experienced or are suspected to have experienced an overdose, it is strongly encouraged to consult with one of the 24-hour poison consultation centers that specialize in providing information specific for veterinary patients. For general information related to overdose and toxin exposures, as well as contact information for poison control centers, refer to ***Appendix***.

Drug Interactions

The following drug interactions have either been reported or are theoretical in humans or animals receiving clonazepam and may be of significance in veterinary patients. Unless otherwise noted, use together is not necessarily contraindicated, but weigh the potential risks and perform additional monitoring when appropriate.

- ANESTHETIC AGENTS (eg, **alfaxalone, dexmedetomidine, isoflurane, propofol**): Additive sedation or respiratory depression may occur.
- ANTICHOLINERGIC AGENTS (eg, **atropine, glycopyrrolate**): Anticholinergic effects may be potentiated.
- ANTIDEPRESSANTS (eg, **amitriptyline, clomipramine, mirtazapine**): Concurrent use may decrease the risk for CNS and/or respiratory depression.
- ANTIHYPERTENSIVE AGENTS (eg, **amlodipine, benazepril, telmisartan**): Concurrent use may increase the risk for hypotension and orthostasis.
- AZOLE ANTIFUNGALS (eg, **itraconazole, ketoconazole**): May increase clonazepam levels
- CANNABIDIOL: Additive CNS depression may occur
- CARBAMAZEPINE: Concurrent use may result in decreased clonazepam concentrations.
- CARBONIC ANHYDRASE INHIBITORS (CAIs; eg, **acetazolamide, dichlorphenamide, methazolamide**): Clonazepam may interfere with the beneficial effects of CAIs by inhibiting responses to hypoxia.
- CIMETIDINE: May decrease metabolism of benzodiazepines
- DANAZOL: Danazol may increase clonazepam concentrations.
- DIGOXIN: Concurrent use may increase digoxin levels, increasing the risk for toxicity. Digoxin levels should be closely monitored and doses adjusted as indicated.
- DILTIAZEM: May increase levels of clonazepam. Monitor for overextension of pharmacologic effect.
- ERYTHROMYCIN: May decrease the metabolism of benzodiazepines
- OPIOIDS (eg, **buprenorphine, fentanyl, methadone, morphine, tramadol**): Concomitant use may result in profound sedation and respiratory depression.
- PHENOBARBITAL: May decrease clonazepam concentrations. Additive CNS depression may occur.
- PHENOTHIAZINES (eg, **acepromazine**): Additive CNS depression may occur
- PHENYTOIN: May decrease clonazepam concentrations
- PROPANTHELINE: Concurrent propantheline use with orally disintegrating clonazepam tablets may decrease clonazepam concentrations.
- RIFAMPIN: May induce hepatic microsomal enzymes and decrease the pharmacologic effects of benzodiazepines
- VALPROIC ACID, DIVALPROEX: Concurrent use may increase risk of teratogenesis and may displace benzodiazepines from protein binding sites and inhibit metabolism. Monitor for excessive sedation and avoid combination in pregnancy.
- YOHIMBINE: May decrease therapeutic effects of anxiolytic drugs

Laboratory Considerations

- Benzodiazepines may decrease the thyroidal uptake of I^{123} or I^{131}.

Dosages

DOGS:

Anxiolytic (extra-label): Dosage recommendations vary considerably. Most range from 0.1 – 1 mg/kg PO up to 2 to 3 times per day, but up to 2.2 mg/kg every 6 hours has also been recommended.[5] In general, dosages are started near the low end and increased if necessary. If discontinuing after long-term use, do so gradually.

Adjunctive treatment of seizures or sleep disorders (extra-label): Most dosage recommendations range from 0.5 – 1 mg/kg PO 2 to 3 times per day, but up to every 6 hours or dosages up to 2 mg/kg PO every 12 hours have also been recommended. In general, dosages are started near the low end and increased if necessary. If discontinuing after long-term use, do so gradually.

CATS:

Anxiolytic (extra-label): Dosage recommendations vary considerably. Most range from 0.02 – 0.25 mg/kg PO up to 2 times a day.[5] In general, dosages are started near the low end and increased if necessary. If discontinuing after long-term use, do so gradually.

Adjunctive treatment of seizures (extra-label): Dosage recommendations vary considerably. Most range from 0.02 – 0.5 mg/kg PO up to 2 times a day. In general, dosages are started near the low end and increased if necessary. If discontinuing after long-term use, do so gradually.

Monitoring

- Efficacy
- Adverse effects
- The therapeutic plasma concentration has been reported as 0.02 to 0.07 μg/mL in humans[6]; therapeutic drug monitoring is not routinely performed in veterinary patients.
- In cats, baseline and periodic liver panel

Client Information

- This drug is used to help control seizures and as a tranquilizer.
- Can cause sedation and/or disorientation, which may impair performance of working animals.
- When using for thunderstorm anxiety or other triggers (eg, owner separation) that upset your animal, try to give clonazepam ≈1 hour before the event or trigger. This medication works best for treating anxiety-related behaviors when given along with behavior therapy.
- When used to treat for seizures, it is very important to give doses regularly.
- May be given with or without food. Food or small treats may be given if your animal vomits or acts sick after receiving the medication on an empty stomach. Contact your veterinarian if vomiting continues.
- Contact your veterinarian immediately if you see yellowing of the skin, gums, or whites of the eyes.
- Sleepiness is the most common side effect, but this drug can change the animal's behavior (eg, hyperactivity, anxiety) in unexpected ways.
- This drug may increase appetite, especially in cats.
- Men or women who are actively trying to conceive, women who are pregnant or may become pregnant, and women who are breast feeding should consider wearing gloves while handling this drug and wash their hands after handling.
- Do not stop treatment abruptly. Contact your veterinarian if you feel the drug should be discontinued.
- Clonazepam is a schedule 4 (C-IV) controlled drug and requires a new written prescription for refills. Use of this medication in animals or humans other than those for whom they are prescribed is illegal.
- This medication is considered to be a hazardous drug as defined by the National Institute for Occupational Safety and Health (NIOSH). Talk with your veterinarian or pharmacist about the use of personal protective equipment when handling this medicine.

Chemistry/Synonyms

Clonazepam, a benzodiazepine anticonvulsant, occurs as an off-white to light-yellow crystalline powder with a faint odor. It is insoluble in water and slightly soluble in alcohol.

Clonazepam may also be known as clonazepamum, Ro-5-4023, *Antelepsin*®, *Clonagin*®, *Clonapam*®, *Clonax*®, *Clonex*®, *Diocam*®, *Epitril*®, *Iktorivil*®, *Kenoket*®, *Klonopin*®, *Kriadex*®, *Neuryl*®, *Paxam*®, *Rivatril*®, *Rivotril*®, or *Solfidin*®.

Storage/Stability

Tablets should be stored in airtight, light-resistant containers at room temperature of 20°C to 25°C (68°F-77°F). For orally disintegrating tablets, excursions to 15°C to 30°C (59°F-86°F) are permitted.

Clonazepam is a schedule 4 (C-IV) controlled substance, clonazepam must be stored in an area that is substantially constructed and securely locked. Follow applicable local, state, and federal rules regarding disposal of unused or wasted controlled drugs.

Compatibility/Compounding Considerations

Compounded preparation stability: Clonazepam oral suspension compounded from commercially available tablets has been published.[7] Triturating 6 clonazepam 2 mg tablets with 60 mL of *Ora-Plus*® and qs ad to 120 mL with *Ora-Sweet*® (or *Ora-Sweet*® *SF*) yields a 0.1 mg/mL suspension that retains greater than 90% potency for 60 days stored at both 5°C (41°F) and 25°C (77°F). Compounded preparations of clonazepam should be protected from light.

Dosage Forms/Regulatory Status

VETERINARY-LABELED PRODUCTS: NONE

The Association of Racing Commissioners International (ARCI) has designated this drug as a class 2 substance. See ***Appendix*** for more information. Use of this drug may not be allowed in certain animal competitions. Check rules and regulations before entering in a competition while this medication is being administered. Contact local racing authorities for further guidance.

HUMAN-LABELED PRODUCTS:

Clonazepam Oral Tablets: 0.5 mg, 1 mg, and 2 mg; *KlonoPIN*®, generic; (Rx; C-IV)

Clonazepam Orally Dispersible (Disintegrating) Tablets: 0.125 mg, 0.25 mg, 0.5 mg, 1 mg, and 2 mg (with mannitol); generic; (Rx; C-IV). **NOTE:** May contain xylitol

Report dispensing to state monitoring programs where required.

References

For the complete list of references, see **wiley.com/go/budde/plumb**

Clonidine

(***klah***-nih-deen) *Catapres*®, *Duraclon*®

Alpha-2-Adrenergic Agonist

Prescriber Highlights

- ► Centrally acting alpha-adrenergic agonist used as a preanesthetic agent, an adjunct analgesia in epidurals, and an adjunctive treatment for some behavioral conditions
- ► Can be used in diagnostic agent testing for growth hormone deficiency or pheochromocytoma in dogs and as an antidiarrheal agent
- ► Limited experience in veterinary species for therapeutic or diagnostic purposes
- ► Potential adverse effects include transient hyperglycemia, dry mouth, constipation, sedation, aggressive behavior, hypotension, collapse, and bradycardia
- ► When discontinuing after prolonged use, reduce dosage over several days.

Uses/Indications

Clonidine may be useful as a preanesthetic medication and as an epidural adjunct, with or without opioids, in dogs[1-3] and cattle.[4]

The use of clonidine as an adjunctive treatment for certain behavioral conditions in dogs has been of interest, but limited evidence supporting its use is available. An open trial using clonidine on an as-needed basis for fear-based behavioral problems suggested that clonidine reduced phobic signs and aggression in most treated dogs.[5] Clonidine combined with fluoxetine appeared effective in dogs with behavioral disorders.[6]

Clonidine may be used as a diagnostic agent to determine growth hormone deficiency or pheochromocytoma in dogs. Clonidine has been used as an antidiarrheal agent in dogs and cats,[7] and as adjunctive treatment of diarrhea-predominant inflammatory bowel disease in dogs.[8]

Pharmacology/Actions

Clonidine acts in the brain stem, stimulating alpha-adrenergic receptors, and results in reduced sympathetic outflow from the CNS and decreased renal vascular resistance, peripheral resistance, cardiac rate, and blood pressure. Renal blood flow and glomerular filtration rates are not affected.

Clonidine causes growth hormone (GH, somatotropin) release from the pituitary gland by stimulating hypothalamic release of GHRH, but this effect does not persist with continued dosing. Clonidine reduces plasma renin activity and aldosterone excretion.

Clonidine possesses central analgesic effects most likely at presynaptic and postjunctional $alpha_2$-adrenoreceptors in the spinal cord, thereby blocking pain signal transmission to the brain. It may also increase seizure threshold, but the clinical significance of this effect is unclear. Clonidine acts on the GI tract to increase fluid and electrolyte absorption. Studies have shown that clonidine reduces renal sympathetic nerve activity, restores vascular sensitivity to phenylephrine and angiotensin II, and results in better preservation of arterial pressure during hypotensive sepsis in sheep.[9]

Pharmacokinetics

Limited information is available on the pharmacokinetics of clonidine in domestic animals. In cats, clonidine exhibits a 2-compartment open model and penetrates into tissues rapidly.

In humans, the drug is well absorbed after oral administration. Peak plasma concentrations occur ≈1 to 3 hours after oral administration. After epidural administration, maximal analgesia occurs within 30 to 60 minutes. Clonidine is apparently widely distributed into body tissues; tissue concentrations are higher than in plasma. Clonidine enters the CSF, but brain concentrations are low compared with other tissues. In humans with normal renal function, clonidine's half-life is 12 to 16 hours. Elimination may be prolonged with higher dosages (dose-dependent elimination kinetics) or in patients with renal dysfunction. Up to 60% of a dose is eliminated unchanged in the urine, but the remainder is metabolized in the liver; 1 active metabolite (p-hydroxyclonidine) has been identified.

Contraindications/Precautions/Warnings

Clonidine is contraindicated in patients known to be hypersensitive to it. It should be used with caution in patients with severe cardiovascular disease, including conduction disturbances or heart failure; lower dosages may be required in patients with renal insufficiency.

Abrupt cessation of oral clonidine use has produced withdrawal-like symptoms (eg, agitation, nervousness, tremor, elevated blood pressure) in humans.[10] Although the veterinary significance is unknown, gradual dose reduction over 2 to 4 days should be considered.

Do not confuse cloNIDine with cloNAZepam, KLONOpin, or QUINidine.

Adverse Effects

Bradycardia and hypotension have been observed following epidural[2,11] and IM[12] administration in dogs. Dogs receiving IV clonidine for the diagnosis of growth hormone deficiency have experienced adverse reactions including sedation, aggressive behavior, hypotension, collapse, and bradycardia (responsive to atropine) lasting for 15 to 60 minutes post-clonidine administration.[13] Marked sedation and ataxia occurred after epidural administration in horses.[14]

Long-term use in rats, but not in humans, has been associated with dose-dependent retinal degeneration.

Reproductive/Nursing Safety

Clonidine crosses the placenta. No teratogenic or embryotoxic effects were found in rabbits, but increased resorption occurred in rats and mice.[10] Because safety has not been established in animal species, this drug should only be used when the maternal benefits outweigh the potential fetal risks.

Clonidine enters human maternal milk and may reach concentrations exceeding that of maternal plasma; severe adverse effects in the nursing infant may occur. Use cautiously in nursing veterinary species or consider milk replacer.

Overdose/Acute Toxicity

Clonidine has a narrow margin of safety. Common clinical signs associated with an overdose mirror the adverse effect profile in dogs and cats and include lethargy/sedation, bradycardia, ataxia, vomiting, and hypotension. In humans, seizures or respiratory depression are rarely seen. The LD_{50} values reported for oral clonidine in rats and mice are 465 mg/kg and 206 mg/kg, respectively.[10]

Treatment for overdoses associated with clinical signs includes GI decontamination using standard protocols. Use of emetics should be considered carefully, as level of consciousness may deteriorate rapidly. Treatment of systemic effects is primarily based on clinical signs and is supportive. Hypotensive effects may be treated, if necessary, using fluids or pressors (eg, dopamine); bradycardia may be treated with IV atropine, if required. Atipamezole or yohimbine may also be used to help reverse the cardiovascular effects, but multiple doses may be required as clinical signs can last up to 48 hours, depending on clonidine dosage.

For patients that have experienced or are suspected to have experienced an overdose, consultation with a 24-hour poison center specializing in providing veterinary-specific information is recommended. For general information related to overdose and toxin exposures, as well as contact information for poison control centers, refer to ***Appendix***.

Drug Interactions

The following drug interactions have either been reported or are theoretical in humans or animals receiving clonidine and may be of significance in veterinary patients. Unless otherwise noted, use together is not necessarily contraindicated, but weigh the potential risks and perform additional monitoring when appropriate.

- Antihypertensive Drugs (eg, **amlodipine, enalapril, hydralazine, sildenafil, telmisartan**): Possible additive hypotensive effects
- Beta-Adrenergic Antagonists (eg, **propranolol**): May enhance bradycardia when given with clonidine. If clonidine is to be discontinued in patients concurrently receiving clonidine and beta-adrenergic antagonists, the beta-adrenergic antagonist should be discontinued prior to clonidine and clonidine gradually discontinued; otherwise, rebound hypertension may occur.
- Calcium Channel Blockers (eg, **diltiazem, verapamil,** but not **amlodipine**): Increased risk of sinus bradycardia and complete AV block; blood pressure and heart rate should be closely monitored.
- CNS Depressant Drugs (eg, **barbiturates, opioids**): Clonidine may exacerbate the actions of other CNS depressant drugs.

- **Digoxin**: Possible additive bradycardia. Blood pressure and heart rate should be closely monitored.
- **Glucocorticoids** (eg, **dexamethasone, prednis(ol)one**): May decrease the antihypertensive effects of clonidine by causing fluid and sodium retention
- **Prazosin**: May decrease the antihypertensive effects of clonidine
- **Stimulants** (eg, **doxapram**): Concurrent use may increase risk of hypertension and tachycardia. Monitor pulse and blood pressure.
- **Tricyclic Antidepressants** (**TCAs**; eg, **amitriptyline, clomipramine**): May block the antihypertensive effects of clonidine and increase risk of severe hypertension. Risk of corneal opacities is increased. Combination should be avoided if possible. If use together is necessary, monitor blood pressure diligently. Withdrawal of either drug should be done gradually.

Laboratory Considerations

- False-positive **Coombs test** has been reported.[10]

Dosages

DOGS:

Adjunctive treatment (with other medications and behavioral therapy) for situational fears, phobias, and separation anxiety (extra-label): 0.01 – 0.05 mg/kg PO up to twice daily; median effective dosage was 0.017 – 0.026 mg/kg PO up to twice daily. The same dose may be used on an as-needed basis ≈1.5 to 2 hours prior to the triggering event.[5]

Epidural analgesia (extra-label):

1. 150 µg/dog (NOT µg/kg) administered immediately after anesthetic induction[1,11]
2. 5 µg/kg with 2.5 mg/kg lidocaine (1%). **NOTE**: Supplemental isoflurane was required.[3]

Premedicant prior to anesthesia (extra-label): 6 – 10 µg/kg IV prior to etomidate/halothane anesthesia[2]

Diagnosing growth hormone deficiency (hyposomatotropism; extra-label): Dosage may vary depending on the laboratory's protocol. Contact laboratory prior to test to determine protocol and sample handling instructions. Usual dose is 10 µg/kg IV.[13] Obtain plasma for growth hormone (GH) concentrations prior to clonidine dosing and again at 15, 30, 45, 60, and 120 minutes. Healthy dogs should demonstrate GH concentrations of 10 ng/mL after clonidine administration.[15]

Adjunctive antidiarrheal therapy for refractory cases of inflammatory bowel disease (extra-label): 5 – 10 µg/kg PO or SC 2 to 3 times daily[7]; can activate alpha-2-receptors in the chemoreceptor trigger zone (CRTZ) and cause vomiting[8,16]

CATS:

Adjunctive antidiarrheal therapy for refractory cases of inflammatory bowel disease (extra-label): As fourth-line therapy after prostaglandin synthetase inhibitors (ie, sulfasalazine, bismuth subsalicylate), opioid agonists (ie, loperamide), and 5-HT_3 serotonergic antagonists (ie, ondansetron) are being used: clonidine 5 – 10 µg/kg 2 to 3 times daily, SC or PO[7,8]

CATTLE:

Epidural analgesia/analgesia (extra-label): 2 – 3 µg/kg diluted to 8 mL with sterile normal saline epidurally. Onset/duration of analgesia is 19 minutes/192 minutes respectively, with a 2 µg/kg dosage. Onset/duration of analgesia is 9 minutes/311 minutes respectively, with a 3 µg/kg dosage. Peak analgesic effects with both dosages occurs at 60 to 180 minutes.[4]

Monitoring

- Baseline and periodic blood pressure, and heart rate and rhythm with chronic use. **NOTE**: Cardiovascular effects usually only persist for 1 hour after dose.
- Clinical efficacy

Client Information

- This medicine may be given with or without food. If your animal vomits or acts sick after receiving this medicine on an empty stomach, try giving the next dose with food or a small treat. If vomiting continues, contact your veterinarian.
- Experience with this drug in dogs or cats is limited. Sleepiness and lowered blood pressure (eg, weakness, collapse) are the most likely side effects. Report unusual effects to your veterinarian.
- When used to treat fear-based behavioral problems, clonidine is usually given 90 minutes to 2 hours before the event. Dosages are started low and then gradually increased, depending on side effects and effectiveness. Sometimes this medicine is used longer term on a regular basis (up to twice daily).
- This medicine is best used with behavioral modification training for fear-based problems.
- When used daily, do not change or skip doses, or discontinue treatment, without your veterinarian's advice.

Chemistry/Synonyms

An imidazoline derivative, clonidine HCl is a centrally acting alpha-adrenergic agonist that occurs as an odorless, bitter, white or almost white crystalline powder. It is soluble in water and alcohol and is considered highly lipid soluble. The commercially available injection for epidural use has an adjusted pH between 5 and 7.

Clonidine may also be known as ST-155 or clonidini hydrochloridum; *Catapres*® and *Duraclon*® are common trade names.

Storage/Stability

Clonidine tablets should be stored in tight, light-resistant containers at room temperature, 25°C (77°F); excursions from 15°C to 30°C (59°F-86°F) are permitted. The preservative-free injection for epidural use should be stored at controlled room temperature, 20°C to 25°C (68°F-77°F). Because it contains no preservative, unused portions of the injection should be discarded.

Compatibility/Compounding Considerations

Clonidine is reportedly **compatible** with 0.9% sodium chloride, and in the same syringe with bupivacaine, fentanyl, heparin, ketamine, lidocaine, and morphine.

Dosage Forms/Regulatory Status

VETERINARY-LABELED PRODUCTS: NONE.

The Association of Racing Commissioners International (ARCI) has designated this drug as a class 3 substance. See ***Appendix*** for more information. Use of this drug may not be allowed in certain animal competitions. Check rules and regulations before entering in a competition while this medication is being administered. Contact local racing authorities for further guidance.

HUMAN-LABELED PRODUCTS:

Clonidine HCl Injection for epidural use: 100 µg/mL and 500 µg/mL (must be diluted before use) preservative-free in 10 mL vials; *Duraclon*®, generic; (Rx)

Clonidine HCl Oral Tablets: 0.1 mg, 0.2 mg, and 0.3 mg; *Catapres*®, generic; (Rx)

Clonidine extended-release tablets and transdermal patches also are available.

References

For the complete list of references, see **wiley.com/go/budde/plumb**

Clopidogrel

(kloe-***pid***-oh-grel) *Plavix®*

Platelet Aggregation Inhibitor

Prescriber Highlights

- Oral, once-daily platelet aggregation inhibitor that may be useful in the treatment of dogs, cats, and horses with hypercoagulable conditions and in the prevention of thromboembolic disease
- Inhibits platelet function for the lifespan of the platelet; clinically normal platelet function gradually returns 3 to 7 days after discontinuation of the medication as new platelets are released
- Appears to be well tolerated, but can potentially cause vomiting or bleeding

Uses/Indications

Clopidogrel, a platelet aggregation inhibitor, may be useful for the prevention of thromboembolic disease in cats and dogs.[1] Clopidogrel appears to reduce recurrent cardiogenic arterial thromboembolism and mortality in cats when administered after arterial thromboembolism.[2] Although aspirin and clopidogrel have historically (and in humans, are commonly) been used together, evidence supporting the combination of these drugs in veterinary patients is scarce.[3,4] Clopidogrel may also improve pelvic limb circulation in cats after a cardiogenic embolic event via a vasomodulating effect secondary to inhibition of serotonin release from platelets.[5]

Clopidogrel has been suggested as a treatment to decrease the chances of arterial thromboembolism in dogs with hypercoagulable conditions, although evidence supporting this recommendation is limited.[4,6] Thromboprophylaxis is recommended in all dogs with immune-mediated hemolytic anemia (IMHA), except those with severe thrombocytopenia (ie, platelet count less than 30,000/µL), in which clopidogrel is preferred to aspirin for antiplatelet therapy.[7]

Clopidogrel inhibits platelet function in healthy adult horses[8-11] but failed to attenuate the clinicopathologic effects of endotoxin infusion or ex vivo equine herpesvirus (EHV)-1-induced platelet activation.[12,13]

Pharmacology/Actions

Clopidogrel is a prodrug and must be hepatically metabolized to form an active, highly unstable thiol compound (commonly referred to as clopidogrel active metabolite [CAM]). This compound binds selectively to the platelet surface adenosine diphosphate (ADP) receptor, $P2Y_{12}$, and irreversibly alters the ADP receptor for the lifespan of the platelet.[14] This receptor alteration reduces activation of the platelet by ADP and inhibits full activation of the glycoprotein GPIIb/IIIa complex (which is responsible for platelet binding to fibrinogen and integration into clots).[15]

In a pharmacodynamic study in healthy dogs, most dogs had significant inhibition of platelet function within 3 hours after the initial oral dose of clopidogrel; inhibition lasted at least 24 hours.[16] In cats, a daily oral dosage of clopidogrel 18.75 mg/cat (NOT mg/kg), inhibited platelet function within 1 day, whereas a lower daily oral dosage of 10 mg/cat (NOT mg/kg) had a delayed effect.[17] Clinically apparent decreases in platelet aggregation persist for 3 to 7 days in dogs and cats.[16-20] Generic clopidogrel had antiplatelet effects comparable with *Plavix®* in cats.[21] Desmopressin acetate (DDAVP) is not effective for reversing the antiplatelet effects of clopidogrel in healthy dogs.[22] In healthy dogs, the combination of clopidogrel and prednisone did not change platelet aggregation responses as compared with dogs receiving clopidogrel alone.[23]

In horses, antiplatelet effects were seen after 3 to 5 days of treatment and lasted for 5 days after discontinuation of the medication.[10]

Pharmacokinetics

Because clopidogrel inactivates platelets for their lifespan, the drug's biological action is not explained by its pharmacokinetic profile.[20]

In dogs, clopidogrel's pharmacokinetics have not been fully elucidated, but onset of clinical effects on platelets may range from 3 hours to 2 days.[16,18] Concentrations of an inactive metabolite peaked between 1 to 2 hours after a single oral dose.[16] The variable time to full inhibition may provide justification for a loading dose when initiating therapy.[18]

In a pilot pharmacokinetic study of clopidogrel in 2 cats, time to peak clopidogrel active metabolite (CAM) concentration was 1.5 to 2 hours, and the elimination half-life was 2.8 to 4.9 hours. An almost 2-fold difference was noted in total CAM exposure (as measured by area under the curve [AUC]).[24] High interindividual variation in CAM formation was determined to be due primarily to genetic polymorphism in CYP2C; however, males were associated with reduced CAM formation.[25] Variability in the *P2RY1* gene may alter the pharmacodynamics of clopidogrel in cats (and likely other species) and may explain the interpatient differences in response to therapy.[26]

In horses, clopidogrel decreased ADP-induced platelet aggregation, but the time to onset and total required dose in horses was greater than in other species.[10] A loading dose inhibited platelet function within hours; platelet function returned to baseline 6 days after cessation of therapy.[8]

In humans, clopidogrel is rapidly absorbed with a bioavailability of ≈50%; food does not alter its absorption. Clopidogrel is highly bound to plasma proteins. It is rapidly and predominantly hydrolyzed to an inactive carboxylic acid derivative (SR 26334) that is excreted via the urine and feces. A small fraction of a dose is transformed to the active intermediate compound (see ***Pharmacology/Actions***), which has a half-life of 30 minutes. Two percent of the administered drug is covalently bound to platelets and has an elimination half-life of ≈11 days.[14]

Contraindications/Precautions/Warnings

Clopidogrel is contraindicated in patients hypersensitive to it or those with active pathologic bleeding or inherited thrombocytopathias. Clopidogrel is relatively contraindicated in patients with thrombocytopenia or coagulopathies, depending on the underlying cause.

In dogs, platelet function does not return to normal until ≈7 days after stopping administration of clopidogrel.[18] Consideration must be taken to assess the patient's risk for thrombosis versus the risk for bleeding during surgical procedures.[27] In dogs and cats at high risk for thrombosis, it is recommended to continue antiplatelet therapy through surgery unless animals are receiving more than one anticoagulant. For dogs and cats at low to moderate risk for thrombosis, it is recommended to discontinue antiplatelet agents 5 to 7 days prior to an elective procedure.[27]

In humans undergoing elective surgery with a major risk for bleeding, it is recommended to withhold clopidogrel 5 days prior to surgery to reduce the antiplatelet effect; platelet transfusion prior to surgery may be considered if clopidogrel withdrawal is not indicated.[14]

Adverse Effects

Clopidogrel appears to be well tolerated in dogs, cats, and horses. Vomiting (dogs and cats), anorexia, or diarrhea may occur; giving the drug with food may alleviate these effects in dogs and cats. Nonregenerative anemia has been reported in some cats receiving long-term clopidogrel treatment.

Clopidogrel alone did not cause GI bleeding or ulceration in dogs and did not appear to increase the incidence of GI ulceration when given in combination with prednisone.[28]

In humans, primary adverse effects have been related to bleeding. Major bleeding events occur in 3.7% of humans receiving clopidogrel and aspirin combination therapy, versus 2.7% incidence with clopidogrel alone.[14] Minor bleeding occurs in 5.1% of patients receiving both clopidogrel and aspirin, versus 2.4% in those receiving aspirin alone.[14] Rashes and GI effects (eg, diarrhea) have also been reported. Thrombotic thrombocytopenic purpura and aplastic anemia are rarely reported.

Reproductive/Nursing Safety

In pregnant rats, doses ≈65 times, and in rabbits doses 78 times, that of the human recommended dose (compared on an mg/m^2 basis) caused no teratogenic effects.[14]

In rats, clopidogrel and its metabolites are distributed into maternal milk.[14]

Because safety of clopidogrel has not been established in animals, this drug should only be used when the maternal benefits outweigh the potential risks to offspring.

Overdose/Acute Toxicity

Limited information is available. Reported lethal oral doses in mice and rats were 1500 mg/kg and 2000 mg/kg (460 times the human adult dose on an mg/m^2 basis), respectively.[14] Acute toxic signs may include bleeding or vomiting. Because clopidogrel irreversibly inhibits platelet function for the lifespan of the platelet, toxic effects may persist for several days. Platelet transfusions have been suggested if rapid reversal is required. Clopidogrel is unlikely to be dialyzable.

For patients that have experienced or are suspected to have experienced an overdose, consultation with a 24-hour poison consultation center specializing in providing veterinary-specific information is recommended. For general information related to overdose and toxin exposures, as well as contact information for poison control centers, refer to ***Appendix***.

Drug Interactions

In humans, clopidogrel is a substrate and inhibitor of CYP2C19 and a strong inhibitor of CYP2C8. The following drug interactions have either been reported or are theoretical in humans or animals receiving clopidogrel and may be of significance in veterinary patients. Unless otherwise noted, use together is not necessarily contraindicated, but weigh the potential risks and perform additional monitoring when appropriate.

- **Aspirin**: Concurrent use may increase the risk for bleeding; however, simultaneous use in humans is common.
- **Azole Antifungals** (eg, **fluconazole, ketoconazole**): Concurrent use may result in decreased efficacy of clopidogrel.
- **Calcium Channel Blockers** (eg, **amlodipine, diltiazem, verapamil**): Concurrent use may result in decreased efficacy of clopidogrel and increased risk for thrombosis.
- **Chloramphenicol**: Concurrent use may decrease efficacy of clopidogrel.
- **Cimetidine**: May decrease the effects of clopidogrel[29]
- **Cyclosporine**: A study in dogs showed that cyclosporine can increase clopidogrel peak concentration, but drug exposure was the same as compared with clopidogrel alone.[30]
- **Heparin; Low Molecular Weight Heparins** (eg, **dalteparin, enoxaparin**): Clopidogrel appears safe to use with heparin (both unfractionated and low molecular weight).
- **Isoniazid**: Concurrent use may reduce formation of the clopidogrel active metabolite.
- **Nonsteroidal Anti-Inflammatory Drugs** (NSAIDs; eg, **carprofen, robenacoxib**): Concurrent use may increase the risk for bleeding; clopidogrel may interfere with NSAID metabolism.
- **Opioids** (eg, **hydromorphone, morphine**): Opioid use may delay and reduce formation of the clopidogrel active metabolite and the drug's antiplatelet effect, possibly by reducing GI motility and drug absorption.
- **Proton Pump Inhibitors** (PPIs; eg, **esomeprazole, omeprazole**): In humans, concurrent use of omeprazole and esomeprazole (but not other PPIs) may decrease the efficacy of clopidogrel and increase the risk for thrombosis; however, a study in dogs found omeprazole combined with clopidogrel did not alter antiplatelet effects in healthy dogs.[31]
- **Rifampin**: May increase the effects of clopidogrel by increasing formation of the clopidogrel active metabolite[29]
- **Rivaroxaban**: Concurrent use may increase the risk for bleeding.
- **Selective Serotonin Reuptake Inhibitors** (SSRIs; eg, **fluoxetine, paroxetine**): Concurrent use may increase the risk for bleeding.
- **Telmisartan**: Concurrent telmisartan use did not alter formation of the inactive clopidogrel metabolite.[30]
- **Torsemide**: Clopidogrel may interfere with metabolism.
- **Warfarin**: Concurrent use may increase the risk for bleeding; clopidogrel may interfere with metabolism of warfarin.

Laboratory Considerations

- None noted

Dosages

NOTE: Because of the drug's extreme bitterness, administering the medication in a gelatin capsule may be considered.

DOGS:

Antiplatelet agent (extra-label): 1 – 4 mg/kg PO once daily.[4,6,16,18,32] A loading dose of 4 – 10 mg/kg PO on the first day of treatment can be considered.[32,33] Experimental evidence suggests efficacy in prevention of arterial thromboembolism, but data are lacking for venous thromboembolism.[33]

CATS:

Aortic thromboembolism (extra-label): Loading dose: 37.5 – 75 mg/cat (NOT mg/kg) PO once after diagnosis.[5,33] Maintenance dose: 18.75 mg/cat (NOT mg/kg) PO every 24 hours

Thrombus prevention; antiplatelet agent (extra-label): 18.75 mg/cat (NOT mg/kg) PO once daily.[2,33] Experimentally in healthy cats, 10 mg/cat (NOT mg/kg) PO once daily had a similar antiplatelet effect as 18.75 mg/cat (NOT mg/kg) PO once daily, although the lower dosage required 2 days for onset of antiplatelet activity as compared with 1 day for the higher dosage.[17]

HORSES:

Antiplatelet agent (extra-label): From experimental studies, loading dose of 4 – 6.5 mg/kg PO once on the first day of treatment[8,11]; maintenance dose: 1.2 – 4 mg/kg PO once daily[8-10]

Monitoring

- Clinical efficacy
- Current guidelines do not provide recommendations for objective monitoring of clopidogrel therapy due to lack of data and the safety of clopidogrel when administered at recommended dosages.[34]
- Platelet aggregometry and modified thromboelastography have been used to evaluate clopidogrel effects in dogs, cats, and horses under experimental conditions.[16,19,20,31,35,36]
- Adverse effects (eg, vomiting, bleeding)

Client Information

- Bleeding is not likely but can occur. If your animal shows any signs of bleeding; bruising; difficulty breathing; blood in vomit (looks like coffee grounds); blood in urine; or black, tarry stools, consult your veterinarian immediately.

- This medicine may be given with or without food, but if vomiting occurs, give with food.

Chemistry/Synonyms

Clopidogrel bisulfate, a thienopyridine, occurs as a white to off-white powder that is practically insoluble in water at a pH of 7 but is freely soluble at a pH of 1.

Clopidogrel may also be known as SR-259990C, PCR-4099, or clopedogreli. A common trade name is *Plavix®*.

Storage/Stability

Clopidogrel tablets should be stored at 25°C (77°F), with excursions permitted to 15°C to 30°C (59°F-86°F).

Compatibility/Compounding Considerations

Compounded preparation stability: Clopidogrel oral suspension compounded from commercially available tablets has been published.[37] Triturating 4 clopidogrel 75 mg tablets with 30 mL of *Ora-Plus®* and qs ad to 60 mL with *Ora-Sweet®* (or *Ora-Sweet® SF*) yields a 5 mg/mL oral suspension that retains greater than 90% potency for 60 days stored at both 5°C (41°F) and 25°C (77°F). Compounded preparations of clopidogrel should be protected from light and may retain a bitter taste.

Dosage Forms/Regulatory Status

VETERINARY-LABELED PRODUCTS: NONE

HUMAN-LABELED PRODUCTS:

Clopidogrel Bisulfate Tablets: 75 mg and 300 mg; *Plavix®*, generic; (Rx)

References

For the complete list of references, see **wiley.com/go/budde/plumb**

Cloprostenol

(kloe-**pros**-te-nol) *Estrumate®*

Prostaglandin $F_{2\text{-alpha}}$

Prescriber Highlights

- ► Synthetic prostaglandin used in many large and small animal species to induce luteolysis and abortion and to treat pyometra and endometritis
- ► Contraindications include pregnancy (when abortion or induced parturition is not desired).
- ► Can cause cholinergic-like adverse effects in dogs
- ► Do not administer IV.
- ► Wear gloves when handling. Pregnant women should not handle the drug and those with asthma and women of childbearing age should handle with caution.

Uses/Indications

Cloprostenol (racemic) is FDA-approved for use in beef or dairy cows and replacement beef and dairy heifers for unobserved or undetected estrus; for the treatment of pyometra, chronic endometritis, or luteal cysts; expulsion of a mummified fetus; to induce abortions; and for estrus synchronization. It is also approved for use with gonadorelin to synchronize estrous cycles for artificial insemination in lactating dairy cows.[1]

Cloprostenol has been used in dogs for pregnancy termination and in dogs and cats for treatment of open pyometra. Cloprostenol has been shown to be ineffective for inducing abortion in cats[2]; however, it has been used successfully in cats for the treatment of open pyometra.[3]

In horses, cloprostenol has been used for luteolysis, inducing abortion, and stimulating uterine contractions.

Cloprostenol has been used in sows to induce farrowing; in sheep and goats for estrus synchronization, inducing parturition, and for pseudopregnancy; and in camelids for luteolysis.

Pharmacology/Actions

Prostaglandin F_{2alpha} and its analogues, cloprostenol and fluprostenol, are powerful luteolytic agents. They cause rapid regression of the corpus luteum to arrest its secretory activity. These prostaglandins also cause uterine smooth muscle contraction with relaxation of the cervix.

In normally cycling animals, estrus generally occurs 2 to 5 days after treatment. In pregnant cattle treated between 10 and 150 days of gestation, abortion will usually occur 2 to 3 days after cloprostenol injection.

Pharmacokinetics

In cows, cloprostenol peaks in the blood within the first hour following IM administration and falls to undetectable levels by 24 hours. The half-life of cloprostenol has been reported to be ≈3 hours, much longer than that of dinoprost tromethamine (9 minutes).

Contraindications/Precautions/Warnings

Should not be administered to pregnant animals unless abortion is the desired outcome.

Wear gloves when handling; cloprostenol is readily absorbed through the skin and must be washed off immediately with soap and water. Women of childbearing age and persons with asthma or other respiratory diseases should use extreme caution when handling cloprostenol, as the drug may induce abortion or acute bronchoconstriction.

Do not administer IV.

Adverse Effects

The manufacturer does not list any adverse effects for this product when used as labeled. If used after the fifth month of gestation, there is an increased risk for dystocia and decreased efficacy.

In dogs, cloprostenol can cause increased salivation, tachycardia, increased urination and defecation, gagging, vomiting, ataxia, and mild depression. Pretreatment with an anticholinergic drug (eg, atropine) may reduce the severity of these effects.

In cats, cloprostenol has been noted to cause diarrhea, vomiting, and vocalization.

In horses, cloprostenol causes uterine contractions for ≈5 hours postdose; higher doses of cloprostenol can cause sweating, cramping, and loose stools, but the incidence of adverse effects is less than with dinoprost tromethamine.

Reproductive/Nursing Safety

Cloprostenol is contraindicated in pregnant animals unless abortion or induced parturition is desired.

Cloprostenol is approved for use in lactating dairy cows.

Overdose/Acute Toxicity

The manufacturer states that at 50 and 100 times the recommended dosages of cloprostenol, cattle may show signs of uneasiness, slight frothing, and milk ejection. In cattle, 200 times the dose of cloprostenol sodium caused only mild and transient diarrhea.

Overdoses of cloprostenol or other synthetic prostaglandin F_{2alpha} analogues in small animals can reportedly result in shock and death.

For patients that have experienced or are suspected to have experienced an overdose, consultation with a 24-hour poison consultation center specializing in providing veterinary-specific information is recommended. For general information related to overdose and toxin exposures, as well as contact information for poison control centers, refer to ***Appendix.***

Drug Interactions

The following drug interactions have either been reported or are theoretical in humans or animals receiving cloprostenol and may be of significance in veterinary patients. Unless otherwise noted, use

together is not necessarily contraindicated, but weigh the potential risks and perform additional monitoring when appropriate.

- **Oxytocin and Related Agents**: Activity of ecbolic agents may be enhanced by cloprostenol.

Laboratory Considerations

None noted

Dosages

DOGS:

Adjunctive treatment of pyometra[4] (extra-label): Cloprostenol 1 µg/kg SC in combination with cabergoline 5 µg/kg PO once daily for 7 days with oral antibiotic therapy and supportive hydration. If no response to treatment, cloprostenol (without cabergoline), along with supportive treatment, can be continued for another 7 days.

Abortifacient (extra-label):

NOTE: Multiple protocols have been published. Combination protocols minimize adverse GI effects associated with the use of cloprostenol as a single agent.

a) 1 – 2.5 µg/kg SC once daily for 4 to 7 days has been successful in terminating pregnancy in dogs after 30 days gestation.[5]
b) 1 – 2.5 µg/kg SC every 48 hours for 3 doses. Higher doses (2.5 µg/kg) appear to be effective starting at 30 days of pregnancy. Anticholinergic drug administration (eg, atropine) 15 minutes prior to dosing appears to lessen adverse effects.
c) Between gestation days 35 and 45: cloprostenol 1 µg/kg SC (after a tenfold dilution with physiologic saline) on days 1 and 3 given at least 8 hours after food, in combination with cabergoline 5 µg/kg PO once daily with food for 7 days.[6] If pregnancy is not terminated by day 8, continue cabergoline (at same dose) until day 12.

CATS:

Adjunctive treatment of open pyometra (extra-label): Cloprostenol 5 µg/kg SC once daily for 3 days in addition to appropriate antibiotic therapy.

CATTLE:

Labeled indications in beef or dairy cows and replacement beef and dairy heifers using cloprostenol as a single agent (label dosage; FDA-approved)[1]:

a) **Unobserved or undetected estrus; treatment of pyometra, chronic endometritis, or luteal cysts; expulsion of a mummified fetus; induced abortions**: cloprostenol 500 µg/cow (NOT µg/kg) IM once.[1] When used for unobserved or non-detected estrus, cows can be inseminated at the usual time after detection of estrus, or twice at ≈72 and 96 hours after injection.
b) **Estrus synchronization**:

NOTE: Controlled breeding programs should be completed by observing animals and re-inseminating, hand mating after returning to estrus, or turning in clean-up bull(s) 5 to 7 days after the last cloprostenol injection to cover any animals returning to estrus.

Single injection method: Use only for animals with a mature corpus luteum. Complete rectal examination to determine corpus luteum maturity, anatomic normality, and lack of pregnancy. Give cloprostenol 500 µg/cow (NOT µg/kg) IM. Estrus should occur in 2 to 5 days. Inseminate at usual time after detecting estrus or inseminate 72 hours after cloprostenol injection; consider repeating insemination 96 hours after injection.

Double injection method: Complete rectal examination to determine corpus luteum maturity, anatomic normality, and lack of pregnancy. Give cloprostenol 500 µg/cow (NOT µg/kg) IM. Repeat dose 11 days later. Estrus should occur in 2 to 5 days after second injection. Inseminate at usual time after detecting estrus or inseminate 72 hours after second cloprostenol injection; consider repeating insemination 96 hours after second injection.

In combination with gonadorelin to synchronize estrous cycles for fixed time artificial insemination in lactating dairy cows (label dosage; FDA-approved): Gonadorelin 86 µg/cow (NOT µg/kg) IM on Day 0, then give cloprostenol 500 µg/cow (NOT µg/kg) IM 6 to 8 days later, then repeat gonadorelin 86 µg/cow (NOT µg/kg) IM 30 to 72 hours after cloprostenol.[7] Inseminate cows 8 to 24 hours after the second gonadorelin injection or using standard herd practices.

HORSES:

Abortifacient (extra-label):

a) For mismating, cloprostenol 100 – 250 µg/mare (NOT µg/kg) IM may be administered as a single injection beginning at day 5 or 6 postovulation.
b) For pregnancy termination, cloprostenol 100 – 250 µg/mare (NOT µg/kg) IM may be administered as a single injection until day 35 of gestation. From day 35 until 100 days of gestation, serial daily injections may be needed to effectively terminate pregnancy.

Luteolysis and to stimulate uterine contractions (extra-label):

a) Cloprostenol 250 µg/horse (NOT µg/kg) IM once. Research has shown that 10% of a dose (25 µg) can cause luteolysis; if this dose is given once or on two consecutive days, adverse effects can be avoided.[8]
b) As an ecbolic: 250 µg /horse (NOT µg/kg) IM every 24 hours. Cloprostenol should not be used more than one day after ovulation because it can affect normal luteal function and risk pregnancy maintenance.

SWINE:

Induce parturition in sows (extra-label): Cloprostenol 175 µg/pig (NOT µg/kg) IM; give 2 days or less before anticipated date of farrowing. Farrowing generally occurs ≈36 hours after injection.[9]

SHEEP/GOATS:

Estrus synchronization (extra-label): During the breeding period, cloprostenol 125 µg/female (NOT µg/kg) IM or SC twice 9 to 10 days apart. Males can be reintroduced 48 hours after the second injection.

Induce parturition in does (extra-label):

a) Cloprostenol 62.5 – 125 µg/female (NOT µg/kg) IM at 144 days of gestation in early morning. Deliveries will peak at 30 to 35 hours after injection. Maintain goat in usual surroundings and minimize disturbances.
b) Toxemia in does: If there is only a partial response to medical therapy, induction of parturition with cloprostenol 250 µg/female (NOT µg/kg) IM can be attempted. Kidding or abortion typically occurs in 30 to 36 hours. A cesarean section may be needed if the animal does not respond quickly to therapy.[10]

Pseudopregnancy |hydrometra | mucometra (extra-label): Cloprostenol 125 µg/female (NOT µg/kg) IM once

CAMELIDS:

Luteolysis (extra-label): *Alpacas:* Cloprostenol 100 to 175 µg/alpaca (NOT µg/kg) IM once. *Llamas:* Cloprostenol 250 µg/llama (NOT µg/kg) IM. Give once or twice 24 hours apart. Luteolysis and abortion can be induced at any stage of pregnancy with 2 to 4 injections of cloprostenol.[11]

Monitoring

- Adverse effects
- Abdominal ultrasound to confirm pregnancy and/or termination of pregnancy

Client Information

- Cloprostenol should only be used by individuals familiar with its use and precautions.
- Pregnant women should not handle this medicine. Asthmatics or persons with other lung conditions should handle this product with extreme caution.
- Wear disposable gloves when handling and any accidental skin exposure should be washed off immediately.

Chemistry/Synonyms

A synthetic prostaglandin of the F class, cloprostenol sodium occurs as a white to off- or almost white, amorphous, hygroscopic powder. It is freely soluble in water and alcohol. Potency of the commercially available product is expressed in terms of cloprostenol.

Cloprostenol sodium may also be known as ICI-80996, *Estrumate*®, or *estroPLAN*®.

Storage/Stability

Cloprostenol sodium should be stored at room temperature (15°C-30°C [59°F-86°F]); protect from light. Use vial within 28 days of first puncture.

Compatibility/Compounding Considerations

No specific information noted

Dosage Forms/Regulatory Status

VETERINARY-LABELED PRODUCTS:

Cloprostenol Sodium Injection equivalent to 250 µg/mL cloprostenol in 20 mL vials; *Estrumate*®, *estroPLAN Injection*; (Rx). FDA-approved for use in beef and dairy cattle. No preslaughter or milk withdrawal is required when used at labeled dosages; no specific tolerances for cloprostenol residues have been published.

HUMAN-LABELED PRODUCTS: NONE

References

For the complete list of references, see **wiley.com/go/budde/plumb**

Clorazepate

(klor-***az***-e-pate) *Tranxene*®

Benzodiazepine

Prescriber Highlights

- ▶ Benzodiazepine anxiolytic, sedative-hypnotic, and anticonvulsant used in dogs and cats
- ▶ Contraindications include hypersensitivity to benzodiazepines, closed-angle glaucoma, or significant liver disease.
- ▶ Use with caution in aggressive animals (especially those with fear-induced aggression).
- ▶ Most prevalent adverse effects include sedation and ataxia
- ▶ DEA Schedule IV (C-IV) controlled substance

Uses/Indications

Clorazepate has been used in dogs both as an adjunctive anticonvulsant (often in conjunction with phenobarbital) and in the treatment of behavior disorders (primarily those that are anxiety or phobia related). It may be used chronically, or for short-term bridging until steady state is reached with primary, long-term therapies (eg, phenobarbital or bromides for seizure control or fluoxetine for anxiety) Clorazepate, along with fluoxetine and behavior modification, was shown to be most effective in treating nonaggressive dogs with anxiety-related disorders; aggressive dogs were less likely to improve or to show worsening of their undesired behavior.[1] Dogs have been reported to develop tolerance to the anticonvulsant effects of clorazepate less rapidly than to clonazepam or diazepam.[2]

Clorazepate has also been used as an anxiolytic or anticonvulsant agent in cats; however, there is little published on its use in this species.

Pharmacology/Actions

The subcortical levels (primarily limbic, thalamic, and hypothalamic) of the CNS are depressed by clorazepate and other benzodiazepines, thus producing the anxiolytic, sedative, skeletal muscle relaxant, and anticonvulsant effects seen. The exact mechanism of action is unknown, but postulated mechanisms include antagonism of serotonin, increased release of and/or facilitation of gamma-aminobutyric acid (GABA) activity, and diminished release or turnover of acetylcholine in the CNS. Benzodiazepine-specific receptors have been located in the mammalian brain, kidney, liver, lungs and heart. In all species studied, receptors are lacking in the white matter.

Pharmacokinetics

In dogs, clorazepate peak serum concentrations generally occur within 1 to 2 hours. Oral volume of distribution is ≈1.8 L/kg after multiple doses.[3] Clorazepate is metabolized to nordiazepam (also a metabolite of diazepam) and other metabolites in humans and dogs.[4] Nordiazepam is active and has a very long half-life (in humans, up to 100 hours), although the nordiazepam half-life after diazepam administration is only 2 to 10 hours.[5-7].

Contraindications/Precautions/Warnings

Clorazepate is contraindicated in patients with acute closed-angle glaucoma and in those that are hypersensitive to it or other benzodiazepines. Benzodiazepines, including clorazepate, should be used cautiously, if at all, in aggressive and fearful patients, as it may disinhibit the anxiety that may help prevent aggressive behavior in these animals.[1] Benzodiazepines have been reported to exacerbate myasthenia gravis. Patients with renal or hepatic dysfunction may require a reduced dosage, closer observation, or both. Because benzodiazepines increase the risk for respiratory depression, they should be used with caution in patients with respiratory disease.

The effect, if any, of clorazepate on the performance of working dogs is unknown. Physical dependence has been demonstrated in dogs and rabbits, and abrupt withdrawal of clorazepate has caused irritability and nervousness in humans and seizures in animals.[8] Withdrawal seizures have been observed in dogs one day after cessation of treatment and was lethal in one dog.[2]

Because the metabolism of clorazepate in cats has not been fully elucidated, cats should be monitored for potential development of acute hepatic necrosis that has been documented in cats receiving diazepam.[4] (See ***Diazepam***)

Do not confuse clorazepate with clonazepam. Consider writing orders and prescriptions using tall man letters: clorazePATE.

Adverse Effects

In dogs, the most commonly seen adverse effects include sedation and ataxia; similar effects may occur in cats. These effects occur infrequently and are mild and usually transient.

Reproductive/Nursing Safety

Nordiazepam, a metabolite of clorazepate, crosses the placenta. No fetal toxicity was noted after oral administration to rabbits given up to 15 mg/kg or rats given up to 150 mg/kg[8]; however, teratogenic effects of similar benzodiazepines have been noted in rabbits and rats. In humans, other benzodiazepines have been implicated in causing congenital abnormalities when administered during the first trimester of pregnancy. Signs of withdrawal have occurred in infants whose mothers chronically took benzodiazepines during pregnancy. The veterinary significance of these effects is unclear, but these agents should only be used during the first trimester of pregnancy, when the benefits clearly outweigh the risks associated with their use.

Benzodiazepines and their metabolites, including nordiazepam, are distributed into milk and may cause CNS effects in nursing neonates. Use with caution in nursing veterinary patients.

Overdose/Acute Toxicity

The oral LD_{50} in rats is 1320 mg/kg.[8] Dogs have tolerated doses up to 75 mg/kg. When clorazepate is used alone, overdoses are generally limited to significant CNS depression (eg, confusion, coma, decreased reflexes). Treatment of significant oral overdoses consists of standard protocols for GI decontamination and supportive systemic measures. Flumazenil may be considered for more serious overdoses; repeated flumazenil doses may be needed. The use of analeptic agents (CNS stimulants such as caffeine, amphetamines) is generally not recommended.

For patients that have experienced or are suspected to have experienced an overdose, consultation with a 24-hour poison consultation center specializing in providing veterinary-specific information is recommended. For general information related to overdose and toxin exposures, as well as contact information for poison control centers, refer to ***Appendix***.

Drug Interactions

The following drug interactions have either been reported or are theoretical in humans or animals receiving clorazepate and may be of significance in veterinary patients. Unless otherwise noted, use together is not necessarily contraindicated, but weigh the potential risks and perform additional monitoring when appropriate.

- **Amiodarone**: Concurrent use may increase bioavailability and pharmacologic effects of benzodiazepines. Monitor for adverse effects and adjust benzodiazepine dose accordingly.
- **Antacids, Oral** (eg, **calcium carbonate, aluminum/magnesium combinations**): May slow the rate, but not the extent, of oral absorption; administer 2 hours apart to avoid this potential interaction.
- **Antihypertensive Agents** (eg, **atenolol, amlodipine, lisinopril**): Concurrent use may increase risk for hypotension and orthostasis. Monitor blood pressure.
- **Carbonic Anhydrase Inhibitors** (CAIs; eg, **dichlorphenamide, methazolamide**): Benzodiazepines may interfere with the beneficial effects of CAIs by inhibiting respiratory responses to hypoxia. Avoid combination.
- **CNS Depressant Agents** (eg, **acepromazine, anesthetic agents, cannabidiol**): Combination may increase the risk of CNS and/or respiratory depression. Monitor and adjust doses accordingly.
- **Digoxin**: Serum digoxin concentrations may be increased with concurrent administration; monitor serum digoxin levels and for clinical signs of toxicity.
- **Flumazenil:** Flumazenil reduces the effects of clorazepate by competing for benzodiazepine receptors. NOTE: This action is an expected outcome when flumazenil is used as a reversal agent.
- **Fluoxetine, Fluvoxamine**: Decreased clorazepate metabolism is possible.
- **Hepatic Enzyme Inducers** (eg, **dexamethasone, carbamazepine, rifampin**): Concurrent use may increase benzodiazepine metabolism. Monitor clinical response and adjust doses accordingly.
- **Hepatic Enzyme Inhibitors** (eg, **cimetidine, erythromycin, isoniazid, ketoconazole, itraconazole**): Metabolism of clorazepate may be decreased, and excessive sedation may occur. Cimetidine reduced nordiazepam half-life by 37%.[9]
- **Ifosfamide:** Concurrent use may increase the risk for ifosfamide-induced neurotoxic effects. Carefully monitor patients and discontinue both drugs if signs of encephalopathy occur.
- **Non-Depolarizing Neuromuscular Blockers** (eg, **atracurium, pancuronium**): Concurrent use of benzodiazepines may potentiate, attenuate, or have no effect on nondepolarizing neuromuscular blockers.
- **Opioids** (eg, **buprenorphine, fentanyl, morphine, tramadol**): Concurrent use may increase the risk for respiratory and/or CNS depression.
- **Phenobarbital:** Concurrent phenobarbital may reduce concentration of clorazepate's active metabolite, nordiazepam.[10] Concurrent use may increase risk for respiratory and/or CNS depression.
- **Theophylline/Aminophylline:** Concurrent use may decrease the levels and effectiveness of benzodiazepines. Withdrawing theophylline from a stable patient may increase risk of benzodiazepine toxicity.
- **Tricyclic Antidepressants** (TCAs; eg, **amitriptyline, clomipramine, imipramine**): Clorazepate may increase plasma concentrations of these drugs; clinical significance is not known. However, concurrent use may increase the risk of CNS and/or respiratory depression. Anticholinergic effects may be additive.
- **Valproic Acid/Divalproex:** Concurrent use may increase risk for teratogenesis and may displace benzodiazepines from protein binding sites and inhibit benzodiazepine metabolism. Monitor for over sedation and avoid combination in pregnancy.
- **Yohimbine:** Limited data indicate that yohimbine may decrease therapeutic effects of anxiolytic drugs.

Laboratory Considerations

- Benzodiazepines may decrease the thyroidal uptake of I^{123} or I^{131}.
- Clorazepate may increase **serum alkaline phosphatase** and **serum cholesterol** levels; clinical significance is unclear.

Dosages

DOGS:

Adjunctive treatment of epilepsy (extra-label): Dosing recommendations vary but consider: 0.5 – 1.5 mg/kg PO every 8 hours or 1 – 2.5 mg/kg PO every 12 hours; generally used in conjunction with phenobarbital (see ***Drug Interactions***).

Adjunctive therapy for treatment of fears and phobias (extra-label):

a) 1 mg/kg PO every 24 hours combined with fluoxetine 1 mg/kg PO once daily and behavior modification therapy[1]; clorazepate was discontinued after 4 weeks.

b) 0.55 – 2.2 mg/kg PO up to every 8 hours

CATS:

Anxiolytic or for treatment of compulsive behaviors (extra-label): 0.2 – 0.5 mg/kg PO every 12 to 24 hours[11]

Alternative drug to phenobarbital for seizures (extra-label): 3.75 – 7.5 mg/cat (NOT mg/kg) PO once to twice daily[4]

Monitoring

- Efficacy based on indication for use (eg, seizure control, improvement in desired behavior)
- Adverse effects (eg, sedation, ataxia)
- Cats: baseline and periodic (eg, after 1 week of treatment and again within one month) liver enzyme measurements[4]

Client Information

- This medicine can be used to prevent fear and anxiety in dogs and cats.
- This medicine may increase appetite, especially in cats.
- When using this medicine for thunderstorm phobias or other triggers (eg, separation anxiety) that upset your animal, give the

clorazepate about an hour before the event or trigger.

- Clorazepate can be given with or without food. If your animal vomits or acts sick after receiving the medicine on an empty stomach, try giving the next dose with food or a small treat. If vomiting continues, contact your veterinarian.
- If your cat stops eating or if you see yellowing of the whites of the eyes, gums, or skin (jaundice), contact your veterinarian immediately.
- Sleepiness is the most common side effect, but sometimes the drug can change behavior or work in a way that's opposite from what is expected.
- Clorazepate is classified as a Schedule IV (C-IV) controlled drug by the federal Drug Enforcement Agency (DEA). Use of this medication in animals or humans other than those for whom they are prescribed is illegal.

Chemistry/Synonyms

A benzodiazepine anxiolytic, sedative-hypnotic, and anticonvulsant, clorazepate dipotassium occurs as a light yellow, fine powder that is very soluble in water and slightly soluble in alcohol.

Clorazepate dipotassium may also be known as Abbott-35616, AH-3232, 4306-CB, clorazepic acid, dipotassium clorazepate, dikalii clorazepas, or potassium clorazepate; many trade names are available.

Storage/Stability

Store clorazepate tablets at room temperature (20°C-25°C [68°F-77°F) and protected from light and moisture.

Clorazepate dipotassium is unstable in the presence of water. Consider keeping the desiccant packets in with the original container and adding a desiccant packet to the prescription vial when dispensing large quantities of tablets to the client.

Follow applicable local, state, and federal rules regarding controlled drug storage, waste, and disposal.

Compatibility/Compounding Considerations

No specific information noted

Dosage Forms/Regulatory Status

VETERINARY-LABELED PRODUCTS: NONE

The Association of Racing Commissioners International (ARCI) has designated this drug as a class 2 substance. Use of this drug may not be allowed in certain animal competitions. Check rules and regulations before entering a competition while this medication is being administered. Contact local racing authorities for further guidance. See ***Appendix*** for more information.

HUMAN-LABELED PRODUCTS:

Clorazepate Dipotassium Tablets: 3.75 mg, 7.5 mg, and 15 mg; *Tranxene® T-tab*, generic; (Rx DEA C-IV). Report prescribing and/or dispensing to state monitoring programs where required.

References

For the complete list of references, see **wiley.com/go/budde/plumb**

Cloxacillin

Cloxacillin Benzathine

Cloxacillin Sodium

(klox-a-***sill***-in) *Dariclox®, Orbenin-DC®, Dry-Clox®*

Anti-Staphylococcal Penicillin

Prescriber Highlights

- ► Intramammary isoxazolyl (anti-staphylococcal) penicillin
- ► Contraindications include hypersensitivity to penicillins
- ► Oral dosage forms of cloxacillin (human) no longer marketed in the United States
- ► Rarely used systemically in veterinary medicine

Uses/Indications

Cloxacillin is used via intramammary infusion in dry and lactating dairy cattle.

The World Health Organization (WHO) has designated cloxacillin as a Highly Important antimicrobial for human medicine.[1] The Office International des Epizooties (OIE) has designated cloxacillin as a Veterinary Critically Important Antimicrobial (VCIA) Agent in bovine, caprine, equine, ovine, and swine species.[2]

Pharmacology/Actions

Cloxacillin, dicloxacillin, and oxacillin have nearly identical spectrums of activity and can be considered therapeutically equivalent when comparing their in vitro activity. These penicillinase-resistant penicillins have a narrower spectrum of activity than the natural penicillins. Their antimicrobial efficacy is aimed directly against penicillinase-producing strains of gram-positive cocci, particularly staphylococcal species, and they are sometimes called anti-staphylococcal penicillins. Cloxacillin is not destroyed by the enzyme penicillinase, and therefore it is active against penicillin-resistant strains of *Staphylococcus aureus*. It is also active against non-penicillinase–producing *Staphylococcus aureus* as well as *Streptococcus agalactiae*. Although this class of penicillins has activity against some other gram-positive and gram-negative aerobes and anaerobes, other antibiotics (penicillins and otherwise) are usually better choices. The penicillinase-resistant penicillins are *not* effective against methicillin-resistant staphylococci, *Rickettsia* spp, mycobacteria, fungi, *Mycoplasma* spp, and viruses.

Pharmacokinetics

Cloxacillin is only available in intramammary dosage forms in the United States. In the nonlactating mammary gland, cloxacillin benzathine provides bactericidal cloxacillin levels for a prolonged period. This prolonged activity is due to the low solubility of the cloxacillin benzathine and to the slow-release oil-gel base. This prolonged contact between the antibiotic and the pathogenic organism enhances the probability of a bacteriologic cure.

Contraindications/Precautions/Warnings

Penicillins are contraindicated in patients with a history of hypersensitivity to them. Use penicillins cautiously in patients that are documented to be hypersensitive to other beta-lactam antibiotics (eg, cephalosporins, cefamycins, carbapenems) because there may be cross-reactivity.

Adverse Effects

Adverse effects with the penicillins are usually not serious and have a relatively low frequency of occurrence.

Hypersensitivity reactions, unrelated to dose, can occur with these agents and can manifest as rashes, fever, eosinophilia, neutropenia, agranulocytosis, thrombocytopenia, leukopenia, anemias, lymphadenopathy, or anaphylaxis. In humans, it is estimated that up to 15% of patients that are hypersensitive to cephalosporins will also be hypersensitive to penicillins.[3] The incidence of cross-reactivity in veterinary patients is unknown.

Reproductive/Nursing Safety

Penicillins have been shown to cross the placenta. Safe use of these drugs during pregnancy has not been firmly established, but neither have there been any documented teratogenic problems associated with these drugs. This class of drugs is likely safe when used via the intramammary route.

Because safety has not been established in animals, this drug should only be used when the maternal benefits outweigh the potential risks to offspring.

Overdose/Acute Toxicity

Overdose of intramammary infusions is unlikely to pose much risk to the patient but may prolong withdrawal times.

Drug Interactions

- No significant interactions are likely when intramammary dosage forms are used as labeled.

Laboratory Considerations

- No specific concerns were noted.

Dosages

CATTLE:

Mastitis (treatment or prophylaxis) caused by susceptible organisms (Label dosage; FDA-approved):

a) Lactating cows (using lactating cow formula; sodium cloxacillin): After milking out completely, clean and disinfect teat(s), then instill contents of one syringe into each affected quarter; massage. Repeat every 12 hours for 3 total doses.[4]

b) Dry (nonlactating) cows (using dry cow formula; cloxacillin benzathine): After last milking (or early in the dry period), clean and disinfect teats, then instill contents of one syringe into each quarter; massage.[5,6]

Monitoring

- Because penicillins usually have minimal toxicity associated with their use, monitoring for efficacy is usually all that is required unless toxic signs develop. Serum levels and therapeutic drug monitoring are not routinely done with these agents.

Client Information

- Prior to administration, be sure to follow all product instructions for milking, cleaning, and disinfecting the udder and teats.
- After administration, gently massage the affected quarter(s) to distribute the medicine
- Lactating cow product (sodium cloxacillin; *Dariclox*®) withdrawal times after last treatment, when used as labeled: milk withdrawal = 48 hours; slaughter withdrawal = 10 days
- Dry cow products (benzathine; *Orbenin-DC*®, *Dry-Clox*®) slaughter withdrawal is 28 or 30 days depending on product used.

Chemistry/Synonyms

Cloxacillin sodium, an isoxazolyl-penicillin, is a semisynthetic, penicillinase-resistant penicillin. It is available commercially as the monohydrate sodium salt that occurs as an odorless, bitter-tasting, white, crystalline powder. It is freely soluble in water and soluble in alcohol and has a pK_a of 2.7. One milligram of cloxacillin sodium contains not less than 825 µg of cloxacillin.

Cloxacillin benzathine occurs as a white or almost white powder that is slightly soluble in water and alcohol. A 1% (10 mg/mL) suspension has a pH from 3 to 6.5.

Cloxacillin sodium may also be known as BRL-1621, sodium cloxacillin, chlorphenylmethyl isoxazolyl penicillin sodium, methylchlorophenyl isoxazolyl penicillin sodium, cloxacilina sodica, cloxacillinum natricum, or P-25; many trade names are available.

Storage/Stability

Unless otherwise instructed by the manufacturer, store cloxacillin benzathine or cloxacillin sodium mastitis syringes at temperatures less than 25°C (77°F).

Compatibility/Compounding Considerations

No specific information was noted.

Dosage Forms/Regulatory Status

VETERINARY-LABELED PRODUCTS:

Cloxacillin Benzathine 500 mg (of cloxacillin) in a peanut-oil gel; 10 mL syringe for intramammary infusion: *Orbenin-DC*®, *Dry-Clox*; (Rx). FDA-approved for use in dairy cows during the dry period (immediately after last milking or early in the dry period). Do not use *Dry-Clox*® within 30 days prior to calving; (28 days for *Orbenin-DC*®). Slaughter withdrawal for *Dry-Clox*® = 30 days; *Orbenin*®-DC = 28 days

Cloxacillin Sodium 200 mg (of cloxacillin) in vegetable oils; 10 mL syringe for intramammary infusion: *Dariclox*®; (Rx). FDA-approved for use in lactating dairy cows. When the drug is used as labeled, milk withdrawal = 48 hours; slaughter withdrawal = 10 days

HUMAN-LABELED PRODUCTS: NONE

References

For the complete list of references, see **wiley.com/go/budde/plumb**

Cobalamin

Cyanocobalamin, Hydroxocobalamin, Methylcobalamin, Vitamin B_{12}

(koe-***bal***-a-min)

Vitamin

Prescriber Highlights

- Used for oral (eg, cyanocobalamin, methylcobalamin) and parenteral (eg, cyanocobalamin, hydroxocobalamin) treatment of cobalamin (ie, vitamin B_{12}) deficiency
- Safe to use
- Cyanocobalamin and hydroxocobalamin have equivalent biologic activity in humans; there are no data available in animals.
- Hydroxocobalamin at very high (mg/kg, NOT µg/kg) doses can be used as a cyanide antidote.

Uses/Indications

Cyanocobalamin is used for the treatment of cobalamin (ie, vitamin B_{12}) deficiencies secondary to GI tract disease or exocrine pancreatic insufficiency (EPI). It is also used for dietary chromium deficiencies (in ruminants) that can be associated with cobalamin dietary deficiencies. As there appears to be a high percentage of dogs and cats with EPI or GI disease that are deficient in cobalamin, there is considerable interest in evaluating serum cobalamin in these patients. Cobalamin supplementation appears to improve overall EPI treatment response.[1] Beagles, border collies, and komondors have a genetic defect (ie, Imerslund-Gräsbeck syndrome) that affects the location of the cobalamin-intrinsic factor receptor, causing cobalamin deficiency.[2-4] Chinese shar-peis in the United States are an overrepresented breed for cobalamin deficiency of undetermined etiology that is likely related to abnormal cobalamin metabolism.[5] Other breeds (eg, giant schnauzers, Australian shepherd dogs)[6,7] have been associated with cobalamin deficiency, but these breeds generally do not have a higher incidence of cobalamin deficiency as compared with other breeds. Dogs with EPI or chronic enteropathy also commonly develop cobalamin deficiency. Hypocobalaminemia at the time of diagnosis has been associated with reduced survival in dogs with

EPI.[8] Oral and parenteral cobalamin supplementation both appear to be effective in dogs[9] and cats.[10]

Hydroxocobalamin may have potential use in dogs with cyanide poisoning.[11] Hydroxocobalamin has shown promise in experimental models of hydrogen sulfide exposure[12] and anecdotally in dogs with smoke inhalation.

Pharmacology/Actions

Cobalamin, a cobalt-containing water-soluble vitamin, serves as an important cofactor for many enzymatic reactions in mammals that are required for normal cell growth, function, and reproduction; nucleoprotein and myelin synthesis; amino acid synthesis; carbohydrate and fat metabolism; and erythropoiesis. Cobalamin is required for folate utilization; cobalamin deficiency can cause functional folate deficiency. Unlike in humans, macrocytic anemias do not appear to be a significant component for cobalamin deficiency in dogs or cats.[13]

In ruminants, cobalamin appears to be synthesized by rumen microbiota and requires dietary cobalt to be present for its formation.

Hydroxocobalamin can be used interchangeably with cyanocobalamin for cobalamin supplementation.[14]

Hydroxocobalamin is used as a cyanide antidote by binding to cyanide and forming cyanocobalamin, which is excreted in the urine.

Pharmacokinetics

After food is consumed in monogastric mammals, gastric proteolytic enzymes cleave cobalamin from dietary proteins. Cobalamin then binds to haptocorrin in the stomach. The haptocorrin–cobalamin complex becomes hydrolyzed by pancreatic proteases in the duodenum. After being separated from the complex, cobalamin binds to intrinsic factor (IF), a protein produced in the stomach in humans and in the exocrine pancreas in dogs and cats.[14] The cobalamin–IF complex is absorbed in the small intestine and binds to cubulin, which facilitates its entry into the portal circulation. Transcobalamin 2 (TCII), a protein, then binds to cobalamin, allowing its entry into target cells. Some cobalamin is rapidly excreted into the bile where enterohepatic recirculation occurs.

In healthy cats, the circulating half-life of cobalamin is ≈13 days; however, in 2 cats with inflammatory bowel disease, the circulating half-life was only 5 days.[15]

After a hydroxocobalamin bolus at 70 mg/kg (NOT µg/kg) IV was given to dogs, the volume of distribution was 0.49 L/kg, clearance was 0.58 L/hour, and elimination half-life was 7.4 hours.[16]

In humans, IM hydroxocobalamin is more slowly absorbed from the injection site and produces a more sustained rise in cobalamin concentrations than cyanocobalamin. Hydroxocobalamin is stored in the liver and undergoes some enterohepatic recirculation. Hydroxocobalamin is excreted in the urine more slowly than cyanocobalamin.

Contraindications/Precautions/Warnings

No contraindications are documented for injectable or oral use in domestic animals. In humans, cyanocobalamin is contraindicated in patients hypersensitive to it, hydroxocobalamin, or cobalt.

In humans, administration by the IV route results in almost all of the dose being lost in the urine.

Do not use cyanocobalamin to treat cyanide toxicity.

Adverse Effects

Cyanocobalamin appears to be very well tolerated when used parenterally in animals. In humans, anaphylaxis has rarely been reported after parenteral use. Pain at the injection site is uncommon with cyanocobalamin but may be more problematic with hydroxocobalamin, as the latter has a lower pH. Skin discoloration, hypotension, and bradycardia may occur when hydroxocobalamin is used at high doses as a cyanide antidote.[17]

Reproductive/Nursing Safety

Serum cobalamin decreases in late pregnancy; it is unclear what, if any, adverse effects result.[18] Cobalamin crosses the placenta. Studies documenting safety during pregnancy have apparently not been done in humans or animals, but cobalamin is likely safe to use. Vitamin B_{12} deficiencies are thought to cause teratogenic effects.

Although cobalamin can be excreted into milk, it is safe for use while nursing.

Overdose/Acute Toxicity

Overdose has not been reported with cyanocobalamin.[19] Hydroxocobalamin LD_{50} is 50 mg/kg when given IV to mice.[20]

Drug Interactions

The following drug interactions have either been reported or are theoretical in humans or animals receiving cobalamin and may be of significance in veterinary patients. Unless otherwise noted, use together is not necessarily contraindicated, but weigh the potential risks and perform additional monitoring when appropriate.

- **Chloramphenicol:** Concurrent use may result in decreased hematologic response.
- **Proton Pump Inhibitors (PPIs**; eg, **omeprazole, pantoprazole**): Long-term use of PPIs may reduce cobalamin absorption in humans; veterinary significance is unknown. Cobalamin deficiency was not detected after 60 days of twice-daily omeprazole administration in 6 healthy cats.[21]

Laboratory Considerations

- Serum samples to be analyzed for cobalamin and/or folate should be protected from bright light and excessive heat.

Dosages

NOTE: Cyanocobalamin and hydroxocobalamin have equivalent biologic activity in humans. Although cost and availability may be obstacles, hydroxocobalamin can be a substitution for veterinary patients that do not readily respond to cyanocobalamin.[14] All dosages are for cyanocobalamin unless otherwise noted.

DOGS:

Cobalamin (ie, vitamin B_{12}) deficiency:

Cyanocobalamin (extra-label):

a) **Injectable**: 25 µg/kg SC, or practically, if body weight is less than 5 kg (11 lb), 250 µg/dog (NOT µg/kg); 5 to 10 kg (11 to 22 lb), 400 µg/dog (NOT µg/kg); 10 to 20 kg (22 to 44 lb), 600 µg/dog (NOT µg/kg); 20 to 30 kg (44 to 66 lb), 800 µg/dog (NOT µg/kg); 30 to 40 kg (66 to 88 lb), 1000 µg/dog (NOT µg/kg); 40 to 50 kg (88 to 110 lb), 1200 µg/dog (NOT µg/kg); greater than 50 kg (110 lb), 1500 µg/dog (NOT µg/kg) once weekly for 4 to 6 weeks, then once monthly. If serum cobalamin concentrations are low after monthly administration, consider reducing dosing interval to every 2 weeks.[14,22]

b) **Oral**: Body weight 1 to 10 kg (2.2 to 22 lb), 250 µg/dog (NOT µg/kg); 10 to 20 kg (22 to 44 lb), 500 µg/dog (NOT µg/kg); greater than 20 kg (44 lb), 1000 µg/dog (NOT µg/kg) PO every 24 hours.[23] Alternatively, dogs less than 20 kg (44 lb), 250 µg/dog (NOT µg/kg); greater than 20 kg (44 lb), 1000 µg/dog (NOT µg/kg) PO every 24 hours.[24] Cyanocobalamin at 1000 µg PO once daily maintained normal clinical status and cellular markers in 3 beagles with Imerslund-Gräsbeck syndrome.[25]

Hydroxocobalamin for chronic enteropathy (extra-label): 0.25 – 1 mg/dog (NOT mg/kg) IM. Administration of hydroxocobalamin at 1 mg/dog (NOT mg/kg) IM every other month controlled clinical signs and laboratory parameters in beagles with Imerslund-Gräsbeck syndrome.[26]

Adjunctive treatment for cyanide poisoning, including sodium nitroprusside toxicity or smoke inhalation (extra-label):

NOTE: Cyanocobalamin should *not* be used for this indication. **Hydroxocobalamin** 75 – 150 mg/kg (NOT µg/kg) IV infusion over 7.5 minutes.[11,17] Intraosseous infusion may be considered.[27]

CATS:

Cobalamin (ie, vitamin B_{12}) deficiency (extra-label):

a) **Injectable**: 250 µg/cat (NOT µg/kg) SC once weekly for 6 weeks, then once every 1 to 2 months based on cobalamin levels

b) **Oral**: 250 µg/cat (NOT µg/kg) PO every 24 hours for 12 weeks[22]; 0.91 mg/m^2 (NOT mg/kg) PO once daily has been reported[10]

HORSES:

Vitamin B_{12} nutritional supplement (label dosage; not FDA-approved): 1000 – 6000 µg/horse (NOT µg/kg) IM or SC; dose may be repeated every 1 to 2 weeks depending on condition and response to treatment.[19,28]

CATTLE, SHEEP:

Vitamin B_{12} nutritional supplement (label dosage; not FDA approved): 1000 – 6000 µg/animal (NOT µg/kg) IM or SC; dose may be repeated every 1 to 2 weeks depending on condition and response to treatment[19,28]

Cobalamin (ie, vitamin B_{12}) deficiency associated with cobalt deficiency in sheep (extra-label):

a) **Adult sheep**: 300 – 1000 µg/sheep (NOT µg/kg) IM or SC once weekly[29]

b) **Lambs**: 100 µg/lamb (NOT µg/kg) IM or SC[29]

Cobalamin (ie, vitamin B_{12}) deficiency in lambs (extra-label): 2000 µg/lamb (NOT µg/kg) SC once; may be repeated every 60 days[30,31]

SWINE:

Vitamin B_{12} nutritional supplement (label dosage; not FDA-approved): 1000 – 6000 µg/pig (NOT µg/kg) IM or SC; dose may be repeated every 1 to 2 weeks depending on condition and response to treatment[19,28]

RABBITS:

Deep vein thrombosis (extra-label): cyanocobalamin (vitamin B_{12}) 500 µg /rabbit (NOT µg/kg) once daily in addition to folic acid (vitamin B_9) 15 mg/rabbit (NOT mg/kg) PO daily.[32] High levels of cobalamin (vitamin B_{12}) and folic acid (vitamin B_9) can improve plasma hyperhomocysteinemia, coagulation indexes, and some pathologic changes seen in deep vein thrombosis of the lower extremity.

Monitoring

- Cobalamin levels (serum cobalamin concentration) are improved by 1 month after initial loading therapy (either daily oral doses or weekly injections) is complete.[9] If the cobalamin concentration is low then increase dosing frequency from weekly to twice weekly.[14]
- In small animal species, folate status (before and after treatment with cyanocobalamin)
- Improvement of clinical signs associated with deficiency
- Baseline and periodic CBC if/when indicated by clinical condition
- Serum methylmalonic acid may be useful for diagnosis of cobalamin deficiency and monitoring treatment response.[24,33,34]

Client Information

- This medication is a vitamin injected under the skin to treat vitamin B_{12} (ie, cobalamin) deficiency. Treatment may be needed for the rest of your animal's life.
- Improvement is often seen after the first 1 to 2 weeks of treatment.
- This medication is very safe; injections may sting on administration.
- Dispose of needles and syringes safely in a sharps container provided by your veterinarian.

Chemistry/Synonyms

Cyanocobalamin occurs as dark red crystals or a crystalline powder. Hydroxocobalamin appears as dark red orthorhombic needles or as an amorphous or crystalline red powder. Cyanocobalamin is sparingly soluble in water and soluble in alcohol, and hydroxocobalamin is moderately water soluble. In the anhydrous form, cyanocobalamin and hydroxocobalamin are very hygroscopic and can absorb substantial amounts of water from the air. The pH range of commercial cyanocobalamin for injection is 4.5 to 7; the pH of hydroxocobalamin for injection is 3.5 to 5. Cyanocobalamin and hydroxocobalamin have equivalent biologic activity in humans.

Vitamin B_{12} may also be known as cobalamin. Cyanocobalamin may also be known as cianocobalamina, cianokobalaminas, cobamin, cyanocobalamine, cyanocobalaminum, or cycobemin; there are many internationally registered trade names.

Storage/Stability

Cyanocobalamin injection should be stored below 40°C (104°F) and protected from light and freezing.

Hydroxocobalamin for injection should be stored protected from light and moisture at controlled room temperature 20°C to 25°C (59°F-77°F). Cyanide antidote kits may experience excursions up to 60°C (140°F) for up to 4 days and freeze/thaw cycles for up to 15 days.

Compatibility/Compounding Considerations

Cyanocobalamin, a USP active pharmaceutical ingredient powder, is magenta in color and often used as a tracer instead of azo dyes when compounding capsules for cats or other patients that cannot tolerate azo dyes found in food colors.

Compatibility is dependent on factors such as pH, concentration, temperature, and diluent used; specialized references or a hospital pharmacist should be consulted for more specific information

Cyanocobalamin injection is reportedly **compatible** with all commonly used IV fluids; it is reported to be **incompatible** with chlorpromazine hydrochloride, phytonadione, prochlorperazine edisylate, warfarin sodium, ascorbic acid, dextrose, heavy metals, oxidizing or reducing agents, and alkaline or strongly acidic solutions.

Hydroxocobalamin is reportedly **incompatible** with ascorbic acid, diazepam, dobutamine, fentanyl, nitroglycerin, pentobarbital, propofol, sodium nitrite, sodium thiosulfate, and thiopental.

Dosage Forms/Regulatory Status

VETERINARY-LABELED PRODUCTS:

Cyanocobalamin Chewable Tablets: 250 µg and 1000 µg tablets; *Cobalequin*®; (OTC); also contains methyltetrahydrofolate. Flavored with hydrolyzed chicken

Cyanocobalamin (Vitamin B_{12}) Injection: 1000, 3000, and 5000 µg/mL in 100 mL, 250 mL, and 500 mL multidose vials depending on source; generic; (Rx). Products may be labeled as cyanocobalamin or vitamin B_{12} and be labeled for use in dogs, cats, cattle, horses, sheep, or swine.

There are many combination products, both oral and injectable, that contain cyanocobalamin as an ingredient. These formulations are not recommended for use when cobalamin deficiency exists.

HUMAN-LABELED PRODUCTS:

Cyanocobalamin (crystalline, Vitamin B_{12}) Injection: 100 µg (0.1 mg)/mL and 1000 µg (1 mg)/mL, vial sizes range from 1 mL single use to 10 mL and 30 mL multidose; generic; (Rx). In addition to generic-labeled products, there are several products available with a variety of trade names, including *Crystamine*®, *Crysti*®, *Cyanoject*®, and *Rubesol*®.

Cyanocobalamin (Vitamin B_{12}) Oral Tablets: 100 µg, 250 µg, 500 µg, 1000 µg, 2000 ug, and 5000 ug; generic; (OTC)

Hydroxocobalamin Injection: 1000 µg/mL in 10 mL vials; generic; (Rx). Hydroxocobalamin is also available as a 2.5 g cyanide antidote kit (*Cyanokit*®).

A nasally administered product, oral lozenges, sustained-release tablets, and oral sublingual tablets are marketed, but there is little to no information regarding their use in dogs or cats. Limited information has shown these formulations to be ineffective in veterinary species.

References

For the complete list of references, see **wiley.com/go/budde/plumb**

Codeine

(***koe***-deen)

Opioid, Antitussive

Prescriber Highlights

- Opioid used for analgesia and cough in dogs and cats
- Oral bioavailability in dogs is very low (high first-pass effect), and analgesic efficacy is unknown.
- Use is often in combination products with acetaminophen; these combination products are *not* for use in cats or ferrets.
- Common adverse effects include sedation, constipation, and respiratory depression (when administered in high doses). Cats may also show CNS stimulation.
- DEA controlled substance. Schedule varies by product used: C-II when used as a sole agent; combination products are either C-III or C-V.

Uses/Indications

In small animal medicine, codeine is potentially useful as an oral analgesic for mild pain or as an antitussive, and possibly as an antidiarrheal agent. Its pharmacokinetic profile raises questions of codeine's efficacy in dogs. Codeine did not provide antinociceptive effects in experimental studies in dogs[1] or cats.[2] A pharmacokinetic study[3] concluded that future studies are needed to assess the antinociceptive effects of oral codeine in dogs to determine if the drug can be effectively used. To date, there are no studies that definitively prove the efficacy of oral codeine formulations for antitussive or antidiarrheal effects in veterinary patients.

In dogs with experimentally induced lameness, carprofen was more effective than acetaminophen/codeine at improving lameness scores.[4] In a different study, acetaminophen/codeine and meloxicam were equally effective as perioperative analgesic in dogs undergoing surgery.[5]

Hydrocodone is more potent than codeine, and commercially available dosage forms of hydrocodone are combined with homatropine to prevent abuse, which is why many clinicians prefer a hydrocodone/homatropine combination versus codeine for use as an antitussive in dogs.

Pharmacology/Actions

Codeine possesses mu-opioid activity similar to other opioids. Codeine's pharmacokinetics and metabolic fate—and hence its efficacy—can vary widely between species. In humans, codeine is an effective antitussive and a mild analgesic that produces similar respiratory depression as compared with morphine at equianalgesic dosages. Although the major metabolite in dogs (ie, codeine-6-glucuronide) has opioid activity, it is not clear how much antinociceptive, antitussive, or antidiarrheal activity it possesses.[3] Codeine, like other opioids, can have immunosuppressive effects, but it is not clear if this is clinically significant.[6]

Pharmacokinetics

In dogs, oral codeine is well absorbed, but its bioavailability is ≈4% to 6%, as it appears to undergo extensive first-pass metabolism (primarily to codeine-6-glucuronide). The volume of distribution is 3.2 L/kg, and the elimination half-life is ≈1.5 hours.[1,3,7] Codeine is metabolized predominantly to codeine-6-glucuronide, and only negligible amounts of morphine are formed.[1,3]

In horses, the time to peak codeine concentration is ≈0.44 hours, and its elimination half-life is 2 hours.[8] The drug undergoes extensive biotransformation, with the primary metabolite being morphine-3-glucuronide; morphine-6-glucuronide and morphine were formed but to lesser extents.

In humans, codeine salts are rapidly absorbed after oral administration. Codeine is about ⅔ as effective after oral administration when compared with parenteral administration. After oral administration, the onset of action is usually within 30 minutes, and analgesic effects persist for 4 to 6 hours. Codeine is metabolized in the liver, primarily by glucuronidation and demethylation, and morphine is an active metabolite. Codeine and metabolites are eliminated in the urine.

Contraindications/Precautions/Warnings

<u>**Do not use the combination product containing acetaminophen in cats or ferrets;**</u> use caution with the combination product in dogs with hepatic insufficiency. Codeine is contraindicated in patients that are hypersensitive to it or other narcotic analgesics; in patients with significant respiratory depression, a known or suspected GI obstruction, or diarrhea caused by toxic ingestion (until the toxin is eliminated from the GI tract); and in patients that are receiving or are within 14 days of receiving monoamine oxidase inhibitors (MAOIs).[9] It should not be used repeatedly in patients with severe inflammatory bowel disease.

All opioids should be used with caution in patients with hypothyroidism, severe renal insufficiency, and hypoadrenocorticism (ie, Addison disease), as well as in geriatric or severely debilitated patients. Because it may obscure the diagnosis or clinical course of these conditions, codeine should be used with caution in patients with head injuries or increased intracranial pressure, seizure disorders, and acute abdominal conditions (eg, colic). Use codeine with extreme caution in patients suffering from respiratory disease or acute respiratory dysfunction (eg, pulmonary edema secondary to smoke inhalation). Dogs experiencing respiratory depression may not be able to efficiently pant and cool themselves in warmer climates.

Opioid analgesics are contraindicated in patients that have been stung by the scorpion species *Centruroides sculpturatus Ewing* or *Centruroides gertschi Stahnke*, as venom may be potentiated.[10] Respiratory depressants should not be used in coral snake envenomation in dogs or cats.[11]

Abrupt discontinuation of codeine after long-term use may lead to clinical signs of withdrawal; gradual tapering of the drug is suggested.

Although other opioids, such as butorphanol, are known to be problematic in dogs with multidrug resistance-1 gene (*MDR1* gene, also known as *ABCB1* gene) polymorphisms, codeine appears to be well tolerated in these dogs.

Some humans have a CYP2D6 genotype that can lead to ultra-rapid metabolism of codeine and the formation of a greater amount of morphine, increasing the risk for respiratory depression. Codeine has a high abuse potential in humans, and diversion from its intended use is possible.

Adverse Effects

Codeine is generally well tolerated, but typical opioid adverse effects are possible, particularly at higher doses or with repeated use. Sedation is the most likely adverse effect. Potential adverse GI effects include anorexia, vomiting, constipation, ileus, and biliary and pancreatic duct spasms. Respiratory depression is generally not noted unless the patient receives high doses or is at an increased risk (see ***Contraindications/Precautions/Warnings***).

In cats, opioids may cause CNS stimulation with hyperexcitability, tremors, and/or seizures.

Reproductive/Nursing Safety

Opioids cross the placenta. Very high doses in mice have caused delayed ossification, and embryo- and fetotoxic effects have occurred in other laboratory animals.[9] Neonatal opioid withdrawal syndrome may occur in humans. Use during pregnancy only when the benefits outweigh the risks, particularly with chronic use. Long-term opioid use may cause reduced fertility.

Codeine enters maternal milk. Breastfeeding is not recommended in women taking codeine-containing products. Because safety has not been established in animals, this drug should only be used when the maternal benefits outweigh the potential risks to offspring.

Overdose/Acute Toxicity

Opioid overdose may produce profound respiratory and/or CNS depression in most species, and airway management is crucial. Other effects can include cardiovascular collapse, hypothermia, and skeletal muscle hypotonia. If an oral overdose occurs, gastric decontamination using standard protocols should be performed. Because rapid changes in CNS status may occur, inducing emesis should be attempted with caution. Naloxone should be used to treat respiratory depression. In cases of massive overdoses, the naloxone dose may need to be repeated, and animals should be closely observed because naloxone's effects may diminish before subtoxic levels of codeine are attained. Mechanical respiratory support should also be considered in cases of severe respiratory depression. Serious overdoses involving opioids should be closely monitored.

For patients that have experienced or are suspected of having experienced an overdose, consultation with a 24-hour poison consultation center specializing in providing veterinary-specific information is recommended. For general information related to overdose and toxin exposures, as well as contact information for poison control centers, refer to ***Appendix.***

Drug Interactions

The following drug interactions have either been reported or are theoretical in humans or animals receiving codeine and may be of significance in veterinary patients. Unless otherwise noted, use together is not necessarily contraindicated, but weigh the potential risks and perform additional monitoring when appropriate.

- Anticholinergic Drugs (eg, **atropine, glycopyrrolate, oxybutynin**): Use with codeine may increase the chances of developing constipation.
- Azole Antifungals (eg, **itraconazole, ketoconazole**): May increase codeine exposure and morphine formation
- Cannabidiol: May potentiate CNS depression
- Clopidogrel: Opioid use may delay and reduce formation of the clopidogrel-active metabolite and the drug's antiplatelet effect, possibly by reducing GI motility and drug absorption.
- CNS Depressants, Other (eg, **anesthetic agents, antihistamines, barbiturates, benzodiazepines, muscle relaxants, phenothiazines**): May cause increased CNS or respiratory depression when used with codeine
- Desmopressin (DDAVP): Increased risk for hyponatremia
- Dexamethasone: May reduce codeine exposure and morphine formation
- Diuretics (eg, **furosemide, hydrochlorothiazide**): Opioids may reduce diuretic efficacy by releasing an antidiuretic hormone.
- Macrolide Antibiotics (eg, **clarithromycin, erythromycin**): May increase codeine exposure and morphine formation
- Monoamine Oxidase Inhibitors (**MAOIs**; eg, **amitraz, linezolid, selegiline**): May potentiate CNS effects; concurrent use or use within 14 days of stopping MAOIs is contraindicated.
- Naloxone: Antagonizes opioid effects. **NOTE**: This action is an expected outcome when naloxone is used as a reversal agent.
- Prokinetic Agents (eg, **cisapride, metoclopramide**): Opioids may decrease the effectiveness of GI prokinetic agents
- Quinidine: May increase codeine exposure and morphine formation
- Serotonergic Drugs, Other (eg, **mirtazapine, trazodone**): May increase the risk for serotonin syndrome
- Selective Serotonin Reuptake Inhibitors (**SSRIs**; eg, **fluoxetine, paroxetine, sertraline**): May increase codeine exposure and morphine formation; there is an increased risk for serotonin syndrome.
- Terbinafine: May increase codeine exposure and morphine formation
- Tricyclic Antidepressants (**eg, amitriptyline, clomipramine**): May increase the risk for serotonin syndrome[12,13]

Laboratory Considerations

- Opioids may increase biliary tract pressure, leading to increased plasma **amylase** and **lipase** values up to 24 hours following opioid administration.

Dosages

DOGS:

Antitussive (extra-label): Codeine 1 – 2 mg/kg PO every 6 to 12 hours

Analgesic (extra-label):

a) **When used alone**: Anecdotal analgesic dosages for codeine are usually 1 – 2 mg/kg PO every 4 to 6 hours, but it has been suggested that doses up to 4 mg/kg may be required. Codeine's pharmacokinetics in dogs may be problematic as it undergoes a high first-pass effect, and it is not clear how much analgesic efficacy the primary metabolite possesses.

b) **When used with the acetaminophen combination products** (eg, *Tylenol® #3*): Calculate the dose to provide acetaminophen 10 – 15 mg/kg PO every 8 hours (every 12 hours if using long-term), then choose the tablet size (eg, *Tylenol® #3 or #4*) to provide codeine 1 – 2 mg/kg. Codeine dosage may be cautiously increased, provided the acetaminophen dose does not exceed 15 mg/kg. For example, the dose when giving 1 tablet of *Tylenol® #4* (acetaminophen 300 mg/codeine 60 mg) PO every 8 hours to a 20 kg (44 lb) dog would be acetaminophen 15 mg/kg and codeine 3 mg/kg. When giving *Tylenol® #3* (acetaminophen 300 mg/codeine 30 mg) to the same dog, the codeine dose would be 1.5 mg/kg.

CATS:

NOTE: Do *not* use the combination product that contains acetaminophen in cats.

Analgesic (extra-label): 0.5 – 2 mg/kg PO every 6 to 8 hours

RABBITS:

Analgesic (extra-label): Using the acetaminophen and codeine elixir, 1 mL in 10 to 20 mL of drinking water (add dextrose to enhance palatability)[14]

Monitoring

- Efficacy
- Adverse effects

Client Information

- This medicine may be given with food or on an empty stomach.

- Sedation (drowsiness) and constipation are the most common side effects. Slowed breathing can occur with higher doses.
- Cats may become overly excited after receiving this medicine.
- **Do not use combination products that contain acetaminophen (eg, *Tylenol® #3* or *Tylenol® #4*) in cats or ferrets.**
- Codeine (alone) is a C-II controlled drug and requires a new written prescription for refills. The use of this medication in animals or humans other than those for whom they are prescribed is illegal.
- Keep this medicine out of reach of children and animals.
- Report any significant changes in behavior, activity level, breathing rate, or gastrointestinal effects (eg, constipation, lack of appetite, vomiting) to your veterinarian.

Chemistry/Synonyms

Codeine, a phenanthrene-derivative opioid agonist, is available as the base and 2 separate salts. Codeine base is slightly soluble in water and freely soluble in alcohol. Codeine phosphate occurs as fine, white, needle-like crystals or as a white, crystalline powder. It is freely soluble in water. Codeine sulfate's appearance resembles codeine phosphate, but it is soluble in water.

Codeine may also be known as codeini or codeinii; many trade names are available.

Storage/Stability

Store codeine sulfate tablets in light-resistant, well-closed containers at room temperature 15°C to 30°C (59°F-86°F).

Codeine is a controlled substance. In accordance with DEA regulations, store it in an area that is substantially constructed and securely locked. Follow applicable local, state, and federal rules regarding the disposal of unused or wasted controlled drugs. Report dispensing to state monitoring programs where required.

Compatibility/Compounding Considerations

Compatibility is dependent on factors such as pH, concentration, temperature, and diluent used; specialized references or a hospital pharmacist should be consulted for more specific information.

Codeine phosphate 3 mg/mL compounded oral suspension has been reported to be stable for 98 days at controlled room temperature (20°C to 25°C [68°F-77°F]) when protected from light.[15] Codeine phosphate injection is reportedly **compatible** with glycopyrrolate or hydroxyzine HCl. It is reportedly **incompatible** with aminophylline, ammonium chloride, heparin sodium, pentobarbital sodium, phenobarbital sodium, phenytoin sodium, sodium bicarbonate, and sodium iodide.

Dosage Forms/Regulatory Status

VETERINARY-LABELED PRODUCTS: NONE

The Association of Racing Commissioners International (ARCI) has designated this drug as a class 1 substance. Use of this drug may not be allowed in certain animal competitions. Check rules and regulations before entering a competition while this medication is being administered. Contact local racing authorities for further guidance. See ***Appendix*** for more information.

HUMAN-LABELED PRODUCTS:

There are many products available containing codeine. The following is a partial listing:

Codeine Sulfate Tablets: 15 mg, 30 mg, and 60 mg; generic; (Rx, C-II)

Codeine Phosphate 7.5 mg (#1), 15 mg (#2), 30 mg (#3), and 60 mg (#4) with Acetaminophen 300 mg tablets; *Tylenol® with Codeine #s 1, 2, 3, 4;* generic; (Rx, C-III); **WARNING**: Do not use in cats or ferrets.

Codeine and Acetaminophen Oral Solution: codeine 12 mg and acetaminophen 120 mg/5 mL (2.4 mg and 24 mg/mL) in 118 mL and 473 mL bottles; generic; (Rx, C-V). Contains 7% alcohol. **WARNING**: Do not use in cats or ferrets

NOTE: Codeine-only products are C-II controlled substances. Combination products with aspirin or acetaminophen are C-III. Codeine-containing cough syrups are either C-III or C-V, depending on the state. Report prescribing and/or dispensing to state monitoring programs where required.

References

For the complete list of references, see **wiley.com/go/budde/plumb**

Colchicine

(***kol***-chi-seen) *Colcrys®*

Anti-inflammatory

Prescriber Highlights

- ▶ Unique anti-inflammatory that has been used for shar-pei fever; occasionally used in dogs for hepatic cirrhosis/fibrosis
- ▶ Contraindications include serious GI or cardiac dysfunction and in those with severe renal or hepatic disease that are also receiving certain concomitant drugs.
- ▶ Use with caution in geriatric or debilitated patients and in those with renal or hepatic insufficiency
- ▶ The most likely adverse effects include GI distress (diarrhea, vomiting; may be an early sign of toxicity), but several serious effects are possible, including myelosuppression.
- ▶ Teratogenic; reduces spermatogenesis
- ▶ The National Institute for Occupational Safety and Health (NIOSH) classifies colchicine as a hazardous drug; use appropriate precautions when handling.

Uses/Indications

Colchicine has been proposed as a treatment in small animal species for amyloidosis and shar-pei fever; however, it must be given early in the course of the disease, and it is ineffective once renal insufficiency has occurred. No conclusive evidence currently exists for its efficacy for these or any other indication in dogs.

Colchicine has also been proposed for treating chronic hepatic fibrosis, presumably by decreasing the formation and increasing the breakdown of collagen, but its efficacy is in question. Because of the lack of proven efficacy and common occurrence of adverse effects, some veterinary specialists do not recommend the use of colchicine in dogs.[1]

A case report[2] using colchicine to treat endotracheal stent granulation stenosis in a dog has been published, and the drug may find a place in therapy for this indication after further investigation.

Colchicine possibly may be beneficial to reduce hyperuricemia in birds with renal disease or amyloidosis, or to reduce renal or hepatic fibrosis. No controlled studies were located to document efficacy for any of these potential uses.

Pharmacology/Actions

Colchicine inhibits cell division during metaphase by interfering with the sol-gel formation and the mitotic spindle. The mechanism for its antifibrotic activity is believed to be secondary to collagenase activity stimulation.

Colchicine apparently blocks the synthesis and secretion of serum amyloid A (SAA; an acute-phase reactant protein) by hepatocytes, thereby preventing the formation of amyloid-enhancing factors and preventing amyloid disposition.

Colchicine is best known in human medicine for its anti-gout activity. The mechanism for this effect is not fully understood, but it is likely related to the drug's ability to reduce the inflammatory response to the disposition of monosodium urate crystals.

Pharmacokinetics

No information was located specifically for domestic animals. The following information is human and laboratory animal data unless otherwise noted. After oral administration, colchicine is absorbed from the GI tract. Some of the absorbed drug is metabolized in the liver (first-pass effect). These metabolites and unchanged drug are re-secreted into the GI tract via biliary secretions where it is reabsorbed. This recycling phenomena may explain the intestinal manifestations noted with colchicine toxicity. Colchicine is distributed into several tissues but is concentrated in leukocytes. The plasma half-life is about 20 minutes, but the leukocyte half-life is ≈60 hours.

Colchicine is deacetylated in the liver and metabolized in other tissues. Although most of a dose (as colchicine and metabolites) is excreted in the feces, some is excreted in the urine. More of the dose may be excreted in the urine of patients with hepatic disease. Patients with severe renal disease may have prolonged half-lives.

Contraindications/Precautions/Warnings

Colchicine is contraindicated in patients with serious GI or cardiac dysfunction. In humans with severe renal or hepatic impairment, colchicine is contraindicated when combined with strong inhibitors of CYP3A and/or P-glycoprotein (see ***Drug Interactions***). Colchicine should be used with caution in geriatric or debilitated patients and in those with renal or hepatic insufficiency; a dose reduction may be warranted.

Colchicine use in veterinary medicine is somewhat controversial, as safety and efficacy have not been well documented.

The National Institute for Occupational Safety and Health (NIOSH) classifies colchicine as a hazardous drug; personal protective equipment (PPE) should be used accordingly to minimize the risk for exposure.[3]

Adverse Effects

There has been only marginal experience with colchicine in domestic animals. Colchicine can cause nausea, vomiting, and diarrhea in dogs, particularly at higher dosages. Rarely, myelosuppression (neutropenia), renal toxicity, and peripheral neuropathy can occur.

In humans, GI effects (eg, abdominal pain, anorexia, vomiting, diarrhea) have been noted and can be an early indication of toxicity; it is recommended to discontinue therapy (in humans) should these occur. Prolonged administration has caused myelosuppression. Colchicine may impair cobalamin (vitamin B_{12}) absorption.

Reproductive/Nursing Safety

Because colchicine has been demonstrated to be teratogenic in laboratory animals (mice and hamsters), it should be used during pregnancy only when its potential benefits outweigh its risks. Colchicine may decrease spermatogenesis.

Colchicine enters maternal milk; use it cautiously in nursing mothers.[4]

Because safety has not been established in animals, this drug should only be used when the maternal benefits outweigh the potential risks to offspring.

Overdose/Acute Toxicity

Colchicine can be a very toxic drug after relatively small overdoses. GI manifestations are usually the presenting signs seen. These can range from anorexia and vomiting to bloody diarrhea or paralytic ileus. Renal insufficiency, hepatotoxicity, pancytopenia, paralysis, shock, and vascular collapse may also occur.[5] In humans, colchicine doses of 0.5 – 0.8 mg/kg presented with significant GI symptoms and myelosuppression[4]; doses exceeding 0.8 mg/kg were uniformly fatal.

There is no specific antidote to colchicine. GI decontamination should be employed when applicable. Because of extensive enterohepatic recycling of the drug, repeated doses of activated charcoal and a saline cathartic may reduce systemic absorption. Other treatment is supportive and based on clinical signs. Dialysis (peritoneal) may be of benefit. One case report in a dog describes successful treatment of a significant colchicine overdose (≈10 times the recommended dose), using aggressive supportive care including activated charcoal, IV lipid emulsion therapy, and N-acetylcysteine.[6]

Drug Interactions

The following drug interactions have either been reported or are theoretical in humans or animals receiving colchicine and may be of significance in veterinary patients. Unless otherwise noted, use together is not necessarily contraindicated, but weigh the potential risks and perform additional monitoring when appropriate.

- **AMPHOTERICIN B:** May increase risk for nephrotoxicity
- **AZOLE ANTIFUNGALS** (eg, **itraconazole, ketoconazole**): Concurrent use may result in increased colchicine plasma concentrations and increased risk for toxicity.[7] The combination is contraindicated in humans.
- **CALCIUM CHANNEL BLOCKERS** (eg, **diltiazem, verapamil** [not amlodipine]): Concurrent use may result in increased colchicine plasma concentration and increased risk for toxicity. The combination is contraindicated in humans with severe renal or hepatic impairment.
- **CHLORAMPHENICOL:** May cause additive myelosuppression or GI effects
- **CYCLOSPORINE:** May increase risk for nephrotoxicity or myelosuppression. The combination is contraindicated in humans with severe renal or hepatic impairment.
- **DIGOXIN:** May increase the risk for rhabdomyolysis
- **FENOFIBRATE/GEMFIBROZIL:** Concurrent use may increase the risk for myopathy or rhabdomyolysis.
- **MACROLIDE ANTIBIOTICS** (eg, **clarithromycin, erythromycin**): May increase colchicine concentrations and risk for toxicity. The combination is contraindicated in humans with severe renal or hepatic impairment.
- **MYELOSUPPRESSIVE AGENTS** (eg, **antineoplastics, azathioprine**): May cause additive myelosuppression or GI effects when used with colchicine
- **P-GLYCOPROTEIN INHIBITORS** (eg, **amiodarone, doxorubicin, spironolactone**): May increase colchicine concentrations and risk for toxicity

Laboratory Considerations

- Colchicine may cause false-positive results when testing for **erythrocytes or hemoglobin in urine.**
- Colchicine may interfere with **17-hydroxycorticosteroid** determinations in urine if using the Reddy, Jenkins, and Thorn procedure.
- Colchicine may cause increased serum values of **alkaline phosphatase (ALP)**.

Dosages

DOGS:

Adjunctive treatment of hepatic cirrhosis/fibrosis, shar-pei fever, amyloidosis (extra-label): Most clinicians recommend 0.03 mg/kg PO once daily. Some clinicians suggest starting at a lower initial dose to determine if the dog will tolerate it (GI adverse effects). As an example, for an adult shar-pei, using the commercially available 0.6 mg tablets: start with ½ tablet (0.3 mg) PO once daily and increase the dose in 0.3 mg increments every 4 to 5 days as tolerated until a target dose of up to 0.6 mg/dog (NOT mg/kg) PO twice daily is reached. In dogs that cannot tolerate a given dose, the dose is reduced, or the drug is temporarily discontinued and restarted at a lower dose.

BIRDS:

Adjunctive treatment of hepatic fibrosis, amyloidosis, or hyperuricemia (extra-label): Recommended anecdotal doses can vary widely from 0.01 – 0.2 mg/kg PO every 12 hours. It is recommended to start at the lower end of the dosage range and increase the dosage gradually.

Monitoring

- Efficacy
- Adverse effects (eg, vomiting, diarrhea, myelosuppression)
- Baseline and periodic CBC, chemistry panel, and urinalysis
- Consider checking cobalamin levels when using colchicine long term

Client Information

- There is limited experience using this medicine in animals; side effects are not well known. Report any suspected side effects to your veterinarian.
- This medicine may be given with or without food.
- Pregnant women should avoid exposure to this medicine or to the waste (eg, urine, feces) of animals receiving it.
- This medication is considered to be a hazardous drug as defined by the National Institute for Occupational Safety and Health (NIOSH). Talk with your veterinarian or pharmacist about the use of personal protective equipment when handling this medicine.

Chemistry/Synonyms

Colchicine is an anti-gout drug that possesses many other pharmacologic effects. It occurs as a pale yellow, amorphous powder or scales. It is soluble in water and freely soluble in alcohol.

Colchicine may also be known as colchicinum or *Colcrys*®, *Gloperba*®, or *Mitigare*®.

Storage/Stability

Store colchicine tablets in tight, light-resistant containers.

Compatibility/Compounding Considerations

No specific information was noted.

Dosage Forms/Regulatory Status

VETERINARY-LABELED PRODUCTS: NONE

The Association of Racing Commissioners International (ARCI) has designated this drug as a class 4 substance. Use of this drug may not be allowed in certain animal competitions. Check rules and regulations before entering in a competition while this medication is being administered. Contact local racing authorities for further guidance. See the ***Appendix*** for more information.

HUMAN-LABELED PRODUCTS:

Colchicine Oral Capsules and Tablets: 0.6 mg (1/100 gr); *Colcrys*®, *Mitigare*®, generic; (Rx)

Colchicine Solution: 0.12 mg/mL (0.6 mg/5 mL); *Gloperba*®; (Rx)

References

For the complete list of references, see **wiley.com/go/budde/plumb**

Corticotropin

(kor-ti-koe-***troe***-pin) *Acthar*®

Hormonal Diagnostic Agent

See also ***Cosyntropin***

Prescriber Highlights

- ► Cosyntropin is more commonly used.
- ► Stimulates cortisol release; used primarily to test for hyper- or hypoadrenocorticism (ACTH-stimulation test)
- ► Use as a screening test for naturally occurring hyperadrenocorticism is becoming less popular than in the past; may also be used to test for iatrogenic hyperadrenocorticism and to monitor therapy when treating with anti-adrenal drugs.
- ► Adverse effects are unlikely unless used chronically.
- ► Commercial formulation contains naturally derived ACTH analogues in a gel for IM administration; do not administer IV.

Uses/Indications

A corticotropin (ACTH) product (*Adrenomone*®) was FDA-approved for use in dogs, cats, and beef or dairy cattle for stimulation of the adrenal cortex (during ACTH-deficient states) and as a therapeutic agent in primary bovine ketosis, but it is no longer commercially available.

In practice, ACTH tends to be used most often in the diagnosis of hypoadrenocorticism (ACTH-stimulation test), iatrogenic hyperadrenocorticism, and to monitor the response to mitotane or trilostane therapy in patients being treated for hyperadrenocorticism. It is less often recommended as a screening test for naturally occurring hyperadrenocorticism in dogs since the test is not as sensitive as the low-dose dexamethasone suppression test.

One reference recommends using the ACTH-stimulation test if the dog has non-adrenal illness, received any form of exogenous glucocorticoids (including topicals) or phenobarbital. When performing the ACTH-stimulation test, cosyntropin is the agent of choice. See ***Cosyntropin***. If the dog has no known non-adrenal illness and moderate to severe clinical signs of hyperadrenocorticism, use the low-dose dexamethasone suppression test.[1]

Pharmacology/Actions

Corticotropin (adrenocorticotropic hormone, ACTH) stimulates the adrenal cortex (principally the zona fasciculata) to produce and release glucocorticoids (primarily cortisol in mammals and corticosterone in birds). ACTH release is controlled by corticotropin-releasing factor (CRF), activated in the hypothalamus via a negative feedback pathway, whereby either endogenous or exogenous glucocorticoids suppress ACTH release.

Pharmacokinetics

Because it is rapidly degraded by proteolytic enzymes in the gut, corticotropin (ACTH) cannot be administered PO. It is not effective if administered topically to the skin or eye.

After IM injection in humans, repository corticotropin injection is absorbed over 8-16 hours. The elimination half-life of circulating ACTH is about 15 minutes but because of the slow absorption after IM injection of the gel, effects may persist up to 24 hours.

Contraindications/Precautions/Warnings

ACTH gel should not be used in patients hypersensitive to porcine proteins.

When used for diagnostic purposes, it is unlikely that increases in serum cortisol levels induced by corticotropin (ACTH) will have significant deleterious effects on conditions where increased cortisol levels are contraindicated (eg, systemic fungal infections, osteoporosis, peptic ulcer disease).

Compounded ACTH preparations may contain ACTH in

amounts that deviate considerably from their labeled potency and may have varying consistency (from watery to solid).[2]

Do not confuse corticotropin with cosyntropin. Corticotropin gel should be administered IM; do not administer by the IV route.

Adverse Effects

Prolonged use may result in fluid and electrolyte disturbances and other adverse effects; potassium supplementation may be required with chronic therapy.[3] Refer to the human literature for an extensive listing of potential adverse reactions if using corticotropin on a chronic basis.

Reproductive/Nursing Safety

Corticotropin (ACTH) may reduce fetal growth and result in preterm birth and may also be embryocidal. Neonates born from mothers receiving ACTH should be observed for signs of adrenocortical insufficiency. It is unknown if ACTH is excreted in milk.[3]

Because safety has not been established in animals, this drug should only be used when the maternal benefits outweigh the potential risks to offspring.

Overdose/Acute Toxicity

When used for diagnostic purposes, acute inadvertent overdoses are unlikely to cause any significant adverse effects. Monitor as required and treat based on clinical signs if necessary.

For patients that have experienced or are suspected to have experienced an overdose, consultation with a 24-hour poison consultation center specializing in providing veterinary-specific information is recommended. For general information related to overdose and toxin exposures, as well as contact information for poison control centers, refer to ***Appendix***.

Drug Interactions

The following drug interactions have either been reported or are theoretical in humans or animals receiving corticotropin (ACTH) for diagnostic purposes and may be of significance in veterinary patients. Unless otherwise noted, use together is not necessarily contraindicated, but weigh the potential risks and perform additional monitoring when appropriate.

- **ANTICHOLINESTERASES** (eg, **pyridostigmine**): ACTH may antagonize the beneficial effects of anticholinesterase therapy in patients with myasthenia gravis and cause a worsening of signs.
- **DIURETICS** (eg, **furosemide**): Long-term administration of ACTH may increase electrolyte loss.

Laboratory Considerations

- Patients should not receive **hydrocortisone** or **cortisone** on test day.
- ACTH may decrease **I^{131} uptake** by the thyroid gland.
- ACTH may suppress **intradermal skin test** reactions.
- ACTH may interfere with **urinary estrogen** determinations.
- Obtain specific information from the laboratory on sample handling and laboratory normals for cortisol when doing ACTH stimulation tests.

Dosages

NOTE: When using compounded ACTH products, it is recommended to get several post-ACTH samples (at a minimum, 1 and 2 hours following injection).[2] **Do not confuse these dosages/protocols with those for cosyntropin.**

DOGS:

ACTH stimulation test (extra-label): Draw baseline blood sample for cortisol determination then administer ACTH gel 2.2 units/kg IM. Draw sample 60 and 120 minutes after injection.[1,4]

HORSES:

ACTH stimulation test (extra-label): Draw baseline blood sample for cortisol determination then administer ACTH gel 1 unit/kg IM between 8 AM and 10 AM; draw post-ACTH cortisol levels at 2 and 4 hours postdose. Horses with a functional adrenal gland should have a 2- to 3-fold increase in plasma cortisol when compared with baseline.[5]

BIRDS:

ACTH Stimulation Test (extra-label): Draw baseline blood sample for corticosterone (not cortisol) determination then administer ACTH gel 16 – 25 units IM. Draw post-ACTH corticosterone levels 1 to 2 hours later. Normal baseline corticosterone levels vary with regard to species, but generally range from 1.5 – 7 ng/mL. After ACTH, corticosterone levels generally increase by 5-10 times those of baseline. Specific values are listed in the reference.[6]

Chemistry/Synonyms

A 39 amino acid polypeptide, corticotropin (ACTH) is secreted from the anterior pituitary. The first 24 amino acids (from the N-terminal end of the chain) define its biologic activity. While human, sheep, cattle, and swine corticotropin have different structures, the first 24 amino acids are the same and, therefore, biologic activity is thought to be identical. Commercial products are extracts obtained from porcine pituitaries that contain the full polypeptide ACTH (amino acids 1-39) and related peptide analogues. One USP unit of corticotropin is equivalent to 1 mg of the international standard.

Corticotropin may also be known as ACTH, adrenocorticotrophic hormone, adrenocorticotrophin, corticotrophin, corticotropinum, *Acethropan®*, *Acortan simplex®*, *Actharn®*, *Acthelea®*, *Acton prolongatum®*, *H.P. Acthar® Gel* or *Cortrophin-Zinc®*.

Storage/Stability

Repository corticotropin injection should be stored in the refrigerator 2°C to 8°C (36°F-46°F) but warmed to room temperature prior to administration. Do not over-pressurize the vial prior to withdrawing the product.

Compatibility/Compounding Considerations

No specific information noted

Dosage Forms/Regulatory Status

VETERINARY-LABELED PRODUCTS: NONE

Compounded ACTH products may be available from compounding pharmacies.

HUMAN-LABELED PRODUCTS:

Corticotropin Repository Injection: 80 units/mL in 5 mL multi-dose vials; *Acthar® Gel*; (Rx) **NOTE:** This product is only available through a specialty pharmacy distribution system and is not available via regular retail pharmacies or drug wholesalers.

References

For the complete list of references, see **wiley.com/go/budde/plumb**

Cortisone

(kor-ti-***zone***)

Corticosteroid

Prescriber Highlights

- Oral glucocorticoid with both glucocorticoid and mineralocorticoid effects; an option to manage hypoadrenocorticism by reducing dosage requirements for mineralocorticoid drugs
- Not commonly used in veterinary medicine; whether it has any clinically significant benefit in dogs over oral prednis(ol)one is controversial
- Similar cautions and adverse effects as with other corticosteroid drugs if used at supra-physiologic replacement doses; otherwise, should be well tolerated

Uses/Indications

Cortisone may be used as an alternative to prednis(ol)one for the oral treatment of hypoadrenocorticism in dogs. In vivo cortisone acetate is rapidly converted to cortisol and therefore could serve as a total replacement therapy for both glucocorticoid and mineralocorticoid deficiencies. Whether cortisone acetate is any more effective than prednis(ol)one for long-term treatment in dogs is controversial, as some clinicians believe that any benefit of the increased mineralocorticoid activity that cortisone has is clinically insignificant.

Pharmacology/Actions

Cortisone is a short-acting corticosteroid with a biologic half-life of 8 to 12 hours. Glucocorticoids have effects on almost every cell type and system in mammals. See ***Glucocorticoid Agents, General Information*** for more details.

Pharmacokinetics

Like other glucocorticoids, cortisone acetate's pharmacokinetics do not correlate with its pharmacodynamic activity. Cortisone acetate is absorbed and converted to cortisol (hydrocortisone) in vivo. Oral bioavailability in humans ranges widely but is ≈50%.

Contraindications/Precautions/Warnings

When used for physiologic replacement in dogs with hypoadrenocorticism, cortisone is contraindicated if the patient is hypersensitive to it. If cortisone is used at supra physiologic dosages, the typical contraindications and warnings for drugs like prednis(ol)one should be followed. See ***Glucocorticoid Agents, General Information*** for more details.

Adverse Effects

Cortisone is usually well tolerated when it is used for physiologic replacement in dogs with hypoadrenocorticism. Potentially, GI effects (vomiting, inappetence, diarrhea) could occur, and hypersensitivity reactions are possible. If used at supra-physiologic dosages, the typical adverse effect profile for drugs like prednis(ol)one is possible. See ***Glucocorticoid Agents, General Information*** for more details.

Reproductive/Nursing Safety

During normal fetal development glucocorticoids may be required for adequate surfactant production, myelin, retinal, pancreatic, and mammary development; however, excessive dosages early in pregnancy may lead to teratogenic effects. Substantial maternal doses of corticosteroids during pregnancy may result in hypoadrenalism in the offspring.[1] Corticosteroid therapy may induce parturition in large animal species during the later stages of pregnancy.

Caution is advised when cortisone is used in nursing dams; glucocorticoids unbound to plasma proteins can enter the milk. High doses or prolonged administration to nursing dams may potentially inhibit growth, interfere with endogenous corticosteroid production, or cause other unwanted effects in nursing offspring.

Because safety has not been established in animals, this drug should only be used when the maternal benefits outweigh the potential risks to offspring.

Overdose/Acute Toxicity

Acute ingestion is rarely a clinical problem and clinical effects are unlikely with an acute overdose. However, neuropsychiatric effects can occur; cardiac arrhythmias and anaphylaxis are possible but rare.

For patients that have experienced or are suspected to have experienced an overdose, consultation with a 24-hour poison consultation center specializing in providing veterinary-specific information is recommended. For general information related to overdose and toxin exposures, as well as contact information for poison control centers, refer to ***Appendix.***

Drug Interactions

The following drug interactions have either been reported or are theoretical in humans or animals receiving cortisone and may be of significance in veterinary patients. Unless otherwise noted, use together is not necessarily contraindicated, but weigh the potential risks and perform additional monitoring when appropriate.

- **AMPHOTERICIN B**: Concomitant administration with glucocorticoid may cause hypokalemia; in humans, there have been cases of CHF and cardiac enlargement reported after using hydrocortisone to treat amphotericin B adverse effects.
- **ANTICHOLINESTERASE AGENTS** (eg, **pyridostigmine, neostigmine**): In patients with myasthenia gravis, concomitant glucocorticoid and anticholinesterase agent administration may lead to profound muscle weakness.
- **ASPIRIN**: Corticosteroids may increase the clearance of salicylates and decrease salicylate serum concentrations; however, there is an increased risk for GI ulceration/bleeding.
- **DIURETICS, POTASSIUM-DEPLETING** (eg, **furosemide, thiazides**): Concomitant administration with glucocorticoids may cause hypokalemia.
- **ESTROGENS**: The effects of hydrocortisone, and possibly other glucocorticoids, may be potentiated by concomitant administration with estrogens.
- **FLUOROQUINOLONES** (eg, **enrofloxacin, marbofloxacin**): Concurrent use may increase the risk for tendon rupture.
- **INSULIN; ANTIDIABETIC AGENTS**: Insulin requirements may increase in patients that are receiving glucocorticoids.
- **MITOTANE**: Mitotane may alter the metabolism of corticosteroids; higher than usual doses of corticosteroids may be necessary to treat mitotane-induced adrenal insufficiency.
- **NONSTEROIDAL ANTI-INFLAMMATORY DRUGS** (**NSAIDs,** eg, **carprofen, meloxicam**): Administration of ulcerogenic drugs with glucocorticoids may increase the risk for GI ulceration.
- **PHENOBARBITAL/PRIMIDONE**: Concurrent use may result in decreased cortisone efficacy.
- **VACCINES, LIVE ATTENUATED**: Patients receiving corticosteroids at immunosuppressive dosages should generally not receive live attenuated virus vaccines as virus replication may be augmented; a diminished immune response may occur after vaccine, toxoid, or bacterin administration in patients receiving glucocorticoids.
- **WARFARIN**: Hydrocortisone may affect PT; monitor.

Laboratory Considerations

- Cortisone cross-reacts with cortisol in **ACTH response test.** This test must be performed before cortisone is administered. (**NOTE**: Dexamethasone does not cross-react.)
- Glucocorticoids may increase **serum cholesterol.**
- Glucocorticoids may increase **urine glucose** concentrations.
- Glucocorticoids may decrease **serum potassium.**
- Glucocorticoids can suppress the release of **thyroid-stimulating hormone (TSH)** and reduce T_3 and T_4 values. Thyroid gland atrophy has been reported after chronic glucocorticoid administration. Uptake of I^{131} by the thyroid may be decreased by glucocorticoids.
- Reactions to **skin tests** may be suppressed by glucocorticoids.
- False-negative results of the **nitroblue tetrazolium** test for systemic bacterial infections may be induced by glucocorticoids.
- Glucocorticoids may cause **neutrophilia** within 4 to 8 hours after dosing and return to baseline within 24 to 48 hours after drug discontinuation.
- Glucocorticoids can cause **lymphopenia** that can persist for weeks after drug discontinuation in dogs.

Dosages

DOGS:

Long-term treatment of hypoadrenocorticism (extra-label):

Initially, 0.5 – 1 mg/kg PO once every 12 to 24 hours. Maintenance: 0.5 mg/kg PO once every 12 to 24 hours usually provides adequate additional glucocorticoid supplementation. Begin cortisone once animal recovers from the acute adrenal crisis, starts eating and drinking, and is changed from parenteral to oral medication. Usually used in conjunction with a semi-selective mineralocorticoid (fludrocortisone). Although some sources advocate for cortisone acetate,[2,3] others recommend prednisone as the glucocorticoid supplement of choice in dogs for treatment of hypoadrenocorticism.[4,5]

Monitoring

Monitoring during cortisone therapy is dependent on its reason for use, dosage, adjunctive mineralocorticoid therapy, dosage schedule (daily vs alternate-day therapy), duration of therapy, and the animal's age and condition. The following list may not be appropriate or complete for all animals; use clinical assessment and judgment should adverse effects be noted:

- Weight, appetite, and/or signs of fluid retention
- Serum and/or urine electrolytes
- Total plasma proteins and albumin
- Blood glucose
- Urine culture
- Growth and development in young animals

Client Information

- Give this medicine with food.
- The goal of treatment is to find the lowest dose possible and use it for the shortest period of time. Follow your veterinarian's instructions on how to give this medicine.
- Many side effects are possible, especially when used long-term or when given in higher doses. The most common side effects are increased appetite, thirst, and need to urinate.
- Make sure your animal has access to plenty of fresh, clean water while taking this medicine. Do not restrict water at any time while your animal is taking this medicine.
- In dogs, stomach or intestinal ulcers, perforation, or bleeding can occur while taking this medicine. Contact your veterinarian right away if your animal stops eating or if you notice a high fever, black tarry stools, or bloody vomit (will look like coffee grounds).
- Do not stop therapy abruptly without your veterinarian's guidance, as serious side effects could occur.
- Be sure to tell your veterinarian what other medications (including vitamins, supplements, or herbal therapies) you give your animal.

Chemistry/Synonyms

Cortisone acetate is a synthetic acetate ester of cortisone. It occurs as a white or practically white, odorless, crystalline powder. It is insoluble in water and slightly soluble in alcohol.

Cortisone acetate may also be known as acetato de cortisona, compound E acetate, acétate de cortisone, cortisoni acetas, or 11-dehydro-17-hydroxycorticosterone acetate.

Storage/Stability

Cortisone acetate tablets should be stored in well-closed containers at a temperature less than 40°C (104°F), preferably at 15°C to 30°C (59°F-86°F).

Compatibility/Compounding Considerations

No specific information noted.

Dosage Forms/Regulatory Status

VETERINARY-LABELED PRODUCTS: NONE

HUMAN-LABELED PRODUCTS:

Cortisone Acetate Oral Tablets: 25 mg; generic; (Rx)

References

For the complete list of references, see **wiley.com/go/budde/plumb**

Cosyntropin
Tetracosactide

(koh-***sin***-troh-pin) *Cortrosyn®*

Hormonal Diagnostic Agent

Prescriber Highlights

- ► Used for adrenal function tests. Similar to but not the same as corticotropin (ACTH)
- ► Stimulates cortisol release; agent used primarily to perform an ACTH-stimulation test to evaluate for hyper- or hypoadrenocorticism and to monitor therapy when treating with antiadrenal drugs.
- ► Best results achieved when drug is given IV.
- ► Do not confuse with corticotropin (ACTH) gel.

Uses/Indications

Cosyntropin is used most often to perform an ACTH-stimulation test for the diagnosis of hypoadrenocorticism and iatrogenic hyperadrenocorticism and to monitor the response to mitotane or trilostane in the treatment of hyperadrenocorticism. It is less often recommended as a screening test for naturally occurring hyperadrenocorticism (ie, pituitary-dependent hyperadrenocorticism, adrenal tumors) in dogs because the test is not as sensitive as the low-dose dexamethasone suppression test.[1] One reference[2] recommends using the ACTH stimulation test if the dog has nonadrenal illness or has received any form of exogenous glucocorticoids (including topicals) or phenobarbital. If the dog has no known nonadrenal illness and moderate to severe clinical signs of hyperadrenocorticism, the low-dose dexamethasone suppression test is preferred.

Cosyntropin can also be used to assess adrenal function in horses (both adults and foals).[3-5]

Pharmacology/Actions

Like endogenous corticotropin, cosyntropin stimulates the adrenal cortex (principally the zona fasciculata) to stimulate the production and release of glucocorticoids (primarily cortisol in mammals and corticosterone in birds). Because of its structure, cosyntropin retains biologic activity but is not as immunogenic as endogenous corticotropin. The bulk of immunogenicity appears to reside in the C-terminal portion of corticotropin (amino acids 22-39), and cosyntropin ends after amino acid 24.

Pharmacokinetics

Cosyntropin must be given parenterally because it is inactivated by GI enzymes.

Cosyntropin administration causes a dose-dependent increase in cortisol response in dogs.[6] In both healthy dogs and dogs with hyperadrenocorticism, peak cortisol concentration occurs 90 minutes after administration of cosyntropin at 5 or 10 µg/kg IV but peaks at 30 minutes at 1 µg/kg IV dose.[7] Cosyntropin administered IM or IV results in equivalent peak cortisol concentration.[8] The 2 commercially available parenteral forms in the United States appear to be bioequivalent in dogs when given IV.[9] Under experimental conditions, intentional perivascular administration resulted in similar cortisol response as IV administration.[10]

In cats, cosyntropin given IM resulted in peak cortisol concentration after 45 minutes, as compared with 75 minutes after IV administration. Cortisol returns to baseline by 2 hours and 4 hours after IM and IV administration, respectively.[11]

In neonatal foals, a 10 µg IV total dose produces a peak cortisol response 30 minutes after administration, with a return to baseline

90 minutes after administration. Higher doses (100 or 250 µg IV total dose) have a peak response of greater magnitude, which occurs after 90 minutes, with a duration of 1.5 to 2.5 hours.[4]

It is unknown how cosyntropin is inactivated or eliminated after parenteral administration.

Contraindications/Precautions/Warnings

Cosyntropin is contraindicated in patients with known hypersensitivity to it. Use with caution in patients that have shown hypersensitive reactions to ACTH in the past, as cross-reactivity could occur.

Do not confuse cosyntropin with corticotropin (ACTH).

Adverse Effects

When cosyntropin is used short term, the primary concern is hypersensitivity reactions.

Reproductive/Nursing Safety

Effects on reproductive capacity, risk for fetal harm, or nursing offspring are unknown. Use only when maternal benefits outweigh risk to offspring.

Overdose/Acute Toxicity

Unlikely to be of clinical consequence if used one time.

For patients that have experienced or are suspected to have experienced an overdose, consultation with a 24-hour poison consultation center specializing in providing veterinary-specific information is recommended. For general information related to overdose and toxin exposures, as well as contact information for poison control centers, refer to ***Appendix***.

Drug Interactions

The following drug interactions have either been reported or are theoretical in humans or animals receiving corticotropin for diagnostic purposes and may be of significance in veterinary patients receiving cosyntropin:

- **Anticholinesterases** (eg, **pyridostigmine**): ACTH may antagonize the beneficial effects of anticholinesterase therapy in patients with myasthenia gravis and cause a worsening of signs.
- **Diuretics** (eg, **furosemide**): Long-term administration of ACTH may increase electrolyte loss.

Laboratory Considerations

- Patients should not receive **hydrocortisone** or **cortisone**[12] on test day; dexamethasone sodium phosphate does not interfere with cortisol assays.[13]
- If using a fluorometric analysis, falsely high cortisol values may be observed if the patient is taking **estrogens** (eg, DES, estriol) or **spironolactone.**
- Falsely high cortisol values may be observed in patients with high **bilirubin** or if free plasma **hemoglobin** is present.

Dosages

NOTES:

1. The following dosages are for the cosyntropin aqueous (either liquid or lyophilized) products available commercially in the US. There is also depot injectable cosyntropin zinc hydroxide (*Synacthen*® Depot) available in some countries which should only be used IM and **not** given IV. Contact your laboratory for specific dosing protocols if using the depot form.
2. Do not confuse these dosages/protocols with those for ***corticotropin (ACTH).***

DOGS:

Testing (screening) for hyperadrenocorticism using ACTH stimulation test (extra-label): Draw pre-ACTH stim serum cortisol level. Give 5 µg/kg IV (with a maximum dose of 250 µg per dog); draw post-ACTH serum cortisol level 60 minutes after dose during peak cortisol concentrations.[1,14]

Testing (screening) for hypoadrenocorticism using ACTH stimulation test (extra-label): Draw pre-ACTH stim serum cortisol level. Give 1 µg/kg IV; draw post-ACTH serum cortisol level 60 minutes after dose during peak cortisol concentrations.[15,16]

Monitoring dogs diagnosed with hyperadrenocorticism and being treated with mitotane or trilostane using an ACTH stimulation test (extra-label): Draw pre-ACTH stim serum cortisol level. Give 1 µg/kg IV; draw post-ACTH stim serum cortisol level 60 minutes after dose to measure peak cortisol concentrations.[14] Cosyntropin 5 µg/kg IV and 1 µg/kg IV were pharmacologically equivalent in dogs being treated with mitotane or trilostane.

CATS:

Testing (screening) adrenal function using ACTH stimulation test (extra-label): Based on a study[17] in healthy cats, draw pre-ACTH stim serum cortisol level. Give 5 µg/kg IV followed by a post-ACTH stim serum cortisol sample at 60 to 75 minutes. Serum cortisol and aldosterone concentrations were equivalent to those achieved following administration of cosyntropin at 125 µg/cat IV (NOT mg/kg), the historical dose for cats.[18,19]

HORSES:

Testing (screening) adrenal function in adult horses (extra-label): 0.1 µg /kg IV resulted in maximum adrenal stimulation, with peak cortisol concentration 30 minutes after cosyntropin administration.[3]

Testing (screening) adrenal function in neonatal foals (extra-label):

1. 100 µg /foal or 250 µg /foal (total dose, NOT µg /kg) IV.[5] Cortisol response may be reduced in critically ill foals.[20,21]
2. 0.1 to 0.25 µg /kg IV, with peak cortisol concentration 20 to 30 minutes after cosyntropin administration[22,23]
3. Paired low dose/high dose ACTH stimulation test: Cosyntropin 10 µg IV (total dose, NOT µg /kg) after baseline blood draw, and Cosyntropin 100 µg IV (total dose, NOT µg/kg) administered immediately 90 minutes later (after blood draw). Collect blood sample to measure baseline cortisol and ACTH, and repeat blood draw for cortisol 30, 90, 120 and 180 minutes later.[4]

Monitoring

- See specific protocols for test procedures.
- Peak cortisol response is dose dependent and typically observed within 30 to 60 minutes in dogs,[6,7] cats,[24] and horses.[3,5]
- It is recommended to perform ACTH stimulation testing at or about the same time after trilostane administration (4 to 6 hours postdosing is recommended[25]).

Chemistry/Synonyms

Cosyntropin is a synthetic polypeptide that mimics the effects of corticotropin (ACTH). It is commercially available as a lyophilized white to off-white powder containing mannitol. Cosyntropin's structure is identical to the first 24 (of 39) amino acids in natural human, canine, and feline corticotropin.[26] Cosyntropin 0.25 mg is equivalent to 25 units of corticotropin.

Cosyntropin may also be known as tetracosactide, alpha(1–24)-corticotrophin, beta(1–24)-corticotrophin, tetracosactido, tetracosactidum, tetracosactrin, tetracosapeptide, *Cortrosina*®, *Cortrosyn*®, *Cosacthen*®, *Nuvacthen*® *Depot, Synacthen*®, *Synacthen*® *Depot, Synacthène Retard,* or *Synacthène.*

Storage/Stability

The lyophilized powder should be stored at room temperature (20°C-25°C [68°F-77°F]). Reconstitute with sterile normal saline and discard any unused portion.

The commercially available injectable solution is labeled to be stored at 15°C to 30°C (59°F-86°F); protect from light and freezing. Discard any unused portion.

One study showed that cosyntropin can be reconstituted and stored frozen (-20°C [-4°F]) in plastic syringes for up to 6 months and still show biologic activity in the dog.[27] It is recommended to freeze in small aliquots as it is unknown what effect thawing and refreezing has on potency. At present, it is recommended to store in plastic containers (eg, tuberculin syringes) as it may bind to glass.

Compatibility/Compounding Considerations

No specific information noted

Dosage Forms/Regulatory Status

VETERINARY-LABELED PRODUCTS: NONE

HUMAN-LABELED PRODUCTS:

Cosyntropin Powder for Injection: 0.25 mg lyophilized (250 µg) in single-dose vials with diluent; *Cortrosyn®*, generic; (Rx)

Cosyntropin Solution for Injection: 0.25 mg/mL (250 µg /mL), preservative-free in 1 mL single-dose vials; generic; (Rx)

NOTE: Corticotropin (compounded ACTH gel for IM or SC use) is not the same as cosyntropin.

References

For the complete list of references, see **wiley.com/go/budde/plumb**

Crofelemer

(cro-***fell***-a-mer) *Canalevia®-CA1*

Antidiarrheal

Prescriber Highlights

- ► Conditionally approved for the treatment of chemotherapy-induced diarrhea in dogs. Due to conditional approval, this drug must only be used as labeled.
- ► Contraindicated in dogs hypersensitive to it
- ► Rule out infections or other causes of diarrhea prior to use.
- ► Appears well tolerated. Adverse effects may include GI effects (eg, abnormal feces, vomiting, reduced appetite), decreased activity, hypoglycemia, and hypocalcemia.

Uses/Indications

Crofelemer is conditionally approved (pending a full demonstration of effectiveness) by the FDA for the treatment of chemotherapy-induced diarrhea in dogs. In one study, crofelemer administration decreased stool frequency and improved stool consistency in healthy beagles receiving neratinib (a tyrosine kinase inhibitor).[1]

As a conditionally approved drug, it is a violation of United States federal law to use crofelemer other than as directed on the label.

Crofelemer is approved in humans for symptomatic relief of noninfectious diarrhea in adult HIV/AIDS patients on retroviral therapy.[2]

Pharmacology/Actions

The mechanism of action of crofelemer in dogs is not fully characterized. In humans, crofelemer inhibits 2 types of chloride channels: (1) cyclic adenosine monophosphate-stimulated cystic fibrosis transmembrane conductance regulator (CFTR) chloride channels; and (2) calcium-activated chloride channels.[3] By inhibiting both types of channels at the luminal membrane of intestinal epithelial cells, crofelemer blocks chloride ion secretion and the accompanying high volume water loss that occurs with diarrhea, thereby normalizing the flow of chloride ions and water in the GI tract.

Pharmacokinetics

In dogs, crofelemer was not absorbed at dosages used clinically.[4] After oral administration to humans, the drug was undetectable in plasma.[2] Standard pharmacokinetic parameters have not been determined due to the absence of systemically available drug. Humans do not appear to metabolize crofelemer, and presumably the drug is eliminated in the feces. See ***Overdose/Acute Toxicity*** for further information.

Contraindications/Precautions/Warnings

Crofelemer is contraindicated in patients that are hypersensitive to it. Rule out other causes of diarrhea (eg, infection, toxicosis) prior to crofelemer use.

Do not confuse with CROfelemer with SEVelamer.

Adverse Effects

Crofelemer appears to be well tolerated by dogs. Adverse effects observed in preapproval studies occurred at rates similar to the control (placebo) group and included abnormal feces (eg, soft, watery, mucoid, discolored feces), vomiting, reduced appetite, decreased activity, upper respiratory signs (eg, coughing, nasal discharge, sneezing, congestion), and urinary system abnormalities (eg, UTI, cystitis, worsened pyuria). Hypoglycemia and hypocalcemia were noted in 8% and 4% of dogs receiving crofelemer, respectively. Increased neutrophils were also observed.[5]

Adverse effects reported by humans receiving crofelemer include upper respiratory tract infections and bronchitis, cough, flatulence, and increased liver enzymes.

Reproductive/Nursing Safety

Safe use of crofelemer has not been evaluated in dogs that are pregnant, lactating, or used for breeding. However, a reasonable degree of safety during pregnancy can be expected because crofelemer is not absorbed into systemic circulation. Crofelemer was not teratogenic in rats or rabbits, and embryofetal toxicity was not observed in rats; increased fetal resorption was demonstrated in rabbits but this may have been due to maternal toxicity.[2]

It is unknown if crofelemer is excreted into milk.[2] As the lack of systemic absorption should preclude delivery of the drug into milk, and any drug that may be excreted is unlikely to be absorbed by the nursing litters, it is expected that crofelemer may be safely administered to nursing animals.

Because safety has not been established in animals, this drug should only be used when the maternal benefits outweigh the potential risks to offspring.

Overdose/Acute Toxicity

Oral LD_{50} in dogs is greater than 1,200 mg/kg.[6] Systemic crofelemer absorption was demonstrated with dosages at or greater than 50 mg/kg PO daily.[4] Dosages up to 600 mg/kg PO daily given for 1 to 9 months to 6- to 7-month-old beagles resulted in decreased food intake, reduced weight gain, vomiting, and black or rust-colored feces, and hematologic changes consistent with microcytic, hypochromic anemia, and thrombocytosis (consistent with GI ulceration and hemorrhage). Pathology changes included red streaks and erosions in the GI tract along with intestinal congestion and inflammation.[7]

For patients that have experienced or are suspected to have experienced an overdose, it is strongly encouraged to consult with one of the 24-hour poison consultation centers that specialize in providing information specific for veterinary patients. For general information related to overdose and toxin exposures, as well as contact information for poison control centers, refer to ***Appendix.***

Drug Interactions

Although in vitro studies suggest that crofelemer has the potential to inhibit CYP3A4 and other transporters in the GI tract, limited studies performed in healthy humans have not demonstrated drug interactions. The following drug interactions have either been reported or are theoretical in humans or animals receiving crofelemer and may be of significance in veterinary patients. Unless otherwise noted, use together is not necessarily contraindicated, but weigh the potential risks and perform additional monitoring when appropriate.

- **Anticholinergic Agents** (eg, **atropine, glycopyrrolate, hyoscyamine, oxybutynin**): Increased risk for constipation or other GI complications
- **Antidiarrheal Agents** (eg, **diphenoxylate, loperamide**): Increased risk for constipation or other GI complications
- **H_1 Receptor Antihistamines** (eg, **diphenhydramine, hydroxyzine**): Increased risk for constipation or other GI complications
- **Opioids** (eg, **butorphanol, fentanyl, morphine, tramadol**): Increased risk for constipation or other GI complications
- **Phenothiazines** (eg, **acepromazine**): Increased risk for constipation or other GI complications

Laboratory Considerations

None were noted.

Dosages

DOGS:

Treatment of chemotherapy-induced diarrhea (label dosage; conditionally approved by FDA): 125 mg/dog (NOT mg/kg) PO twice daily for 3 days for dogs weighing 63.6 kg (140 lb) or less, and 250 mg/dog (NOT mg/kg) PO twice daily for 3 days for dogs weighing over 63.6 kg (140 lb)[5]

Monitoring

- Fecal testing (eg, flotation, antigen, and/or PCR testing) prior to treatment to rule out infectious causes of diarrhea
- Efficacy of treatment based on clinical improvement (eg, resolution of diarrhea, improved appetite and food intake)
- Hydration status, body weight, patient reaction to abdominal palpation
- Adverse effects (eg, worsening of GI signs, abdominal discomfort, lethargy)

Client Information

- This medicine may be given either with food or on an empty stomach. If your animal vomits or acts sick after receiving it on an empty stomach, try giving the next dose with food or a small treat. If vomiting continues, contact your veterinarian.
- Administer tablets whole; do not split, break, or crush. If the tablet is chewed, one additional dose may be administered.

Chemistry/Synonyms

Crofelemer is a proanthocyanidin mixture derived from the red latex of the South American *Croton lechleri* Müll Arg plant. It is composed primarily of monomer units of (+)–catechin, (–)–epicatechin, (+)–gallocatechin, and (–)–epigallocatechin linked in random sequence, with the average degree of polymerization between 5 and 7.5. In solution, crofelemer is reddish-brown in color.[8]

Crofelemer may also be known as SP-303, *Canalevia*®-CA1, and *Mytesi*®.

Storage/Stability

Store crofelemer tablets at 20°C to 25°C (68°F-77°F); excursions are permitted between 15°C and 30°C (59°F-86°F).

Compatibility/Compounding Considerations

No information was available.

Dosage Forms/Regulatory Status

VETERINARY-LABELED PRODUCTS:

Crofelemer Delayed-Release Tablets: 125 mg enteric coated tablets; *Canalevia*®-CA1; (Rx). Conditional Approval Application Number 141-552. Extra-label use of conditionally approved drugs is not permitted by FDA. See ***Conditional Approval Explained: A Resource for Veterinarians*** for more information on conditionally approved drugs.

HUMAN-LABELED PRODUCTS:

Crofelemer Delayed-Release Tablets: 125 mg enteric coated tablets; *Mytesi*®; (Rx)

References

For the complete list of references, see **wiley.com/go/budde/plumb**

Cromolyn (Inhaled)

(***kroh***-mah-lin) *Intal*®

Mast Cell Stabilizer

For ophthalmic use, see ***Cromolyn Ophthalmic.***

Prescriber Highlights

- Inhaled mast cell stabilizer that may be useful adjunctive treatment in preventing respiratory clinical signs and airway obstruction in horses with mild to moderate asthma characterized by an elevated mast cell count or in horses with severe equine asthma
- Not for treatment of acute bronchoconstriction; used as a preventive agent
- May take several days to weeks for efficacy

Uses/Indications

Cromolyn is a mast cell stabilizer that may be useful in reducing or preventing respiratory clinical signs and airway obstruction in horses with mild to moderate asthma characterized by an elevated mast cell count, or in horses with severe equine asthma (formerly known as recurrent airway obstruction, heaves).[1-4] Use of this agent is somewhat controversial; studies have yielded conflicting efficacy results and it is not widely used clinically. Cromolyn was ineffective in preventing exercise-induced pulmonary hemorrhage (EIPH).[5,6]

Pharmacology/Actions

Cromolyn inhibits the release of histamine and leukotrienes from sensitized mast cells found in lung mucosa, nasal mucosa, and eyes. Its exact mechanism of activity is not understood, but it is thought to block indirect entry of calcium ions into cells. Other effects of cromolyn include inhibition of neuronal reflexes in the lung and bronchospasm secondary to tachykinins, and movement of other inflammatory cells (neutrophils, monocytes, eosinophils). Cromolyn also prevents down-regulation of beta-2 adrenergic receptors on lymphocytes. Cromolyn does not have antihistaminic, anticholinergic, antiserotonin, corticosteroid-like, or anti-inflammatory effects.

Pharmacokinetics

Limited information is available for horses. The amount of cromolyn reaching the distal airways is likely variable and dependent on the type of nebulizer used and amount of concurrent bronchoconstriction present.[7] Absorbed cromolyn is eliminated in the urine and via the bile into the feces.

In humans, less than 2% of cromolyn is absorbed from the GI tract after oral dosing. Approximately 8% is absorbed when inhaled into the lung. Absorbed drug is eliminated via the feces and urine as unchanged drug.

Contraindications/Precautions/Warnings

Do not use cromolyn in patients with documented hypersensitivity to it.

Cromolyn is unlikely to be of benefit in treating horses with mild to moderate asthma free of mastocytic inflammation. Cromolyn has no efficacy in treating acute bronchospasm.[8]

Adverse Effects

Adverse effects associated with inhaled cromolyn use in horses are not well documented. Cough and treatment avoidance (possibly due to bad taste) have been reported. It has been proposed that pretreatment with albuterol may reduce the incidence of cough.

Humans can occasionally develop a cough, throat irritation, or report unpleasant taste. Very rarely, bronchoconstriction and anaphylaxis have been reported.

Reproductive/Nursing Safety

Laboratory animal studies have shown no effect on fertility. Teratogenicity studies in mice, rats, and rabbits have not demonstrated any teratogenic effects, and it is likely safe for use during pregnancy.[8]

Extremely low (or undetectable) concentrations have been detected in milk; cromolyn is most likely safe for use during nursing.

Because safety has not been established in animals, this drug should only be used when the maternal benefits outweigh the potential risks to offspring.

Overdose/Acute Toxicity

Because of the drug's low systemic bioavailability after inhalation or oral administration, acute overdoses are unlikely to cause significant morbidity.

For patients that have experienced or are suspected to have experienced an overdose, consultation with a 24-hour poison consultation center specializing in providing veterinary-specific information is recommended. For general information related to overdose and toxin exposures, as well as contact information for poison control centers, refer to ***Appendix.***

Drug Interactions

No notable drug interactions have been reported.

Laboratory Considerations

None have been noted.

Dosages

HORSES:

Adjunctive treatment of equine asthma (extra-label):

a) Using a jet nebulizer, 200 mg/horse (NOT mg/kg) every 12 hours[9]
b) Using an ultrasonic nebulizer, 80 mg/horse (NOT mg/kg) every 24 hours[9]

Monitoring

- Clinical efficacy
- For horses with equine asthma, reductions in mast cell counts in bronchoalveolar lavage (BAL) could help confirm efficacy.

Client Information

- This medication does not treat airway constriction but is used to prevent airway constriction by reducing the release of substances from cells that can cause it. It should not be used to treat acute bronchoconstriction (difficulty breathing).
- This medication must be given once to twice daily and it may take several days to weeks before it can be determined if it is working.
- Be sure you understand how to use the device that delivers the medicine to your animal. Contact your veterinarian if you have questions.

Chemistry/Synonyms

Cromolyn sodium occurs as a white, odorless, hygroscopic crystalline powder that is soluble in water and insoluble in alcohol.

Cromolyn sodium may also be known as cromoglicic acid, cromoglycic acid, sodium cromoglicate, disodium cromoglycate, sodium cromoglycate, DSCG, SCG, FPL-670, or DNSG; there are many international trade names.

Storage/Stability

Cromolyn sodium solution for inhalation should be stored below at 20°C to 25°C (68°F-77°F).[8] Protect from freezing and light. Store the product in a foil pouch until ready for use. Do not use solution if it is cloudy or contains a precipitate. Solution remaining in nebulizers after use should be discarded.

Compatibility/Compounding Considerations

Compatibility is dependent on factors such as pH, concentration, temperature, and diluent used; specialized references or a hospital pharmacist should be consulted for more specific information.

Cromolyn solution is reportedly **compatible** with acetylcysteine, albuterol, epinephrine, isoetherine, isoproterenol, metaproterenol, or terbutaline solutions for up to 60 minutes. It is **incompatible** with bitolterol.

Dosage Forms/Regulatory Status

VETERINARY-LABELED PRODUCTS: NONE IN THE UNITED STATES

HUMAN-LABELED PRODUCTS:

Cromolyn Sodium Solution for Inhalation: 20 mg/2 mL (10 mg/mL) vials or amps; generic; (Rx)

Cromolyn Sodium Ophthalmic Solution: 4% solution; generic; (Rx)

There is also an OTC nasal solution (*Nasalcrom*®, generic), and an oral concentrate (*Gastrocrom*®, generic) indicated for mastocytosis available, but these dosage forms are unlikely to be of use in veterinary medicine.

References

For the complete list of references, see **wiley.com/go/budde/plumb**

Cyclophosphamide

(sye-kloe-***foss***-fa-mide) *Cytoxan*®, *Neosar*®

Antineoplastic

Prescriber Highlights

- ► Antineoplastic agent used in dogs and cats
- ► Metronomic (low-dose, continuous) therapy shows promise for some cancers in dogs, with fewer adverse effects than high-dose treatment.
- ► Contraindications include prior anaphylaxis or history of sterile hemorrhagic cystitis. Use with caution in patients with leukopenia, thrombocytopenia, previous radiotherapy, or impaired hepatic or renal function and in patients for which immunosuppression may be dangerous (eg, infection)
- ► Primary adverse effects include myelosuppression, GI effects, alopecia (especially in poodles and old English sheepdogs), and sterile hemorrhagic cystitis
- ► Vigorous diuresis during administration is recommended to reduce the risk for sterile hemorrhagic cystitis.
- ► Potentially teratogenic and fetotoxic; for sexually intact patients, verify pregnancy status prior to administration
- ► The National Institute for Occupational Safety and Health (NIOSH) classifies cyclophosphamide as a hazardous drug; use appropriate precautions when handling.

Uses/Indications

In veterinary medicine, cyclophosphamide is used primarily in dogs and cats in combination with other drugs as an antineoplastic agent for lymphoma[1] and other hematopoietic tumors, carcinomas,[2,3] and sarcomas.[4]

Most clinicians do not consider cyclophosphamide for initial use as an immunosuppressive agent for treating immune-mediated diseases (eg, immune-mediated hemolytic anemia (IMHA),[5] systemic lupus erythematosus [SLE], immune-mediated thrombocytopenia [ITP], pemphigus-related conditions, rheumatoid arthritis, proliferative urethritis) because alternative treatment options with fewer adverse effects (eg, azathioprine, cyclosporine, mycophenolate mofetil, leflunomide) are available. One review article proposed that cyclophosphamide therapy in dogs be used primarily for cancer treatment, as published efficacy data, although scant, suggest an increased incidence of serious adverse effects (eg, sterile hemorrhagic cystitis, myelosuppression), including death.[6]

Pharmacology/Actions

Cyclophosphamide, an alkylating agent, is a prodrug. One of its primary metabolites, 4-hydroxycyclophosphamide (4-OHCP), is thought to be responsible for the drug's cytotoxic effect. This metabolite enters cells and rapidly decomposes to phosphoramide mustard and acrolein. These alkylating agents interfere with DNA replication and RNA transcription and replication to ultimately disrupt nucleic acid function. The cytotoxic properties of cyclophosphamide are enhanced by its phosphorylating activity.

Cyclophosphamide has marked immunosuppressive activity manifest as decreased WBC and antibody production; the exact mechanisms by which this occurs have not been fully elucidated.

Pharmacokinetics

Peak concentrations of cyclophosphamide and 4-OHCP (active metabolite) were reached in 45 minutes and the elimination half-life of parent and metabolite were between 30 and 60 minutes after oral cyclophosphamide administration in dogs with lymphoma. Area under the curve (AUC) of 4-OHCP was similar after both oral and IV administration. Pharmacokinetics of 4-OHCP in plasma were similar to those of cyclophosphamide after IV or PO dosing, but marked differences were observed in peak concentrations (IV concentration approximately twice as high as PO concentration) and time to reach peak concentrations (IV ≈13 minutes, PO ≈75 minutes). The authors concluded that PO and IV cyclophosphamide can likely be used interchangeably while achieving the same exposure of active metabolite in dogs with lymphoma.[7]

In healthy cats, intraperitoneal (IP) administration resulted in ≈50% lower peak cyclophosphamide concentration and ≈20% lower drug exposure as compared with IV administration, whereas PO administration peak concentration and overall exposure were 80% and ≈50% lower than after IV administration., respectively. The peak concentration and overall exposure of 4-OHCP were similar for all routes of administration. Terminal half-life of cyclophosphamide and 4-OHCP after IV and IP administration were ≈0.6 hours and ≈0.8 hours, respectively, and could not be established after PO administration.[8]

In horses, higher dosages may be necessary to obtain clinically useful concentrations of 4-OHCP.[9]

In humans, cyclophosphamide is well absorbed after PO administration, with peak concentrations of metabolites occurring in 2 to 3 hours. Cyclophosphamide is ≈20% protein bound, and its metabolites are distributed throughout the body, including the CSF (albeit at subtherapeutic concentrations). Cyclophosphamide is metabolized in the liver into several metabolites. Elimination half-life of cyclophosphamide is ≈3 to 12 hours, but drug/metabolites can be detected up to 72 hours after administration. The drug is primarily excreted as metabolites and unchanged drug in the urine.

Contraindications/Precautions/Warnings

Cyclophosphamide should not be used in patients with prior anaphylactic reactions to the drug or in patients with urinary obstruction or a history of sterile hemorrhagic cystitis. Use with caution in patients with impaired hepatic or renal function, patients receiving concurrent radiation, or patients in which immunosuppression may be dangerous (eg, systemic infections). Discontinue cyclophosphamide if sterile hemorrhagic cystitis develops, and further use should be considered contraindicated. Use with caution, if at all, in patients with UTIs or in breeds at risk for developing transitional cell carcinoma (eg, Scottish terriers).

In patients that develop myelosuppression, subsequent doses should be delayed until adequate recovery occurs.

Because of the potential for development of serious adverse effects, cyclophosphamide should be used only in patients that can be adequately and regularly monitored.

Do not confuse cycloPHOSphamide with cycloSPORINE (ciclosporin), or *Cytoxan*® with *Cytotec*®. Consider writing part of the drug's name in uppercase letters on prescriptions/orders to reduce the risk of errors. Additionally, <u>do not write prescriptions for this drug using the abbreviation SID.</u> Many nonveterinary pharmacists are unfamiliar with this abbreviation and could interpret it as another abbreviation (eg, QID).

The National Institute for Occupational Safety and Health (NIOSH) classifies cyclophosphamide as a hazardous drug; personal protective equipment [PPE] should be used accordingly to minimize the risk for exposure.[10]

Adverse Effects

In animals, the primary adverse effects associated with cyclophosphamide are myelosuppression (eg, leukopenia, neutropenia, anemia, thrombocytopenia), gastroenterocolitis (eg, anorexia, especially in cats; nausea; vomiting; diarrhea), renal toxicity (eg, sterile hemorrhagic cystitis, hematuria), and cardiac, hepatic, and pulmonary toxicities. Many dogs receiving chemotherapy will have minor hair coat changes (eg, shagginess, loss of luster). Breeds with continuously growing hair coats (eg, poodles, terriers, Afghan hounds, or old English sheepdogs) are more likely to experience significant alopecia.

The myelosuppressive effects of cyclophosphamide primarily impact the WBC lines but may also affect RBC and platelet production. The nadir for WBCs generally occurs between 5 and 14 days after dosing and may require up to 4 weeks for recovery. When cyclophosphamide is used with other drugs causing myelosuppression, toxic effects may be exacerbated. A study in dogs using recombinant-canine granulocyte colony-stimulating factor (rcG-CSF) at 2.5 μ/kg 3 times a day for 2 to 5 days after cyclophosphamide treatment showed accelerated recovery and reduced severity of neutropenia.[11] Thrombocytopenia occurs occasionally.

Sterile hemorrhagic cystitis induced by cyclophosphamide is thought to be caused by the metabolite acrolein, with an incidence rate of up to 30% of dogs receiving long-term (greater than2 months) cyclophosphamide at standard doses[12,13] and metronomic doses.[14,15] Furosemide administered with cyclophosphamide may reduce the occurrence of this adverse effect.[16-18]

In cats, cyclophosphamide-induced cystitis (CIC) is rare. Initial signs may present as hematuria and dysuria. Because bacterial cystitis is not uncommon in immunosuppressed patients, it must be ruled out by culturing the urine. A negative urine culture with an inflammatory urine sediment on urinalysis is diagnostic for CIC. Because bladder fibrosis and/or transitional cell carcinoma of the bladder are also associated with cyclophosphamide use, these conditions may need to be ruled out via abdominal ultrasonography or other advanced imaging modalities (eg, computed tomography [CT]). The incidence of CIC may be minimized by increasing urine production and frequent voiding. The drug should be given in the morning, and animals should be encouraged to drink and urinate whenever possible. Recommendation for treatment of CIC includes discontinuing cyclophosphamide and beginning therapy with IV fluids, furosemide, and corticosteroids. Refractory cases have been treated by surgical debridement and 1% formalin or 25% DMSO instillation in the bladder.

In a retrospective study in cats, cyclophosphamide was the most likely chemotherapy agent to cause vomiting, anorexia/inappetence, and neutropenia, although adverse effects were noted to occur only infrequently and the severity was typically graded as mild.[19]

Other adverse effects that may be noted with cyclophosphamide therapy include pulmonary infiltrates and fibrosis, depression, hyponatremia, and leukemia. Cardiac toxicity (myocarditis, pericardial effusion, CHF, atrial and ventricular arrhythmias) have occurred in humans.

Reproductive/Nursing Safety

Cyclophosphamide is teratogenic and embryotoxic and may cause fetal harm (neural tube defects; cleft palate; limb, digit, and other skeletal malformation) and miscarriage when administered during pregnancy. Cyclophosphamide may impair fertility.

Cyclophosphamide is distributed in milk and nursing is not recommended when dams are receiving the drug.

For sexually intact female patients, verify pregnancy status prior to administration.

Overdose/Acute Toxicity

Only limited information on acute overdoses of this drug is available, but extensions of adverse effects could be expected. The lethal dose in dogs has been reported as 44 mg/kg IV.[20] In case reports describing cyclophosphamide overdose in dogs, rcG-CSF is often used to help stimulate the bone marrow and hasten the recovery of WBCs in peripheral blood. One case report of a dog with complete recovery after administration of cyclophosphamide 1750 mg PO over 21 days (total exposure 2303 mg/m^2) described use of broad-spectrum antibiotics, whole blood transfusions, rcG-CSF, and tranexamic acid.[21] If an oral overdose occurs, gut emptying should proceed if indicated and the animal should be hospitalized for supportive care. Cyclophosphamide is considered moderately dialyzable.

Common clinical signs associated with overdose in dogs may include neutrophilia, anorexia, hematuria, hyperchloremia, hypernatremia, polydipsia, nystagmus, seizures, tremors, and vomiting.

For patients that have experienced or are suspected to have experienced an overdose, consultation with a 24-hour poison center that specializes in providing information specific to veterinary patients is recommended. For general information related to overdose and toxin exposures, as well as contact information for poison control centers, refer to the ***Appendix***.

Drug Interactions

The following drug interactions have either been reported or are theoretical in humans or animals receiving cyclophosphamide and may be of significance in veterinary patients. Unless otherwise noted, use together is not necessarily contraindicated, but weigh the potential risks and perform additional monitoring when appropriate.

- ALLOPURINOL: May increase risk for myelosuppression
- AMIODARONE: Concurrent use may increase risk for pulmonary toxicity.
- AMPHOTERICIN B: Concurrent use may increase risk for renal toxicity.
- AZATHIOPRINE: Concurrent use may increase risk for hepatic toxicity.
- CARDIOTOXIC DRUGS (eg, **cytarabine, doxorubicin**): May cause potentiation of cardiotoxicity
- CYCLOSPORINE: Reduced cyclosporine concentration may result; additive immunosuppressive effect may also occur.
- DIPYRONE: Increased risk for agranulocytosis and pancytopenia
- IMMUNOSUPPRESSIVE AGENTS (eg, **leflunomide, tacrolimus**): May increase immunosuppressive effect
- MYELOSUPPRESSIVE AGENTS (eg, **carboplatin, vincristine**): May increase risk for neutropenia or other hematologic effects
- THIAZIDE DIURETICS (eg, **hydrochlorothiazide**): May result in increased cyclophosphamide exposure and enhanced myelosuppression
- ONDANSETRON: May decrease cyclophosphamide systemic exposure
- PHENOBARBITAL (or other **barbiturates**): When given chronically, may increase the rate of metabolism of cyclophosphamide to active metabolites via microsomal enzyme induction and increase the likelihood of toxicity development
- VACCINES, LIVE: Cyclophosphamide may diminish vaccine efficacy.
- WARFARIN: May result in increased risk for bleeding

Laboratory Considerations

- **Uric acid** concentrations (blood and urine) may be increased after cyclophosphamide use.
- The immunosuppressant properties of cyclophosphamide may cause false negative **intradermal allergy testing** results for a variety of antigens, including tuberculin, *Candida* spp, and *Trichophyton* spp.

Dosages

NOTES:

1. Because of the potential toxicity of this drug to patients, veterinary personnel, and pet owners, and because chemotherapy indications, treatment protocols, monitoring, and safety guidelines often change, the following dosages should be used only as a general guide. Consultation with a veterinary oncologist and referral to current veterinary oncology references[22-26] are strongly recommended.
2. Cyclophosphamide dosages are commonly listed as mg/m^2 (NOT mg/kg). Do not confuse with citations that list dosages in mg/kg.
3. When dosing in cats or very small dogs, or if using low-dose therapy, compounding pharmacies may be able to compound oral dosage forms containing less than 25 mg.
4. All dosages are extra-label.

DOGS:

Antineoplastic agent: Often used as part of a multidrug chemotherapy protocol (eg, COP, CHOP). Based on formation of the active 4-OHCP metabolite, IV and PO routes can be used interchangeably.[7] Dosages vary considerably depending on the protocol used, and cyclophosphamide is most often dosed by body surface area (mg/m^2).

a. Standard: 250 mg/m^2 (NOT mg/kg) once every 3 to 4 weeks,[27] or 50 mg/m^2 (NOT mg/kg) once a day for 3 to 4 days each week[28]
b. Metronomic: Dosages can range from 10 – 15 mg/m^2 (NOT mg/kg) PO once daily.[14,29-32] 25 mg/m^2 (NOT mg/kg) PO every other day was associated with a higher incidence of adverse effects, including sterile hemorrhagic cystitis in 32% of dogs.[15]

CATS:

Antineoplastic agent: cyclophosphamide 10 mg/kg IV or 200 – 250 mg/m^2 (NOT mg/kg) IV or PO has been noted as part of a multi-agent protocol.[33,34]

HORSES:

NOTE: Research in horses found that cyclophosphamide administered at doses of 400 mg/m^2 (NOT mg/kg) (IV) and 600 mg/m^2 (NOT mg/kg) (PO) did not achieve therapeutic concentrations of 4-OHCP at levels proven for the treatment of malignancies in other species.[9] Consultation with a veterinary oncologist is encouraged before use.

Antineoplastic agent:

a) Doses historically used in horses have been 200 mg/m^2 (NOT mg/kg) (usually 1 g per horse per dose) IV every 1 to 2 weeks.[35]
b) **CAP protocol for generalized lymphoma**: cytarabine (cytosine arabinoside) at an average dose of 1 – 1.2 g per horse (total dose; NOT mg/kg) SC or IM once every 1 to 2 weeks;

cyclophosphamide 1 g per horse (total dose; NOT mg/kg) IV every 2 weeks (alternating with cytarabine); and prednisolone 1 mg/kg PO every other day. Vincristine 2.5 mg per horse (total dose; NOT mg/kg) IV is added on the weeks when the cytarabine is administered if there is no response.[35] See the ***Vincristine*** monograph for more information.

c) **Squamous cell carcinoma**: cyclophosphamide 0.15 mg/kg PO once daily was administered with meloxicam 0.1 mg/kg PO once daily after debulking surgery.[36]

RABBITS:

Antineoplastic agent (eg, lymphoma): 50 mg/m^2 (NOT mg/kg) PO daily for 3 days each week or 100 – 200 mg/m^2 (NOT mg/kg) IV (cephalic or saphenous veins) every 7 days. Consider using a fully implantable vascular access device for IV administration of multiple chemotherapy agents.[37]

FERRETS

Antineoplastic agent (eg, lymphoma):

a) 10 mg/kg PO or SC every 3 weeks as part of a multi-agent, modified COP protocol[38]
b) An alternative multi-agent, non-IV protocol used 250 mg/m^2 (NOT mg/kg) PO every 4 to 5 weeks throughout the 26-week treatment course.[38]

Monitoring

- Efficacy: assessment of remission
- Baseline and periodic CBCs with differential counts
- Baseline and periodic renal profile
- Baseline and periodic urinalysis and urine culture if indicated
- Hydration status and urinary output

Client Information

- Cyclophosphamide is a chemotherapy (anticancer) drug. This drug can be hazardous to other animals and people that come in contact with it. On the day your animal receives the drug, and then for a few days afterward, only handle all bodily waste (urine, feces, litter), blood, or vomit while wearing disposable gloves. Seal the waste in a plastic bag, then place the bag and gloves in the regular trash.
- Cyclophosphamide can cause vomiting and gastrointestinal upset. Giving with food may minimize these side effects.
- Contact your veterinarian immediately if your animal has any bleeding, bruising, signs of infection, fever, or blood in the urine.
- After dosing in dogs, frequent walks to encourage urination is suggested to attempt to lessen the risk for bladder toxicity. In the interest of public safety, do not take your animal to a park or allow your animal to urinate and defecate in public places until your veterinarian tells you that it is okay to do so.
- Your veterinarian will need to perform follow-up examinations and blood tests on your animal after it receives this medication. Do not miss these important follow-up visits.
- Do not give your animal any vaccinations while receiving this drug without consulting your veterinarian first.
- Your animal should not participate in animal competitions while on this drug. Exposure to other animals may put your animal at serious risk of infections during chemotherapy treatment. Talk with your veterinarian about when it is safe to return to these events.
- Many dogs receiving chemotherapy will have minor hair coat changes (eg, shagginess, loss of luster). Breeds with continuously growing hair coats (eg, poodles, terriers, Afghan hounds, or old English sheepdogs) are more likely to experience significant hair loss.
- This medication is considered to be a hazardous drug as defined by the National Institute for Occupational Safety and Health (NIOSH). Talk with your veterinarian or pharmacist about the use of personal protective equipment when handling this medicine.

Chemistry/Synonyms

A nitrogen-mustard derivative, cyclophosphamide occurs as a white, crystalline powder that is soluble in water and alcohol. The commercially available injection has a pH of 3 to 7.5.

Cyclophosphamide may also be known as CPM, CTX, CYT, B-518, ciclofosfamida, cyclophosphamidum, cyclophosphanum, NSC-26271, or WR-138719. *Cytoxan*® is a common trade name.

Storage/Stability

Store cyclophosphamide powder for injection at or below 25°C (77°F) and avoid exposure to excessive heat. Cyclophosphamide capsules should be stored between 20°C and 25°C (68°F-77°F); brief excursions between 15°C and 30°C (59°F-86°F) are allowed.

After dilution with sodium chloride 0.9% or 0.45%, use within 24 hours if stored at room temperature or 6 days if refrigerated. When diluting in D_5W or dextrose 5% in sodium chloride 0.9%, the product is stable for 24 hours at room temperature or 36 hours under refrigeration.[21]

Compatibility/Compounding Considerations

Because of the variable potency and stability of compounded cyclophosphamide capsules,[39,40] dosing forms should be obtained from an experienced compounding pharmacist.

Cyclophosphamide power for injection may be dissolved in aromatic elixir to be used as an oral solution. The solution is stable for 14 days if refrigerated in a glass container.[41]

Compatible with multiple IV solutions and drugs, including D_5W, D_5 in sodium chloride 0.9%, lactated Ringer's injection, sodium chloride 0.9% and 0.45%, and total parenteral nutrition containing amino acids 4.25% and dextrose 25%. **Compatible** in syringes or at Y-sites for brief periods with the following drugs: bleomycin sulfate, cefazolin, cisplatin, doxorubicin HCl, droperidol, filgrastim, fluorouracil, furosemide, heparin sodium, hydroxyzine, leucovorin calcium, methotrexate sodium, metoclopramide HCl, mitomycin, ondansetron HCL, vinblastine sulfate, and vincristine sulfate. Compatibility is dependent on factors such as pH, concentration, temperature, and diluent used; consult specialized references or a hospital pharmacist for more specific information.

Dosage Forms/Regulatory Status

VETERINARY-LABELED PRODUCTS: NONE.

HUMAN-LABELED PRODUCTS:

Cyclophosphamide Capsules: 25 mg and 50 mg; generic; (Rx)

Cyclophosphamide Powder for Injection: 500 mg, 1 g, and 2 g vials; *Cytoxan*®, *Neosar*®, generic; (Rx)

References

For the complete list of references, see **wiley.com/go/budde/plumb**

Cyclosporine (Systemic)

Ciclosporin, Cyclosporine A

(**sye**-kloe-spor-een) *Atopica®, Cyclavance®, Neoral®, Sandimmune®*

Immunosuppressive

See also ***Cyclosporine Ophthalmic***

Prescriber Highlights

- FDA-approved products are available for dogs to control atopic dermatitis and for cats to control allergic dermatitis.
- Often used extra-label for treatment of immune-mediated disorders in dogs and cats, and to prevent rejection of kidney transplants in cats
- GI adverse effects (eg, vomiting, soft stools) are common at the start of treatment but typically resolve within a few weeks.
- Use of microemulsion or "modified" formulations is highly recommended. If using human-labeled products, *Sandimmune®* is not bioequivalent to, and must not be interchanged with, *Atopica®, Cyclavance®, Neoral®*, or *Gengraf®*.
- Counseling pet owners to ensure knowledge of the dispensing system is important when using solutions FDA-approved for animals.
- For indications other than atopic dermatitis, consider therapeutic drug monitoring (pharmacokinetic and pharmacodynamic) to assess efficacy and minimize adverse effect potential.
- Many potential drug interactions
- The National Institute for Occupational Safety and Health (NIOSH) classifies cyclosporine as a hazardous drug; personal protective equipment (PPE) should be used accordingly to minimize the risk for exposure.

Uses/Indications

Cyclosporine is FDA-approved for use in dogs for the control of atopic dermatitis. In cats, it is FDA-approved for the control of feline allergic dermatitis as manifested by excoriations (including facial and neck), miliary dermatitis, eosinophilic plaques, and self-induced alopecia. Therapeutic effect for atopic dermatitis may not be seen in the first few weeks of treatment, and the drug is unsuitable for acute flares of atopic dermatitis.[1] Concurrent treatment with corticosteroids[1,2] or oclacitinib[3] can be considered during this interval to control pruritus.

In dogs, extra-label indications include perianal fistulas (anal furunculosis),[4-7] immune-mediated blood disorders (eg, IMHA),[8] inflammatory bowel disease,[9] idiopathic chronic hepatitis, sebaceous adenitis, sterile nodular panniculitis, sterile granuloma/pyogranuloma complex, neutrophilic dermatosis resembling pyoderma gangrenosum, eosinophilic dermatitis with edema (ie, Wells syndrome), neutrophilic dermatitis (ie, Sweet syndrome), alopecia areata, vasculitis, ulcerative dermatoses of the nasal philtrum, dermatomyositis, contact allergy, chronic pedal furunculosis, metatarsal sinus tracts, refractory cases of juvenile sterile granulomatous dermatitis and lymphadenitis (ie, juvenile cellulitis), reactive histiocytic disorders, proliferative otitis externa, idiopathic keratinization disorders (ie, primary seborrhea in springer spaniels, cairn terriers, and West Highland white terriers and follicular hyperkeratosis in cocker spaniels), autoimmune diseases such as pemphigus foliaceus (controversial results), lupus erythematosus complex, meningoencephalitis of unknown etiology (MUE),[10] erythema multiforme, and uveodermatologic syndrome.[11] Ketoconazole may be concurrently prescribed to reduce cyclosporine dose requirements as a cost-saving measure (see ***Drug Interactions***).

In cats, extra-label indications include feline urticaria pigmentosa, chronic stomatitis,[12] feline acquired alopecia (ie, pseudopelade), pemphigus erythematosus and foliaceus,[13] dirty face syndrome in Persian cats,[11] idiopathic pruritus, allograft transplant rejection,[14] pure red cell aplasia,[15] immune-mediated thrombocytopenia,[16,17] and inflammatory bowel disease.[18]

The microemulsion form, or "modified" version, of oral products (ie, *Atopica®, Cyclavance®, Neoral®*) is highly recommended, as it is better absorbed and provides more consistent peak and trough drug concentrations.[19]

Pharmacology/Actions

Cyclosporine, a calcineurin inhibitor, is an immunosuppressive agent that focuses on cell-mediated immune responses, with some humoral immunosuppressive action. Cyclosporine binds to T-cell cyclophilin and blocks calcineurin-mediated T-cell activation. T-helper lymphocytes are the primary target, but T-suppressor cells are also affected. Cyclosporine can also inhibit cytokine production and release (including IL-2 and interferon-gamma in dogs[20-22] and IL-3, IL-4, and tissue necrosis factor-alpha in humans), thereby affecting the function of eosinophils, mast cells, granulocytes, and macrophages. It may also inhibit antigen-presenting functions of the dermal immune system.[23] It is not considered myelosuppressive. One study suggests that cyclosporine therapy does not affect circulating lymphocyte CD4/CD8 ratio.[24] Cyclosporine appears to increase thromboxane production in dogs,[25,26] and low-dose aspirin inhibits this effect.[27]

Pharmacokinetics

Cyclosporine is a substrate for the P-glycoprotein (P-gp) efflux transporter, resulting in a wide range of bioavailability between patients. **NOTE:** *Neoral®, Gengraf®, Atopica®*, and *Cyclavance®* are **NOT** bioequivalent with *Sandimmune®*. In addition, the human microemulsion product (ie, *Neoral®*) has not been proven to be as equally bioavailable as *Atopica®* in dogs; however, a generic veterinary-modified cyclosporine product (ie, *Cyclavance®*) has demonstrated bioequivalence with *Atopica®*.[28]

In dogs, the veterinary-labeled oral product (ie, cyclosporine modified, *Atopica®*) is rapidly absorbed, and bioavailability is 45% in fasted dogs. Food in the GI tract increases variability of bioavailability and reduces it by ≈20%.[29] Protein binding is ≈90%,[23] and volume of distribution is 7.8 L/kg.[30] Cyclosporine is distributed in high concentrations into the liver, fat, and blood cells (granulocytes, 5% to 12%; lymphocytes, 5% to 9%) and significantly accumulates in the skin.[23] It does not appreciably enter the CNS; this may be because it is a P-glycoprotein efflux transporter substrate.[29] The drug is primarily metabolized in the liver via the cytochrome P450 system (likely CYP3A), excreted into the bile, and eliminated in the feces. Less than 1% of a dose is excreted unchanged into the urine. Elimination half-life in dogs has been reported as ≈5 to 12 hours.[31] Clearance has been consistently found to be 3.66 to 7.1 mL/minute/kg.[29] Dogs with diabetes mellitus demonstrate increased clearance and reduced elimination half-life.[32] Pharmacokinetic parameters were not altered when the veterinary-labeled cyclosporine capsules were stored frozen (-20°C [-4°F]) for 28 days.[33]

In cats, oral cyclosporine (modified) bioavailability is ≈25% and is highly variable, but drug absorption is not significantly altered when administered with or without food.[23,34] Additionally, the bioavailability of subcutaneous cyclosporine was reported to be very good in cats.[35] The drug does not appear to be absorbed transdermally.[36] The product label recommends administering on a consistent schedule (ie, with or without food, time of day).[37] Volume of distribution is 3.3 L/kg, time to maximum absorption (T_{max}) is 1 to 2 hours, and maximum concentration (C_{max}) is 480 ng/mL.[23,34] Hepatic and intestinal metabolism (eg, hydroxylation, demethylation) produce inactive metabolites. Elimination half-life in cats is ≈24 hours but varies considerably, with estimates as short as 6.8 hours to more than 40 hours in some healthy cats. Elimination occurs mainly in the feces.

Contraindications/Precautions/Warnings

Cyclosporine is contraindicated in patients that are hypersensitive to it or any component (eg, polyoxyethylated castor oil) in the products. It is contraindicated in animals with malignant disorders or a history of malignant neoplasia and in cats infected with FeLV or FIV. Safe use has not been established in dogs weighing less than 1.8 kg (4 lb); in cats weighing less than 1.4 kg (3 lb); or in dogs or cats less than 6 months of age.[37,38]

This drug should be used with caution in animals with diabetes mellitus or renal insufficiency, as it may cause elevated levels of serum glucose, creatinine, and/or urea nitrogen.[37,38] Cats should test negative for FeLV and FIV before being treated with this drug. Cats on cyclosporine therapy appear to be at risk for developing systemic toxoplasmosis.[39] High cyclosporine blood concentrations (administered doses of 7.5 mg/kg/day orally) may be associated with a higher risk for developing systemic toxoplasmosis.[40] To avoid infection, cats should be kept indoors, not eat raw meat, and not be allowed to hunt during treatment.[41] Ideally, toxoplasma titers should be evaluated prior to starting cyclosporine in cats.[42] Only use cyclosporine in animals with active infection when the benefits outweigh the risks.[23] Use may increase susceptibility to opportunistic bacterial and fungal infections and development of neoplasia.[43,44] Diminished immune response to vaccinations can occur. Killed vaccines are recommended if vaccination is considered in dogs receiving cyclosporine therapy. The drug's impact on the immune response to modified live vaccines is not known.

Cyclosporine is a P-gp substrate. Historically, reports have not shown increased sensitivity to cyclosporine and dose reductions in dogs with the multidrug resistance (*MDR1*) gene mutation (also known as *ABCB1*-1delta) have not been recommended.[45,46] However, there is a case report of one dog receiving a low dose of cyclosporine (3.3 mg/kg PO every 12 hours) who developed a secondary infection. Subsequent pharmacodynamic testing revealed marked immunosuppression and *MDR1* testing showed that the dog was heterozygous for the *MDR1* gene mutation. The *MDR1* mutation was suspected to have contributed to the excessive immunosuppression experienced in this patient.[47] Careful use with clinical and therapeutic drug monitoring is recommended, especially when the patient is not responding to therapy at recommended dosages, or when secondary infections develop at dosages lower than expected to cause significant immunosuppression.

The National Institute for Occupational Safety and Health (NIOSH) classifies cyclosporine as a hazardous drug (nonantineoplastic agent representing an occupational hazard to healthcare workers); personal protective equipment (PPE) should be used accordingly to minimize the risk for exposure.

Do not confuse cycloSPORINE (ciclosporin) with cycloPHOSphamide.[49] In addition, **do not write prescriptions for this drug using the abbreviation SID**. Many human-medicine pharmacists are not aware of this abbreviation and could interpret it as another abbreviation (eg, QID).

NOTE: *Neoral®*, *Gengraf®*, *Atopica*, and *Cyclavance®* are **NOT** bioequivalent with *Sandimmune®*.

Adverse Effects

In dogs, vomiting, anorexia, soft stools, and diarrhea[50] are the most commonly seen adverse effects. Dogs commonly vomit when starting therapy, but this generally abates with time. GI effects rarely require discontinuation of the drug. Giving the drug with a small amount of food or freezing capsules for 30 to 60 minutes before administration have been suggested to alleviate vomiting.[33]

Gingival hyperplasia, altered glucose metabolism/diabetes mellitus,[51] hypertrichosis, excessive shedding, psoriasiform lichenoid-like dermatosis, and papillomatosis have been reported in dogs. Gingival hyperplasia has been treated with oral and toothpaste forms of azithromycin with limited efficacy.[52] Hepatotoxicity or thromboembolic events have been reported but are believed to be rare. One study showed that low-dose aspirin inhibits cyclosporine-induced thromboxane synthesis.[27] One case series of 6 dogs describes the development of *Burkholderia cepacia* complex deep skin infections while receiving oral cyclosporine.[53] Bacteriuria and UTIs may occur.[54]

In one appraisal study, the prevalence of bacterial infections in 828 dogs with atopic dermatitis receiving anti-allergic dosages of oral cyclosporine was 11%, most commonly affecting the cutaneous and urinary systems and not multiple systems.[55] In 95 dogs receiving higher dosages of cyclosporine for other diseases, the prevalence of bacterial infection was 17%, occurring most often in the GI, urinary, and respiratory systems. The prevalence of bacterial infections in atopic dogs treated with cyclosporine appears to be low and occur most often in the skin. However, when given for immunosuppression, the prevalence of bacterial infections appears to be higher and to affect 1 or more body systems.

In cats, GI effects (including vomiting, diarrhea, hypersalivation, decreased appetite, and anorexia) are often reported during the first month of therapy.[56,57] Resulting weight loss may lead to hepatic lipidosis in this species (rare). Lethargy, malaise, behavior changes, increased hair growth, acute bullous keratopathy,[58] gingival hyperplasia, and flares of latent viral infections have also been noted in cats receiving cyclosporine. Hemolytic uremic syndrome has been reported after renal transplant.[59] Cats developing fatal systemic toxoplasmosis while on cyclosporine therapy have been reported.[39,41,60] Anaphylaxis is rare but possible.

Although nephrotoxicity and hepatotoxicity[61] are potential concerns in dogs and cats, extremely high blood cyclosporine concentrations (ie, greater than 3000 ng/mL) must be present before nephrotoxicity is a significant problem.

Because of the drug's immunosuppressive effects, animals may be more susceptible to opportunistic infections (eg, nocardiosis[62], atypical fungal infections[63,64]). Cyclosporine use may predispose dogs and cats to development of neoplastic diseases; however, evidence is lacking. In humans, this risk is increased with long-term use and when administered in combination with other immunosuppressive agents (eg, steroids).[65]

Because the drug has an unpleasant taste, it has been suggested that oral solutions be placed in gelatin capsules or used with water or taste-masking flavoring agents. In one study, *Cyclavance®* oral solution was shown to be significantly more often accepted by dogs, improving dosing compliance, compared with *Atopica®* capsules, when both were mixed with dry food (99.3% vs 27.1%, respectively).[66]

Reproductive/Nursing Safety

Cyclosporine has been shown to be fetotoxic and embryotoxic in rats and rabbits at doses 2 to 5 times the recommended dose.[65] Reduced fetal weight and growth, skeletal retardation, and premature birth have occurred. The manufacturer does not recommend use in pregnant or breeding dogs or cats. Use during pregnancy only when the risks outweigh the benefits.

Cyclosporine is distributed into maternal milk; the manufacturer does not recommend use in lactating queens or bitches.

Because safety has not been established in animals, this drug should only be used when the maternal benefits outweigh the potential risks to offspring.

Overdose/Acute Toxicity

Oral LD_{50} in rabbits is greater than 320 mg/kg.[65] Single oral doses of 33 mg/kg in dogs and 40 mg/kg in cats have resulted in no clinical signs. Acute overdoses may cause adverse GI effects as well as transient renal or hepatotoxicity. Acute kidney injury requiring hemodialysis and increased liver enzymes was reported in a dog that accidentally received a single 33 mg/kg IV dose.[61] Clinical signs in cats given 40 mg/kg for up to 6 months were extensions of adverse effects. Overdoses may be treated with gastric decontamination (induction of emesis is apparently effective in humans if done within 2 hours of ingestion); treat supportively and according to clinical signs.

For patients that have experienced or are suspected to have experienced an overdose, consultation with a 24-hour poison consultation center specializing in providing veterinary-specific information is recommended. For general information related to overdose and toxin exposures, as well as contact information for poison control centers, refer to ***Appendix***.

Drug Interactions

The following drug interactions have either been reported or are theoretical in humans or animals receiving cyclosporine and may be of significance in veterinary patients. Unless otherwise noted, use together is not necessarily contraindicated, but weigh the potential risks and perform additional monitoring when appropriate. Cyclosporine is a CYP450 and P-glycoprotein substrate and its metabolism can be affected by inhibitors, inducers, and other substrates.

The following drugs may **increase** cyclosporine blood levels and the risk for cyclosporine toxicity:

- **Acetazolamide**
- **Allopurinol**
- **Amiodarone**
- **Amphotericin B Liposome/Lipid complex**
- **Angiotensin Receptor Blockers** (ARBs; eg, **telmisartan, valsartan**)
- **Azole Antifungals** (eg, **fluconazole, itraconazole, ketoconazole**): Ketoconazole significantly increases cyclosporine blood concentration in dogs[67,68]; fluconazole has demonstrated variable effects.[69,70] Itraconazole appears to affect cyclosporine pharmacokinetics in cats[71] but not in dogs. Many clinicians concurrently use ketoconazole in dogs to reduce the dose and resultant cost of cyclosporine treatment, particularly for large dogs. Only use a combination of ketoconazole and cyclosporine with caution and understand that monitoring of cyclosporine levels may be required. Of note, one study found an increase in cyclosporine concentrations up to 75% following a dose of ketoconazole.
- **Bromocriptine**
- **Calcium Channel Blockers** (eg, **amlodipine, diltiazem, verapamil**)
- **Carvedilol**
- **Ceftriaxone**
- **Chloramphenicol**
- **Cimetidine:** May delay absorption but was not found to significantly alter maximum concentrations (C_{max})[72]
- **Cisapride**
- **Clonidine**
- **Colchicine:** Colchicine levels may also increase. This combination is contraindicated in human patients with renal impairment.
- **Corticosteroids:** Methylprednisolone does not appear to affect cyclosporine levels in dogs.
- **Danazol**
- **Digoxin**
- **Estrogens**
- **Fatty Acids (Essential/Omega)**: Fatty acid supplementation may provide a cyclosporine-sparing effect.[73]
- **Fluoroquinolones** (eg, **ciprofloxacin, enrofloxacin, marbofloxacin, orbifloxacin, pradofloxacin**)
- **Fluvoxamine**
- **Glipizide, Glyburide**
- **Grapefruit Juice, Grapefruit Juice Powder**[74]
- **Imipenem**
- **Macrolide Antibiotics** (eg, **azithromycin, clarithromycin,**[75,76] **erythromycin**)
- **Medroxyprogesterone**
- **Metoclopramide:** A study in dogs demonstrated that metoclopramide did not significantly alter cyclosporine pharmacokinetics.[74]
- **Metronidazole**
- **Omeprazole**
- **Sertraline**

The following drugs may **decrease** the blood levels of cyclosporine:

- **Azathioprine**
- **Carbamazepine**
- **Clindamycin:** Clindamycin may decrease cyclosporine bioavailability; however, this interaction does not appear to occur in dogs.
- **Cyclophosphamide**
- **Famotidine**
- **Griseofulvin**
- **Mitotane**
- **Octreotide**
- **Phenobarbital**[77]
- **Rifampin**
- **St. John's Wort:** This interaction appears to be of significance in dogs.[78]
- **Sulfadiazine/Sulfamethoxazole**
- **Sulfasalazine**
- **Terbinafine**
- **Trimethoprim**: May also increase the risk for nephrotoxicity
- **Warfarin**: May also reduce efficacy of warfarin

Additional interactions:

- **ACE Inhibitors** (eg, **benazepril, enalapril**): There have been case reports in humans in which renal function declined.
- **Alprazolam:** Concurrent use may decrease alprazolam bioavailability and pharmacodynamics effects.
- **Darbepoetin:** May cause additive increases in blood pressure. Additionally, may alter cyclosporine blood concentrations, as cyclosporine is bound by red blood cells
- **Digoxin:** Cyclosporine may increase digoxin levels with possible toxicity.
- **Doxorubicin:** Cyclosporine can increase doxorubicin and doxorubicinol (active metabolite) levels.
- **Fentanyl:** Concurrent use may increase the risk for fentanyl toxicity.
- **Furosemide:** Concurrent use may increase the risk for gouty arthritis in humans.
- **Hydrochlorothiazide:** Concurrent use may increase the risk for hyperuricemia.
- **Immunosuppressive Agents** (eg, **azathioprine, corticosteroids**): May increase the risk for infection or malignancy
- **Ivermectin:** Cyclosporine may inhibit P-gp (MDR1) transporter and increase ivermectin concentrations.[23,34]
- **Leflunomide:** Increased risk for leflunomide-induced adverse hematologic effects
- **Melphalan:** Increased risk for renal injury
- **Methotrexate (MTX)**: Cyclosporine may increase MTX concentrations.

- **Midazolam**: Concurrent use may decrease midazolam clearance and increase midazolam plasma concentrations.
- **Morphine**: Combination may increase morphine exposure.
- **Mycophenolate**: Concurrent use may reduce levels of mycophenolate.
- **Nephrotoxic Drugs, Other** (eg, **acyclovir, aminoglycosides, amphotericin B, colchicine, NSAIDs, trimethoprim, vancomycin**): Possible additive nephrotoxicity; avoid combination
- **Oclacitinib:** Although concurrent administration of oclacitinib and cyclosporine appears safe when administered for up to 3 weeks,[3] the combination of cyclosporine and oclacitinib is relatively contraindicated for long-term use, especially in cases in which infection is present, because of the theoretical increased risk for immunosuppression.[1]
- **Omeprazole:** Concurrent use may result in altered cyclosporine concentrations.
- **Potassium Supplements:** Increased risk for hyperkalemia
- **Spironolactone** and other **Potassium-Sparing Diuretics** (eg, **triamterene**): Increased risk for hyperkalemia
- **Vaccinations**: Vaccine response may be delayed or reduced in patients receiving cyclosporine[79]; avoid use of modified live vaccines.
- **Vincristine:** Concurrent use may increase vincristine plasma concentrations.

Laboratory considerations

- **Intradermal allergy testing (IDT):** Drug withdrawal may be recommended for at least 4 weeks prior to intradermal testing if cyclosporine has been administered for longer than 30 days.[80]

Dosages

NOTE: Dosages are for cyclosporine (modified), *Atopica*®, *Cyclavance*®, *Neoral*®, or equivalent; these dosages are not interchangeable with *Sandimmune*® (or equivalent) dosages.

DOGS:

Control of atopic dermatitis:

a) **Label dosage; FDA-approved**: 5 mg/kg (3.3 – 6.7 mg/kg) PO once daily for 30 days in dogs weighing at least 1.8 kg (3.9 lb). Following this initial treatment period, dose may be tapered to every other day, then twice per week until a minimum frequency that will maintain the desired therapeutic effect is reached. Give at least 1 hour before, or 2 hours after, meals.[38] It may take 4 to 6 weeks to observe the full benefits. To reduce the incidence of vomiting in dogs when starting therapy, some clinicians will start at a low dose, give with food, and gradually increase oral doses over the first week or so. In one small study[81], 12 of 21 dogs (57%) were able to be maintained on every-other-day or twice-weekly cyclosporine administration.

b) **Concurrent administration with ketoconazole** (extra-label): In larger dogs, cyclosporine 2.5 – 3 mg/kg PO once daily with ketoconazole 2.5 – 5 mg/kg PO once daily is effective and may reduce cost.[68] Ideally, cyclosporine should be given on an empty stomach, but if it causes GI upset, giving with food may help. One study found similar cyclosporine levels in dogs treated with either cyclosporine (alone) 5 mg/kg PO once daily or cyclosporine 2.5 mg/kg PO once daily with ketoconazole 2.5 mg/kg PO once daily.[67] After control of pruritus is achieved, the cyclosporine dose can gradually be reduced to the lowest effective dose (eg, daily, then switch to giving every second or third day). For less than daily administration (eg, every 48 hours), give ketoconazole only on the days cyclosporine is administered.

Perianal fistulas (Anal furunculosis) (extra-label): Many dosages have been found to be effective. When used alone, cyclosporine 4 – 7.5 mg/kg PO twice daily. Alternatively, cyclosporine 1 – 4 mg/kg PO twice daily with ketoconazole 5 mg/kg PO once daily. After condition is controlled, increase the administration interval to the lowest frequency that controls clinical signs.[4–7]

Immune-mediated hemolytic anemia (extra-label): 5 mg/kg PO every 12 hours as adjunctive treatment to corticosteroids[8]

Sebaceous adenitis,[82] sterile nodular panniculitis, neutrophilic dermatoses resembling pyoderma gangrenosum, alopecia areata, chronic pedal furunculosis, metatarsal sinus tracts, cutaneous histiocytosis, dermatomyositis, proliferative chronic otitis, idiopathic keratinization disorders (extra-label): 5 mg/kg PO once daily. After condition is controlled, increase the administration interval to the lowest frequency that controls clinical signs.

Pemphigus foliaceus, refractory cases (extra-label): Variable results have been reported. Higher doses such as cyclosporine 15 mg/kg PO once daily or cyclosporine 5 – 10 mg/kg PO once daily combined with ketoconazole 5 – 10 mg/kg PO once daily may be helpful.[83]

Discoid lupus erythematosus, vesicular cutaneous lupus erythematosus (extra-label): 5 mg/kg PO once daily

Exfoliative cutaneous lupus erythematosus (extra-label): Cyclosporine 2.5 – 10 mg/kg PO once daily with or without ketoconazole 5 – 7 mg/kg PO once daily

Steroid-refractory inflammatory bowel disease (extra-label): Cyclosporine 5 mg/kg PO once daily demonstrated an improvement in clinical signs in 12 out of 14 dogs.[9] Some clinicians advocate for giving cyclosporine as a divided dose given twice daily for treatment of inflammatory bowel disease.

Idiopathic chronic hepatitis (extra-label): Median dose is 8 mg/kg PO daily, with a range of 2.5 – 12.7 mg/kg/day. Median time to biochemical remission (ie, ALT, less than 1.1 times the upper limit of normal) was 2.5 months. Concurrent hepatoprotectant treatment was not associated with increased likelihood of remission.[84]

Juvenile sterile granulomatous dermatitis and lymphadenitis (juvenile cellulitis), refractory cases (extra-label): 10 mg/kg PO once daily

Immunosuppressant for renal transplant (extra-label): Empirical dosages generally range from 3 – 6 mg/kg PO twice daily or 5 – 7.5 mg/kg once daily. Ketoconazole or grapefruit juice powder have been used to lower cyclosporine dose requirements. To reduce transplant rejection, 10 – 15 mg/kg PO twice daily[85,86] is generally used and therapeutic drug monitoring (blood cyclosporine concentrations) or pharmacodynamic monitoring can be used to assess adequacy of therapy.

Meningoencephalitis of unknown etiology/origin (MUE/MUO; extra-label): 3 – 15 mg/kg PO every 12 hours.[87] A reasonable starting dosage is 5 mg/kg PO every 12 hours.[10]

Primary immune-mediated polyarthritis (IMPA) (extra label): Cyclosporine 5 mg/kg PO every 12 hours with carprofen 2.2 mg/kg PO every 12 hours for 7 days for analgesia was shown in one study to be an effective alternative to prednisone.[88]

Myasthenia gravis: 4 mg/kg PO every 12 hours demonstrated improved clinical signs of 2 dogs in a case report

CATS:

Allergic dermatitis as manifested by excoriations (including facial and neck), miliary dermatitis, eosinophilic plaques, and self-induced alopecia (label dosage; FDA-approved): Initially, 7 mg/kg PO once daily for a minimum of 4 to 6 weeks or until resolution of clinical signs. Following this initial daily treatment period, the dosage may be tapered by decreasing administration to every other day or twice weekly to maintain the desired therapeutic effect. The lowest effective dosing frequency should be used. Administer directly on a small amount of food or orally just after feeding. When possible, administer on a consistent schedule with regard to meals and time of day. If a dose is missed, the next dose should be administered (without doubling) as soon as possible, but administration should be no more frequent than once daily.[37] **NOTE:** In studies,[89,90] ≈75% of cats receiving daily cyclosporine were able to undergo dose reduction. Of those cats, ≈60% were able to be maintained on twice-weekly administration and 15% were maintained on every-other-day administration for the 8-week study period.

Allergic dermatitis (extra-label): 2.5 – 5.0 mg/kg SC once daily to every other day seemed to be an effective alternative therapy for cats that cannot be treated orally.[35]

Pemphigus complex (extra-label): 5 mg/kg PO every 24 hours either alone or in combination with a glucocorticoid[13]

Sebaceous adenitis, idiopathic granulomatous folliculitis and furunculosis (extra-label): 5 mg/kg PO once daily[91]

Immunosuppressant (usually as part of an immunosuppressive protocol) (extra-label): 3 – 4 mg/kg PO every 12 hours or 5 – 7 mg/kg PO once daily. To reduce transplant rejection, twice-daily administration with prednisolone 0.125 – 0.25 mg/kg PO every 12 hours is generally used; therapeutic drug monitoring is recommended. See ***Monitoring***.

Alternative to glucocorticoid therapy for feline asthma (extra-label): 4 mg/kg PO every 12 hours was reported in one case as effective for treatment of feline asthma.[92]

Chronic stomatitis (extra-label): 2.5 mg/kg PO twice daily[12]

Pure red cell aplasia (extra-label): 5 – 10 mg/kg/day PO, although a dosage up to 20 mg/kg/day was noted[15]

Thrombocytopenia purpura (extra-label): 5 mg/kg PO every 12 hours with prednisone 2 mg/kg PO every 12 hours, from a case report[17]

Monitoring

- Therapeutic efficacy
- Adverse effects
- Consider therapeutic drug monitoring (pharmacokinetic and pharmacodynamic) to assess effectiveness of therapy, particularly when response is poor or when adverse effects occur. Therapeutic drug monitoring can also be considered when changing brands or manufacturers, especially if response to therapy changes in the individual patient. Cyclosporine blood concentrations are not typically monitored when treating atopic dermatitis[93] or inflammatory bowel disease[9] because the blood concentrations were found to not correlate with clinical efficacy, but this may be warranted in some cases.[50]
  a) Pharmacokinetic monitoring (or measurement of blood concentrations) should ideally occur no sooner than 60 hours after starting therapy and whole blood (not plasma) should be tested, as cyclosporine concentrates in blood cells.[19] When monitoring blood drug concentrations, therapeutic trough whole-blood concentrations (12 hours after last dose) have been suggested to be between 300 and 500 ng/mL for transplantation and life-threatening disease but may not reliably predict clinical response for immunosuppression.[94] Because different methodologies may yield different results and different conditions are managed with a range of cyclosporine blood concentrations, it is recommended to contact a laboratory for current recommendations.
  b) Pharmacodynamic monitoring can also be used in dogs receiving cyclosporine therapy to provide information on dosing for individual animals. This test is offered to clinicians as a PCR-based assay, with samples being submitted after 1 week of starting or changing therapy.[95,96] When using pharmacodynamic monitoring in dogs, a single peak sample (2 hours post-administration) is recommended for dogs receiving twice-daily administration, whereas both peak and trough (just before the next dose) samples are recommended in dogs receiving once daily therapy.
- Baseline CBC; repeat as clinically relevant (eg, signs of infection)
- Baseline serum chemistry profile, then monthly to every 3 to 6 months has been suggested for most conditions. For treatment of IMHA in dogs, recommendations are to evaluate relevant biochemical variables every 2 to 3 months owing to the risk for hepatotoxicity in a small proportion of dogs.[8]
- Urinalysis and urine culture should also be monitored due to potential risks for UTIs.[54]
- Blood glucose in diabetic patients
- Body weight: Persistent, progressive weight loss that resulted in hepatic lipidosis was reported during field studies in 2 out of 205 cats.

Client Information

- For this medication to work, give it exactly as your veterinarian has prescribed. It is a good idea to always check the prescription label to be sure you are giving the medicine correctly.
- Preferably, dogs should receive the medicine on an empty stomach (at least 1 hour before or 2 hours after a meal). If the dog vomits after receiving the drug, try giving the medication frozen or with a small amount of food. Freezing capsules for 30 to 60 minutes before administration can also be tried.
- Cats can be given the medication with or without food; make sure to give it the same way each day. If giving with food, first mix the medication into a small portion of food to ensure the entire dose is consumed, then offer the remaining food.
- For many conditions, if a dose is missed, the next dose should be given as soon as possible and then the usual schedule should be restarted. For serious conditions (eg, kidney transplant), contact your veterinarian if a dose is missed.
- Vomiting, decreased appetite, soft stools, and diarrhea are the most common side effects. These signs usually get better on their own, but if they worsen or continue, contact your veterinarian.
- Capsules should be stored in their original container until administration.
- Capsules should not be broken or opened.
- If using the oral liquid, do not rinse or clean the syringe between doses.
- It is recommended that you wear gloves when giving capsules or oral solutions to your animal. Wash your hands thoroughly after handling.
- Depending on the condition being treated, it may take up to 4 to 6 weeks to see an improvement in your animal's condition.
- Watch for signs of infection (eg, low energy level, poor appetite) and/or persistent, progressive weight loss; if seen, contact your veterinarian immediately.
- If your animal is taking cyclosporine for immunosuppression, your veterinarian may need to perform blood tests to evaluate how well this medicine is working. Do not miss these important follow-up visits.
- This medication is considered to be a hazardous drug as defined by the National Institute for Occupational Safety and Health (NIOSH). Talk with your veterinarian or pharmacist about the use of personal protective equipment when handling this medicine.

- Cats receiving cyclosporine should be kept indoors and not allowed to hunt or eat raw meat due to the risk for developing an infection called toxoplasmosis.

Chemistry/Synonyms

Cyclosporine (ie, cyclosporin A, ciclosporin, cyclosporin) is a naturally produced immunosuppressant agent. It is a nonpolar, cyclic, polypeptide antibiotic that consists of 11 amino acids and it occurs as a white, fine crystalline powder. It is relatively insoluble in water but generally soluble in organic solvents and oils. Molecular weight is 1202.61.

Because of the difficulties surrounding absorption, many different formulations have been approved over the years. Initial formulations included a vegetable-oil base (ie, *Sandimmune®*), but marked differences in bioavailability led to the approval of a human microemulsion formulation (ie, *Neoral®*) and a veterinary product (ie, *Atopica®*) with better bioavailability as compared with the parent product.[31] Because of the wide differences in formulation, and therefore pharmacokinetics, it is recommended that only the veterinary product (ie, *Atopica®*) be used for veterinary patients.

Cyclosporine is commercially available in several dosage forms, including oral solutions, capsules, and a concentrate for injection. To increase oral absorption, a microemulsion-forming preparation (ie, *Neoral®*) is also available as capsules and an oral liquid. The veterinary products (ie, *Atopica®* and *Cyclavance®*) are microemulsion products equivalent to *Neoral®*. All oral formulations contain ethanol ≈10% to 13% and the injection contains ≈33% ethanol.

Cyclosporine may also be known as ciclosporin, 27-400, ciclosporinum, cyclosporine A, OL-27-400, *Atopica®*, *Cyclavance®*, *Gengraf®*, *Neoral®*, *Sandimmune®*, or *Sigmasporin®*.

Storage/Stability

The veterinary capsules (ie, *Atopica®*) should be stored and dispensed in the original unit-dose container at controlled room temperature (15°C-25°C [59°F-77°F]). One study reported that capsules are stable in the freezer for 28 days.[33] The veterinary oral solutions are labeled to only be dispensed in the original container and stored at controlled room temperature between 15°C to 30°C (59°F-86°F); do not refrigerate. After the container is opened, use contents within 2 months to 12 weeks. Refer to specific product labels for further information.

The human oral liquid and capsules for emulsion (ie, *Neoral®*, *Gengraf®*) should be stored in their original containers at 20°C to 25°C (68°F-77°F). Temperatures below 20°C (68°F) may cause the solution to gel or flocculate. Rewarming to 25°C (77°F) can reverse this process without harm.

The oral liquid and oral capsules (ie, *Sandimmune®*) should be stored in their original containers at temperatures less than 30°C (86°F); protect from freezing and do not refrigerate. After opening the oral liquid, use within 2 months.

Compatibility/Compounding Considerations

Compatibility is dependent on factors such as pH, concentration, temperature, and diluent used; consult specialized references or a hospital pharmacist for more specific information.

Cyclosporine for injection is compatible with lactated Ringer's, sodium chloride 0.9%, and dextrose 5% IV solutions. It is reportedly **Y-site compatible** with amikacin, atropine, buprenorphine, butorphanol, calcium salts, cefazolin, dexamethasone sodium succinate, dexmedetomidine, diphenhydramine, dobutamine, dopamine, doxycycline, epinephrine, erythromycin, famotidine, fentanyl, fluconazole, furosemide, heparin, lidocaine, methadone, methylprednisolone sodium succinate, metoclopramide, metronidazole, morphine, penicillin G, piperacillin/tazobactam, potassium salts, propofol, sodium bicarbonate, vasopressin, and zoledronic acid.

It is **Y-site incompatible** with amphotericin B (lipid-based), ampicillin, cyanocobalamin, diazepam, insulin (regular), ketamine, magnesium sulfate, phenobarbital, sulfamethoxazole/trimethoprim, and voriconazole.

Human preparations of cyclosporine solutions may adhere to plastic and therefore should not be mixed in a plastic cup or with plastic utensils.[65]

Because there are approved oral dosage forms for both dogs and cats, routine compounding for use in these species is discouraged. A study[97] found some compounded cyclosporine solutions deviated by more than 10% from the labeled concentration.

Dosage Forms/Regulatory Status

VETERINARY-LABELED PRODUCTS:

Cyclosporine (Modified) Capsules: 10 mg, 25 mg, 50 mg, and 100 mg; *Atopica®*; (Rx). FDA-approved for use in dogs. NADA #141-218

Cyclosporine (Modified) Oral Solution: 100 mg/mL in 5 mL, 15 mL, 30 mL, and 50 mL vials; *Cyclavance®*; (Rx). FDA-approved for use in dogs. ANADA #200-689

Cyclosporine (Modified) Oral Solution: 100 mg/mL in 5 mL and 17 mL bottles; *Atopica®* for Cats; (Rx). FDA-approved for use in cats. NADA #141-329

HUMAN-LABELED PRODUCTS:

Cyclosporine Modified (Microemulsion) Oral Capsules (Soft-gelatin): 25 and 100 mg; *Neoral®*, *Gengraf®*, generic; (Rx). These products may be bioequivalent with, and *Neoral®* contains the same formulation as, the veterinary-approved product (ie, *Atopica®*).

Cyclosporine Modified Oral Solution (Microemulsion): 100 mg/mL in 50 mL bottles; *Neoral®*, generic; (Rx). This product may be bioequivalent with, and contains the same formulation as, the veterinary-approved product (ie, *Atopica® for Cats*).

Cyclosporine Oral Solution: 100 mg/mL in 50 mL bottles with syringe; *Sandimmune®*; (Rx). This product is <u>*not* bioequivalent</u> with the veterinary-approved product (ie, *Atopica® for Cats*).

Cyclosporine Oral Capsules (Soft gelatin): 25 and 100 mg; *Sandimmune®*; generic; (Rx). These products are <u>*not* bioequivalent</u> with veterinary-approved products (ie, *Atopica®*).

Cyclosporine Concentrated Solution for Injection: 50 mg/mL in 5 mL single-use amps; *Sandimmune®*, generic; (Rx)

References

For the complete list of references, see **wiley.com/go/budde/plumb**

Cyproheptadine

(sip-roe-***hep***-ta-deen) *Periactin®*

First-Generation Antihistamine

Prescriber Highlights

- ▶ Serotonin antagonist antihistamine that can be useful in the management of serotonin-syndrome in small animals and has been used as an appetite stimulant in cats. Limited or no efficacy as an antipruritic/antihistamine in dogs and cats or for asthma in cats
- ▶ In horses, used for photic head shaking and treatment of pituitary pars intermedia dysfunction (PPID).
- ▶ Use with caution in animals with urinary or GI obstruction, severe CHF, or angle-closure glaucoma
- ▶ Adverse effects include CNS depression (cats may demonstrate paradoxical hyperexcitability) and anticholinergic effects.

Uses/Indications

Cyproheptadine may be useful in cats as an appetite stimulant,[1,2] but it is not recommended in the management of hepatic lipidosis.[3,4] It may be useful for urine spraying in male cats.[5] Cyproheptadine use in cats as monotherapy for eosinophilic airway inflammation[6] and asthma[7] is not effective.

Cyproheptadine is indicated for the treatment of histamine-mediated pruritic and allergic skin conditions, including urticaria and insect-bite hypersensitivity in dogs and cats; however, its efficacy for pruritic and allergic diseases is questionable in dogs. In one double-blind, placebo-controlled study, there was no improvement of pruritus in 16 of 16 allergic dogs that were treated with cyproheptadine 0.1 mg/kg PO every 24 hours.[8] Guidelines for atopic dermatitis treatment in dogs indicate that antihistamines have modest efficacy in controlling pruritus associated with atopic dermatitis; for optimal efficacy, cyproheptadine should be given continuously (ie, daily) as preventive therapy. Cyproheptadine is of limited benefit in the management of acute flares.[9]

Historically the drug has been used as adjunctive therapy for canine hyperadrenocorticism. However, one study demonstrated lack of efficacy of cyproheptadine in dogs treated for pituitary dependent hyperadrenocorticism,[10] and more effective medications (eg, trilostane, mitotane) are now available.

Cyproheptadine may be useful as adjunctive treatment in dogs[11,12] or cats[13] with serotonin syndrome or to reduce dysphoria (vocalization, disorientation) associated with baclofen, carisoprodol, selective serotonin reuptake inhibitors (SSRIs), or tricyclic antidepressants (TCAs).

In horses, cyproheptadine has been used for treating photic headshaking[14] and as adjunctive therapy for pituitary pars intermedia dysfunction (PPID) when sole therapy with pergolide fails to control signs. [15]

Pharmacology/Actions

Similar to other H_1-receptor antihistamines, cyproheptadine acts by competing with histamine for H_1-receptor sites on effector cells. Antihistamines do not block histamine release but can antagonize its effects. Cyproheptadine also possesses potent antiserotonin activity, in addition to anticholinergic and calcium channel blocking actions.[16]

Pharmacokinetics

Available data are limited. Cyproheptadine is well absorbed after oral administration; however, its distribution characteristics are not well-described. Cyproheptadine may be almost completely metabolized in the liver, and the metabolites are excreted in the urine; in humans, elimination is reduced in chronic kidney disease.[17] Elimination half-life in cats averages about 13 hours,[18] but there is wide interanimal variability.

Contraindications/Precautions/Warnings

Cyproheptadine is contraindicated in patients hypersensitive to it. In humans, the manufacturer states the drug is contraindicated in newborn or premature infants, and should be used with caution in patients with prostatic hypertrophy, hyperthyroidism, bladder neck obstruction, severe cardiac disease, hypertension, epilepsy, angle-closure glaucoma or increased intraocular pressure, or pyloroduodenal obstruction.[17]

Cyproheptadine increased seizure severity, reduced seizure threshold, and decreased anticonvulsant efficacy in animal models of convulsions.[19]

Adverse Effects

The most likely adverse effects seen with cyproheptadine use in veterinary patients are related to its CNS depressant (eg, sedation) and anticholinergic effects (eg, dry mucous membranes, decreased GI motility, hyperthermia, tachycardia, urine retention).

Polyphagia may be an unwanted effect in dogs[8] and cats[20] when this drug is used for indications other than as an appetite stimulant. A paradoxical agitated state can develop in cats, which resolves with dose reduction or drug discontinuation.

Reproductive/Nursing Safety

Cyproheptadine has been tested in pregnant lab animals in doses up to 32 times higher than the labeled dose without evidence of harm to fetuses. Nevertheless, because safety has not been established in other species, its use during pregnancy should be weighed carefully.

It is not known whether cyproheptadine is distributed into milk. In humans, the drug is contraindicated in nursing mothers because of potential for toxicity in newborns and infants.[17] Because safety has not been established in animals, this drug should only be used when the maternal benefits outweigh the potential risks to offspring.

Overdose/Acute Toxicity

The oral LD_{50} in the rat is 295 mg/kg orally.[17] There are no specific antidotes available. Treat significant overdoses using standard GI decontamination protocols when appropriate and supportive therapy when required. The adverse effects seen with overdoses are an extension of the drug's adverse effects, principally CNS depression (although CNS stimulation may be seen), anticholinergic effects (eg, dry mucous membranes, tachycardia, urinary retention, hyperthermia) and possibly hypotension. Physostigmine may be considered for serious CNS anticholinergic effects; benzodiazepines may be used to treat seizures, if necessary.

For patients that have experienced or are suspected to have experienced an overdose, consultation with a 24-hour poison consultation center specializing in providing veterinary-specific information is recommended. For general information related to overdose and toxin exposures, as well as contact information for poison control centers, refer to ***Appendix***.

Drug Interactions

The following drug interactions have either been reported or are theoretical in humans or animals receiving cyproheptadine and may be of significance in veterinary patients. Unless otherwise noted, use together is not necessarily contraindicated but weigh the potential risks and perform additional monitoring when appropriate.

- Anticholinergic Agents (eg, **amantadine, atropine, glycopyrrolate, oxybutynin**): May have additive anticholinergic effects
- Cholinergic Agonists (eg, **pilocarpine**): Decreased efficacy of cyproheptadine
- CNS Depressant Agents (eg, **acepromazine, anesthetic agents [inhalant, injectable], cannabidiol, diazepam, gabapentin, methocarbamol, phenobarbital**): May increase CNS depression
- Monoamine Oxidase Inhibitors (MAOIs; eg, **amitraz, selegiline**): Prolonged and intensified anticholinergic effects. Combination is considered contraindicated in humans.
- Mirtazapine: Concurrent cyproheptadine and mirtazapine use should be avoided due to antagonistic mechanisms of action.[2]
- Opioids (eg, **buprenorphine, morphine**): May increase anticholinergic and/or CNS depressant effects
- Selective Serotonin Reuptake Inhibitors (eg, **fluoxetine, paroxetine, sertraline**): Cyproheptadine may decrease efficacy.
- Tricyclic Antidepressants (TCAs; eg, **clomipramine, amitriptyline**): Cyproheptadine may decrease TCA efficacy.
- Tramadol: Cyproheptadine may decrease tramadol efficacy.

Laboratory Considerations

- It is recommended that antihistamines be discontinued at least 7 days prior to **intradermal allergy testing (IDT)**.[21]
- Cyproheptadine may increase amylase and prolactin serum levels

when administered with **thyrotropin-releasing hormone**.

- Cyproheptadine can decrease **TSH** secretion.
- Cyproheptadine may cause a false-positive **tricyclic antidepressant** screen.

Dosages

DOGS:

Appetite stimulant (extra-label): 0.2 mg/kg PO every 12 hours; may be dosed less frequently if inappetence is mild.

Adjunctive treatment of dysphoria associated with serotonin syndrome and toxicoses (eg, SSRIs, TCAs, amphetamines, baclofen; extra-label): 1.1 mg/kg PO; doses may be repeated every 1 to 6 hours as needed until signs have resolved.[11,12] In cases where PO dosing is not possible (eg, severe vomiting), crush tablets, mix with saline, and administer rectally.[22]

Antihistamine (extra-label): 0.5 – 2 mg/kg PO every 12 hours; there is little evidence that higher dosages improve efficacy.

CATS:

Appetite stimulant (extra-label): 1 – 4 mg/cat (NOT mg/kg) PO every 12 to 24 hours; alternatively, 0.2 – 1 mg/kg PO every 12 hours.[1,2] Most cats require twice-daily dosing and it may take 3 days to see effect. Before starting treatment, adequate antiemetic and/or analgesic therapy is necessary. Taper drug when discontinuing to prevent rebound anorexia.

Antihistamine (extra-label): 2 – 4 mg/cat (NOT mg/kg) PO every 12 hours.[20] Efficacy was noted within 3 to 10 days of initiating therapy.

Adjunctive treatment of serotonin syndrome (extra-label): 2 – 4 mg/cat (NOT mg/kg) PO; additional doses may be repeated every 4 to 6 hours as needed until clinical signs related to serotonin syndrome have resolved. In cases where PO dosing is not possible (eg, severe vomiting), crush tablets, mix with saline, and administer rectally.[22]

HORSES:

Photic head shaking (extra-label): 0.3 – 0.6 mg/kg PO every 12 hours[14]

Adjunctive therapy for refractory pituitary pars intermedia dysfunction (PPID) (extra-label): Cyproheptadine 0.25 mg/kg PO once to twice daily given concurrently with pergolide[15,23]; may require 4 to 8 weeks to determine efficacy. See ***Pergolide***.

Monitoring

- Appetite
- Body weight
- Adverse effects (eg, CNS depression, anticholinergic effects [eg, dry mucous membranes, tachycardia, urine retention])

Client Information

- Cyproheptadine is an antihistamine that can also be used as an appetite stimulant or as a treatment for certain toxicities.
- Antihistamines should be used on a regular, ongoing basis in animals that respond to them. They work better if used before exposure to an allergen (eg, pollens).
- May be given with or without food. If your animal vomits or acts sick after receiving the drug on an empty stomach, try giving the next dose with food or a small treat. If vomiting continues, contact your veterinarian.
- May cause drowsiness (sleepiness); this effect may lessen with time.
- Cats can become overly excited when receiving this medication.

Chemistry/Synonyms

An antihistamine that also possesses serotonin antagonist properties, cyproheptadine HCl occurs as a white to slightly yellow crystalline powder. Approximately 3.64 mg are soluble in 1 mL of water and 28.6 mg in 1 mL of methanol.

Cyproheptadine HCl may also be known as cyproheptadini hydrochloridum, *Ciplactin®*, *Cyheptine®*, *Cyprogin®*, *Cyprono®*, *Cyprosian®*, *Klarivitina®*, *Nuran®*, *Periactine®*, *Periactinol®*, *Periatin®*, *Peritol®*, *Polytab®*, *Practin®*, *Preptin®*, *Supersan®*, or *Trimetabol®*.

Storage/Stability

Store cyproheptadine HCl tablets and oral solution at room temperature 20° to 25°C (68°F-77°F). Avoid freezing oral syrup (solution).

Compatibility/Compounding Considerations

No specific information noted

Dosage Forms/Regulatory Status

VETERINARY-LABELED PRODUCTS: NONE

The Association of Racing Commissioners International (ARCI) has designated this drug as a class 3 substance. See ***Appendix*** for more information. Use of this drug may not be allowed in certain animal competitions. Check rules and regulations before entering in a competition while this medication is being administered. Contact local racing authorities for further guidance.

HUMAN-LABELED PRODUCTS

Cyproheptadine HCl Oral Tablets: 4 mg; generic; (Rx)

Cyproheptadine HCl Oral Syrup: 2 mg/5 mL (0.4 mg/mL) in 473 mL; generic; (Rx)

References

For the complete list of references, see **wiley.com/go/budde/plumb**

Cytarabine

Cytosine Arabinoside

(sye-***tare***-a-bean) *Cytosar-U®*

Antineoplastic

Prescriber Highlights

- Parenteral immunosuppressant/antineoplastic used in dogs and cats for lymphoreticular neoplasms and leukemias and meningoencephalomyelitis of unknown origin.
- Contraindications include patients with a hypersensitivity to this drug.
- Adverse effects primarily include GI effects and myelosuppression; increased ALT may occur.
- Adequate monitoring is essential.
- Potential embryotoxic and teratogenic effects
- The National Institute for Occupational Safety and Health (NIOSH) classifies cytarabine as a hazardous drug; use appropriate precautions when handling.

Uses/Indications

Cytarabine is used primarily in small animals as adjunctive treatment for lymphoreticular neoplasms (eg, lymphoma), myeloproliferative disease (ie, leukemias), and CNS lymphoma. Its use as a single agent in canine lymphoma demonstrated poor efficacy.[1] Data for use as a single agent or as part of multiagent protocol in cats for the treatment of lymphoma or leukemia are limited. Other studies have shown that rescue protocols containing cytarabine for the treatment of canine lymphoma are effective.[2-6]

Cytarabine can be used in combination with glucocorticoids for treating meningoencephalomyelitis of unknown origin in dogs[7-10] and cats.[11]

Cytarabine has also been used in horses to treat lymphomas, but data are limited to individual case reports.[12,13]

Pharmacology/Actions

Cytarabine is converted intracellularly into aracytidine triphosphate, which competes with deoxycytidine triphosphate to inhibit DNA polymerase, resulting in inhibition of DNA synthesis. Cytarabine is specific to the S phase of the cell cycle (DNA synthesis) and blocks cell progress from the G1 phase to the S phase. Incorporation of cytarabine into DNA is responsible for both drug activity and toxicity.

Acquired resistance to cytarabine has been reported and is thought to be due to several mechanisms.

Pharmacokinetics

Cytarabine has very poor systemic availability after oral administration but can be administered IV, SC, and intrathecally. Doses of 600 mg/m² IV as a bolus or as an IV CRI over 12 hours cross the blood–brain barrier in healthy beagles.[14] In dogs given cytarabine 50 mg/m² SC injections or 25 mg/m² per hour IV CRI for 8 hours, the volume of distribution was 0.67 L/kg. Elimination half-lives were similar (1.35 hours SC; 1.15 hours CRI), as were peak concentrations. Rate of absorption after SC was very rapid, with peak levels occurring less than 1 hour after the dose was administered. It is important to note that SC administration did not achieve steady-state concentrations, as cytarabine was rapidly absorbed and eliminated quickly (t½= 1.35 hours). This study also suggests a CRI may produce prolonged exposure of cytarabine at cytotoxic levels in plasma, but it is not known if this correlates with differences in efficacy or toxicity.[15] Similar pharmacokinetic parameters (V_d = 0.9 L/kg, t ½ = 1.1 hours) in dogs given 50 mg/m² SC injection were noted in a separate study,[9] and cytarabine concentration remained above 1 µg/mL for 2 hours after administration. Overall drug exposure was similar, but cytarabine concentrations were significantly higher for a longer duration (as compared with 50 mg/m² SC every 12 hours for 4 doses) with dosing regimens of 100 mg/m² SC every 12 hours for 2 doses or 200 mg/m² SC as a single dose.[8]

In humans, cytarabine is widely distributed throughout the body. CSF levels can reach ≈40% of the levels found in plasma. Elimination half-life in the CSF is significantly longer than that of serum. Circulating cytarabine is rapidly metabolized by the enzyme cytidine deaminase principally in the liver to the inactive metabolite ara-U (uracil arabinoside). About 80% of the dose is excreted in the urine within 24 hours as both ara-U (≈90%) and unchanged cytarabine (≈10%).

The drug apparently crosses the placenta, but it is unknown if it enters milk.

Contraindications/Precautions/Warnings

Cytarabine can cause severe toxicity, depending on the dose and rate of administration. It should only be used where adequate monitoring and support can be administered. Cytarabine is contraindicated in patients with previous hypersensitivity reactions and should be used with caution in patients with pre-existing bone marrow depression, hepatic or renal dysfunction, or infection. In humans, acute pancreatitis and sudden respiratory distress syndrome have been reported.

Some commercially available products contain benzyl alcohol.

The National Institute for Occupational Safety and Health (NIOSH) classifies cytarabine as a hazardous drug; personal protective equipment (PPE) should be used accordingly to minimize the risk for exposure.[16]

Adverse Effects

In dogs, the most common adverse effects following IV CRI are GI (65%) and hematologic toxicities, with neutropenia (35%) and thrombocytopenia (12%) being the most common.[1,17] Myelosuppressive effects (eg, anemia, neutropenia, thrombocytopenia) are more pronounced with IV versus SC administration. Lower doses in dogs (eg, for inflammatory brain disease) had minimal adverse effects (ie, mild to moderate anemia in less than 1% of patients).[18] Humans experience biphasic leukocyte nadir, first from days 7 to 9 and again at days 15 to 24, with a brief rise in cell count between the nadirs. Platelet decreases begin around day 5, with nadir occurring at ≈days 12 to 15.

GI disturbances include anorexia, nausea, vomiting, diarrhea, and oral ulceration. Neurotoxicity, hepatotoxicity, lethargy, and fever may also occur with cytarabine therapy. Increased ALT was noted in 15% of dogs in a study.[17]

Alopecia and delayed regrowth of shaven hair have been reported in dogs; breeds with a continuously growing hair coat (eg, poodles, terriers, Afghan hounds, old English sheepdogs) are more likely to experience significant hair loss.

Three cases (n = 138) of calcinosis cutis at cytarabine SC injection sites were reported in dogs receiving concurrent prednisolone for treatment of meningoencephalomyelitis of unknown etiology.[19]

In addition, there was 1 case report of suspected drug-induced infiltrative lung disease following a 24-hour cytarabine infusion.[20]

Reproductive/Nursing Safety

Cytarabine is teratogenic in laboratory animals, particularly when administered during the first trimester. Fetal harm has been described following cytarabine administration to pregnant women.

Although it is unknown if cytarabine enters maternal milk, the potential mutagenicity and carcinogenicity of the drug warrants using extreme caution in allowing the dam to continue nursing while receiving cytarabine.

Because safety has not been established in animals, this drug should only be used when the maternal benefits outweigh the potential risks to offspring.

Overdose/Acute Toxicity

The toxicity of cytarabine is dependent on dose and rate of administration. The intravenous LD_{50} in dogs is 172 mg/kg and greater than 7000 mg/kg in mice.[21] Treatment is supportive, as there is no known antidote, but the drug is dialyzable.

For patients that have experienced or are suspected to have experienced an overdose, it is strongly encouraged to consult with one of the 24-hour poison consultation centers that specialize in providing information specific for veterinary patients. For general information related to overdose and toxin exposures, as well as contact information for poison control centers, refer to ***Appendix.***

Drug Interactions

The following drug interactions have either been reported or are theoretical in humans or animals receiving cytarabine and may be of significance in veterinary patients. Unless otherwise noted, use together is not necessarily contraindicated, but weigh the potential risks and perform additional monitoring when appropriate.

- **Flucytosine (5-FC)**: Cytarabine may antagonize the anti-infective activity of flucytosine.
- **Myelosuppressive Agents** (eg, **antineoplastics, immunosuppressants, iron chelators**): Concurrent use with other bone marrow depressant medication may result in additive myelosuppression, avoid combination when possible.
- **Vaccines** (live and inactivated): May diminish vaccine efficacy and enhance adverse effects of live vaccines

Dosages

NOTE: The following dosages should be used only as a general guide because of the potential toxicity of this drug to patients, veterinary staff, and clients and because chemotherapy indications, treatment protocols, monitoring and safety guidelines often change.

Consultation with a veterinary oncologist and referral to current veterinary oncology references[22-26] are strongly recommended.

DOGS:

Antineoplastic agent (extra-label):

Intravenous:

a) 300 mg/m² (NOT mg/kg) as a continuous IV infusion (delivered over 4 to 72 hours) once weekly or as part of the day 1 DMAC multi-agent chemotherapy protocol[17,27,28]

b) 600 mg/m² (NOT mg/kg) as a continuous IV infusion (300 mg/m² given daily over 48 hours)[1]

c) 300 – 600 mg/m² (NOT mg/kg), as a continuous IV infusion (delivered over 5-8 hours) starting on day 1 with an injection of carboplatin chemotherapy, on day 7, and/or day 14 of the treatment cycle[3]

d) 750 mg/m² (NOT mg/kg) as a continuous IV infusion (150 mg/m² given daily for 5 consecutive days, in addition to GMCSF, EPO, and ondansetron injections) as part of a VCAA-based multi-agent chemotherapy protocol[4]

Subcutaneous: (See ***Pharmacokinetics*** regarding SC administration concerns.)

a) Two doses of 100 mg/m² (NOT mg/kg) SC given 2 hours apart (total dose, 200 mg/m²) as part of the DMAC multi-agent chemotherapy protocol[2]

b) 300 mg/m² (NOT mg/kg) SC as a single dose as part of DMAC multi-agent chemotherapy protocol[27,28]

c) 300 – 600 mg/m² (NOT mg/kg) SC split into 3 to 4 daily doses over 3 to 4 days, starting on day 1 along with carboplatin chemotherapy[3]

d) 150 mg/m² (NOT mg/kg) SC every 12 hours for 48 hours was used in a patient with large granular lymphocyte T-cell lymphoma as part of a multi-agent chemotherapy protocol with L-asparaginase, CCNU, and vincristine.[29]

e) 33 mg/m² (NOT mg/kg) SC every 8 hours for 5 days along with bleomycin[6]

Inflammatory brain disease (eg, meningoencephalomyelitis of unknown etiology; extra-label): In combination with glucocorticoid therapy:

Subcutaneous: (see ***Pharmacokinetics*** for SC administration) 50 mg/m² (NOT mg/kg) SC every 12 hours for 48 hours, repeat every 3 weeks[7,8,18,30-32]

Intravenous:

a) 100 mg/m² (NOT mg/kg) as a continuous IV infusion given over 24 hours[33,34]

b) 200 mg/m² (NOT mg/kg) as a continuous IV infusion given over 8 to 24 hours[35] or over 48 hours[36]

CATS:

Antineoplastic agent (extra-label): There are limited data available to support dosing in cats, but cytarabine has been dosed as below:

Subcutaneous: (See ***Pharmacokinetics*** regarding SC administration concerns.)

a) 10 mg/m² (NOT mg/kg) SC every 12 hours for 2 to 4 days[37]

b) 50 mg/m² (NOT mg/kg) SC every 12 hours for 48 hours as part of multi-agent chemotherapy protocol[38]

c) 300 mg/m² (NOT mg/kg) SC has also been used as part of DMAC chemotherapy rescue protocol for feline lymphoma.[5]

Intravenous: 100 mg/m² (NOT mg/kg) IV along with other chemotherapeutic agents[39]

Inflammatory brain disease (eg, meningoencephalomyelitis of unknown etiology; extra-label):

Subcutaneous: (See ***Pharmacokinetics*** regarding SC administration concerns.) 50 mg/m² (NOT mg/kg) SC every 12 hours for 48 hours[11]

HORSES:

Antineoplastic agent (extra-label): Consultation with a veterinary oncologist is encouraged before use; usual doses in horses are 200 – 300 mg/m² (usually 1 – 1.5 g/horse per dose) SC or IM every 1 to 2 weeks.[12,40]

Monitoring

- Adverse effects (eg, inappetence, lethargy, drooling [oral ulcerations], vomiting, diarrhea, fever)
- CBC with platelets (baseline, nadir, prior to subsequent treatments)
- Liver and renal function (baseline and periodic)

Client Information

- Cytarabine is a chemotherapy (ie, cancer) drug. The drug and its byproducts can be hazardous to other animals and people that come in contact with it. On the day your animal gets the drug and then for a few days afterward, all bodily waste (eg, urine, feces, litter), blood, and vomit should only be handled while wearing disposable gloves. Seal the waste in a plastic bag, and then place both the bag and gloves in the regular trash.
- GI toxicity (eg, ulceration, diarrhea, vomiting) can occur. If diarrhea is severe or continues, contact your veterinarian.
- Bone marrow depression can occur. The greatest effects on bone marrow usually occur within a few weeks after treatment. Your veterinarian will do blood tests to watch for this, but if you see bleeding, bruising, fever (indicating an infection), or if your animal becomes very tired easily, contact your veterinarian right away.
- It is important to immediately report any signs associated with toxicity (eg, abnormal bleeding, bruising, urination, depression, infection, shortness of breath).
- Hair loss and delayed regrowth of shaven hair have been reported in dogs; breeds with a continuously growing hair coat (eg, poodles, terriers, Afghan hounds, old English sheepdogs) are more likely to experience significant hair loss.
- This medication is considered to be a hazardous drug as defined by the National Institute for Occupational Safety and Health (NIOSH). Talk with your veterinarian or pharmacist about the use of personal protective equipment when handling this medicine.

Chemistry/Synonyms

Cytarabine, a synthetic pyrimidine nucleoside antimetabolite, occurs as an odorless, white to off-white crystalline powder with a pK_a of 4.35. It is freely soluble in water and slightly soluble in alcohol.

Cytarabine may also be known as 1-beta-D-arabinofuranosylcytosine, arabinosylcytosine, ara-C, cytarabine liposome, cytarabinum, cytosine arabinoside, liposomal cytarabine, NSC-63878, U-19920, U-19920A, WR-28453, ARA-cell®, *Alexan*®, *Arabine*®, *Aracytin*®, *Aracytine*®, *Citab*®, *Citagenin*®, *Citaloxan*®, *Cylocide*, *Cytarbel*®, *Cytarine*®, *Cytosar-U*®, *DepoCyt*®, *DepoCyte*®, *Erpalfa*®, *Ifarab*®, *Larac-it*®, *Medsara*®, *Novutrax*®, *Serotabir*®, *Starasid*®, *Tabine*®, *Tarabine*®, or *Udicil*®.

Storage/Stability

Cytarabine sterile powder for injection should be stored protected from light at 20°C to 25°C (68°F-77°F); store intact vials of solution at 15°C to 30°C (59°F-86°F). After reconstitution with bacteriostatic water for injection, solutions are stable for 48 hours at room temperature, although the manufacturer recommends administration as soon as possible after preparation.

Compatibility/Compounding Considerations

Compatible with 5% dextrose in water, 5% dextrose in sodium chloride (0.2%, 0.9%), 5% dextrose in lactated Ringer's, 10% dextrose in 0.9% sodium chloride, lactated Ringer's, normal saline, Ringer's, and sodium lactate 1/6 M. Cytarabine is **incompatible** with the following for y-site administration: allopurinol, amiodarone, amphotericin B, daptomycin, diazepam, lansoprazole, and phenytoin. **Incompatible** with the following in admixtures and syringes: fluorouracil, heparin, regular insulin, oxacillin, and penicillin G potassium.

Compatibility is dependent on factors such as pH, concentration,

temperature, and diluent used; consult specialized references or a hospital pharmacist for more specific information.

Dosage Forms/Regulatory Status

VETERINARY-LABELED PRODUCTS: NONE

HUMAN-LABELED PRODUCTS:

Cytarabine Injection: 20 mg/mL in 5 mL, 25 mL, and 50 mL single- and multi-dose vials, and 100 mg/mL in 20 mL single-dose vials; generic; (Rx)

Cytarabine Injection, liposomal: 10 mg/mL preservative free (for intrathecal use only) vials; *DepoCyt®*; (Rx). Marketing status is uncertain.

References

For the complete list of references, see **wiley.com/go/budde/plumb**

Dacarbazine (DTIC)

(da-***kar***-ba-zeen)

Antineoplastic

Prescriber Highlights

- ► Parenteral antineoplastic used in dogs for relapsed lymphomas, soft tissue sarcomas, and melanoma
- ► Not recommended for use in cats
- ► Contraindications include hypersensitivity to the drug and pregnancy (potentially teratogenic).
- ► GI adverse effects can be severe and dose-limiting; high emetogenic potential necessitates premedication to reduce acute vomiting. Myelosuppression also may occur.
- ► Solution must be diluted before IV administration; extravasation injuries can be serious.
- ► The National Institute for Occupational Safety and Health (NIOSH) classifies dacarbazine as a hazardous drug; use appropriate precautions when handling.

Uses/Indications

Dacarbazine has been used to treat relapsed canine lymphoma,[1] soft tissue sarcomas, histiocytic sarcoma,[2] and melanoma in dogs. It has also been used in combination with doxorubicin, mitoxantrone, vincristine, or lomustine to treat dogs with relapsed lymphoma[3-6] and hemangiosarcoma.[7,8]

Pharmacology/Actions

Dacarbazine is metabolized by hepatic cytochrome P450 enzymes to methyl-triazeno-imidazole-carboxamide (MTIC), an active metabolite. MTIC spontaneously decomposes to release a methyl diazonium that methylates the O6 and N7 positions of guanine, thereby ceasing DNA replication elongation and causing DNA double-strand breaks. Dacarbazine and MTIC are alkylating agents. Dacarbazine possesses minimal immunosuppressive activity and is probably not a cell cycle-phase specific drug.

Resistance to dacarbazine is mediated by upregulation of O6-methylguanine methyltransferase (MGMT), and potentially through enhancement of several other DNA repair mechanisms.

Pharmacokinetics

No pharmacokinetic data were identified in canines. Dacarbazine is poorly absorbed from the GI tract and must be administered IV. In humans, the drug is only slightly bound to plasma proteins and concentrates in the liver where it is extensively metabolized. It is converted into an active form of the drug (MTIC) in the liver by the cytochrome P450 system. Only limited amounts of the drug cross the blood-brain barrier. It is excreted in the urine via tubular secretion with ≈40% as unchanged drug. Elimination half-life is ≈5 hours.

Contraindications/Precautions/Warnings

Dacarbazine is not recommended for use in cats as it is unknown if cats can adequately metabolize it; however, cats are able to metabolize temozolomide (a similar antineoplastic drug) into the same active metabolite (MTIC).[9]

Dacarbazine is contraindicated in patients with a history of hypersensitivity to it. Dacarbazine can cause life-threatening toxicity and should only be used where adequate monitoring and support can be administered. It should be used with caution in patients with preexisting bone marrow depression, hepatic or renal dysfunction, or infection.

Dacarbazine can cause extensive pain and tissue damage during IV administration. Administer IV following a single, clean venipuncture attempt through an IV catheter (indwelling or butterfly). If clinical signs of extravasation are noted, discontinue infusion immediately at that site and apply moderate, dry heat to the area to help disperse the drug and promote vascular absorption. Dacarbazine should **not** be administered IM or SC due to the risk for extravasation.

The National Institute for Occupational Safety and Health (NIOSH) classifies dacarbazine as a hazardous drug; personal protective equipment (PPE) should be used accordingly to minimize the risk for exposure.

Adverse Effects

In dogs, GI toxicity (including acute vomiting within 24 hours of administration, anorexia, and diarrhea) is commonly seen after administration and is dose-limiting. Dacarbazine is highly emetogenic and pretreatment with an antiemetic (eg, maropitant, ondansetron) is warranted.

Bone marrow toxicity is usually mild and includes anemia, neutropenia, and thrombocytopenia. One study found thrombocytopenia to be the most common hematological toxicity occurred 1 to 2 weeks after treatment.[1] Occasionally severe hematopoietic toxicity can occur with fatal consequences. Other delayed toxic effects can include alopecia, hepatotoxicity, renal impairment, and photosensitivity reactions, but these are rarely seen.

Dacarbazine is considered a vesicant and can cause extensive pain, venous spasm, phlebitis, and tissue damage during IV administration. Pretreatment with dexamethasone and/or butorphanol has been suggested to reduce associated injection site reactions. Dilution is also recommended to reduce the risk for injection site reactions and extravasation.

If signs of extravasation occur, the following has been recommended[10]:

- Stop the infusion immediately and, if possible, withdraw 3 to 5 mL blood to remove some of the drug.
- Remove the infusion needle.
- Delineate the infiltrated area on the patient's skin with a felt tip marker.
- Elevate for 48 hours above heart level using a sling or stockinette dressing with an observation window cut in the dressing.
- Avoid pressure or friction; do not rub the area.
- Observe for signs of increased erythema, pain, or skin necrosis.
- Ensure that no medication is given distal to the extravasation site.
- After 48 hours, encourage the patient to use the extremity normally to promote full range of motion.

Many dogs receiving chemotherapy will have minor hair coat changes (eg, shagginess, loss of luster). Breeds with continuously growing hair coats (eg, poodles, terriers, Afghan hounds, or Old English sheepdogs) are more likely to experience significant alopecia, change in hair coat color or texture, or hyperpigmentation.

Reproductive/Nursing Safety

Dacarbazine is teratogenic in rats at higher than clinically used dosages. For intact female patients, verify pregnancy status prior to administration.

Although it is unknown if dacarbazine enters milk, the potential carcinogenicity of the drug warrants using extreme caution in allowing the mother to continue nursing while receiving this drug.

Because safety has not been established in animals, this drug should only be used when the maternal benefits outweigh the potential risks to offspring.

Overdose/Acute Toxicity

The intravenous LD_{50} in mice is 466 mg/kg.[11] Due to the potential for serious toxicity associated with this agent, dosage calculations should be checked thoroughly to avoid overdosing. Treatment of an overdose is supportive as there is no known antidote.

For patients that have experienced or are suspected to have experienced an overdose, consultation with a 24-hour poison consultation center specializing in providing veterinary-specific information is recommended. For general information related to overdose and toxin exposures, as well as contact information for poison control centers, refer to ***Appendix.***

Drug Interactions

The following drug interactions have either been reported or are theoretical in humans or animals receiving dacarbazine and may be of significance in veterinary patients. Unless otherwise noted, use together is not necessarily contraindicated, but weigh the potential risks and perform additional monitoring when appropriate.

- **CYP1A2 Inducers** (eg, **phenobarbital**, **rifampin**): May increase the metabolism of dacarbazine
- **CYP1A2 Inhibitors, Strong** (eg, **ciprofloxacin, mexiletine**): May decrease the metabolism of dacarbazine, consider therapy modification
- **Immunosuppressive Agents** (eg, **cyclosporine**, **leflunomide**, **mycophenolate**): Concurrent use with other bone marrow depressant medication may result in additive myelosuppression, avoid combination when possible
- **Myelosuppressive Agents** (eg, **antineoplastics**, **iron chelators**): Concurrent use with other bone marrow depressant medication may result in additive myelosuppression, avoid combination when possible.
- **Vaccines** (live and inactivated): May diminish vaccine efficacy and enhance adverse effects of vaccines.

Dosages

NOTE: Because of the potential toxicity of this drug to patients, veterinary personnel, and clients, and because chemotherapy indications, treatment protocols, monitoring and safety guidelines often change, the following dosages should only be used as a general guide. Consultation with a veterinary oncologist and referral to current veterinary oncology references[12-16] are strongly recommended.

DOGS:

Antineoplastic (extra-label): Dacarbazine dosage depends on the protocol being used.

a) 600 – 1000 mg/m^2 (NOT mg/kg) IV over 4 to 8 hours every 2 to 3 weeks[6]

b) 200 – 250 mg/m^2 (NOT mg/kg) once daily IV for 5 days with the treatment cycle repeated every 3 to 4 weeks. Administer as a bolus in a freely running IV solution.

Monitoring

- Efficacy
- Toxicity, including CBC with differential and platelets; renal and hepatic function tests

Client Information

- Dacarbazine is a chemotherapy (anticancer) medicine. This medicine can be hazardous to other animals and people that come in contact with it. On the day your animal receives the medicine and then for a few days afterward, all bodily waste (urine, feces, litter), blood, or vomit should only be handled while wearing disposable gloves. Seal the waste in a plastic bag and then place both the bag and gloves in with the regular trash.
- Gastrointestinal toxicity(eg, ulcers, diarrhea) can occur. If diarrhea is severe or continues, contact your veterinarian.
- Bone marrow suppression can occur which may put your animal at risk for infection. The greatest effects on bone marrow usually occur within a few weeks after treatment. Your veterinarian will do blood tests to watch for this, but if you see bleeding, bruising, fever (indicating an infection), or if your animal tires easily, contact your veterinarian immediately. Do not miss these important follow-up visits.
- This medication is considered to be a hazardous drug as defined by the National Institute for Occupational Safety and Health (NIOSH). Talk with your veterinarian or pharmacist about the use of personal protective equipment when handling this medicine.

Chemistry/Synonyms

An antineoplastic agent, dacarbazine occurs as a colorless to ivory colored crystalline solid. It is slightly soluble in water or alcohol. After reconstituting with sterile water, the injection has a pH of 3 to 4.

Dacarbazine may also be known as dacarbazinum, DIC, DTIC, imidazole carboxamide, dimethyl triazeno imadazol carboxamide, NSC-45388, WR-139007, *Asercit®*, *DTI®*, *DTIC-Dome®*, *Dacarb®*, *Dacarbaziba®*, *Dacatic®*, *Deticene®*, *Detilem®*, *Detimedac®*, *Fauldetic®*, *Ifadac®*, or *Oncocarbil®*.

Storage/Stability

The powder for injection should be protected from light and stored at 2°C to 8°C (36°F-46°F). If exposed to heat, the powder may change color from ivory to pink, indicating some decomposition.

As per the manufacturer, after reconstituting with sterile water for injection, the resultant solution is stable for up to 8 hours at room temperature or 72 hours if kept refrigerated. If further diluted (up to 500 mL) with either 5% dextrose or 0.9% sodium chloride, the solution is stable for 24 hours when refrigerated and 8 hours at room temperature.

Compatibility/Compounding Considerations

Compatibility is dependent on factors such as pH, concentration, temperature, and diluent used; consult specialized references or a hospital pharmacist for more specific information.

Dacarbazine is **compatible** with 5% dextrose in water and 0.9% sodium chloride for dilution.

There are many drugs that are reported to be **Y-site compatible** including bleomycin, cyclophosphamide, cytarabine, dactinomycin, doxorubicin, ondansetron, and vinblastine.

Dosage Forms/Regulatory Status

VETERINARY-LABELED PRODUCTS: NONE

HUMAN-LABELED PRODUCTS:

Dacarbazine Powder for Injection: 100 mg, 200 mg, and 500 mg (may contain mannitol) vials; generic; (Rx)

References

For the complete list of references, see **wiley.com/go/budde/plumb**

Dactinomycin

Actinomycin D

(dak-ti-noe-***mye***-sin) *Cosmegen®*

Antineoplastic

Prescriber Highlights

- ► Antibiotic antineoplastic agent used for treatment of a variety of neoplasms in dogs and cats
- ► Contraindications include hypersensitivity to the drug and pregnancy (teratogenic).
- ► Use caution in patients with pre-existing myelosuppression, hepatic dysfunction, or infection
- ► Primary adverse effects include GI toxicity and myelosuppression (may be life-threatening); adequate monitoring essential
- ► Specific administration techniques required; avoid extravasation injuries
- ► The National Institute for Occupational Safety and Health (NIOSH) classifies dactinomycin as a hazardous drug; use appropriate precautions when handling.

Uses/Indications

Dactinomycin has been used as treatment of lymphoma, bone and soft tissue sarcomas, and carcinomas in small animals.[1] However, limited efficacy has been shown with carcinomas.[2] Its use as a single chemotherapeutic agent has produced mixed efficacy results in relapsed or resistant lymphomas.[3,4] A study in dogs demonstrated that doxorubicin was superior to dactinomycin when used as part of a 'CHOP' protocol to treat lymphoma.[5] Studies have shown efficacy in rescue protocols containing dactinomycin for canine[6] and feline[7] lymphoma, but significant toxicity has been noted.[8]

Pharmacology/Actions

Dactinomycin is an antibiotic with activity against a variety of gram-negative, gram-positive bacteria, and some fungi, but its cytotoxicity prevents it from being clinically useful as an antimicrobial. Dactinomycin forms a complex with DNA, ultimately binding DNA and inhibiting RNA synthesis. Dactinomycin also possesses immunosuppressive and some hypocalcemic activity.

Pharmacokinetics

Because dactinomycin is poorly absorbed, it must be given IV. It is rapidly distributed and high concentrations may be found in bone marrow and nucleated cells but does not cross the blood-brain barrier. In humans, dactinomycin is only minimally metabolized and ≈30% of the drug is excreted unchanged in the bile and urine. The terminal half-life for radioactivity is 36 hours.

Contraindications/Precautions/Warnings

Dactinomycin can cause life-threatening toxicity. It should only be used where adequate monitoring and support can be administered. Dactinomycin is contraindicated in patients with previous hypersensitivity reactions and should be used with caution in patients with preexisting myelosuppression, hepatic dysfunction, or infection.

The P-glycoprotein pump actively transports dactinomycin, and certain breeds susceptible to *MDR1* mutation (also known as *ABCB1*-1delta; eg, collies, Australian shepherds, Shetland sheepdogs, long-haired whippets) are at higher risk for toxicity. *MDR1* gene mutation testing is suggested for susceptible breeds prior to treating.

Care must be taken to avoid perivascular extravasation. Securely placed indwelling IV catheters and close monitoring of IV patency/integrity during infusion are recommended. Dactinomycin should **not** be administered IM or SC due to the risk for extravasation.

Dactinomycin is a high-alert drug in human medicine.[9] Consider using tall man lettering when writing orders for dactinomycin: DACTINomycin. Dosage calculations should be checked thoroughly to avoid overdosing.

The National Institute for Occupational Safety and Health (NIOSH) classifies dactinomycin as a hazardous drug; personal protective equipment (PPE) should be used accordingly to minimize the risk for exposure.

Adverse Effects

In dogs, the two most common adverse effects are GI and hematological toxicities. Bone marrow toxicity is usually mild and includes anemia, neutropenia, and thrombocytopenia. One study found thrombocytopenia to be the most common hematological toxicity.[10] Other adverse effects can include ulcerative stomatitis or other GI ulceration, and hepatotoxicity. Because dactinomycin may increase serum uric acid levels, allopurinol may be required to prevent urate stone formation in susceptible patients.

Dactinomycin is considered a vesicant and can cause extensive pain and tissue damage during IV administration. Administer IV following a single, clean venipuncture attempt through an IV catheter (indwelling or butterfly); administration by IV infusion, or slow IV bolus into a running IV line, is recommended. If clinical signs of extravasation are noted, discontinue infusion and apply ice to the site; in humans it is recommended to apply ice for 15 minutes four times per day for 3 days.[11]

Many dogs receiving chemotherapy will have minor hair coat changes (eg, shagginess, loss of luster). Breeds with continuously growing hair coats (eg, poodles, terriers, Afghan hounds, Old English sheepdogs) are more likely to experience significant alopecia, change in hair coat color or texture, or hyperpigmentation.

Reproductive/Nursing Safety

Dactinomycin crosses the placenta and has been demonstrated to be embryotoxic and teratogenic in rats, rabbits, and hamsters at higher than clinically used dosages.[12] For intact female patients, verify pregnancy status prior to administration.

Although it is unknown if dactinomycin enters maternal milk, the potential mutagenicity and carcinogenicity of the drug warrants using extreme caution in allowing the mother to continue nursing while receiving dactinomycin.

Because safety has not been established in animals, this drug should only be used when the maternal benefits outweigh the potential risks to offspring.

Overdose/Acute Toxicity

The lowest detectable lethal dose in dogs is 0.16 mg/kg IV. The intravenous LD_{50} in mice is 1.025 mg/kg.[13] Due to the potential for serious toxicity associated with this agent, dosage calculations should be checked thoroughly to avoid overdosing. Overdose treatment is supportive as there is no known antidote.

For patients that have experienced or are suspected to have experienced an overdose, consultation with a 24-hour poison consultation center specializing in providing veterinary-specific information is recommended. For general information related to overdose and toxin exposures, as well as contact information for poison control centers, refer to ***Appendix***.

Drug Interactions

The following drug interactions have either been reported or are theoretical in humans or animals receiving dactinomycin and may be of significance in veterinary patients. Unless otherwise noted, use together is not necessarily contraindicated, but weigh the potential risks and perform additional monitoring when appropriate.

- **Myelosuppressive Agents** (eg, **antineoplastics, immunosuppressants, iron chelators**): Concurrent use with other bone marrow depressant medication may result in additive myelosuppression, avoid combination when possible.

- **Vaccines** (live and inactivated): May diminish vaccine efficacy and enhance adverse effects of vaccines

Laboratory Considerations

- Dactinomycin may interfere with determination of antibacterial drug levels if using bioassay techniques.

Dosages

NOTE: Because of the potential toxicity of this drug to patients, veterinary personnel, and clients, and because chemotherapy indications, treatment protocols, monitoring and safety guidelines often change, the following dosages should only be used as a general guide. Consultation with a veterinary oncologist and referral to current veterinary oncology references[13-17] are strongly recommended.

DOGS:

Antineoplastic (extra-label): Depending on the protocol, usual doses for dactinomycin in dogs range from 0.5 – 1 mg/m^2 (NOT mg/kg) IV over 20 minutes; doses may be repeated every 1 to 3 weeks. [1,3,6,10,18]

CATS:

Antineoplastic (extra-label): 0.75 mg/m^2 (NOT mg/kg) IV repeated continuously every 2 weeks as part of a rescue protocol for feline lymphoma.[7]

Monitoring

- CBC with hepatic and renal function tests to monitor for potential toxicities
- Check oral mucous membranes for ulceration.
- Monitor injection site for signs of extravasation.

Client Information

- Dactinomycin is a chemotherapy (anticancer) drug. This medicine can be hazardous to other animals and people that come in contact with it. On the day your animal receives this medicine and then for a few days afterward, all bodily waste (urine, feces, litter), blood, or vomit should only be handled while wearing disposable gloves. Seal the waste in a plastic bag and then place both the bag and gloves in with the regular trash.
- Gastrointestinal toxicity (eg, ulcers, diarrhea) can occur. If diarrhea is severe or continues, contact your veterinarian.
- Bone marrow suppression can occur, which may put your animal at risk for infection. The greatest effects on bone marrow usually occur within a few weeks after treatment. Your veterinarian will do blood tests to watch for this, but if you see bleeding, bruising, fever (indicating an infection), or if your animal becomes very tired easily, contact your veterinarian immediately. Do not miss these important follow-up visits.
- This medication is considered to be a hazardous drug as defined by the National Institute for Occupational Safety and Health (NIOSH). Talk with your veterinarian or pharmacist about the use of personal protective equipment when handling this medicine.

Chemistry/Synonyms

An antibiotic antineoplastic agent, dactinomycin (also known as actinomycin D) occurs as an odorless, bright red, crystalline powder. It is somewhat hygroscopic and soluble in water at 10°C (50°F) and slightly soluble at 37°C (98.6°F). The commercially available preparation is a yellow lyophilized mixture of dactinomycin and mannitol.

Dactinomycin may also be known as ACT, actinomycin C(1), actinomycin D, meractinomycin, NSC-3053, *Ac-De*®, *Bioact-D*®, *Cosmegen*® or *Dacmozen*®.

Storage/Stability

The commercially available powder should be protected from light and stored at 25°C (77°F); excursions permitted to 15°C to 30°C (59°F-86°F). When reconstituting, sterile water for injection without preservatives must be used as preservatives may cause precipitation. After reconstituting, the manufacturer recommends using the solution immediately and discarding any unused portion.[16] IV fluid in-line filters with cellulose ester membranes may partially remove dactinomycin.

Compatibility/Compounding Considerations

Compatibility is dependent on factors such as pH, concentration, temperature, and diluent used; consult specialized references or a hospital pharmacist for more specific information.

A precipitate may form when dactinomycin is added to sterile water that contains preservatives. **Compatible** with 5% dextrose in water and 0.9% sodium chloride for dilution.

Dactinomycin is reported to be **incompatible** for Y-site administration with the following drugs: diazepam, filgrastim, indomethacin, pantoprazole, and phenytoin. Drugs that are reported to be **compatible with dactinomycin when injected at a Y-site** include: granisetron and ondansetron.

Dosage Forms/Regulatory Status

VETERINARY-LABELED PRODUCTS: NONE.

HUMAN-LABELED PRODUCTS:

Dactinomycin Powder for Injection, lyophilized: 0.5 mg with 20 mg mannitol in vials; *Cosmegen*®, generic; (Rx)

References

For the complete list of references, see **wiley.com/go/budde/plumb**

Dalteparin

(***dahl***-tep-ah-rin) *Fragmin*®

Anticoagulant

Prescriber Highlights

- Low molecular weight (fractionated) heparin that may be useful for treatment or prophylaxis of thromboembolic disease
- Preferentially inhibits factor Xa and usually only minimally impacts clotting times
- Hemorrhage unlikely, but possible
- Must be given SC
- Dogs and cats may require very frequent dosing, making outpatient administration unfeasible.
- May be cost-prohibitive, particularly in horses and large dogs

Uses/Indications

Dalteparin may be useful for prophylaxis or treatment of thromboembolic disease.[1] Recent pharmacokinetic work in dogs and cats raised questions on whether the drug can be effectively and practically administered in the long term. In humans, it is also indicated for prevention of ischemic complications associated with unstable angina and non-Q-wave myocardial infarction.

Pharmacology/Actions

By binding to and accelerating antithrombin III, low molecular weight heparins (LMWHs) enhance the inhibition of factor Xa and thrombin. The potential advantage to using these products over standard (unfractionated) heparin is that LMWHs preferentially inhibit factor Xa and only minimally impact clotting times (prothrombin time, thrombin time, and activated partial thromboplastin time).

Pharmacokinetics

In dogs, dalteparin is completely absorbed after SC injection. It has a volume of distribution of 50 to 70 mL/kg and a dose-dependent half-life of ≈1.5 to 3 hours.[2]

After SC administration to cats, dalteparin is completely absorbed, and the half-life is ≈2 hours.[3] Cats appear to have a much shorter duration of activity (anti-Xa) associated with low molecular weight heparins (LMWHs) than humans. To maintain a therapeutic target of anti-Xa activity of 0.5 – 1 units/mL, pharmacokinetic modeling in one study predicted that a dalteparin dose of 150 units/kg SC every 4 hours would be required.[4] A later study reported that all cats receiving 75 units/kg SC every 6 hours achieved target peak anti-Xa activity of 0.5 –1 units/mL when measured 2 hours postdose.[5]

In horses, dalteparin's pharmacokinetics are similar to humans, but a pharmacodynamic study where 50 units/kg SC were used showed that twice-daily dosing kept anti-Xa activity above the thromboprophylactic range, but that once-daily administration did not.[6]

In humans, after SC injection, dalteparin is absorbed rapidly with a bioavailability of ≈87%; peak plasma concentration (activity) occurs in ≈4 hours.[7] Anti-Xa activity persists for up to 24 hours and doses are usually given once to twice a day. Dalteparin is excreted in the urine; elimination half-life is ≈3 to 5 hours. Half-life may be prolonged in patients with renal impairment.

Contraindications/Precautions/Warnings

Dalteparin is contraindicated in patients that are hypersensitive to it, heparin, or pork products. It is also contraindicated in patients with major bleeding heparin-induced thrombocytopenia, or thrombocytopenia associated with positive in vitro tests for antiplatelets in the presence of dalteparin. Use dalteparin cautiously in patients with significant renal dysfunction as drug accumulation could result. It should be used with extreme caution in patients receiving epidural anesthesia or with increased risk for hemorrhage.

Do not administer via IM or IV routes; dalteparin must be given via SC injection only. Dalteparin cannot be used interchangeably with other low molecular weight heparins (LMWHs) or heparin sodium, as dosages differ for each.

Do not confuse dalteparin with darbepoetin.

Adverse Effects

A retrospective study observed that bleeding complications occurred in ≈9% of critically ill dogs receiving dalteparin[1]. Bleeding complications in cats were infrequent with client-administered dalteparin.[8] In humans, adverse effects do not routinely occur, but hemorrhage is a possibility. Injection site hematomas or pain, allergic reactions, and neurologic sequelae secondary to epidural or spinal hematomas have been reported.

Reproductive/Nursing Safety

There was no evidence of embryo-fetal toxicity or teratogenicity when dalteparin sodium was administered to pregnant laboratory animals.[7]

Dalteparin is present in human breastmilk in small amounts. As oral absorption of dalteparin is minimal, it is likely safe to use during nursing.

Because safety has not been established in animals, this drug should only be used when the maternal benefits outweigh the potential risks to offspring.

Overdose/Acute Toxicity

Overdose may lead to hemorrhagic complications. If treatment is necessary, protamine sulfate slow IV may be administered.

Protamine sulfate 1 mg IV can inhibit the effects of 100 units of administered anti-Xa dalteparin. Avoid overdoses of protamine sulfate.

For patients that have experienced or are suspected to have experienced an overdose, consultation with a 24-hour poison consultation center specializing in providing veterinary-specific information is recommended. For general information related to overdose and toxin exposures, as well as contact information for poison control centers, refer to ***Appendix.***

Drug Interactions

The following drug interactions have either been reported or are theoretical in humans or animals receiving dalteparin and may be of significance in veterinary patients. Unless otherwise noted, use together is not necessarily contraindicated, but the potential risks should be weighed, and additional monitoring performed when appropriate.

- **ANTICOAGULANTS, ORAL** (eg, **rivaroxaban, warfarin**): Increased risk for hemorrhage
- **NONSTEROIDAL ANTI-INFLAMMATORY DRUGS** (**NSAIDs**; eg, **carprofen, flunixin, meloxicam, robenacoxib**): Increased risk for hemorrhage
- **PLATELET-AGGREGATION INHIBITORS** (eg, **aspirin, clopidogrel**): Increased risk for hemorrhage
- **SELECTIVE SEROTONIN REUPTAKE INHIBITORS** (**SSRIs**; eg, **fluoxetine, sertraline**): Concurrent use may increase risk for bleeding.

Laboratory Considerations

- Low molecular weight heparins (LMWHs) may cause subclinical, fully reversible increases in **AST** or **ALT**; **bilirubin** is only rarely increased in these patients, therefore, interpret these tests with caution, as increases do not necessarily indicate hepatic damage or dysfunction.

Dosages

DOGS:

Thromboprophylaxis (extra-label): 150 – 175 units/kg SC every 8 hours[9]

CATS:

Thromboprophylaxis (extra-label): 75 – 150 units/kg SC every 6 hours[5,9]

HORSES:

Thromboprophylaxis (extra-label):

a) Adults: 50 units/kg SC twice daily based on a pharmacodynamic study.[6] There was considerable variability in anti-Xa activity between horses, which may indicate the need for more frequent monitoring.

b) Foals: 100 units/kg SC once daily may be effective[10]

Monitoring

- Baseline and periodic CBC with platelet count during therapy
- Urinalysis (free catch)
- Fecal occult blood test (horses)
- Routine coagulation tests (activated partial thromboplastin time [aPTT], PT) are usually insensitive measures of activity and normally not warranted.[11]
- Anti-Xa activity may be useful to guide dosage adjustments, particularly if bleeding occurs or patient has renal dysfunction. A target peak anti-Xa range of 0.5 – 1 units/mL, extrapolated from human literature, has been suggested for use in dogs and cats.[1,5] The suggested thromboprophylactic range for horses is 0.1 – 0.2 units/mL.[6] **NOTE**: To measure peak anti-Xa activity, sample at 2 hours postdose for cats, 3 hours postdose for dogs, and 3 to 4 hours postdose for horses.[12] If an anti-Xa assay is not available, consider activated clotting time, aPTT, thrombin generation, or viscoelastic tests to monitor anticoagulant treatment.[13]

Client Information

- Dalteparin must be injected subcutaneously (SC, under the skin); be sure you understand how to correctly give the injections. Several injections a day may be required, and treatment may be very expensive. Injections may be painful.
- Bleeding is not likely but can occur. Contact your veterinarian immediately if it happens.

- If your animal is listless (lacking energy or interest in things), appears to be having trouble breathing, trouble walking or loses the use of its rear legs, contact your veterinarian immediately, as it may mean blood clots have formed.

Chemistry/Synonyms

A low molecular weight heparin (LMWH), dalteparin sodium is obtained by nitrous acid depolymerization of heparin derived from pork intestinal mucosa. The average molecular weight is ≈5000 and 90% ranges from 2000 to 9000 daltons (heparin sodium has a molecular weight of ≈12,000). 1 mg of dalteparin is equivalent to not less than 110 units and not more than 210 units of anti-factor Xa.

Dalteparin sodium may also be known as: Daltaparinum natricum, Kabi-2165, *Boxol*®, *Fragmine*®, *Ligofragmin*®, or *Low Liquemine*®.

Storage/Stability

The manufacturer of the commercially available injection states the product should be stored at controlled room temperature (20°C-25°C [68°F-77°F]). Do not use if particulate matter or discoloration occur. Once the multi-dose vial is punctured, store at room temperature; discard any unused solution after 2 weeks.

A study showed that commercially available dalteparin solution was stable for up to 30 days when drawn into syringes and stored at room temperature or refrigerated.[14]

Compatibility/Compounding Considerations

Do not mix dalteparin with other compounds.

Dosage Forms/Regulatory Status

VETERINARY-LABELED PRODUCTS: NONE

HUMAN-LABELED PRODUCTS:

Dalteparin Sodium Injection (Anti-factor Xa International Units): Available in a variety of preservative-free single dose syringes that range from 2500 units/0.2 mL to 18,000 units/0.72 mL; these are less likely to be of clinical use in veterinary medicine. A multi-dose vial containing 25,000 units/mL in a 3.8 mL/vial is available; also contains benzyl alcohol; *Fragmin*®; (Rx).

References

For the complete list of references, see **wiley.com/go/budde/plumb**

Danofloxacin

(dan-oh-***floks***-a-sin) *Advocin*®

Fluoroquinolone Antibiotic

Prescriber Highlights

- Parenteral third-generation fluoroquinolone antibiotic labeled for use in beef cattle (excluding dairy or veal) to treat and control bovine respiratory disease (BRD) associated with *Mannheimia (Pasteurella) haemolytica* and *Pasteurella multocida.* May also be of benefit in treating fluoroquinolone-susceptible infections in non-food-producing species (horses, camelids, exotics)
- Labeled in cattle for a single SC injection or 2 SC injections 48 hours apart
- FDA prohibits extra-label use in food animals.

Uses/Indications

Danofloxacin injection is indicated for the treatment of bovine respiratory disease (BRD) associated with *Mannheimia (Pasteurella) haemolytica* and *Pasteurella multocida* in beef cattle and for the control of BRD in beef cattle at high risk for developing BRD associated with the same bacteria. Danofloxacin is not indicated for use in dairy or veal cattle. In other countries, danofloxacin may be labeled for use in other cattle (non-dairy) as well as swine and chickens (non-laying), but in the US, it is illegal to use the drug in an extra-label manner in food-producing species.

Danofloxacin may be of benefit in treating susceptible infections in adult horses, camelids, and other non-food-producing species.

Danofloxacin is classified by the World Health Organization as a Critically Important, Highest Priority antimicrobial.[1] The Office International des Epizooties (OIE) has designated danofloxacin as a Veterinary Critically Important Antimicrobial (VCIA) Agent in avian, bovine, caprine, lagomorph, ovine, and swine species.[2]

Pharmacology/Actions

Danofloxacin is a fluoroquinolone bactericidal antibiotic that inhibits bacterial DNA-gyrase, preventing DNA supercoiling and DNA synthesis. Fluoroquinolones have good activity against many gram-negative bacilli and some gram-positive cocci (*Staphylococcus aureus* and *Staphylococcus pseudintermedius*). It has little activity against anaerobes. In general, fluoroquinolones have a dose- or concentration-dependent effect rather than a time-dependent bactericidal effect.

MIC_{90} values for *Mannheimia (Pasteurella) haemolytica* and *P multocida* average 0.06 µg/mL and 0.015 µg/mL, respectively.[3]

Pharmacokinetics

After SC injection in the neck of cattle, danofloxacin is reportedly rapidly absorbed with high bioavailability (≈90%). Peak serum concentrations occur ≈2 to 3 hours after dosing. Steady-state volume of distribution is ≈2.7 L/kg; lung concentrations exceed those in plasma. Terminal elimination half-life ranges from 3 to 6 hours. In cattle, elimination is primarily unchanged drug into the urine. Other species may metabolize greater percentages of the drug into a desmethyl metabolite (desmethyldanofloxacin). Danofloxacin distributes extensively throughout the body, as evidenced by a steady-state volume of distribution (VDss) in cattle exceeding 1 L/kg. Danofloxacin concentrations in the lung homogenates markedly exceed those observed in plasma, further suggesting extensive distribution to the indicated site of infection. Linear pharmacokinetics has been demonstrated when danofloxacin is administered to cattle by SC injection at doses between 1.25 and 10 mg/kg. One study in calves experimentally infected with *P multocida* showed danofloxacin had a significantly lower clearance rate in 3-week-old calves compared with 6-month-old calves, and a significantly higher AUC in 6-month-old calves than in 3-week-old calves.[4] Plasma protein differences among different ages of calves has not been shown to cause clinically significant changes in danofloxacin pharmacokinetics.[5]

In horses, a research study on the pharmacokinetics of IM, IV, and IG (intragastric) administration of danofloxacin at 1.25 mg/kg to healthy mature horses revealed favorable bioavailability with the IM route at 89% and poor bioavailability of the IG route at 22%.[6] The authors reported good tolerability of the IG route.

In sheep, the drug quickly reaches high tissue concentrations. One hour after IM administration, the concentration peaks in lung tissue and interdigital skin. A study dosing sheep at 1.25 mg/kg IV and IM resulted in similar concentrations for serum, exudates, and transudates.[7]

In goats, a study of danofloxacin administered at 1.25 mg/kg IV or IM revealed similar half-lives of 4.67 and 4.41 hours after IV and IM, respectively.[8] Volume of distribution was high via either route with 100% bioavailability reported after IM administration. The drug's penetration into both exudates and transudates was slightly slower after IM administration[8]. Another study found that goats challenged with *Escherichia coli* endotoxin receiving danofloxacin at 1.25 mg/kg IV or IM had an altered clearance of the drug with significant increases in plasma concentrations and AUC.[9]

In camels, IV administration of the drug at 1.25 mg/kg results in a high volume of distribution, a half-life of 5.37 hours, and rapid clearance.[10] The IM administration of the drug at the same dose resulted in rapid and near complete absorption, with a half-life of 5.71 hours.

In pigs, the drug has been shown to reach a high concentration in lung tissue and GI tissue, including mucosa. In the first 24 hours after an IM dose of 2 mg/kg, 43% of the dose is eliminated in the urine. Elimination half-life in swine is ≈7 hours.

Contraindications/Precautions/Warnings

The FDA prohibits extra-label use of this drug in food animals. The manufacturer cautions use of danofloxacin in animals with known or suspected CNS disorders as quinolones have caused CNS stimulation and seizures (rare). Fluoroquinolones have been shown to produce erosions of cartilage of weight-bearing joints and other signs of arthropathy in immature, rapidly growing animals of various species.[3]

Adverse Effects

Hypersensitivity reactions and lameness have been reported after administration to calves at labeled dosages. Incidence rates are not known, but they are believed to be uncommon. In cattle, SC injections can cause a local tissue reaction that may result in trim loss.

Quinolone-class drugs should be used with caution in animals with known or suspected CNS disorders. In such animals, quinolones have, in rare instances, been associated with CNS stimulation, which may lead to convulsive seizures.

Quinolone-class drugs have been shown to produce erosions of cartilage of weight-bearing joints and other signs of arthropathy in immature, rapidly growing animals of various species.

Reproductive/Nursing Safety

Studies documenting safety during pregnancy in cattle are not available. In studies performed in rats (100 mg/kg/day), mice (50 mg/kg/day), and rabbits (15 mg/kg/day), no teratogenic effects were observed.[3]

Danofloxacin safety during nursing is not known, but it is prohibited from use in lactating dairy cattle where the milk is for human consumption.

Overdose/Acute Toxicity

Limited information is available for cattle. High dosages (18 – 60 mg/kg for 3 to 6 days) administered to feeder calves resulted in arthropathies/lameness (consistent with other fluoroquinolones), CNS stimulation (ataxia, nystagmus, tremors), inappetence, recumbency, depression, and exophthalmos. Some (3/6) 21-day-old calves receiving 18 mg/kg twice 48 hours apart developed nasal pad erythema.

Studies performed in adult dogs given 2.4 mg/kg/day PO for 90 days showed no observable effects.

Drug Interactions

No specific interactions have been reported when danofloxacin is used in cattle. In humans:

- **Corticosteroids** (eg, **dexamethasone, prednis(ol)one**): Concomitant use with fluoroquinolones may increase risk for tendonitis and tendon rupture.
- **Probenecid**: May block renal tubular secretion of danofloxacin and may increase danofloxacin serum level and elimination half-life
- **Theophylline/Aminophylline**: Some injectable fluoroquinolones (eg, ciprofloxacin) can potentially increase serum concentrations; increased monitoring of theophylline concentrations is recommended.

Laboratory Considerations

- None are identified.

Dosages

BEEF CATTLE (EXCLUDING DAIRY CATTLE OR VEAL CALVES):

Label indications (label dosage; FDA-approved): 8 mg/kg SC as a single injection for bovine respiratory disease (BRD) treatment and control in high-risk cattle, or 6 mg/kg SC repeated once ≈48 hours following the first injection as multi-day therapy for BRD treatment.[3] Administered dose volume should not exceed 15 mL per injection site.

REPTILES:

Mycoplasma infections in desert tortoises (extra-label): 6 mg/kg SC (vary injection site) every 48 hours (every other day) for 3 to 6 weeks[11]

Monitoring

- Clinical efficacy

Client Information

- If clients are to administer this product to food animals, they should be advised on correct injection technique and the importance of using the product per the label only.

Chemistry/Synonyms

Danofloxacin mesylate is a synthetic fluoroquinolone that occurs as a white to off-white crystalline powder. Approximately 180 grams are soluble in 1 liter of water. The color of the injectable solution is yellow to amber and does not affect potency.

Danofloxacin may also be known by the following synonyms: CP-76136-27, danofloxacine or danofloxacino. Internationally registered trade names include *Advocin®*, *Advocine®*, *Danocin®*, *Advocid®*, and *Advovet®*.

Storage/Stability

Danofloxacin mesylate for injection should be stored at or below 30°C (86°F) and protected from light and freezing.

Vials of *Advocin®* (danofloxacin) are multiuse vials and should be discarded 28 days after first puncture. Vials should not be punctured more than 7 times (100 mL) or 17 times (250 mL).

Compatibility/Compounding Considerations

Danofloxacin injection for SC use should not be mixed with other medication or diluents. Fluoroquinolone injectable products can be very sensitive to pH changes or chelation with cationic substances (eg, calcium, magnesium, zinc).

Dosage Forms/Regulatory Status

VETERINARY-LABELED PRODUCTS:

Danofloxacin Mesylate: 180 mg/mL (of danofloxacin) in 100 mL and 250 mL multidose vials; *Advocin®*; (Rx). FDA-approved for use in beef cattle only. Not for use in cattle intended for dairy production or calves to be processed for veal. When administered per the label directions, slaughter withdrawal = 4 days from the last treatment.

HUMAN-LABELED PRODUCTS: NONE

References

For the complete list of references, see **wiley.com/go/budde/plumb**

Dantrolene

(***dan***-troe-leen) *Dantrium*®
Skeletal Muscle Relaxant

Prescriber Highlights

- Direct-acting muscle relaxant
- Primary indications: horses: post-anesthesia myositis/acute rhabdomyolysis; dogs and cats: functional urethral obstruction, potentially rhabdomyolysis
- Use with extreme caution in animals with hepatic dysfunction. Caution in patients with severe cardiac dysfunction or pulmonary disease
- Adverse effects: weakness, sedation, increased urinary frequency, GI effects. Hepatotoxicity possible especially with chronic use

Uses/Indications

In humans, oral dantrolene is indicated primarily for the treatment of conditions associated with upper motor neuron disorders (eg, multiple sclerosis, cerebral palsy, spinal cord injuries).[1,2] In veterinary medicine, its proposed indications include prevention and treatment of malignant hyperthermia syndrome in various species, treatment of functional urethral obstruction due to increased external urethral tone in dogs and cats, prevention and treatment of equine post-anesthetic myositis (PAM) and equine exertional rhabdomyolysis. Dantrolene has also been recommended for use in the treatment of bites from black widow spiders in small animals and for the treatment of porcine stress syndrome.

Pharmacology/Actions

Dantrolene exhibits muscle relaxation activity by direct action on muscle. Although the exact mechanism is not well understood, it probably acts on skeletal muscle by interfering with the release of calcium from the sarcoplasmic reticulum. It has no discernible effects on the respiratory or cardiovascular systems, but can cause drowsiness and dizziness; the reasons for these CNS effects are not known.

Pharmacokinetics

After intragastric administration to horses, bioavailability is ≈39%. The drug is slowly absorbed, with peak concentrations occurring within ≈1.5 hours in horses. Oral dantrolene absorption can be affected by food. Although there was considerable interpatient variation in the results, a study concluded that, where possible, feed restriction before nasogastric dantrolene administration should be avoided or should not exceed 4 hours. Oral dantrolene has a half-life of ≈3 to 4 hours in horses.

In the dog, oral administration is well tolerated, and the drug is rapidly absorbed. A 5 mg/kg and 10 mg/kg dose PO had a peak plasma concentration of 0.43 µg/mL and 0.65 µg/mL, respectively and the terminal half-life was 1.26 hours and 1.21 hours, respectively. However, there was large interpatient variability on all parameters.

In humans, bioavailability of dantrolene after oral administration is ≈35%. Peak concentrations occur ≈5 hours after oral administration. The drug is substantially bound to plasma proteins (principally albumin). The elimination half-life in humans is ≈8 hours. Dantrolene is metabolized in the liver and metabolites are excreted in the urine. Only ≈1% of the parent drug is excreted unchanged in the urine and bile.

Contraindications/Precautions/Warnings

Because dantrolene can cause hepatotoxicity, it should be used with extreme caution in patients with preexisting liver disease and with caution in patients with severe cardiac dysfunction or pulmonary disease.

Dantrolene injection has a high pH (9.5 or higher); care must be taken to prevent extravasation at the infusion site.[3]

Adverse Effects

The most significant adverse effect is hepatotoxicity. In humans, this effect is most commonly associated with high-dose chronic therapy but may also be seen after short-term high dose therapy. The incidence of this reaction is unknown in veterinary medicine but monitor for its occurrence.

Hyperkalemia has been reported in dogs and horses receiving dantrolene IV.[4,5]

More common, but less significant, are the CNS associated signs of weakness, sedation, dizziness, headache, and GI effects (diarrhea, nausea, vomiting).[1,2,6] Also seen are increased urinary frequency and, possibly, hypotension.

Reproductive/Nursing Safety

Dantrolene readily crosses the placenta, reaching roughly equivalent fetal and maternal blood concentrations. The drug reduced pup survival in rats and demonstrated embryocidal effects in rabbits.[7]

Dantrolene is distributed into milk; safe use cannot be assured during nursing.[1,2,6]

Because safety has not been established in animals, this drug should only be used when the maternal benefits outweigh the potential risks to offspring.

Overdose/Acute Toxicity

There is no specific antidotal therapy to dantrolene overdoses, therefore, remove the drug from the gut if possible and treat supportively.

For patients that have experienced or are suspected to have experienced an overdose, consultation with a 24-hour poison consultation center specializing in providing veterinary-specific information is recommended. For general information related to overdose and toxin exposures, as well as contact information for poison control centers, refer to ***Appendix.***

Drug Interactions

The following drug interactions have either been reported or are theoretical in humans or animals receiving dantrolene and may be of significance in veterinary patients. Unless otherwise noted, use together is not necessarily contraindicated, but weigh the potential risks and perform additional monitoring when appropriate.

- **BENZODIAZEPINES** (eg, **diazepam, midazolam**): Increased sedation may be seen if tranquilizing agents are used concomitantly with dantrolene.
- **CALCIUM CHANNEL BLOCKERS** (eg, **amlodipine, diltiazem, verapamil**): Rare reports of severe hyperkalemia with cardiovascular collapse in humans; concomitant use with dantrolene during malignant hyperthermia crises not recommended.
- **CNS DEPRESSANTS** (eg, **acepromazine, cannabidiol, dexmedetomidine, methocarbamol, phenobarbital**): Increased sedation may be seen.
- **ESTROGENS** (eg, **diethylstilbestrol [DES], estriol**): Increased risks for hepatotoxicity from dantrolene have been seen in women younger than 35 years of age that are also receiving estrogen therapy; veterinary significance is unknown.
- **OPIOIDS** (eg, **fentanyl, morphine**): Increased sedation may be seen if tranquilizing agents are used concomitantly with dantrolene.
- **VECURONIUM**: Dantrolene may potentiate neuromuscular blockade.

Laboratory Considerations

None noted

Dosages

DOGS:

Canine stress syndrome (CSS), malignant hyperthermia (MH); (extra-label):

a) Acute attack: 0.2 – 3 mg/kg IV
b) MH-like syndrome associated with hops (*Humulus lupulus*) ingestion: 2 – 3 mg/kg IV or 3.5 mg/kg PO as soon as possible after ingestion.

Adjunctive treatment of rhabdomyolysis (extra-label): 1.5 mg/kg PO every 8 hours (from a case report; very intensive drug and supportive therapy used).

Functional urethral obstruction due to increased external urethral tone (extra-label): 1 – 5 mg/kg PO every 8 to 12 hours; limited evidence to support this dosage.

CATS:

Functional urethral obstruction due to increased external urethral tone (extra-label):

a) 1 mg/kg IV as a single dose was effective in male cats under experimental conditions.[8,9] May be given with prazosin[8]
b) 0.5 – 2 mg/kg PO every 12 hours; limited evidence to support this dosage.

HORSES:

Rhabdomyolysis prevention (all dosages are extra-label):

a) Thoroughbreds: 4 mg/kg PO or via NG tube. Feed restriction before nasogastric dantrolene administration should be avoided or should not exceed 4 hours.[10]
b) 800 mg/horse (NOT mg/kg); within 30 minutes prior to administration, mix contents of capsules with 9 mL tap water to make a suspension and given PO one hour before exercise.
c) Several dosage regimens have been recommended, but caution should be used, as use and efficacy are uncertain: 2 mg/kg PO once daily for 3 to 5 days and then every third day for a month has been recommended. Drug is diluted in normal saline and given via stomach tube. Another dosage recommendation is 300 mg/horse (NOT mg/kg) PO once daily (may be preferable because the drug is hepatotoxic). Another recommendation is 500 mg/horse (NOT mg/kg) PO for 3 to 5 days and then 300 mg/horse (NOT mg/kg) PO every third day. Monitor hepatic function and status.

Prevention of post-anesthetic myositis (PAM); (extra-label): To prevent muscle damage in horses undergoing hypotensive anesthesia: 4 – 6 mg/kg enterally (in 2 L of water given via NG tube) 60 to 90 minutes prior to general anesthesia.[11] Dantrolene reduces muscle damage in horses undergoing general anesthesia without inhibiting anesthetic recovery, but because it decreases cardiac output and can precipitate hyperkalemia and arrhythmias, this practice is currently discouraged. If horses susceptible to hyperkalemic paralysis need to be treated before the anesthetic is administered, cardiovascular parameters should be closely monitored.

RABBITS:

Functional urethral obstruction due to increased external urethral tone (extra-label): 10 mg/kg intraperitoneally as soon as possible (preferably within 1 hour) after spinal cord injury, along with 30 mg/kg IV methylprednisolone sodium succinate

Monitoring

- Baseline and periodic liver chemistry panel if to be used chronically or using high dosages
- Serum potassium
- Body temperature for patients with malignant hyperthermia
- Urine volume, frequency, continence

Client Information

- Drowsiness, vomiting, diarrhea,[3] and a greater need to urinate are the most likely side effects.
- Liver toxicity can rarely occur. If your animal shows signs of extreme lack of energy, frequent vomiting (small animals), not eating, bleeding, or yellow discoloration of the whites of the eyes, gums, or skin (jaundice), contact your veterinarian immediately.

Chemistry/Synonyms

A hydantoin derivative that is dissimilar structurally and pharmacologically to other skeletal muscle relaxant drugs, dantrolene sodium is a weak acid with a pK_a of 7.5. It occurs as an odorless, tasteless, orange, fine powder that is slightly soluble in water. It rapidly hydrolyzes in aqueous solutions to the free acid form that precipitates out of solution.

Dantrolene Sodium may also be known by the following synonyms and internationally registered trade names: F-440, F-368, *Danlene*®, *Dantamacrin*®, *Dantralen*®, or *Dantrolen*®.

Storage/Stability

Dantrolene products should be stored at room temperature 20°C to 25°C (68°F-77°F). Dantrolene capsules should be stored in well-closed containers. Dantrolene powder for injection should protected from prolonged exposure to light. After reconstitution with sterile water for injection, the powder for injection should be used within 6 hours when stored at room temperature and should be protected from direct light.

Compatibility/Compounding Considerations

To dose small dogs or cats, it has been suggested to re-encapsulate ⅛ to ¼ of the contents of a 25 mg capsule and place into a size 2 or 4 gelatin capsule.

Dantrolene powder for injection is **incompatible** with either 0.9% sodium chloride or 5% dextrose injection.[1,2]

Dosage Forms/Regulatory Status

VETERINARY-LABELED PRODUCTS:

The Association of Racing Commissioners International (ARCI) has designated this drug as a class 4 substance. Use of this drug may not be allowed in certain animal competitions. Check rules and regulations before entering in a competition while this medication is being administered. Contact local racing authorities for further guidance. See ***Appendix*** for further information.

HUMAN-LABELED PRODUCTS:

Dantrolene Sodium Oral Capsules: 25 mg, 50 mg, and 100 mg; *Dantrium*®, generic; (Rx)

Dantrolene Sodium Powder for Injection Solution: 20 mg/vial (≈0.32 mg/mL dantrolene after reconstitution; with mannitol 3 g/vial) in 70 mL vials; *Dantrium® Intravenous, Revonto*®; (Rx).

Dantrolene Sodium Powder Injectable Suspension: 50 mg/mL in 5 mL vials (250 mg dantrolene sodium per vial); *Ryanodex*®; (Rx).

References

For the complete list of references, see **wiley.com/go/budde/plumb**

Dapsone

Diaminodiphenyl sulfone (DDS)

(*dap*-sone)

Antimycobacterial Antibiotic

Prescriber Highlights

- May be useful for treating protozoal (*Pneumocystis* spp) infections, brown recluse spider bites, and cutaneous vasculitis; however, it is rarely used due to potential for severe adverse effects
- Not recommended for use in cats due to severe adverse effects
- Adverse effects include hepatotoxicity, methemoglobinemia, anemia, thrombocytopenia, neutropenia, GI effects, neuropathies, and cutaneous drug eruptions; photosensitivity reactions are possible.

Uses/Indications

Because of its leukocyte inhibitory characteristics, dapsone may be useful for adjunctive treatment of brown recluse spider (*Loxosceles reclusa*) bites,[1,2] or when an underlying etiology causing cutaneous vasculitis cannot be determined[3,4]; however, it is rarely used in veterinary medicine and little safety or efficacy information is available.

In a foal, dapsone has been used to treat *Pneumocystis jiroveci* (formerly *Pneumocystis carinii*) infection.[5]

In humans, dapsone has been used as a second-line treatment for immune-mediated thrombocytopenia.

The World Health Organization (WHO) has designated dapsone as a Highly Important antimicrobial for human medicine.[6]

Pharmacology/Actions

Dapsone's antimicrobial actions are thought to be due to inhibition of the synthesis of dihydrofolic acid via competition with para-aminobenzoate for the active site of dihydropteroate synthetase. Dapsone also decreases neutrophil chemotaxis, complement activation, antibody production, and lysosomal enzyme synthesis. The mechanisms for these actions are not well understood. Dapsone is both bactericidal and bacteriostatic against *Mycobacterium leprae.*

Pharmacokinetics

After oral administration to dogs, dapsone is rapidly and completely absorbed.[7] Elimination half-life ranges from about 6 to 10 hours. In humans, the monoacetyl metabolite is almost completely bound to plasma proteins, but in dogs, it is only about 60% bound. Dapsone is primarily eliminated via the kidneys as conjugates and unidentified metabolites. Half-life in dogs is ≈6 to 10 hours, and in humans is widely variable and ranges from about 10 to 50 hours.[8]

Contraindications/Precautions/Warnings

Because of increased incidences of neurotoxicity and hemolytic anemia, dapsone is generally not recommended for use in cats.[9]

Dapsone is contraindicated in patients that are hypersensitive to it or other sulfone drugs.[8] It should not be used in patients with severe anemias or other preexisting blood dyscrasias. Because of its potential for causing hepatic toxicity, dapsone should be used with caution in animals with preexisting hepatic dysfunction.

Adverse Effects

Adverse effects include hepatotoxicity, dose-dependent methemoglobinemia, hemolytic anemia, thrombocytopenia, neutropenia, GI effects, and neuropathies.[8] A dog developed a fatal bleeding diathesis after 6 days of dapsone treatment for skin disease, and evidence suggested dapsone-induced destruction of the dog's platelets and megakaryocytes.[10] Cutaneous drug eruptions are due to sensitization to dapsone. Photosensitivity is possible. Dapsone is a potential carcinogen.

Reproductive/Nursing Safety

In pregnant animals, dapsone should be used with caution. Animal studies have apparently not been performed with dapsone to determine its effects during pregnancy.[8]

Dapsone is excreted into milk in concentrations equivalent to those found in plasma,[8] and hemolytic reactions have been seen in human neonates. Consider switching to milk replacer if dapsone is required in a nursing dam.

Because safety has not been established in animals, this drug should only be used when the maternal benefits outweigh the potential risks to offspring.

Overdose/Acute Toxicity

Because of its toxicity potential and species-specific differences in sensitivity and pharmacokinetics, it is recommended to contact an animal poison control center in cases of dapsone overdoses. In humans, dapsone overdoses generally cause nausea, vomiting, and hyperexcitability that can occur within minutes of an overdose. Methemoglobinemia with associated depression, seizures, and cyanosis can occur. Hemolysis may be delayed, occurring from 7 to 14 days after the overdose. Treatment in humans involves removal of the drug from the GI tract including use of activated charcoal, methylene blue for methemoglobinemia, and, sometimes, hemodialysis to enhance removal of the drug and the monoacetyl metabolite.

For patients that have experienced or are suspected to have experienced an overdose, consultation with a 24-hour poison control center specializing in providing veterinary-specific information is recommended. For general information related to overdose and toxin exposures, as well as contact information for poison control centers, refer to ***Appendix.***

Drug Interactions

The following drug interactions either have been reported or are theoretical in humans or animals receiving dapsone and may be of significance in veterinary patients. Unless otherwise noted, use together is not necessarily contraindicated, but weigh the potential risks and perform additional monitoring when appropriate.

- **Clofazimine**: There is weak evidence that suggests dapsone may reduce the anti-inflammatory effects of clofazimine; clinical significance is unclear.
- **Methotrexate**: May increase risk for hematologic reactions occurring with dapsone
- **Probenecid**: May decrease the renal excretion of active metabolites of dapsone
- **Pyrimethamine**: May increase risk for hematologic reactions occurring with dapsone
- **Rifampin**: May decrease plasma dapsone concentrations (7- to 10-fold)
- **Trimethoprim**: May increase plasma concentrations of both drugs and potentially increase each other's toxicity
- **Warfarin**: May increase anticoagulant effects

Laboratory Considerations

- No specific laboratory interactions or considerations are noted.

Dosages

DOGS:

Immunomodulatory agent for cutaneous conditions (eg, **cutaneous vasculitis;** extra-label): 1 – 1.1 mg/kg PO every 8 hours initially.[3,4] May be used in combination with other immunomodulating drugs (eg, prednis(ol)one). Once remission occurs, taper to lowest effective dose frequency (eg, once daily). Evidence is relatively weak to support the use of dapsone in this situation.

Adjunctive treatment of brown recluse spider (*Loxosceles* spp) bite (extra-label): 1 mg/kg PO 3 times daily for 10 to 14 days[1,2]

HORSES:

***Pneumocystis carinii* pneumonia in foals** (extra-label): 3 mg/kg PO every 24 hours. **NOTE**: This dosage is from one case report of a foal treated for 56 days.[5]

Monitoring

- Baseline and periodic CBC with platelets: every 2 to 3 weeks during first 4 months of treatment and then every 3 to 4 months
- Baseline and periodic serum liver chemistry profile during treatment
- Adverse effects (eg, vomiting, diarrhea, cutaneous drug eruptions, neurotoxicity)
- Efficacy based on improvement of clinical condition

Client Information

- Clients should understand that limited experience has occurred with dapsone in animals; serious toxicity is possible.
- Because photosensitivity can occur, exposed skin should be protected from prolonged exposure to sunlight.

Chemistry/Synonyms

A sulfone antimycobacterial/antiprotozoan, dapsone occurs as a white or creamy-white odorless crystalline powder. It is very slightly soluble in water, freely soluble in alcohol, and insoluble in fixed or vegetable oils.

Dapsone may also be known as DADPS, dapsonum, DDS, diaminodiphenylsulfone, NSC-6091, diaphenylsulfone, disulone, sulfonyldianiline, *Avlosulfone*®, *Daps*®, *Dapsoderm-X*®, *Dopsan*®, *Novasulfone*®, *Servidapsone*®, and *Sulfona*®.

Storage/Stability

Dapsone tablets should be stored protected from light at controlled room temperature between 20°C and 25°C (68°F-77°F).

Compatibility/Compounding Considerations

Dapsone tablets may be compounded into a stable liquid dosage form. The simplest method is to use a 1:1 ratio of *Ora-Plus*®:*Ora-Sweet*® and use crushed tablets to make a concentration of 2 mg/mL. This preparation is stable either stored refrigerated or at room temperature for 90 days.[11]

Dosage Forms/Regulatory Status

VETERINARY-LABELED PRODUCTS: NONE

HUMAN-LABELED PRODUCTS:

Dapsone Oral Tablets: 25 mg and 100 mg (scored); generic; (Rx)

Gel formulations for topical application are also available.

References

For the complete list of references, see **wiley.com/go/budde/plumb**

Darbepoetin Alfa

(***dar***-beh-***poe***-eh-tin ***al***-fah) *Aranesp*®

Erythropoiesis-stimulating Agent

Prescriber Highlights

- Biosynthetic erythropoietic agent potentially useful for treating anemia associated with chronic kidney disease in dogs and cats
- May be less immunogenic in dogs and cats than epoetin alfa (epoetin)
- Longer duration of effect as compared with epoetin; initially only dosed once per week
- Considerably more expensive than epoetin, and treatment expense may be formidable

Uses/Indications

Darbepoetin is used to treat normocytic, normochromic non-regenerative anemia associated with chronic kidney disease (CKD) in dogs and cats. Chronic anemia has been shown to be a contributing factor in the progression of CKD and has been associated with conditions related to chronic hypoxia (eg, poor appetite, diminished overall health). It is recommended to initiate darbepoetin therapy in dogs and cats with CKD when clinical signs associated with anemia are present or when PCV is less than 20%.[1,2]

A retrospective study in dogs with CKD found that 85% of treated dogs attained packed cell volumes greater than or equal to 30%.[3] One group with experience of treating over 70 cats with epoetin or darbepoetin reported that only about 60% to 65% of treated cats had an adequate response.[4] Another study describing the use of blood products in dogs and cats was unable to demonstrate a reduction in blood transfusion due to erythropoiesis-stimulating agents.[5]

Darbepoetin has largely replaced the use of epoetin alfa (epoetin) due to a 3-fold longer half-life, allowing for less frequent dosing. Additionally, it may be less immunogenic than epoetin.[6,7]

Pharmacology/Actions

Darbepoetin is a hyperglycosylated synthetic human recombinant erythropoietin analogue. It stimulates erythropoiesis using the same mechanism as endogenous erythropoietin by interacting with progenitor stem cells to increase RBC production. Darbepoetin may be less immunogenic in animals than epoetin,[6,7] secondary to its formulation, which utilizes carbohydrates as part of its structure. Theoretically, carbohydrates may shield the sites on the drug of greatest antigenic potential from immune cell detection.

Carbohydrates also increase the solubility and stability of the compound, causing less aggregate formation and, therefore, potentially less immunogenicity. Additionally, despite a four-fold lower EPO receptor binding activity compared to epoetin, PK studies in dogs and mice show that darbepoetin is 13- to 14-fold more potent allowing for lower dosages.[8]

Pharmacokinetics

In dogs, IV darbepoetin has an elimination half-life of 25 hours, which is 3.5 times that of epoetin, and clearance is also correspondingly reduced.[8] No information has been noted for cats.

In humans with chronic kidney disease, bioavailability after subcutaneous injection is about 37%, and the drug is absorbed slowly with a distribution half-life of about 1.4 hours.[9] It is extensively metabolized, and the terminal elimination half-life averages 21 hours after IV administration and 70 hours following SC dosing.[9] Terminal half-life is approximately 3 times greater than that of epoetin, allowing for less frequent dosing.[8]

Contraindications/Precautions/Warnings

Darbepoetin should not be used in dogs or cats with documented anti-epoetin antibodies. Antibody formation diagnosis is based upon high myeloid:erythroid ratio on bone marrow cytology and exclusion of other causes of anemia. In humans, darbepoetin is contraindicated in patients hypersensitive to it or to excipients in the formulation, in those with uncontrolled hypertension, and in patients in whom pure red cell aplasia begins after treatments with erythropoietin or darbepoetin.[9]

Adequate iron stores are necessary for efficacy. Most clinicians prefer using injectable iron dextran rather than oral iron products for this purpose. Iron deficiency may be most relevant after initiation of darbepoetin treatment because of consumption of iron stores in the therapeutically induced regenerative response.[10]

In humans, darbepoetin use is associated with an increased risk of death, serious cardiovascular events (eg, myocardial infarction, stroke, venous thrombosis), and progression of certain tumors[9]; the relevance of these findings for veterinary patients is uncertain. Using the lowest possible darbepoetin dose to avoid transfusion is recommended. Quality of life and patient well-being have not been demonstrated in humans.

Do not confuse darbepoetin with epoetin alfa or dalteparin.

Adverse Effects

Potential adverse effects include anti-epoetin antibody formation with resultant pure red blood cell aplasia (PRCA), injection site reactions, polycythemia, hypertension, seizures, or iron deficiency. A retrospective study conducted in 33 dogs with chronic kidney disease (CKD) found increased blood pressure (36%), seizures (15%), and vomiting and/or diarrhea (9%). Pure red cell aplasia developed in 2 (6%) treated dogs.[7]

Anecdotally, PRCA is reported to occur less often than with epoetin. One source states that the incidence of PRCA is about 25% to 30% in dogs and cats receiving epoetin and less than 10% with darbepoetin.[6] PRCA can be difficult to treat, but immediate discontinuation of epoetin or darbepoetin is required. Immunosuppressive therapy and blood transfusions can potentially help, but the long-term prognosis is often grave.

Hypertension is reported to occur in up to 50% of dogs and cats treated with darbepoetin. Hypertension may be a result of increased blood viscosity and cardiac output and decreased anemia-mediated vasodilation; it may also be a sequela to CKD in advanced stages. Seizures may occur in response to hypertension.

Reproductive/Nursing Safety

Due to its high molecular weight, darbepoetin is unlikely to cross the placenta or be distributed into milk.

Studies performed in pregnant rats and rabbits demonstrated no overt teratogenicity at daily doses of up to 20 μg/kg IV. However, increased early post-implantation loss was noted with doses of 0.5 mg/kg three times per week. Decreased body weights were noted in some rat pups.

It is unknown if darbepoetin is distributed into milk, but it is unlikely to pose much risk to nursing animals.

Overdose/Acute Toxicity

Little information is available. Humans have received therapeutic dosages of up to 8 μg/kg every week for 12 weeks. Polycythemia and severe hypertension have been reported in humans, and therapeutic phlebotomy may be required; veterinary significance is unclear.

For patients that have experienced or are suspected to have experienced an overdose, consultation with a 24-hour poison consultation center specializing in providing veterinary-specific information is recommended. For general information related to overdose and toxin exposures, as well as contact information for poison control centers, refer to ***Appendix***.

Drug Interactions

The following drug interactions have either been reported or are theoretical in humans or animals receiving epoetin (a related compound) and may be of significance in veterinary patients. Unless otherwise noted, use together is not necessarily contraindicated, but weigh the potential risks and perform additional monitoring when appropriate.

- **ANDROGENS** (eg, **danazol, testosterone**): May increase the sensitivity of erythroid progenitors; this interaction has been used for therapeutic effect. **NOTE**: This effect has not been confirmed in well-controlled studies, nor has the safety of this combination been determined.
- **CYCLOSPORINE:** May cause additive increases in blood pressure. Additionally, may alter cyclosporine blood levels, as cyclosporine is bound by red blood cells.
- **PROBENECID**: Probenecid has been demonstrated to reduce the renal tubular excretion of EPO; clinical significance remains unclear.

Laboratory Considerations

- No specific lab issues have been identified; see ***Contraindications*** and ***Monitoring*** for more information.

Dosages

DOGS:

Stimulate erythropoiesis in anemia associated with CKD (extra-label): 0.5 – 0.8 μg/kg SC weekly (the higher dosage appears to be more effective).[7] Once the target PCV range is met, the dosing frequency can be extended to the longest interval, which maintains a stable maintenance target for PCV (eg, every 14 or every 21 days). A dosing interval greater than 21 days is unlikely to maintain an effective target PCV long-term.[7] Iron supplementation is recommended.[10] See ***Ferrous Sulfate*** or ***Iron Dextran***.

CATS:

Stimulate erythropoiesis in anemia associated with CKD (extra-label): 1 μg/kg SC once weekly.[11,12] Other recommendations have ranged from 0.25 – 1.5 μg/kg SC per week.[13-15] Once the target PCV range is met, the dosing frequency can be extended to the longest interval, which maintains a stable maintenance target for PCV (eg, every 14 or every 21 days). Iron supplementation is recommended. [6,12,13,16-18] ***See Ferrous Sulfate*** or ***Iron Dextran***.

Monitoring

- **PCV.** Check PCV prior to each dose of darbepoetin or at least until PCV is stable, and then once monthly.
  - A PCV greater than or equal to 30% or a greater than or equal to 10% change in PCV from baseline have been suggested as a positive response for dogs.[12]
  - PCV target goals vary; 25% to 35%[19] and 35% to 40%[14] have been suggested. Ideally, an increase in PCV of no more than 3% per week is suggested as greater increases may increase the risks for hypertension.
- Consider performing reticulocyte counts during the induction phase, but it has been reported that reticulocyte counts in cats receiving darbepoetin may not reflect efficacy.[4]
- Measure baseline and periodic serum ferritin concentrations or supplement with iron. See ***Ferrous Sulfate*** or ***Iron Dextran***.
- Baseline and periodic (every 1-2 months) blood pressure

Client Information

- Injectable (subcutaneous; under the skin) medicine used to treat anemia (too few red blood cells) caused by end-stage kidney failure. This medicine may take several weeks to work. Your veterinarian will need to closely monitor your animal while it is receiving this medicine. Do not miss these important follow-up visits.
- This medicine may cause your animal's immune system to interfere with how well this medicine works. Your veterinarian will monitor for this with blood tests during follow-up visits. At home, watch for skin reactions at the site of the shot.
- Contact your veterinarian immediately if your animal has seizures (convulsions), has loss of vision (bumping into furniture), appears unwell, has a low energy level, is unable to walk, or has a poor appetite.

Chemistry/Synonyms

Darbepoetin alfa is a 165 amino acid protein that is produced using recombinant DNA technology in Chinese hamster ovary cells. Two additional N-linked oligosaccharide chains are added to human erythropoietin, yielding a glycoprotein with a molecular weight of ≈37,000.

Darbepoetin may also be known by the following synonyms: NESP, novel erythropoiesis-stimulating protein, darbepoetina, or darbepoetinum. Internationally registered trade names include *Aranesp®* and *Nespo®*.

Storage/Stability

The commercially available injection solutions (polysorbate-based) should be stored in the refrigerator at 2 to 8°C (36°F-46°F) and protected from light. Do not freeze or shake.

Compatibility/Compounding Considerations

No specific information has been noted. Do not dilute or administer with other compounds.

Dosage Forms/Regulatory Status

VETERINARY-LABELED PRODUCTS: NONE

The Association of Racing Commissioners International (ARCI) has designated this drug as a class 1 substance. It is also prohibited on the premises of a racing facility. See ***Appendix*** for more information.

HUMAN-LABELED PRODUCTS:

Darbepoetin Alfa Solution for Injection (preservative-free; albumin-free); *Aranesp®*; (Rx). The needle cover on prefilled syringes contains natural rubber.

10 µg in single-dose prefilled syringes (0.4 mL)

25 µg in single-dose prefilled syringes (0.42 mL) and single-dose vials (1 mL)

40 µg in single-dose prefilled syringes (0.4 mL) and single-dose vials (1 mL)

60 µg in single-dose prefilled syringes (0.3 mL) and single-dose vials (1 mL)

100 µg in single-dose prefilled syringes (0.5 mL) and single-dose vials (1 mL)

150 µg in single-dose prefilled syringes (0.3 mL)

200 µg in single-dose prefilled syringes (0.4 mL) and single-dose vials (1 mL)

300 µg in single-dose prefilled syringes (0.6 mL) and single-dose vials (1 mL)

500 µg in single-dose prefilled syringes (1 mL)

References

For the complete list of references, see **wiley.com/go/budde/plumb**

Decoquinate

(de-koe-***kwin***-ate) *Deccox®*

Antiprotozoal/Coccidiostat

Prescriber Highlights

- Not FDA-approved for dairy animals that produce milk for human consumption or laying chickens that produce eggs for human consumption
- Not effective against the sexual stage of coccidia development
- No effect on clinical coccidiosis; results in treating calves with cryptosporidiosis have been disappointing.

Uses/Indications

Decoquinate is labeled for the prevention of coccidiosis caused by certain pathogenic *Eimeria* spp in cattle (including ruminating and nonruminating calves and veal calves), young goats and sheep, and broiler chickens.

In dogs, decoquinate may be used as adjunctive treatment for hepatozoonosis.[1,2] Decoquinate is being investigated for the treatment of *Sarcocystis neurona* in horses[3] and myositis due to *Sarcocystis* spp in dogs.

Pharmacology/Actions

Decoquinate is a 4-hydroxy quinolone agent that has anticoccidial activity. Decoquinate acts on *Eimeria* spp sporozoites (released from ingested oocysts) and on first-generation meronts to arrest development through disruption of electron transport and respiration in coccidial mitochondria and thus, prevent release of merozoites. The sporozoites can apparently still penetrate the host intestinal cell, but further development is prevented.

Pharmacokinetics

Decoquinate is minimally absorbed from the GI tract of chickens and is primarily eliminated in the feces. The absorbed drug is widely distributed to tissues, in particular skin and adipose tissue. Elimination of absorbed drug is through bile and, to a much lesser extent, urine.

Contraindications/Precautions/Warnings

Decoquinate is not effective for treating clinical coccidiosis and has no efficacy against the sexual stage of coccidia development. Decoquinate is not FDA-approved for use in animals producing milk for human consumption or in laying chickens.

Adverse Effects

No adverse effects listed when given as directed.

Reproductive/Nursing Safety

Decoquinate did not impair fertility in laboratory animals, but embryotoxicity was noted.

Because safety has not been established in animals, this drug should only be used when the maternal benefits outweigh the potential risks to offspring.

Overdose/Acute Toxicity

Decoquinate is considered to have a wide safety margin. Rats receiving single doses up to 5000 mg/kg orally developed no clinical signs of toxicity and had no noted postmortem pathological changes. Pneumonia developed in rats but not beagles receiving 1000 to 2000 mg/kg PO per day in studies lasting up to 2 years, with no other clinical or pathological changes noted.

For patients that have experienced or are suspected to have experienced an overdose, consultation with a 24-hour poison consultation center specializing in providing veterinary-specific information is recommended. For general information related to overdose and toxin exposures, as well as contact information for poison control centers, refer to ***Appendix.***

Drug Interactions

- None noted

Laboratory Considerations

- None noted

Dosages

DOGS:

NOTE: When using decoquinate for dogs, obtain decoquinate 6% (27.2 g/lb) powder. An approximate conversion is ¼ teaspoonful is equivalent to ≈45 mg decoquinate, and 1 teaspoonful (5 mL) is equivalent to ≈180 mg decoquinate.

American canine hepatozoonosis (ACH; *Hepatozoon americanum*) (extra-label): **Initially**, administer a 14-day treatment with **either** ponazuril 10 mg/kg every 12 hours **OR** a triple combination (TCP) of trimethoprim/sulfadiazine 15 mg/kg PO every 12 hours, clindamycin 10 mg/kg PO every 8 hours, and pyrimethamine 0.25 mg/kg PO every 24 hours ***followed by*** 2 years of decoquinate 10 – 20 mg/kg PO twice daily mixed in food.[2] Although this treatment regimen is not curative, it extends life expectancy and improves the quality of life for many ACH patients. Should clinical relapse occur, repeat TCP or ponazuril treatment again followed by long-term decoquinate.[4]

Canine sarcocystosis myositis (from a case report; 2 dogs) (extra-label)**:** From a case report of 2 dogs, decoquinate 10 – 20 mg/kg PO every 12 hours appeared to be effective in 1 dog. The dog also received clindamycin initially (discontinued after 3 months on decoquinate) and tramadol.[5]

CATTLE:

Prevention of coccidiosis in ruminating and nonruminating calves (including veal calves) and cattle caused by *Eimeria bovis* and *Eimeria zuernii* (label dosage; FDA-approved): 0.5 mg/kg PO once daily in milk or mixed in feed.[6] Administer for at least 28 days during periods of coccidiosis exposure or when experience indicates that coccidiosis is likely to be a hazard. Coccidiostats are not indicated for use in adult animals due to continuous previous exposure.

Treatment of coccidiosis in calves (extra-label): 1 mg/kg in feed PO daily for at least 28 days[7,8]

Cryptosporidium in calves (extra-label): 2 mg/kg PO twice daily for 21 days[9]

SHEEP/GOATS:

Prevention of coccidiosis in young sheep caused by *Eimeria ovinoidalis*, *Eimeria crandallis*, *Eimeria parva*, and *Eimeria bakuensis* (label dosage; FDA-approved): 0.5 mg/kg PO per day mixed in feed.[6] Feed for at least 28 days during periods of coccidiosis exposure or when experience indicates that coccidiosis is likely to be a hazard.

Prevention of coccidiosis in young goats caused by *Eimeria christenseni* and *Eimeria ninakohlyakimovae* (label dosage; FDA-approved): 0.5 mg/kg PO per day mixed in feed.[6] Feed for at least 28 days during periods of coccidiosis exposure or when experience indicates that coccidiosis is likely to be a hazard.

Prevention or treatment of coccidiosis in lambs (extra-label): Treatment: 1 mg/kg in feed PO daily for at least 28 days[7,10,11]; Prevention: 0.5 mg/kg in feed PO daily for at least 28 days[11]

Aid in the prevention of abortions and perinatal losses caused by toxoplasmosis in ewes (extra-label)**:** 2 mg/kg daily in feed continuously for 14 weeks prior to lambing[7,10]

CAMELIDS:

Prophylaxis of coccidiosis in llamas (extra-label): 0.5 mg/kg daily in feed for at least 28 days[12]

CHICKENS:

Prevention of coccidiosis in broiler chickens caused by *Eimeria tenella*, *Eimeria necatrix*, *Eimeria acervulina*, *Eimeria mivati*, *Eimeria maxima*, and *Eimeria brunetti* (label dosage; FDA-approved): Thoroughly mix 0.45 kg (1 lb) in each ton of complete ration and feed continuously.[6]

Monitoring

- Efficacy
- Adverse effects

Client Information

- Decoquinate should be administered for at least 4 weeks when it is used for preventing coccidiosis outbreaks.
- When decoquinate is used in dogs for hepatozoonosis, treatment may need to continue for up to 2 years.
- Mix this medicine well into food or milk. When this medicine is mixed into milk, prepare fresh each day, and feed immediately after mixing. Discard unused portions. Not for use in bulk feeding systems.
- Do not feed this medicine to cows, sheep, or goats that produce milk for human consumption, or to laying hens that produce eggs for human consumption.

Chemistry/Synonyms

A coccidiostat, decoquinate occurs as a cream to buff-colored fine amorphous powder with a slight odor. It is insoluble in water and practically insoluble in alcohol.

Decoquinate may also be known as HC-1528, M&B-15497, or *Deccox®*.

Storage/Stability

Follow label storage directions; store in a cool, dry place, preferably in airtight containers.

Compatibility/Compounding Considerations

Compatibility is dependent on factors such as pH, concentration, temperature, and diluent used; specialized references or a hospital pharmacist should be consulted for more specific information.

Decoquinate is reportedly **incompatible** with strong bases or oxidizing material and is **incompatible** with feeds containing bentonite binders. *Deccox®* is labeled as being **compatible** (and cleared for use) with bacitracin zinc (with or without roxarsone), chlortetracycline, and lincomycin.

Dosage Forms/Regulatory Status

VETERINARY-LABELED PRODUCTS:

Decoquinate 6% (27.2 g/lb) Type A Medicated Article (with corn meal, soybean oil, lecithin, and silicon dioxide) in 22.7-kg (50-lb) bags; *Deccox®*; (OTC). FDA-approved for use in cattle, sheep, goats (**DO NOT** feed to cows, goats, or sheep that produce milk for food), and chickens (NOT laying chickens).

Decoquinate 0.5% (2.271 g/lb) Type B Medicated Feed in 22.7-kg (50-lb) bags; *Deccox®-L*; (OTC). FDA-approved for use in ruminating and nonruminating calves and cattle. **DO NOT** feed to cows that produce milk for food.

Decoquinate 0.8% (3.632 g/lb) Medicated Powder for Whole Milk in 2.3-kg (5-lb) and 22.7-kg (50-lb) bags; *Deccox®M*; (OTC). FDA-approved for use in ruminating and nonruminating calves, including veal calves.

Decoquinate (6.8 mg/lb) Medicated Milk Replacer in 22.7-kg (50-lb) bags; *Land O Lakes® Does's Match® Kid Milk Replacer DC Medicated*; (OTC). FDA-approved for use in young goats. **DO NOT** feed to goats that produce milk for food.

Decoquinate (18.15 mg/lb) Type C Medicated Milk Replacer in 11.3-kg (25-lb) and 22.7-kg (50-lb) bags; *Sav-A-Caf® Performance AM DX Calf Milk Replacer Medicated*; (OTC). FDA-approved for use in calves.

HUMAN-LABELED PRODUCTS: NONE

References

For the complete list of references, see **wiley.com/go/budde/plumb**

Deferoxamine

(de-fer-**ox**-a-meen) *Desferal®*

Chelating Agent

Prescriber Highlights

- Used primarily for parenteral treatment of iron intoxication in dogs and cats
- Contraindications include severe chronic kidney disease and anuria, unless used with dialysis.
- Use with caution in pregnant and pediatric patients
- Adverse effects include allergic reactions, auditory neurotoxicity, pain or swelling at injection sites, and GI distress. Urine may turn reddish-brown.
- When used IV, must be given slowly

Uses/Indications

Deferoxamine (DFO) is primarily used for the treatment of acute or chronic iron toxicity.[1] This drug has been evaluated as an iron chelator for adjunctive treatment of acute cardiac ischemia, intracerebral hemorrhage, and as a chelator for aluminum and thallium toxicity.[2–5] Its efficacy in treating reperfusion injuries is disappointing. Additional experimental uses include topical preparations to accelerate wound healing in diabetic rodent models, and local injection to promote angiogenesis and bone formation.[6,7]

Pharmacology/Actions

Deferoxamine (DFO) binds ferric (Fe^{+++}) ions to its 3 hydroxamic groups and forms ferrioxamine, a stable, water-soluble compound that is readily excreted by the kidneys. Approximately 100 mg of DFO will bind 8.5 mg of elemental iron.[8] DFO will not combine with iron already bound to transferrin or hemoglobin but will chelate iron bound to hemosiderin and ferritin.[8] Except aluminum and thallium, DFO does not appear to chelate other trace metals or electrolytes in clinically significant quantities.

Pharmacokinetics

Deferoxamine (DFO) is poorly absorbed from the GI tract and is usually given parenterally. The drug is widely distributed in the body. DFO and ferrioxamine (the chelated compound) are excreted primarily in the urine.

Contraindications/Precautions/Warnings

Deferoxamine (DFO) is contraindicated in patients with severe kidney injury or anuria unless dialysis is used to remove ferrioxamine (the chelated compound). Growth retardation has been associated with use of high doses and the drug should be used with caution in pediatric patients.

Due to increased susceptibility from iron overload, patients infected with *Yersinia enterocolitica* or *Yersinia pseudotuberculosis* should not be treated with DFO. Rare cases in humans have occurred wherein DFO acts as an iron transporter for these organisms, enhancing the susceptibility to infection.[8]

Oral administration of DFO after oral iron ingestions may actually increase the amount of iron absorbed from the gut and use by this route is not recommended.

Fungal infections with mucormycosis have occurred in humans, some fatal; DFO use should be stopped and evaluation of infection should occur if clinical signs are present.[8]

Adverse Effects

Veterinary experience with deferoxamine (DFO) is limited. Potential adverse effects include allergic reactions, auditory neurotoxicity (particularly with long-term, high-dose therapy), changes in visual acuity, renal dysfunction, pain or swelling at injection sites, and GI distress. Respiratory distress syndrome has been reported in humans that have received deferoxamine in very high doses. Rapid IV injection may cause tachycardia, convulsions, hypotension, hives, and wheezing. Ferrioxamine (the chelated compound) will give the urine a reddish-brown color ("vin rosé"), which is innocuous and indicates iron removal.

Reproductive/Nursing Safety

Deferoxamine (DFO) has caused skeletal abnormalities in animals at dosages above those recommended for iron toxicity. It is unknown if deferoxamine enters into milk.

Because safety has not been established in animals, this drug should only be used when the maternal benefits outweigh the potential risks to offspring.

Overdose/Acute Toxicity

See ***Adverse Effects***. Long-term, high-dose use of deferoxamine (DFO) may also lead to hypocalcemia and thrombocytopenia.

For patients that have experienced or are suspected to have experienced an overdose, consultation with a 24-hour poison control center specializing in providing veterinary-specific information is recommended. For general information related to overdose and toxin exposures, as well as contact information for poison control centers, refer to ***Appendix***.

Drug Interactions

The following drug interactions either have been reported or are theoretical in humans or animals receiving DFO and may be of significance in veterinary patients. Unless otherwise noted, use together is not necessarily contraindicated, but weigh the potential risks and perform additional monitoring when appropriate.

- **PROCHLORPERAZINE**: Use with deferoxamine (DFO) may cause temporary impairment of consciousness.
- **VITAMIN C**: May be synergistic with DFO in removing iron, and vitamin C deficiency is common in humans with iron overload. However, concurrent use could lead to increased tissue iron toxicity, especially in cardiac muscle; it should be used with caution, particularly in patients with preexisting cardiac disease.

Laboratory Considerations

- Deferoxamine (DFO) may interfere with colorimetric **iron** assays resulting in falsely low values.
- DFO may falsely elevate total iron binding capacity (**TIBC**) measurements.[9]

Dosages

DOGS & CATS:

Animals at risk for or exhibiting signs of severe iron toxicosis (extra-label): Infuse slowly up to 15 mg/kg/hour IV.[10] Initiate therapy as soon as able, within 12 to 24 hours of ingestion, prior to iron distribution to tissues. More rapid infusion may precipitate arrhythmias or aggravate hypotension, although this dosage has been safely exceeded in critical situations. If IV infusion is unfeasible or unable to monitor patient during infusion, give 40 mg/kg IM every 4 to 8 hours, depending on clinical status. Continue therapy until serum iron levels are below 300 µg/dL and the animal is stable. Some clinicians advise continuing chelation until the urine is clear, but there is little evidence for this.[9] Ideally, limit duration of dosing to 24 hours to maximize effectiveness and minimize adverse pulmonary effects.[9] Following recovery, monitor for signs of GI stricture, which may develop 4 to 6 weeks post-ingestion.

Experimentally, as a ferric ion chelator during treatment of cardiac arrest (extra-label):

a) 5 – 15 mg/kg IV, IM, or SC once[11]

b) 10 mg/kg IV or IM every 2 hours for 2 doses, then 3 times daily for 24 hours[12]

HORSES:

To reduce iron overload after packed red blood cell transfusion

in foals (extra-label): 1 g/foal (NOT mg/kg) diluted to 5 mL and administered SC twice daily for 14 days beginning immediately before transfusion. Results suggest that deferoxamine (DFO) increases urinary iron elimination after blood transfusion and may help prevent hepatotoxic iron overload. Additional studies need to evaluate the effects of DFO on iron elimination in foals with neonatal isoerythrolysis that require multiple transfusions.[13]

Monitoring

- Serum ferritin
- Serum iron
- TIBC no longer recommended in cases of iron poisoning[9]
- Kidney function tests (due to renal excretion, measure prior to dosing or serially in animals with renal disease)
- Serum aluminum if used for aluminum chelation
- Treatment is continued until serum iron concentration decreases below 300 µg/dL and the patient is stable.
- If chronic iron overload: eye examinations (iron intoxication and its subsequent removal may adversely affect vision)
- If used in conjunction with vitamin C, monitor cardiac function.

Client Information

- Deferoxamine (DFO) should only be used in an inpatient setting.
- Given the potential toxicity of DFO and the seriousness of most iron intoxications, this drug should be used with close professional supervision only.
- DFO often turns the urine a reddish-brown ("vin rosé") color, which occurs due to urinary iron excretion.

Chemistry/Synonyms

An iron-chelating agent, deferoxamine (DFO) is a white to off-white powder that is freely soluble in alcohol or water.

Deferoxamine may also be known as desferoxamine mesylate, DFO, Ba-33112, Ba-29837, deferoxamini mesilas, desferrioxamine mesylate, desferrioxamine methanesulphonate, NSC-527604, *Desferal*® or *Desferin*®.

Storage/Stability

Reconstituted product further diluted in compatible solution may be stored up to 24 hours at room temperature when protected from light. Do not refrigerate reconstituted product.

Compatibility/Compounding Considerations

Compatibility is dependent on factors such as pH, concentration, temperature, and diluent used; specialized references or a hospital pharmacist should be consulted for more specific information.

Use sterile water for injection to reconstitute product. Deferoxamine should not be mixed with other drugs. Do not use if solution is turbid. Further dilution in normal saline, lactated Ringer's, or dextrose 5% has been recommended when administering as an IV infusion.

After aseptic reconstitution with sterile water for injection use product immediately.

Dosage Forms/Regulatory Status

VETERINARY-LABELED PRODUCTS: NONE

HUMAN-LABELED PRODUCTS:

Deferoxamine Mesylate Powder for Injection (lyophilized): 500 mg and 2 g in vials; *Desferal*®, generic; (Rx)

References

For the complete list of references, see **wiley.com/go/budde/plumb**

Deracoxib

(***dare***-a-***cox***-ib) *Deramaxx*®

Nonsteroidal Anti-Inflammatory Drug (NSAID) COX-2 Selective

Prescriber Highlights

- FDA-approved for use in dogs for treatment of postoperative pain associated with orthopedic (higher dose, 7 days maximum) and dental surgery (lower dose for 3 days) and treatment for pain and inflammation associated with osteoarthritis (lower dose, ongoing administration).
- May be a useful alternative to piroxicam in adjunctive treatment for transitional cell carcinoma of bladder
- Appears to cause predominantly COX-2 inhibition at therapeutic doses
- Adverse GI and renal effects are possible.
- Not for use in cats

Uses/Indications

Deracoxib is indicated in dogs for the treatment of postoperative pain associated with orthopedic (higher dose, 7 days maximum) and dental (lower dose for 3 days) surgery, and treatment for pain and inflammation associated with osteoarthritis (lower dose, ongoing dosing).

Like piroxicam, deracoxib may be used as adjunctive treatment for transitional cell carcinoma of the bladder.[1] The drug has also shown promise in the treatment of canine splenic hemangiosarcoma.[2,3]

Pharmacology/Actions

Deracoxib is a coxib-class NSAID. It is believed to predominantly inhibit cyclooxygenase-2 (COX-2) and spare COX-1 at therapeutic doses in dogs; this selectivity is lost at higher doses. This action would theoretically inhibit production of the prostaglandins that contribute to pain and inflammation (COX-2) and spare those that maintain normal GI and renal function (COX-1).[4,5] However, COX-1 and COX-2 inhibition studies are done in vitro and do not necessarily correlate perfectly with clinical effects seen in vivo.

Deracoxib's effect on platelet function in dogs is not entirely understood. In one study, healthy dogs given 2 mg/kg PO once daily for 7 days had a decrease in platelet aggregation induced by 50 microM ADP, but deracoxib did not affect results of other platelet function tests; the clinical significance of this finding is not known.[6] Another study concluded that all COX-2 selective NSAIDs evaluated (eg, meloxicam, deracoxib, carprofen) caused significantly prolonged Platelet Function Assay (PFA-100) closure times as measured using collagen plus ADP cartridges, suggesting NSAID-induced alterations in platelet function.[7]

Pharmacokinetics

After oral administration in dogs, bioavailability is greater than 90%; the time to peak serum concentration occurs at ≈2 hours. The presence of food in the gut can enhance bioavailability. The drug has an apparent volume of distribution of 1.5 L/kg in dogs and is at least 90% bound to canine plasma proteins. Deracoxib is metabolized in the liver to 4 primary metabolites. These metabolites, along with unchanged drug, are principally eliminated in the feces. Some excretion of metabolites occurs via renal mechanisms. Terminal elimination half-life in dogs is based on dose. At doses up to ≈8 mg/kg, half-life is ≈3 hours (clearance, ≈5 mL/minute/kg). Half-life at a dose of 20 mg/kg is ≈19 hours (clearance, ≈1.7 mL/minute/kg). Serum half-life is not necessarily a good predictor of duration of effect due to the complex relationship between pharmacokinetics and pharmacodynamics with NSAIDs.

In cats, peak concentrations (0.28 µg/mL) occurred ≈3.6 hours after oral administration. Elimination half-life was ≈8 hours.[8]

In horses, deracoxib has a long half-life of ≈13 hours. Based on dosage simulations and plasma concentrations, authors in a study suggested that dosages of 2 mg/kg PO every 12 to 24 hours be further studied for safety and efficacy.[9]

Contraindications/Precautions/Warnings

Deracoxib is contraindicated in patients known to be hypersensitive to it or other NSAIDs; cross-sensitivity with sulfonamides is possible. This drug should be used with caution in patients with concurrent GI ulcerative diseases; with cardiovascular, renal, or hepatic dysfunction; are dehydrated, hypovolemic, or hypotensive; or are on concomitant diuretic therapy.

The product's label states that it cannot be accurately dosed in dogs weighing less than 5.7 kg (12.5 lb); safe use in dogs younger than 4 months of age has not been established.[10]

Deracoxib is not approved or recommended for use in cats.

Adverse Effects

Deracoxib appears to be well tolerated in the majority of dogs treated, particularly when given as labeled and not in conjunction with other NSAIDs or corticosteroids. However, like other NSAIDs, many adverse effects associated with deracoxib have been reported, including GI (eg, vomiting, anorexia, weight loss, diarrhea, melena, hematemesis, hematochezia, GI ulceration, perforation), urinary (eg, azotemia, polydipsia, polyuria, UTI, hematuria, incontinence, chronic kidney disease), hematologic (eg, anemia, thrombocytopenia), hepatic (eg, increased hepatic enzymes, changes in total protein), neurologic (eg, lethargy, weakness, seizures), cardiovascular/respiratory (eg, tachypnea, bradycardia, cough), and dermatologic/immunologic (eg, fever, facial/muzzle edema, urticaria, dermatitis).

Reproductive/Nursing Safety

There is no information on deracoxib's safety during pregnancy or lactation. Until information is available, this drug cannot be recommended in these animals.

Overdose/Acute Toxicity

This medication is an NSAID. As with any NSAID, overdose can lead to GI and renal effects. Decontamination with emetics and/or activated charcoal is appropriate. For doses in which GI effects are expected, the use of GI protectants is warranted.

There is little data available regarding deracoxib's acute toxicity. A 14-day study in dogs demonstrated no clinically observable adverse effects in dogs that received 10 mg/kg PO. Dogs that received 25 mg/kg, 50 mg/kg, or 100 mg/kg PO per day for up to 14 days survived but showed weight loss, vomiting, and melena; gross GI lesions were noted, but no hepatic or renal lesions were demonstrated.[11] A dose of 16.92 mg/kg PO once daily for 7 days resulted in decreased appetite, diarrhea, increased water intake, and vomiting.[12]

In safety studies performed by the manufacturer,[13] oral deracoxib was well tolerated by dogs when administered for up to 6 months at a variety of doses. Some dogs receiving greater than 6 mg/kg/day (1.5 to 5 times the recommended dose) showed signs of focal renal tubular degeneration/regeneration on histopathology that were dose-dependent. Focal tubular necrosis was seen in 1 out of 10 dogs given 8 mg/kg/day and in 3 out of 10 dogs given 10 mg/kg/day. Clinical pathology findings associated with these lesions included elevated BUN and hyposthenuria.

Common clinical signs include vomiting, diarrhea, lethargy, and elevated creatinine.

In otherwise healthy dogs, the ASPCA APCC recommends GI protectants if deracoxib 15 mg/kg or greater has been ingested; IV fluid diuresis should also be given when ingestions are 30 mg/kg or more.

For patients that have experienced or are suspected to have experienced an overdose, it is strongly encouraged that a 24-hour poison consultation center that specializes in providing information specific for veterinary patients be consulted. For general information related to overdose and toxin exposures, as well as contact information for poison control centers, refer to ***Appendix.***

Drug Interactions

The following drug interactions have either been reported or are theoretical in humans or animals receiving coxib-class NSAIDs and may be of significance in veterinary patients. Unless otherwise noted, use together is not necessarily contraindicated, but weigh the potential risks and perform additional monitoring when appropriate.

- **ACE Inhibitors** (eg, **benazepril, enalapril**): NSAIDs can reduce effects on blood pressure. Because ACE inhibitors can potentially reduce renal blood flow, use with NSAIDs could increase the risk for renal injury.
- **Angiotensin Receptor Blockers** (**ARBs**; eg, **irbesartan, telmisartan**): NSAIDs can reduce effects on blood pressure. Because ARBs can potentially reduce renal blood flow, use with NSAIDs could increase the risk for renal injury.
- **Aspirin**: May increase the risk for GI toxicity (eg, ulceration, bleeding, vomiting, diarrhea)
- **Beta-Adrenergic Blockers** (eg, **atenolol, propranolol**): Concurrent use may result in increased blood pressure.
- **Corticosteroids** (eg, **prednis(ol)one**): May increase the risk for GI toxicity (eg, ulceration, GI perforation, bleeding, vomiting, diarrhea). It is not recommended to use corticosteroids in conjunction with an NSAID.
- **Digoxin**: NSAIDs may increase serum levels.
- **Diuretics** (eg, **furosemide**): Increased risk for deracoxib adverse effects[10]
- **Fluconazole**: Administration has increased plasma levels of celecoxib in humans and could also affect deracoxib levels in dogs.
- **Fluoroquinolones** (eg, **enrofloxacin, marbofloxacin**): Concurrent use may result in an increased risk for seizures.
- **Furosemide**: NSAIDs may reduce saluretic and diuretic effects.
- **Methotrexate**: Serious toxicity has occurred when NSAIDs have been used concomitantly with methotrexate; use together with extreme caution.
- **Nephrotoxic Drugs** (eg, **aminoglycosides, amphotericin B**): May enhance the risk for nephrotoxicity development
- **NSAIDs, Other** (eg, **carprofen**): May increase the risk for GI toxicity (eg, ulceration, bleeding, vomiting, diarrhea). Multiple NSAIDs should not be administered concurrently.
- **Selective Serotonin Reuptake Inhibitors** (**SSRIs**; eg, **fluoxetine**): Concurrent use may increase risk for bleeding.
- **Tramadol:** May increase the risk for GI toxicity (from a case report[14])
- **Tricyclic Antidepressants** (eg, **amitriptyline, clomipramine**): Concurrent use may result in an increased risk for bleeding.

Laboratory Considerations

- No specific laboratory interactions were noted. Deracoxib does not appear to affect thyroid function tests in dogs.

Dosages

DOGS:

NOTE: Manufacturer recommends using the lowest effective dose for the shortest duration possible.

Control of pain and inflammation associated with osteoarthritis (label dosage; FDA-approved): 1 – 2 mg/kg PO once daily as needed[10]

Control of postoperative pain and inflammation associated

with dental surgery (label dosage; FDA-approved): 1 – 2 mg/kg PO once daily for 3 days[10]

Control of postoperative pain and inflammation associated with orthopedic surgery (label dosage; FDA-approved): 3 – 4 mg/kg PO once daily as needed, not to exceed 7 days[10]

Monitoring

- Clinical efficacy
- Adverse effects
- Baseline and periodic physical examination
- Baseline and periodic: CBC, serum chemistry profile (including BUN, creatinine, liver enzymes), urinalysis

Client Information

NOTE: The manufacturer provides a client handout sheet that is recommend to be given each time the drug is dispensed.

- Deracoxib is an NSAID used in dogs for pain and inflammation associated with orthopedic and dental surgery. This medication can be given with or without food, but food may reduce the chances for stomach problems. If your dog vomits or acts sick after receiving this medication on an empty stomach, give with food or small treat to see if this helps. If vomiting continues, contact your veterinarian. Fresh water should always be available.
- Most dogs tolerate deracoxib well, but some dogs rarely develop stomach ulcers or serious kidney and liver problems. Stop giving this medicine and contact your veterinarian immediately if your animal has decreased appetite (ie, eating less than normal), persistent vomiting, diarrhea, changes in behavior or activity levels (ie, more or less active than normal), changes in drinking and urinating habits (ie, frequency, amount consumed), or yellowing of gums, skin, or whites of the eyes (ie, jaundice).
- Store chewable tablets well out of reach of animals and children.
- Keep water readily accessible during treatment and avoid dehydration.
- Periodic laboratory tests are needed to check for liver and kidney side effects. Do not miss these important follow-up visits.
- Other medicines for pain or inflammation should not be used with this medication without the approval of your veterinarian.
- Do not increase or alter the dose without approval from your veterinarian.

Chemistry/Synonyms

Deracoxib is a diaryl-substituted pyrazole that is chemically related to other coxib-class NSAIDs (eg, celecoxib). Its molecular weight is 397.38.

Storage/Stability

The commercially available chewable tablets for dogs should be stored at room temperature between 15°C to 30°C (59°F-86°F).

Compatibility/Compounding Considerations

No specific information noted

Dosage Forms/Regulatory Status

VETERINARY-LABELED PRODUCTS:

Deracoxib Chewable (scored) Tablets: 12 mg, 25 mg, 75 mg, and 100 mg; *Deramaxx*®[10]; generic; (Rx). FDA-approved for use in dogs; NADA # 141-203

The Association of Racing Commissioners International (ARCI) has designated this drug as a class 3 substance. See ***Appendix*** for more information. Use of this drug may not be allowed in certain animal competitions. Check rules and regulations before entering in a competition while this medication is being administered. Contact local racing authorities for further guidance.

HUMAN-LABELED PRODUCTS: NONE

References

For the complete list of references, see **wiley.com/go/budde/plumb**

Desflurane

(dez-***floor***-ane) *Suprane*®

Inhalant Anesthetic

Prescriber Highlights

- ► Inhaled general anesthetic
- ► Primary benefit is when very rapid recoveries are desired
- ► Contraindications include hypersensitivity to desflurane and history of malignant hyperthermia.
- ► Adverse effects include dose-dependent hypotension and respiratory depression.
- ► Requires desflurane-specific vaporizer (electric, heated, pressurized, expensive)

Uses/Indications

Desflurane is a volatile anesthetic that may be of particular use when rapid recoveries are desired.[1] Desflurane has a very high vapor pressure that necessitates the use of an electric, heated, pressurized vaporizer, which can be cumbersome and expensive.

Pharmacology/Actions

Desflurane is a halogenated inhalant anesthetic. It is structurally related to isoflurane, with a fluorine atom substituted for chlorine at the alpha-ethyl carbon. Although the precise mechanism by which inhalant anesthetics exert their general anesthetic effect is not precisely known, inhalant anesthetics may interfere with functioning of nerve cells in the brain by acting at $GABA_A$-R and voltage-gated channels.[2] Desflurane has a very low blood:gas solubility ratio of 0.42 (at 37°C [98.6°F]).

Some of the key pharmacologic effects noted with desflurane include rapid inductions and recoveries[3]; rapid recoveries may be a benefit, but they could also be detrimental, particularly if perioperative analgesics are not used. Desflurane is relatively resistant to biodegradation that may minimize risk for nephrotoxicity.

Pharmacokinetics

Onset of action is very rapid after inhalation; some have described it as "one breath" induction. At body temperature (37°C [98.6°F]), desflurane has a blood/gas coefficient (predicts rate of facemask induction and recovery) of 0.42, an oil/gas coefficient of ≈19, and a brain/blood coefficient of 1.3.

Very little of desflurane is eliminated via hepatic routes, as only 0.02% is recovered as metabolites. In humans, elimination half-life is 2.5 minutes (isoflurane about 9.5 minutes).

Contraindications/Precautions/Warnings

Desflurane is contraindicated in patients that are hypersensitive to it or other halogenated agents, or in those that have a history or predilection towards malignant hyperthermia. It should be used with caution (benefits versus risks) in patients with increased CSF pressure or head injury.

Because of desflurane's rapid action, use caution not to overdose during the induction phase. Because of the rapid recovery associated with desflurane, use caution (and appropriate analgesia and sedation during the recovery phase), particularly with large animals.

Geriatric or critically ill animals may require less inhalation anesthetic.

The National Institute for Occupational Safety and Health (NIOSH) has recommended that no worker should be exposed at ceiling concentrations greater than 2 ppm of any halogenated anesthetic agent over a sampling period not to exceed 1 hour.

Desflurane should only be used in situations in which sufficient monitoring and patient-support capabilities (eg, intubation, ventilation) are available.

Adverse Effects

Desflurane is usually very well tolerated. Hypotension and respiratory depression may occur and are considered dose dependent. Like all halogenated anesthetics, desflurane can cause malignant hyperthermia in susceptible individuals (usually humans or pigs). Desflurane may have a lower incidence rate of this effect than other halogenated anesthetics.

Like isoflurane and sevoflurane, desflurane does not potentiate catecholamine-induced arrhythmias, and like all the inhalant anesthetics, it decreases arterial blood pressure and depresses ventilation in a dose-dependent manner.

Desflurane is a respiratory irritant, has a pungent odor, and is not well suited for mask inductions. When used for mask inductions, desflurane can cause respiratory irritation and cause salivation in dogs and cats. Rapid changes in desflurane concentrations may result in a sympathetic response and can temporarily increase cardiac work.

Reproductive/Nursing Safety

Desflurane appears to be relatively safe to use during pregnancy, but data are limited. Because of its low blood solubility, desflurane may be one of the safest inhalant anesthetics for use during pregnancy. In rats and rabbits, no overt teratogenic effects were observed when exposed at 1 MAC-hour/day during organogenesis (10 to 13 days exposure).

The minimal alveolar concentration (MAC) of inhalation agents is 25% to 40% lower during pregnancy.[4]

Desflurane is likely compatible with nursing, as levels are low in milk and rapidly washout within 24 hours of use; however, safety during nursing has not been established.

Because safety has not been established in animals, this drug should only be used when the maternal benefits outweigh the potential risks to offspring.

Overdose/Acute Toxicity

In the event of an overdose, discontinue desflurane; maintain airway and support respiratory and cardiac function as necessary.

Drug Interactions

The following drug interactions either have been reported or are theoretical in humans or animals receiving desflurane and may be of significance in veterinary patients. Unless otherwise noted, use together is not necessarily contraindicated, but weigh the potential risks and perform additional monitoring when appropriate.

- **ACE Inhibitors or Other Hypotensive Agents**: Concomitant use may increase risks for hypotension. Enalapril caused significant decreases in systolic blood pressure in dogs and cats undergoing isoflurane anesthesia.[5] Similar effects may be expected with desflurane.
- **Acepromazine:** Can decrease minimal alveolar concentration (MAC)
- **Alpha-2 Agonists** (eg, **dexmedetomidine, xylazine**): Can decrease MAC[6]
- **Aminoglycosides:** Use with caution with halogenated anesthetic agents, as additive neuromuscular blockade may occur
- **Anesthetic Agents** (eg, **alfaxalone, ketamine, propofol**): Can decrease MAC
- **Benzodiazepines** (eg, **midazolam**): Can decrease MAC
- **Butorphanol**: Can cause hypotension and decreased ventilation in dogs when given with desflurane[7]
- **Non-Depolarizing Neuromuscular Blocking Agents** (eg, **atracurium**): Additive neuromuscular blockade may occur.
- **Opioids** (eg, **fentanyl**): Can decrease MAC
- **Sympathomimetics** (eg, **dopamine, epinephrine, norepinephrine**): Although desflurane sensitizes the myocardium to the effects of sympathomimetics less so than halothane, arrhythmias may still result. If these drugs are needed, they should be used with caution, and in significantly reduced dosages with intensive monitoring.
- **Succinylcholine**: With inhalation anesthetics, may induce increased incidences of cardiac effects (eg, bradycardia, arrhythmias, sinus arrest, apnea) and, in susceptible patients, malignant hyperthermia

Laboratory Considerations

- Like other halogenated anesthetics, desflurane can cause transient increases in **glucose** and white blood cell count.

Dosages

Approximate minimal alveolar concentration (MAC; %) in oxygen reported for desflurane: dogs = 7 – 10.3; cats = 9.8; horse = 7.23; rabbit = 8.9; alpacas/llamas = 7.8 – 8

General anesthesia (extra-label):

a) Clinically useful concentrations: Induction = 8 – 15%; Maintenance = 5 – 9%[8]

b) Approximate MAC for emergency patients: 6%[9]

c) Following IV induction: The author usually starts with a vaporizer setting of about 8% (around MAC in most animals), increasing the concentration as required.[10]

Monitoring

- Respiratory rate and ventilatory status (eg, $ETCO_2$, SpO_2)
- Heart rate, ECG, blood pressure
- Depth of anesthesia
- Body temperature

Client Information

- Desflurane is only used in an inpatient setting.

Chemistry/Synonyms

Desflurane has the chemical name (±)-2-Difluoromethyl 1,2,2,2-tetrafluoroethyl ether and has a molecular weight of 168. It is a clear, colorless, heavy liquid. It is nonflammable and nonexplosive. At 1 atmosphere, it has a boiling point of 22°C to 23°C (71.6°F-73.4°F), a vapor pressure of 669 mm Hg at 20°C (68°F), and specific gravity of 1.465 at 20°C (68°F). Desflurane is practically insoluble in water, but miscible with anhydrous alcohol.

Halogenated inhalation anesthetics are greenhouse gases. Vaporization of one bottle of desflurane has the same global warming potential as 886 kg of carbon dioxide.[11]

Desflurane may also be known as I-653, desfluraani, desflurano, or desfluranum. A common trade name is *Suprane*®.

Storage/Stability

Desflurane solution should be stored in its original container at 15°C to 30°C (59°F-86°F). Secure cap on bottle tightly after use. Protect this product from light.

Compatibility/Compounding Considerations

No specific information was noted.

Dosage Forms/Regulatory Status

VETERINARY-LABELED PRODUCTS: NONE

HUMAN-LABELED PRODUCTS:

Desflurane Solution for Inhalation Anesthesia in 240 mL bottles; *Suprane*®; (Rx)

References

For the complete list of references, see **wiley.com/go/budde/plumb**

Deslorelin

(dess-*lor*-a-lin) *SucroMate®, Suprelorin® F*

Hormonal Agent

Prescriber Highlights

- Synthetic GnRH analogue indicated to induce ovulation in cyclic estrous mares. It is especially useful in artificial insemination and estrus synchronization programs.
- Deslorelin acetate implants are also prescribed for the management of adrenocortical disease in ferrets.
- Deslorelin acetate implants may be used to induce temporary infertility in intact male dogs.

Uses/Indications

Deslorelin is FDA-approved for inducing ovulation in cyclic estrous mares.[1] In the United States, the deslorelin acetate implant is not approved by the FDA, but legally marketed as an FDA-indexed product for use only in ferrets for the management of adrenocortical disease. Extra-label use of FDA-indexed products is prohibited in the United States.

Deslorelin has been used in an extra-label fashion for inducing ovulation in multiple animal species. Various implants are compounded or approved in countries other than the United States, and have been used for long-term, reversible contraception in a variety of animal species. Studies have investigated the use of deslorelin implants for prostatic disease in male dogs, incontinence in ovariectomized female dogs, suppression of egg laying in birds, aggressive behavior in various species, and in various bovine reproductive management protocols.

Pharmacology/Actions

Deslorelin is a potent GnRH analogue that causes the release of FSH and LH. When deslorelin is administered to cyclic estrous mares with a growing, preovulatory follicle at least 30 mm in diameter, the LH increase in the blood induces follicle maturation and ovulation within 48 hours. Deslorelin acetate implants induce an initial release of FSH and LH but the sustained, prolonged action will eventually downregulate GnRH receptors, a phenomenon that desensitizes and internalizes the GnRH receptors; this leads to a decline in ovarian and testicular function.[2]

Pharmacokinetics

In mares and cows, serum LH is elevated 15 minutes after deslorelin IM administration and peaks at ≈2 to 3 hours in cows and ≈8 hours in mares. In horses, after implantation of a 2.1 mg pellet, concentrations of LH and FSH peak ≈12 hours after implant and return to pretreatment levels ≈3 to 4 days after implantation. Oral dosing of 100 μg/kg to beagles showed no increase in LH or FSH.

Contraindications/Precautions/Warnings

The only label contraindication is to not use in animals with known hypersensitivity to deslorelin acetate.[1,3] Do not administer deslorelin suspension for injection by the IV route.

Implants are biocompatible and do not require removal; however, implants may be surgically removed to end treatment.

Pregnant women and women of childbearing age should exercise caution when handling this product; direct contact with skin should be avoided. The National Institute for Occupational Safety and Health (NIOSH) classifies other GnRH analogues as hazardous drugs; personal protective equipment (PPE) should be used accordingly to minimize the risk for exposure. Refer to the Occupational Safety and Health Association (OSHA) website for more information."

Adverse Effects

The injectable formulation of deslorelin can cause swelling at the site of injection, which generally subsides within 5 days. With the implants, minor local swelling, sensitivity to touch, and elevated skin temperature at the injection site may occur; these effects should resolve within 5 days of implantation.

Deslorelin use may result in a prolonged interovulatory period. To avoid this potential negative effect when using deslorelin acetate implants, the implant should be removed from mares and bitches as soon as ovulation is documented. Extra-label use of the 4.7 mg implant (not available in the United States) to prevent estrus in female dogs has demonstrated (rarely) adverse effects of follicular cysts, prolonged estrus, and pyometra, especially in older dogs.[4]

Reproductive/Nursing Safety

Deslorelin implants are not for use in ferrets intended for breeding.[3] The decline in ovarian and testicular function associated with deslorelin acetate is reversible in all species tested. A case study was reported of a female cat implanted with a 4.7 mg deslorelin implant (*Suprelorin-6®*, not available in the United States), that later delivered 4 healthy kittens but displayed no maternal care and did not adequately lactate.[5]

Because safety has not been established in animals, this drug should only be used when the maternal benefits outweigh the potential risks to offspring.

Overdose/Acute Toxicity

In the original tolerance study (8 mares treated with a single IM injection of deslorelin acetate at 10 times the recommended dose of 1.8 mg), one mare exhibited moderate tremors, hives, and elevated heart and respiratory rates 6 hours after injection.[6] If there is inadvertent administration of an additional implant, it can be removed on detection.

For patients that have experienced or are suspected to have experienced an overdose, consultation with a 24-hour poison consultation center specializing in providing veterinary-specific information is recommended. For general information related to overdose and toxin exposures, as well as contact information for poison control centers, refer to ***Appendix.***

Drug Interactions

- No specific interactions were noted.

Laboratory Considerations

- None were noted.

Dosages

DOGS:

NOTE: There are several deslorelin products licensed and approved for various species; see specific labels for more information.

Contraceptive in male dogs (extra-label): Using the 4.7 mg implant: Implant SC every 6 months.[7] Using the 9.4 mg implant: Implant SC every 12 months.[8] Place implant in loose skin between lower neck and lumbar area; avoid implanting into fat. Pregnant women should not administer the implant. **NOTE**: Extra-label use of the ferret implant product in dogs is prohibited in the United States.

HORSES:

Induction of ovulation within 48 hours in cyclic estrous mares with an ovarian follicle measuring at least 30 mm in diameter (label dosage; FDA-approved): 1.8 mg/mare (NOT mg/kg) IM; administer in the neck[1]

FERRETS:

Management of adrenal gland cortical disease in the male and female domestic ferret (label dosage; FDA-Indexed product): One 4.7 mg implant/ferret SC every 12 months.[3] Place implant in the back midway between the shoulder blades. See label for specific administration instructions.

Contraceptive in male ferrets (extra-label): One 9.4 mg implant/ferret SC up to every 4 years[8]

Monitoring

- Clinical efficacy is based on indication for use.
- In ferrets treated for adrenal gland disease, monitor for effectiveness by improvement of clinical signs.

Client Information

- This medicine is only given by a veterinarian.
- Swelling or inflammation can occur at injection site. Contact your veterinarian if this gets worse.
- Removal of the implant is not required unless it is necessary to stop treatment.

Chemistry/Synonyms

Deslorelin acetate is a synthetic gonadotropin-releasing hormone (GnRH, gonadorelin) analogue. It is a nonapeptide and has chemical modifications in the amino acid composition at positions 6 and 9/10.

Storage/Stability

Deslorelin implants or injectable suspension should be refrigerated (2°C-8°C [36°F-46°F]). Do not freeze deslorelin implants.

Compatibility/Compounding Considerations

No specific information was noted.

Dosage Forms/Regulatory Status

VETERINARY-LABELED PRODUCTS:

Deslorelin Suspension for Injection 1.8 mg/mL in 10 mL multi-dose vials; *SucroMate® Equine*; (Rx). FDA-approved for horses (not intended for food); NADA #141-319

Deslorelin Implants 4.7 mg; *Suprelorin-F®*; not approved by FDA, but legally marketed for use in ferrets only as an FDA Indexed Product under MIF 900-013. Extra-label use is prohibited. This product is not to be used in animals intended for use as food for humans or other animals.

Deslorelin 2.1 mg cylindrical implant with implanter; 5 per box *Ovuplant®*; (Rx). FDA-approved for ovulation induction in mares. Not for use in horses intended for food. This product is FDA-approved in the United States (per FDA Green Book), but it is not currently marketed in the United States.

Other deslorelin products may be licensed for animal use in other countries and compounded preparations may be available.

HUMAN-LABELED PRODUCTS: NONE

References

For the complete list of references, see **wiley.com/go/budde/plumb**

Desmopressin

(des-moe-***press***-in) *DDAVP®*

Synthetic Vasopressin (Antidiuretic Hormone) Analogue, Hemostatic Agent

Prescriber Highlights

- ► Used in the diagnosis and treatment of central diabetes insipidus in dogs, cats, and possibly horses, and type 1 von Willebrand disease in dogs
- ► Contraindications include hypersensitivity to desmopressin and those with type IIB, type III, or platelet-type (pseudo) von Willebrand disease.
- ► Use with caution in patients susceptible to thrombosis.
- ► Adverse effects include eye irritation after conjunctival administration; hypersensitivity possible
- ► Overdoses can cause fluid retention and life-threatening hyponatremia.
- ► Monitor serum sodium concentration closely at the onset of treatment.

Uses/Indications

Desmopressin is useful in the diagnosis and/or treatment of central diabetes insipidus in small animals.[1,2] It may be used perioperatively in dogs with type 1 von Willebrand disease.[3-6] Desmopressin may be useful as a surgical adjuvant perioperatively to reduce lymph node involvement and metastatic disease in canine[7] (not feline[8]) mammary carcinoma or other aggressive tumors,[9] although this is controversial.[10]

Desmopressin has demonstrated an antidiuretic response in horses.[11-14]

Pharmacology/Actions

Desmopressin is related structurally to arginine vasopressin, but it has more antidiuretic activity and less vasopressor properties on a per weight basis. Desmopressin causes a dose-dependent increase in water reabsorption by the collecting ducts in the kidneys, thereby increasing urine osmolality and decreasing net urine production. Therapeutic doses do not directly affect either urinary sodium or potassium excretion.

Desmopressin causes a dose-dependent increase in von Willebrand factor by releasing von Willebrand factor from endothelial cells and macrophages; it also increases plasma factor VIII and causes smaller increases in factor VIII-related antigen and ristocetin cofactor activities.[5,15,16]

Pharmacokinetics

Because desmopressin is destroyed in the GI tract, it is usually given parenterally or topically in the eye or nose. Oral tablets have been used in those dogs that cannot tolerate ophthalmic administration, but bioavailability is very low. In humans, intranasal administration is commonly used, although in veterinary medicine topical administration to the conjunctiva is preferred. The onset of antidiuretic action in dogs usually occurs within 1 hour of administration, peaks in 2 to 8 hours, and may persist for up to 24 hours. Distribution characteristics of desmopressin are not well described. The metabolic fate is also not well understood. Terminal half-life in humans after IV administration is 3 hours but increased to 9 hours in a patient with severe renal impairment.[17]

Contraindications/Precautions/Warnings

Desmopressin is contraindicated in patients hypersensitive to it. In humans, it is contraindicated in patients with moderate to severe renal impairment and in patients with hyponatremia or a history of hyponatremia. Desmopressin should be used with caution in patients susceptible to thrombotic events.

Desmopressin is ineffective in the treatment of nephrogenic diabetes insipidus; it is strongly encouraged to consult with a veterinary endocrinologist or endocrinology textbook when using this drug for treatment of diabetes insipidus. Administration of desmopressin may cause sudden drops in serum sodium concentrations due to water retention, and close monitoring of serum sodium concentrations is required. Institute fluid restriction and/or reduce desmopressin dosage if fluid retention or signs of hyponatremia occur.

Desmopressin should not be used for treatment of type IIB von Willebrand disease (vWD) as platelet aggregation and thrombocytopenia may occur, or for type III vWD due to a lack of therapeutic effect. When desmopressin is used with repeated administration to stimulate von Willebrand factor, tachyphylaxis (progressive lack of efficacy) will occur to a variable extent within 24 hours.

Adverse Effects

Adverse effects in small animals are uncommon. Occasionally eye irritation may occur after conjunctival administration. Sodium decreases of more than 0.5 mEq/hour may result in neurologic signs (eg, nausea, vomiting, obtundation, seizures, coma).

Hypersensitivity reactions are possible. Humans using the drug have complained about increased headache frequency. Rarely, increased blood pressure may occur, and thrombotic events have been reported in humans predisposed to thrombus formation[17]; veterinary significance is unknown.

Reproductive/Nursing Safety

Safe use during pregnancy has not been established; however, doses up to 10 µg/kg/day have been given to rats and rabbits without demonstration of fetal harm.[17]

Desmopressin is likely safe to use during nursing; however, because safety has not been established in animals, this drug should only be used when the maternal benefits outweigh the potential risks to offspring.

Overdose/Acute Toxicity

Oral dosages of 0.2 mg/kg/day have been administered to dogs for 6 months without any significant drug-related toxicity reported. Dosages that are too high may lead to fluid retention and hyponatremia; dosage reduction and fluid restriction may be employed to treat. Adequate monitoring should be performed.

For patients that have experienced or are suspected to have experienced an overdose, consultation with a 24-hour poison consultation center specializing in providing veterinary-specific information is recommended. For general information related to overdose and toxin exposures, as well as contact information for poison control centers, refer to ***Appendix***.

Drug Interactions

The following drug interactions have either been reported or are theoretical in humans or animals receiving desmopressin and may be of significance in veterinary patients. Unless otherwise noted, use together is not necessarily contraindicated, but weigh the potential risks and perform additional monitoring when appropriate.

- **Carbamazepine:** May decrease the antidiuretic response. May increase risk for hyponatremia
- **Chlorpromazine:** May increase risk of hyponatremia
- **Corticosteroids** (eg, **dexamethasone, fludrocortisone, predniso(lo)ne**): May increase risk of hyponatremia
- **Heparin**: May decrease the antidiuretic response
- **Loop Diuretics** (eg, **bumetanide, furosemide, torsemide**): May increase risk for hyponatremia
- **Nonsteroidal Anti-Inflammatory Drugs** (**NSAIDs**; eg, **carprofen, flunixin, meloxicam**): May increase risk for hyponatremia
- **Opioids** (eg, **buprenorphine, morphine**): May increase risk for hyponatremia
- **Oxybutynin:** Seizures have occurred with concurrent use in humans
- **Selective Serotonin Reuptake Inhibitors** (**SSRIs**; eg, **fluoxetine**): May increase risk for hyponatremia
- **Tricyclic Antidepressants** (**TCAs**; eg, **amitriptyline, clomipramine**): May increase risk for hyponatremia
- **Vasopressor Agents** (eg, **dobutamine, norepinephrine**): Increased risk for hypertension

Laboratory Considerations

- See ***Monitoring***

Dosages

NOTE: Dosages listed below that are administered by SC, IV, or ophthalmic routes use the 0.1 mg/mL (0.01%) nasal solution product.

DOGS:

Treatment of confirmed central diabetes insipidus (extra-label):

a) Using 0.1 mg/mL (0.01%) human intranasal desmopressin product:
   - i. Initially, 1 drop/dog (NOT drops/kg or drops/eye) is placed into the conjunctival sac once to twice daily.[18,19] 1 – 2 drops/dog (NOT drops/kg or drops/eye) administered once or twice daily controls clinical signs in most dogs,[20] but up to 4 drops/dog (NOT drops/kg or drops/eye) per dose may be required.[21]
   - ii. 0.1 – 0.2 µg/kg SC once or twice daily.[19]

b) Using oral formulations based on body weight: Evaluate response after 7 days. May increase dosing interval to every 8 hours if clinical signs remain uncontrolled.[1]
   - i. Less than 5 kg: 0.05 mg/dog (NOT mg/kg) PO every 12 hours
   - ii. 5 to 20 kg: 0.1 mg/dog (NOT mg/kg) PO every 12 hours
   - iii. More than 20 kg: 0.2 mg/dog (NOT mg/kg) PO every 12 hours

Differentiate central vs nephrogenic diabetes insipidus (extra-label): ½ to 1 tablet (0.1 or 0.2 mg *DDAVP®* tablet)/dog PO every 8 hours OR, using 0.1 mg/mL (0.01%) human intranasal desmopressin product, 1 – 4 drops/dog (NOT drops/kg or drops/eye) into the conjunctival sac every 12 hours for 5 to 7 days. If central DI, there should be a noticeable decrease in PU/PD and an increase in urine specific gravity (USG) by at least 50% from baselines or if the USG is greater than 1.018 by the end of treatment period.[18,22] **NOTE**: Causes of acquired nephrogenic diabetes insipidus (eg, hyperadrenocorticism) must have been ruled out prior to interpreting the findings from this test.

To improve hemostatic function (extra-label):

a) **Presurgical prophylaxis or treatment of type 1 von Willebrand disease or factor VII deficiency**: 1 µg/kg IV or SC 30 minutes to 1 hour before surgery using the 0.01% intranasal solution.[3-6] Duration of activity is ≈2 hours. Have transfusion capability ready.

b) **Aspirin-induced coagulopathy** (extra-label): 0.3 – 1 µg/kg IV over 15 to 30 minutes,[23] or 3 µg/kg SC.[24] Dramatically shortened buccal mucosal bleeding time measured 15 to 120 minutes after administration and reduced the risk for intraoperative hemorrhage during surgery.[23]

c) **Hemorrhage secondary to canine monocytic ehrlichiosis** (extra-label): 1 µg/kg SC once daily for 3 days[25]; dosage based on a case report with 3 dogs

d) **Hemostatic impairment due to chronic liver disease**: 3 µg/kg SC[24]

Adjunctive treatment of mammary gland tumors (extra-label): 1 µg/kg IV in saline 30 minutes before, and 24 hours after surgery appeared to reduce the spread of, survival of, or numbers of residual malignant cells.[7] However, a more recent study did not prevent metastasis in dogs with mammary carcinoma.[10]

CATS:

Differentiate central vs nephrogenic diabetes insipidus (extra-label): 1 drop/cat (NOT drop/kg or drop/eye) into the conjunctival sac twice daily for 2 to 3 days; a dramatic reduction in water intake or a 50% or greater increase in urine concentration gives strong evidence for a deficiency in ADH production. For treatment of central DI: 1 – 2 drops/ cat (NOT drops/kg or drops/eye) into the conjunctival sac once or twice a day; duration of activity is 8 to 24 hours.[26] Intranasal administration (10 µg/cat [NOT µg/kg]) every 24 hours has also been used.[27]

Treatment of confirmed central diabetes insipidus (extra-label):

a) Using 0.1 mg/mL (0.01%) human intranasal desmopressin product:
   i. 1 – 4 drops/cat (NOT drops/kg or drops/eye) of the intranasal solution in the conjunctival sac once to twice daily[28]
   ii. 2 – 5 µg/cat (NOT µg/kg) SC once to twice daily[28]

b) Using oral formulations: 25 – 50 µg/cat (NOT µg/kg) PO every 8 to 12 hours. Dose and response may be variable[2]

HORSES:

Differentiate central vs nephrogenic diabetes insipidus (extra-label): Using 0.1 mg/mL (0.01%) human intranasal desmopressin product:

a) 20 µg/horse (NOT µg/kg) IV[11,14]
b) Dilute the nasal spray formulation (0.1 mg/mL) in sterile water and administer 0.05 µg/kg IV. Urine specific gravity (SG) should be measured every 2 hours. An increase in SG to 1.025 or greater within 2 to 7 hours is consistent with central DI. No change in urine SG is consistent with nephrogenic DI if medullary washout has been accounted for.[29]
c) 1 drop into each eye, and repeated 2 hours later.[13]

Treatment of confirmed central diabetes insipidus (extra-label): Using 0.1% nasal solution, 25 µg/horse (NOT µg/kg) SC every 24 hours administered in the neck and shoulder area. Response was maintained for at least 5 years. A partial response had been achieved using 3 drops (30 µg)/horse (NOT drops/kg or drops/eye) administered into the conjunctival sac of both eyes every 12 hours, but further dose increase was limited by fluid overflow volume from the eye.[12]

BIRDS:

Treatment of documented central diabetes insipidus in an African Grey parrot (extra-label): 24 µg/kg IM every 12 hours was continued for at least 8 months. Initial treatment with oral desmopressin was ineffective.[30]

Monitoring

***Central diabetes insipidus*:**

- Urine volume; improvement of polyuria, polydipsia
- Serum electrolytes (especially sodium) and urine specific gravity
- Fluid intake
- Patient weight

Von Willebrand disease and other coagulopathies:

- Buccal mucosal bleeding time
- Pre-/post procedure packed cell volume

Client Information

- In dogs and cats, the human nasal spray is usually prescribed; however, it is given by putting drops into the eye instead of the nose.
- This medicine is usually tolerated well as an eye drop though sometimes eye irritation occurs.
- Your veterinarian will need to monitor your animal closely with examinations and blood tests during the initial treatment period while an effective dose is being established. Do not miss these important follow-up visits.
- Contact your veterinarian if your animal begins to drink and urinate excessively again.
- Store this medicine in the refrigerator; discard open bottles after 30 days.

Chemistry/Synonyms

A synthetic polypeptide related to arginine vasopressin (antidiuretic hormone), desmopressin acetate occurs as a fluffy white powder with a bitter taste. The commercially available nasal solution has HCl added, and the pH is ≈4. This preparation also contains chlorobutanol 0.5% as a preservative.

Desmopressin acetate may also be known as 1-Deamino-8-D-Arginine Vasopressin, *DFDAVP®*, *Concentraid®*, *D-Void®*, *Defirin®*, *Desmogalen®*, *Desmospray®*, *Desmotabs®*, *Emosint®*, *Minirin®*, *Minirin/DDAVP®*, *Minrin®*, *Minurin®*, *Nocdurna®*, *Nocutil®*, *Octim®*, *Octostim®*, *Presinex®*, or *Stimate®*.

Storage/Stability

Desmopressin nasal solution storage requirements vary by manufacturer, and the manufacturer's label should be consulted. Some nasal solutions are able to be stored at room temperature 20°C to 25°C (68°F-77°F) whereas others require refrigeration at 2°C to 8°C (36°F-46°F), although the latter are able to be stored at room temperature for up to 3 weeks. Consult product label.

The product for injection should be protected from light and refrigerated at 2°C to 8°C (36°F-46°F); do not freeze.

Compatibility/Compounding Considerations

Parenteral drug products should be inspected visually for particulate matter and discoloration prior to administration. In humans it is recommended that for IV infusion, the appropriate dose of desmopressin acetate be diluted in 10 or 50 mL of 0.9% sodium chloride injection for administration in children weighing 10 kg or less or in adults and children weighing more than 10 kg, respectively; the solution is then infused IV slowly over 15 to 30 minutes. The intranasal solution has been administered SC or diluted and given IV to veterinary patients; however, no specific published safety or stability data were located, and care should be taken to maintain sterility during preparation.

Dosage Forms/Regulatory Status

VETERINARY-LABELED PRODUCTS: NONE

HUMAN-LABELED PRODUCTS:

Desmopressin Acetate Intranasal Spray Solution: 0.1 mg/mL (0.01%; 10 µg/spray) in 5 mL bottle or 2.5 mL rhinal tube delivery system; *DDAVP®*; generic; (Rx).

Desmopressin Acetate Injection Solution: 4 µg/mL in 1 mL single-dose vials and amps and 10 mL multiple dose vials; *DDAVP®*; generic; (Rx)

Desmopressin Acetate Oral Tablets: 0.1 mg and 0.2 mg; *DDAVP®*; generic; (Rx)

Desmopressin Acetate Sublingual Tablets: 55.3 µg (0.0553 mg); *Nocdurna®*; generic; (Rx)

NOTE: Desmopressin Acetate Intranasal Spray: 1.5 mg/mL (0.15% [150 µg/spray]; *Stimate®*) is available but is not used in veterinary medicine.

References

For the complete list of references, see **wiley.com/go/budde/plumb**

Desoxycorticosterone Pivalate (DOCP)

(de-sox-ee-kor-ti-***ko***-ster-ohn ***pih***-vah-late)

Percorten-V®, Zycortal®

Mineralocorticoid

Prescriber Highlights

- ▶ Parenteral mineralocorticoid used to treat hypoadrenocorticism (Addison's disease) in dogs; limited experience with its use in cats due to rare nature of this condition in this species.
- ▶ Adjust dose based on monitoring parameters. Extra-label dosing protocols using either lower desoxycorticosterone pivalate (DOCP) dose or extended dosing interval can be considered.
- ▶ Does not contain any glucocorticoid activity and thus a glucocorticoid must be used concurrently in the treatment of hypoadrenocorticism.
- ▶ Contraindications include congestive heart failure, severe renal disease, primary hepatic failure, or edema; use with caution in pregnant animals.
- ▶ May cause irritation at injection site. Shake vial well prior to withdrawing dose.

Uses/Indications

Desoxycorticosterone pivalate (DOCP) is indicated for the parenteral treatment of primary hypoadrenocorticism (ie, Addison's disease) in dogs. Compared to fludrocortisone, DOCP use resulted in lower prednisolone requirements[1] and more effectively suppressed plasma renin activity.[2] Extra-label lower dosages (ie, lower dose, longer dosing interval, or both) of DOCP can effectively control clinical signs of hypoadrenocorticism and maintain serum electrolytes.[3-5] Oral supplementation with salt (NaCl) is not necessary with animals receiving DOCP.[6]

DOCP has also been used to treat hypoadrenocorticism in cats (extra-label)[7,8]; experience is limited as this condition is rare in this species.

Pharmacology/Actions

Desoxycorticosterone pivalate (DOCP) is a long-acting mineralocorticoid agent that requires a functioning kidney to be effective. The site of action of mineralocorticoids is at the renal distal tubule, where it increases the reabsorption of sodium. Mineralocorticoids also enhance potassium and hydrogen ion excretion in the collecting tubules.

Pharmacokinetics

Little information is available. Desoxycorticosterone pivalate (DOCP) is injected IM or SC as a microcrystalline depot for slow dissolution into the circulation. Duration of action after injection is usually 21 to 30 days.

Contraindications/Precautions/Warnings

Do not use desoxycorticosterone pivalate (DOCP) in patients with documented hypersensitivity reactions to DOCP. Do not administer DOCP IV; acute collapse and shock may result.

DOCP is labeled as contraindicated in dogs suffering from congestive heart failure, severe renal disease, primary hepatic failure, or edema. Animals suffering from an Addisonian crisis (ie, hypovolemia, prerenal azotemia, inadequate tissue perfusion [shock]) must be rehydrated with IV fluid (eg, 0.9% sodium chloride) therapy before starting DOCP therapy.

Animals treated with DOCP for hypoadrenocorticism will also require glucocorticoid supplementation, as DOCP does not have glucocorticoid activity. All animals with hypoadrenocorticism should receive additional glucocorticoids (2-10 times basal) during periods of stress or acute illness. See ***Prednisolone/Prednisone*** monograph.

Ongoing monitoring is required to ensure proper dosing of this drug because individual dosage requirements vary.

Adverse Effects

Occasionally, irritation at the site of injection may occur; injection site abscesses have been reported.

Postapproval reported adverse effects in dogs receiving *Percorten-V®* included (in decreasing frequency) depression and lethargy, vomiting, anorexia, polydipsia, polyuria, diarrhea, facial and muzzle edema, weakness, urticaria, and anaphylaxis. Anemia has been reported following DOCP administration.

Adverse effects in a field safety analysis of *Zycortal®* listed the following (in decreasing frequency): polyuria, polydipsia, depression and lethargy, inappropriate urination, alopecia, decreased appetite/anorexia, panting, vomiting, diarrhea, shaking/trembling, polyphagia, UTI, urinary incontinence, restlessness, urticaria, and facial edema. Postapproval drug experience reporting with *Zycortal®* included reports of anaphylaxis and anemia.

Reproductive/Nursing Safety

The manufacturers state that the drug should not be used in pregnant dogs.

Because safety has not been established in animals, this drug should only be used when the maternal benefits outweigh the potential risks to offspring.

Overdose/Acute Toxicity

Desoxycorticosterone pivalate (DOCP) overdoses may cause polyuria, polydipsia, hypernatremia, hypertension, edema, and/or hypokalemia. Cardiomegaly is possible with prolonged overdoses; weight gain may be indicative of fluid retention. Glomerulonephropathy has occurred with prolonged exposure to doses 3 to 5 times the labeled initial starting dose.[6,9]

Electrolytes should be aggressively monitored; potassium may need to be supplemented. Discontinue DOCP treatment until clinical signs associated with overdose have resolved, then restart the drug at a lower dose (eg, 20% lower).

For patients that have experienced or are suspected to have experienced an overdose, it is strongly encouraged to consult with one of the 24-hour poison consultation centers that specialize in providing information specific for veterinary patients. For general information related to overdose and toxin exposures, as well as contact information for poison control centers, refer to ***Appendix***.

Drug Interactions

The following drug interactions have either been reported or are theoretical in humans or animals receiving desoxycorticosterone pivalate (DOCP) and may be of significance in veterinary patients. Unless otherwise noted, use together is not necessarily contraindicated, but weigh the potential risks and perform additional monitoring when appropriate.

- **AMPHOTERICIN B**: Patients may develop hypokalemia if mineralocorticoids are administered concomitantly with amphotericin B.
- **ASPIRIN**: DOCP may reduce salicylate levels.
- **DIGOXIN**: Because DOCP may cause hypokalemia, it should be used with caution and monitoring should be increased in patients receiving digitalis glycosides.
- **INSULIN**: DOCP could potentially increase the insulin requirements of diabetic patients.
- **POTASSIUM-DEPLETING DIURETICS** (eg, **chlorothiazide, furosemide, hydrochlorothiazide**): Patients may develop hypokalemia if mineralocorticoids are administered concomitantly with potassium-depleting diuretics; because diuretics can cause a loss of sodium, they may counteract the effects of DOCP.

- **Potassium-Sparing Diuretics** (eg, **spironolactone**): Concomitant use of DOCP with potassium-sparing diuretics may counter the effects of DOCP because desoxycorticosterone pivalate and potassium-sparing diuretics exhibit opposing mechanisms of action.

Dosages

DOGS:

Hypoadrenocorticism:

NOTES:

1. Dosage requirements are variable and must be individualized on the basis of the response of the patient to therapy.
2. Many clinicians begin treatment at dosages lower than what is found on the product label (see **Hypoadrenocorticism, lower dosage protocols** for extra-label dosage information).
3. DOCP replaces the mineralocorticoid hormones only. Glucocorticoid replacement (eg, predniso(lo)ne 0.2 – 0.4 mg/kg/day) is necessary. See ***Prednisolone/Prednisone***. Failure to concurrently administer glucocorticoids is the most common reason for treatment failure. Signs of glucocorticoid deficiency include depression, lethargy, vomiting, and diarrhea. Such signs should be treated with high doses of injectable glucocorticoids (prednisolone or dexamethasone), followed by continued oral therapy with predniso(lo)ne 0.2 – 0.4 mg/kg/day. Polyuria and polydipsia (PU/PD) usually indicate excess glucocorticoid but may also indicate DOCP excess. Begin by decreasing the glucocorticoid dose. If PU/PD persists, decrease the DOCP dosage without changing the interval between doses.

Percorten-V® (labeled dose FDA-approved): Begin treatment at a dose of 2.2 mg/kg IM (**NOTE:** *Some administer the drug SC in an extra-label manner—Plumb*) every 25 days. In some patients, the dose may be reduced. Most patients are well controlled with a dosage of 1.65 – 2.2 mg/kg every 21 to 30 days. Serum sodium and potassium levels should be monitored at days 14 and 25 initially and any time there is a dosage change. Well-controlled patients have normal electrolytes at day 14 after administration or may exhibit slight hyponatremia and hyperkalemia. This result needs no additional therapy as long as the patient is active and eating normally. Monitor for depression, lethargy, vomiting, or diarrhea, which indicate a probable glucocorticoid deficiency. Electrolyte results at Day 14 allow assessment of the dose, whereas results at Day 25 allow assessment of dosing interval. At the end of the 25-day dosing interval, the patient should be clinically normal and have normal serum electrolytes; the patient may have slight hyponatremia and slight hyperkalemia. This indicates that the dosage should not be altered. If the dog is not clinically normal or serum electrolytes are abnormal, the dosing interval should be decreased by 2 to 3 days.

Zycortal® (label dose; FDA-approved): Indicated for long-term administration at dosages dependent upon individual response to therapy. Tailor the DOCP dosage and concurrently administered glucocorticoid therapy to the individual dog based on clinical response and normalization of sodium and potassium concentrations. Initial dosage is 2.2 mg/kg SC every 25 days. Re-evaluate the dog and measure the serum sodium/potassium ratio ≈10 days after the first dose, which is the time to maximum concentration of desoxycorticosterone. If the dog's clinical signs have worsened or not resolved, adjust the dose of predniso(lo)ne therapy and/or investigate other causes of the clinical signs.

At ≈25 days after the first dose, re-evaluate the dog and repeat the sodium/potassium ratio:

- If the dog is both clinically normal and has a normal Na+/K+ ratio on Day 25, adjust the dose based on the Day 10 Na+/K+ ratio using the guidelines in the table below.
- If the dog is clinically normal and has a Na+/K+ ratio greater than 32 on Day 25, either adjust the dose based on the Day 10 Na+/K+ ratio according to the table below or delay the dose (see Prolonging the dosing interval below).
- If the dog is either not clinically normal or if the Na+/K+ ratio is abnormal on Day 25, adjust the dose of predniso(lo)ne or *Zycortal®* (see Subsequent doses and long-term management below).

Day 25: Administering the second dose of *Zycortal®* Suspension

If the Day 10 Na+/K+ ratio is:		25 days after the first dose, administer Zycortal® Suspension, as follows:
>34	Do not administer Dose 2 on Day 10.	Decrease dose to 2 mg/kg
>32 to 34	Do not administer Dose 2 on Day 10.	Decrease dose to 2.1 mg/kg
27 to 32	Do not administer Dose 2 on Day 10.	Continue 2.2 mg/kg
24 to <27	Do not administer Dose 2 on Day 10.	Increase dose to 2.3 mg/kg
<24	Do not administer Dose 2 on Day 10.	Increase dose to 2.4 mg/kg

Prolonging the dosing interval: If the dog is clinically normal and the Day 25 Na+/K+ ratio is greater than 32, it is possible to prolong the dosing interval instead of adjusting the dose as described in the above table. Evaluate the electrolytes every 3 to 7 days until the Na+/K+ ratio is less than 32, then administer 2.2 mg/kg of *Zycortal®* Suspension.

Subsequent doses and long-term management: For subsequent doses, use the following guidelines if the dog is not clinically normal and/or has abnormal Na+ or K+ concentrations:

- Clinical signs of polyuria/polydipsia: Decrease the prednisone/prednisolone dose first. If the polyuria/polydipsia persists, decrease the dose of *Zycortal®* Suspension without changing the dosing interval.
- Clinical signs of depression, lethargy, vomiting, diarrhea, or weakness: Increase prednisone/prednisolone dose.
- Hyperkalemia, hyponatremia, or Na+/K+ ratio less than 27: Decrease the *Zycortal®* Suspension dosing interval by 2 to 3 days.
- Hypokalemia or hypernatremia: Decrease the *Zycortal®* Suspension dose.

Hypoadrenocorticism, lower dosage protocols (extra-label): Different options exist; *choose only one* (ie, do not decrease the amount given and increase the dosing interval at the same time).

a) **Lower initial dosage**: In a study evaluating lower initial DOCP dosages for the treatment of canine primary hypoadrenocorticism, dogs were divided into 4 treatment groups (dosage range, median dosage, % of dogs in group): substantially lower than label dosages (0.36 – 0.96 mg/kg, 0.75 mg/kg, 38.8%), moderately lower dosages (1 – 1.47 mg/kg, 1.14 mg/kg, 14.3%), slightly lower dosages (1.76 – 2.19 mg/kg, 2.16 mg/kg, 20.4%), and recommended or higher dosages (2.20 – 3.82 mg/kg, 2.2 mg/kg, 26.5%).[5] All doses were administered IM. Despite the wide range of initial DOCP dosages administered, all dogs had similar responses with no dog developing an Addisonian crisis after diagnosis and beginning therapy. In addition, no dogs, regardless of DOCP dosage, developed persistent or severe electrolyte derangements warranting a dosage adjustment. This retrospective study suggests that lower initial dosages of DOCP may be sufficient.

b) **Dose reduction**: If using the initial recommended starting dosage of DOCP (2.2 mg/kg IM or SC), follow guidelines to allow normalization of sodium and potassium concentrations. Then consider tapering the dose by 10% each month while monitoring the sodium and potassium concentrations prior to each injection. Using this method, ideally the lowest effective dose can be found for the individual patient. Once electrolyte concentrations begin trending outside of the normal reference range prior to the next injection, return to the previous increased dose that allowed normalization of sodium and potassium concentrations for the entire dosing interval.[10]

c) **Extended dosing interval**: Initial dose 2.1 – 2.6 mg/kg IM or SC. Check plasma sodium and potassium concentration after 30 days and every 7 days thereafter until hyponatremia or hyperkalemia developed at a planned evaluation or the dog exhibited clinical signs (eg, vomiting, diarrhea, anorexia, lethargy, trembling, collapse) with concurrent electrolyte concentration outside the reference interval. The duration of action (dosing interval) of DOCP was recorded as the duration of time from DOCP administration to the time that either hyponatremia or hyperkalemia developed. In dogs newly diagnosed with primary hypoadrenocorticism receiving the first DOCP dose (median dose 2.2 mg/kg), the median dosing interval was 56 days (range 41-85 days). Notably, the median dosing interval was 59 days (range 38-90 days) in dogs previously receiving DOCP, but ≈34% of those dogs received a DOCP dose less than 2 mg/kg. The DOCP dosage (mg/kg) did not predict the duration of action.[4]

CATS:

Hypoadrenocorticism (extra-label):

a) 2.2 mg/kg IM or SC every 25 days plus prednisolone 0.25 – 1 mg/cat (NOT mg/kg) PO twice daily. If daily oral dosing is not feasible, consider methylprednisolone acetate 10 mg IM once a month.[11] From 2 case reports,[7,8] 2.2 mg/kg IM plus prednisolone 0.2 mg/kg/day PO. DOCP dosing interval was every 21 days for one cat,[8] and every 35 to 40 days for the other cat.[7]

b) 10 – 12.5 mg/cat (NOT mg/kg) IM per month. Adjust dose based upon follow-up serum electrolyte concentrations monitored every 1 to 2 weeks during initial maintenance period. Normal electrolyte values 2 weeks following injection suggests adequate dosing but does not provide information regarding duration of action. Prednisolone 1.25 mg/cat (NOT mg/kg) PO once a day or methylprednisolone acetate 10 mg/cat (NOT mg/kg) IM once a month provides long-term glucocorticoid supplementation.[12]

Monitoring

- Serum electrolytes (including calculation of sodium/potassium ratio), BUN, creatinine: initially every 1 to 2 weeks, then once stabilized, every 3 to 4 months. See ***Dosages*** section above for details.
- Body weight and physical exam checking for evidence of edema (eg, peripheral, pulmonary)
- Clinical efficacy

Client Information

- Long-acting injection administered into the muscle (IM) or subcutaneous tissues (SC) every 20 to 30 days. Your veterinarian will adjust the dose and times between doses depending on your animal's response.
- Shake vial vigorously before drawing up into syringe.
- Must not be given IV (into the vein).
- For this medication to work, give it exactly as your veterinarian has prescribed. It's a good idea to always check the prescription label to be sure you are giving the drug correctly. If there is difficulty administering the medicine, contact your veterinarian.
- Watch for signs of the dose being too high (greater thirst and need to urinate, swelling/edema, weight gain, pot belly); be sure to contact your veterinarian if you see any of these signs.
- Watch for signs that the dose is too low (muscle weakness, lethargy [lack of energy], shaking, collapsing/fainting, loss of appetite/weight loss, vomiting, diarrhea, slower heartbeat, or painful abdomen). Contact your veterinarian right away if you see any of these signs.
- Regular laboratory testing is essential for monitoring the effectiveness of the therapy. Do not miss these important follow-up visits.

Chemistry/Synonyms

A mineralocorticoid, desoxycorticosterone pivalate (DOCP) occurs as a white or creamy white powder that is odorless and stable in air. It is practically insoluble in water and slightly soluble in alcohol and vegetable oils. The injectable product is a white aqueous suspension and has a pH between 5 and 8.5.

The commercially available injection (*Percorten-V®*) contains (per mL): 25 mg desoxycorticosterone pivalate, 10.5 mg methylcellulose, 3 mg sodium carboxymethylcellulose, 1 mg polysorbate 80, and 8 mg sodium chloride with 0.002% thimerosal added as preservative in water for injection.

The commercially available injection (*Zycortal®*) contains (per mL): 25 mg desoxycorticosterone pivalate, 10.5 mg methylcellulose, 3 mg sodium carboxymethylcellulose, 1 mg polysorbate 60, 8 mg sodium chloride, and 1 mg chlorocresol in water for injection.

Desoxycorticosterone pivalate may also be known as deoxycorticosterone pivalate, deoxycorticosterone trimethyl-acetate, deoxycortone pivalate, deoxycortone trimethylacetate, desoxycorticosterone trimethyl-acetate, *Cortiron®*, *Zycortal®*, or *Percorten-V®*.

Storage/Stability

Store the injectable suspension at room temperature 25°C (77°F), with excursions between 15°C and 30°C (59°F-86°F) permitted. Protect from light or freezing. The *Zycortal®* label states to use within 120 days of first puncture and puncture a maximum of 4 times.

The *Percorten-V®* label states that once the vial is broached, product should be used within 4 months.

Compatibility/Compounding Considerations

Do not mix desoxycorticosterone pivalate (DOCP) with any other agent.

Dosage Forms/Regulatory Status

VETERINARY-LABELED PRODUCTS:

Desoxycorticosterone Pivalate Injectable Suspension: 25 mg/mL in 4 mL vials; *Percorten-V®*, *Zycortal®* Suspension; (Rx). FDA-approved for use in dogs; NADA #141-029 (*Percorten-V®*) and 141-444 (*Zycortal®*).

HUMAN-LABELED PRODUCTS: NONE

References

For the complete list of references, see **wiley.com/go/budde/plumb**

Detomidine

(de-***toe***-ma-deen) *Dormosedan*®

Alpha-2-Adrenergic Agonist

Prescriber Highlights

- Sedative and analgesic used primarily in horses
- Contraindications include pre-existing sinoatrial (SA) or pathologic atrioventricular (AV) block; severe coronary, cerebrovascular, or respiratory disease; and chronic kidney disease
- Use with caution in horses with endotoxic or traumatic shock or approaching shock; advanced hepatic or renal disease; stress caused by temperature extremes, fatigue, or high altitude; with intestinal impactions or suspected colic because detomidine may mask abdominal pain or changes in respiratory and cardiac rates when administered prior to establishing diagnosis
- Handle animals sedated with detomidine as a single agent with caution as they may respond (eg, kick) to external stimuli even when deeply sedated; the addition of opioids may temper this response.
- Adverse effects include decreased GI motility, piloerection, and an initial blood pressure increase with concurrent reflex bradycardia and/or heart block.

Uses/Indications

Detomidine is FDA-approved for use as a sedative analgesic in horses; it is also used clinically (extra-label) in other species (eg, cattle, camelids, sheep, goats). In a comparative study in horses, detomidine delivered as an oral transmucosal (OTM) gel produced sedation (chin to ground) similar to that achieved from IV administration but caused less ataxia.[1] The OTM gel has been used orally in dogs and cats, and in horses, orally and transvaginally.

Pharmacology/Actions

Detomidine, like xylazine, is an alpha-2-adrenergic agonist that reduces norepinephrine-mediated neural impulses, resulting in a dose-dependent sedative and analgesic effect. Detomidine is ≈50 to 100 times more potent than xylazine.

Detomidine effects on the cardiovascular system include an initial increase in peripheral vascular resistance with increased blood pressure followed by a longer period of lowered blood pressures (below baseline). Bradycardia can be seen with some animals developing a second-degree heart block or other arrhythmias. An overall decrease in cardiac output may be seen.

Detomidine effects on respiratory function are usually clinically insignificant, but at high doses it can cause respiratory depression with decreased tidal volumes and respiratory rates, and an overall decreased minute volume. Brachycephalic dogs and horses with upper airway disease may develop dyspnea.

Detomidine causes skeletal muscle relaxation through inhibition of central mediated pathways, and the retractor muscle can be affected. As with other alpha-2-adrenergic agonists, detomidine is emetogenic in species that vomit. Detomidine depresses thermoregulatory mechanisms and either hypo- or hyperthermia is a possibility depending on ambient air temperatures.

Detomidine can increase blood glucose secondary to decreased serum levels of insulin. In nondiabetic animals, there appears to be little clinical significance associated with this effect although an osmotic diuresis may result from transient hyperglycemia.

Pharmacokinetics

In dogs, after receiving an OTM dose of 1 mg/m^2 (NOT mg/kg), median maximum concentration was 7.03 ng/mL, time to maximum concentration was 1 hour, and bioavailability was 34.52%; mean elimination half-life was 0.63 hours.[2]

In horses, onset of sedative effect after IV or IM administration is within 5 minutes, and peaks at ≈5 to 20 minutes; sedative duration is dose-related, lasting 30 to 120 minutes after labeled parenteral doses.[3] Following OTM administration, sedation begins within 40 minutes, peaks at 60 to 80 minutes and is ≈2 hours in duration.

In horses, detomidine is well absorbed after oral administration (ie, swallowed), but because of a high first-pass effect, little drug is available systemically. Bioavailability is 38% with IM administration and 22% after the OTM gel, and the peak concentrations observed after administration of the gel are ≈40% of those observed after IM injection. Following administration, maximum blood concentration is reached ≈2 minutes (IV), 77 minutes (IM), and 1.83 hours (OTM). The drug is 85% protein bound and is rapidly distributed into tissues; the volume of distribution is 0.5 to 1.9 L/kg and is lower at rest (0.47 to 0.59 L/kg) compared to after exercise (1.3 L/kg). Detomidine is extensively metabolized, and elimination half-lives are ≈24 to 66 minutes (IV, at rest), 46 minutes (IV, after exercise), 51 minutes (IM, at rest), and 90 minutes (OTM). Detomidine is a high-extraction drug and clearance (≈12 to 16 mL/minute/kg) can be altered by changes to liver blood flow (eg, with exercise[4]). Metabolites are excreted primarily into the urine.[3,5-10]

When the OTM gel is administered intravaginally in mares, sedation lasts longer than IV detomidine, with a mean maximum plasma concentration of 8.57 ng/mL, time to maximum concentration of 0.37 hour, and bioavailability of 25%.[11]

In cattle, IM administration resulted in peak concentration at ≈16 minutes, bioavailability was 85%, and apparent Vd was 1.9 L/kg. Elimination half-life was 2.6 hours but was 1.3 hours after IV administration.[12]

Contraindications/Precautions/Warnings

Detomidine is contraindicated in horses with preexisting SA block or pathologic AV block, severe coronary insufficiency, cerebrovascular disease, respiratory disease, or chronic renal failure. Use cautiously in animals with endotoxic or traumatic shock or approaching shock, and in patients with advanced hepatic or renal disease. Use with caution in horses that are stressed because of temperature extremes, fatigue, or high altitude; consider using lower dosages. Because this drug may inhibit GI motility, use with caution in patients treated for intestinal impactions. When possible in horses with suspected colic, the use of detomidine analgesia should be used only after confirmation of the diagnosis as it may mask abdominal pain and conceal changes in respiratory and cardiac rates, making diagnosis more difficult.

Although animals may appear to be deeply sedated, some may respond (eg, kick) to external stimuli; use appropriate caution. The addition of opioids (eg, butorphanol) may help temper this effect. To improve the effects of detomidine, allow the horse to stand quietly for 5 minutes prior to injection and for 10 to 15 minutes after injection to improve the effect of the drug.[3] After administering detomidine, protect the animal from temperature extremes.

The OTM gel can be absorbed across human skin; wear impermeable gloves during drug administration or when performing procedures that require contact with the horse's mouth.[10]

In cattle, use of alpha-2-agonists under emergency conditions is discouraged as the risk of profound cardiovascular instability or recumbency exceeds the benefits observed with the use of these drugs.[13]

Adverse Effects

Detomidine can cause an initial and immediate rise in blood pressure followed by reflex bradycardia and AV block. Atropine 0.02 mg/kg IV has been successfully used to prevent or correct the bradycardia that may be seen when detomidine is administered at labeled dosages. However, routine use of anticholinergics is generally not recommended because of the potential for GI motility reduction and hypertension. In addition, detomidine can cause piloerection, sweating, ataxia, salivation, mild muscle tremors, and penile prolapse. Horses may stagger or appear uncoordinated for 3 to 5 minutes following injection. Decreased tear production has also been noted.[14,15]

When compared to xylazine, detomidine causes more pronounced bradycardia and bradyarrhythmias (eg, AV block). Because the sedative and muscle-relaxing effects of detomidine in horses can persist for up to 90 minutes, it may influence the quality of recovery and contribute to postanesthesia ataxia. One study reported that detomidine caused a mild increase in atrial fibrillation cycle length.[16]

Emesis occurred in 100% of cats receiving OTM gel.[17]

Reproductive/Nursing Safety

Detomidine is not recommend for use in breeding animals as the possible effects of detomidine in breeding horses is limited to uncontrolled clinical reports[3] In small studies, administration during the last trimester or the last 3 weeks of pregnancy in healthy mares resulted in no apparent detrimental effects[18,19]; however, in pregnant ruminants, administration of detomidine at recommended doses is considered less likely than xylazine to induce premature parturition.

Overdose/Acute Toxicity

The manufacturer states that detomidine is tolerated by horses at doses 5 times (0.2 mg/kg) the maximum dose level (0.04 mg/kg). Dosages of 0.4 mg/kg given daily for 3 consecutive days produced microscopic foci of myocardial necrosis in 1 of 8 horses tested. Doses at 10 to 40 times the recommended amount may cause severe respiratory and cardiovascular changes that are irreversible and fatal. Atipamezole or tolazoline can be used to reverse some or all the effects of the drug.

Drug Interactions

The following drug interactions have either been reported or are theoretical in humans or animals receiving detomidine and may be of significance in veterinary patients. Unless otherwise noted, use together is not necessarily contraindicated, but weigh the potential risks and perform additional monitoring when appropriate.

- **Alpha-2 Agonists, Other** (eg, **clonidine, dexmedetomidine, romifidine, xylazine**): Not recommended for routine use with detomidine as effects may be additive
- **Sulfonamides, Potentiated** (eg, **trimethoprim/sulfa**): Concurrent use may precipitate fatal dysrhythmias.[3] Combination is contraindicated.

Although the manufacturer warns to use extreme caution combining detomidine with other sedative or analgesic drugs, the preponderance of research studies and clinical experience indicate balanced anesthetic protocols can safely use detomidine in combination with the following agents although lower dosages of detomidine and/or the following agents may be required.

- **Anesthetic Agents** (eg, **alfaxalone, isoflurane, ketamine, propofol**)
- **Benzodiazepines** (eg, **diazepam, midazolam**)
- **Opioids** (eg, **fentanyl, morphine**)
- **Phenothiazines** (eg, **acepromazine**): Alpha-2 effects may be additive and severe hypotension can result.

Dosages

CAUTION: Do not confuse µg/kg or mg/m^2 with mg/kg doses.

DOGS:

Sedation/anxiolytic (extra-label): Using the equine oromucosal gel, 0.35 – 2 mg/m^2 (NOT mg/kg) administered via the oral transmucosal (OTM) route.[2,20,21] Maximum sedation occurred 45 to 75 minutes after administration; effects were reversed with atipamezole 0.1 mg/kg IM.

CATS:

Sedation (extra-label): Using the equine oromucosal gel, 0.25 mg/kg) OTM, all cats vomited within 2 minutes of administration, yet moderate sedation was noted within 30 minutes after administration and duration was 45 to 60 minutes.[17]

HORSES:

Analgesia (label dosages; FDA-approved): Detomidine 0.02 – 0.04 mg/kg IV; allow animal to rest quietly prior to and after injection. Effects generally occur within 2 to 4 minutes of administration. Lower doses will generally provide 30 to 45 minutes of analgesia. The higher dose will provide 45 to 75 minutes of analgesia.

Sedation (label dosages; FDA-approved):

- *Injection*: Detomidine 0.02 – 0.04 mg/kg IV or IM; allow animal to rest quietly prior to and after injection. Effects generally occur within 2 to 4 minutes of administration. Lower dose will generally provide 30 to 90 minutes of sedation. The higher dose will generally provide 90 to 120 minutes of sedation.
- *OTM Gel*: Detomidine 0.04 mg/kg placed beneath the tongue of the horse; not meant to be swallowed. The dosing syringe delivers the product in 0.25 mL (1.9 mg) increments. See dosing tablc[3]

Dosing Table for Detomidine Oral Gel

Approximate body weight (kg [lb])	Range of doses (mg/kg)	Dose volume (mL)
150 to 199 (330-439)	0.051 – 0.038	1
200 to 249 (440-549)	0.047 – 0.038	1.25
250 to 299 (550-659)	0.046 – 0.038	1.5
300 to 349 (660-769)	0.044 – 0.038	1.75
350 to 399 (770-879)	0.043 – 0.038	2
400 to 449 (880-989)	0.043 – 0.038	2.25
450 to 499 (990-1099)	0.042 – 0.038	2.5
500 to 549 (1100-1209)	0.042 – 0.038	2.75
550 to 600 (1210-1320)	0.041 – 0.038	3

Sedation, chemical restraint, analgesia (extra-label):

As a single agent:

a) Detomidine 0.005 – 0.03 mg/kg IV[22]
b) Detomidine 0.022 mg/kg/hr IV CRI
c) **Oral gel formulation**: Detomidine 0.04 mg/kg intravaginally; sedation lasts over 3 hours.[11]
d) **Caudal epidural**: Detomidine 0.06 mg/kg diluted to 10 mL with sterile water and administered as a caudal epidural block[23]; onset of action: ≈5 minutes, duration of analgesia: ≈3 hours.

As a combination:

a) Detomidine 0.01 mg/kg IV in combination with methadone 0.2 mg/kg and administered IV was more antinociceptive than methadone 0.2 mg/kg in combination with acepromazine 0.05 mg/kg IV.[24]
b) Detomidine 0.01 mg/kg slow IV followed by buprenorphine 0.005 mg/kg IV will produce sedation for standing procedures; if sedation is inadequate, doses can be repeated. Horses developed marked ataxia, bradycardia (some with 2nd AV block), and decreased respiratory rates. Sedation lasted 60 minutes.[25]
c) **CRI for standing procedures:**
   i. Begin with acepromazine 0.02 mg/kg IV followed 30

minutes later by detomidine 0.01 mg/kg IV then 5 minutes later by *either* buprenorphine 0.01 mg/kg IV or morphine 0.1 mg/kg IV. Then add detomidine 0.006 mg/kg/minute IV CRI. Both protocols (eg, using buprenorphine or morphine) provided sedation and analgesia; however, more adverse effects were observed with buprenorphine (eg, CNS excitation [box-walking, head bobbing]).[26]

ii. Detomidine 0.005 mg/kg in combination with methadone 0.2 mg/kg IV followed by detomidine 0.0125 mg/kg/hour and methadone 0.05 mg/kg/hour (starting rate) IV CRI produced adequate sedation for standing surgery when combined with locoregional anesthesia.[27]

d) **Caudal epidural**: Detomidine 0.03 mg/kg in combination with morphine 0.2 mg mg/kg and administered as a caudal epidural block[28]; duration of analgesia is greater than 6 hours.

CRI for partial intravenous anesthesia (PIVA; extra-label): Detomidine 0.013 – 0.038 mg/kg/hour IV resulted in a significant MAC reduction.[29]

CRI for total intravenous anesthesia (TIVA; extra-label): Detomidine 10 mg (total amount; NOT mg/kg) and ketamine 500 – 1000 mg (total amount; NOT mg/kg) added to 500 mL of guaifenesin 5%. This drug combination will yield a solution of guaifenesin 50 mg/mL, ketamine 1 – 2 mg/mL, and detomidine 0.02 mg/mL to be infused at a rate of 1.2 – 1.6 mL/kg/hour IV CRI. **NOTE**: If 500 mL of guaifenesin <u>10%</u> is used as the base, the total amounts of detomidine and ketamine to be added should be doubled, which will result in final concentrations that are also doubled, and thus, the infusion rate for this solution will need to be halved to deliver the same CRI rate.[30]

Donkeys, sedation (extra-label):

a) Detomidine 0.0135, 0.017, and 0.02 mg/kg IV increased sedation scores above control in 1 study.[31]

b) Detomidine 0.06 mg/kg in combination with butorphanol 0.05 mg/kg IM sedated miniature donkeys for 38 minutes.[32]

c) Detomidine gel 0.04 mg/kg OTM may be useful for standing sedation prior to painful minor procedures.[33]

CATTLE:

Standing sedation (extra-label): Information regarding the use of detomidine in ruminants is limited. The dosage ranges provided are estimates and should be adjusted based on experience. Administering the IV dose IM further reduces the possibility of recumbency.[34]

a) <u>Tractable cattle</u>: Detomidine 0.002 – 0.005 mg/kg IV or 0.006 – 0.01 mg/kg IM

b) <u>Anxious cattle</u>: Detomidine 0.005 – 0.0075 mg/kg IV or 0.01 – 0.015 mg/kg IM

c) <u>Extremely anxious or unruly cattle</u>: Detomidine 0.01 – 0.015 mg/kg IV or 0.015 – 0.02 mg/kg IM

Analgesia (extra-label): 0.01 mg/kg IV[35]; short (½ hour) duration of action.

Sedation/analgesia for horn disbudding in calves (extra-label): Detomidine 0.03 mg/kg IV or detomidine gel 0.08 mg/kg OTM produced sedation in 11 and 38 minutes, respectively. All recoveries were without complications.[36]

Restraint in free-ranging cattle (extra-label): Detomidine 0.04 mg/kg in combination with tiletamine-zolazepam 0.53 mg/kg and ketamine 0.53 mg/kg IM. Rapid onset and suitable immobilization were achieved for minor procedures. Atipamezole was administered at the end of the procedure to decrease recovery time.[37]

SHEEP, GOATS:

Analgesia (extra-label): Detomidine 0.005 – 0.05 mg/kg IV, IM every 3 to 6 hours[38]

Sedation in sheep (extra-label): Loading dose of detomidine 0.02 mg/kg IV followed by detomidine 0.06 mg/kg/hour IV CRI produces satisfactory sedation for minimally invasive procedures with minimal cardiorespiratory adverse effects.[39]

Anesthesia (extra-label): Detomidine 0.01 mg/kg IM, followed by propofol at 3 – 5 mg/kg IV

Lumbosacral epidural in goats (extra-label): Detomidine 0.02 – 0.04 mg/kg produced analgesia within 1 to 5 minutes of administration, which lasted 70 to 120 minutes.[40,41]

CAMELIDS:

Analgesia (extra-label): Detomidine 0.005 – 0.05 mg/kg IV or IM every 3 to 6 hours (once)[42]

Epidural in calves (extra-label): Detomidine 0.05 mg/kg in combination with lidocaine 0.22 mg/kg administered into the sacro-coccygeal epidural space had reliable sedation and analgesia for 60 to 90 minutes.[43]

BIRDS:

Sedation/analgesia (extra-label): 12 – 15 mg/kg intranasally in parakeets and canaries.[44-46]

Monitoring

- Level of sedation and analgesia; body temperature
- Heart rate and rhythm, blood pressure, respiratory rate, and pulse oximetry

Client Information

- When used parenterally (by injection), detomidine should be used in a professionally supervised setting by individuals familiar with its properties.
- Withhold feed and water until the sedative effects of detomidine have subsided.
- When administering the oromucosal gel, ensure the following:
  a) The lock ring is securely in place at the desired volume mark before administering.
  b) The horse's mouth contains no feed.
  c) The dose is deposited under the horse's tongue.
- When handling the oromucosal gel, wear disposable gloves; avoid contact with human skin.
- If dispensing gel for clients to administer to their animals, give clients the ***Client Information Sheet for Owner/Handler Use and Safety***.

Chemistry/Synonyms

An imidazoline derivative alpha-2-adrenergic agonist, detomidine HCl occurs as a white, crystalline substance that is soluble in water.

Detomidine HCl may also be known as demotidini hydrochloridum, MPV-253-AII, or *Dormosedan*®.

Storage/Stability

Detomidine HCl for injection should be stored at room temperature, 15°C to 30°C (59°F-85°F) and protected from light.

Detomidine gel for sublingual administration should be stored at controlled room temperature, 20°C to 25°C (68°F-77°F); excursions are permitted from 15°C to 30°C (59°F-85°F).

Dosage Forms/Regulatory Status

VETERINARY-LABELED PRODUCTS:

Detomidine HCl for Injection: 10 mg/mL in 5 mL and 20 mL vials; *Dormosedan*®; (Rx). FDA-approved for use in mature horses and yearlings. In cattle, goats, and sheep, the FARAD-suggested withdrawal time[47] for single or multiple doses of detomidine (up to 0.08 mg/kg IM or IV) are 3 days for meat and 72 hours for milk.

Detomidine HCL Oromucosal Gel for Sublingual Administration: 7.6 mg/mL in 3 mL graduated dosing syringes; *Dormosedan Gel®*; (Rx). FDA-approved for use in horses not intended for human consumption. NADA #141-306. Based on times when detomidine was indetectable in blood and urine, 1 study recommended a 72-hour withdrawal time (prior to racing) after a single 40 µg/kg SL dose for horses.[48]

The Association of Racing Commissioners International (ARCI) has designated this drug as a class 3 substance. See ***Appendix*** for more information.

HUMAN-LABELED PRODUCTS: NONE

References

For the complete list of references, see **wiley.com/go/budde/plumb**

Dexamethasone

Dexamethasone Sodium Phosphate

(dex-a-***meth***-a-zone) *Azium®, Dexasone®*

Glucocorticoid

*For more information, see **Glucocorticoid Agents, General Information**.*

Prescriber Highlights

- ► Injectable, oral, and ophthalmic glucocorticoid
- ► Long-acting; 30 times more potent than hydrocortisone; no mineralocorticoid activity. For practical dosing in dogs and cats, determine the dosage of prednis(ol)one needed and divide by 7 to determine the dexamethasone dosage.
- ► Dexamethasone sodium phosphate has an effective dexamethasone concentration of 3 mg/mL.
- ► Contraindications (relative) include systemic fungal infections. Concurrent use with NSAIDS increases the risk for GI ulceration.
- ► Caution is advised for use in animals with active bacterial infections, corneal ulcers, hyperadrenocorticism, diabetes mellitus, osteoporosis, chronic psychotic reactions, predisposition to thrombophlebitis, hypertension, and renal insufficiency.
- ► Goal of therapy should be to use the lowest dose possible for the least amount of time to treat and control patient's condition.
- ► Primary adverse effects with sustained use are Cushingoid in nature, but acute effects (primarily GI related, colon perforation in dogs receiving high doses) can be seen.
- ► Many potential drug and laboratory interactions

Uses/Indications

Although glucocorticoids have been used to treat many conditions in humans and animals, dexamethasone has 5 primary uses with accompanying dosage ranges: 1) as a diagnostic agent to test for hyperadrenocorticism, 2) as a replacement or supplementation (eg, relative adrenal insufficiency associated with septic shock) for glucocorticoid deficiency secondary to hypoadrenocorticism, 3) as an anti-inflammatory agent, 4) for immunosuppression, and 5) as an antineoplastic agent.[1,2]

Glucocorticoids are used in the treatment of endocrine conditions (eg, adrenal insufficiency), autoimmune and immune-mediated diseases (eg, rheumatoid arthritis, systemic lupus, masticatory myositis[3]), severe allergic conditions, anaphylaxis, envenomation, respiratory diseases (eg, asthma), dermatologic diseases (eg, pemphigus, allergic dermatoses), hematologic disorders (eg, thrombocytopenia, autoimmune hemolytic anemia), neoplasias, nervous system disorders (eg, increased CSF pressure), GI diseases (eg, ulcerative colitis exacerbations, inflammatory bowel disease), renal diseases (eg, nephrotic syndrome), and induction of fetal maturation. Some glucocorticoids are used topically on the eye and skin or are injected intra-articularly or intralesionally. This list is not exhaustive. High-dose glucocorticoid use in the treatment of hemorrhagic or hypovolemic shock, head trauma, spinal cord trauma, and/or sepsis is not supported.[4]

In general, when administering glucocorticoids, the following principles should be followed:

- A specific diagnosis is needed before glucocorticoids are administered, as they can mask disease.
- A course of treatment should be determined prior to treatment.
- A therapeutic endpoint should be determined prior to treatment.
- The least potent glucocorticoid should be used at the lowest dose for the shortest amount of time.
- It is important to understand when glucocorticoid use is inappropriate (eg, acute infection, diabetes).[5]

See ***Glucocorticoid Agents, General Information.***

Pharmacology/Actions

Dexamethasone is a long-acting glucocorticoid with a rapid onset. Glucocorticoids have effect on virtually every cell type and system:

- **Cardiovascular system**: Glucocorticoids can reduce capillary permeability and enhance vasoconstriction. Increased blood pressure and a clinically insignificant positive inotropic effect can occur after glucocorticoid administration.
- **Cells**: Glucocorticoids can inhibit fibroblast proliferation, macrophage response to migration inhibiting factor, sensitization of lymphocytes, and cellular response to inflammation mediators; they can also stabilize lysosomal membranes.
- **CNS/autonomic nervous system**: Glucocorticoids can lower seizure threshold, alter mood and behavior, diminish response to pyrogens, stimulate appetite, and maintain α rhythm. Glucocorticoids are necessary for normal adrenergic receptor sensitivity.
- **Endocrine system**: When an animal is not stressed, glucocorticoids suppress the release of corticotropin (adrenocorticotropic hormone [ACTH]) from the anterior pituitary, which reduces or prevents the release of endogenous corticosteroids. Stress factors (eg, renal disease, liver disease, diabetes) may occasionally nullify the suppressing aspects of exogenously administered steroids. The release of thyroid-stimulating hormone (TSH), follicle-stimulating hormone (FSH), prolactin, and luteinizing hormone may be reduced when glucocorticoids are administered at pharmacologic doses. Conversion of thyroxine (T_4) to triiodothyronine (T_3) may be reduced by glucocorticoids, and plasma levels of parathyroid hormone may be increased. Glucocorticoids may inhibit osteoblast function. Vasopressin (antidiuretic hormone [ADH]) activity is reduced at the renal tubules, and diuresis may occur. Glucocorticoids inhibit insulin binding to insulin receptors and the postreceptor effects of insulin.
- **Fluid and electrolyte balance**: Glucocorticoids can increase renal potassium and calcium excretion, sodium and chloride reabsorption, and extracellular fluid volume. Hypokalemia and/or hypocalcemia rarely occur. Diuresis may develop following glucocorticoid administration.
- **GI tract and hepatic system**: Glucocorticoids increase the secretion of gastric acid, pepsin, and trypsin. Glucocorticoids alter the structure of mucin and decrease mucosal cell prolifer-

ation. Iron salts and calcium absorption are decreased, whereas fat absorption is increased. Hepatic changes can include increased fat and glycogen deposits in hepatocytes and increased serum concentrations of alanine aminotransferase (ALT) and gamma-glutamyl transpeptidase (GGT). Significant increases can be seen in serum alkaline phosphatase (ALP) concentrations. Glucocorticoids can cause minor increases in bromosulfophthalein (BSP) retention time.

- **Hematopoietic system**: Glucocorticoids can increase the number of circulating platelets, neutrophils, and red blood cells (RBCs), but platelet aggregation is inhibited. Decreased amounts of lymphocytes (peripheral), monocytes, and eosinophils can be seen, as glucocorticoids sequester these cells in the lungs and spleen and can decrease the release from bone marrow; removal of old RBCs becomes diminished. Glucocorticoids can cause involution of lymphoid tissue.
- **Immune system** (also see ***Cells*** and ***Hematopoietic system***): Glucocorticoids can decrease circulating levels of T lymphocytes; inhibit lymphokines; inhibit neutrophil, macrophage, and monocyte migration; reduce production of interferon; and inhibit phagocytosis, chemotaxis, antigen processing, and intracellular killing. Specific acquired immunity is affected less than nonspecific immune responses. Glucocorticoids can also antagonize the complement cascade and mask clinical signs of infection. Mast cells are decreased in number, and histamine synthesis is suppressed. Many of these effects only occur at high doses, and different species have different responses.
- **Metabolic effects**: Glucocorticoids stimulate gluconeogenesis. Lipogenesis is enhanced in certain areas of the body (eg, abdomen), and adipose tissue can be redistributed away from the extremities to the trunk. Fatty acids are mobilized from tissue, and their oxidation is increased. Plasma levels of triglycerides, cholesterol, and glycerol are increased. Protein is mobilized from most areas of the body (except the liver).
- **Musculoskeletal**: Glucocorticoids can cause muscular weakness, atrophy, and osteoporosis. Bone growth can be inhibited via growth hormone and somatomedin inhibition, increased calcium excretion, and inhibition of vitamin D activation. Resorption of bone can be enhanced. Fibrocartilage growth is also inhibited.
- **Ophthalmic**: Prolonged glucocorticoid use (both systemic or topically to the eye) can cause increased intraocular pressure, glaucoma, cataracts, and exophthalmos.
- **Skin**: Thinning of dermal tissue and skin atrophy can be seen with glucocorticoid therapy. Hair follicles can become distended, and alopecia can occur.

Pharmacokinetics

The pharmacokinetics of dexamethasone do not translate into pharmacologic effects. The half-life of dexamethasone in dogs is ≈2 to 5 hours, but biologic activity can persist for 48 hours or more after administration. In a study, transdermal absorption was *not* demonstrated after dexamethasone 0.25 mg/0.05 mL in PLO was applied to the inner pinna of healthy cats.[6] The half-life in cattle is ≈4.5 to 5 hours.[7,8] In a study of horses, after doses of 0.05 mg/kg PO, IV, IM, or IA, half-life was ≈3.5 hours, and endogenous cortisol concentrations did not return to baseline until 96 to 120 hours (IV, IM, and IA) and 72 hours (PO) after administration.[9] In another study, bioavailability of dexamethasone sodium phosphate injection delivered via nebulization to healthy horses was 4.3%.[10] Application of dexamethasone ophthalmic ointment to equines has been shown to produce anti-inflammatory concentrations only in the anterior parts of the eye, but dexamethasone has been detected in the serum of horses receiving 7 applications per day.[11] Dermal dexamethasone application to horses has been shown to suppress plasma cortisol more than 75% below baseline and blunt cortisol response to ACTH stimulation.[12]

Contraindications/Precautions/Warnings

Because dexamethasone has negligible mineralocorticoid effects, it should generally not be used alone in the treatment of adrenal insufficiency.

The injectable propylene glycol base product should not be administered rapidly IV, as hypotension, collapse, and hemolytic anemia can occur. Many clinicians only use dexamethasone sodium phosphate when administering the drug IV.

Systemic use of glucocorticoids is generally contraindicated in patients with systemic fungal infections (unless used for replacement therapy for Addison's disease), when administered IM in patients with idiopathic thrombocytopenia, and in patients hypersensitive to glucocorticoids. Concurrent use of sustained-release injectable glucocorticoids is contraindicated with chronic corticosteroid therapy in the treatment of systemic diseases. Corticosteroid use may be contraindicated in horses predisposed to laminitis or exhibiting endocrinopathies.

Patients that have received systemic glucocorticoids for more than 2 weeks should be slowly tapered off the drug to allow return of normal endogenous ACTH and corticosteroid function. If the animal undergoes a stressful event (eg, surgery, trauma, illness) during the tapering process and/or before normal adrenal and pituitary functions resume, additional glucocorticoids should be administered.

Animals, particularly cats, at risk for diabetes mellitus (eg, obese patients, patients with hyperadrenocorticism) should receive glucocorticoids with caution due to the potent hyperglycemic effect.

In dogs, dexamethasone can cause more GI complications and bleeding as compared with prednisone, so careful attention to the minimum dose necessary is required. There is a high incidence of GI bleeding and colonic perforation in canine neurosurgical patients treated with dexamethasone (also seen with methylprednisolone sodium succinate); as a result, the dose and duration of therapy should be limited to as short a time as possible, and prednisone or prednisolone should be used instead of dexamethasone when possible.[13] Animals with significantly diminished renal function may be more susceptible to adverse GI effects.

Use dexamethasone with caution in rabbits as serious adverse effects may occur, even after single doses.

Dexamethasone sodium phosphate delivered via nebulization is not an effective treatment for severe equine asthma.[10,14,15] Dexamethasone should be withdrawn at least 14 days prior to intradermal skin testing in horses.[16] Intra-articular dexamethasone administration to horses results in systemic endocrine effects.[9,17]

Adverse Effects

Adverse effects are generally associated with long-term administration of these drugs, especially if the drugs are administered at high doses or not on an alternate-day regimen. Effects typically manifest as clinical signs of hyperadrenocorticism. Glucocorticoids can delay growth when administered to young, growing animals. A list of potential effects is provided in ***Glucocorticoid Agents, General Information***.

In dogs, polyuria (PU), polydipsia (PD), and polyphagia (PP) may occur during short-term burst therapy and on days when the drug is administered during alternate-day maintenance therapy. Adverse effects in dogs can include dull/dry coat, weight gain, panting, vomiting, diarrhea, elevated liver enzymes, GI ulceration/perforation (especially with high parenteral or oral doses), hypercoagulability, hyperlipidemia, activation or worsening of diabetes mellitus, muscle wasting, and behavior changes (eg, depression, lethargy, aggression).[18] Glucocorticoids have been known to delay growth in young animals. Discontinuation of the drug may be necessary; changing to an alternate steroid may also alleviate adverse effects. Adverse effects associated with anti-inflammatory therapy are relatively uncommon, with the exception of PU, PD, and PP. Adverse effects (eg, secondary infections) associated with immunosuppressive doses are more common and potentially more severe.

High dexamethasone doses in dogs with spinal cord injuries have caused fatal colonic perforations.

In a study, topical otic and dermal dexamethasone administration to healthy beagles reduced cortisol and thyroid T_4 and T_3 concentrations.[19]

Cats generally require higher doses than dogs for clinical effects but typically develop fewer adverse effects. Glucocorticoids appear to have a greater hyperglycemic effect in cats than in other species. Occasionally, PU, PD, and PP with weight gain, diarrhea, and/or depression will be present. Long-term, high-dose therapy can lead to Cushingoid effects. Increases in intraocular pressure have been reported after prolonged administration of dexamethasone eye drops.[20]

Administration of dexamethasone or triamcinolone may play a role in the development of laminitis in horses, but this is thought to only occur rarely. In a study of healthy adult horses, hyperglycemia and hyperinsulinemia returned to baseline values within 2 to 3 days of discontinuing dexamethasone, but recovery of insulin secretion was delayed by ≈2 weeks.[21]

In pigeons, dexamethasone at high doses (0.5 mg/kg IV) suppressed the hypothalamic–pituitary–adrenal (HPA) axis for ≈52 hours, and suppression may persist longer as compared with dogs and cats.[22] Birds appear particularly susceptible to immunosuppressive effects.[23]

Reproductive/Nursing Safety

A positive effect of dexamethasone supplementation on preimplantation of in vitro bovine embryos has been reported.[24,25] Pregnancy rate has reportedly been enhanced by dexamethasone injection administered during early lactation[26] or with intrauterine dexamethasone administration at the time of artificial insemination.[25] Corticosteroid therapy may induce parturition in large animal species during the later stages of pregnancy. Dexamethasone administered to pregnant mares has altered foal pancreatic cell function.[27] Use of corticosteroids in pregnant laboratory animals has resulted in cleft palate.[28]

Corticosteroids are present in human breast milk.[29] In humans, single doses of dexamethasone are considered compatible with breastfeeding. Exposure of the nursing offspring to dexamethasone over a longer time period may suppress growth or interfere with endogenous corticosteroid production.[30]

Because safety has not been established in animals, this drug should only be used when the maternal benefits outweigh the potential risks to offspring.

Overdose/Acute Toxicity

When administered in the short term, glucocorticoids are unlikely to cause significant harmful effects, but dogs may be susceptible to GI ulceration/perforation. Should clinical signs occur, supportive treatment should be implemented if necessary.

Chronic glucocorticoid administration can lead to serious adverse effects. Refer to the ***Adverse Effects*** section for more information.

For patients that have experienced or are suspected to have experienced an overdose, consultation with a 24-hour poison consultation center specializing in providing veterinary-specific information is recommended. For general information related to overdose and toxin exposures, as well as contact information for poison control centers, refer to ***Appendix***.

Drug Interactions

The following drug interactions have either been reported or are theoretical in humans or animals receiving dexamethasone and may be of significance in veterinary patients. Unless otherwise noted, use together is not necessarily contraindicated, but the potential risks should be weighed and additional monitoring performed when appropriate.

- **Amphotericin B**: May cause hypokalemia when administered concomitantly with glucocorticoids
- **Anticholinesterase Agents** (eg, **pyridostigmine, neostigmine**): In patients with myasthenia gravis, concomitant glucocorticoid and anticholinesterase agent administration may lead to profound muscle weakness. If possible, anticholinesterase medication should be discontinued at least 24 hours prior to glucocorticoid administration.
- **Aspirin**: Concurrent use with glucocorticoids may reduce salicylate blood concentrations.
- **Azole Antifungals**: May decrease the metabolism of glucocorticoids and increase dexamethasone blood concentrations; ketoconazole may induce adrenal insufficiency when glucocorticoids are withdrawn by inhibiting adrenal corticosteroid synthesis.
- **Cyclophosphamide**: Glucocorticoids may inhibit the hepatic metabolism of cyclophosphamide; cyclophosphamide dosage adjustments may be required.
- **Cyclosporine**: Concomitant administration of glucocorticoids and cyclosporine may increase blood concentrations of each by mutually inhibiting the hepatic metabolism of each other; the clinical significance of this interaction is not clear.
- **Diazepam**: Concurrent use with dexamethasone may decrease diazepam concentrations.
- **Diuretics, Potassium-Depleting** (eg, **furosemide, thiazides**): May cause hypokalemia when administered concomitantly with glucocorticoids
- **Doxorubicin**: Concurrent use with dexamethasone may result in decreased doxorubicin exposure.
- **Ephedrine**: May reduce dexamethasone blood levels and interfere with dexamethasone suppression tests
- **Fentanyl**: Concurrent use with dexamethasone may result in decreased plasma concentrations of fentanyl.
- **Fluoroquinolone Antibiotics** (eg, **enrofloxacin, marbofloxacin**): Concurrent use with glucocorticoids may result in an increased risk for tendon rupture.
- **Insulin**: Insulin requirements may increase in patients receiving glucocorticoids.
- **Ivermectin**: Dexamethasone may alter ivermectin pharmacokinetics by modulating P-glycoprotein.[31] In a study in cattle, concurrent dexamethasone injection impaired ivermectin anthelmintic activity against *Cooperia oncophora* but not *Osteragia ostertagia*.[32]
- **Macrolide Antibiotics** (eg, **erythromycin, clarithromycin**): May decrease the metabolism of glucocorticoids and increase dexamethasone blood concentrations
- **Mitotane**: May alter the metabolism of steroids; higher than usual doses of steroids may be necessary to treat mitotane-induced adrenal insufficiency
- **Nonsteroidal Anti-Inflammatory Drugs (NSAIDs)**: Administration of ulcerogenic drugs with glucocorticoids may increase the risk for GI ulceration.
- **Phenobarbital**: Concurrent use with glucocorticoids may result in decreased dexamethasone efficacy.
- **Praziquantel**: Concurrent use with dexamethasone may significantly decrease praziquantel plasma concentrations.
- **Quinidine**: In a study of dogs, dexamethasone increased quinidine volume of distribution (49% to 78%) and elimination half-life (1.5 to 2.3 times greater than that associated with quinidine use alone).[33]

- **Rifampin**: May increase the metabolism of glucocorticoids and decrease dexamethasone blood concentrations
- **Vaccines, Modified Live**: Patients receiving immunosuppressive doses of glucocorticoids should generally not receive live attenuated-virus vaccines, as virus replication may be augmented; a diminished immune response may occur after vaccine, toxoid, or bacterin administration in patients receiving glucocorticoids.
- **Vincristine**: Concurrent use with dexamethasone may result in decreased vincristine plasma concentrations.

Laboratory Considerations

- Although dexamethasone does not interfere with the cortisol assay, it will start to suppress the hypothalamic–pituitary–adrenal (HPA) axis over a few days and thus suppress endogenous release of cortisol. If dexamethasone is being used to treat patients with suspected hypoadrenocorticism, **ACTH stimulation tests** should be performed as soon as possible. When interpreting the results of the ACTH stimulation test, the effects of dexamethasone on the HPA axis should be considered.
- Glucocorticoids may increase **serum cholesterol**.
- Glucocorticoids may induce **ALP** activity in dogs but not cats.
- Glucocorticoids may increase **urine glucose** concentrations.
- Glucocorticoids may decrease **serum potassium.**
- Glucocorticoids can suppress the release of **thyroid stimulating hormone (TSH)** and reduce T_3 and T_4 values. Thyroid gland atrophy has been reported after chronic glucocorticoid administration. Uptake of I^{-131} by the thyroid may be decreased by glucocorticoids.
- Reactions to **skin tests** may be suppressed by glucocorticoids.
- False negative results of the **nitroblue tetrazolium** test for systemic bacterial infections may be induced by glucocorticoids.
- Glucocorticoids may cause **neutrophilia** within 4 to 8 hours of administration, which can return to baseline within 24 to 48 hours after drug discontinuation.
- Glucocorticoids can cause **lymphopenia** in dogs; this effect can persist for weeks after drug discontinuation.

Dosages

NOTE: All dosages should be titrated to effect to maximize therapeutic benefit but minimize adverse effects. Strong scientific evidence for dose regimens is lacking, and the following serve as guidelines.

DOGS:

NOTE: In general, most clinicians use prednisone or prednisolone when administering a glucocorticoid orally as an anti-inflammatory or immunosuppressive agent in dogs. Despite a short circulating half-life, dexamethasone has a long biologic duration of effect (thought to be greater than 48 hours, whereas the biologic duration of effect of prednisone is 12 to 36 hours). Thus, it is difficult to spare normal adrenal function, even when dexamethasone is administered every other day.[13] The dose of dexamethasone can be extrapolated from standard prednis(ol)one dosages by dividing by 7 (ie, prednis(ol)one 1 mg/kg/day is equivalent to 0.14 mg/kg/day dexamethasone).

Anti-inflammatory; glucocorticoid agent (label dosage; FDA-approved): **NOTE**: The label dosage for dogs is much higher than what is generally used by most clinicians today. Injection: 0.25 – 1 mg/dog (NOT mg/kg) IV or IM[34]; may be repeated for 3 to 5 days. Tablets: 0.25 – 1.25 mg/dog (NOT mg/kg) PO daily in single or 2 divided doses[35]

Anti-inflammatory; glucocorticoid agent (extra-label): 0.1 mg/kg IM or 0.05 – 2 mg/kg PO daily

Initial anti-inflammatory indications (extra-label): 0.07 – 0.14 mg/kg/day[36,37]

Postvaccination reactions (extra-label): 0.1 mg/kg IV once. Dogs that have a mild postvaccination reaction that requires treatment should receive a single, anti-inflammatory dose.[38]

Replacement of glucocorticoid activity in patients with adrenal insufficiency (**NOTE**: Dexamethasone has no mineralocorticoid activity):

a) **Addisonian crisis**: Dexamethasone sodium phosphate 0.1 – 0.2 mg/kg IV as the initial dose. Dexamethasone is not measured on the cortisol assay, so the ACTH stimulation test will be valid after dexamethasone is administered. If the dog is vomiting or inappetent, dexamethasone may be continued at 0.05 – 0.1 mg/kg IV every 12 hours until able to switch to oral predniso(lo)ne as the glucocorticoid replacement (see ***Prednisolone/Prednisone*** for more information).[13]
b) **Addisonian crisis**: Dexamethasone sodium phosphate 0.2 – 0.5 mg/kg IV once; followed by maintenance therapy with prednisone. Dexamethasone, unlike prednisone, will not interfere with cortisol assays.[39]

Immunosuppressive agent (eg, immune-mediated hemolytic anemia; extra-label): 0.2 – 0.4 mg/kg/day IV on a temporary basis if the patient cannot tolerate oral medication.[40] One publication describes injectable and oral dexamethasone for the treatment of masticatory muscle myositis in dogs, with an initial injectable dosage of 0.2 mg/kg followed by an initial oral dosage of ≈0.1 mg/kg that was then tapered over time.[3]

As a chemotherapeutic agent (extra-label):

a) **Parenteral glucocorticoid therapy when oral predniso(lo)ne is not an option**: Anecdotally, calculate prednis(ol)one equivalent dosage (predniso(ol)ne dosage divided by 7) and administer IV until oral prednis(ol)one may be instituted.
b) **Lymphoma rescue protocol (DMAC)**: Dexamethasone 1 mg/kg PO or SC with actinomycin D 0.75 mg/m² IV and cytarabine 300 mg/m² SC or IV as a 4-hour CRI on day 1; followed by dexamethasone 1 mg/kg PO or SC and melphalan 20 mg/m² PO on day 8 of a 14-day cycle. This treatment cycle is repeated every 2 weeks while the dog is in remission (complete or partial) or demonstrates static disease or until signs of relapse or progressive disease occur.[1] It is recommended to consult with a board-certified oncologist or an oncology textbook for further details surrounding chemotherapy protocols.

As a diagnostic agent:

a) **Low-dose dexamethasone suppression (LDDS) test** (extra-label): Plasma samples for cortisol should be obtained before and 4 and 8 hours after administration of dexamethasone 0.01 mg/kg IV. The 8-hour plasma cortisol level is used as a screening test for hyperadrenocorticism; cortisol concentrations above the laboratory cutoff (often greater than 1.4 µg/dL) are consistent with hyperadrenocorticism. The LDDS test is a *screening* test with a sensitivity of 85% to 100% and specificity of 44% to 73%.[41] Approximately 90% of dogs with hyperadrenocorticism have an 8-hour postdexamethasone plasma cortisol concentration greater than 1.4 µg/dL, and another 6% to 8% have values of 0.9 to 1.3 µg/dL. The results of a LDDS test may also aid in discriminating pituitary-dependent hyperadrenocorticism (PDH) from adrenocortical tumor (ACT) using 3 criteria. If a dog has hyperadrenocorticism and it meets any of these 3 criteria, it most likely has PDH: 1) an 8-hour plasma cortisol greater than 1.4 µg/dL but less than 50% of the basal value, 2) a 4-hour plasma cortisol concentration less than 1 µg/dL, and 3) a 4-hour plasma cortisol concentration less than 50% of the basal value. Approximately 65% of dogs with naturally occurring PDH demonstrate suppression as defined by these 3 criteria. A dog with hyperadrenocorticism that fails to meet any of these 3 criteria could have either PDH or ACT. Additional testing with abdominal ultrasonography or high-dose dexamethasone suppression (see below) may be helpful in distinguishing between the 2 conditions; if 2 relatively equal-sized adrenal glands are present on abdominal ultrasonography, the patient most likely has PDH.[42]

b) **High-dose dexamethasone suppression (HDDS) test** (extra-label): Plasma samples for cortisol should be obtained before and 4 and 8 hours after administration of dexamethasone 0.1 mg/kg IV. The HDDS test is a *differentiating* test to discriminate PDH from an ACT; it should only be performed in dogs when a screening test (LDDS or ACTH stimulation test) is diagnostic for hyperadrenocorticism. Dogs with HDDS results that meet any of the following criteria likely have PDH: 1) a 4- or 8-hour plasma cortisol less than 50% of the basal value or 2) a 4- or 8-hour plasma cortisol less than the laboratory cutoff (often ≈1 – 1.5 µg/dL). Approximately 75% of dogs with PDH demonstrate suppression with the HDDS test. Because ≈65% of PDH dogs demonstrate suppression with the LDDS test (consistent with PDH), the HDDS test may only identify an additional 10% of afflicted dogs.[41]

CATS:

NOTE: Generally, most clinicians use prednisolone when a glucocorticoid is administered orally to cats. Approximately 0.75 mg of dexamethasone is equivalent to 5 mg of prednisolone. Doses can be approximated by dividing the prednisolone dose by 7 to obtain the dexamethasone dose.

Anti-inflammatory; glucocorticoid agent (label dosage): Injection: 0.125 – 0.5 mg/cat (NOT mg/kg) IV or IM[34]; may be repeated for 3 to 5 days; Tablets: 0.125 – 0.5 mg/cat (NOT mg/kg) PO daily in a single dose or 2 divided doses[35]

Anti-inflammatory; glucocorticoid agent (extra-label): Injection: 0.1 mg/kg IM. Tablets: 0.05 – 2 mg/kg/day orally

Initial anti-inflammatory indications (extra-label): 0.14 – 0.28 mg/kg/day[36,37]

Hypersensitivity dermatitis (extra-label): Using dexamethasone sodium phosphate (4 mg/mL) *injection*, 0.2 mg/kg/day PO rapidly relieved pruritus and clinical lesions.[43]

Replacement of glucocorticoid activity in patients with adrenal insufficiency (**NOTE**: Dexamethasone has no mineralocorticoid activity): Dexamethasone sodium phosphate 0.1 – 0.2 mg/kg IV or IM as the initial dose.[44] Dexamethasone is not measured on the cortisol assay, so the ACTH stimulation test will be valid after dexamethasone is administered. If the cat is vomiting or inappetent, dexamethasone may be continued every 12 hours until able to switch to oral prednisolone as the glucocorticoid replacement. See ***Prednisolone/Prednisone***.

As a diagnostic agent:

a) **Low-dose dexamethasone suppression (LDDS) test** (extra-label): Test of choice for the initial diagnosis of feline hyperadrenocorticism. **NOTE**: Cats require a higher dexamethasone dosage for this test than dogs. Plasma samples for cortisol should be obtained before and 4 and 8 hours after administration of dexamethasone 0.1 mg/kg IV. A cortisol concentration greater than or equal to 1.4 µg/dL is consistent with a diagnosis of hyperadrenocorticism if the patient is also displaying appropriate clinical signs.[45,46]

b) **High-dose dexamethasone suppression (HDDS) test** (extra-label): Hyperadrenocorticism should be confirmed before performing this test to differentiate PDH from ACT. **NOTE**: Cats require a higher dexamethasone dosage for this test than dogs. Plasma samples for cortisol should be obtained before and 4 and 8 hours after administration of dexamethasone 1 mg/kg IV. Cats with HDDS results that meet any of the following criteria likely have PDH: 1) a 4- or 8-hour plasma cortisol less than 50% of the basal value or 2) a 4- or 8-hour plasma cortisol less than the laboratory cutoff (often ≈1 – 1.5 µg/dL).

c) **HDDS test combined with urine cortisol creatinine ratio (UCCR**; extra-label): For cats with elevated UCCR values *and* clinical signs consistent with hyperadrenocorticism: At home, dexamethasone 0.1 mg/kg PO every 8 hours, with urine samples collected the following morning to perform UCCR.[46] If the postdexamethasone UCCR is less than 50% of the pretest samples, the results are consistent with PDH; results greater than 50% do not discriminate between PDH and ACT.

HORSES:

Anti-inflammatory; glucocorticoid agent (label dosage; FDA-approved): dexamethasone 2.5 – 5 mg/horse (NOT mg/kg) IV or IM[34]; dexamethasone sodium phosphate: 2.5 – 5 mg/horse (NOT mg/kg) IV[47]

Anti-inflammatory; glucocorticoid agent (extra-label): Injection: 0.06 mg/kg IM or IV[48]

Adjunctive treatment of severe equine asthma (extra-label):

a) For a 500 kg (1102.3 lb) horse, dexamethasone 40 mg/horse (NOT mg/kg) IM once every other day for 3 treatments, followed by 35 mg/horse (NOT mg/kg) IM once every other day for 3 treatments, followed by 30 mg/horse (NOT mg/kg) IM once every other day for 3 treatments; continue tapering until horse is weaned off this therapy.[49]

b) For short-term treatment with environmental control: In a study, dexamethasone sodium phosphate was dosed at 0.1 mg/kg IM once daily for 4 days, 0.075 mg/kg IM once daily for 4 days, and 0.05 mg/kg IM once daily for 4 days. Except for bronchoalveolar lavage cytology results, PO prednisolone (1 mg/kg PO for 4 days, 0.75 mg/kg PO for 4 days, 0.5 mg/kg PO for 4 days) was shown to be as effective as IM dexamethasone.[50]

c) In a study, dexamethasone 0.05 mg/kg IM every 24 hours was as effective as inhaled fluticasone in reducing clinical signs, airway inflammatory cells, and bronchoprovocative histamine response.[51]

d) In a study, horses under continuous antigen exposure were given dexamethasone at 0.05 mg/kg PO once daily for 7 days or prednisolone at 2 mg/kg PO once daily for 7 days. Both were effective but dexamethasone more so.[52]

e) In a study, horses received 0.1 mg/kg PO once daily for 3 weeks. The study states: *The VAS (visual analog scale) score (owner scored) improved significantly in dexamethasone but not placebo treated horses. In contrast, the clinician failed to differentiate between dexamethasone and placebo treated animals based on clinical observations, BALF cytology or endoscopic mucus score. Respiratory rate and arterial oxygen pressure (PaO_2) improved with dexamethasone but not placebo. The authors concluded, in the design of clinical trials of airway disease treatments, more emphasis should be placed on owner-assessed VAS than on clinical, cytological and endoscopic observations made during brief examinations by a veterinarian.*[53]

Dexamethasone suppression test to diagnose pituitary pars intermedia dysfunction (extra-label):

a) 20 mg/horse (NOT mg/kg) IM. Normal values: Cortisol levels should decrease by 50% in 2 hours, 70% in 4 hours, and 80% in 6 hours. At 24 hours, cortisol levels should remain depressed by ≈30% of presuppression value.[54] Seasonal variability may affect results.[55]

b) After baseline cortisol (serum or plasma) is collected, dexamethasone 0.04 mg/kg IM can be administered, and a second cortisol sample collected 18 to 20 hours later.[56] Cortisol values greater than 10 µg/mL are diagnostic. Testing performed in autumn is more likely to yield false positive results.[57]

Treatment of arthritis, bursitis, or tenosynovitis (extra-label): 2 – 10 mg/horse (NOT mg/kg) as an intra-articular injection[48]

CATTLE:

Primary bovine ketosis | anti-inflammatory agent (label dosage; FDA-approved): 5 – 20 mg/cow (NOT mg/kg) IV or IM[34]

Anti-inflammatory; glucocorticoid agent (label dosage; FDA-approved): 5 – 10 mg/animal (NOT mg/kg) PO on the first day, then 5 mg/animal (NOT mg/kg) PO daily as required.[58] Administer as a drench or sprinkled on a small amount of feed.

Primary bovine ketosis (extra-label): 0.02 – 0.04 mg/kg IM. Larger doses will be required if the signs have been present for some time or if relapsed animals are being treated[48]

Anti-inflammatory; glucocorticoid agent (extra-label): 0.06 mg/kg IM[48]

Induction of parturition (extra-label): A single injection of 0.04 mg/kg IM after day 260 of pregnancy.[48] Parturition will normally occur within 48 to 72 hours.

SWINE:

Anti-inflammatory; glucocorticoid agent (extra-label): 0.06 mg/kg IM[48]

RABBITS/RODENTS/SMALL MAMMALS:

Mice, rats, gerbils, hamsters, guinea pigs, chinchillas (extra-label): 0.6 mg/kg IM (as an anti-inflammatory)[59]

Monitoring

Monitoring of glucocorticoid therapy is dependent on the reason for use, dosage, agent used (amount of mineralocorticoid activity), dose schedule (daily versus alternate-day therapy), duration of therapy, and the animal's age and condition. The following list may not be appropriate or complete for all animals; clinical assessment and judgment should be used if adverse effects are noted:

- Weight, appetite, and/or signs of fluid retention
- Serum and/or urine electrolytes
- Total plasma protein and albumin
- Blood glucose
- Periodic urine culture especially with chronic use
- GI adverse effects (eg, vomiting, diarrhea, melena)
- Growth and development in young animals

Client Information

- Long-acting glucocorticoid that is best given with food but may be given without. If your animal vomits or acts sick after receiving the drug on an empty stomach, try giving the next dose with food or a small treat. If vomiting continues, contact your veterinarian.
- There are many side effects, especially when the drug is used long term. The most common side effects in dogs are excessive thirst, urinations, and appetite.
- In dogs, stomach or intestinal ulcers, perforation, or bleeding can occur. The risk for this occurring is increased if used with drugs like aspirin, NSAIDs (eg, carprofen) or other cortisone-like drugs (eg, prednisone). If your animal stops eating, or develops a low energy level, black tarry stools, or bloody vomit, contact your veterinarian immediately.
- Do not stop this drug suddenly if your animal has been on the drug for more than a couple of weeks as serious side effects could occur.

Chemistry/Synonyms

Dexamethasone, a synthetic glucocorticoid, occurs as an odorless white to practically white crystalline powder that melts with some decomposition at ≈250°C (482°F). It is practically insoluble in water and sparingly soluble in alcohol. Dexamethasone sodium phosphate occurs as a white to slightly yellow hygroscopic powder and is odorless or has a slight odor. One gram is soluble in ≈2 mL of water; it is slightly soluble in alcohol.

1.3 mg of dexamethasone sodium phosphate is equivalent to 1 mg of dexamethasone. 4 mg/mL of dexamethasone sodium phosphate injection is equivalent to ≈3 mg/mL of dexamethasone.

Dexamethasone may also be known as desamethasone, dexametasone, dexamethasonum, 9-alpha-fluoro-16-alpha-methylprednisolone; hexadecadrol; many trade names are available.

Storage/Stability

Dexamethasone is heat labile and should be stored at room temperature (15°C-30°C [59°F-86°F]) unless otherwise directed by the manufacturer. Dexamethasone sodium phosphate injection should be protected from light. Dexamethasone tablets should be stored in well-closed containers.

Compatibility/Compounding Considerations

Compatibility is dependent on factors such as pH, concentration, temperature, and diluent used; specialized references or a hospital pharmacist should be consulted for more specific information.

Dexamethasone sodium phosphate for injection is reportedly **compatible** with the following drugs: amikacin sulfate, aminophylline, bleomycin sulfate, cimetidine HCl, glycopyrrolate, lidocaine HCl, prochlorperazine edisylate, and verapamil.

Dexamethasone sodium phosphate is reportedly **incompatible** with daunorubicin HCl, doxorubicin HCl, metaraminol bitartrate, and vancomycin.

Dosage Forms/Regulatory Status

VETERINARY-LABELED PRODUCTS:

Dexamethasone Injection: 2 mg/mL; *Azium® Solution*, generic; (Rx). FDA-approved for use in dogs, cats, horses (those not intended for food), and cattle. There are no withdrawal times required for use in cattle. A withdrawal period has not been established for this product in preruminal calves; should not be used in veal calves

Dexamethasone Sodium Phosphate Injection: 4 mg/mL (equivalent to 3 mg/mL dexamethasone), generic; (Rx). FDA-approved for use in horses

Dexamethasone Oral Powder: 10 mg crystalline in 10 mg packets; *Azium® Powder*; (Rx). FDA-approved for use in cattle and horses (not horses intended for food)

Dexamethasone 5 mg and trichlormethiazide 200 mg oral bolus: In boxes of 30 and 100 boluses; *Naquasone® Bolus*; (Rx). FDA-approved for use in cattle. Milk withdrawal = 72 hours

The Association of Racing Commissioners International (ARCI) has designated dexamethasone as a class 4 substance. Use of this drug may not be allowed in certain animal competitions. Check rules and regulations before entering in a competition while this medication is being administered. Contact local racing authorities for further guidance. See the ***Appendix*** for more information.

HUMAN-LABELED PRODUCTS:

Dexamethasone Oral Tablets: 0.5 mg, 0.75 mg, 1 mg, 1.5 mg, 2 mg, 4 mg, and 6 mg; *Decadron®*, generic; (Rx)

Dexamethasone Oral Elixir/Solution: 0.5 mg/5 mL in 100 mL, 237 mL, and 500 mL and UD 5 mL and UD 20 mL; 1 mg/mL (concentrate) in 30 mL with dropper; *Dexamethasone Intensol®*, generic; (Rx)

Dexamethasone Sodium Phosphate Injection: 4 mg/mL (as sodium phosphate solution) in 1 mL, 5 mL, 10 mL, and 30 mL vials, 1 mL syringe and 1 mL fill in 2 mL vials; generic; (Rx); 10 mg/mL (as sodium phosphate solution) in 1 mL and 10 mL vials and 1 mL syringes; generic; (Rx); 20 mg/mL (as sodium phosphate solution) in 5 mL vials (IV); *Hexadrol® Phosphate*; (Rx)

Dexamethasone is also available in topical ophthalmic and inhaled aerosol dose forms.

References

For the complete list of references, see **wiley.com/go/budde/plumb**

Dexmedetomidine

(deks-mee-deh-***toe***-mih-deen) *Dexdomitor®, Sileo®*
Alpha-2-*Adrenergic Agonist*

Prescriber Highlights

- Reversible sedative analgesic used primarily in dogs, cats, small mammals, and exotic species; can also be used as an emetic in cats.
- Contraindications include most forms of cardiac disease, respiratory disorders, shock, severe debilitation, or animals stressed due to heat, cold, or fatigue. It is also contraindicated in liver or kidney disease, although some anesthesiologists consider those contraindications to be relative because dexmedetomidine effects can be reversed.
- Use with caution in geriatric and pediatric animals.
- Adverse effects include bradycardia, occasional AV block, decreased respiratory rate, hypothermia, urination, vomiting, and hyperglycemia. Rarely, prolonged sedation, hypersensitivity, apnea, and death from circulatory failure may occur.
- Systemic and central effects may be reversed with atipamezole; however, analgesia will also be reversed, and additional analgesic agents may be required for adequate pain control.
- Do **NOT** confuse dexmedetomidine with detomidine or medetomidine.
- Gloves should be worn when handling products, particularly the oral transmucosal gel, as the drug is absorbed through the skin, eyes, and mouth.

Uses/Indications

Dexmedetomidine is FDA-approved for dogs and cats for use as a sedative and analgesic to facilitate clinical examinations, clinical procedures, minor surgical procedures, and minor dental procedures and as a preanesthetic to general anesthesia. In cats, the injectable formulation has been used in an extra-label manner as an emetic,[1,2] but hydromorphone may be a better emetic.[3] Dexmedetomidine rapidly controlled clinical signs of sympathetic nervous system stimulation in a 5-month-old kitten that ingested lisdexamphetamine.[4]

The oromucosal gel product (*Sileo®*) is approved for the treatment of noise aversion in dogs and is used extra-label to reduce fear and anxiety during veterinary examinations.[5]

Pharmacology/Actions

Dexmedetomidine is the dextrorotatory enantiomer of the alpha-2-adrenergic agonist medetomidine. The other enantiomer, levomedetomidine, is thought to be pharmacologically inactive[6]; dexmedetomidine is therefore ≈2 times more potent than medetomidine.[7] Dexmedetomidine is more specific than xylazine for alpha-2 receptors versus alpha-1 receptors. The alpha-2 to alpha-1 selectivity of dexmedetomidine and xylazine is 1620:1 and 160:1, respectively.[8]

The pharmacologic effects of dexmedetomidine include depression of CNS (eg, sedation, anxiolysis), GI (eg, decreased secretions, reduced intestinal smooth muscle tone), and endocrine functions (eg, inhibition of insulin release leading to hyperglycemia); peripheral and coronary vasoconstriction; bradycardia; respiratory depression; diuresis; hypothermia; analgesia; muscle relaxation; and blanched or cyanotic mucous membranes. Effects on blood pressure are biphasic, with initial hypertension followed by hypotension; dexmedetomidine can cause hypertension for a longer period than can xylazine. Vomiting is mediated by central alpha-2-adrenergic agonist stimulation.[1,2,9]

Pharmacokinetics

After IM administration to dogs, dexmedetomidine is absorbed (bioavailability 60%) and reaches peak plasma concentrations in ≈35 minutes. Volume of distribution is 0.9 L/kg, and elimination half-life is ≈40 to 50 minutes. The drug is primarily metabolized in the liver via hydroxylation[10,11]; metabolism depends on hepatic blood flow. No metabolites are active, and they are eliminated primarily in the urine and, to lesser extent, in the feces.

The mean bioavailability of the oral transmucosal gel (*Sileo®*) in dogs is 28%. Protein binding is 93%. Peak concentrations occur at ≈0.6 hours, similar to IM administration. Half-life is 0.5 to 3 hours after oromucosal administration.[12,13]

After IM administration in cats, dexmedetomidine is absorbed and reaches peak plasma concentrations of ≈17 ng/mL in ≈15 minutes. Oral transmucosal (OTM [buccal]) administration of dexmedetomidine 0.5 mg/mL injection solution (40 µg/kg) appears to give similar concentrations (extrapolated from clinical effects) as IM administration in cats.[14] Two studies compared OTM versus IM dexmedetomidine 20 µg/kg combined with buprenorphine 20 µg/kg. IM administration resulted in a higher peak dexmedetomidine concentration more quickly than the OTM group,[15] and sedation was more satisfactory with IM administration.[16,17] After administration as a 5-minute IV infusion in isoflurane-anesthetized cats, clearance was 6.3 mL/minute/kg and elimination half-life was 198 minutes.[18] Volume of distribution is 2.2 L/kg and elimination half-life is ≈1 hour. Metabolism occurs via hydroxylation in the liver and is dependent on hepatic blood flow.[19] Metabolites are eliminated primarily in the urine and, to lesser extent, in the feces.

In adult horses given 5 µg/kg IV bolus, elimination half-life was 8.3 minutes; pharmacologic effects (eg, head height, analgesia, bradycardia, reduced ambulation) lasted less than 1 hour.[20] When administered as an IV CRI at 8 µg/kg/hour, volume of distribution at steady-state was 13.7 L/kg, clearance was 0.3 L/minute/kg, and elimination half-life was ≈21 minutes.[21]

In humans, after IV administration, dexmedetomidine is rapidly distributed (volume of distribution ≈1.6 L/kg) and is 94% bound to plasma proteins.[22] It undergoes almost complete biotransformation via both glucuronidation and CYP450 enzyme systems and has a terminal elimination half-life of ≈2 hours. Metabolites are eliminated in the urine and feces. Clearance is reduced in patients with hepatic impairment. CYP450 isoenzymes have, at best, a minor role in dexmedetomidine metabolism.

Contraindications/Precautions/Warnings

Do not use dexmedetomidine in dogs or cats that are hypersensitive to dexmedetomidine or in patients with cardiovascular disease, respiratory disorders, or liver or kidney disease, or in conditions of shock, severe debilitation, stress caused by extreme heat or cold, or fatigue.[23] Because of the pronounced cardiovascular effects of dexmedetomidine, only clinically healthy dogs and cats should be treated; do not use dexmedetomidine in animals with preexisting hypotension, bradycardia, and hypoxia. Although not contraindicated in pediatric or geriatric dogs or cats, the drug's United States label states that the drug has not been evaluated in dogs younger than 16 weeks, in cats younger than 12 weeks, or in geriatric dogs and cats. Geriatric patients should be dosed based on health, not age. Use with caution in pediatric patients, as cardiac output in this population is heart rate dependent.

Dexmedetomidine should only be used in situations in which sufficient monitoring and patient support capabilities (eg, intubation, ventilation) are available.

Because the systemic and CNS effects of dexmedetomidine are reversible, some anesthesiologists consider dexmedetomidine contraindications to be relative, particularly in patients with hepatic or renal disease. Dexmedetomidine may be used in patients with a seizure history; however, it should not be used in patients with severe CNS clinical signs (eg, obtundation). Not all forms of cardiac disease create a contraindication. For instance, medetomidine administered to cats with left ventricular outflow obstruction improved cardiac function secondary to slowed heart rate with subsequent increased ventricular filling.[24]

Although dexmedetomidine can be used as an emetic in cats, sedation may increase the incidence of aspiration of vomitus. More effective emetics (eg, apomorphine, ropinirole) are available for dogs.

The United Kingdom label states not to use dexmedetomidine in puppies younger than 6 months or kittens younger than 5 months or in animals with cardiovascular disorders, with severe systemic disease, that are moribund, or that are known to be hypersensitive to the active substance or any of the excipients.

Although the manufacturer recommends that patients be fasted for 12 hours before use,[23] general recommendations for fast duration are 4 to 6 hours prior to sedation/anesthesia in most patients due to adverse effects of long-duration fasting (eg, decreased gastric pH, decreased intestinal motility).[25] If vomiting could be detrimental to the patient, an antiemetic should be administered at least 1 hour prior to dexmedetomidine administration.

Transient alpha-2-mediated hyperglycemia is a common sequelae with dexmedetomidine administration.[23]

Dexmedetomidine reduces tear flow in dogs and cats.[26-28] Ophthalmic ointment should be used to protect eyes when using this drug.

The oromucosal product for dogs (*Sileo*®) has not been evaluated in dogs younger than 16 weeks of age or in dogs with dental or gingival disease.[13] Avoid feeding or giving treats within 15 minutes after a dose, as this may decrease absorption from the mucous membranes. Drinking water within that time frame may have the same effect. It should not be swallowed, as it may not be effective. If swallowed, the dose should not be repeated for at least 2 hours to eliminate the risk for overdose in the event that some of the drug was absorbed across the mucous membranes.

Dexmedetomidine effects (eg, sedation, physiologic effects, and analgesia) can be reversed with atipamezole; however, the use of additional analgesics may be required for adequate pain control.

In humans, dose reduction may be necessary in patients with hepatic disease.[22]

Do not confuse dexmedetomidine with dexamethasone, detomidine, or medetomidine. Do not interchange dexmedetomidine with medetomidine dosages. On a **mg**/kg basis, dexmedetomidine doses are ≈½ of the medetomidine dose because dexmedetomidine is more potent; however, dexmedetomidine is ½ the concentration of medetomidine so the doses are the same on a **mL**/kg basis.

Adverse Effects

The adverse effects reported with dexmedetomidine are essentially extensions of its pharmacologic effects, including bradycardia, vasoconstriction, muscle contractions or tremors, transient hypertension, reduced tear production, occasional arrhythmias (second-degree AV block, supraventricular tachycardia [SVT], ventricular escape beats, premature ventricular complexes [PVCs]), hypoventilation, dyspnea, hypothermia, urination, vomiting, hyperglycemia, and decreased or absent pupil response. Hypothermia may persist longer than sedation and analgesia[29]; body temperature may need to be externally maintained. In field studies of dexmedetomidine injection, vomiting occurred in 12% to 25% of dogs and 57% to 68% of cats.[23] Ondansetron[9] and maropitant[30] may ameliorate dexmedetomidine-induced emesis, as may combination with butorphanol.[31]

Rare effects include prolonged sedation, paradoxical excitation, defensive reaction from handling or sudden stimuli, hypersensitivity, pulmonary edema, apnea, and death from circulatory failure.[13,23] Adverse effects that require treatment can generally be alleviated with atipamezole; however, it is important to note that analgesic effects will also be reversed.

In dogs, medetomidine causes a significant decrease in tear production whereas dexmedetomidine caused an initial decrease followed by an increase.[32] Intraocular pressure was decreased. In 2 other studies, dexmedetomidine caused a decrease in tear production lasting for ≈8 hours[33] and occurring within 15 minutes of administration when combined with butorphanol.[28] In the latter study, tear production was improved but still below baseline when atipamezole was administered. The cumulative conclusion from these studies was that dexmedetomidine was safe for patients undergoing ocular procedures but that eye lubrication should be used.

In humans, withdrawal-like symptoms (eg, nausea, vomiting, agitation) occurred in 3% to 5% of patients receiving dexmedetomidine infusion for up to 7 days for ICU sedation.[22] The veterinary significance of this finding is uncertain.

Reproductive/Nursing Safety

Although the product label recommends against use in pregnant dogs or those used for breeding purposes due to lack of safety information, **medetomidine and dexmedetomidine combinations with propofol have demonstrated safety in dogs undergoing cesarean section.**[34,35] The parent drug of dexmedetomidine, medetomidine (7 µg/kg IV), combined with propofol (1 – 2 mg/kg IV) was also determined safe for cesarean sections in dogs.[34]

Placental transfer of dexmedetomidine occurred in pregnant rats. No teratogenic effects were observed when rats were given up to 200 µg/kg SC from days 5 to 16 of gestation or when rabbits were given up to 96 µg/kg IV from days 6 to 18 of gestation.

Dexmedetomidine is distributed into the milk of lactating rats[22]; safe use during nursing has not been established.[22,23]

Overdose/Acute Toxicity

Single doses up to 5 times the label-recommended IV dose and 10 times the label-recommended IM dose were tolerated in healthy young dogs, but adverse effects can occur (see ***Adverse Effects***) in a dose-related manner. Doses of 200 µg/kg IM in cats (5 times the label dose) produced prolonged sedation (longer than 8 hours), reduced respiratory rate, hypothermia, bradycardia, and junctional escape arrhythmias. Vomiting occurred in 5 of 6 cats given 400 µg/kg IM. Because of the potential for additional adverse effects (eg, AV block, PVCs, tachycardia), treatment of dexmedetomidine-induced bradycardia with anticholinergic agents (eg, atropine, glycopyrrolate) is usually not recommended if the blood pressure is normal or high but anticholinergics can be used if both the heart rate and the blood pressure are low. Reversal with atipamezole is recommended to treat any dexmedetomidine-induced adverse effects.

For patients that have experienced or are suspected to have experienced an overdose, it is strongly encouraged to consult with one of the 24-hour poison consultation centers that specialize in providing information specific for veterinary patients. For general information related to overdose and toxin exposures, as well as contact information for poison control centers, refer to ***Appendix.***

Drug Interactions

The following drug interactions have either been reported or are theoretical in humans or animals receiving dexmedetomidine or medetomidine (the parent compound of dexmedetomidine) and may be of significance in veterinary patients. Unless otherwise noted, use together is not necessarily contraindicated, but weigh the potential risks and perform additional monitoring when appropriate. **NOTE**: Before attempting combination therapy with dexmedetomidine, it is strongly advised to consult veterinary anesthesia references or veterinary anesthesiologists familiar with the use of this drug.

- **ANGIOTENSIN-CONVERTING ENZYME INHIBITORS** (ACEIs; eg, **enalapril**): Additive hypotensive effects may occur.
- **ACEPROMAZINE**: Effects may be additive; dose reduction of one or both agents may be required. General anesthetic requirements may be reduced by 30% to 60%.
- **AMLODIPINE**: Additive hypotensive effects may occur.
- **ANESTHETICS** (eg, **alfaxalone, isoflurane, ketamine, propofol**): Effects may be additive; dose reduction of one or both agents may be required. General anesthetic requirements may be reduced by 30% to 60%. Dexmedetomidine lowered the seizure threshold in cats undergoing anesthesia with enflurane.[36]
- **ATROPINE, GLYCOPYRROLATE**: The use of atropine (or glycopyrrolate) with dexmedetomidine can significantly increase arterial blood pressure, heart rate, cardiac work, and may increase the risk for arrhythmias; use together is not recommended in dogs (and probably other species).[37]
- **BENZODIAZEPINES** (eg, **diazepam, midazolam**): Effects may be additive; dose reduction of one or both agents may be required. General anesthetic requirements may be reduced by 30% to 60%.
- **BETA-ADRENERGIC RECEPTOR ANTAGONISTS** (eg, **atenolol, esmolol, metoprolol**): AV-blocking and bradycardic effects may be enhanced.
- **EPINEPHRINE**: Because epinephrine possesses alpha-agonist effects and could cause or exacerbate hypertension and arrhythmias, it should not be used to treat cardiac effects caused by dexmedetomidine.
- **OPIOIDS** (eg, **butorphanol, morphine, tramadol**): Effects may be additive; dose reduction of one or both agents may be required. General anesthetic requirements may be reduced by 30% to 60%. Sedation with buprenorphine and dexmedetomidine is less predictable and of slower onset but longer duration than that achieved with butorphanol and dexmedetomidine.[38,39]
- **SILDENAFIL**: Additive hypotensive effects may occur.
- **TELMISARTAN**: Additive hypotensive effects may occur.
- **YOHIMBINE**: Effects may be partially reversed, but atipamezole is preferred for full reversal of dexmedetomidine's effects.

Laboratory Considerations

Dexmedetomidine can inhibit ADP-induced **platelet aggregation** in cats, but this does not appear to be clinically significant.[40]

Dosages

NOTES:

1. Dexmedetomidine dosages depend on the combination of drugs used and the dosage(s) of the other drug(s). Premedication with dexmedetomidine will significantly reduce the dose of the induction agent required and will reduce volatile anesthetic requirements for maintenance anesthesia. All anesthetic agents used for induction or maintenance of anesthesia should be administered to effect.
2. Dose adjustments will also need to be made to account for the degree of desired sedation; type, duration, and pain level of the procedure; and patient temperament and body weight/size.
3. Dosing based on body surface area (BSA; or allometric scaling) is not common in clinical practice but decreases the variability in drug response between giant/large and small/toy breed dogs. See ***Conversion Tables: Body Weight (kg) to Body Surface Area (m²)***.
4. For all dosages, the low end of the dose range is generally appropriate for IV administration, whereas the mid-upper range is most appropriate for IM or SC administration. Higher dosages will provide more profound sedation and analgesia.
5. When SC administration is used, the speed of sedation is slower, and the level of sedation is lighter and inconsistent. For more predictable sedation, IM or IV administration is recommended.
6. The effects of dexmedetomidine can be reversed with atipamezole. It is most often dosed by volume at ½ or the same volume of dexmedetomidine that was administered and given IM. See ***Atipamezole***.

DOGS:

Label dosages (FDA-approved):

a) **Sedation and analgesia**: 375 µg/m² BSA IV; 500 µg/m² BSA IM. The µg/kg dosage decreases as body weight increases. It is recommended that patients be fasted for 12 hours before use.

b) **Preanesthetic agent**: Depending on duration and severity of the procedure and anesthetic regimen: 125 – 375 µg/m² BSA IM. The µg/kg dosage decreases as body weight increases. Accurate dosing is not possible with dogs weighing less than 2 kg (4.4 lb). An extensive dosing table using patient weights is available in the package insert. After injection, allow the animal to rest quietly for 15 minutes; sedation/analgesia occurs within 5 to 15 minutes, with peak effects occurring 30 minutes postdose. When used as a preanesthetic, dexmedetomidine can reduce induction agent dose requirements by 30% to 60% and inhalational anesthetic requirements by 40% to 60%. The anesthetic dose should always be titrated against the response of the patient.[23]

c) **Noise aversion using the oromucosal gel** (*Sileo®*): 125 µg/m² BSA administered onto the oral mucosa between the dog's cheek and gum.[13] The first dose should be administered ≈30 to 60 minutes before the fear and/or anxiety-eliciting noise stimulus, immediately after the dog shows the first signs of anxiety or fear related to noise, or when the owner detects a typical noise stimulus (eg, sound of fireworks) eliciting anxiety or fear in the dog. Dosing should only be performed by an adult wearing disposable, impermeable gloves. The gel must be administered using the accompanying syringe (*Sileo®* dot syringe). The following table can be used to convert a dog's body weight into the appropriate number of dots (•).

Body weight (lb)	Number of dots	Body weight (kg)
4.4 – 12.1	1 •	2 – 5.5
12.2 – 26.5	2 ••	5.6 – 12
26.6 – 44	3 •••	12.1 – 20
44.1 – 63.9	4 ••••	20.1 – 29
64 – 86	5 •••••	29.1 – 39
86.1 – 110.2	6 ••••••	39.1 – 50
110.3 – 137.8	7 •••••••	50.1 – 62.6
137.9 – 166.4	8 ••••••••	62.7 – 75.6
166.5 – 196.2	9 •••••••••	75.7 – 89.2
196.3 – 220.5	10 ••••••••••	89.3 – 100.2

If the dose is more than 6 dots, divide the dose between both sides of the mouth. Avoid feeding or giving treats within 15 minutes after a dose, as this may decrease absorption from the mucous membranes. Drinking water within that time frame may have the same effect. If noise lasts longer than 2 to 3 hours and the dog's signs of fear and/or anxiety reappear, another dose may need to be given. To avoid overdosing, there should always be a pause of at least 2 hours between doses. No more than 5 doses can be given during one noise event. Partially used syringes can be used again within 2 weeks of initial opening, provided there is enough gel to administer a complete dose. To minimize risk for incorrect dosing, a partially used syringe without enough gel for a complete dose should not be used. Make sure to give owner a copy of the client information sheet found on the reverse side of the package insert.[13]

Extra-label dosages:

In combination with an opioid and ketamine (ie, "doggie magic") to provide anesthesia and pain management (extra-label): **NOTE**: Dosing tables for conversion of patient weight to various µg/m² doses of dexmedetomidine (based on depth of sedation needed) have been presented.[41] Opioid concentrations used in the reference are butorphanol 10 mg/mL, hydromorphone 2 mg/mL, morphine 15 mg/mL, and buprenorphine 0.3 mg/mL. Ketamine concentration is 100 mg/mL. As these drugs may be available in other concentrations, only use those products with the above concentrations if using this protocol. For lighter sedation/anesthesia, the ketamine can be omitted from these protocols.

a) **Geriatric dogs and dogs with renal or liver dysfunction as a premedication before propofol induction, followed by maintenance on isoflurane or sevoflurane**: Dexmedetomidine 62.5 µg/m² IM or IV. Combine this dose with equal volumes of one of the opioids noted above and ± an equal dose of ketamine.
b) **For slightly heavier sedation in ASA class II or III dogs requiring sedation for radiographic procedures**: Dexmedetomidine 125 µg/m² IM or IV. Combine this dose with equal volumes of one of the opioids noted above and an equal volume of ketamine.
c) **Dogs undergoing minor surgery, Penn hip, or OFA types of radiographic procedures that require significant muscle relaxation**: Dexmedetomidine 250 µg/m² IM or IV. Combine this dose with equal volumes of one of the opioids noted above and an equal volume of ketamine.
d) **Induction of general anesthesia for OHE, castration, or other abdominal surgery**: Dexmedetomidine at 375 µg/m² IM or IV. Combine with equal volumes of one of the opioids noted above and an equal volume of ketamine. Provides rapid immobilization; lateral recumbency in 5 to 8 minutes. This protocol provides deep enough sedation to allow intubation before maintenance of general anesthesia. Dogs can be intubated and maintained on oxygen. Supplemental low doses of isoflurane (0.5%) or sevoflurane (1%) can be used.
e) **Immobilizing extremely fractious dogs and wolf-hybrid dogs**: Dexmedetomidine 500 µg/m² IM. Combine this dose with equal volumes of one of the opioids noted above and an equal volume of ketamine. **NOTE**: This high dose is rarely required.

In combination with alfaxalone (extra-label): Dexmedetomidine 3 µg/kg in combination with methadone 0.3 mg/kg and alfaxalone 0.5 – 1 mg/kg and administered IM[42]

Postoperative pain management IV CRI in critically ill dogs (extra-label):

a) After surgery, dexmedetomidine 25 µg/m² IV as a loading dose followed by dexmedetomidine 25 µg/m²/hour IV CRI for 24 hours was as effective as morphine 2.5 mg/m² IV loading dose, followed by morphine 2.5 mg/m²/hour CRI.[43]
b) Dexmedetomidine 1 – 2 µg/kg IV as a loading dose followed by 0.72 – 1 µg/kg/hour IV CRI has been used with satisfactory results.[44-47]

Dexmedetomidine/morphine/lidocaine/ketamine (DMLK) (extra-label): Dexmedetomidine 0.5 µg/kg/hour with lidocaine 3 mg/kg/hour, morphine 0.2 mg/kg/hour, and ketamine 0.6 mg/kg/hour admixed in IV fluids and administered as CRI[48]

Dexmedetomidine gel to decrease fear/anxiety prior to veterinary visits (extra-label): 78% of dogs receiving dexmedetomidine 125 µg/m² or 250 µg/m² were easier to handle and had relaxed body posture compared to only 4.3% of the placebo dogs.[5]

CATS:

Sedation, analgesia, and preanesthesia (label dosage; FDA-approved): 40 µg/kg IM. A dosing table is available in the package insert. After injection, allow the animal to rest quietly for 15 minutes; sedation/analgesia occurs within 5 to 15 minutes, with peak effects occurring 30 minutes postdose. When used as a preanesthetic, dexmedetomidine can markedly reduce anesthetic requirements. The anesthetic dose should always be titrated against the response of the patient.[23]

Extra-label dosages:

Sedation/analgesia when dexmedetomidine is used as a sole agent (extra-label): Dosage ranges commonly used to achieve general sedation levels include:

a) **Light sedation (often used for preanesthesia)**: 5 – 15 µg/kg IV, IM, or SC
b) **Moderate sedation (may be used for preanesthesia if deeper sedation is desired or the patient has a high energy or anxiety level)**: 20 – 30 µg/kg IV, IM, or SC
c) **Deep sedation**: 40 µg/kg IV, IM, or SC

CRI (extra-label): For ovariohysterectomy, hydromorphone 0.1 mg/kg IM premedication was followed by anesthesia induction with propofol 4.3 – 7.8 mg/kg IV; during isoflurane anesthesia cats were given dexmedetomidine 0.5 µg/kg IV loading dose followed by dexmedetomidine 0.5 µg/kg/hour IV CRI. Isoflurane maintenance requirements were reduced.[49]

In combination with an opioid and ketamine (ie, "kitty magic", DKT, or Triple Combination) to provide sedation and analgesia (extra-label): Dexmedetomidine concentration is 0.5 mg/mL (500 µg/mL). Opioid concentrations referenced here are butorphanol 10 mg/mL, hydromorphone 2 mg/mL, and buprenorphine 0.3 mg/mL. Ketamine concentration is 100 mg/mL. These drugs may be available in other concentrations, but only the products with these concentrations should be used for this protocol. See the table below for volumes used to attain the desired degree of patient sedation.[50]

Drug Volume of *Each* Drug (Ketamine/Dexmedetomidine*/Opioid) to Be Given IM

Cat body weight	Mild†	Moderate‡	Profound§
2-3 kg (4-7 lb)	0.025 mL	0.05 mL	0.1 – 0.15 mL
3-4 kg (7-9 lb)	0.05 mL	0.1 mL	0.2 – 0.25 mL
4-6 kg (9-13 lb)	0.1 mL	0.2 mL	0.3 – 0.35 mL
6-7 kg (14-15 lb)	0.2 mL	0.3 mL	0.4 – 0.45 mL
7-8 kg (15-18 lb)	0.3 mL	0.4 mL	0.5 – 0.55 mL

*Dexmedetomidine can be reversed immediately with an equal volume (of dexmedetomidine used) of atipamezole.

†For sedation or as a premedication prior to anesthetic induction

‡For castration or minor surgical procedures

§Invasive surgical procedures, including OHE and declawing

In combination with alfaxalone OR ketamine (extra-label): Dexmedetomidine 10 µg/kg and butorphanol 0.2 mg/kg combined with *either* alfaxalone 3 mg/kg OR ketamine 5 mg/kg and administered IM provided adequate analgesia with minor physiologic and anesthetic duration differences when administered to cats undergoing castration.[51]

In combination with buprenorphine: Dexmedetomidine 40 µg/kg in combination with buprenorphine 20 µg/kg administered by either the OTM (buccal cavity) or IM (quadriceps muscle) routes provided equal sedation and antinociceptive scores.[17] Vomiting occurred in both groups; however, dexmedetomidine 20 µg/kg with buprenorphine 20 µg/kg IM provided more reliable sedation than the OTM route.[16]

Induction of emesis: 6 – 18 µg/kg IM[1-3] or 3.5 µg/kg IV[1]

HORSES:

Total IV anesthesia in foals (extra-label): Dexmedetomidine 3 – 7 µg/kg IV to place arterial catheter; alfaxalone 2 mg/kg IV for anesthesia induction; anesthesia maintained with a combination of dexmedetomidine 1 µg/kg/hour, alfaxalone 6 mg/kg/hour, and remifentanil 3 µg/kg/hour IV CRI. Regimen was suitable for laparotomy, although prolonged recovery may occur (time to standing was 46 to 106 minutes after stopping infusion).[52]

Constant rate infusion in adult horses/ponies (extra-label):

a) Dexmedetomidine used for MAC reduction and analgesia example: 3.5 µg/kg dexmedetomidine IV followed by dexmedetomidine 1.75 µg/kg/hour IV CRI reduced sevoflurane MAC by an average of 52% in anesthetized ponies.[53]
b) Dexmedetomidine 3.5 – 5.5 µg/kg combined with butorphanol 30 µg/kg and given IV followed by dexmedetomidine 1.75 – 5.3 µg/kg/hour IV CRI successfully allowed transvenous electrical cardioversion in 5 adult horses with atrial fibrillation.[54]

SMALL MAMMALS:

Rabbits (extra-label): Numerous protocols are published for sedation/anesthesia in rabbits using medetomidine. Dexmedetomidine can be substituted for medetomidine at ½ the dose in mg/kg or same dose in mL/kg.

a) Dexmedetomidine 100 µg/kg, ketamine 15 mg/kg and buprenorphine 30 µg/kg combined in the same syringe and administered SC.[55] Anecdotally, this dosage can also be used IV or IM. If longer duration anesthesia is necessary, inhalants can be administered.
b) Dexmedetomidine 250 µg/kg in combination with ketamine 35 mg/kg ± buprenorphine 30 µg/kg and administered IM[56]

Dwarf rabbits (extra-label):

a) Dexmedetomidine 25 µg/kg in combination with midazolam 0.2 mg/kg and administered IM allowed complete abdominal ultrasonography to be performed, but 3 (33%) required additional doses of the drug combination.[57]
b) Dexmedetomidine 100 µg/kg in combination with butorphanol 0.4 mg/kg and midazolam 2 mg/kg and administered intranasally produced deep sedation and analgesia suitable for minor surgical procedures.[58]

Guinea pigs (extra-label): Dexmedetomidine 250 µg/kg in combination with buprenorphine 0.05 mg/kg and alfaxalone 15 – 20 mg/kg SC yielded sedation within ≈7 to 8 minutes and recumbency for 74 minutes but did not induce anesthesia.[59]

Monitoring

- Level of sedation and analgesia
- Heart rate and rhythm, blood pressure, pulse oximetry
- Respiratory depth and rate, $ETCO_2$
- Body temperature

Client Information

- When given by injection (in the veterinary clinic), dexmedetomidine should be used in a professionally supervised setting by individuals familiar with its properties.
- Withhold feed and water until the sedative effects of dexmedetomidine have subsided.

When using the dexmedetomidine *oromucosal gel*:

- Avoid handling this medicine if pregnant.
- Because this medicine can be absorbed through the skin, mucous membranes (mouth/gums), and eyes, impermeable (eg, latex) disposable gloves should be worn when handling the syringe. If the medicine makes contact with skin, thoroughly wash affected area with soap and water. In case of accidental eye exposure, flush eye(s) with water for 15 minutes. In the case of accidental ingestion, seek medical attention immediately; alert physician about exposure to an alpha-2-adrenergic agonist.
- When dialing the "ring-stop" to the appropriate dose (ie, number of dots), the ring-stop must be locked in place prior to administration. An accidental overdose may occur if the ring-stop is not fully locked.
- Administer the medicine between your dog's cheek and gums. The medicine is intended to be absorbed from the inside of the mouth and may be less effective if swallowed.
- If your veterinarian instructed you to give the medicine more than once, you may give another dose at least 2 hours after the previous dose. Give another dose only if your dog is showing signs of fear or anxiety. Do not give the medicine if your dog is still sleepy from the previous dose. Up to 5 doses (total) may be given to your dog during any one noise event.
- The potential side effects associated with use, particularly in dogs at risk (ie, those that are older or have preexisting conditions) include low-energy level, weakness, sedation, sleepiness, slow heart rate, loss of consciousness, shallow or slow breathing, trouble breathing, impaired balance or incoordination, low blood pressure, and muscle tremors.

Chemistry/Synonyms

Dexmedetomidine is the dextrorotatory enantiomer of medetomidine. It occurs as a white or almost white crystalline substance that is water-soluble.

Dexmedetomidine HCl may also be known as (*S*)-medetomidine, (+)-medetomidine, MPV 1440, MPV 295, or MPV 785. Trade names include *Cepedex*®, *Dexdomitor*®, *Dexvetidine*®, *Precedex*®, *Sedadex*®, and *Sileo*®.

Storage/Stability

Store the injection at room temperature (ie, 15°C-30°C [59°F-86°F]); do not freeze. Discard unused product 90 days after first piercing the vial.

Store the oromucosal gel syringes (unopened or opened) at controlled room temperature of 20°C to 25°C (68°F-77°F), with excursions permitted to 15°C to 30°C (59°F-86°F). Use syringe contents within 4 weeks after opening the syringe.

Compatibility/Compounding Considerations

Information from the manufacturer states that dexmedetomidine 0.5 mg/mL solution for injection can be mixed with butorphanol 2 mg/mL, ketamine 50 mg/mL solution, or with butorphanol 2 mg/mL solution and ketamine 50 mg/mL solution, in the same syringe for up to 2 hours. Anecdotal comments have been noted that buprenorphine, hydromorphone, or morphine can also be mixed with dexmedetomidine.

In humans, dexmedetomidine injection is administered as a 0.004 mg/mL (4 µg/mL) IV infusion. The drug is **compatible** in the following solutions: 0.9% sodium chloride, 5% dextrose, lactated Ringer's, and 20% mannitol. Dexmedetomidine is **incompatible** with amphotericin B, diazepam, pantoprazole and blood or plasma products.

Compatibility is dependent on factors such as pH, concentration, temperature, and diluent used; specialized references or a hospital pharmacist should be consulted for more specific information.

Dosage Forms/Regulatory Status

VETERINARY-LABELED PRODUCTS:

Dexmedetomidine HCl 0.5 mg/mL (500 µg/mL) in 10 mL multidose vials; *Dexdomitor*®; (Rx). FDA-approved for use in dogs and cats. NADA #141-267

Dexmedetomidine HCl 0.1 mg/mL (100 µg/mL) in 10 mL multidose vials; *Dexdomitor*® 0.1; (Rx). FDA-approved for use in dogs and cats. NADA #141-267

Dexmedetomidine Oromucosal Gel 0.09 mg/mL (equivalent to 0.1 mg/mL dexmedetomidine HCl) in 3 mL dosing syringes; *Sileo*® (Rx). FDA-approved for use in dogs. NADA #141-456

HUMAN-LABELED PRODUCTS:

Dexmedetomidine HCl Concentrated Solution for Injection: 100 µg/mL (equivalent to dexmedetomidine hydrochloride 118 µg), in 2 mL single-dose vials and 4 mL multi-dose vials; *Precedex*®, generic; (Rx). Must be diluted prior to administration.

Dexmedetomidine HCl in 0.9% NaCl Solution for Infusion: 4 µg/mL in 20 mL and 50 mL; *Precedex*®, generic; (Rx)

References

For the complete list of references, see **wiley.com/go/budde/plumb**

Dexrazoxane

(dex-ra-***zox***-ane) *Zinecard*®

Antidote

Prescriber Highlights

- May attenuate the cardiotoxic effects of doxorubicin in dogs showing signs of anthracycline cardiotoxicity, that have cardiac disease prior to doxorubicin therapy, or that are at maximum cumulative doses of doxorubicin; also used to treat extravasation injuries associated with doxorubicin
- Contraindications include use in patients receiving non-anthracycline chemotherapy.
- Adverse effects include myelosuppression; this effect is additive with anthracycline-related myelosuppression.
- Administer within 6 hours of extravasation injury to attenuate local tissue damage and necrosis
- The National Institute for Occupational Safety and Health (NIOSH) classifies dexrazoxane as a hazardous drug; use appropriate precautions when handling.

Uses/Indications

Dexrazoxane may be useful to attenuate the cardiotoxic effects of doxorubicin in patients that are showing signs of anthracycline cardiotoxicity, that develop cardiac disease while taking doxorubicin, or that are at maximum cumulative life-time dosage of doxorubicin. Dexrazoxane can also be used to treat extravasation injuries associated with doxorubicin. In a case series involving 4 dogs, it was recommended that because of the importance of timely administration (within 6 hours), veterinarians that administer doxorubicin should have dexrazoxane readily available.[1,2]

Pharmacology/Actions

Dexrazoxane is hydrolyzed to an active metabolite that chelates intracellular iron, which is believed to prevent the formation of an anthracycline-iron complex free radical that is thought to be the primary cause of anthracycline-induced cardiomyopathy and extravasation injury.

Pharmacokinetics

In dogs, dexrazoxane's pharmacokinetics fit a 2-compartment open model.[3] Steady-state volume of distribution is 0.67 L/kg; terminal half-life is about 1.2 hours; and clearance is about 11 mL/kg/minute. Clearance was dose-independent, and the drug showed low tissue and protein binding. Dexrazoxane is primarily excreted in the urine as unchanged drug and metabolites.

Contraindications/Precautions/Warnings

Dexrazoxane should not be used unless an anthracycline antineoplastic agent is being used.

Efficacy and safety of dexrazoxane for use in cats is not known.

The National Institute for Occupational Safety and Health (NIOSH) classifies dexrazoxane as a hazardous drug; personal protective equipment (PPE) should be used accordingly to minimize the risk for exposure. Refer to the Occupational Safety and Health Association (OSHA) website for more information.

Adverse Effects

Dexrazoxane may cause additive myelosuppression when used with other myelosuppressive agents.

Wear gloves when handling this product and use normal procedures for handling and disposing of anticancer medications. If non-reconstituted powder contacts skin or mucous membranes, thoroughly wash the exposed area with soap and water.

Reproductive/Nursing Safety

Dexrazoxane has been shown to cause testicular atrophy in dogs when it is administered at usual doses for 13 weeks.[4] In rats and rabbits, dexrazoxane was teratogenic at doses lower than those administered to humans.

It is unknown if dexrazoxane enters maternal milk; human mothers are advised to discontinue nursing if they are given the drug.

Because safety has not been established in animals, this drug should only be used when the maternal benefits outweigh the potential risks to offspring.

Overdose/Acute Toxicity

Because of the method of administration and drug expense, overdoses of dexrazoxane are unlikely in veterinary medicine. As there is no known antidote, treatment would be supportive. Potentially, the drug could be removed via hemodialysis.

For patients that have experienced or are suspected to have experienced an overdose, consultation with a 24-hour poison control center specializing in providing veterinary-specific information is recommended. For general information related to overdose and toxin exposures, as well as contact information for poison control centers, refer to ***Appendix.***

Drug Interactions

Dexrazoxane does not influence the pharmacokinetics of doxorubicin.

The following drug interactions either have been reported or are theoretical in humans or animals receiving dexrazoxane and may be of significance in veterinary patients. Unless otherwise noted, use together is not necessarily contraindicated, but weigh the potential risks and perform additional monitoring when appropriate.

- **Myelosuppressive Agents, Other**: Additive myelosuppression may occur when dexrazoxane is used with other myelosuppressive agents.

Laboratory Considerations

- No specific laboratory interactions or considerations were noted.

Dosages

DOGS:

Treatment of anthracycline (eg, **doxorubicin, epirubicin) extravasation** (extra-label): **NOTE**: In a retrospective study of 4 dogs, the authors concluded that the most effective dosage and timing of administration are unknown; however, there is evidence to suggest that administration within 6 hours after the event is warranted; further studies are needed.[1]

a) IV administration of dexrazoxane at 10 times the doxorubicin dose within 3 hours (when possible) and again at 24 and 48 hours after extravasation significantly reduces local tissue injury.[1,2,5]

b) Terminate doxorubicin infusion immediately and infuse IV 1000 mg/m^2 of dexrazoxane at a separate (new) infusion site within 6 hours of extravasation and again on day 2. Infuse 500 mg/m^2 IV on day 3. Acute surgical evaluation is performed. **NOTE**: Dosage recommendations are for human patients but may apply to veterinary patients.[6]

Prevention of doxorubicin-induced cardiomyopathy (extra-label): In dogs that met at least one of the following criteria: pre-existing diagnosed clinical heart disease; onset of impaired systolic function during the course of doxorubicin therapy; cumulative dose of doxorubicin of 180 mg/m^2; or cardiac disease as determined by echocardiographic evaluation: 10 minutes prior to doxorubicin infusion, dexrazoxane at a dose of 10 times the administered milligram dose of doxorubicin administered IV over 5 to 10 minutes. Although no information regarding efficacy of cardioprotection could be gleaned, it appears that 1 to 2 doses of dexrazoxane administered with doxorubicin are safe and well tolerated.[7]

Monitoring

- Baseline and periodic CBC
- If used for cardioprotection: serial echocardiogram and ECG

Client Information

- This medication is considered to be a hazardous drug as defined by the National Institute for Occupational Safety and Health (NIOSH). Talk with your veterinarian or pharmacist about the use of personal protective equipment when handling this medicine.

Chemistry/Synonyms

A derivative of EDTA, dexrazoxane occurs as a white crystalline powder that is soluble in water, slightly soluble in ethanol, and practically insoluble in nonpolar organic solvents. It has a pK_a of 2.1 and degrades rapidly at a pH above 7.

Dexrazoxane may also be known as 2,6-Piperazinedione, ADR-529, ICRF-187, NSC-169780, *Zinecard®*, *Cardioxane®* or *Eucardion®*.

Storage/Stability

Unreconstituted dexrazoxane vials should be stored at 25°C (77°F); excursions are permitted to 15°C to 30°C (59°F-86°F). Once reconstituted with the supplied diluent, the product is stable for 6 hours at room temperature or refrigerated.[4] Unused solutions after that time should be discarded. After reconstitution, the resulting solution may be diluted with either 0.9% sodium chloride injection or 5% dextrose in concentrations of 1.3 – 5 mg/mL. Inspect visually for particulate matter and discoloration prior to administering.

Compatibility/Compounding Considerations

Dexrazoxane should not be mixed with any other drug.[4]

Dosage Forms/Regulatory Status

VETERINARY-LABELED PRODUCTS: NONE

HUMAN-LABELED PRODUCTS:

Dexrazoxane Lyophilized Powder for Injection Solution: 250 mg in single-use vials with 25 mL vial of sodium lactate injection; and 500 mg regular and preservative free in single-use vials with 50 mL vial of sodium lactate injection; *Zinecard®*, generic; (Rx)

References

For the complete list of references, see **wiley.com/go/budde/plumb**

Dextran 70

(***dex***-tran)

Synthetic Colloid, Plasma Volume Expander

NOTE: Dextran is also available as Dextran 40. As Dextran 70 has been the most commonly used version in veterinary medicine, the following monograph is limited to Dextran 70.

Prescriber Highlights

- ► Branched polysaccharide plasma volume expander
- ► Limited availability. Other colloids (eg, hydroxyethyl starch) have largely supplanted use.
- ► Contraindicated in patients with preexisting coagulopathies
- ► Use with caution in patients susceptible to circulatory overload (severe heart or chronic kidney disease), or with thrombocytopenia.
- ► Adverse effects are quite rare in dogs and include increased bleeding times, acute kidney injury, and anaphylaxis (very rare).
- ► Must monitor for fluid overload

Uses/Indications

Dextran 70 is a relatively low-cost colloid for the adjunctive treatment of hypovolemic shock. Hydroxyethyl starches are the more commonly employed synthetic colloids in use today.

Pharmacology/Actions

Dextran 70 has osmotic effects similar to albumin. Dextran's colloidal osmotic effect draws fluid into the vascular system from the interstitial spaces, resulting in increased circulating blood volume.

Pharmacokinetics

After IV infusion, circulating blood volume is increased maximally within 1 hour and effects can persist for 24 hours or more.

Approximately 20% to 30% of a given dose remains in the intravascular compartment at 24 hours and it may be detected in the blood 4 to 6 weeks after dosing. Dextran 70 is slowly degraded to glucose by dextranase in the spleen and then metabolized to carbon dioxide and water. A small amount may be excreted directly into the gut and eliminated in the feces.

Contraindications/Precautions/Warnings

Patients overly susceptible to circulatory overload (severe heart or chronic kidney disease) should only receive dextran 70 with great caution. Dextran 70 is contraindicated in patients with severe coagulopathies and should be used with caution in patients with thrombocytopenia, as it can interfere with platelet function. Do not give dextran IM. Patients on strict sodium restriction should receive dextran cautiously as a 500 mL bag contains 77 mEq of sodium.

Adverse Effects

Dextran 70 may increase bleeding time and decrease von Willebrand factor antigen, platelet function, buccal mucosal bleeding time, and factor VIII activity; however, this effect does not usually cause clinical bleeding in dogs.[1,2]

Anaphylactoid reactions to dextran 70 occur rarely in dogs, but at a higher rate than with hetastarch. Unlike dextran 40, dextran 70 has rarely been associated with acute kidney injury. In humans, GI effects (abdominal pain, nausea, vomiting) have been reported with use of dextran 70.

Reproductive/Nursing Safety

Because safety has not been established in animals, this drug should only be used when the maternal benefits outweigh the potential risks to offspring.

Overdose/Acute Toxicity

The drug should be dosed and monitored carefully as volume overload may result.

For patients that have experienced or are suspected to have experienced an overdose, consultation with a 24-hour poison consultation center specializing in providing veterinary-specific information is recommended. For general information related to overdose and toxin exposures, as well as contact information for poison control centers, refer to ***Appendix***.

Drug Interactions

The following drug interactions have either been reported or are theoretical in humans or animals receiving dextran 70 and may be of significance in veterinary patients. Unless otherwise noted, use together is not necessarily contraindicated, but weigh the potential risks and perform additional monitoring when appropriate.

- **Anticoagulants** (eg, **heparins, rivaroxaban, warfarin**): Increased risk for bleeding
- **Anti-Platelet Agents** (eg, **aspirin, clopidogrel**): Increased risk for bleeding

Laboratory Considerations

- Dextran 70 may interfere with **blood cross-matching,** as it can cross-link with red blood cells and appear as rouleaux formation. Isotonic saline may be used to negate this effect.
- **Blood glucose** levels may be increased as dextran is degraded.
- Falsely elevated **bilirubin** levels may be noted; reason unknown

Dosages

DOGS:

Volume resuscitation (extra-label):

a) Small-volume resuscitation techniques are recommended in any dog with closed cavity hemorrhage, head injury, pulmonary contusions or edema, cardiogenic shock, or oliguric acute kidney injury. An initial dose of balanced isotonic crystalloids (10 – 15 mL/kg) is given. Either a hydroxyethyl starch or dextran 70 is then administered (5 mL/kg in dogs) over 1 to 5 minutes. The perfusion parameters are reassessed, and the initial mL/kg bolus is repeated as needed until the end point of resuscitation is reached.[3]

b) 20 mL/kg/day; when acute resuscitation is required, may be given as a slow bolus over 30 to 60 minutes. May also be given as a constant rate infusion (CRI) over a longer period to augment colloid oncotic pressure or decrease the volume of crystalloids infused, thereby reducing hemodilution.[4]

CATS:

Volume resuscitation (extra-label):

a) Small-volume resuscitation techniques are recommended in the hypovolemic cat with closed cavity hemorrhage, head injury, pulmonary contusions or edema, cardiogenic shock, or oliguric acute kidney injury. An initial dose of balanced isotonic crystalloids (5 – 10 mL/kg) is given. Either hetastarch or dextran 70 is then administered (2 – 5 mL/kg) over 1 to 5 minutes. The perfusion parameters are reassessed, and the initial mL/kg bolus repeated as needed until the end point of resuscitation is reached.[3]

b) 10 mL/kg/day; when acute resuscitation is required. May be given as a slow bolus over 30 to 60 minutes. May also be given as a CRI over a longer period to augment colloid oncotic pressure or decrease the volume of crystalloids infused, thereby reducing hemodilution[4]

CATTLE:

Volume resuscitation in calves with dehydration due to diarrhea (extra-label): Administered as 6% dextran 70 in 7.2% sodium chloride. To prepare this solution, add 31.6 g sodium chloride crystals into the barrel of a 60 mL syringe. Draw 60 mL of 6% dextran 70 in 0.9% sodium chloride from the bag/bottle and use to dissolve the sodium chloride crystals. Using a 0.22 µm filter, reinject the dissolved solution into the 6% dextran 70 in 0.9% sodium chloride bag/bottle to produce a 6% dextran 70 in 7.2% sodium chloride solution. Resultant solution may be refrigerated for up to 3 months. Inject 4 – 5 mL/kg IV of the prepared solution over 4 to 5 minutes, followed immediately by oral administration of isotonic electrolyte solution. Give dextran 70 solution only once or hypernatremia may result; following up with isotonic fluids (oral or IV) is critical. [5]

Monitoring

- Hydration status and signs of fluid overload (eg, increased respiratory rate and effort, pulmonary edema)
- Clinical signs of anaphylactic-like reactions, including worsening signs of shock and pruritus
- Renal chemistry panel and urine output
- Serum electrolytes, acid-base balance
- Colloid oncotic pressure
- Blood pressure, central venous pressure
- Coagulation parameters, particularly in high-risk patients or when using high doses of dextran 70

Chemistry/Synonyms

A branched polysaccharide, dextran 70 occurs as a white to light yellow amorphous powder. It is freely soluble in water and insoluble in alcohol. Dextran 70 contains (on average) molecules of 70,000 daltons. Each 500 mL of the commercially available 6% dextran 70 in normal saline provides 77 mEq of sodium. Dextran 70 in normal saline has a viscosity of 3.68 centipoise (blood is 3 centipoise) and a colloid osmotic pressure of 62 mm Hg (canine plasma is ≈20 mm Hg).

Dextran 70 may also be known as dextranum 70, polyglucin, *Dextran 70®*, *Fisiodex 70®*, *Gentran 70®*, *Hyskon®*, *Lomodex 70®*, *Longasteril 70®*, *Macrodex®*, *Macrohorm 70®*, *Neodextril 70®*, *Plander®*, *RescueFlow®*, or *Solplex 70®*.

Storage/Stability

Dextran 70 injection should be stored at room temperature, preferably in an area with little temperature variability. Although only clear solutions should be used, dextran flakes can form but may be resolubilized by heating the solution in a boiling water bath until clear or autoclaving at 110°C (230°F) for 15 minutes.

Compatibility/Compounding Considerations

Compatibility is dependent on factors such as pH, concentration, temperature, and diluent used; specialized references or a hospital pharmacist should be consulted for more specific information.

Dextran 70 is **compatible** with many other solutions and drugs; refer to specialized references or a hospital pharmacist for more information.

Dosage Forms/Regulatory Status

VETERINARY-LABELED PRODUCTS: NONE

HUMAN-LABELED PRODUCTS:

Dextran 70: 6% in 5% dextrose in 500 mL; generic; (Rx). Not available in all countries

References

For the complete list of references, see **wiley.com/go/budde/plumb**

Dextromethorphan

(***dex***-troe-meth-***or***-fan) *Delsym*®

N-Methyl-D-Aspartate (NMDA) Receptor Antagonist

Prescriber Highlights

- May reduce self-directed behaviors in dogs with atopic dermatitis and cribbing in horses
- Oral use in dogs is limited by poor absorption and short half-life.
- PK studies in horses suggest significant interpatient variability with drug metabolism.
- GI effects (eg, vomiting, diarrhea) and ataxia are possible.

Uses/Indications

Dextromethorphan may be useful in reducing compulsive[1] or self-injurious behavior in dogs[2] and cribbing in horses.[3]

In humans, dextromethorphan is used primarily as an antitussive for the short-term control of coughing. In dogs, however, it is not a first-line medication for management of coughing. When other therapies have failed, dextromethorphan may be useful for some animals. The dosage for this indication is unknown.

Pharmacology/Actions

Dextromethorphan and its active metabolite dextrorphan are noncompetitive N-methyl-D-aspartate (NMDA) receptor antagonists. Sustained or repetitive NMDA activation by the excitatory amino acids glutamate and aspartate appears to sensitize neurons, stimulate C-fibers, and cause neurotoxicity. The resulting effects include reduced opioid efficacy, allodynia, wind-up pain, and secondary pain. By blocking the NMDA receptor, dextromethorphan and dextrorphan may potentiate the effects of other analgesics.[4]

In the medullary cough center, dextromethorphan stimulates σ-1 receptors, which inhibit glutamate transmission, and interferes with the cough impulse and reduces cough receptor sensitivity. Although dextromethorphan is structurally similar to codeine (see ***Chemistry/Synonyms***), its affinity for the mu, delta, and kappa opioid receptors is weak, even at excessive doses following abuse or overdose. Naloxone does not block the drug's antitussive effect, but it can reverse some effects associated with toxicity.

Dextromethorphan weakly inhibits serotonin reuptake, leading to the potential for drug interactions with other serotonergic agents.

Pharmacokinetics

In a randomized crossover study of 6 dogs, oral bioavailability was 11%. Volume of distribution and elimination half-life after IV dextromethorphan administration were 5.1 L/kg and 2 hours, respectively. Dextrorphan (the active metabolite) was not detected. Ex vivo treatment of plasma samples indicated the drug was conjugated.[4]

In horses given dextromethorphan 2 mg/kg PO once,[5,6] peak concentration was reached 30 minutes to 1 hour after administration, and elimination half-life was between 12 and 18 hours. Significant interpatient variability in pharmacokinetic parameters was attributed to differences in CYP2D50 metabolic activity, with horses classified as ultrarapid metabolizers ($n = 3$), extensive metabolizers ($n = 19$), and poor metabolizers ($n = 1$).[5] The highest dextrorphan exposure (AUC) was observed in the ultrarapid metabolizers, and the lowest exposure occurred in the poor metabolizer.[5] Free and glucuronidated dextrorphan were identified in plasma.[6] Dextrorphan was identified in urine as the primary form of excretion.[6]

In humans, peak concentration is reached 2 to 3 hours after administration, and antitussive effects typically last less than 6 hours. Metabolism depends on CYP2D6 enzyme expression; humans can be poor metabolizers or extensive metabolizers. The drug is hepatically metabolized to the active form, dextrorphan. Demethylation by CYP2D6 occurs in the liver; CYP3A subfamilies also have a minor role. Elimination half-life averages 11 hours but can range from 2 to 4 hours (in extensive CYP2D6 metabolizers) to 24 hours (in poor CYP2D6 metabolizers).

Contraindications/Precautions/Warnings

Dextromethorphan should not be used in patients hypersensitive to it. Dextromethorphan should be used with caution in patients with hepatic impairment. Use of the drug has been associated with histamine release in humans, and it should be used with caution in atopic patients, as it is unknown if this effect occurs in animals.

In humans, dextromethorphan should be used with caution in patients with a chronic cough or a cough due to excessive secretions.

Dextromethorphan should not be confused with dextromethorphan/quinidine, which is approved for use in humans with pseudobulbar affect. Caution should be used when referring clients to purchase OTC dextromethorphan products, because many of these products contain other drugs or ingredients (eg, xylitol) that are not appropriate for use in veterinary medicine.

Adverse Effects

Adverse effects in dogs receiving oral dextromethorphan appear uncommon, likely due to the drug's poor and erratic absorption in this species. In a blinded study of 14 dogs, lethargy was noted in 1 dog receiving oral dextromethorphan 2 mg/kg twice daily.[2] Sedation, diarrhea, vomiting, excitement, loss of balance, disorientation, lethargy, and decreased rate of breathing have been observed.[7] In a randomized crossover study of 6 dogs, dextromethorphan caused muscle rigidity, ataxia, sedation, and ptyalism after IV administration.[4]

Adverse effects from oral dextromethorphan were not observed in single-dose pharmacokinetic study in horses.[6]

In humans, adverse effects (eg, GI distress [eg, nausea, anorexia, constipation[8]], dizziness, drowsiness) may limit therapy. Case studies have shown fixed drug eruption after therapeutic doses of dextromethorphan. Respiratory distress may occur rarely. Doses greater than 100 mg may cause euphoria, hallucinations, dissociation, and coma.[9]

Reproductive/Nursing Safety

In humans, dextromethorphan is considered safe for use during pregnancy at standard doses.[10,11]

Because safety has not been established in animals, this drug should only be used when the maternal benefits outweigh the potential risks to offspring.

Overdose/Acute Toxicity

The LD_{50} of IV dextromethorphan in dogs is 22 mg/kg. The LD_{50} of oral dextromethorphan in mice and rats is 210 mg/kg and 116 mg/kg, respectively, and the LD_{50} of IV dextromethorphan in rats is 16.3 mg/kg.[12] Nausea, vomiting, CNS effects (eg, ataxia, hyperexcitability, dystonia, nystagmus, stupor), respiratory depression, hypertension, tachycardia, and seizures are possible.

For overdoses in veterinary patients, treatment is based on clinical signs and is supportive. Gut decontamination can be considered. Naloxone may reverse some manifestations of toxicity.

For patients that have experienced or are suspected to have experienced an overdose, consultation with a 24-hour poison consultation center specializing in providing veterinary-specific information is recommended. For general information related to overdose and toxin exposures, as well as contact information for poison control centers, refer to ***Appendix.***

Drug Interactions

Dextromethorphan is a CYP2D6 substrate in humans. Canine polymorphism of CYP2D15 is recognized,[13] but relation to dextromethorphan metabolism in this species is unknown. Polymorphism of equine CYP2D50, as well as variability of dextromethorphan metabolism (ie, poor, extensive, and ultrarapid metabolizers), has been demonstrated.[5] The following drug interactions have been reported or are theoretical in humans or animals receiving dextromethorphan and may be of significance in veterinary patients; unless otherwise noted, use together may not be contraindicated, but the potential risks should be weighed and additional monitoring performed when appropriate:

- **CYP2D6 Inhibitors** (eg, **amiodarone, fluoxetine, paroxetine, terbinafine**): Concurrent use may increase detromethorphan exposure via inhibition of cyp2d6.
- **Monoamine Oxidase Inhibitors** (MAOIs; eg, **amitraz, methylene blue, selegiline**): Concurrent use should be avoided. The MAOI should be discontinued 2 weeks prior to dextromethorphan use.
- **Naloxone**: Naloxone does not block antitussive effect of dextromethorphan in humans.
- **Opioids** (eg, butorphanol, hydrocodone, hydromorphone, morphine): Concurrent use may increase risk for serotonin syndrome.
- **Quinidine**: Concurrent use may result in 20-fold increases in dextromethorphan levels and exposure. Concurrent use should be avoided.
- **Serotonergic Agents** (eg, **clomipramine, metoclopramide, mirtazapine, ondansetron, SSRIs** [eg, **fluoxetine, paroxetine**], **tramadol, trazodone**): Concurrent use may increase risk for serotonin syndrome.

Laboratory Considerations

- In humans, dextromethorphan can cause false-positive results for **phencyclidine (PCP)** on **urine drug screening tests**; it may also cause false-positive results for **opioids**.[14]

Dosages

DOGS:

Reduction of self-directed scratching, biting, or chewing in dogs with allergic dermatitis (extra-label): 2 mg/kg PO twice daily reduced pruritus score and modestly reduced time engaged in self-injurious behavior in a blinded study of 14 dogs.[2]

CATS:

Adjunctive pain management (extra-label): Anecdotally, 0.5 – 2 mg/kg PO every 6 to 8 hours provides mild to moderate analgesia.[15]

HORSES:

Reduction of cribbing (extra-label): 1 mg/kg IV reduced cribbing rate (bites/minute) in 4 of 9 horses. Effect lasted ≈35 to 60 minutes. Cribbing rate increased in 1 horse.[3]

Monitoring

- Clinical efficacy
- Adverse effects

Client Information

- GI effects (eg, vomiting, loose stools, diarrhea) or lethargy may occur. Contact your veterinarian if these become serious or persist.
- Contact your veterinarian if your animal's condition worsens.

Chemistry/Synonyms

Dextromethorphan is the methyl ether of d-levorphanol. Commercial formulations contain dextromethorphan hydrobromide, which occurs as a white or crystalline powder. It is sparingly soluble in water and freely soluble in alcohol.

Dextromethorphan may also be known as dextromethorphan hydrobromide, dextromethorphan polistirex, d-Methorphan, DM, *Cough-Tabs*®, or *Delsym*®. Many other trade names exist.

Storage/Stability

Store dextromethorphan at controlled room temperature (20°C-25°C [68°F-77°F]).

Compatibility/Compounding Considerations

- Dextromethorphan is **incompatible** with penicillins, tetracyclines, salicylates, phenobarbital sodium, and high concentrations of sodium or potassium iodide.[16]

Dosage Forms/Regulatory Status

VETERINARY-LABELED PRODUCTS:

Dextromethorphan and Guaifenesin Tablets: Dextromethorphan 10 mg and Guaifenesin 100 mg tablets; *Cough Tabs for Dogs and Cats*®, generic; (OTC). Note: This drug has not been found by FDA to be safe and effective, and this labeling has not been approved by FDA.

The Association of Racing Commissioners International (ARCI) has designated dextromethorphan as a class 4 substance. See ***Appendix*** for more information. Use of this drug may not be allowed in certain animal competitions. Check rules and regulations before entering in a competition while this medication is being administered. Contact local racing authorities for further guidance.

HUMAN-LABELED PRODUCTS:

NOTE: Some products may contain xylitol; label should be checked to avoid toxicity in dogs.

Dextromethorphan Hydrobromide GelCaps: 15 mg; generic; (OTC)

Dextromethorphan Hydrobromide Syrup: 1 mg/mL, 1.33 mg/mL, 2 mg/mL in 118 mL, 120 mL, 236 mL, and 354 mL bottles; generic; (OTC)

Dextromethorphan Polistirex Extended Release Suspension: 6 mg/mL in 89 mL and 148 mL bottles; *Delsym*®, *Robitussin 12 Hour Cough Relief*®, generic; (OTC). Contains dextromethorphan polistirex equivalent to dextromethorphan hydrobromide 6 mg/mL

Dextromethorphan is also available as a spray, lozenge, chewable tablet, orally disintegrating film or strip, and oral granules or powder, in a variety of strengths and sizes. Many products that combine dextromethorphan with guaifenesin, analgesics, antihistamines, and/or decongestants are available, but these are generally inappropriate for use in animal patients because of the potential for unpredictable adverse effects.

References

For the complete list of references, see **wiley.com/go/budde/plumb**

Dextrose 50% Injection

D-glucose

*(**deks**-trose)*

Glucose Elevating Agent

Prescriber Highlights

- ▶ Used primarily to treat acute hypoglycemia
- ▶ Used concomitantly with IV insulin for treatment of severe hyperkalemia
- ▶ Diluting dextrose to 10% or less for administration to dogs and cats decreases the risk for phlebitis.
- ▶ Glucose levels should be monitored during therapy.

Uses/Indications

IV dextrose is indicated in emergency treatment of hypoglycemia caused by various conditions (eg, neonatal/juvenile hypoglycemia, hepatic insufficiency or failure, hypoadrenocorticism, insulin overdose, sepsis, insulinoma, glycogen storage disease, pregnancy, xylitol toxicity). Buccal administration increased blood glucose concentration in healthy dogs; however, the effect was not observed until 15 minutes after administration and may be too slow for more severely hypoglycemic patients.[1]

In veterinary patients, IV dextrose is given IV concomitantly with regular insulin to treat hyperkalemia.[2] In dogs and cats, ECG changes seen in critical patients with hyperkalemia may be affected by concurrent metabolic derangements (eg, metabolic acidosis, hypermagnesemia, hypocalcemia) and thus may not typify the expected ECG changes (eg, bradyarrhythmias, loss of P wave, wide QRS complexes, peaked T waves) previously described for hyperkalemia.[3] In humans, treatment for hyperkalemia is recommended when serum potassium is greater than 5.5 mEq/L if there are ECG changes or when serum potassium is greater than 6 mEq/L, regardless of ECG findings.[4]

Dextrose may also be used as adjunctive therapy for nutritional support and as part of fluid therapy for some patients with diabetic ketoacidosis (see ***Insulin, General Information***).

Pharmacology/Actions

Dextrose solution provides a source of water and glucose. The solution restores blood glucose levels; it is thought to aid in minimizing liver glycogen depletion and to exert a protein-sparing effect.

Pharmacokinetics

No pharmacokinetic data in animals were located. In humans, serum glucose levels cannot be quantitatively predicted after a single IV bolus. Dextrose is metabolized to carbon dioxide and water with the release of energy (ie, ATP).

Contraindications/Precautions/Warnings

IV dextrose supplementation is contraindicated in patients with severe hyperglycemia or with CNS hemorrhage. Avoid IV dextrose boluses in patients with suspected insulinoma (or other insulin-like analogue secreting tumors) as additional insulin can be secreted, leading to rebound hypoglycemia. Use with caution in patients with head trauma or intracranial edema as hyperglycemia can worsen neurologic injury.[5]

Dextrose 50% is a hypertonic solution and can cause severe phlebitis when administered IV; diluting with a sterile isotonic (eg, lactated Ringer's solution, 0.9% sodium chloride) or hypotonic solution (eg, 0.45% sodium chloride) reduces this risk. Dextrose concentrations 10% or greater are best administered via a central line; if a peripheral line is used, administer slowly.

Dextrose-only IV fluids (eg, dextrose 5%) should not be used as sole fluid therapy for prolonged periods as hyponatremia and water intoxication may occur.

Adverse Effects

The primary adverse effect caused by IV administration of dextrose is hyperglycemia. Hyperosmolar syndrome can occur if dextrose is administered too rapidly; clinical signs can include neurologic changes (eg, decreased mentation, weakness, ataxia, abnormal pupillary light reflexes, seizure activity). Administration site reactions (eg, phlebitis, infection) are possible especially when administered through a peripheral vein; avoid extravasation.

Fluid overload is a risk if large volumes are administered. Fluid overload may occur in patients with cardiac or chronic kidney disease, even at recommended dosages.

In humans, IV dextrose 50% may increase histamine release and has rarely caused a febrile response or anaphylaxis.

Reproductive/Nursing Safety

When used in humans during breastfeeding, risk to the infant cannot be ruled out. Available evidence and/or expert consensus is inconclusive or is inadequate for determining infant risk.

Potential benefits versus risk should be weighed when considering use of dextrose in pregnant or lactating animals.

Overdose/Acute Toxicity

There are no data available on overdose in veterinary patients. However, an overdose will likely result in hyperglycemia, phlebitis, neurologic changes, or fluid overload. Discontinue or reduce dextrose dose if hyperglycemia occurs. Monitor clinical signs and blood glucose concentrations. Treat supportively; rapid-/short-acting insulin (eg, regular insulin) may be considered.

Drug Interactions

No drug interactions were noted.

Laboratory Considerations

None

Dosages

DOGS/CATS:

Emergency treatment of hypoglycemia (extra-label):

1. Dextrose 50% 0.5 – 1 mL/kg (0.25 – 0.5 g/kg) is diluted 1:2 – 1:4 in a sterile fluid and administered slowly as bolus (usually over 5 minutes).[6] Follow with dextrose 2.5% to 5% (or more) IV CRI as needed in isotonic fluids.[6-8] Administration via a central IV line is strongly encouraged. Solution should be administered very slowly (eg, 3 mL/minute) in the rare instance when dextrose 50% cannot be diluted or if clinical situation requires administration via a peripheral linc (see ***Adverse Effects***).[9]
2. 0.5 – 1 g/kg slow bolus IV followed by IV CRI of dextrose ranging from 1.25% to 10% in crystalloid fluid[10]
3. **Buccal administration**: 1 g/kg administered in the buccal vestibule followed by gentle lip massage. Increase in blood glucose may not be observed until 15 minutes after administration.[1]

Adjunctive treatment of hyperkalemia with corresponding ECG changes (extra-label): Redistribution of serum potassium can be achieved with dextrose and regular insulin. Dextrose 50% 1 mL/kg (0.5 g/kg) can be given as an IV bolus slowly (eg, 3 mL/minute). Regular insulin can be given at the same time at 0.25 – 0.5 units/kg slow IV. When using insulin and dextrose, it is imperative that dextrose be supplemented in the fluids at 2.5% to 5% to prevent secondary hypoglycemia.[11]

HORSES:

Hypoglycemia (label dosage; not FDA-approved): 100 – 500 mL IV.[12] Warm solution to body temperature and administer slowly.

Short-term caloric source for foals with diarrhea: 0.25 – 0.5 g/kg added to resuscitation fluids for 24 to 48 hours[13]

CATTLE:

Uncomplicated primary ketosis or hypoglycemia (label dosages; not FDA-approved):

1. 100 – 500 mL IV, depending on size and condition of animal. Solution should be warmed to body temperature and administered slowly.[14]
2. 1.1 mL/kg IV (50 mL per 45 kg [100 lb] body weight[15]), every 8 to 10 hours. Warm solution to body temperature and administer slowly.

SHEEP & SWINE:

Hypoglycemia (label dosage; not FDA-approved): 30 – 100 mL IV.[12] Warm solution to body temperature and administer slowly.

Monitoring

- Blood glucose concentrations should be assessed immediately after initiating dextrose and periodically thereafter to maintain euglycemia.
- Hydration status
- Electrolytes

Client Information

- If clients are to administer this product to food animals, they should be advised on correct injection technique and the importance of using the product per the label only.
- Unused vial or bottle portions should be discarded and not be saved for reuse.

Chemistry/Synonyms

Each 1 mL contains 0.5 g dextrose (hydrous), which delivers 3.4 kcal/g. The injection may contain hydrochloric acid or sodium hydroxide for pH adjustment. Dextrose 50% has an osmolarity of 2.5 mOsmol/mL and a pH of 3.2 to 6.5. Dextrose is also known as D-glucose.

Storage/Stability

Avoid excessive heat. Protect from freezing. Storage requirements vary by manufacturer; products intended for use in cattle typically are stored at 15°C to 30°C (59°F-86°F). The solution does not contain a preservative and is intended for single use only. Do not use cloudy solutions. Discard any unused portion.

Compatibility/Compounding Considerations

Dextrose 50% is compatible with isotonic fluids such as 0.9% sodium chloride (saline), lactated Ringer's solution, *PlasmaLyte*®, and *Normosol*®.

Examples of how to add dextrose to crystalloid solutions:

- 2.5% dextrose in a crystalloid solution: remove 50 mL of crystalloid fluid from a 1000 mL bag then add 50 mL of 50% dextrose to the bag
- 5% dextrose solution in a crystalloid solution: remove 100 mL of crystalloid fluid from a 1000 mL bag then add 100 mL of 50% dextrose to the bag

Dextrose should not be simultaneously administered with blood through the same infusion set because there is a possibility of pseudoagglutination of red blood cells.

Dosage Forms/Regulatory Status

VETERINARY-LABELED PRODUCTS:

Dextrose 50% Solution: 500 mL bottle; generic, (OTC and Rx). Not an FDA approved product

HUMAN-LABELED PRODUCTS:

Dextrose 50% Solution: 50 mL syringes, 10 mL, 20 mL, and 50 mL vials, and 500 mL and 1000 mL bottles/bags; generic; (Rx). Some products may not be approved by the FDA.

References

For the complete list of references, see **wiley.com/go/budde/plumb**

Diazepam

(dye-**az**-e-pam) *Valium*®, *Diastat*®

Benzodiazepine

Prescriber Highlights

- ▶ Benzodiazepine used for a variety of indications (eg, anxiolytic, muscle relaxant, hypnotic, appetite stimulant, anticonvulsant, anesthetic adjunct, behavioral modifier) in several species
- ▶ In dogs, long-term use results in tolerance to anticonvulsant effects, making the drug less useful when treating status epilepticus.
- ▶ Contraindications include hypersensitivity to benzodiazepines, significant liver disease (especially in cats), and in cats exposed to chlorpyrifos. Oral use in cats should be avoided.
- ▶ Caution is advised with hepatic or renal disease; aggressive behavior; debilitated or geriatric patients; and patients in coma, in shock, or with significant respiratory depression. May be teratogenic. Withdraw slowly after long-term dosing
- ▶ Adverse effects of sedation and ataxia are most prevalent. Dogs: CNS excitement, increased appetite. Cats: Hepatic failure (with oral administration) or behavior changes. Horses: Muscle fasciculations, ataxia
- ▶ IV injections should be administered slowly to prevent hypotension. IM injections cause pain and result in unpredictable absorption.
- ▶ DEA schedule IV (C-IV) controlled substance
- ▶ Effects are reversible with flumazenil.

Uses/Indications

Diazepam is used clinically for its anxiolytic, muscle relaxant, hypnotic, appetite stimulant, and anticonvulsant effects. It is also used in preanesthetic and/or anesthetic induction protocols for neuroleptanesthesia and to decrease the amount of induction agents required to induce general anesthesia. Diazepam has been shown to significantly decrease the amount of anesthetic (ie, alfaxalone, propofol) required for endotracheal intubation.[1-3] Diazepam is commonly used with ketamine to prevent ketaminemediated excitement and muscle rigidity.

Benzodiazepines are drugs of choice for treating status epilepticus and cluster seizures in dogs. Although diazepam can be used, it is relatively short-acting, and midazolam may be preferred. In a study, intranasal midazolam appeared to control status epilepticus better than did rectal diazepam.[4] Long-term administration of benzodiazepines usually results in the animal developing a tolerance to the drug's anticonvulsant effects.[5] In addition, long-term use of this class of drugs in dogs may prevent effective use for emergency treatment of seizures. In cats, diazepam has a longer elimination half-life, and tolerance is not a major concern.

Pharmacology/Actions

Diazepam and other benzodiazepines depress CNS subcortical levels (primarily limbic, thalamic, and hypothalamic), thereby producing anxiolytic, sedative, skeletal muscle relaxation, and anticonvulsant effects. Diazepam binds to gamma-aminobutyric acid type A ($GABA_A$) receptors and increases the affinity of the receptor for GABA, a major CNS inhibitory neurotransmitter, which results in increased chloride conductance and hyperpolarization of the postsynaptic cell membrane. Other postulated mechanisms include antagonism of serotonin, increased release of GABA, and diminished release or turnover of acetylcholine in the CNS. Benzodiazepine-specific receptors have been located in the mammalian brain, kidney, liver, lung, and heart; receptors are lacking in the white matter of all species studied.

Pharmacokinetics

Diazepam is rapidly absorbed following oral administration. Peak plasma concentrations occur within 30 minutes to 2 hours after oral dosing. As compared with PO administration, diazepam is slowly and incompletely absorbed following IM administration. The rectal bioavailability of diazepam (parent drug) in dogs is less than 10%,[6] but bioavailability increases to 50% to 80% when considering diazepam plus its metabolites (eg, desmethyldiazepam, oxazepam).[6,7] Bioavailability is ≈80% when diazepam is administered intranasally to dogs.[8]

Diazepam is highly lipid-soluble and is widely distributed throughout the body. It readily crosses the blood–brain barrier and is highly bound to plasma proteins. In horses, 87% of the drug is bound to plasma proteins when the diazepam serum concentration was 75 ng/mL.[9] In humans, this value has been reported to be 98% to 99%.

Diazepam is metabolized in the liver to several metabolites, including desmethyldiazepam (nordiazepam), temazepam, and oxazepam, which are pharmacologically active. Diazepam metabolites are conjugated with glucuronide and eliminated primarily in urine in most species.[10] In horses, CYP3A is largely responsible for temazepam formation.[11] In 4-day-old foals, the diazepam half-life, clearance, and volume of distribution were significantly lower as compared with 21-day-old foals.[12] Because of the active metabolites, serum values of diazepam are not useful in predicting efficacy.

Serum Half-Lives (Approximated) for Diazepam and Metabolites in Dogs, Cats, and Horses

Metabolite	Dogs[10,13,14] (hours)	Cats[10] (hours)	Horses[15] (hours)	Humans (hours)
Diazepam	1-3.2	3.5-5.5	7-13	20-50
Nordiazepam	2-10	21.3	12	30-200
Temazepam	3	4.5	No data found	10-20
Oxazepam	3-6	No data found	18-28	3-21

Contraindications/Precautions/Warnings

Diazepam should not be used in patients that are hypersensitive to it or that have severe hepatic disease.[16] Fulminant hepatic failure has occurred in cats receiving oral diazepam,[17] and PO administration is best avoided in cats. Diazepam should be used cautiously, if at all, in aggressive patients and, if used, it should always be paired with another sedative drug (eg, alpha-2 agonist). Some clinicians believe that benzodiazepines are contraindicated in aggressive dogs, as anxiety may restrain the animal from aggressive tendencies; however, this remains controversial.[18] Diazepam may impair the performance of working animals.

Caution is advised when using in animals that have hepatic or renal disease, that are comatose or in shock, that have respiratory depression, or that are debilitated, obese, or geriatric. Although uncommon, cardiovascular or respiratory support may be necessary if diazepam is being administered IV.

Rapid injection of diazepam IV in small-sized animals or neonates may cause hypotension or cardiotoxicity secondary to propylene glycol in the formulation. Slow IV injection is recommended, particularly when using a small vein for access or in small-sized animals, because diazepam may cause significant phlebitis. Intracarotid artery injections must be avoided.

Other than in debilitated patients, diazepam used as a premedicant is unlikely to provide sedation and may cause paradoxical excitement, especially in young healthy patients. Thus, if used as a premedicant, diazepam should always be combined with an opioid or a true sedative. Diazepam is more commonly used during induction.

Long-term use of diazepam may induce physical dependence, and if the drug is to be discontinued, the dose must be gradually decreased (tapered) over several weeks.[19]

As compared with dosages for humans, diazepam dosages for dogs are very high; human pharmacists may be unaware that these are appropriate.

Using diazepam to control adverse effects related to toxicities should be approached with caution to avoid exacerbating clinical signs. It is recommended not to use diazepam for seizure control in cats exposed to chlorpyrifos because organophosphate toxicity may be potentiated.[16] Animals with toxicity from ingesting amphetamines or human sleep aids, such as zolpidem (*Ambien*®) or eszopiclone (*Lunesta*®), should not receive diazepam or other benzodiazepines to treat paradoxical CNS stimulation, as these drugs also increase GABA activity; IV phenothiazines (eg, acepromazine, chlorpromazine) or phenobarbital are recommended instead.

Do not confuse diazePAM with dilTIAZem or diaZOXide.

Adverse Effects

Rapid IV administration of diazepam can potentially cause hypotension; IV administration should be done slowly (5 mg/minute), and the IV catheter should be flushed with fluids after administration to help prevent phlebitis. IM injection may cause pain at the injection site.

Adverse effects reported in dogs include sedation, increased appetite, agitation, ataxia, and aggression. In addition, dogs may exhibit a contradictory response (eg, in ≈30% of dogs, CNS excitement was described as increased activity or agitation) following administration of diazepam; doses greater than or equal to 0.8 mg/kg are more likely to cause this effect.[20] Because sedation and tranquilization in dogs can be variable, diazepam may not be an ideal sedating agent, particularly when used alone. Diazepam used alone or in combination with ketamine increases intraocular pressure in dogs.[21,22]

Cats may exhibit changes in behavior (eg, irritability, depression, aberrant demeanor) after receiving diazepam. Anesthetic recovery from diazepam/ketamine was more active and unsettled as compared with alfaxalone as a sole agent.[23] There have been sporadic reports of cats developing idiosyncratic hepatic failure after receiving oral (but not injectable) diazepam (not dose-dependent) for several days.[17] Clinical signs (eg, anorexia, lethargy, increased ALT/AST, hyperbilirubinemia) occurred 5 to 11 days after beginning oral therapy, and 10 out of 11 patients died or were euthanized within 15 days. Slow biotransformation and inhibition of the efflux of bile, resulting in accumulation of bile acids in the hepatocytes, might contribute to the liver injury observed in cats that received repeated doses of oral diazepam.[10]

In horses, diazepam may cause muscle fasciculations, weakness, and ataxia at doses sufficient to cause sedation. Doses greater than 0.2 mg/kg may induce recumbency as a result of muscle relaxant properties and general CNS depressant effects. Diazepam is not recommended as a sole agent for sedation in this species.

Adverse effects can be reversed with flumazenil. See ***Flumazenil.***

Reproductive/Nursing Safety

In humans, diazepam has been implicated in causing congenital abnormalities when it is administered during the first trimester of pregnancy. Infants born to mothers who were given large doses of benzodiazepines shortly before delivery have been reported to suffer from apnea, impaired metabolic response to cold stress, difficulty in feeding, hyperbilirubinemia, and hypotonia. Withdrawal symptoms have occurred in infants whose mothers took benzodiazepines long-term during pregnancy. The veterinary significance of these effects is unclear, but these agents should only be used during the first trimester of pregnancy when the benefits clearly outweigh the risks associated with their use.

Benzodiazepines and their metabolites are distributed into milk and may cause CNS effects in nursing neonates. In humans, diazepam use is not recommended while breastfeeding.[24]

Because safety has not been established in animals, this drug should only be used when the maternal benefits outweigh the potential risks to offspring.

Overdose/Acute Toxicity

When diazepam is administered alone, overdose effects are generally limited to significant CNS depression (eg, confusion, coma, decreased reflexes). In rare circumstances, hypotension, respiratory depression, and cardiac arrest have been reported in human patients.

Treatment of acute toxicity consists of standard protocols for removing and/or binding the drug in the gut if diazepam is administered orally; provide supportive systemic therapies as needed. Use of analeptic agents (ie, CNS stimulants such as caffeine) is generally not recommended. Flumazenil may be considered for adjunctive treatment of benzodiazepine overdose.

Successful treatment of a cat with hepatic necrosis included the use of lactulose, metronidazole, vitamin K, N-acetylcysteine, and Sadenosylmethionine, along with supportive care.[25]

For patients that have experienced or are suspected of having experienced an overdose, consultation with a 24-hour poison consultation center specializing in providing veterinary-specific information is recommended. For general information related to overdose and toxin exposures, as well as contact information for poison control centers, refer to ***Appendix***.

Drug Interactions

The following drug interactions have either been reported or are theoretical in humans or animals receiving diazepam and may be of significance in veterinary patients. Unless otherwise noted, use together is not necessarily contraindicated, but weigh the potential risks and perform additional monitoring when appropriate.

- **Amiodarone**: Concurrent use may increase the bioavailability and pharmacologic effects of benzodiazepines; monitoring and adjustment of benzodiazepine dose are needed.
- **Antacids, Aluminum-, Calcium- and Magnesium-Containing**: May slow the rate, but not the extent, of oral absorption; administration 2 hours apart may avoid this potential interaction.
- **Antidepressants** (eg, **amitriptyline**, **clomipramine**, **mirtazapine**): Concurrent use increases the risk for CNS and/or respiratory depression.
- **Antihypertensive Agents** (eg, **amlodipine**, **atenolol**, **enalapril**): Concurrent use may increase the risk for hypotension and orthostasis. Blood pressure monitoring is necessary.
- **Azole Antifungals** (eg, **itraconazole, ketoconazole**[11]): Metabolism of diazepam may be decreased, and excessive sedation may occur.
- **Carbonic Anhydrase Inhibitors** (eg, **acetazolamide, methazolamide**): Benzodiazepines may interfere with the beneficial effects of carbonic anhydrase inhibitors by inhibiting respiratory responses to hypoxia; this combination should be avoided.
- **CNS Depressant Agents** (eg, **barbiturates, opioids, anesthetics**): Combination may increase the risk for CNS and/or respiratory depression; monitoring and adjustment of dosages are needed.
- **Digoxin**: Serum levels may be increased; monitoring of serum digoxin levels and clinical signs of toxicity is needed.
- **Fluoxetine, Fluvoxamine**: Increased benzodiazepine levels are possible.
- **Hepatic Enzyme Inducers** (eg, **glucocorticoids, mitotane, rifampin, phenobarbital**[26]): Concurrent use may decrease benzodiazepine levels; monitoring of clinical response and adjustment of doses are necessary.
- **Hepatic Enzyme Inhibitors** (eg, **cimetidine, isoniazid**): Metabolism of diazepam may be decreased, and excessive sedation may occur.
- **Ifosfamide**: Concurrent use may increase the risk for ifosfamide-induced neurotoxic effects. Careful monitoring is needed, and discontinuation of both drugs may be necessary if signs of encephalopathy occur.
- **Macrolide Antibiotics** (eg, **clarithromycin, erythromycin**): Metabolism of diazepam may be decreased, and excessive sedation may occur.
- **Macrocyclic Lactones** (eg, **ivermectin, milbemycin oxime**): Benzodiazepine effects may be potentiated by concurrent macrocyclic lactone use.
- **Melatonin**: Increased risk for CNS depression and prolonged diazepam effects
- **Non-Depolarizing Neuromuscular Blockers** (eg, **atracurium, pancuronium**): Concurrent use may potentiate, attenuate, or have no effect; monitoring of respiratory status is necessary.
- **Propranolol**: May slow diazepam metabolism
- **Theophylline, Aminophylline**: Concurrent use may decrease the concentrations and effectiveness of benzodiazepines. Withdrawing theophylline from a stable patient may increase the risk for benzodiazepine toxicity; monitoring for adverse effects is needed, and dosages must be adjusted accordingly.
- **Yohimbine**: Limited data indicate that yohimbine may decrease the therapeutic effects of anxiolytic drugs.

Laboratory Considerations

- Patients receiving diazepam may show false-negative **urine glucose** results if *Diastix*® or *Clinistix*® tests are used.
- Secondary to propylene glycol in IV diazepam, patients may show a false-positive **ethylene glycol** test.
- Benzodiazepines may decrease the thyroidal uptake of $\mathbf{I^{123}}$ or $\mathbf{I^{131}}$.

Dosages

DOGS:

Cluster seizures or status epilepticus (extra-label):

Rectal: Using diazepam parenteral solution, diazepam 0.5 – 2 mg/kg rectally[27,28]; if the patient is receiving phenobarbital, diazepam 2 mg/kg rectally can be used.[26] Administer at the onset of a seizure and up to 3 times in a 24-hour period.[28] If the client is administering, they should stay with the dog for 1 hour after administration. Because diazepam is inactivated by light and adheres to plastic, it is best to dispense the drug in the original glass vial and instruct the client to draw the required amount into a syringe when needed. A rubber catheter or teat cannula is then placed on the syringe for rectal administration. A study found that compounded 2 mg rectal suppositories did not achieve plasma levels of diazepam/nordiazepam sufficient for emergency treatment of seizures in dogs.[14] **NOTE**: Intranasal midazolam appears superior to rectal diazepam for controlling status epilepticus.[4]

Intranasal: Based on a pharmacokinetic study, diazepam may also be given intranasally (at home or in the clinic) at 0.5 mg/kg. Dogs on chronic phenobarbital therapy may require higher doses (1 – 2 mg/kg).[29]

IV (bolus): Diazepam 0.5 – 1 mg/kg IV; may be repeated every 10 minutes up to 3 times[16]

IV (CRI): Diazepam 0.1 – 2 mg/kg/hour IV CRI. Caution is advised, as diazepam can crystallize in solution and adsorb to PVC tubing. (See ***Compatibility/Compounding Considerations*** and ***Storage/Stability***)

Functional urethral obstruction/urethral sphincter hypertonus (extra-label): Diazepam 2 – 10 mg/dog (NOT mg/kg) PO every 8 hours[30]

Short-term management of skeletal muscle spasms (extra-label): Diazepam 0.5 – 2 mg/kg IV[31]

Psychotherapeutic agent (extra-label):

a) **Situational anxiety**: Diazepam 0.5 – 2 mg/kg PO PRN; preferably 30 minutes to 1 hour in advance of the anticipated event.[32] **NOTE**: As compared with humans, diazepam dosages for dogs are very high; human pharmacists may be unaware that these are appropriate.
b) **In combination with fluoxetine and behavior modification therapy for anxiety-related disorders**: Diazepam 0.3 mg/kg PO once daily for 4 weeks; it should be initiated at the same time as fluoxetine 1 mg/kg PO once daily.[33]

Adjunctive treatment of metronidazole toxicity (extra-label): 0.43 mg/kg IV as an initial bolus, followed by 0.43 mg/kg PO every 8 hours for 3 days[34]

Strychnine poisoning (extra-label): Diazepam 1 mg/kg IV slowly, followed by 1 mg/kg IM[35]

Anesthetic premedication in combination with other sedatives (extra-label): Diazepam 0.1 – 0.5 mg/kg IV. Combination with opioids or alpha-2 agonists is highly recommended to decrease drug dosages, minimize paradoxical excitation, and achieve a more profound, predictable level of sedation and muscle relaxation.[36] A slightly higher dose of diazepam 0.2 – 0.6 mg/kg IV is approved for products available in other countries.[31,37] Diazepam is more commonly used as part of induction rather than as a premedicant.

In combination with an induction agent for anesthesia (extra-label): Diazepam 0.1 – 0.3 mg/kg IV. Can be combined with ketamine to counteract the muscle rigidity caused by ketamine and reduce the dose of ketamine. Diazepam is also used with propofol or alfaxalone to reduce the amount of these induction agents, which decreases dose-dependent cardiovascular and respiratory depression caused by many induction drugs.[38-42]

CATS:

NOTE: Because of concerns associated with oral diazepam and rare idiosyncratic hepatic failure in cats, oral use in cats is not recommended; safer alternatives are available.

Anesthetic premedication in combination with other sedatives (extra-label): Diazepam 0.1 – 0.3 mg/kg IV. Combination with opioids or alpha-2 agonists is highly recommended to decrease drug dosages, minimize paradoxical excitation, and achieve a more profound, predictable level of sedation and muscle relaxation. A slightly higher dose of diazepam (0.2 – 0.6 mg/kg IV) is approved in a UK product.[16,31] Diazepam 0.5 mg/cat (NOT mg/kg) in combination with ketamine 10 mg/cat (NOT mg/kg) given IV was deemed effective and safe to assist physical restraint for blood sampling.[43] Diazepam is more commonly used as part of induction rather than as a premedicant.

In combination with an induction agent for anesthesia (extra-label): Diazepam 0.1 – 0.3 mg/kg IV. Can be combined with ketamine to counteract the muscle rigidity caused by ketamine and reduce the dose of ketamine. Diazepam is also used with propofol or alfaxalone to reduce the amount of these induction agents, which decreases dose-dependent cardiovascular and respiratory depression caused by many induction drugs.[38-42]

EQUINE:

Anticonvulsant in foals (extra-label): 0.1 – 0.4 mg/kg slow IV and repeated as necessary[17]

Field anesthesia (extra-label):

a) The following protocol was used for field castration in ponies with good results: After premedication with detomidine 20 µg/kg IV and phenylbutazone 4.4 mg/kg IV, anesthesia was induced with diazepam 0.06 mg/kg combined with ketamine 2.2 mg/kg IV. Midazolam can be substituted for diazepam at the same dosage.[44]
b) Preanesthetic: Diazepam 0.13 mg/kg IM 20 minutes prior to xylazine and ketamine[37]
c) Total IV anesthesia in mules: Following sedation with xylazine 1.3 mg/kg IV, induce anesthesia with diazepam 0.03 mg/kg and ketamine 2.2 mg/kg IV, lateral recumbency and normal gait occurred at 1.8 and 32.8 minutes, respectively; duration of anesthesia was 15.3 minutes.[45]
d) Tranquilization in donkeys: Diazepam 0.1 mg/kg with acepromazine 0.1 mg/kg IV decreased the latency period and enhanced tranquilization compared with acepromazine alone.[46]

SHEEP/GOATS:

Sedation/tranquilization (extra-label): Diazepam 0.2 – 0.5 mg/kg IV or 0.5 – 1 mg/kg IM.[47] Lower doses (ie, 0.1 – 0.2 mg/kg IV) of diazepam have also been recommended.[48,49]

Anesthesia (extra-label):

a) Diazepam 0.15 – 0.5 mg/kg IV in combination with ketamine 5 – 10 mg/kg IV is one of the most common anesthetic protocols.[47,50-54]
b) Diazepam 0.4 mg/kg IM in combination with ketamine 22 mg/kg IM[55]; however, this combination provided longer time to onset and inadequate anesthetic depth during the most painful portion of the surgery when compared to IM ketamine combined with xylazine.

NEW WORLD CAMELIDS:

Field anesthesia in alpacas (extra-label): Diazepam 0.2 mg/kg with ketamine 4 mg/kg IV[56]

BIRDS:

Adjunctive therapy of pain control (with analgesics); (extra-label): Diazepam 0.5 – 2 mg/kg IV or IM[57]

Sedation/induction (extra-label):

a) Diazepam 0.5 – 2 mg/kg IV or IM. Dosage applies to small pet birds and medium-sized parrots. Adjustments need to be made for large-sized parrots or wild species, such as raptors.[58]
b) Diazepam 0.5 mg/kg IM with ketamine 10 mg/kg IM as premedication reduced induction time and sevoflurane requirements in parrots.[59]
c) Intranasal sedation with diazepam 13.6 mg/kg produced adequate sedation in budgerigars; midazolam had a faster onset (1.3 vs 2.8 minutes, respectively) but shorter duration (71 vs 165 minutes).[60]

FERRETS:

Premedication/sedation (extra-label):

Diazepam 0.5 mg/kg IM or IV (IV preferred)

Diazepam 0.2 mg/kg (IV assumed) if using in combination with ketamine 2 – 5 mg/kg[58]

RABBITS/RODENTS/SMALL MAMMALS (extra-label):

Rabbits: *Sedation*: Diazepam 0.5 – 2 mg/kg IV, IM, or intranasally[61,62] (IV preferred; intranasal may cause tissue irritation – midazolam is preferred for this route). *Anesthesia:* Diazepam 0.5 – 1 mg/kg in combination with ketamine 20 – 35 mg/kg IM or IV[58]

Hedgehogs: *Long anesthesia:* Diazepam 0.5 – 2 mg/kg in combination with ketamine 5 – 20 mg/kg IM[58]

Hamsters, gerbils, mice, rats: Diazepam 3 – 5 mg/kg IM

Guinea pigs: Diazepam 0.5 – 3 mg/kg IM[63]

Monitoring

- CNS: signs of sedation or paradoxical excitement
- Cardiovascular system: blood pressure—can cause hypotension if administered rapidly IV

- Respiratory system: respiratory rate, $ETCO_2$, and SpO_2—mild respiratory depression can occur, with a more moderate impact if other respiratory depressants (eg, opioids) are administered.
- Horses should be observed carefully for ataxia.
- Clinical response to treatment

Client Information

- This medicine may cause sedation and/or disorientation, which may impair the performance of working animals.
- When using this medicine for thunderstorm phobias or other triggers (eg, separation anxiety), give the medicine to your animal about an hour before the event or trigger.
- This medicine may be given with or without food. If your animal vomits or acts sick after receiving the medication on an empty stomach, give the medicine with food or small treats. Contact your veterinarian if vomiting continues.
- Contact your veterinarian immediately if your animal develops yellowing of the skin, gums, or whites of the eyes (*jaundice*).
- Sleepiness is the most common side effect. This medicine can change your animal's behavior (eg, hyperactivity, anxiety) in unexpected ways.
- This medicine may increase your animal's appetite, especially in cats.
- Contact your veterinarian immediately if your animal stops eating or seems depressed.

Chemistry/Synonyms

Diazepam, a benzodiazepine, is a white-to-yellow, practically odorless, crystalline powder with a melting point between 131°C (267.8°F) and 135°C (275°F) and pK_a of 3.4. Diazepam is tasteless initially but develops a bitter aftertaste. One gram of diazepam is soluble in 333 mL of water or 25 mL of alcohol and is sparingly soluble in propylene glycol. The pH of the commercially prepared injectable solution is 6.2 to 6.9. It consists of a 5 mg/mL solution with 40% propylene glycol, 10% ethanol, 5% sodium benzoate/benzoic acid buffer, and 1.5% benzyl alcohol as a preservative.

Diazepam may also be known as diazepamum, LA-III, NSC-77518, or Ro-5-2807; many trade names are available.

Storage/Stability

Store all diazepam products at room temperature (15°C to 30°C [59°F-86°F]). Keep the injection from freezing temperatures and protect from light. Store the oral forms (eg, tablets, capsules) in tightly closed containers and protect them from light.

Because diazepam may adsorb to plastic, it should not be stored in plastic syringes but can be drawn up in syringes if intended to be administered within 4 hours. The drug may also significantly adsorb to IV solution plastic (eg, PVC) bags and infusion tubing. This adsorption appears to be dependent on several factors (eg, temperature, drug concentration, flow rates, line length).

Consider the following to minimize the adsorption of diazepam. Use glass or polyolefin containers; if you use PVC bags, select the lowest possible surface:volume ratio and minimize the storage time. The use of non-PVC administration sets will reduce loss. If you use PVC tubing, it should be the shortest possible length with a small diameter, and the set should not contain a burette chamber. More rapid flow rates (consistent with safe clinical use) will also reduce the loss of diazepam.[64]

Compatibility/Compounding Considerations

Compatibility is dependent on factors such as pH, concentration, temperature, and diluent used; specialized references or a hospital pharmacist should be consulted for more specific information.

The manufacturers of injectable diazepam do not recommend the drug be mixed with any other medication or IV diluent, and diluting for infusion cannot be recommended. Although some studies have shown that dilution in some IV solutions at low concentrations may not exhibit visible precipitates, microcrystal formation could not be ruled out. Because there is continued interest in IV infusions of diazepam, some studies indicate that diazepam injection may be **compatible** with various drugs and IV fluids (eg, diluted to a concentration of 5 mg/50 mL to 5 mg/100 mL with 0.9% sodium chloride, 5% dextrose, Ringer's, or lactated Ringer's injection).

Mixing ketamine with diazepam in the same syringe or IV bag has been suggested but is not recommended, as precipitation may occur. Although there are many anecdotal reports of mixing ketamine with diazepam in the same syringe just prior to injection, there does not appear to be any published information documenting the stability of the drugs after mixing. Use should be avoided if a visible precipitate forms.

Dosage Forms/Regulatory Status

VETERINARY-LABELED PRODUCTS: NONE IN THE UNITED STATES

The Association of Racing Commissioners International (ARCI) has designated this drug as a class 2 substance. Use of this drug may not be allowed in certain animal competitions. Check rules and regulations before entering a competition while this medication is being administered. Contact local racing authorities for further guidance. See ***Appendix*** for more information.

The International Federation for Equestrian Sports (FEI) lists this drug as a *prohibited substance–controlled substance.*

HUMAN-LABELED PRODUCTS:

Diazepam Injection: 5 mg/mL in 2 mL *Carpuject®* cartridges; generic; (Rx, C-IV)

Diazepam Oral Tablets: 2 mg, 5 mg, and 10 mg; *Valium®*, generic; (Rx, C-IV)

Diazepam Oral Solution: 1 mg/mL in 500 mL, and 5 mg and 10 mg patient cups; generic; (Rx, C-IV); Concentrated oral solution: 5 mg/mL in 30 mL with dropper; *Diazepam Intensol®*; (Rx, C-IV)

Diazepam Rectal Gel: 2.5 mg, 10 mg, and 20 mg; *Diastat®*, generic; (Rx, C-IV)

References

For the complete list of references, see **wiley.com/go/budde/plumb**

Diazoxide

(di-az-***ok***-side) *Proglycem®*

Direct Vasodilator/Hyperglycemic

Prescriber Highlights

- Orally administered drug used in the management of insulinomas in small animal species
- Contraindications include functional hypoglycemia or hypoglycemia secondary to insulin overdose (diabetics) and hypersensitivity to thiazide diuretics.
- Use with caution in patients with congestive heart failure or renal insufficiency
- Most common adverse effects include anorexia, vomiting, and/or diarrhea (may be reduced by giving with food).
- Availability and expense may be problematic. May need to be compounded
- Bitter taste may make administration difficult.

Uses/Indications

Oral diazoxide has been used for the treatment of hypoglycemia secondary to hyperinsulin secretion (eg, insulinoma) in patients refractory to glucocorticoid and dietary therapy.

Pharmacology/Actions

Although related structurally to the thiazide diuretics, diazoxide does not possess any appreciable diuretic activity. By directly causing a vasodilatory effect on the smooth muscle in peripheral arterioles, diazoxide reduces peripheral resistance and blood pressure.

Diazoxide exhibits hyperglycemic activity by directly inhibiting pancreatic insulin secretion, stimulating hepatic gluconeogenesis and glycogenolysis, and stimulating the beta-adrenergic system to cause epinephrine release and inhibit tissue use of glucose. Diazoxide's inhibition of insulin release may be a result of the drug's ability to decrease the intracellular release of ionized calcium, thus preventing release of insulin from beta cell insulin granules. Diazoxide does not apparently affect the synthesis of insulin, nor does it possess any antineoplastic activity.

Pharmacokinetics

The serum half-life of diazoxide has been reported to be ≈5 hours in dogs; other pharmacokinetic parameters in dogs appear to be unavailable. In humans, serum diazoxide levels (dosed at 10 mg/kg PO) peaked at ≈12 hours after dosing with capsules. It is unknown what blood levels are required to obtain hyperglycemic effects. Highest concentrations of diazoxide are found in the kidneys with high levels also found in the liver and adrenal glands. Approximately 90% of the drug is bound to plasma proteins and it crosses the placenta and into the CNS. It is not known if diazoxide is distributed into milk. Diazoxide is partially metabolized in the liver and is excreted as both metabolites and unchanged drug by the kidneys. Serum half-life of the drug is prolonged in patients with renal impairment.

Contraindications/Precautions/Warnings

Diazoxide should not be used in patients with functional hypoglycemia or for treating hypoglycemia secondary to insulin overdose in diabetic patients. Unless the potential advantages outweigh the risks, do not use in patients hypersensitive to thiazide diuretics.

Because diazoxide can cause sodium and water retention, use cautiously, and consider dose reductions in patients with congestive heart failure or renal insufficiency.

Do not confuse diaZOXide with DIAZepam or diltiazem.

Adverse Effects

When used to treat insulinomas in dogs, the most common adverse effects include hypersalivation, anorexia, vomiting, and/or diarrhea. Other effects that may be seen include tachycardia, hematologic abnormalities (eg, agranulocytosis, aplastic anemia, thrombocytopenia), pancreatitis, diabetes mellitus, cataracts, and sodium and water retention.

Administering the drug with meals or temporarily reducing the dosage may alleviate the GI side effects. Because diazoxide is metabolized in the liver, adverse effects may be more readily noted in dogs with concurrent hepatic disease.

Adverse effects reported in ferrets include inappetence, vomiting, diarrhea, malaise, and myelosuppression.

Reproductive/Nursing Safety

Diazoxide crosses the placenta.[1] Fetal islet cell degeneration has been demonstrated in animals. In addition, fetal resorption has been observed in rats, and fetal skeletal and cardiac malformations or teratogenicity have been observed in rabbits. Diazoxide may cause cessation of uterine contractions when administered during labor.

It is unknown if diazoxide enters milk.

Because safety has not been established in animals, this drug should only be used when the maternal benefits outweigh the potential risks to offspring.

Overdose/Acute Toxicity

Oral doses of up to 500 mg/kg have been tolerated in dogs.[1] The oral LD_{50} is over 5000 mg/kg in rats and 219 mg/kg in guinea pigs. An acute overdose may result in severe hyperglycemia and ketoacidosis. Treatment should include insulin (see specific ***Insulin*** monographs), fluids, and electrolytes. Intensive and prolonged monitoring is recommended.

For patients that have experienced or are suspected to have experienced an overdose, consultation with a 24-hour poison consultation center specializing in providing veterinary-specific information is recommended. For general information related to overdose and toxin exposures, as well as contact information for poison control centers, refer to ***Appendix.***

Drug Interactions

The following drug interactions have either been reported or are theoretical in humans or animals receiving diazoxide and may be of significance in veterinary patients. Unless otherwise noted, use together is not necessarily contraindicated, but weigh the potential risks and perform additional monitoring when appropriate.

- **Alpha-Adrenergic Agents** (eg, **phenoxybenzamine**): May decrease the effectiveness of diazoxide by increasing glucose levels
- **Glucocorticoids** (eg, **dexamethasone, prednis(ol)one**): If used in combination with diazoxide, may enhance hyperglycemic effects
- **Hypotensive Agents, Other** (eg, **amlodipine, hydralazine, prazosin, telmisartan**): Diazoxide may enhance the hypotensive actions of other hypotensive agents.
- **Phenothiazines** (eg, **acepromazine, chlorpromazine**): May enhance the hyperglycemic effects of diazoxide
- **Thiazide diuretics**: May potentiate the hyperglycemic effects of oral diazoxide.[1] Some clinicians have recommended using hydrochlorothiazide in combination with diazoxide, if diazoxide alone is ineffective to increase blood glucose levels. Caution: hypotension may occur.

Laboratory Considerations

- Diazoxide will cause a false negative insulin response to the **glucagon-stimulation** test.
- Diazoxide may displace **bilirubin** from plasma proteins.

Dosages

DOGS:

Adjunctive treatment of hypoglycemia secondary to insulin-secreting islet cell or non-islet cell tumors (extra-label): Initially 5 mg/kg PO twice daily.[2] May gradually increase to effect up to a maximum dosage of 30 mg/kg PO twice daily. If diazoxide alone is ineffective, may consider using hydrochlorothiazide (1 – 2 mg/kg PO every 12 hours) in combination with diazoxide.

FERRETS:

Hypoglycemia secondary to insulin-secreting islet cell tumors (extra-label): After surgical resection of pancreatic nodules or partial pancreatectomy: Prednisone 0.5 – 2 mg/kg PO every 12 hours will usually control mild to moderate clinical signs. Begin at lowest dose and gradually increase as needed. Add diazoxide when clinical signs cannot be controlled with prednisone alone. Begin diazoxide 5 – 10 mg/kg PO every 12 hours. Prednisone dosage may need to be lowered at the same time. If the initial dosage does not control clinical signs, the dosage can be gradually increased to a maximum of 30 mg/kg PO every 12 hours.

SMALL MAMMALS:

Guinea pigs; Hypoglycemia secondary to insulin-secreting islet cell tumors (extra-label): Based on a single case report: Initially, 5 mg/kg PO every 12 hours. Based on the blood glucose curve, dosage was gradually increased to 25 mg/kg PO every 12 hours.

Monitoring

- Blood (serum) glucose. The goal of therapy is to identify a dosage that reduces or eliminates hypoglycemia and its associated clinical signs. The ideal dosage would also avoid hyperglycemia (glucose greater than 180 mg/dL). The dosage should be adjusted, starting with lower dosages and titrating upwards, until the lowest dosage is found to produce the desired clinical and laboratory results.

- Baseline and periodic (at least every 3 to 4 months) CBC
- Physical examination (monitor for adverse effects)

Client Information

- This medicine is used to increase blood sugar levels.
- Give this medicine with food to decrease the gastrointestinal side effects (drooling, vomiting, diarrhea, loss of appetite).
- If you have difficulty getting your animal to take the medicine, contact your veterinarian or pharmacist for tips to help with dosing and reducing the stress of medication time. Diazoxide has a bitter taste and taste-masking agents (preferably sugar-free) may be useful in increasing acceptance of this medication.
- Shake suspensions well.
- Watch for signs of high blood sugar (*hyperglycemia*) such as drinking more than normal, needing to urinate more, increased appetite, lack of energy, muscle weakness, depression, or severe vomiting. These signs may indicate the dose of the medicine may need to be adjusted.
- Contact your veterinarian if you notice your animal has signs of low blood sugar (*hypoglycemia*) such as seizures, muscle weakness, collapse, muscle twitching, low energy level/depression, or unsteadiness. These signs may indicate the dose of the medicine may need to be adjusted.

Chemistry/Synonyms

Related structurally to the thiazide diuretics, diazoxide occurs as an odorless white to creamy-white crystalline powder with a melting point of ≈165°C (330°F). It is practically insoluble to sparingly soluble in water and slightly soluble in alcohol.

Diazoxide may also be known as diazoxidum, NSC-64198, Sch-6783, SRG-95213, *Eudemine®*, *Glicemin®*, *Hypertonalum®*, *Hyperstat IV®*, *Proglycem®*, *Proglicem®*, *Sefulken®*, or *Tensuril®*.

Storage/Stability

Diazoxide capsules and oral suspensions should be stored protected from light at 25°C (77°F), with excursions permitted from 15°C to 30°C (59°F-86°F).[1] Protect solutions and suspensions from freezing. Do not use darkened solutions/suspensions, as they may be subpotent.

Compatibility/Compounding Considerations

Diazoxide has a very bitter taste and taste-masking agents (preferably sugar-free) may be useful in increasing patient acceptance of this medication.

Dosage Forms/Regulatory Status

VETERINARY-LABELED PRODUCTS: NONE.

The Association of Racing Commissioners International (ARCI) has designated this drug as a class 3 substance. Use of this drug may not be allowed in certain animal competitions. Check rules and regulations before entering in a competition while this medication is being administered. Contact local racing authorities for further guidance. See the ***Appendix*** for more information.

HUMAN-LABELED PRODUCTS:

Diazoxide Oral Suspension: 50 mg/mL with sorbitol in 30 mL calibrated dropper; *Proglycem®*; (Rx). Available in chocolate-mint flavor.

References

For the complete list of references, see **wiley.com/go/budde/plumb**

Dichlorphenamide

(dye-klor-***fen***-a-mide) *Keveyis®*

Carbonic Anhydrase Inhibitor

Prescriber Highlights

- ► Oral agent used primarily for open-angle glaucoma when topical carbonic anhydrase inhibitors cannot be used
- ► Contraindicated in patients with significant hepatic, renal, pulmonary, or adrenocortical insufficiency; hyponatremia; hypokalemia; hyperchloremic acidosis; or electrolyte imbalance
- ► Adverse effects include panting, GI disturbances, alteration of CNS state, and rashes.
- ► Give oral doses with food if GI upset occurs.
- ► Monitor for glaucoma with tonometry; check electrolytes
- ► Limited product availability; may need to be obtained from a compounding pharmacy

Uses/Indications

Dichlorphenamide is used for the medical treatment of glaucoma. Because of availability issues and toxic effects associated with systemic therapy, topical carbonic anhydrase inhibitors (eg, dorzolamide, brinzolamide) are preferred over those administered orally.

Pharmacology/Actions

The carbonic anhydrase inhibitors act by a noncompetitive, reversible inhibition of the enzyme carbonic anhydrase. This reduces the formation of hydrogen and bicarbonate ions from carbon dioxide and reduces the availability of these ions for active transport into body secretions.

Pharmacologic effects of the carbonic anhydrase inhibitors include decreased formation of aqueous humor and thus reduced intraocular pressure; increased renal tubular secretion of sodium and potassium and, to a greater extent, bicarbonate, leading to increased urine alkalinity and volume; and anticonvulsant activity, which is independent of its diuretic effects (mechanism not fully understood, but may be due to carbonic anhydrase or a metabolic acidosis effect).

Pharmacokinetics

The pharmacokinetics of this agent have apparently not been studied in domestic animals. In small animal species, onset of action is 30 minutes, maximal effect occurs in 2 to 4 hours, and duration of action is 8 to 12 hours.

Contraindications/Precautions/Warnings

Carbonic anhydrase inhibitors are contraindicated in patients with significant hepatic disease (may precipitate hepatic coma), renal or adrenocortical insufficiency, hyponatremia, hypokalemia, hyperchloremic acidosis, or electrolyte imbalance. They should not be used in patients with severe pulmonary obstruction that are unable to increase alveolar ventilation or those that are hypersensitive to them.

Adverse Effects

Adverse effects that may be encountered include panting, GI disturbances (eg, inappetence, vomiting, diarrhea), CNS effects (eg, sedation, depression, excitement), hematologic effects (eg, myelosuppression), renal effects (eg, crystalluria, dysuria, renal colic, polyuria), metabolic acidosis, hypokalemia, hyperglycemia, hyponatremia, hyperuricemia, hepatic insufficiency, dermatologic effects (rash), and hypersensitivity reactions.

Reproductive/Nursing Safety

Teratogenicity has been demonstrated in rats given dichlorphenamide at 17 times the maximum recommended human dose.[1] It is unknown if dichlorphenamide enters into milk. Because safety has not been established in animals, this drug should only be used when the maternal benefits outweigh the potential risks to offspring.

Overdose/Acute Toxicity

Information regarding overdose of this drug is not readily available. It is suggested to monitor serum electrolytes, blood gases, volume status, and CNS status during an acute overdose. Treat clinical signs supportively.

For patients that have experienced or are suspected to have experienced an overdose, consultation with a 24-hour poison consultation center specializing in providing veterinary-specific information is recommended. For general information related to overdose and toxin exposures, as well as contact information for poison control centers, refer to ***Appendix.***

Drug Interactions

The following drug interactions have either been reported or are theoretical in humans or animals receiving dichlorphenamide and may be of significance in veterinary patients. Unless otherwise noted, use together is not necessarily contraindicated, but weigh the potential risks and perform additional monitoring when appropriate.

- **Amantadine**: Increased amantadine concentrations may occur.
- **Antidepressants, Tricyclic**: Alkaline urine caused by dichlorphenamide may decrease excretion.
- **Aspirin** (or other **salicylates**): Increased risk for dichlorphenamide accumulation and toxicity; increased risk for metabolic acidosis; dichlorphenamide may result in elevated salicylate levels. This combination is contraindicated in human patients.
- **Digoxin**: Increased risk for toxicity, as dichlorphenamide may cause hypokalemia
- **Famotidine**: Increased famotidine exposure may occur.
- **Insulin**: Rarely, carbonic anhydrase inhibitors interfere with the hypoglycemic effects of insulin.
- **Methenamine Compounds**: Dichlorphenamide may negate antiseptic effects in the urine.
- **Methotrexate**: May increase methotrexate exposure and risk for methotrexate toxicity. Avoid combination if possible.
- **Mexiletine**: Dichlorphenamide may reduce mexiletine excretion and increase risk for mexiletine toxicity.
- **Potassium, Drugs Affecting** (eg, **amphotericin B, corticosteroids, corticotropin,** or other **diuretics**): Concomitant use may exacerbate potassium depletion.
- **Phenobarbital**: Dichlorphenamide increases urinary excretion of phenobarbital and may reduce phenobarbital levels.
- **Primidone**: Decreased primidone concentrations
- **Quinidine**: Alkaline urine caused by dichlorphenamide may decrease excretion.

Laboratory Considerations

- By alkalinizing the urine, carbonic anhydrase inhibitors may cause false positive results in determining **urine protein** using bromophenol blue reagent (*Albustix*®, *Albutest*®, *Labstix*®), sulfosalicylic acid (*Bumintest*®, Exton's Test Reagent), nitric acid ring test, or heat and acetic acid test methods.
- Carbonic anhydrase inhibitors may decrease **iodine uptake** by the thyroid gland in hyperthyroid or euthyroid patients.

Dosages

DOGS:

Adjunctive glaucoma treatment (extra-label): 2 – 5 mg/kg PO every 8 to 12 hours[2-4]

CATS:

Adjunctive glaucoma treatment (extra-label): 0.5 – 2 mg/kg PO every 8 to 12 hours[3,5]

Monitoring

- Intraocular pressure measurement (ie, tonometry)
- Baseline and periodic serum electrolytes and acid-base status
- Baseline and periodic CBC with differential when used long term
- Adverse effects (eg, GI signs, rash, panting, altered CNS status)

Client Information

- Give this medicine as directed by your veterinarian. If your animal vomits or acts sick after receiving the medicine on an empty stomach, try giving the next dose with food or a small treat. If vomiting continues, contact your veterinarian.
- Notify your veterinarian if you notice abnormal bleeding or bruising, vomiting, diarrhea, abnormal behavior, tremors, or a rash.

Chemistry/Synonyms

A carbonic anhydrase inhibitor, dichlorphenamide occurs as a white or nearly white crystalline powder with a melting range of 235-240°C, and pK_as of 7.4 and 8.6. It is very slightly soluble in water and soluble in alcohol.

Dichlorphenamide may also be known as diclofenamidum, *Antidrasi*®, *Daranide*®, *Fenamide*®, *Glaucol*®, *Glauconide*®, *Glaumid*®, *Keveyis*®, *Oralcon*®, *Oratrol*®, or *Tensodilen*®.

Storage/Stability

Store tablets in well-closed containers and at room temperature (20°C-25°C [68°F-77° F]).

Compatibility/Compounding Considerations

No specific information was noted.

Dosage Forms/Regulatory Status

VETERINARY-LABELED PRODUCTS: NONE

HUMAN-LABELED PRODUCTS:

Oral Tablet: 50 mg; *Keveyis*®; (Rx)

References

For the complete list of references, see **wiley.com/go/budde/plumb**

Diclazuril

(dye-***klaz***-yoor-il) *Protazil*®, *Clinacox*®

Antiprotozoal

Prescriber Highlights

- ► FDA-approved for equine protozoal myeloencephalitis (EPM) in horses and as a coccidiostat in broiler chickens and growing turkeys
- ► Appears to be well tolerated

Uses/Indications

In the United States, diclazuril is FDA-approved for the treatment of equine protozoal myeloencephalitis (EPM) caused by *Sarcocystis neurona*[1] and as a coccidiostat in broiler chickens and growing turkeys.[2] Diclazuril prevents *S neurona* infection in foals that live in high exposure areas.[3]

In the United Kingdom, oral diclazuril suspension is approved for the treatment and prevention of coccidial infections in lambs, caused in particular by the more pathogenic *Eimeria* spp, *Eimeria crandallis,* and *Eimeria ovinoidalis,* and in calves as an aid in the control of coccidiosis caused by *Eimeria bovis* and *Eimeria zuernii.* Studies comparing diclazuril and toltrazuril have shown that both are effective in reducing oocyte shedding in calves, whereas toltrazuril appears to be more effective than diclazuril in lambs.[4-7]

Diclazuril could potentially be useful in treating coccidiosis, *Neospora caninum,* and *Toxoplasma* spp infections in dogs or cats.

Pharmacology/Actions

The triazine class of antiprotozoals is believed to target the plastid body, an organelle found in the members of the Apicomplexa phylum, including *Sarcocystis neurona*. The actual mechanism of action is not well described. In vitro levels required to inhibit (95%) *S neurona* are about 1 ng/mL.[1]

Pharmacokinetics

In horses, oral bioavailability is about 5%. CSF concentrations are ≈5% of those found in plasma. Elimination half-life is prolonged (43 to 65 hours).[1] Doses of 1 mg/kg/day should give mean steady-state plasma concentrations of about 2 – 2.5 mg/mL, with corresponding CSF concentrations of 20 – 70 ng/mL, which is in excess of the in vitro IC_{95} (1 ng/mL).[8] A dosage of 0.5 mg/kg/day given to adult horses resulted in CSF concentrations of 26 ng/mL, compared with 25 ng/mL in horses that received 1 mg/kg/day.[9]

Contraindications/Precautions/Warnings

Diclazuril is contraindicated in patients that are known to be hypersensitive to it.

Do not feed diclazuril to breeding turkeys or to birds that produce eggs for human consumption.[2]

Adverse Effects

Diclazuril appears to be well tolerated in horses. In field trials, no adverse effects could be ascribed to the drug.[1,8]

On rare occasions, highly susceptible lambs may develop severe diarrhea (scour) after dosing; fluid therapy is required, and antibiotics may be necessary.

Reproductive/Nursing Safety

The manufacturer states that the safe use of diclazuril in horses used for breeding purposes, during pregnancy, or in lactation has not been evaluated.[1] Because safety has not been established in animals, this drug should only be used when the maternal benefits outweigh the potential risks to the offspring.

Overdose/Acute Toxicity

Limited information is available, but diclazuril appears to have a large safety margin in animals. Normal horses dosed up to 50 mg/kg/day (50 times the label dosage) for 42 days developed only marginal adverse effects (decreased grain intake, decreased weight gain, increases in creatinine and BUN).[1] Single doses of up to 60 times the label dosage in lambs and calves did not cause any demonstrable adverse effects.[10]

For patients that have experienced or are suspected to have experienced an overdose, consultation with a 24-hour poison consultation center specializing in providing veterinary-specific information is recommended. For general information related to overdose and toxin exposures, as well as contact information for poison control centers, refer to ***Appendix.***

Drug Interactions

- None were noted. The safety of diclazuril with concomitant therapies in horses has not been evaluated.[1]

Laboratory Considerations

- None were noted.

Dosages

DOGS/CATS

***Cystoisospora* spp (Coccidiosis) infection** (extra-label):

a) 25 mg/kg PO once[11,12]

b) Kittens: 1 mL (2.5 mg) of the sheep solution per 4 kg (8.8 lb) PO[13]

c) 2.5 – 5 mg/kg PO once, using product labeled for mammals[14]

HORSES:

Treatment of equine protozoal myeloencephalitis | *Sarcocystis neurona* (label dosage; FDA-approved): Using the oral pellets and provided cup: Top-dress at the rate of 1 mg/kg/day for 28 days.[1] If horse's bodyweight is in between 2 graduations on the dosing cup, fill the cup to the higher of the 2 marks. **NOTE**: Although the label lists the duration of treatment as 28 days, most horses will require longer periods of therapy (ie, 6 to 8 weeks or longer); endpoint of therapy is determined by sustained improvement of neurologic signs.[15]

Prevention of equine protozoal myeloencephalitis (*S neurona*) in foals (extra-label): Using the oral pellets, top-dress at daily ration of 0.5 mg/kg. Begin at 4 weeks of age; study duration was 12 months.[3]

Prevention of equine protozoal myeloencephalitis (*S neurona*) in adult horses (extra-label): 0.5 mg/kg twice weekly (every 3 or 4 days). Horses maintained serum diclazuril concentration above 1 ng/mL throughout the study period.[16]

CATTLE (CALVES):

Aid to control coccidiosis (extra-label): 1 mg/kg PO as a single dose, 14 days after moving into a potentially high-risk environment.[10] It is good practice to ensure the cleanliness of calf housing. Recommended to treat all calves in pen.

SHEEP (LAMBS):

Coccidiosis (extra-label):

a) Treatment: 1 mg/kg PO once[10]

b) Prevention: 1 mg/kg PO once at about 4 to 6 weeks of age at the time that coccidiosis can normally be expected on the farm.[10] May repeat one time ≈3 weeks after the first dosing if conditions of high infection pressure exist. Recommended to treat all lambs in flock.

BROILER CHICKENS:

Prevention of coccidiosis caused by *Eimeria tenella, Eimeria necatrix, Eimeria acervulina, Eimeria brunetti, Eimeria mitis (mivati),* and *Eimeria maxima* (label dosage; FDA-approved). The Type A medicated feed article must be mixed per manufacturer's directions to result in a Type B (and ultimately a Type C) medicated feed to be fed directly to broilers.[2]

GROWING TURKEYS:

For the prevention of coccidiosis caused by *Eimeria adenoeides, Eimeria gallopavonis,* and *Eimeria meleagrimitis* (label dosage; FDA-approved). The Type A medicated feed article must be mixed per manufacturer's directions to result in a Type B (and ultimately a Type C) medicated feed to be fed directly to turkeys.[2]

RABBITS:

Coccidiosis (extra-label): Add to drinking water at 10 ppm (0.01 mg/mL) for 48 hours[17]

Monitoring

- Clinical efficacy
- In horses with equine protozoal myeloencephalitis (EPM): neurologic examinations

Client Information

- Diclazuril is an antiprotozoal medication that is used for treating equine protozoal myeloencephalitis (EPM) in horses. It is also used to treat coccidiosis in dogs, cats, chickens, and other species.
- In dogs and cats, this medicine may be given with or without food. If your animal vomits or acts sick after receiving the drug on an empty stomach, give the medicine with food or a small treat to see if that helps. If vomiting continues, contact your veterinarian.
- For horses, this medicine is used as a "top-dress" over feed. This medicine must be given daily. It is important that your horse eats the entire dose.
- It is recommended to treat all animals in a pen or flock. Be sure to keep housing and pens clean.
- This medicine appears to be tolerated well, but you should report any side effects to your veterinarian.

Chemistry/Synonyms

Diclazuril occurs as a white to light-yellow powder. It is practically insoluble in water and alcohol.

Diclazuril may also be known as diclazurilo; diclazurilum; R 64433; and by the trade names, *Clinacox*®, *Protazil*®, and *Vecoxan*®.

Compatibility/Compounding Considerations

No specific information was noted.

Storage/Stability

Diclazuril pellets should be stored at room temperature (15-30°C [59°-86°F]). Store diclazuril granules at or below 25°C (77°F), excursions permitted to 40°C (104°F).

Dosage Forms/Regulatory Status

VETERINARY-LABELED PRODUCTS:

Diclazuril Oral Pellets 1.56% in 1.1 kg (2.4 lb) and 4.5 kg (10 lb) containers: *Protazil*®; (Rx). FDA-approved for use in horses not intended for food. One 1.1 kg (2.4 lb) bucket will treat a 577.9 kg (1274 lb) horse for 28 days; a 4.5 kg (10 lb) bucket treats five 500 kg (1100 lb) horses for 28 days.

Diclazuril 0.2% Type A Medicated Feed Article in 11.3 kg (25 lb) containers; *Clinacox*®; (OTC). FDA-approved for use in broiler chickens and growing turkeys; do not feed to breeding turkeys or birds producing eggs for human consumption. When used as labeled, no withdrawal time is required in the United States.

In the United Kingdom and other countries, diclazuril may be available as an oral suspension containing 2.5 mg/mL diclazuril.

HUMAN-LABELED PRODUCTS: NONE

References

For the complete list of references, see **wiley.com/go/budde/plumb**

Diclofenac, Topical

(dye-***kloe***-fen-ak) *Surpass*®

Nonsteroidal Anti-Inflammatory Agent (NSAID)

Prescriber Highlights

- ► Topical NSAID FDA-approved for control of joint pain and inflammation in horses
- ► Use with caution in horses that are dehydrated or have preexisting GI, cardiac, or renal disease.
- ► Adverse effects (uncommon) may include local inflammation at the site of application, GI ulceration, diarrhea, weight loss, and renal toxicity.
- ► Avoid concurrent use with other NSAIDs and with glucocorticoids; use cautiously with diuretics.
- ► Wear gloves when handling this product.

Uses/Indications

Diclofenac topical cream is labeled for control of pain and inflammation associated with osteoarthritis in tarsal (hock), carpal (knee), metacarpophalangeal (forelimb fetlock), metatarsophalangeal (hindlimb fetlock), and proximal interphalangeal (pastern) joints in horses for up to 10 days. Topical administration has been shown to reduce lameness regardless of the severity or chronicity of the clinical condition.[1] Application of topical diclofenac reduced inflammation at the injection site of an amikacin IV regional limb perfusion.[2]

In a case report, topically applied diclofenac 3% gel resulted in clinical resolution of actinic keratosis in a rabbit.[10]

Pharmacology/Actions

Diclofenac is a nonspecific inhibitor of cyclooxygenase (COX1 and COX2) and may also have some inhibitory effects on lipoxygenase. By inhibiting COX2 enzymes, diclofenac reduces the production of prostaglandins associated with pain, hyperpyrexia, and inflammation.

Pharmacokinetics

Diclofenac 1% liposomal cream administered topically to horses is absorbed locally, but specific bioavailability data was not located. Peak concentrations in transudate obtained from tissue cages were ≈80 ng/mL; drug concentrations stay increased from 6 to at least 18 hours after administration. At the dosages recommended for the topical cream, most of the drug remains in the tissues local to the administration point, but detectable drug concentrations in systemic circulation may occur.[3] In humans, diclofenac is more than 99% bound to plasma proteins. It is metabolized in the liver, and the metabolites are excreted primarily in the urine.

Contraindications/Precautions/Warnings

Topical diclofenac should not be used in horses hypersensitive to it or any component of the cream. According to the manufacturer's label, diclofenac topical has not been evaluated in horses younger than 1 year of age; however, repeated applications (every 12 hours for 7 days) on the tarsometatarsal region were well tolerated in neonatal foals.[4]

Exceeding the recommended dosage (ie, applying a strip longer than 5 inches or treating multiple joints) may increase plasma concentrations of diclofenac and the risk of adverse effects.

The risk for developing renal toxicity is increased in patients that are dehydrated or with renal, cardiovascular, or hepatic dysfunction.

Diclofenac has been implicated in causing death in vultures,[5,6] and toxicity has been observed in other avian species.[7,8]

Caretakers should wear disposable, impermeable (eg, rubber) gloves during application of this medicine to prevent dermal exposure.[9]

Adverse Effects

In horses, the topical cream appears to be well-tolerated. Adverse effects may include weight loss, gastric ulcers, diarrhea, colic, icterus, renal toxicity, uterine discharge, and local dermatologic reactions (eg, erythema, swelling, alopecia). During the field study for FDA approval, 1 horse developed colic on day 4 of therapy and responded to supportive care.[9]

Reproductive/Nursing Safety

Reproductive safety has not been investigated in breeding, pregnant, or lactating horses.

Because safety has not been established in animals, this drug should only be used when the maternal benefits outweigh the potential risks to offspring.

Overdose/Acute Toxicity

Clinical signs associated with topical overdose of diclofenac in horses reflect the adverse effect profile and include renal toxicity, weight loss, glandular gastric ulcers, colic, diarrhea, and uterine discharge; treatment is supportive based on clinical presentation.

Enteral overdose of diclofenac cream may cause GI ulceration and renal toxicity. For horses with recent ingestion, consider placing a nasogastric tube for gastric lavage followed by administration of mineral oil. For species that can vomit (eg, dogs, cats), GI decontamination with emesis induction and activated charcoal is appropriate in situations of recent ingestion. For doses in which GI adverse effects are expected, use of GI protectants (eg, proton pump inhibitors, sucralfate) is warranted. If renal adverse effects are also expected, IV fluid diuresis is warranted in all species.

Diclofenac ingestion has caused death in vultures that ingested carcasses of animals that received diclofenac.[5,6]

For patients that have experienced or are suspected to have experienced an overdose, consultation with a 24-hour poison center specializing in providing veterinary-specific information is recommended. For general information related to overdose and toxin exposures, as well as contact information for poison control centers, refer to ***Appendix***.

Drug Interactions

When used topically at recommended dosages, there are no reported drug interactions in horses. The following drug interactions have either been reported or are theoretical in humans or animals receiving diclofenac and may be of significance in veterinary patients. Unless otherwise noted, use together is not necessarily contraindicated, but weigh the potential risks and perform additional monitoring when appropriate.

- CORTICOSTEROIDS (eg, **dexamethasone, prednis(ol)one**): Use with corticosteroids may increase the risk for adverse GI effects (eg, gastric ulceration); concurrent use is not recommended.
- DIURETICS (eg, **furosemide**): Concurrent diuretic therapy may increase the risk for renal toxicity.
- NONSTEROIDAL ANTI-INFLAMMATORY DRUGS (NSAIDs, OTHER; eg, **firocoxib, flunixin, phenylbutazone**): Use with other NSAIDs may increase the risk for adverse GI effects (eg, gastric ulceration); concurrent use is not recommended.

Laboratory Considerations

- No specific laboratory interactions or considerations were noted.

Dosages

HORSES:

Control of pain and inflammation associated with osteoarthritis in tarsal (hock), carpal (knee), metacarpophalangeal (forelimb fetlock), metatarsophalangeal (hindlimb fetlock), and proximal interphalangeal (pastern) joints (label dosage; FDA-approved): Apply a 12.7-cm (5-in) ribbon twice daily over the affected joint for up to 10 days.[9] Wear impermeable rubber gloves and rub cream thoroughly into the hair covering the joint until cream disappears.

Monitoring

- Efficacy
- Adverse effects, including weight loss, gastric ulcers, diarrhea, icterus, uterine discharge, and dermatologic inflammation at application site
- Baseline and periodic serum chemistry profile as needed during therapy

Client Information

- The manufacturer-provided Client Information Sheet should be included with the medication at the time of dispension.
- This medicine is a topical nonsteroidal anti-inflammatory drug (NSAID) cream used to treat horses for joint pain and inflammation for up to 10 days. It may take several applications before your horse's condition improves.
- For this medication to work, give it exactly as your veterinarian has prescribed. Always check the prescription label to ensure you are giving the drug correctly. Do not use more cream than your veterinarian recommends.
- Horses usually tolerate this medicine well; loss of hair or mild swelling at the application site is possible.
- Discontinue and immediately contact your veterinarian if you see signs of loss of appetite, weight loss, colic, diarrhea, yellowing of the skin, eyes, gums (ie, jaundice).
- Manufacturer warns against using this medicine on more than 1 joint or using more than a 12.7-cm (5-in) ribbon, as this may cause side effects.
- Wear rubber or other disposable impermeable gloves and rub cream thoroughly into the hair covering the joint until cream disappears. Wash hands immediately with soap and water in case of direct skin contact.

Chemistry/Synonyms

Diclofenac sodium, a phenylacetic acid derivative NSAID, occurs as a white to off-white hygroscopic crystalline powder. It is sparingly soluble in water, soluble in alcohol, and practically insoluble in chloroform and ether. The commercial (equine) cream is formulated in a liposomal base.

Diclofenac may also be known as GP-45840, diclofenacum, or diclophenac; many trade names are available for diclofenac products outside the United States.

Storage/Stability

The commercially available 1% cream should be stored at temperatures up to 25°C (77°F); protect from freezing.

Compatibility/Compounding Considerations

No specific information noted

Dosage Forms/Regulatory Status

VETERINARY-LABELED PRODUCTS:

The Association of Racing Commissioners International (ARCI) has designated this drug as a class 4 substance. See ***Appendix*** for more information. Use of this drug may not be allowed in certain animal competitions. Check rules and regulations before entering in a competition while this medication is being administered. Contact local racing authorities for further guidance.

Diclofenac sodium (liposomal) 1% (1 g contains 10 mg diclofenac sodium) topical cream in 124 g tubes; *Surpass*®; (Rx). FDA-approved for use in horses. NADA #141-186

Injectable forms of this medication are available in some countries.

HUMAN-LABELED PRODUCTS:

Diclofenac Topical Patch, Extended Release: 1.3%; *Flector*®; (Rx)

Diclofenac Sodium Gel: 1% (1 g contains 10 mg diclofenac sodium) and 3% (1 g contains 30 mg diclofenac sodium) with benzyl alcohol in 25 g and 50 g; *Voltaren Gel*®, *Solaraze*®, *Diclo Gel*®, *Diclozor*®, generic; (Rx)

Diclofenac Sodium Topical Solution: 1.5%; *Klofensaid* II®, *Pennsaid*®, *Xrylix*®, generic; (Rx)

Diclofenac Sodium Topical Spray: 3%; generic; (Rx)

Diclofenac sodium is also FDA-approved as a topical ophthalmic agent (see ***Diclofenac Ophthalmic***).

Diclofenac is also available in a variety of oral dosage forms (eg, tablets, capsule, oral powder), including in combination with misoprostol.

References

For the complete list of references, see **wiley.com/go/budde/plumb**

Dicloxacillin

(di-klox-a-***sill***-in) *Dicloxin®, Dynapen®*
Anti-Staphylococcal Penicillin

Prescriber Highlights

- Oral anti-staphylococcal penicillin
- Contraindicated in patients hypersensitive to it; do not use oral medications in critically ill patients.
- Use with caution in patients with known hypersensitivity to other beta-lactam antibiotics.
- Adverse effects may include GI disturbances, CNS disturbances, elevated liver values, and cardiorespiratory disturbances (tachypnea, tachycardia).
- Rarely used in veterinary medicine as it has no apparent advantages over approved veterinary products, and administering doses every 6 to 8 hours may be challenging for owners.

Uses/Indications

The veterinary use of dicloxacillin has been primarily in the PO treatment of bone, skin, and other soft tissue infections in small animals when penicillinase-producing *Staphylococcus* spp have been isolated. Because of its low oral bioavailability and short half-life, other drugs with good staphylococcal coverage are usually employed.

The World Health Organization has designated dicloxacillin as a Highly Important antimicrobial for human medicine.[1] The Office International des Epizooties (OIE) has designated dicloxacillin as a Veterinary Critically Important Antimicrobial (VCIA) Agent in avian, bovine, caprine, ovine, and swine species.[2]

Pharmacology/Actions

Penicillins are beta-lactam antimicrobials that disrupt bacterial cell wall synthesis by binding penicillin-binding proteins (PBPs) within the bacterial cell wall, which inhibits peptidoglycan synthesis. This results in a defective barrier and an osmotically unstable spheroplast. The number and type of PBPs vary between different bacteria, as do the different affinities for various beta-lactams. This helps explain the differences in spectrums of activity the drugs have, which are not explained by the influence of beta-lactamases. Penicillins are timedependent antimicrobials, usually bactericidal, and like other beta-lactam antibiotics, they are generally considered more effective against actively growing bacteria.

Cloxacillin, dicloxacillin, and oxacillin have nearly identical spectrums of activity and can be considered therapeutically equivalent when comparing *in vitro* activity. These penicillinase-resistant penicillins have a narrower spectrum of activity than the natural penicillins. Their antimicrobial efficacy is aimed directly against penicillinase-producing strains of gram-positive cocci, particularly *Staphylococcus* spp. They are sometimes called anti-staphylococcal penicillins. They are ineffective against methicillin-resistant staphylococci. While this class of penicillins has activity against some other gram-positive and gram-negative aerobes and anaerobes, other antibiotics (penicillins and others) are usually better choices. The penicillinase-resistant penicillins are inactive against *Rickettsia* spp, mycobacteria, fungi, *Mycoplasma* spp, and viruses.

Pharmacokinetics

Dicloxacillin is only available in oral dosage forms. Dicloxacillin sodium is resistant to acid inactivation in the gut but is only partially absorbed. The bioavailability after oral administration in dogs is only about 23%,[3] and in humans has been reported to range from 35% to 76%. If given with food, both the rate and extent of absorption are decreased.

The drug is distributed to the liver, kidneys, bone, bile, pleural, and synovial fluids. Five or more doses are required before clinically therapeutic concentrations of the drug are achieved in ascitic fluid.[4] As with the other penicillins, only minimal amounts are distributed into the CSF. In dogs, dicloxacillin is 90% protein-bound,[4] whereas in humans, ≈95 *to* 99% of the drug is bound to plasma proteins.

Dicloxacillin is partially metabolized to both active and inactive metabolites. These metabolites and the parent compound are rapidly excreted in the urine via both glomerular filtration and tubular secretion mechanisms. A small amount of the drug is also excreted in the feces via biliary elimination. The serum half-life in humans with normal renal function ranges from about 24 to 48 minutes. In dogs, the elimination half-life is 0.8 to 2.6 hours,[3,4] and in cats the half-life is ≈0.9 hours.[5]

Contraindications/Precautions/Warnings

Penicillins are contraindicated in patients with a history of hypersensitivity to them. Because there may be cross-reactivity, use penicillins cautiously in patients that have documented hypersensitivity to other beta-lactam antibiotics (eg, cephalosporins, cephamycins, carbapenems).

Do not administer systemic antibiotics orally in patients with septicemia, shock, or other grave illnesses as absorption of the medication from the GI tract may be significantly delayed or diminished. Parenteral (preferably IV) routes should be used for these cases.

Do not confuse dicloxacillin with doxycycline.

Adverse Effects

Adverse effects with the penicillins are usually not serious and have a relatively low frequency of occurrence.

Hypersensitivity reactions, unrelated to dose, can occur with these agents and can manifest as rashes, fever, eosinophilia, neutropenia, agranulocytosis, thrombocytopenia, leukopenia, anemias, lymphadenopathy, or anaphylaxis. In humans, it is estimated that 1% to 15% of patients hypersensitive to cephalosporins will also be hypersensitive to penicillins. The incidence of cross-reactivity in veterinary patients is unknown.

When given orally, penicillins may cause GI effects (eg, anorexia, vomiting, diarrhea). Because the penicillins may also alter gut flora, antibiotic-associated diarrhea can occur and allow the proliferation of resistant bacteria in the colon (superinfections).

Neurotoxicity (eg, ataxia in dogs) has been associated with high doses or prolonged use. Although the penicillins are not considered hepatotoxic, elevated liver enzymes have been reported. Other effects reported in dogs include tachypnea, dyspnea, edema, and tachycardia.

Reproductive/Nursing Safety

Penicillins cross the placenta, but there have not been any documented teratogenic problems associated with these drugs.

Dicloxacillin is distributed into milk in very small amounts. Although it may alter neonatal gut flora or cause hypersensitivity, it is unlikely to pose much risk to nursing offspring. Penicillins are considered compatible with breastfeeding.[6]

Because safety has not been established in animals, this drug should only be used when the maternal benefits outweigh the potential risks to offspring.

Overdose/Acute Toxicity

Acute oral penicillin overdoses are unlikely to cause significant problems other than GI distress, but other effects are possible (see ***Adverse Effects***). In humans, very high dosages of parenteral penicillins, especially in patients with renal disease, have induced CNS effects.

For patients that have experienced or are suspected to have experienced an overdose, consultation with a 24-hour poison control center specializing in providing veterinary-specific information is recommended. For general information related to overdose and

toxin exposures, as well as contact information for poison control centers, refer to ***Appendix***.

Drug Interactions

The following drug interactions either have been reported or are theoretical in humans or animals receiving dicloxacillin and may be of significance in veterinary patients. Unless otherwise noted, use together is not necessarily contraindicated, but weigh the potential risks and perform additional monitoring when appropriate.

- **Aminoglycosides**: In vitro evidence of synergism with dicloxacillin against *S aureus* strains
- **Cyclosporine**: Dicloxacillin may reduce levels.
- **Methotrexate**: May increase methotrexate concentration and risk of toxic effects
- **Mycophenolate**: May reduce formation of the active mycophenolate metabolite, possibly decreasing mycophenolate efficacy
- **Probenecid**: Competitively blocks the tubular secretion of dicloxacillin, thereby increasing serum levels and serum half-lives
- **Tetracyclines**: Theoretical antagonism; use together usually not recommended
- **Warfarin**: Dicloxacillin may cause decreased warfarin efficacy.

Laboratory Considerations

- As penicillins and other beta-lactams can inactivate aminoglycosides in vitro (and in vivo in patients with renal insufficiency), serum concentrations of aminoglycosides may be falsely decreased if the patient is also receiving beta-lactam antibiotics and the serum is stored prior to analysis. It is recommended that if the assay is delayed, samples be frozen and, if possible, drawn at times when the beta-lactam antibiotic is at a trough.

Dosages

DOGS/CATS:

Pyoderma due to sensitive penicillinase-producing staphylococci in dogs (label dosage; FDA-approved): 11 – 22 mg/kg PO three times daily; in severe cases, up to 55 mg/kg PO three times daily may be used.[7] **NOTE**: The lower end of the label dosage range is considered to be less than what is currently recommended.

Susceptible infections (extra-label): 20 – 40 mg/kg PO every 8 hours[8]

Monitoring

- Efficacy (ie, resolution of clinical signs)
- Culture and susceptibility as indicated for clinical condition being treated
- Adverse effects including hypersensitivity reactions and GI disturbances (ie, vomiting, diarrhea, inappetence)
- Serum levels and therapeutic drug monitoring are not routinely done with this drug.

Client Information

- Give dicloxacillin to animals on an empty stomach. If GI side effects (not eating, vomiting, diarrhea) occur, give with a small meal or treat.
- The most common side effects are diarrhea, vomiting, and loss of appetite.
- It is important to give this medication exactly as prescribed and to complete the full course of treatment, even if your animal seems better. Missing doses or stopping treatment early may result in treatment failure.

Chemistry/Synonyms

An isoxazolyl-penicillin, dicloxacillin sodium is a semisynthetic, penicillinase-resistant penicillin. It is available commercially as the monohydrate sodium salt that occurs as a white to off-white crystalline powder that is freely soluble in water and has a pK_a of 2.7 to 2.8.

One mg of dicloxacillin sodium contains not less than 850 micrograms of dicloxacillin.

Dicloxacillin sodium may also be known as sodium dicloxacillin, dichlorphenylmethyl isoxazolyl penicillin sodium, methyldichlorophenyl isoxazolyl penicillin sodium, dicloxacilina sodica, dicloxacillinum natricum, or P-1011; many trade names are available.

Storage/Stability

Dicloxacillin sodium capsules should be stored at temperatures at 20°C to 25°C (68°F-77°F).

Compatibility/Compounding Considerations

No specific information noted

Dosage Forms/Regulatory Status

VETERINARY-LABELED PRODUCTS:

No products currently marketed in the United States; however, the FDA's Green Book still lists *Dicloxin®* capsules as approved for use in dogs.

HUMAN-LABELED PRODUCTS:

Dicloxacillin Sodium Capsules: 250 mg and 500 mg; generic; (Rx)

References

For the complete list of references, see **wiley.com/go/budde/plumb**

Diethylstilbestrol (DES)

(dye-ethel-stil-***bes***-tral)

Hormonal Agent

Prescriber Highlights

- ► Synthetic estrogen used in dogs primarily for estrogen-responsive urinary incontinence and other estrogen indications (eg, prostatic hypertrophy, estrus induction). FDA approval of estriol for dogs has made diethylstilbestrol (DES) use controversial, particularly in dogs starting estrogen therapy for urinary incontinence.
- ► Prohibited for use in food animals (potential carcinogen)
- ► Many potential adverse effects: blood dyscrasias, GI effects, cystic endometrial hyperplasia and pyometra (nonspayed females), feminization (males), neoplasia
- ► Teratogenic and carcinogenic
- ► The National Institute for Occupational Safety and Health (NIOSH) classifies DES as a hazardous drug; use appropriate precautions when handling.
- ► Availability issues; must be obtained from a compounding pharmacy

Uses/Indications

Diethylstilbestrol (DES) has been used in estrogen-responsive urinary incontinence in spayed female dogs and for medical treatment of benign prostatic hypertrophy in male dogs. DES is no longer the first drug of choice for benign prostatic hypertrophy because of risk of squamous metaplasia, the availability of finasteride,[1] and poor efficacy.[2] It has also been used for the prevention of pregnancy after mismating in female dogs and cats but is typically no longer recommended because of serious adverse effects.

Pharmacology/Actions

Estrogens are necessary for the normal growth and development of the female sex organs and in some species contribute to the development and maintenance of secondary female sex characteristics. Estrogens cause increased cell height and secretions of the cervical mucosa, thickening of the vaginal mucosa, endometrial proliferation, and increased uterine tone.

Estrogens affect the skeletal system by increasing calcium deposition, accelerating epiphyseal closure, and increasing bone formation. Estrogens have a mild anabolic effect and can increase sodium and water retention.

Estrogens affect the release of gonadotropins from the pituitary gland, which can inhibit lactation, ovulation, and androgen secretion.

Excessive estrogen will delay the transport of the ovum and prevent it from reaching the uterus at the appropriate time for implantation. DES also possesses antineoplastic activity against some types of neoplasias (perianal gland adenoma and prostatic hyperplasia). It affects mRNA and protein synthesis in the cell nucleus and is cell cycle nonspecific.

The mechanism of action of DES in patients with estrogen-responsive urinary incontinence is thought to be caused by increased sphincter sensitivity to norepinephrine.

Pharmacokinetics

Diethylstilbestrol (DES) is well absorbed from the GI tract of monogastric animals. It is slowly metabolized by the liver, primarily to a glucuronide form, and then excreted in the urine and feces.

Contraindications/Precautions/Warnings

Diethylstilbestrol (DES) is prohibited by the FDA for use in food animals.

DES is contraindicated in patients hypersensitive to it, and in females with estrogen-sensitive neoplasms. Because of its potential effects on bone marrow, DES should be used with extreme caution in patients with preexisting anemias or leukopenias (refer to the ***Adverse Effects*** section for more information). Use with caution in patients with hepatic impairment.

The National Institute for Occupational Safety and Health (NIOSH) classifies DES as a hazardous drug; personal protective equipment [PPE] should be used accordingly to minimize the risk of exposure. Because of the potential for danger to the public health, DES must not be used in animals intended for human consumption.

Adverse Effects

Although adverse effects with estrogen therapy can be serious (see below) in small animals, when used for estrogen-responsive incontinence at the lowest effective dose, it is usually well tolerated.

In cats and dogs, estrogens are considered toxic to the bone marrow and can cause blood dyscrasias. Blood dyscrasias are more prevalent in older animals and when higher dosages are used. Initially, a thrombocytosis and/or leukocytosis may be noted, but thrombocytopenia and/or leukopenias will gradually develop. Changes in a peripheral blood smear may be apparent within 2 weeks after estrogen administration. Chronic estrogen toxicity may be characterized by a normocytic, normochromic anemia; thrombocytopenia; and neutropenia. Bone marrow depression may be transient and begin to resolve within 30 to 40 days or may persist or progress to a fatal aplastic anemia. Dosages of 2.2 mg/kg per day have caused death in cats secondary to bone marrow toxicity.

In females, signs of estrus may occur and persist for 7 to 10 days. Estrogens may cause cystic endometrial hyperplasia and pyometra in intact females; an open-cervix pyometra may be noted 1 to 6 weeks after initiation of therapy.

When used chronically long-term in male animals, feminization and squamous metaplasia may occur.

Estrogens have been documented to be carcinogenic at low concentrations in some laboratory animals. Estrogens may induce mammary neoplasias. Experimental administration of DES to female dogs as young as 8 months of age have induced malignant ovarian adenocarcinomas. Doses ranging from 60 – 495 mg/dog (NOT mg/kg) given over 1 month to 4 years were implicated in causing these tumors.

In cats, daily administration of DES has resulted in pancreatic, hepatic, and cardiac lesions.

In humans (females), estrogen use may cause GI distress, increased liver enzymes, glucose intolerance, increased risk of thromboembolic events, and menstrual irregularities.

Reproductive/Nursing Safety

Diethylstilbestrol (DES) is contraindicated during pregnancy, as it can cause fetal malformations of the genitourinary system. Chronic use in males may lead to feminization.

Estrogens are found in breast milk; therefore, consider use of milk replacer for nursing offspring.

Overdose/Acute Toxicity

Acute estrogen overdose in humans has resulted in nausea, vomiting, and withdrawal bleeding in women. No information was located regarding acute overdose in veterinary patients; however, the reader is referred to the warnings and adverse effects listed above.

For patients that have experienced or are suspected to have experienced an overdose, it is strongly encouraged to consult with one of the 24-hour poison consultation centers that specialize in providing information specific for veterinary patients. For general information related to overdose and toxin exposures, as well as contact information for poison control centers, refer to ***Appendix***.

Drug Interactions

The following drug interactions have either been reported or are theoretical in humans or animals receiving DES and may be of significance in veterinary patients. Unless otherwise noted, use together is not necessarily contraindicated, but weigh the potential risks and perform additional monitoring when appropriate.

- **Azole Antifungals** (eg, **itraconazole, ketoconazole**): May increase estrogen concentrations
- **Cimetidine**: May decrease metabolism of estrogens
- **Corticosteroids** (eg, **dexamethasone, prednis(ol)one**): Enhanced glucocorticoid effects may result if estrogens are used concomitantly with corticosteroid agents. It has been postulated that estrogens may either alter the protein binding of corticosteroids and/or decrease their metabolism. Corticosteroid dosage adjustment may be necessary when estrogen therapy is either started or discontinued.
- **Erythromycin, Clarithromycin**: May decrease the metabolism of estrogens
- **Estrogens, Other** (eg, **diethylstilbestrol** [DES]): Possible additive effects. Do not use with other estrogens; concomitant use with other estrogens has not been evaluated.
- **Levothyroxine**: Estrogens may diminish the therapeutic effect of levothyroxine, and an increase in levothyroxine dose may be needed. Monitor thyroid status when using these drugs in combination and adjust levothyroxine dose accordingly. See ***Monitoring*** in ***Levothyroxine***.
- **Phenobarbital**: May decrease estrogen concentrations
- **Rifampin**: May induce hepatic microsomal enzymes and decrease estrogen concentrations
- **Tricyclic Antidepressants** (TCAs; eg, **amitriptyline, clomipramine**): Concurrent use may attenuate TCA efficacy and toxicity.
- **Warfarin**: Oral anticoagulant activity may be decreased if estrogens are administered concurrently; increases in anticoagulant dosage may be necessary if adding estrogens.

Laboratory Considerations

- Estrogens in combination with progestins (eg, oral contraceptives) have been demonstrated in humans to increase **thyroxine-binding globulin (TBG)** with resultant increases in total circulating **thyroid hormone**. Decreased T_3 resin uptake also occurs, but **free** T_4 concentrations are unaltered.

Dosages

DOGS:

Primary urethral sphincter mechanism incompetence (idiopathic urinary incontinence, hormone-responsive urinary incontinence); (extra-label): 0.1 – 1 mg/dog (total dose; NOT mg/kg) (0.02 mg/kg; maximum total dose of 1 mg/dog [total dose; NOT mg/kg]) for 3 to 5 days as an induction dose and then periodically decreased to the lowest dose that will maintain continence (typically 1 to 3 doses per week). In difficult cases, may be used with phenylpropanolamine[3,4]

Monitoring

When therapy is either at high dosages or chronic:

- Baseline and (at least) monthly CBC with platelet count
- Serum chemistry profile at baseline and 1 month after therapy begins; repeat in 2 months after cessation of therapy if results are abnormal.

Client Information

- **Pregnant women should avoid handling diethylstilbestrol (DES)**; wear gloves and wash hands after handling.
- May be given with or without food. If your animal vomits or acts sick after receiving the drug on an empty stomach, try giving the next dose with food or a small treat. If vomiting continues, contact your veterinarian.
- Although DES can cause serious side effects, when used to treat urinary incontinence at the lowest effective dose, itis usually well-tolerated in dogs.
- Your veterinarian will need to do blood tests to watch for serious side effects. Do not miss these important follow-up visits.
- Contact your veterinarian if your animal has weakness, diarrhea, vomiting, bruising, abnormal discharge from the vulva, abnormal growth or swelling near the teats (nipples), excessive water consumption and urination, or abnormal bleeding.

Chemistry/Synonym

A synthetic nonsteroidal estrogen agent, diethylstilbestrol (DES) occurs as an odorless white crystalline powder with a melting range of 169°C to 175°C (336°F-347°F). It is practically insoluble in water and soluble in alcohol or fatty oils.

Diethylstilbestrol may also be known as DES, diethylstilbestrolum, diethylstilboestrol, NSC-3070, stilbestrol, stilboestrol, *Apstil®*, *Boestrol®*, *Destilbenol®*, or *Distilbene®*.

Storage/Stability

Diethylstilbestrol should be stored at room temperature between 15°C and 30°C (59°F-86°F) in well-closed containers unless otherwise specified by the compounding pharmacy.

Compatibility/Compounding Considerations

No specific information noted. It is recommended that when compounding diethylstilbestrol (DES), it be treated as a cytotoxic agent with appropriate safety precautions to prevent exposure to humans.

Dosage Forms/Regulatory Status

VETERINARY-LABELED PRODUCTS: NONE

HUMAN-LABELED PRODUCTS: NONE

No commercially available regular oral diethylstilbestrol (DES) products are available in the United States. Compounded preparations may be available from compounding pharmacies. Use of DES in food producing animals is prohibited by the FDA.

References

For the complete list of references, see **wiley.com/go/budde/plumb**

Digoxin

(di-***jox***-in) *Lanoxin®*

Cardiac Glycoside

Prescriber Highlights

- ► Oral and parenteral cardiac glycoside used primarily for supraventricular tachycardia (SVT)
- ► Contraindications include ventricular fibrillation, digitalis intoxication. Many veterinary cardiologists feel that digoxin is relatively contraindicated in cats with hypertrophic cardiomyopathy.
- ► Use extreme caution in patients with renal disease and heart failure, with frequent and/or complex ventricular arrhythmias, or with subaortic stenosis (SAS).
- ► Adverse effects usually associated with high or toxic blood digoxin concentrations. Cardiac adverse effects may include almost every type of cardiac arrhythmia described with a resultant worsening of clinical signs associated with heart failure. Extracardiac adverse effects include mild GI upset, anorexia, weight loss, vomiting, or diarrhea.
- ► Vesicant, avoid extravasation
- ► Many drug interactions possible
- ► Monitoring of digoxin blood concentrations highly recommended

Uses/Indications

Digoxin is used in the treatment of congestive heart failure (CHF), atrial fibrillation or flutter, and supraventricular tachycardia. Presently, digoxin use (often combined with diltiazem) is generally limited to dogs for the management of rapid atrial fibrillation with concurrent CHF caused by either dilated cardiomyopathy or myxomatous mitral valve disease (MMVD) without evidence of renal insufficiency. Digoxin therapy is more controversial for treating heart failure in dogs or cats without accompanying supraventricular arrhythmias and its use for this indication has diminished. Today, most cardiologists no longer use digoxin as a first line therapy for heart failure in dogs and cats and its use as a positive inotropic agent has been supplanted by pimobendan. In a review of the pharmacologic management of MMVD in dogs,[1] the authors state: *Digoxin has little role in veterinary cardiology other than for heart rate control in atrial fibrillation or as an inotrope in patients whose owners have financial constraints.*

In horses, digoxin is still used in the management of CHF, particularly when complicated by atrial arrhythmias, as other oral inotropic drugs are not feasible. It has also been used as adjunctive therapy for CHF in ferrets, and for supraventricular tachycardia in cattle.

Pharmacology/Actions

Digoxin causes the following effects in patients with a failing heart: increased myocardial contractility (inotropism) with increased cardiac output; increased diuresis with reduction of edema secondary to a decrease in sympathetic tone; reduction in heart size, heart rate, blood volume, and pulmonary and venous pressures; and (usually) no net change in myocardial oxygen demand.

Digoxin has several electrocardiac effects, including decreased conduction velocity through the atrioventricular (AV) node and a prolonged effective refractory period (ERP), ECG changes include prolonged PR interval, shortened QT interval, and ST segment depression.

The exact mechanism of action of these agents has not been fully described, but they are thought to increase the availability of Ca^{++} to myocardial fibers and inhibit Na^+-K^+-ATPase with resultant increased intracellular Na^+ and reduced K^+.

Pharmacokinetics

Absorption following oral administration occurs in the small intestine and is variable dependent upon the oral dosage form used (see ***Dosage Forms/Regulatory Status***). The bioavailability of digoxin in veterinary species has only been studied in a limited manner, with oral bioavailability for tablets ≈58% and oral elixir ≈71 % in dogs,[2] but in horses only ≈20% of an intragastric dose of crushed oral tablets was bioavailable.[3] The bioavailability of digoxin formulations in humans: IV 100%, IM ≈80%, oral tablets ≈60%, and oral elixir ≈75%. Food may delay, but not alter, the extent of absorption in most species studied; however, food reportedly decreases the amount absorbed by 50% in cats after tablet administration. Peak serum concentration generally occurs within 45 to 60 minutes after oral elixir and ≈90 minutes after oral tablet administration. In patients receiving an initial oral dose of digoxin, peak effects may occur 6 to 8 hours after the dose.

The drug is distributed widely throughout the body with highest concentrations found in kidneys, heart, intestine, stomach, liver, and skeletal muscle. Lowest concentrations are found in the brain and plasma. Digoxin does not significantly enter ascitic fluid, so dosage adjustments may be required in animals with ascites. At therapeutic levels, ≈20% to 30% of the drug is bound to plasma proteins. Because only small amounts are found in fat, dosing calculations should be based on lean body weight.

Digoxin is metabolized slightly, but the primary method of elimination is renal excretion both by glomerular filtration and tubular secretion. As a result, dosage adjustments must be made in patients with significant renal disease. Values reported for the elimination half-life of digoxin in dogs and cats have been highly variable, with values reported from 30 to 42 hours for dogs[2,4] and 33 hours for cats.[5] Approximate elimination half-lives reported in other species include sheep, 7 hours[6]; horses, 17 to 29 hours[3,7-9]; and cattle, 8 hours.[10]

Contraindications/Precautions/Warnings

Digoxin is contraindicated in patients hypersensitive to it, in those with ventricular fibrillation, or in digitalis intoxication. Digoxin is contraindicated in patients with third-degree AV block without implantation of a permanent pacemaker. In cattle, it is also contraindicated in monensin toxicosis.[11] Digoxin should be used with extreme caution in patients with renal dysfunction, frequent or complex ventricular tachycardia, heart failure, or with subaortic stenosis (SAS). Digoxin should be used with caution in patients with severe pulmonary disease, hypoxia, acute myocarditis, myxedema, or acute myocardial infarction, frequent ventricular premature contractions, chronic constrictive pericarditis, preexisting sinus node disease, or second-degree AV block.

When used to treat atrial fibrillation or flutter prior to administration with an antiarrhythmic agent that has anticholinergic activity (eg, quinidine, procainamide, disopyramide), digoxin will reduce but not eliminate the increased ventricular rates that may be produced by those agents. Because digoxin may cause increased vagal tone, they should be used with caution in patients with increased carotid sinus sensitivity.

Elective cardioversion of patients with atrial fibrillation should not be attempted in patients with signs of digoxin toxicity.

The p-glycoprotein pump actively transports digoxin. Washington State University clinical pharmacology laboratory does not recommend any dose reductions in dogs with *MDR1* genetic mutations; however, they recommend therapeutic drug monitoring.[12] One case of digoxin toxicity in a collie with the *MDR1* mutation has been described.[13]

Digoxin is relatively contraindicated in cats with hypertrophic cardiomyopathy as it may worsen dynamic outflow tract obstruction and increase ventricular arrhythmogenesis.

Principally eliminated by the kidneys, digoxin should be used with caution in patients with renal disease. In these patients, therapy should be initiated at ¼ to ½ the normal dose, and serum digoxin concentrations should be monitored. Animals that are hypernatremic, hypokalemic, hypercalcemic, hypomagnesemic, hyperthyroid, or hypothyroid may require lower doses; monitor carefully. Hypokalemia and hypomagnesemia, in particular, should be corrected prior to digoxin therapy. Digoxin competes for the same ATPase binding site as potassium, whereas magnesium is a cofactor of the sodium-potassium ATPase pump; depletion of either electrolyte makes digoxin toxicity more likely, even with normal blood concentrations of the drug.

As digoxin does not distribute well into ascitic fluid or fat, dosing is generally based on lean body weight. Underweight patients may be at increased risk for digoxin toxicity.

As digoxin is a vesicant, IV doses should be injected slowly to reduce extravasation risk.

Do not confuse digoxin with doxepin.

Adverse Effects

Adverse effects of digoxin are usually associated with high or toxic serum concentrations and are categorized into cardiac and extracardiac adverse effects. There are also species differences with regard to the sensitivity to digoxin's toxic effects; cats are relatively sensitive to digoxin, whereas dogs tend to be more tolerant of high serum digoxin concentrations.

Cardiac effects may include almost every type of cardiac arrhythmia described with a resultant worsening of heart failure clinical signs. More common arrhythmias or ECG changes observed include complete or incomplete AV block, ventricular bigeminy, ST segment changes, paroxysmal ventricular or atrial tachycardias with concurrent AV block, and multifocal premature ventricular complexes. Because these effects can also be caused by worsening heart disease, it may be difficult to determine if they are a result of the disease process or digitalis intoxication. If in doubt, monitor serum digoxin concentrations or stop digoxin therapy temporarily.

Extracardiac clinical signs most commonly seen in veterinary medicine include mild GI upset or colic, anorexia, weight loss, and diarrhea. Vomiting has been associated with IV injections. Ocular and neurologic effects are routinely seen in humans but are not prevalent in animals or are not detected.

Reproductive/Nursing Safety

Digoxin crosses the placenta, but studies in animals have not been conducted. Studies have shown that digoxin concentrations in a mother's serum and milk are similar; however, it is unlikely to have any pharmacological effect on nursing offspring.[14]

Because safety has not been established in animals, this drug should only be used when the maternal benefits outweigh the potential risks to offspring.

Overdose/Acute Toxicity

Clinical signs of chronic toxicity are discussed above. In dogs, the acute toxic dose after IV administration has been reported to be 0.2 mg/kg IV and 0.3 mg/kg PO.[15] Cats given 0.11 mg/kg IV (≈10-fold overdose) experienced salivation, vomiting, anorexia, and depression prior to ECG changes (increased PR interval, elevated ST segment, bradycardia), and plasma digoxin concentration was 4.5 – 12 ng/mL,[16] although toxicity also has been observed with concentrations at or above 2.4 ng/mL.[5]

Treatment of chronic digoxin toxicity is dictated by the severity of the clinical signs. Many patients do well after temporarily stopping the drug and reevaluating the dosage regimen.

If an acute ingestion has recently occurred and no cardiotoxic or neurologic signs (eg, coma, seizures) have manifested, emptying the stomach may be indicated, followed with activated charcoal administration. Because digoxin can be slowly absorbed and there is some enterohepatic recirculation of the drug, repeated charcoal administration may be beneficial even if the ingestion occurred well before treatment. Anion-exchange resins such as colestipol or cholestyramine have been suggested to reduce the absorption and enterohepatic circulation of digoxin.

Dependent on the type of cardiotoxicity, supportive therapy based on clinical signs should be implemented. Serum electrolyte concentrations, serum digoxin concentrations (if available on a stat basis), and continuous ECG monitoring should be instituted. Careful attention is required to correct fluid and electrolyte imbalances (particularly hypokalemia and hypomagnesemia), acid-base disturbances, and hypoxia. The use of potassium in normokalemic patients is controversial and should only be attempted with constant monitoring and clinical expertise.

The use of specific antiarrhythmic agents in treating life-threatening digitalis-induced arrhythmias may be necessary. Lidocaine is most commonly employed for ventricular arrhythmias, and phenytoin also may be used. Atropine may be used to treat sinus bradycardia, sinoatrial arrest, or second- and third-degree AV block.

Digoxin immune Fab (a digoxin-specific IgG antibody that binds to and directly inactivates the drug) is a potential treatment for life-threatening digoxin toxicity. Although veterinary experience with digoxin immune Fab is extremely limited, it has been successfully used for the treatment of oleander (glycoside-containing plant) toxicosis in a dog.[17] Digoxin is not removed by dialysis.

For patients that have experienced or are suspected to have experienced an overdose, consultation with a 24-hour poison consultation center specializing in providing veterinary-specific information is recommended. For general information related to overdose and toxin exposures, as well as contact information for poison control centers, refer to ***Appendix***.

Drug Interactions

There are many potential drug interactions associated with digoxin and the following list is not necessarily all-inclusive. Because of the narrow therapeutic index associated with the drug, consider enhanced monitoring when these drugs (or those in the same class) are added to patients stabilized on digoxin.

The following drug interactions have either been reported or are theoretical in humans or animals receiving digoxin and may be of significance in veterinary patients. Unless otherwise noted, use together is not necessarily contraindicated, but weigh the potential risks and perform additional monitoring when appropriate.

- **Beta-Blockers** (eg, **atenolol, carvedilol, propranolol**): Can have additive negative effects on AV conduction, complete heart block possible
- **Calcium**: Concurrent use may result in a serious risk for arrhythmia and cardiovascular collapse. Oral calcium administration may reduce oral digoxin absorption.
- **Calcium-Channel Blockers** (eg, **diltiazem, verapamil,** but not **amlodipine**): Can have additive negative effects on AV conduction. Data are conflicting. Safe and effective diltiazem use has been demonstrated in dogs.[18]
- **Colchicine**: Concurrent use with digoxin may enhance the adverse effects of colchicine in humans.
- **Penicillamine**: May decrease serum levels of digoxin independent of route of digoxin dosing
- **Potassium/Electrolyte Balance, Drugs Affecting** (eg, **amphotericin B, dextrose/insulin infusions, diuretics, furosemide, glucagon, glucocorticoids, high dose IV dextrose, laxatives, sodium polystyrene sulfonate, thiazides**): May predispose the patient to digitalis toxicity
- **Spironolactone**: May enhance or decrease the toxic effects of digoxin
- **Thyroid Supplements**: Patients on digoxin that receive thyroid replacement therapy may need their digoxin dosage adjusted.

The following drugs or plants/herbs may **reduce digoxin serum concentration**:

- **Aminosalicylic acid**
- **Albuterol, Systemic**
- **Aluminum Hydroxide**
- **Aluminum or Magnesium Containing Oral products**
- **Chloramphenicol** (dogs)[19]
- **Cholestyramine**
- **Metoclopramide**
- **Neomycin, Oral**
- **Phenobarbital**[4]
- **Phenytoin**
- **St John's Wort**
- **Sucralfate** (oral digoxin only)
- **Sulfasalazine**

The following drugs or herbs may **increase serum concentration, decrease the elimination rate, or enhance the toxic effects of digoxin**:

- **Amiodarone**
- **Angiotensin-Converting Enzyme Inhibitors (ACEIs;** eg, **benazepril, enalapril**)
- **Anticholinergics** (eg, **atropine, glycopyrrolate, oxybutynin**)
- **Benzodiazepines** (specifically **alprazolam, diazepam**)
- **Clonidine**
- **Coleus**
- **Cyclosporine**
- **Furosemide**: Not significantly altered in cats receiving furosemide and aspirin[20]
- **Gentamicin**
- **Hawthorn**
- **Ketoconazole; Itraconazole**
- **Macrolide antibiotics** (eg, **azithromycin, clarithromycin, erythromycin**)
- **NSAIDs** (eg, **carprofen, meloxicam**)
- **Octreotide**
- **PPIs** (eg, **omeprazole, pantoprazole**)
- **Quinidine**: If used together, the rule of thumb is to decrease digoxin dose by 50%.
- **Reserpine**
- **Spironolactone**
- **Succinylcholine**
- **Telmisartan**
- **Tetracyclines** (eg, **minocycline, oxytetracycline**)
- **Thiazide Diuretics** (eg, **hydrochlorothiazide**)
- **Trazodone**
- **Trimethoprim**

Laboratory Considerations

- No specific laboratory test concerns

Dosages

NOTE: Do not confuse µg/kg, mg/kg, and µg/m^2 doses. **Always double-check calculations.**

DOGS:

Atrial fibrillation and CHF with normal renal function (extra-label): Initially, 0.0025 – 0.005 mg/kg PO every 12 hours[21] (alternatively in dogs weighing more than 20 kg [44 lb], use digoxin/body surface area at 0.22 mg/m²). Median dosage in one study was 0.004 mg/kg PO every 12 hours.[22] Can increase up to 0.011 mg/kg if warranted. Do not exceed 0.25 mg/dog (NOT mg/kg) (regardless of size) twice daily. Monitor for signs of toxicity and efficacy and measure serum digoxin concentrations to adjust dose (see ***Monitoring***). One study[18] demonstrated that digoxin 0.005 mg/kg PO every 12 hours and diltiazem used together had a more effective ventricular rate reduction in dogs with secondary atrial fibrillation than when either was given alone, but it still remains unknown if this translates into decreased morbidity or mortality.

Dilated cardiomyopathy (extra-label): 0.003 mg/kg PO every 12 hours with an ACE-inhibitor (eg, enalapril) and furosemide.[23] Doses of 0.008 – 0.011 mg/kg per day PO also have been used.[24,25]

CATS:

Dilated cardiomyopathy or atrial fibrillation (**NOTE**: digoxin is generally contraindicated for feline hypertrophic cardiomyopathy); (extra-label): The starting dose for healthy cats weighing less than 3 kg (6.6 lb), ¼ of a 0.125 mg tablet PO every other day; for cats weighing 3 to 6 kg (6.6 – 13.2 lb), ¼ of a 0.125 mg tablet PO once daily; for cats weighing more than 6 kg (13.2 lb), ¼ of a 0.125 mg tablet PO once daily to every 12 hours. Tablets are better tolerated than the alcohol-based elixir.[26]

HORSES:

Supraventricular tachycardia (extra-label):

1. 0.0022 mg/kg IV every 12 hours or 0.011 mg/kg PO every 12 hours.[27,28] If unsuccessful, propranolol 0.03 mg/kg IV may be tried.[29]
2. Loading dosage: 0.0022 mg/kg IV given slowly every 12 hours for 2 doses. Use loading dose with caution due to risk for digoxin toxicity. Maintenance dosage: 0.0022 mg/kg slow IV every 24 hours or 0.011 mg/kg PO every 12 hours.[30] Maintain trough serum digoxin concentrations between 0.8 – 1.2 ng/mL.[31]

Adjunct to quinidine cardioversion of atrial fibrillation (extra-label): If cardioversion has not occurred after 24 hours of quinidine therapy, digoxin 0.0055 - 0.011 mg/kg PO every 12 hours may be added for 24 to 48 hours.[11,30] If digoxin is continued beyond 24 hours, use the lower end of the dosing range and monitor digoxin serum digoxin concentration. See ***Drug Interactions***.

CATTLE:

Supraventricular tachycardia (extra-label): Loading dosage: 0.022 mg/kg slow IV; followed by maintenance dosage (choose one): 0.011 mg/kg slow IV 3 times daily,[27] 0.00086 mg/kg/hour (0.86 µg/kg/hour) IV CRI,[10] *or* 0.0034 mg/kg slow IV every 4 hours[10]

FERRETS:

Adjunctive therapy for heart failure associated with dilated cardiomyopathy (extra-label): 0.005 – 0.01 mg/kg PO once daily initially (use oral liquid). May increase to twice daily if necessary. Furosemide and an ACE-inhibitor are also commonly employed.

Monitoring

- Serum digoxin concentrations: Because of significant interpatient pharmacokinetic variation and narrow therapeutic index seen with this drug, it is strongly recommended to monitor serum digoxin concentrations to help guide therapy. Unless the patient received an initial loading dose, at least 3 to 6 days should pass after beginning therapy to monitor serum concentrations to allow levels to approach steady-state.[7,32] Usually a trough measurement (just before next dose or at least 8 to 10 hours after the last dose[32]) is recommended. Historically, suggested therapeutic serum concentrations in the dog have ranged widely, but most now believe that concentrations above 1.2 ng/mL are potentially toxic. Serum trough digoxin concentration of 0.5 – 1.2 ng/mL have been suggested for dogs.[21,33] Therapeutic concentrations in cats are reported to be between 0.9 – 2 ng/mL.[34] Therapeutic concentrations in the horse are reported as 0.8 – 1.2 ng/mL.[30] Concentrations at the higher end of the suggested range may be necessary to treat some atrial arrhythmias but may also result in greater incidence of adverse effects.
- Appetite and body weight
- Baseline and periodic heart rate and rhythm (ECG), chest radiographs, echocardiography, pulse oximetry as indicated
- Baseline and periodic BUN, creatinine, and electrolytes
- Resting respiratory rate
- Improved clinical signs related to underlying heart disease (eg, cough, energy level)

Client Information

- Digoxin can be given with or without food. If your animal vomits or acts sick after receiving this medication on an empty stomach, try giving the next dose with food or a small treat. If vomiting continues, contact your veterinarian.
- Digoxin side effects usually occur when the dose is too high. Signs that may be observed include gastrointestinal effects (eg, lack of appetite, vomiting, diarrhea), lack of energy, behavior changes, and collapse. Digoxin toxicity can be very serious. Contact your veterinarian immediately if your animal develops any of these signs.
- Regular monitoring of blood digoxin levels and electrolytes helps detect problems. Do not miss these important follow-up visits with your veterinarian.

Chemistry/Synonyms

The cardiac glycosides (or digitalis glycosides), including digoxin, are derived from the foxglove plant *Digitalis purpura*. Digoxin occurs as bitter tasting, clear to white crystals or as a white crystalline powder. It is practically insoluble in water, slightly soluble in diluted alcohol, and very slightly soluble in 40% propylene glycol solution. Above 235°C (455°F), it melts with decomposition. The commercial injection consists of a 40% propylene glycol, 10% alcohol solution, and has a pH of 6.6 to 7.4.

Digoxin may also be known as digoxinum or digoxosidum. Cardiac glycosides maybe be referred to as digitalis glycosides; digoxin occasionally may be described as digitalis.

Storage/Stability

Digoxin tablets, elixir, and injection should be stored at room temperature 20°C to 25°C (68°F-77°F) and protected from light.

At pH of 5 to 8, digoxin is stable, but in solutions with a pH of less than 3, it is hydrolyzed.

Compatibility/Compounding Considerations

The injectable product is **compatible** with most commercially available IV solutions, including lactated Ringer's, D5W, and normal saline. To prevent the possibility of precipitation occurring, one manufacturer recommends that the injection be diluted by a volume at least 4 times with either sterile water, D5W, or normal saline. Digoxin injection has been demonstrated to be **compatible** with bretylium tosylate, cimetidine HCl, lidocaine HCl, and verapamil HCl.

Digoxin is **incompatible** with dobutamine HCl, acids, and alkalies. The manufacturer does not recommend mixing digoxin injection with other medications. Compatibility is dependent upon factors such as pH, concentration, temperature, and diluent used; consult specialized references or a hospital pharmacist for more specific information.

Dosage Forms/Regulatory Status

There are bioavailability differences between dosage forms and in tablets produced by different manufacturers. It is recommended that tablets be used from a manufacturer that the clinician has confidence in and that brands not be routinely interchanged. Should a change in dosage form be desired, bioavailability differences (see ***Pharmacokinetics***) can be used as guidelines in altering the dose for monogastric animals.

VETERINARY-LABELED PRODUCTS:

The veterinary-labeled products are no longer commercially available in the US.

The Association of Racing Commissioners International (ARCI) has designated this drug as a class 4 substance. See the ***Appendix*** for more information.

HUMAN-LABELED PRODUCTS:

Digoxin Solution for Injection: 250 µg/mL (0.25 mg/mL), Pediatric solution for Injection: 100 µg/mL (0.1 mg/mL) in 1 mL amps; *Lanoxin*®, generic, (Rx)

Digoxin Oral Tablets: 125 µg (0.125 mg), and 250 µg (0.25 mg); *Lanoxin*®, generic; (Rx)

Digoxin Oral Solution: 50 µg/mL (0.05 mg/mL) and 100 µg/mL (0.1 mg/mL); generic; (Rx)

References

For the complete list of references, see **wiley.com/go/budde/plumb**

Diltiazem

(dil-***tye***-a-zem) *Cardizem*®, *Dilacor XR*®

Calcium Channel Blocker

Prescriber Highlights

- Calcium channel blocker used in dogs, cats, and ferrets for supraventricular tachycardias (SVT) and as adjunctive therapy for systemic or pulmonary hypertension; also used historically in cats and ferrets for hypertrophic cardiomyopathy. May prove useful in horses with atrial fibrillation during quinidine therapy to control ventricular response rate
- Contraindications include severe hypotension, sinus node dysfunction, high grade atrioventricular (AV) block, concurrent radiographically documented pulmonary congestion or edema, acute myocardial infarction, hypersensitivity.
- Use with caution in geriatric patients or in those with controlled heart failure (particularly if also receiving beta-blockers), hepatic or renal impairment.
- Several extended-/sustained-release products available; ensure prescriptions are sufficiently clear and clients understand how to administer.
- Many drug interactions are possible.

Uses/Indications

Diltiazem may be useful in dogs with tachyarrhythmias originating above the atrioventricular (AV) node (broadly termed supraventricular tachycardias [SVTs]) such as focal atrial tachycardia, focal junctional tachycardia, atrial flutter, atrial fibrillation, or AV-reciprocating tachycardia. For the tachyarrhythmias listed here, the primary effect of diltiazem is slowing of AV nodal conduction and improved control of the ventricular response rate. One study demonstrated that when digoxin and diltiazem were used together, they resulted in more effective ventricular rate reduction in dogs with secondary atrial fibrillation than when either was given alone.[1] Although not proving a causal benefit of rate control in dogs with atrial fibrillation, another study demonstrated that a lower 24-hour mean heart rate in a dog with atrial fibrillation was associated with longer survival.[2] In cats, diltiazem has historically been used for the treatment of feline hypertrophic cardiomyopathy and some clinicians continue this practice, but enthusiasm for its use for this indication has waned, and a recent expert consensus panel did not advise use of diltiazem in feline cardiomyopathy.[3] Diltiazem potentially could be used as third-line therapy for systemic arterial hypertension or pulmonary arterial hypertension, although other medications are more targeted (amlodipine for systemic arterial hypertension, sildenafil for pulmonary arterial hypertension) and are often used first.

The injectable formulation can be used in animals for acute therapy of hemodynamically unstable SVT.

Pharmacology/Actions

Diltiazem is a calcium channel blocker and a class IV antiarrhythmic. There are 3 subclasses of calcium channel blockers: benzothiazepines (eg, diltiazem), dihydropyridines (eg, amlodipine), and phenylalkylamines (eg, verapamil). Although all calcium channel blockers inhibit the transmembrane influx of extracellular calcium ions into cardiac and vascular smooth muscle cells, they show different affinities, and the relative actions of each class differ. The dihydropyridines act primarily on vascular smooth muscle with a primary effect of smooth muscle vasodilation and reduced total peripheral resistance. The nondihydropyridines (eg, diltiazem) act predominately on nodal cells to prolong the refractory period and slow conduction. All calcium channel blockers can have effects on cardiac contractility, although diltiazem is typically associated with weak negative inotropic effects compared with other calcium channel blockers.

Diltiazem affects cardiac conduction; it slows atrioventricular (AV) node conduction, prolongs PQ interval, and prolongs refractory times. Diltiazem rarely affects sinoatrial node activity, but in patients with sinus node dysfunction (sick sinus syndrome), diltiazem is contraindicated as resting heart rates may be reduced.

Diltiazem does not appear to affect plasma renin, aldosterone, glucose, or insulin concentrations.

Pharmacokinetics

In dogs, bioavailability of tablet forms may only be ≈25%.[4] Volume of distribution is ≈8 L/kg and ≈97% of the drug is bound to serum proteins. Elimination half-life is ≈2 to 4 hours, but up to 8 hours has been reported. Time to peak plasma concentration in dogs is ≈3 hours after oral administration of immediate-release tablets.[4,5]

Bioavailability of immediate-release tablets in cats is reported to range from 50% to 80% with peak concentrations occurring ≈45 minutes after oral dosing.[6] Protein binding is ≈50%. Half-life is ≈1-2 hours.

Pharmacokinetics of a long-acting product (*Cardizem*® *CD*) given at 10 mg/kg PO once daily to healthy cats were noted as follows: bioavailability was 22% to 59%; peak concentrations were achieved in 4 to 8 hours; protein binding was ≈40%; and half-life was ≈7 hours.[6]

In horses, elimination half-life is ≈90 minutes. The distribution half-life was 12 minutes after IV administration, total plasma clearance was 14.4 mL/kg/minute, and the volume of distribution at steady-state was 1.84 L/kg.[7]

Diltiazem is rapidly and almost completely metabolized by the liver into several metabolites, including some that are active.[5]

In humans after an oral dose, ≈80% of the dose is absorbed rapidly from the gut, but because of a high first-pass effect, only about half of the absorbed drug reaches the systemic circulation; elimination half-life ranges from 3 to 9 hours.[5]

Contraindications/Precautions/Warnings

Diltiazem is contraindicated in patients hypersensitive to it or those with severe hypotension (less than 90 mm Hg systolic), sinus node dysfunction (eg, sick sinus syndrome), high-grade atrioventricular

(AV) block (unless a functioning artificial pacemaker is in place), or radiographically documented pulmonary congestion.

Diltiazem should be used with caution in geriatric patients or in those with heart failure (particularly if also receiving beta-blockers) or with hepatic or renal impairment.

When diltiazem is administered IV, it should be given slowly over at least 2 minutes.[8]

Adverse Effects

Diltiazem appears to be well tolerated at recommended doses. One feline study found that the 60 mg sustained-release pellet (9.3 to 14.8 mg/kg) was associated with lethargy, GI disturbances, and weight loss in 36% of treated cats.[9] GI disturbances were recognized within one week, and weight loss was detected after 2 to 6 months of treatment.[9] Lethargy, GI distress (anorexia), hypotension, atrioventricular (AV) block and other rhythm disturbances, CNS effects, rashes, and elevations in liver function tests could potentially occur in any species.

Reproductive/Nursing Safety

High doses in rodents have resulted in increased embryolethality, fetal deaths, and skeletal abnormalities.[10,11] Use during pregnancy only when the benefits outweigh the potential risks.

Diltiazem is excreted in milk and concentrations may approximate those found in the plasma; therefore, it should be used with caution when nursing.

Overdose/Acute Toxicity

The oral LD_{50} in dogs has been reported as greater than 50 mg/kg.[11] Clinical signs noted after an overdose may include GI signs (eg, inappetence, vomiting, diarrhea), atrioventricular (AV) block, bradycardia, hypotension, and heart failure.[12] A dog that ingested ≈100 mg/kg PO of a sustained-release product developed bradycardia, hypotension, CNS depression, second-degree AV block with ventricular escape, and GI effects. Ultimately the dog required a temporary transvenous pacemaker for 19 hours, but recovered.[13]

Treatment for calcium channel blocker intoxication can be complicated and treatment modalities are evolving. GI decontamination (including emesis or activated charcoal) should be considered in subclinical cases (particularly with recent exposure of less than 2 hours), along with supportive care based on clinical signs, including IV fluids and calcium supplementation IV.[12] Atropine may be used to treat bradycardias and second- or third-degree AV blocks. Patients that are not responsive to atropine can be administered glucagon or may require temporary artificial pacemaker implantation. Inotropic agents (eg, glucagon, dobutamine, dopamine) and vasopressors (eg, dopamine, norepinephrine) may be required to treat heart failure and hypotension. IV lipid emulsion (ILE) and high-dose insulin have been suggested as potential therapies for severe diltiazem toxicity; a successful case report using this treatment in a 4-year-old Pomeranian has been published.[14]

For patients that have experienced or are suspected to have experienced an overdose, consultation with a 24-hour poison control center specializing in providing veterinary-specific information is recommended. For general information related to overdose and toxin exposures, as well as contact information for poison control centers, refer to ***Appendix***.

Drug Interactions

The following drug interactions have either been reported or are theoretical in humans or animals receiving diltiazem and may be of significance in veterinary patients. Unless otherwise noted, use together is not necessarily contraindicated, but weigh the potential risks and perform additional monitoring when appropriate.

- **AMIODARONE**: Concurrent use may result in bradycardia, atrioventricular (AV) block, or sinus arrest.
- **ANESTHETICS, GENERAL** (eg, **isoflurane, propofol**): May increase cardiac depressant effects of diltiazem
- **AZOLE ANTIFUNGALS** (eg, **fluconazole, ketoconazole, itraconazole**): Concurrent use may increase diltiazem exposure and risk for toxicity.
- **BENZODIAZEPINES** (eg, **diazepam, midazolam**): Diltiazem may increase benzodiazepine concentrations.
- **BETA-ADRENERGIC ANTAGONISTS** (eg, **atenolol, esmolol, propranolol**): Diltiazem may increase the likelihood of bradycardia, AV block, or congestive heart failure developing in patients also receiving beta-blockers (including **ophthalmic beta-blockers (eg, timolol)**); additionally, diltiazem may substantially increase the bioavailability of propranolol.
- **BUSPIRONE**: Diltiazem may increase buspirone concentrations.
- **CANNABIDIOL**: Diltiazem may increase cannabidiol concentration.
- **CLONIDINE**: Increased risk for bradycardia
- **CLOPIDOGREL**: Concurrent use may result in decreased antiplatelet effects and increased risk for thrombotic events.
- **CIMETIDINE/RANITIDINE**: Cimetidine may increase plasma diltiazem concentrations; increased monitoring of diltiazem's effects is warranted. Ranitidine may also affect diltiazem concentrations but to a lesser extent.
- **CYCLOSPORINE**: Diltiazem may increase serum cyclosporine concentrations; increased monitoring and dosage adjustments may be required.
- **DEXAMETHASONE**: Concurrent use may result in increased plasma dexamethasone concentrations and enhanced adrenal-suppressant effects.
- **DIGOXIN**: Although data conflict regarding whether diltiazem affects digoxin pharmacokinetics, diligent monitoring of serum digoxin concentrations should be performed.
- **MACROLIDE ANTIBIOTICS** (eg, **clarithromycin, erythromycin**): Concurrent use may result in an increased risk for cardiotoxicity.
- **METHYLPREDNISOLONE**: Concurrent use may result in increased plasma methylprednisolone concentrations and enhanced adrenal-suppressant effects.
- **OPIOIDS** (eg, **buprenorphine, fentanyl, hydrocodone, morphine, methadone**): Concurrent use may increase opioid exposure and risk for increased or prolonged effects.
- **QUINIDINE**: Diltiazem may increase serum quinidine concentrations; increased monitoring and dosage adjustments may be required.
- **RIFAMPIN**: May decrease diltiazem concentrations
- **TACROLIMUS**: Concurrent use may increase tacrolimus trough concentrations and risk for tacrolimus toxicity.
- **THEOPHYLLINE**: Concurrent use may result in increased serum theophylline concentrations and risk for theophylline toxicity.
- **VINCRISTINE**: Concurrent use may increase plasma vincristine concentrations.

Dosages

NOTE: See *Dosage Forms/Regulatory Status* for important information related to different formulations of diltiazem as they are not interchangeable.

DOGS:

Supraventricular tachyarrhythmias (extra-label): **NOTE**: Dosage recommendations can vary significantly and evidence supporting any dosage recommendation is not strong. The following information is adapted from multiple sources[15-18]:

Acute treatment of supraventricular tachycardia:

a) 0.05 – 0.1 mg/kg IV administered over 2 minutes; this dose may be repeated up to 2 times with 5 minutes between doses.
b) 0.25 mg/kg IV administered over 2 to 5 minutes; if required, dosage may be carefully increased up to a total dose of 0.5 mg/kg IV.
c) 2 – 6 µg/kg/minute IV CRI has been described when the arrhythmia recurs before oral dosing is feasible.
d) 0.5 mg/kg PO followed by 0.25 mg/kg PO every hour until conversion or a total oral dose of 1.5 – 2 mg/kg has been given.[15-17]

Chronic treatment of supraventricular tachycardia: Initially, 1 mg/kg PO every 8 hours and titrated upward to a maximum of 3 mg/kg PO every 8 hours. Doses exceeding 2.5 mg/kg every 8 hours should probably not be given to dogs that have severe myocardial failure or with significant cardiac compromise.

Decreasing ventricular rate associated with atrial fibrillation (extra-label):
a) Using immediate-release tablets, initially 0.5 – 2 mg/kg PO 3 times daily. Titrate upward if necessary. Total daily dose of 7 – 9 mg/kg is often necessary for adequate ventricular rate control.
b) Using a sustained-release product, initially 2 – 4 mg/kg PO twice daily. Dosage may carefully be titrated upward if required. Total daily dose required is similar to the regular tablets but divided twice, rather than 3 times, daily.
c) Diltiazem administered either as extended-release 3 mg/kg PO every 12 hours *OR* immediate-release tablet 1 mg/kg PO every 8 hours in combination with digoxin (0.003 – 0.006 mg/kg PO every 12 hours) had a more effective ventricular rate reduction than either agent given alone.[1, 19]

CATS:

Acute treatment of supraventricular tachyarrhythmias (extra-label): 0.125 – 0.25 mg/kg IV over 2 minutes with subsequent boluses at 15-minute intervals until conversion to a normal sinus rhythm or to a cumulative dose of 0.75 mg/kg IV.[16]

Adjunctive treatment of hypertrophic cardiomyopathy; supraventricular tachyarrhythmias (extra-label): Dosage recommendations can vary significantly and evidence supporting any dosage is not strong. If using the immediate-release tablets, dose at 7.5 – 15 mg/cat (NOT mg/kg) PO 2 to 3 times daily. If using a sustained-release product, 30 – 45 mg/cat (NOT mg/kg) PO once daily.

HORSES:

Ventricular rate control in atrial fibrillation and interruption of nodal-dependent supraventricular tachyarrhythmias (extra-label): 0.125 mg/kg IV over 2 minutes, repeated every 10 minutes to effect, up to 1.25 mg/kg cumulative dose.[20]

FERRETS:

Hypertrophic cardiomyopathy (extra-label): 1.5 – 7.5 mg/kg PO every 12 hours[21]

SMALL MAMMALS (RABBITS, RODENTS):

Supraventricular tachyarrhythmias (extra-label): 0.5 – 1 mg/kg PO every 12 to 24 hours[22]

Monitoring

- Baseline and periodic heart rate, ECG, and blood pressure
- Adverse effects

Client Information

- Diltiazem is used in animals to treat heart rhythm problems and, in cats and ferrets, heart muscle disease.
- Be sure your animal receives all doses. It is important to not skip any treatments.
- This medicine may be given with or without food. If your animal vomits or acts sick after getting it on an empty stomach, give with food or small treat to see if this helps. If vomiting continues, contact your veterinarian.
- Common side effects include vomiting (cats), poor appetite, diarrhea, and a slowed heart rate.
- Your veterinarian will need to monitor your animal while they are receiving this medicine. Do not miss these important follow-up visits.
- Extended-release capsules may need to be opened and only a partial amount of the capsule contents administered per dose. Follow your veterinarian's instructions closely.

Chemistry/Synonyms

A benzothiazepine calcium channel blocker, diltiazem HCl occurs as a white to off-white crystalline powder with a bitter taste. It is soluble in water and alcohol. Potencies may be expressed in terms of base (active moiety) and the salt. Dosages are generally expressed in terms of the salt.

Diltiazem may also be known as CRD-401, diltiazemi hydrochloridum, latiazem hydrochloride, and MK-793; many trade names are available.

Storage/Stability

Diltiazem oral products should be stored at room temperature in tight, light-resistant containers.

The powder for injection should be stored between 15°C to 30°C (59°F-86°F). Discard 24 hours after reconstituting. Diltiazem solution for injection should be refrigerated at 2°C to 8°C (36°F-46°F). It may be stored at room temperature for up to one month but must be discarded after 30 days if stored in this manner; do not freeze.

Compatibility/Compounding Considerations

Compatibility is dependent on factors such as pH, concentration, temperature, and diluent used; specialized references or a hospital pharmacist should be consulted for more specific information.

Diltiazem is **compatible** with D5W and sodium chloride 0.9%, digoxin, bumetanide, dobutamine, dopamine, epinephrine, lidocaine, morphine, nitroglycerin, potassium chloride, sodium nitroprusside, and vasopressin. It is **incompatible** with diazepam, furosemide, phenytoin, and thiopental.

Dosage Forms/Regulatory Status

NOTE: Oral diltiazem is available in several human dosage forms, including different types of sustained-release products. There is only limited information available on the pharmacokinetics of these sustained-release products in dogs or cats.[6, 9, 23] There are multiple trade names and strengths, and 4 basic groups: immediate-release tablets, sustained-release capsules containing coated beads, sustained-release compressed tablets containing coated beads, and sustained-release capsules containing multiples of 60 mg pellets. Sustained-release products for use in small animals are most commonly reformulated (compounded) capsules using the coated beads or pellets – in some formulations (eg, *Dilacor XR*), clients should be advised to remove the pellets from the sustained-release capsule to provide the prescribed dosage if obtained from a human pharmacy (eg, the 240 mg capsules contain four 60 mg pellets; the dosage should be clearly defined, such as "*open capsule and administer one 60 mg pellet twice daily*" and not a 240 mg capsule). For cats, when using sustained-release capsules, compound capsules made from the coated beads, or ½ of a 60-mg pellet is preferred over the use of the sustained-release diltiazem tablets.

VETERINARY-LABELED PRODUCTS: NONE

The Association of Racing Commissioners International (ARCI) has designated this drug as a class 4 substance. See the ***Appendix*** for more information. Use of this drug may not be allowed in certain animal competitions. Check rules and regulations before entering in a competition while this medication is being administered. Contact local racing authorities for further guidance.

HUMAN-LABELED PRODUCTS:

Diltiazem Oral Tablets: 30 mg, 60 mg, 90 mg, and 120 mg; *Cardizem*®, generic; (Rx)

Diltiazem Tablets and Capsules Extended/Sustained Release: 60 mg, 90 mg, 120 mg, 180 mg, 240 mg, 300 mg, 360 mg, and 420 mg; *Cardizem CD*® and *LA*®, *Cartia XT*®, *Dilacor XR*®, *Dilt-XR*®, *Taztia XT*®, *Tiazac*®, generic; (Rx)

Diltiazem Injection: 5 mg/mL in 5 mL, 10 mL, and 25 mL vials; Powder for Injection: 25 mg in single-use containers (carton of 6 Lyo-Ject® syringes with diluent); *Cardizem*®, generic; (Rx)

References

For the complete list of references, see **wiley.com/go/budde/plumb**

Dimenhydrinate

(dye-men-***hye***-dri-nate) *Dramamine*®, *Gravol*®

Antihistamine; Antiemetic

Prescriber Highlights

- Antihistamine used primarily for prevention of motion sickness in dogs and as an antiemetic in dogs (less so in cats)
- Contraindications include hypersensitivity to it or others in its class. Caution: Angle closure glaucoma, GI or urinary obstruction, COPD, hyperthyroidism, seizure disorders, cardiovascular disease or hypertension; may mask clinical signs of ototoxicity
- Adverse effects include CNS depression and anticholinergic effects. GI effects (eg, diarrhea, vomiting, anorexia) are less common.

Uses/Indications

In veterinary medicine, dimenhydrinate is used primarily for its antiemetic effects and in the prophylactic treatment of motion sickness (eg, vestibular disease) in dogs. Because histamine is thought to not be an important mediator of vomiting in cats, other agents such as NK-1 antagonists (eg, maropitant) or M_1-cholinergic antagonists (eg, prochlorperazine, chlorpromazine, meclizine) may be better choices for treating motion sickness or vomiting in cats.[1]

Pharmacology/Actions

Dimenhydrinate has antihistaminic (H_1), antiemetic, anticholinergic, CNS depressant, and local anesthetic effects; it is a combination of diphenhydramine and 8-chlorotheophylline. These principal pharmacologic actions are thought to be a result of only the diphenhydramine moiety. Used most commonly for its antiemetic/motion sickness effects, dimenhydrinate's exact mechanism of action for this indication is unknown, but the drug does inhibit vestibular stimulation. The anticholinergic actions of dimenhydrinate may play a role in blocking acetylcholine stimulation of the vestibular and reticular systems. Tolerance to the CNS depressant effects can ensue after a few days of therapy and antiemetic effectiveness may also diminish with prolonged use.

In humans, the 8-chlorotheophylline component is intended to offset the sedating effect of diphenhydramine.

Pharmacokinetics

In beagles, oral bioavailability was 22% and peak diphenhydramine concentration (124 ng/mL) was reached 1 hour after administration.[1] C_{max} and bioavailability were ≈3 times higher with dimenhydrinate compared to an equivalent oral diphenhydramine dose. Diphenhydramine apparent volume of distribution was ≈180 L/kg and elimination half-life was 11.5 hours. An inactive metabolite (N-desmethyl diphenhydramine) is formed. 8-Chlorotheophyline peak concentration occurred 1.5 hours after administration, and elimination half-life was 21 hours.

In humans, the drug is well absorbed after oral administration, with antiemetic effects occurring within 30 minutes of administration. Antiemetic effects occur almost immediately after IV injection. The duration of effect is usually 3 to 6 hours. Diphenhydramine is metabolized in the liver, and the majority of the drug is excreted as metabolites into the urine. The terminal elimination half-life in adult humans ranges from 2.4 to 9.3 hours.

Contraindications/Precautions/Warnings

Dimenhydrinate is contraindicated in patients that are hypersensitive to it or to other antihistamines in its class. Because of their anticholinergic activity, antihistamines should be used with caution in patients with angle closure glaucoma, prostatic hypertrophy, pyloroduodenal or bladder neck obstruction, and COPD and asthma if mucosal secretions are a problem. Additionally, they should be used with caution in patients with hyperthyroidism, seizure disorders, cardiovascular disease, or hypertension. It may mask the clinical signs of ototoxicity[2] (eg, head tilt, hearing loss, ataxia) and should therefore be used with this knowledge when concomitantly administering ototoxic drugs.

The sedative effects of antihistamines may adversely affect the performance of working dogs.

In humans, pediatric patients are more susceptible to the adverse CNS effects of antihistamines, and it is recommended to avoid use in neonates.

Do not confuse dimenhyDRINATE with diphenhydrAMINE.

Adverse Effects

Most common adverse effects seen are CNS depression (eg, lethargy, somnolence) and anticholinergic effects (eg, dry mouth, urinary retention). GI effects (eg, diarrhea, vomiting, anorexia) are less common, but have been noted. Anecdotally, the sedative effects of antihistamines may diminish with time.

Because dimenhydrinate contains diphenhydramine, paradoxical excitement or agitation may occur in some animals (particularly cats).

Reproductive/Nursing Safety

Dimenhydrinate is the 8-chlorotheophylline salt of diphenhydramine. Diphenhydramine crosses the placenta. No evidence of impaired fertility, reproductive performance, or fetal harm have been noted in rats or rabbits.[2] Theophylline crosses the placenta and has been shown to reduce uterine contractions; relevance for 8-chlorotheophylline is uncertain.

Small amounts of dimenhydrinate are excreted in milk. Use is contraindicated in breastfeeding women, particularly those feeding neonates and/or premature infants. Theophylline is distributed into milk; relevance for 8-chlorotheophylline is uncertain.

Because safety has not been established in animals, this drug should only be used when the maternal benefits outweigh the potential risks to offspring.

Overdose/Acute Toxicity

Overdose may cause CNS stimulation (excitement to seizures) or depression (lethargy to coma), anticholinergic effects, respiratory depression, and death. Treatment consists of GI decontamination, including induction of emesis if the patient is alert and CNS status is stable. Administration of a saline cathartic and/or activated charcoal may be given after emesis or gastric lavage. Treatment of other clinical signs should be performed using symptomatic and supportive therapies.

For patients that have experienced or are suspected to have expe-

rienced an overdose, consultation with a 24-hour poison consultation center specializing in providing veterinary-specific information is recommended. For general information related to overdose and toxin exposures, as well as contact information for poison control centers, refer to ***Appendix.***

Drug Interactions

The following drug interactions have either been reported or are theoretical in humans or animals receiving dimenhydrinate and may be of significance in veterinary patients. Unless otherwise noted, use together is not necessarily contraindicated, but weigh the potential risks and perform additional monitoring when appropriate.

- **ANTICHOLINERGIC DRUGS** (eg, **atropine, glycopyrrolate**): Dimenhydrinate may potentiate the anticholinergic effects of other anticholinergic drugs.
- **CNS DEPRESSANT DRUGS**: Increased sedation can occur if dimenhydrinate is combined with other CNS depressant drugs.
- **MONOAMINE OXIDASE INHIBITORS (MAOIs**; eg, **amitraz, selegiline**): MAOIs may potentiate anticholinergic effects.
- **TRICYCLIC ANTIDEPRESSANTS (TCAs**; eg, **amitriptyline, clomipramine**): TCAs may potentiate anticholinergic effects.

Laboratory Considerations

- **Intradermal allergy testing (IDT)**: Whereas antihistamines may suppress IDT results,[3] dimenhydrinate did not demonstrate an effect on wheal formation despite reaching plasma diphenhydramine concentration believed to be therapeutic.[1]
- Dimenhydrinate may falsely elevate theophylline concentrations (see ***Chemistry/Synonyms***).

Dosages

DOGS/CATS:

Antiemetic/Antihistamine (particularly for prevention and treatment of motion sickness in dogs) (extra-label): 4 – 8 mg/kg PO, IM, IV every 8 hours.[4] When given IV, each 50 mg dimenhydrinate must be diluted with 10 mL 0.9% saline solution and administered over 2 minutes.[2]

Vomiting and nausea due to vestibular disease (extra-label): 25 – 50 mg/dog (NOT mg/kg) PO 3 times daily[2]

Monitoring

- Clinical efficacy
- Adverse effects (eg, sedation, anticholinergic signs)

Client Information

- Use only products that contain dimenhydrinate as a single active ingredient. Any other ingredients (eg, pain relievers, decongestants) found in human-label combination products can be toxic to animals.
- Antihistamine (related to diphenhydramine [*Benadryl*®]) that is used for prevention of motion sickness.
- When used for motion sickness, it is best to administer at least 30 to 60 minutes prior to travel.
- May cause drowsiness/sleepiness, which can be a beneficial effect when used to treat motion sickness.
- This medicine can be given on an empty stomach or with a small amount of food.

Chemistry/Synonyms

An ethanolamine derivative antihistamine, dimenhydrinate contains ≈54% diphenhydramine and ≈46% 8-chlorotheophylline. Hence, it is sometimes called "½ strength diphenhydramine." It occurs as an odorless, bitter-tasting and numbing, white crystalline powder with a melting range of 102°C to 107°C (215°F-225°F). Dimenhydrinate is slightly soluble in water and is freely soluble in propylene glycol or alcohol. The pH of the commercially available injection ranges from 6.4 to 7.2.

Dimenhydrinate may also be known as chloranautine, dimenhydrinatum, diphenhydramine teoclate, and diphenhydramine theoclate; many trade names are available, a common name is *Dramamine*®.

Storage/Stability

Dimenhydrinate products should be stored at room temperature 20°C to 25°C (68°F-77°F); avoid freezing of oral and injectable solutions. Store tablets in air-tight containers.

Compatibility/Compounding Considerations

Dimenhydrinate injection is reportedly physically **compatible** with all commonly used IV replenishment solutions and the following drugs: amikacin sulfate, atropine sulfate, calcium gluconate, chloramphenicol sodium succinate, corticotropin, diphenhydramine HCl, fentanyl citrate, ketamine, metoclopramide, morphine sulfate, norepinephrine bitartrate, oxytetracycline HCl, penicillin G potassium, phenobarbital sodium, scopolamine HBr, vancomycin HCl, and vitamin B complex with vitamin C.

The following drugs are either physically **incompatible** or **compatible only in certain concentrations** with dimenhydrinate: aminophylline, ammonium chloride, midazolam, oxytocin, pantoprazole sodium, pentobarbital sodium, prochlorperazine edisylate, potassium chloride, promazine HCl, promethazine HCl, and tetracycline HCl.

Compatibility is dependent upon factors such as pH, concentration, temperature, and diluent used; consult a hospital pharmacist or specialized references for more specific information.

Dosage Forms/Regulatory Status

VETERINARY-LABELED PRODUCTS: NONE

HUMAN-LABELED PRODUCTS:

Dimenhydrinate Oral Tablets: 50 mg (regular and chewable); *Dramamine*®, *Driminate*®, *Travtabs*®, *Triptone*®, generic; (OTC)

Dimenhydrinate Injection: 50 mg/mL in 1 mL and 10 mL vials; generic; (Rx). Some preparations may contain benzyl alcohol and propylene glycol.

References

For the complete list of references, see **wiley.com/go/budde/plumb**

Dimercaprol (BAL)

(dye-mer-***kap***-role) *BAL in Oil*®

Heavy Metal Chelator

Prescriber Highlights

- ▶ Chelating agent for arsenicals; less frequently used for lead, mercury, and gold compounds
- ▶ Contraindications include patients with impaired hepatic function (unless secondary to acute arsenic toxicosis), and iron, cadmium, or selenium toxicosis.
- ▶ Use caution in patients with impaired renal function.
- ▶ Adverse effects are usually transient and may include vomiting, seizures with higher dosages, increased blood pressure, and tachycardia. Injection site pain may occur; injecting deeply IM may decrease this.
- ▶ Alkalinize urine to ensure optimal clearance of chelated compound.

Uses/Indications

The principal use of dimercaprol in veterinary medicine is to treat intoxications caused by arsenical compounds. Due to the risk for nephrotoxicity, succimer is preferred in small animals and sodium thiosulfate in large animals.[1] Dimercaprol has historically been used for the treatment of lead (with edetate calcium disodium [CaEDTA]), mercury, and gold intoxication although use has waned with development of safer chelators.

Pharmacology/Actions

Sulfhydryl groups found on dimercaprol form heterocyclic ring complexes with heavy metals, principally arsenic, lead, mercury, and gold. This binding prevents or reduces heavy metal binding to sulfhydryl-dependent enzymes. Different metals have differing affinities for both dimercaprol and sulfhydryl-dependent enzymes and the drug is relatively ineffective in chelating some metals (eg, selenium). Chelation to dimercaprol is reversible as metals can dissociate from the complex when dimercaprol concentrations decrease, as in an acidic environment or with oxidation. The dimercaprol-metal complex is excreted via renal and fecal routes.

Pharmacokinetics

After IM injection, peak serum/plasma concentrations occur in 30 to 60 minutes. Dimercaprol is slowly absorbed through the skin after topical administration.

Dimercaprol is distributed throughout the body, including the brain. The highest tissue concentrations are found in the liver and kidneys.

Non-metal bound drug is rapidly metabolized to inactive compounds and excreted in the urine, bile, and feces. The duration of action in humans is ≈4 hours with complete drug elimination within 6 to 24 hours.

Contraindications/Precautions/Warnings

Dimercaprol is contraindicated in patients with impaired hepatic function, unless secondary to acute arsenic toxicosis. The drug is also contraindicated in iron, cadmium, and selenium toxicosis, as the chelated complex can be more toxic than the metal alone, nor is it recommended for methylmercury intoxication due to redistribution of mercury to the brain.[2]

Because dimercaprol is potentially nephrotoxic, it should be used cautiously with impaired renal function. To protect the kidneys, the urine should be alkalinized to prevent chelated drug from dissociating in urine. Animals with diminished renal function, or that develop renal dysfunction during therapy, should have the dosage adjusted or discontinue therapy dependent on the clinical situation.

Some dosage forms may contain benzyl alcohol as a preservative. In human newborns, drug formulations containing benzyl alcohol and derivatives should be used with caution as they can potentially displace bilirubin from protein binding sites.

Adverse Effects

Injection site pain may occur, particularly if not administered deeply IM[3]; other injection sites reactions (eg, hematoma) are possible. Most systemic adverse effects are transient in nature as the drug is eliminated rapidly. Transient increases in blood pressure with concomitant tachycardia have been reported.[4] Vomiting and seizures can occur with higher dosages. In humans, the frequency of adverse effects is related to the dose and frequency of administration.

Dimercaprol is potentially nephrotoxic.

Reproductive/Nursing Safety

Safe use of dimercaprol during pregnancy has not been determined. It is unknown if dimercaprol is excreted in milk.

Because safety has not been established in animals, this drug should only be used when the maternal benefits outweigh the potential risks to offspring.

Overdose/Acute Toxicity

Clinical signs of dimercaprol overdose in animals include vomiting, seizures, tremors, coma, and death. No specific doses were located to correspond with these clinical signs in veterinary species.

For patients that have experienced or are suspected to have experienced an overdose, consultation with a 24-hour poison consultation center specializing in providing veterinary-specific information is recommended. For general information related to overdose and toxin exposures, as well as contact information for poison control centers, refer to ***Appendix***.

Drug Interactions

The following drug interactions have either been reported or are theoretical in humans or animals receiving dimercaprol and may be of significance in veterinary patients. Unless otherwise noted, use together is not necessarily contraindicated, but weigh the potential risks and perform additional monitoring when appropriate.

- **IRON** or **SELENIUM**: Because dimercaprol forms a toxic complex with certain metals (**cadmium, selenium, uranium, iron**), do not administer with iron or selenium salts. Wait 24 hours after the last dimercaprol dose before starting iron or selenium therapy.

Laboratory Considerations

- **Iodine[131] thyroidal uptake** values may be decreased during or immediately following dimercaprol therapy as dimercaprol interferes with normal iodine accumulation by the thyroid.[5]

Dosages

DOGS & CATS:

Note: It is highly recommended to contact an animal poison center before treating heavy metal poisonings.

Arsenic toxicosis (extra-label)[6]: 2.5 – 5 mg/kg IM every 4 hours for the first 2 days of treatment and then every 12 hours until recovery. 5 mg/kg doses are typically only given on the first day of treatment and only to acutely affected patients. Provide aggressive supportive therapy if indicated.

RUMINANTS:

Arsenic, lead, or mercury toxicosis (extra-label): 2.5 – 5 mg/kg IM every 4 hours for 2 days. Withdrawal information is not available in food animals. Efficacy is questionable unless dimercaprol is given before signs appear or very early in the clinical course. FDA has not exempted this drug for compounding from bulk supplies.[5]

HORSES:

Arsenic toxicosis (extra-label): 5 mg/kg IM initially, followed by 3 mg/kg IM every 6 hours for the remainder of the first day, then 1 mg/kg IM every 6 hours for 2 or more additional days, as needed. Dimercaprol therapy in horses is challenging because of the large amounts of dimercaprol that are required, the necessity to inject the drug IM, and the requirement to administer it as soon as possible after exposure because any substantial delays in treatment significantly decrease its effectiveness.[7]

Monitoring

- Liver enzymes
- BUN, Creatinine
- CBC
- Hydration and cardiovascular status
- Electrolytes and acid/base status
- Urine pH

Client Information

- Dimercaprol should only be used with close professional supervision due to the potential toxicity of this agent and the seriousness of most heavy metal intoxications.
- Dimercaprol can cause bad breath.

Chemistry/Synonyms

A dithiol chelating agent, dimercaprol occurs as a colorless or nearly colorless, viscous liquid that is soluble in alcohol, vegetable oils, and water, but unstable in aqueous solutions. It has a disagreeable mercaptan-like odor. The commercially available injection is a peanut oil and benzyl benzoate solution. The solution may be turbid or contain small amounts of flocculent material or sediment, this does not mean that the solution is deteriorating.

Dimercaprol may also be known as BAL, British Anti-Lewisite, dimercaptopropanol, dithioglycerol dimercaprolum, *BAL in Oil®*, or *Sulfactin Homburg®*.

Storage/Stability

Dimercaprol injection should be stored below 40°C (104°F); preferably at room temperature (15°C-30°C [59°F-86°F]).

Compatibility/Compounding Considerations

Dimercaprol is not on the FDA's GFI #256 list of drugs allowed to be compounded from bulk supplies.[8]

Dosage Forms/Regulatory Status

VETERINARY-LABELED PRODUCTS: NONE

HUMAN-LABELED PRODUCTS:

Dimercaprol Injection: 100 mg/mL (10%); (for IM use only) in 3 mL amps, *BAL in Oil®*; (Rx)

References

For the complete list of references, see **wiley.com/go/budde/plumb**

Dimethyl Sulfoxide

(dye-***meth***-el sul-***fox***-ide) *Domoso®*

Free Radical Scavenger

Prescriber Highlights

- Free radical scavenger that has anti-inflammatory, cryopreservative, anti-ischemic, and radioprotective effects
- Use with caution in patients with mast cell tumors, dehydration, and shock; may mask existing pathology
- May cause localized burning when administered topically
- Administer IV to horses slowly and at concentrations of ≈10%; may occasionally cause diarrhea, tremors, and colic.
- Handle cautiously; will be absorbed through skin and can carry toxic compounds across skin. Use of impervious gloves is recommended.
- Strong, offensive odor may be an issue.

Uses/Indications

The purported uses for dimethyl sulfoxide (DMSO) are rampant, but the only FDA-approved veterinary indication for DMSO is as a topical application to reduce acute swelling due to trauma.[1] Other possible indications for DMSO include adjunctive treatment in transient ischemic conditions; CNS trauma and cerebral edema; calcinosis cutis; endometritis; skin ulcers; wounds; burns; adjunctive therapy in intestinal surgeries; analgesia for postoperative or intractable pain; amyloidosis in dogs; reduction of mammary engorgement in the nursing bitch; enhancement of antibiotic penetration in mastitis in cattle; treatment of cyclophosphamide-induced hemorrhagic cystitis in dogs[2]; and limitation of tissue damage following extravasation injuries secondary to chemotherapeutic agents.[3] DMSO plus calcium chloride intratesticular injections have been used for chemical castration in dogs and cats.[4,5]

Although the potential indications for DMSO are many, the lack of well-controlled studies leaves many more questions than answers regarding this drug.

Pharmacology/Actions

The pharmacologic effects of dimethyl sulfoxide (DMSO) are diverse. DMSO traps free radical hydroxide, and its metabolite (dimethyl sulfide [DMS]) traps free radical oxygen. It appears that these actions help to explain some of the anti-inflammatory, cryopreservative, anti-ischemic, and radioprotective qualities of DMSO.

DMSO easily penetrates the skin. It serves as a carrier agent in promoting the percutaneous absorption of other compounds (including drugs and toxins) that normally would not penetrate. Drugs such as insulin, heparin, phenylbutazone, and sulfonamides may all be absorbed systemically when they are mixed with DMSO and applied to the skin. DMSO has been shown to increase the rate of oral absorption of the triazine antiprotozoal drugs, diclazuril, and toltrazuril in horses.[6]

DMSO has weak antibacterial activity and possibly has some clinical efficacy as an antifungal when it is used topically. The mechanism for these antimicrobial effects has not been elucidated.

The anti-inflammatory/analgesic properties of DMSO have been thoroughly investigated. DMSO appears to be more effective as an anti-inflammatory agent when it is used for acute inflammation versus chronic inflammatory conditions. The analgesic effects of DMSO have been compared with those produced by narcotic analgesics. It can be efficacious for both acute and chronic musculoskeletal pain.

DMSO decreases platelet aggregation, but reports regarding its effects on coagulability and the myocardium have been conflicting. DMSO has diuretic activity independent of the method of administration. It provokes histamine release from mast cells, which likely contributes to the local vasodilatory effects seen after topical administration.

DMSO also apparently has some anticholinesterase activity and enhances prostaglandin E, but blocks the synthesis of prostaglandins E_2, F_2-alpha, H_2, and G_2. DMSO inhibits the enzyme alcohol dehydrogenase, which is responsible for not only the metabolism of alcohol, but also the metabolism of ethylene glycol into toxic metabolites.

Pharmacokinetics

Dimethyl sulfoxide (DMSO) is well absorbed after topical administration, especially at concentrations between 80% and 100%. It is extensively and rapidly distributed to virtually every area of the body. After IV administration to horses, the serum half-life is ≈9 hours. In dogs, the elimination half-life is ≈1.5 days. DMSO is metabolized to dimethyl sulfide (DMS) and primarily excreted by the kidneys, although biliary and respiratory excretion also takes place.

In cattle, the drug is eliminated quite rapidly and after 20 days, no detectable drug or metabolites are found in milk, urine, blood, or tissues.

Contraindications/Precautions/Warnings

Wear impervious gloves when applying dimethyl sulfoxide (DMSO) topically and apply this product with clean or sterile cotton to minimize the chances for contamination with potentially harmful substances. Only apply this product to clean, dry areas, to avoid carrying other chemicals into the systemic circulation. Do not apply DMSO topically mixed with compounds (eg, heavy metals) that could be toxic if absorbed systemically.[7] The topical DMSO application site should be dry before other topical medications or treatments are applied to that area.

DMSO may mask existing pathology with its anti-inflammatory and analgesic activity.

Because DMSO may degranulate mast cells, animals with mast cell tumors should only receive DMSO with extreme caution. DMSO should be used cautiously in animals that are suffering from dehydration or shock, as its diuretic and peripheral vasodilatory effects may exacerbate these conditions.

Because DMSO is absorbed transdermally and may carry with it potentially toxic chemicals into the systemic circulation, it is recommended that staff and caregivers wear impervious gloves while handling DMSO products.

Adverse Effects

When dimethyl sulfoxide (DMSO) is used as labeled, it appears to be an extremely safe drug. Local effects (burning, erythema, vesiculation, dry skin, local allergic reactions) and garlic or oyster-like breath odor are the most likely adverse effects. These effects are transient and quickly resolve when therapy is discontinued. Lenticular changes, which may result in myopia, have been noted, primarily in dogs and rabbits, when DMSO is used chronically at high doses. These effects are slowly reversible after the drug is discontinued.

When DMSO is administered IV to horses, it may cause hemolysis and hemoglobinuria. Although older dosage references often recommended concentrations of 20% or less for IV use in horses, 10% solutions, which are likely safer, are more commonly recommended today.[8] Slow IV administration may reduce adverse effects. Other adverse effects can include diarrhea, muscle tremors, and colic.

Hepatotoxicity and renal toxicity have been reported for various species and dosages. These conditions occur fairly rarely, and some clinicians actually believe DMSO has a protective effect on is chemically insulted renal tissue.

Reproductive/Nursing Safety

At high doses, dimethyl sulfoxide (DMSO) has been shown to be teratogenic in hamsters, mice, rats, and rabbits[9]; weigh the risks versus benefits when using in pregnant animals.

It is not known whether this drug is excreted in milk; use in nursing dams with caution.

Because safety has not been established in animals, this drug should only be used when the maternal benefits outweigh the potential risks to offspring.

Overdose/Acute Toxicity

The reported LD_{50} following IV dosage is ≈200 mg/kg in cats and ≈2.5 g/kg in dogs.[10] Signs of toxicity include sedation and hematuria at non-lethal doses; coma, seizures, opisthotonus, dyspnea, and pulmonary edema at higher dosages. Should an acute overdose be encountered, treat the patient supportively.

For patients that have experienced or are suspected to have experienced an overdose, consultation with a 24-hour poison consultation center specializing in providing veterinary-specific information is recommended. For general information related to overdose and toxin exposures, as well as contact information for poison control centers, refer to ***Appendix.***

Drug Interactions

The following drug interactions either have been reported or are theoretical in humans or animals receiving DMSO and may be of significance in veterinary patients. Unless otherwise noted, use together is not necessarily contraindicated, but weigh the potential risks and perform additional monitoring when appropriate.

- **Alcohol**: Effects may be potentiated by dimethyl sulfoxide (DMSO).
- **Atropine**: Effects may be potentiated by DMSO.
- **Corticosteroids**: Effects may be potentiated by DMSO.
- **Insulin**: Effects may be potentiated by DMSO.
- **Organophosphates** (or other cholinesterase inhibitors): Avoid use with DMSO.

Dosages

DOGS:

Reduce acute swelling due to trauma (label dosage; FDA-approved): Apply topically to the skin over the affected area 3 to 4 times daily.[11] Total daily dosage should not exceed 20 g (or mL of liquid) and therapy should not exceed 14 days.

Calcinosis cutis (extra-label): Clinical recommendations generally are to treat each lesion with topical dimethyl sulfoxide (DMSO; gel is preferred if available) once daily. If there are many sites, or a large area is involved, treat ⅓ of the lesions (or ⅓ of the affected areas) each day. There are differing recommendations to 1) either rotate these sites each day, or 2) add new treatment areas as the treated sites improve. Dogs reportedly appear ill if large areas are treated initially, but usually do not become hypercalcemic. Wear impervious gloves when applying. Treatment may require several weeks and not all cases resolve. Most clinicians recommend periodic monitoring of serum calcium.

Bladder instillation to treat persistent cases of hemorrhagic cystitis (secondary to cyclophosphamide treatment): 10 mL of DMSO medical-grade 50% solution is diluted with 10 mL of water and instilled into bladder and removed after 20 minutes.[2]

Doxorubicin extravasation: See the ***Doxorubicin*** monograph for more information.

HORSES:

Reduce acute swelling due to trauma; topical application (label dosage; FDA-approved): Liberal application should be administered topically to the skin over the affected area 2 to 3 times daily.[11] Total daily dosage should not exceed 100 g (or mL of liquid) and therapy should not exceed 30 days.

Anti-inflammatory/hydroxyl radical scavenger (IV administration) (extra-label): 0.5 – 2 g/kg via slow IV infusion as a 10% solution (diluted in a polyionic solution) every 12 to 24 hours.[8] **NOTE**: Although DMSO has been used IV for many years in horses for a variety of purposes, actual evidence demonstrating its efficacy is slim.

Chronic endometritis; abnormal mucous (extra-label): 30% solution as an intrauterine infusion daily; up to 5 days during estrus. To prepare a 30% solution using 90% DMSO, 33 mL of a 90% DMSO solution is added to 64 mL of sterile saline.[12]

Monitoring

- Efficacy
- Check for hemoglobinuria with urinalysis
- Hematocrit, if indicated
- Ophthalmic examinations with high dosages or chronic use in dogs

Client Information

- Use only medical-grade dimethyl sulfoxide (DMSO), as other products may contain harmful impurities.
- Wear rubber gloves when applying this medicine topically. Use medicine in well-ventilated area; avoid inhalation and contact with eyes.
- Apply with clean or sterile cotton to reduce chances for contaminating DMSO with other substances. Apply only to clean, dry skin.
- Do not mix DMSO with other drugs or chemicals without your veterinarian's approval. Keep the lid tightly closed on the container when the medicine is not in use.
- DMSO can cause garlic or oyster-like breath odor or local skin reactions.

Chemistry/Synonyms

Dimethyl sulfoxide (DMSO) is a clear, colorless to straw-yellow liquid. It is dipolar, aprotic (acts as a Lewis base) and extremely hygroscopic. It has a melting/freezing point of 18.5°C (65.3°F), boiling point of 189°C (372.2°F), and a molecular weight of 78.1. It is miscible with water (heat is produced), alcohol, acetone, chloroform, ether, and many organic solvents. A 2.15% solution in water is isotonic with serum.

Dimethyl sulfoxide may also be known as dimethyl sulphoxide, dimethylis sulfoxidum, DMSO, methyl sulphoxide, NSC-763, SQ-9453, sulfonylbismethane, *Domoso®*, *Kemsol®*, *Rheumabene®*, *Rimso®*, or *Synotic®*.

Storage/Stability

This product must be stored in airtight containers away from light. As dimethyl sulfoxide (DMSO) may react with some plastics, it should be stored in glass or in the container provided by the manufacturer. If DMSO is allowed to contact room air it will self-dilute to a concentration of 66% to 67%.

Compatibility/Compounding Considerations

Dimethyl sulfoxide (DMSO) is compatible with many compounds, but because of the chances for accidental percutaneous absorption of potentially toxic compounds, the admixing of DMSO with other compounds is not to be done casually.

Dosage Forms/Regulatory Status

VETERINARY APPROVED PRODUCTS:

Dimethyl Sulfoxide Veterinary Gel 90%: *Domoso® Gel* 90% (medical grade) in 60 g and 120 g tubes, and 425 g containers. FDA-approved (NADA #47-925) for use in dogs and horses. Do not administer to horses that are to be used for food.

Dimethyl Sulfoxide Veterinary Solution 90%: *Domoso® Solution* 90% (medical grade) in 1 pint and 1 gallon bottles. FDA-approved (NADA #32-168) for use in canines and equines. Do not administer to horses that are to be used for food. Marketing status is uncertain.

Dimethyl Sulfoxide Veterinary Solution: 99% in 1 pint and 1 gallon bottles; generic. Not FDA-approved

The Association of Racing Commissioners International (ARCI) has designated this drug as a class 5 substance. Use of this drug may not be allowed in certain animal competitions. Check rules and regulations before entering in a competition while this medication is being administered. Contact local racing authorities for further guidance. See the ***Appendix*** for more information.

NOTE: Topical otic products, *Synotic®* that contains DMSO 60% and fluocinolone acetonide 0.01% and *Synsac®*, which is DMSO 20% and fluocinolone 0.01%, are also available for veterinary use. Supplied in 8 mL and 60 mL dropper bottles.

HUMAN APPROVED PRODUCTS:

Dimethyl Sulfoxide Solution: 50% aqueous solution in 50 mL; *Rimso-50®*; (Rx)

References

For the complete list of references, see **wiley.com/go/budde/plumb**

Diminazene

(dye-***min***-ah-zeen) *Berenil® RTU*

Antiprotozoal

Prescriber Highlights

- Antiprotozoal agent used in several species for trypanosomiasis, babesiosis, or cytauxzoonosis
- Usually administered once; repeat doses may increase risk for toxicity
- Available in several countries, but not in United States

Uses/Indications

Diminazene is used to treat trypanosomiasis in dogs and livestock (eg, sheep, goats, cattle), *Babesia* spp infections in dogs and horses, cytauxzoonosis and babesiosis in cats, and leishmaniasis in humans. A prospective, unmasked study in dogs with *Babesia gibsoni* infection comparing atovaquone/azithromycin (AA) with a protocol using clindamycin, diminazene, and imidocarb (CDI) found that CDI had higher recovery and lower relapse rates, albeit longer therapy duration and slower reduction in parasite numbers, than AA. The authors concluded that CDI was effective for initial therapy and when the *M121I* gene in *B gibsoni* had mutated.[1] A study in naturally infected cats with chronic *Cytauxzoon felis* parasitemia found no difference in parasite burden between diminazene (3 mg/kg IM; 2 doses 7 days apart) and placebo-treated cats.[2] A dose-intensified treatment (diminazene 4 mg/kg IM once daily for 5 consecutive days) failed to reduce parasite burden and was accompanied by frequent side effects.[3]

Diminazene is not commercially available in the United States but is available and used in many countries.

Pharmacology/Actions

Diminazene's exact mechanism of action is not well understood. With *Babesia* spp, it is thought to interfere with aerobic glycolysis and DNA synthesis.

Diminazene may not completely eradicate the organism, but, because it is slowly metabolized, suppression of recurring clinical signs or prophylaxis can be attained for several weeks after a single dose.

Pharmacokinetics

Diminazene's pharmacokinetics have been investigated in several species. The drug is rapidly absorbed and distributed after IM administration in target species studied. High concentrations can be found in the liver and kidney. The drug appears to enter the CSF but at concentrations significantly lower than that found in plasma in healthy animals. CSF concentrations are higher in dogs infected with African trypanosomiasis, probably due to meningeal inflammation. Diminazene apparently is metabolized somewhat in the liver, but identification of these metabolites and whether they possess antiprotozoal activity is not known.

Reported elimination half-lives are widely variable. Values range from 5 to 30 hours in dogs, goats, and sheep to over 200 hours in one study for cattle. Elimination half-life in cats is short, with an average of ≈1.7 hours.[4] Differences in assay methodology and study design may account for some of this variation, but even within one individual study in dogs using a modern assay (HPLC), wide interpatient variability was noted.

Contraindications/Precautions/Warnings

Camels appear highly susceptible to the toxic effects of diminazene, and product labels[5] may state the drug is contraindicated in camelids.

CNS toxic effects in dogs may be associated with cumulative dosages of diminazene, and repeated dosing must be carefully considered. One reference states, *the dose cannot be repeated with this or another diaminidine-derivative within a 6-week period.*[6,7]

Adverse Effects

At usual dosages in domestic livestock, diminazene is reportedly relatively free of adverse effects. Adverse effects associated with therapeutic dosages of diminazene in dogs may include vomiting and diarrhea, pain and swelling at the injection site, and transient decreases in blood pressure. Very rarely (less than 0.1%), ataxia, seizures, or death have been reported.

Reproductive/Nursing Safety

Little information is available. Rats given diminazene up to 1 g/kg PO on days 8 to 15 demonstrated no teratogenic effects, but decreased body weights and increased resorptions were noted at the highest dose.

Diminazene is distributed into milk; safety for nursing offspring has not been established.

Because safety has not been established in animals, this drug should only be used when the maternal benefits outweigh the potential risks to offspring.

Overdose/Acute Toxicity

Little information is available. Diminazene appears most toxic in dogs and camels. Dosages greater than 7 mg/kg can be very toxic to camels; dosages above 10 mg/kg IM in dogs can cause severe GI, respiratory, nervous system, or musculoskeletal effects.

For patients that have experienced or are suspected to have experienced an overdose, consultation with a 24-hour poison consultation center specializing in providing veterinary-specific information is recommended. For general information related to overdose and toxin exposures, as well as contact information for poison control centers, refer to ***Appendix.***

Drug Interactions

- No significant drug interactions were identified.

Laboratory Considerations

- No issues were noted.

Dosages

NOTE: There is a multitude of protozoal diseases worldwide that may respond to diminazene. Depending on the infective agent and species of the patient treated, there may be local specific recommendations for treatment and prevention. The following should be used as general guidelines only.

DOGS:

***Babesia* spp infections** (extra-label):

a) Large or small *Babesia* spp (extra-label): 3.5 mg/kg IM once. Variable efficacy and unpredictable toxicity (CNS signs may be severe)[8]

b) Babesiosis when the *M121I* gene in *Babesia gibsoni* has mutated (based on a prospective, unmasked study): Clindamycin 30 mg/kg PO every 12 hours with diminazene aceturate 3.5 mg/kg IM once on the day of presentation and imidocarb dipropionate 6 mg/kg SC once on the day after the diminazene was administered[1]

African trypanosomiasis (extra-label): 3.6 – 7 mg/kg IM every 2 weeks as needed to control relapse or reinfection[9,10]

HORSES, CATTLE, SHEEP, GOATS:

Susceptible protozoal (trypanosomes, *Babesia* spp) infections (extra-label): 3.5 mg/kg IM once. In some jurisdictions the label states that, depending on susceptibility, the dose can be increased to 8 mg/kg. See ***Overdose/Acute Toxicity***. Regardless of the dosage used, do not exceed 4 grams total dose per animal.[5,11]

RABBITS:

***Trypanosoma evansi* infections** (extra-label): 3.5 mg/kg IM[12]

Monitoring

- For *Babesia* spp infections in dogs, monitoring should include surveillance for potential adverse effects of diminazene and signs of clinical efficacy, including baseline and periodic CBCs. Severe cases may have elevated BUN or liver enzymes and hypokalemia.
- Current recommendation for determining clearing of the organism (*Babesia gibsoni*) is to perform a PCR test at 60 and 90 days posttherapy.

Client Information

- Clients should understand that depending on the species treated, parasites may not be completely eradicated and that retreatment may be required.

Chemistry/Synonyms

Diminazene aceturate is an aromatic diamidine derivative chemically related to pentamidine. One gram of diminazene is soluble in ≈14 mL of water and it is slightly soluble in alcohol.

Diminazene aceturate may also be known as diminazene diaceturate or diminazeno; many international trade names are available.

Storage/Stability

Read and follow label directions for storage and preparation of each product used; diminazene powder, granules, or packets for reconstitution for injection should generally be stored in a dry, cool place out of direct sunlight. Once reconstituted, the solution's stability is temperature dependent: up to 14 days when refrigerated, up to 5 days at 20°C (68°F) and only for 24 hours at temperatures above 50°C (122°F).

Compatibility/Compounding Considerations

No specific information noted

Dosage Forms/Regulatory Status

VETERINARY-LABELED PRODUCTS: NONE IN THE UNITED STATES

Diminazene aceturate is available in many countries either alone or in combination products (eg, with antipyrine), with the following trade names: *Azidin®*, *Berenil®* RTU, *Dimesol®*, *Demin®*, *Diminicin RTU®*, *Veriben®*, or *Veriben® B12 LA.*

Withdrawal times may vary depending on the product, dosage, and the country where it is used; check local regulations.

HUMAN-LABELED PRODUCTS: NONE

References

For the complete list of references, see **wiley.com/go/budde/plumb**

Dinoprost

Prostaglandin F2-alpha

(***dye***-noe-prost) *Lutalyse®*

Prostaglandin

Prescriber Highlights

- Naturally occurring prostaglandin F2alpha used as a luteolytic agent for estrus induction and synchronization, pyometra treatment, and parturition induction; also used as an abortifacient
- Contraindicated during pregnancy (when abortion or induced parturition are not wanted). Dinoprost has been associated with serious toxicity and death in camelids.
- Do not administer IV; use with extreme caution in elderly or debilitated animals.
- Adverse effects in dogs and cats include abdominal pain, emesis, defecation, urination, pupillary dilation followed by constriction, tachycardia, restlessness, anxiety, fever, hypersalivation, dyspnea, and panting; death is possible (especially in dogs).
- Adverse effects in cattle include infection at injection site, salivation, and hyperthermia.
- Adverse effects in swine include erythema, pruritus, urination, defecation, mild ataxia, hyperpnea, dyspnea, nesting behavior, abdominal muscle spasms, tail movements, increased vocalization, and salivation.
- Adverse effects in horses include body temperature changes and/or sweating. Less frequent effects include increased respiratory and heart rates, ataxia, abdominal pain, and lying down; more adverse effects are observed with prostaglandin F2alpha than with cloprostenol.
- The National Institute for Occupational Safety and Health (NIOSH) classifies dinoprost as a hazardous drug; use appropriate precautions when handling.
- Pregnant women should not handle dinoprost; humans with asthma and women of childbearing age should handle with caution.

Uses/Indications

Dinoprost (ie, prostaglandin F2alpha; PGF2alpha) is a luteolytic agent labeled for use in cattle for treatment of estrus synchronization, unobserved (ie, silent) estrus in lactating dairy cattle, pyometra, and abortion in feedlot and nonlactating dairy cattle. This drug is labeled in swine to act as a parturient-inducing agent. Dinoprost is labeled for use in cycling mares as a luteolytic agent to control the time of estrus and to assist in inducing estrus in mares that are difficult to breed.

In small animals, dinoprost is used extra-label as an abortifacient agent and as adjunctive medical therapy treatment for pyometra. Combination therapies (eg, dinoprost with cabergoline) allow lower doses of dinoprost to be used, reducing or eliminating GI adverse effects that may occur when dinoprost is used alone.

Although dinoprost is not FDA-approved, it is also used in sheep and goat reproductive medicine.

A review of the evidence for the therapeutic efficiency of antibiotics and dinoprost in postpartum dairy cows with clinical endometritis concluded that no scientific evidence supports the effectiveness of dinoprost as a treatment for clinical endometritis in postpartum dairy cows.[1]

Pharmacology/Actions

Dinoprost has several pharmacologic effects on the female reproductive system, including stimulation of myometrial activity, relaxation of the cervix, and inhibition of steroidogenesis by corpora lutea. Dinoprost can potentially lyse corpora lutea.

Pharmacokinetics

In studies done in rodents, dinoprost was demonstrated to distribute very rapidly into tissues after injection. In cattle, the serum half-life of dinoprost has been stated to be only minutes long.[2]

Contraindications/Precautions/Warnings

Unless dinoprost is being used as an abortifacient or to induce parturition, it should not be used in any species during pregnancy. Dinoprost is contraindicated in animals with bronchoconstrictive respiratory disease (eg, asthma, recurrent airway obstruction [RAO] in horses). This drug should not be administered IV.

According to the manufacturer, dinoprost is contraindicated in mares with acute or subacute disorders of the vascular system, GI tract, respiratory system, or reproductive tract.

Dinoprost should be used with extreme caution, if at all, in dogs or cats older than 8 years of age or with pre-existing cardiopulmonary or other serious disease (eg, liver, kidney, sepsis, peritonitis). Some clinicians regard closed-cervix pyometra as a relative contraindication to the use of dinoprost.

Dinoprost has been associated with acute toxicity and death in camelids.

The National Institute for Occupational Safety and Health (NIOSH) classifies the human-labeled drug dinoprostone as a hazardous drug; personal protective equipment (PPE) should be used accordingly to minimize the risk of exposure.[3] Dinoprost should be handled in the same manner as dinoprostone. It has been recommended that dinoprost should not be dispensed for client administration due to the risk of adverse effects in the patient as well as the risk associated with potential human exposure.[4]

Adverse Effects

Bacterial infections at the injection site and limited salivation have been reported. If administered IV, increased heart rates have been noted.

In mares, transient decreased body (rectal) temperature and sweating are most often reported. Less frequently, increased respiratory and heart rates, ataxia, abdominal pain, and lying down have also been noted. These effects are generally seen within 15 minutes of administration and resolve within 1 hour.

In swine, dinoprost has caused erythema and pruritus, urination, defecation, slight ataxia, hyperpnea, dyspnea, nesting behavior, abdominal muscle spasms, tail movements, increased vocalization, and salivation. Although these effects may last up to 3 hours, they are not detrimental to the animal.

In dogs and cats, dinoprost can cause abdominal pain, emesis, defecation, urination, pupillary dilation followed by constriction, tachycardia, restlessness, anxiety, fever, hypersalivation, dyspnea, and panting. Cats may also exhibit increased vocalization and intense grooming behavior. Severity of effects is generally dose dependent. Defecation can be seen with very low doses. Signs generally appear 5 to 120 minutes after administration and may persist for 20 to 30 minutes. Death has occurred (especially in dogs) after receiving this drug. Dogs and cats should be monitored for cardiorespiratory effects, especially after receiving higher doses.

When used as an abortifacient in humans, dinoprost causes nausea, vomiting, and diarrhea in ≈50% of patients.

Reproductive/Nursing Safety

Pregnancy status should be determined prior to use. Unless being used as an abortifacient or parturition inducer, dinoprost should not be used in any species during pregnancy. In swine, dinoprost should not be administered prior to 3 days of normal predicted farrowing, as increased neonatal mortality may result.

Because safety has not been established in nursing animals, this drug should only be used when the maternal benefits outweigh the potential risks to offspring.

Overdose/Acute Toxicity

Dogs are apparently more sensitive to the toxic effects of dinoprost than are other species. The LD_{50} in the bitch has been reported as 5.13 mg/kg after SC injection,[5] which may be only 5 times greater than the recommended dosage given by some clinicians.

Increased body temperature has been reported when dinoprost is administered to cattle in overdose quantities (5-10 times recommended doses). Vomiting may be seen in swine given 10 times the recommended dosage. In any species, if clinical signs are severe and require treatment, supportive therapy is recommended.

For patients that have experienced or are suspected to have experienced an overdose, it is strongly encouraged to consult with one of the 24-hour poison consultation centers that specialize in providing information specific for veterinary patients. For general information related to overdose and toxin exposures, as well as contact information for poison control centers, refer to ***Appendix.***

Drug Interactions

The following drug interactions have either been reported or are theoretical in humans or animals receiving dinoprost and may be of significance in veterinary patients. Unless otherwise noted, use together is not necessarily contraindicated, but weigh the potential risks and perform additional monitoring when appropriate.

- **Other Oxytocic Agents**: Activity may be enhanced by dinoprost. Reduced effect of dinoprost would be expected with concomitant administration of a progestin.

Dosages

DOGS:

Abortifacient (extra-label):

a) After day 25 or 30, dinoprost SC injections must be given at least twice daily using a maximum dose of 80 – 100 µg/kg, starting with half the dose the first day (or first 2 administrations). Treatment must initially be administered under the supervision of a clinician and adverse effects carefully (monitored) after the first injection, after which the bitch can be sent home (with subsequent dose administered by owner). Treatment must continue (for 6 days or longer) until verification with ultrasound or palpation.[6]

b) Combination therapies may allow for a lower dinoprost dose to be used and minimize adverse effects as compared with dinoprost used alone.
   i. Starting on day 25, give dinoprost 0.025 mg/kg SC every other day with cabergoline 5 µg/kg PO once daily until termination of pregnancy.[7]
   ii. After day 27, give dinoprost 0.03 mg/kg IM once daily with cabergoline 5 µg/kg PO once daily until termination of pregnancy (6-9 days).[8]
   iii. Once pregnancy is confirmed with ultrasound, treatment should be started no sooner than 30 days after breeding. Give dinoprost 0.1 mg/kg SC 3 times daily for 3 days, then 0.2 mg/kg SC 3 times daily to effect in conjunction with misoprostol 1 – 3 µg/kg intravaginally once daily.[9]

Pyometra (extra-label): Use is restricted to bitches 6 years of age or younger that have an open cervix, are not critically ill, do not have significant concurrent illness, and have an owner adamant about saving the animal's reproductive potential.

a) Day 1, dinoprost 0.1 mg/kg SC once daily; day 2, 0.2 mg/kg SC once daily; days 3 to 7, 0.25 mg/kg SC once daily. Use antibiotics (effective against *E coli*) concurrent with dinoprost treatment and for 14 days beyond completion of the 7-day dinoprost regimen. Reevaluate the patient at 7 and 14 days after being treating with dinoprost. Re-treat at 14 days if purulent discharge persists or fever, increased WBC, and fluid-filled uterus persist.[10]
b) Dinoprost 0.1 mg/kg SC once daily for 7 days along with supportive therapy showed resolution of pyometra in all 7 dogs, with recurrence occurring in 3 dogs and successful subsequent pregnancies in 4 dogs.[10]
c) Dinoprost 250 µg/kg SC every 12 hours until the uterus reduces to near normal size (typically, 3-5 days).[4]
d) Dinoprost 150 µg/kg intravaginal infusion once or twice daily for 3-12 days along with antibiotics (amoxicillin or gentamicin administered IM). No adverse effects from dinoprost were observed.[11]
e) Combination therapy: Dinoprost 0.025 – 0.03 mg/kg SC or IM with cabergoline 5 µg/kg PO once daily; combination may allow for a lower dinoprost dose to be used and minimize adverse effects as compared with dinoprost used alone.

CATS:

Abortifacient (extra-label): 2 mg (total dose) per cat (NOT mg/kg) IM once daily beginning at day 33. Adverse effects include prostration, vomiting, and diarrhea.[6]

Pyometra (extra-label): Initially, 0.1 mg/kg SC on the first day, then 0.25 mg/kg SC once daily for 5 days.[12] Give bactericidal antibiotics concurrently. Not recommended in animals older than 8 years of age or in severely ill animals. Closed-cervix pyometra is a relative contraindication. Re-evaluate in 2 weeks; re-treat for 5 more days if necessary.[13,14]

HORSES:

Labeled indications; as a luteolytic agent to control the timing of estrus in estrous cycling and clinically anestrous difficult-to-breed mares that have a corpus luteum (FDA approved): Evaluate the reproductive status of the mare. Administer a single injection of dinoprost 1 mg/45 kg (1 mg/100 lb) IM. Observe for signs of estrus by means of daily teasing with a stallion, and evaluate follicular changes on the ovary by palpation of the ovary per rectum. Some clinically anestrus mares will not express estrus but will develop a follicle that will ovulate. These mares may become pregnant if inseminated at the appropriate time relative to rupture of the follicle. Breed mares in estrus in a manner consistent with normal management.[2]

Estrus synchronization in normally cycling mares (extra-label): Choose one.

1) **Two-injection method**: On days 1 and 16, give dinoprost 5 mg IM. Most mares (60%) will begin estrus 4 days after the second injection and ≈90% will show estrus behavior by the sixth day after the second injection. Breed using artificial insemination every second day during estrus or inseminate at predetermined times without estrus detection. Alternatively, add an injection of hCG (2500 – 3300 IU) IM on the first or second day (usually day 21) of estrus to hasten ovulation. Breed using artificial insemination on days 20, 22, 24, and 26. This protocol may be of more benefit when used early in the breeding season.
2) **Progestogen/prostaglandin method**: Give altrenogest 0.44 mg/kg PO for 8 to 12 days. On the last day of altrenogest therapy (usually day 10) give dinoprost IM (dose is not noted, but it is suggested to use the same dose as the two-injection method listed above). The majority of mares will show estrus 2 to 5 days after their last treatment. Inseminate every 2 days after detection of estrus. Synchronization may be improved by giving hCG 2500 IU IM on the first or second day of estrus or 5 to 7 days after altrenogest is withdrawn.
3) On day 1, inject progesterone 150 mg and 17-beta-estradiol 10 mg daily for 10 days. On the last day, also give dinoprost IM (dose is not noted, but it is suggested to use the same dose as the two-injection method listed above). Perform artificial insemination on alternate days after estrus detection or on days 19, 21, and 23.[15]

Abortifacient (extra-label):

a) Prior to the twelfth day of pregnancy: dinoprost 5 mg IM. After the fourth month of pregnancy, give 1 mg/45 kg (1 mg/100 lb) body weight daily until abortion takes place.[16]
b) From day 80 to 300: dinoprost 2.5 mg IM every 12 hours; ≈4 injections are required on average to induce abortion.[17]

CATTLE:

Labeled indications as a luteolytic agent (FDA approved): Dinoprost is effective only in cattle with a corpus luteum (ie, those that ovulated at least 5 days prior to treatment). Future reproductive performance of animals that are not cycling will be unaffected by injection of dinoprost.

Management considerations: Many factors contribute to success and failure of reproduction management; these factors are also important when the time of breeding is to be regulated with dinoprost sterile solution. Some of these factors are: (a) cattle must be ready to breed—they must have a corpus luteum and be healthy; (b) nutritional status must be adequate, as this has a direct effect on conception and the initiation of estrus in heifers or return of estrous cycles in cows following calving; (c) physical facilities must be adequate to allow cattle handling without being detrimental to the animal; (d) estrus must be detected accurately if timed artificial insemination is not employed; and (e) highly fertile semen must be used and inseminated properly. A successful breeding program can employ dinoprost effectively, but a poorly managed breeding program will continue to be poor when dinoprost is employed unless other management deficiencies are remedied first. Cattle expressing estrus following dinoprost are receptive to breeding by a bull. Using bulls to breed large numbers of cattle in heat following dinoprost will require proper management of bulls and cattle.

a) **Estrus synchronization in beef cattle and nonlactating dairy heifers**: Dinoprost is used to control the timing of estrus and ovulation in estrous cycling cattle that have a corpus luteum. Inject dinoprost 25 mg IM once, dose may be repeated 10 to 12 days later. Dose may be administered SC if using high-concentration dinoprost product. With the single injection, cattle should be bred at the usual time relative to estrus. If receiving 2 injections of dinoprost, cattle can be bred after the second injection either at the usual time relative to detected estrus or at ≈80 hours after the second injection. Estrus is expected to occur 1 to 5 days after injection if a corpus luteum was present. Cattle that do not become pregnant to breeding at estrus on days 1 to 5 after injection will be expected to return to estrus in ≈18 to 24 days.

b) **Estrus synchronization in suckled beef cows, replacement beef and dairy heifers**: Using high-concentration dinoprost product: 25 mg IM or SC. Used in combination with progesterone vaginal insert[18]; see dinoprost product label for administration schedule.[2,19]

c) **Estrus synchronization in lactating dairy cows**: Dinoprost 25 mg IM. Used in combination with progesterone vaginal insert[18]; see dinoprost product label for administration schedule.[2,19] Dose may be administered SC if using high-concentration dinoprost product.

d) **Estrus synchronization in lactating dairy cows to allow fixed-time artificial insemination**: Dinoprost 25 mg IM. Used in combination with gonadorelin injection; see dinoprost product label for administration schedule.[2,19] Dose may be administered SC if using high-concentration dinoprost product.

e) **Unobserved (silent) estrus in lactating dairy cows with a corpus luteum**: Dinoprost 25 mg IM. If the cow returns to estrus, breed at the usual time relative to estrus. If estrus has not been observed by 80 hours after injection, breed at 80 hours. Dose may be administered SC if using high-concentration dinoprost product.

f) **Pyometra (chronic endometritis)**: Dinoprost 25 mg IM. Dose may be administered SC if using high-concentration dinoprost product.

g) **Abortifacient for feedlot and other nonlactating cattle during the first 100 days of gestation**: Dinoprost 25 mg IM. Cattle that abort will do so within 35 days of injection.[2] Dose may be administered SC if using high-concentration dinoprost product.

Induce parturition (extra-label): 25 – 30 mg IM; delivery will occur in ≈72 hours.[20]

Increase fertility during artificial insemination (extra-label): 10 mg IM given concurrently with timed artificial insemination significantly increased the conception rate in lactating dairy cows in a study.[21]

Cystic ovarian disease in dairy cows (extra-label): 25 mg IM. The response to dinoprost was greater in cows with luteal cysts than in those with follicular cysts.[22]

SWINE:

Parturition induction in swine when injected within 3 days of normal predicted farrowing (label dose; FDA approved): 10 mg (2 mL) IM[2]

Management considerations: The product must be administered at a relatively specific time (there is an increased chance of piglet mortality if treatment is given earlier than 3 days prior to normal predicted farrowing). It is important that adequate records be maintained on (1) the average length of gestation period for the animals on a specific location and (2) the breeding and projected farrowing dates for each animal.

Parturition induction in swine (extra-label): 5 mg IM injected into the vulva-cutaneous junction, with a second dose administered 6 hours after the first dose, will result in most sows farrowing during the next working day.[23]

Estrus synchronization (grouping) (extra-label): At gestation day 15 to 55, give dinoprost 15 mg IM followed by dinoprost 10 mg IM 12 hours later. Animals will abort and return to estrus in 4 to 5 days. Close observation of estrus over several days is needed.[24]

SHEEP/GOATS:

Estrus synchronization in cycling ewes and does (extra-label):

a) **Ewes**: Dinoprost 8 mg IM on day 5 of the estrous cycle, and repeat in 11 days. Estrus will begin ≈2 days after the last injection.

b) **Does**: Dinoprost 8 mg IM on day 4 of the estrous cycle, and repeat in 11 days. Estrus will begin ≈2 days after the last injection.[24]

Pseudopregnancy (hydrometra, mucometra) in goats (extra-label): dinoprost 5 mg IM once[25]

Abortifacient (extra-label):

a) **Does**: Dinoprost 5 – 10 mg IM once; effective throughout the entire pregnancy; abortion takes place in 4 to 5 days.

b) **Ewes**: Dinoprost 10 – 15 mg IM once; effective during the first 2 months of pregnancy; abortion takes place within 72 hours.[20]

Induce parturition in does (extra-label): Dinoprost 2.5 – 20 mg on days 144 to 149. Higher dose (20 mg) yields a more predictable interval from injection to delivery (ie, ≈32 hours).[26]

Monitoring

- Adverse effects
- Abdominal ultrasound to confirm pregnancy and/or termination of pregnancy

Client Information

- Dinoprost should be used only by individuals familiar with its use and precautions.
- Pregnant women, people with asthma, or other persons with bronchial diseases should handle this product with extreme caution. Dinoprost may be absorbed through the skin; in the event of accidental exposure, wash the affected area immediately and contact a physician.

Chemistry/Synonyms

Dinoprost tromethamine, the tromethamine (THAM) salt of naturally occurring prostaglandin F2alpha, occurs as a white to off-white, very hygroscopic, crystalline powder with a melting point of ≈100°C (212°F). One gram is soluble in ≈5 mL of water. Dinoprost tromethamine 1.3 µg is equivalent to dinoprost 1 µg.

Dinoprost and dinoprost tromethamine may also be known as PGF(2alpha), prostaglandin F(2alpha), idinoprostum trometamoli, PGF(2-alpha) THAM, prostaglandin F(2-alpha) trometamol, U-14583E, U-14583, *Amtech Prostamate®*, *Dinolytic®*, *Enzaprost®*, *Glandin®*, *In-Synch®*, *Lutalyse®*, *Minprostin F(2)alpha®*, *Noroprost®*, *Oriprost®*, *Prostamate®*, *Prostarmon F®*, *Prostin®*, *Prostin F2®*, *Prostin F2 Alpha®*, or *Prostine F(2) Alpha®*.

Storage/Stability

Dinoprost for injection should be stored at room temperature (20°C-25°C [68°F-77°F]). Protect from freezing. Dinoprost is relatively insensitive to heat, light, and alkalis. Vials may be punctured no more than 20 times, and unused portions should be discarded 12 weeks after the first vial puncture.

Compatibility/Compounding Considerations

No specific information is noted. This drug should not be compounded by pregnant humans.

Dosage Forms/Regulatory Status

VETERINARY-LABELED PRODUCTS:

Dinoprost for Injection, equivalent to 5 mg/mL of dinoprost in 30 mL and 100 mL vials; *Lutalyse*®; (Rx). FDA-approved for use in beef and nonlactating dairy cattle, horses, and swine. No preslaughter withdrawal or milk withdrawal is required when used as labeled; no specific tolerance for dinoprost residues has been published. Dinoprost is not for use in horses intended for food. NADA #108-901

Dinoprost for Injection, equivalent to 12.5 mg/mL of dinoprost in 20 mL, 100 mL, and 250 mL vials; *Lutalyse® HighCon*; (Rx). For use in cattle only; no preslaughter withdrawal or milk withdrawal is required when used as labeled. NADA #141-442

HUMAN-LABELED PRODUCTS: NONE

References

For the complete list of references, see **wiley.com/go/budde/plumb**

Diphenhydramine

(dye-fen-***hye***-dra-meen) *Benadryl*®

First-Generation Antihistamine

Prescriber Highlights

- Antihistamine that is used primarily for its antihistaminic effects, but it also has additional indications (eg, motion sickness prevention, sedative, antiemetic)
- Should be used with caution in patients with angle-closure glaucoma, GI or urinary obstruction, chronic obstructive pulmonary disease, hyperthyroidism, seizure disorders, cardiovascular disease, and/or hypertension. In humans, diphenhydramine may mask ototoxicity signs.
- Adverse effects can include CNS depression and anticholinergic effects. GI effects (eg, diarrhea, vomiting, anorexia) are less common.
- Its use in neonates should be avoided.

Uses/Indications

Diphenhydramine is used primarily for its antihistaminic effects. In dogs and cats, diphenhydramine may be used to manage allergic and pruritic conditions, including urticaria, angioedema, and insect bite hypersensitivity. There is no conclusive evidence regarding the efficacy of oral, first-generation antihistamines in the treatment of chronic and acute flares of canine atopic dermatitis, with only highly variable therapeutic efficacy reported anecdotally.[1,2] Additionally, a randomized, double-blind crossover study found that diphenhydramine did not have an inhibitory effect on cutaneous allergic reactions in dogs.[3]

Diphenhydramine may be more effective in mildly pruritic animals and in preventing flares rather than treating them after clinical signs have occurred.[2] It has also been used as a steroid-sparing agent and with essential fatty acids to improve potential efficacy; however, no difference in measured outcomes was observed between dogs treated with diphenhydramine alone versus those treated with glucocorticoid and diphenhydramine in a population of dogs with uncomplicated allergic reactions.[4]

Diphenhydramine may also be used as adjunctive therapy for mast cell tumors to help prevent the local effects of histamine release from mast cells during surgical excision of mast cell tumors. However, diphenhydramine had no clear clinical cardiorespiratory benefits as compared with a placebo in isoflurane-anesthetized dogs undergoing mast cell tumor excision.[5]

This drug has also been used in the treatment and prevention of motion sickness and as an antiemetic in small animals.[6] Diphenhydramine was not effective in preventing motion-induced emesis in cats,[6] and NK_1 antagonists (eg, maropitant) or M_1-cholinergic antagonists (eg, prochlorperazine, chlorpromazine) may be better choices in the treatment of motion sickness or vomiting in this species. Diphenhydramine did not offer significantly different sedative effects as compared with a saline placebo when used as a sole sedative at single IM doses in healthy dogs,[7] although sedation may be observed in dogs when diphenhydramine is administered orally.

Pharmacology/Actions

Diphenhydramine has antihistaminergic (H1), antiemetic, anticholinergic, CNS depressant, and local anesthetic effects. Diphenhydramine did not suppress wheal response after intradermal histamine administration.[3,8] In one study, diphenhydramine was shown to have more potent growth-inhibitory effects in primary neoplastic mast cell tumors when compared to other H1-receptor antagonists.[9]

Pharmacokinetics

In a study of dogs, diphenhydramine had low oral bioavailability (2.8% to 7.8%),[8,10] whereas bioavailability after IM administration was 88%.[11] IV and IM administration in dogs rapidly resulted in plasma concentrations that exceeded therapeutic concentrations in humans. In dogs, the volume of distribution after a single IV dose was 7.6 L/kg, and the terminal half-life was 4.2 hours.[11] Terminal half-lives after oral and IM administration were 5 hours[8] and 6.8 hours,[11] respectively. In another study, oral absorption of diphenhydramine in healthy dogs was ≈3 times greater, with a longer half-life, when administered as the combination product, dimenhydrinate (*Dramamine*®, a combination of diphenhydramine with 8-chlorotheophylline). Mean oral bioavailability of diphenhydramine and dimenhydrinate was 7.8% and 22%, respectively, whereas mean peak plasma concentrations were 36 (±20) ng/mL and 124 (±46) ng/mL, respectively. Terminal elimination half-lives of diphenhydramine and dimenhydrinate were 5 (±7.1) hours and 11.6 (±17.7) hours, respectively.[8] One dog in this study was considered an outlier, with oral diphenhydramine bioavailability 9 times higher than other dogs, peak plasma concentration 5.5 times higher than other dogs, and an elimination half-life of 288 hours.[8]

In horses that received diphenhydramine 0.625 mg/kg IV, the volume of distribution (steady-state) was 6 L/kg, and the elimination half-life was 6.1 hours.[12]

In humans, diphenhydramine is well absorbed after oral administration, but due to a relatively high first-pass effect, only ≈40% to 60% reaches systemic circulation. The volume of distribution is 14 to 22 L/kg. Diphenhydramine is ≈80% bound to plasma proteins. Diphenhydramine is metabolized in the liver, and most of the drug is excreted as metabolites in urine. Terminal elimination half-life in adult humans ranges from 2.4 to 9.3 hours.

Contraindications/Precautions/Warnings

Diphenhydramine is contraindicated in patients that are hypersensitive to it or other antihistamines in its class. Because of their anticholinergic activity, antihistamines should be used with caution in patients with angle-closure glaucoma, prostatic hypertrophy, pyloroduodenal or bladder neck obstruction, and asthma or chronic obstructive pulmonary disease if mucosal secretions are a problem. In addition, antihistamines should be used with caution in patients with hyperthyroidism, cardiovascular disease, seizure disorders, or hypertension. In humans, it has been shown that diphenhydramine may also mask the clinical signs of ototoxicity (eg, head tilt, hearing loss, ataxia) and should therefore be used with caution when concomitantly administering ototoxic drugs.

The sedative effects of antihistamines may adversely affect the performance of working dogs.

In humans, pediatric patients are more susceptible to the adverse CNS effects of antihistamines, including paradoxical CNS excitation (eg, hallucinations, seizures); antihistamines are contraindicated in neonates.

DiphenhydrAMINE should not be confused with dimenhyDRINATE.

Adverse Effects

The most common adverse effects are CNS depression (eg, lethargy, sedation) and anticholinergic effects (eg, constipation, dry mouth, urinary retention). The sedative effects of antihistamines may be dose-dependent and diminish with chronic administration. GI effects (eg, diarrhea, vomiting, anorexia) are also possible. Oral diphenhydramine had no effect on tear production or intraocular pressure in healthy dogs.[13,14]

Diphenhydramine may cause paradoxical excitement or agitation, particularly in cats.

Liquid formulations are unpalatable, may contain alcohol, and may not be easily administered. SC injections may cause local necrosis.

Reproductive/Nursing Safety

Diphenhydramine crosses the placenta. No evidence of impaired fertility, reproductive performance, or fetal harm has been noted in rats or rabbits.

Diphenhydramine is excreted in milk. Use is contraindicated in breastfeeding women, particularly those feeding neonates and/or premature infants.

Because safety has not been established in animals, this drug should only be used when the maternal benefits outweigh the potential risks to offspring.

Overdose/Acute Toxicity

Reported LD_{50} in rats following IV, SC, and PO dosing was 35 mg/kg,[15] 201 mg/kg,[16] and 500 mg/kg,[17] respectively.

Overdose with diphenhydramine can cause CNS stimulation (eg, excitement, seizures) or depression (eg, lethargy, coma), anticholinergic effects, cardiovascular abnormalities, respiratory depression, and death. Treatment consists of GI decontamination, including induction of emesis if the patient is alert and CNS status is stable. Administration of saline cathartic and/or activated charcoal may be given after emesis or gastric lavage. Other clinical signs should be treated using supportive therapies.

Of 621 dogs with diphenhydramine toxicosis reported between 2008 and 2013, 146 developed clinical signs (eg, lethargy, hyperactivity, agitation, hyperthermia, ataxia, tremors, fasciculations, tachycardia), and 3 dogs died.[18] Supportive treatment based on clinical signs has been suggested.

For patients that have experienced or are suspected of having experienced an overdose, consultation with a 24-hour poison consultation center specializing in providing veterinary-specific information is recommended. For general information related to overdose and toxin exposures, as well as contact information for poison control centers, refer to ***Appendix***.

Drug Interactions

The following drug interactions have either been reported or are theoretical in humans or animals receiving diphenhydramine and may be of significance in veterinary patients. Unless otherwise noted, use together is not necessarily contraindicated, but weigh the potential risks and perform additional monitoring when appropriate.

- **Acetylcholinesterase Inhibitors** (eg, **neostigmine, pyridostigmine**): Diphenhydramine may reduce the efficacy of acetylcholinesterase inhibitors.
- **Anticholinergic Drugs** (eg, **atropine, glycopyrrolate**): Diphenhydramine may potentiate anticholinergic effects.
- **CNS Depressant Agents** (eg, **anesthetics [inhalant and injectable], barbiturates, benzodiazepines, opioids**): Increased CNS depression can occur. Consider lower initial doses of CNS depressants.
- **Monoamine Oxidase Inhibitors (MAOIs**; eg, **amitraz, linezolid, selegiline**): MAOIs may potentiate anticholinergic effects.
- **Potassium Supplements**: Diphenhydramine's anticholinergic effects may reduce GI motility, increasing the risk for focal upper GI injury from solid oral potassium formulations (ie, tablets, capsules).
- **Prokinetic Agents** (eg, **cisapride, metoclopramide**): Diphenhydramine may diminish the therapeutic effect of prokinetic agents.
- **Tricyclic Antidepressants (TCAs**; eg, **amitriptyline, clomipramine**): TCAs may potentiate anticholinergic effects.

Laboratory Considerations

- **Intradermal allergy testing (IDT)**: Although antihistamines may suppress IDT results,[19] diphenhydramine did not demonstrate an effect on wheal formation in dogs despite reaching a plasma diphenhydramine concentration believed to be therapeutic in humans.[3] A 7-day withdrawal prior to IDT is considered optimal; a 2-day withdrawal should be considered the minimum.[19]
- Diphenhydramine may cause false-positive screening results for **TCAs** (serum) and **methadone** (urine).

Dosages

DOGS/CATS:

Antihistamine (eg, adjunctive treatment of allergic pruritus or reactions, including angioedema, urticaria, insect bite hypersensitivity, and atopic dermatitis, in addition to anaphylaxis, mast cell tumors, vaccine or transfusion reactions; extra-label):

a) 2 – 4 mg/kg PO every 8 to 12 hours

b) 0.5 – 2 mg/kg IM, SC, or IV. **NOTE**: In humans, it is recommended to avoid the SC route due to risk for tissue necrosis, and IV administration should occur at a rate not exceeding 25 mg/minute with undiluted diphenhydramine or as an infusion over 10 to 15 minutes. Relevance in veterinary patients is not known.

Prevention of motion sickness/antiemetic (extra-label): 2 – 4 mg/kg PO or IM every 8 hours. Usually not very effective in cats

HORSES:

Antihistamine (extra-label):

a) 1 – 2 mg/kg PO every 8 to 12 hours

b) 0.5 – 1 mg/kg IV or IM every 6 to 8 hours[20]

CATTLE:

a) **Adjunctive therapy for anaphylaxis** (extra-label): 0.5 – 1 mg/kg IM or IV[20]; used in combination with epinephrine and glucocorticoids[21]

b) **Adjunctive therapy for aseptic laminitis during the acute phase** (extra-label): 0.55 – 1.1 mg/kg IV or IM every 6 to 8 hours[20] in combination with corticosteroids[22]

BIRDS:

Adjunctive treatment of pruritus causing feather picking in psittacines (extra-label): 2 mg/kg PO every 12 hours[23]

FERRETS:

Prevaccination (extra-label): 2 mg/kg PO, IM, or IV 10 minutes before vaccination[24]

Pretreatment before doxorubicin (extra-label): 5 mg/ferret (NOT mg/kg) IM

RABBITS/RODENTS/SMALL MAMMALS:

Guinea pigs (extra-label): 7.5 mg/kg PO[25]

Rabbits (extra-label): 1 – 2 mg/kg PO every 12 hours as an antihistamine.[26,27] 2 mg/kg IV before blood transfusion[28]

Monitoring

- Clinical efficacy (trial periods to determine an individual antihistamine's efficacy are usually 1 to 2 weeks long)
- Adverse effects (eg, lethargy, sedation, constipation, urinary retention, vomiting, diarrhea, anorexia)

Client Information

- Use antihistamines on a regular, ongoing basis in animals that respond to them. They work better if used before exposure to an allergen or an allergy flare-up.
- When used for motion sickness, it is best to give this medicine at least 30 to 60 minutes prior to travel.
- May cause drowsiness/sleepiness. This effect may lessen with long-term use.
- Rarely, cats may become excited when given this medication.
- Discontinue medication in animals that develop severe drowsiness or agitation.
- Discuss with your veterinarian if your animal becomes constipated, has difficulty urinating, or develops redness or discharge from the eyes.
- Use caution with over-the-counter formulations of this medicine, as other potentially toxic ingredients may be combined in the products (eg, decongestants, such as pseudoephedrine or acetaminophen). Be sure the product used only contains diphenhydramine as the active ingredient. Alcohol-free formulations may be more palatable.
- This medicine can be given either with or without food, but if an animal vomits or drools after receiving the medication on an empty stomach, try giving it with food. If vomiting continues, contact your veterinarian.

Chemistry/Synonyms

Diphenhydramine HCl, an ethanolamine-derivative antihistamine, occurs as an odorless white crystalline powder that slowly darkens when exposed to light. It has a melting range between 167°C and 172°C (332.6°F and 341.6°F). One gram is soluble in ≈1 mL of water or 2 mL of alcohol. Diphenhydramine HCl has a pK_a of ≈9; the pH of the commercially available injection is adjusted to 5 to 6.

Diphenhydramine HCl may also be known as chloranautine, dimenhydrinatum, diphenhydramine teoclate, and diphenhydramine theoclate; many trade names exist.

Storage/Stability

Store the preparations containing diphenhydramine away from light at room temperature 20°C to 25°C (68°F to 77°F); protect solutions from freezing. Keep tablets, oral solutions, capsules, and elixir in airtight containers.

Compatibility/Compounding Considerations

Compatibility is dependent on factors, such as pH, concentration, temperature, and diluent used; specialized references or a hospital pharmacist should be consulted for more specific information.

Diphenhydramine for injection is reportedly physically **compatible** with all commonly used IV solutions and the following drugs: amikacin sulfate, ascorbic acid injection, atropine sulfate, buprenorphine HCl, butorphanol tartrate, calcium gluconate, ciprofloxacin, clindamycin phosphate, cyclosporine, dobutamine HCl, erythromycin lactobionate, famotidine, fentanyl citrate, glycopyrrolate, hydromorphone HCl, hydroxyzine HCl, iothalamate meglumine/sodium, ketamine HCl, lidocaine HCl, meperidine HCl, metoclopramide, midazolam HCl, morphine sulfate, ondansetron HCl, penicillin G potassium/sodium, piperacillin/tazobactam, potassium chloride, propofol, ranitidine, tetracycline HCl, and vitamin B complex with vitamin C.

Diphenhydramine is reportedly physically **incompatible** with the following drugs: amphotericin B, ampicillin sodium, most cephalosporins, dexamethasone sodium phosphate, diazepam, furosemide, hydrocortisone sodium succinate, insulin (regular), nitroprusside sodium, pantoprazole, phenobarbital sodium, and pentobarbital sodium.

Dosage Forms/Regulatory Status

VETERINARY-LABELED PRODUCTS:

NOTE: Diphenhydramine tablets labeled for veterinary use have not been found by FDA to be safe or effective.

Diphenhydramine HCl Chewable Tablets (liver-flavored): 10 mg and 30 mg; *Vetadryl*®; (OTC).

Diphenhydramine HCl Tablets: 25 mg; generic; (OTC).

Diphenhydramine HCl Capsules: 25 mg; *Calmatrol*®; (OTC).

Various topical formulations containing diphenhydramine are available. See ***Diphenhydramine, Topical*** for more information.

The Association of Racing Commissioners International (ARCI) has designated this drug as a class 3 substance. Use of this drug may not be allowed in certain animal competitions. Check rules and regulations before entering a competition while this medication is being administered. Contact local racing authorities for further guidance. See ***Appendix*** for more information.

The International Federation for Equestrian Sports (FEI) lists this drug as a *prohibited substance – controlled medication*.[29]

For guidance in determining the use and associated withdrawal times, contact FARAD (see ***Important Contact Information*** in ***Appendix***).

HUMAN-LABELED PRODUCTS:

NOTE: ONLY products containing diphenhydramine as a single agent should be used in veterinary species.

Diphenhydramine Capsules and Tablets: 12.5 mg (as hydrochloride, chewable), 25 mg (as either hydrochloride or tannate, chewable), and 50 mg (as hydrochloride). There are many trade name products that contain diphenhydramine. *Benadryl*®, *Banophen*®, and *Diphenhist*® are commonly seen; generic; (OTC, Rx).

Diphenhydramine Orally Disintegrating Tablets: 12.5 mg and 25 mg; *Benadryl*®, *Unisom Sleep*®, generic; (OTC)

Diphenhydramine Orally Disintegrating Strips: 12.5 mg (as hydrochloride); *Triaminic*® *Children's Allergy*; (OTC)

Diphenhydramine Oral Liquid, Solution, Suspension, Elixir, or Syrup: 12.5 mg/5 mL (as hydrochloride) in 30 mL, 118 mL, 120 mL, 236 mL, 237 mL, 473 mL, and 3.8 L; 31.25 mg/5 mL (as HCl); 25 mg/5 mL (as tannate) in 118 mL. There are many trade name products, including *Benadryl*®, *Diphenhist*®, *Banophen*®, *Hydramine Cough* (various), generic; (OTC, Rx). Some products may contain alcohol; consult the label before prescribing.

Diphenhydramine Injection: 50 mg/mL (as hydrochloride); generic; (Rx)

Topical creams, gels, solutions, and sprays are also available.

References

For the complete list of references, see **wiley.com/go/budde/plumb**

Diphenoxylate/Atropine

(dye-fen-***ox***-i-late/***at***-roe-peen) *Lomotil®*

Opioid Agonist/Anticholinergic

Prescriber Highlights

- ▶ Opioid GI motility modifier with antitussive properties that is used primarily in dogs
- ▶ Contraindications include known hypersensitivity to opioids, partial or complete biliary obstruction, diarrhea caused by an infectious agent or toxic ingestion, and intestinal obstruction.
- ▶ Use with caution in patients with respiratory disease, CNS depression, uncontrolled hypothyroidism (myxedema), renal insufficiency, Addisonian crisis, and acute GI conditions; use in patients with acute abdominal conditions (eg, hemoabdomen, splenic torsion) may obscure the diagnosis or worsen the clinical course.
- ▶ Adverse effects include constipation, bloating, and sedation; cats may exhibit excitable behaviors. Potential for paralytic ileus, toxic megacolon, pancreatitis, and CNS depression
- ▶ Drug interactions possible with other CNS depressants. Avoid concurrent use with monoamine oxidase inhibitors.
- ▶ DEA Schedule V (C-V) controlled substance

Uses/Indications

Diphenoxylate is an opioid that is commercially available in a fixed-dose combination with atropine. It is used primarily in dogs for its antidiarrheal and antitussive properties. Diphenoxylate/atropine may also be used for medical management in dogs with tracheal collapse.[1,2]

Many clinicians do not recommend using this drug in cats.[3]

Pharmacology/Actions

Among other effects, opioids inhibit GI motility and propulsion. They decrease intestinal secretions induced by cholera toxin and prostaglandin E_2 and alleviate diarrhea caused by factors in which calcium is the second messenger (noncyclic AMP/GMP mediated). Opioids may also enhance intestinal mucosal absorption.

In dogs, diphenoxylate directly affects the smooth muscle in the GI tract by enhancing segmentation contractions and results in prolongation of GI transit time.[4]

Atropine is present in drug formulations in subtherapeutic amounts to deter human abuse of diphenoxylate for its narcotic effects. Atropine is not expected to have a clinical effect at therapeutic diphenoxylate doses.

Pharmacokinetics

In dogs, ≈72% of an oral dose is eliminated in the feces within 5 days of administration.[5] No other pharmacokinetic information in veterinary species was located.

In humans, diphenoxylate is rapidly absorbed after administration of either the tablets or oral solution; bioavailability of the tablets is ≈90% of the solution's bioavailability. Generally, onset of action occurs within 45 to 60 minutes after administration and is sustained for 3 to 4 hours. Diphenoxylate is metabolized into diphenoxylic acid, an active metabolite. The serum half-lives of diphenoxylate and diphenoxylic acid are ≈2.5 hours and 4 to 14 hours, respectively.[4,6]

Contraindications/Precautions/Warnings

Opioid antidiarrheals are contraindicated in patients who are hypersensitive to narcotic analgesics, with partial or complete biliary obstruction, intestinal obstruction, and with diarrhea caused by an infectious agent or toxic ingestion.

Opioid antidiarrheals should be used with extreme caution in patients with respiratory disease or acute respiratory dysfunction (eg, pulmonary edema secondary to smoke inhalation) and in patients with conditions that cause CNS depression (eg, traumatic head injuries, hepatic encephalopathy, increased intracranial pressure) as this may exacerbate CNS depression to the point of coma or death. All opioids should be used with caution in patients with renal insufficiency, uncontrolled hypothyroidism (myxedema), Addisonian crisis, and in debilitated patients.

Use of opioid antidiarrheals in patients with acute abdominal conditions (eg, hemoabdomen, splenic torsion) may obscure the diagnosis or worsen the clinical course of these conditions.

Many clinicians recommend not using diphenoxylate or loperamide in dogs weighing less than 10 kg (22 lb), but this is likely a result of the potency of the tablet or capsule forms and the resultant difficulty in accurately dosing the medication. Dosage titration using the liquid forms may allow safer, more accurate dosing in small dogs when indicated.

Adverse Effects

In dogs, constipation, bloat, and sedation are the most likely adverse effects encountered when recommended dosages are used; paralytic ileus, toxic megacolon, vomiting, pancreatitis, and CNS depression (ie, sedation) may also be seen. Constipation can be managed with dietary changes, stool softeners, or laxatives.[2] Reduced GI motility may delay or prolong nutrient absorption.

Because opioids prolong GI transit time, use in animals with acute infectious diarrhea may contribute to bacterial overgrowth and delay expulsion of the pathogen and/or enterotoxins from the GI tract, thus increasing the risk for sepsis and/or prolonged recovery.

Use of antidiarrheal opioids in cats is controversial; this species may react with excitatory behavior.

Reproductive/Nursing Safety

Safety of diphenoxylate/atropine has not been clearly established in pregnant animals. Reduced maternal weight gain and fertility in rats were noted at 20 mg/kg/day.[4] Teratogenic effects were not noted in laboratory animals given oral doses of 0.4 – 20 mg/kg/day.

Diphenoxylic acid may be, and atropine is, excreted in maternal milk. Exercise caution when administering diphenoxylate/atropine to nursing animals.

Because safety has not been established in animals, this drug should only be used when the maternal benefits outweigh the potential risks to offspring.

Overdose/Acute Toxicity

Acute overdose of opioid antidiarrheals could result in CNS, cardiovascular, GI, or respiratory toxicity. GI decontamination and supportive therapy should be employed with recent ingestions. Naloxone may reverse the opioid effects.

Massive overdoses of diphenoxylate/atropine sulfate may induce atropine toxicity. Refer to ***Atropine*** for more information.

For patients that have experienced or are suspected to have experienced an overdose, consultation with a 24-hour poison center specializing in providing veterinary-specific information is recommended. For general information related to overdose and toxin exposures, as well as contact information for poison control centers, refer to ***Appendix***.

Drug Interactions

The following drug interactions have either been reported or are theoretical in humans or animals receiving opioid antidiarrheals and may be of significance in veterinary patients. Unless otherwise noted, use together is not necessarily contraindicated, but weigh the potential risks and perform additional monitoring when appropriate.

- ANTICHOLINERGIC AGENTS (eg, **glycopyrrolate, oxybutynin**): Additive anticholinergic effects (eg, dry mucous membranes, tachycardia, constipation, urinary retention) may occur.
- ANTIHISTAMINE H1 RECEPTOR ANTAGONISTS, FIRST GENERATION (eg, **chlorpheniramine, diphenhydramine**): Concurrent use may increase risk of CNS depression and have additive anticholinergic effects.

- **CNS Depressant Drugs** (eg, **anesthetic agents, barbiturates, cannabidiol**): Concurrent use may cause increased CNS or respiratory depression when used with opioid antidiarrheal agents.
- **Digoxin**: Concurrent use may result in increased serum digoxin concentrations.
- **Laxatives** (eg, **oral magnesium salts, polyethylene glycol 3350**): Concurrent use may decrease efficacy of diphenoxylate.
- **Monoamine Oxidase Inhibitors** (MAOIs; eg, **amitraz, linezolid, methylene blue, selegiline**): Opioid antidiarrheal agents are contraindicated in human patients receiving systemic MAOIs for at least 14 days after receiving MAOIs because of an increased risk of a hypertensive crisis.
- **Opioids** (eg, **buprenorphine, morphine, tramadol**): Therapeutic duplication. Concurrent use may increase risk of CNS or respiratory depression and have additive anticholinergic effects.
- **Phenothiazines** (eg, **acepromazine, chlorpromazine**): Concurrent use may increase risk of CNS depression and have additive anticholinergic effects.
- **Potassium Salts, Oral**: Reduced GI motility may increase the risk for GI irritation and ulceration caused by potassium salts. The use of solid oral forms of potassium concurrently with drugs that decrease GI motility is contraindicated in humans; consider use of liquid/gel potassium formulations.
- **Prokinetic Agents** (eg, **cisapride, erythromycin, metoclopramide**): Concurrent use may result in decreased efficacy of both agents.
- **Tricyclic Antidepressants** (eg, **amitriptyline, clomipramine**): Concurrent use may increase risk of CNS depression and have additive anticholinergic effects.

Laboratory Considerations

- Opioids may increase biliary tract pressure, resulting in increased plasma **amylase** and **lipase** values up to 24 hours following their administration.

Dosages

DOGS:

Antidiarrheal agent (extra-label): Dosage is based on the diphenoxylate component:

a) 0.05 – 0.1 mg/kg PO 3 to 4 times daily [7-9]

b) 0.1 – 0.2 mg/kg PO every 12 hours

Antitussive agent (extra-label): 0.2 – 0.5 mg/kg PO every 8 to 12 hours[2]

CATS:

Antidiarrheal agent (extra-label): 0.08 – 0.1 mg/kg PO every 12 hours[10]; **NOTE**: Not usually recommended for cats.

Monitoring

- Clinical efficacy: as antidiarrheal, decrease in volume and frequency of diarrhea; for tracheal collapse, improved cough suppression
- Monitor hydration and serum electrolytes in patients with severe diarrhea
- Adverse effects: respiratory and CNS depression, constipation, vomiting

Client Information

- This medicine may be used to treat diarrhea or as a cough suppressant.
- May be given with or without food. If your animal vomits or acts sick after receiving the drug on an empty stomach, try giving the next dose with food or a small treat. If vomiting continues, contact your veterinarian.
- Constipation and sleepiness are the most common side effects in dogs.
- Must use cautiously in cats as they can get overly excited
- This medicine is a controlled drug in the United States. It is against federal law to use, give away, or sell this medication to others than for whom it was prescribed.
- Contact your veterinarian if diarrhea does not improve or if your animal appears listless.

Chemistry/Synonyms

Structurally related to meperidine, diphenoxylate HCl is a synthetic phenylpiperidine-derivative opioid agonist. It occurs as an odorless, white, crystalline powder that is slightly soluble in water and sparingly soluble in alcohol. Commercially available preparations also contain a small amount of atropine sulfate as a bittering agent to discourage abuse of diphenoxylate for its narcotic effects; at therapeutic doses, the atropine component has no clinical effect in humans.

This combination may be known as co-phenotrope in the United Kingdom and elsewhere. Other synonyms include R 1132, NIH 7562, or difenoxilato. A commonly used trade name is *Lomotil*®.

Compatibility/Compounding Considerations

No specific information is noted.

Storage/Stability

Diphenoxylate/atropine tablets should be stored at room temperature of 20°C to 25°C (68°F-77°F). Diphenoxylate/atropine oral solution should be stored at room temperature of 20°C to 25°C (68°F-77°F); avoid freezing.

Follow applicable local, state, and federal rules regarding controlled drug storage, waste, and disposal.

Dosage Forms/Regulatory Status

VETERINARY-LABELED PRODUCTS: NONE

HUMAN-LABELED PRODUCTS:

Diphenoxylate HCl and Atropine Sulfate Tablets: Diphenoxylate 2.5 mg and Atropine 0.025 mg; *Lomotil*®, generic; (Rx, C-V)

Diphenoxylate HCl and Atropine Sulfate Liquid: Diphenoxylate 2.5 mg and Atropine Sulfate 0.025 mg per 5 mL; *Lomotil*®, generic; (Rx, C-V)

Report prescribing and/or dispensing to state monitoring programs where required.

References

For the complete list of references, see **wiley.com/go/budde/plumb**

Dipyrone

Metamizole

(***dye***-purr-own) *Zimeta*®

Nonsteroidal Anti-Inflammatory Drug (NSAID)

Prescriber Highlights

- ▶ Approved for short-term (up to 3 days) control of pyrexia in horses
- ▶ Not approved for use in food-producing animals in the United States
- ▶ May also be useful for analgesia in dogs and cats
- ▶ Use with caution in horses at risk for hemorrhage or those receiving nephrotoxic drugs (eg, aminoglycosides).
- ▶ Do not administer concurrently with other NSAIDs or with corticosteroids.
- ▶ Adverse effects include increased serum sorbitol dehydrogenase, hypoalbuminemia, and gastric ulcers. Prolongation of coagulation parameters (eg, PT, aPTT) may occur.

Uses/Indications

Dipyrone injection is indicated for the control of pyrexia in horses.

The drug was deemed effective (decrease of rectal temperature by more than 1.1°C [2°F] or return to normothermia by 6 hours after drug administration) in ≈75% of treated horses.[1]

Historically, dipyrone was FDA-approved for use in humans but was withdrawn from the market in 1977 due to reports of agranulocytosis. Dipyrone had been used in a variety of veterinary species as an analgesic, antipyretic, and muscle relaxant. An unapproved dipyrone product continued to be sold for equine use until 1996 when the FDA removed the product due to concerns of use in food-producing animals. Veterinary use of compounded dipyrone formulations increased after its withdrawal. A commercially prepared formulation for use in horses is now available and is strongly recommended over use of a compounded product.

In countries outside the United States, dipyrone may be approved for use in other species as an analgesic and/or antipyretic. Dipyrone has demonstrated analgesic properties in dogs.[2–5] In cats, dipyrone may be useful for postoperative analgesia[6] but efficacy is unclear.[7]

Pharmacology/Actions

Dipyrone is an NSAID. It is a prodrug that is rapidly hydrolyzed to the active compound 4-methylaminoantipyrine (4-MAA).[8]

Dipyrone is thought to inhibit peripheral cyclooxygenase COX-1 and COX-2 mediated production of prostaglandins. Dipyrone also inhibits cyclooxygenase (COX-3) within the CNS[9] and may have agonist activity on cannabinoid and opioid systems. In addition to its antipyretic effects, the drug has analgesic and weak anti-inflammatory properties. It may also have antispasmodic activity on bradykinin-induced spasms on the intestinal tract without appreciably altering spontaneous intestinal motility.[10–12]

Dipyrone inhibits platelet aggregation in dogs.[13] In horses, it prolongs coagulation parameters (eg, PT, aPTT) at higher doses.[8]

Pharmacokinetics

Dipyrone circulates only briefly before rapid hydrolysis into the active primary metabolite 4-methylaminoantipyrine (4-MAA). In humans, 4-MAA is hepatically metabolized to 4-aminoantypyrine (4-AA) and other inactive end metabolites that are renally excreted.[8] 4-MAA and 4-AA are both considered active metabolites in humans and therefore pharmacokinetic studies focus primarily on 4-MAA and 4-AA. In veterinary species, it is unknown if 4-AA contributes to analgesic activity as plasma concentrations are very low compared with 4-MAA.[14,15]

In healthy dogs, peak 4-MAA concentration occurs ≈2 hours after oral dosing and ≈0.6 hours after IM injection. Volume of distribution is ≈5 to 7.5 L/kg, clearance is 552 to 921 mL/kg/hour, and elimination half-life is ≈6 hours. Plasma 4-MAA concentrations remain at or above human inhibitory concentrations (IC50) for COX-1 and COX-2 enzymes for ≈12 and 8 hours, respectively.[15,16] Rectal administration produces low levels of 4-MAA and is likely the least effective route in dogs.[15]

In healthy cats, oral absorption is high with maximum concentrations achieved ≈6 hours after dosing. Volume of distribution is ≈1 to 1.4 L/kg, clearance is ≈92 to 131 mL/kg/hour, and half-life is ≈6 to 7 hours. Low absorption was seen after IM administration compared to both IV and PO routes.[17]

In healthy horses receiving dipyrone, 4-MAA elimination half-life is reported as 3 to 5 hours and clearance is 230 to 285 mL/kg/hour.[14,18] 4-MAA has a large volume of distribution (1 to 1.9 L/kg), moderate protein binding (low compared with other NSAIDs), and readily penetrates into the CNS.[10] When dipyrone was given IM, time to peak concentration was ≈1.2 hours and the maximum concentration was lower than when given IV, but otherwise the pharmacokinetic profiles were similar between routes.[14] When dipyrone was given to horses at the labeled dose every 12 hours, minimal accumulation was seen after 9 days. However, higher doses and more frequent dosing did result in drug accumulation and increases in trough concentrations and AUC that were not proportional to increases in dose alone, which suggests the possibility of nonlinear pharmacokinetics at higher doses.[19]

In healthy donkeys, 4-MAA volume of distribution is 0.5 to 0.8 L/kg, clearance is 160 to 300 mL/kg/hour, and elimination half-life is ≈1.9 hours.[20]

Contraindications/Precautions/Warnings

Dipyrone is contraindicated in patients that are hypersensitive to it. Safe use in horses younger than 3 years has not been evaluated.[8] Due to the potential for prolongation of PT, dipyrone should not be given more frequently than every 12 hours.[8]

The drug should be used with caution in horses at risk for hemorrhage and those that are dehydrated, receiving diuretics, or with preexisting renal, cardiac, or hepatic dysfunction. Use with caution in animals with a history of or current hematologic or bone marrow abnormalities.

In humans, a significant decrease in clearance was seen in patients with liver cirrhosis. In humans with renal impairment, elimination of end metabolites was impaired, but 4-MAA clearance was not significantly altered.[21] It is unclear how this translates to veterinary species, but dipyrone should be used with caution in animals with renal or hepatic dysfunction.

Do not use dipyrone in horses intended for human consumption or in any food-producing animal.[8]

Due to risk for agranulocytosis in humans, those preparing or administering the drug should avoid direct contact with skin or accidental injection.[8]

Do not confuse meTAMizole with meTHIMazole. Do not confuse ZImeta (dipyrone) with ZOmeta (zoledronic acid).

Adverse Effects

Adverse effects associated with administration of dipyrone to horses during an FDA field study were elevated serum sorbitol dehydrogenase (SDH; an acute marker of hepatocellular injury) (5%), hypoalbuminemia (3%), and gastric ulcers (2%).[8] In addition, one of each of the following occurred in different horses: hyperemic mucosa right dorsal colon, prolonged aPTT, elevated creatinine, injection site reaction, and anorexia. Bloody nasal discharge and death occurred in one horse during a safety study. Clinical signs associated with NSAID intolerance may include colic, diarrhea, and decreased appetite.[8]

Reported adverse effects in dogs and cats include vomiting and salivation.[15,17] In dogs, dipyrone has been shown to inhibit platelet aggregation.[22]

Experience in EU countries suggests the drug is well tolerated in horses at approved dosages.[23] Historically, the occurrence of agranulocytosis and leukopenia was associated with high doses and prolonged treatment.

In humans, dipyrone seems to have a lower risk for GI bleeding as compared with other NSAIDs such as piroxicam and aspirin.[24]

Reproductive/Nursing Safety

Safe use in horses used for breeding, or in pregnant or lactating horses has not been evaluated. Because safety has not been established in animals, this drug should only be used when the maternal benefits outweigh the potential risks to offspring.

Decreased pup survival was observed in rats treated with 250 – 625 mg/kg/day prior to and throughout pregnancy.[23]

Overdose/Acute Toxicity

Dipyrone 30 mg/kg given every 8 hours did not demonstrate an adequate margin of safety due to prolongation of PT and aPTT, clinical signs of coagulopathy, and hepatotoxicity (increased bilirubin and liver weight). In healthy horses receiving 60 mg/kg or 90 mg/kg IV 3 times daily, the following adverse effects were noted: cough, depression, tachypnea or dyspnea, epistaxis, nasal discharge, inappetence, loose manure, colic, and fever. PT was prolonged in both treatment groups and minimal or mild renal tubular dilation was noted; however, there were no clinical signs of renal dysfunction. Two horses receiving 90 mg/kg IV developed epistaxis and pneumonia, and one died.

Treatment of an overdose consists of supportive therapy based on clinical signs. Monitor for coagulopathy.

Drug Interactions

The following drug interactions have either been reported or are theoretical in humans or animals receiving dipyrone and may be of significance in veterinary patients. Unless otherwise noted, use together is not necessarily contraindicated, but weigh the potential risks and perform additional monitoring when appropriate.

- ACETAMINOPHEN: Combined use may increase risk for hepatocellular injury.
- ANTICOAGULANTS (eg, **clopidogrel, heparins, rivaroxaban, warfarin**): Risk for bleeding may be increased.
- CHLORAMPHENICOL: Combined use may increase risk for myelosuppression.
- CHLORPROMAZINE: Concurrent use may cause profound hypothermia.[25] Effect of other phenothiazines (eg, **acepromazine**) is uncertain.
- CORTICOSTEROIDS: Concomitant use of dipyrone with corticosteroids should be avoided.[8]
- DIURETICS (eg, **furosemide**): Concurrent use increases risk for adverse renal effects.
- NALOXONE: May block antinociceptive effect of dipyrone
- NEPHROTOXIC DRUGS (eg, **amphotericin B, aminoglycosides, cyclosporine, trimethoprim**): Concurrent use with nephrotoxic drugs should be avoided.[8]
- NSAIDs (eg, **flunixin, phenylbutazone**): Concomitant use of dipyrone with NSAIDs should be avoided.[8] Consider appropriate washout time when switching between NSAIDs. Concomitant administration of dipyrone and meloxicam resulted in more prolonged inhibition of platelet function than dipyrone alone[13]; however, this combination has been used clinically in dogs.[5]
- SELECTIVE SEROTONIN REUPTAKE INHIBITORS (SSRIs; eg, **fluoxetine**): Risk for bleeding may be increased.
- TRICYCLIC ANTIDEPRESSANTS (TCAs, eg, **amitriptyline, clomipramine**): Risk for bleeding may be increased.

Laboratory Considerations

- None noted

Dosages

DOGS:

Analgesic (extra-label): 25 mg/kg IV prior to[2] or immediately following[4] surgery. The results of one study suggest that dipyrone should not be used as the sole analgesic in the perioperative period.[26]

CATS:

Analgesic (extra-label): 25 mg/kg IV every 24 hours and 12.5 mg/kg IV every 12 hours have been reported for postoperative analgesia.[6]

HORSES:

Control of pyrexia (label dosage; FDA-approved): 30 mg/kg IV once or twice daily (at 12-hour intervals) for up to 3 days. Under field conditions, pyrexia was controlled in most horses with once-daily treatment.[8]

Monitoring

- Body temperature
- Level of pain control
- Hydration status
- Baseline and periodic CBC and serum chemistry profile
- Adverse effects
- Signs of coagulopathy

Client Information

- The manufacturer's client information sheet should be provided to the person(s) treating the animal or providing care.
- Dipyrone can cause bone marrow suppression in humans. Avoid contact with skin. Immediately wash skin with soap and water in case of accidental contact. Seek medical care urgently in cases of self-injection.
  - Side effects include colic, decreased appetite, depression, and diarrhea. If serious side effects occur, discontinue treatment, and contact your veterinarian.
  - Check with your veterinarian before administering any other medications.
  - Overdoses can be very serious; measure liquid doses very carefully and keep out of reach of children or animals.

Chemistry/Synonyms

A pyrazolone derivative, dipyrone occurs as an odorless, bitter, white or yellowish-white crystalline powder. One gram of dipyrone is very soluble in water and soluble in alcohol. The commercial solution for injection is preserved with benzyl alcohol.

Dipyrone may also be known as metamizole sodium, dipyronium, methamizole, and methampyrone. Many trade names exist, including *Analate®*, *Analgin®*, *Myovin®*, *Novin®*, *Novalgin®*, *Vetalgin®*, and *Zimeta®*.

Storage/Stability

Store dipyrone injection protected from light, at controlled room temperature of 20°C to 25°C (68°F-77°F) with excursions permitted between 15°C to 30°C (59°F-86°F). Use multi-dose vial within 30 days of first puncture.

Compatibility/Compounding Considerations

Compounding of dipyrone is no longer necessary given the availability of an FDA-approved dipyrone formulation (as well as the availability of therapeutically equivalent drugs such as flunixin).

Dosage Forms/Regulatory Status

VETERINARY-LABELED PRODUCTS:

Dipyrone Injection: 500 mg/mL in 100 mL multi-dose vial; *Zimeta®*, (Rx). NADA #141-513. Not for use in horses intended for human consumption or in food-producing animals

The Association of Racing Commissioners International (ARCI) has designated dipyrone as a drug class 4 substance. See ***Appendix*** for more information. Use of this drug may not be allowed in certain animal competitions. Check rules and regulations before entering in a competition while this medication is being administered. Contact local racing authorities for further guidance.

In some countries, dipyrone may be found in combination with butylscopolamine (*Buscopan® Compositum* solution for injection).

HUMAN-LABELED PRODUCTS: NONE

References

For the complete list of references, see **wiley.com/go/budde/plumb**

Dobutamine

(**doe**-byoo-ta-meen) *Dobutrex*®
Beta-Adrenergic Inotrope

Prescriber Highlights

- ► Parenteral, rapid-acting inotropic agent used in a variety of species to improve cardiac output
- ► Contraindications in humans (may not be applicable to animals) include patients with known hypersensitivity to the drug or to the preservative (sodium bisulfite); patients with idiopathic hypertrophic subaortic stenosis (IHSS).
- ► Use with caution in patients with pre-existing arrhythmias.
- ► Animals with atrial fibrillation should receive a digoxin preparation prior to dobutamine administration.
- ► Most common adverse effects include facial twitching (dogs), tachycardia; CNS effects (eg, tremors, seizures) may be seen in cats receiving higher doses.
- ► Dobutamine should be used in critical care settings with continuous monitoring of heart rate/rhythm and blood pressure.

Uses/Indications

Dobutamine is an injectable, rapid-onset positive inotropic agent for short term adjunctive treatment (usually less than 72 hours) of congestive heart failure. It is also useful in shock patients when fluid therapy alone does not restore acceptable arterial blood pressure, cardiac output, or tissue perfusion. Dobutamine is also used to treat hypotension caused by decreased cardiac contractility in patients undergoing general anesthesia.

Dobutamine is administered as an IV CRI and should be used only in critical care settings where adequate monitoring (eg, continuous BP, ECG, cardiac output, pulmonary capillary wedge pressure) can be provided.

Pharmacology/Actions

Dobutamine is considered a direct beta-1-adrenergic agonist. At therapeutic doses, it also has mild beta-2- and alpha-1-adrenergic effects, which balance each other and cause little direct effect on the systemic vasculature. In contrast to dopamine, dobutamine does not cause the release of norepinephrine. Dobutamine has relatively mild chronotropic, arrhythmogenic, and vasodilative effects, but higher doses can cause tachycardia.

Increased myocardial contractility and stroke volumes result in increased cardiac output. However, increased myocardial contractility may increase myocardial oxygen demand and coronary blood flow. Blood pressure and heart rate generally are mildly increased because of increased cardiac output.

Pharmacokinetics

Because dobutamine is rapidly metabolized in the GI tract and is not systemically absorbed after oral administration, dobutamine is only administered intravenously as a constant rate infusion (CRI). After IV administration, the onset of action generally occurs within 2 minutes and peaks within 10 minutes.

Dobutamine is metabolized rapidly in the liver and other tissues and has a plasma half-life of ≈2 minutes in humans. The drug's effects diminish rapidly after cessation of therapy.

Pharmacokinetic data for domestic animals is unavailable.

Contraindications/Precautions/Warnings

Dobutamine is contraindicated in patients with known hypersensitivity to the drug or its preservative, sodium bisulfite, which has been documented to cause allergic-type reactions in humans. Dobutamine is also contraindicated in humans with idiopathic hypertrophic subaortic stenosis (IHSS).

Adequate vascular volume is required for dobutamine use; hypovolemic states must be corrected before use.

Use with extreme caution in patients with ventricular tachyarrhythmias or atrial fibrillation because dobutamine can enhance atrioventricular conduction. In animals with atrial fibrillation, digoxin (ie, digitalization) is recommended before dobutamine administration to slow AV nodal conduction. In horses that will receive electrocardioversion for atrial fibrillation, dobutamine should be stopped for at least 5 minutes before shock delivery.[1]

Do not confuse DOBUTamine with DOPamine. Writing part of the drug's name in upper case on prescriptions/orders may reduce the risk of errors.

Adverse Effects

Adverse effects reported in dogs include tachycardia, facial twitching, and seizures. Infusions greater than 20 µg/kg/minute IV may cause tachycardia. One published study has reported dobutamine-induced bradycardia.[2] Tachyphylaxis (a rapid decrease in drug response; increased dosages may be required to achieve the desired effect) may occur, and in dogs, can become apparent within 48 to 72 hours of starting dobutamine therapy.

In cats, doses greater than 5 µg/kg/minute may cause CNS effects such as tremors or seizures. In this species, dobutamine can be administered under general anesthesia but should be discontinued before recovery.

Dobutamine is a weaker proarrhythmic drug than most other catecholamines, and arrhythmias observed at 3 – 5 µg/kg/minute in horses are usually limited to bradyarrhythmias, second-degree atrioventricular blocks, premature atrial complexes, and isorhythmic atrioventricular dissociation. Use parasympatholytics (eg, atropine) with caution, as the risk for tachyarrhythmias[3] and ileus is increased.

In humans, the most commonly reported adverse effects are increased heart rate (5 to 15 bpm) and increased blood pressure (10 to 20 mm Hg). Ectopic beats, chest pain, and palpitations may also occur. At usual doses, these effects are generally mild and will not necessitate halting therapy; modify dose as clinically indicated. Other, less common, adverse effects reported include nausea, headache, hypotension, vomiting, hypokalemia, leg cramps, paresthesia, and dyspnea. Phlebitis and infusion-site reactions may occur.

Reproductive/Nursing Safety

Fetal toxicity was not demonstrated in rats or rabbits at doses used clinically. It is unknown if dobutamine crosses the placenta or enters maternal milk. Because safety has not been established in animals, this drug should only be used when the maternal benefits outweigh the potential risks to offspring.

Overdose/Acute Toxicity

Clinical signs reported with excessive doses include tachycardia, hypertension, nervousness, vomiting, fatigue, tremor, and seizures. Because of the drug's short duration of action, temporarily halting therapy usually reverses these effects. Tachyarrhythmias may be treated with propranolol or lidocaine.

For patients that have experienced or are suspected to have experienced an overdose, consultation with a 24-hour poison consultation center specializing in providing veterinary-specific information is recommended. For general information related to overdose and toxin exposures, as well as contact information for poison control centers, refer to the ***Appendix***.

Drug Interactions

The following drug interactions have either been reported or are theoretical in humans or animals receiving dobutamine and may be of significance in veterinary patients. Unless otherwise noted, use together is not necessarily contraindicated, but weigh the potential risks and perform additional monitoring when appropriate.

- **Anticholinergics** (eg, **atropine; butylscopolamine, glycopy-**

rrolate): May increase the risk for tachyarrhythmias in horses; use with caution.

- **Beta-Adrenergic Receptor Antagonists** (eg, **atenolol, metoprolol, propranolol**): May antagonize the cardiac effects of dobutamine and result in a preponderance of alpha-adrenergic effects and increased total peripheral resistance
- **Nitroprusside**: Synergistic effects (increased cardiac output and reduced wedge pressure) can result if dobutamine is used with nitroprusside.

Laboratory Considerations

- None

Dosages

NOTE: Dobutamine is administered as an IV CRI and should be used only in critical care settings where adequate monitoring (eg, continuous BP, ECG, cardiac output, pulmonary capillary wedge pressure) can be provided.

DOGS:

Short-term treatment of low cardiac output and acute congestive heart failure (CHF; extra-label): Dosages are usually started on the low end and titrated upward. Most recommendations fall in the 2 – 15 µg/kg/minute IV CRI range,[4-7] but suggested lower end dosages ranging from 1 – 5 µg/kg/minute and upper end dosages of up to 40 µg/kg/minute can be found.

CHF associated with myxomatous mitral valve disease (MMVD; extra-label):

Acute management of patients in stage C heart failure (either current or past clinical signs of heart failure): Start with dobutamine 2.5 µg/kg/minute IV CRI and increase as needed up to 10 µg/kg/minute.[8] Dobutamine should be used in addition to other treatments to improve the left ventricular function in patients that fail to respond adequately to diuretics, pimobendan, sedation, oxygen, and comfort care measures.

Acute management of patients in stage D heart failure (end-stage, in which clinical signs of heart failure are refractory to standard treatment): Start with dobutamine 1 µg/kg/minute IV CRI and up-titrate every 15 to 30 minutes to a maximum of ≈10 – 15 µg/kg/minute.[8] May be administered concomitantly with nitroprusside to provide afterload reduction. Use for 12 to 48 hours to improve hemodynamics and refractory cardiogenic pulmonary edema.

Hypotension during general anesthesia (extra-label):

a) 5 µg/kg/minute IV CRI during propofol anesthesia[9]
b) 2 – 12 µg/kg/minute during isoflurane anesthesia[10]

CATS:

Short-term treatment of low cardiac output and acute congestive heart failure (extra-label): 1 – 5 µg/kg/minute IV CRI.[7] Dosage suggestions tend to be lower for cats (than dogs). Dosages are usually started on the low end and titrated upward. Titrate dose to effect, but doses above 5 µg/kg/minute have anecdotally been associated with seizures.

Hypotension during general anesthesia (extra-label): 2 – 20 µg/kg/minute IV CRI[11]

HORSES:

Cardiovascular support in anesthetized horses (extra-label):

a) 1 – 1.5 µg/kg/minute IV CRI, arterial blood pressure increases, but cardiac output is marginally affected. At higher rates, both cardiac output and arterial blood pressure are increased, but the risk for arrhythmias is increased.[3]
b) **Hypotension during inhalant anesthesia** (extra-label): Doses between 0.5 – 3 µg/kg/minute IV CRI have been used to treat hypotension caused by inhalational agents (ie, isoflurane and sevoflurane). At these doses, an increase in blood pressure, right atrial pressure, stroke volume, jejunum and colon blood flow, cardiac output, oxygen content, and oxygen delivery is noted.[12-15]

Foals (after volume repletion) (extra-label): 2 – 20 µg/kg/minute IV CRI[16]

BIRDS:

Isoflurane-induced severe hypotension in Hispaniolan Amazon parrots (extra-label): In the study, dobutamine CRI at 15 µg/kg/minute caused the greatest increases in arterial blood pressure of the 3 tested dobutamine infusions (5, 10, or 15 µg/kg/minute).[17]

Monitoring

- Blood pressure, heart rate and rhythm, including continuous ECG
- Mucous membrane color, capillary refill time, hydration status
- Serum potassium
- Baseline and periodic renal parameters (eg, BUN, creatinine) as needed for underlying problem being treated
- Urine output
- Ideally, measurement of central venous or pulmonary capillary wedge pressures and cardiac output

Client Information

- Dobutamine should only be administered by professionals familiar with its use and in a setting in which adequate patient monitoring can be performed.

Chemistry/Synonyms

Dobutamine HCl is a synthetic inotropic agent related structurally to dopamine. It occurs as a white, to off-white, crystalline powder with a pK_a of 9.4. Dobutamine is sparingly soluble in water and alcohol.

Dobutamine HCl may also be known as 46236, compound 81929, dobutamini hydrochloridum, and LY-174008; many trade names are available.

Storage/Stability

Dobutamine injection should be stored at room temperature, 20°C to 25°C (68°F-77°F); diluted solutions should be used within 24 hours.

Compatibility/Compounding Considerations

To prepare solution: The solution for injection must be further diluted to a concentration no greater than 5 mg/mL (total of at least 50 mL of diluent/20 mL of dobutamine) before administering.

Generally, dobutamine is added to D_5W, normal saline (if animal not severely sodium restricted), or other compatible IV solutions. The following approximate concentrations will result if 1 vial (250 mg) is added to 250 mL, 500 mL, or 1000 mL IV solutions: 250 mL: ≈1000 µg/mL; 500 mL: ≈500 µg/mL; 1000 mL: ≈250 µg/mL.

A mechanical fluid administration control device (eg, fluid pump) should be used to administer dobutamine. To calculate a dobutamine CRI[18]: 6 times body weight (in kg) = the number of mg (NOT mL) of dobutamine added to a sufficient quantity of 0.9% NaCl to obtain a total volume of 100 mL. When this solution is delivered at 1 mL/hour IV, 1 µg/kg/min is administered.

Compatibility is dependent on factors such as pH, concentration, temperature, and diluent used; specialized references or a hospital pharmacist should be consulted for more specific information.

Dobutamine is physically **compatible** with the following IV solutions: D_5W, sodium chloride 0.45% and 0.9%, dextrose-saline combinations, and lactated Ringer's. Dobutamine is physically **compatible** with the following drugs: amiodarone, atropine sulfate, dopamine, epinephrine, hydralazine, isoproterenol, lidocaine, meperidine, morphine sulfate, nitroglycerin, norepinephrine, phentolamine, phenylephrine, procainamide, propranolol, and verapamil.

Dobutamine may be physically **incompatible** with the following agents: aminophylline, bumetanide, calcium chloride, calcium gluconate, diazepam, digoxin, furosemide, heparin (inconsistent results), regular insulin, magnesium sulfate, phenytoin sodium, potassium chloride (at high concentrations [160 mEq/L] only), potassium phosphate, and sodium bicarbonate.

Dosage Forms/Regulatory Status

VETERINARY-LABELED PRODUCTS: NONE

The Association of Racing Commissioners International (ARCI) has designated dobutamine as a class 2 substance. See the ***Appendix*** for more information. Use of this drug may not be allowed in certain animal competitions. Check rules and regulations before entering in a competition while this medication is being administered. Contact local racing authorities for further guidance.

HUMAN-LABELED PRODUCTS:

Dobutamine HCl Injection Concentrated Solution: 12.5 mg/mL in 20 mL and 40 mL single-use vials; generic; (Rx)

Dobutamine HCL Solution for Injection: 250 mg/250 mL (1 mg/mL) preservative free in 250 mL single-use containers; 500 mg/250 mL (2 mg/mL) preservative free in 250 mL single-use containers and 1000 mg/250 mL (4 mg/mL) preservative free in 250 mL single-use containers Dobutamine Hydrochloride in 5% Dextrose Injection; (Rx)

References

For the complete list of references, see **wiley.com/go/budde/plumb**

Docusate

Dioctyl Sodium Sulfosuccinate (DSS)

(***dok***-yoo-sate) *Colace®*

Surfactant Stool Softener

Prescriber Highlights

- Used to soften and ease passage of hard stools in a variety of species
- Use with caution in patients with fluid/electrolyte abnormalities. Overdoses can be fatal in horses.
- Adverse effects include cramping, diarrhea, and GI mucosal damage.

Uses/Indications

Docusate is used in small animal species when feces are hard or dry, or with anorectal conditions when passing firm feces would be painful or detrimental. Docusate can be used alone or in combination with mineral oil in treating fecal impactions in horses, although one study found docusate to be as effective as water[1] and that psyllium is the preferred treatment (over docusate) in cases of sand accumulation.[2] Docusate can be used for partial defaunation in sheep to increase voluntary food intake and increase digestion and absorption of nutrients.[3,4]

Pharmacology/Actions

Docusate salts reduce surface tension and allow water and fat to penetrate the ingesta and formed feces thereby softening the stool. Recent in vivo studies have demonstrated that docusate also increases cAMP concentrations in colonic mucosal cells that may increase both ion secretion and fluid permeability from these cells into the colon lumen.

Pharmacokinetics

It is unknown how much docusate is absorbed after oral administration, but it is believed that some is absorbed from the small intestine and then excreted into the bile.

Contraindications/Precautions/Warnings

Docusate is contraindicated in patients hypersensitive to it. Use with caution in patients with preexisting fluid or electrolyte abnormalities and in those at risk for aspiration.

Adverse Effects

At usual doses, clinically significant adverse effects should be rare. Cramping, diarrhea, and intestinal mucosal damage are possible. The liquid preparations may cause throat irritation if administered by mouth. Docusate sodium is bitter tasting.

Severe gastric and esophageal changes have been reported in snakes.[5]

Reproductive/Nursing Safety

It is not known whether docusate crosses the placenta or is excreted in milk, but it is unlikely to be of concern.

Overdose/Acute Toxicity

Overdoses in horses may be serious.[6] In healthy horses, single doses of 0.65 – 1 g/kg have caused dehydration, intestinal mucosal damage, and death.[6] Maximum therapeutic dosages up to 0.2 g/kg have been reported. Signs of overdoses in horses can begin within 1 to 2 hours of dosing with initial signs including restlessness and increased intestinal sounds; increases in respiratory and cardiac rates can follow. Abdominal pain, watery diarrhea, and dehydration can occur with horses deteriorating over hours to several days to lateral recumbency and death. Because high dose docusate can cause secretory effects, hydration and electrolyte status should be monitored and treated if necessary. Treatment is supportive; GI protectants, correct fluid and electrolyte imbalances, analgesics, and antiendotoxemic agents (eg, corticosteroids or NSAIDs) have been suggested.

For patients that have experienced or are suspected to have experienced an overdose, consultation with a 24-hour poison consultation center specializing in providing veterinary-specific information is recommended. For general information related to overdose and toxin exposures, as well as contact information for poison control centers, refer to ***Appendix***.

Drug Interactions

The following drug interactions have either been reported or are theoretical in humans or animals receiving docusate and may be of significance in veterinary patients. Unless otherwise noted, use together is not necessarily contraindicated, but weigh the potential risks and perform additional monitoring when appropriate.

Mineral Oil: Theoretically, mineral oil should not be given with docusate (DSS) as enhanced mineral oil absorption could occur; however, this interaction does not appear to be of significant clinical concern with large animal species. It is less clear whether this could be of significance with small animals; therefore the concurrent use of these agents in dogs or cats cannot be recommended. If it is deemed necessary to use both docusate and mineral oil in small animal species, separate doses by at least 2 hours.

Dosages

DOGS:

Stool softener (extra-label): 25 – 100 mg/dog (depending on dog size; NOT mg/kg) PO once to twice daily. May give up to 240 mg or 250 mg once daily to very large dogs

CATS:

Stool softener (extra-label): 50 mg/cat (NOT mg/kg) PO once daily

HORSES:

Large colon impaction (extra-label): 6 – 12 g/500 kg (1102 lb) diluted in 2 to 4 liters of water by nasogastric tube every 12 to 24 hours[7]

Cecal impaction (extra-label): 10 – 20 mg/kg in 8 L water and administered via NG tube[8]

SHEEP:

Partial defaunation (extra-label): 0.8 – 1.2 g/kg of diet (NOT per kg body weight)[3,4]

Monitoring

- Clinical efficacy
- Hydration and serum electrolyte status, if indicated

Client Information

- Used to treat constipation caused by hard or dry stools
- Generally well tolerated with few side effects
- Should be given on an empty stomach; 1 hour before or 2 hours after a meal
- Docusate is available OTC (over the counter; without a prescription), but do **NOT** give it (or any other laxatives or medications) to your animal without first consulting your veterinarian.

Chemistry/Synonyms

Docusate is available in sodium and calcium salts. They are anionic, surface-active agents and possess wetting and emulsifying properties.

Docusate sodium (also known as dioctyl sodium succinate, DSS, or DOSS) occurs as a white, wax-like plastic solid with a characteristic odor. One gram is soluble in ≈70 mL of water and it is freely soluble in alcohol and glycerin. Solutions are clear and have a bitter taste.

Docusate calcium (also known as dioctyl calcium succinate) occurs as a white, amorphous solid with a characteristic odor (octyl alcohol). It is very slightly soluble in water, but freely soluble in alcohol.

Docusate sodium may also be known as dioctyl sodium sulphosuccinate, dioctyl sodium sulfosuccinate, docusatum natricum, DSS, and sodium dioctyl sulphosuccinate; many trade names are available; *Colace*® is the most commonly known sodium salt product and *Surfak*® is the most commonly known calcium salt product.

Storage/Stability

Capsules of salts of docusate should be stored in tight containers at room temperature. Temperatures above 30°C (86°F) can soften or melt soft gelatin capsules. Docusate sodium solutions should be stored in tight containers and the syrup should be stored in tight, light-resistant containers.

Compatibility/Compounding Considerations

No specific information noted

Dosage Forms/Regulatory Status

VETERINARY APPROVED PRODUCTS:

There are several docusate products marketed for veterinary use; their FDA-approval status is unknown, and no entries were found in the FDA Green Book, searchable at AnimalDrugs@FDA. Commercially available products may include:

Docusate Sodium Bloat Preparation: 240 mg/30 mL in 360 mL containers; (OTC). Labeled milk withdrawal = 96 hours; slaughter withdrawal = 3 days.

Docusate Sodium Enema: 5% water miscible solution in 1-gallon containers; *Dioctynate*®; (OTC)

Docusate Sodium Enema: 250 mg in 12 mL syringes; *Pet-Enema*®, *Enema SA*®, *Docu-Soft*® *Enema*; (OTC or RX)

Docusate Sodium Oral Liquid 5% in gallons; various; generic. May also be called Veterinary Surfactant (OTC)

HUMAN-LABELED PRODUCTS:

There are many trade name products for docusate. The two most commonly known are *Colace*® (sodium salt) and *Surfak*® (calcium salt).

Docusate Sodium Oral Tablets: 100 mg; (OTC)

Docusate Sodium Oral Capsules and Soft-gel Capsules: 50 mg, 100 mg, and 250 mg; generic; (OTC)

Docusate Sodium Oral Syrup/Liquid: 50 mg/5 mL (10 mg/mL); (OTC)

Docusate Calcium Capsules: 240 mg (regular and soft gel); (OTC)

References

For the complete list of references, see **wiley.com/go/budde/plumb**

Dolasetron

(dole-***a***-se-tron) *Anzemet*®

Antiemetic Agent; 5-HT_3 Receptor Antagonist

Prescriber Highlights

- 5-hydroxytryptamine$_3$ (5-HT_3) receptor antagonist antiemetic particularly useful for chemotherapy-related nausea and vomiting in small animals
- Once-daily administration
- Usually well tolerated; may cause dose-related ECG changes
- Oral human tablets not easily dosed in small animals due to strength sizes; must be reformulated for PO use in cats
- Expense and availability may be issues.

Uses/Indications

Dolasetron may be effective in treating severe nausea and vomiting in dogs and cats, particularly if it is caused by chemotherapy drugs. Because dolasetron is given once daily, it is often preferred over ondansetron (a similarly effective antiemetic). However, for oral use in small animals, dolasetron tablets are too large (50 and 100 mg) to be practically administered. In a study, dolasetron did not prevent xylazine-induced emesis in cats.[1]

Pharmacology/Actions

Dolasetron exerts its antinausea and antiemetic actions by selectively antagonizing 5-hydroxytryptamine$_3$ (5-HT_3) receptors. These receptors are found primarily in the CNS chemoreceptor trigger zone, on vagal nerve terminals, and on enteric neurons in the GI tract. Chemotherapy-induced vomiting is believed to be caused principally by serotonin release from the mucosal enterochromaffin cells in the small intestine. Dolasetron does not have prokinetic activity.

Pharmacokinetics

After dolasetron is administered IV to dogs, its half-life is only minutes long, as it is rapidly reduced via carbonyl reductase to hydrodolasetron (also called reduced dolasetron or red-dolasetron), and it is presumed that, as in humans, hydrodolasetron is primarily responsible for the drug's pharmacologic effect. Oral dolasetron is rapidly absorbed and converted to hydrodolasetron, although oral bioavailability of dolasetron is only 7%. Hydrodolasetron's apparent volume of distribution in dogs is 8.5 L/kg; total body clearance is 25 mL/minute/kg and half-life is about 4 hours.[2]

In humans, dolasetron is rapidly absorbed and converted to hydrodolasetron, which is ≈100 times more potent as a serotonin antagonist than its precursor. Oral bioavailability is ≈75%. Hydrodolasetron's half-life in humans is ≈7 to 8 hours. The drug is partially metabolized in the liver, but 50% *to* 60% is excreted unchanged into the urine. Clearance may be reduced in patients with severe renal or hepatic impairment.[3]

Contraindications/Precautions/Warnings

Dolasetron is contraindicated in patients that are hypersensitive to it, with second- and third-degree atrioventricular block, or with markedly prolonged QT interval. It should be given with caution to patients with (or who are susceptible to developing) prolongation of cardiac conduction intervals. Use this drug with caution in patients with congenital QT syndrome, hypokalemia, hypomagnesemia; patients receiving anti-arrhythmic drugs or diuretics that affect electrolyte levels; or patients with high cumulative doses of anthracycline (eg, doxorubicin) chemotherapy.

Adverse Effects

Dolasetron appears to be well tolerated in the limited numbers of small animal patients that have received it. In humans, it has been associated with dose-related ECG interval (PR, QT) prolongation and QRS widening. Other adverse effects that have been reported in humans using dolasetron during chemotherapy include headache, dizziness, and increased appetite.[3]

Reproductive/Nursing Safety

Teratogenicity studies in laboratory animals failed to demonstrate any teratogenic effects.

It is unknown if the drug enters milk; the manufacturer urges caution.

Because safety has not been established in animals, this drug should only be used when the maternal benefits outweigh the potential risks to offspring.

Overdose/Acute Toxicity

There are limited data available. One human patient who received 13 mg/kg of dolasetron developed severe hypotension and dizziness and was treated with vasopressors and IV fluids. The patient's blood pressure returned to baseline 3 hours after the dose was administered. It is suggested to manage overdoses with supportive therapy. The lethal IV doses in mice and rats were 160 mg/kg and 140 mg/kg, respectively.[4] This is equivalent to 6 to 12 times the human recommended dose when comparing equivalent body surface areas.

For patients that have experienced or are suspected to have experienced an overdose, consultation with a 24-hour poison control center specializing in providing veterinary-specific information is recommended. For general information related to overdose and toxin exposures, as well as contact information for poison control centers, refer to ***Appendix***.

Drug Interactions

The following drug interactions either have been reported or are theoretical in humans or animals receiving dolasetron and may be of significance in veterinary patients. Unless otherwise noted, use together is not necessarily contraindicated, but weigh the potential risks and perform additional monitoring when appropriate.

- **AMIODARONE**: Concurrent use may increase risk for QT interval prolongation.
- **APOMORPHINE**: Emetics and antiemetics counteract the effects of each other. 5-hydroxytryptamine$_3$ (5-HT$_3$) antagonists may enhance the hypotensive effect of apomorphine. In humans, it is recommended to avoid this combination.
- **ATENOLOL**: May reduce the clearance and increase blood levels of hydrodolasetron
- **AZOLE ANTIFUNGALS** (eg, **ketoconazole, itraconazole**): May reduce the clearance and increase blood levels of hydrodolasetron
- **BUPRENORPHINE**: Concurrent use may increase risk for serotonin syndrome.
- **CISAPRIDE**: Concurrent use may increase risk for QT interval prolongation.
- **FLUOROQUINOLONE ANTIBIOTICS** (eg, **ciprofloxacin, moxifloxacin**): Concurrent use may increase risk for QT interval prolongation.
- **MACROLIDE ANTIBIOTICS** (eg, **erythromycin, clarithromycin**): Concurrent use may increase risk for cardiotoxicity.
- **METRONIDAZOLE**: Concurrent use may increase risk for QT interval prolongation.
- **PHENOBARBITAL**: Can reduce hydrodolasetron blood levels
- **PHENOTHIAZINES** (eg, **acepromazine**): Concurrent use may increase risk for cardiotoxicity.
- **QUINIDINE**: Concurrent use may increase risk for QT interval prolongation.
- **SOTALOL**: Concurrent use may increase risk for QT interval prolongation.

Laboratory Considerations

- None are noted.

Dosages

DOGS/CATS:

Antiemetic (extra-label): 0.6 mg/kg PO once daily (every 24 hours). Some clinicians recommend giving higher dosages up to 1 mg/kg to treat active vomiting disorders.

Monitoring

- Efficacy
- ECG in at-risk patients

Client Information

- This medicine is often used to prevent or treat chemotherapy-induced nausea and vomiting.
- Side effects are uncommon.

Chemistry/Synonyms

A 5-hydroxytryptamine$_3$ (5-HT$_3$) receptor antagonist antiemetic, dolasetron mesylate occurs as a white to off-white powder. It is freely soluble in water or propylene glycol, and slightly soluble in 0.9% sodium chloride solution or alcohol.

Dolasetron may also be known as *Anzemet*®, *Anemet*® or *Zamanon*®.

Storage/Stability

The commercially available tablets should be stored at room temperature 20°C to 25°C (68°F -77°F) and protected from light.

Compatibility/Compounding Considerations

Dolasetron 10 mg/mL oral suspension prepared with a 1:1 mixture of *Ora-Plus*® and *Ora-Sweet*® was stable for at least 90 days when stored at room temperature or refrigerated.[5]

Dosage Forms/Regulatory Status

VETERINARY-LABELED PRODUCTS: NONE

HUMAN-LABELED PRODUCTS:

Dolasetron Tablets: 50 mg; *Anzemet*®; (Rx)

References

For the complete list of references, see **wiley.com/go/budde/plumb**

Domperidone

(dohm-***pare***-i-dohne) *Equidone*®, *Motilium*®

Dopamine-2 Antagonist

Prescriber Highlights

- ► D$_2$ dopamine antagonist used in horses for prevention of fescue toxicosis, treatment of agalactia/hypogalactia in periparturient mares, and as a diagnostic agent for pituitary pars intermedia dysfunction (PPID). Potential treatment for leishmaniasis in dogs
- ► Galactorrhea and gynecomastia are the most likely adverse effects.

Uses/Indications

Domperidone is FDA-approved in the United States for prevention of fescue toxicosis in periparturient mares. Domperidone has been shown to increase plasma ACTH in horses with equine pituitary pars intermedia dysfunction (PPID, equine hyperadrenocorticism), and has been considered for use in the diagnosis of this condition.[1] However, the thyrotropin-releasing hormone (TRH) stimulation test appears to be more accurate for the diagnosis of PPID.[2]

Domperidone appears ineffective as a GI prokinetic and antiemetic agent in small animals. A study and follow-up report in dogs showed that domperidone may have some efficacy in both preventing and treating mild to moderate canine leishmaniasis.[3-5]

Pharmacology/Actions

Domperidone's apparent efficacy for the treatment of fescue toxicosis in pregnant mares is related to the fact that tall fescue toxicosis causes decreased prolactin levels. Dopamine is involved in the reduction of prolactin secretion, and it is postulated that the alkaloids found in tall fescue act as dopaminergic agonists. Domperidone ostensibly blocks this effect.

Domperidone is a dopamine antagonist (D_2 receptors) with similar actions as metoclopramide. It does not readily cross into the CNS, but CNS adverse effects in overdose situations are common, and extrapyramidal adverse effects have been reported in some human patients. In dogs and cats, metoclopramide appears to have more prokinetic effects on gastric emptying than domperidone. Domperidone does not appreciably affect small intestinal transit time but may increase lower esophageal sphincter tone. Horses that received 5 mg/kg PO (4.5 times the normal dose) demonstrated increased rate of gastric emptying, without changes in GI contractility or overall transit time.[6]

Domperidone antagonizes dopamine in the GI tract and chemoreceptor trigger zone, which is thought to be the primary cause of its prokinetic and antiemetic effects. It also is an antagonist for alpha-2 and beta-2-adrenergic receptors in the stomach, which may contribute to the drug's pharmacological actions.

Domperidone may have effects on cell-mediated immunity possibly due to its stimulation of prolactin. Prolactin has been classified as a pro-inflammatory lymphocyte-derived cytokine, and a study done in healthy dogs found that domperidone induced a statistically significant increase in the percentages of activated phagocytes in the treated group during and for up to one month after treatment.[7]

Pharmacokinetics

Domperidone is absorbed from the GI tract, but its bioavailability in dogs is only about 20%, presumably due to a high first pass effect. Peak serum concentrations occur about 2 hours after oral dosing and the drug is highly bound (93%) to serum proteins. Domperidone is primarily metabolized and is a substrate of the cytochrome P450 3A4 family. Metabolites are excreted in the feces and urine.

Domperidone is poorly absorbed in horses. It is widely distributed throughout the body but does not readily cross the blood-brain barrier or placenta. The average terminal half-life in horses is 6 hours.

Contraindications/Precautions/Warnings

Domperidone should not be used in animals with known hypersensitivity to it, or when GI hemorrhages, perforations, or obstructions are present or suspected. Do not use domperidone in pregnant mares more than 15 days prior to their expected foaling date (see ***Reproductive/Nursing Safety***). In horses, failure of passive transfer of immunoglobulins (IgG) may occur even in the absence of leakage of colostrum or milk. All foals born to mares treated with domperidone should be tested for serum IgG concentrations.

Because domperidone is potentially a neurotoxic substrate of P-glycoprotein, it should be used with caution in those herding breeds (eg, Collies) that may have the multidrug sensitivity gene (*MDR-1*) gene mutation (also known as *ABCB1*-1delta) that causes a nonfunctional protein. Also see ***Drug Interactions***.

Domperidone is contraindicated in human patients with hepatic failure. Prolongation of the QT interval prompted removal of the human product in the US; use cautiously in patients receiving other drugs that prolong the QT interval or inhibit domperidone metabolism. Also see ***Drug Interactions***.

Adverse Effects

Because plasma prolactin levels may be increased, galactorrhea or gynecomastia may result. In horses, the most commonly reported adverse effects are premature lactation (dripping of milk prior foaling) and failure of transfer of passive immunity. Foals of mares treated with domperidone may experience loose stools or diarrhea. Injectable products (no longer available) have been associated with arrhythmias in human patients with heart disease or hypokalemia. Rarely, somnolence or dystonic reactions have occurred in humans.

Reproductive/Nursing Safety

Accurate breeding date(s) and an expected foaling date are needed for the safe use of domperidone.[8] When administered more than 15 days prior to the expected foaling date, domperidone may lead to premature birth, low birth weight foals, or foal morbidity. The safety of domperidone has not been evaluated in stallions or in breeding, pregnant, and lactating mares other than in the last 45 days of pregnancy and the first 15 days of lactation. The long-term effects on foals born to mares treated with domperidone have not been evaluated.

Domperidone has been shown to have teratogenic effects when it is used at high doses in mice, rats, and rabbits. The drug's effect of causing prolactin release may impact fertility in both female and male patients.

Domperidone has been used to increase milk supply in humans. In rats, it enters milk in small amounts with ≈1/500th of the adult dose reaching the pups.

Because safety has not been established in animals, this drug should only be used when the maternal benefits outweigh the potential risks to offspring.

Overdose/Acute Toxicity

There is no specific antidote for domperidone overdose. Methemoglobinemia has been reported in humans. Use standard decontamination procedures and treat supportively.

For patients that have experienced or are suspected to have experienced an overdose, consultation with a 24-hour poison control center specializing in providing veterinary-specific information is recommended. For general information related to overdose and toxin exposures, as well as contact information for poison control centers, refer to ***Appendix***.

Drug Interactions

The following drug interactions either have been reported or are theoretical in humans or animals receiving domperidone and may be of significance in veterinary patients. Unless otherwise noted, use together is not necessarily contraindicated, but weigh the potential risks and perform additional monitoring when appropriate.

- AZOLE ANTIFUNGALS (eg, **itraconazole, ketoconazole**): May increase domperidone concentrations
- ANTACIDS, ALUMINUM- CALCIUM- OR MAGNESIUM-CONTAINING: May decrease domperidone bioavailability
- ANTICHOLINERGIC DRUGS (eg, **atropine, diphenhydramine, hyoscyamine**): May reduce the efficacy of domperidone
- BROMOCRIPTINE/CABERGOLINE: Domperidone may antagonize effects on prolactin.
- CIMETIDINE: May decrease domperidone bioavailability and decrease domperidone metabolism
- DRUGS THAT PROLONG QT INTERVAL (eg, **ciprofloxacin, chlorpromazine, cisapride, methadone, ondansetron, quinidine**): May increase risk for QT prolongation
- H_2-RECEPTOR ANTAGONISTS (eg, **ranitidine**): May decrease domperidone bioavailability
- MACROLIDE ANTIBIOTICS (eg, **erythromycin, clarithromycin**): May increase domperidone concentrations and may increase risk of QT prolongation.

- **Opioids** (eg, **morphine**): May reduce the efficacy of domperidone
- **Pergolide**: May reduce the efficacy of domperidone
- **Proton Pump Inhibitors** (**PPIs**; eg, **omeprazole, pantoprazole**): May decrease domperidone bioavailability
- **Sustained-Release** or **Enteric-Coated Oral Medications**: Domperidone may alter the absorptive characteristics of these drugs by decreasing GI transit times.

Laboratory Considerations

- Domperidone may increase **serum prolactin** concentrations.
- Domperidone may increase **ALT** and **AST.**
- Domperidone may cause a false positive result on the **milk calcium** test used to predict foaling.

Dosages

DOGS:

Alternative treatment for leishmaniasis in dogs with mild to moderate clinical signs (extra-label): In the initial study, dogs received 1 mg/kg PO twice daily for 30 days. In the short-term follow-up report, dosages reported were 0.5 mg/kg PO once daily (every 24 hours) for 30 days.[3,4] In one study, domperidone 0.5 mg/kg PO was administered once daily for 4 weeks was followed by 3 months without treatment and which time domperidone 0.5 mg/kg PO was administered once daily for another 4-week treatment.[9]

Prevention of leishmaniasis (extra-label): 0.5 mg/kg PO once daily for 30 days, every 4 months[5] for dogs living in endemic areas

HORSES:

Fescue toxicity (label dosage; FDA-approved): 1.1 mg/kg PO once daily starting 10 to 15 days prior to expected foaling date (EFD).[8] Treatment may be continued for up to 5 days after foaling if mares are not producing adequate milk after foaling.

Assisting in the diagnosis of pituitary par intermedia dysfunction (PPID) | domperidone response test (extra-label): Collect EDTA plasma for endogenous ACTH level at 8 AM. Administer domperidone, 3.3 mg/kg PO. Collect additional EDTA plasma for endogenous ACTH levels at 2 hours and 4 hours after domperidone administration. A 2-fold increase in plasma ACTH concentration suggests PPID. Higher doses (5 mg/kg PO) may improve response. The 2-hour sample is more diagnostic in the summer and autumn, and the 4-hour sample is best in the winter and spring.[1,10]

Monitoring

- Clinical efficacy

Client Information

- Equine gel: Be sure you understand the proper use of the multi-dose dosing syringe, including how to set the dial ring for accurate dosing after the first dose.
- This medicine should not be given to mares more than 15 days before their expected foaling date, as premature birth can occur.
- In mares, premature lactation (dripping of milk prior to foaling) and failure of the mare's milk to pass on immunoglobulins to the foal are the most common side effects.
- In dogs, this medicine may be given with or without food. Do not give this medicine to your animal at the same time as antacids while it is receiving this medication. If your animal vomits or acts sick after receiving this medicine on an empty stomach, try giving the medicine with food or small treat to see if this helps. If vomiting continues, contact your veterinarian.
- Pregnant or nursing women should use caution when handling this medication.

Chemistry/Synonyms

Domperidone maleate occurs as a white or almost white powder that exhibits polymorphism. It is very slightly soluble in water or alcohol.

Domperidone may also be known as domperidonum and R-33812. Common trade names include *Motilium®* or *Equidone®*, but many trade names are available internationally.

Storage/Stability

Domperidone gel should be stored at controlled room temperature 25°C (77°F) with excursions between 15°C to 30°C (59°F-86°F) permitted. Recap the container after each use. Domperidone tablets should be stored at room temperature and protected from light and moisture.

Compatibility/Compounding Considerations

No specific information is noted.

Dosage Forms/Regulatory Status

VETERINARY-LABELED PRODUCTS:

Domperidone Oral Gel 11% (110 mg/mL) in 25 mL multi-dose oral syringes; *Equidone® Gel*; (Rx). FDA-approved for use in horses. Do not use in horses intended for human consumption. NADA #141-314.

An FDA Indexed Product (MIF 900-001) also containing salmon gonadotropin releasing hormone is available for use in ornamental finfish.

HUMAN-LABELED PRODUCTS: NONE IN THE UNITED STATES

In Canada (10 mg tablet only) and in Europe, human oral tablets of 10 mg; suppositories and oral suspension may be available.

References

For the complete list of references, see **wiley.com/go/budde/plumb**

Dopamine

(***doe***-pa-meen) *Intropin®*

Adrenergic/Dopaminergic Inotrope

Prescriber Highlights

- ► Parenteral, rapid-acting inotrope used primarily in dogs and cats
- ► Catecholamine that increases systemic peripheral resistance to raise blood pressure and can be considered for treatment of hypotension associated with poor cardiac contractility and/or vasodilation.
- ► There is no evidence that dopamine increases GFR or improves outcome in the treatment of oliguric or anuric renal failure; therefore, dopamine is not recommended as a treatment modality to increase GFR and urine output.
- ► Contraindications include pheochromocytoma, ventricular fibrillation, and uncorrected tachyarrhythmia.
- ► Administered dose should be substantially reduced in patients receiving monoamine oxidase inhibitors (MAOIs).
- ► Adverse effects include nausea/vomiting, ectopic beats, tachycardia, hypotension, hypertension, dyspnea, and vasoconstriction.
- ► Dopamine should be used in critical care settings with continuous monitoring of heart rate/rhythm and blood pressure.

Uses/Indications

Dopamine is an injectable rapid-onset positive inotrope used to correct hypotension associated with low cardiac output in patients with shock after adequate fluid volume replacement and as adjunctive therapy for acute congestive heart failure. Dopamine is also used to treat hypotension in patients under general anesthesia. In rabbits, however, this treatment is not recommended because hypotension in New Zealand white rabbits anesthetized with isoflurane did not improve when given 5, 10, 15, 20, or 30 µg/kg/minute IV.[1]

Dopamine is administered as an IV CRI and should be used only in critical care settings where adequate monitoring (eg, continuous blood pressure, ECG, cardiac output, pulmonary capillary wedge pressure) can be provided.

In humans with oliguric acute kidney injury, low-dose dopamine does not effectively improve GFR[2]; this use is unproven and somewhat controversial in dogs. In cats, low-dose dopamine reportedly does not cause renal vasodilation. Generally, for dogs and cats with acute kidney injury, a dopamine CRI is not recommended as part of therapy to increase GFR and urine output.

Pharmacology/Actions

Dopamine is a precursor to norepinephrine and acts directly and indirectly (by releasing norepinephrine) on alpha and beta receptors. Dopamine also has peripheral dopaminergic effects. In dogs and cats, dopamine 5 – 10 µg/kg/minute IV CRI will have predominantly beta-1 effects, exerting positive cardiac inotropic activity (eg, increased contractility, cardiac output, heart rate); a CRI of 10 to 15 µg/kg/minute IV will have both alpha-1 and beta-1 effects,[3-6] although alpha-1 effects (eg, increased systemic and pulmonary vascular resistance, increased venous return) predominate in a dose-dependent fashion.

Pharmacokinetics

Because dopamine is rapidly metabolized in the GI tract and is not systemically absorbed after oral administration, dopamine is only administered as an IV CRI. After IV administration, onset of action is usually within 5 minutes and persists for less than 10 minutes after infusion has stopped.

Dopamine is widely distributed in the body but does not cross the blood-brain barrier in appreciable quantities.

Plasma half-life is ≈2 minutes. The drug is metabolized in the kidney, liver, and plasma by monoamine oxidase (MAO) and catechol-O-methyltransferase (COMT) to inactive compounds. Up to 25% of a dose of dopamine is metabolized to norepinephrine in the adrenergic nerve terminals. In humans receiving MAO inhibitors, dopamine's duration of activity can be as long as 1 hour. Inactive metabolites are eliminated renally.

Contraindications/Precautions/Warnings

Dopamine is contraindicated in patients with pheochromocytoma, ventricular fibrillation, and uncorrected tachyarrhythmias and is not a substitute for adequate fluid, electrolyte, or blood product replacement therapy. Dopamine should be used with caution in patients with ischemic heart disease or occlusive vascular disease. Decrease dose or discontinue the drug if clinical signs occur that implicate dopamine as the cause of reduced circulation to the extremities or the heart and if arrhythmias (eg, PVCs) occur.

Cats with oliguric acute kidney injury are unlikely to benefit from low-dose dopamine therapy, and treatment may be detrimental.

Do not confuse DOPamine with DOBUTamine or *Dopram®* (doxapram). Writing part of the drug›s name in upper case on prescriptions/orders may reduce the risk for errors.

Adverse Effects

The most frequent adverse effects include nausea and vomiting, ectopic beats, tachycardia, hypotension, hypertension, dyspnea, and vasoconstriction. Ventricular arrhythmias were noted in 2 cats receiving dopamine.[7] A stepwise dose reduction leading to discontinuation can reduce risk for hypotension.

Two dogs with hypotension that were given dopamine 7 µg/kg/minute IV CRI while under isoflurane general anesthesia had a profound decrease in heart rate (ie, 40 to 45 beats per minute) and blood pressure.[8] Dopamine was discontinued, and atropine was given to one of the dogs. Heart rate and blood pressure returned to normal values in both patients. This demonstrates how dopamine can cause an increase in cardiac contractility and initiate the Bezold-Jarisch reflex, which is an inhibitory reflex that causes hypopnea, bradycardia, and hypotension.

Extravasation injuries, including necrosis and sloughing of surrounding tissue, have occurred rarely with dopamine use in humans. Administration through large veins is recommended, and the infusion site should be closely monitored.

Reproductive/Nursing Safety

It is not known whether dopamine crosses the placenta or is excreted into milk. Decreased pup survival resulted from dopamine administration to pregnant rats.[9] Because safety has not been established in animals, this drug should only be used when the maternal benefits outweigh the potential risks to offspring.

Overdose/Acute Toxicity

Accidental overdose is manifested by excessive blood pressure elevation (see ***Adverse Effects***). Treatment consists of temporarily discontinuing therapy because dopamine's short duration of action. If the patient fails to stabilize, phentolamine can be used.

For patients that have experienced or are suspected to have experienced an overdose, consultation with a 24-hour poison center specializing in providing veterinary-specific information is recommended. For general information related to overdose and toxin exposures, as well as contact information for poison control centers, refer to ***Appendix***.

Drug Interactions

The following drug interactions have either been reported or are theoretical in humans or animals receiving dopamines and may be of significance in veterinary patients. Unless otherwise noted, use together is not necessarily contraindicated, but weigh the potential risks and perform additional monitoring when appropriate.

- **Alpha-Adrenergic Receptor Antagonists** (eg, **prazosin**): May antagonize the vasoconstrictive properties of dopamine (high-dose)
- **Anesthetics, Inhalant** (eg, **halothane, isoflurane**): Use of halothane with dopamine may result in increased incidences of ventricular arrhythmias.
- **Bromocriptine**: Concurrent use may result in severe hypertension and tachycardia
- **Beta-Blockers** (eg, **metoprolol**, **propranolol**): May antagonize the cardiac effects of dopamine
- **Digoxin**: Concurrent use may increase risk for arrhythmias.
- **Haloperidol**: May inhibit dopaminergic renal and mesenteric vasodilation
- **Hypotensive Agents, Other** (eg, **amlodipine, enalapril, telmisartan**): May antagonize the vasoconstrictive properties of dopamine
- **Monoamine Oxidase Inhibitors** (MAOIs; eg, **amitraz, linezolid, selegiline**): MAOIs can significantly prolong and enhance the effects of dopamine. Reduce dopamine dose by up to 90%.
- **Oxytocin**: May cause severe hypertension when used with dopamine
- **Phenothiazines** (eg, **acepromazine, prochlorperazine**): May inhibit dopaminergic renal and mesenteric vasodilation
- **Tricyclic Antidepressants** (eg, **amitriptyline, clomipramine**): May potentiate the arrhythmogenic and hypertensive effect of dopamine
- **Vasopressors/Vasoconstrictors**: Use with dopamine may cause severe hypertension

Laboratory Considerations

Dopamine may:

- Suppress **serum prolactin** secretion from the pituitary

- Suppress **thyrotropin** secretion from the pituitary
- Suppress **growth hormone** secretion from the pituitary

Dosages

NOTE: Dopamine is administered as an IV CRI only in a critical care setting. Use an IV pump or other flow-controlling device to increase precision in dosing. A stepwise dose reduction prior to discontinuation can reduce the risk for hypotension.

DOGS/CATS:

Severe hypotension/shock caused by poor cardiac contractility and/or peripheral vasodilation (extra-label): 5 – 20 µg/kg/minute IV.[10] Initially, 2.5 – 5 µg/kg/minute is recommended and then should be titrated upward to effect. Adequate volume replacement is required before use. A study in cats noted an initial CRI of 10 µg/kg/minute IV, with increases in increments of 2.5 – 5 µg/kg/minute IV.[7]

Isoflurane-induced hypotension: 7 – 10 µg/kg/minute IV[11,12]

Monitoring

- Blood pressure, heart rate and rhythm, including continuous ECG
- Mucous membrane color, capillary refill time, hydration status
- Ideally, measurement of central venous or pulmonary capillary wedge pressures and cardiac output
- Baseline and periodic renal parameters (eg, BUN, creatinine) as needed for underlying problem being treated
- Urine output
- IV infusion site for signs of inflammation related to extravasation

Client Information

- Dopamine should be used only in an intensive care setting or settings in which adequate monitoring is possible.

Chemistry/Synonyms

Dopamine (as the HCl salt), an endogenous catecholamine that is the immediate precursor to norepinephrine, occurs as a white to off-white crystalline powder. It is freely soluble in water and soluble in alcohol. The injectable concentrated solution has a pH of 2.5 to 5.5 and may contain an antioxidant (sodium bisulfate). The pH of the ready-to-use injectable products in dextrose range from 3 to 5.

Dopamine HCl may also be known as ASL-279, dopamini hydrochloridum, and 3-hydroxytyramine hydrochloride; many trade names are available.

Storage/Stability

Dopamine injectable products should be protected from light. Solutions that are pink, yellow, brown, or purple indicate decomposition of the drug. Solutions that are darker than a light yellow should be discarded. Dopamine solutions should be stored at room temperature of 20°C to 25°C (68°F-77°F).

After dilution in a common IV solution (NOT 5% bicarbonate), dopamine is stable for at least 24 hours at room temperature, but it is recommended to dilute the drug just prior to use. Dopamine is stable in solutions with a pH of less than 6.4 and most stable at a pH less than 5. It is oxidized at alkaline pH.

Compatibility/Compounding Considerations

To prepare solution: Add contents of the dopamine vial to 250 mL, 500 mL, or 1000 mL of normal saline, D_5W, lactated Ringer's injection, or other compatible IV fluid. If adding a 200 mg vial (5 mL; 40 mg/mL) to a 1 L bag, the resultant solution concentration will be ≈200 µg/mL.

A mechanical fluid administration control device (fluid pump) should be used to administer dopamine. If using a mini-drip IV set (60 drops/mL), each drop will contain ≈3.3 µg. To calculate a dopamine CRI[6]: 6 times body weight (in kg) = the number of mg (NOT mL) of dopamine added to a sufficient quantity of 0.9% NaCl to obtain a total volume of 100 mL. When this solution is delivered at 1 mL/hour IV, 1 µg/kg/minute is administered.

Compatibility is dependent on factors such as pH, concentration, temperature, and diluent used; specialized references or a hospital pharmacist should be consulted for more specific information.

Dopamine is physically **compatible** with the following IV solutions: D_5 in LRS, D_5 in half-normal saline, D_5 in normal saline, D_5W, mannitol 20% in water, lactated Ringer's solution, normal saline, and $^1/_6$ molar sodium lactate. Dopamine is reported to be physically **compatible** with the following drugs: aminophylline, calcium chloride, chloramphenicol sodium succinate, dobutamine HCl, gentamicin sulfate (gentamicin potency retained for only 6 hours), heparin sodium, hydrocortisone sodium succinate, lidocaine HCl, methylprednisolone sodium succinate, potassium chloride, tetracycline HCl, and verapamil HCl.

Dopamine is reported to be physically **incompatible** with amphotericin B, ampicillin sodium, iron salts, metronidazole with sodium bicarbonate, penicillin G potassium, and sodium bicarbonate.

Dosage Forms/Regulatory Status

VETERINARY-LABELED PRODUCTS: NONE

The Association of Racing Commissioners International (ARCI) has designated dopamine as a class 2 substance. Use of this drug may not be allowed in certain animal competitions. Check rules and regulations before entering in a competition while this medication is being administered. Contact local racing authorities for further guidance. See ***Appendix*** for more information.

HUMAN-LABELED PRODUCTS:

Dopamine HCl for Concentrated Solution for Injection: 40 mg/mL, 80 mg/mL, and 160 mg/mL in 5 mL and 10 mL vials; generic; (Rx). Dilute prior to administration.

Dopamine HCl in Dextrose 5% Injection Solution: 200 mg/250 mL (0.8 mg/mL); 400 mg/500 mL (0.8 mg/mL); 400 mg/250 mL (1.6 mg/mL); 800 mg/500 mL (1.6 mg/mL); and 800 mg/250 mL (3.2 mg/mL) in premixed single-use containers; generic; (Rx)

References

For the complete list of references, see **wiley.com/go/budde/plumb**

Doramectin

(dor-a-***mek***-tin) *Dectomax®*

Avermectin Antiparasitic

Prescriber Highlights

- Injectable (cattle, swine) and topical (cattle only) avermectin ecto- and endoparasiticide
- Manufacturer warns about extra-label use in other species.
- IM injections may cause muscle blemishes.
- Not labeled for female dairy cattle 20 months or older
- Relatively long slaughter withdrawal times

Uses/Indications

Doramectin injection is indicated for the treatment and control of the following endo- and ectoparasites in cattle: GI roundworms (adults and some fourth-stage larvae)—*Ostertagia ostertagi* (including inhibited larvae), *Ostertagia lyrata, Haemonchus placei, Trichostrongylus axei, Trichostrongylus colubriformis, Trichostrongylus longispicularis, Cooperia oncophora, Cooperia pectinata, Cooperia punctata, Cooperia surnabada* (syn. *Cooperia mcmasteri*), *Bunostomum phlebotomum, Strongyloides papillosus, Oesophagostomum radiatum, Trichuris* spp; lungworms (adults and fourth-stage larvae)—*Dictyocaulus viviparus*; eyeworms (adults)—*Thelazia* spp; grubs (parasitic stages)—*Hypoderma bovis, Hypoderma lineatum*; sucking lice—*Haematopinus eurysternus, Linognathus vituli, Solenopotes capillatus*; and mange mites—*Psoroptes bovis, Sarcoptes scabiei*.[1] The manufacturer states doramectin protects cattle against infection or reinfection with *Cooperia oncophora* and *Haemonchus placei* for 14 days, *Ostertagia ostertagi* for up to 21 days, and *Cooperia punctata, Oesophagostomum radiatum*, and *Dictyocaulus viviparus* for 28 days after treatment. Doramectin topical (pour-on) is FDA-approved for the treatment and control in cattle of a similar spectrum of endo- and ectoparasites, but also includes horn flies (*Haematobia irritans*) and biting lice (*Bovicola [Damalinia] bovis*).[2]

In swine, the injection is labeled for the treatment and control of GI roundworms (adults and some fourth-stage larvae)—*Ascaris suum, Oesophagostomum dentatum, Oesophagostomum quadrispinolatum, Strongyloides ransomi*, and *Hydrostrongylus rubidus*; lungworms (adults)—*Metastrongylus* spp; kidney worms (adults)—*Stephanurus dentatus*; mange mites (adults and immature stages)—*Sarcoptes scabiei* var. *suis*); and sucking lice (adults and immature stages)—*Haematopinus suis*.[1]

Injectable doramectin has been used in an extra-label manner orally or as an SC injection for treating a variety of nematode and arthropod parasites in companion animals, including generalized demodicosis in dogs and cats.[3-5] However, isoxazolines (eg, fluralaner, sarolaner) have supplanted avermectins for the treatment of demodicosis.[6-9] Based on an open, clinical study in 38 dogs, 72% with generalized demodicosis and 89% with localized demodicosis showed remission after a mean of 11.4 weeks (generalized) and 7.8 weeks (localized). In a retrospective review of 232 dogs with generalized demodicosis, remission was achieved in 94.8% of patients that completed treatment with weekly doramectin injections; the average treatment duration was 7.1 weeks.[3]

Pharmacology/Actions

The primary mode of action of avermectins like doramectin is to affect chloride ion channel activity in the nervous system of nematodes and arthropods. Doramectin binds to receptors that increase membrane permeability to chloride ions. This inhibits the electrical activity of nerve cells in nematodes and muscle cells in arthropods and causes paralysis and the death of the parasites. Avermectins also enhance the release of gamma-aminobutyric acid (GABA) at presynaptic neurons. GABA acts as an inhibitory neurotransmitter and blocks the post-synaptic stimulation of the adjacent neuron in nematodes or the muscle fiber in arthropods.

Avermectins are generally not toxic to mammals as they do not have glutamate-gated chloride channels, and these compounds do not readily cross the blood–brain barrier where mammalian GABA receptors occur.

Pharmacokinetics

After subcutaneous injection, the time to peak plasma concentration in cattle is about 5 days. Bioavailability is, for practical purposes, equal with SC and IM injections in cattle.

In llamas and alpacas given doramectin 0.5 mg/kg topically, peak plasma concentration of ≈4 ng/mL was reached ≈5.5 hours after administration, and half-life was 9 days.[10] When doramectin 0.2 mg/kg SC was given to alpacas, peak concentration of 6 ng/mL was reached ≈ 4 hours after administration and half-life was 6 days.[11]

Contraindications/Precautions/Warnings

Doramectin should not be used in other animal species as severe adverse reactions, including fatalities in dogs, may result.[1,2]

Although extra-label use is not advised in small animal species, if it is used, it is recommended to test all dogs for the *MDR1* mutation (also known as *ABCB1*-1delta) before treatment; use only in dogs tested negative for heartworm microfilariae or heartworm infection. If this testing is not possible: 1) Use alternative treatments in untested dogs of breeds susceptible to *MDR1* mutation (collies, Australian shepherds, shelties, long-haired whippet) as they are at higher risk for toxicity; 2) Obtain informed consent from the owner.

Adverse Effects

Doramectin appears to be well-tolerated in cattle and swine when administered at label dosages. IM injections may have a higher incidence of injection site blemishes at slaughter than do SC injections. Short-term fiber discoloration was noted in llamas and alpacas after application of the pour-on formulation.[10]

When doramectin is used to treat demodicosis in dogs (not recommended), adverse effects are uncommon but may include pupil dilation, lethargy, blindness, or coma.

Reproductive/Nursing Safety

In studies performed in breeding animals (bulls and boars, as well as sows and cows in early and late pregnancy), 3 times the recommended dose had no effect on breeding performance.[1,2] Doramectin administration (0.3 mg/kg, route not stated) to inexperienced male rats resulted in a diminution of the appetitive and consummatory phases of sexual behavior.[12] Safety in neonatal calves and piglets treated with up to 3 times the recommended dose has also been demonstrated.

Overdose/Acute Toxicity

In field trials, no toxic signs were seen in cattle given up to 25 times the recommended dose of the injectable product.[1,2]

Doramectin toxicity may be alleviated with the use of IV lipid emulsion therapy.

For patients that have experienced or are suspected of having experienced an overdose, consultation with a 24-hour poison consultation center specializing in providing veterinary-specific information is recommended. For general information related to overdose and toxin exposures, as well as contact information for poison control centers, refer to ***Appendix***.

Drug Interactions

- None noted

Dosages

DOGS:

NOTE: Caution is warranted when administering doramectin to dogs with the *MDR1* mutation (also known as *ABCB1*-1delta). See ***Contraindications/Precautions/Warnings*** before using doramectin in dogs.

Ectoparasiticide: **NOTE**: isoxazolines (eg, fluralaner, sarolaner) have supplanted avermectins for ectoparasite management.

Adjunctive treatment of generalized demodicosis (extra-label): Based on retrospective reviews and open clinical studies, 600 µg/kg (0.6 mg/kg) PO or SC once weekly; continue treatment until remission of clinical signs and no evidence of mites on 2 successive skin scrapings 2 weeks apart.[4,13,14] Giving an initial dose of 300 µg/kg (0.3 mg/kg) has been suggested to minimize adverse effects.[4] Twice weekly doses of 300 µg/kg (0.3 mg/kg) SC may be better tolerated than 600 µg/kg (0.6 mg/kg) once weekly.[15]

Sarcoptic mange (extra-label): 400 µg/kg (0.4 mg/kg) SC once weekly[16]

***Spirocerca lupi* infections** (extra-label): 400 µg/kg (0.4 mg/kg) SC every 14 days. Treatment duration has ranged from 3[17] to 6[18] treatments followed by 400 µg/kg (0.4 mg/kg) SC once monthly until clinical resolution.

CATS:

Follicular demodicosis (extra-label): 400 – 600 µg/kg (0.4 – 0.6 mg/kg) SC once weekly for 4 weeks past 2 consecutive negative skin scrapings 4 to 6 weeks apart[15]

Notoedric mange (extra-label): 200 – 300 µg/kg (0.2 – 0.3 mg/kg) SC as a single dose or once weekly for 2 to 3 treatments[15]

CATTLE:

Label indications for injectable product (label dosage; FDA-approved): 200 µg/kg (1 mL/50 kg [110 lb] body weight) SC or IM.[1] Injections should be given using 16- to 18-gauge needles. Subcutaneous injections should be administered under the loose skin in front of or behind the shoulder. Intramuscular injections should be administered into the muscular region of the neck. Beef Quality Assurance guidelines recommend subcutaneous administration as the preferred route.

Label indications for pour-on product (label dosage; FDA-approved): 500 µg/kg (1 mL/10 kg [22 lb] body weight) applied topically along the mid-line of the back in a narrow strip between the withers and tailhead[2]

SWINE:

Label indications (label dosage; FDA-approved): 300 µg/kg (1 mL/ 34 kg [75 lb] body weight) IM.[1] Injections should be made using 16 g x 1.5 inch needles for sows and boars and 18 g x 1 inch needles for young animals. Use a tuberculin syringe and a 20 g x 1 inch needle for piglets. IM injections should be administered into the muscular region of the neck. See the label for a recommended treatment program for sows, gilts, boars, feeder pigs, weaners, growers, and finishers.

EQUINE:

Control of strongylid (large and small strongyles) infections (extra-label): 200 µg/kg (0.2 mg/kg) SC had 99.6% efficacy against large strongyles at 14 days after injection, 82.4% at 28 days, and 47.8% at 58 days; small strongyle infections were eradicated from 83.3% horses at 14 days.[19]

NEW WORLD CAMELIDS

Control of susceptible parasites in alpacas (extra-label):

a) 200 – 300 µg/kg (0.2-0.3 mg/kg) IM, SC once[20]

b) 500 µg/kg (0.5 mg/kg) applied topically once[21]

RABBITS:

***Psoroptes cuniculi* infestations** (extra-label): 200 µg/kg (0.2 mg/kg) IM once[22]

Monitoring

- Efficacy
- Adverse effects

Client Information

- Use this medicine only as directed by your veterinarian.
- As an antiparasite medication in cattle and swine: Carefully read and follow all instructions and drug residue withdrawal times listed on the product label. Do not apply pour-on product to the backline if covered with mud or manure.
- The pour-on product is flammable. Store away from sources of ignition. Do not smoke while handling this product.

Chemistry/Synonyms

Doramectin, an avermectin antiparasitic compound, is isolated from fermentations from the soil organism *Streptomyces avermitilis*.

Doramectin may also be known as Doramectina, Doramectine, Doramectinum, Doramektiini, Doramektin, UK-67994, or *Dectomax®*.

Storage/Stability

The commercially available injectable solution is colorless to pale yellow, sterile solution. Store the injectable solution below 30°C (86°F). Discard vial 90 days after first puncture, and puncture vial no more than 25 times.[1]

The topical pour-on solution is flammable; store it below 30°C (86°F) and protect it from light.[2] Wear protective clothing when administering the topical pour-on solution.[2]

Compatibility/Compounding Considerations

No specific information was noted.

Dosage Forms/Regulatory Status

VETERINARY-LABELED PRODUCTS:

Doramectin Injectable Solution: 10 mg/mL in 100 mL, 200 mL, and 500 mL multi-dose vials; *Dectomax®*; (OTC). FDA-approved for use in cattle and swine. When used at labeled doses: Slaughter withdrawal: cattle = 35 days, swine = 24 days. Do not use it in female dairy cattle 20 months of age or older or in calves to be used for veal. A withdrawal period has not been established in pre-ruminating calves.

Doramectin Pour-On Solution: 5 mg/mL in 250 mL, 1 L, 2.5 L, and 5 L multi-dose containers; *Dectomax® Pour-On*, generic; (OTC). FDA-approved for use in cattle. Slaughter withdrawal = 45 days. Not for use in female dairy cattle 20 months of age or older. A withdrawal period has not been established in pre-ruminating calves. Do not use it in calves to be used for veal.

HUMAN-LABELED PRODUCTS: NONE

References

For the complete list of references, see **wiley.com/go/budde/plumb**

Doxapram

(***docks***-a-pram) *Dopram-V®*

CNS/Respiratory Stimulant

Prescriber Highlights

- ► CNS stimulant usually used to initiate respirations in newborns or after anesthesia. Also used for assessment of laryngeal function in small animals. Use in small animal neonates is controversial.
- ► Not a substitute for aggressive artificial (mechanical) ventilatory support
- ► Possible contraindications include patients with hypersensitivity to doxapram, seizure disorders, head trauma, cerebrovascular accident (CVA), significant cardiovascular impairment (eg, decompensated heart failure, severe hypertension), mechanical disorders of ventilation (eg, neuromuscular disorders or blockade, airway obstruction, pulmonary embolism or fibrosis, pneumothorax, acute asthma, dyspnea, or whenever hypoxia is not associated with hypercapnia) and those receiving mechanical ventilation.
- ► Use with caution in patients with a history of asthma, arrhythmias, or tachycardias. Use extreme caution in patients with cerebral edema or increased CSF pressure, pheochromocytoma, or hyperthyroidism.
- ► Avoid IV extravasation or using a single injection site for a prolonged period.
- ► Adverse effects include hypertension, arrhythmias, seizures, and hyperventilation (leading to respiratory alkalosis).

Uses/Indications

Doxapram is FDA-approved for use in horses, cats, and dogs to stimulate the respiratory center during and after anesthesia to speed awakening and the return of reflexes.[1] It is also approved for use in neonatal dogs and cats to initiate respiration following dystocia or caesarean section. Use of doxapram to initiate ventilation by stimulation of the respiratory center in newborns is controversial, as the drug has been shown in experimental animals to increase myocardial oxygen demand and reduce cerebral blood flow. Many no longer recommend its use for this purpose, and some state that the drug is contraindicated in situations of respiratory arrest. In humans, routine use of doxapram in neonatal infants is no longer recommended.[2]

Doxapram has been used for treatment of CNS depression in many species and has been suggested as a treatment for respiratory depression in small animal species caused by reactions to radiopaque contrast media[3] or adverse effects from CNS-depressing drugs (eg, acepromazine). See ***Contraindications/Precautions/Warnings***

Doxapram has been shown to be useful to offset suppression of general anesthetic agents when laryngeal function is being assessed.[4-7]

Pharmacology/Actions

Doxapram appears to directly stimulate peripheral chemoreceptors within the carotid bodies leading to subsequent release of catecholamines and other neurotransmitters. As doses increase, the central respiratory center is also stimulated, as are other parts of the brain and spinal cord, leading to general CNS stimulation.[8] Respiratory stimulation leads to an increase in tidal volume with a slight increase in rate of respirations with resultant increased oxygen consumption and carbon dioxide production. Doxapram has been associated with an increased release of catecholamines.

Doxapram can antagonize opioid-induced respiratory depression without affecting analgesia in humans.[8] However, the mu-receptor antagonist naloxone is more commonly used in humans to reverse opioid-induced respiratory depression due to high receptor affinity as well as ease of use. Doxapram does not reverse respiratory depression caused by barbiturates such as pentobarbital.[9]

Pharmacokinetics

There are little published pharmacokinetic data available for dogs and cats. The onset of effect in humans and animals after IV injection usually occurs within 2 minutes. Doxapram is well-distributed into tissues. In dogs, doxapram is rapidly metabolized and most is excreted as metabolites in the urine and feces within 24 to 48 hours after administration. Small quantities of metabolites may be excreted up to 120 hours after dosing.[10]

Doxapram administered IV to horses, protein binding was 76% to 85%, median volume of distribution at steady-state was 1.2 L/kg, median biologic half-life was ≈2-3 hours, and median plasma clearance was 10.6 to 10.9 mL/minute/kg.[11] Following administration of 2.5 mg/kg IV doxapram in newborn lambs (2 to 6 days old), the terminal half-life was 5.2 hours, clearance was 9 mL/kg/minute, C_{max} was 3.1 mg/L, and apparent Vd was 1.2 L/kg.[12]

Contraindications/Precautions/Warnings

Doxapram is contraindicated for patients with a history of hypersensitivity to it or that are receiving mechanical ventilation.; doxapram should not be used as a substitute for aggressive artificial (mechanical) ventilatory support in instances of severe respiratory depression. Use to stimulate respiration in newborns is controversial, and some state it is contraindicated in apnea.

Doxapram has been reported as contraindicated in premature calves or other patients with clinical signs indicative of lung immaturity, as effects are only minimal. In addition, its use could lead to increased pulmonary blood pressure with fetal circulation persisting resulting from a right-to-left shunt via the patent ductus and foramen ovale.[13]

Doxapram should be used with caution in patients with a history of asthma, arrhythmias, or tachycardias. It should be used with extreme caution in patients with cerebral edema or increased CSF pressure, pheochromocytoma, or hyperthyroidism. Impaired hepatic or renal function may alter response to doxapram. Vomiting may occur, and airway protection may be required.

Avoid using a single IV injection site for a prolonged period to minimize risk for thrombophlebitis.[8] Ensure IV catheter patency before administering to avoid extravasation. Rapid IV infusion of doxapram can result in hemolysis.

Repeated IV doses in neonates should be done with caution, as the product contains benzyl alcohol.[8]

Contraindications from the human literature include seizure disorders, head trauma, cardiovascular impairment (eg, decompensated heart failure, severe hypertension), respiratory failure secondary to neuromuscular disorders, airway obstruction, pulmonary embolism, pulmonary fibrosis, and pneumothorax.

Do not confuse doxapram with doxazosin or doxepin or confuse *Dopram®* with dopamine.

Adverse Effects

Doxapram has a narrow margin of safety when used in humans. Hypertension, arrhythmias, seizures, and hyperventilation (leading to respiratory alkalosis) have been reported. These effects appear most probable with repeated or high doses. Depth of anesthesia may be reduced when doxapram is used intraoperatively.

Doxapram has been shown in experimental animals to increase myocardial oxygen demand and reduce cerebral blood flow.

Reproductive/Nursing Safety

Although adverse effects have not been observed in animal reproduction studies, the safety of doxapram has not been established in pregnant animals. No evidence of fetal harm was noted in rats given doses up to 1.6 times the human label dose.[8] It is not known whether doxapram is excreted in milk.

Because safety has not been established in animals, this drug should only be used when the maternal benefits outweigh the potential risks to offspring.

Overdose/Acute Toxicity

Reported LD_{50} for IV administration in dogs and cats is 40 – 100 mg/kg.[8,10] Clinical signs of an overdose include respiratory alkalosis, hypertension, skeletal muscle hyperactivity, tachycardia, vomiting, diarrhea, and generalized CNS excitation including seizures. Treatment is supportive (eg, oxygen, anticonvulsants) based on clinical signs.

For patients that have experienced or are suspected to have experienced an overdose, consultation with a 24-hour poison consultation center specializing in providing veterinary-specific information is recommended. For general information related to overdose and toxin exposures, as well as contact information for poison control centers, refer to ***Appendix***.

Drug Interactions

The following drug interactions have either been reported or are theoretical in humans or animals receiving doxapram and may be of significance in veterinary patients. Unless otherwise noted, use together is not necessarily contraindicated, but weigh the potential risks and perform additional monitoring when appropriate.

- **Anesthetics, Inhalant** (eg, **halothane**, but not **isoflurane**): Doxapram may increase epinephrine release; therefore, use should be delayed for ≈10 minutes after discontinuation of anesthetic agents that have been demonstrated to sensitize the myocardium to catecholamines (eg, **halothane**).
- **Monoamine Oxidase Inhibitors** (MAOIs; eg, **amitraz, linezolid, selegiline**): Additive pressor effects may occur.
- **Muscle Relaxants** (eg, **guaifenesin, methocarbamol**): Doxapram may mask the effects of muscle relaxant drugs.
- **Neuromuscular Blockers** (eg, **pancuronium, vercuronium**): Doxapram may temporarily mask residual effects of neuromuscular blockers.
- **Sympathomimetic Agents** (eg, **dopamine, epinephrine, phenylpropanolamine**): Additive pressor effects may occur.
- **Theophylline, Aminophylline**: Additive skeletal muscle activity, agitation, and hyperactivity may occur.

Dosages

DOGS/CATS:

To stimulate respirations during and after general anesthesia; to speed awakening and return of reflexes after anesthesia (label dosage; FDA-approved): 1.1 mg/kg (when used with gas anesthesia) or 5.5 – 11 mg/kg (when used with barbiturate anesthesia) IV; adjust dose based on depth of anesthesia, tidal volume and respiratory rate.[1] Dosage may be repeated in 15 to 20 minutes if necessary.

To initiate or stimulate respirations in neonates after cesarean section or dystocia (label dosage; FDA-approved): *Kittens*: 1 – 2 mg/kitten (NOT mg/kg) SC or sublingually (SL); *Puppies*: 1 – 5 mg/puppy NOT mg/kg) SC, SL, or via the umbilical vein.[1] Dosage may be repeated in 15 to 20 minutes if necessary. **NOTE**: In humans, routine use of doxapram in neonatal infants is no longer recommended.[2]

Stimulate respiratory function in neonates (extra-label): 0.1 mL (2 mg)/neonate (NOT mL/kg) IV, IM, SL; most likely to be beneficial to increase efforts in neonates with a low-frequency, gasping, and erratic pattern of breathing after receiving oxygen therapy.[14] **NOTE**: In humans, routine use of doxapram in neonatal infants is no longer recommended.[2]

Assess laryngeal function (extra-label): 0.25 – 2.5 mg/kg IV to stimulate respiration and increase intrinsic laryngeal motion.[6,7,15-18] Premedicating dogs permits lower doses of anesthetic induction drugs to be used, which improves the diagnostic utility of the procedure.[18]

To reduce sedative effects of acepromazine (extra-label): doxapram 1.25 mg/kg IV given 30 minutes after acepromazine 0.05 mg/kg IM significantly reduced sedation in a study with 10 dogs.[19]

HORSES:

Stimulate respiration during and after general anesthesia and speed awakening and return of reflexes after anesthesia (label dosage; FDA-approved): 0.44 mg/kg (for inhalant anesthesia) or 0.55 mg/kg (for barbiturate anesthesia) IV; adjust dosage for depth of anesthesia, respiratory volume, and rate.[1] Dose may be repeated in 15 to 20 minutes if necessary.

Adjunctive treatment to stimulate respirations in foals with sepsis or hypoxic-ischemic encephalopathy/neonatal maladjustment syndrome (extra-label): 0.02 – 0.05 mg/kg/hour IV CRI[20,21]; foals with significant hypercapnia and hypoxia, despite O_2 treatment, require positive pressure ventilation.

CATTLE & SWINE:

Primary apnea in asphyxic calves when intubation and mechanical ventilation are not feasible (extra-label): 2 mg/kg IV[13,22]

BIRDS:

Emergency treatment of respiratory depression (extra-label):

a) 5 – 10 mg/kg IM or IV
b) 5 – 20 mg/kg IM, IV, IO, or IT[23]

FERRETS/RABBITS/RODENTS/SMALL MAMMALS:

Emergency treatment of respiratory depression (extra-label): Suggested anecdotal dosages range from 1 – 10 mg/kg.[24,25] Suggested routes of administration include IV, SL, IO, IP, SC, and intratracheally.

REPTILES:

Stimulate respiration after general anesthesia (extra-label): 5 mg/kg IV, IO[26-28]

Monitoring

- Respiratory rate and depth
- Cardiac rate and rhythm, blood pressure, pulse oximetry
- Arterial blood gas if available and indicated
- CNS level of excitation; deep tendon reflexes

Client Information

- This drug should only be used in an inpatient setting (ie, in a veterinary clinic) or with direct professional supervision.

Chemistry/Synonyms

Doxapram HCl is a white to off-white, odorless, crystalline powder that is stable in light and air. It is soluble in water, sparingly soluble in alcohol, and practically insoluble in ether. Injectable products have a pH from 3.5 to 5. Benzyl alcohol or chlorobutanol is added as a preservative agent in the commercially available injections.

Doxapram HCl may also be known as AHR-619, doxaprami hydrochloridum, *Docatone*®, *Dopram*®, *Doxapril*®, or *Respiram*®.

Storage/Stability

Store at room temperature 20°C to 25°C (68°F-77°F) and avoid freezing.

Compatibility/Compounding Considerations

Compatibility is dependent on factors such as pH, concentration, temperature, and diluent used; specialized references or a hospital pharmacist should be consulted for more specific information.

Doxapram is physically **compatible** with D_5W or normal saline.[1]

Do not mix with alkaline solutions (eg, thiopental, aminophylline, sodium bicarbonate). Doxapram is also **incompatible** with ascorbic acid, cefoperazone, cefotaxime, cefotetan, cefuroxime, folic acid, dexamethasone disodium phosphate, diazepam, hydrocortisone sodium phosphate, methylprednisolone sodium, minocycline, and hydrocortisone sodium succinate.[1]

Dosage Forms/Regulatory Status

VETERINARY-LABELED PRODUCTS:

Doxapram HCl for Injection: 20 mg/mL; 20 mL multi-dose vial; *Dopram-V*®, *Respiram*®; (Rx). FDA-approved for use in dogs, cats, and horses. Although this drug is still listed in the FDA's Green Book of approved animal drugs, it may not be commercially available.

The Association of Racing Commissioners International (ARCI) has designated this drug as a class 2 substance. See the ***Appendix*** for more information. Use of this drug may not be allowed in certain animal competitions. Check rules and regulations before entering in a competition while this medication is being administered. Contact local racing authorities for further guidance.

HUMAN-LABELED PRODUCTS:

Doxapram HCl for Injection: 20 mg/mL in 20 mL multi-dose vials; *Dopram*®, (Rx)

References

For the complete list of references, see **wiley.com/go/budde/plumb**

Doxepin

(**dox**-e-pin) *Sinequan® Sinequan**

Tricyclic Antidepressant, Antihistamine

Prescriber Highlights

- ► Used primarily in small animal species for adjunctive therapy of pruritus associated with atopic dermatitis and psychogenic dermatoses, particularly those that have an anxiety component; also has anticholinergic, alpha-1-adrenergic, and antihistaminic (H1, H2) properties
- ► Contraindications include prior sensitivity to tricyclic antidepressants (TCAs) and concomitant use with monoamine oxidase inhibitors (MAOIs).
- ► Use with extreme caution in patients with urinary retention or glaucoma.
- ► Common adverse effects include hyperexcitability, GI distress, or lethargy.

Uses/Indications

The primary use for doxepin in veterinary medicine is for the adjunctive therapy of pruritus associated with atopic dermatitis and psychogenic dermatoses, particularly those that include an anxiety component (eg, tail biting, flank sucking, anal licking, acral lick dermatitis, excessive grooming, psychogenic alopecia, feather plucking). Its efficacy as an antihistamine for atopic dermatitis is in question[1,2]; however, it may be beneficial in dogs to prevent acute flares of mild pruritus associated with atopic dermatitis[3] and concurrent behavior abnormalities. Anecdotally, doxepin has also been used to improve clinical signs in animals with canine laryngeal paralysis, but in one study its use did not improve quality of life.[3]

Pharmacology/Actions

Doxepin is a tricyclic antidepressant. In the CNS, doxepin inhibits the reuptake of norepinephrine and serotonin (5-HT) by the presynaptic neuronal membrane, thereby increasing their synaptic concentrations. Doxepin is considered a moderate inhibitor of norepinephrine and weak inhibitor of serotonin. Doxepin also has anticholinergic, alpha-1-adrenergic, and potent antihistamine effects.

Pharmacokinetics

Pharmacokinetic information in veterinary species is lacking. In humans, doxepin appears to be well-absorbed after oral administration and is extensively metabolized in the liver.

Contraindications/Precautions/Warnings

Doxepin is contraindicated if prior sensitivity to any other tricyclic antidepressant (TCA) has been noted. Monoamine oxidase inhibitors should be discontinued at least 14 days prior to starting doxepin. Doxepin should be used with extreme caution in patients with urinary retention or glaucoma. Use with caution or avoid use in patients with cardiovascular disease. Use with caution in patients with a history of seizures, as it may lower seizure threshold.

In humans who have taken doxepin chronically, it is recommended to withdraw the drug slowly; this caution likely applies to veterinary patients.

Do not confuse DOXepin with DIGoxin, doxaPRAM or doxycycline.

Adverse Effects

In dogs, doxepin may cause hyperexcitability, GI distress, constipation, urine retention, or lethargy. Although doxepin has less potential for cardiac adverse effects than many other TCAs, it can cause ventricular arrhythmias, particularly after overdose. In humans, common adverse effects include CNS depression, tremor, weakness, blurred vision, dry eyes, hypotension, tachycardia, constipation, urinary retention, and blood dyscrasias.

Reproductive/Nursing Safety

Reproduction studies in rats, rabbits, monkeys, and dogs indicate no evidence of fetal harm.

Doxepin and its N-demethylated active metabolite are distributed into milk in concentrations that are roughly equivalent to that of plasma. Exercise caution when using in a nursing patient.

Overdose/Acute Toxicity

Overdoses with TCAs can quickly become life-threatening. Manifestations may include arrhythmias, profound hypotension, cardiorespiratory collapse, seizures, and coma. Airway support, antiarrhythmics, and anticonvulsants often are required; inducing emesis is contraindicated. Doxepin toxicity may be amenable to activated charcoal and IV lipid emulsion (ILE) treatments.[4]

For patients that have experienced or are suspected to have experienced an overdose, consultation with a 24-hour poison consultation center specializing in providing veterinary-specific information is recommended. For general information related to overdose and toxin exposures, as well as contact information for poison control centers, refer to ***Appendix***.

Drug Interactions

The following drug interactions have either been reported or are theoretical in humans or animals receiving doxepin and may be of significance in veterinary patients. Unless otherwise noted, use together is not necessarily contraindicated, but weigh the potential risks and perform additional monitoring when appropriate.

- Anticholinergic Agents (eg, **atropine, oxybutynin**): Because of additive effects, use with doxepin cautiously.
- Antihistamines (eg, **diphenhydramine, hydroxyzine, meclizine**): Potential for increased sedation
- Antiplatelet Agents (eg, **aspirin, clopidogrel**): Increased risk for bleeding
- Cannabidiol: Additive CNS depression is possible.
- Cimetidine: May inhibit tricyclic antidepressant metabolism and increase the risk for toxicity
- Hypotensive Agents (eg, **amlodipine, enalapril, prazosin, telmisartan**): Additive blood pressure reduction is possible
- Dextromethorphan: Increased risk for serotonin syndrome.
- Monoamine Oxidase Inhibitors (**MAOIs**; eg, **amitraz, linezolid,** possibly **selegiline**): Concomitant use (within 14 days) of tricyclics with monoamine oxidase inhibitors is generally contraindicated due to risk for serotonin syndrome.
- Nonsteroidal Anti-Inflammatory Drugs (**NSAIDs**; eg, **carprofen, meloxicam, robenacoxib**): Increased risk for bleeding
- Opioids (eg **buprenorphine, morphine**): Additive CNS depression and anticholinergic effects may occur. The risk for serotonin syndrome may be increased when doxepin is used concurrently with opioids with greater serotonergic activity (eg, **meperidine, tramadol**).
- Phenobarbital: May reduce doxepin concentration
- Prokinetic Agents (eg, **bethanechol, cisapride, metoclopramide**): Doxepin may decrease prokinetic effects.
- QT Prolongation Agents (eg, **amiodarone, chlorpromazine, cisapride, fluconazole, fluoxetine, ketoconazole, methadone, ondansetron, quinidine, sotalol**): May increase risk for QT prolongation
- Serotonergic Agents (eg, **buspirone, fluoxetine, mirtazapine, trazodone**): Increased risk for serotonin syndrome
- Sympathomimetic Agents (eg, **albuterol, phenylpropanolamine**): Use in combination with tricyclic agents may increase the risk for cardiac effects (eg, arrhythmias, hypertension, hyperpyrexia).
- Tramadol: Increased risk for serotonin syndrome

Laboratory Considerations

- Tricyclics can widen QRS complexes, prolong PR intervals, and invert or flatten T-waves on **ECG**.
- Tricyclics may alter (increase or decrease) **blood glucose** levels.
- **Intradermal allergy testing (IDT)**: Antihistamines may suppress IDT results. It is recommended to discontinue antihistamine 1 week prior to testing; a 2-day withdrawal should be considered the minimum.[5,6]

Dosages

DOGS:

Pruritus associated with atopic dermatitis | Antihistamine (extra-label):

a) 0.5 – 1 mg/kg PO every 12 hours, then titrate upward to maximum as for psychogenic dermatoses (above). There is little evidence to support any dosage recommendation.[7]

b) Apply doxepin 5% cream to affected areas up to 4 times daily.[8-10]

Psychogenic dermatoses (extra-label): 3 – 5 mg/kg (maximum dose 50 mg/dog [NOT mg/kg]) PO every 12 hours. Generally, start at the low end of the dosing range and increase in increments of 1 mg/kg every 12 hours every two weeks to the maximum (5 mg/kg or 50 mg/dog [NOT mg/kg]). If no effect is seen after 4 weeks, wean to the starting dose in increments of 1 mg/kg every 12 hours every two weeks before discontinuing. There is little evidence to support any dosage recommendation.[6,11]

CATS:

Psychogenic dermatoses and allergies (extra-label): 0.5 – 1 mg/kg PO every 12 to 24 hours. May titrate slowly upward if cat tolerates, but many cats become profoundly sedated and ataxic at higher dosages. There is little evidence to support any dosage recommendation.[4,5]

HORSES:

Antihistamine (extra-label): 0.5 – 0.75 mg/kg PO every 12 hours[12]

BIRDS:

Anxiety, pruritus-caused feather plucking in psittacines (extra-label): 0.5 – 2 mg/kg PO every 12 hours[13]

Monitoring

- Efficacy
- Adverse effects

Client Information

- When used as an antihistamine, doxepin should be used on a regular, ongoing basis in animals that respond to it. This medicine works better if used before exposure to an allergen (eg, pollens).
- When doxepin is used for behavior modification, it may take several days to several weeks to determine if the drug is effective.
- This medicine may be given with or without food. If your animal vomits or acts sick after receiving this medicine on an empty stomach, try giving the next dose with food or small treat. If vomiting continues, contact your veterinarian.
- Most common side effects are sleepiness, dry mouth, and constipation. Be sure your animal has access to plenty of fresh, clean water.
- Rare side effects that can be serious (contact veterinarian immediately) include abnormal bleeding, fever, seizures, collapse, or profound sleepiness.
- Overdoses (in animals and in humans) can be very serious; keep out of the reach of animals and children.
- Certain flea and tick collars should not be used on your animal while it is receiving this medicine. Let your veterinarian know if your animal has worn a flea and tick collar in the past 2 weeks.

Chemistry/Synonyms

A dibenzoxazepine derivative tricyclic antidepressant, doxepin HCl occurs as a white powder that is freely soluble in water and alcohol.

Doxepin may also be known as doxepini hydrochloridum, NSC-108160, P-3693A, *Adapin®*, *Anten®*, *Aponal®*, *Deptran®*, *Desidoxepin®*, *Doneurin®*, *Doxal®*, *Doxepia®*, *Gilex®*, *Mareen®*, *Quitaxon®*, *Sinequan®*, *Triadapin®*, *Xepin®*, and *Zonalon®*.

Compatibility/Compounding Considerations

No specific information noted

Storage/Stability

Store doxepin products protected from direct sunlight in tight, light-resistant containers at room temperature (20°C-25°C [68°F-77°F]).

Dosage Forms/Regulatory Status

VETERINARY-LABELED PRODUCTS: NONE

The Association of Racing Commissioners International (ARCI) has designated this drug as a class 2 substance. See the ***Appendix*** for more information. Use of this drug may not be allowed in certain animal competitions. Check rules and regulations before entering in a competition while this medication is being administered. Contact local racing authorities for further guidance.

HUMAN-LABELED PRODUCTS:

Doxepin Capsules: 10 mg, 25 mg, 50 mg, 75 mg, 100 mg and 150 mg, generic; (Rx)

Doxepin Tablets: 3 mg and 6 mg; *Silenor®*; (Rx)

Doxepin Oral Solution Concentrate: 10 mg/mL in 120 mL; generic; (Rx)

Doxepin Hydrochloride 5% Cream: 45 gram; generic; (Rx)

References

For the complete list of references, see **wiley.com/go/budde/plumb**

Doxorubicin

(dox-oh-***roo***-bi-sin) *Adriamycin®*

Antineoplastic

Prescriber Highlights

- Injectable antibiotic antineoplastic used alone or in combination chemotherapy protocols in small animal species
- Relatively contraindicated in patients with myelosuppression, with impaired cardiac function, or that have reached the total cumulative dose of doxorubicin
- Caution is recommended in patients with hyperuricemia, hyperuricuria, or impaired hepatic function; dosage adjustments may be necessary.
- Monitor cardiac status carefully or avoid use in breeds predisposed to developing cardiomyopathy (eg, Doberman pinschers, Great Danes, rottweilers, boxers).
- Adverse effects include myelosuppression, cardiac toxicity (dogs), nephrotoxicity (cats), alopecia, gastroenteritis (eg, vomiting, diarrhea), and stomatitis.
- Immediate hypersensitivity has been reported (primarily in dogs).
- Avoid extravasation; vesicant injuries can be severe.
- Teratogenic and embryotoxic. Handle and administer drug carefully.
- The National Institute for Occupational Safety and Health (NIOSH) classifies doxorubicin as a hazardous drug; use appropriate precautions when handling.

Uses/Indications

Doxorubicin is perhaps the most widely used antineoplastic agent in small animal medicine. In dogs and cats, it may be useful in the treatment of a variety of lymphomas, leukemias, carcinomas, and sarcomas, either as a single agent or in combination protocols.

Pharmacology/Actions

Although doxorubicin possesses antimicrobial properties, its cytotoxic effects preclude its use as an anti-infective agent. The drug causes inhibition of DNA synthesis, DNA-dependent RNA synthesis, and protein synthesis by inhibiting DNA and RNA polymerases and impairing topoisomerase II, as well as through generation of free radicals. Doxorubicin alters transcription and replication by intercalating with DNA base pairs.[1] The drug acts throughout the cell cycle and also possesses some immunosuppressant activity. Rapidly proliferating normal cells (eg, bone marrow, hair follicles in anagen, GI mucosa) are affected by the drug.

Pharmacokinetics

Doxorubicin must be administered IV, as it is not absorbed from the GI tract, and is extremely irritating to tissues if administered SC or IM. After IV injection, the drug is rapidly and widely distributed, but it does not appreciably enter the CSF. Doxorubicin is highly bound to tissue and plasma proteins, probably crosses the placenta, and is distributed into milk.

Doxorubicin is extensively metabolized in the liver and other tissues by aldo-keto reductase, primarily to form doxorubicinol (active) and other inactive metabolites. Doxorubicin and its metabolites are excreted mostly in bile and feces. Only ≈5% of the drug is excreted in the urine within 5 days of dosing. Doxorubicin is eliminated in a triphasic manner. During the first phase (half-life, ≈0.6 hours), doxorubicin is rapidly metabolized via the first pass effect; a second phase (half-life, ≈3.3 hours) follows. The third phase has a slower elimination half-life (doxorubicin, ≈17 hours; metabolites, ≈32 hours), presumably due to the slow release of the drug from tissue proteins.

Contraindications/Precautions/Warnings

Only clinicians who have the experience and resources to monitor the toxicity of this agent should administer this drug. Doxorubicin is contraindicated in patients hypersensitive to it or other anthracyclines, with pre-existing myelosuppression or impaired cardiac function, or that have reached the total cumulative dose concentration of doxorubicin or other anthracyclines.[2]

Doxorubicin is contraindicated in cats with pre-existing renal insufficiency.

Doxorubicin should be used with caution in patients with hyperuricemia, hyperuricuria, or impaired hepatic function. Dosage reductions are necessary in patients with severe hepatic impairment.

Extreme care must be taken to avoid perivascular extravasation. Securely placed indwelling IV catheters and close monitoring of IV patency/integrity during infusion are recommended. Automated fluid pumps should not be used. Doxorubicin should be administered IV slowly over at least 10 to 15 minutes in a free-flowing line.

Breeds predisposed to developing dilated cardiomyopathy (eg, Doberman pinschers, Great Danes, rottweilers, boxers) should be monitored carefully (see ***Monitoring***) while receiving doxorubicin therapy.

Doxorubicin is actively transported by the p-glycoprotein pump. Certain breeds that are susceptible to mutation in the *MDR1* gene (also known as *ABCB1*; including but not limited to collies, Australian shepherds, Shetland sheepdogs, and long-haired Whippets) may be at higher risk for toxicity. In dogs with the *MDR1* mutation, myelosuppression (particularly neutropenia) and GI toxicity (eg, anorexia, vomiting, diarrhea) are more likely to occur at normal dosages. If a mutant/normal dog must receive doxorubicin, a reduced dose should be given to decrease the likelihood of severe toxicity.[3] Doxorubicin should be avoided in mutant/mutant dogs.[4]

After treatment, doxorubicin drug residues may be found in a treated dog's urine for up to 21 days and in feces for several days.[5]

The National Institute for Occupational Safety and Health (NIOSH) classifies doxorubicin as a hazardous drug; personal protective equipment (PPE) should be used accordingly to minimize the risk for exposure.

Do not confuse conventional doxorubicin formulations with liposomal doxorubicin. Do not confuse DOXOrubicin with doxapram.

Adverse Effects

Doxorubicin may cause myelosuppression, cardiac toxicity, alopecia, gastroenteritis (eg, vomiting, diarrhea), and stomatitis. After administration, nausea and vomiting most commonly occur within the first 72 hours, diarrhea can occur in ≈4 to 5 days, and neutrophil and platelet nadirs are generally observed after 7 to 10 days. Systemic doxorubicin exposure, as measured by AUC, demonstrates a relationship to neutrophil nadir and the degree of neutropenia; however, the clinical application of this finding is unclear.[7]

In dogs, administration of maropitant 2 mg/kg PO daily for 5 days immediately followed by doxorubicin has been shown to reduce the frequency and severity of vomiting and diarrhea the first week after treatment.[8]

An immediate histamine-mediated hypersensitivity reaction characterized by urticaria, facial swelling, vomiting, arrhythmias, and/or hypotension may be seen (particularly in dogs). The rate of infusion can have a direct impact on this effect; generally, IV infusions should be administered no faster than over 10 minutes. Pretreatment with a histamine$_1$ antagonist (eg, diphenhydramine 1 – 2 mg/kg IM) or a glucocorticoid (eg, dexamethasone 0.1 – 0.2 mg/kg IV or IM) have been used to reduce or prevent histamine-mediated effects.

Cardiac toxicity of doxorubicin falls into 2 categories: acute and cumulative. Acute cardiac toxicity may occur during IV administration or several hours after the drug is given. This toxicity is manifested by ECG changes (eg, T-wave flattening, S-T depression, voltage reduction, arrhythmias), and in humans, may include cardiac arrest. Acute cardiac toxicity does not preclude further use of the drug, but additional treatment should be delayed. Administration of diphenhydramine and/or glucocorticoids before doxorubicin may prevent these effects.

Doxorubicin-iron complex free radicals are thought to be the primary cause of cardiomyopathy and extravasation injury. Cumulative cardiotoxicity can be extremely serious and necessitates halting any further therapy. Diffuse cardiomyopathy, with severe congestive heart failure refractory to traditional therapies, is generally noted. It is believed that the risk for cardiac toxicity is greatly increased in dogs when the cumulative doxorubicin dose exceeds 180 – 240 mg/m^2 (NOT mg/kg); however, cardiac toxicity may be seen at cumulative doses as low as 90 mg/m^2 (NOT mg/kg), particularly in dog breeds predisposed to dilated cardiomyopathy. In dogs, the safety of concurrent administration of the cardioprotective agent dexrazoxane has been documented,[9,10] but the benefit of such therapy in preventing cardiotoxicity in this species has not yet been prospectively evaluated.

Doxorubicin-associated alopecia in dogs may be generalized or local and may include loss of whiskers[11]; cats may lose whiskers and guard hairs.

In cats, doxorubicin is a potential nephrotoxin; renal chemistry values (eg, BUN, creatinine) should be monitored both before and during therapy.[12,13] The incidence of cardiotoxicity or the dosage ceiling for doxorubicin in cats is unknown.

Extravasation injuries secondary to perivascular administration of doxorubicin can be serious, with severe tissue ulceration and necrosis and subsequent tissue sloughing possible. If extravasation occurs, dexrazoxane can be administered (through a new IV catheter placed in a different vein) at 10 times the doxorubicin dosage immediately (within 3-6 hours of extravasation), with doses repeated at 24 hours and at 48 hours in most cases (see ***Dexrazoxane***).[10,14,15] In addition, ice compresses should be applied to the affected area for 15 minutes every 6 hours for 48 hours.

Reproductive/Nursing Safety

For sexually intact patients, verify pregnancy status prior to administration.

Doxorubicin is abortifacient, teratogenic, and embryotoxic in laboratory animals given doses lower than the clinical dose. Other effects include decreased fertility in females, as well as testicular atrophy and oligospermia in males.

Doxorubicin is excreted in milk in concentrations that may exceed those found in plasma. Because of risks to nursing offspring, consider using milk replacer if the dam is receiving doxorubicin.

Overdose/Acute Toxicity

Acute overdose may manifest as exacerbations of the adverse effects. In dogs, a lethal dose has been reported to be 72 mg/m^2 (NOT mg/kg).[16] Supportive therapy in response to clinical signs (eg, antiemetics, antidiarrheals, GI protectants, broad-spectrum antibacterial coverage, filgrastim) are suggested in cases of overdose.[10]

For patients that have experienced or are suspected to have experienced an overdose, it is strongly encouraged to consult with one of the 24-hour poison consultation centers that specialize in providing information specific for veterinary patients. For general information related to overdose and toxin exposures, as well as contact information for poison control centers, refer to ***Appendix.***

Drug Interactions

The following drug interactions have either been reported or are theoretical in humans or animals receiving doxorubicin and may be of significance in veterinary patients. Unless otherwise noted, use together is not necessarily contraindicated, but weigh the potential risks and perform additional monitoring when appropriate.

- CALCIUM CHANNEL BLOCKERS (eg, **diltiazem, verapamil**): Potential increased risk for cardiotoxicity associated with doxorubicin
- CISPLATIN: Increased risk for toxicity (eg, myelosuppression); carefully weigh the risks versus the benefits.
- CYCLOPHOSPHAMIDE: May increase doxorubicin blood concentrations (AUC) and prolong hematologic toxicity; coma and seizures have been reported in humans. A study in dogs, in which 1 of the treatment protocols combined doxorubicin and cyclophosphamide, did not find a significant difference in the prevalence of toxicity.[17]
- CYCLOSPORINE: Cyclosporine can increase doxorubicin and doxorubicinol (active metabolite) concentrations. Avoid use together.
- GLUCOSAMINE: May reduce doxorubicin effectiveness; use together not recommended in humans
- KETOCONAZOLE: Can increase doxorubicin and doxorubicinol (active metabolite) concentrations and lead to toxicity. Avoid use together.
- LEFLUNOMIDE: May have additive adverse hematologic toxicity
- MORPHINE: Concurrent use may increase morphine exposure.
- PHENOBARBITAL: May increase elimination and reduce blood concentrations of doxorubicin
- QUINIDINE: Concurrent use may result in increased doxorubicin exposure.
- SPINOSAD: Can increase doxorubicin and doxorubicinol (active metabolite) concentrations and lead to toxicity. Avoid use together.
- STREPTOZOCIN: May inhibit doxorubicin metabolism
- VACCINES. Live or live-attenuated vaccines may result in active infections in immunocompromised patients.
- WARFARIN: Increased risk for bleeding
- ZIDOVUDINE: Increased risk for neutropenia

Laboratory Considerations

- Doxorubicin may significantly increase both blood and urine concentrations of **uric acid.**

Dosages

NOTE: Because of the potential toxicity of this drug to patients, veterinary staff, and pet owners and because chemotherapy indications, treatment protocols, monitoring, and safety guidelines often change, the following dosages should be used only as a general guide. Consultation with a veterinary oncologist and referral to current veterinary oncology references[18-22] are strongly recommended. All dosages are extra-label. **When administering doxorubicin, do NOT flush IV catheters with heparin or heparinized saline; use sterile saline** (See ***Compatibility/Compounding Considerations***).

DOGS:

Chemotherapeutic agent (extra-label): 30 mg/m^2 (NOT mg/kg) IV every 2 to 3 weeks, depending on the protocol used. Smaller patients (eg, less than 10-15 kg [22-33 lb]) may be dosed at 1 mg/kg IV. The maximum cumulative dose is 180 – 240 mg/m^2 (NOT mg/kg) depending on breed and risk factors.

CATS:

Chemotherapeutic agent (extra-label):

a) 20 – 25 mg/m^2 (NOT mg/kg) IV every 3 weeks
b) 1 mg/kg IV every 3 weeks

FERRETS:

Chemotherapeutic agent (extra-label):

a) 20 mg/m^2 (NOT mg/kg) IV[23,24]; premedicate with diphenhydramine 1 – 2 mg/kg IM 30 minutes before doxorubicin administration
b) 2 mg/kg IV[24]; premedicate with diphenhydramine 1 – 2 mg/kg IM 30 minutes before doxorubicin administration

Rescue therapy (extra-label): 1 – 2 mg/kg IV[23]; premedicate with diphenhydramine 1 – 2 mg/kg IM 30 minutes before doxorubicin administration

HORSES:

Chemotherapeutic agent (extra-label): 70 mg/m^2 (NOT mg/kg) IV every 3 weeks. Adjunctive treatment with antihistamines and NSAIDs should be used to control hypersensitivity.[25,26]

Monitoring

- Baseline CBC, serum chemistry profile, urinalysis
- Prior to each chemotherapy, check CBC, BUN, creatinine, and USG
- Dogs with pre-existing heart disease should be monitored with echocardiography;[27] baseline and every 60 – 90 mg/m^2 (NOT mg/kg) cumulative dose increments could be considered. Cardiac troponin I can be a sensitive tool for detecting doxorubicin cardiotoxicity.[28]
- Efficacy/response to therapy

Client Information

- Doxorubicin is a chemotherapy (anticancer) drug. The drug and its byproducts can be hazardous to other animals and humans. On the day your animal receives the drug and for ≈72 hours after, all bodily waste (eg, urine, feces, litter), blood, or vomit should be handled only while wearing disposable gloves. Seal the waste in a plastic bag, then place both the bag and gloves in the regular trash. Pregnant women SHOULD NOT handle any waste or items used to clean the waste while your animal is on this drug.

- Doxorubicin has a maximum total amount that can be given to a patient over its lifetime. Exceeding this limit greatly increases the chance that your animal will develop heart damage from the drug. Your veterinarian will be keeping track of how much doxorubicin your animal has received.
- Your veterinarian will need to perform examinations and lab work on your animal after it receives this medication. Do not miss these important follow-up visits.
- Your animal should not receive vaccines containing live (or modified live) viruses while receiving this medication.
- In the interest of safety to other animals and humans, don't take your dog to a dog park or allow your animal to urinate and defecate in public places until your veterinarian tells you that it is okay to do so.
- Your animal should not participate in animal competitions while on this drug. Exposure to other animals may put your animal at serious risk of infections during chemotherapy treatment. Talk with your veterinarian about when itis safe to return to these events.
- Immediately report any signs associated with toxicity (eg, abnormal bleeding, bruising, infection, fever, gastrointestinal upset, injection site irritation).
- It is normal for urine to appear red for 1 to 2 days after administration.
- This medication is considered to be a hazardous drug as defined by the National Institute for Occupational Safety and Health (NIOSH). Talk with your veterinarian or pharmacist about the use of personal protective equipment when handling this medicine.

Chemistry/Synonyms

Doxorubicin HCl, an anthracycline glycoside antibiotic antineoplastic, occurs as a lyophilized, red–orange powder that is freely soluble in water, slightly soluble in normal saline, and very slightly soluble in alcohol. The commercially available powder for injection also contains lactose and methylparaben to aid dissolution. After reconstituting, the solution has a pH of 3.8 to 6.5. The commercially available solution for injection has a pH of ≈3.

Doxorubicin HCl may also be known as cloridrato de doxorrubicina, doxorubicini hydrochloridum, NSC-123127, *Adriamycin RDF®*, *Adriblastin®*, *Adriblastina®*, *Adriblastine®*, *Adrim®*, *Adrimedac®*, *Biorrub®*, *DOXO-cell®*, *Doxolem®*, *Doxorbin®*, *Doxorubin®*, *Doxotec®*, *Doxtie®*, *Farmiblastina®*, *Fauldoxo®*, *Flavicina®*, *Ifadox®*, *Neoxan®*, *Ribodoxo-L®*, and *Rubex®*.

Storage/Stability

Lyophilized powder for injection should be stored away from direct sunlight and in a dry place. After reconstituting with sodium chloride 0.9%, the single-use lyophilized powder product is reportedly stable for 24 hours at room temperature and 48 hours when refrigerated. The manufacturer recommends protecting from sunlight, not freezing the product, and discarding any unused portion. However, one study found that powder reconstituted with sterile water to a concentration of 2 mg/mL lost only ≈1.5% of its potency per month over 6 months when stored in the refrigerator. When frozen at -20°C (-68°F), no potency loss after 30 days was detected, and sterility was maintained by filtering the drug through a 0.22-micron filter before injection.

The manufacturer states that after reconstitution, the multidose vials may be stored for up to 7 days at room temperature in normal room light and up to 15 days in the refrigerator.

The commercially available solution for injection is stable for 18 months when stored in the refrigerator at 2°C to 8°C (36°F-46°F) and protected from light.

Compatibility/Compounding Considerations

Do not flush IV catheters with heparin or heparinized saline; use sterile saline.

Doxorubicin HCl is reportedly physically **compatible** with the following IV solutions and drugs: dextrose 3.3% in sodium chloride 3%, D_5W, *Normosol® R* (pH 7.4), lactated Ringer's injection, and sodium chloride 0.9% and in syringes with bleomycin sulfate, cisplatin, cyclophosphamide, droperidol, fluorouracil, leucovorin calcium, methotrexate sodium, metoclopramide HCl, mitomycin, and vincristine sulfate. The drug is physically **compatible during Y-site injection** with bleomycin sulfate, cisplatin, cyclophosphamide, droperidol, fluorouracil, leucovorin calcium, methotrexate sodium, metoclopramide HCl, mitomycin, and vincristine sulfate.

Doxorubicin HCl **compatibility information conflicts** or is dependent on diluent or concentration factors with the following drugs or solutions: vinblastine sulfate (in syringes and as an IV additive). Compatibility is dependent on factors such as pH, concentration, temperature, and diluent used; consult specialized references or a hospital pharmacist for more specific information.

Doxorubicin HCl is reportedly physically **incompatible** with the following solutions or drugs: aminophylline, dexamethasone sodium phosphate, diazepam, fluorouracil (as an IV additive only), furosemide, heparin sodium, and hydrocortisone sodium succinate.

Dosage Forms/Regulatory Status

VETERINARY-LABELED PRODUCTS: NONE

HUMAN-LABELED PRODUCTS:

Doxorubicin HCl (Conventional) Lyophilized Powder for Injection, (conventional): 10 mg and 150 mg vials; *Adriamycin RDF®*, generic; (Rx). Reconstitute with appropriate amount of 0.9% sodium chloride for final concentration of 2 mg/mL.

Doxorubicin HCl (Conventional) Injection (aqueous): 2 mg/mL in 5 mL, 10 mL, 25 mL, and 100 mL; *Adriamycin PFS®*, generic; (Rx)

References

For the complete list of references, see **wiley.com/go/budde/plumb**

Doxycycline

(dox-i-**sye**-kleen) *Vibramycin®*, *Doxy 100®*

Tetracycline Antibiotic

Prescriber Highlights

- ▶ Oral and parenteral tetracycline antibiotic
- ▶ Bone and teeth abnormalities are possible but much less likely to occur than with other tetracyclines; ensure benefits outweigh potential risks in pregnant and pediatric animals.
- ▶ May be used in patients with renal insufficiency
- ▶ Not for IV injection in horses. Should not be given IM or SC to any species due to injection site adverse effects
- ▶ Most common adverse effects are GI, but increased liver enzymes can occur.
- ▶ Esophagitis and strictures are possible, particularly in cats. Oral doses must be followed with sufficient fluid to minimize the risk for medication becoming lodged in the esophagus.
- ▶ Drug interactions with mineral-containing antacids, iron products, and other antibiotics are well documented.

Uses/Indications

Although there are no FDA-approved systemic veterinary doxycycline products available, the drug's efficacy, favorable pharmacokinetic parameters (ie, longer half-life, wide volume of distribution, higher CNS penetration), and safety profile, as compared with tetracycline or oxytetracycline, make it the preferred choice in small animal species when a tetracycline is indicated, particularly in azotemic patients.

Doxycycline is commonly used in small animals to treat a variety of infections caused by several different microorganisms, including *Borrelia* spp, *Leptospira* spp, *Rickettsia* spp, *Anaplasma* spp, *Ehrlichia* spp, *Chlamydia* spp, *Mycoplasma* spp, *Bartonella* spp, and *Bordetella* spp. In a study, use of doxycycline to treat *A phagocytophilum* infection resulted in clinical resolution in all infected dogs ($n = 16$)[1], all of which became blood PCR-negative 30 and 60 days after treatment onset. Hematologic abnormalities (ie, leukopenia, eosinophilia, lymphopenia) persisted in 4 dogs. A small study suggested that a combination of doxycycline, clindamycin, and metronidazole may be an effective alternative treatment for canine babesiosis caused by *Babesia gibsoni* in dogs that fail first-line therapy (atovaquone and azithromycin).[2]

Doxycycline therapy is part of the American Heartworm Society's recommended canine heartworm treatment protocol.[3,4] *Dirofilaria immitis* harbors *Wolbachia* spp organisms as endosymbiotic bacteria. The presence of *Wolbachia* spp—even in very low numbers—appears necessary for filarial embryogenesis. In addition, *Wolbachia* spp organisms contribute to pulmonary and renal inflammation of filarial disease.[3] Doxycycline greatly reduces *Wolbachia* spp organisms in filarial nematodes, which can result in amicrofilaremia for up to 12 months.[3,4] Antibiotic resistance has been noted in heartworm-treated dogs receiving adjunctive doxycycline therapy,[5] but this data should not prevent doxycycline use in dogs requiring adulticidal therapy.

In a study, 6 dogs were given subantimicrobial doses of systemic doxycycline to treat experimentally induced periodontitis,[6] which was effectively treated, and antimicrobial resistance did not appear to be induced[7]; however, systemic use of antimicrobial drugs for nonantimicrobial uses is discouraged.[7]

In foals with mild to moderate bronchopneumonia, the combination of doxycycline and azithromycin appears effective in treating *Rhodococcus equi*.[8] In horses, doxycycline use for synovial infection may be a suitable first-line treatment of synovial sepsis while culture and susceptibility results are pending,[9] but a negative effect on return to function following doxycycline use has also been demonstrated.[10] The usefulness of doxycycline will likely depend on regional susceptibility of expected pathogens.

In avian species, doxycycline may be a suitable first-line choice for oral treatment of chlamydiosis.[11,12]

The World Health Organization (WHO) has designated doxycycline as a Highly Important antimicrobial in human medicine.[13] The Office International des Epizooties (OIE) has designated doxycycline as a Veterinary Critically Important Antimicrobial (VCIA) Agent in avian, bovine, camelid, caprine, equine, lagomorph, ovine, piscine, and swine species.[14]

Pharmacology/Actions

Tetracyclines are time-dependent bacteriostatic antibiotics that inhibit protein synthesis by reversibly binding to 30S ribosomal subunits of susceptible organisms, thereby preventing aminoacyl transfer-RNA binding to those ribosomes. Tetracyclines also alter cytoplasmic membrane permeability in susceptible organisms. In high concentrations, tetracyclines can also inhibit protein synthesis by mammalian cells.

Doxycycline generally has similar activity as other tetracyclines against susceptible organisms, but some strains of bacteria, including methicillin resistant *Staphylococcus pseudintermedius* (MRSP), may be more susceptible to doxycycline or minocycline; additional in vitro testing may be required.

Tetracyclines have activity against most *Mycoplasma* spp, spirochetes (including *Borrelia burgdorferi*, the causative agent for Lyme disease), *Chlamydia* spp, and *Rickettsia* spp. For gram-positive bacteria, tetracyclines have activity against some strains of staphylococci and streptococci, but resistance by these organisms is increasing.[15]

Staphylococcal resistance to tetracyclines occurs via the *tet*(K) and *tet*(M) genes. *tet*(K) confers resistance to tetracycline but not doxycycline or minocycline, whereas *tet*(M) confers resistance to tetracycline, doxycycline, and minocycline. Tetracycline susceptibility indicates doxycycline susceptibility; however, the reverse is not true. Tetracycline-resistant bacteria can be susceptible to doxycycline, necessitating doxycycline susceptibility testing.

Other gram-positive bacteria that are usually susceptible to tetracyclines include *Actinomyces* spp, *Bacillus anthracis, Clostridium perfringens, C tetani, Listeria monocytogenes*, and *Nocardia* spp. Tetracyclines usually have in vitro and in vivo activity against some gram-negative bacteria, including *Bordetella* spp, *Brucella* spp, *Bartonella* spp, *Haemophilus* spp, *Pasteurella multocida, Shigella* spp, and *Yersinia pestis*. Many or most strains of *Escherichia coli, Klebsiella* spp, *Bacteroides* spp, *Enterobacter* spp, *Proteus* spp, and *Pseudomonas aeruginosa* are resistant to tetracyclines.[16]

Minocycline and doxycycline have significant inhibitory properties against the activity of matrix metalloproteinases (eg, collagenase, gelatinase) and can act as a disease-modifying agent for osteoarthritis. In a pharmacokinetic study, doxycycline at 5 mg/kg PO every 48 hours significantly decreased synoviocyte matrix metalloproteinase (MMP)-13 concentration and gene expression in healthy horses.[17] The clinical relevance of this is unclear.

Doxycycline did not impair olfactory function in explosives detection dogs.[18]

Pharmacokinetics

In most species, doxycycline is well absorbed after oral administration. Bioavailability after PO administration is 90% to 100% in humans, and the drug is thought to be readily absorbed in most monogastric animals. Unlike tetracycline or oxytetracycline, doxycycline absorption in humans may only be reduced by 20% by either a high-fat meal or dairy products in the gut. However, in horses, oral administration of doxycycline in the fed state may reduce bioavailability, possibly because of the high fiber content in most equine diets.[19]

Tetracyclines are generally widely distributed to the heart, kidneys, lungs, muscle, pleural fluid, bronchial secretions, sputum, bile, synovial fluid, and ascitic fluid in most species. Doxycycline is more lipid soluble and penetrates body tissues and fluids better than tetracycline or oxytetracycline, including into the CSF, prostate, and eye. Although CSF concentrations are generally insufficient to treat most bacterial infections, doxycycline has been shown to be efficacious in the treatment of CNS effects associated with *Borrelia burgdorferi* infection in humans. Doxycycline (10 mg/kg PO every 12 hours) given to horses did not yield appreciable concentrations in the aqueous or vitreous humor,[20] but 20 mg/kg every 24 hours resulted in an aqueous humor concentration that was 10% to 75% that of plasma.[21] Drug concentration in tear film did not appear to be dose-related[22]; the tear:serum ratio in cats and dogs was 12% and 16%, respectively.[23] In horses, doxycycline has been shown to penetrate into the synovial fluid with an AUC synovial fluid-to-plasma factor of 4.6 and is eliminated from synovial fluid more slowly than plasma.[24]

The volume of distribution at steady state in dogs is ≈1.5 L/kg. Doxycycline is bound to plasma proteins in varying amounts depending on the species. The drug is ≈25% to 93% bound to plasma proteins in humans, 75% to 86% in dogs, 82% in horses, and ≈93% in cattle and pigs. Cats have higher binding to plasma proteins as compared with dogs. Doxycycline accumulates intracellularly and concentrates in equine polymorphonuclear neutrophils (PMNs).[21]

Doxycycline's elimination from the body is relatively unique. The drug is primarily excreted into the feces via nonbiliary routes in an inactive form. The drug is thought to be partially inactivated in the intestine by chelate formation and excreted into the intestinal lumen; in dogs, ≈75% of a dose is processed in this manner. Renal excretion of doxycycline can only account for ≈25% of a dose in dogs, and biliary excretion can only account for less than 5%.[25] The serum half-life of doxycycline in dogs is ≈10 to 12 hours, and clearance is ≈1.7 mL/kg/minute[25]; similar pharmacokinetic values are found in calves. In horses, elimination half-life is 9 to 12 hours,[21,26] and estimated clearance is ≈0.7 mL/kg/minute.[27] Doxycycline does not accumulate in patients with renal dysfunction.

Contraindications/Precautions/Warnings

Doxycycline is contraindicated in patients that are hypersensitive to it. Because tetracyclines can retard fetal skeletal development, discolor deciduous teeth, and lead to enamel hypoplasia; tetracyclines should only be used in the last half of pregnancy when the benefits outweigh the fetal risks; however, doxycycline is much less likely to cause these abnormalities than other more water-soluble tetracyclines (eg, tetracycline, oxytetracycline). Unlike oxytetracycline or tetracycline, doxycycline can be used in patients with renal insufficiency. Because increases in hepatic enzymes have been documented in some dogs after doxycycline treatment, this drug should be used with caution in dogs that have significant liver dysfunction. Tetracycline therapy (especially long-term) may result in overgrowth (ie, superinfections) of nonsusceptible bacteria or fungi. In humans, tetracyclines can cause photosensitivity; limit sun exposure for patients with thin or light-colored coats.

Doxycycline use has been associated with the development of esophageal stricture, particularly in cats.[28-32] If using oral tablets in cats, pilling should be followed by at least 5 mL of water or food.[32] Dry pilling should be avoided. Oral doxycycline monohydrate may have a lower risk for causing esophagitis than the hyclate salt, as it is much less acidic and slower to dissolve in neutral solutions[32]; however, it is recommended that all oral formulations administered to cats should be followed by a water or food swallow, regardless of the salt used.[32,33]

In horses, IV injection of even relatively low doses of doxycycline has been associated with cardiac arrhythmias, collapse, and death.[34] Until further studies are performed to document the safety of IV doxycycline in horses, the parenteral route of administration should be considered contraindicated in horses.

Doxycycline is a P-glycoprotein substrate; however, the Washington State University Clinical Pharmacology Laboratory has reported no increased sensitivity to doxycycline in dogs with the multidrug sensitivity (*MDR1*; ie, *ABCB1*) gene mutation and does not recommend any dose alterations in these dogs.[35]

Adverse Effects

The most commonly reported adverse effects of oral doxycycline therapy in dogs and cats are vomiting, diarrhea, and anorexia. Giving the drug with food may help alleviate these GI effects without significantly reducing drug absorption. Doxycycline monohydrate may be less likely to cause GI adverse effects and esophagitis/strictures than doxycycline hyclate,[33] but comparative data in animals are lacking. Increased ALT and ALP have been reported in up to 40% of dogs and 19% of cats.[36] This increase does not appear to be clinically significant in dogs.[37]

Oral doxycycline has been implicated in causing esophagitis and esophageal strictures, particularly in cats. See ***Contraindications/Precautions/Warnings*** for more information.

In goats, IM injection has led to severe edema and pain at the injection site.[38]

In humans, doxycycline and other tetracyclines have also been associated with photosensitivity reactions and, rarely, hepatotoxicity or blood dyscrasias. In humans, IV administration should occur over a minimum of 1 hour, and the SC or IM routes should not be used.[39]

Reproductive/Nursing Safety

Tetracyclines cross the placenta; they are embryotoxic when used early in pregnancy and can retard fetal skeletal growth and permanently discolor teeth. A litter of puppies with midline and congenital cardiac defects was born to a dam treated with doxycycline, prednisone, and tramadol at 21 days gestation.[40]

Tetracyclines are excreted in milk. Milk:plasma ratios vary between 0.25 and 1.5. Dams that require doxycycline should not nurse their young.

Because safety has not been established in animals, this drug should only be used when the maternal benefits outweigh the potential risks to offspring.

Overdose/Acute Toxicity

With the exception of IV administration in horses (see ***Adverse Effects***), doxycycline is apparently safe in most mild overdose cases. Oral overdoses most commonly cause GI disturbances (eg, vomiting, anorexia, diarrhea). Increased serum cardiac troponin 1 was found in 3 calves receiving doxycycline 32.5 mg/kg/day PO.[41]

Although doxycycline is less vulnerable to chelation with cations than other tetracyclines, oral administration of divalent or trivalent cation antacids may bind some of the drug and reduce GI distress. If a patient develops severe emesis or diarrhea, fluids and electrolytes should be monitored and replaced if necessary.

Rapid IV injection of doxycycline has induced transient collapse in horses[34] and cats[34,42] and cardiac arrhythmias in horses, presumably due to chelation with intravascular calcium ions. These effects may be more pronounced if overdose quantities are inadvertently administered.

For patients that have experienced or are suspected to have experienced an overdose, consultation with a 24-hour poison consultation center specializing in providing veterinary-specific information is recommended. For general information related to overdose and toxin exposures, as well as contact information for poison control centers, refer to ***Appendix***.

Drug Interactions

The following drug interactions have either been reported or are theoretical in humans or animals receiving doxycycline and may be of significance in veterinary patients. Unless otherwise noted, use together is not necessarily contraindicated, but the potential risks should be weighed and additional monitoring performed when appropriate.

- **Aluminum, Calcium,** and **Magnesium-Containing Oral Products**: When orally administered, tetracyclines can chelate divalent or trivalent cations that can then decrease the absorption of the tetracycline or the other drug if it contains these cations. Oral products that contain aluminum, calcium, or magnesium cations are most commonly associated with this interaction. Although doxycycline has a relatively low affinity for calcium ions, it is recommended that all oral tetracyclines be given at least 1 to 2 hours before or after any cation-containing product.
- **Ascorbic Acid** (ie, **Vitamin C**): May result in decreased doxycycline efficacy
- **Avermectins** (eg, **doramectin, ivermectin**): Doxycycline inhibited P-glycoprotein in an experimental model of the blood–brain barrier in alpacas. This interaction may have clinical rele-

vance in treating meningeal worms.[43]

- **Bismuth Subsalicylate**: May reduce absorption of tetracyclines; it is recommended that all oral tetracyclines be given at least 1 to 2 hours before or after bismuth subsalicylate.
- **Enrofloxacin**: Concurrent doxycycline use reduced and delayed enrofloxacin in vitro activity against *Escherichia coli*. Bactericidal effects were better with concomitant administration than when separated by 12 hours.[44]
- **Iron, Oral**: Oral iron products are associated with decreased tetracycline absorption, and administration of iron salts should preferably be 3 hours before or 2 hours after the tetracycline dose.
- **Kaolin/Pectin**: May reduce absorption of tetracyclines; it is recommended that all oral tetracyclines be given at least 1 to 2 hours before or after kaolin/pectin.
- **Penicillins**: Bacteriostatic drugs (eg, tetracyclines) may interfere with bactericidal activity of penicillins, cephalosporins, and aminoglycosides. The actual clinical significance, if any, of this interaction has likely been overstated.[45]
- **Phenobarbital**: May decrease doxycycline half-life and reduce concentrations
- **Proton Pump Inhibitors (PPIs)** (eg, **omeprazole, pantoprazole**): May reduce oral bioavailability of doxycycline
- **Sucralfate**: Concomitant sucralfate significantly reduces peak doxycycline concentration and overall exposure in dogs. No interaction occurred when sucralfate was administered 2 hours after doxycycline.[46]
- **Warfarin**: Tetracyclines may depress plasma prothrombin activity, and patients receiving anticoagulant (eg, warfarin) therapy may need a dosage adjustment.
- **Zinc**: When orally administered, tetracyclines can chelate divalent or trivalent cations that can then decrease the absorption of tetracycline or the other drug if it contains zinc; it is recommended that all oral tetracyclines be given at least 1 to 2 hours before or after the zinc-containing product.

Laboratory Considerations

- Tetracyclines (not minocycline) may cause falsely elevated values of **urine catecholamines** when fluorometric methods of determination are used.
- Tetracyclines can reportedly cause false positive **urine glucose** results if the cupric sulfate method of determination (Benedict's reagent, *Clinitest*®) is used; however, this may be the result of ascorbic acid that is found in some parenteral formulations of tetracyclines. Tetracyclines have also reportedly caused false-negative **urine glucose** results when the glucose oxidase method (*Clinistix*®, *Tes-Tape*®) is used.

Dosages

DOGS:

Susceptible bacterial infections (extra-label): 5 – 10 mg/kg PO every 12 to 24 hours. Treatment durations vary, but 7 to 14 days is commonly recommended.

a) **Acute respiratory infections** (extra-label): 5 mg/kg PO every 12 hours or 10 mg/kg PO every 24 hours; treat for 7 to 10 days[47]
b) **Adjunctive treatment for canine heartworm disease** (extra-label): In combination with an approved heartworm preventive, doxycycline 10 mg/kg PO every 12 hours for 4 weeks (days 1 through 28 of the American Heartworm Society protocol)[48]
c) **Leptospirosis** (extra-label): 5 mg/kg PO or IV every 12 hours for 2 weeks is recommended. For dogs that experience significant GI signs (eg, vomiting, anorexia, diarrhea) while receiving doxycycline PO, an alternative antibiotic (eg, ampicillin, penicillin G) should be considered. Once GI signs resolve, dogs should then receive doxycycline at the recommended dosage to eliminate organisms from the renal tubules. Duration of antibiotic therapy appears uncertain; most recommend a 2-week regimen of doxycycline.[49] If given IV, doxycycline should be administered as a slow IV infusion. In humans, 100 mg diluted to 0.5 mg/mL is given over at least 1 hour. Doxycycline IV is not recommended unless GI adverse effects prevent PO administration and other antimicrobials cannot be used.
d) **Granulocytic anaplasmosis (*Anaplasma phagocytophilum*)** (extra-label): 5 mg/kg PO every 12 hours for 14 days; most dogs show clinical improvement in 24 to 48 hours.[50]
e) **Borreliosis (ie, *Borrelia burgdorferi* [Lyme disease])** (extra-label): 10 mg/kg PO every 12 to 24 hours for 30 days[51]
f) **Ehrlichiosis** (extra-label): 10 mg/kg PO every 24 hours for 28 days[52,53]
g) **Rickettsial diseases (eg, *Rickettsia rickettsii* [Rocky Mountain spotted fever])** (extra-label): 5 mg/kg PO every 12 hours[54]
h) **Alternative treatment for *Babesia gibsonii* after atovaquone and azithromycin failed to eliminate infection on PCR test**: doxycycline 5 mg/kg PO once daily in combination with clindamycin 25 mg/kg PO twice daily and metronidazole 15 mg/kg PO twice daily and for 30 to 90 days[2]

Periodontitis (subantimicrobial regimen) (extra-label): 2 mg/kg PO once daily appeared to be an appropriate dose and may be suitable for treatment of gelatinolytic inflammatory diseases (eg, periodontitis).[6,55] **NOTE**: Systemic use of antimicrobial drugs at subantimicrobial doses for nonantimicrobial uses is discouraged.

CATS:

WARNING: Cats should not be dry pilled with doxycycline PO; administration should be followed with at least 5 mL of water. Alternatively, a compounded slurry (eg, "triple fish" or similar) can be used to administer the dose (see ***Compatibility/Compounding Considerations***).

Susceptible infections (extra-label): 5 mg/kg PO twice daily or 10 mg/kg PO once daily is generally recommended.

a) **Acute respiratory infections** (extra-label): 5 mg/kg PO every 12 hours or 10 mg/kg PO every 24 hours; treat for 7 to 10 days[47]
b) ***Mycoplasma felis* upper respiratory tract infections** (extra-label): Shelter cats were given 10 mg/kg PO (as oral liquid) once daily for either 7 or 14 days.[56] Authors concluded that the 14-day course produced superior microbiologic, but not clinical, results.
c) ***Mycoplasma haemofelis* (ie, hemotropic mycoplasmosis, hemoplasmosis, or feline infectious anemia)** (extra-label): 10 mg/kg PO once daily or 5 mg/kg PO every 12 hours for 2 to 4 weeks.[57-59] An alternate antimicrobial (eg, marbofloxacin) should be considered if bacteremia persists.[57]
d) **Ehrlichiosis or anaplasmosis** (extra-label): 5 – 10 mg/kg PO every 12 hours for 21 days[60,61]
e) **Bartonellosis** (extra-label): 10 mg/kg PO every 12 to 24 hours[62]
f) **Clinical *Toxoplasma gondii*** (extra-label): 5 – 10 mg/kg PO every 12 hours for 4 weeks[63]
g) **Susceptible mycobacterial, L-forms, or mycoplasma infections** (extra-label): 5 – 10 mg/kg PO every 12 hours[64]
h) ***Nocardia* spp (eg, *N nova*) infections** (extra-label): doxycycline 5 mg/kg or higher PO twice daily in combination

with amoxicillin 20 mg/kg PO twice daily; clarithromycin 62.5 – 125 mg/cat (NOT mg/kg) PO twice daily can also be added [65]

i) **Feline chlamydial infections (eg, *Chlamydia felis*)** (extra-label): 10 mg/kg PO every 24 hours for a minimum of 3 to 4 weeks; additional topical ocular treatment may reduce ocular discomfort[66–68]

HORSES:

WARNING: Doxycycline IV in horses has been associated with fatalities. Until this drug's safety has been further demonstrated, it cannot be recommended for parenteral use in this species. Commercially available PO doxycycline hyclate or monohydrate has low bioavailability in horses and treating Lyme disease or anaplasmosis may be problematic. Food appears to significantly reduce absorption in horses, and administration on an empty stomach is recommended.

Borreliosis (ie, *Borrelia burgdorferi* [Lyme disease]) (extra-label): 10 mg/kg PO every 12 hours. Treatment for 2 weeks may be adequate for early-stage infections, whereas treatment for 1 to 2 months may be required for patients with neuroborreliosis or ocular involvement.[26,69]

Equine granulocytic ehrlichiosis (EGE; anaplasmosis) as an alternative to oxytetracycline (extra-label): 10 mg/kg PO every 12 hours for 10 to 14 days[70]

***Rhodococcus equi* bronchopneumonia in foals** (extra-label): Doxycycline 10 mg/kg in combination with azithromycin 5 mg/kg PO twice daily for a minimum of 41 days; continue treatment until resolution of clinical signs and no evidence of pulmonary consolidation is seen on thoracic ultrasound. The efficacy of this combination was similar rifampin/azithromycin.[8]

RABBITS/RODENTS/SMALL MAMMALS:

***Mycoplasma* spp pneumonia (mice, rats)** (extra-label): Doxycycline 5 mg/kg PO twice daily with enrofloxacin 10 mg/kg PO twice daily[71]

Chinchillas, gerbils, guinea pigs, hamsters, mice, rats (extra-label): 2.5 – 5 mg/kg PO every 12 hours. Doxycycline should not be used in young or pregnant animals

BIRDS:

Psittacosis (*Chlamydia psittaci*) (extra-label):

a) 25 – 50 mg/kg PO once a day is the recommended starting dosage for unstudied avian species[72–74]; split and give twice daily if regurgitation occurs. May be administered orally via liquid/suspension, or by medicated feed (doxycycline hyclate 1 g per kg feed [corn, beans, rice, oatmeal]).
b) **Cockatiels, Senegal parrots, blue-fronted Amazon parrots, and orange-winged Amazon parrots**: 40 – 50 mg/kg PO once daily.[72,73] In a study of experimentally infected cockatiels, doxycycline 35 mg/kg PO was given once daily for 21 days, which was as effective as a 45-day treatment. The drug was administered via a metallic feeding tube into the crop using the commercially available human oral suspension (*Vibramycin®*).[12]
c) **African grey parrots, Goffin's cockatoos, blue and gold macaws, and green-winged macaws**: 25 mg/kg PO once daily[72]
d) Using the injectable product (*Vibaravenos®*—may not be available commercially in the United States): 25 – 50 mg/kg IM every 5 to 7 days for 45 days[74]; **NOTE**: May cause muscle necrosis

REPTILES:

Susceptible infections (extra-label):

Chelonians: 10 mg/kg PO once daily for 4 weeks. Useful for bacterial respiratory infections in tortoises with suspected *Mycoplasma* spp infections

In most species: 10 mg/kg PO once daily for 10 to 45 days[75]

Monitoring

- Clinical efficacy
- Adverse effects (eg, vomiting, diarrhea, anorexia)
- Renal and hepatic function during long-term use

Client Information

- This medicine *must* be given with a moist treat or a small amount of liquid to ensure it reaches the stomach; this is especially important for cats. Doxycycline can cause ulcers in the throat and esophagus if it gets stuck before reaching the stomach. If your animal has trouble swallowing or eating while taking this medicine, contact your veterinarian immediately.
- This medicine may cause stomach upset. Give with a small amount of food that does not contain iron or dairy products.
- Do not give multivitamins, calcium supplements, antacids, or laxatives 2 hours before or after giving doxycycline as these products can reduce effectiveness of the medicine.
- This medicine may make your animal's skin more sensitive to sunlight and increase the risk for sunburn on hairless areas such as the nose and around the eyelids and ears. Tell your veterinarian if you notice any reddening of the skin (sunburn) while your animal is on this medication.
- Complete the entire course of this medication (even if your animal seems back to normal) unless directed otherwise by your veterinarian.

Chemistry/Synonyms

Doxycycline is a semisynthetic tetracycline that is derived from oxytetracycline. It is available as hyclate, calcium, and monohydrate salts. The hyclate salt is used in the injectable dosage form, oral tablets, and oral capsules. It occurs as a yellow crystalline powder that is soluble in water and slightly soluble in alcohol. After reconstitution with sterile water, the hyclate injection has a pH between 1.8 and 3.3. Doxycycline hyclate may also be known as doxycycline hydrochloride.

The monohydrate salt is found in the oral powder for reconstitution. It occurs as a yellow crystalline powder that is very slightly soluble in water and sparingly soluble in alcohol. The calcium salt is formed in situ during manufacturing. It is found in the commercially available oral syrup and other oral dosage forms.

Doxycycline may also be known as doxycycline monohydrate, doxycyclinum, and GS-3065; many trade name products are available.

Storage/Stability

Doxycycline hyclate tablets and capsules should be stored in tight, light-resistant containers below 30°C (86°F), preferably at controlled room temperature (15°C to 30°C [59°F-86°F]). After being reconstituted with water, the monohydrate oral suspension is stable for 14 days when stored at room temperature.

When reconstituted with a suitable diluent (eg, 5% dextrose, Ringer's injection, 0.9% sodium chloride, *Plasma-Lyte® 56* in 5% dextrose) to a concentration of 0.1 to 1 mg/mL, the hyclate injection may be stored for 72 hours if refrigerated. Infusions should be completed within 12 hours of removal from the refrigerator. Frozen reconstituted solutions (10 mg/mL in sterile water) are stable for at least 8 weeks if kept at -20°C (-4°F) but should not be refrozen once thawed. For diluted solutions stored at room temperature, different manufacturers give different recommendations regarding stability, ranging from 12 to 48 hours. Refer to product label for specific information.

Compatibility/Compounding Considerations

Compatibility is dependent on factors such as pH, concentration, temperature, and diluent used; specialized references or a hospital pharmacist should be consulted for more specific information.

Doxycycline hyclate for injection is reportedly physically **compatible** with the following IV infusion solutions and drugs: 5% dextrose, Ringer's injection, lactated Ringer's injection, 0.9% sodium chloride, *Plasma-Lyte® 56* in 5% dextrose, *Plasma-Lyte® 148* in 5% dextrose, *Normosol-M* in 5% dextrose, *Normosol-R* in 5% dextrose, invert sugar 10%, acyclovir sodium, amikacin sulfate, aminophylline, amiodarone HCl, atracurium, atropine sulfate, azithromycin, buprenorphine HCl, butorphanol tartrate, calcium chloride, calcium gluconate, cefotaxime, ceftriaxone, clindamycin, cyanocobalamin, cyclosporine, dexmedetomidine HCl, digoxin, diltiazem HCl, diphenhydramine HCl, dopamine HCl, ephedrine sulfate, famotidine, fentanyl citrate, fluconazole, gentamicin sulfate, hydromorphone HCl, insulin regular, lorazepam, magnesium sulfate, meperidine HCl, methadone HCl, metoclopramide HCl, metronidazole, midazolam HCl, morphine sulfate, multiple vitamins injection, mycophenolate mofetil HCl, naloxone HCl, norepinephrine bitartrate, ondansetron HCl, oxytocin, pantoprazole sodium, phenylephrine HCl, polymyxin B sulfate, potassium chloride, propofol, propranolol HCl, ranitidine HCl, voriconazole, and zoledronic acid.

It is **incompatible** with aminocaproic acid, amphotericin B (conventional and liposomal), ampicillin, cefazolin, ceftazidime, chloramphenicol, dexamethasone sodium phosphate, diazepam, erythromycin lactobionate, furosemide, heparin sodium, hydrocortisone sodium succinate, ketorolac tromethamine, methylprednisolone sodium succinate, penicillin G sodium/potassium, phenobarbital sodium, piperacillin sodium, and sodium bicarbonate.

One study examining doxycycline blood concentrations in birds following injection of a commercially available (not in United States) IM formulation (*Vibravenos®*; Pfizer CH) and 2 concentrations of a pharmacist-compounded product showed variable blood concentrations and a high incidence of localized tissue reactions, including necrosis, with the compounded products.[11]

Doxycycline 250 – 300 ppm administered to budgerigars in a hulled seed diet has been shown to maintain concentrations sufficient for treatment of chlamydiosis.[76]

An oral extended-release formulation that combined doxycycline with acrylic acid and polymethacrylate produced a longer release time and a favorable pharmacokinetic–pharmacodynamic relationship in healthy dogs.[77]

The commercially available syrup (*Vibramycin®*) and powder for oral suspension should be used when possible. Compounded doxycycline oral suspensions should be refrigerated, protected from light, and used within 7 days. Although some compounding pharmacies claim stability of 6 months for compounded doxycycline suspensions, others have demonstrated that compounded aqueous doxycycline suspensions degrade rapidly after 7 to 14 days, even when refrigerated.[78] A study evaluating compounded aqueous oral suspensions made from 100 mg doxycycline tablets at concentrations of 33.3 and 166.7 mg/mL concluded that stability cannot be assured beyond 7 days.[79] Another study demonstrated that doxycycline tablets mixed with water or foods (eg, milk, pudding, yogurt, applesauce, jellies) lose more than 10% potency after 24 hours.[80] Compounded doxycycline formulations (ie, chews, aqueous- and oil-based suspensions) had variable doxycycline content, and no formulation met US Pharmacopeia standards after 21 days of storage under recommended conditions.[81]

Dosage Forms/Regulatory Status

VETERINARY-LABELED PRODUCTS:

None for systemic use

Doxycycline gel (*Doxirobe®*) is FDA-approved for subgingival application for the prevention and treatment of periodontal disease in dogs.

HUMAN-LABELED PRODUCTS:

Doxycycline (as hyclate) Tablets and Capsules: 20 mg, 50 mg, and 100 mg; *Periostat®*, *Alodox® Convenience Kit*, *Vibramycin®*, *Vibra-Tabs®*, *Oraxyl®*, generic; (Rx)

Doxycycline (as hyclate) Delayed-Release Tablets and Capsules: 75 mg, 100 mg, and 150 mg; 40 mg (30 mg immediate release and 10 mg delayed release); *Doryx®*, *Oracea®*; (Rx)

Doxycycline (as monohydrate) Tablets and Capsules: 50 mg, 75 mg, 100 mg, and 150 mg; *Monodox®*, *Adoxa®*, generic; (Rx)

Doxycycline Capsules (coated pellets; as hyclate): 75 mg and 100 mg; *Doryx®*, generic; (Rx)

Doxycycline (as monohydrate) Powder for Oral Suspension: 5 mg/mL after reconstitution in 60 mL; *Vibramycin®*, generic; (Rx)

Doxycycline (as calcium salt) Oral Syrup: 10 mg/mL in 473 mL; *Vibramycin®*; (Rx)

Doxycycline Injection: 42.5 mg (as hyclate, 10%) in vials; *Atridox®*; (Rx)

Doxycycline (as hyclate) Lyophilized Powder for Injection: 100 mg and 200 mg with 300 mg and 600 mg mannitol, respectively, in vials; *Doxy®-100* and *-200*, generic; (Rx)

References

For the complete list of references, see **wiley.com/go/budde/plumb**

Edetate Calcium Disodium (CaEDTA)

(***ed***-a-tayt ***kal***-see-um dye-***so***-dee-um)

Calcium Disodium Versenate

Antidote

Prescriber Highlights

- Heavy metal chelator used primarily for lead and zinc toxicities
- Contraindications include patients with anuria, renal disease, or lead still in the GI tract; use extreme caution in patients with decreased renal function.
- Recommend using the SC route when treating small animals; do not administer orally.
- Adverse effects include pain on injection and renal toxicity (renal tubular necrosis). May cause depression and GI signs in dogs
- Do not confuse calcium disodium edetate with sodium edetate (edetate disodium).

Uses/Indications

Edetate calcium disodium (CaEDTA) is a chelating agent used in the treatment of lead and zinc toxicities. Oral succimer is more commonly recommended today for treating lead poisoning in dogs and cats, but CaEDTA can be considered when oral therapy is not practical.

CaEDTA may be used in combination with dimercaprol treatment.

Pharmacology/Actions

The calcium in edetate calcium disodium (CaEDTA) can be displaced by divalent or trivalent metals to form a stable, water-soluble complex that is excreted in the urine. One gram of CaEDTA can theoretically bind 620 mg of lead, but in reality, only about 5 mg of lead per gram of CaEDTA is actually excreted into the urine of patients that are treated for lead toxicity. In addition to chelating lead, CaEDTA readily chelates and eliminates zinc from the body. CaEDTA also binds cadmium, copper, iron, and manganese, but does not facilitate removal of those metals from the body.[1] CaEDTA is relatively ineffective for use in treating mercury, gold, or arsenic toxicities.

There is some evidence that thiamine supplementation may increase the clinical efficacy of CaEDTA in treating acute lead poisoning in cattle.

Pharmacokinetics

Edetate calcium disodium (CaEDTA) is poorly absorbed from the GI tract but is well absorbed after either IM or SC administration. It is distributed primarily in the extracellular fluid. Unlike dimercaprol, CaEDTA does not penetrate erythrocytes or enter the CNS in appreciable amounts. The drug is rapidly excreted renally, either as an unchanged drug or chelated with metals. Changes in urine pH or urine flow do not significantly alter the rate of excretion. In humans with normal renal function, the average elimination half-life of CaEDTA is 20 to 60 minutes after IV administration.[1] Decreased renal function can cause accumulation of CaEDTA and can increase its nephrotoxic potential.

Contraindications/Precautions/Warnings

Edetate calcium disodium (CaEDTA) is contraindicated in patients with anuria. It should be used with extreme caution in patients with diminished renal function; reduced doses are necessary in these patients.

Most small animal clinicians recommend using the SC route when treating small animals. Rapid IV administration of CaEDTA has been associated with abrupt increases in intracranial pressure and death in patients with lead encephalopathy and cerebral edema.

Termination of lead or zinc exposure is essential in the management of toxicities. Ideally, lead or zinc material should be removed from the GI tract before using CaEDTA. Do not administer CaEDTA orally as it may increase the amount of lead absorbed from the GI tract.

Do not confuse edetate CALCIUM disodium with sodium edetate (edetate disodium), which should **not** be used for lead poisoning as it may cause fatal hypocalcemia.[2]

Adverse Effects

The most serious adverse effect associated with this compound is dose-dependent renal toxicity (renal tubular necrosis resulting in nephrosis). Glycosuria, proteinuria, and microscopic hematuria may occur. This effect may be reduced by ensuring adequate diuresis prior to initiating therapy. In dogs, edetate calcium disodium (CaEDTA) can cause depression, vomiting, and diarrhea. GI clinical signs may be alleviated by zinc supplementation. Injection site pain and thrombophlebitis may occur after IV infusion. Fever, transient hypotension, mild increases in hepatic enzymes, tremor, and rash have been reported in humans. Prolonged administration of CaEDTA at high doses may produce transient bone marrow depression and skin and mucous membrane lesions, but these adverse effects usually resolve on discontinuation of the drug.

No evidence of muscle damage, nephrotoxicity, or hepatotoxicity was seen when administered IM to falcons.

Long-term therapy may lead to zinc deficiency; zinc supplementation should be considered in these animals.

Reproductive/Nursing Safety

Safe use of edetate calcium disodium (CaEDTA) during pregnancy has not been established. It is not known whether this drug is excreted in milk.

Because safety has not been established in animals, this drug should only be used when the maternal benefits outweigh the potential risks to offspring.

Overdose/Acute Toxicity

The oral LD_{50} in dogs is 12 g/kg; refer to ***Adverse Effects*** for more information.

For patients that have experienced or are suspected to have experienced an overdose, consultation with a 24-hour poison consultation center specializing in providing veterinary-specific information is recommended. For general information related to overdose and toxin exposures, as well as contact information for poison control centers, refer to ***Appendix***.

Drug Interactions

The following drug interactions have either been reported or are theoretical in humans or animals receiving edetate calcium disodium (CaEDTA) and may be of significance in veterinary patients. Unless otherwise noted, use together is not necessarily contraindicated, but weigh the potential risks and perform additional monitoring when appropriate.

- **Glucocorticoids** (eg, **dexamethasone, prednis(ol)one**): Concurrent administration of CaEDTA with glucocorticoids may increase the risk for renal toxicity.
- **Insulin** (eg, **NPH, PZI**): Concurrent administration of CaEDTA with zinc insulin preparations (NPH, PZI) will decrease the sustained action of the insulin preparation.
- **Nephrotoxic Drugs** (eg, **aminoglycosides, amphotericin B**): Use with caution with other nephrotoxic compounds
- **Nonsteroidal Anti-Inflammatory Drugs** (**NSAIDs**; eg, **carprofen, meloxicam, robenacoxib**): Concurrent administration of CaEDTA with NSAIDs may increase the risk for renal toxicity.

Laboratory Considerations

- May increase **urine glucose** values
- Inverted T waves on **ECG** are possible.

Dosages

NOTES:

1. It is imperative that the source of lead/zinc is removed from the animal (eg, GI decontamination).
2. The manufacturer of the injectable (human) product recommends diluting the total daily dose with 250 to 500 mL of either 0.9% sodium chloride or 5% dextrose when used IV.
3. Maintain adequate hydration throughout edetate calcium disodium (CaEDTA) treatment.
4. Consider zinc supplementation when treating for lead poisoning.

DOGS/CATS:

Lead and zinc toxicities (extra-label):

a) Dogs: 25 mg/kg (diluted in 5% dextrose to a concentration of 10 mg/mL) SC 4 times a day for 5 days.[3] Some sources say not to exceed 2 g per animal per day.[4] Repeat course of treatment if required.

b) Cats: 27.5 mg/kg diluted in 15 mL of 5% dextrose and administered SC every 6 hours for 5 days.[3,4] Repeat course of treatment if required.

Lead poisoning (extra-label): 75 mg/kg IV slowly as a 5% (50 mg/mL) solution in 0.9% sodium chloride or 5% dextrose. Total daily CaEDTA dose for dogs not to exceed 2000 mg. Administer calculated dose in 4 equally divided doses per day (ie, every 6 hours) for 2 to 5 days. Repeat the treatment course after 2 to 3 days, as necessary, if signs of lead poisoning are still present.[5]

HORSES:

Lead poisoning (extra-label): If severely affected, administer CaEDTA 75 mg/kg IV slowly in 5% dextrose or 0.9% sodium chloride daily for 4 to 5 days (may divide daily dose into 2 to 3 administrations per day). Stop therapy for 2 days, then repeat for another 4 to 5 days.[6]

FOOD ANIMALS:

Lead poisoning (extra-label):

a) 110 mg/kg per day; administer calculated dose in 3 to 4 divided doses; dilute CaEDTA solution to 1 g/mL in 5% dextrose. Administer the first dose IV, then subsequent doses are given SC[7]

b) Cattle: 67 mg/kg slow IV twice daily for 2 days; withhold dose for 2 days and then give again for 2 days. Cattle may require 10 to 14 days to recover and may require several series of treatments.[8]

c) Cattle (extra-label): 75 mg/kg as 5% (50 mg/mL) solution in saline or glucose; give IV slowly. Administer in 4 equally divided doses per day (ie, every 6 hours) for 2 to 5 days. Repeat the treatment course after 2 to 3 days, as necessary, if signs of lead poisoning are still present.[5]

CAMELIDS:

Lead poisoning (extra-label): 110 mg/kg (route not specified) for 5 days[9]

BIRDS:

Lead and zinc toxicities (extra-label):

a) 30 – 35 mg/kg IM every 12 hours for 3 to 5 days, off 3 to 5 days, may repeat same treatment and/or use another chelator. Can be used IV short term (48 hours) at 20 – 35 mg/kg diluted in 0.9% sodium chloride. Many published regimens[10]

b) Raptors (falcons): In this study, 25% CaEDTA was given undiluted IM at a dose of 100 mg/kg every 12 hours for 5 to 25 consecutive days.[11] Falcons were treated for 5-day courses if blood lead level was greater than 65 µg/dL until blood lead level was less than 20 µg/dL. No evidence of muscle damage, nephrotoxicity, or hepatotoxicity was seen.

c) Raptors: 35 – 50 mg/kg IM (diluted with saline and given as a 6.6% solution) SC every 8 or 12 hours for 5 days. Repeat after 2 to 3 days if indicated by blood lead levels. Higher dosages, up to 100 mg/kg, have been used.[12]

RABBITS:

Lead poisoning (extra-label): 27 – 30 mg/kg SC every 12 hours for 5 to 7 days[13,14]

Monitoring

- Serial blood lead or zinc levels; monitor during treatment and for 1 to 2 weeks after treatment
- Urinalysis (including urine sediment), hydration status, and urine output daily or every other day during treatment
- Baseline and periodic serum chemistry panel that includes renal values and phosphorus and calcium
- Blood levels of zinc, iron, and copper when treating for lead intoxication, as levels may be affected during treatment
- Heart rate and rhythm (ECG) when using IV route for edetate calcium disodium (CaEDTA) treatment

Client Information

- Because of the potential toxicity of this agent and the seriousness of most heavy metal intoxications, this drug should only be used with close professional supervision.

Chemistry/Synonyms

Edetate calcium disodium (CaEDTA), a heavy metal chelating agent, occurs as an odorless, white, crystalline powder or granules and is a mixture of dihydrate and trihydrate forms. It has a slightly saline taste and is slightly hygroscopic. CaEDTA is freely soluble in water and very slightly soluble in alcohol. The commercially available injection (human) has a pH of 6.5 to 8 and has ≈5.3 mEq of sodium per gram of CaEDTA.

Edetate calcium disodium may also be known as sodium calcium edetate, calcium disodium edathamil, calcium disodium edetate, calcium disodium ethylenediaminetetra-acetate, calcium disodium versenate, calcium EDTA, disodium calcium tetracemate, E385, natrii calcii edetas, sodium calciumedetate, *Calcium Vitis®*, *Calciumedetat-Heyl®*, *Chelante®*, *Chelintox®*, or *Ledclair®*.

Storage/Stability

Store edetate calcium disodium CaEDTA at 25°C (77°F); excursions to 15°C to 30°C (59°F-86°F) are permitted. Dilute the injection with either normal saline or 5% dextrose.

Compatibility/Compounding Considerations

Commercially available CaEDTA injection is usually diluted to a 1% solution with 5% dextrose for SC administration in small animals. CaEDTA is **incompatible** with Ringer's solution, lactated Ringer's solution, amphotericin B, and 10% dextrose.

To minimize pain from the IM injection, CaEDTA can be mixed in equal quantities with lidocaine hydrochloride 1% (eg, 1 mL of lidocaine 1% for each 1 mL of CaEDTA).

Dosage Forms/Regulatory Status

NOTES:

1) Edetate calcium disodium (CaEDTA) should not be confused with SODIUM edetate (edetate disodium), which should **not** be used for lead poisoning, as it may cause fatal hypocalcemia.[2]
2) FARAD recommends 2-day meat and milk withdrawal time after use in food animals.[15]

VETERINARY-LABELED PRODUCTS:

None; may be available from compounding pharmacies

HUMAN-LABELED PRODUCTS:

Edetate Calcium Disodium Injection Solution: 200 mg/mL in 5 mL ampules (1 g/amp); *Calcium Disodium Versenate*; (Rx)

References

For the complete list of references, see **wiley.com/go/budde/plumb**

Edrophonium

(ed-roe-***foe***-nee-um) *Tensilon®, Enlon®*

Anticholinesterase (Cholinergic) Agent

Prescriber Highlights

- Short-acting parenteral cholinergic used primarily to test for myasthenia gravis (MG).
- Secondary indications are to reverse nondepolarizing neuromuscular blocking agents (NMBAs) and to treat some supraventricular tachycardias (SVTs).
- Relatively contraindicated for use in patients that have asthma or mechanical urinary or intestinal tract obstruction
- Use with caution in patients that have bradycardia or atrioventricular blocks.
- Overdoses can cause cholinergic crisis; atropine for IV injection and ventilatory support should be readily available.
- Commercial availability may limit use.

Uses/Indications

The primary use for edrophonium is in the diagnostic workup for myasthenia gravis (MG). The edrophonium response test for MG is not specific or sensitive and has limitations, but a dramatic positive response is suggestive of MG. Both false-positive and false-negative results can occur; therefore, it is best to use while awaiting results from a more specific, sensitive test (eg, acetylcholine receptor antibody test).

In patients that do not have good control of clinical signs, edrophonium can be used to assess the efficacy of longer-acting anticholinesterase inhibitors by providing immediate amelioration of weakness if the dose of the long-acting agent is too low.

Edrophonium can also be used for the reversal of nondepolarizing neuromuscular blocking agents (NMBAs; eg, pancuronium, metocurine, atracurium, cisatracurium, rocuronium, or tubocurarine). Because of its short duration of action, the clinical usefulness of edrophonium for this indication is questionable since longer-acting drugs such as neostigmine or pyridostigmine may be more useful.

Edrophonium, in a controlled intensive care-type setting, may also be useful in the diagnosis and treatment of some supraventricular tachycardias (SVTs), particularly when other more traditional treatments are ineffective.

Pharmacology/Actions

Edrophonium is a relatively short-acting anticholinesterase agent. It inhibits acetylcholinesterase by reversible electrostatic attachment to the enzyme, thereby blocking its hydrolytic activity on acetylcholine. By blocking acetylcholinesterase, acetylcholine accumulates in the synaptic cleft to prolong cholinergic stimulation. Cholinergic effects result in miosis, increased skeletal muscle tone, intestinal hyperperistalsis, bronchoconstriction, ureter constriction, salivation, sweating (in animals with sweat glands), and bradycardia, and possibly sinus arrest (overdose). For these reasons, it is recommended to administer an anticholinergic (eg, atropine or glycopyrrolate) immediately before administering edrophonium. Compared to other drugs used to reverse nondepolarizing (NMBAs; eg, neostigmine and pyridostigmine), the effects of edrophonium on muscarinic receptors are mild. Edrophonium is a better choice in species where anticholinergics should be avoided (eg, horses).

Pharmacokinetics

Edrophonium is only effective when given parenterally. After IV administration, it begins to have effects on skeletal muscle within one minute, persisting up to 10 minutes. Myasthenic patients may have effects persisting longer after the first dose. In humans, ≈30% of edrophonium is metabolized in the liver to an inactive metabolite, edrophonium glucuronide, and renal excretion is responsible for the elimination of the remainder of the drug.

Contraindications/Precautions/Warnings

Edrophonium is contraindicated in patients that are hypersensitive to it or other acetylcholinesterase inhibitors. Edrophonium is considered relatively contraindicated in patients with bronchial asthma or mechanical urinary or intestinal tract obstruction. This drug should be used with caution (with adequate monitoring and treatment available) in patients with bradycardia or atrioventricular blocks.

It is recommended to have atropine injection (0.02 – 0.04 mg/kg IV) and ventilatory support readily available before administering edrophonium.

Adverse Effects

Adverse effects associated with edrophonium are generally dose-related and cholinergic in nature (eg, urination, lacrimation, vomiting, defecation, bradycardia, sinus arrest, and bronchospasm). Although the effects are usually mild and easily treated with time, pretreatment or treatment with an anticholinergic drug (eg, atropine, glycopyrrolate) can help prevent or alleviate these effects. Severe adverse effects are possible with large overdoses (see ***Overdose/Acute Toxicity***).

Reproductive/Nursing Safety

Edrophonium is a quaternary ammonium chloride that is ionized at physiologic pH and therefore would not be expected to cross the placenta in significant amounts. However, the drug's safety profile during pregnancy has not been established.

It is unknown whether edrophonium enters maternal milk.

Because safety has not been established in animals, this drug should only be used when the maternal benefits outweigh the potential risks to offspring.

Overdose/Acute Toxicity

Overdose of edrophonium may induce a cholinergic crisis. Clinical signs of cholinergic toxicity include GI effects (nausea, vomiting, diarrhea), salivation, sweating (in animals able to do so), respiratory effects (increased bronchial secretions, bronchospasm, pulmonary edema, respiratory paralysis), ophthalmic effects (miosis, blurred vision, lacrimation), cardiovascular effects (bradycardia or tachycardia, hypotension, cardiac arrest), muscle cramps, and weakness.

Treatment of edrophonium overdose consists of both ventilatory and cardiac supportive therapy and atropine injection (0.02 to 0.04 mg/kg IV) if necessary. Refer to ***Atropine*** for more information on its use for cholinergic toxicity.

For patients that have experienced or are suspected of having experienced an overdose, consultation with a 24-hour poison consultation center specializing in providing veterinary-specific information is recommended. For general information related to overdose and toxin exposures, as well as contact information for poison control centers, refer to ***Appendix.***

Drug Interactions

The following drug interactions have either been reported or are theoretical in humans or animals receiving edrophonium and may be of significance in veterinary patients. Unless otherwise noted, use together is not necessarily contraindicated, but weigh the potential risks and perform additional monitoring when appropriate.

- **Atropine**: Atropine will antagonize the muscarinic effects of edrophonium. Although some clinicians routinely use the 2 medications together, caution is advised, as atropine can mask the early clinical signs of cholinergic crisis.
- **Dexpanthenol**: Theoretically, dexpanthenol may have additive effects when it is used with edrophonium.
- **Digoxin**: Edrophonium's cardiac effects may be increased in patients receiving digoxin; excessive slowing of heart rate may occur.
- **Muscle Relaxants**: Edrophonium may prolong the Phase I block of depolarizing muscle relaxants (eg, **succinylcholine, decamethonium**), and edrophonium antagonizes the actions of nondepolarizing neuromuscular blocking agents (eg, **pancuronium, tubocurarine, gallamine, vecuronium, atracurium**).

Dosages

DOGS:

Presumptive diagnosis of myasthenia gravis (MG)| Edrophonium response test (extra-label): Place indwelling IV catheter and flush with sterile saline. The patient is gently exercised, or if nonambulatory, they are encouraged to rise until fatigued. Administer edrophonium 0.1 – 0.2 mg/kg IV[1] In patients with focal MG, such as facial muscle weakness, the palpebral reflex may be assessed after edrophonium is given.[2,3] **NOTE**: Be sure to have atropine (0.02 – 0.04 mg/kg IV) readily available in the event cholinergic signs (eg, salivation, lacrimation, urination, defecation, GI distress, emesis ["SLUDGE"]) develop.

Reversal of nondepolarizing neuromuscular blocking agents (NMBAs; extra-label): 0.25 – 0.5 mg/kg IV.[4] Start with a low dose first; repeat if necessary. **NOTE**: Administration of atropine 0.02 – 0.04 mg/kg IV immediately prior to edrophonium is recommended.[5]

CATS:

Presumptive diagnosis of MG | Edrophonium response test (extra-label): Place indwelling IV catheter and flush with sterile saline. The patient is gently exercised, or if nonambulatory, they are encouraged to rise until fatigued. Administer edrophonium

0.2 – 0.5 mg/cat (NOT mg/kg) IV.[1,6] In patients with focal MG, such as facial muscle weakness, the palpebral reflex may be assessed after edrophonium is given.[2,3] **NOTE**: Be sure to have atropine (0.02 – 0.04 mg/kg IV) readily available in the event cholinergic signs (eg, salivation, lacrimation, urination, defecation, GI distress, emesis ["SLUDGE"]) develop.

Reversal of NMBAs (extra-label): 0.25 – 0.5 mg/kg IV.[7] Start with a low dose first and repeat if necessary. **NOTE**: Administration of atropine 0.02 – 0.04 mg/kg IV immediately prior to edrophonium is recommended.

HORSES:

Reversal of NMBAs (extra-label): 0.1 – 0.5 mg/kg IV have been commonly used.[7,8] Because edrophonium can increase acetylcholine concentrations, parasympathetic tone may increase, causing bradycardia, bronchospasm, and increased salivation. Slow IV administration using low doses helps to minimize this effect.

Monitoring

- Cholinergic adverse effects: salivation, lacrimation, urination, defecation, GI distress, emesis ("SLUDGE")
- Improvement (for ≈1 to 15 minutes) of paresis is consistent with but not definitive for the diagnosis of myasthenia gravis (MG).

Client Information

- Edrophonium is a medicine that is only given to your animal in the veterinary clinic.

Chemistry/Synonyms

Edrophonium chloride, a synthetic quaternary ammonium cholinergic (parasympathomimetic) agent, occurs as a white crystalline powder having a bitter taste. Approximately 2 g are soluble in 1 mL of water. The injection has a pH of ≈5.4.

Edrophonium chloride may also be known as edrophonii chloridum, *Anticude*®, *Camsilon*®, *Enlon*®, *Reversol*®, or *Tensilon*®.

Storage/Stability

Store edrophonium chloride injection at room temperature.

Compatibility/Compounding Considerations

Compatibility is dependent on factors, such as pH, concentration, temperature, and diluent used; specialized references or a hospital pharmacist should be consulted for more specific information.

Edrophonium is reportedly physically **compatible** at Y-site injections with heparin sodium, hydrocortisone sodium succinate, potassium chloride, and vitamin B complex with C.

Dosage Forms/Regulatory Status

VETERINARY-LABELED PRODUCTS: NONE

HUMAN-LABELED PRODUCTS:

Edrophonium Chloride Solution for Injection: 10 mg/mL in 10 mL and 15 mL vials; *Enlon*®; (Rx)

Edrophonium Chloride/Atropine Sulfate for Injection: 10 mg/mL with 0.14 mg/mL atropine sulfate in 5 mL single-dose amps and 15 mL multi-dose vials; *Enlon-Plus*®; (Rx)

NOTE: Edrophonium appears to no longer be manufactured, and no commercially available dosage forms could be located.

References

For the complete list of references, see **wiley.com/go/budde/plumb**

Emodepside/Praziquantel

(ee-moe-***dep***-side with pra-zi-***kwon***-tel) *Profender*®

Topical Antiparasitic (Nematocide; Cestocide)

Prescriber Highlights

- Topical formulation is FDA-approved for use in cats weighing more than 1 kg (2.2 lb) and that are at least 8 weeks of age for the treatment of roundworms, hookworms, and tapeworms; it may also be used extra-label for the treatment of lungworms.
- Emodepside may be considered for oral use in dogs with confirmed multidrug-resistant hookworm infections; however, efficacy is still being established for this indication, and safety is a major concern in this species.
- Use with caution in cats with a history of an adverse reaction to MDR1 substrates (eg, ivermectin). Dogs with the *MDR1* gene mutation (also known as *ABCB1*-1delta) are more susceptible to emodepside toxicity.
- Emodepside has a microfilaricidal effect; use with caution in heartworm-positive dogs and cats.

Uses/Indications

Emodepside/praziquantel topical solution is FDA-approved for use in cats to treat and control roundworm (*Toxocara cati*), hookworm (*Ancylostoma tubaeforme*), and tapeworm (*Dipylidium caninum*, *Taenia taeniaeformis*) infections.[1]

Emodepside/praziquantel has also demonstrated effectiveness against *Toxascaris leonina*, *Echinococcus multilocularis*, and *Echinococcus granulosus*, as well as lungworm infections caused by *Troglostrongylus brevior*, *Aelurostrongylus abstrusus*, and *Capillaria aerophila* (*Eucoleus aerophagia*).[2-8] Emodepside/praziquantel can be administered to queens in late pregnancy to prevent lactogenic *T cati* transmission to kittens.[5,9]

In dogs, emodepside/praziquantel combinations are not FDA-approved; however, tablet formulations are available in other countries to treat dogs with roundworms, hookworms, whipworms, and tapeworms.[8] In the US, the feline *topical* product has been used *orally* in an extra-label manner in dogs for cases in which there is multidrug resistance from all 3 major anthelmintic classes (nicotinic agonists [eg, pyrantel], benzimidazoles [eg, fenbendazole], and avermectin/milbemycin endectocides [eg, moxidectin]), as confirmed by fecal egg count reduction testing.[10,11]

The topical emodepside/praziquantel formulation may also be of use for treating other species (eg, reptiles, rodents) in which oral dosing may be challenging.[12,13]

Pharmacology/Actions

Emodepside has a unique mode of action as compared with other antiparasitic compounds. In the parasite, the drug attaches presynaptically at the neuromuscular junction to a latrophilin-like receptor, resulting in increased intracellular calcium and diacylglycerol concentrations. At the end of the signal transduction cascade, vesicles containing inhibitory neuropeptide fuse with presynaptic membranes. Inhibitory neuropeptides (eg, PF-1, PF-2-like receptors) are then released into the synaptic cleft. When these peptides bind to postsynaptic receptors, there is an inhibition of pharyngeal pumping and locomotion of the nematode. The end result is flaccid paralysis and death of the parasite.

Emodepside also has activity against microfilaria, including in vitro activity against dirofilarial fourth-stage larvae and microfilaria.[1,14,15]

Praziquantel's exact mechanism of action against cestodes has not been determined. It may be the result of interacting with phospholipids in the integument of the parasite, causing ion fluxes of sodium, potassium, and calcium. At low concentrations in vitro, the drug appears to impair the function of mouth parts and stimulates the worm's motility. At higher concentrations in vitro, praziquantel increases the contraction (irreversibly at very high concentrations) of the worm's strobila (ie, chain of proglottids). In addition, praziquantel causes irreversible focal vacuolization and subsequent cestodal disintegration at specific sites within the cestodal integument.

A synergistic effect against nematodes has been suggested when emodepside is used with diethylcarbamazine.[16,17]

Pharmacokinetics

Following dermal application of the emodepside/praziquantel product to cats, both drugs are absorbed through the skin and into the systemic circulation. Absorption of both active ingredients through the skin is relatively rapid, with serum concentrations detectable within 2 hours for emodepside and 1 hour for praziquantel. Peak concentrations occur within 6 hours for praziquantel and 2 days for emodepside. After a single application, both emodepside and praziquantel were detectable for up to 28 days following treatment.

In dogs, peak concentrations of emodepside and praziquantel were reached 2 hours after administration, and half-life was ≈1.5 hours for both agents.[8]

A study looking at topical absorption in a variety of reptiles found variability in blood concentrations associated with skin thickness.[18]

Contraindications/Precautions/Warnings

Do not use emodepside/praziquantel in animals that are hypersensitive to emodepside or praziquantel.[1] Safe use has not been evaluated in cats younger than 8 weeks of age, weighing less than 1 kg (2.2 lb), used for breeding, or during pregnancy or in lactating queens. Use with caution in sick, debilitated, or heartworm-positive cats.

Dogs with the *MDR1* gene mutation (also known as *ABCB1*-1delta) may be susceptible to emodepside toxicity; vomiting, mydriasis, ataxia, muscle tremors, and seizures have been reported.[19-22] It is advisable to test susceptible breeds of dogs before using emodepside-containing products. Cats with *MDR1* gene mutations may also experience neurotoxicity,[23] and emodepside/praziquantel should be used with caution in cats with a history of adverse reaction to MDR1 substrates (eg, ivermectin).

Oral administration of emodepside or emodepside/praziquantel to dogs should be only to fasted dogs as administration with food increases the incidence and severity of adverse reactions; no food should be given until 4 hours after treatment.[8]

Emodepside is microfilaricidal at label dosages and should be used with caution in heartworm-positive animals.[1,15] See ***Adverse Effects***.

Adverse Effects

In pre-approval efficacy studies for emodepside/praziquantel topical solution, the most common adverse effects observed in cats were dermal and GI related. In a field study, adverse reactions reported by cat owners included licking and excessive grooming (3%), scratching treatment site (2.5%), salivation (1.7%), lethargy (1.7%), alopecia (1.3%), agitation and nervousness (1.2%), vomiting (1%), diarrhea (0.5%), eye irritation (0.5%), respiratory irritation (0.2%), and shaking/tremors (0.2%)[1]; all adverse reactions were self-limiting. The following additional adverse events were reported voluntarily during post-approval use of the product in markets outside the US: pyoderma, edema, erythema, dehydration, ataxia, loss of appetite, facial swelling, rear leg paralysis, seizures, hyperesthesia, twitching, and death. A case report of one cat developing a morphea-like (ie, scleroderma) lesion after application has been reported.[24]

In a study of cats artificially infected with heartworms then treated with topical emodepside/praziquantel, adverse effects consistent with a microfilaricidal effect included salivation, labored breathing, and lethargy.[1,14]

In dogs, adverse effects documented to have occurred following oral administration of emodepside/praziquantel tablets include hypersalivation, vomiting, tremors, and incoordination.[8] These effects are described as rare, transient, and mild but may be more common and more severe in dogs with the MDR1 mutation (also known as *ABCB1*-1delta). Heartworm-positive dogs treated with emodepside exhibited adverse effects consistent with dead or dying circulating microfilariae (eg, lethargy, tremors, ataxia, hypersalivation) within 2 hours of dosing.[15] Oral administration without fasting may increase the risk for adverse effects. Adverse effects associated with extra-label oral administration of the topical formulation in dogs are unknown.

Reproductive/Nursing Safety

Emodepside/praziquantel topical solution can be safely used in late pregnancy in queens to prevent lactogenic *Toxocara* cati transmission.[5,9,25] Studies performed in laboratory animals (eg, rats, rabbits) suggest that emodepside may interfere with fetal development in those species.[1]

Overdose/Acute Toxicity

Emodepside 200 mg/kg PO was tolerated in rats without mortalities. The oral LD_{50} in rats is greater than 500 mg/kg and in mice is greater than 2500 mg/kg. The acute dermal toxicity dose of emodepside in rats is high; a dose of 2000 mg/kg was tolerated without mortality.[26,27]

Praziquantel has a wide margin of safety. In rats and mice, the oral LD_{50} is at least 2000 mg/kg. An oral LD_{50} could not be determined in dogs because vomiting was induced at doses greater than 200 mg/kg. Parenteral doses of 50 to 100 mg/kg in cats caused transient ataxia and depression; parenteral doses of 200 mg/kg were lethal.

Kittens ≈8 weeks of age were treated topically with the combination product up to emodepside 15 mg/kg and praziquantel 60 mg/kg (5 times the labeled dose) at 2-week intervals for 6 treatments.[1] Clinical signs of transient salivation and/or tremors were observed in the group receiving 5 times the labeled dose. All clinical signs in this group were self-limiting. Cats 7 to 8 months of age treated with the topical solution at emodepside 30 mg/kg and praziquantel 120 mg/kg (10 times the labeled dose) developed transient salivation, tremors, and lethargy.

The combination product administered orally to cats caused salivation, vomiting, anorexia, tremors, abnormal respiration, and ataxia.[1] Adverse effects resolved without treatment.

For patients that have experienced or are suspected to have experienced an overdose, consultation with a 24-hour poison consultation center specializing in providing veterinary-specific information is recommended. For general information related to overdose and toxin exposures, as well as contact information for poison control centers, refer to ***Appendix***.

Drug Interactions

The following drug interactions have either been reported or are theoretical in humans or animals receiving emodepside/praziquantel and may be of significance in veterinary patients. Unless otherwise noted, use together is not necessarily contraindicated, but weigh the potential risks and perform additional monitoring when appropriate.

- **P-Glycoprotein Substrates Or Inhibitors** (eg, **ivermectin**, **erythromycin**, **prednisolone**, **cyclosporine**): Emodepside is a substrate for P-glycoprotein.[20,22,28] Concurrent use with other drugs that are P-glycoprotein substrates or inhibitors could cause pharmacokinetic drug interactions.[5]
- **CYP3A4 Inducers** (eg, **dexamethasone**, **phenobarbital**, **rifampin**): Concurrent use may decrease praziquantel concentrations and efficacy, and concurrent use is contraindicated in humans. A 4-week washout period is recommended in humans following rifampin treatment.
- **CYP3A4 Inhibitors** (eg, **itraconazole**, **ketoconazole**): May increase praziquantel concentrations. Monitor for praziquantel toxicity.

Laboratory Considerations

None

Dosages

DOGS:

NOTE: Dogs should be fasted overnight prior to oral administration and for 4 hours after treatment.

Treatment of susceptible ascarids, hookworms (including MDR hookworms[10]), whipworms[8,29], and tapeworms[5,8] (extra-label): Minimum dose of emodepside 1 mg/kg and praziquantel 5 mg/kg PO once rounding up to the nearest tablet size (tablet formulation not available in the US).[30]

Treatment of multidrug-resistant hookworms (extra-label): Emodepside 1 mg/kg and praziquantel 4 mg/kg PO once using topical formulation administered orally. As the safety and efficacy of this protocol have not been evaluated, its use should be reserved for cases in which resistance to drugs from all 3 other major anthelmintic classes (ie, nicotinic agonists [eg, pyrantel], benzimidazoles [eg, fenbendazole], and avermectin/milbemycin endectocide [eg, moxidectin]) as confirmed by the fecal egg count reduction test.

CATS:

Treatment and control of susceptible roundworms, hookworms, and tapeworms (label dosage; FDA approved): Minimum dose is emodepside 3 mg/kg and praziquantel 12 mg/kg applied to the skin on the back of the neck as a single topical dose (see ***Table*** for dose information).[1] A second treatment should not be necessary; however, if re-infection occurs, the product can be re-applied after 30 days.

Cat weight kg (lb)	Topical solution size	Volume (mL)	Emodepside (mg)	Praziquantel (mg)
1-2.5 (2.2-5.5)	Small	0.35	7.5	30
2.5-5 (5.5-11)	Medium	0.7	15	60.1
5-8 (11-17.6)	Large	1.12	24	96.1
More than 8 (17.6)	Use appropriate number of tube sizes			

Susceptible lungworms (*Troglostrongylus brevior, Aelurostrongylus abstrusus, Capillaria aerophilia* [aka *Eucoleus aerophilius*]; extra-label): Emodepside 3 mg/kg and praziquantel 12 mg/kg topically, repeat dose 14 days after initial treatment[2,4,6,7]

REPTILES:

Ascarids, oxyurids, and rhabditids in various reptile species (extra-label): Topical absorption varies between species, but 4 drops/100 g body weight appears to be effective. Aquatic species must be kept in a dry place for 48 hours after treatment. Caution is advised until further studies verify safety and efficacy, particularly in sick animals.[18]

Oxyurids in tortoises (extra-label): Emodepside 21.5 mg/kg and praziquantel 85.5 mg/kg (1 mL/kg) applied to the prefemoral fossa may be considered as an alternative to oral treatment.[12]

Monitoring

- Clinical efficacy: fecal flotation, fecal antigen testing, fecal egg count reduction test
- Adverse effects: GI effects (salivation, vomiting, diarrhea), topical reactions (pruritis, alopecia), neurologic effects (tremors, incoordination), particularly when using the topical solution orally in dogs.
- Prior to treatment: consider heartworm antigen testing with microfilaria check (dogs and cats) and MDR1 testing (dogs)

Client Information

- Topical (spot-on) medication is for treatment of roundworms, hookworms, and tapeworms in cats. Re-application usually is not necessary but can be administered after 30 days if reinfection occurs. More than one treatment may be needed when treating for lungworm infections.
- To apply the product, part the hair on the back of the cat's neck at the base of the head, place the tip of the tube on the skin, and squeeze the entire contents directly onto the skin.
- This medication is typically well-tolerated.
- Do not apply to broken skin or if hair coat is wet.
- Do not get topical product in the cat's mouth or eyes and do not allow the animal to lick the application site for 1 hour. Oral exposure to cats can cause salivation and vomiting; treatment at the base of the head minimizes the opportunity for ingestion.
- In households with multiple pets, keep them separated to prevent licking of the application site.
- Avoid direct human contact with the application site while it is wet. Avoid prolonged contact (eg, sleeping) with treated cats for 24 hours after application. In case of accidental spillage onto human skin, immediately wash off using soap and water.
- Your veterinarian may recommend *oral* administration of the *feline topical* product for dogs with resistant hookworm infections. Side effects may include salivation, vomiting, loss of appetite, tremors, abnormal breathing, and abnormal gait. Because this treatment is a new way to use this product, it is important to monitor your dog for any unusual signs not mentioned here and report them to your veterinarian if you have concerns.

Chemistry/Synonyms

Emodepside is an N-methylated 24-membered cyclooctadepsipeptide that consists of 4 alternating residues of N-methyl-L-leucine, 2 residues of D-lactate, and 2 residues of D-phenylacetate.

Praziquantel occurs as a white to practically white, hygroscopic, bitter tasting, crystalline powder that is either odorless or has a faint odor. It is very slightly soluble in water and freely soluble in alcohol. Available formulation is a clear yellow ready-to-use solution.

Emodepside may also be known as BAY44-4400 or PF1022-221. Praziquantel may also be known as EMBAY-8440 or praziquantelum.

Storage/Stability

Store product at or below 25°C (77°F); do not allow product to freeze.

Compatibility/Compounding Considerations

No specific information noted.

Dosage Forms/Regulatory Status

VETERINARY-LABELED PRODUCTS:

Emodepside (1.98% w/w; 21.4 mg/mL)/Praziquantel (7.94% w/w; 85.8 mg/mL) Topical Solution in 0.35 mL (cats, 1 to 2.5 kg [2.2 to 5.5 lb]), 0.7 mL (cats, 2.5 to 5 kg [5.5 to 11 lb]), and 1.12 mL (cats, 5 to 8 kg [11 to 17.6 lb]) tubes; *Profender*®; (Rx). NADA #141-275

An oral product for dogs (ie, *Profender*® for Dogs) is available in many countries but is not FDA-approved in the US. A combination oral suspension for dogs and cats that contains emodepside and toltrazuril (ie, *Procox*®) is also available in some markets.

HUMAN-LABELED PRODUCTS: NONE

References

For the complete list of references, see **wiley.com/go/budde/plumb**

Enalapril

Enalaprilat

(e-***nal***-a-pril) *Enacard®, Vasotec®*

Angiotensin-Converting Enzyme (ACE) Inhibitor

Prescriber Highlights

- ▶ Used to treat congestive heart failure (CHF), hypertension, chronic kidney disease (CKD), and proteinuria in dogs and cats
- ▶ Not recommended for acute kidney injury
- ▶ Should be used with caution in animals with dehydration, increased creatinine, hyperkalemia, hyponatremia, systemic lupus erythematosus (SLE), and hematologic disorders
- ▶ Adverse effects are uncommon. GI disturbances are the most likely adverse effects, but hypotension, renal dysfunction, and hyperkalemia are also possible.
- ▶ Use during pregnancy should be avoided.

Uses/Indications

Enalapril may be useful in the adjunctive treatment of congestive heart failure (CHF) in dogs and cats. Enalapril has been approved for use in dogs, and published studies have found therapeutic benefits in dogs with CHF[1,2]; however, concerns about those studies, coupled with a lack of prospective, controlled studies in cats, have raised questions regarding enalapril's value in small animals with CHF. Despite these concerns and the ongoing debate, ACE inhibitors continue to be used by many veterinary cardiologists to treat CHF in cats and dogs.[3] According to the 2019 ACVIM consensus guidelines for the treatment of degenerative mitral valve disease in dogs, use of an ACE inhibitor is recommended in the chronic management of dogs with stage C and stage D heart failure.[1] In the 2020 ACVIM consensus guidelines for the treatment of CHF in cats with cardiomyopathy, the use of an ACE inhibitor was not encouraged.[4]

Recommendations for ACE inhibitor use in dogs with the early stages of degenerative mitral valve disease (eg, prior to the onset of clinical signs) are mixed, with only half of the ACVIM panelists recommending its use in this stage.[1] Prior prospective, placebo-controlled clinical trials in dogs with subclinical degenerative mitral valve disease receiving enalapril failed to show a significant delay in the onset of CHF compared to placebo.[5,6] In another study, dogs with mitral regurgitation receiving enalapril 0.5 mg/kg/day for 14 days had increased cardiac parasympathetic tone and decreased sympathetic tone, which may theoretically lead to a reduction in cardiac preload and afterload.[7] The benefit, or lack of benefit, for ACE inhibitors in dogs with heart disease may relate to dose, with a retrospective study suggesting a twice-daily dosing of ACE inhibitors was predictive of improved 2 year survival compared to a once daily dosing.[8]

In a study of 26 Doberman pinschers with occult dilated cardiomyopathy, enalapril at a dosage of 10 mg/dog (NOT mg/kg) PO every 12 hours for 1 week, followed by 20 mg/dog (NOT mg/kg) PO every 12 hours showed a *statistically* significant increase in serum magnesium, serum potassium, and BUN from baseline when used in combination with spironolactone, carvedilol, and mexiletine. However, these changes were small and not *clinically* significant, suggesting this medication combination appears to be safe at the studied dosages.[9]

Because ACE inhibitors can decrease efferent glomerular resistance, can reduce proteinuria, and have renoprotective effects,[10] they are used for adjunctive treatment of idiopathic glomerulonephritis, CKD, and protein-losing nephropathies (PLNs) in small animals. There is stronger evidence for ACE inhibitor efficacy in dogs with PLN as compared with animals that have CKD without severe PLN. Enalapril at 0.5 mg/kg PO every 12 hours, in combination with a renal diet, further ameliorates proteinuria.[11] However, one study found that the angiotensin receptor blocker telmisartan was superior to enalapril in reducing proteinuria.[12]

Although ACE inhibitors are a mainstay in the treatment of hypertension in humans, they have not been particularly useful when used alone in the treatment of hypertension in cats.[13] In experimental models of renal insufficiency in dogs, enalapril at 0.5 mg/kg PO every 12 hours lowered mean arterial blood pressure.[14] ACE inhibitors are considered first-line treatment for hypertension in dogs due to the high prevalence of CKD in this population.[15] Combining ACE inhibitors with amlodipine ± an angiotensin receptor blocker (eg, telmisartan) can be considered for blood pressure management in dogs with CKD.[16]

Pharmacology/Actions

Enalapril is converted in the liver to the active compound enalaprilat. Enalaprilat prevents the formation of angiotensin-II, a potent vasoconstrictor, by competing with angiotensin-I for the ACE. ACE appears to have a much higher affinity for enalaprilat than for angiotensin-I. Because angiotensin-II concentrations are decreased, aldosterone secretion is reduced, and plasma renin activity is increased (due to the negative feedback mechanism). However, aldosterone breakthrough (elevated secretion of aldosterone) has been consistently documented in dogs receiving enalapril, which may be due to angiotensin-II reactivation, alternative renin-angiotensin-aldosterone pathways, or overriding effects in patients with activated ACE.[17]

The cardiovascular effects of enalaprilat in patients with CHF include decreased total peripheral and pulmonary vascular resistance, mean arterial and right atrial pressures, and pulmonary capillary wedge pressure; unchanged or decreased heart rate; and increased cardiac index and output, stroke volume, and exercise tolerance.

ACE inhibitors increase renal blood flow and decrease glomerular efferent arteriole resistance. In animals with glomerular disease, ACE inhibitors may decrease proteinuria and may help to preserve renal function. In healthy dogs, enalapril partially blocks activation of the renin-angiotensin-aldosterone system (RAAS) caused by amlodipine[18] and furosemide[17,19] Aldosterone breakthrough from ACE inhibition is independent of dose.[19]

Pharmacokinetics

Enalapril and enalaprilat have different pharmacokinetic properties as compared with captopril (ACE inhibitor) in dogs. Enalapril has a slower onset of action (4 to 6 hours) but a longer duration of action (12 to 14 hours) than captopril. In dogs, enalapril is readily absorbed and subsequently hydrolyzed to the active metabolite enalaprilat. Approximately 95% of enalaprilat is cleared via renal routes; reduced renal function can impact elimination rates.

In a study of horses, after administration of enalapril 0.5 mg/kg IV or PO, elimination half-lives of enalapril and enalaprilat were 0.59 and 1.25 hours, respectively.[20] After PO administration, enalapril and enalaprilat were not detectable in the serum. ACE activity had a tendency to decrease 40 to 120 minutes after enalapril PO administration, but ACE suppression was never greater than 16%. Serum concentrations of potassium, magnesium, serum creatinine, BUN, venous blood gases, and lactate did not change.[20]

In a different study, horses were given enalapril 0.5 mg/kg IV and 0.5 mg/kg, 1 mg/kg, and 2 mg/kg PO.[21] After IV administration, elimination half-lives of enalapril and enalaprilat were 0.67 and 2.76 hours, respectively. After PO administration, enalapril was below the limits of detection. Maximum mean ACE inhibition from baseline was 88.38% following IV administration and 21.69%, 26.11%, and 30.19% following the respective PO doses. Blood pressure and concentrations of BUN, serum creatinine, and electrolytes remained unchanged.[21]

In humans, enalapril is well absorbed after oral administration, but enalaprilat is not. Approximately 60% of an oral dose of enalapril is bioavailable, and food does not alter bioavailability. Both enalapril and enalaprilat are distributed poorly in the CNS. Enalaprilat is ≈50% bound to plasma proteins. In humans, the half-life of enalapril is ≈2 hours and the half-life of enalaprilat is ≈11 hours. Half-lives are increased in patients with CKD or severe CHF. The drug is renally eliminated.

Contraindications/Precautions/Warnings

Enalapril and enalaprilat administration is contraindicated in patients that have demonstrated hypersensitivity to ACE inhibitors. It is also contraindicated in humans with hereditary or idiopathic angioedema; veterinary clinical significance is unknown.

Enalapril should be used with caution and under close supervision in patients with renal insufficiency; doses may need to be reduced. One recommendation for an empiric dose reduction in cats with CKD is to start the daily administration at 50% of the usual total daily dose of 0.5 mg/kg every 12 hours when serum creatinine is greater than 2.3 mg/dL (roughly equivalent to creatinine clearance greater than 0.4 mL/kg/minute).[22] Although there are no specific dose adjustment recommendations for dogs, the same empiric approach would likely apply. Use of ACE inhibitors in critically ill patients with acute kidney injury (AKI) is generally not recommended because of their potential negative effects on glomerular filtration rate (GFR). Before receiving this class of drugs, patients should be stable after recovering from AKI.

Enalapril and enalaprilat should also be used with caution in patients with hyponatremia or sodium depletion, dehydration, pre-existing hematologic abnormalities, and/or collagen vascular disease (eg, SLE).

Dogs given enalapril at 0.5 mg/kg PO every 12 hours under isoflurane general anesthesia experienced significant hypotension and required more interventions as compared with dogs that did not receive the drug.[23] As such, withholding enalapril on the day of general anesthesia is advisable.

Liver disease does not appear to alter drug effects or dosing. Hepatic failure due to administration of enalapril has rarely been reported in humans.

Adverse Effects

Enalapril's primary adverse effect in dogs is GI distress (eg, anorexia, vomiting, diarrhea). Weakness and hypotension can also occur. In a study of Doberman pinschers with cardiomyopathy treated with enalapril, carvedilol, and spironolactone, elevated concentrations of magnesium, potassium, and BUN were noted but deemed clinically insignificant.[9] Polydipsia and polyuria have also been observed.

Adverse effects associated with enalapril in cats include lethargy and inappetence.

Because enalapril lacks a sulfhydryl group (unlike captopril), there is less likelihood that immune-mediated reactions will occur, but rashes, neutropenia, and agranulocytosis have been reported in humans. In humans, ACE inhibitors can commonly cause coughing, but this reaction is rare in dogs and cats.

Reproductive/Nursing Safety

Enalapril and enalaprilat cross the placenta, and the human label has a black box warning to discontinue enalapril as soon as possible when pregnancy is detected.[24] Veterinary-labeled enalapril is contraindicated in pregnant dogs in the United Kingdom.[25] High doses in rodents have caused decreased fetal weights and increases in fetal and maternal death rates; teratogenic effects have not been reported.

Enalapril and enalaprilat are excreted in milk, and use is not recommended in nursing animals.

Overdose/Acute Toxicity

In a study of dogs, administration of 200 mg/kg (400 times recommended dose) was reported to be lethal, but 100 mg/kg (200 times recommended dose) was not.[26] No adverse effects were noted in dogs given 15 mg/kg/day for up to one year.[26] In overdose situations, the primary concern is hypotension; supportive treatment with volume expansion using normal saline is recommended to correct blood pressure. Because of the drug's long duration of action, prolonged monitoring and treatment may be required. Acute overdoses should be managed by using gut-emptying protocols when warranted. The drug is removed by dialysis.

For patients that have experienced or are suspected to have experienced an overdose, consultation with a 24-hour poison consultation center specializing in providing veterinary-specific information is recommended. For general information related to overdose and toxin exposures, as well as contact information for poison control centers, refer to ***Appendix***.

Drug Interactions

The following drug interactions have either been reported or are theoretical in humans or animals receiving enalapril or enalaprilat and may be of significance in veterinary patients. Unless otherwise noted, use together is not necessarily contraindicated, but the potential risks should be weighed and additional monitoring performed when appropriate.

- Anesthetic Agents, Inhalant and Injectable (eg, **alfaxalone, etomidate, isoflurane, propofol**): Concurrent use may increase risk for hypotension. Dogs given enalapril 0.5 mg/kg PO every 12 hours under isoflurane general anesthesia experienced significant hypotension and required more interventions as compared with dogs that did not receive enalapril.[23]
- Angiotensin Receptor Blockers (ARBs; eg, **telmisartan**): Concurrent use of an ACE inhibitor with an angiotensin II receptor antagonist may cause additive effects on the renin-angiotensin system causing hyperkalemia, hypotension, syncope, and acute kidney injury.
- Antacids, Aluminum-, Calcium-, or Magnesium-Containing: Reduced oral absorption of enalapril may occur if administered concomitantly with antacids; administration should be separated by at least 2 hours.
- Antihypertensive Agents and Vasodilators (eg, **amlodipine, hydralazine, nitrates, prazosin**): Concurrent use may increase the risk for hypotension and other adverse effects; doses should be titrated carefully.
- Buspirone: Concurrent use may increase the risk for hypotension.
- Cabergoline: Concurrent use may lead to additive hypotension.
- Cimetidine: Concurrent use with ACE inhibitors has caused neurologic dysfunction in 2 human patients.
- Corticosteroids (eg, **dexamethasone, fludrocortisone, prednis(ol)one**): May decrease the antihypertensive effects of ACE inhibitors
- Dalteparin, Enoxaparin: Concurrent use may increase the risk for hyperkalemia.
- Darbepoetin Alfa; Epoetin Alfa: ACE inhibitors may interfere with erythropoietin.
- Digoxin: Digoxin concentration may increase by 15% to 30% when an ACE inhibitor is added; automatic dose reduction is not recommended but monitoring of serum digoxin concentration should be performed.
- Diphenhydramine: Concurrent use may increase the risk for hypotension.
- Disopyramide: Hypoglycemic effects may be enhanced.

- **Diuretics** (eg, **furosemide**): Concomitant diuretics may cause hypotension if used with enalapril; doses should be titrated carefully.
- **Doxepin**: Concurrent use may increase the risk for hypotension.
- **Glycerin, Oral**: Concurrent use may increase the risk for hypotension.
- **Heparin**: Concurrent use may increase the risk for hyperkalemia.
- **Lanthanum**: Reduced oral absorption of enalapril may occur if administered concomitantly; administration should be separated by at least 2 hours.
- **Lithium**: May increase risk for lithium toxicity
- **Nonsteroidal Anti-Inflammatory Drugs (NSAIDs**; eg, **carprofen, meloxicam, robenacoxib**): Potentially could increase the risk for nephrotoxicity and/or reduce efficacy of the ACE inhibitor in animals with cardiac or renal disease[27,28]; monitoring is advised.
- **Opioids** (eg, **butorphanol, hydrocodone, morphine**): Concurrent use may increase the risk for hypotension.
- **Potassium** Or **Potassium-Sparing Diuretics** (eg, **spironolactone**): Hyperkalemia may develop. The UK label states that combination with veterinary-labeled enalapril is contraindicated.
- **Probenecid**: Can decrease renal excretion of enalapril and possibly enhance the clinical and toxic effects of probenecid
- **Sildenafil**: Concurrent use may increase risk for hypotension.

Laboratory Considerations

- When iodohippurate sodium I-123/I-134 or technetium-99m pentetate is used for **renal imaging** in patients with renal artery stenosis, ACE inhibitors may cause a reversible decrease in localization and excretion of these agents in the affected kidney, which may lead to confusion in test interpretation.

Dosages

DOGS:

NOTE: Dehydration should be corrected prior to initiating therapy.

Adjunctive treatment of heart failure (label dosage; FDA-approved): 0.5 mg/kg PO once daily initially with or without food; if after 2 weeks the response is inadequate, dose can be increased to a maximum of 0.5 mg/kg every 12 hours. Diuretics should be administered at least 1 day prior to starting enalapril.[26] **NOTE**: Many consider the labeled starting dose to be too low; an initial dose of 0.5 mg/kg PO every 12 hours has been recommended.[3]

Adjunctive treatment of proteinuria (extra-label):

NOTE: Therapeutic goal is to reduce the urine protein:creatinine ratio by at least half—ideally, into the normal range (ie, UP:C less than 0.5).[29]

a) Nonazotemic patients: 0.25 – 1 mg/kg PO every 12 hours. Most initially treat at ≈0.5 mg/kg PO every 12 hours.[29,30]

b) Azotemic patients: 0.25 mg/kg PO every 12 hours. If azotemia does not worsen after 7 days of therapy, enalapril can be increased to 0.5 mg/kg PO every 12 hours with continued monitoring. See ***Monitoring***. **NOTE**: No conclusive data support a specific dose adjustment based on degree of azotemia. Higher dosages (eg, 2 mg/kg twice daily) may reduce progression of CKD in dogs.[31,32]

Systemic hypertension in dogs with CKD (extra-label): Initially 0.5 mg/kg PO every 12 hours. Dose can be increased (as tolerated) up to 2 mg/kg PO every 12 hours until target blood pressure is reached.[15] If this treatment regimen does not adequately control blood pressure, adding a second antihypertensive agent (eg, amlodipine, telmisartan) could be considered to achieve blood pressure management goals.[16]

CATS:

NOTE: Dehydration should be corrected prior to initiating therapy.

Chronic adjunct treatment for congestive heart failure (extra-label): 0.25 – 0.5 mg/kg PO every 24 hours. Practically given as 1.25 – 2.5 mg/cat (NOT mg/kg) PO every 24 hours[33]

Adjunctive treatment of proteinuria (extra-label):

NOTE: The therapeutic goal is to reduce the urine protein:creatinine ratio by at least half or, ideally, into the normal range (ie, UP:C less than 0.4).

a) Nonazotemic patients: 0.25 – 0.5 mg/kg PO every 12 to 24 hours. Most initially treat at ≈0.25 mg/kg PO every 12 hours.

b) Azotemic patients: 0.25 mg/kg PO every 12 to 24 hours. See ***Monitoring***. **NOTE**: No conclusive data support a specific dose adjustment based on degree of azotemia.[16,31,34,35]

Systemic hypertension (extra-label): Most recommend using amlodipine as the first-line agent in cats; however, for patients with hypertension that cannot be controlled with amlodipine alone or those with concurrent proteinuria, enalapril can be added at 0.5 mg/kg PO every 24 hours.[15]

FERRETS:

Adjunctive therapy for heart failure (extra-label):

a) 0.25 – 0.5 mg/kg PO every 48 hours; can be increased to every 24 hours as tolerated by the patient[36]

b) Dilated cardiomyopathy: 0.5 mg/kg PO every 24 to 48 hours[37]

BIRDS:

Adjunctive therapy for heart failure (extra-label):

a) 1.25 mg/kg PO every 8 to 12 hours[38]

b) 0.25 – 0.5 mg/kg PO every 24 to 48 hours in combination with furosemide[39]

Monitoring

- Clinical signs of CHF (eg, exercise intolerance, cough, increased resting respiratory rate and effort)
- Renal function (serum creatinine, BUN, urine protein:creatinine ratio) and electrolytes (in particular, potassium): These parameters should be measured prior to starting enalapril therapy and within 1 to 2 weeks of starting therapy or changing dose. These parameters should be rechecked every 3 months if the patient is stable. Large or progressive increases in serum creatinine should prompt reassessment of therapy. If serum creatinine increases by more than 0.2 mg/dL, a dose decrease is recommended.[34] ACE inhibitor doses should be cautiously increased to maximize impact on degree of proteinuria yet minimize the impact on renal function. Hyperkalemia or anorexia may also limit dose increases.
- Periodic CBCs are performed on humans receiving enalapril; this test may not be necessary in veterinary patients unless the patient's underlying condition warrants it.
- Blood pressure: baseline and periodic (eg, 7 to 10 days after initiating treatment [sooner if patient develops clinical signs associated with hypotension or if target organ damage is present in hypertensive animals]) or after dosage changes

Client Information

- Enalapril is used to treat heart failure, high blood pressure, and some forms of kidney disease in dogs and cats.
- This medicine is usually well tolerated but vomiting and diarrhea can occur. It may be given with or without food. If your animal vomits, stops eating, or acts sick after getting enalapril on an empty stomach, give with food or a small treat to see if this helps. If vomiting continues, contact your veterinarian.

- If a rash or signs of infection (eg, fever) occur, contact your veterinarian immediately.
- Very important to give this medicine as prescribed by your veterinarian. Do not stop or change the amount of medicine you give your animal without talking to your veterinarian first.
- Your animal will need to be monitored with blood tests and blood pressure checks while on this medication. Do not miss these important follow-up visits.

Chemistry/Synonyms

As ACE inhibitors, enalapril maleate and enalaprilat are derivatives of an alanine-proline dipeptide. Enalapril is a prodrug and is converted in vivo by the liver to enalaprilat. Enalapril maleate occurs as a white to off-white crystalline powder; 25 mg is soluble in 1 mL of water. Enalaprilat occurs as a white to off-white crystalline powder and is slightly soluble in water.

Enalapril maleate may also be known as enalaprili maleas and MK-421; many trade names are available. Enalaprilat may also be known as enalaprilic acid, MK-422, *Enacard®*, *Enalfor®*, *Epaned®*, *Glioten®*, *Lotrial®*, *Pres®*, *Renitec®*, *Reniten®*, *Vasotec®*, and *Xanef®*.

Storage/Stability

Enalapril tablets should be stored at temperatures less than 30°C (86°F) in tight containers. Enalapril solution should be stored under refrigeration at 2°C to 8°C (36°F-46°F) in tightly closed containers; avoid freezing or excessive heat. Enalapril solution may be stored at room temperature (20°C-25°C [68°F-77°F]) but must be discarded after 60 days.

Enalaprilat injection should be stored at 25°C (77°F), with excursions permitted between 15°C and 30°C (59°F-86°F). After dilution with D5W, normal saline, normal saline in D5W, or D5W in lactated Ringer's solution, the injectable formulation is stable for up to 24 hours at room temperature.

Compatibility/Compounding Considerations

Enalaprilat has been documented to be physically **incompatible** with amphotericin B, diazepam, and phenytoin sodium. Enalaprilat has **uncertain compatibility** with ampicillin, ampicillin/sulbactam, hydralazine, pantoprazole, and sulfamethoxazole/trimethoprim. Many other medications have been noted to be **compatible** with enalaprilat at various concentrations.

Compatibility is dependent on factors such as pH, concentration, temperature, and diluent used; specialized references or a hospital pharmacist should be consulted for more specific information.

Compounded preparation stability: Enalapril oral suspension compounded from commercially available tablets has been published.[40] Triturating 6 enalapril 20 mg tablets with 60 mL of *Ora-Plus®* and qs ad to 120 mL with *Ora-Sweet®* (or *Ora-Sweet® SF*), yields a 1 mg/mL oral suspension that retains greater than 90% potency for 60 days stored at both 5°C (41°F) and 25°C (77°F). Degradation of enalapril is pH dependent, with maximum stability at a pH of 3 and increased decomposition above a pH of 5. Compounded preparations of enalapril should be protected from light.

Dosage Forms/Regulatory Status

VETERINARY-LABELED PRODUCTS:

Enalapril Maleate Tablets: 1 mg, 2.5 mg, 5 mg, 10 mg, and 20 mg; *Enacard®*; (Rx). FDA approved for use in dogs. Although this product is still listed as approved at AnimalDrugs@FDA, it is no longer marketed in the United States. It is licensed for use in dogs in Canada, the United Kingdom, Australia, and other countries.

The Association of Racing Commissioners International (ARCI) has designated this drug as a class 3 substance. Use of this drug may not be allowed in certain animal competitions. Check rules and regulations before entering in a competition while this medication is being administered. Contact local racing authorities for further guidance. See ***Appendix*** for more information.

HUMAN-LABELED PRODUCTS:

Enalapril Maleate Tablets: 2.5 mg, 5 mg, 10 mg, and 20 mg; *Vasotec®*, generic; (Rx)

Enalapril Oral Solution: 1 mg/mL; *Epaned®*; (Rx)

Enalaprilat Injection: (for IV use) equivalent to 1.25 mg/mL in 1 mL and 2 mL vials; generic; (Rx)

Enalapril also is available in combination with hydrochlorothiazide.

References

For the complete list of references, see **wiley.com/go/budde/plumb**

Enoxaparin

(en-***ocks***-a-par-in) *Lovenox®*

Anticoagulant

Prescriber Highlights

- ► Low molecular weight (fractionated) heparin that may be useful for treatment or prophylaxis of thromboembolic disease
- ► Preferentially inhibits factor Xa and only minimally impacts clotting times
- ► Hemorrhage unlikely, but possible
- ► Must be given SC; uncertainty about effective dosing requirements for dogs or cats

Uses/Indications

Enoxaparin may be useful for prophylaxis or treatment of thromboembolic disease, including use in dogs with primary immune-mediated hemolytic anemia[1,2]; however, for dogs and cats, there is little published data to support its use in clinical patients, and it is still not known if it is safe and effective as well as economically viable for veterinary patients. Enoxaparin has also been used in horses to prevent laminitis following colic surgery.[3] In humans, enoxaparin is also indicated for prevention of ischemic complications associated with unstable angina and non-Q-wave myocardial infarction.[4]

Pharmacology/Actions

By binding to and accelerating antithrombin, low molecular weight heparins (LMWHs) enhance the inhibition of factor Xa and thrombin. The potential advantage to using these products over standard (unfractionated) heparin is that LMWHs preferentially inhibit factor Xa and only minimally impact clotting times (prothrombin time, thrombin time, and activated partial thromboplastin time). Recent studies in cats suggest that inhibition of factor Xa activity may not be an accurate indicator for predicting antithrombotic activity, as there may not be an association between the pharmacokinetics and pharmacodynamics in vivo.[5]

Pharmacokinetics

It is unclear if enoxaparin's pharmacokinetics directly relate to its antithrombotic actions in animals. In dogs after SC administration, enoxaparin has a shorter duration of inhibitory activity on factor Xa than in humans and therefore likely requires more frequent dosing in dogs. A study examining enoxaparin dose response (based on inhibition of factor Xa) in healthy greyhounds showed that enoxaparin 0.8 mg/kg SC every 6 hours was required to effectively and consistently inhibit factor Xa activity.[6] A subsequent study evaluating enoxaparin 0.8 mg/kg SC every 6 hours in healthy beagles demonstrated transient inhibition of factor Xa activity in only 3 of 8 dogs, and suggested that assumptions regarding pharmacodynamic effects of enoxaparin cannot be generalized across breeds.[7]

Cats appear to have a much shorter duration of factor Xa inhibitory activity associated with low molecular weight heparins (LMWHs) than do humans. To maintain a therapeutic target of factor Xa inhibitory activity of 0.5 – 1 IU/mL, 1.5 mg/kg enoxaparin SC every 6 hours is required.[8] However, a recently published study suggests that factor Xa inhibitory activity may not be an accurate determiner for antithrombotic activity of enoxaparin in cats. In their venous stasis model, antithrombotic activity persisted well beyond the expected therapeutic time for factor Xa inhibition.[5] A different study found that following a single enoxaparin SC injection, C_{max} was 0.83 anti-Xa IU/mL with a T_{max} of 110 minutes. The total clearance for enoxaparin was 23.4 mL/kg/hour, and the terminal half-life was 2.27 hours.[9]

A study investigating the pharmacokinetic variables of enoxaparin in horses demonstrated that the drug has similar activity (effect, duration) as in humans and the once daily SC injections may be useful for anticoagulant therapy.[10]

After SC injection in humans, enoxaparin is absorbed rapidly, with a bioavailability of ≈92%; peak plasma concentrations occur in 3 to 5 hours. Activity against factor Xa persists for up to 24 hours; doses are usually given once to twice a day. Enoxaparin is metabolized in the liver and excreted in the urine as both unchanged drug and metabolites; elimination half-life is ≈4 to 5 hours.

Contraindications/Precautions/Warnings

Enoxaparin is contraindicated in patients that are hypersensitive to it, other low molecular weight heparins (LMWHs), heparin, or porcine products. Its use is contraindicated in patients with active major bleeding and heparin-induced thrombocytopenia.[4] It should be used with extreme caution in patients receiving epidural anesthesia or with increased risk for hemorrhage, such as with a congenital or acquired bleeding disorder. In humans, it is recommended to use enoxaparin with caution in patients with bleeding diathesis, uncontrolled arterial hypertension, or history of recent GI ulceration, or diabetic retinopathy. Use enoxaparin cautiously in patients with hepatic impairment or significant renal dysfunction as drug accumulation could result.

Do **not** administer via IM or IV routes; enoxaparin must be given via SC injection only. Enoxaparin cannot be used interchangeably with other LMWHs or heparin sodium products as the dosages differ for each.

Adverse Effects

Minor hemorrhage was reported in ≈10% of dogs with immune-mediated hemolytic anemia receiving enoxaparin.[11]

In humans, adverse effects do not routinely occur with enoxaparin. Hemorrhage is a possibility and has been reported in 13% of patients in one study.[4] Injection site pain, ecchymosis, erythema, and hematoma are possible. Anemia, thrombocytopenia, nausea, and fever have also been reported.

Reproductive/Nursing Safety

No evidence of teratogenicity or fetotoxicity was observed when enoxaparin was given to pregnant laboratory animals.[4]

It is unclear whether enoxaparin enters milk.[4] As the drug is not absorbed orally, effects on nursing offspring would be unlikely.

Because safety has not been established in animals, this drug should only be used when the maternal benefits outweigh the potential risks to offspring.

Overdose/Acute Toxicity

Overdose may lead to hemorrhagic complications. If treatment is necessary, protamine sulfate may be administered at 1 mg IV slowly for each 1 mg of enoxaparin given within the past 8 hours.[4] If enoxaparin administration occurred greater than 8 hours previously, or if a second protamine dose is needed (eg, if activated partial thromboplastin time (aPTT) remains prolonged 2 to 4 hours after first protamine dose), an infusion of protamine 0.5 mg IV slowly may be administered for every 1 mg enoxaparin given. Avoid overdoses of protamine sulfate.

For patients that have experienced or are suspected to have experienced an overdose, consultation with a 24-hour poison consultation center specializing in providing veterinary-specific information is recommended. For general information related to overdose and toxin exposures, as well as contact information for poison control centers, refer to ***Appendix.***

Drug Interactions

The following drug interactions have either been reported or are theoretical in humans or animals receiving enoxaparin and may be of significance in veterinary patients. Unless otherwise noted, use together is not necessarily contraindicated, but weigh the potential risks and perform additional monitoring when appropriate.

- **Anticoagulants, Oral** (eg, **warfarin**): Increased risk for hemorrhage
- **Nonsteroidal Anti-Inflammatory Drugs** (**NSAIDs**; eg, **carprofen, flunixin, meloxicam, robenacoxib**): Increased risk for hemorrhage
- **Platelet-Aggregation Inhibitors** (eg, **aspirin, clopidogrel**): Increased risk for hemorrhage
- **Selective Serotonin Reuptake Inhibitors** (**SSRIs**; eg, **fluoxetine, sertraline**): Increased risk for hemorrhage
- **Thrombolytic Agents**: Increased risk for hemorrhage

Laboratory Considerations

Low molecular weight heparins (LMWHs) may cause subclinical, fully reversible increases in **AST** or **ALT**[4]; bilirubin is only rarely increased in these patients. Therefore, interpret these tests with caution; increased values do not necessarily indicate hepatic damage or dysfunction.

Dosages

DOGS:

Thromboprophylaxis (extra-label): At present, there is no substantial evidence to support any dosage, but based on pharmacokinetics and inhibition of Xa activity in dogs, suggested dosages are:

a) 0.8 – 1 mg/kg SC every 6 to 8 hours[1,2]

b) 0.8 mg/kg SC every 6 hours[12]; dosage was found to be safe and well tolerated in dogs but may not achieve anti-Xa concentrations considered therapeutic in all breeds.

CATS:

Thromboprophylaxis (extra-label): 0.75 – 1 mg/kg SC every 6 to 12 hours[12]; every-6-hour administration provided the most consistent anti-Xa activity.[9]

HORSES:

Thromboprophylaxis (extra-label): 0.35 mg/kg SC every 24 hours was used in horses to prevent laminitis after colic surgery.[13] **NOTE**: The drug's expense may be problematic for use in this species.

Monitoring

- Baseline and periodic CBC with platelet count during treatment
- Urinalysis (free catch)
- Routine coagulation tests (activated partial thromboplastin time [aPTT], ACT, PT) are insensitive measures of enoxaparin's effect and usually not warranted.[14]
- Anti-Xa activity (available at Cornell University, Animal Health Diagnostic Center) may be useful to guide dosage adjustments, particularly if bleeding occurs or patient has renal dysfunction. A

target anti-Xa peak range of 0.5 to 1 IU/mL, extrapolated from human literature, has been suggested for use in dogs and cats. The suggested thromboprophylactic range for horses is 0.1 – 0.2 IU/mL.[15]

NOTE: To measure peak anti-Xa activity, sample at 2 hours postdose for cats, 3 hours postdose for dogs, and 3 to 4 hours postdose for horses.[16] If an anti-Xa assay is not available, consider activated clotting time, aPTT, thrombin generation, or viscoelastic tests to monitor anticoagulant treatment.[1,17]

Client Information

- This medicine must be injected subcutaneously (under the skin). Be sure you understand how to correctly give the injections. Several injections a day may be required, and treatment can be very expensive. Administration of the injections may be painful for your animal.
- Bleeding is not likely, but if it does occur, contact your veterinarian immediately.
- If your animal is very listless (lacking energy), appears to be having trouble breathing, trouble walking, or loses the use of its rear legs, contact your veterinarian immediately, as it may mean blood clots have formed.

Chemistry/Synonyms

A low molecular weight heparin (LMWH), enoxaparin sodium is obtained by alkaline depolymerization of heparin derived from pork intestinal mucosa. The average molecular weight is ≈4500 and ranges from 3500 to 5500 (heparin sodium has a molecular weight of ≈12,000); 1 mg of enoxaparin is equivalent to 100 units of anti-factor Xa.

Enoxaparin sodium may also be known as Enoxaparinum natricum, PK-10169, RP-54563, *Clexane®*, *Decipar®*, *Klexane®*, *Lovenox®*, *Plaucina®*, and *Trombenox®*.

Storage/Stability

The commercially available injection should be stored at room temperature (25°C [77°F]); excursions permitted to 15°C to 30°C (59°F-86°F).

One study showed that diluting the 100 mg/mL commercially available solution with sterile water to 20 mg/mL resulted in a product that was stable for 4 weeks when stored in a glass vial or in plastic syringes at room temperature or refrigerated.[18]

Compatibility/Compounding Considerations

Do not mix or coadminister enoxaparin with other medications.[4]

Dosage Forms/Regulatory Status

VETERINARY-LABELED PRODUCTS: NONE

HUMAN-LABELED PRODUCTS:

Enoxaparin Sodium for Injection: 30 mg/0.3 mL, 40 mg/0.4 mL, 60 mg/0.6 mL, 80 mg/0.8 mL, 100 mg/1 mL, 120 mg/0.8 mL, and 150 mg/1 mL preservative-free in single-dose prefilled syringes; 300 mg/3 mL containing 15 mg/mL benzyl alcohol in 3 mL multidose vials; *Lovenox®*, generic; (Rx)

References

For the complete list of references, see **wiley.com/go/budde/plumb**

Enrofloxacin

(en-roe-***flox***-a-sin) *Baytril®*, *Zobuxa®*

Fluoroquinolone Antibiotic

Prescriber Highlights

- ► Effective against a variety of pathogens except for anaerobes
- ► In dogs, oral bioavailability is greater and more predictable than with ciprofloxacin.
- ► When possible, use should be avoided in young, growing animals because of the potential negative impact on cartilage development.
- ► Caution is advised in patients with hepatic or renal insufficiency or dehydration.
- ► Higher doses (greater than 5 mg/kg/day) not recommended in cats; may cause blindness
- ► Adverse effects include GI distress, CNS stimulation, crystalluria, or hypersensitivity.
- ► Oral administration to dogs and cats ideally should be on an empty stomach (unless vomiting occurs).
- ► Many potential drug interactions
- ► FDA prohibits extra-label use in food animals.

Uses/Indications

Enrofloxacin is FDA-approved for use in dogs (by oral[1] and IM[2] routes) and cats (oral[2] only) for the management of bacterial infections susceptible to enrofloxacin. Because of the feline dose restriction (5 mg/kg/day) and because better options are usually available for cats, enrofloxacin is generally used in this species to treat only the most susceptible bacterial infections or if an injectable fluoroquinolone is needed and where enrofloxacin is the only injectable option.

Enrofloxacin is FDA-approved for use in beef and nonlactating dairy cattle for the treatment and control of bovine respiratory disease (BRD).[3] It is conditionally approved for the treatment of clinical anaplasmosis associated with *Anaplasma marginale* in replacement dairy heifers under 20 months of age, in all classes of beef cattle except beef calves less than 2 months of age, and in beef bulls of any age that are intended for breeding.[4] Enrofloxacin is also FDA-approved for use in pigs for the treatment and control of swine respiratory disease (SRD) and as second-line therapy for the control of colibacillosis in groups or pens of weaned pigs.[3]

The World Health Organization (WHO) has designated fluoroquinolones as Critically Important, Highest Priority antimicrobials for human medicine.[5] The Office International des Epizooties (OIE) has designated enrofloxacin as a Veterinary Critically Important Antimicrobial (VCIA) Agent in veterinary species.[6]

Pharmacology/Actions

Enrofloxacin has broad-spectrum coverage. Enrofloxacin has good activity against many gram-negative bacilli and cocci, including most species and strains of *Pseudomonas aeruginosa, Klebsiella* spp, *Escherichia coli, Enterobacter* spp, *Campylobacter* spp, *Shigella* spp, *Salmonella* spp, *Aeromonas* spp, *Haemophilus* spp, *Proteus* spp, *Yersinia* spp, *Serratia* spp, and *Vibrio* spp. Other organisms that are generally susceptible include *Brucella* spp, *Chlamydia trachomatis,* staphylococci (including penicillinase-producing and methicillin-resistant strains), *Mycoplasma* spp, and some *Mycobacterium* spp (but not the etiologic agent for Johne's disease).

Fluoroquinolones have variable activity against most streptococci and are not usually recommended for use in these infections. Enrofloxacin is contraindicated with *Streptococcus canis* infections (or when it has not been ruled out) because of the potential for drug-induced necrotizing fasciitis.[7] This adverse effect does not appear to be a problem with other fluoroquinolones. Enrofloxacin has weak activity against enterococci and is not recommended in the treatment of enterococcal infections. Enrofloxacin is generally ineffective in treating anaerobic infections.

Development of bacterial resistance is an ongoing concern with many different bacteria, particularly staphylococci, Enterobacterales (eg, *E coli*), and *Pseudomonas* spp. Resistance occurs by mutation, particularly with *P aeruginosa, Klebsiella pneumoniae, Acinetobacter* spp, and enterococci, but plasmid-mediated resistance is not thought to commonly occur. *E coli* resistance was demonstrated in enrofloxacin-treated weaner pigs as well as untreated pigs housed with treated animals.[8]

The bactericidal activity of enrofloxacin is concentration-dependent (antibacterial activity improves with high peak concentrations), and susceptible bacteria cell death occurs within 20 to 30 minutes of exposure. Enrofloxacin's mechanism of action is believed to be inhibition of bacterial DNA gyrase (a type II topoisomerase), thereby preventing DNA supercoiling and DNA synthesis.

Enrofloxacin has demonstrated a significant postantibiotic effect for both gram-negative and gram-positive bacteria and is active in stationary and growth phases of bacterial replication. In vitro kill assays for enrofloxacin and its active metabolite, ciprofloxacin, have demonstrated an additive response (effect equal to the combined action of each of the drugs used separately) in dog and cat isolates of *E coli, Staphylococcus pseudintermedius,* and *P aeruginosa*.[9] Methicillin-resistant *S pseudintermedius* present within biofilm have higher MICs, indicating reduced susceptibility to enrofloxacin.[10]

In vitro synergic antibacterial effects were not observed when enrofloxacin was combined with amikacin.[11]

Pharmacokinetics

Enrofloxacin is well absorbed after oral administration in most species. In dogs, enrofloxacin's bioavailability (≈80%) is approximately twice that of ciprofloxacin after oral administration. Oral bioavailability in horses is between 60% and 80%.[12,13] Fifty percent of peak plasma concentration (C_{max}) is reportedly attained within 15 minutes of administration and C_{max} occurs within 1 hour of administration. In sheep, oral enrofloxacin bioavailability is ≈90% or higher[14] and 83% after IM administration.[15] Presence of food in the stomach generally delays the rate but not the extent of absorption; however, foods with increased divalent or trivalent cation concentrations (eg, milk) can reduce bioavailability. Enrofloxacin is rapidly absorbed after IM administration in dogs (peak concentrations in ≈30 minutes).[2]

Enrofloxacin is widely distributed throughout the body. Volume of distribution in dogs is ≈3 to 4 L/kg. Only ≈27% is bound to canine plasma proteins. Highest concentrations are found in the bile, kidney, liver, lungs, and reproductive system (including prostatic fluid and tissue). Enrofloxacin reportedly concentrates in macrophages. Therapeutic concentrations are also attained in bone, synovial fluid, skin, muscle, aqueous humor, and pleural fluid. Low concentrations are found in the CSF; concentrations may only reach 6% to 10% of those found in serum. In hospitalized horses, volume of distribution was ≈1.25 L/kg. After mechanical disruption of the blood–aqueous humor barrier in horses, enrofloxacin (7.5 mg/kg IV) produced concentrations in the aqueous humor sufficient to treat *Leptospira pomona*.[16] Enrofloxacin concentration in bronchoalveolar fluid of calves was higher than plasma 1 hour and 2 hours after SC injection.[17] After SC administration to steers, enrofloxacin penetrated GI tissue better than ciprofloxacin.[18] The volume of distribution was 1.5 to 2.3 L/kg in sheep[15] and ≈1.5 L/kg in cattle.

Enrofloxacin is eliminated via renal and hepatic mechanisms. Approximately 15% to 50% of the drug is eliminated unchanged into the urine by tubular secretion and glomerular filtration. Enrofloxacin is metabolized to various metabolites, most of which are less active than the parent compounds. Approximately 10% to 40% of circulating enrofloxacin is metabolized to ciprofloxacin in most species, including, dogs, cats, adult horses, cattle, turtles, snakes, and humans. Foals, pigs, and some lizards convert little, if any, enrofloxacin to ciprofloxacin. Enrofloxacin metabolites are eliminated in the urine and feces. Because of the dual elimination routes (renal and hepatic), dogs with moderately impaired renal function may have slightly prolonged half-lives and higher serum concentrations but may not require any dosage adjustment. Approximate elimination half-lives in various species are in dogs, 2 to 5 hours[19,20]; cats, 6 hours; calves, 9 hours[18]; sheep and goats, 1.5 to 4.5 hours[15,21]; horses, 5 to 10 hours[12,22]; turtles, 18 hours; and alligators, 55 hours. After SC administration to calves, fecal enrofloxacin and ciprofloxacin concentrations were ≈ 115 and ≈50 times higher than their respective plasma concentrations.

Contraindications/Precautions/Warnings

Enrofloxacin is labeled as contraindicated in patients that are hypersensitive to it as well as in small- and medium-breed dogs aged 2 to 8 months. Bubble-like changes in articular cartilage have been noted when the drug was given at 2 to 5 times the recommended dosage for 30 days, although clinical signs have only been seen at 5 times the recommended dosage. To avoid cartilage damage, treatment for large- and giant-breed dogs may need to wait until 12 and 18 months of age, respectively. Enrofloxacin at concentrations greater than 1 mg/mL was toxic to equine chondrocytes.[23] Enrofloxacin is not recommended in cats with impaired renal function or at doses above 5 mg/kg/day due to increased risk for retinal degeneration.[24]

Because ciprofloxacin has occasionally been reported to cause crystalluria in humans, animals should not be allowed to become dehydrated during fluoroquinolone therapy. Enrofloxacin may cause CNS stimulation and should be used with caution in patients with seizure disorders. Patients with severe renal or hepatic impairment may require dosage interval adjustments to prevent drug accumulation.

Use of the canine injectable products in cats or dogs via non-FDA–approved parenteral routes (eg, IV, SC) is controversial and may result in significant adverse effects. Because of the high pH (≈11) of the solution, SC administration in any species may cause pain and tissue damage. Rapid or undiluted IV administration to dogs increases risk for cardiac arrhythmias, hypotension, vomiting, and mast cell degranulation (ie, release of histamine and other inflammatory mediators). See ***Compatibility/Compounding Considerations***.

Dilution and extra-label use of the large animal product (100 mg/mL; 10%) in small animal species via any route is strongly discouraged.

Enrofloxacin should not be used in foals, as they appear to be highly susceptible to the fluoroquinolone's arthropathic effects. Although there has been much discussion regarding the potential for cartilage abnormalities or other arthropathies in horses, objective data are lacking. In horses, IV administration should be slow as ataxia and other neurologic effects may occur when given rapidly. Intrauterine infusion and IM injections are not recommended in horses, as localized tissue reactions (eg, endometrial ulceration, necrosis, fibrosis, inflammation, hemorrhage) can occur.[25]

Extra-label use of fluoroquinolones is prohibited in food animals.

Enrofloxacin and ciprofloxacin cannot be considered equivalent due to pharmacokinetic differences (see ***Pharmacokinetics***).

Enrofloxacin should not be used in humans; it may cause hallucinations, vivid dreams, and/or headaches.

Adverse Effects

When enrofloxacin is used as labeled, its adverse effect profile is usually limited to GI distress (eg, vomiting, diarrhea, anorexia). In dogs, rare incidences of elevated hepatic enzymes, ataxia, seizures, depression, lethargy, and nervousness have also been reported[1,2]; dogs may vomit after IV administration. Hypersensitivity reactions or crystalluria could occur.

In cats, ocular toxicity has been reported, characterized by mydriasis, retinal degeneration, and blindness.[24,26] These effects were generally seen at higher dosage ranges and have necessitated a maximum dosage of 5 mg/kg/day in cats. Mydriasis may be an indication of impending or existing retinal changes. Retinal toxicity in cats appears to be caused by amino acid changes in the ABCG2 transporter in the blood–retina barrier, which allows photoreactive fluoroquinolones to accumulate in the feline retina.[27] Other rare adverse effects seen in cats can include vomiting, anorexia, elevated hepatic enzymes, diarrhea, ataxia, seizures, depression/lethargy, vocalization, and aggression.

Articular cartilage abnormalities have been noted in young, rapidly growing animals given fluoroquinolones (see ***Contraindications/Precautions/Warnings***).[1,2,4]

Fluoroquinolones may cause photosensitization and prolonged exposure of bare skin (eg, nose) to direct sunlight should be avoided.

Enrofloxacin 100 mg/mL injection can be irritating to the mouth when given orally to horses. This effect may be alleviated by coating the liquid with molasses or preparing a gel (see ***Compatibility/Compounding Considerations***) and rinsing the horse's mouth with water after administration. The prevalence of antibiotic-associated diarrhea due to enrofloxacin use in horses is ≈5%.[28]

In humans, fluoroquinolones may alter cardiac conduction and cause prolongation of the QT interval, especially in those with a history of QT interval prolongation, electrolyte disorders, cardiac disease, or are taking other QT interval prolonging medications.

Reproductive/Nursing Safety

The safety of enrofloxacin use in pregnant dogs has been investigated; breeding, pregnant, and lactating dogs receiving up to 15 mg/kg/day have demonstrated no treatment-related adverse effects.[1,2] However, because of the risk for cartilage abnormalities in young animals, fluoroquinolones are not generally recommended for use during pregnancy unless the benefits of therapy clearly outweigh the risks. Limited studies in male dogs at various dosages have indicated no effects on male breeding performance.

Safety in breeding, pregnant, or lactating cats has not been established.[1]

Enrofloxacin administration to mares during pregnancy resulted in detectable concentrations of enrofloxacin and ciprofloxacin in fetal fluids and cartilage.[29] Fetal abnormalities were not detected after enrofloxacin administration to pregnant mares for 2 weeks during early pregnancy (gestation days 46 to 60).[30] Enrofloxacin administration during late pregnancy did not result in clinical lameness or cartilage lesions in the foals[31]; however, the small sample sizes (6 or 7 horses per treatment arm) of these studies cannot be taken as an indication of no risk to the fetus.

The effects of enrofloxacin on cattle and swine reproductive performance, pregnancy, and lactation have not been adequately determined. Enrofloxacin and its metabolite ciprofloxacin are actively secreted into bovine milk.[32]

No teratogenic effects were observed in rabbits given a dose of 25 mg/kg or rats given a dose of 50 mg/kg.[3]

Overdose/Acute Toxicity

The oral LD_{50} for enrofloxacin in laboratory rats was greater than 5000 mg/kg. Dogs receiving 50 mg/kg/day for at least 14 days developed only vomiting and anorexia, but signs associated with an overdosage of 125 mg/kg/day for 11 days (in decreasing frequency) included vomiting, anorexia, depression, difficult locomotion, and death.[1,2]

In cats, an overdose can be serious (eg, blindness, seizures); a dose of 20 mg/kg or more can cause retinopathy and blindness,[1] which can be irreversible. Enrofloxacin 20 or 50 mg/kg/day for 3 weeks resulted in salivation, vomiting, and depression.[1]

For patients that have experienced or are suspected to have experienced an overdose, consultation with a 24-hour poison consultation center specializing in providing veterinary-specific information is recommended. For general information related to overdose and toxin exposures, as well as contact information for poison control centers, refer to ***Appendix.***

Drug Interactions

In pigs, enrofloxacin induced expression and activity of CYP1A2 and inhibited CYP2E1 and CYP3A4.[33] In hepatic microsomes from healthy beagles, enrofloxacin and ciprofloxacin inhibited CYP1A activity, but clinically relevant drug interactions were more likely with ciprofloxacin than with enrofloxacin.[34] The following drug interactions have either been reported or are theoretical in humans or animals receiving ciprofloxacin or enrofloxacin and may be of significance in veterinary patients. Unless otherwise noted, use together is not necessarily contraindicated, but the potential risks must be weighed, and additional monitoring performed when appropriate.

- ALUMINUM-, CALCIUM-, AND MAGNESIUM-CONTAINING ORAL PRODUCTS: May bind to enrofloxacin and prevent its oral absorption; doses of these products should be separated from enrofloxacin by at least 2 hours.
- ANTIBIOTICS, OTHER (eg, **aminoglycosides, third-generation cephalosporins** [eg, **cefpodoxime, ceftiofur**], **doxycycline, extended-spectrum penicillins**): Synergism may occur against some bacteria (particularly *Pseudomonas aeruginosa*), but this is unpredictable.[35] Although enrofloxacin and ciprofloxacin have minimal activity against anaerobes, in vitro synergy has been reported when these drugs are used with clindamycin against strains of *Peptostreptococcus* spp, *Lactobacillus* spp, and *Bacteroides fragilis*.
- BLOOD GLUCOSE LOWERING AGENTS (eg, **insulins, sulfonylureas** [eg, **glipizide, glyburide**]): Fluoroquinolones may enhance the hypoglycemic effect of blood glucose lowering agents.
- CORTICOSTEROIDS (eg, **dexamethasone, prednis(ol)one**): Concomitant use with fluoroquinolones may increase risk for tendonitis and tendon rupture.
- CYCLOSPORINE, SYSTEMIC: Fluoroquinolones may exacerbate nephrotoxicity and reduce the metabolism of cyclosporine.
- DOXORUBICIN: Enrofloxacin may increase doxorubicin exposure.
- FLUNIXIN: In dogs, flunixin has been shown to increase the area under the curve (AUC) and elimination half-life of enrofloxacin, and enrofloxacin increases the AUC and elimination half-life of flunixin; it is unknown whether other NSAIDs interact with enrofloxacin in dogs.
- IRON, ZINC (**oral**): Concomitant administration may decrease fluoroquinolone absorption; doses should be separated by at least 2 hours.
- LEVOTHYROXINE: Ciprofloxacin may decrease levothyroxine efficacy.
- MYCOPHENOLATE MOFETIL: Ciprofloxacin may decrease mycophenolic acid exposure.
- METHOTREXATE (MTX): Concomitant administration may increase MTX concentrations and increase risk for toxicity.
- NITROFURANTOIN: May antagonize the antimicrobial activity of fluoroquinolones; concomitant use of these drugs is not recommended.
- PROBENECID: May block renal tubular secretion of ciprofloxacin and may increase ciprofloxacin serum concentration and elimination half-life; monitor for increased enrofloxacin adverse effects (nausea, diarrhea)

- **QT Interval Prolongation Drugs** (eg, **azithromycin, chlorpromazine, cisapride, fluconazole, fluoxetine, ketoconazole, methadone, ondansetron, quinidine, sotalol**): Combination with ciprofloxacin may increase risk for QT prolongation; concurrent use of cisapride and ciprofloxacin is contraindicated in humans. These interactions may also apply to enrofloxacin.
- **Sildenafil**: Concomitant use with ciprofloxacin may increase sildenafil serum concentrations and adverse effects.
- **Sucralfate**: In dogs, sucralfate can affect absorption of ciprofloxacin but does not appear to affect enrofloxacin absorption.[36]
- **Theophylline, Aminophylline**: Enrofloxacin may increase theophylline blood concentrations; in dogs, theophylline concentrations may be increased by ≈30% to 50%.[37]
- **Tilmicosin**: May decrease enrofloxacin metabolism[38]
- **Warfarin**: Concomitant use may increase anticoagulant effects of warfarin.

Laboratory Considerations

- Enrofloxacin may cause false positive **urine glucose** determinations when cupric sulfate solution (Benedict's solution, *Clinitest*®) is used. Tests using glucose oxidase (*Tes-Tape*®, *Clinistix*®) are not affected by enrofloxacin.
- In some humans, fluoroquinolones caused increases in **liver enzymes, BUN**, and **serum creatinine** and decreases in **hematocrit**. The clinical relevance of these changes in veterinary patients is unknown.

Dosages

DOGS:

Susceptible infections (label dosage; FDA-approved):

Oral tablets: 5 – 20 mg/kg PO once daily for at least 2 to 3 days beyond resolution of clinical signs.[1] Selection of a dose from this range is based on clinical experience, severity of infection, susceptibility of the pathogen. If no improvement is seen within 5 days, diagnosis should be reevaluated. Maximum duration of therapy is 30 days.

Injectable solution 2.27% (22.7 mg/mL): 2.5 mg/kg IM once, followed by oral enrofloxacin therapy[2]

Susceptible infections (extra-label): Using the 2.27% (22.7 mg/mL) injection, 10 – 20 mg/kg every 24 hours IM, SC (must be diluted), or slow IV based on the susceptibility, site, and severity of the infection. See ***Compatibility/Compounding Considerations.***

Lower UTIs (extra-label):

a) 10 – 20 mg/kg PO every 24 hours. Use of this drug should be reserved for cystitis cases caused by bacteria resistant to other antibiotics (eg, amoxicillin). Enrofloxacin has limited efficacy against *Enterococcus* spp.[39]

b) Sporadic bacterial cystitis: 18 – 20 mg/kg PO every 24 hours for 3 days was shown to be as effective as a 14-day treatment with amoxicillin plus clavulanate.[40]

Pyelonephritis (extra-label): 20 mg/kg PO every 24 hours; good first-line choice for treatment of pyelonephritis[39]

Enteric infections (extra-label):

a) **Enrofloxacin-sensitive *E coli* in dogs with granulomatous colitis** (extra-label): 10 mg/kg PO every 24 hours for 8 weeks[41]

b) **Campylobacteriosis**: 10 mg/kg PO every 24 hours. Resistance can develop during treatment.[42]

Bacterial skin infections (extra-label): 5 – 20 mg/kg PO every 24 hours.[43] Administration of this drug at the high end of the dose range may be required for treatment of *Pseudomonas* spp infections. Most clinicians consider enrofloxacin to be a second-line drug for the treatment of deep pyoderma in dogs; use is only recommended if culture and susceptibility results indicate first-line drugs will not be effective.

CATS:

Susceptible infections (label dosage; FDA-approved): 5 mg/kg PO every 24 hours or divided and given every 12 hours; continue for at least 2 or 3 days beyond cessation of clinical signs to a maximum of 30 days.[1] **NOTE**: Because enrofloxacin is a concentration-dependent antibiotic, once-daily administration is recommended. For serious infections that require a higher dose, consider using a different fluoroquinolone (eg, pradofloxacin).

Susceptible infections (extra-label): 5 mg/kg (or less) every 24 hours IM or IV using the canine injectable product (2.27%, 22.7 mg/mL). For IV administration, see ***Compatibility/Compounding Considerations.***

HORSES:

Susceptible infections (extra-label):

a) 5 – 7.5 mg/kg PO or IV every 24 hours.[44] Respiratory infections should be treated with the high end of the dose range.[45]

b) 7.5 mg/kg PO as a compounded gel every 24 hours. See ***Compatibility/Compounding Considerations.*** Horses should have feed withheld for 11 to 14 hours before and 1 to 2 hours after administration. The horse's mouth should be rinsed with water after administration to reduce the risk for oral ulceration.[46]

CATTLE:

Single day treatment of bovine respiratory disease (BRD) associated with *Mannheimia haemolytica, Pasteurella multocida, Histophilus somni,* and *Mycoplasma bovis* in beef and nonlactating dairy cattle (label dosage; FDA-approved): 7.5 – 12.5 mg/kg SC once.[3]

Multiple day treatment of BRD associated with *M haemolytica, P multocida, H somni,* and *M bovis* in beef and nonlactating dairy cattle (label dosage; FDA-approved): 2.5 – 5 mg/kg SC every 24 hours for 3 days; additional daily treatments may be given to animals that have shown improvement but not complete recovery.[3]

Control of BRD in beef and nonlactating dairy cattle at high risk for developing BRD associated with *M haemolytica, P multocida, H somni, and M bovis* (label dosage; FDA-approved): 7.5 – 12.5 mg/kg SC once[3]

Clinical anaplasmosis associated with *Anaplasma marginale* in replacement dairy heifers under 20 months of age, all classes of beef cattle except beef calves less than 2 months of age, and beef bulls (of any age) intended for breeding (label dosage; conditionally approved by FDA): 12.5 mg/kg SC once; do not administer more than 20 mL per injection site.[4]

NEW WORLD CAMELIDS:

Susceptible infections in alpacas (extra-label): 5 mg/kg SC or 10 mg/kg PO every 24 hours[47]

SWINE:

Treatment and control of swine respiratory disease (SRD) associated with *Actinobacillus pleuropneumoniae, P multocida, Haemophilus parasuis, Streptococcus suis, Bordetella bronchiseptica,* and *Mycoplasma hyopneumoniae* and control of colibacillosis in groups or pens of weaned pigs where colibacillosis associated with *E coli* has been diagnosed (label-dosage; FDA-approved): 7.5 mg/kg IM or SC (behind the ear) once; do not administer more than 5 mL per injection site.[3]

BIRDS:

NOTE: Compounding the liver-flavored tablets with grape syrup

(*Syrpalta*®) may improve acceptance when enrofloxacin is administered PO.[48]

Susceptible gram-negative infections in Psittacines (extra-label):

a) Stable, immune-competent birds: 20 mg/kg PO every 24 hours
b) Debilitated, immune-competent birds: 15 – 20 mg/kg SC in fluid pocket every 24 hours
c) Debilitated, immunocompromised birds: 15 – 20 mg/kg SC in fluid pocket every 12 hours

FERRETS:

Susceptible infections (extra-label): 10 – 20 mg/kg PO, IM, or SC every 24 hours.[49] **NOTE**: If parenteral administration is required, it is recommended to dilute the solution to avoid injection site tissue necrosis.

RABBITS, RODENTS, & SMALL MAMMALS:

NOTE: All dosages are extra-label.

Rabbits:

a) For *Pasteurella* spp upper respiratory infection: 15 – 20 mg/kg PO every 12 hours for a minimum of 14 days in mild cases and up to several months for chronic infections; first dose may be given SC. Subsequent doses should NOT be given SC, as severe tissue reactions can occur.[50]
b) 5 mg/kg PO, SC, IM, or IV every 12 hours for 14 days. Enrofloxacin is the drug of choice for treatment of *Pasteurella* spp infections. Dilution is suggested if administering SC, as skin may slough. Injectable product should not be given PO because it is unpalatable.[51] See ***Compatibility/Compounding Considerations***.

Hedgehogs: 5 – 10 mg/kg PO or SC every 12 hours[52]

Chinchillas: 5 – 10 mg/kg PO or IM every 12 hours[53]

Chinchillas, gerbils, guinea pigs, hamsters, mice, rats: 5 – 10 mg/kg PO or IM every 12 hours or 5 – 20 mg/kg PO or SC every 24 hours. 50 – 200 mg/L for 14 days in drinking water. Not for use in young animals[54]

Rats: Chronic respiratory disease: 10 – 25 mg/kg PO every 12 hours[55]

REPTILES:

Susceptible respiratory infections for most species (extra-label): 5 mg/kg IM every 5 days for 25 days

Chronic respiratory infections (extra-label):

a) **Tortoises**: 15 mg/kg IM every 72 hours for 5 to 7 treatments[56]
b) **Bearded dragons**: 10 mg/kg IM once blood concentrations are high enough to kill susceptible bacteria[57]

Monitoring

- Clinical efficacy
- Adverse effects
- In cats, mydriasis and/or retinal changes may indicate retinal toxicity.

Client Information

- Enrofloxacin is best given on an empty stomach without food; however, if your animal vomits or acts sick, give with food or a small treat (no dairy products, antacids, or anything containing iron). If vomiting continues, contact your veterinarian.
- Do not crush film-coated tablets, as the drug is bitter, which may cause difficulty when getting your animal to take it.
- Do not give this medicine at the same time with other drugs or vitamins that contain certain minerals (eg, calcium, iron, magnesium, aluminum, zinc), as these products can reduce the amount of drug absorbed.
- This medicine may cause joint abnormalities if used in young, pregnant, or nursing animals.
- Most common side effects are vomiting, nausea, or diarrhea.
- Do not exceed prescribed dose in cats, as blindness can result. If your cat develops large pupils, contact your veterinarian immediately.

Chemistry/Synonyms

Enrofloxacin, a fluoroquinolone antibiotic, occurs as a pale-yellow crystalline powder. It is slightly soluble in water, but solubility is pH-dependent and altering the pH of the commercially available injections can cause precipitation. Enrofloxacin is related structurally to the human FDA-approved drug ciprofloxacin (enrofloxacin has an additional ethyl group on the piperazinyl ring).

Enrofloxacin may also be known as enrofloksasiini, enrofloxacine, enrofloxacino, enrofloxacinum, Bay-Vp-2674, *Baytril*®, *Baytril*® *100*, *Baytril*® *100-CA1*, *Enroflox*®, *Enroflox*®*-100*, *Enroquin*®, *Enrosite*®, or *Zobuxa*®.

Storage/Stability

Unless otherwise directed by the manufacturer, enrofloxacin tablets should be stored in tight containers at temperatures less than 25°C (77°F); excursions to 30°C (86°F) may be permitted for some products.

The canine FDA-approved injectable solution (2.27%) for IM injection should be stored protected from light at or below 25°C (77°F)[2]; do not freeze. Discard unused product 90 days from first vial puncture or after puncturing vial a maximum of 20 times.

The FDA-approved injectable solution (10%) for cattle and swine should be stored protected from sunlight at 20°C to 30°C (68°F-86°F), with excursions permitted to 40°C (104°F).[3,4] It should not be refrigerated or frozen. If exposed to cold temperatures, precipitation may occur; to redissolve, warm the solution, then shake the vial. Discard unused solution 30 days after first vial puncture, or after vial is punctured a maximum of 30 times with a needle or 4 times with a dosage delivery device.

Compatibility/Compounding Considerations

Compatibility is dependent on factors such as pH, concentration, temperature, and diluent used; specialized references or a hospital pharmacist should be consulted for more specific information.

Enrofloxacin 100 mg/mL injection may be diluted with sterile water for injection prior to IM or SC administration; use diluted solution within 24 hours of mixing.[3] Injectable enrofloxacin (both 22.7 mg/mL and 100 mg/mL) has been demonstrated to be physically **incompatible** with 1:1 dilution with 0.9% sodium chloride, lactated Ringer's solution (LRS), *Plasma-Lyte*® *A*, hydroxyethyl starch (HES) 6%, and potentially any drugs that have been reconstituted or diluted with those solutions (eg, ampicillin/sulbactam).[58] It must NOT be mixed with or come into contact with any IV solution containing calcium or magnesium (eg, *Normosol*®*-R*, *Plasma-Lyte*®*-R*, *-A*, or *-56*); morbidity and mortality secondary to microprecipitants lodging in patients' lungs have been reported.

Because physical incompatibilities may not be readily apparent to the naked eye or may develop 15 to 60 minutes after admixture or dilution (ie, during an infusion), it has been recommended to administer enrofloxacin injection only via labeled routes. If IV route must be used and suitable alternatives to enrofloxacin are not available, consider administration of undiluted enrofloxacin through a separate line.

For horses, an oral gel formulated from the bovine injectable product has been described[46]: 100 mL of the 100 mg/mL bovine injection (*Baytril*® *100*) is used. Stevia (0.35 g) is mixed with ≈15 mL of liquid enrofloxacin until dissolved. Apple flavoring (0.6 mL) is added until dissolved. Sodium carboxymethylcellulose (2 g) should be sprinkled over the mixture and stirred until incorporated, with immediate gradual addition of the remaining enrofloxacin (85 mL) before the mixture solidifies. The resulting concentration is ≈100 mg/mL. The compounded gel should be stable for up to 84 days if kept refrigerated and protected from light.

For exotic animals, 3 compounded oral suspension preparations were shown to be stable for up to 56 days when stored at room temperature in amber-colored containers[59]:

1. Formulation A was made starting with 40 mL of corn syrup and 40 mL of distilled water mixed together; 30 mL of this solution was placed in a small mortar. Then, 27 film-coated tablets (68 mg) of commercially available enrofloxacin were added to the mortar and allowed to sit for 15 minutes. Once the film coating was dissolved, the tablets were pulverized in the mortar with a pestle until a homogeneous paste was formed. The mixture was then carefully transferred to a plastic amber-colored, 8 oz (240 mL) dispensing vial (bottle). Another 30 mL of the corn syrup-distilled water mixture was poured into the mortar and carefully stirred to facilitate the transfer of any remaining enrofloxacin residue in the mortar to the vial. A sufficient quantity of the corn syrup-distilled water vehicle was then added to the vial to bring the final volume of the suspension to 80 mL, which resulted in a final concentration of 22.95 mg/mL.
2. Formulation B was made following the same steps as Formulation A, but a 50:30 mixture of 50 mL of cherry syrup and 30 mL distilled water was used, which resulted in a final concentration of 22.95 mg/mL.
3. Formulation C was made using 40 mL of the 2.27% (22.7 mg/mL) injectable product and 40 mL of a liquid sweetener (*Ora-Sweet®*), which resulted in a final concentration of 11.35 mg/mL.

The authors concluded subjectively that although all 3 compounds were stable as described above, the cherry syrup mixture (Formulation B) best masked the smell and taste of enrofloxacin.

Enrofloxacin was found to elute from calcium sulfate hemihydrate (ie, plaster of Paris) beads over 30 days in experimental conditions.[60]

Enrofloxacin 2% in poloxamer 409 gel has been used as a safe and effective option for superficial corneal ulceration in California sea lions.[61] An in situ forming gel was prepared with poloxamers 407 and 188 and was bioavailable when administered IM to dogs.[62] The potency and stability of these formulations were not reported.

Dosage Forms/Regulatory Status

VETERINARY-LABELED PRODUCTS:

Enrofloxacin Tablets Oral Flavored Tablets, and Soft Chewable Tablets: 22.7 mg, 68 mg, and 136 mg; *Baytril®* Taste Tabs, *Zobuxa®* generic; (Rx). FDA-approved for use in dogs and cats

Enrofloxacin Tablets (film-coated): 22.7 mg, 68 mg, and 136 mg; *Baytril®*, (Rx). NADA #140-441. FDA-approved for use in dogs and cats

Enrofloxacin Injection: 22.7 mg/mL (2.27%) in 20 mL vials; *Baytril®*, generic; (Rx). NADA #140-913. FDA-approved for use in dogs only

Enrofloxacin Injection: 100 mg/mL in 100 mL and 250 mL bottles; *Baytril® 100*, generic; (Rx). FDA-approved for use in swine and cattle only. Not for use in calves to be processed for veal or for female dairy cattle 20 months or older, including dry dairy cows. Any extra-label use in food animals is banned by the FDA. Slaughter withdrawal in cattle is 28 days when used as labeled. A withdrawal period has not been established in preruminating calves. Slaughter withdrawal in swine is 5 days when the drug is used as labeled.

Enrofloxacin Injection: 100 mg/mL in 250 mL bottles; *Baytril® 100-CA1*;(Rx). Conditionally approved by the FDA pending a full demonstration of effectiveness under application number 141-527 for use in replacement dairy heifers under 20 months of age, all classes of beef cattle except beef calves less than 2 months of age, and beef bulls intended for breeding (any age). Not for use in any other class of dairy cattle, including dry dairy cows, or in veal calves. Slaughter withdrawal in cattle is 28 days; a withdrawal period has not been established in preruminating calves. Extra-label use of conditionally approved drugs, or of fluoroquinolones in food producing animals, is not permitted by the FDA.

There is also an otic preparation containing enrofloxacin and silver sulfadiazine: *Baytril® Otic*; (Rx). See ***Antibacterials, Otic*** for more information.

HUMAN-LABELED PRODUCTS: NONE

References

For the complete list of references, see **wiley.com/go/budde/plumb**

Ephedrine

(e-***fed***-rin)

Sympathomimetic Bronchodilator/Vasopressor

Prescriber Highlights

- ► Sympathomimetic used parenterally as a vasopressor agent for anesthesia-associated hypotension in dogs, cats, and horses.
- ► Contraindications include severe cardiovascular disease, especially with arrhythmias.
- ► Should be used with caution in patients with glaucoma, prostatic hypertrophy, hyperthyroidism, diabetes mellitus, cardiovascular disorders, or hypertension
- ► Adverse effects include CNS stimulation, arrhythmias, tachycardia, hypertension, vomiting, or anorexia.
- ► Crosses the placenta and is excreted into milk

Uses/Indications

Ephedrine can be used parenterally as a vasopressor agent in the treatment of anesthesia-associated hypotension in dogs, cats, and horses. In a study in horses with isoflurane-induced hypotension, ephedrine increased mean arterial pressure by increasing the cardiac index and systemic vascular resistance.[1] The authors concluded that ephedrine would be preferable to phenylephrine for this indication because ephedrine increases both blood flow and blood pressure. Mean arterial pressure, cardiac index, and systemic vascular resistance have also been shown to increase in isoflurane-anesthetized dogs treated with ephedrine.[2]

Ephedrine has been used in dogs and cats for the treatment of urinary incontinence due to urethral sphincter hypotonus, but the lack of available oral dosage forms limits the use of ephedrine for this indication.

Pharmacology/Actions

Ephedrine is a noncatecholamine that directly acts as an alpha- and beta-adrenergic receptor agonist and indirectly causes endogenous release of norepinephrine from sympathetic neurons[3, 4] and decreases the metabolism of norepinephrine by inhibiting the action of monoamine oxidase on norepinephrine.[5] Prolonged use or excessive dosing frequency can deplete norepinephrine from its storage sites and tachyphylaxis may ensue.[4] Tachyphylaxis has not been documented in dogs or cats when used for urethral sphincter hypotonus.

Pharmacologic effects of ephedrine include increased vasoconstriction, heart rate, coronary blood flow, and blood pressure; mild CNS stimulation; and decreased bronchoconstriction, nasal congestion, and appetite. Ephedrine can also increase urethral sphincter tone and produce closure of the neck of the urinary bladder.

Pharmacokinetics

Ephedrine is rapidly absorbed after oral and parenteral administration. In humans, ephedrine is thought to cross the blood–brain barrier by some researchers[6] and not others.[7-9] In dogs, ephedrine undergoes rapid N-demethylation to norephedrine, which suggests that the activity of ephedrine is largely mediated through its metabolite.[10]

Ephedrine and norephedrine are both eliminated in the urine and urine pH may significantly alter excretion characteristics. In humans, at urine pH of 5, half-life is ≈3 hours; at urine pH of 6.3, half-life is ≈6 hours.

Compared with other vasopressor agents, IV ephedrine has a longer duration of action. When it is used to treat anesthesia-associated hypotension, it is recommended to administer as a bolus rather than as a CRI.

Contraindications/Precautions/Warnings

Ephedrine is contraindicated in patients with severe cardiovascular disease, particularly with arrhythmias. Ephedrine should be used with caution in patients with glaucoma, prostatic hypertrophy, hyperthyroidism, diabetes mellitus, or cardiovascular disorders. In humans, there is an increased risk of hypertension if ephedrine is used prophylactically.[4]

Tachyphylaxis secondary to depleted stores of endogenous norepinephrine can occur with repeated ephedrine doses.[4]

Renal impairment may increase elimination half-life and result in prolonged therapeutic or adverse effects.[4]

When this drug is administered as an IV bolus to humans, the drug concentration should be ≈5 – 10 mg/mL (see ***Compounding/Compatibility***);[4] it is assumed that this information also applies to veterinary patients.

Do not confuse ePHEDrine with EPINEPHrine.

Adverse Effects

The most common adverse effects include restlessness, irritability, tachycardia, or hypertension; nausea and vomiting may occur.[4] Anorexia may be a problem in some animals.

Reproductive/Nursing Safety

Limited data are available on the effects of ephedrine on fertility, pregnancy, and fetal safety. Use with caution during pregnancy. Ephedrine crosses the placental barrier and may have an effect on the fetuses.[4, 11] In humans, cases of potential metabolic acidosis in newborns at delivery with maternal ephedrine exposure have been reported.[4]

In humans, ephedrine is excreted in milk.[4] If ephedrine is absolutely necessary for the dam, consider using a milk replacer.

Because safety has not been established in animals, this drug should only be used when the maternal benefits outweigh the potential risks to offspring.

Overdose/Acute Toxicity

Clinical signs of overdose result from sympathomimetic excess and may consist of an exacerbation of the adverse effects listed above or, with large overdoses, severe cardiovascular (hypertension to rebound hypotension, bradycardias to tachycardias, and cardiovascular collapse) and CNS effects (stimulation to coma).[12]

In acute oral overdoses, perform GI decontamination using the usual precautions and administer charcoal and a cathartic. Monitor blood pressure and treat clinical signs supportively (eg, antihypertensive agents).

For patients that have experienced or are suspected to have experienced an overdose, consultation with a 24-hour poison consultation center specializing in providing veterinary-specific information is recommended. For general information related to overdose and toxin exposures, as well as contact information for poison control centers, refer to ***Appendix.***

Drug Interactions

The following drug interactions have either been reported or are theoretical in humans or animals receiving ephedrine and may be of significance in veterinary patients. Unless otherwise noted, use together is not necessarily contraindicated, but weigh the potential risks and perform additional monitoring when appropriate.

- Alpha-Adrenergic Antagonists (eg, **phentolamine, prazosin**): May inhibit the therapeutic effects of ephedrine
- Alpha-2 Adrenergic Agonists (eg, **clonidine, dexmedetomidine, xylazine**): May augment the pressor effects of ephedrine
- Atropine: May augment the pressor effects of ephedrine
- Beta-Adrenergic Receptor Antagonists (eg, **atenolol, propranolol**): Concomitant use with ephedrine may diminish the effects of both drugs.
- Cardiac Glycosides (eg, **digoxin**): Concurrent use of cardiac glycosides with ephedrine may increase risk for arrhythmias.
- Epidural Anesthesia: Ephedrine may decrease the efficacy of epidural anesthesia.
- Monoamine Oxidase Inhibitors (**MAOIs**; eg, **amitraz, selegiline**): Ephedrine should not be given within 2 weeks of a patient receiving MAOIs as severe hypertension and hyperpyrexia are possible.
- Oxytocin: May result in additive hypertensive effect
- Phenothiazines (eg, **acepromazine**): Phenothiazines may antagonize effects of ephedrine.[13] Ephedrine may decrease neuroleptic effects of phenothiazines and may increase risk for cardiac arrhythmias, including QT interval prolongation and torsade de pointes. Combination should be avoided.
- Propofol: May augment the pressor effects of ephedrine
- Quinidine: May diminish the effects of both drugs
- Reserpine: May inhibit the pressor effects of ephedrine
- Sodium Bicarbonate: Concurrent use of ephedrine with sodium bicarbonate may result in ephedrine toxicity.
- Sympathomimetic Agents (eg, **phenylpropanolamine**): Ephedrine should not be administered with other sympathomimetic agents as increased toxicity may result.
- Theophylline/Aminophylline: Concurrent use of ephedrine with theophylline may increase the risk for GI and CNS toxicity.
- Tricyclic Antidepressants (eg, **amitriptyline, clomipramine**): May decrease the pressor effects of ephedrine
- Urinary Alkalinizers (eg, **carbonic anhydrase inhibitors** [eg, methazolamide], **citrates**): May reduce the urinary excretion of ephedrine and prolong its duration of activity. Dosage adjustments may be required to avoid toxic clinical signs.
- Vasopressin: May result in additive hypertensive effect

Laboratory Considerations

- Ephedrine may cause a false-positive **amphetamine** when using EMIT assay.[14]

Dosages

DOGS:

Hypotension associated with anesthesia (extra-label):

a) For relatively short procedures in ASA I or II patients with hypotension nonresponsive to 1 or 2 crystalloid boluses: 0.1 – 0.25 mg/kg IV[2, 15]; dilute ephedrine and administer incremental IV boluses until desirable blood pressure achieved (see ***Compatibility/Compounding Considerations***). Duration of action is ≈15 to 60 minutes after a single bolus.

b) 5 – 10 µg/kg/minute IV CRI[16]

Urinary incontinence responsive to adrenergic drugs (extra-label): 1.5 mg/kg PO every 12 hours.[17, 18] **NOTE**: Commercial oral dosage forms have been discontinued in the United States.

CATS:

Hypotension associated with anesthesia (extra-label):

a) 0.15 – 0.25 mg/kg diluted into 5 mL of a balanced electrolyte solution or saline and administer small increment IV boluses until desirable blood pressure achieved (see ***Compatibility/ Compounding Considerations***)[16]

b) 5 – 10 µg/kg/minute IV CRI[16]

HORSES:

Hypotension associated with anesthesia (extra-label):

a) 0.06 mg/kg IV as a bolus[19, 20]

b) 0.02 mg/kg/minute IV CRI[1]

Monitoring

- Clinical effectiveness including resolution of hypotension or stabilization of blood pressure
- Adverse effects including CNS stimulation, arrhythmias, tachycardia, hypertension, vomiting, or anorexia, particularly in patients with impaired renal function
- Consider electrolyte monitoring in susceptible patients as beta-adrenergic agonists may decrease serum potassium concentrations.
- C-section neonates should be monitored for signs of metabolic acidosis.[4]

Client Information

- Ephedrine will be given to your animal by your veterinarian at the veterinary clinic. Effects of this medicine should wear off before your animal is sent home.
- Contact your veterinarian if you have any concerns about your animal's condition.

Chemistry/Synonyms

A sympathomimetic alkaloid, ephedrine sulfate occurs as fine, odorless, white crystals or powder. Approximately 770 mg are soluble in 1 mL of water. The commercially available injection has a pH of 4.5 to 7.[4]

Ephedrine sulfate may also be known as ephedrine sulphate. Many trade names are available.

Storage/Stability

Store ephedrine sulfate products at room temperature 25°C (77°F) with excursions permitted to 15°C to 30°C (59°F-86°F).[4] Discard unused portion.

Compatibility/Compounding Considerations

Compatibility is dependent on factors such as pH, concentration, temperature, and diluent used; specialized references or a hospital pharmacist should be consulted for more specific information.

If using the 50 mg/mL product, it can be diluted 1:10 in 5% dextrose, 0.9% sodium chloride, or lactated Ringer's solution. Do not dilute the premixed 5 mg/mL product.

Ephedrine is **Y-site incompatible** with amphotericin B conventional form, diazepam, and pantoprazole.

Dosage Forms/Regulatory Status

VETERINARY-LABELED PRODUCTS: NONE

The Association of Racing Commissioners International (ARCI) has designated this drug as a class 2 substance. See ***Appendix*** for more information. Use of this drug may not be allowed in certain animal competitions. Check rules and regulations before entering in a competition while this medication is being administered. Contact local racing authorities for further guidance.

HUMAN-LABELED PRODUCTS:

Ephedrine Sulfate Injection: 50 mg/mL in 1 mL single-dose vials and ampules; generic; (Rx)

Ephedrine Sulfate Injection: 47 mg/mL in 1 mL vials; 4.7 mg/mL and 9.4 mg/mL in 5 mL vials; *Rezipres*®; (Rx)

Ephedrine Sulfate Injection: 5 mg/mL in 10 mL single-dose vials; *Emerphed*®; (Rx)

Oral ephedrine dosage forms have been discontinued in the United States, although oral combinations with guaifenesin (OTC) are available. The herbal supplement ma huang contains ephedrine as one of many active components.

References

For the complete list of references, see **wiley.com/go/budde/plumb**

Epinephrine

(ep-i-***nef***-rin) *Adrenalin*®, *Epi-Pen*®

Alpha-Adrenergic Agonist; Beta-Adrenergic Agonist

Prescriber Highlights

- ► Alpha- and beta-adrenergic agonist agent used systemically for treatment of anaphylaxis, cardiac resuscitation, and for refractory hypotension, as well as to prolong local effects of local anesthetic agents
- ► No absolute contraindications in life-threatening situations. Relative contraindications include closed-angle glaucoma, hypersensitivity to epinephrine, shock due to nonanaphylactic causes, during general anesthesia with inhalant anesthetics, during parturition (may delay the second stage), dilated cardiomyopathy or coronary insufficiency, thyrotoxicosis, acute or uncontrolled diabetes or hypertension, and toxemia of pregnancy.
- ► Use extreme caution in patients with a prefibrillatory cardiac rhythm. Caution is advised in patients with hypovolemia; this drug is not a substitute for adequate volume replacement.
- ► Do not inject into small appendages of the body (eg, toes, ears) either directly or combined with local anesthetic agents, as this may cause tissue necrosis and sloughing.
- ► Adverse effects include anxiety, tremors, excitability, vomiting, hypertension, tachycardia, pulmonary edema, arrhythmias, and lactic acidosis (with prolonged use or overdose situations).
- ► Do not confuse 1 mg/mL (formerly 1:1000) with 0.1 mg/mL (1:10,000) concentrations.
- ► Many drug interactions are possible.

Uses/Indications

In veterinary medicine, epinephrine is primarily used as treatment for anaphylaxis and cardiac resuscitation. Because of its vasoconstrictive properties, epinephrine can be added to local anesthetic agents to delay systemic absorption and prolong the local anesthetic effect. Epinephrine administered by IV continuous rate infusion may also be considered for the treatment of anesthetic-induced hypotension that is nonresponsive to other inotropic support.

Epinephrine has been used in reptiles to decrease recovery time after receiving inhalant anesthesia.[1,2]

Pharmacology/Actions

Epinephrine is an endogenous adrenergic agent with alpha- and beta-receptor activity. It relaxes smooth muscles in the bronchi and iris, antagonizes the effects of histamine, increases glycogenolysis, and raises blood sugar. If given IV at a low dose (0.01 mg/kg), epinephrine directly stimulates cardiac beta-1 receptors to cause increased heart rate and contractility with resultant increased cardiac output. As a result of these effects, myocardial work and oxygen consumption also increase. In the periphery, epinephrine activates beta-2 receptors, causing a decrease in peripheral vascular resistance, which lowers diastolic blood pressure. When administered at higher dosages (0.1 mg/kg), peripheral vascular resistance increases due to alpha-1-adrenergic effects.

Pharmacokinetics

Epinephrine is well-absorbed following IM or SC administration. IM injections are absorbed slightly faster than via the SC route; absorption can be expedited by massaging the injection site. The IM or SC routes are not used during cardiovascular resuscitation due to poor peripheral perfusion. Epinephrine is not effective when given PO, as it is rapidly metabolized in the GI tract and liver. Following SC injection, the onset of action is generally within 5 to 10 minutes. The onset of action following IV administration is immediate and intense.

Epinephrine does not cross the blood–brain barrier.

Epinephrine is metabolized in the liver and other tissues by monoamine oxidase (MAO) and catechol-O-methyltransferase (COMT) to inactive metabolites (3-methoxy-4-hydroxymandelic acid and metanephrine) that are then excreted in the urine after conjugation with glucuronic acid or sulfates.

Contraindications/Precautions/Warnings

In life-threatening situations there are no absolute contraindications to epinephrine use.

In nonemergent circumstances, epinephrine is contraindicated in patients with closed-angle glaucoma, hypersensitivity to epinephrine, shock due to nonanaphylactic causes, during general anesthesia with inhalant anesthetics, during parturition (may delay the second stage), and cardiac dilatation or coronary insufficiency. Epinephrine should not be injected either directly or with local anesthetics into small appendages of the body (eg, toes, ears) because of the degree of vasoconstriction that may lead to tissue necrosis and sloughing; administration through a central line is recommended.

Epinephrine should be used with extreme caution in patients with a prefibrillatory cardiac rhythm because of its excitatory effects on the heart. Epinephrine should be used with caution in patients in with thyrotoxicosis, acute or uncontrolled hypertension or diabetes, and toxemia of pregnancy. Use epinephrine with caution in patients with hypovolemia; this drug should not be used as a substitute for adequate fluid resuscitation.

Do not confuse EPINEPHrine with ePHEDrine or the 2 concentrations of commercially available epinephrine injection: 1 mg/mL (formerly labeled as 1:1000) and 0.1 mg/mL (formerly labeled as 1:10,000).

Adverse Effects

Epinephrine can induce tremors, excitability, vomiting, hypertension, tachycardia, other arrhythmias (especially if patient has organic heart disease or has received another drug that sensitizes the heart to arrhythmias), pulmonary edema, hyperglycemia, behavior changes (eg, anxiety, excitability), and lactic acidosis (with prolonged acute use or overdose situations). This information is largely extrapolated from the human label; application to veterinary species is assumed to be accurate. Repeated SC injections at or around the same site can cause tissue necrosis and sloughing at the injection site.[3] Administer through a central line, if possible, as administration through a peripheral vein may lead to local tissue necrosis if extravasation occurs. Phentolamine can be used locally for the treatment of extravasation.[4]

Reproductive/Nursing Safety

Epinephrine crosses the placenta but should not be withheld during life-threatening situations for the dam.

Although small amounts of epinephrine may be excreted into milk, it is unlikely to affect nursing offspring because it is rapidly destroyed in the GI tract and unlikely to be absorbed.

Overdose/Acute Toxicity

Clinical signs seen with overdose or inadvertent IV administration of SC or IM doses include cardiac arrhythmias, pulmonary edema and dyspnea, vomiting, and sharp rises in systolic, diastolic, and venous blood pressures.[3] Cerebral hemorrhages may result because of increased blood pressure. Renal failure, metabolic acidosis, and cold skin may also result.

Because epinephrine has a relatively short duration of effect, overdose treatment is mainly supportive.[3] If necessary, use of an alpha-adrenergic antagonist (eg, **phentolamine**) or a beta-adrenergic antagonist (eg, **propranolol**) can be considered for treatment of severe hypertension and cardiac arrhythmias. Prolonged periods of hypotension may follow, possibly requiring treatment with norepinephrine.

For patients that have experienced or are suspected to have experienced an overdose, consultation with a 24-hour poison control center specializing in providing veterinary-specific information is recommended. For general information related to overdose and toxin exposures, as well as contact information for poison control centers, refer to ***Appendix***.

Drug Interactions

The following drug interactions have either been reported or are theoretical in humans or animals receiving epinephrine and may be of significance in veterinary patients. Unless otherwise noted, use together is not necessarily contraindicated, but weigh the potential risks and perform additional monitoring when appropriate.

- Alpha-2 Adrenergic Agonists (eg, **detomidine, dexmedetomidine, medetomidine, xylazine**): Epinephrine possesses alpha agonist effects; thus, it should **NOT** be used to treat cardiac effects caused by alpha-2-adrenergic agonists.
- Alpha-Adrenergic Antagonists (eg, **phenoxybenzamine, phentolamine, prazosin**): May reverse the pressor effects of epinephrine due to alpha-1 blockade by the phenothiazine (ie, epinephrine reversal).
- Anesthetics, Halogenated Inhalant (eg, **isoflurane, sevoflurane**): An increased risk for developing arrhythmias can occur if epinephrine is administered to patients that have received a halogenated anesthetic agent; propranolol may be administered in these cases.
- Antihistamines: Certain antihistamines (eg, **chlorpheniramine, diphenhydramine**) may potentiate the effects of epinephrine.
- Beta-Adrenergic Antagonist (eg, **atenolol, propranolol, sotalol**): may potentiate hypertension and antagonize epinephrine's cardiac and bronchodilating effects by blocking the beta effects of epinephrine.
- Digoxin: An increased risk for arrhythmias may occur if epinephrine is used concurrently with digitalis glycosides.
- Levothyroxine: May potentiate the effects of epinephrine
- Monoamine Oxidase Inhibitors (MAOIs; eg, **amitraz, selegiline**): May potentiate the pressor effects of epinephrine
- Nitrates (eg, **nitroglycerin**): May reverse the pressor effects of epinephrine
- Oxytocic Agents: Hypertension may result if epinephrine is used with oxytocic agents.
- Phenothiazines (eg, **acepromazine**): May reverse the pressor effects of epinephrine due to alpha-1 blockade by the phenothiazine (ie, epinephrine reversal)
- Reserpine: May potentiate the pressor effects of epinephrine
- Sympathomimetic Agents, Other (eg, **albuterol, dobutamine, isoproterenol, phenylpropanolamine, terbutaline**): Epinephrine should not be administered with other sympathomimetic agents as increased toxicity may result.
- Tricyclic antidepressants (eg, **amitriptyline, clomipramine**): May potentiate the effects of epinephrine

Dosages

NOTE: Epinephrine concentrations were formerly expressed using ratios (ie, 1:1000 and 1:10,000 strengths), but in 2017 the FDA mandated that ratios be removed from all labeling to reduce the risk for medication errors. Be certain when preparing the injection not to confuse 1 mg/mL (formerly 1:1000) with 0.1 mg/mL (1:10,000) concentrations.

DOGS/CATS:

Anaphylactoid shock (label-dosage; not FDA-approved): 0.1 – 0.5 mL (total dose, NOT mg/kg) IM or SC using epinephrine 1 mg/mL solution[5]

Cardiopulmonary resuscitation | asystole (extra-label): **NOTE:** Clinicians are strongly encouraged to obtain the *RECOVER CPR Initiative*, Part 7[6] available as open access via the Veterinary Emergency and Critical Care Society website (veccs.org); this publication (summarized directly below) includes more detailed information including treatment algorithms and drug dosage tables.

a) *Low-dose* epinephrine 0.01 mg/kg IV, IO administered every 3 to 5 minutes early in CPR is recommended. In order to minimize under- or overdosing during CPR, epinephrine should be administered during every other cycle of basic life support (BLS; 1 cycle is 2 minutes uninterrupted compression/ventilation). Administration of vasopressin 0.8 units/kg IV, IO every other cycle alternating with epinephrine may be considered (see ***Vasopressin***).
b) *High-dose* epinephrine 0.1 mg/kg IV, IO may be considered after prolonged CPR (greater than 10 minutes).
c) *In patients in which IV or IO access is not possible*, the intratracheal (IT) route may be considered. Dilute epinephrine with saline or sterile water and administer via a catheter longer than the endotracheal tube. Optimal dosages are not known, but dosages up to 10 times the standard have been recommended for IT administration. (In a subsequent reference, the IT dose is listed as 0.02 mg/kg for the low dose and 0.2 mg/kg for the high dose.[6,7]) **NOTE:** Blind intracardiac (IC) administration of resuscitation drugs is not recommended.

Anaphylaxis (extra-label): Initially, epinephrine 0.01 mg/kg IM using a 1 mg/mL solution; maximum dose of 0.3 mg (total dose; NOT mg/kg) in patients weighing less than 40 kg (88.2 lb) and 0.5 mg (total dose; NOT mg/kg) in patients weighing more than 40 kg (88.2 lb). Depending on episode severity and response to the initial injection, the dose can be repeated every 5 to 15 minutes as needed. However, if shock has already developed, epinephrine 0.05 µg/kg/minute should be given by slow IV infusion, ideally with the dose titrated to clinical response.[8] The SC route should be avoided.[9]

Hypotension associated with anesthesia (extra-label): 0.125 – 2 µg/kg/minute CRI[10]; **NOTE:** Because epinephrine can cause increased tissue oxygen demand and severe splanchnic vasoconstriction, it should be considered only when other interventions have failed.

Prolongation of local anesthetic effect (extra-label): Epinephrine may be added to local anesthetic formulations at a very low concentration (eg, epinephrine 5 µg/mL local anesthetic) to cause vasoconstriction at the site of administration, thereby reducing the rate of systemic absorption of the local anesthetic. Practically, remove 0.1 mL from 20 mL of local anesthetic solution and add 0.1 mL of 1 mg/mL epinephrine solution.

HORSES:

Anaphylactoid shock (label-dosage; not FDA-approved): 0.022 mg/kg (1 mL/100 lb) IM or SC using epinephrine 1 mg/mL solution[5]

Anaphylaxis (extra-label): 0.01 – 0.02 mg/kg IM, SC as a single dose; or 0.1 – 0.2 mg/kg IM, SC as a single dose[11,12]

Cardiopulmonary resuscitation of newborn foals (extra-label): 0.01 – 0.02 mg/kg IV every 3 minutes until return of spontaneous circulation. If given IT, 0.1 – 0.2 mg/kg[13,14]

RUMINANTS, SWINE:

Anaphylactoid shock (label-dosage; not FDA-approved): 0.022 mg/kg (1 mL/100 lb) IM or SC using epinephrine 1 mg/mL solution[5]

Anaphylaxis (extra-label): 0.01 – 0.02 mg/kg SC or IM; if using IV, dilute solution 10-fold; may be repeated at 15-minute intervals.[15]

BIRDS:

Cardiopulmonary resuscitation (extra-label):

a) mg/kg IV, IO[16]
b) 0.01 mg/kg using 1 mg/mL epinephrine diluted to 2 – 4 mL with saline or sterile water and administered via a catheter down the trachea. If there is tracheal obstruction, a sterile endotracheal tube needs to be inserted and stitched into the left abdominal air sac.[17,18]

SMALL MAMMALS

Cardiopulmonary resuscitation in small herbivores (eg, chinchillas, guinea pigs, rabbits; extra-label): 0.2 – 0.4 mg/kg IM, IV (bolus), or IT[19]

REPTILES:

Hasten recovery time after inhalant anesthesia (extra-label): 0.1 mg/kg IM significantly decreased the recovery time in American alligators[1] and common snapping turtles.[2]

Monitoring

- Heart rate, ECG, blood pressure; central venous pressure, if possible
- Respiratory rate and thoracic auscultation
- Urine production, if possible
- Blood gases
- Neurologic status (eg, mentation, pupillary light reflexes)
- If epinephrine is administered in a peripheral vein, monitor the site for signs of localized tissue necrosis

Client Information

- Note to pharmacist or veterinarian: Be sure to discuss clinical signs associated with anaphylaxis. Review proper use of using the injector including determining dosage (if required) and injection technique using manufacturer's patient insert. Incorrect device usage can lead to inadvertent human injection. In case of accidental human injection, seek emergency medical care immediately.
- Administering epinephrine is not a substitute for immediate veterinary care. Seek veterinary care as soon as possible after administering this medication.
- The best treatment for a severe allergic reaction is avoidance of situations that predispose your animal to triggers (eg, keep away from flowers if your animal has a severe allergy to bees).
- When avoidance cannot be prevented or when it happens unexpectedly, learn to recognize the early signs of a severe allergic reaction: collapse, pale gums, difficulty breathing (cats), noisy breathing (that is unusual for your animal), swelling of the face, vomiting, or diarrhea.
- Always have this medication easily accessible. Consider attaching it to the leash, crate, or something that always travels with your animal.
- Administer medication exactly as instructed by your veterinarian; refer to instructions that came with the product. Familiarize yourself with how the injector works before you need to use it.
- Absorption can be sped up by gently massaging the site of the shot.
- Store pre-filled injector pens in carrier tube at room temperature;

do not refrigerate. Do not store medication in a car where storage temperatures can be extreme. Do not use if liquid is discolored (pinkish or dark yellow) or particles are seen floating in it. Check expiration date and refill before expiration date.

- Contact your veterinarian or pharmacist for more information on safe disposal of used or expired epinephrine autoinjectors or needles.

Chemistry/Synonyms

Epinephrine, an endogenous catecholamine, occurs as white to nearly white, microcrystalline powder or granules. It is only very slightly soluble in water, but it readily forms water-soluble salts (eg, HCl) when combined with acids. Both the commercial products and endogenous epinephrine are in the levo-form, which is about 15 times more active than the dextro-isomer. The pH of the commercial injection ranges from 2.5 to 5.

Epinephrine is commonly called adrenalin.

Storage/Stability

Epinephrine HCl for injection should be stored 15°C to 30°C (59°F – 86°F) in tight containers protected from light. Epinephrine will darken (oxidation) when exposed to light and air. Do not use the injection if it is pink or brown or contains a precipitate. The stability of the injection depends on the form and the preservatives present and may vary among manufacturers. Epinephrine is rapidly destroyed by alkalis or oxidizing agents.

A study[20] investigated epinephrine stability when pre-drawn in syringes. Epinephrine 1 mg/mL solution containing sodium metabisulfite (antioxidant) was drawn under room air into 1 mL plastic syringes. Syringes were stored at 38°C with needles left attached and recapped. Epinephrine potency was maintained for 2 months when stored under low (15%) humidity and 4 months at high (95%) humidity.

Compatibility/Compounding Considerations

Epinephrine HCl is reported to be physically **compatible** with the following IV solutions and drugs: dextran 6% in dextrose 5%, dextran 6% in 0.9% sodium chloride, dextrose/Ringer's combinations, dextrose/lactated Ringer's combinations, dextrose/saline combinations, dextrose 2.5%, dextrose 5% (becomes unstable at a pH greater than 5.5), dextrose 10%, Ringer's injection, lactated Ringer's injection, 0.9% sodium chloride, sodium lactate 1/6 M, amikacin sulfate, cimetidine HCl, dobutamine HCl, and verapamil HCl.

Epinephrine HCl is reported to be physically **incompatible** with the following IV solutions and drugs: Ionosol-D-CM, Ionosol-PSL (Darrow's), Ionosol-T with dextrose 5% (**NOTE**: other Ionosol products are compatible), sodium chloride 5%, sodium bicarbonate 5%, aminophylline, hyaluronidase, sodium bicarbonate, and warfarin sodium.

Compatibility is dependent on factors such as pH, concentration, temperature, and diluent used; consult specialized references or a hospital pharmacist for more specific information.

Dosage Forms/Regulatory Status

NOTE: Epinephrine concentrations were formerly expressed using ratios (ie, 1:1000 and 1:10,000 strengths), but in 2017 the FDA mandated that ratios be removed from all labeling to reduce the risk for medication errors. Be certain when preparing the injection not to confuse 1 mg/mL (formerly 1:1000) with 0.1 mg/mL (1:10,000) concentrations.

VETERINARY-LABELED PRODUCTS:

Epinephrine HCl for Injection 1 mg/mL in 1 mL amps and syringes and 10 mL, 30 mL, 50 mL, and 100 mL vials; generic; (Rx). Labeled for use in dogs, cats, cattle, horses, sheep, and swine.

The Association of Racing Commissioners International (ARCI) has designated this drug as a class 2 substance. See ***Appendix*** for more information. Use of this drug may not be allowed in certain animal competitions. Check rules and regulations before entering in a competition while this medication is being administered. Contact local racing authorities for further guidance.

HUMAN-LABELED PRODUCTS:

Epinephrine HCl Solution for Injection: 1 mg/mL in 1 mL ampules and 1 mL, 10 mL, and 30 mL vials; generic; (Rx)

Epinephrine HCl Solution for Injection: 0.1 mg/mL 10 mL syringes and vials; generic; (Rx)

Epinephrine HCl Solution for Injection: 0.3 mg/0.3 mL; in prefilled single-dose syringes or in dual-dose autoinjectors; *EpiPen®*, *Twinject®*, *Adrenaclick®*, *Auvi-Q®*; *Symjepi®*; generic; (Rx)

Epinephrine HCl Solution for Injection: 0.15 mg /0.15 mL in single-dose or dual-dose autoinjectors; *Twinject®*, *Adrenaclick®*, *Auvi-Q®*, generic; (Rx)

Epinephrine HCl Solution for Injection: 0.15 mg/0.3 mL; *EpiPen Jr®*, *Symjepi®*; (Rx)

Epinephrine bitartrate is available as a powder form (aerosol) for inhalation, topical solution, and solution for nebulization; ophthalmic preparations are available.

References

For the complete list of references, see **wiley.com/go/budde/plumb**

Epirubicin

(ep-ee-***roo***-bi-sin) *Ellence®*

Antineoplastic

Prescriber Highlights

- ▶ Injectable anthracycline antineoplastic agent that potentially could be used as a replacement for doxorubicin in dogs and cats.
- ▶ Limited published information is available for its use in animal patients.
- ▶ Adverse effect profile for animals is not well documented compared to doxorubicin. It may have less cardiotoxicity potential but more GI adverse effects. Otherwise, similar cautions and caveats as doxorubicin apply.
- ▶ Dexrazoxane may be used to manage extravasation or for prevention of cardiac toxicity.
- ▶ The National Institute for Occupational Safety and Health (NIOSH) classifies epirubicin as a hazardous drug; use appropriate precautions when handling.

Uses/Indications

Epirubicin could potentially be used as a replacement for doxorubicin in dogs and cats, but there is much less published on it for veterinary use compared to doxorubicin. Retrospective studies have evaluated epirubicin use in dogs for the adjuvant treatment of splenic hemangiosarcoma,[1] as part of a multi-agent protocol for lymphoma,[2] and in combination with lomustine or as a single agent rescue drug for histiocytic sarcoma;[3] another study specifically assessed epirubicin toxicity.[4] From this work, it appears that epirubicin has similar efficacy as doxorubicin and the potential for less cardiotoxicity but may have a higher incidence of adverse GI effects.

Epirubicin demonstrated tumor- and disease-free survival in cats with injection-site sarcoma.[4]

Pharmacology/Actions

Epirubicin has a similar mode of action as doxorubicin; it causes inhibition of DNA synthesis, DNA-dependent RNA synthesis, and protein synthesis, but the precise mechanisms for these effects are not well understood. The drug acts throughout the cell cycle and also possesses some immunosuppressant activity.

Pharmacokinetics

No published data on epirubicin pharmacokinetics or pharmacodynamics in dogs or cats were located. Epirubicin, like doxorubicin, must be administered IV as it is not absorbed from the GI tract and is extremely irritating to tissues if administered SC or IM.

In humans after IV injection, epirubicin is rapidly and widely distributed but does not appreciably enter the CSF. It is marginally bound (77%) to tissue and plasma proteins and concentrates in red blood cells.

Epirubicin is metabolized extensively by the liver and other tissues via aldo-keto reductase primarily to epirubicinol, which is active, but only at 10% of the parent compound's activity; other inactive metabolites are also formed. Epirubicin and its metabolites are primarily excreted in the bile and feces, with lesser amounts excreted into the urine. Epirubicin is eliminated in a triphasic manner. In humans, average half-lives for the three elimination phases are the first phase (3 minutes), the second phase (2.5 hours), and the third phase (33 hours).

Contraindications/Precautions/Warnings

In humans, and likely in dogs as well, epirubicin is contraindicated or relatively contraindicated (measure risk vs benefit) in patients with myelosuppression (neutrophil count less than 1500 cells/μL), severe myocardial insufficiency, cardiomyopathy and/or heart failure, recent myocardial infarction, severe arrhythmias, or those already having received maximum cumulative anthracycline (eg, doxorubicin) doses. Epirubicin should be used with caution in patients with hyperuricemia, hyperuricuria, or impaired hepatic function. Dosage adjustments may be necessary for patients with hepatic impairment.

Epirubicin, like doxorubicin, should be administered IV slowly (over at least 3 to 5 minutes) in a free flowing IV line. Extreme care must be taken to avoid perivascular infusion (extravasation). IM or SC dosages are contraindicated.

Breeds predisposed to developing cardiomyopathy (eg, Doberman pinschers, Great Danes, rottweilers, boxers) should be monitored carefully while receiving epirubicin therapy.

P-glycoprotein actively transports doxorubicin and possibly epirubicin, and certain breeds susceptible to the *MDR1* mutation (also known as *ABCB1-1delta*; eg, collies, Australian shepherds, shelties, long-haired Whippets) may be at higher risk for toxicity. Bone marrow suppression (decreased blood cell counts, particularly neutrophils) and GI toxicity (anorexia, vomiting, diarrhea) are more likely to occur at normal doxorubicin dosages in dogs with the *MDR1* mutation. To reduce the likelihood of severe toxicity in these dogs (mutant/normal or mutant/mutant), the Veterinary Clinical Pharmacology Laboratory at Washington State University recommends reducing doxorubicin doses by 25% to 30% and carefully monitoring these patients.[5] A similar empiric dosage modification strategy should be considered for epirubicin.

Because epirubicin can be irritating to the skin, gloves should be worn when administering or preparing the drug. Ideally, doxorubicin injection should be prepared in a biological safety cabinet using standard chemotherapy preparation procedures. If accidental skin or mucous membrane contact occurs, wash the area immediately using soap and copious amounts of water. Spills or leakage of epirubicin solutions should be diluted with sodium hypochlorite solutions (with 1% available chlorine), preferably by soaking, and then diluted further with water.

Do not confuse EPIrubicin with DOXOrubicin or DAUNOrubicin.

The National Institute for Occupational Safety and Health (NIOSH) classifies epirubicin as a hazardous drug; personal protective equipment (PPE) should be used accordingly to minimize the risk for exposure.

Adverse Effects

Epirubicin can cause several adverse effects similar to doxorubicin, including bone marrow suppression, cardiac toxicity, alopecia, gastroenteritis (vomiting, diarrhea), and stomatitis. Cardiotoxic effects may be less likely to occur than with doxorubicin, based upon preclinical toxicity studies.[6] After administration of doxorubicin in dogs (and probably epirubicin), nausea and vomiting commonly occur within the first 72 hours; diarrhea can occur within ≈4 to 5 days, and myelosuppression nadirs are generally seen 7 to 10 days after treatment. Many dogs receiving chemotherapy will have minor hair coat changes (eg, shagginess, loss of luster). Breeds with continuously growing hair coats (eg, poodles, terriers, Afghan hounds, or old English sheepdogs) are more likely to experience significant alopecia.

An immediate histamine-mediated hypersensitivity reaction may be seen characterized by urticaria, facial swelling, vomiting, arrhythmias (see below), and/or hypotension. The rate of infusion can have a direct impact on this effect, and generally, IV infusions should be administered no faster than over 10 to 20 minutes. Pretreatment with a histamine H_1 blocker such as diphenhydramine or an IV glucocorticoid may also reduce or eliminate these effects. This reaction has also been reported in one cat.[7]

For more information on cardiac toxicity of anthracycline antineoplastics, refer to the ***Doxorubicin*** monograph.

In cats, doxorubicin (and potentially epirubicin) is a potential nephrotoxin, and renal function should be monitored both before and during therapy.

Extravasation injuries secondary to perivascular administration of epirubicin can be quite serious, with severe tissue ulceration and necrosis possible. Prevention of extravasation should be a priority, and animals should be frequently checked during the infusion. Should extravasation occur, it is suggested to treat as per the recommendations for humans. There are currently two treatments recommended for doxorubicin (and epirubicin) extravasation injuries. Both have been shown to be effective, but no comparative trials have been published. **1)** Apply dimethyl sulfoxide (DMSO) 99% by saturating a gauze pad and painting on twice the area of the extravasation.[8] Allow the site to air dry and repeat the application every 6 hours for 14 days. Do not cover the area with a dressing. **2)** Dexrazoxane is FDA-approved for the treatment of extravasation resulting from anthracycline IV therapy; refer to the ***Dexrazoxane*** monograph for more information. Additionally, ice compresses applied to the affected area for 15 minutes every 6 hours for 3 days may be useful.

Reproductive/Nursing Safety

Epirubicin is teratogenic and embryotoxic in laboratory animals. It may reduce male and female fertility.[9] For sexually intact patients, verify pregnancy status prior to administration.

Epirubicin is excreted in milk in concentrations that may exceed those found in plasma. Because of risks to nursing offspring, consider using milk replacer if the dam is receiving epirubicin. In humans, nursing is contraindicated in patients receiving the drug.

Overdose/Acute Toxicity

Inadvertent acute overdose may be manifested by exacerbations of the adverse effects outlined above. For dogs, a lethal dose of epirubicin is not publicly available; however, 6-week daily repeated IV dose toxicity studies conducted in research dogs identified 0.4 mg/kg/day as the Lowest Observed Adverse Effect Level (LOAEL) with the kidney being the target organ.[10] Supportive and symptomatic therapy is suggested should an overdose occur. ***Dexrazoxane*** may be useful to help prevent cardiac toxicity.

For patients that have experienced or are suspected of having experienced an overdose, consultation with a 24-hour poison consultation center specializing in providing veterinary-specific information is recommended. For general information related to overdose and toxin exposures, as well as contact information for poison control centers, refer to ***Appendix***.

Drug Interactions

The following drug interactions have either been reported or are theoretical in humans or animals receiving doxorubicin or epirubicin and may be of significance in veterinary patients. Unless otherwise noted, use together is not necessarily contraindicated, but weigh the potential risks and perform additional monitoring when appropriate.

- **Antineoplastic Agents, Other**: May potentiate the toxic effects of doxorubicin
- **Calcium Channel Blockers** (eg, **amlodipine, diltiazem**): May result in an increased risk for heart failure
- **Cimetidine**: Can increase epirubicin levels; avoid using together
- **Cyclosporine**: Cyclosporine can increase doxorubicin and doxorubicinol (active metabolite) levels. Avoid using together.
- **Glucosamine**: May reduce doxorubicin effectiveness; use together is not recommended in humans.
- **Immunosuppressive Agents, Other** (eg, **leflunomide, tacrolimus**): Immunosuppressant effects may be enhanced.
- **Ketoconazole**: Can increase doxorubicin and doxorubicinol (active metabolite) levels and lead to toxicity. Avoid using together.
- **Paclitaxel**: Can increase epirubicin toxicity
- **Phenobarbital**: May increase elimination and reduce blood levels of doxorubicin
- **Spinosad**: Can increase doxorubicin and doxorubicinol (active metabolite) levels and lead to toxicity. Avoid using together.
- **Streptozocin**: May inhibit doxorubicin metabolism
- **Vaccines**: Live or live-attenuated vaccines may result in active infections in immunocompromised patients.
- **Verapamil**: May increase doxorubicin levels
- **Warfarin**: Increased risk for bleeding
- **Zidovudine**: Increased risk for neutropenia

Laboratory Considerations

- Epirubicin may significantly increase both blood and urine concentrations of **uric acid.**
- Handling of blood samples should pose no health hazard after 7 days.[11] **NOTE**: Reference pertains to doxorubicin; epirubicin not determined.

Dosages

NOTE: Because of the potential toxicity of this drug to patients, veterinary personnel, and clients, and since chemotherapy indications, treatment protocols, monitoring, and safety guidelines often change, the following dosages should be used only as a general guide. Consultation with a veterinary oncologist and referral to current veterinary oncology references[12–16] are strongly recommended.

DOGS:

Depending on the protocol used, epirubicin is usually dosed similarly to doxorubicin at 30 mg/m² (**NOT** mg/kg) IV[17] in a free-flowing line over at least 3 to 5 minutes. Smaller patients (eg, less than 10 kg [22 lb]) may be dosed at 1 mg/kg IV. The maximum cumulative epirubicin dose is probably similar to doxorubicin at 240 mg/m² (**NOT** mg/kg).

Lymphoma (extra-label): In a retrospective study, either a modified Wisconsin-Madison continuous chemotherapy protocol (CEOP-C; vincristine, prednisolone, cyclophosphamide, asparaginase, and epirubicin): Epirubicin 30 mg/m² (**NOT** mg/kg) or 1 mg/kg IV on weeks 4 and 9, followed by vincristine, chlorambucil, and methotrexate weeks 11 to 17, OR a modified Wisconsin-Madison discontinuous chemotherapy protocol (CEOP-25) used; same epirubicin dosage and frequency[2]

Splenic hemangiosarcoma (extra-label): In a retrospective study, after splenectomy, treated dogs received epirubicin at 30 mg/m² (**NOT** mg/kg) IV every 3 weeks for up to 4 to 6 treatments.[1]

Histiocytic sarcoma (extra-label): In a retrospective study, used in combination with lomustine or as a single-agent rescue drug, epirubicin was dosed at 25 – 30 mg/m² (**NOT** mg/kg), and in dogs less than 10 kg (22 lb) in weight, the drug was dosed at 1 mg/kg.[3]

CATS:

Injection site sarcoma: In one study, cats received 25 mg/m² (**NOT** mg/kg) IV every 21 days for 3 doses before undergoing surgical resection.[4]

Monitoring

- Efficacy
- CBC with platelet count. Neutrophil counts of less than 1500/µL generally require a delay in dosing.
- Dogs with pre-existing heart disease should be monitored with regular ECGs (insensitive to early toxic changes) and/or echocardiogram or surrogate biomarkers, such as cardiac troponin I.
- Evaluate hepatic function prior to therapy.
- Urinalysis, BUN, and creatinine in cats

Client Information

- Clients must be briefed on the possibilities of severe toxicity developing from this drug, including drug-related mortality. Clients should contact the veterinarian if the animal exhibits any clinical signs of profound depression, abnormal bleeding (including bloody diarrhea), and/or bruising.
- Epirubicin may cause urine to be colored orange to red for 1 to 2 days after dosing; although uncommon in animals, it is not harmful if it occurs.
- Mild anorexia and occasional vomiting are commonly seen 2 to 5 days posttherapy.
- Avoid skin contact with urine or feces of treated animals. After treatment, doxorubicin drug residues may be found in the treated dog's urine up to 21 days and feces for several days.[18]
- Although it is unknown how much drug is in the saliva of treated animals, do not allow treated animals to lick human skin while receiving chemotherapy treatment.
- This medication is considered to be a hazardous drug as defined by the National Institute for Occupational Safety and Health (NIOSH). Talk with your veterinarian or pharmacist about the use of personal protective equipment when handling this medicine.
- Laboratory work must be monitored periodically while your animal is being treated with epirubicin; do not miss these important follow-up visits with your veterinarian.

Chemistry/Synonyms

Epirubicin (4-epidoxorubicin) is a semisynthetic stereoisomer of the anthracycline doxorubicin antibiotic antineoplastic and occurs as a red-orange powder soluble in water and methyl alcohol, slightly soluble in alcohol, and practically insoluble in acetone. The commercially available solution for injection has a pH of ≈3. CAS Registry: 56420-45-2 (epirubicin); 56390-09-1 (epirubicin hydrochloride); ATC: L01DB03.

Epirubicin HCl may also be known as 4-epidoxorubicin, 4-epi-adriamycin HCl, IMI-28, or pidorubicin HCl. A common trade name is *Ellence*®.

Storage/Stability

Store lyophilized powder for injection at 25°C (77°F); excursions are permitted to 15°C to 30°C (59°F-86°F). Reconstituted solutions are stable for 24 hours when stored at 2°C to 8°C (36°F-46°F) and protected from light or 25°C (77°F) in normal lighting conditions. Discard any unused portion.

Store the commercially available solution in a refrigerator between 2°C and 8°C (36°F and 46°F). Do not freeze. Store protected from light, but no light protection is needed when administering the drug. The manufacturer recommends using the solution within 24 hours of removal from the refrigerator or first penetration of the rubber stopper and discarding any unused solution. When reconstituted, the solution should be clear and red in color. Do not use the solution if precipitation or significant discoloration is present.

Studies have shown that 2 mg/mL concentrations in sterile water for injection are stable for at least 43 days at 4°C (39°F) in plastic syringes.

Compatibility/Compounding Considerations

Compatibility is dependent on factors such as pH, concentration, temperature, and diluent used; specialized references or a hospital pharmacist should be consulted for more specific information.

To reconstitute the lyophilized powder: Reconstitute 50 mg vial with 25 mL sterile water for injection, to a final concentration of 2 mg/mL. Shake vigorously; it may take up to 4 minutes for the mixture to completely dissolve. Epirubicin can be further diluted with sterile water for injection.

Epirubicin can be used in combination with other chemotherapy agents but should not be mixed with other drugs in the same syringe. Prolonged contact with any alkaline solution should be avoided as hydrolysis can occur. Epirubicin should not be mixed with heparin or fluorouracil due to chemical incompatibility that may lead to precipitation.

Epirubicin HCl is reportedly physically **compatible** with the following IV solutions and drugs: 3.3% dextrose in 0.3% sodium chloride, 5% dextrose, lactated Ringer's injection, 0.9% sodium chloride, and ifosfamide.

Dosage Forms/Regulatory Status

VETERINARY-LABELED PRODUCTS: NONE

HUMAN-LABELED PRODUCTS:

Epirubicin HCl for Injection: 2 mg/mL in 25 mL and 100 mL vials; *Ellence*®, generic; (Rx)

References

For the complete list of references, see **wiley.com/go/budde/plumb**

Epoetin Alfa
Erythropoietin (EPO)
Recombinant Human Erythropoietin (rHuEPO)

(eh-***poe***-ee-tin ***al***-fah) *Epogen*®, *Procrit*®

Erythropoietic Agent

Prescriber Highlights

- ► Hormone that regulates erythropoiesis; used for anemia associated with chronic kidney disease and myelosuppressive disorders.
- ► Concurrent iron supplementation is necessary for most patients.
- ► Contraindications include patients with uncontrolled hypertension or patients that are hypersensitive to the drug. Do not use in patients that have a history of forming autoantibodies with treatment.
- ► Adverse effects include autoantibody development that causes resistance to treatment, vomiting, hypertension, seizures, uveitis, iron depletion, local reactions at injection sites, fever, arthralgia, pure red cell aplasia (PRCA), and mucocutaneous ulcers.
- ► Adequate monitoring is vital.
- ► Because of decreased potential for development of antibodies and more favorable kinetics, darbepoetin is often recommended as a first-choice treatment for dogs and cats with anemia associated with chronic kidney disease as compared with erythropoietin.

Uses/Indications

Epoetin alfa, or recombinant human erythropoietin (rHuEPO), has been used for treatment of dogs and cats with anemia associated with end-stage chronic kidney disease (CKD) and myelosuppressive disorders. One group with experience treating more than 70 CKD cats with epoetin or darbepoetin reported that only ≈60% to 65% of cats had an adequate response.[1] Epoetin has also been used as part of a treatment regimen in cats and dogs with myelodysplasia, although evidence is limited to a small retrospective case study.[2] Because of concerns associated with expense and adverse effects (eg, pure red cell aplasia [PRCA]), most specialists do not recommend starting therapy in dogs or cats until there is development of clinical signs associated with the anemia (eg, lethargy, exercise intolerance), or when the packed cell volume (PCV) is less than 20% to 22%. It is hoped that canine and feline recombinant products will become commercially available in the future to reduce the risks for autoantibody formation.[3,4]

Many clinicians choose darbepoetin (instead of epoetin) because it may be less immunogenic and may require less frequent dosing compared with epoetin; however, the prohibitive cost of darbepoetin may preclude its use.

Pharmacology/Actions

Erythropoietin (EPO) is a hormone produced in the kidneys that regulates erythropoiesis. Under conditions of anemia and hypoxemia, EPO is secreted by interstitial cells surrounding renal tubules to promote erythrocyte precursor proliferation, maturation, and viability. The result is an increase in red blood cell mass and oxygen carrying capacity in the blood.[5]

Epoetin alfa (recombinant human EPO [rhEPO]) has an identical amino acid sequence as endogenous human EPO.

Pharmacokinetics

Epoetin alfa is only absorbed after parenteral administration. The drug's metabolic fate is unknown. In patients with chronic kidney disease, half-lives are prolonged ≈20% over those with normal renal function.

In healthy dogs, epoetin alfa has an elimination half-life of ≈7 hours, which is ≈3 times shorter than darbepoetin.[6] The T_{max} of epoetin alfa appears to be ≈4 hours with otherwise variable kinetics. Correction of hematocrit may require 2 to 8 weeks, depending on initial hematocrit and dosage used.

Contraindications/Precautions/Warnings

Epoetin alfa is contraindicated in patients with uncontrolled hypertension or those that are hypersensitive to it (see ***Adverse Effects***); it should also not be used in patients that develop pure red cell aplasia (PRCA) after starting treatment with epoetin alfa or other erythropoietin (EPO) protein drug products. In animals with moderate to severe hypertension, epoetin alfa therapy should be started with caution or withheld until BP is controlled.

Adequate iron stores are necessary for efficacy; iron deficiency should be corrected prior to starting therapy with epoetin alfa. Providing iron supplementation concomitantly with epoetin alfa treatment is recommended[7] (some say it is imperative[8]); injectable iron dextran is preferable to oral iron products for this purpose because it has fewer adverse GI effects (eg, inappetence, vomiting, diarrhea).

Adverse Effects

The 2 most common adverse effects that occur in dogs and cats receiving epoetin alfa therapy are systemic hypertension (40% to 50% of patients[9]) and development of neutralizing antibodies to epoetin alfa, which could lead to a sudden worsening of anemia and/or pure red cell aplasia (PRCA).

Hypertension may be a result of increased blood viscosity and cardiac output and decreased anemia-mediated vasodilation. One study reported 40% of dogs and 50% of cats developed hypertension while being treated with EPO.[10] Targeting a quicker rise in PCV increases the risk for hypertension; a target of 1% to 3% PCV increase has been reported to balance clinical improvement while lowering the risk for adverse effects.[1] This finding echoes the risk described in humans—epoetin alfa has a black box warning from the FDA alerting prescribers to the increased risk for death, myocardial infarction, stroke, venous thromboembolism, and other serious cardiovascular events, especially when targeting a hemoglobin concentration greater than 11 g/dL.[11] In addition, underlying cardiac disease may be a result of, or compounded by, chronic kidney disease and hypertension. Seizures may be in response to hypertension.

An estimated 70% of dogs and cats receiving epoetin alfa (recombinant human erythropoietin [rHuEPO]) develop anti-rHuEPO antibodies, and up to 30% of all patients develop sufficient antibodies to cause PRCA with resultant profound anemia, arrest of erythropoiesis, and transfusion dependency.[9] A bone marrow aspirate should be considered in patients that develop refractory anemia while receiving adequate epoetin alfa doses and have normal iron metabolism. A myeloid:erythroid ratio of greater than 4 predicts significant autoantibody formation and contraindicates further EPO therapy.[8,9,12] Some clinicians believe that epoetin alfa should be withdrawn if packed cell volume (PCV) starts to decline while the patient is receiving therapy. Of note, some commercially available epoetin alfa contains 2.5 mg/mL human albumin, and, anecdotally, PRCA is reported to occur less often with darbepoetin, which does not contain human albumin. One study states that the incidence of PRCA is ≈25% to 30% in dogs and cats receiving epoetin alfa compared with less than 10% in those receiving darbepoetin.[1] Studies indicate that the incidence of PRCA can be seen in 25% to 40% of cats receiving epoetin alfa therapy.[1,7,9] Treatment of PRCA includes immediate discontinuation of epoetin, and immunosuppressive therapy and blood transfusions; however, the long-term prognosis once EPO antibodies have developed is grave regardless of these interventions.

Other adverse effects reported include high blood viscosity, polycythemia, seizures, and iron depletion. Local reactions at injection sites (which may be a predictor of antibody formation), fever, anorexia, cellulitis, arthralgia, and mucocutaneous ulcers are also possible.

Therapy should be discontinued if any of the above adverse effects occur.[13]

Reproductive/Nursing Safety

Little information is available for dogs and cats; it is unclear whether the drug crosses the placenta or enters milk. Some teratogenic effects (eg, decrease in body weight gain, delayed ossification) and implantation losses have been noted in pregnant rats given epoetin alfa 100 units/kg/day (which approximates initial human dosages).[11] Rabbits receiving 500 mg/kg IV during days 6 to 18 of gestation and rats receiving 500 mg/kg IV during days 7 to 17 of gestation showed no untoward effects on offspring. Use during pregnancy only when benefits outweigh the potential risks.

It is not known whether epoetin alfa is excreted in milk, but it is unlikely to pose much risk to nursing offspring due to digestion in the GI tract.

Overdose/Acute Toxicity

Acute overdoses do not appear to cause significant adverse or toxic effects. In humans, single doses of up to 1600 units/kg demonstrated no signs of toxicity. Chronic overdoses may lead to hypertension or polycythemia. Treatment includes drug discontinuation, cautious phlebotomy (if polycythemia occurs), and/or control of systemic hypertension.

For patients that have experienced or are suspected to have experienced an overdose, consultation with a 24-hour poison consultation center specializing in providing veterinary-specific information is recommended. For general information related to overdose and toxin exposures, as well as contact information for poison control centers, refer to ***Appendix***.

Drug Interactions

The following drug interactions have either been reported or are theoretical in humans or animals receiving epoetin alfa and may be of significance in veterinary patients. Unless otherwise noted, use together is not necessarily contraindicated, but weigh the potential risks and perform additional monitoring when appropriate.

- **ANDROGENS** (eg, **danazol**): May increase the sensitivity of erythroid progenitors; this interaction has been used for therapeutic effect. **NOTE**: Neither this effect nor the safety of this combination has been confirmed in well-controlled studies.
- **CYCLOSPORINE**: May cause additive increases in blood pressure and may alter cyclosporine blood levels, as cyclosporine is bound by RBCs
- **DESMOPRESSIN**: Use with epoetin alfa can decrease bleeding times.
- **PROBENECID**: Probenecid has been demonstrated to reduce the renal tubular excretion of epoetin alfa; clinical significance of this remains unclear.

Laboratory Considerations

- No laboratory interactions of major clinical importance have been described.

Dosages

DOGS/CATS:

Adjunctive therapy for anemia associated with end-stage chronic kidney disease (extra-label):

a) *Initial dosage*: 100 units/kg SC 3 times per week[8,9]; continue this dose until the target packed cell volume (PCV) is reached, typically within 3 to 4 weeks. Taking the RBC lag phase (ie, time for RBC maturation in bone marrow) into account, do not adjust dose more frequently than once every 3 weeks. Adjust the dose and frequency as necessary to find the lowest dose needed to control anemia. If adequate control is not achieved within 8 to 12 weeks, the dose can be increased by an additional 25 – 50 units/kg every 3 to 4 weeks while maintaining a dosing interval of 3 times per week.

b) *Maintenance dosage*: 50 – 100 units/kg once to twice weekly. Continue monitoring the PCV and If animal requires greater than 145 units/kg 3 times a week, evaluate for epoetin resistance.[1,12,16,17] Iron supplementation is highly recommended. See ***Iron Dextran***.

FERRETS:

Adjunctive therapy for anemia (extra-label): 50 – 150 units/kg IM 3 times weekly; may decrease to once weekly once PCV improves to desired range[18]

RABBITS/RODENTS/SMALL MAMMALS:

Adjunctive therapy anemia in rabbits (extra-label): 50 – 150 units/kg SC every 2 to 3 days until desired PCV is reached, then reduce to once weekly for at least 4 weeks[19]

Monitoring

- Baseline and periodic CBC with reticulocyte count to identify response to treatment.
- Baseline and periodic (weekly or every other week) packed cell volume (PCV) for the first 2 to 4 months of therapy. Target PCV is an increase by more than 10% or exceeds 30% for dogs,[8,14,15] and greater than 25% for cats.[7,8] Once the PCV is stable and a maintenance dose is established, recheck PCV every 1 to 3 months (frequency will depend on patient's clinical condition).
- Baseline and periodic renal serum chemistry
- Baseline and periodic blood pressure; begin with weekly, then every 1 to 3 months[1] (frequency will depend on patient's clinical condition)
- Baseline and periodic iron testing (eg, serum ferritin, total iron-binding capacity [TIBC]) during therapy to ensure adequate iron availability

Client Information

- Epoetin alfa is an injectable medication used to treat anemia (too few red blood cells) caused by chronic kidney disease.
- If you are giving this medicine at home, be sure you understand how and where to administer the shots. It may take several weeks before it works.
- Contact your veterinarian immediately if you notice skin reactions at the site of the shot, seizures (convulsions), low energy level, joint pain (difficulty walking), mouth ulcers (may appear as excessive drooling), or loss of appetite.
- Ongoing examinations and blood work are necessary while your animal receives this drug. Do not miss these important follow-up visits.

Chemistry/Synonyms

Epoetin alfa is a biosynthetic form of the glycoprotein human hormone erythropoietin with an identical amino acid sequence as endogenous human erythropoietin (EPO) but with different carbohydrate moieties. It is commercially available as a sterile, colorless solution adjusted for tonicity and pH (7 to 7.5). Commercial products may contain human albumin (2.5 mg/mL) or be formulated in an amino acid solution. Canine and feline EPO have an 81.3% and 83.3% amino acid homology, respectively, compared with human EPO. The relative conservation of amino acid sequencing allows for binding of recombinant human EPO to canine and feline EPO receptors.[1]

Epoetin may also be known as erythropoietin, rHuEPO, BI-71.052 (epoetin gamma), BM-06.019 (epoetin beta), EPO (epoetin alfa), EPOCH (epoetin beta), *Epogen®*, *Eprex®*, *Procrit®*, and *Retacrit*.

Storage/Stability

The injectable solution should be stored in the refrigerator at 2°C to 8°C (36°F-46°F); do not freeze. Do not use the product if there is discoloration or particulate matter present. Do not shake the solution, as denaturation of the protein with resultant loss of activity may occur. Protect from light; if light exposure is limited to 24 hours or less, no effects on potency should occur. Do not mix with other drugs or use the same IV tubing when other drugs are running.

Compatibility/Compounding Considerations

A method of diluting the Amgen product to facilitate giving very small dosages has been described.[20] Use of a 1:20 dilution (1 part *Epogen®* to 19 parts bacteriostatic normal saline) does not require any additional albumin to prevent binding of the drug to container. No data are available commenting on this dilution's stability.

Dosage Forms/Regulatory Status

VETERINARY-LABELED PRODUCTS: NONE

The Association of Racing Commissioners International (ARCI) has designated this drug as a class 2 substance; it is also prohibited on the premises of a racing facility. See ***Appendix*** for more information.

HUMAN-LABELED PRODUCTS:

Epoetin Alfa, Solution for Injection (preserved; contains human albumin): 10,000 units/mL in 2 mL multi-dose vials and 20,000 units/mL in 1 mL multi-dose vials; *Epogen, Procrit*; (Rx)

Epoetin Alfa, Solution for Injection (preservative free; contains human albumin): 2000 units/mL, 3000 units/mL, 4000 units/mL, 10,000 units/mL, and 40,000 units/mL in 1 mL vials; *Epogen, Procrit*; (Rx)

Epoetin Alfa-epbx, Solution for Injection (preserved; contains amino acids): 10,000 units/mL in 2 mL multi-dose vials and 20,000 units/mL in 1 mL multi-dose vials; *Retacrit*; (Rx)

Epoetin Alfa-epbx, Solution for Injection (preservative free; contains amino acids): 2000 units/mL, 3000 units/mL, 4000 units/mL, 10,000 units/mL, and 40,000 units/mL in 1 mL vials; *Retacrit*; (Rx)

References

For the complete list of references, see **wiley.com/go/budde/plumb**

Eprinomectin/Praziquantel

(e-pri-no-***mek***-tin/pra-zi-***kwon***-tel) *Centragard®*

Topical Avermectin and Anticestodal Combination

Antiparasitic Agent

Prescriber Highlights

- ▶ Topical feline heartworm preventive, also treats and controls roundworms, hookworms, and tapeworms
- ▶ For use in cats and kittens 7 weeks and older and 0.8 kg (1.8 lb) or greater
- ▶ Usually well tolerated. Salivation may occur if cats lick the application site.

Uses/Indications

Eprinomectin/praziquantel transdermal solution is indicated for the prevention of heartworm disease caused by *Dirofilaria immitis*, and for the treatment and control of roundworms (adult and fourth-stage larval *Toxocara cati*), hookworms (adult and fourth-stage larval *Ancylostoma tubaeforme*; adult *Ancylostoma braziliense*), and tapeworms (adult *Dipylidium caninum* and *Echinococcus multilocularis*) in cats and kittens 7 weeks of age and older and 0.8 kg (1.8 lb) or greater. However, because the prepatent period for *E multilocularis* may be as short as 26 days, cats treated at the labeled monthly intervals may become reinfected and shed eggs between treatments.

Eprinomectin/praziquantel transdermal solution also has demonstrated activity in cats against *Toxascaris leonina*,[1] *Joyeuxiella* spp,[2] lungworms,[3-5] and bladder worms,[6] and is approved for several of these indications in countries outside of the United States.[7] Efficacy against GI nematodes and cestodes is comparable to the topical combination of emodepside/praziquantel.[8]

Pharmacology/Actions

Eprinomectin binds selectively to glutamate-gated chloride ion channels that occur in invertebrate nerve and muscle cells. This leads to an increase in cell membrane permeability to chloride ions, causing paralysis and death of the parasite. Like ivermectin, eprinomectin enhances the release of gamma aminobutyric acid (GABA) at presynaptic neurons. GABA acts as an inhibitory neurotransmitter and blocks the postsynaptic stimulation of the adjacent neuron in nematodes or the muscle fiber in arthropods. These compounds are generally not toxic to mammals, as they do not have glutamate-gated chloride channels and do not readily cross the blood–brain barrier.

Praziquantel's exact mechanism of action against cestodes has not been determined, but it may be the result of interaction with phospholipids in the integument, causing ion fluxes of sodium, potassium, and calcium. At low concentrations in vitro, the drug appears to impair sucker function and stimulates the worm's motility. At higher concentrations in vitro, praziquantel increases (irreversibly at very high concentrations) the contraction of the worm's strobilla (chain of proglottids). In addition, praziquantel causes irreversible focal vacuolization with subsequent cestodal disintegration at specific sites of the cestodal integument.

In schistosomes and trematodes, praziquantel directly kills the parasite, possibly by increasing calcium ion flux into the worm. Focal vacuolization of the integument follows, and the parasite is phagocytized by the host.

Pharmacokinetics

Following eprinomectin 0.4 mg/kg IV to cats, the average maximum plasma concentration (C_{max}) of eprinomectin $B1_a$ was 503 ng/mL. The drug distributed widely, with a steady-state volume of distribution of 2.39 L/kg and protein binding greater than 99%. Terminal elimination half-life (t½) was 23.1 hours. Eprinomectin was not conjugated in liver microsomal incubates, and although metabolism appeared to correlate with relative CYP3A4 activity, the drug undergoes minimal biotransformation and is excreted primarily in the feces as unchanged drug. In cats receiving eprinomectin 0.5 mg/kg in a multi-component transdermal solution, C_{max} averaged 20.1 ng/mL and was reached on average after 24 hours. Slow topical absorption prolonged its terminal half-life (114 hours). Topical bioavailability was 31%. Total drug exposure after topical application was proportionate to the dose administered.[9] An in vitro study determined that eprinomectin interacts with P-glycoprotein similar to ivermectin.[10]

Praziquantel is distributed throughout the body. It crosses the intestinal wall and blood–brain barrier into the CNS. Praziquantel is metabolized in the liver via CYP3A enzymes to metabolites of unknown activity. It is excreted primarily in the urine; elimination half-life is ≈3 hours in dogs.

Contraindications/Precautions/Warnings

Eprinomectin/praziquantel transdermal solution is contraindicated in patients with a known hypersensitivity to eprinomectin or praziquantel. The manufacturer does not recommend using eprinomectin/praziquantel transdermal solution in cats or kittens less than 7 weeks old or weighing less than 0.8 kg (1.8 lb). Do not administer the transdermal solution orally. In humans, praziquantel is contraindicated in patients that are hypersensitive to the drug, and it should not be administered to patients with a history of epilepsy.

Adverse Effects

Eprinomectin/praziquantel transdermal solution appears to be well tolerated. Vomiting, inappetence, and lethargy have been noted. Excessive salivation commonly occurs if cats lick the application site. Skin reactions (eg, itching, hair clumping, hair loss) may occur uncommonly after application of eprinomectin/praziquantel transdermal solution but are usually mild and temporary. Transient ataxia, disorientation, lethargy, and pupil dilation also have been noted at higher doses.

In cats, adverse effects were quite rare (less than 2%) in field trials using oral praziquantel, with salivation and diarrhea being reported.

Reproductive/Nursing Safety

Safe use of eprinomectin/praziquantel transdermal solution in breeding or pregnant cats has not been tested; however, praziquantel is considered safe to use during pregnancy. Praziquantel did not impair fertility or reproductive performance in rats at doses up to 300 mg/kg/day. The same dosage produced no harm to rabbit or rat fetuses.[11]

Safe use of eprinomectin/praziquantel transdermal solution in lactating cats has not been tested. Praziquantel appears in maternal milk at a concentration of ≈25% of that in maternal serum, and in humans it is recommended that women avoid nursing on the day of treatment and the subsequent 72 hours.[11]

Because safety has not been established in animals, this drug should only be used when the maternal benefits outweigh the potential risks to offspring.

Overdose/Acute Toxicity

Kittens that were exposed to 3 times and 5 times the eprinomectin/praziquantel transdermal solution label doses experienced ataxia, disorientation, lethargy, and pupil dilation that lasted 12 to 24 hours before recovering completely. Cats receiving 3 times the label dose orally immediately exhibited excessive salivation; vomiting and lethargy also were noted. Safety was also demonstrated when a similar transdermal solution was given to kittens at up to 15 times the label dose every 4 weeks for 6 treatments, and in adult cats receiving 5 times the label dose every 2 weeks for 3 treatments.[7]

Praziquantel has a wide margin of safety. In rats and mice, the oral LD_{50} is at least 2 g/kg. An oral LD_{50} could not be determined in dogs, as at doses greater than 200 mg/kg, the drug induced vomiting. Parenteral doses of 50 – 100 mg/kg in cats caused transient ataxia and depression; injected doses at 200 mg/kg were lethal in cats.

For patients that have experienced or are suspected to have experienced an overdose, consultation with a 24-hour poison control center specializing in providing veterinary-specific information is recommended. For general information related to overdose and toxin exposures, as well as contact information for poison control centers, refer to ***Appendix***.

Drug Interactions

Eprinomectin is a P-glycoprotein substrate and inhibitor.[10] Praziquantel is a substrate of CYP 3A4 in humans. The following drug interactions either have been reported or are theoretical in humans or animals receiving eprinomectin or praziquantel and may be of significance in veterinary patients. Unless otherwise noted, use together is not necessarily contraindicated, but veterinarians should weigh the potential risks and perform additional monitoring when appropriate.

- **ALBENDAZOLE**: Praziquantel may increase albendazole sulphoxide concentration.
- **CIMETIDINE**: May increase the serum concentration of praziquantel
- **CYP3A4 INDUCERS** (eg, **dexamethasone, phenobarbital, rifampin**): May decrease eprinomectin and/or praziquantel concentrations. In humans, it is recommended to discontinue rifampin 4 weeks prior to praziquantel administration.

- **CYP3A4 Inhibitors** (eg, **amiodarone, clarithromycin, fluoxetine, itraconazole, ketoconazole, verapamil**): May increase eprinomectin and/or praziquantel concentrations
- **Grapefruit Juice**: Can significantly increase praziquantel serum concentrations in beagles.[12] May increase eprinomectin concentrations
- **P-Glycoprotein Inhibitors** (eg, **amiodarone, cyclosporine, digoxin, itraconazole, spironolactone**): May increase eprinomectin concentrations
- **P-Glycoprotein Substrates** (eg, **cyclosporine, doxorubicin, mitoxantrone, phenothiazines, vinca alkaloids**): Eprinomectin may inhibit P-glycoprotein and increase exposure to P-glycoprotein substrates.

Laboratory Considerations

- None noted

Dosages

CATS:

Prevention of heartworm disease, and for the treatment and control of roundworms, hookworms, and tapeworms (label dosage; FDA-approved): A minimum of 0.12 mL/kg (0.055 mL/lb), which delivers a minimum dose of eprinomectin 0.5 mg/kg (0.23 mg/lb) and praziquantel 10 mg/kg (4.55 mg/lb), is administered topically.[13] For the treatment of roundworms, hookworms, and tapeworms, administer once. For heartworm prevention, and for the control of roundworms, hookworms, and tapeworms, apply once monthly. Follow dosing table (see below) provided by the manufacturer. Part the hair and apply the entire applicator contents directly on the skin in 1 spot on the midline of the neck between the base of the skull and the shoulder blades. Cats weighing greater than 7.5 kg (16.5 lb) will require application of more than 1 unit.

Body weight in kg (lb)	Volume (mL)	Eprinomectin (mg)	Praziquantel (mg)
0.8-2.5 (1.8-5.5)	0.3	1.2	24.9
2.5-7.5 (5.6-16.5)	0.9	3.6	74.7
7.5-10 (16.6-22)	0.3 + 0.9	4.8	99.6
10-15 (22.1-33)	0.9 + 0.9	7.2	149.4

Monitoring

- Clinical efficacy; adverse effects

Client Information

- Dead tapeworms are typically not seen in feces after treatment.
- For heartworm prevention: This medicine may be administered year-round, or, at a minimum, treatment should start 1 month before the cat's first expected exposure to mosquitoes and continue at monthly intervals until at least 1 month after the cat's last exposure to mosquitoes. If a dose is missed and a 30-day interval between doses is exceeded, administer immediately and resume the monthly dosing schedule.
- Cats commonly scratch or groom the application site. Ingested product can cause excessive salivation or drooling, vomiting, and lack of energy.
- Apply this medicine directly to the skin, between the base of the skull and the shoulder blades where the cat cannot lick. Part the hair and place the tip of the applicator against the cat's skin during application. If 2 applicators are required, apply both in the same spot. Prevent treated cat and other cats in the household from grooming the application site. Avoid contact of the medicine with the cat's eyes.
- Caregivers should avoid contact with the application site for 5 hours following treatment and wash their hands after applying the product. If the product accidentally gets into the eyes, flush thoroughly with water. In case of accidental ingestion, or if skin or eye irritation occurs, contact a poison control center or physician for treatment advice.

Chemistry/Synonyms

Eprinomectin is a member of the avermectin class of antiparasitic agents, and the transdermal solution contains a mixture of eprinomectin $B1_a$ and $B1_b$. It is also known as MK-397, ML-635, or 4-epi-acetylamino-4-deoxy-avermectin B1.

A prazinoisoquinoline-derivative anthelmintic, praziquantel occurs as a white to practically white, hygroscopic, bitter tasting crystalline powder, either odorless or having a faint odor. It is very slightly soluble in water and freely soluble in alcohol. Praziquantel may also be known as EMBAY-8440 or praziquantelum, and it is sold under many trade names.

Eprinomectin/praziquantel transdermal solution is also known as *Centragard*®. In other countries, transdermal solutions containing eprinomectin/praziquantel combinations include *BROADLINE*® (also contains fipronil and S-methoprene and may be known as ML-635) and *NexGard*® *Combo* (also contains esafoxolaner).

Storage/Stability

Eprinomectin/praziquantel transdermal solution should be stored protected from light at or below 30°C (86°F) with excursions permitted to 40°C (104°F). Keep out of reach of children.

Compatibility/Compounding Considerations

No information noted

Dosage Forms/Regulatory Status

VETERINARY-LABELED PRODUCTS:

Eprinomectin/Praziquantel Transdermal Solution: Eprinomectin 4 mg/mL and praziquantel 83 mg/mL in 0.3- and 0.9-mL applicators; *Centragard*®; (Rx). For use on cats and kittens 7 weeks of age or older weighing at least 0.8 kg (1.8 lb). NADA #141-492

HUMAN-LABELED PRODUCTS: NONE

References

For the complete list of references, see **wiley.com/go/budde/plumb**

Eprinomectin

(e-pri-no-***mek***-tin) *Eprinex®; LongRange®*

Avermectin Antiparasitic Agent

Prescriber Highlights

- Topically applied (pour-on) or extended-release injection (for cattle on pasture only) avermectin antiparasiticide
- When pour-on is used as labeled, there are no milk or meat withdrawal times required.
- Injectable product has a 48-day slaughter withdrawal and specific syringe compatibilities. It must be administered SC in front of the shoulder (not for IV or IM use).
- Adverse effects of the pour-on product are rare but may include anorexia, hypogalactia, pruritus, and alopecia.
- Adverse effects of the injectable product include injection site reactions including granulomas and necrosis.

Uses/Indications

In cattle, topical eprinomectin is indicated for the treatment and control of the following:

- GI roundworms: *Haemonchus placei* (adult and L4 stages), *Ostertagia ostertagi* (L4), *Trichostrongylus axei, Trichostrongylus colubriformis, Trichostrongylus longispicularis* (adults only), *Cooperia oncophora, Cooperia punctate, Cooperia surnabada, Nematodirus helvetianus, Oesophagostomum radiatum, Bunostomum phlebotomum, Strongyloides papillosus* (adults only), and *Trichuris* spp (adults only)

- Cattle grubs: *Hypoderma lineatum, Hypoderma bovis* (all parasitic stages)
- Lungworms: *Dictyocaulus viviparus* (adults and L4, for 21 days after treatment)
- Lice: *Damalinia bovis, Linognathus vituli, Haematopinus eurysterus, Solenopotes capillatus*
- Mange mites: *Chorioptes bovis, Sarcoptes scabiei*
- Horn flies: *Haematobia irritans* (for 7 days after treatment)

The extended-release eprinomectin 5% injection is indicated for the treatment and control of internal and external parasites (eg, susceptible GI roundworms, grubs, lungworms, mites) in cattle on pasture with persistent effectiveness. It has also shown efficacy for controlling *Rhipichephalus microplus* ticks.[1,2] Although one study reported the efficacy of SC eprinomectin in pastured dairy heifers,[3] it is not approved for use in female dairy cattle 20 months of age or older, including dry dairy cows, calves to be processed for veal, breeding bulls, calves less than 3 months of age, or cattle managed in feedlots or under intensive rotational grazing.

Various eprinomectin products are approved for use in sheep and goats in other countries. Topical eprinomectin has demonstrated efficacy against GI nematodes in lactating and nonlactating goats.[4–6] However, high variability in pharmacokinetic parameters and low bioavailability from this route of administration causes concern for suboptimal efficacy at recommended doses. SC administration in nonlactating goats at 0.2 mg/kg and 0.4 mg/kg had over 97.8% efficacy against *Haemonchus contortus and Trichostrongylus colubriformis*.[7] Eprinomectin has also shown efficacy against pulmonary and GI nematodes in sheep.[8] Small studies have shown a beneficial effect on milk yield when given SC at 0.2 mg/kg[9] or topically at 1 mg/kg.[10]

Topical eprinomectin may be useful in an extra-label manner for the topical treatment of psoroptic mange (*Psoroptes equi*) in horses or ear mites (*Psoroptes cuniculi*) in rabbits. One small study (6 subjects) showed a partial response when rabbits were dosed at 5 mg/kg topically, twice at 14-day intervals.[11]

Pharmacology/Actions

Eprinomectin binds selectively to glutamate-gated chloride ion channels that occur in invertebrate nerve and muscle cells. This leads to an increase in cell membrane permeability to chloride ions, causing paralysis and the death of the parasite. Like ivermectin, eprinomectin enhances the release of gamma-aminobutyric acid (GABA) at presynaptic neurons. GABA acts as an inhibitory neurotransmitter and blocks the postsynaptic stimulation of the adjacent neuron in nematodes or the muscle fiber in arthropods. These compounds are generally not toxic to mammals as they do not have glutamate-gated chloride channels and do not readily cross the blood–brain barrier.

Pharmacokinetics

When the injectable product is injected in cattle as labeled, a polymeric PLGA matrix is formed, allowing a gradual release of eprinomectin into the systemic circulation. Effective plasma concentrations may persist for at least 100 days, with an initial maximum eprinomectin concentration (C_{max}) reached within a few days after injection, followed by a second C_{max} ≈90 days later. A study comparing eprinomectin pharmacokinetic parameters of topical and long-acting injection administered to nonlactating dairy cattle demonstrated higher maximum eprinomectin concentration (C_{max}), longer half-life ($t_{½}$), and a greater area under the concentration-time curve with the long-acting injection. New world camelids experience a similar bi-phasic C_{max}. Administration of the pour-on formulation to goats prevented from grooming resulted in systemic absorption, with time to C_{max} noted at 1.1 days and $t_{½}$ of 4.18 days. Topical administration results in significantly lower systemic bioavailability in goats compared with cattle and has high variability between individuals.

Contraindications/Precautions/Warnings

The pour-on product must only be applied topically; do not give the pour-on orally or IV.

The injectable product's label states that "this product should not be used in other animal species" and that it is "not for intravenous or intramuscular use."

Underdosing and/or subtherapeutic concentrations of extended-release anthelmintic products are likely to encourage the development of parasite resistance. Resistance has been confirmed in *Haemonchus contortus* in geographic regions worldwide. Eprinomectin adversely affects fish and aquatic organisms; dispose of properly in an approved landfill or by incineration.[12–14]

Adverse Effects

Although no adverse reactions are listed in the pour-on product label, the FDA's Cumulative Adverse Drug Experience database for topical administration on cattle lists the 3 most common adverse effects as ineffective parasite control, anorexia, and udder hypogalactia.[15] It must be noted that incidence rates are not listed, and a causal effect is not established for listings in this database. Foreign labels report very rare incidences of pruritis and alopecia.[14]

The injectable product is likely to cause tissue damage at the site of injection, including possible granulomas and necrosis. Reactions have disappeared without treatment. Local tissue reaction may result in trim loss of edible tissue at slaughter. Observe cattle for injection site reactions.[13]

Reproductive/Nursing Safety

The label states that the injection is not for use in bulls, as reproductive safety testing has not been conducted in males intended for breeding or males actively breeding. Eprinomectin should not be used in calves less than 3 months of age because safety testing has not been conducted in calves in this age group. Administration at 3 times the recommended therapeutic dose had no adverse reproductive effects on beef cows at all stages of breeding, their pregnancy, or on their calves.

It is likely safe to use in nursing animals, but it is not approved for use in lactating dairy cattle.

Overdose/Acute Toxicity

For the pour-on formulation, calves given up to 5 times the recommended dosage showed no signs of adverse effects. One subject (of 6) showed signs of mydriasis when given 10 times the normal dose. The sustained-release injectable given at 3 to 5 times the recommended dose resulted in a statistically significant reduction in average weight gain when compared with the group tested at label dose. Treatment-related lesions observed in most cattle administered the product included swelling, hyperemia, or necrosis in the SC tissue of the skin.

For patients that have experienced or are suspected of having experienced an overdose, consultation with a 24-hour poison consultation center specializing in providing veterinary-specific information is recommended. For general information related to overdose and toxin exposures, as well as contact information for poison control centers, refer to ***Appendix.***

Drug Interactions

The following drug interactions either have been reported or are theoretical in humans or animals receiving eprinomectin and may be of significance in veterinary patients. Unless otherwise noted, use together is not necessarily contraindicated, but weigh the potential risks and perform additional monitoring when appropriate.

- **Meloxicam**: Coadministration of eprinomectin and meloxicam in sheep resulted in increased systemic meloxicam concentrations due to the inhibition of ABCG2 transporters.[16]
- **P-Glycoprotein Inhibitors** (eg, **doxycycline**[17]): Eprinomectin has high affinity for P-glycoprotein. Use caution when administering with known P-gp inhibitors.

Dosages

HORSES:

Psoroptic (*Psoroptes equi*) mange (extra-label): 0.5 mg/kg topically once weekly for 4 treatments. The study authors suggest getting informed consent before use.[18]

CATTLE:

Labeled indications (pour-on; FDA-approved): 0.5 mg/kg (1 mL per 10 kg [22 lb]) applied topically along the backline in a narrow strip from the withers to the tailhead. For most effective results against grubs, treat cattle as soon as possible after the end of the heel fly (ie, warble fly) season.[19]

Labeled indications (extended-release injection; FDA-approved): 1 mg/kg (1 mL per 50 kg [110 lb]) SC under the loose skin in front of the shoulder. Divide doses greater than 10 mL between 2 injection sites. Inject using a 16- or 18-gauge, ½- to ¾-inch needle. See additional information on syringe compatibility and automatic syringes in the ***Compatibility/Compounding Considerations*** section below.[13] For most effective results against grubs, treat cattle as soon as possible after the end of the heel fly (ie, warble fly) season.

SHEEP/GOATS:

GI nematodes in nonlactating goats (extra-label): 0.2 – 0.4 mg/kg SC[7]

GI and pulmonary nematodes in sheep and goats (injection; extra-label): 0.2 mg/kg SC[20,21]

GI and pulmonary nematodes in sheep and goats (pour-on; extra-label): 1 mg/kg topically in a narrow strip from the withers to the tailhead[8]

NOTE: This dose may be suboptimal in goats due to high variability and low bioavailability of topical formulations.[22]

CAMELIDS:

Chorioptic mange (extra-label): Data conflict: 0.5 mg/kg topically once weekly for 4 weeks was effective in one field study,[23] but another study found a 10-week treatment to be ineffective.[24]

Client Information

For the pour-on formulation:

- When eprinomectin is used as labeled, there are no milk or meat withdrawal times required.
- Weather conditions (including rainfall) during administration do not affect efficacy.
- Do not apply this medicine to the backline if the animal is covered with mud or manure.
- Dispose of containers in an approved landfill or by incineration; do not contaminate water, as eprinomectin may adversely affect fish and aquatic organisms.

For the injectable formulation:

- 48-day withdrawal time
- Several restrictions on use. Eprinomectin is not approved for bulls, veal calves, or dairy cattle.
- Specific syringes required. Must be administered under the skin in front of the shoulder. Sanitize the injection site and administer with clean, properly disinfected needles.
- Observe for injection site reactions. If suspected, consult your veterinarian.

Chemistry/Synonyms

Eprinomectin is a member of the avermectin class of antiparasitic agents. It is also known as MK-397 or 4-epi-acetylamino-4-deoxy-avermectin B1.

Storage/Stability

Store the commercially available pour-on product at 30°C (86°F) or less, protected from light. Brief excursions up to 40°C (104°F) are permitted but should be minimized.

Store the injectable at 25°C (77°F) with excursions permitted between 15°C and 30°C (59°F and 86°F). Protect it from light. Do not store in automatic syringe equipment.

Compatibility/Compounding Considerations

For the injectable formulation: 100 mL bottle: Use only polypropylene syringes with the 100 mL bottle size. Not for use with polycarbonate syringe material. If syringe material is not known, contact the syringe manufacturer prior to use for identification. Do not use beyond 3 months after the stopper has been punctured. Discard bottle after 15 stopper punctures.

250 mL and 500 mL bottle sizes: Use only automatic syringe equipment provided by Merial. To obtain **compatible** equipment, contact Merial at 1-888-637-4251 or your veterinarian; should not be stored (left) in automatic syringe equipment. Automatic syringe equipment should be thoroughly cleaned after each use. Discard bottle after one stopper puncture with a draw-off spike. No special handling or protective clothing is necessary.

Dosage Forms/Regulatory Status

VETERINARY-LABELED PRODUCTS:

Eprinomectin Topical (Pour-On) Solution: 5 mg/mL in 250 mL/8.5 fl oz and 1 L/33.8 fl oz bottle with a squeeze-measure-pour-system, or a 2.5 L/84.5 fl oz and 5 L/169 fl oz collapsible pack or 20 L/ 676 oz container for use with appropriate automatic dosing equipment; *Eprinex*®, generic; (OTC). FDA-approved for use in beef or dairy cattle of all ages; not for use in calves to be processed for veal.

Eprinomectin 5% (50 mg/mL) Sustained-release Injectable: In 100, 250, and 500 mL bottles; *LongRange*®; (Rx). FDA-approved for use in cattle on pasture with persistent effectiveness. It is not approved for use in female dairy cattle 20 months of age or older, including dry dairy cows; calves to be processed for veal; breeding bulls; calves less than 3 months of age; or cattle managed in feedlots or under intensive rotational grazing. Animals intended for human consumption must not be slaughtered within 48 days of the last treatment. A withdrawal period has not been established for pre-ruminating calves. NADA #141-327

HUMAN-LABELED PRODUCTS: NONE

References

For the complete list of references, see **wiley.com/go/budde/plumb**

Epsiprantel

(ep-si-***pran***-tel) *Cestex*®

Anticestodal Antiparasitic Agent

Prescriber Highlights

- ► Anticestodal for dogs and cats 7 weeks of age and older
- ► Limited oral absorption results in high concentration of the drug within the GI tract (ie, at the site of action).
- ► Adverse effects are uncommon due to limited oral absorption.
- ► Resistance to epsiprantel has been demonstrated in *Dipylidium caninum*.

Uses/Indications

Epsiprantel is FDA-approved for the removal of *Dipylidium caninum* and *Taenia pisiformis* in dogs, and *Dipylidium caninum* and *Taenia taeniaeformis* in cats. For *D caninum*, flea and louse control are mandatory, or tapeworm reinfestation is likely. Epsiprantel has demonstrated extra-label efficacy against adult stages of *Echinococcus* spp in dogs and cats.[1-3]

Pharmacology/Actions

Epsiprantel's exact mechanism of action against cestodes has not been determined. The tapeworm's ability to regulate calcium is apparently affected, causing tetany and disruption of attachment to the host. Alteration to the integument makes the worm vulnerable to digestion by the host animal. Isolated cases of resistance to epsiprantel have been demonstrated in *Dipylidium caninum*.[4]

Pharmacokinetics

Epsiprantel is absorbed poorly after oral administration. The bulk of the drug remains within the GI tract and is eliminated unchanged in the feces. Less than 0.1% of the drug is recovered in the urine after dosing. No metabolites have been identified.

Contraindications/Precautions/Warnings

There are no labeled contraindications to this drug. Epsiprantel should be considered contraindicated in patients hypersensitive to it. Do not use in puppies or kittens less than 7 weeks of age.

Adverse Effects

Adverse effects appear to be rare when epsiprantel is used at the labeled dosage.

Reproductive/Nursing Safety

Safety for use in pregnant, lactating, or breeding animals has not been determined, but adverse effects to the offspring would be highly unlikely because the drug is so poorly absorbed.

Overdose/Acute Toxicity

Acute toxicity resulting from an inadvertent overdose is highly unlikely. Dosages of up to 500 mg/kg (≈90 times recommended dose) given to dogs once daily for 14 days resulted in isolated instances of vomiting, increased alkaline phosphatase (ALP), and leukopenia. Dosages as high as 110 mg/kg (20 times recommended dose) given once daily for 4 days resulted in trembling and vomiting in some of the kittens tested. Dosages of 16.5 mg/kg (3 times recommended dose) given once daily for 3 days produced no adverse effects in adult greyhounds or in 7-week-old puppies. Dosages up to 13.75 mg/kg (2.5 times recommended dose) given once daily for 3 days produced no adverse effects in cats 4 to 5 months of age.[5]

For patients that have experienced or are suspected to have experienced an overdose, consultation with a 24-hour poison consultation center specializing in providing veterinary-specific information is recommended. For general information related to overdose and toxin exposures, as well as contact information for poison control centers, refer to ***Appendix***.

Drug Interactions

- None reported; theoretically, prokinetic agents or fast-acting laxatives may reduce the drug's efficacy.

Laboratory Considerations

- None reported

Dosages

DOGS:

Treatment (removal) of tapeworms – *Dipylidium caninum* and *Taenia pisiformis* (label dosage; FDA-approved): 5.5 mg/kg PO once; round up to the next larger tablet size. For dogs over 46 kg (101 lb), round up to the next whole tablet combination.[5]

Treatment (removal) of *Echinococcus* spp (extra-label): 5 – 7.5 mg/kg PO once.[1-3] In one study,[3] total worm clearance occurred only in dogs given the higher dose.

CATS:

Treatment (removal) of tapeworms – *Dipylidium caninum* and *Taenia taeniaeformis* (label dosage; FDA-approved): 2.75 mg/kg PO once. Cats up to 4.5 kg (10 lb) should receive one 12.5 mg tablet; cats weighing 4.9 kg to 9 kg (11 to 20 lb) should receive one 25 mg tablet[5]

Treatment (removal) *Echinococcus multiocularis* (extra-label): 2.7 – 5.5 mg/kg PO once[2]

Monitoring

- Clinical efficacy

Client Information

- Oral medicine for treating tapeworms in dogs and cats
- Give this medicine with food
- Adverse effects are rare.
- Because the tapeworm may be partially or completely digested, worm fragments may not be seen in the feces after treatment.
- A single dose is usually effective. Talk with your veterinarian about measures (such as flea protection) that can be taken to prevent reinfection.

Chemistry/Synonyms

A pyrazino-benzazepine oral cestocide, epsiprantel occurs as a white powder that is sparingly soluble in water.

Epsiprantel may also be known as BRL-38705 or *Cestex*®.

Storage/Stability

Tablets should be stored at room temperature 20°C to 25°C (68°F-77°F) with excursions between 15°C to 30°C (59°F-86°F).

Compatibility/Compounding Considerations

No specific information noted

Dosage Forms/Regulatory Status

VETERINARY-LABELED PRODUCTS:

Epsiprantel Oral Tablets (film-coated): 12.5 mg, 25 mg, 50 mg, and 100 mg; *Cestex*®; (Rx). NADA #140-893

HUMAN-APPROVED PRODUCTS: NONE

References

For the complete list of references, see **wiley.com/go/budde/plumb**

Ergocalciferol

Vitamin D2

(er-goh-kal-***sif***-er-ole) *Drisdol*®

Vitamin D Analogue

Prescriber Highlights

- ► May be used to treat hypocalcemia associated with hypoparathyroidism, but calcitriol usually recommended first
- ► Less expensive than dihydrotachysterol (DHT) or calcitriol, but large initial doses are required, effects take longer to be seen, and if hypercalcemia develops, it takes longer (up to 18 weeks) to recover from

Uses/Indications

Ergocalciferol is sometimes used in dogs or cats to treat hypocalcemia secondary to parathyroid gland failure, particularly when dihydrotachysterol or calcitriol are too expensive for the owner. As compared with those agents, ergocalciferol takes longer to have a maximal effect on serum calcium. Additionally, if hypercalcemia should develop, ergocalciferol's effects persist longer than either calcitriol or dihydrotachysterol.

Pharmacology/Actions

Ergocalciferol is first hydroxylated in the liver to 25-hydroxyvitamin D (has some activity) and then activated in the kidneys to 1,25-dihydroxyvitamin D, the primary active form of the drug. Vitamin D is considered a hormone and, in conjunction with parathormone (PTH) and calcitonin, regulates calcium homeostasis in the body. Active analogues (or metabolites) of vitamin D enhance calcium and phosphate absorption from the GI tract, promote reabsorption of calcium by the renal tubules, and increase the rate of accretion and resorption of minerals in bone. Ergocalciferol has ≈1/10 the activity of cholecalciferol for enhancing intestinal calcium absorption.

Pharmacokinetics

Specific pharmacokinetic values for dogs and cats were not located. The following information (human-based) generally applies: In the presence of bile salts, ergocalciferol is absorbed from the small intestine; after conversion to its 25-hydroxylated form in the liver and kidneys, it is stored in the liver and fat. Cats do not appear to convert ergocalciferol to its 25-hydroxylate form as well as cholecalciferol. Several days of therapy may be required until steady-state volume of distribution is achieved. In dogs and cats, maximal effect on calcium homeostasis is usually noted from 5 to 21 days after treatment begins; effects may persist for up to 18 weeks once treatment is discontinued.[1]

Contraindications/Precautions/Warnings

Ergocalciferol, at therapeutic dosages, is contraindicated in patients with hypercalcemia, vitamin D toxicity, malabsorption syndrome, or abnormal sensitivity to the effects of vitamin D. It should be used with extreme caution in patients with hyperphosphatemia. As patients with kidney dysfunction may not convert ergocalciferol into the primary active metabolite, calcitriol or DHT would be preferred because they do not require activation by the kidney. Chronic therapy should not be initiated unless owners are willing to commit to ongoing patient monitoring.

Adverse Effects

The primary concern with using ergocalciferol is exceeding the dosage with resultant hypercalcemia and, potentially, hyperphosphatemia or nephrocalcinosis. Hypercalcemia can persist for weeks to months.

Reproductive/Nursing Safety

Hypervitaminosis D in pregnant females has been implicated in causing teratogenic effects in animals and infants. Potential benefits of therapy must be weighed against the risks if considering use in pregnant dogs or cats.

As large doses of vitamin D can be excreted into milk, consider using milk replacer in offspring of dams receiving therapeutic dosages of ergocalciferol.

Because safety has not been established in animals, this drug should only be used when the maternal benefits outweigh the potential risks to offspring.

Overdose/Acute Toxicity

Because of the potential serious ramifications of overdoses, contacting an animal poison control center is strongly recommended. The toxic acute oral dose of ergocalciferol in dogs is reported as 4 mg/kg (160,000 units/kg).[2]

Acute ingestions should be managed using established protocols for GI decontamination if done within 6 hours of ingestion. Orally administered mineral oil may reduce absorption and enhance fecal elimination. Cholestyramine may also be beneficial.

Hypercalcemia secondary to chronic dosing of ergocalciferol should be treated by first temporarily discontinuing the drug and exogenous calcium therapy. If hypercalcemia is severe, furosemide, calcium-free IV fluids (eg, normal saline), urine acidification, bisphosphonates, and corticosteroids may be employed. Because of the long duration of action of ergocalciferol (potentially up to 18 weeks), hypercalcemia may persist. Restart ergocalciferol therapy (if desired) at a reduced dosage only when serum calcium concentrations return to the normal range. Diligent monitoring (eg, serum PTH, ionized calcium, phosphorus, vitamin D concentrations, renal function) is required.

For patients that have experienced or are suspected to have experienced an overdose, consultation with a 24-hour poison consultation center specializing in providing veterinary-specific information is recommended. For general information related to overdose and toxin exposures, as well as contact information for poison control centers, refer to ***Appendix***.

Drug Interactions

The following drug interactions have either been reported or are theoretical in humans or animals receiving ergocalciferol and may be of significance in veterinary patients. Unless otherwise noted, use together is not necessarily contraindicated, but weigh the potential risks and perform additional monitoring when appropriate.

- CIMETIDINE: May result in decreased vitamin D exposure
- CHOLESTYRAMINE: May decrease vitamin D absorption
- CORTICOSTEROIDS (eg, **dexamethasone, prednis(ol)one**): Can reduce the effects of vitamin D
- DIGOXIN or VERAPAMIL: Patients on these drugs are sensitive to the effects of hypercalcemia; intensified monitoring is required
- MINERAL OIL: May reduce the amount of ergocalciferol absorbed
- PHENOBARBITAL: May result in decreased systemic vitamin D exposure
- THIAZIDE DIURETICS (eg, **hydrochlorothiazide**): May cause hypercalcemia when given in conjunction with vitamin D

Laboratory Considerations

- **Serum cholesterol** levels may be falsely elevated by vitamin D analogues when using the Zlatkis-Zak reaction for determination.

Dosages

DOGS/CATS:

Maintenance therapy of parathyroid failure after using parenteral calcium to control hypocalcemic tetany (extra-label): Calcitriol is generally preferred due to a more rapid effect and a risk of overshooting the ergocalciferol dosage leading to persistent hypercalcemia; however, ergocalciferol can be a less expensive option. The ergocalciferol dosage is 4000 – 6000 units/kg PO once daily. Effect is usually seen between 5 and 14 days after initiation of treatment. After 1 to 5 days, parenteral calcium can usually be discontinued. Patient should remain hospitalized until serum calcium concentration remains between 8 and 10 mg/dL without parenteral calcium support. Continue ergocalciferol but administer every other day. Weekly serum calcium concentrations should be measured and ergocalciferol dosage adjusted to maintain serum calcium concentrations between 8 and 9.5 mg/dL. Maintenance dosages usually range from 1000 – 2000 units/kg PO once daily to once weekly. Goal is to prevent hypocalcemic tetany, but not induce hypercalcemia.[3] Once animal is stable, monthly rechecks for 6 months are strongly advised; then every 2 to 3 months thereafter.[1,3]

Monitoring

- See dosage information above.

Client Information

- Using vitamin D products may require lifelong treatment and regular laboratory monitoring.

- Although this agent can be used to treat low calcium concentrations, excessive ergocalciferol doses can cause calcium concentrations in the blood to become too high. This effect can last for many weeks, even after the medication is discontinued.

Chemistry/Synonyms

Ergocalciferol is obtained by irradiating (with ultraviolet light) ergosterol, a sterol present in fungi and yeasts. It occurs as white or almost white crystals or yellowish crystalline powder and is practically insoluble in water but is soluble in fatty oils. One mg of ergocalciferol provides 40,000 units of vitamin D activity.

Ergocalciferol may be known as calciferol, vitamin D_2, viosterol, activated ergosterol, or irradiated ergosterol; there are many international trade names.

Storage/Stability

Ergocalciferol is sensitive to light, heat, and air. Store capsules or liquid at room temperature (15°C-30°C [59°F-86°F]) and protect from light.

Compatibility/Compounding Considerations

No specific information noted

Dosage Forms/Regulatory Status

VETERINARY-LABELED PRODUCTS: NONE

HUMAN-LABELED PRODUCTS:

Calciferol® Drops, generic; (OTC)

Ergocalciferol Oral Capsules: 50,000 units (1.25 mg); *Drisdol®*, generic; (Rx)

Ergocalciferol Oral Tablets: 400 units and 2000 units; generic; (Rx)

Ergocalciferol Oral Solution: 8000 units/mL in 60 mL bottles; generic; (Rx)

References

For the complete list of references, see **wiley.com/go/budde/plumb**

Ertapenem

(er-ta-***pen***-um) *Invanz®*

Carbapenem Antibiotic

Prescriber Highlights

- Carbapenem antibiotic similar to imipenem and meropenem but with a narrower spectrum of activity
- Not effective against *Pseudomonas* spp or *Acinetobacter* spp
- Rarely used in veterinary medicine; must be considered investigational, as there is limited information available for use in dogs and cats
- Use in veterinary medicine is controversial because of the drug's importance in human medicine. Veterinary infectious disease specialists should be consulted prior to treatment. Use should be reserved for infections with confirmed susceptibility that are resistant to lower-tier options.

Uses/Indications

Because ertapenem is used for multidrug-resistant infections in humans, its use in veterinary medicine should be reserved for confirmed infections where culture and susceptibility testing demonstrate resistance to all other options, the infection is considered treatable, and consultation with an infectious disease expert has concluded that ertapenem is a viable and reasonable treatment.[1,2] Empirical use should be discouraged. If a carbapenem is required, the use of meropenem or imipenem would be preferred because of greater information available regarding the use of these antibiotics in animals.

Ertapenem may be useful in treating resistant gram-negative bacterial infections, particularly when aminoglycoside use would be risky (eg, renal failure) or not effective (eg, resistance or CNS infections). Although ertapenem has a broad spectrum of antibacterial activity, it is not active against *Pseudomonas aeruginosa*. It potentially could be useful against mixed anaerobic and gram-negative aerobic infections when *Pseudomonas spp* is not considered a likely pathogen.

The World Health Organization (WHO) has designated ertapenem as a Critically Important, High Priority antimicrobial for human medicine.[3]

Pharmacology/Actions

Ertapenem is a carbapenem antibiotic similar to imipenem and meropenem. Like other beta-lactams, it inhibits bacterial cell wall synthesis, is time-dependent, and is usually bactericidal.

Ertapenem has a broad antibacterial spectrum similar to that of imipenem, but it is more active against Enterobacteriaceae and anaerobes. It has equivalent activity against gram-positive bacteria and minimal activity against *Pseudomonas aeruginosa* and *Acinetobacter* spp. Methicillin-resistant *Staphylococcus* spp and *Enterococcus faecium* are resistant to the effects of ertapenem. Because ertapenem (like meropenem) is more stable than imipenem to renal dehydropeptidase I, it does not require the addition of cilastatin to inhibit that enzyme.

Pharmacokinetics

No pharmacokinetic data have been published for dogs or cats. Anecdotally, it has been reported that the pharmacokinetics in dogs and cats do not mimic those values seen in humans.

In humans, ertapenem must be administered parenterally as it is not appreciably absorbed after oral administration. Intramuscular bioavailability is about 90%, and peak plasma concentrations occur in ≈2.3 hours.[2] Ertapenem exhibits concentration-dependent binding to human plasma proteins. At plasma concentrations of less than 100 µg/mL, it is 95% bound; at 300 µg/mL, it is 85% bound. Ertapenem biotransformation is not dependent on hepatic mechanisms, as the major metabolite (inactive) is formed by hydrolysis of the beta-lactam ring. Approximately 80% of an IV dose is excreted in the urine, evenly split between inactive metabolites and an unchanged drug. Approximately. 10% is excreted in the feces. In young, healthy adults, the elimination half-life is about 4 hours and about 2.5 hours in pediatric patients.[2]

Contraindications/Precautions/Warnings

Ertapenem is contraindicated in patients that are hypersensitive to it and other carbapenems and in those patients that have developed anaphylaxis after receiving any beta-lactam antibiotic.[2] It is contraindicated in patients that are hypersensitive to lidocaine or other amide-type local anesthetics (if used IM with 1% lidocaine as the diluent).[2]

Consider the use of ertapenem investigational since it has not been widely used clinically in veterinary medicine and has little published information for its use in dogs or cats. See ***Uses/Indications***.

Adverse Effects

The adverse effect profile for ertapenem in dogs or cats is unknown. In humans, IV injection site reactions and diarrhea are the most common adverse effects.[2] Other GI effects (eg, nausea, vomiting), headache, or tachycardia have occasionally been reported. Rarely, hypersensitivity or CNS effects (eg, hallucinations, agitation, seizures) have been seen.

Reproductive/Nursing Safety

Ertapenem has been shown to cross the placenta in rats, but no teratogenic effects have been reported.[2]

Ertapenem is distributed into breast milk.

Because safety has not been established in animals, this drug should only be used when the maternal benefits outweigh the potential risks to offspring.

Overdose/Acute Toxicity

Clinical signs as a result of an overdose are unlikely. Humans receiving ertapenem 3 g IV had an increased incidence of nausea and diarrhea.[2] If an overdose occurs and adverse effects are noted, treat supportively.

For patients that have experienced or are suspected to have experienced an overdose, consultation with a 24-hour poison control center specializing in providing veterinary-specific information is recommended. For general information related to overdose and toxin exposures, as well as contact information for poison control centers, refer to ***Appendix.***

Drug Interactions

The following drug interactions have either been reported or are theoretical in humans or animals receiving ertapenem and may be of significance in veterinary patients. Unless otherwise noted, use together is not necessarily contraindicated, but weigh the potential risks and perform additional monitoring when appropriate.

- **Probenecid**: In humans, coadministration of ertapenem with probenecid can increase ertapenem AUC by 25% and the elimination half-life by about 20%.[2] Because of these relatively small effects, the manufacturer does not recommend using probenecid to extend the half-life of ertapenem.

Laboratory Considerations

- No specific laboratory interactions or concerns were noted.

Dosages

DOGS/CATS:

IMPORTANT: Because ertapenem is used for multidrug-resistant infections in humans, its use in veterinary medicine should be reserved for confirmed infections where culture and susceptibility testing demonstrate resistance to all other options, the infection is considered treatable, and consultation with an infectious disease expert has concluded that ertapenem is a viable and reasonable treatment.[1,2] Empirical use should be discouraged. If a carbapenem is required, the use of meropenem or imipenem would be preferred because of greater information available regarding the use of these antibiotics in animals.

Susceptible infections (extra-label): Anecdotally, 30 mg/kg IV or SC every 8 hours

Monitoring

- Clinical efficacy
- Adverse effects (eg, GI, neurotoxicity, hypersensitivity)
- In humans receiving ertapenem for a prolonged period, hepatic, hematopoietic, and renal function tests are suggested for periodic assessment.[2]

Client Information

- This medicine must be injected into a vein (*intravenous* [IV]; only done in the hospital) or under the skin (*subcutaneously [SC]*).
- Your veterinarian or pharmacist will give you all of the items you need to give the shots (eg, needles, syringes, diluent). If there is a need to mix the medicine before you give it, mix it exactly as your veterinarian or pharmacist tells you.
- Because of the need to inject this medicine, be sure you understand the correct amount to give the shot (*injection*), where to give it, and how to give it. Injections may sting when given. If your animal objects too much, your veterinarian may be able to give you something to mix with the liquid to help it sting less.

Chemistry/Synonyms

Ertapenem sodium is a synthetic 1-(beta) methyl carbapenem antibiotic that occurs as a white to off-white, hygroscopic, crystalline powder. It is soluble in water and normal saline. The 1 g injectable product contains ≈6 mEq of sodium and 175 mg of sodium bicarbonate (as an excipient).

Ertapenem may also be known as L-749345, ML-0826, ZD-4433, ertapenemum, or *Invanz*®.

Storage/Stability

Store unreconstituted ertapenem vials at temperatures at or below 25°C (77°F).[2] Once reconstituted and diluted in 0.9% sodium chloride for IV use, ertapenem is stable at room temperature for 6 hours. If refrigerated, it can be stored for 24 hours and used within 4 hours after removal from the refrigerator. Do not freeze reconstituted solutions.

Compatibility/Compounding Considerations

For IV use, reconstitute vial contents with 10 mL of water for injection, bacteriostatic water for injection, or 0.9% sodium chloride injection. After shaking to dissolve the powder, immediately transfer to a 50 mL bag of 0.9% sodium chloride. Do not use diluents containing dextrose.

The manufacturer advises to avoid mixing ertapenem with other medications or using IV solutions containing dextrose. Ertapenem is **compatible** with lactated Ringer's solution. Ertapenem is **Y-site compatible** with some medications; please consult a hospital pharmacist or an appropriate pharmacy reference for further information about Y-site compatibility of ertapenem.

Dosage Forms/Regulatory Status

VETERINARY-LABELED PRODUCTS: NONE

HUMAN-LABELED PRODUCTS:

Ertapenem Sodium Lyophilized Powder for Injection: 1 g (as 1.045 g ertapenem) in single-dose vials; *Invanz*®, generic; (Rx)

References

For the complete list of references, see **wiley.com/go/budde/plumb**

Erythromycin

(er-ith-roe-***mye***-sin) *Gallimycin*®

Macrolide Antibiotic; Prokinetic

*For ophthalmic use, refer to **Erythromycin, Ophthalmic***

Prescriber Highlights

- ► Prokinetic agent; effect occurs at doses much lower than required for treating bacterial infections
- ► May be used in combination with rifampin for treatment of *Rhodococcus equi* infections in foals
- ► Contraindications include use in rabbits, gerbils, guinea pigs, and hamsters; oral use in ruminants and adult horses at antimicrobial doses; and animals with a hypersensitivity to erythromycin or related drugs (eg, azithromycin, clarithromycin).
- ► Adverse effects include GI distress (with oral administration), pain on IM injection, thrombophlebitis (with IV administration), and hyperthermia in foals. Erythromycin may cause neurologic signs in dogs with *MDR1* mutation (also known as *ABCB1-1delta*).
- ► Many documented drug interactions

Uses/Indications

Erythromycin may be used for treatment of susceptible infections and as a prokinetic agent to increase gastric emptying. In healthy cats, erythromycin and metoclopramide demonstrated similar shortening of gastric emptying time.[1] Erythromycin may also be beneficial in treating reflux esophagitis, especially in cats,[2] and colonic motility disorders in dogs[3] and horses.[4, 5]

Erythromycin in combination with rifampin is used to treat foals with *Rhodococcus equi* infections. Erythromycin estolate[6] and a microencapsulated base[7] appear to be the most efficacious form of the drug in foals due to better absorption and less frequent adverse effects. Other macrolides (ie, clarithromycin or azithromycin ± rifampin/rifampicin)[8, 9] are more commonly used because they are better tolerated, have more favorable pharmacokinetics (eg, bioavailability, tissue penetration, half-life). The combination of clarithromycin/rifampin appears to be more effective than erythromycin/rifampin or azithromycin/rifampin for treating *R equi* infections in foals.[8]

Erythromycin is uncommonly used systemically because of its narrow spectrum of activity, high risk for adverse effects in hindgut fermenters (eg, adult horses, rabbits, hamsters), and increasing resistance in target bacteria.

A previously available injectable erythromycin product was approved for treatment of infections caused by susceptible organisms in cats, dogs, and cattle; however, it is no longer commonly used for this purpose in these species.

The World Health Organization (WHO) has designated erythromycin as a Critically Important, Highest Priority antimicrobial for human medicine. The Office International des Epizooties (OIE) has designated macrolides as Veterinary Critically Important Antimicrobial (VCIA) Agents in veterinary species.[10]

Pharmacology/Actions

Erythromycin, a time-dependent antibiotic, is usually a bacteriostatic agent, but it may be bactericidal at high concentrations or against highly susceptible organisms (eg, streptococci). Macrolides (eg, erythromycin, tylosin) are believed to act by binding to the 50S ribosomal subunit of susceptible bacteria, thereby inhibiting peptide bond formation and protein synthesis.

Erythromycin has in vitro activity predominantly against gram-positive cocci (eg, staphylococci, streptococci), gram-positive bacilli (eg, *Bacillus anthracis, Corynebacterium* spp, *Clostridium* spp, [not *C difficile*], *Listeria* spp, *Erysipelothrix* spp), and some strains of gram-negative bacilli (eg, *Campylobacter* spp, *Haemophilus* spp, *Pasteurella* spp, *Bartonella* spp, *Brucella* spp). Some strains of *Actinomyces* spp, *Mycoplasma* spp, *Chlamydia* spp, *Ureaplasma* spp, and rickettsial organisms are also inhibited by erythromycin. Most strains of the Enterobacteriaceae family (eg, *Pseudomonas* spp, *Escherichia coli, Klebsiella* spp) are intrinsically resistant to erythromycin and acquired erythromycin resistance occurs frequently in methicillin-resistant staphylococci. Tolerance (ie, increasing minimum inhibitory concentrations [MICs]) by *Rhodococcus equi* to both erythromycin and rifampin is problematic, and resistance has been documented in some isolates. One study suggests biofilm formation as a cause of *R equi* erythromycin resistance.[11]

Like other macrolides, antimicrobial activity is reduced at lower pH, in abscesses, and in necrotic tissues.

At subantimicrobial doses, erythromycin mimics the effects of motilin (in cats, humans, and rabbits) and 5-hydroxytryptophan type 3 (5-HT$_3$) (in dogs) and can stimulate migrating motility complexes and antegrade peristalsis.[12] By inducing antral contractions, gastric emptying is enhanced. Erythromycin also increases lower esophageal sphincter pressure and could be useful in treating cats (and possibly dogs) with gastroesophageal reflux and reflux esophagitis. Erythromycin is reported to stimulate colonic activity in dogs and horses but not in cats. Erythromycin's prokinetic mechanism of action in dogs is not completely understood but is probably via activation of 5-HT$_3$ receptors. Erythromycin increases abomasal motility and emptying rate in calves and adult cattle.[13-15] Prokinetic activity may diminish with chronic use (tachyphylaxis). It has been suggested that combining erythromycin with metoclopramide could lessen this effect.[16]

Pharmacokinetics

Erythromycin is absorbed after oral administration in the upper small intestine. Several factors can influence the bioavailability of erythromycin, including salt form, dosage form, GI acidity, presence of food in the stomach, and gastric emptying time. Both the erythromycin base and stearate are susceptible to acid degradation; enteric coatings are often used to alleviate this. In most species, ethylsuccinate and estolate forms are dissociated in the upper small intestine and then absorbed, but a study in cats found that oral administration of erythromycin ethylsuccinate tablets or suspension did not result in measurable serum concentrations.[17] Fasting increases oral bioavailability in foals, and estolate[6] and a microencapsulated base[7] formulations appear to be better absorbed than other formulations.[7] After IM or SC injection of the polyethylene-based veterinary product in cattle, absorption was very slow. Bioavailability is ≈40% after SC injection and 65% after IM injection.

Erythromycin is distributed throughout the body into most fluids and tissues including the prostate, macrophages, and leukocytes. CSF concentrations are poor. In foals, erythromycin concentrations in bronchiolar lavage cells are equivalent to those found in the serum, but concentrations in pulmonary epithelial lining fluid are lower. Protein binding of erythromycin and the estolate salt are 73% to 81%, and 96%, respectively. The volume of distribution for erythromycin is reportedly 2 L/kg in dogs, 3.7 to 7.2 L/kg in foals, 2.3 L/kg in mares, 2.34 L/kg in cats, and 0.8 to 1.6 L/kg in cattle. In lactating dairy cattle, the milk:plasma ratio is 6:7.

Erythromycin is primarily excreted unchanged in the bile but is also partly metabolized by the liver via N-demethylation to inactive metabolites. Some of the drug is reabsorbed after biliary excretion. Only ≈2% to 5% of a dose is excreted unchanged in the urine.

The reported elimination half-life of erythromycin in various species is 60 to 90 minutes in dogs[18] and cats,[17] 60 to 70 minutes in foals and mares,[19, 20] and 190 minutes in cattle.[21]

Contraindications/Precautions/Warnings

Erythromycin is contraindicated in patients that are hypersensitive to it. In humans, erythromycin should be used with caution in patients with hepatic dysfunction or pre-existing liver disease; repeated courses or prolonged treatment with the estolate form have been rarely associated with the development of reversible cholestatic hepatitis. This effect has not been reported in veterinary species, but given the availability of other salt formulations, the estolate should probably be avoided in patients with pre-existing liver dysfunction. Erythromycin rarely causes prolongation of the QT interval and development of ventricular arrhythmias in humans, including atypical ventricular tachycardia (torsades de pointes). Caution is advised when using erythromycin in patients with pre-existing arrhythmias or in conjunction with other QT prolongation drugs. See ***Drug Interactions***.

Many clinicians consider erythromycin contraindicated in adult horses (see ***Adverse Effects***). Unless *Rhodococcus equi* is confirmed, erythromycin should be used with caution in horses older than 4 months of age.[22] In foals with *R equi* infections, prolonged monotherapy could potentially induce *R equi* resistance; treatment with concomitant rifampin is recommended. Because erythromycin is implicated in causing hyperthermia and fatal respiratory distress in foals treated during hot weather,[23, 24] provision of shade and close observation is advised, or an alternate macrolide should be used.

Oral erythromycin should not be used in ruminants, as severe diarrhea may result. Erythromycin and other macrolides are contraindicated in rabbits, gerbils, guinea pigs, and hamsters, as toxic enterocolitis may be induced.

Although erythromycin can be used to improve GI motility, the use of antimicrobial agents for noninfectious indications is discouraged.[25]

As a P-glycoprotein substrate, erythromycin should be used with caution in patients with confirmed *MDR1* gene mutation (also known as *ABCB1-1delta*).[26]

Adverse Effects

When erythromycin is injected IM, local reactions and pain at the injection site may occur. Oral erythromycin may cause GI disturbances (eg, diarrhea, anorexia, vomiting). IV injections must be given slowly (ie, over 20 to 60 minutes), as they may cause thrombophlebitis.[27]

Hyporexia; bruxism; and a mild, self-limiting diarrhea can occur in foals treated with erythromycin. These effects generally resolve after treatment is temporarily stopped. However, severe enterocolitis is possible. Erythromycin may induce anhidrosis, which alters temperature homeostasis in foals.[24] Foals 2 to 4 months of age have reportedly developed hyperthermia with associated respiratory distress and tachypnea.[23] Physically cooling off these animals has been successful in controlling this effect. Mares of treated foals can develop clostridial enterocolitis, presumably via ingestion of the foal's feces.[28]

Adult horses may develop severe, sometimes fatal, diarrhea, making use of erythromycin in adults controversial.

Erythromycin used as a prokinetic agent may increase clinical signs of intestinal distress because it can stimulate emptying of larger food particles into the intestine than is normal. Rectal edema and partial anal prolapse have been associated with erythromycin in swine.[29]

Reproductive/Nursing Safety

Erythromycin crosses the placenta, with fetal serum concentrations being 5% to 20% of maternal concentrations. Erythromycin fed to rats did not reveal evidence of impaired fertility.[30] Although erythromycin has not demonstrated teratogenic effects in rats, and the drug is not thought to possess serious teratogenic potential, it should only be used during pregnancy when the benefits outweigh the risks.

Erythromycin is excreted in milk in small amounts, with an observed milk:plasma ratio of 0.5 in humans; it is considered compatible with breastfeeding.

Overdose/Acute Toxicity

Except in the situations listed in ***Adverse effects***, erythromycin is relatively nontoxic; however, shock reactions have been reported in neonatal pigs receiving erythromycin overdoses.

For patients that have experienced or are suspected to have experienced an overdose, consultation with a 24-hour poison center specializing in providing veterinary-specific information is recommended. For general information related to overdose and toxin exposures, as well as contact information for poison control centers, refer to ***Appendix***.

Drug Interactions

The following drug interactions have either been reported or are theoretical in humans or animals receiving erythromycin and may be of significance in veterinary patients. Unless otherwise noted, use together is not necessarily contraindicated, but weigh the potential risks and perform additional monitoring when appropriate.

- **ANTIARRHYTHMIC AGENTS** (eg, **amiodarone, procainamide, quinidine, sotalol**): Concurrent use may increase plasma concentration of antiarrhythmic agents and also enhance QT prolonging effect. In humans, cases of adverse cardiovascular events including cardiac arrest and arrythmias have been reported. Avoid combination.
- **CISAPRIDE**: Erythromycin can inhibit the metabolism of cisapride, and the manufacturer states that use of these drugs together (in humans) is contraindicated; however, in one study in dogs, erythromycin did not alter the pharmacodynamics of cisapride.[31]
- **CLINDAMYCIN, LINCOMYCIN**: In vitro evidence of antagonism
- **COLCHICINE**: Erythromycin may inhibit P-glycoprotein and increase the serum colchicine concentration.
- **DIGOXIN**: Erythromycin may inhibit P-glycoprotein and increase the serum digoxin concentration.
- **LOPERAMIDE**: Loperamide may reduce promotility effects of erythromycin. Erythromycin may inhibit P-gp, theoretically increasing the risk for loperamide toxicity in dogs homozygous for the *MDR1* genetic mutation (also known as *ABCB1-1delta*).
- **SUCRALFATE**: May reduce absorption of erythromycin; separate doses by 2 hours if possible

Erythromycin is a potent CYP3A4 inhibitor that can inhibit the metabolism of other drugs that use the CYP3A subfamily of the cytochrome P450 enzyme system. Depending on the therapeutic index of the drug(s) involved, therapeutic drug monitoring and/or dosage reduction may be required if the drugs must be used together. These drugs include:

- **ANTICOAGULANTS** (eg, **rivaroxaban, warfarin**)
- **AZOLE ANTIFUNGALS** (eg, **fluconazole, itraconazole, ketoconazole**): Possible increased erythromycin concentrations and increased risk for QT interval prolongation and cardiac arrhythmias
- **BENZODIAZEPINES** (eg, **alprazolam, midazolam, triazolam**)
- **BROMOCRIPTINE**
- **BUSPIRONE**
- **CALCIUM CHANNEL BLOCKERS** (eg, **amlodipine, diltiazem, verapamil**)
- **CANNABIDIOL**
- **CARBAMAZEPINE**
- **CYCLOSPORINE**
- **DISOPYRAMIDE**: Risk for increased QT interval
- **DOXORUBICIN**
- **MAROPITANT**
- **METHYLPREDNISOLONE**
- **OPIOIDS** (eg, **alfentanil, fentanyl, methadone, morphine**)
- **QUINIDINE**: Risk for prolonged QT interval
- **SILDENAFIL**: Erythromycin may increase the serum concentration of sildenafil. Consider therapy modification and monitor pulmonary arterial hypertension.
- **TACROLIMUS, SYSTEMIC**
- **THEOPHYLLINE/AMINOPHYLLINE**
- **VINCA ALKALOIDS** (eg, **vinblastine, vincristine, vinorelbine**)

Laboratory Considerations

- Erythromycin may cause falsely elevated values of **AST** and **ALT** when using colorimetric assays.
- Fluorometric determinations of **urinary catecholamines** can be altered by concomitant erythromycin administration.

Dosages

NOTE: IV injections should be given slowly (ie, over 20-60 minutes). See ***Adverse Effects***.

DOGS:

Susceptible infections (extra-label): 10 – 20 mg/kg PO every 8 to 12 hours

Prokinetic agent (extra-label): 0.5 – 1 mg/kg PO, IV every 8 hours[32-34]

CATS:

Susceptible infections (extra-label): 10 – 20 mg/kg PO every 8 to 12 hours

Prokinetic agent (extra-label): 0.5 – 1 mg/kg PO or IV every 8 hours[32, 33] has been suggested; however, erythromycin does not appear to have colonic motility stimulating effects in cats.

HORSES:

***Rhodococcus equi* infections in foals** (extra-label): Most clinicians recommend using the estolate or enteric-coated (base) forms of erythromycin 20 – 25 mg/kg PO every 8 hours with rifampin 5 mg/kg PO every 12 hours or 10 mg/kg PO once daily (every 24 hours).[9] Treatment may be required for 1 to 3 months. Early diagnosis and treatment may reduce treatment duration.

Proliferative enteropathy caused by *Lawsonia intracellularis* infections in foals (extra-label): Erythromycin estolate 25 mg/kg PO every 6 to 8 hours with rifampin 10 mg/kg PO every 12 hours for a minimum of 21 days[35]

Regional limb perfusion (extra-label): 2000 mg administered via catheter inserted into cephalic or saphenous vein[36]

Prokinetic agent (extra-label):

a. 0.1 - 1 mg/kg diluted in saline and administered IV over 1 hour[37, 38]
b. 1 mg/kg IV every 6 to 8 hours[39]

CATTLE:

Bovine respiratory disease (ie, shipping fever complex, bacterial pneumonia) associated with *Pasteurella multocida* organisms susceptible to erythromycin in beef and dairy (not breeding age) cattle (label dosage; FDA-approved): 4 mL/100-lb body weight (4 mg/lb or 8.8 mg/kg) once daily for up to 5 days as needed. Administer via deep IM injection (no more than 10 mL per site) into the heavy neck muscles or, if necessary for alternating injection sites, into the heavy muscular portion of the hind legs (semitendinosus muscles). In calves weighing less than 90 kg (200 lb), no more than 4 mL/site deep IM injection into the heavy muscles of the hind legs only. Use a 1- to 2-inch, 16- or 18-gauge needle, depending on the animal's size. Do not use in female dairy cattle older than 20 months of age or in calves to be processed for veal.[40]

Prokinetic agent (extra-label):

Calves: 8.8 mg/kg IM or 20 mg/kg PO as a single dose[15, 41, 42]
Adults: 8.8 – 10 mg/kg IM once daily for up to 3 days[43]

BIRDS:

Susceptible infections (extra-label): Oral suspension, 60 mg/kg PO every 12 hours[44]

FERRETS:

Susceptible infections (extra-label): 10 mg/kg PO 4 times daily[45]

Monitoring

- Clinical efficacy
- Culture and susceptibility testing when used for antimicrobial indications
- Adverse effects
- Baseline and periodic hepatic enzymes (eg, ALT, AST, ALP) for patients receiving erythromycin estolate long-term

Client Information

- The intramuscular 100 mg/mL (*Erythro-100®*) product has specific instructions on where and how to inject the drug in cattle. Refer to the label directions or package insert for more information before using.
- When administering the medicine orally to small animal species, give it on an empty stomach. If gastrointestinal signs (eg, vomiting, lack of appetite, diarrhea) occur, then give medicine with food. Administer the medicine to foals prior to offering hay.
- If gastrointestinal side effects are severe or persist, contact your veterinarian.

Chemistry/Synonyms

Erythromycin, a macrolide antibiotic produced from *Streptomyces erythreus*, is a weak base that is available commercially in several salts and esters and has a pK_a of 8.9. Erythromycin base occurs as a bitter-tasting, odorless or practically odorless, white to slight yellow, crystalline powder. Approximately 1 mg is soluble in 1 mL of water; it is soluble in alcohol.

Erythromycin estolate occurs as a practically tasteless and odorless, white, crystalline powder. It is practically insoluble in water and ≈50 mg is soluble in 1 mL of alcohol. Erythromycin estolate may also be known as erythromycin propionate lauryl sulfate.

Erythromycin ethylsuccinate occurs as a practically tasteless and odorless, white to slight yellow, crystalline powder. It is very slightly soluble in water and freely soluble in alcohol.

Erythromycin lactobionate occurs as white to slightly yellow crystals or powder. It may have a faint odor and is freely soluble in water and alcohol.

Erythromycin may also be known as eritromicina and erythromycinum; many trade names are available.

Storage/Stability

Erythromycin (base) capsules and tablets should be stored in airtight containers at room temperature of 15°C to 30°C (59°F-86°F). Erythromycin estolate preparations should be protected from light. To retain palatability, the oral suspensions should be refrigerated.

Erythromycin ethylsuccinate tablets and powder for oral suspension should be stored in airtight containers at room temperature. The commercially available oral suspension should be stored in the refrigerator to preserve palatability. After dispensing, the oral suspensions are stable for at least 14 days at room temperature, but individual products may have longer labeled stabilities.

Erythromycin lactobionate powder for injection should be stored at room temperature. For initial reconstitution (vials), use only sterile water for injection. After reconstitution, the drug is stable for 24 hours at room temperature and for 2 weeks if refrigerated. To prepare for administration via continuous or intermittent infusion, the drug is further diluted in 0.9% sodium chloride, lactated Ringer's solution, or *Normosol®-R*. Other infusion solutions may be used but first must be buffered with 4% sodium bicarbonate injection (1 mL per 100 mL of solution). At a pH of less than 5.5, the drug is unstable and loses potency rapidly.

Compatibility/Compounding Considerations

Many drugs are physically **incompatible** with erythromycin lactobionate. Compatibility is dependent on factors such as pH, concentration, temperature, and diluent used; specialized references or a hospital pharmacist should be consulted for more specific information.

Dosage Forms/Regulatory Status

VETERINARY-LABELED PRODUCTS:

Although many products continue to be listed in the FDA Green Book, there are currently no approved veterinary products available.

HUMAN-LABELED PRODUCTS:

Erythromycin Base Delayed-release Oral Tablets enteric-coated: 250 mg, 333 mg, and 500 mg; *Ery-Tab®*; (Rx)

Erythromycin Base Tablets Film-coated: 250 mg and 500 mg; generic; (Rx)

Erythromycin Base Delayed-release Oral Capsules enteric-coated pellets: 250 mg; *ERYC®*, generic; (Rx)

Erythromycin Stearate Film-coated Tablets: 250 mg; generic; (Rx)

Erythromycin Ethylsuccinate Tablets: 400 mg; *E.E.S. 400®*, generic; (Rx)

Erythromycin Ethylsuccinate Powder for Oral Suspension: 200 mg/5 mL (40 mg/mL) when reconstituted 100 mL and 200 mL; *EryPed®* 200 and 400, *E.E.S. Granules®*; (Rx)

Erythromycin Ethylsuccinate Powder for Oral Suspension: 400 mg/5 mL (80 mg/mL) in 100 mL; *EryPed*®; (Rx)

Erythromycin Lactobionate Lyophilized Powder for Injection Solution: 500 mg (as lactobionate) vial; *Eythrocin*®; (Rx)

Erythromycin and Sulfisoxazole Granules for Oral Suspension: erythromycin ethylsuccinate (equivalent to 200 mg erythromycin activity) and sulfisoxazole acetyl (equivalent to sulfisoxazole 600 mg/5 mL [120 mg/mL] when reconstituted in 100 mL, 150 mL, and 200 mL); *Eryzole*®, *Pediazole*®, generic; (Rx)

Topical and ophthalmic preparations are also available.

References

For the complete list of references, see **wiley.com/go/budde/plumb**

Esmolol

(***ess***-moe-lol) *Brevibloc*®

Beta-1-Adrenergic Blocker

Prescriber Highlights

- Ultra-short-acting beta-1 blocker used IV for short-term treatment of supraventricular tachycardias or to determine if beta-blockers are effective for controlling arrhythmias
- Beta-blocker of choice for use under general anesthesia
- Contraindications include patients with overt cardiac failure, second- or third-degree AV block, sinus bradycardia, or cardiogenic shock.
- Use caution in patients with congestive heart failure (CHF), bronchoconstriction, or diabetes mellitus.
- Adverse effects: hypotension and bradycardia are most common
- Many possible drug interactions

Uses/Indications

Esmolol may be used as a test drug to indicate whether beta-blocker therapy is warranted, as an antiarrhythmic agent (particularly in cats with hypertrophic cardiomyopathy), or as an infusion in the short-term treatment of supraventricular tachyarrhythmias (eg, atrial fibrillation/flutter, sinus tachycardia). Esmolol may also be used to manage hyperdynamic right ventricular outflow tract obstruction following balloon valvuloplasty in dogs with pulmonary valve stenosis.[1]

Pharmacology/Actions

Esmolol is classified as a class II antiarrhythmic drug. It primarily blocks beta-1-adrenergic receptors in the myocardium. At clinically used doses, esmolol does not have any intrinsic sympathomimetic activity (ISA) and, unlike propranolol, does not possess membrane-stabilizing effects (quinidine-like) or bronchoconstriction. Cardiovascular effects secondary to esmolol include negative inotropic and chronotropic activity that can lead to reduced myocardial oxygen demand. Systolic and diastolic blood pressures are reduced at rest and during exercise.[2] The antiarrhythmic effect is thought to be due to its blockade of adrenergic stimulation of the cardiac pacemaker potential. Esmolol increases sinus cycle length, slows AV node conduction, and prolongs sinus node recovery time.[3]

Esmolol is considered the beta-blocker of choice in animals under general anesthesia that might develop hypertension and supraventricular tachycardia due to inappropriate sympathetic activity.

Pharmacokinetics

After IV injection, esmolol is rapidly and widely distributed but not appreciably to the CNS, spleen, and testes.[4] The distribution half-life is ≈2 minutes. Steady-state blood concentrations occur in ≈5 minutes if a loading dose is given or ≈30 minutes without it. Esmolol is rapidly metabolized in the blood by esterases to a practically inactive metabolite. Renal or hepatic dysfunction does not appreciably alter elimination characteristics. Terminal half-life is ≈10 minutes and duration of action after discontinuing IV infusion is usually ≈20 minutes postinfusion in dogs.

Contraindications/Precautions/Warnings

Esmolol is contraindicated in patients with overt cardiac failure, second- or third-degree AV block, sinus bradycardia, or in cardiogenic shock. It should be used with caution (weigh benefit vs risk) in patients with CHF, bronchoconstriction, or diabetes mellitus.

In humans with tachycardia secondary to pheochromocytoma, it is recommended that esmolol be given in combination with (or after) an alpha-blocker, or a paradoxical increase in blood pressure can occur secondary to attenuation of beta-mediated vasodilation in skeletal muscle.[5]

Adverse Effects

At usual dosages, adverse effects are uncommon and generally an extension of the pharmacologic effects. Hypotension (with resultant clinical signs) and bradycardia are the most likely adverse effects seen. These usually prove to be mild and transient in nature. Esmolol may mask certain clinical signs of developing hypoglycemia (such as increased heart rate or blood pressure).

Reproductive/Nursing Safety

It is unknown whether esmolol crosses the placenta. Studies done in rats and rabbits demonstrated no teratogenic effects at doses up to 3 times the maximum human maintenance dose (MHMD). Higher doses (8 times or more than the MHMD) demonstrated some maternal death and fetal resorption.

It is unknown if esmolol is excreted in milk.

Because safety has not been established in animals, this drug should only be used when the maternal benefits outweigh the potential risks to offspring.

Overdose/Acute Toxicity

The IV LD_{50} in dogs is ≈32 mg/kg. Dogs receiving 2 mg/kg/minute for 1 hour showed no adverse effects; doses of 3 mg/kg/minute for 1 hour produced ataxia and salivation; and 4 mg/kg/minute for 1 hour caused muscular rigidity, tremors, seizures, ptosis, vomiting, hyperpnea, vocalizations, and prostration. These effects all resolved within 90 minutes of the end of infusion. Because of the short duration of action of the drug, discontinuation or dosage reduction may be all that is required; otherwise, clinical and supportive treatment may be initiated.

For patients that have experienced or are suspected to have experienced an overdose, consultation with a 24-hour poison consultation center specializing in providing veterinary-specific information is recommended. For general information related to overdose and toxin exposures, as well as contact information for poison control centers, refer to ***Appendix.***

Drug Interactions

The following drug interactions have either been reported or are theoretical in humans or animals receiving esmolol and may be of significance in veterinary patients. Unless otherwise noted, use together is not necessarily contraindicated, but weigh the potential risks and perform additional monitoring when appropriate.

- Acetylcholinesterase Inhibitors (eg, **physostigmine**): Concurrent use may increase risk for severe bradycardia.
- Alpha-2 Agonists (eg, **dexmedetomidine**): Concurrent use may increase risk for AV block.
- Amiodarone: Concurrent use may result in bradycardia, hypotension, sinus arrest, and AV block.
- Anesthetic Agents, General: Additive myocardial depression may occur with the concurrent use of propranolol and myo-

cardial depressant anesthetic agents.

- **Anticholinergics** (eg, **atropine**): May negate bradycardic effects of beta-blockers
- **Beta-2-Adrenergic Agonists** (eg, **albuterol, terbutaline**): At higher doses, atenolol may impair bronchodilation.
- **Calcium Channel Blockers** (eg, **diltiazem, verapamil**): Myocardial depressant effects of both classes of agents may be potentiated. IV administration in close proximity is contraindicated. Monitor cardiac function and adjust therapy as needed. Generally, drugs such as diltiazem can be safely administered 30 minutes after esmolol administration has been discontinued.
- **Digoxin**: Esmolol may increase serum digoxin levels up to 20%; concurrent use increases the risk for bradycardia.
- **Hypotensive Agents** (eg, **amlodipine, enalapril, telmisartan**): Concurrent use may result in increased risk for hypotension.
- **Monoamine Oxidase Inhibitors (MAOIs)**: Concurrent use of MAOIs with esmolol is not recommended due to potential risk for hypertension.
- **Morphine**: Titrate esmolol dosage carefully in patients also receiving morphine, as it may increase steady-state esmolol serum concentrations up to 50%.
- **Phenothiazines** (eg, **acepromazine, chlorpromazine**): May increase risk for hypotension
- **Reserpine**: May see additive effects (eg, hypotension, bradycardia) if used with esmolol
- **Theophylline, Aminophylline**: Esmolol may cause severe bronchospasm and reduce the therapeutic effects of theophylline.
- **Vasoconstrictors and Inotropes** (eg, **dopamine, epinephrine, norepinephrine**): If systemic vascular resistance is high, there is an increased risk for blocked cardiac contractility; esmolol is not recommended to control supraventricular tachycardias in patients receiving these drugs.

Laboratory Considerations

- None noted

Dosages

DOGS/CATS:

Ultra-short-acting beta-blocker (for treating or assisting in treatment of ventricular arrhythmias) (extra-label): Dosage recommendations vary somewhat and there does not appear to be clear evidence supporting any dosage. Often an initial IV loading dose of 0.25 – 0.5 mg/kg (250 – 500 μg/kg) is administered IV over 2 to 5 minutes and then a CRI of 10 – 200 μg/kg/minute IV is started.[6-9] Some clinicians recommend initial dosages as low as 0.05 – 0.1 mg/kg (50 – 100 μg/kg) with intermittent IV bolus doses of 0.05 – 0.1 mg/kg (50 – 100 μg/kg) administered every 5 minutes up to a maximum dose of 0.5 mg/kg (500 μg/kg). If esmolol is to be used in animals with severe heart failure or mitral regurgitation, it is best dosed without an initial bolus and at the lower end of the CRI rates. CRI can be adjusted upwards every 10 minutes while the patient is continuously monitored.

Monitoring

- Blood pressure
- ECG
- Heart rate

Client Information

- Esmolol should only be used in an inpatient setting where appropriate monitoring is available.

Chemistry/Synonyms

A short-acting beta-1-adrenergic blocker, esmolol occurs as a white or off-white crystalline powder. It is not as lipophilic as either labetalol or propranolol but is comparable to acebutolol. 650 mg is soluble in 1 mL of water, and 350 mg is soluble in 1 mL of alcohol.

Esmolol HCl may also be known as ASL-8052, *Brevibloc*®, or *Miniblock*®.

Storage/Stability

The concentrate for injection should be stored at room temperature 25°C (77°F), with excursions permitted to 15°C to 30°C (59°F-86°F). Do not freeze; protect this product from excessive heat. It is a clear, colorless to light yellow solution.

After dilution to a concentration of 10 mg/mL, esmolol HCl is stable (at refrigeration temperatures or room temperature) for at least 24 hours in commonly used IV solutions.

Compatibility/Compounding Considerations

Compatibility is dependent upon factors such as pH, concentration, temperature, and diluent used; consult specialized references or a hospital pharmacist for more specific information.

Esmolol may be diluted in standard 5% dextrose, lactated Ringer's solution, or saline (or combinations thereof) IV fluids. At 10 mg/mL, esmolol is reportedly physically **compatible** with digoxin, dopamine, fentanyl, lidocaine, morphine sulfate, nitroglycerin, and nitroprusside.

Dosage Forms/Regulatory Status

VETERINARY-LABELED PRODUCTS: NONE

The Association of Racing Commissioners International (ARCI) has designated this drug as a class 3 substance. See the ***Appendix*** for more information. Use of this drug may not be allowed in certain animal competitions. Check rules and regulations before entering in a competition while this medication is being administered. Contact local racing authorities for further guidance.

HUMAN-LABELED PRODUCTS:

Esmolol HCl Injection: 10 mg/mL regular and preservative free in 10 mL vials; 20 mg/mL preservative free in 100 mL bags; *Brevibloc*®; generic; (Rx)

References

For the complete list of references, see **wiley.com/go/budde/plumb**

Esomeprazole

(ess-oh-***meh***-prah-zahl) *NexIUM*®

Proton Pump Inhibitor

Prescriber Highlights

- ► Used for GI ulcers and erosions; limited information on its use in veterinary species
- ► Available in oral capsules and suspensions as well as IV forms
- ► Oral doses should be given on an empty stomach (preferably 1 hour before food).
- ► Adverse effects: Small animal species: Likely to be well tolerated; potentially GI distress (eg, anorexia, colic, nausea, vomiting, flatulence, diarrhea), hematologic abnormalities, UTIs, proteinuria, or CNS disturbances. Horses: Unlikely; potential hypersensitivity

Uses/Indications

Esomeprazole, the S-enantiomer of omeprazole, is a proton pump inhibitor (PPI) that is potentially useful in treating both gastroduodenal ulcer disease and to prevent and treat gastric erosions caused by ulcerogenic drugs (eg, aspirin).

A study to determine whether preanesthetic IV administration of esomeprazole alone or esomeprazole with cisapride increased esophageal pH and decreased frequency of GI reflux (GER) in anesthetized dogs found that although esomeprazole alone increased gastric and esophageal pH, it did not alter the incidence of GER as compared with the control group.[1] In the study, gastric and esophageal pH was measured in anesthetized dogs at 12 to 18 hours before induction and again 1 to 1.5 hours before induction. The combination of esomeprazole and cisapride significantly increased pH and reduced reflux events.[1] Esomeprazole also increased intragastric pH after SC and PO administration in dogs.[2] In a study evaluating the efficacy of three acid-suppressing medications over 72 hours of treatment in 9 healthy beagles (esomeprazole 1 mg/kg IV every 12 hours; pantoprazole 1 mg/kg IV every 12 hours; famotidine loading dose of 1 mg/kg IV followed by 8 mg/kg IV CRI), significant increases in mean intragastric pH were noted over time for all 3 treatments; however, only esomeprazole and famotidine CRI achieved the goals for treatment of gastroduodenal ulcers in humans.[3] The conclusions were that the famotidine CRI and IV esomeprazole might be superior acid suppressants compared with standard doses of pantoprazole for the first 72 hours of treatment.

In a study evaluating the efficacy of 3 oral acid-suppressing medications in 12 healthy cats (esomeprazole 1 mg/kg every 12 hours; lansoprazole 1 mg/kg every 12 hours; dexlansoprazole 6 mg/kg every 12 hours), only esomeprazole achieved the established goals for treatment of gastroduodenal ulcers in humans.[4] Orally administered esomeprazole may be a superior acid-suppressant in cats compared with PO lansoprazole or PO dexlansoprazole.

Two studies in horses (PO/NGT and IV) found that esomeprazole caused significant increases in gastric pH.[5,6] It has been shown that both dosage (0.5 mg/kg/day vs 2 mg/kg/day) and diet (high grain with low fiber vs ad libitum hay) had an inconsistent effect on gastric pH in horses.[7] A study evaluating oral enteric-coated esomeprazole paste (0.5 mg/kg once daily) with oral enteric omeprazole paste (1 mg/kg once daily) in 9 adult standardbred horses found both treatments were equally effective in increasing gastric pH, with no difference in mean pH between treatments, and that enteric-coated esomeprazole may be a therapeutic alternative to omeprazole for prevention of gastric ulcers in horses.[8]

An advantage of esomeprazole is the large variety of dosage forms (eg, oral capsules, oral suspensions, IV) and strengths that are commercially available.

Pharmacology/Actions

Esomeprazole is a substituted benzimidazole proton pump inhibitor (PPI). It binds irreversibly at the secretory surface of parietal cells to the enzyme H^+/K^+ ATPase, where it inhibits hydrogen ion transport into the stomach. Esomeprazole reduces acid secretion during both basal and stimulated conditions. There is a lag time between administration and efficacy in most species, but it appears that in both dogs and horses, effects can be rapid. Esomeprazole may also inhibit some hepatic cytochrome P450 oxidase system isoenzymes (see ***Drug Interactions*** below).

Pharmacokinetics

In dogs, after administration of 1 mg/kg IV, terminal elimination half-life, systemic plasma clearance, and steady state volume of distribution were 0.73 hours, 0.3 L/hour/mL, and 0.27 L/kg, respectively. When the same dose was administered SC and PO, time until maximum concentration, peak plasma concentration, terminal elimination half-life, and bioavailability were 0.38 hours (SC) and 1.81 hours (PO), 2.62 µg/mL (SC) and 1.34 µg/mL (PO), 0.9 hours (SC) and 0.98 hours (PO), and 106% (SC) and 71.4% (PO), respectively.[2]

In humans, oral esomeprazole is well absorbed when taken on an empty stomach, but the presence of food can reduce bioavailability from ≈90% to ≈50%. Peak concentrations occur ≈1.5 hours after dosing. Esomeprazole is 97% bound to human plasma proteins and in healthy human adults, the apparent volume of distribution at steady state is ≈16 L. Esomeprazole is predominantly metabolized in the liver by the cytochrome P450 (CYP-450) enzyme system with the isoenzyme CYP2C19 forming the majority of metabolites (hydroxy and desmethyl forms) and, to a lesser extent, the CYP3A4 isoenzyme forming the sulphone metabolite. Plasma elimination half-life of esomeprazole in humans is ≈1 to 1.5 hours. Less than 1% of the parent drug is excreted in the urine unchanged with ≈80% of the dose excreted into the urine as metabolites. The remainder is excreted in the feces as unabsorbed drug or its metabolites.

Contraindications/Precautions/Warnings

Esomeprazole is contraindicated in patients that are hypersensitive to it. In patients with severe hepatic disease, the drug's half-life may be prolonged and dosage adjustment may be necessary. In humans, hypomagnesemia is rarely reported with prolonged treatment. Cutaneous lupus erythematosus and systemic lupus erythematosus have also been reported in patients taking proton pump inhibitors (PPIs) and have occurred both as new onset and as an exacerbation of existing autoimmune disease.[9]

Do not confuse ESOmeprazole with omeprazole or other similar-sounding PPIs.

Adverse Effects

There is little clinical experience or published data on the safety of esomeprazole in animal patients, but it is likely to be well tolerated, similar to other proton pump inhibitors (PPIs). Vomiting has been observed after oral and parenteral administration. Potentially, other GI signs (eg, anorexia, colic, nausea, flatulence, diarrhea, *Clostridium difficile* infection) could occur, as well as hematologic abnormalities (rare in humans), UTI, proteinuria, increased liver enzymes, or CNS disturbances.[10]

Reproductive/Nursing Safety

Esomeprazole did not demonstrate teratogenicity in laboratory animals.[10] Reduced body weight, neurodevelopmental delays, and embryolethality were observed in rats receiving doses 17 to 34 times the human dose.

It is not known whether esomeprazole is excreted in maternal milk. For humans, because of the potential for serious adverse effects in nursing infants, and the potential for tumorigenicity shown in rat carcinogenicity studies, nursing is discouraged if the drug is required.

Because safety has not been established in animals, this drug should only be used when the maternal benefits outweigh the potential risks to offspring.

Overdose/Acute Toxicity

Little information is available on acute toxicity. The LD_{50} of esomeprazole in rats after oral administration is reportedly more than 4 g/kg. Humans have tolerated oral dosages of 360 mg/day of esomeprazole without significant toxicity. If a massive overdose occurs, treat symptomatically and supportively.

For patients that have experienced or are suspected to have experienced an overdose, consultation with a 24-hour poison consultation center specializing in providing veterinary-specific information is recommended. For general information related to overdose and toxin exposures, as well as contact information for poison control centers, refer to ***Appendix.***

Drug Interactions

The following drug interactions have either been reported or are theoretical in humans or animals receiving esomeprazole and may be of significance in veterinary patients. Unless otherwise noted, use together is not necessarily contraindicated, but weigh the potential risks and perform additional monitoring when appropriate.

- **Azole Antifungals** (eg, **itraconazole, ketoconazole**): Esomeprazole can reduce absorption, and azoles can potentially increase esomeprazole exposure.
- **Benzodiazepines** (eg, **diazepam**): Esomeprazole may potentially alter benzodiazepine metabolism and prolong CNS effects.

- **Cefpodoxime, Cefuroxime**: Esomeprazole may decrease cefpodoxime or cefuroxime absorption; consider use of an alternative antibiotic.
- **Clarithromycin**: Increased concentrations of esomeprazole, clarithromycin, and 14-hydroxyclarithromycin are possible.
- **Clopidogrel**: In humans, concurrent use of omeprazole and esomeprazole (but not other proton pump inhibitors [PPIs]) may decrease the efficacy of clopidogrel and increase the risk for thrombosis[10]; however, a study in dogs found omeprazole combined with clopidogrel did not alter antiplatelet effects in healthy dogs.[11]
- **Cyanocobalamin** (oral form): Esomeprazole may decrease oral absorption.
- **Cyclosporine**: Esomeprazole may reduce cyclosporine metabolism.
- **Digoxin**: Esomeprazole may increase digoxin concentrations.
- **Diuretics (loop or thiazides)**: Increased risk for hypomagnesemia; increased monitoring suggested, particularly in susceptible patients
- **Iron, Oral**: Esomeprazole may decrease iron absorption.
- **Levothyroxine**: May result in increased TSH concentrations
- **Methotrexate**: Esomeprazole may increase and prolong methotrexate (and its metabolite) concentrations.
- **Mycophenolate**: Esomeprazole may reduce mycophenolic acid (MPA; active metabolite) concentrations.
- **Propranolol**: May result in increased propranolol exposure
- **Sucralfate**: May inhibit absorption of esomeprazole; stagger doses
- **Tacrolimus**: May result in increased tacrolimus exposure
- **Warfarin**: Esomeprazole may increase anticoagulant effect.

Laboratory Considerations

- Esomeprazole will increase **serum gastrin** concentration early in therapy, potentially interfering with secretin stimulation test.[10]

Dosages

DOGS:

Reduce gastric acid production (extra-label):

a) 0.5 – 1 mg/kg IV slowly over 3 minutes every 12 hours[3,12]

b) 1 mg/kg PO once daily on an empty stomach[2]

Reduce gastroesophageal reflux events during anesthesia (extra-label): 1 mg/kg IV over 3 minutes in combination with cisapride 1 mg/kg IV administered 1 to 1.5 hours prior to induction[1]

CATS:

Reduce gastric acid production (extra-label): 1 mg/kg PO every 12 hours[4]

HORSES:

Reduce gastric acid production (extra-label):

a) 40 – 80 mg/horse (NOT mg/kg) PO once daily[5]

b) 0.5 – 2 mg/kg PO once daily[7]

c) 0.5 mg/kg IV once daily[6]

Monitoring

- Efficacy
- Adverse effects (eg, GI distress)

Client Information

- This medicine is best given on an empty stomach, preferably in the morning 1 hour before feeding.
- Do not crush capsules unless instructed to. Capsules may be opened, and the contents mixed with applesauce or similar foods. Be sure to give the medicine to your animal immediately after preparing.
- If you have difficulty getting your animal to take the medicine, contact your veterinarian or pharmacist for tips to help with dosing and reduce the stress of medication time for both you and your animal.

Chemistry/Synonyms

A substituted benzimidazole proton pump inhibitor, esomeprazole is the S-isomer of omeprazole and is available commercially as 2 primary salts: magnesium (PO use) and sodium (IV use). Esomeprazole magnesium (CAS Registry: 217087-09-7; ATC: A02BC05) occurs as a white to slightly colored powder. It is slightly soluble in water, soluble in methyl alcohol, and practically insoluble in heptane. Esomeprazole sodium (CAS Registry: 161796-78-7; ATC: A02BC05) commercially available injection is a lyophilized powder with edetate disodium 1.5 mg and sodium hydroxide added to adjust pH (9 to 11) during manufacturing.

NexIUM® 20 and 40 mg capsules contain sugar spheres. *NexIUM*® 2.5, 5, 10, 20, and 40 mg powder for oral suspension also contains dextrose.

Esomeprazole may also be known as (*S*)-omeprazole, H199/18I, or perprazole. A common trade name is *NexIUM*®.

Storage/Stability

Oral capsules should be stored in tightly closed containers at 25°C (77°F) and may be exposed to 15°C-30°C (59°F-86°F) in tightly closed containers.

Intact vials of esomeprazole sodium for injection should be stored at controlled room temperature and protected from light. After reconstitution and dilution with 0.9% sodium chloride, it should be administered within 12 hours when stored at room temperature. The manufacturer states that refrigeration is not required. Stability of esomeprazole sodium in solution is strongly dependent on pH; stability of the drug decreases with decreasing pH.

Compatibility/Compounding Considerations

Compatibility is dependent on factors such as pH, concentration, temperature, and diluent used; specialized references or a hospital pharmacist should be consulted for more specific information.

Esomeprazole sodium for injection should be reconstituted only with sterile 0.9% sodium chloride when being administered as an IV injection over 3 minutes, although lactated Ringer's injection, or dextrose 5% may be used when administering as an IV infusion over 10 to 30 minutes (see ***Storage/Stability*** above). Flushing the administration line with sodium chloride 0.9%, Ringer's injection, lactated Ringer's, or dextrose 5% is required both before and after administering the drug. Mixing or giving with other drugs is not recommended.

If mixing capsule contents with food, only cold or room temperature applesauce is recommended, and administration should occur immediately after mixing.

Use of the esomeprazole delayed-release oral suspension packets: Empty the contents of a 2.5 mg or 5 mg packet into a container with 5 mL of water; empty the contents of a 10 mg, 20 mg, or 40 mg packet into a container with 15 mL of water. Stir, then leave for 2 to 3 minutes to thicken. Stir and drink within 30 minutes. If any material remains after drinking, add more water, stir, and drink immediately. In cases where there is a need to use 2 packets, they may be mixed in a similar way by adding twice the required amount of water or follow the mixing instructions provided.

Nasogastric/gastric tube administration: Add 5 mL of water to a catheter-tipped syringe and then add the contents of a 2.5 mg or 5 mg packet; for the 10 mg, 20 mg, or 40 mg packet, the volume of water in the syringe should be 15 mL. It is important to only use a catheter-tipped syringe when administering esomeprazole through a nasogastric or gastric tube. Immediately shake the syringe and leave for 2 to 3 minutes to thicken. Shake the syringe and inject through the nasogastric or gastric tube (French size 6 or larger) into the stomach within 30 minutes. Refill the syringe with an equal amount of water (5 or 15 mL). Shake and flush any remaining contents from the nasogastric or gastric tube into the stomach.

Dosage Forms/Regulatory Status

VETERINARY-LABELED PRODUCTS: NONE

HUMAN-LABELED PRODUCTS:

Esomeprazole Magnesium Oral Delayed-Release Capsules (containing enteric-coated granules): 20 mg and 40 mg; *NexIUM®*; generic; (Rx)

Esomeprazole Magnesium Oral Delayed-Release Tablets: 20 mg; *NexIUM® 24HR*; generic; (OTC)

Esomeprazole Magnesium Powder for Oral Delayed-Release Suspension (containing enteric-coated granules): 2.5 mg, 5 mg, 10 mg, 20 mg, and 40 mg packets. *NexIUM®*; (Rx)

Esomeprazole Strontium Oral Delayed-Release Capsules: 24.65 mg and 49.3 mg; generic; (Rx)

Esomeprazole Sodium for Injection: 20 mg and 40 mg; *NexIUM I.V.®*; generic; (Rx)

There is also an oral product combined with naproxen, but it is not appropriate for veterinary use.

References

For the complete list of references, see **wiley.com/go/budde/plumb**

Estradiol

(ess-tra-***dye***-ole) *ECP®*

Hormonal Agent (Estrogen)

Prescriber Highlights

- Natural estrogen salt used primarily to induce estrus; has been used as an abortifacient (rarely recommended today)
- Contraindicated during pregnancy; do not use in ferrets because of the risk for myelosuppression.
- Adverse effects in cats and dogs include myelotoxicity, cystic endometrial hyperplasia, pyometra, feminization in males, and signs of estrus in females.
- Feminization may occur in male animals; in female animals, signs of estrus may occur.
- Use of estradiol in food animals is prohibited by the FDA.
- The National Institute for Occupational Safety and Health (NIOSH) classifies estrogens as group II hazardous drugs; use appropriate precautions when handling.

Uses/Indications

Estradiol is used to enhance estrus behavior and receptivity in noncycling or ovariectomized mares and to hasten the onset of ovulation in transitional mares. It is also used in mares to synchronize estrus (when used in combination with progesterone), to induce lactation (when used in combination with domperidone), and to treat placentitis[1] and estrogen-responsive urinary incontinence.[2]

Historically, estradiol has been used to treat estrogen-responsive urinary incontinence in dogs, but safer estrogens (eg, diethylstilbestrol [DES], estriol) are now preferred; its use as an abortifacient in small animal species is no longer recommended.

Estradiol has previously been used as an abortifacient agent in cattle; however, the manufacturing and compounding of estradiol for use in food-producing animals is now prohibited by the FDA.

Pharmacology/Actions

Estradiol is the most active endogenous estrogen. Estrogens are necessary for the normal growth and development of female sex organs and, in some species, contribute to the development and maintenance of secondary female sex characteristics. Estrogens cause increased cell height and secretions of the cervical mucosa, thickening of the vaginal mucosa, endometrial proliferation, and increased uterine tone.

Estrogens also have effects on the skeletal system; they increase calcium deposition, accelerate epiphyseal closure, and increase bone formation. Estrogens have a slight anabolic effect and can increase sodium and water retention. Estrogens affect the release of gonadotropins from the pituitary gland, which can cause inhibition of lactation, ovulation, and androgen secretion.

Pharmacokinetics

No specific information was located regarding the pharmacokinetics of estradiol in veterinary species. In humans, estrogen in oil solutions after IM administration is absorbed promptly and absorption continues over several days. Esterified estrogens (eg, estradiol) have delayed absorption after IM administration. Estrogens are distributed throughout the body and accumulate in adipose tissue. Elimination of steroidal estrogens occurs principally by hepatic metabolism. Estrogens and their metabolites are primarily excreted in the urine, but they are also excreted into bile and undergo enterohepatic recirculation.

Contraindications/Precautions/Warnings

Estradiol is contraindicated in patients hypersensitive to the drug formulation and during pregnancy, as it can cause fetal malformations of the genitourinary system and induce bone marrow depression in the fetus. In humans, the drug is contraindicated in patients with abnormal genital bleeding of unknown etiology, breast cancer or estrogen-dependent neoplasia, hepatic dysfunction or disease, or with a history of arterial or deep vein thrombosis or pulmonary embolism. Use with caution in patients with diabetes mellitus or hypoparathyroidism.

Estradiol should not be used to treat estrogen-responsive incontinence in small animals; other estrogens (eg, diethylstilbestrol [DES], estriol) are less toxic.

When estradiol is used for treatment of a prolonged corpus luteum, a thorough uterine examination should be completed to determine if endometritis or a fetus is present.

In ferrets, estradiol is reportedly extremely toxic to bone marrow; therefore, estradiol should be avoided in this species.

The National Institute for Occupational Safety and Health (NIOSH) classifies estrogens as hazardous drugs representing an occupational hazard to healthcare workers; personal protective equipment (PPE) should be used accordingly to minimize the risk for exposure.[3]

Do not confuse estriol with estrADiol.

Adverse Effects

Estrogens have been associated with severe adverse effects in small animals. In cats and dogs, estrogens are considered toxic to the bone marrow and can cause blood dyscrasias. Blood dyscrasias are more prevalent in older animals and when higher dosages are used. Initially, a thrombocytosis and/or leukocytosis may be noted, but thrombocytopenia and leukopenia will gradually develop. Changes in a peripheral blood smear may be apparent within 2 weeks after estrogen administration. Chronic estrogen toxicity is characterized by a normochromic, normocytic anemia; thrombocytopenia; and neutropenia. Myelosuppression may be transient and begin to resolve within 30 to 40 days after discontinuation, or it may persist and progress to a fatal aplastic anemia.

Estrogens may cause cystic endometrial hyperplasia and pyometra.[4-6] After therapy is initiated, an open-cervix pyometra may be noted 1 to 6 weeks after therapy.

Estrogens have been shown to induce mammary neoplasia.[7,8]

When estradiol is used chronically in male animals, feminization may occur. In females, signs of estrus may occur and persist for 7 to 10 days. In cattle, prolonged estrus, genital irritation, decreased milk flow, precocious development, and follicular cysts may develop after estrogen therapy. These effects may be secondary to overdose; dosage adjustment may reduce or eliminate them.

Reproductive/Nursing Safety

Estradiol is contraindicated during pregnancy. Estrogens are present in breast milk and have been shown to decrease the quantity and quality of maternal milk.

Because safety has not been established in animals, this drug should only be used when the maternal benefits outweigh the potential risks to offspring.

Overdose/Acute Toxicity

Dogs exposed to estrogens at excessive doses may develop myelotoxicity characterized by normocytic, normochromic anemia; thrombocytopenia; and leukocytosis. Common clinical signs associated with overdose include inappetence, pallor, exercise intolerance, vulvar edema, vaginal bleeding, respiratory distress, hematuria, melena, fever, epistaxis, and petechiation of the skin or mucous membranes.[9] Treatment is supportive including cessation of estrogen therapies, correction of anemia and thrombocytopenia, and administration of antibiotics if the patient is severely leukopenic.

For patients that have experienced or are suspected to have experienced an overdose, consultation with a 24-hour poison consultation center specializing in providing veterinary-specific information is recommended. For general information related to overdose and toxin exposures, as well as contact information for poison control centers, refer to ***Appendix***.

Drug Interactions

The following drug interactions have either been reported or are theoretical in humans or animals receiving estradiol and may be of significance in veterinary patients. Unless otherwise noted, use together is not necessarily contraindicated, but weigh the potential risks and perform additional monitoring when appropriate.

- **Anticoagulants** (eg, **heparins, rivaroxaban, warfarin**): Concurrent use may diminish anticoagulant effect.
- **Ascorbic Acid**: Ascorbic acid may increase estrogen concentration.
- **Azole Antifungals** (eg, **fluconazole, itraconazole, ketoconazole**): May increase estrogen concentration
- **Corticosteroids** (eg, **dexamethasone, prednis(ol)one**): Enhanced glucocorticoid effects may result if estrogens are used concomitantly with corticosteroid agents. It has been postulated that estrogens may either alter the protein binding of corticosteroids and/or decrease their metabolism; corticosteroid dosage adjustment may be necessary when estrogen therapy is either started or discontinued.
- **Cyclosporine**: Estrogens may increase cyclosporine serum cyclosporine concentration.
- **Estrogens, Other** (eg, **diethylstilbestrol [DES]**): Possible additive effects. Do not use with other estrogens; concomitant use with other estrogens has not been evaluated.
- **Hypoglycemic Agents** (eg, **glipizide, insulin, metformin**): Estrogens may increase blood glucose concentration.
- **Levothyroxine**: Estrogens may diminish the therapeutic effect of levothyroxine, and an increase in levothyroxine dose may be needed. Monitor thyroid status when using these drugs in combination and adjust levothyroxine dose accordingly. See ***Monitoring*** in ***Levothyroxine***.
- **Macrolide Antibiotics** (eg, **clarithromycin, erythromycin**): May increase estrogen concentration
- **Mitotane**: May decrease estrogen concentration if administered concomitantly
- **Phenobarbital**: May decrease estrogen concentration if administered concomitantly
- **Rifampin**: May decrease estrogen concentration if administered concomitantly
- **St. John's Wort**: May decrease estrogen concentration if administered concomitantly
- **Theophylline, Aminophylline**: Estrogens may increase theophylline concentration.
- **Thyroid Hormones**: Possible alteration of thyroxine and thyrotropin serum concentrations
- **Ursodiol**: Estrogens may diminish ursodiol efficacy.

Laboratory Considerations

- Estrogens have been demonstrated to increase **thyroxine-binding globulin (TBG)** in humans, with resultant increases in total circulating thyroid hormone. Decreased T_3 resin uptake also occurs, but **free T_4** concentration is unaltered. It is unclear if estradiol affects these laboratory tests in veterinary patients.
- Estrogens may decrease the diagnostic effect of **cosyntropin**[10] and **metyrapone**.[11]

Dosages

HORSES:

NOTE: All dosages are for estradiol cypionate (ECP) unless otherwise noted.

Estrus synchronization (extra-label): Estradiol 50 mg/mare (NOT mg/kg) in combination with progesterone 150 mg/mare (NOT mg/kg) IM once daily for 10 days. Concurrently, administer dinoprost 5 mg/mare (NOT mg/kg) SC as a single dose on the last treatment day.[12]

Enhance estrus behavior and receptivity in ovariectomized mares (extra-label): 5 – 10 mg/horse (NOT mg/kg) IM once[13]

Induction of ovulation in anovulatory mares (extra-label):

a) Estradiol 50 mg/horse (NOT mg/kg) IM once on January 21; sulpiride 3 g/horse (NOT mg/kg) SC was administered on the 5th and 12th days after ECP injection[14,15]
b) Estradiol benzoate: 11 mg/mare (NOT mg/kg) IM every other day (beginning January 11) for a total of 10 injections. On the day after the 6th estradiol dose, begin sulpiride 250 mg/mare (NOT mg/kg) SC daily; continue sulpiride until the mare ovulates or for 35 doses (whichever occurs first)[16]

Ascending placentitis (extra-label): 10 mg/horse (NOT mg/kg) IM every 3 days for 3 treatments was beneficial under experimental conditions[1]

Induction of lactation in nonpregnant mares (extra-label): Estradiol 50 mg/mare (NOT mg/kg) in combination with progesterone 150 mg (NOT mg/kg) IM once daily for 7 days; administer dinoprost 5 mg/mare (NOT mg/kg) IM as a single dose on treatment day 7. Throughout treatment, also administer sulpiride 500 mg/mare (NOT mg/kg) IM twice daily for 10 days.

Mares with estrogen-responsive urinary incontinence (extra-label): 5 – 12 µg/kg IM daily for 3 days and then every other day.[2,17] Some mares will improve, but treatment does not cure the condition.

Monitoring

When therapy is chronic or used at high doses, perform baseline and periodic (eg, monthly):

- CBC: The frequency of monitoring with chronic therapy depends on the underlying clinical presentation.
- Hepatic enzymes (eg, ALT, AST, ALP)

Client Information

- Injectable estrogen should only be administered by a veterinarian. Estrogen hormone is used in mares to induce estrus (heat) and for long-term treatment of urinary incontinence.
- This hormone may be used (rarely) in dogs and cats as a mismate treatment to avoid pregnancy.
- Avoid use in pregnant animals as this medicine will cause loss of pregnancy.
- Contact your veterinarian immediately if your animal develops a decrease in appetite, pale gums, lethargy, vaginal bleeding or other vaginal discharge, swelling of the vulva, difficulty breathing, bloody urine, dark stool, fever, bloody nose, and bruising on the skin or gums.
- Pregnant women and those who are breastfeeding should use caution when handling this medicine. Wear disposable gloves when handling this drug.
- Estradiol use in food-producing animals is illegal.
- Your veterinarian will need to periodically examine your animal and perform blood tests while your animal is on this treatment. Do not miss these important follow-up visits.
- This medication is considered to be a hazardous drug as defined by the National Institute for Occupational Safety and Health (NIOSH). Talk with your veterinarian or pharmacist about the use of personal protective equipment when handling this medicine.

Chemistry/Synonyms

Estradiol cypionate is a naturally occurring steroidal estrogen. Estradiol cypionate is produced by esterifying estradiol with cyclopentanepropionic acid and occurs as a white to off-white, crystalline powder. It is either odorless or has a slight odor and has a melting range of 149°C to 153°C (300°F-307°F). Less than 0.1 mg/mL is soluble in water, and 25 mg/mL is soluble in alcohol. Estradiol cypionate is sparingly soluble in vegetable oils.

Estradiol may also be known as beta-oestradiol, dihydrofolliculin, dihydrotheelin, dihydroxyoestrin, estradiolum, NSC-9895, NSC-20293 (α-estradiol), and oestradiol; many trade names are available.

Estradiol cypionate may also be known as oestradiol cyclopentylpropionate, oestradiol cypionate, *Delestrogen®*, *Depo-Estradiol®*, *DepoGen®*, *Dura-Estrin®*, *ECP®*, *E-Cypionate®*, *Estra-D®*, *Estrace®*, *Estro-Cyp®*, *Estroject®*, *depGynogen®*, *Femtrace®*, or *Gynodiol®*.

Storage/Stability

Estradiol cypionate should be stored in light-resistant containers at controlled room temperature (20°C-25°C [68°F-77° F]); avoid freezing.

Commercially available injectable solutions of estradiol cypionate are sterile solutions in a vegetable oil (usually cottonseed oil); they may contain chlorobutanol as a preservative.

Compatibility/Compounding Considerations

Do not mix estradiol cypionate with other medications.

Dosage Forms/Regulatory Status

VETERINARY-LABELED PRODUCTS:

Several estradiol-containing implants are available for use in beef cattle, but in 2006, the FDA stated that the use of estradiol cypionate (ECP) in food-producing animals is illegal, and manufacturing and compounding of ECP for such use is illegal. In the United States, it is illegal to compound estradiol for use in food-producing animals.

HUMAN-LABELED PRODUCTS:

Estradiol Cypionate in Oil for Injection: 5 mg/mL in 5 mL vials; *Depo-Estradiol®*; (Rx)

Estradiol Valerate in Oil for Injection: 10 mg/mL, 20 mg/mL, and 40 mg/mL in 5 mL multidose vials; *Delestrogen®*, generic; (Rx)

References

For the complete list of references, see **wiley.com/go/budde/plumb**

Estriol

(ess-***trye***-ole) *Incurin®*

Hormonal Agent (Estrogen)

Prescriber Highlights

- ► Short-acting estrogen approved for treating estrogen-responsive urethral sphincter mechanism incompetence (USMI) in ovariohysterectomized female dogs
- ► Not dosed by animal's weight. Dosage should be tapered to the lowest effective dose.
- ► Use is contraindicated in male dogs, intact female dogs, dogs less than 1 year of age, pregnant or lactating dogs, dogs that have polyuria and polydipsia (PU/PD), dogs that are pregnant or lactating, or dogs receiving other estrogen medications.
- ► Use caution in dogs with liver disease or when using in combination with glucocorticoids.
- ► Most common adverse effects are GI (eg, hyporexia, vomiting) and estrogen-related (eg, swollen vulva); myelotoxicity risk appears to be low.
- ► The National Institute for Occupational Safety and Health (NIOSH) classifies estrogens as hazardous drugs; use appropriate precautions when handling.

Uses/Indications

Estriol tablets are FDA-approved for control of estrogen-responsive urethral sphincter mechanism incompetence (USMI) in ovariohysterectomized female dogs. At present, estriol is the only estrogen approved in the US for this use.

No clinical studies were found that compared efficacy or adverse effects of estriol with other estrogens (eg, diethylstilbestrol) or α-adrenergic drugs (eg, phenylpropanolamine) in female dogs with USMI. Some have proposed that using an estrogen with an α-adrenergic may be more effective[1] and allow dosage reductions for both drugs; however, one study compared use of estriol alone with use of estriol in combination with phenylpropanolamine in female dogs with USMI and showed no difference in urethral resistance.[2]

Pharmacology/Actions

Estriol is a short-acting estrogenic drug. By binding to estrogen receptors in the female canine lower urinary tract, estriol can improve urinary continence in ovariohysterectomized dogs. This effect is thought to occur through enhanced urethral sphincter tone via increased sensitivity of urethral smooth muscle receptors to norepinephrine and thus, increased smooth muscle contractility. In comparison to other estrogen analogues (eg, 17 beta-estradiol, diethylstilbestrol [DES]), estriol binds to estrogen receptors for a much shorter period but still yields therapeutic effects and apparently reduces the risk for tumorigenic effects and myelotoxicity.

Pharmacokinetics

After oral administration, estriol is nearly completely absorbed from the GI tract, and peak plasma concentrations occur in about one hour. Absorbed estriol is highly, but weakly, bound to plasma proteins, which partly explains its short acting duration. In dogs, it is not known how the drug is biotransformed, but in other species it is oxidated, sulfated, and glucuronidated in the liver. Half-life is roughly 8 to 12 hours but is difficult to determine as most pharmacokinetic studies produce multiple concentration peaks, suggesting that enterohepatic recirculation occurs. Estriol and its conjugated forms are excreted in the urine.

Contraindications/Precautions/Warnings

Estriol is contraindicated in animals that are hypersensitive to it and in animals receiving other estrogens (eg, diethylstilbestrol [DES]).

In some countries, estriol is labeled as contraindicated in male dogs, intact female dogs, dogs less than one year of age, pregnant or lactating dogs, or dogs with signs of polyuria and polydipsia (PU/PD).[3,4]

Estriol should be used with caution in dogs with liver disease or when used in combination with glucocorticoids as the safety has not been established.[5]

The National Institute for Occupational Safety and Health (NIOSH) classifies estrogens as hazardous drugs representing an occupational hazard to healthcare workers; personal protective equipment (PPE) should be used accordingly to minimize the risk for exposure.[6]

Do not confuse estriol with estrADiol.

Adverse Effects

Estriol may cause adverse GI effects (eg, anorexia, vomiting) and adverse estrogenic effects (eg, swollen vulva [most common],[7] vulvovaginitis, mammary hyperplasia, behavioral changes, and enhanced attractiveness to male dogs).[5] Rarely, polydipsia, lethargy, hyperactivity, aggression, and local alopecia have been reported. Very rarely, blood dyscrasias, vaginal bleeding, and an increased incidence of seizures have been noted. Most adverse effects are reversible by lowering the dose of estriol.

Estrogens may increase the risk of mammary tumors and may cause myelotoxicity[8]; the risk for these effects in dogs at recommended dosages of estriol appears to be low, likely owing to its relatively short duration of action.[5] No hematologic abnormalities were associated with estriol therapy in a study with 114 dogs.[9]

Reproductive/Nursing Safety

Exogenously administered estrogens are contraindicated for use during pregnancy. Some estrogens (eg, diethylstilbestrol [DES]) have been associated with significant fetal malformations or tumorigenic effects in humans.

Exogenous estrogen administration during nursing is generally not recommended because of the potential for milk transmission and reduction in milk quality and quantity.

Because safety has not been established in animals, this drug should only be used when the maternal benefits outweigh the potential risks to offspring.

Overdose/Acute Toxicity

Acute oral overdoses may cause emesis or other GI effects. Estrogenic effects (see ***Adverse Effects***) are possible in both males (ie, feminization) and females. Clinical signs in female beagles given estriol for 6 months at up to 10 mg/day included estrogenic effects; pathology showed vulvar and vaginal tissue with a proestrus-like appearance with or without lymphoplasmacytic infiltrate and urothelial hyperplasia of the renal pelvis.[10] Increased white blood cell and platelet counts were observed in dogs receiving 6 mg/day and 10 mg/day doses.[5] In 2 acute toxicity trials performed in rats, LD_{50} after oral administration was greater than 2 g/kg,[11] suggesting that an acute overdose is unlikely to cause mortality.

Long-term (26 weeks) overdoses of 6 to 10 mg/day (3 to 5 times the recommended dose) demonstrated redness and swelling of the vulva, vulvar discharges, mammary hyperplasia, and higher white blood cell counts.[12]

For patients that have experienced or are suspected to have experienced an overdose, consultation with a 24-hour poison consultation center specializing in providing veterinary-specific information is recommended. For general information related to overdose and toxin exposures, as well as contact information for poison control centers, refer to the ***Appendix***.

Drug Interactions

The following drug interactions have either been reported or are theoretical in humans or animals receiving oral estrogens and potentially could be of significance in veterinary patients:

- ANTICOAGULANTS (eg, **heparins, rivaroxaban, warfarin**): Concurrent use may diminish anticoagulant effect.
- ASCORBIC ACID: Ascorbic acid may increase estrogen concentration.
- AZOLE ANTIFUNGALS (eg, **fluconazole, itraconazole, ketoconazole**): May increase estrogen concentration
- CIMETIDINE: May increase estrogen concentration
- CYCLOSPORINE: Estrogens may increase serum cyclosporine concentration.
- HYPOGLYCEMIC AGENTS (eg, **glipizide, insulin, metformin**): Estrogens may increase blood glucose concentration.
- ESTROGENS, OTHER (eg, **diethylstilbestrol [DES]**): Possible additive effects. Do not use with other estrogens; concomitant use with other estrogens has not been evaluated.[5]
- LEVOTHYROXINE: Estrogens may diminish the therapeutic effect of levothyroxine, and an increase in levothyroxine dose may be needed. Monitor thyroid status when using these drugs in combination and adjust levothyroxine dose accordingly. See ***Monitoring*** in ***Levothyroxine***.
- MACROLIDE ANTIBIOTICS (eg, **clarithromycin, erythromycin**): May increase estrogen concentration
- MITOTANE: May decrease estrogen concentration if administered concomitantly
- PHENOBARBITAL: May decrease estrogen concentration if administered concomitantly
- RIFAMPIN: May decrease estrogen concentration if administered concomitantly
- THEOPHYLLINE, AMINOPHYLLINE: Estrogens may increase theophylline concentration.
- THYROID HORMONES: Possible alteration of thyroxine and thyrotropin serum concentrations
- URSODIOL: Estrogens may diminish ursodiol efficacy.

Laboratory Considerations

- In humans, estrogens have been demonstrated in humans to increase **thyroxine-binding globulin** (**TBG**) concentrations with resultant increases in total circulating thyroid hormone. Decreased T_3 resin uptake also occurs, but **free T_4** concentration is unaltered. It is unclear if estradiol affects these laboratory tests in veterinary patients.
- Estrogens may decrease the diagnostic effect of **cosyntropin**[13] and **metyrapone.**[14]

Dosages

DOGS:

Estrogen-responsive urinary incontinence in ovariohysterectomized female dogs (label dosage; FDA approved): Initially, 2 mg/dog (NOT mg/kg) PO once daily for a minimum of 14 days.[5] After urinary incontinence is controlled, decrease the dose to 1 mg/dog (NOT mg/kg) PO once daily, then 0.5 mg/dog (NOT mg/kg) PO once daily, then 0.5 mg/dog (NOT mg/kg) PO every other day until the lowest effective dose is determined. Allow a minimum of 7 days between each dose adjustment. The maximum daily dose is 2 mg/dog (NOT mg/kg). If the dog does not respond to this dosage, the diagnosis should be re-assessed.

Hormone-dependent urinary incontinence caused by sphincter mechanism incompetence in ovariohysterectomized female dogs (extra-label): Initially, 1 mg/dog (NOT mg/kg) PO once daily for 7 to 14 days.[3,4]

- If 1 mg/dog (NOT mg/kg) PO once daily is *effective*, decrease to 0.5 mg/dog (NOT mg/kg) PO once daily. When the lowest effective daily dose is determined, treatment every other day may be tried. Seven days should be allowed between dosage adjustments before judging the full effect of the dosage change. Ensure the dosage used to achieve the therapeutic effect is as low as possible; dosage should not be less than 0.5 mg/dog (NOT mg/kg) per day.
- If 1 mg/dog (NOT mg/kg) PO once daily was *ineffective*, increase dosage to 2 mg/dog (NOT mg/kg) PO once daily. The maximum dosage should not exceed 2 mg/dog (NOT mg/kg) per day. If 2 mg/dog (NOT mg/kg) per day is successful, reduce dosage to 2 mg/dog (not mg/kg) PO every other day. If treatment with 2 mg/dog (NOT mg/kg) PO once daily is ineffective, reassess diagnosis.[3,15]

Monitoring

- Clinical efficacy
- Adverse effects (eg, inappetence, vomiting, polydipsia, swollen vulva, vulvovaginitis, mammary hyperplasia, behavioral changes)
- Baseline CBC and urinalysis; recheck CBC after 1 month of therapy[16]

Client Information

- Estriol is used in dogs to treat estrogen-responsive urinary incontinence.
- The most common side effects include lack of appetite, vomiting, greater thirst, and swollen vulva.
- This medicine may be given with or without food. If your dog vomits or acts sick after getting estrogen on an empty stomach, give with food or a small treat to see if this helps. If vomiting continues, contact your veterinarian.
- Treatment will likely continue for the remainder of the life of the dog.
- Your veterinarian will need to monitor your dog with periodic examinations and laboratory testing. Do not miss these important follow-up visits.
- Pregnant women and those who are breastfeeding should use caution when handling. Wash your hands with soap and water thoroughly after administration to avoid exposure to the drug.
- This medication is considered to be a hazardous drug as defined by the National Institute for Occupational Safety and Health (NIOSH). Talk with your veterinarian or pharmacist about the use of personal protective equipment when handling this medicine.

Chemistry/Synonyms

Estriol is a natural estrogenic sex hormone that occurs as a white to off-white, odorless, crystalline powder. It is insoluble in water; sparingly soluble in alcohol; and soluble in acetone, chloroform, dioxan, ether, and vegetable oils. Its molecular weight is 288.4 g/mol.

The commercially available veterinary tablets contain amylopectin, magnesium stearate, potato starch, and anhydrous lactose.

Estriol may also be known as E3, oestriol, follicular hormone hydrate, theelol, or *Incurin*®.

Storage/Stability

Store estriol tablets at or below 25°C (77°F) with excursions permitted to 40°C (104°F). Protect from light.

Compatibility/Compounding Considerations

No specific information has been noted.

Dosage Forms/Regulatory Status

VETERINARY-LABELED PRODUCTS:

Estriol Tablets: 1 mg scored tablets in 30- or 90-count foil-sealed blister packs; *Incurin*®; (Rx). FDA-approved for oral use in dogs. NADA #141-325

Estriol should not be used in food-producing animals.

HUMAN-LABELED PRODUCTS: NONE

References

For the complete list of references, see **wiley.com/go/budde/plumb**

Ethambutol

(e-***tham***-byoo-tole) *Myambutol*®

Antimycobacterial Agent

Prescriber Highlights

- ► Can be used as part of an antimycobacterial drug combination protocol for dogs, cats, and birds
- ► Treating *Mycobacterium tuberculosis* complex infections in veterinary species is controversial because of potential risk for public health.
- ► Contraindicated in patients hypersensitive to the drug
- ► Caution is advised in patients with renal disease and preexisting optic neuritis.
- ► Adverse effects include optic neuritis, peripheral neuritis, and neurotoxicity.

Uses/Indications

In combination with other antimycobacterial drugs, ethambutol may be useful in treating mycobacterial infections caused by *Mycobacterium bovis, Mycobacterium tuberculosis, Mycobacterium genavense, Mycobacterium avium-intracellulare* complex (MAC) in dogs or cats, particularly when the organism is resistant to treatment with other drug combinations (eg, rifampin, fluoroquinolones, macrolides). In birds, ethambutol has been used in combination with other agents for treating mycobacterial (eg, *M avium*) infections.

Because of public health risks, particularly in the face of increased populations of immunocompromised humans, and the possible contribution to development of antimicrobial resistance, treatment of *Mycobacterium tuberculosis* complex infections (eg, *M bovis, M tuberculosis, Mycobacterium microti,* among others) in domestic or captive animals is controversial.

The World Health Organization has designated ethambutol as a Critically Important, High Priority antimicrobial for human medicine.[1]

Pharmacology/Actions

A synthetic, bacteriostatic, antimycobacterial agent, ethambutol only acts against actively dividing mycobacteria. It enters mycobacterial cells and interferes with RNA synthesis and appears to interfere with the incorporation of mycolic acid into cell walls, allowing other antimycobacterial agents to penetrate the cell wall. Ethambutol does not have appreciable activity against other bacteria or fungi. Resistance can occur and is thought to develop in a stepwise manner; resistance is more likely with monotherapy. Cross-resistance with other antimycobacterial agents has not been reported.

Pharmacokinetics

Pharmacokinetic values for cats or birds were not located. In dogs, ethambutol is reported to have a volume of distribution of 3.8 L/kg, a total body clearance of 13.2 mL/minute/kg, and an elimination half-life of 4.1 hours. Nephrectomized dogs had an elimination half-life of 5 hours.

In humans, ethambutol is rapidly absorbed after PO administration and bioavailability is around 75%. The drug is distributed widely in the body, but CSF concentrations only range from 10% to 50% of those found in serum. Erythrocyte concentrations are about twice that of the serum and can serve as a depot for the drug. About 15% of absorbed drug is hepatically metabolized to inactive metabolites. The majority of the drug is eliminated both by tubular secretion and glomerular filtration as unchanged drug in the urine. Elimination half-life in humans with normal renal function is about 3 to 4 hours; up to 8 hours if renal function is impaired.

Contraindications/Precautions/Warnings

Ethambutol should not be used in patients with a history of prior hypersensitivity reactions to it. In humans, the drug is contraindicated in patients with optic neuritis.

Patients with markedly reduced renal function may need dosage adjustment.

To help ensure human health, it is recommended to contact local public health authorities and obtain their recommendations before treating *Mycobacterium tuberculosis* complex infections in companion animals.

Adverse Effects

Well-described adverse effect profiles for ethambutol in dogs, cats, or birds are not available. Because ethambutol is used in combination with other medications, adverse effects associated with treatment may not be a result of ethambutol. In pre-clinical studies, some dogs receiving ethambutol over prolonged periods developed non-dose related degenerative changes in the central nervous system. In toxicology studies, dogs receiving large, prolonged doses developed signs of myocardial toxicity and depigmentation of the tapetum lucidum of the eyes. However, dosages as large as 400 mg/kg/day for 4 weeks in dogs demonstrated no significant abnormalities in electroretinogram or visual evoked potential. In humans, optic neuritis (usually reversible after drug discontinuation) causing decreased visual acuity has been reported; optic neuritis may respond to treatment with vitamin B_{12} injections.

Hepatotoxicity, sometimes fatal, has been noted in humans taking ethambutol. Peripheral neuritis, blood dyscrasias, and hyperuricemia also have occurred.

Because antimycobacterial therapy involves multiple drugs for extended periods of time, bacterial or fungal overgrowth infections can occur. Antifungal medications may be required.

Reproductive/Nursing Safety

Ethambutol crosses the placenta; fetal levels are reported to range from 30% to 75% of that found in maternal serum. Teratogenic effects associated with ethambutol have not been reported in humans, but studies in mice, rats, and rabbits given high doses yielded a variety of abnormalities in offspring.

Ethambutol is excreted into milk in levels approximating those found in maternal serum. In humans, ethambutol is considered compatible with pregnancy.[2]

Because safety has not been established in animals, this drug should only be used when the maternal benefits outweigh the potential risks to offspring.

Overdose/Acute Toxicity

Very limited information exists. Acute overdoses of greater than 10 grams in humans have caused optic neuritis. Other adverse effects noted with human overdoses include CNS effects (confusion, visual hallucinations), abdominal pain, nausea, fever, and headache; treatment is supportive.

For patients that have experienced or are suspected to have experienced an overdose, consultation with a 24-hour poison control center specializing in providing veterinary-specific information is recommended. For general information related to overdose and toxin exposures, as well as contact information for poison control centers, refer to ***Appendix***.

Drug Interactions

The following drug interactions either have been reported or are theoretical in humans or animals receiving ethambutol and may be of significance in veterinary patients. Unless otherwise noted, use together is not necessarily contraindicated, but weigh the potential risks and perform additional monitoring when appropriate.

- **Aluminum-containing Antacids**: In humans, it has been documented that coadministration can reduce oral absorption of ethambutol; it is suggested to separate dosing by at least 4 hours if both drugs are necessary.

Laboratory Considerations

- No specific concerns; in humans, increased **serum uric acid** levels have been noted.

Dosages

DOGS:

Disseminated *Mycobacterium tuberculosis* (extra-label): Ethambutol 10 – 25 mg/kg PO once daily, in combination with rifampin 5 – 10 mg/kg PO every 12 to 24 hours (maximum of 600 mg/day) and isoniazid 10 – 20 mg/kg PO once daily (maximum of 300 mg/day). May also add pyrazinamide 15 – 40 mg/kg PO once daily. Treatment must continue for more than 9 months.[3] **NOTE**: Pyrazinamide is ineffective for *Mycobacterium bovis*.

CATS:

Mycobacterial infections (extra-label): 10 – 25 mg/kg PO once daily, in combination with 1 or preferably 2 antimycobacterial drugs (eg, rifampin, isoniazid, clarithromycin or azithromycin, marbofloxacin or pradofloxacin).[4] **NOTE**: Ethambutol is not recommended in the current guidelines for treating *Mycobacterium tuberculosis* complex infections in cats.[5]

BIRDS:

***Mycobacterium avium* infections in caged birds** (extra-label): Several protocols have been used, but controlled trials have not been performed. Combination therapy and treatment for 6 to 12 months is required.

Protocol 1: Ciprofloxacin 20 mg/kg PO every 12 hours or enrofloxacin 15 mg/kg PO or IM (**NOTE**: Repeated IM injections can cause muscle necrosis) for 10 days; clofazimine 1.5 mg/kg PO once daily; cycloserine 5 mg/kg PO every 12 hours; and ethambutol 20 mg/kg PO every 12 hours

Protocol 2: Clofazimine 6 mg/kg PO once daily; ethambutol 30 mg/kg PO once daily; rifampin 45 mg/kg PO once daily

Protocol 3: Ciprofloxacin 80 mg/kg PO once daily or enrofloxacin 30 mg/kg PO once daily; ethambutol 30 mg/kg PO once daily; rifampin 45 mg/kg PO once daily or rifabutin 15 mg/kg PO once daily[6]

Protocol 4: Clarithromycin 61 mg/kg, moxifloxacin 25 mg/kg and ethambutol 60 mg/kg administered by crop gavage every 12 hours for 18 weeks[7]

Monitoring

- Clinical efficacy
- With long-term therapy, consider periodic monitoring of CBC, liver enzymes, and renal parameters.
- Routine ophthalmologic examinations are recommended for humans taking this medication long term.
- Monitor for fungal or bacterial overgrowth infections

Client Information

- Animals that have certain forms of mycobacterial infections may be contagious to humans. Discuss this with your veterinarian and your physician for more information.

- The length of treatment with ethambutol may be very long (months to years). Be sure to give all of the medication that is prescribed as directed and until it is all gone.
- This medication can be administered with or without food.
- Report any changes noted with your animal's eyes or vision, or any other new concerns to your veterinarian.
- Periodic monitoring of bloodwork and response to treatment is recommended. Do not miss important follow up visits with your veterinarian.

Chemistry/Synonyms

Ethambutol HCl occurs as a white, crystalline powder that is freely soluble in water and soluble in alcohol.

Ethambutol may also be known as: CL-40882, etambutol, or ethambutoli; there are many trade names for international products.

Storage/Stability

Ethambutol tablets should be stored at 20°C to 25°C (68°F-77°F) in well-closed, light-resistant containers.

Compatibility/Compounding Considerations

No specific information was noted.

Dosage Forms/Regulatory Status

VETERINARY-LABELED PRODUCTS: NONE

HUMAN-LABELED PRODUCTS:

Ethambutol HCl Tablets: 100 mg and 400 mg (scored); *Myambutol®*, generic; (Rx)

References

For the complete list of references, see **wiley.com/go/budde/plumb**

Ethanol

Ethyl Alcohol

(***eth***-a-nol)

Antidote

Prescriber Highlights

- Used as second-line treatment of ethylene glycol (EG) toxicity for dogs and cats (fomepizole recommended as first-line)
- Adverse effects include CNS and respiratory depression, hypoglycemia, diuresis, as well as pain and infection at the injection site.
- No absolute contraindications when used for treatment of ethylene glycol toxicity; use caution in animals with CKD and hepatic disease
- Avoid extravasation. Monitor fluid, electrolyte, and respiratory status; consider measuring alcohol and toxin levels (if possible).
- No FDA-approved products exist; must be compounded

Uses/Indications

The principal use of ethanol in veterinary medicine is for the treatment of ethylene glycol toxicity. Although fomepizole (4-methylpyrazole; 4 MP) is the treatment of choice for ethylene glycol poisoning, ethanol is more readily available and a more economical alternative when patients present within a few hours after ingestion.

Ethanol is used in the management of methanol poisoning in humans but is not recommended for methanol toxicity in dogs and cats as it exacerbates CNS depression and prolongs toxicity by delaying methanol elimination.[1]

Percutaneous injection of ethanol 95% to 96% has been used successfully to treat canine[2] and feline[3] hyperparathyroidism. Percutaneous injection of 96% ethanol has also been used for feline hyperthyroidism with varying results. In one study of 4 cats with unilateral thyroid nodules, percutaneous ethanol injection (PEI) successfully decreased serum total T_4 concentrations, which remained within or below the reference range for 12 months.[4] Another study of 7 cats with bilateral thyroid nodules showed only transient decreases in serum total T_4.[5]

In horses, ethanol has been used in aerosol form as a mucokinetic agent and for intraarticular administration to promote distal tarsal joint ankylosis with osteoarthritis.

Pharmacology/Actions

Ethanol competitively inhibits alcohol dehydrogenase, preventing the conversion of ethylene glycol to its toxic metabolites (glycoaldehyde, glycolate, glyoxylate, and oxalic acid). This inhibition allows ethylene glycol to be principally excreted in the urine unchanged. For ethanol to be effective, it must be given early after ethylene glycol ingestion, ideally sooner than 4 to 8 hours after ingestion. It is seldom useful if started 8 hours after significant ingestion.

When injected into a thyroid or parathyroid mass, ethanol causes necrosis of the nodule tissue.

Pharmacokinetics

Alcohol is well absorbed orally, but it is administered intravenously for toxicity treatment. It rapidly distributes throughout the body and crosses the blood–brain barrier.

Contraindications/Precautions/Warnings

As ethylene glycol intoxication is life-threatening, there are no absolute contraindications to ethanol's use for this indication. Use it with caution in animals with chronic kidney disease, as the unmetabolized parent compound will not be eliminated unless hemodialysis is available. Ethanol may exacerbate hepatic disease.

Prior to ethanol ablation in cats, laryngeal function should be assessed and should be normal due to the possibility of laryngeal paralysis.[5,6]

The use of ethanol with fomepizole is usually contraindicated; see ***Drug Interactions*** for more information.

Adverse Effects

General adverse effects associated with ethanol are CNS depression and respiratory depression. A high risk for hypothermia and respiratory arrest is associated with high blood levels. Ethanol's effects on antidiuretic hormone (ADH; vasopressin) may enhance diuresis. As ethylene glycol may also cause diuresis, fluid and electrolyte therapy requirements need to be monitored and managed. Hypoglycemia, hypocalcemia, and metabolic acidosis may be seen; pulmonary edema can also occur. Orally administered ethanol is a gastric irritant, and vomiting may result. The risk of aspiration is increased due to ethanol's inhibitory effect on the epiglottis.

Following ethanol treatment for ethylene glycol exposure, animals will be depressed and lethargic during recovery. Other adverse effects include pain and infection at the injection site, phlebitis, and intravascular hemolysis. Extravasation should be watched for and avoided; use of a central catheter may reduce this risk.

Dysphonia can occur following ethanol ablation in dogs and cats. In humans, transient injection site pain has been reported.

When aerosolized in horses, irritation and bronchoconstriction may result. With intraarticular administration in horses, mild swelling at the injection site can occur; severe swelling with secondary cellulitis and fibrosis occurs rarely.

Reproductive/Nursing Safety

Alcohol crosses the placenta. Alcohol's safety during pregnancy has not been established for short-term use. Use only when necessary.

Alcohol passes freely into milk to levels that approximate maternal serum levels.

Because safety has not been established in animals, this drug should only be used when the maternal benefits outweigh the potential risks to offspring.

Overdose/Acute Toxicity

The lowest lethal IV dose in dogs is 1600 mg/kg.[7] The oral lethal dose of ethanol in dogs is 5 – 8 g/kg. If clinical signs of overdose occur (lateral nystagmus, hypothermia, respiratory depression, profound obtundation), either slow the infusion or discontinue temporarily. Alcohol blood levels may be used to monitor both the efficacy and toxicity of alcohol.

For patients that have experienced or are suspected of having experienced an overdose, consultation with a 24-hour poison consultation center specializing in providing veterinary-specific information is recommended. For general information related to overdose and toxin exposures, as well as contact information for poison control centers, refer to ***Appendix***.

Drug Interactions

The following drug interactions have either been reported or are theoretical in humans or animals receiving ethanol and may be of significance in veterinary patients. Unless otherwise noted, use together is not necessarily contraindicated, but weigh the potential risks and perform additional monitoring when appropriate.

- **Bromocriptine**: Alcohol may increase the severity of adverse effects seen with bromocriptine.
- **Charcoal, Activated**: Will inhibit the absorption of orally administered ethanol; do not use activated charcoal if administering ethanol orally for methanol or ethylene glycol intoxication.
- **CNS Depressant Drugs** (eg, **barbiturates, benzodiazepines, phenothiazines, opioid analgesics, antihistamines, tricyclic antidepressants**): Alcohol may cause additive CNS depression when used with other CNS depressant drugs.
- **Fomepizole** (**4-methylpyrazole; 4-MP**): Inhibits alcohol dehydrogenase; ethanol metabolism is reduced significantly, and alcohol poisoning (CNS depression, coma, death) can occur. Use together is generally not recommended, but if both drugs are used, monitoring of ethanol blood levels is mandatory.
- **Insulin**: Alcohol may affect glucose metabolism and the actions of insulin or oral antidiabetic agents.
- **Sulfonylureas** (eg, **glipizide, glyburide**): Increased risk for hypoglycemia
- **Chlorpropamide and Metronidazole**: A disulfiram reaction (increased acetaldehyde with tachycardia, vomiting, weakness) may occur if alcohol is used concomitantly with these drugs.
- **Antihypertensive Agents** (eg, **amlodipine, enalapril, telmisartan**): Ethanol may enhance the hypotensive effect of antihypertensive drugs.

Laboratory Considerations

Ethylene Glycol Testing Kits: Ethanol may cause false-positive reports on ethylene glycol screening tests. Refer to the label of the testing kit for more information.

Dosages

DOGS:

Ethylene glycol poisoning (extra-label): **NOTE**: Fomepizole is generally preferred, but availability and/or cost may be an issue.

When using ethanol, a CRI is preferred as it results in more stable blood ethanol concentrations.[8] **See *Compatibility/Compounding Considerations*** **for detailed ethanol dilution instructions.**

a) Using a 20% ethanol solution: give 5.5 mL/kg dose over 1 hour IV every 4 hours for 5 treatments, then every 6 hours for four additional treatments (each treatment is dosed as a CRI over 1 hour).[9,10,11]

b) Using a 7% ethanol solution: give 8.6 mL/kg slowly IV, followed by 1.43 mL/kg/hour IV CRI for at least 36 hours (48 hours of treatment is optimal). If the EG test was positive initially, then check it before stopping treatment. Discontinue treatment when it converts to negative.[12]

c) If IV administration is not possible, ethanol can be given orally (via an indwelling nasogastric tube). Using a 40% ethanol solution (80 proof), a typical dosage is ≈1 – 1.4 mL/kg PO. The solution can be diluted as gastric irritation may result in vomiting.[13]

Percutaneous ultrasound-guided ethanol ablation of presumed functional parathyroid nodules (extra-label): 95% ethanol injected into the center of the nodule; target injected volume equal to the measured volume of the nodule. Hypercalcemia resolved in 85% of cases; 22% of treated cases developed hypocalcemia, but only 1 was symptomatic.[2]

CATS:

Ethylene glycol poisoning (extra-label): **NOTE**: High-dose fomepizole is generally preferred, but availability and/or cost may be an issue.

When using ethanol, a CRI is preferred as it will result in more stable blood ethanol concentrations.[8] **See *Compatibility/Compounding Considerations*** **for detailed ethanol dilution instructions.**

a) Using a 20% ethanol solution[11]; give 5 mL/kg dose over 1 hour IV every 6 hours for 5 treatments, then every 8 hours for four additional treatments (each treatment is dosed as a CRI over 1 hour).[9,10]

b) Using a 7% ethanol solution: give 8.6 mL/kg slowly IV, followed by 1.43 mL/kg/hour IV CRI for at least 36 hours (48 hours of treatment is probably better). If the EG test was positive initially, then check it before stopping treatment. Discontinue treatment when it converts to negative.[12]

c) If IV administration is not possible, ethanol can be given orally (via an indwelling nasogastric tube). Using a 40% solution (80 proof), a typical dosage is ≈1 – 1.4 mL/kg PO. The solution can be diluted as gastric irritation may result in vomiting.[13]

Percutaneous ultrasound-guided ethanol ablation of hyperplastic thyroid nodule (extra-label): 96% ethanol injected into the nodule. Injected ethanol volume is based on nodule size; 50% to 100% of the calculated nodule volume has been used as targets. If bilateral nodules are present, only one nodule should be treated at a time.[4,5]

HORSES:

Promote ankylosis in horses with distal tarsal joint osteoarthritis (extra-label): In the study, joints were treated if there was no contrast-mediated radiographic evidence of communication with the proximal intertarsal joint (PITJ). The same needle was kept in the joint space, and either 70% ethanol solution in sterile water or 100% ethanol was injected until minor resistance was felt (2 to 4 mL). In their conclusion, the authors stated: *...findings of this study support the use of 70% ethanol solution for treatment of distal tarsal joint OA in cases that do not respond to corticosteroid medication. Careful case selection and accurate contrast-facilitated injection technique are mandatory to minimize potential complications of this treatment.*[14]

Monitoring

- Alcohol blood levels (and ethylene glycol or methanol levels). **NOTE**: In humans, blood ethanol levels should be maintained at 100 – 130 (some say up to 200) mg/dL (21.7 – 28.2 milliMoles/L). It is safer to maintain a blood ethanol concentration greater than 130 mg/dL than to have it fall below 100 mg/dL. (*POISINDEX® Managements*, Thompson; *MICROMEDEX®* Healthcare Series, 2007)
- Degree of CNS and respiratory depression (eg, respiratory rate,

SpO2, venous CO_2 if available)

- Body temperature
- Fluid, electrolyte, acid/base, and blood glucose status

Client Information

- Give systemically administered alcohol in a controlled clinical environment.
- There are no FDA-approved ethanol products. Emergencies may require the use of non-pharmaceutical-grade ethanol.

Chemistry/Synonyms

Ethanol is a transparent, colorless, volatile liquid having a characteristic odor and a burning taste. Ethyl alcohol is miscible with water and many other solvents.

"Proof" is considered 2 times the percentage of ethanol. For example, 100 proof vodka is 50% ethanol; 80 proof vodka is 40% ethanol. In some states, pure grain alcohol (often called "Everclear"), which is a 95% ethanol (190 proof) product, can be purchased.

Ethanol may also be known as aethanolum, alcohol, grain alcohol, ethanolum, and ethyl alcohol.

Storage/Stability/Preparation

Protect alcohol from extreme heat or freezing. Do not use it unless the solution is clear. Alcohol may precipitate many drugs; do not administer other medications in the alcohol infusion solution unless compatibility is documented (consult specialized references or a hospital pharmacist for more specific information).

Compatibility/Compounding Considerations

Compatibility is dependent on factors such as pH, concentration, temperature, and diluent used; specialized references or a hospital pharmacist should be consulted for more specific information.

NOTE: Since alcohol infusions are generally only used in veterinary medicine for the treatment of ethylene glycol and methanol toxicities, obtaining medical/pharmaceutical grade or laboratory-grade alcohol can be difficult in an emergency. One improvised method that has been successful, albeit not pharmaceutically elegant, is to use commercially available vodka (40% [80 proof] or 50% [100 proof]) or grain alcohol ("Everclear"; 95% [190 proof]) diluted in an appropriate IV solution (eg, 5% dextrose or 0.9% sodium chloride).

To make an ethanol dilution:

1. Determine the volume of ethanol to dilute:

volume of stock ethanol needed=

$$\left(\frac{\textbf{\% desired}}{\textbf{\% stock}}\right) \times \textbf{total} \text{ volume desired}$$

2. Remove the volume determined in Step 1 from the fluid bag before adding the ethanol to the diluent

Example: make a 20% ethanol solution using 80 proof vodka (40% ethanol) in a one-liter bag of fluids

1. Determine the volume of vodka to dilute:

$$\textit{Volume of vodka needed} = \left(\frac{20\%}{40\%}\right) \times 1000\ mL$$

2. Volume of vodka needed is 500 mL. Remove 500 mL from 1 L bag of fluids, then add 500 mL of vodka.

Use an in-line filter to administer IV. The client should give informed consent regarding the use of this non-pharmaceutical product before use.

Dosage Forms/Regulatory Status

VETERINARY-LABELED PRODUCTS: NONE

The Association of Racing Commissioners International (ARCI) has designated this drug as a class 2 substance. Use of this drug may not be allowed in certain animal competitions. Check rules and regulations before entering a competition while this medication is being administered. Contact local racing authorities for further guidance. See ***Appendix*** for more information.

HUMAN-LABELED PRODUCTS: NONE

Alcohol (ethanol) 5% and 10% in dextrose 5% IV solutions that were commercially available have been discontinued.

For information on obtaining tax-free alcohol for medicinal purposes, contact a regional office of the Bureau of Alcohol, Tobacco, and Firearms.

In the UK: Dehydrated Alcohol (absolute alcohol) BP for Injection, Ethanol BP 100% v/v; 2 mL, 5 mL, 10 mL, 20 mL, and 50 mL ampules. (Martindale Pharma)

References

For the complete list of references, see **wiley.com/go/budde/plumb**

Etodolac

(ee-toe-***doe***-lak) *EtoGesic®, Lodine®*

Nonsteroidal Anti-inflammatory Agent (NSAID)

Prescriber Highlights

- ► A second-generation NSAID used in dogs; uncommonly used today. The veterinary-approved dosage forms of etodolac are not commercially available.
- ► Contraindicated in patients that are hypersensitive to it or other NSAIDs. Use this drug with caution in patients with preexisting or occult GI, hepatic, renal, cardiovascular, or hematologic abnormalities.
- ► Adverse effects include vomiting, diarrhea, lethargy, surgical bleeding, hypoproteinemia, keratoconjunctivitis sicca (KCS), and localized pain and tissue reactions at the injection site.
- ► Many potential drug interactions

Uses/Indications

Etodolac is labeled for the management of pain and inflammation associated with osteoarthritis in dogs. Etodolac appeared to provide analgesia to chronically lame horses with navicular syndrome.[1]

Pharmacology/Actions

Like other NSAIDs, etodolac has analgesic, anti-inflammatory, and antipyretic activity. Etodolac appears to be more selective for inhibition of cyclooxygenase-2 than cyclooxygenase-1, but studies conflict on this, and a definitive answer is not presently agreed upon. It may be better to describe etodolac as a COX-1–sparing drug rather than a COX-2–selective drug. In dogs, etodolac dosage affects whether the drug causes GI (COX-1 related) adverse effects. Dosages as little as 2.7 times the labeled dose can produce GI lesions.[2] Etodolac is also thought to inhibit macrophage chemotaxis, which may explain some of its anti-inflammatory activity.

In horses, etodolac does not exhibit much COX-2 selectivity.

Pharmacokinetics

The S(+) enantiomer is thought to provide the bulk of the pharmacologic activity, but the drug is supplied as a racemic mixture. Pharmacokinetic studies that measure both forms as one are not clinically relevant. After oral administration to healthy dogs, etodolac is rapidly and nearly completely absorbed.[2] The presence of food may alter the rate, but not the extent, of absorption. Peak serum concentrations occur 1 to 2 hours postdosing. Etodolac is highly bound to serum proteins. The drug is primarily excreted via the bile into the feces.[2] Glucuronide conjugates have been detected in the bile but not the urine. Elimination half-life in dogs varies depending on whether food is present in the gut, which may affect the rate of enterohepatic circulation of the drug.[2] These values range from about 8 hours (fasted) to 12 hours (non-fasted). Serum half-life is not necessarily a good predictor for the duration of efficacy, possibly due to the drug's high protein binding.

In horses, etodolac has an oral bioavailability of about 77%.[3] After

IV dosing, the volume of distribution was 0.29 L/kg, and the clearance was 235 mL/kg/hour. Elimination half-life (after IV dosing) was ≈2.5 to 3 hours.

Contraindications/Precautions/Warnings

Etodolac is contraindicated in dogs that are hypersensitive to it. It should be used with caution in dogs with preexisting or occult GI, hepatic, cardiovascular, or hematologic abnormalities (eg, von Willebrand disease or receiving anticoagulant therapy), as NSAIDs may exacerbate these conditions. Patients may be more susceptible to renal injury from etodolac if they are dehydrated, on diuretics, or have preexisting renal, hepatic, or cardiovascular dysfunction.

Safety of etodolac has not been established in dogs less than 12 months of age.

Adverse Effects

In clinical field studies, etodolac's primary adverse effects were vomiting and regurgitation,[4-6] and these effects were reported in about 5% of dogs tested.[2] Diarrhea, lethargy, and hypoproteinemia have also been reported in dogs. Urticaria, behavioral changes, and inappetence were reported in less than 1% of dogs treated. Hepatotoxicity and/or nephrotoxicity are possible but are not well-documented problems in dogs.

Therapy with etodolac should be terminated if inappetence, vomiting, fecal abnormalities, or anemia are observed.[2]

Etodolac injection may cause localized pain or tissue reactions at the injection site.

Etodolac may decrease total serum T_4 in some dogs.[7] However, its clinical significance is unclear.[8]

Etodolac appears to have less impact on clotting times than some other canine FDA-approved NSAIDs, but bleeding during surgery has been reported.

Cases have been reported of dogs developing keratoconjunctivitis sicca (KCS) after receiving etodolac treatment,[9] and the incidence rate is unknown at this time.

GI distress is the primary adverse effect of etodolac in horses.[10]

Reproductive/Nursing Safety

Safe use has not been established in breeding, pregnant, or lactating dogs.

Most NSAIDs are excreted in the milk; use with caution.

Because safety has not been established in animals, this drug should only be used when the maternal benefits outweigh the potential risks to offspring.

Overdose/Acute Toxicity

Limited information is available, but in a safety study where dogs were given 40 mg/kg/day (2.7 times the label dosage), GI ulcers, weight loss, emesis, and fecal occult blood were noted.[2] Dosages of 80 mg/kg/day (5.3 times the label dosage) caused 6 of 8 dogs to either die or become moribund secondary to GI ulceration. It should be noted that these were not single-dose overdoses; however, they demonstrate that there is a relatively narrow therapeutic window for the drug in dogs and that dosages should be carefully determined (ie, do not confuse mg/kg dosages with mg/lb).

Common clinical signs include acute renal failure, anorexia, collapse, hyperkalemia, and hypersalivation. As with any NSAID, overdosage can lead to GI and renal effects. GI decontamination with emetics and/or activated charcoal may be appropriate. For doses where GI effects are expected, the use of GI protectants is warranted. If renal effects are also expected, fluid diuresis is warranted.

For patients that have experienced or are suspected to have experienced an overdose, consultation with a 24-hour poison consultation center specializing in providing veterinary-specific information is recommended. For general information related to overdose and toxin exposures, as well as contact information for poison control centers, refer to ***Appendix***.

Drug Interactions

NOTE: Although the manufacturer does not list any specific drug interactions in the package insert, it does caution to avoid or closely monitor etodolac's use with other drugs, especially those that are also highly protein bound. It also recommends close monitoring or avoiding **using etodolac with any other ulcerogenic drugs** (eg, **corticosteroids, other NSAIDs**). Although some clinicians advocate a multi-day washout period when switching from one NSAID to another (not aspirin—see below), there does not appear to be any substantial evidence that this is required. Until there is more evidence, consider starting the new NSAID when the next dose would be due for the old one.

The following drug interactions have either been reported or are theoretical in humans or animals receiving etodolac and may be of significance in veterinary patients. Unless otherwise noted, use together is not necessarily contraindicated, but weigh the potential risks and perform additional monitoring when appropriate.

- ACE INHIBITORS (eg, **enalapril, benazepril**): Etodolac may reduce the antihypertensive effects of ACE inhibitors. Because ACE inhibitors potentially reduce renal blood flow, use with NSAIDs could increase the risk for renal injury
- AMINOGLYCOSIDES (eg, **gentamicin, amikacin**): Concurrent use may increase the risk for nephrotoxicity.
- ANGIOTENSIN RECEPTOR BLOCKERS (ARB; eg, **telmisartan**): Etodolac may reduce the antihypertensive effects of ARBs. Because ARBs potentially reduce renal blood flow, use with NSAIDs could increase the risk for renal injury
- ANTICOAGULANTS (eg, **heparin, LMWH, rivaroxaban, warfarin**): Concurrent use may increase the risk for bleeding.
- ASPIRIN: Concurrent use may increase the risk for GI ulceration.
- BISPHOSPHONATES (eg, **alendronate**): Concurrent use may increase the risk for GI ulceration and nephrotoxicity.
- CHOLESTYRAMINE: May reduce etodolac absorption
- CISPLATIN: Etodolac may potentiate the renal toxicity of cisplatin when it is used in combination with cisplatin.
- CLOPIDOGREL: Concurrent use may increase the risk for bleeding.
- CORTICOSTEROIDS (eg, **dexamethasone, fludrocortisone, prednis(ol)one**): Concomitant administration with NSAIDs may significantly increase the risk for GI adverse effects.
- CYCLOSPORINE: Concurrent use may result in an increased risk for cyclosporine nephrotoxicity.
- DIGOXIN: Concurrent use may result in increased serum concentration of digoxin and prolonged digoxin half-life.
- DIURETICS (eg, **furosemide**): Concurrent use may result in reduced diuretic efficacy and possible nephrotoxicity.
- METHOTREXATE: Serious toxicity has occurred when NSAIDs have been used concomitantly with methotrexate; use together with caution.
- NEPHROTOXIC AGENTS (eg, **amphotericin B, aminoglycosides, cisplatin**): Potential for increased risk for nephrotoxicity if used with NSAIDs
- NONSTEROIDAL ANTI-INFLAMMATORY DRUGS (NSAIDs), OTHER: Concurrent use of multiple NSAIDs should be avoided.
- PHENOBARBITAL: Concurrent use may increase the metabolism of etodolac in dogs.
- PROBENECID: May cause a significant increase in serum levels and half-life of etodolac
- SELECTIVE SEROTONIN REUPTAKE INHIBITORS (SRIs; eg, **fluoxetine**): Concurrent use with etodolac may result in an increased risk for bleeding.

- **TACROLIMUS**: Concurrent use with etodolac may result in acute renal failure.
- **TIGILANOL TIGLATE**: Because tigilanol tiglate must be used concomitantly with a glucocorticoid medication, NSAIDs must be avoided.

Laboratory Considerations

- Etodolac may cause false-positive determinations of **urine bilirubin**.
- Etodolac therapy may alter **thyroid function tests** and their interpretation; falsely low values may occur in dogs receiving etodolac.

Dosages

DOGS:

Treatment of pain and inflammation associated with osteoarthritis (labeled-dose; FDA-approved):

Oral tablets: 10 – 15 mg/kg PO once daily[2]. Dogs less than 5 kg (11 lb) cannot be accurately dosed with *EtoGesic*® tablets. Adjust the dose to obtain a satisfactory response, but do not exceed 15 mg/kg.[2] For long-term therapy, reduce dose level to minimum effective dosage.

Injection: 10 – 15 mg/kg SC as a single dorsoscapular injection. If needed, daily dosing with tablets may begin 24 hours after the last injectable treatment.

HORSES:

Navicular pain (extra-label): 23 mg/kg PO every 24 hours[11]

Monitoring

- Baseline (especially in geriatric dogs, dogs with chronic diseases, or those where prolonged treatment is likely): physical examination, CBC, serum chemistry panel (including liver enzymes and renal values), and urinalysis. It is recommended to reassess liver enzymes after 1 week of therapy. If liver enzyme elevations occur, recommend discontinuing the drug.
- Schirmer tear test prior to and periodically during therapy
- Clinical efficacy
- Signs of potential adverse reactions: inappetence, diarrhea, mucoid feces, vomiting, melena, polyuria, polydipsia, anemia, jaundice, lethargy, behavior changes, ataxia, or seizures
- Long-term therapy: Consider repeating CBC, urinalysis, and serum chemistries on an ongoing basis

Client information

- This medicine can be given with or without food; however, giving medicine with food may reduce the chances for stomach problems. If your animal vomits or acts sick after getting it on an empty stomach, give your animal the medicine with food or with a small treat to see if this helps. If vomiting continues, contact your veterinarian.
- Most dogs usually tolerate etodolac well, but rarely, some dogs will develop ulcers or serious kidney and liver problems. Watch for the following signs: not eating (as much as usual), vomiting, changes in bowel movements; changes in behavior or activity levels (more or less active than normal), incoordination (eg, stumbling, clumsiness), seizures (convulsions), or aggression; yellowing of gums, skin, or whites of the eyes (jaundice); changes in drinking (frequency, amount consumed) or urination habits (frequency, color, or smell).
- Periodic laboratory tests to check for liver and kidney side effects are required; do not miss important follow up visits with your veterinarian.

Chemistry/Synonyms

Etodolac is an indole acetic acid derivative and an NSAID that occurs as a white, crystalline compound that is insoluble in water but soluble in alcohol or DMSO. Etodolac has a chirally active center with a corresponding S (+) enantiomer and an R (-) enantiomer. The commercially available product is supplied as a racemic mixture of the forms.

Etodolac may also be known as AY-24236, etodolacum, etodolic acid, *Acudor*®, *Articulan*®, *Dualgan*®, *Eccoxolac*®, *Edolan*®, *Elderin*®, *EtoGesic*®, *Etonox*®, *Etopan*®, *Flancox*®, *Hypen*®, *Lodot*®, *Lonine*®, *Metazin*®, *Sodolac*®, *Todolac*®, *Ultradol*®, and *Zedolac*®.

Storage/Stability

Store the commercially available veterinary tablets at controlled room temperature (15°C to 30°C [59°F to 86°F]).

Store the commercially available injection at or below 25°C (77°F).

Compatibility/Compounding Considerations

No specific information was noted.

Dosage Forms/Regulatory Status

VETERINARY-LABELED PRODUCTS:

The Association of Racing Commissioners International (ARCI) has designated this drug as a class 4 substance. Use of this drug may not be allowed in certain animal competitions. Check rules and regulations before entering a competition while this medication is being administered. Contact local racing authorities for further guidance. See ***Appendix*** for more information.

NOTE: Although etodolac is still listed in FDA's Green Book of approved animal drugs, it is not commercially available in the United States.

Etodolac Scored Tablets: 150 mg, 300 mg and 500 mg; *EtoGesic*®; (Rx). FDA-approved for use in dogs. Do not use in cats. NADA #141-108

Etodolac Injection 10% (100 mg/mL); *EtoGesic*® *Injectable*; (Rx). FDA-approved for use in dogs. NADA #141-274

HUMAN-LABELED PRODUCTS:

Etodolac Tablets: 400 and 500 mg; extended-release tablets: 400, 500, and 600 mg; capsules: 200 and 300 mg; generic; (Rx)

References

For the complete list of references, see **wiley.com/go/budde/plumb**

Etomidate

(ee-***tom***-i-date) *Amidate*®

Injectable Anesthetic

Prescriber Highlights

- ► Injectable nonbarbiturate anesthetic agent that may be useful as an alternative to alfaxalone or propofol for induction of general anesthesia, particularly in patients with preexisting cardiac dysfunction, or that are critically ill
- ► Can inhibit cortisol production; may need to supplement corticosteroids in critically ill patients
- ► Not a controlled substance
- ► Relatively expensive, especially for large-sized dogs

Uses/Indications

Etomidate may be useful as an alternative to alfaxalone or propofol for anesthetic induction in small animals, particularly in patients with preexisting cardiac dysfunction, or those that are critically ill.

Pharmacology/Actions

Etomidate acts at the GABA receptor in the CNS to increase chloride conductance, causing hyperpolarization of postsynaptic neurons and resulting in hypnosis and CNS depression.[1] Etomidate causes minimal hemodynamic changes and little effect on the cardiovascular system as compared with other injectable anesthetic agents. At clinical doses, etomidate has little effect on respiratory rate or rhythm.[2] Etomidate decreases cerebral blood flow and oxygen consumption.[2] It usually lowers intraocular pressure (IOP) and causes slight decreases in intracranial pressure[2,3]; however, when combined with other drugs, IOP may increase.[4] Etomidate reportedly does not induce malignant hyperthermia, but can speed its onset in susceptible patients secondary to a triggering agent.[5]

The reported therapeutic index (toxic dose/therapeutic dose) for etomidate is 26.[6] For comparison, therapeutic indexes for propofol and thiopental are ≈3 and 5, respectively.

When comparing etomidate to propofol for inductions in dogs, patients receiving etomidate had higher systolic arterial pressures and mean arterial pressures, but etomidate caused longer and poorer recoveries than propofol.[7]

Pharmacokinetics

No specific information on the pharmacokinetics of etomidate in domesticated animals was located. In humans, after IV injection, etomidate is rapidly distributed into the CNS and then rapidly cleared from the brain back into systemic tissues. Duration of hypnosis is short (3 to 5 minutes) and is dependent on dose. Recovery from anesthesia appears to be as fast as with thiopental, but slower than propofol. Etomidate is 75% bound to plasma proteins. The drug is rapidly metabolized in the liver, primarily via hydrolysis or glucuronidation to inactive metabolites. The majority of the drug and metabolites are excreted into the urine. Elimination half life ranges from 1.25 to 5 hours.

Contraindications/Precautions/Warnings

Etomidate is contraindicated in patients that are known to be hypersensitive to it.[8]

Etomidate can inhibit adrenocortical function[9-11]; it should not be used for purposes other than induction. Use with caution in patients with impaired adrenocortical function, particularly those with septic shock. Exogenous glucocorticoid administration may be considered in severely compromised animals.

Etomidate does not provide analgesia.[8]

Limited studies in patients with impaired hepatic or renal function have shown that elimination half-lives may be significantly increased in these patients, and the propylene glycol carrier in the injection may be problematic in patients with liver dysfunction.

A study in dogs concluded that etomidate/midazolam induction of anesthesia be used with caution in dogs undergoing ocular surgery, as it caused clinically relevant miosis, significant increases in intraocular pressure (IOP), and commonly caused ptyalism, gagging, and abdominal heaving.[12]

Do not confuse etomidate with etidronate. Etomidate is considered a high-alert medication (medication that requires special safeguards to reduce the risk for errors).[13] Consider instituting practices such as redundant drug dosage and volume checking, and special alert labels.

Adverse Effects

Common adverse effects include pain at IV injection site, phlebitis, vomiting, regurgitation, hypersalivation, skeletal muscle movements (myoclonus), eye movements, apnea, tachypnea, pigmenturia, and postoperative retching.[14,15] Preanesthetic medications administered prior to etomidate can decrease these effects.

Some hemolysis may occur due to the propylene glycol content of the injection, especially in cats.[16] Anecdotally, it may be beneficial to dilute etomidate (eg, inject into a running IV line) to decrease the pain associated with injection and, potentially, reduce hemolysis. Hemoglobinuria and intravascular hemolysis occurred in 2 dogs receiving etomidate infusion.[17]

Although etomidate causes minimal cardiopulmonary depression, a brief period of hypoventilation and decreased arterial blood pressure can occur after administration.

Apnea, laryngospasm, hiccups, hyperventilation, hypoventilation, hypertension, hypotension, lactic acidosis, arrhythmias, and postoperative vomiting have been reported in humans that have received etomidate.[8] Seizures have been reported in a few humans receiving etomidate; this adverse effect may be reduced if an opioid premedication is administered prior to etomidate.

Reproductive/Nursing Safety

Etomidate has caused embryocidal effects in rats and maternal toxicity in rabbits and rats.[8]

Some etomidate is excreted into maternal milk; use with caution in nursing patients.

Because safety has not been established in animals, this drug should only be used when the maternal benefits outweigh the potential risks to offspring.

Overdose/Acute Toxicity

Acute overdoses would be expected to cause enhanced pharmacologic effects of the drug. Treatment would be supportive (eg, mechanical ventilation), until the effects of the medication are diminished.

Drug Interactions

The following drug interactions have either been reported or are theoretical in humans or animals receiving etomidate and may be of significance in veterinary patients. Unless otherwise noted, use together is not necessarily contraindicated, but weigh the potential risks and perform additional monitoring when appropriate.

- **CNS and Respiratory Depressants** (eg, **barbiturates, opiates, anesthetics**): Additive pharmacological effects can occur if etomidate is used concurrently with other drugs that depress CNS or respiratory function.
- **Verapamil**: Has been associated with potentiating the anesthetic and respiratory depressant effects of etomidate

Laboratory Considerations

- The effects of etomidate on inhibiting cortisol may invalidate **ACTH stimulation** and **glucose tolerance** tests. Cortisol function may be affected for 2 to 6 hours in dogs, and up to 5.5 hours in cats after etomidate administration.

Dosages

DOGS & CATS:

Induction agent (extra-label): Dosing recommendations vary somewhat but generally range from 0.5 – 2 mg/kg IV,[7,14,18-23] although dosages up to 4 mg/kg IV have been noted.[23] A suitable premedication is required and can help reduce the incidence and severity of vomiting and myoclonic tremors. A benzodiazepine (eg, midazolam) ± low-dose ketamine administered prior to use can further reduce adverse effects and potentially allow lower etomidate induction dosages of 0.25 – 1 mg/kg.[24] Some clinicians also recommend administering a short-acting IV glucocorticoid to help offset etomidate's effects on cortisol production.

FERRETS:

Induction agent in the cardiovascular unstable patient (extra-label): Etomidate 1 – 2 mg/kg IV after diazepam 0.5 mg/kg IV[25]

SMALL MAMMALS:

Induction agent (extra-label):

a) **Rabbits**: As an induction agent in the cardiovascular unstable patient, etomidate 1 – 2 mg/kg IV after diazepam 0.5 mg/kg IV[25]

b) 1 – 2 mg/kg IV; must use with a benzodiazepine to prevent seizures[26]

Monitoring

- Depth of anesthesia and CNS effects (eg, seizures, paddling, myoclonus)

- Respiratory depression (eg, respiratory rate, pulse oximetry, end-tidal CO_2 ($ETCO_2$)
- Cardiovascular status (eg, cardiac rate and rhythm; blood pressure)

Client Information

- Etomidate is a potent sedative-hypnotic that should only be used by professionals in a setting where adequate patient monitoring is available.

Chemistry/Synonyms

An injectable, carboxylic imidazole anesthetic, etomidate occurs as a white or almost white powder. It is very slightly soluble in water and freely soluble in alcohol. The commercially available injection has a pH of 8.1, contains 35% propylene glycol, and is hyperosmolar (4640 mosm/L).

Etomidate may also be known as R-16659, *Amidate®*, *Hypnomidate®*, *Radenarcon®*, or *Sibul®*.

Storage/Stability

Unless otherwise labeled, store etomidate injection at room temperature and protected from light.

Compatibility/Compounding Considerations

No specific information was noted.

Dosage Forms/Regulatory Status

VETERINARY-LABELED PRODUCTS: NONE

HUMAN-LABELED PRODUCTS:

Etomidate Injection: 2 mg/mL in 10 mL and 20 mL single-dose vials; 10 mL and 20 mL ampules; and 20 mL *Abboject®* syringes; *Amidate®*; generic; (Rx)

References

For the complete list of references, see **wiley.com/go/budde/plumb**

Euthanasia Agents with Pentobarbital

(yoo-thon-***ayzh***-ya; pen-toe-***barb***-i-tal) *Beuthanasia-D®*

*See **Pentobarbital** monograph for therapeutic uses (other than euthanasia)*

Prescriber Highlights

- Used for humane euthanasia in animals not intended for food purposes
- Store product separately and securely so it is not confused with therapeutic agents.
- Use care in handling filled syringes; avoid accidental injection and any contact with open wounds. Dispose of used needles and syringes properly.
- A sedative, analgesic, and/or anesthetic agent may be required prior to injection with this agent in painful, distressed, or fractious animals.
- Minor muscle twitching, agonal breathing, urination, defecation, vocalization, and dysphoria can occur during and after injection.
- Pentobarbital is a DEA schedule II (C-II) controlled substance when used as a single agent; pentobarbital with phenytoin is a DEA schedule III (C-III) controlled substance.

Uses/Indications

Euthanasia agents with pentobarbital can be used for rapid, humane euthanasia in animals not intended for food purposes. Individual products may be labeled for use in specific species. Euthanasia induced by pentobarbital occurs rapidly, smoothly, and is relatively painless, particularly when administered IV (preferred).[1] See ***Dosages.***

Pharmacology/Actions

Pentobarbital administered at high doses causes rapid loss of consciousness with simultaneous collapse of the animal. This stage rapidly progresses to deep anesthesia with concomitant reduction in blood pressure. Subsequent depression of the medullary respiratory center terminates breathing; encephalographic activity becomes isoelectric, indicating cerebral death; and then cardiac activity ceases.

Some euthanasia solutions contain phenytoin for its cardiac depressant effects, which hastens cessation of cardiac electrical activity.

Contraindications/Precautions/Warnings

Euthanasia agents with pentobarbital must not be used in animals intended for food purposes (human or animal consumption); care must be taken to prevent scavenging wildlife from consuming carcasses. Contact the US Fish and Wildlife Service for additional advice for prevention of relay pentobarbital toxicity in wildlife.

Use extreme care in handling filled syringes and properly disposing of used injection equipment. Avoid accidental injection and any contact with open wounds.

Death may be delayed in animals with cardiac or circulatory deficiency[2]; death may be delayed or not accomplished if injection is given perivascularly. Prior use of a sedative, analgesic, and/or anesthetic agent may be required in painful, distressed, or fractious animals. Do not combine neuromuscular blockers with pentobarbital-containing injection, as paralysis may occur prior to onset of unconsciousness.[3]

Dosage forms of pentobarbital-containing euthanasia solutions are not indicated or formulated (eg, denatured, nonsterile) for therapeutic use.

Do not confuse PHENObarbital with PENTObarbital.

Adverse Effects

Minor muscle twitching may occur after injection. Reflex responses may cause motor activity to continue; however, the unconscious animal does not experience pain or distress because the cerebral cortex is not functioning. In a study of dogs euthanized with pentobarbital-phenytoin combination,[4] the incidence of muscle activity was 14%. Other reported adverse events included agonal breaths (≈10%), urination (≈8%), vocalization (5%), and dysphoria (4%).[4]

Reproductive/Nursing Safety

Pentobarbital readily crosses the placenta and fetal depression occurs following administration of pentobarbital euthanasia; however, it is not considered a viable method of fetal euthanasia.[1]

Dosages

NOTES:

1. For a thorough discussion of the use of pentobarbital (and other methods) for humane euthanasia in a variety of species, refer to the most recent version of the AVMA Guidelines for the Euthanasia of Animals.[3]
2. Because different products may contain different concentrations of pentobarbital, refer to the specific information provided with the product being used.
3. IV injection is the preferred route for euthanasia of dogs, cats, other small animals, and horses.[3] Intraperitoneal or intracoelomic injection may be used in situations when an IV injection would be distressful, dangerous, or difficult because of small patient size. Administration of pentobarbital via intraorgan routes (eg, intraosseous, intracardiac, intrahepatic, intrarenal) generally should be performed only in unconscious or anesthetized animals.
4. Because of the viscous nature of these compounds, many cli-

nicians dilute the euthanasia solution with commonly used isotonic fluids (eg, lactated Ringer's solution, 0.9% sodium chloride). No studies have confirmed the stability of these dilutions; administration should occur immediately after mixing.

DOGS:

Humane euthanasia:

a) **Pentobarbital with phenytoin** (label dosage; FDA-approved): pentobarbital 390 mg with phenytoin 50 mg (1 mL) for each 4.5 kg (10 lb) of body weight IV[5]

b) **Pentobarbital as a single agent** (label dosage; not FDA-approved): pentobarbital 390 mg (1 mL) for each 4.5 kg (10 lb) of body weight IV[6]

CATS:

Humane euthanasia:

a) **Pentobarbital sodium as a single agent** (label dosage; not FDA-approved): pentobarbital 390 mg (1 mL) for each 4.5 kg (10 lb) of body weight IV[6]

b) **Pentobarbital with phenytoin** (extra-label): pentobarbital 390 mg with phenytoin 50 mg (1 mL) for each 4.5 kg (10 lb) of body weight IV[5]

LARGE ANIMALS:

Humane euthanasia:

a) **Pentobarbital as a single agent** (label-dosage; not FDA-approved): pentobarbital 390 mg [or 6 grains] (1 mL) for each 4.5 kg (10 lb) of body weight IV[6,7]

b) **Pentobarbital with phenytoin**(extra-label): pentobarbital 390 mg with phenytoin 50 mg (1 mL) for each 4.5 kg (10 lb) of body weight IV.[6] Use of an IV catheter is suggested due to the large volume to be injected.[3] **NOTE**: This drug must not be used in animals to be consumed by humans or other animals.

Monitoring

Verification of death in some species (eg, reptiles, amphibians) can be challenging; species-specific references should be consulted. Using a combination of criteria to confirm death is recommended[1] and may include:

- The absence of respirations and heart sounds
- Graying of mucous membranes
- Fixed, dilated pupils
- Rigor mortis

Client Information

- Administration of euthanasia agents must only be performed by authorized veterinary professionals.
- Clients should be forewarned about the possibility of agonal breathing, muscle twitching, dysphoria during injection, elimination of bodily fluids, and eyes not closing once unconscious. The animal is unconscious and not experiencing any pain during these events.
- Euthanized animals must be properly disposed of (eg, by deep burial; local laws and regulations may apply) to prevent toxicity to scavenging animals that may consume carcass material.

Storage/Stability

Unless stated otherwise on the product label, store pentobarbital euthanasia agents at controlled room temperature of 20°C to 25°C (68°F-77°F) with excursions of 15°C to 30°C (59°F-86°F).

Euthanasia agents with pentobarbital are schedule 2 (C-II) or schedule 3 (C-III) controlled substances that should be stored in an area that is substantially constructed and securely locked. Follow applicable local, state, and federal laws regarding disposal of unused or wasted controlled drugs. Euthanasia agents should be stored separately in a manner that will not be confused with therapeutic agents. Diversion of euthanasia solution for suicide has occurred.[8,9]

Dosage Forms/Regulatory Status

Information on lower concentration products used therapeutically can be found in ***Pentobarbital***. Pentobarbital-only products have not been approved by the FDA.

VETERINARY-LABELED PRODUCTS:

NOTE: Report dispensing to state monitoring programs as required. Properly dispose of euthanized animals. Renderers may not accept carcasses euthanized with pentobarbital.

Pentobarbital Sodium 390 mg/mL and Phenytoin Sodium 50 mg/mL for Injection (Euthanasia) in 100 mL vials; nonsterile; *Beuthanasia*®-D Special,[5] generic; (Rx, C-III). FDA-approved for use in dogs. NADA #119-807

Pentobarbital Sodium Powder for Reconstitution and Injection: 392 mg/mL when constituted with 250 mL of water; nonsterile; *Fatal-Plus® Powder*[10]; (Rx, C-II). Labeled for use in animals regardless of species.

Pentobarbital Sodium for Injection: 390 mg/mL_in 250 mL vials; nonsterile; *Socumb*®[7]; *Fatal-Plus® Solution*[6]; (Rx, C-II). Some products labeled for use in animals regardless of species.

HUMAN-LABELED PRODUCTS: NONE

References

For the complete list of references, see **wiley.com/go/budde/plumb**

Exenatide

(ex-**en**-a-tide) *Bydureon®, Byetta®*

Glucagon-like Peptide-1 (GLP-1) Receptor Agonist

Prescriber Highlights

- ► An incretin mimetic that is administered SC for adjunctive management of diabetes mellitus in cats
- ► Exenatide is NOT an insulin substitute and cannot be used to treat diabetic ketoacidosis; it should not be used as monotherapy to manage type 1 diabetes mellitus.
- ► Contraindications include hypersensitivity, severe GI disease, severe or end-stage renal disease, medullary thyroid carcinoma, and multiple endocrine neoplasia syndrome type 2.
- ► Use with caution in patients with impaired renal function or history of renal transplant, history of pancreatitis, or drug-induced immune-mediated thrombocytopenia (DIIMT); occurrence of pancreatitis or DIIMT precludes further exenatide use.
- ► Adverse effects include nausea, vomiting, diarrhea, anorexia, and weight loss. Hypoglycemia is unlikely unless exenatide is used in conjunction with other hypoglycemic agents (eg, insulin).
- ► The National Institute for Occupational Safety and Health (NIOSH) has determined that exenatide meets the definition of a hazardous drug; use appropriate precautions when handling.
- ► Obtaining doses for cats from exenatide formulations intended for use in humans may prove challenging.
- ► Exenatide immediate-release (IR) solution is not interchangeable with exenatide extended-release (ER) formulation.

Uses/Indications

Exenatide is used for the adjunctive treatment of uncomplicated diabetes mellitus in cats. In studies using exenatide immediate-release (IR) solution, median or average changes in study parameters (eg, fasting blood glucose, insulin concentration) in obese or diabetic cats were not significant but tended toward improvement, and positive responses were apparent in individual cats.[1,2] When exenatide extended-release (ER) was administered with glargine insulin to newly diagnosed diabetic cats, glucose variability was reduced, and remission rates and metabolic control appeared improved compared with cats that received only glargine; however, these results were significant only at interim study analyses, and were not statistically different from placebo at the study conclusion.[3,4]

Pharmacology/Actions

Exenatide is an incretin mimetic. As a glucagon-like peptide-1 (GLP-1)–receptor agonist, exenatide augments glucose-dependent insulin synthesis and secretion, enhances pancreatic endocrine beta-cell proliferation and survival, and inhibits glucagon secretion (without impeding glucagon secretion in response to hypoglycemia).[5] The drug improves insulin sensitivity in muscles and reduces hepatic gluconeogenesis.[6] Exenatide efficacy depends on an adequate mass of functional pancreatic endocrine beta cells.[7] Because exenatide amplifies the insulin response to food within the lumen of the GI tract, the risk for hypoglycemia is low.

Exenatide immediate-release (IR) was administered to healthy cats and increased insulin secretion in response to glucose,[8–10] and one study noted variable effects on glucagon secretion.[10] No significant changes in glucose, insulin, or glucagon concentrations were observed in obese[1] or diabetic[2] cats.

In healthy cats that received exenatide extended-release (ER), fasting blood glucose and glucagon concentration were reduced, and insulin secretion increased (including first-phase insulin response).[10,11] After a single dose of exenatide ER, readings from continuous glucose monitors were below baseline at 2 and 6 weeks after injection.[11] However, studies returned conflicting results for glucose, insulin, and glucagon responses to meals.[10,11] At the time of writing, no publications describing the effects of exenatide ER on glucose, insulin, or glucagon concentrations in diabetic cats were located.

GLP-1 activity in the CNS may help regulate satiety.[6] In the GI tract, GLP-1 agonists delay gastric emptying and reduce GI motility, an effect that may help attenuate postprandial hyperglycemia.[6] Exenatide delays gastric emptying in cats,[12] and has resulted in colic in alpacas.[13,14]

Pharmacokinetics

Exenatide concentration peaked 45 minutes after SC administration of exenatide immediate-release (IR) to healthy fasted cats and was no longer significantly different from baseline after 90 minutes.[8]

Exenatide extended-release (ER) formulation was administered to healthy cats and resulted in measurable exenatide concentrations after 15 minutes. An initial peak exenatide concentration was noted after 1 hour; a second, higher peak occurred 4 weeks after injection. Exenatide concentration was no longer significantly different from baseline 6 weeks after injection.[11]

In humans, exenatide is renally eliminated, undergoing glomerular filtration and proteolytic degradation. The half-life of exenatide IR solution is 2.4 hours,[5] whereas the ER formulation has a half-life of ≈14 days. Unlike endogenous glucagon-like peptide-1 (GLP-1), dipeptidyl peptidase-4 (DPP-4) is not involved in exenatide metabolism.

Contraindications/Precautions/Warnings

Exenatide is NOT an insulin substitute and cannot be used to treat diabetic ketoacidosis; it should not be used as monotherapy for treatment of type 1 diabetes mellitus. Because exenatide use in cats is emerging, the safety profile is still being studied; current information for use in cats is limited to small sample-size studies and extrapolation from known human information.

Exenatide is contraindicated in patients with known hypersensitivity to it or any components of the formulation. Exenatide extended-release (ER) is contraindicated for use in humans with medullary thyroid carcinoma or multiple endocrine neoplasia syndrome type 2.[15] In humans, exenatide immediate-release (IR) should not be used in patients with severe GI disease (eg, gastroparesis, inflammatory bowel disease), or with severe or end-stage renal disease.[5] In humans, development of either pancreatitis or drug-induced immune-mediated thrombocytopenia is considered a contraindication to continued exenatide use.[5,15] Pancreatitis is more likely to occur in humans with concurrent risk factors (eg, cholelithiasis, hypertriglyceridemia).

Acute kidney injury has occurred in humans taking exenatide.[5,15] The drug should be used with caution in patients with impaired renal function or in renal transplant recipients.

Absorption of orally administered medication may be impacted (eg, delayed time to peak concentration) as exenatide may slow GI transit times. Orally administered medication should be administered at least one hour prior to exenatide administration.

Exenatide ER caused dose- and duration-dependent thyroid C-cell tumors in rats.[15] The National Institute for Occupational Safety and Health (NIOSH) has determined this carcinogenicity meets the definition of a hazardous drug, and personal protective equipment (PPE) should be used accordingly to minimize the risk for exposure.

Adverse Effects

Exenatide may cause adverse GI effects (eg, diarrhea, vomiting, anorexia) in cats; obese cats had a reduced appetite, as noted by owners using a 5-point assessment scale.[1] Weight loss (≈0.7 kg[1.5 lb]) has been documented in healthy,[9] obese,[1] and diabetic[2] cats that have received exenatide immediate-release (IR); however, when exenatide extended-release (ER) was administered with glargine insulin to newly diagnosed diabetic cats, it had a variable effect on weight and no effect on body condition score.[3] Although subclinical hypoglycemia occurred in 63% of diabetic cats that were treated with exenatide IR and glargine insulin,[2] hypoglycemia rates were similar in diabetic cats that received either glargine insulin alone or in combination with exenatide ER.[3]

Injection site reactions are common in humans but have not been reported in cats with either exenatide formulation.[2,3,8,11,16] Increased aggression during injection of exenatide IR was noted in one study of obese cats,[1] and increased sleeping and hiding in dark places were noted in newly diagnosed diabetic cats treated with exenatide ER and glargine insulin.[3] Exenatide-induced pancreatitis or increased feline pancreatic lipase has not been identified in cats, although the number of cats with exposure to exenatide formulations remains small.

In humans, severe hypersensitivity reactions (eg, angioedema and anaphylaxis) are rare, whereas less severe reactions (eg, rash, urticaria, pruritus) are more common.[5] Antibodies to exenatide developed in 44% to 49% of patients who were treated with either exenatide formulation.[5,15] In most of the patients, antibodies occurred at low levels and did not impact glycemic control; however, 6% of patients had high antibody titers associated with an attenuated glycemic response.

Reproductive/Nursing Safety

Exenatide is unlikely to cross the placenta.[17] However, administration of high doses (12 to 390 times the recommended human dose) of exenatide immediate-release (IR) to pregnant mice and rabbits during periods of fetal organogenesis resulted in skeletal abnormalities, cleft palate, and reduced fetal and neonatal growth. Neonatal deaths were observed in mice receiving 6 µg/kg/day (≈3 times the recommended human dose).[5] Exenatide extended-release (ER) administered to rats during organogenesis reduced fetal growth and delayed fetal ossification.[15]

Exenatide is excreted in the maternal milk of mice with concentrations in milk 2.5% that of maternal plasma.[5] Because exenatide is not orally absorbed, the risk to nursing offspring is likely negligible.[17]

Because safety has not been established in animals, this drug should only be used when the maternal benefits outweigh the potential risks to offspring.

Overdose/Acute Toxicity

An overdose of exenatide may result in severe nausea, vomiting, and hypoglycemia. Based on pharmacokinetic data,[8,11] clinical signs caused by overdoses of exenatide immediate-release (IR) would be expected to be short-lived, whereas overdoses of exenatide extended-release (ER) could have effects for many weeks. Patients should be treated supportively based on clinical signs.

For patients that have experienced or are suspected to have experienced an overdose, it is strongly encouraged to consult with one of the 24-hour poison consultation centers that specialize in providing information specific for veterinary patients. For general information related to overdose and toxin exposures, as well as contact information for poison control centers, refer to ***Appendix.***

Drug Interactions

The following drug interactions have either been reported or are theoretical in humans or animals receiving exenatide and may be of significance in veterinary patients. Unless otherwise noted, use together is not necessarily contraindicated, but weigh the potential risks and perform additional monitoring when appropriate.

- **Beta-Adrenergic Receptor Antagonists** (eg, **atenolol, propranolol**): Can have variable effects on glycemic control and can mask the signs associated with hypoglycemia
- **Clonidine**: Can mask the signs associated with hypoglycemia
- **Digoxin**: Peak concentration may be delayed and reduced but overall steady-state digoxin exposure (AUC) is unchanged.[5]
- **Orally Administered Medications**: By slowing gastric emptying, exenatide may change the rate and extent of absorption of all concomitantly administered oral medications. Oral medications should be administered at least 1 hour prior to exenatide.
- **Reserpine**: Can mask the signs associated with hypoglycemia
- **Warfarin**: Concurrent use may prolong prothrombin time.

The following drugs or drug classes may potentiate exenatide hypoglycemic activity:

- **Anabolic Steroids** (eg, **boldenone, stanozolol, testosterone**)
- **Angiotensin II Receptor Blockers** (ARBs; eg, **telmisartan**)
- **Angiotensin Converting Enzyme Inhibitors** (ACEIs; eg, **benazepril, enalapril**)
- **Disopyramide**
- **Fenofibrate**
- **Fluoroquinolones** (eg, **ciprofloxacin, enrofloxacin, pradofloxacin**)
- **Fluoxetine**
- **Hypoglycemics, Oral** (eg, **acarbose, glipizide, metformin**)
- **Monoamine Oxidase Inhibitors** (MAOIs; eg, **amitraz, linezolid, selegiline**)
- **Pentoxifylline**
- **Salicylates** (eg, **aspirin, bismuth subsalicylate**)
- **Somatostatin Derivatives** (eg, **octreotide**)
- **Sulfonamides** (eg, **sulfadimethoxine, sulfamethoxazole**)

The following drugs or drug classes may diminish exenatide hypoglycemic activity:

- **Alpha-2-Adrenergic Receptor Agonists** (eg, **dexmedetomidine, xylazine**): May cause hyperglycemia and temporarily interfere with glycemic control
- **Beta-Adrenergic Receptor Agonists** (eg, **albuterol, terbutaline**)
- **Corticosteroids** (eg, **dexamethasone, prednis[ol]one**)
- **Cyclosporine**
- **Danazol**
- **Diazoxide**
- **Diuretics** (eg, **furosemide, hydrochlorothiazide**)
- **Estrogens** (eg, **diethylstilbestrol [DES], estriol**)
- **Isoniazid**
- **Leuprolide**
- **Niacin**
- **Phenothiazines** (eg, **acepromazine, chlorpromazine**)
- **Progestins** (eg, **megestrol**)
- **Sympathomimetic Agents** (eg, **epinephrine, phenylpropanolamine**)
- **Thyroid Hormones**: Can elevate blood glucose levels in diabetic patients when thyroid hormone therapy is first initiated

Laboratory Considerations

- None noted

Dosages

NOTE: Exenatide immediate-release (IR) and exenatide extended-release (ER) are NOT interchangeable.

CATS:

Adjunctive therapy for diabetes mellitus (extra-label):

- Using exenatide IR: 1 µg/kg SC twice daily in combination with twice-daily glargine insulin and a low-carbohydrate diet.[2] Administer *before* feeding; do not administer after a meal. Injecting exenatide into the same body region as insulin injection is acceptable as long as injection sites are not adjacent (ie, separate injections by 1 inch or more if possible[18]). Glargine dose reduction of 25% to 50% was required in some cats.
- Using exenatide ER: 200 µg/kg SC every 7 days in combination with twice-daily glargine insulin and a low-carbohydrate diet[3]

Monitoring

The overarching goal when monitoring diabetic patients is control of clinical signs related to hyperglycemia (eg, polyuria, polydipsia) while avoiding hypoglycemia.[19] All monitoring strategies should be interpreted based on clinical signs. Results from the monitoring options listed below may conflict in regard to achieving good glycemic and clinical control. Diabetic patients should be closely monitored.

- Patient status and control of clinical signs: Body weight, appetite, fluid intake, urine output
- Blood glucose curve. It is encouraged to refer to additional information on regulating diabetic patients and insulin adjustments. Flash glucose monitoring systems (eg, *FreeStyle Libre* system) are easy to apply, are user-friendly, and provide useful information surrounding glycemic control when the patient is in the hospital or home environment.[20-23] A blood glucose curve can be considered at the following times[19]:
    - After the first dose of a new insulin type
    - 7 to 14 days after starting insulin or an insulin dose change
    - At least every 3 months, even in animals with well-controlled diabetes
    - Any time clinical signs recur in an animal with previously well-controlled diabetes
    - When hypoglycemia is suspected
- Urine glucose monitoring is typically only helpful for documenting prolonged hypoglycemia (eg, persistently negative urine glucose testing when monitoring for diabetic remission in cats). Because most diabetic patients spend time above the renal threshold for urinary glucose spillage, even patients with well-controlled diabetes may be intermittently glucosuric throughout the day.
- Fructosamine or glycosylated hemoglobin can be measured if

available and warranted.

- Pancreatitis, acute kidney injury, and drug-induced immune-mediated thrombocytopenia (DIIMT) are uncommon but significant concerns in humans. It is recommended to monitor feline pancreatic lipase immunoreactivity (fPLI) concentration, BUN, creatinine, and CBC with platelet count.
- Injection sites, for local reactions
- As exenatide may slow GI transit and alter oral drug absorption, response to orally administered medication should be monitored closely for intended effect.
- For patients that have experienced or are suspected to have experienced repeated or unexplained hypoglycemia, it is strongly encouraged to consult with a veterinary emergency and critical care and/or endocrinology specialist or reference text that specializes in providing information specific for treatment of hypoglycemia.

Client Information

- Exenatide is administered by injection under the skin (subcutaneous). Your veterinarian should demonstrate and allow practice of correct injection techniques.
- Always double-check the dose in the syringe before you inject your animal.
- The injection site should be frequently changed, with the main sites being the back of the neck or shoulder area.
- Nausea, vomiting, and lack of appetite are common side effects. Report significant or prolonged changes in appetite, abnormal feces, or weight loss to your veterinarian.
- This medication requires frequent monitoring by your veterinarian, including blood work. Do not miss these important follow-up visits.
- When using exenatide immediate-release (IR) solution:
  - The pen device requires priming before the first use.
  - The needle must be removed before storing to prevent leakage.
  - Store refrigerated until first use; once in use, it may be stored in the refrigerator or at room temperature. Discard 30 days after first use.
  - Do not freeze; the drug must be discarded if it freezes.
  - Missed doses should be omitted, and the next dose resumed at the scheduled time.
- When using exenatide extended-release (ER) solution:
  - Store refrigerated until ready to use; allow it to come to room temperature prior to injection. Exenatide ER may be stored at room temperature for up to 4 weeks. Do not freeze; the drug must be discarded if it freezes.
  - Wear gloves and eye protection when preparing and administering. Wash hands thoroughly after administration.
  - Vials are single-use only and any unused portion must be discarded.
- Use a new needle for each dose. Place used needles and syringes in a puncture-resistant ("sharps") disposal container immediately after use, making sure you do not attempt to disconnect the needle from the syringe or recap the needle. Your veterinarian or pharmacist can help you obtain these containers.
- This medicine is considered to be a hazardous drug as defined by the National Institute for Occupational Safety and Health (NIOSH). Talk with your veterinarian or pharmacist about the use of personal protective equipment when handling this medicine.

Chemistry/Synonyms

Exenatide is a synthetic 39-amino-acid protein originally identified in the saliva of the Gila monster (*Heloderma suspectum*). It has a molecular weight of 4187. The amino acid sequence has 53% similarity to mammalian glucagon-like peptide-1 (GLP-1). Exenatide immediate-release (IR) is clear and colorless with a pH of 4.5. Exenatide extended-release (ER) contains exenatide incorporated into a microsphere polymer formulation that appears as a white to off-white powder and requires reconstitution with the manufacturer-provided diluent. After reconstitution, exenatide ER is cloudy and white to off-white.

Exenatide may also be known as AC 2993, LY2148568, exendin-4, *Bydureon*®, and *Byetta*®.

Storage/Stability

Store all unused exenatide products refrigerated at 2°C to 8°C (36°F-46°F). Protect from light and freezing; discard exenatide if it has been frozen.

After first use, store exenatide immediate-release (IR) between 2°C and 25°C (36°F-77°F); do not store pen device with a needle attached as the solution may leak from the device and air bubbles may form. The manufacturer states that exenatide IR is to be discarded 30 days after first use.

Exenatide extended-release (ER) may be stored unmixed at room temperature for no more than 4 weeks. Once reconstituted, it must be administered immediately.

Compatibility/Compounding Considerations

Do not mix exenatide immediate-release (IR) with insulin.[5]

Studies have described dilution of exenatide IR with saline or with a diluent composed of the same excipients as commercial exenatide solution.[1,9] Despite plasma exenatide being measurable in the participants of one study,[1] dilution of exenatide IR is not recommended as potency and stability were not assessed. Exenatide IR was diluted 1:10 using a diluent composed of the same excipients as commercial exenatide solution and stored at room temperature for a maximum of 30 days.[1] Despite plasma exenatide being measurable in the study participants,[1] dilution of exenatide IR is not recommended as potency and stability analyses were not performed. Another study used a 1:10 to 1:100 dilution of exenatide IR with 0.9% sodium chloride, which was mixed prior to each dose (dilution technique and storage [if any] was not described).[9]

Dosage Forms/Regulatory Status

VETERINARY-LABELED PRODUCTS: NONE

HUMAN-LABELED PRODUCTS:

Exenatide Immediate-Release (IR) Injection: 250 µg/mL in prefilled pens that deliver 60 doses of either 5 µg (1.2 mL total) or 10 µg (2.4 mL total); *Byetta*®; (Rx)

Needles for pen device are sold separately.

Exenatide Extended-Release (ER) Injection: 2 mg single-dose vial in a kit with a prefilled syringe containing 0.65 mL diluent, a vial connector, and custom needles specific to the delivery system; 4 vial-diluent pairs per unit; *Bydureon*®; (Rx). It is also available as a pen device containing 2 mg exenatide and 0.65 mL diluent in separate compartments, and as an autoinjector (*Bydureon*® *BCise*); however, these presentations are not practical for feline dosages.

References

For the complete list of references, see **wiley.com/go/budde/plumb**

Famciclovir

(fam-***sye-kloe***-veer) *Famvir®*

Antiviral (Herpes)

Prescriber Highlights

- ► May be effective in treating feline herpes (FHV-1) infections and equine herpesvirus myeloencephalopathy (EHM). Dosage recommendations still in flux
- ► Appears to be well tolerated when used short-term (2 to 3 weeks)
- ► May administer without regard to meals
- ► Dosage reduction recommended for human patients with renal impairment; veterinary significance is uncertain

Uses/Indications

Famciclovir improved clinical signs and reduced viral shedding in cats experimentally infected with herpesvirus type 1 (FHV-1),[1] and in a retrospective case series of cats with naturally occurring FHV-1, 85% of owners reported improved clinical signs.[2] However, in shelter cats neither a single dose[3] nor a 7-day course of famciclovir[4] improved clinical signs following shelter admission, but the 7-day treatment reduced conjunctival FHV-1 shedding.[4]

Famciclovir may also prove beneficial in horses with equine herpesvirus-1 (EHV-1) myeloencephalopathy, but additional research is needed before it can be confidently recommended.

Pharmacology/Actions

In most species, famciclovir is rapidly converted in vivo to penciclovir. In cells infected with susceptible herpesvirus or varicella zoster virus, viral thymidine kinase phosphorylates penciclovir to penciclovir monophosphate. Cellular kinases further convert penciclovir monophosphate to penciclovir triphosphate, which inhibits herpesvirus DNA polymerase via competition with deoxyguanosine triphosphate, thereby selectively inhibiting viral DNA synthesis. Famciclovir is considered a virostatic agent and therefore does not affect latent virus and doesn't necessarily clear the virus.

Viral resistance can occur by mutation of viral thymidine kinase or DNA polymerase.

Pharmacokinetics

Famciclovir is deacetylated in the intestinal wall and blood and then oxidized via aldehyde oxidase in the liver to the active compound, penciclovir. Although deacetylation occurs rapidly and completely, cats are deficient in aldehyde oxidase and extrapolating pharmacokinetic data from other species to cats is not reliable because of this. Pharmacokinetics are non-linear in cats probably due to saturation of biotransformation enzymatic systems.[5]

Oral administration of 40 mg/kg or 90 mg/kg famciclovir to cats demonstrated variable famciclovir absorption and low bioavailability of penciclovir (7%-13%).[6] Food may reduce oral bioavailability. Both dosages had similar peak concentrations of penciclovir (C_{max}, ≈1.3 µg/mL) and peak times (T_{max}, 3 hours). Penciclovir elimination half-life was between 4 and 5 hours at both doses. Penciclovir administered IV demonstrated a volume of distribution that approximated the total body water of cats.[6]

In another pharmacokinetic study in cats given 40 mg/kg and 90 mg/kg oral doses, plasma penciclovir C_{max} was 2 µg/mL and 2.7 µg/mL respectively and elimination half-life was ≈4 to 5 hours at both doses.[5] Penciclovir concentration in tears was significantly higher with 90 mg/kg dosages, and C_{max} in tears was ≈25% that of plasma.

In horses, after oral famciclovir doses of 20 mg/kg, peak plasma penciclovir concentrations occurred ≈1 hour after dosing with peak concentrations of ≈3 µg/mL. Elimination was biphasic with a slow terminal half-life of ≈33 hours.[7]

In humans, famciclovir is well absorbed after oral administration, but undergoes extensive first-pass metabolism (not by CYP enzymes). Food can decrease peak concentrations but does not significantly impact clinical efficacy. Penciclovir is only marginally bound to plasma proteins. In humans, penciclovir elimination half-life is ≈2 to 3 hours; excretion is primarily via renal mechanisms. Intracellular half-lives of penciclovir in infected cells are significantly longer.

Contraindications/Precautions/Warnings

Famciclovir is contraindicated in patients known to be hypersensitive to it or penciclovir.

It should be used with caution (and dosage adjustment) in patients with renal dysfunction. Dosage adjustments are recommended in human patients with creatinine clearance less than 60 mL/min; significance in veterinary species is unclear.

Do not confuse famciclovir with acyclovir.

Adverse Effects

One study[2] noted adverse effects in 17% of cats receiving famciclovir, including diarrhea (7%), polydipsia (5%), weight loss (1.7%), vomiting (1.7%), and hiding behavior (1.7%). Urethral obstruction occurred in one cat receiving 90 mg/kg every 8 hours for 3 days, but the investigators determined the obstruction was not caused by famciclovir.[5]

In a small ($n = 4$) pharmacokinetic study in horses, adverse effects were not observed following a single oral dose of 20 mg/kg.[7]

In humans, famciclovir can cause nausea, vomiting, diarrhea, pruritus, and headache. Neutropenia, electrolyte disturbances, and increased liver transaminases have been reported and renal failure can occur, particularly when doses are not adjusted in patients with renal dysfunction.

Reproductive/Nursing Safety

In laboratory animals, doses up to 1000 mg/kg/day did not cause any observed effects on developing embryos or fetuses.[8] Dose-related testicular toxicity (reduced and abnormal sperm, seminiferous tubule atrophy) and reduced male fertility was observed in laboratory animals; no effect on females was observed.

Famciclovir (as penciclovir) is excreted in the milk of rats at concentrations 8 times higher than in plasma. Recommendations for humans is to avoid famciclovir use in nursing mothers.[9]

Because safety has not been established in animals, this drug should only be used when the maternal benefits outweigh the potential risks to offspring.

Overdose/Acute Toxicity

Little information is available. Supportive treatment has been recommended. Penciclovir can be removed by hemodialysis.

For patients that have experienced or are suspected to have experienced an overdose, consultation with a 24-hour poison consultation center specializing in providing veterinary-specific information is recommended. For general information related to overdose and toxin exposures, as well as contact information for poison control centers, refer to the ***Appendix***.

Drug Interactions

The following drug interactions have either been reported or are theoretical in humans or animals receiving famciclovir and may be of significance in veterinary patients. Unless otherwise noted, use together is not necessarily contraindicated, but weigh the potential risks and perform additional monitoring when appropriate.

- Probenecid: Can reduce the amount of penciclovir excreted by the kidneys and increase penciclovir plasma concentrations

Laboratory Considerations

- No specific information found.

Dosages

CATS:

Feline herpesvirus type 1 (FHV-1; extra-label): 90 mg/kg PO every 12 hours may be most reliable at achieving therapeutic active metabolite (penciclovir) concentrations in the superficial cornea; dosages ranging from 30 – 90 mg/kg PO every 8 to 12 hours have been studied.[2,4-6,10,11] Treatment duration recommendations can vary somewhat with 2 to 4 week durations often suggested. Kittens (at least 5 days old) may only require treatment for 2 weeks. Available human oral dosage forms may limit options for doses that can be practically administered. Treatment with famciclovir may preclude the need for topical ocular antiviral medications; however, other topical drugs such as an antibacterial agents or mucinomimetic artificial tear replacement may be critical.[12]

Monitoring

- Clinical efficacy
- Adverse effects most frequently seen in cats include diarrhea, polydipsia, inappetence, and vomiting.
- Baseline CBC, electrolytes, and renal panel with periodic recheck examinations if the drug is being administered chronically

Client Information

- Medicine used to control, but not cure, herpesvirus infections in cats
- Try giving medicine without food, but if your cat vomits or acts sick after getting the medicine, give with a small amount of food. Because there is limited experience with this medicine in veterinary medicine, be sure to report any concerns about your cat to your veterinarian while your cat is taking it.
- Usually well tolerated.

Chemistry/Synonyms

A prodrug, famciclovir is a purine-derived, synthetic, acyclic purine nucleoside analogue. It is white to pale-yellow solid, freely soluble in acetone and methanol, and sparingly soluble in ethanol and isopropanol. At 25°C famciclovir is freely soluble (greater than 25% w/v) in water initially, but rapidly precipitates.

Famciclovir may also be known as AV 42810, BRL 42810, famciclovirum, or by the trade name *Famvir*®.

Storage/Stability

Famciclovir tablets should be stored at room temperature (20°C-25°C [68°F-77°F]) in an airtight, light-resistant container.

Compatibility/Compounding Considerations

The film-coated tablets may be split.

Dosage Forms/Regulatory Status

VETERINARY-LABELED PRODUCTS: NONE

HUMAN-LABELED PRODUCTS:

Famciclovir Oral Tablets (film-coated): 125 mg, 250 mg, and 500 mg; *Famvir*®, generic; (Rx)

References

For the complete list of references, see **wiley.com/go/budde/plumb**

Famotidine

(fa-***moe***-ti-deen) *Pepcid*®

H_2-Receptor Antagonist

Prescriber Highlights

- Used to reduce gastric acid production. Studies in dogs and cats suggest omeprazole is superior to famotidine for increasing gastric pH.
- Longer duration of action and fewer drug interactions than cimetidine
- Adverse effects include possible bradycardia with rapid IV infusion. Potential for GI effects or dry mouth or skin; rare idiopathic intravascular hemolysis anecdotally reported when given IV to cats

Uses/Indications

Famotidine may be useful for the treatment and/or routine prophylaxis of gastric, abomasal, and duodenal ulcers; stress-related or drug-induced erosive gastritis; esophagitis; duodenal gastric reflux; and esophageal reflux. However, oral omeprazole provided superior gastric acid suppression as compared with oral famotidine,[1] and omeprazole was also deemed superior to famotidine when used to prevent exercise-induced gastritis in racing Alaskan sled dogs.[2] Coadministration of famotidine and pantoprazole in dogs was not superior to pantoprazole alone for increasing intragastric pH, so combining these drugs is likely not necessary.[3] A recent study reported diminished effect on intragastric pH in dogs when oral famotidine 1 mg/kg was repeatedly administered every 12 hours for 14 days.[4]

Famotidine could be considered for immediate relief of signs when used on an as needed basis, and when used in the short term (eg, prevention of esophageal reflux under anesthesia[5,6]).[7]

In dogs, famotidine did not improve outcomes (eradication) of *Helicobacter* spp infections when added to triple antibiotic therapy.[8]

When famotidine was administered to cats for 14 days, a diminished effect on intragastric pH was observed, indicating decreased effectiveness with prolonged administration.[9]

In cattle, famotidine significantly increased the pH of abomasal outflow fluid for up to 4 hours after a single dose. When famotidine was administered every 8 hours for 3 doses, tachyphylaxis appeared to occur, as the duration of increased pH progressively diminished after each dose. The total time of increased pH was ≈7 hours (30% of a 24 hour period).[10]

Pharmacology/Actions

At the H_2 receptors of the parietal cells, famotidine competitively inhibits histamine, thereby reducing gastric acid output, both during basal conditions and when stimulated by food, pentagastrin, histamine, or insulin. Gastric emptying time, pancreatic or biliary secretion, and lower esophageal pressures are not altered by famotidine. By decreasing the amount of gastric juice produced, H_2 blockers reduce the amount of pepsin secreted. Famotidine leads to transient increases in serum gastrin, which returns to baseline concentrations a week after discontinuation.[11]

Pharmacokinetics

Famotidine is not completely absorbed after oral administration but undergoes minimal first-pass metabolism. In humans, systemic bioavailability is ≈40% to 50%. Distribution characteristics are not well described. In rats, only ≈15% to 20% is bound to plasma proteins; the drug does not cross the blood–brain barrier or the placenta. When the drug is administered orally, ≈⅓ is excreted unchanged in the urine, and the remainder is primarily metabolized in the liver and then excreted in the urine. After IV dosing, ≈⅔ is excreted unchanged.

The pharmacokinetics of famotidine, ranitidine, and cimetidine have been investigated in horses.[12] After administration of a single IV dose, elimination half-lives of famotidine, ranitidine, and cimetidine ranged from 2 to 3 hours and were not significantly different. Bioavailability of each of the drugs was low in horses (ie, famotidine, 13%; ranitidine, 13.5%; cimetidine, 30%).

After administration of a single famotidine dose (0.4 mg/kg IV) to adult steers, the half-life was 3.33 hours.[10]

Contraindications/Precautions/Warnings

Famotidine is contraindicated in patients with known hypersensitivity to the drug.

Consider dosage reduction in patients with significant renal dysfunction.

Do not confuse famotidine with fluoxetine or furosemide.

Adverse Effects

Rapid IV infusion may cause bradycardia. H_2 blockers have been demonstrated to be relatively safe and exhibit minimal adverse effects. In humans, agranulocytosis, pancytopenia, and leukopenia have been rarely reported.[13,14] Other reported rare to infrequent adverse effects in humans include fever, fatigue, vomiting, nausea, headache, dizziness, constipation, diarrhea, abdominal discomfort, arrhythmias, hypotension, AV block, elevated liver enzymes, elevated bilirubin, hypersensitivity skin reactions, and CNS signs (confusion, agitation).

There have been rare anecdotal reports of famotidine causing intravascular hemolysis when given IV to cats. A retrospective study evaluating IV famotidine in 56 hospitalized cats did not show any evidence of hemolysis. The authors concluded that IV famotidine appeared safe in cats when administered over 5 minutes.[15]

Reproductive/Nursing Safety

In laboratory animal studies, famotidine demonstrated no detectable harm to offspring.[13,14] Large doses could affect the mother's food intake and weight gain during pregnancy, which could indirectly be harmful to developing fetuses.

Famotidine enters into milk. It is unclear if there is any clinical significance for nursing offspring.

Because safety has not been established in animals, this drug should only be used when the maternal benefits outweigh the potential risks to offspring.

Overdose/Acute Toxicity

The minimum acute lethal dose in dogs is reported to be more than 2 g/kg for oral doses and ≈300 mg/kg for IV doses.[13,14] In dogs, IV doses of 5 – 200 mg/kg caused vomiting, restlessness, mucous membrane pallor, and redness of the mouth and ears. Higher doses caused hypotension, tachycardia, and collapse.

Because of the wide margin of safety associated with the drug, most overdoses should require only monitoring. In massive oral overdoses, gut-emptying protocols should be considered, and supportive therapy should be initiated when warranted.

For patients that have experienced or are suspected to have experienced an overdose, consultation with a 24-hour poison consultation center specializing in providing veterinary-specific information is recommended. For general information related to overdose and toxin exposures, as well as contact information for poison control centers, refer to ***Appendix***.

Drug Interactions

Unlike cimetidine or ranitidine, famotidine does not appear to inhibit hepatic cytochrome P450 enzyme systems, and dosage adjustments of other drugs (eg, warfarin, theophylline, diazepam, procainamide) that are metabolized by these metabolic pathways are usually not required.

The following drug interactions have either been reported or are theoretical in humans or animals receiving famotidine and may be of significance in veterinary patients. Unless otherwise noted, use together is not necessarily contraindicated, but the potential risks should be weighed and additional monitoring performed when appropriate.

- **AZOLE ANTIFUNGALS** (eg, **fluconazole, itraconazole, ketoconazole**): By increasing gastric pH, famotidine may decrease the absorption of these agents; if both drugs are required, the azole should be administered 1 hour before famotidine.
- **CEFPODOXIME, CEFUROXIME**: Famotidine may decrease the absorption of these cephalosporins; separating doses by 2 hours may alleviate this effect.
- **DICHLORPHENAMIDE**: Increased famotidine exposure may occur.
- **IRON SALTS, ORAL**: Famotidine may decrease the absorption of oral iron; iron should be administered at least 1 hour before famotidine.

Laboratory Considerations

- H_2 blockers may antagonize the effects of **histamine** and **pentagastrin** in the evaluation of gastric acid secretion.
- A study in dogs showed that famotidine only had transient effects on **serum gastrin** concentrations. The authors concluded that in dogs with clinical features consistent with gastrinomas, chronic famotidine administration would likely not contribute to increases in serum gastrin concentration.[16]
- After use of allergen extract **skin tests**, H_2 antagonists may inhibit histamine responses. It is recommended that H_2 blockers be discontinued at least 24 hours before these tests are performed.

Dosages

DOGS & CATS:

Reduce gastric acid production (extra-label):

a) 1 mg/kg IV slowly (over at least 5 minutes) as a loading dose followed by 8 mg/kg/day IV as a CRI may provide the best antacid efficacy in dogs.[17,18]

b) 1 mg/kg PO, SC, or IV (slowly over at least 5 minutes) every 12 hours. Rounding oral doses up to the nearest 5 mg increment (eg, 5 mg/cat [NOT mg/kg]) is reasonable. Once daily administration should be considered in patients with significantly diminished renal function.

HORSES:

Adjunct in ulcer treatment (extra-label): 0.23 mg/kg IV every 8 hours or 0.35 mg/kg IV every 12 hours; 1.88 mg/kg PO every 8 hours or 2.8 mg/kg PO every 12 hours[12]

CATTLE:

Reduce gastric acid production (extra-label): From a pharmacokinetic study in 4 adult steers: 0.4 mg/kg IV every 8 hours for 3 doses increased abomasal outflow fluid pH for 3 hours, 2 hours, and 1 hour after each respective dose.[10] Further studies are needed to support clinical efficacy.

FERRETS:

Stress-induced ulcers (extra-label): 0.25 – 0.5 mg/kg PO or IV every 24 hours[19]

In combination with antibiotics for *Helicobacter* spp treatment (extra-label): 0.25 – 0.5 mg/kg PO or IV every 24 hours[20]

SMALL MAMMALS:

Rabbits: Stress-induced ulcer prevention once critically ill animal has stabilized (extra-label): 1 mg/kg IV every 24 hours[21]

Monitoring

- Clinical efficacy (dependent on reason for use); monitored by decrease in signs, endoscopic examination, blood in feces
- Adverse effects, if noted

Client Information

- This medicine is used to treat or prevent stomach ulcers. Give this medicine as directed by your veterinarian. Clinical signs may recur if doses are missed.
- This medicine works best if given before the first meal of the day. If your animal vomits or appears sick after giving this medicine on an empty stomach, give it with food or a small treat. If vomiting continues, contact your veterinarian.
- Famotidine is available over the counter (ie, without a prescription), but you should only give it to your animal if your veterinarian recommends its use.

Chemistry/Synonyms

Famotidine is an H_2-receptor antagonist. It occurs as a white to pale yellow crystalline powder and is odorless but has a bitter taste. 740 µg are soluble in 1 mL of water.

Famotidine may also be known as famotidinum, L-643341, MK-208, and YM-11170; many trade names are available.

Storage/Stability

Tablets should be stored in well-closed, light-resistant containers at room temperature (20°C-25°C [68°F-77°F]).[14]

The oral suspension dry powder and suspension should be stored in well-closed, light-resistant containers at 25°C (77°F); excursions permitted to 15°C to 30°C (59°F-86°F). After reconstitution, the resultant suspension is stable for 30 days when stored at temperatures below 30°C (86°F); do not freeze.

Famotidine injection should be stored in the refrigerator at 2°C to 8°C (36°F-46°F).[13]

Compatibility/Compounding Considerations

Commercially available famotidine tablets can be split or crushed but have a bitter taste.

Famotidine for injection is physically **compatible** with most commonly used IV infusion solutions and is stable for 48 hours at room temperature when diluted in these solutions.

Compounded preparation stability: Famotidine oral suspension compounded from commercially available tablets has been published.[22] Triturating 24 famotidine 40 mg tablets with 60 mL of *Ora-Plus*® and qs ad to 120 mL with *Ora-Sweet*® (or *Ora-Sweet® SF*) brought to a favorable pH of 5.8 yields an 8 mg/mL oral suspension that retains more than 90% potency for 95 days when stored at 25°C (77°F). Famotidine is stable in buffered solutions at a pH of 4 to 6, but rapid and extensive drug degradation occurs at a pH less than 2.

Another recipe to make a 4 mg/mL flavored, oral aqueous-based suspension from 10 mg tablets: To make a 30 mL suspension: Pulverize twelve (12) 10 mg tablets (0.12 g; 120 mg) to a fine powder in a mortar and pestle. Wet with glycerin (1 – 2 mL) to make a thick paste. Add up to 1 mL of a water-soluble flavoring agent. Add enough oral suspending vehicle (OSV; eg, *Ora-Plus*®, *Ora-Sweet*®) and mix to allow transfer to an amber prescription bottle. This process may need to be repeated several times to wash the mortar; qs ad to 30 mL with additional OSV. Shake well before use; store in the refrigerator and dispose of any unused amount after 30 days.

Dosage Forms/Regulatory Status

VETERINARY-LABELED PRODUCTS: NONE

The Association of Racing Commissioners International (ARCI) has designated this drug as a class 5 substance. See ***Appendix*** for more information. Use of this drug may not be allowed in certain animal competitions. Check rules and regulations before entering in a competition while this medication is being administered. Contact local racing authorities for further guidance.

HUMAN-LABELED PRODUCTS:

Famotidine Oral Tablets (plain, film-coated, chewable): 10 mg and 20 mg, gelcaps 40 mg; *Pepcid*®, *Pepcid® AC*®, and *Pepcid RPD*®, generic; (Rx and OTC)

Famotidine Powder for Oral Suspension: 8 mg/mL when reconstituted in 400 mg bottles; *Pepcid*®, generic; generic; (Rx)

Famotidine Injection: 10 mg/mL in 1 mL and 2 mL single-dose vials and 4 mL, 20 mL, and 50 mL multidose vials (may contain mannitol or benzyl alcohol); generic; (Rx)

References

For the complete list of references, see **wiley.com/go/budde/plumb**

Fatty Acids, Omega-3

Nutritional Supplement

Prescriber Highlights

- Most commonly used orally for adjunctive treatment of pruritus associated with a variety of inflammatory skin conditions in dogs and cats; may be useful as an anti-inflammatory associated with other chronic conditions (eg, chronic kidney disease, osteoarthritis).
- In horses, may also be used for adjunctive therapy for chronic lower airway inflammation associated with equine asthma.
- Safety in pregnancy has not been established.
- May affect platelet function and bleeding times in dogs and cats; use caution in patients with primary or secondary hemostatic disorders or in those patients concurrently receiving medication to alter these systems.
- Adverse effects include GI distress with high doses; rarely, some dogs may become lethargic or more pruritic.

Uses/Indications

Fatty acid products are often used for the adjunctive treatment of pruritus associated with atopy, idiopathic seborrhea, miliary dermatitis, and eosinophilic granuloma complex; however, it is important to note that they are not helpful to treat acute flares of pruritis as prolonged periods (ie, weeks to months) are required for their actions to take effect.[1] Omega-3 fatty acids may be added to commercial veterinary diets to improve coat quality, as well as to commercial veterinary prescription diets specifically formulated for a variety of inflammatory conditions (eg, osteoarthritis; cardiac, liver, and kidney disease; neurologic conditions).

Polyunsaturated fatty acids (PUFA n-3s), eicosapentaenoic acid (EPA), and docosahexaenoic acid (DHA) are commonly found in higher concentrations in fish oil-containing products and are often chosen for their anti-inflammatory properties, which may be beneficial as adjunctive treatment for chronic kidney disease, arthritis (both degenerative and autoimmune), cardiovascular disease (hypercoagulable states, heart failure, dysrhythmias, boxer dogs with arrhythmogenic right ventricular cardiomyopathy[2]), inflammatory bowel disease, hepatic fibrosis, steatosis, and some neoplastic diseases. Omega-3 fatty acid supplementation may also reduce the incidence of lipemic aqueous in miniature schnauzers.[3]

Essential fatty acids may provide benefit when used as adjunctive therapy in dogs with atopic dermatitis.[4-6] When they are used for pruritus, significant therapeutic effects may be noted in only 25% to 50% of treated patients. Several months of treatment are required before evaluating efficacy.[1] Antihistamine and fatty acid therapy may be synergistic for treatment of pruritus.

One study in dogs with chronic osteoarthritis fed a diet supplemented with fish oil omega-3 fatty acids suggested that carprofen dosage reductions could be possible.[7] In another study, dogs with osteoarthritis fed a diet with a high omega-3 to omega-6 ratio (compared with the control diet, omega-3 levels were 31 times greater, and omega-6 levels were 34 times lower) had significantly lower serum levels of arachidonic acid and owners reported subjective improvement in arthritic condition.[8]

A supplement containing omega-3 fatty acids, magnesium citrate, and zinc sulfate reduced behavioral disorders in dogs.[9]

Dietary supplementation with omega-3 polyunsaturated fatty acids or feeding animals a diet that has a reduced omega-6:omega-3 ratio that is close to 5:1 (as found in most commercially available renal diets) is expected to alter the long-term course of renal injury and decrease the magnitude of proteinuria.[10,11]

In a study of horses with chronic lower airway disease, addition of an omega-3 PUFA supplement resulted in clinically significant improvement in pulmonary function, airway inflammation, and clinical signs compared with the control group. All horses in the study also were fed a low-dust pelleted diet.[12]

Pharmacology/Actions

The most commonly supplemented fatty acids are eicosapentaenoic acid (EPA) and docosahexaenoic acid (DHA), which, along with α-linoleic acid, are considered essential fatty acids. They are an integral part of the cellular framework of all cells and help to maintain normal cellular function; however, it remains difficult to ascertain which compounds may be responsible for their proposed efficacy, particularly when considering the combination nature of the commercial products being marketed. The therapeutic benefits and optimal ratios of EPA versus DHA remain unclear.

Omega-3 fatty acids affect arachidonic acid concentrations in plasma lipids and cellular membranes, and affect the degree of inflammatory prostaglandins, leukotrienes, and thromboxane production in the body.

Contraindications/Precautions/Warnings

Most commercial pet foods contain a source of omega-3 fatty acids. Before supplementation, determine the amount of omega-3 fatty acids already in the animal's diet to determine the appropriate amount to be supplemented.

Fatty acids should be used with caution in dogs that have had previous bouts of pancreatitis or protracted diarrhea.[13]

Because of potential effects on platelet function and bleeding times, use with caution in patients with primary or secondary hemostatic disorders or in those receiving medications to alter these systems.[13,14]

Adverse Effects

At high dosages, GI disturbances (eg, belching, vomiting, diarrhea) may be seen.[13] Rarely, some dogs become lethargic, have impaired wound healing, or become more pruritic. Omega-3 fatty acids may alter immune function, but any clinical significance of these effects is not clearly known. Omega-3 fatty acids may decrease platelet activity and increase the risk of bleeding.

Reproductive/Nursing Safety

In humans, women are encouraged to consume omega-3 fatty acids during pregnancy. Omega-3 fatty acid supplements are considered compatible with pregnancy and during lactation[15]; the relevance of this recommendation for veterinary patients is unclear.

Overdose/Acute Toxicity

Acute ingestions may produce clinical signs that mirror omega-3 fatty acid adverse effects. Acute toxicosis may result after accidental overdoses of fatty acid products containing vitamin A. See ***Vitamin A*** for more information.

For patients that have experienced or are suspected to have experienced an overdose, consultation with a 24-hour poison consultation center specializing in providing veterinary-specific information is recommended. For general information related to overdose and toxin exposures, as well as contact information for poison control centers, refer to ***Appendix***.

Drug Interactions

The following drug interactions have either been reported or are theoretical in humans or animals receiving omega-3 fatty acids and may be of significance in veterinary patients. Unless otherwise noted, use together is not necessarily contraindicated, but weigh the potential risks and perform additional monitoring when appropriate.

- **Anticoagulants** (eg, **aspirin, clopidogrel, warfarin, heparin**): Because of potential effects on bleeding times, use with caution in patients receiving anticoagulant medication. Omega-3 fatty acids have been shown to augment the antiplatelet effect of aspirin.[14]
- **Corticosteroids** (eg, **prednis(ol)one**): May have a steroid-sparing effect in dogs with atopic dermatitis[5]
- **Cyclosporine**: May have a cyclosporine-sparing effect in dogs with atopic dermatitis[4]
- **Nonsteroidal Anti-inflammatory Drugs (NSAIDs**; eg, **carprofen, meloxicam, robenacoxib**): May increase the risk of bleeding

Laboratory Considerations

None

Dosages

NOTE: Fish oil should contain vitamin E as an antioxidant; however, to avoid toxicities, supplements that contain other nutrients are not recommended. Cod liver oil and flax oil should not be used.[13,16,17]

DOGS:

Omega-3 nutritional supplement (extra-label): The National Research Council (NRC) recommended daily allowances (indicating safe upper limits) and suggested dosages for therapeutic use are determined using metabolic weight (not actual body weight) and the *combined* weight of eicosapentaenoic acid (EPA) and docosahexaenoic acid (DHA). To calculate this, first convert the dog's body weight in kg to the metabolic body weight by taking the actual weight in kg and raising it to the power of 0.75. For example, a dog weighing 10 kg would convert to 5.62. (***Plumb's note****: Those not adept at using a scientific calculator for this purpose can use a calculator that has a square root function key. In the example above of a dog weighing 10 kg; cube the bodyweight in kg [10 x 10 x 10 = 1000], then take the square root of 1000 twice = 5.62.)* This value is then multiplied by the recommended dosage for a particular condition. Consider the amount of EPA/DHA already present in the diet when determining daily dose. The following are suggested daily dosages of *combined* EPA/DHA per metabolic weight:

- **NRC recommended daily allowance**: 30 mg/kg$^{0.75}$ PO
- **NRC safe upper limit**: 370 mg/kg$^{0.75}$ PO

Idiopathic hyperlipidemia (extra-label):

a) 120 mg/kg$^{0.75}$ PO once daily
b) Alternatively, 200 – 300 mg/kg PO once daily, with a suggested upper limit of 4 – 5 g daily[18]

Kidney disease (extra-label):

a) 140 mg/kg$^{0.75}$ PO; may be increased to the NRC safe upper limit
b) **Adjunctive treatment of glomerular disease**: In combination with a diet containing a reduced omega-6:omega-3 polyunsaturated fatty acids (PUFA) ratio, approximating 5:1. Where dietary supplementation with an omega-3 PUFA is used to alter this ratio, a dosage of EPA in combination with DHA 250 – 500 mg/kg of should be considered appropriate for most canine diets.[10]
b) **Proteinuria** (extra-label): Anecdotal dosage extrapolated from human data suggest a minimum of omega-3 fatty acids

1 g/4.55 kg body weight PO every 24 hours.[19]

Cardiovascular disorder (extra-label): EPA 40 mg/kg in combination with DHA 25 mg/kg PO once daily[17]

Osteoarthritis (extra-label):

a) 310 mg/kg$^{0.75}$ PO; may be increased to the NRC safe upper limit

b) EPA 90 mg/kg in combination with DHA 20 mg/kg PO once daily significantly improved indicators of pain and quality of life.[20]

Inflammatory or immunologic disorders (eg, inflammatory bowel disease, atopy; extra-label): 125 mg/kg$^{0.75}$ PO[21,22]

Cyclosporine-sparing effect in atopic dermatitis (extra-label): EPA 36 mg/kg in combination with DHA 25 mg/kg PO once daily resulted in ≈35% reduction in the median daily cyclosporine dosage over the 12-week study period.[4] Pruritus also was improved. The product used in this study also contained α-linolenic acid, linoleic acid, and docosapentaenoic acid.

Symmetrical lupoid onychodystrophy (extra-label): EPA 82.5 mg/kg in combination with DHA 53 mg/kg (average dosage) PO once daily was equivalent to cyclosporine in improving the number of healthy claws and long-term hunting abilities; note that the study sample size was limited to 6 dogs per treatment arm.[23]

CATS:

NOTE: There is less evidence supporting safety and efficacy use of omega-3 fatty acids in cats than in dogs; optimal dosages are not yet known. Dosages greater than EPA + DHA 75 mg/kg$^{0.67}$ per day should be used with caution and under veterinary supervision until further evaluations of long-term safety are performed.[21]

Kidney disease | Proteinuria (extra-label): anecdotal dosage extrapolated from human data suggest a minimum of omega-3 fatty acids 1 g/4.55 kg body weight PO every 24 hours[19]

Adjunctive treatment of CHF (extra-label): EPA 40 mg/kg in combination with DHA 25 mg/kg PO once daily has been recommended. Practically, capsules that contain EPA ≈180 mg in combination with DHA 120 mg DHA can be administered at a dose of 1 capsule/4.5 kg (10 lb) body weight.[16,17]

HORSES:

Chronic lower airway inflammatory disease (extra-label): 30 g or 60 g omega-3 fatty acid feed supplement added to pellet-only diet for 2 months improved cough and lung function in horses with severe equine asthma (SEA; formerly known as recurrent airway obstruction) and inflammatory airway disease.[12]

Monitoring

- Efficacy for treated indication
- Adverse effects (eg, vomiting, diarrhea)

Client Information

- Omega-3 fatty acids are also known as fish oils.
- This medicine may be given with or without food.
- Often used in addition to other treatments for controlling skin diseases, arthritis, and some heart conditions
- When this medicine is used to control itching, treatment may require 2 to 3 months to see if it will be effective.
- Usually tolerated well. Upset stomach and loose stools/diarrhea are the most common side effects, especially when higher doses are used. Some animals may bruise or bleed more easily. If this occurs, contact your veterinarian.
- Be sure to read product labels closely as fatty acid content varies widely between products. It is recommended to purchase a product from a reputable manufacturer. Consult your veterinarian or pharmacist to find a safe and reliable product selection for your animal.

Chemistry/Synonyms

The commercially available veterinary products generally contain a combination of eicosapentaenoic acid [EPA] and docosahexaenoic acid (DHA) derived from fish oil and vegetable oil (gamma-linolenic acid) that serve as essential fatty acids. They may also contain vitamin E (d-α-tocopherol) and vitamin A.

Storage/Stability

Because fatty acids are susceptible to oxidation and breakdown by exposure to elevated temperatures, light, and air, products should be stored in an airtight container in a cool, dry place, protected from heat.

Compatibility/Compounding Considerations

No specific information has been noted.

Dosage Forms/Regulatory Status

NOTE: Fish oil supplements should contain vitamin E as an antioxidant. Use of a high-quality product, preferably one certified free of heavy metals or other environmental contaminants, is suggested.[13]

VETERINARY-LABELED PRODUCTS:

There are many combination products available without prescription having various trade names, including (partial listing): *Dermapet Eicosderm®, Dermapet OFA plus EZ-C Caps®, F.A. Caps®, F.A. Caps ES®, Omega EFA® Capsules, Omega EFA® Capsules XS, Performer® OFA Gel Capsules Extra Strength, Aliera®.*

HUMAN-LABELED PRODUCTS:

There are many fish oil capsules available without prescription having various trade names.

References

For the complete list of references, see **wiley.com/go/budde/plumb**

Felbamate

(***fell***-ba-mate) *Felbatol®*

Anticonvulsant

Prescriber Highlights

- ► Second- or third-line antiepileptic medication for dogs
- ► Contraindicated in patients hypersensitive to it or other carbamates
- ► Use caution in patients with pre-existing hepatic dysfunction or blood dyscrasias.
- ► Adverse effects may include KCS, liver enzyme induction, tremors, limb rigidity, salivation, restlessness, and agitation; use in dogs appears to be relatively safe, but because of limited use, adverse effect profile and incidence may be incomplete.
- ► Cost and accessibility may be issues.

Uses/Indications

Felbamate is an anticonvulsant agent that may be useful for treating seizure disorders (generalized seizures, but especially complex partial seizures) in dogs. A potential advantage of felbamate therapy is that when used alone or in combination with phenobarbital and/or bromides, it does not appear to cause additive sedation.

Pharmacology/Actions

Felbamate's anticonvulsant activity is thought to be due to its ability to reduce excitatory neurotransmission; its exact mechanism is unknown, but it is believed to increase activation of sodium channels, thereby decreasing sustained high-frequency firing of action potentials.

Pharmacokinetics

Felbamate is well absorbed after oral administration in dogs. Felbamate is both excreted unchanged and as metabolites in the urine. The half-life in adult dogs averages around 4 to 6 hours. Because the drug can induce liver enzyme induction, half-lives may decrease with time, and dosages may need adjustment.

Contraindications/Precautions/Warnings

Felbamate is contraindicated in patients hypersensitive to it or other carbamates (eg, meprobamate). In humans, felbamate has caused aplastic anemia and acute hepatic failure, and should not be used in patients with a history of blood dyscrasias or hepatic dysfunction.

Adverse Effects

Adverse reactions in the dog include keratoconjunctivitis sicca (KCS), liver enzyme induction, tremor, limb rigidity, salivation, restlessness, and agitation (at high doses). Sedation is not reported in the dog when used as a monotherapy, but excitability does occur at high doses. In humans, aplastic anemia and hepatic necrosis have been noted and could be a factor in canine medicine. There apparently have not been any case reports yet of aplastic anemia in dogs, but blood dyscrasias (thrombocytopenia, lymphopenia, and leukopenia) have anecdotally been reported. Additionally, sedation, vomiting, and nausea have been reported in dogs but usually in those receiving other anticonvulsants as well.

Reproductive/Nursing Safety

Felbamate crosses the placenta. Teratogenicity was not documented in pregnant laboratory animals exposed to felbamate.[1]

The drug is excreted into maternal milk. Decreased pup weight and increased pup death were observed in rats during lactation.[1]

Because safety has not been established in animals, this drug should only be used when the maternal benefits outweigh the potential risks to offspring.

Overdose/Acute Toxicity

Limited information is available. One human subject taking 12 g over 12 hours only developed mild gastric distress and a slightly increased heart rate.

For patients that have experienced or are suspected of having experienced an overdose, consultation with a 24-hour poison consultation center specializing in providing veterinary-specific information is recommended. For general information related to overdose and toxin exposures, as well as contact information for poison control centers, refer to ***Appendix***.

Drug Interactions

The following drug interactions have either been reported or are theoretical in humans or animals receiving felbamate and may be of significance in veterinary patients. Unless otherwise noted, use together is not necessarily contraindicated, but weigh the potential risks and perform additional monitoring when appropriate.

- **Clopidogrel**: Concurrent use may result in a reduction in the clinical efficacy of clopidogrel.
- **Phenobarbital, Primidone**: When felbamate is added to patients taking phenobarbital, it may cause increases in phenobarbital levels. When phenobarbital is added to patients taking felbamate, felbamate levels may decrease.
- **QTc Prolonging Drugs** (eg, **amiodarone, cisapride, quinidine, sotalol**): Concurrent use may increase the risk for QT-interval prolongation.
- **Valproate**: Felbamate can cause increases in valproic acid levels.

Dosages

DOGS:

Seizure control[2]; second- to third-line agent; (extra-label): Felbamate is not commonly used, but it can be considered as an add-on drug when acceptable seizure control is not attained or adverse effects are not tolerated with other standard treatments. Evidence supporting any dosage regimen was not located. Most recommend using initially at 15 – 20 mg/kg PO every 8 hours, with gradual dosage increases of ≈15 mg/kg PO every 2 weeks, if required and tolerated. Some start at lower dosages 5 – 10 mg/kg PO every 12 hours and titrate to every 8 hours. Upper limits of 60 – 70 mg/kg PO every 8 hours have been noted.

Monitoring

- CBC, chemistry panel; baseline and regularly during treatment
- Therapeutic drug levels for felbamate in dogs are not known but appear to be in the 25 – 100 µg/mL range. The usefulness of monitoring serum levels is uncertain.

Client Information

- Anticonvulsant that may be useful to treat seizure disorders (eg, epilepsy) in dogs. Limited experience using it in veterinary medicine. It usually does not cause sleepiness or sedation.
- May be given with or without food. If your animal vomits or acts sick after getting it on an empty stomach, give it with food or a small treat to see if this helps. If vomiting continues, contact your veterinarian.
- Appears to be relatively safe in dogs, but report anything out of the ordinary to your veterinarian. Possible side effects include tremors, shaking, stiff legs, excessive salivation (drooling), restlessness, agitation, dry eyes, or increases in liver enzymes.
- Requires dosing several times a day. It will not be effective if dosages are missed.
- While your animal is taking this medication, it is important to return to your veterinarian for periodic monitoring of lab work. Do not miss these important follow-up visits.

Chemistry/Synonyms

Felbamate is a unique dicarbamate anticonvulsant agent that is slightly soluble in water.

Felbamate may also be known as AD-03055, W-554, *Felbamyl*®, *Felbatol*®, and *Taloxa*®.

Storage/Stability

Store felbamate preparations at room temperature 20°C to 25°C (68°F-77°F) in tight containers. Shake the suspension well before use.

Compatibility/Compounding Considerations

No specific information has been noted.

Dosage Forms/Regulatory Status

VETERINARY-LABELED PRODUCTS: NONE

Association of Racing Commissioners International (ARCI) Uniform Classification Guidelines for Foreign Substances (UCGFS) Class 3 Drug). Use of this drug may not be allowed in certain animal competitions. Check rules and regulations before entering in a competition while this medication is being administered. Contact local racing authorities for further guidance. See ***Appendix*** for more information.

HUMAN-LABELED PRODUCTS:

Felbamate Tablets: 400 and 600 mg; *Felbatol*®, generic; (Rx).

Felbamate Suspension: 120 mg/mL in 240 and 960 mL; *Felbatol*®, generic; (Rx).

References

For the complete list of references, see **wiley.com/go/budde/plumb**

Fenbendazole

(fen-**ben**-da-zole) *Panacur®, Safe-Guard®*
Antiparasitic Agent

Prescriber Highlights

- ► Anthelmintic useful for reduction and removal of nematode and protozoal parasites in a variety of species
- ► Adverse effects are uncommon; vomiting can occur infrequently in dogs and cats. Hypersensitization reactions caused by antigen release from dying parasites are possible, particularly at high doses.
- ► Generally safe to use during pregnancy
- ► In dogs, this drug should be given with food to increase bioavailability.

Uses/Indications

In dogs, fenbendazole is labeled for removal of the following parasites: roundworms (*Toxocara canis, Toxascaris leonina*), hookworms (*Ancylostoma caninum, Uncinaria stenocephala*), whipworms (*Trichuris vulpis*), and tapeworms (*Taenia pisiformis*). It is not effective against *Dipylidium caninum*. Fenbendazole has also been used clinically to treat *Eucoleus aerophilus* (formerly known as *Capillaria aerophila*), *Filaroides hirthi*, and *Paragonimus kellicotti* infections in dogs; it may be useful in combination with praziquantel for some cases of subclinical schistosomiasis caused by *Heterobilharzia americana*.[1,2]

Fenbendazole has been used extra-label in domestic cats, sheep, camelids, small mammals, pet birds, and reptiles and may be approved in countries outside the United States for these species. See ***Dosages*** for more information.

In horses, fenbendazole is labeled for removal of the following parasites: large strongyles (*Strongylus edentatus, Strongylus equinus, S vulgaris, Triodontophorus* spp), small strongyles (also known as cyathostomes; eg, *Cylicocyclus* spp, *Cylicostephanus* spp, *Cylicodontophorus* spp), ascarids (*Parascaris equorum*), and pinworms (*Oxyuris equi*). Benzimidazole resistance is a concern when treating horses for cyathostomes.[3-6]

In cattle, fenbendazole is labeled for removal of the following parasites in their adult forms (and most immature stages): *Haemonchus contortus, Ostertagia ostertagi, Trichostrongylus axei, Bunostomum phlebotomum, Nematodirus helvetianus, Cooperia* spp, *Trichostrongylus colubriformis, Oesophagostomum radiatum*, and *Dictyocaulus viviparus*. In beef cattle only, fenbendazole is FDA-approved for removal and control of *Moniezia* spp and arrested fourth-stage forms of *O ostertagi*.

In nonlactating goats, fenbendazole is labeled for removal of adult stomach worms (*H contortus, Teladorsagia circumcincta*).

In swine, fenbendazole is labeled for removal of the following parasites: large roundworms (*Ascaris suum*), lungworms (*Metastrongylus apri, Metastrongylus pudendotectus*), nodular worms (*Oesophagostomum dentatum, Oesophagostomum quadrispinulatum*), small stomach worms (*Hyostrongylus rubidus*), whipworms (*Trichuris suis*), and kidney worms (*Stephanurus dentatus*; both mature and immature).

In broiler chickens and replacement chickens intended to become breeding chickens, fenbendazole is indicated for the treatment and control of adult *Ascaridia galli* and in breeding chickens for the treatment and control of adult *A galli* and *Heterakis gallinarum*.

Fenbendazole is approved for control of ascarids in big cats (eg, lions, leopards, tigers) and in bears; in some of those species, it is also labeled for control of hookworms and/or tapeworms.

Fenbendazole resistance is a growing concern for canine hookworms,[7-10] and *Ostertagia* spp.[11-13]

Pharmacology/Actions

Benzimidazole antiparasitic agents have a broad spectrum of activity against a variety of pathogenic internal parasites. In susceptible parasites, their mechanism of action disrupts intracellular microtubular transport systems by binding tubulin, preventing tubulin polymerization, and inhibiting microtubule formation. Benzimidazoles are also believed to act at higher concentrations to disrupt metabolic pathways within the helminth, and inhibit metabolic enzymes, including malate dehydrogenase and fumarate reductase.

Benzimidazoles may be considered time-dependent antiparasitic agents.

Fenbendazole has activity against adult life cycle stages of susceptible parasites and may have larvicidal and ovicidal activity against certain parasites.[14,15]

Benzimidazoles appear to exert anticancer effects through multiple mechanisms. In vitro and preclinical studies have demonstrated that benzimidazoles destabilize microtubules, increase the stability of p53 tumor suppressor proteins, induce apoptosis, and reduce glucose uptake in cancer cells.[16-18] Additional research is required to determine clinical relevance.

Pharmacokinetics

Fenbendazole is only marginally absorbed after oral administration in dogs.[19] The amount absorbed from the gut is associated more with the solubility of the drug and not the dosage given. In dogs, when administered doses ranged from 25 – 100 mg/kg, the area under the curve (AUC) was similar. Bioavailability is increased in dogs when fenbendazole is administered with food; the fat content of the food does not significantly alter bioavailability.[20] The absorbed drug is sequentially converted to sulfoxide (active) and sulfone (inactive) metabolites. Fenbendazole and metabolites are excreted in the feces.

After PO administration in calves and horses, peak blood concentrations of 0.11 µg/mL and 0.07 µg/mL, respectively, were measured. After 10 mg/kg PO in sheep and goats, maximum concentrations were 128 and 146 µg/mL, respectively.[21] Absorbed fenbendazole is metabolized to the active compound, oxfendazole (sulfoxide), and sulfone (inactive). In cattle, sheep, and pigs, 44% to 50% of a dose of fenbendazole is excreted unchanged in the feces and less than 1% in the urine.

Contraindications/Precautions/Warnings

Fenbendazole is not FDA-approved for use in horses intended for food purposes.

Adverse Effects

At labeled dosages, fenbendazole does not typically cause any adverse effects. Hypersensitivity reactions secondary to antigen release by dying parasites may occur, particularly at high doses. Salivation, vomiting, and diarrhea may infrequently occur in dogs or cats that have been given fenbendazole. Pancytopenia was reported in 1 dog.[22] Fenbendazole may cause intestinal problems and myelosuppression in some birds.[23,24]

Reproductive/Nursing Safety

Fenbendazole is considered generally safe to use in all species during pregnancy and is the drug of choice for treatment of giardiasis in pregnant animals.[25] Fenbendazole administered to males and pregnant and nonpregnant females (including *Felidae* and *Ursidae*) at 10 times the recommended dose for twice the recommended treatment period did not have an effect on reproduction.[26] Fenbendazole may interfere with implantation in pigs during early pregnancy.[27]

Fenbendazole should only be used when the maternal benefits outweigh the potential risks to offspring.

Overdose/Acute Toxicity

Fenbendazole is well tolerated at doses up to 100 times what is recommended. The LD_{50} in laboratory animals exceeds 10 g/kg when administered PO.[28] It is unlikely that an acute overdose will lead to clinical signs.

For patients that have experienced or are suspected to have experienced an overdose, consultation with a 24-hour poison consultation center specializing in providing veterinary-specific information is recommended. For general information related to overdose and toxin exposures, as well as contact information for poison control centers, refer to ***Appendix.***

Drug Interactions

The following drug interactions with fenbendazole have either been reported or are theoretical in humans or animals and may be of significance in veterinary patients. Unless otherwise noted, use together is not necessarily contraindicated, but the potential risks must be weighed and additional monitoring performed when appropriate.

- **Bromsalan Flukicides** (eg, **dibromsalan, tribromsalan**; not available in the United States): Oxfendazole or fenbendazole should not be given concurrently with bromsalan flukicides; abortions in cattle and death in sheep have been reported when these compounds are used together.
- **Methimazole:** In sheep, methimazole has increased fenbendazole (parent) concentration and delayed the formation of sulfoxide and sulfone metabolites.[29]
- **Triclabendazole:** In an in vitro study, triclabendazole reduced the rate of oxfendazole formation but increased oxfendazole accumulation.[30]

Laboratory Considerations

None were noted.

Dosages

DOGS:

Treatment and control of roundworms (*Toxocara canis, Toxascaris leonina*), hookworms (*Ancylostoma caninum, Uncinaria stenocephala*), whipworms (*Trichuris vulpis*), and tapeworms (*Taenia pisiformis*) (label dosage; FDA approved): 50 mg/kg PO daily for 3 consecutive days. It is recommended to give with food. Puppies (6 weeks or older) should be dewormed at ages 6, 8, 10, and 12 weeks. The dam should be treated at the same time as the puppies.[26,31]

Dosing Table for Premeasured Powder Packets[31]

Body weight kg (lb)	Packet size (222 mg/g)*
4.5 (10)	1 g
5-9.1 (11-20)	2 g
9.5-13.6 (21-30)	1 g + 2 g
14.1-18.2 (31-40)	4 g
18.6-22.7 (41-50)	1 g + 4 g
23.2-27.3 (51-60)	2 g + 4 g
27.7-36.4 (61-80)	Two 4 g
Over 36.4 (80)	Combinations should be used to obtain recommended daily dose.

**Packet size is the daily dose. The dog must be given this dose for 3 consecutive days.*

Alternative dosages for the labeled indications above (extra-label):

a) **Treatment of *T vulpis*:** Some clinicians suggest treatment be repeated after 2 weeks and then after 3 months.
b) 100 mg/kg PO once for adult dogs[32]

Treatment for a variety of other parasites (extra-label):

a) **Slow adulticide kill of *Angiostrongylus vasorum*:** For animals in which severe clinical signs and pulmonary hypertension have occurred: 50 mg/kg PO every 24 hours for 3 to 5 days, discontinue for a few days, then repeat course of fenbendazole 50 mg/kg PO every 24 hours for 3 to 5 days.[33]
b) ***Crenosoma vulpis*:** 25 – 50 mg/kg PO every 24 hours for 3 to 14 days[34]
c) ***Eucoleus* spp (formerly *Capillaria* spp):** 50 mg/kg PO every 24 hours for 10 days[34]
d) ***Filaroides* spp:** 50 mg/kg PO every 24 hours for 14 to 21 days or 100 mg/kg PO every 24 hours for 7 days[34]
e) ***Giardia* spp:** 50 mg/kg PO every 24 hours for 3 to 5 days[32,35,36]
f) ***Mesocestoides* spp:** 100 mg/kg PO every 12 hours for at least 4 weeks[37]
g) ***Oslerus osleri*:** 50 mg/kg PO every 24 hours for 7 to 14 days[32,34]
h) ***Paragonimus kellicotti*:** 50 mg/kg PO every 24 hours for 10 to 14 days[38]
i) ***Physaloptera* spp:** Fenbendazole 75 – 90 mg/kg PO every 24 hours for 5 days in combination with pyrantel pamoate 7.5 mg/kg PO once; repeat in 3 weeks[39]
j) ***Heterobilharzia americana*:** Fenbendazole 24 mg/kg PO every 24 hours for 7 days in combination with praziquantel 10 mg/kg PO every 8 hours for 2 days[1,2]
k) **Persistent or suspected resistant *A caninum* using a 3-drug regimen:** fenbendazole 50 mg/kg PO once daily for 3 days in combination with pyrantel 5 mg/kg PO once and moxidectin 2.5 mg/kg topically[40]

Preventing transplacental and transmammary transmission of somatic *T canis* and *A caninum* (extra-label):

a) 50 mg/kg PO every 24 hours from day 40 of gestation to day 14 of lactation[41]
b) 25 mg/kg PO once daily from day 40 of gestation to 2 days postwhelping[32]

CATS:

Treatment for a variety of parasites (extra-label):

a) **Ascarids (*Toxocara* spp), *Ancylostoma* spp, *Trichuris* spp, *Uncinaria* spp, and *Taenia* spp** (extra-label): Cats older than 6 months and pregnant cats: 100 mg/kg PO once.[32] Kittens younger than 6 months: 50 mg/kg PO every 24 hours for 3 days[32]
b) ***Aelurostrongylus abstrusus*** (extra-label): 50 mg/kg PO every 24 hours for 3 days[32]; longer treatments (ie, 10 to 14 days) may be required[42]
c) ***Eurytrema procyonis* (pancreatic fluke;** extra-label): 30 mg/kg PO every 24 hours for 6 days[43]
d) ***Giardia* spp** (extra-label): 50 mg/kg PO once daily for 5 to 7 days[44,45]
e) ***Strongyloides* spp** (extra-label): 50 mg/kg PO every 24 hours for 3 to 5 days
f) ***Paragonimus kellicotti, Pearsonema feliscati* (formerly *Capillaria feliscati*), or *Eucoleus aerophilus* (formerly *Capillaria aerophila*) infections** (extra-label): 25 – 50 mg/kg PO every 12 hours for 10 or more days

HORSES:

Control of large strongyles (*Strongylus edentatus, Strongylus equinus, Strongylus vulgaris, Triodontophorus* spp), small strongyles (*Cyathostomum* spp, *Cylicocyclus* spp, *Cylicostephanus* spp, *Cylicodontophorus* spp), pinworms (*Oxyuris equi*), and ascarids (*Parascaris equorum*) (label dosage; FDA-approved): Adult horses: 10 mg/kg PO for ascarids, 5 mg/kg PO for all other indications; regular deworming at intervals of 6 to 8 weeks may be required because of the possibility of reinfection. Foals and weanlings younger than 18 months, in which ascarids are a common problem: 10 mg/kg PO; regular deworming at intervals of 6 to 8 weeks may be required because of the possibility of reinfection.[28]

Treatment of encysted early third-stage, late third-stage, and fourth-stage cyathostome larvae as well as fourth-stage *S vulgaris* larvae (label dosage; FDA-approved): 10 mg/kg PO once daily for 5 consecutive days. In the case of fourth-stage larvae *S vulgaris*, treatment and re-treatment should be based on life cycle and epidemiology. Treatment should be initiated in the spring and repeated in the fall after a 6-month interval.[28,46]

CATTLE:

Removal and control of lungworms (*Dictyocaulus viviparus*); adult stomach worms (ie, brown stomach worms [*Ostertagia ostertagi*]); adult and fourth-stage larvae stomach worms (ie, Barber's pole worms [*Haemonchus contortus* and *Haemonchus placei*]); small stomach worms (*Trichostrongylus axei*); adult and fourth-stage larvae intestinal worms (ie, hookworm [*Bunostomum phlebotomum*], thread-necked intestinal worms [*Nematodirus helvetianus*], small intestinal worms [*Cooperia punctata* and *Cooperia oncophora*], bankrupt worms [*Trichostrongylus colubriformis*], and nodular worms [*Oesophagostomum radiatum*]) (label dosage; FDA-approved): 5 mg/kg PO once. Re-treatment may be necessary after 4 to 6 weeks.[47]

Removal and control of stomach worms (fourth-stage inhibited larvae; *O ostertagi*) and tapeworms (*Moniezia benedeni*) in beef cattle *only* (label dosage; FDA-approved): 10 mg/kg PO once. Should not be used in dairy cattle at 10 mg/kg.[46]

***Giardia* spp in calves** (extra-label): 15 mg/kg/day PO for 3 consecutive days; animals should then be moved to a pen that has been thoroughly cleaned and disinfected with ammonia 10%.[48]

GOATS:

Removal and control of adult stomach worms (*H contortus* and *Teladorsagia circumcincta*) in nonlactating goats (label dosage; FDA-approved): 5 mg/kg PO; re-treatment may be necessary after 4 to 6 weeks.[46]

Removal and control of adult stomach worms in nonlactating goats (extra-label): 10 mg/kg; extended withdrawal times required.

CAMELIDS:

Susceptible parasites in new world camelids (extra-label): 10 – 20 mg/kg PO for 3 to 5 days[49]

Adjunctive treatment of meningeal worm infestation (*Parelaphostrongylus tenuis*) (extra-label): 50 mg/kg PO once daily for 5 days with ivermectin at 0.3 mg/kg SC for 5 days. Fluids, nutritional support, prophylactic treatment (ranitidine, omeprazole), and anti-inflammatories (flunixin, dexamethasone, dimethylsulfoxide [DMSO]) should also be used for stress ulcers.[50]

SWINE:

NOTE: There are also medicated feed/premix products labeled for use in swine.

Large roundworms (*Ascaris suum*), lungworms (*Metastrongylus apri, Metastrongylus pudendotectus*), nodular worms (*Oesophagostomum dentatum, Oesophagostomum quadrispinulatum*), small stomach worms (*Hyostrongylus rubidus*), whipworms (*Trichuris suis*), and kidney worms (*Stephanurus dentatus*; both adult and larvae) (label dosage; FDA-approved): Must be administered PO to swine via drinking water at 2.2 mg/kg/day for 3 consecutive days. Not for use in nursing piglets.[51] Alternatively, 9 mg/kg PO (as a 20% medicated feed/premix) can be fed as a sole ration for 3 to 12 consecutive days.[52]

A suum (extra-label): 2.5 mg/kg PO in drinking water once daily for 2 consecutive days 1 week after arriving at fattening mill; treatment course repeated 6 weeks after arriving at fattening mill.[53]

Whipworms in potbellied pigs (extra-label): 10 mg/kg PO once daily for 3 days[54,55]

BIRDS:

NOTE: Fenbendazole may cause severe toxicity in some birds.

Routine deworming (extra-label):

a) **Labeled indications in breeding, broiler, and replacement chickens** (FDA-approved): 1 mg/kg PO daily in drinking water for 5 consecutive days. The required daily volume of fenbendazole suspension is calculated from the total estimated body weight (kg) of the entire group of chickens to be treated. Formula on product label contains calculations for daily requirements and mixing instructions.[51]
b) **Raptors**: 20 mg/kg PO every 24 hours for 5 days[56]
c) **Psittacines, passerines**: 20 mg/kg PO every 24 hours for 3 days[56]
d) **Pigeons**: 10 mg/kg PO once daily for 3 days[56]

FERRETS:

Routine deworming (extra-label): 20 mg/kg PO every 24 hours for 5 days, repeated every 3 months[56]

SMALL MAMMALS & RODENTS:

a) **Mice, rats, gerbils, hamsters, guinea pigs, chinchillas** (extra-label): 20 – 50 mg/kg PO every 24 hours for 5 days; the higher end of the dose range is needed for *Giardia* spp[57]
b) **Rabbits:**
   i. **Treatment and prevention of *Encephalitozoon cuniculi*** (extra-label): 20 mg/kg PO every 24 hours for 28 days; single treatment course only[58]
   ii. **Routine deworming** (extra-label): 20 mg/kg PO once daily for 9 days, repeated 2 to 4 times per year[58]
c) ***Giardia* spp in chinchillas** (extra-label): 25 mg/kg PO every 24 hours for 3 days[59]
d) **Nematodes in hedgehogs** (extra-label): 25 mg/kg PO, repeated at 14 and 28 days[60]
e) **Nematodes, Tapeworms in sugar gliders** (extra-label): 20 – 50 mg/kg every 24 hours for 3 days, repeated in 14 days[61]

REPTILES:

Routine deworming (extra-label):

a) 25 mg/kg PO once daily for 3 days
b) **Tortoises**: 50 mg/kg PO once[56]

Nematodes (extra-label): 50 – 100 mg/kg PO, repeated in 2 weeks

Trematodes (extra-label): 100 mg/kg repeated in 2 weeks[62]

BIG CATS/EXOTIC CATS:

Susceptible parasites (label dosage; FDA-approved): 10 mg/kg PO every 24 hours for 3 consecutive days[26]

BEARS (*URSIDAE*):

Susceptible parasites (label dosage; FDA-approved): 10 mg/kg PO every 24 hours for 3 consecutive days[26]

Monitoring

- Efficacy via fecal flotation, fecal egg count (FEC), fecal egg count reduction test (FECRT)

Client Information

- This oral dewormer is used in many species.
- This medicine may need to be given for several days to be effective. Follow the instructions from your veterinarian and do not miss doses or stop giving it to your animal early.

- This medicine is best given with food in small animals.
- Although there are usually no side effects, gastrointestinal effects (eg, vomiting, drooling, diarrhea) can occur. Rarely, allergic reactions can develop.

Chemistry/Synonyms

Fenbendazole, a benzimidazole anthelmintic, occurs as a white crystalline powder. It is only slightly soluble in water.

Fenbendazole may also be known as Hoe-881V, *Panacur®*, and *Safe-Guard®*.

Storage/Stability

Fenbendazole products should be stored at room temperature.

Compatibility/Compounding Considerations

No specific information was noted.

Dosage Forms/Regulatory Status

VETERINARY-LABELED PRODUCTS:

Fenbendazole Granules: 222 mg/g (22.2%) in 0.18 oz and 1 g, 2 g, and 4 g packets and 1 lb jars; *Panacur® Granules 22.2%*; (Rx). *Safe-guard® Canine Dewormer, Panacur® C* (OTC). FDA-approved for use in dogs, horses, large exotic cats (eg, lions), and bears (eg, black bears, polar bears)

Fenbendazole Suspension: 100 mg/mL (10%); there are products labeled for use in horses, cattle, and goats: *Panacur® Suspension*, (Rx). FDA-approved for use in horses (not intended for food) and cattle. Slaughter withdrawal is 8 days and milk withdrawal is 48 hours in cattle. *Safe-Guard® Suspension*; (OTC). FDA-approved for use in beef and dairy cattle and nonlactating goats. Cattle must not be slaughtered within 8 days following treatment; there is no milk withdrawal in cattle for this product. A withdrawal period has not been established for this product in preruminating calves. Should not be used in calves to be processed for veal. Goats must not be slaughtered for food within 6 days following treatment. Because a withdrawal time in milk has not been established, this drug should not be used in lactating goats.

Fenbendazole Paste: 100 mg/g (10%); available in both equine and bovine labeled products and sizes. *Panacur® Paste; Safe Guard® Paste;* (OTC). FDA-approved for use in horses not intended for food and in cattle. Slaughter withdrawal for cattle at labeled dosages is 8 days; milk withdrawal time at labeled dosages is 96 hours.

Fenbendazole Pellets: *Safe-Guard® 0.5% Alfalfa-Based Pellets*; (OTC). FDA-approved for use in beef and dairy cattle and swine. There is no milk withdrawal time at labeled dosages; slaughter withdrawal time at labeled dosages for cattle is 13 days and 0 days for swine (no withdrawal period for swine).

Fenbendazole Pellets: *Safe-Guard® Equi-Bits* 0.5% (OTC)

Fenbendazole Suspension: 200 mg/mL in 1 L bottles. *Safe-Guard® AquaSol*; (OTC). For use in swine and in breeding and broiler chickens and replacement chickens intended to become breeding chickens. Withdrawal period for swines is 2 days. Not for use in nursing piglets. No withdrawal period required for chickens when used according to label.

Fenbendazole Premix 20% Type A (200 mg/g): *Safe-Guard® Premix*; (OTC). FDA-approved for use in swine, growing turkeys, dairy and beef cattle, and zoo and wildlife animals. Slaughter withdrawal for cattle is 13 days; no milk withdrawal time is noted. There is no slaughter withdrawal for turkey or swine at labeled dosages. Wildlife animal slaughter (hunting) withdrawal is 14 days at labeled dosages.

There may also be Type B and C medicated feeds available.

HUMAN-LABELED PRODUCTS: NONE

References

For the complete list of references, see **wiley.com/go/budde/plumb**

Fenofibrate

(fen-oh-***fye***-brate) *TriCor®*

Fibric acid derivative; anti-lipemic agent

Prescriber Highlights

- May be useful as adjunctive therapy, along with a low-fat diet, to treat hypertriglyceridemia in dogs
- Limited experience and no published clinical studies in cats; efficacy or safety is not established
- Avoid use in patients with preexisting gallbladder disease, severe renal impairment, or active liver disease
- Many preparations are available; not bioequivalent.

Uses/Indications

Fenofibrate could be useful to lower triglycerides in dogs when diet modifications alone have been unsuccessful. In dogs with hypertriglyceridemia, triglycerides were normalized in 86% to 100% of dogs treated with fenofibrate.[1,2] After 3 to 4 weeks of initiating fenofibrate treatment, a 73% to 88% median reduction in triglycerides and a 10% to 20% reduction in total cholesterol were observed. Under experimental conditions, fenofibrate reduced both total cholesterol and triglycerides in obese beagles by ≈30% after 1 to 2 weeks of use[3]; dogs with the highest pretreatment values experienced the greatest reductions.

In humans, fenofibrate is used as adjunctive therapy to lifestyle changes in the management of dyslipidemia primarily to reduce triglycerides; with treatment, HDL-cholesterol concentrations are typically increased, and reductions in total- and LDL-cholesterol may occur. It is recommended to discontinue treatment in humans if an adequate response is not achieved with 2 to 3 months.[4]

Pharmacology/Actions

Fenofibric acid, the active form of fenofibrate, activates peroxisome proliferator-activated receptors, which increases lipoprotein lipase concentrations and activity. The resulting increased clearance of very low-density lipoproteins and triglycerides causes LDL-cholesterol to be less atherogenic and more easily eliminated. Fenofibrate also increases urinary uric acid excretion. Increased biliary cholesterol saturation contributes to the increased risk for cholelithiasis.

Pharmacokinetics

Fenofibrate is a prodrug that must be converted to its active form, fenofibric acid, but dogs may produce other metabolites.[5] The oral bioavailability varies by dosage form and fed state; fenofibrate nanocrystal tablets have a bioavailability of ≈30% in dogs.[6] In dogs receiving radiolabeled fenofibrate (5 mg/kg PO once), 9% of the dose was eliminated in urine and 81% in feces, primarily within 24 hours of administration.[7]

In humans, peak concentrations occur 4 to 6 hours after administration. Certain preparations must be given with food to increase absorption, whereas others may be taken without regard to meals. Fenofibrate is completely hydrolyzed to its active form, fenofibric acid. Protein binding is 99%, primarily to albumin. The drug is renally eliminated (≈60%), and elimination half-life is ≈20 hours with normal renal function.

Contraindications/Precautions/Warnings

Fenofibrate is contraindicated in patients that are hypersensitive to it or fenofibric acid and with current liver disease or preexisting gallbladder disease.

In humans, hypersensitivity reactions (eg, toxic epidermal

necrolysis, Stevens-Johnson syndrome) have been reported, as have increased liver enzymes, hepatitis, pancreatitis, cholelithiasis, and increased serum creatinine.[8] Serious drug-induced liver injury has been reported. The risk for muscle toxicity (eg, myopathy, rhabdomyolysis) may be increased in geriatric patients and those with diabetes mellitus, hypothyroidism, or renal disease. A paradoxical reduction in HDL-cholesterol may occur.

The role and safety of fenofibrate in humans with preexisting hepatobiliary disease are not clear, and data in dogs are absent. Fenofibrate may contribute to the progression of cholelithiasis in humans with preexisting choleliths; however, its use has been recommended in humans with primary biliary cirrhosis. Fenofibrate should be used with care in dogs with gallbladder mucocele. There is an association between hypercholesterolemia and gallbladder mucocele that could be ameliorated by decreasing serum cholesterol; however, fenofibrate may also increase secretion of cholesterol into the bile, which could contribute to cholelith or mucocele formation. Fenofibrate should be discontinued if liver enzymes persistently exceed 3 times the upper limit of normal, if choleliths are found, or if myopathy or myositis occurs.

Fenofibrate is contraindicated in humans with severe renal impairment, and dosage reduction should be considered in the presence of decreased renal function. Renal elimination is minimal in dogs, but safety in patients with preexisting renal disease has not been determined. Until further research demonstrates safe use of fenofibrate in dogs with preexisting renal disease, this drug should be used with caution in these patients (see ***Monitoring***).

There are several fenofibrate/fenofibric acid preparations, all of which are not bioequivalent. Be sure to specify the intended product when ordering fenofibrate (see ***Dosage Forms/Regulatory Status***).

Adverse Effects

Diarrhea and flatulence have been reported in dogs that received fenofibrate; however, these effects are reduced by temporarily withholding the drug, followed by reinstating at a lower dose for 1 week before resuming the full dose.[2] Increased ALT (2.5 times normal) was noted in 1 dog, and 2 dogs experienced increased creatine kinase.[1]

In humans, adverse effects include nausea, reduced appetite, headache, malaise, back pain, and myalgia.[8] Increases in liver enzymes and serum creatinine are possible. Cholelithiasis and pancreatitis have been reported. Mild or moderate reductions in hemoglobin and white blood cells may occur, as may thrombocytopenia and agranulocytosis.

Reproductive/Nursing Safety

Administration of fenofibrate to pregnant laboratory animals during periods of organogenesis did not result in embryo- or fetal toxicity.[8]

Fenofibrate is contraindicated in nursing women due to the potential to disrupt lipid metabolism in the infant.[8] In veterinary patients, use of milk replacer can be considered if the drug must be continued.

Because safety has not been established in animals, this drug should only be used when the maternal benefits outweigh the potential risks to offspring.

Overdose/Acute Toxicity

No information found. The drug is not removed by dialysis.

For patients that have experienced or are suspected to have experienced an overdose, consultation with a 24-hour poison consultation center specializing in providing veterinary-specific information is recommended. For general information related to overdose and toxin exposures, as well as contact information for poison control centers, refer to ***Appendix.***

Drug Interactions

In humans, fenofibrate may inhibit CYP2C9; it is not a CYP isoenzyme substrate. The following drug interactions either have been reported or are theoretical in humans or animals receiving fenofibrate or fenofibric acid and may be of significance in veterinary patients; unless otherwise noted, use together is not necessarily contraindicated, but the potential risks should be weighed and additional monitoring should be performed when appropriate.

- **Cannabidiol**: Concurrent use may increase cannabinoid exposure.
- **Cholestyramine**: Administer fenofibrate 1 hour before or 4 to 6 hours after cholestyramine.
- **Colchicine**: Concurrent use may increase risk for serious muscle toxicity.
- **Cyclosporine**: Concurrent use may increase risk for nephrotoxicity in humans. Fenofibrate may decrease serum concentrations of cyclosporine.
- **HMG CoA Reductase Inhibitors** (**"statins"**; eg, **atorvastatin, lovastatin**): Concurrent use may increase risk for serious myopathy.
- **Mycophenolate**: Concurrent use may increase risk for neutropenia and other adverse effects of mycophenolate.
- **Omeprazole**: Concurrent omeprazole with fenofibric acid preparations may modestly increase fenofibric acid exposure.
- **Sulfonylureas** (eg, **glipizide**): Concurrent fenofibrate may increase sulfonylurea exposure and risk for hypoglycemia.
- **Ursodiol**: Concurrent fenofibrate may increase biliary cholesterol secretion and reduce ursodiol effectiveness.
- **Warfarin**: Concurrent use may potentiate anticoagulant effect and risk for bleeding.

Laboratory Considerations

No specific laboratory interactions or considerations were noted.

Dosages

NOTE: There are many fenofibrate/fenofibric acid preparations that, except for generic equivalents, are not bioequivalent (ie, they cannot be interchanged/substituted). Be sure to specify the intended product when ordering fenofibrate.

DOGS:

Reduce serum triglycerides (extra-label): 6.5 – 10 mg/kg PO once daily with the first meal of the day.[1-3,9] Fenofibrate nanocrystal tablets were used in one study,[1] while the other studies used fenofibrate tablets.

Monitoring

- Fasting cholesterol panel (including triglyceride measurement)
- Adverse effects, including signs of muscle toxicity and gallbladder disease (eg, weakness, exercise intolerance, lethargy, appetite loss, vomiting, or diarrhea)
- Baseline and periodic serum chemistry panel to include evaluation of renal, liver, and muscle parameters (eg, BUN, creatinine, AST, ALT, bilirubin, CK)

Client Information

- *Fenoglide*®, *Lofibra*®, *Lipofen*®, and their generic equivalents must be taken with food. All other preparations may be taken without regard to food or meals.
- *Antara*®, *Fenoglide*®, *Lipofen*®, *Trilipix*®, and their generic equivalents should be administered whole, without crushing or chewing.
- Report to your veterinarian any vomiting, diarrhea, yellowing of the eyes or skin, and significant lethargy (weakness) or change in activity level.

Chemistry/Synonyms

Fenofibrate occurs as a white to almost-white, solid, nonhygroscopic, odorless, nonbitter-tasting substance. It is practically insoluble in water.

Storage/Stability

Store fenofibrate protected from light and moisture at controlled room temperature (25°C [77°F]) with excursions of 15°C to 30°C (59°F-86°F) permitted.

Compatibility/Compounding Considerations

No specific information was noted.

Dosage Forms/Regulatory Status

VETERINARY-LABELED PRODUCTS: NONE

HUMAN-LABELED PRODUCTS:

NOTE: There are several fenofibrate/fenofibric acid preparations which are not bioequivalent. Be sure to specify the intended product when prescribing fenofibrate.

Fenofibrate Oral Tablets: 35 mg, 40 mg, 50 mg, 54 mg, 105 mg, 120 mg, and 160 mg; *Fenoglide®*, *Fibricor®*, *Lipofen®*, *Lofibra®*, *Triglide®*, generic; (Rx)

Fenofibrate Oral Tablets (nanocrystal): 48 mg and 145 mg; *Tricor®*, generic; (Rx)

Fenofibrate Oral Capsules: 30 mg, 43 mg, 50 mg, 67 mg, 90 mg, 130 mg, 134 mg, 150 mg, and 200 mg; *Antara®*, *Lipofen®*, *Lofibra®*, generic; (Rx)

Fenofibrate Oral Capsules (micronized): 43 mg, 67 mg, 130 mg, 134 mg, and 200 mg; *Antara®*, *Lofibra®*, generic; (Rx)

Fenofibric Acid Delayed-Release Oral Capsules: 45 mg and 135 mg; *Trilipix®*;(Rx)

Fenofibric Acid Capsules: 30 mg, 35 mg, 90 mg, and 105 mg; *Antara®*, *Fibricor®*

References

For the complete list of references, see **wiley.com/go/budde/plumb**

Fenoldopam

(fe-***nol***-doe-pam) *Corlopam®*

Dopamine Agonist (D_1); Antihypertensive

Prescriber Highlights

- May be useful in treating hypertensive emergencies in dogs and cats and nonpolyuric acute kidney injury in dogs, cats, and foals.
- No known contraindications; it can cause tachycardia and hypokalemia.
- Blood pressure, heart rate, urine output, and serum electrolytes should be monitored closely.
- Must be administered as a CRI with an accurate infusion pump; it must not be given as an IV bolus.

Uses/Indications

Fenoldopam may be used for the management of hypertensive emergencies in dogs and cats.[1] It is also used as adjunctive treatment of nonpolyuric acute kidney injury (AKI) in dogs, cats, and foals.

In healthy, anesthetized dogs with experimentally-induced hypovolemia, fenoldopam was shown to be renoprotective and helped to maintain renal blood flow, glomerular filtration rate, and natriuresis without causing hypotension.[2,3] However, in a prospective study of dogs with heatstroke, fenoldopam did not demonstrate a clinically relevant effect on the occurrence of acute kidney injury, kidney function parameters, or mortality.[4] An experimental study in young, healthy cats, a 2-hour infusion of 0.5 µg/kg/minute induced diuresis (delayed effect) and natriuresis, with creatinine clearance significantly increasing 6 hours after the infusion was stopped.[5] A retrospective study of 62 dogs and cats with AKI receiving fenoldopam demonstrated that the treatment was safe but there was no improvement in length of hospital stay, survival to discharge, or renal biochemical parameters compared to those that did not receive fenoldopam.[6]

In normotensive neonatal foals, low-dosage fenoldopam (0.04 µg/kg/min IV CRI) had no significant effects on systemic hemodynamics, creatinine clearance, sodium, chloride, or potassium excretion, but it did significantly increase urine output. High-dosage fenoldopam (0.4 µg/kg/min IV CRI) increased heart rate, decreased systemic arterial blood pressure, and had no significant effects on renal function. The authors concluded that low-dosage fenoldopam had a potential clinical application for prophylaxis or treatment of acute kidney injury in neonatal foals, but additional studies were warranted.[7]

In humans, fenoldopam is labeled for the treatment of severe hypertension; it is also used as a renoprotectant following cardiovascular surgery to improve GI oxygen flow in hypovolemic patients.[8] Due to its selectivity and lower risk for adverse effects, fenoldopam has largely replaced dopamine for adjunctive treatment of acute kidney injury. No beneficial effect on renal function has been noted in human patients with severe chronic kidney disease, heart failure, or hepatic disease.

Pharmacology/Actions

Fenoldopam is a selective postsynaptic dopamine agonist at D_1-receptors, resulting in peripheral arterial vasodilation, increased mesenteric and renal blood flow, diuresis, and reduced total peripheral resistance and systemic blood pressure. In humans, it has been shown to be renoprotective after cardiovascular surgery. Heart rates can increase secondary to a reflex-response to vasodilatory effects. Fenoldopam causes dose-related increases in renal plasma flow, decreases in renal vascular resistance, and produces diuresis, natriuresis, and kaliuresis without significantly affecting the glomerular filtration rate.

Fenoldopam antagonizes alpha-receptors (alpha$_2$ greater than alpha$_1$) at dosages higher than those that activate D_1-receptors, which also contributes to vasodilation. Fenoldopam has no affinity for D_2-receptors, beta-adrenergic receptors, serotonin receptors, or muscarinic receptors.

Pharmacokinetics

A pharmacokinetic study, conducted in 6 healthy beagles given fenoldopam 0.8 µg/kg/minute IV CRI for 3 hours, showed highly variable values of plasma concentrations and clearance, but the drug achieved steady-state plasma concentrations within 10 minutes of the infusion start and was rapidly eliminated with the drug becoming undetectable within 10 minutes of discontinuation. The authors suspected fenoldopam undergoes complete first-pass hepatic elimination in dogs and may undergo additional extra-hepatic clearance, including metabolism and/or renal excretion of unchanged drug.[9]

Six healthy cats given fenoldopam 0.8 µg/kg/minute IV CRI for 2 hours showed a pharmacokinetic profile similar to humans with the volume of distribution, clearance, and half-life of 198 mL/kg, 46 mL/kg/minute, and 3 minutes, respectively.[9]

In humans, fenoldopam has a rapid onset of action, with the antihypertensive effect occurring within 15 minutes. It is about 88% bound to plasma proteins, and almost no drug crosses the blood–brain barrier. The duration of action is ≈1 hour, and the elimination half-life is ≈5 minutes. Fenoldopam is metabolized in the liver with an extensive first-pass effect. The majority of a dose is excreted into the urine, primarily as the inactive glucuronide metabolite.

Contraindications/Precautions/Warnings

There are no known contraindications, but fenoldopam should be used with caution in patients with a history of sulfite sensitivity and glaucoma as increased intraocular pressure has been reported.[8] Additionally, cases of tachycardia and hypokalemia have been reported.

The drug must not be given as an IV bolus. Some preparations contain propylene glycol.

Adverse Effects

The adverse effect profile for fenoldopam is not well documented in animals. The majority of experimental studies were conducted in healthy dogs and cats and did not show any overt adverse effects.[3,5] Foals administered high-dose fenoldopam (0.4 µg/kg/minute) had significantly higher heart rates compared to low-dose fenoldopam or baseline values; 3/6 foals showed signs of restlessness.[7]

In humans, fenoldopam has caused tachycardia (dose-related), headache, flushing, nausea, vomiting, hypotension, and hypokalemia.

Reproductive/Nursing Safety

Fenoldopam was not teratogenic or fetotoxic when administered orally to laboratory animals during periods of organogenesis.[8] Fenoldopam is excreted in milk, but its effects on offspring have not been determined.

Because safety has not been established in animals, this drug should only be used when the maternal benefits outweigh the potential risks to offspring.

Overdose/Acute Toxicity

Overdoses of fenoldopam would likely produce hypotension and reflex tachycardia. The drug effects are generally short-lived (up to 1 hour). Monitoring heart rate, blood pressure, and electrolytes are mandatory. Data suggests it is unlikely to be removed via dialysis.

For patients that have experienced or are suspected of having experienced an overdose, consultation with a 24-hour poison consultation center specializing in providing veterinary-specific information is recommended. For general information related to overdose and toxin exposures, as well as contact information for poison control centers, refer to ***Appendix.***

Drug Interactions

The following drug interactions have either been reported or are theoretical in humans or animals receiving fenoldopam and may be of significance in veterinary patients. Unless otherwise noted, use together is not necessarily contraindicated, but weigh the potential risks and perform additional monitoring when appropriate.

- Beta-Adrenergic Receptor Antagonists (eg, **atenolol, propranolol**): Can inhibit sympathetic reflex response to fenoldopam; concurrent use is not recommended.
- Hypotensive Drugs (eg, **amlodipine, hydralazine, nitroprusside, telmisartan**): Hypotensive effects of fenoldopam may be enhanced.

Laboratory Considerations

None noted

Dosages

NOTES:

1. Do NOT administer fenoldopam as an IV bolus; it must be diluted with 0.9% sodium chloride or 5% dextrose to a concentration of 40 to 60 µg/mL and administered IV as a CRI. See ***Compatibility/Compounding Considerations.***
2. CRI administration should be done with a calibrated, mechanical infusion pump.
3. Fenoldopam infusions can be discontinued abruptly or slowly withdrawn.

DOGS:

Adjunctive treatment of acute, nonpolyuric kidney injury (extra-label): 0.8 µg/kg/minute IV CRI for 5 hours has been suggested.[3,10]

Hypertensive emergency (extra-label): 0.1 µg/kg/minute IV CRI; monitor blood pressure carefully, and increase dosage by 0.1 µg/kg/minute every 15 minutes until the desired systolic blood pressure is reached, or to a maximum of 1.6 µg/kg/minute.[1]

CATS:

Adjunctive treatment of acute kidney injury (oliguric, anuric) (extra-label): 0.1 – 1 µg/kg/minute IV CRI for 2 hours has been recommended.[11] In a study in healthy cats, 0.5 µg/kg/minute IV CRI documented an increase in urine output.[5]

Hypertensive emergency (extra-label): 0.1 µg/kg/minute IV CRI; monitor BP carefully, and increase dosage by 0.1 µg/kg/minute every 15 minutes until the desired systolic blood pressure is reached, or to a maximum of 1.6 µg/kg/minute.[1]

FOALS:

Adjunctive treatment of acute kidney injury (extra-label): 0.04 – 0.4 µg/kg/minute IV CRI for 30 minutes has been used.[7]

Monitoring

- Blood pressure, heart rate
- Urine output
- Serum electrolytes, especially potassium. Infusions of fenoldopam have caused hypokalemia in human patients receiving infusions lasting less than 6 hours.

Client Information

Use fenoldopam only in an inpatient setting.

Chemistry/Synonyms

Fenoldopam mesylate (CAS Registry: 67227-56-9 fenoldopam, 67227-57-0 fenoldopam mesylate; ATC: C01CA190) occurs as a white to off-white powder and is soluble in water. The injectable solution contains propylene glycol and sodium metabisulfite. Unlike nitroprusside, fenoldopam is not degraded by light, nor does it cause thiocyanate toxicity.

Fenoldopam mesylate may also be known as fenoldopam mesilate, SKF-82526-j, or *Corlopam®*.

Storage/Stability

Store ampules and vials at 2°C to 30°C (36°F-86°F). Following dilution, discard solution after 4 hours at room temperature or 24 hours under refrigeration.

Compatibility/Compounding Considerations

Compatibility is dependent on factors, such as pH, concentration, temperature, and diluent used; specialized references or a hospital pharmacist should be consulted for more specific information.

Before administration, the 10 mg/mL injectable concentrate should be diluted and is **compatible** with 0.9% sodium chloride injection or 5% dextrose injection for dilution. To dilute to 60 µg/mL (the usual dilution guideline for human pediatric patients and recommended for small animal species to reduce the risk for volume overload): add fenoldopam 30 mg (3 mL of concentrate) to 500 mL 0.9% sodium chloride or 5% dextrose, or add fenoldopam 15 mg (1.5 mL of concentrate) to 250 mL 0.9% sodium chloride or 5% dextrose. Fenoldopam should be administered as an IV CRI using a calibrated, mechanical infusion pump.

Drugs that are **Y-site compatible** with fenoldopam infusions include alfentanil, amikacin, atracurium, atropine, butorphanol, calcium gluconate, dexmedetomidine, diltiazem, diphenhydramine, dolasetron, epinephrine, fentanyl, heparin, hydrocortisone sodium succinate, hydromorphone, mannitol, naloxone, ondansetron, potassium chloride, and propofol.[12]

Drugs that are **Y-site incompatible** with fenoldopam infusions include ampicillin sodium, bumetanide, dexamethasone sodium phosphate, diazepam, fosphenytoin, furosemide, methylprednisolone sodium succinate, and sodium bicarbonate.[13]

Dosage Forms/Regulatory Status

VETERINARY-LABELED PRODUCTS: NONE

The Association of Racing Commissioners International (ARCI) has designated this drug as a class 3 substance. Use of this drug may not be allowed in certain animal competitions. Check rules and regulations before entering a competition while this medication is being administered. Contact local racing authorities for further guidance. See ***Appendix*** for more information. The FEI (International Federation for Equestrian Sports) lists this drug as a "prohibited substance - banned".

HUMAN-LABELED PRODUCTS:

Fenoldopam injection solution: 10 mg/mL in 1 or 2 mL single-use ampules or vials; *Corlopam®*; (Rx)

References

For the complete list of references, see **wiley.com/go/budde/plumb**

Fentanyl, Injection

(***fen***-ta-nil) *Sublimaze®*

Opioid

Prescriber Highlights

- ► Opioid analgesic used parenterally in small animals; potentially useful as a CRI in horses
- ► Contraindications: scorpion stings; use extreme caution when additional respiratory or CNS depression would be detrimental.
- ► Use caution in geriatric, ill, or debilitated patients and in those with GI obstruction, pre-existing respiratory problems, or renal or hepatic impairment.
- ► Adverse effects include dose-dependent respiratory, CNS, and circulatory depression (eg, bradycardia); urine retention; constipation; dysphoria; and agitation.
- ► Schedule II controlled substance in the United States
- ► See also ***Fentanyl, Transdermal Patch***

Uses/Indications

In veterinary medicine, fentanyl injection is used primarily in dogs and cats for the adjunctive control of postoperative pain and in the control of severe pain associated with nonspecific, widespread pain (eg, associated with cancer, pancreatitis, aortic thromboemboli, peritonitis). Perioperative injectable fentanyl may also reduce the requirements for inhalational anesthetics during surgery, which could be particularly advantageous in patients with compromised cardiac function. In healthy beagles, fentanyl decreased isoflurane and sevoflurane MAC by ≈40%.[1,2] Because of its short duration of action, fentanyl CRIs are particularly useful in critically ill or postsurgical patients, as it can be adjusted to meet the analgesia needs of the patient, minimize adverse effects, and be temporarily halted to assess neurologic status. Injectable fentanyl may be particularly useful in cats for perioperative pain control, especially when higher analgesic doses are required, as it appears to have fewer adverse effects in this species than either hydromorphone or morphine.

Pharmacology/Actions

Fentanyl is a mu-opioid agonist that is short acting and ≈80 to 100 times more potent than morphine. Mu receptors are found primarily in the pain-regulating areas of the brain, dorsal horn of the spinal cord, and different peripheral tissues; they are thought to contribute to the analgesia, euphoria, respiratory depression, physical dependence, miosis, and hypothermic actions of opioids. Receptors for opioid analgesics are found in high concentrations in the limbic system, spinal cord, thalamus, hypothalamus, striatum, and midbrain; they are also found in tissues such as the GI tract, urinary tract, and other smooth muscles.

Pharmacokinetics

Fentanyl used via a single dose IV injection has a relatively short duration of effect in most species.

In dogs, a fentanyl 10 µg/kg IV bolus rapidly distributes and exhibits a large volume of distribution (ie, 5 L/kg). The terminal elimination half-life is ≈45 minutes; total clearance is 78 mL/min/kg. After dogs received a fentanyl 10 µg/kg IV bolus followed by a fentanyl 10 µg/kg/hour IV CRI, fentanyl blood concentrations were maintained ≈1 ng/mL, which is the assumed but not verified therapeutic analgesic level for this species.[3]

In cats, an elimination half-life of 2.4 hours, mean systemic clearance of 1.4 L/kg/hour, and an apparent volume of distribution of 4.42 L/kg were recorded after administration of a 5 µg/kg IV bolus, followed by 5 µg/kg/hour IV CRI for 2 hours.[4]

One study looked at pharmacokinetics of IV fentanyl in foals at 6 to 8, 20 to 22, and 41 to 42 days of age.[5] In this study, the average volumes of distribution were 3.55, 1.53, and 1.82 L/kg, respectively. The elimination half-lives were 49.3 minutes, 25.8 minutes, and 33.7 minutes, respectively.

Contraindications/Precautions/Warnings

Fentanyl is contraindicated in patients with known hypersensitivity to it or other opioids.

Because of its potency, fentanyl injection should be used only by those familiar with its use and when patients can be adequately monitored and supported.

Use with extreme caution in patients with CNS or respiratory depression or when using in conjunction with other CNS, respiratory, or cardiac depressants; adequate monitoring should be used. Use cautiously in geriatric, ill, or debilitated patients and in those with GI obstruction, pre-existing respiratory problems, or renal or hepatic impairment.

Opioid analgesics are contraindicated in patients stung by scorpions (eg, *Centruroides* spp), as it may potentiate venom effects.[6]

Opioids may cause mydriasis in cats. Approach patients slowly so as not to startle them, and keep patients out of bright light while pupils are dilated.

Do not confuse fentaNYL with ALFentanil, CARFentanil, REMIFentanil, or SUFentanil.

Adverse Effects

The primary adverse effects are dose-related respiratory (eg, bradypnea, hypercapnia), CNS (eg, sedation), and circulatory depression (eg, bradycardia, hypotension). Hypothermia is possible in dogs. Anticholinergic agents may be required to treat bradycardia when fentanyl is used intraoperatively. Dogs and cats appear to be susceptible, but less prone than humans, to opioid-induced respiratory depression. In a study[7] in healthy, young-adult dogs, concurrent administration of fentanyl and isoflurane resulted in significant decreases in mean arterial blood pressure, heart rate, cardiac index, and a significant increase in partial pressure of carbon dioxide ($PaCO_2$); all of which, except $PaCO_2$ returned to pretreatment levels over time. Dysphoria has been reported in ≈25% of dogs treated with fentanyl IV CRI postoperatively.[8] Fentanyl-induced asystole has been reported in 2 dogs under isoflurane anesthesia.[9] Data regarding fentanyl's effect on intraocular pressure in dogs are conflicting.[10,11]

Some patients exhibit dysphoria or agitation after receiving fentanyl; acepromazine or other mild tranquilizers may alleviate these effects.

In horses, fentanyl, like morphine, can initially stimulate then inhibit cecocolic activity. Horses heterozygous for the G57C polymorphism of the mu-opioid receptor had an increased locomotor response to fentanyl in one study.[12]

In humans, fentanyl can cause a rare syndrome called wooden chest, which is characterized by chest wall rigidity[13,14]; however, this syndrome has never been reported in dogs.[15]

Reproductive/Nursing Safety

Opioids cross the placenta. Embryocidal effects and reduced pup survival have been noted in rats.[16]

Most narcotic agonist analgesics are excreted into milk, but effects on nursing offspring may not be significant.

Overdose/Acute Toxicity

Overdoses may produce profound respiratory and/or CNS depression in most species. Newborns may be more susceptible to these effects than adult animals. Other toxic effects may include hypersalivation, ataxia, bradycardia, hypothermia, diarrhea, cardiovascular collapse, tremors, neck rigidity, and seizures.

Naloxone is the agent of choice when treating fentanyl-related respiratory and circulatory depression. In massive overdoses, naloxone may need to be repeated; mechanical respiratory support should be considered in patients with severe respiratory depression. Patients should be closely observed, as naloxone's effects sometimes diminish before subtoxic levels of fentanyl are attained.

Drug Interactions

The following drug interactions have either been reported or are theoretical in humans or animals receiving fentanyl and may be of significance in veterinary patients. Unless otherwise noted, use together is not necessarily contraindicated, but weigh the potential risks and perform additional monitoring when appropriate.

- **ACE Inhibitors** (eg, **enalapril**): Concurrent use may increase the risk for bradycardia, hypotension, and orthostasis.
- **Alfaxalone**: Fentanyl reduced alfaxalone dosage requirements in dogs.[17,18]
- **Anesthetic, Inhalant**: Isoflurane anesthesia reduced fentanyl clearance in horses, and increased mean arterial pressure was noted.[19] Fentanyl reduces MAC by ≈40%.[1,2] Combination increases the risk for bradycardia or hypotension.
- **Anticholinergic Agents** (eg, **acepromazine, amitriptyline, atropine, clomipramine, hyoscyamine**): Concurrent use may increase the risk for urinary retention, constipation, and CNS and respiratory depression.
- **Angiotensin Receptor Blockers** (ARBs, eg, **telmisartan**): Concurrent use may increase the risk for bradycardia, hypotension, and orthostasis.
- **Azole Antifungals** (eg, **fluconazole, itraconazole, ketoconazole**): May increase the half-life and decrease the clearance of fentanyl, leading to prolonged effects and an increased risk of respiratory depression. However, a study in dogs showed that ketoconazole did not significantly alter the elimination of fentanyl.[20]
- **Barbiturates** (eg, **pentobarbital, phenobarbital**): Concurrent use may increase the risk for CNS and/or respiratory depression. Monitor, and adjust doses accordingly.
- **Benzodiazepines** (eg, **diazepam, midazolam**): Concurrent use may increase the risk for CNS and/or respiratory depression. Monitor, and adjust doses accordingly.
- **Beta-Blockers** (eg, **atenolol, esmolol, propranolol**): May produce bradycardia or hypotension if used concurrently with fentanyl
- **Bethanechol**: Concurrent use may antagonize the beneficial effects of bethanechol on GI motility; avoid combination of these drugs.
- **Calcium Channel Blockers** (eg, **amlodipine, diltiazem**): Concurrent use may increase the risk for bradycardia, hypotension, and orthostasis. Diltiazem may increase the half-life and decrease the clearance of fentanyl, leading to prolonged effects and an increased risk for respiratory depression.
- **Cannabidiol**: Concurrent use may increase the risk for CNS depression.
- **Cimetidine**: May increase the half-life and decrease the clearance of fentanyl, leading to prolonged effects and an increased risk for respiratory depression.
- **Desmopressin**: Concurrent use may increase levels of oral desmopressin and increase the risk for water intoxication and/or hyponatremia, which can progress to seizures, coma, respiratory arrest, and death. Monitor electrolytes and renal function.
- **Dextromethorphan**: Concurrent use may increase the risk for serotonin syndrome.
- **Diuretics** (eg, **furosemide**): Opioids may decrease therapeutic effects of diuretics.
- **Domperidone**: Concurrent use may antagonize the GI effects of domperidone.
- **Hepatic Enzyme Inducers** (eg, **griseofulvin, mitotane, phenobarbital**): Concurrent use may decrease levels of fentanyl. Monitor clinical response and adjust doses accordingly.
- **Grapefruit Juice**: May increase the half-life and decrease the clearance of fentanyl, leading to prolonged effects and an increased risk for respiratory depression
- **Ifosfamide**: Concurrent use may increase the risk for neurotoxicity, including somnolence, confusion, hallucinations, blurred vision, urinary incontinence, seizures, and coma. Use cautiously and monitor.
- **Iohexol**: Concurrent use of opioids with intrathecal iohexol may increase the risk for seizures. Opioids should be withheld for 48 hours before and 24 hours after intrathecal administration of iohexol.
- **Loperamide**: Concurrent use may increase the risk for constipation.
- **Macrolide Antibiotics** (eg, **clarithromycin, erythromycin**): May increase the half-life and decrease the clearance of fentanyl, leading to prolonged effects and an increased risk for respiratory depression.
- **Monoamine Oxidase Inhibitors** (MAOIs; eg, **amitraz, selegiline**): Concurrent use may increase the risk for anxiety, confusion, hypotension, respiratory depression, cyanosis, and coma. MAOIs inhibitors should be withheld for 14 days prior to administration of opioids; avoid combination of these drugs.
- **Metoclopramide**: Concurrent use may antagonize the prokinetic effects of metoclopramide.
- **Neuromuscular Blocking Agents** (eg, **atracurium, pancuronium**): Concurrent use may increase the risk for tachycardia, bradycardia, and/or hypotension. Use cautiously and monitor.
- **Propofol**: Increased risk for CNS and cardiorespiratory depression
- **Serotonergic Agents** (eg, **fluoxetine, ondansetron**): Concurrent use may increase the risk for serotonin syndrome; avoid combination of these drugs.
- **Tramadol**: Concurrent use may increase the risk for seizures, serotonin syndrome, urine retention, and constipation. The risk for CNS and respiratory depression may be additive.

Laboratory Considerations

- Because opioids may increase biliary tract pressure, plasma **amylase** and **lipase** values can be increased up to 24 hours following drug administration.

Dosages

NOTES:

1. **Adequate patient monitoring is essential. Be sure to have naloxone readily available when administering fentanyl.**
2. Do not confuse dosages listed as µg/kg or mg/kg; CRI dosages may be reported as mg/kg/hour, µg/kg/hour, or µg/kg/minute.

3. Always double-check dosages and resulting volumes when using injectable fentanyl.
4. All dosages are extra-label.

DOGS/CATS:

Perioperative analgesia: Fentanyl 10 µg/kg IV loading dose, followed by fentanyl 10 µg/kg/hour IV CRI may be a guideline during general anesthesia to provide analgesia in dogs.[3] Others have recommended loading doses ranging from 2 – 10 µg/kg IV, followed by 2 – 10 µg/kg/hour IV CRI for dogs.[21] In cats, fentanyl 5 µg/kg IV loading dose followed by 5 µg/kg/hour IV CRI.[22] If bolus IV, IM, or SC doses (usually 5 – 8 µg/kg) are administered without a follow-up CRI, duration of action is very short and re-administration may need to be repeated at 1 to 2 hour intervals.

Severe pain in the emergent patient: Fentanyl 10 – 50 µg/kg IV titrated to effect; use the effective dose as an hourly IV CRI. Give CRI in conjunction with NSAIDs when they are not contraindicated. Ketamine 4 mg/kg IV as a bolus can be used with fentanyl to provide additional analgesia. In addition, the following can be added: _in dogs_, lidocaine 2 – 4 mg/kg IV bolus, followed by lidocaine 2 – 4mg/kg/hour IV CRI; _in cats_, lidocaine 0.25 – 1 mg/kg IV bolus, followed by lidocaine 0.5 – 2 mg/kg/hour IV CRI. Use caution to avoid toxicity if local anesthetics have been administered by means of a different route. Consider combining this regimen with other analgesic modalities (eg, epidural analgesia, local nerve blocks), or anesthetize the patient while attempting to find or treat the inciting cause.[23]

Epidural analgesia: Fentanyl 4 µg/kg, diluted with 0.2 mL preservative-free saline or local anesthetic, and placed in the epidural space. This has predominantly supraspinal effects, with onset occurring in less than 10 minutes, with a ½-hour duration.[24]

Anesthetic agent: Fentanyl 20 – 40 µg/kg IV (or SC, IM) bolus has been noted when used a sole agent; decrease the dose if using with other cardio- or respiratory depressant agents. Dosages are generally higher than those used for analgesia but, like all anesthetic agents, vary depending on comorbidities, patient response, and other coadministered drugs and anesthetic agents. To reduce MAC and provide intraoperative pain control, fentanyl may then be administered as a CRI. CRI dosage recommendations vary considerably, but usually are in the 5 – 20 µg/kg/hour (up to 40 µg/kg/hour in dogs) range.

FERRETS:

Perioperative analgesia and adjunctive anesthetic agent: fentanyl 5 – 10 µg/kg IV preoperatively followed by fentanyl 10 – 20 µg/kg/hour IV CRI with ketamine 0.3 – 0.4 mg/kg/hour IV CRI intraoperatively. Postoperatively, fentanyl 2 – 5 µg/kg/hour IV CRI with ketamine 0.3 – 0.4 mg/kg/hour IV CRI.[25]

RABBITS/RODENTS/SMALL MAMMALS:

Perioperative analgesia: 5 – 20 µg/kg IV bolus for a 30 to 60 minute duration.[26] In rabbits, fentanyl has been shown to reduce isoflurane MAC when used intraoperatively.[27]

HORSES:

Analgesia: 10 µg/kg IV over 5 minutes produced analgesia for up to 30 minutes.[28]

Partial intravenous anesthesia (PIVA) protocol: A study in anesthetized horses showed that a fentanyl IV CRI ranging from 6 – 8 µg/kg/hour (plasma concentration 13 ng/mL) must be administered to decrease the MAC of isoflurane by 18%.[29] In another study, the authors used a loading dose of fentanyl 4 – 8 µg/kg IV over 12 minutes, followed by fentanyl 6 – 12 µg/kg/hour IV CRI (plasma concentration was 13 – 24 ng/mL).[30] These doses did not significantly decrease the MAC of isoflurane. Several horses showed undesirable and potentially injurious behavior during recovery. The authors concluded that the study results did not support use of fentanyl as an anesthesia adjuvant.

SHEEP/GOATS:

Anesthetic agent: One study determined that 5 µg/kg/hour IV CRI did not reduce isoflurane MAC.[31] Another study suggested that 10 µg/kg/hour IV CRI with isoflurane in oxygen reduced the isoflurane requirements without clinically affecting the cardiorespiratory stability or postoperative recovery.[32] In goats, dosages of 15 µg/kg/hour IV CRI or greater have been associated with severe excitatory behavior.[33]

Epidural analgesia: fentanyl 4 µg/kg with bupivacaine 0.25 mg/kg for lumbosacral epidural provided analgesia for 180 minutes.[34]

Monitoring

- Analgesic efficacy
- Heart rate, blood pressure, pulse oximetry, respiratory rate, $ETCO_2$
- CNS effects (eg, sedation, dysphoria, excitement)

Chemistry/Synonyms

Fentanyl citrate, a potent opioid agonist, occurs as a white crystalline powder. It is sparingly soluble in water and soluble in alcohol. It is odorless and tasteless (not recommended for taste test because of extreme potency) with a pK_a of 8.3 and a melting point between 147°C to 152°C (296.6°F-305.6°F). Fentanyl citrate injection has a pH between 4 to 7.5.

Fentanyl and fentanyl citrate may also be known as fentanylum, fentanyli citras, McN-JR-4263-49, phentanyl citrate, R-4263, or *Sublimaze®*.

Storage/Stability

Fentanyl injection should be stored protected from light at controlled room temperature. It is hydrolyzed in an acidic solution.

Fentanyl is a schedule 2 (C-II) controlled substance that should be stored in an area that is substantially constructed and securely locked. Follow applicable local, state, and federal rules regarding disposal of unused or wasted controlled drugs.

Compatibility/Compounding Considerations

The injection is **compatible** with normal saline and D_5W. Fentanyl citrate injection is reported to be **compatible** with clonidine, bupivacaine, ropivacaine, and ketamine.

Dosage Forms/Regulatory Status

VETERINARY-LABELED PRODUCTS: NONE

The Association of Racing Commissioners International (ARCI) has designated this drug as a class 1 substance. See the ***Appendix*** for more information.

HUMAN-LABELED PRODUCTS:

Fentanyl Injectable: 0.05 mg/mL (50 µg/mL) in 1 mL, 2 mL, 5 mL, 10 mL, 20 mL, and 50 mL preservative-free ampules and vials; *Sublimaze®*, generic; (Rx, C-II)

All fentanyl products are schedule 2 controlled substances. Report dispensing to state monitoring programs where required.

References

For the complete list of references, see **wiley.com/go/budde/plumb**

Fentanyl, Transdermal Patch

(**fen**-ta-nil) *Duragesic®, Ionsys®*

Opioid

See also ***Fentanyl, Injection***

Prescriber Highlights

- ► Opioid analgesic used transdermally (extra-label) in veterinary patients
- ► Contraindications include scorpion stings; use extreme caution when additional respiratory or CNS depression would be detrimental.
- ► Use caution in geriatric, ill, febrile, or debilitated patients and in those with GI obstruction, pre-existing respiratory problems, or renal or hepatic impairment.
- ► Adverse effects include dose-dependent respiratory, CNS, and circulatory depression (eg, bradycardia); rashes at the patch site; urine retention; constipation; dysphoria; and agitation.
- ► Delayed onset of analgesia (eg, 6 hours in cats, 12 to 24 hours in dogs) precludes use for acute pain.
- ► Body temperature and application site influence transdermal absorption of fentanyl; inadequate patch adherence increases risk for detachment or ingestion.
- ► Schedule II controlled substance in the United States

Uses/Indications

In veterinary medicine, transdermal patches are used primarily in dogs[1,2] and cats[3] and have been shown to be useful for the adjunctive control of postoperative pain, severe pain associated with chronic pain, and nonspecific, widespread pain (eg, associated with cancer, pancreatitis, aortic thromboemboli, peritonitis).

Overall, transdermal fentanyl is thought to be clinically effective and has not demonstrated substantial adverse effects. A noncontrolled study in 10 dogs following spinal surgery measured plasma fentanyl concentrations after transdermal patch application (mean patch concentration, 4.1 ± 0.8 µg/kg/hour) and concluded that fentanyl patches may represent a valid aid for pain relief in small animals and can contribute to the postoperative well-being of patients undergoing major surgery.[1] However, one study in dogs comparing transdermal (patch) fentanyl with morphine IM for pain control during the first 24 hours after orthopedic surgery did not show any significant pain control benefit from the patch, which is considerably more expensive than morphine IM.[4]

In humans, significant respiratory depression with fentanyl patches after surgery has precluded postoperative use, but this has not been a significant problem in veterinary medicine.

Pharmacology/Actions

Fentanyl is a mu-opioid agonist that is short acting and ≈80 to 100 times more potent than morphine. Mu receptors are found primarily in the pain-regulating areas of the brain, dorsal horn of the spinal cord, and different peripheral tissues; they are thought to contribute to the analgesia, euphoria, respiratory depression, physical dependence, miosis, and hypothermic actions of opioids. Receptors for opioid analgesics are found in high concentrations in the limbic system, spinal cord, thalamus, hypothalamus, striatum, and midbrain; they are also found in tissues such as the GI tract, urinary tract, and other smooth muscles.

Pharmacokinetics

There have been limited pharmacokinetic studies performed with transdermal fentanyl patches in dogs, cats, horses, sheep, chickens, rabbits, goats, alpacas, and ball pythons. Although therapeutic concentrations of fentanyl are usually attained, there is significant interpatient variability for both the time to achieve therapeutic concentrations and the concentrations themselves. Some animals may not achieve serum concentrations thought to be therapeutic (ie, 0.6 – 1 ng/mL). In an in vitro study of canine skin, fentanyl penetrated skin from the groin region more rapidly and with a shorter lag time than skin from the neck and thorax.[5] In dogs, the patch should be applied 24 hours in advance of need if possible, with a minimum of 12 hours before the patch is needed; for continued use, patches may need to be changed every 48 to 72 hours. Cats tend to achieve therapeutic concentrations faster than dogs. Most cats attain therapeutic benefit ≈6 hours after application; duration of action persists for at least 72 hours (usually for at least 104 hours). Duration of action is generally longer in cats than in dogs.

In horses, fentanyl from patches is rapidly absorbed, with therapeutic concentrations (thought to be 0.6 – 1 ng/mL) achieved ≈6 hours after application and persisting for 48 hours or more; however, in ≈⅓ of the horses, plasma concentrations never reached greater than 1 ng/mL.[6]

In sheep, patches applied at a mean dose of 2.05 µg/kg/hour had an average T_{max} of 12 hours (range, 4-24 hours) and a C_{max} of 1.3 ng/mL (range, 0.62 – 2.73 ng/mL); concentrations remained above 0.5 ng/mL for 40 hours after application.[7] A study showed that fentanyl patches delivering 1.1 – 1.4 µg/kg/hour did not affect thermal or mechanical nociceptive threshold in sheep.[8] A more recent study suggested that a 2 µg/kg/hour patch should be applied 24 to 36 hours prior to surgery.[9]

In goats, a target dose of 2.5 µg/kg/hour resulted in a peak fentanyl concentration 12 hours after application, and concentrations were maintained above 0.5 ng/mL for 40 hours.[10]

Contraindications/Precautions/Warnings

Fentanyl is contraindicated in patients with known hypersensitivity to it, other opioids, or any component of the product (including the adhesive for the patch).

Absorption and efficacy can be highly variable between patients wearing transdermal patches; injectable rescue analgesia should be available.

Use with extreme caution in patients with CNS or respiratory depression or when using with other CNS, respiratory, or cardiac depressants; adequate monitoring should be used. Doses of other opioids may need to be reduced when given in conjunction with transdermal fentanyl, particularly several hours after application of the patch. Transdermal fentanyl should be used cautiously in geriatric, ill, or debilitated patients and in those with GI obstruction, pre-existing respiratory problems, or renal or hepatic impairment. Febrile patients may have increased absorption of fentanyl and will require increased monitoring.

Opioid analgesics are contraindicated in patients stung by scorpions (eg, *Centruroides* spp), as it may potentiate venom effects.[11]

Opioids may cause mydriasis in cats. Approach these patients slowly in order to not startle them, and keep the patient out of bright light while pupils are dilated.

In a study, 4 out of 7 calves displayed adverse cardiac and behavioral effects after application of patches with 1 – 2 µg/kg/hour; 2 calves required reversal with naloxone.[12]

Previously, fentanyl patches were only available in a gel-matrix form that could not be cut. Although brands are now available that potentially can be cut, it is recommended to prescribe appropriately sized patches that do not require cutting. Consult a veterinary pharmacist before cutting patches.

Increased body temperature increases fentanyl absorption. Consider removing the patch if the patient develops a fever; if the patch is left in place, the patient must be closely monitored for adverse effects. Do not allow an applied fentanyl patch to be exposed to exogenous heat sources (eg, heating pads). Increased drug release and absorption have occurred with fatal results.

Used fentanyl patches must be disposed of safely, as they can contain significant amounts of residual drug and can pose a risk for intoxication of exposed humans, especially children, if placed in the regular trash.[13] To avoid this risk, and the risk of diversion, the FDA recommends that used patches be disposed of promptly via a drug take-back program or be flushed down the toilet.

Do not confuse fentanyl with ALFentanil, CARFentanil, REMIFentanil, or SUFentanil.

Adverse Effects

The primary adverse effects of most concern are respiratory (eg, bradypnea), CNS (eg, sedation), and circulatory depression (eg, bradycardia, hypotension); however, the incidence of these effects has not been widespread when fentanyl patches are used alone (ie, without other opioids or respiratory and cardiac depressant medications). Rashes at the patch site have been reported. If a rash occurs, the patch should be removed, and a different application site should be chosen if an additional patch is warranted. Urine retention and constipation may occur. Consider removing the patch in patients that develop a fever after application, as fentanyl absorption may increase. Some patients exhibit dysphoria or agitation after application; acepromazine or other mild tranquilizers may alleviate these effects.

Reproductive/Nursing Safety

Opioids cross the placenta. Embryocidal effects and reduced pup survival have been noted in rats.[14] Prolonged opioid use during pregnancy may result in neonatal withdrawal symptoms. Fentanyl may reduce fertility in males and females.

Most narcotic agonist analgesics are excreted into milk, but effects on nursing offspring may not be significant.

Overdose/Acute Toxicity

Overdoses may produce profound respiratory and/or CNS depression in most species. Neonates may be more susceptible to these effects than adult animals. Other toxic effects may include hypersalivation, ataxia, bradycardia, hypothermia, diarrhea, cardiovascular collapse, tremors, neck rigidity, and seizures.

Naloxone is the agent of choice when treating respiratory and circulatory depression. In massive overdoses, naloxone may need to be repeated; mechanical respiratory support should be considered in patients with severe respiratory depression. Patients should be closely observed, as naloxone's effects sometimes diminish before subtoxic levels of fentanyl are attained.

Drug Interactions

In humans, fentanyl is a substrate of CYP3A4. The following drug interactions have either been reported or are theoretical in humans or animals receiving fentanyl and may be of significance in veterinary patients. Unless otherwise noted, use together is not necessarily contraindicated, but weigh the potential risks and perform additional monitoring when appropriate.

- Anticholinergic Agents (eg, **acepromazine, amitriptyline, atropine, clomipramine, hyoscyamine**): Concurrent use may increase the risk for urinary retention, constipation, and CNS and respiratory depression.
- Anesthetic Agents (eg, **isoflurane, propofol**): May produce bradycardia or hypotension
- Angiotensin Receptor Blockers (ARBs, eg, **telmisartan**): Concurrent use may increase the risk for bradycardia, hypotension, and orthostasis
- Azole Antifungals (eg, **fluconazole, itraconazole, ketoconazole**): May increase the half-life and decrease the clearance of fentanyl, leading to prolonged effects and an increased risk for respiratory depression. However, a study in dogs showed that ketoconazole did not significantly alter the elimination of fentanyl.[15]
- Barbiturates (eg, **pentobarbital, phenobarbital**): Concurrent use may increase the risk for CNS and/or respiratory depression. Monitor, and adjust doses accordingly.
- Benzodiazepines (eg, **diazepam, midazolam**): Concurrent use may increase the risk for CNS and/or respiratory depression. Monitor, and adjust doses accordingly.
- Beta Blockers (eg, **atenolol, esmolol, propranolol**): May produce bradycardia or hypotension if used concurrently with fentanyl
- Bethanechol: Concurrent use may antagonize the beneficial effects of bethanechol on GI motility; avoid combination of these drugs.
- Calcium Channel Blockers (eg, **amlodipine, diltiazem**): Concurrent use may increase the risk for bradycardia, hypotension, and orthostasis. Diltiazem may increase the half-life and decrease the clearance of fentanyl, leading to prolonged effects and an increased risk for respiratory depression.
- Cannabidiol: Concurrent use may increase the risk for CNS depression.
- Cimetidine: May increase the half-life and decrease the clearance of fentanyl, leading to prolonged effects and an increased risk for respiratory depression.
- Desmopressin: Concurrent use may increase levels of oral desmopressin and increase the risk for water intoxication and/or hyponatremia, which can progress to seizures, coma, respiratory arrest, and death. Monitor electrolytes and renal function.
- Dextromethorphan: Concurrent use may increase the risk for serotonin syndrome.
- Diuretics (eg, **furosemide**): Opioids may decrease therapeutic effects of diuretics.
- Domperidone: Concurrent use may antagonize the GI effects of domperidone.
- Hepatic Enzyme Inducers (eg, **griseofulvin, mitotane, phenobarbital**): Concurrent use may decrease levels of fentanyl. Monitor clinical response and adjust doses accordingly.
- Grapefruit Juice: May increase the half-life and decrease the clearance of fentanyl, leading to prolonged effects and an increased risk for respiratory depression.
- Ifosfamide: Concurrent use may increase the risk for neurotoxicity, including somnolence, confusion, hallucinations, blurred vision, urinary incontinence, seizures, and coma. Use cautiously and monitor.
- Iohexol: Concurrent use of opioids with intrathecal iohexol may increase the risk for seizures. Opioids should be withheld for 48 hours before and 24 hours after intrathecal administration of iohexol.
- Loperamide: Concurrent use may increase the risk for constipation.
- Macrolide Antibiotics (eg, **clarithromycin, erythromycin**): May increase the half-life and decrease the clearance of fentanyl, leading to prolonged effects and an increased risk of respiratory depression
- Monoamine Oxidase Inhibitors (MAOIs; eg, **amitraz, selegiline**): Concurrent use may increase the risk for anxiety, confusion, hypotension, respiratory depression, cyanosis, and coma. MAOIs should be withheld for 14 days prior to administration of opioids; avoid combination of these drugs.
- Metoclopramide: Concurrent use may antagonize the prokinetic effects of metoclopramide.
- Neuromuscular Blocking Agents (eg, **atracurium, pancuronium**): Concurrent use may increase the risk for tachycardia, bradycardia, and/or hypotension. Use cautiously and monitor.

- **Serotonergic Agents** (eg, **fluoxetine, ondansetron**): Concurrent use may increase the risk for serotonin syndrome; avoid combination of these drugs.
- **Tramadol**: Concurrent use may increase the risk for seizures, serotonin syndrome, urinary retention, and constipation. The risk for CNS and respiratory depression may be additive.

Laboratory Considerations

- Because opioids may increase biliary tract pressure, serum **amylase** and **lipase** values can be increased up to 24 hours following drug administration.

Dosages

NOTES:

1. Do not confuse total amount of fentanyl per patch with the fentanyl delivery rate (eg, 75 mcg/hr patches contains 7.65 mg fentanyl).
2. Always double-check dosages when using fentanyl.
3. Human-labeled fentanyl patches are used in an extra-label manner in all veterinary species.

Postoperative pain control or palliative short-term control of cancer pain: There is significant interspecies and interpatient variability of response to the transdermal product. Application prior to surgery is advised when used as the primary analgesic for postoperative pain, as many hours may be required for therapeutic concentrations to be achieved. In general, therapeutic concentrations may be reached in 12 to 24 hours in dogs, 6 to 24 hours in cats, and 12 hours in horses. Patches used for short-term cancer pain control generally need to be replaced every 4 to 5 days in dogs and cats.

To transition from fentanyl infusions to a fentanyl patch in cats: Adjust fentanyl IV CRI rate to reach optimal effect before patch is applied; after patch application, the infusion should then be tapered and discontinued over the next 8 to 24 hours and the patient response observed. Failure of the patch is suspected if the patient responds well on the infusion but poorly on the patch. In cats, fentanyl delivery from the patch is highly variable. A 25 µg patch provides ≈10 µg/hour.[16]

Dosage range recommendations are typically 2 – 2.5 µg/kg/hour but may range from 1 – 5 µg/kg/hour. The following table can be used as a general guide:

Species	Body weight	Dose, patch size (µg/hour)	Patch location
Cats	Less than 4 kg[17] (11 lb)	12 (a 25 µg/hour patch may be used in larger cats)	Lateral thorax, inguinal area, metatarsal/carpal areas, or base of tail. Cervical area is not recommended, as the patch tends to fall off.
Dogs	Less than 5 kg (11 lb)	12 µg/hour	Thorax, inguinal area, metatarsal/carpal areas, or base of tail. Dorsal or lateral cervical area has been used, but leashes must not be placed around the neck if fentanyl patches are in place.
Dogs	5-10 kg (11-22 lb)	25 µg/hour	Thorax, inguinal area, metatarsal/-carpal areas, or base of tail. Dorsal or lateral cervical area has been used, but leashes must not be placed around the neck if fentanyl patches are in place.
Dogs	10-20 kg (22-44 lb)	50 µg/hour	Thorax, inguinal area, metatarsal/-carpal areas, or base of tail. Dorsal or lateral cervical area has been used, but leashes must not be placed around the neck if fentanyl patches are in place.
Dogs	20-30 kg (44-66 lb)	75 µg/hour	Thorax, inguinal area, metatarsal/-carpal areas, or base of tail. Dorsal or lateral cervical area has been used, but leashes must not be placed around the neck if fentanyl patches are in place.
Dogs	Greater than 30 kg (66 lb)	100 µg/hour	Thorax, inguinal area, metatarsal/-carpal areas, or base of tail. Dorsal or lateral cervical area has been used, but leashes must not be placed around the neck if fentanyl patches are in place.
Horses	350-500 kg (772-1102 lb)	Two 100 µg/hour applied simultaneously	Neck, antebrachium (foals), thorax (adults)
Pigs	17-30 kg (38-66 lb)	50 - 100 µg/hour	Lateral thorax
Sheep	55-70 kg (121-154 lb)	50 – 100 µg/hour	Abdomen, cervical, antebrachial area
Goats	20-40 kg (44-88 lb)	50 – 100 µg/hour	Abdomen, cervical, antebrachial area
Alpacas	60 kg (132 lb)	100 + 25 µg/hour	Antebrachium
Rabbits	3.5-4 kg (7.7-8.8 lb)	12 – 25 µg/hour	Lateral thorax
Chickens	2.2-3.6 kg (4.8-7.9 lb)	25 µg/hour	Iliopsoas muscle, feathers plucked from 4 cm^2 area[18]

PATCH APPLICATION

NOTE: Direct patch contact with heating pads can significantly increase fentanyl absorption and the risk for toxicity. The patch should be kept dry.

1) Carefully shave or closely clip the site. DO NOT use depilatory (ie, hair removal) agents in preparation of the site. Clip at least a 1- to 2-cm margin around the patch.
2) Gently wipe (do not scrub) the site with a damp cloth (use water only) to remove hair and any debris; allow the skin to completely dry. This step is absolutely necessary, or the patch will not stick to the skin. DO NOT wipe the area with alcohol or surgical scrub solution, as they may remove surface lipids from the skin and alter drug absorption.
3) Place the patch on the skin and hold it in place with the palm of your hand for 2 to 3 minutes. The heat of your hand will help the adhesive bond to the skin. Failure to perform this step will result in the patch falling off. Fentanyl will not be absorbed properly if the patch is not fully adhered to the skin.
4) Although not required, patches may be secured in place with a transparent adhesive film dressing or first aid tape *around the edges only*; never cover fentanyl patches with any other bandage or tape.[19] If *Bioclusive*® is used, apply the fentanyl patch as described above, then spray around the perimeter and over the patch with medical adhesive spray (eg, *Medical Adhesive*®), place *Bioclusive*® over the site, and press it down firmly. Be sure to clip an area large enough so *Bioclusive*® can adhere to the patch and the skin. If *Bioclusive*® only adheres to the patch and fur without good adherence to the skin, the patch tends to peel up and dislodge.
5) Using a permanent marker, label the patch with the patch size (eg, 12, 25, 50, 75, 100 µg/hour) and the date and time the patch was placed. Patches have been shown to release effective fentanyl levels for up to 5 days in cats, 3 days in dogs, and 2 days in horses. Patches can potentially be left on longer, especially in dogs.
6) The person applying or removing the patch must thoroughly wash their hands with soap and water to remove any drug residue. Surgical gloves may be worn to place or remove patches, as skin contact does occur when handling the adhesive edges.
7) Dispose of used patches by flushing them down the toilet if drug take-back programs are not available.

Monitoring

- Analgesic efficacy
- Heart rate and respiratory rate
- CNS effects (eg, sedation, dysphoria, excitement)
- Security of patch placement

Client Information

Explain carefully to owners how to apply (if applicable), remove, and dispose of patches. Consider making application, removal, and disposal an outpatient procedure, thereby bypassing owner concerns.

- This drug is a narcotic pain reliever in the form of a topical patch. It may take several hours after application before the drug starts working. Pain relief may be provided for 3 to 5 days in dogs and cats.
- Fentanyl is a C-II controlled drug and requires a new written prescription for refills. Use of this medication in animals or humans other than those for whom they are prescribed is illegal.
- This drug is usually tolerated well by animals. High doses can cause sedation, dysphoria (eg, howling, whining), slowed heart rate, constipation, and slow breathing. Contact your veterinarian if you feel your animal is too sedated or if you notice skin irritation or redness in the area of the patch application.
- Increased body temperature (eg, fever, overheating, warm compresses) may cause your pet to receive too much of this medicine at one time and increase the risk for side effects and toxicity. Use caution with warming blankets, increased exercise, and exposure to hot surrounding temperatures.
- Patches (new, on the animal, or used) must be kept away from children; use cautiously in households in which young children or animals could remove, ingest, or be exposed to patches. If human skin comes into contact with the patch, wash the area with water only (do not use soap).
- Dispose of the patch using a drug take-back program (preferred) or by flushing the patch down the toilet if a take-back program is not available.

Chemistry/Synonyms

Fentanyl citrate, a very potent opioid agonist, occurs as a white crystalline powder. It is sparingly soluble in water and soluble in alcohol. It is odorless and tasteless (not recommended for taste test because of extreme potency) with a pK_a of 8.3 and a melting point between 147°C to 152°C (296.6°F-305.6°F).

Fentanyl and fentanyl citrate may also be known as fentanylum, fentanyli citras, McN-JR-4263-49, phentanyl citrate, R-4263, *Actiq*®, *Fenodid*®, *Fenta-Hameln*®, *Fentabbott*®, *Fentanest*®, *Fentax*®, *Fentora*®, *Haldid*®, *Ionsys*®, *Leptanal*®, *Nafluvent*®, *Sintenyl*®, *Sublimaze*®, *Tanyl*®, or *Trofentyl*®.

Storage/Stability

Fentanyl transdermal patches should be stored at temperatures less than 25°C (77°F) and applied immediately after being removed from the individually sealed package. Do not freeze. Do not cut patches without first verifying the patch matrix.

Fentanyl is a schedule 2 (C-II) controlled substance that should be stored in an area that is substantially constructed and securely locked. Follow applicable local, state, and federal rules regarding disposal of unused or wasted controlled drugs.

Compatibility/Compounding Considerations

Most modern transdermal fentanyl patches can be cut, but it is advised to obtain the opinion of a pharmacist before doing so.

Dosage Forms/Regulatory Status

VETERINARY-LABELED PRODUCTS: NONE

The Association of Racing Commissioners International (ARCI) has designated this drug as a class 1 substance. See the ***Appendix*** for more information. Use of this drug may not be allowed in certain animal competitions. Check rules and regulations before entering in a competition while this medication is being administered. Contact local racing authorities for further guidance.

HUMAN-LABELED PRODUCTS:

Fentanyl Transdermal System (Patch):

Fentanyl delivery rate (µg/hour)	Patch physical size (varies by manufacturer [cm²])	Total fentanyl content (varies by manufacturer [mg])
12.5	3.1-5.4	1.3-1.5
25	6.25-10.7	2.5-3.1
37.5	9.4-16.4	3.8-4.1
50	12.5-21.4	5-6.9
62.5	15.6-26.8	6.4-6.9
75	15.7-32.1	7.5-9.3
87.5	18.8-37.5	8.9-9.7
100	25-42.8	10-12.4

Duragesic®-12, - 25, -50, -75 and *-100*; generic; (Rx, C-II) Patch dimensions and fentanyl content vary by manufacturer.

The following human product is available, but there is currently no information on their clinical usefulness or safety in animals:

Fentanyl Iontophoretic Transdermal System: 40 **µg**/dose fentanyl hydrochloride (equivalent to 44.4 **µg** of fentanyl) delivered over a 10-minute period after each activation of the dose button. Each system contains fentanyl hydrochloride 10.8 mg; *Ionsys®*; (Rx; C-II)

All fentanyl products are schedule II controlled substances. Report dispensing to state monitoring programs where required.

References

For the complete list of references, see **wiley.com/go/budde/plumb**

Ferrous Sulfate

(***fair***-us sul-***fayte***)

Nutritional, Hematinic

Prescriber Highlights

- Oral iron supplement for the treatment of iron deficiency anemia or as an iron supplement
- The most common adverse effect is GI upset.
- Overdoses can be life-threatening.
- A wide variety of products exist, and none are FDA-approved; use caution when choosing a product.

Uses/Indications

Ferrous sulfate can be used to treat iron deficiency anemia in dogs due to chronic blood loss, as iron is a necessary trace element in all hemoglobin-utilizing animals. Additionally, it has been used as adjunctive therapy in dogs or cats when receiving epoetin (erythropoietin) or darbepoetin therapy.

Pharmacology/Actions

Iron is necessary for the formation of hemoglobin and myoglobin and for the transport and utilization of oxygen. If an iron deficiency exists, iron administration will correct physical signs of iron deficiency and will correct decreased hemoglobin concentrations secondary to iron deficiency. Iron will not stimulate erythropoiesis or correct hemoglobin abnormalities that are not caused by iron deficiency.

Ferrous sulfate is one of many available iron salts. Ferrous sulfate contains 20% elemental iron by weight (325 mg ferrous sulfate = 65 mg elemental iron).

Pharmacokinetics

Oral absorption of iron salts is complex and determined by a variety of factors, including diet, iron stores present, degree of erythropoiesis, and dose. Iron is thought to be absorbed throughout the GI tract but is primarily absorbed in the duodenum and proximal jejunum. Food in the GI tract may reduce the amount absorbed but can help manage GI upset.

After absorption, the ferrous iron is immediately bound to transferrin, transported to the bone marrow, and eventually incorporated into hemoglobin. Iron metabolism occurs in a nearly closed system. Because iron liberated by the destruction of hemoglobin is reused by the body and only small amounts are lost by the body via hair and nail growth, normal skin desquamation, and GI tract sloughing, normal dietary intake usually is sufficient to maintain iron homeostasis.

Contraindications/Precautions/Warnings

Ferrous sulfate and other oral iron products are considered contraindicated in patients with known hypersensitivity to any component of the product and should be used with caution in patients with hemosiderosis, hemochromatosis, or hemolytic anemia. Due to its GI-irritating properties, oral iron products are not used by some clinicians in patients with GI ulcerative diseases.

No FDA-approved products exist; use caution when choosing a product. Some preparations contain alcohol and propylene glycol.

Adverse Effects

Adverse effects are usually limited to mild GI upset, including discomfort, constipation, nausea, and diarrhea. Division of the daily dose or administration with food may reduce this effect, but dose reduction may be necessary for some animals.

Reproductive/Nursing Safety

Iron requirements increase during pregnancy, and oral iron supplements may be used to correct iron deficiency in pregnant females.

Breast milk naturally contains iron, but the level does not appear to correspond with maternal iron status. In women, ferrous sulfate is considered compatible with breastfeeding.[1]

Overdose/Acute Toxicity

Ingestion of iron-containing products may result in serious toxicity, and acute intoxication should be considered an emergency. As little as 400 mg of elemental iron is potentially fatal in a child, and the reported LD_{50} of ferrous sulfate in dogs following IV administration was 79 mg/kg.[2] Initial clinical signs of acute iron poisoning usually present with an acute onset of GI irritation and distress (vomiting—possibly hemorrhagic, abdominal pain, diarrhea). The onset of these effects may be seen within 30 minutes of ingestion but can be delayed several hours. Peripheral vascular collapse may rapidly follow with clinical signs of depression, weak and/or rapid pulse, hypotension, cyanosis, ataxia, and coma possible. Some patients do not exhibit this phase of toxicity and may be subclinical for 12 to 48 hours after ingestion, when another critical phase may occur. This phase may be exhibited by pulmonary edema, vasomotor collapse, cyanosis, pulmonary edema, fulminant hepatic failure, coma, and death. Animals that survive this phase may exhibit long-term sequelae (including gastric scarring, contraction) and have persistent digestive disturbances.

Because the acute onset of gastroenteritis may be associated with a multitude of causes, diagnosis of iron intoxication may be difficult unless the animal has been observed ingesting the product or physical evidence suggests ingestion. Ferrous sulfate (and gluconate) tablets are radiopaque and often can be observed on abdominal radiographs. Serum iron levels and total iron-binding capacity (TIBC) may also be helpful in determining the diagnosis but must be done on an emergency basis to have any clinical benefit.

Deferoxamine is useful in chelating iron that has been absorbed. See ***Deferoxamine*** for further information.

In addition to chelation therapy, other supportive measures may be necessary, including treatment of acidosis, prophylactic antibiotics, oxygen, treatment for shock, coagulation abnormalities, seizures, and/or hyperthermia. After the acute phases have been resolved, dietary evaluation and management may be required.

For patients that have experienced or are suspected of having experienced an overdose, consultation with a 24-hour poison consultation center specializing in providing veterinary-specific information is recommended. For general information related to overdose and toxin exposures, as well as contact information for poison control centers, refer to ***Appendix***.

Drug Interactions

The following drug interactions have either been reported or are theoretical in humans or animals receiving ferrous sulfate and may be of significance in veterinary patients. Unless otherwise noted, use together is not necessarily contraindicated, but weigh the potential risks and perform additional monitoring when appropriate.

- **ALENDRONATE**: Oral iron may reduce the absorption of oral bisphosphonates; administer at least 2 hours apart.

- **Antacids, Aluminum- or Magnesium- Containing**: May bind and decrease oral iron absorption; administer at least 2 hours apart
- **Calcium Supplements, Antacids**: May bind and decrease oral iron absorption; administer at least 2 hours apart
- **Chloramphenicol**: May delay the response to iron administration; avoid the use of chloramphenicol in patients with iron deficiency anemia
- **Fluoroquinolones** (eg, **enrofloxacin, marbofloxacin**): Iron may reduce the absorption of oral fluoroquinolones; administer 2 to 4 hours apart.
- **H_2-Receptor Antagonists** (eg, **famotidine, ranitidine**): May decrease iron absorption
- **Levothyroxine**: Oral iron may reduce the absorption of levothyroxine; administer at least 4 hours apart.
- **Mycophenolic Acid**: Concurrent use may result in decreased mycophenolate efficacy; separate administration by at least 2 hours.
- **Penicillamine**: Oral iron can decrease the absorption of penicillamine; administer at least 1 hour apart.
- **Proton Pump Inhibitors** (eg, **omeprazole**): May decrease iron absorption
- **Tetracyclines**: Oral iron preparations can bind to orally administered tetracyclines, thereby decreasing the absorption of both compounds.
- **Vitamin C**: May enhance the absorption of iron

Laboratory Considerations

- Large doses of oral iron can color the feces black and cause false positives with the **guaiac test** for occult blood in the feces.

Dosages

CAUTION: Use caution when dosing oral iron products; some authors state dosages in terms of the iron salt (ferrous sulfate), and some state doses in terms of elemental iron. Dosages below are for ferrous sulfate, <u>not</u> elemental iron.

DOGS:

Iron deficiency anemia or patients treated with epoetin or darbepoetin (extra-label): Oral ferrous sulfate may be considered, although injectable iron dextran is more commonly used. Recommended dosages are 11 mg/kg or 100 – 300 mg/dog PO once daily.[3,4] If underlying blood loss is the cause of iron deficiency, it must be corrected before treatment.

CATS:

Iron deficiency anemia or patients treated with epoetin or darbepoetin (extra-label): Oral ferrous sulfate may be considered, although injectable iron dextran is more commonly used, as cats do not tolerate oral iron products well. Usual recommended dosages are 50 – 100 mg/cat PO once daily,[5] but doses range from 30 – 200 mg/cat/day PO.[3] If underlying blood loss is the cause for iron deficiency, it must be corrected before treatment.

Monitoring

- Baseline and periodic CBC, including RBC indices (eg, MCV, MCHC). **NOTE**: RBC indices may take months to normalize.[6]
- Serum iron parameters (eg, ferritin) can be measured to monitor and approximate total body iron concentrations.[6]
- Adverse reactions

Client Information

- This medicine can be given with food to minimize GI upset, but do not give with dairy products, including cheese.
- Side effects can include constipation, diarrhea, vomiting, or nausea. In case of black tarry stools or bloody vomit, contact your veterinarian immediately.
- Keep this medicine out of reach from other animals and children, as accidental overdoses can be very toxic.

Chemistry/Synonyms

Ferrous sulfate, an orally available iron supplement, occurs as odorless, pale-bluish-green crystals or granules having a saline, styptic taste. In dry air, the drug is efflorescent.

If exposed to moisture or moist air, the drug is rapidly oxidized to a brownish-yellow ferric compound that should not be used medicinally. Exposure to light or an alkaline medium will enhance the conversion from the ferrous to the ferric state.

Ferrous sulfate is available commercially in 2 forms: regular and dried. Regular ferrous sulfate contains 7 molecules of water of hydration and is freely soluble in water and insoluble in alcohol. Ferrous sulfate contains ≈200 mg of elemental iron per gram. Dried ferrous sulfate consists primarily of the monohydrate with some tetrahydrate. It is slightly soluble water. Dried ferrous sulfate contains 300 mg of elemental iron per gram. Ferrous sulfate, dried may also be known as ferrous sulfate, exsiccated.

Ferrous sulfate may also be known as eisen(II)-sulfat, ferreux (sulfate), ferrosi sulfas heptahydricus, ferrous sulphate, ferrum sulfuricum oxydulatum, iron (II) sulphate heptahydrate, iron sulphate; many trade names are available.

Storage/Stability

Unless otherwise instructed, store ferrous sulfate preparations in tight, light-resistant containers. Store tablets at 15°C to 30°C (59°F-86°F). Store liquid preparations at 20°C to 25°C (68°F-77°F).

Compatibility/Compounding Considerations

None were noted.

Dosage Forms/Regulatory Status

VETERINARY-LABELED PRODUCTS: NONE

There are many available multivitamin products containing iron.

HUMAN-LABELED PRODUCTS:

There are no ferrous sulfate products regulated by the FDA. To ensure that the product contains the labeled amount of ferrous sulfate and does not contain contaminants, look for third-party verification marks, such as USP or NSF, on the bottle.

Ferrous Sulfate Oral Tablets: several strengths available, most commonly as 325 mg (65 mg elemental iron); *Feosol®*, *FeroSul®*, generic; (OTC)

Ferrous Sulfate Oral Elixir/Liquid: 220 mg/5 mL (44 mg iron/5 mL) and 300 mg/5 mL (60 mg iron/5 mL); generic; (OTC)

Ferrous Sulfate Oral Drops: 15 mg iron/mL and 5 mg iron/20 mL; *Enfamil Fer-In-Sol®*, *Fer-Gen-Sol®*, generic; (OTC)

Many other oral iron salts are available that contain different percentages of elemental iron, such as ferrous fumarate and ferrous gluconate. Exercise caution when choosing iron products.

References

For the complete list of references, see **wiley.com/go/budde/plumb**

Fexofenadine

(fex-oh-***FEN***-ah-deen) *Allegra®*
Antihistamine, Second Generation

Prescriber Highlights

- May be useful in treating or preventing allergy-related conditions
- Limited published data to support use
- Incidence of adverse effects appears minimal, but sedation, CNS depression, and GI effects are possible
- Do not confuse with, or use combination products containing, pseudoephedrine (*Allegra-D®*). Human fexofenadine oral suspension contains xylitol, which is toxic to dogs.

Uses/Indications

Fexofenadine is a second-generation, nonsedating antihistamine. It may be useful in small animal species for controlling clinical signs associated with histamine-mediated conditions, including atopic dermatitis, allergic pruritus, and rhinitis. However, limited scientific evidence exists to support antihistamines for these uses in animals, or the use of any one antihistamine over another. Oral H_1-antihistamines might be of some benefit in dogs with mild signs of atopic dermatitis; however, there is insufficient evidence in favor of or against recommending H_1-antihistamines to treat active or chronic atopic dermatitis in dogs.[1-3] Antihistamines appear to be more effective if given consistently and before dogs become moderately pruritic.[1,4] One small, randomized controlled noninferiority trial suggested consistent benefit from fexofenadine in treated dogs with atopic dermatitis[5,6]; however, this study was likely underpowered.[7]

Pharmacology/Actions

Fexofenadine, a second-generation H_1-antihistamine, is a selective peripheral histamine$_1$-receptor antagonist. Second-generation antihistamines are more lipophobic than first-generation antihistamines (eg, diphenhydramine, chlorpheniramine). Therefore, they do not readily cross into the CNS and do not cause sedation or have substantial anticholinergic effects. Fexofenadine may have other anti-inflammatory effects, including mast cell stabilization, and effects on inflammatory mediators such as leukotrienes and prostaglandins that are associated with allergic responses.

Fexofenadine is an active metabolite of terfenadine, which was withdrawn from the market secondary to concerns that it could prolong QTc intervals in humans. Fexofenadine did not prolong the QTc interval in dogs at plasma concentrations many times higher than those seen after administration of recommended dosages.[8]

Pharmacokinetics

Fexofenadine is a P-glycoprotein substrate drug and theoretically could have altered bioavailability in dogs with deficient P-glycoprotein function (*MDR-1* mutation); however, it is unclear if fexofenadine pharmacokinetics are altered in these dogs. One study found that plasma concentrations of fexofenadine were significantly higher at 4 and 8 hours postdose in *MDR-1* dogs,[9] but the results are in question as dogs also received famotidine (another P-glycoprotein substrate) 1 hour before dosing and additional P-glycoprotein/CYP-3A substrates (quinidine, loperamide) were administered at the same time as fexofenadine.[10]

A pharmacokinetic study in horses[11] showed low oral bioavailability (median = 2.6% alone; 1.5% when ivermectin was given PO 12 hours prior), a volume of distribution (steady-state) of 0.8 L/kg, plasma clearance of 0.75 mL/hour/kg, and a terminal half-life of 5 hours after oral administration. The authors concluded that despite fexofenadine having antihistaminic effects in the horse at low plasma concentrations, extended studies are needed to determine its therapeutic value. Low bioavailability in horses may mean that oral treatment is not suitable.

In humans, fexofenadine is rapidly absorbed following oral administration, with peak concentrations occurring between 2 and 3 hours after dosing.[12] Elimination half-life is ≈14.4 hours when dosed twice daily. Approximately 5% of the total dose is eliminated by hepatic metabolism. The majority of an oral dose is eliminated in the feces, which may be due to low oral absorption or biliary excretion. Dose adjustments are recommended for moderate to severe renal function impairment, as plasma concentrations can increase by 100% or more.

Contraindications/Precautions/Warnings

Do not use fexofenadine in patients hypersensitive to it.

In humans, dosage adjustment is recommended in patients with severe renal impairment.

Adverse Effects

Although there has been limited clinical experience with fexofenadine in veterinary patients, adverse effects are not common. Sedation, CNS depression, and GI effects are possible.

Reproductive/Nursing Safety

No evidence of teratogenicity was seen in rats or rabbits given 300 mg/kg doses; however, dose-related decreases in implantation and an increased incidence of postimplantation losses have been noted in rats,[13] and rats given dosages of 3 times the recommended human dose were associated with decreased pup weights and survival rates. In humans, other second-generation antihistamines have more available information regarding use in pregnant or nursing patients and are therefore preferred over fexofenadine.[14,15]

It is unknown if fexofenadine is excreted into milk, but it is unlikely to pose much risk to nursing offspring. In humans, it is recommended that infants exposed to fexofenadine through nursing be monitored closely for irritability or drowsiness.[14,15]

Because safety has not been established in animals, this drug should only be used when the maternal benefits outweigh the potential risks to offspring.

Overdose/Acute Toxicity

In laboratory studies, dogs receiving oral doses up to 2 g/kg (300 times the maximum recommended adult human oral daily dose) showed no evidence of toxicity. QT intervals were not prolonged in dogs receiving 30 mg/kg PO twice daily for 5 days, despite fexofenadine plasma concentrations being ≈9 times those of humans receiving the maximum recommended dose (180 mg/day).[8]

Clinical signs associated with a fexofenadine overdose may include lethargy, facial edema, and vomiting; CNS depression may also occur. Because fexofenadine may be found in combination with other drugs (eg, pseudoephedrine), it is important to determine what product was actually ingested.

For patients that have experienced or are suspected to have experienced an overdose, consultation with a 24-hour poison consultation center specializing in providing veterinary-specific information is recommended. For general information related to overdose and toxin exposures, as well as contact information for poison control centers, refer to ***Appendix.***

Drug Interactions

The following drug interactions have either been reported or are theoretical in humans or animals receiving fexofenadine and may be of significance in veterinary patients. Unless otherwise noted, use together is not necessarily contraindicated, but weigh the potential risks and perform additional monitoring when appropriate.

- **Antacids Containing Aluminum** or **Magnesium**: Reduced oral bioavailability of fexofenadine; separate dosing by at least one hour

- **Erythromycin, Ketoconazole**: May increase fexofenadine concentrations by enhancing its absorption. This effect is unlikely to be clinically significant due to the wide margin of safety of fexofenadine.
- **Fruit Juices**: In humans, grapefruit, apple, or orange juice may reduce bioavailability; therefore, it is recommended that fexofenadine be taken with water.
- **Ivermectin**: In a small pharmacokinetic study in horses, oral ivermectin decreased the oral bioavailability of fexofenadine.[16]

Laboratory Considerations

- **Allergy testing (intradermal tests)**: Most veterinary dermatologists recommend discontinuing oral antihistamines 1 to 2 weeks prior to intradermal skin tests in dogs or cats; however, one pharmacokinetic/pharmacodynamic study with hydroxyzine and cetirizine in dogs[17] suggests that when tests cannot be delayed, a minimum wait time of 2 days may be acceptable for some drugs in dogs.[7]
- **Allergy testing (IgE serological tests)**: Withdrawal of antihistamines prior to testing is theoretically not necessary, but this has not been proven.[7]

Dosages

DOGS:

Antihistamine for treatment of allergic (histamine-mediated) conditions (extra-label): 2 – 5 mg/kg PO every 12 to 24 hours. Higher doses have been recommended, including one study that used 18 mg/kg PO once daily and reported positive results in dogs with atopic dermatitis.[6] Practically, because of available tablet dosage forms, initial doses should be rounded to the nearest multiple of 15 mg (small dogs) and 30 mg (large dogs). As with other antihistamines, patient response is individualized and unpredictable. When evaluating efficacy for any antihistamine, a minimum trial period of 2 weeks has been recommended.[4] In patients exhibiting benefit, response may be improved when used prior to allergen exposure and on a regular, ongoing basis.

CATS:

Antihistamine for treatment of allergic (histamine-mediated) conditions (extra-label): 10 – 15 mg/cat (NOT mg/kg) PO every 12 to 24 hours. Higher dosages up to 30 mg/cat (NOT mg/kg) PO every 12 hours have been recommended. The oral 30 mg disintegrating tablets may be a useful dosage form for cats as they dissolve rapidly inside the mouth. When splitting tablets of this dosage form, protect remaining tablet from moisture.

Monitoring

- Improvement of clinical signs related to allergies (eg, pruritis, rhinitis)
- Adverse effects (eg, sedation, GI effects)

Client Information

- Antihistamines should be used on a regular, ongoing basis in animals that respond to them. They work better if they are given to your animal before exposure to an allergen or allergy flare.
- This medicine may take several days to 2 weeks to determine if it is effective.
- Fexofenadine may be given with or without food. If your animal vomits or acts sick after getting it on an empty stomach, give with food or small treat to see if this helps. If vomiting continues, contact your veterinarian.
- This medicine is less likely to cause drowsiness (sleepiness) than some other antihistamines, but it can still occur.
- Use caution with over-the-counter formulations of this medicine, as other potentially toxic ingredients may be combined in the products (eg, decongestants, such as pseudoephedrine or acetaminophen). Be sure the product used only contains fexofenadine as the active ingredient. Liquid formulation of this product may contain xylitol, an artificial sweetener, which can be toxic to animals.

Chemistry/Synonyms

Fexofenadine HCl (CAS Registry: 138452-21-8; ATC: R06AX26) occurs as a white to off-white powder. It is slightly soluble in water, freely soluble in ethanol, and very slightly soluble in acetone.

Fexofenadine may also be known as terfenadine carboxylate hydrochloride or MDL-16455A. A common trade name is *Allegra®* or *Telfast®*.

Storage/Stability

Fexofenadine tablets, orally dispersible (disintegrating) tablets, and oral suspension should be stored at room temperature (20°C-25°C [68°F-77°F]).

Orally dispersible tablets should be protected from moisture and are recommended for use immediately after opening individual tablet blisters.

Compatibility/Compounding Considerations

No specific information noted

Dosage Forms/Regulatory Status

VETERINARY-LABELED PRODUCTS: NONE

The Association of Racing Commissioners International (ARCI) has designated this drug as a class 4 substance. See the ***Appendix*** for more information.

HUMAN-LABELED PRODUCTS:

Oral Tablets: 60 mg and 180 mg; *Allegra Allergy®*, generic; (OTC)

Oral Disintegrating Tablets (ODT): 30 mg; *Allegra Allergy Children's®*; (OTC). **NOTE**: The orally disintegrating tablet is designed to disintegrate on the tongue and may be of use in animals difficult to pill.

Oral Gelcaps (Gel Coated Tablets): 180 mg; *Allegra Allergy®*, generic; (OTC)

Oral Suspension: 30 mg/5 mL (6 mg/mL); *Allegra Allergy Children's®*; (OTC). **CAUTION**: Oral suspensions contain xylitol; do not use in dogs.

There are also fexofenadine/pseudoephedrine combination products available (eg, *Allegra D®*), but they are **NOT** recommended for use in animal patients.

References

For the complete list of references, see **wiley.com/go/budde/plumb**

Filgrastim (Granulocyte Colony Stimulating Factor; GCSF)

(fill-***grass***-stim) *Neupogen®*

Cytokine Hematopoietic Agent

Prescriber Highlights

- ▶ Cytokine that, in the bone marrow, primarily increases the proliferation, differentiation, and activation of progenitor cells in the neutrophil-granulocyte line
- ▶ Human origin product; antibodies may form that can cause prolonged neutropenia
- ▶ Biosimilar products are available, but are not considered interchangeable by the FDA; intended product must be specified on the prescription

Uses/Indications

Filgrastim may be of benefit in managing neutropenic complications (eg, infections) in dogs, cats, horses, and alpacas. It should only be used when the intrinsic response to endogenously produced cytokines is thought to be inadequate and when there is evidence that granulocyte precursors are available in the bone marrow. The use of filgrastim in veterinary medicine is controversial because of the drug's cost, potential for antibody development, and the lack of evidence for its efficacy in reducing mortality versus using antibiotic therapy alone.

Pharmacology/Actions

Filgrastim is a hematopoietic agent that primarily affects bone marrow to increase the proliferation, differentiation, and activation of progenitor cells in the neutrophil-granulocyte line. Filgrastim increases neutrophil precursor cells, neutrophil production rate, and shortens maturation time. A dose-dependent increase in neutrophil counts is observed within a few hours of filgrastim administration and persists for the duration of filgrastim exposure. Chemotherapy-induced neutropenia is shortened in duration and severity.[1] Although derived from human DNA, the product is not species-specific for its bone marrow effects.

Pharmacokinetics

After subcutaneous injection, filgrastim is rapidly absorbed and distributed with highest concentrations found in the bone marrow, liver, kidneys, and adrenal glands. The elimination half-life is ≈3.5 hours in humans. Filgrastim undergoes non-hepatic metabolism and renal elimination.

Contraindications/Precautions/Warnings

Filgrastim is contraindicated in patients hypersensitive to it. Animals that have developed antibodies to filgrastim with resultant neutropenia, or animals that experienced severe allergic reactions to filgrastim should probably not receive it in the future. Filgrastim may support or accelerate acute leukemia and myelodysplastic syndromes, and its use in these patients is considered controversial.

Filgrastim should not be given in the 24 hours before or after chemotherapy administration.

Do not confuse filgrastim with pegfilgrastim, tbo-filgrastim, or sargramostim. Biosimilar filgrastim products have not been determined to be interchangeable.

Adverse Effects

Because the human DNA origin product can be immunogenic to other species, some patients may develop severe neutropenia by mounting an immune response against both endogenously produced and exogenously administered G-CSF. Studies in cats have demonstrated that short pulse doses of filgrastim for 3 to 5 days, during the time of neutropenia, may be safe and may minimize development of neutrophil neutralizing antibodies. Preliminary studies using canine origin G-CSF have not demonstrated autoantibody formation in either dogs or cats.

Additionally, there are concerns that exogenously administered filgrastim can cause undesirable responses in other tissues, including myelofibrosis and medullary histiocytosis.

Occasionally, irritation at the injection site may occur. Bone or musculoskeletal pain, splenomegaly (including splenic rupture), glomerulonephritis, capillary leak syndrome, and hypotension have been reported in humans.

Reproductive/Nursing Safety

Adverse effects in females and offspring have been demonstrated after filgrastim was administered to pregnant laboratory animals at high doses. Interpretation of this data for use in a clinical setting is difficult, but filgrastim should only be used in pregnant females when the benefits of treating outweigh the potential risks.

Filgrastim is excreted in milk, but as the drug is not absorbed orally it is unlikely to pose significant risk to nursing offspring.

Because safety has not been established in animals, this drug should only be used when the maternal benefits outweigh the potential risks to offspring.

Overdose/Acute Toxicity

Limited information is available. Filgrastim has limited acute toxic potential and clinically significant overdoses are unlikely.

For patients that have experienced or are suspected to have experienced an overdose, consultation with a 24-hour poison consultation center specializing in providing veterinary-specific information is recommended. For general information related to overdose and toxin exposures, as well as contact information for poison control centers, refer to ***Appendix.***

Drug Interactions

The following drug interactions have either been reported or are theoretical in humans or animals receiving filgrastim and may be of significance in veterinary patients. Unless otherwise noted, use together is not necessarily contraindicated, but weigh the potential risks and perform additional monitoring when appropriate.

- **Antineoplastic Agents**: Although filgrastim was developed primarily to prevent neutropenia associated with some chemotherapeutic agents, avoid filgrastim use within 24 hours before or after antineoplastic drugs.[1]
- **Bleomycin**: Concurrent use may increase the risk for pulmonary toxicity.
- **Cyclophosphamide**: Concurrent use may increase the risk for pulmonary toxicity.
- **Vincristine**: Concurrent use may increase the risk for peripheral neuropathy.

Laboratory Considerations

- Positive **bone imaging** changes have been noted due to increased hematopoietic activity.

Dosages

NOTE: To avoid the development of autoantibody formation, most clinicians that prescribe this agent in dogs or cats recommend a pulse therapy of no more than 5 days in duration.

DOGS/CATS:

Adjunctive treatment of neutropenia (extra-label): No consensus or evidence was located on any dosing strategy for this agent in animals. Most commonly, a dosage of 5 – 10 µg/kg SC daily is recommended.[2]

HORSES:

Neutropenia in foals (extra-label): From a retrospective study (abstract) of 13 foals dosed with filgrastim 5 µg/kg SC, 8 were discharged and 5 died or were euthanized. From the data, the authors concluded that the use of filgrastim in foals was safe; adverse effects were not observed. Leukopenic foals treated with filgrastim that survived to discharge tended to have higher mean WBC counts, higher percentages of neutrophils, and lower percentages of band neutrophils than the foals that did not survive.[3]

Adjunctive treatment for the prevention of shipping fever in yearlings (extra-label): 0.23 µg/kg SC given once prior to transportation sustained neutrophil counts within the reference range for 48 hours during long-distance transportation; however, no cases of shipping fever developed in either treatment or control groups.[4]

CAMELIDS:

Adjunctive treatment of neutropenia in alpaca (extra-label): 5 µg/kg SC daily for 3 days given to healthy alpacas increased neutrophil counts within 24 hours of the first dose and returned to pretreatment values 72 hours after the last dose.[5]

Monitoring

- Baseline and periodic CBC with platelets as indicated by clinical condition

Client Information

- Clients should be informed of the cost of filgrastim as well as the possibility that it may cause antibodies to form against endogenously produced G-CSF, thereby causing a potentially life-threatening neutropenia.

Chemistry/Synonyms

Prepared via recombinant DNA technology from human DNA, filgrastim is a single chain polypeptide consisting of G-CSF plus a N-terminal methionine. Its 175 amino acids are not glycosylated, and it has a molecular weight of ≈18,800 daltons. The commercially available injection occurs as a clear solution buffered to a pH of ≈4. Filgrastim 10 µg is equivalent to 1 million units.

Filgrastim may also be known as: granulocyte colony-stimulating factor, G-CSF, XM-02; *Filgen*®, *Gran*®, *Granulen*®, *Granulokine*®, *Neupogen*®, *Nivestym*® (filgrastim-aafi), *Releuko*® (filgrastim-ayow), *Neutromax*®, and *Zarxio*® (filgrastim-sndz).

Storage/Stability

Filgrastim injection should be stored in the refrigerator (2°C-8°C [36°F-46°F]), and at room temperature for up to 24 hours. Do not freeze or shake contents of vial; protect from light.

Compatibility/Compounding Considerations

If necessary, filgrastim may be diluted into 5% dextrose for injection, but if diluted to concentrations between 5 and 15 µg/mL, it is recommended that albumin be added to the solution to a concentration of 2 mg/mL to reduce adsorption to plastic IV tubing. It is not recommended to dilute to concentrations of less than 5 µg/mL. Filgrastim should never be diluted with saline as a precipitate may form.

Dosage Forms/Regulatory Status

VETERINARY-LABELED PRODUCTS: NONE

HUMAN-LABELED PRODUCTS:

Filgrastim Injection: 300 µg/mL preservative free in 1 mL and 1.6 mL single dose vials; 300 µg/0.5 mL preservative free in 0.5 mL and 0.8 mL prefilled syringes; *Neupogen*®; biosimilar;(Rx). FDA-approved biosimilar products are available but not considered interchangeable. Please refer to the FDA's Purple Book for more information about FDA-licensed biologics, including biosimilar and interchangeable products.

References

For the complete list of references, see **wiley.com/go/budde/plumb**

Finasteride

(fi-***nass***-ter-ide) *Proscar*®, *Propecia*®

5-Alpha-Reductase Inhibitor

Prescriber Highlights

- Potentially useful for dogs with benign prostatic hypertrophy and in ferrets with adrenal disease
- Can be used in breeding males without requiring castration and without affecting libido or spermatogenesis
- Contraindications include hypersensitivity to finasteride, sexually developing animals, and sexually mature females.
- Use with caution in patients with significant hepatic impairment
- Adverse effects include GI and possible minor sexual adverse effects.

Uses/Indications

Finasteride may be useful in treating benign prostatic hypertrophy in canine patients, particularly those used for breeding, as it allows successful treatment without castration and does not affect libido or spermatogenesis.[1] Because of the long duration of therapy required for response (up to 8 weeks), its usefulness may be limited in veterinary medicine.[2,3]

It may also be useful in the adjunctive treatment of adrenal disease in ferrets.[4]

Pharmacology/Actions

Finasteride competitively inhibits 5-alpha-reductase, the enzyme responsible for metabolizing testosterone to dihydrotestosterone (DHT) in the prostate, liver, and skin. DHT is a potent androgen and the primary hormone responsible for the development of the prostate. In dogs with BPH, clinical effects may be noted in as little as one week, but full efficacy may require up to 8 weeks of treatment.

Pharmacokinetics

In humans, finasteride exhibits 65% bioavailability following oral administration, reaches peak plasma concentration in 1 to 2 hours, and is approximately 90% protein bound. The presence of food does not affect absorption. It is distributed across the blood-brain barrier and is found in seminal fluid. Finasteride is extensively metabolized in the liver. Elimination half-life is 5 to 6 hours, and its metabolites are excreted in the urine and feces. In humans, a single daily dose suppresses DHT concentrations for 24 hours.

Contraindications/Precautions/Warnings

Finasteride is contraindicated in sexually developing animals, sexually mature females, and in patients with a history of hypersensitivity to the drug. It should be used with caution in patients with significant hepatic impairment as metabolism of the drug may be reduced.

Finasteride-induced reduction in prostate size is maintained only while the drug is being administered; prostate volume can be expected to increase after finasteride is discontinued.[5]

The National Institute for Occupational Safety and Health (NIOSH) classifies finasteride as a hazardous drug. Personal protective equipment (PPE) should be used accordingly to minimize the risk for exposure. Cutting, crushing or otherwise manipulating tablets will increase risk of exposure.[2] Because finasteride can be absorbed through the skin, women should avoid contact with crushed or broken tablets.[6]

Adverse Effects

One study in dogs reported no adverse effects after treating for 21 weeks at 1 mg/kg.[5] Finasteride may reduce semen volume while maintaining semen quality in breeding dogs.[1,5] Reduced clinical benefit is seen one week after therapy discontinuation.

Adverse effects reported in humans have been very limited, mild, and transient; decreased libido, decreased ejaculate volume, and impotence have been reported.

Reproductive/Nursing Safety

Finasteride is not indicated for use in female patients, and it is unknown whether finasteride is excreted in milk. Breeding males retain fertility while taking finasteride, but ejaculate volume may be decreased.[5]

Overdose/Acute Toxicity

The reported LD_{50} in dogs following oral administration is greater than 1 g/kg and resulted in GI effects including nausea or vomiting. Recommended treatment is supportive as there is no known antidote and it is unlikely to be removed via dialysis.

For patients that have experienced or are suspected to have experienced an overdose, consultation with a 24-hour poison control center specializing in providing veterinary-specific information is recommended. For general information related to overdose and toxin exposures, as well as contact information for poison control centers, refer to ***Appendix***.

Drug Interactions

The following drug interactions either have been reported or are theoretical in humans or animals receiving finasteride and may be of significance in veterinary patients. Unless otherwise noted, use together is not necessarily contraindicated, but weigh the potential risks and perform additional monitoring when appropriate.

- **Anticholinergic Drugs**: May precipitate or aggravate urinary retention.

Dosages

DOGS:

Benign prostatic hypertrophy (BPH) (extra-label): Finasteride 0.1 – 0.5 mg/kg PO once daily has shown benefit.[1,7] Because of commercially available dosage forms, dosages are often rounded to the nearest full or half tablet; 5 mg is generally the maximum dose. Anecdotally, dose frequency may be able to be decreased to every other day after 3 to 4 months of therapy. Because finasteride's effects on prostate size are reversible, treatment is often continued for the life of the dog. To increase ejaculate volume, intact males used for breeding purposes should have finasteride discontinued several days in advance of breeding; the drug is resumed afterward.

FERRETS:

Adjunctive treatment of adrenal disease (extra-label): 5 mg/ferret (NOT mg/kg) PO once daily[4]

Monitoring

- Prostate examination in dogs and monitor for relief from clinical signs (eg, improved urine and fecal elimination)
- Prostatic ultrasound before starting therapy to obtain baseline measurements of the prostate; recheck prostatic ultrasound 6 to 8 weeks after starting therapy to monitor for decrease in prostate size.

Laboratory Considerations

- None

Client Information

- This medicine may be given with or without food. If your animal vomits or acts sick after receiving finasteride on an empty stomach, give it with food or small treats. If vomiting continues, contact your veterinarian.
- This medicine may take several weeks to determine if it is working. Do not skip doses.
- Pregnant or women of childbearing potential should use caution when handling this medication. This medicine is considered to be a hazardous drug as defined by the National Institute for Occupational Safety and Health (NIOSH). Talk with your veterinarian or pharmacist about the use of personal protective equipment when handling this medicine.

Chemistry/Synonyms

Finasteride is a 4-azasteroid synthetic drug that inhibits 5-alpha-dihydroreductase (DH) and has a molecular weight of 372.55.

Finasteride may also be known as: finasteridum, MK-0906, and MK-906; many trade names are available.

Storage/Stability

Store tablets below 30°C (86°F) in tight containers and protected from light.

Compatibility/Compounding Considerations

No specific information noted.

Dosage Forms/Regulatory Status

VETERINARY-LABELED PRODUCTS: NONE

HUMAN-LABELED PRODUCTS:

Finasteride Oral Tablets: 1 mg and 5 mg; *Proscar®*, *Propecia®*, generic; (Rx)

References

For the complete list of references, see **wiley.com/go/budde/plumb**

Firocoxib

(feer-oh-***koks***-ib) *Previcox®, Equioxx®*

Nonsteroidal Anti-Inflammatory Drug (NSAID), COX-2 Selective

Prescriber Highlights

- ► FDA-approved for use in dogs and horses for the control of pain and inflammation associated with osteoarthritis and in dogs for the control of pain and inflammation following orthopedic and soft-tissue surgery
- ► GI effects (eg, vomiting, anorexia) are the most likely adverse effects in dogs; renal and hepatic adverse effects are also possible.
- ► Adverse effects in horses include mouth ulcers, facial skin lesions, and excitation (rare).
- ► Appears to cause predominantly COX-2 inhibition at therapeutic doses
- ► Extra-label use in cats is not recommended, as the large tablet size makes safe administration difficult.

Uses/Indications

Firocoxib is indicated in dogs and horses for the control of pain and inflammation associated with osteoarthritis and in dogs for the control of postoperative pain and inflammation associated with orthopedic surgery. Like other NSAIDs, firocoxib can be useful for treatment of pyrexia, pain, and/or inflammation associated with other conditions.

In dogs with transitional cell carcinoma, firocoxib had antitumor effects and significantly enhanced the antitumor activity of cisplatin. Firocoxib could potentially be useful as a palliative treatment.[1]

Firocoxib may also be useful in other species, but information is limited regarding its safety and efficacy. One study[2] in cats evaluated firocoxib in treatment of experimentally induced pyrexia and demonstrated that the a single oral dose was effective in preventing or attenuating pyrexia. The drug also controlled postoperative pain in cats undergoing ovariohysterectomy.[3]

Pharmacology/Actions

Firocoxib is a coxib-class NSAID. It is believed to predominantly inhibit cyclooxygenase-2 (COX-2) and spare COX-1 at therapeutic dosages. This effect would theoretically inhibit production of the prostaglandins that contribute to pain and inflammation (COX-2) and spare those that maintain normal GI, platelet, and renal function (COX-1).[4,5] However, COX-1 and COX-2 inhibition studies are done in vitro and do not necessarily correlate perfectly with clinical effects seen in vivo.

Pharmacokinetics

In dogs, firocoxib absorption after oral administration varies individually. Oral bioavailability with the chewable tablets is ≈38% on average. Food will delay, but not affect the amount absorbed. Peak concentrations occur ≈1 hour after administration if the dog is fasted and 5 hours if the dog is fed. Volume of distribution at steady state is ≈3 L/kg; it is 96% bound to plasma proteins. Biotransformation occurs predominantly via dealkylation and glucuronidation in the liver; elimination is principally in the bile and feces. Elimination half-life in dogs is ≈6 to 8 hours.

In horses, oral availability after receiving the paste is ≈79%. The equine chewable tablet provides a similar peak concentration and AUC as the paste formulation. Peak concentrations occur 4 to 12 hours after administration. Volume of distribution at steady state is ≈1.7 to 2.3 L/kg and it is 98% bound to plasma proteins. Biotransformation in horses occurs primarily via decyclopropylmethylation and then glucuronidation. Metabolites are primarily excreted in the urine. Elimination half-life is ≈30 to 40 hours. In neonatal foals, firocoxib 0.1 mg/kg PO every 24 hours for 9 consecutive days was rapidly absorbed and a maximum plasma concentration was reached 30 minutes after the first dose. Estimated terminal elimination half-life was ≈11 hours after the last dose.[6] One study reported significantly lower maximum plasma concentrations in ponies during late pregnancy as compared with early postpartum mares.[7]

Pharmacokinetics of firocoxib have only been reported in 2 cats.[2] Oral bioavailability after administering an oral suspension was ≈60% and the volume of distribution was 2 to 3 L/kg. Elimination half-life averaged ≈10 hours.

Contraindications/Precautions/Warnings

Firocoxib should not be used in animals hypersensitive to it or other NSAIDs. The drug should be used with caution and enhanced monitoring performed in patients with pre-existing renal, hepatic, or cardiovascular dysfunction and in those that are dehydrated, hypovolemic, hypotensive, or on concomitant diuretic therapy. Because many geriatric patients have reduced renal function and firocoxib is often used for treatment of osteoarthritis in these patients, ongoing monitoring for adverse effects is strongly recommended.

Because all NSAIDs can potentially cause GI toxicity, firocoxib is relatively contraindicated in dogs with active GI ulcerative conditions.

A chronic dosing study (ie, 5 mg/kg for 6 months) performed in puppies 10 to 13 weeks of age showed subclinical periportal hepatic fatty changes in half the puppies. Higher doses (ie, 15 – 25 mg/kg, which is 3-5 times the label recommendation) in this age range caused increased rates of hepatic fatty changes; some puppies died or were euthanized due to moribund conditions. The manufacturer package insert states, *Use of this product at doses above the recommended 5 mg/kg in puppies less than 7 months of age has been associated with serious adverse reactions, including death* and … *Due to tablet sizes and scoring, dogs weighing less than 12.5 lb (5.7 kg) cannot be accurately dosed.*[8] The UK label states the drug should not be used in dogs younger than 10 weeks of age.[9]

If changing NSAIDs due to lack of efficacy, consider a washout period between agents.

In horses, the manufacturer's label states that the safety of firocoxib in horses younger than 1 year of age, horses used for breeding, and pregnant or lactating mares has not been established, and treatment should be discontinued if signs such as inappetence, colic, abnormal feces, or lethargy are observed. Firocoxib's long half-life should be considered when switching from firocoxib to another NSAID and may necessitate a longer drug withdrawal for horses that are subject to drug testing (eg, race or performance horses).

Adverse Effects

In pre-approval studies in which 128 dogs were treated, vomiting and decreased appetite/anorexia were the most common adverse effects with an approximate incidence rate of 4% and 2%, respectively. Adverse effects reported postapproval included GI effects (eg, diarrhea, GI ulceration, hematemesis, hematochezia), renal effects (eg, azotemia, proteinuria, urinary incontinence, kidney failure), lethargy/depression, elevated liver enzymes (ALP, ALT) and bilirubin, anemia, tachycardia, pruritus, and dermatitis. It should be noted that the postapproval data reflect voluntary reporting to the FDA and do not reflect actual incidence rates nor is causation necessarily proven. Of note, one study in dogs did not show any changes in platelet aggregation.[10]

In pre-approval studies in horses treated for 14 days, diarrhea and loose stools were seen in ≈2% of horses; excitation was rarely detected (ie, less than 1%). In safety studies, oral lesions/ulcers were seen in some horses after receiving 1 to 5 times the recommended label dose.[11]

In a small study in cats (n = 8), 1 cat experienced vomiting and 2 cats developed reversible azotemia with significant increases in BUN and creatinine.[3]

Reproductive/Nursing Safety

Information on the safety of firocoxib in breeding, pregnant, or lactating dogs and horses is not available. Studies performed in pregnant rabbits given doses approximating those given to dogs demonstrated maternotoxic and fetotoxic effects.

Overdose/Acute Toxicity

Limited information is available for acute overdose in animals. The reported oral LD_{50} for rats is greater than 2 g/kg. Use of gastric decontamination protocols and supportive treatment (eg, IV fluids, oral sucralfate) may be useful.

For patients that have experienced or are suspected to have experienced an overdose, consultation with a 24-hour poison consultation center that specializes in providing veterinary-specific information is recommended. For general information related to overdose and toxin exposures, as well as contact information for poison control centers, refer to ***Appendix***.

Drug Interactions

The following drug interactions have either been reported or are theoretical in humans or animals receiving firocoxib and may be of significance in veterinary patients. Unless otherwise noted, use together is not necessarily contraindicated, but weigh the potential risks and perform additional monitoring when appropriate.

- **ACE Inhibitors** (eg, **benazepril, enalapril**): Some NSAIDs can reduce effects on blood pressure.
- **Aspirin**: May increase the risk for GI toxicity (eg, ulceration, bleeding, vomiting, diarrhea)
- **Corticosteroids** (eg, **dexamethasone, prednis(ol)one**): May increase the risk for GI toxicity (eg, ulceration, bleeding, vomiting, diarrhea)
- **Digoxin**: NSAIDS may increase serum levels.
- **Fluconazole**: Administration has increased plasma levels of celecoxib in humans and could potentially also affect firocoxib levels in dogs.
- **Furosemide**: NSAIDs may reduce the saluretic and diuretic effects.
- **Highly Protein Bound Drugs** (eg, **oral anticoagulants, phenytoin, salicylates, sulfonamides, sulfonylurea antidiabetic agents, valproic acid**): Because firocoxib is highly bound to plasma proteins (greater than 95%), it could theoretically displace other highly bound drugs; a temporary increase in serum levels may occur. These interactions have not been shown to be of clinical concern.
- **Methotrexate**: Serious toxicity has occurred when NSAIDs have been used concomitantly with methotrexate; use together with extreme caution.
- **Nephrotoxic Drugs** (eg, **aminoglycosides, amphotericin B, furosemide**): May enhance the risk for nephrotoxicity development
- **Nonsteroidal Anti-inflammatory Drugs (NSAIDs;** eg, **carprofen, meloxicam, phenylbutazone**): May increase the risk for GI toxicity (eg, ulceration, bleeding, vomiting, diarrhea)

Laboratory Considerations

- No specific laboratory concerns

Dosages

DOGS:

Control of pain and inflammation associated with osteoarthritis and control of postoperative pain and inflammation associated with soft-tissue and orthopedic surgery in dogs (labeled dosage; FDA-approved): 5 mg/kg (2.27 mg/lb) PO once daily as needed for osteoarthritis and for 3 days as needed for postoperative pain and inflammation associated with soft-tissue and orthopedic surgery. Firocoxib tablets may be administered ≈2 hours prior to surgery. Dose should be calculated in half-tablet increments and can be administered with or without food. Use the lowest effective dose for the shortest duration consistent with individual response.[8,12,13]

Adjunctive treatment for transitional cell carcinoma of the urinary bladder (extra-label): Firocoxib 5 mg/kg PO every 24 hours used alone and in combination with cisplatin (60 mg/m^2 IV every 21 days)[1]

Adjunctive treatment for inflammatory colorectal polyps (extra-label): From a case series of miniature dachshunds, firocoxib 5 mg/kg PO once daily with chlorambucil 1.5 – 3.1 mg/m^2 (not mg/kg) PO daily. Median doses were 6.1 mg/kg/day and 1.8 mg/m^2/day respectively.[14]

HORSES:

Control of pain and inflammation associated with osteoarthritis (labeled dosage; FDA-approved):

Oral (Paste): 0.1 mg/kg (0.045 mg/lb) PO with or without food daily for up to 14 days[15]

Oral (Tablets): For horses weighing 364 to 591 kg (800-1300 lb): one 57 mg tablet (total dose; NOT mg/kg) PO once daily for up to 14 days; may be given with or without food[15]

Parenteral: 0.09 mg/kg (0.04 mg/lb) IV once daily for up to 5 days. If further treatment is needed, the oral paste can be used at 0.1 mg/kg PO once daily for an additional 9 days. Overall duration of treatment with injection and oral paste will be dependent on the response observed, but should not exceed 14 days.[15]

Monitoring

- Clinical efficacy
- Adverse effects
- Baseline and periodic physical examination
- Baseline and periodic: CBC, serum chemistry panel with electrolytes, and urinalysis.

Client Information

NOTE: The manufacturer provides a client handout that is recommended to be distributed each time the drug is dispensed.

- For dogs: This medicine is used for pain and inflammation associated with arthritis and surgery. It can be given with or without food, but food may reduce the chances for stomach problems (eg, poor appetite, nausea, vomiting). If your dog vomits or acts sick after receiving this medication on an empty stomach, give with food or small treat to see if this helps. If vomiting continues, contact your veterinarian.
- Most dogs tolerate firocoxib well, but some dogs rarely develop stomach ulcers or serious kidney and liver problems. Stop giving this medicine and contact your veterinarian immediately if your animal has decreased appetite (ie, eating less than normal), persistent vomiting, diarrhea, changes in behavior or activity levels (ie, more or less active than normal), changes in drinking and urinating habits (ie, frequency, amount consumed), or yellowing of gums, skin, or whites of the eyes (ie, jaundice).
- Store chewable tablets well out of reach of animals and children.
- Keep water readily accessible during treatment and avoid dehydration.
- For dogs: Periodic laboratory tests are needed to check for liver and kidney side effects. Do not miss these important follow-up visits.
- For horses, contact your veterinarian if your horse develops ulcers or sores on the tongue or in the mouth, sores on facial skin or lips, diarrhea/loose stools, changes in behavior/activity, changes in feed or water consumption, or yellowing of the whites of the eyes or gums (ie, jaundice).
- Other medicines for pain or inflammation should not be used with this medication without the approval of your veterinarian.
- When using the equine paste, ensure the lock ring is secured to the nearest appropriate 50 lb weight notch.
- Do not increase or alter the dose without approval from your veterinarian.

Chemistry/Synonyms

Firocoxib occurs a white crystalline powder. The commercially available injection occurs as a colorless to pale-yellow solution.

Firocoxib may also be known as 3-(cyclopropylmethoxy)-5,5-dimethyl-4-(4-methylsulfonyl) phenylfuran-2(5H)-on; ML-1,785,713; *Equioxx*®; and *Previcox*®.

Storage/Stability

Commercially available tablets and oral paste should be stored at room temperature (15°C-30°C [59°F-86°F]); brief excursions are permitted up to 40°C (104°F). The injection should be stored at 20°C to 25°C (68°F-77°F), with excursions between 15°C to 30°C (59°F-86°F) permitted.

Compatibility/Compounding Considerations

The injection is a nonaqueous solution and should not be mixed with aqueous solutions. Do not flush through IV lines using aqueous flush solutions.

Dosage Forms/Regulatory Status

VETERINARY-LABELED PRODUCTS:

Firocoxib Chewable Tablets (scored): 57 mg and 227 mg; *Previcox*®; (Rx). FDA-approved for use in dogs; NADA #141-230

Firocoxib Oral Paste: 0.82% w/w (8.2 mg firocoxib per gram of paste) in a 6.93 g oral syringe (total of 56.8 mg of firocoxib per syringe); *Equioxx Oral Paste*®; (Rx). FDA approved for use in horses; NADA #141-253.

Firocoxib Chewable Tablets (scored): 57 mg; *Equioxx*® Tablets; (Rx). FDA-approved for use in horses; NADA #141-458. Not to be used in horses intended for food.

Firocoxib Injection: 20 mg/mL in 25 mL vials; *Equioxx*® Injection; (Rx). FDA-approved for use in horses; NADA #141-313. Do not use in horses intended for human consumption.

The Association of Racing Commissioners International (ARCI) has designated this drug as a class 4 substance. Use of this drug may not be allowed in certain animal competitions. Check rules and regulations before entering in a competition while this medication is being administered. Contact local racing authorities for further guidance. See ***Appendix*** for more information.

HUMAN-LABELED PRODUCTS: NONE

References

For the complete list of references, see **wiley.com/go/budde/plumb**

Florfenicol

(flor-**fen**-i-col) *NuFlor®*
Antibiotic
For topical formulations containing florfenicol, please see ***Corticosteroid/Antimicrobial Preparations.***

Prescriber Highlights

- Broad-spectrum antibiotic FDA-approved for use in cattle, swine, and fish
- Do **NOT** give IV. Not for use in veal calves or cattle of breeding age
- Adverse effects in cattle include anorexia, decreased water consumption, diarrhea, and injection site reactions, which may result in trim loss. IM injection may be painful in small animal species. Florfenicol does not appear to have the same risk for aplastic anemia as chloramphenicol.
- Slaughter withdrawals in cattle depend on route of administration (eg, IM shorter than SC).

Uses/Indications

In cattle, injectable florfenicol is FDA-approved for the treatment and control of bovine respiratory disease (BRD) associated with *Mannheimia haemolytica*, *Pasteurella multocida*, and *Histophilus somni* and for the treatment of bovine interdigital phlegmon (eg, foot rot, acute interdigital necrobacillosis, infectious pododermatitis) associated with *Fusobacterium necrophorum* and *Bacteroides melaninogenicus*.[1]

An oral solution is FDA-approved for the treatment of swine respiratory disease (SRD) associated with *Actinobacillus pleuropneumoniae, Pasteurella multocida, Salmonella choleraesuis,* and *Streptococcus suis*. An injectable solution is also FDA-approved in swine for the same indications with an increased spectrum that also includes *Bordetella bronchiseptica* and *Glaesserella (Haemophilus) parasuis*.

Because florfenicol has activity against a wide range of microorganisms, it may also be useful for extra-label treatment of other infections in cattle (or other species), but specific data are limited.

Anecdotally, the injectable formulation has been used orally in dogs, but efficacy data are lacking and a short half-life after oral absorption may limit clinical use. Dosing regimens are not established in dogs or cats.

The combination product containing florfenicol and flunixin is FDA-approved for SC use in beef and nonlactating dairy cattle (not veal calves) for treatment of BRD associated with *Mannheimia haemolytica, Pasteurella multocida, Histophilus somni, Mycoplasma bovis,* and to control BRD-associated pyrexia.[2]

The World Health Organization (WHO) has designated florfenicol as a Highly Important antimicrobial for human medicine.[3] The Office International des Epizooties (OIE) has designated florfenicol as a Veterinary Critically Important Antimicrobial (VCIA) Agent in avian, bovine, caprine, equine, lagomorph, ovine, and swine species.[4]

Pharmacology/Actions

Like chloramphenicol, florfenicol is a time-dependent, broad-spectrum antibiotic that has activity against many aerobic and anaerobic gram-negative and gram-positive bacteria. Florfenicol acts by binding to the 50S ribosome, thereby inhibiting bacterial protein synthesis. Florfenicol is primarily bacteriostatic but is bactericidal against certain bacteria.

Pharmacokinetics

After IM injection in feeder calves, ≈79% of the dose is bioavailable.[1,5] The drug appears to be well-distributed throughout the body, including therapeutic levels in the CSF. In cattle, the volume of distribution is ≈0.7 L/kg, and only ≈13% is bound to serum proteins. Mean serum half-life is 18 hours, but wide interpatient variation exists. When administered at 40 mg/kg IM, serum concentrations are above the MIC_{90} (1 µg/mL) for *Mannheimia haemolytica* for 72 hours and above the MIC_{90} (0.5 µg/mL) for *Pasteurella multocida* and *Histophilus somni* for 96 hours.

Oral absorption is variable (24% to 97%) after gavage dosing in swine. Volume of distribution is ≈1 L/kg, and half-life is 2.2 hours.[6]

In dogs, florfenicol is absorbed poorly after SC injection and has an elimination half-life of less than 5 hours. After IV administration, total body clearance is ≈1 L/kg/hour. PO administration results in good bioavailability (ie, 95%), but the drug is eliminated rapidly (elimination half-life, 1.25 hours).[7]

Cats have high absorption of a 100 mg/mL solution administered IM or PO and an elimination half-life of less than 5 hours. In cats, time duration above an MIC of 2 mg/mL is 12 hours (IM) and 18 hours (PO); time duration above an MIC of 8 mg/mL is 10 hours (IM) and 6 hours (PO), respectively.

In sheep, florfenicol elimination half-life is ≈9 hours and has a mean residence time of ≈20 hours for its major metabolite (ie, FFC-a). Based on these values, a calculated withdrawal time of 42 days was determined.[8,9]

Contraindications/Precautions/Warnings

Do **NOT** give this drug IV. Florfenicol is contraindicated in animals hypersensitive to it and is not for use in animals intended for breeding. The effects of florfenicol on bovine reproductive performance, pregnancy, and lactation have not been determined. See residue warnings in ***Dosage Forms/Regulatory Status***.

Do not use this drug in female dairy cattle 20 months of age or older or in calves to be processed for veal.

Do not use in nursing piglets and swine of reproductive age intended for breeding.

Florfenicol is not recommended for use in equines, as administration resulted in loose stools and elevated bilirubin regardless of route (PO, IV, or IM).[10]

Florfenicol formulations contain an inactive ingredient that has been shown to cause reproductive and developmental toxicities in laboratory animals following high, repeated exposures; those who are pregnant should wear gloves when handling or avoid handling when possible.[11]

Adverse Effects

Noted transient adverse effects in cattle include anorexia, decreased water consumption, and diarrhea.[1] Injection site reactions after IM administration may persist for longer than 28 days and may result in trim loss. Reactions may be more severe if injected at sites other than the neck. Anaphylaxis and collapse have been reported in cattle.

GI effects, including severe diarrhea, are possible when this drug is used in other mammalian species.

Reproductive/Nursing Safety

Testicular degeneration and atrophy associated with florfenicol use has been observed in dogs, mice, and rats.[1] Safety or adverse effects of using this drug in breeding cattle or swine, during pregnancy, or during lactation are unknown; the manufacturer states florfenicol is not for use in cattle of breeding age or swine intended for breeding.[1,6]

Because safety has not been established in animals, this drug should only be used when the maternal benefits outweigh the potential risks to offspring.

Overdose/Acute Toxicity

In dogs administered florfenicol 30 or 100 mg/kg/day orally over 13 weeks, CNS vacuolation, hematopoietic toxicity, and renal tubule dilation were seen.[12]

In toxicology studies in which feeder calves were injected with up to 10 times the recommended dosage, increased serum liver and muscle enzymes (lactate dehydrogenase [LDH], gamma-glutamyl transferase [GGT], ALT, AST) and anorexia, decreased water consumption, weight loss, and diarrhea were seen—these effects were generally transient in nature.[12] Long-term (ie, 43 days) standard dosage studies showed a transient decrease in feed consumption, but no long-term negative effects were noted.[12]

In swine receiving up to 10 times the recommended dosage, constipation and anal swelling, reduced feed and water intake, decreased body weight, and increased urine specific gravity were noted.[13]

A case report documented severe bone marrow suppression resulting in death in a gazelle that was administered 2 doses that were 10 times higher than intended.[14]

Because of the potential for serious bone marrow toxicity noted in some species, overdoses of oral florfenicol should be handled with gastric decontamination using standard protocols.

For patients that have experienced or are suspected to have experienced an overdose, consultation with a 24-hour poison control center specializing in providing veterinary-specific information is recommended. For general information related to overdose and toxin exposures, as well as contact information for poison control centers, refer to ***Appendix***.

Drug Interactions

No specific drug interactions for florfenicol were located, but florfenicol may behave similarly to chloramphenicol. If so, florfenicol could antagonize the bactericidal activity of **penicillins** or **aminoglycosides**. This antagonism has not been demonstrated in vivo, and these drug combinations have been used successfully many times clinically. Other antibiotics that bind to the 50S ribosomal subunit of susceptible bacteria (eg, **erythromycin, clindamycin, lincomycin, tylosin**) may potentially antagonize the activity of chloramphenicol or vice versa, but the clinical significance of this potential interaction has not been determined. For other drug interactions that florfenicol may share with chloramphenicol, see ***Chloramphenicol***.

In studies done in chickens[15] and rabbits,[16] CYP3A and p-glycoproteins are involved in the pharmacokinetics of florfenicol and may result in drug interactions with substrates, inducers, or inhibitors of CYP3A and p-glycoproteins.

Dosages

CATTLE:

Treatment of bovine respiratory disease (BRD) associated with *Mannheimia haemolytica, Pasteurella multocida*, and *Histophilus somni* or bovine interdigital phlegmon (ie, foot rot) associated with *Fusobacterium necrophorum* and *Bacteroides melaninogenicus* (label dosage; FDA-approved): 20 mg/kg IM (in neck muscle only); repeat after 48 hours.[1] Alternatively, a single 40 mg/kg SC dose (in neck) may be used. **NOTE**: 20 mg/kg equates to 3 mL of the injection per 45.4 kg (100 lb) body weight. Do not exceed 10 mL per injection site.

Control of respiratory disease in cattle at high risk for developing BRD associated with *Mannheimia haemolytica, Pasteurella multocida*, and *Histophilus somni* (label dosage; FDA-approved): 40 mg/kg SC once.[1] Do not administer more than 10 mL at each site. Injection should be given only in the neck.

Florfenicol in combination with flunixin for treatment of bovine respiratory disease (BRD) associated with *Mannheimia haemolytica, Pasteurella multocida*, and *Histophilus somni*, and control of BRD-associated pyrexia in beef and non-lactating dairy cattle (label dosage; FDA-approved): flunixin 2.2 mg/kg with florfenicol 40 mg/kg (6 mL/100 lb where each mL contains flunixin 16.5 mg with florfenicol 300 mg) SC once.[2] Do not administer more than 10 mL at each site. The injection should be administered only in the neck. Injection sites other than the neck have not been evaluated.

Infectious bovine keratoconjunctivitis (**IBK**; extra-label): 20 mg/kg IM in neck, repeated after 48 hours, or 40 mg/kg SC in neck once[17]

SHEEP/GOATS:

Respiratory disease complex in kids (extra-label): 20 mg/kg IM once daily for 2 days[18,19]

SWINE:

Treatment of swine respiratory disease associated with *Actinobacillus pleuropneumoniae, Pasteurella multocida, Salmonella choleraesuis*, and *Streptococcus suis* (label dosage; FDA-approved): In water at a concentration of 400 mg/gallon (100 ppm)[20]; use as only source of drinking water for 5 days.[6] For bulk tank, add 1 gallon of concentrate to 128 gallons of water, with proportioner set to 1:128 (0.8%).

Treatment of swine respiratory disease associated with *Actinobacillus pleuropneumoniae, Pasteurella multocida, Salmonella choleraesuis, Streptococcus suis, Bordetella bronchiseptica*, and *Glaesserella* (*Haemophilus*) *parasuis* (label dosage; FDA-approved): 15 mg/kg IM[11]; administer a second dose 48 hours later

CAMELIDS:

Susceptible pathogens (extra-label): 20 mg/kg IM once daily[18,21]

Monitoring

- Clinical efficacy
- Injection site reactions

Client Information

- Florfenicol is administered by injection into the muscle (intramuscular, IM) or under the skin (subcutaneous, SC). Your veterinarian will instruct which route is appropriate to use for your animal(s). Do NOT inject into the vein (IV).
- Injections into the muscle may result in local tissue reaction that persists beyond 28 days; this may result in trim loss at slaughter. Tissue reaction at injection sites other than the neck is likely to be more severe.
- US residue warnings: When florfenicol is administered as labeled, slaughter withdrawal in cattle is 28 days postinjection if injecting into the muscle (IM), and 38 days postinjection if injecting under the skin (SC); and slaughter withdrawal in swine (in drinking water) is 16 days.
- This medicine should not be used in female dairy cattle 20 months of age or older
- A withdrawal period has not been established for this medicine in preruminating calves. Do not use this medicine in calves to be processed for veal.
- Those who are pregnant should wear gloves when handling this medicine or avoid handling when possible.

Chemistry/Synonyms

Florfenicol, a fluorinated analogue of thiamphenicol, is commercially available as a light-yellow to straw-colored injectable solution that also contains n-ethyl-2-pyrolidone, propylene glycol, and polyethylene glycol. The commercially available products range from a bright yellow to straw color. Color does not affect potency.

Florfenicol may also be known as Sch-25298, *Aquaflor*®, *Florcon*®, *Florvio*®, *Longcor*®, *Norfenicol*®, *NuFlor*®, and *NuFlor-S*®.

Storage/Stability

Florfenicol injection storage requirements vary by manufacturer, but vials generally should be stored between 2°C to 30°C (36°F-86°F). Discard dates after first use range from 30 days to 6 months, and some products list a maximum number of times the vial may be punctured. Refer to individual product label for specific information.

The oral solution (swine) should be stored between 2°C to 26°C (36°F-77°F).

The combination product with flunixin should not be stored above 30°C (86°F) and should be used within 28 days. The 500 mL vial should not be punctured more than 20 times.

Compatibility/Compounding Considerations

No specific information has been noted.

Dosage Forms/Regulatory Status

VETERINARY-LABELED PRODUCTS:

Florfenicol Injection: 300 mg/mL in 100 mL, 250 mL, and 500 mL multi-dose vials; *NuFlor®*; (Rx). FDA-approved for use in cattle. Slaughter withdrawal (at label dosages) is 28 days (IM) and 38 days (SC). Do not use in female dairy cattle 20 months of age or older. A withdrawal period has not been established in preruminating calves. Do not use in calves to be processed for veal.

Florfenicol Injection: 300 mg/mL in multi-dose vials; *NuFlor®-S*; (Rx). FDA-approved for swine. Slaughter withdrawal (at label dosages) is 11 days (IM). Do not use in nursing piglets and swine of reproductive age intended for breeding.

Florfenicol Injection: 300 mg/mL (also contains 2-pyrrolidone 300 mg and triacetin qs) in 100 mL, 250 mL, and 500 mL vials; *Nuflor Gold®*; (Rx). FDA-approved for use in beef and nonlactating dairy cattle; NADA #141-265. Do not slaughter within 44 days of last treatment. Do not use in female dairy cattle 20 months of age or older. Use may cause milk residues. A withdrawal period has not been established in preruminating calves. Although this product is listed in the FDA Green Book, its marketing status is uncertain.

Florfenicol 2.3% (23 mg/mL) Concentrate Solution in 2.2 L bottles; *NuFlor® Concentrate Solution, Florcon®, Florvio®*; (Rx). FDA-approved for use in swine. Slaughter withdrawal (at label dosages) is 16 days.

There are florfenicol products for addition to catfish or salmonid feeds (*Aquaflor®*); (VFD) and swine feed additives (*Nuflor® Type A Medicated Article*); (VFD)

Florfenicol 300 mg/mL with Flunixin 16.5 mg/mL Injection in 100 mL, 250 mL, and 500 mL vials; *Resflor Gold®*; (Rx). FDA-approved for use in beef and nonlactating dairy cattle; NADA #141-299. Do not slaughter within 38 days of last treatment. Not for use in female dairy cattle 20 months of age or older or in calves to be processed for veal. Use may cause milk residues. A withdrawal period has not been established in preruminating calves.

For topical formulations containing florfenicol, please see ***Corticosteroid/Antimicrobial Preparations.***

HUMAN-LABELED PRODUCTS: NONE

References

For the complete list of references, see **wiley.com/go/budde/plumb**

Fluconazole

(floo-***kon***-a-zole) *Diflucan®*

Antifungal, Azole

Prescriber Highlights

- ▶ Oral or parenteral antifungal particularly useful for CNS infections. Systemic mycoses may require treatment over several months.
- ▶ Similar efficacy as itraconazole; however, fluconazole does not require an acidic environment for PO absorption. Can be given with or without food
- ▶ Caution is advised in patients with chronic kidney disease, pregnancy, and hepatic failure.
- ▶ Adverse effects include occasional GI effects (eg, inappetence, vomiting, diarrhea) in cats and dogs; increased liver enzyme activity; and, rarely, severe hepatotoxicity.
- ▶ Many drug interactions are possible.
- ▶ The National Institute for Occupational Safety and Health (NIOSH) classifies fluconazole as a hazardous drug; use appropriate precautions when handling.

Uses/Indications

Fluconazole is used in the treatment of systemic mycoses, including cryptococcal meningitis, blastomycosis, histoplasmosis, and coccidioidomycosis. Because of the drug's unique pharmacokinetic qualities, it is likely more useful for treating CNS or urinary tract fungal infections than other azole derivatives. Unlike ketoconazole, fluconazole does not have appreciable effects on steroid hormone synthesis and may have fewer adverse effects in small animal species. Similarly, fluconazole impairs hepatic drug metabolism to a lesser extent than ketoconazole.

A retrospective study in dogs with blastomycosis found there was no significant difference in efficacy between fluconazole and itraconazole,[1] and although treatment with fluconazole was longer than with itraconazole (ie, median of 183 vs 138 days), fluconazole treatment costs were ≈⅓ less than itraconazole. Similarly, another retrospective study found no difference in efficacy between fluconazole and itraconazole in dogs with histoplasmosis.[2]

In dogs, fluconazole is effective for the treatment of *Malassezia* spp dermatitis,[3] but ketoconazole or itraconazole are preferred.[4]

Pharmacology/Actions

Fluconazole is a fungistatic triazole compound that inhibits a fungal CYP450-dependent demethylation enzyme that produces ergosterol in the fungal cell membrane. The resultant intracellular accumulation of methylated sterols weakens the cellular membranes of susceptible fungi, thereby increasing membrane permeability and allowing leakage of cellular contents and impairing uptake of purine and pyrimidine precursors. Fluconazole has efficacy against a variety of pathogenic fungi including yeasts and dermatophytes, although fluconazole's MIC against *Malassezia pachydermatis* is significantly higher than other azole antifungals.[4] In vivo studies using laboratory models have shown that fluconazole has fungistatic activity against some strains of *Candida* spp, *Coccidioides* spp, *Cryptococcus* spp, *Histoplasma* spp, and *Blastomyces* spp. Results from in vivo studies of efficacy against *Aspergillus* spp have been conflicting, and fluconazole is not considered a first-choice agent for these infections. Fluconazole and terbinafine combination treatment may have synergistic antifungal effects against *Candida albicans*.

Fluconazole resistance in *Candida* spp may be caused by overexpression of the target enzyme, reduced target enzyme affinity for fluconazole, or overexpression of efflux pumps.

In addition to its antifungal effects, fluconazole (similarly to other azoles) has been shown to have anti-inflammatory properties by reducing IL-4 production, increasing production of interferon-gamma in *Candida albicans*-infected mice, and inhibiting the production of leukotriene B4 in vitro.[3] Fluconazole also inhibited neurogenic inflammation in mouse models, suggesting an additional antipruritic activity.[3]

Pharmacokinetics

In dogs, fluconazole oral bioavailability was 100%, and peak plasma concentration was reached 4 hours after oral administration. Volume of distribution was 0.7 to 0.8 L/kg, and plasma protein binding was low (11%). Elimination half-life was 13 to 15 hours. Plasma clearance was ≈0.65 mL/kg/minute. Approximately 70% of the fluconazole dose was excreted unchanged in urine.[5]

In cats, fluconazole was completely absorbed, with peak concentration reached 2.6 hours after oral administration. Volume of distribution was 1 L/kg. Mean ratios of fluid:serum fluconazole concentrations were 0.88 and 0.79 for CSF and aqueous humor, respectively, and 1.2 for epithelial lining fluid. Clearance was 0.6 to 0.9 mL/kg/minute and elimination half-life was ≈13 to 25 hours.[6,7]

In horses, fluconazole was completely absorbed after oral administration, with peak concentration reached after 2 hours. Volume of distribution was 1.2 L/kg, and the drug was found in CSF, synovial fluid, and aqueous humor at concentrations 35% to 50% that of plasma; urine concentration was almost twice that of plasma. Clearance was 0.02 L/kg/minute and elimination half-life was ≈38 to 42 hours.[8]

In cockatiels receiving fluconazole orally, peak concentration was reached ≈5 hours after oral administration, and elimination half-life was 19 hours. Pharmacokinetic data were similar when fluconazole was administered in drinking water.[9]

In humans, fluconazole is rapidly and nearly completely absorbed (ie, 90%) after oral administration.[10] Gastric pH or the presence of food does not appreciably alter fluconazole's oral bioavailability. It has low protein binding and is widely distributed throughout the body; however, protein binding may be altered in renal disease states associated with increased alpha-1-acid glycoprotein (AAG) concentrations.[11] The drug readily penetrates into bodily fluids, including into the CSF, eye, and peritoneal fluid. Fluconazole is eliminated primarily via the kidneys as unchanged drug and achieves high concentrations in the urine. Fluconazole's serum half-life is ≈30 hours in patients with normal renal function. Patients with impaired renal function may have significantly extended half-lives and dosage adjustments may be required. Because of its long half-life, fluconazole does not reach steady-state plasma concentrations for 6 to 14 days after beginning therapy, unless loading doses are given. Administration of a loading dose (2 times the labeled daily dose) on the first day of treatment results in plasma concentrations close to steady-state by the second day.[10]

Contraindications/Precautions/Warnings

Fluconazole should not be used in patients that are hypersensitive to it or other azole antifungal agents. As fluconazole may cause hepatotoxicity (rarely, and less than itraconazole or ketoconazole), this drug should only be used in patients with hepatic impairment when the potential benefits outweigh the risks. Because fluconazole is eliminated primarily by the kidneys, dosages may need to be adjusted in patients with renal impairment.

Fluconazole has been associated with prolongation of the QT interval and should be used with caution in patients at increased risk for arrhythmias (eg, structural heart disease, heart failure, electrolyte imbalance). In humans, fluconazole is contraindicated in patients receiving drugs that both prolong the QTc interval and are metabolized by cytochrome P450 3A4; significance in animals is unknown. See ***Drug Interactions***.

Fluconazole is reportedly both ineffective and highly toxic to budgerigars at typical doses.[12]

The National Institute for Occupational Safety and Health (NIOSH) classifies fluconazole as a hazardous drug; personal protective equipment (PPE) should be used accordingly to minimize the risk for exposure.

Do not confuse fluconazole with flecaine, fluoxetine, or furosemide.

Adverse Effects

Fluconazole is well tolerated in the majority of dogs and cats. Inappetence, vomiting, soft stools, and diarrhea have occasionally been reported, but these may be mild and transient and not require cessation of therapy. Other adverse effects reported include focal alopecia, hypoadrenocorticism, ocular discharge, dry skin, and malaise.[14] Hepatotoxicity is possible and ≈15% to 20% of dogs receiving long-term treatment may have increased ALT activity; with continued monitoring of liver enzymes, most dogs were able to complete treatment without dose reduction or discontinuation of therapy.[1,2] There can also be an increase in ALT in cats.[14]

In humans, adverse effects have been generally limited to occasional GI effects (eg, vomiting, diarrhea, anorexia, nausea) and headaches.[10] Increased liver enzymes and hepatotoxicity, adrenal insufficiency, exfoliative skin disorders, and thrombocytopenia have been reported in humans (rarely). Humans receiving fluconazole for 28 days for treatment of coccidioidomycosis experienced adverse effects (eg, dry skin, alopecia, fatigue, and nausea and vomiting), with ≈⅔ requiring therapy changes.[15]

Reproductive/Nursing Safety

Fluconazole did not affect fertility in rats.[10] High-dose fluconazole resulted in congenital abnormalities in laboratory animals and women receiving fluconazole during pregnancy. In humans, it is recommended to avoid use of prolonged or high-dose therapy during pregnancy, except in patients with severe or life-threatening fungal infections in which the benefits to the mother outweigh potential risk to the fetus.[16,17]

Fluconazole is excreted into maternal milk at concentrations similar to plasma. Use with caution in lactating animals; consider milk replacer.

Overdose/Acute Toxicity

There is limited information available on the acute toxicity of fluconazole. Rats and mice survived doses of 1 g/kg but died within several days after receiving 1 – 2 g/kg.[18] Rats and mice receiving higher dosages demonstrated respiratory depression, salivation, lacrimation, urinary incontinence, and cyanosis. If a massive overdose occurs, consider gastric decontamination and give supportive therapy as required. Fluconazole may be removed by hemodialysis or peritoneal dialysis. In humans, a 3-hour hemodialysis decreases fluconazole plasma concentrations by ≈50%.[10]

For patients that have experienced or are suspected to have experienced an overdose, consultation with a 24-hour poison consultation center specializing in providing veterinary-specific information is recommended. For general information related to overdose and toxin exposures, as well as contact information for poison control centers, refer to ***Appendix***.

Drug Interactions

In humans, fluconazole is a potent CYP2C and moderate CYP3A inhibitor. The following drug interactions have either been reported or are theoretical in humans or animals receiving fluconazole and may be of significance in veterinary patients. Unless otherwise noted, use together is not necessarily contraindicated, but weigh the potential risks and perform additional monitoring when appropriate.

- **Amphotericin B**: Laboratory animal studies have shown that fluconazole used concomitantly with amphotericin B may be antagonistic against *Aspergillus* spp or *Candida* spp; the clinical importance of these findings is unclear.

- **Benzodiazepines** (eg, **alprazolam, diazepam, midazolam**): Increased benzodiazepine concentrations and subsequent adverse effects (eg, sedation) are possible. Fluconazole decreased midazolam clearance by 50% in dogs,[19] and prolonged clinical effects (eg, time to standing, heart rate) and recovery times have been noted in horses.[20]
- **Buspirone**: Plasma buspirone concentrations may be elevated.
- **Calcium Channel Blocking Agents** (eg, **amlodipine, diltiazem**): Fluconazole may increase exposure of calcium channel blockers.
- **Cannabidiol**: May increase cannabidiol concentration
- **Cimetidine**: May reduce fluconazole concentrations
- **Cisapride**: In humans, concomitant use is contraindicated, as it may increase cisapride plasma concentration and the risk for QT prolongation; significance in animals is unknown.
- **Colchicine**: Increased colchicine concentrations and adverse effects are possible. Contraindicated in humans with hepatic or renal impairment
- **Corticosteroids** (eg, **dexamethasone, prednis(ol)one**): Fluconazole may inhibit the metabolism of corticosteroids; potential for increased adverse effects
- **Cyclophosphamide**: Fluconazole may inhibit the metabolism of cyclophosphamide and its metabolites; potential for increased toxicity
- **Cyclosporine**: Fluconazole increases cyclosporine concentrations without changing half-life. In healthy dogs, fluconazole 5 mg/kg PO once daily decreased cyclosporine dosages by ≈50% to achieve similar therapeutic trough concentrations.[21,22] In renal transplant dogs (also on mycophenolate), fluconazole decreased cyclosporine dose requirements by 33% on average.[23]
- **Diuretics, Thiazides** (eg, **hydrochlorothiazide**): Increased fluconazole concentrations are possible.
- **Fentanyl/Alfentanil**: Fluconazole may increase fentanyl concentrations.
- **Ketamine**: Fluconazole decreased ketamine clearance by 50% and prolonged clinical effects (eg, time to standing, heart rate) in dogs.[19] Prolonged recovery was noted in horses.[20]
- **Losartan**: Increased losartan effects are possible; increased monitoring of blood pressure is recommended.
- **Macrolide Antibiotics** (eg, **clarithromycin, erythromycin**): Concomitant use may increase the risk for QT prolongation; concurrent therapy is contraindicated in humans. Interaction may not apply to azithromycin.
- **Methadone**: Fluconazole significantly increases methadone exposure in dogs.[24] In humans, concomitant use is contraindicated, as it may also increase the risk for QT prolongation; significance in animals is unknown.
- **Nonsteroidal anti-inflammatory drugs (NSAIDs**; eg, **carprofen, flunixin, meloxicam, phenylbutazone, robenacoxib**): Fluconazole may increase plasma concentrations of some agents; increased risk for adverse effects
- **Quinidine**: May reduce quinidine metabolism, increasing the risk for cardiotoxicity. Concurrent therapy is contraindicated in humans.
- **QT prolonging Agents** (eg **amiodarone, disopyramide, ondansetron, procainamide, sotalol**): Increased risk for arrhythmias
- **Rifampin**: May decrease fluconazole exposure and efficacy; fluconazole may increase rifampin concentrations
- **Sildenafil**: Increased sildenafil exposure
- **Sulfonylurea Antidiabetic Agents** (eg, **glipizide, glyburide**): Fluconazole may increase concentrations; hypoglycemia is possible.
- **Theophylline/Aminophylline**: Increased theophylline concentrations are possible.
- **Tramadol**: In dogs, fluconazole increased tramadol and its M1 metabolite by 31 and 39 times, respectively.[25]
- **Tricyclic Antidepressants** (TCAs; eg, **amitriptyline, clomipramine**): Fluconazole may exacerbate the effects of tricyclic antidepressants.
- **Vincristine/Vinblastine**: Fluconazole may inhibit vinca alkaloid metabolism.
- **Warfarin**: Fluconazole may cause increased prothrombin times in patients receiving warfarin or other coumarin anticoagulants.
- **Zidovudine**: Increased zidovudine concentration and exposure

Laboratory Considerations

None were noted.

Dosages

DOGS:

Systemic mycosis for fluconazole-sensitive organisms (potentially cryptococcosis,[26] blastomycosis,[1] histoplasmosis[2]) (extra-label): 5 – 10 mg/kg PO, IV every 12 to 24 hours. Infections involving the CNS and eyes may require dosages up to 15 mg/kg twice daily. IV doses should be administered over 1 to 2 hours. Treatment may be required for 4 to 8 months and should continue for 2 months after resolution of clinical signs with accompanying decline in antigen titers.

Urinary candidiasis (extra-label): 5 – 10 mg/kg PO every 24 hours for 3 to 5 weeks

***Coccidioides* osteomyelitis** (extra-label): Average initial dosage was 18 mg/kg/day PO; clinical signs improved rapidly, but long-term treatment was required.[27]

Systemic treatment for *Malassezia* dermatitis, dermatophytosis, onychomycosis (extra-label): 2.5 – 5 mg/kg PO every 24 hours. Continue treatment for at least 1 week after complete resolution of clinical signs (for *Malassezia* dermatitis) or until 2 negative skin cultures (taken 2 weeks apart) are obtained (for dermatophytosis and onychomycosis).[28,29] Ketoconazole or itraconazole are preferred.[4]

CATS:

Systemic mycosis for fluconazole-sensitive organisms (potentially cryptococcosis,[30,31] blastomycosis,[32,33] histoplasmosis,[34] coccidioidomycosis[35]) (extra-label): 10 mg/kg PO every 12 hours,[7] practically administered as one 50 mg tablet/cat (NOT mg/kg) PO every 12 hours. Rapidly progressing or severely disseminated infections may require 100 mg/cat (NOT mg/kg) PO every 12 hours. Tablets may be crushed. Treatment is usually required for several months and should continue for 1 to 3 months after resolution of clinical signs or negative antigen test results on serum and CSF.

Anterior uveitis due to cryptococcosis (extra-label): 10 – 15 mg/kg PO every 24 hours, continuing for 2 months after resolution of clinical signs with accompanying decline in antigen titers[26]

Systemic treatment for *Malassezia* dermatitis, dermatophytosis, onychomycosis (extra-label): 5 mg/kg PO every 12 hours. Continue treatment for at least 1 week after complete resolution of signs (for *Malassezia* dermatitis) or until 2 negative skin cultures (taken 2 weeks apart) are obtained (for dermatophytosis and onychomycosis).[36] Itraconazole is preferred.[4]

HORSES:

Susceptible fungal infections (extra-label): Loading dose of 14 mg/kg PO followed by 5 mg/kg PO once daily.[8] This dosage is supported by several case reports for a variety of topical[37-39] and systemic[40-42] fungal infections.

Cutaneous pythiosis: 10 mg/kg PO once as a loading dose followed by 5 mg/kg PO once daily[43]

***Coccidioides immitis* infection or *Candida* spp bacteremia** (extra-label): Loading dose of 14 mg/kg PO followed by 5 mg/kg PO once daily. There have been anecdotal reports of successful treatment of fungal keratitis using fluconazole 1 mg/kg PO every 24 hours.[44]

Infectious endometritis caused by susceptible fungal organisms of *Candida* spp (extra-label): Based on plasma and endometrial tissue concentrations, giving a 14 mg/kg PO loading dose and a maintenance dose of 5 mg/kg PO every 24 hours will result in endometrial tissue concentrations near the accepted MIC values for most *Candida* spp and surpass the MIC for *Candida albicans* in the reproductive tract of mares.[45]

BIRDS:

Candidiasis (extra-label): Fluconazole pharmacokinetics were determined in Goffin's cockatoos. Timneh African grey parrots and orange-winged Amazon parrots showed fluconazole 20 mg/kg PO every 24 to 48 hours or 10 mg/kg PO every 24 hours would likely be effective for treatment of *C albicans*.[46,47] This dose may be too low for treatment of *Candida glabrata* and *Candida parapsilosis*.

Candidiasis in cockatiels (extra-label): 10 mg/kg PO suspension and 100 mg/mL fluconazole-treated drinking water both maintained plasma concentrations above the MIC for most strains of *C albicans*. Computer modeling predicted 5 mg/kg PO once daily or 10 mg/kg PO every other day would also maintain plasma concentration above MIC or AUC:MIC ratio.[48]

Alternative treatment of aspergillosis (extra-label): 5 – 10 mg/kg PO once daily for up to 6 weeks, with or after amphotericin B treatment and/or surgical debridement[49,50]

RABBITS/RODENTS/SMALL MAMMALS:

Rabbits (extra-label): 25 – 43 mg/kg IV slowly every 12 hours[51]

REPTILES:

Dermatophytosis in iguanas (extra-label): 5 mg/kg PO once daily

Monitoring

- Clinical efficacy
- GI adverse effects
- Fungal antigen testing and/or fungal cultures when indicated
- Baseline and periodic chemistry panel (eg, ALT, ALP) are recommended with long-term therapy.

Client Information

- This medicine may be given with or without food. If your animal vomits or acts sick after receiving fluconazole on an empty stomach, give with food or a small treat. If vomiting continues, contact your veterinarian.
- The most likely side effects are gastrointestinal (eg, lack of appetite, vomiting, diarrhea). Liver toxicity is possible but is very rare.
- Do not skip doses.

Chemistry/Synonyms

Fluconazole, a synthetic triazole antifungal agent, occurs as a white crystalline powder. It is slightly soluble in water. Solutions for injection have a pH of 4 to 8.

Fluconazole may also be known as fluconazolum, flukonatsoli, or UK-49858; many trade names are available, including *Diflucan*®.

Storage/Stability

Fluconazole tablets and the powder for oral suspension should be stored at temperatures less than 30°C (86°F) in tight containers. Fluconazole injection should be stored at temperatures of 5°C to 30°C (41°F-86°F); varies by manufacturer, refer to product label); avoid freezing. After reconstitution, fluconazole oral suspension should be stored at temperatures of 5°C to 30°C (41°F-86°F); avoid freezing. Discard unused portions of reconstituted oral suspension after 2 weeks.

Compatibility/Compounding Considerations

Compatibility is dependent on factors such as pH, concentration, temperature, and diluent used; consult specialized references or a hospital pharmacist for more specific information.

Do not add additives to the injection. The following drugs have been reported to be **Y-site compatible** with fluconazole: amikacin, azithromycin, buprenorphine, butorphanol, cefazolin, dexamethasone sodium phosphate, dexmedetomidine, diltiazem, diphenhydramine, dobutamine, famotidine, fentanyl, gentamicin, heparin, hydrocortisone sodium succinate, insulin (regular), lactated Ringer's solution, lidocaine, magnesium sulfate, meropenem, metoclopramide, metronidazole, midazolam, morphine, nitroprusside, ondansetron, penicillin G, piperacillin/tazobactam, potassium chloride, and sodium bicarbonate.

The following drugs have been reported to be completely or variably **incompatible** with fluconazole: ampicillin, amphotericin B (all formulations), ceftazidime, clindamycin, dantrolene, diazepam, furosemide, hydroxyzine, pantoprazole, and sulfa-/trimethoprim.

In one study, compounded fluconazole suspension concentration varied by 74% to 95% of the labeled concentration.[52]

Dosage Forms/Regulatory Status

VETERINARY-LABELED PRODUCTS: NONE

HUMAN-LABELED PRODUCTS:

Fluconazole Oral Tablets: 50 mg, 100 mg, 150 mg, and 200 mg; *Diflucan*®; generic; (Rx)

Fluconazole Powder for Oral Suspension: 10 mg/mL and 40 mg/mL (when reconstituted) in 35 mL; *Diflucan*®; generic; (Rx); orange flavored

Fluconazole in Sodium Chloride 0.9% Injection: 2 mg/mL in 100 mL and 200 mL bottles or bags; *Diflucan*®; generic; (Rx)

References

For the complete list of references, see **wiley.com/go/budde/plumb**

Flucytosine

(floo-***sye***-toe-seen) *Ancobon®*

Antifungal

Prescriber Highlights

- ▶ Antifungal used only in combination with other drugs for serious fungal infections. CNS penetration is excellent, and high urinary concentrations are attainable.
- ▶ Extreme caution is advised in patients with renal impairment, preexisting myelosuppression, hematologic diseases, or receiving other bone marrow suppressant drugs. Caution is advised in patients with hepatic disease.
- ▶ Not recommended for dogs, as they may develop severe cutaneous and/or mucocutaneous reactions
- ▶ Teratogenic in rats
- ▶ The most common adverse effects are GI effects (eg, inappetence, vomiting, diarrhea). Other potential effects include, dose-dependent myelosuppression, cutaneous eruption, oral ulceration, increased hepatic enzymes, and CNS effects (cats).

Uses/Indications

Flucytosine is active against *Cryptococcus* spp, *Candida* spp, and *Aspergillus* spp. It is used in combination with other antifungals (eg, azoles, amphotericin B). When flucytosine is used as a single agent, resistance can develop rapidly, particularly with *Cryptococcus* spp. Because it penetrates relatively well into the CNS, flucytosine has been used for the treatment of CNS cryptococcosis. Some cases of SC and systemic chromomycosis (chromoblastosis) may also respond to flucytosine.

Pharmacology/Actions

Flucytosine penetrates fungal cells where it is deaminated by cytosine deaminase to fluorouracil. Fungi lacking cytosine deaminase are not susceptible to flucytosine. Fluorouracil acts as an antimetabolite by competing with uracil, thereby interfering with pyrimidine metabolism and eventually RNA and protein synthesis. It is thought that fluorouracil is subsequently converted to fluorodeoxyuredylic acid that inhibits thymidylate synthesis and, ultimately, DNA synthesis.

In human cells, cytosine deaminase is apparently not present or only has minimal activity. Rats metabolize some of the drug to fluorouracil, which may explain the teratogenic effects seen in this species. It is unclear how much cytosine deaminase activity dog and cat cells possess. GI bacteria may deaminate small amounts of flucytosine to fluorouracil.

Flucytosine can have synergistic efficacy when used with amphotericin B.

Pharmacokinetics

Flucytosine is well absorbed after oral administration. The rate, but not extent, of absorption will be decreased if given with food.

Flucytosine is distributed widely throughout the body. CSF concentrations may be 60% to 100% of those found in the serum. In healthy humans, the volume of distribution is about 0.7 L/kg. Only about 2% to 4% of the drug is bound to plasma proteins. It is unknown if flucytosine is distributed into milk.

Flucytosine is excreted basically unchanged in the urine via glomerular filtration. The elimination half-life of flucytosine is ≈2.7 hours in dogs.[1] In humans, the half-life is about 3 to 6 hours in patients with normal renal function but may be significantly prolonged in patients with renal dysfunction.

Contraindications/Precautions/Warnings

Flucytosine is contraindicated in patients that are hypersensitive to it.

Flucytosine should be used with extreme caution in patients with renal impairment. Some clinicians recommend monitoring serum flucytosine concentrations in these patients and adjusting the dose (or dosing interval) to maintain peak serum concentration less than 100 µg/mL. One recommendation is to divide the flucytosine dose by the serum creatinine level if azotemia develops.[2]

Use flucytosine with extreme caution in dogs, as mucocutaneous or cutaneous drug eruptions can develop rapidly (within 10 to 20 days) but may occur as late as 6 weeks after beginning treatment.[1,3] Lesions may be localized to the nasal planum, lips, eyelids, and scrotum.

Use flucytosine with extreme caution in patients with preexisting myelosuppression, hematologic diseases, or in those receiving other bone marrow suppressant drugs. Flucytosine should also be used cautiously (with enhanced monitoring) in patients with hepatic disease.

Because resistance can develop rapidly when flucytosine is used alone, it should only be used in combination with other antifungal drugs.

Do not confuse flucytosine with fluorouracil.

Adverse Effects

The most common adverse effects seen with flucytosine are GI disturbances (eg, nausea, vomiting, diarrhea). Other potential adverse effects include a dose-dependent myelosuppression (eg, anemia, leukopenia, thrombocytopenia), oral ulceration, and increased liver enzymes. Dogs receiving flucytosine often develop a severe drug reaction (ie, mucocutaneous or cutaneous eruption with depigmentation, ulceration, exudation and crust formation, primarily seen on the scrotum and nasal planum) that typically appears within 10 to 20 days of initiating treatment.[1,3] Lesions should resolve within 2 to 3 weeks of stopping treatment and were less severe with immediate discontinuation of flucytosine.

Reports of aberrant behavior and seizures in a cat without concurrent CNS infection have been noted after flucytosine use. There are anecdotal reports of toxic epidermal necrolysis occurring in cats treated with flucytosine.

Reproductive/Nursing Safety

The effects of flucytosine on fertility and reproductive effects have not been well studied. Flucytosine crosses the placenta and has caused teratogenic effects in rats, but not in rabbits or mice.[4] It should be used in pregnant animals only when the benefits of therapy outweigh the risks.

It is not known whether flucytosine is excreted in milk. Because there are potential serious adverse reactions in nursing offspring, consider using milk replacer.

Overdose/Acute Toxicity

Limited information on the acute toxicity of flucytosine is available. It is suggested that a substantial overdose be handled with gut emptying, administration of activated charcoal, and a cathartic unless contraindicated. Flucytosine can be removed by dialysis.

For patients that have experienced or are suspected of having experienced an overdose, consultation with a 24-hour poison consultation center specializing in providing veterinary-specific information is recommended. For general information related to overdose and toxin exposures, as well as contact information for poison control centers, refer to ***Appendix***.

Drug Interactions

The following drug interactions have either been reported or are theoretical in humans or animals receiving flucytosine and may be of significance in veterinary patients. Unless otherwise noted, use together is not necessarily contraindicated, but weigh the potential risks and perform additional monitoring when appropriate.

- **Antacids, Aluminum- or Magnesium-Containing**: May delay the absorption of flucytosine[5]

- **Amphotericin B**: When used with amphotericin B, synergism against *Cryptococcus* spp and *Candida* spp has been demonstrated in vitro. However, if amphotericin B induces renal dysfunction, the toxicity of flucytosine may be enhanced if it accumulates. If clinically significant renal toxicity develops, flucytosine dosage may need to be adjusted.
- **Cytarabine**: Impaired flucytosine activity may occur due to competition by cytarabine for fungal sites of action.
- **Myelosuppressive Drugs** (eg, **antineoplastics, azathioprine, chloramphenicol, methimazole**): Additive myelosuppression may occur.
- **Zidovudine**: Increased risk for neutropenia

Laboratory Considerations

- When determining **serum creatinine** using the ***Ektachem***® analyzer, false elevations in levels may be noted if patients are also taking flucytosine.

Dosages

DOGS:

NOTE: Because of potentially serious toxicity, flucytosine is usually **not recommended** for use in dogs.

Cryptococcosis (extra-label): 50 – 75 mg/kg PO every 8 hours; treatment requires 1 to 12 months. Flucytosine must be given with amphotericin B or azole antifungal agent.[6]

CATS:

Cryptococcosis (extra-label): Must be used with another antifungal (amphotericin B or an azole). 30 mg/kg PO every 6 hours or 50 mg/kg PO every 8 hours or 75 mg/kg PO every 12 hours, or 250 mg/cat (NOT mg/kg) every 6 to 8 hours. Treatment requires 1 to 9 months.[6]

Candidiasis (extra-label): 25 – 50 mg/kg PO every 6 hours or 50 – 65 mg/kg PO every 8 hours for 42 days. Flucytosine must be given with amphotericin B or azole antifungal agent.[7]

Monitoring

- Renal function (at least twice weekly if also receiving amphotericin B)
- CBC with platelets
- Hepatic enzymes at least monthly
- In humans, dosage adjustments should target peak flucytosine concentration of less than 100 µg/mL and trough flucytosine concentration of 20 – 40 µg/mL to minimize toxicity.[8]

Client Information

- Clients should report any clinical signs associated with hematologic toxicity (eg, abnormal bleeding, bruising).
- If vomiting occurs, give flucytosine with food or a small treat.
- Pregnant women should take precautions handling this medication. It has caused birth defects in laboratory animals.

Chemistry/Synonyms

Flucytosine, a fluorinated pyrimidine antifungal agent, occurs as a white to off-white, crystalline powder that is odorless or has a slight odor with pK_as of 2.9 and 10.71. Flucytosine has a molecular weight of 129.09. It is sparingly soluble in water and slightly soluble in alcohol. Flucytosine may also be known as 5-FC, 5-fluorocytosine, flucitozin, flucytosinum, Ro-2-9915, *Alcobon*®, and *Ancotil*®.

Storage/Stability

Store flucytosine capsules in tight, light-resistant containers at 25°C (77°F); excursions permitted to 15°C to 30°C (59°F-86°F).

Flucytosine may decompose to fluorouracil if stored at higher temperatures.

Compatibility/Compounding Considerations

Compounded preparation stability: Flucytosine oral suspension compounded from commercially available capsules has been published.[9] Triturating four (4) flucytosine 250 mg capsules with 50 mL of *Ora-Plus*® and *qs ad* to 100 mL with *Ora-Sweet*® (or *Ora-Sweet® SF*) yields a 10 mg/mL oral suspension that retains greater than 95% potency for 60 days stored at both 5°C (41°F) and 25°C (77°F).

Dosage Forms/Regulatory Status

VETERINARY-LABELED PRODUCTS: NONE

HUMAN-LABELED PRODUCTS:

Flucytosine Oral Capsules: 250 mg and 500 mg; *Ancobon*®, generic; (Rx)

References

For the complete list of references, see **wiley.com/go/budde/plumb**

Fludrocortisone

(flue-droe-***kor***-ti-sone) *Florinef*®

Mineralocorticoid

Prescriber Highlights

- ► Oral mineralocorticoid alternative to DOCP for treating hypoadrenocorticism in small animal species
- ► Although fludrocortisone has some glucocorticoid activity that could cause adverse effects, some patients may require supplemental glucocorticoid therapy (eg, prednis[ol]one).
- ► Adverse effects are dose-related and include polyuria, polydipsia, GI upset, hypertension, edema, and hypokalemia.
- ► May be given without regard to food unless GI upset is noted

Uses/Indications

Fludrocortisone is used primarily for its mineralocorticoid effects in the treatment of hypoadrenocorticism (Addison's disease) in small animal species. One study assessing plasma renin activity of hypoadrenocorticism in dogs suggests that desoxycorticosterone pivalate (DOCP) may be more effective at suppressing renin activity (which is increased with hypoadrenocorticism due to decreased aldosterone production) than fludrocortisone.[1] Further studies are needed to understand the clinical significance of this difference, especially when measurement of renin activity is limited in veterinary patients.

In humans, fludrocortisone has also been used for severe postural hypotension and salt-losing, congenital adrenal hyperplasia.

Pharmacology/Actions

Fludrocortisone acetate is a potent corticosteroid that possesses both glucocorticoid and mineralocorticoid activity. It is ≈10 to 15 times as potent a glucocorticoid agent as hydrocortisone but is a much more potent mineralocorticoid (125 times that of hydrocortisone). It is only used clinically for its mineralocorticoid effects. Mineralocorticoids increase sodium reabsorption at the renal distal tubule and enhance potassium and hydrogen ion excretion in the collecting tubule.

The site of action of mineralocorticoids is at the renal distal tubule, where they increase the absorption of sodium and enhance urinary potassium and hydrogen ion excretion.

Pharmacokinetics

In humans, fludrocortisone is well-absorbed from the GI tract, with peak concentrations occurring in ≈1.7 hours. Plasma half-life is ≈3.5 hours, but biologic activity persists for 18 to 36 hours.[2]

Contraindications/Precautions/Warnings

Fludrocortisone is contraindicated in patients known to be hypersensitive to it and in patients with systemic fungal infections.

Some dogs or cats may require additional supplementation with a glucocorticoid agent on an ongoing basis. All animals with hypoadrenocorticism should receive additional glucocorticoids (at least 2 times basal) during periods of stress or acute illness. Because fludrocortisone has glucocorticoid properties, it should be withdrawn slowly if therapy is discontinued.

Long-term corticosteroid administration causes immunosuppression and increases risk for infection. The risk for glaucoma and cataract development may also be increased.

Use with caution in patients with cardiac or renal disease, as fludrocortisone causes fluid retention and may lead to electrolyte imbalances and hypertension. Use corticosteroids cautiously in patients with fresh intestinal anastomoses, active or latent peptic ulcer, osteoporosis, or myasthenia gravis.[2]

Adverse Effects

Adverse effects of fludrocortisone are generally a result of chronic, excessive dosage (see ***Overdose/Acute Toxicity***) or if withdrawal is too rapid. Because fludrocortisone also possesses glucocorticoid activity, it can cause the adverse effects associated with those compounds, such as polyuria/polydipsia, polyphagia, and panting. (See ***Glucocorticoid Agents, General Information***)

Reproductive/Nursing Safety

Specific information on fludrocortisone effects in pregnant or lactating animals is lacking. Corticosteroids have been shown to be teratogenic (eg, reduced fetal growth, cleft palate, deformed forelegs, phocomelia, anasarca).

Corticosteroids may be excreted in clinically significant quantities in milk. Puppies or kittens of mothers receiving fludrocortisone should receive milk replacer after colostrum is consumed.

Because safety has not been established in animals, this drug should only be used when the maternal benefits outweigh the potential risks to offspring.

Overdose/Acute Toxicity

Overdose may cause hypertension, edema, and hypokalemia. Electrolytes should be aggressively monitored, and potassium may need to be supplemented. The drug should be discontinued until clinical signs associated with overdose have resolved, then restarted at a lower dosage.

For patients that have experienced or are suspected to have experienced an overdose, consultation with a 24-hour poison consultation center specializing in providing veterinary-specific information is recommended. For general information related to overdose and toxin exposures, as well as contact information for poison control centers, refer to ***Appendix.***

Drug Interactions

The following drug interactions have either been reported or are theoretical in humans or animals receiving fludrocortisone and may be of significance in veterinary patients. Unless otherwise noted, use together is not necessarily contraindicated, but weigh the potential risks and perform additional monitoring when appropriate.

- **AMPHOTERICIN B**: Concomitant administration may increase risk for hypokalemia.
- **ASPIRIN**: Concomitant administration may reduce salicylate levels and may also increase risk for GI adverse effects.
- **CALCITRIOL**: Concomitant administration may decrease the therapeutic effect of calcitriol.
- **CHOLESTYRAMINE**: May decrease fludrocortisone bioavailability
- **CORTICOSTEROIDS** (eg, **dexamethasone, prednis(ol)one**): Concomitant administration may increase risk for corticosteroid side effects.
- **COSYNTROPIN**: Concomitant administration may decrease diagnostic effects of cosyntropin.
- **DESMOPRESSIN**: Concomitant administration may increase risk for hyponatremia from desmopressin.
- **DIGOXIN**: By lowering potassium, fludrocortisone may increase the risk for digoxin toxicity.
- **DIURETICS, POTASSIUM-DEPLETING** (eg, **thiazides, furosemide**): Concomitant administration may increase risk for hypokalemia. Diuretics also cause a loss of sodium and may counteract the effects of fludrocortisone.
- **HYPOGLYCEMIC AGENTS** (eg, **glipizide, insulin, metformin**): Fludrocortisone may increase blood glucose, reducing antidiabetic effect.
- **I^{131}**: Uptake of I^{131} by thyroid tissue may be decreased by glucocorticoids.
- **IMMUNOSUPPRESSIVE AGENTS** (eg, **leflunomide, mycophenolate, tacrolimus**): Concomitant administration may increase risk for immunosuppression and subsequent infection.
- **NONSTEROIDAL ANTI-INFLAMMATORY DRUGS** (NSAIDs; eg, **carprofen, meloxicam**): Concomitant administration may increase risk for GI adverse effects.
- **PHENOBARBITAL**: Concomitant administration may result in decreased fludrocortisone efficacy.
- **RIFAMPIN**: Concomitant administration may result in decreased fludrocortisone efficacy.
- **VACCINES**: Fludrocortisone may result in inadequate immunological response to the vaccine due to its immunosuppressive effects.

Laboratory Considerations

- Glucocorticoids may <u>increase</u> serum **cholesterol** and **urine glucose** levels.
- Glucocorticoids may <u>decrease</u> serum **potassium.**
- Glucocorticoids can <u>suppress</u> the release of thyroid stimulating hormone (TSH) and reduce T_3 and T_4 values. Thyroid gland atrophy has been reported after chronic glucocorticoid administration.
- Fludrocortisone suppressed serum **aldosterone** in healthy adult cats.[3]
- False-negative results of the **nitroblue tetrazolium test for systemic bacterial infections** may be induced by glucocorticoids.
- **Intradermal allergy testing (IDT)**: Suppression of IDT results may persist for 1 to 2 weeks after discontinuation of fludrocortisone. It is recommended that treatment be discontinued at least 2 weeks prior to testing.[4]

Dosages

DOGS:

Maintenance therapy for hypoadrenocorticism (extra-label): Initially, 0.01 – 0.02 mg/kg PO as either a single dose or divided and given twice daily. Dosages are adjusted in 0.05 – 0.1 mg increments (½ to one 0.1 mg tablet) every 5 days based on assessment of serum electrolyte concentrations. Once dose is stabilized, some dogs can be transitioned to once daily dosing. Most dogs will eventually require 0.02 – 0.03 mg/kg per day. Approximately 50% of dogs will require supplemental prednis(ol)one, and owners should have supplemental prednis(ol)one on hand and be instructed to use it when animal undergoes stress or illness (eg, veterinary visits, boarding). See ***Prednisolone/Prednisone.*** In dogs that develop signs of hyperadrenocorticism (eg, polyuria, polydipsia) while being treated with fludrocortisone, first withdraw any additional glucocorticoid supplementation. If clinical signs persist, the signs may be due to the glucocorticoid activity of fludrocortisone. In dogs in which electrolyte concentrations cannot be effectively normalized with fludrocortisone, consider switching mineralocorticoid supplementation to desoxycorticosterone pivalate (DOCP).[5-9,10]

CATS:

Maintenance therapy for hypoadrenocorticism (extra-label): 0.05 – 0.1 mg/cat (NOT mg/kg) PO twice daily with prednisolone 2.5 – 5 mg/cat (NOT mg/kg) PO per day added as needed.[5] Taper prednisolone to the minimum dosage that controls clinical signs.

Possible diagnostic tool in the diagnosis of feline primary hyperaldosteronism (PHA)[11] (extra-label):

1. Urine aldosterone:creatinine ratio (UACR) is measured before and after administration of fludrocortisone 0.05 mg/kg PO every 12 hours for 4 days.[3,12]
2. Serum aldosterone:creatinine ratio is measured before and after administration of fludrocortisone 0.05 mg/kg PO every 12 hours for 3 doses.[3]

FERRETS:

Maintenance therapy for hypoadrenocorticism (extra-label): 0.05 – 0.1 mg/kg PO once daily (every 24 hours) or divided every 12 hours for animals that still exhibit signs of hypoadrenocorticism despite prednis(ol)one therapy[13]

Monitoring

- Prior to beginning treatment and following a dosage change, measure serum electrolyte concentrations, then measure again every 5 to 7 days until sodium and potassium concentrations have normalized.[14] Once dose is stabilized, recheck electrolytes every 3 to 6 months.
- Body weight, physical examination to check for edema (peripheral and pulmonary)
- Baseline and periodic blood pressure
- Signs of glucocorticoid excess (eg, polyuria, polydipsia)

Client Information

- This medicine may be given with or without food. If your animal vomits or acts sick after getting it on an empty stomach, give medicine with food or small treat to see if this helps. If vomiting continues, contact your veterinarian.
- Side effects are unlikely, but if the dose is too high (long-term), your animal may develop changes in fur, abdominal swelling, hair loss. Contact your veterinarian as soon as possible if your animal shows signs of weakness, depression, lack of appetite, vomiting, and/or diarrhea, as these signs may mean the dose is too low.
- Surgery or stress (eg, trauma, illness) requires administration of additional glucocorticoids (eg, prednisolone). A supply of prednisolone should always be kept on hand.
- Do not stop this medicine suddenly or serious side effects could occur.

Chemistry/Synonyms

A synthetic glucocorticoid with significant mineralocorticoid activity, fludrocortisone acetate occurs as hygroscopic, fine, white to pale yellow powder or crystals. It is odorless or practically odorless. Fludrocortisone is insoluble in water and slightly soluble in alcohol.

Fludrocortisone acetate may also be known as fluohydrisone acetate, fluohydrocortisone acetate, 9alpha-fluorohydrocortisone acetate, fludrocortisoni acetas, 9alpha-fluorohydrocortisone 21-acetate, *Astonin*®, *Astonin H*®, *Florinef*®, *Florinefe*®, and *Lonikan*®.

Storage/Stability

Fludrocortisone acetate tablets should be stored at room temperature 20°C to 25°C (68°F-77°F) in well-closed containers; avoid excessive heat. The drug is relatively stable in light and air.

Compatibility/Compounding Considerations

No specific information noted

Dosage Forms/Regulatory Status

VETERINARY-LABELED PRODUCTS: NONE

HUMAN-LABELED PRODUCTS:

Fludrocortisone Acetate Tablets: 0.1 mg; generic; (Rx)

References

For the complete list of references, see **wiley.com/go/budde/plumb**

Flumazenil

(floo-***maz***-eh-nill) *Romazicon*®

Benzodiazepine Antagonist

Prescriber Highlights

- ▶ Used in a variety of species to reverse benzodiazepine overdose (OD) or adverse effects caused by intentional doses or when rapid recovery is required. May also have efficacy in ODs of non-benzodiazepine agonists of the benzodiazepine receptor (eg, zolpidem)
- ▶ Contraindications include known hypersensitivity, treatment with benzodiazepines for life-threatening conditions (eg, status epilepticus, increased intracranial pressure [ICP]), and tricyclic antidepressant OD treatment. Use extreme caution in mixed overdoses.
- ▶ Adverse effects in dogs occur primarily at higher dosages and include salivation, shivering, seizures, howling, hacking coughs, and opisthotonos. Injection-site reactions, vomiting, cutaneous vasodilatation, vertigo, and/or ataxia may also occur.

Uses/Indications

Flumazenil may be useful for reversal of the effects of benzodiazepines used in sedation or anesthetic protocols when adverse benzodiazepine effects arise or when rapid recovery is required. Flumazenil may also be used to reverse the anesthetic effects of tiletamine/zolazepam in dogs[1,2]; however, the effects of tiletamine (which are not reversible) may persist and be undesirable. Flumazenil also is used in the management of benzodiazepine overdoses and has shown benefit in the treatment of overdoses of nonbenzodiazepine agonists (eg, zolpidem[3]) of the benzodiazepine receptor.

In horses, flumazenil reversed the effect of midazolam/ketamine induction and midazolam CRI in two 2-hour total IV anesthesia protocols (ketamine/xylazine/midazolam and ketamine/dexmedetomidine/midazolam) with good to excellent recovery quality and improved respiratory function.[4,5]

Pharmacology/Actions

Flumazenil is a competitive neutral antagonist of benzodiazepines at benzodiazepine receptors on the $GABA_A$ receptor in the CNS. It antagonizes the sedative and amnestic qualities of benzodiazepines.

Pharmacokinetics

The therapeutic effect of flumazenil may occur within 1 to 2 minutes of IV administration.[6] It is rapidly distributed and almost completely metabolized in the liver. In humans, the average half-life is ≈1 hour. Half-life is prolonged in patients with liver dysfunction. This prolongs flumazenil effects but does not alter dosage requirements.

Contraindications/Precautions/Warnings

Flumazenil is contraindicated in patients hypersensitive to it or other benzodiazepines or in patients in which benzodiazepines are being used to treat a potentially life-threatening condition (eg, status epilepticus, increased intracranial pressure [ICP]).[6] Flumazenil should not be used, or should be used with extreme caution, in patients with mixed overdoses, particularly those receiving cyclic antidepressants (eg, clomipramine), as reversal of the benzodiazepine may lead to seizures or other complications (eg, cardiac dysrhythmias) that may emerge once the benzodiazepine effects are removed.[6,7] Flumazenil should be used with caution in patients with head trauma, as it may precipitate seizures and alter cerebral blood flow.[6]

Although flumazenil has been investigated as treatment for overdoses of both baclofen and carisoprodol, it can cause worsening of clinical signs and thus may be contraindicated.[8]

In humans, flumazenil only antagonizes benzodiazepine effects without altering benzodiazepine pharmacokinetics.[6] Effects of long-acting benzodiazepines may recur after flumazenil's effects subside, and additional flumazenil doses may be needed.

Routine use of flumazenil as a benzodiazepine reversal agent is not advised as rare but serious adverse reactions, (including cardiac arrhythmias, seizures, and sudden death) have been reported in humans and experimental canine studies.

Adverse Effects

Adverse effects reported in dogs receiving higher doses (eg, 0.08 – 0.16 mg/kg) of flumazenil for the reversal of tiletamine/zolazepam include salivation, shivering, seizures, howling, hacking coughs, and opisthotonos. These effects are likely attributed to the effects of flumazenil on the CNS and the continued effects of tiletamine.[1] Muscle rigidity has been observed in miniature pigs.[9]

In humans, the risk for seizures is higher in patients with severe hepatic impairment and in patients receiving benzodiazepines chronically to control seizures.[6] Other adverse effects reported in humans include vomiting, cutaneous vasodilatation, arrhythmias, vertigo, agitation, increased muscle tone, ataxia, and blurred vision. Injection site reactions have occurred, and administration through a freely running infusion in a large vein is recommended. Deaths have been associated with flumazenil use in humans with serious underlying diseases.

Reproductive/Nursing Safety

Teratogenicity was not observed in rabbits or rats at oral doses up to 150 mg/kg, but embryocidal effects occurred in rabbits at doses exceeding 15 mg/kg IV.

It is unknown whether flumazenil is passed in milk.[6]

Because safety has not been established in animals, this drug should only be used when the maternal benefits outweigh the potential risks to offspring.

Overdose/Acute Toxicity

Large IV overdoses in the absence of a benzodiazepine have rarely caused symptoms in otherwise healthy humans. In humans, seizures, if precipitated, have been successfully managed with barbiturates, phenytoin, or benzodiazepines at high doses.

For patients that have experienced or are suspected to have experienced an overdose, consultation with a 24-hour poison consultation center specializing in providing veterinary-specific information is recommended. For general information related to overdose and toxin exposures, as well as contact information for poison control centers, refer to ***Appendix***.

Drug Interactions

The following drug interactions have either been reported or are theoretical in humans or animals receiving flumazenil and may be of significance in veterinary patients. Unless otherwise noted, use together is not necessarily contraindicated, but weigh the potential risks and perform additional monitoring when appropriate.

- **Cyclic** (tri-, tetra-) **Antidepressants** (eg, **clomipramine, amitriptyline**): Increased risk for seizures; use is contraindicated in patients experiencing a cyclic antidepressant overdose.[7]
- **Neuromuscular Blocking Agents**: Not recommended to use flumazenil until neuromuscular blockade has been fully reversed[6]

Laboratory Considerations

None noted

Dosages

DOGS/CATS:

Antagonist for benzodiazepine effects or toxicity (eg, respiratory depression) and for imidazopyridine sleep-aid drugs (eg, zolpidem) toxicity (extra-label): Most sources recommend an initial dose of 0.01 – 0.2mg/kg IV (or IO)[10]; start at the lower end of the dosage range (0.01 mg/kg) and repeat as needed to reverse sedation. If the high end of the dosage range does not elicit a reversal response, be sure to reverse any other drugs that were given and address other problems that could be contributing to the clinical situation (eg, hypothermia). Intratracheal administration has been suggested in an emergency situation when venous access is not possible. 0.04 – 0.06 mg/kg IV can be used to reverse tiletamine/zolazepam anesthesia.[1]

HORSES:

Reversal of benzodiazepine effects as part of multi-modal anesthesia (extra-label): 0.01 – 0.02 mg/kg IV over 10 minutes; administer 20 minutes after terminating TIVA.[5,11]

BIRDS

Reversal of intranasal midazolam sedation (extra-label): 0.05 mg/kg administered intranasally reversed the effects of intranasal midazolam within 10 minutes.[12]

REPTILES

Reversal of sedation protocols containing midazolam (extra-label)

1. **Snakes**: 0.08 mg/kg IM in the cranial third of the body. Re-sedation was observed in all snakes 3 hours after flumazenil administration.[13]
2. **Green iguanas**: 0.05 mg/kg IM[14]
3. **Leopard geckos**: 0.05 mg/kg SC craniodorsal to the contralateral thoracic limb where midazolam was administered[15]

Monitoring

- Efficacy at resolving respiratory depression and recovery from sedation
- Re-sedation may occur in patients that have received large doses of benzodiazepines, or multiple anesthetic agents and neuromuscular antagonists. Re-sedation may be more common in snakes.[13]
- Monitor for seizures in susceptible patients, particularly those with pre-existing hepatic dysfunction or neurologic disease.

Client information

- This drug is administered in a veterinary clinic to reverse the effects of certain sedating drugs.
- If your animal has received flumazenil, monitor for re-emergence of sedation.

Chemistry/Synonyms

A benzodiazepine antagonist, flumazenil is a 1,4-imidazobenzodiazepine derivative. It occurs as a white to off-white crystalline compound that is insoluble in water but slightly soluble in acidic aqueous solutions.

Flumazenil may also be known as: flumazenilum, flumazepil, Ro-15-1788, Ro-15-1788/000, *Anexate®*, *Fadaflumaz®*, *Flumage®*, *Flumanovag®*, *Flumazen®*, *Fluxifarm®*, *Lanexat®*, and *Romazicon®*.

Storage/Stability

Store flumazenil at 25°C (77°F). Excursions are permitted from 15°C to 30°C (59°F-86°F).[6] Once drawn into a syringe or mixed with the solutions listed below, discard after 24 hours.

Compatibility/Compounding Considerations

Compatibility is dependent on factors such as pH, concentration,

temperature, and diluent used; specialized references or a hospital pharmacist should be consulted for more specific information.

Flumazenil is physically **compatible** with lactated Ringer's, dextrose 5%, and normal saline solutions.

Dosage Forms/Regulatory Status

VETERINARY-LABELED PRODUCTS: NONE

HUMAN-LABELED PRODUCTS:

Flumazenil Injection: 0.1 mg/mL in 5 mL and 10 mL vials; generic; (Rx)

References

For the complete list of references, see **wiley.com/go/budde/plumb**

Flumethasone

(floo-***meth***-a-sone) *Flucort®*

Glucocorticoid

Prescriber Highlights

- ▶ Injectable and oral long-acting glucocorticoid. No longer commonly used in small animal species
- ▶ 15 times more potent than hydrocortisone; no appreciable mineralocorticoid activity
- ▶ Therapy goal is to use as much as is required and as little as possible for as short an amount of time as possible.
- ▶ Primary adverse effects are Cushingoid in nature with sustained use.
- ▶ Many potential drug and laboratory interactions

Uses/Indications

Flumethasone injection is available commercially as a free steroid alcohol solution. Although flumethasone does not work as rapidly as the corticosteroid phosphate and succinate esters (methylprednisolone sodium succinate, prednisolone sodium succinate, or dexamethasone sodium phosphate), it can be given either IM or IV and is useful for acute reactions, such as insect bite hypersensitivity or vaccine reactions.[1]

Flumethasone injection is labeled in horses as indicated for: 1) Musculoskeletal conditions due to inflammation, where permanent structural changes do not exist, such as bursitis, carpitis, osselets, and myositis. Following therapy, an appropriate period of rest should be instituted to allow a more normal return to function of the affected part. 2) Allergic states, such as urticaria (hives) and insect bites

Flumethasone injection is labeled in dogs as indicated for: 1) Musculoskeletal conditions due to inflammation of muscles or joints and accessory structures, where permanent structural changes do not exist, such as arthritis, osteoarthritis, intervertebral disc syndrome, and myositis. In septic arthritis, appropriate antibacterial therapy should be concurrently administered. 2) Certain acute and chronic dermatoses of varying etiology to help control the pruritus, irritation, and inflammation associated with these conditions. The drug has proven useful in otitis externa in conjunction with topical medication for similar reasons. 3) Allergic states, such as urticaria and insect bites.

Flumethasone injection is labeled in cats as indicated for certain acute and chronic dermatoses of varying etiology to help control the pruritus, irritation, and inflammation associated with these conditions.

Pharmacology/Actions

Flumethasone is considered a long-acting glucocorticoid agent with a duration of effect of 36 to 48 hours. Flumethasone is ≈15 times more potent than hydrocortisone; 1.3 mg of flumethasone is equivalent to ≈5 mg of prednisone. It does not have significant mineralocorticoid activity and is not suitable for every-other-day dosing.

For more information, refer to the ***Glucocorticoid Agents, General Information*** monograph.

Pharmacokinetics

Following IV administration to exercised horses, the volume of distribution (steady state) was 5.9 L/kg, systemic clearance was 30.7 mL/kg/min, and elimination half-life was 4.8 hours.[2]

Contraindications/Precautions/Warnings

Flumethasone is contraindicated during the last trimester of pregnancy. Systemic use of glucocorticoids is generally considered contraindicated in systemic fungal infections (unless used for replacement therapy in patients with hypoadrenocorticism) when administered IM in patients with idiopathic thrombocytopenia and in those hypersensitive to a particular compound. Use of sustained-release, injectable glucocorticoids is contraindicated for chronic corticosteroid therapy of systemic diseases.

Animals that have received glucocorticoids systemically, other than with burst therapy, should be tapered off the drugs. Patients that have received the drugs chronically should be tapered off slowly as endogenous ACTH and corticosteroid function may return slowly. Should the animal undergo a stressor (eg, surgery, trauma, illness) during the tapering process or until normal adrenal and pituitary function resume, additional glucocorticoids should be administered.

Adverse Effects

Adverse effects are generally associated with long-term administration of these drugs, especially if given at high dosages or not on an alternate day regimen. Effects generally manifest as clinical signs of hyperadrenocorticism. When administered to young, growing animals, glucocorticoids can retard growth. Many of the potential effects, adverse and otherwise, are outlined in the ***Pharmacology*** section of the ***Glucocorticoid Agents, General Information*** monograph.

In dogs, GI effects (including GI ulceration) can occur with acute dosing. Polydipsia (PD), polyphagia (PP), and polyuria (PU) may be seen with short-term burst therapy. Adverse effects in dogs can include dull, dry haircoat, weight gain, panting, vomiting, diarrhea, increased liver enzymes, pancreatitis, GI ulceration, dyslipidemias, activation or worsening of diabetes mellitus, muscle wasting, and behavioral changes (depression, lethargy, viciousness). Discontinuation of the drug may be necessary; changing to an alternate-day steroid may also alleviate the problem. With the exception of PU/PD/PP, adverse effects associated with anti-inflammatory therapy are relatively uncommon. Adverse effects associated with immunosuppressive dosages are more common and potentially more severe.

Cats generally require higher dosages than dogs for clinical effect but tend to develop fewer adverse effects. Occasionally, polydipsia, polyuria, polyphagia with weight gain, diarrhea, or depression can be seen. However, long-term, high-dose therapy can lead to Cushingoid effects.

Reproductive/Nursing Safety

Corticosteroid therapy may induce parturition in large animal species during the latter stages of pregnancy. Corticosteroids administered orally or by injection to animals may induce the first stage of parturition if used during the last trimester of pregnancy and may precipitate premature parturition followed by dystocia, fetal death, retained placenta, and metritis.[3] In addition, corticosteroids administered to dogs, rabbits, and rodents during pregnancy have resulted in other congenital anomalies, including deformed forelegs, phocomelia, and anasarca

Caution is advised when using in nursing dams; glucocorticoids unbound to plasma proteins can enter milk. High doses or prolonged administration to nursing dams may potentially inhibit growth, interfere with endogenous corticosteroid production, or cause other unwanted effects in nursing offspring.

Because safety has not been established in animals, this drug should only be used when the maternal benefits outweigh the potential risks to offspring.

Overdose/Acute Toxicity

Glucocorticoids, when given short-term, are unlikely to cause harmful effects, even in massive doses. One incidence of a dog developing acute CNS effects after accidental ingestion of glucocorticoids has been reported. Should clinical signs occur, use supportive treatment if required.

For patients that have experienced or are suspected of having experienced an overdose, consultation with a 24-hour poison consultation center specializing in providing veterinary-specific information is recommended. For general information related to overdose and toxin exposures, as well as contact information for poison control centers, refer to ***Appendix.***

Drug Interactions

The following drug interactions have either been reported or are theoretical in humans or animals receiving flumethasone and may be of significance in veterinary patients. Unless otherwise noted, use together is not necessarily contraindicated, but weigh the potential risks and perform additional monitoring when appropriate.

- **Amphotericin B**: Concomitant administration with glucocorticoids may cause hypokalemia.
- **Anticholinesterase Agents** (eg, **pyridostigmine, neostigmine**): In patients with myasthenia gravis, concomitant glucocorticoid and anticholinesterase agent administration may lead to profound muscle weakness. If possible, discontinue anticholinesterase medication at least 24 hours prior to corticosteroid administration.
- **Aspirin**: Glucocorticoids may reduce salicylate blood concentration and increase the risk for GI ulceration/bleeding.
- **Azole Antifungals** (eg, **ketoconazole**): May decrease the metabolism of glucocorticoids and increase flumethasone blood concentration; ketoconazole may induce adrenal insufficiency when glucocorticoids are withdrawn by inhibiting adrenal corticosteroid synthesis.
- **Cyclophosphamide**: Glucocorticoids may inhibit the hepatic metabolism of cyclophosphamide; dosage adjustments may be required.
- **Cyclosporine**: Concomitant administration of glucocorticoids and cyclosporine may increase the blood concentration of each by mutually inhibiting the hepatic metabolism of the other; the clinical significance of this interaction is not clear.
- **Diazepam**: Flumethasone may decrease diazepam concentration.
- **Diuretics, Potassium-Depleting** (eg, **furosemide, thiazides**): Concomitant administration with glucocorticoids may cause hypokalemia.
- **Ephedrine**: May increase glucocorticoid metabolism, thereby reducing flumethasone blood concentration
- **Estrogens**: May potentiate the effects of glucocorticoids
- **Insulin**: Insulin requirements may increase in patients receiving glucocorticoids.
- **Macrolide Antibiotics** (eg, **erythromycin, clarithromycin**): May decrease the metabolism of glucocorticoids and increase flumethasone blood concentration
- **Mitotane**: May alter the metabolism of steroids; higher than usual doses of steroids may be necessary to treat mitotane-induced adrenal insufficiency.
- **Nonsteroidal Anti-Inflammatory Drugs (NSAIDs**; eg, **carprofen, flunixin, meloxicam, phenylbutazone**): Administration of ulcerogenic drugs with glucocorticoids may increase the risk for GI ulceration.
- **Rifampin**: May increase the metabolism of glucocorticoids and decrease flumethasone blood concentration
- **Phenobarbital, Primidone**: May increase the metabolism of glucocorticoids and decrease flumethasone blood concentration
- **Vaccines, Live Attenuated**: Patients receiving corticosteroids at immunosuppressive dosages should generally not receive live attenuated-virus vaccines as virus replication may be augmented; a diminished immune response may occur after the vaccine, toxoid, or bacterin administration in patients receiving glucocorticoids.

Laboratory Considerations

- Glucocorticoids may increase **serum cholesterol** and **urine glucose** concentration.
- Glucocorticoids may decrease **serum potassium.**
- Glucocorticoids can suppress the release of thyroid-stimulating hormone (TSH) and reduce T_3 and T_4 values. Thyroid gland atrophy has been reported after chronic glucocorticoid administration. The uptake of I^{131} by the thyroid may be decreased by glucocorticoids.
- Reactions to **intradermal skin tests** may be suppressed by glucocorticoids.
- False-negative results of the **nitroblue tetrazolium** test for systemic bacterial infections may be induced by glucocorticoids.
- Glucocorticoids may cause **neutrophilia** within 4 to 8 hours after dosing and return to baseline within 24 to 48 hours after drug discontinuation.
- Glucocorticoids can cause **lymphopenia**, which can persist for weeks after drug discontinuation in dogs.

Dosages

DOGS:

Musculoskeletal conditions due to inflammation; certain acute and chronic dermatoses when given orally, and also for allergic states or shock when given intravenously (label dosage; FDA-approved): Treat and adjust the dosage on an individual basis.

a) 0.0625 – 0.25 mg/dog (NOT mg/kg) PO daily in divided doses.[4] Dosage is dependent on the size of the animal, stage, and severity of the disease. **NOTE**: *Tablets no longer marketed in the United States.*
b) Parenterally: 0.0625 – 0.25 mg/dog (NOT mg/kg) IV, IM, SC daily[5]; dose may be repeated
c) Intra-articularly: 0.166 – 1 mg/dog (NOT mg/kg) depending on the severity of the condition and the size of the involved joint[5]
d) Intra-lesionally: 0.125 – 1 mg/dog (NOT mg/kg) depending on the size and location of the lesion[5]

CATS:

Certain acute and chronic dermatoses to control associated pruritus, irritation, and inflammation (label dosage; FDA-approved): Treat and adjust the dosage on an individual basis:

a) 0.03125 – 0.125 mg/cat (NOT mg/kg) PO daily in divided doses.[4] **NOTE**: *Tablets no longer marketed in the United States.*
b) Parenterally: 0.03125 – 0.125 mg/cat (NOT mg/kg) IV, IM, or SC[5]; dose may be repeated.

HORSES:

Musculoskeletal conditions due to inflammation, where permanent changes do not exist; also for allergic states, such as hives, urticaria, and insect bites (label dosage; FDA-approved): 1.25 – 2.5 mg/horse (NOT mg/kg) daily by IV, IM, or intra-articular injection[5]; dose may be repeated.

Monitoring

Monitoring of glucocorticoid therapy is dependent on its reason for use, dosage, the agent used (amount of mineralocorticoid activity), dosage schedule (daily versus alternate day therapy), duration of therapy, and the animal's age and condition. The following list may not be appropriate or complete for all animals; use clinical assessment and judgment should adverse effects be noted:

- Weight, appetite, signs of edema
- Serum and/or urine electrolytes
- Total plasma proteins and albumin
- Blood glucose
- Urine culture
- Growth and development in young animals

Client Information

- Goal is to find the lowest dose possible and use for the shortest period of time. Carefully follow your veterinarian's instructions for how to give this medicine to your animal. Do not stop giving this medicine to your animal without talking to your veterinarian first, as serious side effects could occur.
- There might be side effects with this medicine. Contact your veterinarian should these effects become severe or progress. In dogs, stomach or intestinal ulcers, perforation, and/or bleeding can occur. Contact your veterinarian immediately if your dog stops eating or you notice a high fever, black tarry stools, or bloody vomit (will look like coffee grounds).
- This medicine may be given with (preferred) or without food. If your animal vomits or acts sick after receiving the medication on an empty stomach, give with food or small treat to see if this helps. If vomiting continues, contact your veterinarian.
- Be sure to tell your veterinarian about what other medications (including vitamins, supplements, or herbal therapies) you give your animal.

Chemistry/Synonyms

Flumethasone occurs as an odorless, white to creamy white, crystalline powder. Its chemical name is 6alpha, 9alpha-difluoro-16alpha methylprednisolone.

Flumethasone may also be known as flumetasone, glumetasoni pivalas, NSC-107680, *Anaprime*®, *Cerson*®, *Flucort*®, *Fluosmin*®, *Locacorten*®, *Locacortene*®, *Locorten*®, *Locortene*®, and *Lorinden*®.

Storage/Stability

Store flumethasone injection at room temperature; avoid freezing. Store flumethasone tablets at room temperature.

Dosage Forms/Regulatory Status

VETERINARY-LABELED PRODUCTS:

NOTE: Although this product is still listed in FDA's Green Book of approved animal drugs, it may no longer be commercially available in the United States.

The Association of Racing Commissioners International (ARCI) has designated this drug as a class 4 substance. Use of this drug may not be allowed in certain animal competitions. Check rules and regulations or contact local racing authorities for further guidance before entering in a competition while this medication is being administered. See ***Appendix*** for more information.

Flumethasone Injection: 0.5 mg/mL in 100 mL vials; *Flucort*® *Solution*; (Rx). FDA-approved for use in dogs, cats, and horses. NADA #030-414

Flumethasone Suspension: 2 mg/mL; *Anaprime*® Suspension; (Rx). FDA-approved for intra-articular use in horses. NADA #036-211

Flumethasone Tablets: 0.0625 mg; *Flucort*®; (Rx). FDA-approved for use in dogs and cats. NADA #030-415

Flumethasone Suspension: 2 mg/mL; *Fluosmin*® Suspension; (Rx). FDA-approved for use in dogs. (NADA #036-212)

HUMAN-LABELED PRODUCTS: NONE

References

For the complete list of references, see **wiley.com/go/budde/plumb**

Flunixin

(floo-***nix***-in) *Banamine*®

Nonsteroidal Anti-Inflammatory Agent

Prescriber Highlights

- ▶ Veterinary-only NSAID used primarily in large-animal species
- ▶ Use with caution in patients with pre-existing GI ulcers or renal, hepatic, or hematologic diseases; in horses with colic, flunixin may mask the behavior and cardiopulmonary signs associated with endotoxemia or intestinal devitalization.
- ▶ Use in small animal species has been largely supplanted by FDA-approved agents or those with better adverse effect profiles in target species.
- ▶ If first dose is ineffective for pain control, subsequent doses are unlikely to be of benefit.
- ▶ Adverse effects in horses and cattle: rare anaphylaxis (especially after rapid IV administration); IM injections (extra-label in food animals) may cause pain and swelling; myonecrosis reported in some horses

Uses/Indications

In the United States, flunixin is FDA-approved for use in horses, cattle, and swine; it is approved for use in dogs in other countries. FDA-approved indications for its use in horses include alleviation of inflammation and pain associated with musculoskeletal disorders and alleviation of visceral pain associated with colic. In cattle, the injectable form of flunixin is FDA-approved for the control of pyrexia associated with bovine respiratory disease (BRD), endotoxemia, and acute bovine mastitis and for the control of inflammation in endotoxemia. The transdermal flunixin formulation is FDA-approved to control pyrexia associated with BRD and control of pain associated with foot rot in steers, beef heifers, beef cows, beef bulls intended for slaughter, and replacement dairy heifers under 20 months of age. In swine, flunixin is FDA-approved for controlling pyrexia associated with swine respiratory disease. In ruminants, there is anecdotal evidence that flunixin is a better analgesic for visceral pain rather than for musculoskeletal pain.

Flunixin has also been suggested for many other indications in horses including foal diarrhea, shock, colitis, respiratory disease, postrace treatment, and pre- and postophthalmic and general surgery. In cattle, it may be used to treat acute respiratory disease, acute coliform mastitis with endotoxic shock, and pain (eg, downer cow); in swine, it may be used to treat agalactia/hypogalactia, lameness, and piglet diarrhea. In dogs and cats, flunixin has been used historically for analgesia and as an antipyretic, and in dogs undergoing ophthalmic surgery[1,2]; however, this therapy is no longer recommended with the availability of approved NSAIDs for these species. There may still be a limited use for flunixin in dogs undergoing ophthalmic surgery; use with caution.

The combination product containing florfenicol and flunixin is FDA-approved for SC use in beef and nonlactating dairy cattle (not veal calves) for treatment of BRD associated with *Mannheimia haemolytica*, *Pasteurella multocida*, *Histophilus somni*, *Mycoplasma bovis*, and to control BRD-associated pyrexia.[3]

The combination product containing oxytetracycline and flunixin is FDA-approved for SC or IM use in beef and nonlactating dairy cattle for the treatment of bacterial pneumonia associated with *Pasteurella* spp and for the control of associated pyrexia.[4]

Pharmacology/Actions

Flunixin is a potent inhibitor of cyclooxygenase and, like other NSAIDs, it exhibits analgesic, anti-inflammatory, and antipyretic activity. Flunixin does not appreciably alter GI motility in horses and may improve hemodynamics in animals with septic shock.

Pharmacokinetics

In the horse, flunixin is rapidly absorbed following oral administration, with an average bioavailability of 80% and peak serum levels in 30 minutes. Oral bioavailability is good when the injection is mixed with molasses and given orally. The onset of action is generally within 2 hours; peak response occurs between 12 to 16 hours, and the duration of action lasts up to 30 hours. Flunixin is highly bound to plasma proteins (ie, greater than 99% in cattle, 92% in dogs, 87% in horses). Volume of distribution ranges from ≈0.15 L/kg in horses to 0.78 L/kg in cattle, and flunixin persists in inflammatory tissue. Elimination in horses is primarily via hepatic routes by biliary excretion. Serum half-lives after IV administration have been determined as follows: dogs, ≈3.7 hours; horses, ≈1.6 to 4.2 hours; cattle, ≈3.1 to 8.1 hours; and swine, ≈6 to 8 hours. Flunixin is detectable in equine urine for at least 48 hours after a dose.

In cattle, absorption of flunixin transdermal solution is highly dependent on environmental temperature; higher temperatures can increase absorption, although dosage adjustments are not necessary.[5] The manufacturer states that treating cattle when the hide is wet or may get wet within 6 hours after dosing may affect absorption. Under experimental conditions with calves, rain was shown to reduce absorption of flunixin when administered within 30 minutes of light rain or within 4 hours of heavy rain.[6]

One study suggested that the pharmacokinetics and elimination of IV flunixin in milk differed between healthy cows and those with mastitis. The study also indicated that an extended withdrawal time may be needed in cows with mastitis.[7]

Flunixin transdermal solution in cattle has an average half-life of 8 hours in non-licking cattle compared to 9 hours in licking cattle.[5] Elimination of flunixin occurs through biliary excretion.

Contraindications/Precautions/Warnings

The only contraindication the manufacturer lists for flunixin use in horses is for patients with a history of hypersensitivity reactions to the drug. It is suggested, however, that flunixin be used cautiously in animals with renal, hepatic, or hematologic diseases, and in animals with suspected preexisting gastric erosions or ulcerations. When used to treat colic, flunixin may mask the behavioral and cardiopulmonary signs associated with endotoxemia or intestinal devitalization and must be used with caution.

Do not inject intra-arterially.

In horses with known or suspected equine gastric ulcer syndrome (EGUS), use should be avoided; single doses of flunixin will likely not result in catastrophic consequences, but repeated doses can exacerbate gastric ulcers.[8]

In cattle, the drug is contraindicated in animals that have shown hypersensitivity reactions. The IM route causes injection site muscle damage[9] and is extra-label in cattle; this route of administration has resulted in violative residues in the edible tissues of cattle sent to slaughter. Longer withdrawal times are required after IM use. Flunixin should not be used to move cattle to be shipped for slaughter. Cattle may lick the transdermal product; however, no dose adjustment is needed to account for this behavior. Do not treat cattle if hide is wet or may get wet within 6 hours after dosing.

Flunixin is not recommended in dogs and cats since safer, FDA-approved products are available.

Use of flunixin in birds is generally avoided as flunixin can have significant effects on renal function in some species.

Adverse Effects

When flunixin is used for pain, if the animal does not respond to an initial dose, additional doses will unlikely be effective and may increase the chance for toxicity. Following IM injection in horses, especially in the neck, localized swelling and tissue necrosis, induration, stiffness, and sweating have been reported; clinical signs are transient and generally do not require any treatment. Do not inject intra-arterially, as flunixin may cause CNS stimulation (hysteria), ataxia, hyperventilation, and muscle weakness. Flunixin appears to be a relatively safe agent for use in horses, but the potential exists for GI intolerance, hypoproteinemia, and hematologic abnormalities.

Horses have developed oral and gastric ulcers, anorexia, and depression when given high doses for prolonged periods (greater than 2 weeks). Although gastric ulceration is frequently observed in adult horses and foals, evidence of an association between this disease and administration of NSAIDs such as flunixin at recommended dosages is lacking. Giving prophylactic antiulcer medications to horses receiving therapeutic doses of NSAIDs is probably unnecessary in animals that are otherwise at low risk for gastric ulceration.[10]

In horses and cattle, rare anaphylactic-like reactions have been reported, primarily after rapid IV administration.[11] IM injections may rarely be associated with clostridial myonecrosis. Flunixin transdermal solution has been shown to irritate the skin and can potentially cause irreversible eye damage.

In swine, IM injection may result in local tissue damage,[12] which can persist for 28 days postinjection and result in trim loss at slaughter.

In dogs, GI distress is the most likely adverse reaction. Clinical signs may include vomiting, diarrhea, and ulceration with high doses or chronic use. There have been anecdotal reports of flunixin causing renal shutdown in dogs when used preoperatively at higher dosages.

In birds, flunixin has been shown to cause significant dose-related renal ischemia and nephrotoxicity.

Reproductive/Nursing Safety

Although reports of teratogenicity, effects on breeding performance, or gestation length have not been noted, flunixin should be used cautiously in pregnant animals.[11] Flunixin may delay parturition and prolong labor, increasing the risk of stillbirth. Flunixin use within 24 hours after parturition may lead to placental retention and metritis. Estrus may be delayed if flunixin is administered during the prostaglandin phase of the estrous cycle. Flunixin improved pregnancy rate in embryo-transfer beef cows without affecting return to estrus in nonpregnant cows.[13] While flunixin is not recommended for use in breeding bulls (lack of reproductive safety data), data in breeding stallions have shown no detrimental effect on spermatogenesis.

Flunixin is contraindicated within 48 hours of expected parturition, as it can delay parturition or increase the risk for stillbirth due to prolonged labor.

Overdose/Acute Toxicity

No clinical case reports of flunixin overdoses were discovered. Minimal toxicity was noted in horses or cattle at up to 5 times the labeled dosage. It is suggested that acute overdoses be handled using established protocols of GI decontamination (if oral ingestion and procedure is practical or possible) and treating the patient supportively.

Gastric ulceration is a distinct possibility in horses that have received overdoses of flunixin. Consider using antiulcer medications in overdosed horses.

Hematuria and occult fecal blood were observed in 6-month-old beef cattle receiving up to 5 times the label dose of the transdermal product for 3 consecutive days (3 times the label frequency).[5] These findings were also noted on occasion in cattle given 3 and 5 times the label injectable dose for 9 days.[11] Dose-related dermal and epidermal necrosis occurred at topical application sites; abomasal erosions and ulceration were noted on pathology.[5]

For patients that have experienced or are suspected to have experienced an overdose, it is strongly encouraged to consult with one of the 24-hour poison consultation centers that specialize in providing information specific for veterinary patients. For general information related to overdose and toxin exposures, as well as contact information for poison control centers, refer to ***Appendix***.

Drug Interactions

Drug/drug interactions have not been appreciably studied for flunixin, and the label does not mention any drug interactions. However, the following drug interactions have either been reported or are theoretical in humans or animals receiving other NSAIDs and may be of significance in veterinary patients receiving flunixin.

- **ACE Inhibitors** (eg, **benazepril, enalapril**): Some NSAIDs can reduce effects on blood pressure.
- **Aspirin**: When aspirin is used concurrently with NSAIDs, plasma levels of the NSAID could decrease, and the likelihood of GI adverse effects (eg, blood loss) could increase.
- **Corticosteroids** (eg, **dexamethasone, prednis(ol)one**): Concurrent use may increase the risk for GI toxicity.
- **Cyclosporine**: NSAIDs may increase cyclosporine blood levels and increase the risk for nephrotoxicity.
- **Digoxin**: NSAIDs may increase serum levels of digoxin; use with caution in patients with severe cardiac failure.
- **Fluoroquinolones**: Enrofloxacin has been shown in dogs to increase the area under the curve (AUC) and elimination half-life of flunixin, and flunixin increases the AUC and elimination half-life of enrofloxacin.[14] Enrofloxacin and flunixin did not interact in rabbits.[15] Flunixin significantly increased moxifloxacin elimination half-life and total drug exposure (AUC). Applicability to other fluoroquinolones is unknown.[16]
- **Loop Diuretics** (eg, **furosemide**): NSAIDs may reduce the saluretic and diuretic effects of furosemide.
- **Methotrexate**: Serious toxicity has occurred when NSAIDs have been used concomitantly with methotrexate; use together with caution.
- **Nephrotoxic Agents** (eg, **aminoglycosides, amphotericin B, cisplatin**): Potential for increased risk for nephrotoxicity if used with NSAIDs
- **Oxytetracycline**: Flunixin increased clearance of oxytetracycline in dairy goats.[17]
- **Phenylbutazone**: Phenylbutazone administration 24 hours prior to flunixin increased flunixin clearance. Flunixin administration prior to phenylbutazone prolonged suppression of prostaglandin E2 and thromboxane B2.[18]
- **Probenecid**: May cause a significant increase in serum levels and half-life of some NSAIDs
- **Warfarin**: Use with NSAIDs may increase the risk for bleeding.

Dosages

HORSES:

Alleviation of inflammation and pain associated with musculoskeletal disorders and alleviation of visceral pain associated with colic (label dosage; FDA-approved):

a) Injectable: 1.1 mg/kg IV or IM once daily for up to 5 days.[11] For colic cases, use IV route; may re-dose when necessary.
b) Oral paste: 1.1 mg/kg PO (see markings on syringe—calibrated in 250 lb weight increments) once daily.[19] One syringe will treat a 453 kg (1000 lb) horse for 3 days. Do not exceed 5 days of consecutive therapy.

Decreasing pain, inflammation, and edema in laminitis (extra-label): 0.5 – 1.1 mg/kg IV or PO every 8 to 12 hours. A dose of 0.25 mg/kg can be administered IV every 8 hours to interrupt eicosanoid production associated with endotoxemia.[20]

Adjunctive treatment of uveitis in foals (extra-label): 0.5 – 1 mg/kg (route not noted) twice daily[21]

CATTLE:

Flunixin as a single agent (label dosage; FDA-approved):

a) **Control of pyrexia associated with respiratory disease, endotoxemia, and acute bovine mastitis and for the control of inflammation associated with endotoxemia (injectable)**: 1.1 – 2.2 mg/kg (0.5 – 1 mg/lb, 1 – 2 mL/100 lb) given slow IV either once a day as a single dose or divided into 2 doses every 12 hours for up to 3 days.[11] Avoid rapid IV administration.
b) **Control of pyrexia associated with bovine respiratory disease and the control of pain associated with foot rot (transdermal)**: Single application of 3.3 mg/kg (1.5 mg/lb, 3 mL/100 lb) topically in a narrow strip along the dorsal midline from withers to tailhead.[5] Round doses up to the nearest weight increment on dosing chamber located on the product.

Flunixin in combination with florfenicol for treatment of bovine respiratory disease (BRD) associated with *Mannheimia haemolytica, Pasteurella multocida,* and *Histophilus somni,* and control of BRD-associated pyrexia in beef and nonlactating dairy cattle (label dosage; FDA-approved): flunixin 2.2 mg/kg with florfenicol 40 mg/kg (6 mL/100 lb where each mL contains flunixin 16.5 mg with florfenicol 300 mg) SC once.[3] Do not administer more than 10 mL at each site. The injection should be given only in the neck. Injection sites other than the neck have not been evaluated.

Flunixin in combination with oxytetracycline for treatment of bacterial pneumonia associated with *Pasteurella* spp and for the control of associated pyrexia in beef and nonlactating dairy cattle (label dosage; FDA-approved): 1 mL/10 kg (22 lb) equals flunixin 2 mg/kg (0.9 mg/lb) with oxytetracycline 30 mg/kg (13.6 mg/lb) IM or SC once.[4] Do not administer more than 10 L/injection site (1-2 mL/site in small calves). Drug combination recommended where re-treatment of calves and yearlings is impractical because of husbandry conditions, such as cattle on range, or where repeated restraint is inadvisable.

Analgesic using flunixin as a single agent (extra-label): 1.1 – 2.2 mg/kg IV every 6 to 12 hours; recommend 72-hour milk withdrawal at this dose rate.[22]

SHEEP, GOATS:

Analgesic (extra-label): 1 – 2 mg/kg IV once daily (every 24 hours); oral paste has also been used at 1 – 4 mg/kg PO once daily[23]

SWINE:

Controlling pyrexia associated with swine respiratory disease (label dosage; FDA-approved): 2.2 mg/kg IM once, only in the neck musculature with a maximum of 10 mL/site[12]

FERRETS:

Analgesic/anti-inflammatory (extra-label): 0.5 – 2 mg/kg PO or IM once daily[24]

RABBITS, RODENTS, & SMALL MAMMALS:

a) Rabbits: 1.1 mg/kg SC, IM, or IV every 12 to 24 hours[25]
b) Rabbits: 1.1 mg/kg SC or IM every 12 hours; Rodents: 2.5 mg/kg SC or IM every 12 hours[26]
c) Chinchillas: 1 – 3 mg/kg SC every 12 hours; Guinea pigs: 2.5 – 5 mg/kg SC every 12 hours; Gerbils, mice, rats, hamsters: 2.5 mg/kg SC every 12 to 24 hours[27]

Monitoring

- Analgesic/anti-inflammatory effects

- Body temperature
- GI effects in dogs
- Periodic CBC and fecal occult blood testing with chronic use in horses

Client Information

- If injecting IM, do not inject into neck muscles (except swine).
- The IM route is extra-label in cattle and has resulted in violative residues in the edible tissues of cattle sent to slaughter. Longer withdrawal times are required after IM use.
- Flunixin should not be used in cattle to be shipped for slaughter.
- Flunixin transdermal solution should not be used if hide is wet or may get wet in the 6 hours after dosing.
- Dosage adjustment of the transdermal solution for environmental temperatures is not necessary. Cattle may be permitted to lick the solution without compromising its effectiveness or increasing the risk for side effects.
- Flunixin transdermal solution may cause severe and potentially irreversible eye damage or skin irritation. Users should wear gloves and appropriate eye protection, as well as clothing that will prevent skin contact with the transdermal solution. In case of accidental eye contact, flush eyes immediately with water and seek medical attention. In case of accidental skin contact, wash skin thoroughly with soap and water. Wash hands after use.

Chemistry/Synonyms

Flunixin meglumine, a nonsteroidal anti-inflammatory agent, is a highly substituted derivative of nicotinic acid, and is unique structurally when compared to other NSAIDs. It occurs as a white to off-white powder that is soluble in water and alcohol. The chemical name for flunixin is 3-pyridine-carboxylic acid.

Flunixin may also be known as 3-pyridine-carboxylic acid, flunixin meglumine, Sch-14714, *Banamine*®, *Flumeglumine*®, *Finadyne*®, *Flu-Nix*®*D*, *Flunixamine*®, *Flunixiject*®, *Flunizine*®, *Prevail*®, *Suppressor*®, and *Vedagesic*®.

Storage/Stability

All flunixin products should be stored between 2°C and 30°C (36°F-86°F). Flunixin transdermal solution should be used within 6 months of first opening. Vials for injection should be used within 28 days of first puncture, punctured a maximum of 10 times.

The combination product with florfenicol (*Resflor Gold*®) should not be stored above 30°C (86°F). Once the vial is entered, it should be used within 28 days. The 500 mL vial should not be punctured more than 10 times.

Compatibility/Compounding Considerations

It has been recommended that flunixin meglumine injection not be mixed with other drugs because of unknown compatibilities.

Dosage Forms/Regulatory Status

VETERINARY-LABELED PRODUCTS:

NOTE: Individual products may be FDA-approved and labeled for different species, lactation status, different routes of administration (IV, IM). Refer to the specific product label for more information. The ARCI (Racing Commissioners International) has designated flunixin as a class 4 substance. See ***Appendix*** for more information. Use of this drug may not be allowed in certain animal competitions. Check rules and regulations before entering in a competition while this medication is being administered. Contact local racing authorities for further guidance.

Flunixin Meglumine for Injection: 50 mg/mL in 50 mL, 100 mL, and 250 mL vials; *Banamine*®, generic; (Rx). Products may be FDA-approved for use in horses (not for use in horses intended for food) and beef and dairy cattle (IV use only; not for use in dry dairy cows or veal calves). Depending on product, when used as labeled, withdrawal in cattle occurs as follows: Milk: 36 hours; Slaughter: 4 days (US).

Flunixin Meglumine Oral Paste: 1500 mg/syringe in 30 g syringes in boxes of 6; *Banamine*® *Paste*; (Rx). FDA-approved for use in horses

Flunixin Meglumine for Injection: 50 mg/mL in 100 mL vials; *Banamine*®*-S*; (Rx). FDA-approved for IM use in swine; slaughter withdrawal = 12 days

Flunixin Transdermal Solution: 50 mg/mL in 100 mL, 250 mL, and 1 L multiple-dose bottles; *Banamine*® *Transdermal;* (Rx). FDA-approved for topical use in cattle/steers, beef heifers, beef cows, beef bulls intended for slaughter, and replacement dairy heifers under 20 months of age. Do not slaughter within 8 days of last treatment. Not for use in female dairy cattle 20 months of age or older, including dry dairy cows. Use in these cattle may cause drug residues in milk and/or in calves born to these cows or heifers. Not for use in suckling beef calves, dairy calves, and veal calves. A withdrawal period has not been established in preruminating calves.

Combination Products:

Flunixin 16.5 mg/mL with Florfenicol 300 mg/mL injection in 100 mL, 250 mL, and 500 mL vials; *Resflor Gold*®; (Rx). FDA-approved for use in beef and nonlactating dairy cattle. Do not slaughter within 38 days of last treatment. Not for use in female dairy cattle 20 months of age or older or calves to be processed for veal. Use may cause milk residues. A withdrawal period has not been established in preruminating calves.

Flunixin 20 mg/mL (as flunixin meglumine) with oxytetracycline 300 mg/mL in 100 mL, 250 mL, and 500 mL vials; *Hexasol*®; (Rx). FDA-approved in beef and nonlactating dairy cattle. Do not slaughter within 21 days of last treatment. Not for use in female dairy cattle 20 months of age or older, including dry dairy cows. Use may cause milk residues. A withdrawal period has not been established for this product in preruminating calves.

HUMAN-LABELED PRODUCTS: NONE

References

For the complete list of references, see **wiley.com/go/budde/plumb**

Fluorouracil

(flure-oh-***yoor***-a-sill) *Adrucil*®

Antineoplastic Agent

For ophthalmic uses, refer to ***Ophthalmic***

Prescriber Highlights

- Used in dogs for susceptible tumors, including GI adenocarcinoma, anal sac adenocarcinoma, nasal adenocarcinoma, and sun-induced squamous cell carcinoma. This agent can also be given intralesionally or topically to horses with skin tumors.
- Contraindications: Do **NOT** use fluorouracil in any form with cats or in patients with known hypersensitivity, poor nutritional states, bone marrow suppression, or serious infections.
- Known teratogen
- Adverse effects include dose-dependent myelosuppression, GI toxicity, and neurotoxicity
- The National Institute for Occupational Safety and Health (NIOSH) classifies fluorouracil as a hazardous drug; use appropriate precautions when handling.

Uses/Indications

Fluorouracil is a chemotherapeutic agent that has been used for canine mammary carcinoma (in combination with doxorubicin and cyclophosphamide—AC or FAC protocol), dermal squamous cell carcinoma, and GI tract tumors. One study described the use of fluorouracil in combination with carboplatin in dogs for various carcinomas; the overall response rate was 43%.[1] It is also used topically and for intralesional injection with epinephrine for certain skin neoplasms (squamous cell carcinoma, melanoma, sarcoid) in horses. Use of fluorouracil in horses with cutaneous and nonperiocular SCC and sarcoids haves demonstrated efficacy with repeated intralesional injections and topical administration.[2–4]

Pharmacology/Actions

Fluorouracil is a pyrimidine analogue antimetabolite. The drug is converted via intracellular mechanisms to active monophosphate and triphosphate metabolites which interfere with DNA and RNA synthesis, inhibit cell growth, and promote cell death.[5]

Pharmacokinetics

Following IV administration, fluorouracil is rapidly removed from the systemic circulation (plasma half-life is about 15 minutes in humans) and primarily distributed into tumor cells, intestinal mucosa, liver, and bone marrow. The drug is predominantly metabolized by the liver and is excreted via the lungs and urine, while ≈15% of the dose is excreted unchanged into the urine.

Contraindications/Precautions/Warnings

Fluorouracil has a very narrow therapeutic index and should be used only by clinicians with experience using cancer chemotherapeutic agents. Fluorouracil is contraindicated in patients with known hypersensitivity, poor nutritional states, bone marrow suppression, or concurrent serious infections. It should be used with caution in patients with severe renal or hepatic impairment.

Cats develop a severe, potentially fatal neurotoxicity when given fluorouracil. Do **NOT** use in cats in any form. Severe, life-threatening toxicities have developed when pets have licked areas of topical application.

The National Institute for Occupational Safety and Health (NIOSH) classifies fluorouracil as a hazardous drug; personal protective equipment (PPE) should be used accordingly to minimize the risk for exposure.

Do not confuse fluorouracil with flucytosine. Fluorouracil is considered a high alert medication (medication that requires special safeguards to reduce the risk for errors).[6] Consider instituting practices such as redundant drug dosage and volume checking and special alert labels.

Adverse Effects

In dogs, fluorouracil causes dose-dependent myelosuppression, GI toxicity (diarrhea, GI ulceration/sloughing, stomatitis), and neurotoxicity (seizures). Fluorouracil has a very narrow therapeutic index and should be used only by clinicians with experience using cancer chemotherapeutic agents. Additionally, cases of heart failure, severe mucositis/stomatitis/esophagopharyngitis, and hyperammonemic encephalopathy in the absence of liver disease have developed in humans following fluorouracil treatment.[7]

In humans, fluorouracil can increase cellular thiamine metabolism, inducing or exacerbating thiamine deficiency[8]; application to veterinary patients is unknown.

Reproductive/Nursing Safety

The drug is a known teratogen and has demonstrated fetal malformations (eg, cleft palate, skeletal defects) and embryolethality in laboratory animals. Its use during pregnancy should be weighed against any risks to offspring.

It is not known whether fluorouracil is excreted in milk. Because fluorouracil inhibits DNA, RNA, and protein synthesis, milk replacer should be considered if the dam requires fluorouracil.

Overdose/Acute Toxicity

Oral ingestions of topical products have occurred in dogs and cats. Toxic doses in dogs can be as little as 5 mg/kg, and doses greater than or equal to 40 mg/kg are reported to be uniformly fatal.[9] The LD_{50} in dogs following IV fluorouracil administration is 31.5 mg/kg. Signs at lower doses include mild GI irritation and vomiting. Seizures and death have been reported at doses as low as 10.3 mg/kg, and survival in dogs may be as low as 25%. The fatality rate in dogs was 65% following toxic exposure to flururacil.[10]

Very small ingestions can reportedly cause death in cats. Clinical signs may be seen within 30 minutes to 6 hours after ingestion; death has been reported in 7 hours. Clinical signs include acute nausea, vomiting, hemorrhagic diarrhea, abdominal pain, GI sloughing, ataxia, severe and non-responsive seizures, and severe dose-dependent myelosuppression affecting all cell lines. Severe metabolic acidosis and signs of multi-organ failure can also be seen.[11]

Should oral ingestion occur, aggressive GI decontamination with GI protection is recommended but may not be effective due to the rapid onset of toxicity. Treatment is primarily supportive and can include antiemetics, anticonvulsants, and fluid support. Seizure control with benzodiazepines, levetiracetam, or general anesthesia is often required.[12,13] Pain relief and body temperature control are important. Use broad-spectrum antibiotics to prevent secondary bacterial infections, and if bone marrow suppression develops, colony growth stimulating factors (eg, ***Filgrastim***) can be considered to stimulate stem cell proliferation in dogs. Complete blood counts should be routinely performed every 3 to 4 days for at least 18 days, as it may take up to 3 weeks before all cell lines return to normal.[11] Patients given an accidental parenteral overdose should undergo intensive hematologic monitoring for at least 4 weeks and be supported as required.

Uridine triacetate has been used as a successful antidote in humans, but it is not used in veterinary medicine due to the cost and administration requirements. Fluorouracil is dialyzable, but the rapid onset of toxicity limits its effectiveness.

For patients that have experienced or are suspected of having experienced an overdose, consultation with a 24-hour poison consultation center specializing in providing veterinary-specific information is recommended. For general information related to overdose and toxin exposures, as well as contact information for poison control centers, refer to ***Appendix.***

Drug Interactions

The following drug interactions have either been reported or are theoretical in humans or animals receiving fluorouracil and may be of significance in veterinary patients. Unless otherwise noted, use together is not necessarily contraindicated, but weigh the potential risks and perform additional monitoring when appropriate.

- **CYP2C9 Substrates** (eg, **diclofenac**): Fluorouracil may decrease the metabolism of CYP2C9 substrates.
- **Folic Acid/Leucovorin**: May increase the toxic effects of fluorouracil
- **Leflunomide**: Concurrent or sequential use of leflunomide without following a washout procedure may increase risk for myelosuppression and infections; avoid combination when possible.
- **Metronidazole**: May increase fluorouracil concentration and risk for toxicity
- **Myelosuppressive Agents** (eg, **antineoplastics, immunosuppressants, iron chelators**): Concurrent use with other bone marrow depressant medications may result in additive myelosuppression; avoid combination when possible.
- **Vaccines** (live and inactivated): Fluorouracil may diminish vaccine efficacy and enhance adverse effects of vaccines.

Laboratory Considerations

Fluorouracil may cause increases in **alkaline phosphatase, serum transaminase, serum bilirubin**, and **lactate dehydrogenase**.

Dosages

NOTE: Because of the potential toxicity of this drug to patients, veterinary personnel, and clients, and since chemotherapy indications, treatment protocols, and monitoring and safety guidelines often change, the following dosages should be used only as a general guide. Consultation with a veterinary oncologist and referral to current veterinary oncology references[14–18] are strongly recommended. All doses are extra-label.

DOGS:

NOTE: Do not confuse mg/m² with mg/kg dosages.

Canine mammary carcinoma (in combination with cyclophosphamide and/or doxorubicin AC or FAC protocol), dermal squamous cell carcinoma, GI adenocarcinoma, anal sac adenocarcinoma, and nasal adenocarcinoma: 150 mg/m² IV weekly, or 5 – 10 mg/kg IV weekly[19–24]

Mesothelioma: Initially, 150 – 200 mg/m² IV weekly for 4 weeks, then 150 – 200 mg/m² IV every 2 weeks[25]

Canine soft tissue sarcoma; postsurgical, incisional injection: 150 mg/m² was injected along the surgical scar or in different parallel sites of the open wound to provide uniform distribution, using a 22-gauge needle attached to a 5-mL Luer lock syringe. Multiple injections may be needed to cover the treatment field.[26]

In combination with carboplatin to treat various carcinomas: Fluorouracil 150 mg/m² IV as a slow push followed by carboplatin 200 mg/m² IV over 10 minutes 1 hour after fluorouracil administration.[1]

HORSES:

Intralesional injection for squamous cell carcinoma (SCC), melanomas, sarcoids:

a) Fluorouracil can be injected intralesionally at doses of 1 – 3 mL per tumor site depending on the size of the tumor. Epinephrine is typically added to the injection at a ratio of 1 part epinephrine to 10 parts fluorouracil. It can also be mixed with sterile sesame seed oil (1:1) immediately prior to injection. Generally, this combination can be successful for the resolution of small sarcoids and SCC but is often ineffective for melanoma. The maximum systemic dosage is ≈750 mg (15 mL of 50 mg/mL fluorouracil injection) for an average horse.[27,28]
b) 50 mg/cm³ injected intralesionally a single time[2] or every 2 weeks until resolution occurs[4]

Cutaneous neoplasia using a topical formulation (extra-label): Fluorouracil 5% cream administered topically to affected area once daily for 4 to 6 weeks[3]

Monitoring

- Baseline and periodic CBC with platelet counts (in humans, nadirs usually occur between days 9 and 14 with recovery by day 30)
- Baseline and periodic serum chemistry profiles
- GI and CNS adverse effects

Client Information

- Fluorouracil is a chemotherapy (anticancer) drug. The drug can be hazardous to other animals and people that come in contact with it. On the day your animal gets the drug and then for a few days afterward, handle all bodily waste (urine, feces, litter), blood, or vomit only while wearing disposable gloves. Seal the waste in a plastic bag and then place both the bag and gloves in with the regular trash.
- If applying fluorouracil to the skin of your animal, wear disposable gloves, and wash your hands immediately after each use. Take care to avoid contact with the administration site.
- Fluorouracil must NEVER be used in cats.
- Bone marrow depression can occur. The greatest effects on bone marrow usually occur within a few weeks after treatment. Your veterinarian will do blood tests to watch for this, but if you see bleeding, bruising, fever (indicating an infection), or if your animal becomes tired easily, contact your veterinarian right away.
- Clients must understand the importance of immediately reporting any signs associated with toxicity (eg, abnormal bleeding, bruising, depression, infection, shortness of breath, changes in urination). Fluorouracil can be very toxic to the nervous system (seizures, convulsions) and to the gastrointestinal tract (vomiting and gastrointestinal upset).
- This medicine is considered to be a hazardous drug as defined by the National Institute for Occupational Safety and Health (NIOSH). Talk with your veterinarian or pharmacist about the use of personal protective equipment when handling this medicine.

Chemistry/Synonyms

Fluorouracil (5-FU), a pyrimidine antagonist antineoplastic agent, occurs as a white, practically odorless, crystalline powder. It is sparingly soluble in water and slightly soluble in alcohol. The commercially available injection's pH is adjusted to 8.6 to 9.4 and may be colorless or slightly yellow in color.

Fluorouracil may also be known as 5-fluorouracil, fluorouracilo, fluorouracilum, 5-FU, NSC-19893, Ro-2-9757, and WR-69596; many trade names are available, including *Adrucil*®, *Carac*®, *Efudex*®, *Fluoroplex*®, *Tolak*®.

Storage/Stability

Store the injection between 20°C and 25°C (68°F and 77°F); avoid freezing and exposure to light.

Compatibility/Compounding Considerations

Slight color changes in the solution can occur during storage. If a precipitate forms, the solution can be gently heated to 60°C (140°F) to dissolve. Cool to body temperature before administering. If unsuccessful in dissolving the precipitate, discard. According to the manufacturer, vials should be used within 4 hours of initial entry, and solutions for infusion should be administered immediately. However, available data suggest that both undiluted and diluted solutions remain stable for longer periods.[29,30]

Dosage Forms/Regulatory Status

VETERINARY-LABELED PRODUCTS: NONE

HUMAN-LABELED PRODUCTS:

Fluorouracil Solution for Injection: 50 mg/mL in 10 mL, 20 mL, 50 mL, and 100 mL vials; *Adrucil*®; generic; (Rx).

Fluorouracil Cream: 0.5%, 1% and 5% in 30g and 40 g tubes; generic; (Rx)

Fluorouracil is also available in topical solutions.

References

For the complete list of references, see **wiley.com/go/budde/plumb**

Fluoxetine

(***floo-ox**-e-teen*) *Prozac®, Reconcile®*

Selective Serotonin Reuptake Inhibitor (SSRI)

Prescriber Highlights

- ▶ FDA-approved for use in dogs, and used extra-label in cats and horses for a variety of behavior disorders
- ▶ Contraindicated in animals with a known hypersensitivity to the drug and in those receiving monoamine oxidase inhibitors (MAOIs)
- ▶ Use with caution in animals with diabetes mellitus or seizure disorders; dose may need to be reduced for animals with severe hepatic impairment
- ▶ Most common adverse effects in dogs include anorexia, lethargy, GI effects, anxiety/restlessness, and vocalization. Seizures and aggressive behavior have been reported. Cats may show behavior changes (eg, anxiety, irritability, sleep disturbances, anorexia, changes in elimination patterns).
- ▶ Many potential drug interactions

Uses/Indications

Fluoxetine is a veterinary FDA-approved product labeled for treatment of canine separation anxiety in conjunction with a behavior modification plan.[1] Fluoxetine may be beneficial for treatment of canine (and feline) aggression,[2-4] stereotypic behaviors (and other compulsive behaviors),[5,6] and anxiety.[7-9] It also may be useful for treatment of inappropriate elimination in cats.[10-12]

Pharmacology/Actions

Fluoxetine is a highly selective inhibitor of the presynaptic reuptake of serotonin in the CNS with negligible effects on other neurotransmitters (eg, dopamine, norepinephrine). In dogs and cats, fluoxetine has anxiolytic and anticompulsive effects and may reduce aggressive behaviors by decreasing reactivity.

Pharmacokinetics

In dogs, fluoxetine is well absorbed after oral administration, and the bioavailability is 72% to 88%.[1,13] Fluoxetine chewable tablets caused 15% greater fluoxetine exposure (area under the curve [AUC]) as compared with fluoxetine-filled gelatin capsules.[1] The presence of food altered the rate, but not the extent, of absorption. Oral capsules and liquid are bioequivalent.

Fluoxetine and its principal metabolite, norfluoxetine (active), are distributed throughout the body, with the highest concentrations found in the lungs and liver. CNS concentrations can be detected within 1 hour of administration. Fluoxetine is primarily metabolized in the liver by CYP450 to a variety of metabolites, including norfluoxetine (active). Fluoxetine and norfluoxetine are eliminated slowly. In dogs, the average elimination half-life for fluoxetine and norfluoxetine is 6 to 18 hours and 49 hours, respectively.[1,13] Renal impairment does not significantly affect elimination rates, but liver impairment can decrease clearance rates.

In cats, the elimination half-life of fluoxetine and norfluoxetine is 47 and 52 hours, respectively, after oral administration.[14] When fluoxetine was applied transdermally (15% in a PLO gel) to cats, bioavailability was ≈10% of the oral route.[14] An alternative transdermal preparation (lipoderm base) produced significantly lower fluoxetine and norfluoxetine concentrations as compared with oral fluoxetine, and the authors theorized that the limited surface area on a cat's pinnae may limit the amount of drug that can be delivered by the transdermal route.[15]

In horses, the time to reach maximum concentration was 1.5 hours and half-life was 15.6 hours; norfluoxetine was not detected in any sample.[16]

In humans, fluoxetine is ≈95% bound to plasma proteins. The elimination half-life of fluoxetine and norfluoxetine is ≈2 to 3 days and ≈7 to 9 days, respectively.

Contraindications/Precautions/Warnings

The manufacturer states that fluoxetine should not be used in dogs with epilepsy or a history of seizures and should not be given in combination with drugs that lower the seizure threshold (eg, acepromazine, chlorpromazine). **NOTE**: No published evidence exists to support the claim that phenothiazines alone lower the seizure threshold.[17] It is not known if the use of fluoxetine in combination with this class of drugs may lower the seizure threshold, and SSRIs are recommended for treatment of anxiety and depression in humans with epilepsy.[18]

Fluoxetine is contraindicated in animals with a known hypersensitivity to it and in those receiving monoamine oxidase inhibitors (MAOIs; see ***Drug Interactions***). Although the veterinary label states that fluoxetine should not be used in the treatment of aggressive dogs, fluoxetine has safely and effectively reduced aggression in dogs.[2-4] Safe use has not been established in dogs younger than 6 months.

Fluoxetine should be used with caution in animals with diabetes mellitus because it may alter blood glucose concentrations.[1] Doses may need to be reduced in animals with severe hepatic impairment.

Because norfluoxetine has a long half-life, tapering the drug may only be necessary when an animal has been on the drug long term (ie, longer than 8 weeks)[19]; tapering the drug over a 3- to 5-week period has been recommended.[7] Because of its long half-life, the manufacturer recommends a 6-week washout after discontinuing fluoxetine and before starting medications that have significant interactions with fluoxetine or norfluoxetine.[1]

In humans, it is recommended to use a lower or less frequent dose in elderly patients due to risk for significant hyponatremia.[20]

Do not to confuse FLUoxetine with famotidine, FluVOXamine, or PARoxetine.

Adverse Effects

In multisite field trials in dogs, seizures were reported in some of the dogs treated with fluoxetine (0.4% to 2.5%); the absolute causality and incidence rate was not determined. Fluoxetine may cause lethargy (33%), vomiting (17%), diarrhea (10%), tremors (11%), restlessness (7%), and excessive vocalization (6%).[1] Anorexia (27%) and weight loss (30%) have occurred in dogs[1] but are usually transient and may be negated by starting the dog on a low dose and titrating up, which can temporarily increase the palatability of food. Some dogs have persistent anorexia that precludes further fluoxetine treatment. Aggressive behavior occurred in dogs at a rate similar to that in dogs that received a placebo.[1] Reducing the dose may eliminate or reduce the severity of adverse effects; returning to full dose may be tolerated following a dose reduction. Other reported adverse effects include mydriasis, panting, confusion, incoordination, and hypersalivation.

Cats may exhibit behavior changes (eg, anxiety, irritability, sleep disturbances), anorexia, and diarrhea or changes in elimination patterns. Skin irritation was noted with 2 different transdermal fluoxetine preparations.[14,15]

In humans, potential adverse effects are extensive and diverse, but those most commonly noted include anxiety, nervousness, insomnia, drowsiness, fatigue, dizziness, anorexia, nausea, rash, diarrhea, and sweating; seizures, hyponatremia, or hepatotoxicity are also possible. Epidemiology studies have noted an association between SSRI use and bleeding reactions, particularly when combined with other drugs (eg, NSAIDs, anticoagulants) that increase the risk for bleeding.[20] Approximately 15% of human patients discontinue treatment because of adverse effects.

Reproductive/Nursing Safety

Fluoxetine's safety during pregnancy has not been established. Studies to determine the effects of fluoxetine in breeding, pregnant, or lactating dogs or in animals younger than 6 months have not been conducted.[1] Fluoxetine crosses the placenta. Preliminary studies in rats demonstrated no overt teratogenic effects. In humans, SSRI use during the third trimester of pregnancy has been associated with neonatal complications.[20]

Fluoxetine is excreted in human milk (20% to 30% of plasma concentrations), and caution is advised in nursing patients. Clinical implications for nursing offspring are not clear.

Because safety has not been established in animals, this drug should only be used when the maternal benefits outweigh the potential risks to offspring.

Overdose/Acute Toxicity

The LD_{50} for rats is 452 mg/kg and for dogs is greater than 100 mg/kg, but a median dose of 15.9 mg/kg is reported to cause clinical signs of SSRI toxicosis in dogs.[21] In a study, 5 out of 6 dogs given an oral toxic dose developed seizures that immediately stopped after the dogs received diazepam IV. A retrospective study in cats found doses as low as 3.7 mg/kg caused clinical signs of toxicity.[22] In cats with SSRI toxicosis, only 24% exhibited clinical signs, including vomiting, diarrhea, agitation, and tremors. Approximately half the cats were hospitalized for a mean duration of 15 hours, and all cats survived.[22]

Common clinical signs associated with overdose include vomiting, hypersalivation, mydriasis, and vocalization.

Treatment for fluoxetine overdose consists of providing treatment based on clinical signs and supportive therapy. Gut-emptying techniques should be used when warranted and not contraindicated. Diazepam should be considered to treat seizures. Cyproheptadine can be used as a serotonin antagonist.

For patients that have experienced or are suspected to have experienced an overdose, consultation with a 24-hour poison consultation center specializing in providing veterinary-specific information is recommended. For general information related to overdose and toxin exposures, as well as contact information for poison control centers, refer to ***Appendix.***

Drug Interactions

The following drug interactions have either been reported or are theoretical in humans or animals receiving fluoxetine and may be of significance in veterinary patients. Unless otherwise noted, use together is not necessarily contraindicated, but the potential risks must be weighed and additional monitoring performed when appropriate.

- **ALPRAZOLAM**: Fluoxetine can increase alprazolam concentrations.
- **ANTICOAGULANTS** (eg, **clopidogrel, heparin, warfarin**): Concurrent use with fluoxetine has been associated with an increased risk for bleeding in humans.
- **ANTIPLATELET AGENTS** (eg, **aspirin, clopidogrel**): In humans, concurrent use with fluoxetine has been associated with an increased risk for bleeding.
- **BUSPIRONE**: Increased risk for serotonin syndrome
- **CYPROHEPTADINE**: May decrease or reverse the effects of SSRIs
- **DEXTROMETHORPHAN**: Serotonin syndrome-like adverse effects are possible.
- **DIAZEPAM**: Fluoxetine can prolong diazepam half-life.
- **DIURETICS**: Increased risk for hyponatremia
- **INSULIN**: May alter insulin requirements
- **ISONIAZID (INH)**: Increased risk for serotonin syndrome
- **MONOAMINE OXIDASE INHIBITORS** (**MAOIs**; eg, **amitraz, linezolid,** and, potentially, **selegiline**): High risk for serotonin syndrome; concurrent use is contraindicated in dogs. A 6-week washout period is required after fluoxetine is discontinued, and a 2-week washout period is needed if the MAOI is first discontinued.[1]
- **METHADONE**: In dogs, concurrent oral administration of fluoxetine may increase peak methadone concentration and exposure (AUC).[23]
- **NONSTEROIDAL ANTI-INFLAMMATORY DRUGS** (**NSAIDs**; eg, **carprofen, meloxicam, robenacoxib**): SSRIs may increase the risk for GI ulceration and bleeding.
- **PENTAZOCINE**: Serotonin syndrome-like adverse effects are possible.
- **PROPRANOLOL, METOPROLOL**: Fluoxetine may increase the plasma concentration of these beta-blockers; atenolol may be safer to use if fluoxetine is required.
- **ST. JOHN'S WORT**: Increased risk for serotonin syndrome
- **TRAMADOL**: SSRIs can inhibit the metabolism of tramadol to active metabolites, which may decrease its efficacy and increase the risk for toxicity (eg, serotonin syndrome, seizures).
- **TRICYCLIC ANTIDEPRESSANTS** (**TCA**; eg, **clomipramine, amitriptyline**): Fluoxetine may increase TCA blood concentrations and the risk for serotonin syndrome.
- **TRAZODONE**: Increased plasma concentrations of trazodone are possible; increased risk for serotonin syndrome

Laboratory Considerations

None were noted.

Dosages

DOGS:

Treatment for canine separation anxiety in conjunction with a behavior modification plan (label dosage; FDA-approved): 1 – 2 mg/kg PO once daily in conjunction with a behavior modification plan[1]

Adjunctive treatment for behavior disorders (eg, noise aversion, compulsive disorder, stereotypic behaviors, aggression) (extra-label): 1 – 2 mg/kg PO every 24 hours; doses as high as 4 mg/kg every 24 hours have been noted. **NOTE**: It may take 4 to 8 weeks before efficacy can be fully assessed.

CATS:

Adjunctive treatment for behavior disorders (eg, urine marking, separation anxiety, aggression) (extra-label): Recommended dosage in cats is typically 0.5 – 1.3 mg/kg PO every 24 hours[11,24]; treatment may be required for up to 8 weeks before full determination of efficacy. When using fluoxetine to treat urine marking, after 8 to 12 weeks of successful treatment, dose may be reduced gradually (≈25%) per week. If urine marking returns, dose can be increased to the last effective dose.

HORSES:

Facilitating stall rest or treatment of behavior-related problems (extra-label): 0.25 mg/kg PO once daily was reported by owners to be successful in facilitating stall rest and for anxious or fractious behaviors. Daily doses ranged from 0.15 – 0.54 mg/kg.[25]

Monitoring

- Efficacy (eg, control of unwanted behaviors)
- Adverse effects, including appetite (weight)

Client Information

- This medication should be used along with a behavior modification plan. Some improvement may be seen in the first week, but it may take several weeks to reach full effect and determine if this medicine is working.
- This medicine may be given with or without food. If your ani-

mal vomits or acts sick after receiving this medicine on an empty stomach, give future doses with food or a small treat. If vomiting continues, contact your veterinarian.

- Do not suddenly stop giving this medicine to your animal without your veterinarian's guidance.
- The most common side effects are drowsiness or sleepiness and reduced appetite. Rare serious side effects can include seizures and aggression. Contact your veterinarian immediately if these are noted.
- Overdoses can be serious. Keep fluoxetine out of reach of other animals and children.
- Tell your veterinarian if your animal has worn a flea and tick collar in the past 2 weeks. Do not use a flea and tick collar on your animal while this medicine is being administered without first talking to your veterinarian.

Chemistry/Synonyms

Fluoxetine, part of the phenylpropylamine-derivative antidepressant group, differs structurally and pharmacologically from the tricyclic and monoamine oxidase inhibitor antidepressants. Commercial forms contain fluoxetine hydrochloride and potency is expressed in mg fluoxetine. Fluoxetine HCl occurs as a white to off-white crystalline solid. Approximately 50 mg are soluble in 1 mL of water.

Fluoxetine may also be known as fluoxctini hydrochloridum and/or LY-110140; many trade names are available.

Storage/Stability

Store capsules and tablets in well-closed containers at room temperature (20°C-25°C [68°F-77°F]); excursions are permitted between 15°C to 30°C (59°F-86°F). Do not remove desiccant from the chewable tablet bottle. The oral liquid should be stored in tight, light-resistant containers at room temperature.

Compatibility/Compounding Considerations

Fluoxetine has been compounded into transdermal formulations, but studies demonstrating efficacy and safety are lacking.[14,15]

Dosage Forms/Regulatory Status

VETERINARY-LABELED PRODUCTS:

Fluoxetine Chewable Tablets: 8 mg, 16 mg, 32 mg, and 64 mg; *Reconcile*®; (Rx). FDA-approved (NADA # 141-272) for use in dogs.

The Association of Racing Commissioners International (ARCI) has designated this drug as a class 2 substance. Use of this drug may not be allowed in certain animal competitions. Check rules and regulations before entering in a competition while this medication is being administered. Contact local racing authorities for further guidance. See ***Appendix*** for more information.

HUMAN-LABELED PRODUCTS:

Fluoxetine HCl Oral Tablets: 10 mg and 20 mg; generic; (Rx)

Fluoxetine HCl Oral Capsules: 10 mg, 20 mg, and 40 mg; *Prozac*®, generic; (Rx)

Fluoxetine HCl Oral Delayed-release Capsules: 90 mg; generic; (Rx)

Fluoxetine HCl Oral Solution: 20 mg/5 mL (4 mg/mL; may contain alcohol, sucrose, benzoic acid) in 120 mL and 473 mL; *Prozac*®; generic; (Rx)

References

For the complete list of references, see **wiley.com/go/budde/plumb**

Fluralaner

(***floor***-ah-lan-er) *Bravecto*®

Isoxazoline Ectoparasiticide

Prescriber Highlights

- ► Insecticide and acaracide FDA-approved for use in dogs and cats
- ► Effective for 8 to 12 weeks against labeled parasites
- ► Chewable tablets should be administered with food.
- ► Adverse effects may include vomiting, diarrhea, inappetence, and lethargy.
- ► The FDA has warned that drugs in the isoxazoline class have the potential to cause neurologic adverse effects (eg, muscle tremors, ataxia, seizures) in dogs and cats. Use caution in animals with a history of seizures or other neurologic disorders.

Uses/Indications

For dogs and puppies 6 months of age and older weighing at least 2 kg (4.4 lb), fluralaner chewable tablets and topical solution (*Bravecto*®) are FDA-approved for the treatment and prevention of flea (*Ctenocephalides felis*) infestations; the treatment and control of tick infestations (*Ixodes scapularis* [black-legged tick], *Dermacentor variabilis* [American dog tick], and *Rhipicephalus sanguineus* [brown dog tick]) for 12 weeks; and for the treatment and control of *Amblyomma americanum* (Lone Star tick) infestations for 8 weeks.[1,2] Fluralaner chewable tablets that provide protection for 1 month (ie, *Bravecto*®*-1 Month*) for the same parasites and indications are FDA-approved for dogs and puppies weighing at least 2 kg (4.4 lb) and that are 8 weeks of age (6 months for *A americanum)* and older.[3] Fluralaner is effective as part of the treatment and control of flea allergy dermatitis in dogs.[4-6] Flea egg production is reduced by 100% within 48 hours of oral administration to dogs.[7] In other countries, fluralaner is also labeled for the treatment of flea (*C felis* and *Ctenocephalides canis*) and tick (*Ixodes ricinus, Rhipicephalus sanguineus,* and *Dermacentor reticulatus*) infestations in dogs.[8]

Fluralaner has been shown to be effective against generalized demodicosis in dogs, with studies showing no mites detectable at 56 and 84 days following a single oral dose[9] or following one or several doses for treatment of either adult- or juvenile-onset demodicosis.[8,10,11] Single oral or topical fluralaner treatment in dogs with naturally acquired *Sarcoptes scabiei* var *canis* infestation has resulted in a 100% reduction in mite counts 28 days posttreatment[12] and in clinical improvement within 14 to 21 days after a single oral dose.[8,11,13] Fluralaner has demonstrated efficacy in dogs against *Ixodes holocyclus*,[14] *Linognathus setosus*,[15] and *Otodectes cynotis*.[16] Fluralaner administered PO or topically has been shown to prevent transmission of *Babesia canis* from *D variabilis* ticks to dogs,[17,18] and *Ehrlichia canis* by *R sanguineus* ticks.[19]

A single dose of oral fluralaner killed greater than 99% of the insect *Triatoma infestans*, the vector of *Trypanosoma cruzi* (ie, Chagas disease, American trypanosomiasis), regardless of life stage, through 7 to 8 weeks posttreatment[20,21]; another study reported that 100% efficacy was demonstrated for up to 7 months.[22]

For cats and kittens 6 months of age and older weighing at least 1.2 kg (2.6 lb), fluralaner topical solution (*Bravecto*®) is FDA-approved for the treatment and prevention of flea infestations (*C felis*), for the treatment and control of *I scapularis* (black-legged tick) infestations for 12 weeks, and for the treatment and control of *D variabilis* (American dog tick) infestations for 8 weeks.[23] In other countries, fluralaner is also labeled for the treatment of *I ricinus* tick infestations in cats.[8] Fluralaner has also been used to treat *O cynotis*,[16] *Demodex gatoi*,[24] and *Demodex cati*[25] infestations in cats and maintained efficacy for 12 weeks (6 weeks for *Lynxacarus radovsky* infestations).[26]

Fluralaner in combination with moxidectin topical solution (*Bravecto® Plus*) is FDA-approved for cats and kittens 6 months of age and older weighing at least 1.2 kg (2.6 lb) for the prevention of heartworm disease caused by *Dirofilaria immitis, the* treatment of intestinal roundworms (*Toxocara cati*) and hookworms (*Ancylostoma tubaeforme), the* treatment and prevention of flea infestations (*C felis*), and the treatment and control of tick infestations (*I scapularis* [black-legged tick] and *D variabilis* [American dog tick]) for 2 months.[27]

Pharmacology/Actions

Fluralaner is an isoxazoline acaricide/insecticide that inhibits gamma-aminobutyric acid (GABA)- and glutamate-gated chloride channels with significant selectivity for insect neurons over mammalian neurons.[28] Inhibition induces uncontrolled neuronal activity with resultant paralysis and death of fleas and ticks. In dogs, onset of action is within 8 hours of fleas feeding[21,23] and within 12 hours of ticks feeding.[24-26] In cats, onset of action is within 12 hours of fleas feeding and within 48 hours of ticks feeding.[6]

Pharmacokinetics

The bioavailability of fluralaner following oral and topical administration is ≈25%[29]; giving chewable tablets with food increases bioavailability by ≈2 to 2.5 times.[30] Peak fluralaner concentrations are achieved between 7 and 42 days following topical administration in dogs, and the elimination half-life ranges between 14 and 29 days.[1,8] After oral administration in dogs, elimination half-life averages 9 to 16 days. The drug is not appreciably metabolized, and unchanged fluralaner is excreted in the feces.

Peak fluralaner concentrations are achieved between 7 and 21 days following topical administration in cats, and the elimination half-life ranges between 11 and 13 days. Fluralaner is highly bound to plasma proteins in cats. The drug is not appreciably metabolized, and the hepatic extraction ratio is estimated to be low (0.3%). Unchanged fluralaner is excreted in the feces.[1,8,31,32]

Contraindications/Precautions/Warnings

No contraindications have been listed for fluralaner and fluralaner combination products.[1-3,23,27] For topical applications, do not allow the animal to lick the site of application for 30 minutes after application; wait 3 days before bathing the animal.[33]

Use fluralaner and fluralaner combination products with caution in dogs and cats with a history of seizures or epilepsy. The FDA has warned that drugs in the isoxazoline class have the potential to cause neurologic adverse effects (eg, muscle tremors, ataxia, seizures) in dogs and cats.[34] These effects have also been noted in patients without a history of neurologic disorders.

No adverse effects were noted in a study after 3 times fluralaner labeled doses were administered to collies homozygous for the *MDR1* gene mutation (also known as *ABCB1-1delta*).[35]

Because ticks must feed on the host to become exposed to fluralaner, the risk of transmission of vector-borne diseases cannot be excluded.[36] This particularly applies to infections that have a shorter transmission time (eg, *Anaplasma phagocytophilum, Ehrlichia canis*); however, there is evidence that even in these cases fluralaner reduces this risk.[37]

For fluralaner/moxidectin combination products, use caution in cats with an unknown heartworm status or that are heartworm positive.

Adverse Effects

In preapproval field trials for dogs receiving fluralaner chewable tablets (*Bravecto®*), vomiting was the most common adverse effect reported; decreased appetite, hypersalivation, lethargy, and diarrhea were also reported.[1] Reported adverse effects in dogs receiving the fluralaner topical solution (*Bravecto®*) included vomiting, alopecia, diarrhea, and lethargy.[2] Adverse effects reported in dogs receiving the one-month fluralaner chewable tablets (*Bravecto® 1-Month*) included pruritus, vomiting, diarrhea and decreased appetite.[3]

Isoxazolines, including fluralaner, have been associated with neurologic adverse effects (eg, muscle tremors, ataxia, seizures) even in dogs with no known history of neurologic problems.[1-3,23,27]

Reported adverse effects in cats receiving the fluralaner topical solution (*Bravecto®*) included vomiting, pruritus, diarrhea, alopecia, decreased appetite, and lethargy; ataxia and tremors were also reported in field studies.[23] Adverse effects reported in preapproval field trials for cats receiving the fluralaner/moxidectin combination topical solution (*Bravecto® Plus*) included vomiting, alopecia, pruritus, diarrhea, lethargy, dry skin, elevated ALT (greater than twice the upper reference range of 100 IU/L in the absence of clinical signs).[27]

In both dogs and cats, adverse events were reported at a rate similar to control groups. Hypersalivation was noted in most dogs and cats that received topical fluralaner products orally at the maximum topical dose under experimental conditions.[1,23]

Reproductive/Nursing Safety

The United States product labels have no specific cautions regarding use in breeding, pregnant, or lactating dogs[1,3]; however, safe use in breeding and pregnant dogs has been established in other jurisdictions.[8,36] A reproductive safety study in beagles receiving the chewable tablet at doses up to 3 times the recommended dose found no clinically relevant effects on body weight, food consumption, reproductive performance, semen analysis, litter data, gross necropsy (in adult dogs), or histopathology findings (in adult dogs and puppies).[1] However, abnormalities were noted in 7 puppies from 2 of the 10 dams in the treated group: limb deformity (4 puppies), enlarged heart (2 puppies), enlarged spleen (3 puppies), and cleft palate (2 puppies).

The safety of fluralaner topical solutions for cats, either as a single agent or in combination with moxidectin, has not been evaluated in breeding, pregnant, and lactating cats.[8,23,27,38]

No information regarding fluralaner's distribution in maternal milk was located, but concentrations would be expected to be very low.

Because safety has not been firmly established, this drug should only be used when the maternal benefits outweigh the potential risks to offspring.

Overdose/Acute Toxicity

Some puppies (8 to 9 weeks old) receiving up to 5 times the labeled dose of fluralaner tablets developed diarrhea with mucoid and bloody feces[1]; tremors were observed on the day of administration. No adverse reactions were noted in ≈12-week-old kittens that received up to 5 times the label dose topically at 8-week intervals.[8,23] If clinical signs occur after an overdose, treat supportively.

For patients that have experienced or are suspected to have experienced an overdose, it is strongly encouraged to consult with a 24-hour poison consultation center that specializes in providing information specific for veterinary patients. For general information related to overdose and toxin exposures, as well as contact information for poison control centers, refer to ***Appendix.***

Drug Interactions

In field trials, dogs and cats received concurrent vaccines, anthelmintics, antibiotics, and steroids without observed adverse reactions.[1-3,23] Fluralaner has been safely administered to dogs concurrent with milbemycin oxime/praziquantel[39] and deltamethrin collar.[40] In cats, concurrent use of fluralaner with emodepside/praziquantel combination has been determined to be safe.[41] The following drug interactions with fluralaner either have been reported or are theoretical in humans or animals and may be of significance in veterinary patients. Unless otherwise noted, use together is not necessarily contraindicated, but weigh the potential risks, and perform additional monitoring when appropriate.

- **Highly Protein Bound Drugs** (eg, **maropitant, NSAIDs, warfarin**): Concurrent use of fluralaner with other highly protein bound drugs may cause a transient increase in serum concentrations of each drug. These interactions are unlikely to be of clinical concern because increased free drug concentrations will equilibrate through increased clearance.[8]

Dosages

DOGS:

Labeled indications (label dosage; FDA-approved): A minimum dose of 25 mg/kg (11.4 mg/lb) PO with food or topically every 12 weeks (8 weeks for *Amblyomma americanum* ticks).[1,2] Dosage forms deliver fluralaner 25 – 50 mg/kg. Dosed according to body weights listed in the table below.

Bravecto® chewable tablets and topical solution for dogs

Body weight in kg (lb)	Fluralaner (mg)	Number of tablets/ tubes to administer
2-4.5 (4.4-9.9)	112.5	1
More than 4.5-10 (9.9-22)	250	1
More than 10-20 (22-44)	500	1
More than 20-40 (44-88)	1000	1
More than 40-55.8 (88-123)	1400	1
More than 55.8 (123)	--	Appropriate combination of tablets/tubes

Labeled indications (label dosage; FDA-approved): A minimum dose of 10 mg/kg (4.5 mg/lb) PO with food every month.[3] Dosage form delivers fluralaner 10 – 22.5 mg/kg. Dosed according to body weights listed in the table below.

Bravecto® 1-Month chewable tablets for dogs

Body weight in kg (lb)	Fluralaner (mg)	Number of tablets to administer
2-4.5 (4.4-9.9)	45	1
More than 4.5-10 (9.9-22)	100	1
More than 10-20 (22-44)	200	1
More than 20-40 (44-88)	400	1
More than 40-55.8 (88-123)	560	1
More than 55.8 (123)	--	Appropriate combination of tablets

Demodicosis, generalized (extra-label): 25 mg/kg PO as a single dose.[9,42] Number of mites on skin scraping were reduced by greater than 99% by 28 days posttreatment.

Ixodes holocyclus (extra-label): 25 mg/kg PO as a single dose has prevented tick infestation for at least 115 days[14]

Linognathus setosus (extra-label): 25 mg/kg PO as a single dose has eliminated infestation within 28 days and led to complete dermatologic recovery[15]

Otodectes cynotis (extra-label): 25 mg/kg PO or topically as a single dose achieved clinical and parasitological cure within 14 to 28 days under experimental conditions[16]

***Sarcoptes scabiei* var *canis* infestation** (extra-label): 25 mg/kg PO or topically as a single dose.[12,13] Skin scrapings were negative for mites by 14 days posttreatment.[12]

***Triatoma infestans* (vector of *Trypanosoma cruzi*;** extra-label): 25 mg/kg PO as a single dose[20-22]

CATS:

Labeled indications using fluralaner as a single agent (label dosage; FDA-approved): A minimum dose of 40 mg/kg (18.2 mg/lb) topically every 12 weeks (8 weeks for *Dermacentor variabilis* ticks).[23] Dosage forms deliver fluralaner 40 – 90 mg/kg. Dosed according to body weights listed in the table below.

Bravecto® topical solution for cats

Body weight in kg (lb)	Fluralaner (mg)	Number of tubes to administer
1.2-2.8 (2.6-6.2)	112.5	1
More than 2.8-6.3 (6.2-13.8)	250	1
More than 6.3-12.5 (13.8-27.5)	500	1

Demodex gatoi, Demodex cati (extra-label): 26 – 34 mg/kg PO (a single 112.5-mg tablet/cat) as a single dose[24,25]

Lynxacarus radovsky (extra-label): 25 – 50 mg/kg PO as a single dose eliminated 100% of mites within 28 days of administration, with clinical improvement noted by day 14[26]

Otodectes cynotis (extra-label): 40 mg/kg applied topically as a single dose achieved clinical and parasitological cure within 14 to 28 days under experimental conditions.[16]

Ixodes holocyclus (extra-label): 40 mg/kg applied topically as a single dose has been shown to kill 100% of ticks within 48 hours and maintain efficacy for 84 days[43]

Labeled indications using fluralaner/moxidectin combination product (label dosage; FDA-approved): A minimum dose of 40 mg/kg (18.2 mg/lb) of fluralaner and a minimum dose of 2 mg/kg (0.9 mg/lb) of moxidectin topically every 8 weeks.[27] Dosage forms deliver fluralaner 40 – 95 mg/kg and moxidectin 2 – 4.7 mg/kg. Dosed according to body weights listed in the table below.

Bravecto® Plus topical solution for cats

Body weight in kg (lb)	Fluralaner (mg)	Moxidectin (mg)	Number of tubes to administer
1.2-2.8 (2.6-6.2)	112.5	5.6	1
More than 2.8-6.3 (6.2-13.8)	250	12.5	1
More than 6.3-12.5 (13.8-27.5)	500	25	1

RABBITS:

Psoroptes cuniculi (extra-label): 25 mg/kg PO as a single dose yielded clinical and parasitological cure 12 days after administration and was maintained for the remainder of the 90-day study period[44]

HEDGEHOGS:

Caparinia tripilis (extra-label): 10 mg/kg PO as a single dose killed mites between 7 and 14 days after administration in an African pygmy hedgehog[45]

Monitoring

- Efficacy based on clinical signs and diagnostic testing (eg, fecal flotation, heartworm antigen testing [combination product only], external parasite elimination)
- For demodicosis, clinical signs and monthly skin scrapings;

continue treatment for 4 weeks beyond 2 negative monthly skin scrapings
- Adverse effects (eg, decreased appetite, vomiting, diarrhea)

Client Information
- Keep this medicine and all medicines out of the reach of other animals and children. Keep the product in the original packaging until use to prevent unintended exposure.
- Chewable tablets should be administered with a meal.
- For the topical dog product, avoid bathing or swimming for 3 days after application.
- Do not apply this medicine to irritated skin. Do not contact the application site or allow children to contact the application site until dry. Skin irritation has been reported in humans after close contact with the application site within 4 days of application. Contact a physician if there are any concerns. Be sure to have the product label available when calling.
- Do not eat, drink, or smoke while handling the topical products. The topical products are flammable. Keep away from heat, open flames, sparks, or other sources of ignition.
- Wash your hands thoroughly with soap and water immediately after use.
- Report any side effects, including adverse neurologic effects such as tremors, difficulty walking, or seizures, to your veterinarian.

Chemistry/Synonyms
Fluralaner is an isoxazoline-substituted benzamide derivative insecticide and acaracide. It has a molecular weight of 556.29 and an octanol/water partition coefficient of 5.35. The spot-on solution is colorless to yellow. ATCvet code is QP53BX, and trade name is *Bravecto*®.

Storage/Stability
Do not store fluralaner chewable tablets above 30°C (86°F) or topical solutions above 25°C (77°F). Store in the original packaging to protect from moisture. The topical solution is highly flammable. Keep away from heat, sparks, open flame, or other sources of ignition.

Compatibility/Compounding Considerations
No specific information noted

Dosage Forms/Regulatory Status
VETERINARY-LABELED PRODUCTS:

Fluralaner Chewable Tablets for Dogs: 112 mg, 250 mg, 500 mg, 1000 mg, and 1400 mg; *Bravecto*®; (Rx). FDA-approved. NADA #141-426

Fluralaner Chewable Tablets for Dogs: 45 mg, 100 mg, 200 mg, 400 mg, and 560 mg; *Bravecto® 1-Month*; (Rx). FDA-approved. NADA #141-532

Fluralaner 280 mg/ml Topical Solution for Dogs: 112 mg, 250 mg, 500 mg, 1000 mg, and 1400 mg; *Bravecto® topical solution for dogs*; (Rx). FDA-approved. NADA #141-459

Fluralaner 280 mg/ml Topical Solution for Cats: 112.5 mg, 250 mg, and 500 mg; *Bravecto® topical solution for cats*; (Rx). FDA-approved. NADA #141-459

Fluralaner 28% (280 mg/mL) and Moxidectin 1.4% (14 mg/mL) Topical Solution for Cats: 0.4 mL, 0.9 mL, and 1.8 mL tubes; *Bravecto® Plus* topical solution for cats; (Rx). FDA approved. NADA #141-518

HUMAN-LABELED PRODUCTS: NONE

References
For the complete list of references, see **wiley.com/go/budde/plumb**

Fluticasone

(floo-***ti***-ca-sone) *Flovent*®

Glucocorticoid, Inhaled

Prescriber Highlights
- ► Glucocorticoid used most commonly in veterinary medicine as an inhaled aerosol as local treatment of a condition while minimizing systemic adverse effects
- ► Has shown efficacy in the treatment of feline asthma, as well as chronic inflammatory airway disease in dogs and horses
- ► Adverse effects include possible suppression of HPA axis and secondary nasal demodicosis.
- ► Must be used with a species-appropriate delivery device
- ► Expense may be an issue.

Uses/Indications
The inhaled aerosol formulation of fluticasone is used for treatment of canine chronic bronchitis, feline asthma and chronic bronchitis, and equine asthma. The optimal dosing of inhaled corticosteroids is unknown, and currently there are no studies specifically showing any advantages of inhaled corticosteroids over oral prednisolone in dogs and cats with naturally occurring airway disease.[1] In an 8-week study in cats ($n = 9$) with naturally occurring lower airway disease that compared oral prednisolone with fluticasone administered via inhalation twice daily, the authors concluded both treatments were effective in eliminating clinical signs and reducing airway eosinophilia; oral glucocorticoids were associated with more robust improvement in airway resistance and static compliance.[2]

The authors in one study[3] concluded that the benefits of using inhaled corticosteroids in the treatment of severe equine asthma (SEA) include a more rapid effect on lung function and airway smooth muscle remodeling as compared with antigen avoidance alone, without inducing detectable adverse effects with prolonged use. However, antigen avoidance leads to better control of inflammation and has additional beneficial effects on pulmonary function of inhaled corticosteroid-treated horses, even when clinical signs are apparently controlled by medication.

Pharmacology/Actions
Like other glucocorticoids, fluticasone has potent anti-inflammatory activity. Fluticasone has an affinity 18 times more than dexamethasone for human glucocorticoid receptors.[4] In a feline study, inhaled fluticasone significantly reduced airway eosinophilia.[5] For a more thorough discussion of glucocorticoid effects, refer to ***Glucocorticoid Agents, General Information***.

Pharmacokinetics
In humans administered inhaled fluticasone aerosol via the lungs, ≈30% is absorbed into systemic circulation; a dose of 880 µg showed peak plasma concentrations of 0.1 to 1 ng/mL. Volume of distribution averages 4.2 L/kg and is 91% bound to plasma proteins. Fluticasone is metabolized via CYP 3A4 isoenzymes to a metabolite with negligible pharmacologic activity. Following IV administration, terminal elimination half-life is ≈8 hours, with most of the drug excreted in the feces as parent drug and metabolites.

Medication administered via metered-dose inhalers was confirmed to deposit in the respiratory tract of dogs breathing tidally both with and without sedation; significantly more drug is deposited with nebulization.[6]

Contraindications/Precautions/Warnings
Fluticasone is contraindicated in patients hypersensitive to it, and is not indicated for treatment of acute bronchospasm (eg, status asthmaticus); cases of fluticasone-induced paradoxical bronchospasm have been reported in humans.[4]

When transitioning patients from systemic steroid therapy to inhaled steroids, wean slowly off systemic therapy to avoid acute adrenal insufficiency. During this transition period, patients should receive supplemental systemic steroid therapy during periods of acute stress or if severe asthma attacks occur during the withdrawal stage.

Adverse Effects

In humans, the most likely adverse effects are pharyngitis and upper respiratory infection. Although inhaled steroids generally cause significantly fewer adverse effects than injectable or oral therapy, suppression of the HPA axis can occur.

One study comparing ACTH-stimulated cortisol concentrations in healthy beagles, found that inhaled budesonide did not significantly affect cortisol concentrations, but oral prednisolone 1 mg/kg/day and inhaled fluticasone 250 µg twice daily did have a significant effect on cortisol concentrations after 35 days of treatment.[7] Evidence of pituitary-adrenal axis inhibition was identified in 2 dogs; 1 dog developed signs of iatrogenic hyperadrenocorticism (eg, weight gain, PU/PD, alopecia, skin thinning, abdominal distension, hepatomegaly, panting).[8]

A study in cats given different dosages of inhaled fluticasone did not show significant HPA axis suppression at 44 µg, 110 µg, or 220 µg every 12 hours.[5] Cats treated with inhaled corticosteroids may develop localized demodicosis on the muzzle/nasal planum.[9,10]

Another study in horses demonstrated that long-term inhaled fluticasone did not cause detectable effects on innate and adaptive (both humoral and cell-mediated) immune parameters studied.[11] Suppression of serum cortisol has been documented in horses treated long-term with inhaled fluticasone.[12]

Reproductive/Nursing Safety

Fluticasone given SC to laboratory animals caused a variety of teratogenic effects, including growth delays, cleft palate, omphalocele, and delayed cranial ossification.[4] See ***Glucocorticoid Agents, General Information.***

It is not known if the drug enters maternal milk; use with caution in nursing dams.

Because safety has not been established in animals, this drug should only be used when the maternal benefits outweigh the potential risks to offspring.

Overdose/Acute Toxicity

An acute overdose of this medication is unlikely, but there have been reported cases of dogs puncturing canisters of albuterol and developing adverse effects. A similar occurrence with fluticasone would unlikely require treatment. Chronic overdoses could result in significant HPA axis suppression and adverse effects related to iatrogenic hyperadrenocorticism.

For patients that have experienced or are suspected to have experienced an overdose, consultation with a 24-hour poison consultation center specializing in providing veterinary-specific information is recommended. For general information related to overdose and toxin exposures, as well as contact information for poison control centers, refer to ***Appendix.***

Drug Interactions

Although the manufacturer states that due to the low systemic plasma concentrations associated with inhalational therapy clinically significant drug interactions are unlikely, use caution when fluticasone is used in conjunction with other drugs that can inhibit CYP3A4 isoenzymes (eg, **ketoconazole**); theoretically, fluticasone concentrations could be increased.

Laboratory Considerations

- **Intradermal skin testing** (IDST) for allergens: A related inhaled corticosteroid (ie, budesonide) in cats (for 1 month) eliminated skin reactivity in 3 out of 6 cats tested.[13] The authors suggested a 2-week withdrawal if using IDST, but withdrawal may not be necessary if using serum IgE testing for allergies. This same effect may apply to inhaled fluticasone.

Dosages

NOTES:

1. Optimal dosing of inhaled corticosteroids is unknown, and there have been no studies specifically demonstrating advantages of inhaled glucocorticoids over oral prednisone/prednisolone in patients with naturally occurring airway disease.
2. When using inhalant therapy, dogs and cats must take 7 to 10 breaths (3 to 5 breaths for horses) (with the appropriate delivery device [eg, *AeroDawg, AeroKat, AeroHippus*] still placed) after each time the metered dose inhaler (MDI) has been actuated to ensure the maximal dose is inhaled.

DOGS:

NOTE: Most commonly, when starting fluticasone, oral glucocorticoid therapy is continued for 10 to 14 days with a tapering overlap.[14]

Adjunctive treatment for chronic tracheobronchial disease (extra-label): Using 110 – 220 µg/puff MDI, administer 1 puff 2 to 4 times daily via an appropriate delivery device.[15-17] Adjust dose based on clinical response.

Eosinophilic bronchopneumopathy (extra-label): 100 – 250 µg/puff MDI twice daily[8,15]; dose can be adjusted based on clinical response.

CATS:

NOTE: Most commonly, when starting fluticasone, oral glucocorticoid therapy is continued for 10 to 14 days with a tapering overlap.[14]

Chronic bronchitis, feline asthma (extra-label):

1. Initially, 44 µg/puff or 110 µg/puff MDI, 1 puff every 12 hours[5]
2. 110 µg/puff MDI, 1 puff twice daily. Cats with more serious disease may require fluticasone 220 µg MDI.[18,19]
3. 250 µg MDI once daily[20] (**NOTE**: In the United States, the 250 microgram/puff concentration is labeled as 220 µg/puff; see ***Dosage Forms***)

Feline idiopathic chronic rhinitis; (extra-label): 220 µg/puff MDI, 2 puffs every 12 hours in combination with oral prednisolone. Once fluticasone therapy has been comfortably implemented, begin dose reductions of oral prednisolone (typically, 25% every 2 weeks) while monitoring clinical signs.[21,22]

HORSES:

Severe equine asthma (SEA; formerly known as recurrent airway obstruction [RAO], heaves; extra-label):

1. 2000 µg MDI every 12 hours for 1 month, then adjust dosages (2000 – 3000 µg every 12 to 24 hours) to control clinical signs[3,11]
2. 6000 µg MDI every 12 hours *prevented* acute exacerbations of SEA but did not treat acute SEA exacerbations as well as dexamethasone IV.[23]

Monitoring

- Efficacy: control of cough and/or other respiratory signs (eg, exercise intolerance, tachypnea, wheezing)
- Clinical signs of iatrogenic hyperadrenocorticism (eg, polyuria/polydipsia, polyphagia)

Client Information

- Shake the inhaler well before using. Do not puncture or incinerate the can. This product must be used with a spacer device appropriate for the species being treated.
- When using inhaled fluticasone with an appropriate spacer/facemask (eg, *AeroDawg, AeroKat*) in dogs and cats, the following tips

have been recommended[24]:

1. Allow the cat to get used to the device over several days, letting it investigate (eg, leaving the device by food bowl).
2. Reward (ie, praise, food, catnip, stroking) fearless approaches to the device, and start placing it near the cat's face.
3. Practice putting the mask over the cat's face without anything in the chamber.
4. Make sure the mask is placed snugly over the muzzle.
5. With the mask on, actuate the MDI and allow the animal to take 7 to 10 breaths before removing.
6. Container will last ≈2 months when used at 1 puff twice per day.

- When using inhaled fluticasone with an appropriate spacer/facemask (eg, *AeroHippus*) in horses, the following tips have been recommended:
  1. Slowly introduce the *AeroHippus* Chamber. Start with the mask only, getting your horse used to the feel of it.
  2. Reward your horse with treats before and/or after treatment.
  3. If your horse does not respond well to the sound of the inhaler, depress the inhaler behind your back before bringing the *AeroHippus* Chamber forward and placing mask over horse's nostril.
  4. With the mask over the nostril, allow the horse to take 3 to 5 breaths for each puff (actuation) from the MDI.

Chemistry/Synonyms

Fluticasone propionate, a trifluorinated glucocorticoid, occurs as a white to off-white powder that is practically insoluble in water and slightly soluble in ethanol.

Fluticasone may also be known as CCI-18781, fluticasoni propionas, *Advair Diskus*®, *Cutovate*®, *Flixotide*®, *Flixonase*®, *Flovent*®, and *Flutivate*®.

Storage/Stability

Fluticasone propionate aerosol for inhalation (*Flovent® HFA*) should be stored between 59°F to 86°F (15°C to 30°C); protect from freezing and direct sunlight, and do not store near heat or open flame. Store canister with the mouthpiece down.

Compatibility/Compounding Considerations

No specific information noted

Dosage Forms/Regulatory Status

VETERINARY-LABELED PRODUCTS: NONE

NOTE: The Association of Racing Commissioners International (ARCI) has designated fluticasone as a class 4 substance. Use of this drug may not be allowed in certain animal competitions. Check rules and regulations before entering in a competition while this medication is being administered. Contact local racing authorities for further guidance. See ***Appendix*** for more information.

HUMAN-LABELED PRODUCTS:

Fluticasone Propionate Aerosol for Inhalation: 44 µg/actuation, 110 µg/actuation, and 220 µg/actuation in 10.6-g and 12-g canisters with actuator. Each canister contains 120-metered inhalations; *Flovent® HFA*; (Rx). **NOTE**: In countries outside the United States, *Flovent® HFA* canister concentrations may be listed as 50 µg, 125 µg, and 250 µg per actuation; the difference in labeling relates to where the drug concentration is measured (eg, metering valve [eg, 50 µg] vs actuator nozzle [44 µg]). There are also breath-activated dry powder inhalers (ie, *Flovent® Diskus*, *Advair Diskus®* [with salmeterol]), but they are not suitable for veterinary use.

Fluticasone is also available commercially in combination as:

Fluticasone Propionate/Salmeterol Aerosol for Inhalation: fluticasone propionate 45 µg/salmeterol 21 µg/actuation; fluticasone propionate 115 µg/salmeterol 21 µg/actuation; and fluticasone propionate 230 µg/salmeterol 21 µg/actuation equivalent to salmeterol xinafoate 30.45 µg in 12-g pressurized canisters containing 120-metered inhalations.

Nasal solutions, topical creams, and ointments containing fluticasone are also available.

References

For the complete list of references, see **wiley.com/go/budde/plumb**

Fluvoxamine

(floo-***vox***-a-meen) *Luvox*®

Selective Serotonin Reuptake Inhibitor (SSRI)

Prescriber Highlights

- ▶ Uncommonly used selective serotonin reuptake inhibitor (SSRI) antidepressant similar to fluoxetine; can be used in dogs and cats for a variety of behavior disorders, but little information available to recommend its use in place of more commonly prescribed SSRIs
- ▶ Contraindications include patients with known hypersensitivity or who are receiving monoamine oxidase inhibitors (MAOIs).
- ▶ Use with caution in patients with severe cardiac, renal, or hepatic disease; dosages may need to be reduced in patients with severe renal or hepatic impairment.
- ▶ May take up to 8 weeks before efficacy can be fully assessed
- ▶ Adverse effect profile not well established. Possible adverse effects in dogs include anorexia, lethargy, GI effects, anxiety, irritability, insomnia, hyperactivity, or panting, as well as aggressive behavior in previously nonaggressive dogs. Cats may exhibit sedation, decreased appetite/anorexia, vomiting, diarrhea, behavior changes (eg, anxiety, irritability, sleep disturbances), and changes in elimination patterns.
- ▶ Many possible drug interactions. Coadministration of more than one serotonergic drug is not recommended due to the risk for the development of serotonin syndrome.

Uses/Indications

Fluvoxamine may be considered for use in treating a variety of behavior-related disorders in dogs and cats, including aggression and stereotypic behaviors (and other obsessive-compulsive behaviors). Because of a lack of published information documenting its safety and efficacy in animals, it is not commonly prescribed.

Pharmacology/Actions

Fluvoxamine is a highly selective inhibitor of the reuptake of serotonin in the CNS, thereby potentiating the pharmacologic activity of serotonin. Fluvoxamine has little effect on dopamine or norepinephrine and apparently no effect on other neurotransmitters.

Pharmacokinetics

There are limited data on the pharmacokinetics of fluvoxamine in domestic animals. In dogs, fluvoxamine appears to be completely absorbed; only about 10% of a dose is excreted unchanged in the urine.[1,2] The half-life appears to be similar to humans (15 hours).[1] No pharmacokinetic information for cats was located.

In humans, fluvoxamine is absorbed after oral administration, but bioavailability is only around 50%. Peak plasma concentrations occur between 3 and 8 hours postdose. Food does not appear to affect the absorptive characteristics of the drug. Fluvoxamine is widely distributed in the body and about 80% bound to plasma proteins. The drug is extensively metabolized in the liver to nonactive metabolites and eliminated in the urine. The plasma half-life is about 15 hours.

Contraindications/Precautions/Warnings

Fluvoxamine is contraindicated in patients hypersensitive to it or any selective serotonin reuptake inhibitor (SSRI) or if the patient is receiving a monoamine oxidase inhibitor (MAOI) or cisapride. Consider using a lower dosage in patients with hepatic impairment or in geriatric patients.

Do not confuse FLUVoxamine with fluOXetine.

Adverse Effects

The adverse effect profile of fluvoxamine in dogs or cats has not been well established. In dogs, selective serotonin reuptake inhibitors (SSRIs) can cause lethargy, adverse GI effects, anxiety, irritability, insomnia/hyperactivity, or panting. Anorexia is a common adverse effect in dogs, which is usually transient and may be negated by temporarily increasing the palatability of food and/or hand feeding. Some dogs have persistent anorexia that precludes further treatment. Aggressive behavior in previously nonaggressive dogs has been reported. SSRIs in cats can cause sedation, decreased appetite/anorexia, vomiting, diarrhea, behavior changes (eg, anxiety, irritability, sleep disturbances), and changes in elimination patterns.

In humans, common adverse reactions (greater than 10%) include sexual adverse effects (eg, abnormal ejaculation, anorgasmia), agitation/nervousness, insomnia, nausea, dry mouth, constipation/diarrhea, dyspepsia, dizziness, headache, and somnolence. Hyponatremia and abnormal bleeding also have been noted.

Reproductive/Nursing Safety

In rats, fluvoxamine reportedly increased embryofetal death and pup mortality at birth and was associated with fetal abnormalities and decreased birth weights.[3]

Although fluvoxamine enters maternal milk, it is not expected to cause adverse effects to the offspring.[4]

Because safety has not been established in animals, this drug should only be used when the maternal benefits outweigh the potential risks to offspring.

Overdose/Acute Toxicity

Limited data exist for animals. Reportedly, any dose over 10 mg/kg can cause tremors and lethargy. A case of a dog developing clinical signs (CNS depression) after ingesting 1.5 mg/kg has been reported.[5] Other signs associated with overdoses may include nausea, salivation, vomiting, diarrhea, hypotension, heart rate and rhythm disturbances (bradycardia/tachycardia, ECG changes), hyperthermia, tremors, ataxia, muscle rigidity, somnolence/coma, and seizures.[6]

Fatalities have been reported in human overdoses; the highest reported dose where the patient survived was 10,000 mg. Treatment recommendations include standard protocols for drug adsorption and removal from the GI tract for potentially dangerous overdoses and supportive care based on clinical signs. Serotonin effects may be negated somewhat by administration of cyproheptadine. See ***Cyproheptadine***. Seizures or other neurologic signs may be treated with diazepam. See ***Diazepam***.

For patients that have experienced or are suspected of having experienced an overdose, consultation with a 24-hour poison consultation center specializing in providing veterinary-specific information is recommended. For general information related to overdose and toxin exposures, as well as contact information for poison control centers, refer to ***Appendix.***

Drug Interactions

The following drug interactions have either been reported or are theoretical in humans or animals receiving fluvoxamine and may be of significance in veterinary patients. Unless otherwise noted, use together is not necessarily contraindicated, but weigh the potential risks and perform additional monitoring when appropriate.

- **Benzodiazepines** (eg, **alprazolam, diazepam, midazolam**): May increase benzodiazepine concentrations
- **Buspirone**: May paradoxically decrease the clinical efficacy of buspirone and increase the risk for serotonin syndrome
- **Cisapride**: Fluvoxamine may increase plasma concentrations of cisapride, leading to toxicity.
- **Cyproheptadine**: May decrease or reverse the effects of selective serotonin reuptake inhibitors (SSRIs)
- **Diltiazem**: May increase the effects of diltiazem; bradycardia has been reported in humans taking this drug combination.
- **Fentanyl**: May increase the risk for serotonin syndrome
- **Monoamine Oxidase Inhibitors** (MAOIs; eg, **amitraz, linezolid, selegiline**): High risk for serotonin syndrome; use together is contraindicated. In humans, a 5-week washout period is required after discontinuing fluvoxamine and a 2-week washout period if the MAOI is discontinued first.
- **Methadone**: May increase plasma concentrations of methadone, leading to toxicity; concurrent use may increase the risk for serotonin syndrome.
- **Metoclopramide**: May enhance adverse/toxic effects of SSRIs and increase the risk for serotonin syndrome
- **Mexiletine**: SSRIs may decrease the metabolism of mexiletine.
- **Propranolol, Metoprolol**: Fluvoxamine may increase these beta-blockers' plasma levels; atenolol may be safer to use if fluvoxamine is required.
- **Serotonergic Agents** (eg, **mirtazapine, ondansetron, trazodone**): Concurrent use may increase the risk for serotonin syndrome.
- **Theophylline, Aminophylline**: May increase plasma concentrations of theophylline
- **Tramadol**: SSRIs can inhibit the metabolism of tramadol to the active metabolites, thereby decreasing its efficacy and increasing the risk for toxicity (serotonin syndrome, seizures).
- **Tricyclic Antidepressants** (TCAs; eg, **amitriptyline, clomipramine**): May increase TCA blood concentrations and increase the risk for serotonin syndrome
- **Warfarin**: Fluvoxamine may increase the risk for bleeding.

Laboratory Considerations

- No fluvoxamine-related laboratory interactions were noted.

Dosages

NOTE: Fluvoxamine is available commercially as both regular tablets and extended-release capsules. Although the contents of the extended-release capsules could be compounded into smaller strengths for use in veterinary patients, there does not appear to be any information available to support this practice.

DOGS:

Adjunctive treatment of behavioral disorders (extra-label): 1 – 2 mg/kg PO once daily.[7] Treatment for 3 to 8 weeks may be required before assessing efficacy. If discontinuing therapy after this time, wean off over several weeks.

CATS:

Adjunctive treatment of behavioral disorders (extra-label): 0.25 – 0.5 mg/kg PO once daily.[7] Treatment for 3 to 8 weeks may be required before assessing efficacy. If discontinuing therapy after this time, wean off over several weeks. The smallest practical dosage available (without compounding) is ¼ of a 25 mg tablet (≈6 mg), which may be too high for the suggested dosage listed above.

Monitoring

- Efficacy
- Adverse effects (eg, hyporexia/anorexia, lethargy, and monitor for signs of serotonin syndrome [eg, nausea, vomiting, mydriasis, hy-

persalivation, and hyperthermia])

Client Information

- This medicine may be given with or without food. If your animal vomits or acts sick after getting it on an empty stomach, give the medicine with food or a small treat to see if this helps. If vomiting continues, contact your veterinarian.
- This medication is most effective when used with a behavior modification program. It may take several days to weeks to determine if the medicine is working.
- Do not stop this medication abruptly without talking to your veterinarian first.
- The most common side effects of fluvoxamine are drowsiness/sleepiness and decreased appetite. Rarely, more serious side effects (eg, seizures, aggression) may occur. Contact your veterinarian immediately if these signs occur.
- Overdoses can be very serious. Keep this and all other medicines out of the reach of animals and children.
- If your animal has worn a flea and tick collar in the past two weeks, let your veterinarian know. Do not use one on your animal while it's getting this medicine without first talking to your veterinarian.

Chemistry/Synonyms

Fluvoxamine maleate is a selective serotonin reuptake inhibitor (SSRI) that occurs as a white to almost white crystalline powder. It is freely soluble in alcohol and sparingly soluble in water.

Fluvoxamine may also be known as DU-23000, desifluvoxamin, and *Luvox®*.

Storage/Stability

Store the commercially available tablets and extended-release capsules in tight, light-resistant containers at room temperatures 20°C to 25°C (68°F-77°F); excursions permitted to 15°C to 30°C (59°F-86°F); protect from high humidity.

Compatibility/Compounding Considerations

No specific information was noted.

Dosage Forms/Regulatory Status

VETERINARY-LABELED PRODUCTS: NONE

The Association of Racing Commissioners International (ARCI) has designated this drug as a class 2 substance. Use of this drug may not be allowed in certain animal competitions. Check rules and regulations before entering a competition while this medication is being administered. Contact local racing authorities for further guidance. See the ***Appendix*** for more information.

HUMAN-LABELED PRODUCTS:

Fluvoxamine Oral Tablets: 25 mg, 50 mg, and 100 mg; generic; (Rx)

Fluvoxamine Oral Extended-release (24-hour for humans) Capsules: 100 mg and 150 mg; *Luvox CR®*, generic; (Rx)

References

For the complete list of references, see **wiley.com/go/budde/plumb**

Folic Acid

Folate, Folacin, Vitamin B_9

(***foe***-lik ***ass***-id)

B Vitamin

Prescriber Highlights

- ► B vitamin necessary for nucleoprotein synthesis and normal erythropoiesis.
- ► Used for oral and parenteral treatment of folic acid (vitamin B_9) deficiency caused by small intestinal inflammatory disease, chronic administration of dihydrofolate reductase inhibitor drugs, or dietary deficiency.

Uses/Indications

Folic acid is used to treat folic acid deficiency in dogs, cats, horses, and other animal species, often due to small intestinal disease. GI malabsorption may lead to low serum folate concentrations, although hypocobalaminemia is more common than hypofolatemia in dogs and cats with chronic small intestinal disease or exocrine pancreatic insufficiency.[1,2] The incidence of clinically significant folic acid deficiency is unknown, although an association between hypofolatemia and hyperhomocysteinemia has been demonstrated in greyhounds.[3] Chronic administration of dihydrofolate reductase inhibiting drugs, such as pyrimethamine, ormetoprim, or trimethoprim, can lead to reduced activated folic acid (tetrahydrofolic acid); folic acid supplementation may be prescribed to prevent or treat hypofolatemia in these cases. Folic acid supplementation during pregnancy has been shown to reduce the occurrence of lip and/or palate cleft in pug and Chihuahua puppies,[4] but similar results were not observed in a colony of guide dogs.[5]

Pharmacology/Actions

Folic acid is required for several metabolic processes. It is reduced via dihydrofolate reductase in the body to tetrahydrofolate (5-methyltetrahydrofolate), which acts as a coenzyme in the synthesis of purine and pyrimidine nucleotides necessary for DNA synthesis. Folic acid is also required for the maintenance of normal erythropoiesis.

Pharmacokinetics

Folic acid is primarily absorbed in the proximal small intestine via carrier-mediated diffusion. In humans, synthetic folic acid is nearly completely absorbed after oral administration, while bioavailability of folate from dietary sources is about 50%. Peak concentrations are reached within 1 hour. Folic acid is converted to its active form, tetrahydrofolic acid, principally in the liver and plasma. Folate is distributed widely throughout the body and stored in the liver. Erythrocyte and CSF concentrations can be significantly higher than those found in serum. It can undergo enterohepatic recirculation and is excreted primarily in the urine either as metabolites or unchanged drug when administered in excess of body requirements.

Contraindications/Precautions/Warnings

Folic acid supplementation is contraindicated when known hypersensitivity to the drug is documented. In humans, cobalamin (B_{12}) levels may be reduced with megaloblastic anemias, and folic acid therapy may mask the signs associated with it. Folic acid supplementation should not be given until pernicious anemia (anemia associated with vitamin B_{12} deficiency) has been ruled out. As dogs may have increased, normal, or decreased folate levels associated with enteropathies, do not administer therapeutic doses until folate and cobalamin levels have been determined.

Parenteral products may contain aluminum and/or benzyl alcohol.

Adverse Effects

Folic acid has a wide safety margin and should not cause significant adverse effects. Rarely in humans, folic acid tablets or injections have reportedly caused hypersensitivity reactions or GI effects. Very high oral doses in humans (15 mg/day) have occasionally caused CNS effects (eg, difficulty sleeping, excitement, confusion).

Reproductive/Nursing Safety

Folic acid is safe to use during pregnancy. In humans, it is routinely prescribed as part of prenatal vitamin supplementation as folate deficiency can increase the risk for fetal neural tube defects.

Folic acid is distributed into milk but is safe. Folic acid requirements may be increased in lactating animals.

Overdose/Acute Toxicity

Folic acid is relatively non-toxic, and no treatment should be required if an inadvertent overdose occurs. The excess drug is metabolized or rapidly excreted unchanged in the urine.

Drug Interactions

The following drug interactions have either been reported or are theoretical in humans or animals receiving folic acid and may be of significance in veterinary patients. Unless otherwise noted, use together is not necessarily contraindicated, but weigh the potential risks and perform additional monitoring when appropriate.

- Chloramphenicol: May delay response to folic acid
- Methotrexate, Trimethoprim, Ormetoprim, Pyrimethamine (drugs that inhibit dihydrofolate reductase): May interfere with folic acid utilization
- Phenobarbital: May decrease phenobarbital serum levels; monitor therapy.
- Primidone: May increase risk for folate deficiency
- Sulfasalazine, Primidone: May increase risk for folate deficiency

Laboratory Considerations

- **Serum samples** to be analyzed for cobalamin and/or folate should be protected from bright light and excessive heat.
- **Hemolysis** can cause falsely elevated serum concentrations of folate.
- Decreased **serum cobalamin levels** (B_{12}) can occur in patients receiving prolonged folic acid supplementation.

Dosages

DOGS/CATS:

Folate deficiency associated with inflammatory bowel disease and pancreatic insufficiency (extra-label): Dosage recommendations vary, and there is little evidence to support any specific dosage recommendation. Suggested PO dosages for small animal species generally range from 400 µg to 1 mg/dog or cat (NOT mg/kg) once daily, although doses of 2 – 5 mg/dog (NOT mg/kg) PO once daily have been noted. When used for IBD, many recommend using with cobalamin (B_{12}).

Cats on long-term use of high dose sulfa-/trimethoprim (for treating *Nocardia* spp infections) (extra-label): 2 mg/cat (NOT mg/kg) PO once daily has been recommended.[6]

HORSES:

Prolonged therapy with antifolate medications (eg, trimethoprim, pyrimethamine); (extra-label): Some recommend folic acid at 20 – 40 mg/horse (NOT mg/kg) PO daily. Pregnant mares should routinely receive folic acid supplementation during treatment with antifolates.[7]

RABBITS:

Deep vein thrombosis (extra-label): Folic acid (vitamin B_9) 15 mg/rabbit (NOT mg/kg) in combination with cobalamin (vitamin B_{12}) 500 µg/rabbit (NOT µg/kg) PO once daily.[8] High levels of cobalamin (vitamin B_{12}) and folic acid (vitamin B_9) can improve plasma hyperhomocysteinemia, coagulation indexes, and some pathologic changes seen in deep vein thrombosis of the lower extremity.

Monitoring

- Small animal species: serum folate and cobalamin levels before, during, and after treatment
- Clinical signs associated with folate deficiency
- Baseline and periodic CBC

Client Information

- This medicine may be given with or without food. If your animal vomits or acts sick after receiving the medication on an empty stomach, give with food or a small treat. If vomiting continues, contact your veterinarian.
- When used to treat folate deficiency associated with a small intestinal disease or pancreatic insufficiency, lifelong monitoring and periodic replacement therapy may be required. Do not miss important follow-up visits with your veterinarian.

Chemistry/Synonyms

Folic acid occurs as a yellow, yellow-brownish, or yellowish-orange, odorless crystalline powder. It is very slightly soluble in water and insoluble in alcohol. Commercially available folic acid is obtained synthetically.

Folic acid may also be known as folate, folacin, vitamin B_9, acidumfolicum, pteroylglutamic acid, pteroylmonoglutamic acid, *Folvite®*, and vitamin B_{11}.

Storage/Stability

Store folic acid tablets in well-closed containers between 20°C and 25°C (68°F and 77°F); protect from light and moisture. Store the injection protected from light between 20°C and 25°C (68°F and 77°F). Do not freeze.

Compatibility/Compounding Considerations

Compatibility is dependent on factors such as pH, concentration, temperature, and diluent used; specialized references or a hospital pharmacist should be consulted for more specific information.

To compound a 1 mg/mL oral solution, bring 90 mL of purified water to near boiling. Dissolve methylparaben 200 mg and propylparaben 20 mg in the heated water. Allow it to cool to room temperature. Crush one hundred 1 mg tablets and dissolve in the solution. Using sodium hydroxide 10%, adjust pH to 8 to 8.5, *qs ad* to 100 mL with purified water, and mix well. The solution is stable for 30 days at room temperature.[9]

To compound a 0.05 mg/mL folic acid oral solution, mix 1 mL of injectable folic acid (5 mg/mL) with 90 mL of purified water. Using sodium hydroxide 10%, adjust pH to 8 to 8.5, *qs ad* to 100 mL with purified water, and mix well. The solution is stable for 30 days at room temperature.[10]

Dosage Forms/Regulatory Status

VETERINARY-LABELED PRODUCTS:

None, but there are many available products containing folic acid. If using one of these products, verify the folic acid content is enough to treat folate deficiency without overdosing fat-soluble vitamins (A, D, E, K).

HUMAN-LABELED PRODUCTS:

Folic Acid Tablets: 0.4 mg, 0.8 mg, and 1 mg; generic; (OTC); 1 mg; generic; (Rx).

Folic Acid Capsules: 0.8 mg, 5 mg, and 20 mg; generic; (OTC).

Folic Acid Injection: 5 mg/mL in 10 mL vials; generic; (Rx).

References

For the complete list of references, see **wiley.com/go/budde/plumb**

Fomepizole

4-Methylpyrazole (4-MP)

(foe-***me***-pi-zole) *Antizol-Vet®*

Antidote

Prescriber Highlights

- ► Synthetic alcohol dehydrogenase inhibitor used to treat dogs and cats with ethylene glycol toxicosis
- ► Has been shown to be efficacious in dogs if treated within 8 hours of ethylene glycol ingestion, and in cats at high dosages if given within 3 hours of ethylene glycol ingestion
- ► Monitor and treat acid/base, fluid, and electrolyte imbalances
- ► May inhibit or exacerbate elimination of ethanol
- ► Expensive and limited availability

Uses/Indications

Fomepizole (4-methylpyrazole; 4-MP) is used for the treatment of known or suspected ethylene glycol toxicosis in dogs if given within 8 hours of ingestion.[1] At high doses, it may be efficacious in treating recent ingestion (within 3 hours) of ethylene glycol in cats.[2,3] Ethanol treatment has previously been recommended as the drug of choice for ethylene glycol toxicosis in cats, but high-dose fomepizole was more effective.[3]

Pharmacology/Actions

Ethylene glycol is metabolized primarily by alcohol dehydrogenase into glycoaldehyde, which in turn forms glycolate, glyoxalic acid, and oxalic acid. The metabolic acidosis and renal tubular necrosis that result from these compounds can be fatal. Fomepizole is a competitive inhibitor of alcohol dehydrogenase, which allows ethylene glycol to be excreted, primarily unchanged, in the urine, decreasing the morbidity and mortality associated with ethylene glycol ingestion.

Pharmacokinetics

Fomepizole exhibits a dose-dependent accumulation over time due to saturable elimination; therefore, a reduction in subsequent doses can safely occur.

Contraindications/Precautions/Warnings

There are no labeled contraindications to fomepizole's use. In dogs, fomepizole treatment may be successful as late as 8 hours postingestion, but if azotemia is noted, treatment is less successful, and the prognosis is poor. Treatment should still be considered up to 36 hours postingestion, as fomepizole can potentially prevent further renal damage and some dogs may survive with dialysis and supportive therapy.[1]

Fomepizole has been shown to be effective in treating ethylene glycol toxicosis in cats, but a higher dose is required (6 times the dose in dogs or humans) and treatment should be started within 3 hours of ethylene glycol ingestion.[2,3]

Use of fomepizole alone without adequate monitoring and adjunctive supportive care (eg, correction of acid/base, fluid, and electrolyte imbalances) may lead to therapeutic failure; however, as fomepizole may increase serum bicarbonate (HCO_3), it has been recommended that correction of severe metabolic acidosis in cats, and presumably dogs, be treated with appropriate IV fluid therapy and fomepizole before consideration of HCO_3 administration.[4] If the animal is presented within 1 to 2 hours of ethylene glycol ingestion, consider inducing emesis and/or gastric lavage with activated charcoal to prevent further absorption.

Fomepizole does not prevent the CNS depression caused by unmetabolized ethylene glycol and could prolong it.

Adverse Effects

Fomepizole appears to be well tolerated. Cats receiving high-dose fomepizole may experience mild sedation.[3] Giving concentrated drug by rapid IV infusion may cause phlebitis and phlebosclerosis. Dilute as directed according to label instructions.

During clinical trials, one dog developed anaphylaxis.[1]

Cats may develop mild sedation, ataxia, and hypothermia when receiving fomepizole. Breath and urine may have the distinctive smell of fomepizole up to a week after dosing.[3]

Fomepizole may increase serum bicarbonate concentrations in dogs and cats. See ***Contraindications/Precautions/Warnings***.

Reproductive/Nursing Safety

Fomepizole's safe use during pregnancy, lactation, or in breeding animals has not been established; however, because of the morbidity and mortality associated with ethylene glycol toxicosis, the benefits of fomepizole generally outweigh its risks.

It is not known whether this drug is excreted in milk. Because safety has not been established in animals, this drug should only be used when the maternal benefits outweigh the potential risks to offspring.

Overdose/Acute Toxicity

Overdoses may cause significant CNS depression. Monitor closely and treat supportively. Fomepizole is dialyzable.

For patients that have experienced or are suspected to have experienced an overdose, consultation with a 24-hour poison consultation center specializing in providing veterinary-specific information is recommended. For general information related to overdose and toxin exposures, as well as contact information for poison control centers, refer to ***Appendix.***

Drug Interactions

The following drug interactions have either been reported or are theoretical in humans or animals receiving fomepizole and may be of significance in veterinary patients. Unless otherwise noted, use together is not necessarily contraindicated, but weigh the potential risks and perform additional monitoring when appropriate.

- ETHANOL: Fomepizole inhibits alcohol dehydrogenase; ethanol metabolism is reduced significantly and alcohol poisoning (eg, CNS depression, coma, death) can occur. Use together is generally not recommended, but if both drugs are used, monitoring of ethanol blood concentration is mandatory.

Laboratory Considerations

Ethylene Glycol Testing Kits: Fomepizole may cause false readings on ethylene glycol screening tests. Refer to the product used for more information.

Dosages

NOTES:

1. A non-polycarbonate syringe must be used to withdraw fomepizole from the vial.
2. In humans, the drug should be diluted in at least 100 mL of 0.9% sodium chloride or 5% dextrose and infused over 30 minutes.[5] It is assumed these are relevant to veterinary patients.

DOGS:

Ethylene glycol toxicosis (extra-label): Initially, fomepizole 20 mg/kg IV; 12 hours after the initial dose, give 15 mg/kg IV; 24 hours after initial dose, give another 15 mg/kg IV; and 36 hours after initial dose, give 5 mg/kg IV; may give additional 5 mg/kg IV doses as necessary (eg, if animal has not recovered or has additional ethylene glycol in blood).[6]

CATS:

Ethylene glycol toxicosis (extra-label): Evidence from an experimental study and naturally occurring ethylene glycol intoxication (3 cats). Initially, 125 mg/kg slow IV; then at 12, 24, and 36 hours after initial dose, give 31.25 mg/kg IV. In addition, treat supportively with supplemental IV fluids. Cats must be treated within 3 hours of ingestion. Cats that began treatment 4 hours after ethylene glycol ingestion had 100% mortality with either fomepizole or ethanol therapy.[3,4]

Monitoring

- Baseline ethylene glycol blood concentration to document diagnosis followed by intermittent testing to determine if therapy can be discontinued after 36 hours of treatment
- Hydration status
- Urine output
- Renal function tests (eg, BUN, serum creatinine, urinalysis)
- Blood gases and serum electrolytes
- Cats: body temperature

Client Information

- Clients should be informed that treatment of serious ethylene glycol toxicosis is an intensive care admission, and appropriate monitoring and therapy can be quite expensive, particularly when fomepizole is used in large dogs.
- Because time is critical, clients will need to make an informed decision rapidly. Dogs treated within 8 hours of ingestion have a significantly better prognosis than those treated after 10 to 12 hours. Cats must be treated within 3 hours of ingestion.

Chemistry/Synonyms

A synthetic alcohol dehydrogenase inhibitor, fomepizole is commonly called 4-methylpyrazole (4-MP). Its chemical name is 4-methyl-1H-pyrazole. It has a molecular weight of 81; it is soluble in water and highly soluble in ethanol.

Fomepizole may also be known as: 4-methylpyrazole, 4-MP, fomepisol, fomepizolum, and *Antizol*®.

Storage/Stability

Commercially available solutions should be stored at room temperature. The concentrate for injection may solidify at temperatures less than 25°C (77°F). Should this occur, resolubolize by running warm water over the vial. Solidification or resolubolization does not affect drug potency or stability.

Store reconstituted vials at room temperature and discard after 72 hours.

Compatibility/Compounding Considerations

Fomepizole diluted in 5% dextrose or 0.9% sodium chloride injection is stable for at least 24 hours when stored at room temperature or refrigerated.[5]

Dosage Forms/Regulatory Status

VETERINARY-LABELED PRODUCTS:

None. *Antizol-Vet*® was withdrawn from the US market in 2015.

HUMAN-LABELED PRODUCTS:

Fomepizole Injection Concentrate: 1 g/mL in 1.5 mL vials; *Antizol*®, generic; (Rx)

References

For the complete list of references, see **wiley.com/go/budde/plumb**

Fosfomycin

(fos-foe-***my***-sin) *Monurol*®

Phosphonic Acid Antimicrobial

Prescriber Highlights

- ► Uncommonly used in dogs for treatment of multidrug-resistant bacterial UTIs; may be useful for systemic infections with some multidrug-resistant bacteria, but data supporting clinical use are lacking.
- ► Nephrotoxic in cats; do not use in this species.
- ► Adverse effects in dogs are primarily GI related (eg, diarrhea, anorexia).

Uses/Indications

Fosfomycin is an antibacterial agent that may be useful for treating multidrug-resistant UTIs in dogs; use should be limited to infections with documented resistance to other antibiotics and involving bacterial species typically susceptible to fosfomycin.[1] It may also be useful for other multidrug-resistant genitourinary infections (eg, prostatitis), although data and experience are limited.[1]

The World Health Organization (WHO) has designated fosfomycin as a Critically Important (High Priority) antimicrobial in human medicine.[2] The Office International des Epizooties (OIE) has designated fosfomycin as a Veterinary Highly Important Antimicrobial Agent in avian, bovine, and swine species.[3]

Pharmacology/Actions

Fosfomycin is a synthetic phosphonic acid derivative antibacterial agent. It irreversibly inhibits bacterial phosphoenolpyruvate transferase, an enzyme that catalyzes the formation of uridine diphosphate-N-acetylmuramic acid, which is the first step of microbial cell wall peptidoglycan synthesis. Additionally, it reduces adherence of bacteria to uroepithelial cells.[4]

Fosfomycin is a time-dependent antibacterial agent.[5] At therapeutic dosages, this antibiotic is rapidly bactericidal in urine. It has generally good activity against *Escherichia coli, Enterococcus faecalis,* and *Proteus* spp, typically including strains that are resistant to many other antimicrobials. It can also be effective against other bacteria such as staphylococci, *Enterococcus faecium, Klebsiella* spp, and *Enterobacter* spp.

Cross-resistance apparently does not occur with beta-lactams or aminoglycosides. Acquired (plasmid-mediated) resistance is currently uncommon in most areas[6,7] but has been identified in humans and companion animals, with potential transfer between humans and companion animals.[8-10]

Pharmacokinetics

Fosfomycin tromethamine is rapidly converted to the free acid fosfomycin after absorption.[11] Fosfomycin is distributed into the kidneys, bladder wall, and prostate, and crosses the placenta. The primary route of elimination is as unchanged drug in urine (38% of an oral dose in humans).

In dogs, following oral administration of fosfomycin disodium (compounded product) peak concentration occurs at ≈2 hours, bioavailability is ≈29%, and terminal half-life is ≈2 hours.[12] In the same study, following IV administration of fosfomycin disodium to dogs the volume of distribution (steady-state) is ≈0.7 L/kg with minimal protein binding, and clearance is ≈15 mL/kg/hour.[12]

The commercially available oral product is the tromethamine salt. Dogs receiving 80 mg/kg PO of this product showed high (≈100%) oral bioavailability when it was given with food. Fasted bioavailability was lower and averaged 66%. Elimination half-life was ≈2.5 hours. Serum concentrations exceeded the MIC_{90} reported for multidrug-resistant *Escherichia coli* (1.5 µg/mL) for 12 hours.[5,13] In healthy dogs receiving 80 mg/kg fosfomycin tromethamine PO, fosfomycin half-life in the urine was 10 hours, and urinary concentrations were above 660 micrograms/mL for the entire 12-hour observation window.[14]

In horses, SC bioavailability of fosfomycin disodium is ≈85%. Peak concentrations occur ≈3.25 hours after SC dosing. Mean volume of distribution (steady-state) is 0.21 L/kg; clearance is 16 to 24 mL/kg/hour; and terminal half-life is ≈1.3 hours.[15]

Contraindications/Precautions/Warnings

Fosfomycin is contraindicated in patients with a known hypersensitivity to this antibiotic.

Because fosfomycin has been documented to be nephrotoxic in cats, it should also be considered contraindicated in this species.[16,17] In one study, cats were given fosfomycin (as the calcium or sodium salt) 20 mg/kg PO or IV twice daily for 3 days, and all cats (n = 25) that were given the drug had significant increases in serum creatinine.[17] Tubular necrosis, disappearance of tubular cells, and rearrangement of eosinophilic nonstructural material were observed in the kidneys of all the treated cats.

In humans, renal impairment can substantially increase half-life and dose reductions are recommended.[18] No data are available for specific recommendations when using fosfomycin in veterinary patients with impaired renal function.

Do not confuse fosfomycin with aminoglycoside antibacterials (eg, gentamicin).

Adverse Effects

There is little information available on this drug's adverse effect profile in animals. Mild to moderate diarrhea is the most common adverse effect seen in dogs treated with fosfomycin[13]; anecdotally, hyporexia and anorexia have also been reported.

In humans, the most common adverse effect is diarrhea (9%), with vaginitis (5%), nausea (4%), and headache (4%) also reported.[11]

Reproductive/Nursing Safety

Fosfomycin crosses the placental barrier in humans. Teratogenic effects were not observed in rats receiving up to 1000 mg/kg.[11]

It is unknown if fosfomycin is distributed into milk following oral administration[11]; following IM injection in pregnant sows, fosfomycin was found in to cross into milk.[19]

Because safety has not been established in animals, this drug should only be used when the maternal benefits outweigh the potential risks to offspring.

Overdose/Acute Toxicity

In most species, overdoses would most likely cause GI effects. In dogs, single oral overdoses up to 5 g/kg caused diarrhea and anorexia 2 to 3 days after administration.[11]

For patients that have experienced or are suspected to have experienced an overdose, consultation with a 24-hour poison consultation center specializing in providing veterinary-specific information is recommended. For general information related to overdose and toxin exposures, as well as contact information for poison control centers, refer to ***Appendix***.

Drug Interactions

The following drug interactions have either been reported or are theoretical in humans or animals receiving fosfomycin and may be of significance in veterinary patients. Unless otherwise noted, use together is not necessarily contraindicated, but weigh the potential risks and perform additional monitoring when appropriate.

- **Prokinetic Gastrointestinal (GI) Agents** (eg, **metoclopramide**): Can decrease serum and urine concentrations of fosfomycin.[11] Although no interactions have been reported, drugs that can increase GI motility (eg, **bethanechol, cisapride, domperidone, metoclopramide, ranitidine, laxatives**) may have a similar effect. Separating administration may help minimize interaction.

Laboratory Considerations

- No specific concerns noted

Dosages

DOGS:

Bacterial cystitis caused by multidrug-resistant bacteria documented to be resistant to other antibiotics and involving bacterial species with confirmed susceptibility to fosfomycin (extra-label): 40 – 80 mg/kg PO (with food) every 12 hours.[1,14] Treatment for 3 to 5 days is likely to be sufficient for most infections, although longer treatment (eg, 7-14 days) may be needed for persistent or relapsing infections.[1]

Tissue-associated infections (eg, prostatitis, pyelonephritis; extra-label): 40 mg/kg PO (with food) every 8 hours[1]

Monitoring

- Clinical efficacy: resolution of clinical signs associated with UTI[1]
- Recheck urinalysis and aerobic bacterial urine culture 5 to 7 days after cessation of antimicrobials[1]
- Adverse effects: GI signs (eg, diarrhea, loss of appetite)

Client Information

- There is little clinical experience with this drug in animals; report any possible side effects to your veterinarian immediately. The most common side effects are diarrhea and loss of appetite.
- It is important to give this medication exactly as prescribed and to complete the full course of therapy, even if your animal seems better. Missing doses or stopping treatment early may result in the treatment not working.
- Give this medicine to your animal with food.
- After your animal finishes taking this medicine, it is important to return to your veterinarian for recheck testing 5 to 7 days after the last dose. Do not miss this important follow-up visit.
- This medicine should not be given to cats.

Chemistry/Synonyms

Fosfomycin is an antibacterial agent originally isolated from *Streptomyces fradiae*, now exclusively produced by chemical synthesis. It occurs as a white or almost white, hygroscopic powder that is very soluble in water, slightly soluble in alcohol or methyl alcohol, and practically insoluble in acetone. A 5% solution in water has a pH of 3.5 to 5.5.

Fosfomycin may also be known as MK-955, phosphomycin, phosphonomycin, fosfomicina, fosfomycine, fosfomycinum, or fosfomysiini. Its chemical name is cis-1, 2-epoxyphosphonic acid.

Storage/Stability

Fosfomycin tromethamine granules should be stored at room temperature (25°C [77°F]) with excursions permitted to 15°C to 30°C (59°F-86°F).[11]

Compatibility/Compounding Considerations

To reconstitute, pour the entire contents of a single-dose sachet of fosfomycin into 90 to 120 mL of water (½ cup) and stir to dissolve. Do not use hot water. Fosfomycin should be taken immediately after dissolving in water.[11]

Dosage Forms/Regulatory Status

VETERINARY-LABELED PRODUCTS: NONE

HUMAN-LABELED PRODUCTS:

Fosfomycin Tromethamine 3 g per packet (for dilution and oral use); *Monurol*®; (Rx)[11]

Fosfomycin sodium for injection may be available in countries outside the United States.

References

For the complete list of references, see **wiley.com/go/budde/plumb**

Frunevetmab

(froo-neh-***vet***-mab) *Solensia®*

Feline antinerve growth factor monoclonal antibody

Prescriber Highlights

- ▶ Feline-specific biologic agent approved for the control of pain associated with osteoarthritis in cats
- ▶ Contraindications include hypersensitivity to it, breeding cats, and pregnant or lactating queens. Product is not intended for use in any other species.
- ▶ Appears to be well-tolerated. Injection site pain, injection site reactions, and GI effects are possible.
- ▶ Pregnant or breastfeeding women, as well as those trying to conceive, should exercise extreme caution to avoid accidental self-injection; use appropriate precautions when handling.

Uses/Indications

Frunevetmab is approved for the control of pain associated with osteoarthritis in cats.[1,2] A single injection provided significant pain relief and increased activity for up to 6 weeks in cats with degenerative joint disease.[3] Up to 76% of cats that received 3 doses of frunevetmab were considered a treatment success based on objective owner assessments.[4] The analgesic effect of frunevetmab became apparent ≈2 to 3 weeks after administration.[3-5]

It is unknown whether frunevetmab is effective or safe for use in cats with immune-mediated arthropathies or with pain from other causes (eg, visceral pain, orthopedic surgery, fracture, metastatic cancer).

Pharmacology/Actions

Frunevetmab is a felinized immunoglobulin G (IgG) monoclonal antibody (mAb) that binds to nerve growth factor (NGF). NGF is essential for peripheral neuronal survival, particularly in early (prenatal and early postnatal) life, but in mature animals, NGF also modulates nociceptive neural activity.[6] NGF is one of many chemical mediators released in response to noxious stimuli and produces peripheral sensitization, neurogenic inflammation, and increased perception of pain. NGF is elevated in osteoarthritic joints. NGF receptors (tropomyosin receptor kinase A [TrkA] and $p75^{NTR}$) are found in many cell types (eg, immune and endothelial cells, synoviocytes, chondrocytes) as well as on peripheral nerves. Frunevetmab binds NGF, which subsequently inhibits the binding of NGF to its receptors and results in decreased release of other chemical mediators of pain and inflammation as well as reduced cellular signal transduction in cell types involved in pain.[6]

Frunevetmab does not bind to other neurotrophins (eg, feline neurotrophin-4, human neurotrophin -3 or -4, brain-derived neurotrophic factor).

Pharmacokinetics

Frunevetmab bioavailability following SC injection was 60% to 73% in cats with osteoarthritis (OA).[2,7] In healthy cats, peak frunevetmab concentration (C_{max}, ≈43 µg/mL) occurred 3.5 days after SC administration.[2] However, C_{max} was lower (26.1 µg/mL) and was reached later (3 to 7 days) in cats with OA.[7] Monoclonal antibodies have a volume of distribution roughly equal to the plasma volume and typically do not cross the blood–brain barrier.[8] Steady-state frunevetmab concentrations are reached after 2 doses.[2] Monoclonal antibodies undergo peptide degradation.[9] Frunevetmab half-life is ≈10 to 12 days.[2,7]

Contraindications/Precautions/Warnings

Frunvetmab is contraindicated in patients hypersensitive to it, in breeding cats, and in pregnant or lactating queens.[2] See ***Reproductive/Nursing Safety***. Hypersensitivity reactions, including delayed hypersensitivity, may occur with frunevetmab use and necessitates discontinuation. Frunevetmab is a feline-specific product; it has not been evaluated in cats less than 7 months old or 2.5 kg (5.5 lb) and should not be used in any other species.

Cats may form anti-frunevetmab antibodies, with resulting loss of effectiveness.[2]

Nerve growth factors play an important role in the normal development of the nervous system. The manufacturer cautions that women who are pregnant, trying to conceive, or breastfeeding should use extreme caution to avoid accidental self-injection. Use of personal protective equipment to minimize the risk for exposure is recommended.

Adverse Effects

In cats receiving frunevetmab, local reactions at the injection site (scabbing, dermatitis, alopecia, pruritus, swelling) were reported in ≈3% to 6% of cats and were reported more frequently with frunevetmab than placebo.[2] GI signs (vomiting, diarrhea, and anorexia) and injection site pain were reported in ≈7% to 14% of cats and occurred with similar/equivalent frequency in cats receiving frunevetmab and placebo. Worsening of existing renal insufficiency (6.6%), dehydration (4.4%), weight loss (3.3%), and gingival disorders (2.2%) also were reported in cats receiving frunevetmab.

Treatment-emergent immunogenicity was identified in 1.5% of cats treated with frunevetmab and in 2.3% of placebo-treated cats.[7]

The safety and immunogenicity of long-term (administered over many months or years) frunevetmab use are not yet known.

In humans, the use of antinerve growth factor monoclonal antibodies for knee or hip osteoarthritis pain has resulted in mild to moderate, dose-dependent peripheral or extremity pain and neurosensory symptoms (paresthesia, hypoesthesia, or hyperesthesia)[6]; these effects typically were transient and/or reversible.[10] Rapidly progressive osteoarthritis (RPOA) and osteonecrosis in nontarget joints were also observed; the incidence of RPOA was increased with concurrent NSAID use.[11,12] The significance of these findings for veterinary patients is uncertain.

Reproductive/Nursing Safety

Frunevetmab is contraindicated in breeding cats or in pregnant or lactating queens.[2] Fetal abnormalities, increased rates of stillbirths, and increased postpartum fetal mortality have been noted in rodents and primates receiving anti-NGF mAbs.

Overdosage/Acute Toxicity

Clinical signs in cats receiving up to 14 mg/kg every 28 days (5 times the maximum label dose) included GI (vomiting, diarrhea) and dermatologic (abrasions, alopecia, scabbing) signs.[2] Bilirubinuria was observed in 1 cat receiving 2.8 mg/kg, 1 cat receiving 8.4 mg/kg, and 1 receiving 14 mg/kg (3 cats total).

For patients that have experienced or are suspected of having experienced an overdose, it is strongly encouraged to contact a 24-hour poison consultation center that specializes in providing information specific for veterinary patients. For general information related to overdose and toxin exposures, as well as contact information for poison control centers, refer to ***Appendix.***

Laboratory Considerations

None noted

Drug Interactions

Frunevetmab has not been studied in combination with other medications, including NSAIDs. The following drug interactions have either been reported or are theoretical in humans or animals receiving similar medications and may be of significance in veterinary patients. Unless otherwise noted, use together is not necessarily contraindicated, but weigh the potential risks and perform additional monitoring when appropriate.

- MONOCLONAL ANTIBODIES, OTHER (eg, **lokivetmab**): Concurrent use of frunevetmab with other monoclonal antibodies has not been evaluated.[2]

- **Nonsteroidal Anti-Inflammatory Drugs** (**NSAIDs**; eg, **meloxicam, robenacoxib**): In humans, the incidence of rapidly progressing osteoarthritis (RPOA) is increased in patients that received a humanized antinerve growth factor concurrent with long-term NSAID use.[11,12] The significance of this finding for veterinary patients is uncertain, and RPOA has not been reported in cats.
- **Vaccines**: Administer vaccines at a different site than frunevetmab.[1]

Dosages

CATS:

Control of pain associated with osteoarthritis in cats (label dosage; FDA approved): Cats weighing 2.5 to 7 kg (5.5 to 15.4 lb): 1 vial (7 mg, 1 mL)/cat (NOT mg/kg) SC once per month; cats weighing 7.1 to 14 kg (15.5 to 30.8 lb): 2 vials (14 mg, 2 mL)/cat (NOT mg/kg) SC once monthly.[2] The entire contents of 1 or 2 vials is administered with a target dosage range of 1 – 2.8 mg/kg.

Body weight in kg (lb)	Monthly dose (mg)	Volume (mL)	Number of vials (entire contents)
2.5 to 7 kg (5.5 to 15.4 lb)	7	1	1
7.1 to 14 kg (15.5 to 30.8 lb)	14	2	2

Monitoring

- Clinical efficacy
- Pain scale or rating system
- Adverse effects, including injection site reactions

Client Information

- This medicine is given by injection under the skin once each month to relieve pain caused by osteoarthritis in cats.
- Frunevetmab should not be given to cats used for breeding, pregnant or lactating queens, or cats less than 7 months old.
- This medicine has not been studied in cats receiving other medications. Be sure to check with your veterinarian before giving your cat any other medication(s).
- Side effects are uncommon, but pain upon giving the injection, local skin reactions at the injection site, or vomiting are possible.
- Frunevetmab was developed specifically for cats. Do not use it in any other species (eg, dogs).
- This medicine is considered to be a hazardous drug as defined by the National Institute for Occupational Safety and Health (NIOSH). Talk with your veterinarian or pharmacist about the use of personal protective equipment when handling this medicine.

Chemistry/Synonyms

Frunevetmab is a felinized immunoglobulin G monoclonal antibody. It is derived from murine antibodies in which mouse antibody regions have been replaced by feline counterparts except for the complementarity-determining regions and is manufactured through recombinant techniques in Chinese hamster ovary (CHO) cells.[13] The commercial solution is clear to slightly opalescent, has a pH of 6, and contains no preservatives.

Frunevetmab may also be known as anti-NGF mAb or *Solensia*®.

Storage/Stability

Protect frunevetmab from light and refrigerate at 2°C to 8°C (35°F-46°F); do not freeze. Store vials in an upright position; avoid shaking or foaming the solution. Use contents immediately once the vial is punctured.

Compatibility/Compounding Considerations

None noted

Dosage Forms/Regulatory Status

VETERINARY-LABELED PRODUCTS:

Frunevetmab Injection: 7 mg/mL in 1 mL single-use vials supplied in cartons of 1, 2, or 6 vials; *Solensia*®; (Rx). NADA #141-546

HUMAN-LABELED PRODUCTS: NONE

References

For the complete list of references, see **wiley.com/go/budde/plumb**

Furazolidone

(fyoor-a-**zoe**-li-done) *Furoxone*®

Antibacterial/Antiprotozoal

Prescriber Highlights

- ► Antibacterial/antiprotozoal nitrofuran that has been used in dogs and cats; not available in the United States
- ► Contraindicated in animals with known hypersensitivity
- ► Adverse effects include GI effects (eg, anorexia, vomiting, cramping, diarrhea) and innocuous discoloration of urine to a dark yellow or brown color.
- ► Many potential drug interactions
- ► Extra-label use is prohibited in food animals.

Uses/Indications

Furazolidone is usually a second-line choice for treatment of enteric infections in small animal species caused by susceptible bacteria and protozoa (see ***Pharmacology***). It is no longer commercially available in the United States.

Pharmacology/Actions

Furazolidone interferes with susceptible bacterial enzyme systems and is bactericidal. Its mechanism against susceptible protozoa is not well determined. Furazolidone has activity against *Giardia* spp, *Vibrio cholerae, Trichomonas* spp, *Coccidia* spp, and many strains of *Escherichia coli, Enterobacter* spp, *Campylobacter* spp, *Salmonella* spp, and *Shigella* spp. Not all strains are sensitive, but resistance is usually limited and develops slowly. Furazolidone metabolites inhibit monoamine oxidase.

Pharmacokinetics

Published information on the absorption characteristics of furazolidone is conflicting. Pigmented metabolites in the urine indicate that it is absorbed to some extent; however, because furazolidone is used to treat enteric infections, absorption only becomes important regarding the adverse effect profile and drug interactions. Reportedly, furazolidone distributes into the CSF. Absorbed furazolidone is rapidly metabolized in the liver, and the majority of the absorbed drug is eliminated in the urine.

Contraindications/Precautions/Warnings

Furazolidone is contraindicated in patients that are hypersensitive to it.

Because furazolidone also inhibits monoamine oxidase, it may potentially interact with several other drugs and foods (see ***Drug Interactions*** below). The clinical significance of these interactions remains unclear, especially in the presence of poor absorption.

Extra-label use of furazolidone in food animals is prohibited.

Adverse Effects

Adverse effects noted with furazolidone are usually minimal. Anorexia, vomiting, cramping, and diarrhea may occasionally occur.

Hypersensitivity has been reported in some humans.

Reproductive/Nursing Safety

Although no teratogenic effects of furazolidone have been located, the safe use of furazolidone during pregnancy has not been established. One reference states that furazolidone should not be used in pregnant queens.[1] It is unknown if furazolidone enters maternal milk.

Because safety has not been established in animals, this drug should only be used when the maternal benefits outweigh the potential risks to offspring.

Overdose/Acute Toxicity

No information was located, but moderate overdoses are unlikely to cause significant toxicity. GI decontamination may be considered for large overdoses.

For patients that have experienced or are suspected to have experienced an overdose, consultation with a 24-hour poison consultation center specializing in providing veterinary-specific information is recommended. For general information related to overdose and toxin exposures, as well as contact information for poison control centers, refer to ***Appendix.***

Drug Interactions

The following drug interactions have either been reported or are theoretical in humans or animals receiving furazolidonc and may be of significance in veterinary patients. Unless otherwise noted, use together is not necessarily contraindicated, but weigh the potential risks and perform additional monitoring when appropriate.

- ETHANOL: Concomitant administration may cause a disulfiram-like reaction.

Because furazolidone inhibits monoamine oxidase, its use concurrently with the following drugs is not recommended because dangerous hypertension could occur:

- AMITRAZ
- BUSPIRONE
- LINEZOLID
- METHYLENE BLUE
- SELEGILINE
- SEROTONERGIC AGENTS (eg, **cyproheptadine, fluoxetine, mirtazapine, sertraline, trazodone**)
- SYMPATHOMIMETIC AMINES (eg, **phenylpropanolamine, ephedrine**)
- TRICYCLIC ANTIDEPRESSANTS (eg, **amitriptyline, clomipramine**)
- TYRAMINE-CONTAINING FOODS (eg, **fish, poultry, smoked meats, aged cheeses**)

Laboratory Considerations

- Furazolidone may cause a false-positive **urine glucose** determination when using the cupric sulfate solution test (eg, *Clinitest*®).

Dosages

CATS:

Giardiasis (extra-label): 4 mg/kg PO every 12 hours for 7 to 10 days; if re-treatment is required, higher doses or longer treatment duration may provide better results.[2,3]

Monitoring

- Efficacy (stool exams for parasitic infections)

Client Information

- Although this medicine may discolor your animal's urine to a dark yellow to brown color, it does not cause harm and will go away once the medicine is stopped.
- Contact your veterinarian if your animal has continued serious vomiting or diarrhea or loss of an appetite to your veterinarian.

Chemistry/Synonyms

Furazolidone, a synthetic nitrofuran-derivative antibacterial/antiprotozoal, occurs as a bitter-tasting, yellow, crystalline powder. It is practically insoluble in water.

Furazolidone may also be known as nifurazolidonum, *Enterolidon*®, *Exofur*®, *Furasian*®, *Furion*®, *Furoxona*®, *Fuxol*®, *Giarcid*®, *Giardil*®, *Giarlam*®, *Neo Furasil*®, *Nifuran*®, *Novafur*®, *Salmocide*®, and *Seforman*®.

Storage/Stability

Store this product protected from light in tight containers.

Compatibility/Compounding Considerations

No specific information was noted.

Dosage Forms/Regulatory Status

VETERINARY-LABELED PRODUCTS: NONE

Extra-label use of furazolidone is prohibited in food-producing animals.

HUMAN-LABELED PRODUCTS:

None; the human product *Furoxone*® has been withdrawn from the United States market. Preparations may be available from compounding pharmacies.

References

For the complete list of references, see **wiley.com/go/budde/plumb**

Furosemide

(fur-***oh***-se-mide) *Disal*®, *Lasix*®, *Salix*®

Loop Diuretic

Prescriber Highlights

- ► A loop diuretic commonly used in many species for treatment of congestive heart failure, pulmonary edema, udder edema, hypercalcemia, and acute kidney injury. Used as adjunctive therapy in hyperkalemia and rarely as an antihypertensive agent. Used in racehorses to prevent/reduce exercise-induced pulmonary hemorrhage (EIPH)
- ► Contraindications include patients with anuria, hypersensitivity, dehydration, or serious electrolyte depletion.
- ► Use with caution in patients with preexisting electrolyte or water balance abnormalities, impaired hepatic function, progressive renal disease, and/or diabetes mellitus.
- ► Adverse effects include fluid and electrolyte (especially hyponatremia/hypochloremia) abnormalities, acid-base disturbances (metabolic alkalosis), ototoxicity, GI distress, hematologic effects, weakness, and restlessness. SC injection may cause ulcerative skin lesions in dogs and other species.
- ► Prerenal azotemia is possible if dehydration occurs.
- ► Normal food and water intake should be encouraged.

Uses/Indications

Furosemide is used for its diuretic activity in all species. It is used in small animals for the treatment of congestive heart failure (CHF), pulmonary edema, hypercalcemia, acute kidney injury, as adjunctive therapy in hyperkalemia, and, rarely, as an antihypertensive agent. It can be used to decrease the incidence of sterile hemorrhagic cystitis associated with cyclophosphamide administration in dogs.[1-4]

In cattle, furosemide is FDA-approved for the treatment of postparturient udder edema.[5]

Furosemide has also been used to help prevent or reduce the severity of epistaxis (ie, exercise-induced pulmonary hemorrhage; EIPH) in racehorses.[6,7] An American College of Veterinary Internal Medicine consensus statement declared that, based on the research done on EIPH in horses, there is high-quality evidence that furosemide is effective in the prophylaxis of this disease.[8] The panel makes a weak recommendation for its use in management of racehorses with EIPH because of regulation of this issue by racing jurisdictions. The panel also found high-quality evidence that furosemide is associated with improved performance by thoroughbred and standardbred racehorses.

Pharmacology/Actions

Furosemide can reduce the absorption of electrolytes in the medullary portion of the thick ascending loop of Henle by impairing the activity of the NA^+-K^+-$2Cl^-$ cotransporter. It also decreases the reabsorption of both sodium and chloride, increases the excretion of potassium in the distal renal tubule, and directly affects electrolyte transport in the proximal tubule. It has no effect on carbonic anhydrase and does not antagonize aldosterone. In dogs and cats, furosemide is considered to have a potency of $1/10^{th}$ to $1/20^{th}$ that of torsemide, the other loop diuretic commonly used in veterinary medicine.[9-11]

Furosemide can increase renal excretion of water, sodium, potassium, chloride, calcium, magnesium, hydrogen, ammonium, and bicarbonate. In dogs, excretion of potassium is affected much less than sodium; hyponatremia may be more of a concern than hypokalemia and hypochloremia is common. Furosemide causes some renal vendilation and transiently increases glomerular filtration rates (GFR). Renal blood flow is increased (so long as profound dehydration does not develop) and decreased peripheral vascular resistance may occur. Although furosemide increases renin secretion, because of its other effects on the nephron, increases in sodium and water retention do not occur.[12,13] Furosemide can cause hyperglycemia, but to a lesser extent than the thiazide diuretic agents.

Doses of 1 – 4 mg/kg IV or PO decreased, in a dose-proportional manner, left atrial pressure in dogs with experimentally induced mitral regurgitation.[14] It has been shown that in dogs, doses lower than 1 mg/kg can produce diuresis with only mild activation of the renin–angiotensin–aldosterone system.[15] In a study of healthy dogs, furosemide was diluted with 2.4% hypertonic saline and administered as a CRI for 5 hours. The results showed no intravascular volume expansion and a reduced activation of the renin–angiotensin–aldosterone system. The authors concluded that dilution of furosemide with hypertonic saline may be beneficial in dogs with heart failure.[16] At high doses (10 – 12 mg/kg), thoracic duct lymph flow is increased in dogs.[17] In horses, furosemide has some bronchodilatory effects.[18] Cats are reportedly more sensitive to the diuretic effects of furosemide as compared with other species.

In horses with recurrent obstructive pulmonary disease, furosemide administered by aerosol or IV at 1 mg/kg may significantly reduce pulmonary resistance and increase dynamic compliance.[18-20] This effect can persist for at least 5 hours, but it is abolished by flunixin meglumine.[20]

The efficacy of furosemide in reptiles, birds, and fish has been questioned because of these species' lack of a loop of Henle. However, furosemide seems to have other effects on the nephron and has been shown to reduce body weight and/or pulmonary blood volume, even when diuresis does not occur.[21]

Pharmacokinetics

In dogs, the oral bioavailability is ≈77%. It has a rapid onset of action of ≈5 minutes when administered IV, 30 minutes when administered IM, and 30 to 60 minutes when administered PO. The drug is highly (more than 90%) protein bound. Its duration of action is 3 to 6 hours, and the elimination half-life is ≈1 to 1.5 hours in dogs and cats, up to 2.7 hours in cattle,[22] and up to 3.2 hours in horses.[6] In healthy dogs, when administered IV, SC, and PO, the urine output peaked at 1 hour (IV), 1 hour (SC), and 2 hours (PO) and returned to baseline levels at 2, 4, and 6 hours, respectively. The total urine output was similar for all 3 routes of administration.[23]

The pharmacokinetics of furosemide were studies in healthy cats.[24] After oral administration, bioavailability was ≈50%, and half-life was ≈1.2 hours. After IV administration, the volume of distribution was 227 mL/kg, clearance was 149 mL/kg/hour, and elimination half-life was 2.25 hours.

In sheep, the time to peak concentration after IM and SC administration was 20 minutes and 25 minutes, respectively, with considerably different bioavailability of 97.9% after IM administration and 38% after SC, suggesting IM or IV as the preferred parenteral routes of administration in sheep. The elimination half-life was 0.8 hours by all routes of administration (IV, IM, SC) in sheep. The mean total clearance and volume of distribution at steady state following IV administration were 0.24 L/hour/kg and 0.17 L/kg, respectively.[25]

In humans, furosemide is 60% to 75% absorbed following oral administration. The diuretic effect takes place within 5 minutes after IV administration and within 1 hour after oral administration. Peak effects occur ≈30 minutes after IV administration and 1 to 2 hours after oral administration. The drug is ≈95% bound to plasma proteins in both azotemic and normal patients. The serum half-life is ≈2 hours but is prolonged in patients with chronic kidney disease, uremia, or CHF, and in neonates.

Contraindications/Precautions/Warnings

Furosemide is contraindicated in patients with anuria or hepatic coma and those that are hypersensitive to the drug. The manufacturer states that the drug should be discontinued in patients with progressive renal disease if increasing azotemia and oliguria occur during therapy.

Furosemide should be used with caution in patients with preexisting electrolyte or water balance abnormalities, impaired hepatic function (may precipitate hepatic coma), progressive renal disease, or diabetes mellitus. Patients with conditions that may lead to electrolyte or water balance abnormalities (eg, vomiting, diarrhea) should be monitored carefully. Patients hypersensitive to sulfonamides may also be hypersensitive to furosemide (not documented in veterinary species).

Furosemide should be used cautiously with other drugs that can cause renal toxicity or ototoxicity (eg, aminoglycoside antibiotics), as furosemide may potentiate these toxic effects.

Adverse Effects

Furosemide may induce fluid and electrolyte abnormalities. Patients should be monitored for hydration status and electrolyte imbalances (particularly potassium, sodium, and chloride, as well as calcium and magnesium). Prerenal azotemia may result if moderate to severe dehydration occurs. Hypochloremia is commonly encountered, and hyponatremia is likely the greatest concern, but hypocalcemia, hypokalemia, and hypomagnesemia may all occur. Animals with normal food and water intake are much less likely to develop water and electrolyte imbalances than those without.

Other potential adverse effects include ototoxicity, especially in cats receiving high-dose IV therapy.[26] Dogs reportedly require doses greater than 22 mg/kg IV to cause hearing loss.[27] Other effects include GI disturbances (eg, nausea, vomiting, diarrhea), weakness, and restlessness.

A case of a dermatologic reaction (ulcerative lesions) at the injection sites after SC administration of furosemide in a dog has been reported.[28] This dog had received injections from 2 separate formulations from different manufacturers. The product suspected of causation had a pH between 8.66 and 9.05, whereas the product that did not cause a reaction had a pH between 7.2 and 7.47 (although none of the tested lots were used in the patient). The authors concluded that veterinarians should exercise caution when prescribing furosemide SC and consider the potential effects of the furosemide formulation (eg, pH) in their choice when prescribing this route.

Reproductive/Nursing Safety

Furosemide may cause fetal abnormalities and its use is contraindicated in pregnant animals and stallions used for breeding.[29,30] Unexplained maternal deaths and abortion occurred in the second trimester in rabbits receiving furosemide at 10 to 25 times the recommended average dose of 2 mg/kg for dogs, cats, horses, and cattle[5,31]; and fetal hydronephrosis has been noted in laboratory animals.[29,31] Although the United Kingdom product label states that furosemide can be used during pregnancy and lactation,[22] the United States product labels state that the drug is either not recommended during the second trimester of pregnancy[5,31] or that the drug is contraindicated in pregnant animals.[29,30] Clinicians should consider the risks versus benefits when using furosemide in a pregnant animal, as there is conflicting information between the United States and United Kingdom product labels.

Caution should be used in reproductively active hens, as furosemide has been shown to decrease eggshell thickness and inhibit calcium transport in the shell gland mucosa, which could lead to dystocia.[32]

Furosemide appears in milk; clinical significance to nursing offspring is unknown. Because safety has not been established in animals, this drug should only be used when the maternal benefits outweigh the potential risks to offspring.

Overdose/Acute Toxicity

The LD_{50} in dogs is greater than 1000 mg/kg after oral administration and 300 mg/kg after IV injection.[31] Chronic overdosing at 10 mg/kg for 6 months in dogs has led to mild dehydration and development of calcification and scarring of the renal parenchyma.[31] Temporary deafness may occur, particularly after rapid IV administration of high doses. See ***Adverse Effects***.

Acute overdoses may cause electrolyte and water imbalances, neurologic effects (eg, lethargy, coma, seizures), and cardiovascular collapse.

Treatment consists of standard protocols to empty the gut after acute oral ingestion. Concomitant cathartics should not be used, as they may exacerbate fluid and electrolyte imbalances. Electrolyte and water balance abnormalities should be aggressively monitored and treated supportively. Respiratory, neurologic, and cardiovascular status should also be monitored and treated as clinically indicated.

Drug Interactions

The following drug interactions have either been reported or are theoretical in humans or animals receiving furosemide and may be of significance in veterinary patients. Unless otherwise noted, use together is not necessarily contraindicated, but the potential risks should be weighed and additional monitoring performed when appropriate.

- ANGIOTENSIN CONVERTING ENZYME INHIBITORS (ACEIs; eg, **benazepril, enalapril**): Increased risk for hypotension, particularly in patients that are volume- or sodium-depleted secondary to diuretics
- AMINOGLYCOSIDES (eg, **amikacin, gentamicin**): Increased risk for nephrotoxicity and ototoxicity (including complete deafness, even with use of typical drug dosages)
- AMPHOTERICIN B: Loop diuretics may increase the risk for nephrotoxicity and hypokalemia.
- CEPHALOSPORINS (eg, **cefazolin, cefovecin**): Increased risk for nephrotoxicity
- CISPLATIN: Increased risk for nephrotoxicity and ototoxicity (including complete deafness, even with use of typical drug dosages)
- CORTICOSTEROIDS (eg, **fludrocortisone, prednisone**): Increased risk for GI ulceration; hypokalemia
- CYCLOSPORINE: Increased risk for hyperuricemia
- DESMOPRESSIN: Increased risk for hyponatremia
- DIGOXIN: Furosemide-induced hypokalemia may increase the potential for digoxin toxicity.
- INSULIN: Furosemide may alter insulin requirements.
- NONDEPOLARIZING MUSCLE RELAXANTS (eg, **atracurium, tubocurarine**): Furosemide may prolong neuromuscular blockade.
- NONSTEROIDAL ANTI-INFLAMMATORY DRUGS (NSAIDs; eg, **carprofen, firocoxib, flunixin, meloxicam, phenylbutazone**): Increased risk for acute kidney injury
- OXYTETRACYCLINE: Increased risk for nephrotoxicity
- POLYMYXIN B: Increased risk for acute kidney injury
- PROBENECID: Furosemide can reduce uricosuric effects.
- SALICYLATES (eg, **aspirin**): Loop diuretics can reduce excretion of salicylates.
- SUCCINYLCHOLINE: Furosemide may potentiate effects.
- THEOPHYLLINE/AMINOPHYLLINE: Pharmacologic effects of theophylline may be enhanced when used with furosemide.

Laboratory Considerations

- **Free thyroxine (fT_4)**: Furosemide can result in an increased fT_4 fraction; furosemide inhibits T_4 binding to canine serum in vitro.

Dosages

NOTE: Watch units closely when calculating doses. Do not confuse CRI dosages using mg/kg/hour with µg/kg/minute.

DOGS:

Label dosages (FDA-approved):

Treatment of edema (pulmonary congestion, ascites) associated with cardiac insufficiency and acute noninflammatory tissue edema:

- Injection: 2.75 – 5.5 mg/kg IV or IM once or twice daily after a 6- to 8-hour interval[5,29-31]
- PO: 2.2 – 5.5 mg/kg PO once or twice daily with a 6- to 8-hour interval between doses[30,31]

The dose should be adjusted to the individual animal's response.[5,31] In refractory or severe edematous cases, the dose may be doubled or increased by increments of 2.2 mg/kg of body weight to establish the effective dose. The established effective dose should be administered once or twice daily. The daily schedule can be timed for the convenience of the pet owner or veterinarian. Diuretic therapy should be discontinued after reduction of edema or, when necessary, maintained after determining a programmed dose schedule to prevent recurrence.

Extra-label dosages:

Acute cardiogenic or pulmonary edema (parenteral administration):

a) **Congestive heart failure from stage C myxomatous mitral valve disease**: Initial dose, furosemide 2 mg/kg IV (or IM), followed by 2 mg/kg IV or IM hourly until the patient's respiratory signs are substantially improved or a total of 8 mg/kg has been reached over 4 hours.[33] For life-threatening pulmonary edema, furosemide may also be administered as a CRI (see below).

b) Bolus dosing: Initially, 1 – 4 mg/kg IV, IM, or SC (use SC route with caution, see ***Adverse Effects***) is administered, then adjusted and repeated every 1 to 2 hours until respiratory rate and/or respiratory character improves. A maximum daily dose of 12 mg/kg has been noted.[33,34] **NOTE**: SC furosemide administration produced similar total urine output as compared with IV and PO doses.[23]

c) **CRI**: 0.66 – 1 mg/kg/hour IV CRI after the furosemide initial bolus[35,36] may produce greater diuresis, natriuresis, and less kaliuresis.[16,33,34,37] One study noted lower cumulative furosemide use when given by CRI (median dosage, 0.99 mg/kg/hour; range 0.025 – 3.73 mg/kg/hour) as compared with IV bolus (median, 1.19 mg/kg/hour; range 0.027 – 7.14 mg/kg/hour) with a trend toward longer hospitalization in the IV bolus group.[37] Another study found similar diuresis when furosemide was diluted to a final concentration of 2.2 mg/mL with 5% dextrose solution (1.5 mL/kg) or 2.4% hypertonic saline solution (1 mL/kg of 5% dextrose + 0.5 mL/kg of 7.2% sodium chloride).[16] Prolonged CRI administration (beyond 12 to 24 hours) should be performed cautiously as severe volume depletion may occur.

Adjunctive treatment of CHF (oral administration): Oral dosage recommendations can vary widely and are tailored for each patient. In general, the goal is to give the lowest effective dose of furosemide. Dogs with mild heart failure signs may initially be controlled with 1 mg/kg PO every 24 hours, whereas dogs with severe heart failure may require doses as high as 5 mg/kg PO every 8 hours. A common oral starting dosage in dogs with stage C myxomatous mitral valve disease when treating chronically at home is 2 mg/kg orally every 12 hours with the dose adjusted to effect to maintain patient comfort.[33]

Adjunctive treatment of dogs with glomerular disease and pulmonary edema or hyperkalemia: Furosemide may be administered at an initial dosage of 1 mg/kg every 6 to 12 hours IV or IM, with incremental increases of 0.5 – 1 mg/kg every 6 to 12 hours or conversion into 2 – 15 µg/kg/minute IV after an initial loading dose of 2 mg/kg IV in animals with insufficient response.[38]

Adjunctive treatment of moderate to severe hypercalcemia: Volume expansion is necessary before use of furosemide; 2 – 4 mg/kg every 8 to 12 hours, IV, SC, or PO.[39] Use SC route with caution, see ***Adverse Effects.***

Adjunctive therapy for systemic hypertension: 1 – 4 mg/kg PO every 8 to 24 hours. Loop diuretics can be considered as adjunctive treatment for systemic hypertension in dogs with edema that are not responding adequately to standard combination therapy (ie, amlodipine with ACE inhibitor or angiotensin receptor blocker).[40]

Oliguric acute kidney injury: Furosemide can increase urine output so that IV fluid therapy can correct acid-base and electrolyte imbalances, but it does not improve GFR or necessarily affect clinical outcome. Two basic dose protocols have been recommended:

a) 0.5 – 1 mg/kg/hour IV. If furosemide administration fails to increase urine production, osmotic diuresis (mannitol) can be attempted.
b) Initial bolus 1 – 2 mg/kg IV (up to 4 mg/kg in dogs if no response seen within 30 to 60 minutes), followed by 0.1 – 2 mg/kg/hour IV, adjusted depending on patient's response

Prevent sterile hemorrhagic cystitis (SHC) caused by cyclophosphamide treatment: 0.5 – 2.2 mg/kg PO and IV every 24 hours during the course of chemotherapy reduced the incidence of or prevented SHC.[1-3] 0.5 mg/kg PO every 12 hours is also effective.[4]

CATS:

Label Dosages (FDA-approved):

Treatment of edema (pulmonary congestion, ascites) associated with cardiac insufficiency and acute noninflammatory tissue edema:

- Injection: 2.75 – 5.5 mg/kg IV or IM once or twice daily with a 6- to 8-hour interval between doses[5]
- PO: 2.2 – 5.5 mg/kg PO once or twice daily with a 6- to 8-hour interval between doses[31]

The dose should be adjusted to the individual animal's response. In refractory or severe edematous cases, the dose may be doubled or increased by increments of 2.2 mg/kg to establish the effective dose. The established effective dose should be administered once or twice daily on an intermittent daily schedule. Diuretic therapy should be discontinued after reduction of edema or, when necessary, maintained after determining a programmed dose schedule to prevent recurrence.[5,31]

Extra-Label Dosages:

Severe acute cardiogenic or pulmonary edema (parenteral administration): 1 – 3 mg/kg IV, IM, or SC (use SC route with caution, see ***Adverse Effects***), then dose is adjusted and repeated every 1 to 2 hours until respiratory rate and/or respiratory character improves. In general, slightly lower doses of furosemide should be given to cats as compared to standard doses for dogs. Cats that can tolerate IV injection may benefit from a faster onset of action (5 minutes when given IV as compared with 30 minutes when given IM). The dose may be repeated within 1 to 2 hours. To avoid severe dehydration, dose must be reduced sharply once respiratory rate starts to decrease.[34]

Adjunctive treatment of CHF (oral administration): Oral dosage recommendations can vary widely in cats and are tailored for each patient. In general, the goal is to give the lowest effective dose of furosemide. Dosages tend to be slightly lower than that for dogs and range from 1 mg/kg PO every 2 to 3 days to 2 mg/kg PO every 8 to 12 hours for most patients. Dosages up to 7 mg/kg every 12 hours have been noted. Practically, many cats receive increments of 6.25 mg (½ of a 12.5 mg tablet).[41]

Oliguric acute kidney injury: Furosemide can increase urine output so that IV fluid therapy can correct acid-base and electrolyte imbalances, but it does not improve GFR or necessarily affect clinical outcome. Two basic dosing protocols have been recommended:

a) 0.25 – 1 mg/kg/hour IV. If furosemide administration fails to increase urine production, osmotic diuresis (mannitol) can be attempted.
b) Bolus of 1 – 2 mg/kg IV and, if an effect is seen, 0.25 to 1 mg/kg/hour IV CRI is started and adjusted based on patient's response.

HORSES:

Label Dosages (FDA-approved):

Edema (pulmonary congestion, ascites) associated with cardiac insufficiency and acute noninflammatory tissue edema: 250 – 500 mg/horse (NOT mg/kg) IM or IV once or twice daily at 6- to 8-hour intervals. Should not be used in horses intended for human consumption[5]

Acute noninflammatory tissue edema: 1 mg/kg IV or IM once or twice daily at 6- to 8-hour intervals or on an intermittent daily (eg, every other day) administration schedule[29]

Extra-Label Dosages:

Adjunctive therapy for CHF: Initially, 1 – 3 mg/kg IM or IV every 6 to 12 hours to control edema, which may be followed by a 0.12 mg/kg/hour IV CRI until improvement in clinical signs. Long-term therapy: 0.5 – 2 mg/kg PO or IM every 8 to 12 hours[42,43]

Adjunctive therapy of acute kidney injury:

a) 1 – 2 mg/kg IV every 2 hours up to 4 times[44]
b) 1 mg/kg IV every 8 hours[45]
c) Loading dose of furosemide 0.12 mg/kg IV followed by 0.12 mg/kg/hour IV CRI[45]

Epistaxis and to lessen the severity of exercise-induced pulmonary hemorrhage (EIPH; NOT racehorses): 0.5 – 1 mg/kg administered IV 4 hours before strenuous exercise has been shown to decrease the severity and incidence of EIPH. Consult applicable local, state, and/or federal rules prior to any competition (including performance horses).

Epistaxis and to lessen the severity of EIPH (racehorses): If the horse to be raced is on the furosemide list, the furosemide administered dose must be between 150 mg and 500 mg/horse (NOT mg/kg) given IV as a single injection. Administration must be given *not less than 4 hours prior to scheduled post time of the race for which a horse is entered to compete.* Consult applicable local, state, and/or federal rules prior to competition, as some United States tracks may have restrictions on the use of this drug in racing horses.

CATTLE:

Physiologic parturient edema of the mammary gland and associated structures (label dosage; FDA-approved): 500 mg/cow (NOT mg/kg) IM or IV once daily or 250 mg/cow (NOT mg/kg) IV or IM twice daily at 12-hour intervals; treatment should not exceed 48 hours postparturition.[5]

BIRDS:

Cardiopulmonary disorders (edema, pericardial effusion) (extra-label): Recommended dosages ranging from 0.15 – 2 mg/kg/day PO or IM.[46] **NOTE**: Lories are very sensitive to this agent and can be easily overdosed.[47]

Oliguria/anuria in patients with renal failure (extra-label): 1 mg/kg IM[48]

FERRETS:

Adjunctive therapy for fulminant congestive heart failure (extra-label): Initially 1 – 4 mg/kg IV or IM every 8 to 12 hours; repeated after 30 minutes if there is no improvement. Once the patient is stabilized, dosage is transitioned to 1 – 2 mg/kg PO every 12 hours.[46,49,50]

RABBITS, RODENTS, & SMALL MAMMALS:

NOTE: Dosages are primarily extrapolated from those recommended for dogs and cats with similar disease states. Use furosemide with caution when administering SC (see ***Adverse Effects***), as local tissue reactions can occur.

Rabbits (extra-label):

a) **CHF**: 2 – 5 mg/kg PO, SC, IM, or IV every 12 hours

b) **Pulmonary edema**: 1 – 4 mg/kg IV or IM every 4 to 6 hours[51]

Mice, rats, gerbils, hamsters, guinea pigs, chinchillas (extra-label): 5 – 10 mg/kg every 12 hours[52]

REPTILES:

Edema and pulmonary congestion (extra-label): 5 mg/kg PO, IM, IV every 12 to 24 hours[46]

FISH:

Edema and ascites (extra-label): 2 – 5 mg/kg IM every 12 to 72 hours[53]

Monitoring

- Serum electrolytes, acid-base balance (ie, venous blood gas), BUN, creatinine, glucose
- Hydration status (eg, serial body weight measurements, PCV/TP)
- Sleeping/resting respiratory rate
- Blood pressure and thoracic radiographs, if indicated by underlying disease
- Clinical signs of edema, (eg, increased resting respiratory rate, distal limb swelling, girth measurements)
- Evaluation of ototoxicity (hearing loss most common), particularly with prolonged treatment in cats

Client Information

- Furosemide may be given with or without food. If your animal vomits or acts sick after receiving this medicine on an empty stomach, try giving the next dose with food or a small treat. If vomiting continues, contact your veterinarian.
- Your animal will need to urinate more often than normal while taking this medication. Be sure that your animal always has ready access to fresh, clean water. Never withhold water to lessen the times your animal needs to urinate.
- Your veterinarian may ask you to keep a record of your animal's respiratory rate to help monitor for early signs of heart problems. Be sure to follow your veterinarian's instructions about how to measure your animal's respiratory rate and information about when to call your veterinarian.
- Your animal will need to be monitored closely by your veterinarian while it is taking this medicine. Do not miss these important follow-up visits.
- Contact your veterinarian immediately if you notice your animal has weakness, hearing loss, collapse, a head tilt, lack of urination, or a racing heartbeat.

Chemistry/Synonyms

Furosemide is an anthranilic acid derivative structurally related to the sulfonamides. It occurs as an odorless, practically tasteless, white to slightly yellow, fine crystalline powder. Furosemide has a melting point between 203°C and 205°C (397°F-401°F), with decomposition and a pK_a of 3.9. It is practically insoluble in water, sparingly soluble in alcohol, and freely soluble in alkaline solutions. The veterinary injectable products use either the diethanolamine or monoethanolamine salts of furosemide. Diethanolamine salts have a pH of 7 to 7.8 and monoethanolamine salts have a pH of 8 to 9.3; pH may be adjusted with NaOH or HCl.

Furosemide may also be known as frusemide, furosemidum, and LB-502; many trade names are available.

Storage/Stability

Store furosemide protected from light at room temperature up to 25°C (77°F). Furosemide tablets should be protected from moisture and stored in light-resistant, well-closed containers. Tablets may discolor with exposure to light, and discolored tablets should be discarded. The oral solution should be stored at room temperature and protected from light and freezing; discard opened bottles after 90 days.

Furosemide injection should be stored at room temperature. A precipitate may form if the injection is refrigerated, but it will resolubilize when warmed without alteration in potency. The human injection (10 mg/mL) should not be used if it has a yellow color. The veterinary injection (50 mg/mL) normally has a slight yellow color. Furosemide is unstable at an acid pH but is very stable under alkaline conditions. One manufacturer warns to discard the product after 32 vial punctures.

Compatibility/Compounding Considerations

Compatibility is dependent on factors such as pH, concentration, temperature, and diluent used; specialized references or a hospital pharmacist can be consulted for more specific information.

Furosemide injection (10 mg/mL) is reportedly physically **compatible** with all commonly used IV solutions and with the following drugs (depending on concentration): amikacin sulfate, atropine sulfate, cefazolin, cyclosporine, dexamethasone sodium phosphate, dexmedetomidine, digoxin, epinephrine, heparin, lidocaine, mannitol, pamidronate, penicillin G, potassium chloride, ranitidine, sodium bicarbonate, sodium nitroprusside, tobramycin sulfate, vasopressin, verapamil, and zoledronic acid. Refer to a specialized reference or consult a hospital pharmacist for additional information.

Furosemide is reported to be physically **incompatible** with the following agents: ascorbic acid solutions, atracurium, butorphanol tartrate, ciprofloxacin, diazepam, diphenhydramine, dobutamine HCl, esmolol, gentamicin sulfate, glycopyrrolate, hydralazine, ketamine, metoclopramide, mycophenolate mofetil, ondansetron, pantoprazole, potassium phosphates, thiamine, and tetracyclines. It should generally not be mixed with antihistamines, local anesthetics, alkaloids, hypnotics, or opiates.

Dosage Forms/Regulatory Status

VETERINARY-LABELED PRODUCTS:

NOTE: Consult applicable local, state, and/or federal rules prior to competition, as some United States tracks may have restrictions on the use of this drug in racing animals.

Furosemide Tablets: 12.5 mg and 50 mg; *Salix*®, *Disal*®, generic; (Rx). Products may be FDA-approved for use in dogs and cats. Additional tablet strengths may be available in other countries.

Furosemide Oral Solution (Syrup): 10 mg/mL in 60 mL; generic; (Rx). FDA-approved for use in dogs

Furosemide for Injection: 50 mg/mL (5%) in 50 mL and 100 mL vials; *Disal*® *Injection*, *Salix*® *Injection*, generic; (Rx). Products may be FDA-approved for use in dogs, cats, horses, and cattle. Not for use in horses intended for human consumption. FDA milk/meat withdrawal periods in cattle are 48 hours; slaughter withdrawal for cattle is 28 days in the United Kingdom.

HUMAN-LABELED PRODUCTS:

Furosemide Oral Tablets: 20 mg, 40 mg, and 80 mg; *Lasix*®, generic; (Rx)

Furosemide Oral Solution: 10 mg/mL and 40 mg/5 mL (8 mg/mL); generic; (Rx)

Furosemide Injection: 10 mg/mL in 2 mL (20 mg), 4 mL (40 mg), and 10 mL (100 mg) single-dose vials or prefilled syringes; generic, (Rx)

References

For the complete list of references, see **wiley.com/go/budde/plumb**

Gabapentin

(gab-ah-***pen***-tin) *Neurontin*®

Anticonvulsant; Anxiolytic; Neuropathic Pain Analgesic

Prescriber Highlights

- May be useful in dogs and cats as adjunctive therapy for refractory or complex partial seizures and in many species for the treatment of chronic pain (especially neuropathic pain)
- Appears beneficial in cats for reducing fear responses associated with handling and examination, and in dogs for storm phobia
- Use of xylitol-containing oral liquid should be avoided in dogs.
- Sedation or ataxia are the most likely adverse effects in small animal species.
- Administration 3 times a day (ie, every 8 hours) in dogs or cats is likely the most effective regimen but may be problematic for pet owners.

Uses/Indications

Gabapentin may be useful as adjunctive therapy for refractory or complex partial seizures. As an analgesic, gabapentin has been demonstrated to be useful in treating chronic pain, particularly neuropathic pain, in small animals. Gabapentin has improved the quality of life in dogs[1] (but not in cats[2]) with chronic pain conditions. In the cat study, quality of life deteriorated in both the gabapentin and placebo group, leading the authors to state that the osteoarthritis in all cats was likely worsening.[2] Cats receiving gabapentin did have improved owner-identified impaired activities.

Gabapentin does not appear to be effective for treating acute pain, but it may be of benefit when given preemptively (eg, before surgery) for acute pain when it is used with other analgesics.[3] Research has shown that, when used preoperatively, gabapentin reduced the amount of opioids needed postoperatively in dogs undergoing mastectomy.[4] Gabapentin has been proposed for further study in horses to determine its efficacy as an adjunctive treatment for laminitis pain[5] and in cattle for treating neuropathic pain.[6]

Gabapentin has been used in cats to decrease fear responses and anxiety associated with transport and veterinary examinations[7-9] and in dogs for control of storm phobia.[10]

It appears that when used in combination with meloxicam, gabapentin can reduce the severity of lameness in calves.[11]

Pharmacology/Actions

Gabapentin has analgesic effects and can prevent allodynia (ie, sensation of pain resulting from a normally non-noxious stimulus) or hyperalgesia (ie, exaggerated response to painful stimuli). It also has anticonvulsant activity. The mechanism of action of gabapentin for either its anticonvulsant, analgesic, or anxiolytic actions is not fully understood, but it appears to bind to CaV alpha2delta, a subunit of the voltage-gated calcium channels. By decreasing calcium influx, the release of excitatory neurotransmitters (eg, substance P, glutamate, norepinephrine) is inhibited. Although gabapentin is structurally related to gamma-aminobutyric acid type A (GABA), it does not appear to alter GABA binding, reuptake, or degradation or to serve as a GABA agonist in vivo.

Pharmacokinetics

In dogs, oral bioavailability is ≈80% at a dose of 50 mg/kg. Peak plasma concentrations occur ≈1 to 2 hours after administration. Thirty-four percent of a gabapentin dose is metabolized to *N*-methyl-gabapentin; elimination is primarily via renal routes. Elimination half-life is ≈2 to 4 hours.[12-14]

In cats, gabapentin bioavailability was 90% to 95% after oral administration, with significant interpatient variation (50% to 120%) possible. Peak concentrations occurred 65 to 100 minutes after a single dose and at 45 minutes with repeated doses. Apparent volume of distribution at steady state was relatively low at 0.65 L/kg. Clearance was 2.7 to 3 mL/minute/kg, and the mean elimination half-life of 2.8 to 3.7 hours was similar to that of dogs.[15,16] Cats with IRIS stage 2 or 3 CKD had significantly higher serum gabapentin concentrations than healthy cats; gabapentin concentration correlated with serum creatinine and symmetric dimethylarginine.[17]

In 4 horses given single oral doses of 5 mg/kg, gabapentin was rapidly absorbed, with peak concentrations noted within 2 hours (mean, 1.4 hours). Plasma elimination half-life was ≈3.4 hours.[18] Another study in 6 horses showed that oral gabapentin had a low bioavailability (≈16%), and peak concentrations occurred ≈1 hour after administration. Elimination half-life was ≈7 to 8 hours. Gabapentin is cleared almost entirely by the kidneys.[19]

In ruminating calves, oral gabapentin (with or without meloxicam) at 10 or 15 mg/kg yielded plasma gabapentin concentrations of more than 2 µg/mL for up to 15 hours. The elimination half-life was ≈8 to 10 hours; the authors speculated that a decreased rate of oral absorption in ruminant calves prolonged half-life.[6]

One study in Hispaniolan Amazon parrots showed oral bioavailability of 80% to 89%.[20] IV half-life was 2.9 hours and oral half-life was 7.7 hours.[20]

In humans, gabapentin bioavailability decreases as dosage increases.[21] For example, at dosages of 900 mg/day, 60% of the dose is absorbed; however, at 4800 mg/day, only a minimum of 27% of the dose is absorbed. Limited data suggest that this effect may occur in dogs[14] and horses,[22] but it did not occur in Hispaniolan Amazon parrots.[20] The presence of food only marginally alters absorption rate and extent of absorption.[21] Gabapentin is only minimally bound to plasma proteins; CSF concentrations are ≈20% of those in plasma. The drug is not significantly metabolized and is almost exclusively excreted unchanged in the urine. Elimination half-lives in humans are ≈5 to 7 hours.

An extended-release tablet formulation (gabapentin enacarbil) is available for humans, but no pharmacokinetic information for this product is noted for veterinary species.

Contraindications/Precautions/Warnings

Gabapentin is considered contraindicated in patients that are hypersensitive to it. Because gabapentin is eliminated via renal routes (practically 100% in humans), it should be used with caution in patients with renal insufficiency; if required, dosage adjustment should be considered. In dogs, the drug is also metabolized (30% to 40% of a dose), so dosage adjustment may not be required in dogs with mild to moderate renal dysfunction. However, one reference recommends that dosages be reduced and/or dose intervals increased in dogs and cats when serum creatinine clearance is 0.7 mL/kg/minute or less.[23]

In general, use of commercially available human oral solutions containing xylitol should be avoided in dogs. Because the threshold dose of xylitol that can cause hypoglycemia in dogs is ≈100 mg/kg, doses of gabapentin up to 15 mg/kg in dogs using the solution should be safe, but further data are needed to confirm this. In addition, xylitol may be hepatotoxic in dogs. Doses of 500 mg/kg of xylitol are currently thought to be the threshold for this toxicity, but there have been anecdotal reports of it occurring at much lower doses. In cats, at the dosages presently used for gabapentin oral solution, xylitol toxicity does not appear to be a problem, but the solution should be used with caution.[24]

Abrupt discontinuation of the drug after chronic use has led to withdrawal-precipitated seizures. In humans, it is recommended to wean off the drug when it is used for epilepsy treatment, and similar advice for animal patients seems prudent.

Adverse Effects

Sedation and ataxia are the most likely adverse effects seen in small animals. Starting the dose at the lower end of the range and increasing with time may alleviate these effects. One study in cats noted hypersalivation and vomiting, both of which resolved within 8 hours of administration.[8] In humans, the most common adverse effects associated with gabapentin therapy are dizziness, somnolence, and peripheral edema.[21]

Gabapentin was associated with an increased rate of pancreatic adenocarcinoma in male rats.[21] It is unknown if this effect occurs in other species.

Reproductive/Nursing Safety

At high doses (ie, at or above human maximum doses), gabapentin was associated with a variety of fetotoxic and teratogenic effects (eg, delayed ossification, hydronephrosis, fetal loss) in rats, mice, and rabbits.[21]

Gabapentin enters maternal milk. It has been calculated that a nursing human infant could be exposed to a maximum dosage of 1 mg/kg/day. This is 5% to 10% of the usual pediatric (older than 3 years) therapeutic dose. In veterinary patients, this appears unlikely to be of significant clinical concern.

Overdose/Acute Toxicity

In humans, doses up to 49 g have been reported without fatality. The most likely effects include ataxia, lethargy, somnolence, and diarrhea.[21] Common clinical signs associated with gabapentin overdose include ataxia, lethargy, and vomiting; cats may present with lethargy, sedation, and/or ataxia.

The commercially available oral solution contains xylitol 300 mg/mL; xylitol-containing gabapentin solution dosages of 0.33 mL/kg may cause hypoglycemia or liver toxicity in dogs.

Treatment is supportive, with general decontamination procedures including emesis, activated charcoal, and cathartics. Gabapentin can be removed with hemodialysis. If xylitol toxicity is suspected, secondary to the human-labeled liquid formulation, an animal poison control center should be contacted for further guidance. See ***Appendix***.

For patients that have experienced or are suspected to have experienced an overdose, consultation with a 24-hour poison consultation center specializing in providing veterinary-specific information is recommended. For general information related to overdose and toxin exposures, as well as contact information for poison control centers, refer to ***Appendix***.

Drug Interactions

The following drug interactions have either been reported or are theoretical in humans or animals receiving gabapentin and may be of significance in veterinary patients. Unless otherwise noted, use together is not necessarily contraindicated, but the potential risks should be weighed and additional monitoring performed when appropriate.

- **ANTACIDS (ALUMINUM-, MAGNESIUM-, CALCIUM-CONTAINING)**: Oral antacids given concurrently with gabapentin may decrease oral bioavailability by 20%; if antacids are required, administration should be separated from gabapentin administration by at least 2 hours. High doses of IV or epidural magnesium may increase the risk for sedation associated with gabapentin.
- **CANNABIDIOL**: May result in an increased risk for sedation
- **HYDROXYZINE**: May result in an increased risk for sedation
- **MINOCYCLINE**: May result in an increased risk for sedation
- **MIRTAZAPINE**: May result in an increased risk for sedation
- **OPIOID ANALGESICS**: May result in an increased risk for sedation. Concurrent administration of gabapentin and hydrocodone may increase the area under the curve (AUC) of gabapentin and increase its efficacy and/or adverse effects. Gabapentin can reduce the AUC of hydrocodone, potentially reducing the drug's effectiveness. Morphine may increase gabapentin concentrations.

Laboratory Considerations

- There are reports of gabapentin causing false positive **urine protein** readings on *Ames N-Multistix® SG* dipstick tests in humans. Use of a sulfosalicylic acid precipitation test to determine presence of urine protein is recommended for patients receiving gabapentin.

Dosages

DOGS:

Ancillary therapy of refractory seizures (extra-label):

a) Evidence to support use is relatively weak; suggested dosages range from 10 – 20 mg/kg PO every 8 hours. Some clinicians recommend starting therapy at 10 mg/kg PO every 8 hours to reduce potential for oversedation; some clinicians suggest that dosages up to 30 mg/kg PO every 8 hours or administration every 6 hours may be required for efficacy.

b) A study in dogs with uncontrolled seizures (at least 2 per month and at least 6 over the past 3 months) when phenobarbital and potassium bromide concentrations were therapeutic or subtherapeutic but had unacceptable adverse effects. Dogs received gabapentin at ≈10 mg/kg PO every 8 hours for 3 months. Six of 11 dogs had a minimum of 50% reduction in seizures per week.[25]

Adjunctive analgesic (extra-label): Evidence to support use has strengthened in recent years, and the drug may be effective in some dogs, particularly for treatment of chronic pain conditions with a neuropathic component. Dosage recommendations are 10 – 20 mg/kg PO every 12 hours, but similar doses as for seizures (10 – 20 mg/kg PO every 8 hours) may be considered. Based on pharmacokinetics, dosing every 8 hours is likely more effective than twice daily dosing.[26] A single oral dose of gabapentin 20 mg/kg 2 hours prior to isoflurane anesthesia produced a 20% MAC-sparing effect.[27]

Storm phobia (extra-label): 25 – 30 mg/kg PO administered 90 minutes before exposure reduced fear behavior.[10]

CATS:

Ancillary therapy of refractory seizures (extra-label): Evidence to support use is weak, but anecdotal initial dosages of 5 – 10 mg/kg PO every 8 to 12 hours have been noted. A recently published review article on epilepsy in cats lists an anecdotal dosage of 5 – 20 mg/kg PO every 6 to 12 hours.[28] Some clinicians have suggested initially giving the drug every 24 hours and then giving more often as necessary.

Adjunctive analgesic (extra-label): Evidence to support use is weak, but anecdotally it has been reported to be effective in some cats, particularly for chronic pain conditions with a neuropathic component. There is no strong evidence to support one dosage recommendation over another, and suggested initial dosages range from 3 mg/kg PO every 24 hours titrated up to 5 – 10 mg/kg PO every 12 hours (if required). Others start at 5 – 10 mg/kg PO every 8 to 12 hours. Based on pharmacokinetics, dosing every 8 hours is likely more effective than twice daily dosing.[26]

Transdermal analgesia (extra-label): 10 mg/kg transdermally to the pinna every 8 hours. Gabapentin was compounded in the proprietary base *Lipoderm*®; the drug was measurable in the serum, and lower pain scores were documented at some, but not all, study points.[29]

Postoperative analgesia following ovariohysterectomy (extra-label): 50 mg/cat (NOT mg/kg) PO 12 hours and 1 hour prior to surgery in addition to buprenorphine at the time of induction[3]

Osteoarthritis (extra-label): 10 mg/kg PO every 12 hours improved osteoarthritic cats overall as assessed by accelerometer and client questionnaire; quality of life was not changed as compared with placebo.[2]

Reduce fear responses and anxiety associated with veterinary examinations (extra label): 50 – 200 mg/cat (NOT mg/kg) PO (equating to 9 to ≈48 mg/kg) reduced fear responses in confined community cats without measurable sedation over 3 hours post-administration.[7-9] In cats with IRIS stage 2 or 3 CKD, 10 mg/kg PO resulted in improved compliance with handling 3 hours after administration.[17]

BIRDS:

Adjunctive analgesic for neuropathic pain in Hispaniolan Amazon parrots (extra-label): One study suggested 15 mg/kg PO every 8 hours as a reasonable starting point.[20]

Monitoring

NOTE: Gabapentin serum concentrations are usually not monitored; therapeutic concentrations are thought to be 4 – 16 µg/mL. When monitoring concentrations in dogs, samples should be taken when peak concentrations occur (≈2 hours postdose). Subsequent concentrations should be drawn at consistent times after administration.

- Clinical efficacy and adverse effects

Client Information

- This medicine may be given with or without food. If your animal vomits or acts sick after receiving the medicine on an empty stomach, give it with food or a small treat. If vomiting continues, contact your veterinarian.
- Drowsiness and loss of coordination are the most common side effects.
- The oral liquid made for humans should not be given to dogs as it contains xylitol, which is toxic to dogs.

Chemistry/Synonyms

Gabapentin occurs as a white to off-white crystalline solid that is freely soluble in water. It has a pK_{a1} of 3.7 and a pK_{a2} of 10.7. It is structurally related to GABA.

Gabapentin may also be known as CI-945, GOE-3450, *Aclonium*®, *Equipax*®, *Gantin*®, *Gabarone*®, *Neurontin*®, *Neurostil*®, and *Progresse*®.

Storage/Stability

The commercially available capsules and tablets should be stored at room temperature (25°C [77°F]); excursions are permitted between 15°C and 30°C (59°F-86°F). The oral liquid should be stored in the refrigerator between 2°C and 8°C (36°F-46°F).

Compatibility/Compounding Considerations

Compounded preparation stability: Commercially available gabapentin solutions contain xylitol, which may be toxic to canine patients. Gabapentin oral suspension compounded from commercially available tablets has been published.[30] Triturating 20 gabapentin 600 mg tablets with 60 mL of *Ora-Plus*® and qs ad to 120 mL with *Ora-Sweet*® (or *Ora-Sweet*® *SF*) yields a 100 mg/mL oral suspension that retains more than 90% potency for 56 days stored at both 4°C (39.2°F) and 25°C (77°F). Liquid formulations of gabapentin are most stable in the pH range of 5.5 to 6.5.

Dosage Forms/Regulatory Status

VETERINARY-LABELED PRODUCTS: NONE

The Association of Racing Commissioners International (ARCI) has designated this drug as a class 4 substance. Use of this drug may not be allowed in certain animal competitions. Check rules and regulations before entering in a competition while this medication is being administered. Contact local racing authorities for further guidance. See ***Appendix*** for more information.

HUMAN-LABELED PRODUCTS:

Gabapentin Oral Capsules and Tablets: 100 mg, 300 mg, and 400 mg; 600 mg and 800 mg (film-coated); *Neurontin*®, generic; (Rx)

Gabapentin Oral Solution: 250 mg/5 mL (50 mg/mL) in 470 mL; *Neurontin*®, generic; (Rx). **NOTE**: May contain xylitol; label should be checked, and drug should be used cautiously in dogs.

Gabapentin Enacarbil Oral Extended-Release Tablets: 300 mg and 600 mg; *Horizant*®; (Rx). **NOTE**: No information on pharmacokinetics or clinical usage in dogs and cats is noted.

References

For the complete list of references, see **wiley.com/go/budde/plumb**

Gamithromycin

(gah-***mith***-roe-my-sin) *Zactran®*

Macrolide (Azalide) Antibiotic

Prescriber Highlights

- ▶ Injectable azalide-class macrolide antibiotic FDA-approved for treatment of BRD in beef and nonlactating dairy cattle; potentially useful in horses, foals, swine, and goats
- ▶ Not for use in female dairy cattle 20 months of age or older or in calves to be processed for veal
- ▶ Most common adverse effect is pain and swelling at injection site; colic and lameness have been reported in foals
- ▶ 35-day slaughter withdrawal (United States label)

Uses/Indications

Gamithromycin is FDA-approved for the treatment of bovine respiratory disease (BRD) associated with *Mannheimia haemolytica, Pasteurella multocida, Histophilus somni,* and *Mycoplasma bovis* in beef and nonlactating dairy cattle.[1] It is also indicated for the control of respiratory disease in beef and nonlactating dairy cattle at high risk for developing BRD associated with *Mannheimia haemolytica* and *Pasteurella multocida.*

Gamithromycin could be useful in other species as well. One study in foals showed that IM doses of 6 mg/kg every 7 days would maintain pulmonary epithelial lining fluid (PELF) concentrations above the MIC_{90} for susceptible isolates of *Streptococcus equi* subsp *zooepidemicus* and phagocytic cell concentrations above the MIC_{90} for susceptible isolates of *Rhodococcus equi.*[2]

A single IM gamithromycin dose is effective for the treatment of swine respiratory disease (SRD) and infectious pododermatitis (foot rot) in sheep.[3]

The World Health Organization (WHO) has designated gamithromycin as a Critically Important, Highest Priority antimicrobial for human medicine.[4] The Office International des Epizooties (OIE) Antimicrobial Classification has designated gamithromycin as a Veterinary Critically Important antimicrobial for bovines.[5]

Pharmacology/Actions

Like other macrolides, gamithromycin penetrates bacterial cell membranes and binds to the 50s ribosomal subunit, thereby inhibiting protein synthesis. It inhibits the translocation process between 30S and 50s ribosomes, causing premature detachment of incomplete peptide chains.

The macrolide antimicrobials, as a class, are weak bases and as such, concentrate in some cells (such as pulmonary leukocytes). Prolonged exposure of extracellular pulmonary pathogens to macrolides appears to reflect the slow release of drug from its intracellular reservoir to the site of action, the pulmonary epithelial lining fluid (PELF). It is the drug concentration in the PELF that is relevant to the successful treatment and control of BRD. Gamithromycin is primarily bacteriostatic at therapeutic concentrations. Macrolides typically exhibit substantially higher concentrations in the alveolar macrophages and PELF as compared to concentrations observed in plasma.[1] Gamithromycin concentrations in the PELF and PELF cells exceed the concentrations observed in the plasma.

Significant increases in MIC can occur in *P multocida* and *M haemolytica* with the *msr*(E)-*mph*(E) gene.[6]

Pharmacokinetics

In cattle, after a 6 mg/kg SC (in neck) dose, gamithromycin absorption is complete and peak plasma concentrations occur in ≈1 hour. Volume of distribution is very high (≈25 L/kg) and only 26% of drug in plasma is bound to plasma proteins. Based on plasma and lung homogenate data, the terminal half-life ($T_{1/2}$) of gamithromycin is ≈3 days. Clearance is 712 mL/kg/hour and elimination half-life is ≈51 hours. The primary route of elimination is biliary excretion of unchanged drug. After a single (6 mg/kg) dose, gamithromycin concentrations in PELF, bronchiolar lavage fluid (BAL) cells, and lung tissue can persist above reported MIC_{90} for labeled organisms for 7 days (PELF) to 10 to 15+ days (BAL cells and lung tissue).[7-10]

In foals after a 6 mg/kg IM dose, peak plasma concentrations occur in ≈1 hour and elimination half-life is ≈39 hours. Gamithromycin concentrations in PELF were above the MIC_{90} for susceptible isolates of *S zooepidemicus* and phagocytic cell concentrations above the MIC_{90} for susceptible isolates of *R equi* for ≈7 days.[2]

Contraindications/Precautions/Warnings

Gamithromycin is contraindicated in animals that are hypersensitive to it. Potentially, animals hypersensitive to other azalide or macrolide antibiotics could also react to gamithromycin. Subcutaneous injection may cause a temporary local tissue reaction in some animals that may result in trim loss of edible tissues at slaughter.

Cross-resistance may occur with other macrolide/azalide antibiotics (eg, tulathromycin, tilmicosin).

Adverse Effects

Pain and swelling at the injections site are common. Swelling and local inflammation at injection site usually resolves within 3 to 14 days but has been reported to persist up to 35 days postinjection.[3]

In foals being treated for bronchopneumonia with IM gamithromycin, colic and hind limb lameness were observed in 45% and 40% of foals, respectively.[11]

Reproductive/Nursing Safety

Although gamithromycin is not labeled for use in pregnant animals, the product's material safety data sheet (MSDS) notes that none of the ingredients are considered to be a reproductive, teratogenic, or developmental toxin. The UK label reads: *Based on laboratory animal data, gamithromycin has not produced any evidence of selective developmental or reproductive effects. The safety of gamithromycin during pregnancy and lactation has not been evaluated in cattle. Use only according to the risk-benefit assessment by the responsible veterinarian.*[3]

Because safety has not been established in animals, this drug should only be used when the maternal benefits outweigh the potential risks to offspring.

Overdose/Acute Toxicity

Subcutaneous injections of gamithromycin 18 mg/kg and 30 mg/kg (3 times and 5 times the label dose, respectively) given every 5 days for 3 doses to 6-month-old beef cattle caused swelling and pain at the injection site (neck twisting, attempts to scratch or lick the injection site, and pawing at the ground).[12] Other clinically relevant treatment-related effects were not observed.

For patients that have experienced or are suspected to have experienced an overdose, consultation with a 24-hour poison consultation center specializing in providing veterinary-specific information is recommended. For general information related to overdose and toxin exposures, as well as contact information for poison control centers, refer to ***Appendix.***

Drug Interactions

The following drug interactions have either been reported or are theoretical in humans or animals receiving gamithromycin and may be of significance in veterinary patients. Unless otherwise noted, use together is not necessarily contraindicated, but weigh the potential risks and perform additional monitoring when appropriate.

- **RIFAMPIN:** Decreased gamithromycin clearance and increased gamithromycin exposure (AUC) in foals[13]

Laboratory Considerations

None noted

Dosages

HORSES:

Mild-moderate bronchopneumonia due to *Rhodococcus equi* (extra-label): 6 mg/kg bodyweight IM in the semimembranosus/semitendinosus muscles once a week for a minimum of 40 days; efficacy was similar to the combination of azithromycin with rifampin but had a much higher frequency of adverse effects.[14] Criteria for discontinuation of treatment were resolution of clinical signs and no evidence of consolidation upon thoracic ultrasonography for 2 consecutive weeks after a minimum of 40 days of treatment. The use of a diluted, IV administration of gamithromycin (6 mg/kg diluted with water to 50 mL final volume and injected IV over 2 to 3 minutes) has been reported.[15]

CATTLE:

Treatment of bovine respiratory disease (BRD) associated with *Mannheimia haemolytica, Pasteurella multocida, Histophilus somni*, and *Mycoplasma bovis* in beef and nonlactating dairy cattle; also indicated for the control of respiratory disease in beef and nonlactating dairy cattle at high risk for developing BRD associated with *Mannheimia haemolytica* and *Pasteurella multocida* (label dosage; FDA-approved): 6 mg/kg (2 mL/110 lb) bodyweight (BW) SC in the neck (in front of the shoulder) once.[1] If the total dose exceeds 10 mL, divide the dose so that no more than 10 mL is administered at each injection site. Animals should be appropriately restrained to achieve the proper route of administration.

SHEEP:

Elimination of footrot due to *Dichelobacter nodosus* (extra-label): 6 mg/kg SC administered cranial to the shoulder[3], or in the axilla[16]

GOATS:

Naturally occurring pneumonia in kids (extra-label): 6 mg/kg IM once[17]

SWINE:

Bacterial swine respiratory disease (extra-label): 6 mg/kg IM once in the neck[3,18,19]

***Bordetella bronchiseptica*-associated respiratory disease in piglets** (extra-label): 6 mg/kg IM once[20]

Monitoring

- Clinical response: In field trials, animals that responded to therapy did so within 24 hours of injection.

Client Information

- Understand and follow use restrictions and withdrawal times for food animals.
- Reactions (pain, swelling) at the administration site are common but usually resolve within a few days.
- Humans with a known drug allergy to macrolide antibiotics (eg, erythromycin, clarithromycin) should avoid contact with this medicine.
- In case of skin or eye exposure, wash and flush area with clean water. If accidental self-injection, seek medical advice immediately and show the product label to the physician.

Chemistry/Synonyms

Gamithromycin is a 7a-azalide macrolide antibiotic (CAS Registry: 145435-72-9). It differs structurally from other macrolides by having a 15-membered semisynthetic lactone ring with an alkylated nitrogen at the 7a-position. The commercially available injectable solution contains per mL: 150 mg of gamithromycin as the free base, 1 mg of monothioglycerol, and 40 mg of succinic acid in a glycerol formal vehicle.

Gamithromycin may also be known as ML-1,709,460 or UNII-ZE856183S0. A trade name is *Zactran*®.

Storage/Stability

The injection should be stored at or below 25°C (77°F) with excursions permitted between 15°C and 30°C (59°F-86°F). Use within 18 months of first puncture (United States label); once opened, use within 28 days (UK label). Viscosity of the injectable solution may increase at sub-freezing temperatures but should not affect syringability.[7]

Compatibility/Compounding Considerations

Compatibility is dependent on factors such as pH, concentration, temperature, and diluent used; specialized references or a hospital pharmacist should be consulted for more specific information.

No information was noted on the label (United States) or in other references, but the UK label states: Do not mix with any other veterinary medicinal product. In one study, gamithromycin injection was diluted with water to a final volume of 50 mL immediately prior to IV administration (over 2 to 3 minutes).[15]

Dosage Forms/Regulatory Status

VETERINARY-LABELED PRODUCTS:

Solution for Injection: 150 mg/mL in 100 mL, 250 mL, and 500 mL bottles. *Zactran*®; (Rx). FDA-approved for use in beef and nonlactating dairy cattle. NADA #141-328

Withdrawal times/restrictions in the United States: Do not treat cattle within 35 days of slaughter. Do not use in female dairy cattle 20 months of age or older, or in calves to be processed for veal.

Withdrawal times/restrictions in the UK: Meat and offal withdrawal period: cattle, 64 days; sheep, 29 days; swine, 16 days. Not authorized for use in lactating animals producing milk for human consumption. In pregnant animals which are intended to produce milk for human consumption, do not use within 2 months (cows, heifers) or 1 month (sheep) of expected parturition.

HUMAN-LABELED PRODUCTS: NONE

References

For the complete list of references, see **wiley.com/go/budde/plumb**

Gemcitabine

(jem-***site***-ah-ben) *Gemzar*®

Antineoplastic

Prescriber Highlights

- ► Antineoplastic agent potentially useful for treatment of several cancer types in dogs and cats as a single agent or part of chemotherapy protocol, or for tumors in which standard of care has not been definitively established
- ► Adverse effects: GI effects and myelosuppression (neutropenia) are most likely.
- ► The National Institute for Occupational Safety and Health (NIOSH) classifies gemcitabine as a hazardous drug; use appropriate precautions when handling.

Uses/Indications

Gemcitabine is an antineoplastic agent that has demonstrated limited clinical efficacy when used as a single agent in dogs with solid tumors.[1,2] However, no benefit was found when it was used in dogs with lymphoma[3] or nonresectable hepatocellular carcinoma,[4] or as an adjuvant to surgical removal of aggressive malignant mammary tumors.[5] The assessment of gemcitabine's additive or synergistic activities in combination have not been definitively confirmed. Similarly, studies that assessed gemcitabine combination therapy in dogs have produced mixed results.[6–8]

A retrospective study in cats with exocrine pancreatic carcinoma showed that 82% of cats treated with gemcitabine (± carboplatin) had decreased clinical signs associated with their malignancies, but due to the retrospective nature of the study, any determination of actual improvement of quality of life was questionable.[9]

Gemcitabine has been used as a radiosensitizer for nonresectable tumors.[10] However, safe and effective dosing regimens have not been established and life-threatening toxicities have been reported with concurrent use in humans.[11] In one study, gemcitabine was given IV twice weekly as a radiosensitizing agent to 10 cats with oral squamous cell carcinoma and 15 dogs with nasal carcinoma undergoing radiotherapy.[12] The average dose was 50 mg/m^2 and 25 mg/m^2 in dogs and cats, respectively. Twelve of 15 dogs (80%) and 5 of 10 cats (50%) required chemotherapy dose reduction or postponement because of hematologic or normal tissue toxicity.

Based on documented significant toxicities, the use of gemcitabine at the studied dose and schedule is not recommended as a radiosensitizer.[12] In contrast, one small pilot study with 8 cats found that gemcitabine combined with palliative radiation was tolerable and produced exceptional response rates (75%) in cats with oral squamous cell carcinoma.[10]

In humans, gemcitabine, in combination with other chemotherapeutic agents, has shown efficacy in treating breast, pancreatic, small-cell lung, and ovarian cancers.

Pharmacology/Actions

Gemcitabine exhibits cell phase specificity, acting primarily on the S phase killing cells undergoing DNA synthesis and inhibiting cell progression through the G1/S-phase boundary.

Gemcitabine is metabolized intracellularly to diflurodeoxycytidine monophosphate (dFdCMP), which is then converted into diphosphate (dFdCDP) and triphosphate (dFdCTP) forms, the metabolites that give the drug its activity. The diphosphate inhibits ribonucleotide reductase. The triphosphate competes with deoxycytidine triphosphate (dTCP; the "normal nucleotide") for incorporation into DNA strands. DNA polymerase epsilon is unable to recognize the abnormal nucleotide (gemcitabine) and repair the DNA strand, which results in a prolonged intracellular half-life of gemcitabine compared with other nucleoside analogues.

Pharmacokinetics

In dogs, gemcitabine exhibits first-order elimination and has a terminal half-life of ≈1.5 to 3.2 hours. Volume of distribution (steady-state) is ≈1 L/kg. Approximately 80% of the drug is excreted in the urine within 24 hours of dosing, primarily as the uracil metabolite.[4]

In humans, gemcitabine pharmacokinetics were significantly influenced by gender and duration of infusion.[11] For infusions lasting less than 70 minutes versus longer infusions, volume of distribution was ≈50 L/m^2 and 370 L/m^2, respectively. Protein binding is negligible and less than 10% of the drug is excreted unchanged in the urine.

Contraindications/Precautions/Warnings

Gemcitabine is contraindicated in patients with a history of hypersensitivity to it and should be used with caution in patients with diminished renal or hepatic function.

In humans, infusions lasting longer than 60 minutes or administration more frequent than once weekly resulted in increased toxicities. Doses should be reduced or postponed in animals with severe myelosuppression.[11] Pulmonary toxicity has been reported in humans and can occur up to 2 weeks after the last dose; gemcitabine should be discontinued if unexplained new or worsening dyspnea or any other pulmonary symptoms occur. Life-threatening toxicities have occurred in humans receiving gemcitabine within 7 days of radiation therapy.

The National Institute for Occupational Safety and Health (NIOSH) classifies gemcitabine as a hazardous drug; personal protective equipment (PPE) should be used accordingly to minimize the risk for exposure.

Adverse Effects

Myelosuppression is usually the dose-limiting toxicity of gemcitabine and can include neutropenia, anemia, and thrombocytopenia, but neutrophils and platelets appear to be most affected. Neutrophil nadirs usually occur 3 to 7 days after treatment. GI effects have been reported but are usually mild to moderate.[2,8] Retinal hemorrhage could occur in animals receiving gemcitabine.[2]

In humans, the most common adverse effects are nausea and vomiting, anemia, hepatic transaminitis, neutropenia, increased alkaline phosphatase, proteinuria, fever, hematuria, rash, thrombocytopenia, dyspnea, and peripheral edema.[11]

Reproductive/Nursing Safety

Gemcitabine was teratogenic, embryotoxic, and fetotoxic in mice and rabbits.[11]

For sexually intact patients, verify pregnancy status prior to administration.

It is unknown whether gemcitabine is excreted in maternal milk.

Because safety has not been established in animals, this drug should only be used when the maternal benefits outweigh the potential risks to offspring.

Overdose/Acute Toxicity

There is no known antidote to gemcitabine. In humans following a single dose of 5700 mg/m^2, myelosuppression, paresthesia, and severe rash were reported.[11] It is unknown if the drug is dialyzable, and the recommended treatment is supportive.

For patients that have experienced or are suspected of having experienced an overdose, consultation with a 24-hour poison consultation center specializing in providing veterinary-specific information is recommended. For general information related to overdose and toxin exposures, as well as contact information for poison control centers, refer to ***Appendix***.

Drug Interactions

The following drug interactions have either been reported or are theoretical in humans or animals receiving gemcitabine and may be of significance in veterinary patients. Unless otherwise noted, use together is not necessarily contraindicated, but weigh the potential risks and perform additional monitoring when appropriate.

- **Immunosuppressive Agents** (eg, **azathioprine, high-dose glucocorticoids, leflunomide, pyrimethamine**): Concurrent use may result in additive immunosuppression.
- **Myelosuppressive Agents** (eg, **antineoplastics**, **chloramphenicol, iron chelators**): Concurrent use with other bone marrow depressant medication may result in additive myelosuppression; avoid combination when possible.
- **Vaccines** (live and inactivated): Gemcitabine may diminish vaccine efficacy and enhance adverse effects of vaccines.

Laboratory Considerations

- None were noted.

Dosages

NOTE: Because of the potential toxicity of this drug to patients, veterinary personnel, and clients, and because chemotherapy indications, treatment protocols, monitoring and safety guidelines often change, the following dosages should only be used as a general guide. Consultation with a veterinary oncologist and referral to current veterinary oncology references[13–17] are strongly recommended.

DOGS/CATS:

Antineoplastic agent (extra-label): Relatively safe and effective dosages for gemcitabine in veterinary patients with potentially susceptible tumors are not known. Depending on the study, clinician, and protocol, dosages for dogs and cats have ranged widely from 45 mg/m² – 900 mg/m² (NOT mg/kg), usually given IV over 30 to 60 minutes every 7 to 14 days. Some studies combining gemcitabine with carboplatin in dogs and cats have used 2 mg/kg IV over 20 to 30 minutes no more than once every 7 days.

- 400 mg/m² (NOT mg/kg) weekly in dogs with lymphoma; dose reduction or treatment delay required due to significant decreases in neutrophils and platelets.[18]
- 675 mg/m² (NOT mg/kg) every 2 weeks in dogs; demonstrated minimal and acceptable toxicity[1]
- 800 – 950 mg/m² (NOT mg/kg) in dogs; efficacy was demonstrated at the maximum tolerated dose of 900 mg/m² (NOT mg/kg).[1]

Monitoring

- CBC before each treatment
- Fundic examination weekly while on therapy
- Prior to therapy, baseline renal and hepatic function and periodically thereafter

Client Information

- Gemcitabine is a chemotherapy (anticancer) drug. The drug can be hazardous to other animals and people that come in contact with it. On the day your animal gets the drug and then for a few days afterward, all bodily waste (eg, urine, feces, litter), blood, or vomit should only be handled while wearing disposable gloves. Seal the waste in a plastic bag, then place both the bag and gloves in the regular trash.
- This medication is considered to be a hazardous drug as defined by the National Institute for Occupational Safety and Health (NIOSH) because it may affect the reproductive ability of men or women actively trying to conceive, women who are pregnant or may become pregnant, and women who are breastfeeding. It is recommended that you wear gloves when administering this medication to your animal and wash your hands thoroughly afterwards. If you have questions about this medication's hazards, please speak with your veterinarian or pharmacist.
- Bone marrow suppression can occur. The greatest effects on bone marrow usually occur within a few weeks after treatment. Your veterinarian will do blood tests to watch for this, but if you see bleeding, bruising, fever (indicating an infection), or if your animal becomes tired easily, contact your veterinarian right away.
- Monitor for and immediately report any signs associated with toxicity (eg, abnormal bleeding, bruising, urination, depression, infection, shortness of breath).
- While your animal is taking this medication, it is important to return to your veterinarian for laboratory work. Do not miss these important follow-up visits.

Chemistry/Synonyms

A synthetic pyrimidine nucleoside cytarabine analogue antineoplastic agent, gemcitabine HCl occurs as white to off-white solid. It is soluble in water and practically insoluble in ethanol or polar organic solvents. Its chemical name is 2,2'-difluorodeoxycytidine.

Gemcitabine may also be known as: dFdC, LY-288022, *Abine*®, *Antoril*®, *Gemcite*®, or *Gemtrol*®, and *Gemzar*®.

Storage/Stability

Store gemcitabine solution refrigerated at (2°C-8°C [36°F-46°F]). Store unreconstituted gemcitabine lyophilized powder at controlled room temperature (20°C-25°C [68°F-77°F]). After reconstitution with 0.9% sodium chloride injection without preservatives, the resulting solution may be stored at room temperature for up to 24 hours.[11] Do not refrigerate, as crystallization may occur. Reconstituted solution concentration should not be greater than 40 mg/mL (at least 5 mL of diluent for 200 mg vial; 25 mL diluent for 1 gram vial). Additional diluent may be added to yield concentrations as low as 0.1 mg/mL. Discard all unused portions.

Compatibility/Compounding Considerations

Compatibility is dependent on factors such as pH, concentration, temperature, and diluent used; specialized references or a hospital pharmacist should be consulted for more specific information.

Gemcitabine injection is reportedly physically **incompatible** with the following medications when used via Y-site injection: acyclovir, amphotericin B, cefoperazone, cefotaxime sodium, furosemide, imipenem, methotrexate, methylprednisolone sodium succinate, mitomycin, piperacillin, and prochlorperazine.

Dosage Forms/Regulatory Status

VETERINARY-LABELED PRODUCTS: NONE

HUMAN-LABELED PRODUCTS:

Gemcitabine HCl Lyophilized Powder for Injection: 200 mg, 1 g, and 2 g in single-use vials; generic; (Rx)

Gemcitabine Injection: 200 mg/5.26 mL, 1 g/26.3 mL, and 2 g/52.6 mL in single use vials; generic; (Rx)

References

For the complete list of references, see **wiley.com/go/budde/plumb**

Gemfibrozil

(jem-***fih***-broh-zil) *Lopid*®

Oral Antihyperlipidemic

Prescriber Highlights

- May be useful as adjunctive therapy, along with a low-fat diet, to treat hypertriglyceridemia in dogs and cats
- Limited experience in veterinary medicine and no published clinical studies in dogs or cats. Safety and efficacy are not established; dosages are anecdotal.
- Contraindications in dogs and cats are extrapolated from human data and include hypersensitivity to gemfibrozil, hepatic dysfunction, severe renal dysfunction, and pre-existing gallbladder disease.
- Adverse effects may include GI effects (eg, vomiting, diarrhea, abdominal pain, decreased appetite) and abnormal liver function tests.

Uses/Indications

Gemfibrozil may be useful in dogs and cats with hypertriglyceridemia to reduce serum triglycerides when diet modifications alone have been unsuccessful. The addition of drug therapy to maintain fasting serum triglyceride concentration below 400 mg/dL has been suggested.[1] Another recommendation is to add gemfibrozil to dietary therapy in dogs when dietary therapy alone fails to lower triglyceride levels below 5.65 mmol/L (500 mg/dL).[2] Some canine patients reportedly do not respond well to treatment with gemfibrozil.[3,4]

Pharmacology/Actions

Gemfibrozil inhibits lipoprotein lipase lipolysis in adipose tissue and reduces hepatic uptake of plasma-free fatty acids, causing reduced production of triglycerides and reduced serum triglyceride concentrations. Secondarily, gemfibrozil inhibits the synthesis of very-low-density lipoprotein (VLDL) carrier apolipoprotein B, which reduces VLDL production and incorporation of long-chain fatty acids into triglycerides. Gemfibrozil increases high density lipoprotein (HDL) cholesterol but has only a modest effect on LDL or total cholesterol.[5]

Pharmacokinetics

No pharmacokinetic data for dogs or cats were found. In humans, gemfibrozil is rapidly and completely absorbed from the GI tract and undergoes enterohepatic recirculation. The rate and extent of absorption are greatest when administered 30 minutes before a meal. It is highly bound to plasma proteins, and the highest concentrations are found in the liver and kidneys. In the liver, 4 major metabolites are formed in humans, which are primarily excreted in the urine. The elimination half-life is ≈1.5 hours.[5] Reductions in plasma VDL concentrations are noted within 5 days; peak reductions occur about 4 weeks after starting therapy.

Contraindications/Precautions/Warnings

Gemfibrozil is contraindicated in dogs or cats that are hypersensitive to it. In humans, gemfibrozil is contraindicated in patients with hepatic dysfunction, severe renal dysfunction, or preexisting gallbladder disease.[5] Gemfibrozil is not recommended in humans with elevations of LDL only or with low HDL only.

Long-term studies done in rats that were administered at 1.7 times the labeled human dosage demonstrated increased rates of neoplasia (hepatic and testicular interstitial cell)[5]; gemfibrozil should only be used when the benefits outweigh the potential risks.

Use with caution in dogs and cats as very limited safety data are available for this medication.

Adverse Effects

Because no clinical studies have been published regarding gemfibrozil use in dogs and cats and clinical use has been quite limited, the accurate adverse effect profile is not known. Anecdotal reports indicate that gemfibrozil is well tolerated in the small population of patients that have received it. Reported adverse effects include abdominal pain, vomiting, diarrhea, and decreased appetite.[3,4]

In humans, the most common adverse effects reported are GI related (dyspepsia, nausea, vomiting, diarrhea) and CNS related (headache, paresthesias, somnolence, dizziness, fatigue). Other reported adverse effects include myositis, taste alterations, blurred vision, eczema, and decreased libido (impotence). Rarely, hypersensitivity reactions, myelosuppression, cholelithiasis, and increases in liver enzymes and function test values (AST, ALT, ALP, bilirubin) have been reported.[5]

Reproductive/Nursing Safety

Gemfibrozil administered to female rats prior to and during gestation at 0.6 to 2 times the human dose showed decreased fertility rates, and their offspring had an increased incidence of skeletal abnormalities. When given to pregnant rabbits at 1 to 3 times the human dose, litter sizes were decreased, and at the highest dose (3 times the labeled dose), parietal bone variations were noted.[5]

It is not known if gemfibrozil enters milk, and safe use during nursing cannot be assured. Because safety has not been established in animals, this drug should only be used when the maternal benefits outweigh the potential risks to offspring.

Overdose/Acute Toxicity

Limited information is available. One 7-year-old child ingested up to 9 g of gemfibrozil and recovered with supportive treatment.[5] The reported LD_{50} (oral) in rats is 3160 mg/kg. Consider GI decontamination protocols for acute, large oral ingestions and support as required. Monitor for dehydration and electrolyte imbalance if vomiting and/or diarrhea is severe or persists. Monitor liver enzymes and function tests.

For patients that have experienced or are suspected to have experienced an overdose, consultation with a 24-hour poison consultation center specializing in providing veterinary-specific information is recommended. For general information related to overdose and toxin exposures, as well as contact information for poison control centers, refer to ***Appendix.***

Drug Interactions

The following drug interactions have either been reported or are theoretical in humans or animals receiving gemfibrozil and may be of significance in veterinary patients. Unless otherwise noted, use together is not necessarily contraindicated, but weigh the potential risks and perform additional monitoring when appropriate.

- **Amiodarone**: May increase amiodarone exposure
- **Beta-Adrenergic Receptor Antagonists** (eg, **atenolol, propranolol**): May increase triglyceride concentrations
- **Colchicine**: Increased risk for myopathy
- **Estrogens**: May increase triglyceride concentrations
- **Glipizide, Glyburide, and Glimeperide**: May result in hypoglycemia
- **Insulin**: May increase risk for hypoglycemia
- **Loperamide**: Concurrent use may result in increased loperamide plasma concentrations
- **Statins** (eg, **atorvastatin, simvastatin**): Increased risk for myopathy and rhabdomyolysis; concurrent use is contraindicated in humans
- **Thiazide Diuretics**: May increase triglyceride concentrations
- **Ursodiol**: May reduce the effectiveness of gemfibrozil
- **Warfarin**: Gemfibrozil may potentiate anticoagulant effects.

Laboratory Considerations

- No specific concerns associated with gemfibrozil; see ***Monitoring*** section below.

Dosages

DOGS/CATS:

Hypertriglyceridemia that has not been controlled with diet alone (extra-label): There is little information published on the safety and efficacy of this agent in dogs or cats. Anecdotal dosage recommendations for dogs are 10 mg/kg PO every 12 hours[1,4] or 150 – 300 mg/dog (NOT mg/kg) PO twice daily and for cats 7.5 – 10 mg/kg PO twice daily.[1] Based on human data, gemfibrozil should be given ≈30 minutes prior to meals.[5]

Monitoring

- Fasting plasma triglycerides; the realistic goal for therapy is 400 mg/dL or less.
- Baseline and periodic CBC
- Baseline and periodic serum liver enzymes and function tests
- Adverse effects (vomiting, diarrhea, appetite)
- If treatment is less effective than expected, ensure that clients have adhered to prescribed diet and dosing schedule before altering the dosage.

Client Information

- The use of this medicine in animals is investigational. Although it is FDA-approved for use in humans, there is little information about its use in dogs or cats.
- For this medicine to work, it is important to use gemfibrozil with the dietary recommendations made by your veterinarian.
- Give this medication 30 minutes before meals, as food can interfere with how well this medicine works.
- Report any significant side effects to your veterinarian, including changes in behavior, activity level, gastrointestinal effects (vomiting, diarrhea, lack of appetite), or yellowing of the eyes, skin, or gums (*jaundice*).

Chemistry/Synonyms

Gemfibrozil is a fibric acid derivative that occurs as a waxy, crystalline solid that is practically insoluble in water but soluble in alcohol.

Gemfibrozil may also be known as CI-719, gemfibrozilo, or gemfibrozilium; many international trade names are available.

Storage/Stability

Store gemfibrozil tablets or capsules below 30°C (86°F) in tight containers.

Dosage Forms/Regulatory Status

VETERINARY-LABELED PRODUCTS: NONE

HUMAN-LABELED PRODUCTS:

Gemfibrozil Oral Tablets: 600 mg; *Lopid*®, generic; (Rx). **NOTE:** 300 mg capsules are available in Canada.

References

For the complete list of references, see **wiley.com/go/budde/plumb**

Gentamicin, Systemic

(jen-ta-***mye***-sin) *Gentocin*®, *Garamycin*®

Aminoglycoside Antibiotic

See also ***Gentamicin Ophthalmic***

Prescriber Highlights

- Parenteral aminoglycoside antibiotic that is active against a variety of bacteria, predominantly gram-negative aerobic bacilli but also many staphylococci
- Intravitreal injection may be used to manage equine recurrent uveitis (ERU) and for management of uncontrolled elevated intraocular pressure (IOP) associated with end-stage glaucoma.
- Reserved for serious infections because of potential adverse effects (nephrotoxicity, ototoxicity, and neuromuscular blockade)
- Cats may be more sensitive to toxic effects, especially vestibular effects.
- Risk factors for nephrotoxicity include preexisting renal disease, age (both neonatal and geriatric), fever, treatment duration, hypokalemia, sepsis, hypotension, dehydration, and concurrent use with other potentially nephrotoxic drugs (eg, furosemide).

Uses/Indications

Although gentamicin is considered a first line agent in horses, the potential for toxicity of aminoglycosides limits their systemic (parenteral) use in other species to the treatment of serious infections when there is either a documented lack of susceptibility to other less toxic antibiotics or when the clinical situation dictates immediate treatment of a presumed gram-negative infection before culture and susceptibility results can be reported.

Various gentamicin products are FDA-approved for parenteral use in dogs, cats, swine, chickens, and turkeys, although the injectable products for small animal species are no longer marketed. Although routinely used parenterally in horses, gentamicin is only FDA-approved for intrauterine infusion in this species. Oral products are FDA-approved for GI infections in swine and turkeys.

Intravitreal injection of gentamicin may be beneficial for managing end-stage glaucoma[1] and equine recurrent uveitis (ERU).[2,3]

The World Health Organization has designated gentamicin as a Critically Important, High Priority antimicrobial for human medicine.[4] The Office International des Epizooties (OIE) has designated gentamicin as a Veterinary Critically Important Antimicrobial (VCIA) Agent in avian, bovine, camelid, caprine, equine, lagomorph, and ovine species.[5]

Pharmacology/Actions

Gentamicin has a mechanism of action and spectrum of activity (primarily gram-negative aerobes) similar to the other aminoglycosides covering *Escherichia coli*, *Klebsiella*, *Proteus*, *Pseudomonas*, *Salmonella*, *Enterobacter*, *Serratia*, *Shigella*, *Mycoplasma*, and *Staphylococcus*. Strains of *Pseudomonas aeruginosa*, *Proteus*, and *Serratia* that are resistant to gentamicin may still be susceptible to amikacin. Although gentamicin has in vitro activity against *Rhodococcus equi*, its water-soluble nature does not allow it to penetrate intracellularly, but liposomal forms show promise. Gentamicin acts on susceptible bacteria presumably by irreversibly binding to the 30S ribosomal subunit, thereby inhibiting protein synthesis. It is considered a bactericidal concentration-dependent antibiotic. A ratio of 10 or greater for peak plasma concentration to MIC is believed to be optimal for antibacterial efficacy.

Antimicrobial activity of the aminoglycosides is enhanced in an alkaline environment. The presence of pus, necrotic tissue, or cellular debris reduce aminoglycoside efficacy.

The aminoglycoside antibiotics are not active against fungi, viruses, and most anaerobic bacteria, although gentamicin has demonstrated in vitro activity against *Malassezia pachydermatis*.[6]

Intravitreal injection of gentamicin chemically ablates the ciliary body, thus reducing production of aqueous humor and lowering intraocular pressure (IOP).[1]

Pharmacokinetics

Gentamicin, like other aminoglycosides, is not appreciably absorbed after oral or intrauterine administration, but is absorbed from local administration (not skin or urinary bladder) when it is used in irrigations during surgical procedures, regional limb perfusion, or when impregnated into materials that are administered locally (eg, PMMA beads, collagen sponges, gels). Patients receiving oral aminoglycosides with hemorrhagic or necrotic enteritises may absorb appreciable quantities of the drug. After IM administration to dogs and cats, peak concentrations occur in 30 minutes to 1 hour. SC injection results in slightly delayed peak concentrations and more variability than after IM injection. Bioavailability from extravascular injection (IM or SC) is greater than 90%.

After absorption, aminoglycosides are distributed primarily in the extracellular fluid. They are found in ascitic, pleural, pericardial, peritoneal, synovial, and abscess fluids and high concentrations are found in sputum, bronchial secretions, and bile. Aminoglycosides are minimally protein bound (less than 20%) to plasma proteins. Aminoglycosides do not readily cross the blood-brain barrier or penetrate ocular tissue. CSF concentrations are unpredictable and range from 0% to 50% of those found in the serum. Therapeutic concentrations are found in the bone, heart, gallbladder, and lung tissues after parenteral dosing. Aminoglycosides tend to accumulate in certain tissues, such as the inner ear and kidneys, which may explain their toxicity. Volumes of distribution have been reported to be 0.15 to 0.3 L/kg in adult dogs and cats, and 0.26 – 0.58 L/kg in horses. Volumes of distribution may be significantly larger in neonates and juvenile animals due to their higher extracellular fluid fractions. Elimination of aminoglycosides after parenteral administration occurs almost entirely by glomerular filtration. The elimination half-lives for gentamicin have been reported to be 1.82 to 3.25 hours in horses, 2.2 to 2.7 hours in calves, 2.4 hours in sheep, 1.8 hours in cows, 1.9 hours in swine, 1 hour in rabbits, and 0.5 to 1.5 hours in dogs and cats. Patients with decreased renal function can have significantly prolonged half-lives. In humans with normal renal function, elimination rates can be highly variable with the aminoglycoside antibiotics.

Contraindications/Precautions/Warnings

Aminoglycosides are contraindicated in patients that are hypersensitive to them. Because these drugs are often the only effective agents in severe gram-negative and staphylococcal infections, there are no other absolute contraindications to their use. However, they should be used with extreme caution in patients with preexisting renal disease, with concomitant monitoring and dosage interval adjustments made. Other risk factors for the development of toxicity include age (both neonatal and geriatric patients), fever, hypokalemia, treatment duration, sepsis, hypotension, and dehydration.

Monitor renal function prior to and during therapy. If signs of acute kidney injury (eg, renal casts in urine sediment, glucosuria, low urine-specific gravity, azotemia) are noted, therapy should be halted if possible, and alternative antibiotic therapy should be instituted.

Dosing adjustments (ie, prolonging dosing interval) can be used in situations where the risks for ongoing treatment outweigh renal concerns. Dosing is best based on measurement of peak and trough drug levels.

When administering gentamicin by intravitreal injection, it is recommended to use a preservative-free formulation.

Because aminoglycosides can cause irreversible ototoxicity, they should be used with caution in working or service dogs (eg, seeing-eye, herding, dogs for the hearing impaired) and should be avoided for treatment of otitis if an intact tympanic membrane is not known to be present. Gentamicin is considered more ototoxic than amikacin.[7]

Aminoglycosides should be used with caution in patients with neuromuscular disorders (eg, myasthenia gravis) because of their neuromuscular blocking activity. They should not be used in animals with botulism.

Sighthound dogs may require reduced dosages of aminoglycosides, as they have significantly smaller volumes of distribution.

Because aminoglycosides are eliminated primarily through renal mechanisms, they should be used cautiously, preferably with serum monitoring and dosage adjustment in neonatal or geriatric animals.

IM injections in horses have caused muscle irritation and IV injections are preferred. IV administration may be associated with allergic and anaphylactic reactions in horses. The injection should be pre-warmed and administered slowly. If clinical signs occur, corticosteroid treatment may be necessary. The risk for antibiotic-associated diarrhea/colitis in horses caused by gentamicin is thought to be low, but gentamicin may enhance beta-2 toxin production by *Clostridium perfringens* and may increase the severity of colitis.[8]

The American Association of Bovine Practitioners discourages extra-label aminoglycoside use in bovines.

Adverse Effects

Aminoglycosides' nephrotoxic and ototoxic effects are well known. The nephrotoxic (tubular necrosis) mechanisms of these drugs are not completely understood but are likely related to accumulation in the renal convoluted tubules, interfering with phospholipid metabolism in the lysosomes of proximal renal tubular cells, and resulting in leakage of proteolytic enzymes into the cytoplasm. Nephrotoxicity is usually recognized by azotemia and decreases in urine-specific gravity and creatinine clearance. Proteinuria and cells or casts may also be seen in the urine. Nephrotoxicity is usually reversible once the drug is discontinued, but development of oliguric acute kidney injury portends a poor prognosis. Although gentamicin may be more nephrotoxic than some other aminoglycosides, the risk for nephrotoxicity with all systemic aminoglycosides requires equal caution and monitoring. Strategies to reduce the potential for nephrotoxicity in animals with uncompromised renal function include once-daily administration, renal function monitoring, hydration and electrolyte balance, avoidance of other nephrotoxic drugs, and employment of therapeutic drug monitoring to adjust dosages and/or dosing intervals to maintain low trough concentrations (preferably less than 1 – 2 µg/mL). One study in rats showed that concurrent administration of ampicillin prevented nephrotoxicity, presumably by having a higher affinity than gentamicin for the renal tubule system.[9]

Aminoglycoside ototoxicity (eighth cranial nerve toxicity) can manifest by either auditory and/or vestibular clinical signs and may be irreversible. Vestibular clinical signs are more frequent with streptomycin, gentamicin, or tobramycin. Auditory clinical signs are more frequent with amikacin, neomycin, or kanamycin, but other forms can occur with any of the drugs.[7] Cats are apparently very sensitive to the vestibular effects of the aminoglycosides and can exhibit signs of vertigo, head tilt, ataxia, impaired righting reflex, and post-rotatory righting reflex.

Aminoglycosides can also cause neuromuscular blockade, facial edema, pain and inflammation at the injection site, peripheral neuropathy, and hypersensitivity reactions. Rarely, GI clinical signs, hematologic, and hepatic effects have been reported.

It has been anecdotally reported that some horses, after IV gentamicin administration, have colic-like symptoms including groaning, flehmen response, heavy sweating, pawing, tachypnea, tachycardia, laying down, rolling, shivering, and muscle tremors. These symptoms may indicate an allergic/anaphylactic reaction. In most cases, effects have been temporary, with full recovery occurring in a short time. Pre-warming the injection and injecting slowly may possibly prevent this reaction. Corticosteroid treatment may be necessary.

Although causation has not been proven, intravitreal gentamicin injections for ciliary body ablation may be linked to the development of intraocular tumors in dogs and cats.[10,11] Cataract formation and diffuse retinal degeneration have been reported in horses following intravitreal injection of low-dose gentamicin for management of equine recurrent uveitis (ERU).[3]

Reproductive/Nursing Safety

Aminoglycosides can cross the placenta and, although rare, may cause eighth cranial nerve toxicity or nephrotoxicity in fetuses. Because the drug should only be used in serious infections, the benefits of therapy may exceed the potential risks. One study showed no detectable levels in foals when gentamicin was administered to mares at term.[12] In other species, fetal concentrations range from 15% to 50% of those found in maternal serum.

Although small amounts of gentamicin may be excreted into milk, the risk to nursing offspring appears minimal.

Because safety has not been established in animals, this drug should only be used when the maternal benefits outweigh the potential risks to offspring.

Overdose/Acute Toxicity

No toxic effects were observed in cats receiving 10 mg/kg/day for 40 days,[13] but respiratory paralysis and neuromuscular blockade have been reported in cats receiving doses of 40 mg/kg.[14]

If an inadvertent overdose is given, dialysis can be used to reduce serum gentamicin concentrations. Hemodialysis effectively reduces serum gentamicin concentrations[14] but is not a viable option for most veterinary patients. Peritoneal dialysis also will reduce serum gentamicin concentrations but is much less effective.

For patients that have experienced or are suspected to have experienced an overdose, consultation with a 24-hour poison consultation center specializing in providing veterinary-specific information is recommended. For general information related to overdose and toxin exposures, as well as contact information for poison control centers, refer to ***Appendix.***

Drug Interactions

The following drug interactions either have been reported or are theoretical in humans or animals receiving gentamicin and may be of concern in veterinary patients. Unless otherwise noted, use together is not necessarily contraindicated, but weigh the potential risks and perform additional monitoring when appropriate.

- **Beta-Lactam Antibiotics** (eg, **penicillins, cephalosporins**): May have synergistic effects against some bacteria; there is some potential for inactivation of aminoglycosides when admixed or when administered together in patients with renal failure.
- **Cephalosporins**: The concurrent use of aminoglycosides with cephalosporins is somewhat controversial. Potentially, cephalosporins could cause additive nephrotoxicity when used with aminoglycosides, but this interaction has only been well documented with cephaloridine and cephalothin (both no longer marketed).
- **Diuretics, Loop** (eg, **furosemide, torsemide**): Concurrent use with loop diuretics may increase the nephrotoxic or ototoxic potential of the aminoglycosides.
- **Diuretics, Osmotic** (eg, **mannitol**): Concurrent use of osmotic diuretics may increase the nephrotoxic or ototoxic potential of the aminoglycosides.
- **Nephrotoxic Drugs, Other (eg, cisplatin, amphotericin B, cyclosporine, polymyxin B, vancomycin)**: Potential for increased risk for nephrotoxicity
- **Neuromuscular-Blocking Agents and Anesthetics, General**: Concomitant use with general anesthetics or neuromuscular-blocking agents could potentiate neuromuscular blockade.

Laboratory Considerations

- **Gentamicin serum concentrations** may be falsely decreased if the patient is also receiving beta-lactam antibiotics and the serum is stored prior to analysis. It is recommended that if assay is delayed, samples be frozen and, if possible, be drawn at times when the beta-lactam antibiotic is at a trough.

Dosages

NOTE: Most infectious disease clinicians agree that aminoglycosides should be dosed once a day in most patients (mammals) with uncompromised renal function. This dosing regimen yields higher peak levels with resultant greater bacterial kill, and as aminoglycosides exhibit a postantibiotic effect, surviving susceptible bacteria generally do not replicate as rapidly even when antibiotic concentrations are below MIC. Periods where levels are low may decrease the adaptive resistance (bacteria take up less drug in the presence of continuous exposure) that can occur. Once-daily dosing may also decrease the toxicity of aminoglycosides, as lower urinary concentrations may mean less uptake into renal tubular cells.

DOGS:

Susceptible infections (extra-label):

- Normal renal function: 9 – 14 mg/kg IV, IM, or SC once a day is reasonable for most breeds and infections. Use the higher end of dosing range for life-threatening infections, or in immunocompromised or neutropenic patients.
- Reduced renal function: If gentamicin use cannot be avoided, the following dosage modifications can be considered[15]:
  - ClCr 0.4 – 0.7 mL/kg/minute (serum creatinine ≈2.3 to 4 mg/dL): 9 – 14 mg/kg IV, IM, SC every 36 to 48 hours
  - ClCr 0.15 – 0.4 mL/kg/minute (serum creatinine ≈ 4.9 to 5.5 mg/dL): 9 – 14 mg/kg IV, IM, SC every 48 hours
  - ClCr less than 0.15 mg/kg/minute (serum creatinine ≈8.5 mg/dL or more): Use is not recommended
- Greyhounds, other sighthounds: 6 mg/kg IV once daily or 9 mg/kg SC/IM once daily[16]

Aerosolized treatment of *Bordetella bronchiseptica* (extra-label): 4 mg/kg nebulized over 10 minutes every 12 hours for 3 to 4 weeks[17]

Chemical ciliary body ablation (extra-label): 0.25 – 0.5 mL of gentamicin sulfate 100 mg/mL injection into the vitreous humor

CATS:

Susceptible infections (extra-label): 5 – 8 mg/kg IV, IM, or SC once daily

- Reduced renal function: If gentamicin use cannot be avoided, the following dosage modifications can be considered[15]:
  - ClCr 0.4 – 0.7 mL/kg/minute (serum creatinine ≈2.3 to 4 mg/dL): 5 – 8 mg/kg IV, IM, SC every 36 to 48 hours
  - ClCr 0.15 – 0.4 mL/kg/minute (serum creatinine ≈4.9 to 5.5 mg/dL): 5 – 8 mg/kg IV, IM, SC every 48 hours
  - ClCr less than 0.15 mg/kg/minute (serum creatinine ≈8.5 mg/dL or more): Use is not recommended

Chemical ciliary body ablation (extra-label): 0.25 – 0.5 mL of gentamicin sulfate 100 mg/mL injection into the vitreous humor

HORSES:

WARNING: IV administration may be associated with allergic and anaphylactic reactions in horses. The injection should be prewarmed and administered slowly. If clinical signs occur, corticosteroid treatment may be necessary.

Susceptible uterine infections via intrauterine infusion:

- Label Dosage (FDA-approved): 2 – 2.5 g (20 – 25 mL) diluted in 200 – 500 mL sterile normal saline and infused aseptically into uterus once daily for 3 to 5 days during estrus[13]
- Extra-label: Irrigate uterus for 2 to 3 days prior to antibiotic infusion to remove inflammatory debris. Gentamicin dosed at 1 – 2 g intrauterine infusion. Buffer with bicarbonate (equal volume of 7.5% bicarbonate and diluted in saline) or large volume (200 mL) of saline. Mares with bacterial endometritis should be treated with IU antibiotics once daily for 3 to 7 days. Treatment length is dependent on history, chronicity of infection, bacteria isolated, and mare's ability to clear uterine fluid.[18]

Susceptible infections (extra-label):

- Adults: 7.7 – 9.7 mg/kg IV once daily.[19] Historically, 6.6 mg/kg IV every 24 hours had been used and remains a viable option for ambulatory practices where isolate MICs may be lower.[20,21] IM administration may cause muscle irritation.
- Foals:
  - Less than 2 weeks old: 12 mg/kg IV every 36 hours
  - Greater than 2 weeks old: 6.6 mg/kg IV once daily (every 24 hours) should be adequate.[22]

Septic arthritis (extra-label): Direct intra-articular (IA) administration gentamicin 500 mg has been used, as well as IA continuous infusion of 0.17 mg/kg/hour using a CRI pump.[23] Regional intravenous limb perfusion (RILP) administration has also been used, under sedation in standing horses, using gentamicin 500 mg diluted in 40 mL 0.9% NaCl.[24]

Management of recurrent uveitis (extra-label): 4 or 6 mg/eye (total dose, NOT mg/kg) given as an intravitreal injection[2,3,25]

SWINE:

Susceptible infections (label dosage; FDA-approved):

- Colibacillosis in neonates: 5 mg/piglet (NOT mg/kg) PO or IM once[26,27]
- Weanlings and other swine[28]:
  - Colibacillosis: 1.1 mg/kg/day in drinking water (concentration of 25 mg/gallon) for 3 days
  - Swine dysentery (*Brachyspira hyodysenteriae*): 2.2 mg/kg per day in drinking water (concentration of 50 mg/gallon) for 3 days

BIRDS:

Susceptible infections (extra-label): 5 – 10 mg/kg IM every 12 hours[29,30]

FERRETS:

Susceptible infections (extra-label): 5 – 8 mg/kg IV, IM, or SC once daily

RABBITS/RODENTS/SMALL MAMMALS:

Rabbits (extra-label): 5 – 8 mg/kg daily dose (may divide into every 8 to 24 hours) SC, IM, or IV. Increased efficacy and decreased toxicity if given once daily. If given IV, dilute into 4 mL/kg of saline and give over 20 minutes.[31] Aminoglycosides adversely affect the GI flora balance in these animals; use with caution.

Chinchillas, gerbils, guinea pigs, hamsters, mice, rats (extra-label): 2 – 4 mg/kg SC or IM every 8 to 24 hours[32]

REPTILES:

Susceptible infections (extra-label):

Bacterial shell diseases in turtles: 5 – 10 mg/kg daily in water turtles, every other day in land turtles and tortoises for 7 to 10 days. Used commonly with a beta-lactam antibiotic. Recommend beginning therapy with 20 mL/kg fluid injection. Maintain hydration and monitor uric acid levels when possible.[33]

Monitoring

- Efficacy (cultures, clinical signs associated with infection)
- Renal toxicity; baseline urinalysis, serum creatinine/BUN. Casts in the urine are often the initial sign of impending nephrotoxicity. Decreasing urine-specific gravity is an earlier indicator than azotemia. Casts, urine-specific gravity, or increased serum creatinine may not be good markers in neonates. Frequency of monitoring during therapy is unclear. There is no contraindication to daily monitoring with urinalysis (cytological examination for casts and assessment of specific gravity) and serum creatinine but monitoring every 3 to 5 days at the start of treatment may be more practical in lower-risk cases (eg, adults, animals with no underlying renal disease or concerns about dehydration or hypotension).
- Gross monitoring for vestibular or auditory toxicity is recommended, especially in cats.
- Therapeutic drug monitoring (TDM) when possible in patients with uncompromised renal function; highly recommended for patients with risk factors for nephrotoxicity. Peak and trough levels are determined through samples collected 30 minutes after administration (peak) and immediately before administration of the next dose (trough). Generally, peak levels (≈30 to 60 minutes post IV dose) should be greater than 32 µg/mL and trough levels less than 1 – 2 µg/mL.[34] A clinical laboratory may be able to assist in sample-time determination and dosage amount and frequency adjustment.

Client Information

- To treat infections in the body, gentamicin must be injected; it is only given orally (by mouth) to reduce the amount of bacteria in animals' intestines before intestinal surgery.
- Gentamicin can be given once daily either in the vein (by your veterinarian), in a muscle, or under the skin (subcutaneously). If injecting at home, be sure you understand how to properly inject it.
- This drug can damage nerves, hearing, and kidneys. Cats may be more likely to have damage to their hearing.
- This drug can be used topically for ear, skin, or eye infections.

Chemistry/Synonyms

An aminoglycoside obtained from cultures of *Micromonospora purpurea*, gentamicin sulfate occurs as a white to buff powder that is soluble in water and insoluble in alcohol. The commercial product is a combination of gentamicin sulfate C_1, C_2, and C_3, but all these compounds apparently have similar antimicrobial activities. Commercially available injections have a pH from 3 to 5.5.

Gentamicin may also be known as gentamicin sulphate, gentamicini sulfas, NSC-82261, and Sch-9724; many trade names are available.

Storage/Stability

Gentamicin sulfate for injection and the oral solution should be stored at room temperature (15°C-30°C [59°F-86°F]); freezing or temperatures above 40°C (104°F) should be avoided. The soluble powder should be stored from 2°C to 30°C (46°F-86°F). Do not store or offer medicated drinking water in rusty containers or the drug may be destroyed.

Compatibility/Compounding Considerations

Although the manufacturer does not recommend that gentamicin be mixed with other drugs, it is reportedly physically **compatible** and stable in all commonly used IV solutions and with the following drugs: bleomycin sulfate, cefoxitin sodium, cimetidine HCl, clindamycin phosphate, metronidazole (with and without sodium bicarbonate), penicillin G sodium, and verapamil HCl.

The following drugs or solutions are reportedly physically **incompatible** or only compatible in specific situations with gentamicin: amphotericin B, ampicillin sodium, dopamine HCl, furosemide, and heparin sodium. In vitro inactivation of aminoglycoside antibiotics by beta-lactam antibiotics is well documented. Gentamicin is very susceptible to this effect, and it is recommended to avoid mixing with these compounds.

Compatibility is dependent upon factors such as pH, concentration, temperature, and diluent used; consult specialized references or a hospital pharmacist for more specific information.

Dosage Forms/Regulatory Status

VETERINARY-LABELED PRODUCTS:

The American Association of Bovine Practitioners and the American Veterinary Medical Association discourages extra-label aminoglycoside use in bovines.

Gentamicin Sulfate Solution (for intrauterine infusion): 100 mg/mL in 100 mL and 250 mL vials; multiple trade names, generic; (Rx); FDA-approved for horses

Gentamicin Sulfate Injection: 100 mg/mL (poultry only) in 100 mL vials; *Garasol® Injection*, *Gentapoult®*; (OTC). For use only in day-old chickens (slaughter withdrawal = 5 weeks) and 1- to 3-day-old turkeys (slaughter withdrawal = 9 weeks)

Gentamicin Sulfate Injection: 5 mg/mL in 250 mL vials; *Garacin® Piglet Injection*; (OTC). FDA-approved for use in piglets up to 3 days of age. Slaughter withdrawal (when used as labeled) = 40 days

Gentamicin Sulfate Oral Solution: 5 mg/mL in 118 mL bottles with pump applicator; generic; (Rx). FDA-approved for use in neonatal swine only. Slaughter withdrawal = 14 days

Gentamicin Soluble Powder: 333.33 mg/g in 360 g jars. FDA-approved for use in weanling swine. Slaughter withdrawal = 10 days. *Gen-Gard® Soluble Powder*; (OTC)

Gentamicin Sulfate Soluble Powder: 2 g gentamicin/30 g of powder in 360 g jar; *Garacin® Soluble Powder*; (OTC). FDA-approved for use in swine. Slaughter withdrawal (when used as labeled) = 10 days

Veterinary FDA-approved injections for chickens and turkeys plus a water additive for egg dipping may also be available. Ophthalmic, otic, and topical preparations are available with veterinary labeling.

HUMAN-APPROVED PRODUCTS:

Partial listing:

Gentamicin Sulfate Injection: 10 mg/mL and 40 mg/mL (as sulfate) in vials and cartridge-needle units and in various concentrations

(0.8 – 1.6 mg/mL) pre-mixed in saline in 50 mL and 100 mL single-dose containers; generic; (Rx)

Topical-, otic-, and ophthalmic-labeled products are also available.

References

For the complete list of references, see **wiley.com/go/budde/plumb**

Glipizide

(*glip*-i-zide) *Glucotrol®*

Sulfonylurea Antidiabetic Agent

Prescriber Highlights

- ▶ Human oral type II antidiabetic agent that may be useful in cats with nonketotic diabetes mellitus with mild to moderate signs and that are in good physical condition and able to be closely monitored.
- ▶ It may take 4 to 8 weeks before full effects are seen.
- ▶ Glipizide is NOT recommended in dogs.
- ▶ Contraindications include hypersensitivity, absolute insulin deficiency, and diabetic ketosis or ketoacidosis.
- ▶ Use with caution in patients with untreated adrenal or pituitary insufficiency, thyroid, renal, or hepatic function impairment, prolonged vomiting, high fever, malnourishment, other debilitating conditions, and patients with hypersensitivity to other sulfonamide derivatives.
- ▶ Adverse effects in cats include GI effects (eg, anorexia, vomiting), hypoglycemia, and liver toxicity.
- ▶ Do not confuse glipizide with glimepiride or glyburide.

Uses/Indications

Glipizide may be of benefit in treating cats with type II diabetes if there is existing pancreatic beta cell function. Glipizide has been reported to be beneficial in ≈30%[1] to 40%[2] of cats, but there is no way to predict which cats will benefit in advance of a trial. Glipizide should only be used in cats that have nonketotic diabetes mellitus with mild to moderate signs and that are in good physical condition and able to be closely monitored[1]; it should only be used in situations when owners refuse insulin therapy and only in combination with dietary therapy.[2] Insulin therapy is considered superior to glipizide therapy and should be the initial recommendation in newly diagnosed diabetic cats, as insulin therapy has an increased possibility for diabetic remission.[1,2]

A glipizide trial may also be appropriate when a cat appears to be relatively well controlled on small doses of insulin, and the owner would strongly prefer to no longer give insulin.[3]

Glipizide should not be used in dogs.[2] Although glipizide could theoretically be useful in treating canine patients with type II or III diabetes, dogs are typically absolutely or relatively insulinopenic by the time they present with hyperglycemia, and glipizide would therefore be ineffective.

Pharmacology/Actions

Glipizide is a second-generation sulfonylurea. Sulfonylureas lower blood glucose concentrations in both diabetic and non-diabetic patients. The exact mechanism of action is not known, but these agents are thought to exert the effect primarily by stimulating the beta cells in the pancreas to secrete additional endogenous insulin. Extrapancreatic effects include enhanced tissue sensitivity of circulating insulin. Ongoing use of the sulfonylureas appears to enhance peripheral sensitivity to insulin and reduce the production of hepatic basal glucose. The mechanisms causing these effects are yet to be fully explained.

Prolonged hyperglycemia may cause beta cell exhaustion with permanent damage, leading to cell death. It has been suggested that by treating all cats initially with insulin to rapidly reduce hyperglycemia, increases in beta cell sensitivity and insulin release may occur with time and potentially increase success using glipizide.[4]

Pharmacokinetics

Glipizide is rapidly and practically completely absorbed after oral administration. The absolute bioavailability reported in humans ranges from 80% to 100%. Food will alter the rate, but not the extent, of absorption. Transdermal administration on cats does not appear to be as adequately absorbed compared to oral administration but did lower blood glucose over time. Further studies are warranted to evaluate long-term use and topical effects of transdermal glipizide before it should be recommended for use.[5] Glipizide is highly bound to plasma proteins.[6] It is primarily biotransformed in the liver to inactive metabolites that are then excreted by the kidneys. In humans, the half-life is ≈2 to 4 hours.[6] Effects on insulin concentrations in cats tend to be short-lived. Effects peak in about 15 minutes and return to baseline after about 60 minutes.

Contraindications/Precautions/Warnings

Glipizide is contraindicated in patients hypersensitive to it. Glipizide is contraindicated in cats with an absolute insulin deficiency or that have diabetic ketosis or ketoacidosis. Glipizide should be used with caution in cats with untreated adrenal or pituitary insufficiency, thyroid, renal, or hepatic dysfunction, prolonged vomiting, high fever, malnourishment, or other debilitating conditions. Use with caution in cats that are allergic to other sulfonamide derivatives, as they may also develop an allergic reaction to glipizide.

Sulfonylureas have the potential to produce severe hypoglycemia. Although glipizide may initially be effective, it may become ineffective in weeks to months after starting therapy; insulin will then be required. Glipizide does not appear to be effective in cats demonstrating insulin resistance.

Some patients with type II or type III diabetes may have their disease complicated by the production of excessive amounts of cortisol or growth hormone, which may antagonize insulin's effects. These underlying causes should be ruled out before initiating oral antidiabetic therapy.

In humans, the use of oral antihyperglycemic medications has been reportedly associated with increased cardiovascular mortality compared to treatment with diet or diet plus insulin.[6]

Do not confuse glipiZIDE with glyBURIDE or gliMEPIRIDE. Consider writing part of the drug's name in uppercase letters (tall-man designations) on prescriptions/orders to reduce the risk of errors.

Adverse Effects

GI adverse effects (eg, anorexia, vomiting) occur in ≈15% of cats receiving glipizide. Vomiting typically occurs shortly after dosing and subsides in 2 to 5 days. If persistent or severe, decrease dose or frequency; discontinue if necessary.

Some cats receiving glipizide have developed hypoglycemia, but severe hypoglycemia appears to be rare. If hypoglycemia occurs, discontinue glipizide and recheck blood glucose in one week; if hyperglycemia recurs, glipizide may be restarted at a lower dose or dosing frequency.

Increased amyloid deposit formation can occur with glipizide, which can potentially cause further destruction of functional beta cells.[7]

Hepatic adverse effects have been reported, and ≈8% of cats treated with glipizide may develop cholestatic jaundice with increased liver enzymes. Discontinue glipizide in cats with elevated enzymes if they develop lethargy, anorexia, vomiting, or if ALT exceeds 500 IU/L. If icterus occurs, discontinue glipizide and restart at a lower dose once icterus resolves; discontinue use if icterus reoccurs.

Other adverse effects reported in humans include allergic skin reactions and myelosuppression.[6]

Reproductive/Nursing Safety

Safe use during pregnancy has not been established. Glipizide was found to be mildly fetotoxic in rats when given at doses at 5 to 50 mg/kg; however, no other teratogenic effects were noted.[6] Use in pregnancy only when benefits outweigh potential risks.

It is unknown if glipizide enters milk. Because safety has not been established in animals, this drug should only be used when the maternal benefits outweigh the potential risks to offspring.

Overdose/Acute Toxicity

Oral LD_{50} values are greater than 4 g/kg in all animal species tested. Profound hypoglycemia is the greatest concern after an overdose. GI decontamination protocols should be employed when warranted. Because of its shorter half-life, prolonged hypoglycemia is less likely with glipizide, but blood glucose monitoring and treatment with parenteral glucose may be required for several days. Massive overdoses may also require additional monitoring (blood gases, serum electrolytes) and supportive therapy.

For patients that have experienced or are suspected to have experienced an overdose, consultation with a 24-hour poison consultation center specializing in providing veterinary-specific information is recommended. For general information related to overdose and toxin exposures, as well as contact information for poison control centers, refer to ***Appendix.***

Drug Interactions

The following drug interactions have either been reported or are theoretical in humans or animals receiving glipizide and may be of significance in veterinary patients. Unless otherwise noted, use together is not necessarily contraindicated, but weigh the potential risks and perform additional monitoring when appropriate.

- Azole Antifungals (eg, **fluconazole, itraconazole, ketoconazole**): May increase plasma levels of glipizide
- Beta-Adrenergic Receptor Antagonists (eg, **atenolol, propranolol**): May potentiate the hypoglycemic effect
- Chloramphenicol: May displace glipizide from plasma proteins
- Cimetidine: May potentiate the hypoglycemic effect
- Corticosteroids: May reduce the efficacy of glipizide
- Diuretics, Thiazide: May reduce hypoglycemic efficacy
- Ethanol: A disulfiram-like reaction (anorexia, nausea, vomiting) has been reported in humans who have ingested alcohol within 48 to 72 hours of receiving glipizide.
- Fluoroquinolones (eg, **ciprofloxacin, enrofloxacin**): May increase risk for hypoglycemia or hyperglycemia
- Isoniazid: May reduce hypoglycemic efficacy
- Monoamine Oxidase Inhibitors (MAOIs; eg, **amitraz, linezolid, selegiline**): May potentiate the hypoglycemic effect
- Niacin: May reduce hypoglycemic efficacy
- Phenothiazines (eg, **acepromazine, chlorpromazine**): May reduce hypoglycemic efficacy
- Probenecid: May potentiate the hypoglycemic effect
- Sulfonamides: May displace glipizide from plasma proteins
- Sympathomimetic Agents: May reduce hypoglycemic efficacy
- Thyroid Agents: May reduce the hypoglycemic effect
- Warfarin: May displace glipizide from plasma proteins

Dosages

CATS:

NOTE: Glipizide is rarely recommended (see ***Uses/Indications***), and evidence to support any dosage regimen is low.

Diabetes mellitus (extra-label): Recommended initial dose is 2.5 mg/cat (NOT mg/kg) PO twice daily with food. The dose can be increased to 5 mg/cat (NOT mg/kg) PO twice daily with food if an inadequate response is seen after 2 weeks and no adverse effects are seen.[1,2] If no response is seen after 4 to 6 weeks, insulin therapy should be instituted. If the cat appears to be clinically responsive, the glipizide trial can continue for 12 weeks to assess response to therapy. If euglycemia or hypoglycemia develops, the dosage may be tapered down or discontinued. Re-evaluate blood glucose concentrations 1 week later to assess the need for the drug. If hyperglycemia recurs, increase or reinitiate glipizide at a lower maintenance dose.[8]

Monitoring

- Physical examinations and body weight weekly during the first month of treatment, then periodically
- Urine glucose and ketones weekly during the first month of treatment
- Blood glucose weekly during the first month of therapy, then periodically; some recommend blood glucose measurements every 3 to 4 hours for the first 12 to 18 hours of therapy to check for hypoglycemia. Blood glucose curves help to monitor therapeutic response.[6]
- Baseline and periodic CBC
- Regular serum chemistry profiles should be performed to screen for liver toxicity; every 1 to 2 weeks initially, then periodically[6]
- Adverse effects (eg, anorexia, vomiting, icterus)

Client Information

- Give this medicine with meals as directed by your veterinarian.
- About 15% of cats will throw up after starting this medicine, but this usually improves after a few days.
- This medicine can take 1 to 2 months to see if it is working properly.
- Rarely, glipizide can cause yellowing of the skin, gums, or eyes (*jaundice*) or cause blood sugar to be too low (*hypoglycemia*). Watch for signs of low blood sugar, such as seizures (convulsions), collapsing/fainting, rear leg weakness or paralysis, muscle twitching, unsteadiness, lack of energy, or depression.

Chemistry/Synonyms

Glipizide, a sulfonylurea antidiabetic agent, occurs as a whitish powder. It is practically insoluble in water and has a pK_a of 5.9.

Glipizide may also be known as CP-28720, glipizidum, glydiazinamide, or K-4024; many international trade names are available.

Storage/Stability

Store glipizide tablets in tight, light-resistant containers at controlled room temperature.

Dosage Forms/Regulatory Status

VETERINARY-LABELED PRODUCTS: NONE

HUMAN-LABELED PRODUCTS:

Glipizide Oral Tablets: 5 mg and 10 mg; generic (Rx).

Glipizide Oral Extended-Release Tablets: 2.5 mg, 5 mg, and 10 mg; *Glucotrol XL®*, generic; (Rx). **NOTE:** This product is generally not used in veterinary medicine.

Also available in fixed-dose combinations of glipizide with metformin.

References

For the complete list of references, see **wiley.com/go/budde/plumb**

Glucagon

(***gloo***-ka-gon) *GlucaGen®*

Hormonal Agent

Prescriber Highlights

- ► Hormone to increase blood glucose that may be useful for treating hypoglycemia in small animals and potentially fatty liver syndrome in transition dairy cows
- ► May be effective in treating beta-blocker or calcium channel blocker overdoses, or when patients being treated for anaphylaxis have received beta-blockers
- ► Use extreme caution in patients with pheochromocytoma; use caution in patients with cardiac disease.
- ► Not indicated for hypoglycemia due to starvation, adrenal insufficiency, or chronic hypoglycemia
- ► Must be parenterally administered
- ► When used as CRI, must be in a setting where blood glucose can be monitored.
- ► Possible adverse effects include sedation, nausea, vomiting, and diarrhea.

Uses/Indications

In small animals, the primary use for glucagon is to increase blood glucose in patients with excessive insulin levels, either endogenously produced (insulinoma) or exogenously administered (insulin overdose). There is significant interest in its potential SC use in emergency home treatment of hypoglycemia in small animals.[1]

In human medicine and potentially for veterinary patients, glucagon can be used in treating the cardiac manifestations of beta-blocker, calcium channel blocker, and tricyclic antidepressant overdoses. One study in dogs, however, demonstrated insulin to be superior to glucagon in treating experimental propranolol overdoses.[2] Glucagon can also be used in conjunction with epinephrine for treating anaphylaxis in patients that have received beta-blockers, and it has potential in the treatment of fatty liver syndrome in dairy cattle.

Glucagon is used to treat steakhouse syndrome (ie, food bolus lodged in the esophagus) in human patients by relaxing the esophagus so that food can pass into the stomach.

Pharmacology/Actions

Glucagon's main pharmacologic activities are to increase blood glucose and relax smooth muscles of the GI tract. It primarily increases blood glucose by stimulating hepatic glycogenolysis but can also increase glucose via hepatic gluconeogenesis from available amino acid substrates. Glucagon does not stimulate the reactive release of insulin or cause rebound hypoglycemia. In healthy dogs, glucagon can overcome the inhibitory activity of insulin on hepatic glucose production; IV (not SC) glucagon can also cause transient increases in ACTH and cortisol.[3]

During radiologic examinations, glucagon has been used to prevent GI motility and is thought to act by relaxing the smooth muscles of the stomach. At higher doses (greater than 1 mg in a human adult), contractility of the duodenum and jejunum can be seen, which is most likely attributable to nausea and diarrhea that can be caused by glucagon administration.[4] The exact mechanisms of action for its GI effects are not well understood.

Glucagon increases lipolysis and decreases lipid synthesis in cow hepatocytes.[5]

Pharmacokinetics

Glucagon must be administered parenterally; it is destroyed in the gut after oral dosing. In healthy beagles, 1 mg given SC caused plasma glucose to increase significantly within 10 minutes and peak at 20 minutes. Glucose levels were still ≈60% above baseline at 30 minutes. After IV injection, maximum glucose levels were attained ≈20 minutes later.[3]

Glucagon is degraded in the plasma, liver, and kidneys. In humans, hyperglycemic effects persist up to 90 minutes after dosing, and plasma half-life is around 10 minutes.

Contraindications/Precautions/Warnings

Glucagon should usually not be given to patients with pheochromocytoma, as catecholamines may be released, leading to hypertension. When glucagon is used for insulinoma, it must be in a setting where blood glucose can be closely monitored. Although glucagon may be useful for blood glucose elevation in insulinoma patients, its use for this indication in humans is cautioned, as it can stimulate insulin production, leading to greater hypoglycemia once the drug is discontinued.

Use with caution in patients with known cardiac disease, as glucagon increases myocardial oxygen demand. For glucagon treatment to reverse hypoglycemia, there must be adequate amounts of glycogen stored in the liver. Glucagon is of little or no help in states of starvation, adrenal insufficiency, or chronic hypoglycemia. Hypoglycemia in these conditions should be treated with glucose.[6]

Adverse Effects

Glucagon is usually well tolerated, but sedation and injection site reactions may occur. Potentially, nausea, vomiting, and diarrhea soon after administration are possible, which is increased if doses greater than 1 mg are administered.[4] Hypokalemia and hypersensitivity reactions (very rare) are unlikely but possible.

Reproductive/Nursing Safety

As an endogenously produced hormone, glucagon is unlikely to cause significant risk to offspring.

It is unknown if glucagon enters maternal milk, but it is unlikely to cause harm to nursing offspring.

Because safety has not been established in animals, this drug should only be used when the maternal benefits outweigh the potential risks to offspring.

Overdose/Acute Toxicity

Adverse effects seen with overdose include nausea, vomiting, diarrhea, gastric hypotonicity, and, possibly, hypokalemia. Because glucagon's elimination half-life is so short, treatment may not be necessary and would be symptomatic in nature. If the patient is also receiving beta-blockers, greater increases in blood pressure and heart rate may be seen.

For patients that have experienced or are suspected of having experienced an overdose, consultation with a 24-hour poison consultation center specializing in providing veterinary-specific information is recommended. For general information related to overdose and toxin exposures, as well as contact information for poison control centers, refer to ***Appendix.***

Drug Interactions

The following drug interactions have either been reported or are theoretical in humans or animals receiving glucagon and may be of significance in veterinary patients. Unless otherwise noted, use together is not necessarily contraindicated, but weigh the potential risks and perform additional monitoring when appropriate.

- Anticholinergic Agents (eg, **amitriptyline, atropine, diphenhydramine, glycopyrrolate**): May enhance GI adverse effects of glucagon
- Beta-Blockers (eg, **atenolol, propranolol**): Glucagon may transiently increase heart rate and blood pressure.
- Glucose-Lowering Agents (eg, **exenatide**, **glipizide, metformin**): Glucagon may decrease efficacy of glucose-lowering agents.
- Indomethacin: May diminish the effect of glucagon

- **Insulin**: Glucagon and insulin have opposing effects on blood glucose.
- **Warfarin**: Anticoagulant effect may be increased when glucagon is concurrently administered; this effect may be delayed. It is suggested to monitor for bleeding and prothrombin activity if glucagon is necessary.

Laboratory Considerations

- No glucagon-related laboratory interactions were noted.

Dosages

DOGS/CATS:

IV dosing for severe hypoglycemia (extra-label): There are 2 primary recommended dosing regimens; the available evidence does not support one over the other:

Regimen 1: Glucagon 1 mg (NOT mg/kg) is reconstituted per manufacturer directions and then added to 1000 mL of 0.9% sodium chloride; this results in a 1000 nanogram/mL solution. [**NOTE**: Some references state not to mix or dilute with saline solutions but use 5% dextrose only.] Initially, give a 50 nanogram/kg IV bolus and then administer at a CRI using a suitable pump at a rate of 10 – 15 nanograms/kg/minute. The rate may need to be increased up to 40 nanograms/kg/minute to maintain euglycemia.

Regimen 2: Prepare solution as above, but give as an IV CRI at an initial infusion rate of 5 – 10 nanograms/kg/minute and adjust as needed to maintain the blood glucose concentration between 60 and 100 mg/dL.[7] An average initial dosage of 11.8 nanograms/kg per minute also has been used.[8] When discontinuing glucagon therapy, the dose should be gradually decreased over 1 to 2 days, and the blood glucose concentration should be monitored for recurrence of severe hypoglycemia.

CATTLE:

Fatty liver in early lactation dairy cows older than 3.5 years (extra-label): Glucagon 5 mg (NOT mg/kg) in 60 mL of normal saline SC every 8 hours (15 mg/day) for 14 days[9]

Fatty liver in multiparous cows (extra-label): Glucagon 10 mg/cow/day (NOT mg/kg) diluted in 480 mL sodium chloride and given as continuous IV infusion at 20 mL/hour using a volumetric pump for 14 days[10]

Prevention of fatty liver development in postpartum dairy cows (extra-label): Glucagon 5 mg/cow (NOT mg/kg) diluted in 60 mL 0.9% sodium chloride and administered SC between the fifth and seventh intercostal space 3 times daily for 14 days. The dose is started on day 2 postpartum.[11]

FERRETS:

IV dosing for severe hypoglycemia (extra-label): Evidence is limited, but glucagon has been shown to be effective in a case study treating a ferret with hypoglycemia subsequent to insulinoma. The dose was as follows: Glucagon 1 mg (NOT mg/kg) reconstituted with 0.9% sodium chloride, diluted in 1000 mL 5% dextrose and administered at a rate of 15 nanograms/kg/minute IV CRI. If needed, the rate may be increased to 40 nanograms/kg/minute.[12]

Monitoring

- Blood glucose
- Serum potassium if used other than for acute treatment

Client Information

- Could potentially use glucagon for outpatient emergency initial treatment of hypoglycemia, but oral glucose is probably more appropriate (and cheaper) for use.

Chemistry/Synonyms

Glucagon is a hormone secreted by the alpha-2 cells of the pancreas. It is a straight-chain polypeptide that contains 29 amino acids whose sequence is consistent throughout mammalian species. It has a molecular weight of 3483. When in crystalline form, it is a white- to off-white powder that is relatively insoluble in water at physiologic pH but is soluble at a pH of less than 3 and greater than 9.5. Glucagon may be expressed in terms of international units (IU) or by weight. One IU is equivalent to one milligram of glucagon. Commercially available glucagon is now obtained via recombinant DNA sources.

Glucagon may also be known as glucagonum or HGF and *GlucaGen®*.

Storage/Stability

Store the commercially available powder for reconstitution at room temperature between 20°C and 25°C (68°F-77°F); avoid freezing and protect from light. Once reconstituted with the supplied diluent, ensure the solution is clear with a water-like consistency and use immediately; discard any unused portion. Discard the solution if it contains any gel formation or particles.

Compatibility/Compounding Considerations

Compatibility is dependent on factors such as pH, concentration, temperature, and diluent used; specialized references or a hospital pharmacist should be consulted for more specific information.

To prepare for a CRI, dilute glucagon 1 mg with the supplied diluent or sterile water; gently roll until dissolved, and this may then be further diluted in 5% dextrose. It may be given through a Y-tube or 3-way stopcock if a dextrose solution is running.

Dosage Forms/Regulatory Status

VETERINARY-LABELED PRODUCTS: NONE

HUMAN-LABELED PRODUCTS:

Glucagon (human rDNA-origin) Powder for Injection: 1 mg (1 unit) with 1 mL diluent in vials and syringes; *GlucaGen Diagnostic®*, *GlucaGen HypoKit®*, *Glucagon Emergency Kit*, generic; (Rx)

References

For the complete list of references, see **wiley.com/go/budde/plumb**

Glucosamine/Chondroitin Sulfate

(gloo-***kose***-a-meen/kon-***droy***-tin ***sul***-fayt) *Cosequin®*

Nutritional Supplement

Prescriber Highlights

- Dietary supplement (not an FDA-approved drug) that may be useful as an adjunctive treatment for osteoarthritis or other painful conditions in dogs, cats, and horses
- Well tolerated, but efficacy is uncertain
- Not a regulated drug; therefore, choose products carefully. There is a large variation in commercially available products.

Uses/Indications

Compounds containing glucosamine and/or chondroitin sulfate may be useful in treating osteoarthritis or other painful conditions in domestic animals, but large, well-designed controlled clinical studies proving efficacy were not located. Additionally, because there is no FDA approval process or oversight for these products, product quality and bioavailability are highly variable.

Studies have shown variable efficacy of glucosamine and/or chondroitin for improvement of osteoarthritis in veterinary patients. One study in dogs[1] showed some positive effect, but this study was not placebo-controlled and compared responses with carprofen. Other placebo-controlled, blinded studies in dogs failed to demonstrate statistically significant improvement after 60 days[2] and 90 days[3] of treatment. An article reviewing the quality of evidence supporting the use of glucosamine-based dietary supplements in equine joint disease concluded that …*the quality of these studies is generally low.*[4] A systematic review of articles published from 2004 to 2014 dealing with dietary supplements and their efficacy in treatment of osteoarthritis in dogs came to the conclusion that the existing studies suffer from major limitations and/or bias.[5] Another review came to a similar conclusion that it is difficult to draw meaningful conclusions about efficacy because available trials used different products, salt forms, doses, and dosing regimens.[6] Based on available literature, the benefit of glucosamine/chondroitin for osteoarthritis is still questionable. However, studies have revealed that there are few adverse effects and therefore it can be administered long-term, even to dogs with comorbidities, unlike other treatments for osteoarthritis such as NSAIDs. Combining glucosamine/chondroitin with a veterinary NSAID appears beneficial.[7,8]

Glucosamine and chondroitin improved mobility and lameness scores in cats with osteoarthritis.[9] The potential benefit of N-acetyl-d-glucosamine has been tested in cats with feline lower urinary tract disease (FLUTD) but results have been conflicting.[10,11]

Glucosamine alone or with chondroitin has shown some benefit in horses with arthritis or reduced mobility.[12–14]

Pharmacology/Actions

Cartilage cells use glucosamine to produce glycosaminoglycans and hyaluronan, which form articular cartilage. Glucosamine supplementation is thought to provide the glycosaminoglycan building blocks required to strengthen existing cartilage. Glucosamine also regulates synthesis of collagen and proteoglycans in cartilage and has mild anti-inflammatory effects due to its inhibition of nuclear factor kappaB (NF-κB). Chondrocytes normally produce ample quantities of glucosamine from glucose and amino acids, but this ability may diminish with age, disease, or trauma. Exogenously administered glucosamine appears to be able to be used by chondrocytes. Glycosaminoglycans form part of the protective layer of the urinary tract.

Chondroitin sulfate possesses several pharmacologic effects. It appears to inhibit destructive enzymes in joint fluid and cartilage. In joint cartilage, chondroitin sulfate stimulates the production of glycosaminoglycans and proteoglycans and has a slight anti-inflammatory action. Thrombus formation in microvasculature may be reduced. It has been shown in vitro that glucosamine does not affect equine or canine platelet aggregation.[15]

Although in vitro evidence exists, there is no solid evidence that using these compounds together improves clinical effect over either alone, but in vivo studies are ongoing. Onset of any clinical efficacy may require 2 to 6 weeks of treatment.

Pharmacokinetics

The pharmacokinetics of these compounds are difficult to evaluate because of the different salts, lack of manufacturing or regulatory standards, and variability in product purity. Both glucosamine hydrochloride (HCl) and glucosamine sulfate can be absorbed in the gut after the salt is cleaved in the stomach, but bioavailability may be very low. One study in 6 mature horses that were fed diets with pure glucosamine and chondroitin top-dressed on their feed did not detect any absorption into plasma.[16] A study of oral absorption of tablet, chewable, and liquid formulations of glucosamine revealed there is a difference in pharmacokinetic parameters among these formulations; however, conclusions could not be drawn as to whether differences in these parameters impacted efficacy of the product.[17] Controversy exists as to whether one salt of glucosamine is superior to the other. Most clinical studies in veterinary species have been done with the HCl salt. Of the available OTC formulations, crystalline glucosamine sulfate has been shown to produce the highest plasma and synovial joint concentrations.[18] A study in rats and dogs concluded that addition of chitosan, a product derived from the shells of sea crustaceans, enhanced oral bioavailability of glucosamine.[19]

Contraindications/Precautions/Warnings

No absolute contraindications were located for these compounds. As hypersensitivity reactions are a theoretical possibility, animals demonstrating prior hypersensitivity reactions to these compounds should not receive them.

In humans, glucosamine may exacerbate symptoms associated with asthma. Although this has not yet been reported in veterinary patients, caution is advised in patients with bronchoconstrictive conditions.

Some glucosamine sulfate products contain significant amounts of potassium. Patients on a potassium-restricted diet should be given a glucosamine/chondroitin product that is low in potassium.

Adverse Effects

These products appear to be well tolerated in dogs, cats, and horses. Adverse effects could potentially include some minor GI effects (flatulence, stool softening). Because these products are often derived from natural sources including shellfish, hypersensitivity reactions could occur.

Reproductive/Nursing Safety

No studies on the safety of these compounds in pregnant or lactating animals have been performed.

Because safety has not been established in animals, this drug should only be used when the maternal benefits outweigh the potential risks to offspring.

Overdose/Acute Toxicity

Oral overdose is unlikely to cause significant problems. The LD_{50} for the combined compound in rats is greater than 5 g/kg.[20] GI effects may result. Changes in coagulation parameters could occur but have not been documented to date.

Products that contain manganese could lead to manganese toxicity if given in very high dosages (above label recommendations) chronically.

For patients that have experienced or are suspected to have experienced an overdose, consultation with a 24-hour poison consultation center specializing in providing veterinary-specific information is recommended. For general information related to overdose and toxin exposures, as well as contact information for poison control centers, refer to ***Appendix***.

Drug Interactions

The following drug interactions have either been reported or are theoretical in humans or animals receiving glucosamine and/or chondroitin and may be of significance in veterinary patients. Unless otherwise noted, use together is not necessarily contraindicated, but the potential risks must be weighed and additional monitoring performed when appropriate.

- ANTICOAGULANTS (eg, **heparin, rivaroxaban, warfarin**): A high dose of chondroitin sulfate and/or glucosamine potentially could enhance the effects of drugs that affect coagulation.
- ANTIDIABETIC AGENTS (eg, **glipizide, insulin, metformin**): Glucosamine may decrease the efficacy of hypoglycemic agents.
- DOXORUBICIN: Glucosamine may induce resistance by reducing inhibition of topoisomerase II.

Laboratory Considerations

- None noted

Dosages

NOTE: Because of the variability in products available, lack of controlled studies clearly documenting efficacy, or FDA approval, use of these products for controlling chronic pain conditions is controversial. If a therapy trial is undertaken, it is recommended to choose a product that has been tested in the species for which it is marketed. Consult the product's label for specific label information.

DOGS/CATS:

Adjunctive treatment of chronic pain conditions (extra-label): Anecdotal recommendations are to treat initially at 15 – 30 mg/kg (of the chondroitin component). After 4 to 6 weeks, if a positive response is seen, dosage may be halved or given every other day.

Feline idiopathic cystitis (extra-label): N-acetyl glucosamine 250 mg/cat (NOT mg/kg) PO once daily[21]

HORSES:

Adjunctive treatment of chronic pain conditions (extra-label): Glucosamine 9.96 g with chondroitin 2 g and methylsufonyl methane (MSM) 2.5 g/500 kg (1102 lb) body weight (NOT mg/kg) PO once daily[12]

Monitoring

- Clinical efficacy

Client Information

- This supplement may be given with or without food. If your animal vomits or acts sick after getting it on an empty stomach, give the medicine with food or a small treat to see if this helps. If vomiting continues, contact your veterinarian.
- It may take 2 to 6 weeks (or longer) of treatment to see if this supplement is helping.
- Do not switch brands from what is prescribed without first con tacting your veterinarian.
- Side effects are unlikely, but mild gastrointestinal upset (eg, decreased appetite) has been reported.

Chemistry/Synonyms

Glucosamine is most often available as either glucosamine HCl or glucosamine sulfate. It is an amino sugar that is synthesized in vivo by animal cells from glucose and glutamine. Commercial preparations of glucosamine are primarily derived from crustaceans.[22]

Glucosamine (HCl or sulfate) may also be known as chitosamine, NSC-758, 2-amino-2-deoxy-beta-D-glucopyranose, G6SD-glucosamine, glucose-6-phosphate, or amino monosaccharide.

Chondroitin sulfate is an acid mucopolysaccharide/glycosaminoglycan that is found in most cartilaginous tissues. It is a long-chain compound that contains units of galactosamine and glucuronic acid.

Chondroitin sulfate may also be known as chondroitin 4-sulfate, chondroitin sulfate A, chondroitin sulfate B, chondroitin sulfate C, chondroitin sulfate sodium, CSA, sodium chondroitin sulfate, chondroitin polysulfate, CDA, CSCSC, GAG, or galactosaminoglucono-glycan sulfate.

Storage/Stability

Because of the multiple products and product formulations available, check label for storage and stability (expiration date) information. Chondroitin sulfate is an extremely hygroscopic compound and, generally, these products should be stored in tight containers at room temperature. Avoid storing in direct sunlight and keep away from moisture.

Compatibility/Compounding Considerations

No specific information was noted; refer to the product label for more information.

Dosage Forms/Regulatory Status

VETERINARY-LABELED PRODUCTS:

None as pharmaceuticals. Supplements are available from a wide variety of sources, and dosage forms include tablets, capsules, and powder in a variety of concentrations. There are specific products marketed for use in animals, including *Cosequin®*, *Glycoflex®*, *NutriVet®*, *Next Level®*, *AniFlex®*, *Phycox®*, *Restor-A-Flex®*, *OsteO-3®*, *Arthri-Nu®*, *ProMotion®*, *Seraquin®*, *Oste-O-Guard®*, *Caniflex®*, *Equi-Phar Flex®*.

Glucosamine and chondroitin sulfate are considered dietary supplements by the FDA. No standards have been accepted for potency, purity, safety, or efficacy by regulatory bodies. Bioequivalence between products cannot be assumed and independent analysis has shown a wide variation in products.

HUMAN-LABELED PRODUCTS:

None as pharmaceuticals but a variety of OTC nutraceuticals are available.

References

For the complete list of references, see **wiley.com/go/budde/plumb**

Glyburide

(***glye***-byoor-ide) *DiaBeta®, Micronase®*

Sulfonylurea Antidiabetic Agent

Prescriber Highlights

- ► Oral antidiabetic agent that may be useful in cats with type 2-like diabetes
- ► Glipizide is used more often when oral hypoglycemics are tried; glyburide may be useful if glipizide is unavailable or if once-daily dosing is important.
- ► Contraindications include hypersensitivity, diabetic ketoacidosis, and insulin-dependent diabetes.
- ► Use caution with renal or hepatic insufficiency, elderly or malnourished patients, and adrenal or pituitary insufficiency.
- ► Adverse effects include vomiting, hypoglycemia, and liver toxicity.
- ► Do not confuse glyBURIDE with glipiZIDE or gliMEPERIDE.

Uses/Indications

Glyburide is an oral treatment for type 2-like diabetes mellitus in cats with mild diabetes, or for use as add-on therapy or when owners cannot or will not administer insulin.[1] Although there are more data supporting the use of glipizide, glyburide can be used if glipizide is unavailable or if twice-daily administration of glipizide is not tolerated (by cat or owner). Insulin therapy for cats with diabetes is generally preferred over oral treatments.

Pharmacology/Actions

Like glipizide and other oral sulfonylureas, glyburide lowers blood glucose concentrations in both diabetic and normal patients. Glyburide stimulates the release of insulin from the pancreas; therefore, functioning pancreatic beta cells are required for efficacy. Although the insulin secretory response generally declines over time, the blood glucose-lowering effect persists. The mechanism of blood glucose lowering with long-term administration is not precisely known but may be related to enhanced insulin activity at post-receptor sites and reduced basal hepatic glucose production.[2]

Pharmacokinetics

Glyburide appears to be well absorbed, but bioavailability data are lacking. Food apparently does not have an effect on the absorptive characteristics of the drug. Glyburide is distributed throughout the body, including into the brain and across the placenta. Glyburide is apparently completely metabolized, presumably in the liver. Metabolites are excreted in both the feces and urine. Although glyburide's elimination half-life in cats is not known, it is known to be a longer-acting sulfonylurea, so once-daily dosing appears to be effective in cats with noninsulin-dependent diabetic mellitus.[3]

Contraindications/Precautions/Warnings

Glyburide is contraindicated in patients that are hypersensitive to it, patients with diabetic ketoacidosis, or patients with insulin-dependent diabetes.[2] Animals that are allergic to other sulfonamide derivatives may develop an allergic reaction to glyburide as well.

Renal or hepatic insufficiency may cause increased drug levels and increase the risk for severe hypoglycemia. Use glyburide with caution in elderly patients, malnourished patients, and patients with adrenal or pituitary insufficiency, as they may be more susceptible to hypoglycemia.

Glyburide tablets (eg, *DiaBeta*®, *Micronase*®) are not bioequivalent to glyburide micronized tablets (*Glynase*® generic equivalent). Monitor blood glucose if switching between forms.[2]

Glyburide requires functioning pancreatic beta cells for efficacy. Some patients with type 2 diabetes may have their disease complicated by the production of excessive amounts of cortisol or growth hormone that may antagonize insulin's effects. These causes should be ruled out before initiating oral antidiabetic therapy.

Do not confuse glyBURIDE with glipiZIDE or gliMEPIRIDE.

Adverse Effects

Experience with glyburide is limited in veterinary medicine. Hypoglycemia, vomiting, icterus, and increased ALT (SGPT) levels are all potentially possible. If adverse effects develop, a lower dose may be attempted after clinical signs resolve.

Other adverse effects reported in humans include allergic skin reactions (eg, pruritis, erythema, urticaria), other allergic reactions (eg, angioedema, arthralgia, myalgia, vasculitis), bone marrow suppression, cholestatic jaundice, liver function abnormalities, nausea, heartburn, photosensitivity, and blurred vision.

Glyburide may not be effective in cats demonstrating insulin resistance.

Reproductive/Nursing Safety

Studies in mice have shown that glyburide is a substrate of the BCRP transporter, which is expressed in placental tissue. BCRP plays an active role in preventing glyburide exposure to the fetus, which makes glyburide a possible therapeutic option in pregnancy. Caution needs to be taken when considering glyburide during pregnancy due to potential exposure to the fetus if BCRP inhibitors are present or if a genetic mutation exists where BCRP is not expressed in the animal.[4] Prolonged and severe hypoglycemia has occurred in human infants born of mothers receiving a sulfonylurea at the time of birth, and discontinuing glyburide 2 weeks prior to expected delivery date is recommended.[2]

In humans, glyburide was found to be excreted in breast milk after large doses (85 mg/day) of glyburide were given.[5] It is unknown the extent of glyburide that appears in breast milk after normal doses. There are still conflicting data as to whether or not glyburide should be used during lactation.

Because safety has not been established in animals, this drug should only be used when the maternal benefits outweigh the potential risks to offspring.

Overdose/Acute Toxicity

Profound hypoglycemia is the greatest concern after an overdose. In humans, severe hypoglycemia has occurred at relatively low dosages. GI decontamination protocols should be employed when warranted. Because its half-life is longer than glipizide, prolonged hypoglycemia may occur, and blood glucose monitoring and treatment with parenteral glucose may be required for several days. Massive overdoses may also require additional monitoring (eg, blood gases, serum electrolytes) and supportive therapy.

For patients that have experienced or are suspected of having experienced an overdose, consultation with a 24-hour poison consultation center specializing in providing veterinary-specific information is recommended. For general information related to overdose and toxin exposures, as well as contact information for poison control centers, refer to ***Appendix.***

Drug Interactions

The following drug interactions have either been reported or are theoretical in humans or animals receiving glyburide and may be of significance in veterinary patients. Unless otherwise noted, use together is not necessarily contraindicated, but weigh the potential risks and perform additional monitoring when appropriate.

- **ACE Inhibitors**: May increase the risk for hypoglycemia
- **Alcohol**: A disulfiram-like reaction (eg, anorexia, nausea, vomiting) is possible.
- **Antifungals, Azole** (eg, **ketoconazole, itraconazole, fluconazole**): May increase plasma levels of glyburide
- **Beta-Blockers**: May potentiate the hypoglycemic effect
- **Chloramphenicol**: May displace glyburide from plasma proteins
- **Cimetidine**: May potentiate the hypoglycemic effect
- **Ciprofloxacin** (and potentially **other quinolones**): May potentiate the hypoglycemic effect of glyburide
- **Corticosteroids** (eg, **dexamethasone, fludrocortisone, predniso(lo)ne**): May reduce glyburide efficacy
- **Diuretics, Thiazide** (eg, **hydrochlorothiazide**): May reduce hypoglycemic efficacy
- **Fluoxetine**: May potentiate the hypoglycemic effect
- **Isoniazid**: May reduce hypoglycemic efficacy
- **Monoamine oxidase Inhibitors (MAOIs)**: May potentiate the hypoglycemic effect
- **Niacin**: May reduce hypoglycemic efficacy
- **nonsteroidal anti-inflammatory drugs (NSAIDs**; eg, **meloxicam, robenacoxib**): Highly protein-bound; may displace glyburide and potentiate hypoglycemic effect
- **Phenothiazines**: May reduce hypoglycemic efficacy
- **Probenecid**: May potentiate the hypoglycemic effect
- **Rifampin**: May reduce hypoglycemic efficacy by increasing glyburide metabolism
- **Sulfonamides**: May displace glyburide from plasma proteins
- **Sympathomimetic agents** (eg, **epinephrine**): May reduce hypoglycemic efficacy
- **Thyroid Agents**: May reduce the hypoglycemic effect
- **Warfarin**: May displace each other from plasma proteins; closely monitor both PT and blood glucose

Dosages

CATS:

Noninsulin-dependent diabetes mellitus (extra-label): There is little information published on using this medication in cats, and evidence to support clinical use is very weak. Using regular (ie, not micronized) glyburide tablets, 2 anecdotal dosage suggestions have been noted:

a) Initial dose at 0.625 mg/cat (NOT mg/kg) PO twice daily; may increase to 1.25 mg/cat (NOT mg/kg) twice daily. Once-daily administration may be suitable for some cats.[1,6]

b) 2.5 mg/cat (NOT mg/kg) PO twice a day for cats that are generally well, not ketoacidotic, and do not have peripheral neuropathy[7]

Monitoring

- Weekly examinations during the first month of therapy, including PE, body weight, urine glucose/ketones, and several types of blood glucose examinations
- Adverse effects (eg, vomiting, icterus) and occasional liver enzymes and CBC

Client Information

- May be useful for treating diabetes in cats; limited experience in veterinary medicine

- Give medicine with food around the same time each day. If severe or persistent vomiting occurs, contact your veterinarian.
- Watch for signs of blood sugar that is too low (ie, hypoglycemia; uncommon), seizures (ie, convulsions), collapsing/fainting, rear leg weakness or paralysis, muscle twitching, unsteadiness, lack of energy, or depression. If you see any of these signs, contact your veterinarian right away.
- This medicine has not been in use in many cats, so other side effects could occur. Report anything unusual to your veterinarian.
- While your animal is taking this medication, it is important to return to your veterinarian for examinations and bloodwork. Do not miss these important follow-up visits.

Chemistry/Synonyms

Glyburide is an oral sulfonylurea antidiabetic agent that occurs as a white or nearly white, odorless or almost odorless, crystalline powder. As pH increases, solubility increases. At a pH of 4, solubility in water is about 4 µg/mL, and at a pH of 9, solubility is 600 µg/mL. Glyburide has a pK_a of 6.8.

Glyburide may also be known as glibenclamide, glibenclamidum, glybenclamide, glybenzcyclamide, HB-419, and U-26452; many trade names are available, including *DiaBeta*®, *Glynase*®, and *Micronase*®.

Storage/Stability

Store glyburide oral tablets in well-closed containers at room temperature 20°C to 25°C (68°F-77°F).

Compatibility/Compounding Considerations

No specific information was noted.

Dosage Forms/Regulatory Status

VETERINARY-LABELED PRODUCTS: NONE

HUMAN-LABELED PRODUCTS:

Glyburide Oral Tablets: 1.25 mg, 2.5 mg, and 5 mg; micronized tablets: 1.5 mg, 3 mg, 4.5 mg, and 6 mg; *Glynase*® *PresTab*, *DiaBeta*®; generic; (Rx)

Glyburide/metformin tablets: 1.25 mg glyburide/250 mg metformin, 2.5 mg glyburide/500 mg metformin, and 5 mg glyburide/500 mg metformin; *Glucovance*®; generic; (Rx). **NOTE**: This product is unlikely to be of benefit to veterinary patients.

References

For the complete list of references, see **wiley.com/go/budde/plumb**

Glycerin, Oral

(***gli***-ser-in) *Glycerol, Osmoglyn*®

Osmotic Agent

Prescriber Highlights

- Oral osmotic agent that reduces intraocular and CSF pressures
- Contraindicated in patients with known hypersensitivity, well-established anuria, severe dehydration, severe cardiac decompensation, acute pulmonary edema
- Use caution in patients with compromised blood–aqueous barrier, hypovolemia, cardiac disease, or diabetes.
- Most common adverse effect is vomiting

Uses/Indications

Oral glycerin is used primarily for the short-term (up to 12 hours) reduction of intraocular pressure (IOP) in small animals with acute glaucoma. It may also be considered to reduce increased CSF pressure.

The IOP-lowering effect of glycerin may be more variable than with mannitol, but because glycerin may be given orally, it may be more advantageous to use in certain cases.

Pharmacology/Actions

Glycerin, in therapeutic oral doses, increases the osmotic pressure of plasma so that water from extracellular spaces is drawn into the blood to decrease intraocular pressure (IOP). The amount of decrease in IOP is dependent on the dose of glycerin, and the cause and extent of increased IOP. Glycerin also decreases extracellular water content from other tissues and can cause dehydration and decreased CSF pressure.

Pharmacokinetics

Glycerin is rapidly absorbed from the GI tract and decreases in intraocular pressure (IOP) can be seen within 30 minutes; peak serum concentrations generally occur within 90 minutes and maximum decreases in IOP usually occur within an hour of dosing and persist for 5 to 12 hours. Glycerin is distributed throughout the blood and is primarily metabolized by the liver. Approximately 10% of the drug is excreted unchanged in the urine. Serum half-life in humans is ≈30 to 45 minutes.

Contraindications/Precautions/Warnings

Glycerin is contraindicated in patients hypersensitive to it. It is also contraindicated in patients with well-established anuria, severe dehydration, severe cardiac decompensation, or with acute pulmonary edema. Glycerin may increase blood glucose,[1] and should be used with caution in dogs with diabetes mellitus.

Glycerin should be used with caution in animals when the blood–ocular barrier is not intact (hyphema, uveitis), and in those patients with hypovolemia, cardiac disease, or diabetes.[2] Another reference considers heart failure a contraindication and its use should be avoided in patients with chronic renal failure or compromised renal function.[3]

Adverse Effects

Vomiting after dosing is the most common adverse effect seen with glycerin use in animals. In humans, headache, nausea, thirst, and diarrhea have also been reported.

Reproductive/Nursing Safety

The safety of this drug in pregnant or lactating animals is unknown.

Because safety has not been established in animals, this drug should only be used when the maternal benefits outweigh the potential risks to offspring.

Overdose/Acute Toxicity

No specific information was located, but cardiac arrhythmias, nonketotic hyperosmolar coma, and severe dehydration have been reported with the drug.

For patients that have experienced or are suspected to have experienced an overdose, consultation with a 24-hour poison consultation center specializing in providing veterinary-specific information is recommended. For general information related to overdose and toxin exposures, as well as contact information for poison control centers, refer to ***Appendix.***

Drug Interactions

The following drug interactions have either been reported or are theoretical in humans or animals receiving glycerin and may be of significance in veterinary patients. Unless otherwise noted, use together is not necessarily contraindicated, but weigh the potential risks and perform additional monitoring when appropriate.

- **CARBONIC ANHYDRASE INHIBITORS** (eg, **acetazolamide, dichlorphenamide**): Concomitant administration of carbonic anhydrase inhibitors may prolong the intraocular pressure (IOP)-reducing effects of glycerin.
- **MIOTIC AGENTS, TOPICAL**: Concomitant administration of topical miotic agents may prolong the IOP-reducing effects of glycerin.

Dosages

DOGS & CATS:

Acute glaucoma as an emergency drug in place of aqueous centesis to rapidly reduce intraocular pressure (IOP) (extra-label): Most recommend using 1 – 2 g/kg PO. This would be ≈1.1 – 2.2 mL/kg of the 90% solution. To reduce the risk for vomiting, glycerin is recommended to be diluted to a 45% to 50% concentration with water, milk, or ice cream. In patients where it would not be contraindicated, withholding water or fluids for 3 to 4 hours after administering can increase efficacy.[2-5]

Monitoring

- Intraocular pressure (IOP)
- Urine output
- Hydration status

Chemistry/Synonyms

A trihydric alcohol, glycerin occurs as a clear, sweet, syrupy, hygroscopic liquid that has a characteristic odor. It is miscible with water and alcohol, but not miscible in oils. Glycerin solutions are neutral to litmus.

Glycerin may also be known as E422, glycerol, glicerol, glycerine, and glycerolum; many trade names are available.

Storage/Stability

Glycerin oral solution should be stored in tight containers at room temperature; protect from freezing.

Compatibility/Compounding Considerations

90% glycerin USP can be mixed into water, milk, or ice cream to reduce the potential for vomiting and improve palatability. To convert 90% glycerin to a 50% concentration, 1 mL of 90% glycerin can be diluted to a 50% concentration by the addition of 0.8 mL of diluent.

Practically, many clinicians will dilute with equal parts of diluent to obtain a 45% concentration.

Dosage Forms/Regulatory Status

VETERINARY-LABELED PRODUCTS: NONE

HUMAN-LABELED PRODUCTS: NONE FOR SYSTEMIC USE

USP glycerin 90% could be used for oral use in small animals (see ***Compatibility/Compounding Considerations***).

Glycerin is also available in a topical ophthalmic solution and as suppositories or liquid for rectal laxative use.

References

For the complete list of references, see **wiley.com/go/budde/plumb**

Glycopyrrolate

(glye-koe-***pye***-roe-late) *Robinul®*

Anticholinergic (Antimuscarinic)

Prescriber Highlights

- ▶ Synthetic antimuscarinic agent similar to atropine and available both orally and parenterally; used for a variety of indications including bradycardia and as an antidote
- ▶ Contraindicated in conditions where anticholinergic effects would be detrimental (eg, narrow-angle glaucoma, tachycardia, ileus, urinary obstruction). Not recommended for use in treating bradycardia secondary to dexmedetomidine
- ▶ Adverse effects are dose related and anticholinergic in nature, including dry secretions; initial bradycardia, then tachycardia; slowing of gut and urinary tract motility; and mydriasis and cycloplegia.
- ▶ Many potential drug interactions

Uses/Indications

Glycopyrrolate injection is FDA-approved for use in dogs and cats as a preanesthetic anticholinergic agent. Glycopyrrolate may be of benefit in neonatal animals when cardiac output is dependent on heart rate or when potent opioids are used. The drug is also used in an extra-label manner to prevent perioperative bradycardia, treat sinus bradycardia, sinoatrial arrest, second-degree AV block, and when anticholinergic therapy may be beneficial. When cholinergic agents such as neostigmine or pyridostigmine are used to reverse neuromuscular blockade due to non-depolarizing muscle relaxants, glycopyrrolate may be administered immediately prior to the reversal to prevent the peripheral muscarinic effects of the cholinergic agent.

Pharmacology/Actions

Glycopyrrolate is an antimuscarinic with similar actions as atropine. It is a quaternary ammonium compound, and unlike atropine, glycopyrrolate does not appreciably cross the blood-brain and blood-placenta barriers. Therefore, CNS adverse effects and clinical effects in the fetus/newborn should not be exhibited. Antimuscarinic agents competitively inhibit acetylcholine or other cholinergic stimulants at postganglionic parasympathetic neuroeffector sites. High doses may block nicotinic receptors at the autonomic ganglia and at the neuromuscular junction. Pharmacologic effects are dose related. At low doses, salivation, bronchial secretions, and sweating (not in horses) are inhibited. At moderate systemic doses, glycopyrrolate increases heart rate. High doses decrease GI and urinary tract motility. Very high doses can inhibit gastric acid secretion.

Pharmacokinetics

In dogs, following IV administration, the onset of action is generally within a few minutes (ie, slower than atropine). After IM or SC administration, peak effects occur ≈30 to 45 minutes postinjection, and after IM administration they last for ≈1 hour.[1] The vagolytic effects persist for 2 to 3 hours, and the antisialagogue (reduced salivation) effects persist for up to 7 hours. Quaternary anticholinergic agents are incompletely absorbed after oral administration, but quantitative data reporting the rate and extent of absorption of glycopyrrolate are not available. After oral administration, the anticholinergic effects of glycopyrrolate may persist for 8 to 12 hours.

Little information is available regarding glycopyrrolate's distribution characteristics. Being a quaternary ammonium compound, it is completely ionized and therefore has poor lipid solubility and does not readily penetrate into the CNS or eye. Glycopyrrolate crosses the placenta only marginally; it is unknown if it is excreted into milk.

For horses, the pharmacokinetics of IV glycopyrrolate have been described. After 1 mg (1.72 – 1.93 µg/kg) was given IV, the following median values were reported: volume of distribution (SS), 1.43 L/kg; clearance, 14.2 mL/kg/minute; and terminal half-life, 7.4 hours. Plasma clearance of the drug in horses appears to be similar to hepatic blood flow.[2]

In humans, glycopyrrolate is eliminated rapidly from the serum after IV administration and virtually no drug remains in the serum 30 minutes to 3 hours after dosing. Only a small amount is metabolized; the majority is eliminated unchanged in the feces and urine.

Contraindications/Precautions/Warnings

Glycopyrrolate is contraindicated in patients that are hypersensitive to it.

Antimuscarinic agents should be used with extreme caution in patients with known or suspected GI obstruction or infections. Glycopyrrolate and other antimuscarinic agents decrease GI motility and prolong retention of the causative agent(s) or toxin(s), resulting in prolonged clinical signs.[3,4] Antimuscarinic agents must also be used with extreme caution in patients with autonomic neuropathy. Anticholinergic agents such as atropine or glycopyrrolate are not recommended to treat bradycardias secondary to dexmedetomidine;

the reversal agent atipamezole is preferred.

Antimuscarinic agents should be used with caution in geriatric patients and in patients with hepatic or renal disease, hyperthyroidism, hypertension, hypertrophic cardiomyopathy, congestive heart failure, tachyarrhythmias, prostatic hypertrophy, or esophageal reflux. These drugs can produce sinus tachycardia and predispose hypotensive patients to cardiac arrhythmias (including ventricular fibrillation).

Alpha-2 agonist-mediated bradycardia is primarily a reflex secondary to alpha-2-mediated vasoconstriction with a resultant increase in blood pressure. Administration of anticholinergic agents in dogs or cats at the same time or after alpha-2 agonists leads to adverse cardiovascular effects (secondary tachycardia, prolonged hypertension, and cardiac arrhythmias).[5-7] The routine use of anticholinergics simultaneously with, or after, dexmedetomidine in dogs or cats is neither recommended nor necessary because blood pressure is generally normal to high. During anesthesia, if both the heart rate AND the blood pressure are low, an anticholinergic drug (atropine or glycopyrrolate) can be used as part of blood pressure support.[8] Another treatment option is reversal of the alpha-2 agonist (see ***Atipamezole***).

Antimuscarinics (eg, atropine, glycopyrrolate) are not routinely administered to reptiles, as they can cause increased viscosity of respiratory tract secretions with resultant risks for airway obstruction or endotracheal tube occlusion.

Adverse Effects

With the exceptions of rare CNS adverse effects and being slightly less arrhythmogenic, glycopyrrolate can be expected to have a similar adverse effect profile as atropine, which generally includes dose-related extensions of the drug's pharmacologic effects. At usual doses, adverse effects tend to be mild in relatively healthy patients. The more severe effects listed tend to occur with high or toxic doses. GI effects include dry mouth (xerostomia), increased viscosity of secretions, dysphagia, constipation, vomiting, and thirst. Genitourinary effects include urinary retention or hesitancy. Ocular effects, including blurred vision, pupil dilation, cycloplegia, and photophobia, are possible but less likely than with atropine. In dogs, glycopyrrolate 0.01 mg/kg IM decreased tear production but did not have any effects on intraocular pressure or pupil diameter.[9] Cardiovascular effects include sinus tachycardia (at higher doses), increased myocardial work and oxygen consumption, bradycardia (initially, or at very low doses), hypertension, hypotension, arrhythmias (ectopic complexes), and circulatory failure.

The veterinary drug label only lists mydriasis, tachycardia, and xerostomia as adverse effects in dogs and cats at labeled doses.

Reproductive/Nursing Safety

Glycopyrrolate only marginally crosses the placenta, and teratogenicity was not observed in rabbits that received IM glycopyrrolate.[10]

No specific lactation safety information was found; however, it is unlikely to be excreted into milk in substantial quantities because of its quaternary structure.

Because safety has not been established in animals, this drug should only be used when the maternal benefits outweigh the potential risks to offspring.

Overdose/Acute Toxicity

Signs of glycopyrrolate toxicity are an extension of its pharmacologic activity. GI effects can include dry mouth (ie, xerostomia), increased viscosity of secretions, dysphagia, constipation, and vomiting. Genitourinary effects may include urinary retention. CNS effects may include stimulation, drowsiness, ataxia, seizures, and respiratory depression; however, because of its quaternary structure, it would be expected that minimal CNS effects would occur after an overdose of glycopyrrolate when compared with atropine. Ophthalmic effects include mydriasis, cycloplegia, photophobia, and an increase in intraocular pressure. Cardiovascular effects include sinus tachycardia (at higher doses), increased myocardial oxygen consumption, bradycardia (initially, or at very low doses), hypertension, hypotension, tachyarrhythmia (eg, premature ventricular complexes [PVCs], ventricular tachycardia), and circulatory failure. In dogs, the LD_{50} for glycopyrrolate is reported to be 25 mg/kg IV. Glycopyrrolate doses of 2 mg/kg IV daily for 5 days per week for 4 weeks demonstrated no signs of toxicity. In cats, the LD_{50} after IM injection is 283 mg/kg.[11]

For patients that have experienced or are suspected to have experienced an overdose, consultation with a 24-hour poison consultation center specializing in providing veterinary-specific information is recommended. For general information related to overdose and toxin exposures, as well as contact information for poison control centers, refer to ***Appendix***.

Drug Interactions

Glycopyrrolate would be expected to have a similar drug interaction profile as atropine. The following drug interactions either have been reported or are theoretical in humans or animals receiving atropine or glycopyrrolate and may be of significance in veterinary patients. Unless otherwise noted, use together is not necessarily contraindicated, but weigh the potential risks and perform additional monitoring when appropriate.

- **Acetylcholinesterase Inhibitors** (AChI, eg, **neostigmine**): May reduce glycopyrrolate effects. Glycopyrrolate may intentionally be administered immediately prior to AChI to prevent peripheral muscarinic effects.
- **Alpha-2 Agonists** (eg, **dexmedetomidine, medetomidine, xylazine**): Use of glycopyrrolate with alpha-2 agonists may significantly increase arterial blood pressure, heart rate, and the incidence of arrhythmia.[12,13] Clinical use of atropine or glycopyrrolate to prevent or treat bradycardia caused by alpha-2 agonists is controversial and use together is discouraged; this may be particularly important when using higher doses of the alpha-2 agonist. See ***Contraindications/Precautions/Warnings***.
- **Amitraz**: Glycopyrrolate may aggravate some signs seen with amitraz toxicity, leading to hypertension and further inhibition of peristalsis.
- **Antacids (Aluminum-, Magnesium-, Calcium-Containing)**: May decrease oral glycopyrrolate absorption; give oral glycopyrrolate at least 1 hour prior to oral antacids.
- **Beta-Blockers** (eg, **atenolol, propranolol**): Glycopyrrolate may increase oral bioavailability.
- **Bethanechol**: Concurrent use of cholinergic agonists and antagonists should be avoided.
- **Digoxin (tablets)**: Glycopyrrolate may increase serum digoxin concentrations; use oral liquid.
- **Domperidone**: Glycopyrrolate may reduce domperidone efficacy.
- **Potassium Chloride, Oral (solid dosage forms)**: Concurrent use with glycopyrrolate may significantly increase the amount of potassium absorbed. This combination may also increase risk for GI lesions and is contraindicated in humans.
- **Promotility Agents** (eg, **cisapride, metoclopramide**): Concurrent use with glycopyrrolate may antagonize promotility effects.

The following drugs may enhance the activity or toxicity of glycopyrrolate:

- **Amantadine**
- **Anticholinergic Agents (Other)** (eg, **atropine, hyoscyamine**)
- **Anticholinergic Muscle Relaxants** (eg, **dantrolene, methocarbamol**)

- **Antihistamines** (eg, **diphenhydramine**)
- **Opioids** (eg, **fentanyl, morphine, oxymorphone**)
- **Phenothiazines** (eg, **acepromazine**)
- **Procainamide**
- **Primidone**
- **Tricyclic Antidepressants** (eg, **amitriptyline, clomipramine**)

Dosages

DOGS/CATS:

Adjunct to anesthesia:

a) Label dosage (FDA-approved): 0.011 mg/kg IV, IM, or SC[14]

b) Extra-label dosage: Not routinely used but may be of benefit in pediatric patients or when using potent opioids. When used, it is usually as part of a premedication dosed at 0.005 – 0.01 mg/kg IV, IM, or SC, but doses as low as 0.003 mg/kg have been noted.

Vagolytic agent for bradyarrhythmias (extra-label):

a) To determine if increased vagal tone is contributing to a bradyarrhythmia: 0.01 mg/kg IV

b) To treat vagally induced bradyarrhythmias, glycopyrrolate is usually dosed at 0.005 – 0.01 mg/kg IV. If given IM or SC, slightly higher dosages (up to 0.02 mg/kg) may be considered.

Adjunctive treatment of muscarinic signs associated with carbamate or organophosphate intoxication (extra-label): 0.01 – 0.02 mg/kg IV; repeat as necessary

HORSES:

Treatment of bradyarrhythmias (extra-label): 0.00175 – 0.0025 mg/kg (1.7 – 2.5 μg/kg) IV[2,15-19]

Controlling muscarinic adverse effects associated with imidocarb therapy (extra-label): 0.0025 mg/kg IV[16]

RUMINANTS:

Bradycardia, reduce salivary secretions (extra-label): 0.005 – 0.001 mg/kg IM, or 0.002 – 0.005 mg/kg IV[20]

FERRETS:

Premedication (extra-label): 0.01 – 0.02 mg/kg IM, SC, or IV

RABBITS/RODENTS/SMALL MAMMALS:

Preanesthetic (extra-label): **Rodents**: 0.01 – 0.02 mg/kg SC or IM. **Rabbits**: 0.01 – 0.1 mg/kg IM or SC. As part of an injectable anesthesia protocol in rabbits: acepromazine (0.2 mg/kg) with oxymorphone (0.1 mg/kg) and glycopyrrolate (0.01 mg/kg) IM[21]

Adjunctive drug for CPR in rabbits (extra-label): A retrospective study found the median dose used was 0.01 mg/kg IV.[22]

REPTILES:

Treatment of bradycardia (prolonged or profound) associated with anesthesia (extra-label): 0.01 mg/kg IM, IV, or IC (intracoelemic)[23]

Monitoring

Dependent on dose and indication:

- Heart rate and rhythm
- Blood pressure
- GI motility (via auscultation) in horses and potentially in ruminants
- Urination, defecation capability
- Hydration; dry mouth and secretions (eg, respiratory)

Client Information

- Injectable glycopyrrolate administration is best performed by professional staff at a veterinary clinic where adequate cardiac monitoring is available.
- If your animal is receiving glycopyrrolate tablets, provide access to water, and encourage drinking if dry mouth is a problem. The medicine can be given with or without food. If your animal vomits or acts sick after receiving it on an empty stomach, give the medicine with food or a small treat to see if this helps. If vomiting continues, contact your veterinarian.

Chemistry/Synonyms

A synthetic quaternary ammonium antimuscarinic agent, glycopyrrolate occurs as a bitter-tasting, practically odorless, white, crystalline powder with a melting range of 193 °C to 198°C (379°F-388 °F). One gram is soluble in 20 mL of water; 30 mL of alcohol. The commercially available injection is adjusted to a pH of 2 to 3 and contains 0.9% benzyl alcohol as a preservative.

Glycopyrrolate may also be known as glycopyrronium bromide, AHR-504, *Acpan®*, *Gastrodyn®*, *Glycostigmin®*, and *Robinul®*.

Storage/Stability

Glycopyrrolate tablets should be stored in tight containers and both the injection and tablets should be stored at room temperature (15°C -30°C [59°F-86°F]).

Glycopyrrolate is stable under ordinary conditions of light and temperature. It is most stable in solution at an acidic pH and undergoes ester hydrolysis at pH above 6.

Compatibility/Compounding Considerations

Compatibility is dependent on factors such as pH, concentration, temperature, and diluent used; consult specialized references or a veterinary hospital pharmacist for more specific information. Although stability information was not located, glycopyrrolate injection has been mixed in syringes with acepromazine, buprenorphine, morphine, and ketamine.

Glycopyrrolate injection is physically **stable** in the following IV solutions: D_5W, D_5/half normal saline, Ringer's injection, and normal saline. Glycopyrrolate may be administered via the tubing of an IV running lactated Ringer's, but rapid hydrolysis will occur if it is added to an IV bag of LRS. The following drugs are reportedly physically **compatible** with glycopyrrolate: atropine sulfate, chlorpromazine HCl, codeine phosphate, diphenhydramine HCl, hydromorphone, hydroxyzine HCl, lidocaine HCl, meperidine HCl, morphine sulfate, neostigmine methylsulfate, oxymorphone HCl, procaine HCl, prochlorperazine HCl, promazine HCl, promethazine HCl, pyridostigmine Br, and scopolamine HBr.

The following drugs are reportedly physically **incompatible** with glycopyrrolate: chloramphenicol sodium succinate, dexamethasone sodium phosphate, diazepam, dimenhydrinate, methohexital sodium, methylprednisolone sodium succinate, pentazocine lactate, pentobarbital sodium, sodium bicarbonate, and thiopental sodium. Other alkaline drugs (eg, thiamylal) would also be **expected to be incompatible** with glycopyrrolate.

Dosage Forms/Regulatory Status

VETERINARY-LABELED PRODUCTS:

Glycopyrrolate for Injection: 0.2 mg/mL; (Rx). Although approved products for dogs and cats are still listed in the FDA Green Book, they may not be commercially marketed.

The Association of Racing Commissioners International (ARCI) has designated this drug as a class 4 substance. See the ***Appendix*** for more information. Use of this drug may not be allowed in certain animal competitions. Check rules and regulations before entering in a competition while this medication is being administered. Contact local racing authorities for further guidance.

HUMAN-LABELED PRODUCTS:

Glycopyrrolate Tablets: 1 mg and 2 mg; *Robinul®* and *Robinul Forte®*, generic; (Rx)

Glycopyrrolate Oral Solution: 1 mg/5 ml (0.2 mg/mL); *Cuvposa®*; (Rx)

Glycopyrrolate Injection: 0.2 mg/mL in 1 mL, 2 mL, 5 mL, and 20 mL vials; *Robinul®*, generic; (Rx)

References

For the complete list of references, see **wiley.com/go/budde/plumb**

Gonadorelin

GnRH

(goe-***nad***-oe-rell-in)

Hormonal Agent

Prescriber Highlights

- Hypothalamic hormone used to treat ovarian cysts and other reproductive disorders in a variety of species. In cattle, FDA restricts use for fixed time artificial insemination (FTAI) in combination with prostaglandins to specific approved products.
- Duration of action is very short (minutes).
- No contraindications and adverse effects have been reported.
- No slaughter or milk withdrawal when used as labeled

Uses/Indications

Gonadorelin (GnRH) is indicated (FDA-approved) for the treatment of ovarian follicular cysts in cattle, which reduces the number of days to first estrus. It also is approved for use with cloprostenol or dinoprost to synchronize estrous cycles to allow for fixed time artificial insemination (FTAI) in cattle. In manufacturer field studies, pregnancy rates were approximately doubled with use of gonadorelin compared to the prostaglandin only. One study comparing two different GnRH products (gonadorelin hydrochloride and gonadorelin diacetate tetrahydrate) demonstrated equivalent pregnancy rates.[1]

Additionally, gonadorelin has been used in cattle to reduce the time interval from calving to first ovulation and to increase the number of ovulations within the first 3 months after calving. This may be particularly important in increasing fertility in cows with retained placenta.

In dogs, gonadorelin has been used experimentally to help diagnose reproductive disorders or to identify intact animals versus castrated ones by maximally stimulating FSH and LH production. It has also been used experimentally in dogs to induce estrus through pulsatile dosing. Although apparently effective, specialized administration equipment is required for this method. Other uses in dogs may include enhancement of libido and treatment of oligospermia in male dogs and induction of ovulation or treatment of ovarian cysts in bitches.

Gonadorelin has been used as an alternate therapy to FSH or hCG to induce estrus or ovulation in cats with prolonged anestrus.

In other species, gonadorelin has been used to enhance sexual behavior in breeding stallions, for estrus synchronization in sheep and goats, and to induce ovulation in alpacas.

In human medicine, gonadorelin has been used for the diagnosis of hypothalamic-pituitary dysfunction, cryptorchidism, and depression secondary to prolonged severe stress.

Pharmacology/Actions

Gonadorelin is a synthetic form of GnRH and it stimulates the production and release of FSH and LH from the anterior pituitary. Secretion of endogenous GnRH from the hypothalamus is thought to be controlled by several factors, including circulating sex hormones. Synthetic gonadorelin administered IV or IM also causes the release of endogenous LH or FSH from the anterior pituitary.[2] Synthetic gonadorelin is physiologically and chemically identical to the endogenous bovine hypothalamic releasing factor.

Gonadorelin causes a surge of FSH and LH after a single injection. In cows and ewes, this can induce ovulation, but not in estrus mares. A constant infusion of gonadorelin will initially stimulate LH and FSH release, but after a period of time, LH and FSH concentrations will return to baseline.

Pharmacokinetics

After IV injection in pigs, gonadorelin is rapidly distributed to extracellular fluid, with a distribution half-life of ≈2 minutes. The elimination half-life of gonadorelin is ≈13 minutes in the pig.

After IV injection in humans, gonadorelin has a plasma half-life of 10 to 40 minutes. Within one hour, approximately ½ the dose is excreted in the urine as metabolites. It is not absorbed after oral administration.

Contraindications/Precautions/Warnings

None are noted on the label.

Adverse Effects

Adverse effects, including injection site reactions, were reported at the same rate as placebo in manufacturer field studies. Synthetically prepared gonadorelin should not cause any hypersensitivity reactions. This may not be the case with pituitary-obtained LH preparations or hCG.

Reproductive/Nursing Safety

Administration of 60 µg/kg/day of gonadorelin diacetate tetrahydrate to pregnant rats and rabbits during organogenesis did not cause embryotoxic or teratogenic effects.[3]

No specific lactation safety information was listed for this drug.

Overdose/Acute Toxicity

In doses up to 120 µg/kg, no adverse effects were noted in several species of test animals.[3] The LD_{50} in rats and dogs is 60 mg/kg and 600 µg/kg, respectively. Gonadorelin is unlikely to cause significant adverse effects after inadvertent overdosage.

For patients that have experienced or are suspected to have experienced an overdose, consultation with a 24-hour poison consultation center specializing in providing veterinary-specific information is recommended. For general information related to overdose and toxin exposures, as well as contact information for poison control centers, refer to ***Appendix.***

Drug Interactions

None noted

Dosages

DOGS:

GnRH stimulation test to differentiate castration from cryptorchidism (extra-label): Take preinjection blood sample, administer 50 µg/dog (NOT µg/kg) IM, 2 to 3 hours later take postinjection blood sample. Neutered dogs have testosterone concentrations less than 0.1 ng/mL; GnRH does not stimulate testosterone production.[4]

Increasing libido in male dogs (extra-label): 50 µg IM weekly for 4 to 6 weeks may improve libido.[5]

Improvement in semen quality (extra-label): 1 – 3 µg/kg IM once, or once weekly[6]

Cystic ovarian disease (extra-label): 3.3 µg/kg IM once daily for 3 days. An elevated progesterone concentration (more than 2 ng/mL) measured 1 to 2 weeks posttreatment verifies success.[7]

CATS:

Infertility, reduced libido, testis descent in male cats (extra-label): 1 µg/kg every 2 to 3 days[8]

Detection of ovarian remnants after ovariohysterectomy (extra-label): 25 µg/cat (NOT µg/kg). A progesterone concentration more than 1 ng/mL measured 1 to 2 weeks posttreatment verifies presence of ovarian tissue in the abdomen.[7]

CATTLE:

Treatment of ovarian cysts (label dosage; FDA-approved): 86 or 100 µg gonadorelin *base* (depends on product)/cow (NOT µg/kg) IM or IV. **NOTE:** *Factrel*® is labeled for IM use only.

Using with dinoprost tromethamine to synchronize estrous cycles to allow fixed-time artificial insemination (FTAI) in lactating dairy cows (label dosage; FDA approved): 100 – 200 µg/cow (NOT µg/kg) IM at Day 0. Administer dinoprost 25 mg/cow (NOT mg/kg) (as dinoprost tromethamine) IM 6 to 8 days after the first dose of gonadorelin. Administer a second dose of gonadorelin 30 to 72 hours after dinoprost. Perform fixed-time artificial insemination (FTAI) 0 to 24 hours after the second dose of gonadorelin or inseminate cows on detected estrus using standard herd practices.[9]

Using with cloprostenol sodium to synchronize estrous cycles to allow fixed-time artificial insemination (FTAI) in beef and/or lactating dairy cows (label dosage for *Cystorelin*®, *GONABreed*®, *OvaCyst*® and *Fertagyl*®; FDA-approved): Administer 86 µg/cow (NOT µg/kg) IM (2 mL; *Fertagyl*® or *Cystorelin*®) or 100 µg/cow (NOT µg/kg) IM (1 mL; *GONABreed*®) at Day 0. Administer cloprostenol (as cloprostenol sodium) 500 µg/cow (NOT µg/kg) IM 6 to 8 days after the first gonadorelin dose. Administer a second gonadorelin dose (*Fertagyl*® or *Cystorelin*® 2 mL OR *GONABreed*® 1 mL) 30 to 72 hours after cloprostenol. Perform FTAI 0 to 24 hours after the second gonadorelin dose or inseminate cows on detected estrus using standard herd practices. See table below. (Adapted from labels; *Cystorelin*®, *Fertagyl*®, *GONABreed*®, *OvaCyst*®)

Gonadorelin product	First Gonadorelin dose at Day 0 of cycle	Cloprostenol dose (day of cycle)	Second Gonadorelin dose 30 to 72 hours after Cloprostenol	FTAI timing
Fertagyl®	86 µg/cow (NOT µg/kg) (2 mL) IM	500 µg/cow (NOT µg/kg) IM (Day 6 to 8)	86 µg/cow (NOT µg/kg) (2 mL) IM	0 to 24 hours after the second gonadorelin dose for beef cattle, 8 to 24 hours for lactating dairy cattle or on detected estrus using standard herd practices
Cystorelin®, *OvaCyst*®	86 µg/cow (NOT µg/kg) (2 mL) IM	500 µg/cow (NOT µg/kg) IM (Day 6 to 8)	86 µg/cow (NOT µg/kg) (2 mL) IM	0 to 24 hours after the second gonadorelin dose or on detected estrus using standard herd practices
GONABreed®	100 µg/cow (NOT µg/kg) (1 mL) IM	500 µg/cow (NOT µg/kg) IM (Day 6 to 8)	100 µg/cow (NOT µg/kg) (1 mL) IM	0 to 24 hours after the second gonadorelin dose or on detected estrus using standard herd practices

Monitoring

- Dependent on reason for use; efficacy

Client Information

- In small animals, gonadorelin is best administered by a veterinarian.

Chemistry/Synonyms

A hormone produced by the hypothalamus, gonadorelin is obtained from natural sources or is synthetically produced. It is a decapeptide that occurs as a white or faintly yellowish-white powder. One gram is soluble in 25 mL of water or in 50 mL of methyl alcohol. 50 µg of gonadorelin acetate is equivalent to ≈31 units.

Gonadorelin may also be known as follicle stimulating hormone-releasing factor, GnRH, gonadoliberin, gonadorelinum, gonadotrophin-releasing hormone, Hoe-471, LH/FSH-RF, LH/FSH-RH, LH-RF, LH-RH, luliberin, luteinising hormone-releasing factor, *Cystorelin*®, *Factrel*®, *Fertagyl*®, *GONABreed*®, and *OvaCyst*®.

Storage/Stability

Most gonadorelin products (*Factrel*®, *Fertagyl*®, and *GONABreed*®) should be refrigerated at 2°C to 8°C (36°F to 46°F) for long-term storage. One product (*Cystorelin*®) should be stored at or below 25°C (77°F), with brief excursions to 30°C (86°F) permitted. Discard dates for in-use vials vary by manufacturer:

- *Cystorelin*®: discard after 6 months
- *Factrel*®: 1 month after first puncture
- *Fertagyl*®: within 28 days of first use, but the 100 mL vial should not be punctured more than 10 times; see product label for further details
- *GONABreed*®: 180 days after first use, and in-use vials may be stored at temperatures up to 25°C (77°F)
- *OvaCyst*®: 3 months after first use

There is very little information available on the stability of gonadorelin.

Compatibility/Compounding Considerations

There is very little information available on the compatibility of gonadorelin.

Dosage Forms/Regulatory Status

VETERINARY-LABELED PRODUCTS:

NOTE: Because the FDA does not consider estrous control and synchrony a "therapeutic purpose" under the requirements of extra-label drug use in food-producing animals, using a drug in an extra-label manner for estrous control in cattle is not permissible.[10]

Gonadorelin (diacetate tetrahydrate) for Injection: 43 µg/mL gonadorelin (equivalent to 50 µ/mL gonadorelin diacetate tetrahydrate suitable for IM or IV administration according to the indication) in 10 mL, 30 mL, 50 mL, and 100 mL multidose vials; *Cystorelin*®; (Rx). FDA-approved for the IV or IM treatment of ovarian follicular cysts in dairy cattle, and IM with cloprostenol sodium to synchronize estrous cycles to allow for fixed time artificial insemination (FTAI) in lactating dairy cows and synchronize estrous cycles to allow for FTAI in beef cows. *Ovacyst*®; (Rx). FDA-approved for the IM treatment of ovarian follicular cysts in dairy cattle, in 36 mL multidose vials. There are no withdrawal times required for either milk or slaughter.

Gonadorelin (acetate) for Injection: 43 µg/mL (gonadorelin) available in 20 mL and 100 mL multidose vials; *Fertagyl*®; (Rx). FDA-approved IV or IM for the treatment of ovarian follicular cysts in dairy cattle, and IM with cloprostenol to synchronize estrous cycles to allow for FTAI in beef cows. There are no withdrawal times required for either milk or slaughter.

Gonadorelin (acetate) for Injection: 100 µg/mL (gonadorelin) in 20 mL and 100 mL multidose vials; *GONABreed*®; (Rx). FDA-approved for the treatment of ovarian follicular cysts in dairy cattle (IM or IV) and in combination with cloprostenol sodium to synchronize estrous cycles to allow for FTAI in lactating dairy and beef cows (IM only). No withdrawal period required.

Gonadorelin HCl Solution for Injection: 50 µg/mL (gonadorelin) 20 and 50 mL multidose vials; *Factrel®*; (Rx). FDA-approved for the IM treatment of ovarian follicular cysts in in lactating dairy cows, beef cows, and replacement dairy and beef heifers and in combination with dinoprost tromethamine to synchronize estrous cycles to allow FTAI in lactating dairy cows. No withdrawal period required.

HUMAN-LABELED PRODUCTS: NONE

References

For the complete list of references, see **wiley.com/go/budde/plumb**

Granisetron

(gran-***iss***-eh-tron) *Kytril®*

5-HT_3 Antagonist Antiemetic

Prescriber Highlights

- ► Used for the treatment of severe vomiting or emesis prophylaxis before chemotherapy.
- ► It appears safe, but it is not commonly used in veterinary medicine.

Uses/Indications

Granisetron is an alternative to other 5-HT_3 receptor antagonists (eg, ondansetron or dolasetron) for the treatment of severe vomiting or prophylaxis before administering antineoplastic drugs, such as cisplatin, that can cause severe vomiting.

Pharmacology/Actions

Granisetron, like ondansetron or dolasetron, exerts its antinausea and antiemetic actions by selectively antagonizing 5-hydroxytryptamine$_3$ (5-HT_3; serotonin$_3$) receptors. These receptors are found primarily in the CNS chemoreceptor trigger zone, on vagal nerve terminals, and enteric neurons in the GI tract. Chemotherapy-associated vomiting in cats is believed primarily due to activation of 5-HT_3 receptors in the chemoreceptor trigger zone (CTZ), but in dogs, enteric and vagal receptors may be more important. Granisetron did not prevent apomorphine-induced vomiting in beagles.[1]

Pharmacokinetics

No pharmacokinetic data for dogs or cats were located. In humans, granisetron is rapidly absorbed after oral dosing, and peak concentrations occur in about 2 hours. Oral bioavailability is only 60% due to first-pass metabolism in the liver. The presence of food can decrease AUC by 5% but increase peak concentrations by 30%. Granisetron has a volume of distribution of about 3 L/kg, and plasma protein binding is ≈65%. The drug is metabolized in the liver, primarily via demethylation and oxidation and then conjugation. Less than 20% is excreted unchanged in the urine; the remainder is eliminated in the urine and feces as metabolites. Elimination half-life varies considerably, with reported values from about 1 to 30 hours. Cancer patients appear to have longer elimination half-lives compared to healthy adults.

Contraindications/Precautions/Warnings

There are no known contraindications to using this medication in dogs or cats. In humans, granisetron is contraindicated in patients hypersensitive to it, and it should not be used to treat vomiting associated with apomorphine (see ***Drug Interactions***).

No dosage adjustments are required in elderly patients or those with impaired renal or hepatic function. Granisetron may mask signs associated with progressive ileus and/or gastric distention; it should not replace required nasogastric suction.

Adverse Effects

Because of limited use in dogs and cats, a comprehensive adverse effect profile for granisetron is not known; however, it appears to be tolerated well.

In humans, the most common adverse effect reported is headache. Other adverse effects that may occur include abdominal pain, constipation or diarrhea, asthenia, or somnolence. Rarely, hypersensitivity reactions or cardiovascular effects (arrhythmias, chest pain, hypotension) have been reported.

Reproductive/Nursing Safety

Safety in pregnancy is not clearly established, but high-dose studies in rodents and rabbits did not demonstrate overt fetal toxicity or teratogenicity.

It is not known if granisetron enters milk.

Because safety of granisetron has not been established in animals, this drug should only be used when the maternal benefits outweigh the potential risks to offspring.

Overdose/Acute Toxicity

Limited information is available. An overdose of 38.5 mg in a human caused only a slight headache. Observation and, if required, supportive treatment are suggested.

For patients that have experienced or are suspected of having experienced an overdose, consultation with a 24-hour poison consultation center specializing in providing veterinary-specific information is recommended. For general information related to overdose and toxin exposures, as well as contact information for poison control centers, refer to ***Appendix.***

Drug Interactions

The following drug interactions have either been reported or are theoretical in humans or animals receiving granisetron and may be of significance in veterinary patients. Unless otherwise noted, use together is not necessarily contraindicated, but weigh the potential risks and perform additional monitoring when appropriate.

- APOMORPHINE: Profound hypotension can occur.
- BUPRENORPHINE: Concurrent use may increase the risk for serotonin syndrome.
- CISAPRIDE: Concurrent use may result in increased risk for QT-interval prolongation. This combination is contraindicated in humans.
- FLUCONAZOLE: Concurrent use may result in increased risk for QT-interval prolongation. This combination is contraindicated in humans.
- FLUOROQUINOLONE ANTIBIOTICS (eg, **enrofloxacin**): Concurrent use may increase the risk for QT interval prolongation.
- KETOCONAZOLE: May inhibit the metabolism of granisetron and increase the risk for QT-interval prolongation
- MACROLIDE ANTIBIOTICS (eg, **clarithromycin**): Concurrent use may increase the risk for QT interval prolongation.
- METRONIDAZOLE: Concurrent use may increase the risk for QT interval prolongation.
- MONOAMINE OXIDASE INHIBITORS (MAOIs; eg, **amitraz, linezolid, selegiline**): Increased risk for serotonin syndrome
- PHENOBARBITAL: Can induce the metabolism of granisetron
- SEROTONERGIC AGENTS, OTHER (eg, **clomipramine, fentanyl, fluoxetine, mirtazapine, tramadol, trazodone**): Increased risk for serotonin syndrome

Laboratory Considerations

- No specific laboratory concerns are associated with granisetron.

Dosages

DOGS/CATS:

Antiemetic (extra-label): Little is published on the clinical use of this drug in animals; single doses of 0.02 – 0.4 mg/kg IV have demonstrated efficacy in dogs,[2,3] and dosages of 0.1 – 0.5 mg/kg PO or IV every 12 hours to 24 hours have been suggested. IV administration may be more effective than PO. In cats, 1 mg/kg IM 3 times daily also has been reported.[4]

Monitoring

- Clinical efficacy

Client Information

- This drug is usually used on an inpatient basis or during outpatient visits for chemotherapy.
- If used orally on an outpatient basis, be sure to contact your veterinarian for further instructions in case of uncontrolled vomiting or if the dose is vomited up after administering.

Chemistry/Synonyms

Granisetron HCl occurs as a white or almost white powder that is freely soluble in water. Dosages are expressed in terms of the base; 1.12 mg of granisetron HCl is equivalent to 1 mg of granisetron base.

Granisetron may also be known as granistroni, granisetrono, or BRL-43694A, *Aludal®*, *Eumetic®*, *Granicip®*, *Granitron®*, *Kytril®*, *Kevatril®*, *Rigmoz®*, or *Setron®*.

Storage/Stability

Store granisetron products at room temperature (20°C to 25°C [68°F-77°F]) in tight containers and protected from light. Do not freeze the solution for injection. Upon penetration of the multi-dose vial, use it within 30 days.

Compatibility/Compounding Considerations

Compatibility is dependent on factors such as pH, concentration, temperature, and diluent used; specialized references or a hospital pharmacist should be consulted for more specific information.

The injectable solution is **compatible** with 0.9% sodium chloride, 5% dextrose in 0.45% or 0.9% sodium chloride, and 5% dextrose in water. It is **compatible** with many drugs at intravenous Y-sites, but it is **incompatible** with amphotericin B.

Dosage Forms/Regulatory Status

VETERINARY-LABELED PRODUCTS: NONE

HUMAN-LABELED PRODUCTS:

Granisetron Oral Tablets: 1 mg (1.12 mg as HCl); generic; (Rx)

Granisetron Injection Solution: 0.1 mg/mL (0.112 mg/mL as HCl) preservative-free, may contain sodium chloride 9 mg in 1 mL single-use vials; 1 mg/mL (1.12 mg/mL as HCl), regular and preservative-free, in 1 mL single-dose and 4 mL multi-dose vials; generic; (Rx)

Granisetron transdermal patch and extended-release subcutaneous injection solution also are available, although there is no information about the use of these products in veterinary species.

References

For the complete list of references, see **wiley.com/go/budde/plumb**

Grapiprant

(**gra**-pi-prant) *Galliprant®*

Prostaglandin E_2 EP4-Receptor Antagonist

Prescriber Highlights

- ► Used for the treatment of osteoarthritis (OA) pain in dogs
- ► Contraindicated in dogs hypersensitive to it
- ► Adverse GI effects (eg, vomiting; loose, mucoid, watery, or bloody stool) are possible.
- ► Dogs homozygous for the MDR1 gene mutation (also known as *ABCB1*-1delta) likely require lower dosages.

Uses/Indications

Grapiprant is approved for the control of pain and inflammation associated with osteoarthritis (OA) in dogs.[1] In the UK and Europe, grapiprant is specifically indicated for use in dogs with mild to moderate OA.[2]

Grapiprant has demonstrated an antinociceptive effect in rabbits under experimental conditions[3]; further study is warranted before the drug is used clinically in this species.

Pharmacology/Actions

Grapiprant is a prostaglandin E_2 (PGE_2) EP4-receptor antagonist NSAID; it does not inhibit cyclooxygenase like other commonly prescribed NSAIDs.

EP4 receptors are found in a wide range of tissues (eg, hematopoietic tissues, GI tract, cardiovascular system, bones, kidneys) and are the most widely expressed PGE_2 receptors.[4] EP4 receptors impact GI homeostasis and renal function[4]; they have also been shown to be upregulated during arthritic states.[5] The EP4 receptor is the sole PGE_2-mediated receptor for stimulation of acid secretion in the stomach, bicarbonate secretion in the duodenum, and mucus secretion in the duodenum and large intestine.[1,4] The EP4 receptor can mediate the antinatriuretic effects of PGE_2 by stimulating release of renin in the kidney.[4,6] EP4 receptors are abundantly expressed in the hearts of dogs[1,7]; however, the clinical significance of this is not yet known.

By inhibiting the EP4 receptor, grapiprant decreases the inflammatory effects of PGE_2 and therefore lessens pain transmission at sensory neurons.[1,8] Grapiprant may also inhibit PGE_2-mediated small intestine motility and cytokine expression in the large intestine.[9]

EP4 receptors are not involved with causing pyrexia.

Pharmacokinetics

Grapiprant tablets are rapidly absorbed after oral administration, with peak concentrations (C_{MAX}) of up to 1600 ng/mL occurring ≈1 to 2 hours postadministration in fasted dogs.[10] The presence of food can significantly delay time to peak concentrations and reduce C_{MAX} (4-fold) and area under the curve (AUC; 2-fold).[1,11] AUC in fasted dogs was 2.8 micrograms*hour/mL following a single 2 mg/kg PO dose.[1] The US label does not recommend administering grapiprant in the fasted state,[1] whereas the UK label states to administer on an empty stomach and at least 1 hour prior to the next meal.[2] A plasma concentration of 164 ng/mL has been reported to be effective for analgesia.[12] Plasma protein-binding is ≈95%.[2,12] Elimination half-life can range from ≈4.5 to 6 hours.[1,12,13] Biotransformation and elimination processes have not been fully described, but hydroxylated and *N*-oxidated metabolites have been detected in urine and feces.[1,11,14] Excretion is predominantly fecal (≈65%) and renal (≈20%).[2]

In collies homozygous for the multidrug sensitivity gene (*MDR1* gene, also known as *ABCB1* gene) receiving the label dose, C_{MAX} was 4600 to 5200 ng/mL, AUC_{0-24} was 15.2 to 17.3 micrograms*hour/mL, and half-life was 4.3 hours.[15] While the reported half-life is similar to that of "normal" dogs, the values for C_{MAX} and

AUC are substantially higher.

In cats given 3 mg/kg PO once daily for 28 days, peak concentrations of ≈1100 ng/mL occurred 1.2 to 1.7 hours after administration.[16] Elimination half-life was 3.1 to 14.1 hours.[16] Following single 2 mg/kg doses given IV or PO, oral bioavailability was 40%, steady state volume of distribution was 0.9 L/kg, clearance was 173 mL/kg/hour, and half-life was 5.5 hours.[17]

In fasted, exercised thoroughbreds given a single 2 mg/kg PO dose, a peak serum concentration of 31.1 ng/mL was reached within 90 minutes of administration. Elimination half-life was 5.9 hours.[18] In fasted mixed-breed mares, the peak plasma concentrations ranged from 71 to 149 ng/mL (mean 106 ng/mL) reached 30 minutes after administration.[19]

Contraindications/Precautions/Warnings

Grapiprant is contraindicated in dogs that are hypersensitive to it or that are currently taking other NSAIDs or corticosteroids.

Safety has not been evaluated in dogs younger than 9 months or weighing less than 3.6 kg (8 lb). Grapiprant use in dogs with cardiac disease has not been studied.[1] The UK label states to *use with caution in dogs suffering from pre-existing liver, cardiovascular, or renal dysfunctions or from gastrointestinal disease.*[2]

Grapiprant is a methylbenzenesulfonamide, and it is not known if dogs with a history of hypersensitivity to sulfonamide drugs will react to grapiprant.[1]

Adverse Effects

Adverse effects in dogs include vomiting; diarrhea or soft stools; decreased appetite; lethargy; mucoid, watery, or bloody stool; increases in alkaline phosphatase and alanine aminotransferase; and decreases in serum albumin and total protein.[1] A preapproval efficacy study of 131 dogs given labeled doses also reported increased calcium concentrations.[14] These adverse effects were deemed mild and transient by the authors.[20] In collies homozygous for the multidrug sensitivity gene (*MDR1* gene, also known as *ABCB1* gene), 25% experienced vomiting, and one dog had slight decreases in serum albumin and total protein; CNS effects were not observed.[15]

In a study, grapiprant was tolerated in cats receiving up to 15 mg/kg/day orally for 28 days; no adverse effects or histopathologic changes were detected.[16]

Reproductive/Nursing Safety

Safe use has not been established in breeding, pregnant, or lactating dogs.[1]

Because safety has not been established in animals, this drug should only be used when the maternal benefits outweigh the potential risks to offspring.

Overdose/Acute Toxicity

In a preapproval safety study, grapiprant was administered at 50 mg/kg PO every 24 hours in a methylcellulose suspension to healthy 9-month-old beagles.[20] Because the bioavailability of the suspension is significantly less than that of the tablet's and feeding status can impact bioavailability, this dose equates to ≈5 to 10 times that of the labeled dose.[21] All (n = 12) dogs survived the study. GI signs included vomiting and loose, watery, bloody, and/or mucoid stools were observed in 67% to 100% of dogs. Mildly decreased albumin, total protein, and/or calcium concentrations were observed in some treated dogs.[20] Overdoses should be treated with supportive care based on presenting clinical signs.[2]

For patients that have experienced or are suspected to have experienced an overdose, consultation with a 24-hour poison center specializing in providing veterinary-specific information is recommended. For general information related to overdose and toxin exposures, as well as contact information for poison control centers, refer to ***Appendix***.

Drug Interactions

NOTE: The manufacturer warns that concomitant use of grapiprant with other anti-inflammatory drugs (eg, COX-inhibiting NSAIDs, corticosteroids) should be avoided, as concurrent use has not been studied. An appropriate washout period has been suggested when switching from corticosteroids or COX-inhibiting NSAIDs to grapiprant.[1]

Grapiprant does not inhibit metabolism pathways mediated by cytochrome P450 1A2 isozyme (CYP1A2), CYP2C9, CYP2C19, CYP2D6, or CYP3A4.[1] Grapiprant is a substrate of P-glycoprotein transport, but no clinically relevant drug interactions have been identified.

Although the following drug interactions have either been reported or are theoretical in humans or animals receiving NSAIDs, their significance in veterinary patients is unknown. Unless otherwise noted, use together is not necessarily contraindicated, but the potential risks must be weighed and additional monitoring performed when appropriate.

- **Angiotensin Converting Enzyme Inhibitors (ACEIs**; eg, **benazepril, enalapril**): NSAIDs may decrease effectiveness of ACE inhibitors by reducing renal vasodilatory prostaglandins. Interaction may apply to grapiprant.
- **Aspirin or Other NSAIDs** (eg, **carprofen, meloxicam**): Concurrent administration with grapiprant may increase the risk for toxicity (eg, GI ulceration).
- **Corticosteroids** (eg, **dexamethasone, fludrocortisone, prednis(ol)one**): Concomitant administration with grapiprant may increase the risk for GI adverse effects.
- **Highly Protein Bound Drugs** (eg, **oral anticoagulants, other anti-inflammatory agents, salicylates, sulfonamides, sulfonylurea antidiabetic agents**): Because grapiprant is highly bound to plasma proteins (95%), it could theoretically displace other highly bound drugs causing a transient increase in serum concentrations of each drug. These interactions are unlikely to be of clinical concern because increased free drug concentrations will equilibrate through increased clearance. Monitor for adverse effects of each drug when using this combination.
- **Loop Diuretics** (eg, **furosemide**): Concurrent use of NSAIDs and loop diuretics may increase the risk for renal damage secondary to decreased renal blood flow. Interaction may apply to grapiprant.

Laboratory Considerations

- Some dogs receiving grapiprant may develop **decreased serum albumin** and **total protein** concentrations. Laboratory test relevance, if any, is not known.
- Increased **alkaline phosphatase** and **alanine aminotransferase** have been reported.

Dosages

DOGS:

Control of pain and inflammation associated with osteoarthritis (labeled dosage; FDA-approved): 2 mg/kg (0.9 mg/lb.) PO every 24 hours.[1] Tablets are scored (except the 100 mg size), and the dose should be calculated in half-tablet increments (see table below). The lowest effective dose should be used for the shortest duration consistent with individual response. Dogs weighing less than 3.6 kg (8 lb) cannot be accurately dosed. The "Information for Dog Owners" sheet should be provided with the prescription. According to the UK label, the drug should be administered on an empty stomach at least 1 hour before the next meal, and if no clinical improvement is noted after 14 days, grapiprant should be discontinued and other treatment options explored.[2]

Patient weight in kg (lb)	Number of 20 mg tablets	Number of 60 mg tablets	Number of 100 mg tablets
3.6 - 6.8 (8 – 15)	0.5		
6.9 - 13.6 (15.1 – 30)	1		
13.7 - 20.4 (30.1 – 45)		0.5	
20.5 – 34 (45.1 – 75)		1	
34.1 – 68 (75.1 – 150)			1
Greater than 68(150)	Use a combination of half and full tablets to achieve the appropriate dose		

Control of pain and inflammation associated with osteoarthritis in dogs homozygous or heterozygous for the multidrug sensitivity gene (*MDR1* gene, also known as *ABCB1* gene) (extra-label): 1 mg/kg (50% dose reduction) PO once daily (homozygous) or 1.5 mg/kg (25% dose reduction) PO once daily (heterozygous) has been suggested.[15] The dose could then be increased as tolerated to the full 2 mg/kg/day dose. Alternatively, for dogs with more severe pain and inflammation, the full dose could be administered with close monitoring for adverse effects and recheck of plasma protein concentration 4 to 6 weeks after the first administration.

Monitoring

- Clinical efficacy
- Appetite; vomiting
- Stool characteristics (eg, presence of blood or mucus; changes in consistency)
- Although no mention is made on the product label, a baseline CBC, serum chemistry profile and urinalysis should be considered before prescribing. For dogs receiving this drug long term, monitoring these laboratory values at regular intervals may be helpful to detect development of problems. Frequency of monitoring is not known at this time. More frequent monitoring should be considered in patients with underlying problems or in patients with clinical signs; less frequent monitoring can be considered in healthy patients with no apparent adverse effects.

Client Information

- This medicine may be given with or without food. Try giving the medicine with food if vomiting occurs.
- Side effects can include vomiting, diarrhea, and decreased appetite. Contact your veterinarian if your animal's appetite decreases or if your animal vomits or develops abnormal stool (eg, watery, presence of blood or mucus).
- Store this medicine well out of reach of animals and children.

Chemistry/Synonyms

Grapiprant is a methylbenzenesulfonamide in the piprant class of NSAIDs. It has a molecular weight of 491.6 daltons. It appears as a white to off-white crystalline powder and is poorly soluble in water. The commercially available flavored tablets contain desiccated pork liver as a flavoring agent.

Grapiprant may also be known as AT-001, grapiprantrum, UNII-J9F5ZPH7NB, MR10A7, CJ-023423, RQ-00000007, 415903-37-6, or *Galliprant*®.

Storage/Stability

Store tablets at or below 30°C (86°F) and out of reach of other animals and children.

Compatibility/Compounding Considerations

No specific information noted

Dosage Forms/Regulatory Status

VETERINARY-LABELED PRODUCTS:

Grapiprant Flavored Tablets (scored): 20 mg, 60 mg, and 100 mg; *Galliprant*®; (Rx). FDA-approved for use in dogs (NADA #141-455). The 20 mg and 60 mg tablets are scored; the 100 mg tablets are not scored and the manufacturer states that these tablets should not be broken in half, as the amount of drug in each half of the tablet cannot be guaranteed.[1]

HUMAN-LABELED PRODUCTS: NONE

References

For the complete list of references, see **wiley.com/go/budde/plumb**

Griseofulvin

(gri-see-oh-***ful***-vin) *Fulvicin*®, *Gris-PEG*®

Antifungal Agent

Prescriber Highlights

- ► Fungistatic antibiotic used to treat dermatophytosis; it has no effect on other fungi. Azole antifungal agents and terbinafine have largely supplanted griseofulvin use for treating small animal species.
- ► Contraindications include known hypersensitivity, hepatocellular failure, and pregnancy (known teratogen in cats).
- ► Use with caution in cats with FIV and in kittens, as they may be overly sensitive to the drug.
- ► Adverse effects include anorexia, vomiting, diarrhea, anemia, neutropenia, leukopenia, thrombocytopenia, depression, ataxia, hepatotoxicity, or dermatitis/photosensitivity.
- ► Only new hair and nail growth are resistant to dermatophytes after treating.
- ► Dosing is different for microsize and ultramicrosize forms.

Uses/Indications

Griseofulvin has been FDA-approved for use in dogs and cats to treat dermatophytic fungal infections of the skin, hair, and claws. In horses, griseofulvin is FDA-approved to treat dermatophyte infections caused by *Trichophyton equinum* and *Microsporum gypseum.*

The oral tablets (FDA-approved for dogs and cats) are no longer marketed in the United States, but human dosage forms are available. Due to the availability of more effective and less toxic drugs such as azole antifungals, griseofulvin is infrequently recommended today for use in small animal species, especially cats.[1]

In horses, griseofulvin has also been shown to be effective for dermatophyte isolates *T mentagrophytes* and *T verrucosum.*[2]

Griseofulvin has also been used to treat dermatophytic fungal infections in laboratory animals and ruminants.

Pharmacology/Actions

Griseofulvin acts on susceptible fungi by disrupting the structure of the cell's mitotic spindle, arresting the metaphase of cell division, and inhibiting nucleic acid synthesis. Griseofulvin has activity against species of *Trichophyton, Microsporum,* and *Epidermophyton.* Because griseofulvin is deposited only in new hair and nail growth, response time depends on rate of keratinization and time required to desquamate infected structures. It has no antibacterial activity and is not clinically useful against other pathogenic fungi, including *Malassezia* spp.

Pharmacokinetics

Griseofulvin is a weak water-soluble drug that is poorly absorbed in the GI tract.[3] The microsize formulations have variable absorption (25% to 70%); dietary fat will enhance absorption. The ultramicrosize form of the drug has the best absorption and is absorbed 1.5 times as well as the microsize form for a given patient.

Griseofulvin is concentrated in skin, hair, nails, fat, skeletal muscle, and the liver, and can be found in the stratum corneum within 4 hours of dosing.

Griseofulvin is metabolized by the liver via oxidative demethylation and glucuronidation to 6-desmethylgriseofulvin, which is not active.[3] In humans, the half-life is 9 to 24 hours. A serum half-life of 47 minutes has been reported for dogs. Less than 1% of the drug is excreted unchanged in the urine.

In humans, topically applied griseofulvin does not penetrate keratinized tissue.

Contraindications/Precautions/Warnings

Griseofulvin is contraindicated in patients that are hypersensitive to it or with hepatocellular failure.[3] The drug is considered contraindicated during pregnancy.

Because kittens may be overly sensitive to the adverse effects associated with griseofulvin, they should be monitored carefully if treatment is instituted. Cats should be tested for FIV before using griseofulvin because of the possible neutropenic or panleukopenic effects of the drug.

In humans, use of griseofulvin is not considered justified for minor infections that will respond to topical treatment.

Do not confuse griseofulvin microsize and ultramicrosize formulations, as dosages are not interchangeable.

Adverse Effects

Griseofulvin can cause anorexia, vomiting, diarrhea, anemia, neutropenia, leukopenia, thrombocytopenia, depression, ataxia, hepatotoxicity, dermatitis, photosensitivity, and toxic epidermal necrolysis. The drug has a disagreeable taste so dosing may be difficult. With the exception of GI clinical signs, adverse effects are uncommon in dogs at usual doses. Cats, particularly kittens, may be more susceptible to adverse effects (eg, bone marrow depression) than other species. Cats with FIV are at increased risk for neutropenia and bone marrow suppression associated with griseofulvin administration.[4] This effect could be due to this species' propensity to more slowly form glucuronide conjugates and thus metabolize the drug at a slower rate than either dogs or humans.

Reproductive/Nursing Safety

Griseofulvin is contraindicated during pregnancy.[3] For sexually intact females, verify pregnancy status before administration. It is a known teratogen in dogs,[3,5] cats, mice, and rats and likely horses as well. Dosages of 35 mg/kg given to cats during the first trimester caused cleft palate and other skeletal and brain malformations in kittens. Administration of griseofulvin to pregnant cats for treatment of dermatomycosis has resulted in anophthalmos or microphthalmos in their kittens.[6] Griseofulvin may also inhibit spermatogenesis and decrease sperm counts; however, in one study, therapeutic dosage of griseofulvin had no deleterious effect on the semen quality in dogs.[7] Griseofulvin has been used in mares during the later stages of pregnancy without noted ill effect.[8]

Safety during lactation has not been established.

Because safety has not been established in animals, this drug should only be used when the maternal benefits outweigh the potential risks to offspring.

Overdose/Acute Toxicity

No specifics regarding griseofulvin overdosage or acute toxicity were located. It is suggested that significant overdoses be handled with GI decontamination, charcoal, and cathartic administration unless contraindicated.

Cats that received griseofulvin 110 – 145 mg/kg for 11 weeks did not have any changes in liver enzymes, bone marrow aspirates, or ACTH stimulation tests.[9]

Cats with FIV received 80 – 147 mg/kg developed fever, anorexia, diarrhea, and depression with increased risk for neutropenia.[4]

Horses have received 100 mg/kg PO for 20 days without apparent ill effect.

For patients that have experienced or are suspected to have experienced an overdose, consultation with a 24-hour poison control center specializing in providing veterinary-specific information is recommended. For general information related to overdose and toxin exposures, as well as contact information for poison control centers, refer to ***Appendix.***

Drug Interactions

The following drug interactions either have been reported or are theoretical in humans or animals receiving griseofulvin and may be of significance in veterinary patients. Unless otherwise noted, use together is not necessarily contraindicated, but weigh the potential risks and perform additional monitoring when appropriate.

- ALCOHOL (ETHANOL): Griseofulvin may potentiate the effects of alcohol.
- ASPIRIN: Griseofulvin may decrease salicylate concentrations.
- CYCLOSPORINE: Griseofulvin may decrease cyclosporine concentrations.
- ESTROGENS (eg, **estriol**): Griseofulvin may decrease estrogen concentrations.
- PHENOBARBITAL: Decreased griseofulvin blood concentrations
- PROGESTINS (eg, **medroxyprogesterone, megestrol**): Griseofulvin may decrease progestin concentrations.
- THEOPHYLLINE, AMINOPHYLLINE: In some patients, griseofulvin may decrease theophylline half-life and concentrations.
- WARFARIN: Anticoagulant activity may be reduced.

Dosages

DOGS:

Dermatophytosis (label dosage; FDA-approved):

a) Daily dosing given as a single dose or divided[10]:
- For animals weighing up to 2.7 kg (6 lb): 62.5 mg
- For animals weighing 2.7 to 8.2 kg (6 to 18 lb): 125 mg
- For animals weighing 8.2 to 16.4 kg (18 to 36 lb): 250 mg
- For animals weighing 16.4 kg to 21.8 kg (36 to 48 lb): 375 mg
- For animals weighing 21.8 kg to 34.1 kg (48 to 75 lb): 500 mg

b) Weekly dose[10]: Dose is administered at intervals of 7 to 10 days; amount to be given at each interval is calculated as 10 mg/lb of body weight times the number of days between treatments. Adjust dose according to response. Administer additional dose after animal is free of infection.

Dermatophytosis (extra-label): Griseofulvin is not frequently recommended today and dosage forms suitable for dogs may be difficult to obtain. Dosage recommendations have usually been: *Microsize forms*: 50 mg/kg PO once daily or divided and given twice daily. *Ultramicrosize forms*: 5 – 10 mg/kg PO once daily. Both forms should be given with or immediately following a fatty meal. Treat for at least 2 weeks following clinical cure and 2 negative skin cultures taken at least 1 week apart. Treatment may be required for many months.

HORSES:

Dermatophytosis caused by *T equinum* and *M gypseum* (label dosage; FDA-approved): Using griseofulvin (microsize) powder sachets: adults, 1 packet (2.5 g griseofulvin) daily; yearlings, ½ to 1 packet (1.25 – 2.5 g) daily; foals, ½ packet (1.25 g) daily.[11] Treat for at least 10 days and continue until all affected areas are confirmed negative.

Dermatophytosis (extra-label): Using the microsize (not ultramicrosize) products: 5 mg/kg PO once daily. Smaller doses (1.25 g) should be used for foals or ponies. If using ultramicrosize (human) formulations, the dose should be reduced by 50%.[8]

RABBITS/RODENTS/SMALL MAMMALS:

Dermatophytosis in small exotic mammals (extra-label): 25 – 100 mg/kg/day PO divided into 2 to 3 doses for 2 to 4 weeks[12]

Monitoring

- Clinical efficacy; dermatophyte culture
- Adverse effects
- Baseline and periodic (every 1 to 3 weeks) CBC during therapy
- Baseline and periodic chemistry panel as indicated during therapy

Client Information

- Follow your veterinarian's instructions for how to clean up the animal's environment to minimize the risk for reinfection.
- This medicine should be given with fatty foods or oils (eg, cheese, cream, butter, corn oil).
- Contact your veterinarian if your animal has a lack of appetite (eating less or not at all), vomiting, and/or diarrhea.
- Pregnant women should not handle this medicine, as it has caused birth defects in animals and may do so in humans.
- Your veterinarian will need to monitor your animal while it is taking this medicine. Do not miss these important follow-up visits.

Chemistry/Synonyms

A fungistatic antibiotic produced by species of penicillium (primarily *P griseofulvum*), griseofulvin occurs as an odorless or nearly odorless, bitter tasting, white to creamy white powder. It is very slightly soluble in water and sparingly soluble in alcohol.

Two forms of the drug are available commercially. Microsize griseofulvin contains particles with a predominant size of 4 micrometers in diameter, while the ultramicrosize form particle size averages less than 1 micron in diameter.

Griseofulvin may also be known as curling factor, griseofulvina, and griseofulvinum; many trade names are available.

Storage/Stability

Griseofulvin products should be stored at 20° to 25°C (68°F-77°F).[3] Griseofulvin suspension should be stored in tight, light-resistant containers. Microsize tablets and capsules should be stored in tight containers; the ultramicrosize tablets should be stored in well-closed containers.

Compatibility/Compounding Considerations

If obtaining compounded dosage forms, understand which form (microsize or ultramicrosize) of griseofulvin is being supplied and adjust dosage accordingly.

Dosage Forms/Regulatory Status

VETERINARY-LABELED PRODUCTS:

Griseofulvin (Microsize) Powder: 2.5 g griseofulvin in 15 g sachets; generic; (Rx). FDA-approved for use in horses not intended for food. Marketing status is unknown.

The FDA's Green Book still lists several other veterinary FDA-approved griseofulvin products, but it does not appear they are presently being marketed.

HUMAN-LABELED PRODUCTS:

Griseofulvin Microsize Tablets: 250 mg and 500 mg; generic; (Rx)

Griseofulvin Ultramicrosize Tablets: 125 mg and 250 mg; generic; (Rx)

Griseofulvin Microsize Oral Suspension: 125 mg/5 mL (25 mg/mL) in 120 mL bottles; generic; (Rx)

References

For the complete list of references, see **wiley.com/go/budde/plumb**

Guaifenesin, Intravenous

(gwye-***fen***-e-sin) *GG, Guailaxin®*

Parenteral Muscle Relaxant

Prescriber Highlights

- ▶ Used as adjunctive therapy for anesthesia in horses, camelids, and small ruminants
- ▶ No contraindications noted. Must be used with caution in induction protocols.
- ▶ Adverse effects include a mild hypotensive effect and thrombophlebitis; concentration-dependent hemolysis is possible.
- ▶ Availability is an issue; must be obtained from a compounding pharmacy.

Uses/Indications

In veterinary medicine, guaifenesin is used to induce muscle relaxation and as an adjunct to anesthesia for short procedures (30 to 60 minutes) in horses, camelids, and small ruminants. There are oral products containing guaifenesin that treat respiratory conditions in horses.

Pharmacology/Actions

Although the exact mechanism of action for the muscle relaxant effect is not known, it is believed that guaifenesin acts centrally by depressing or blocking nerve impulse transmission at the internuncial neuron level of the subcortical areas of the brain, brainstem, and spinal cord. It relaxes both the laryngeal and pharyngeal muscles, thus allowing easier intubation. Guaifenesin produces muscle relaxation but has no clinically relevant intrinsic analgesic effects.

After adequate sedation, guaifenesin combined with ketamine causes an excitement-free induction and recovery from anesthesia in horses. It produces relaxation of the skeletal muscles but does not affect diaphragmatic function and has little, if any, effect on respiratory function at commonly used dosages. Possible effects on the cardiovascular system include transient mild decreases in blood pressure without changes in heart rate. GI motility may be increased, but generally no issues are seen with this effect.

Guaifenesin can potentiate the activity of preanesthetic and anesthetic agents.

Pharmacokinetics

The pharmacokinetics of guaifenesin have not been thoroughly studied in most species. After oral administration to horses, peak concentrations were reached at 15 minutes, and elimination half-life averaged 2.6 hours. In 3 horses, guaifenesin was detectable in serum longer than 48 hours after the last dose.[1] After IV administration (≈130 mg/kg in donkeys and 210 mg/kg in horses), the volume of distribution was 678 mL/kg and 794 mL/kg, and the clearance was 546 mL/kg/hour and 313 mL/kg/hour in donkeys and horses, respectively.[2]

When guaifenesin is administered alone to horses IV, recumbency usually occurs within 2 minutes, and light (not surgical level) restraint persists for about 6 minutes. Muscle relaxation reportedly persists for 10 to 20 minutes after a single dose.

Guaifenesin is conjugated in the liver and excreted into the urine. A gender difference in the elimination half-life of guaifenesin in ponies has been demonstrated, with a half-life of ≈85 minutes in male ponies and a half-life of about 60 minutes in female ponies.[3] Guaifenesin reportedly crosses the placenta, but adverse effects in newborns of mothers who received guaifenesin have not been described.

Contraindications/Precautions/Warnings

When guaifenesin is used as part of an induction protocol in horses, appropriate numbers of personnel and equipment (eg, induction swing-gate) should be available. Muscle relaxation and ataxia can occur dramatically, and timing of the administration of a drug like ketamine is critical. These concerns have led some clinicians to NOT use guaifenesin as part of induction for field anesthesia.[4] Although guaifenesin has some sedative effects, it must be used intraoperatively with other suitable anesthetic and analgesic agents.

Because guaifenesin can cause significant tissue damage if given perivascularly, it should always be administered through an IV catheter.

Adverse Effects

At usual doses, adverse effects with guaifenesin are transient and generally minor. A mild decrease in blood pressure can be seen. Thrombophlebitis has been reported after IV injection; perivascular administration may cause tissue reaction. Hemolysis may occur in solutions containing greater than a 5% concentration of guaifenesin, although some sources state this is insignificant at even a 15% concentration.[4,5] Hemolysis may be more of an issue in ruminants than in horses.[6]

Reproductive/Nursing Safety

Guaifenesin crosses the placenta, with neonatal plasma guaifenesin concentration ≈30% that of maternal plasma.[7] It is not known whether guaifenesin is excreted in milk.

Because safety has not been established in animals, this drug should only be used when the maternal benefits outweigh the potential risks to offspring.

Overdose/Acute Toxicity

The margin of safety with guaifenesin is reportedly 3 times the usual dose. Clinical signs associated with toxic levels of parenteral guaifenesin include opisthotonus, apneustic breathing, nystagmus, hypotension, and contradictory muscle rigidity. If any of these signs occur, it is recommended to stop the infusion and give supportive care as needed.

No specific antidote is available. It is suggested that treatment be supportive until the drug is cleared to sub-toxic levels.

Drug Interactions

Drug interactions with parenteral guaifenesin are not well studied. The following drug interactions either have been reported or are theoretical in animals receiving guaifenesin and may be of significance in veterinary patients. Unless otherwise noted, use together is not necessarily contraindicated, but weigh the potential risks and perform additional monitoring when appropriate.

- **PHYSOSTIGMINE**: The veterinary label states that physostigmine is contraindicated in horses receiving guaifenesin but does not elucidate on the actual interaction. It may be logical to assume that other anticholinesterase agents (eg, **neostigmine**, **pyridostigmine**, **edrophonium**) may also be contraindicated; however, anecdotal reports suggest that concurrent use appears to be tolerated.

Dosages

NOTE: Various protocols combining guaifenesin with other drugs are too numerous to list in this reference. The following listings are examples for horses, small ruminants, and new world camelids. Additional protocols for other drug combinations and species can be found in other anesthesia references. Referring to these references or consulting with a veterinary anesthesiologist is highly recommended when considering using this agent as an anesthetic adjunct.

HORSES:

Part of induction protocols (extra-label): **NOTE**: Use with caution; this protocol is not recommended for field anesthesia without an IV catheter in place. The following is one example using xylazine as the alpha-2 agonist in the protocols. There are numerous others that use different alpha-2 agonists (eg, detomidine, romifidine), butorphanol, and/or acepromazine. See equine anesthesia references for additional information.[8]

a) For normal healthy animals: Premedicate with xylazine 0.44 – 0.66 mg/kg IV (or 200 – 300 mg/450 kg [992 lb] horse [NOT mg/kg]). Wait for sedation and muscle relaxation to occur (≈5 minutes), then rapidly infuse guaifenesin 5% solution (50 mg/mL) IV using pressurization until marked sedation and muscle relaxation is achieved, generally a total dose of 30 – 50 mg/kg. Administer ketamine 2.2 mg/kg IV (or 1000 mg/450 kg [992 lb] horse [NOT mg/kg]) at a point that allows for slow onset to occur without the animal becoming excessively weak and collapsing from the effects of guaifenesin. Recumbency generally occurs ≈45 to 60 seconds following ketamine administration. The slow administration of guaifenesin (described below) can also be used in normal healthy animals in place of a supplemental dose of xylazine when the level of initial sedation is inadequate.

b) For compromised animals: Premedicate with xylazine 0.22 – 0.44 mg/kg IV (or 100 – 200 mg/450 kg [992 lb] horse [NOT mg/kg]), depending on the status and demeanor of the animal, to minimize cardiovascular effects in compromised animals. Slow IV administration of guaifenesin 5% solution can be used initially to gradually achieve the desired level of sedation. It is still important to allow adequate time for centralization of cardiac output to progress sufficiently prior to initiating the rapid phase of guaifenesin administration. Guaifenesin has a slow onset of action when used to augment the level of pre-induction sedation, and it is important to control drug administration rate to avoid creating an overly weak and ataxic patient while waiting for centralization to progress sufficiently. Guaifenesin is then rapidly infused using pressurization until marked sedation and muscle relaxation is achieved, generally a total dose of 30 – 50 mg/kg IV. To induce anesthesia, decrease the ketamine dose as the degree of compromise increases: ketamine 1.34 – 1.55 mg/kg (or 600 – 700 mg/450 kg [992 lb] horse [NOT mg/kg]) IV for extremely compromised animals at a point that allows slow onset to occur without the animal becoming excessively weak and collapsing from the growing effects of guaifenesin. Experience may be required to get the timing right. Recumbency takes longer (up to a couple minutes) when the ketamine dose is reduced in compromised patients.[9]

Total IV anesthesia:

a) **Guaifenesin/ketamine/xylazine (GKX) | "triple-drip"** (extra-label): Guaifenesin 50 mg/mL, ketamine 1 – 2 mg/mL (2 mg/mL concentration used for more painful or noxious procedures), and xylazine 0.5 mg/mL. To prepare this mixture, add ketamine 10 mL (100 mg/mL) for 1 mg/mL (add 20 mL ketamine for 2 mg/mL) and xylazine 5 mL (100 mg/mL) to a 1000 mL bag of guaifenesin 5%. Most clinicians prefer to induce with xylazine/ketamine or xylazine/midazolam/ketamine and then use GKX for maintenance. Use GKX 1.5 – 2.2 mL/kg/hour IV CRI, depending on the procedure, animal response, and ketamine concentration.

b) **Guaifenesin/ketamine/detomidine (GKD)**: In ponies sedated with detomidine 0.02 mg/kg IM and induced with ketamine 2 mg/kg IV: Guaifenesin 100 mg/mL, ketamine 4 mg/mL, and detomidine 0.04 mg/mL at 0.8 mL/kg/hour IV CRI for the first hour and 0.6 mL/kg/hour IV CRI for the final 30 minutes.[10,11] To prepare this mixture, add ketamine 40 mL (100 mg/mL) and detomidine 4 mL (10 mg/mL) to a 1000 mL bag of guaifenesin 10%.

Muscle relaxant as part of a general anesthesia after induction (extra-label): **NOTE**: When used as part of total IV anesthetic protocols, guaifenesin is used in triple-drip ("GKX") mixtures that also contain an alpha-agonist (eg, xylazine, detomidine, romifidine) and ketamine. These mixtures can be particularly useful for field use with short procedures (up to 60 minutes). Additional information can be found in anesthesia references.[8,12] The following is an example of a dosage recommendation:

Augmentation of muscle relaxation in horses that are too light or too tense after alpha-2 agonist + ketamine ± benzodiazepine induction, and do not respond sufficiently to additional increments of alpha-2 agonist or ketamine: Guaifenesin 5% dosed at ≈25 – 50 mg/kg (250 – 500 mL) IV

SHEEP, GOATS:

General anesthesia (extra-label):

a) **Using "GK" (or "double-drip") for induction and maintenance**: Add ketamine 1000 mg to 1000 mL of guaifenesin 5% (50 mg/mL). Induce with this combination 1.7 – 2.2 mL/kg IV. Maintain with ≈ 2.6 mL/kg/hour IV CRI (adjust rate as needed).[13]

b) **Using "GKX" for induction and maintenance**:

1. Mix 1000 mL of guaifenesin 5% (50 mg/mL) with ketamine 1000 mg and xylazine 0 – 100 mg. Induce with 2.2 mL/kg IV (calculate dose carefully to avoid an overdose). Maintain with ≈2.2 mL/kg/hour IV CRI (adjust rate as needed).[14]
2. To a 500 mL bag of guaifenesin 5%, add xylazine 50 mg and ketamine 500 mg. Administer at a rate of 2 – 4 mL/kg IV. It is given rapidly until animal is recumbent and then slowed to maintain desired anesthesia plane.[15]
3. To a 500 mL bag of guaifenesin 5%, add xylazine 50 mg and ketamine 500 mg. Induce at a rate of 1 – 1.5 mL/kg IV; in small ruminants, administer via syringe to minimize risk for overdose. Maintain anesthesia at 2.6 mL/kg/hour IV CRI.[13]

CAMELIDS:

General anesthesia using "GKX" for induction/maintenance (extra-label): Mix 1000 mL of guaifenesin 5% (50 mg/mL) with ketamine 1000 mg ± xylazine 200 mg. Induce with 2.2 mL/kg IV (calculate dose carefully to avoid an overdose). Maintain with ≈2.2 mL/kg/hour IV CRI (adjust rate as needed).[14]

Monitoring

Monitoring patients during general anesthesia is vital, and guaifenesin-based injectable anesthesia can affect multiple systems. Monitoring depth of anesthesia, muscle relaxation, respiratory rates/oxygenation, heart rate, and blood pressure are all warranted.

Refer to specific anesthesia references for more information.

Client Information

Injectable guaifenesin must be given by your veterinarian.

Chemistry/Synonyms

Formerly known as glyceryl guaiacolate, guaifenesin occurs as a white to slightly gray, crystalline powder that may have a characteristic odor. It is nonhygroscopic and melts between 78°C to 82°C (172.4°F-179.6°F). One gram is soluble in 50 mL water at room temperature, but it is much more soluble in hot water; it is soluble in alcohol, propylene glycol, and glycerin.

Guaifenesin may also be known as GG, glyceryl guaiacolate, glycerylguayacolum, guaiacol glycerol ether, guaiacyl glyceryl ether, guaifenesina, guaifenesinum, guaiphenesin, and guajacolum glycerolatum; many trade names are available.

Storage/Stability

Guaifenesin is stable in light and heat (less than melting point). Parenteral guaifenesin prepared by compounding pharmacies should be stored as specified on the product label.

When guaifenesin is dissolved into aqueous solutions, it may slightly precipitate out of solution when the temperature is less than 22°C (72°F). Slight warming and agitation generally resolubilizes the drug. A microwave oven has been suggested for heating and dissolving the drug. It is recommended that the solution be prepared freshly before use, but a 10% solution (in sterile water) may apparently be stored safely at room temperature for up to one week with only slight precipitation occurring.

Compatibility/Compounding Considerations

Guaifenesin is physically **compatible** with sterile water or D_5W. It is also reportedly **compatible** with ketamine, pentobarbital, thiamylal, thiopental, and xylazine.

"Triple drip" and similar mixtures should be prepared at the time of administration and promptly discarded after discontinuation.

As there are no commercially available formulations being marketed in the US, compounding an injection product from a USP grade powder may be the only way to obtain a parenteral dosage form. Compounding pharmacies with appropriate facilities, equipment, and procedures may be able to prepare a sterile product. The commercially available products contained per mL: Guaifenesin 50 mg, dextrose (anhydrous) 50 mg, propylene glycol 20 mg, dimethyl acetamide 50 mg, edetate disodium 0.75 mg, water for injection *qs*. For stability, it is highly recommended that the compounding pharmacy use this or another validated formula.

Dosage Forms/Regulatory Status

VETERINARY-LABELED PRODUCTS:

Guaifenesin Injection: 50 mg/mL in 500 mL and 1000 mL. There are several guaifenesin 5% injection products still listed as FDA-approved in the FDA Green Book, but there are no products presently being marketed. Compounding pharmacies may be available to provide (see ***Compatibility/Compounding Considerations*** above).

Guaifenesin is available in oral formulations labeled for use as an expectorant in horses.

The Association of Racing Commissioners International (ARCI) has designated guaifenesin as a class 4 substance. Use of this drug may not be allowed in certain animal competitions. Check rules and regulations before entering in a competition while this medication is being administered. Contact local racing authorities for further guidance. See ***Appendix*** for more information.

HUMAN-LABELED PRODUCTS:

No parenteral preparations are FDA-approved. There are many OTC oral expectorant/cough preparations on the market. Many of these contain additional active ingredients that are not appropriate for use in dogs or cats.

References

For the complete list of references, see **wiley.com/go/budde/plumb**

Hemoglobin Glutamer-200 (Bovine)

(hee-moe-***gloe***-bin ***gloo***-ta-mer) *Oxyglobin®*

Semi-Synthetic Hemoglobin Replacer; Colloid

Prescriber Highlights

- ▶ Polymerized hemoglobin product of bovine origin that is FDA-approved for the treatment of anemia in dogs
- ▶ Typing and crossmatching not required prior to use
- ▶ Contraindications include advanced cardiac disease and renal impairment with oliguria or anuria.
- ▶ Many potential adverse effects, including discoloration of mucous membranes and skin, arrhythmias, bradycardia, vomiting and diarrhea, dyspnea, pulmonary edema, pleural effusion, and peripheral edema
- ▶ Carefully monitor for volume overload
- ▶ Many drug-laboratory effects
- ▶ Not available in the United States

Uses/Indications

Hemoglobin glutamer-200 (HG-200) is FDA-approved for the treatment of anemia in dogs, regardless of the cause of anemia (eg, hemolysis, blood loss, or ineffective erythropoiesis). HG-200 increases systemic oxygen content and improves clinical signs associated with anemia for at least 24 hours.[1] It is likely more valuable in dogs with regenerative anemias than those with nonregenerative anemias. It has also been used as a colloid for treating hypotension in dogs and cats.

Its primary benefit is for the patient that is anemic and difficult to transfuse due to unavailability of blood, or when no suitable donors are identified on crossmatch.[2]

Dogs with gastric dilatation-volvulus resuscitated with HG-200 reached resuscitation end points more rapidly and required significantly smaller volumes of crystalloids and colloids than those resuscitated with hetastarch 6%.[3]

Pharmacology/Actions

Hemoglobin glutamer-200 (HG-200) is a plasma volume expander with colloidal properties similar to dextran 70 and hetastarch. It is a bovine hemoglobin-based oxygen-carrying fluid that increases arterial oxygen content. The bovine hemoglobin in the product is polymerized into larger molecules to increase safety, efficacy, and intravascular persistence; it is shipped in a deoxygenated state and becomes oxygenated once circulated through the lungs. HG-200 does not contain red blood cells (RBCs) and is stroma free. HG-200 releases oxygen to tissue in a mechanism similar to endogenous hemoglobin, thereby increasing plasma and total hemoglobin concentrations and systemic oxygen carrying capacity. Because of its small size in comparison to normal RBCs, it may better deliver oxygen to cells supplied by severely constricted arteries. HG-200 shifts the oxygen dissociation curve to the right, so oxygen is transferred to tissues more easily.

Pharmacokinetics

In dogs receiving hemoglobin glutamer-200 (HG-200) at a dose of 15 mL/kg, peak hemoglobin concentrations increased by ≈2.5 g/dL; at a dose of 30 mL/kg, concentrations increased by ≈4 g/dL. Duration of effect continues for at least 24 hours. The half-life in dogs at labeled dosages is ≈18 to 43 hours, and HG-200 can be detected in plasma for 5 to 7 days after a single dose.

As with endogenous hemoglobin, HG-200 is metabolized and eliminated by the reticuloendothelial system. Small amounts of destabilized hemoglobin (less than 5%) may be excreted through the kidneys, causing a red discoloration of the urine.

Contraindications/Precautions/Warnings

Hemoglobin glutamer-200 (HG-200) is labeled as a single-dose treatment and should not be used in patients that have previously been treated with it. Administration of any foreign protein has the potential to cause immunologic reactions. Although low concentrations of IgG antibodies have been detected after administration of multiple doses, only rare, anecdotal reports of anaphylactic reactions have been reported. Plasma expanders such as HG-200 are generally contraindicated in dogs with advanced cardiac disease (ie, congestive heart failure) or renal impairment with oliguria or anuria. Safety and efficacy have not been evaluated in dogs with disseminated intravascular coagulation, thrombocytopenia with active bleeding, hemoglobinemia, hemoglobinuria, or autoagglutination.

HG-200 is a potent colloid and can cause vasoconstriction. In experimentally induced hypovolemic shock in dogs, HG-200 caused severe vasoconstriction and decreased cardiac output.[4] Because of its vasoconstrictive properties, the amount of HG-200 required for fluid resuscitation in trauma patients is ≈⅓ that of hetastarch.[5] Exercise caution to prevent volume-overloading patients when giving this drug, as hydrostatic pressures may be increased and cause pulmonary overload (eg, pleural effusion, pulmonary edema). Cats are particularly vulnerable to fluid overload, and slower infusion rates are recommended.

If an acute hypersensitivity reaction occurs, immediately discontinue the infusion and administer appropriate treatment. If a delayed hypersensitivity reaction occurs, immunosuppressant therapy is recommended.

Oxidative damage to HG-200 occurs after removal from the foil wrapper, leading to formation of methemoglobin. Toxic concentrations of methemoglobin can occur.[6] Therefore, HG-200 should be discarded 24 hours after removing from the foil wrapper.[7]

Adverse Effects

Adverse effects that occur in more than 4% of dogs treated with HG-200 include discoloration of mucous membranes, sclera (yellow, red, brown), urine (orange, red, brown), and skin (yellow); increased central venous pressure; ventricular arrhythmias (eg, AV block, tachycardia, premature ventricular contractions); ecchymoses/petechiae; bradycardia; vomiting; diarrhea; anorexia; tachypnea; dyspnea; pulmonary edema; harsh lung sounds/crackles; pleural effusion; fever; peripheral edema; hemoglobinuria; dehydration; and death.

Coughing, disseminated intravascular coagulopathy, melena, nasal discharge/crusts (red), peritoneal effusion, respiratory arrest, and weight loss (5% to 7% body weight) have been reported in ≈4% of dogs treated with HG-200.

Adverse effects occurring in less than 2% of dogs treated with HG-200 include abdominal discomfort on palpation, acidosis, cardiac arrest, cardiovascular volume overload (by echocardiography), collapse, cystitis, dark stool, discolored soft stool (red-brown) and tongue (purple), focal hyperemic areas on gums, forelimb cellulitis/lameness, hematemesis or hemoptysis (unable to differentiate), hypernatremia, hypotension, hypoxemia, lack of neurologic responses, left forebrain signs, nystagmus, pancreatitis, pendulous abdomen, polyuria, pulmonary thromboembolism, ptosis, reddened pinnae with papules/head shaking, reduction in heart rate, worsening thrombocytopenia, and venous thrombosis.

Increases in AST and ALT (not associated with histopathologic changes in the liver), increase in serum total protein, and hemoglobinuria may also be seen.

Following infusion, small amounts of unstabilized hemoglobin (less than 5%) may be excreted through the kidneys, resulting in transient red discoloration of the urine. This urine discoloration should not be interpreted as being caused by intravascular hemolysis and has no effect on renal function.

Cats are particularly susceptible to pulmonary edema and pleural effusion; rapid infusion and larger doses increase this risk. A retrospective study using low doses in 44 cats with hypotension reported respiratory changes (8), vomiting (2), and pigmented serum (30).[8] Most adverse effects were not considered to be clinically significant.

Reproductive/Nursing Safety

Safe use in breeding dogs and pregnant or lactating bitches has not been determined.

Because safety has not been established in animals, this drug should only be used when the maternal benefits outweigh the potential risks to offspring.

Overdose/Acute Toxicity

In healthy dogs given 2 doses of hemoglobin glutamer-200 (HG-200) up to 90 mL/kg (3 times the recommended dose) 3 days apart, clinical signs included yellow-orange discoloration of skin, ear canals, pinnae, mucous membranes, and sclera, red-dark-green-black discoloration of feces, brown-black discoloration of urine, red spotting of skin and/or lips (less common), decreased appetite and thirst, vomiting, diarrhea, and decreased skin elasticity. The frequency and/or intensity of these signs increased with repeated and increasing doses. All dogs survived.

Overdoses or rapid infusions (ie, more than 10 mL/kg/hour) may result in circulatory overload.

For patients that have experienced or are suspected to have experienced an overdose, consultation with a 24-hour poison consultation center specializing in providing veterinary-specific information is recommended. For general information related to overdose and toxin exposures, as well as contact information for poison control centers, refer to ***Appendix.***

Drug Interactions

No specific drug interactions have been noted. See ***Compatibility/Compounding Considerations***.

Laboratory Considerations

- Hemoglobin-based oxygen carriers (HBOCs) can impact several laboratory tests.
- The presence of hemoglobin glutamer-200 (HG-200) in serum may cause artifactual increases or decreases in the results of **serum chemistry tests**, depending on the type of analyzer and reagents used. May cause false increases in AST or creatinine. May cause false decreases in LDH. May cause unacceptable interference with GGT, albumin, or bilirubin
- There is reportedly no interference with directly measured hemoglobin tests, but due to the dilutional effects of HG-200, PCV and RBC count are not accurate measures of the degree of anemia for 24 hours following administration. **Prothrombin time** (PT) and **activated partial thromboplastin time** (aPTT) determined using methods that are mechanical, magnetic, and light scattering are accurate, but optical methods are not reliable while HG-200 is present.
- **Urine dipstick** measurements (eg, pH, glucose, ketones, protein) are inaccurate while urine is grossly discolored.

Dosages

DOGS:

Anemia, regardless of the cause (hemolysis, blood loss, or ineffective erythropoiesis) (label dosage; FDA-approved): One-time dose of 10 – 30 mL/kg IV at a rate of up to 10 mL/kg/hour.[9] Administer using aseptic technique via a dedicated standard IV infusion set and catheter through a central or peripheral vein. May be warmed to 37°C (98.6°F) prior to administration. Blood transfusions are not contraindicated in dogs that receive HG-200, nor is HG-200 contraindicated in dogs that have previously received a blood transfusion. Typing or crossmatching is not required prior to use.

Providing oxygen-carrying capacity until immunosuppressive drugs take effect in dogs with IMHA after a blood transfusion reaction (extra-label): 7 – 10 mL/kg IV every 12 hours can maintain hemoglobin concentrations above 3.5 g/dL; higher doses of 30 mL/kg may provide oxygen-carrying support for 48 to 72 hours.[10]

Trauma/resuscitation (extra-label):

a) Resuscitation of trauma patients in shock, with or without hemorrhage: Empirically, 3 – 5 mL/kg IV with concurrent crystalloid at ½ to 2 times maintenance fluid rate.[11] See ***Compatibility/Compounding Considerations***.
b) Provide oxygen-carrying capacity in the trauma patient: 10 – 15 mL/kg IV given over several hours. Care must be taken not to cause fluid overload.[12]
c) As a vasopressor once there is adequate intravascular volume in trauma patients: 3 – 5 mL/kg IV[5]

CATS:

Hypotension (extra-label): From a retrospective study of 44 cases, the average IV bolus dose and administration time was 3.1 mL/kg and 25 minutes.[8] Mean increase of systemic arterial pressure more than 20 mm Hg after the bolus. Most patients also received CRIs after bolus with a mean volume administered of 0.8 ± 0.5 mL/kg/hour. Mean SAP during CRI was 92 ± 18 mm Hg.

Provide oxygen-carrying capacity in the trauma patient (extra-label): 5 – 10 mL/kg IV given over several hours. Care must be taken not to cause fluid overload.[12] Rates of 0.5 to 2 mL/kg/hour have been recommended.[6]

Monitoring

- Hemoglobin
- Clinical signs of adequate tissue oxygenation
- Respiratory rate and character; thoracic auscultation
- Physical examination to check for adverse effects[6]
- Attitude and demeanor[6]
- Central venous pressure

Client Information

- This medicine is used to treat anemia. It is expensive and has many potential side effects. Your veterinarian will go over the cost and risks versus benefits for this agent before use.
- This medicine must be administered by your veterinarian.

Chemistry/Synonyms

Hemoglobin glutamer-200 ((HG-200; bovine) is a sterile, clear, dark purple solution containing 13 g/dL purified, polymerized hemoglobin of bovine origin in a modified lactated Ringer's solution. It has an osmolality of 300 mOsm/kg and a pH of 7.8. Less than 5% of the hemoglobin are unstabilized tetramers, and ≈50% have a molecular weight between 65 and 130 kD, with no more than 10% having a molecular weight more than 500 kD. The product contains less than the detectable concentration of 3.5 µg/mL free-glutaraldehyde and 0.05 EU/mL endotoxin.

Hemoglobin glutamer-200 (bovine) may also be known as HBOC-301, HB-200, HG-200, or *Oxyglobin®*.

Storage/Stability

The product remains stable at room temperature or refrigerated (2°C-30°C [36°F-86°F]) for up to 3 years; expiration date is printed on the bag. Do not freeze. It must remain in its overwrap during storage. Use the product within 24 hours of removing the overwrap. The foil overwrap serves as an oxygen barrier, protecting the hemoglobin from conversion to methemoglobin.

Compatibility/Compounding Considerations

Hemoglobin glutamer-200 should not be mixed with other solutions or medications in the bag. Other IV solutions and medications should be administered via a separate site and line. Do not combine the contents of more than one bag.

Dosage Forms/Regulatory Status

VETERINARY-LABELED PRODUCTS:

Hemoglobin Glutamer-200 (bovine) in 60 mL and 125 mL ready-to-use infusion bags; *Oxyglobin*®; (Rx). FDA-approved for use in dogs. Not currently available in the United States; may be available in Europe

The Association of Racing Commissioners International (ARCI) has designated this drug as a class 2 substance. Use of this drug may not be allowed in certain animal competitions, and it is prohibited to be at racing premises. Check rules and regulations before entering in a competition while this medication is being administered. Contact local racing authorities for further guidance. See ***Appendix*** for more information.

HUMAN-LABELED PRODUCTS: NONE

References

For the complete list of references, see **wiley.com/go/budde/plumb**

Heparin

Unfractionated Heparin (UFH)

(***hep***-ah-rin)

Anticoagulant

Prescriber Highlights

- Parenteral anticoagulant used for thromboprophylaxis in dogs, cats, and horses as adjunctive treatment for thromboembolic disease
- Contraindications include known hypersensitivity, severe thrombocytopenia, or uncontrollable bleeding.
- The most common adverse effect is bleeding.
- Protamine may be used to reverse effects.
- Monitoring is necessary; however, specific guidelines are not yet clear for veterinary patients. Anti-Xa monitoring has been recommended during heparin treatment in dogs.

Uses/Indications

Heparin is primarily used for thromboprophylaxis in the adjunctive treatment for immune-mediated hemolytic anemia (IMHA), pulmonary thromboembolism, and other thromboembolic diseases. Prophylactic heparin can reduce the incidence of developing macrovascular thromboembolism in high-risk patients.

Thromboprophylaxis is recommended for all dogs with IMHA, except those with severe thrombocytopenia (ie, less than 30,000 platelets/μL).[1] Although heparin, aspirin, and clopidogrel have been used for thromboprophylaxis in dogs with IMHA, lack of validated therapeutic endpoints and lack of controlled studies make it difficult to determine the efficacy of one drug over another or effect on survival.[2]

Heparin use in patients with disseminated intravascular coagulation (DIC) is controversial. Heparin may be indicated in patients to prevent the formation of microthrombi during the hypercoagulable phase, in patients with evidence of arterial or venous thromboembolic disease, or in patients that do not have signs of hemorrhage but are judged to be at risk for thromboembolism due to severe systemic inflammation.[3]

In horses, heparin has been used in the treatment of jugular vein thrombophlebitis, DIC, and to prevent development of laminitis; however, there are no controlled, prospective studies that demonstrate efficacy for these indications. Heparin has also been administered systemically or as part of a lavage solution administered intraperitoneally to prevent intra-abdominal adhesion formation after surgery, but its efficacy is uncertain.[4-8] Heparin may prevent equine herpesvirus myeloencephalopathy during an equine herpesvirus-1 outbreak.[9]

The use of heparin to prevent clotting in peripheral IV catheters in human medicine has largely been replaced by flushing fluid lines with 0.9% sodium chloride. A study in dogs concluded that over 48 hours, peripheral catheter maintenance with 0.9% saline was equally effective as flushing with heparinized saline.[10] Heparin lock solution, which contains high concentrations of heparin, has been used as a dwell solution to prevent clot formation in long-term central venous catheters such as those used for hemodialysis. When these solutions are used, the catheter should be clearly labeled, and the dwell solution aspirated and discarded prior to catheter use. See ***Laboratory Considerations***.

Pharmacology/Actions

Heparin binds to antithrombin (AT), causing a conformational change that accelerates the binding of AT to several activated clotting factors, particularly factor Xa and factor IIa (thrombin). This binding inactivates their procoagulant activity in the clotting cascade.[11] Heparin also inhibits the activation of factor XIII (fibrin stabilizing factor), preventing the formation of stable fibrin clots. Heparin does not have fibrinolytic activity and will not lyse existing clots.

Heparin causes increased release of lipoprotein lipase, thereby increasing the clearance of circulating lipids and boosting plasma concentrations of free fatty acids.

Pharmacokinetics

Anticoagulant activity begins immediately after direct IV bolus injection but may take up to 1 hour after SC injection. When heparin is given by IV CRI, an initial bolus can be administered to rapidly achieve full anticoagulant activity. Even though heparin is not systemically absorbed when given orally, an anticoagulant effect is possible after oral administration.[12] Preliminary work with inhaled heparin in dogs has been unsuccessful.[13]

In healthy dogs, bioavailability after SC injection is ≈50%. Heparin is extensively protein bound, primarily to fibrinogen, low-density lipoproteins, and globulins. It does not appreciably cross the placenta or enter milk.

The metabolism of heparin is not completely understood. The drug is apparently partially metabolized by the liver and also inactivated by the reticuloendothelial system. Peak anti-factor Xa activity and anticoagulant effects are seen in healthy dogs 2 to 3 hours after a single dose of 300 units/kg SC.[14] In these dogs, plasma heparin concentrations were in the therapeutic range between 1 and 6 hours after administration.[15] In healthy cats, a dose of 250 units/kg SC achieved a target anti-Xa activity 4 hours following injection, and had sustained anti-Xa activity at trough time points.[16,17]

Contraindications/Precautions/Warnings

Heparin is contraindicated in patients that are hypersensitive to it and in patients with severe thrombocytopenia or coagulopathy.[3,11] Because heparin is derived from bovine or porcine tissues, hypersensitivity reactions may be possible.

Individual anticoagulant response to a given dose of heparin may vary based on antithrombin concentrations and severity of underlying condition being treated; monitoring is recommended. Use with caution in patients at an increased risk for hemorrhage.

Do not administer heparin IM, as it may cause hematoma formation. Hematomas, pain, and irritation may occur after SC dosing.

In humans, resistance to heparin is possible in patients with fever, thrombosis, thrombophlebitis, cancer, antithrombin deficiency, and in postsurgical patients.[11]

Medication errors can be fatal. Medication errors have occurred due to use of incorrect heparin sodium strength when preparing patient doses. Confirm correct product prior to preparation and administration. The word "unit" should be written out on all doses to avoid errors, as a "U"may easily be mistaken for a zero.

Adverse Effects

Bleeding is the most common adverse effect associated with heparin and can result in anemia and thrombocytopenia. Patients with hypertension, GI ulcers, hepatic disease, thrombocytopenia, and older patients may be at an increased risk for hemorrhage.[11] Pain at injection site is also possible.

In humans, additional adverse effects reported include elevated AST and ALT; cutaneous necrosis; rebound hyperlipidemia; hyperkalemia; delayed, transient alopecia; suppressed aldosterone synthesis; injection site reactions; pain on injection; and priapism.[11,18] Osteoporosis has been reported after long-term, high-dose administration, and vasospastic reactions several days after initiation of therapy have rarely been reported.

In humans, heparin-induced thrombocytopenia (HIT) is a serious antibody-mediated reaction that can occur with heparin treatment.[11] HIT has not yet been reported in animals.

Reproductive/Nursing Safety

Although heparin does not cross the placenta and is generally the anticoagulant of choice during pregnancy, its safe use in pregnancy has not been firmly established.[11] Heparin is unlikely to be excreted into milk because of its large molecular weight and negative charge[11,19]; however, preservative-free heparin is recommended for use during lactation, as the benzyl alcohol preservative may enter the milk.[11]

Because safety has not been established in animals, this drug should only be used when the maternal benefits outweigh the potential risks to offspring.

Overdose/Acute Toxicity

Bleeding is the primary effect of a heparin overdose. Hematuria, tarry stools, petechiae, and bruising may be seen before frank bleeding occurs. Protamine can reverse the effects of heparin; see ***Protamine*** for more information.

For patients that have experienced or are suspected to have experienced an overdose, consultation with a 24-hour poison consultation center specializing in providing veterinary-specific information is recommended. For general information related to overdose and toxin exposures, as well as contact information for poison control centers, refer to ***Appendix.***

Drug Interactions

The following drug interactions have either been reported or are theoretically possible in humans or animals receiving heparin and may be of significance in veterinary patients. Unless otherwise noted, use together is not necessarily contraindicated, but weigh the potential risks and perform additional monitoring when appropriate.

- **ASPIRIN**: May increase the risk for hemorrhage
- **CLOPIDOGREL**: May increase the risk for hemorrhage
- **DEXTRAN OR HETASTARCH**: May increase the risk for hemorrhage
- **NONSTEROIDAL ANTI-INFLAMMATORY DRUGS**: May increase the risk for hemorrhage
- **SELECTIVE SEROTONIN REUPTAKE INHIBITORS (SSRIs; eg, fluoxetine, sertraline)**: May increase the risk for hemorrhage
- **WARFARIN**: May increase the risk for hemorrhage

The following drugs may partially counteract heparin's anticoagulant effects:

- **ANTIHISTAMINES**
- **NITROGLYCERIN** (IV)
- **PROPYLENE GLYCOL**
- **DIGOXIN**
- **TETRACYCLINES**

Laboratory Considerations

- The presence of heparin in samples obtained from indwelling catheters can alter the results of coagulation tests such as prothrombin time (PT) and activated partial thromboplastin time (aPTT). To avoid sample contamination in patients receiving a continuous infusion of heparin, a dedicated IV catheter should be used or a large presample should be removed prior to sampling.
- When heparin is used as an anticoagulant in vitro (eg, in **blood collection containers**), white cell counts should be performed within 2 hours of collection. Do not use heparinized blood for platelet counts, erythrocyte sedimentation rates, erythrocyte fragmentation tests, or for any tests involving complement or isoagglutinins. Errors in blood gas determinations for CO_2 pressure, bicarbonate concentration, or base excess may occur if heparin encompasses 10% or more of the blood sample.
- Heparin can interfere with the results of the **BSP** (sulfobromophthalein, bromosulfophthalein) test by changing the color intensity of the dye and shifting the absorption peak from 580 nm to 595 nm.
- Heparin can cause falsely elevated values of serum **thyroxine** if using competitive protein binding methods of determination. Radioimmunoassay (RIA) and protein bound iodine methods are apparently unaffected by heparin.
- Heparin may cause increases in **AST** and **ALT**. It is unclear if this is due to interference with the laboratory test or to hepatotoxicity.

Dosages

DOGS:

NOTE: In critically ill animals, an IV CRI is more likely to result in consistent anticoagulation effects and prolongation of aPTT.

Thromboprophylaxis in patients with immune-mediated hemolytic anemia (IMHA) (extra-label):

a) 150 – 300 units/kg SC every 6 hours.[1,2] Individual responses are highly variable; in one study, dosages ranging from 150 – 566 units/kg SC every 6 hours were required to reach target anti-factor Xa activity.[20]

b) 100 units/kg IV bolus, then 900 units/kg/day IV CRI[1]

c) Loading dose of 100 units/kg IV followed by 20 – 50 units per kg/hour IV CRI.[21] In critically ill animals, an IV CRI is more likely to result in consistent anticoagulation and prolongation of aPTT. Small dose changes can result in large changes in aPTT; starting at a low dose and slowly titrating in increments of 5 units/kg/hour is recommended. When discontinuing, taper the dose gradually (eg, decrease by 50 units/kg/day over 3 to 4 days) to help prevent rebound hypercoagulability.[22]

Thromboprophylaxis (extra-label):

a) 100 units/kg IV bolus, then 480 – 900 units/kg/day IV CRI[23]

b) 150 – 300 units/kg SC every 6 hours[23]

Arterial thromboembolic disease (extra-label): 200 – 300 units/kg IV initially followed by 200 – 250 units/kg SC every 6 to 8 hours[24]

Disseminated intravascular coagulopathy (extra-label): 75 – 100 units/kg SC every 8 hours; however, use is controversial and optimal dosing regimens are unknown.[25]

CATS:

Thromboprophylaxis for feline arterial thromboembolism (FATE) (extra-label): No outcome-based studies have evaluated any heparin dose for FATE, and dosage recommendations are highly variable. **NOTE**: Only the SC route has been studied in cats.

a) 50 – 100 units/kg (low-dose) or 200 – 300 units/kg (high-dose)

SC every 6 to 8 hours.[26,27] There is wide individual variation in heparin pharmacokinetics with FATE, and some cats may require doses up to 475 units/kg.[28]

b) 250 – 375 units/kg IV initially followed by 150 – 250 units/kg SC every 6 to 8 hours[24]

Thromboprophylaxis (extra-label): 250 units/kg SC every 6 hours[23]

HORSES:

Thromboprophylaxis (extra-label): 40 – 100 units/kg SC or IV every 6 hours have been noted[29,30] but are not well established and recommendations range widely.

Prevention of abdominal adhesions (extra-label): 30,000 – 50,000 units of heparin in 10 L of lavage fluid (warm LRS) administered intraperitoneally via a 32 French fenestrated trocar catheter placed in the right ventral abdomen at the time of surgery. Lavage should be performed at 12, 18, 36, and 48 hours post-surgery and allowed to drain through a Heimlich valve. Remove drain after final lavage to prevent occlusion.[4]

Monitoring

NOTE: Appropriate monitoring in veterinary patients receiving heparin is controversial; no outcome-based guidelines have been accepted. Anti-factor Xa activity, activated clotting time (ACT), prothrombin time (PT), and activated partial thromboplastin times (aPTT) may all be used to monitor therapy.

- Anti-factor Xa activity: Target of 0.35 – 0.7 units/mL in dogs.[23] Although there is insufficient evidence for a strong target recommendation in cats, 0.35 – 0.7 units/mL may be reasonable until more evidence is available.[31] The suggested thromboprophylactic range for horses is 0.1 – 0.2 units/mL. Anti-Xa activity may be more reliable than aPTT and may improve survival during heparin treatment for IMHA.[20,32] It may be particularly useful if bleeding occurs or for patients with renal dysfunction.
- Activated partial thromboplastin time (aPTT): Monitoring parameter most often recommended for dogs; less reliable monitoring parameter for cats but may still be recommended.[33] Target is prolongation of aPTT by 1.5 to 2 times baseline value (1.3 – 1.5 sometimes used); however, aPTT may not correlate with anti-Xa activity in dogs, especially those with inflammatory diseases.
- Thromboelastography (TEG): Modified thromboelastography has been significantly correlated to both anti-activated factor X activity and aPTT and could potentially be used to monitor dogs treated with heparin; however, this test is often not readily available.[34]
- Baseline and periodic CBC with platelet counts as needed based on clinical condition
- Baseline and periodic physical examinations to check for signs of bleeding (eg, hematuria, hematochezia, melena, epistaxis, bleeding from the gums)

Client Information

- This medicine must be injected under the skin (subcutaneously). Be sure you understand how to correctly give the injection. Several injections may be required each day.
- Watch for signs of bleeding, such as blood in the urine or stool or bleeding from the nose or gums. If you see any signs of bleeding, contact your veterinarian immediately.
- If your animal is listless (lacking energy or interest in things), appears to be having trouble breathing, has trouble walking, or loses the use of its rear legs, contact your veterinarian immediately.

Chemistry/Synonyms

Heparin is an anionic, heterogeneous sulfated glycosaminoglycan molecule with an average molecular weight of 12,000 daltons that is found naturally in mast cells. It is available commercially as the sodium salt and is obtained from either porcine intestinal mucosa or bovine lung tissue (sodium salt only). Heparin sodium occurs as a white, amorphous, hygroscopic powder having a faint odor. It is soluble in water and practically insoluble in alcohol; the commercial injections have a pH of 5 to 7.5. Heparin potency is expressed in terms of USP heparin units, and values are obtained by comparing against a standard reference from the USP. The USP requires that potencies be not less than 180 units/mg on a dried basis for heparin derived from lung tissue, and 140 units/mg when derived from all other tissue sources.

Heparin sodium may also be known as heparinum natricum, sodium heparin, and soluble heparin; many trade names are available.

Storage/Stability

Heparin solutions should be stored at room temperature (15°C-30°C [59°F-86°F]) and not frozen. Avoid excessive exposure to heat.

Compatibility/Compounding Considerations

Compatibility is dependent on factors such as pH, concentration, temperature, and diluent used; consult specialized references or a hospital pharmacist for more specific information.

Heparin sodium is reportedly physically **compatible** with the following IV solutions and drugs: amino acids 4.25%-dextrose 25%, dextrose-Ringer's combinations, dextrose-lactated Ringer's solutions, fat emulsion 10%, Ringer's injection, *Normosol®-R*, aminophylline, amphotericin B lipid complex, ascorbic acid injection, bleomycin sulfate, buprenorphine HCl, butorphanol tartrate, calcium gluconate, cefazolin sodium, chloramphenicol sodium succinate, clindamycin phosphate, dimenhydrinate, dexamethasone sodium phosphate, dexmedetomidine, dopamine HCl, erythromycin gluceptate, famotidine, fentanyl citrate, isoproterenol HCl, lidocaine HCl, magnesium sulfate, metoclopramide, metronidazole with sodium succinate, norepinephrine bitartrate, potassium chloride, prednisolone sodium succinate, propofol, ranitidine HCl, sodium bicarbonate, verapamil HCl, and vitamin B-complex with or without vitamin C.

Heparin **compatibility information conflicts** or is dependent on diluent or concentration factors with the following drugs or solutions: dextrose-saline combinations, dextrose in water, lactated Ringer's injection, saline solutions, ampicillin sodium, amphotericin B (conventional), atracurium besylate, diltiazem HCl, diphenhydramine HCl, dobutamine HCl, hydrocortisone sodium succinate, methylprednisolone sodium succinate, midazolam HCl, oxytetracycline HCl, penicillin G sodium/potassium, pantoprazole sodium, and tetracycline HCl.

Heparin sodium is reported physically **incompatible** when mixed with the following solutions or drugs: sodium lactate 1/6 M, amikacin sulfate, chlorpromazine HCl, ciprofloxacin, codeine phosphate, cytarabine, daunorubicin HCl, diazepam, dolasetron HCl, doxorubicin HCl, doxycycline hyclate, erythromycin lactobionate, gentamicin sulfate, hyaluronidase, hydroxyzine HCl, hydromorphone HCl, ketamine HCl, levorphanol bitartrate, meperidine HCl, methadone HCl, mitoxantrone, morphine sulfate, pentazocine lactate, phenytoin sodium, polymyxin B sulfate, and vancomycin HCl.

Dosage Forms/Regulatory Status

VETERINARY-LABELED PRODUCTS: NONE

HUMAN-LABELED PRODUCTS:

NOTE: To minimize risk for medication errors, product labels for heparin sodium list the strength of the entire container followed closely by the strength per mL (eg, heparin 10,000 USP units/10 mL, 1000 USP units/mL). Always read product labels carefully.

Heparin Sodium Injection: 1000 units/mL, 5000 units/mL, 10,000 units/mL, and 20,000 units/mL in 0.5 mL, 1 mL, 2 mL, 4 mL, 5 mL, 10 mL, and 30 mL vials; generic; (Rx)

Heparin Unit-Dose Sodium Injection: 1000 units/dose, 2500 units/dose, 5000 units/dose, 10,000 units/dose and 20,000 units/dose in 0.5 mL and 1 mL single-dose vials; *Tubex*®, *Carpuject*®; generic; (Rx)

Heparin Sodium and 0.9% Sodium Chloride Injection: 250 units in 250 mL; 1000 units in 500 mL; 2000 units, 4000 units, 5000 units, 10,000 units and 30,000 units in 1000 mL; generic; (Rx)

Heparin Sodium and 0.45% Sodium Chloride Injection: 2500 units in 250 mL; 4000 units in 1000 mL; 12,500 in 250 mL and 25,000 units in 250 mL and 500 mL, respectively; 25,000 units in 250 mL and 500 mL; generic; (Rx)

Heparin Sodium and 5% Dextrose Injection: 2500 units in 250 mL; 20,000 units in 500 mL; 12,500 units in 250 mL and 25,000 units in 500 mL; 10,000 units in 100 mL and 25,000 units in 250 mL; generic; (Rx)

Heparin Sodium Lock Flush (IV use) Injection: 10 units/mL in 5 mL prefilled syringes; 100 units/mL in 3 mL and 5 mL prefilled syringes; generic; (Rx)

References

For the complete list of references, see **wiley.com/go/budde/plumb**

Hyaluronate
Hyaluronan

(hy-al-yoo-***ron***-nate) *Hyalovet*®, *Hyvisc*®, *Legend*®

Mucopolysaccharide

Prescriber Highlights

- ▶ Parenteral, high-viscosity mucopolysaccharide used for synovitis
- ▶ No contraindications listed on the product label
- ▶ Adverse effects vary by route of administration
- ▶ Different products have different dosages; check label before using.

Uses/Indications

Hyaluronate is useful in the treatment of synovitis not associated with severe degenerative joint disease. It may be helpful for treatment of secondary synovitis in conditions where full-thickness cartilage loss exists.

The choice of a high molecular weight product (molecular weight more than $1x10^6$) versus a low molecular weight one is controversial. One author states ...*low molecular weight products (which tend to be less expensive) can be equally efficacious in ameliorating signs of joint disease. When synovial adhesions and pannus are to be avoided (as in most surgeries for carpal and fetlock fracture fragment removal), higher molecular weight preparations are recommended because they inhibit proliferation of synovial fibroblasts.*[1] However, there are no controlled studies directly comparing the various products for treating joint disease and product choice is primarily a result of a clinician's personal preference.

There is considerable interest in oral hyaluronate administration for treatment of equine joint disease. One blinded, controlled study found that the use of an oral gel nutraceutical significantly reduced synovial effusion in tarsocrural joints postarthroscopic surgery for osteochondritis dissecans (OCD).[2]

In dogs, one study looked at using an oral supplement (*Hyaloral*®) containing hyaluronic acid, hydrolyzed collagen, glucosamine, chondroitin sulfate, and gamma oryzanol to prevent elbow dysplasia. The number of dogs (Labradors) developing elbow dysplasia was significantly lower in the treated group compared to the control, but the study had several limitations, including lack of blinding, radiographic evaluation (not CT or MRI) only, and using a fixed dose combination product where determining which components were responsible for the effect was not possible.[3]

Pharmacology/Actions

Hyaluronate is found naturally in the connective tissue of both humans and animals and is chemically identical regardless of species. Highest concentrations are found in the synovial fluid, vitreous of the eye, and umbilical cord. Surfaces of articular cartilage are covered with a thin layer of a protein-hyaluronate complex; hyaluronate is also found in synovial fluid and the cartilage matrix. The net effects in joints include a cushioning effect, reduction of protein and cellular influx into the joint, and lubrication. Hyaluronate has a direct anti-inflammatory effect in joints by scavenging free radicals and suppressing prostaglandins.

Pharmacokinetics

In the equine joint, the half-life of hyaluronate has been reported to be 96 hours.[4]

Contraindications/Precautions/Warnings

No contraindications to the use of hyaluronate are noted on the product labels. Hyaluronate should not be used as a substitute for adequate diagnosis; radiographic examinations should be performed to rule out severe fractures. Do not perform intra-articular injections through skin that has recently been fired or blistered, or that has excessive scurf and counterirritants on it. Administer hyaluronate only by routes listed on the product label.

Adverse Effects

The following adverse effects are based on voluntary post-approval reporting. IV administration: occasional depression, lethargy, and fever. Intra-articular administration: transient lameness, joint effusion, joint or injection-site swelling, joint pain, and synovial sepsis.[5] Effects generally subside within 24 to 48 hours; some animals may require up to 96 hours for resolution. No treatments for these effects are recommended. When used in combination with other drugs, incidence of flares may be higher. No systemic adverse effects have been noted.

Reproductive/Nursing Safety

Although hyaluronate is unlikely to cause problems, safe use in breeding animals has not been established and most manufacturers caution against its use in these animals.

Because safety has not been established in animals, this drug should only be used when the maternal benefits outweigh the potential risks to offspring.

Overdose/Acute Toxicity

Acute toxicology studies performed in horses have demonstrated no systemic toxicity associated with overdoses.

Drug Interactions

- None were noted.

Laboratory Considerations

- None were noted.

Dosages

HORSES:

Joint dysfunction of the carpus or fetlock due to noninfectious synovitis associated with osteoarthritis (label dosage; FDA-approved):

NOTE: Because of the differences in the commercially available products, see each individual product's label for specific dosing information.

- *Hyvisc*®: 22 mg/joint (NOT mg/kg) IA in small or medium joints (eg, carpal, fetlock), 44 mg/joint IA in larger joints (eg, hock); treatment may be repeated weekly for a total of 3 treatments

- *Hyalovet®*: 20 mg/joint (NOT mg/kg) IA in small or medium joints (eg, carpal, fetlock); more than 1 joint may be treated at the same time. Treatment may be repeated after 1 or more weeks, but do not exceed 2 injections each week for a total of 4 weeks.
- *Legend®*:
  a) 20 mg IA in the carpus or fetlock. Treatment may be repeated weekly for a total of 3 treatments.
  b) 40 mg IV slowly into the jugular vein. Treatment may be repeated weekly for a total of 3 treatments.
- *NexHA®*: 40 mg IV slowly into the jugular vein at weekly intervals for a total of 3 treatments

Reducing joint effusion postarthroscopic surgery for osteochondritis dissecans (OCD) (extra-label): 100 mg/horse (NOT mg/kg) PO (as an oral gel [*Conquer®*]) once daily for 30 days[2]

DOGS:

Adjunctive treatment of synovitis not associated with damaged articular cartilage (extra-label): Using a high molecular weight compound: 5 – 15 mg/joint (NOT mg/kg) IA once,[6-8] or 5 mg/joint (NOT mg/kg) IA weekly for 3 to 5 weeks[8]

Monitoring

- Efficacy
- Adverse effects

Client Information

- Hyaluronate should only be administered by your veterinarian.

Chemistry/Synonyms

Hyaluronate sodium (HS) is the sodium salt of hyaluronic acid, which is a naturally occurring high-viscosity mucopolysaccharide. Many of the commercially available hyaluronic acid products are derived from the combs of roosters.

Hyaluronate sodium may also be known as HA, sodium hyaluronate, hyaluronan, hyaluronic acid, and natrii hyaluronas; many trade names are available.

Storage/Stability

Store at room temperature or refrigerate depending on the product label. Do not freeze. Protect from light. Discard unused portion.

Compatibility/Compounding Considerations

Do not mix with other drugs unless the product's label states otherwise.

Dosage Forms/Regulatory Status

VETERINARY-LABELED PRODUCTS:

Hyaluronate Sodium: 10 mg/mL or 11 mg/mL in 2 mL vials or prefilled syringes; *Hyalovet®*, *Hyvisc®*; (Rx) FDA-approved for IA use in horses not intended for food.

Hyaluronate Sodium: 10 mg/mL in 2 mL or 4 mL single-dose vials and 20 mL multi-dose vials; *Legend®*; (Rx). FDA approved for IV or intra-articular administration for use in horses not intended for food.

Hyaluronate Sodium: 10 mg/mL in 4 mL single-dose vials; *NexHA®*; (Rx). FDA-approved for IV use only for use in horses not intended for food.

There may also be other hyaluronate products marketed as topical solutions, semen extenders, and oral supplements. These products are not necessarily approved by the FDA. Products that are approved as devices (ie, semen extenders, wound management products) should not be used in place of FDA-approved drug products.

HUMAN-LABELED PRODUCTS: NONE

References

For the complete list of references, see **wiley.com/go/budde/plumb**

Hydralazine

(hye-***dral***-a-zeen) *Apresoline®*
Vasodilator

Prescriber Highlights

- ► Vasodilator drug used primarily for systemic hypertension or adjunctive treatment of congestive heart failure
- ► Contraindications include known hypersensitivity, hypovolemia, or pre-existing hypotension.
- ► Use caution in patients with severe renal disease, intracranial bleeding, or pre-existing autoimmune diseases.
- ► Adverse effects include hypotension, reflex tachycardia, sodium/water retention, or GI distress (eg, vomiting, diarrhea).

Uses/Indications

The primary uses of hydralazine in veterinary medicine have been as an afterload reducer in patients with congestive heart failure (CHF) or aortic valve disease. By reducing peripheral vascular resistance, hydralazine promotes forward left ventricular stroke volume and reduces the mitral regurgitant fraction. Hydralazine is not particularly useful in treating heart failure when myocardial disease is present. Additionally, it may be useful in dogs and cats with large septal defects or severe aortic regurgitation. When used to treat systemic hypertension, hydralazine may be used in combination with other drugs (eg, beta-blockers) to offset hydralazine's tendency to cause reflex tachycardia and fluid retention.

Pharmacology/Actions

Hydralazine is a direct systemic arterial vasodilator, which acts upon vascular smooth muscle and reduces peripheral resistance and blood pressure (BP). Hydralazine is a semicarbazide-sensitive amine oxidase (SSAO) inhibitor. It is believed that hydralazine alters cellular calcium metabolism in smooth muscle, thereby interfering with calcium movements and preventing the initiation and maintenance of the contractile state. Hydralazine has more effect on arterioles than on veins.

In patients with congestive heart failure (CHF), hydralazine significantly increases cardiac output and decreases systemic vascular resistance. Cardiac rate may be slightly increased or unchanged, while BP, pulmonary venous pressure, and right atrial pressure may be decreased or unchanged.

When hydralazine is used to treat primary or secondary systemic hypertension, increased heart rate, cardiac output, and stroke volume can be noted. Hydralazine may activate the renin-angiotensin system, and in humans, the drug has been documented to increase sodium and water retention if not given with diuretics. Sodium and water retention has not been documented in veterinary medicine, but careful monitoring is recommended.

Parenteral hydralazine administration can cause respiratory stimulation.

Pharmacokinetics

Specific pharmacokinetic parameters for this drug in veterinary species are limited, but in dogs, hydralazine is rapidly absorbed after oral administration with an onset of action within 1 hour and peak effects at 3 hours.[1] Food decreases oral bioavailability in dogs by about 63%.[2] At lower doses, there is a relatively high first-pass effect, but this is apparently a saturable process as bioavailability increases with the dose.[2] Duration of action of hydralazine in dogs after oral administration is reportedly 11 to 13 hours. N-acetylation is a primary enzymatic pathway for hydralazine metabolism, and this pathway is mostly absent in dogs, leading to concerns for increased risks for toxicity.

Hydralazine is widely distributed in body tissues. In humans,

≈85% of the drug in the blood is bound to plasma proteins. Hydralazine crosses the placenta, and small amounts are excreted into the milk. Hydralazine is extensively metabolized in the liver, and ≈15% is excreted unchanged in the urine. The half-life in humans is usually 2 to 4 hours but may be as long as 8 hours.

Contraindications/Precautions/Warnings

Hydralazine is contraindicated in patients that are hypersensitive to it. The drug is listed as contraindicated in human patients with mitral valvular rheumatic disease, but it has been recommended for use in small animal patients with myxomatous mitral valve disease. It is not recommended to use the drug in patients with hypovolemia or pre-existing hypotension.

Hydralazine doses need to be titrated upwards carefully, as severe hypotension can result.

Hydralazine should be used with caution in patients with renal disease. Secondary to reduced renal blood flow, hydralazine can activate the renin-angiotensin-aldosterone system (RAAS) and exacerbate renal injury.

In humans, a syndrome resembling systemic lupus erythematosus has been documented after hydralazine use. Although this syndrome has not been documented in veterinary patients, the drug should be used with caution in patients with pre-existing autoimmune diseases.

Do not confuse hydrALAzine with hydrOXYzine.

Adverse Effects

The most prevalent adverse effects seen in small animals are hypotension, weakness, lethargy, and syncope, particularly when doses are increased too fast. Reflex tachycardia, sodium and water retention, and GI distress (eg, vomiting, diarrhea) can also occur. Reflex sinus tachycardia may be treated with beta-blockers; however, caution must be exercised due to the risk for reduced cardiac performance. Hydralazine can increase creatinine levels due to decreased renal perfusion. Other adverse effects documented in humans that could occur include systemic lupus erythematosus-like syndrome, lacrimation, conjunctivitis, blood dyscrasias, urinary retention, constipation, and hypersensitivity reactions. Peripheral neuritis may occur and appears to be due to hydralazine-induced pyridoxine deficiency.[3]

Reproductive/Nursing Safety

Hydralazine crosses the placenta and teratogenic effects (eg, cleft palate, facial and cranial bone malformations) have been noted in mice.

Hydralazine is excreted in milk. According to the American Academy of Pediatrics, hydralazine is compatible with breastfeeding, but exercise caution.[4]

Because safety has not been established in animals, this drug should only be used when the maternal benefits outweigh the potential risks to offspring.

Overdose /Acute Toxicity

Overdoses may be characterized by severe hypotension, tachycardia or other arrhythmias, skin flushing, and myocardial ischemia. Cardiovascular system support is the primary treatment modality. Evacuate gastric contents and administer activated charcoal using standard precautionary measures if the ingestion was recent and cardiovascular status has been stabilized. Treat shock using volume expanders without using pressor agents if possible. If a pressor agent is required to maintain blood pressure (BP), the use of a minimally arrhythmogenic agent (eg, phenylephrine) is recommended. Monitor BP and renal function diligently.

For patients that have experienced or are suspected of having experienced an overdose, consultation with a 24-hour poison consultation center specializing in providing veterinary-specific information is recommended. For general information related to overdose and toxin exposures, as well as contact information for poison control centers, refer to ***Appendix***.

Drug Interactions

The following drug interactions have either been reported or are theoretical in humans or animals receiving hydralazine and may be of significance in veterinary patients. Unless otherwise noted, use together is not necessarily contraindicated, but weigh the potential risks and perform additional monitoring when appropriate.

- **ACE INHIBITORS** (eg, **enalapril**): May cause an additive hypotensive effect; may be used for therapeutic advantage
- **DIAZOXIDE**: May cause profound hypotension
- **DIURETICS**: May cause an additive hypotensive effect; usually used for therapeutic advantage
- **FUROSEMIDE**: Hydralazine may increase furosemide's renal effects.
- **MONOAMINE OXIDASE INHIBITORS** (MAOIs; eg, **amitraz, linezolid, selegiline**): May cause an additive hypotensive effect
- **PROPRANOLOL**: Concurrent use may increase the risk for propranolol adverse effects, such as bradycardia, fatigue, and bronchospasm. With concomitant oral administration, hydralazine increased propranolol bioavailability, peak concentration, and AUC.[5]
- **SILDENAFIL**: May cause an additive hypotensive effect
- **SYMPATHOMIMETICS** (eg, **epinephrine**). Hydralazine may cause decreased pressor effect and additive tachycardia.

Laboratory Considerations

- None were noted.

Dosages

Because of the sodium and water retention associated with this drug, it is often used concurrently with a diuretic when used for adjunctive treatment of heart failure. When used to treat systemic hypertension, a diuretic may not be required.

DOGS:

Adjunctive therapy in the treatment of heart failure secondary to valve disease (extra-label): Published high-level evidence is not available to support any dosage, but many cardiologists believe the drug may be useful in certain circumstances, particularly in dogs with refractory CHF. The following dosage regimen is one example:

The effective dose is 0.5 – 3 mg/kg PO every 12 hours. The dose must be titrated, starting with a low dose and titrating upwards in 0.5 mg/kg increments.

In dogs that are not receiving ACE inhibitors: Establish initial baseline parameters (eg, mucous membrane color, capillary refill time, murmur intensity, cardiac size on radiographs, and severity of pulmonary edema). Starting dose is 1 mg/kg PO every 12 hours, and repeat assessments are made in 12 to 48 hours. If no response is identified, increase the dosage to 2 mg/kg every 12 hours. Repeat assessments as above and increase to 3 mg/kg PO every 12 hours if there is no response. Hydralazine can be titrated with or without blood pressure (BP) monitoring. If BP cannot be monitored, titration is performed more slowly while clinical and radiographic signs are monitored.

If BP measurement is available, dosage titration can be made more rapidly than above. Measure baseline BP. Administer the drug 1 mg/kg PO. Repeat BP measurement in 1 to 2 hours, and if BP has decreased by at least 15 mm Hg, administer every 12 hours from then on. If the response is inadequate, give another 1 mg/kg dose and repeat BP measurement in 1 to 2 hours. This may be repeated until a cumulative dose of 3 mg/kg has been given within a 12-hour period. The resulting cumulative dose becomes the dosage to be given every 12 hours.

In dogs that are receiving ACE inhibitors: Give hydralazine with caution as severe hypotension may occur if the dosage is not titrated carefully. Begin dosing at 0.5 mg/kg PO every 12 hours with BP monitoring and increase in 0.5 mg/kg increments until a response is identified to a maximum of 3 mg/kg within a 12-hour period. Consider referral to a board-certified cardiologist.

For dogs with acute, fulminant heart failure due to severe mitral regurgitation and not receiving ACE inhibitors: 2 mg/kg PO every 12 hours along with IV furosemide. Monitor BP closely.[6,7]

Systemic hypertension (extra-label): For severe, acute hypertension, hydralazine can be considered as an alternative to nitroprusside. Parenteral doses of 0.5 – 3 mg/kg IV every 12 hours or a 0.1 mg/kg IV loading dose, followed by 1.5 – 5 µg/kg/minute IV CRI, have been noted.[8] Oral dosages of 0.5 – 3 mg/kg PO every 12 hours to effect have also been reported and are commonly used. For long-term use, 0.5 – 2 mg/kg PO every 12 hours[9]

CATS:

Adjunctive therapy in the treatment of heart failure (extra-label): See the dog dosage above for heart failure but start titration at 2.5 mg/cat (NOT mg/kg), and, if necessary, increase up to 10 mg/cat (NOT mg/kg).[10]

Systemic hypertension (extra-label): For severe, acute hypertension: Parenteral doses of 1 – 2.5 mg/cat (NOT mg/kg) SC; may be repeated in 15 to 30 minutes if systolic BP has not decreased; or 0.1 mg/kg IV loading dose, followed by 1.5 – 5 µg/kg/minute IV CRI, have been noted.[9] Oral dosages of 2.5 mg/cat PO every 12 hours to effect have also been recommended. For long-term treatment of hypertension in cats, hydralazine is usually considered as a third- or fourth-step drug after amlodipine, ACE inhibitors, and possibly spironolactone. Hydralazine is usually dosed at 2.5 mg/cat (NOT mg/kg) PO every 12 to 24 hours.[9]

HORSES:

Adjunctive therapy in the treatment of heart failure (afterload reducer); (extra-label): Not commonly used in horses. One dosage recommendation is 0.5 mg/kg IV; for long-term therapy, use 0.5 – 1.5 mg/kg PO every 12 hours.[11]

Monitoring

- Baseline thoracic radiographs
- Clinical signs of CHF (eg, exercise intolerance, cough, increased resting respiratory rate and effort, mucous membrane color)
- Hydration status, urine output
- Serum electrolytes
- If possible, arterial blood pressure and venous PO_2. A mean arterial pressure (MAP) of between 60 and 80 mm Hg has been recommended when used in dogs for the short-term treatment of CHF secondary to valve disease.[12]
- Because blood dyscrasias have been noted in humans, consider monitoring CBC.

Client Information

- Give this medication with food.
- When starting your animal on this medication, your veterinarian may start with a low dose and gradually increase it over time. Be sure you are giving your animal the right dose.
- If the initial dose is too large, hydralazine may cause low blood pressure (BP) and cause your animal's condition to worsen. Loss of appetite, depression, lack of energy, or muscle weakness can indicate that BP is too low.

Chemistry/Synonyms

Hydralazine HCl, a phthalazine-derivative antihypertensive and vasodilating agent, occurs as an odorless, white to off-white crystalline powder with a melting point between 270°C and 280°C (518°F-536°F) and a pK_a of 7.3. One gram is soluble in ≈25 mL of water or 500 mL of alcohol. The commercially available injection has a pH of 3.4 to 4.

Hydralazine may also be known as apressinum, hydralazini, hydrallazine, idralazina, *or Apresoline®*.

Storage/Stability

Store the hydralazine tablets in tight, light-resistant containers at room temperature. Store the injectable product at room temperature; avoid refrigeration or freezing.

When hydralazine is mixed with most infusion solutions, a color change can occur, which does not necessarily indicate a loss in potency (if occurred over 8 to 12 hours).

Compatibility/Compounding Considerations

Compatibility is dependent on factors such as pH, concentration, temperature, and diluent used; specialized references or a hospital pharmacist should be consulted for more specific information.

Hydralazine is reported to be physically **compatible** with the following infusion solutions and drugs: dextrose-Ringer's combinations, dextrose-saline combinations, Ringer's injection, lactated Ringer's injection, sodium chloride solutions, and dobutamine HCl.

Hydralazine is reported to be physically **incompatible** when mixed with 10% dextrose or fructose and is reported to be physically **incompatible** when mixed with the following drugs: aminophylline, ampicillin sodium, chlorothiazide sodium, edetate calcium disodium, hydrocortisone sodium succinate, phenobarbital sodium, and verapamil HCl.

Dosage Forms/Regulatory Status

VETERINARY-LABELED PRODUCTS: NONE

The Association of Racing Commissioners International (ARCI) has designated this drug as a class 3 substance. Use of this drug may not be allowed in certain animal competitions. Check rules and regulations before entering a competition while this medication is being administered. Contact local racing authorities for further guidance. See ***Appendix*** for more information.

HUMAN-LABELED PRODUCTS:

Hydralazine HCl Oral Tablets: 10 mg, 25 mg, 50 mg, and 100 mg; generic; (Rx)

Hydralazine Injection: 20 mg/mL in 1 mL vials; generic; (Rx)

References

For the complete list of references, see **wiley.com/go/budde/plumb**

Hydrochlorothiazide

(hye-***droe***-klor-oh-***thye***-a-zide) *HydroDIURIL®, Microzide®*

Thiazide Diuretic

Prescriber Highlights

- ► Thiazide diuretic used for nephrogenic diabetes insipidus, hypertension, calcium oxalate urolith prevention, hypoglycemia, and as a diuretic for heart failure
- ► Contraindications include hypersensitivity, anuria, and pregnancy (relative contraindication).
- ► Use extreme caution in patients with severe renal disease, pre-existing electrolyte and water imbalances, concurrent high-dose administration of loop diuretics, impaired hepatic function, hyperuricemia, SLE, and diabetes mellitus.
- ► Adverse effects include hypokalemia, hypochloremic metabolic alkalosis, other electrolyte imbalances, hyperuricemia, and GI effects.
- ► Many possible drug interactions and laboratory test interactions

Uses/Indications

In veterinary medicine, furosemide has largely supplanted the use of thiazides as a general diuretic. Thiazides are still used for the treatment of ascites, hypermagnesemia, nephrogenic diabetes insipidus, to help prevent recurrence of calcium oxalate uroliths in dogs (potentially also in cats), and as adjunctive therapy (eg, in combination with a loop diuretic[1]) in advanced cases of congestive heart failure. Thiazides are also a diuretic choice in avian species with cavitary effusion or heart failure. In horses, hydrochlorothiazide may be used as an alternative to acetazolamide for hyperkalemic periodic paralysis (HyPP) when dietary therapy alone does not control episodes.

Pharmacology/Actions

Thiazide diuretics act by interfering with the transport of sodium ions across renal tubular epithelium, possibly by altering the metabolism of tubular cells. The principal site of action is at the cortical diluting segment of the nephron. This results in enhanced excretion of sodium, chloride, and water. Thiazides increase the excretion of potassium, magnesium, phosphate, iodide, and bromide and decrease the glomerular filtration rate (GFR). Plasma renin and resulting aldosterone levels are increased, which contribute to the hypokalemic effects of thiazides. Bicarbonate excretion is increased, but effects on urine pH are usually minimal. Thiazides initially have a hypercalciuric effect, although with continued treatment, calcium excretion is significantly decreased. Uric acid excretion is decreased by thiazides. Thiazides can cause or exacerbate hyperglycemia in diabetic patients or induce diabetes mellitus in prediabetic patients.

In nephrogenic diabetes insipidus, the administration of a thiazide diuretic can result in a paradoxical decrease in urine output. The proposed mechanism for this effect is related to sodium reduction. Thiazide diuretics reduce the reabsorption of sodium and chloride in the distal tubule of the nephron, initially resulting in sodium loss and extracellular volume contraction. Over time, this results in increased reabsorption of sodium and water in the proximal tubule, then less filtrate is presented to the distal nephron, collecting duct, and subsequently excreted as urine.[2]

The antihypertensive effects of thiazides are well known, and these agents are used extensively in human medicine for treating essential hypertension. The exact mechanism for this effect has not been established.

Pharmacokinetics

The pharmacokinetics of thiazides have apparently not been studied in domestic animals. In humans, hydrochlorothiazide is ≈65% to 75% absorbed after oral administration. The onset of diuretic activity occurs 2 hours after administration and peaks at 4 to 6 hours. The serum half-life is ≈5.6 to 14.8 hours, and the duration of activity is 6 to 12 hours. The drug is not metabolized and is excreted unchanged in the urine. Like all thiazides, the antihypertensive effects of hydrochlorothiazide may take several days to occur.

Contraindications/Precautions/Warnings

Hydrochlorothiazide is contraindicated in patients with anuria or in patients that are hypersensitive to any thiazide. Although many sources state that thiazides are contraindicated in patients that are hypersensitive to sulfonamides, clear evidence for cross-reactivity has not been established in humans or animals.[3] In humans, use is inappropriate during pregnancy in women who are otherwise healthy and have only mild edema.

Do not use hydrochlorothiazide in dogs with absorptive (intestinal) hypercalciuria, as hypercalcemia may result.

Thiazides should be used with extreme caution, if at all, in patients with severe renal disease (may worsen azotemia) or with a pre-existing electrolyte (including hypercalcemia) or water imbalance, impaired hepatic function (may precipitate hepatic coma), hyperuricemia, lupus (SLE), or diabetes mellitus. Patients with conditions that may lead to an electrolyte or water imbalance (eg, vomiting, diarrhea) should be monitored carefully.

Do not confuse hydroCHLOROthiazide with hydrocortisONE, hydrALAZIne, or hydrOXYzine.

Adverse Effects

Hydrochlorothiazide may cause electrolyes disturbances, including hypokalemia, dilutional hyponatremia, and hypomagnesemia. Hypochloremic metabolic alkalosis (with hypokalemia) may develop, especially if there are other causes of potassium and chloride loss (eg, vomiting, diarrhea, potassium-losing nephropathies, concurrent use of loop diuretics) or the patient has cirrhotic liver disease. Hyperuricemia can occur but is usually subclinical. Hyperparathyroid-like effects of hypercalcemia and hypophosphatemia have been reported in humans, but have not led to effects such as nephrolithiasis, bone resorption, or peptic ulceration. GI effects (eg, vomiting, diarrhea) are possible and may be more prevalent in animals with mild azotemia. Other possible adverse effects include hypersensitivity and dermatologic reactions, GU reactions (polyuria), hematologic toxicity, hyperglycemia, hyperlipidemias, and orthostatic hypotension.

Reproductive/Nursing Safety

Hydrochlorothiazide crosses the placenta; no evidence of fetal harm occurred when it was administered to pregnant mice or rats during periods of organogenesis.[4]

Thiazides enter human breastmilk,[4] but hydrochlorothiazide is considered compatible with breastfeeding in humans.[5]

Because safety has not been established in animals, this drug should only be used when the maternal benefits outweigh the potential risks to offspring.

Overdose/Acute Toxicity

Acute overdose may cause an electrolyte and water imbalance, CNS effects (lethargy to coma and seizures), and GI effects (eg, hypermotility, GI distress). Transient increases in BUN have been reported.

Treatment consists of GI decontamination after recent oral ingestion using standard protocols. Avoid giving concomitant cathartics, as they may exacerbate the fluid and electrolyte imbalances that may ensue. Monitor and treat electrolyte and water imbalances supportively. Additionally, monitor respiratory, CNS, and cardiovascular status; treat signs supportively if required.

For patients that have experienced or are suspected to have experienced an overdose, consultation with a 24-hour poison consultation center specializing in providing veterinary-specific information

is recommended. For general information related to overdose and toxin exposures, as well as contact information for poison control centers, refer to ***Appendix***.

Drug Interactions

The following drug interactions have either been reported or are theoretical in humans or animals receiving hydrochlorothiazide and may be of significance in veterinary patients. Unless otherwise noted, use together is not necessarily contraindicated, but weigh the potential risks and perform additional monitoring when appropriate.

- **Amphotericin B**: Use with thiazides can lead to an increased risk for severe hypokalemia.
- **Bromides**: May enhance the excretion of bromides, thereby affecting seizure control and dosage requirements
- **Calcium-Containing Products**: Hypercalcemia may be exacerbated if thiazides are concurrently administered.
- **Cholestyramine**: May reduce hydrochlorothiazide absorption
- **Corticosteroids, Corticotropin**: Use with thiazides can lead to an increased risk for severe hypokalemia.
- **Diazoxide**: Increased risk for hyperglycemia, hyperuricemia, and hypotension
- **Digoxin**: Thiazide-induced hypokalemia, hypomagnesemia, and/or hypercalcemia may increase the likelihood of digitalis toxicity.
- **Hypotensive Agents** (eg, **amlodipine, enalapril, telmisartan**): May have additive hypotensive effects
- **Insulin**: Thiazides may increase insulin requirements.
- **Loop Diuretics** (eg, **furosemide, torsemide**): May have additive hypotensive, hypovolemic, and electrolyte effects. Concurrent use may be considered in cases of advanced heart failure.[1]
- **Methenamine**: Thiazides can alkalinize urine and reduce methenamine effectiveness.
- **Myelosuppressive Agents** (eg, **cyclophosphamide, methotrexate**): May increase exposure and enhance myelosuppression
- **Nonsteroidal Anti-Inflammatory Drugs** (**NSAIDs;** eg, **carprofen, meloxicam, robenacoxib**): Thiazides may increase risk for renal toxicity, and NSAIDs may reduce diuretic actions of thiazides.
- **Neuromuscular Blocking Agents**: May increase the response or duration of effect of tubocurarine or other nondepolarizing neuromuscular blocking agents
- **Probenecid**: Blocks thiazide-induced uric acid retention (used to therapeutic advantage)
- **Quinidine**: Half-life may be prolonged by thiazides (thiazides can alkalinize the urine).
- **Vitamin D**: Hypercalcemia may be exacerbated if thiazides are concurrently administered.

Laboratory Considerations

- **Acetaminophen**: May falsely increase acetaminophen levels
- **Amylase**: Thiazides can increase serum amylase values in subclinical patients and those in the developmental stages of acute pancreatitis (humans).
- **Cortisol**: Thiazides can decrease the renal excretion of cortisol.
- **Estrogen, urinary**: Hydrochlorothiazide may falsely decrease total urinary estrogen when using a spectrophotometric assay.
- **Histamine**: Thiazides may cause false negative results when testing for pheochromocytoma.
- **Hydroxycorticosteroids**: Thiazides may decrease urinary corticosteroid values by interfering in vitro with the absorbance in the modified Glenn-Nelson technique for urinary 17-hydroxycorticosteroids.
- **Parathyroid-function tests**: Thiazides may elevate serum calcium; it is recommended to discontinue thiazides prior to testing.
- **Phenolsulfonphthalein (PSP)**: Thiazides can compete for secretion at proximal renal tubules.
- **Phentolamine test**: Thiazides may give false negative results.
- **Protein-bound iodine**: Thiazides may decrease values.
- **Triiodothyronine resin uptake test**: Thiazides may slightly reduce uptake.
- **Tyramine**: Thaizides can cause false negative results when testing for pheochromocytoma.

Dosages

DOGS:

Prevention of recurrent calcium oxalate uroliths with renal hypercalcuria (extra-label): Usually added when dietary treatment does not adequately control calcium oxalate crystalluria. Most clinicians recommend 2 – 2.2 mg/kg PO twice daily.[6]

Diuretic agent (extra-label):

a) Adjunctive treatment of heart failure when patients become refractory to loop diuretics alone: 0.2 – 0.84 mg/kg PO daily.[1] Other dosage regimens have recommended 0.5 to 4 mg/kg PO once or twice daily.[7] For dogs already on loop diuretic therapy to achieve sequential nephron blockade, low starting doses should be selected with frequent monitoring of renal values and electrolytes as the dose is escalated pending clinical response. The fixed-dose (1:1) combination with spironolactone (*Aldactazide*®) can be considered for dogs already receiving spironolactone.

b) Ascites in patients with liver disease using the fixed-dose (1:1) combination with spironolactone (*Aldactazide*®): Dosed empirically based on the spironolactone content at 0.5 – 1 mg/kg PO twice daily[8]

Systemic hypertension (extra-label): 2 – 4 mg/kg PO once or twice daily as an alternate agent to calcium channel blockers or renin-angiotensin-aldosterone blocking drugs.[9] Other reports suggest 1 mg/kg PO once to twice daily that may be combined with spironolactone 1 – 2 mg/kg PO twice daily to reduce potassium loss.[10]

Nephrogenic diabetes insipidus (extra-label):

a) 2 mg/kg PO twice daily with a low sodium diet[11]

b) 2.5 – 5 mg/kg PO twice daily[12]

Hypoglycemia secondary to insulinoma (extra-label): 1 – 2 mg/kg PO twice daily in conjunction with diazoxide if diazoxide alone does not adequately increase blood glucose.[13]

CATS:

Diuretic agent (extra-label):

a) For heart failure in combination with furosemide in patients that have become refractory to furosemide alone: 1 – 2 mg/kg PO twice daily.[14,15] As in dogs, low starting doses should be selected with frequent monitoring of renal values and electrolytes as the dose is escalated pending clinical response. The fixed-dose (1:1) combination with spironolactone (*Aldactazide*®) can be considered for cats already receiving spironolactone.

b) For ascites in patients with liver disease using the fixed-dose (1:1) combination with spironolactone (*Aldactazide*®): Dosed empirically based on the spironolactone content at 0.5 – 1 mg/kg PO twice daily[8]

Reduce calcium oxalate saturation in urine (extra-label): 1 mg/kg PO twice daily.[16] **NOTE**: Study was done in healthy cats; it is unknown what effect hydrochlorothiazide will have in cats with spontaneously occurring calcium oxalate urolithiasis.

Nephrogenic diabetes insipidus (extra-label): 2.5 – 5 mg/kg PO twice daily[12]

Central diabetes insipidus (extra-label): 12.5 mg/cat (NOT mg/kg) PO twice daily[17,18]

HORSES:

Adjunctive therapy of hyperkalemic periodic paralysis (HyPP) (extra-label): 0.5 – 1 mg/kg PO every 12 hours when diet adjustment does not control episodes[19]

BIRDS:

Diuretic agent for heart failure treatment, using the fixed-dose (1:1) combination with spironolactone (*Aldactazide*®) (extra-label): Hydrochlorothiazide 1 mg/kg PO twice daily[20]

Monitoring

- Serum electrolytes, BUN, creatinine, glucose
- Hydration status
- Blood pressure, if indicated
- CBCs, if indicated

Client Information

- When beginning this medicine, your animal may urinate more often than normal.
- This medicine may be given with or without food. Allow access to water at all times and encourage normal food intake. If your animal vomits or acts sick after getting the medicine on an empty stomach, give with food or small treat to see if this helps. If vomiting continues, contact your veterinarian.
- Because this drug can change electrolytes (salts) in the blood, your veterinarian will recommend more frequent monitoring.
- Contact your veterinarian immediately if excessive thirst, muscle weakness, collapsing or fainting, head tilt, lack of urination, or a racing heartbeat is noticed.

Chemistry/Synonyms

Hydrochlorothiazide occurs as a practically odorless, slightly bitter, white or practically white crystalline powder with pK_as of 7.9 and 9.2. It is slightly soluble in water and soluble in alcohol.

Hydrochlorothiazide may also be known as HCTZ, hidroclorotiazida, or hydrochlorothiazidum; many trade names are available.

Storage/Stability

Hydrochlorothiazide capsules and tablets should be stored at room temperature (20°C-25°C [68°F-77°F]) in tight, light-resistant containers.

Compatibility/Compounding Considerations

Compounded preparation stability: A method for compounding a spironolactone/hydrochlorothiazide oral suspension from commercially available tablets has been published.[21] Triturate 24 spironolactone/hydrochlorothiazide 25/25 mg tablets with 60 mL of *Ora-Plus*® and make up to 120 mL with *Ora-Sweet*® (or *Ora-Sweet*® *SF*). This yields a 5 mg/mL suspension of both spironolactone and hydrochlorothiazide that retains more than 90% potency for 60 days stored at both 5°C (41°F) and 25°C (77°F). Compounded preparations of hydrochlorothiazide should be protected from light.

Dosage Forms/Regulatory Status

VETERINARY-LABELED PRODUCTS: NONE

The Association of Racing Commissioners International (ARCI) has designated this drug as a class 4 substance. See ***Appendix*** for more information. Use of this drug may not be allowed in certain animal competitions. Check rules and regulations before entering in a competition while this medication is being administered. Contact local racing authorities for further guidance.

HUMAN-LABELED PRODUCTS:

Hydrochlorothiazide Oral Tablets: 12.5 mg, 25 mg, and 50 mg; generic; (Rx)

Hydrochlorothiazide Oral Capsules: 12.5 mg; *Microzide*® *Capsules*; generic; (Rx)

Spironolactone/Hydrochlorothiazide Oral Tablets: 25 mg/25 mg and 50 mg/50 mg; *Aldactazide*®; generic; (Rx)

There are other fixed-dose combinations with hydrochlorothiazide, including (partial list) with: amlodipine, benazepril, candesartan, enalapril, irbesartan, lisinopril, losartan, metoprolol, telmisartan, and triamterene.

References

For the complete list of references, see **wiley.com/go/budde/plumb**

Hydrocodone Combinations

(hye-droe-***koe***-done) *Hycodan*®, *Vicodin*®

Opioid Agonist; Anti-tussive Agent

Prescriber Highlights

- Immediate-release product available in combination with homatropine or acetaminophen, or ibuprofen
- Prescriptions must specify which combination is to be dispensed.
- Used primarily as an antitussive in dogs; efficacy as an oral analgesic for moderate pain in dogs has been disappointing.
- Contraindicated in patients with hypersensitivity to narcotic analgesics, receiving monoamine oxidase inhibitors (MAOIs), or presented with diarrhea due to toxic ingestion. Any combination with acetaminophen should **NOT** be used in cats or ferrets.
- Additional monitoring may be required in patients with hypothyroidism, severe renal or hepatic insufficiency, hypoadrenocorticism, head injuries or increased intracranial pressure, and acute abdominal conditions, as well as in geriatric or severely debilitated patients. Extreme caution should be exercised in patients with increased respiratory secretions or with nebulized treatments.
- Potential adverse effects include sedation, constipation (with long-term therapy), vomiting, other GI disturbances (eg, gastroesophageal reflux, regurgitation), and respiratory depression.
- May mask the clinical signs of respiratory disease (eg, cough)
- All products are DEA Schedule II (C-II) controlled substances

Uses/Indications

Hydrocodone is used principally in dogs as an antitussive for cough secondary to conditions such as collapsing trachea, bronchitis, or canine infectious respiratory disease complex (CIRDC; also known as kennel cough, canine infectious tracheobronchitis). Hydrocodone use is generally reserved for harsh, dry, nonproductive coughs.

Hydrocodone is more potent than codeine, and commercially available dosage forms of hydrocodone are combined with homatropine to prevent abuse, which is why many clinicians prefer a combination hydrocodone/homatropine versus codeine for use as an antitussive in dogs.

Hydrocodone has not proved to be a useful analgesic. Neither extended-release hydrocodone tablets (single agent)[1] nor a combination product containing hydrocodone and acetaminophen[2] provided acceptable postoperative analgesia in dogs following tibial plateau leveling osteotomy (TPLO).

Pharmacology/Actions

Opioid receptors are found in high concentrations in the limbic system, spinal cord, thalamus, hypothalamus, striatum, and midbrain. The GI tract, urinary tract, and other smooth muscle tissues also contain opiate receptors. Hydrocodone has primary activity at mu receptors, with some activity at kappa and delta receptors at higher doses, and binding at these CNS receptors results in reduced neuronal excitability.

Primary pharmacologic effects of opioids include analgesia, antitussive activity, respiratory depression, sedation, and GI effects (eg, vomiting, constipation).

Secondary pharmacologic effects include CNS: sedation, excitatory effects (disinhibition); cardiovascular: bradycardia due to central vagal stimulation, syncope, decreased peripheral resistance, and baroreceptor inhibition; urinary: increased bladder sphincter tone can induce urinary retention; endocrine: inhibited secretion of glucagon, insulin, somatostatin, and vasopressin.

Although hydrocodone exhibits the characteristics of other opioid agonists, it tends to have a slightly greater antitussive effect than codeine (on a weight basis) because of direct suppression of the cough reflex in the medullary cough center. Hydrocodone tends to have a drying effect on respiratory mucosa, and the viscosity of respiratory secretions may be increased; the addition of homatropine methylbromide (in *Hycodan®* and others) may enhance this effect.

Pharmacokinetics

Hydrocodone oral bioavailability is ≈40% in dogs.[3] In healthy greyhounds (n = 6), oral doses of ≈0.5 mg/kg hydrocodone bitartrate (in combination with acetaminophen) produced peak concentrations of hydrocodone in ≈45 minutes and hydromorphone, the active metabolite, in ≈1.5 hours. Plasma concentrations of hydromorphone remained greater than 1.6 ng/mL through the 8 hours of the study; this value is greater than the concentration thought to be antinociceptive. Mean elimination half-life (t½) of hydrocodone was 1.6 to 1.8 hours.[4,5] In a study of postoperative client-owned dogs,[6] time to hydrocodone peak concentration and elimination half-life was 3.5 hours and 16 hours, respectively. The hydrocodone data in this study could not be fit into a pharmacokinetic model, and the 16-hour value for t½ (which exceeds the 8-hour study interval) was not robust. The authors speculate that reduced GI transit due to anesthesia or preoperative morphine may have altered drug absorption. In addition, hydromorphone was isolated in only 3 of 24 dogs. Dogs hepatically metabolize hydrocodone via *N*- and *O*-demethylation pathways, and hydromorphone is an active metabolite.[4,7,8]

The antitussive and analgesic actions of hydrocodone are thought to persist for 6 to 12 hours, but pharmacokinetic/pharmacodynamic studies correlating oral hydrocodone's antinociceptive effects in dogs are not currently available. Extrapolating data from hydromorphone, drug concentration did not correlate with analgesic activity in cats[9] and horses.[10,11]

In humans, hydrocodone is well absorbed after oral administration, and absorption is not affected by food. The drug is hepatically metabolized by several pathways, including *N*- and *O*-demethylation and glucuronidation and has a serum half-life of ≈3.8 hours. The antitussive effect usually lasts 4 to 6 hours in adults.

Information regarding the pharmacokinetics of the extended-release (ER) formulation of hydrocodone in veterinary patients is not available.

Contraindications/Precautions/Warnings

Hydrocodone is contraindicated in patients hypersensitive to it or with marked respiratory depression, GI obstruction, or diarrhea caused by a toxic ingestion (until the toxin is eliminated from the GI tract). Because opioids may impact the CNS, cardiac, respiratory, and GI systems, animals with underlying conditions affecting these systems (eg, hypothyroidism, severe renal or hepatic insufficiency, seizure disorders, hypoadrenocorticism, GI obstruction or reduced motility, geriatric or severely debilitated) should be monitored closely for adverse effects related to these systems.[12,13]

Commercially marketed hydrocodone products in the United States are available only as extended-release or combination products. Combinations containing acetaminophen (eg, *Vicodin®*) should **NOT** be used in cats or ferrets, and products containing ibuprofen should not be used in dogs or cats. Because of available dosage form concerns and lack of evidence supporting hydrocodone use in cats for any purpose, it cannot be recommended for feline patients.

Because hydrocodone may obscure the diagnosis or clinical course, this drug should be used with caution in patients with head injuries or increased intracranial pressure and acute abdominal conditions. The drug should be used with extreme caution in patients with respiratory disease, with increased respiratory secretions, or nebulized treatments.

Hydrocodone may impair the performance of service or working dogs.

Hydrocodone products have a high abuse potential in humans, and diversion from its intended use is possible.

Do not confuse hydroCODone, hydroMORPHone, and hydroCORTisone.

Adverse Effects

Adverse effects in dogs include sedation, constipation (with long-term therapy), vomiting, or other GI disturbances. Hydrocodone may mask the clinical signs (eg, cough) of respiratory disease and should not replace appropriate specific treatments for the underlying cause of cough.

Long-term opioid use has been associated with dysfunction of the hypothalamic-pituitary-adrenal axis in humans.[14]

Reproductive/Nursing Safety

Skeletal malformations and reductions in fetal weight, survival rate, and litter size occurred following hydrocodone exposure to pregnant laboratory animals, usually at higher doses (2 to 15 times the recommended dose).[14] Long-term opioid use may cause reduced fertility in both male and females.[14]

Hydrocodone and its hydromorphone metabolite enter breast milk in humans.

Because safety has not been established in animal species, this drug should only be used when the maternal benefits outweigh the potential fetal risks.

Overdose/Acute Toxicity

The initial concern with a hydrocodone overdose is CNS, cardiovascular, and respiratory depression secondary to opioid effects. Common clinical signs associated with overdose may include lethargy/sedation, vocalizing, hyperactivity, ataxia, and vomiting.

If ingestion was within 2 to 3 hours of presentation, gastric decontamination using standard protocols should be performed, and treatment with naloxone instituted as necessary. The homatropine ingredient may give rise to anticholinergic effects that can complicate the clinical picture, but its relatively low toxicity may not require treatment. For further information on handling opioid or anticholinergic overdoses, see ***Meperidine*** and ***Atropine***, respectively. Refer to ***Acetaminophen*** for toxicosis associated with acetaminophen combination products.

For patients that have experienced or are suspected to have experienced an overdose, consultation with a 24-hour poison consultation center specializing in providing veterinary-specific information is recommended. For general information related to overdose and toxin exposures, as well as contact information for poison control centers, refer to ***Appendix***.

Drug Interactions

The following drug interactions have been reported or are theoretical in humans or animals receiving hydrocodone and may be of significance in veterinary patients. Unless otherwise noted, use together is not necessarily contraindicated, but weigh the potential risks and perform additional monitoring when appropriate.

- Anticholinergic Drugs (eg, **atropine, glycopyrrolate**): May cause additive anticholinergic effects and increased risk for urinary retention, constipation, or paralytic ileus; risk is likely greater with hydrocodone/homatropine combinations
- Benzodiazepines (eg, **alprazolam, diazepam, midazolam**): May result in additive CNS and respiratory depressant effects
- Clopidogrel: May reduce the efficacy of clopidogrel in humans
- CNS Depressants, Other (eg, **anesthetic agents, antihistamines, phenothiazines**): May cause increased CNS or respiratory depression
- Desmopressin: May result in increased risk for hyponatremia
- Diuretics (eg, **furosemide**): May decrease diuretic efficacy because opioids can induce antidiuretic hormone (ADH) secretion
- GI Agents, Prokinetic (eg, **cisapride, metoclopramide**): May antagonize the GI motility effects of these agents
- Macrolide Antibiotics (eg, **clarithromycin, erythromycin**): May increase serum hydrocodone concentration and risk for toxicity
- Monoamine Oxidase Inhibitors (MAOIs; eg, **amitraz, selegiline**): May potentiate CNS and respiratory adverse effects; not recommended (in humans) with concurrent MAOI use, or if MAOI has been used within 14 days
- Ondansetron: May increase risk for serotonin syndrome
- Naloxone: Antagonizes opioid effects. **NOTE**: This action is an expected outcome when naloxone is used as a reversal agent.
- Opioid Mixed Agonists/Antagonists (eg, **butorphanol, buprenorphine**): May reduce the efficacy of hydrocodone
- Rifampin: May induce hydrocodone metabolism and decrease hydrocodone serum concentration
- Phenobarbital/Primidone: May increase risk for CNS and respiratory depression; may induce hydrocodone metabolism and decrease hydrocodone serum concentration
- Quinidine: May result in reduced analgesic and antitussive effects
- Serotonin Modulators (eg, **fluoxetine, mirtazapine, trazodone**): May result in psychomotor impairment and increase risk for serotonin syndrome
- Skeletal Muscle Relaxants (eg, **dantrolene, methocarbamol**): May enhance CNS depressant effects
- Tricyclic Antidepressants(eg, **amitriptyline, clomipramine**): May have additive CNS depressant and anticholinergic effects

Laboratory Considerations

- Opioids may increase pressure on the biliary tract, leading to increased plasma **lipase** and **amylase** activity for up to 24 hours following opioid administration.

Dosages

NOTE: All prescriptions for hydrocodone combinations must specify the strength of both hydrocodone and the combination drug (eg, hydrocodone 5 mg/homatropine 1.5 mg tablet).

DOGS:

Antitussive (extra-label): 0.2 – 0.5 mg/kg PO every 6 to 12 hours is usually recommended, but doses up to 1 mg/kg PO every 6 hours have been noted. The goal of therapy is to suppress cough without excessive sedation.[15]

Analgesic (extra-label): Pharmacokinetic studies[4,6] suggest hydrocodone may be an effective analgesic for mild to moderate pain in dogs, but clinical trials do not support analgesic efficacy following orthopedic surgery.[1,2] If using the combination product that contains hydrocodone with acetaminophen, calculate the dose to provide **hydrocodone** 0.5 – 0.6 mg/kg and **acetaminophen** 15 mg/kg PO every 8 hours.[2,16] Fixed-dose combinations of hydrocodone and acetaminophen make it difficult to administer less than 15 mg/kg of the acetaminophen component every 8 hours.

Monitoring

- Adverse effects (eg, vomiting, constipation, excessive sedation)
- Clinical efficacy for condition being treated (eg, improved cough suppression, improved analgesia)

Client Information

- Any product that also contains acetaminophen (eg, *Tylenol*®, APAP, *Vicodin*®) should **NEVER** be used in cats or ferrets. If you are unsure whether a product containing hydrocodone is safe for use in your animal, ask your veterinarian.
- This medicine can be given with or without food. If your animal vomits or acts sick after receiving hydrocodone on an empty stomach, give with food or a small treat to see if this helps. If vomiting continues, contact your veterinarian.
- Sedation (ie, sleepiness, fatigue) and constipation are the most likely side effects. Watch for side effects and contact your veterinarian immediately if your animal stops eating, if the whites of the eyes become yellowish, if the animal continues to vomit or has diarrhea, or if blood is seen in vomit or stool.
- Contact your veterinarian if you are concerned that your animal's condition is not improving on this medication.
- Do **NOT** give more to your animal than your veterinarian prescribes. Unless your veterinarian instructs, do **NOT** give other pain, cough, or fever medication at the same time as using hydrocodone.
- Hydrocodone in combination with acetaminophen or homatropine is a controlled substance in the United States and requires a new written prescription for refills. Use of this medication in animals or humans other than those for whom they were prescribed is illegal.

Chemistry/Synonyms

Hydrocodone, a phenanthrene-derivative opiate agonist, is a hydrogenated ketone derivative of codeine. Hydrocodone bitartrate occurs as fine, white crystals or crystalline powder. It is susceptible to photodegradation. One gram is soluble in ≈16 mL of water; it is slightly soluble in alcohol.

Hydrocodone bitartrate may also be known as hydrocodone tartrate, dihydrocodeinone acid tartrate, hydrocodone acid tartrate, or hydrocodoni bitartras.

Storage/Stability

Products should be protected from light and stored at room temperature (20°C-25°C [68°F-77°F]); excursions from 15°C to 30°C (59°F-86°F) may be permitted for some products.

Hydrocodone is a Schedule II controlled substance. In accordance with DEA regulations, it must be stored in an area that is substantially constructed and securely locked. Follow applicable local, state, and federal rules regarding disposal of unused or wasted controlled drugs. Report dispensing to state monitoring programs where required.

Compatibility/Compounding Considerations

No specific information was noted.

Dosage Forms/Regulatory Status

VETERINARY-LABELED PRODUCTS: NONE

The Association of Racing Commissioners International (ARCI) has designated this drug as a class 1 substance. Use of this drug may not be allowed in certain animal competitions. Check rules and regulations before entering in a competition while this medication is being administered. Contact local racing authorities for further guidance. See ***Appendix*** for more information.

HUMAN-LABELED PRODUCTS:

Hydrocodone Bitartrate Oral Tablets: 5 mg with Homatropine MBr 1.5 mg; *Tussigon*®, *Hycodan*®, generic; (Rx, C-II)

Hydrocodone Bitartrate Oral Syrup: 5 mg with Homatropine MBr 1.5 mg (per 5 mL) in 473 mL; *Hydromet*® Syrup, *Hycodan*® Syrup, generic (Rx, C-II). Hydrocodone 1 mg/mL syrup is available in Canada; Narcotic (CDSA I)

Hydrocodone Bitartrate Extended-Release Oral Tablets: 10 mg, 15 mg, 20 mg, 30 mg, 40 mg, 50 mg, 60 mg, 80 mg, 100 mg, and 120 mg; *Hysingla ER*®, *Zohydro ER*®; (Rx, C-II)

The following products are representative oral dosage forms containing hydrocodone and acetaminophen and include those most likely to be of benefit (higher ratios of hydrocodone to acetaminophen) in treating dogs and that are usually stocked at human pharmacies. **WARNING**: These products should **NOT** be used in cats or ferrets.

Hydrocodone/Acetaminophen Oral Tablets: 5 mg/300 mg, 5 mg/325 mg, 7.5 mg/300 mg, 7.5 mg/325 mg, 10 mg/300 mg, and 10 mg/325 mg. A commonly used trade name is *Vicodin*®; generic; (Rx, C-II)

Hydrocodone/Acetaminophen Oral Solution: Hydrocodone 2.5 mg/5 mL (0.67 mg/mL) in combination with acetaminophen 100 mg/5 mL (20 mg/mL). generic; (Rx, C-II)

Combination products with hydrocodone/ibuprofen are also available: 5 mg/200 mg, 7.5 mg/200 mg, and 10 mg/200 mg under the commonly used trade name *Vicoprofen*® and generics; (Rx, C-II). **NOTE**: This product is not recommended for use in dogs or cats.

Oral liquids with hydrocodone are also available in combination with chlorpheniramine and/or pseudoephedrine. Some of these products have 2 or more active ingredients; (Rx, C-II)

Report dispensing to state monitoring programs where required.

References

For the complete list of references, see **wiley.com/go/budde/plumb**

Hydrocortisone

Hydrocortisone Sodium Succinate

(hye-droe-***kor***-ti-zone) *Cortef*®, *Solu-Cortef*®

Glucocorticoid

Prescriber Highlights

- Benchmark injectable, oral, and topical glucocorticoid. The IV form (sodium succinate salt) is most commonly used when immediate glucocorticoid and mineralocorticoid activity is desired (eg, Addisonian crisis, critical illness-related corticosteroid insufficiency [CIRCI]).
- Contraindications include systemic fungal infections and idiopathic thrombocytopenia (IM use).
- Primary adverse effects occur with sustained use and include clinical signs of hyperadrenocorticism.
- Tapering required after chronic use
- Many potential drug interactions and laboratory interactions

Uses/Indications

Hydrocortisone is used in dogs and cats for acute treatment of hypoadrenocorticism (Addisonian crisis) and for long-term maintenance therapy for hypoadrenocorticism. Because of its rapid effect and relatively high mineralocorticoid effect, IV hydrocortisone sodium succinate is the most commonly used form of this medication when an acute glucocorticoid/mineralocorticoid effect is desired (eg, acute adrenal insufficiency; critical illness-related corticosteroid insufficiency [CIRCI]). While oral forms are available, they are not routinely used in veterinary patients.

Pharmacology/Actions

Glucocorticoids have effects on virtually every cell type and system in mammals. See the ***Glucocorticoid Agents, General Information*** monograph for more information.

Pharmacokinetics

In humans, hydrocortisone is readily absorbed after oral administration, and hydrocortisone sodium succinate is rapidly absorbed after IM administration. Duration of activity is 8 to 12 hours.

Contraindications/Precautions/Warnings

Hydrocortisone products are contraindicated in patients with known hypersensitivity to those particular products or their constituents. Glucocorticoid agents used systemically are generally considered contraindicated in systemic fungal infections (unless used for replacement therapy in patients with Addison's disease). IM administration is contraindicated in patients with idiopathic thrombocytopenia. Intrathecal administration is contraindicated.[1] In humans, epidural administration of glucocorticoids has resulted in serious neurologic events including spinal cord infarction, cortical blindness, and death.

Some formulations contain benzyl alcohol and are contraindicated in neonatal patients.[1]

Patients that have received the drug chronically should be tapered off slowly until normal adrenal and pituitary function resume, as endogenous ACTH and corticosteroid function may return slowly. If the animal undergoes a stressful event (eg, surgery, trauma, illness) during the tapering process, additional glucocorticoids should be administered.

Do not confuse hydroCORTIsone with hydroCODONE, hydroCHLOROthiazide, or hydroxyCHLOROquine. Do not confuse Solu-CORTEF with SOLU-Medrol. Consider writing part of the drug's name in uppercase letters (tall-man designations) on prescriptions/orders to reduce the risk of errors.

Adverse Effects

Adverse effects are generally associated with long-term administration of glucocorticoids, especially if given at high dosages or on a daily basis. Effects generally manifest as clinical signs of hyperadrenocorticism. Glucocorticoids can delay growth when administered to young, growing animals. A complete list of potential adverse effects is provided in ***Glucocorticoid Agents, General Information.***

The adverse effect profile for IV hydrocortisone in dogs and cats for acute hypoadrenocorticism or CIRCI is not well described. In humans in the ICU setting (CIRCI), potential important adverse effects include immune suppression with increased risk for infection, impaired wound healing, hyperglycemia, myopathy, hypokalemic metabolic acidosis, psychosis, and HPA axis and glucocorticoid receptor suppression.[2]

Reproductive/Nursing Safety

Excessive glucocorticoid doses early in pregnancy may lead to teratogenic effects. When administered in the latter stages of pregnancy, exogenous steroids may induce parturition, including premature parturition followed by dystocia, fetal death retained placenta and metritis. Cleft palate, foreleg deformities, phocomelia, and anasarca have occurred in offspring of dogs that received corticosteroids during pregnancy.[3] In horses and ruminants, exogenous steroid administration may induce parturition when administered in the latter stages of pregnancy.

Glucocorticoids not bound to plasma proteins will enter milk.

High doses or prolonged administration to mothers may potentially inhibit the growth of nursing newborns.

Because safety has not been established in animals, this drug should only be used when the maternal benefits outweigh the potential risks to offspring.

Overdose/Acute Toxicity

Glucocorticoids, when given short-term, are unlikely to cause harmful effects, even in massive doses. One incidence of a dog developing acute CNS effects after accidental ingestion of glucocorticoids has been reported. If clinical signs occur, use supportive treatment as necessary.

For patients that have experienced or are suspected to have experienced an overdose, consultation with a 24-hour poison consultation center specializing in providing veterinary-specific information is recommended. For general information related to overdose and toxin exposures, as well as contact information for poison control centers, refer to ***Appendix.***

Drug Interactions

The following drug interactions have either been reported or are theoretical in humans or animals receiving hydrocortisone and may be of significance in veterinary patients. Unless otherwise noted, use together is not necessarily contraindicated, but weigh the potential risks and perform additional monitoring when appropriate.

- **Amphotericin B**: Administered concomitantly with glucocorticoids may cause hypokalemia; in humans, there have been cases of CHF and cardiac enlargement reported after using hydrocortisone to treat amphotericin B adverse effects.
- **Anticholinesterase Agents** (eg, **neostigmine, pyridostigmine**): In patients with myasthenia gravis, concomitant glucocorticoid and anticholinesterase agent administration may lead to profound muscle weakness. If possible, discontinue anticholinesterase medication at least 24 hours prior to hydrocortisone administration.
- **Aspirin**: Glucocorticoids may reduce salicylate blood levels and increase the risk for GI ulceration/bleeding.
- **Azole Antifungals** (eg, **ketoconazole**): May decrease the metabolism of glucocorticoids and increase hydrocortisone blood levels; ketoconazole may induce adrenal insufficiency when glucocorticoids are withdrawn by inhibiting adrenal corticosteroid synthesis.
- **Barbiturates** (eg, **phenobarbital**): May increase the metabolism of glucocorticoids and decrease hydrocortisone blood levels
- **Cyclophosphamide**: Glucocorticoids may inhibit the hepatic metabolism of cyclophosphamide; dosage adjustments may be required.
- **Cyclosporine**: Concomitant administration of glucocorticoids and cyclosporine may increase the blood levels of both drugs by mutually inhibiting the hepatic metabolism of each other; the clinical significance of this interaction is not clear.
- **Diuretics, Potassium-Depleting** (eg, **furosemide, thiazides**): When administered concomitantly with glucocorticoids, may cause hypokalemia
- **Ephedrine**: May reduce hydrocortisone blood levels
- **Estrogens**: The effects of hydrocortisone and, possibly, other glucocorticoids may be potentiated by concomitant administration with estrogens.
- **Insulin**: Insulin requirements may increase in patients receiving glucocorticoids.
- **Macrolide Antibiotics** (eg, **clarithromycin, erythromycin**): May decrease the metabolism of glucocorticoids and increase hydrocortisone blood levels
- **Mitotane**: May alter the metabolism of steroids; higher than usual doses of steroids may be necessary to treat mitotane-induced adrenal insufficiency.
- **Nonsteroidal Anti-Inflammatory Drugs** (NSAIDs; eg, **carprofen, meloxicam**): Administration of ulcerogenic drugs with glucocorticoids may increase the risk for GI ulceration.
- **Rifampin**: May increase the metabolism of glucocorticoids and decrease hydrocortisone blood levels
- **Vaccines**: Patients receiving corticosteroids at immunosuppressive dosages should generally not receive live attenuated-virus vaccines as virus replication may be augmented; a diminished immune response may occur after the vaccine, toxoid, or bacterin administration in patients receiving glucocorticoids.
- **Warfarin**: Hydrocortisone may affect coagulation status; monitor

Laboratory Considerations

- Hydrocortisone can cross-react with **cortisol** in the ACTH response test. This test must be performed before hydrocortisone is administered or 24 hours after the last dose of hydrocortisone. NOTE: Dexamethasone does not cross-react.
- Glucocorticoids may increase **serum cholesterol.**
- Glucocorticoids may increase **urine glucose** levels.
- Glucocorticoids may decrease **serum potassium.**
- Glucocorticoids can suppress the release of thyroid-stimulating hormone (TSH) and reduce $\mathbf{T_3}$ **and** $\mathbf{T_4}$ values. Thyroid gland atrophy has been reported after chronic glucocorticoid administration. The uptake of $\mathbf{I^{131}}$ by the thyroid may be decreased by glucocorticoids.
- Reactions to **skin tests** may be suppressed by glucocorticoids.
- False-negative results of the **nitroblue tetrazolium** test for systemic bacterial infections may be induced by glucocorticoids.
- Glucocorticoids may cause **neutrophilia** within 4 to 8 hours after dosing and return to baseline within 24 to 48 hours after drug discontinuation.
- Glucocorticoids can cause **lymphopenia** that can persist for weeks after drug discontinuation in dogs.
- Glucocorticoids can cause elevations in **ALT, ALP, and GGT** in dogs.

Dosages

DOGS/CATS:

Adjunctive therapy for acute adrenocortical insufficiency (extra-label): After completion of the ACTH stimulation test, most recommendations are hydrocortisone sodium succinate 0.3 – 0.5 mg/kg/hour IV CRI or 2 – 4 mg/kg IV every 6 to 8 hours. Once GI function has returned and the patient is eating and drinking normally, therapy can be changed to oral steroid supplementation.

Long-term treatment of hypoadrenocorticism (extra-label): In the changeover period, as animals recover from an acute crisis and start to eat and drink, glucocorticoid supplementation is changed from parenteral to an oral dosage form. Traditionally, treatment is initially started with a mineralocorticoid (fludrocortisone or DOCP) combined with a glucocorticoid (eg, cortisone acetate, hydrocortisone, or prednisolone). The mineralocorticoid can be discontinued in some patients after 1 to 2 months. When using oral hydrocortisone tablets, most dogs are started on an anecdotal dose of 0.4 – 0.8 mg/kg PO once to twice a day. Once stable, generally, a dose of hydrocortisone 0.4 mg/kg PO once to twice a day provides adequate additional glucocorticoid supplementation.

Relative adrenal insufficiency (RAI); critical illness-related corticosteroid insufficiency (CIRCI); (extra-label): At present, there is no strong evidence for the use of any corticosteroid in veterinary patients for these indications, and no consensus guidelines have been published; however, based upon research done in critically ill humans, it is reasonable to consider hydrocortisone. One recommended dosage is hydrocortisone sodium succinate 1 – 4.3 mg/kg/day divided into 4 equal doses and given IV every 6 hours or as a CRI. Because the HPA dysfunction in CIRCI is thought to be transient, lifelong therapy with corticosteroids is not required, and dosage is tapered by 25% each day after resolution of critical illness. An ACTH stimulation test should be repeated to confirm the return of normal adrenocortical function following the resolution of critical illness and discontinuation of corticosteroid supplementation.[4] Human data suggest that CRIs may provide better glycemic control but may cause greater HPA axis suppression than when given episodically.

Post-CPR resuscitation (extra-label): Routine administration of corticosteroids is not recommended. Use may be considered in patients that remain hemodynamically unstable despite administration of fluids and positive inotropes and vasopressors. Hydrocortisone sodium succinate 1 mg/kg IV, followed by either 1 mg/kg every 6 hours IV or 0.15 mg/kg/hour IV CRI, then tapered as the patient's condition allows.[5]

Monitoring

Monitoring of glucocorticoid therapy is dependent on its reason for use, dosage, dosage schedule (daily versus alternate day therapy), duration of therapy, and the animal's age and condition. The following list may not be appropriate or complete for all animals; use clinical assessment and judgment when adverse effects occur.

- Body weight, appetite, signs of edema
- Serum and/or urine electrolytes
- Total plasma proteins and albumin
- Blood glucose
- Urine culture

Client Information

- If using oral tablets at home, carefully follow the dosage instructions and do not discontinue the medicine abruptly without consulting with your veterinarian beforehand.
- Give oral tablets with food to help prevent stomach upset.

Chemistry/Synonyms

Hydrocortisone, also known as compound F or cortisol, is secreted by the adrenal gland. Hydrocortisone occurs as an odorless, white to practically white, crystalline powder. It is very slightly soluble in water and sparingly soluble in alcohol. Hydrocortisone is administered orally.

Hydrocortisone sodium succinate occurs as an odorless, white to nearly white, hygroscopic, amorphous solid. It is very soluble in both water and alcohol. Hydrocortisone sodium succinate injection is administered via IM or IV routes.

Hydrocortisone may also be known as an anti-inflammatory hormone, compound F, cortisol, hydrocortisonum, 17-hydroxycorticosterone, and NSC-10483; many trade names are available.

Storage/Stability

Store hydrocortisone sodium succinate in intact containers at controlled room temperatures of 20°C to 25°C (68°F-77°F). After reconstitution, solutions are stable if protected from light and kept at or below controlled room temperature. Use the solution only if it is clear; discard unused solutions after 3 days. Hydrocortisone sodium succinate is heat labile and cannot be autoclaved. Reconstituted HSS 500 mg/4 mL solution kept frozen for 4 weeks showed no loss of potency.

Store hydrocortisone tablets in well-closed containers at room temperature (15°C to 30°C [59°F-86°F]).

Compatibility/Compounding Considerations

Compatibility is dependent upon factors such as pH, concentration, temperature, and diluent used; consult specialized references or a hospital pharmacist for more specific information.

Hydrocortisone sodium succinate is reportedly physically **compatible** with the following solutions and drugs: dextrose-Ringer's injection combinations, dextrose-Ringer's lactate injection combinations, dextrose-saline combinations, dextrose injections, Ringer's injection, lactated Ringer's injection, sodium chloride injections, amikacin sulfate, aminophylline, amphotericin B (limited quantities), calcium chloride/gluconate, chloramphenicol sodium succinate, clindamycin phosphate, corticotropin, daunorubicin HCl, dopamine HCl, erythromycin gluceptate, erythromycin lactobionate, lidocaine HCl, mephentermine sulfate, metronidazole with sodium bicarbonate, penicillin G potassium/sodium, piperacillin sodium, polymyxin B sulfate, potassium chloride, prochlorperazine edisylate, sodium bicarbonate, vancomycin HCl, verapamil HCl, and vitamin B-complex with C.

Hydrocortisone sodium succinate is reportedly physically **incompatible** when mixed with the following solutions and drugs: ampicillin sodium, bleomycin sulfate, dimenhydrinate, diphenhydramine HCl, doxorubicin HCl, ephedrine sulfate, heparin sodium, hydralazine HCl, oxytetracycline HCl, pentobarbital sodium, phenobarbital sodium, promethazine HCl, and tetracycline HCl.

Dosage Forms/Regulatory Status

VETERINARY-LABELED PRODUCTS:

There are no products containing hydrocortisone (or its salts) known for systemic use. There are a variety of hydrocortisone veterinary products for topical use. A 10 ppb tolerance has been established for hydrocortisone (as the succinate or acetate) in milk.

The Association of Racing Commissioners International (ARCI) has designated this drug as a class 4 substance. Use of this drug may not be allowed in certain animal competitions. Check rules and regulations before entering a competition while this medication is being administered. Contact local racing authorities for further guidance.

See the ***Appendix*** for more information.

HUMAN-LABELED PRODUCTS:

Hydrocortisone Oral Tablets: 5 mg, 10 mg, and 20 mg; *Cortef®*, generic; (Rx)

Hydrocortisone Oral Sprinkle: 0.5 mg, 1 mg, 2 mg, and 5 mg; *Alkindi Sprinkle®*; (Rx)

Hydrocortisone Sodium Succinate Injection: 100 mg/vial, 250 mg/vial, 500 mg/vial, and 1000 mg/vial; *Solu-Cortef®*, *A-Hydrocort®*; (Rx)

There are many OTC and Rx topical and anorectal products are available in a variety of dosage forms.

References

For the complete list of references, see **wiley.com/go/budde/plumb**

Hydrogen Peroxide 3% (Oral)

(***hye***-droe-jen per-***oks***-ide)

Oral Emetic

NOTE: Also refer to the ***Overdose and Toxin Exposure Decontamination Guidelines*** in the ***Appendix***

Prescriber Highlights

- Topical antiseptic that is used orally as a home-administered emetic in dogs when clients cannot transport the patient to a veterinary hospital in a timely manner or when other emetics have failed or are unavailable.
- Can cause esophageal irritation or other gastric effects; aspiration is possible
- Not recommended for use in cats
- Many contraindications for use as an emetic
- Do not use hydrogen peroxide solutions greater than 3%; solution should not be expired

Uses/Indications

Hydrogen peroxide 3% solution can be used as an orally administered emetic in dogs, pigs, and ferrets. It is reserved primarily for those cases when animals cannot be transported to a veterinary hospital promptly and immediate emesis is required; it may also be used in a clinic setting when other emetics have failed or are unavailable. A prospective observational study found that hydrogen peroxide 3% solution successfully induced emesis in 90% of treated dogs and was equally as effective as apomorphine at 94%.[1]

Hydrogen peroxide is not recommended in cats because of its unreliability as an emetic and because of potentially life-threatening adverse effects (eg, hemorrhagic gastritis,[2] acute respiratory failure[3,4]).

Apomorphine or ropinirole for dogs and alpha-adrenergic agonists (eg, dexmedetomidine) or hydromorphone for cats are preferred emetic agents for administration in a veterinary clinic.

Pharmacology/Actions

Orally administered hydrogen peroxide 3% solution induces a vomiting reflex via direct irritant effects of the oropharynx and gastric lining. Emesis typically ensues within 10 to 15 minutes following oral administration to dogs.[1,5] It is estimated that an average ≈50% of ingested contents are recovered after inducing emesis with either apomorphine or hydrogen peroxide.[1]

Pharmacokinetics

No pharmacokinetic information located. Emetic effects may persist up to ≈2 hours after administering PO to dogs.[1]

Contraindications/Precautions/Warnings

Emesis with hydrogen peroxide should only be considered if preferred methods (eg, apomorphine, ropinirole) are not available and the benefits of decontamination outweigh the risks of its use.[2] Before inducing emesis, obtain a complete history of the ingestion and ensure that vital signs are stable.

If home administration of hydrogen peroxide is necessary, be sure that clients use only the 3% medical-grade solution and not another, more concentrated hydrogen peroxide product. Do not induce emesis with solutions that contain greater than 3% hydrogen peroxide, or that contain other active ingredients (eg, "accelerated" solutions, teat dips).

Emetics can be an important aspect in the treatment of orally ingested toxins, but they must be used judiciously. Most emetics are effective only if given within 2 hours of ingestion. Emetics should not be used in horses, rodents, or rabbits because these patients are either unable to vomit or do not have stomach walls strong enough to tolerate emesis. Emetics are also contraindicated in patients that are hypoxic, have evidence of cardiovascular shock or respiratory distress, are actively having seizures, and/or lack normal pharyngeal reflexes (ie, laryngeal paralysis). The risks and benefits of administering an emetic should also be considered for animals with a recurrent history of aspiration pneumonia or with recent abdominal surgery, seizures, coma, severe CNS depression or deteriorating CNS function, or extreme physical weakness. Emetics should also be withheld in patients that have previously vomited repeatedly. Because of the risk for additional esophageal or gastric injury with emesis, emetics are contraindicated in patients that have ingested a sharp object, strong acids, alkalis, or other caustic agents. Because of the risk for aspiration, emetics are usually contraindicated after petroleum distillate ingestion but may be employed when the risk for toxicity of the compound is greater than the risk for aspiration. Use of emetics after ingestion of strychnine or other CNS stimulants may precipitate seizures.

Emetics generally do not remove more than 80% of the material in the stomach (usually 40% to 60%) and significant quantities of the ingested drug/toxin may remain or may have already been absorbed. Successful induction of emesis does not signal the end of appropriate monitoring or therapy.

Because aspiration and/or bradycardia are possible, animals should be closely observed after administration. Suctioning, respiratory support, and cardiovascular support (eg, atropine) should be available. Do not allow animal to re-ingest vomitus.

Adverse Effects

In dogs, diarrhea, lethargy, and protracted nausea and vomiting are possible[1]; antiemetic agents administered after desired emesis occurs may alleviate nausea and vomiting in severely affected dogs. Hydrogen peroxide solution may be aspirated during administration or after inducing emesis. In an experimental study, significant visual and histopathologic gastric lesions occurred following administration of hydrogen peroxide 3% solution to dogs; less severe duodenal lesions were seen.[2] Gastric ulcers and gastric degeneration and necrosis were evident at 4 and 24 hours. Most gastroduodenal lesions were present for up to 1 week and resolved by 2 weeks. Gastric dilatation-volvulus in dogs has been reported following hydrogen peroxide administration.

Cats can be particularly susceptible to hemorrhagic gastritis or esophagitis.[6] Aspiration with life-threatening lung injury and acute respiratory failure has also been reported in a cat.[4]

Reproductive/Nursing Safety

No specific information was located. Although orally administered hydrogen peroxide 3% solution is unlikely to cause reproductive harm, this drug should only be used when the maternal benefits outweigh the potential risks to offspring.

Overdose/Acute Toxicity

Hydrogen peroxide 3% solution can cause significant injury to the GI tract (see ***Adverse Effects***) after oral ingestion. Hydrogen peroxide in concentrations of 10% or greater can be very corrosive (causing severe burns to oral/gastric mucosa) and in humans, can induce oxygen emboli after oral ingestion.[7]

For patients that have experienced or are suspected to have experienced an overdose, consultation with a 24-hour poison center specializing in providing veterinary-specific information is recommended. For general information related to overdose and toxin exposures, as well as contact information for poison control centers, refer to ***Appendix.***

Drug Interactions

The following drug interactions have either been reported or are theoretical in humans or animals receiving hydrogen peroxide and may be of significance in veterinary patients. Unless otherwise noted, use

together is not necessarily contraindicated, but weigh the potential risks and perform additional monitoring when appropriate.

- **Acetylcysteine, Oral**: Hydrogen peroxide can oxidize acetylcysteine in the GI tract and, although clinical significance is unclear, alternative emetics (eg, apomorphine, hydromorphone, xylazine) are preferred to induce emesis in patients with acetaminophen overdoses.[8]
- **Antiemetics** (eg, **maropitant, ondansetron**): Pre-administration or ingestion of these products may negate the emetic effects of hydrogen peroxide.

Laboratory Considerations

- No specific concerns were noted.

Dosages

NOTE: All dosages use hydrogen peroxide 3% solution. The solution should not be expired.

DOGS:

Emetic (extra-label): 1 – 2.2 mL/kg PO (recommended maximum 50 mL/dog [NOT mL/kg][9]) once; a subsequent dose may be given after 10 to 15 minutes if emesis is not achieved.[1,10] Results are improved if there is a small amount of food in the stomach.[5,11]

POT-BELLIED PIGS:

Emetic (extra-label): 1 – 2 mL/kg PO not to exceed 50 mL/pig (NOT mL/pig). Mix with a small amount of milk to encourage voluntary ingestion.[12]

FERRETS:

Emetic (extra-label): 0.45 – 1.4 mL/kg PO, which can be repeated once if necessary. Results are improved if there is food in the stomach.[13,14]

Monitoring

- Efficacy (ie, emesis)
- Adverse effects (eg, prolonged nausea or vomiting, respiratory distress)
- Heart rate and respiratory rate/character, including thoracic auscultation after emesis
- Clinical signs associated with toxicity of the substance ingested
- Blood toxicant concentrations if applicable

Client Information

- Use only under the direct instructions of your veterinarian or an animal poison control center.
- Only use hydrogen peroxide 3% solution; stronger concentrations can be very toxic. Do not use expired solutions.
- Do not shake bottle. Carefully administer to avoid your animal unintentionally inhaling the liquid.
- Monitor your animal after giving hydrogen peroxide. Do not allow your animal to re-ingest the vomited material.
- Save all vomited fluid and material for your veterinarian to examine.
- Your animal should be seen by your veterinarian as soon as possible.

Chemistry/Synonyms

Hydrogen peroxide 3% solution is a clear, colorless liquid containing 2.5% to 3.5% w/v hydrogen peroxide. Up to 0.05% of the liquid may contain preservatives.

Hydrogen peroxide 3% solution may also be known as dilute hydrogen peroxide solution, hydrogen peroxide solution 10-volume (**NOTE**: **NOT** 10%), or hydrogen peroxide topical solution.

Storage/Stability

Store hydrogen peroxide 3% solutions in airtight containers at controlled room temperature between 15°C to 30°C (59°F-86°F) and protected from light. If hydrogen peroxide is allowed to become alkaline or it comes into contact with oxidizable organic matter, it will decompose. Do not shake bottle.

Hydrogen peroxide 3% solution can deteriorate with time; outdated or improperly stored products may not be effective as an emetic.

Compatibility/Compounding Considerations

No specific information noted. Any compounded emetic for home use should be made from hydrogen peroxide 3% solution and not stronger concentrations.

Dosage Forms/Regulatory Status

VETERINARY-LABELED PRODUCTS:

Hydrogen peroxide 3% solution in 473 mL bottles and 3.8 L (1 gallon) jugs; generic; (OTC). Not reviewed or approved by the FDA

HUMAN-LABELED PRODUCTS:

Hydrogen peroxide 3% solution is readily available OTC from a variety of manufacturers. Not reviewed or approved by the FDA. It is usually sold in pint bottles.

References

For the complete list of references, see **wiley.com/go/budde/plumb**

Hydromorphone

(hye-droe-***mor***-fone) *Dilaudid®*

Opioid Agonist

Prescriber Highlights

- ► Injectable opioid used as a sedative/restraining agent, analgesic, and preanesthetic agent. May be used as an emetic
- ► Adverse effects in dogs include nausea, vomiting, defecation, panting, vocalization, and sedation. CNS depression, respiratory depression, and bradycardia are possible; decreased GI motility with resultant constipation may occur with chronic use.
- ► Nausea is a common adverse effect in cats. Ataxia, hyperesthesia, hyperthermia, and behavior changes (without concomitant tranquilization) are also possible.
- ► Many drug interactions are possible.
- ► DEA Schedule II controlled substance

Uses/Indications

Hydromorphone is used in dogs and cats as a sedative/restraining agent, analgesic, and preanesthetic agent. Hydromorphone may be useful as an analgesic in horses and other species. In dogs, equipotent doses of hydromorphone and morphine cause similar degrees of sedation.[1] In dogs and cats, hydromorphone usually causes minimal histamine release after IV administration, and rarely causes vasodilation or hypotension. Hydromorphone may be useful as an emetic, but this effect may be more reliable in cats than in dogs.[2]

Pharmacology/Actions

Opioid receptors are found in high concentrations in the limbic system, spinal cord, thalamus, hypothalamus, striatum, and midbrain. The GI tract, urinary tract, and other smooth muscle tissue also contain opioid receptors.

Hydromorphone is ≈5 times more potent an analgesic on a per weight basis as compared with morphine and similar in potency as compared with oxymorphone. Morphine-like agonists (eg, morphine, meperidine, fentanyl, oxymorphone, hydromorphone) have primary activity at mu receptors and some activity at delta receptors. The precise mechanism of action is unknown but appears to reduce neuronal excitability in the CNS.

Primary pharmacologic effects include analgesia, antitussive activity, respiratory depression, sedation, physical dependence, and intestinal effects (eg, emesis, constipation/defecation, reduced secretions). Analgesic effects in dogs and cats begin ≈1 to 5 minutes after IV injection and usually persist for 2 to 4 hours, depending on dose and pain severity. Duration of analgesia has not been shown to correlate with plasma hydromorphone concentration in cats[3] or horses.[4]

Secondary pharmacologic effects include:

CNS: Euphoria, sedation, and confusion; excitatory effects (ie, disinhibition) can occur, possibly through reduction in the release of inhibitory neurotransmitters (eg, gamma-aminobutyric acid [GABA]), and may be mediated by a glucuronide metabolite.

Cardiovascular: Bradycardia due to central vagal stimulation, peripheral vasodilation from depressed alpha-adrenergic receptors but not histamine release,[5] decreased peripheral resistance, and baroreceptor inhibition. Orthostatic hypotension and syncope may occur.

Urinary: Increased bladder sphincter tone can induce urinary retention.

Endocrine: Inhibited secretion of glucagon, insulin, somatostatin, and vasopressin. Hydromorphone administered to healthy dogs after mask induction reduced isoflurane minimum alveolar concentration (MAC) by 33% to 50% for up to 4.5 hours after administration.[6]

Various species may exhibit contradictory effects from hydromorphone. For example, horses, cattle, swine, and cats may develop excitement, and dogs may defecate after hydromorphone injections. These effects are in contrast to the expected effects of sedation and constipation. Dogs and humans may develop miosis, and other species, particularly cats, may develop mydriasis.

Hydromorphone-associated sedation in dogs is often reported as an attribute/adverse effect (see ***Adverse Effects***). A prospective, randomized, blinded, controlled trial found that clinically normal dogs receiving hydromorphone (alone) 0.1 mg/kg IM did not have significantly higher sedation scores as compared with placebo, whereas acepromazine (alone) and acepromazine/hydromorphone caused significant levels of sedation.[7]

Respiratory depression can occur, especially in debilitated, neonatal, or geriatric patients. Bradycardia, slight decrease in cardiac contractility, and/or decrease in blood pressure may occur. Like oxymorphone, hydromorphone initially increases respiratory rates (panting in dogs), and oxygenation may decrease and blood CO_2 concentrations may increase by 10 mm Hg or more. Gut motility decreases with resultant increases in gastric emptying times. Unlike morphine or meperidine, IV hydromorphone rarely causes mild histamine release in dogs or cats. Unlike morphine and fentanyl, hydromorphone does not appear to affect the immune system or stimulate the hypothalamic-pituitary-adrenal (HPA) axis or cortisol release.[8]

Horses have marked variation in response. Opioids can induce eating behavior at low doses and dose-dependent locomotor activity with incoordination at high doses.[9]

Pharmacokinetics

Hydromorphone is absorbed via IM, SC, and rectal routes. It is rapidly absorbed following oral administration, but extensive first-pass metabolism limits bioavailability. Peak concentrations occur 10 to 30 minutes after SC administration in dogs. The volume of distribution in dogs is high (more than 4 L/kg) with IV and SC administration.[1] In a study of cats, bioavailability was 22% following buccal (OTM) administration.[10] Protein binding is negligible.

Hydromorphone is metabolized in the liver by glucuronidation. The terminal half-life is short and appears to be route- and dose-dependent; half-life in dogs receiving 0.1 mg/kg IV is ≈30 to 50 minutes and ≈60 to 80 minutes at higher doses (0.2 – 0.5 mg/kg IV)[1,11], and SC dosing extends half-life ≈10% to 15%.[11] In a study of cats, elimination half-life was 99 minutes,[3] possibly due to reduced capacity for glucuronidation. The glucuronidated metabolite is excreted by the kidneys.

After IM administration (0.04 mg/kg) in horses, bioavailability was high.[12] Volume of distribution is 1.1 – 2.2 L/kg, and clearance is 66-92 mL/minute/kg.[4,12] In horses receiving IV hydromorphone, elimination half-life appeared to be dose-dependent: 0.01 mg/kg, 18.1 minutes; 0.04 mg/kg, 34 minutes; 0.08 mg/kg, 41 minutes.[4] After IM administration (0.04 mg/kg), elimination half-life was 27 minutes.[12]

Contraindications/Precautions/Warnings

Hydromorphone is contraindicated in patients hypersensitive to it or other narcotic analgesics and in patients that have significant respiratory depression, asthma, or other airway hyperresponsiveness. Due to the adverse effect of vomiting, hydromorphone as a preanesthetic medication in animals with suspected gastric dilatation volvulus, ileus, or intestinal obstruction is usually considered contraindicated. Opioid analgesics are contraindicated in patients that have been stung by the scorpion species *Centruroides sculpturatus Ewing* or *C gertschi Stahnke*, as they may potentiate the scorpion's venom.[13] Hydromorphone is generally considered contraindicated in humans if a monoamine oxidase inhibitor (MAOI; eg, selegiline) has been used in the past 14 days due to unpredictable CNS effects with concurrent therapy.

Hydromorphone should be used with extreme caution in patients with head injuries, increased intracranial and ocular pressure, or deep corneal ulcers, as reduced respiration and resulting CO_2 retention may exacerbate the underlying conditions. Hydromorphone should also be used with extreme caution in patients suffering from respiratory disease or acute respiratory dysfunction (eg, pulmonary edema secondary to smoke inhalation). However, opioids may be used in animals that are anesthetized and ventilated. Consider having a narcotic antagonist (eg, naloxone) readily available if use of hydromorphone in high-risk patients cannot be avoided. Use with caution in animals with acute abdominal conditions (eg, colic), as it may obscure the diagnosis or clinical course of these conditions.

Opioids should be used with caution in patients with hypothyroidism, seizure disorders, hypotension, and/or hypoadrenocorticism (Addison's disease). Opioids should also be used with caution in patients with moderate to severe hepatic or renal insufficiency, and a dose reduction of 25% to 50% is recommended in humans with hepatic or renal impairment. All opioids should be avoided in patients with diarrhea caused by a toxic ingestion until the toxin is eliminated from the GI tract.

Hydromorphone can cause bradycardia and therefore should be used cautiously in patients with pre-existing bradyarrhythmias. Hypotension resulting in decreased cardiac output can occur with hydromorphone.

Neonatal, debilitated, or geriatric patients may be more susceptible to the effects of hydromorphone and may require lower dosages.

Hyperthermia has been reported in cats with hydromorphone use, and some recommend avoiding use in cats.[14-16] If hydromorphone is used in cats at high dosages, it has been recommended to give concurrently with a tranquilizing agent (eg, acepromazine), as hydromorphone can produce unpredictable behavior changes in this species.

For humans, there is an FDA black-box warning to emphasize the risk for respiratory depression, abuse, and medication errors associated with prescribing hydromorphone.

Hydromorphone may impair the performance of service or working dogs.

Adverse Effects

Hydromorphone has an adverse effect profile that is similar to oxymorphone and morphine in dogs and cats. In dogs, vomiting, sedation, panting, whining/vocalization, and defecation can be noted. Studies in dogs have concluded that hydromorphone-induced vomiting can be prevented by maropitant (SC given 15 to 45 minutes prior or PO given at least 2 hours prior to hydromorphone).[17-21] Vomiting, nausea, and defecation may occur more frequently after SC administration as compared with IV administration. CNS depression may be greater than desired, particularly when treating moderate to severe pain. In dogs, CRIs administered at greater than 0.05 mg/kg/hour IV for more than 12 hours may cause sedation and adverse effects severe enough to require reducing the rate.[14] In a study, acupuncture at pericardium 6 reduced the incidence of vomiting in dogs receiving hydromorphone.[22]

Dose-related respiratory depression is possible and more likely to occur with general anesthesia. Panting may occur more often with hydromorphone than with oxymorphone. Cough suppression can occur and may be a benefit of therapy.

Hydromorphone can cause bradycardia secondary to enhanced vagal tone to the same degree as with morphine, and can be treated with an anticholinergic (eg, atropine, glycopyrrolate). QT interval prolongation has been documented in dogs.[23]

Hydromorphone may cause histamine release that may be significant in critically ill animals, although this is generally significantly less than what is seen with morphine and usually clinically insignificant.[5]

Constipation is possible with prolonged administration.

In cats, hydromorphone may increase body temperature following anesthesia.[15,24] One study in 8 cats showed that hydromorphone, morphine, butorphanol, and buprenorphine all similarly cause an equivalent increase in body temperature.[24,25] The increased body temperature in all of the experimental treatments was self-limiting, and most returned to normal within 5 hours. No apparent morbidity or mortality was noted. Administration of ketamine or isoflurane in addition to hydromorphone did not produce a clinically relevant increase in body temperature as compared with hydromorphone alone.[25] Naloxone can be used to reverse hydromorphone to rapidly reduce body temperature in cats if hyperthermia occurs. As an alternative, if analgesia is still required, low doses of dexmedetomidine can be administered. One study documented dysphoria in 2 of 6 cats.[16]

Increased heart rate, respiratory rate, and body temperature have been noted in healthy horses given hydromorphone under experimental conditions.[4] Hydromorphone does not appear to increase the incidence of postanesthesia signs of colic in horses.[26]

Reproductive/Nursing Safety

Following hydromorphone exposure in pregnant laboratory animals, reduced postnatal survival, neural tube defects, and skeletal and soft tissue abnormalities were noted.[27] Reduced fertility (both male and female) has been noted in laboratory animals. Hypogonadism has occurred in humans.

Hydromorphone is excreted in breastmilk but minimal effects in the nursing offspring would be expected as oral hydromorphone is poorly bioavailable.

Because safety has not been established in animals, this drug should only be used when the maternal benefits outweigh the potential risks to offspring.

Overdose/Acute Toxicity

Massive overdoses may produce profound respiratory and/or CNS depression in most species. Other effects may include cardiovascular collapse, hypothermia, and skeletal muscle hypotonia. Mania may be seen in cats. Naloxone is the agent of choice in the treatment of respiratory or circulatory depression. In overdoses, naloxone doses may need to be repeated and animals observed closely, as naloxone's effects can diminish before subtoxic concentrations of hydromorphone are attained. Mechanical ventilatory support should be considered in cases of severe respiratory depression.

For patients that have experienced or are suspected to have experienced an overdose, consultation with a 24-hour poison consultation center specializing in providing veterinary-specific information is recommended. For general information related to overdose and toxin exposures, as well as contact information for poison control centers, refer to ***Appendix***.

Drug Interactions

The following drug interactions have either been reported or are theoretical in humans or animals receiving hydromorphone and may be of significance in veterinary patients. Unless otherwise noted, use together is not necessarily contraindicated, but the potential risks should be weighed and additional monitoring performed when appropriate.

- **Anticholinergic Agents** (eg, **atropine, glycopyrrolate**): Medications with anticholinergic properties may increase the risk for urinary retention and constipation when combined with opioids.
- **Antihistamines** (eg, **diphenhydramine, hydroxyzine**): Additive CNS depressant effects possible
- **Benzodiazepines** (eg, **alprazolam, diazepam, midazolam**): Additive CNS and respiratory depressant effects are possible.
- **Buprenorphine**: Concurrent high-concentration buprenorphine and hydromorphone did not provide additive antinociception, and the combination had a shorter duration of effect as compared with high-concentration buprenorphine used alone.[28]
- **Butorphanol**: Butorphanol has been shown to decrease the duration of analgesia in dogs and cats and may be considered a partial antagonist.[29,30]
- **Clopidogrel**: Opioid use may delay and reduce formation of the clopidogrel active metabolite and the drug's antiplatelet effect, possibly by reducing GI motility and drug absorption.
- **Desmopressin**: Opioids may increase the risk for water intoxication or hyponatremia when combined.
- **Diuretics** (eg, **furosemide**): Opioids may decrease efficacy in heart failure patients.
- **Gabapentin**: Additive CNS depressant effects possible
- **Gastrointestinal Agents, Prokinetic** (eg, **metoclopramide, cisapride**): Opioids may antagonize the GI motility effects of these agents.
- **Local Anesthetic Agents** (eg, **bupivacaine, lidocaine, ropivacaine**): Additive cardiorespiratory depressant effects possible
- **Magnesium Sulfate**: The CNS effects of hydromorphone may be increased, more likely with higher magnesium doses or IV magnesium therapy.
- **Monoamine Oxidase Inhibitors** (MAOIs; eg, **amitraz, linezolid, selegiline**): Severe and unpredictable opioid potentiation may be seen; not recommended in humans if MAOIs have been given within 14 days.
- **Ondansetron**: Increased risk for serotonin syndrome
- **Phenobarbital**: Additive CNS depressant effects possible
- **Phenothiazines** (eg, **acepromazine**): Some phenothiazines may antagonize analgesic effects and increase the risk for hypotension.
- **Serotonin Modulators** (eg, **fluoxetine, mirtazapine, trazodone**): CNS depression may occur when combined with hydromorphone and increase the risk for serotonin syndrome.
- **Sevoflurane**: Sevoflurane enhanced hydromorphone-induced QT prolongation in dogs.[23]
- **Skeletal Muscle Relaxants** (eg, **dantrolene, methocarbamol**): Hydromorphone may enhance CNS depressant effects.

- **Succinylcholine**: Opioids combined with succinylcholine may enhance the bradycardic effects of opioids.
- **Trazodone**: Additive CNS depressant effects possible
- **Tricyclic Antidepressants** (eg, **amitriptyline, clomipramine**): Hydromorphone may exacerbate the effects of tricyclic antidepressants.

Laboratory Considerations

- Opioids may increase biliary tract pressure, resulting in increased plasma **amylase** and **lipase** values up to 24 hours following their administration.

Dosages

DOGS:

Analgesic (extra-label): Recommendations vary but are generally 0.05 – 0.2 mg/kg IV, IM, or SC every 2 to 4 hours. May be given as a CRI with an initial dose of 0.025 – 0.05 mg/kg IV followed by 0.03 mg/kg/hour IV CRI[31]

Sedative or premedication prior to painful procedures (extra-label): Used in combination with another agent:

Young, healthy patients:

a) Hydromorphone 0.1 mg/kg in combination with acepromazine 0.02 – 0.05 mg/kg and administered IM, although acepromazine has been used at higher (0.1 mg/kg)[7] and lower doses (0.005 mg/kg).[32]

b) Hydromorphone 0.1 mg/kg IM combined with dexmedetomidine 3.5 µg/kg IM. Injection into the semimembranosus and cervical muscle sites had a faster onset of sedation compared to gluteal and lumbar sites.[33]

Sedative/restraint agent for fractious or aggressive dogs: Hydromorphone 0.1 – 0.2 mg/kg combined with acepromazine 0.05 mg/kg and administered IM. Maximal effect usually reached in ≈15 minutes but waiting another 15 minutes may be necessary in some dogs.

Alternative induction method (especially in critical patients): Hydromorphone 0.05 – 0.2 mg/kg IV slowly to effect, followed by diazepam 0.02 mg/kg IV (do NOT mix together). Endotracheal intubation may be possible after administration; if not, use an induction agent (eg, propofol [IV]; ketamine or alfaxalone [IV or IM]). Controlled ventilation will likely be necessary.[34]

Anesthesia (extra-label):

a) **During surgical sterilization**: Hydromorphone 0.09 mg/kg combined with medetomidine 40 µg/kg and ketamine 4.5 mg/kg and administered IM.[35]

b) Hydromorphone 0.1 mg/kg IV bolus followed by 0.02 – 0.1 mg/kg/hour IV CRI with isoflurane.[36]

Emetic (extra-label): 0.1 mg/kg IM. Apomorphine and ropinirole may be more reliable emetics in dogs.

CATS:

Analgesic (extra-label): Recommendations vary but are generally 0.05 – 0.1 mg/kg IV, IM, or SC every 2 to 6 hours. May be given as an IV CRI with an initial dose of 0.025 mg/kg IV followed by 0.01 – 0.05 mg/kg/hour IV CRI (starting at low end of range).

Sedation (extra-label): Hydromorphone 0.1 mg/kg combined with alfaxalone 1.5 mg/kg and midazolam 0.2 mg/kg and administered IM.[37]

Premedication prior to moderately painful procedures (extra-label):

Young, healthy patients: Hydromorphone 0.1 mg/kg combined with acepromazine 0.05 – 0.2 mg/kg and administered IM

Alternative induction method (especially in critical patients): Hydromorphone 0.05 – 0.2 mg/kg IV slowly to effect, followed by diazepam 0.02 mg/kg IV (do not mix together). Endotracheal intubation may be possible after administration; if not, delivery of an inhalant by facemask will give a greater depth of anesthesia. Positive pressure ventilation will likely be necessary.[34]

Anesthesia (extra-label): Hydromorphone 0.05 – 0.1 mg/kg combined with dexmedetomidine 15 – 20 µg/kg, and ketamine 5 – 8 mg/kg and administered IM.[38,39] Doses at the high end of these ranges have been used for female cats being sterilized.[38] Once intubated, alfaxalone or inhalant anesthesia can be added to maintain general anesthesia as needed for longer procedures.

Epidural (extra-label): 0.05 mg/kg provided analgesia for up to 3 hours in healthy cats without causing hyperthermia.[40]

Emetic (extra-label): 0.1 mg/kg SC; hydromorphone causes less sedation as compared with dexmedetomidine when used as an emetic.[2]

HORSES:

Analgesia (extra-label): 0.04 mg/kg IV or IM.[4,12,41] Analgesia and an increase in thermal threshold persisted for 8 to 12 hours in healthy horses under experimental conditions.[4,12]

Epidural (extra-label): 0.04 mg/kg administered epidurally increased avoidance threshold to noxious stimuli for 250 minutes after administration to 6 healthy horses.[42]

FERRETS:

Analgesic (extra-label):

a) 0.05 – 0.2 mg/kg IV, IM, or SC every 6 to 8 hours[43]

b) 0.05 mg/kg IV loading dose, followed by 0.05 – 0.1 mg/kg per hour IV CRI[43]

SMALL MAMMALS:

Analgesia for moderate to severe pain (extra-label): 0.05 – 0.2 mg/kg SC or IM every 6 to 8 hours[43]

Chinchillas (extra-label): 2 mg/kg SC was effective for short-term analgesia but caused transient decreases in food intake and fecal output.[44]

Rabbits (extra-label): Hydromorphone 0.1 mg/kg combined in the same syringe with dexmedetomidine 5 µg/kg and alfaxalone 5 – 7 mg/kg and administered IM facilitated orotracheal intubation.[45]

REPTILES:

Analgesic (extra-label): Most clinicians recommended dosages are 0.5 – 1 mg/kg SC or IM every 24 hours.

Monitoring

- Respiratory rate and depth, $ETCO_2$, pulse oximetry (SpO_2)
- Heart rate
- CNS level of depression/excitation
- Blood pressure (especially with IV use)
- Analgesic efficacy
- Body temperature

Client Information

- Use injectable hydromorphone in an in-patient setting or with direct veterinary professional supervision.
- Hydromorphone is classified as a schedule II (C-II) controlled drug by the federal Drug Enforcement Agency (DEA). Use of this medication in animals or humans other than those for whom they are prescribed is illegal.

Chemistry/Synonyms

Hydromorphone HCl, a semisynthetic phenanthrene-derivative opioid related to morphine, occurs as a white to off-white, fine, crystalline powder. It is freely soluble in water and very slightly soluble in ethanol. The commercial injection has a pH of 3.5 to 5.5.

Hydromorphone may also be known as dihydromorphinone hydrochloride. *Dilaudid®* is a common trade name.

Storage/Stability

The injection should be stored protected from light at room temperature (20°C-25°C [68°F-77°F]); excursions are permitted between 15°C and 30°C (59°F-86°F). A slight yellowish tint to the solution for injection may occur but does not indicate loss of potency. The injection remains stable for at least 24 hours when mixed with commonly used IV fluids if protected from light.

Hydromorphone tablets should be stored at room temperature (20°C-25°C [68°F-77°F]) in tight, light-resistant containers. Refrigerate suppositories and protect from light.

Hydromorphone is a DEA Schedule II-controlled substance that should be stored in an area that is substantially constructed and securely locked. Follow applicable local, state, and federal rules regarding disposal of unused or wasted controlled drugs.

Compatibility/Compounding Considerations

Compatibility is dependent on factors such as pH, concentration, temperature, and diluent used; specialized references or a hospital pharmacist should be consulted for more specific information.

Hydromorphone injection is **compatible** with commonly used IV fluids (for 24 hours when protected from light at 25°C [77°F]) and with atracurium, atropine, dexmedetomidine, glycopyrrolate, mannitol, metoclopramide, midazolam, ondansetron, potassium chloride, and propofol. Hydromorphone injection mixed in the same syringe with atropine and medetomidine for use as a preoperative agent in dogs prior to sevoflurane or propofol anesthesia has been described.[46]

Hydromorphone is **incompatible** with ampicillin, cefazolin, dantrolene, diazepam, ketamine, pantoprazole, phenobarbital, sodium bicarbonate, and thiopental.

Dosage Forms/Regulatory Status

VETERINARY-LABELED PRODUCTS: NONE

HUMAN-LABELED PRODUCTS:

Hydromorphone HCl Injection: 1 mg/mL in 0.5 mL syringes; 1 mg/mL in 1 mL ampules and syringes; 2 mg/mL in 1 mL vials, ampules, and syringes; 2 mg/mL in 20 mL vials; 4 mg/mL in 1 mL ampules and syringes; 10 mg/mL in 1 mL and 5 mL ampules and syringes; and 10 mg/mL in 50 mL vials; *Dilaudid®*, generic; (Rx, C-II). Preservative-free formulations available

Hydromorphone HCl Oral Tablets: 2 mg, 4 mg, and 8 mg; generic; (Rx, C-II)

Hydromorphone HCl Oral Tablets (extended-release): 8 mg, 12 mg, 16 mg, and 32 mg; generic; (Rx, C-II)

Hydromorphone HCl Oral Liquid: 1 mg/1 mL in 473 mL bottle (may contain sodium metabisulfite); *Dilaudid®*, generic; (Rx, C-II)

Hydromorphone Suppositories: 3 mg; generic; (Rx, C-II)

Report dispensing to state monitoring programs where required.

References

For the complete list of references, see **wiley.com/go/budde/plumb**

Hydroxychloroquine

(hye-***drox***-ee-***klor***-oh-kwin) *Plaquenil®*

Antimalarial; Immunomodulator

Prescriber Highlights

- Oral antimalarial and immunomodulating drug with potential to treat variants of canine lupus erythematosus
- Contraindications include hypersensitivity to it or other 4-aminoquinolones.
- Adverse effect profile is not well established because of lack of experience in veterinary medicine, but may include lethargy, vomiting, diarrhea, and sensitivity to the sun.
- Little clinical experience or published evidence for veterinary use; use with caution

Uses/Indications

There is limited information available on the safety and efficacy of this agent in dogs, but case reports suggest hydroxychloroquine may be useful for treating variants of canine exfoliative cutaneous lupus erythematosus[1,2] and generalized discoid lupus erythematosus.[3] Only a few case reports have been published to date, and while the drug may prove beneficial, its use at present must be considered experimental.

Pharmacology/Actions

Hydroxychloroquine is an orally administered aminoquinoline with antimalarial and immunomodulatory properties. The exact immunomodulatory mechanism is unknown, but it is thought to inhibit neutrophil phagocytosis and superoxide production, chemotaxis, and toll-like receptor (TLR)-9 stimulation. Other actions that may contribute to its effects for treating lupus erythematosus include decreasing ultraviolet light sensitivity, and antiplatelet and antihyperlipidemic effects.

Hydroxychloroquine is active against the erythrocytic forms of chloroquine-sensitive strains of *Plasmodium* spp, but not against exoerythrocytic forms and gametocytes. The drug appears to concentrate in parasite digestive vacuoles; antimalarial activity may result from impairment of the parasite's ability to metabolize and utilize erythrocyte hemoglobin.

Pharmacokinetics

No information was located for dogs. In humans, hydroxychloroquine has an oral bioavailability of 74%. It is extensively metabolized by the liver. Elimination half-life is very long (40 days).

Contraindications/Precautions/Warnings

Hydroxychloroquine is contraindicated in patients hypersensitive to the drug or to other 4-aminoquinoline compounds (eg, amodiaquine, chloroquine). In humans, it is recommended to use hydroxychloroquine with caution in pediatric patients and in patients with pre-existing cardiac abnormalities (eg, cardiomyopathy, rhythm disturbances), psoriasis or other dermatoses, porphyria, myopathy, neuropathy, and renal or hepatic disease. Application of this information to animals is unknown.

Avoid excessive sun exposure in dogs with thin hair coats.

In humans, irreversible retinopathy has been noted, particularly in association with higher dosages, duration of treatment greater than 5 years, concurrent macular disease, and reduced renal function.

Do not confuse hydroxyCHLORoquine with hydroxyUREA or hydroCORTisone.

Adverse Effects

There is not enough clinical experience of this drug's use in dogs to fully characterize an adverse effect profile. In the limited numbers of dogs treated, it generally has been tolerated well. Lethargy and GI effects (eg, vomiting, diarrhea) have been noted.[5]

In humans, common adverse effects include ocular effects (eg, retinal damage), myopathy or neuromyopathy, GI effects (eg, anorexia, diarrhea, nausea, abdominal cramps, vomiting), CNS effects (eg, headache, dizziness, decreased seizure threshold), dermatologic effects, and hypoglycemia. Children appear especially prone to adverse effects. The risk for retinal changes in humans is low when dosages are 6.5 mg/kg per day or less.

Reproductive/Nursing Safety

Hydroxychloroquine readily crosses the placenta. Embryonic death and fetal ophthalmic toxicity (eg, anophthalmia, microphthalmia) have been demonstrated in mice. In humans, when used at antimalarial dosages, the CDC considers the drug safe for use during pregnancy, but it is unknown if it is safe at higher doses. Manufacturers state its use during pregnancy should be avoided except in the suppression or treatment of malaria.

Hydroxychloroquine is excreted into milk. While one source considers the drug compatible with nursing,[6] use cautiously during nursing as pediatric patients appear particularly sensitive to the effects of hydroxychloroquine.

Because safety has not been established in animals, this drug should only be used when the maternal benefits outweigh the potential risks to offspring.

Overdose/Acute Toxicity

Overdoses can be very serious and toxic quinidine-like effects can be noted within 30 minutes of ingestion. Signs of overdose and toxicity in humans include headache, drowsiness, visual disturbances, seizures, severe hypokalemia, rhythm, and conduction disorders (eg, QT prolongation, torsades de pointes, ventricular tachycardia, ventricular fibrillation) followed by sudden, potentially fatal, respiratory and cardiac arrest.

For patients in which the potential hydroxychloroquine overdose is large, consider GI decontamination. Acidification of the urine may increase urinary excretion.

For patients that have experienced or are suspected of having experienced an overdose, consultation with a 24-hour poison consultation center specializing in providing veterinary-specific information is recommended. For general information related to overdose and toxin exposures, as well as contact information for poison control centers, refer to ***Appendix***.

Drug Interactions

The following drug interactions have either been reported or are theoretical in humans or animals receiving hydroxychloroquine and may be of significance in veterinary patients. Unless otherwise noted, use together is not necessarily contraindicated, but weigh the potential risks and perform additional monitoring when appropriate.

- **ANTACIDS** (eg, **aluminum hydroxide, calcium carbonate, magnesium hydroxide**): Reduced hydroxychloroquine absorption may occur; separate dosing by 4 hours.
- **CIMETIDINE**: Potentially increases pharmacological effects of hydroxychloroquine; dosage adjustment may be required.
- **CYCLOSPORINE**: Increased serum levels of cyclosporine possible
- **DAPSONE**: Combination may increase risk for hematologic toxicity
- **DIGOXIN**: Increased digoxin levels and effects possible
- **HEPATOTOXIC DRUGS**: (eg, **androgens, azole antifungals [fluconazole, itraconazole, ketoconazole], estrogens, NSAIDs**): Increased risk for hepatotoxicity
- **HYPOGLYCEMIC AGENTS** (eg, **glipizide, insulin**): Enhanced glucose-lowering effects may occur.
- **KAOLIN**: May reduce hydroxychloroquine absorption; separate dosages by at least 4 hours.
- **METOPROLOL**: Hydroxychloroquine may increase effects.
- **PRAZIQUANTEL**: Reduced praziquantel absorption may occur.
- **QT PROLONGING DRUGS** (eg, **amiodarone, cisapride, sotalol**): May increase risk for QT prolongation
- **RABIES VACCINE**: In human patients, hydroxychloroquine may decrease immune response. Veterinary significance is not known.

Laboratory Considerations

- No specific information noted

Dosages

DOGS:

Adjunctive treatment of canine exfoliative cutaneous lupus erythematosus (extra-label): There is little information available on doses, efficacy, or adverse effects. The following is derived from two case reports of 4 dogs total (German shorthaired pointers [$n = 3$], Chinese crested dog [$n = 1$]): 5 – 10 mg/kg PO once daily.[1,2]

Adjunctive treatment of canine generalized discoid lupus erythematosus (extra-label): From a report on the treatment of 3 dogs that received 5 mg/kg PO once daily along with topical tacrolimus 0.1% ointment applied twice daily, 2 dogs experienced complete remission; the third dog had 75% partial remission.[3]

Monitoring

- Efficacy
- Because there is little information on the safety of this drug in dogs, consider regular monitoring with eye examinations, CBC, serum chemistry profiles (including creatine kinase [CK]).
- Consider ECG and cardiac examinations in dogs with pre-existing cardiac abnormalities.
- Adverse effects include lethargy, GI disturbance, muscle pain, weakness.

Client Information

- Give this medicine with food.
- Not much experience when used in animals, report any side effects to your veterinarian.
- Keep away from children and other animals; overdoses can be very serious.
- While your animal is taking this medication, it is important to return to your veterinarian for examinations and lab work. Do not miss these important follow-up visits.

Chemistry/Synonyms

Hydroxychloroquine is a 4-aminoquinoline antimalarial agent that occurs as a white or practically white, odorless, crystalline powder. It exists in 2 forms: one form (usually used as the pharmaceutical) melts at about 240°C (464°F) and the other form melts at about 198°C (388.4°F). It is freely soluble in water and practically insoluble in alcohol, chloroform, and ether. Solutions in water have a pH of about 4.5. Hydroxychloroquine sulfate is a colorless crystalline solid, soluble in water to at least 20%. Hydroxychloroquine sulfate 200 mg is equivalent to 155 mg hydroxychloroquine.

Hydroxychloroquine sulfate may also be known as WIN-1258-2. A common trade name is *Plaquenil®*.

Storage/Stability

Hydroxychloroquine tablets can be stored at room temperature between 20°C and 25°C (68°F-77°F) in light-resistant containers with child-resistant closures. Medication should be stored out of reach of children and pets.

Compatibility/Compounding Considerations

Tablets may be split. Dogs weighing less than 5 kg (11 lb) require the dosage form to be compounded for accurate dosing (¼ tablet is

≈50 mg; upper end of suggested dosage is 10 mg/kg).

Dosage Forms/Regulatory Status

VETERINARY-LABELED PRODUCTS: NONE

HUMAN-LABELED PRODUCTS:

Hydroxychloroquine Sulfate Oral Tablets: 200 mg; *Plaquenil®*, generic; (Rx). Dosages for animals may need to be compounded.

References

For the complete list of references, see **wiley.com/go/budde/plumb**

Hydroxyethyl Starch (HES) Colloids

Hetastarch

Pentastarch

Tetrastarch

(***hye***-drox-ee ***eth***-il starch) *Hespan®, Vetstarch®*

Colloid Volume Expander

Prescriber Highlights

- Used to treat hypovolemia when colloidal therapy is required
- Contraindicated in patients with heart failure, pulmonary edema, intracranial bleeding, severe bleeding disorders, severe hypernatremia or hyperchloremia, and/or oliguric or anuric renal failure. Caution recommended in patients with thrombocytopenia or severe liver disease and patients undergoing CNS surgery
- May cause volume overload; use with caution in patients with cardiac or renal dysfunction.
- Adverse effects include the following: coagulopathies possible; rapid administration to small animal species (especially cats) may cause nausea and/or vomiting; hypersensitivity reactions are possible but very rare.
- Available hydroxyethyl starch (HES) colloids differ in their molecular weight (MW), degree of substitution, and concentration; nomenclature for these products can be confusing.

Uses/Indications

Hydroxyethyl starch (HES) colloids are used in the adjunctive treatment of hypovolemia and states of low oncotic pressure (ie, hypoalbuminemia) in small and large animal species.[1] They can be used to increase and support colloid osmotic pressure (COP). HES therapy can be considered when crystalloid therapy is not sufficiently improving or maintaining blood volume, when there is a need to prolong the duration of fluid resuscitation effects, or if crystalloids cannot be delivered fast enough to resuscitate a patient. They may also be chosen if edema develops during fluid resuscitation, when hypovolemia is due to blood loss but blood products are not deemed necessary, or to provide oncotic support in patients with decreased oncotic pressure (ie, total protein is less than 3.5 g/dL or albumin is less than 1.5 g/dL) where crystalloid therapy will cause hemodilution and promote further drops in oncotic pressure.[2]

Colloids (in combination with crystalloids) may also be considered in patients with traumatic brain injury.[3,4]

In experimental isoflurane-induced hypotension in dogs, hetastarch administration was found to be superior to lactated Ringer's solution (LRS) for restoration of blood pressure.[5]

In horses, hetastarch may be useful in increasing plasma oncotic pressure and volume expansion in hypoproteinemic conditions (eg, acute colitis); however, it has been shown that plasma may be superior to treat horses with enterocolitis when compared with hetastarch.[6] A study in anesthetized horses found that administration of hetastarch 6% at 2.5 mL/kg IV over 1 hour in combination with LRS failed to attenuate the decrease in COP typically seen during anesthesia with crystalloid administration alone.[7] Hetastarch 10 mL/kg and plasma 10 mL/kg both comparatively increased plasma COP in healthy horses for up to 48 hours.[8]

Pharmacology/Actions

Hydroxyethyl starch (HES) colloid acts as a plasma volume expander by increasing the oncotic pressure within the intravascular space similarly to either dextran or albumin. Maximum volume expansion occurs within a few minutes of the completion of infusion.

Duration of effect is variable but may persist for 24 hours or more for hetastarch (HES 450/0.7)[9] and ≈12 hours for tetrastarch (HES 130/0.4).

Pharmacokinetics

Lower molecular weight (MW) molecules (less than 50 kDa) are rapidly excreted by the kidneys; larger molecules are slowly degraded enzymatically to a size where they then can be excreted.[9] In a human pharmacokinetic study, 33% of a single 500 mL dose of 6% hydroxyethyl starch (HES) colloids 450/0.7 was excreted in the first 24 hours after infusion and after 2 weeks, more than 90% of the drug was excreted. In hypoproteinemic horses, colloidal pressure may be increased up to 24 hours after dosing. A study in healthy llamas found that administration of 15 mL/kg of HES 450/0.7 during a 60-minute IV infusion significantly increased plasma COP for 96 hours.[10]

Contraindications/Precautions/Warnings

The veterinary-labeled product (6% hydroxyethyl starch [HES] colloid 130/0.4) lists the following contraindications: known hypersensitivity to hydroxyethyl starch, fluid overload (eg, pulmonary edema, congestive heart failure), renal failure with oliguria or anuria not related to hypovolemia, patients receiving dialysis treatment, severe hypernatremia or hyperchloremia, or intracranial bleeding.[1] In severely dehydrated patients a crystalloid solution should be given prior to HES administration.[1]

Because of the danger of volume overload, use of HES for the treatment of shock that is not accompanied by hypovolemia or in the face of renal dysfunction or cardiac insufficiency may be hazardous. Additionally, administration of HES to animals with sepsis, systemic inflammatory response syndrome (SIRS), or severe trauma may cause extravasation of fluids into the lungs to cause or worsen pulmonary edema. See ***Monitoring***.

It is believed that significant bleeding can occur if HES colloids are used in animals with compromised coagulation systems (eg, von Willebrand disease, severe liver disease, thrombocytopenia), and therefore should be used with caution in these patients.[1,11,12] Because of their effect on platelets, HES should also be used with extreme caution in patients undergoing CNS surgery.

As they have no oxygen carrying capacity, HESs are not a replacement for whole blood or red blood cells.

In humans, there is a risk for acute kidney injury (AKI) with HES, particularly in acute sepsis patients.[9,13] The risk for AKI in animals remains under investigation.[14-17]

Nomenclature for these products can be confusing. Be certain when using HES products that you are familiar with the specific product and its respective cautions and uses. See ***Chemistry/Synonyms***.

Adverse Effects

Hydroxyethyl starch (HES) colloids can affect platelet function and coagulation times and alter factor VIII and von Willebrand factor. At recommended dosages, HES may cause changes in clotting times and platelet counts due to direct (precipitation of factor VIII) and dilutional causes.[1,9] A retrospective study in dogs showed that hetastarch can significantly increase PTT, but did not affect patient survival rates.[18] Tetrastarch did not impair primary hemostasis and induced transient dilutional coagulopathy comparable with lactated Ringer's solution in hemorrhaged dogs.[19] Clinically, all these effects may be insignificant, but patients with pre-existing coagulopathies or severe liver disease may be predisposed to further bleeding. Dosages of HES 450/0.7 exceeding 20 mL/kg/day are more likely to cause coagulation abnormalities.[11,20] Potentially, tetrastarch (HES 130/0.4) may have less effect on coagulation than hetastarch (HES 450/0.7 or HES 670/0.75). One in vitro study found that HES 130/0.4 affected canine platelet function, but the authors concluded that the clinical relevance of these in vitro findings is not obvious.[21] Another study found that HES 200/0.5, but not HES 130/0.4, significantly increased platelet closure time beyond the dilutional effect.[22] An in vivo study in dogs found that HES 670/0.75 at clinically relevant dosages prolonged closure time for up to 24 hours.[23]

HESs are less antigenic than dextrans, but they can cause sensitivity reactions and interfere with antigen-antibody testing. Anaphylactic reactions and severe coagulopathies can occur.[1] Pruritus has been observed in dogs.

When it is given via rapid infusion to cats, hetastarch may cause signs of nausea and vomiting[24]; if administered over 15 to 30 minutes, these signs are eliminated.

Circulatory overload leading to pulmonary edema is possible, particularly when large doses are administered to patients with diminished cardiac or renal function.[1] Do not give HES intramuscularly, as bleeding, bruising, or hematomas may occur.

When HES infusions are stopped, colloid that has leaked into interstitial spaces can pull additional fluid from the intravascular space.[25]

Administration of HES can cause hemodilution with resulting decreases in hematocrit and plasma protein concentration.[1]

Reproductive/Nursing Safety

Hydroxyethyl starch colloid (HES) 130/0.4 was not teratogenic in rabbits or rats, but embryolethality and fetal retardation have been observed.[1] It is not known whether HES are excreted in milk.[9]

Because safety has not been established in animals, this drug should only be used when the maternal benefits outweigh the potential risks to offspring.

Overdose/Acute Toxicity

An overdose could result in volume overload (eg, pulmonary edema) in susceptible patients. Monitor fluid status carefully. In case of volume overload, the infusion should be stopped immediately and, if necessary, a diuretic should be administered.[1]

For patients that have experienced or are suspected to have experienced an overdose, consultation with a 24-hour poison consultation center specializing in providing veterinary-specific information is recommended. For general information related to overdose and toxin exposures, as well as contact information for poison control centers, refer to ***Appendix***.

Drug Interactions

The following drug interactions have either been reported or are theoretical in humans or animals receiving HES colloids and may be of significance in veterinary patients. Unless otherwise noted, use together is not necessarily contraindicated, but weigh the potential risks and perform additional monitoring when appropriate.

- ANTICOAGULANTS (eg, **heparins, rivaroxaban, warfarin**): High doses of hydroxyethyl starch colloid (HES) may increase risk for bleeding; use together with caution
- ANTI-PLATELET AGENTS (eg, **aspirin, clopidogrel**): High doses of HES may increase risk for bleeding; use together with caution
- ANGIOTENSIN CONVERTING ENZYME INHIBITORS (ACEIs; eg, **enalapril**): Potential for increased serum potassium if used with HES in lactated electrolytes; increased monitoring warranted
- ANGIOTENSIN RECEPTOR BLOCKERS (ARBs; eg, **irbesartan, telmisartan**): Potential for increased serum potassium if used with HES in lactated electrolytes; increased monitoring warranted
- POTASSIUM-SPARING DIURETICS (eg, **spironolactone**): Potential for increased serum potassium if used with HES in lactated electrolytes; increased monitoring warranted
- CEFTRIAXONE: In human neonates, use with calcium-containing IV fluids (eg, HES in lactated Ringer's solution) is contraindicated.

Laboratory Considerations

- Administration of 6% hydroxyethyl starch colloid (HES) 130/0.4 in dogs has been found to cause an overestimation of total plasma protein when assessed via refractometry for at least 3 hours after treatment.[26]
- HES can falsely elevate **urine specific gravity** in dogs.[27]
- In humans, **serum amylase** concentrations may be increased for 3 to 5 days and interfere with pancreatitis diagnosis.[9]
- Increased **indirect bilirubin** concentration has been observed in humans for up to 96 hours following infusion of HES 450/0.7.
- At high doses, the dilutional effects may result in decreased concentrations of **coagulation factors**, other **plasma proteins,** and a decrease in **hematocrit.**[1,9]

Dosages

NOTE: Rate of administration is determined by individual patient requirements (ie, blood volume, indication, and patient response); adequate monitoring for successful treatment of shock is mandatory. The initial 10 – 20 mL should be infused slowly, keeping the patient under close observation due to possible anaphylactic-like reactions.[1] See ***Monitoring***. The following dosages should be used as general guidelines for treatment.

DOGS/CATS:

Plasma volume substitute: The daily dose and rate of infusion depend on the patient's blood loss, on the maintenance or restoration of hemodynamics, and on the hemodilution (dilution effect); can be administered repetitively over several days. The following dosages should be used as general guidelines for treatment.

a) **Using 6% HES 130/0.4 | *Vetstarch*®** (label dosage; not FDA-approved): As a general recommendation, up to 20 mL/kg/day in small animal patients[1]

b) **Using 6% HES 450/0.7 | *Hespan*®** (extra-label): Recommenations vary somewhat. In general, shock bolus (resuscitation): 10 – 20 mL/kg in dogs and 5 – 10 mL/kg in cats IV usually over 15 to 30 minutes. A CRI can follow at 1 – 2 mL/kg/hour IV; not to exceed 20 mL/kg/day (some clinicians recommend not exceeding 10 mL/kg/day in cats).

HORSES:

Plasma volume substitute (extra-label):

Adult horses:

a) 3 – 10 mL/kg IV bolus using hetastarch or tetrastarch. Total daily doses of 10 mL/kg should not be exceeded due to risk for coagulopathies.[28]

b) 10 mL/kg/hour IV bolus OR 8 – 10 mL/kg/day IV; maximum of 10 mL/kg/day[29]

c) 0.5 – 1 mL/kg/hour IV CRI; maximum of 10 mL/kg/day[29]

Neonatal foals: From a study using healthy foals, tetrastarch 20 mL/kg IV increased colloid osmotic pressure for up to 3 hours post-infusion.[30]

CAMELIDS:

Plasma volume substitute (extra-label): A study done in healthy llamas showed that 15 mL/kg IV significantly increased colloid oncotic pressure for up to 96 hours. Transient, mild hemodilution, and mild increases in PT and PTT were noted.[10]

BIRDS:

Plasma volume substitute (extra-label): 10 – 15 mL/kg IV over 20 to 40 minutes, up to 4 times daily, OR 10 – 15 mL/kg bolus over 20 to 40 minutes followed by 1 – 2 mL/kg/hour IV CRI. Recommended maximum dosage is 20 mL/kg/day, but the author notes that she has exceeded this dosage with no adverse effects noted.[31]

Small volume replacement/CPCR resuscitation (extra-label): For debilitated patients in shock, administer hypertonic saline 3 – 5 mL/kg IV over 5 minutes, followed by hetastarch 3 – 5 mL/kg IV over 5 minutes. Follow with small boluses of crystalloid fluids (eg, lactated Ringer's solution, *Plasma-Lyte*® 15 – 20 mL/kg IV) in combination with hetastarch 3 – 5 mL/kg IV over 15 minutes and reassess the bird every 15 minutes. The crystalloids and hetastarch can be combined in the same syringe or fluid bag. This process is repeated every 15 to 20 minutes until temperature normalizes and blood pressure is over 120 mm Hg.[31]

Monitoring

- Hydration status and signs of fluid overload (eg, increased respiratory rate and effort, pulmonary edema)[1]
- Clinical signs of anaphylactic-like reactions, including worsening signs of shock and pruritus
- Renal chemistry panel and urine output[1]
- Serum electrolytes, acid-base balance[1]
- Colloid oncotic pressure
- Blood pressure, central venous pressure
- Coagulation parameters particularly in high-risk patients or when using high doses of hydroxyethyl starch colloid (HES)[1]

Client Information

- As these fluids are used in an inpatient setting only, factors to consider when communicating with owners are the drug's cost, the reasons for using colloid therapy, and potential adverse effects of therapy.

Chemistry/Synonyms

A synthetic polymer derived from a waxy starch, hydroxyethyl starch colloid (HES) is composed primarily of amylopectin. Hetastarch occurs as a white powder. It is very soluble in water and insoluble in alcohol.

To avoid degradation by serum amylase, hydroxyethyl ether groups are added to the glucose units. Commercially available HES solutions are classified by their mean molecular weight (MW) and degree of substitution (DS). The DS refers to the average number of hydroxyethyl groups per glucose unit within the branched-chain polymer.

A commonly used HES solution is 6% HES 450/0.7 in 0.9% sodium chloride (*Hespan*®), which has an average MW of 450 kD and a DS of 0.75. Although the average MW is 450 kD, commercial HES solutions contain a wide variation in molecule sizes, ranging from a few thousand to a few million Daltons distributed in a concentration/size ratio that is more or less a bell-shaped curve. The commercially available colloidal solution appears as a clear, pale yellow to amber solution. The 500 mL-commercial preparation (containing 6% HES 450/0.7 and 0.9% sodium chloride) contains sodium 77 mEq and chloride 77 mEq with an osmolality of 310 mOsm/L and a pH of ≈5.5.

The high-MW product 6% HES 670/0.75 in lactated electrolyte solution (*Hextend*®) contains sodium 143 mEq/L, chloride 124 mEq/L, lactate 28 mEq/L, calcium 5 mEq/L, potassium 3 mEq/L, magnesium 0.9 mEq/L, and dextrose 0.99 g/L. These values approximate what is found in human plasma.

The low-MW product 6% HES 130/0.4 in 0.9% sodium chloride (*Vetstarch*®, *Voluven*®) has an average MW of 130 kD, a DS of 0.4 (range 0.38-0.45), and a pH of 4 to 5.5. Each 500 mL bag contains sodium 77 mEq and chloride 77 mEq. Calculated osmolarity is 308.

Pentastarch 10% in 0.9% sodium chloride (*Pentaspan*®) MW ranges from 200 to 300 kD, has a DS range of 0.4 to 0.5, and a pH of ≈5. Calculated osmolarity is 326.

Hetastarch may also be known by the following synonyms: etherified starches, synthetic colloid, HES, and hydroxyethyl starch; many trade names are available.

Storage/Stability

Hetastarch 6% in 0.9% sodium chloride or lactated electrolyte should be stored at room temperature (15°C-25°C [59°F-77°F]); freezing and excessive heat should be avoided. Exposure to temperature extremes may result in formation of a crystalline precipitate or a color change to a turbid deep brown; do not use this product if this occurs.[9]

Compatibility/Compounding Considerations

Compatibility is dependent on factors such as pH, concentration, temperature, and diluent used; specialized references or a hospital pharmacist should be consulted for more specific information.

The following drugs are reported **compatible** at Y-sites with hetastarch (6% HES 450/0.7 in 0.9% sodium chloride): cimetidine, diltiazem, enalaprilat, and ertapenem. For *Hextend*®: Do not administer this product simultaneously with blood products through the same administration set, as there is a risk for coagulation.

Dosage Forms/Regulatory Status

VETERINARY-LABELED PRODUCTS:

The Association of Racing Commissioners International (ARCI) has designated plasma expanders including hydroxyethyl starch colloid (HES) as class 3 substances with no legitimate use in racehorses. Use of this drug may not be allowed in certain animal competitions. Check rules and regulations before entering in a competition while this medication is being administered. Contact local racing authorities for further guidance. See the ***Appendix*** for more information.

Tetrastarch Injection: 6% (6 g/100 mL) HES 130/0.4 in 0.9% sodium chloride injection in 250 mL and 500 mL polyolefin bags; *Vetstarch*®[1]; (Rx). This product is not FDA-approved for use in animals, but the label information has been approved by FDA.

HUMAN-LABELED PRODUCTS:

Hetastarch Injection 6% (6 g/100 mL) HES 450/0.7 in 0.9% sodium chloride in 500 mL IV infusion bottles, polyolefin bags, and single-dose containers; *Hespan*®; generic; (Rx)

Hetastarch Injection 6% (6 g/100 mL) HES 670/0.75 in lactated electrolyte in 500 mL IV infusion single-dose containers; *Hextend*®, generic; (Rx)

Tetrastarch Injection: 6% (6 g/100 mL) HES 130/0.4 in 0.9% sodium chloride in 500 mL polyolefin bags; *Voluven*®; (Rx). In some countries (not in the United States): Pentastarch 10% in 0.9% sodium chloride in 250 mL and 500 mL plastic bags; *Pentaspan*®; (Rx)

References

For the complete list of references, see **wiley.com/go/budde/plumb**

Hydroxyurea

(hye-*drox*-ee-yor-*ee*-a) *Hydrea®, Droxia®, Mylocel®*
Antineoplastic

Prescriber Highlights

- ▶ Used for the treatment of polycythemia vera, mast cell tumor, meningioma, and leukemias in dogs and cats
- ▶ Use with caution in patients that have anemia, myelosuppression, history of urate stones, infection, impaired renal function, or in patients receiving other chemotherapy or radiotherapy.
- ▶ Adverse effects include myelosuppression, GI-related (eg, anorexia, vomiting, diarrhea), stomatitis, sloughing of nails, alopecia, and dysuria.
- ▶ Proven teratogen; the National Institute for Occupational Safety and Health (NIOSH) classifies hydroxyurea as a hazardous drug; use appropriate precautions when handling it.

Uses/Indications

Hydroxyurea may be useful in the treatment of polycythemia vera, mast cell tumors, meningioma (as a single agent or combined with radiation therapy),[1,2] and leukemias in dogs and cats. A prospective, open-label study in dogs with mast cell tumors found an overall response rate of 28%.[3] It has also been used to treat dogs with chronic myelogenous leukemia that is no longer responsive to busulfan, and for the adjunctive medical treatment (to reduce hematocrit) of right to left shunting patent ductus arteriosus or tetralogy of Fallot. Hydroxyurea may also be of benefit in the treatment of feline hypereosinophilic syndrome.[4]

Pharmacology/Actions

Although the exact mechanism of action for hydroxyurea has not been determined, it appears to interfere with DNA synthesis without interfering with RNA or protein synthesis. Hydroxyurea apparently inhibits thymidine incorporation into DNA and may directly damage DNA. It is an S-phase inhibitor but may also arrest cells at the G_1-S border.

Hydroxyurea inhibits urease but is less potent than acetohydroxamic acid. Hydroxyurea can stimulate the production of fetal hemoglobin.

Pharmacokinetics

In humans, hydroxyurea is well absorbed after oral administration, reaching C_{max} in 1 to 4 hours. It crosses the blood–brain barrier and has a volume of distribution similar to total body water. Approximately 50% of an absorbed dose is excreted unchanged in the urine, and about 50% is metabolized in the liver and then excreted in the urine.

Contraindications/Precautions/Warnings

Risk versus benefit should be considered before using hydroxyurea in patients with the following conditions: anemia, bone marrow depression, history of urate stones, current infection, impaired renal function, or in patients that have received previous chemotherapy or radiotherapy (resulting in bone marrow dysfunction).

The National Institute for Occupational Safety and Health (NIOSH) classifies hydroxyurea as a hazardous drug; personal protective equipment (PPE) should be used accordingly to minimize the risk for exposure.

Do not confuse hydroxyUREA with hydroxyZINE, hydroxychloroquine, or hydrochlorothiazide.

Adverse Effects

Potential adverse effects include GI effects (eg, anorexia, vomiting, diarrhea), stomatitis, sloughing of nails,[5] alopecia, and dysuria. Many dogs receiving chemotherapy will have minor hair coat changes (eg, shagginess, loss of luster). Breeds with continuously growing hair coats (eg, poodles, terriers, Afghan hounds, or old English sheepdogs) are more likely to experience significant alopecia. Although hydroxyurea can cause vomiting, it is usually not severe. In humans, the most serious adverse effects associated with hydroxyurea are myelosuppression (eg, anemia, thrombocytopenia, leukopenia) and pulmonary fibrosis. If myelotoxicity occurs, it is recommended to halt therapy until values return to normal.

Macrocytosis has been reported in a dog receiving hydroxyurea therapy.[6]

In a case series of cats treated for primary erythrocytosis, 3 of 10 cats that were treated with hydroxyurea developed methemoglobinemia.[7] These cats had received hydroxyurea at greater than 100 mg/kg per dose, with clinical signs (eg, dyspnea, tachypnea, and cyanosis) seen after administration of the first dose.

Reproductive/Nursing Safety

Hydroxyurea is a teratogen. Use only during pregnancy when the benefits to the mother outweigh the risks to the offspring. Hydroxyurea can suppress gonadal function; the arrest of spermatogenesis has been noted in dogs. For sexually intact patients, verify pregnancy status prior to administration.

Hydroxyurea is distributed into milk, and nursing puppies or kittens should receive milk replacer when the dam is receiving hydroxyurea.

Overdose/Acute Toxicity

The reported LD_{50} in dogs following PO and IV administration was greater than 2 g/kg and greater than 1 g/kg, respectively. Cats given hydroxyurea in doses greater than 500 mg (total) may develop methemoglobinemia.

The most common clinical signs associated with an overdose include vomiting, ataxia, methemoglobinemia, tachycardia, lethargy, and hypothermia.

Because of the potential toxicity of the drug, overdoses should be treated aggressively with GI decontamination protocols employed when possible. Acetylcysteine or methylene blue (not for cats) has been suggested for treating methemoglobinemia.[8] For patients that have experienced or are suspected to have experienced an overdose, consultation with a 24-hour poison consultation center specializing in providing veterinary-specific information is recommended. For general information related to overdose and toxin exposures, as well as contact information for poison control centers, refer to ***Appendix***.

Drug Interactions

The following drug interactions have either been reported or are theoretical in humans or animals receiving hydroxyurea and may be of significance in veterinary patients. Unless otherwise noted, use together is not necessarily contraindicated, but weigh the potential risks and perform additional monitoring when appropriate.

- Immunosuppressive Agents (eg, **glucocorticoids, leflunomide**): Additive immunosuppressant effects may increase the risk for infection.
- Myelosuppressive Agents (eg, **other antineoplastics, chloramphenicol, iron chelators**): Concurrent use with other myelosuppressive medications may result in additive myelosuppression; avoid combination when possible.
- Vaccines (live and inactivated): Hydroxyurea may diminish vaccine efficacy and enhance adverse effects of vaccines.

Laboratory Considerations

- Hydroxyurea may raise serum **uric acid** concentrations; drugs such as allopurinol may be required to control hyperuricemia.

Dosages

NOTE: Hydroxyurea is not commonly used in veterinary medicine, and published dosage recommendations can vary widely. Because of the potential toxicity of this drug to patients, veterinary personnel, and clients, and because chemotherapy indications, treatment protocols, monitoring, and safety guidelines often change, the following dosages should be used only as a general guide.[9]

DOGS:

Polycythemia vera (PV) | Chronic myelogenous leukemia | mast cell tumors (extra-label): Dosage recommendations vary considerably. Generally, initial dosages of 30 – 60 mg/kg PO once daily (or divided twice daily) for 1 to 2 weeks (for PV, until hematocrit is below 60%) and then every other day (for PV, taper to lowest effective dosing frequency).[10]

Meningioma (extra-label): 50 mg/kg PO every 48 to 72 hours[1,2,11]

CATS:

PV | Chronic myelogenous leukemia (extra-label): Dosage recommendations vary considerably. Generally, initial dosages of 30 mg/kg PO once daily or 10 – 15 mg/kg PO twice daily for 1 to 2 weeks (for PV, until hematocrit is below 60%) and then every other day (for PV, taper to lowest effective dosing frequency). In one report, the median maintenance dosage for treatment of primary erythrocytosis was 22 mg/kg PO every 48 hours.[7]

Monitoring

NOTE: Cats may require more frequent monitoring than dogs.

- Baseline CBC with platelets followed by periodic evaluation at least every 1 to 2 weeks until stable, then every 3 months
- Baseline BUN and creatinine, then every 3 to 4 months
- Monitor for signs of methemoglobinemia (dyspnea, tachypnea, and cyanosis).

Client Information

- Hydroxyurea is a type of chemotherapy (anticancer). This medicine can be hazardous to other animals and people that come in contact with it. On the day your animal gets the medicine, and then for a few days afterward, handle all bodily waste (ie, urine, feces, litter), blood, or vomit only while wearing disposable gloves. Seal the waste in a plastic bag, then place both the bag and gloves in with the regular trash.
- This medicine affects your animal's ability to fight infection. This effect will be greatest within a few weeks after treatment. Your veterinarian will monitor your animal for this problem. Do not miss important recheck appointments.
- Contact your veterinarian immediately if you see bleeding, bruising, fever (indicating an infection), difficulty breathing, or if your animal becomes tired easily.
- Hydroxyurea can be toxic to the gastrointestinal tract, causing vomiting, diarrhea, ulcers, and stomach upset. Giving the medicine to your animal with food may decrease these side effects.
- Hydroxyurea can cause loss of toenails and fur.
- This medication is considered to be a hazardous drug as defined by the National Institute for Occupational Safety and Health (NIOSH). Talk with your veterinarian or pharmacist about the use of personal protective equipment when handling this medicine.

Chemistry/Synonyms

Structurally similar to urea and acetohydroxamic acid, hydroxyurea occurs as a white, crystalline powder that is freely soluble in water. It is moisture labile.

Hydroxyurea may also be known as hydroxycarbamide, hydroxycarbamidum, NSC-32065, SQ-1089, WR-83799, *Dacrodil*®, *Droxiurea*®, *Hydrea*®, *Droxia*®, *Hydrine*®, *Litalir*®, *Medroxyurea*®, *Neodrea*®, *Onco-Carbide*®, *Oxeron*®, *Siklos*®, and *Syrea*®.

Storage/Stability

Protect hydroxyurea capsules and tablets from light and store at 20°C to 25°C (68°F-77°F); keep bottle tightly closed.

Compatibility/Compounding Considerations

Because of limited available dosage forms, compounded preparations may be necessary to accurately dose small animals.

Compounded preparation stability:

A 40 mg/mL oral suspension has been prepared with eight 500 mg capsules and a 1:1 mixture of *OraSweet*® and *OraPlus*®, or a 1:1 mixture of methylcellulose 1% and simple syrup NF *qs ad* to 100 mL. Suspension is stable for 14 days at room temperature or refrigerated.[12]

Additionally, triturating ten hydroxyurea 500 mg capsules with room temperature water, stirring, filtering, and bringing to a final volume of 50 mL with *Syrpalta*® yields a 100 mg/mL suspension that retains greater than 95% potency for 180 days when stored at 25°C (77°F).[13]

Suspensions of hydroxyurea heated to 41°C (106°F) result in an immediate 40% loss of drug potency. Compounded preparations of hydroxyurea should be protected from light.

Dosage Forms/Regulatory Status

VETERINARY-LABELED PRODUCTS: NONE

HUMAN-LABELED PRODUCTS:

Hydroxyurea Oral Capsules: 200 mg, 300 mg, 400 mg, and 500 mg; *Hydrea*®, *Droxia*®, generic (500 mg only); (Rx)

Hydroxyurea Oral Tablets: 100 mg and 1 g; *Siklos*®; (Rx)

References

For the complete list of references, see **wiley.com/go/budde/plumb**

Hydroxyzine
Hydroxyzine Hydrochloride
Hydroxyzine Pamoate

(hye-***drox***-i-zeen) *Atarax*®, *Vistaril*®

Antihistamine, First-Generation

Prescriber Highlights

- Used principally for antihistaminic, antipruritic, and sedative or tranquilization qualities; should be given on a regular basis when prescribed for adjunctive therapy of atopic dermatitis
- Contraindications include hypersensitivity to hydroxyzine or cetirizine (metabolite of hydroxyzine).
- Caution is advised with narrow-angle glaucoma, hypertension, GI or urinary obstruction, hyperthyroidism, seizures, and cardiovascular disease.
- Sedation is the most common adverse effect. Tremors and/or seizures can occur in dogs (rare); polydipsia, depression, and/or behavioral changes can occur in cats.

Uses/Indications

Hydroxyzine is a first-generation antihistamine that may be useful in dogs, cats, and horses for the adjunctive treatment of histamine-mediated pruritic and allergic conditions (eg, urticaria, insect bite hypersensitivity) and atopic dermatitis. It also has sedative and tranquilization effects. Guidelines for atopic dermatitis treatment in dogs state that antihistamines have modest efficacy; hydroxyzine should be given continuously (ie, daily) as preventive therapy before an acute flare.[1,2]

The response to hydroxyzine, as with other antihistamines in dogs and cats, is individualized and not predictable. One patient may respond to one antihistamine but not another. Better results might be obtained if hydroxyzine is combined with chlorpheniramine, as this combination has been reported to be effective in reducing the clinical signs of canine atopic dermatitis in ≈1 of 3 treated dogs,[3] and pruritus improved by more than 25% in 10 of 17 dogs.[4]

This class of drugs may also be used as adjunctive therapy for mast cell tumors and to prevent local histamine release during surgical excision of mast cell tumors.

Because of its CNS depressant effects, hydroxyzine may also be of benefit as a mild sedative in small animal species.

Pharmacology/Actions

H_1-receptor antagonist antihistamines competitively inhibit histamine H_1 receptors; they do not inactivate or prevent the release of histamine but can prevent histamine's action on the cell. In addition to its antihistaminic effects, hydroxyzine has anticholinergic, sedative, tranquilizing, antispasmodic, local anesthetic, mild bronchodilative, and antiemetic effects.

Pharmacokinetics

In dogs, hydroxyzine (pamoate) has an oral bioavailability of ≈70% but with high interpatient variability. Peak concentrations occur ≈3 hours after administration, and elimination half-life is ≈18 hours. Hydroxyzine is rapidly converted to the active metabolite, cetirizine, which has an elimination half-life of ≈11 hours. Area under the curve (AUC) for cetirizine was ≈10 times that for hydroxyzine.[5]

In a study with 12 horses, peak plasma concentration was reached ≈45 minutes after a single 500 mg oral dose of hydroxyzine hydrochloride was given. Elimination half-life was 7.4 hours. Hydroxyzine AUC was roughly double that of cetirizine.[6]

Contraindications/Precautions/Warnings

Hydroxyzine is contraindicated in patients hypersensitive to it or its active metabolite, cetirizine. Because of its anticholinergic activity, hydroxyzine should be used with caution in patients with prostatic hypertrophy, bladder neck obstruction, severe cardiac failure, angle-closure glaucoma, prolonged QT interval, pulmonary diseases with minimal mucosal secretions, or pyeloduodenal obstruction. Avoid or use with caution in patients with a history of seizures.

Pediatric human patients are more susceptible to the adverse CNS effects of antihistamines; it is recommended to avoid use in neonates.

Hydroxyzine is a vesicant; injections should only be administered IM, preferably into a large muscle. Injection by any other route (eg, IV, SC) is contraindicated in humans.

Do not confuse hydrOXYzine with hydrALAZINE, HYDROmorphone, hydroxychloroquine, or hydroxyurea.

Adverse Effects

The most likely adverse effect associated with hydroxyzine is sedation. In dogs, this is usually mild and transient and may diminish with repeated doses. Antihistamines may cause paradoxical excitement, and fine rapid tremors, whole body tremors, and seizures (rare) are possible in dogs. Anticholinergic effects (eg, dry mouth, urine and fecal retention) are possible.

Local reactions (including significant tissue damage) may occur after administration of hydroxyzine injection. Tissue necrosis and abscesses have occurred after SC injection.

The sedative effects of antihistamines may adversely affect the performance of working dogs and horses.

Reproductive/Nursing Safety

Hydroxyzine crosses the placenta. The drug has been shown to be teratogenic in laboratory animals at doses substantially greater than those used therapeutically.[7] Use during the first trimester of pregnancy is contraindicated in humans.[7]

It is unknown if hydroxyzine enters maternal milk. In breastfeeding women that require an antihistamine, second-generation agents (eg, cetirizine) are preferred.[8]

Because safety has not been established in animals, this drug should only be used when the maternal benefits outweigh the potential risks to offspring.

Overdose/Acute Toxicity

Overdoses would be expected to cause increased sedation and hypotension (possible). Coma and apnea were reported in a dog with a large oral exposure.[9] At high doses, common signs can include lethargy, hyperthermia, tremors, tachycardia, ataxia, and seizures.

Treatment consists of GI decontamination (if ingestion was oral) using standard protocols. Induce emesis if the animal is alert and CNS status is stable. Administration of a saline cathartic and/or activated charcoal may be given after emesis or gastric lavage. Treatment should be performed using supportive therapy based on clinical signs.

For patients that have experienced or are suspected to have experienced an overdose, consultation with a 24-hour poison consultation center specializing in providing veterinary-specific information is recommended. For general information related to overdose and toxin exposures, as well as contact information for poison control centers, refer to ***Appendix***.

Drug Interactions

The following drug interactions have either been reported or are theoretical in humans or animals receiving hydroxyzine and may be of significance in veterinary patients. Unless otherwise noted, use together is not necessarily contraindicated, but weigh the potential risks and perform additional monitoring when appropriate.

- ACETYLCHOLINESTERASE INHIBITORS (eg, **neostigmine, pyridostigmine**): Hydroxyzine may reduce effects of acetylcholinesterase inhibitors.
- ANTICHOLINERGIC AGENTS (eg, **atropine, glycopyrrolate, oxybutynin**): Additive anticholinergic effects may occur when hydroxyzine is used concomitantly with other anticholinergic agents.
- BENZODIAZEPINES (eg, **alprazolam, diazepam, midazolam**): Additive CNS depression may occur.
- CIMETIDINE: Cimetidine increased hydroxyzine serum concentration and area under the curve (AUC) as well as prolonging the duration of IDT wheal suppression in rabbits.[10]
- CNS DEPRESSANT DRUGS, OTHER (eg, **acepromazine, ketamine, methocarbamol, mirtazapine, phenobarbital, trazodone**): Additive CNS depression may occur if hydroxyzine is combined with other CNS depressant medications.
- EPINEPHRINE: Hydroxyzine may inhibit or reverse the vasopressor effects of epinephrine; use norepinephrine or metaraminol instead.
- OPIOIDS (eg, **buprenorphine, fentanyl, hydromorphone, methadone, morphine, tramadol**): Additive CNS depression and anticholinergic effects may occur. In humans, hydroxyzine may have an opioid-sparing effect.
- POTASSIUM SALTS, ORAL: Hydroxyzine may reduce GI motility, which can enhance the ulcerogenic effects of oral solid potassium dosage forms.
- PROKINETIC AGENTS (eg, **cisapride, erythromycin, metoclopramide**): The anticholinergic effects of hydroxyzine may decrease the effects of prokinetic agents.
- QT PROLONGING AGENTS (eg, **amiodarone, cisapride, ondansetron, quinidine, sotalol**): May have additive arrhythmogenic effects
- TRICYCLIC ANTIDEPRESSANTS (eg, **amitriptyline, clomipramine, doxepin**): Additive CNS depression and anticholinergic effects may occur.

Laboratory Considerations

- False increases have been reported in **17-hydroxycorticosteroid** urine values after hydroxyzine use.

- **Intradermal allergy testing (IDT)**: Suppression of IDT results may persist for 3 to 5 days after discontinuation of the drug but was as long as 9 days in some dogs.[11] It is recommended to discontinue hydroxyzine at least 1 to 2 weeks prior to testing in dogs[12] and 7 days in horses.[13]

Dosages

DOGS:

Antipruritic/antihistamine (extra-label): Based on a pharmacokinetic study,[5] 2 mg/kg PO every 12 hours. 3 mg/kg PO twice daily has also been used.[11] Data suggest that increasing dose or frequency of administration would not result in greater histamine inhibition. Antihistamines appear to be more useful when used routinely (ie, before a flare) in dogs with mild atopic dermatitis.[1]

CATS:

Antipruritic/antihistamine (extra-label): 5 – 10 mg/cat (NOT mg/kg) PO every 12 hours; 2 mg/kg PO every 12 hours

HORSES:

Antipruritic/antihistamine (extra-label):

a) 0.5 – 1 mg/kg IM or PO twice daily[14]
b) Using the pamoate salt: 500 mg/horse (NOT mg/kg) PO twice daily[13]

BIRDS:

Pruritus associated with allergies, feather-picking, or self-mutilation (extra-label):

a) 2 mg/kg PO every 8 hours PO; adjust dose to minimize drowsiness and maximize effect[15]
b) 1.5 – 2 mg/4 oz (≈120 mL) of drinking water (NOT mg/kg) PO daily; adjust dose to minimize drowsiness and maximize effect.[15]
c) 2 mg/kg PO every 12 hours[16]

FERRETS:

Antipruritic/antihistamine (extra-label): 2 mg/kg PO 2 or 3 times daily[17,18]

RABBITS:

Antipruritic/antihistamine (extra-label): 2 mg/kg PO every 8 to 12 hours[18]

Monitoring

- Clinical efficacy; trial periods to determine an antihistamine's efficacy are usually 1 to 2 weeks long
- Adverse effects

Client Information

- Antihistamines are normally used on a regular, ongoing basis in animals that respond well to them. Antihistamines work better when used before an animal has been exposed to an allergen or before an allergy flare-up occurs.
- The most common side effect is drowsiness/sleepiness, which may be helpful in some animals.
- Dry mouth, decreased gastrointestinal activity (including constipation), and urine retention (less frequent urinations) are possible.
- This medicine may be given with or without food. If your animal drools, vomits, or acts sick after receiving this medicine on an empty stomach, give with food or a small treat to see if this helps. If vomiting continues, contact your veterinarian.

Chemistry/Synonyms

Hydroxyzine HCl, a piperazine-derivative antihistamine, occurs as a white, odorless powder. It is very soluble in water and freely soluble in alcohol. Hydroxyzine pamoate occurs as a light yellow, practically odorless powder. It is practically insoluble in water or alcohol. Hydroxyzine oral syrup/solution has a pH of 2.8 to 4.3.

Hydroxyzine may also be known as hydroxyzine embonate, hydroxyzine HCl, hydroxyzine pamoate, hydroxyzini HCl, *Atarax®*, *Hyzine®*, *Masmoran®*, *Neucalm®*, *Vistacot®*, *Vistaril®*, or *Vistazine®*.

Storage/Stability

Hydroxyzine oral products should be stored in tight, light-resistant containers at room temperature 20°C to 25°C (68°F-77°F). Hydroxyzine injection should be stored protected from light at room temperature 20°C to 25°C (68°F-77°F) with excursions permitted to 15°C to 30°C (59°F-86°F). Avoid freezing all liquid products.

Compatibility/Compounding Considerations

Compatibility is dependent on factors such as pH, concentration, temperature, and diluent used; consult specialized references or a hospital pharmacist for more specific information.

Hydroxyzine injection has been reported to be physically **compatible** with the following drugs when mixed in syringes: atropine, buprenorphine, butorphanol, diphenhydramine, doxapram, droperidol, fentanyl, glycopyrrolate, hydromorphone, lidocaine, meperidine, metoclopramide, midazolam, morphine, and oxymorphone.

Hydroxyzine injection has been reported to be physically **incompatible** with cefazolin sodium, clindamycin, furosemide, heparin, pantoprazole, penicillin G potassium, phenobarbital, and sodium bicarbonate.

Dosage Forms/Regulatory Status

VETERINARY-LABELED PRODUCTS: NONE

The Association of Racing Commissioners International (ARCI) has designated this drug as a class 2 substance. Use of this drug may not be allowed in certain animal competitions. Check rules and regulations before entering in a competition while this medication is being administered. Contact local racing authorities for further guidance. See ***Appendix*** for more information.

HUMAN-LABELED PRODUCTS:

Hydroxyzine HCl Oral Tablets: 10 mg, 25 mg, and 50 mg; *Atarax®*, generic; (Rx)

Hydroxyzine HCl Oral Syrup/Solution: 10 mg/5 mL (2 mg/mL) in 118 mL and 473 mL bottles (may contain alcohol, propylene glycol, and flavoring); *Atarax®*, generic; (Rx)

Hydroxyzine HCl Injection:25 mg/mL (may contain benzyl alcohol) in 1 mL and 2 mL vials and 50 mg/mL (may contain benzyl alcohol) in 1 mL, 2 mL, and 10 mL vials; generic; (Rx)

Hydroxyzine Pamoate Oral Capsules (equivalent to hydroxyzine HCl): 25 mg, 50 mg, and 100 mg (as pamoate); *Vistaril®*, generic; (Rx)

References

For the complete list of references, see **wiley.com/go/budde/plumb**

Hyoscyamine

(hye-oh-***sye***-ah-meen or hye-***ah***-ska-meen) *Levsin®*

Anticholinergic

Prescriber Highlights

- May be useful for treating hypermotile GI conditions such as irritable bowel syndrome, bradycardia, or AV block in dogs
- Limited use or experience in veterinary medicine
- Based on human data, hyoscyamine is contraindicated in patients with glaucoma, intestinal obstruction, toxic megacolon, intestinal atony, severe ulcerative colitis, obstructive uropathy, or acute hemorrhage.
- Use with caution in patients with renal dysfunction, tachyarrhythmias, cardiac valve disease, congestive heart failure, or myasthenia gravis.
- Adverse effects may include mydriasis, xerostomia, constipation, urinary retention, and xerophthalmia.

Uses/Indications

Although not commonly used in veterinary medicine, hyoscyamine may be useful in dogs as an alternative to other anticholinergic drugs (eg, glycopyrrolate) for treating bradycardia or AV block that is associated with clinical signs when pacemaker implantation is not possible.[1] In dogs, it may also be useful for short-term treatment of hypermotile GI conditions such as chronic idiopathic large bowel disease.[2] It potentially could be useful for treating hypersalivation, urinary spasms, vomiting, or reducing secretions perioperatively; however, little is known regarding safety and efficacy in animals when used for these conditions.

In humans, hyoscyamine is used primarily for its effects in reducing GI tract motility or to decrease pharyngeal, bronchial, and tracheal secretions.[3] It can also be used for acetylcholinesterase inhibitor poisoning.

Pharmacology/Actions

Hyoscyamine is an anticholinergic agent, and the levo-isomer of atropine. Therefore, it is more potent than atropine in its central and peripheral effects. It inhibits acetylcholine at tissues innervated by postganglionic nerves and on smooth muscles that respond to acetylcholine but do not have cholinergic innervation. It does not have action on autonomic ganglia. Pharmacologic effects include dose-related reductions in secretions, GI and urinary tract motility, mydriasis, and increased heart rate.

Pharmacokinetics

No pharmacokinetic data were located for veterinary species. In humans, hyoscyamine is rapidly and nearly completely absorbed after oral or sublingual administration.[3] Extended-release oral dosage forms may have somewhat reduced oral bioavailability. Hyoscyamine is distributed throughout the body, enters the CNS, and crosses the placenta. Hyoscyamine is partially hydrolyzed in the liver to tropic acid and tropine. The majority of the drug is excreted unchanged in the urine. Elimination half-life is about 3.5 hours; about 7 hours for the sustained-release product (*Levsinex®*). Average duration of action in humans is ≈4 to 6 hours.

Contraindications/Precautions/Warnings

Hyoscyamine is contraindicated in patients hypersensitive to it. Patients sensitive to one belladonna alkaloid or derivative may be sensitive to another. In humans, contraindications include glaucoma (narrow or wide angle), unstable cardiac disease in acute hemorrhage, intestinal obstruction, toxic megacolon, intestinal atony, severe ulcerative colitis, obstructive uropathy, or myasthenia gravis.[3]

Use hyoscyamine with caution in patients with renal dysfunction as hyoscyamine elimination may be reduced. Carefully consider use of anticholinergics in patients with tachyarrhythmias, cardiac valve disease, or congestive heart failure.

Do not confuse hyosCYAmine with hyosCINE.

Adverse Effects

Adverse effects can include mydriasis, xerostomia, constipation, urinary retention, tachycardia, and xerophthalmia. Higher doses may cause CNS depression or excitation.

Reproductive/Nursing Safety

There is limited information available on the drug's use during pregnancy. Although hyoscyamine crosses the placenta, reproductive studies in animals have not been performed. Two limited studies (322 and 281 pregnancies) in humans have been published evaluating hyoscyamine safety during pregnancy. One study showed no increase in congenital malformations, but the other showed a slight increase above normally expected malformations in infants.

Only traces of hyoscyamine are detected in milk. Although no problems have been reported, risk to offspring cannot be ruled out.

Because safety has not been established in animals, this drug should only be used when the maternal benefits outweigh the potential risks to offspring.

Overdose/Acute Toxicity

The LD_{50} for hyoscyamine in rats is 375 mg/kg.[3] Significant overdoses in animals may be serious and contacting an animal poison control center is advised. Toxicity is exhibited by intensified and prolonged anticholinergic effects including tachycardia, CNS effects (behavior changes, depression, seizures), urinary retention, decreased gut sounds/motility, and mydriasis. Protocols to decrease oral absorption should be considered in acute overdoses. Severe anticholinergic effects can be treated with physostigmine or neostigmine, but it is suggested to do so only under the guidance of an animal poison control center. In humans, delirium or excitement has been treated with small doses of short-acting barbiturates or benzodiazepines. Hyoscyamine can be removed by hemodialysis.

For patients that have experienced or are suspected to have experienced an overdose, consultation with a 24-hour poison consultation center specializing in providing veterinary-specific information is recommended. For general information related to overdose and toxin exposures, as well as contact information for poison control centers, refer to ***Appendix.***

Drug Interactions

The following drug interactions have either been reported or are theoretical in humans or animals receiving hyoscyamine and may be of significance in veterinary patients. Unless otherwise noted, use together is not necessarily contraindicated, but weigh the potential risks and perform additional monitoring when appropriate.

- **ANTACIDS containing magnesium, aluminum,** or **calcium salts**: May interfere with hyoscyamine absorption
- **ANTICHOLINERGICS, OTHER** (eg, **atropine, glycopyrrolate**): Additive actions and adverse effects can occur.
- **ANTIHISTAMINES, FIRST GENERATION** (eg, **diphenhydramine**): Additive actions and adverse effects can occur.
- **KETOCONAZOLE**: Hyoscyamine may decrease serum concentration of ketoconazole; separate administration by at least 2 hours.
- **POTASSIUM CHLORIDE, POTASSIUM CITRATE (ORAL)**: Anticholinergic agents may enhance ulcerogenic effect of oral potassium chloride or citrate; combination is contraindicated in humans.
- **PROKINETIC AGENTS** (eg, **cisapride, metoclopramide**): Hyoscyamine may counteract their prokinetic effects.

Laboratory Considerations

- No specific concerns noted with hyoscyamine

Dosages

DOGS:

NOTE: The following doses are assumed to be for the immediate release oral dosage forms. Extended-release tablets or capsules may be effective and reduce dosing frequency, but no data were located.

Antimuscarinic for irritable bowel syndrome (extra-label): 3 – 6 μg/kg (0.003 – 0.006 mg/kg) PO every 8 to 12 hours[2]

Sinus node dysfunction, atrioventricular block (extra-label): 3 – 6 μg/kg (0.003 – 0.006 mg/kg) PO every 8 hours[4]

Monitoring

- Clinical efficacy (eg, heart rate, syncopal episodes, exercise tolerance, GI signs)
- Adverse effects (eg, tachycardia and bowel or urinary elimination difficulties)

Client Information

- This medicine may be given with or without food. If your animal vomits or acts sick after getting it on an empty stomach, give it with food or small treat to see if this helps. If vomiting continues, contact your veterinarian.
- Common side effects include dry mouth, dry eyes, constipation, trouble urinating, and faster heartbeat.
- Be sure animal has access to water at all times.
- Contact your veterinarian immediately if seizures (convulsions), collapsing/fainting or large changes in behavior (eg, hyperexcitability (overly excited) or depression) occur.
- If using a sustained-release capsule or tablet, do not split, crush, or allow the animal to chew it.

Chemistry/Synonyms

Hyoscyamine sulfate is a tertiary amine that occurs as white, odorless crystals or crystalline powder. One gram is soluble in 0.5 mL of water or in 1 mL of alcohol. It is practically insoluble in ether.

Hyoscyamine may also be known as daturin, duboisine, tropine-L-tropate. International trade names include: *Egazil Duretter*® and *Neo-Allospasmin*®.

Storage/Stability

Unless otherwise advised by the manufacturer, hyoscyamine sulfate oral products should be stored at room temperature, in tight containers, and protected from light. The injectable product should be stored at room temperature and protected from freezing.

Compatibility/Compounding Considerations

No specific information noted.

Dosage Forms/Regulatory Status

VETERINARY-LABELED PRODUCTS:

None as single ingredient products

HUMAN-LABELED PRODUCTS:

Hyoscyamine Oral Tablets: 0.125 mg (regular and chewable) and 0.15 mg; many trade names are available including: *Anaspaz*®, *ED-SPAZ*®, *HyoMax*®, *Levsin*®, *Cystospaz*®, generic; (Rx)

Hyoscyamine Orally Disintegrating Tablets: 0.125 mg and 0.25 mg; *Neosol*®, *NuLev*®, *Symax FasTab*®, *Mar-Spas*®; (Rx)

Hyoscyamine Sublingual Oral Tablets: 0.125 mg; *Levsin/SL*®, *Symax-SL*®, generic; (Rx)

Hyoscyamine Extended/Sustained-Release Oral Tablets: 0.25 mg (0.125 mg immediate-release) and 0.375 mg; *Levbid*®, *Symax-SR*® and *Symax Duotab*®, generic; (Rx)

Hyoscyamine Extended/Timed-Release Oral Capsules: 0.375 mg; *Levsinex*®, generic; (Rx)

Hyoscyamine Oral Solution: 0.125 mg/mL in 15 mL; generic; (Rx)

Hyoscyamine Oral Elixir: 0.025 mg/mL (0.125mg/5mL) in pint bottles; generic; (Rx)

Hyoscyamine Oral Spray: 0.125 mg/spray in 30 mL; *IB-Stat*®; (Rx)

Hyoscyamine Injection: 0.05 mg/mL in 1 mL ampules and 10 mL vials; *Levsin*®; (Rx)

References

For the complete list of references, see **wiley.com/go/budde/plumb**

Hypertonic Saline (7% to 7.5%)

Sodium Chloride 7% to 7.5%

(hye-per-***ton***-ik ***say***-leen)

Prescriber Highlights

- Hypertonic saline (HTS) can provide immediate intravascular expansion in hypovolemic shock and reduce intracranial pressure in traumatic brain injury.
- Must be administered IV slowly; prolonged infusions are not recommended. Follow with isotonic crystalloids to replenish body water
- Contraindicated in patients with hypernatremia, hyperosmolality, hyperchloremia, hypokalemia, or intravascular overload
- Use caution in patients that are dehydrated, coagulopathic, thrombocytopenic, or have platelet dysfunction.
- Veterinary-labeled product is not an FDA-approved drug. If compounding from concentrated sodium chloride, use extreme caution.

Uses/Indications

Hypertonic saline (HTS) solutions with concentrations of 7% to 7.5% are most commonly used in veterinary medicine. HTS is used as an alternative to isotonic crystalloids for resuscitation in previously normovolemic healthy patients with intravascular hypovolemic shock, and in patients with burns or hypovolemic traumatic brain injury (TBI). HTS is particularly useful in conditions where large fluid volumes of crystalloids can cause interstitial edema (eg, traumatic brain injury, spinal cord trauma, pancreatitis, burns). HTS is also used as a hyperosmolar agent for intracranial pressure reduction after TBI or to reduce spinal edema after spinal cord trauma. In patients with increased intracranial pressure and systemic hypotension, HTS is preferred to mannitol because hypotension after HTS administration is less likely to occur due to sodium redistribution within the body and the diuretic effect.

Use in combination with a synthetic colloid (eg, dextran, hydroxyethyl starch) is somewhat controversial. Duration of extravascular expansion can be significantly prolonged, but in 2 studies of experimental controlled hemorrhagic shock in dogs, HTS-colloid solutions were shown to be inferior for improving systemic and regional tissue oxygenation as compared with either lactated Ringer's or hydroxyethyl starch alone (both given in various ratios with shed blood).[1,2]

A study in horses comparing isotonic saline versus HTS (7.2%) for fluid resuscitation after an endurance ride found that HTS-treated horses had greater decreases in PCV, total protein, albumin and globulin concentrations, and had a shorter time to urination with lower urine specific gravity.[3]

Calves with noninfectious diarrhea and metabolic acidosis treated with HTS (7.5%) and an oral PO isotonic electrolyte solution had faster decreases in hematocrit, total protein and albumin concentrations, BUN, increased plasma volume, and faster increases in blood pH, bicarbonate concentration, and central venous pressure than calves treated with oral PO isotonic electrolyte solution alone.[4]

Pharmacology/Actions

Small bolus doses of hypertonic saline (HTS) can cause immediate intravascular volume expansion. High sodium concentration increases plasma osmolarity, causing movement of water from the interstitial space into the intravascular space. Intravascular volume expansion can be in excess of the amount of HTS infused. Equilibrium between the intravascular and interstitial spaces is restored by intracellular water moving into the interstitial space.

HTS may have additional benefits when it is used for trauma resuscitation, including positive immunomodulatory effects due to alterations of neutrophil-endothelial interactions, albumin leakage, and endothelial cell swelling reduction, improvement of cardiac function and microcirculation, and reduction of edema formation.

Pharmacokinetics

Volume expansion occurs immediately and is highest at the end of the infusion. Volume expansion effects are relatively transient and may only persist for 30 minutes to 3 hours. Effects may last longer than 3 hours if combined with a colloid (eg, dextran or hydroxyethyl starch).

Contraindications/Precautions/Warnings

Hypertonic saline (HTS) is contraindicated in patients with significant hypernatremia, hyperosmolality, hyperchloremia, hypokalemia, or intravascular overload. It must be used with extreme caution in dehydrated patients, and isotonic crystalloid therapy is required after HTS infusion to replenish interstitial and intracellular water.

Adequate patient monitoring is mandatory as the effects of HTS are transient and critically ill patients can rapidly decompensate.

HTS can improve perfusion, but it is not a replacement for blood products.

Use HTS with caution, especially at higher than recommended dosages in patients with coagulopathies, thrombocytopenia, or platelet dysfunction.[5-7] Until further evaluation, prolonged infusions of HTS are not recommended.[8]

HTS is a high-risk medication, and mistakenly administering HTS instead of isotonic crystalloids can be extremely hazardous. To ensure patient safety in human hospitals, the following controls have been recommended: limiting the available concentrations, standardizing dosing and monitoring, keeping the solution separate from other fluids in controlled-access cabinets, colored labeling, and oversight by pharmacists.[9]

Adverse Effects

When used at dosages less than 5 mL/kg IV and at infusion rates not greater than 1 mL/kg/minute IV, hypertonic saline (HTS) is considered relatively safe in patients where it is not contraindicated. If infused at a higher rate (infusion time less than 1 minute, or infusion rate greater than 1 mL/kg/minute), arteriolar vasodilation with transient reductions in mean arterial pressure and vagally mediated bradycardia can occur.

Fluid and electrolyte disturbances (eg, hypokalemia, hypernatremia, hyperchloremia) are possible, especially when used repeatedly, at high doses, or if adequate fluid replenishment is not administered.

At concentrations less than 10%, infused at recommended rates into peripheral veins, HTS is not likely to cause phlebitis. Consider administering via a central line if available.

In vitro studies have shown that HTS infusions exceeding 5 mL/kg may prolong clotting or cause clinical coagulopathies.[5-7]

Reproductive/Nursing Safety

When used appropriately in critically ill patients, use of hypertonic saline (HTS) in pregnant animals should not be a clinical concern.

Overdose/Acute Toxicity

Inadvertent overdose can cause electrolyte imbalance (eg, hypernatremia, hyperchloremia, hypokalemia), edema, and aggravation of existing acidosis.

For patients that have experienced or are suspected to have experienced an overdose, consultation with a 24-hour poison consultation center specializing in providing veterinary-specific information is recommended. For general information related to overdose and toxin exposures, as well as contact information for poison control centers, refer to ***Appendix***.

Drug Interactions

- No specific drug interactions were noted.

Laboratory Considerations

- No specific concerns were noted.

Dosages

DOGS/CATS:

NOTE: All dosages are for hypertonic saline (sodium chloride) 7% to 7.5%. Many clinicians use the veterinary labeled 7.2% product, but there is no evidence to suggest that using concentrations from 7% to 7.5% is unacceptable.

Low-volume resuscitation using hypertonic saline (HTS) alone (extra-label): Using HTS 7% to 7.5%, 4 – 6 mL/kg IV infusion at a rate not to exceed 1 mL/kg/minute is recommended; however, dosages ranging from 2 – 8 mL/kg IV have been noted. Some clinicians suggest that cats should receive dosages at the low end of the range. Follow with crystalloid therapy to maintain adequate tissue hydration.

Low-volume resuscitation using HTS with a colloid (extra-label): Mix concentrated sodium chloride 23.4% solution with hetastarch in a 1:2 ratio (1 part sodium chloride 23.4% to 2 parts hetastarch 6%); administer 4 – 5 mL/kg IV over 5 minutes.

Neurologic trauma using HTS alone (extra-label): Dosage recommendations vary but 3 – 5 mL/kg IV over 15 to 20 minutes has been noted.[10] Follow with crystalloids. Do not use in hyponatremic patients and monitor sodium concentrations.

Symptomatic hyponatremia refractory to mannitol and furosemide treatment (extra-label): For patients with plasma sodium of 120 mEq/L or lower, sodium correction should not exceed 2 mEq/L/hour (maximum increase of 15 mEq/L in the first 24 hours). The sodium deficit, which will determine the amount of HTS to be administered, is calculated using the following formula Na^+ deficit = (target Na^+ - patient Na^+) × (0.6 × lean body weight in kg). The target Na^+ should be no higher than 10% to 15% of the current patient's sodium. Administer as a HTS 3% solution.[11]

HORSES:

Small-volume resuscitation (extra-label): In the study (after an endurance ride), treated horses received an initial IV bolus of 2 liters/horse (NOT L/kg) of HTS 7.2% and 5 liters/horse (NOT L/kg) of lactated Ringer's solution (also contained 250 mL of 23% calcium gluconate) followed with additional LRS as deemed necessary by the treating veterinarian.[3]

CATTLE:

Adjunctive treatment of neonatal diarrhea in calves (extra-label): Using HTS 7.2%, 5 mL/kg IV over 3 to 10 minutes along with 60 mL of an isotonic electrolyte solution PO (repeated twice at 8 and 16 hours)[4]

BIRDS:

Small-volume replacement/CPR resuscitation (extra-label): For the shocky debilitated patient, hypertonic saline is administered 3 – 5 mL/kg over 5 minutes, followed by hetastarch 3 – 5 mL/

kg over 5 minutes. This combination prior to crystalloid administration enables fluids to stay within the vascular space. Blood pressure should be monitored closely. Follow with small boluses of crystalloid fluids (LRS, *Plasma-Lyte*® at 15 – 20 mL/kg) along with hetastarch 3 – 5 mL/kg over 15 minutes; reassess the bird every 15 minutes. The crystalloids and hetastarch can be combined in the same syringe or bag. This process is repeated every 15 to 20 minutes until temperature normalizes and blood pressure is over 120 mm Hg.[12]

Monitoring

- Efficacy: blood pressure, central venous pressure (if possible), and clinical parameters (eg, heart rate, pulse quality, mucous membrane color, capillary refill time, mental acuity, body temperature)
- Serum electrolytes (ie, sodium, potassium, chloride), serum osmolality, urine output, hematocrit

Client Information

- Hypertonic saline should only be used in an inpatient setting with appropriate monitoring.

Chemistry/Synonyms

7.2% sodium chloride for injection solution contains 1232 mEq/liter (1.23 mEq/mL) of sodium and 1232 mEq/liter (1.23 mEq/mL) of chloride. Osmolarity is 2464 mOsm/L. Colloid osmotic pressure (COP) is 0.

Storage/Stability

Sodium chloride 7.2% injection should be stored at controlled room temperature between 15°C and 30°C (59°F-86°F). It does not contain a preservative and is appropriate for single use only. Discard any unused solution.

Sodium chloride 14.6% and 23.4% (both for additive use) should be stored at controlled room temperature and protected from excessive heat and freezing.

Compatibility/Compounding Considerations

Compatibility is dependent on factors such as pH, concentration, temperature, and diluent used; specialized references or a hospital pharmacist should be consulted for more specific information.

The veterinary labeled 7.2% product does not contain a preservative and is appropriate for one-time use only.

Concentrated sodium chloride solutions for IV additive use (14.6% and 23.4%) are thought to be compatible with hydroxyethyl starch compounds.

Dosage Forms/Regulatory Status

VETERINARY-LABELED PRODUCTS:

Hypertonic Saline (sodium chloride 7.2%) Injection Solution: in 1000 mL bottles; generic; (Rx). Contains no preservative and is labeled for single use. Labeled (not FDA-approved) for use in horses and cattle.

HUMAN-LABELED PRODUCTS:

Sodium Chloride Solution Concentrate 14.6%, 23.4%; generic; (Rx). For IV additive use only; must be diluted before use.

References

For the complete list of references, see **wiley.com/go/budde/plumb**

Ifosfamide

(eye-***foss***-fa-mide) *Ifex*®

Antineoplastic

Prescriber Highlights

- Alkylating agent that may be useful in treating lymphomas and sarcomas in dogs and cats
- Limited veterinary experience to date
- Cat dose is much greater than dog dose
- Contraindications include patients with severe myelosuppression, urinary outflow obstruction, active hemorrhagic cystitis, and patients that are hypersensitive to ifosfamide.
- Significant toxicities (eg, myelosuppression, nephrotoxicity, bladder toxicity, neurotoxicity, GI toxicity) may occur.
- Must be given with saline diuresis and mesna, an injectable bladder-protective agent; do not use in patients that are unable to tolerate forced saline diuresis (eg, severe heart disease)
- The National Institute for Occupational Safety and Health (NIOSH) classifies ifosfamide as a hazardous drug; use appropriate precautions when handling.

Uses/Indications

In small animal species, ifosfamide may be beneficial in combination chemotherapy protocols for a variety of neoplasms. Limited efficacy has been demonstrated with ifosfamide in the treatment of lymphomas and soft tissue sarcomas in dogs and cats. It appears to be inferior to single-agent treatment for lymphoma. A phase II study in cats with vaccine-associated sarcoma demonstrated a measurable response in 41% of treated cats.[1]

Ifosfamide has been evaluated in alternating cycles with doxorubicin in dogs with soft tissue sarcomas and hemangiosarcoma. Although ifosfamide was well tolerated, no significant survival advantage was conferred.[2] Minor anti-tumor activity against metastatic canine osteosarcoma has been documented.[3]

In humans, ifosfamide is used in various treatment protocols for neoplasias of the urinary bladder, cervix, ovaries, and some types of lymphomas.

Pharmacology/Actions

Ifosfamide is an alkylating antineoplastic agent. Its chemical reactivity is nonspecific, but the primary cytotoxic effect is thought to be due to alkylation of cancer cell DNA strands resulting in cross-linking and inhibition of tumor growth, DNA replication, RNA transcription, and protein synthesis.

Pharmacokinetics

The pharmacokinetics of ifosfamide are complex. Although ifosfamide is normally given IV, it is well absorbed after SC injection or oral administration; bioavailability via these routes is 90% or greater. Ifosfamide and its metabolites are widely distributed and enter bone and CNS, although not in therapeutic concentrations. Ifosfamide, a prodrug, is metabolized primarily via oxidative pathways found in the liver and, to a smaller extent, in the lungs. It then is catalyzed into the primary active alkylating agent, ifosfamide mustard. In humans, ifosfamide's half-life and excretion is dose dependent, but its metabolites are primarily excreted via the kidney into urine.

Contraindications/Precautions/Warnings

Because of its toxicity, ifosfamide should only be used by clinicians that are experienced with the use of cytotoxic agents and able to adequately monitor the effects of therapy. Ifosfamide is contraindicated in patients with a history of hypersensitivity, severe myelosuppression, urinary outflow obstruction, or active hemorrhagic cystitis. Ifosfamide should be used with extreme caution in patients with impaired renal function. Do not use ifosfamide in patients that are unable to tolerate forced saline diuresis (eg, severe heart disease).

Ifosfamide must be used in conjunction with mesna, an injectable detoxifying agent, to reduce the risk for hemorrhagic cystitis. If secondary UTIs occur, it has been recommended that ifosfamide (or cyclophosphamide) must not be used again in that patient, even after clinical resolution.

The National Institute for Occupational Safety and Health (NIOSH) classifies ifosfamide as a hazardous drug; personal protective equipment (PPE) should be used accordingly to minimize the risk for exposure.

Adverse Effects

Dose-related neutropenia generally occurs at 5 to 7 days posttreatment but may be delayed (14 to 21 days), particularly with repeated dosing. Nadirs in cats are seen typically at day 7 or 8. Platelets can also be significantly impacted.

Ifosfamide can damage urinary bladder epithelium and cause nephrotoxicity with resultant electrolyte abnormalities. Renal toxicity is primarily focused on proximal and distal tubular damage, but glomerular effects may occur. To reduce the incidence of nephrotoxicity and urinary bladder toxicity, saline diuresis is required, and mesna is given concomitantly to reduce urinary bladder epithelial toxicity; however, volume overload and pulmonary edema may result, particularly in patients with pre-existing cardiac disease. GI effects including nausea, drooling, and vomiting have been reported, especially during drug administration. Treatment with antiemetics may be required. Other adverse effects may include hypersensitivity reactions, anorexia, neurotoxicity (eg, somnolence to confusion, coma, encephalopathy), alopecia, and increased hepatic enzymes.

In cats, doses of 900 mg/m^2 or less resulted in neutrophil counts less than 1000 cells/μL in ≈33% of treated cats, but no secondary infections were noted. Some cats demonstrated mild, self-limiting GI effects, including lack of appetite, vomiting, and diarrhea. Signs of nausea during IV infusion were seen in ≈⅓ of treated cats. Pulmonary edema and hypersensitivity were each seen in 1 cat, and nephrotoxicity was seen in 2 cats.[1,4]

Administering mesna with ifosfamide significantly reduces the incidence and severity of ifosfamide-induced hemorrhagic cystitis. Mesna interacts with metabolites of ifosfamide that cause this toxicity. Because mesna is hydrophilic, it does not enter most cells and therefore does not appear to significantly reduce the anti-tumor efficacy of ifosfamide. Mesna does not prevent or reduce the incidence of other adverse effects associated with ifosfamide (eg, myelosuppression, GI effects, neurotoxicity, renal toxicity).

Many dogs receiving chemotherapy will have minor hair coat changes (eg, shagginess, loss of luster). Breeds with continuously growing hair coats (eg, poodles, terriers, Afghan hounds, or old English sheepdogs) are more likely to experience significant alopecia.

Reproductive/Nursing Safety

Teratogenic and fetotoxic effects have been demonstrated at usual dosages in humans and laboratory animals; treatment is not recommended during pregnancy. For sexually intact patients, verify pregnancy status prior to administration.

Ifosfamide is excreted in maternal milk. If this drug is being used in lactating mothers, consider using milk replacer.

Overdose/Acute Toxicity

The lowest reported lethal dose in dogs following IV administration was 66 mg/kg, resulting in acute pulmonary edema and hemorrhage.[5]

The drug is dialyzable, but no data are available regarding use during overdose. No specific antidote is known, and treatment is supportive. Methylene blue (50 mg in a 1%-2% aqueous solution IV over 5 minutes) has been suggested to treat ifosfamide-induced encephalopathy in humans.

For patients that have experienced or are suspected to have experienced an overdose, consultation with a 24-hour poison consultation center specializing in providing veterinary-specific information is recommended. For general information related to overdose and toxin exposures, as well as contact information for poison control centers, refer to ***Appendix.***

Drug Interactions

The following drug interactions have either been reported or are theoretical in humans or animals receiving ifosfamide and may be of significance in veterinary patients. Unless otherwise noted, use together is not necessarily contraindicated, but weigh the potential risks and perform additional monitoring when appropriate.

- **Azole Antifungals** (eg, **ketoconazole**): Concomitant use may decrease metabolism of ifosfamide to its active metabolites, resulting in reduced ifosfamide efficacy.
- **Cisplatin**: Ifosfamide may enhance cisplatin-induced ototoxicity and nephrotoxicity.
- **Maropitant**: In humans, NK1-receptor antagonists similar to maropitant are thought to increase concentrations of toxic metabolites of ifosfamide; monitor for clinical signs of ifosfamide neurotoxicity.
- **Myelosuppressive Agents** (eg, **antineoplastics, immunosuppressants, iron chelators**): Concurrent use with other bone marrow depressant medications may result in additive myelosuppression; avoid combination when possible.
- **Vaccines** (live and inactivated): Ifosfamide may diminish vaccine efficacy and enhance adverse effects of vaccines.

Laboratory Considerations

- None were noted.

Dosages

NOTE: Because of the potential toxicity of this drug to patients, veterinary personnel, and clients, and because chemotherapy indications, treatment protocols, monitoring and safety guidelines often change, the following dosages should be used only as a general guide. Consultation with a veterinary oncologist and referral to current veterinary oncology references[6-10] are strongly recommended.

DOGS:

Adjunctive treatment of lymphomas and sarcomas (extra-label):

a) Saline diuresis is required prior to ifosfamide administration. Administer 0.9% sodium chloride IV at a fluid rate of 6 times the maintenance dose over 30 minutes. Mesna 75 mg/m^2 (NOT mg/kg) should then be administered immediately prior to ifosfamide. Ifosfamide 375 mg/m^2 (NOT mg/kg) should be diluted to 20 mg/mL or less and given IV over 20 minutes, followed by 0.9% sodium chloride IV diuresis at 6 times maintenance over 5 hours. Mesna dose is repeated 2 hours and 5 hours after ifosfamide. This therapy may be repeated on a 21-day basis.[11] **NOTE**: Some sources say treatment can be repeated every 2 to 3 weeks.[12]

b) Administer 0.9% sodium chloride IV at 18.3 mL/kg/hour for 6 hours. After 30 minutes of the saline infusion, administer ifosfamide 350 mg/m^2 (NOT mg/kg) IV over 30 minutes for patients less than 10 kg (22 lb) or 375 mg/m^2 (NOT mg/kg) IV over 30 minutes for patients greater than 10 kg (22 lb). Administer mesna (20% of ifosfamide dose) as an IV bolus at the start of the ifosfamide infusion, and again 2 hours and 5 hours after the ifosfamide infusion is complete. Repeat treatment regimen every 3 weeks.[13] **NOTE**: Some sources say treatment can be repeated every 2 to 3 weeks.

CATS:

Adjunctive treatment of lymphomas and sarcomas (extra-label):

a) Based on a phase I safety study and a phase II trial for vaccine-related sarcomas, the authors recommend ifosfamide 900 mg/m² (NOT mg/kg) IV every 3 weeks. Before ifosfamide administration, give mesna bolus (20% of ifosfamide dose) and begin diuresis with 0.9% sodium chloride 18.3 mL/kg per hour IV CRI over 30 minutes prior to ifosfamide; continue saline diuresis for 5 hours after completion of ifosfamide administration.[1,4]

b) Administer 0.9% sodium chloride IV at a fluid rate of 6 times the maintenance dose over 30 minutes, then administer ifosfamide 900 mg/m² (NOT mg/kg) diluted to 20 mg/mL or less IV over 20 minutes, followed by diuresis with 0.9% sodium chloride at 6 times the maintenance dose over 5 hours. Administer mesna (20% of ifosfamide dose) immediately before ifosfamide administration and repeat 2 hours and 5 hours after ifosfamide. This treatment regimen may be repeated every 21 days.[11]

Monitoring

- Baseline and periodic (ie, before each dose):
  - Complete blood count with platelet count
  - Serum chemistry panel and electrolytes
  - Urinalysis
- Adverse effects: volume overload/pulmonary edema, neurotoxicity, GI toxicity
- Efficacy of therapy

Client Information

- Ifosfamide is a chemotherapy (anticancer) drug. This medicine can be hazardous to other animals and humans that come in contact with it. On the day your animal gets this medicine and then for a few days afterward, all bodily waste (eg, urine, feces, litter), blood, or vomit should only be handled while wearing disposable gloves. Seal the waste in a plastic bag and then place both the bag and gloves in with the regular trash.
- Bone marrow suppression can occur. The greatest effects on bone marrow usually occur within a week or 2 after treatment. Your veterinarian will do blood tests to watch for this problem. Do not miss these important follow-up visits.
- If you see bleeding, bruising, fever (indicating an infection), shortness of breath, or if your animal becomes tired easily, it is important that you contact your veterinarian right away.
- This medicine is considered a hazardous drug as defined by the National Institute for Occupational Safety and Health (NIOSH). Talk with your veterinarian or pharmacist about the use of personal protective equipment when handling this medicine.

Chemistry/Synonyms

Ifosfamide is an alkylating agent that is structurally related to cyclophosphamide and occurs as a white, crystalline powder with a melting point of 40°C (104°F). It is freely soluble in water and very soluble in alcohol. A 10% solution in water has a pH between 4 and 7.

Ifosfamide may also be known as MJF-9325, NSC-109724, Z-4942, and *Ifex*®.

Storage/Stability

Ifosfamide powder for injection should be stored at 20°C to 25°C (68°F-77°F). It should be protected from temperatures greater than 30°C (86°F), as the drug may liquefy at temperatures greater than 35°C (95°F). Once reconstituted with sterile water for injection or bacteriostatic water for injection, the solution is stable for 24 hours when refrigerated (2°C-8°C [36°F-46°F]).

Compatibility/Compounding Considerations

The reconstituted drug is **compatible** for dilution with 5% dextrose, 0.9% sodium chloride, or lactated Ringer's and is stable for up to 24 hours when refrigerated. Ifosfamide is compatible and stable when mixed with mesna in 5% dextrose or lactated Ringer's.

Dosage Forms/Regulatory Status

VETERINARY-LABELED PRODUCTS: NONE

HUMAN-LABELED PRODUCTS:

Ifosfamide Injection: 1 g/20 mL and 3 g/60 mL in single-dose vials; generic; (Rx)

Ifosfamide Powder for injection: 1 g and 3 g in single dose vials; *Ifex*®, generic; (Rx)

References

For the complete list of references, see **wiley.com/go/budde/plumb**

Imepitoin

(ih-meh-pi-***toyn***) *Pexion*®

$GABA_A$ receptor partial agonist

Prescriber Highlights

- ▶ Approved in the United States for the treatment of noise aversion in dogs
- ▶ Licensed in the United Kingdom and European Union as an anticonvulsant for idiopathic epilepsy in dogs and for the reduction of anxiety and fear associated with noise phobia
- ▶ Contraindications include hypersensitivity to imepitoin, severely impaired hepatic function, severe renal disease, and severe cardiovascular disorders.
- ▶ Use imepitoin with caution in animals weighing less than 2 kg (4.4 lb) and in animals less than 5 months of age, as there are limited safety data.
- ▶ Adverse effects may include ataxia, increased appetite, lethargy, and emesis; hyperactivity also has been observed.
- ▶ Disinhibition of fear-based behavior may lead to aggression; observe the patient carefully during treatment.

Uses/Indications

Imepitoin is approved in the United States to treat noise aversion in dogs. FDA approval was based on the results of a clinical field trial using New Year's Eve fireworks as the test noise event.[1] Another study found imepitoin to be effective for storm phobia but also showed a high incidence of mild-to-moderate adverse effects.[2]

This drug is also available in the United Kingdom and European Union, where it is indicated in dogs for the reduction of anxiety and fear associated with noise phobia, as well as initial therapy for generalized seizures due to idiopathic epilepsy.[3] The safety or efficacy of imepitoin as an add-on drug is uncertain.

A study comparing imepitoin and phenobarbital efficacy and adverse effects in dogs with idiopathic epilepsy found imepitoin's efficacy comparable with phenobarbital; however, imepitoin had significantly fewer adverse effects (ie, somnolence/sedation, polydipsia, increased appetite).[4] In contrast, another study found that phenobarbital had a significantly higher reduction in seizure frequency. Although this was a smaller cohort study rather than a randomized trial, phenobarbital resulted in a significantly lower seizure frequency than imepitoin and had a similar frequency of persistent adverse effects. After 3 years, 70% of dogs discontinued imepitoin due to poor seizure control or adverse effects, compared with zero in the phenobarbital group.[5] There are also conflicting studies regarding imepitoin's ability to reduce or prevent the development of cluster seizures.[5,6] A clinical consensus statement on seizure management in dogs has identified imepitoin as having Level IA evidence for monotherapy and Level IIIC evidence for add-on treatment.[7]

One small study in cats demonstrated that imepitoin was well tolerated at 30 mg/kg twice daily for 30 days, with no serious adverse effects reported.[8] This study also demonstrated that imepitoin showed preliminary efficacy for idiopathic epilepsy in cats,[8] but further studies are needed.

Pharmacology/Actions

Imepitoin is a low-affinity partial agonist at benzodiazepine binding sites of the $GABA_A$ receptor. Affinity at the site is ≈600 times less than for diazepam. When compared with full agonists, imepitoin may cause less severe adverse effects and have a lower risk for tolerance and dependence development.[9] $GABA_A$–receptor-mediated inhibitory effects on neurons are potentiated, thereby preventing seizures. In addition, a weak inhibition of neuronal calcium channels may contribute to its anticonvulsant activity. Imepitoin also possesses anxiolytic effects.

Pharmacokinetics

In dogs, imepitoin demonstrates linear kinetics over the therapeutic dosing range. It is slowly but well absorbed after oral administration. Peak concentrations occur ≈2 hours after dosing. The presence of food does not significantly affect peak concentrations or time to peak. Bioavailability under fasting conditions is ≈92%, but administration with food may reduce the total AUC by 20%. The volume of distribution ranges from 0.6 to 1.6 L/kg; protein binding is relatively low (60% to 70%). It is extensively metabolized via oxidative mechanisms in the liver to 4 major inactive metabolites. Clearance ranges from 260 to 570 mL/hour/kg. The elimination half-life is ≈1.5 to 2 hours.[1] The majority of a dose is eliminated via fecal routes. Although imepitoin absorption is greater in a fasted state, clinical field studies support imepitoin efficacy for noise aversion when administered in either a fed or fasted state.[1]

Following rectal administration, imepitoin is slowly and poorly absorbed, and drug delivery by this route is not recommended.[10]

Contraindications/Precautions/Warnings

Imepitoin is contraindicated in patients that are hypersensitive to it, patients that have severely impaired hepatic function, or in patients that have severe renal or cardiovascular disorders. Safety has not been tested in dogs weighing less than 2 kg (4.4 lb); dogs younger than 5 months of age; or in dogs with renal, liver, cardiac, GI, or another disease.[3,11,12]

Imepitoin may lead to disinhibition of fear-based behaviors and may result in a change in aggression level.[1]

In dogs receiving imepitoin for seizures, mild behavioral or muscular signs may be observed upon abrupt termination of treatment. Consider withdrawing the drug gradually if appropriate. One taper schedule reduced the dosage to 20 mg/kg twice daily for 1 month, then 10 mg/kg twice daily for 1 month, then 10 mg/kg once daily for 1 month.[13]

Adverse Effects

Common adverse effects include ataxia, increased appetite, lethargy, emesis, hyperactivity, aggression, somnolence, and hypersalivation.[1] Ataxia has occurred in up to 60% of dogs receiving the drug.[2] Other reported adverse effects include polyphagia (especially at the beginning of treatment), decreased appetite, polyuria, polydipsia, apathy, diarrhea, prolapsed nictitating membrane, and decreased sight and sensitivity to sound.

Mild elevations in plasma creatinine and cholesterol levels were noted but did not exceed normal reference ranges and were not associated with clinically significant observations or events. Elevation of liver enzymes has been noted.[2]

Skin lesions were noted after a dose increase in a dog that had been receiving imepitoin for 5 months.[14]

In cats, emesis, lethargy, and decreased appetite were the most common adverse effects reported. Hypersalivation was common at higher doses.[8]

Reproductive/Nursing Safety

Reproductive safety or safety during nursing is not known; imepitoin is not recommended in male breeding dogs or in female dogs during pregnancy and lactation.[3,11,12] In male dogs receiving 10 times the recommended dosage, diffuse atrophy of seminiferous tubules in the testes and associated decreased sperm counts were observed.

Because safety has not been established in animals, this drug should only be used when the maternal benefits outweigh the potential risks to offspring.

Overdose/Acute Toxicity

The acute toxicity of imepitoin was assessed in rats and mice after oral administration; no mortality was noted in either species up to 2105 mg/kg.[15] The TD_{50} for motor impairment in the rotarod test was ≈1 g/kg PO in rats.[16]

In dogs receiving repeated overdoses of up to 5 times the highest recommended dose, CNS effects (eg, loss of righting reflex, decreased activity, eyelid closure, lacrimation, dry eye, tremors, nystagmus), GI effects (eg, vomiting, diarrhea, salivation), and reversible prolongation of the QT interval were noted. These effects are not usually life-threatening and generally resolve within 24 hours with supportive and symptomatic treatment. Weight gain was noted and was greater in dogs receiving 3 times the highest recommended dose as compared with the group receiving 5 times the highest recommended dose. Daily administration of the labeled dosage (30 mg/kg PO twice daily) for 6 months was generally well tolerated.[1]

The benzodiazepine antagonist flumazenil could potentially be used to reverse severe CNS effects associated with an overdose and to eliminate the drug's anticonvulsant action.

For patients that have experienced or are suspected to have experienced an overdose, consultation with a 24-hour poison consultation center specializing in providing veterinary-specific information is recommended. For general information related to overdose and toxin exposures, as well as contact information for poison control centers, refer to ***Appendix***.

Drug Interactions

The United Kingdom product label states, *The product [imepitoin] has been used in combination with phenobarbital in a small number of cases and no harmful clinical interactions were observed.*[11] Imepitoin has a very low drug interaction potential, and interactions with highly protein-bound or enzyme-inducing drugs are not expected.[17] The following drug interactions have either been reported or are theoretical in humans or animals receiving imepitoin and may be of significance in veterinary patients; unless otherwise noted, use together is not necessarily contraindicated, but the potential risks should be weighed, and additional monitoring should be performed when appropriate.

- FLUMAZENIL: Could antagonize the anxiolytic and anticonvulsant effects of imepitoin[16]

Laboratory Considerations

- No specific laboratory interactions or considerations were noted.

Dosages

DOGS:

Noise aversion (label dosage; FDA-approved): 30 mg/kg PO every 12 hours. Initiate therapy starting 2 days prior to the day of the expected noise event and continue through the noise event.[12]

Storm anxiety (extra-label): 30 mg/kg PO every 12 hours (continuously, not as needed)[2]

Generalized seizures due to idiopathic epilepsy (extra-label): Initially, 10 mg/kg PO twice daily (≈12 hours apart).[3,11] If the frequency of seizures is not adequately reduced following a minimum of 1 week of treatment at the current dose, the dose may be increased in 50% to 100% increments to a maximum of 30 mg/kg twice daily.[11]

CATS:

Idiopathic epilepsy (extra-label): 30 mg/kg PO every 12 hours has been reported in cats and appears well tolerated, but data are limited.[8]

Monitoring

- Clinical efficacy
- Adverse effects including ataxia, change in appetite, polyuria/polydipsia, lethargy, and somnolence
- If imepitoin is being used long term, consider baseline and intermittent renal and hepatic analyte testing.

Client Information

- This medicine is best given on an empty stomach about 12 hours apart; however, if the animal vomits after receiving the drug, try giving it with food.
- To be effective, the drug must be given on a regular basis as instructed by your veterinarian.
- Possible side effects in dogs include abnormal gait, increased appetite and thirst, increased urination, increased drooling, vomiting, and changes in behavior or activity level. Contact your veterinarian if these effects are severe or continue.

Chemistry/Synonyms

Imepitoin, an imidaolinone, occurs as a white to almost-white, solid, nonhygroscopic, odorless, non-bitter–tasting substance. It is practically insoluble in water.

Imepitoin may also be known as AWD 131–138, ELB 138, or 1-(4-chlorophenyl)-4-morpholino-imidazolin-2-one. The canine product trade name is *Pexion*®.

Storage/Stability

Store at 20°C to 25°C (68°F-77°F), excursions are permitted between 15°C to 30°C (59°F-86°F).

Compatibility/Compounding Considerations

No specific information was noted.

Dosage Forms/Regulatory Status

VETERINARY-LABELED PRODUCTS:

Imepitoin Oral Tablets (scored): 100 mg and 400 mg; *Pexion*®; (Rx). FDA-approved in the United States, but not yet commercially marketed; NADA 141-509. This product is also available in the United Kingdom, Australia, New Zealand, and the European Union.

HUMAN-LABELED PRODUCTS: NONE

References

For the complete list of references, see **wiley.com/go/budde/plumb**

Imidacloprid, Systemic

(eye-mi-da-***kloe***-prid) *advantus*®

Oral Insecticide

See also ***Imidacloprid/Imidacloprid Combinations, Topical*** and ***Moxidectin/Moxidectin Combination Products*** for imidacloprid combination products containing moxidectin

Prescriber Highlights

- ► Rapid-acting oral medication used for short-term treatment of acute flea infestations in dogs or puppies 10 weeks of age and older and weighing 1.8 kg (4 lb) or greater; it does not protect against ticks or mosquitoes.
- ► Flea kill begins within 1 hour; 97% of fleas are killed within 4 hours.
- ► **Not for use in cats**
- ► Use with caution in debilitated, aged, pregnant, or nursing animals.
- ► Adverse effects include decreased appetite, vomiting, diarrhea, lethargy, and difficulty walking.
- ► Does not treat the environment; separate environmental treatments are required for treatment of infestations.
- ► All pets in a household must be treated with a flea preventive to help resolve flea infestations.

Indications/Actions

Imidacloprid is indicated for treatment of flea infestations in dogs and puppies 10 weeks of age and older and weighing 1.8 kg (4 lb) or greater.[1] Postadministration, 30% of fleas are killed within 1 hour and 97% within 4 hours. Worldwide, *Ctenocephalides felis* ("cat flea," the most common flea found on dogs) susceptibility to imidacloprid remains high.[2]

Pharmacology/Actions

Imidacloprid acts on nicotinic acetylcholine receptors on the postsynaptic membrane, causing CNS impairment and death. This is a different mechanism of action than other insecticidal agents (eg, organophosphates, pyrethrins, carbamates, insect growth regulators, insect development inhibitors). The nicotinic acetylcholine receptors of insect species have higher affinity for imidacloprid than the receptors of vertebrate species.[3]

Pharmacokinetics

In healthy dogs given imidacloprid soft chewable tablets under laboratory conditions, maximum imidacloprid concentration was reached after 1.3 hours, and terminal half-life was 2.2 hours.[4] Under experimental conditions, imidacloprid given in combination with either methoprene or pyriproxyfen displayed synergistic insecticidal activity against *Ctenocephalides felis* second and third instars.[5]

Contraindications/Precautions/Warnings

Do not use in puppies younger than 10 weeks of age or weighing less than 1.8 kg (4 lb).[1] The manufacturer of topical imidacloprid combination products recommends to use it with caution in sick, debilitated, or underweight animals.[6,7]

Do not confuse imidaCLOPRID with imidoCARB.

Adverse Effects

Adverse effects are unlikely at the label dosage. Vomiting, decreased appetite, decreased energy, soft stools, and difficulty walking have been noted.[1] Imidacloprid may be a contributing or exacerbating factor for gallbladder mucocele formation in Shetland sheepdogs.[8]

Reproductive/Nursing Safety

Oral imidacloprid has not been tested in pregnant or nursing dogs. Because safety has not been established in animals, this drug should only be used when the maternal benefits outweigh the potential risks to offspring.

Overdoses/Acute Toxicity

In dogs given 18.7 mg/kg/day (4.5 times the labeled dose), no adverse effects were noted clinically or on laboratory, histology, or necropsy examinations.[4] No adverse effects were observed in dogs that received a single oral dose of 30 mg/kg.[9]

Most adverse effects are seen following oral administration of *topical* imidacloprid products. Signs include hypersalivation and vomiting; oral ulcers have been rarely reported in cats. See ***Imidacloprid/Imidacloprid Combinations, Topical.***

For patients that have experienced or are suspected to have experienced an overdose, consultation with a 24-hour poison consultation center specializing in providing veterinary-specific information is recommended. For general information related to overdose and toxin exposures, as well as contact information for poison control centers, refer to ***Appendix***.

Drug Interactions

Oral imidacloprid chewable tablets may be used together with other products, including heartworm preventives, corticosteroids, antibiotics, vaccines, deworming medications, and shampoos.[1]

Laboratory Considerations

- None noted

Dosages

DOGS:

Flea infestation in dogs or puppies (label dosage; FDA-approved): Administer the appropriate tablet size based on body weight (see table below).[1] Dose may be repeated as often as once daily; do not exceed more than 1 tablet/day. Field studies used a dose range of 0.7 – 4 mg/kg PO once.[4]

Body weight in kg (lb)	Imidacloprid (mg)	Number of tablets
1.8 – 10 (4-22)	7.5	1
10.5 – 50 (23-110)	37.5	1
More than 50 (110)	--	Appropriate combination of tablets

Monitoring

- Clinical efficacy (ie, absence of adult fleas after dosing)
- Adverse effects (eg, vomiting, diarrhea, lethargy, difficulty walking)

Client Information

- This medicine is used to treat flea infestations on dogs only. It does not protect against ticks or mosquitoes.
- Weigh your dog before administration of this medicine to make sure the correct amount is given.
- Make sure your dog swallows the medicine.
- Fleas begin to die within 1 hour of administration, and most fleas die within 4 hours.
- This medicine does not treat fleas living in the environment, and reinfestation is possible if the environment is not treated at the same time.
- All pets in a household must be treated with a flea preventive to help resolve flea infestations.

Chemistry/Synonyms

Imidacloprid occurs as a colorless to beige powder or crystals with a slight characteristic odor. It is freely soluble in water.

Systemic imidacloprid may be known as *advantus*®. Imidacloprid is widely used as a pesticide for agricultural purposes.

Storage/Stability

Imidacloprid soft chews should be stored at temperatures between 20°C to 25°C (68°F-77°F) out of reach of children and pets.

Dosage Forms/Regulatory Status

VETERINARY-LABELED PRODUCTS:

Imidacloprid tablet, chewable: 7.5 mg and 37.5 mg soft chewable tablets in 7- or 30-count bottles; *advantus*®; OTC. NADA #141-435. Chewable tablets do not contain any animal proteins and are suitable for dogs with animal protein food allergies.[10]

Imidacloprid is also available in topical formulations (eg, spot-on, collar) alone or in combination with other antiparasitic agents. See ***Imidacloprid/Imidacloprid Combinations, Topical*** and ***Moxidectin/Moxidectin Combination Products*** for imidacloprid combination products containing moxidectin.

HUMAN-LABELED PRODUCTS: NONE

References

For the complete list of references, see **wiley.com/go/budde/plumb**

Imidapril

(ih-***mid***-a-pril) *Prilium*®

Angiotensin-Converting Enzyme (ACE) Inhibitor

Prescriber Highlights

- ► Veterinary ACE inhibitor (not presently available in the United States) labeled in the United Kingdom for dogs to treat moderate to severe heart failure caused by mitral regurgitation or dilated cardiomyopathy.
- ► Contraindications include hypersensitivity to ACE inhibitors, hypotension, acute renal insufficiency, congenital heart disease, obstructive hypertrophic cardiomyopathy, and patients with hemodynamically relevant stenoses (aortic stenosis, mitral valve stenosis, pulmonic stenosis).
- ► Use with caution in patients with renal insufficiency (doses may need to be reduced), patients with hyponatremia, coronary or cerebrovascular insufficiency, pre-existing hematologic abnormalities, or a collagen vascular disease (eg, SLE).
- ► Adverse effects may include GI distress (eg, anorexia, vomiting, diarrhea), and, less commonly, weakness, hypotension, renal dysfunction, and hyperkalemia.

Uses/Indications

Imidapril is labeled in the United Kingdom for use in dogs to treat moderate to severe heart failure by mitral regurgitation or by dilated cardiomyopathy.[1] When compared to other ACE inhibitors in dogs, imidapril has similar clinical efficacy and safety profile in dogs with congestive heart failure.[2,3] Like other ACE inhibitors, it could also be useful for treating dogs with protein-losing nephropathy.

Pharmacology/Actions

Like enalapril, imidapril is a prodrug and is converted in the liver to the active compound imidaprilat. Imidaprilat prevents the formation of angiotensin-II (a potent vasoconstrictor) by competing with angiotensin-I for the enzyme angiotensin-converting enzyme (ACE). ACE has a much higher affinity for imidaprilat than for angiotensin-I. Because angiotensin-II concentrations are decreased, aldosterone secretion is reduced, and plasma renin activity is increased by negative feedback mechanisms.

The cardiovascular effects of ACE inhibitors in patients with CHF include decreased total peripheral resistance, pulmonary vascular resistance, mean arterial and right atrial pressures, and pulmonary capillary wedge pressure; no change or decrease in heart rate; and increased cardiac index and output, stroke volume, and exercise tolerance.

ACE inhibitors increase renal blood flow and decrease glomerular efferent arteriole resistance. In animals with glomerular disease, ACE inhibitors decrease proteinuria and may help to preserve renal function. Imidapril partially blocks amlodipine's activation of the renin-angiotensin-aldosterone system (RAAS) in dogs.[4]

Pharmacokinetics

Following oral administration in the dog, imidapril is rapidly absorbed, but bioavailability is decreased by the presence of food.[1] Maximum plasma concentration occurs less than one hour after dosing, and elimination half-life is about 2 hours. Imidapril is mainly hydrolyzed in the liver and kidney to its active metabolite, imidaprilat. Peak imidaprilat plasma concentrations occur in about 5 hours; elimination half-life is more than 10 hours. Protein binding of imidapril and imidaprilat is moderate (85% and 53%, respectively). After oral administration of radiolabeled imidapril, about 40% of total radioactivity is excreted in urine and about 60% in feces. After multiple dosing, plasma imidaprilat concentrations are about 3 times higher after the second dose than after the first, but no additional increase is observed with subsequent doses.

Contraindications/Precautions/Warnings

The product label has several contraindications for use in dogs, including hypersensitivity to ACE inhibitors, low blood pressure, acute renal insufficiency, congenital heart disease, obstructive hypertrophic cardiomyopathy, and those with hemodynamically relevant stenoses (aortic stenosis, mitral valve stenosis, pulmonic stenosis).

Use ACE inhibitors with caution in patients with hypovolemia or dehydration, hyponatremia or sodium depletion, coronary or cerebrovascular insufficiency, pre-existing hematologic abnormalities, or a collagen vascular disease (eg, SLE). Patients with severe CHF should be monitored very closely upon initiation of therapy.

Adverse Effects

Imidapril's adverse effect profile in dogs is not well described. The product label states, *Diarrhea, hypotension and related symptoms such as fatigue, dizziness or anorexia can occur in rare cases. Vomiting can also occur in very rare cases. In such cases treatment should be discontinued until the patient's condition has returned to normal. The use of ACE inhibitors in dogs with hypovolemia/dehydration can lead to acute hypotension. In such cases the fluid and electrolyte balance should be restored immediately, and treatment suspended until it has been stabilized. Parameters used for monitoring renal function should be checked at the beginning of the treatment and at regular time intervals thereafter.*

Other ACE inhibitors' primary adverse effect in dogs is GI distress (eg, anorexia, vomiting, diarrhea). Potentially, weakness, hypotension, renal dysfunction, and hyperkalemia could occur. Because it lacks a sulfhydryl group (unlike captopril), there is less likelihood that immune-mediated reactions will occur, but rashes, neutropenia, and agranulocytosis have been reported in humans with other ACE inhibitors. No signs of toxicity were noted in cats receiving 0.5 mg/kg/day PO for 3 months.[5]

Reproductive/Nursing Safety

The product label states, *Laboratory studies in rats and rabbits did not produce any evidence of teratogenic, embryotoxic or maternotoxic effects, or effects on reproductive performances, when imidapril was administered at the therapeutic dose. In the absence of data, do not use in pregnant or lactating bitches or in breeding dogs.* Other ACE Inhibitors cross the placenta and are associated with decreased fetal weights and increases in fetal and maternal death rates. Human product labels contain black box warnings to discontinue ACE inhibitor treatment as soon as possible when pregnancy is detected.

It is not known if imidapril/imidaprilat enters maternal milk. Other ACE Inhibitors are excreted in milk, and safe use of imidapril during nursing cannot be assumed.

Because safety has not been established in animals, this drug should only be used when the maternal benefits outweigh the potential risks to offspring.

Overdose/Acute Toxicity

In dogs, doses up to 5 mg/kg (20 times label dose) of imidapril PO have been well-tolerated in healthy dogs. Hypotension may occur as a clinical sign of overdose with signs of apathy and ataxia; treatment is symptomatic.

For patients that have experienced or are suspected of having experienced an overdose, consultation with a 24-hour poison consultation center specializing in providing veterinary-specific information is recommended. For general information related to overdose and toxin exposures, as well as contact information for poison control centers, refer to ***Appendix***.

Drug Interactions

The following drug interactions have either been reported or are theoretical in humans or animals receiving ACE inhibitors and may be of significance in veterinary patients receiving imidapril. Unless otherwise noted, use together is not necessarily contraindicated, but the potential risks should be weighed and additional monitoring performed when appropriate.

- **Anesthetic Agents, Inhalant and Injectable** (eg, **alfaxalone, etomidate, isoflurane, propofol**): Concurrent use may increase the risk for hypotension.
- **Antacids, Aluminum-, Calcium-, or Magnesium-Containing**: Reduced oral absorption of ACE inhibitors may occur if given concomitantly with antacids; it is suggested to separate dosing by at least two hours.
- **Angiotensin Receptor Blockers** (ARBs; eg, **telmisartan**): Concurrent use of an ACE inhibitor with an angiotensin II receptor antagonist may cause additive effects on the renin-angiotensin system causing hyperkalemia, hypotension, syncope, and acute kidney injury.
- **Antihypertensive Agents/Vasodilators** (eg, **amlodipine, hydralazine, prazosin, sildenafil**): Concurrent use may increase the risk for hypotension and other adverse effects.
- **Baclofen**: Concurrent administration may increase the risk for hypotension.
- **Buspirone**: Concurrent use may increase the risk for hypotension.
- **Cabergoline**: Concurrent use may lead to additive hypotension.
- **Cimetidine**: Concurrent use with ACE inhibitors has caused neurologic dysfunction in two human patients.
- **Corticosteroids** (eg, **dexamethasone, fludrocortisone, prednis(ol)one**): May decrease the antihypertensive effects of ACE inhibitors
- **Darbepoetin alfa; Epoetin Alfa**: ACE inhibitors may interfere with erythropoiesis.
- **Digoxin**: Levels may increase 15% to 30% when an ACE inhibitor is added; automatic reduction in dosage is not recommended but monitoring of serum digoxin levels should be performed.
- **Diphenhydramine**: Concurrent use may increase the risk for hypotension.
- **Disopyramide**: Hypoglycemic effects may be enhanced.
- **Diuretics** (eg, **furosemide, torsemide**): Concomitant diuretics may cause hypotension if used with ACE inhibitors; titrate dosages carefully.
- **Doxepin**: Concurrent use may increase the risk for hypotension.
- **Glycerin, Oral**: Concurrent use may increase the risk for hypotension.
- **Heparin, Low Molecular Weight Heparins** (eg, **dalteparin, enoxaparin**): Concurrent use may increase the risk for hyperkalemia

- **Nonsteroidal Anti-inflammatory Agents** (NSAIDs, eg, **carprofen, meloxicam, robenacoxib**): May reduce the clinical efficacy of ACE inhibitors when it is being used as an antihypertensive agent
- **Opioids** (eg, **butorphanol, hydrocodone, morphine**): Concurrent use may increase the risk for hypotension.
- **Potassium** or **Potassium Sparing Diuretics** (eg, **spironolactone**): Hyperkalemia may develop.
- **Probenecid**: Can decrease renal excretion of ACE inhibitors and possibly enhance the clinical and toxic effects of the drug

Laboratory Considerations

- When using iodohippurate sodium I^{123}/I^{134} or Technetium Tc^{99} pentetate **renal imaging** in patients with renal artery stenosis, ACE inhibitors may cause a reversible decrease in localization and excretion of these agents in the affected kidney, which may lead to confusion in test interpretation.

Dosages

DOGS:

Adjunctive treatment of moderate to severe heart failure by mitral regurgitation or by dilated cardiomyopathy[1] (extra-label): 0.25 mg/kg PO once daily

Heart failure: 0.25 mg/kg PO once daily; dosage may be increased to 0.25 mg/kg every 12 hours[2]

Monitoring

- Clinical signs of CHF
- Serum electrolytes, creatinine, BUN, urine protein:creatinine ratio
- CBC with differential, periodic
- Blood pressure (if treating hypertension or clinical signs associated with hypotension arise)

Client Information

- Use imidapril to treat heart failure, high blood pressure, and some forms of kidney disease in dogs and cats.
- Usually well tolerated but vomiting and diarrhea can occur. Imidapril is best given on an empty stomach. However, if your animal vomits, stops eating, or acts sick after getting it on an empty stomach, give it with food or a small treat to see if this helps. If vomiting continues, contact your veterinarian.
- If a rash or signs of infection occur (eg, fever), contact your veterinarian immediately.
- Very important to give as prescribed. Do not stop or reduce the dosage without your veterinarian's guidance.
- Your animal will need to have blood pressure and lab tests performed regularly.

Chemistry/Synonyms

Imidapril and imidaprilat, angiotensin-converting enzyme (ACE) inhibitors, are structurally related to captopril. Imidapril is a prodrug and is converted in vivo by the liver to imidaprilat. Imidapril occurs as a fine, white powder. After reconstitution, the resulting solution is clear and colorless.

Imidapril may also be known as imidaprilum. *Tanatril*® and *Prilium*® are two trade names.

Storage/Stability

Before reconstitution, do not store this product above 25°C (77°F). After reconstitution, store at 2°C to 8°C (36°F-46°F; in the refrigerator) for up to 77 days.

Compatibility/Compounding Considerations

Preparation of the oral solution: Remove the nipple and the stopper of the vial containing the powder and fill with tap water up to the 30 mL mark that is indicated by a raised ring around the body of the bottle; place the childproof cap on the bottle and screw on tightly.

Dosage Forms/Regulatory Status

VETERINARY-LABELED PRODUCTS:

None in the United States. In the United Kingdom and some other countries: Imidapril Powder for Oral Solution: 2.5 mg/mL (75 mg per bottle), and 5 mg/mL (150 mg per bottle); *Prilium*®; POM-V (United Kingdom)

HUMAN-LABELED PRODUCTS: NONE

References

For the complete list of references, see **wiley.com/go/budde/plumb**

Imidocarb

(i-***mid***-oh-karb) *Imizol*®

Antiprotozoal

Prescriber Highlights

- ► Antiprotozoal with activity for *Babesia* spp and related parasites
- ► Contraindications include patients exposed to cholinesterase-inhibiting drugs (eg, pyridostigmine), pesticides, or chemicals.
- ► Use caution in patients with impaired lung, hepatic, or renal function; safety in puppies, pregnant, lactating, or breeding animals has not been established.
- ► Adverse effects: The most common effects are pain during injection and mild cholinergic signs (eg, salivation, nasal drip, and brief episodes of vomiting); less common effects include panting, diarrhea, injection site inflammation (rarely ulceration), and restlessness. Cholinergic effects may be lessened with antimuscarinic drugs.
- ► Not for IV administration

Uses/Indications

Imidocarb is FDA-approved for use in dogs to treat *Babesia canis* infections (babesiosis), but the drug may also be efficacious against other *Babesia* spp (eg, *Babesia conradae* and North Carolina *Babesia* spp). Imidocarb appears to be more effective against *B canis* than *Babesia gibsoni*.[1] A prospective, unmasked study in dogs with *B gibsoni* comparing atovaquone/azithromycin (AA) with a protocol using clindamycin, diminazene, and imidocarb (CDI) found that CDI had higher recovery and lower relapse rates, albeit longer therapy duration and slower reduction in parasite numbers than AA. The authors concluded that CDI was effective for initial therapy and when the M121I gene in *B gibsoni* had mutated.[2] Imidocarb has been used to treat canine ehrlichiosis (*Ehrlichia canis*), but one study found that, when used alone, it did not clear the organism.[3] Imidocarb appears to be effective in treating hepatozoonosis (*Hepatozoon canis*) in dogs, but without eliminating gamonts.[4] It has also been suggested as a treatment for American canine hepatozoonosis (*Hepatazoon americanum*), but it does not clear the encysted stage.

In cats, imidocarb therapy has been recommended for treating cytauxzoonosis (*Cytauxzoon felis*), but currently AA is the treatment of choice.[5]

In horses, imidocarb dipropionate is considered to be the most effective treatment for piroplasmosis, including *Babesia caballi* and *Theileria equi* (formerly *Babesia equi*), currently causing infections in horses in the United States.[6]

Imidocarb may be of benefit in treating *Babesia* spp and related parasitic diseases in a variety of other domestic and exotic animals.

Pharmacology/Actions

Imidocarb is thought to act by combining with nucleic acids of DNA in susceptible organisms, causing the DNA to unwind and denature. This damage to DNA is believed to inhibit cellular repair and replication. It also appears to alter the parasite's ability to regulate glucose. Imidocarb has cholinergic properties that contribute to its toxicity profile.

Pharmacokinetics

Imidocarb is poorly absorbed after oral administration. After IM injection of imidocarb dipropionate in horses, imidocarb rapidly distributes and is not detected in plasma 12 hours after dosing. However, urine concentrations are similar to peak plasma concentrations up to 36 hours, and the drug is detectable in feces up to 10 days, suggesting that it is rapidly sequestered into tissues. Imidocarb undergoes little metabolism and is primarily eliminated from the body as an unchanged drug.

Contraindications/Precautions/Warnings

Do not use imidocarb in patients that have been exposed to cholinesterase-inhibiting drugs, pesticides, or chemicals. The manufacturer states to consider risks versus benefits before treating dogs with impaired lung, hepatic, or renal function. Donkeys and mules appear to be more sensitive to the toxic effects of the drug than are horses.

Do **NOT** give imidocarb IV. In cats, puppies, and debilitated dogs, pretreatment with atropine or glycopyrrolate has been advised. See warnings in ***Dosages***.

Do not use imidocarb in horses less than 1 year of age[7] or in horses intended for food. See ***Reproductive/Nursing Safety.***

Imidocarb is not intended for use in humans. In the event of human exposure, it is recommended to immediately contact a local poison control center.

Do not confuse imidocarb with imidacloprid.

Adverse Effects

The most commonly reported adverse effects in dogs include pain during injection and mild cholinergic signs (eg, salivation, nasal drip, and brief episodes of vomiting). Less commonly reported effects include panting, diarrhea, restlessness, and injection site inflammation (more common after the second dose and rarely may ulcerate). Hypoglycemia has been reported. Rarely, severe renal tubular or hepatic necrosis and severe cholinergic signs have occurred. Adverse effects in cats include salivation, lacrimation, vomiting, diarrhea, muscle tremors, restlessness, tachycardia, and dyspnea. Cholinergic adverse effects can be treated with an antimuscarinic (eg, atropine, glycopyrrolate) agent if necessary.

Horses given therapeutic dosages (2.4 mg/kg) can show signs of abdominal pain/colic, diarrhea, lacrimation, sweating, and serous nasal discharge after treatment. Antimuscarinic agents (eg, atropine, glycopyrrolate, or butylscopolamine) have been used to mitigate these effects.

Imidocarb has reportedly caused an increased incidence of tumor formation in rats.

Reproductive/Nursing Safety

Imidocarb can cross the placenta. Safety in puppies, pregnant, lactating, or breeding animals has not been established.[8] Imidocarb should not be used in equids in near-term pregnancies.[7]

Imidocarb is detectable in mare's milk 2 hours after a single dose of 2.4 mg/kg IM. Safety has not been established for nursing foals. Because safety has not been established in animals, this drug should only be used when the maternal benefits outweigh the potential risks to offspring.

Overdose/Acute Toxicity

Dogs receiving a dosage of 9.9 mg/kg (1.5 times the labeled dose) showed signs of liver injury (slightly increased liver enzymes), pain and swelling at the injection site, and vomiting.[8] Overdoses or chronic toxicity may present with cholinergic signs (eg, anorexia, vomiting, weakness, lethargy, salivation) or adverse changes in liver, kidney, lung, or intestinal function. Treatment with atropine may be useful to treat cholinergic signs associated with imidocarb.

The LD_{50} in horses is reportedly 16 mg/kg. Deaths in cattle have been reported at 5 times the labeled dose.

For patients that have experienced or are suspected of having experienced an overdose, consultation with a 24-hour poison consultation center specializing in providing veterinary-specific information is recommended. For general information related to overdose and toxin exposures, as well as contact information for poison control centers, refer to ***Appendix.***

Drug Interactions

The manufacturer warns not to use imidocarb in patients exposed to **cholinesterase-inhibiting drugs** (eg, **neostigmine, pyridostigmine**), **pesticides,** or **chemicals.**

Laboratory Considerations

- Imidocarb IM injections may cause significant increases in **creatine kinase** (**CK**).

Dosages

DOGS:

WARNINGS:

1. Do NOT administer imidocarb by the IV route.
2. Some references recommend using atropine 0.5 mg/kg SC as a pre-medication to mitigate the muscarinic effects of imidocarb in dogs. This is a decimal point error that can lead to tachycardia and other antimuscarinic effects. A more reasonable dose would be 0.02 – 0.05 mg/kg SC.[9-11]

Babesiosis:

Label Dosage (FDA-approved): 6.6 mg/kg IM or SC; repeat dose in 2 weeks[8]

Extra-label Dosages:

a) ***Babesia canis***: Dosage recommendations vary somewhat and range from 5 – 7.5 mg/kg IM or SC; repeat in 2 weeks. Some clinicians will re-treat in 7 days if the dog is doing poorly clinically.
b) ***Babesia gibsoni* when the *M121I* gene has mutated** (extra-label): Based on a prospective, unmasked study, clindamycin 30 mg/kg PO every 12 hours with diminazene aceturate 3.5 mg/kg IM once on the day of presentation and imidocarb dipropionate 6 mg/kg SC once on the day after administration of diminazene[2]

Ehrlichiosis (extra-label): In particularly severe cases, imidocarb 5 mg/kg SC (in a single injection, or 2 injections 15 days apart) in combination with doxycycline 10 mg/kg PO every 24 hours for 28 days.[12] Use is generally reserved for when doxycycline or minocycline are demonstrated to be ineffective. A study has demonstrated that imidocarb alone was not effective in clearing *Ehrlichia canis* from the blood of experimentally infected dogs.[3]

Hepatozoonosis (*Hepatozoon canis*) (extra-label): Most clinicians recommend 5 – 6 mg/kg IM or SC, every 14 days until gamonts clear from blood smears and remain absent for 2 to 3 consecutive months.[13] However, PCR or buffy-coat smears are much more sensitive to detect the presence of parasitemia for *H canis* than blood smears.[14] The prognosis for dogs with low levels of parasitemia is usually good with repeated injections, but the prognosis is guarded in dogs with higher levels of parasitemia.

CATS:

Cytauxzoon felis (extra-label): At present, treatment with atovaquone with azithromycin is considered superior to treatment with imidocarb. If therapy is attempted with imidocarb, 5 mg/kg IM once and repeated in 14 days. Consider pretreatment with atropine or another antimuscarinic agent. Aggressive supportive therapy (eg, IV fluids, prophylactic heparin, nutritional and nursing care, analgesia, and potentially transfusion) is required.[5]

Feline babesiosis (large babesia) (extra-label): Primaquine is usually the drug choice. Imidocarb 2.5 mg/kg IM once alone or with co-administration with doxycycline may be effective for treating *B canis* subsp *presentii* and *Babesia herpailuri*. Does not appear to have efficacy against *Babesia felis*[15]

Feline hemoplasmosis (Nomenclature is in flux: *Haemobartonella felis, Mycoplasma haemofelis; Candidatus Mycoplasma, Candidatus Mycoplasma turicensis)* (extra-label): Doxycycline is preferred, but in cats that are intolerant to it, marbofloxacin, enrofloxacin, or orbifloxacin may be effective. Alternatively, imidocarb 5 mg/kg IM every 2 weeks for at least 2 injections was used successfully in the management of 5 naturally infected cats that had failed treatment with other drugs. Blood transfusion should be given if clinically indicated. Most drug protocols have failed to eliminate infection, and so at this time, there is no clinical utility to repeat PCR testing. The owners should be warned that recurrence might occur.[16,17]

EQUIDS (HORSES/ZEBRAS):

Babesia caballi (label dosage; FDA-approved): 2 mg/kg IM, repeating dosage once after 24 hours.[7] Administer IM in the neck region.

Theleria (Babesia) equi (label dosage; FDA-approved): 4 mg/kg IM, repeating dosage 4 times at 72 hour intervals.[7] Administer IM in the neck region.

Equine piroplasmosis | *B caballi; T equi* (extra-label): Reported dosages for alleviation of clinical signs vary; most sources indicate that 2.2 – 4.4 mg/kg given IM once are effective. If necessary, lower dosages can be repeated at 24- to 72-hour intervals for 2 to 3 treatments. In nonendemic areas where chemotherapeutic clearance of the organism is desired, animals infected with *B caballi* or *T equi* can be cleared with a dose of 4.4 mg/kg IM every 72 hours for 4 treatments.[6]

CATTLE:

Treatment bovine babesiosis | *Babesia divergens* (extra-label): 0.85 mg/kg SC once[18]; do not administer IM or IV and do not exceed 10 mL per injection site.

Prevention of bovine babesiosis/*Babesia divergens* (extra-label): 2.125 mg/kg SC once[18]; do not administer IM or IV and do not exceed 10 mL per injection site.

Monitoring

- Efficacy. Usually via blood smear in patients with acute infections; however, PCR tests are more sensitive for detecting the presence of the parasite when organism numbers are low.[19]
- Adverse effect profile
- Baseline and periodic renal and hepatic function tests after treatment until stable

Client Information

Imidocarb should only be administered by your veterinarian. Possible side effects after a dose include:

- Dogs: Common: salivation/drooling, nasal drip, and brief episodes of vomiting. Less common: panting, diarrhea, injection site inflammation (rarely ulceration), and restlessness
- Cats: salivation/drooling, lacrimation, tearing, vomiting, diarrhea, muscle tremors, restlessness, fast heart rate, and difficulty breathing
- Horses: abdominal pain/colic, diarrhea, lacrimation, tearing, sweating, and nasal discharge
- Your veterinarian may give your animal another medicine to counteract some of these side effects if they are severe.

Chemistry/Synonyms

Imidocarb dipropionate is a diamidine of the carbanalide series of antiprotozoal compounds.

Imidocarb may also be known as 4A65 (imidocarb hydrochloride) and *Imizol*®.

Storage/Stability

Store the injection between 2°C and 25°C (36°F-77°F) and protected from light.

Compatibility/Compounding Considerations

Do not mix imidocarb injection with other medications.

Dosage Forms/Regulatory Status

VETERINARY-LABELED PRODUCTS:

Imidocarb Dipropionate for IM or SC Injection: 120 mg/mL in 10 mL multi-dose vials; *Imizol*®; (Rx). FDA-approved for use in dogs. A formulation approved for use in horses and zebras (100 mg/mL, *Imizol® Equine*) is still listed in FDA's Green Book of approved animal drugs but does not appear to be commercially available in the United States. Some countries have a product (85 mg/mL) approved for single-dose use in cattle (check the label or consult FARAD for withdrawal times). Imidocarb should not be used in horses intended for food.

HUMAN-LABELED PRODUCTS: NONE

References

For the complete list of references, see **wiley.com/go/budde/plumb**

Imipenem/Cilastatin Sodium

(ih-me-***peh***-nem sye-la-***sta***-tin) *Primaxin*®

Carbapenem Antibiotic

Prescriber Highlights

- ► Parenteral broad-spectrum carbapenem antibiotic and deactivating enzyme inhibitor combination used for serious, multidrugresistant infections
- ► Contraindications/Cautions: Patients hypersensitive to it or other beta-lactams, patients with renal impairment (dosage adjustment may be required), or patients with CNS disorders (eg, seizures, head trauma)
- ► Adverse Effects: GI effects, CNS toxicity (seizures, tremors), hypersensitivity, and infusion reactions (thrombophlebitis)
- ► Rapid IV infusions may cause GI or CNS toxicity.

Uses/Indications

Imipenem may be useful in rare situations in equine or small animal medicine to treat serious infections caused by multidrug-resistant bacteria when lower tier antibiotics are ineffective or have unacceptable adverse effect profiles. The most common uses of carbapenems are for the treatment of extended-spectrum beta-lactamase (ESBL) producing Enterobacterales or *Pseudomonas* spp. However, when a carbapenem is indicated, meropenem is most often used as meropenem is generally more active against gram negatives and is amenable to SC administration. The carbapenems (eg, imipenem, meropenem) can be valuable when treating serious gram-negative infections, particularly when multidrug-resistant bacteria are documented to be susceptible to imipenem. *Because this antibiotic is used for multidrug-resistant infections in humans, its use in veterinary medicine should be reserved for confirmed infections where culture and susceptibility testing demonstrates resistance to all other options, the infection is considered treatable, and consultation with an infectious disease expert has concluded that meropenem is a viable and reasonable treatment.*[1,2]

The World Health Organization classifies carbapenems, including imipenem, as a Critically Important, High Priority antimicrobial for human medicine.[3]

Pharmacology/Actions

This fixed combination of a carbapenem antibiotic (imipenem) and an inhibitor of dehydropeptidase I (DHP I) (cilastatin) has a very broad spectrum of activity. Imipenem is generally considered to be a time-dependent bactericidal agent but may be bacteriostatic against some bacteria. As it is a beta-lactam, it has an affinity for and binds to most penicillin-binding protein sites, thereby inhibiting bacterial cell wall synthesis.

Imipenem has activity against a wide variety of bacteria, including gram-positive aerobic cocci (including some bacteriostatic activity against some enterococci), gram-positive aerobic bacilli (including static activity against *Listeria* spp), gram-negative aerobic bacteria (*Haemophilus* spp, Enterobacterales, many strains of *Pseudomonas aeruginosa*), and anaerobes (including some strains of *Bacteroides* spp). *Enterococcus faecium* has inherent carbapenem resistance. Methicillin-resistant staphylococci are resistant to imipenem. Acquired imipenem resistance is currently rare in animals but has been identified and is an increasingly serious problem in human medicine.

Cilastatin inhibits the metabolism of imipenem by DHP I on the brush borders of renal tubular cells. This serves 2 functions: it allows higher imipenem urine concentrations and may protect against proximal renal tubular necrosis that can occur when the imipenem is used alone.

Pharmacokinetics

Neither drug is absorbed appreciably from the GI tract, and, therefore, they are given parenterally. In dogs, the bioavailability of imipenem after SC injection is complete, and the elimination half-life is about an hour.[4]

In cats, 5 mg/kg (using the IV form) SC and IM bioavailability was high (greater than 90%). The elimination half-life is between 1 and 2 hours after IV, SC, or IM administration.[5]

In horses, the elimination half-life is about 70 minutes. When used for regional limb perfusion, the concentration of imipenem in the synovial fluid remained above the MIC of most susceptible pathogens for ≈6 hours.[6]

Imipenem is distributed widely throughout the body, with the exception of the CSF. When given with cilastatin, imipenem is eliminated by both renal and non-renal mechanisms. ≈75% of a dose is excreted in the urine, and about 25% is excreted by unknown non-renal mechanisms. Half-lives in patients with normal renal function range from 1 to 3 hours on average.

Contraindications/Precautions/Warnings

The potential risks versus benefits should be carefully weighed before using imipenem/cilastatin in patients hypersensitive to it or other beta-lactam antibiotics (eg, penicillins or cephalosporins) as partial cross-reactivity may occur. Patients with impaired renal function may require dose reductions or increased dose intervals, as severe renal impairment can increase the risk for seizures. Caution in patients with CNS disorders (eg, seizures, head trauma), as CNS adverse effects are more likely.

Serious and sometimes fatal hypersensitivity reactions have been reported in humans. Use in the absence of a proven or strongly suspected infection or for a prophylactic indication can increase the risk for bacterial resistance and is not recommended.[7]

Do not give this drug via rapid IV infusion, as seizures are possible. In humans, it is recommended to give doses of 500 mg or less over 20 to 30 minutes and doses over 500 mg over 40 to 60 minutes.

Adverse Effects

Potential adverse effects include GI effects (eg, vomiting, anorexia, diarrhea), CNS toxicity (seizures, tremors), hypersensitivity (pruritus, fever to anaphylaxis), and infusion reactions (thrombophlebitis; too rapid IV infusions may cause GI or CNS toxicity). Rapid IV infusion or multiple high doses to animals with reduced renal function (including neonates and geriatric animals) may increase the risk for seizures.

SC or IM administration may cause severe pain at the injection site and neurovascular damage. There was a separate IM form available, but that product has been discontinued. Rarely, hypotension, tachycardia, or transient increases in renal (BUN or serum creatinine values) function tests and/or hepatic (AST/ALT/ALP) enzymes may be noted.

Reproductive/Nursing Safety

Imipenem crosses the placenta and is distributed into milk. While no teratogenic or reproductive effects have been noted in animal studies, safe use during pregnancy has not been firmly established. While imipenem enters milk, no adverse effects attributable to it have been noted in nursing offspring.

Because safety has not been established in animals, this drug should only be used when the maternal benefits outweigh the potential risks to offspring.

Overdose/Acute Toxicity

Little information is available. The LD_{50} of imipenem/cilastatin in a 1:1 ratio in mice and rats is ≈1 g/kg/day. At that dosage, ataxia and clonic convulsions and death occurred within 1 hour. Acute overdoses should be handled by halting therapy then treating supportively and symptomatically.

For patients that have experienced or are suspected of having experienced an overdose, consultation with a 24-hour poison consultation center specializing in providing veterinary-specific information is recommended. For general information related to overdose and toxin exposures, as well as contact information for poison control centers, refer to ***Appendix***.

Drug Interactions

The following drug interactions have either been reported or are theoretical in humans or animals receiving imipenem/cilastatin and may be of significance in veterinary patients. Unless otherwise noted, use together is not necessarily contraindicated, but weigh the potential risks and perform additional monitoring when appropriate.

- **Aminoglycosides**: Additive effects or synergy may result when aminoglycosides are added to imipenem/cilastatin therapy, particularly against *Enterococcus* spp, *Staphylococcus aureus*, and *Listeria monocytogenes*. There is apparently neither synergy nor antagonism when used in combination against Enterobacteriaceae or *Pseudomonas aeruginosa*.
- **Beta-Lactam Antibiotics**: Antagonism may occur when used in combination with other beta-lactam antibiotics against several Enterobacteriaceae or *Pseudomonas aeruginosa*. The clinical importance of this interaction is unclear, but at present, it is **not** recommended to use imipenem in conjunction with other beta-lactam antibiotics.
- **Chloramphenicol**: May antagonize the antibacterial effects of imipenem (in vitro evidence)
- **Cyclosporine**: Increased cyclosporine levels and potential for CNS effects
- **Ganciclovir**: Increased risk for seizures
- **Probenecid**: May increase concentrations and the elimination half-life of cilastatin, but not imipenem; concurrent use not recommended.
- **Theophylline**: May result in theophylline toxicity
- **Trimethoprim/Sulfa**: Synergy may occur against *Nocardia*

asteroides when imipenem is used in combination with trimethoprim/sulfa.

Laboratory Considerations

- Imipenem may cause a false-positive **urine glucose** determination when using the cupric sulfate solution test (eg, *Clinitest*®), Benedict's solution, or Fehling's solution. Enzymatic glucose oxidase-based tests are not affected (eg, *Tes-Tape, Clinistix*®).

Dosages

NOTES:

1. Dosages are for imipenem alone, not the combined drugs.
2. Reconstituted imipenem solution should be further diluted in a compatible IV solution and infused over 20 to 60 minutes.

DOGS/CATS:

Susceptible infections (extra-label): 5 – 10 mg/kg IV every 6 to 8 hours

HORSES:

Susceptible infections (extra-label):

Adult horses[8]: 10 – 20 mg/kg via slow IV (over a 10-minute period) every 6 hours; alternatively, 16 µg/kg/minute (0.016 mg/kg per minute) IV CRI should maintain synovial concentrations greater than 1 µg/mL (0.01 mg/mL)[9]

Foals: 10 – 15 mg/kg slow IV every 6 to 12 hours; IM if diluted into lidocaine 1%. May give 0.4 – 0.8 mg/kg/hour IV CRI[10]

Intravenous regional limb perfusion (extra-label): Based on a pharmacokinetic study, 500 mg (diluted in 0.9% sodium chloride to 100 mL total) injected into the cephalic or saphenous vein of standing horses with a 30-minute tourniquet time; concentrations above the MIC of most susceptible pathogens were maintained for ≈6 hours.[6]

Monitoring

- Efficacy
- Adverse effects, including vomiting, diarrhea, anorexia, seizures, tremors, pruritus, and fever
- Renal and liver values in cases of prolonged treatment or pre-existing renal or liver disease

Client Information

- Your veterinarian must administer imipenem/cilastatin in an inpatient setting.

Chemistry/Synonyms

Imipenem monohydrate is a carbapenem antibiotic that occurs as a white or off-white, non-hygroscopic, crystalline compound. At room temperature, 11 mg are soluble in 1 mL of water. Cilastatin sodium, an inhibitor of dehydropeptidase I (DHP I), occurs as an offwhite to yellowish, hygroscopic, amorphous compound. More than 2 g are soluble in 1 mL of water.

The commercially available injections are available in a 1:1 fixed-dose ratio. The solutions are clear to yellowish in color; pH after reconstitution ranges from 6.5 to 7.5. These products have sodium bicarbonate added as a buffer.

Imipenem may also be known as N-formimidoyl thienamycin, imipemide, MK-787, and MK-0787; multi-ingredient preparations: *Imipem*®, *Klonam*®, *Primaxin*®, *Tenacid*®, *Tienam*®, *Tracix*®, and *Zienam*®.

Storage/Stability

Store the commercially available sterile powders for injection at room temperature (less than 25°C [77°F]). After reconstitution, the solution is stable for 4 hours at room temperature; 24 hours when refrigerated. If other diluents are used, stability times may be reduced (see package insert). Do not freeze solutions. The manufacturer does not recommend admixing with other drugs.

Compatibility/Compounding Considerations

Vials should be reconstituted with 10 mL of an appropriate diluent: normal saline, 5% or 10% dextrose, 5% dextrose with 0.9% sodium chloride, 5% dextrose with 0.225% or 0.45% saline, 5% dextrose with 0.15% potassium chloride, and 5% or 10% mannitol. Reconstituted solutions can range from clear to yellow, but the potency is the same within this color range. The solution must be further diluted before administration (see package insert).

Compatibility is dependent on factors such as pH, concentration, temperature, and diluent used; specialized references or a hospital pharmacist should be consulted for more specific information.

Imipenem is **compatible** with 5% dextrose and 0.9% sodium chloride, depending on concentration. The following drugs are reportedly **compatible** with imipenem/cilastatin for an IV infusion at a Y-site: aztreonam, buprenorphine, butorphanol, cefazolin, cefepime, ceftazidime, clindamycin, dexamethasone HCl and SP, diltiazem, famotidine, furosemide, insulin, metoclopramide, ondansetron, propofol, and voriconazole.

Dosage Forms/Regulatory Status

VETERINARY-LABELED PRODUCTS: NONE

HUMAN-LABELED PRODUCTS:

Imipenem/Cilastatin Powder for Injection: imipenem 500 mg equivalent and cilastatin 500 mg equivalent (1.6 mEq sodium); *Primaxin*®, generic; (Rx)

References

For the complete list of references, see **wiley.com/go/budde/plumb**

Imipramine

(im-***ip***-ra-meen) *Tofranil*®

Tricyclic Antidepressant

Prescriber Highlights

- ▶ Used primarily in dogs and cats for urinary incontinence, narcolepsy, and behavior disorders. It may be useful for the adjunctive treatment of chronic pain. In horses, imipramine has been tried for treatment of narcolepsy and ejaculatory dysfunction.
- ▶ May reduce seizure thresholds in epileptic animals
- ▶ Can be very toxic in overdoses
- ▶ May take a few weeks to see clinical effects; taper dose when discontinuing.
- ▶ Most likely adverse effects include sedation and anticholinergic effects (tachycardia, hyperexcitability, tremors)
- ▶ Many possible drug interactions

Uses/Indications

In dogs and cats, imipramine has been used for urinary incontinence, narcolepsy, and tricyclic-responsive behavior disorders. Like other tricyclic antidepressant agents, it may be useful for the adjunctive treatment of chronic pain. In horses, imipramine has been used to treat narcolepsy[1] and ejaculatory dysfunction.[2,3]

Pharmacology/Actions

Imipramine and its active metabolite, desipramine, have a complicated pharmacologic profile, including inhibition of serotonin and norepinephrine reuptake at the neuronal membrane, thereby increasing neurotransmitter concentrations; sedation; and central and peripheral anticholinergic activity. Although not completely understood, it is thought that the antienuretic activity of imipramine is related to its anticholinergic effects, but imipramine may also have some alpha-1-adrenergic receptor antagonist activity. Imipramine also antagonizes the histamine H1 receptor. In animals, tricyclic antidepressants have similar pharmacologic actions to the phenothiazines with respect to altering avoidance behaviors.

Pharmacokinetics

Imipramine is rapidly absorbed from both the GI tract and parenteral injection sites. Peak concentrations occur within 1 to 2 hours after oral dosing. Imipramine and desipramine enter the CNS and maternal milk in concentrations equal to that found in maternal serum. The drug is metabolized in the liver to several metabolites, including desipramine, which is active. In humans, the terminal half-life is ≈8-16 hours.

Contraindications/Precautions/Warnings

Imipramine is contraindicated if prior sensitivity has been noted with any other tricyclic antidepressant. Concomitant use (or use within 14 days before or after treatment) with monoamine oxidase inhibitors (MAOIs) is generally contraindicated.[4]

Use with caution in patients with seizure disorders as imipramine may lower the seizure threshold.[4] Because of its anticholinergic effects, use imipramine with caution in animals with decreased GI motility, urinary retention, cardiovascular disease (especially cardiac rhythm disturbances), narrow angle glaucoma, or increased intraocular pressure. Use with caution in patients with thyroid, renal or hepatic disease.

If discontinuing imipramine, the dose should be slowly tapered over 2 to 3 weeks to minimize the risk for signs of withdrawal.

Adverse Effects

The most predominant adverse effects seen with the tricyclic antidepressants are related to their anticholinergic (dry mouth, constipation, tachycardia, hyperexcitability, tremors) and sedative properties. They have been shown to cause CNS stimulation with the potential to lead to seizures. Adverse effects may also affect the following systems: cardiac (dysrhythmias), hematologic (bone marrow suppression), GI (diarrhea, vomiting), endocrine (glycemic changes, hyponatremia), and renal (delayed micturition).

Reproductive/Nursing Safety

Imipramine crosses the placenta. Studies in rats have shown systemic and embryotoxic potential, and isolated reports of limb reduction abnormalities have been noted.[4]

Imipramine is excreted into milk in low concentrations (approximate milk:plasma ratio of 0.4 to 1.5).

Because safety has not been established in animals, this drug should only be used when the maternal benefits outweigh the potential risks to offspring.

Overdose/Acute Toxicity

The oral LD_{50} for dogs is 100 – 215 mg/kg.[4] Overdoses of tricyclic antidepressants can be life-threatening (arrhythmias, cardiorespiratory collapse, seizures, CNS depression and coma).

Overdoses should be treated with standard decontamination measures if appropriate for the animal. IV lipid emulsion therapy has been used successfully in humans and may be beneficial in veterinary patients as well.[5]

For patients that have experienced or are suspected to have experienced an overdose, consultation with a 24-hour poison consultation center specializing in providing veterinary-specific information is recommended. For general information related to overdose and toxin exposures, as well as contact information for poison control centers, refer to ***Appendix.***

Drug Interactions

The following drug interactions have either been reported or are theoretical in humans or animals receiving imipramine and may be of significance in veterinary patients. Unless otherwise noted, use together is not necessarily contraindicated, but weigh the potential risks and perform additional monitoring when appropriate.

- Alpha-2-Adrenergic Agonists (eg, **clonidine, dexmedetomidine, xylazine**): Increased risk for CNS and respiratory depression, hypertension, and bradycardia. Tricyclic antidepressants (TCAs) may interfere with the antihypertensive effects of alpha-2 agonists. Use cautiously in combination
- Antihypertensive Agents (eg, **amlodipine, enalapril, telmisartan**): Increased risk for hypotension
- Albuterol: Concurrent use may increase risk for cardiotoxicity.
- Alprazolam: Concurrent use may result in increased imipramine plasma concentrations.
- Anticholinergic Agents (eg, **atropine, glycopyrrolate, oxybutynin**): Because of additive effects, use with imipramine cautiously.
- Antihistamines (eg, **cetirizine, chlorpheniramine, diphenhydramine, hydroxyzine**): Concurrent use may increase risk for CNS depression and additive anticholinergic effects. Avoid combination or monitor for sedation, tachycardia, ileus, mydriasis, or constipation.
- Azole Antifungals (eg, **itraconazole, ketoconazole**): Concurrent use may increase the risk for QT-interval prolongation.
- Cimetidine: May inhibit tricyclic antidepressant metabolism and increase the risk for toxicity
- CNS Depressants (eg, **cannabidiol, diazepam, methocarbamol, pregabalin**): Because of additive effects, use with imipramine cautiously.
- Cyclobenzaprine: Concurrent use may result in increased risk for serotonin syndrome.
- Cyproheptadine: May antagonize the serotonergic effects of tricyclic antidepressants
- Dextromethorphan: Increased risk for serotonin syndrome
- Flumazenil: Flumazenil use in animals suspected of TCA overdose may increase the risk for seizures and arrhythmias.[6]
- Metoclopramide: Concurrent use may result in an increased risk for extrapyramidal reactions or neuroleptic malignant syndrome. This combination is considered contraindicated in humans.
- Mirtazapine: Increased risk for constipation, urinary retention, CNS depression and serotonin syndrome
- Monoamine Oxidase Inhibitors (eg, **amitraz, linezolid,** and possibly **selegiline**): Concomitant use (within 14 days) with monoamine oxidase inhibitors is generally contraindicated (serotonin syndrome).
- Nonsteroidal Anti-Inflammatory Drugs (NSAIDs; eg, **carprofen, meloxicam**): Concurrent use may result in an increased risk for bleeding.
- Opioids (eg, **buprenorphine, butorphanol, fentanyl, methadone, morphine, tramadol**): Concurrent use may increase the risk for urinary retention, constipation and paralytic ileus, CNS and respiratory depression, and serotonin syndrome.
- Phenobarbital: May decrease tricyclic antidepressant concentrations
- Phenothiazines (eg, **acepromazine**): Concurrent use may result in an increased risk for cardiotoxicity.
- QT Prolonging Agents (eg, **amiodarone, cisapride, procainamide, quinidine, sotalol**): Increased risk for QTc interval prolongation and tricyclic antidepressant adverse effects
- Rifampin: May decrease tricyclic antidepressant blood concentrations
- Selective Serotonin Reuptake Inhibitors (SSRIs; eg, **fluoxetine, paroxetine, sertraline**): Increased risk for serotonin syndrome; avoid concurrent use

- **Sympathomimetic Agents** (eg, **epinephrine, phenylpropanolamine**): Use with sympathomimetic agents may increase the risk for cardiac effects (arrhythmias, hypertension) and hyperpyrexia.
- **Thyroid Agents**: May increase risk for cardiac arrhythmias

Laboratory Considerations

- **ECG**: Tricyclic antidepressants can widen QRS complexes, prolong PR intervals, and invert or flatten T-waves on ECG.
- **Glucose, blood**: Tricyclic antidepressants may alter (increase or decrease) blood glucose levels.

Dosages

DOGS:

Urethral incompetence (extra-label): No controlled studies were noted documenting efficacy; most clinicians recommend 5 – 15 mg/dog (NOT mg/kg) PO every 12 hours; some recommend dosages up to 20 mg/dog (NOT mg/kg) twice daily.

Adjunctive therapy for narcolepsy (extra-label):

a) 0.5 – 1 mg/kg PO 2 to 3 times a day (every 8 to 12 hours); titrate dose based on clinical effect.[7]

b) 0.45 – 2.2 mg/kg PO every 8 to 12 hours was used in narcoleptic dogs with cataplexy[8]

Behavior-related conditions (extra-label): Not often recommended as clomipramine (FDA-approved) or amitriptyline are most commonly used when a tricyclic antidepressant is employed. One recommended dosage for adjunctive treatment of separation anxiety or other tricyclic antidepressant-responsive behavior disorders: 2.2 – 4.4 mg/kg PO once to twice daily.[9]

Adjunctive treatment of chronic pain (extra-label): No controlled studies located documenting efficacy. Recommended dosage is 0.5 – 1 mg/kg PO every 8 hours.

CATS:

Urethral incompetence or adjunctive treatment of chronic pain (extra-label): No controlled studies were noted documenting efficacy; most clinicians recommend 2.5 – 5 mg/cat (NOT mg/kg) PO every 12 hours.

HORSES:

NOTE: The injectable product is no longer marketed in the United States. Compounded preparations may be available.

Pharmacologic induced ejaculation (extra-label):

a) 2 mg/kg IV followed 10 minutes later by xylazine 0.3 mg/kg IV[10]

b) 3 mg/kg PO followed 2 hours later by xylazine 0.66 mg/kg IV.[2] Imipramine doses as low as 100 mg/stallion (NOT mg/kg) PO have been noted.[3]

Narcolepsy and cataplexy (extra-label): 0.55 mg/kg IV or 250 – 750 mg/horse (NOT mg/kg) PO.[1] PO administration produces inconsistent results.[11]

Monitoring

- Efficacy
- Adverse effects
- Baseline CBC, serum chemistry profile, urinalysis, and baseline thyroid testing (eg, tT_4, thyroid panel) prior to therapy, 1 month after initial therapy, and yearly, thereafter.
- Baseline ECG is recommended prior to therapy. TCAs can widen QRS complexes, prolong PR intervals, and invert or flatten T-waves on ECG; significance in animals is not fully understood.

Client Information

- This medicine may be given with or without food. If your animal vomits or acts sick after receiving it on an empty stomach, give with food or small treat to see if this helps. If vomiting continues, contact your veterinarian.
- It may take several days to weeks to determine if the medicine is working.
- The most common side effects are drowsiness/sleepiness, dry mouth, and constipation. Be sure your animal has access to fresh water at all times.
- Rare side effects that can be serious: abnormal bleeding or fever, seizures, very fast or irregular heartbeat. Contact your veterinarian immediately if you see any of these.
- Overdoses can be very serious. Keep this medicine out of reach of animals and children.
- If your animal has worn a flea and tick collar in the past two weeks, let your veterinarian know. Do not use one of these collars on your animal while it's getting this medicine without first talking to your veterinarian.

Chemistry/Synonyms

A tricyclic antidepressant agent, imipramine is available commercially in either the hydrochloride or pamoate salts. Imipramine HCl occurs as an odorless or practically odorless, white to off-white crystalline powder that is freely soluble in water or alcohol. Imipramine pamoate occurs as a fine yellow powder that is practically insoluble in water, but soluble in alcohol. The HCl injection has a pH of 4 to 5.

Imipramine HCl may also be known as imipramini chloridum, imipramini hydrochloridum, imizine, and *Tofranil*®.

Storage/Stability

Imipramine HCl tablets and the pamoate capsules should be stored in tight, light-resistant containers, preferably at room temperature. The HCl injection should be stored at temperatures less than 40°C (104°F) and freezing should be avoided. Expiration dates for oral HCl products are from 3 to 5 years after manufacture; for the pamoate, 3 years.

Imipramine HCl will turn yellow to reddish on exposure. Slight discoloration will not affect potency but marked changes in color are associated with a loss of potency.

Compatibility/Compounding Considerations

No specific information noted.

Dosage Forms/Regulatory Status

VETERINARY-LABELED PRODUCTS: NONE

The Association of Racing Commissioners International (ARCI) has designated this drug as a class 2 substance. Use of this drug may not be allowed in certain animal competitions. Check rules and regulations before entering in a competition while this medication is being administered. Contact local racing authorities for further guidance. See ***Appendix*** for more information.

HUMAN-LABELED PRODUCTS:

Imipramine HCl Tablets: 10 mg, 25 mg, and 50 mg; *Tofranil*®, generic; (Rx)

Imipramine Pamoate Capsules: 75 mg, 100 mg, 125 mg, and 150 mg; *Tofranil®-PM*, generic; (Rx)

References

For the complete list of references, see **wiley.com/go/budde/plumb**

Immune Globulin (Human), Intravenous

(im-***myoon glob***-yoo-lin) *IGIV, IVIG, hIVIG*

Immune Serum

Prescriber Highlights

- ► Potentially useful for refractory cases of canine immune-mediated diseases (eg, immune-mediated hemolytic anemia [IMHA], immune-mediated thrombocytopenia [ITP]), and immune-mediated dermatopathies
- ► Limited experience in veterinary medicine; limited studies to support use
- ► Hypersensitivity reactions possible. Potentially could increase the risk for thrombosis in dogs with IMHA
- ► Very expensive. Can be difficult to obtain. May require obtaining from human hospitals

Uses/Indications

Human intravenous immune globulin (IVIG) has been used in veterinary medicine for immune-mediated hemolytic anemia (IMHA), immune-mediated thrombocytopenia (ITP), Evans syndrome, myasthenia gravis, sudden acquired retinal degeneration syndrome (SARDS),[1] and dermatologic autoimmune diseases. However, available studies have demonstrated mixed results. Definitive studies evaluating the safety and efficacy in veterinary patients are not available and are unlikely to be done in the foreseeable future due to the high cost of IVIG. There is some question whether the drug should be used at all in veterinary patients since supply is limited and some countries ration its use for humans. Current literature suggests it might be most beneficial when used as an adjust therapy for ITP and dermatologic autoimmune diseases in dogs.[1]

Although IVIG has been used for IMHA, there is no substantial evidence to support its use. A prospective, randomized, double-blinded, controlled trial of IVIG (with glucocorticoids) in 28 dogs with recently diagnosed IMHA found no statistically significant differences between the treated and placebo groups in survival, length of hospitalization, time to hematocrit stabilization, and transfusion requirements.[2] Although the study population was relatively small, the authors concluded that the cost of the treatment does not lend support to its use as an early intervention treatment in dogs.[2] The ACVIM consensus statement on the treatment of IMHA recommends the use of IVIG only as salvage therapy in dogs that are not responding to treatment with 2 immunosuppressive agents.[3]

Studies suggest that IVIG may be most useful in treating primary immune-mediated thrombocytopenia in dogs. In 1 prospective study, dogs receiving a single dose of IVIG 6% at 0.5 g/kg IV over 6 to 12 hours were compared with dogs receiving corticosteroids alone.[4] The authors concluded that adjunctive emergency therapy of a single IVIG infusion was safe and associated with a significant reduction in platelet count recovery time and duration of hospitalization without increasing the expense of medical care.[4] However, a prospective, randomized study in 20 dogs with ITP comparing vincristine versus IVIG found that there were no significant differences between both groups in median platelet recovery time (2.5 days) or median hospitalization time for dogs that survived (4 days).[5] Seven of 10 dogs in the IVIG group and 10 of 10 in the vincristine group survived to discharge. There were no significant differences in survival at discharge, 6 months, and 1 year. No adverse effects were reported in either group. The authors concluded that vincristine should be the first-line adjunctive treatment for the acute management of canine ITP because of its lower cost and ease of administration.

There have also been case reports of IVIG used for Evans syndrome[6]; SARDS; cancer-associated retinopathy[7]; "stiff dog syndrome"[8]; and dermatologic autoimmune diseases, including Stevens-Johnson syndrome,[9] pemphigus foliaceus,[10] and erythema multiforme,[11,12] but there are no controlled studies for these uses. Although case reports exist, IVIG is not considered first-line therapy for dermatologic autoimmune diseases in dogs.

In humans, IVIG has been used for a variety of immune system–related conditions, including primary and secondary immunodeficiencies, graft vs host disease, Guillain-Barré syndrome, chronic inflammatory demyelinating polyneuropathy, autoimmune hemolytic anemia, juvenile idiopathic arthritis, myasthenia gravis, toxic epidermal necrolysis, systemic vasculitis, and sepsis.

Pharmacology/Actions

Immunoglobulins are produced by B lymphocytes as part of the humoral response to foreign antigens. The actions of intravenous immune globulin (IVIG) antibodies in autoimmune disease are poorly understood and likely multifactorial and modulate the immune system by Fc receptor disruption, pathologic autoantibody neutralization, complement inhibition, Fas-Fas ligand (FasL) binding interference, and cytokine synthesis downregulation.[1] Other actions may include negative feedback and downregulation of antibody production; binding to CD5, interleukin (IL)-1a, IL-6, tumor necrosis factor-alpha, and T-cell receptors; and suppressing pathogenic cytokines and phagocytes.

Pharmacokinetics

Elimination half-life in dogs is reported to be 7 to 9 days. In humans, the onset of action is rapid. Immunoglobulins are primarily eliminated by catabolism, and the mean half-life is about 3 weeks. Fever or infection may decrease antibody half-life because of increased catabolism or consumption.

Contraindications/Precautions/Warnings

Dogs that have had prior hypersensitivity reactions after receiving human albumin should not receive intravenous immune globulin (IVIG). Trace amounts of human albumin may be found in IVIG.

In humans, many adverse reactions are associated with administering IVIG at rates higher than recommended. Follow infusion rate guidelines carefully. At doses used in dogs (0.5 – 1.5 g/kg), IVIG is generally infused over a 6- to 12-hour period. A study in healthy dogs showed that IVIG promoted hypercoagulability and an inflammatory state, which raises concerns about using it in dogs with immune-mediated hemolytic anemia (IMHA).[13]

The FDA has placed a boxed warning on the labeling of IVIG for use in humans, as it has been associated with thrombosis, renal dysfunction, acute renal failure, osmotic nephrosis, and death. For patients at risk for thrombosis or renal failure, IVIG should be administered at the lowest possible dose and infusion rate. Ensure adequate hydration before administration. Higher rates of renal failure are associated with IVIG products containing sucrose.[14]

Adverse Effects

In dogs, intravenous immune globulin (IVIG) can cause increased blood pressure. Local reactions at or near the injection site are possible. Anecdotal reports of anaphylaxis have been reported in dogs receiving IVIG. IVIG can contain trace amounts of human albumin that has been associated with hypersensitivity reactions in dogs. As IVIG can have colloid-like properties, volume overload is possible. In patients with underlying heart disease, careful consideration for dosing and rate of delivery must take place. Thrombotic events have been reported in humans and are possible in dogs. One study done in healthy dogs demonstrated that IVIG promoted hypercoagulability and an inflammatory state.[13]

In humans, adverse effects of IVIG are relatively uncommon, and most are transient and self-limiting, including fever, chills, facial flushing, fatigue, headache, and nausea. Thrombotic events have been reported. Rarely, acute renal failure, acute tubular necrosis, osmotic nephrosis, and proximal tubular nephropathy have been reported in humans. Increases in creatinine and BUN have been seen as soon as 1 to 2 days following infusion. Hypersensitivity reactions, including anaphylaxis, have been reported but are rare in human patients. Rarely, aseptic meningitis syndrome has been reported in humans, especially with a rapid infusion or high doses. Other rare adverse effects seen in human medicine can include hemolytic anemia as well as transfusion-related acute lung injury (TRALI).

Reproductive/Nursing Safety

Although maternal antibodies cross the placenta, it is unknown whether human intravenous immune globulin (IVIG) crosses the placenta in veterinary species. The drug appears to be safe for use during lactation and nursing.

Because safety has not been established in animals, this drug should only be used when the maternal benefits outweigh the potential risks to offspring.

Overdose/Acute Toxicity

Fluid volume overload is possible. Other reactions could include pain and tenderness at the injection site.

For patients that have experienced or are suspected of having experienced an overdose, consultation with a 24-hour poison consultation center specializing in providing veterinary-specific information is recommended. For general information related to overdose and toxin exposures, as well as contact information for poison control centers, refer to ***Appendix***.

Drug Interactions

The following drug interactions have either been reported or are theoretical in humans or animals receiving intravenous immune globulin (IVIG) and may be of significance in veterinary patients. Unless otherwise noted, use together is not necessarily contraindicated, but weigh the potential risks and perform additional monitoring when appropriate.

- **Vaccines, Live**: IVIG may interfere with immune response and efficacy.

Laboratory Considerations

- **Blood Glucose**: Falsely elevated blood glucose measurements can occur when using the glucose dehydrogenase pyrroloquinoline quinone (GDH-PQQ)–based test. Consider using tests that are not affected, including the glucose oxidase, glucose dehydrogenase nicotine adenine dinucleotide (GDH-NAD), or glucose dehydrogenase flavin adenine dinucleotide (GDH-FAD) methods.
- **Coombs Test**: In humans, the transitory rise of the various passively transferred antibodies may cause positive serological testing results, potentially altering the test's results and interpretation.

Dosages

DOGS:

NOTES:

1. Intravenous immune globulin (IVIG) should be administered through a separate line. The line may be flushed with saline or dextrose prior to administration. An inline filter is recommended during administration. Before administration, IVIG should be allowed to warm to room temperature. Recommendations are to begin infusions slowly (eg, 0.01 mL/kg/minute) and gradually increase the rate, not to exceed ≈0.08 mL/kg per minute, with comprehensive monitoring during the infusion.[1]
2. Various dosages have been used in dogs ranging from 0.5 – 2.2 g/kg, with 1 g/kg being the most commonly used dosage.[1]

Immune-mediated hemolytic anemia (IMHA) in dogs refractory to other immunosuppressive therapies (extra-label): 0.5 – 1.5 g/kg IV over 4 to 12 hours.[15] ACVIM recommends 0.5 – 1 g/kg as salvage therapy in dogs not responding to 2 immunosuppressive drugs.[3] **NOTE**: See ***Contraindications/Precautions/Warnings*** regarding hypercoagulability.

Primary immune-mediated thrombocytopenia (ITP) (extra-label): The optimal dose of IVIG for ITP remains to be identified, and a wide variety of doses have been reported, ranging from 0.28 – 1.3 g/kg.[16] Vincristine is likely a better first-line adjunctive treatment for the acute management of canine ITP due to similar efficacy, but lower cost and ease of administration compared to IVIG.[5]

Evans syndrome, sudden acquired retinal degeneration syndrome (SARDS) (extra-label): 0.5 – 1.3 g/kg doses have been used in case reports.[6,17]

Refractory cases of erythema multiforme, pemphigus foliaceus, Stevens-Johnson syndrome, toxic epidermal necrolysis, and other cutaneous adverse drug reactions (extra-label): No controlled studies were located, and dosage recommendations are based on case reports. One suggested dosage is a 5% to 6% solution given at 0.5 – 1 g/kg IV over a 4- to 6-hour period, 1 to 2 times, 24 hours apart. This treatment may need to be repeated for 3 to 4 days in a row. Further study is needed.[18]

Monitoring

- Blood pressure and TPR prior to infusion and frequently during administration
- Lung auscultation to assess for volume overload
- Renal function tests and urine output
- Clinical efficacy and subsequent monitoring depend on the purpose for use.

Client Information

- Clients should understand that the use of this drug in veterinary medicine is not common, plus the costs and risks associated with its use.
- Monitor for side effects after your animal gets intravenous immune globulin (IVIG), such as difficulty breathing, not eating, vomiting, and lethargy.
- While your animal is taking this medication, it is important to return to your veterinarian for examinations and laboratory work. Do not miss these important follow-up visits.

Chemistry/Synonyms

Intravenous immune globulin (IVIG) consists of fractionated immunoglobulins and is primarily intact IgG. It is obtained from human plasma pooled from thousands of donors. It may also contain trace amounts of IgM, IgA, soluble CD4, CD8, and HLA molecules, and some cytokines. Further processing is performed to inactivate viruses and remove IgG aggregates and other contaminants. Stabilizing agents can include polyethylene glycol, glycine, sorbitol, polysorbate 80, and sugars (ie, maltose, glucose, sucrose).

Immune globulin (human) may also be known as hIVIG, IVIG, IGIV, immunoglobulin, immunglobuline, or immunoglobulinas.

Storage/Stability

Intravenous immune globulin (IVIG) storage requirements vary with each product; refer to the label. Do not freeze these products. Discard unused portions.

Compatibility/Compounding Considerations

Compatibility is dependent on factors such as pH, concentration, temperature, and diluent used; specialized references or a hospital pharmacist should be consulted for more specific information.

Each product may have differing instructions for mixing and dilution. Refer to the product label for specific directions. Generally, intravenous immune globulin (IVIG) should not be mixed with other medications. Some product labels (eg, *Gammaked*®, *Privigen*®) state they can be diluted with 5% dextrose if necessary. Lyophilized products can usually be reconstituted with sterile water, 5% dextrose, or sterile saline. Do not shake; excessive shaking will cause foaming. Any undissolved particles should respond to careful rotation of the bottle; avoid foaming.

Dosage Forms/Regulatory Status

VETERINARY-LABELED PRODUCTS: NONE

HUMAN-LABELED PRODUCTS:

Immune Globulin (Human) Injection: 5% (50 mg/mL) preservative-free in 10 mL, 20 mL, 50 mL, 100 mL, and 200 mL (0.5 g, 1 g, 2.5 g, 5 g, and 10 g—depending on the product) single-use bottles; *Flebogamma*®, *Gammaplex*® 5%, *Octagam*®; (Rx)

Immune Globulin (Human) Injection: 10% (100 mg/mL) preservative-free in 10 mL, 20 mL, 50 mL, 100 mL, and 200 mL (1 g, 2 g, 10 g, and 20 g—depending on the product) single-use bottles; *Flebogamma*®, *Gamunex-C*®, *Gammagard*® *Liquid*, *Gammaked*®, *Gammaplex*® 10%, *Bivigam*®, *Privigen*®, *Panzyga*®, *Octagam*® 10%; (Rx)

Immune Globulin (Human) SC Injection: 10% (100 mg/mL) preservative-free in 10 mL, 25 mL, 50 mL, 100 mL, 200 mL and 300 mL (1 g, 2.5 g, 5 g, 10 g, 20 g, and 30 g) single-use vials; *Gammagard*® *Liquid*, *Hyqvia*® (also contains recombinant human hyaluronidase); (Rx)

Immune Globulin (Human) SC Injection: 20% (200 mg/mL) preservative-free in 5 mL, 10 mL, 20 mL, and 50 mL (1 g, 2 g, 4 g, and 10 g) single-use vials or prefilled syringes; *Cuvitru*®, *Hizentra*®, *Xembify*®; (Rx)

Immune Globulin (Human) IM Injection: 15% to 18% (150 to 180 mg/mL); preservative-free in 2 mL and 10 mL single-use vials; *Gamastan*®; (Rx)

Immune Globulin (Human) Lyophilized Powder for Solution: 5 g and 10 g kits; *Gammagard S/D*®; (Rx). A 5% or 10% solution can be prepared.

References

For the complete list of references, see **wiley.com/go/budde/plumb**

Insulin, Aspart

(***inn***-suh-lin, ***ass***-part) *NovoLog*®

Insulin, Rapid/Short-Acting

NOTE: Insulin preparations available to clinicians are in a constant state of change. To maximize the efficacy of therapy and reduce the chance for errors, it is highly recommended to review current references or sources of information pertaining to insulin therapy for dogs and cats.

For additional information, see ***Insulin, General Information.***

Prescriber Highlights

- Rapid/short-acting insulin used to treat diabetic ketoacidosis (DKA); can be used in place of regular insulin
- There are no absolute contraindications, except during episodes of hypoglycemia.
- Adverse effects include hypoglycemia, hypokalemia, hypophosphatemia (DKA only), insulin-induced rebound hyperglycemia (ie, Somogyi effect), and local reactions to the "foreign" proteins.
- Do not confuse insulin types, strengths, and syringes. Insulin aspart is a U100 human product; use only U100 insulin syringes to measure a dose.
- Many potential drug interactions

Uses/Indications

Insulin aspart is a rapid, or short-acting, insulin used in diabetic emergencies (eg, diabetic ketoacidosis [DKA]). As an insulin analogue similar in action to regular insulin (ie, rapid/short acting), insulin aspart could be considered for the same indications as regular insulin (eg, hyperkalemia) if regular insulin is not an option, although evidence in veterinary species is lacking. IV insulin administration is recommended in patients with poor tissue perfusion, shock, or cardiovascular collapse, as well as in those that require adjunct therapy for hyperkalemia.

Retrospective studies have shown that early administration (ie, within 6 hours of presentation) of insulin aspart as an IV CRI to canine DKA patients led to resolution of hyperglycemia, acidemia, and ketonemia while being safe and well tolerated.[1] When compared with an intensive SC glargine administration protocol, insulin aspart administered as an IV CRI to cats in the early stages of treatment for diabetes mellitus was shown to decrease long-term insulin requirements and increase remission rates.[2]

In patients with DKA, initial aggressive fluid replacement therapy is of paramount importance to restore tissue perfusion and begin correcting electrolyte or acid-base derangements. Once the patient is stabilized, longer-acting insulin products can be started for maintenance insulin therapy. It is strongly encouraged to consult a veterinary emergency and critical care and/or endocrinology specialist or reference when treating this complex condition.

Insulin aspart has also been used in combination with 50% dextrose to treat hyperkalemia in diarrheic calves.[3]

Pharmacology/Actions

The primary action of insulin is to regulate glucose metabolism. Insulin and its analogues lower blood glucose by increasing glucose uptake in peripheral tissues, especially by skeletal muscle and fat. In the liver, insulin increases glucose storage (ie, glycogen) while also inhibiting gluconeogenesis. Insulin's anabolic actions also enhance fatty acid and protein synthesis while inhibiting lipolysis and proteolysis.

For additional information, see ***Insulin, General Information***.

Pharmacokinetics

Insulin formulations contain insulin polymers (aggregates of multiple insulin molecules). Insulin is absorbed from the administration site only after insulin polymers break down into insulin monomers or dimers. Insulin aspart is less likely to form hexamers, and its rapid absorption results in a fast onset and short duration of effect.

After SC and IM administration in healthy cats, onset was within 0.25 hours and duration of action was 2.5 to 3 hours.[4] Higher plasma concentrations were achieved following SC administration. Onset, duration of action, and time to peak insulin effect did not differ based on route of administration. Elimination half-life was ≈1.25 hours after SC administration.

In humans, hypoglycemic effect begins within ≈0.25 hours of SC administration, peak effect is between 1 to 3 hours, and duration of effect is 3 to 5 hours. Protein binding is less than 10%. Clearance is 1.2 L/kg/hour.

Contraindications/Precautions/Warnings

Because there are no alternatives for insulin when it is used for diabetic indications, there are no absolute contraindications to its use except during episodes of hypoglycemia. If animals develop hypersensitivity (local or otherwise) or if insulin resistance develops, a change in type or species source (eg, human, bovine, porcine) of insulin should be considered after other etiologies for poor control (eg, expired insulin, concurrent disease, or medication interference) have been ruled out. See ***Insulin, General Information***.

For obese patients, dose calculations should be based on the patient's ideal body weight to avoid inadvertent insulin overdose.

In humans, long-term repeated SC/IM injections of insulin at the same site may cause lipodystrophic reactions, which could interfere with insulin absorption[5]; however, there have been no specific reports of this reaction occurring in dogs or cats.

Similar to regular insulin and other insulin analogue solutions (eg, lispro, glulisine), insulin aspart may be given IV or IM; however, insulin aspart administered IM is limited to anecdotal experience. In patients with moderate to severe dehydration, poor tissue perfusion necessitates insulin aspart be given IM or IV as absorption of SC injections is likely to be impaired or delayed. Short-acting insulin analogues administered IV offer little therapeutic or pharmacokinetic advantage over regular insulin.

Insulin aspart is U100 strength. It is crucial for patient safety to only use U100 syringes when measuring and administering U100 insulin. Calculations can be done to convert to U40 syringes or TB syringes, but these conversions are not recommended due to the potential for introducing dosing errors. See ***Insulin, General Information***.

When writing prescriptions, do not abbreviate units as "U", as this has been shown to increase the rate of transcription and dosage errors. In human medicine, insulin is considered a "high alert" medication (ie, medications that require special safeguards to reduce the risk for errors). Consider instituting practices such as redundant drug dosage and volume checking and special alert labels.

Do not confuse insulin aspart (clear solution that may be administered by a variety of routes) with insulin aspart protamine/insulin aspart mixture (cloudy solution that may be administered only by the SC route). *Fiasp®* is an insulin aspart formulation that also contains niacinamide, which, in humans, promotes a faster onset of action than *NovoLog®*.[6] It is suggested to avoid interchanging these insulins until more is known about the use of *Fiasp®* or insulin aspart protamine/insulin aspart mixtures in animals.

Adverse Effects

Adverse effects of insulin aspart therapy may include hypoglycemia (see ***Overdose/Acute Toxicity***), hypokalemia, hypophosphatemia (diabetic ketoacidosis [DKA] only), insulin-induced rebound hyperglycemia (ie, Somogyi effect), and local or allergic reactions to the "foreign" proteins.

Reproductive/Nursing Safety

Insulin aspart given during organogenesis to pregnant laboratory animals did not result in developmental effects; however, maternal hypoglycemia may result in pre- and postimplantation losses and visceral or skeletal abnormalities.[5]

In humans, insulin is considered compatible while nursing.[7]

Overdose/Acute Toxicity

Insulin overdose can lead to various degrees of hypoglycemia. Signs may include weakness, shaking, head tilt, lethargy, ataxia, seizures, blindness, bizarre behavior, and coma. Other signs may include restlessness, hunger, and muscle fasciculations. Electrolyte disturbances, including hypokalemia, may occur. Prolonged hypoglycemia can result in permanent brain damage or death.

Mild hypoglycemia can be treated by offering the animal its usual food. More serious signs (eg, seizures) should be treated with oral dextrose solutions (eg, *Karo®* syrup) applied to the buccal mucosa (if the animal is seizing, use caution to avoid being bit or injured) or by IV injections of 50% dextrose solutions (small amounts—usually 2 – 15 mL [0.5 – 1 mL/kg], diluted, and slowly administered[8]; see ***Dextrose 50% Injection***). For in-clinic management, glucagon may also be considered on an as-needed basis for an insulin overdose. See ***Glucagon***. Once the animal's hypoglycemia is alleviated (response usually occurs within 1 to 2 minutes), it should be closely monitored (both by physical observation and serial blood glucose concentrations) to prevent a recurrence of hypoglycemia (especially with the slower-absorbed/longer-acting products) and to prevent hyperglycemia from developing. Future insulin dosages or feeding regimens should be evaluated or adjusted based on consultation with the clinician to prevent further occurrences of hypoglycemia.

For patients that have experienced or are suspected of having experienced an overdose, consultation with a 24-hour poison consultation center specializing in providing veterinary-specific information is recommended. For general information related to overdose and toxin exposures, as well as contact information for poison control centers, refer to ***Appendix***.

Drug Interactions

The following drug interactions have either been reported or are theoretical in humans or animals receiving insulin and may be of significance in veterinary patients. Unless otherwise noted, use together is not necessarily contraindicated, but weigh the potential risks and perform additional monitoring when appropriate.

- BETA-ADRENERGIC ANTAGONISTS (eg, **atenolol, propranolol**): Can have variable effects on glycemic control and can mask the signs associated with hypoglycemia
- CLONIDINE: Can mask the signs associated with hypoglycemia
- DIGOXIN: Because insulin can reduce serum potassium concentrations, patients receiving concomitant digoxin therapy—especially in patients receiving concurrent diuretic therapy—should be closely monitored.
- DIURETICS (eg, **furosemide, hydrochlorothiazide**): Insulin shifts extracellular potassium into the intracellular space; serum potassium concentration should be closely monitored in patients receiving concomitant diuretic therapy. Diuretics may also decrease the hypoglycemic activity of insulin (ie, increase insulin requirements).
- RESERPINE: Can mask the signs associated with hypoglycemia

The following drugs or drug classes may potentiate the hypoglycemic activity of insulin (ie, decrease insulin requirements):

- ANABOLIC STEROIDS (eg, **boldenone, stanozolol, testosterone**)
- ANGIOTENSIN II RECEPTOR BLOCKERS (ARBs; eg, **telmisartan**)
- ANGIOTENSIN CONVERTING ENZYME INHIBITORS (ACEIs; eg, **benazepril, enalapril**)

- **Disopyramide**
- **Ethanol**
- **Fenofibrate**
- **Fluoroquinolones** (eg, **ciprofloxacin, enrofloxacin**)
- **Fluoxetine**
- **Hypoglycemics, Oral** (eg, **acarbose, glipizide, metformin**)
- **Monoamine Oxidase Inhibitors** (MAOIs; eg, **amitraz, linezolid, selegiline**)
- **Pentoxifylline**
- **Salicylates** (eg, **aspirin, bismuth subsalicylate**)
- **Somatostatin Derivatives** (eg, **octreotide**)
- **Sulfonamides** (eg, **sulfadimethoxine, sulfamethoxazole**)

The following drugs or drug classes may decrease the hypoglycemic activity of insulin (ie, increase insulin requirements):

- **Alpha-2-Adrenergic Agonists** (eg, **dexmedetomidine, medetomidine, xylazine**): May cause hyperglycemia and temporarily interfere with glycemic control
- **Beta-2-Adrenergic Agonists** (eg, **albuterol, terbutaline**)
- **Corticosteroids** (eg, **dexamethasone, prednis(ol)one**)
- **Danazol**
- **Diazoxide**
- **Estrogens** (eg, **diethylstilbestrol [DES], estriol**)
- **Isoniazid**
- **Niacin**
- **Phenothiazines** (eg, **acepromazine, chlorpromazine**)
- **Progestins** (eg, **megestrol**)
- **Thyroid Hormones**: Can elevate glucose concentrations in diabetic patients when thyroid hormone therapy is first initiated

Laboratory Considerations

- None

Dosages

NOTES:

1. Treatment of diabetes mellitus and, in particular, diabetic ketoacidosis (DKA) is complex. Insulin is only one component of therapy; treatment may require fluid and electrolyte replacement, management of acid/base disturbances, dietary adjustments, and antimicrobial therapy. Adequate patient monitoring is mandatory. It is strongly encouraged to refer to more thorough discussions of treatment in veterinary endocrinology or internal medicine references.
2. For obese patients, dose calculations should be based on the individual patient's estimated ideal body weight to avoid inadvertent insulin overdose.
3. Insulin aspart given by IV CRI appears to be a safe and effective alternative when regular insulin is not an option or is unavailable.
4. All dosages are extra-label.

DOGS:

Adjunctive treatment of DKA using an IV CRI: To prepare a CRI that delivers 0.1 units/kg/hour: 2.2 units/kg insulin aspart is added to 240 mL (**NOTE**: Many clinicians add insulin directly to a 250 mL bag without removing the 10 mL of fluid) of 0.9% sodium chloride.[1] Run ≈50 mL of the insulin-containing fluid through the drip set prior to administration (see ***Adsorption*** in ***Compatibility/Compounding Considerations***). The initial administration rate is 10 mL/hour in a separate line to that used for fluid therapy. When starting initial therapy for DKA, serum potassium concentrations must be taken into account and therapy adjusted accordingly to avoid hypokalemia. Adjust infusion rate based on blood glucose concentrations taken every 2 hours. An hourly reduction in blood glucose by 50 – 100 mg/dL is ideal.[9] Once blood glucose approaches 250 mg/dL, adjust fluid type and rate based on periodic measurement of blood glucose concentration (see table) with a goal of keeping blood glucose in the 150 – 300 mg/dL range and continuing the insulin IV infusion at a decreased rate until it can be exchanged for a longer-acting product.

Blood glucose concentration (mg/dL [mmol/L])	Maintenance IV fluid	Rate of insulin IV CRI administration (mL/hour)	Dose of insulin administered (units/kg/hour)*
Greater than 250 (13.8)	0.9% sodium chloride	10	0.09
200-250 (11.1-13.8)	0.45% sodium chloride + 2.5% dextrose	7	0.064
150-199 (8.3-11)	0.45% sodium chloride + 2.5% dextrose	5	0.045
100-149 (5.5-8.2)	0.45% sodium chloride + 5% dextrose	5	0.045
Less than 100 (5.5)	0.45% sodium chloride + 5% dextrose	0 (Stop insulin administration)	0 (Stop insulin administration)

Table adapted from Walsh ES, Drobatz KJ, Hess RS. Use of intravenous insulin aspart for treatment of naturally occurring diabetic ketoacidosis in dogs. *J Vet Emerg Crit Care.* 2016;26(1):101-107.

*CRI prepared by adding insulin aspart 2.2 units/kg to 240 mL of 0.9% sodium chloride

CATS:

Adjunctive treatment of DKA using an IV CRI: Insulin aspart 12.5 units was added to 250 mL of 0.9% sterile sodium chloride for injection. The initial infusion rate was 0.05 units/kg/hour (1 mL/kg/hour) IV CRI and adjusted up to every 15 to 30 minutes in increments of 0.025 – 0.05 units/kg/hour to achieve a target glucose concentration range of 90 – 180 mg/dL.[2] Cats were transitioned to SC glargine on the seventh day at ¼ the total Day 6 insulin aspart dose.

CATTLE:

Adjunctive treatment of hyperkalemia using an IV CRI: In calves with diarrhea, insulin aspart 0.25 units/kg SC along with dextrose 50% 1 mL/kg IV over 5 minutes; sodium bicarbonate 1.3% (40 mL/kg/hour) and IV fluids were administered prior to insulin.[3]

Monitoring

- Diabetic patients should be closely monitored. Each patient requires an individualized treatment plan, frequent reassessment, and adjustments of the plan based on the response of the patient. It is encouraged to review a veterinary endocrinology reference text or consult with a veterinary emergency and critical care and/or endocrinology specialist for further information related to regulating diabetic patients and insulin adjustments. The overarching goal for monitoring diabetic patients is control of clinical signs related to hyperglycemia (eg, polyuria, polydipsia) while avoiding hypoglycemia.[10] Interpret all monitoring strategies in light of clinical signs. Results from the below monitoring options may conflict in regard to achieving good glycemic control and good clinical control.

- Patient status and control of clinical signs: body weight, appetite, fluid intake, urine output
- Glucose (blood or interstitial). Because of how often glucose needs to be checked in sick diabetic patients, consider a central line or continuous interstitial glucose monitoring system in dogs and cats. Experience with continuous interstitial glucose monitoring in dogs and cats is that these devices are easy to apply, user friendly, and provide useful information surrounding glycemic control while the patient is in the clinic or home environment.[9,11-15]
  - For patients that have experienced or are suspected to have experienced repeated or unexplained hypoglycemia, it is strongly encouraged to consult a veterinary emergency and critical care and/or endocrinology specialist or review a reference text that specializes in providing information specific for treatment of hypoglycemia.
- Additional monitoring for patients with diabetic ketoacidosis (DKA)[9]:
  - Glucose measurement every 1 to 2 hours initially; adjust insulin therapy and begin dextrose infusion when glucose decreases below 250 mg/dL (14 mmol/L). See ***Dosages***.
  - Hydration status, respiration, pulse every 2 to 4 hours
  - Serum electrolyte (eg, magnesium, phosphorous, potassium), plasma ketones, and total venous CO_2 concentrations every 4 to 8 hours
  - Urine output, glycosuria, and urine ketones every 4 to 8 hours
  - Body weight, packed cell volume, temperature, and blood pressure every 6 to 8 hours
  - Additional monitoring as applicable to address concurrent disease

Chemistry/Synonyms

All commercial preparations of human-labeled insulin currently manufactured in the United States are supplied in solution or suspension at a concentration of 100 units/mL, which is ≈3.5 mg of insulin/mL. Likewise, 1 unit of insulin is ≈35 µg of insulin, and 1 mg insulin is ≈28.8 units.

Insulin aspart injection, USP (rDNA origin) is a rapid-acting human insulin analogue that is produced by recombinant human DNA technology using a genetically modified strain of *Saccharomyces cerevisiae.* It is identical to human insulin, except aspartic acid is substituted for proline at the B chain amino acid position 28. The sterile solution consists of insulin aspart in a clear, colorless aqueous fluid.

Insulin aspart protamine/insulin aspart contains 70% insulin aspart protamine crystals and 30% soluble insulin aspart. It provides biphasic hypoglycemic effects, with an early onset and a second effect of intermediate duration.

Insulin aspart may also be known as aspart, B-28 aspart insulin, insulin aspart protamine, insulin X14, or *NovoLog®*.

For additional information, see ***Insulin, General Information***.

Storage/Stability

Unopened insulin aspart products should be stored in the refrigerator at 2°C to 8°C (36°F-46°F) and protected from temperature extremes and direct sunlight. Do not freeze.[5]

***In-use** vials* may be used for 28 days after first use and can be stored at room temperature or in the refrigerator.[5] Store ***in-use** pens/devices* at room temperature; do not refrigerate.

Freezing (less than 2°C [36°F]) insulin aspart products may alter the protein structure and decrease potency. Particle aggregation and crystal damage may be visible to the naked eye. Higher temperatures (greater than 30°C [86°F]) and direct exposure to sunlight (as might occur when insulin is stored in a car or on a windowsill) may produce insulin transformation products and fibril formation.

Although manufacturers recommend discarding opened bottles of insulin after 4 to 6 weeks (or expiration date, whichever comes first), studies support that insulin potency and stability are maintained for longer durations.[16,17] Veterinary internal medicine specialists indicate that the vial may be used for 3 to 6 months after opening and possibly beyond the expiration date as long as it is handled carefully, stored in the refrigerator, and the solution does not develop discoloration, flocculent precipitates, or changes in consistency. If a lack of diabetes regulation is noted when using the product beyond the expiration date (3 to 6 months after starting therapy), it may be prudent to replace with new insulin prior to adjusting insulin therapy.[10]

Compatibility/Compounding Considerations

Diluting insulin: Other than for immediate use, insulin aspart should only be diluted using product-specific sterile diluent, which is supplied by the manufacturer on request. Diluted insulin (10 units/mL) prepared in this manner is stable for 4 weeks and should be stored in the refrigerator, although refrigeration is not required.[5] For immediate use, insulin can be diluted with normal saline for injection, but the potency cannot be predicted after 24 hours.

Adsorption: Insulin aspart adsorbs to infusion materials,[5] although details are lacking. The adsorption of regular insulin to the surfaces of IV infusion solution containers, glass and plastic (including PVC, ethylene vinyl acetate, polyethylene, and other polyolefins), tubing, and filters has been demonstrated.[18] Estimates of loss of regular insulin potency due to adsorption range from 20% to 80%, although reports of 20% to 30% are more common.[19-22] The percent adsorbed is inversely proportional to the concentration of the insulin and may include other factors (eg, amount of container surface area, fill volume of the solution, type of solution, type and length of administration set, temperature, previous exposure of tubing to insulin, presence of other drugs or blood).[20-22] The adsorption process is instantaneous, with the bulk of insulin adsorption occurring within the first 30 to 60 minutes. To saturate binding sites and deliver a more predictable dose to the patient through an IV infusion, it is recommended that the first 50 mL be run through the IV tubing and discarded.

Insulin syringes: Syringes are designed for use with a specific strength of insulin, with the needle covers color-coded according to strength. U100 syringes are available in 0.3 mL, 0.5 mL, and 1 mL size. Measuring U100 insulin to the 1 unit mark in a U100 syringe will contain 1 unit of insulin. Some brands of 0.3 mL syringes include ½ unit markings. Insulin syringes should not be reused.

Dosage Forms/Regulatory Status

VETERINARY-LABELED PRODUCTS: NONE

HUMAN-LABELED PRODUCTS:

Insulin Aspart Injection Solution Human (rDNA): 100 units/mL in 10 mL vials and 3 mL *Penfill®* cartridges, *FlexPen®*, and *FlexTouch®*; *NovoLog®*; (Rx). **CAUTION**: *Fiasp®* is not interchangeable with *NovoLog®*.

References

For the complete list of references, see **wiley.com/go/budde/plumb**

Insulin, Detemir

(***inn***-suh-lin, ***deh***-tih-meer) *Levemir®*

Insulin, Long-Acting

NOTE: Insulin preparations available to clinicians are in a constant state of change. To maximize the efficacy of therapy and reduce the chance for errors, it is highly recommended to review current references or sources of information pertaining to insulin therapy for dogs and cats.

For additional information, see ***Insulin, General Information.***

Prescriber Highlights

- Modified long-acting insulin used for treatment in dogs and cats newly diagnosed with diabetes mellitus and for long-term maintenance therapy
- Starting dose for dogs is a much lower dose than with other insulins.
- Animals presented with ketoacidosis, anorexia, lethargy, and/or vomiting should first be stabilized with appropriate therapy, including short-acting insulin.
- There are no absolute contraindications, except during episodes of hypoglycemia.
- Adverse effects include hypoglycemia, hypokalemia, insulin-induced rebound hyperglycemia (ie, Somogyi effect), and local reactions to the "foreign" proteins.
- Do not confuse insulin types, strengths, and syringes: insulin detemir is a U100 human product; only use U100 syringes to measure the dose.
- Many potential drug interactions

Uses/Indications

Insulin detemir is a long-acting insulin preparation that can be used in dogs and cats for initial treatment and long-term management of uncomplicated diabetes mellitus. In cats, insulin detemir appears to have a similar profile to glargine insulin in terms of blood glucose control and remission rates; however, cats often require a lower dose of insulin detemir for glycemic control as compared with glargine insulin. Insulin detemir could be considered for use in dogs in which the duration of activity of porcine insulin zinc (lente) or NPH insulin is too short. Compared with humans and cats, dogs show a stronger hypoglycemic response with insulin detemir and should start treatment at a much lower dose than other insulins.[1,2]

Pharmacology/Actions

The primary action of insulin is to regulate glucose metabolism. Insulin and its analogues lower blood glucose by increasing glucose uptake in peripheral tissues, especially by skeletal muscle and fat. In the liver, insulin increases glucose storage (ie, glycogen) while also inhibiting gluconeogenesis. Insulin's anabolic actions also enhance fatty acid and protein synthesis while inhibiting lipolysis and proteolysis.

For additional information, see ***Insulin, General Information.***

Pharmacokinetics

Insulin formulations contain insulin polymers (aggregates of multiple insulin molecules). Insulin is absorbed from the administration site only after insulin polymers break down into insulin monomers or dimers.

After SC injection, insulin detemir both strongly self-associates and binds protein at the injection site, slowing absorption and prolonging the hypoglycemic effect with no pronounced peak in humans.[3] In circulation, it is 98% protein-bound to albumin and has an elimination half-life of ≈6 hours.[3] A comparison study[4] of 10 healthy young cats given insulin glargine and insulin detemir showed that following administration of 0.5 units/kg SC, the onset of action was 1.8 ± 0.8 and 1.3 ± 0.5 hours for insulin detemir and insulin glargine, respectively. The end of action was 13.5 ± 3.5 hours and 11.3 ± 4.5 hours for insulin detemir and insulin glargine, respectively. Time-to-peak action was 6.9 ± 3.1 hours and 5.3 ± 3.8 hours for insulin detemir and insulin glargine, respectively. The time–action curves for both insulin analogues varied between relatively flat curves in some cats and peaked curves in others. In dogs, blood glucose nadir occurred ≈8 hours after SC administration (range, 4-10 hours).[2,5,6] The duration of action was ≈9 to 15 hours.[6]

Contraindications/Precautions/Warnings

Because there are no alternatives for insulin when it is used for diabetic indications, there are no absolute contraindications to its use except during episodes of hypoglycemia. If animals develop hypersensitivity (local or otherwise) or if insulin resistance develops, a change in type or species source (eg, human, bovine, porcine) of insulin should be considered after other etiologies for poor control (eg, expired insulin, concurrent disease, or medication interference) have been ruled out. See ***Insulin, General Information***.

Insulin detemir is not an appropriate insulin choice for patients presenting with severe ketoacidosis, anorexia, lethargy, and/or vomiting or other conditions when treatment with short-acting insulin (eg, regular insulin) is indicated.

For obese patients, dose calculations should be based on the individual patient's ideal body weight to avoid inadvertent insulin overdose.

In humans, long-term repeated SC/IM injections of insulin at the same site may cause lipodystrophic reactions, which could interfere with insulin absorption[3]; however, there have been no specific reports of this reaction occurring in dogs or cats.

The high molar insulin concentration of the insulin detemir formulation elicits a greater hypoglycemic response in dogs when compared to humans, necessitating a lower starting dose of insulin detemir for dogs.[5] Without the availability of an insulin detemir-specific diluent, the use of this type of insulin in dogs weighing less than 10 to 15 kg (22 to 33 lb) is not recommended.[2]

Insulin detemir is U100 strength insulin. It is crucial for patient safety to only use U100 syringes when measuring and administering U100 insulin. Calculations can be done to convert to U40 syringes or tuberculin (TB) syringes, but these conversions are not recommended because of the potential for introducing dosing errors. See ***Insulin, General Information***.

When writing prescriptions, do not abbreviate units as "U," as this has been shown to increase the rate of transcription and dosage errors. In human medicine, insulin is considered a "high alert" medication (ie, medications that require special safeguards to reduce the risk for errors). Consider instituting practices such as redundant drug dosage and volume checking and special alert labels.

Adverse Effects

Adverse effects of insulin therapy may include hypoglycemia (see ***Overdose/Acute Toxicity***), hypokalemia, insulin-induced rebound hyperglycemia (ie, Somogyi effect), and local or allergic reactions to the "foreign" proteins. In dogs administered insulin detemir, hypoglycemia was present on 22% of blood glucose curves,[2] and 4 out of 10 dogs experienced clinically relevant hypoglycemia, including 3 episodes that were considered severe.

Injection site reactions have not been reported in published studies in dogs or cats receiving insulin detemir, although the number of animals enrolled in studies has been relatively small.

Reproductive/Nursing Safety

Insulin detemir is considered safe for use during human pregnancy and while nursing[7]; the same is assumed to be true for veterinary patients. In humans, insulin is considered a treatment of choice for gestational diabetes.[8]

Overdose/Acute Toxicity

Insulin overdose can lead to various degrees of hypoglycemia. Signs may include weakness, shaking, head tilt, lethargy, ataxia, seizures, blindness, bizarre behavior, and coma. Other signs may include restlessness, hunger, and muscle fasciculations. Electrolyte disturbances, including hypokalemia, may occur. Prolonged hypoglycemia can result in permanent brain damage or death.

Mild hypoglycemia can be treated by offering the animal its usual food. More serious signs (eg, seizures) should be treated with oral dextrose solutions (eg, *Karo*® syrup) applied to the buccal mucosa (if the animal is seizing, use caution to avoid being bit or injured) or by IV injections of 50% dextrose solutions (small amounts—usually 2 –15 mL [0.5 – 1 mL/kg], diluted, and slowly administered).[9] See ***Dextrose 50% injection.*** For in-hospital management, glucagon may also be considered on an as-needed basis for an insulin overdose. See ***Glucagon.*** Once the animal's hypoglycemia is alleviated (response usually occurs within 1 to 2 minutes), the animal should be closely monitored (both by physical observation and serial blood glucose levels) to prevent a recurrence of hypoglycemia (especially with the slower-absorbed/longer-acting products) and to prevent hyperglycemia from developing. Future insulin dosages or feeding regimens should be evaluated or adjusted based on consultation with the clinician to prevent further occurrences of hypoglycemia.

For patients that have experienced or are suspected of having experienced an overdose, consultation with a 24-hour poison consultation center specializing in providing veterinary-specific information is recommended. For general information related to overdose and toxin exposures, as well as contact information for poison control centers, refer to ***Appendix.***

Drug Interactions

The following drug interactions have either been reported or are theoretical in humans or animals receiving insulin and may be of significance in veterinary patients. Unless otherwise noted, use together is not necessarily contraindicated, but weigh the potential risks and perform additional monitoring when appropriate.

- **Beta-Adrenergic Antagonists** (eg, **atenolol, propranolol**): Can have variable effects on glycemic control and can mask the signs associated with hypoglycemia
- **Clonidine**: Can mask the signs associated with hypoglycemia
- **Digoxin**: Because insulin can reduce serum potassium levels, patients receiving concomitant digoxin therapy—especially those receiving concurrent diuretic therapy—should be closely monitored.
- **Diuretics** (eg, **furosemide, hydrochlorothiazide**): Insulin shifts extracellular potassium into the intracellular space; serum potassium concentration should be closely monitored in patients receiving concomitant diuretic therapy. Diuretics may also *decrease* the hypoglycemic activity of insulin (ie, increase insulin requirements).
- **Reserpine**: Can mask the signs associated with hypoglycemia

The following drugs or drug classes may potentiate the hypoglycemic activity of insulin (ie, decrease insulin requirements):

- **Anabolic Steroids** (eg, **boldenone, stanozolol, testosterone**)
- **Angiotensin II Receptor Blockers** (ARBs; eg, **telmisartan**)
- **Angiotensin-Converting Enzyme Inhibitors** (ACEIs; eg, **benazepril, enalapril**)
- **Disopyramide**
- **Ethanol**
- **Fenofibrate**
- **Fluoroquinolones** (eg, **ciprofloxacin, enrofloxacin**)
- **Fluoxetine**
- **Hypoglycemic Agents, Oral** (eg, **acarbose, glipizide, metformin**)
- **Monoamine Oxidase Inhibitors** (MAOIs; eg, **amitraz, linezolid, selegiline**)
- **Pentoxifylline**
- **Salicylates** (eg, **aspirin, bismuth subsalicylate**)
- **Somatostatin Derivatives** (eg, **octreotide**)
- **Sulfonamides** (eg, **sulfadimethoxine, sulfamethoxazole**)

The following drugs or drug classes may decrease the hypoglycemic activity of insulin (ie, increase insulin requirements):

- **Alpha-2-Adrenergic Agonists** (eg, **dexmedetomidine, medetomidine, xylazine**): May cause hyperglycemia and temporarily interfere with glycemic control
- **Beta-Adrenergic Agonists** (eg, **albuterol, terbutaline**)
- **Corticosteroids** (eg, **dexamethasone, prednis(ol)one**)
- **Danazol**
- **Diazoxide**
- **Estrogens** (eg, **diethylstilbestrol [DES], estriol**)
- **Isoniazid**
- **Niacin**
- **Phenothiazines** (eg, **acepromazine, chlorpromazine**)
- **Progestins** (eg, **megestrol**)
- **Thyroid Hormones**: Can elevate glucose levels in diabetic patients when thyroid hormone therapy is first initiated

Laboratory Considerations

- None

Dosages

NOTES:

1. Treatment of diabetes mellitus is complex. Insulin is only one component of therapy; treatment may require fluid electrolyte replacement, management of acid/base disturbances, dietary adjustments, and antimicrobial therapy. Adequate patient monitoring is mandatory. It is strongly encouraged to refer to more thorough discussions of treatment in veterinary endocrinology or internal medicine references for additional information.
2. For obese patients, dose calculations should be based on the individual patient's estimated ideal body weight to avoid inadvertent insulin overdose.
3. Key goals of therapy are control of clinical signs associated with diabetes mellitus and avoidance of hypoglycemia.[1,10]
4. All dosages are extra-label.

DOGS:

Initial insulin treatment of uncomplicated diabetes mellitus:

NOTE: Insulin detemir doses in dogs are much lower than for other species and other insulins. See ***Monitoring.***

a) 0.1 unit/kg SC every 12 hours[1]
b) Initial dose, 1 unit/dog (NOT unit/kg) SC every 12 hours, regardless of the size of the dog. In a study, dose adjustments were made in 0.5 – 1 unit/dog (NOT unit/kg) increments. The average insulin detemir dose at study completion was 0.12 unit/kg (range, 0.05 – 0.34 unit/kg).[2]

CATS:

Initial insulin treatment of uncomplicated diabetes mellitus: 0.5 unit/kg SC every 12 hours if blood glucose is more than 360 mg/dL (on initial presentation) or 0.25 unit/kg SC every 12 hours if blood glucose is less than 360 mg/dL (on initial presentation). For a starting dose, round down to the nearest unit, which is generally less than or equal to 2 units/cat every 12 hours regardless of weight.[1,11,12] See ***Monitoring.***

Monitoring

Each patient requires an individualized treatment plan, frequent reassessment, and adjustments of the plan based on the response of the patient. It is encouraged to consult a veterinary endocrinology reference text or with a veterinary emergency and critical care and/or endocrinology specialist for further information related to regulating diabetic patients and insulin adjustments. The overarching goal when monitoring diabetic patients is control of clinical signs related to hyperglycemia (eg, polyuria, polydipsia) while avoiding hypoglycemia. A so-called "loose-control" (ie, managing clinical signs while avoiding hypoglycemia and reducing frequency of hospitalizations for glucose curves) approach to diabetes management in cats using insulin detemir has also been described.[11] Interpret all monitoring strategies based on clinical signs. Results from the monitoring options below may conflict in regard to achieving good glycemic control and good clinical control.

- Patient status and control of clinical signs: body weight, appetite, fluid intake, and urine output
- Glucose (blood or interstitial) curve. Experience with continuous interstitial glucose monitoring in dogs and cats is that these devices are easy to apply, user friendly, and provide useful information surrounding glycemic control while the patient is in the clinic or home environment.[13-16] A glucose curve can be considered at the following times[1]:
  - After the first dose of a new insulin type—blood glucose can be checked every 2 hours after administration. The goal for monitoring following the first dose of insulin would be solely to identify hypoglycemia. The insulin dose should NOT be increased based on the first-day blood glucose evaluation. If blood glucose falls below 150 mg/dL during the glucose curve, the frequency of monitoring should increase to hourly until blood glucose is greater than 150 mg/dL.[1] Although the insulin detemir dose should never be increased on the first day of therapy, the dose should be decreased by 10% to 50% in dogs, and 50% in cats if blood glucose is less than 150 mg/dL at any time during the day.[1] Repeat glucose curves on subsequent days (and decrease insulin dose if necessary) until nadir is greater than 150 mg/dL.
  - 7 to 14 days after starting insulin or an insulin dose change
  - At least every 3 months, even in animals with well-controlled diabetes. In well-controlled patients, it may be possible to use clinical signs, body weight, +/- serum fructosamine measurements to determine frequency of glucose curve evaluations.[11]
  - Any time clinical signs related to hyperglycemia (eg, polyuria, polydipsia) recur in an animal with previously well-controlled diabetes
  - When hypoglycemia is a concern. **NOTE**: For patients that have experienced or are suspected of having experienced repeated or unexplained hypoglycemia, it is strongly encouraged to consult with a veterinary emergency and critical care and/or endocrinology specialist or reference text that specializes in providing information specific for the treatment of hypoglycemia.
- Urine glucose monitoring is typically only helpful for documenting prolonged hypoglycemia (eg, persistently negative urine glucose testing when monitoring for diabetic remission in cats). As most diabetic patients spend time above the renal threshold for urinary glucose spillage, even patients with well-controlled diabetes may be intermittently glucosuric throughout the day.
- Fructosamine or glycosylated hemoglobin can be evaluated if available and warranted.

Client Information

NOTES for veterinarian:

1. Correct injection techniques should be taught and practiced with the client before the animal's discharge.
2. Emphasis should be placed on matching the appropriate syringe and insulin concentration (eg, do not interchange U40 insulin and syringes with U100 insulin and syringes) and correct needles with pens/devices.

- For this medication to work safely, give the insulin ***exactly*** as your veterinarian has prescribed. Do not give this medicine and contact your veterinarian for guidance if your animal is not eating.
- Your veterinarian will teach you proper injection technique. ***Only*** use U100 insulin syringes with insulin detemir.
- Always double-check the dose in the syringe or pens/devices before you inject your animal. Overdoses may be fatal.
- Prior to using, visually inspect the insulin container. Insulin detemir solutions should be clear and colorless, without visible particles. Do not use insulin if you see crystals on the inside of the vial. There should never be clumps or unexpected particles in the vial.
- After measuring the dose into a syringe, allow the contents to come to room temperature (if the vial is stored in the refrigerator) before giving the injection.
- The injection site should be frequently changed, with the main sites being the back of the neck, side of the animal, or shoulder area.
- Place the used needles and syringes in a sharps disposal container immediately after use, making sure you do not attempt to disconnect the needle from the syringe or recap the needle. Your veterinarian or pharmacist will help you obtain these containers.
- Do not reuse needles or syringes.
- Keep insulin products out of temperature extremes.
- Signs of low blood sugar include weakness, depression, lack of energy, sluggishness, staggering gait (ie, stumbling) when walking, behavior changes, muscle twitching, seizures (convulsions), or coma. **If your animal is unconscious or having a seizure, this is a medical emergency.** Take your animal to your veterinarian immediately. **If your animal is conscious and able to swallow**, rub ≈1 tablespoon of corn syrup (*Karo®*) or honey on your animal's gums until it is alert enough to eat. Feed the usual meal and contact your veterinarian for recommendations. Some animals may not show any obvious physical signs of low blood sugar. If your animal is not acting normally, contact your veterinarian to make sure your animal's blood sugar levels are in a safe range.
- Contact your veterinarian at your earliest convenience if you notice excessive thirst, increased frequency of urination, or increased appetite in your animal, as these signs may indicate the insulin dose needs to be adjusted.
- When traveling, do not leave insulin in carry-on luggage that will pass through airport surveillance equipment. Generally, insulin stability is not affected by a single pass through surveillance equipment; however, longer than normal exposure or repeated passes through surveillance equipment may alter insulin potency.
- Do not stop giving this medication to your animal unless instructed to do so by your veterinarian.
- Your veterinarian will need to closely monitor your animal during treatment. Do not miss these important follow-up visits.

Chemistry/Synonyms

Insulin detemir is a U100 (ie, 100 units/mL) insulin that contains 14.2 mg insulin detemir insulin/mL. In contrast, all other commercial preparations of U100 human-labeled insulin currently manufactured in the United States contain ≈3.5 mg of insulin/mL.[3]

Insulin detemir is a long-acting human insulin analogue produced by recombinant DNA technology using a genetically modified strain *of Saccharomyces cerevisiae*. Insulin detemir differs from human insulin in that the amino acid threonine in position B30 has been omitted and that a C14 fatty acid chain has been attached to the amino acid B29. The fatty acid slows absorption from the injection site. It is a clear, colorless, aqueous solution.

Insulin detemir may also be known as NN-304 or *Levemir*®.

Storage/Stability

Unopened insulin detemir *vials* and *pens/devices* should be stored in the manufacturer's carton in the refrigerator at 2°C to 8°C (36°F-46°F).[3] Do not freeze; discard if the product is frozen. Unused product may be stored unrefrigerated if kept below 30°C (86°F) and out of direct heat and sunlight but must be discarded after 42 days.

In-use insulin detemir *vials* may be refrigerated or stored at room temperature; discard 42 days after first use. ***In-use*** *pens/devices* should be stored at room temperature only (do not refrigerate) and discard 42 days after first use.

Discard insulin detemir vials or pens/devices if the solution is discolored, cloudy, or contains visible particles.

Although manufacturers recommend discarding opened bottles of insulin after 4 to 6 weeks (or expiration date, whichever comes first), studies[17,18] support that insulin potency and stability is maintained for longer durations. Veterinary internal medicine specialists indicate that the vial may be used for 3 to 6 months after opening and possibly beyond the listed expiration date as long as it is handled carefully, stored in the refrigerator, and the solution does not develop discoloration, flocculent precipitates, or changes in consistency. If a lack of diabetes regulation is noted when using the product beyond the expiration date (3 to 6 months after starting therapy), it may be prudent to replace it with new insulin prior to adjusting insulin therapy.[1]

Compatibility/Compounding Considerations

Diluting insulin: Insulin detemir requires a specific diluent that is not readily available. Because dogs require a lower dose of this insulin, it is not recommended to use insulin detemir in dogs weighing less than 10 to 15 kg (22 to 33 lb).[2]

Insulin syringes: Syringes are designed for use with a specific strength of insulin, and needle covers are color-coded for each insulin strength. U100 syringes are available in 0.3 mL, 0.5 mL, and 1 mL size. Drawing U100 insulin to the 1 unit mark in a U100 syringe will result in 1 unit of insulin. Some brands of 0.3 mL syringes include ½ unit markings. Insulin syringes should not be reused.

Dosage Forms/Regulatory Status

VETERINARY-LABELED PRODUCTS: NONE

HUMAN-LABELED PRODUCTS:

Insulin Detemir Injection Human (rDNA) 100 units/mL in 10 mL vials and 3 mL prefilled pen system; *Levemir*®; (Rx)

References

For the complete list of references, see **wiley.com/go/budde/plumb**

Insulin, Glargine

(***inn***-suh-lin, ***glar***-jeen) *Lantus*®

Insulin, Long-Acting

NOTE: Insulin preparations available to clinicians are in a constant state of change. To maximize the efficacy of therapy and reduce the chance for errors, it is highly recommended to review current references or sources of information pertaining to insulin therapy for dogs and cats.

For additional information, see ***Insulin, General Information.***

Prescriber Highlights

- ▶ Long-acting insulin used for treatment in patients newly diagnosed with diabetes mellitus and for long-term maintenance therapy. Although short-acting insulins (ie, regular insulin) are typically used to stabilize cats with diabetic ketoacidosis (DKA), insulin glargine can also be considered for management of cats with DKA.
- ▶ There are no absolute contraindications, except during episodes of hypoglycemia.
- ▶ Adverse effects include hypoglycemia, hypokalemia, hypophosphatemia (DKA only), insulin-induced rebound hyperglycemia (ie, Somogyi effect), and local reactions to "foreign" proteins.
- ▶ Do not confuse insulin types, strengths, and/or syringes. Insulin glargine is available in 2 strengths, U100 and *U300*. Only use U100 syringes with U100 glargine and the appropriate needle for the *U300* insulin pen to measure dose.
- ▶ Many potential drug interactions

Uses/Indications

Insulin glargine is a long-acting insulin preparation that can be used for initial treatment and long-term management of diabetes mellitus, especially in cats. U100 insulin glargine is recommended as a first-choice insulin in newly diagnosed diabetic cats.[1] Intermediate-acting insulins (eg, porcine insulin zinc [ie, lente], neutral protamine Hagedorn [NPH]) are considered first-choice insulin therapies in dogs with uncomplicated diabetes mellitus[1]; however, glargine can also be considered if these insulins do not have a long enough duration of activity. Data are emerging regarding the role of *U300* glargine in dogs and cats,[2-5] and it has demonstrated safety and efficacy in client-owned diabetic cats.[6]

In a study evaluating U100 glargine versus regular insulin for feline DKA, glargine administration was found to be an effective and safe alternative to the current standard regular insulin CRI protocol for the management of DKA in cats.[7]

U100 insulin glargine can also be considered for treatment of diabetes mellitus in ferrets,[8] horses,[9] and guinea pigs.[10]

Pharmacology/Actions

The primary action of insulin is to regulate glucose metabolism. Insulin and its analogs lower blood glucose by increasing glucose uptake in peripheral tissues, especially skeletal muscle and fat. In the liver, insulin increases glucose storage (ie, glycogen) while also inhibiting gluconeogenesis. Insulin's anabolic actions also enhance fatty acid and protein synthesis while inhibiting lipolysis and proteolysis.

For additional information, see ***Insulin, General Information***.

Pharmacokinetics

Insulin formulations contain insulin polymers (aggregates of multiple insulin molecules). Insulin is absorbed from the administration site only after insulin polymers break down into insulin monomers or dimers.

After SC injection of insulin glargine, the acidic solution is neutralized, and microprecipitates that slowly release small amounts of insulin glargine are formed, resulting in a relatively constant concentration/time profile over 24 hours, with no pronounced peak in humans. Microprecipitates are not formed when glargine is diluted or administered either IM or IV; thus, a rapid reduction of blood glucose—similar to regular insulin—is produced.[4,11]

In diabetic dogs receiving SC U100 insulin glargine, a hypoglycemic effect was noted 2 hours after administration and persisted for 12 hours. There was no significant difference between mean minimum and maximum blood glucose concentrations.[12] In healthy, nondiabetic dogs given *U300* insulin glargine, the peak effect occurred at 6.3 hours, and the duration was 16.3 hours.[2] In beagles with induced diabetes mellitus receiving *U300* insulin glargine, day-to-day variability of interstitial glucose was ≈20% to 30%.[5] In humans, cleavage of the insulin glargine B-chain N terminus occurs at the injection site and this results in 2 active metabolites (M1 and M2),[13] whereas dogs only form the M1 metabolite.[4]

A small study of 9 healthy cats compared equal doses of U100 insulin glargine, protamine zinc insulin (PZI; mixed beef/pork), and purified pork lente insulin.[14] Results showed no significant difference in onset of action (0.8 to 1.8 hours) or nadir glucose concentrations among different insulin types; time to reach nadir glucose concentration was longer for insulin glargine (≈14 hours) versus PZI insulin (≈4 hours) and lente insulin (≈5 hours). Duration was significantly shorter for lente insulin (10 hours) than for insulin glargine (22 hours) or PZI (21 hours), with glargine and PZI not appearing to be significantly different. This study also showed definite peaks in glargine concentration and in its glucose-lowering effects. In healthy, nondiabetic cats, the onset and duration of effect for *U300* insulin glargine is nearly identical to that of U100 glargine (≈2 hours, and 12 to 17 hours, respectively)[3,15]; however, *U300* glargine resulted in a more evenly distributed metabolic effect over a 24-hour period.[15]

Contraindications/Precautions/Warnings

Because there are no alternatives for insulin when it is used for diabetic indications, there are no absolute contraindications to its use except during episodes of hypoglycemia. If animals develop hypersensitivity (local or otherwise) or if insulin resistance develops, a change in type or species source (eg, human, bovine, porcine) of insulin should be considered after other etiologies for poor control (eg, expired insulin, concurrent disease or medication interference) have been ruled out. See ***Insulin, General Information***.

For obese patients, dose calculations should be based on the patient's ideal body weight to avoid inadvertent insulin overdose.

In humans, long-term repeated SC/IM injections of insulin at the same site may cause lipodystrophic reactions, which could interfere with insulin absorption[16]; however, there have been no specific reports of this reaction occurring in dogs or cats.

It is crucial for patient safety to only use U100 syringes when measuring and administering U100 insulin. Calculations can be done to convert to U40 syringes or TB syringes, but these conversions are not recommended due to the potential for introducing dosing errors. See ***Insulin, General Information***. Do not confuse U100 insulin glargine (*Lantus*®, *Basaglar*®, *Semglee*®) with *U300* insulin glargine (*Toujeo*®).

When writing prescriptions, do not abbreviate units as "U," as this has been shown to increase the rate of transcription and dosage errors. In human medicine, insulin is considered a "high alert" medication (ie, medications that require special safeguards to reduce the risk for errors). Consider instituting practices such as redundant drug dosage and volume checking and special alert labels.

Adverse Effects

Adverse effects of insulin therapy may include hypoglycemia (see ***Overdose/Acute Toxicity***), hypokalemia, hypophosphatemia (DKA only), insulin-induced rebound hyperglycemia (ie, Somogyi effect), weight gain, and local or allergic reactions to the "foreign" proteins.

Clinical signs associated with hypoglycemia were not observed in diabetic cats receiving *U300* insulin glargine, although biochemical hypoglycemia was detected in 12.5% of blood glucose curves.[6]

In a case report, a cat was initially treated with insulin glargine for diabetes mellitus and went into remission, at which time insulin glargine was discontinued.[17] Approximately 36 months later, the diabetes recurred, and insulin glargine therapy was restarted. Within 2 to 3 minutes of the first injection, the cat experienced a hypersensitivity reaction, including collapse, vomiting, diarrhea, facial swelling, and diffuse erythema. This cat recovered with aggressive supportive care. An intradermal skin challenge 6 months later confirmed a hypersensitivity reaction to insulin glargine. This cat was switched to PZI insulin and became well regulated for its diabetes.

Reproductive/Nursing Safety

Insulin glargine is considered safe for use during human pregnancy and while nursing[18]; the same is assumed to be true for veterinary patients. In humans, insulin is considered a treatment of choice for gestational diabetes.[19]

Overdose/Acute Toxicity

Insulin overdose can lead to various degrees of hypoglycemia. Signs may include weakness, shaking, head tilt, lethargy, ataxia, seizures, blindness, bizarre behavior, and coma. Other signs may include restlessness, hunger, and muscle fasciculations. Electrolyte disturbances, including hypokalemia, may occur. Prolonged hypoglycemia can result in permanent brain damage or death.

Mild hypoglycemia can be treated by offering the animal its usual food. More serious signs (eg, seizures) should be treated with oral dextrose solutions (eg, *Karo*® syrup) applied to the buccal mucosa (if the animal is seizing, use caution to avoid being bit or injured) or by IV injections of 50% dextrose solutions (small amounts—usually 2 - 15 mL [0.5 - 1 mL/kg]), diluted and slowly administered[20]; see ***Dextrose 50% injection***. For inhospital management, glucagon may also be considered on an as-needed basis for an insulin overdose. See ***Glucagon***. Once the animal's hypoglycemia is alleviated (response usually occurs within 1 to 2 minutes), the animal should be closely monitored (both by physical observation and serial blood glucose concentrations) to prevent a recurrence of hypoglycemia (especially with the slower absorbed/longer-acting products) and to prevent hyperglycemia from developing. Future insulin dosages or feeding habits should be evaluated or adjusted based on consultation with the clinician to prevent further occurrences of hypoglycemia.

For patients that have experienced or are suspected of having experienced an overdose, consultation with a 24-hour poison consultation center specializing in providing veterinary-specific information is recommended. For general information related to overdose and toxin exposures, as well as contact information for poison control centers, refer to ***Appendix***.

Drug Interactions

The following drug interactions have either been reported or are theoretical in humans or animals receiving insulin and may be of significance in veterinary patients. Unless otherwise noted, use together is not necessarily contraindicated, but weigh the potential risks and perform additional monitoring when appropriate.

- Beta-Adrenergic Antagonists (eg, **atenolol, propranolol**): Can have variable effects on glycemic control and can mask the signs associated with hypoglycemia
- Clonidine: Can mask the signs associated with hypoglycemia

- **Digoxin**: Because insulin can reduce serum potassium concentrations, patients receiving concomitant digoxin therapy—especially those receiving concurrent diuretic therapy—should be closely monitored.
- **Diuretics** (eg, **furosemide, hydrochlorothiazide**): Insulin shifts extracellular potassium into the intracellular space; serum potassium concentration should be closely monitored in patients receiving concomitant diuretic therapy. Diuretics may also decrease the hypoglycemic activity of insulin (ie, increase insulin requirements).
- **Reserpine**: Can mask the signs associated with hypoglycemia

The following drugs or drug classes may potentiate the hypoglycemic activity of insulin (ie, decrease insulin requirements):

- **Anabolic Steroids** (eg, **boldenone, stanozolol, testosterone**)
- **Angiotensin II Receptor Blockers** (ARBs; eg, **telmisartan**)
- **Angiotensin Converting Enzyme Inhibitors** (ACEIs; eg, **benazepril, enalapril**)
- **Disopyramide**
- **Ethanol**
- **Fenofibrate**
- **Fluoroquinolones** (eg, **ciprofloxacin, enrofloxacin**)
- **Fluoxetine**
- **Hypoglycemic Agents, Oral** (eg, **acarbose, glipizide, metformin**)
- **Monoamine Oxidase Inhibitors** (MAOIs; eg, **amitraz, linezolid, selegiline**)
- **Pentoxifylline**
- **Salicylates** (eg, **aspirin, bismuth subsalicylate**)
- **Somatostatin Derivatives** (eg, **octreotide**)
- **Sulfonamides** (eg, **sulfadimethoxine, sulfamethoxazole**)

The following drugs or drug classes may decrease the hypoglycemic activity of insulin (ie, increase insulin requirements):

- **Alpha-2-Adrenergic Agonists** (eg, **dexmedetomidine, medetomidine, xylazine**): May cause hyperglycemia and temporarily interfere with glycemic control
- **Beta-Adrenergic Agonists** (eg, **albuterol, terbutaline**)
- **Corticosteroids** (eg, **dexamethasone, prednis(ol)one**)
- **Danazol**
- **Diazoxide**
- **Estrogens** (eg, **diethylstilbestrol [DES], estriol**)
- **Isoniazid**
- **Niacin**
- **Phenothiazines** (eg, **acepromazine, chlorpromazine**)
- **Progestins** (eg, **megestrol**)
- **Thyroid Hormones**: Can elevate glucose concentrations in diabetic patients when thyroid hormone therapy is first initiated

Laboratory Considerations

- None

Dosages

NOTES:

1. Treatment of diabetes mellitus and, in particular DKA, is complex. Insulin is only one component of therapy; treatment may require fluid electrolyte replacement, management of acid/base disturbances, dietary adjustments, and antimicrobial therapy. Adequate patient monitoring is mandatory. It is strongly encouraged to refer to more thorough discussions of treatment in veterinary endocrinology or internal medicine references.
2. For obese patients, dose calculations should be based on the patient's estimated ideal body weight to avoid inadvertent insulin overdose.
3. Key goals of therapy are control of clinical signs associated with diabetes mellitus and avoidance of hypoglycemia or other complications (eg, DKA).[1,21]
4. All dosages refer to U100 glargine unless otherwise specified and are extra-label.

DOGS:

Initial insulin treatment of uncomplicated diabetes mellitus (extra-label):

a) 0.3 unit/kg SC every 12 hours[1]
b) 0.25 – 0.5 unit/kg SC every 12 hours[12,22]

CATS:

Initial insulin treatment of uncomplicated diabetes mellitus (extra-label): Using either U100 or *U300* glargine insulin: 0.5 unit/kg SC every 12 hours if blood glucose is more than 360 mg/dL or 0.25 unit/kg SC every 12 hours if blood glucose is less than 360 mg/dL.[1,6,21,23] This dosing regimen often equates to 1 – 2 units/cat (NOT units/kg) SC every 12 hours. The initial dose should not exceed 2 unit/cat (NOT unit/kg) SC every 12 hours regardless of the size of the cat. Most cats are well regulated at an average dosage of 0.5 units/kg SC every 12 hours. See ***Monitoring***.

Transitioning poorly controlled cats to *U300* insulin (extra-label): The *U300* insulin glargine starting dose was the same as the last dose of the patient's previously used insulin.[6]

Adjunctive therapy for diabetic ketoacidosis:

a) **Combined IM/SC protocol** (extra-label):
   i. 1 – 2 units/cat (NOT unit/kg) IM in combination with 1 – 3 units/cat (NOT unit/kg) SC initially.[24] Blood glucose was monitored every 2 to 4 hours, and insulin glargine 0.5 – 1 units/cat (NOT unit/kg) IM was administered to maintain blood glucose between 180 – 252 mg/dL. Insulin glargine 1 – 2 units/cat (NOT unit/kg) SC was continued every 12 hours. The median time to second IM insulin glargine dose was 14 hours when the insulin glargine IM/SC combination was used and 4 hours with IM insulin glargine alone.[24] No cats developed hypoglycemia during the stabilization period. The median time for all cats to be managed with insulin glargine SC as their sole insulin therapy was 24 hours (range, 18 to 72 hours).
   ii. 2 units/cat (NOT units/kg) SC initially while starting rehydration.[7] Then 1 unit/cat (NOT unit/kg) IM 2 hours later. IM injections at 1 unit/cat (NOT unit/kg) were subsequently repeated every 4 hours if the glucose was greater than 250 mg/dL, and SC insulin glargine was continued every 12 hours with 0.25 units/kg (based on ideal body weight) rounded to the next half or whole unit. Once the blood glucose was less than 250 mg/dL, glucose containing solutions were used in addition to insulin therapy to maintain the blood glucose between 180 and 250 mg/dL. Insulin was decreased or stopped (at the discretion of the clinician) when the blood glucose was less than 80 mg/dL.
b) **Glargine in combination with regular insulin** (extra label): insulin glargine 0.25 units/kg SC every 12 hours and regular insulin 1 unit/cat (NOT unit/kg) IM up to every 6 hours for a blood glucose concentration greater than 250 mg/dL[25]

HORSES:

Diabetes mellitus (extra label): From a case report, glargine 0.2 – 0.4 units/kg SC every 24 hours after stabilization with rapid-/short-acting insulin.[9]

FERRETS:

Diabetes mellitus (extra label): 0.5 units/ferret (NOT units/kg) SC between the scapulae every 12 hours if urine dipstick test is positive for glucose[8]

GUINEA PIGS:

Diabetes mellitus, type 1 (extra label): 0.5 units/guinea pig (NOT units/kg) SC once daily administered on the right or left side of the abdomen or thorax[10]

Monitoring

Each patient requires an individualized treatment plan, frequent reassessment, and adjustments of the plan based on the response of the patient. It is encouraged to consult a veterinary endocrinology reference text or with a veterinary emergency and critical care and/or endocrinology specialist for further information related to regulating diabetic patients and insulin adjustments. The overarching goal when monitoring diabetic patients is control of clinical signs related to hyperglycemia (eg, polyuria, polydipsia) while avoiding hypoglycemia.[1] Interpret all monitoring strategies based on clinical signs. Results from the monitoring options below may conflict in regards to achieving good glycemic and clinical control. Diabetic patients should be closely monitored—especially during the first month of insulin therapy.

- Patient status and control of clinical signs: body weight, appetite, fluid intake, urine output
- Glucose (blood or interstitial) curve. Experience with continuous interstitial glucose monitoring in dogs and cats is that these devices are easy to apply, user friendly, and provide useful information surrounding glycemic control while the patient is in the clinic or home environment.[26-29] A glucose curve can be considered at the following times[1]:
  - After the first dose of a new insulin type. If performing a glucose curve, glucose can be checked every 3 to 4 hours for 10 to 12 hours after administration. The goal for monitoring following the first dose of insulin would be solely to identify hypoglycemia. The insulin dose should NOT be increased based on first-day glucose evaluation. If glucose falls below 150 mg/dL during the glucose curve, frequency of monitoring should increase to hourly until glucose is greater than 150 mg/dL.[1] Although the glargine dose should never be increased on the first day of therapy, the dose should be decreased by 10% to 50% in dogs and by 0.5 units (total) in cats if glucose is less than 150 mg/dL at any time during the day.[1] Repeat glucose curves on subsequent days (and decrease insulin dose if necessary) until nadir is greater than 150 mg/dL.
  - 7 to 14 days after starting insulin or an insulin dose change
  - At least every 3 months, even in animals with well-controlled diabetes
  - Any time clinical signs recur in an animal with previously well-controlled diabetes
  - When hypoglycemia is suspected. For patients that have experienced or are suspected to have experienced repeated or unexplained hypoglycemia, it is strongly encouraged to consult with a veterinary emergency and critical care and/or endocrinology specialist or reference text that specializes in providing information specific for treatment of hypoglycemia.
- Urine glucose monitoring is typically only helpful for documenting prolonged hypoglycemia (eg, persistently negative urine glucose testing when monitoring for diabetic remission in cats). As most diabetic patients spend time above the renal threshold for urinary glucose spillage, even patients with well-controlled diabetes may be intermittently glucosuric throughout the day.
- Fructosamine or glycosylated hemoglobin can be measured if available and warranted.
- Additional monitoring for patients with DKA[30]:
  - Gucose measurement every 1 to 2 hours initially; adjust insulin therapy and begin dextrose infusion when blood glucose decreases below 250 mg/dL (14 mmol/L)
  - Hydration status, respiration, pulse every 2 to 4 hours
  - Serum electrolyte (eg, magnesium, phosphorous, potassium), plasma ketones, and total venous CO_2 concentrations every 4 to 8 hours
  - Urine output, glycosuria, and urine ketones every 4 to 8 hours
  - Body weight, packed cell volume, temperature, and blood pressure every 6 to 8 hours
  - Additional monitoring as applicable to address concurrent disease

Client Information

NOTES for veterinarian:

1. Correct injection techniques should be taught and practiced with the client before the animal's discharge.
2. Emphasis should be placed on matching the appropriate syringe and insulin concentration (eg, do not interchange U40 insulin and syringes with U100 insulin and syringes) and correct needles with pens/devices.
3. Both veterinary-approved insulins have owner information sheets, client-friendly handouts, and websites to provide client support on administration and use of insulin.

- For this medication to work safely, give the insulin *exactly* as your veterinarian has prescribed. Do not give this medicine and contact your veterinarian for guidance if your animal is not eating.
- Your veterinarian will teach you the correct injection technique. ***Only*** use U100 insulin syringes with U100 insulin glargine.
- Always double-check the dose in the syringe or pens/devices before you inject your animal. Overdoses may be fatal.
- Prior to using, visually inspect the insulin container prior to use. Glargine solutions should be clear and colorless, without visible particles. Do not use insulin if crystals are seen. Mixing or shaking the insulin is not needed prior to use.
- After measuring the U100 insulin glargine dose into a syringe, allow the contents to come to room temperature (if the product is stored in the refrigerator) before injection.
- The injection site should be frequently changed, with the main sites being the back of the neck, side of the animal, or shoulder area.
- Place the used needles and syringes in a sharps disposal container immediately after use, making sure you do not attempt to disconnect the needle from the syringe or recap the needle. Your veterinarian or pharmacist will help you obtain these containers.
- Do not reuse needles or syringes.
- Keep insulin products out of temperature extremes. Follow the label instructions for storage of the insulin vial and pens/devices.
- Signs of low blood sugar include weakness, depression, lack of energy, sluggishness, staggering gait (ie, stumbling) when walking, behavior changes, muscle twitching, seizures (convulsions), or coma. **If your animal is unconscious or having a seizure, this is a medical emergency.** Take your animal to the veterinarian immediately. **If your animal is conscious and able to swallow**, rub ≈1 tablespoon of corn syrup (*Karo*®) or honey on your animal's gums until it is alert enough to eat. Feed the usual meal and contact your veterinarian for recommendations. Some animals may not show any obvious physical signs of low blood sugar. If your animal is not acting normally, contact your veterinarian to make sure your animal's blood sugar levels are in a safe range.
- Contact your veterinarian at your earliest convenience if you

notice excessive thirst, increased frequency of urination, or increased appetite in your animal, as these signs may indicate the insulin dose needs to be adjusted.

- When traveling, insulin should not be left in carry-on luggage that will pass through airport surveillance equipment. Generally, insulin stability is not affected by a single pass through surveillance equipment; however, longer than normal exposure or repeated passes through surveillance equipment may alter insulin potency.
- Do not stop giving this medication to your animal unless instructed to do so by your veterinarian.
- Your veterinarian will need to closely monitor your animal during treatment. Do not miss these important follow-up visits.

Chemistry/Synonyms

All commercial preparations of human-labeled insulin currently manufactured in the United States are supplied in solution or suspension at a concentration of 100 units/mL, which is ≈3.5 mg of insulin/mL. Likewise, 1 unit of insulin equals ≈35 µg of insulin, and 1 mg of insulin is ≈28.8 units.

Glargine is a long-acting human insulin analogue produced by recombinant DNA technology using a nonpathogenic laboratory strain of *Escherichia coli*. Glargine differs from human insulin in that the amino acid asparagine in position A21 has been replaced by glycine, and 2 arginines added to the C-terminus of the B chain. The solutions for injection consist of glargine dissolved in a clear aqueous fluid with a pH ≈4.

Insulin glargine may also be known as HOE901, glargine, *Lantus*®, *Abasaglar*®, *Basaglar*®, *Lusduna*®, *Rezvoglar*® (insulin glargine-aglr), *Semglee*® (insulin glargine-yfgn), *Soliqua*®, *Suliqua*®, or *Toujeo*®.

Storage/Stability

Unopened *vials* and *pens/devices* should be stored in the manufacturer's carton in the refrigerator at 2°C to 8°C (36°F-46°F). Do not freeze; discard if product has been frozen. Unused product may be stored unrefrigerated if kept below 30°C (86°F) and out of direct heat and sunlight but must be discarded after 28 days.[16,31]

In-use insulin glargine *vials* may be refrigerated or stored at room temperature; discard 28 days after first use.[16]

In use U100 insulin glargine *pens/devices* should be stored at room temperature **only** (do not refrigerate); discard 28 days after first use.[16]

In-use *U300* insulin glargine *pens/devices* should be stored at room temperature **only** (do not refrigerate); discard 56 days after first use.[31]

Discard glargine vials or pens/devices if the solution is discolored, cloudy, or contains visible particles.

Although manufacturers recommend discarding opened bottles of insulin after 4 to 6 weeks (or expiration date, whichever comes first), studies support that insulin potency and stability is maintained for longer durations.[32,33] Veterinary internal medicine specialists indicate that the vial may be used for 3 to 6 months after opening and possibly beyond the expiration date as long as it is handled carefully, stored in the refrigerator, and the solution does not develop discoloration, flocculent precipitates, or changes in consistency. If a lack of diabetes regulation is noted when using the product beyond the expiration date (3 to 6 months after starting therapy), it may be prudent to replace it with new insulin prior to adjusting insulin therapy.[1]

Compatibility/Compounding Considerations

Diluting insulin: The prolonged action of glargine depends on its pH. Insulin glargine must <u>not</u> be diluted or mixed with any other insulin or solution, as the resulting pH change transforms glargine into a rapid-acting insulin.

Insulin syringes: Syringes are designed for use with a specific strength of insulin, with the needle covers color-coded according to strength. U100 syringes are available in 0.3 mL, 0.5 mL, and 1 mL size. Measuring U100 insulin to the 1 unit mark in a U100 syringe will result in 1 unit of insulin. Some brands of 0.3 mL syringes include ½ unit markings. Insulin syringes should not be reused. *U300* glargine was successfully administered to diabetic cats using the manufacturer's pen system, which can accurately deliver a 1 unit dose.[6]

Dosage Forms/Regulatory Status

VETERINARY-LABELED PRODUCTS: NONE

HUMAN-LABELED PRODUCTS:

Insulin Glargine Injection Human (rDNA) 100 units/mL in 10 mL vials and/or 3 mL prefilled pen system; *Basaglar*®, *Lantus*®, *Rezvoglar*®, *Semglee*®; (Rx). **NOTE**: Insulins are FDA-licensed (approved) biological products, and *Semglee*® (insulin glargine-yfgn) has been licensed as an interchangeable biosimilar (ie, it can be expected to produce the same clinical result) with *Lantus*®. Please refer to the FDA's Purple Book for more information about FDA-approved biologics, including biosimilar and interchangeable products.

Insulin Glargine Injection Human (rDNA) 300 units/mL in a 1.5 mL and 3 mL prefilled pen system; *Toujeo*®; (Rx). The 1.5 mL pen can dispense a minimum dose increment of 1 unit.

References

For the complete list of references, see **wiley.com/go/budde/plumb**

Insulin, Lente

Porcine Zinc Insulin

(***inn***-suh-lin, ***lenn***-tay) *vetsulin*®

Insulin, Intermediate-Acting

NOTE: Insulin preparations available to clinicians are in a constant state of change. To maximize the efficacy of therapy and reduce the chance for errors, it is highly recommended to review current references or sources of information pertaining to insulin therapy for dogs and cats.

For additional information, see ***Insulin, General Information.***

Prescriber Highlights

- FDA-approved intermediate-acting insulin for the treatment of hyperglycemia and associated clinical signs caused by diabetes mellitus in dogs and cats.
- Animals presented with ketoacidosis, anorexia, lethargy, and/or vomiting should first be stabilized with appropriate therapy, including short-acting insulin.
- Contraindicated during episodes of hypoglycemia, and in dogs and cats with a systemic allergy to pork, or pork products
- Adverse effects include hypoglycemia, hypokalemia, insulin-induced rebound hyperglycemia (ie, Somogyi effect), and local reactions to the "foreign" proteins.
- Do not confuse insulin types, strengths, and syringes: lente insulin is a U40-approved veterinary product; only use U40 insulin syringes when measuring doses from a vial.
- Must shake insulin vials and cartridges vigorously to resuspend prior to administration
- Many potential drug interactions

Uses/Indications

Lente insulin is an FDA-approved intermediate-acting preparation used for initial treatment and long-term management of uncomplicated diabetes mellitus in dogs and cats. In a study comparing lente and NPH insulins, glycemic control in newly diagnosed, uncomplicated diabetic dogs was similar[1]; lente and NPH insulins are the first-choice recommended insulins in dogs with uncomplicated diabetes mellitus.[2] Although the FDA label recommends initiating lente insulin once daily in diabetic dogs, many experts recommend initiating use with this insulin twice daily.

Although lente insulin is FDA-approved for the treatment of diabetes mellitus in cats; either protamine zinc insulin (ie, PZI; FDA-approved for cats) or insulin glargine is recommended as first-choice insulin therapy.[2-6]

Pharmacology/Actions

The primary action of insulin is to regulate glucose metabolism. Insulin and its analogues lower blood glucose by increasing glucose uptake in peripheral tissues, especially by skeletal muscle and fat. In the liver, insulin increases glucose storage (ie, glycogen) while also inhibiting gluconeogenesis. Insulin's anabolic actions also enhance fatty acid and protein synthesis while inhibiting lipolysis and proteolysis.

For additional information, see ***Insulin, General Information***.

Pharmacokinetics

Insulin formulations contain insulin polymers (aggregates of multiple insulin molecules). Insulin is absorbed from the administration site only after insulin polymers break down into insulin monomers or dimers.

Lente insulin has 2 peaks of activity following SC administration in diabetic dogs: the first is at 2 to 6 hours, and the second is at 8 to 14 hours.[7] The duration of activity varies between 14 and 24 hours. The peak(s), duration of activity, and the dose required to adequately control diabetic signs vary among dogs.

In cats, lente insulin has peak activity between 1.5 and 8 hours after administration.[7] Duration of activity varies between 8 and 12 hours, which may be too short for most cats.

Contraindications/Precautions/Warnings

Lente insulin should not be used during episodes of hypoglycemia and in animals known to have a systemic allergy to pork or pork products. If animals develop hypersensitivity (local or otherwise) or if insulin resistance develops, a change in type or species source (eg, human, bovine, porcine) of insulin should be considered after other etiologies for poor control (eg, expired insulin, concurrent disease, or medication interference) have been ruled out. See ***Insulin, General Information***.

Lente insulin is not an appropriate insulin choice for patients presenting with severe ketoacidosis, anorexia, lethargy, and/or vomiting or other conditions when treatment with short-acting insulin (eg, regular insulin) is indicated.

For obese patients, dose calculations should be based on the patient's ideal body weight to avoid inadvertent insulin overdose.

In humans, long-term repeated SC/IM injections of insulin at the same site may cause lipodystrophic reactions, which could interfere with insulin absorption[8]; however, there have been no specific reports of this reaction occurring in dogs or cats.

Lente insulin is U40 strength. It is crucial for patient safety to only use U40 syringes when measuring and administering U40 insulin. Calculations can be done to convert to U100 syringes or TB syringes, but these conversions are not recommended because of the potential for introducing dosing errors. See ***Insulin, General Information***. The pen delivery system requires the use of needles designed specifically for that product.

When writing prescriptions, do not abbreviate units as "U," as this has been shown to increase the rate of transcription and dosage errors. In human medicine, insulin is considered a "high alert" medication (ie, medications that require special safeguards to reduce the risk for errors). Consider instituting practices such as redundant drug dosage and volume checking and special alert labels.

Do not confuse PORCINE zinc insulin (ie, lente insulin) with PROTAMINE zinc insulin (PZI).

Adverse Effects

Adverse effects of insulin therapy may include hypoglycemia (see ***Overdose/Acute Toxicity***), hypokalemia, insulininduced rebound hyperglycemia (ie, Somogyi effect), weight gain, and local reactions to the "foreign" proteins.

Reproductive/Nursing Safety

There is limited information regarding the safe use of veterinary-labeled lente insulin (ie, *vetsulin*®) in breeding, pregnant, and lactating animals.[7] A case series reports that lente has been used to manage gestational diabetes in dogs.[9] In humans, insulin is considered a treatment of choice for gestational diabetes.[10]

Overdose/Acute Toxicity

Insulin overdose can lead to various degrees of hypoglycemia. Signs may include weakness, shaking, head tilt, lethargy, ataxia, seizures, blindness, bizarre behavior, and coma. Other signs may include restlessness, hunger, and muscle fasciculations. Electrolyte disturbances, including hypokalemia, may occur. Prolonged hypoglycemia can result in permanent brain damage or death.

Mild hypoglycemia can be treated by offering the animal its usual food. More serious signs (eg, seizures) should be treated with oral dextrose solutions (eg, *Karo*® syrup) applied to the buccal mucosa (if the animal is seizing, use caution to avoid being bit or injured) or by IV injections of 50% dextrose solutions (small amounts—usually 2 to 15 mL [0.5 to 1 mL/kg], diluted and slowly administered[11]; see ***Dextrose 50% injection***). For inhospital management, glucagon may also be considered on an as-needed basis for an insulin overdose. See ***Glucagon.*** Once the animal's hypoglycemia is alleviated (response usually occurs within 1 to 2 minutes), the animal should be closely monitored (both by physical observation and serial blood glucose levels) to prevent a recurrence of hypoglycemia (especially with the slower-absorbed/longer-acting products) and to prevent hyperglycemia from developing. Future insulin dosages or feeding habits should be evaluated or adjusted based on consultation with the clinician to prevent further occurrences of hypoglycemia.

For patients that have experienced or are suspected of having experienced an overdose, consultation with a 24-hour poison consultation center specializing in providing veterinary-specific information is recommended. For general information related to overdose and toxin exposures, as well as contact information for poison control centers, refer to ***Appendix.***

Drug Interactions

The following drug interactions have either been reported or are theoretical in humans or animals receiving insulin and may be of significance in veterinary patients. Unless otherwise noted, use together is not necessarily contraindicated, but weigh the potential risks and perform additional monitoring when appropriate.

- Beta-Adrenergic Antagonists (eg, **atenolol, propranolol**): Can have variable effects on glycemic control and can mask the signs associated with hypoglycemia
- Clonidine: Can mask the signs associated with hypoglycemia
- Digoxin: Because insulin can reduce serum potassium levels, patients receiving concomitant digoxin therapy—especially those receiving concurrent diuretic therapy—should be closely monitored.
- Diuretics (eg, **furosemide, hydrochlorothiazide**): Insulin shifts extracellular potassium into the intracellular space; serum potassium concentration should be closely monitored in patients receiving concomitant diuretic therapy. Diuretics may also decrease the hypoglycemic activity of insulin (ie, increase insulin requirements).
- Reserpine: Can mask the signs associated with hypoglycemia

The following drugs or drug classes may potentiate the hypoglycemic activity of insulin (ie, decrease insulin requirements):

- ANABOLIC STEROIDS (eg, **boldenone, stanozolol, testosterone**)
- ANGIOTENSIN II RECEPTOR BLOCKERS (ARBs; eg, **telmisartan**)
- ANGIOTENSIN-CONVERTING ENZYME INHIBITORS (ARBs; eg, **benazepril, enalapril**)
- DISOPYRAMIDE
- ETHANOL
- FENOFIBRATE
- FLUOROQUINOLONES (eg, **ciprofloxacin, enrofloxacin**)
- FLUOXETINE
- HYPOGLYCEMIC AGENTS, ORAL (eg, **acarbose, glipizide, metformin**)
- MONOAMINE OXIDASE INHIBITORS (eg, **amitraz, linezolid, selegiline**)
- PENTOXIFYLLINE
- SALICYLATES (eg, **aspirin, bismuth subsalicylate**)
- SOMATOSTATIN DERIVATIVES (eg, **octreotide**)
- SULFONAMIDES (eg, **sulfadimethoxine, sulfamethoxazole**)

The following drugs or drug classes may decrease the hypoglycemic activity of insulin (ie, increase insulin requirements):

- ALPHA-2-ADRENERGIC AGONISTS (eg, **dexmedetomidine, medetomidine, xylazine**): May cause hyperglycemia and temporarily interfere with glycemic control
- BETA-ADRENERGIC AGONISTS (eg, **albuterol, terbutaline**)
- CORTICOSTEROIDS (eg, **dexamethasone, prednis(ol)one**)
- DANAZOL
- DIAZOXIDE
- ESTROGENS (eg, **diethylstilbestrol [DES], estriol**)
- ISONIAZID
- NIACIN
- PHENOTHIAZINES (eg, **acepromazine, chlorpromazine**)
- PROGESTINS (eg, **megestrol**)
- THYROID HORMONES: Can elevate glucose levels in diabetic patients when thyroid hormone therapy is first initiated

Laboratory Considerations

- None

Dosages

NOTES:

1. Treatment of diabetes mellitus is complex; insulin is only one component of therapy; treatment may require fluid electrolyte replacement, management of acid/base disturbances, dietary adjustments, and antimicrobial therapy. Adequate patient monitoring is mandatory. It is strongly encouraged to refer to more thorough discussions of treatment in veterinary endocrinology or internal medicine references for additional information.
2. For obese patients, dose calculations should be based on the patient's estimated ideal body weight to avoid inadvertent insulin overdose.
3. Key goals of therapy are control of clinical signs associated with diabetes mellitus and avoidance of hypoglycemia.[2,12]

DOGS:

Reduction of hyperglycemia and hyperglycemia-associated clinical signs (label dosage; FDA-approved): 0.5 units/kg SC once daily concurrent with or right after a meal.[7] Twice-daily administration should be initiated if the duration of insulin action is determined to be inadequate with once-daily administration. If twice-daily administration is initiated, the 2 doses should each be ≈25% less than the once-daily dose required to attain an acceptable glucose nadir. For example, if a dog receiving 20 units SC once daily has an acceptable nadir but inadequate duration of activity, the dose should be changed to 15 units SC twice daily.

Initial insulin treatment of uncomplicated diabetes mellitus (extra-label): 0.25 – 0.5 units/kg SC every 12 hours; give equal-sized meals at the time of insulin injection.[2]

CATS:

Reduction of hyperglycemia and hyperglycemia-associated clinical signs (label dosage; FDA-approved): Starting dose, 1 – 2 units/cat (NOT units/kg) SC twice daily at ≈12-hour intervals.[7] For cats fed twice daily, injections should be given concurrently with or right after each meal. For cats fed ad libitum, no change in the feeding schedule is needed.

Initial insulin treatment of uncomplicated diabetes mellitus (extra-label): 0.25 – 0.5 units/kg SC every 12 hours; starting dose should not exceed 3 units/cat (NOT units/kg).[2]

Monitoring

Each patient requires an individualized treatment plan, frequent reassessment, and adjustments to the plan based on the response of the patient. It is encouraged to consult a veterinary endocrinology reference text or with a veterinary emergency and critical care and/or endocrinology specialist for further information related to regulating diabetic patients and insulin adjustments. The overarching goal when monitoring diabetic patients is the control of clinical signs related to hyperglycemia (eg, polyuria, polydipsia) while avoiding hypoglycemia. Interpret all monitoring strategies based on clinical signs. Results from the monitoring options below may conflict in regards to achieving good glycemic control and good clinical control.

- Patient status and control of clinical signs: body weight, appetite, fluid intake, urine output
- Glucose (blood or interstitial) curve. Experience with continuous interstitial glucose monitoring in dogs and cats is that these devices are easy to apply, user friendly, and provide useful information surrounding glycemic control while the patient is in the clinic or home environment.[13-16] A glucose curve can be considered at the following times[2]:
  - After the first dose of a new insulin type—glucose can be checked every 2 hours after administration. The goal for monitoring following the first dose of insulin would be solely to identify hypoglycemia. The insulin dose should NOT be increased based on the first-day glucose evaluation. If glucose falls below 150 mg/dL during the glucose curve, the frequency of monitoring should increase to hourly until glucose is greater than 150 mg/dL.[2] Although the lente insulin dose should never be increased on the first day of therapy, the dose should be decreased by 10% to 50% in dogs and 50% in cats if glucose is less than 150 mg/dL at any time during the day.[2] Repeat glucose curves on subsequent days (and decrease insulin dose if necessary) until nadir is greater than 150 mg/dL.
  - 7 to 14 days after starting insulin or an insulin dose change
  - At least every 3 months, even in animals with well-controlled diabetes
  - Any time clinical signs related to hyperglycemia (eg, polyuria, polydipsia) recur in an animal with previously well-controlled diabetes
  - When hypoglycemia is a concern. **NOTE**: For patients that have experienced or are suspected of having experienced repeated or unexplained hypoglycemia, it is strongly encouraged that pet owners consult with a veterinary emergency and critical care and/or endocrinology specialist or reference text that specializes in providing information specific for the treatment of hypoglycemia.
- Urine glucose monitoring is typically only helpful for documenting prolonged hypoglycemia (eg, persistently negative urine glu-

cose testing when monitoring for diabetic remission in cats). As most diabetic patients spend time above the renal threshold for urinary glucose spillage, even patients with well-controlled diabetes may be intermittently glucosuric throughout the day.

- Fructosamine or glycosylated hemoglobin can be monitored if available and warranted.

Client Information

NOTES for veterinarian:

1. Correct injection techniques should be taught and practiced with the client before the animal's discharge.
2. Emphasis should be placed on matching the appropriate syringe and insulin concentration (eg, do not interchange U40 insulin and syringes with U100 insulin and syringes) and correct needles with pens/devices.
3. Both veterinary-approved insulins have owner information sheets, client-friendly handouts, and websites to provide client support on administration and use of insulin.

- For this medication to work safely, give the insulin *exactly* as your veterinarian has prescribed. Do not give this medicine and contact your veterinarian for guidance if your animal is not eating.
- Your veterinarian will teach you proper injection technique. ***Only*** use U40 syringes with lente insulin. When using the *VetPen*® device, only use matching pen needles.
- Always double-check the dose in the syringe before you inject your animal. Overdoses may be fatal.
- Shake lente insulin vials thoroughly until a uniform, milky suspension is formed. Prior to using, visually inspect the insulin bottle prior to use. Do not use if clumps or white particles persist after mixing.
- After measuring the dose into a syringe, allow the contents to come to room temperature before giving the injection.
- The injection site should be frequently changed, with the main sites being the back of the neck, side of the animal, or shoulder area.
- Place the used needles and syringes in a sharps disposal container immediately after use, making sure you do not attempt to disconnect the needle from the syringe or recap the needle. Your veterinarian or pharmacist will help you obtain these containers.
- Do not reuse needles or syringes.
- Signs of low blood sugar include weakness, depression, lack of energy, sluggishness, staggering gait (ie, stumbling) when walking, behavior changes, muscle twitching, seizures (convulsions), or coma. **If your animal is unconscious or having a seizure, this is a medical emergency.** Take your animal to your veterinarian immediately. **If your animal is conscious and able to swallow**, rub ≈1 tablespoon of corn syrup (*Karo*®) or honey on your animal's gums until it is alert enough to eat. Feed the usual meal and contact your veterinarian for recommendations. Some animals may not show any obvious physical signs of low blood sugar. If your animal is not acting normally, contact your veterinarian to make sure your animal's blood sugar level is in a safe range.
- Contact your veterinarian at your earliest convenience if you notice excessive thirst, increased frequency of urination, or increased appetite in your animal, as these signs may indicate the insulin dose needs to be adjusted.
- When traveling, do not leave insulin in carry-on luggage that will pass through airport surveillance equipment. Generally, insulin stability is not affected by a single pass through surveillance equipment; however, longer than normal exposure or repeated passes through surveillance equipment may alter insulin potency.
- Do not stop giving this medication to your animal unless instructed to do so by your veterinarian.
- Your veterinarian will need to closely monitor your animal during treatment. Do not miss these important follow-up visits.

Chemistry/Synonyms

Porcine zinc (lente) insulin is a sterile aqueous suspension of purified pork insulin that consists of 35% amorphous zinc insulin and 65% crystalline zinc insulin. Lente insulin is supplied at a concentration of 40 units/mL; it is a cloudy or milky suspension of a mixture of characteristic crystals and particles with no uniform shape. One unit of insulin is equivalent to ≈35 µg of insulin, and 1 mL of U40 insulin contains 1.38 mg insulin, and 1 mg of porcine insulin is ≈28.8 units.

Lente insulin may also be known as *Caninsulin*®, porcine zinc insulin, or *vetsulin*®.

Storage/Stability

Store ***unopened*** and ***in-use*** lente insulin *vials* and *pens/devices* in the manufacturer's carton in the refrigerator at 2°C to 8°C (36°F-46°F). Do not freeze; discard if product has been frozen. Store vials upright; may store pens/devices on their sides. Discard *vials* and *pens/devices* 42 days after first use.

Although manufacturers recommend discarding opened bottles of insulin after 4 to 6 weeks (or expiration date, whichever comes first), studies support that insulin potency and stability is maintained for longer durations.[17,18] Veterinary internal medicine specialists indicate that the vial may be used for 3 to 6 months after opening and possibly beyond the expiration date as long as it is handled carefully, stored in the refrigerator, and the solution does not develop discoloration, flocculent precipitates, or changes in consistency. If a lack of diabetes regulation is noted when using the product beyond the expiration date (3 to 6 months after starting therapy), it may be prudent to replace it with new insulin prior to adjusting insulin therapy.[2]

Compatibility/Compounding Considerations

Diluting *vetsulin*® is not recommended, as dilution alters the balance of amorphous and crystalline insulin, thereby changing the hypoglycemic effects.[19]

Insulin syringes: Syringes are designed for use with a specific strength of insulin, with the needle covers color-coded according to strength. U40 syringes are available in 0.3 mL, 0.5 mL, and 1 mL size. Drawing U40 insulin to the 1 unit mark in a U40 syringe will contain 1 unit of insulin. Some brands of 0.3 mL and 0.5 mL syringes include ½ unit markings. Insulin syringes should not be reused.

Dosage Forms/Regulatory Status

VETERINARY-LABELED PRODUCTS:

Porcine Zinc [Lente] Insulin Suspension: 40 units/mL in 10 mL vials; also available in 2.7 mL cartridges for use in an insulin pen system: *Vetpen*®*8* delivers a dose between 0.5 to 8 units in 0.5 unit increments; *Vetpen*®*16* delivers a dose between 1 and 16 units, in 1 unit increments; *vetsulin*®; (Rx). FDA-approved for use in dogs and cats; NADA# 141-236

HUMAN-LABELED PRODUCTS: NONE

References

For the complete list of references, see **wiley.com/go/budde/plumb**

Insulin, Lispro

(***inn***-suh-lin, ***liss***-pro) *Humalog®*

Insulin, Rapid/Short-Acting

NOTE: Insulin preparations available to clinicians are in a constant state of change. To maximize the efficacy of therapy and reduce the chance for errors, it is highly recommended to review current references or sources of information pertaining to insulin therapy for dogs and cats.

For additional information, see ***Insulin, General Information.***

Prescriber Highlights

- Rapid/short-acting insulin used to treat diabetic ketoacidosis (DKA); can be used in place of regular insulin. There is limited clinical experience in dogs and cats with this insulin.
- There are no absolute contraindications, except during episodes of hypoglycemia.
- Adverse effects include hypoglycemia, hypokalemia, hypophosphatemia (DKA only), insulin-induced rebound hyperglycemia (ie, Somogyi effect), and local reactions to the "foreign" proteins.
- Do not confuse insulin types, strengths, and syringes. Insulin lispro is a U100 human product; use only U100 insulin syringes to measure a dose. Other insulin lispro formulations (ie, U200, insulin lispro combinations) have not been evaluated in veterinary patients.
- Many potential drug interactions

Uses/Indications

Insulin lispro is a rapid, or short-acting, insulin used for diabetic emergencies (eg, diabetic ketoacidosis [DKA]) and for control of the complicated diabetic patient. As an insulin analogue similar in action to regular insulin (ie, rapid/short-acting), insulin lispro could be considered for the same indications as regular insulin (eg, hyperkalemia) if regular insulin is not an option, although evidence in veterinary species is lacking. IV insulin administration is recommended in patients with poor tissue perfusion, shock, cardiovascular collapse, or in those that require adjunct therapy for hyperkalemia.

Insulin lispro is not commonly used for maintenance insulin therapy in diabetic dogs and cats; however, it could be considered in complicated diabetic patients that cannot be regulated using more standard insulin preparations, particularly those in which a profound postprandial hyperglycemic response exists.[1] It is strongly encouraged to consult an endocrinology specialist or reference when using insulin lispro as part of a protocol for long-term maintenance insulin therapy.

Insulin lispro administered as an IV CRI appears to be safe and as effective as regular insulin in dogs[2] and cats with DKA.[3,4] One study describes the safe and effective use of insulin lispro IM for the management of DKA in dogs.[5] In patients with DKA, initial aggressive fluid replacement therapy is of paramount importance to restore tissue perfusion and begin correcting electrolyte or acid-base derangements. Early administration (ie, within 6 hours of presentation) of insulin to patients with DKA leads to earlier resolution of hyperglycemia, acidemia, and ketonemia while being safe and well tolerated.[6] Once the patient is stabilized, longer-acting insulin products can be started for maintenance of insulin therapy. It is strongly encouraged to consult a veterinary emergency and critical care and/or endocrinology specialist or reference when treating this complex condition.

Pharmacology/Actions

The primary action of insulin is to regulate glucose metabolism. Insulin and its analogues lower blood glucose by increasing glucose uptake in peripheral tissues, especially by skeletal muscle and fat. In the liver, insulin increases glucose storage (ie, glycogen) while also inhibiting gluconeogenesis. Insulin's anabolic actions also enhance fatty acid and protein synthesis while inhibiting lipolysis and proteolysis.

For additional information, see ***Insulin, General Information***.

Pharmacokinetics

Insulin formulations contain insulin polymers (aggregates of multiple insulin molecules). Insulin is absorbed from the administration site only after insulin polymers break down into insulin monomers or dimers. Insulin lispro is less likely to form hexamers, and its rapid absorption results in a fast onset and short duration of effect.

The hypoglycemic response of insulin lispro administered by continuous IV infusion appears similar to that of regular insulin in cats and dogs.[1,2] Although published studies are lacking, the pharmacokinetics of insulin lispro given IV to dogs and cats appear to be comparable with that of humans. After SC administration in diabetic dogs, the onset of hypoglycemic effect is within 0.5 hours, and the peak effect occurs over 1 to 3 hours.[7]

Contraindications/Precautions/Warnings

Because there are no alternatives for insulin when it is used for diabetic indications, there are no absolute contraindications to its use except during episodes of hypoglycemia. If animals develop hypersensitivity (local or otherwise) or if insulin resistance develops, a change in type or species source (eg, human, bovine, porcine) of insulin should be considered after other etiologies for poor control (eg, expired insulin, concurrent disease, or medication interference) have been ruled out. See ***Insulin, General Information***.

For obese patients, dose calculations should be based on the patient's ideal body weight to avoid inadvertent insulin overdose.

In humans, long-term repeated SC/IM injections of insulin at the same site may cause lipodystrophic reactions, which could interfere with insulin absorption[8]; however, there have been no specific reports of this reaction occurring in dogs or cats.

Similar to regular insulin and other insulin analogue solutions (eg, aspart, glulisine), insulin lispro may be given IV or IM; however, insulin lispro administered IM is limited to anecdotal experience. In patients with moderate to severe dehydration, poor tissue perfusion necessitates regular insulin to be given IM or IV as absorption of SC injections is likely to be impaired or delayed. Short-acting insulin analogues administered IV offer little therapeutic or pharmacokinetic advantage over regular insulin.

Insulin lispro is U100 strength. It is crucial for patient safety to only use U100 syringes when measuring and administering U100 insulin. Calculations can be done to convert to U40 syringes or TB syringes, but these conversions are not recommended because of the potential for introducing dosing errors. See ***Insulin, General Information***.

When writing prescriptions, do not abbreviate units as "U," as this has been shown to increase the rate of transcription and dosage errors. In human medicine, insulin is considered a "high alert" medication (medications that require special safeguards to reduce the risk for errors). Consider instituting practices such as redundant drug dosage and volume checking and special alert labels.

Do not confuse insulin lispro (a clear solution that may be administered by a variety of routes) with insulin lispro protamine/insulin lispro mixture (a cloudy solution that may be administered only by the SC route). *Lyumjev®* is an insulin lispro formulation that produces a different hypoglycemic response in humans (slower onset and longer duration) than *Humalog®*.[9] It is suggested to avoid interchanging these insulins until more is known about the use of *Lyumjev®* in animals.

Adverse Effects

Adverse effects of insulin therapy may include hypoglycemia

(see ***Overdose/Acute Toxicity***), hypokalemia, hypophosphatemia (diabetic ketoacidosis [DKA] only), insulin-induced rebound hyperglycemia (ie, Somogyi effect), and local or allergic reactions to the "foreign" proteins.

Reproductive/Nursing Safety

Insulin lispro given at clinically effective doses to pregnant laboratory animals did not result in developmental effects; however, fetal growth retardation was noted at a dosage of 20 units/kg/day.[8]

In humans, insulin is considered compatible with nursing.[10]

Overdose/Acute Toxicity

Insulin overdose can lead to various degrees of hypoglycemia. Signs may include weakness, shaking, head tilt, lethargy, ataxia, seizures, blindness, bizarre behavior, and coma. Other signs may include restlessness, hunger, and muscle fasciculations. Electrolyte disturbances, including hypokalemia, may occur. Prolonged hypoglycemia can result in permanent brain damage or death.

Mild hypoglycemia can be treated by offering the animal its usual food. More serious signs (eg, seizures) should be treated with oral dextrose solutions (eg, *Karo*® syrup) applied to the buccal mucosa (if the animal is seizing, use caution to avoid being bit or injured) or by IV injections of 50% dextrose solutions (small amounts—usually 2 – 15 mL [0.5 –1 mL/kg], diluted, and slowly administered[11]). See ***Dextrose 50% Injection.*** For inhospital management, glucagon may also be considered on an as-needed basis for an insulin overdose. See ***Glucagon.*** Once the animal's hypoglycemia is alleviated (response usually occurs within 1 to 2 minutes), it should be closely monitored (both by physical observation and serial blood glucose levels) to prevent a recurrence of hypoglycemia (especially with the slower-absorbed/longer-acting products) and to prevent hyperglycemia from developing. Future insulin dosages or feeding regimens should be evaluated or adjusted based on consultation with the clinician to prevent further occurrences of hypoglycemia.

For patients that have experienced or are suspected of having experienced an overdose, consultation with a 24-hour poison consultation center specializing in providing veterinary-specific information is recommended. For general information related to overdose and toxin exposures, as well as contact information for poison control centers, refer to ***Appendix.***

Drug Interactions

The following drug interactions have either been reported or are theoretical in humans or animals receiving insulin and may be of significance in veterinary patients. Unless otherwise noted, use together is not necessarily contraindicated, but weigh the potential risks and perform additional monitoring when appropriate.

- Beta-Adrenergic Blockers (eg, **atenolol, propranolol**): Can have variable effects on glycemic control and can mask the signs associated with hypoglycemia
- Clonidine: Can mask the signs associated with hypoglycemia
- Digoxin: Because insulin can reduce serum potassium levels, patients receiving concomitant digoxin therapy—especially patients receiving concurrent diuretic therapy—should be closely monitored.
- Diuretics (eg, **furosemide, hydrochlorothiazide**): Insulin shifts extracellular potassium into the intracellular space; serum potassium concentration should be closely monitored in patients receiving concomitant diuretic therapy. Diuretics may also decrease the hypoglycemic activity of insulin (ie, increase insulin requirements).
- Reserpine: Can mask the signs associated with hypoglycemia

The following drugs or drug classes may potentiate the hypoglycemic activity of insulin (ie, decrease insulin requirements):

- Anabolic Steroids (eg, **boldenone, stanozolol, testosterone**)
- Angiotensin II Receptor Blockers (ARBs; eg, **telmisartan**)
- Angiotensin-Converting Enzyme Inhibitors (ACEIs; eg, **benazepril, enalapril**)
- Disopyramide
- Ethanol
- Fenofibrate
- Fluoroquinolones (eg, **ciprofloxacin, enrofloxacin**)
- Fluoxetine
- Hypoglycemics, Oral (eg, **acarbose, glipizide, metformin**)
- Monoamine Oxidase Inhibitors (MAOIs; eg, **amitraz, linezolid, selegiline**)
- Pentoxifylline
- Salicylates (eg, **aspirin, bismuth subsalicylate**)
- Somatostatin Derivatives (eg, **octreotide**)
- Sulfonamides (eg, **sulfadimethoxine, sulfamethoxazole**)

The following drugs or drug classes may decrease the hypoglycemic activity of insulin (ie, increase insulin requirements):

- Alpha-2-Adrenergic Agonists (eg, **dexmedetomidine, medetomidine, xylazine**): May cause hyperglycemia and temporarily interfere with glycemic control
- Beta-2-Adrenergic Agonists (eg, **albuterol, terbutaline**)
- Corticosteroids (eg, **dexamethasone, prednis(ol)one**)
- Danazol
- Diazoxide
- Estrogens (eg, **diethylstilbestrol [DES], estriol**)
- Isoniazid
- Niacin
- Phenothiazines (eg, **acepromazine, chlorpromazine**)
- Progestins (eg, **megestrol**)
- Thyroid Hormones: Can elevate glucose levels in diabetic patients when thyroid hormone therapy is first initiated

Laboratory Considerations

- None

Dosages

NOTES:

1. Treatment of diabetes mellitus and, in particular, diabetic ketoacidosis (DKA) is complex. Insulin is only one component of therapy; treatment may require fluid and electrolyte replacement, management of acid/base disturbances, and antimicrobial therapy. Adequate patient monitoring is mandatory. It is strongly encouraged to refer to more thorough discussions of treatment in veterinary endocrinology or internal medicine references.
2. For obese patients, dose calculations should be based on the individual patient's estimated ideal body weight to avoid inadvertent insulin overdose.
3. Insulin lispro given by IV CRI appears to be a safe and effective alternative when regular insulin is not an option or is unavailable.
4. All dosages are extra-label.

DOGS:

Adjunctive therapy of DKA using an IV CRI: To prepare an infusion that delivers 0.09 units/kg/hour: 2.2 units/kg insulin lispro is added to 240 mL (**NOTE**: Many clinicians add insulin directly to a 250 mL bag without removing the 10 mL of fluid) of 0.9% sodium chloride. Run ≈50 mL of the insulin-containing fluid through the drip set prior to administration (see ***Adsorption*** in ***Compatibility/Compounding Considerations***). The initial administration rate is 10 mL/hour in a separate line to that used for fluid therapy.[2,12] When starting initial therapy for DKA, potassium levels must be taken into account and therapy adjusted accordingly to avoid hypokalemia. Adjust infusion rate based on blood glucose determinations taken every 2 hours. An hourly reduction in blood glucose by 50 – 100 mg/dL is recommended.[12] Once blood glucose approaches 250 mg/dL, adjust the fluid type and rate based on the periodic measurement of blood glucose concentration (see table) with a goal of keeping the blood glucose in the 150 – 300 mg/dL range and continuing the insulin IV infusion at a decreased rate until it can be exchanged for a longer-acting product.

Blood glucose concentration (mg/dL [mmol/L])	Maintenance IV fluid	Rate of insulin IV CRI administration (mL/hour)	Dose of insulin administered (units/kg/hour)*
Greater than 250 (13.8)	0.9% sodium chloride	10	0.09
200-250 (11.1-13.8)	0.45% sodium chloride + 2.5% dextrose	7	0.064
150-200 (8.3-11)	0.45% sodium chloride + 2.5% dextrose	5	0.045
100-150 (5.5-8.2)	0.45% sodium chloride + 5% dextrose	5	0.045
Less than 100 (5.5)	0.45% sodium chloride + 5% dextrose	0 (Stop insulin administration)	0 (Stop insulin administration)

Table adapted from Sears KW, Drobatz KJ, Hess RS. Use of lispro insulin for treatment of diabetic ketoacidosis in dogs. *J Vet Emerg Crit Care.* 2012;22(2):211-218.

*CRI prepared by adding insulin lispro 2.2 units/kg to 240 mL 0.9% sodium chloride.

Adjunctive therapy of DKA using an IM protocol:

a) **Glucose greater than 250 mg/dL at the time of diagnosis:** Insulin lispro initial dose of 0.25 units/kg IM with glycemia monitored hourly with a goal of dropping at least 10% in blood glucose between 1 hour and the next.[5] If the goal was *not* achieved, the insulin dose was repeated hourly. If the goal was achieved, the insulin dose was not repeated up to a maximum of 3 hours, after which the insulin dose was repeated anyway. When blood glucose reached 250 mg/dL, the insulin dose was decreased to 0.125 units/kg IM every 3 hours, and the IV fluids were changed to dextrose, starting with a 2.5% solution, and adjusted up to 5% or 7.5% solution as needed in order to keep the blood glucose between 150 and 300 mg/dL until resolution of DKA. If the blood glucose was less than 80 mg/dL or the dog became clinical for hypoglycemia, 0.25 to 0.5 g/kg of 50% dextrose was administered IV, and the insulin therapy was discontinued.
b) **Glucose less than or equal to 250 mg/dL at the time of diagnosis**: Insulin lispro 0.125 units/kg IM every 3 hours, with supplementation of dextrose as described above

Combination with NPH for patients experiencing significant postprandial hyperglycemia on standard insulin protocols: Insulin lispro 0.1 units/kg SC every 12 hours therapy was added to patients ($n = 6$) already receiving NPH treatment but experiencing postprandial hyperglycemia.[1] The median glucose concentrations at 1 hour and 1.5 hours postprandial and serum fructosamine were significantly lower with this combination therapy.[1]

CATS:

Adjunctive therapy of DKA using an IV CRI:

a) Insulin lispro 1.1 units/kg added to 48 mL of 0.9% sodium chloride for CRI. The initial infusion rate of 1 – 2 mL/hour was determined by the cat's blood glucose concentration and adjusted every 1 to 2 hours (see table).[4] When starting initial therapy for DKA, serum potassium levels must be taken into account and therapy adjusted accordingly to avoid hypokalemia. Efficacy and safety were similar to treatment with regular insulin CRI. **NOTE:** Because of the small volume prepared, the insulin solution was allowed to saturate the IV tubing for 30 minutes, then was run through the IV line and discarded. A fresh solution was then prepared and administered.[4]

Blood glucose concentration (mg/dL [mmol/L])	Maintenance IV fluid*	Rate of insulin IV CRI administration (mL/hour)	Dose of insulin administered (units/kg/hour)*
Greater than 250 (13.9)	0.9% sodium chloride	2	0.045
200-250 (11.1-13.9)	0.9% sodium chloride + 2.5% dextrose	1.5	0.032
150-199 (8.4-11)	0.9% sodium chloride + 2.5% dextrose	1.5	0.032
100-149 (5.6-8.3)	0.9% sodium chloride + 5% dextrose	1	0.023
Less than 100 (5.5)	0.9% sodium chloride + 5% dextrose	0 (Stop insulin administration)	0 (Stop insulin administration)

Table adapted from Malerba E, Mazzarino M, Del Baldo F, et al. Use of lispro insulin for treatment of diabetic ketoacidosis in cats. *J Feline Med Surg.* 2019;21(2):115-123.

*CRI prepared by adding insulin lispro 1.1 units/kg to 48 mL 0.9% sodium chloride or lactated Ringer's solution.

b) To prepare a CRI with an initial administration rate of 0.09 units/kg/hour: prepare solution by adding insulin lispro 2.2 units/kg per 240 mL of 0.9% sodium chloride/sterile saline. Run ≈50 mL of the insulin-containing fluid through the drip set prior to administration (see **Adsorption** in ***Compatibility/Compounding Considerations***).[3] Insulin infusions should be run through a fluid line that is separate from that used for fluid therapy.[12] The initial administration rate is 10 mL/hour to deliver insulin at 0.09 units/kg/hour. When starting initial therapy for DKA, serum potassium levels must be taken into account and therapy adjusted accordingly to avoid hypokalemia. Adjust infusion rate based on blood glucose determinations taken every 2 hours. Once blood glucose approaches 300 mg/dL, adjust the fluid type and rate based on periodic measurement of blood glucose concentration (see table) with a goal of keeping the blood glucose in the 150 – 300 mg/dL range and continuing the insulin IV infusion at a decreased rate until it can be exchanged for a longer-acting product.

Blood glucose concentration (mg/dL [mmol/L])	Maintenance IV fluid	Rate of insulin IV CRI administration (mL/hour)	Dose of insulin administered (units/kg/hour)*
Greater than 300 (16.7)	0.9% sodium chloride	10	0.09
200-300 (11.1-16.7)	0.9% sodium chloride + 2.5% dextrose	7	0.064
150-199 (8.3-11)	0.9% sodium chloride + 2.5% dextrose	5	0.045
100-149 (5.5-8.2)	0.9% sodium chloride + 5% dextrose	5	0.045
Less than 100 (5.5)	0.9% sodium chloride + 5% dextrose	0 (Stop insulin administration)	0 (Stop insulin administration)

Table adapted from Anderson JD, Rondeau DA, Hess RS. Lispro insulin and electrolyte supplementation for treatment of diabetic ketoacidosis in cats. *J Vet Intern Med.* 2019;33(4):1593-1601.

*CRI prepared by adding insulin lispro 2.2 units/kg to 240 mL 0.9% sodium chloride.

Monitoring

- Diabetic patients should be closely monitored. Each patient requires an individualized treatment plan, frequent reassessment, and adjustments of the plan based on the response of the patient. It is encouraged to review a veterinary endocrinology reference text or consult with a veterinary emergency and critical care and/or endocrinology specialist for further information related to regulating diabetic patients and insulin adjustments. The overarching goal for monitoring diabetic patients is control of clinical signs related to hyperglycemia (eg, polyuria, polydipsia) while avoiding hypoglycemia.[13] Interpret all monitoring strategies in light of clinical signs. Results from the below monitoring options may conflict in regards to achieving good glycemic control and good clinical control.
- Patient status and control of clinical signs: body weight, appetite, fluid intake, urine output
- Glucose (blood or interstitial). Because of how often glucose needs to be checked in sick diabetic patients, consider a central line or continuous interstitial glucose monitoring system in dogs and cats. Experience with continuous interstitial glucose monitoring in dogs and cats is that these systems are easy to apply, user friendly, and provide useful information surrounding glycemic control while the patient is in the clinic or home environment.[14-17]
  - For patients that have experienced or are suspected to have experienced repeated or unexplained hypoglycemia, it is strongly encouraged to consult a veterinary emergency and critical care and/or endocrinology specialist or reference text that specializes in providing information specific for treatment of hypoglycemia.
- Additional monitoring for patients with diabetic ketoacidosis (DKA)[18]:
  - Glucose measurement every 1 to 2 hours initially; adjust insulin therapy and begin dextrose infusion when glucose decreases below 250 mg/dL (14 mmol/L). See ***Dosages***.
  - Hydration status, respiration, pulse every 2 to 4 hours
  - Serum electrolyte (eg, magnesium, phosphorous, potassium), plasma ketones, and total venous CO_2 concentrations every 4 to 8 hours
  - Urine output, glycosuria, and urine ketones every 4 to 8 hours
  - Body weight, packed cell volume, temperature, and blood pressure every 6 to 8 hours
  - Additional monitoring as applicable to address concurrent disease

Client Information

NOTES for veterinarian:

1. Correct injection techniques should be taught and practiced with the client before the animal's discharge.
2. Emphasis should be placed on matching the appropriate syringe and insulin concentration (eg, do not interchange U40 insulin and syringes with U100 insulin and syringes) and correct needles with pens/devices.
3. Both veterinary-approved insulins have owner information sheets, client-friendly handouts, and websites to provide client support on administration and use of insulin.

- For this medication to work safely, give the insulin *exactly* as your veterinarian has prescribed. Do not give this medicine and consult your veterinarian for guidance if your animal is not eating.
- Your veterinarian will teach you proper injection technique. ***Only*** use U100 syringes with insulin lispro.
- Always double-check the dose in the syringe before you inject your animal. Overdoses may be fatal.
- Prior to using, visually inspect the insulin bottle. Insulin lispro should appear as a clear, colorless solution. Do not use insulin solutions if you see crystals on the inside of the vial. There should never be clumps or unexpected particles in the vial.
- After measuring the dose into a syringe, allow the contents to come to room temperature (if the vial is stored in the refrigerator) before injection.
- The injection site should be frequently changed, with the main sites being the back of the neck or shoulder area.
- Place the used needles and syringes in a sharps disposal container immediately after use, making sure you do not attempt to disconnect the needle from the syringe or recap the needle. Your veterinarian or pharmacist will help you obtain these containers.
- Do not re-use needles or syringes.
- Keep insulin products out of temperature extremes. Follow the label instructions for storage of the insulin vial and pens/devices.
- Signs of low blood sugar include weakness, depression, lack of energy, sluggishness, staggering gait (ie, stumbling) when walking, behavior changes, muscle twitching, seizures (convulsions), or coma. **If your animal is unconscious or having a seizure, this is a medical emergency.** Take your animal to your veterinarian immediately. **If your animal is conscious and able to swallow**, rub ≈1 tablespoon of corn syrup (*Karo*®) or honey on your animal's gums until it is alert enough to eat. Feed the usual meal and contact your veterinarian for recommendations. Some animals may not show any obvious physical signs of low blood sugar. If your animal is not acting normally, contact your veterinarian to make sure your animal's blood sugar levels are in a safe range.
- Contact your veterinarian at your earliest convenience if you notice excessive thirst, increased frequency of urination, or increased appetite in your animal, as these signs may indicate the insulin dose needs to be adjusted.
- When traveling, do not leave insulin in carry-on luggage that will pass through airport surveillance equipment. Generally, insulin stability is not affected by a single pass through surveillance equipment; however, longer than normal exposure or repeated passes through surveillance equipment may alter insulin potency.

- Do not stop giving this medication to your animal unless instructed to do so by your veterinarian.
- Your veterinarian will need to closely monitor your animal during treatment. Do not miss these important follow-up visits.

Chemistry/Synonyms

All commercial preparations of human-labeled insulin currently manufactured in the United States are supplied in solution or suspension at a concentration of 100 units/mL or greater. U100 insulins contain ≈3.5 mg of insulin/mL. Likewise, 1 unit of insulin is ≈35 µg of insulin, and 1 mg of insulin is ≈28.8 units.

Insulin lispro injection, USP (rDNA origin) is a rapid-acting human insulin analogue that is synthesized in a special nonpathogenic laboratory strain of *Escherichia coli*. It is created by the reversal of the lysine and proline amino acids at positions 28 and 29 on the B chain. The sterile solution consists of zinc-insulin lispro crystals dissolved in buffered water for injection.

Insulin lispro may also be known as LY-275585, insulin lispro protamine, insulin lispro-aabc, *Admelog®*, *HumaLOG®*, and *Lyumjev®*. See ***Contraindications/Precautions/Warnings*** as these products are not all considered equivalent.

Storage/Stability

Unopened insulin lispro vials and pens/devices should be stored in the refrigerator at 2°C to 8°C (36°F-46°F) and protected from temperature extremes and direct sunlight. Do not freeze. Discard after 28 days if unopened containers are stored at room temperature below 30°C (86°F).

In-use *vials* may be used for 28 days after first use and should be stored at room temperature or in the refrigerator. Store ***in-use*** *pens/devices* at room temperature (do not refrigerate) and discard 28 days after first use.

Freezing (less than 2°C [36°F]) insulin lispro products may alter the protein structure and decrease potency. Particle aggregation and crystal damage may be visible to the naked eye. Higher temperature (greater than 30°C [86°F]) extremes and direct exposure to sunlight (as might occur when insulin is stored in a car or on a windowsill) may produce insulin transformation products and fibril formation.

Although manufacturers recommend discarding opened bottles of insulin after 4 to 6 weeks (or expiration date, whichever comes first), studies support that insulin potency and stability is maintained for longer durations.[19,20] Veterinary internal medicine specialists indicate that the vial may be used for 3 to 6 months after opening and possibly beyond the expiration date as long as it is handled carefully, stored in the refrigerator, and the solution does not develop discoloration, flocculent precipitates, or changes in consistency. If a lack of diabetes regulation is noted when using the product beyond the expiration date (3 to 6 months after starting therapy), it may be prudent to replace it with new insulin prior to adjusting insulin therapy.[13]

Compatibility/Compounding Considerations

Diluting insulin: Other than for immediate use, insulin lispro should only be diluted using a product-specific sterile diluent, which is supplied by the manufacturer upon request. Diluted insulin (10 units/mL) prepared in this manner is stable for 4 weeks and should be stored in the refrigerator, although refrigeration is not required.

Adsorption: The adsorption of insulin lispro to the surfaces of IV syringes and infusion sets has been demonstrated and appears similar to that of regular insulin.[21] Less than 10% adsorption occurs in syringes, and adsorption occurs within 5 to 10 minutes. Up to 50% loss occurred in IV bags. The percent adsorbed is inversely proportional to the concentration of the insulin. To saturate binding sites and deliver a more predictable dose to the patient through an IV infusion, it is recommended that the first 20 mL be run through the IV tubing over 1 minute and discarded, although allowing the solution to sit in the tubing for 15 minutes resulted in reaching steady-state more quickly than the 1-minute flush.[21]

Insulin syringes: Syringes are designed for use with a specific strength of insulin, with the needle covers color-coded according to strength. U100 syringes are available in 0.3 mL, 0.5 mL, and 1 mL size. Measuring U100 insulin to the 1 unit mark in a U100 syringe will contain 1 unit of insulin. Some brands of 0.3 mL syringes include ½ unit markings. Insulin syringes should not be reused.

Dosage Forms/Regulatory Status

VETERINARY-LABELED PRODUCTS: NONE

HUMAN-LABELED PRODUCTS:

Insulin Lispro Injection Human (rDNA): 100 units/mL in 3 mL prefilled pen system and 10 mL vials, and 200 units/mL in 3 mL prefilled pen system. *HumaLOG®*, *Admelog®*, generic; (Rx)

References

For the complete list of references, see **wiley.com/go/budde/plumb**

Insulin, NPH
Insulin, Neutral Protamine Hagedorn
Insulin, Isophane

(***inn***-suh-lin, N-P-H) *Humulin® N, Novolin® N*

Insulin, Intermediate-Acting

NOTE: Insulin preparations available to clinicians are in a constant state of change. To maximize the efficacy of therapy and reduce the chance for errors, it is highly recommended to review current references or sources of information pertaining to insulin therapy for dogs and cats.

For additional information, see ***Insulin, General Information.***

Prescriber Highlights

- ► Modified intermediate-acting insulin used for treatment in patients newly diagnosed with diabetes mellitus and for long-term maintenance therapy
- ► Not recommended for use in cats because of its short duration of action in that species
- ► Animals presented with ketoacidosis, anorexia, lethargy, and/or vomiting should first be stabilized with appropriate therapy, including short-acting insulin.
- ► There are no absolute contraindications except during episodes of hypoglycemia.
- ► Adverse effects include hypoglycemia, hypokalemia, insulin-induced rebound hyperglycemia (ie, Somogyi effect), and local reactions to "foreign" proteins.
- ► Do not confuse insulin types, strengths, and/or syringes: NPH insulin is a U100 human product; use only U100 syringes to measure a dose.
- ► Insulin vials and pens need to be gently rolled prior to administration.
- ► Many potential drug interactions

Uses/Indications

Neutral protamine Hagedorn (NPH) insulin is an intermediate-acting insulin preparation that can be used for initial treatment and long-term management of diabetes mellitus, especially in dogs. In a study comparing lente and NPH insulins, glycemic control in newly diagnosed, uncomplicated diabetic dogs was similar[1]; lente and NPH insulins are the first-choice recommended insulins in dogs with uncomplicated diabetes mellitus.[2] NPH insulin can also be considered for the treatment of diabetes mellitus in horses, camelids, ferrets, and guinea pigs; it is not recommended for use in cats because of its short duration of action.[2]

Pharmacology/Actions

The primary action of insulin is to regulate glucose metabolism. Insulin and its analogues lower blood glucose by increasing glucose uptake in peripheral tissues, especially by skeletal muscle and fat. In the liver, insulin increases glucose storage (ie, glycogen) while also inhibiting gluconeogenesis. Insulin's anabolic actions also enhance fatty acid and protein synthesis while inhibiting lipolysis and proteolysis.

For additional information, see ***Insulin, General Information.***

Pharmacokinetics

Insulin formulations contain insulin polymers (aggregates of multiple insulin molecules). Insulin is absorbed from the administration site only after insulin polymers break down into insulin monomers or dimers.

Neutral protamine Hagedorn (NPH) insulin is only administered by the SC route. Following SC administration of NPH (porcine source) in normal dogs, the onset of hypoglycemic effect is 0.5 hours, peak effect occurs after 1 to 2 hours, and duration is 6 to 10 hours.[3] Following SC administration of NPH to 10 diabetic dogs, the median onset of effect was 1.5 hours, median peak effect was 4 hours, and median duration was 8.5 hours.[4] In normal cats given NPH insulin (bovine/porcine source), peak insulin concentration is reached ≈1.5 hours after SC injection, and insulin concentration returned to baseline ≈6 to 8 hours postinjection.[5]

Contraindications/Precautions/Warnings

Neutral protamine Hagedorn (NPH) should not be used during episodes of hypoglycemia. If animals develop hypersensitivity (local or otherwise) or if insulin resistance develops, a change in type or species source (eg, human, bovine, porcine) of insulin should be considered after other etiologies for poor control (eg, expired insulin, concurrent disease, or medication interference) have been ruled out. See ***Insulin, General Information.***

NPH insulin is not an appropriate insulin choice for patients presenting with severe ketoacidosis, anorexia, lethargy, and/or vomiting or other conditions when treatment with short-acting insulin (eg, regular insulin) is indicated.

For obese patients, dose calculations should be based on the individual patient's ideal body weight to avoid inadvertent insulin overdose.

In humans, long-term repeated SC/IM injections of insulin at the same site may cause lipodystrophic reactions, which could interfere with insulin absorption[6]; however, there have been no specific reports of this reaction occurring in dogs or cats.

NPH insulin is U100 strength. It is crucial for patient safety to only use U100 syringes when measuring and administering U100 insulin. Calculations can be done to convert to U40 syringes or TB syringes, but these conversions are not recommended because of the potential for introducing dosing errors. See ***Insulin, General Information.***

When writing prescriptions, do not abbreviate units as "U," as this has been shown to increase the rate of transcription and dosage errors. In human medicine, insulin is considered a "high alert" medication (ie, medications that require special safeguards to reduce the risk for errors). Consider instituting practices such as redundant drug dosage and volume checking and special alert labels.

Do not confuse trade names that use letters to identify insulin types (eg, do not confuse *Humulin® N* with *Humulin® R*). Anecdotally, loss of glycemic control has been attributed to changing the NPH insulin product used (eg, switching from *Novolin® N* to *Humulin® N*), although published evidence of this is lacking.

Adverse Effects

Adverse effects of insulin therapy may include hypoglycemia (see ***Overdose/Acute Toxicity***), hypokalemia, insulin-induced rebound hyperglycemia (ie, Somogyi effect), weight gain, and local reactions to the "foreign" proteins.

Reproductive/Nursing Safety

A case series reports that neutral protamine Hagedorn (NPH) insulin has been used to manage gestational diabetes in dogs.[7] NPH is considered safe for use during human pregnancy and while nursing[8]; this is also assumed to be true for veterinary patients.

Overdose/Acute Toxicity

Insulin overdose can lead to various degrees of hypoglycemia. Signs may include weakness, shaking, head tilting, lethargy, ataxia, seizures, blindness, bizarre behavior, and coma. Other signs may include restlessness, hunger, and muscle fasciculations. Electrolyte disturbances, including hypokalemia, may occur. Prolonged hypoglycemia can result in permanent brain damage or death.

Mild hypoglycemia can be treated by offering the animal its usual food. More serious signs (eg, seizures) should be treated with oral dextrose solutions (eg, *Karo®* syrup) applied to the buccal mucosa (if the animal is seizing, use caution to avoid being bit or injured) or by IV injections of 50% dextrose solutions (small amounts—usually 2 to 15 mL [0.5 to 1 mL/kg], diluted, and slowly administered[9]; see ***Dextrose 50% injection***). For inhospital management, glucagon may also be considered on an as-needed basis for an insulin overdose. See ***Glucagon.*** Once the animal's hypoglycemia is alleviated (response usually occurs within 1 to 2 minutes), the animal should be closely monitored (both by physical observation and serial blood glucose levels) to prevent a recurrence of hypoglycemia (especially with the slower-absorbed/longer-acting products) and to prevent hyperglycemia from developing. Future insulin dosages or feeding regimens should be evaluated and adjusted based on consultation with the clinician to prevent further occurrences of hypoglycemia.

For patients that have experienced or are suspected of having experienced an overdose, consultation with a 24-hour poison consultation center specializing in providing veterinary-specific information is recommended. For general information related to overdose and toxin exposures, as well as contact information for poison control centers, refer to ***Appendix.***

Drug Interactions

The following drug interactions have either been reported or are theoretical in humans or animals receiving insulin and may be of significance in veterinary patients. Unless otherwise noted, use together is not necessarily contraindicated, but weigh the potential risks and perform additional monitoring when appropriate.

- **Beta-Adrenergic Blockers** (eg, **atenolol, propranolol**): Can have variable effects on glycemic control and can mask the signs associated with hypoglycemia
- **Clonidine**: Can mask the signs associated with hypoglycemia
- **Digoxin**: Because insulin can reduce serum potassium levels, patients receiving concomitant digoxin therapy—especially those receiving concurrent diuretic therapy—should be closely monitored.
- **Diuretics** (eg, **furosemide, hydrochlorothiazide**): Insulin shifts extracellular potassium into the intracellular space; serum potassium concentration should be closely monitored in patients receiving concomitant diuretic therapy. Diuretics may also *decrease* the hypoglycemic activity of insulin (ie, increase insulin requirements).
- **Reserpine**: Can mask the signs associated with hypoglycemia

The following drugs or drug classes may potentiate the hypoglycemic activity of insulin (ie, decrease insulin requirements):

- **Anabolic Steroids** (eg, **boldenone, stanozolol, testosterone**)
- **Angiotensin II Receptor Blockers** (ARBs; eg, **telmisartan**)
- **Angiotensin-Converting Enzyme Inhibitors** (ACEIs; eg, **benazepril, enalapril**)
- **Disopyramide**
- **Ethanol**
- **Fenofibrate**
- **Fluoroquinolones** (eg, **ciprofloxacin, enrofloxacin**)
- **Fluoxetine**
- **Hypoglycemics, Oral** (eg, **acarbose, glipizide, metformin**)
- **Monoamine Oxidase Inhibitors** (MAOIs; eg, **amitraz, linezolid, selegiline**)
- **Pentoxifylline**
- **Salicylates** (eg, **aspirin, bismuth subsalicylate**)
- **Somatostatin Derivatives** (eg, **octreotide**)
- **Sulfonamides** (eg, **sulfadimethoxine, sulfamethoxazole**)

The following drugs or drug classes may decrease the hypoglycemic activity of insulin (ie, increase insulin requirements):

- **Alpha-2-Adrenergic Agonists** (eg, **dexmedetomidine, medetomidine, xylazine**): May cause hyperglycemia and temporarily interfere with glycemic control
- **Beta-Adrenergic Agonists** (eg, **albuterol, terbutaline**)
- **Corticosteroids** (eg, **dexamethasone, prednis(ol)one**)
- **Danazol**
- **Diazoxide**
- **Estrogens** (eg, **diethylstilbestrol [DES], estriol**)
- **Isoniazid**
- **Niacin**
- **Phenothiazines** (eg, **acepromazine, chlorpromazine**)
- **Progestins** (eg, **megestrol**)
- **Thyroid Hormones**: Can elevate glucose levels in diabetic patients when thyroid hormone therapy is first initiated

Laboratory Considerations

- None

Dosages

NOTES:

1. Treatment of diabetes mellitus is complex. Insulin is only one component of therapy; treatment may require fluid electrolyte replacement, management of acid/base disturbances, dietary adjustments, and antimicrobial therapy. Adequate patient monitoring is mandatory. It is strongly encouraged to refer to more thorough discussions of treatment in veterinary endocrinology or internal medicine references for additional information.
2. For obese patients, dose calculations should be based on the individual patient's estimated ideal body weight to avoid inadvertent insulin overdose.
3. Key goals of therapy are control of clinical signs associated with diabetes mellitus and avoidance of hypoglycemia.[2,10]
4. All dosages are extra-label.

DOGS:

Initial insulin treatment of uncomplicated diabetes mellitus (extra-label): 0.25 – 0.5 units/kg SC every 12 hours.[2] Consider starting with the lower end of the dosing range for larger dogs and the higher end for smaller dogs.

Combination with insulin lispro for patients experiencing significant postprandial hyperglycemia on standard insulin protocols: Lispro 0.1 units/kg SC every 12 hours was administered to patients ($n = 6$) already receiving neutral protamine Hagedorn (NPH) treatment (median dosage, 0.5 – ≈1 unit/kg SC every 12 hours) but experiencing postprandial hyperglycemia.[11] Fructosamine and the median glucose concentrations at 1 hour and 1.5 hours postprandial were significantly lower with this combination therapy.[11]

HORSES:

Diabetes mellitus: 0.2 – 0.4 units/kg SC every 24 hours[12]

NEW WORLD CAMELIDS:

Severe hyperlipemia: Based on a single-dose study, 0.4 units/kg SC produced a peak effect 4.7 hours after administration; the mean duration of effect was 15.4 hours.[13]

BIRDS:

Diabetes mellitus: 0.067 – 3.3 units/kg IM every 12 to 24 hours. In most cases, twice-daily injections are necessary.[14]

FERRETS:

Diabetes mellitus:

a) 0.5 – 1 units/ferret (NOT unit/kg) SC twice daily[15]

b) 0.1 – 0.5 units/kg IM or SC twice daily to start; adjust to optimal dose. May require insulin to be diluted[16]

SMALL MAMMALS:

Diabetes mellitus in Guinea pigs: 1 unit/Guinea pig (NOT unit/kg) SC every 12 hours. Monitor urine for glucose and ketones, and adjust the dose if needed.[17]

Monitoring

Each patient requires an individualized treatment plan, frequent reassessment, and adjustments to the plan based on the response of the patient. It is encouraged to consult a veterinary endocrinology reference text or with a veterinary emergency and critical care and/or endocrinology specialist for further information related to regulating diabetic patients and insulin adjustments. The overarching goal when monitoring diabetic patients is the control of clinical signs related to hyperglycemia (eg, polyuria, polydipsia) while avoiding hypoglycemia.[2] Interpret all monitoring strategies based on clinical signs. Results from the monitoring options below may conflict in regards to achieving good glycemic and clinical control.

- Patient status and control of clinical signs: body weight, appetite, fluid intake, urine output
- Glucose (blood or interstitial) curve. Experience with continuous interstitial glucose monitoring in dogs and cats is that these devices are easy to apply, user friendly, and provide useful information surrounding glycemic control while the patient is in the clinic or home environment.[18–21] A glucose curve can be considered at the following times[2]:
  - After the first dose of a new insulin type, glucose can be checked every 2 hours after administration. The goal for monitoring following the first dose of insulin would be solely to identify hypoglycemia. The insulin dose should NOT be increased from the first-day glucose evaluation. If glucose falls below 150 mg/dL during the glucose curve, the frequency of monitoring should increase to hourly until glucose is greater than 150 mg/dL. Although the neutral protamine Hagedorn (NPH) insulin dose should never be increased on the first day of therapy, the dose should be decreased by 10% to 50% in dogs if the glucose is less than 150 mg/dL at any time during the day. Repeat glucose curves on subsequent days (and decrease insulin dose if necessary) until nadir is greater than 150 mg/dL.
  - 7 to 14 days after starting insulin or an insulin dose change
  - At least every 3 months, even in animals with well-controlled diabetes
  - Any time clinical signs recur in an animal with previously well-controlled diabetes
  - When hypoglycemia is suspected. For patients that have ex-

periencedorare suspected of having experienced repeated or unexplained hypoglycemia, it is strongly encouraged that pet owners consult with a veterinary emergency and critical care and/or endocrinology specialist or reference text that specializes in providing information specific for the treatment of hypoglycemia.

- Urine glucose monitoring is typically only helpful for documenting prolonged hypoglycemia (eg, persistently negative urine glucose testing when monitoring for diabetic remission in cats). As most diabetic patients spend time above the renal threshold for urinary glucose spillage, even patients with well-controlled diabetes may be intermittently glucosuric throughout the day.
- Fructosamine or glycosylated hemoglobin can be monitored if available and warranted.

Client Information

NOTES for veterinarian:

1. Correct injection techniques should be taught and practiced with the client before the animal's discharge.
2. Emphasis should be placed on matching the appropriate syringe and insulin concentration (eg, do not interchange U40 insulin and syringes with U100 insulin and syringes) and correct needles with pens/devices.
3. Both veterinary-approved insulins have owner information sheets, client-friendly handouts, and websites to provide client support on administration and use of insulin.

- For this medication to work safely, give the insulin *exactly* as your veterinarian has prescribed. Do not give this medicine and contact your veterinarian for guidance if your animal is not eating.
- Your veterinarian will teach you proper injection technique. ***Only*** use U100 syringes with neutral protamine Hagedorn (NPH) insulin.
- Always double-check the dose in the syringe before you inject your animal. Overdoses may be fatal.
- To avoid bubbles and the potential for inaccurate dosing, NPH suspensions should be rolled gently until thoroughly mixed, not shaken. Prior to using, visually inspect the insulin bottle prior to use. NPH solutions should appear as uniform milky suspensions. Do not use insulin suspensions if clumps or white particles persist after mixing.
- After measuring the dose into a syringe, allow the contents to come to room temperature (if the vial is stored in the refrigerator) before giving the injection.
- The injection site should be frequently changed, with the main sites being the back of the neck, side of the animal, or shoulder area.
- Place the used needles and syringes in a sharps disposal container immediately after use, making sure you do not attempt to disconnect the needle from the syringe or recap the needle. Your veterinarian or pharmacist will help you obtain these containers.
- Do not reuse needles or syringes.
- Keep insulin products out of temperature extremes. Follow the label instructions for storage of the insulin vial and pens/devices.
- Signs of low blood sugar include weakness, depression, lack of energy, sluggishness, staggering gait (ie, stumbling) when walking, behavior changes, muscle twitching, seizures (convulsions), or coma. **If your animal is unconscious or having a seizure, this is a medical emergency.** Take your animal to your veterinarian immediately. **If your animal is conscious and able to swallow**, rub ≈1 tablespoon of corn syrup (*Karo®*) or honey on your animal's gums until it is alert enough to eat. Feed the usual meal and contact your veterinarian for recommendations. Some animals may not show any obvious physical signs of low blood sugar. If your animal is not acting normally, contact your veterinarian to make sure your animal's blood sugar level is in a safe range.
- Contact your veterinarian at your earliest convenience if you notice excessive thirst, increased frequency of urination, or increased appetite in your animal, as these signs may indicate the insulin dose needs to be adjusted.
- When traveling, do not leave insulin in carry-on luggage that will pass through airport surveillance equipment. Generally, insulin stability is not affected by a single pass through surveillance equipment; however, longer than normal exposure or repeated passes through surveillance equipment may alter insulin potency.
- Do not stop giving insulin to your animal unless instructed to do so by your veterinarian.
- Your veterinarian will need to closely monitor your animal during treatment. Do not miss these important follow-up visits.

Chemistry/Synonyms

Neutral protamine Hagedorn (NPH) insulin is an intermediate-acting, sterile suspension of human insulin, zinc, and protamine sulfate in buffered water for injection. NPH insulin is produced using recombinant DNA technology via a nonpathogenic *Escherichia coli* strain (*Humulin® N*) or using *Saccharomyces cerevisiae* (*Novolin® N*) and is available only as a U100 insulin concentration containing ≈3.6 mg of insulin/mL.

NPH insulin may also be known as isophane, neutral protamine Hagedorn, *Humulin® N*, or *Novolin® N*.

Storage/Stability

Store ***unopened*** neutral protamine Hagedorn (NPH) *vials* and *pens/devices* in the manufacturer's carton in the refrigerator at 2°C to 8°C (36°F-46°F). Do not freeze; discard if product has been frozen.[6] Freezing (less than 2°C [36°F]) may alter the protein structure and decrease potency. Particle aggregation and crystal damage may be visible to the naked eye or may require microscopic examination.

Unopened NPH *vials* may be stored unrefrigerated if kept below 25°C to 30°C (77°F-86°F) and out of direct heat and sunlight but must be discarded after 31 days (*Humulin® N*) or 42 days (*Novolin® N*). Higher temperature extremes (more than 30°C [86°F]) and direct exposure to sunlight (eg, stored in a car or on a windowsill) may produce insulin transformation products and fibril formation, thereby further shortening the insulin shelf-life.

Unopened NPH *pens/devices* may be stored unrefrigerated if kept below 25°C to 30°C (77°F-86°F) and out of direct heat and sunlight but must be discarded after 14 days (*Humulin® N*) or 28 days (*Novolin® N*).

In-use storage requirements vary by manufacturer:

- *Humulin® N vials* can be kept for 31 days refrigerated (2°C to 8°C [36°F-46°F]) or at room temperature (below 30°C [86°F]); *pens/devices* can be kept 14 days at room temperature (below 30°C [86°F]).
- *Novolin® N vials* can be kept 42 days at room temperature (below 25°C [77°F]); *pens/devices* can be kept 28 days at room temperature (below 30°C [86°F]). Do not refrigerate in-use *Novolin® N* products.

Although manufacturers recommend discarding opened bottles of insulin after 4 to 6 weeks (or expiration date, whichever comes first), studies support that insulin potency and stability is maintained for longer durations.[22,23] Veterinary internal medicine specialists indicate that the vial may be used for 3 to 6 months after opening and possibly beyond the listed expiration date as long as it is handled carefully, stored in the refrigerator, and the solution does not develop discoloration, flocculent precipitates, or changes in consistency. If a lack of diabetes regulation is noted when using the product beyond the expiration date (3 to 6 months after starting therapy), it may be prudent to replace it with new insulin prior to adjusting insulin therapy.[2]

Compatibility/Compounding Considerations

Insulin syringes: Syringes are designed for use with a specific strength of insulin, with the needle covers color-coded according to strength. U100 syringes are available in 0.3 mL, 0.5 mL, and 1 mL size. Measuring U100 insulin to the 1 unit mark in a U100 syringe will contain 1 unit of insulin. Some brands of 0.3 mL syringes include ½ unit markings. Insulin syringes should not be reused.

Dosage Forms/Regulatory Status

VETERINARY-LABELED PRODUCTS: NONE

HUMAN-LABELED PRODUCTS:

NPH Insulin (Isophane or Neutral Protamine Hagedorn) Human (rDNA): 100 units/mL in 3 mL vials and prefilled pen system and in 10 mL vials; *Humulin® N, Novolin® N* (OTC in humans; requires prescription under extra-label provisions of AMDUCA when used in animals). *Humulin®*- or *Novolin®*-brand insulins may be rebranded and sold by large retailers under different trade names.

Mixtures of short-acting insulins combined with intermediate-acting insulins are available.

References

For the complete list of references, see **wiley.com/go/budde/plumb**

Insulin, Protamine Zinc

Protamine Zinc Recombinant Human Insulin (rPZI)

(***inn***-suh-lin, ***pro***-ta-meen zeenk) *ProZinc®*

Insulin, Long-Acting

NOTE: Insulin preparations available to clinicians are in a constant state of change. To maximize the efficacy of therapy and reduce the chance for errors, it is highly recommended to review current references or sources of information pertaining to insulin therapy for dogs and cats.

For additional information, see ***Insulin, General Information.***

Prescriber Highlights

- Long-acting insulin for treatment in dogs and cats newly diagnosed with diabetes mellitus and for long-term maintenance therapy
- Animals that are presented with ketoacidosis, anorexia, lethargy, and/or vomiting should first be stabilized with appropriate therapy, including short-acting insulin.
- There are no absolute contraindications, except during episodes of hypoglycemia.
- Adverse effects include hypoglycemia, hypokalemia, insulin-induced rebound hyperglycemia (ie, Somogyi effect), and local reactions to the "foreign" proteins.
- Do not confuse insulin types, strengths, and syringes: protamine zinc insulin is a U40 approved veterinary product; only use U40 insulin syringes to measure dose.
- Many potential drug interactions

Uses/Indications

Protamine zinc recombinant human insulin (rPZI) is a long-acting insulin preparation FDA-approved for use in dogs and cats for initial treatment and long-term management of diabetes mellitus. rPZI is a first-choice recommended insulin in newly diagnosed diabetic cats.[1] rPZI and intermediate-acting insulins (eg, porcine insulin zinc [ie, lente]) are considered first-choice insulin therapies in newly diagnosed diabetic dogs.[1,2]

rPZI can also be considered for treatment of hyperlipemia in camelids and ponies, as well as for treatment of ketosis in cattle.[3]

Pharmacology/Actions

The primary action of insulin is to regulate glucose metabolism. Insulin and its analogues lower blood glucose by increasing glucose uptake in peripheral tissues, especially skeletal muscle and fat. In the liver, insulin increases glucose storage (ie, glycogen) while also inhibiting gluconeogenesis. Insulin's anabolic actions also enhance fatty acid and protein synthesis while inhibiting lipolysis and proteolysis.

For additional information, see ***Insulin, General Information.***

Pharmacokinetics

Insulin formulations contain insulin polymers (aggregates of multiple insulin molecules); protamine zinc recombinant human insulin (rPZI) is composed of hexamers. Insulin is absorbed from the administration site only after insulin polymers break down into insulin monomers or dimers.

After SC administration of rPZI 0.8 units/kg to healthy (ie, nondiabetic) dogs, median onset of action was 3.5 hours (0.5 to 10 hours), time to glucose nadir was 14 hours (5 to 24 hours), and duration was less than 24 hours (16 to 24 hours).[4] After SC administration to cats (nondiabetic and diabetic), onset of activity was 0.5 to 1.5 hours; peak effect was 4 to 9 hours, and duration of effect was 7 to 18 hours.[5,6]

Contraindications/Precautions/Warnings

Protamine zinc recombinant human insulin (rPZI) is contraindicated in animals that are hypersensitive to human insulin and during episodes of hypoglycemia. If animals develop hypersensitivity (local or otherwise) or if insulin resistance develops, a change in type or species source (eg, human, bovine, porcine) of insulin should be considered after other etiologies for poor control have been ruled out (eg, expired insulin, concurrent disease, or medication interference). See ***Insulin, General Information***.

PZI insulin is not an appropriate insulin choice for patients presenting with severe ketoacidosis, anorexia, lethargy, and/or vomiting or other conditions when treatment with short-acting insulin (eg, regular insulin) is indicated.

For obese patients, dose calculations should be based on the patient's ideal body weight to avoid inadvertent insulin overdose.

In humans, long-term repeated SC/IM injections of insulin at the same site may cause lipodystrophic reactions, which could interfere with insulin absorption[7,8]; however, there have been no specific reports of this reaction occurring in dogs or cats.

rPZI is a U40-strength insulin. It is crucial for patient safety to only use U40 syringes when measuring and administering U40 insulin. Calculations can be done to convert to U100 syringes or TB syringes, but these conversions are not recommended due to the potential for introducing dosing errors. See ***Insulin, General Information***.

When writing prescriptions, do not abbreviate units as "U," as this has been shown to increase the rate of transcription and dosage errors. In human medicine, insulin is considered a "high alert" medication (ie, medications that require special safeguards to reduce the risk for errors). Consider instituting practices such as redundant drug dosage, volume checking, and special alert labels.

Do not confuse PROTAMINE zinc insulin (PZI) with PORCINE zinc insulin (ie, lente insulin).

Adverse Effects

Adverse effects of insulin therapy may include hypoglycemia (see ***Overdose/Acute Toxicity***), hypokalemia, insulin-induced rebound hyperglycemia (ie, Somogyi effect), insulin antagonism and resistance, rapid insulin metabolism, and local or allergic reactions to the "foreign" proteins.

Lethargy, anorexia, hypoglycemia, vomiting, seizures, shaking, diarrhea, and ataxia were reported in an FDA field study in dogs treated with PZI.[9] Half of the hypoglycemic episodes did not have clinical signs. Injection site reactions occurred in 2.5% of dogs and 1.7% of cats.[10]

Reproductive/Nursing Safety

The safe use of PZI in breeding, pregnant, or lactating animals has not been studied[10]; however, in humans, insulin is considered a treatment of choice for gestational diabetes,[11] and insulin is known to be compatible with nursing.[12]

Overdose/Acute Toxicity

Insulin overdose can lead to various degrees of hypoglycemia. Signs may include weakness, shaking, head tilt, lethargy, ataxia, seizures, blindness, bizarre behavior, and coma. Other signs may include restlessness, hunger, and muscle fasciculations. Electrolyte disturbances, including hypokalemia, may occur. Prolonged hypoglycemia can result in permanent brain damage or death.

Mild hypoglycemia can be treated by offering the animal its usual food. More serious signs (eg, seizures) should be treated with oral dextrose solutions (eg, *Karo*® syrup) applied to the buccal mucosa (if the animal is seizing, use caution to avoid being bit or injured) or by IV injections of 50% dextrose solutions (small amounts—usually 2 - 15 mL [0.5 - 1 mL/kg], diluted, and slowly administered)[13]; see ***Dextrose 50% injection***. For inhospital management, glucagon may also be considered on an as-needed basis for an insulin overdose. See ***Glucagon.*** Once the animal's hypoglycemia is alleviated (response usually occurs within 1 to 2 minutes), the animal should be closely monitored (both by physical observation and serial blood glucose concentrations) to prevent a recurrence of hypoglycemia (especially with the slower-absorbed/longer-acting insulin products) and to prevent hyperglycemia from developing. Future insulin dosages or feeding regimens should be evaluated or adjusted based on consultation with the clinician to prevent further occurrences of hypoglycemia.

For patients that have experienced or are suspected to have experienced an overdose, consultation with a 24-hour poison consultation center specializing in providing veterinary-specific information is recommended. For general information related to overdose and toxin exposures, as well as contact information for poison control centers, refer to ***Appendix.***

Drug Interactions

The following drug interactions have either been reported or are theoretical in humans or animals receiving insulin and may be of significance in veterinary patients. Unless otherwise noted, use together is not necessarily contraindicated, but weigh the potential risks and perform additional monitoring when appropriate.

- **Beta-Adrenergic Antagonists** (eg, **atenolol, propranolol**): Can have variable effects on glycemic control and can mask the signs associated with hypoglycemia
- **Clonidine**: Can mask the signs associated with hypoglycemia
- **Digoxin**: Because insulin can reduce serum potassium concentrations, patients receiving concomitant digoxin therapy—especially those receiving concurrent diuretic therapy—should be closely monitored.
- **Diuretics** (eg, **furosemide, hydrochlorothiazide**): Insulin shifts extracellular potassium into the intracellular space; serum potassium concentration should be closely monitored in patients receiving concomitant diuretic therapy. Diuretics may also *decrease* the hypoglycemic activity of insulin (ie, increase insulin requirements).
- **Reserpine**: Can mask the signs associated with hypoglycemia

The following drugs or drug classes may potentiate the hypoglycemic activity of insulin (ie, decrease insulin requirements):

- **Anabolic Steroids** (eg, **boldenone, stanozolol, testosterone**)
- **Angiotensin II Receptor Blockers** (ARBs; eg, **telmisartan**)
- **Angiotensin Converting Enzyme Inhibitors** (ACEIs; eg, **benazepril, enalapril**)
- **Disopyramide**
- **Ethanol**
- **Fenofibrate**
- **Fluoroquinolones** (eg, **ciprofloxacin, enrofloxacin**)
- **Fluoxetine**
- **Hypoglycemics, Oral** (eg, **acarbose, glipizide, metformin**)
- **Monoamine Oxidase Inhibitors** (MAOIs; eg, **amitraz, linezolid, selegiline**)
- **Pentoxifylline**
- **Salicylates** (eg, **aspirin, bismuth subsalicylate**)
- **Somatostatin Derivatives** (eg, **octreotide**)
- **Sulfonamides** (eg, **sulfadimethoxine, sulfamethoxazole**)

The following drugs or drug classes may decrease the hypoglycemic activity of insulin (ie, increase insulin requirements):

- **Alpha-2-Adrenergic Agonists** (eg, **dexmedetomidine, medetomidine, xylazine**): May cause hyperglycemia and temporarily interfere with glycemic control
- **Beta-Adrenergic Agonists** (eg, **albuterol, terbutaline**)
- **Corticosteroids** (eg, **dexamethasone, prednis(ol)one**)
- **Danazol**
- **Diazoxide**
- **Diuretics** (eg, **furosemide, hydrochlorothiazide**)
- **Estrogens** (eg, **diethylstilbestrol [DES], estriol**)
- **Isoniazid**
- **Niacin**
- **Phenothiazines** (eg, **acepromazine, chlorpromazine**)
- **Progestins** (eg, **megestrol**)
- **Thyroid Hormones**: Can elevate glucose concentrations in diabetic patients when thyroid hormone therapy is first initiated

Laboratory Considerations

- None

Dosages

NOTES:

1. Treatment of diabetes mellitus is complex; treatment may require fluid electrolyte replacement, management of acid/base disturbances, dietary adjustments, and antimicrobial therapy. Adequate patient monitoring is mandatory. It is strongly encouraged to refer to more thorough discussions of treatment in veterinary endocrinology or internal medicine references for additional information.
2. For obese patients, dose calculations should be based on the individual's estimated ideal body weight to avoid inadvertent insulin overdose.
3. Key goals of therapy are control of clinical signs associated with diabetes mellitus and avoidance of hypoglycemia or other complications (diabetic ketoacidosis).[1,14]

DOGS:

Reduction of hyperglycemia and hyperglycemia-associated clinical signs (label dosage; FDA-approved): 0.5 - 1 unit/kg SC once daily, concurrent with or right after a meal.[10] The recommended starting dose for insulin-naive dogs is at the lower end of the dosage range, but poorly controlled diabetic dogs or those transitioning from another insulin product could begin at the mid to higher end of the range. When transitioning from another insulin, protamine zinc recombinant human insulin (rPZI) should be started once daily regardless of the frequency of the previous insulin. Twice-daily administration should be considered if the duration of insulin action is determined to be inadequate with once-daily administration. If twice-daily administration is initiated, the 2 doses should each be ≈25% less than the once-daily dose required to attain an acceptable glucose nadir (eg, 10 units SC once daily becomes 7 units SC twice daily). In field efficacy studies, the mean successful insulin dose was 1.4 units/kg/day.[2]

Initial insulin treatment of uncomplicated diabetes mellitus (extra-label): 0.25 – 0.5 units/kg SC every 12 hours.[1] A starting dose of 0.25 units/kg SC every 12 hours is often used; more potentially challenging cases may require the higher starting dose. Some clinicians have found 0.5 units/kg to be a more effective starting dose. Once-daily administration may be possible in some dogs.[1,15]

CATS:

Reduction of hyperglycemia and hyperglycemia-associated clinical signs (label dosage; FDA-approved): 0.2 – 0.7 units/kg SC every 12 hours, given concurrently with or right after a meal

Initial insulin treatment of uncomplicated diabetes mellitus (extra-label): 1 – 2 units/cat (NOT units/kg) SC every 12 hours.[1] The initial starting dose in cats should not exceed 2 units/cat (NOT units/kg) SC every 12 hours regardless of the size of the cat.

HORSES:

Hyperlipemia in ponies (extra-label):

a) 200 kg (440 lb) pony: 30 units/animal (NOT units/kg) IM every 12 hours on odd days (given with 100 g glucose PO once daily); 15 units/animal (NOT units/kg) IM every 12 hours on even days (given with 100 g glucose PO once daily) until hyperlipemia resolves[16]
b) 0.4 units/kg SC or IM every 24 hours[17]
c) 0.1 – 0.3 units/kg SC or IM every 12 to 24 hours[3,18]

CATTLE:

Adjunctive treatment of ketosis (extra-label): 200 – 300 units per animal (NOT units/kg) SC every 24 to 48 hours[3]

NEW WORLD CAMELIDS:

Severe hyperlipemia (extra-label): 0.2 – 0.4 units/kg SC with glucose every 12 to 24 hours. Duration of effect is generally 8 to 16 hours.[19]

Monitoring

Each patient requires an individualized treatment plan, frequent reassessment, and adjustments of the plan based on the response of the patient. It is encouraged to consult a veterinary endocrinology reference text or with a veterinary emergency and critical care and/or endocrinology specialist for further information related to regulating diabetic patients and insulin adjustments. The overarching goal when monitoring diabetic patients is control of clinical signs related to hyperglycemia (eg, polyuria, polydipsia) while avoiding hypoglycemia. A so-called "loose-control" (ie, managing clinical signs while avoiding hypoglycemia and reducing frequency of hospitalizations for glucose curves) approach to diabetes management in cats using PZI has also been described.[20] Interpret all monitoring strategies based on clinical signs. Results from the monitoring options below may conflict in regard to achieving good glycemic control and good clinical control.

- Patient status and control of clinical signs: body weight, appetite, fluid intake, and urine output
- Glucose (blood or interstitial) curve. Experience with continuous interstitial glucose monitoring in dogs and cats is that these devices are easy to apply, user friendly, and provide useful information surrounding glycemic control while the patient is in the clinic or home environment.[21-24] A glucose curve can be considered at the following times[1]:
  - After the first dose of a new insulin type. If performing a glucose curve, glucose can be checked every 2 to 4 hours for 10 to 12 hours after administration. The goal for monitoring following the first dose of insulin would be solely to identify hypoglycemia. The insulin dose should NOT be increased based on first-day glucose evaluation. If glucose falls below 150 mg/dL during the glucose curve, frequency of monitoring should increase to hourly until glucose is greater than 150 mg/dL.[1] Although the PZI dose should never be increased on the first day of therapy, the dose should be decreased by 10% to 50% in dogs and 0.5 units (total) in cats if glucose is less than 150 mg/dL at any time during the day.[1] Repeat glucose curves on subsequent days (and decrease insulin dose if necessary) until nadir is greater than 150 mg/dL.
  - 7 to 14 days after starting insulin or after an insulin dose change
  - At least every 3 months, even in well-controlled diabetics. In well-controlled patients, it may be possible to use clinical signs, body weight, +/- serum fructosamine measurements to determine frequency of glucose curve evaluations.[20]
  - Any time clinical signs recur in an animal with previously well-controlled diabetes
  - When hypoglycemia is suspected. For patients that have experienced or are suspected to have experienced repeated or unexplained hypoglycemia, it is strongly encouraged to consult with a veterinary emergency and critical care and/or endocrinology specialist or reference text that specializes in providing information specific for treatment of hypoglycemia.
- Urine glucose monitoring is typically only helpful for documenting prolonged hypoglycemia (eg, persistently negative urine glucose testing when monitoring for diabetic remission in cats). As most diabetic patients spend time above the renal threshold for urinary glucose spillage, even patients with well-controlled diabetes may be intermittently glucosuric throughout the day.
- Fructosamine or glycosylated hemoglobin if available and warranted

Client Information

NOTES for veterinarian:

1. Correct injection techniques should be taught and practiced with the client before the animal's discharge.
2. Emphasis should be placed on matching the appropriate syringe and insulin concentration (eg, do not interchange U40 insulin and syringes with U100 insulin and syringes) and correct needles with pens/devices.
3. Both veterinary-approved insulins have owner information sheets, client-friendly handouts, and websites to provide client support on administration and use of insulin.

- For this medication to work safely, give the insulin ***exactly*** as your veterinarian has prescribed. Do not give this medicine and contact your veterinarian for guidance if your animal is not eating.
- Your veterinarian will teach you the correct injection technique. ***Only*** use U40 insulin syringes with PZI insulin.
- Always double-check the dose in the syringe before you inject your animal. Overdoses may be fatal.
- Gently roll the vial to mix the contents; do not shake. Once mixed, the suspension has a white, cloudy appearance. Do not use this product if clumps or visible white particles persist after gently rolling the vial.
- After measuring the dose into a syringe, allow the contents to

come to room temperature before giving the injection.

- The injection site should be frequently changed, with the main sites being the back of the neck, side of the animal, or shoulder area.
- Place the used needles and syringes in a sharps disposal container immediately after use, making sure you do not attempt to disconnect the needle from the syringe or recap the needle. Your veterinarian or pharmacist will help you obtain these containers.
- Do not reuse needles or syringes.
- Keep insulin products out of temperature extremes. Unused and opened vials of PZI insulin should be stored in the refrigerator.
- Signs of low blood sugar include weakness, depression, lack of energy, sluggishness, staggering gait (ie, stumbling) when walking, behavior changes, muscle twitching, seizures (convulsions), or coma. **If your animal is unconscious or having a seizure, this is a medical emergency.** Take your animal to the veterinarian immediately. **If your animal is conscious and able to swallow**, rub ≈1 tablespoon of corn syrup (*Karo*®) or honey on your animal's gums until it is alert enough to eat. Feed the usual meal and contact your veterinarian for recommendations. Some animals may not show any obvious physical signs of low blood sugar. If your animal is not acting normally, contact your veterinarian to make sure your animal's blood sugar concentrations are in a safe range.
- Contact your veterinarian at your earliest convenience if you notice excessive thirst, increased frequency of urination, or increased appetite in your animal, as these signs may indicate the insulin dose needs to be adjusted.
- When traveling, do not leave insulin in carry-on luggage that will pass through airport surveillance equipment. Generally, insulin stability is not affected by a single pass through surveillance equipment; however, longer than normal exposure or repeated passes through surveillance equipment may alter insulin potency.
- Do not stop giving insulin to your animal unless instructed to do so by your veterinarian.
- Your veterinarian will need to closely monitor your animal during treatment. Do not miss these important follow-up visits.

Chemistry/Synonyms

Protamine zinc recombinant human insulin (rPZI) is a sterile aqueous protamine zinc suspension of recombinant human insulin produced with recombinant DNA technology in the yeast *Pichia pastoris.* PZI is available only as a U40 insulin concentration and is a cloudy or milky suspension.

Protamine zinc insulin may also be known as PZI, rhPZI, protamine zinc recombinant human insulin, PZIR, or *ProZinc*®.

Storage/Stability

Unopened and ***in-use*** protamine zinc recombinant human insulin (rPZI) vials should be refrigerated at 2°C to 8°C (36°F-46°F). Do not freeze; discard if product has been frozen. Vials should be stored upright and protected from light. Discard within 60 days (10 mL vial) or 80 days (20 mL vial) of first use.

Although the manufacturer recommends discarding opened bottles of rPZI after 60 days (10 mL vial) or 80 days (20 mL vial), studies support that insulin potency and stability are maintained for longer durations.[25,26] Veterinary internal medicine specialists indicate that the vial may be used for 3 to 6 months after opening and possibly beyond the listed expiration date as long as it is handled carefully, stored in the refrigerator, and the solution does not develop discoloration, flocculent precipitates, or changes in consistency. If a lack of diabetes regulation is noted when using the product beyond the expiration date (3 to 6 months after starting therapy), it may be prudent to replace with new insulin prior to adjusting insulin therapy.[1]

Compatibility/Compounding Considerations

Insulin syringes: Syringes are designed for use with a specific strength of insulin, and needle covers are color-coded for each insulin strength. Use only U40 syringes with protamine zinc recombinant human insulin (rPZI). U40 syringes are available in 0.3 mL, 0.5 mL, 1 mL, and 2 mL sizes. Drawing U40 insulin to the 1 unit mark in a U40 syringe will result in 1 unit of insulin. Insulin syringes should not be reused.

Dosage Forms/Regulatory Status

VETERINARY-LABELED PRODUCTS:

Protamine Zinc (rDNA) Insulin (PZI) Aqueous Suspension 40 units/mL in 10 mL and 20 mL vials; *ProZinc*®; (Rx). FDA-approved for use in dogs and cats. NADA# 141-297

HUMAN-LABELED PRODUCTS: NONE

References

For the complete list of references, see **wiley.com/go/budde/plumb**

Insulin, Regular (Crystalline Zinc)

(***inn***-suh-lin, ***reh***-gyoo-ler) *Humulin® R, Novolin® R*

Insulin, Rapid/Short-Acting

NOTE: Insulin preparations available to clinicians are in a constant state of change. To maximize the efficacy of therapy and reduce the chance for errors, it is highly recommended to review current references or sources of information pertaining to insulin therapy for dogs and cats.

For additional information, see ***Insulin, General Information.***

Prescriber Highlights

- Rapid/short-acting insulin used to treat diabetic ketoacidosis (DKA) and as adjunctive therapy to treat hyperkalemia
- There are no absolute contraindications, except during episodes of hypoglycemia.
- Adverse effects include hypoglycemia, hypokalemia, hypophosphatemia (DKA only), insulin-induced rebound hyperglycemia (ie, Somogyi effect), and local reactions to the "foreign" proteins.
- Do not confuse insulin types, strengths, and syringes. Regular insulin is a U100 human product; use only U100 insulin syringes to measure a dose.
- Many potential drug interactions

Uses/Indications

Regular insulin is a rapid, or short-acting, insulin that is commonly used for diabetic emergencies (eg, diabetic ketoacidosis [DKA]). It is administered by IM or SC injection or IV infusion. IV insulin administration is recommended in patients with poor tissue perfusion, with shock, with cardiovascular collapse, or in those that require adjunct therapy for hyperkalemia.

Regular insulin is the rapid/short-acting insulin most often used in diabetic emergencies (ie, DKA). When regular insulin is not an option, safe and effective alternatives for cats include insulin glargine (SC or IM),[1-3] and for dogs include insulin lispro[4,5] or insulin aspart[6] administered as an IV CRI. Once the patient is stabilized, longer-acting insulin products can be given SC for maintenance insulin therapy.

In patients with DKA, initial aggressive fluid replacement therapy is of paramount importance to restore tissue perfusion and begin correcting electrolyte or acid-base derangements. In one study, early administration (ie, within 6 hours of presentation) of insulin to patients with DKA leads to earlier resolution of hyperglycemia, acidemia, and ketonemia while being safe and well tolerated.[7] It is strongly encouraged to consult a veterinary emergency and critical care and/or endocrinology specialist or reference when treating this condition.

Regular insulin may also be given IV concomitantly with dextrose IV to treat hyperkalemia.[8] In dogs and cats, ECG changes seen in critical patients with hyperkalemia may be affected by concurrent metabolic derangements (eg, metabolic acidosis, hypermagnesemia, hypocalcemia) and thus may not typify the expected ECG changes (eg, bradyarrhythmias, loss of P wave, wide QRS complexes, peaked T waves) previously described for hyperkalemia.[9] In humans, treatment for hyperkalemia is recommended when serum potassium is greater than 5.5 mEq/L if there are ECG changes or when serum potassium is greater than 6 mEq/L, regardless of ECG findings.[10]

Pharmacology/Actions

The primary action of insulin is to regulate glucose metabolism. Insulin and its analogues lower blood glucose by increasing glucose uptake in peripheral tissues, especially by skeletal muscle and fat. In the liver, insulin increases glucose storage (ie, glycogen) while also inhibiting gluconeogenesis. Insulin's anabolic actions also enhance fatty acid and protein synthesis while inhibiting lipolysis and proteolysis.

For additional information, see ***Insulin, General Information***.

Pharmacokinetics

Insulin formulations contain insulin hexamers (aggregates of 6 insulin molecules). Insulin is absorbed from the administration site only after insulin hexamers break down into insulin monomers or dimers. The rate of hexamer breakdown is largely responsible for differences of time to peak effect and duration of activity of the various insulin types.

When the recombinant human insulin product is given IV to dogs and cats, it has an immediate onset of action, with maximum effects occurring at 15 minutes; duration of action is 1 to 4 hours. After SC administration, onset is generally 10 to 30 minutes, peak is 1 to 2 hours, and duration is 5 to 6 hours. Half-life is 16 to 18 minutes.[11,12] Following IM administration, onset is 10 to 30 minutes, peak is 1 to 4 hours, and duration is 3 to 8 hours.

In alpacas, regular insulin has an immediate onset of action, but the duration of action is less than 1 hour.[13]

Although the kinetics of each insulin product vary markedly among species, regular insulin appears to have the most consistent pharmacokinetics.

Contraindications/Precautions/Warnings

Because there are no alternatives for insulin when it is used for diabetic indications, there are no absolute contraindications to its use except during episodes of hypoglycemia. If animals develop hypersensitivity (local or otherwise) or if insulin resistance develops, a change in type or species source (eg, human, bovine, porcine) of insulin should be considered after other etiologies for poor control (eg, expired insulin, concurrent disease, or medication interference) have been ruled out. See ***Insulin, General Information***.

For obese patients, dose calculations should be based on the patient's ideal body weight to avoid inadvertent insulin overdosing.

In humans, long-term repeated SC/IM injections of insulin at the same site may cause lipodystrophic reactions, which could interfere with insulin absorption[14]; however, there have been no specific reports of this reaction occurring in dogs or cats.

In patients with moderate to severe dehydration, poor tissue perfusion necessitates regular insulin be given IM or IV as absorption of SC injections is likely to be impaired or delayed.

Regular insulin is U100 strength. It is crucial for patient safety to only use U100 syringes when measuring and administering U100 insulin. Calculations can be done to convert to U40 syringes or TB syringes, but these conversions are not recommended due to the potential for introducing dosing errors. See ***Insulin, General Information***.

When writing prescriptions, do not abbreviate units as "U," as this has been shown to increase the rate of transcription and dosage errors. In human medicine, insulin is considered a "high alert" medication (ie, medications that require special safeguards to reduce the risk for errors). Consider instituting practices such as redundant drug dosage and volume checking and special alert labels.

Do not confuse trade names that use letters to identify insulin types (eg, do not confuse *Humulin® R* with *Humulin® N*).

Adverse Effects

Adverse effects of insulin therapy may include hypoglycemia (see ***Overdose/Acute Toxicity***), hypokalemia, hypophosphatemia (diabetic ketoacidosis [DKA] only), insulin-induced rebound hyperglycemia (ie, Somogyi effect), and local or allergic reactions to the "foreign" proteins.

Reproductive/Nursing Safety

In humans, regular insulin is considered compatible with pregnancy and nursing[15]; the same is assumed to be true for veterinary patients.

Overdose/Acute Toxicity

Insulin overdose can lead to various degrees of hypoglycemia. Signs may include weakness, shaking, head tilting, lethargy, ataxia, seizures, blindness, bizarre behavior, and coma. Other signs may include restlessness, hunger, and muscle fasciculations. Electrolyte disturbances, including hypokalemia, may occur. Prolonged hypoglycemia can result in permanent brain damage or death.

Mild hypoglycemia can be treated by offering the animal its usual food. More serious signs (eg, seizures) should be treated with oral dextrose solutions (eg, *Karo®* syrup) applied to the buccal mucosa (if the animal is seizing, use caution to avoid being bit or injured) or by IV injections of 50% dextrose solutions (small amounts—usually 2 - 15 mL [0.5 - 1 mL/kg], diluted, and slowly administered[16]; see ***Dextrose 50% injection***). For in-clinic management, glucagon may also be considered on an as needed basis for an insulin overdose. See ***Glucagon.*** Once the animal's hypoglycemia is alleviated (response usually occurs within 1 to 2 minutes), it should be closely monitored (both by physical observation and serial blood glucose concentrations) to prevent a recurrence of hypoglycemia (especially with the slower-absorbed/longer-acting products) and to prevent hyperglycemia from developing. Future insulin dosages or feeding regimens should be evaluated or adjusted based on consultation with the clinician to prevent further occurrences of hypoglycemia.

For patients that have experienced or are suspected of having experienced an overdose, consultation with a 24-hour poison consultation center specializing in providing veterinary-specific information is recommended. For general information related to overdose and toxin exposures, as well as contact information for poison control centers, refer to ***Appendix.***

Drug Interactions

The following drug interactions have either been reported or are theoretical in humans or animals receiving insulin and may be of significance in veterinary patients. Unless otherwise noted, use together is not necessarily contraindicated, but weigh the potential risks and perform additional monitoring when appropriate.

- **Beta-Adrenergic Antagonists** (eg, **atenolol**, **propranolol**): Can have variable effects on glycemic control and can mask the signs associated with hypoglycemia
- **Clonidine**: Can mask the signs associated with hypoglycemia
- **Digoxin**: Because insulin can reduce serum potassium concentrations, patients receiving concomitant digoxin therapy—especially in patients receiving concurrent diuretic therapy—should be closely monitored.

- **Diuretics** (eg, **furosemide, hydrochlorothiazide**): Insulin shifts extracellular potassium into the intracellular space; serum potassium concentration should be closely monitored in patients receiving concomitant diuretic therapy. Diuretics may decrease the hypoglycemic activity of insulin (ie, increase insulin requirements).
- **Reserpine**: Can mask the signs associated with hypoglycemia

The following drugs or drug classes may potentiate the hypoglycemic activity of insulin (ie, decrease insulin requirements):

- **Anabolic Steroids** (eg, **boldenone, stanozolol, testosterone**)
- **Angiotensin II Receptor Blockers** (**ARBs**; eg, **telmisartan**)
- **Angiotensin Converting Enzyme Inhibitors** (**ACEIs**; eg, **benazepril, enalapril**)
- **Disopyramide**
- **Ethanol**
- **Fenofibrate**
- **Fluoroquinolones** (eg, **ciprofloxacin, enrofloxacin**)
- **Fluoxetine**
- **Hypoglycemics, Oral** (eg, **acarbose, glipizide, metformin**)
- **Monoamine Oxidase Inhibitors** (**MAOIs**; eg, **amitraz, linezolid, selegiline**)
- **Pentoxifylline**
- **Salicylates** (eg, **aspirin, bismuth subalicylate**)
- **Somatostatin Derivatives** (eg, **octreotide**)
- **Sulfonamides** (eg, **sulfadimethoxine, sulfamethoxazole**)

The following drugs or drug classes may decrease the hypoglycemic activity of insulin (ie, increase insulin requirements):

- **Alpha-2-Adrenergic Agonists** (eg, **dexmedetomidine, medetomidine, xylazine**): May cause hyperglycemia and temporarily interfere with glycemic control
- **Beta-2-Adrenergic Agonists** (eg, **albuterol, terbutaline**)
- **Corticosteroids** (eg, **dexamethasone, prednis(ol)one**)
- **Danazol**
- **Diazoxide**
- **Estrogens** (eg, **diethylstilbestrol [DES], estriol**)
- **Isoniazid**
- **Niacin**
- **Phenothiazines** (eg, **acepromazine, chlorpromazine**)
- **Progestins** (eg, **megestrol**)
- **Thyroid Hormones**: Can elevate glucose concentrations in diabetic patients when thyroid hormone therapy is first initiated

Laboratory Considerations

- None

Dosages

NOTES:

1. Treatment of diabetes mellitus and, in particular, diabetic ketoacidosis (DKA) is complex. Insulin is only one component of therapy; treatment may require fluid and electrolyte replacement, management of acid/base disturbances, dietary adjustments, and antimicrobial therapy. Adequate patient monitoring is mandatory. It is strongly encouraged to refer to more thorough discussions of treatment in veterinary endocrinology or internal medicine references for additional information.
2. For obese patients, dose calculations should be based on the individual patient's estimated ideal body weight to avoid inadvertent insulin overdose.
3. Insulin aspart or insulin lispro given by IV CRI appear to be safe and effective alternatives when regular insulin is not an option or is unavailable.
4. All dosages are extra-label.

DOGS:

Adjunctive therapy of diabetic ketoacidosis: Using regular insulin, choose *either* the intermittent IM technique or constant low-dose IV infusion technique.

a) **Intermittent IM protocol**: Initial dose: 0.1 – 0.2 units/kg IM into muscles of the pelvic limbs; repeat dose of 0.1 units/kg IM every 1 to 2 hours. Initial doses (first 2 to 3 injections) may be reduced by 25% to 50% if hypokalemia is a concern[17]; refer to specific endocrinology references for more information. When small doses are required, regular insulin may be diluted 1:10 with insulin diluents (preferred method) or sterile saline and administered via 0.3 mL U100 insulin syringes. Goal is to slowly lower blood glucose to 200 – 250 mg/dL over a 6- to 10-hour period; an hourly reduction in blood glucose by 50 – 100 mg/dL is ideal.[17] As blood glucose approaches 250 mg/dL, switch to IM regular insulin every 4 to 6 hours or SC (if hydration status is good) every 6 to 8 hours, with an initial dosage of 0.1 – 0.3 units/kg IM or SC, and adjust based on response to therapy. The goal is to keep blood glucose in the 150 – 300 mg/dL range.[17]

b) **Constant low-dose infusion technique**: To prepare an infusion that delivers 0.1 units/kg/hour: 2.2 units/kg regular insulin is added to 240 mL (**NOTE**: Many clinicians add insulin directly to a 250 mL bag without removing the 10 mL of fluid) of 0.9% sodium chloride. Run ≈50 mL of the insulin-containing fluid through the drip set prior to administration (see ***Adsorption*** in ***Compatibility/Compounding Considerations***). The initial administration rate is 10 mL/hour in a separate line to that used for fluid therapy.[17] When starting initial therapy for DKA, the potassium concentration must be taken into account and therapy adjusted accordingly to avoid hypokalemia. Adjust infusion rate based on hourly blood glucose determinations. An hourly reduction in blood glucose by 50 – 100 mg/dL is ideal.[17] Once blood glucose approaches 250 mg/dL, options include switching to IM regular insulin every 4 to 6 hours or SC (if hydration status is good) every 6 to 8 hours, with an initial dosage of 0.1 – 0.3 units/kg for either IM or SC administration, as described for the IM protocol or continuing the IV infusion at a decreased rate (see table) until exchanged for a longer-acting product[17] with a goal of keeping blood glucose in the 150 – 300 mg/dL range.

Blood glucose concentration (mg/dL [mmol/L])	Maintenance IV fluid	Rate of insulin CRI administration (mL/hour)	Dose of insulin administered (units/kg/hour)*
Greater than 250 (13.8)	0.9% sodium chloride	10	0.09
200-250 (11.1-13.8)	0.45% sodium chloride + 2.5% dextrose	7	0.064
150-200 (8.3-11)	0.45% sodium chloride + 2.5% dextrose	5	0.045
100-150 (5.5-8.2)	0.45% sodium chloride + 5% dextrose	5	0.045
Less than 100 (5.5)	0.45% sodium chloride + 5% dextrose	0 (Stop insulin infusion)	0 (Stop fluid administration)

Table adapted from Macintire DK. Treatment of diabetic ketoacidosis in dogs by continuous low-dose intravenous infusion of insulin. *J Am Vet Med Assoc.* 1993 Apr 15;202(8):1266-72.

*CRI prepared by adding regular insulin 2.2 units/kg to 250 mL 0.9% sodium chloride

Adjunctive treatment of hyperkalemia: NOTE: When using either of these protocols, it is imperative that 2.5% to 5% dextrose also be added to the concurrently given maintenance IV fluids to prevent secondary hypoglycemia.[18] See ***Dextrose 50% Injection*** for more information on administering dextrose.

a) 0.25 – 0.5 units/kg slow IV bolus followed by dextrose 50% (4 mL/unit of administered insulin)[8,18]

b) 0.5 – 1 units/kg in parenteral fluids plus 2 g dextrose (eg, 4 mL of dextrose 50%) per unit insulin administered.[19,20]

CATS:

Adjunctive therapy of diabetic ketoacidosis:

a) **Intermittent IM protocol:** Initial dose, 0.1 – 0.2 units/kg IM; repeat dose of 0.1 units/kg IM every 1 to 2 hours. Initial doses (first 2 to 3 injections) may be reduced by 25% to 50% if hypokalemia is a concern[17]; refer to specific endocrinology references for more information.

b) **Constant low-dose infusion technique:** 0.05 – 0.1 units/kg per hour IV CRI.[3,17,21-23] To prepare the solution, add the appropriate amount of regular insulin (1.1 or 2.2 units/kg) directly to 250 mL 0.9% sodium chloride/sterile saline. Run ≈50 mL of the insulin-containing fluid through the drip set prior to administration. Use the same IV CRI administration protocol as described above for dogs.

c) **Regular insulin plus glargine:** Regular insulin 1 unit/cat (NOT unit/kg) IM up to every 6 hours while the blood glucose concentration is greater than 250 mg/dL; used in combination with glargine 0.25 units/kg SC every 12 hours.[2]

Adjunctive treatment of hyperkalemia: When using either of these protocols, it is imperative that dextrose be provided to prevent secondary hypoglycemia[18]; this can be accomplished by adding 2.5% or 5% dextrose to the maintenance fluids. See ***Dextrose 50% Injection*** for more information on administering dextrose.

a) 0.5 – 1 units/kg IM with dextrose 2 g (eg, 4 mL of dextrose 50%)/insulin unit administered as a slow IV bolus.[24]

b) 0.25 – 0.5 units/kg with dextrose 0.5 g/kg slow IV bolus[8,18]

HORSES:

Diabetes mellitus:

a) 0.1 units/kg IM every 6 to 12 hours or 0.1 unit/kg/hour IV CRI. Once stabilized, transition therapy to a longer-acting insulin.[25]

b) 0.05 – 0.1 units/kg IV every 8 to 12 hours[26]

Management of hyperglycemia in critically ill foals during parenteral nutrition support:

a) **Continuous IV infusion:** 0.01 – 0.07 units/kg/hour IV CRI.[27,28] If blood glucose is more than 150 mg/dL after 2 hours, increase CRI by 50% at 2-hour intervals until blood glucose is below 150 mg/dL. Adding regular insulin 20 units to 500 mL 0.9% sodium chloride is one recommended method to prepare the insulin infusion.[28] Run ≈50 mL of the insulin-containing fluid through the drip set prior to administration (see ***Adsorption*** in ***Compatibility/Compounding Considerations***).

b) **Intermittent SC or IM technique:** Dosages have varied widely, from 0.01 – 0.1 units/kg IV or SC every 6 to 24 hours[29] to 0.1 – 0.5 units/kg SC.[28] Some clinicians have suggested intermittent injections are not recommended due to risk for hypo- or hyperglycemia being greater than with CRI.[30]

NEW WORLD CAMELIDS:

Severe hyperlipemia: 0.2 units/kg IV with dextrose every 6 hours (more frequently if needed, up to a maximum frequency every hour).[31] Administration of 0.2 units/kg SC had peak effect at ≈4.7 hours, and duration was 8.5 hours.[32]

BIRDS:

Diabetes mellitus: 0.1 – 0.2 units/kg SC or IM.[33] Insulin therapy is sometimes hindered by the highly variable dose needed for individual birds, development of insulin resistance, and development of pancreatic atrophy/insufficiency. Adjust insulin dose every 1 to 2 hours until blood glucose concentration is maintained within normal range. Once stabilized, NPH insulin can be started for long-term therapy.

Monitoring

- Diabetic patients should be closely monitored. Each patient requires an individualized treatment plan, frequent reassessment, and adjustments of the plan based on the response of the patient. It is encouraged to consult a veterinary endocrinology reference text or with a veterinary emergency and critical care and/or endocrinology specialist for further information related to regulating diabetic patients and insulin adjustments. The overarching goal for monitoring diabetic patients is control of clinical signs related to hyperglycemia (eg, polyuria, polydipsia) while avoiding hypoglycemia.[34] Interpret all monitoring strategies in light of clinical signs. Results from the below monitoring options may conflict in regard to achieving good glycemic control and good clinical control.
- Patient status and control of clinical signs: body weight, appetite, fluid intake, urine output
- Glucose (blood or interstitial). Because of how often glucose needs to be checked in sick diabetic patients, consider a central line or continuous interstitial glucose monitoring system in dogs and cats. Experience with continuous interstitial glucose monitoring in dogs and cats is that these devices are easy to apply, user friendly, and provide useful information surrounding glycemic control while the patient is in the clinic or home environment.[35-38]
  - For patients that have experienced or are suspected to have experienced repeated or unexplained hypoglycemia, it is strongly encouraged to consult a veterinary emergency and critical care and/or endocrinology specialist or reference text that specializes in providing information specific for treatment of hypoglycemia.
- Additional monitoring for patients with diabetic ketoacidosis (DKA)[39]:
  - Glucose measurement every 1 to 2 hours initially; adjust insulin therapy and begin dextrose infusion when glucose decreases below 250 mg/dL (14 mmol/L). See ***Dosages***.
  - Hydration status, respiration, pulse every 2 to 4 hours
  - Serum electrolyte (eg, magnesium, phosphorous, potassium), plasma ketones, and total venous CO_2 concentrations every 4 to 8 hours
  - Urine output, glycosuria, and urine ketones every 4 to 8 hours
  - Body weight, packed cell volume, temperature, and blood pressure every 6 to 8 hours
  - Additional monitoring as applicable to address concurrent disease

Chemistry/Synonyms

All commercial preparations of human-labeled insulin currently manufactured in the United States are supplied in solution or suspension at a concentration of 100 units/mL, which is ≈3.5 mg of insulin/mL. Likewise, 1 unit of insulin equals ≈35 µg of insulin, and 1 mg insulin equals ≈28.8 units.

Regular insulin human injection, USP (rDNA origin), is structurally identical to human insulin and is synthesized through rDNA technology in a special nonpathogenic laboratory strain of *Escherichia coli* bacteria (*Humulin® R*) or *Saccharomyces cerevisiae* yeast (*Novolin® R*). It is a rapid-acting, sterile, clear, and colorless or almost colorless solution. Discoloration, turbidity, or unusual viscosity indicates deterioration or contamination.

Regular insulin may also be known as crystalline zinc insulin, regular human insulin, insulin human, recombinant human insulin, *Humulin® R*, and *Novolin® R*.

Storage/Stability

Unopened regular insulin *vials* and pens/devices should be stored in the refrigerator at 2°C to 8°C (36°F-46°F) and protected from temperature extremes and direct sunlight. Do not freeze.

In-use *vials* or *pens/devices*:

- Regular insulin: *Humulin® R* should be stored for 31 days refrigerated or at room temperature. *Novolin® R* vials should be stored for 42 days, and *Novolin® R* pens/devices should be stored for 28 days. *Novolin® R* vials and pens/devices should be stored at room temperature only; do not refrigerate.
- Regular insulin may be stored in plastic or glass syringes refrigerated or at room temperature for 28 days without loss of potency; however, the antibacterial preservatives in the insulin formulations may be lost if stored at room temperature.[40] It is generally accepted that syringes of insulin can be stored for 28 days refrigerated without loss of potency.

Freezing (less than 2°C [36°F]) may alter the protein structure and decrease potency. Particle aggregation and crystal damage may be visible to the naked eye. Higher temperature (greater than 30°C [86°F]) extremes and direct exposure to sunlight (as might occur when insulin is stored in a car or on a windowsill) may produce insulin transformation products and fibril formation.

Although manufacturers recommend discarding opened bottles of insulin after 4 to 6 weeks (or expiration date, whichever comes first), studies[41,42] support that insulin potency and stability is maintained for longer durations. Veterinary internal medicine specialists indicate that the vial may be used for 3 to 6 months after opening and possibly beyond the listed expiration date as long as it is handled carefully, stored in the refrigerator, and the solution does not develop discoloration, flocculent precipitates, or changes in consistency. If a lack of diabetes regulation is noted when using the product beyond the expiration date (3 to 6 months after starting therapy), it may be prudent to replace with new insulin prior to adjusting insulin therapy.[34]

Compatibility/Compounding Considerations

Compatibility is dependent on factors such as pH, concentration, temperature, and diluent used; consult specialized references for more specific information.

Regular insulin is reportedly physically **compatible** with the following drugs/solutions: 0.9% sodium chloride, TPN solutions (4% amino acids, 25% dextrose with electrolytes and vitamins; must occasionally shake bag to prevent separation), ascorbic acid, atropine, bumetanide, calcium gluconate, cefazolin, cimetidine, esmolol, fentanyl, hydromorphone, lidocaine, mannitol, metoclopramide, metronidazole, oxytetracycline, penicillin G potassium/sodium, potassium chloride, sodium bicarbonate, and verapamil. Regular insulin may be mixed with other insulin products (except for glargine) used in veterinary medicine (eg, NPH, PZI). If mixing 2 insulin products in the same syringe, regular insulin should be drawn into the syringe first.

Regular insulin is reportedly physically **incompatible** when mixed with the following drugs/solutions: aminophylline, ampicillin, butorphanol, chlorothiazide, cytarabine, diazepam, dobutamine, famotidine, furosemide, gentamicin, glycopyrrolate, ketamine, pantoprazole, pentobarbital, phenobarbital, piperacillin/tazobactam, polymyxin B, propranolol, quinidine, and thiopental.

Diluting insulin: Other than for immediate use, regular insulin should only be diluted using product-specific sterile diluent, which is supplied by the manufacturer upon request. Diluted insulin (10 units/mL) prepared in this manner is stable for 4 weeks and should be stored in the refrigerator, although refrigeration is not required. For immediate use, regular insulin can be diluted with normal saline for injection, but the potency cannot be predicted after 24 hours.

Adsorption: The adsorption of regular insulin to the surfaces of IV infusion solution containers, glass and plastic (including PVC, ethylene vinyl acetate, polyethylene, and other polyolefins), tubing, and filters has been demonstrated. Estimates of loss of potency range from 20% to 80%, although reports of 20% to 30% are more common.[43-46] The percent adsorbed is inversely proportional to the concentration of the insulin,[43] and may include other factors (eg, amount of container surface area, fill volume of the solution, type of solution, type and length of administration set, temperature, previous exposure of tubing to insulin, presence of other drugs or blood).[44-46] The adsorption process is instantaneous, with the bulk of insulin adsorption occurring within the first 30 to 60 minutes. To saturate binding sites and deliver a more predictable dose to the patient through an IV infusion, it is recommended that the first 50 mL be run through the IV tubing and discarded.

Insulin syringes: Syringes are designed for use with a specific strength of insulin, with the needle covers color-coded according to strength. U100 syringes are available in 0.3 mL, 0.5 mL, and 1 mL sizes. Measuring U100 insulin to the 1 unit mark in a U100 syringe will result in 1 unit of insulin. Some brands of 0.3 mL syringes include ½ unit markings. Insulin syringes should not be reused.

Dosage Forms/Regulatory Status

VETERINARY-LABELED PRODUCTS: NONE

HUMAN-LABELED PRODUCTS:

Insulin, Regular Injection Human (rDNA): 100 units/mL in 3 mL vials and pens/devices, and 10 mL vials; *Humulin® R*, *Novolin® R*; (OTC in humans; requires prescription under extra-label provisions of AMDUCA when used in animals). A 500 units/mL concentration is available, as is a 1 unit/mL premixed solution. Most clinics have little need for the 500 units/mL concentration, and the 1 unit/mL solution is not conducive for use in established diabetic ketoacidosis (DKA) protocols. If stocked, adequate safeguards should be implemented to prevent the significant harm that could result from inadvertent use of these strengths.

References

For the complete list of references, see **wiley.com/go/budde/plumb**

Interferon Alfa, Human Recombinant

(in-ter-***feer***-on ***al***-fah) *Intron-A®*

Immunomodulator

See also ***Interferon Omega, Feline Origin***

Prescriber Highlights

- Cytokine used to alleviate clinical effects of certain viral diseases; little solid evidence available to document safety and efficacy in small animals
- Adverse effects: In cats, adverse effects are apparently uncommon with PO dosing; higher dosages given parenterally may cause malaise, fever, allergic reactions, myelotoxicity, and myalgia.

Uses/Indications

Interferon alfa has primarily been used in cats to treat a variety of virus-induced diseases using either SC or oral/buccal administration. Despite rapid antibody development when injected parenterally and little, if any, absorption after oral administration, the drug does appear to have some efficacy for certain diseases, either via direct antiviral action or, more likely, an immunomodulatory effect. Interferon-alfa has been used in dogs and cats for the adjunctive treatment of a wide variety of viral- or immunosuppression-related conditions (eg, papillomas, keratoconjuntivitis sicca), but the strength of the evidence to support most indications is either weak or absent.[1] Cats naturally infected with feline immunodeficiency virus (FIV) or feline leukemia virus (FeLV) demonstrated favorable clinical and biopathological response to long-term oral interferon alfa.[2,3]

Feline interferon-omega is available in several countries, and it may be useful in treating viral diseases in both cats and dogs. See ***Interferon Omega, Feline Origin***.

Pharmacology/Actions

There are at least 25 subtypes of interferon alfa, each possessing similar but not identical biological activity. The pharmacologic effects of the interferons are widespread and complex. Suffice it to say that interferon alfa has antiviral, antiproliferative, and immunomodulating effects. Its antiproliferative and antiviral activities are thought to be due to its effects on the synthesis of RNA, DNA, and cellular proteins (oncogenes included). The mechanisms for its antineoplastic activities are not well understood but are probably related to these effects as well.

Pharmacokinetics

Interferon alfa is poorly absorbed after oral administration due to its degradation by proteolytic enzymes, and studies have not detected measurable levels in the systemic circulation; however, there may be some absorption in the upper GI mucosa. It may have some immunomodulating effect via stimulation of local lymphoid tissues.

Interferon alfa is widely distributed throughout the body, although it does not penetrate into the CNS well. It is unknown if it crosses the placenta. Interferon alfa is freely filtered by the glomeruli and is absorbed by the renal tubules, where it is metabolized by brush border enzymes of lysosomes. Hepatic metabolism is of minor importance. The plasma half-life in cats has been reported as 2.9 hours.[4]

Contraindications/Precautions/Warnings

When interferon alfa is used parenterally, consider the risks versus benefits in patients with pre-existing autoimmune disease, severe cardiac disease, pulmonary disease, hard-to-control (brittle) diabetes, severe hepatic disease, herpes infections, hypersensitivity to the drug, or CNS disorders.

Adverse Effects

When interferon alfa is used orally in cats, adverse effects are apparently uncommon. Higher dosages given parenterally to cats may cause malaise, fever, allergic reactions, myelotoxicity, and myalgia. Injection site reactions (eg, discomfort, redness) are possible. Cats given human interferon-alfa parenterally may develop significant antibodies to it after 3 to 7 weeks of treatment with resultant loss of efficacy.[4]

When interferon alfa is used systemically in humans, adverse effects are common and include anemia, leukopenias, thrombocytopenia, hepatotoxicity, neurotoxicity, vision loss, hypothyroidism, taste sensation changes, anorexia, nausea, vomiting, diarrhea, dizziness, influenza-like symptoms, transient blood pressure changes, hair loss, skin rashes, hypertriglyceridemia, and dry mouth.[5] Except for the flu-like syndrome, most adverse effects are dose-related and may vary depending on the condition treated. Depression of mild to moderate severity has been noted in up to 25% of humans receiving interferon alfa; it is unclear how this relates to veterinary patients.

Reproductive/Nursing Safety

Interferon alfa did not impair fertility in laboratory animals, although decreased estrogen and progesterone levels and changes to the menstrual cycle were noted in rhesus monkeys. Safety during pregnancy has not been established; high parenteral doses in monkeys did not cause teratogenic effects but did increase abortifacient activity.

It is not known whether this drug is excreted in milk. Studies in mice have shown that mouse interferons are excreted into the milk.

Because safety has not been established in animals, this drug should only be used when the maternal benefits outweigh the potential risks to offspring.

Overdose/Acute Toxicity

Decreased food consumption, weight loss, vascular leakage, and bone marrow suppression were observed in laboratory animals receiving up to 11 to 100 times the FDA-approved human dose. Determine dosages carefully.

For patients that have experienced or are suspected of having experienced an overdose, consultation with a 24-hour poison consultation center specializing in providing veterinary-specific information is recommended. For general information related to overdose and toxin exposures, as well as contact information for poison control centers, refer to ***Appendix.***

Drug Interactions

The following drug interactions have either been reported or are theoretical in humans or animals receiving interferon alfa and may be of significance in veterinary patients. Unless otherwise noted, use together is not necessarily contraindicated, but weigh the potential risks and perform additional monitoring when appropriate.

- **ACYCLOVIR, VIDARABINE, ZIDOVUDINE**: Additive or synergistic antiviral effects may occur when interferon alfa is used in conjunction with zidovudine (AZT) or acyclovir. This effect does not appear to occur with vidarabine, although increased toxicities may occur. The veterinary significance of these potential interactions is unclear.
- **COLCHICINE**: Reduced interferon effectiveness
- **THEOPHYLLINE**: Doubling of theophylline concentration has been noted in humans.

Dosages

NOTE: All dosages are extra-label, and evidence for safety and efficacy is relatively weak. All dosages are for human interferon alfa-2b as interferon alfa-2a is no longer marketed.

DOGS:

Cutaneous T-cell lymphoma and severe cases of oral/cutaneous papillomas: 1.5 – 2 million units/m^2 (NOT units/kg) SC every other day or 3 times weekly until clinical resolution[6,7]

Immunostimulant for the adjunctive treatment of certain dermatologic conditions (eg, pododermatitis, papillomas, digital keratomas): 1000 units PO once daily (given as 1000 unit/mL solution)[8]

Canine transmissible venereal tumor: 1.5 million units/dog (NOT units/kg) as an intra-lesional injection once weekly, along with vincristine 0.025 mg/kg IV, was found to shorten the duration of treatment when compared with vincristine alone.[9]

CATS:

Feline immunodeficiency virus (FIV)- +/- feline leukemia virus (FeLV)-infected cats: Low-dose oral: Using an experimentally produced interferon alfa product, 10 units/kg PO once daily resulted in clinical improvement and prolonged survival.[10] Using recombinant human interferon alfa, 60 units/cat (NOT units/kg), PO or buccally once daily, treated 7 days on, 7 days off[3,11]

Feline calicivirus or feline herpesvirus-1: High-dose SC injection: 10,000 units/kg (diluted in saline) SC once daily for up to 14 days has led to clinical resolution of disease in some cats.[12,13] Low-dose oral: 50 units/cat (NOT units/kg) PO once daily[14]

Monitoring

- Baseline and periodic CBC with platelets and chemistry panel should be performed during treatment.
- Consider measurement of serum triglycerides and thyroid panel, as abnormalities have been noted in humans
- Baseline and periodic ophthalmic examinations to monitor for improvement or progression of ocular effects caused by viral infection
- Efficacy and adverse effects

Client Information

- Owners must be aware of the investigational nature of this compound and understand that efficacy and safety are not necessarily known.
- For oral use: Compounded liquid is given orally (by mouth) or inside the cheek (buccally). It is best not to mix it with food. If your animal vomits or acts sick after getting it on an empty stomach, give the drug with food or a small treat to see if this helps. If vomiting continues, contact your veterinarian.
- It is usually well tolerated.

Chemistry/Synonyms

Prepared from genetically engineered cultures of *Escherichia coli* with genes from human leukocytes, interferon alfa-2b is commercially available as a sterile solution or sterile powder. Human interferon alfa is a complex protein that contains 165 or 166 amino acids.

Interferon may also be known as huIFN-alfa, IFN-alpha, interferon-alpha, or Sch-30500 (interferon alfa-2b); there are many internationally registered trade names available.

Storage/Stability

Store commercially available products in the refrigerator; do not freeze. Do not expose solutions to room temperature for longer than 24 hours. Do not vigorously shake solutions. Avoid exposure to direct sunlight.

An article proposing using this product in cats for the treatment of FeLV states that after dilution of 3 million units in 1 L of sterile saline, the resultant solution remains active for years if frozen or for months if refrigerated; however, data corroborating this were not located.

Compatibility/Compounding Considerations

Interferon alfa products supplied as powder should be reconstituted with the accompanying diluent and swirled gently to dissolve the powder; manufacturers recommend discarding unused portions of reconstituted interferon alfa.

Preparation of solution for 30 units/mL oral administration: Using the 6 million unit vial (see below), dilute the entire contents into a 1 L bag of sterile normal saline; mix well. The resulting solution contains ≈6000 units/mL. Divide into aliquots of either 1 mL or 10 mL and freeze. By diluting further 200-fold (1 mL of 6000 units/mL solution with 200 mL of sterile saline, or 5 mL with 1000 mL of sterile saline), a 30 units/mL solution will result. Some clinicians have advised aliquoting the diluted solution into 1 mL volumes for freezing up to a year; defrost as necessary. Once defrosted, the drug can be refrigerated for up to one week. Freezing the most dilute solutions is associated with loss in the activity unless protein such as albumin (see above) is added during dilution.[12]

Dosage Forms/Regulatory Status

VETERINARY-LABELED PRODUCTS: NONE

Interferon Alfa-2a (*Roferen® A*) that was used in veterinary medicine has been discontinued.

HUMAN-LABELED PRODUCTS:

Interferon Alfa-2b (human recombinant) (IFN-alpha$_2$; rIFN-a2; a-2-interferon) Powder for Injection: 10 million units/vial, 18 million units/vial, and 50 million units/vial in vials with diluent; *Intron A®*; (Rx)

Interferon Alfa-2b (human recombinant) (IFN-alpha$_2$; rIFN-a2; a-2-interferon) Injection: 6 million units/mL in 3.6 mL vials and 10 million units/mL in 3.2 mL vials; *Intron A®*; (Rx)

References

For the complete list of references, see **wiley.com/go/budde/plumb**

Interferon Omega, Feline Origin

(in-ter-***feer***-on oh-***may***-ga) *Virbagen® Omega*

Immunomodulator

See also ***Interferon Alfa, Human Recombinant***

Prescriber Highlights

- Immunomodulating cytokine approved in Europe for treating feline leukemia virus (FeLV) and feline immunodeficiency virus (FIV) in cats and enteral parvovirus in dogs
- Appears to be well tolerated; adverse effects include hyperthermia, vomiting, diarrhea (cats), and fatigue (cats).
- Increases in ALT and decreases in RBC, WBC, and platelet counts have been seen.
- Not commercially available in the United States; treatment may be expensive.

Uses/Indications

Interferon omega is labeled in the EU for dogs 1 month of age or older for the reduction in mortality and clinical signs associated with the enteric form of parvovirus. In cats 9 weeks of age or older, it is labeled for treating feline leukemia virus (FeLV) and/or feline immunodeficiency virus (FIV) in nonterminal clinical stages. It may be of benefit in treating canine distemper, acute feline calicivirus infections, and FIP. In an open-label study of 16 naturally infected cats with FIV/FeLV given labeled doses of interferon omega, improved clinical signs and decreased concurrent virus excretion were noted.[1] Similarly, interferon omega improved clinical signs and reduced viral shedding in cats with feline chronic gingivitis-stomatitis (FCGS) and were infected with feline calicivirus (FCV).[2,3]

Interferon omega may also be of benefit topically for feline herpetic keratitis, but data are still being gathered to document efficacy. Interferon omega treatment has been noted to produce some clinical benefit in dogs with atopic dermatitis, including inconsistent and mild improvement in skin lesions and pruritus.[4]

Pharmacology/Actions

Omega interferon is a type 1 interferon related to interferon alpha. Its principal action is not as a direct anti-viral agent but by inhibiting host mRNA and translation proteins in virusinfected cells, thereby inhibiting viral replication. It may also nonspecifically enhance immune defense mechanisms.

Pharmacokinetics

Omega interferon pharmacokinetics in dogs and cats appear to be similar to that of human interferons. After IV injection, omega interferon is rapidly bound to specific receptor sites on a variety of cells. The highest tissue concentrations are found in the liver and kidneys. Interferon is filtered in the renal glomeruli and catabolized in the kidneys. In dogs, the volume of distribution at steady state is about 0.1 L/kg. Biphasic elimination occurs with an alpha half-life of 3.14 hours and a beta half-life of 0.24 hours. Total body clearance is

6.9 mL/minute/kg. Pharmacologic effects of interferon omega persist after its disappearance from plasma.

Contraindications/Precautions/Warnings

The manufacturer cautions against vaccinating dogs currently being treated with omega interferon and not to vaccinate until the patient appears to have recovered from infection. As both feline leukemia virus (FeLV) and feline immunodeficiency virus (FIV) infections are known to be immunosuppressive, the manufacturer states that cat vaccinations are contraindicated during and after omega interferon treatment.

There are several different interferons available for use in humans (several subtypes of alpha, beta, or gamma interferon); one cannot be substituted for another.

Adverse Effects

In cats and dogs, hyperthermia (3 to 6 hours postdose) and vomiting have been reported. Slight decreases in RBCs, platelets, and WBCs and increased ALT have been observed, but, reportedly, these indices return to normal within a week of the last injection.
Additionally, soft feces and mild diarrhea and transient fatigue may be noted in cats. IV administration to cats may cause increased incidence and severity of adverse effects, but adverse effects occur uncommonly in this species.

Dogs may develop antibodies to interferon omega if treatment is prolonged (beyond labeled dosage period) or repeated.

Reproductive/Nursing Safety

Safety during pregnancy or lactation has not been established.

Because safety has not been established in animals, this drug should only be used when the maternal benefits outweigh the potential risks to offspring.

Overdose/Acute Toxicity

Overdoses of 10 times the labeled dose in dogs and cats caused mild lethargy, somnolence, slight hyperthermia, and slight increases in respiratory and heart rates. In animals tested, signs resolved within 7 days, and no treatment was required.

For patients that have experienced or are suspected of having experienced an overdose, consultation with a 24-hour poison consultation center specializing in providing veterinary-specific information is recommended. For general information related to overdose and toxin exposures, as well as contact information for poison control centers, refer to ***Appendix***.

Drug Interactions

The following drug interactions have either been reported or are theoretical in humans or animals receiving interferon omega and may be of significance in veterinary patients. Unless otherwise noted, use together is not necessarily contraindicated, but weigh the potential risks and perform additional monitoring when appropriate.

- Hepatotoxic Agents (eg, **lomustine, NSAIDs, rifampin**): Increased risk for hepatotoxicity
- Myelosuppressive Agents (eg, **antineoplastics, chloramphenicol, zidovudine**): Concurrent use may result in additive myelosuppression.
- Vaccines: Vaccine administration is contraindicated during interferon omega treatment.

Laboratory Considerations

- None are noted.

Dosages

DOGS:

Parvovirus (extra-label): 2.5 million units/kg IV once daily for 3 days.[5] The earlier the dog is treated, the more likelihood of success.

Atopic dermatitis (extra-label): 1 – 5 million units/kg SC 3 times per week for 4 weeks, then once monthly[4,6]

CATS:

Feline leukemia virus (FeLV) or feline immunodeficiency virus (FIV) (extra-label): 1 million units/kg SC once daily for 5 days.[5] Three separate 5-day treatments performed at day 0, day 14, and day 60

FIV (extra-label): 100,000 units/cat (NOT units/kg) PO once daily for 90 days[7]

Feline herpesvirus-1 (FHV-1) facial dermatitis (extra-label): From a case report treating a cat with FHV-1 facial dermatitis: Day 0: 1.5 million units/kg injected, half of which was injected peri-lesionally and intradermally and the other half SC on the lateral thorax. Days 2 and 9: 1.5 million units/kg injected SC on the lateral thorax. On days 19, 21, and 23: 0.75 million units/kg injected peri-lesionally and intradermally as well as 0.75 million units/kg SC on the lateral thorax. The cat was sedated when each peri-lesional and intradermal injection was made.[8]

Feline chronic gingivostomatitis syndrome (FCGS; extra-label): 100,000 units/cat (NOT units/kg) PO once daily for 90 days[2,3,9]

Adjunctive treatment of cowpox virus-associated pneumonia and dermatitis (extra-label): From a case series of 5 cats, all received broad-spectrum antibacterial therapy along with other supportive treatments, and 4 cats received interferon omega, with 3 cats administered 1 million units/kg IV or SC every 24 and 1 cat given 2.5 million units/kg SC every 48 hours. The 2 cats that received interferon and lived were felt to have been diagnosed and treated earlier in the disease course.[10]

Monitoring

- Efficacy
- Baseline and periodic CBC, chemistry panel

Client Information

- Your veterinarian must administer this drug on an inpatient basis to provide the observation and support the animal may need.

Chemistry/Synonyms

Interferon omega of feline origin is a type 1 recombinant interferon obtained from silkworms after inoculation with a recombinant baculovirus. It is provided commercially as a lyophilisate powder with a separate solvent (saline).

Interferon omega may also be known as recombinant omega interferon of feline origin, omega interferon, interferon-omega, IFN-omega, IFN-omega (feline recombinant), rFelFN-omega, and *Virbagen® Omega*.

Storage/Stability

Store the commercial veterinary product in its original carton refrigerated (2°C-6°C [36°F-43°F]); protect from freezing.[5] It has a designated shelf life of 2 years when properly stored. Once reconstituted with the supplied isotonic sodium chloride solution, use it immediately as it contains no preservative; however, there are anecdotal reports that the solution is stable for at least 3 weeks when refrigerated. No data were located on the stability of the reconstituted solution when frozen.

Compatibility/Compounding Considerations

Interferon omega should not be mixed with any other vaccine/immunological product, except the solvent supplied for use with the product.[5]

Dosage Forms/Regulatory Status

VETERINARY-LABELED PRODUCTS:

None in the United States

Recombinant Omega Interferon of Feline Origin: 10 million units/vial; *Virbagen® Omega*; (Rx); licensed for dogs and cats in the EU only. A 5 million unit vial may be available in some countries.

HUMAN-LABELED PRODUCTS: NONE

References

For the complete list of references, see **wiley.com/go/budde/plumb**

Iodide (Potassium-, Sodium-)

(**eye**-oh-dide) *SSKI®, Iodoject®*

Antifungal, Nutritional Supplement

Prescriber Highlights

- Iodides have been used for actinomycosis/actinobacillosis in ruminants and sporotrichosis in dogs, cats, and horses.
- Contraindications include iodide hypersensitivity, lactating animals, hyperthyroidism, renal failure, or dehydration. May cause abortion in cattle
- Metallic taste, patient acceptance can be problematic
- Do not inject IM; in horses, give IV slowly and with caution, as severe generalized reactions have been reported.
- Adverse effects include iodism (signs include excessive tearing, vomiting, anorexia, nasal discharge, muscle twitching, cardiomyopathy, scaly haircoats/dandruff, hyperthermia, decreased milk production, weight gain, coughing, inappetence, and diarrhea).
- Cats may be more prone to developing toxicity.

Uses/Indications

The primary use for sodium iodide is in the treatment of actinobacillosis and actinomycosis in cattle. Although sodium iodide 20 mg/kg PO achieved presumed therapeutic iodine concentrations in calves,[1,2] it was not effective at preventing bovine respiratory disease.[1] It has been used as an expectorant with little success in a variety of species, and occasionally as a supplement for iodine deficiency disorders. Iodide has been used as adjunctive therapy for pythiosis in horses, but clinical studies are lacking.[3-6] In dogs, cats, and horses, oral sodium or potassium iodide has been used in the treatment of sporotrichosis.

Use in cats is controversial, as they may be prone to developing adverse effects; cats may require other antifungal (eg, itraconazole) therapy. A study using oral potassium iodide (alone) for sporotrichosis reported a cure rate of 48% and a treatment failure rate of 37%.[7]

Pharmacology/Actions

Although the exact mode of action for their efficacy in treating actinobacillosis is unknown, iodides likely have some effect on the granulomatous inflammatory process. Iodides have little, if any, in vitro antibiotic activity.

Pharmacokinetics

Little published information appears to be available. When given orally to humans, iodide salts are converted into iodine and transported to the thyroid gland. The majority of any remaining iodine is eliminated in the urine. Therapeutic efficacy of IV sodium iodide for actinobacillosis is rapid, with beneficial effects usually seen within 48 hours of therapy.

Contraindications/Precautions/Warnings

Sodium iodide injection labels state that it should not be given to pregnant animals, lactating animals, or those with hyperthyroidism. Do not inject iodide IM.

Animals vary in their susceptibility to iodides; give them with caution until tolerance is determined.[8] Iodides given parenterally should be administered slowly IV and with caution to horses; severe generalized reactions have been reported.

Iodide should not be used in animals in renal failure or in those that are severely dehydrated.

Adverse Effects

In ruminants, the adverse effect profile is related to excessive iodine (see ***Overdose/Acute Toxicity*** below). Young animals may be more susceptible to iodism than adults.

Long-term use or overdoses may cause iodism. Cats are apparently more prone to developing this than other species. Signs can include vomiting, inappetence, depression/lethargy, twitching, hypothermia, and cardiovascular failure. One study reported that 27% of treated cats had increased liver enzymes, and about half of those cats exhibited signs of hepatotoxicity.[7]

The taste of the liquid is unpleasant, so animals may avoid dosing. Administering iodide with food or a fatty liquid (eg, whole milk, ice cream) may improve palatability and reduce nausea and vomiting. Cats reportedly tolerate the taste of sodium iodide better than potassium iodide. Potassium iodide oral tablets 130 mg (available OTC for reducing risk for thyroid cancer after radioactive isotope exposure) or compounded capsules may be useful in small dogs or cats that cannot tolerate oral solutions.

Reproductive/Nursing Safety

Iodides readily cross the placenta and may cause goiter or abnormal thyroid function in the neonate.[9] Anecdotal reports that iodides can cause abortion in cattle persist. Clearly, potential risks versus benefits of therapy must be weighed.

Iodides are excreted in milk. If iodides are required in the nursing dam, switch to milk replacer. Foals have developed goiters when mares have been excessively supplemented.

Because safety has not been established in animals, this drug should only be used when the maternal benefits outweigh the potential risks to offspring.

Overdose/Acute Toxicity

Excessive iodine in animals can cause excessive tearing, vomiting, anorexia, diarrhea, nasal discharge, muscle twitching, cardiomyopathy, scaly haircoats/dandruff, hyperthermia, decreased milk production and weight gain, coughing, inappetence, and diarrhea.

Refer to the ***Potassium (-Acetate, -Chloride, -Gluconate)*** monograph for discussion of potassium overdoses.

For patients that have experienced or are suspected to have experienced an overdose, consultation with a 24-hour poison consultation center specializing in providing veterinary-specific information is recommended. For general information related to overdose and toxin exposures, as well as contact information for poison control centers, refer to ***Appendix***.

Drug Interactions

The following drug interactions have either been reported or are theoretical in humans or animals receiving iodide and may be of significance in veterinary patients. Unless otherwise noted, use together is not necessarily contraindicated, but weigh the potential risks and perform additional monitoring when appropriate.

- **ACE Inhibitors** (eg, **enalapril**): Concurrent use with potassium iodide increases the risk for hyperkalemia.
- **Angiotensin Receptor Blockers** (**ARBs**; eg, **telmisartan**): Concurrent use with potassium iodide increases the risk for hyperkalemia.
- **Antithyroid Medications** (eg, **carbimazole, methimazole**): Iodides may decrease the efficacy of antithyroid medications.
- **Potassium Sparing Diuretics** (eg, **triamterene, spironolactone**): Concurrent use with potassium iodide increases the risk for hyperkalemia.
- **Potassium Supplements**: Concurrent use with potassium iodide increases the risk for hyperkalemia.
- **Thyroid Supplements** (eg, **levothyroxine**): Iodides may enhance the efficacy of thyroid medications.

Dosages

DOGS:

Sporotrichosis (extra-label): Using potassium iodide (*SSKI®*),

40 mg/kg PO every 12 hours with food; using itraconazole for treatment of sporotrichosis is less likely to have adverse effects.[10]

CATS:

Sporotrichosis (extra-label): Generally, azole antifungal agents are recommended, but as a low-cost alternative treatment (from an observational cohort study): using potassium iodide compounded into capsules, initially 2.5 mg/kg PO every 24 hours. Doses were progressively increased at each 5-day period until a clinical response was achieved or signs of toxicity appeared: 5 mg/kg, 10 mg/kg, 15 mg/kg, and 20 mg/kg every 24 hours. Cats with mild adverse clinical effects had therapy suspended for 7 days and resumed 2.5 mg/kg dose increments until the highest dose that did not induce toxicity was attained.[7]

Sporotrichosis (extra-label): Using potassium iodide (KI), 2.5 – 20 mg/kg PO once daily *in combination with* itraconazole 100 mg/day. KI dose escalated in 2.5 mg/kg per day increments every 30 days until a maximum dose of 20 mg/kg per day was reached. Treatment continued until 4 weeks after cats were clinically cured.[11]

HORSES:

Sporotrichosis (extra-label):

a) Sodium Iodide: Loading dose of 20 – 40 mg/kg IV slowly once daily for 2 to 5 days, then 20 – 40 mg/kg PO once daily for at least 3 weeks after all clinical lesions disappear. May administer via oral syringe or mixed in sweet feed. Topical hot packs of 20% sodium iodide may be used on open wounds.[12,13]

b) Organic iodides (eg, ethylene diamine dihydroiodide): 1 – 2 mg/kg of the active ingredient mixed with a small amount of grain once or twice daily for the first week, then reduced to 0.5 – 1 mg/kg once daily for the remainder of the treatment. Treatment should be continued for at least 1 month beyond the complete resolution of all cutaneous nodules. Proven to be superior in efficacy to the inorganic iodides (sodium or potassium iodide).[14]

Conidiobolomycosis (extra-label): From a case report: A mare with *Conidiobolus coronatus* granulomatous tracheitis was successfully treated with 20% sodium iodide at 44 mg/kg IV for 7 days, followed by ethylenediamine dihydroiodide (iodide powder, granules) 1.3 mg/kg PO every 12 hours for 4 months, then every 24 hours for 1 year, then once per week. Excessive lacrimation was occasionally noted but resolved if the drug was held for 1 day.[15]

CATTLE:

Actinomycosis | Lump jaw; actinobacillosis | Woody tongue; necrotic stomatitis (label dosage; not FDA-approved): Sodium Iodide 20%, 66 mg/kg IV slowly. May be repeated at weekly intervals if necessary[8]

Actinobacillosis | Woody tongue (extra-label): Potassium iodide 70 mg/kg IV slowly, given as a 10% or 20% solution; repeat at least one more time at a 7-to 10-day interval. Refractory cases may require more frequent (2- to 3-day interval) treatment. Severe, generalized, or refractory cases may require adjunctive treatment with antibiotics (eg, sulfas, aminoglycosides, or tetracyclines).[16]

SHEEP & GOATS:

Actinobacillosis | Woody tongue (extra-label): Potassium iodide 70 mg/kg IV slowly given as a 10% or 20% solution; repeat at least 1 more time at a 7- to 10-day interval. Refractory cases may require more frequent (2- to 3-day interval) treatment. Severe, generalized, or refractory cases may require adjunctive treatment with antibiotics (eg, sulfas, aminoglycosides, or tetracyclines).[16]

Monitoring

- Clinical efficacy
- Signs of iodism (eg, excessive tearing, nasal discharge, scaly haircoats/dandruff, hyperthermia, decreased milk production and weight gain, coughing, inappetence, and diarrhea)
- Thyroid function tests
- Liver enzymes

Client Information

- Nausea and vomiting (dogs, cats), unpleasant taste (which may make your animal difficult to give the medicine to) occurs commonly, especially if given on an empty stomach. Give the medicine with cream or high fat food. Compounded capsules may be easier to administer in some animals. Excessive tearing (lacrimation/tearing); may need to skip a dose if this is a problem.
- Long-term use or high doses can cause iodide toxicity (*iodism*), which may manifest as vomiting, inappetence, depression/lethargy, twitching, hypothermia, and heart failure. Contact your veterinarian if your animal shows any of these signs.
- Do not use if medicine turns brownish yellow.

Chemistry/Synonyms

Sodium iodide occurs as colorless, odorless crystals, or white crystalline powder. It develops a brown tint upon degradation. Approximately 1 g is soluble in 0.6 mL of water and 2 mL of alcohol.

Potassium iodide occurs as a clear to white granular powder. Approximately 1 g is soluble in 0.7 mL of water. One gram (one mL) of *SSKI®* contains 6 mEq of potassium.

Potassium iodide oral solution may also be known as *SSKI®* (super saturated potassium iodide), or *Pima®*.

Storage/Stability

Commercially available veterinary injectable products should generally be stored at room temperature (15°C-30°C [59°F-86°F]).

Super saturated potassium iodide (*SSKI®*) solution should be stored below 40°C (104°F) and preferably between 15°C and 30°C (59°F-86°F) in a tight, light-resistant container; protect from freezing. Crystallization can occur, particularly if stored at low temperatures; re-warming the contents and shaking will usually redissolve the crystals. If oxidation occurs, the solution will turn brownish yellow in color; discard if this occurs.

Compatibility/Compounding Considerations

Compatibility is dependent on factors such as pH, concentration, temperature, and diluent used; specialized references or a hospital pharmacist should be consulted for more specific information.

Sodium iodide injection is reportedly physically **incompatible** with injectable vitamins B and C.

Dosage Forms/Regulatory Status

VETERINARY-LABELED PRODUCTS:

Sodium Iodide Injection: 20 g/100 mL (20%; 200 mg/mL) in 250 mL vials—available as multi- or single-use vials; generic; (Rx). Labeled for use in nonlactating cattle

Oral iodide powders/granules for addition to feeds are available. Active ingredient is ethylenediamine dihydroiodide.

HUMAN-LABELED PRODUCTS:

Potassium Iodide Solution: 1 g potassium iodide/mL (*SSKI®*); generic; (Rx)

Potassium Iodide Oral Syrup: 62.5 mg potassium iodide/mL (325 mg/5 mL) in pints and gallons; *Pima®*; (Rx)

Potassium Iodide Oral Tablets 65 mg and 130 mg; *Thyrosafe®*, *losat®*; (OTC)

There are also radioactive iodine compounds available for thyroid diagnostic and treatment.

References

For the complete list of references, see **wiley.com/go/budde/plumb**

Iohexol

(eye-oh-***hex***-ol) *Omnipaque®*
Contrast Agent

Prescriber Highlights

- ▶ Nonionic, iodinated contrast agent used in medical imaging and to estimate GFR
- ▶ Contraindications include prior hypersensitivity to iohexol or other iodine-based contrast agents.
- ▶ Some formulations are contraindicated for intrathecal use; select product for intrathecal use carefully.
- ▶ Use with caution in animals with renal or hepatic impairment, cardiovascular disease, pheochromocytoma, hyperthyroidism, monoclonal gammopathy, or a history of seizures.
- ▶ Adverse effects associated with intravascular use may include hypersensitivity and nephrotoxicity; oral use may cause nausea, vomiting, and diarrhea.
- ▶ Ensure animals are well hydrated prior to iohexol administration.

Uses/Indications

Iohexol, when used as a contrast agent, can be administered (depending on product and procedure) via intravascular (ie, arterial, venous), intrathecal, intracavitary, subcutaneous, or oral routes.

Iohexol can be used as a marker agent for calculating glomerular filtration rates (GFR),[1,2] although the technique requires inputting results from limited-sample iohexol testing into mathematical formulae that have been suggested for dogs[3,4] and cats.[5] Using iohexol clearance to estimate GFR may be useful for the diagnosis of chronic kidney disease (CKD) before the onset of azotemia and when other indicators of renal function (eg, creatinine, symmetric dimethylarginine [SDMA]) are borderline or inconclusive.[6] It may also be used to monitor progression of CKD, especially in those with sarcopenia for which serum creatinine measurements may not accurately reflect declines in GFR. Iohexol clearance tests may also help inform dosage adjustments for nephrotoxic drugs (eg, carboplatin, aminoglycosides).

Pharmacology/Actions

Iohexol is a near-ideal marker for measuring glomerular filtration rate and, thereby, renal function. Its protein binding is negligible; it is nearly 100% excreted unchanged in the urine within 24 hours and can be measured in plasma using a variety of assays.

When used as a radio-contrast agent, organic iodine is relatively radiopaque and can help define adjacent structures.

Iohexol has a lower osmolality when compared with conventional (ionic) radio-contrast agents and, in humans, has been associated with a lower incidence of adverse effects, such as pain, heat sensations, adverse hemodynamic changes, electrocardiographic changes, and endothelial and erythrocyte damage.

Pharmacokinetics

After intravascular administration, iohexol is rapidly distributed throughout the circulation. Protein binding is very low (less than 1%). Within 24 hours, nearly 100% of a dose is excreted in the urine in patients with normal renal function. In dogs, mean pharmacokinetic parameters reported include volume of distribution (Vdss), 221 mL/kg; clearance in dog: about 2.5 – 2.9 mL/kg/minute; mean residence time, 82 minutes; and elimination half-life, 75 minutes.[3,7] Mean clearances of iohexol in cats reported include 2.3 mL/kg/minute[8] and 2.75 mL/kg/minute.[7]

Iohexol has an elimination half-life of about 2 hours in humans.

Contraindications/Precautions/Warnings

Iohexol is contraindicated in patients with a prior hypersensitivity reaction to it.[9] Use with caution in patients with severe renal or hepatic impairment, severe cardiovascular disease, hyperthyroidism, monoclonal gammopathy, or pheochromocytoma.[9] In humans, patients with allergy-mediated disease (eg, asthma, food allergies) may be at increased risk for idiosyncratic reactions to iohexol. Caution is advised for administration in humans with a history of seizures. Use of contrast medium volumes greater than 8 mL and injection into the cerbellomedullary cistern should be avoided in large dogs undergoing myelography.[10,11]

Patients should be well hydrated prior to and following iohexol administration.

Adverse Effects

When used intravascularly, iohexol appears to be well tolerated in animals, but data are limited. In humans, iohexol is considered one of the least toxic contrast agents, rarely causing nephrotoxicity or hypersensitivity reactions. The oral products have been associated with diarrhea, nausea, and vomiting in humans; data are lacking in veterinary species. In dogs, it has been shown that seizures are more likely to be precipitated when large volumes (but not concentration[12]) of iohexol are administered, contrast agent is injected into the cerebellomedullary cistern, and in large breed dogs with cervical lesions.[11]

Reproductive/Nursing Safety

Iohexol use in laboratory animals has not impaired fertility or demonstrated evidence of fetal harm.[6]

Iohexol is distributed into milk in very low quantities, but no adverse effects have been seen in breastfeeding infants whose mothers received iohexol; iohexol is usually compatible with breastfeeding.[13]

Because safety has not been established in animals, this drug should only be used when the maternal benefits outweigh the potential risks to offspring.

Overdose/Acute Toxicity

The adverse effects of IV overdose can be serious and life-threatening and primarily affect the pulmonary and cardiovascular systems. Clinical signs can include cyanosis, bradycardia, acidosis, pulmonary hemorrhage, convulsions, coma, and cardiac arrest[9]; treatment is supportive.

For patients that have experienced or are suspected to have experienced an overdose, consultation with a 24-hour poison consultation center specializing in providing veterinary-specific information is recommended. For general information related to overdose and toxin exposures, as well as contact information for poison control centers, refer to ***Appendix***.

Drug Interactions

The following drug interactions have either been reported or are theoretical in humans or animals receiving iohexol and may be of significance in veterinary patients. Unless otherwise noted, use together is not necessarily contraindicated, but weigh the potential risks and perform additional monitoring when appropriate.

- Beta-Adrenergic Receptor Antagonists (eg, **atenolol, propranolol**): Concurrent use reduces the threshold for and increases the severity of contrast reactions. Use together cautiously.
- CNS Stimulants (eg, **caffeine**, **doxapram**): Concurrent use with iohexol (especially when used intrathecally) may increase the risk for lowering seizure threshold.
- Iodine Isotopes: Iohexol may alter binding to thyroid tissue for up to two weeks.
- Metformin: Injection of iodinated contrast materials in metformin-treated human patients has been associated with lactic acidosis and can lead to acute renal failure.
- Monoamine Oxidase Inhibitors (MAOIs; eg, **amitraz, linezolid, selegiline**): Concurrent use with iohexol (especially when used intrathecally) may increase the risk for lowering seizure threshold.

- **Phenothiazines** (eg, **acepromazine, chlorpromazine**): Concurrent use with iohexol (especially when used intrathecally) may increase the risk for lowering seizure threshold.
- **QT Prolongation Drugs** (eg, **amiodarone, cisapride, procainamide, quinidine, sotalol**): Iohexol may cause additive prolongation of QT interval.
- **Tricyclic Antidepressants** (**TCAs**; eg, **amitriptyline, clomipramine**): Concurrent use with iohexol (especially when used intrathecally) may increase the risk for lowering seizure threshold.

Laboratory Considerations

- **Thyroid Function Tests**: If iodine-containing isotopes are to be used for diagnosing thyroid disease, prior use of iohexol can reduce the iodine-binding capacity of thyroid tissue for up to 2 weeks.[9] Thyroid function tests that do not depend on iodine estimation are not affected.

Dosages

NOTES:

1. Do not confuse dosages listed as mg/kg iohexol with mg/kg iodine content.
2. Iohexol concentrations of 180 mg/mL or 240 mg/mL are most commonly recommended. See *Chemistry/Synonyms*.
3. Ensure animals are well hydrated prior to iohexol administration.

DOGS:

Estimating glomerular filtration rate (extra-label):

a) A study done in healthy dogs uses an iohexol solution containing 300 mg iodine/mL. Administered doses varied from 129 – 658 mg/kg of iohexol IV over ≈1 minute. Using the 2-sample method, samples were obtained at 2 and 3 hours postdose; with the 3-sample method, samples were obtained at 2, 3, and 4 hours postdose.[3]

b) Iohexol 64.7 mg/kg IV administered over 1 minute.[4] Samples were obtained for the 1-, 2-, or 3- sample method at 60, 90, and 180 minutes, respectively; samples were obtained for the 5-sample method at 5, 15, 60, 90, and 180 minutes.

c) In a study, dogs were administered iohexol at a dose of 90 mg iodine content/kg in nonazotemic animals and 45 mg iodine content/kg in azotemic animals IV. Three samples were drawn at 120, 180, and 240 minutes in non-azotemic animals; 120, 240, and 360 minutes in azotemic animals[7]

GI contrast agent (extra-label):

a) **Suspected GI perforation**: Using iohexol solution containing 240 mg iodine/mL administered at 700 – 875 mg iodine/kg PO; best administered via orogastric tube (dogs). Radiographs should be obtained immediately following administration of contrast material; additional sets of radiographs can be obtained at 15, 30, and 60 minutes.[14]

b) **Dual-purpose contrast medium for radiography and ultrasonography**: Using iohexol 647 mg/mL, iohexol 1.5 mL/kg combined with carboxymethylcellulose 0.5% 8.5 mL/kg and administered PO, provided radiographic contrast enhancement of the small intestines without interfering with ultrasonographic assessment of the small intestines.[15]

CATS

Estimating GFR (extra-label):

a) Using a 3-sample method to estimate iohexol clearance: In the study, animals were administered iohexol at a dose of 90 mg iodine content/kg in non-azotemic animals and 45 mg iodine content/kg in azotemic animals IV. Three samples were drawn (at 120, 180, and 240 minutes in non-azotemic animals; 120, 240, and 360 minutes in azotemic animals).[16]

b) 647 mg/kg iohexol IV followed by 1 mL of saline (0.9% NaCl) solution administered to 20 healthy adult and geriatric cats, and a formula for correcting slope-intercept plasma iohexol clearance to estimate GFR was derived.[5]

Contrast agent for patients with suspected GI perforation (extra-label): The recommended dose is a 1:3 dilution of iohexol 240 at 10 mL/kg of body weight; best administered via nasogastric/nasoesophageal tube. Radiographs should be obtained immediately following the administration of contrast material; additional sets of radiographs can be obtained at 15, 30, and 60 minutes.[14]

HORSES

Estimating GFR (extra-label): 75.5 mg/kg iohexol IV rapid bolus over 1 minute, with plasma iohexol samples measured at 5, 30, and 90 minutes after administration[17]

BIRDS:

Contrast agent (extra-label):

a) 2 – 3 mL/kg IV over 3 to 5 seconds[18,19]

b) In mid-size psittacines using iohexol 240, administer 25 – 30 mL/kg into the crop; solution may be diluted 1:1 with water.[20]

Intestinal permeability (extra-label): 1 mL/kg PO using iohexol 755 mg/mL solution; plasma iohexol concentration was measured 45, 90, and 180 minutes after administration.[21]

RABBITS:

Contrast agent (extra-label): 64.7 mg/kg iohexol (0.1 mL/kg using 300 mg/mL organic iodine) IV rapid bolus over 1 minute[22]

REPTILES

Estimating GFR in green iguanas (extra-label): 75 mg/kg iohexol given IV[23]; blood samples to measure plasma iohexol concentrations are collected at 4, 8, and 24 hours postinjection.

Monitoring

- No specific monitoring outside of adverse effects and hypersensitivity reactions

Client Information

- Only veterinarians administer this medication.
- Patients should be well hydrated prior to and following iohexol administration.

Chemistry/Synonyms

Iohexol is a nonionic iodinated contrast agent that occurs as a white to off-white, hygroscopic, odorless powder; it is very soluble in water and methyl alcohol; it is practically insoluble or insoluble in chloroform and ether. Commercial products list the concentration of the product as organic iodine concentration per mL. For example, *Omnipaque® 180* contains iohexol 288 mg/mL, equivalent to 180 mg/mL of organic iodine content. Iohexol's molecular weight is 821 g/mol. Physical properties of iohexol injection include:

Concentration (mg/mL) organic iodine	Osmolality (mOsm/kg H_2O)	Viscosity (cp) @20°C (68°F)	Viscosity (cp) @37°C (98.6°F)	Specific gravity (g/mL) @37°C (98.6°F)
180	408	3.1	2	1.209
210	460	4.2	2.5	1.244
240	520	5.8	3.4	1.280
300	672	11.8	6.3	1.349
350	844	20.4	10.4	1.406

Iohexol may also be known as WIN-39424, iohexolum, ioheksoli, or ioheksolis. A common trade name is *Omnipaque®*.

Storage/Stability

Store iohexol at room temperature (20-25°C [68-77°F]); excursions permitted between 15°C and 30°C (59°F-86°F). Protect from light; do not freeze. Product may be stored in a contrast media warmer for up to one month at 36° to 38°C (96.8° to 100.4°F).

Compatibility/Compounding Considerations

Compatibility is dependent on factors such as pH, concentration, temperature, and diluent used; specialized references or a hospital pharmacist should be consulted for more specific information.

Depending on the concentration, the following drugs are reported **compatible** with iohexol: ampicillin, chloramphenicol sodium succinate, cimetidine, diazepam, diphenhydramine, epinephrine, gentamicin, heparin, hydrocortisone sodium succinate, lidocaine, methylprednisolone sodium succinate, nitroglycerin, protamine, and vasopressin.

Dosage Forms/Regulatory Status

VETERINARY-LABELED PRODUCTS: NONE

HUMAN-LABELED PRODUCTS:

Iohexol Injection (preservative-free; concentrations are listed as organic iodine content per mL): 140 mg/mL, 180 mg/mL, 240 mg/mL, 300 mg/mL, and 350 mg/mL in 10 mL, 20 mL, 30 mL, 50 mL, 75 mL, 100 mL, 125 mL, 150 mL, 200 mL, and 500 mL vials or bottles (depending on concentration); *Omnipaque®*; (Rx).

References

For the complete list of references, see **wiley.com/go/budde/plumb**

Ipratropium

(eye-prah-***troh***-pee-um) *Atrovent®*

Inhaled Antimuscarinic

Prescriber Highlights

- Inhaled antimuscarinic agent for adjunctive treatment of bronchoconstrictive conditions
- Contraindications include hypersensitivity to it or other atropine derivatives.
- Use caution in animals with narrow-angle glaucoma, bladder neck obstruction, or prostatic hypertrophy.
- Little information available for use in veterinary species
- Likely safe; because medication is inhaled, systemic absorption is minimal.
- May need to be administered quite often; duration of activity is relatively short.

Uses/Indications

Locally administered (inhaled) ipratropium bromide can be used for the adjunctive treatment of bronchospastic conditions (recurrent airway obstruction [RAO]; heaves). Although ipratropium has been shown to have bronchodilatory effects in experimentally induced bronchoconstriction in cats[1-3] and may prove beneficial for the short-term treatment of bronchospasm, additional research is required to determine its role for clinical use. A combination of ipratropium and albuterol (salbutamol) had greater bronchodilatory effects than ipratropium alone.[2,4]

Ipratropium had little or no effect on exercise capacity in healthy horses or horses with equine asthma.[5,6]

Pharmacology/Actions

Ipratropium inhibits vagally mediated reflexes by antagonizing acetylcholine. Increases in intracellular concentrations of cyclic guanosine monophosphate (cyclic GMP) secondary to acetylcholine are prevented, thereby reducing bronchial smooth muscle constriction. Unlike atropine, ipratropium does not reduce mucociliary clearance.

Pharmacokinetics

Because the medication is inhaled, minimal drug is absorbed in the systemic circulation. In humans, elimination half-life is about 2 hours. In healthy cats, with experimentally induced bronchospasm, inhaled (nebulized) ipratropium gave maximal efficacy for about 4 hours. When combined with albuterol (salbutamol), increased efficacy resulted.[3] In horses, onset of action is ≈30 minutes and duration of effect is ≈4 to 6 hours.

Contraindications/Precautions/Warnings

Ipratropium is contraindicated in patients that are hypersensitive to it or other atropine derivatives.

It should be used with caution in other conditions where antimuscarinics may be harmful, including narrow-angle glaucoma, bladder-neck obstruction, or prostatic hypertrophy.

Adverse Effects

Adverse effects are unlikely to be significant. Tracheal or bronchial irritation (coughing) has been reported on occasion. Allergic responses are possible, and some patients develop systemic anticholinergic effects.

Reproductive/Nursing Safety

Large oral dosages in laboratory animals did not cause teratogenic effects.

Ipratropium is likely to be safe to use during nursing.

Overdose/Acute Toxicity

Overdose is unlikely to be a cause for concern. The drug is not well absorbed orally or after inhalation and oral LD_{50} values for laboratory animals were greater than 1 g/kg.

For patients that have experienced or are suspected to have experienced an overdose, consultation with a 24-hour poison consultation center specializing in providing veterinary-specific information is recommended. For general information related to overdose and toxin exposures, as well as contact information for poison control centers, refer to ***Appendix***.

Drug Interactions

The following drug interactions have either been reported or are theoretical in humans or animals receiving ipratropium and may be of significance in veterinary patients. Unless otherwise noted, use together is not necessarily contraindicated, but weigh the potential risks and perform additional monitoring when appropriate.

- **ANTICHOLINERGIC DRUGS** (eg, **atropine**): May cause additive antimuscarinic effects
- **BETA-ADRENERGIC AGONISTS** (eg, **albuterol**): May have additive therapeutic effects[2,4]

Laboratory Considerations

- No specific concerns were noted.

Dosages

HORSES:

Adjunctive treatment of RAO, heaves (mild to moderate disease) (extra-label): For adult horses, most recommend 180 µg aerosol per horse (NOT µg/kg) inhaled via an equine specific mask every 6 hours (range every 4 to 8 hours). A study in 6 adult horses with heaves were given ipratropium 0.3 mg (300 µg) per horse (NOT µg/kg) via inhalation. Results indicated that some indices of airway function were improved for between 6 to 24 hours after ipratropium administration; however, clinical scores for breathing effort were not clinically significant.[7]

Severe bronchospasm in foals with pneumonia (extra-label): 2 – 3 µg/kg via aerosol every 6 to 8 hours in addition to inhaled albuterol[8]

SMALL MAMMALS:

Bronchodilator in rats (extra-label): One puff (17 µg/puff) into nebulization chamber twice daily[9]

Monitoring

- Clinical efficacy

Client Information

- If using the aerosol metered dose inhalers, do not use after dose indication reaches 0, even if there appears to be medication remaining; active ingredient cannot be assured; do not shake the canister before using.
- Normally given as an aerosol into the lungs, often with other drugs, to help your animal breathe better. Special masks for dogs, cats, and horses are usually used.
- Ipratropium is usually safe but irritation of the throat and lungs can occur.
- No need to shake aerosol before each use. Prime (2 sprays) before first using or if not used in past 3 days.
- Do not store aerosol canister in hot places or dispose of it by burning it.

Chemistry/Synonyms

Ipratropium bromide has a quaternary ammonium structure and occurs as a white or almost white crystalline powder. It is soluble in water and slightly soluble in alcohol. The pH of a 1% solution is between 5 to 7.5.

Ipratropium bromide may also be known as Sch-1000; many trade names are available including *Atrovent®*.

Storage/Stability

The solution for inhalation should be stored at room temperature and protected from light. Keep in foil pouch until time of use. The metered dose inhalers should be stored at room temperature.

Compatibility/Compounding Considerations

The solution for nebulization may be mixed with albuterol or metaproterenol if used within 1 hour.

Dosage Forms/Regulatory Status

VETERINARY-LABELED PRODUCTS: NONE

HUMAN-LABELED PRODUCTS:

Ipratropium Bromide Solution for Inhalation: 0.02% (500 µg/vial) preservative free in 25, 30, and 60 unit-dose vials (2.5 mL UD "nebs"); generic; (Rx)

Ipratropium Bromide Aerosol for Inhalation: each actuation delivers 17 µg from the mouthpiece in 12.9 g metered dose inhaler w/mouthpiece (approx. 200 inhalations); *Atrovent® HFA*; (Rx)

Available in combination with albuterol for nebulization (*DuoNeb®*; Rx), and as a metered dose inhaler (*Combivent®* HFA; Rx)

Nasal sprays also are available.

References

For the complete list of references, see **wiley.com/go/budde/plumb**

Irbesartan

(ihr-beh-***sar***-tan) *Avapro®*

Angiotensin-II Receptor Blocker (ARB)

Prescriber Highlights

- ► May be useful in the treatment of dogs and cats with hypertension secondary to renal disease
- ► Limited experience in veterinary medicine
- ► Contraindicated for use during pregnancy
- ► Adverse effect profile is not established in dogs and cats, but GI effects, somnolence, hypotension, or activity changes are possible based on adverse effects in humans.

Uses/Indications

Irbesartan may be useful in dogs and cats for the treatment of hypertension associated with renal insufficiency or for proteinuria associated with glomerular disease in combination with an ACE inhibitor; however, experience in veterinary medicine is limited. It may be effective in the adjunctive treatment of heart failure when dogs are unable to tolerate ACE inhibitors, but documentation for this use is lacking. One study, using high irbesartan dosages (60 mg/kg PO twice daily) in dogs with subacute mitral regurgitation, demonstrated no improvement in left ventricular function or prevention of left ventricular remodeling.[1] An experimental study in cats showed that irbesartan at 2 mg/kg, 6 mg/kg, or 10 mg/kg significantly reduced blood pressure associated with exogenously administered angiotensin at 90 minutes.[2]

Pharmacology/Actions

Irbesartan is an angiotensin-II receptor blocker (ARB). By selectively blocking the AT_1-receptor, aldosterone synthesis and secretion is reduced causing vasodilation, decreased potassium excretion, and increased sodium excretion. Although plasma concentrations of renin and angiotensin-II are increased, this does not counteract the blood pressure lowering effects of irbesartan. Irbesartan does not interfere with substance P or bradykinin responses.

Unlike losartan, another ARB, irbesartan does not need to be converted to an active metabolite.

Pharmacokinetics

After single 30 mg/kg oral doses of irbesartan in dogs with experimentally induced renal hypertension, peak concentrations occurred between 3 and 4 hours and elimination half-life was ≈9 hours. After 30 mg/kg doses PO once daily for 8 days, the elimination half-life was ≈21 hours.[3]

A pharmacokinetic/pharmacodynamic study in healthy beagles concluded that irbesartan 5 mg/kg is more appropriate than 2 mg/kg to obtain a hypotensive effect in beagles, but further studies are needed.[4]

In humans, absorption is rapid and bioavailability ranges from 60% to 80%.[5] Peak concentrations occur in ≈1.5 to 2 hours. Bioavailability is not altered by the presence of food. The drug is 90% bound to plasma proteins and weakly crosses the blood–brain barrier and placenta in small quantities. Irbesartan is metabolized in the liver via glucuronidation and oxidation; metabolites are not active. Both metabolites and unchanged drug are eliminated primarily in the feces and, to a lesser extent, urine. Terminal elimination half-life ranges from 11 to 15 hours. Dosages do not need to be adjusted in patients with renal dysfunction.

Contraindications/Precautions/Warnings

Patients that are volume- or sodium-depleted should have these corrected before starting therapy.[5] Do not use in hypotensive patients or patients hypersensitive to it. It should not be used during pregnancy (see ***Reproductive/Nursing Safety***).

Adverse Effects

Adverse effect profiles for dogs and cats are not known due to its limited veterinary use. In humans, the most commonly reported adverse effects include diarrhea, dyspepsia, fatigue, orthostatic dizziness, and hypotension.[5]

Reproductive/Nursing Safety

Irbesartan is not safe to use during pregnancy.[5] Studies in pregnant rats given high doses demonstrated a variety of fetal abnormalities (renal pelvic cavitation, hydroureter, absence of renal papilla). Smaller doses in rabbits caused increased maternal death and spontaneous abortion. In humans, the drug is considered teratogenic, particularly during the second and third trimesters.

Because small amounts of irbesartan have been detected in rat milk and there is significant concern about the safety of the drug in neonates, it is not recommended for use in nursing women.

Overdose/Acute Toxicity

Rats and mice survived acute oral overdoses in excess of 2000 mg/kg.[5] Likely effects seen in an overdose situation include hypotension and either bradycardia or tachycardia; treatment is supportive.

For patients that have experienced or are suspected to have experienced an overdose, consultation with a 24-hour poison consultation center specializing in providing veterinary-specific information is recommended. For general information related to overdose and toxin exposures, as well as contact information for poison control centers, refer to ***Appendix***.

Drug Interactions

The following drug interactions have either been reported or are theoretical in humans or animals receiving irbesartan and potentially could be of significance in veterinary patients. Unless otherwise noted, use together is not necessarily contraindicated, but weigh the potential risks and perform additional monitoring when appropriate.

- **Angiotensin Converting Enzyme Inhibitors** (**ACEIs**; eg, **benazepril, enalapril**): Increased risk for adverse effects (eg, hypotension, hyperkalemia, renal function changes); increased monitoring may be warranted. Combination is not recommended in humans.[5,6]
- **Aspirin**: Possible reduced antihypertensive effect of irbesartan and increased risk for renal impairment; increased monitoring may be warranted
- **Baclofen**: Concurrent use may have additive blood pressure lowering effects.
- **Benzodiazepines** (eg, **diazepam, lorazepam**): Concurrent use may increase risk for hypotension.
- **Buspirone**: Concurrent use may increase risk for hypotension.
- **Cabergoline**: Concurrent use may increase risk for hypotension.
- **Corticosteroids** (eg, **betamethasone, dexamethasone**): May decrease the antihypertensive effects of ARBs
- **Dexmedetomidine**: Concurrent use may result in additive effects on blood pressure and heart rate.
- **Diazoxide**: Concurrent use may increase risk for hypotension.
- **Dichlorphenamide**: Concurrent use may increase risk for hypotension.
- **Digoxin**: Concurrent use may increase digoxin concentrations. Closely monitor digoxin concentrations and therapeutic effects.
- **Diphenhydramine**: Concurrent use may increase risk for hypotension.
- **Doxepin**: Concurrent use may increase risk for hypotension.
- **Fluconazole**: Concurrent use may increase the concentration of irbesartan. Other azole antifungals (eg, itraconazole, ketoconazole) do not appear to have this effect.
- **Insulin**: Concurrent use may increase risk for hypoglycemia.
- **Lithium**: Concurrent use may increase risk for lithium toxicity.
- **Low Molecular Weight Heparins** (eg, **dalteparin, enoxaparin**): Concurrent use may increase risk for hyperkalemia.
- **Nonsteroidal Anti-Inflammatory Drugs** (**NSAIDs**; eg, **carprofen, meloxicam**): Possible reduced antihypertensive effects of irbesartan and increased risk for renal impairment; increased monitoring may be warranted
- **Opioids** (eg, **buprenorphine, butorphanol**): Concurrent use may increase risk for hypotension.
- **Potassium Preparations**: Increased risk for hyperkalemia; increased monitoring of serum potassium may be warranted.
- **Potassium-Sparing Diuretics** (eg, **spironolactone**): Increased risk for hyperkalemia; increased monitoring of serum potassium may be warranted.
- **Yohimbine**: Concurrent use may decrease the efficacy of ARBs.

Laboratory Considerations

- No specific concerns noted

Dosages

DOGS/CATS:

Hypertension, proteinuria, and heart failure (extra-label): 5 mg/kg PO every 12 to 24 hours has been recommended anecdotally for dogs. Dosages for cats are still mostly unknown although the drug does seem to have efficacy for angiotensin-induced hypertension.[2]

Monitoring

- Blood pressure, heart rate
- Baseline and periodic serum electrolytes, BUN, and creatinine
- Adverse effects, possibly including GI effects, somnolence, or activity changes

Client Information

- This medicine may be given with or without food. If your animal vomits or acts sick after getting it on an empty stomach, give it with food or a small treat to see if this helps. If vomiting continues, contact your veterinarian.
- Because this medicine has not been used often in dogs or cats, watch carefully for any side effects and report them to your veterinarian. Possible side effects include diarrhea, vomiting, lack of appetite, fatigue (tiredness), and low blood pressure. Signs of low blood pressure may include fainting, muscle weakness, or exercise intolerance.
- This medicine has caused birth defects and should not be used in pregnant animals. Pregnant women should wear disposable gloves when handling and wash hands after administering this medication.

Chemistry/Synonyms

Irbesartan is a nonpeptide angiotensin-II antagonist and occurs as a white to off-white, crystalline powder. It is practically insoluble in water and slightly soluble in alcohol.

Irbesartan may also be known as BMS 186295, SR 47436, Irbesartanum, *Aprovel*®, *Arbit*®, *Avalide*®, *Avapro*®, *Cavapro*®, *Coaproval*®, *Ecard*®, *Ibsan*®, *Irban*®, *Irbes*®, *Iretensa*®, *Irovel*®, *Irvell*®, *Isart*®, and *Karvea*®.

Storage/Stability

Irbesartan tablets should be stored at room temperature (15°C-30°C [59°F-86°F]).

Compatibility/Compounding Considerations

No specific information noted

Dosage Forms/Regulatory Status

VETERINARY-LABELED PRODUCTS: NONE

The Association of Racing Commissioners International (ARCI) has designated this drug as a class 3 substance. Use of this drug may not be allowed in certain animal competitions. Check rules and regulations before entering in a competition while this medication is being administered. Contact local racing authorities for further guidance.

HUMAN-LABELED PRODUCTS:

Irbesartan Tablets: 75 mg, 150 mg, and 300 mg; *Avapro*®, generic; (Rx)

Irbesartan 150 mg with Hydrochlorothiazide 12.5 mg tablets and Irbesartan 300 mg with Hydrochlorothiazide 12.5 mg or 25 mg tablets; *Avalide*®, generic; (Rx)

Irbesartan is also available in fixed dose combinations with hydrochlorothiazide.

References

For the complete list of references, see **wiley.com/go/budde/plumb**

Iron Dextran

(***eye***-urn ***dex***-tran)

Iron preparation; Hematinic

Prescriber Highlights

- Iron supplement that may be used alone or with hematopoietic agents in small animals
- Contraindications include known hypersensitivity to iron dextran, and the presence of any anemia other than iron deficiency anemia.
- Use with caution in patients with significant hepatic impairment, during the acute phase of infectious kidney disease, or in conjunction with oral iron supplements.
- Adverse effects include pain with IM injection, prostration, muscular weakness, and anaphylactic-type reactions.
- Do not give IV or SC.
- High doses may cause increased incidences of teratogenicity and embryotoxicity.
- Piglets born from vitamin E- or selenium-deficient sows may demonstrate nausea, vomiting, and sudden death within 1 hour of injection.
- IM use in pigs beyond 4 weeks of age may cause muscle tissue staining.

Uses/Indications

Iron dextran is used in the treatment and prophylaxis of iron deficiency anemia, primarily in neonatal food-producing animals. It is also administered when dogs or cats receive erythropoiesis-stimulating agents, such as epoetin (EPO) or darbepoetin (DPO).

Pharmacology/Actions

Iron is necessary for myoglobin and hemoglobin in the transport and utilization of oxygen. During iron deficient states, iron supplementation restores total body iron and hemoglobin concentrations to improve clinical signs associated with the deficiency; however, it does not stimulate erythropoiesis or correct hemoglobin abnormalities.

Ionized iron is a component of the cytochrome oxidase, succinic dehydrogenase, and xanthine oxidase enzymes.

Pharmacokinetics

After IM injection, iron dextran is slowly absorbed primarily via the lymphatic system. About 60% of the iron is absorbed within 3 days of injection, and up to 90% of the dose is absorbed after 1 to 3 weeks; the remaining iron may be absorbed slowly over several months.

After absorption, the reticuloendothelial cells of the liver, spleen, and bone marrow gradually clear the iron from plasma. The dextran component is cleaved and then metabolized or excreted, and the iron component is made available to form hemosiderin, ferritin, or transferrin.

Iron is not readily eliminated from the body. Iron liberated by the destruction of hemoglobin is reused by the body, and only small amounts are lost by the body via hair and nail growth, normal skin desquamation, and GI tract sloughing. Accumulation and potential iron overload can occur with repeated dosing as only trace amounts of iron are eliminated in the feces, bile, or urine.

Contraindications/Precautions/Warnings

Iron dextran is contraindicated in patients with known hypersensitivity to it or with any anemia other than iron deficiency anemia. In humans, it is recommended to not use iron dextran in patients in the acute phase of pyelonephritis. Use with caution in patients with significant hepatic impairment or evidence of iron overload. Patients with significant allergies and/or asthma may be at higher risk for hypersensitivity reactions.[1] Parenteral iron supplementation should not be used concurrently with oral iron supplements.

Iron dextran should only be administered IM; do not administer SC (poor absorption). While IV administration is performed in human patients, safe use of iron dextran IV has not been documented in veterinary patients.

Observe the patient after dosing as rarely anaphylactic-type reactions can occur. See ***Monitoring***.

Adverse Effects

Prostration and muscular weakness may occasionally occur in pigs after iron dextran injection. Iron dextran used in pigs born from vitamin E- or selenium-deficient sows may demonstrate nausea, vomiting, and sudden death within 1 hour of injection. Iron dextran injected IM in pigs beyond 4 weeks of age may cause muscle tissue staining.

Pain on IM injection can occur.[1] Anaphylactic-type reactions (that may result in death) are rare but can occur. Chronic overdoses can cause iron overload and hemosiderosis.

Repeated IM doses (large or small) in the same injection site have been associated with the development of sarcomas in laboratory animals (eg, rabbits, mice, rats, hamsters).[1]

Reproductive/Nursing Safety

Iron crosses the placenta but in what form is unknown. High doses (≈3 times the recommended human dose) may cause increased incidences of teratogenicity and embryotoxicity.[1] Traces of unmetabolized iron dextran are excreted in milk.[1]

Because safety has not been established in animals, this drug should only be used when the maternal benefits outweigh the potential risks to offspring.

Overdose/Acute Toxicity

Overdose of iron dextran is unlikely to cause acute manifestations; however, it may lead to hemosiderosis.[1] Chelation therapy may be required depending on the extent of the overdose. See ***Deferoxamine***. Iron dextran is not dialyzable.[2]

For patients that have experienced or are suspected to have experienced an overdose, consultation with a 24-hour poison consultation center specializing in providing veterinary-specific information is recommended. For general information related to overdose and toxin exposures, as well as contact information for poison control centers, refer to ***Appendix***.

Drug Interactions

The following drug interactions have either been reported or are theoretical in humans or animals receiving iron and may be of significance in veterinary patients. Unless otherwise noted, use together is not necessarily contraindicated, but weigh the potential risks and perform additional monitoring when appropriate.

- **Angiotensin-Converting Enzyme Inhibitors** (ACEIs; eg, **benazepril, enalapril**): In humans, concurrent use of ACE Inhibitors may increase the risk for anaphylactic-type reactions[1]; veterinary significance is uncertain.
- **Chloramphenicol**: Because chloramphenicol may delay the response to iron administration, avoid using it in patients with iron deficiency anemia.
- **Dimercaprol (BAL)**: Concurrent use may increase the risk for nephrotoxicity.
- **Mycophenolate**: Concurrent use may result in decreased efficacy of mycophenolate mofetil.

Laboratory Considerations

- Large doses of injectable iron may discolor the serum to brown and result in falsely elevated **serum bilirubin** values and falsely decreased **serum calcium** values.
- After large doses of iron dextran, **serum iron** values may not be meaningful for up to 3 weeks.

Dosages

DOGS:

Iron supplementation in association with erythropoiesis-stimulating agents (EPO, DPO; extra-label): 10-20 mg/kg IM,[3] to a maximum of 300 mg/dog, at the time EPO or DPO therapy is initiated; generally, no more than once monthly administration is needed.

Iron deficiency anemia: 10 – 20 mg/kg once IM.[3-5] Iron dextran may be repeated at weekly intervals or administered once and followed by oral therapy with ferrous sulfate (see ***Ferrous Sulfate***).[4,6]

CATS:

Iron supplementation in association with erythropoiesis-stimulating agents (EPO, DPO; extra-label): At the time EPO or DPO therapy is initiated, most recommend a single injection of 50 mg/cat (NOT mg/kg) IM[5,7,8] (≈10 mg/kg); generally, no more than once monthly administration is needed.

Prevention of transient neonatal iron deficiency anemia (extra-label): 50 mg/kitten (NOT mg/kg) IM at 18 days of age[6]

Iron deficiency anemia: 50 mg/cat (NOT mg/kg) IM every 3 to 4 weeks[3]

SWINE:

Prevention or treatment of iron deficiency anemia in baby pigs; (label dosage; FDA-approved):

- Using 100 mg of elemental iron/mL solution: 100 mg/piglet (NOT mg/kg) IM at 2 to 4 days of age[9]; inject into the back of the ham. For treatment of iron deficiency anemia, dose may be repeated in ≈10 days.[9]
- Using 200 mg of elemental iron/mL solution: 200 mg/piglet (NOT mg/kg) IM at 1 to 3 days of age; inject into the back of the ham to a depth of at least ½ inch. For treatment of iron deficiency anemia, administer 200 mg/piglet (NOT mg/kg) IM at the first signs of anemia.[10]

BIRDS:

Iron deficiency anemia or following hemorrhage (extra-label): 10 mg/kg IM; repeat in 7 to 10 days if indicated[11]

FERRETS:

Iron deficiency anemia (extra-label): 10 mg/kg IM once weekly[12]

Monitoring

- Baseline and periodic CBC including RBC indices (eg, MCV, MCHC). **NOTE**: RBC indices may take months to normalize.[4]
- Serum iron parameters (eg, ferritin) can be measured to monitor and approximate total body iron concentrations.[4]
- Adverse reactions

Client Information

- In small animal species (eg, dogs, cats), veterinarians administer iron dextran.
- In pigs, inject into the muscle to a depth of at least ½ inch in the back of the ham.
  - Use of this product beyond 4 weeks of age may result in staining of the ham muscle.
  - Disinfect vial stopper prior to use.

Chemistry/Synonyms

Iron dextran is a complex of ferric oxyhydroxide and low molecular weight partially hydrolyzed dextran derivative. The commercially available injection occurs as a dark brown, slightly viscous liquid that is completely miscible with water or normal saline and has a pH of 5.2 to 6.5.

Iron dextran may also be known as iron-dextran complex, *Cosmofer®*, *DexFerrum®*, *Dexiron®*, *Driken®*, *Fercayl®*, *Ferrocel®*, *Ferroin®*, *Ferrum Hausmann®*, *Fexiron®*, *Imferdex®*, *Imferon®*, *InFeD®*, *Uniferon®*, and *Infufer®*.

Storage/Stability

Store iron dextran injection at room temperature (15°C to 30°C [59°F-86°F]); avoid freezing. Discard vials 60 days after first use. The maximum allowable number of vial punctures varies by product and manufacturer -- consult product label.

Compatibility/Compounding Considerations

Iron dextran injection is reportedly physically **incompatible** when mixed with oxytetracycline HCl and sulfadiazine sodium.

Dosage Forms/Regulatory Status/Withdrawal Times

VETERINARY-LABELED PRODUCTS:

Iron Dextran Injection: 100 mg of elemental iron/mL in 100 mL vials and 200 mg of elemental iron/mL in 100 mL or 250 mL vials; *Uniferon®*, generic; (OTC). FDA-approved for use in swine; NADA #106-772 (100 mg/mL), 134-708 (200 mg/mL). No slaughter withdrawal time required.

HUMAN-LABELED PRODUCTS:

Iron Dextran Injection: 50 mg of elemental iron/mL (as dextran) in 2 mL single-dose vials; *InFeD®*; (Rx)

References

For the complete list of references, see **wiley.com/go/budde/plumb**

Isoflupredone

(eye-so-***floo***-preh-dohn) *Predef 2X®*

Injectable Glucocorticoid

For topical or otic use of isoflupredone, see ***Isoflupredone, Topical*** and ***Corticosteroid/Antimicrobial Preparations***

Prescriber Highlights

- ► Injectable glucocorticoid labeled for use in horses, cattle, and swine for anti-inflammatory and immunosuppressive effects
- ► Less likely to cause early parturition than dexamethasone or betamethasone, but avoid use in pregnancy
- ► May have mineralocorticoid effects in horses and cattle; hypokalemia has been noted

Uses/Indications

Isoflupredone acetate is a potent glucocorticoid and, like other glucocorticoids, can be used for its anti-inflammatory or immunosuppressive effects. Labeled indications for isoflupredone include adjunctive treatment of bovine ketosis, alleviating pain and lameness associated with musculoskeletal conditions, acute hypersensitivity reactions, adjunctive treatment of overwhelming infections with severe toxicity (eg, critical pneumonia, peritonitis, endometritis, septic mastitis), shock, supportive therapy in the treatment of stress conditions (eg, surgery), dystocia, retained placenta, inflammatory ocular conditions, snakebite, and parturient paresis.

A study evaluating the effects of isoflupredone in dairy cows, with or without insulin (ultralente 100 units), on energy metabolism, milk production, and overall health during the early lactation phase showed that isoflupredone, with or without insulin, *offered no metabolic, production, or reproductive benefits in lactating dairy cattle.*[1] A study evaluating oxytetracycline, with or without isoflupredone acetate, for treating experimentally induced bronchopneumonia in heifers found that only animals receiving the combination prevented a reduction in dry matter intake and average daily gain (ADG).[2] However, the author of that study has subsequently stated that *Based on the existing literature, it is currently still not possible to fully determine* whether corticosteroids have *a clinical application in managing BRD. Differences in treatment outcomes between the limited corticosteroids that have been studied thus far may reflect the method used for BRD diagnosis in the feedlot setting, timing of medical intervention with respect to onset of infection, involvement of multiple respiratory pathogens in naturally occurring respiratory disease, or simply effects specific to the corticosteroids used.*[3]

In horses, isoflupredone has been used parenterally to reduce inflammation associated with recurrent airway obstruction (RAO; eg, heaves, COPD) as well as intra-articularly for treatment of joint inflammation.

Although the drug could be used in small animals, it is recommended to instead use other more common glucocorticoid agents that are FDA-approved for use in dogs and cats.

Pharmacology/Actions

Isoflupredone's anti-inflammatory potency is ≈17 times that of hydrocortisone (cortisol). The label states that the glucocorticoid activity of isoflupredone is 50 times that of hydrocortisone and 10 times that of prednisolone as measured by liver glycogen deposition in rats. Isoflupredone reportedly has some mineralocorticoid effects and can cause hypokalemia.

For more information on the pharmacologic actions associated with glucocorticoids, see ***Glucocorticoid Agents, General Information***.

Pharmacokinetics

No specific pharmacokinetic values were located. The manufacturer states that gluconeogenic activity persists for 48 hours after dosing in cattle.

Contraindications/Precautions/Warnings

Systemic use of glucocorticoids is generally considered contraindicated in systemic fungal infections (unless used for replacement therapy in patients with hyperadrenocorticism), when administered IM in patients with idiopathic thrombocytopenia, and in patients that are hypersensitive to a particular compound. Because of their ulcerogenic potential, glucocorticoids should be used with extreme caution in patients with active GI ulcers or those susceptible to them. Use this medicine cautiously in patients with diabetes mellitus.

Because isoflupredone can cause hypokalemia, it should not be used in downer cows or animals susceptible to the effects of hypokalemia.

Long-term use in young, growing animals must be undertaken cautiously, as decreased growth may occur.

Adverse Effects

Adverse effects are generally associated with long-term administration of glucocorticoids, particularly if given at higher dosages; these effects generally manifest as signs of hyperadrenocorticism. The drug can cause hypokalemia in dairy cattle, even from a single dose.[4,5] Potential adverse effects include reduced milk production, hypokalemia, delayed wound healing, GI ulceration, increased infection rates, diabetes mellitus exacerbation/hyperglycemia, pancreatitis, hepatopathy, renal dysfunction, osteoporosis, laminitis (horses), hypothyroidism, and hyperlipidemia. When administered to young, growing animals, glucocorticoids can delay growth.

Reproductive/Nursing Safety

Avoid using isoflupredone during pregnancy. Glucocorticoids can induce abortion or early parturition in the later stages of pregnancy; most commonly seen in ruminants. Although isoflupredone (like hydrocortisone, prednisolone, and triamcinolone) appears to have a much lower abortifacient potential than glucocorticoids such as dexamethasone, betamethasone, or flumethasone, it may induce premature parturition with retained placenta, and its use should generally be avoided during the later stages of pregnancy.

Glucocorticoids used during the first trimester have been linked to a variety of teratogenic effects in dogs and laboratory animals.[6]

Glucocorticoid administration may reduce milk production. Glucocorticoids unbound to plasma proteins will enter milk. High dosages or prolonged administration to mothers may potentially inhibit the growth of nursing newborns.

Because safety has not been established in animals, this drug should only be used when the maternal benefits outweigh the potential risks to offspring.

Overdose/Acute Toxicity

A single overdose of isoflupredone is unlikely to cause harmful effects. If clinical signs require intervention, use supportive treatment.

Long-term use of glucocorticoids can lead to serious adverse effects, which mainly manifest as signs of hyperadrenocorticism. Refer to ***Adverse Effects*** for additional details.

For patients that have experienced or are suspected to have experienced an overdose, consultation with a 24-hour poison consultation center specializing in providing veterinary-specific information is recommended. For general information related to overdose and toxin exposures, as well as contact information for poison control centers, refer to ***Appendix***.

Drug Interactions

The following drug interactions have either been reported or are theoretical in humans or animals receiving isoflupredone or other glucocorticoids and may be of significance in veterinary patients. Unless otherwise noted, use together is not necessarily contraindicated, but weigh the potential risks and perform additional monitoring when appropriate.

- DIGITALIS GLYCOSIDES (eg, **digoxin**): Increased chance of digitalis toxicosis may occur should hypokalemia develop; diligent monitoring of potassium and digitalis glycoside concentrations is recommended.
- FLUOROQUINOLONE ANTIBIOTICS (eg, **enrofloxacin, marbofloxacin**): Concurrent use with glucocorticoids may result in an increased risk for tendon rupture.
- INSULIN: Insulin requirements may increase in patients receiving glucocorticoids.
- POTASSIUM-DEPLETING DIURETICS (eg, **furosemide, thiazides**): Concomitant use may cause hypokalemia.
- SALICYLATES: Glucocorticoids may reduce salicylate blood concentrations.
- ULCEROGENIC DRUGS (eg, **NSAIDs**): Glucocorticoids may increase the risk for GI ulceration when given concomitantly.

- **Vaccines, Toxoids, Bacterins**: A diminished immune response may occur after vaccine, toxoid, or bacterin administration; patients receiving glucocorticoids at immunosuppressive dosages should generally not receive live attenuated-virus vaccines, as virus replication may be augmented.

Laboratory Considerations

- Glucocorticoids may increase **serum cholesterol**, and **serum** and **urine glucose** concentrations.
- Isoflupredone may decrease **serum potassium** concentration.
- Glucocorticoids can suppress the release of thyroid-stimulating hormone (TSH) and reduce $\mathbf{T_3}$ and $\mathbf{T_4}$ values; thyroid gland atrophy has been reported after long-term glucocorticoid administration.
- Reactions to **skin tests** may be suppressed by glucocorticoids.
- Glucocorticoids may cause false negative results of the **nitroblue tetrazolium test** for systemic bacterial infections.

Dosages

HORSES:

Labeled indications (label dosage; FDA-approved):

a. Systemic administration: 5 – 20 mg/horse (NOT mg/kg) IM, repeated as necessary[6]
b. Administration into joint cavity, tendon sheath or bursa: 5 – 20 mg or more (total dose, NOT mg/kg) depending on the size of the joint cavity.[6] Do not use in horses that are intended for human consumption.

Intra-articular administration (extra-label): 4 – 20 mg/joint (NOT mg/kg); has a short to medium duration of action[7]

Recurrent airway obstruction (RAO) (extra-label): In the study, 0.03 mg/kg IM once daily was used.[8] Patients were treated for 14 days; significant decreases in serum potassium concentration occurred.

CATTLE:

Labeled systemic indications (label dosage; FDA-approved): 10 – 20 mg/cow (NOT mg/kg) IM, according to the body size of the animal and severity of the condition. The dose may be repeated in 12 to 24 hours if indicated. See ***Compatibility/Compounding Considerations***.

SWINE:

Labeled systemic indications (label dosage; FDA-approved): 5 mg/136 kg (300 lb) pig (NOT mg/kg) IM.[6] Adjust dose proportionally for a smaller or larger animal.

Monitoring

- Single injections may not require monitoring beyond observation of the patient for efficacy and adverse effects but consider evaluating serum potassium concentration.
- Ongoing use requires enhanced monitoring including renal value and liver enzyme testing, CBC, blood glucose, and serum electrolytes.
- ACTH stimulation tests may be indicated to determine extent of HPA axis suppression.
- Consider thyroid hormone monitoring if use is prolonged or patient exhibits signs associated with thyroid hormone deficiency.

Client Information

- If this medication is used in dairy cattle, warn producer that milk production may be affected.
- If owners are to administer the medication, caution them to only administer as their veterinarian directs.
- Side effects become more likely the longer it is used and when given at higher dosages.

Chemistry/Synonyms

Isoflupredone acetate is a fluorinated synthetic corticosteroid with a molecular weight of 420.5. The commercial injection is in an aqueous suspension that also contains sodium citrate, polyethylene glycol 3350, and povidone.

Isoflupredone acetate may also be known as U-6013, 9-alpha-fluoroprednisolone acetate, and *Predef 2x*®.

Storage/Stability

The injection should be stored at controlled room temperature (20°C-25°C [68°F-77°F]).

Compatibility/Compounding Considerations

Compatibility is dependent on factors such as pH, concentration, temperature, and diluent used; specialized references or a hospital pharmacist should be consulted for more specific information.

Isoflupredone suspensions are **incompatible** with calcium-containing solutions (eg, lactated Ringer's solution).

Dosage Forms/Regulatory Status

VETERINARY-LABELED PRODUCTS:

The Association of Racing Commissioners International (ARCI) has designated this drug as a class 4 substance. Use of this drug may not be allowed in certain animal competitions. Check rules and regulations before entering in a competition while this medication is being administered. Contact local racing authorities for further guidance. See ***Appendix*** for more information.

Isoflupredone acetate 2 mg/mL aqueous suspension for injection in 100 mL vials; *Predef 2x*®; (Rx). In the United States, *Predef 2x*® is FDA-approved for use in cattle, horses, and swine.

Meat withdrawal time is 7 days; it is not to be used in calves to be processed for veal. A withdrawal period has not been established for this product in preruminating calves. There is no milk withdrawal time for isoflupredone in the United States, but in Canada a 72-hour withdrawal time is specified.

Isoflupredone is also found in some topical and otic products. For more information see ***Isoflupredone, Topical*** and ***Corticosteroid/Antimicrobial Preparations***.

HUMAN-LABELED PRODUCTS: NONE

References

For the complete list of references, see **wiley.com/go/budde/plumb**

Isoflurane

(eye-soe-***flure***-ane) *Isoflo*®, *Iso-Thesia*®

General Anesthetic, Inhalant

Prescriber Highlights

- Inhalant general anesthetic commonly used in a wide range of veterinary species
- Contraindications include a history of or predilection to malignant hyperthermia.
- Use with caution in patients with increased intracranial pressure, head injury, or myasthenia gravis.
- Adverse effects include dose-related hypotension, respiratory depression, and GI effects (eg, nausea, vomiting, ileus); cardiodepression is generally minimal at doses causing surgical planes of anesthesia. Arrhythmias are rare.

Uses/Indications

Isoflurane is an inhalant anesthetic commonly used in veterinary medicine. When compared with older anesthetics (eg, halothane, methoxyflurane), isoflurane has fewer myocardial depressant and catecholamine-sensitizing effects, and it can be used in patients with hepatic or renal disease. The newer inhalant anesthetics, sevoflurane (ability to change depth of anesthesia faster, not as irritating to respiratory system) and desflurane (very fast onset, faster recoveries), have some advantages over isoflurane, but are more expensive. Isoflurane with oxygen can be used for refractory status epilepticus in dogs that are refractory to benzodiazepine boluses; however, isoflurane can increase intracranial pressure.

Pharmacology/Actions

The precise mechanism of how inhalant anesthetics produce their general anesthetic effects is not known. They may interfere with the functioning of nerve cells in the brain by acting at $GABA_A$ receptors and voltage-gated channels.[1] Some key pharmacologic effects noted with isoflurane include CNS depression, depression of body temperature–regulating centers, increased cerebral blood flow, respiratory depression, vasodilatation (hypotension), myocardial depression (less so than with halothane), and muscular relaxation.

Minimum alveolar concentrations (MAC; %) in oxygen reported for isoflurane in various species include the following: dog = 1.3 to 1.4; cat = 1.3 to 1.9; horse = 1.3 to 1.6; cow = 1.1; goat = 1.2 to 1.5; sheep = 1.6; pig = 1.5 to 2; rabbit = 2 to 2.1; and human = 1.2.[2] MAC may be altered by several factors (metabolic acidosis, hypo- and hypernatremia, hypo- and hyperthermia, other CNS depressants and stimulants, age, severe hypotension/hypoxemia/hypercarbia, and pregnancy).

Pharmacokinetics

Isoflurane is rapidly absorbed from the alveoli due to its low blood solubility or blood–gas partition coefficient (1.4). It is rapidly distributed into the CNS and crosses the placenta. The vast majority of the drug is eliminated via the lungs; only ≈0.2% is metabolized in the liver, and only a small amount of inorganic fluoride is formed.

Contraindications/Precautions/Warnings

Isoflurane is contraindicated in patients with a history of, or who are predisposed to, malignant hyperthermia. Isoflurane should only be used in situations in which sufficient monitoring and patient-support capabilities (eg, intubation, ventilation) are available. It should be used with caution in patients with increased intracranial pressure or head injury, or myasthenia gravis. If used in patients with increased intracranial pressure, it is recommended to closely monitor and maintain the expiratory end-tidal isoflurane below 1 to 1.5 minimum alveolar concentration (MAC) (1 MAC = 1.4%) and end-tidal carbon dioxide ($ETCO_2$) level between 35 and 40 mm Hg.[3]

Because of its respiratory depressant effects, intermittent positive pressure ventilation may be required to achieve anesthesia and normocapnia, particularly in horses.

The National Institute for Occupational Safety and Health (NIOSH) has recommended that no worker should be exposed at ceiling concentrations greater than 2 ppm of any halogenated anesthetic agent over a sampling period not to exceed 1 hour.

Adverse Effects

At recommended concentrations, dose-related hypotension secondary to vasodilation may occur. As compared with an equipotent propofol total IV anesthesia (TIVA), isoflurane seems to cause more vasodilation.[4] Hypotension usually responds to fluids, but profound hypotension may require the use of positive inotropic and/or vasopressor drugs. Although cardiodepression (ie, decreased heart rate and contractility) is usually not clinically significant in most species and healthy subjects, it can occur at doses used for surgical anesthetic planes. Arrhythmias have rarely been reported and, in horses, the incidence of intraoperative cardiac arrests has decreased since isoflurane and sevoflurane have replaced halothane.[5] Cats appear to be more sensitive to the cardiovascular effects of inhaled anesthetics than dogs.[6]

Dose-dependent respiratory depression has been reported. GI effects (eg, nausea, vomiting, ileus) may occur; administration of pre-anesthetic antiemetic agents can be considered for use in species that vomit. Providing food to horses before elective procedures may maintain GI motility and decrease the risk for postanesthetic colic.[7]

Malignant hyperthermia has been reported in dogs, horses,[8] pigs, and humans.[9]

Reproductive/Nursing Safety

Isoflurane readily crosses the placenta and maternal-to-fetal equilibration is rapid.[10] Increased postimplantation losses and reduced live birth index occurred in mice and rats given isoflurane for 2 hours every day during periods of organogenesis; fetal malformations were not observed.[11] However, with close monitoring, isoflurane can be safely used in pregnant animals when heart rate, minute ventilation, and blood pressure are maintained within a physiologic range.

The minimum alveolar concentration (MAC) of inhalation agents is 25% to 40% lower during pregnancy; the onset of isoflurane anesthesia is more rapid in pregnant animals.[12]

Because safety has not been established in animals, this drug should only be used when the maternal benefits outweigh the potential risks to offspring.

Drug Interactions

The following drug interactions have either been reported or are theoretical in humans or animals receiving isoflurane and may be of significance in veterinary patients. Unless otherwise noted, use together is not necessarily contraindicated, but weigh the potential risks and perform additional monitoring when appropriate.

- **Antihypertensive Agents** (eg, **amlodipine, enalapril, telmisartan**): Concomitant use may increase risks for hypotension. Enalapril caused significant decreases in systolic blood pressure in dogs and cats undergoing isoflurane anesthesia.[13,14]
- **Acepromazine**: May enhance the hypotensive effects of isoflurane in dogs[15]
- **Aminoglycosides** (eg, **amikacin, gentamicin**): Use with caution with halogenated anesthetic agents, as additive neuromuscular blockade may occur.
- **Benzodiazepines** (eg, **midazolam**): May reduce MAC requirements
- **Beta-Adrenergic Receptor Antagonists** (eg, **propranolol**): May enhance the cardiovascular depressant effects of isoflurane
- **Dexmedetomidine**: May worsen cardiovascular depression in cats.[6] May reduce minimum alveolar concentration (MAC) requirements in dogs
- **Ketamine**: May reduce MAC requirements in dogs
- **Lidocaine**: May reduce MAC requirements in dogs and rabbits
- **Lincosamides** (eg, **clindamycin**): Use with caution with halogenated anesthetic agents, as additive neuromuscular blockade may occur.
- **Nondepolarizing Neuromuscular Blocking Agents** (eg, **atracurium**): Additive neuromuscular blockade may occur.
- **Opioids** (eg, **buprenorphine, fentanyl, hydromorphone**): Intraoperative opioids can reduce MAC requirements in dogs.
- **Succinylcholine**: With inhalation anesthetics, may induce increased incidences of cardiac effects (eg, bradycardia, arrhythmias, sinus arrest, and apnea) and, in susceptible patients, malignant hyperthermia.
- **Sympathomimetic Agents** (eg, **dopamine, epinephrine, norepinephrine, ephedrine, metaraminol**): Although isoflurane sensitizes the myocardium to the effects of sympathomimetics less so than halothane, arrhythmias may still occur. If these drugs are needed, they should be used with significantly reduced initial doses and with intensive monitoring.

Laboratory Considerations

- **ACTH:** May reduce mean plasma ACTH concentrations collected from the cavernous sinus of anesthetized horses for determining the success of partial pituitary ablation[16]

Dosages

Approximate minimum alveolar concentrations (MAC; %) in oxygen reported for isoflurane in various species include the following: dog = 1.5; cat = 1.2; horse = 1.31; sheep = 1.5; rabbit = 1.92; and human = 1.2. MAC may be altered by several factors (metabolic acidosis, hypo- and hypernatremia, hypo- and hyperthermia, other CNS depressants and stimulants, age, severe hypotension/hypoxemia/hypercarbia, and pregnancy).

NOTES:

1. General anesthesia using inhalants must be performed with adequate monitoring and support and cannot be dosed in a purely textbook fashion.
2. MAC is affected by many variables, including:
   a) Type and location of stimulus
   b) Concurrent administration of MAC-reducing drugs
   c) Type of ventilation, type of breathing system
   d) Age of the animal (younger cats had higher MAC values)
3. Isoflurane should be used with well-maintained anesthetic machines with proper scavenging equipment and in areas with adequate ventilation to prevent escape of gases that could result in exposure of veterinary personnel to anesthetic vapors.

DOGS:

General anesthesia (label dosage; FDA-approved): Induction: 2% – 2.5% isoflurane alone with oxygen following an injectable anesthetic induction agent is usually employed.[17] **NOTE:** Mask induction of anesthesia is highly discouraged due to the level of stress and excitement produced and possible personnel exposure to gas anesthetics. Maintenance: Surgical levels of anesthesia may be sustained with a 1.5% –1.8% concentration of isoflurane in oxygen.[17]

General anesthesia (extra-label): Induction: 3% – 5% isoflurane with relatively rapid oxygen flow rates (3 to 4 L/minute) and using a non-rebreathing circuit. Maintenance: 1% – 3% isoflurane (typically, 1% – 1.5%) in oxygen adjusted to desired anesthetic depth; vaporizer settings will vary with the patient's condition, the type of breathing circuit used, and the fresh gas flow rate.[2,18]

CATS:

General anesthesia (extra-label): MAC for isoflurane ranged from 1.20 ± 0.13% to 2.22 ± 0.35%, and the average MAC was 1.71 ± 0.07%.[19]

HORSES:

General anesthesia (label dosage; FDA-approved): Induction: 3% – 5% isoflurane alone with oxygen following an injectable anesthetic induction agent are usually employed. **NOTE:** Mask induction of anesthesia is highly discouraged due to the level of stress and excitement produced and possible personnel exposure to gas anesthetics. Maintenance: Surgical levels of anesthesia may be sustained with a 1.5% – 1.8% concentration of isoflurane in oxygen.[17]

SMALL RUMINANTS:

General anesthesia (extra-label): Inhalational anesthesia is seldom feasible in the field but is a viable option in situations that can provide suitable accommodations (eg, sterile field, patient positioning) for small ruminants. Isoflurane is a preferred agent for debilitated, pregnant, very young or aged animals, or for prolonged (ie, more than 1 hour) and complicated surgical procedures. Vaporizer should be set to 1% – 3% during maintenance. Oxygen flow rate should be 10 to 20 mL/kg/minute during maintenance anesthesia.[20]

BIRDS:

General anesthesia (extra-label): Induction occurs within 1 to 2 minutes at a concentration of 3% – 5% delivered by mask. After intubation, maintenance at 1.5% – 2% is adequate for most birds. Recovery is rapid; most patients are standing and cage-safe within 5 minutes after anesthesia is discontinued, but there seems to be a direct relationship between anesthesia time and recovery time.[21]

FERRETS/SMALL MAMMALS:

General anesthesia of mice, rats, gerbils, hamsters, guinea pigs, chinchillas, ferrets, rabbits, prairie dogs (extra-label): Premedication with injectables drugs is recommended prior to induction of general anesthesia. In most cases, IV or IM injectable induction agents are preferred; however, face mask induction with isoflurane can be used after adequate sedation. In most cases, 2% – 3% isoflurane in oxygen delivered via a tight-fitting face mask is adequate. Maintenance of anesthesia can be achieved by delivering 1% – 2% of isoflurane, depending on concurrent drugs administered and type of procedure.[22-27]

REPTILES:

General anesthesia (extra-label): It is preferable to induce reptiles with injectable agents and then maintain anesthesia with inhalant gases. For maintenance of general anesthesia, most reptiles require 2% – 3% of isoflurane.

Monitoring

- Ventilatory status
- Cardiac rate and rhythm; blood pressure (particularly with higher anesthetic risk patients)
- Anesthetic depth

Client Information

Isoflurane is used for general anesthesia only by veterinarians.

Chemistry/Synonyms

Isoflurane is an inhalant general anesthetic agent that occurs as a colorless, nonflammable, stable liquid. It has a characteristic mildly pungent, musty, ethereal odor. At 20°C (68°F), isoflurane's specific gravity is 1.496 and vapor pressure is 238 mm Hg. Its boiling point is 48.5°C (119.3°F), and solubility coefficients include blood–gas partition coefficient of 1.4 and oil–gas partition coefficient of 91.

Halogenated inhalation anesthetics are greenhouse gases. Vaporization of isoflurane for 1 hour has the same global warming potential as driving an automobile for 12 miles.[28]

Isoflurane may also be known as compound 469, isofluranum, *AErrane®*, *Forene®*, *Forenium®*, *Forthane®*, *Isoflo®*, *Isofor®*, *Isoforine®*, *Isosol®*, *Isothane®*, *Iso-Thesia®*, *Lisorane®*, *Sofloran®*, *Tensocold®*, *Terrell®*, and *Zuflax®*.

Storage/Stability

Isoflurane should be stored at room temperature; it is relatively unaffected by exposure to light, but should be stored in a tight, light-resistant container. Isoflurane does not attack aluminum, brass, tin, iron, or copper.

Compatibility/Compounding Considerations

No specific information was noted.

Dosage Forms/Regulatory Status

VETERINARY-LABELED PRODUCTS:

Isoflurane for Inhalation: 99.9%/mL in 100 mL and 250 mL; *Aerrane®*, *Isoflo®*, *Isosol®*, generic; (Rx). Products may be FDA-approved for use in horses (those not intended for food) and dogs.

HUMAN-LABELED PRODUCTS:

Isoflurane Liquid for Inhalation in 100 mL and 250 mL; *Forane®*, *Terrell®*, generic; (Rx)

References

For the complete list of references, see **wiley.com/go/budde/plumb**

Isoniazid (INH)

(eye-so-***nye***-ah-zid) *Laniazid®, Nydrazid®*

Antimycobacterial

Prescriber Highlights

- ▶ May be used for chemoprophylaxis of *Mycobacterium bovis* or *Mycobacterium tuberculosis* in small animal species
- ▶ Has also been used in cattle for paratuberculosis (*Mycobacterium avium* subsp *paratuberculosis* [MAP]; Johne's disease)
- ▶ Treating active infections is controversial because of potential public health risks associated with the infections
- ▶ Contraindicated in patients with acute liver disease and in those that are hypersensitive to it
- ▶ Isoniazid has a narrow therapeutic index; hepatotoxicity and neurotoxicity are possible.

Uses/Indications

Isoniazid (INH) is sometimes used for chemoprophylaxis in small animal species living in households with a human that has tuberculosis. It can potentially be used in combination with other antimycobacterial drugs to treat infections of *Mycobacterium bovis* or *Mycobacterium tuberculosis* in dogs or cats. Because of the public health risks of tuberculosis, particularly in the face of increased populations of immunocompromised humans, treatment of mycobacterial infections in domestic or captive animals is controversial due to the potential for zoonotic infection.[1]

Isoniazid, alone or in combination, has been used to treat *Mycobacterium avium* subsp. *paratuberculosis* (MAP; Johne's disease) in cattle that are of significant economic, genetic, or sentimental value[2]; however, there is no cure for MAP and treatment is aimed at reducing clinical signs. As treatment does not prevent shedding of the organism but may extend survival time, treatment may therefore increase the risk for environmental contamination from that animal.[3]

In humans, INH is routinely used alone to treat latent tuberculosis infections (positive tuberculin skin test) and in combination with other antimycobacterial agents to treat active disease.

Pharmacology/Actions

Isoniazid inhibits the synthesis of mycolic acids, a component of mycobacterial cell walls; its exact mechanism is not well understood. It is most active against mycobacteria that are dividing and affects both extracellular and intracellular mycobacteria. It is bactericidal against dividing mycobacteria and bacteriostatic against dormant or semi-dormant stages.

Isoniazid is only active against *Mycobacterium tuberculosis, Mycobacterium bovis,* and some strains of *Mycobacterium kansasii*. In humans, resistance develops rapidly if used alone against active clinical disease, but not when used for treatment of latent infection.

Isoniazid has an inhibitory effect on monoamine oxidase.

Pharmacokinetics

No information was located on the pharmacokinetics of isoniazid (INH) in dogs or cats. It is reported that INH is absorbed after oral administration to ruminants.[3,4]

In humans, INH is rapidly absorbed after oral or IM administration; food can decrease absorption somewhat and INH may undergo significant first pass metabolism. The drug is highly distributed in the body and crosses into the CSF and caseous material. It is distributed into milk and crosses the placenta. It is only slightly (10%) bound to plasma proteins. In humans, the drug is initially primarily acetylated in the liver. The N-acetylated form is then further biotransformed to isonicotinic acid and monoacetylhydrazine. INH's hepatotoxicity is due to monoacetylhydrazine, which must undergo its own acetylation to become nontoxic. As with some humans, dogs lack N-acetyltransferase, so there is an increased potential for INH toxicity in this species. Elimination half-life in humans that are fast acetylators is 0.5 to 1.6 hours, and half-life is 2 to 5 hours in slow acetylators. Patients with acute or chronic liver disease or severe renal impairment may have substantially longer half-lives, up to 2 times normal. The drug is mostly eliminated in the urine as inactive metabolites.

Contraindications/Precautions/Warnings

Isoniazid (INH) is contraindicated in patients with acute liver disease or those that developed hepatopathy while taking the medication in the past. It is contraindicated in patients that are hypersensitive to it. INH has a narrow therapeutic index and toxicity is a concern (see ***Adverse Effects***). It should be used with caution in patients with decreased hepatic function or severe renal disease.

Adverse Effects

The primary adverse effect associated with INH in dogs is hepatotoxicity manifested by increased serum liver enzymes. Additional adverse effects reported in dogs include CNS stimulation, peripheral neuropathy, and thrombocytopenia. Adverse effects reported in cats include hepatotoxicity and peripheral neuritis.

In cattle, toxic signs (eg, refusal to eat, decreased milk production, rear leg stiffness) can be noted at 30 mg/kg PO. At 60 mg/kg PO, severe ataxia can be seen, and death can occur at doses of 100 mg/kg PO.

In humans, urticaria, hepatotoxicity, and peripheral neuropathy are commonly reported; rarely, blood dyscrasias, systemic lupus erythematous-like syndrome, and seizures have been reported.[5] Hepatotoxicity usually occurs within the first 3 months of treatment, and risk increases with increasing age, and in the postpartum period.

Reproductive/Nursing Safety

Isoniazid (INH) crosses the placenta and has been found to be embryocidal in some laboratory species, but teratogenic effects have not been detected in mice, rabbits, or rats.[5] In humans, concomitant administration of pyridoxine to prevent peripheral neuropathy is recommended for pregnant women receiving INH therapy.

INH can potentially induce abortion in cattle.

INH is excreted in milk in low concentrations (≈1% to 2% of maternal serum concentrations in humans) and it is thought to be safe to use during nursing. Ingested concentrations via milk are not high enough to serve as prophylaxis for tuberculosis in nursing infants.

Because safety has not been established in animals, this drug should only be used when the maternal benefits outweigh the potential risks to offspring. In humans, INH treatment is generally recommended during pregnancy, as the risks of untreated active tuberculosis outweigh the risks of INH therapy.[5]

Overdose/Acute Toxicity

Overdoses of isoniazid (INH) can be very serious. In dogs, the reported LD_{50} is 50 mg/kg; serious toxicity can occur with ingestion of as little as one 300 mg tablet. Ataxia, seizures, myocardial necrosis, metabolic acidosis, rhabdomyolysis, salivation, diarrhea, vomiting, and arrhythmias have been reported after overdoses in dogs. Treatment may include enterogastric lavage, activated charcoal, and benzodiazepines or phenobarbital to control seizures; however, seizures may be difficult to treat. Fluids and acidemia may need correction. Hemodialysis may be indicated.

Pyridoxine (vitamin B_6) can help treat seizures and other CNS effects, as well as acidosis. It has been suggested that pyridoxine be administered IV (preferably over 30 to 60 minutes) on a mg per mg of INH-ingested basis. Pyridoxine is commercially available as a 100 mg/mL, 1 mL vial, but it may be difficult to obtain in an emergency situation. A local human hospital may stock it.

For patients that have experienced or are suspected to have experienced an overdose, consultation with a 24-hour poison consultation center specializing in providing veterinary-specific information is strongly recommended. For general information related to overdose and toxin exposures, as well as contact information for poison control centers, refer to ***Appendix***.

Drug Interactions

The following drug interactions have either been reported or are theoretical in humans receiving INH and may be of significance in veterinary patients. Unless otherwise noted, use together is not necessarily contraindicated, but weigh the potential risks and perform additional monitoring when appropriate.

- ACETAMINOPHEN: May increase risk for hepatotoxicity
- ALFENTANIL: Prolonged alfentanil duration of action
- AMIODARONE: Increased amiodarone exposure
- ANTACIDS (especially those containing **aluminum**): Decreased INH absorption
- BENZODIAZEPINES: Isoniazid (INH) may reduce benzodiazepine metabolism.
- CLOPIDOGREL: INH may reduce antiplatelet effect.
- CORTICOSTEROIDS (eg, **dexamethasone, prednis(ol)one**): May reduce INH efficacy
- KETOCONAZOLE, ITRACONAZOLE: INH may reduce ketoconazole/itraconazole serum concentrations; does not appear to affect other azole antifungals
- OTHER HEPATOTOXIC DRUGS (eg, **azole antifungals, methimazole, phenothiazines, sulfonamides, estrogens**): Increased risk for hepatotoxicity
- OTHER NEUROTOXIC DRUGS: Increased risk for neurotoxicity
- PYRIDOXINE: INH may antagonize or increase the excretion of pyridoxine and reduce formation of the active form. Increased pyridoxine may be required; increased peripheral neuritis may occur secondary to pyridoxine/INH interaction.
- RIFAMPIN: Increased risk for hepatotoxicity
- THEOPHYLLINE: Increased risk for theophylline toxicity
- WARFARIN: Increased risk for bleeding
- FOOD INTERACTIONS: In humans, INH may interfere with metabolism of tyramine and histamine found in **cheese** (eg, Swiss, Cheshire) or **fish** (eg, tuna, sardines).

Laboratory Considerations

- Isoniazid (INH) may cause false positive **urine glucose determinations** when using cupric sulfate solution (Benedict's solution, *Clinitest*®); tests utilizing glucose oxidase (*Tes-Tape*®, *Clinistix*®) are not affected.

Dosages

NOTE: It is recommended to contact local veterinary or public health authorities before treating any animal with a confirmed mycobacterial infection.

DOGS:

***Mycobacterium tuberculosis* chemoprophylaxis** (extra-label): 10 mg/kg PO once daily; dose is extrapolated from human data. Treatment of active *M tuberculosis* or *Mycobacterium bovis* infections in dogs is controversial due to zoonotic potential.[1]

CATS:

Second-line treatment (reserved for resistant infections) for feline tuberculosis (extra-label): 10 – 20 mg/kg PO once daily.[6] Treatment of active *M tuberculosis* or *M bovis* infections in cats is controversial due to zoonotic potential.[1]

CATTLE/RUMINANTS:

Attempting to induce clinical remission of paratuberculosis (MAP; Johne's disease) in cattle or other ruminants that are of significant economic, genetic, or sentimental value (extra-label): 11 – 25 mg/kg PO once daily. Treatment typically must be maintained for the life of the animal and treated animals usually continue to shed MAP. Owner must be fully informed about the implications of keeping an animal with clinical MAP on the premises. Strongly advise having owner sign a document stating that the milk and meat from the animal will never be used for human consumption.[2]

Monitoring

- Baseline and periodic physical examination to evaluate for clinical efficacy
- Adverse effects
- Baseline and periodic CBC and chemistry profile

Client Information

- This medicine is best given on an empty stomach. If your animal vomits or acts sick after receiving the medicine on an empty stomach, try giving the next dose with food or a small treat. If vomiting continues, contact your veterinarian.
- Do not skip any doses. This medicine must be given regularly as directed to be effective.
- If a dose is missed, do not double the next dose.
- Store this medicine well out of reach of other animals and children as overdoses can be very serious.
- Contact your veterinarian if your animal has any of the following signs: vomiting; decreased appetite; weight loss; diarrhea or loose stools; changes in behavior or activity; yellowing of whites of eyes, gums, or skin (jaundice); or difficulty going up or down stairs.

Chemistry/Synonyms

Isoniazid occurs as colorless, or white, odorless crystals. It is freely soluble in water and sparingly soluble in alcohol.

Isoniazid may also be known as INH, INAH, isonicotinic acid hydrazide, isonicotinylhydrazide, isonicotinylhydrazine, or tubazid. INH is available as many trade names throughout the world; some of the more commonly used names include *Isotamine*®, *Laniazid*®, or *Nydrazid*®. CAUTION: *Isopyrin*® is one isoniazid trade name that, in some countries, contains ramifenazone (an NSAID) and *not* isoniazid.

Storage/Stability

Isoniazid (INH) tablets, the oral syrup, and the injection should be stored at temperatures below 40°C (104°F), preferably between 15°C and 30°C (59°F-86°F), in tight, light-resistant containers. The oral syrup and the injection should be protected from freezing. At low temperatures, crystals may form in the injectable solution; crystals should redissolve on warming to room temperature.

Compatibility/Compounding Considerations

It is recommended not to use sugars such as glucose, fructose, or sucrose in compounded oral solutions, as a condensation product may form that can impair absorption. Sorbitol and glycerin are acceptable vehicles. Isoniazid (INH) for injection is intended for IM administration; no information on compatibility with other parenteral drugs was found.

Dosage Forms/Regulatory Status

VETERINARY-LABELED PRODUCTS: NONE

HUMAN-LABELED PRODUCTS:

Isoniazid Oral Tablets: 100 mg and 300 mg; generic; (Rx)

Isoniazid Oral Syrup: 10 mg/mL (50 mg/5 mL) in pints; generic; (Rx)

Isoniazid Injection Solution: 100 mg/mL in 10 mL multidose vials; generic; (Rx)

Fixed dose combination products with rifampin are also available:

Tablets: Rifampin 120 mg with Isoniazid 50 mg and Pyrazinamide 300 mg; *Rifater*®; (Rx)

Capsules: Rifampin 300 mg with Isoniazid 150 mg; *IsonaRif*®, *Rifamate*®; (Rx)

References

For the complete list of references, see **wiley.com/go/budde/plumb**

Isoproterenol

Isoprenoline

(eye-soe-proe-***ter***-e-nole) *Isuprel*®

Beta-Adrenergic Agonist

Prescriber Highlights

- Nonselective beta-adrenergic agonist used for acute bronchial constriction, cardiac arrhythmias (complete AV block), and as adjunctive therapy in shock or heart failure; its use in veterinary medicine is uncommon.
- Contraindications include tachyarrhythmias, ventricular arrhythmias that do not require increased inotropic activity, and tachycardia or AV block caused by cardiac glycoside intoxication.
- Use caution in patients with coronary insufficiency, hyperthyroidism, renal disease, hypertension, or diabetes; not a substitute for adequate fluid replacement in shock
- Adverse effects include tachycardia, hypotension, anxiety, tremors, excitability, headache, weakness, and vomiting; more arrhythmogenic than dopamine or dobutamine
- Short duration of activity (including adverse effects)

Uses/Indications

Isoproterenol is infrequently used in veterinary medicine. It can be used in the treatment of acute bronchial constriction, cardiac arrhythmias (complete AV block), and, occasionally, as adjunctive therapy in shock or heart failure (limited use because of resulting increases in heart rate and ventricular arrhythmogenicity).

Pharmacology/Actions

Isoproterenol is a synthetic beta-1 and beta-2-adrenergic agonist that has no appreciable alpha-adrenergic activity at therapeutic doses. It is thought that isoproterenol's beta-adrenergic activity is a result of stimulating cyclic-AMP production. Its primary actions are increased inotropism and chronotropism, relaxation of bronchial smooth muscle, and peripheral vasodilation. Isoproterenol may increase perfusion to skeletal muscle (at the expense of vital organs in shock). Isoproterenol inhibits the antigen-mediated releases of histamine and slow releasing substance of anaphylaxis (SRS-A).

Hemodynamic effects include decreased total peripheral resistance, increased cardiac output, increased venous return to the heart, and increased rate of discharge by cardiac pacemakers. Isoproterenol can increase myocardial oxygen requirements while also decreasing coronary perfusion.

Pharmacokinetics

After oral administration, isoproterenol is rapidly inactivated by the GI tract and metabolized by the liver. Sublingual administration is not reliably absorbed and effects may take up to 30 minutes to be seen. IV administration results in immediate effects, but these only persist for a few minutes after discontinuation.

The pharmacologic actions of isoproterenol are ended primarily through tissue uptake. Isoproterenol is metabolized in the liver and other tissues by catechol-O-methyltransferase (COMT) to a weakly active metabolite.

Contraindications/Precautions/Warnings

Isoproterenol is contraindicated in patients with tachyarrhythmias, ventricular arrhythmias that do not require increased inotropic activity, and tachycardia or AV block caused by cardiac glycoside intoxication.

Use isoproterenol with caution in patients with coronary insufficiency, hyperthyroidism, renal disease, hypertension, or diabetes mellitus. Isoproterenol is not a substitute for adequate fluid replacement in shock.

Adverse Effects

Isoproterenol can cause tachycardia, hypotension, anxiety, tremors, excitability, headache, weakness, and vomiting. Because of isoproterenol's short duration of action, adverse effects are usually transient and do not require cessation of therapy, but may require lowering the dose or infusion rate. Isoproterenol is considered more arrhythmogenic than either dopamine or dobutamine, so it is rarely used in the treatment of heart failure.

Reproductive/Nursing Safety

Safe use of isoproterenol during pregnancy has not been established. Beta-adrenergic agonists have a tocolytic effect and may interfere with uterine contractions at parturition.

It is unknown if isoproterenol is distributed into milk; however, as isoproterenol is rapidly deactivated in the gut, it is unlikely to pose much risk to nursing offspring.

Because safety has not been established in animals, this drug should only be used when the maternal benefits outweigh the potential risks to offspring.

Overdose/Acute Toxicity

In addition to the signs listed in the ***Adverse Effects*** section, high doses may cause an initial hypertension, followed by hypotension as well as tachycardia and other arrhythmias. High doses are associated with cardiac necrosis.[1] Under experimental conditions, lethal doses of isoproterenol were 10 – 50 μ/kg IV in hypoxic dogs.[2]

Besides halting administration or reducing the drug dosage, treatment is considered to be supportive. If tachycardia persists, a beta-blocker (eg, propranolol) could be considered for treatment (if patient does not have a bronchospastic disease).

For patients that have experienced or are suspected to have experienced an overdose, consultation with a 24-hour poison consultation center specializing in providing veterinary-specific information is recommended. For general information related to overdose and toxin exposures, as well as contact information for poison control centers, refer to ***Appendix***.

Drug Interactions

The following drug interactions have either been reported or are theoretical in humans or animals receiving isoproterenol and may be of significance in veterinary patients. Unless otherwise noted, use together is not necessarily contraindicated, but weigh the potential risks and perform additional monitoring when appropriate.

- ANESTHETICS, INHALANT (eg, **isoflurane, sevoflurane**): An increased risk for arrhythmias if isoproterenol is administered to patients that have received cyclopropane or a halogenated hydrocarbon anesthetic agent. Propranolol may be administered should an arrhythmia occur.
- BETA-BLOCKERS (eg, **atenolol, propranolol**): May antagonize isoproterenol's cardiac, bronchodilating, and vasodilating effects by blocking the beta effects of isoproterenol. Beta-blockers may be administered to treat the tachycardia associated with isoproterenol use, but use with caution in patients with bronchospastic disease.
- DIGOXIN: An increased risk for arrhythmias may occur if isoproterenol is used concurrently with digitalis glycosides.

- **Linezolid**: Increased hypertensive effects possible
- **Oxytocin**: Increased risk for hypertension
- **Selegiline**: Increased hypertensive effects possible
- **Sympathomimetic agents, Other** (eg, **phenylpropanolamine**): Isoproterenol should not be administered with other sympathomimetic agents as increased toxicity may result.
- **Theophylline, Aminophylline**: Isoproterenol may reduce theophylline levels.

Laboratory Considerations

- None noted

Dosages

NOTE: Because of the cardiostimulatory properties of isoproterenol, its parenteral use in human medicine for the treatment of bronchospasm has been largely supplanted by beta-2-adrenergic selective drugs (eg, terbutaline) and administration methods (nebulization). Use with care.

DOGS/CATS:

Sinoatrial arrest, sinus bradycardia, complete AV block, or as an alternative to atropine for calcium channel blocker overdose (extra-label):

a) Dilute injection as described for IV infusion (see ***Compatibility/Compounding Considerations***). Infuse solution to effect at a rate of 0.04 – 0.08 μg/kg/minute IV CRI.[3]

b) Isoproterenol increases heart rate and cardiac output and decreases blood pressure. If administered carefully with close monitoring of blood pressure, it can provide potent augmentation of forward blood flow and tissue perfusion. Dose is 0.02 – 0.5 μg/kg/minute IV.[4]

Monitoring

- Cardiovascular status: heart rate and rhythm; blood pressure; central venous pressure; cardiac output
- Respiratory rate and thoracic auscultation during anaphylaxis
- Urine output
- Blood gases

Client Information

- Isoproterenol for injection should be used only by trained personnel in a setting where adequate monitoring can be performed.

Chemistry/Synonyms

Isoproterenol HCl is a synthetic beta-adrenergic agent that occurs as a white to practically white, crystalline powder that is freely soluble in water and sparingly soluble in alcohol. The pH of the commercially available injection is 3.5 to 4.5.

Isoproterenol HCl may also be known as isoprenaline hydrochloride, isopropylarterenol hydrochloride, isopropylnoradrenaline hydrochloride, *Imuprel*®, *Isolin*®, *Isoprenaline Macure*®, *Isuprel*®, *Lenoprel*®, *Norisodrine Aerotrol*®, *Proterenal*®, *Saventrine*®, and *Vapo-iso*®.

Storage/Stability

Store isoproterenol protected from light at room temperature 20°C to 25°C (68°F-77°F). Isoproterenol salts will darken with time on exposure to air, light, or heat. Sulfites or sulfur dioxide may be added to preparations as an antioxidant. Solutions may become pink or brownish-pink if exposed to air, alkalis, or metals. Do not use solutions that are discolored pink or darker, or contain a precipitate. If isoproterenol is mixed with other drugs or fluids that result in a solution with a pH greater than 6, it is recommended that it be used immediately.

Compatibility/Compounding Considerations

Compatibility is dependent on factors such as pH, concentration, temperature, and diluent used; specialized references or a hospital pharmacist should be consulted for more specific information.

Isoproterenol for injection is reported to be physically **compatible** with all commonly used IV solutions (except sodium bicarbonate 5%), and the following drugs: calcium chloride/gluceptate, cimetidine HCl, dobutamine HCl, heparin sodium, magnesium sulfate, multivitamin infusion, oxytetracycline HCl, potassium chloride, succinylcholine chloride, tetracycline HCl, verapamil HCl, and vitamin B complex with C.

It is reported to be physically **incompatible** when mixed with aminophylline or sodium bicarbonate.

Commercially available as 0.2 mg/mL injection. For direct IV injection, dilute 1 mL of the commercially available injection to a volume of 10 mL with 0.9% sodium chloride injection or 5% dextrose injection. For IV infusion, solutions may be prepared by diluting 1 to 10 mL of the 0.2 mg/mL injection with 500 mL of 5% dextrose, 0.9% sodium chloride, or LRS injection to provide infusion solutions containing 0.4 – 4 μg/mL. For example, 5 mL (1 mg) of the 0.2 mg/mL injection in 500 mL of 5% dextrose would yield a concentration of 2 μg/mL. As the injection concentrate contains no bacteriostatic or antimicrobial agent, each vial/ampule is intended for single use only; any unused solution should be discarded.

Dosage Forms/Regulatory Status

VETERINARY-LABELED PRODUCTS: NONE

HUMAN-LABELED PRODUCTS:

Isoproterenol HCl for Injection: 0.2 mg/mL in 1 mL and 5 mL ampules or single-dose vials; *Isuprel*®, generic; (Rx)

References

For the complete list of references, see **wiley.com/go/budde/plumb**

Isotretinoin

(eye-so-***tret***-i-noyn) *Accutane*®

Retinoid, Synthetic, Second-generation

Prescriber Highlights

- ► May be useful in treatment of a variety of dermatologic conditions associated with epithelial cell proliferation and differentiation
- ► Isotretinoin is a known teratogen and is absolutely contraindicated during pregnancy.
- ► Caution in patients with hypertriglyceridemia, severe renal or hepatic dysfunction, or hypersensitivity
- ► The most common adverse effect in dogs is keratoconjunctivitis sicca (KCS). Other potential adverse effects in small animal species include GI effects (anorexia, vomiting, abdominal distention), CNS effects (lassitude, hyperactivity, collapse), pruritus, erythema of feet and mucocutaneous junctions, polydipsia, and swollen tongue.
- ► Obtaining the medication for veterinary patients may be difficult and cost may be prohibitive.
- ► The National Institute for Occupational Safety and Health (NIOSH) classifies isotretinoin as a hazardous drug. **Pregnant women must avoid contact with this medication**; isotretinoin should NOT be dispensed to households with pregnant women.

Uses/Indications

Isotretinoin may be useful for the treatment of a variety of dermatologic conditions in dogs, including follicular abnormalities such as follicular dysplasias (eg, color dilution alopecia), lamellar ichthyosis, intracutaneous cornifying epitheliomas, multiple epidermal inclusion cysts, idiopathic seborrhea, sebaceous adenitis, keratoacanthoma, benign pilomatrixomas, comedo syndrome in schnauzers, and as palliative treatment for cutaneous T-cell lymphoma. There is little scientific evidence available to support its use in veterinary patients; however, a recent study showed that isotretinoin 9-cis, in combination with surgery, significantly increased the survival rate and prolonged the time to tumor recurrence of thyroid carcinoma in dogs, as compared with doxorubicin-treated or untreated dogs.[1]

Use of isotretinoin in cats is more limited; with potential use for actinic keratosis, solar-induced squamous cell carcinoma, Bowen's disease (ie, multicentric in situ squamous cell carcinoma), sebaceous adenitis, and acne.

Because of the concerns of teratogenic effects in humans, availability to veterinarians may be difficult as it may be restricted by manufacturers and drug distributors.

Pharmacology/Actions

Isotretinoin is a retinoid that appears to regulate epithelial cell proliferation and differentiation, although its exact mechanism of action is unknown. It affects monocyte and lymphocyte function, which can cause changes in cellular immune responses. The effects on skin include reduction of sebaceous gland size and activity, thereby reducing sebum production. It also has anti-keratinization and anti-inflammatory activity and may indirectly reduce bacterial populations in sebaceous pores.

Pharmacokinetics

Isotretinoin is rapidly absorbed from the GI tract once the capsule disintegrates and the drug is dispersed in the GI contents, which may require up to 2 hours after dosing. Animal studies have shown that only ≈25% of a dose reaches the systemic circulation, and food or milk in the GI tract increases the amount of drug absorbed. Isotretinoin is distributed into many tissues, but it is not stored in the liver (unlike vitamin A). It crosses the placenta and is highly bound to plasma proteins. It is unknown if it enters milk. Isotretinoin is metabolized in the liver and is excreted in the urine and feces. Isotretinoin metabolites possess retinoid activity, but it is unclear if or how they contribute to the drug's efficacy or toxicity. In humans, terminal half-life is ≈10 to 20 hours.

Contraindications/Precautions/Warnings

Isotretinoin is contraindicated in pregnancy. Isotretinoin is a known teratogen. Major anomalies have been reported in children of women taking the medication, and it should not be used to treat animals that live in households with pregnant women.

Isotretinoin should be used with caution in patients with hypertriglyceridemia, severe renal or hepatic disease, or sensitivity to isotretinoin, and should only be used when potential benefits outweigh the risks.

Avoid excessive exposure to sunlight, as the effects of UV lights are enhanced by retinoids.

The National Institute for Occupational Safety and Health (NIOSH) classifies isotretinoin as a hazardous drug. Pregnant women must avoid contact with the medication and it should not be dispensed to households with pregnant women.

Adverse Effects

There is limited experience with isotretinoin in veterinary medicine; however, there appears to be a low incidence of adverse effects, particularly in dogs. The most common adverse effect seen in dogs is KCS, which is not seen in cats. Other potential adverse effects in dogs include GI effects (anorexia, vomiting, diarrhea, abdominal distention), CNS effects (lassitude, hyperactivity, behavioral changes, collapse), stiffness of limbs, pruritus, exfoliative dermatitis, erythema of feet and mucocutaneous junctions, cheilitis, polydipsia, and swollen tongue.

Incidence of adverse effects may be higher in cats. Reported adverse effects include blepharospasm, periocular crusting, erythema, diarrhea and, especially, weight loss secondary to anorexia. If adverse effects occur, the time between doses may be extended (eg, instead of giving daily, alternate between giving daily for 1 week and giving every other day for 1 week) to reduce total amount given.

Adverse effects in humans include pancreatitis, osteoporosis, corneal opacities and cataracts, arthralgia, and inflammatory bowel syndrome.

Reproductive/Nursing Safety

Isotretinoin is a known teratogen. Major anomalies have been reported in children of women taking the medication. It is absolutely contraindicated in pregnant veterinary patients as well. Isotretinoin also appears to inhibit spermatogenesis.

It is not known whether this drug is excreted in breast milk. At this time, it is not recommended for use in nursing mothers.

Overdose/Acute Toxicity

A common finding in dogs after overdose is hypersalivation. Because of the drug's potential adverse effects, GI decontamination protocols should be considered with acute isotretinoin overdoses when warranted.

For patients that have experienced or are suspected to have experienced an overdose, consultation with a 24-hour poison consultation center specializing in providing veterinary-specific information is recommended. For general information related to overdose and toxin exposures, as well as contact information for poison control centers, refer to ***Appendix***.

Drug Interactions

The following drug interactions have either been reported or are theoretical in humans or animals receiving isotretinoin and may be of significance in veterinary patients. Unless otherwise noted, use together is not necessarily contraindicated, but weigh the potential risks and perform additional monitoring when appropriate.

- **Vitamin A** or **Other Retinoids**: Isotretinoin used with other retinoids (eg, **etretinate, tretinoin**, or **vitamin A**) may cause additive toxic effects.
- **Corticosteroids** (eg, **dexamethasone, prednis(ol)one**): Concomitant use may further increase risk for osteoporosis.
- **Cyclosporine**: Isotretinoin may increase cyclosporine concentrations.
- **Tetracyclines**: Use with tetracyclines may increase the potential for the occurrence of pseudotumor cerebri (cerebral edema and increased CSF pressure).

Laboratory Considerations

- Increases in serum **triglyceride** and **cholesterol** concentrations may be noted, which can be associated with corneal lipid deposits.
- **Platelets** may be increased.
- **ALT** (SGOT), **AST** (SGPT), and **LDH** concentrations may be increased.

Dosages

DOGS:

Sebaceous adenitis, schnauzer comedo syndrome, keratoacanthoma, pilomatrixoma, idiopathic seborrhea, ichthyosis, and sebaceous gland hyperplasia and adenoma (extra-label): Dosage can vary, and there are no prospective, well-controlled, clinical studies to support any dosage regimen. Most recommend an initial dose of 1 mg/kg PO once or twice daily, given with food. Clinical efficacy may not be seen for 6 to 8 weeks. If efficacy is noted, dose may be decreased to 0.5 mg/kg, or the time between doses may be extended to every other day. Long-term treatment may be required.

Epitheliotropic lymphoma; palliative treatment (extra-label): 3 – 4 mg/kg PO once daily or divided twice daily has been suggested

CATS:

Feline acne (extra-label): 5 – 10 mg/cat (NOT mg/kg) PO once daily has been suggested

Epitheliotropic lymphoma; palliative treatment (extra-label): 10 mg/cat (NOT mg/kg) once daily has been suggested

Monitoring

- Efficacy and adverse effects
- Baseline and periodic (eg, 1 to 2 months later if clinical signs appear) liver enzymes
- Dogs: baseline and monthly Schirmer tear tests—especially in older dogs and KCS-susceptible breeds
- Cats: body weight

Client Information

- **Pregnant women must not be exposed to isotretinoin.** It should not be handled by pregnant women and should not be used in households with pregnant women, as severe birth defects can result.
- This medicine is best given with food but should be given the same way (with food or without) each time. If your animal vomits or acts sick after getting it on an empty stomach, give with food or a small treat to see if this helps. If vomiting continues, contact your veterinarian.
- Dogs tolerate this medication better than cats. The most common side effect in dogs is dry eye syndrome (KCS). In cats, gastrointestinal effects (eg, loss of appetite, diarrhea, weight loss) may limit use.

Chemistry/Synonyms

A synthetic retinoid, isotretinoin occurs as a yellow-orange to orange, crystalline powder. It is insoluble in both water and alcohol. Commercially, it is available in soft gelatin capsules as a suspension in soybean oil.

Isotretinoin may also be known as isotretinoinum, 13-cis-retinoic acid, Ro-4-3780, and *Accutane*®.

Storage/Stability

Capsules should be stored at room temperature in tight, light-resistant containers. The drug is photosensitive and will degrade with light exposure. Expiration dates of 2 years are assigned after manufacture.

Compatibility/Compounding Considerations

No specific information noted

Dosage Forms/Regulatory Status

VETERINARY-LABELED PRODUCTS: NONE

HUMAN-LABELED PRODUCTS:

Isotretinoin Oral Capsules: 10 mg, 20 mg, 25 mg, 30 mg, 35 mg, and 40 mg (regular and soft gel); *Absorica*®, *Accutane* ®, *Amnesteem*®, *Claravis*®, *Sotret*®, *Myorisan*®; Rx

NOTE: Because of the known teratogenic effects, availability is restricted by manufacturers and drug distributors; obtaining the medication for veterinary patients may be difficult.

References

For the complete list of references, see **wiley.com/go/budde/plumb**

Isoxsuprine

(eye-***sox***-suh-preen) *Vasodilan*®

Vasodilator

Prescriber Highlights

- ► Peripheral vasodilator that may have some efficacy in the treatment of navicular disease in horses; efficacy after oral administration is questionable
- ► No commercially available products in the United States; must be compounded
- ► Contraindicated immediately postpartum or in the presence of arterial bleeding
- ► Adverse effects are unlikely after oral administration.

Uses/Indications

Isoxsuprine is used principally for the treatment of navicular disease, sesamoiditis, and laminitis in horses; however, results of clinical trials using the drug are mixed.[1] Although some equine studies appear to show an improvement in lameness scores, there are minimal changes in laminar blood flow to explain the effect. Dosages that cause vasodilation in horses are likely to only be achieved with IV dosing; however, IV formulations are not commercially available and may induce neurologic adverse effects.

There have been anecdotal reports of isoxsuprine being helpful for treating dogs with a Raynaud's-like syndrome (periodic digital cyanosis, onychogryphosis)[2] and improving microcirculation in birds.[3]

Isoxsuprine has been used in humans for the treatment of cerebral vascular insufficiency, dysmenorrhea, and premature labor, but efficacies are unproven for these indications.

Pharmacology/Actions

Isoxsuprine causes direct vascular smooth muscle relaxation, primarily in skeletal muscle. Although it stimulates beta-adrenergic receptors, it is believed that this action is not required for vasodilation to occur. In horses with navicular disease, isoxsuprine raises distal limb temperatures significantly. Isoxsuprine relaxes uterine smooth muscle and may have positive inotropic and chronotropic effects on the heart. At high doses, isoxsuprine decreases blood viscosity and reduces platelet aggregation. Isoxsuprine does not appear to possess significant analgesic properties in horses.[4]

Pharmacokinetics

In humans, isoxsuprine is almost completely absorbed from the GI tract, but in horses, bioavailability is low after oral administration (2.2%), probably due to a high first-pass effect. Despite plasma concentrations of isoxsuprine being undetectable after a single oral dose and less than 5 ng/mL after repeated oral dosing, glucuronide metabolites are detectable in plasma and urine after a single oral dose.[5-7] After IV administration in horses, the elimination half-life is between 2 and 3 hours, with a large volume of distribution (6.8 to 10.5 L/kg) and high plasma clearance (43 to 53.8 mL/minute/kg).

Contraindications/Precautions/Warnings

Isoxsuprine should not be administered to animals immediately postpartum or in the presence of arterial bleeding.

Adverse Effects

After parenteral administration, horses may show signs of CNS stimulation (uneasiness, hyperexcitability, nose-rubbing), tachycardia, increased cardiac output, or sweating. Signs are typically short-lived. Adverse effects are unlikely after oral administration, but hypotension, tachycardia, and GI effects (eg, hyporexia, diarrhea) are possible.

Reproductive/Nursing Safety

No specific lactation safety information was found.

Because safety has not been established in animals, this drug should only be used when the maternal benefits outweigh the potential risks to offspring.

Overdose/Acute Toxicity

Serious toxicity is unlikely in horses after an inadvertent oral overdose, but signs listed in the ***Adverse Effects*** section could be seen. Treat clinical signs supportively if necessary. CNS hyperexcitability may be treated with diazepam and hypotension with IV fluids.

For patients that have experienced or are suspected to have experienced an overdose, consultation with a 24-hour poison consultation center specializing in providing veterinary-specific information is recommended. For general information related to overdose and toxin exposures, as well as contact information for poison control centers, refer to ***Appendix***.

Drug Interactions

No clinically significant drug interactions have been reported for this agent.

Laboratory Considerations

- None were noted.

Dosages

HORSES:

Orthopedic conditions, such as navicular disease (extra-label): 1.2 mg/kg PO every 8 to 12 hours initially, then decrease frequency to once a day, then to every other day. **NOTE**: Efficacy is controversial.

BIRDS:

Frostbite (extra-label): 10 mg/kg PO once daily[8]

Monitoring

- Clinical efficacy
- Adverse effects (eg, tachycardia, GI disturbances, CNS stimulation)

Client Information

- This medicine may be given with or without food.
- Tablets may be crushed and made into a slurry, suspension, or paste by adding corn or cherry syrup just before administration.
- This medicine may cause gastrointestinal effects (eg, lack of appetite, diarrhea). Fast heart rates, low blood pressure, and stimulatory effects (eg, uneasiness, nose-rubbing, overly excited) are possible but not common.

Chemistry/Synonyms

Isoxsuprine, a peripheral vasodilating agent, occurs as an odorless, bitter-tasting, white, crystalline powder with a melting point of about 200°C (392°F). It is slightly soluble in water and sparingly soluble in alcohol.

Isoxsuprine HCl may also be known as Caa-40, isoxsuprini hydrochloridum, phenoxyisopropylnorsuprifen, *Dilum®*, *Duvadilan®*, *Fadaespasmol®*, *Fenam®*, *Inibina®*, *Isodilan®*, *Isotenk®*, *Uterine®*, *Vadosilan®*, *Vasodilan®*, *Vasolan®*, *Vasosuprina Ilfi®*, *Voxsuprine®*, and *Xuprin®*.

Storage/Stability

Store tablets in tightly closed containers at room temperature (15°C to 30°C [59°F-86°F]).

Compatibility/Compounding Considerations

No specific information was noted.

Dosage Forms/Regulatory Status

VETERINARY-LABELED PRODUCTS: NONE

The Association of Racing Commissioners International (ARCI) has designated this drug as a class 4 substance. Use of this drug may not be allowed in certain animal competitions. Check rules and regulations before entering a competition while this medication is being administered. Contact local racing authorities for further guidance. See ***Appendix*** for more information.

HUMAN-LABELED PRODUCTS:

Isoxsuprine HCl Tablets: 10 mg and 20 mg; no longer commercially available in the United States

Isoxsuprine HCl oral powder is available for compounding.

References

For the complete list of references, see **wiley.com/go/budde/plumb**

Itraconazole

(it-ruh-***kon***-uh-zohl) *Itrafungol®*, *Sporanox®*

Antifungal, Azole

Prescriber Highlights

- Oral triazole antifungal approved for treatment of *Microsporum canis* in cats; also used for systemic and cutaneous mycoses in a variety of species
- Avoid compounded oral itraconazole dosage forms, as they may not be absorbed.
- Contraindications include hypersensitivity to this drug or other azole antifungal agents, hepatic or renal impairment, and pregnancy.
- Adverse effects in dogs include anorexia, hepatotoxicity, ulcerative skin lesions, edema, and vasculitis. Rarely, erythema multiforme or toxic epidermal necrolysis may occur.
- Adverse effects in cats are dose-related and include GI effects (eg, anorexia, weight loss, vomiting), hepatotoxicity, and depression.
- Many potential drug interactions

Uses/Indications

In cats, itraconazole is indicated for the treatment of dermatophytosis caused by *Microsporum canis*. Itraconazole has been used in dogs and cats in the treatment of non-life-threatening systemic mycoses that do not involve the CNS, including aspergillosis, cryptococcal meningitis,[1] blastomycosis,[2-4] coccidioidomycosis,[5] sporotrichosis,[6] and histoplasmosis.[5,7,8] It can also be useful as adjunctive treatment for pythiosis,[9-12] lagenidiosis, zygomycosis, phaeohyphomycosis, and hyalohyphomycosis. Itraconazole may reach therapeutic concentrations in ocular or CNS tissue if there is associated inflammation and compromise of the barriers[13]; fluconazole may work better for some systemic mycoses (eg, cryptococcosis) affecting these systems. Itraconazole may also be useful for the treatment of fungal osteomyelitis,[14] onychomycosis, and *Malassezia* spp dermatitis.

In horses, itraconazole may be useful in the treatment of sporotrichosis and *Coccidioides immitis* osteomyelitis.

Pharmacology/Actions

Itraconazole is a fungistatic triazole compound that inhibits a fungal CYP450-dependent demethylation enzyme that produces ergosterol in the fungal cell membrane. The resultant intracellular accumulation of methylated sterols weakens the cellular membranes of susceptible fungi, thereby increasing membrane permeability and allowing leakage of cellular contents and impairing uptake of purine and pyrimidine precursors. Itraconazole has efficacy against a variety of pathogenic fungi, including yeasts and dermatophytes. In vivo studies using laboratory models have shown that itraconazole has fungistatic activity against many strains of *Candida* spp, *Aspergillus* spp, *Cryptococcus* spp, *Histoplasma* spp, *Blastomyces* spp, and *Trypanosoma cruzi*. Itraconazole and terbinafine combination treatment may have synergistic antifungal effects against *Candida albicans.*

Itraconazole has anti-inflammatory activities that, although poorly understood, likely occur via suppression of T-lymphocyte proliferation, inhibition of calcium-dependent proinflammatory activities by neutrophils, and inhibition of leukotriene B_4. Itraconazole demonstrated antiviral activity in a cellular model of type I feline coronavirus infection.[15]

Pharmacokinetics

Itraconazole absorption is highly dependent on gastric pH and the presence of food.

Oral liquid dosage forms:

In cats, bioavailability of the commercial oral solution (human and feline labels) was 78%.[16] The veterinary-labeled oral solution can be administered to cats with or without food; giving with food increases itraconazole exposure (area under the curve [AUC]) by 30% but results in a delayed and lower peak concentration. Absorption characteristics differ between itraconazole oral solution (human- and feline-labeled products) and capsules.[17] In cats, brand-name liquid formulations have increased absorption as compared with capsules,[18] but this does not appear to apply to dogs.[17] The human-labeled oral solution has adequate oral bioavailability in dogs, cats, and other species, and it is suggested to be given *without* food for optimal absorption.[17] Suspensions compounded from bulk powders will likely not be absorbed.[18]

Oral solid dosage forms:

The commercially available capsules are specially formulated to increase oral bioavailability. Capsules compounded from bulk powders are not absorbed to a significant extent.[19] Bioavailability may be 50% or less when human-labeled itraconazole capsules are given to humans on an empty stomach; when given with food, bioavailability may approach 100%.[17,20] The human-labeled itraconazole tablet formulation is best absorbed when given with a high-fat meal. In humans, oral absorption of itraconazole capsules is reduced when administered concurrently with agents that decrease gastric acid secretion (eg, famotidine, omeprazole).[21] In dogs[19,22] and cats[22], studies comparing the pharmacokinetics of generic versus brand-name itraconazole capsules concluded that generic itraconazole is bioequivalent to the drug's innovator (ie, *Sporanox*®).

Itraconazole has high protein binding (eg, 99% in cats[23] and humans[21]) and is widely distributed throughout the body. In dogs, volume of distribution is 17 L/kg.[24] Skin, sebum, the female reproductive tract, and pus all have concentrations of itraconazole greater than those found in serum. Only minimal concentrations are found in CSF,[24] urine, aqueous humor, and saliva.

Itraconazole is metabolized by the liver to many different metabolites, including hydroxyitraconazole, which is active. Itraconazole's metabolism is a saturable process. In cats, administration of the veterinary-labeled oral solution resulted in a half-life of 12 hours after 1 dose and 36 hours after daily administration for 7 days.[23] In dogs, half-life is 33 to 58 hours,[17,24] and clearance is 234 mL/kg/hour after IV administration.[24] In humans, itraconazole's serum half-life ranges from 21 to 64 hours. Because of its long half-life, itraconazole does not reach steady-state plasma concentrations for at least 6 days after the start of therapy. If loading doses are given, steady-state concentrations will be approached sooner. Itraconazole may persist in tissue for several weeks to months after its discontinuation. The drug is eliminated primarily in the feces and, to a lesser extent, in the urine.

In horses, the oral itraconazole solution appears to be better absorbed than capsules. Volume of distribution of the oral solution was 6.3 L/kg, and protein binding was 99%. Elimination half-life was 11.3 hours. Oral absorption of capsules was 33% of the oral solution.[25]

Contraindications/Precautions/Warnings

Itraconazole should not be used in patients that are hypersensitive to it or other azole antifungal agents.

Itraconazole may have a negative inotropic effect,[26] particularly at higher dosages, and should be used with caution in animals with reduced cardiac function.

Itraconazole should only be used in patients with hepatic or renal impairment when the potential benefits outweigh the risks.

Neuropathy has occurred in humans receiving long-term itraconazole therapy[21,27]; veterinary significance is uncertain.

African grey parrots appear to be highly sensitive to itraconazole and can develop anorexia and depression. Other antifungals or reduced dosages of itraconazole are recommended in this species.[28]

Compounding capsules from bulk powders may not yield a dosage form that is well absorbed. Itraconazole absorption may be impaired in patients with achlorhydria (or hypochlorhydria) and could result in therapeutic failure.

Adverse Effects

In dogs, anorexia and hepatotoxicity are the most common adverse effects observed, especially at higher doses.[3] Anorexia is often the clinical marker for toxicity; it is commonly dose-dependent and occurs in the second month of treatment. Approximately 10% of dogs receiving 10 mg/kg/day and 5% of dogs receiving 5 mg/kg/day developed hepatic toxicosis (as determined by increased ALT activity) serious enough to discontinue treatment, at least temporarily.[2,3] Some dogs (ie, 7% or more) given itraconazole may develop ulcerative skin lesions, vasculitis, or limb edema requiring drug discontinuation.[3,29] These signs generally resolve after stopping the drug. Re-exposure after dermal lesions have resolved is not recommended because these types of reactions are likely idiosyncratic, not dose-dependent, and may cause more severe clinical signs. Rarely, serious erythema multiforme or toxic epidermal necrolysis reactions have been noted.

In cats, adverse effects appear to be dose dependent.[29] GI effects (eg, anorexia, diarrhea, hypersalivation, vomiting), hepatotoxicity (eg, increased ALT activity, jaundice), weight loss, and depression have been noted. Increased ALT activity occurred in 13% of cats, although in one report of 21 shelter cats, no cats experienced an increase of ALT activity outside the upper limit of normal.[30] As in dogs, doses above 10 mg/kg may be associated with a greater frequency of adverse effects, including hepatotoxicity. In one retrospective review of cats receiving dosages as high as 27 mg/kg/day, 31% cats experienced GI adverse effects.[31]

If adverse effects occur and ALT activity is markedly increased, the drug should be discontinued. Increased liver enzymes in the absence of other signs does not necessarily mandate dose reduction or drug discontinuation. Once ALT activity returns to normal and other adverse effects have resolved, the drug may be restarted at a lower dose or by using longer dosing intervals with intense monitoring.

Itraconazole (unlike ketoconazole) does not have appreciable effects on hormone synthesis and likely has fewer adverse effects than ketoconazole in small animal species.

Other adverse effects reported in humans include nausea, vomiting, diarrhea, fatigue, skin rash, edema, hypokalemia, and hypertension.[21]

Reproductive/Nursing Safety

Itraconazole did not impair fertility in rats. In laboratory animals, itraconazole has caused dose-related maternotoxicity, fetotoxicity, and teratogenicity at high doses (ie, 5 to 20 times the labeled dose). In a repeated dose study, 16 pregnant queens receiving itraconazole 5 mg/kg PO for a total of 21 days (7 days on alternate weeks) during gestation or lactation showed a high frequency of fetal resorption, abnormal fetuses, and abnormal maternal behaviors.

Itraconazole enters maternal milk. Use with caution in lactating animals; consider milk replacer.

Because safety has not been established in animals, this drug should only be used when the maternal benefits outweigh the potential risks to offspring.

Overdose/Acute Toxicity

Limited information on the acute toxicity of itraconazole is available. Itraconazole dosages up to 25 mg/kg/day given on alternate weeks to healthy cats resulted in hypersalivation and increased liver enzyme activity. Inflammatory lesions were also seen in the lungs and kidneys of some cats and were believed to be caused by a component of the liquid vehicle (hydroxypropyl-beta-cyclodextrin [HP-beta-CD]). Administration of oral antacids may help reduce absorption. If a large overdose occurs, gastric decontamination should be considered, and supportive therapy provided as required. Itraconazole is not removed by dialysis, but dialysis would remove HPbetaCD in cases in which the oral solution was ingested.[32] Itraconazole effects may be reversed by IV lipid emulsion therapy.

For patients that have experienced or are suspected to have experienced an overdose, consultation with a 24-hour poison consultation center specializing in providing veterinary-specific information is recommended. For general information related to overdose and toxin exposures, as well as contact information for poison control centers, refer to ***Appendix***.

Drug Interactions

In humans, itraconazole is a potent inhibitor of CYP3A4 and P-glycoprotein and is metabolized by CYP3A4; veterinary significance is uncertain. The following drug interactions have either been reported or are theoretical in humans or animals receiving itraconazole and may be of significance in veterinary patients. Unless otherwise noted, use together is not necessarily contraindicated, but the potential risks should be weighed and additional monitoring should be performed when appropriate.

- **Amphotericin B**: Laboratory animal studies have shown that itraconazole used concomitantly with amphotericin B may be antagonistic against *Aspergillus* spp or *Candida* spp; the clinical importance of these findings is not clear.
- **Antacids, Oral** (eg, **aluminum, calcium and magnesium containing**): May reduce oral absorption of itraconazole, which should be administered at least 1 hour before or 2 hours after antacids
- **Histamine H_2-Blockers** (eg, **famotidine, ranitidine**): Increased gastric pH may reduce itraconazole absorption.
- **Highly Protein Bound Drugs** (eg, **NSAIDs, phenytoin, salicylates, sulfonamides, sulfonylurea antidiabetic agents** [eg, **glipizide, glyburide**], **warfarin**): Because itraconazole is highly bound to plasma proteins (ie, 99%), it could theoretically displace other highly bound drugs; a temporary increase in serum concentrations may occur. These interactions have not been shown to be of clinical concern.
- **Isoniazid**: May decrease itraconazole concentrations
- **Macrolide Antibiotics** (eg, **clarithromycin, erythromycin**): May increase itraconazole concentrations; itraconazole may increase macrolide antibiotic concentrations
- **Meloxicam**: Itraconazole may decrease peak meloxicam concentrations and reduce meloxicam exposure.
- **Phenobarbital, Primidone**: May decrease itraconazole concentrations
- **Proton Pump Inhibitors** (**PPIs**; eg, **omeprazole, pantoprazole**): Increased gastric pH may reduce itraconazole absorption.
- **Rifampin**: May decrease itraconazole concentrations; itraconazole may increase rifampin concentrations; concurrent use or use within 2 weeks of discontinuing itraconazole is contraindicated.[33]
- **Sucralfate**: May reduce itraconazole absorption
- **Toceranib**: Increased toceranib or itraconazole concentrations may occur

Itraconazole may increase the absorption and/or reduce the metabolism of the following drugs (increasing plasma concentrations or exposure with resulting increased risk for toxicity):

- **Benzodiazepines** (eg, **alprazolam, diazepam, oral midazolam**): Itraconazole may increase benzodiazepine concentrations. In humans, concurrent use with oral midazolam is contraindicated.[21,27]
- **Buspirone**: Itraconazole may increase plasma concentrations of buspirone.
- **Busulfan**: Itraconazole may increase busulfan concentrations.
- **Calcium-Channel Blocking Agents** (eg, **amlodipine, diltiazem**): Itraconazole may increase concentrations and the risk for toxicity. Increased itraconazole concentrations may occur. Negative inotropic effects may be potentiated. Use this combination cautiously in patients with heart failure.
- **Cannabidiol**
- **Ciprofloxacin**: May result in increased itraconazole exposure
- **Cisapride**: Itraconazole may increase cisapride concentrations and the risk for toxicity; in humans, concurrent use or use within 2 weeks of discontinuing itraconazole is contraindicated.[21,27]
- **Colchicine**: In humans, concurrent use or use within 2 weeks of discontinuing itraconazole is contraindicated in patients with hepatic or renal impairment.[21,27]
- **Corticosteroids** (eg, **dexamethasone, predniso(lo)ne**): Itraconazole may inhibit the metabolism of corticosteroids; increased hepatotoxic and GI adverse effects are possible.
- **Cyclophosphamide**: Itraconazole may inhibit the metabolism of cyclophosphamide and its metabolites; increased toxicity can occur.
- **Cyclosporine**: Itraconazole increases cyclosporine concentrations and decreases cyclosporine dose requirements.[34]
- **Digoxin**: Itraconazole may increase digoxin concentrations.
- **Disopyramide**: Use together (in humans) is contraindicated.
- **Doxorubicin**: Itraconazole increases doxorubicin exposure.
- **Ergot Alkaloids** (eg, **bromocriptine, cabergoline, pergolide**): Itraconazole increases ergot alkaloid concentrations; use together (in humans) is contraindicated.
- **Fentanyl/Alfentanil**: Itraconazole may increase fentanyl or alfentanil concentrations; in humans, concurrent use or use within 2 weeks of discontinuing itraconazole is contraindicated.
- **Ivermectin**: Itraconazole may increase the risk for neurotoxicity.
- **Loperamide**
- **Methadone**: In humans, concurrent use or use within 2 weeks of discontinuing itraconazole is contraindicated.
- **Praziquantel**: Increased plasma concentrations of praziquantel
- **Quinidine**: Increased risk for quinidine toxicity; use together (in humans) is contraindicated.
- **Rivaroxaban**: Increased risk for rivaroxaban toxicity; in humans, concurrent use or use within 2 weeks of discontinuing itraconazole is contraindicated.
- **Sildenafil**: Itraconazole increases sildenafil exposure.
- **Sulfonylurea Antidiabetic Agents** (eg, **glipizide, glyburide**): Itraconazole may increase concentrations of these agents; hypoglycemia is possible.
- **Tamsulosin**: Increased risk for tamsulosin toxicity; in humans, concurrent use or use within 2 weeks of discontinuing itraconazole is contraindicated.
- **Tricyclic Antidepressants** (**TCAs**; eg, **amitriptyline, clo-**

mipramine): Itraconazole may decrease metabolism and increase TCA concentrations.

- **Vincristine/Vinblastine**: Itraconazole may inhibit vinca alkaloid metabolism and increase concentrations; in humans, concurrent use or use within 2 weeks of discontinuing itraconazole is contraindicated.
- **Warfarin**: Itraconazole may cause increased prothrombin times in patients receiving warfarin or other coumarin anticoagulants.

Laboratory Considerations

None

Dosages

NOTE: Because commercial itraconazole solutions yield higher peak serum concentrations and overall drug exposure than commercial itraconazole capsules in cats, lower doses can be used with solutions.[18] This does not appear to be the case with dogs.[17] Capsules should be administered with food to maximize absorption. Compounded formulations should be avoided.

DOGS:

Susceptible systemic mycoses (extra-label): Typically, 5 – 10 mg/kg PO once daily (or divided and given every 12 hours) with food; recommendations for treatment duration vary and are determined by the infective agent and site of infection. In general, treatment for systemic mycoses should be maintained for at least 30 to 60 days after clinical resolution. Infections such as pythiosis, lagenidiosis, zygomycosis, phaeohyphomycosis, or hyalohyphomycosis may require 10 – 15 mg/kg PO once daily for many months, as well as surgical resection and additional antifungal agents (eg, terbinafine). **NOTE**: Itraconazole dosages greater than or equal to 10 mg/kg/day are associated with an increased risk for adverse effects.

Blastomycosis (extra-label): 5 mg/kg PO once daily for 1 month beyond resolution of clinical signs.[2–4] Dosages up to 10 mg/kg per day may be used, but the risk for adverse effects increases with higher doses. One study found equivalent results in dogs treated with fluconazole.[2]

Histoplasmosis (extra-label): Median dosage was 10 mg/kg/day PO, but dosages ranged from 4.3 – 33.8 mg/kg/day.[8]

Dermatophytosis, onychomycosis (extra-label): 5 – 10 mg/kg PO once daily[35]; treatment should continue until mycologic cure (2 negative skin cultures taken 2 weeks apart)

***Malassezia* spp dermatitis** (extra-label):

a) **Daily**: 5 mg/kg PO every 24 hours and continued for 1 week after complete resolution of clinical signs[36,37]
b) **Pulse therapy**: 5 mg/kg PO every 24 hours for 2 consecutive days per week[36,37]

***Trypanosoma cruzi* infection (American trypanosomiasis [ie, Chagas disease])** (extra-label): 10 mg/kg PO once daily with amiodarone 7.5 mg/kg PO once daily (with or without amiodarone loading dosage protocol). **NOTE**: Itraconazole 100 mg (total dose; NOT mg/kg) PO every 48 hours was administered to dogs with low body weight; itraconazole dose was rounded down to the nearest 100 mg increment dose.[38]

Pythiosis (extra-label): 5 – 10 mg/kg PO once daily in combination with terbinafine 6 – 12 mg/kg PO once daily.[9–12] This combination may be used in conjunction with mefenoxam 4 mg/kg PO every 12 hours[9–11] or prednisone.[12]

CATS:

Dermatophytosis caused by *Microsporum canis* (label dosage; FDA-approved): 5 mg/kg PO (with or without food) once daily for 7 days given on alternating weeks for 3 treatment cycles. Cats must be treated during weeks 1, 3, and 5 and left untreated during weeks 2 and 4.

Generalized dermatophytosis in shelter cats (extra-label): 5 mg/kg PO once daily for 21 days with concurrent twice-weekly lime sulfur rinses. Treating otherwise healthy cats without biochemical monitoring is reasonable and cost effective; however, if cats become depressed or anorexic, biochemical monitoring is indicated.[30,39]

***Malassezia* spp dermatitis** (extra-label):

a) **Daily**: 5 – 10 mg/kg PO once daily and continued for 1 week after complete resolution of clinical signs[35,37,40]
b) **Pulse therapy**: 5 mg/kg PO once daily for 2 consecutive days per week[36,37]

Susceptible systemic mycoses (extra-label):

a) 5 – 10 mg/kg PO once daily (or divided and given every 12 hours) with food. Treatment duration may be months (ie, 2 or more), and treatment is generally recommended to continue for at least 30 to 60 days after clinical resolution of signs. Certain infections may require additional surgical treatment or additional antifungals (eg, amphotericin B, terbinafine).
b) In a pharmacokinetics study, 100 mg/cat (NOT mg/kg) PO every 48 hours resulted in serum concentrations that should be safe and effective.[41]
c) **Fungal osteomyelitis**: From 2 case reports, 1 cat received itraconazole 10 mg/kg PO every 12 hours for at least 5 weeks and showed marked improvement prior to being lost to follow-up.[14] A second cat received itraconazole 12.8 mg/kg PO every 12 hours with amphotericin B 0.55 mg/kg as a twice-weekly SC infusion. Itraconazole caused inappetence and vomiting, and the itraconazole dose was reduced to 9 mg/kg PO every 12 hours and continued until the patient was seronegative twice, 1 month apart (≈2 years).[42]
d) **Cryptococcosis**: From a retrospective study, 50 – 100 mg/cat (NOT mg/kg) PO once daily. Fluconazole appeared to have greater efficacy with a shorter treatment duration.[1]

Sporotrichosis (extra-label):

a) **Monotherapy**: 10 mg/kg PO every 24 hours for 2 to 3 months, or 1 month after clinical cure, has been recommended.[43–46] Other dosages have included 8.3 – 27.7 mg/kg PO daily[31] or 50 – 100 mg/cat (NOT mg/kg) PO with food every 24 hours.[6] Treatment resulted in 38% to 71% of cats being clinically cured; nasal mucosal involvement, respiratory signs, and high fungal loads in skin lesions were predictors of treatment failure.[6,31] In one study, itraconazole was more effective and better tolerated than ketoconazole.[31]
b) **Combination therapy**:
    i. Itraconazole 100 mg/cat/day PO (NOT mg/kg) in combination with potassium iodide initially, 2.5 mg/kg/day PO, increased by 2.5 mg/kg/day every 30 days until clinical cure was attained or the dosage reached 20 mg/kg/day. This combination cured 96% of treatment-naive cats; the median potassium iodide dosage was 3.1 mg/kg/day, and median time of treatment was 14 weeks (range, 8 to 30 weeks).[47] Itraconazole 100 mg/cat (NOT mg/kg) PO once daily in combination with potassium iodide 5 mg/kg/day PO was effective in cats that failed to respond to itraconazole monotherapy.[48]
    ii. Itraconazole 100 mg/cat/day PO (NOT mg/kg) in combination with intralesional amphotericin B (conventional) resulted in clinical remission in 85% of patients. Amphotericin B was reconstituted with 10 mL 1% lidocaine and multidirectionally directly infiltrated into each lesion until swelling occurred.[49]

HORSES:

Guttural pouch mycosis, mycotic rhinitis, or osteomyelitis (extra-label): Using the oral solution, 5 mg/kg PO every 24 hours should be sufficient for treatment.[50] **NOTE**: Itraconazole oral solution is better absorbed than capsules,[25] and compounded formulations may not be absorbed (see ***Compatibility/Compounding Considerations***).

BIRDS:

NOTE: All dosages are extra-label.

a) 5 – 10 mg/kg PO every 12 to 24 hours. Use with caution in African grey parrots.[51]

b) Aspergillosis: 5 – 10 mg/kg PO once daily in Amazon parrots; 2.5 – 5 mg/kg PO once daily in African grey parrots[52]

RABBITS, RODENTS, SMALL MAMMALS:

Mice (extra-label): Blastomycosis: 50 – 150 mg/kg every 24 hours

Hedgehogs (extra-label): Dermatophytosis: 10 mg/kg PO twice daily using a commercial oral solution[53]

Rats (extra-label): Vaginal candidiasis: 2.5 – 10 mg/kg every 24 hours

Guinea pigs (extra-label): Systemic candidiasis: 5 mg/kg every 24 hours[54]

Rabbits (extra-label): Dermatophytosis: 5 – 10 mg/kg PO once daily

REPTILES:

Susceptible fungal diseases (extra-label):

a) 10 – 20 mg/kg PO every 24 hours[55]

b) 10 mg/kg PO every 48 hours for 14 days or 10 mg/kg every 24 hours for 7 days followed by every 48 hours for 7 days[56]

Monitoring

- Clinical efficacy
- With long-term therapy, periodic laboratory monitoring of renal and hepatic markers is recommended.
- Fungal cultures (eg, Dermatophyte Test Media [DTM]) for dermatophytosis
- Urine antigen testing for systemic mycoses
- Consider monitoring itraconazole serum trough concentrations (when available) with prolonged treatment of systemic infections.
- GI signs (eg, inappetence, vomiting, diarrhea)
- Itraconazole is contraindicated in humans with evidence of ventricular dysfunction. It is unknown if this applies to animals; consider monitoring cardiac function in animals with pre-existing heart disease.
- Physical assessment for ulcerative skin lesions in dogs

Client Information

- Give this medicine as directed by your veterinarian.
- Use the syringe provided with the FDA-approved oral solution for cats. Do not invert the bottle when withdrawing the solution. Rinse and dry the syringe after administration and screw the cap tightly onto the bottle.
- The veterinary-labeled oral solution may be given to cats with or without food. Preferably, give the oral solution to other mammals on an empty stomach. Give capsules or capsule contents with a fatty food (eg, butter, cream, ice cream, cheese).
- This medicine interacts with many others. Do not give your animal other medications without first talking to your veterinarian or veterinary pharmacist.
- Vomiting and loss of appetite are the most common side effects seen in dogs and cats. Liver toxicity and serious skin effects are also possible.

Chemistry/Synonyms

Itraconazole, a synthetic triazole antifungal, is structurally related to fluconazole. It occurs as a white or almost-white powder. It is practically insoluble in water, very slightly soluble in alcohol, and highly lipophilic. The log-P octanol/water partition coefficient is 5.66.[24] The human-labeled commercial oral solution has a pH of 2.

Itraconazole may also be known as itraconazolum, oriconazole, R-51211, or *Sporanox*®; many other trade names are available.

Storage/Stability

Itraconazole capsules should be stored between 15°C and 25°C (59°F-77°F) and protected from light and moisture.

Veterinary-labeled itraconazole solution should be stored upright at 20°C to 25°C (68°F-77°F), with excursions permitted between 15°C to 30°C (59°F-86°F). Human-labeled itraconazole oral solution should be stored at temperatures less than 25°C (77°F) and protected from freezing.

Compatibility/Compounding Considerations

Compounding capsules or solutions from bulk chemicals or powders likely will not yield dosage forms that are absorbed. The oral bioavailability and solubility of itraconazole are dependent on complexation with acidified high-molecular weight polyethylene glycol (PEG) or cyclodextrin molecules,[24] a technology used in the brand name (ie, *Itrafungol*®, *Sporanox*®) and generic commercially produced human drug products for itraconazole, but typically not in compounded dosage forms. Studies have demonstrated that itraconazole compounded from the bulk chemical produces inferior blood concentrations as compared with FDA-approved itraconazole products.[18,22,57,58] Inferior blood concentrations of itraconazole may contribute to treatment failure and fatality if compounded itraconazole is used in life-threatening infections (eg, blastomycosis, pythiosis). Compounded itraconazole products should NOT be used unless they have been prepared from FDA-approved commercial capsules or documented bioavailability and stability data are provided.

Dosage Forms/Regulatory Status

VETERINARY-LABELED PRODUCTS:

Itraconazole Oral Solution: 10 mg/mL in 52 mL; *Itrafungol*®; (Rx). Labeled for use in cats. NADA# 141-474. Cherry–caramel flavor

HUMAN-LABELED PRODUCTS:

Itraconazole Capsules: 100 mg; *Sporanox*®; generic; (Rx)

Itraconazole Oral Solution: 10 mg/mL in 150 mL; *Sporanox*®; (Rx). Cherry–caramel flavor

References

For the complete list of references, see **wiley.com/go/budde/plumb**

Ivermectin

(eye-ver-**mek**-tin) *Heartgard®, Ivomec®*

Antiparasitic

Prescriber Highlights

- Used in dogs and cats to prevent heartworm disease by eliminating tissue stages of heartworm larvae, as well as in cats to remove and control hookworms
- Used in horses, cattle, and sheep as a broad-spectrum ecto- and endoparasiticide. Best used as part of a comprehensive parasite management program that includes fecal egg count reduction testing to treat only those animals with high endoparasite burden
- Also used as an antiparasiticide in a wide variety of other species
- Contraindications include animals that are hypersensitive to it and in chelonians, indigo snakes, crocodilians, and skinks.
- Use of doses higher than those used for heartworm prevention should be undertaken with caution in breeds susceptible to *MDR1* mutation (also known as *ABCB1*-1delta) because they are at higher risk for CNS toxicity.
- Use very cautiously (or avoid use) with other drugs that affect P-glycoprotein (P-gp).
- Use as a microfilaricide in dogs should be avoided, as dogs may exhibit a shock-like reaction that is presumably a result of dying microfilaria.
- Adverse effects in horses include swelling and pruritus at the ventral midline, which can be seen »24 hours after ivermectin administration due to a hypersensitivity reaction to dead *Onchocerca* spp microfilaria.
- In cattle, ivermectin should only be administered via SC route and not by IM or IV routes; ivermectin can induce serious adverse effects by killing parasitic larvae in vital areas of the body; it may also cause discomfort or transient swelling at the injection site.

Uses/Indications

In dogs, ivermectin is FDA-approved only for use as a heartworm preventive. In cats, ivermectin is FDA-approved for heartworm prevention and removal and control of hookworms. This drug has also been used in dogs and cats in an extra-label manner as a broad-spectrum endo- and ectoparasiticide, although isoxazolines are active effective against a wider spectrum of ectoparasites. Ivermectin and doxycycline individually suppress embryogenesis in parasites and weaken adult heartworms; when these drugs are used together as adulticide pretreatment, they provide more rapid adulticidal activity and reduce pulmonary pathology caused by heartworm death. The combination is also more effective at reducing *Wolbachia* spp numbers than doxycycline alone. The American Heartworm Society does **NOT** recommend using macrocyclic lactones in dogs at prophylactic doses as a slow-kill adulticide method for *Dirofilaria immitis*[1]; however, in cats, monthly ivermectin for 2 years may be used to reduce worm burdens.[2]

In horses, ivermectin is FDA-approved for the control of large strongyles (adults), small strongyles (adults, fourth-stage larvae), pinworms (adults, fourth-stage larvae), ascarids (adults, third- and fourth-stage larvae), hairworms (adults), large-mouth stomach worms (adults), neck threadworms (microfilariae), bots (oral and gastric stages), lungworms (adults, fourth-stage larvae), intestinal threadworms (adults), and summer sores (cutaneous third-stage larvae) secondary to *Habronema* spp or *Draschia* spp. For a list of individual species covered, refer to specific product information.[3]

In cattle, ivermectin is FDA-approved for the treatment and control of GI roundworms (adults, fourth-stage larvae), lungworms (adults, fourth-stage larvae), cattle grubs (parasitic stages), sucking lice, mites, and horn flies. For a list of individual species covered, refer to specific product information.[4,5]

In swine, ivermectin is FDA-approved for the treatment and control of GI roundworms (adults, fourth-stage larvae), somatic roundworm larvae, lungworms (adults), lice, and mange mites. For a list of individual species covered, refer to specific product information.[4]

In sheep, ivermectin is FDA-approved for the treatment and control of GI roundworms (adults, fourth-stage larvae), lungworms (adults, fourth-stage larvae), and nasal bots (larval stages). For a list of individual species and life cycles covered, refer to specific product information.[6]

In reindeer, ivermectin is FDA-approved for the treatment and control of warbles.

In American bison, ivermectin is FDA-approved for the treatment and control of grubs.

Pharmacology/Actions

Ivermectin binds glutamate-gated chloride ion channels within invertebrate nerve and muscle cells, increasing cell permeability to chloride ions. The resulting cell hyperpolarization causes paralysis and death of the parasite. Mammals lack glutamate-gated chloride ion channels, and ivermectin has low affinity for other chloride ion channels. Ivermectin may also have activity at gamma-aminobutyric acid (GABA)-gated chloride channels.

Ivermectin kills third- and fourth-larval stage *Dirofilaria immitis* and microfilariae and reduces the life span of adult heartworms. Resistance by *D immitis* to macrocyclic lactones is a concern. The American Heartworm Society has stated: *It is now generally accepted that isolated instances of resistant heartworms have been identified. The extent, the degree of spread, and the reasons for resistance are not well understood and are controversial. . . . The data suggest that owner compliance is the biggest factor in the 'failure' of preventives.*[1]

Studies have shown that ivermectin has some antitumor properties[7-9] and the potential to reverse drug resistance in cancer cells[10], but clinical significance[11] is not yet established.

Although structurally similar to macrolide antibiotics, avermectins have no antibacterial properties.

Pharmacokinetics

In monogastric animals, ivermectin is up to 95% absorbed after oral administration. Oral absorption is reduced in ruminants as the drug may bind to solid material in the rumen. In a variety of species, SC administration results in greater bioavailability and overall drug exposure (AUC), but absorption after oral administration is more rapid.[12] Ivermectin is absorbed after transdermal administration, but results in lower overall exposure than parenteral and oral routes.

Ivermectin is highly bound to plasma proteins (≈90%). Ivermectin is well distributed to most tissues but does not readily penetrate into the CSF. Animals with the *MDR1* mutation (also known as *ABCB1*-1delta; eg, dogs, cats, mice) produce a defective P-glycoprotein (P-gp) transporter,[13] allowing ivermectin to enter into the CNS and increasing the risk for neurotoxicity.

Ivermectin has a long terminal half-life in most species (see below). It is metabolized in the liver via oxidative pathways and is primarily excreted in the feces. In humans, ivermectin is metabolized principally by cytochrome CYP3A4 and, to a lesser extent, by CYP2D6 and CYP2E1. Less than 5% of the drug (as parent compound or metabolites) is excreted in the urine.

Pharmacokinetic parameters of ivermectin have been reported for various species.[12]

- Dogs: Bioavailability was 95%, volume of distribution was 2.5 to 5.3 L/kg, and elimination half-life was 2 to 4 days.[14] Plasma ivermectin concentrations in collies with ivermectin toxicosis were similar to those of nonsensitive dogs.[15]

- Cats: After SC administration, volume of distribution was 9.8 L/kg, and elimination half-life was 2.5 days.[16]
- Horses: After oral administration, the half-life was ≈3 to 4 days.[17] Ivermectin pharmacokinetics may differ between horse breeds.[18]
- Cattle: SC bioavailability was 33 to 55%, volume of distribution was 1.2 – 3.4 L/kg, elimination half-life was 4 to 6 days, and total body clearance was 0.3 to 0.5 L/kg/day. Compared with other routes, topical (pour-on) administration resulted in a lower overall AUC; half-life was ≈5 days in one study.[19]
- Sheep: Bioavailability was 100% with intra-abomasal administration and 25% with intraruminal administration; volume of distribution was ≈5 to 13 L/kg, and elimination half-life was 2 to 7 days.[20]
- Goats: AUC following topical (pour-on) administration was 40% lower than with oral administration;[21] elimination half-life was ≈4 to 6 days and varied by breed.[22]
- Swine: Volume of distribution was 2 to 4 L/kg and elimination half-life was ≈1.5 to 3.5 days.

Contraindications/Precautions/Warnings

Ivermectin is contraindicated in animals with hypersensitivity to it and in chelonians, indigo snakes, crocodilians, and skinks.[23]

Ivermectin is not recommended for use in puppies younger than 6 weeks of age or in dogs without a current negative heartworm test. Secondary to a defect in the P-glycoprotein transport mechanism, dogs with the *MDR1* mutation (also known as *ABCB1*-1delta) can show adverse neurologic effects after receiving a single dose greater than 120 µg/kg and can develop life-threatening neurologic toxicity at doses of 300 µg/kg.[24] Ivermectin should not be used extra-label in breeds susceptible to the *MDR1* mutation (eg, collies, shelties, Australian shepherds) unless the dog has been tested and found to not have the genetic defect; see ***Appendix*** for more information. At higher doses, neurotoxicity can occur (rare) in dogs tested normal/normal, so it is advised to continually monitor for adverse effects. When ivermectin is used at labeled heartworm preventive dosages, toxicity is not observed regardless of the *MDR1* status. It is recommended that if any adverse effects occur at any dose amount, ivermectin should be discontinued.

The injectable products for use in cattle and swine should be given SC only; do **NOT** give IM or IV.

Products should not be used off-label when a labeled product is available for the target species. If using a product in a species for which it is not labeled (ie, extra-label), be certain of the dosage and/or dilutions. There are many reports of overdoses in small animals that received incorrectly diluted large animal injectable products.

Adverse Effects

Neurotoxicity is possible in dogs, particularly in those with the *MDR1* mutation (also known as *ABCB1*-1delta), which is seen most commonly in certain collie-type breeds. There are also case reports of dogs without the *MDR1* mutation developing neurotoxicity after receiving ivermectin at high doses (eg, to treat demodicosis).[25] Heartworm-positive dogs may exhibit a shock-like reaction if ivermectin is used at microfilaricide doses, presumably due to a reaction associated with the dying microfilariae. Vomiting and diarrhea are possible but rare.

In horses, swelling and pruritus at the ventral midline can be seen ≈24 hours after ivermectin administration due to a hypersensitivity reaction to dead *Onchocerca* spp microfilariae. This reaction is preventable by administering a glucocorticoid just prior to and 1 to 2 days after ivermectin administration. If untreated, swelling usually subsides within 7 to 10 days and pruritus resolves within 3 weeks. There are case reports of horses developing neurotoxicity after receiving recommended oral dosages.[26]

When used to treat *Hypoderma* spp larvae (ie, cattle grubs) in cattle, ivermectin can induce serious adverse effects when larvae die in vital areas of the body. Larvae killed in the vertebral canal (*Hypoderma bovis*) can cause paralysis and staggering, and those killed around the esophagus (*Hypoderma lineatum*) can induce salivation and bloat. These adverse effects can be avoided by treating for grubs immediately after the heel fly (ie, warble fly) season, before the larvae migrate into these vital areas. Cattle may experience discomfort or transient swelling at the injection site. Using a maximum of 10 mL at any one injection site can help minimize these effects.

In mice and rats, ivermectin may cause neurologic toxicity at doses slightly more than usually prescribed (less than 0.5 mg/kg).[27]

In birds, death, lethargy, or anorexia may be seen. Orange-cheeked waxbill finches and budgerigars may be more sensitive to ivermectin than other species.

For additional information, refer to ***Overdose/Acute Toxicity***.

Reproductive/Nursing Safety

Ivermectin is considered safe to use during pregnancy. Teratogenicity has been noted in rats and rabbits at doses of 4.5 and 8 times the maximum recommended dose, respectively.[28] However, adverse fetal effects have not been demonstrated in dogs, horses, cattle, or swine. Testicular hypoplasia was noted on pathology in dogs receiving doses 3 times and 5 times the labeled doses of an ivermectin/pyrantel pamoate/praziquantel combination product monthly for 6 months.[29] A separate study of the same product demonstrated a dose-related decrease in testicular maturation in beagle puppies as compared with control. Reproductive performance in adult male animals is apparently unaltered.

Ivermectin is excreted in milk in low concentrations; it is unlikely to pose significant risk for nursing offspring.

Overdose/Acute Toxicity

Common clinical signs associated with an overdose may include ataxia, mydriasis, blindness, tremors, vomiting, seizures, and cardiovascular and respiratory depression.

In dog breeds without the *MDR1* mutation (also known as *ABCB1*-1delta), signs of acute toxicity rarely occur at single doses of 1 mg/kg (1000 µg/kg) or less. Mydriasis occurs at 2.5 mg/kg, and tremors occur at 5 mg/kg. At doses of 10 mg/kg, severe tremors and ataxia are seen. Deaths occurred when doses exceeded 40 mg/kg, but LD_{50} is 80 mg/kg.[30] Beagles receiving 0.5 mg/kg/day PO for 14 weeks developed no signs of toxicity but developed mydriasis and had some weight loss when given 1 – 2 mg/kg/day for the same time period. Half of the dogs receiving 2 mg/kg/day for 14 weeks developed signs of depression, tremors, ataxia, anorexia, and dehydration.

In dog breeds with the *MDR1* mutation, ivermectin enters the CNS at much higher concentrations than unaffected dogs. Doses of 60 µg/kg (10 times the recommended heartworm prophylaxis dose) demonstrated no signs of toxicity in sensitive collies.[31] Dogs with the *MDR1* mutation can show adverse neurologic effects after receiving a single dose greater than 120 µg/kg and develop life-threatening neurologic toxicity at doses of 300 µg/kg.[24] In cases of overdoses, signs of neurotoxicity can develop within 4 hours in breeds homozygous for the *MDR1* mutation.

Dogs that receive an overdose of ivermectin or develop signs of acute toxicity should receive supportive therapy for treatment of clinical signs. Gastric decontamination should be considered for acute massive oral ingestions in dogs or cats. For both oral and injected ivermectin overdoses, the use of repeated activated charcoal doses can interrupt enterohepatic recirculation.

Ivermectin has a large safety margin in cats. Kittens receiving doses of at least 110 µg/kg and adult cats receiving at least 750 µg/kg showed no adverse effects. The margin of safety is narrower in kittens, as significant clinical signs have been seen at 300 μg/kg. Acute toxic signs associated with massive overdoses in cats will appear within 10 hours of ingestion. Signs may include agitation, vocalization, anorexia, mydriasis, rear limb paresis, tremors, and disorientation. Blindness, head pressing, wall climbing, absence of oculomotor menace reflex, and a slow and incomplete response to pupillary light may also be seen. Neurologic signs usually diminish over several days and most animals completely recover within 2 to 4 weeks. Supportive care is recommended.

In horses, doses of 1.8 mg/kg PO (9 times the recommended dose) did not produce signs of toxicity, but doses of 2 mg/kg caused signs of visual impairment, depression, and ataxia.[30,32]

In cattle, toxic effects generally do not appear until doses of 30 times the recommended dose are injected.[33] At 8 mg/kg SC, cattle showed signs of ataxia, listlessness, and, occasionally, death. An oral drench of 4 mg/kg elicited an acute toxic syndrome.[30]

Sheep have shown signs of ataxia and depression at ivermectin doses of 4 mg/kg; the propylene glycol vehicle may have contributed to the toxic signs.[30]

Swine have shown signs of toxicosis (eg, lethargy, ataxia, tremors, lateral recumbency, mydriasis) at doses of 30 mg/kg.[30] Neonatal pigs may be more susceptible to ivermectin overdoses, presumably due to a more permeable blood–brain barrier. Accurate dosing practices are recommended.

IV lipid emulsion has been successfully used to treat dogs, cats, ponies, and an African lion with neurotoxicity and retinopathy/blindness caused by large ivermectin overdoses.[34–46]

For patients that have experienced or are suspected to have experienced an overdose, consultation with a 24-hour poison consultation center specializing in providing veterinary-specific information is recommended. For general information related to overdose and toxin exposures, as well as contact information for poison control centers, refer to ***Appendix***.

Drug Interactions

In humans, ivermectin is a substrate of CYP3A4. The following drug interactions have either been reported or are theoretical in humans or animals receiving ivermectin and may be of significance in veterinary patients. Unless otherwise noted, use together is not necessarily contraindicated, but weigh the potential risks and perform additional monitoring when appropriate.

NOTE: Combined treatment with any of the drugs listed below when ivermectin is used as a single treatment or as heartworm prophylaxis is unlikely to be of clinical significance.

- **BENZODIAZEPINES**: Effects may be potentiated by ivermectin; use together is not advised in humans.
- **GABAPENTIN**: Effect may be potentiated by ivermectin; use together is not advised in humans.
- **KETAMINE**: It has been recommended not to use ivermectin in reptiles within 10 days of administering ketamine.[47]
- **MITOTANE**: May decrease ivermectin exposure and efficacy
- **PHENOBARBITAL**: Effect may be potentiated by ivermectin; use together is not advised in humans. Phenobarbital reduced the ivermectin plasma concentration and overall drug exposure.[48]
- **PREGABALIN**: Effect may be potentiated by ivermectin; use together is not advised in humans.
- **WARFARIN**: Concurrent ivermectin use may increase prothrombin time/INRs.

Caution is advised if using other drugs that can inhibit **P-glycoprotein (P-gp)**. Dogs at risk for the *MDR1* mutation (also known as *ABCB1*-1delta; eg, collies, Australian shepherds, shelties, long-haired whippets, breeds with "white feet") should not receive ivermectin above heartworm preventive doses with the following drugs unless they are tested as normal. Many P-gp inhibitors also inhibit CYP3A4 in humans and may alter ivermectin metabolism. Drugs and drug classes involved include the following:

- **AMIODARONE**
- **AZITHROMYCIN**
- **BROMOCRIPTINE**
- **CARVEDILOL**
- **CETIRIZINE**: In horses, pretreatment (12 hours before cetirizine, but not 1.5 hours) with ivermectin significantly increased cetirizine plasma AUC, mean residence time, and terminal half-life.[49] However, because of cetirizine's large therapeutic index, clinical significance is not likely.
- **CLARITHROMYCIN, ERYTHROMYCIN**
- **CYCLOSPORINE**
- **DILTIAZEM**
- **FLUOXETINE**
- **GRAPEFRUIT JUICE**
- **ITRACONAZOLE, KETOCONAZOLE**: At least one reference states that ivermectin should never be used with ketoconazole in dogs.[50]
- **METHADONE, PENTAZOCINE**
- **QUINIDINE**
- **PAROXETINE**
- ***SOLANUM* spp** (nightshades): Horses ingesting nightshades and receiving oral ivermectin developed neurotoxicity.[51] The authors suggest that *Solanum* spp may alter P-gp in horses or other mammals.
- **SPINOSAD**: Spinosad is a potent inhibitor of canine P-gp. It has been recommended that spinosad should not be used with high extra-label doses of ivermectin.[52] In healthy beagles, spinosad has been shown to alter ivermectin pharmacokinetics and may alter blood–brain barrier permeability and increase the risk for neurotoxicity.[53]
- **SPIRONOLACTONE**
- **ST. JOHN'S WORT**
- **TACROLIMUS**
- **VERAPAMIL**

Laboratory Considerations

- At doses of 50 μg/kg or higher, ivermectin may yield false negative Knott's test results in animals with occult heartworm infection.

Dosages

For combination products, refer to the product label for specific approved dosage suggestions.

DOGS:

NOTE: When using ivermectin for prophylaxis or treatment of dirofilariasis, it is recommended to review the most recently published guidelines provided by the American Heartworm Society.[1]

Heartworm prevention (label dosage; FDA-approved): Minimum dosage of 6 μg/kg (0.006 mg/kg) PO per month.[31] For maximum effectiveness, heartworm prophylaxis should be given year-round; however, if seasonal treatment is chosen, administration should begin at least 1 month prior to the anticipated start of heartworm transmission and should continue for up to 6 months after transmission typically ceases.[1]

Adjunctive treatment for adult heartworm infection (extra-label): Approved heartworm preventives are given at labeled doses on day 1 of the treatment protocol and repeated every 30 days.[1]

Microfilarial keratitis (extra-label): 100 – 300 μg/kg (0.1 – 0.3 mg/kg) PO once per month. Additional treatment included prednisone 1 mg/kg/day PO for 5 to 6 days in conjunction with ivermectin and cyclosporine ophthalmic ointment applied twice daily chronically.[54]

Ectoparasiticide (miticide): **WARNING**: Do not use the dosing regimens listed below in dogs with the *MDR1* **mutation** (also known as *ABCB1*-1delta), or susceptible breeds unless they test as normal/normal. If normal/normal, a drug reaction is unlikely but still possible; continue to monitor for adverse effects. **NOTE**: Isoxazolines (eg, fluralaner, sarolaner) have largely supplanted avermectins for the treatment of demodicosis[55–57] and other ectoparasite indications.

a) **Generalized demodicosis** (extra-label): The usual recommended target dose is 600 µg/kg (0.6 mg/kg) PO once daily until 4 weeks after 2 negative skin scrapings taken 4 to 6 weeks apart. Start at a low dose and increase as follows: **Day 1**: 50 µg/kg (0.05 mg/kg) PO; **Day 2**: 100 µg/kg (0.1 mg/kg) PO; **Day 3**: 150 µg/kg (0.15 mg/kg) PO; **Day 4**: 200 µg/kg (0.2 mg/kg) PO; **Day 5**: 300 µg/kg (0.3 mg/kg) PO. Then increase by 100 µg/kg (0.1 mg/kg) every 3 to 7 days until the final target dose is reached. Treatment may be required for several months. If the animal does not have a reaction at a lower but therapeutic dose (above 300 µg/kg [0.3 mg/kg]), it may be attempted to treat at that lower dose but on an alternate-day treatment schedule to avoid adverse effects at higher doses.[50,58,59]

b) **Sarcoptic mange, cheyletiellosis** (extra-label):
<u>SC</u>: If skin scrapings are positive, 200 – 400 µg/kg (0.2 – 0.4 mg/kg) SC every 2 weeks for 3 treatments. If skin scrapings are not taken or are negative and a therapeutic trial is performed, or if there are positive results after the second injection, give a third injection. If there is no response after the second injection, reconsider diagnosis.
Alternatively, a <u>PO dose</u> for sarcoptic mange can be considered: 200 – 400 µg/kg (0.2 – 0.4 mg/kg) PO once weekly for 4 treatments[58]

c) **Otodectic acariosis** (extra-label): 300 µg/kg (0.3 mg/kg) SC every 2 weeks or topical application of 0.5 mL (using 100 µg/mL [0.1 mg/mL] concentration) per ear for 1 to 2 treatments.[58] Refer to ***Antiparasitic Preparations, Otic*** for alternative dosage forms.

d) **Nasal mites** (extra-label): 300 µg/kg (0.3 mg/kg) SC every 1 to 2 weeks for 2 to 3 treatments[58]

CATS:

NOTE: When using ivermectin for prophylaxis or treatment of dirofilariasis, it is recommended to review the most recently published guidelines provided by the American Heartworm Society.[60]

Heartworm prevention and control of hookworms (label dosage; FDA-approved): The individual minimum monthly prophylactic dose of ivermectin is 24 µg/kg (0.024 mg/kg).[61] Preventives should be started in kittens at 8 weeks of age and administered to all cats in heartworm endemic areas during the heartworm season. Use is not precluded by antibody or antigen seropositivity.[60]

HORSES:

Large and small strongyles, pinworms, ascarids, hairworms, large-mouth stomach worms, neck threadworms, bots, lungworms, intestinal threadworms, and summer sores (label dosage; FDA-approved): 200 µg/kg (0.2 mg/kg) PO. Treat foals initially at 6 to 8 weeks of age. Continue treatment, as appropriate, as part of an overall internal parasite control program.[62]

BOVINE:

GI roundworms (including inhibited stage of *Ostertagia ostertagi* in cattle), lungworms, grubs, sucking lice, and mange mites: (label dosage; FDA-approved):

a) **Injection**: 200 µg/kg (0.2 mg/kg) SC under the loose skin in front of or behind the shoulder. For most effective results against grubs, treat cattle as soon as possible after the end of the heel fly (ie, warble fly) season.[4]

b) **Topical pour-on**: 500 µg/kg (0.5 mg/kg) topically as a narrow strip from withers to tailhead[5]

Treatment and control of grubs (*Hypoderma bovis*) in American bison (label dose; FDA-approved): 200 µg/kg (0.2 mg/kg) SC under the loose skin in front of or behind the shoulder[4]

SHEEP/GOATS:

GI roundworms; lungworms; and nasal bots in sheep (label dosage; FDA-approved): Using the approved oral drench for sheep, 200 µg/kg (0.2 mg/kg) PO.[63]

Adjunctive treatment of meningeal worm (*Parelaphostrongylus tenuis*) (extra-label): To prevent further migration: ivermectin 300 µg/kg (0.3 mg/kg) SC once daily for 5 days with fenbendazole 50 mg/kg PO once daily for 5 days[64]

REINDEER:

Treatment and control of warbles (*Oedemagena tarandi*) (label dose; FDA-approved): 200 µg/kg (0.2 mg/kg) SC under the loose skin in front of or behind the shoulder[4]

CAMELIDS:

GI helminths (extra-label): In new world camelids: 200 µg/kg (0.2 mg/kg) PO once[65]

Adjunctive treatment of meningeal worm (*Parelaphostrongylus tenuis*) (extra-label): To prevent further migration: ivermectin 300 µg/kg (0.3 mg/kg) SC once daily for 5 days with fenbendazole 50 mg/kg PO once daily for 5 days. Camelids are very susceptible to GI ulcers; give prophylaxis or treat with omeprazole or ranitidine.[66]

Sarcoptic mange (extra-label): 200 – 400 µg/kg (0.2 – 0.4 mg/kg) SC every 15 days for 3 treatments[67]

SWINE:

Susceptible parasites (eg, GI roundworms, lungworms, lice, mange mites) (label dosage, FDA-approved): 300 µg/kg (0.3 mg/kg) SC in the neck immediately behind the ear[4]

GI nematodes (*Strongyloides ransomi, Ascaris suum, Metastrongylus salmi, Hyostrongylus rubidus, Trichuris suis*) (extra-label): 100 µg/kg (0.1 mg/kg) PO daily for 7 days[68]

BIRDS:

Susceptible parasites (all are extra-label):

a) **Ascarids, *Capillaria* spp, and other intestinal worms; *Knemidokoptes pilae* (eg, scaly face and leg mites)**: Dilute ivermectin to a 2000 µg/mL (2 mg/mL) concentration. After diluting product, use immediately.
   - **Most birds**: 220 µg/kg (0.22 mg/kg) IM[69]
   - **Amazons**: 100 µg /bird (0.1 mg/bird; NOT mg/kg) IM
   - **Macaws**: 200 µg /bird (0.2 mg/bird; NOT mg/kg) IM
   - **Finches**: 20 µg /bird (0.02 mg/bird; NOT mg/kg) IM

b) **Ascarids, *Coccidia* spp, and other intestinal nematodes; *Oxyspirura* spp, gapeworms, *Knemidokoptes pilae* (eg, scaly face and leg mites)**: Dilute bovine preparation (10 mg/mL) 1:4 with propylene glycol
   - **Most species**: 200 µg/kg (0.2 mg/kg) IM or orally, repeat in 10 to 14 days
   - **Budgerigars**: 12.5 µg/bird (0.0125 mg/bird [0.01 mL of diluted product]; NOT mg/kg), IM or PO[70]

c) **Ectoparasites**: ≈200 µg/kg (0.2 mg/kg) topically.[71,72] For routine prevention of common ectoparasites, this dose should be repeated monthly. For the treatment of an existing infestation, repeat doses are required 2 and 4 weeks after the initial application.

FERRETS:

Heartworm prevention (extra-label): 20 µg/kg (0.02 mg/kg) PO once monthly[73]

Heartworm infection (extra-label): 50 μg/kg (0.05 mg/kg) PO once monthly[74]

RABBITS/RODENTS/SMALL MAMMALS:

NOTE: All are extra-label.

Rabbits:

a) ***Sarcoptes scabiei, Notoedres cati***: 300 – 400 μg/kg (0.3 – 0.4 mg/kg) SC, repeat in 14 days[75]

b) **Ear mites**: 200 μg/kg (0.2 mg/kg) SC, repeat in 2 weeks. All rabbits in the colony should be treated and cages cleaned and disinfected.[76] Similarly, 200 – 440 μg /kg (0.2 – 0.44 mg/kg) PO or SC, repeat in 8 to 18 days[75]

c) **Cheyletiellosis**: From a retrospective study, 200 – 480 μg/kg (0.2 – 0.48 mg/kg) SC; 2 or 3 doses were administered at a mean interval of 11 days[77]

Rodents and lagomorphs for treatment of sarcoptoid and some fur mites: 200 – 250 μg/kg (0.2 – 0.25 mg/kg) SC. Cages should be thoroughly cleaned and disinfected.[76]

Mice, rats, gerbils, guinea pigs, chinchillas: 200 μg/kg (0.2 mg/kg) SC or PO every 7 days for 3 weeks

Hamsters: 200 – 500 μg/kg (0.2 – 0.5 mg/kg) SC or PO every 14 days for 3 weeks[78]

Guinea pigs for treatment of *Trixacarus caviae* mites: 400 μg/kg (0.4 mg/kg) SC, every 10 days for 4 injections[79]

Ectoparasites in rabbits, rodents, guinea pigs, and ferrets: 200 – 400 μg/kg (0.2 – 0.4 mg/kg) topically[72]

Ectoparasites in hamsters, gerbils, mice, rats, and guinea pigs weighing 50 to 300 g (0.11 to 0.66 lb) (extra label): 500 – 1000 μg/kg (0.5 – 1 mg/kg) topically.[80] Treatment can be repeated after 4 weeks if necessary.

REPTILES:

Most nematodes, ectoparasites (extra-label): For lizards, snakes, and alligators: 200 μg/kg (0.2 mg/kg) IM, SC, or PO once; repeat in 2 weeks. A third treatment can be given if still positive after the second treatment. **NOTE**: Ivermectin is toxic to chelonians, indigo snakes, and skinks.[81,82]

Monitoring

- Clinical efficacy
- Adverse effects/toxicity (especially lethargy, ataxia, tremors, mydriasis, blindness, hypersalivation and vomiting)
- Antiparasitic resistance in horses and livestock (ie, fecal egg count reduction [FECR] test)[83]

Client Information

- The manufacturer of large animal ivermectin products recommends washing hands prior to eating. Avoid contact with eyes.
- Liquid products are flammable; use in a well-ventilated area and do not smoke around the product.
- Pour-on products should be applied along the midline of the back in a narrow strip between the withers and tailhead. Do not apply when the hair or hide is wet. Efficacy may be reduced if rain occurs within 2 hours of administration.
- Chewable tablets should be administered in a manner that encourages the animal to chew the tablet. Chewables may be broken into pieces for animals that normally swallow treats whole.
- Heartworm preventives must be administered every 30 days; late or missed doses may cause treatment failure.
- May be given with or without food. If your animal vomits or acts sick after receiving the drug on an empty stomach, give with food or a small treat. If vomiting continues, contact your veterinarian.
- Overdose can be serious. Do not use in species for which the product is not intended (eg, do not administer a horse product to dogs). Measure medicine carefully; for horse pastes, ensure the ring is placed at the prescribed weight and locked in place. Keep flavored chewable tablets out of reach of children and animals.
- This drug is usually tolerated well. If your animal shows signs of lethargy, weakness, stumbling, blindness, seizures, excessive drooling, vomiting, and/or other unusual behavior, contact your veterinarian immediately.
- Dispose of unused product carefully, as it can be toxic to fish and wildlife.
- To minimize antiparasitic resistance, ivermectin treatment in grazing species (eg, horses, cattle, small ruminants) should be part of a comprehensive internal parasite control program.

Chemistry/Synonyms

Ivermectin, an avermectin anthelmintic, occurs as an off-white to yellowish powder. It is very poorly soluble in water (4 μg/mL) but is soluble in ethanol, propylene glycol, polyethylene glycol, and vegetable oils.

Ivermectin may also be known as ivermectina, ivermectine, ivermectinum, or MK 933; many trade names are available.

Storage/Stability

Ivermectin is photolabile in solution; protect from light. Unless otherwise specified by the manufacturer, store ivermectin products at room temperature (20°C-25°C [68°F-77°F]); excursions between 15°C to 30°C (59°F-86°F) are permitted for most products. Solutions are flammable and must be stored away from heat, sparks, open flame, or other sources of ignition.

Environmental exposure to ivermectin may adversely affect fish and other waterborne organisms. Dispose of unused ivermectin by incineration or in an approved landfill. Use caution during treatment to prevent feedlot water runoff from entering lakes, streams, and ground water.

Ivermectin 1% oral solution (equine tube wormer product) is stable at 1:20 and 1:40 dilutions with water for 72 hours when stored in a tight container, at room temperature, and protected from light.

Compatibility/Compounding Considerations

Compatibility is dependent on factors such as pH, concentration, temperature, and diluent used; specialized references or a hospital pharmacist should be consulted for more specific information.

If compounding from the concentrated injectable forms, institute multiple check systems to reduce the chance for overdose.

Dosage Forms/Regulatory Status

VETERINARY PRODUCTS:

NOTE: Because milk withdrawal times have not been established, the drug is not FDA-approved for use in lactating dairy animals or females of breeding age.

Ivermectin Oral Tablets (Plain or Chewable): 68 μg, 136 μg, and 272 μg with 6 doses per carton; *Heartgard®*, generic; (Rx). FDA-approved for use in dogs 6 weeks of age and older. NADA# 140-886

Ivermectin Oral Chewable Tablets: 55 μg and 165 μg with 6 doses per carton; *Heartgard® for Cats*; (Rx). FDA-approved for use in cats 6 weeks of age and older. NADA# 141-078

Ivermectin for Injection: 10 mg/mL (1%) in 50 mL, 100 mL, 200 mL, 250 mL, 500 mL, and 1000 mL bottles; *Ivomec® 1% Injection for Cattle* and *Swine*; generic; (OTC). FDA-approved for use in cattle (not female dairy cattle of breeding age) and swine. Slaughter withdrawal time (when used as labeled): cattle = 35 days, swine = 18 days, reindeer = 56 days, and bison = 56 days. No milk withdrawal time has been established. Do not use in calves to be processed for veal. NADA# 128-409

Ivermectin 1.87% Oral Paste in 6.08 g syringes (sufficient to treat one 566 kg (1250 lb) horse); *Eqvalan*®; (OTC). FDA-approved for use in horses not intended for food purposes. NADA# 134-314

Ivermectin Oral Solution: 0.08% in 240 mL, 960 mL, 1000 mL, and 5000 mL containers; *Ivomec*® *Drench for Sheep*; (OTC). FDA-approved for use in sheep. Slaughter withdrawal time is 11 days. NADA# 131-392

Ivermectin Topical Parasiticide Pour-on for Cattle: 5 mg/mL in 250 mL and 1000 mL squeeze-pour system, 2500 mL and 5000 mL collapsible containers, and 20 L pack; *Ivomec*® *Pour-on for Cattle*; generic; (OTC). FDA-approved for use in cattle (not female dairy cattle of breeding age). Slaughter withdrawal time is 48 days; milk withdrawal has not been established. NADA# 140-841

Ivermectin Spot-on Solution: 50 µg and 450 µg/pipette; *Xeno*® *50-Mini, Xeno*® *450*; (SAES product). Not for use in animals intended for human consumption, including eggs from treated birds.

Combination Products:

Ivermectin for Injection: 10 mg/mL (1%) and Clorsulon 100 mg/mL; *Ivomec*® *Plus Injection for Cattle*; generic; (OTC). FDA-approved for use in cattle (not female dairy cattle of breeding age). Slaughter withdrawal at labeled doses is 40 days. No milk withdrawal has been established. For further information, see ***Ivermectin/Clorsulon***. NADA# 140-833

Ivermectin/Pyrantel Oral Tablets: 68 µg/57 mg, 136 µg/114 mg, and 272 µg/227 mg; *Heartgard*® *Plus Chewables*; generic; (Rx). FDA-approved for use in dogs 6 weeks of age and older. In dogs over 45 kg (100 lb), use the appropriate combination of these chewable tablets. NADA# 140-971

Ivermectin/Pyrantel/Praziquantel Oral Tablets:
34 µg/28.5 mg/28.5 mg, 68 µg/57 mg/57 mg, 136 µg/114 mg/114 mg, and 272 µg/228 mg/228 mg; *Iverhart Max*®; generic; (Rx). FDA-approved for use in dogs 8 weeks of age and older. In dogs over 45 kg (100 lb), use the appropriate combination of these chewable tablets. NADA# 141-441

Ivermectin 1.87% and Praziquantel 14.03% Oral Paste in 6.42 g oral syringes (sufficient to treat one 598.7 kg (1320 lb) horse); *Equimax*®; (OTC). FDA-approved for use in horses or ponies 4 weeks of age and older and not intended for food purposes. NADA# 141-215

Ivermectin 1.55% and Praziquantel 7.75% in 7.35 g oral syringes; *Zimecterin*® *Gold*; (OTC). FDA-approved for use in horses or ponies 8 weeks of age and older and not intended for food purposes. NADA# 141-214

HUMAN-LABELED PRODUCTS:

Ivermectin Tablets: 3 mg; *Stromectol*®; (Rx)

Ivermectin 0.5% Topical Lotion (*Sklice*®) is available as a pediculocide; Ivermectin 1% Topical Cream (*Soolantra*®) is indicated for treatment of acne rosacea.

References

For the complete list of references, see **wiley.com/go/budde/plumb**

Ivermectin/Clorsulon

(***klor***-su-lon) *Ivomec*® *Plus*

Internal/External Antiparasitic and Flukicide

Prescriber Highlights

- ▶ Combination injectable internal/external antiparasitic with an adult flukicide (*Fasciola hepatica*) for cattle only
- ▶ For SC use only; not for IV or IM use
- ▶ Usually well tolerated; injection site discomfort or swelling is possible
- ▶ Not for use in female dairy cattle of breeding age or in calves to be used for veal
- ▶ Use in species other than cattle may result in severe adverse reactions and/or death.
- ▶ Slaughter withdrawal is 21 days.

Uses/Indications

Ivermectin, in combination with clorsulon, is FDA-approved for the effective treatment and control of internal parasites, including GI roundworms (adults and fourth-stage larvae), lungworms (adults and fourth-stage larvae), adult liver flukes (*Fasciola hepatica*), and external parasites, including cattle grubs (parasitic stages), sucking lice, and mange mites (cattle scab).[1]

Pharmacology/Actions

In infected hosts, adult *Fasciola hepatica* ingests clorsulon-bound erythrocytes. Clorsulon causes a concentration-dependent inhibition of glucose uptake. It inhibits the glycolytic enzymes 3-phosphoglycerate kinase and phosphoglyceromutase, thereby blocking the Embden-Meyerhof glycolytic pathway; the fluke is deprived of its main metabolic energy source and dies. Clorsulon 7 mg/kg PO is effective against immature and adult *F hepatica* 14 weeks postinfection[2-4]; however, clorsulon 2 mg/kg SC is effective only against adult flukes (14 weeks postinfection).

For information on ***Ivermectin***, refer to that specific monograph.

Pharmacokinetics

After oral administration in cattle, the drug is absorbed rapidly, with peak concentrations occurring in about 4 hours. ≈75% of the circulating drug is found in plasma and 25% in erythrocytes. At 8 to 12 hours after administration, clorsulon levels peak in the fluke. SC injections in cattle result in maximum plasma levels 6 hours after administration, with a plasma half-life of ≈26 hours.

Contraindications/Precautions/Warnings

Must be administered SC only; do not give IV or IM. Adequate animal restraint is required to ensure proper route of administration. This product is only for use in cattle, as severe reactions, including fatalities in dogs, may occur.

Divide doses greater than 10 mL between 2 injection sites to reduce occasional discomfort or site reaction. Different injection sites should be used for other parenteral products.[1]

Adverse Effects

Discomfort and local swelling may occur at injection sites.[1]

Reproductive/Nursing Safety

Clorsulon is considered safe for use in pregnant or breeding animals. Use of ivermectin/clorsulon commercial products at recommended dosages in breeding bulls and cows showed no effect on breeding performance.[1]

Overdose/Acute Toxicity

Refer to the ***Ivermectin*** monograph for further information.

For patients that have experienced or are suspected of having experienced an overdose, consultation with a 24-hour poison consulta-

tion center specializing in providing veterinary-specific information is recommended. For general information related to overdose and toxin exposures, as well as contact information for poison control centers, refer to ***Appendix***.

Drug Interactions/Laboratory Considerations

None identified when used as directed.

Dosages

CATTLE:

Susceptible roundworms, lungworms, adult liver flukes, cattle grubs, sucking lice, and mange mites (label dosage; FDA-approved): ivermectin 200 µg/kg and clorsulon 2 mg/kg SC behind the shoulder.[1] Divide doses greater than 10 mL between 2 injection sites. For most effective results against grubs, treat cattle as soon as possible after the end of the heel fly (ie, warble fly) season.

Monitoring

- Clinical efficacy
- Fecal egg count reduction testing (FECRT) and fecal sedimentation for fluke recovery

Client Information

- Follow withdrawal times for slaughter (21 days for *Ivermax® Plus*).
- Do not use in female dairy cattle of breeding age.
- Do not use in pre-ruminating calves or those to be processed for veal.
- Do not allow water runoff from feedlots to enter lakes, streams, or ponds, as free ivermectin may adversely affect fish.
- The viscosity of the product increases when ambient temperature is at or below 5°C (41°F), making administration of the product difficult. In such conditions it is suggested warm the product and injection equipment to a temperature of about 15°C (59°F).

Chemistry/Synonyms

Ivermectin, an avermectin anthelmintic, occurs as an off-white to yellowish powder. It is very poorly soluble in water (4 µg/mL) but is soluble in ethanol, propylene glycol, polyethylene glycol, and vegetable oils. Although structurally similar to macrolide antibiotics, avermectins have no antibacterial properties.

Ivermectin may also be known as ivermectina, ivermectine, ivermectinum, or MK 933; many trade names are available.

Clorsulon, a benzenesulfonamide, has a chemical name of 4-amino-6-(trichloroethenyl)-1,3-benzenedisulfonamide. It is a white to off-white powder that is slightly soluble in water and freely soluble in methyl alcohol. Clorsulon may also be known as clorsulone, clorsulonum, MK-401, or *Curatrem®*.

Storage/Stability

Unless otherwise instructed by the manufacturer, store clorsulon at room temperature (15°C to 30°C [59°F-86°F]) and protected from light. Consult the product label for storage duration of in-use vials and the maximum number of vial punctures allowed.

Compatibility/Compounding Considerations

Compatibility is dependent on factors such as pH, concentration, temperature, and diluent used; specialized references or a hospital pharmacist should be consulted for more specific information.

The viscosity of the product increases in cool temperatures.[1] Administration in temperatures at or below 5°C (41°F) may be difficult and warming the product and injection equipment to a temperature of about 15°C (59°F) is recommended.

Dosage Forms/Regulatory Status

VETERINARY-LABELED PRODUCTS:

Clorsulon 10% (100 mg/mL) and Ivermectin 1% (10 mg/mL) Injection in 50 mL, 200 mL, 500 mL, and 1000 mL; *Ivomec® Plus*, generic; (OTC). FDA-approved for SC injection use in cattle. Do not use within 21 days of slaughter; do not use in female dairy cattle of breeding age or in pre-ruminating calves or those intended for veal. NADA #140-833

NOTE: Clorsulon 8.5% (85 mg/mL) Oral Drench; *Curatrem®*; (OTC) is no longer in production. It was FDA-approved for use in cattle with a slaughter withdrawal of 8 days when used as labeled. Clorsulon drench was not FDA-approved for use in female dairy cattle of breeding age, and a milk withdrawal was not established.

HUMAN-LABELED PRODUCTS: NONE

References

For the complete list of references, see **wiley.com/go/budde/plumb**

Kaolin/Pectin

(***kay***-oh-lin/***pek***-tin) *Kaopectolin®*

GI Adsorbent/Protectant

Prescriber Highlights

- ► Adsorbent for treatment of diarrhea and GI toxins; no studies to support efficacy
- ► Most products marketed in the United States contain bismuth subsalicylate, which may be contraindicated in some species.
- ► Should not be relied on to control severe diarrheas or replace adequate fluids and electrolytes in severe or chronic diarrheas
- ► Adverse effects include transient constipation.

Uses/Indications

Although its efficacy is in question, kaolin/pectin is used primarily in veterinary medicine as an oral antidiarrheal agent. It has also been used as an adsorbent agent following the ingestion of certain toxins. Administration may be difficult due to the large oral volumes that may be necessary. No studies documenting the clinical efficacy of this combination in either human or veterinary species were located.

Pharmacology/Actions

Kaolin/pectin is thought to possess adsorbent and protective qualities. Presumably, bacteria and toxins are adsorbed in the gut, and the coating action of the suspension may protect inflamed GI mucosa. The pectin component decreases pH in the intestinal lumen by forming galacturonic acid. Kaolin/pectin can improve stool consistency within 24 to 48 hours, but it does not reduce the ions or amount of fluid lost from the GI tract.[1]

Pharmacokinetics

Neither kaolin nor pectin is absorbed after oral administration. Up to 90% of the pectin administered may be decomposed in the gut.

Contraindications/Precautions/Warnings

There are no absolute contraindications to kaolin/pectin therapy, but it should not be relied on to control severe diarrheas.

Kaolin/pectin should not replace adequate fluid and electrolyte monitoring or replacement therapy in severe or chronic diarrheas.

Branded products that previously contained kaolin/pectin (eg, *Kaopectate®*) may now contain other active ingredients (eg, bismuth subsalicylate). Read product label carefully. Because of the potential for adverse effects caused by the salicylate component, this drug should be used cautiously, if at all, in cats.

Adverse Effects

Kaolin/pectin generally has no adverse effects. Constipation may occur but is usually transient and associated with high dosages. High dosages in debilitated or very old or young patients may rarely cause fecal impaction. In rats, kaolin/pectin has been demonstrated to increase fecal sodium and potassium loss in diarrhea.[1]

In humans, kaolin/pectin is recommended for use only under the direct supervision of a physician in patients less than 3 years of age or if it must be used longer than 48 hours.

Reproductive/Nursing Safety

Adsorbent antidiarrheal products should be safe to use during pregnancy and lactation. The addition of other active ingredients (eg, opioids) may alter this recommendation.

Because safety has not been established in animals, this drug should only be used when the maternal benefits outweigh the potential risks to offspring.

Overdose/Acute Toxicity

Kaolin/pectin is highly insoluble and is not absorbed systemically. Overdose is unlikely to cause any serious effects, but constipation requiring treatment may occur.

Drug Interactions

The following drug interactions have either been reported or are theoretical in humans or animals receiving kaolin/pectin and may be of significance in veterinary patients. Unless otherwise noted, use together is not necessarily contraindicated, but weigh the potential risks and perform additional monitoring when appropriate.

- **Digoxin**: Some evidence exists that kaolin/pectin may impair the oral absorption of digoxin. Separate doses by at least 2 hours.
- **Clindamycin, Lincomycin**: Kaolin/pectin may inhibit oral absorption. If kaolin is to be used with either of these antibiotics, administer kaolin/pectin at least 2 hours before or 3 to 4 hours after the antibiotic dose.
- **Penicillamine**: Kaolin/pectin may inhibit oral absorption. Separate doses by at least 2 hours.
- **Sulfa-/Trimethoprim**: Kaolin/pectin may inhibit oral absorption. Separate doses by at least 2 hours.

Laboratory Considerations

None noted

Dosages

NOTE: Evidence to support the efficacy of kaolin/pectin is weak. All dosages are anecdotal and extra-label as no products have undergone the FDA approval process for use in animals.

DOGS/CATS:

Noninfectious diarrhea (label dosage; not FDA-approved): 1 to 3 tablespoonsful (15 – 45 mL)/animal (NOT tablespoonsful [mL]/kg) PO as needed at the first sign of diarrhea and after each loose bowel movement[2]

Diarrhea (label dosage; not FDA-approved): 2.3 – 6.8 kg (5 – 15 lb): 1 teaspoonful (5 mL) PO; 7.3 – 22.7 kg (16 – 50 lb): 2 teaspoonsful (10 mL) PO; over 23.2 kg (51 lb): 1 tablespoonful (15 mL) PO. Administer dose once daily[3] or every 12 hours,[4]

Diarrhea and loose stools (extra-label): 1 – 2 mL/kg PO 4 to 6 times daily as needed

HORSES:

Noninfectious diarrhea (extra-label): After the first sign of diarrhea and after each loose bowel movement, administer: Adults: 6 – 10 fl oz (180 – 300 mL)/horse (NOT fl oz [mL]/kg) PO; Foals: 3 – 4 fl oz (90 – 120 mL)/foal (NOT fl oz[mL]/kg)[2]

Diarrhea and loose stools (extra-label):

1. 2 – 4 quarts/450 kg (992 lb) body weight PO twice daily[5]
2. 1 fl oz/8 kg (17.6 lb) body weight PO 3 to 4 times daily[6]
3. 2 – 4 mL/kg PO every 8 to 12 hours[7]
4. Foals: 3 – 4 oz/foal PO every 6 to 8 hours (authors believe that bismuth subsalicylate is superior)[8]

CATTLE:

Noninfectious diarrhea (extra-label): After the first sign of diarrhea and after each loose bowel movement, administer: Adults: 6 – 10 fl oz (180 – 300 mL)/animal (NOT fl oz [mL]/kg]) PO; calves: 3 – 4 fl oz (90 – 120 mL)/calf (NOT fl oz[mL]/kg)[2]

Diarrhea and loose stools (extra-label): 0.25 – 1 mL/kg PO every 4 hours[7]

SHEEP/GOATS:

Diarrhea and loose stools (extra-label): 0.25 – 1 ml/kg PO every 4 hours[7]

SWINE:

Diarrhea and loose stools (extra-label): 0.2 mL/kg PO every 4 hours[9]

BIRDS: ALL DOSAGES LISTED ARE EXTRA-LABEL.

1. **Canary or parakeet**: 1 drop/bird (NOT drop/kg) PO twice daily; or 1-½ droppersful/bird (NOT droppersful/kg) placed in ⅔ oz drinking water
2. **Medium-sized birds**: 0.5 mL/bird (NOT mL/kg) PO
3. **Large birds**: 1 mL/bird (NOT mL/kg) PO 1 to 4 times daily[10]
4. 2 mL/kg PO 2 to 4 times daily[11]

FERRETS:

Diarrhea and loose stools (extra-label): 1 – 2 mL/kg PO 3 to 4 times daily[12]

RABBITS/RODENTS/SMALL MAMMALS:

Diarrhea and loose stools in guinea pigs (extra-label): 0.2 mL/animal (NOT mL/kg) PO 3 to 4 times daily[13]

Monitoring

- Clinical efficacy
- Fluid and electrolyte status in severe diarrhea

Client Information

- This medicine is used as an aid in the treatment of noninfectious diarrhea, upset stomach, or nausea.
- Kaolin is very safe when used as directed.
- Constipation is the most common side effect.
- Shake suspensions well before measuring the dose.
- If diarrhea persists or if the animal appears listless or develops a high fever, contact your veterinarian.
- When using this medicine in cats, be sure to check the product label to make sure it does not contain bismuth subsalicylate, as this substance is toxic to cats.

Chemistry/Synonyms

Kaolin is a naturally occurring hydrated aluminum silicate that is powdered and refined for pharmaceutical use. Kaolin is a white/light, odorless, almost tasteless powder that is practically insoluble in water. Light kaolin is preferred for use in pharmaceutical preparations.

Pectin is a carbohydrate polymer consisting primarily of partially methoxylated polygalacturonic acids. Pectin is a course or fine, yellowish-white, almost odorless with a mucilaginous flavor. It is obtained from the inner rind of citrus fruits or apple pomace. One gram of pectin is soluble in 20 mL of water and forms a viscous, colloidal solution.

In the United States, kaolin and pectin are generally used together in an oral suspension formulation in most proprietary products.

Kaolin may also be known as bolus alba, E559, hydrated aluminum silicate, China clay, porcelain clay, white bole, argilla, weisser ton, *Kaopectolin*®, *Kao-Pec*®, *Kao-Pect*®, *Kao-Pront*®, *Kaogel*®; many multi-ingredient trade names are available.

Storage/Stability

Store kaolin/pectin in airtight containers at room temperature between 15°C and 30°C (59°F-86°F); protect from freezing. Shake well before using.

Compatibility/Compounding Considerations

It is physically **incompatible** when mixed with alkalis, heavy metals, salicylic acid, tannic acid, or strong alcohol. If using raw kaolin powder, wear an appropriate particulate mask as pneumonitis can occur if inhaled.

Dosage Forms/Regulatory Status

There are a variety of kaolin/pectin products available over the counter (OTC) without a prescription. Several products are labeled for veterinary use but are not FDA-approved. Many products that formerly contained kaolin (eg, *Kaopectate®*) no longer contain kaolin. In the United States, *Kaopectate®* now contains bismuth subsalicylate as its active ingredient.

VETERINARY-LABELED PRODUCTS:

Kaolin/Pectin: kaolin 5.8 g/pectin 0.268 g/fl oz (30 mL, 2 tablespoonsful) in 1 quart and 1 gallon containers; generic, (OTC). Products may be labeled for use in horses, cattle, dogs, and cats.

Kaolin/Pectin: kaolin 5.8 g/pectin 0.13 g/fl oz (30 mL, 2 tablespoonfuls) in 960 mL and 1 gallon containers; generic; (OTC)

Kaolin/Pectin: kaolin 800 mg/pectin 80 mg/teaspoonful (5 mL) in 118 mL and 237 mL bottles; generic; (OTC)

Kaolin/Pectin: kaolin 900 mg/pectin 50 mg/teaspoonful (5 mL) in 118 mL bottles; generic; (OTC)

HUMAN-LABELED PRODUCTS:

Kaolin/Pectin Antidiarrheal Suspension: kaolin 90 g/pectin 2 gm per 30 mL in 180 mL, 360 mL, 473 mL, and UD 30 mL; *Kaopectolin®* (various), generic; (OTC)

References

For the complete list of references, see **wiley.com/go/budde/plumb**

Ketamine

(***kee***-ta-meen) *Ketaset®, Ketaflo®, Vetalar®*

Dissociative General Anesthetic; NMDA-Receptor Antagonist

Prescriber Highlights

- ► Dissociative general anesthetic that also inhibits N-methyl-D-aspartate (NMDA) receptors and may be for adjunctive therapy to control pain
- ► Contraindications include animals with prior hypersensitivity reactions, animals to be used for human consumption, or using this product as the sole agent for general anesthesia. Relative contraindications include significant blood loss; malignant hyperthermia; increased intraocular pressure or open globe injuries; and procedures involving the pharynx, larynx, or trachea. Caution is advised in animals with significant hypertension, heart failure, arterial aneurysm, hypertrophic cardiomyopathy, hyperthyroidism, hepatic or renal insufficiency, or seizure disorder.
- ► Adverse effects include hypertension, hypersalivation, respiratory depression, hyperthermia, emesis, vocalization, erratic and prolonged recovery, dyspnea, myoclonus, seizures, muscular tremors, hypertonicity, opisthotonos, and cardiac arrest, as well as pain with IM injection.
- ► Animals' eyes remain open after ketamine administration, so ocular protection (eg, lubricants, towel) should be used.
- ► Exposure to handling or loud noises should be minimized during the recovery period.
- ► Dosages should be determined carefully. Care should be taken to not confuse CRI dosages (ie, mg/kg/hour vs µg/kg/minute).

Uses/Indications

Ketamine is FDA-approved for use in humans, subhuman primates, and cats; however, it has also been used in many other species. The FDA-approved indications for cats include *for restraint, or as the sole anesthetic agent for diagnostic, or minor, brief, surgical procedures that do not require skeletal muscle relaxation. . . and in subhuman primates for restraint.*[1]

Ketamine is used to induce general anesthesia in many species and as a CRI to provide analgesia and decrease the amount of inhalant used to maintain a surgical plane of anesthesia. It has been used intranasally in combination with midazolam in cats to induce sedation.[2]

Ketamine can decrease the "wind-up" pain effect. There is increasing interest in using ketamine to prevent exaggerated pain associated with surgery and chronic states of pain in animals.

Pharmacology/Actions

Ketamine is a rapid-acting, general anesthetic that has significant analgesic activity and a relative lack of cardiovascular depressant effects in healthy animals. Ketamine depresses the thalamoneocortical system, dissociating it from the limbic system, which is activated. Ketamine binds the phencyclidine-binding site of the N-methyl-D-aspartate (NMDA) receptors, reducing receptor activity and release of glutamate, an excitatory neurotransmitter. It is unclear whether muscarinic antagonism or inhibition of catecholamine reuptake is responsible for some of ketamine's clinical effects (eg, tachycardia, bronchodilation).[3]

In healthy animals, the effects of ketamine on the cardiovascular system include increased cardiac output, heart rate, mean aortic pressure, pulmonary artery pressure, and central venous pressure. The effects on total peripheral resistance are described as being variable. Cardiovascular effects are secondary to increased sympathetic tone; ketamine has negative inotropic effects if the sympathetic system is blocked or in sick animals experiencing depletion of catecholamines.

Ketamine can cause apneustic breathing (ie, rapid breaths followed by breath holding). This drug does not cause significant respiratory depression at usual doses, but it can cause respiratory rates to decrease at higher doses. Ketamine can cause bronchodilation and decreased airway resistance in humans with asthma.

Ketamine possesses analgesic effects at subanesthetic doses. Analgesia is secondary to effects on NMDA excitatory glutamate receptors through decreases in the activity of areas in the CNS that respond to pain-invoking stimuli. The analgesic effects of ketamine can be synergistic with other analgesics. Ketamine's actions on the NMDA receptors also impact opioid and monoaminergic receptors, which contributes to the antinociceptive effects of this drug.

At standard doses, ketamine generally either causes no change in muscle tone or increased muscle tone. Ketamine does not impede pinnal and pedal, photic, corneal, laryngeal, or pharyngeal reflexes. Muscle tone may decrease with high doses. Changes in body temperature correspond with muscle tone, with hypothermia accompanying hypotonia at higher doses. In cats, ketamine causes a slight hypothermic effect, as body temperature decreases (on average) by 1.6°C (33.9°F) after high anesthetic doses (ie, ≈20 mg/kg).

In some species, ketamine has demonstrated anti-inflammatory effects.[4] In response to endotoxin stimulation in dogs, ketamine caused reductions in tumor necrosis factor-alpha activity; however, it had minimal effects on stabilizing blood pressure.[5]

Pharmacokinetics

Ketamine undergoes significant first-pass metabolism, limiting absorption after oral administration. Peak concentrations occur ≈10 minutes after IM injection in cats. A ketamine spray sublingually to cats appears to be absorbed enough to have pharmacologic action.[6] Ketamine is distributed into all body tissues rapidly, with the highest concentrations found in the brain, liver, lungs, and fat. Plasma protein binding is ≈50% in dogs[7] and horses,[8] and 40% to 50% in cats.[9]

In most species, ketamine is metabolized in the liver principally by demethylation and hydroxylation. These metabolites, along with unchanged ketamine, are eliminated in the urine. In dogs, CYP2B11 plays an active role in metabolizing ketamine. One active metabolite (norketamine) has 10% to 30% of the activity of the parent compound. In cats, ketamine is almost exclusively excreted unchanged in the urine. The elimination half-life in cats, horses, and calves is ≈1 hour and is 2 to 3 hours in humans. Similar to thiobarbiturates, redistribution of ketamine out of the CNS is more likely to determine the duration of anesthesia than is elimination half-life. In horses, S-ketamine is eliminated faster than the racemic mixture.

The duration, but not intensity, of anesthesia can be prolonged by increasing the ketamine dose.

Contraindications/Precautions/Warnings

Ketamine is contraindicated in animals that have exhibited prior hypersensitivity reactions to it and in animals to be used for human consumption. Use of ketamine in animals with significant hypertension, heart failure, or arterial aneurysms could be dangerous. The manufacturer warns against its use in animals with hepatic or renal insufficiency; in humans with renal insufficiency, the duration of action is not prolonged. Because ketamine does not provide good muscle relaxation, it is contraindicated when used alone for major surgery.[1]

Ketamine should only be used in situations in which sufficient monitoring and patient-support capabilities (eg, intubation, ventilation) are available.

It was believed that ketamine can cause increases in intracranial pressure (ICP) and should not be used in animals with elevated ICP or if head trauma has occurred. More recent studies in human medicine have shown that ketamine, when administered with gamma-aminobutyric acid (GABA) agonists to mechanically ventilated animals, does not increase ICP. In humans[10] and animals[3,11,12] with head injuries that have increased ICP, ketamine decreased ICP pressure and improved cerebral perfusion pressure.

Because of its epileptogenic potential, ketamine should generally not be used (unless used with caution) in animals with pre-existing seizure disorders. Some contrast agents used during myelography can induce seizures, so ketamine should be used with caution in animals undergoing this procedure. Ketamine may be beneficial in treating self-sustaining status epilepticus (SSSE) in humans[13] and dogs.[14]

Ketamine is considered to be relatively contraindicated in animals with increased intraocular pressure or open globe injuries and for procedures involving the pharynx, larynx, or trachea. Animals that have lost significant amounts of blood may require significantly reduced ketamine doses.

Ketamine can increase heart rate, blood pressure, and myocardial oxygen consumption; its use should be avoided in cats with hypertrophic cardiomyopathy (HCM) and in animals in which increased heart rate, blood pressure, or myocardial oxygen consumption can be detrimental (ie, result in shock or congestive heart failure). Ketamine's effects on respiratory function may be enhanced in animals with unstable cardiopulmonary function. Use ketamine with caution in animals with pulmonary disease. Because of ketamine's tendencies to increase sympathetic tone (increased norepinephrine release), it should be used with caution in animals in which increased sympathetic tone concurrently exists (eg, pheochromocytoma, hyperthyroidism). Humans with hyperthyroidism and those receiving exogenous thyroid replacement may be susceptible to developing severe hypertension and tachycardia when given ketamine. The veterinary significance of this potential problem is unknown.

Animals' eyes can remain open after receiving ketamine, so an ophthalmic lubricating ointment should be applied to prevent injury or excessive drying of the cornea. Additionally, during field anesthesia, the animal's eyes should also be protected (eg, covered with a towel) from damage from the sun.

It is recommended to minimize handling and loud noises during the recovery period to reduce the incidences of emergence reactions during anesthetic recovery; however, vital signs should also be monitored during the recovery phase.

In horses, it has been recommended to avoid excessive ketamine doses close to time of recovery to reduce the potential for muscle rigidity or CNS excitement.[15]

Because ketamine can increase blood pressure, careful control of postsurgical (eg, declawing) hemorrhage should be managed.

In human medicine, ketamine is considered a high-alert medication (ie, medications that require special safeguards to reduce the risk for errors). Consider instituting practices such as redundant drug dosage and volume checking with special alert labels.

Adverse Effects

At lower doses, adverse effects are generally minimal in most species. Emesis, salivation, and vocalization may occur. Other reported effects include hyperthermia, nystagmus, erratic and prolonged recovery, dyspnea, and cardiac arrest. Musculoskeletal effects may include tremors, myoclonus, hypertonicity, and convulsions. Respiratory depression has been noted at high doses. The manufacturer suggests myoclonic jerking and/or tonic/clonic convulsions can be controlled by ultrashort-acting barbiturates or acepromazine.[1]

When used alone, ketamine may induce seizures. Seizures have been reported in up to 20% of cats that receive ketamine (alone) at therapeutic dosages. Diazepam is suggested if treatment for seizures is necessary. Ketamine has been reported to rarely cause blindness[16] or death. In cats, ketamine administered at 5 - 10 mg/kg has been documented to cause mild, self-limiting hyperthermia[17,18]; low doses of acepromazine 0.01 – 0.02 mg/kg IV may alleviate this effect. Anecdotal reports of ketamine causing acute congestive heart failure in cats with mild to moderate heart disease have been reported.

Pain after IM injection may occur.

Ketamine has been shown to have a confounding effect on the psychomotor subscale of the feline pain scale.[19]

Atropine or glycopyrrolate can sometimes be administered to reduce the incidence of hypersalivation and other autonomic signs.

Increased liver enzymes and hepatotoxicity have occurred in humans receiving repeated doses or prolonged ketamine infusions.[20–22]

Reproductive/Nursing Safety

Ketamine crosses the placenta. Developmental delays and increased fetal resorption have been noted in laboratory animals.[23] This drug may stimulate uterine contractions.

Because safety has not been established in animals, this drug should only be used when the maternal benefits outweigh the potential risks to offspring.

Overdose/Acute Toxicity

Ketamine is considered to have a wide therapeutic index (ie, ≈5 times greater as compared with pentobarbital). When ketamine is given too rapidly or in excessive doses, significant respiratory depression may occur. It is recommended that ketamine overdoses be treated using mechanically assisted respiratory support versus analeptic agents (eg, doxapram). Although there is no specific reversal agent for ketamine, in cats, yohimbine with 4-aminopyridine has been suggested for use as a partial antagonist.[24]

For patients that have experienced or are suspected of having experienced an overdose, it is strongly encouraged to consult with one of the 24-hour poison consultation centers that specialize in providing information specific for veterinary patients. For general information related to overdose and toxin exposures, as well as contact information for poison control centers, refer to ***Appendix.***

Drug Interactions

The following drug interactions have either been reported or are theoretical in humans or animals receiving ketamine and may be of significance in veterinary patients. Unless otherwise noted, use together is not necessarily contraindicated, but weigh the potential risks and perform additional monitoring when appropriate.

- ALPHA-2 AGONISTS (eg, **dexmedetomidine, medetomidine, xylazine**): In dogs, medetomidine can potentially reduce the metabolism of ketamine via inhibition of CYB2B11 (in vitro).[25] Dexmedetomidine (used in dogs) may reduce this drug interaction risk considerably. Xylazine reduced norketamine formation in canine and equine liver microsomal preparations.[26]
- BARBITURATES (eg, **pentobarbital, phenobarbital**): May prolong the recovery time after ketamine anesthesia; lower doses of each agent may be needed
- BENZODIAZEPINES (eg, **diazepam, midazolam**): May prolong the recovery time after ketamine anesthesia; lower doses of each agent may be needed
- HALOTHANE: When ketamine is used with halothane, recovery rates may be prolonged, and the cardiac stimulatory effects of ketamine may be inhibited.
- IVERMECTIN: It has been recommended that ivermectin not be used in reptiles that have received ketamine within 10 days.[27]
- NEUROMUSCULAR BLOCKERS (eg, **succinylcholine, tubocurarine**): May cause enhanced or prolonged respiratory depression
- OPIOIDS (eg, **buprenorphine, fentanyl, hydromorphone, morphine**): May prolong the recovery time after ketamine anesthesia; lower doses of each agent may be needed
- THEOPHYLLINE, AMINOPHYLLINE: In humans, ketamine may lower the seizure threshold; veterinary significance is unknown.
- THYROID HORMONES: When given concomitantly with ketamine, thyroid hormones have induced hypertension and tachycardia in humans; beta-blockers (eg, propranolol) may be beneficial in the treatment of these effects.

Laboratory Considerations

- Ketamine increases plasma cortisol, which limits the use of cortisol as a biomarker for pain.[28–30]

Dosages

NOTES:

1. Ketamine is used in many different combinations with other agents. The following are representative, but not necessarily inclusive; it is suggested to refer to a recent veterinary anesthesia reference for more information.[31,32]
2. Do not confuse IV CRI dosages listed as <u>mg/kg/*HOUR*</u> with those listed as <u>µg/kg/*MINUTE*</u>.

DOGS:

Adjunct to anesthesia (extra-label):

a) **High-volume surgical sterilization program under field conditions**: Ketamine 4.5 mg/kg, medetomidine 0.04 mg/kg, and hydromorphone 0.09 mg/kg combined and given IM. Meloxicam 0.2 mg/kg IM given after surgery[33]

b) **In combination with an opioid and dexmedetomidine (ie, doggie magic) to provide anesthesia and pain management[34]**: Reference contains tables for conversion of animal weight to various µg/m² <u>doses of dexmedetomidine using the 0.5 mg/mL concentration</u>; opioid concentrations used are butorphanol 10 mg/mL, hydromorphone 2 mg/mL, and buprenorphine 0.3 mg/mL. Ketamine concentration is 100 mg/mL. These drugs may be available in other concentrations, but only the products with these concentrations should be used for this protocol. To reverse the dexmedetomidine portion of these drug combinations, give atipamezole IM at the same volume as the amount of dexmedetomidine given.

   i. **Geriatric dogs or dogs with renal or liver dysfunction as a premedication prior to propofol, followed by maintenance on isoflurane or sevoflurane**: Dexmedetomidine 62.5 µg/m² IM or IV; combine with equal volumes of one of the opioids noted above and ketamine.

   ii. **Slightly heavier sedation in American Society of Anesthesiologists (ASA) class II or III dogs for radiography**: Dexmedetomidine 125 µg/m² IM or IV; combine with equal volumes of one of the opioids noted above and ketamine.

   iii. **Dogs undergoing minor surgery with PennHip or Orthopedic Foundation for Animals (OFA)-types of radiography that require significant muscle relaxation**: Dexmedetomidine 250 µg/m² IM or IV; combine with equal volumes of one of the opioids noted above and ketamine.

   iv. **Inducing a surgical plane of anesthesia for ovariohysterectomy (OHE), castration, or other abdominal surgery**: Dexmedetomidine 375 µg/m² IM or IV; combine with equal volumes of one of the opioids noted above and ketamine. Provides rapid immobilization; lateral recumbency occurs in 5 to 8 minutes. Dogs can be intubated and maintained on oxygen. Supplemental low doses of isoflurane (0.5%) or sevoflurane (1%) can be used.

   v. **Immobilizing extremely fractious and wolf-hybrid dogs**: Dexmedetomidine 500 µg/m² IM; combine with equal volumes of one of the opioids noted above and ketamine—this dose is rarely required.

Premedication before surgery or for anesthesia induction (extra-label):

a) **Ketamine/benzodiazepine combinations**:
   i. Ketamine 5.5 mg/kg combined with diazepam 0.28 mg/kg IV[35]
   ii. Ketamine 10 mg/kg combined with midazolam 0.5 mg/kg IV[35]

b) Ketamine 3 mg/kg in combination with dexmedetomidine 15 µg/kg, and *either* buprenorphine 40 µg/kg, butorphanol 0.2 mg/kg, OR hydromorphone 0.05 mg/kg as a single IM injection was given to dogs undergoing castration.[36] Some dogs required intubation and supplemental isoflurane when anesthesia was considered inadequate during surgery. The combination using buprenorphine was deemed most suitable by the authors. Administration of atipamezole postoperatively shortened recovery times.

c) Ketamine 15 mg/kg IM immediately following xylazine 1 mg/kg IM. Onset is within 3 to 7 minutes; duration is ≈24 minutes.[37]

d) Ketamine 5 – 7.5 mg/kg IM in combination with medetomidine 40 µg/kg IM. Onset is within 7 to 11 minutes; duration is 30 to 50 minutes. A higher ketamine dose provides faster onset and longer duration. Do not reverse with atipamezole.[37]

e) Premedicate with medetomidine 25 µg/kg IM in combination with butorphanol 0.1 mg/kg IM. Fifteen minutes after premedication, ketamine 5 mg/kg IM can be given. Onset of sedation is ≈6 minutes after ketamine administration; pedal reflex is lost after ≈14 minutes and returns after ≈53 minutes. Dogs became sternally recumbent and standing 35 minutes and ≈1 hour, respectively, after pedal reflex returns. Do not reverse with atipamezole.[37]

Adjunctive pain control (extra-label): **NOTE**: Do NOT confuse IV CRI dosages listed as mg/kg/*HOUR* with those listed as µg/kg per *MINUTE*.

a) Ketamine 0.5 mg/kg IV loading dose, followed by ketamine 0.1 – 0.6 mg/kg/*HOUR* IV CRI[38]

b) **Intraoperative use**: If anesthesia was induced with a drug other than ketamine, give a loading dose of ketamine 0.5 mg/kg IV, ketamine 10 – 20 µg/kg/*MINUTE* IV CRI.

c) **Postoperative analgesia**: Ketamine 2 – 10 µg/kg/*MINUTE* IV CRI[39]

d) **Ketamine/lidocaine**: Ketamine 0.5 – 3 mg/kg in combination with lidocaine 1.5 – 2 mg/kg IV followed by ketamine 0.03 – 0.1 mg/kg/*MINUTE* with lidocaine 25 – 100 µg/kg per *MINUTE* with IV CRI[40-42]

e) **Ketamine/lidocaine/dexmedetomidine**: Ketamine 1 mg/kg in combination with lidocaine 2 mg/kg and dexmedetomidine 1 µg/kg IV followed by ketamine 40 µg/kg/*MINUTE*, lidocaine 100 µg/kg/*MINUTE*, and dexmedetomidine 3 µg/kg/*HOUR* IV CRI during surgery. At the conclusion of surgery, IV CRI rates were reduced to ketamine 10 µg/kg/*MINUTE*, lidocaine 25 µg/kg/*MINUTE*, and dexmedetomidine 1 µg/kg/*HOUR* and continued for an additional 4 hours.[43,44]

f) **Ketamine/lidocaine/fentanyl**: Ketamine 0.6 mg/kg/*HOUR* in combination with lidocaine 3 mg/kg/*HOUR* and fentanyl 3.6 µg/kg/*HOUR* IV CRI (no loading dose was used in this study).[45]

g) **Morphine/lidocaine/ketamine | MLK**: Morphine 3.3 – 4 µg/kg/*MINUTE*, lidocaine 50 µg/kg/*MINUTE*, and ketamine 10 µg/kg/*MINUTE* admixed in IV fluids and administered as an IV CRI.[46-49] Refer to ***Compatibility/Compounding Considerations*** for more information.

h) **Dexmedetomidine/morphine/lidocaine/ketamine | DMLK**: Dexmedetomidine 0.5 µg/kg/*HOUR*, morphine 0.2 mg/kg per *HOUR*, lidocaine 3 mg/kg/*HOUR*, and ketamine 0.6 mg/kg per *HOUR* admixed in IV fluids and administered as an IV CRI.[50] Refer to ***Compatibility/Compounding Considerations*** for more information.

Refractory status epilepticus (extra-label): 5 mg/kg IV bolus. Although ketamine was usually administered as a single agent, it may be used in conjunction with other anticonvulsants (eg, diazepam, levetiracetam) to manage status epilepticus.[51]

CATS:

Combination as a premedication or immobilizing agent:

a) **Label dosage** (FDA-approved): 11 mg/kg IM for restraint; 22 – 33 mg/kg IM for diagnostic or minor surgical procedures not requiring skeletal muscle relaxation.[1] Anesthetic duration is ≈30 to 45 minutes; recovery usually occurs in 4 to 5 hours but may be as long as 24 hours with higher doses.

b) **Ketamine/benzodiazepine combinations** (extra-label): Ketamine 5 mg/kg combined with diazepam 0.25 mg/kg IV[52]

c) **In combination with an opioid and dexmedetomidine (ie, kitty magic, DKT, or triple combination) to provide sedation and analgesia** (extra-label): Ketamine concentration is 100 mg/mL. Opioid concentrations used in the reference are butorphanol (10 mg/mL), hydromorphone (2 mg/mL), and buprenorphine (0.3 mg/mL). Dexmedetomidine concentration is 0.5 mg/mL. These drugs may be available in other concentrations, but only the products with these concentrations should be used for this protocol.[34] See the table below for volumes used to attain the desired degree of patient sedation.

Total Volume (NOT mL/kg) of *Each* Drug (Ketamine/Dexmedetomidine*/Opioid) to Be Given IM

Cat body weight	Mild†	Moderate‡	Profound§
2-3 kg (4-7 lb)	0.025 mL	0.05 mL	0.1 – 0.15 mL
3-4 kg (7-9 lb)	0.05 mL	0.1 mL	0.2 – 0.25 mL
4-6 kg (9-13 lb)	0.1 mL	0.2 mL	0.3 – 0.35 mL
6-7 kg (14-15 lb)	0.2 mL	0.3 mL	0.4 – 0.45 mL
7-8 kg (15-18 lb)	0.3 mL	0.4 mL	0.5 – 0.55 mL

*Dexmedetomidine can be reversed immediately with an equal volume (of dexmedetomidine used) of atipamezole.[34]

†For sedation or as a premedication prior to anesthetic induction

‡For castration or minor surgical procedures

§Invasive surgical procedures, including OHE and declawing

d) **Combining ketamine with an opioid and dexmedetomidine** (extra-label):
   i. Ketamine 3 mg/kg in combination with dexmedetomidine 25 µg/kg and either butorphanol 0.2 mg/kg OR hydromorphone 0.05 mg/kg given as a single IM injection (with or without reversal by atipamezole) in cats undergoing castration.[53] Cats were also given meloxicam 0.2 mg/kg SC immediately prior to the conclusion of surgery. Supplemental isoflurane was given when the level of anesthesia was considered inadequate during surgery.
   ii. Ketamine 5 mg/kg in combination with dexmedetomidine 10 µg/kg and butorphanol 0.2 mg/kg as a single IM injection showed that this combination was suitable for castration, but recovery was better in the group that received dexmedetomidine, alfaxalone 3 mg/kg, and butorphanol.[54]
   iii. Ketamine 3 mg/kg in combination with dexmedetomidine 15 µg/kg and methadone 0.3 mg/kg IM provided anesthesia and analgesia and was suitable for cats undergoing ovariec-

tomy with comfortable and reliable recoveries.[55]

e) **Combining ketamine, butorphanol, midazolam, and medetomidine for OHE** (extra-label): Ketamine 60 mg/m² (≈3 mg/kg), midazolam 3 mg/m² (≈0.2 mg/kg), medetomidine 600 µg/m² (≈30 µg/kg), and *either* butorphanol 6 mg/m² (≈0.4 µg/kg) *OR* buprenorphine 180 µg/m² (≈9 µg/kg), and give as a single IM injection in the quadricep muscles 10 minutes prior to surgery.[56] In addition, *either* carprofen 4 mg/kg *OR* meloxicam 0.3 mg/kg can be given SC for additional analgesia.

f) **Combining ketamine with butorphanol and midazolam** (extra-label): Ketamine 3 mg/kg, butorphanol 0.4 mg/kg, and midazolam 0.4 mg/kg IM.[57] Substituting dexmedetomidine 5 µg/kg for ketamine produced excellent sedation and recovery but caused more cardiovascular depression and hematologic changes.

Combining ketamine with an opioid, medetomidine, and midazolam to immobilize cats requiring more sedation (extra-label): ketamine 1 – 5 mg/kg in combination with butorphanol 0.2 mg/kg, medetomidine 0.015 – 0.02 mg/kg, and midazolam 0.05 – 0.2 mg/kg and given IM. For painful procedures, consider also adding buprenorphine 0.02 – 0.04 mg/kg *OR* substituting butorphanol and buprenorphine with *either* morphine 0.5 mg/kg IM *OR* hydromorphone 0.1 mg/kg IM.

Highly aggressive cats (extra-label): Spray ketamine 1 mL into the open mouth or directed into the cat's mouth using a feline urethral catheter from a distance. The drug should be sprayed quickly so the cat does not chew and/or swallow the catheter.[58]

Adjunctive analgesia (extra-label):

a) Ketamine 0.5 mg/kg IV loading dose, followed by ketamine 0.1 – 0.6 mg/kg/*HOUR* IV CRI[38]

b) **Intraoperative use**: If anesthesia was induced with a drug other than ketamine, give a loading dose of ketamine 0.5 mg/kg IV followed by ketamine 10 – 20 µg/kg/*MINUTE* IV CRI; CRI rate can be decreased to 2 – 10 µg/kg/*MINUTE* for postoperative analgesia.[39]

c) **Morphine/lidocaine/ketamine (MLK) combination**: To a 500 mL bag of lactated Ringer's solution, add morphine sulfate 10 mg, lidocaine 120 mg, and ketamine 100 mg. Infuse IV at 10 mL/kg/*HOUR* CRI, which will provide morphine 0.2 mg/kg/*HOUR*, lidocaine 40 µg/kg/*MINUTE*, and ketamine 2 mg/kg/*HOUR*. Dexmedetomidine can be added to this mixture if needed.[59]

HORSES:

NOTE: Preferred agents for a short-term anesthesia induction protocol (ie, 20 minutes or less) include xylazine, first administered as a sedative, followed by a combination of ketamine and diazepam.[60] However, other alpha-2 agonists (eg, detomidine, romifidine) or benzodiazepines (eg, midazolam) have been substituted. For longer procedures requiring anesthesia (ie, more than 30-minute duration), protocols most commonly used a combination of guaifenesin, ketamine, and xylazine (GKX) or isoflurane. Thorough discussions of balanced, partial, and total IV anesthesia for horses can be found in the literature.[15,61]

The following dosages are some examples of published protocols:

Field anesthesia: (extra-label):

a) Sedate with xylazine 1 mg/kg IV or 2 mg/kg IM given 5 to 10 minutes (longer for IM route) before induction of anesthesia with ketamine 2 mg/kg IV. Horses must be adequately sedated (ie, head to knees) before receiving ketamine, which can cause muscle rigidity and seizures. If adequate sedation does not occur, do ***ONLY ONE*** of the following:

  i. Re-administer xylazine at up to half the original dose.

  ii. Add butorphanol 0.02 – 0.04 mg/kg IV. Butorphanol can be given with the original xylazine dose if there is suspicion the horse will be difficult to tranquilize (eg, high-strung thoroughbreds), or it can be added before induction with ketamine. This combination will improve induction, increase analgesia, and increase recumbency time by ≈5 to 10 minutes.

  iii. Add diazepam 0.03 mg/kg to the ketamine dose and give IV. This combination will improve induction when sedation is marginal, improve muscle relaxation during anesthesia, and prolong anesthesia by ≈5 to 10 minutes.

  iv. Administer IV guaifenesin 5% solution to effect to increase sedation and muscle relaxation.[62]

b) Premedicate with xylazine 0.7 mg/kg, butorphanol 0.025 mg/kg, and acepromazine at 0.05 mg/kg IV. Induce anesthesia with ketamine 5 mg/kg and diazepam 0.03 mg/kg IV. This combination produced rapid induction, more favorable surgical conditions, and improved recovery quality as compared with the same regimen using a lower ketamine dose of 2.2 mg/kg.[63]

c) **Field castration of ponies**:

  i. Premedicate with detomidine 0.02 mg/kg IV; induce with ketamine 2.2 mg/kg IV and midazolam 0.06 mg/kg IV[64]

  ii. Premedicate with butorphanol 0.05 mg/kg IV and romifidine 0.1 mg/kg IV, then ketamine 2.2 mg/kg or 3 mg/kg IV with diazepam 0.02 mg/kg IV.[65] Additional ketamine doses of 0.5 mg/kg IV were administered when anesthesia was deemed inadequate during surgery.

Part of induction protocols (extra-label): **NOTE**: Use with caution; this is not recommended for field anesthesia.

a) For healthy animals: Premedicate with xylazine 0.44 – 0.66 mg/kg IV (OR 200 – 300 mg/450 kg [992 lb] horse [NOT mg/kg]). Wait for sedation and muscle relaxation to occur (≈5 minutes), then rapidly infuse guaifenesin 5% solution (50 mg/mL) IV using pressurization until marked sedation and muscle relaxation is achieved, generally a total dose of 30 – 50 mg/kg. Administer ketamine 2.2 mg/kg IV (or 1000 mg/450 kg [992 lb] horse [NOT mg/kg]) at a point that allows for slow onset to occur without the animal becoming excessively weak and collapsing from the effects of guaifenesin. Recumbency generally occurs ≈60 seconds following ketamine administration. The slow administration of guaifenesin can also be used in healthy animals in place of a supplemental dose of xylazine when the level of initial sedation is inadequate.

For compromised animals: Premedicate with xylazine 0.22 – 0.44 mg/kg IV (or 100 – 200 mg/450 kg [992 lb] horse [NOT mg/kg]) depending on the status and demeanor of the animal to minimize cardiovascular effects in compromised animals. Slow IV administration of guaifenesin 5% solution (50 mg/mL) can be used initially to gradually achieve the desired level of sedation (see ***Guaifenesin, Intravenous*** monograph for additional details on administration), then rapidly infuse guaifenesin using pressurization until marked sedation and muscle relaxation is achieved, generally a total dose of 30 – 50 mg/kg IV. To induce anesthesia, decrease the ketamine dose as the degree of compromise increases: ketamine 1.34 – 1.55 mg/kg (or 600 – 700 mg/450 kg [992 lb] horse [NOT mg/kg]) IV for extremely compromised animals at a point that allows slow onset to occur without the animal becoming excessively weak and collapsing from the growing effects of guaifenesin. Experience may be required to get the timing right.

Recumbency takes longer (up to a couple minutes) when the ketamine dose is reduced in compromised animals.[66]

b) Using ketamine and propofol after xylazine sedation:

i. In a retrospective study (n = 100), horses were sedated with xylazine 0.99 ± 0.2 mg/kg IV.[67] Some horses also received butorphanol IV. After visually apparent sedation, a combination of propofol 0.40 ± 0.1 mg/kg and ketamine 2.8 ± 0.3 mg/kg were given (separately or in combination) via IV bolus. Following induction, 6 horses required a single administration of additional ketamine 0.7 ± 0.4 mg/kg. Anesthesia was maintained with guaifenesin in 34 horses and with isoflurane and oxygen in 66 horses.

ii. In a smaller study under experimental conditions, premedication occurred with xylazine 1 mg/kg IV, and anesthesia was induced with propofol 0.5 mg/kg IV followed by ketamine 3 mg/kg IV.[68] Anesthesia was maintained with isoflurane.

Partial IV anesthesia | PIVA (extra-label): Ketamine 0.4 – 3 mg/kg/hour IV CRI IV CRI (**NOTE**: ketamine 0.5 – 2 mg/kg/hour IV CRI is more commonly used). IV CRI should be discontinued 20 to 30 minutes before the inhalant anesthetic is turned off and the horse is moved to the recovery stall. This drug combination can also be combined with lidocaine and alpha-2 agonist (eg, dexmedetomidine, xylazine) CRIs.[69,70]

Total IV anesthesia:

a) **Guaifenesin/ketamine/xylazine | GKX | "Triple-drip"** (extra-label): Guaifenesin 50 mg/mL, ketamine 1 – 2 mg/mL (2 mg/mL concentration used for more painful or noxious procedures), and xylazine 0.5 mg/mL. To prepare this mixture, add ketamine (100 mg/mL) 10 mL for 1 mg/mL *OR* 20 mL ketamine for 2 mg/mL and xylazine (100 mg/mL) 5 mL to a 1000 mL bag of guaifenesin 5%. Most clinicians prefer to induce with ketamine/xylazine or ketamine/xylazine/diazepam and then use GKX for maintenance. Use GKX 1.5 – 2.2 mL/kg/*HOUR* IV CRI depending on the procedure, animal response, and ketamine concentration.

b) **Guaifenesin/ketamine/detomidine | GKD** (extra-label): In ponies sedated with detomidine 0.02 mg/kg IM and induced with ketamine 2 mg/kg IV: Guaifenesin 100 mg/mL, ketamine 4 mg/mL, and detomidine 0.04 mg/mL at 0.8 mL/kg/*HOUR* IV CRI for the first hour and 0.6 mL/kg/*HOUR* IV CRI for the final 30 minutes.[71,72] To prepare this mixture, add ketamine (100 mg/mL) 40 mL and detomidine (10 mg/mL) 4 mL to a 1000 mL bag of guaifenesin 10%.

c) **Ketamine/medetomidine/midazolam** (extra-label):

i. Premedicate with medetomidine 7 µg/kg IV then induce general anesthesia with ketamine 2.2 mg/kg IV followed by ketamine 3 mg/kg/*HOUR*, medetomidine 5 µg/kg/*HOUR*, and midazolam 0.1 mg/kg/*HOUR* IV CRI.[73]

ii. Alternatively, premedicate with acepromazine 0.01 – 0.02 mg/kg IV, medetomidine 7 µg/kg IV, and methadone 0.1 mg/kg IV; induce general anesthesia with ketamine 2.2 mg/kg IV and midazolam 0.06 mg/kg IV; maintain anesthesia with ketamine 3 mg/kg/*HOUR*, medetomidine 5 µg/kg/*HOUR*, and midazolam 0.1 mg/kg/*HOUR* IV CRI.[74]

d) **Ketamine/midazolam/xylazine** (extra-label): Premedicate with xylazine 1 mg/kg IV; induce with ketamine 2.2 mg/kg IV. The total intravenous anesthesia (TIVA) regimen consisted of ketamine 0.03 mg/kg/*MINUTE*, midazolam 0.002 mg/kg/*MINUTE*, xylazine 0.016 mg/kg/*MINUTE* IV CRI.[75] Additional ketamine was required in 50% of horses, and the regimen was deemed inferior to those in which midazolam was replaced with propofol 0.05 – 0.1 mg/kg per *MINUTE* IV CRI. In a retrospective review, the average doses were ketamine 0.045 mg/kg/*MINUTE*, xylazine 0.024 mg/kg/*MINUTE*, and midazolam 0.002 mg/kg/*MINUTE* IV CRI. Premedication included an alpha-2 agonist, but the specific agent and dose, other premedication, and anesthesia induction protocol were not standardized. During anesthesia, 33% of horses received a ketamine bolus.[76]

CATTLE/RUMINANTS:

Chemical restraint (mild sedation of standing animals to semi-anesthetized recumbency | Ketamine stun (extra-label): **NOTE**: The following are abbreviated suggested initial dosages. A thorough discussion including dosages for other combinations using ketamine and redosing recommendations is available.[77] Use in combination with local anesthetic blockade improves level of sedation.

a) Ketamine stun; IV recumbent (for short procedures requiring a high level of systemic analgesia and/or animal cooperation [eg, castration, biopsy, flushing joints, casting]): Ketamine 0.3 – 0.5 mg/kg with xylazine 0.025 – 0.05 mg/kg and butorphanol 0.05 – 0.1 mg/kg combined in one syringe and given IV. The upper end of the dosage range is used anecdotally unless contraindicated.[77] Duration of sedation is ≈15 to 25 minutes.

b) Ketamine stun; IM, SC recumbent: Ketamine 0.1 mg/kg with butorphanol 0.025 mg/kg and xylazine 0.05 mg/kg combined in one syringe and given IM or SC. Duration of sedation is ≈45 minutes with SC administration.

c) Ketamine stun; IV standing: Sedate with xylazine 0.02 – 0.0275 mg/kg IV, then ketamine 0.05 – 0.1 mg/kg IV slowly. An opioid (eg, butorphanol 0.05 – 0.1 mg/kg IV or IM [small ruminants], butorphanol 0.02 – 0.05 mg/kg IV or IM [larger ruminants], or morphine 0.05 – 0.1 mg/kg IV or IM) can be added to improve analgesia and level of sedation.

d) Ketamine stun; IM, SC standing: Ketamine 0.04 mg/kg with butorphanol 0.01 mg/kg and xylazine 0.02 mg/kg combined in one syringe and given IM or SC. In a 500 kg (≈1100 lb) cow, this combination equates to butorphanol 5 mg, xylazine 10 mg, and ketamine 20 mg (ie, 5–10–20 technique).

Injectable anesthesia (extra-label): Several protocols have been discussed using ketamine in combination with other anesthetic and analgesic compounds (including IM, IV, and IV CRI protocols).[77] The reader is referred to the full article for details on ketamine use for this purpose.

Adjunctive analgesia (extra-label):

a) Ketamine 0.4 – 1.2 mg/kg/*HOUR* IV CRI[78]

b) Ketamine/lidocaine/fentanyl in goats: IV premedication: fentanyl 10 µg/kg, lidocaine 2 mg/kg, and ketamine 1.5 mg/kg. Induce with propofol 3 mg/kg IV, then begin ketamine 3 mg/kg/*HOUR* with lidocaine 3 mg/kg/*HOUR* and fentanyl 10 µg/kg/*HOUR* all via IV CRI in addition to either propofol or isoflurane to maintain anesthesia.[79]

CAMELIDS (IE, LLAMAS/ALPACAS):

Anesthetic agent (extra-label):

a) **Alpacas**: Ketamine 0.2 – 0.5 mg/kg with butorphanol 0.05 – 0.1 mg/kg and xylazine 0.2 – 0.5 mg/kg combined in one syringe and given IM[80]

b) **Llamas**: Ketamine 0.2 – 0.3 mg/kg with butorphanol 0.07 – 0.1 mg/kg and xylazine 0.2 – 0.3 mg/kg combined in one syringe and given IV[80]

Procedural pain (eg, castrations) when recumbency (up to 30

minutes) is desired (extra-label):

a) **Alpacas**: Ketamine 4.6 mg/kg with butorphanol 0.046 mg/kg and xylazine 0.46 mg/kg combined in one syringe and given IM[78]

b) **Llamas**: Ketamine 3.7 mg/kg with butorphanol 0.037 mg/kg and xylazine 0.37 mg/kg combined in one syringe and given IM.[78] During anesthesia, 50% of the original ketamine and xylazine dose may be administered in order to prolong the effect up to 15 minutes.

NOTE: If performing mass castrations on 3 or more animals, a bottle using the following drug combination can be made: ketamine 1 g, butorphanol 10 mg, and xylazine 100 mg. Give this mixture at 1 mL/18 kg (40 lb) for alpacas, and 1 mL/22 kg (50 lb) for llamas. Handle the animal quietly and allow plenty of time before starting the procedure. Expect 20 minutes of surgical time. The animal should stand 45 minutes to 1 hour after injection of this drug combination.[78]

SWINE:

Injectable anesthesia (extra-label):

a) Administer atropine, then ketamine 11 mg/kg IM. To prolong anesthesia and increase analgesia, administer additional ketamine 2 – 4 mg/kg IV. Injection of local anesthetic agents at the surgical site (eg, lidocaine 2%) may enhance analgesia.[81]

b) Ketamine 22 mg/kg with acepromazine 1.1 mg/kg combined in one syringe and given IM[82]

c) Ketamine 4.4 mg/kg IM or IV after sedation[83]

d) Ketamine 8 mg/kg with detomidine 0.18 mg/kg and butorphanol 0.3 mg/kg combined in one syringe and given IM.[84] Tolazoline reversal shortened the duration of recovery without compromising recovery quality.

BIRDS:

Injectable anesthesia:

a) **Ketamine as a single agent** (extra-label): Birds weighing as follows (**NOTE**: Be aware of units when calculating doses. Birds weighing less than 250 g [0.6 lb] require a higher dose per kg than birds weighing more than 250 g [0.6 lb]):

  i. Less than 100 g (0.2 lb) (eg, canaries, finches, budgies): 0.1 – 0.2 mg/g IM

  ii. 250 g to 500 g (0.6 to 1.1 lb) (eg, parrots, pigeons): 0.05 – 0.1 mg/g IM

  iii. 500 g to 3 kg (1.1 to 6.6 lb) (eg, chickens, owls, hawks): 0.02 – 0.1 mg/g IM

  iv. More than 3 kg (6.6 lb) (eg, ducks, geese, swans): 0.02 – 0.05 mg/g IM[85]

b) **In combination with acepromazine** (extra label): Ketamine 25 – 50 mg/kg combined with acepromazine 0.5 – 1 mg/kg and administered IM[86]

c) **In combination with diazepam** (extra label): Ketamine 10 – 50 mg/kg with diazepam 0.5 – 2 mg/kg combined in a syringe and given IM or IV; doses can be split in half for IV use.

d) **In combination with xylazine** (extra label): Ketamine 10 – 30 mg/kg with xylazine 2 – 6 mg/kg combined in a syringe and administered IM. Xylazine is not recommended to be used in debilitated birds because of its cardiodepressant effects.

FERRETS:

Injectable anesthesia (extra-label): Ketamine 5 mg/kg with butorphanol 0.1 mg/kg and medetomidine 80 µg/kg combined in one syringe and given IM.[87] Maintenance of anesthesia may require supplementation with isoflurane (0.5% to 1.5%) during abdominal surgery.

Adjunctive postoperative analgesia (extra-label): Ketamine 0.3 – 0.4 mg/kg/*HOUR* IV CRI in combination with fentanyl 2.5 – 5 µg/kg/*HOUR* IV CRI[88]

RABBITS/RODENTS/SMALL MAMMALS:

Chemical restraint (extra-label):

Mice:

a) Ketamine 50 – 100 mg/kg IM or intraperitoneal (IP); 50 mg/kg IV

b) **In combination with diazepam**: Ketamine 200 mg/kg with diazepam 5 mg/kg IM or IP

c) **In combination with xylazine**: Ketamine 100 mg/kg with xylazine 5 – 15 mg/kg IM or IP[89]

Rats:

a) Ketamine 50 – 100 mg/kg IM or IP; 40 – 50 mg/kg IV

b) **In combination with diazepam**: Ketamine 40 – 60 mg/kg with diazepam 5 – 10 mg/kg IP

c) **In combination with xylazine**: Ketamine 40 – 75 mg/kg with xylazine 5 – 12 mg/kg IM or IP[89]

Hamsters/gerbils:

a) Ketamine 100 mg/kg IM

b) **In combination with diazepam**: Ketamine 50 mg/kg with diazepam 5 mg/kg IM

c) **In combination with xylazine**: Not recommended[89]

Guinea pigs:

a) Ketamine 10 – 30 mg/kg IM

b) **In combination with diazepam**: Ketamine 60 – 100 mg/kg with diazepam 5 – 8 mg/kg IM

c) **In combination with xylazine**: Ketamine 85 mg/kg with xylazine 12 – 13 mg/kg IM[89]

Rabbits:

a) Ketamine 20 – 60 mg/kg IM or IV

  In combination with diazepam: Ketamine 60 – 80 mg/kg with diazepam 5 – 10 mg/kg IM

  In combination with xylazine: Ketamine 10 mg/kg with xylazine 3 mg/kg IV[89] or ketamine 6 mg/kg with xylazine 0.6 mg/kg IV[90]; another reference does not recommend xylazine for pet rabbits.[91]

b) Ketamine 20 – 50 mg/kg IM or 15 – 20 mg/kg IV

  In combination with diazepam for induction: Diazepam 5 – 10 mg/kg IM, after 30 minutes give ketamine 20 – 40 mg/kg IM or diazepam 0.2 – 0.5 mg/kg and ketamine 10 – 15 mg/kg IV to effect

  In combination with diazepam for anesthesia without inhalants: Diazepam 5 – 10 mg/kg IM, after 30 minutes give ketamine 60 – 80 mg/kg IM

Injectable anesthesia (extra label):

Rodents: Ketamine 100 mg/kg with midazolam 5 mg/kg and buprenorphine 0.05 mg/kg combined in one syringe and given IP

Rabbits:

a) Ketamine 10 mg/kg with midazolam 0.05 mg/kg and buprenorphine 0.03 mg/kg combined in one syringe and given IM[92]

b) Following premedication with acepromazine 0.1 mg/kg and buprenorphine 0.02 mg/kg IM, anesthesia was induced with propofol 2 mg/kg IV and ketamine 1 mg/kg IV; anesthesia was maintained with propofol 0.8 mg/kg/*MINUTE* IV CRI and ketamine 0.1 – 0.2 mg/kg/*MINUTE* IV CRI.[93]

c) Ketamine 1 – 5 mg/kg IV combined with propofol 1 – 5 mg/kg IV can be administered together in a 1:1 mg/kg ratio; higher doses had faster anesthesia onset and longer duration.[94]

d) Medetomidine 0.1 mg/kg with ketamine 10 mg/kg administered intranasally into 2 nares over 30 seconds using a syringe and catheter prior to isoflurane anesthesia.[95] When the rabbits swallowed during intubation, half of the initial induction dose was repeated. Onset of anesthesia was within 5 minutes. Intranasal administration during dorsal recumbency caused dyspnea in all rabbits, and 2 rabbits died; administration during sternal recumbency was better tolerated, with no fatalities.

REPTILES:

NOTE: Reversal of all reptile dosages with atipamezole is 4 to 5 times the medetomidine dose.[96]

Anesthesia (extra-label): Ketamine 22 – 88 mg/kg IM[97]

Medium to small land tortoises (extra-label): Ketamine 5 – 10 mg/kg with medetomidine 100 – 150 µg/kg combined and given IV or IM

Freshwater turtles (extra-label): Ketamine 10 – 20 mg/kg with medetomidine 150 – 300 µg/kg combined and given IV or IM

Chelonians (extra-label): Ketamine 4 – 10 mg/kg with butorphanol 0.5 – 1 mg/kg and medetomidine 40 – 50 µg/kg IM[98]

Iguanas (extra-label): Ketamine 5 – 10 mg/kg with medetomidine 100 – 150 µg/kg combined and given IV or IM

Monitoring

- Depth of anesthesia and analgesia
- Ventilation (eg, $ETCO_2$)
- Cardiovascular status (eg, heart rate and rhythm, blood pressure, pulse oximetry)
- Monitor eyes to prevent drying out or injury
- Body temperature

Chemistry/Synonyms

Ketamine HCl, a phencyclidine derivative, occurs as white, crystalline powder. It has a melting point of 258°C to 261°C (496°F-501°F), emits a characteristic odor, and will precipitate as the free base at high pH. One gram is soluble in 5 mL of water and in 14 mL of alcohol. The commercially available injections are racemic mixtures of R- and S- ketamine, with a pH between 3.5 to 5.5. Ketamine 1 mg is equivalent to ketamine hydrochloride 1.15 mg.

Ketamine HCl may also be known as CI-581, CL-369, CN-52372-2, ketamini hydrochloridum, *Amtech*®, *Brevinaze*®, *Calypsol*®, *Cost*®, *Inducmina*®, *Keta*®, *Keta-Hameln*®, *Ketaject*®, *Ketalin*®, *Ketanest*®, *Ketaset*®, *Ketasthesia*®, *Keta-sthetic*®, *Ketava*®, *Ketina*®, *Ketmin*®, *Ketolar*®, *Narketan*®, *Velonarcon*®, *VetaKet*®, or *Vetalar*®.

Storage/Stability

Ketamine injection should be stored between 15°C to 30°C (59°F-86°F) and protected from light. The discard dates after first vial puncture vary by manufacturer; refer to the specific product label for further information.

The solution may darken with prolonged exposure to light; this does not affect the drug's potency. Do not use this product if precipitates appear.

Ketamine may be mixed with sterile water for injection, 5% dextrose, and 0.9% sodium chloride for diluent purposes.

A human-labeled ketamine product (50 mg/mL) maintained over 90% potency when stored in polypropylene syringes for 180 days.[99]

Compatibility/Compounding Considerations

Ketamine may be mixed with sterile water for injection, 5% dextrose, and 0.9% sodium chloride for diluent purposes. Ketamine is physically **compatible in the same syringe** with xylazine, cefazolin, diphenhydramine, fentanyl, hydromorphone, lidocaine, midazolam, and morphine.

Mixing ketamine with barbiturates or diazepam in the same syringe or IV bag is *not* recommended, as precipitation may occur. Although there are many anecdotal reports of mixing ketamine with diazepam or midazolam in the same syringe just prior to injection, there does not appear to be any published information documenting the drugs' stability after combining. Do not use if a visible precipitate forms.

A study in laboratory rodents, evaluating the stability, sterility, pH, particulate formation, and efficacy of compounded ketamine, acepromazine, and xylazine (KAX) supported the finding that the drugs are stable and efficacious for at least 180 days after mixing if stored in the dark at room temperature.[100]

The manufacturer states that dexmedetomidine 0.5 mg/mL solution for injection can be mixed with butorphanol 2 mg/mL or ketamine 50 mg/mL solution in the same syringe and possesses no pharmacologic risk.[101]

Ketamine is **Y-site compatible** with cefazolin, diphenhydramine, dobutamine, epinephrine, magnesium sulfate, morphine, penicillin G potassium/sodium, potassium chloride, propofol, and ranitidine.

Ketamine appears to be **Y-site incompatible** with ampicillin sodium, dexamethasone sodium phosphate, furosemide, heparin, insulin (regular), and sodium bicarbonate.

- **Morphine/Lidocaine/Ketamine ("MLK") Recipe**:

NOTE: When preparing solutions, be certain that you are **<u>NOT</u>** using the lidocaine product that contains epinephrine.

To prepare IV infusion solution using the veterinary lidocaine 2% solution, add 1 gram (50 mL) to 1 liter of compatible solution (eg, 0.9% sodium chloride, 5% dextrose). This solution will give an approximate lidocaine concentration of 1 mg/mL (1000 µg/mL). When using a mini-drip (60 drops/mL) IV set, each drop will contain ≈17 µg of lidocaine. In small dogs and cats, a less concentrated solution may be used for greater dosage accuracy.

A combination IV infusion for analgesia and sedation in postoperative patients (dogs, **<u>NOT</u>** cats) that require sedation to sleep the night after surgery is described[102]: For this technique, plan on adding the drugs to a bag of fluids for which the administration rate will not change, which usually means picking a fluid and administration rate calculated to provide maintenance needs for water. For example, to calculate a drug plan for a 20 kg dog that is to receive morphine, lidocaine, ketamine, and medetomidine for the first 8 to 24 hours postoperatively, drug doses to consider might include:

<u>Morphine</u>: 0.1 mg/kg/hour x 20 kg = 2 mg/hour
<u>Lidocaine</u>: 2.5 mg/kg/hour x 20 kg = 50 mg/hour
<u>Ketamine</u>: 0.1 mg/kg/hour x 20 kg = 2 mg/hour
<u>Medetomidine</u>: 2 µg/kg/hour x 20 kg = 40 µg/hour (**NOTE**: This is **<u>NOT</u>** the dose for dexmedetomidine; see the ***Dexmedetomidine*** monograph for use as a CRI).

The maintenance fluid administration rate for a 20 kg dog lying quietly in a cage is roughly 800 mL/day or 33 mL/hour. Therefore, a 1 L bag contains ≈30 hours of treatment, and to a 1 L bag one must add:

<u>Morphine</u>: 2 mg/hour x 30 hours = 60 mg = 6 mL (when using 10 mg/mL morphine)
<u>Lidocaine</u>: 50 mg/hour x 30 hours = 1500 mg = 75 mL (when using 2% [20 mg/mL] lidocaine)
<u>Ketamine</u>: 2 mg/hour x 30 hours = 60 mg = 0.6 mL (when using 100 mg/mL ketamine)
<u>Medetomidine</u>: 40 µg/hour x 30 hours = 1200 µg= 1.2 mL (when using 1000 µg/mL medetomidine)

If the drugs are added to a 1 L bag of fluid, the final volume is greater than 1 liter—in this case 1083 mL. Therefore, 83 mL should be removed from the bag *before* addition of the medications.[102]

Dosage Forms/Regulatory Status

VETERINARY-LABELED PRODUCTS:

Ketamine HCl for Injection: 100 mg/mL in 10 mL vials; *Ketaject*®, *Ketaset*®, *Keta-sthetic*®, *VetaKet*®, *Vetalar*®; generic; (Rx, C-III). FDA-approved for use in cats and subhuman primates

The Association of Racing Commissioners International (ARCI) has designated this drug as a class 2 substance. Use of this drug may not be allowed in certain animal competitions. Check rules and regulations before entering in a competition while this medication is being administered. Contact local racing authorities for further guidance. See ***Appendix*** for more information.

Food Animal Residue Avoidance Databank (FARAD) recommends a 3-day meat and 2-day milk withdrawal for ketamine in cattle, goats, and sheep.[103] The recommended meat withdrawal time for ketamine in swine is 2 days. **NOTE**: FARAD withdrawal intervals are dosage-dependent; consult FARAD website for further information.

HUMAN-LABELED PRODUCTS:

Ketamine HCl Injection: 10 mg/mL in 20 mL vials, 50 mg/mL in 10 mL vials, and 100 mg/mL in 10 mL vials; *Ketalar*®; generic; (Rx, C-III)

References

For the complete list of references, see **wiley.com/go/budde/plumb**

Ketoconazole, Systemic

(kee-toe-***kah***-na-zole) *Nizoral*®

Antifungal, Azole

Prescriber Highlights

- Oral imidazole antifungal historically used for systemic mycoses, but newer agents are generally preferred
- Contraindications include known hypersensitivity and liver disease; additionally, some clinicians believe ketoconazole is contraindicated in cats.
- Use caution in thrombocytopenia.
- Potentially teratogenic and embryotoxic
- Adverse effects: GI effects (eg, anorexia, vomiting, and/or diarrhea) are most common; hepatic toxicity, thrombocytopenia, reversible lightening of haircoat, transient dose-related suppressant effect on gonadal and adrenal steroid synthesis
- Many drug interactions are possible.

Uses/Indications

Because of ketoconazole's comparative lack of toxicity as compared with amphotericin B, easy oral administration, and relatively good efficacy, it has been used to treat several types of fungal infections in dogs, cats, and other small species. However, other antifungal agents (eg, fluconazole, itraconazole) are usually preferred, as they have less toxicity, less expense (ie, fluconazole), and/or have enhanced efficacy. In humans, ketoconazole is indicated only for systemic fungal infections in patients who have failed or are intolerant to other options.

In dogs, ketoconazole or itraconazole are recommended when systemic therapy is required for the treatment of *Malassezia* dermatitis. Itraconazole may be preferred due to improved tolerability, but availability and cost may dictate treatment.[1]

Use of ketoconazole in cats is controversial due to its potential for causing hepatotoxicity; some clinicians consider it contraindicated in cats.

Ketoconazole has also been used historically for the medical treatment of hyperadrenocorticism in dogs, but other treatments (mitotane or trilostane) are now recommended.

Ketoconazole interferes with the metabolism of drugs by CYP450 3A isoenzymes, including cyclosporine. This drug interaction has been used in dogs to reduce cyclosporine dosage/cost.[2,3]

Pharmacology/Actions

At usual doses and serum concentrations, ketoconazole is fungistatic against susceptible fungi. At higher concentrations for prolonged periods of time or against very susceptible organisms, ketoconazole may be fungicidal. It is believed that ketoconazole inhibits a fungal cytochrome P450-dependent demethylation enzyme that produces ergosterol in the cell membrane. The resultant intracellular accumulation of methylated sterols weakens the cellular membranes of susceptible fungi, increasing membrane permeability and allowing leakage of cellular contents and impairing uptake of purine and pyrimidine precursors.

Ketoconazole has activity against most pathogenic fungi, including *Blastomyces dermatitidis, Coccidioides immitis, Cryptococcus neoformans, Histoplasma capsulatum, Microsporum* spp, and *Trichophyton* spp. Higher concentrations are necessary to treat most *Aspergillus* spp and *Sporothrix* spp. Resistance to ketoconazole has been documented for some strains of *Candida albicans*.

Ketoconazole has in vitro activity against *Staphylococcus aureus* and *Staphylococcus epidermidis, Nocardia* spp, enterococci, herpes simplex virus types 1 and 2, and some protozoa. The clinical implications of this activity are unknown, but synergism between imidazole antifungal and antimicrobials against susceptible bacteria has been demonstrated.[4]

Via inhibition of 5-lipooxygenase, ketoconazole possesses some anti-inflammatory activity. The drug can suppress the immune system, likely by suppressing T-lymphocyte proliferation.

Ketoconazole also has endocrine effects; steroid synthesis is directly inhibited by blocking several P450 enzyme systems. Measurable reductions in testosterone or cortisol synthesis can occur at dosages used for antifungal therapy, but higher dosages are generally required to reduce concentrations of testosterone or cortisol to be clinically useful in the treatment of prostatic carcinoma or hyperadrenocorticism. Effects on mineralocorticoids are negligible. Other P450 effects include inhibition of vitamin D activation.

Pharmacokinetics

Although it is reported that ketoconazole is well absorbed after oral administration, oral bioavailability of ketoconazole tablets in dogs is highly variable. One study in 6 healthy dogs found the bioavailability ranged from 4% to 89% after ketoconazole 400 mg (19.5 – 25.2 mg/kg) was administered to fasted dogs.[5] Peak serum concentrations ranged from 1.1 to 45.6 µg/mL and occurred 1 to 4.25 hours after dosing. This wide interpatient variation may have significant clinical implications from both a toxicity and efficacy standpoint, particularly because ketoconazole is often used in life-threatening infections and assays for measuring serum concentrations are not readily available. Administration of ketoconazole with food may increase absorption.

Oral absorption of tablets in horses is poor. Single doses of ketoconazole compounded in corn syrup (30 mg/kg) yielded nondetectable drug concentrations in blood, but when given via NG tube in a 0.2 normal hydrochloric acid solution, bioavailability increased to 23% and a peak serum concentration of 3.8 µg/mL was reached 1.5 to 2 hours after administration.[6] Ketoconazole distributed into synovial and peritoneal fluids, endometrial tissue, and into the urine.

Ketoconazole absorption is enhanced in an acidic environment, and drugs that raise gastric pH may lessen absorption (see ***Drug Interactions***). The decision whether to administer ketoconazole with meals or during a fasted state to maximize absorption is controversial. The manufacturer recommends giving ketoconazole with food in human patients. Dogs or cats that develop anorexia and/or vomiting during therapy may benefit from administration with meals.

After absorption, ketoconazole is distributed into the bile, cerumen, saliva, urine, and synovial fluid. Ketoconazole unreliably reaches CSF in humans; CSF concentrations are generally less than 10% of those found in the serum but may be increased if the meninges are inflamed. High concentrations of the drug are found in the liver, adrenals, and pituitary gland, whereas more moderate concentrations are found in the kidneys, lungs, bladder, bone marrow, and myocardium. At usual doses (10 mg/kg), drug concentrations attained are likely inadequate in the brain, testes, and eyes to treat most infections; higher dosages are required. Ketoconazole is 84% to 99% bound to plasma proteins.

Ketoconazole is metabolized into several inactive metabolites by the liver; its metabolism may be saturable as mean residence time increases with repeated doses.[7] These metabolites are excreted primarily into the feces via the bile. Approximately 13% of a given dose is excreted in the urine, and only 2% to 4% of the drug is excreted unchanged in the urine. Half-life in dogs is ≈1 to 6 hours (average of 2.7 hours).

Contraindications/Precautions/Warnings

Ketoconazole is contraindicated in patients with known hypersensitivity to it and in animals with acute or chronic liver disease. It should be used with caution in patients with thrombocytopenia. Because of its effects on cortisol synthesis, it should be used with caution in dogs undergoing stressful events (eg, surgery, trauma, critical illness).

Use in cats is controversial, as anorexia, weight loss, and hepatotoxic effects are possible.

Many potential drug interactions are possible with ketoconazole. It is a potent inhibitor of CYP3A12 (and possibly other isoenzymes) and can inhibit P-glycoprotein. Certain drug combinations are contraindicated (see ***Drug Interactions***).

Long-term use of ketoconazole in small animal species has been associated with development of cataracts.[8]

Adverse Effects

GI signs (eg, anorexia, vomiting, diarrhea, weight loss) are the most common adverse effects seen with ketoconazole therapy and are more prevalent in cats. Dividing the dose and/or giving it with meals may minimize these adverse effects. Appetite stimulants such as mirtazapine (cats) or capromorelin (dogs) may also be of benefit.

Hepatotoxicity manifesting as cholangiohepatitis and increased liver enzymes has been reported with ketoconazole and may be either idiosyncratic in nature or a dose-related phenomenon. Anorexia and lethargy are often the clinical marker for toxicity[9]; hepatotoxicity is commonly dose-dependent and may occur at any time during treatment.[9] Cats may be more prone than dogs to developing hepatotoxicity. If adverse effects occur and ALT activity is markedly increased or hyperbilirubinemia occurs, the drug should be discontinued. Increased liver enzymes (ie, ALT, ALP) in the absence of other signs does not necessarily mandate dose reduction or drug discontinuation. Once ALT activity returns to normal and other adverse effects have resolved, the drug may be restarted at a lower dose or using longer dosing intervals with intense monitoring.

A retrospective study reviewed liver histopathology reports from 15 dogs with probable hepatotoxicity associated with therapeutic ketoconazole dosages.[9] Clinical signs included lethargy, anorexia, and vomiting, and liver enzymes were elevated in all dogs. Because many dogs that received ketoconazole were also receiving other drugs (eg, corticosteroids, phenobarbital), there was an array of liver pathology ranging from hepatocellular cholestasis to chronic hepatitis; the most consistent finding in each of the liver biopsy samples was an accumulation of ceroid-lipofuscin-laden macrophages, which are nonspecific changes associated with historic hepatocyte injury (a finding similar to that in humans with ketoconazole hepatotoxicity). Within the group of 15 dogs evaluated in this study, 7 died from liver injury: fulminant hepatic failure (n = 3), progressive chronic hepatitis (n = 3; pyogranulomatous [n = 2] and lymphoplasmacytic [n = 1]), and 1 was euthanized due to postoperative complications from a surgical liver biopsy with a presumed poor prognosis.

Uncommon adverse effects that have also been reported include thrombocytopenia, ataxia, and behavior changes (eg, anxiety).[10] A reversible lightening of the haircoat may also occur in patients treated with ketoconazole. Cataracts in dogs, anecdotally attributed to ketoconazole therapy, has been reported.[11]

Ketoconazole has a transient dose-related suppressant effect on adrenal steroid synthesis. Doses of 30 mg/kg/day have been demonstrated to suppress serum cortisol concentrations in dogs with hyperadrenocorticism (see ***Dosages***).[12] Dogs undergoing high dose antifungal therapy may need additional glucocorticoid support during periods of acute stress.[13] There are case reports of ketoconazole-induced hypoadrenocorticism in dogs receiving antifungal treatment with ketoconazole, which resolved after discontinuation of ketoconazole.[13,14]

Reproductive/Nursing Safety

Ketoconazole is a known teratogen and embryotoxin in rats, and dystocia has occurred with ketoconazole administration in the third trimester.[15] There have been reports of mummified fetuses and stillbirths in dogs that have been treated. Ketoconazole may cause infertility in male dogs by decreasing testosterone synthesis. Doses as low as 10 mg/kg depressed serum testosterone concentrations in dogs within 3 to 4 hours after administration but concentrations returned to normal within 10 hours.[12] Testosterone production rebounds once the drug is discontinued. In one dog treated with ketoconazole for 3 months, infertility occurred with decreased testosterone and azoospermia. Testosterone concentration and sperm quality were restored 100 days after discontinuing ketoconazole.[13]

Ketoconazole is excreted in milk. In humans, mothers who are under treatment with ketoconazole are advised not to breast feed.[15] Consider use of milk replacer if ketoconazole must be used in a lactating animal.

Because safety has not been established in animals, this drug should only be used when the maternal benefits outweigh the potential risks to offspring.

Overdose/Acute Toxicity

No reports of acute toxicity associated with overdose were located. The oral LD_{50} in dogs after oral administration is greater than 500 mg/kg. If an acute overdose occurs in humans, the manufacturer recommends employing supportive measures, including gastric lavage with activated charcoal within the first hour after ingestion.[15] Administration of oral antacids may help reduce absorption.

Chronic toxicity occurred in dogs given 20 – 40 mg/kg/day for up to 1 year. Signs included decreased food consumption, emesis, and, most notably, liver toxicity. Increased liver enzymes and histopathological changes in the liver were seen. These changes were reversible on discontinuation of ketoconazole. Jaundice and death occurred after 2 to 4 weeks of 80 mg/kg/day doses.[16]

For patients that have experienced or are suspected to have experienced an overdose, it is strongly encouraged to consult with one of the 24-hour poison consultation centers that specialize in providing information specific for veterinary patients. For general information related to overdose and toxin exposures, as well as contact information for poison control centers, refer to ***Appendix***.

Drug Interactions

Ketoconazole is a potent inhibitor of CYP2B11, 2C21/41, 2D15, and 3A12 in dogs[17]; in humans it inhibits CYP3A4 and P-glycoprotein. The following drug interactions have either been reported or are theoretical in humans or animals receiving ketoconazole and may be of significance in veterinary patients. Unless otherwise noted, use together is not necessarily contraindicated, but weigh the potential risks and perform additional monitoring when appropriate.

- **Alcohol**: Ethanol may interact with ketoconazole and produce a disulfiram-like reaction (vomiting).
- **Antacids** (eg, **aluminum, calcium,** and **magnesium contain-**

ing): May reduce oral absorption of ketoconazole; administer ketoconazole at least 1 hour before or 2 hours after

- **Antiarrhythmics** (eg, **amiodarone, disopyramide, quinidine**[18]): Ketoconazole may reduce metabolism and increase risk for ventricular arrhythmia and other adverse effects. Concurrent use is contraindicated in humans.
- **Benzodiazepines** (eg, **diazepam, midazolam**): Ketoconazole may increase benzodiazepine concentrations. A study in greyhounds showed that ketoconazole significantly decreased the elimination of midazolam.[7] Concurrent oral use is contraindicated in humans.
- **Bromocriptine**: Plasma concentrations of bromocriptine may be elevated.
- **Buprenorphine**: Ketoconazole may increase opioid concentrations and risk for toxicity.
- **Buspirone**: Plasma concentrations of buspirone may be elevated.
- **Busulfan**: Ketoconazole may increase busulfan concentrations.
- **Calcium Channel Blockers** (eg, **amlodipine, diltiazem, verapamil**): Ketoconazole may increase concentrations of this class of drug.
- **Cannabidiol**: Ketoconazole may increase cannabidiol concentrations.
- **Cisapride**: Ketoconazole may increase cisapride concentrations and possibility for ventricular arrhythmia; use together is contraindicated in humans.
- **Colchicine**: Increased risk for colchicine toxicity.[19] Concurrent use is contraindicated in humans with renal or hepatic impairment and not recommended in other patients.
- **Corticosteroids** (eg, **dexamethasone, predniso(lo)ne**): Ketoconazole may inhibit the metabolism of corticosteroids; potential for increased adverse effects.[20]
- **Cyclophosphamide**: Ketoconazole may inhibit the metabolism of cyclophosphamide and its metabolites; potential for increased toxicity.[21]
- **Cyclosporine**: Increased cyclosporine concentrations; this interaction has been used in dogs to reduce cyclosporine dosage and cost.[3]
- **Digoxin**: Ketoconazole may increase digoxin concentrations.
- **Doxorubicin**: Increased doxorubicin exposure
- **Fentanyl/Alfentanil**: Ketoconazole may increase fentanyl or alfentanil concentrations.
- **Fluoroquinolones** (eg, **ciprofloxacin, enrofloxacin**): Increased risk for QT prolongation
- **Fluoxetine**: Increased risk for QT prolongation; increased fluoxetine peak concentrations and exposure; clinical significance is unclear[22]
- **Haloperidol**: Increased haloperidol concentrations and increased risk for QT prolongation
- **H_2-Receptor Antagonist** (eg, **famotidine, ranitidine**): Increased gastric pH may reduce ketoconazole absorption.
- **Hepatotoxic Drugs, Other** (eg, **androgens, estrogens, NSAIDs**): Because ketoconazole can cause hepatotoxicity, it should be used cautiously with other hepatotoxic agents.
- **Hydroxyzine**: May increase risk for QT prolongation
- **Isoniazid**: May reduce ketoconazole concentrations and efficacy; concomitant use is not recommended in humans.
- **Ivermectin**: Ketoconazole increases ivermectin concentration and residence time, and may increase risk for neurotoxicity.[23,24] One reference states that ivermectin should never be used with ketoconazole in dogs.[25]
- **Macrolide Antibacterials** (eg, **azithromycin, clarithromycin, erythromycin**): May increase ketoconazole concentrations
- **Maropitant**: In humans, ketoconazole can increase plasma concentrations of NK_1-receptor antagonists, the class of antiemetics maropitant belongs to.
- **Methadone**: Increased plasma methadone concentrations and risk for ventricular arrhythmia; concurrent use is contraindicated in humans
- **Metronidazole**: May increase risk for QT prolongation
- **Mirtazapine**: Ketoconazole may increase mirtazapine concentrations, increasing risk for QT prolongation and ventricular arrhythmias.
- **Mitotane**: Mitotane and ketoconazole are not recommended for use together to treat hyperadrenocorticism, as the adrenolytic effects of mitotane may be inhibited by ketoconazole's inhibition of cytochrome P450 enzymes.
- **Ondansetron**: Increased risk for cardiotoxicity
- **Phenobarbital**: May decrease ketoconazole concentrations
- **Praziquantel**: Increased plasma concentrations of praziquantel; concurrent use is not recommended in humans.
- **Proton Pump Inhibitors** (PPIs; eg, **omeprazole, pantoprazole**): Increased gastric pH may reduce ketoconazole absorption.
- **Rifampin**: May decrease ketoconazole concentrations; ketoconazole may increase rifampin concentrations; increased potential for hepatotoxicity.
- **Rivaroxaban**: Increased rivaroxaban concentrations or exposure may occur; concurrent use is not recommended in humans.
- **Sildenafil**: May increase sildenafil exposure
- **Sotalol**: Increased risk for QT prolongation
- **Sucralfate**: May reduce absorption of ketoconazole
- **Sulfonylureas** (eg, **glipizide, glyburide**): Ketoconazole may increase concentrations; hypoglycemia is possible.
- **Tamsulosin**: Increased tamsulosin concentration is possible; concurrent use is not recommended in humans.
- **Theophylline**: Ketoconazole may decrease serum theophylline concentrations in some patients; theophylline concentrations should be monitored.
- **Toceranib**: May increase toceranib or ketoconazole concentrations via CYP3A4 inhibition
- **Tramadol**: May increase tramadol exposure[26]
- **Trazodone**: May substantially increase trazodone concentrations
- **Tricyclic Antidepressants** (eg, **amitriptyline, clomipramine**): Ketoconazole may reduce metabolism and increase adverse effects.
- **Vinca Alkaloids** (eg, **vinblastine, vincristine, vinorelbine**): Ketoconazole may inhibit vinca alkaloid metabolism and increase concentrations.
- **Warfarin**: Ketoconazole may cause increased prothrombin times in patients receiving warfarin or other coumarin anticoagulants.

Laboratory Considerations

- Ketoconazole can reduce serum cortisol concentrations and affect adrenal function tests. After stopping ketoconazole, cortisol concentrations usually return to baseline within 24 hours.

Dosages

NOTE: All dosages are extra-label.

DOGS:

NOTE: Oral ketoconazole has been used historically to treat various systemic mycoses, including blastomycosis and histoplasmosis. However, to obtain efficacy comparable to itraconazole alone, ketoconazole must be combined with amphotericin B.[27] Triazole antifungals (eg, itraconazole, fluconazole) are now generally recommended. Ketoconazole may be considered for these infections when drug cost determines whether treatment occurs. Ketoconazole continues to be a low-cost and effective treatment for *Malassezia* dermatitis.[28]

***Malassezia* dermatitis**: 5 – 10 mg/kg PO once daily.[1,29] Most clinicians recommend treatment for 3 to 4 weeks, until complete resolution of clinical signs. Use in combination with topical treatments (eg, miconazole/chlorhexidine shampoo) is recommended.[1,24]

Onychomycosis: 5 – 10 mg/kg PO every 12 hours, continued for 1 to 3 months beyond regrowth of healthy claws[30]

Reducing the dosage requirements of cyclosporine (**CSA**; consider monitoring cyclosporine concentrations): 2.5 – 10 mg/kg PO once daily.[2,31-33] Cyclosporine dosage reduction by ketoconazole occurs in a dose-dependent fashion (ie, higher ketoconazole doses result in a greater cyclosporine dosage reduction).[2,32,33]

Systemic mycoses: 5 – 10 mg/kg PO every 12 to 24 hours.[34-36] Treatment duration can vary but generally should continue for at least 1 month after complete resolution of clinical signs. Other azole antifungals (eg, fluconazole, itraconazole) have a more favorable efficacy and safety profile.

CATS:

NOTE: Use is controversial, and some clinicians recommend against using ketoconazole in cats because of its toxic potential. Consider using other antifungals (eg, fluconazole, itraconazole) instead, especially for dermatophytosis.

Systemic mycoses: Ketoconazole 10 mg/kg (or 50 mg/cat [NOT mg/kg]) PO with food every 12 to 24 hours.[37-39] Treatment may be required for many months. Other azole antifungals (eg, fluconazole, itraconazole) have a more favorable efficacy and safety profile.

HORSES:

Susceptible yeasts and *Aspergillus* spp: Using the commercial oral solution (**NOTE**: Not marketed in the United States): 5 mg/kg PO once daily

***Scopulariopsis* spp pneumonia**: Oral ketoconazole tablets may be administered via NG tube by mixing them with 0.2 normal hydrochloric acid and dosed at 30 mg/kg every 12 hours.[40,41]

BIRDS:

Susceptible fungal infections: 20 – 30 mg/kg PO twice daily (based on the kinetics determined in a single trial of Moluccan cockatoos)[42]

Severe refractory candidiasis in psittacines:

a) 5 – 10 mg/kg as a gavage twice daily for 14 days. For local effect in crop, dissolve ¼ of a 200 mg tablet (50 mg) in 0.2 mL of 1 normal hydrochloric acid and add 0.8 mL of water. Solution turns pale pink when dissolved. Add mixture to food for gavage.
b) To add to water for most species: 200 mg/L for 7 to 14 days. As drug is not water soluble at neutral pH, dissolve in acid prior to adding to water (see above).
c) To add to feed for most species: 10 – 20 mg/kg for 7 to 14 days. Add to favorite food or add to mash.[43]

RABBITS/RODENTS/SMALL MAMMALS:

Rabbits: 10 – 40 mg/kg per day PO for 14 days[44]

Hamsters, gerbils, mice, rats, guinea pigs, chinchillas: For systemic mycoses/candidiasis: 10 – 40 mg/kg per day PO for 14 days[30]

REPTILES:

Susceptible fungal infections in most species: 15 – 30 mg/kg PO once daily for 2 to 4 weeks[45]

Monitoring

- Liver biochemistry panel: Evaluate prior to therapy, then after 1 week and 1 month of the initial treatment period[9]; continue to monitor monthly for 3 to 6 months, then every 2 to 3 months thereafter.
- CBC with platelets
- Efficacy
- Signs of adrenal insufficiency (eg, lethargy, decreased appetite, vomiting, diarrhea)
- Adverse effects including vomiting, diarrhea, inappetence, lethargy, and jaundice

Client Information

- Give with food, especially foods high in fat (eg, cream, cheese, butter)
- Gastrointestinal effects (eg, lack of appetite, vomiting) are the most likely side effect seen (especially in cats).
- Liver toxicity is possible; watch for severe vomiting; no appetite; or yellowing of gums, skin, or whites of the eyes (jaundice). If seen, stop giving the medicine and contact your veterinarian immediately.
- May cause birth defects in animals and reduce fertility in males; use only when absolutely necessary in pregnant or breeding animals. Pregnant women should use caution when handling this medicine.

Chemistry/Synonyms

An imidazole antifungal agent, ketoconazole occurs as a white to slightly beige powder with pK_as of 2.9 and 6.5. It is practically insoluble in water.

Ketoconazole may also be known as ketoconazolum and R-41400; many trade names are available.

Storage/Stability

Ketoconazole tablets should be stored at room temperature 20°C to 25°C (68°F-77°F) in well-closed containers, protected from moisture.

Compatibility/Compounding Considerations

Compounded preparation stability: Ketoconazole oral suspension compounded from the commercially available tablets has been published.[46] Triturating twelve (12) ketoconazole 200 mg tablets with 60 mL of *Ora Plus*® and *qs ad* to 120 mL with *Ora Sweet*® or *Ora-Sweet-SF*® yields a 20 mg/mL ketoconazole oral suspension that retains greater than 95% potency for 60 days when stored at both 5°C (41°F) and 25°C (77°F) and protected from light.

Dosage Forms/Regulatory Status

VETERINARY-LABELED PRODUCTS: NONE FOR SYSTEMIC USE

Ketoconazole is available in topical formulations (eg, spray, shampoo, medicated wipe, otic flush); all formulations also contain an antibacterial agent and may have additional therapeutic ingredients; generic; (OTC).

HUMAN-LABELED PRODUCTS:

Ketoconazole Tablets: 200 mg (scored); generic; (Rx)

Topical forms are also available.

References

For the complete list of references, see **wiley.com/go/budde/plumb**

Ketoprofen

(kee-toe-***proe***-fen) *Ketofen®*

Nonsteroidal Anti-Inflammatory Drug (NSAID)

Prescriber Highlights

- Nonsteroidal anti-inflammatory agent approved for use in horses and cattle; used extra-label in other species for anti-inflammatory, analgesic, and antipyretic purposes
- Use with caution in patients that have GI ulceration or bleeding, hypoproteinemia, breeding animals (especially late in pregnancy), renal or hepatic impairment; may mask signs of infection (inflammation, hyperpyrexia)
- Adverse effects include gastric mucosal damage and GI ulceration, renal crest necrosis, hepatitis; may cause vomiting and anorexia. Do not administer intra-arterially and avoid SC injections in horses.

Uses/Indications

Ketoprofen is FDA-approved for use in horses for the alleviation of inflammation and pain associated with musculoskeletal disorders.[1] It is also approved for control of pyrexia associated with bovine respiratory disease in beef heifers, beef steers, beef calves 2 months of age and older, beef bulls, replacement dairy heifers, and dairy bulls. Like other NSAIDs, ketoprofen is used extra-label in a variety of species and conditions. Historically, ketoprofen was used for short-term analgesia in dogs and cats, but the availability of NSAIDs labeled in the United States for administration to those species has decreased its use.

Pharmacology/Actions

Similar to other NSAIDs, ketoprofen possesses antipyretic, analgesic, and anti-inflammatory activity. Its mechanism of action is the nonselective, reversible inhibition of cyclooxygenase (COX-1 and COX-2) catalysis of arachadonic acid to prostaglandin precursors (endoperoxides), thereby inhibiting the synthesis of prostaglandins in tissues. Ketoprofen purportedly has inhibitory activity on lipoxygenase, but the evidence for this action is weak as in vitro studies have not confirmed lipoxygenase activity in studied species.

Ketoprofen is a racemic mixture of S(+) and R(-) enantiomers. The S(+) enantiomer is associated with antiprostaglandin activity and toxicity and the R(-) form is associated with analgesia.

In cats, ketoprofen significantly reduced serum prostaglandin E2 (inflammatory marker) concentrations for up to 36 hours and serum thromboxane B2 (platelet inhibition marker) concentrations after SC administration in one study.[2] The S(+) enantiomer was responsible for COX inhibition.

Pharmacokinetics

In rats, dogs, and humans, ketoprofen is rapidly and nearly completely absorbed after oral administration. The presence of food or milk decreases oral absorption.

Oral absorption is poor in horses. It has been reported that when comparing IV vs IM injections in horses, the areas under the curve are relatively equivalent. Volume of distribution is low in adult horses. Volume of distribution is reportedly higher in foals and doses may need to be higher (1.5 times) with longer durations between doses in neonates.[3] The drug enters synovial fluid and is highly bound to plasma proteins (99% in humans, and ≈93% in horses). In horses, the manufacturer reports that the onset of activity is within 2 hours and peak effects 12 hours postdose.[1]

One study in eight thoroughbred horses also showed different pharmacokinetic parameters for the R(-) and S(+) enantiomers. After IV administration, mean systemic clearance was 0.345 L/kg/hour for R(-) and 0.167 L/kg/hour for S(+), mean steady-state volume of distribution was 0.344 L/kg for R(-) and 0.298 L/kg for S(+), and mean elimination half-life was 2.49 hours for R(-) and 2.86 hours for S(+). Oral bioavailability was calculated at 69.5% for R(-) and 88.2% for S(+) when the injectable formulation was used and 53% for both R(-) and S(+) when a paste was used.[4]

Ketoprofen is eliminated via the kidneys, both as a conjugated metabolite (primarily glucuronidation in horses) and as unchanged drug.

After SC administration to calves, peak concentration was reached 1.5 hours after administration, while after IV/IM administration to cattle peak concentration was reached at 0.75 hours. Half-life is 2 to 3 hours.[1,5]

After IM administration of racemic ketoprofen to 6-day-old piglets, S(+) ketoprofen was rapidly absorbed and had a relatively short half-life (3.5 hours).[6]

One study in loggerhead turtles compared IV and IM administration and found slightly different parameters for the R(-) and S(+) enantiomers.[7] After IM administration, mean bioavailability was 75% for R(-) and 64% for S(+), mean volume of distribution (adjusted for bioavailability) was 0.13 L/kg for R(-) and 0.09 L/kg for S(+), mean time to peak concentration was 0.19 hours for R(-) and 0.35 hours for S(+), and mean peak concentration was 6.94 µg/mL for R(-) and 10.07 µg/mL for S(+). Area under the curve for the S(+) enantiomer was more than twice that for the R(-) enantiomer. After IV administration, mean volume of distribution was 0.11 L/kg for R(-) and 0.07 L/kg for S(+), mean systemic clearance was 0.04 L/kg/hour for R(-) and 0.01 L/kg/hour for S(+), and mean elimination half-life was 2.12 hours for R(-) and 3.6 hours for S(+). Area under the curve for the S(+) enantiomer was more than twice that for the R(-) enantiomer.

Contraindications/Precautions/Warnings

Ketoprofen is contraindicated in patients with a known hypersensitivity to it and in those with impaired renal function or are dehydrated.[1,5] Use ketoprofen with caution in patients that are dehydrated, on concomitant diuretic therapy, or have pre-existing gastric ulcers, renal, cardiovascular, and/or hepatic dysfunction as they are at greatest risk for toxicity.[1] In these cases, ketoprofen should be used only when the potential benefits outweigh the risks. Ketoprofen may mask the clinical signs of infection (eg, signs of inflammation, pyrexia).

Avoid intra-arterial injection,[1] and avoid SC injections in horses.

Because there are approved NSAIDs for use in dogs and cats in the US, extra-label use of ketoprofen is not recommended.

Adverse Effects

In horses, ketoprofen appears to have low toxicity, and reports indicate that it appears relatively safe to use and may have a lower incidence of adverse effects as compared with phenylbutazone or flunixin.[8,9] Gastric mucosal damage and GI ulceration, renal crest necrosis, and mild hepatitis may occur.

Although not labeled for IM use in horses, it is reportedly effective when administered IM[5] and may only cause occasional inflammation at the injection site.

In dogs or cats, ketoprofen may cause vomiting, anorexia, and GI ulcers. When used perioperatively in dogs, ketoprofen can decrease platelet aggregation but this may not have clinical significance.[10] In healthy dogs receiving 2 mg/kg PO daily for 10 days, reduced creatinine clearance was noted in the dogs receiving ketoprofen.[11] Reducing the dose to 1 mg/kg SC then 0.25 mg/kg PO daily effectively eliminated all renal adverse effects and reduced incidence of GI bleeding in another study of long-term administration to dogs, suggesting that these effects were dose-dependent. In cats treated with 2 mg/kg SC daily for 3 days, fewer GI effects were observed in younger cats (less than 3 months old) as compared with older cats (more than 6 months old), suggesting that effects may also be age dependent.[12]

Reproductive/Nursing Safety

The manufacturer cautions against ketoprofen use in breeding horses because effects on fertility, pregnancy, or fetal health have not been established; it also states that, in cattle, the effects of ketoprofen on bovine reproductive performance, pregnancy, lactation, or on animals of reproductive age intended for breeding has not been investigated.[13] However, rat and mice studies have not demonstrated increased teratogenicity or embryotoxicity.[14] Rabbits receiving maternally toxic doses exhibited increased embryotoxicity, but not teratogenicity. Because nonsteroidal anti-inflammatory agents inhibit prostaglandin synthesis, thus adversely affecting neonatal cardiovascular systems (premature closure of patent ductus), ketoprofen should not be used late in pregnancy. Studies in male rats demonstrated no changes in fertility.[14]

It is presently unknown whether ketoprofen enters equine milk. Ketoprofen does enter canine[14] and bovine[15] milk; use with caution.

Because safety has not been established in animals, this drug should only be used when the maternal benefits outweigh the potential risks to offspring.

Overdose/Acute Toxicity

The LD_{50} in dogs after oral ingestion has been reported to be 2000 mg/kg, but exposures as low as 0.44 mg/kg in dogs have caused GI ulcers. Cats have developed renal toxicity at doses as low as 0.7 mg/kg. Horses given ketoprofen at doses up to 11 mg/kg administered IV once daily for 15 days exhibited no signs of toxicity.[1] Severe laminitis was observed in a horse given 33 mg/kg/day (15 times over label dosage) for 5 days. Anorexia, depression, icterus, and abdominal swelling were noted in horses given 55 mg/kg/day (25 times over label dosage) for 5 days, and necropsy findings included gastritis, nephritis, and hepatitis.[1]

As with any NSAID, overdose can lead to GI and renal effects. Decontamination with emetics and/or activated charcoal is appropriate.[14] The use of GI protectants (eg, omeprazole, famotidine, sucralfate) can be considered. If renal effects are suspected, fluid diuresis is warranted.

For patients that have experienced or are suspected to have experienced an overdose, consultation with a 24-hour poison consultation center specializing in providing veterinary-specific information is recommended. For general information related to overdose and toxin exposures, as well as contact information for poison control centers, refer to ***Appendix***.

Drug Interactions

The following drug interactions have either been reported or are theoretical in humans or animals receiving ketoprofen and may be of significance in veterinary patients. Unless otherwise noted, use together is not necessarily contraindicated, but weigh the potential risks and perform additional monitoring when appropriate.

- **Angiotensin Converting Enzyme Inhibitors** (ACEIs; eg, **benazepril, enalapril**): May result in renal dysfunction and/or increased blood pressure
- **Aminoglycosides** (eg, **gentamicin, amikacin**): May increase risk for nephrotoxicity
- **Angiotensin II Receptor Blockers** (ARBs; eg, **telmisartan**): May result in renal dysfunction and/or increased blood pressure
- **Anticoagulants** (eg, **heparin, enoxaparin, warfarin**): May increase risk for bleeding
- **Aspirin**: May increase risk for GI adverse effects or risk for bleeding
- **Beta-Adrenergic Receptor Antagonists** (eg, **atenolol, propranolol**): May increase blood pressure
- **Bisphosphonates** (eg, **alendronate**): May increase risk for GI ulceration
- **Clopidogrel**: May increase risk for bleeding
- **Corticosteroids** (eg, **dexamethasone, prednis(ol)one**): May significantly increase the risk for GI, platelet, or renal adverse effects, especially in dogs
- **Cyclosporine**: May increase risk for nephrotoxicity
- **Desmopressin**: May increase risk for hyponatremia
- **Digoxin**: May result in increased serum concentration of digoxin and a prolonged half-life of digoxin
- **Diuretics** (eg, **furosemide, spironolactone**): May increase risk for renal toxicity and reduce diuretic efficacy
- **Highly Protein Bound Drugs** (eg, **aspirin, phenytoin, valproic acid, oral anticoagulants, sulfonamides, sulfonylurea antidiabetic agents** [eg, **glipizide**]): Because ketoprofen is highly bound to plasma proteins (99%), it could theoretically displace other highly bound drugs and cause a transient increase in serum concentrations of each drug. These interactions are unlikely to be of clinical concern because increased free drug concentrations will equilibrate through increased clearance.
- **Methotrexate**: Severe toxicity has occurred in humans when NSAIDs have been used concurrently with methotrexate; use together with extreme caution.
- **Nonsteroidal Anti-Inflammatory Agents** (NSAIDs; eg, **carprofen, flunixin, robenacoxib, phenylbutazone**): Use of other NSAIDs significantly increases risk for NSAID-related adverse effects.
- **Probenecid**: Probenecid reduces plasma clearance of ketoprofen and decreases its protein binding, causing a significant increase in serum concentrations and half-life of ketoprofen; concurrent use is not recommended.
- **Selective Serotonin Reuptake Inhibitors** (SSRIs; eg, **fluoxetine, paroxetine, sertraline**): May increase risk for bleeding
- **Trazodone**: May increase risk for bleeding
- **Tricyclic Antidepressants** (TCAs; eg, **amitriptyline, clomipramine**): May increase risk for bleeding

Laboratory Considerations

Ketoprofen may cause:

- Falsely elevated **blood glucose** values when using the glucose oxidase and peroxidase method using ABTS as a chromogen
- Falsely elevated **serum bilirubin** values when using DMSO as a reagent
- Falsely elevated **serum iron** concentrations when the Ramsey method is used or falsely decreased serum iron concentrations when bathophenanthroline disulfonate is used as a reagent

Dosages

DOGS:

Anti-inflammatory/analgesic (extra-label): **NOTE**: Use of an NSAID labeled for dogs is recommended.

Acute pain:

a) 2 mg/kg SC, IM, or IV once; may repeat once daily for up 3 days[16]

b) 1 mg/kg PO once daily for 3 to 5 days[17]

Chronic pain:

a) For extended parenteral use, 0.5 mg/kg SC, IM, or IV once daily[16]

b) 0.25 mg/kg PO once daily[17]

CATS:

Anti-inflammatory/analgesic (extra-label): **NOTE**: Use of an NSAID labeled for cats is recommended.

Acute pain:

a) 2 mg/kg SC once daily for up 3 consecutive days[16]

b) 1 mg/kg PO once daily for 3 to 5 days[17]

Chronic pain: 0.25 mg/kg PO once daily[17]

HORSES:

Alleviation of inflammation and pain associated with musculoskeletal disorders (label dosage; FDA-approved): 2.2 mg/kg IV once daily for up to 5 days[1]

Alleviation of inflammation and pain associated with musculoskeletal disorders (extra-label): 2 mg/kg IV, IM once a day for up to 5 days[5]

CATTLE:

Control of pyrexia associated with bovine respiratory disease (BRD) in beef heifers, beef steers, beef calves 2 months of age and older, beef bulls, replacement dairy heifers, and dairy bulls (label dosage; FDA-approved): 3 mg/kg SC once daily for up to 3 days if pyrexia persists

Treatment of clinical signs related to fever, pain, and inflammation associated with a variety of conditions (eg, mastitis, musculoskeletal injury, respiratory tract infections (extra-label): 3 mg/kg IV or IM once daily for up to 3 days[5]

SHEEP:

Postoperative analgesic (extra-label): 3 mg/kg IV or IM as a single dose[18,19]

GOATS:

Anti-inflammatory/analgesic/antipyretic (extra-label):

a) 3 mg/kg IV or IM once daily

b) 2.5 mg/kg IV, may be repeated after 12 hours.[20] Dosage determined based on a pharmacokinetic study, and the safety and efficacy of this dosage have not been evaluated.

SWINE:

Reducing pyrexia in respiratory tract disorders and supportive treatment of postpartum dysgalactiae syndrome (MMA syndrome—mastitis, metritis, agalactia) in conjunction with antibiotic therapy (extra-label): 3 mg/kg deep IM once daily for up to 3 days[21]

BIRDS:

Anti-inflammatory/analgesic (extra-label): 2 mg/kg IM or SC every 8 to 24 hours[22]

FERRETS:

Postoperative analgesic (extra-label): 1 – 3 mg/kg SC, IM every 12 to 24 hours[23]

RABBITS:

Anti-inflammatory/analgesic (extra-label): 1 – 3 mg/kg IM every 12 to 24 hours[23-25]

RATS/MICE:

Analgesic (extra-label): 5 mg/kg SC, IM every 12 to 24 hours[23,26]

Monitoring

- Efficacy: level of analgesia, evidence of decreased inflammation, resolution of pyrexia
- Adverse effects (eg, vomiting, diarrhea, decreased appetite, hematemesis, hematochezia, melena)
- Baseline physical exam, CBC, serum chemistry panel (including renal and liver parameters), urinalysis; consider fecal occult blood testing when clinically appropriate. Repeat after the first few weeks of treatment, and periodically with long-term use.

Client information

- Do not inject this drug into an artery or under the skin (subcutaneously, SC) in horses.
- This medicine must only be used for a few days in cats to reduce risk of developing severe side effects.
- Most common side effects are gastrointestinal-related (eg, reduced appetite, vomiting, diarrhea in small animals). Ulcers, bleeding, and/or liver and kidney problems can also occur. If bloody vomit or stools are observed, discontinue the medication immediately and contact your veterinarian.
- While your animal is taking this medication, it is important to return to your veterinarian for regular examinations and monitoring. Do not miss these important follow-up visits.

Chemistry/Synonyms

Ketoprofen is a propionic-acid derivative NSAID that occurs as an off-white to white, fine to granular powder. It is practically insoluble in water but freely soluble in alcohol at 20°C (68°F). Ketoprofen has a pK_a of 5.9 in a 3:1 methanol:water solution. Ketoprofen has both an S(+) enantiomer and R(-) enantiomer. The commercial product contains a racemic mixture of both. The S(+) enantiomer has greater anti-inflammatory potency than the R(-) form.

Ketoprofen may also be known as *Anafen®*, *Ketofen®*, ketoprofenum and RP-19583; many trade names are available.

Storage/Stability

Ketoprofen injection should be stored below 25°C (77°F), with brief excursions permitted between 0°C and 40°C (32°F-104°F) and used within 4 months of first vial puncture.[13]

Ketoprofen oral capsules should be stored at room temperature (20°C-25°C [68°F-77°F]) in tight, light-resistant containers.[14]

Compatibility/Compounding Considerations

Compatibility is dependent on factors such as pH, concentration, temperature, and diluent used; specialized references or a hospital pharmacist should be consulted for more specific information.

Dosage Forms/Regulatory Status

VETERINARY-LABELED PRODUCTS:

The Association of Racing Commissioners International (ARCI) has designated this drug as a class 4 substance. See ***Appendix*** for more information. Use of this drug may not be allowed in certain animal competitions. Check rules and regulations before entering in a competition while this medication is being administered. Contact local racing authorities for further guidance.

Ketoprofen Injection: 100 mg/mL in 50 mL and 100 mL multidose vials; *Ketofen®*, generic; (Rx). FDA-approved for use in horses not intended for food. Slaughter withdrawal, 48 hours; not for use in female dairy cattle 1 year of age or older, including dry dairy cows; in beef calves less than 2 months of age, or in dairy or veal calves. A withdrawal period has not been established for this product in pre-ruminating calves. NADA #141-269.

A combination solution for injection containing ketoprofen 120 mg/mL with tulathromycin 100 mg/mL (*Draxxin® KP*) is also available for the treatment of bovine respiratory disease. See also ***Tulathromycin***.

HUMAN-LABELED PRODUCTS:

Ketoprofen Capsules: 50 mg and 75 mg; generic; (Rx)

Ketoprofen Extended-Release Capsules: 200 mg; generic; (Rx)

References

For the complete list of references, see **wiley.com/go/budde/plumb**

Ketorolac

(**kee**-toe-role-ak) *Toradol®*
Nonsteroidal Anti-inflammatory Drug (NSAID)

Prescriber Highlights

- NSAID used primarily for short-term analgesia. It is also used topically as an ophthalmic (see ***Ketorolac, Ophthalmic***).
- Contraindications include active or historical GI bleeding or ulcers, prior hypersensitivity reactions, concurrent NSAIDS or aspirin, bleeding disorders, suspected or confirmed cerebrovascular bleeding, and advanced renal or hepatic dysfunction.
- Use with caution in animals with pre-existing hematologic, renal, or hepatic disease; animals with CHF; and geriatric animals.
- Adverse effects may include GI ulcers and perforation; hepatic and renal toxicity; and inhibition of platelet aggregation. Consider co-dosing with misoprostol and/or sucralfate in dogs to reduce risk for GI ulcers.
- Long-term use is not recommended.

Uses/Indications

Ketorolac is used primarily for its analgesic effects for short-term treatment of mild to moderate pain in dogs[1,2] and rodents. Because of the availability of approved, safer, and longer-acting NSAIDs, ketorolac's use in dogs is questionable.

Safe and effective ketorolac use has been demonstrated in healthy horses,[3,4] but it was not superior to phenylbutazone or flunixin.

Pharmacology/Actions

Like other NSAIDs, ketorolac exhibits analgesic, anti-inflammatory, and antipyretic activity, probably through its inhibition of cyclooxygenase with the resultant impediment of prostaglandin synthesis. Ketorolac may exhibit a more potent analgesic effect than some other NSAIDs. It inhibits both COX-1 and COX-2 receptors.

Pharmacokinetics

After 0.5 mg/kg IV injection in dogs, ketorolac's volume of distribution is ≈1 L/kg, and the elimination half-life averages about 11 hours.[2] After oral administration, ketorolac is rapidly absorbed; in dogs, peak concentrations occur in ≈50 minutes, and oral bioavailability is ≈50% to 75%. The duration of analgesic effect in dogs is ≈6 hours.[1,2]

Ketorolac is distributed marginally through the body. It does not appear to cross the blood–brain barrier and is highly bound to plasma proteins (99%). The volume of distribution in dogs is reported to be ≈0.33 to 0.42 L/kg (similar in humans). The drug does cross the placenta.

In one study, horses received 0.5 mg/kg IV, IM, and PO. The drug was rapidly absorbed after IM and PO administration with 71% IM bioavailability and 57% oral bioavailability.[5]

Ketorolac is primarily metabolized via glucuronidation and hydroxylation. Both the unchanged drug and metabolites are excreted mainly in the urine. Patients with the diminished renal function will have longer elimination times than normal. In normal dogs, the elimination halflife is between 4 and 8 hours.

In a small, single-dose study of juvenile loggerhead sea turtles, 0.25 mg/kg ketorolac injected intramuscularly achieved what is presumed to be effective concentrations for ≈ 7 hours.[6] In another small study in Eastern box turtles, 0.25 mg/kg injected intramuscularly maintained presumed effective concentrations for 24 hours.[7]

Contraindications/Precautions/Warnings

Ketorolac is contraindicated in animals with active or recent GI ulcers or bleeding, advanced renal disease or at risk for renal failure due to volume depletion, a history of hypersensitivity to the drug, or suspected or confirmed cerebrovascular bleeding or bleeding disorder. It is relatively contraindicated in animals with a history of hematologic, renal, or hepatic disease, heart failure (may cause fluid retention), and in geriatric patients. In humans, ketorolac can cause serious skin adverse effects, such as Stevens-Johnson syndrome.

Because ketorolac has a tendency to cause gastric erosion and ulcers in dogs, long-term use (greater than 3 days) is not recommended in this species. In humans, combined parenteral and oral dosing should not exceed 5 days.[8] The minimum effective dose should be used.

Do not confuse ketoROLAC with ketAMine or ketoPROFEN.

Adverse Effects

Ketorolac use is limited in domestic animals because of its adverse effect profile and a lack of veterinary-labeled products. The primary issue in dogs is ketorolac's GI toxicity. GI ulceration can be common if the drug is used chronically. Most clinicians who have used this medication in dogs limit treatment to less than 3 days and give misoprostol with or without sucralfate concurrently. Like with other NSAIDs, platelet inhibition and renal and hepatic toxicity are possible with this drug as well. Transient azotemia was observed in 20% of clinically normal dogs that received ketorolac prior to ovariohysterectomy.[9]

In humans, common adverse effects include abdominal pain, dyspepsia, nausea, vomiting, and constipation or diarrhea.[8]

Reproductive/Nursing Safety

Ketorolac does cross the placenta. The use of NSAIDs during late pregnancy is typically avoided in humans due to the possibility of premature closure of the ductus arteriosus. In rats, administration of ketorolac caused dystocia and higher pup mortality.[8]

Most NSAIDs are excreted in milk. Ketorolac was detected in human breast milk at maximum milk:plasma ratio of 0.037. It is unlikely to pose a great risk to nursing offspring.

Because safety has not been established in animals, this drug should only be used when the maternal benefits outweigh the potential risks to offspring.

Overdose/Acute Toxicity

Limited information is available. Cats have developed renal toxicity at doses as low as 0.7 mg/kg. The oral LD_{50} is 200 mg/kg in mice. GI effects, including GI ulceration, are likely in overdoses in small animals. Metabolic acidosis was reported in 1 human patient. Consider GI emptying in large overdoses; patients should be monitored for GI bleeding. Treat ulcers with sucralfate; consider giving misoprostol early.

For patients that have experienced or are suspected of having experienced an overdose, consultation with a 24-hour poison consultation center specializing in providing veterinary-specific information is recommended. For general information related to overdose and toxin exposures, as well as contact information for poison control centers, refer to ***Appendix***.

Drug Interactions

The following drug interactions have either been reported or are theoretical in humans or animals receiving ketorolac and may be of significance in veterinary patients. Unless otherwise noted, use together is not necessarily contraindicated, but weigh the potential risks and perform additional monitoring when appropriate.

- **ACE Inhibitors** (eg, **enalapril**): Increased risk for nephrotoxicity
- **Alprazolam**: Hallucinations reported in some human patients taking with ketorolac
- **Aminoglycosides** (eg, **gentamicin, amikacin**): Increased risk for nephrotoxicity
- **Angiotensin Receptor Blockers** (ARBs; eg, **telmisartan**): Increased risk for nephrotoxicity
- **Anticoagulants** (eg, **heparin, LMWH, warfarin**): Increased risk for bleeding possible

- **Aspirin**: Increased likelihood of GI adverse effects (blood loss); this combination is contraindicated in humans
- **Bisphosphonates, Oral** (eg, **alendronate**): May increase the risk for GI ulceration
- **Corticosteroids** (eg, **dexamethasone, predniso(lo)ne**): Concomitant administration with NSAIDs may significantly increase the risks for GI adverse effects.
- **Cyclosporine**: May increase the risk for nephrotoxicity
- **Digoxin**: May increase the digoxin serum concentration and half-life
- **Diuretics** (eg, **furosemide**): May decrease diuretic efficacy and increase the risk for nephrotoxicity
- **Fluconazole**: May increase NSAID levels
- **Methotrexate**: Serious toxicity has occurred when NSAIDs have been used concomitantly with methotrexate; use together with extreme caution.
- **Muscle relaxants, Nondepolarizing** (eg, **atracurium**): Ketorolac may potentiate effects.
- **NSAIDs** (eg, **carprofen**): Therapeutic duplication; increased risk for adverse effects. This combination is contraindicated in humans.
- **Pentoxifylline**: May increase the risk for bleeding; this combination is contraindicated in humans.
- **Probenecid**: May cause a significant increase in serum levels and half-life of ketorolac. This combination is contraindicated in humans.
- **SSRIs** (eg, **fluoxetine**): Increased risk for bleeding

Dosages

DOGS:

NOTE: An NSAID that is FDA-approved for use in dogs is recommended.

Postoperative analgesic (extra-label): 0.5 mg/kg IV or IM preoperatively, may repeat every 6 hours.[1,2] Because ketorolac had limited efficacy during the intraoperative period, consider using only postoperatively.[2]

RABBITS/RODENTS/SMALL MAMMALS:

Analgesic (extra-label): **Mice**: 0.7 – 10 mg/kg PO once daily. **Rats**: 3 – 5 mg/kg PO 1 to 2 times a day; 1 mg/kg IM 1 to 2 times a day[10]

Monitoring

- Analgesic and anti-inflammatory efficacy
- GI: appetite, feces (occult blood, diarrhea)
- CBC and serum chemistry prior to use; repeat if adverse effects associated with GI, renal, or hepatic toxicity are noted after use.

Client Information

- Human NSAID that can be useful for the short-term treatment of pain in dogs or small mammals. Not for use in cats
- Give this medicine with food to decrease risk for upset stomach, vomiting and diarrhea.
- Gastrointestinal side effects (eg, vomiting, ulcers, bleeding) are highly possible if this medicine is used for more than a few days. Liver, kidney, and blood problems can also occur.
- Notify your veterinarian if signs of gastrointestinal distress (lack of appetite, vomiting, diarrhea, black feces, or blood in stool) occur or if your animal becomes depressed.

Chemistry/Synonyms

Ketorolac tromethamine, a carboxylic acid derivative and an NSAID agent, occurs as an off-white crystalline powder with a pK_a of 3.54 (in water). More than 500 mg are soluble in 1 mL of water at room temperature. The commercially available injection is a clear, slightly yellow solution with a pH of 6.9 to 7.9. Sodium chloride is added to make the solution isotonic.

Ketorolac tromethamine may also be known as RS-37619-00-31-3; many trade names are available.

Storage/Stability

Store both the tablets and injection protected from light at room temperature 20°C to 25°C (68°F-77°F). Protect the tablets from excessive humidity. The injection is stable for at least 48 hours in commonly used IV solutions.

Compatibility/Compounding Considerations

Do not mix with other drugs in the same syringe.

Dosage Forms/Regulatory Status

VETERINARY-LABELED PRODUCTS: NONE

The Association of Racing Commissioners International (ARCI) has designated this drug as a class 3 substance. Use of this drug may not be allowed in certain animal competitions. Check rules and regulations before entering in a competition while this medication is being administered. Contact local racing authorities for further guidance. See the ***Appendix*** for more information.

HUMAN-LABELED PRODUCTS:

Ketorolac Tromethamine Tablets: 10 mg; generic; (Rx)

Ketorolac Tromethamine Injection: 15 mg/mL and 30 mg/mL in 1 mL and 2 mL single-dose vials and 10 mL multiple-dose vials; generic; (Rx)

A topical ophthalmic preparation is also available; see ***Ketorolac, Ophthalmic*** for further information.

References

For the complete list of references, see **wiley.com/go/budde/plumb**

L-Theanine

***(el thee**-ah-neen)* *Anxitane®, Composure®*

Nutritional Anxiolytic Agent

Prescriber Highlights

- ► Used as a calming (anxiolytic) agent in dogs and cats. Limited evidence documenting efficacy
- ► Nutraceutical; not an FDA-approved drug
- ► Appears to be tolerated well

Uses/Indications

L-theanine is a nutritional supplement that is used as an anxiolytic for dogs and cats. There are limited published data that document efficacy in animals. In a study in beagles with anxiety towards humans, the 5 beagles treated with L-theanine showed greater human interaction and approach than the 5 beagles in the placebo control group.[1] L-theanine also reduced storm-related anxiety in dogs.[2] Open-label studies in cats conclude that L-theanine improves anxiety-related emotional disorders.[3] After chronic twice-daily administration in cats, improvement in stress parameters was seen as soon as 15 days, with continued improvement by 30 days.[4]

For human use, *Natural Standard*[5] has assigned the following grades (A to F scale) of scientific evidence for common/studied uses for L-theanine: Anxiety = C, Blood pressure control = C, Mood = C, Cognition = D.

Pharmacology/Actions

L-theanine is thought to increase nutritional serotonin, dopamine, and gamma-aminobutyric acid (GABA) levels in the CNS. Rat studies have found that L-theanine significantly lowered levels of 5-hydroxyindole in the brain and that it may inhibit glutamic acid excitotoxicity.[5] In humans, L-theanine has been shown to increase alpha waves in the brain that indicate a relaxed state.[6]

Pharmacokinetics

Only pharmacokinetic data for laboratory animals were located. The L-form of theanine is preferentially absorbed from the intestine with peak concentrations occurring ≈1 to 2 hours postdose. In rats, it is hydrolyzed by phosphate-independent glutaminase in kidneys to glutamic acid and ethylamine. No drug is detectable after 24 hours.

Contraindications/Precautions/Warnings

L-theanine is contraindicated in patients hypersensitive to it. A veterinary-labeled product (*Anxitane®*) warns: *Not intended for use in animals with severe phobias, separation anxiety or in animals with a known history of aggression.*

Do not confuse L-THEAnine with L-THREOnine.

Adverse Effects

L-theanine is relatively safe and adverse effects are not frequently reported in animals or humans. Some human patients taking L-theanine have reported headaches, reduced blood pressure, or alterations in cognition.

Reproductive/Nursing Safety

Product label states *safe use in pregnant animals or animals intended for breeding has not been proven.*

Because safety has not been established in animals, this drug should only be used when the maternal benefits outweigh the potential risks to offspring.

Overdose/Acute Toxicity

Limited information is available, but it is likely relatively non-toxic. A 13-week study in rats determined no-observed-adverse-effect-level (NOAEL) of 4000 mg/kg/day, the highest dose tested.[7] Products containing L-theanine may contain other ingredients that may have toxic potential.

For patients that have experienced or are suspected to have experienced an overdose, consultation with a 24-hour poison consultation center specializing in providing veterinary-specific information is recommended. For general information related to overdose and toxin exposures, as well as contact information for poison control centers, refer to ***Appendix***.

Drug Interactions

The following drug interactions have either been reported or are theoretical in humans or animals receiving L-theanine and may be of significance in veterinary patients. Unless otherwise noted, use together is not necessarily contraindicated, but weigh the potential risks and perform additional monitoring when appropriate.

- **Antihypertensive Agents**: L-theanine potentially can reduce blood pressure and cause additive effects.
- **D-Theanine; D,L-Theanine**: Can reduce the absorption of L-theanine

Dosages

DOGS/CATS:

Reduction of mild to moderate anxiety (extra-label):

a) Dogs: Based on the size of the dog, 10 – 100 mg/dog (not mg/kg) PO twice daily. Consult label of product being used for specific dosage. Use in conjunction with behavior therapy.

b) Cats: 10 – 25 mg/cat (not mg/kg) PO once or twice daily. Consult label of product being used for specific dosage. Use in conjunction with behavior therapy.

Monitoring

- Efficacy; reduction in stress indicators

Client Information

- Follow label directions or give as your veterinarian has recommended.
- Shake liquid well before use.

Chemistry/Synonyms

Theanine is a nonprotein amino acid found primarily in tea leaves. Younger and fresher tea leaves tend to be richer in caffeine, while older, drier leaves may have higher theanine levels. The L-form is used in nutritional supplements, as it appears to be better absorbed from the gut. Standardized methods for quantifying L-theanine have not been established.

L-theanine may also be known as glutamylethylamide, or L-N-ethylglutamine. *Suntheanine®* is common trade name.

Storage/Stability

Store bulk powder, tablets, or capsules at room temperature away from moisture. Keep chewable tablets away from children or animals. The *Anxitane®* label states to keep tablets in original blister pack until used.

Compatibility/Compounding Considerations

No information noted

Dosage Forms/Regulatory Status

VETERINARY-LABELED PRODUCTS:

The following are considered nutritionals by the FDA and are not approved drugs. Other products containing L-theanine may be marketed for use in dogs and cats.

L-theanine Tablets (chewable): 50 mg and 100 mg; *Anxitane® S* (50 mg) and *M&L* (100 mg); (OTC). Chicken flavor

L-theanine Tablets (chewable): 205 mg (with extracts of *Magnolia officinalis* and *Phellodendron amurense* 450 mg and dried whey protein concentrate 100 mg); *Solliquin®* (OTC)

L-theanine Tablets (soft chews): 35 mg (with extracts of *Magnolia officinalis* and *Phellodendron amurense* 75 mg and dried whey protein concentrate 25 mg); *Solliquin®* (OTC)

L-theanine Tablets (chewable): 10.5 mg (with thiamine 67 mg and colostrum calming complex 11 mg) and 21 mg (with thiamine 134 mg and colostrum calming complex 22 mg); *Composure®* (*Mini*; 10.5 mg) and (regular; 21 mg) *Bite-sized Chews*; (OTC)

Liquid: L-theanine 21 mg/2.5 mL (with thiamine 134 mg/2.5 mL and colostrum calming complex 22 mg/2.5 mL); *Composure® Max Liquid*; (OTC)

HUMAN-LABELED PRODUCTS:

No FDA-approved products noted. Nutritional supplements as bulk powder or capsules containing 100 mg, 150 mg, or 200 mg of L-theanine are available. *Suntheanine®* is a common trade name.

References

For the complete list of references, see **wiley.com/go/budde/plumb**

Lactulose

(*lak*-tyoo-lose) *Cephulac®, Kristalose®*
Ammonia Detoxicant/Osmotic Laxative

Prescriber Highlights

- ▶ Nonabsorbable disaccharide laxative used to reduce blood ammonia concentrations and to manage constipation
- ▶ Avoid use in patients with GI obstruction. Patients with gut dysbiosis may have reduced response.
- ▶ Use with caution in diabetic patients and those with pre-existing fluid or electrolyte imbalances
- ▶ Adverse effects include flatulence, gastric distention, and cramping; diarrhea and dehydration are signs of overdose.
- ▶ Cats dislike the taste of lactulose liquid, so administration may be difficult; lactulose crystals mixed into cat food may be more accepted.

Uses/Indications

Lactulose is used primarily as an adjunctive treatment to reduce ammonia blood concentrations in the prevention and treatment of hepatic encephalopathy (HE; also known as portosystemic encephalopathy [PSE]) in small animal species, pet birds, and, potentially, horses. It results in improvement in clinical signs but does not alter the underlying disease. In small animal species, it is also used as a laxative.

Pharmacology/Actions

Lactulose is a disaccharide (galactose/fructose) that is not hydrolyzable by the gut enzymes of mammals and, potentially, birds. On reaching the colon, lactulose is metabolized by resident bacteria, resulting in the formation of lactic, formic, and acetic acids, as well as carbon dioxide (CO_2). The production of these free fatty acids increases osmotic pressure in the bowel, drawing in water for a laxative effect and acidifying colonic contents. This acidification causes ammonia (NH_3) to migrate from the blood into the colon, where it is trapped as the ammonium ion (NH_4^+) and expelled with the feces. By forming free fatty acids, lactulose can also be considered a prebiotic. Reversible changes in fecal microflora (increased number of Firmicutes and Actinobacteria, and decreased numbers of Bacteroidetes and Fusobacteria) have been demonstrated in healthy dogs following lactulose administration.[1]

Pharmacokinetics

In humans, less than 3% of an oral dose of lactulose is absorbed in the small intestine. The absorbed drug is not metabolized and is excreted unchanged in the urine within 24 hours.

Contraindications/Precautions/Warnings

Lactulose syrup contains some free lactose and galactose and may alter the insulin requirements in diabetic patients. In patients with pre-existing fluid and electrolyte imbalances, lactulose may exacerbate these conditions if it causes diarrhea and should therefore be used cautiously. Lactulose should not be given to patients with intestinal obstruction. Patients with gut dysbiosis (potentially including antibiotic-induced dysbiosis) may experience reduced effectiveness because the effects of lactulose depend on GI bacterial degradation.

Adverse Effects

Signs of flatulence, gastric distention, and cramping may occur early in therapy but generally abate with time. Excessive doses can also lead to diarrhea with potential dehydration, hypokalemia, and hypernatremia; in these cases, the dose should be reduced. Cats dislike the taste of lactulose syrup, and administration may be difficult. Lactulose granules (crystals) have been more successfully administered after being mixed in food.

Reproductive/Nursing Safety

Lactulose does not impair fertility in laboratory animals and has no known teratogenic or mutagenic effects.

It is unknown if lactulose is excreted in milk, but it would be unexpected.

Overdose/Acute Toxicity

Excessive doses may cause flatulence, diarrhea, cramping, and dehydration. Fluids and electrolytes should be replaced, if necessary.

For patients that have experienced or are suspected to have experienced an overdose, it is strongly encouraged to consult with a 24-hour poison consultation center that specialize in providing information specific for veterinary patients. For general information related to overdose and toxin exposures, as well as contact information for poison control centers, refer to ***Appendix***.

Drug Interactions

The following drug interactions have either been reported or are theoretical in humans or animals receiving lactulose and may be of significance in veterinary patients. Unless otherwise noted, use together is not necessarily contraindicated, but the potential risks should be weighed and additional monitoring performed when appropriate.

- **Antacids, Oral** (eg, **aluminum, calcium, magnesium**): Nonabsorbable antacids may reduce the colonic acidification effects (and thus, efficacy) of lactulose.
- **Antidiarrheal Agents** (eg, **kaolin/pectin, loperamide**): May counteract laxative effect and reduce ammonia-lowering effect
- **Anti-Infective Agents, Oral** (eg, **amoxicillin, cephalexin, clindamycin, tylosin**): Theoretically, orally administered antibiotics could eliminate the bacteria responsible for metabolizing lactulose, thereby reducing its efficacy.
- **Diuretics** (eg, **furosemide**): May have additive effects on serum electrolytes
- **Glutamine**: May antagonize the ammonia lowering effects of lactulose
- **Laxatives, Other** (eg, **polyethylene glycol 3350, psyllium**): Lactulose should not be used with other laxatives, as the loose stools that are formed can be falsely attributed to the lactulose with resultant inadequate therapy for hepatic encephalopathy.
- **Neomycin**: Theoretically, neomycin could eliminate the bacteria responsible for metabolizing lactulose, thereby reducing its efficacy. However, some data suggest that synergy may occur when lactulose is used with neomycin for the treatment of hepatic encephalopathy.

Laboratory Considerations

- None noted

Dosages

DOGS:

NOTE: If using the crystals for oral solution: One gram of the crystals is equivalent to 1.5 mL of the liquid.

Hepatic encephalopathy (extra-label):

a) Orally: 1 – 3 mL/10 kg (NOT mL/kg) PO every 6 to 8 hours; adjust dose to achieve 3 to 4 soft stools per day.[2]

b) Retention enema for acute hepatic encephalopathy: 1 – 10 mL/10 kg (NOT mL/kg). After administering a cleansing enema, administer diluted lactulose solution (1 part lactulose to 2 to 3 parts warm water) as a retention enema for 30 minutes.[2-4]

Constipation (extra-label): 0.25 – 0.5 mL/kg PO every 6 to 8 hours. Alternatively, 2.5 – 15 mL/dog (NOT mL/kg) PO every 8 to 12 hours. Adjust dosage to obtain the stool quality desired.

CATS:

NOTE: If using the crystals for oral solution: One gram of the crystals is equivalent to 1.5 mL of the liquid.

Hepatic encephalopathy (extra-label):

a) Orally: 1 – 3 mL/10 kg (NOT mL/kg) PO every 6 to 8 hours; adjust dose to achieve 3 to 4 soft stools per day.[2]

b) Retention enema for acute hepatic encephalopathy: 1 – 10 mL/10 kg (NOT mL/kg). After administering a cleansing enema, administer diluted lactulose solution (1 part lactulose to 2 to 3 parts warm water) as a retention enema for 30 minutes.[2–4]

Constipation (extra-label):

a) Liquid: 0.5 mL/kg (usually 2 – 3 mL/cat) PO every 8 to 12 hours; adjust dosage to obtain the stool quality desired. For acute, severe constipation, can also be administered as an enema as listed above for hepatic encephalopathy.[5]

b) Crystals: ¼ – ½ teaspoonful/cat (≈1.25 – 2.5 mL/cat) twice daily mixed with food is commonly recommended; adjust dosage to obtain the stool quality desired.

HORSES:

Reduction of ammonia (extra-label): From a study in healthy horses, 333 mg/kg PO 3 times daily for 11 days significantly reduced blood ammonia.[6] One horse developed laminitis.

BIRDS:

Hepatic encephalopathy; to stimulate appetite, improve intestinal flora (extra-label):

Cockatiel: 0.03 mL/bird (NOT mL/kg) PO 2 to 3 times a day[7]

Amazon: 0.1 mL/bird (NOT mL/kg) PO 2 to 3 times a day. Reduce dosage if diarrhea develops. May be used for weeks

REPTILES:

Laxative (extra-label): **Green Iguana**: 0.3 mL/kg PO every 12 hours[8]

Hepatic lipidosis (extra-label): **Bearded dragons, leopard geckos, tortoises**: 0.5 mL/kg PO every 24 hours[9–11]

Monitoring

- Clinical efficacy (2 to 3 soft stools per day) and serum ammonia concentrations when used for HE
- Postenema: Measure pH of enema effluent and repeat if pH is greater than 6[2]
- In long-term use (ie, months) or in patients with pre-existing fluid/electrolyte problems, serum electrolytes should be periodically monitored.
- According to the product label, glucose control should be evaluated in diabetic patients. Although disruption of glycemic control is primarily theoretical, it seems prudent to monitor for glycemic control in the initial stages of treatment.

Client Information

- This medicine is used to treat constipation or to reduce ammonia concentrations in small animal species and birds with liver disease.
- Lactulose is generally well tolerated, although diarrhea, abdominal pain, or cramping may occur, particularly early in treatment. Contact your veterinarian if your animal develops diarrhea.
- Lactulose may be mixed in food or other liquids to improve palatability, but make sure the entire dose is consumed.
- When lactulose is used for problems related to liver disease (*hepatic encephalopathy*), contact your veterinarian if signs worsen or fewer than 2 to 3 soft stools are produced each day.

Chemistry/Synonyms

A synthetic derivative of lactose, lactulose is a disaccharide containing one molecule of galactose and one molecule of fructose. It occurs as a white powder that is very slightly soluble in alcohol and very soluble in water. The commercially available solutions are viscous, sweet liquids with an adjusted pH of 3 to 7.

One gram of the lactulose crystals for oral solution (*Kristalose*®) is equivalent to 1.5 mL of the liquid.

Lactulose may also be known as lactulosum; many trade names are available, including *Constulose*®, *Enulose*®, *and Kristalose*®.

Storage/Stability

Lactulose syrup should be stored protected from light in tight containers, preferably at room temperature (20°C-25°C [68°F-77°F]); avoid freezing. Darkening of the solution may occur, but this does not affect drug potency. Exposure to heat or light may cause extreme darkening or cloudiness; these solutions should be discarded. Lactulose solutions may precipitate; crystals dissolve with gentle reheating.

Compatibility/Compounding Considerations

For use as a retention enema, some human references recommend mixing 300 mL lactulose solution with 700 mL water or physiologic saline.

Dosage Forms/Regulatory Status

VETERINARY-LABELED PRODUCTS: NONE

HUMAN-LABELED PRODUCTS:

Lactulose Solution: 1 g/1.5 mL (labeled as 10 g/15 mL or 20 g/30 mL); (per 10 g contains less than 1.6 g galactose, less than 1.2 g lactose, and less than or equal to 1.2 g of other sugars); *Generlac*®, *Constulose*®, and *Enulose*®, generic; (Rx)

Lactulose Crystals for Oral Solution: Lactulose (less than 0.3 g galactose and lactose/10 g) in 10 g and 20 g packets; *Kristalose*®; (Rx)

References

For the complete list of references, see **wiley.com/go/budde/plumb**

Lanthanum

(***lan***-tha-num) *Fosrenol*®, *Lantharenol*®

Oral Phosphate Binding Agent

Prescriber Highlights

- ▶ Orally administered phosphate binder
- ▶ May be useful when aluminum or calcium containing phosphate binders cannot be used
- ▶ Limited experience and relatively little published in veterinary literature; products labeled for use in cats in some countries
- ▶ Contraindications include ileus, GI obstruction, and fecal impaction.
- ▶ Use caution in animals that have GI ulcers.
- ▶ Appears safe; adverse effects may include vomiting, nausea, and inappetence.
- ▶ Chewable tablets should be crushed prior to administration.
- ▶ Expense is a limiting factor.

Uses/Indications

Lanthanum carbonate is potentially useful as an orally administered phosphate binding agent for patients with chronic kidney disease. While phosphorous dietary restrictions are the mainstay of controlling hyperphosphatemia in small animals, binding agents such as aluminum, sevelamer, or lanthanum can be considered for use in patients whose phosphate levels are not controlled with diet alone or that will not consume very-low phosphorous diets. Lanthanum has a potential advantage over calcium or aluminum containing phosphate binders in that it does not appear to be absorbed, even at high doses or with continued use, though palatability can be an issue.

Pharmacology/Actions

Lanthanum carbonate's mechanism of action to reduce hyperphosphatemia is by dissociating in the acid environment of the upper GI tract to release lanthanum ions. These ions bind to dietary phosphate and form highly insoluble lanthanum phosphate complexes that are then eliminated in the feces.

Pharmacokinetics

Following oral doses, lanthanum bioavailability is very low (less than 0.002%). In humans, the small amount of systemically available lanthanum is very highly bound to plasma proteins (greater than 99%). Studies in dogs, mice, and rats have shown that lanthanum concentrations in tissues increase over time and can be several orders of magnitude higher than that found in the plasma. Highest tissue concentrations are found in the GI tract, bone, and liver; it does not cross the blood–brain barrier. Terminal half-life is ≈36 hours but is increased in patients with kidney disease. In rats, absorbed lanthanum is cleared primarily via biliary excretion into the feces. In dogs, mean recovery of an oral dose of lanthanum averages 94%.

Contraindications/Precautions/Warnings

Lanthanum carbonate is contraindicated in patients with bowel obstruction, ileus, or fecal impaction. It should be used with caution in patients where the GI tract is not intact (eg, GI ulcers, colitis) as there is an increased chance for oral absorption. While on this drug, the risk for GI obstruction is greater in patients with reduced GI motility or alterations in GI anatomy (eg, history of GI surgery, diverticula). Tablets should be crushed completely prior to administration to reduce the risk for serious adverse GI events.[1]

Adverse Effects

Limited information is available for dogs and cats, but it appears that lanthanum is well tolerated. Vomiting has been reported in some cats and food avoidance can occur when lanthanum carbonate is mixed into food.

Healthy cats given 1 g/kg PO over 3 months did not show any bone histological changes.[2]

In humans, adverse effects most commonly reported include nausea, vomiting, and diarrhea. These are generally self-limiting and usually abate with continued use.

Reproductive/Nursing Safety

Lanthanum carbonate did not impact fertility or reproductive performance in rats. Administration to pregnant rabbits at 5 times the maximum human labeled daily dose resulted in reduced fetal weight, delayed ossification, and increased postimplantation loss. In pregnant rats, it led to underweight and sexually under-developed offspring.

It is unknown if lanthanum is excreted into milk; use with caution in nursing dams.

Because safety has not been established in animals, this drug should only be used when the maternal benefits outweigh the potential risks to offspring.

Overdose/Acute Toxicity

No specific information was located. It is likely that an acute overdose would be tolerated, with the chance that it might cause GI effects. Only supportive treatment should be required. In a poster presentation of a dose escalation study in cats, cats tolerated oral dosages up to 1 g/kg but vomited repeatedly after receiving 2 g/kg.[3]

For patients that have experienced or are suspected to have experienced an overdose, consultation with a 24-hour poison consultation center specializing in providing veterinary-specific information is recommended. For general information related to overdose and toxin exposures, as well as contact information for poison control centers, refer to ***Appendix***.

Drug Interactions

The following drug interactions with lanthanum have either been reported or are theoretical in humans or animals receiving lanthanum and may be of significance in veterinary patients. Unless otherwise noted, use together is not necessarily contraindicated, but weigh the potential risks and perform additional monitoring when appropriate.

Lanthanum carbonate may **decrease** the amount absorbed or the pharmacologic effect of the drugs listed below; separate oral doses of lanthanum and these drugs by 2 hours to help reduce the potential for this interaction.

- **ACE Inhibitors** (eg, **enalapril**)
- **Allopurinol**
- **Antacids** (eg, **aluminum, magnesium, calcium** preparations): May form insoluble complexes, reducing efficacy
- **Chloroquine**
- **Corticosteroids** (eg, **dexamethasone, predniso(lo)ne**)
- **Digoxin**
- **Ethambutol**
- **Fluoroquinolones** (eg, **enrofloxacin**)
- **H_2-Receptor Antagonists** (eg, **famotidine**)
- **Iron Salts**
- **Isoniazid**
- **Levothyroxine**
- **Penicillamine**
- **Phenothiazines** (eg, **acepromazine**)
- **Tetracyclines** (eg, **doxycycline**)

Laboratory Considerations

- Lanthanum has radiopaque properties that may interfere with abdominal radiographic imaging.

Dosages

DOGS:

NOTE: If tablets are used, they should be crushed completely prior to administration.

Phosphate binder (extra-label): 5 – 20 mg/kg PO every 12 hours; titrate to effect[4]

IRIS treatment recommendations for reduction of phosphate intake in dogs with chronic kidney disease (CKD) [if plasma phosphate concentration is above 1.6 mmol/L (5 mg/dL) after dietary restriction]; (extra-label): starting dose of 30 – 60 mg/kg/day in divided doses given with each meal. Dose required will vary based on dietary phosphate intake and stage of kidney disease. Titrate to effect.[5]

CATS:

Phosphate binder (extra-label): Initially, 30 mg/kg/day PO divided 2 to 3 times a day and administered on or in food. A common dose is 200 mg PO twice daily. **NOTE:** Dosage is to effect.[6,7] Dosages as high as 95 mg/kg/day PO have been noted.[8,9]

IRIS treatment recommendations for reduction of phosphate intake in CKD [if plasma phosphate concentration is above 1.5 mmol/L (4.6 mg/dL) after dietary restriction]; (extra-label): starting dose of 30 – 60 mg/kg/day in divided doses given with each meal. Dose required will vary based on dietary phosphate and stage of kidney disease. Titrate to effect.[10]

Monitoring

- Serum phosphorous. For chronic kidney disease (CKD), most clinicians recommend a target phosphorous range of 0.9 to 1.5 mmol/L (2.7 to 4.6 mg/dL). For stage 3 CKD a more realistic upper limit might be 1.6 mmol/L (5.0 mg/dL). For stage 4 CKD, a more realistic upper limit might be 1.9 mmol/L (6.0 mg/dL).
- Other electrolytes such as potassium, calcium, bicarbonate, chloride, and calcium–phosphate product
- GI motility

Client Information

- Used to bind up phosphorous found in food and prevent it from being absorbed. Only helpful if your animal is eating.
- Administer this medicine at mealtimes. Mix this medicine into or sprinkle on top of food. If using tablets, crush them completely

before mixing into food. Do not give as intact tablet. Entire dose should be immediately consumed.

- Sometimes can cause vomiting.
- While your animal is taking this medication, it is important to return to your veterinarian for lab work. Do not miss these important follow-up visits.

Chemistry/Synonyms

Lanthanum is a chemical element with the symbol La and atomic number 57. When used pharmacologically, it is administered as lanthanum carbonate. Lanthanum carbonate occurs as a white to off-white powder that is insoluble in water.

Lanthanum carbonate may also be known as Bay-78-1887, and by the trade names *Lantharenol*®, *Renalzin*®, and *Fosrenol*®.

Storage/Stability

Store tablets at room temperature (25°C [77°F]); excursions are permitted to 15°C-30°C (59°F-86°F). Protect from moisture.

Compatibility/Compounding Considerations

No specific information noted

Dosage Forms/Regulatory Status

VETERINARY-LABELED PRODUCTS: NONE IN THE UNITED STATES

A lanthanum carbonate (octa-hydrate), kaolin, and vitamin E labeled product (*Renalzin*®) for use in cats had been available in several countries (not United States) but appears to be no longer marketed. It had been reported that 1 mL contained 200 mg of lanthanum carbonate.

HUMAN-LABELED PRODUCTS:

Lanthanum Carbonate Oral Chewable Tablet: 500 mg, 750 mg, and 1000 mg; *Fosrenol*®; (Rx)

Lanthanum Carbonate Oral Powder: 750 mg and 1000 mg; *Fosrenol*®; (Rx). Contains ≈ 357 mg lanthanum carbonate per g of powder.

References

For the complete list of references, see **wiley.com/go/budde/plumb**

Leflunomide

(le-***floo***-noh-myde) *Arava*®

Immunomodulator

Prescriber Highlights

- Immunomodulating drug used in small animal medicine as an immunosuppressant, particularly in patients refractory to treatment with conventional medications or when glucocorticoids are contraindicated
- Appears to be well tolerated by dogs and cats, but numbers treated are low
- Teratogenic and carcinogenic
- The National Institute for Occupational Safety and Health (NIOSH) classifies leflunomide as a hazardous drug; use appropriate precautions when handling.

Uses/Indications

Leflunomide is an immunomodulating drug used as an immunosuppressant in small animal medicine, particularly in patients that are refractory to treatment with conventional medications or when glucocorticoids are contraindicated. Leflunomide has been used in dogs to treat immune-mediated blood disorders (eg, IMHA,[1] IMT,[2] Evans syndrome[3]), systemic and cutaneous reactive histiocytosis, immune-mediated polyarthritis,[2,4,5] inflammatory bowel disease,[2] pancytopenia,[2] vasculitis,[2] and granulomatous meningoencephalitis. Clinical response to leflunomide is noted within 1 to 3 weeks of initiating therapy.[2]

Leflunomide has been used with methotrexate to treat rheumatoid arthritis in cats.[6,7]

A leflunomide analogue (FK778) has been used in transplant rejection protocols in dogs.[8]

Pharmacology/Actions

Leflunomide is a pyrimidine synthesis inhibitor that inhibits autoimmune T-cell proliferation and autoantibody production by B cells. Leflunomide acts almost exclusively via its primary active metabolite, teriflunomide (A77 1726), which reversibly inhibits the mitochondrial enzyme dihydroorotate dehydrogenase. The disruption of this enzyme prevents formation of ribonucleotide uridine monophosphate (rUMP), resulting in decreased DNA and RNA synthesis, inhibition of cell proliferation, and G1 cell cycle arrest. These cytostatic effects occur primarily in lymphocytes, sparing GI, hematopoietic,[9] and other rapidly dividing cells. Leflunomide also has antiviral and tyrosine kinase inhibiting properties, the importance of which is unclear. An antiplatelet effect also has been demonstrated.[10]

Pharmacokinetics

In healthy dogs (n = 4), after a single dose of leflunomide 4 mg/kg PO, the following mean values for teriflunomide were reported: time to peak concentration (T_{max}), 5 hours; peak concentration (C_{max}), 5 µg/mL; elimination half-life, 21.3 hours; and mean residence time (MRT), 27 hours. It is not understood why the apparent half-life for dogs is so much shorter (≈1 day) than it is for humans (15 days).[11] In another study, healthy dogs received leflunomide 4 mg/kg PO as a single dose, and teriflunomide values were reported as T_{max}, 1.4 hours; C_{max}, 18.9 µg/mL; t1/2, 25 hours; and MRT, 175 hours.[12]

In healthy cats (n = 6), after a single dose of teriflunomide (A77 1726) 4 mg/kg IV, the following mean values were reported: volume of distribution (Vd_{ss}), 97 mL/kg; clearance, 1.1 mL/kg/hour; and elimination half-life, 71.8 hours. After a single dose of leflunomide 4 mg/kg PO, bioavailability was 100%; peak teriflunomide concentration occurred ≈8 hours after dosing, and elimination half-life was 59 hours.[13]

In humans, leflunomide is rapidly converted to the active metabolite teriflunomide (A77 1726; M1) in the GI mucosa and liver. Peak concentrations of A77 1726 occur between 6 and 12 hours after an oral dose. The presence of food in the gut does not appear to affect oral bioavailability. Teriflunomide is highly bound to albumin (greater than 99%). It is further degraded in the liver as glucuronides and an oxalinic acid compound that are excreted in the urine and bile. Half-life is ≈15 days, but teriflunomide (A77 1726) can be detected in patients up to 2 years after it is discontinued.

Contraindications/Precautions/Warnings

Leflunomide is contraindicated in patients hypersensitive to it and in patients with severe hepatic impairment. It should be used with extreme caution in patients with severe immunodeficiency and in patients with significant renal impairment, bone marrow dysplasia, or active infection. Use leflunomide with additional (close) monitoring when needed in patients receiving other immunosuppressive drugs, or drugs known to be hepatotoxic.

The National Institute for Occupational Safety and Health (NIOSH) classifies leflunomide as a hazardous drug; *personal protective equipment (PPE) should be used accordingly* to minimize the risk of exposure.[14]

Adverse Effects

Adverse effects of leflunomide appear to be dose-related.[1,2] In a retrospective analysis, leflunomide was discontinued in 8 of 92 dogs because of adverse effects.[2] Across studies, reported adverse effects in dogs include diarrhea, decreased appetite, lethargy, vomiting, respiratory signs (ie, dyspnea, cough), increased liver enzymes, unexplained hemorrhage, leukocytopenia, lymphopenia, thrombocytopenia, hypercholesterolemia, and anemia.[1,2,15,16] Vomiting and lethargy have been reported in cats.[13]

In humans, GI effects (eg, diarrhea, nausea), alopecia, and rash are reported most commonly. Serious adverse effects have included hematologic toxicity, dermatologic effects (eg, TEN, Stevens-Johnson), peripheral neuropathy, interstitial lung disease, hypertension, and severe hepatotoxicity.

Reproductive/Nursing Safety

Leflunomide is contraindicated during pregnancy. Embryo lethality and a variety of teratogenic effects in laboratory animals have been detailed at or below doses used clinically. For sexually intact females, verify pregnancy status prior to administration.

Leflunomide is excreted in milk in rats; milk replacer should be used if the dam is receiving the drug.

Overdose/Acute Toxicity

Acute toxicologic studies in mice and rats have demonstrated that the minimally toxic dose is 200 mg/kg and 100 mg/kg, respectively. The LD_{50} in rabbits is 132 mg/kg. Cholestyramine or activated charcoal is recommended to accelerate elimination.

For patients that have experienced or are suspected to have experienced an overdose, consultation with a 24-hour poison center specializing in providing veterinary-specific information is recommended. For general information related to overdose and toxin exposures, as well as contact information for poison control centers, refer to ***Appendix***.

Drug Interactions

Leflunomide acts almost exclusively via its primary active metabolite, **teriflunomide**. The following drug interactions have either been reported or are theoretical in humans or animals receiving leflunomide and may be of significance in veterinary patients. Unless otherwise noted, use together is not necessarily contraindicated, but weigh the potential risks and perform additional monitoring when appropriate.

- **Charcoal, Activated**: Can increase elimination and decrease teriflunomide drug concentrations; may be used when more rapid elimination is desirable
- **Cholestyramine**: Can increase elimination and decrease teriflunomide drug concentrations; may be used when more rapid teriflunomide elimination is desirable (eg, toxic ingestion, severe toxicity)
- **Furosemide**: May increase furosemide exposure
- **Hepatotoxic Agents, Other**: Increased risk for toxicity
- **Immunosuppressants, Other** (eg, **antineoplastic agents, azathioprine, cyclosporine, high-dose glucocorticoids**): May have additive immune suppressing effect
- **Loperamide**: May inhibit loperamide metabolism
- **Methotrexate**: Increased adverse effects and increased ALT activity possible
- **Mitoxantrone**: May increase mitoxantrone exposure
- **Rifampin**: Can increase teriflunomide peak concentrations
- **Terbinafine**: May inhibit terbinafine metabolism
- **Theophylline**: May decrease theophylline concentrations
- **Vaccines, Modified Live Virus**: Live virus vaccines should be used with caution, if at all, during leflunomide therapy.
- **Warfarin**: Leflunomide may increase or decrease prothrombin time.
- **Zidovudine**: May increase zidovudine exposure

Dosages

DOGS:

Immune-mediated hemolytic anemia (IMHA) (extra-label): 2 mg/kg PO once daily.[1] Most recommendations for initial dosages range from 3 – 4 mg/kg PO once daily,[4,5] although 2 mg/kg PO once daily may also be effective.[1,2]

Immune-mediated polyarthritis (extra-label): 3 – 4.5 mg/kg PO once daily for at least 6 weeks. Adjust dose based on cytologic evaluation of synovial fluid and clinical signs.[4,5]

CATS:

Immunosuppressive agent (extra-label): Based on limited PK/PD information, an initial dosage of 2 – 3 mg/kg (practical dosage 10 mg per cat [NOT mg/kg]) PO once daily is reasonable.[13] Depending on the indication for use and response to treatment, dosage reduction (or increased time between dosages) can be considered over time once a positive clinical response occurs.

Adjunctive therapy for rheumatoid arthritis (extra-label): Initially, leflunomide 10 mg/cat (NOT mg/kg) PO once daily with methotrexate 2.5 mg/cat (NOT mg/kg) PO 3 times on 1 day per week (ie, methotrexate 7.5 mg/cat [NOT mg/kg] is divided and given as 3 separate 2.5 mg doses over 1 day). When significant improvement occurs, reduce leflunomide dosage to 10 mg/cat (NOT mg/kg) PO twice weekly and methotrexate to 2.5 mg/cat (NOT mg/kg) PO once weekly.[6,7]

Monitoring

- Clinical efficacy
- Adverse effects: GI effects (eg, vomiting, diarrhea, inappetence), infection (eg, fever, lethargy)
- Check CBC prior to starting therapy, then every 2 weeks for the first 2 months of therapy, then every 1 to 2 months (sooner if patient condition warrants) thereafter until therapy is complete.[1]
- Liver enzymes (ie, ALP, ALT) every 2 weeks for the first 2 months of treatment; consider checking values every 1 to 2 months (sooner if patient condition warrants) for the duration of therapy as long as patient is doing well.[1] In humans, it is recommended to check at baseline, at least monthly for the first 6 months, then every 6 to 8 weeks chronically.
- Trough concentrations of teriflunomide (active metabolite of leflunomide) may be considered[1]; concentrations between 20 to 30 µ/mL has been suggested for dogs with spontaneous immune-mediated disease. Based on pharmacokinetic data, it is reasonable to measure drug concentrations 1 to 2 weeks after initiating therapy or dosage changes, with samples obtained at any time within the dosing interval (ie, trough measurement is not required).

Client Information

- Use caution when handling this medication. Pregnant women must use caution when handling leflunomide, as this drug can cause birth defects.
- It may take 1 to 3 weeks to determine if leflunomide is effective.
- This medicine may be given with food or on an empty stomach. Give with food if animal vomits or acts sick after getting a dose.
- Side effects can include decreased appetite, lethargy (tiredness), vomiting, and diarrhea.
- Contact your veterinarian right away if you see bleeding or signs of infection (eg, fever, extreme tiredness, not wanting to eat).
- Your veterinarian will need to do periodic blood tests while your animal is taking leflunomide. Do not miss these important follow-up visits.
- This medication is considered to be a hazardous drug as defined by the National Institute for Occupational Safety and Health (NIOSH). Talk with your veterinarian or pharmacist about the use of personal protective equipment when handling this medicine.

Chemistry/Synonyms

Leflunomide is an isoxazole immunomodulator with a melting point of 165°C to 166°C (329°F-331°F). It occurs as a white or almost white powder. It is poorly soluble in water (21 mg/L).

Leflunomide may also be known as HWA 486, RS 34821, or SU 101; a common trade name is *Arava*®.

Storage/Stability

Leflunomide tablets should be stored at room temperature (15°C-30°C [59°F-86°F]) and protected from light.

Compatibility/Compounding Considerations

No specific information noted

Dosage Forms/Regulatory Status

VETERINARY-LABELED PRODUCTS: NONE

HUMAN-LABELED PRODUCTS:

Leflunomide Tablets: 10 mg and 20 mg; *Arava*®, generic; (Rx)

References

For the complete list of references, see **wiley.com/go/budde/plumb**

Leucovorin

Folinic Acid

(loo-koe-**vor**-in)

Folic Acid Derivative

Prescriber Highlights

- ► Primarily used in dogs, cats, and horses to help reverse neurotoxicity or hematologic toxicity associated with dihydrofolate reductase inhibitors (eg, pyrimethamine, trimethoprim, or ormetoprim)
- ► Leucovorin does not require conversion by dihydrofolate reductase for it to be active.

Uses/Indications

Leucovorin calcium is the calcium salt of folinic acid and is used as an antidote for toxicity from folic acid antagonists (eg, methotrexate, pyrimethamine, trimethoprim, ormetoprim). In dogs, cats, and horses, it is more commonly used to help reverse or prevent hematologic toxicity associated with pyrimethamine, trimethoprim, or ormetoprim. In humans, it is used routinely as a rescue agent following high-dose methotrexate chemotherapy

Pharmacology/Actions

Reduced folates act as coenzymes in the synthesis of purine and pyrimidine nucleotides necessary for DNA synthesis. Folates are also required for maintenance of normal erythropoiesis.

Leucovorin is a reduced form of folic acid that, unlike folic acid, does not require dihydrofolate reductase conversion for it to become biologically active. It is further converted to active reduced forms, of which 5-methyltetrahdyrofolate (5-methyl THF) is predominantly responsible for its activity. Although, leucovorin is a mixture of diastereoisomers, only the (-)-L-isomer (citrovorum factor) becomes biologically active.

Leucovorin inhibits thymidylate synthase by stabilizing the binding of fluorodeoxyuredylic acid to the enzyme. This effect can potentiate the activity, but also the toxicity, of fluorouracil (5-FU).

Leucovorin has a protective effect against methotrexate-induced chromosomal damage.

Pharmacokinetics

There is limited information available on the pharmacokinetics of leucovorin in animals. In dogs, the elimination half-life of the active L-isomer of leucovorin is ≈50 minutes. It is extensively metabolized and excreted into the urine. The inactive D-form elimination half-life is ≈2.5 hours. Apparent volume of distribution for both forms is 0.6 L/kg.

In humans, oral bioavailability of leucovorin following a 25 mg dose is 97%, but bioavailability decreases as dose is increased above 25 mg; doses of 50 mg and 100 mg have bioavailabilities of 75% and 37%, respectively. IM bioavailability is similar to IV. Oral doses of 25 mg yield peak leucovorin concentrations in ≈60 minutes, and peaks of the active reduced folates occur between 1.7 and 2.4 hours after dosing. After IV administration, peak total reduced folate concentrations occur in ≈10 minutes. Approximately 50% of oral body stores of reduced folates are found in the liver. Elimination occurs in the urine, primarily as 10-formyl-THF or 5,10-methyl-THF. Elimination half-life is ≈5.7 hours for total reduced folates.

Contraindications/Precautions/Warnings

Leucovorin is contraindicated in patients that are hypersensitive to it.[1] It should be used with caution in patients with megaloblastic anemia due to reduced cobalamin concentrations, as folinic acid therapy may mask the associated clinical signs.

Use with extreme caution in patients receiving systemic fluorouracil. See ***Drug Interactions***.

Large IV doses of leucovorin should be given as a slow infusion rather than a bolus due to the calcium content.

Do not confuse leucovorin with *Leukeran*® (chlorambucil); do not confuse foLINIC acid with foLIC acid, or foLINATE with foLATE.

Adverse Effects

Adverse effects have not been noted when leucovorin has been used in animals. In humans, adverse GI effects can be seen after oral administration; seizures and hypersensitivity reactions have rarely been reported. Pyrexia may occur after parenteral administration.

Reproductive/Nursing Safety

Leucovorin had no effect on the outcome of pregnancy in experimental studies in rabbits.[2] It is not known if leucovorin enters milk.[1] Because leucovorin is a biologically active form of folic acid, and folic acid supplementation is used before and during pregnancy in humans, leucovorin may be safe to administer during pregnancy or nursing.

Because safety has not been established in animals, this drug should only be used when the maternal benefits outweigh the potential risks to offspring.

Overdose/Acute Toxicity

Except in situations where drug interactions are possible, an inadvertent overdose is typically not concerning; however, excessive doses of leucovorin may reduce the effect of folic acid antagonists.

For patients that have experienced or are suspected to have experienced an overdose, consultation with a 24-hour poison consultation center specializing in providing veterinary-specific information is recommended. For general information related to overdose and toxin exposures, as well as contact information for poison control centers, refer to ***Appendix***.

Drug Interactions

The following drug interactions have either been reported or are theoretical in humans or animals receiving leucovorin and may be of significance in veterinary patients. Unless otherwise noted, use together is not necessarily contraindicated, but weigh the potential risks and perform additional monitoring when appropriate.

- **BARBITURATES, PRIMIDONE, PHENYTOIN**: Large doses of leucovorin may reduce the antiseizure efficacy of these agents by decreasing blood concentrations of the antiepileptic drugs.
- **DIHYDROFOLATE REDUCTASE INHIBITORS** (eg, **ormetoprim, pyrimethamine, trimethoprim**): Leucovorin may reduce therapeutic effect.
- **FLUOROURACIL (5-FU), CAPECITABINE (5-FU PRODRUG)**: Leucovorin may increase both the antineoplastic efficacy and toxicity of 5-FU.

Laboratory Considerations

- None noted

Dosages

DOGS/CATS:

Folate deficiency and myelosuppression associated with pyrimethamine, trimethoprim, ormetoprim (extra-label): Extrapolating from human dosages, 0.1 – 0.3 mg/kg PO once daily could be considered. A practical dose would be to round up to the nearest ½ tablet.

Methotrexate overdose (extra-label):

NOTE: Leucovorin is most effective if given within 48 hours of an overdose.

a) The dose of leucovorin is dependent on the serum methotrexate concentration. Administer leucovorin 25 – 200 mg/m^2 (NOT mg/kg) parenterally every 6 hours until methotrexate concentrations are less than 1×10^{-8} M.[3]

b) A case report in 2 dogs described leucovorin administration when MTX assay was unavailable. GI decontamination was performed (apomorphine; charcoal/sorbitol times 3 over 6 hours), followed by leucovorin calcium 200 mg/m^2 (NOT mg/kg) IV every 6 hours for 8 doses. Forced alkaline diuresis and N-acetylcysteine (IV) were also administered.[4]

c) 20 mg IV every 6 hours for 6 doses was given to a 13-kg dog after ingestion of methotrexate 7.7 mg/kg and a blood concentration of 0.09 µmol/L at 12 hours. GI decontamination, gastroprotectants, IV fluids, and antibiotics were also given. The dog developed no signs of toxicosis.[5]

HORSES:

Macrocytic anemia and neutropenia associated with pyrimethamine and/or trimethoprim (especially in pregnant mares; extra-label): 0.1 – 0.3 mg/kg PO once daily, although administration of green hay or pasture, which have high tetrahydrofolate concentrations, may be more practical.[6]

Monitoring

- CBC at baseline and prior to each treatment
- Methotrexate serum concentrations (contact a local human hospital) if used for methotrexate overdoses

Client Information

- If being used for methotrexate (chemotherapy) toxicity, this medication should only be administered in an inpatient setting.
- Oral leucovorin may be given with or without food.
- Give this medicine as directed by your veterinarian. It is very important to not miss any doses.
- Your veterinarian will need to monitor your animal while it is taking this medicine. Do not miss these important follow-up visits.

Chemistry/Synonyms

Leucovorin calcium occurs as a yellowish-white or yellow, odorless powder. It is very soluble in water and practically insoluble in alcohol. It is a mixture of diastereoisomers of 5-formyl tetrahydrofolic acid.

Leucovorin calcium may also be known as folinic acid, citrovorum factor, 5-formyl tetrahydrofolate, citrovorin, folidan, folinic, FTHF, NSC-3590, calcium folinate, calcifolin, calfonat, folinic acid calcium salt, or leucovorin calcium; many international trade names are available.

Storage/Stability

Leucovorin calcium tablets should be stored at 20°C to 25°C (68°F-77°F) in a sealed container protected from light.

Leucovorin powder for reconstitution and injection should be stored at 20°C to 25°C (68°F-77°F) protected from light.

Compatibility/Compounding Considerations

Compatibility is dependent on factors such as pH, concentration, temperature, and diluent used; specialized references or a hospital pharmacist should be consulted for more specific information.

The powder for injection is reconstituted by adding 5 or 10 mL of bacteriostatic water for injection or sterile water for injection. As bacteriostatic water for injection contains benzyl alcohol, it is not recommended in neonates or very small animals. If reconstituting with sterile water for injection, the resulting solution should be administered immediately; solutions made with bacteriostatic water for injection are stable up to 7 days.

Leucovorin calcium is **compatible** for dilution with lactated Ringer's, Ringer's, or 0.9% sodium chloride. Leucovorin calcium is **incompatible** with solutions containing fluorouracil.

A 5 mg/mL oral suspension can be compounded using twenty-four 25 mg tablets, crushed and mixed with 30 mL *Cologel®* and a 2:1 mix of simple and wild cherry syrups *qs ad* to 120 mL. This suspension is stable for 28 days under refrigeration.[7]

Dosage Forms/Regulatory Status

VETERINARY-LABELED PRODUCTS: NONE

HUMAN-LABELED PRODUCTS:

NOTE: Strengths listed are in terms of leucovorin base.

Leucovorin Calcium Oral Tablets: 5 mg, 10 mg, 15 mg, and 25 mg tablets; generic; (Rx)

Leucovorin Calcium Injectable Solution: 10 mg/mL single use vial; generic; (Rx)

Leucovorin Calcium Powder for Injection: 50 mg, 100 mg, 200 mg, 350 mg, and 500 mg in single use vials; generic; (Rx)

References

For the complete list of references, see **wiley.com/go/budde/plumb**

Leuprolide

(loo-***proe***-lide) *Lupron®*

GnRH-analogue Agonist

Prescriber Highlights

- Used for treatment of adrenal associated endocrinopathy in ferrets and to suppress gonadal activity in birds
- Doses listed are for depot formulation; do not confuse with daily injectable formulation.
- At studied doses in birds and ferrets the duration of effect is generally 4 to 6 weeks.
- Contraindicated in pregnancy (teratogenic) and in animals with uterine bleeding
- Use with caution in lactating animals
- Extremely costly (especially for ferrets); may be obtained in smaller aliquots from compounding pharmacies
- The National Institute for Occupational Safety and Health (NIOSH) classifies leuprolide as a hazardous drug; use appropriate precautions when handling.

Uses/Indications

The primary use for leuprolide is for treatment of adrenal associated endocrinopathy in ferrets. Vulvar swelling, pruritus, dysuria, and aggression can be reduced within days to weeks while hair regrowth can take 1 to 2 months.[1] Leuprolide may be more effective earlier in the disease process than later and when treating ferrets with adrenal hyperplasia or adenomas rather than adenocarcinoma.

In captive birds, 30-day depot leuprolide can suppress gonadal activity for 2 to 3 weeks.[2] Leuprolide has been used to treat malignant ovarian neoplasias in birds.

In dogs and cats, leuprolide has been used experimentally to induce estrus and treat hormone-responsive incontinence.

Commercial product labels may include the dosing interval (eg, "for administration every 6 months") but the duration of effect in veterinary patients is seldom that long.

Pharmacology/Actions

Leuprolide is a gonadotropin-releasing hormone (GnRH) agonist. GnRH is also known as luteinizing hormone-releasing hormone. GnRH agonists such as leuprolide act via negative feedback to inhibit release of the gonadotropins, luteinizing hormone (LH), and follicle stimulating hormone (FSH) from the pituitary gland. Decreased LH and FSH lead to decreased serum estrogen and androgen concentrations.

Pharmacokinetics

No veterinary pharmacokinetic data are available. The depot formulation appears to have sustained effects in birds and ferrets.

Duration of effect in ferrets varies when using the 30-day formulation. Clinical effects can persist from 1.5 to 8 months.[1]

In birds, when using the 30-day formulation, the duration of clinical effects may be up to 3 weeks.[3]

Contraindications/Precautions/Warnings

Leuprolide is contraindicated in any veterinary patient hypersensitive to leuprolide or any other gonadotropin-releasing hormone agonist, with uterine bleeding, and during pregnancy.

Prolonged QT intervals may occur in humans receiving leuprolide, increasing risk for cardiac arrhythmias including torsades de pointes. Use caution when combined with other medications that may prolong QT intervals. Hyperglycemia and increased risk for developing diabetes have been reported in humans. Seizures have also been reported.

The National Institute for Occupational Safety and Health (NIOSH) classifies leuprolide as a hazardous drug; personal protective equipment (PPE) should be used accordingly to minimize the risk for exposure.

Adverse Effects

Little information is available on the adverse effect profile of leuprolide in birds. Currently, this drug appears safe at recommended doses. There is a case report of a suspected anaphylactic reaction and death in 2 elf owls (*Micrathene whitneyi*).[3]

In ferrets, adverse effects reported include pain and irritation at injection site, dyspnea, and lethargy. Tolerance (higher dosages required over time to obtain the same effect) has been reported.

In humans, the most common adverse effects include general pain, hot flashes, GI signs (eg, nausea, vomiting), decreased sleep, and edema.

Reproductive/Nursing Safety

Leuprolide is contraindicated in pregnancy. Major fetal abnormalities may result.

It is not known whether leuprolide is excreted in milk; use with caution.

Overdose/Acute Toxicity

Due to expense and dosing method, acute overdose is unlikely. Studies in lab animals at dosages of up to 5 g/kg IM produced no untoward effects.

For patients that have experienced or are suspected to have experienced an overdose, consultation with a 24-hour poison consultation center specializing in providing veterinary-specific information is recommended. For general information related to overdose and toxin exposures, as well as contact information for poison control centers, refer to ***Appendix***.

Drug Interactions

The following drug interactions have either been reported or are theoretical in humans or animals receiving leuprolide and may be of significance in veterinary patients. Unless otherwise noted, use together is not necessarily contraindicated, but weigh the potential risks and perform additional monitoring when appropriate.

- **Antidiabetic Agents** (eg, **glipizide, insulin**): Leuprolide may worsen glycemic control and diminish the effectiveness of antidiabetic agents.
- **QT Prolonging Agents** (eg, **amiodarone, cisapride, procainamide, sotalol**): Leuprolide may prolong QT intervals. This effect may be increased with agents that also prolong QT intervals; use with caution with other QT prolonging agents.

Laboratory Considerations

- Diagnostic tests measuring **pituitary gonadotrophic** and **gonadal functions** may be misleading during and for several months after discontinuing therapy.

Dosages

Note: The doses listed are for the **depot** injection; do not confuse with the daily injection formulation.

BIRDS:

GnRH-agonist (extra-label): The <u>30-day depot formulation</u> is used most frequently in avian medicine; duration of effect in birds is generally less than 4 weeks. A wide range of dosages have been reported for birds, ranging from 100 µg/kg (0.1 mg/kg) to 1.2 mg/kg. For palliative treatment of ovarian neoplasias in cockatiels or macro-orchidism, very high dosages (1.5 – 3.5 mg/kg) have been recommended. However, most recommend dosages between 400 and 1000 µg/kg (0.4 – 1 mg/kg) IM repeated every 2 to 3 weeks.[2,4,5]

FERRETS:

Adrenal associated endocrinopathy (extra-label): Dosages are for the <u>30-day depot formulation</u> and vary by the source. No published evidence currently supports one dosage over another. Initially, 100 – 200 µg/ferret (0.1 – 0.2 mg/ferret [NOT per kg]) (some references recommend 100 µg/ferret (0.1 mg/ferret) (NOT µg/kg) in females or those under 1 kg (2.2 lb) and 200 µg/ferret (0.2 mg/ferret [NOT µg/kg]) in males or those greater than 1 kg (2.2 lb) IM every 4 to 6 weeks. All patients may require 200 µg/ferret (0.2 mg/ferret [NOT µg/kg]) in time and some become refractory to treatment at any dosage.[1,6]

GUINEA PIGS:

Ovarian cysts (extra-label): Leuprolide acetate depot 100 – 300 µg/kg (0.1 – 0.3 mg/kg) SC or IM every 3 to 4 weeks as needed to control clinical signs has been tried,[7] but another source states that the treatment is unproven and personal experience has been unrewarding.[8]

Monitoring

- Clinical effects in birds: decreased egg-laying
- Clinical effects in ferrets: decreased vulvar swelling, pruritus, undesirable sexual behaviors, aggression, and increased hair regrowth
- Adverse effects

Client Information

- Leuprolide is a treatment and will not cure adrenal diseases in ferrets. Life-long treatment is necessary.
- This medication is considered to be a hazardous drug as defined by the National Institute for Occupational Safety and Health (NIOSH). Talk with your veterinarian or pharmacist about the use of personal protective equipment when handling this medicine.

Chemistry/Synonyms

A synthetic nonapeptide analogue of GnRH (gonadotropin-releasing hormone, gonadorelin, luteinizing hormone-releasing hormone), leuprolide acetate occurs as a white to off-white powder. In water more than 250 mg are soluble in 1 mL.

Leuprolide may also be known as leuproprelin, leuprorelinum, abbott-43818, leuprolide acetate, TAP-144, *Carcinil®*, *Daronda®*, *Eligard®*, *Elityran®*, *Enanton®*, *Enantone®*, *Enantone-Gyn®*, *Ginecrin®*, *Lectrum®*, *Leuplin®*, *Lucrin®*, *Lupride®*, *Lupron®*, *Procren®*, *Procrin®*, *Prostap®*, *Reliser®*, *Trenantone®*, *Uno-Enantone®*, and *Viadur®*.

Storage/Stability

Store the injection formulation at room temperatures less than 30°C (86°F); do not freeze and protect from light (store in carton until use).

Store the depot formulation at room temperatures less than 30°C (86°F). After reconstituting the depot suspension use immediately or discard it within 2 hours (no preservative).

Compatibility/Compounding Considerations

Compatibility is dependent on factors such as pH, concentration, temperature, and diluent used; specialized references or a hospital pharmacist should be consulted for more specific information.

Whether the solution containing microspheres (depot formulation) can be frozen for later use is controversial. Some have frozen the solution and state it is still effective. The manufacturer states the depot form is not to be frozen as the microspheres are destroyed. No studies are known that support the stability of the depot activity when frozen and thawed. Some compounding pharmacies may divide the lyophilized powder into individual dosages in vials. If freezing is desirable, recommend putting individual aliquots into tuberculin syringes before freezing; do not re-freeze once thawed.

Dosage Forms/Regulatory Status

VETERINARY-LABELED PRODUCTS: NONE

HUMAN-LABELED PRODUCTS:

Leuprolide Acetate Injection: 1 mg/0.2 mL (2.8 mL multi-dose vial); generic; (Rx)

Leuprolide Acetate for SC Injection (kits): 7.5 mg (regular—30 day), 22.5 mg, 30 mg, and 45 mg; *Eligard®*, *Fensolvi®*; (Rx)

Leuprolide Acetate Microspheres for IM Injection (kits): 3.75 mg, 7.5 mg, 11.25 mg (regular—30 day and 3 month), 15 mg, 22.5 mg, 30 mg, and 45 mg; *Lupron® Depot* and *Lupron® Depot-Ped* and *Lupron® Depot-3, -4,* or *-6 Month*; (Rx)

References

For the complete list of references, see **wiley.com/go/budde/plumb**

Levamisole

(leh-***vam***-i-sole) *LevaMed®*

Antiparasitic

Prescriber Highlights

- ► Antinematodal parasiticide labeled for nematode infections in cattle, sheep, and swine
- ► Not approved for use in milk-producing animals
- ► Use with caution in severely debilitated animals; animals with significant hepatic impairment; or in cattle that are stressed due to vaccination, dehorning, long-distance transport, or castration.
- ► Adverse effects in large animal species include muzzle foaming, lip licking, head shaking, and excitement or tremor.
- ► Many adverse effects reported in small animal species, including GI upset and neurotoxicity

Uses/Indications

Levamisole is a broad-spectrum anthelmintic that is FDA-approved for use in nematode infections in various species, although use today in veterinary medicine is limited. Many products for oral use are no longer commercially marketed ostensibly due to increased resistance and the potential for adverse effects. Depending on the product, levamisole is indicated for the treatment of many nematodes in cattle, sheep, goats, swine, and poultry.

Levamisole has historically been used in dogs as a microfilaricide to treat *Dirofilaria immitis* infection but is rarely used today. It has also garnered some interest as an immunostimulant in the adjunctive therapy of various neoplasms or in combination with glucocorticoids for treating systemic lupus erythematosus.

Levamisole is not generally used in horses as an antiparasitic agent because of its narrow margin for safety and limited efficacy against many equine parasites; however, it has been tried as an immune stimulant. In horses with equine protozoal myeloencephalitis, levamisole may be useful for the control of clinical signs secondary to inflammation after treatment with antiprotozoal therapy. Anecdotal reports of beneficial effects in the treatment of nasal viral papillomas and chronic obstructive pulmonary disease have also been suggested.[1]

In cattle and sheep, levamisole has relatively good activity against abomasal nematodes, small intestinal nematodes (not particularly good against *Strongyloides* spp), large intestinal nematodes (not *Trichuris* spp), and lungworms. Adult forms of species that are usually covered by levamisole include *Haemonchus* spp, *Trichostrongylus* spp, *Teladorsagia* spp, *Osteragia* spp, *Cooperia* spp, *Nematodirus* spp, *Bunostomum* spp, *Oesophagostomum* spp, *Chabertia* spp, and *Dictyocaulus vivapurus*. Levamisole is less effective against the immature forms of these parasites and generally ineffective in cattle against arrested larval forms but has shown efficacy against arrested larval forms of *Teladorsagia* (formerly *Ostertagia) circumcincta* and *Haemonchus contortus* in sheep.[2]

In swine, levamisole is indicated for the treatment of *Ascaris suum*, *Oesophagostomum* spp, *Strongyloides* spp, and *Metastrongylus* spp.

Pharmacology/Actions

Levamisole stimulates the parasympathetic and sympathetic ganglia in susceptible worms. At higher concentrations, levamisole interferes with nematode carbohydrate metabolism by blocking fumarate reduction and succinate oxidation. The net effect is a paralyzing effect on the worm that is then expelled alive. Levamisole's effects are considered to be nicotine-like in action.

Levamisole's mechanism of action for its immune-stimulating effects is not well understood. It is believed that levamisole restores cell-mediated immune function in peripheral T lymphocytes and stimulates phagocytosis by monocytes. Its immune-stimulating effects appear to be more pronounced in animals that are immunocompromised.

Pharmacokinetics

Levamisole is absorbed from the gut after oral dosing and through the skin after dermal application, although bioavailabilities are variable. It is reportedly distributed throughout the body. Levamisole is primarily metabolized with less than 6% excreted unchanged in the urine. Plasma elimination half-life is 1.8 to 4 hours in dogs, 4 to 6 hours in cattle, and 3.5 to 6.8 hours in swine. Metabolites are excreted in both the urine (primarily) and feces.

Contraindications/Precautions/Warnings

Do not use levamisole in dairy animals of breeding age.[3] It should be used cautiously in animals that are severely debilitated and in animals with significant hepatic impairment. If possible, delay use in cattle that are stressed due to vaccination, dehorning, long-distance transport, or castration.[4] Use levamisole with caution if delaying treatment is not possible.

It is important to accurately assess body weight prior to dosing, as underdosing can lead to ineffective treatment and may encourage the development of parasite resistance.[3]

Levamisole use in goats is somewhat controversial, as there is evidence that it is toxic in fiber-producing goats. Oral routes are preferred but some clinicians have administered it SC; IM administration is contraindicated.

Avoid administering levamisole IM to birds.

One reference states that levamisole is contraindicated in cats with FIV or FIP and likely ineffective in cats with FeLV.[5]

Do not confuse levamisole with leucovorin, levETIRAacetam, or levOCARNitine.

Adverse Effects

Adverse effects that may be seen in dogs include GI disturbances (eg, vomiting, diarrhea), neurotoxicity (eg, panting, shaking, agitation, or other behavioral changes), immune-mediated anemia, agranulocytosis, dyspnea, pulmonary edema, immune-mediated skin eruptions (eg, erythroedema, erythema multiforme, toxic epidermal necrolysis), and lethargy.

Adverse effects seen in cats include hypersalivation, excitement, mydriasis, and vomiting.

Adverse effects that may be seen in cattle can include muzzle foaming or hypersalivation, excitement or trembling, lip licking, and head shaking.[3] These effects are generally noted with higher than recommended doses or if levamisole is used concomitantly with organophosphates. Signs generally subside within 2 hours.

In sheep, levamisole may cause transient excitability in some animals after dosing. In goats, levamisole may cause depression, hyperesthesia, and salivation.

In swine, levamisole may cause salivation or muzzle foaming. Swine infected with lungworms may develop coughing or vomiting.[6]

Reproductive/Nursing Safety

There is little information available regarding the safety of this drug in pregnant animals. Levamisole has been implicated in causing an abortion in goats. Although levamisole is considered relatively safe to use in large animals that are pregnant, use it only if the potential benefits outweigh the risks.

Levamisole is excreted in cows' milk; do not administer to dairy animals of breeding age.[3]

Because safety has not been established in animals, this drug should only be used when the maternal benefits outweigh the potential risks to offspring.

Overdose/Toxicity

Signs of levamisole toxicity often mimic those of organophosphate toxicity. Signs may include hypersalivation, hyperesthesias, irritability, clonic seizures, CNS depression, dyspnea, defecation, urination, and collapse. These effects are best treated by supportive means as animals generally recover within hours of dosing. An acute levamisole overdose can result in death due to respiratory failure. If respiratory failure occurs, artificial ventilation with oxygen should be instituted until recovery occurs. Cardiac arrhythmias may also be seen. If the ingestion was oral, GI decontamination protocols and/or administration of charcoal with cathartics may be indicated.

In pet birds (eg, cockatoos, budgerigars, Mynah birds, parrots), 40 mg/kg has been reported as a toxic dose when administered SC. IM injections may cause more severe toxicity. Depression, ataxia, leg and wing paralysis, mydriasis, regurgitation, and death may be seen after a toxic dose in birds.

In humans, the active metabolite of levamisole, aminorex, has amphetamine-like effects. Dosages of 50 – 200 mg daily can cause agranulocytosis.[7]

For patients that have experienced or are suspected to have experienced an overdose, consultation with a 24-hour poison consultation center specializing in providing veterinary-specific information is recommended. For general information related to overdose and toxin exposures, as well as contact information for poison control centers, refer to ***Appendix.***

Drug Interactions

The following drug interactions have either been reported or are theoretical in humans or animals receiving levamisole and may be of significance in veterinary patients. Unless otherwise noted, use together is not necessarily contraindicated, but weigh the potential risks and perform additional monitoring when appropriate.

- **ALBENDAZOLE AND IVERMECTIN**: After intraruminal combined administration of albenazole, ivermectin, and levamisole to parasitized lambs, reduced albendazole-sulfoxide and enhanced ivermectin systemic exposure were noted.[8]
- **ANTICHOLINESTERASES** (eg, **neostigmine, organophosphates**): Could theoretically enhance the toxic effects of levamisole; use together with caution
- **ASPIRIN**: Levamisole may increase salicylate concentrations.
- **CHLORAMPHENICOL**: Fatalities have been reported after concomitant levamisole and chloramphenicol administration; avoid using these agents together.
- **NICOTINIC DRUGS** (eg, **diethylcarbamazine, morantel, pyrantel**): Could theoretically enhance the toxic effects of levamisole; use together with caution
- **WARFARIN**: Increased risk for bleeding

Dosages

DOGS:

Adjunctive therapy for systemic lupus erythematosus (extra-label): 2 – 5 mg/kg (maximum of 150 mg/dog; NOT mg/kg) PO every 48 hours in combination with prednisone 0.5 – 1 mg/kg PO every 12 hours. Taper prednisone dose over 1 to 2 months. Continue levamisole for 4 months or longer if a relapse occurs.[9]

HORSES:

Adjunctive treatment for equine protozoal myeloencephalitis (extra-label):

a) Anecdotally, 1 mg/kg PO every 12 hours for the first 2 weeks in conjunction with antiprotozoal treatment and for the first week of each month thereafter[10]
b) 2.2 mg/kg PO every 24 hours for 3 days, then off for 4 days, repeated for a period of 4 to 6 weeks[1]
c) 1 – 2 mg/kg PO daily[11]

CATTLE:

Susceptible nematodes (label dosage; FDA-approved):

a) **Using the 46.8 g powder packet**:
   i. Standard oral drench: Place the contents of one packet in a 1 quart (960 mL; 32 fl oz) container, fill with water, and swirl until dissolved. Administer as a single oral drench dose of 15 mL/90.7 kg (200 lb) body weight, which provides an 8 mg/kg dose.[3]
   ii. Concentrated drench solution (for use with a 20 mL automatic syringe): Place the contents of one packet in a standard household measuring container and add water to the 8 ¾ fl oz (260 mL) level. Swirl until dissolved. Administer as a single oral drench dose of 2 mL/45.4 kg (100 lb) body weight, which provides an 8 mg/kg dose.[3]
b) **Using the 362.7 g bottle**: When ready to use, add water to the powder in the bottle up to the fill line located on the bottle. Swirl to mix thoroughly before using. Administer as a single oral drench dose of 2 mL/45.4 kg (100 lb) body weight, which provides an 8 mg/kg dose.[3]
c) **Using the 544.5 g bottle**: When ready to use, add water to the powder in the bottle up to the 3 L mark. Swirl to mix thoroughly before using. Administer as a single oral drench dose of 2 mL/45.4 kg (100 lb) body weight, which provides an 8 mg/kg dose.[3]

SWINE:

Susceptible nematodes (label dosage; FDA-approved): Reconstitute bottle to 500 mL and agitate thoroughly before using. Add 10 mL of stock solution to 1 gallon water and mix thoroughly. Offer as the sole source of drinking water, resuming use of regular water once all medicated water has been consumed. Allow 1 gallon of medicated water for each 45.4 kg (100 lb) body weight of pigs to be treated.[6]

SHEEP:

Susceptible nematodes (label dosage; FDA-approved):

a) **Using the 46.8 g powder packet**
   i. Standard oral drench: Place the contents of one packet in a 1 gallon (128 fl oz) container, fill with water, and swirl until dissolved. Administer as a single oral drench dose of 15 mL/22.7 kg (50 lb) body weight, which provides an 8 mg/kg dose.
   ii. Concentrated drench solution (for use with a 20 mL automatic syringe): Place the contents of one packet in a standard household measuring container and add water to the 17 ½ fl oz (520 mL) level. Swirl until dissolved. Administer as a single oral drench dose of 2 mL/22.7 kg (50 lb) body weight, which provides an 8 mg/kg dose.

b) **Using the 362.7 g bottle**: When ready to use, add water to the powder in the bottle up to the fill line located on the bottle. Swirl to mix thoroughly before using. Administer as a single oral drench dose of 1 mL/22.7 kg (50 lb) body weight, which provides an 8 mg/kg dose.[3]

c) **Using the 544.5 g bottle**: When ready to use, add water to the powder in the bottle up to the 3 L mark. Swirl to mix thoroughly before using. Administer as a single oral drench dose of 1 mL/22.7 kg (50 lb) body weight, which delivers an 8 mg/kg dose.[3]

GOATS:

Anthelmintic (extra-label): Use 1.5 times the sheep dosage (ie, 12 mg/kg PO once)[12–14]

REPTILES:

Anthelmintic (extra-label):

a) **Nematodes**: 5 – 10 mg/kg PO; repeat in 2 weeks followed by a fecal examination 14 days after the second dose. If the fecal examination is positive, a third dose is given.

b) **Acanthocephalans or pentastomes**: As stated above, but may also be given SC or intracoelomic[15]

Monitoring

- Clinical efficacy (eg, fecal flotation, fecal egg count reduction test)
- Adverse effects and toxicity observation

Client Information

- This medicine can be very toxic if too much is given. Follow directions on the product label unless otherwise directed by your veterinarian. Careful estimation of the body weight of the animal is essential to minimize the chance of overdose or underdose.
- The most common side effects seen in large animal species include foaming at the mouth, salivation, lip licking, and excitement or trembling.
- The most common side effects seen in small animal species include vomiting, enlarged pupils, diarrhea, drooling, and lack of energy. When this medicine is given by mouth to dogs, giving with food may help prevent vomiting.
- Serious side effects can occur. Report any concerns to your veterinarian.
- Avoid skin contact with liquid forms of this medicine, as it can be absorbed through the skin.
- Levamisole is not approved for use in dairy animals of breeding age.

Chemistry/Synonyms

Levamisole is the levo-isomer of dl-tetramisole, and it has a greater safety margin than does the racemic mixture. Levamisole hydrochloride occurs as a white to pale, cream-colored, odorless or nearly odorless crystalline powder. One gram is soluble in 2 mL of water.

Levamisole HCl may also be known as cloridrato de levamizol, ICI-59623, levamisoli hydrochloridum, NSC-177023, R-12564, RP-20605, l-tetramisole hydrochloride, *Amtech®*, *Ascaridil®*, *Decaris®*, *Ergamisol®*, *Immunol®*, *Ketrax®*, *LevaMed®*, *Levasole®*, *Meglum®*, *Prohibit®*, *Solaskil®*, *Vermisol®*, and *Vizole®*.

Storage/Stability

Store levamisole hydrochloride products at room temperature (15°C to 30°C [59°F-86°F]) unless otherwise instructed by the manufacturer; avoid temperatures greater than 40°C (104°F). Store levamisole phosphate injection at temperatures at or below 21°C (70°F); refrigeration is recommended and avoid freezing. Once mixed with water, levamisole drench solution may be stored in closed containers for up to 90 days.[3]

Compatibility/Compounding Considerations

Compounded preparation stability: Levamisole oral solution compounded from the commercially available tablets and active pharmaceutical ingredient powder has been published.[16] Triturating 2500 mg (2.5 g) of levamisole hydrochloride powder with 100 mL sterile water yields a 25 mg/mL levamisole hydrochloride oral solution that retains greater than 97% potency for 90 days when stored at both 4°C (39°F) and 25°C (77°F) and protected from light.

Dosage Forms/Regulatory Status

VETERINARY-LABELED PRODUCTS:

The Association of Racing Commissioners International (ACRI) has designated this drug as a class 2 substance. Use of this drug may not be allowed in certain animal competitions. Check rules and regulations before entering in a competition while this medication is being administered. Contact local racing authorities for further guidance. See ***Appendix*** for more information.

NOTE: FDA's Green Book still lists many approved levamisole products, but most are no longer marketed. The following products may be available:

Levamisole Hydrochloride Soluble Drench Powder: 46.8 g packet; 362.7 and 544.5 g bottle. *LevaMed®* (OTC). FDA-approved for use in cattle and sheep. Slaughter withdrawal at label dosages is 48 hours in cattle and 72 in hours sheep. Not indicated for dairy animals of breeding age.

Levamisole Hydrochloride Soluble Powder: 18.15 g bottle; *LevaMed®* Soluble Pig Dewormer (OTC); FDA-approved for use in swine. Slaughter withdrawal at labeled dosages is 72 hours.

HUMAN-LABELED PRODUCTS: NONE

References

For the complete list of references, see **wiley.com/go/budde/plumb**

Levetiracetam

(lee-ve-tye-***ra***-see-tam) *Keppra*®
Anticonvulsant

Prescriber Highlights

- ► Levetiracetam is a broad-spectrum anticonvulsant that can be used as adjunct therapy for canine epilepsy or when phenobarbital or bromides are not tolerated. Dogs may become refractory to therapy over time.
- ► In cats, levetiracetam may be used as a second-line drug when phenobarbital alone does not control seizures but can also be tried as sole therapy when phenobarbital is not tolerated.
- ► Appears to be well tolerated; adverse effects may be transient and can include sedation in dogs, and lethargy, decreased appetite, and ataxia in cats
- ► In dogs, phenobarbital may cause significant drug interactions with levetiracetam.
- ► Owner compliance with dosing frequency (every 8 hours) of immediate-release tablets and oral solution may be problematic.
- ► Do not confuse immediate-release and extended-release tablets; use caution when prescribing and dispensing.

Uses/Indications

Levetiracetam can be useful as adjunct therapy to phenobarbital and bromides in patients with canine epilepsy. Convincing evidence for efficacy of levetiracetam monotherapy is lacking.[1-3] Levetiracetam has been shown to be useful in the treatment of status epilepticus and acute repetitive seizures (ie, cluster seizures) in dogs.[4] It has been used at home for oral pulse therapy to abort seizure activity,[5] and SC administration at home may be useful in dogs that develop status epilepticus or acute repetitive seizures that do not always respond sufficiently to benzodiazepine (via rectal and/or intranasal administration).[4] A small open-label study found that the addition of rectal levetiracetam to standard treatment (rectal/IV diazepam and IV phenobarbital) significantly increased response rate for dogs with cluster seizures compared to the standard treatment alone.[6] In addition, in a study, IV levetiracetam was used successfully to treat refractory seizures in a dog that ingested a lethal dose of fluorouracil (5-FU).[7] In one case report, levetiracetam was successfully used to manage a dog with paroxysmal exertion-induced dyskinesia.[8] Another study found levetiracetam to be effective for reactive seizures that were thought to be due to exogenous toxicity.[9] Levetiracetam may have reduced efficacy in dogs over time (ie, "honeymoon effect"), and there have been reports that phenobarbital can significantly affect levetiracetam pharmacokinetics in dogs.[3,10] Lack of efficacy has also been noted when levetiracetam was used as adjunct therapy in dogs with refractory epilepsy.[11]

Levetiracetam appears to be useful as add-on therapy in cats when phenobarbital does not control seizures or as sole therapy in cats that are unable to tolerate phenobarbital.[12] Studies have shown levetiracetam to be more effective than phenobarbital and well tolerated as a monotherapy agent in cats with myoclonic seizures.[13]

Pharmacokinetic data in horses suggest that levetiracetam may be efficacious when given orally.[14-16]

Pharmacology/Actions

The exact mechanism of levetiracetam's antiseizure activity is not well understood. Levetiracetam appears to affect the release of neurotransmitters in the CNS by selective binding to the presynaptic protein SV2A on synaptic vesicles, and it may selectively prevent hypersynchronization of epileptiform burst-firing and propagation of seizure activity.[17] It does not affect normal neuronal excitability.

Pharmacokinetics

In dogs, levetiracetam (immediate-release tablet or oral solution) is rapidly and almost completely absorbed after oral administration. Volume of distribution is 0.5 to 0.7 L/kg.[18-20] Protein binding is minimal, and ≈90% of a dose is renally eliminated.[21] Peak concentration (C_{max}, ≈34 µg/mL; range, 9.2 to 60 µg/mL) occurs 0.6 to 2.2 hours after a single dose of immediate-release tablets, and elimination half-life (T½) is 2.2 to 4.4 hours.[18,22,23] Concurrent phenobarbital reduces C_{max} and T½.[24-26] Repeat oral doses do not appreciably alter pharmacokinetic values.[24,26] In a study, peak concentrations occurred 40 minutes after IM administration; the drug was completely absorbed, and peak concentration was similar to IV administration.[27] SC levetiracetam (60 mg/kg, undiluted) yielded drug concentrations between 65 µg/mL and 114 µg/mL, 15 to 420 minutes after administration.[28] In fasted dogs given an extended-release tablet formulation at 30 mg/kg PO, maximum plasma drug concentration, time to reach maximum plasma concentration, disappearance half-life, and bioavailability were 27 µg/mL, 3.4 hours, 4.4 hours, and 100%, respectively. Pharmacokinetics were similar when dogs were fed, with the exception of the time to reach maximum plasma concentration, which was longer (6.6 hours), and bioavailability, which was greater (126%).[29] Data from different studies suggest that administering extended-release tablets every 12 hours should maintain therapeutic levels in dogs.[22,23,29,30] In a study in dogs, when levetiracetam solution for injection was administered rectally at 40 mg/kg, the maximum serum concentration was 36 µg/mL and time to reach maximum serum concentration was 1.5 to 1.7 hours. Presence of feces may limit absorption.[31,32] Bioequivalence of generic extended-release tablets to *Keppra XR*® has been demonstrated in dogs.[22]

In cats, oral bioavailability of immediate-release levetiracetam is ≈100%, and elimination half-life is ≈3 hours. The authors concluded that 20 mg/kg administered IV or PO every 8 hours should be adequate in most cats.[33] Similar pharmacokinetic values were reported in cats concurrently receiving phenobarbital.[12] In healthy cats receiving a single 500 mg tablet dose of extended-release levetiracetam, serum concentrations remained above 5 µg/mL for 21 hours, with an average peak concentration of ≈90 µg/mL.[34] CSF concentrations appear to parallel serum concentrations, suggesting adequate CSF concentrations are attained after oral administration in cats.[35] With daily administration of extended-release levetiracetam tablets for 7 days, median peak and trough serum concentrations were 92.3 µg/mL and 7 µg/mL, respectively. In a small pilot study, a compounded liposomal levetiracetam cream was administered to the inner pinna at 60 mg/kg every 8 hours for 6 days, which resulted in serum concentrations above 5 µg/mL.[36]

In 1- to 10-day-old foals receiving levetiracetam (32 mg/kg PO and IV as single doses), oral absorption was ≈100%. Peak concentration (38.3 µg/mL) occurred after 0.9 hours, and elimination half-life was 7.8 hours.[15] In adult horses, terminal half-life and volume of distribution at steady-state after IV administration of levetiracetam at 20 mg/kg were 6.22 hours and 630 mL/kg, respectively. When immediate-release and extended-release tablets were crushed and administered orally at 30 mg/kg, maximum plasma concentration, terminal half-life, bioavailability, clearance/bioavailability, and time to peak concentration were 50.72 µg/mL and 53.58 µg/mL, 6.38 hours and 7.07 hours, 96% and 98%, 76.8 mL/kg/hour and 76.8 mL/kg/hour, and 0.66 hours and 0.64 hours, respectively.[14,37] No difference was found between these formulations; however, the extended-release tablets were crushed, which may have affected its pharmacokinetic profile. The authors concluded that oral administration of 30 mg/kg of either the regular or extended-release tablets in healthy adult horses is likely to achieve therapeutic concentrations for at least 12 hours.[14] In another study, generic immediate-release levetiracetam tablets administered to healthy adult horses resulted in equivalent pharmacokinetic parameters as branded levetiracetam.[38] Healthy adult horses receiving levetiracetam 30 mg/kg PO every 12 hours achieved trough levetiracetam CSF and serum concentrations of 33.7 µg/mL and 28.8 µg/mL, respectively, after 4 days.[16]

In humans, levetiracetam is rapidly and nearly completely absorbed after oral administration. Peak levels occur ≈60 minutes after administration. The presence of food in the gut delays the rate but not the extent of drug absorbed, and the drug can be administered regardless of feeding status. Less than 10% of the drug is bound to plasma proteins. Although not extensively metabolized, the drug's acetamide group is enzymatically hydrolyzed to the carboxylic acid metabolite that is apparently not active. Hepatic CYP450 isoenzymes are not involved. In humans, half-life is ≈7 hours and ≈66% of a given dose is excreted unchanged via renal mechanisms, primarily glomerular filtration and active tubular secretion. Clearance can be significantly reduced in patients with impaired renal function.

Contraindications/Precautions/Warnings

Levetiracetam is contraindicated in patients that have previously exhibited hypersensitivity to it or any of its components. Respiratory failure and cardiac arrest were reported in a dog with cluster seizures that received an undiluted levetiracetam injection of 60 mg/kg IV.[39]

Levetiracetam should be used with caution in patients with renal impairment; changes in dose or frequency should be considered. One small retrospective study found that dogs with chronic kidney disease (CKD) had a higher incidence of adverse effects from levetiracetam than dogs without CKD.[40] In humans, renal elimination of levetiracetam correlates with creatinine clearance; total clearance is reduced by 40% in patients with mild renal impairment and up to 60% in patients with severe renal impairment.[17,41]

Anecdotally, it has been reported that extended-release tablets may not fully disintegrate in the canine GI tract. Some neurologists have had experience with this situation and found that these patients still had levetiracetam concentrations within the therapeutic range. The presumption amongst many neurologists is that what is found in the stool is the matrix of the pill and that the medication is still being absorbed.[42]

Discontinuation should be done gradually to decrease risk for withdrawal seizures.

LevETIRAcetam should not be confused with levOCARNitine or levOFLOXacin. Do not confuse immediate-release tablets with extended-release tablets; use caution when prescribing or dispensing. Immediate-release prescriptions can be written as "levetiracetam" or "levetiracetam IR" (immediate-release). "Levetiracetam ER" or "Levetiracetam XR" refers to extended-release tablets.

Adverse Effects

Levetiracetam appears to be well tolerated in dogs and cats. The most common adverse effects reported include sedation and ataxia in dogs and reduced appetite, ataxia, hypersalivation, and lethargy in cats. These effects may be transient. Changes in behavior and GI effects (eg, vomiting) can occur.[43] Transient head-lowering has been observed in horses.[14]

In a study, IM administration produced less muscle inflammation in dogs than the saline control solution.[27] In another study, SC administration of undiluted levetiracetam solution for injection was well-tolerated, but the sample size was small (n = 4 healthy dogs).[28]

A systematic review and meta-analysis of adverse effects of antiepileptic drugs in dogs showed a strong level of evidence for levetiracetam's safety profile as monotherapy and adjunct therapy. Only type I adverse effects (ie, dose-dependent, predictable) were reported and these included vomiting and sedation, followed by ataxia and hyperactivity. Less common adverse effects included anorexia, polyphagia, and polydipsia, followed by polyuria, diarrhea, aggression, disobedience, and attention-seeking.[44]

In humans, adverse effects include sedation, asthenia, anxiety, and headache. Neuropsychiatric adverse effects (eg, aggression, agitation, irritability, depression) have also been reported. It is recommended to withdraw the drug slowly to prevent withdrawal seizures.

Reproductive/Nursing Safety

In pregnant dogs or cats, levetiracetam should be used with caution. At high dosages, levetiracetam has caused increased embryofetal mortality in rabbits and rats. At doses equivalent to the maximum human therapeutic dose, levetiracetam has caused minor skeletal abnormalities and retarded offspring growth in rats.[45]

Levetiracetam is excreted into maternal milk, and its safety in nursing offspring is unknown. Levetiracetam should be used with caution in nursing patients.

Because safety has not been established in animals, this drug should only be used when the maternal benefits outweigh the potential risks to offspring.

Overdose/Acute Toxicity

Levetiracetam is a relatively safe agent. Dogs receiving 1200 mg/kg/day (≈20 times the therapeutic dose) developed only salivation and vomiting.[46] Other clinical signs seen with overdose in dogs include lethargy, hyperthermia, and recumbency. Human patients receiving 6000 mg/kg during drug testing developed only drowsiness.[45] Other effects noted in human overdoses (doses not specified) after the drug was released included depressed levels of consciousness, agitation, aggression, and respiratory depression.

Treatment is supportive based on clinical signs; levetiracetam can be removed with hemodialysis.

For patients that have experienced or are suspected of having experienced an overdose, consultation with a 24-hour poison consultation center specializing in providing veterinary-specific information is recommended. For general information related to overdose and toxin exposures, as well as contact information for poison control centers, refer to ***Appendix***.

Drug Interactions

The following drug interactions have either been reported or are theoretical in humans or animals receiving levetiracetam and may be of significance in veterinary patients. Unless otherwise noted, use together is not necessarily contraindicated, but the potential risks should be weighed and additional monitoring performed when appropriate.

- **Carbamazepine**: Concurrent use may result in signs of carbamazepine toxicity (eg, nystagmus, ataxia, dizziness).
- **CNS Depressants** (eg, **antihistamines**, **benzodiazepines**, **gabapentin**, **opioids**): May increase risk for CNS depression
- **Methotrexate**: May increase methotrexate concentrations and risk for toxicity
- **Phenobarbital**: In dogs, ongoing (21 days in the study) phenobarbital use significantly increased levetiracetam clearance and reduced half-life; levetiracetam dose adjustments (increases) may be required.[24,25] Pharmacokinetic values of levetiracetam appear unchanged in cats concurrently receiving phenobarbital.[12]

Laboratory Considerations

- No specific laboratory interactions or considerations were noted.

Dosages

DOGS:

Refractory epilepsy (extra-label):

a) Using immediate-release tablets: 20 mg/kg PO every 8 hours,[10] although recommendations up to 30 mg/kg PO every 8 hours have been noted. Because of the drug's safety, doses may be increased (every 1 to 2 weeks; up to 60 mg/kg PO every 8 hours) further until efficacy is achieved, adverse effects become apparent, or drug cost becomes prohibitive. If using as an add-on to phenobarbital therapy, levetiracetam exposure is reduced and half-life may be shortened; levetiracetam dose adjustment (increase) may be necessary.[24,25,47]

b) Using extended-release tablets: Begin with 30 mg/kg PO with or without food every 12 hours. Because of the drug's safety, doses may be increased (up to 60 mg/kg PO every 12 hours) further until efficacy is achieved, adverse effects become apparent, or drug cost becomes prohibitive. Administering every 24 hours may be acceptable in some dogs. Tablets should not be split or crushed. The smallest extended-release tablet is 500 mg, so it cannot be practically administered in small dogs.[22,23,29] Higher doses may be needed if using concurrently with phenobarbital.[24]

Prevention of seizures following surgical correction of portosystemic shunt (extra-label): 20 mg/kg PO every 8 hours for a minimum of 24 hours prior to surgery may decrease the likelihood of seizures after portosystemic shunt ligation,[48] although another study found that perioperative use did not reduce postattenuation neurologic signs or seizures.[49]

Status epilepticus or acute repetitive (cluster) seizures (extra-label):

a) **IV use**: 30 mg/kg or 60 mg/kg IV were considered safe and effective in 56% of treated dogs.[4] In healthy dogs from a single-dose pharmacokinetic study, a 60 mg/kg IV bolus dose of levetiracetam was well tolerated and achieved plasma drug concentrations within or above the therapeutic range reported for humans for at least 8 hours after administration.[19] IV doses should be administered over 5 to 15 minutes.

b) **Rectal use**: 40 mg/kg rectally using a 200 mg/mL suspension compounded with levetiracetam powder and sterile water in combination with benzodiazepine and IV phenobarbital.[32] A study in healthy dogs reported that levetiracetam at 40 mg/kg (using commercial levetiracetam 100 mg/mL solution for injection) administered rectally achieved target concentrations in the target range within 10 minutes of administration.[31]

c) **Home administration as pulse therapy for cluster seizures**: 30 mg/kg PO every 8 hours until seizure-free for 24 hours[50]

d) **Home administration in dogs that do not always respond sufficiently to benzodiazepine (rectal and/or intranasal administration)**: 60 mg/kg SC; based on a pilot study in healthy dogs[28]

Reactive seizures (extra-label): From one open-label study, 60 mg/kg IV loading dose followed by maintenance dosage of 20 mg/kg PO every 8 hours until reaching a 6-month seizure-free period. Levetiracetam may then be tapered slowly and discontinued.[9]

CATS:

Epilepsy (extra-label):

a) Based on the drug's pharmacokinetics in cats and the presumed therapeutic levels for the drug, 20 mg/kg IV or PO every 8 hours. Doses up to 40 mg/kg PO every 8 hours may be necessary.[33]

b) As an add-on to phenobarbital treatment: Initially, 20 mg/kg PO every 8 hours. If ineffective, levetiracetam dose should be increased in 20 mg/kg increments.[12,51]

c) Using extended-release tablets: 500 mg/cat (NOT mg/kg) PO once daily[52]

Myoclonic seizures (extra-label): 60 – 75 mg/kg PO divided every 8 hours achieved a reduction greater than or equal to 50% in the number of myoclonic seizure days in 100% of patients.[13]

HORSES:

Anticonvulsant (extra-label): Based on pharmacokinetic studies and presumed therapeutic levels: 30 mg/kg PO every 12 hours using immediate-release tablets.[14,16] Crushing extended-release tablets has yielded similar serum concentrations (see ***Pharmacokinetics***) but may be cost-prohibitive.

Monitoring

- The levetiracetam therapeutic range for animals has not been specifically determined, but it is thought to be similar to humans at 5 – 45 µg/mL. Because the drug appears to be very safe, therapeutic drug monitoring is usually unnecessary but can be considered to establish individual patient variation in drug absorption or half-life.[53]
- Owners should be encouraged to keep a record of seizure activity (eg, seizure frequency, severity, and duration; severity and duration of any postictal signs) to document efficacy and report any potential levetiracetam-associated adverse effects.

Client Information

- This medicine may be given with or without food. If your animal vomits or acts sick after getting it on an empty stomach, give the medicine with food or small treat to see if this helps. If vomiting continues, contact your veterinarian.
- Give this medicine as directed by your veterinarian.
- Lethargy (ie, tiredness, lack of energy) and reduced appetite are the most common side effects.
- Do not crush or allow your pet to chew the extended-release tablets. The matrix of the extended-release tablets may not fully disintegrate in the GI tract and is sometimes seen in the dog's feces. However, the medication is still being absorbed.
- Do not discontinue therapy without talking with your veterinarian first as withdrawal seizures or severe neurologic side effects may result.

Chemistry/Synonyms

Levetiracetam, a pyrrolidone-derivative antiepileptic agent, occurs as an odorless, bitter-tasting, white to off-white crystalline powder. It is very soluble in water and soluble in ethanol. It is a chiral molecule with one asymmetric carbon atom. Levetiracetam is not related chemically to other antiseizure medications.

Levetiracetam may also be known as S-Etiracetam, UCB-22059, UCB-L059, and *Keppra*®.

Storage/Stability

Levetiracetam tablets and oral solution should be stored at 25°C (77°F); excursions between 15°C and 30°C (59°F-86°F) are permitted.

Compatibility/Compounding Considerations

A levetiracetam 50-mg/mL oral suspension prepared with immediate-release levetiracetam tablets crushed and suspended in *Ora-Blend*® was determined to be stable when stored at either 4°C (39.2°F) or 25°C (77°F) in plastic prescription bottles for 91 days.[54]

Extended-release tablets should be taken whole; do not split or crush tablets or allow animal to chew it. In a study, a 200 mg/mL rectal suspension was prepared by mixing levetiracetam powder with sterile water; a new suspension was prepared every month, and it was stored at room temperature and away from direct sunlight; analysis of potency and stability was not reported.[32]

Dosage Forms/Regulatory Status

VETERINARY-LABELED PRODUCTS: NONE

HUMAN-LABELED PRODUCTS:

Levetiracetam Oral Tablets (film-coated, scored): 250 mg, 500 mg, 750 mg, and 1000 mg; *Keppra*®, generic; (Rx)

Levetiracetam Extended-Release Oral Tablets (film-coated): 500 mg and 750 mg; *Keppra XR*®, generic; (Rx). Do not crush or split.

Levetiracetam Oral Solution: 100 mg/mL in 473 mL, 480 mL, and

500 mL; *Keppra*®, generic; (Rx). May also contain acesulfame K, ammonium glycyrrhizinate, or maltitol

Levetiracetam Concentrate for Injection: 100 mg/mL in 5 mL single-use vials, 5 mg/mL in 100 mL, 15 mg/mL in 100 mL, and 10 mg/mL in 100 mL; *Keppra*®, generic; (Rx)

References

For the complete list of references, see **wiley.com/go/budde/plumb**

Levothyroxine

(lee-voe-thye-***rox***-een)

Thyro-Tabs® Canine, Leventa®, Synthroid®

Thyroid Hormone

Prescriber Highlights

- ▶ Used for the treatment of hypothyroidism in all species
- ▶ Contraindications include thyrotoxicosis and untreated adrenal insufficiency.
- ▶ Use with caution in geriatric animals and those with concurrent hypoadrenocorticism (treated), cardiac disease, and diabetes mellitus.
- ▶ Adverse effects are associated with iatrogenic hyperthyroidism (eg, tachycardia, polyphagia, polyuria/polydipsia, excitability, nervousness, and excessive panting); some cats may appear apathetic.
- ▶ Review drug–drug and drug–laboratory interactions prior to prescribing.
- ▶ Should not be confused with liothyronine or desiccated thyroid

Uses/Indications

Levothyroxine is indicated for the treatment of hypothyroidism in all species. In horses, it has been used as an adjunct therapy to treat equine metabolic syndrome (EMS).[1]

Pharmacology/Actions

Levothyroxine is a synthetic form of thyroxine (T_4), which is the principal hormone released by the thyroid. Levothyroxine is mainly converted (deiodinated) to triiodothyronine (T_3) peripherally in the human body. In humans, T_3 is the primary hormone responsible for activity. Approximately 80% of T_3 found in the peripheral tissues is derived from T_4.

Thyroid hormones affect the rate of many physiologic processes, including increasing fat, protein, and carbohydrate metabolism, protein synthesis, gluconeogenesis, cellular metabolism, oxygen consumption, body temperature, heart rate and cardiac output, blood volume, enzyme system activity, and growth and maturity. Thyroid hormones also promote mobilization and utilization of glycogen stores. The thyroid hormone is particularly important for adequate development of the CNS. Although the exact mechanisms of how thyroid hormones exert their effects are not fully understood, it is known that thyroid hormones (primarily triiodothyronine) act at the cellular level by controlling DNA transcription and protein synthesis.

Pharmacokinetics

In dogs, orally administered levothyroxine has relatively low bioavailability (ie, 10% to 20%) and short elimination half-life as compared with humans. Peak serum concentrations reportedly occur 4 to 6 hours after oral administration and the serum half-life is ≈10 to 14 hours. However, there can be wide interpatient variability in pharmacokinetic parameters. Elimination in the feces may account for 50% of a dose.

An oral liquid formulated for dogs (*Leventa*®, not approved in the United States) appears to be better absorbed than tablet formulations. When comparing oral tablets given at 200 µg twice daily with oral liquid given at 200 µg once daily, the relative bioavailability of the liquid was 206% (median) that of the tablets.[2]

Studies in dogs have shown that levothyroxine absorption is affected by delivery with food; administration with food causes less medication to be absorbed and delays time to full absorption.[2] Because absorption of levothyroxine is affected by food at different rates and the levothyroxine dose is titrated individually to each animal, it is important that owners give this medication to their animal at the same time each day, in a consistent manner relative to food, and that the same method of delivery is used each time.

Contraindications/Precautions/Warnings

Levothyroxine (and other replacement thyroid hormones) are contraindicated in animals with thyrotoxicosis or untreated adrenal insufficiency. It should be used with caution, and at a lower initial dosage, in animals with concurrent hypoadrenocorticism (treated), cardiac disease, diabetes mellitus, or in senior animals. For these animals, the recommendation for reduction in the initial levothyroxine dose varies and ranges from 25% to 75% of the usual dose. Because levothyroxine can cause an increased basal metabolic rate that may exacerbate electrolyte disturbances, dogs with hypoadrenocorticism should receive replacement mineralocorticoid and glucocorticoid therapy before receiving levothyroxine.

Do not confuse levothyroxine with liothyronine or desiccated thyroid.

Adverse Effects

The most commonly reported adverse effects include anorexia, dermatitis, vomiting, otitis externa, lethargy, polydipsia, diarrhea, leukocytosis, pruritus, tachypnea, polyuria, hyperactivity, and seborrhea.[3] Case reports of rare incidences of fixed drug eruptions and erythema multiforme have been reported in dogs treated with levothyroxine.

Hypersensitivity to 2 inactive ingredients, magnesium stearate and polyvinylpyrrolidone, found in certain levothyroxine products has been observed in dogs. Reactions include cutaneous reactions that resolve after medication has been discontinued. Dogs that experienced this reaction were then treated with levothyroxine products that did not contain magnesium stearate or polyvinylpyrrolidone and tolerated the medication well.[4]

Reproductive/Nursing Safety

Levothyroxine is considered safe for use during pregnancy, as thyroid hormone is essential for fetal development.[5] In humans, levothyroxine is considered the drug of choice for hypothyroidism during pregnancy.

Levothyroxine requirements may increase during pregnancy. In humans, increasing levothyroxine dose on confirmation of pregnancy is recommended.[6] In hypothyroid bitches, one small study found that standard levothyroxine supplementation was adequate to maintain a euthyroid state during pregnancy[7]; however, thyroid status should be monitored regularly throughout pregnancy and in the postparturient period.

Minimal amounts of thyroid hormones are excreted in milk and should not affect nursing offspring. The World Health Organization (WHO) considers levothyroxine to be compatible with breastfeeding.[8]

Overdose/Acute Toxicity

Long-term overdoses produce signs of hyperthyroidism, including tachycardia, polyphagia, chronic vomiting and diarrhea, weight loss, polyuria/polydipsia, excitability, nervousness, and excessive panting. The dose should be reduced and/or temporarily withheld until signs subside. Some cats (≈10%) may exhibit signs of apathy (eg, listlessness, anorexia).[9] Toxicosis occurred in a dog that routinely consumed the feces of a housemate receiving levothyroxine.

A single, acute overdose in small animals is less likely to cause severe thyrotoxicosis as compared with long-term overdoses. Vomiting, diarrhea, hyperactivity to lethargy, hypertension, tachycardia, tachypnea, dyspnea, and abnormal pupillary light reflexes may be noted in dogs and cats 1 to 9 hours after ingestion. If ingestion occurred within 2 hours, treatment to reduce absorption of the drug should be accomplished using standard protocols (eg, emetics, cathartics, charcoal) unless contraindicated by the animal's condition. Treatment is supportive based on clinical signs. Oxygen, artificial ventilation, cardiac glycosides, beta-blockers (eg, propranolol), fluids, dextrose, and antipyretic agents have all been suggested if necessary. One case of a healthy dog that ingested up to 10 g/kg was managed with gut decontamination, and the dog had normal T_3 concentrations 6 days postingestion and normal T_4 concentrations after 36 days.[10]

For patients that have experienced or are suspected to have experienced an overdose, consultation with a 24-hour poison consultation center specializing in providing veterinary-specific information is recommended. For general information related to overdose and toxin exposures, as well as contact information for poison control centers, refer to ***Appendix.***

Drug Interactions

The following drug interactions have either been reported or are theoretical in humans or animals receiving levothyroxine and may be of significance in veterinary patients. Unless otherwise noted, use together is not necessarily contraindicated, but the potential risks must be weighed and additional monitoring performed when appropriate.

- AMIODARONE: May decrease the metabolism of T_4 to T_3
- ANTACIDS, ORAL (eg, **aluminum, calcium,** or **magnesium salts**): May reduce levothyroxine absorption; doses should be separated by 4 hours
- ANTIDIABETIC AGENTS (eg, **insulin, oral agents**): Levothyroxine may increase requirements for insulin or oral agents.
- ANTITHYROID AGENTS (eg, **carbimazole, methimazole**): Decreased conversion of T_4 to T_3
- CHOLESTYRAMINE: May reduce levothyroxine absorption; doses should be separated by 4 hours
- CORTICOSTEROIDS, HIGH-DOSE (eg, **dexamethasone, fludrocortisone, prednis(ol)one**): Decreased conversion of T_4 to T_3
- DIGOXIN: Potential for reduced digoxin concentrations and/or therapeutic response
- ESTRIOL: May decrease serum free thyroxine concentration
- FERROUS SULFATE: May reduce levothyroxine absorption; doses should be separated by 4 hours
- FIBER SUPPLEMENTS (eg, **psyllium**), HIGH FIBER DIET: May reduce levothyroxine absorption
- KETAMINE: May cause tachycardia and hypertension
- LANTHANUM: May reduce levothyroxine absorption; doses should be separated by 4 hours
- PHENOBARBITAL: Possible increased metabolism of thyroxine; dosage adjustments may be needed
- PROTON PUMP INHIBITORS (PPIs; eg, **omeprazole, pantoprazole**): Reduced gastric acid may reduce levothyroxine absorption.
- RIFAMPIN: Possible increased clearance of thyroxine; dosage adjustments may be needed.
- SERTRALINE: May increase levothyroxine requirements; likely applies to other SSRIs
- SEVELAMER: May reduce levothyroxine absorption; doses should be separated by 4 hours
- SODIUM POLYSTYRENE SULFONATE: May reduce levothyroxine absorption; doses should be separated by 4 hours
- SUCRALFATE: May reduce levothyroxine absorption; doses should be separated by 4 hours
- SYMPATHOMIMETICS (eg, **epinephrine, norepinephrine**): Levothyroxine can potentiate effects.
- THEOPHYLLINE, AMINOPHYLLINE: Levothyroxine may decrease theophylline concentration.
- TRICYCLIC ANTIDEPRESSANTS (eg, **amitriptyline, clomipramine**): Increased risk for CNS stimulation and cardiac arrhythmias
- WARFARIN: Thyroid hormones increase the catabolism of vitamin K-dependent clotting factors that may increase the anticoagulation effects in animals on warfarin.

Laboratory Considerations

- **Renal function tests**: Hypothyroid dogs can have a decreased glomerular filtration rate (GFR); restoration to a euthyroid state can increase GFR and reduce serum creatinine concentrations.

The following drugs may have effects on thyroid function tests; results should be evaluated accordingly.

- **Effects on serum total T_4 (TT_4)**: *Decreases* may be caused by aminoglutethimide, anabolic steroids/androgens, antithyroid drugs (eg, propylthiouracil [PTU], carbimazole, methimazole), asparaginase, barbiturates, corticosteroids, danazol, diazepam, heparin, methadone, mitotane, nitroprusside, phenylbutazone, phenytoin, salicylates (large doses), sulfonamides, and sulfonylureas; *increases* may be caused by estrogens (**NOTE**: Estrogens may have no effect on canine T_3 or T_4 concentrations), fluorouracil, insulin, and propranolol.
- **Effects on serum total T_3**: *Decreases* may be caused by antithyroid drugs (eg, PTU, carbimazole, methimazole), barbiturates, corticosteroids, heparin, propranolol, salicylates (large doses), and sulfonamides; *increases* may be caused by estrogens, fluorouracil, and thiazides.
- **Effects on T_3 uptake resin**: *Decreases* may be caused by antithyroid drugs (eg, PTU, carbimazole, methimazole), estrogens, and fluorouracil; *increases* may be caused by anabolic steroids/androgens, asparaginase, corticosteroids, danazol, heparin, phenylbutazone, and salicylates (large doses).
- **Effects on serum TSH**: *Decreases* may be caused by corticosteroids, danazol; *increases* may be caused by aminoglutethimide, antithyroid drugs (eg, PTU, carbimazole, methimazole), sulfonamides, and toceranib.[11]
- **Effects on serum free T_4**: *Decreases* may be caused by antithyroid drugs (eg, PTU, methimazole), barbiturates, corticosteroids, and NSAIDs; *increases* may be caused by furosemide and heparin.

Dosages

DOGS:

Hypothyroidism:

Oral therapy:

a) **Replacement therapy for diminished thyroid function** (label dosage; FDA-approved): The initial recommended daily dose is 0.022 mg/kg (22 µg/kg) PO in single or divided doses. The dosage is then adjusted by monitoring serum TT_4 concentrations 4 to 6 hours after a dose is given, every 4 to 8 weeks until an adequate maintenance dose is established. In field studies, the majority of dogs required at least one dosage adjustment, and most dogs were maintained on an oral dosage of 0.018 – 0.026 mg/kg/day (18 – 26 µg/kg/day). Administer consistently, with or without food.[3]

b) <u>Oral tablets</u> (extra-label): **NOTE**: Initial dosages vary. There is inadequate published evidence or general consensus supporting one recommendation over another. Initial dosages of 0.01 – 0.02 mg/kg (10 – 20 µg/kg) PO every 12 to 24 hours are typical. A maximum initial dosage of 0.8 mg/dog (NOT mg/kg) every 12 hours is often recommended. Lower doses (eg, 25% reduction) are recommended in dogs with certain concurrent conditions (see ***Contraindications/Precautions/***

Warnings). Average maintenance dosage was ≈0.017 mg/kg (≈17 μg/kg) PO every 12 or 24 hours.[12] If it is not possible to give on an empty stomach, give with consistent timing with regard to food intake.

c) Oral solution (extra-label): 0.02 mg/kg (20 μg/kg) PO every 24 hours resulted in euthyroid status in ≈80% to 90% of dogs[13,14]

Myxedema crisis (extra-label): 0.001 – 0.009 mg/kg (1 – 9 μg/kg) IV[15]; median dosage was 0.005 mg/kg (5 μg/kg) IV every 12 hours. **NOTE**: In humans, it is recommended to administer doses no faster than 0.1 mg/minute (100 μg/minute) during crises. Consider giving a lower dose in dogs with underlying heart disease or heart failure. If administration of parenteral levothyroxine is not possible, can attempt to give oral solution or crushed/slurried tablets via nasoesophageal or orogastric tube. Begin PO therapy after the animal is stabilized and can swallow.[16,17]

CATS:

Hypothyroidism (extra-label): 0.05 – 0.15 mg/cat (50 – 150 μg/cat; NOT mg/kg or μg/kg) PO once daily.[18,19] The dosage is then adjusted in 50% increments based on serum TT_4 and TSH concentrations every 4 to 8 weeks until an adequate maintenance dose is established.

Post-antithyroid medication, thyroidectomy, or radioiodine treatment (extra-label): Cats with hyperthyroidism and chronic kidney disease (IRIS stages 2 and 3) treated with radioiodine that received levothyroxine 0.1 mg/cat (100 μg/cat; NOT mg/kg or μg/kg) PO once daily had significantly lower increases in serum creatinine and BUN over the next 12 months than nontreated cats.[20]

HORSES:

Correction of conditions associated with low circulating thyroid hormone | Hypothyroidism (label dosage; NOT FDA-approved):

a) 0.01– 0.06 mg/kg (10 – 60 μg/kg) PO once daily or divided[21]; adjust dosage to maintain thyroid hormone concentrations in the normal range

b) 0.02 mg/kg (20 μg/kg) PO once daily has been recommended as a starting dose, but 0.05 – 0.1 mg/kg (50 – 100 μg/kg) PO once daily may be well tolerated.[22] Horses were administered levothyroxine in a small meal of grain, which may have affected absorption. Dose may vary based on whether the drug is given to fasted horses or whether it is fed with a meal. Adjust dosage to maintain thyroid hormone concentrations in the normal range.

Adjunctive treatment for equine metabolic syndrome (EMS) (extra-label): High doses of levothyroxine can be administered to induce weight loss in horses with EMS. Recommended dosage is 0.1 mg/kg (100 μg/kg) PO once daily for 3 to 6 months.[23] In horses that weigh 450 to 525 kg (992 to 1157 lb), it is recommended that the dose be rounded to 48 mg/horse/day (NOT mg/kg). A further increase in dose by 50% (to 0.15 mg/kg [150 μg/kg]) may be contemplated if there has been negligible impact on body condition after 3 months. When target body condition has been achieved, the dose is decreased to 0.05 mg/kg (50 μg/kg) for 2 weeks and then 0.025 mg/kg (25 μg/kg) for an additional 2 weeks before withdrawal to allow restoration of the suppressed thyroid axis. This therapy is used in combination with daily calorie restrictions and exercise. Levothyroxine has been shown to cause hyperphagia in horses, so open pasture grazing should be avoided.[23,24]

BIRDS:

Hypothyroidism (extra-label): One 0.1 mg (100 μg) tablet in 30 – 120 mL of water daily; stir water and offer for 15 minutes and remove. Use high dose for budgerigars and low dose for water drinkers.[25]

REPTILES:

Hypothyroidism in tortoises (extra-label): 0.02 mg/kg (20 μg/kg) PO every other day[26]

Monitoring

Levothyroxine monitoring in dogs varies but is generally done 1 to 2 months after initiation of therapy or dose changes, or as needed based on clinical signs. Dose adjustments should be based on both clinical response and thyroid concentrations. Once a therapeutic dose is established, consider monitoring 1 to 2 times per year. The following are general recommendations:

- **Clinical response**: The goal of therapy is to have resolution of clinical signs caused by hypothyroidism. Improvement in activity should be evident within the first 1 to 2 weeks of treatment; weight loss should be evident within 8 weeks. Achievement of a normal hair coat may take several months, and the coat may initially appear worse as telogen hairs are shed. Neurologic deficits improve rapidly after treatment, but complete resolution may take 8 to 12 weeks.[18]
- **Serum TT_4**: A minimum of 6 to 8 weeks should pass after starting therapy or changing the dosage before measuring TT_4. Peak serum TT_4 should be measured 4 to 6 hours after dose administration and should be within the upper half of the reference range.[18] Concentrations slightly above reference range are acceptable in the absence of adverse effects; concentrations slightly below reference range are acceptable if clinical response is adequate and serum TSH is within reference range.
- **Serum TSH**: May be useful if TSH was abnormal prior to therapy, or if TT_4 concentrations are out of range. Concentrations are not dependent on the timing of sampling relative to the timing of dose administration.[18]
- **Medication regimen**: If concentrations are unexpectedly out of range, consider asking owner about administration patterns (eg, missed doses), if the brand of levothyroxine was changed, whether new medications were started or previous medications were stopped, and/or levothyroxine expiration date.

Client Information

- Dogs require a higher dose of thyroid hormone than humans. Cats may require a similar dose as an adult human.
- Side effects most often occur when too much of the medicine is given. Dogs may have a fast or racing heart rate; vomiting; diarrhea; increased appetite, thirst, and urination; excitability/nervousness; and panting. Cats may appear withdrawn or apathetic (uncaring).
- This medicine should ideally be given without food and must always be given the same way. It is important to follow your veterinarian's directions.
- The animal should have improved activity within the first 1 to 2 weeks of treatment. Weight loss should start to occur within 8 weeks of starting therapy. The hair coat may initially appear worse but should be normal in several months. Neurologic signs improve rapidly after treatment, but complete resolution may take 8 to 12 weeks.
- Your veterinarian will need to monitor your animal closely while it is taking this medicine. Do not miss these important follow-up visits.

Chemistry/Synonyms

Levothyroxine sodium is prepared synthetically for commercial use and is the levo isomer of thyroxine that is the primary secretion of the thyroid gland. It occurs as an odorless, light yellow to buff-colored, tasteless, hygroscopic powder that is very slightly soluble in water and slightly soluble in alcohol. The commercially available powders for injection also contain mannitol.

100 μg of levothyroxine is approximately equivalent to 65 mg (1 grain) of desiccated thyroid.

Levothyroxine sodium may also be known as T_4, T_4 thyroxine sodium, levothyroxin natrium, levothyroxinum natricum, 3,5,3',5'-tetra-iodo-L-thyronine sodium, thyroxine sodium, L-thyroxine sodium, thyroxinum natricum, tirossina, and tiroxina sodica. Many trade names are available in other countries, and had been available in the United States until 2016, when some products were removed from the market after the FDA issued warning letters to manufacturers of unapproved products, including *Thyforon®*, *Thyrosyn®*, *Soloxine®*, *Levocrine®*, *Thyromed®*, *Thyroid Chewable Tablets®*, *Thyrokare®*, *Thyroxine L®*, *Leventa®*, *Thyrozine®*, *Nutrived®*, *Levoxine®*, *Thyro-Tabs® Canine*, and *Thyro-L®*.

Storage/Stability

Levothyroxine is unstable when exposed to light, heat, and moisture. Levothyroxine sodium tablets should be stored in tight containers protected from light and moisture at a controlled room temperature of 20°C to 25°C (68°F-77°F), with excursions allowed between 15°C to 30°C (59°F-86°F). The injectable product should be stored protected from light at 20°C to 25°C (68°F-77°F) and reconstituted immediately before use; unused injection should be discarded after reconstituting. Stored levothyroxine oral solutions (not available in the United States) should be refrigerated (2°C-8°C [36°F-46°F]); unused solution should be discarded 6 months after first opening.

Levothyroxine sodium is reportedly unstable in aqueous solutions. If using a commercial liquid preparation, it is suggested to obtain validated stability data for the product.

Compatibility/Compounding Considerations

Levothyroxine sodium injection should **NOT** be mixed with other drugs or IV fluids.

Dosage Forms/Regulatory Status

VETERINARY-LABELED PRODUCTS:

Levothyroxine Sodium Tablets, USP: 0.1 mg, 0.2 mg, 0.3 mg, 0.4 mg, 0.5 mg, 0.6 mg, 0.7 mg, 0.8 mg, and 1 mg; *Thyro-Tabs Canine®*; (Rx). Approved for use in dogs. NADA# 141-448. Unapproved products were removed from the market subsequent to January 2016 FDA warning letter.

Levothyroxine Sodium Powder (Veterinary): 0.22% (1 g of T_4 in 454 g of powder): One level teaspoonful contains 12 mg of T_4. Available in 0.45 kg (1 lb) and 4.5 kg (10 lb) containers; many trade name products may be available and include *Thyrozine Powder®*, *Levoxine® Powder*; *Thyro-L®*, *Thyrosyn Powder®*, *Thyrokare® Powder*; (Rx). Labeled for use in horses. **NOTE**: These products are not FDA-approved.

Levothyroxine Sodium Oral Solution (not available in the United States) 1 mg/mL (1000 µg/mL) in 30 mL bottles; *Leventa®*; (POM-V). Contains ≈50% ethanol.

HUMAN-LABELED PRODUCTS:

Levothyroxine Sodium Tablets: 0.025 mg (25 µg), 0.05 mg (50 µg), 0.075 mg (75 µg), 0.088 mg (88 µg), 0.1 mg (100 µg), 0.112 mg (112 µg), 0.125 mg (125 µg), 0.137 mg (137 µg), 0.15 mg (150 µg), 0.175 mg (175 µg), 0.2 mg (200 µg), and 0.3 mg (300 µg); *Synthroid®*, *Levoxyl®*, *Levothroid®*, *Unithroid®*, generic; (Rx)

Levothyroxine Sodium Liquid-filled Oral Capsules: 0.013 mg (13 µg), 0.025 mg (25 µg), 0.05 mg (50 µg), 0.075 mg (75 µg), 0.088 mg (88 µg), 0.1 mg (100 µg), 0.112 mg (112 µg), 0.125 mg (125 µg), 0.137 mg (137 µg), 0.15 mg (150 µg), and 0.2 mg (200 µg); *Tirosint®*, generic; (Rx)

Levothyroxine Sodium Oral Solution (per mL): 0.013 mg (13 µg), 0.025 mg (25 µg), 0.0375 mg (37.5 µg), 0.044 mg (44 µg), 0.05 mg (50 µg), 0.0625 mg (62.5 µg), 0.075 mg (75 µg), 0.088 mg (88 µg), 0.1 mg (100 µg), 0.112 mg (112 µg), 0.125 mg (125 µg), 0.137 mg (137 µg), and 0.15 mg (150 µg), 0.175 mg (175 µg) and 0.2 mg (200 µg) in 1 mL ampules; *Tirosint®-Sol*; (Rx)

Levothyroxine Sodium Oral Solution: 20 µg/mL in 100 mL bottles; *Thyquidity®*; (Rx)

Levothyroxine Powder for Injection lyophilized: 0.1 mg (100 µg), 0.2 mg (200 µg), and 0.5 mg (500 µg) in 5 mL vials; generic; (Rx)

Levothyroxine Solution for Injection: 20 µg/mL, 40 µg/mL, 100 µg/mL in 5 mL vials; generic; (Rx)

Levothyroxine tablet combinations with liothyronine (T_3) are also available.

References

For the complete list of references, see **wiley.com/go/budde/plumb**

Lidocaine, Local Anesthetic

Lignocaine

(***lye***-doe-kane) *Xylocaine®*

Local Anesthetic

This monograph discusses the use of lidocaine for local anesthesia only. For information regarding lidocaine's use as an antiarrhythmic, systemic analgesic, and prokinetic, please refer to ***Lidocaine, Systemic****.*

Prescriber Highlights

- Local anesthetic with a quick onset (5 minutes) and short duration of action (1 hour)
- Indicated for infiltration, nerve block, and epidural anesthesia in dogs, cats, cattle, and horses
- Local anesthetics are absorbed from the site of administration; significant systemic absorption or unintended systemic administration can lead to severe CNS and cardiac adverse effects, including death.
- Cats appear to be more sensitive to the adverse effects of lidocaine.
- Adverse effects are unlikely when the correct administration technique is used. Clinicians should be knowledgeable in the diagnosis and management of local anesthetic toxicity, and resources for treating acute emergencies must be readily available.

Uses/Indications

Lidocaine is indicated for epidural, nerve block, and infiltration anesthesia in dogs, cats, cattle, and horses. It is also used IV for systemic analgesia and to treat ventricular arrhythmias (see ***Lidocaine, Systemic***). Local analgesia can have a MAC-sparing effect on inhalant anesthesia and leads to better postoperative recovery.[1-6]

Topical application of lidocaine to the mucosa of the laryngeal cartilages of dogs and cats reduces cough response on intubation[7-9]; it is likely that this use is also applicable to other species. Fentanyl IV also reduces coughing in dogs,[10] and lidocaine may not be needed when fentanyl is included in the anesthetic plan in this species.

Topical application of ophthalmic lidocaine formulations to the eye reduces corneal sensitivity in dogs and horses.[11,12]

Some clinicians prefer a combination of lidocaine (faster onset) and bupivacaine (longer duration) but studies in a variety of species suggest the onset of effect is similar to that of either lidocaine or bupivacaine alone[13-16] and the duration of analgesia is shorter than bupivacaine alone (but longer than lidocaine alone).[13,15,17-20] To achieve a faster onset but longer duration nerve block, use only lidocaine prior to the procedure and repeat the block at the end of the procedure using only bupivacaine.

An extensive description of the most common local blocks and epidural/spinal injection in small animals can be found in other reference texts.[21-24]

Pharmacology/Actions

Local anesthetics block sodium ion channels on the nerve cell membrane, thereby altering electrical excitability, depolarization, and action potential propagation. They block the generation and conduction of impulses in motor, sensory, and autonomic nerve fibers around the site of application. Nerve fiber diameter, conduction velocity, and myelination determine loss of nerve function. Clinically, the progressive loss of nerve function occurs in the following order: pain, temperature, touch, proprioception, and skeletal muscle tone. Anesthetic effect is lost in reverse order.

Lidocaine as a sole agent (without adjuvants) produces local anesthesia typically within 3 to 5 minutes after administration and persists for ≈1 hour. Compared to bupivacaine, lidocaine has a faster onset and shorter duration of action.

Pharmacokinetics

Local anesthetics are absorbed from their site of administration into the systemic circulation. The rate and extent of systemic absorption increases with the dose and volume given,[25] repeated administration, administration in the head and neck region, and administration into highly vascularized sites.

In dogs receiving lidocaine 5 – 10 mg/kg administered intra-articularly, peak serum concentrations of 0.5 to 3 µg/mL occurred after 30 minutes. Elimination half-life was ≈73 minutes.[26] In a separate study by the same authors with similar methodology, addition of epinephrine 10 µg/mL solution to lidocaine 2%, a lower peak concentration occurred after 70 minutes, with an elimination half-life of ≈2.6 hours.[27] Although not the same as tissue infiltration, bioavailability after IM administration to dogs was 92% and half-life was ≈1 hour.[28]

Epinephrine may be added to lidocaine formulations at a very low concentration (5 or 10 µg/mL) to cause vasoconstriction at the site of administration, thereby reducing the rate of systemic absorption. Epinephrine increases the speed of analgesia onset, prolongs the duration of action at the site of administration, and minimizes systemic lidocaine toxicity.

Sodium bicarbonate added to lidocaine injection will alkalinize the solution, which increases the non-ionized fraction of the drug. This shortens the onset and increases the duration of action of the solution.

Opioids (eg, buprenorphine) and alpha-2 adrenergic agonists (eg, dexmedetomidine) can also be added to lidocaine to enhance duration and sensory analgesia of the local block.

Refer to the ***Lidocaine, Systemic*** monograph for further pharmacokinetic information on systemic administration.

Contraindications/Precautions/Warnings

Lidocaine is contraindicated in patients with a known hypersensitivity to it or to another amide-type local anesthetic agent. Although risk is low with correct administration technique, use with caution in patients with hepatic or renal disease, atrioventricular (AV) block, or other conduction abnormalities, or impaired cardiovascular function as inadvertent systemic administration may cause adverse effects. Chondrolysis has occurred in humans receiving intra-articular infusions of local anesthetics, and intra-articular lidocaine has demonstrated chondrotoxicity in horses.[29,30]

Injections should be made aseptically, aspirating frequently and relocating the needle if blood is aspirated. Check anesthetic depth before beginning manipulations.

Cats tend to be more sensitive to the adverse effects of lidocaine if inadvertently given systemically; use with caution.

Lidocaine may be included in some IM injections to reduce pain upon administration; verify compatibility prior to mixing.

In humans, epidural use should be undertaken with extreme caution in patients with severe CNS disease.[31] Epidural injections should be administered incrementally, with aspiration prior to injection. Local anesthetics with preservatives should not be used for epidural or caudal anesthesia.

Lidocaine formulations that contain epinephrine should be used with caution, if at all, in patients with cardiovascular disease or hyperthyroidism, or for anesthesia of the digits, ears, nose, or penis. Avoid lidocaine/epinephrine when nerve integrity or collateral circulation is compromised as it causes intense vasoconstriction and diminished blood flow; ischemic injury could result.

Adverse Effects

Local anesthetics are generally well tolerated when administered correctly. The most common adverse effects reported after local administration are dose-related and mild. CNS signs include drowsiness, depression, ataxia, and muscle tremors. Nausea and vomiting may occur but are usually transient. Adverse effects are related to high plasma concentrations (greater than or equal to 6 µg/mL), which may result from the dose or lidocaine concentration used, rapid absorption from the injection site, and/or unintentional intravascular injection.

Epidural administration may cause hypotension, urinary retention, and/or ataxia; other adverse cardiac and neurologic effects are uncommon and generally only occur at high plasma lidocaine concentrations (eg, unintentional subarachnoid injection) and are usually associated with PR and QRS interval prolongation and QT interval shortening. Lidocaine may increase ventricular rates if used in patients with atrial fibrillation. Uncommon but severe reactions include seizures, coma, respiratory arrest, and even death.

Lidocaine formulations that contain epinephrine may cause tachycardia and hypertension. Addition of sodium bicarbonate to lidocaine injection reduces pain ('sting') on administration. (See ***Pharmacokinetics***)

Reproductive/Nursing Safety

Lidocaine crosses the placenta. No fetal toxicity was observed in rats receiving up to 6.6 times the labeled human dose. Maternal and fetal toxicity have occurred with lidocaine use during labor and delivery in women.[32]

Although local anesthetics are excreted in breastmilk, lidocaine is excreted in concentrations of ≈40% of that found in the serum and it is considered unlikely to pose significant risk to nursing offspring.

Because safety has not been established in animals, this drug should only be used when the maternal benefits outweigh the potential risks to offspring.

Overdose/Acute Toxicity

Toxic blood levels are most likely to occur after unintended intravascular administration. To avoid this, ALWAYS aspirate before injecting the local anesthetic. Toxic effects may occur rapidly and simultaneously. Cardiac conduction and excitability are depressed and may lead to AV block, ventricular arrhythmias, and cardiac arrest; arrhythmias may be refractory to treatment. In addition, myocardial contractility is depressed and peripheral vasodilation occurs, leading to decreased cardiac output and arterial blood pressure. CNS stimulation (eg, nystagmus, restlessness, tremors, and shivering progressing to convulsions) may precede CNS depression, coma, and respiratory arrest. Tremors occurred in dogs with a serum lidocaine concentration of 2.7 µg/mL,[33] and seizures occurred in dogs with a mean serum concentration of ≈8 to 10 µg/mL,[34] but another study provoked seizures at 47 µg/mL.[35] The mean cumulative dose that induced seizures in dogs was 21 – 22 mg/kg IV,[35,36] and the cumulative lethal dose was 80 mg/kg IV.[37] The mean convulsive dose in cats was 11.7 mg/kg IV and the mean cardiotoxic dose was 47.3 mg/kg IV.[38]

If signs of overdose are present, management must begin with delivery of oxygen via a patent airway as successful oxygen delivery may prevent convulsions caused by toxicity. Cardiovascular support should be provided and may include IV fluids and vasopressor drugs (eg, dobutamine, norepinephrine). Prolonged resuscitative efforts may be required. Lipid emulsion 20% 1.5 mL/kg IV over 30 minutes can be beneficial in lidocaine toxicity.[39,40] See ***Fat Emulsion, Intravenous***.

Drug Interactions

Drug interactions in animals receiving lidocaine as a local anesthetic are unlikely when administered correctly. The following drug interactions have either been reported or are theoretical in humans or animals receiving lidocaine (systemically) and may be of significance in veterinary patients after unintended intravascular administration. Unless otherwise noted, use together is not necessarily contraindicated, but weigh the potential risks and perform additional monitoring when appropriate.

- ALPHA-2-ADRENERGIC AGONISTS (eg, **dexmedetomidine, xylazine**): Systemic absorption of lidocaine may increase the ataxic effects of alpha 2 agonists in horses.
- ANESTHETICS, INHALANT (eg, **isoflurane, sevoflurane**): Lidocaine infusions perioperatively have been shown to reduce MAC requirements in dogs,[41] horses,[42,43] and cats.[44] In dogs and horses, this effect may be of benefit, but in cats, additive cardiodepression has been shown.[44] However, in horses, lidocaine with inhalant anesthetics can cause tremors and ataxia and affect the quality of anesthetic recovery; it has been recommended to discontinue lidocaine CRIs at least 30 minutes before the start of the recovery period.[45]
- ANTIARRHYTHMICS, OTHER (eg, **procainamide, propranolol, quinidine**): If systemically absorbed, lidocaine may cause additive or antagonistic cardiac effects and toxicity may be enhanced.
- BETA-ADRENERGIC ANTAGONISTS (eg, **atenolol, esmolol, propranolol, sotalol**): Lidocaine levels or effects may be increased.
- KETAMINE: If systemically absorbed, lidocaine may increase ataxic effects in horses.

Severe, prolonged hypertension may result when using lidocaine/epinephrine combination products with the following:

- ERGOT ALKALOIDS
- MONOAMINE OXIDASE INHIBITORS (MAOIs; eg, **amitraz, linezolid, selegiline**)
- TRICYCLIC ANTIDEPRESSANTS (eg, **amitriptyline, clomipramine**)
- VASOPRESSORS (eg, **dobutamine, norepinephrine**)

Laboratory Considerations

- Lidocaine administered intramuscularly may increase **creatine phosphokinase** levels.
- Lidocaine may falsely increase serum **creatinine**.

Dosages

NOTES:

1. Lidocaine formulation concentration, administration volume, site of administration, administration technique (eg, aspiration prior to injection), and underlying patient condition(s) are important interrelated factors that determine lidocaine's safe and effective use.
2. All dosages below use 2% lidocaine (20 mg/mL) unless otherwise specified.

DOGS:

Epidural and infiltration anesthesia (label dosage; not FDA-approved): *Epidural*: 1 mL/4.5 kg (10 lb) of body weight (4.4 mg/kg); *Infiltration*: dilute to 0.5% concentration (for each 1 mL of lidocaine 2% solution, dilute with 3 mL sterile water)

Local anesthesia | Tissue infiltration (line block): (extra-label):

a) 1 – 5 mg/kg is a generally recommended dose for local block[46]
b) 4 – 6 mg/kg. For larger areas, an equal or lower volume of 0.9% sodium chloride may be used to expand the volume.[47]

Regional anesthesia (extra-label):

a) **Regional IV anesthesia (Bier block) of the forelimb**: 3 mg/kg, using 0.5% lidocaine solution, IV in the cephalic vein provided local anesthesia for ≈20 to 30 minutes after tourniquet removal.[48] Prior to using this technique, it is encouraged to review the details of this procedure found in the citation to understand the safe use of the tourniquet and minimize potential for unintentional systemic administration with resulting adverse effects.
b) **CRI via peritoneal wound catheter**: 2 mg/kg/*hour* delivered via infusion or elastomeric pump[49]
c) **Retrobulbar and sub-Tenon injections**: Under general anesthesia, 2 mL of lidocaine 2% is administered in the retrobulbar space or under Tenon's capsule; an additional 1 mL is given if ocular akinesia is not achieved within 10 minutes. Compared to retrobulbar injection, results from sub-Tenon's administration were faster, longer, and more reliable.[50,51]

Epidural anesthesia (extra-label): **NOTE**: only use preservative-free formulations

a) Morphine 0.1 mg/kg combined with lidocaine 2% solution to bring total volume to 0.2 mL/kg[52]
b) Lidocaine 6 mg/kg. Morphine 0.1 mg/kg OR tramadol 1 mg/kg (not available in US) can be added to further reduce pain scores and prolong the duration of analgesia.[53]

Cough suppression prior to endotracheal intubation (extra-label): 0.4 mg/kg topically applied to laryngeal cartilages after induction of general anesthesia[7]

CATS:

Epidural and infiltration anesthesia (label dosage; not FDA-approved): *Epidural*: using lidocaine solution 2%, 1 mL per 4.5 kg (10 lb) of body weight (4.4 mg/kg); *Infiltration*: dilute to 0.5% concentration (each 1 mL of lidocaine 2% solution diluted with 3 mL sterile water)[54]

Local anesthesia | Tissue infiltration (line block): (extra-label): 2 – 4 mg/kg. For larger areas, an equal or lower volume of 0.9% sodium chloride may be used to expand the volume.[47]

Caudal (sacrococcygeal or coccygeal, or low) epidural anesthesia (extra-label):

a) Lidocaine 4 mg/kg administered lumbosacrally with EITHER morphine 0.1 mg/kg OR methadone 0.3 mg/kg delayed the need for rescue analgesia for up to 18 hours compared to lidocaine alone.[55]
b) Coccygeal epidural: 0.1 – 0.2 mL/kg of lidocaine 2% (without epinephrine). The needle is inserted between the first 2 coccygeal vertebrae and directed at a 30° to 45° angle.[56]

Cough suppression prior to endotracheal intubation (extra-label): 4 mg (0.2 mL of Lidocaine 2%)/cat (NOT mg/kg)[9]

HORSES:

Epidural, nerve block, and infiltration anesthesia (label dosage; not FDA-approved): *Epidural*: Lidocaine 2%, 5 – 15 mL; *Nerve block*: Lidocaine 2%, 5 – 20 mL; *Infiltration:* Dilute to 0.5% concentration (each 1 mL of lidocaine 2% solution diluted with 3 mL sterile water).

Local anesthesia, palmar nerve block (extra-label): 1.5 mL injected SC immediately palmar to the medial and lateral neurovascular bundles and immediately proximal to the collateral cartilages of the foot.[57]

Caudal (sacrococcygeal or coccygeal, or low) epidural anesthesia and analgesia (extra-label):

a) Lidocaine 0.2 mg/kg provided analgesia for ≈60 to 80 minutes.[58] Addition of neostigmine (1 µg/kg) extended analgesia to 150 minutes in a separate study.[59]
b) Caudal epidural in donkeys: Lidocaine 0.4 mg/kg administered into Co2-Co3 produced analgesia within 4 minutes and lasted 75 minutes. A dose of lidocaine 0.2 mg/kg combined

with tramadol 0.5 mg/kg (not available in US) produced analgesia within 6 minutes and lasted 180 minutes.[60]

Regional IV anesthesia (or Bier block): 1.3 mg/kg, using lidocaine 2% diluted with saline solution 0.9% to a total volume of 60 mL and administered into the cephalic vein. It provides local anesthesia until the tourniquet is removed (30 minutes).[61]

CATTLE:

Epidural, nerve block, and infiltration anesthesia (label dosage; not FDA-approved): *Epidural*: Lidocaine 2%, 5 – 15 mL; *Nerve block*: Lidocaine 2%, 5 – 20 mL; *Infiltration*: Dilute to 0.5% concentration (each 1 mL of lidocaine 2% solution diluted with 3 mL sterile water).[54]

Local anesthesia (extra-label): 3 mg/kg infiltrated subcutaneously[62]

Caudal epidural anesthesia and analgesia (extra-label): 0.22 – 0.5 mg/kg[63]

SHEEP/GOATS:

Local anesthesia (extra-label):

a) 5 mg/kg; analgesia duration ≈80 to 100 minutes[64,65]
b) Paravertebral anesthesia: Using lidocaine 2% solution, 3 mL infiltrated around each paravertebral nerve. Addition of epinephrine (5 µg/mL) extended duration of analgesia from 65 minutes to 95 minutes.[66] Refer to ***Compatibility/Compounding Considerations*** below.

Epidural anesthesia in **goats** (extra-label): 2.86 mg/kg, analgesia onset was 3 minutes, duration was 85 minutes. Ataxia occurred in all patients.[67]

CAMELIDS:

Local anesthesia (extra-label): Incisional and intratesticular block: 2 mL injected into each testicle and 2 mL SC along the prescrotal incision site (6 mL total, not exceeding 4 mg/kg)[68]

Epidural anesthesia (extra-label): 0.22 mg/kg (0.01 mL/kg of 2% solution) provides analgesia for ≈70 minutes. When the same dose is combined with xylazine 0.17 mg/kg, the duration of analgesia increases to 5.5 hours.[69]

SMALL MAMMALS:

Sciatic-femoral nerve block in rabbits (extra-label): 1 mg/kg per nerve guided by nerve stimulator[70]

REPTILES:

Intrathecal anesthesia in red-eared slider turtles (extra-label): 4 mg/kg provides regional anesthesia of the tail, cloaca, and hind limbs for ≈1 hour.[71]

Monitoring

- Adequacy of analgesia and anesthesia
- Cardiovascular and respiratory function as well as state of consciousness, after each injection
- Plasma lidocaine concentrations greater than or equal to 6 µg/mL are associated with increased risk for adverse effects.

Client Information

- This medication causes temporary loss of feeling. The area where it was injected may not have usual function for several hours.
- This drug should only be used by or on the order of a licensed veterinarian familiar with its use and in a setting where adequate patient monitoring can be performed.

Chemistry/Synonyms

Lidocaine hydrochloride is an amide-class local anesthetic. It occurs as a white or almost white, odorless, slightly bitter tasting crystalline powder with a melting point between 74°C (165.2°F) and 79°C (174.2°F) and a pK_a of 7.86. It is very soluble in water and alcohol.

Lidocaine hydrochloride is also known as lignocaine hydrochloride and lidocaini hydrochloridum. Many trade names are available including *Xylocaine*® and *Lignol*®.

Storage/Stability

Lidocaine should be stored at room temperature, at 15°C to 30°C (59°F-86°F).

Lidocaine stored under field conditions for equine use was found to maintain pH and potency without microbial contamination in a variety of storage conditions and with repeated vial use over 12 months.[72]

Compatibility/Compounding Considerations

Compatibility is dependent on factors such as pH, concentration, temperature, and diluent used; consult specialized references or a hospital pharmacist for more specific information.

Lidocaine HCl is **compatible** with D_5W, lactated Ringer's, and 0.9% sodium chloride solutions, and combinations of these solutions. It is also **compatible** with the following drugs (partial list): bupivacaine, buprenorphine, butorphanol tartrate, dexamethasone sodium phosphate, epinephrine, fentanyl citrate, hydromorphone, methadone, midazolam, and morphine sulfate.

Lidocaine HCl is reported to be **variably compatible** with propofol and sodium bicarbonate. Lidocaine solutions to which sodium bicarbonate have been added (to reduce pain on infiltration) should be used immediately and promptly discarded.

The recommended final concentration of epinephrine is 5 µg/mL. To reach this concentration, add 0.1 mL of epinephrine 1 mg/mL to 20 mL of local anesthetic. Lidocaine solution to which epinephrine has been added should be used immediately and promptly discarded.

Dosage Forms/Regulatory Status

VETERINARY-LABELED PRODUCTS:

Lidocaine HCl for Injection: 2% (20 mg/mL) in 100 mL and 250 mL multiuse vials; (contains preservatives); generic; (Rx). Information regarding its use in food-producing species is conflicting; when using in a food animal, it is suggested to contact FARAD (see ***Appendix***). The ARCI (Association of Racing Commissioners International) has designated this drug as a class 2 substance. See ***Appendix*** for more information. Use of this drug may not be allowed in certain animal competitions. Check rules and regulations before entering in a competition while this medication is being administered. Contact local racing authorities for further guidance.

HUMAN-LABELED PRODUCTS:

Lidocaine HCl injection: 0.5%, 1%, 1.5%, 2%, and 4% in 5 mL, 10 mL, 20 mL, 30 mL, and 50 mL single- and multidose vials, 2 mL and 5 mL amps, 5 mL syringes and cartridges; *Xylocaine*® and *Xylocaine mpf*®, generic; (Rx)

Lidocaine HCl with Epinephrine Injection: All are (Rx).

Lidocaine 0.5% with Epinephrine 5 µg/mL in 50 mL multidose vials

Lidocaine 1% with Epinephrine 5 µg/mL in 10 mL and 30 mL single-dose vials

Lidocaine 1% with Epinephrine 10 µg/mL in 20 mL, 30 mL, and 50 mL multidose vials

Lidocaine 1.5% with Epinephrine 5 µg/mL in 5 mL, 10 mL, and 30 mL single-dose vials

Lidocaine 2% with Epinephrine 5 µg/mL in 10 mL and 20 mL single-dose vials

Lidocaine 2% with Epinephrine 10 µg/mL in 20 mL, 30 mL, and 50 mL multidose vials

Topical liquids, patches, ointment, cream, lotion, gel, spray, and jelly are also available.

References

For the complete list of references, see **wiley.com/go/budde/plumb**

Lidocaine (Intravenous; Systemic)

Lignocaine

(**lye**-doe-kane) *Xylocaine®*

Antiarrhythmic, Analgesic, Prokinetic

For other uses of lidocaine, see ***Lidocaine, Local Anesthetic***; ***Lidocaine, Ophthalmic***; ***Lidocaine, Topical***

Prescriber Highlights

- Local anesthetic and antiarrhythmic (ventricular tachyarrhythmias) agent; may be useful as an IV anesthetic/analgesic adjunct
- Contraindications include known hypersensitivity to the amide-class local anesthetics; severe degree of SA, AV, or intraventricular heart block (if not being artificially paced); or Adams-Stokes syndrome.
- Use with caution in cats as they appear to be more sensitive to the cardiodepressant and CNS effects of lidocaine; many clinicians avoid anesthetic use of lidocaine IV in cats. Use with caution in patients with liver disease, congestive heart failure, shock, hypovolemia, severe respiratory depression, marked hypoxia, bradycardia, or incomplete heart block with PVCs, unless the heart rate is first accelerated.
- Most common adverse effects reported are dose-related (serum concentration) and mild. CNS signs include drowsiness, depression, ataxia, muscle tremors; GI signs include nausea, and vomiting (usually transient); adverse cardiac effects usually occur only at high plasma concentrations in most species, but cats are more susceptible.
- When an IV bolus is given too rapidly, dose-dependent hypotension may occur; consider starting with a lower dose. Seizures are possible.
- Do **NOT** use the product containing epinephrine IV.

Uses/Indications

Besides its use as a local, regional, and topical anesthetic agent, lidocaine is frequently used to treat ventricular arrhythmias (eg, ventricular tachycardia, premature ventricular complexes [PVCs]) in all species. Lidocaine is indicated as an antiarrhythmic agent when PVCs are frequent and/or polymorphic (ie, 2 or more different abnormal QRS-T configurations can be identified), when PVCs appear in runs of more than 2 or 3, when there is marked tachycardia such that there are signs of diminished diastolic filling time and cardiac output (eg, pale mucous membranes, prolonged CRT, hypotension, weak pulses, pulse deficits), or when R on T phenomenon is seen on the ECG.[1,2]

Lidocaine may also have benefit in dogs to terminate supraventricular tachycardia in the presence or absence of an accessory pathway and paroxysmal atrial fibrillation initiated by elevated vagal tone in dogs with normal cardiac function.[3-5] In critically ill dogs, lidocaine may be beneficial secondary to its free radical scavenging abilities, analgesic effects, and antiarrhythmic properties. A retrospective study in dogs undergoing laparotomy for septic peritonitis found that dogs that received lidocaine (50 µg/kg/MINUTE) in addition to an opioid during surgery had significantly increased short-term (48 hour) survival rates versus dogs that received an opioid alone.[6] IV lidocaine could potentially be useful in dogs with gastric dilation volvulus (GDV) to reduce cardiac arrhythmias, acute kidney injury, and hospitalization times.[7]

Cats may be more sensitive to the cardiovascular and CNS effects of the drug[8,9] and most clinicians do not use it IV in this species as an analgesic.[10]

In horses, lidocaine has been used as part of partial intravenous anesthesia (PIVA) protocols for its analgesic, anti-inflammatory, and prokinetic effects. It may be useful to prevent postoperative ileus and reperfusion injury and for the adjunctive treatment of endotoxemia. It appears to increase survival rate in horses undergoing exploratory celiotomy for small intestinal disease.[11]

Low-dose IV lidocaine infusions for hyperalgesia and neuropathic pain states induced by trauma or surgical procedures have been documented to be useful. It has MAC-sparing effects in dogs,[12-14] horses,[15,16] and small ruminants[17,18] but does not reduce propofol requirements in dogs.[19-21]

Intrathecal administration of high-dose lidocaine is an acceptable secondary method for euthanasia in animals under anesthesia when other euthanasia agents or methods are unavailable, cost-prohibitive, or unwarranted due to environmental concerns.[22]

Pharmacology/Actions

Lidocaine is considered to be a class IB antiarrhythmic agent (membrane-stabilizing that shortens the myocardial cell action potential). Lidocaine acts by combining with inactive fast sodium channels, which inhibits recovery after repolarization. Class IB agents demonstrate rapid rates of attachment and dissociation to sodium channels in ventricular conducting tissue more so than atrial tissue. At therapeutic concentrations, lidocaine causes phase 4 diastolic depolarization attenuation, decreased automaticity, and either a decrease or no change in membrane responsiveness and excitability. These effects will occur at serum concentrations that will not inhibit the automaticity of the SA node, and will have little effect on AV node conduction or His-Purkinje conduction.

The systemic analgesic effects are not well understood but are likely via several mechanisms, including reducing ectopic activity of damaged afferent neurons, action at different molecular sites, such as Na^+, Ca^{2+}, and K^+ channels and N-methyl-D-aspartate (NMDA) receptors.

Lidocaine does not demonstrate GI prokinetic effects in dogs[23,24]; however, it apparently has some enhancing effects on intestinal motility in rabbits[25] and in horses with postoperative ileus.[26-28] The mechanism for this effect is not well understood, but probably involves more than just blocking increased sympathetic tone. The results of the prokinetic action of lidocaine in horses undergoing colic surgery are controversial, but they suggest that lidocaine could be used as an analgesic that does not impair GI motility.[29] In a cohort study, the administration of lidocaine to horses undergoing colic surgery due to small intestine lesions did not affect the prevalence, volume, and duration of reflux and did not improve the survival rate.[30]

Systemic and topical lidocaine reduces cough response on intubation.[31,32]

Lidocaine has been shown to inhibit reactive oxygen species (ROS) formation and lipid peroxidation, which may improve clinical outcomes in dogs with gastric dilatation and volvulus.[33]

Pharmacokinetics

Lidocaine is not effective orally, as it has a high first-pass effect. If high oral doses are given, toxic signs occur (possibly due to active metabolites) before therapeutic concentrations can be reached. Following a therapeutic IV bolus dose, the onset of action is generally within 2 minutes and has a duration of action of 10 to 20 minutes. If a constant rate infusion (CRI) is started without an initial IV bolus, it may take up to an hour for therapeutic concentrations to be reached. IM injections may be given every 1.5 hours in dogs, but because monitoring and adjusting doses are difficult with this route of administration, it should be avoided; administration by the IO route can be considered if IV is not possible.

After injection, the drug is rapidly redistributed from the plasma into highly perfused organs (kidney, liver, lungs, heart) and distributed widely throughout body tissues. It has a high affinity for adipose tissue and is bound to plasma proteins, primarily alpha$_1$-acid glycoprotein. It has been reported that lidocaine binding to this protein is highly variable and concentration-dependent in dogs and may be higher in dogs with inflammatory disease. The apparent volume of distribution (V_d) has been reported to be 4.5 L/kg in dogs, 1.9 L/kg in cats,[34] and ≈2.5 L/kg in horses.[35]

Lidocaine is rapidly metabolized in the liver to active metabolites (monoethylglycinexylidide [MEGX] and glycinexylidide [GX]). The terminal half-life of lidocaine has been reported to be 0.9 hours in dogs, 1.7 hours in cats,[34] and ≈1 hour in horses.[35] Lidocaine clearance in horses exceeds hepatic blood flow, suggesting metabolism also occurs at extra-hepatic sites.[36] Lidocaine, MEGX, and GX concentrations may progressively increase with prolonged infusions, and dosage modification may be required.[37-39] The half-lives of lidocaine and MEGX may be prolonged in patients with cardiac failure or hepatic disease. Less than 10% of a parenteral dose is excreted unchanged in the urine.

In healthy beef cattle, elimination half-life after IV administration of 1.5 mg/kg was ≈1 hour.[40] Following a 2 mg/kg IV bolus and 100 µg/kg/*MINUTE* IV CRI in calves, plasma lidocaine concentrations ranged from 1.85 to 2.06 µg/mL.[41] Following an inverted L epidural nerve block in healthy Holstein cows, lidocaine elimination half-life in serum was 4.2 hours and mean residence time was 5.1 hours[42]; in milk, the time to maximum concentration occurred 1.75 hours after administration, and the time of the last detectable milk concentration was 32.5 hours.

In humans, lidocaine is readily absorbed after oral administration, but bioavailability is only 35% due to extensive first-pass metabolism. Absorption from injection sites, including muscle, is rapid. Protein binding is ≈66% to alpha$_1$-acid glycoprotein, with considerable variability. It is widely distributed, including into the CNS and breast milk. Lidocaine is extensively and rapidly metabolized, with an elimination half-life of 1 to 2 hours.

Contraindications/Precautions/Warnings

Lidocaine is contraindicated in patients with known hypersensitivity to the amide-class local anesthetics, a severe degree of SA, AV, or intraventricular heart block (if not being artificially paced), Adams-Stokes syndrome, and Wolff-Parkinson-White (WPW) syndrome.

Cats tend to be more sensitive to the CNS and cardiodepressant effects of lidocaine; use with caution especially in cats with concurrent illnesses or under general anesthesia. Most clinicians avoid the use of IV lidocaine in cats for anesthetic/analgesic purposes. Lidocaine IV CRI does not appear to affect thermal antinociception in cats.[43] When administered to cats anesthetized with isoflurane, lidocaine causes greater cardiovascular depression than an equipotent dose of isoflurane alone and thus, lidocaine is not recommended as part of a balanced anesthesia protocol.[43,44]

Lidocaine should be used with caution in patients with liver disease, congestive heart failure, shock, hypovolemia, severe respiratory depression, or marked hypoxia. Consider reducing doses by 30% to 50% in animals with liver dysfunction. It should also be used with caution in patients with bradycardia or incomplete heart block having PVCs unless the heart rate is first accelerated.[45]

If an IV bolus is given too rapidly, dose-dependent hypotension may occur; consider starting with a lower dose as this effect is dose-dependent.[46] In humans, it is recommended to administer IV bolus injections over 2 to 4 minutes. Sedation and vomiting also may occur during IV bolus administration, which may increase the risk for aspiration, particularly in patients with brachycephalic obstructive airway syndrome. When preparing lidocaine for IV injection, be certain of the concentration and do NOT use products containing epinephrine. The veterinary label lidocaine injection (local anesthetic) contains propylene glycol, which is known to cause hypotension with IV administration.[47]

In human medicine, lidocaine is considered a high-alert medication (ie, medication that requires special safeguards to reduce the risk for errors).[48] Consider instituting practices such as redundant drug dosage and volume checking, and special alert labels.

Adverse Effects

At usual doses, and if the serum concentration remains within the proposed therapeutic range (1 – 5 µg/mL), serious adverse effects are rare. The most common adverse effects reported are dose-related and mild. CNS signs include drowsiness, depression, ataxia, and muscle tremors. Nausea and vomiting may occur but are usually transient; the combination of sedation and vomiting may increase the risk for aspiration.

Adverse cardiac effects generally only occur at high plasma concentrations and are usually associated with PR and QRS interval prolongation and QT interval shortening. Lidocaine may increase ventricular rates if used in patients with atrial fibrillation. Horses are less sensitive than other species to lidocaine's adverse cardiovascular effects but appear more sensitive to the drug's CNS effects. Ataxia and a tendency for poor recovery were noted in horses given lidocaine infusion until the end of surgery, compared to horses in which the infusion was stopped 30 minutes before the end of surgery.[49]

Reproductive/Nursing Safety

Lidocaine crosses the placenta. No fetal harm was demonstrated in rats given 5 to 6.6 times the maximum recommended human dose. In humans, lidocaine is considered compatible with pregnancy.[50]

Lidocaine is excreted into milk at concentrations of ≈40% of that found in the serum and would be unlikely to pose significant risk to nursing offspring. In humans, it is considered compatible with breastfeeding.[51]

Because safety has not been established in animals, this drug should only be used when the maternal benefits outweigh the potential risks to offspring.

Overdose/Acute Toxicity

In dogs, toxicity may result if serum concentrations of greater than 8 µg/mL are attained, although one study noted muscle tremors at concentrations of ≈1.8 – 3.4 µg/mL with corresponding doses of 10 – 13 µg/kg.[52] The lethal dose in dogs is thought to be 16 to 28 mg/kg.[52] Clinical signs related to lidocaine toxicity may include ataxia, nystagmus, depression, seizures, bradycardia, hypotension, and, at very high concentrations, circulatory collapse.

Because lidocaine is rapidly metabolized, cessation of therapy or reduction in infusion rates with monitoring may be all that is required for minor signs. Seizures or excitement may be treated with benzodiazepines. If circulatory depression occurs, treat with fluids, vasopressor agents (eg, dobutamine, norepinephrine), and, if necessary, begin CPR. IV lipid emulsion 20% can be beneficial for the treatment of lidocaine toxicity.[53-55] See ***Fat Emulsion, Intravenous***.

For patients that have experienced or are suspected to have experienced an overdose, it is strongly encouraged to consult with one of the 24-hour poison consultation centers that specialize in providing information specific for veterinary patients. For general information related to overdose and toxin exposures, as well as contact information for poison control centers, refer to ***Appendix***.

Drug Interactions

Lidocaine is a substrate of CYP 1A and 3A in humans. The following drug interactions have either been reported or are theoretical in humans or animals receiving lidocaine and may be of significance in veterinary patients. Unless otherwise noted, use together is not necessarily contraindicated, but weigh the potential risks and perform additional monitoring when appropriate.

- **Alpha-2 Receptor Agonists** (eg, **dexmedetomidine, xylazine**): Lidocaine may increase the ataxic effects of $alpha_2$ agonists in horses.
- **Anesthetics, Inhalant** (eg, **isoflurane, sevoflurane**): Lidocaine infusions perioperatively have been shown to reduce MAC requirements in dogs,[12] horses,[15,16] and cats.[8] In dogs and horses, this effect may be of benefit, but in cats, additive cardiodepression has been shown.[8] In horses, lidocaine with inhalant anesthetics can cause tremors and ataxia and affect the quality of anesthetic recovery; it has been recommended to discontinue lidocaine CRIs at least 30 minutes before the start of the recovery period.[49]
- **Antiarrhythmics, Other** (eg, **procainamide, propranolol, quinidine**): When administered with lidocaine, may cause additive or antagonistic cardiac effects and toxicity may be enhanced
- **Beta-Blockers** (eg, **atenolol, esmolol, propranolol, sotalol**): Lidocaine concentration or effects may be increased.
- **Ceftiofur**: May reduce lidocaine protein binding, increasing free lidocaine concentration, which may increase risk for lidocaine toxicity[37]
- **Cimetidine**: Lidocaine concentration or effects may be increased.
- **Diuretics** (eg, **furosemide**): Hypokalemia may reduce the antiarrhythmic effects of lidocaine.
- **Ketamine**: Lidocaine may increase ataxic effects in horses.
- **Mitotane**: May decrease lidocaine concentration
- **Neuromuscular Blockers** (eg, **atracurium, succinylcholine**): Large doses of lidocaine may prolong succinylcholine-induced apnea.
- **Phenobarbital**: May decrease lidocaine concentration.

Laboratory Considerations

- Lidocaine may cause increased **creatine kinase (CK)** and **serum creatinine** concentrations.

Dosages

NOTES:

1. **Monitoring for adverse effects is critical**.
2. Do not confuse CRI dosages listed as µg/kg/<u>*MINUTE*</u> with those listed as mg/kg/<u>*HOUR*</u>.

DOGS:

Antiarrhythmic agent (extra-label):

Ventricular tachycardia: initial boluses of 2 mg/kg slowly IV, up to 8 mg/kg; or rapid IV infusion at 0.8 mg/kg/*MINUTE* IV CRI; if effective, then 25–80 µg/kg/*MINUTE* IV CRI; can also be used intratracheally for CPR.[2]

Refractory ventricular fibrillation (VF)/pulseless ventricular tachycardia (VT): The treatment of choice is electrical defibrillation, but patients with VF refractory to defibrillation may benefit from treatment with amiodarone. If amiodarone is not available, lidocaine 2 mg/kg slow IV/intraosseous push may be of benefit[56]; however, this should be done with caution, as lidocaine has been shown to increase proarrhythmia activity when used with monophasic defibrillating shocks.[57,58]

Cardioversion of orthodromic atrioventricular reciprocating tachycardia (OAVRT): With continuous ECG recording, 2 mg/kg IV over 20 to 30 seconds, repeated every 2 minutes to a cumulative dose of 8 mg/kg. Median lidocaine dose to cardiovert was 2 mg/kg. Maintenance of cardioversion with a lidocaine CRI 25 – 60 µg/kg/*MINUTE* IV CRI was required in some dogs.[59]

Adjunctive treatment of GDV or other critical illnesses (eg, septic peritonitis) to decrease arrhythmias and minimize risk for acute kidney injury: Loading dose of 1 – 2 mg/kg IV, then 17 – 50 µg/kg/*MINUTE* (1 – 3 mg/kg/*HOUR*) IV CRI.[6,7,60] In one study, lidocaine infusion continued for at least 3 hours following GDV surgery.[60]

Adjunctive systemic analgesia under general anesthesia (extra-label):

NOTE: For additional information on morphine/lidocaine/ketamine (MLK)-type CRIs, refer to other anesthesia-specific references.

a) **Lidocaine as a single agent**: 1 – 2 mg/kg IV followed by 25 – 50 µg/kg/*MINUTE* IV CRI.[61–63]
b) **Lidocaine/dexmedetomidine**: Lidocaine 2 mg/kg IV with dexmedetomidine 2 µg/kg IV followed by lidocaine 3 mg/kg/*HOUR* IV CRI with dexmedetomidine 3 µg/kg/*HOUR* IV CRI during surgery.[64]
c) **Lidocaine/dexmedetomidine/ketamine**: Lidocaine 2 mg/kg with dexmedetomidine 1 µg/kg and ketamine 1 mg/kg IV followed by lidocaine 100 µg/kg/*MINUTE* IV CRI with dexmedetomidine 3 µg/kg/*HOUR* IV CRI and ketamine 40 µg/kg/*MINUTE* IV CRI during surgery. At the conclusion of surgery, rates were reduced to lidocaine 25 µg/kg/*MINUTE* IV CRI, dexmedetomidine 1 µg/kg/*HOUR* IV CRI, and ketamine 10 µg/kg/*MINUTE* IV CRI and continued for an additional 4 hours.[65,66]
d) **Lidocaine/fentanyl/ketamine**: Lidocaine 3 mg/kg/*HOUR* IV CRI combined with fentanyl 3.6 µg/kg/*HOUR* IV CRI and ketamine 0.6 mg/kg/*HOUR* IV CRI (no loading dose was used in this study).[67]
e) **Lidocaine/ketamine**: Lidocaine 1.5 – 2 mg/kg with ketamine 0.5 – 3 mg/kg IV followed by lidocaine 25 – 100 µg/kg/*MINUTE* IV CRI with ketamine 0.03 – 0.1 mg/kg/*MINUTE* IV CRI[68–70]
f) **Morphine/lidocaine/ketamine (MLK)**: Lidocaine 50 µg/kg per *MINUTE*, morphine 3.3 – 4 µg/kg/*MINUTE*, and ketamine 10 µg/kg/*MINUTE* admixed in IV fluids and administered as an IV CRI.[71–74] Refer to ***Compatibility/Compounding Considerations*** for more information.
g) **Dexmedetomidine/morphine/lidocaine/ketamine (DMLK)**: Lidocaine 3 mg/kg/*HOUR*, dexmedetomidine 0.5 µg/kg per *HOUR*, morphine 0.2 mg/kg/*HOUR*, and ketamine 0.6 mg/kg per *HOUR* admixed in IV fluids and administered IV as CRI.[75] Refer to ***Compatibility/Compounding Considerations*** for more information.

CATS:

CAUTION: Cats are reportedly very sensitive to the CNS effects of lidocaine and can develop cardiovascular depression. There are several sources that state that lidocaine should not be used in cats as an injectable analgesic. If using in cats, monitor carefully.

Antiarrhythmic: Initially, 0.2 – 0.7 mg/kg IV slowly, may repeat once or twice.[76] Alternatively, 0.25 – 0.5 mg/kg IV slowly, can repeat at 0.15 – 0.25 mg/kg IV over 5 to 20 minutes; if effective, 10 – 20 µg/kg/*MINUTE* (0.6 – 1.2 mg/kg/*HOUR*) IV CRI.[77]

HORSES:

Ventricular tachyarrhythmias: 0.25 – 0.5 mg/kg IV slowly; can repeat in 5 to 10 minutes. The sum total of IV boluses should not exceed 2 mg/kg. If multiple boluses are required, begin lidocaine 50 µg/kg/*MINUTE* (3 mg/kg/*HOUR*) IV CRI.[1]

Postoperative ileus/colic: Initially, IV bolus of lidocaine 1.3 – 1.4 mg/kg followed by lidocaine 30 – 50 µg/kg/*MINUTE* (1.8 – 3 mg/kg/*HOUR*) IV CRI for 24 hours (for postoperative ileus).[26,27,78,79]

Adjunctive systemic analgesia under general anesthesia:

a) **Lidocaine alone**: 1.5 – 5 mg/kg IV loading dose administered over 15 minutes followed by 25 – 100 μg/kg/*MINUTE* IV CRI.[80,81] One study determined the loading dose did not confer additional advantage.[82]

b) **Lidocaine/ketamine**: Loading doses: ketamine 3 mg/kg IV, followed by lidocaine 2 mg/kg administered IV over 10 minutes; maintenance dosage: lidocaine 3 mg/kg/*HOUR* with ketamine 3 mg/kg/*HOUR* IV CRI. Xylazine 1.1 mg/kg IV was given prior to loading doses. Addition of morphine did not provide additional benefit.[83] Another study demonstrated efficacy with a lidocaine (only) loading dose of 1.5 mg/kg IV over 10 minutes followed by lidocaine 2.4 mg/kg/*HOUR* with ketamine 3.6 mg/kg/*HOUR* IV CRI.[84]

c) **Lidocaine/ketamine/medetomidine**: A loading dose of lidocaine 1.5 mg/kg administered IV over 10 minutes was followed by a combination of lidocaine 2 mg/kg/*HOUR* with ketamine 2 mg/kg/*HOUR* and medetomidine 3.6 μg/kg/*HOUR* IV CRI. After 50 minutes, lidocaine and ketamine CRI rates were reduced to 1.5 mg/kg/*HOUR*, and medetomidine was reduced to 2.75 μg/kg/*HOUR*.[85] Refer to ***Compatibility/Compounding Considerations*** for more information.

d) **Lidocaine/xylazine**: A loading dose of lidocaine 1.3 mg/kg IV over 5 minutes with xylazine 0.55 mg/kg IV over 1 minute were followed by lidocaine 1.5 mg/kg/*HOUR* with xylazine 1.1 mg/kg/*HOUR* IV CRI. A higher lidocaine CRI rate caused significant ataxia.[86]

Partial IV Anesthesia (PIVA): Based on the drug's pharmacokinetics, lidocaine 1.5 – 5 mg/kg IV followed by lidocaine 75 μg/kg per *MINUTE* (4.5 mg/kg/*HOUR*) IV CRI should yield a plasma concentration of 3000 ng/mL (3 μg/mL) and provide an ≈30% reduction in MAC. The rate of administration of the loading dose has varied in studies ranging from 1 to 20 minutes, with 10 to 15 minutes being most common. Administration rate is more relevant in conscious horses but is less so in anesthetized horses because the neurologic effects (ataxia, vision disturbances) are blunted and not observed. Discontinue the CRI at least 30 minutes prior to the start of recovery to minimize risk for rough recovery. Has been used in PIVA protocols with ketamine, medetomidine, or morphine.[80]

Total IV anesthesia (TIVA): After induction with propofol, lidocaine 1 mg/kg IV bolus over 1 minute followed by lidocaine 50 μg/kg/*MINUTE* IV CRI in combination with propofol 0.1 mg/kg/*MINUTE*, medetomidine 3.5 μg/kg/*HOUR*, and butorphanol 24 μg/kg/*HOUR* IV CRI.[87]

CATTLE:

Analgesia: In an experimental study, beginning 40 minutes after induction of general anesthesia, lidocaine 2 mg/kg IV bolus was followed by 100 μg/kg/*MINUTE* IV CRI.[41]

GOATS:

Analgesia:

a) **Lidocaine alone**: 2.5 mg/kg IV over 3 minutes followed by lidocaine 100 μg/kg/*MINUTE* IV CRI[88]

b) **Lidocaine/ketamine**: Lidocaine 2.5 mg/kg with ketamine 1.5 mg/kg IV over 3 minutes followed by lidocaine 100 μg/kg per *MINUTE* with ketamine 50 μg/kg/*MINUTE* IV CRI[88]

Total IV anesthesia (TIVA): Lidocaine 1 mg/kg combined with alfaxalone 2 mg/kg and administered IV over 10 minutes to induce general anesthesia[18]; anesthesia maintained with lidocaine 3 mg/kg/*HOUR* and alfaxalone 9.6 mg/kg/*HOUR* IV CRI.

SHEEP:

Analgesia: Anesthesia was induced with ketamine 3.3 mg/kg and midazolam 0.1 mg/kg IV followed by morphine 1 mg/kg IM.[17] Lidocaine 20 μg/kg/*MINUTE* with ketamine 10 μg/kg/*MINUTE* IV CRI was then started.

SMALL MAMMALS:

Analgesia in rabbits: Lidocaine 2 mg/kg IV over 5 minutes followed by 50 – 100 μg/kg/*MINUTE* IV CRI.[89] Following ovariohysterectomy, rabbits receiving lidocaine 100 μg/kg/*MINUTE* IV CRI for 2 days had better GI motility, food intake, fecal output, and number of normal behaviors than rabbits receiving only buprenorphine.[25]

Ventricular arrhythmias in rabbits and guinea pigs: Under emergency situations, lidocaine 1 – 4 mg/kg IV bolus is relatively safe.[90]

Monitoring

- ECG, blood pressure, heart rate, pulse quality, pulse oximetry
- Signs of toxicity (eg, depression, vomiting, nausea, ataxia, muscle tremors, PR and QRS interval prolongation, QT interval shortening, bradycardia, hypotension)
- If available and indicated, serum lidocaine concentrations may be monitored. Therapeutic concentrations are considered to range from 1 to 6 μg/mL.

Client Information

- Lidocaine should only be used by professionals familiar with its use and in a setting where adequate patient monitoring can be performed.

Chemistry/Synonyms

A potent local anesthetic and antiarrhythmic agent, lidocaine HCl occurs as a white, odorless, slightly bitter, crystalline powder with a melting point between 74°C and 79°C (165.2°F-174.2°F) and a pK_a of 7.86. It is very soluble in water and alcohol. The pH of the commercial injection is adjusted to 5 to 7, and the pH of the commercially available infusion in dextrose 5% is adjusted to 3.5 to 6.

Lidocaine may also be known as lidocaini hydrochloridum, and lignocaine hydrochloride; many trade names are available; a common trade name is *Xylocaine*® (Astra).

Storage/Stability

Lidocaine for injection should be stored at 20°C to 25°C (68°F-77°F); avoid freezing. Temperatures up to 40°C (104°F) may be tolerated.

Compatibility/Compounding Considerations

Compatibility is dependent on factors such as pH, concentration, temperature, and diluent used; consult specialized references or a hospital pharmacist for more specific information.

Lidocaine is physically **compatible** with most commonly used IV infusion solutions, including 5% dextrose, lactated Ringer's, 0.9% sodium chloride, and combinations of these. It is also reportedly physically **compatible** with: aminophylline, atropine, buprenorphine, butorphanol, calcium salts, chloramphenicol sodium succinate, clindamycin, dexamethasone sodium phosphate, dexmedetomidine, digoxin, diphenhydramine, dobutamine, doxycycline, epinephrine, erythromycin, famotidine, fentanyl, furosemide, glycopyrrolate, heparin, hydrocortisone sodium succinate, hydromorphone, hydroxyzine, ketamine, insulin (regular), mannitol, metoclopramide, midazolam, morphine, ondansetron, oxytetracycline, penicillin G potassium, phenylephrine, potassium chloride, procainamide, propranolol, sodium bicarbonate, sodium lactate, verapamil, and Vitamin B-Complex with C.

Lidocaine **may not be compatible** with dopamine, epinephrine, isoproterenol, or norepinephrine as these require low pH for stability. Lidocaine is reportedly physically **incompatible** when mixed with ampicillin, cefazolin, diazepam, pantoprazole, pentobarbital, or sulfa-/trimethoprim.

- **"MLK" Recipe**:

  NOTE: When preparing solutions, be certain that you are not using the lidocaine product that contains epinephrine.

To prepare IV infusion solution using the veterinary lidocaine 2% solution, add 1 g (50 mL) to 1 L of compatible solution (eg, 0.9% sodium chloride, Dextrose 5%). This solution will give an approximate lidocaine concentration of 1 mg/mL (1000 µg/mL). When using a mini-drip (60 drops/mL) IV set, each drop will contain ≈17 µg of lidocaine. In small dogs and cats, a less concentrated solution may be used for greater dosage accuracy.

A combination IV infusion for analgesia and sedation in postoperative patients (dogs, NOT cats) that require sedation to sleep the night after surgery is described[91]: For this technique, plan on adding the drugs to a bag of fluids for which the administration rate will not change, which usually means picking a fluid and administration rate calculated to provide maintenance needs for water. For example, to calculate a drug plan for a 20 kg dog that is to receive morphine, lidocaine, ketamine, and medetomidine for the first 8 to 24 hours postoperatively, drug doses to consider might include:

Morphine: 0.1 mg/kg/HOUR x 20 kg = 2 mg/HOUR
Lidocaine: 2.5 mg/kg/HOUR x 20 kg = 50 mg/HOUR
Ketamine: 0.1 mg/kg/HOUR x 20 kg = 2 mg/HOUR
Medetomidine: 2 µg/kg/HOUR x 20 kg = 40 µg/HOUR (**NOTE**: This is not the dose for dexmedetomidine).

The maintenance fluid administration rate for a 20 kg dog lying quietly in a cage is roughly 800 mL/day or 33 mL/hour. Therefore, a 1 L bag contains ≈30 hours of treatment, and to a 1 L bag one must add:

Morphine: 2 mg/HOUR x 30 hours = 60 mg = 6 mL (when using 10 mg/mL morphine)
Lidocaine: 50 mg/HOUR x 30 hours = 1500 mg = 75 mL (when using 2% [20 mg/mL] lidocaine)
Ketamine: 2 mg/HOUR x 30 hours = 60 mg = 0.6 mL (when using 100 mg/mL ketamine)
Medetomidine: 40 µg/HOUR x 30 hours = 1200 µg = 1.2 mL (when using 1000 µg/mL medetomidine)

If the drugs are added to a 1 L bag of fluid, the final volume is greater than 1 L—in this case 1083 mL. Therefore, 83 mL should be removed from the bag *before* addition of the medications.[91]

Dosage Forms/Regulatory Status

VETERINARY-LABELED PRODUCTS:

There are injectable lidocaine products labeled for use in veterinary medicine (dogs, cats, horses, and cattle) as an injectable anesthetic, but it is not FDA-approved for use as an antiarrhythmic agent. Information regarding its use in food-producing species is conflicting; when using lidocaine in a food animal, it is suggested to contact the Food Animal Residue Avoidance Databank (FARAD). See ***Appendix*** for more information.

The Association of Racing Commissioners International (ARCI) has designated this drug as a class 2 substance. Use of this drug may not be allowed in certain animal competitions. Check rules and regulations before entering in a competition while this medication is being administered. Contact local racing authorities for further guidance. See ***Appendix*** for more information.

Lidocaine HCl for Injection: 2% (20 mg/mL) in 100 mL and 250 mL multi-use vials; (contains preservatives and propylene glycol); generic; (Rx)

HUMAN-LABELED PRODUCTS:

Lidocaine Hydrochloride Injection: 0.5%, 1%, 1.5%, 2%, and 4% in 5 mL, 10 mL, 20 mL, 30 mL, and 50 mL single- and multi-dose vials; 2 mL and 5 mL ampules; 5 mL syringes and cartridges; *Xylocaine®* and *Xylocaine MPF®*, generic; (Rx)

Lidocaine Hydrochloride with Dextrose Injection: 1.5% with 7.5% dextrose and 5% with 7.5 % dextrose in 2 mL ampules and single-dose amps; *Xylocaine MPF®*, generic; (Rx)

Premixed with 5% dextrose for IV infusion in concentrations of 4 mg/mL and 8 mg/mL; injections with epinephrine, topical liquids, patches, ointment, cream, lotion, gel, spray, and jelly available.

References

For the complete list of references, see **wiley.com/go/budde/plumb**

Lincomycin

(lin-koe-***mye***-sin) *Lincocin®, Lincomix®*
Lincosamide Antibiotic

Prescriber Highlights

- Antibiotic similar to clindamycin, with a broad spectrum against many anaerobes, gram-positive aerobic cocci, and *Toxoplasma* spp
- Contraindications include in horses, rodents, ruminants, and lagomorphs; hypersensitivity to lincosamides.
- Use caution in liver or renal dysfunction; consider reducing dosage if severe.
- Adverse effects include gastroenteritis, pain at the injection site if given IM; rapid IV administration can cause hypotension and cardiopulmonary arrest.

Uses/Indications

Lincomycin is FDA-approved in dogs and cats for infections caused by susceptible gram-positive organisms, particularly streptococci and staphylococci.[1] It is also approved in swine for the treatment of infectious arthritis and mycoplasma pneumonia. Lincomycin is also FDA-approved to control American foulbrood in honey bees.

Lincomycin is considered a first-tier antimicrobial for the treatment of bacterial dermal infections in dogs.[2] However, clindamycin is generally better absorbed, more active, likely less toxic, and has largely supplanted the use of lincomycin for oral and injectable therapy in small animals.

The World Health Organization (WHO) has designated lincomycin as a Highly Important antimicrobial for human medicine.[3] The Office International des Epizooties (OIE) Antimicrobial Classification has designated lincomycin as a Veterinary Highly Important Antimicrobial Agent.[4]

Pharmacology/Actions

The lincosamide antibiotics, lincomycin and clindamycin, share mechanisms of action and have similar spectrums of activity, although lincomycin is usually less active. Complete cross-resistance occurs between the 2 drugs, and at least partial cross-resistance occurs between the lincosamides and erythromycin. They may act as bacteriostatic or bactericidal agents, depending on the concentration of the drug at the infection site and the susceptibility of the organism. Lincosamides can accumulate in cells (eg, leukocytes, macrophages). They are believed to act by binding to the 50S ribosomal subunit of susceptible bacteria, thereby inhibiting peptide formation and protein synthesis for the bacteria's cell wall.

Most aerobic gram-positive cocci, including staphylococci and streptococci, are susceptible to the lincosamides. Enterococci are inherently resistant. Many strains of *Staphylococcus pseudintermedius* are resistant. Other organisms that are generally susceptible include *Corynebacterium diphtheriae, Nocardia asteroides, Erysepelothrix* spp, and *Mycoplasma* spp. Anaerobic bacteria are generally susceptible to the lincosamides, although there is a low prevalence of resistance in the *Bacteroides fragilis* group.

Pharmacokinetics

In cats, after IV or oral doses of 15 mg/kg, the following pharmacokinetic parameters (means) were reported: Bioavailability (oral): 82%; volume of distribution (steady-state): 0.98 L/kg; clearance: 0.17 L/kg/hour; elimination half-life: 4.2 hours. The skin to plasma ratio 2 hours postdose was about 2:1.[5] Protein binding in cats is low (less than 20%). IM dosage of 10 mg/kg had a mean bioavailability of 83%. Bone to serum ratio measured 30 to 45 minutes after IM dosing was ≈0.7:1.[6]

In dogs, lincomycin is well absorbed after PO and IM administration. Serum levels peak within 0.5 to 2 hours of administration. Biliary and fecal excretion accounts for 40% to 75% of the dose in dogs. The elimination half-life of lincomycin is reportedly 3 to 4 hours in small animals.

In humans, lincomycin is rapidly absorbed from the gut, but only ≈30% to 40% of the total dose is absorbed. Food both decreases the extent and the rate of absorption. Peak serum levels are attained ≈2 to 4 hours after oral dosing. IM administration gives peak levels about double those reached after oral dosing and peak at ≈30 minutes postinjection.

Lincomycin is distributed into most tissues. Therapeutic levels are achieved in bone, synovial fluid, bile, pleural fluid, peritoneal fluid, skin, and heart muscle. CNS levels may reach 40% of those in the serum if meninges are inflamed but may be inadequate to treat meningitis. Lincomycin is 57% to 72% bound to plasma proteins, depending on the drug's concentration. The drug crosses the placenta and can be distributed into milk at concentrations equal to those found in plasma.

Lincomycin is partially metabolized in the liver. The unchanged drug and metabolites are excreted in the urine, feces, and bile. Half-life (about 5.5 hours) can be 2 to 3 times longer in patients with renal or hepatic dysfunction.

Contraindications/Precautions/Warnings

Although there have been case reports of parenteral administration of lincosamides to horses, cattle, and sheep, the lincosamides are considered **contraindicated** for use in **horses, ruminants, rabbits, hamsters**, and **guinea pigs** because of serious GI effects that may occur, including death.

Lincomycin is contraindicated in patients with known hypersensitivity to it or to clindamycin or patients having a pre-existing monilial (ie, candidiasis) infection.

Lincomycin is generally not recommended for use in neonatal animals because of its effects on gut flora. It should be used with caution in patients with a history of GI disease (eg, colitis), and in patients with a history of asthma or significant allergies.

In patients with hepatic or renal insufficiency, consider dose reduction or using alternative drugs.

Cross-resistance has been demonstrated between clindamycin and lincomycin.

Adverse Effects

Adverse effects reported in dogs and cats include gastroenteritis, emesis, and loose stools, and, infrequently, bloody diarrhea in dogs. IM injections reportedly cause pain at the injection site. Rapid IV administration can cause hypotension and cardiopulmonary arrest.

Swine may develop GI disturbances while receiving the medication. Fatal colitis can occur in horses.

In humans, adverse effects include stomatitis, nausea, vomiting, neutropenia, leukopenia, and skin rashes.

Reproductive/Nursing Safety

In rats exposed to lincomycin, there were no observed effects on fertility, breeding performance, or survival of offspring from birth to weaning. Lincomycin crosses the placenta, and cord blood concentrations are ≈25% of those found in maternal serum. Safe use during pregnancy has not been established, but the drug has not been implicated in causing teratogenic effects.

Because lincomycin is distributed into milk, nursing animals of mothers given lincomycin may develop diarrhea.

Because safety has not been established in animals, this drug should only be used when the maternal benefits outweigh the potential risks to offspring.

Overdose/Acute Toxicity

There is little information available regarding lincomycin overdose. In dogs, oral doses of up to 300 mg/kg/day for up to 1 year or parenterally at 60 mg/kg/day SC for 30 days did not result in toxicity or pathologic findings at necropsy.

For patients that have experienced or are suspected of having experienced an overdose, consultation with a 24-hour poison consultation center specializing in providing veterinary-specific information is recommended. For general information related to overdose and toxin exposures, as well as contact information for poison control centers, refer to ***Appendix.***

Drug Interactions

The following drug interactions have either been reported or are theoretical in humans or animals receiving lincomycin and may be of significance in veterinary patients. Unless otherwise noted, use together is not necessarily contraindicated, but weigh the potential risks and perform additional monitoring when appropriate.

- **CYCLOSPORINE**: Lincomycin may reduce levels.
- **ERYTHROMYCIN**: In vitro antagonism when used with lincomycin; concomitant use should likely be avoided
- **KAOLIN**: Kaolin (found in several over-the-counter antidiarrheal preparations) has been shown to reduce the oral absorption of lincomycin by up to 90% if both are given concurrently; if both drugs are necessary, separate doses by at least 2 hours.
- **NEUROMUSCULAR BLOCKING AGENTS** (eg, **pancuronium**): Lincomycin possesses intrinsic neuromuscular blocking activity and should be used cautiously with other neuromuscular blocking agents.

Laboratory Considerations

- Slight increases in **liver biochemical analytes** (ie, AST, ALT, ALP) may occur; no apparent clinical significance associated with these increases.

Dosages

DOGS:

Susceptible infections (label dosage; FDA-approved): Skin infections (eg, pustular dermatitis, abscesses, infected wounds [including bite and fight wounds]), upper respiratory tract infections (eg, tonsillitis, laryngitis), metritis, and secondary bacterial infections associated with the canine distemper-hepatitis complex: 15.4 mg/kg PO every 8 hours or 22 mg/kg PO every 12 hours; 11 mg/kg every 12 hours or 22 mg/kg every 24 hours IV (diluted in 0.9% sodium chloride or 5% dextrose and administered as a slow infusion) or IM. Treatment may continue for periods as long as 12 days.[1,7,8] **NOTE**: Some clinicians have given the drug SC in an extra-label manner.

Pyoderma (susceptible staphylococci) (extra-label): Although uncommonly recommended and used, 20 – 30 mg/kg PO every 12 hours has been used.

CATS:

Susceptible infections (label dosage; FDA-approved): Localized infections, such as abscesses, pneumonitis, and feline rhinotracheitis: 15.4 mg/kg PO every 8 hours or 22 mg/kg PO every 12 hours; 11 mg/kg every 12 hours or 22 mg/kg every 24 hours IV (diluted in 0.9% sodium chloride or 5% dextrose and administered as a slow infusion) or IM. Treatment may continue for periods as long as 12 days. **NOTE**: Some clinicians have given the drug SC in an extra-label manner.

Skin infections (extra label): Based on pharmacokinetic values and reported MICs, a dosage of 15 mg/kg PO every 12 hours is supported for treating skin infections.[5]

SWINE:

Mycoplasmal pneumonia or infectious arthritis caused by susceptible bacteria (label dosage; FDA-approved): 11 mg/kg IM once daily for 3 to 7 days, or added to drinking water at a rate of 250 mg/gallon (average of 8.36 mg/kg/day)[8]

BIRDS:

Pododermatitis (bumblefoot) (extra-label): 50 mg/kg PO twice daily[9]

FERRETS:

Susceptible infections (extra-label): 10 – 15 mg/kg PO 3 times daily; 10 mg/kg IM twice daily[10]

HONEY BEES:

Control of American foulbrood (label dosage; FDA-approved): For each hive, mix 100 mg lincomycin with 20 g confectioners' sugar and dust over the top bars of the brood chamber once weekly for 3 weeks.[11] Feed the drug in the spring or late fall, and complete treatment at least 4 weeks before main honey flow.

Monitoring

- Clinical efficacy
- Adverse effects, particularly severe diarrheas
- Hepatic and renal function

Client Information

- Use this medicine for infections of skin, wounds, and bone.
- Report severe, continued, or bloody diarrhea to your veterinarian immediately.
- Do **NOT** give this medicine to horses, cattle, sheep, goats, deer, rabbits, mice, rats, hamsters, or guinea pigs, as it may cause fatal diarrhea.
- This medicine is best given on an empty stomach, but do not "dry pill," or it may cause throat burns. Give a small amount of food or a small amount of water (a little over a teaspoonful) after pilling.
- Bitter taste: may require disguising in food to get the animal to take it

Chemistry/Synonyms

Lincomycin is an antibiotic obtained from cultures of *Streptomyces lincolnensis* that is available commercially as the monohydrate hydrochloride. It occurs as a white to off-white, crystalline powder that is freely soluble in water. The powder may have a faint odor and has a pK_a of 7.6. The commercially available injection has a pH of 3 to 5.5 and occurs as a clear to slightly yellow solution.

Lincomycin may also be known as U-10149, NSC-70731, *Lincomix®*, or *Lincocin®*.

Storage/Stability

Store lincomycin capsules, tablets, and soluble powder at room temperature (20°C-25°C [68°F-77°F]) in tight containers. Store lincomycin injectable products at room temperature; avoid freezing.

Compatibility/Compounding Considerations

Compatibility is dependent on factors such as pH, concentration, temperature, and diluent used; specialized references or a hospital pharmacist should be consulted for more specific information.

Lincomycin HCl for injection is reportedly physically **compatible** for at least 24 hours in the following IV infusion solutions and drugs: 5% dextrose, 5% dextrose in 0.9% sodium chloride, 10% dextrose, 0.9% sodium chloride, lactated Ringer's injection, amikacin sulfate, chloramphenicol sodium succinate, cimetidine HCl, cytarabine, heparin sodium, penicillin G potassium (4 hours only), polymyxin B sulfate, tetracycline HCl, and vitamin B complex with C.

Drugs that are reportedly physically **incompatible** when mixed with lincomycin, data conflicts, or compatibility is concentration and/or time-dependent include ampicillin sodium, carbenicillin disodium, and phenytoin sodium.

Dosage Forms/Regulatory Status

VETERINARY-LABELED PRODUCTS:

Lincomycin Oral Solution: 50 mg/mL in 20 mL dropper bottles; *Lincocin® Aquadrops*; (Rx). FDA-approved for use in dogs and cats

Lincomycin Sterile Injection: 100 mg/mL in 20 mL vials; *Lincocin®*; (Rx). FDA-approved for use in dogs and cats

Lincomycin Sterile Injection: 25 mg/mL, 50 mg/mL, 100 mg/mL, and 300 mg/mL in 100 mL vials; FDA-approved for use in swine. Slaughter withdrawal (when used as labeled) = 48 hours. *Lincocin® Sterile Solution*, *Lincomix® Injectable*, generic; (OTC). Not all strengths appear to be marketed.

Lincomycin Soluble Powder (*Lincomix®*, generic; [Rx]) is FDA-approved for use in honey bees. The withholding period for the honey super is 49 days.[12]

There are also several lincomycin feed/water additive products for use in swine and/or poultry.

HUMAN-LABELED PRODUCTS:

Lincomycin Injection: 300 mg (as hydrochloride)/mL in 2 mL and 10 mL vials; *Lincocin®*, generic; (Rx)

References

For the complete list of references, see **wiley.com/go/budde/plumb**

Linezolid

(lih-***neh***-zoh-lid) *Zyvox®*

Oxazolidinone Antibiotic

Prescriber Highlights

- Use of linezolid in veterinary medicine should be very limited because of this antibiotic's importance in human medicine. Veterinary infectious disease specialists should be consulted prior to treatment initiation.
- Antibiotic reserved for multidrug-resistant gram-positive infections with documented resistance to other antibiotics
- Excellent oral bioavailability with PK parameters similar to IV administration
- Most common adverse effects are GI-related, but myelosuppression has been documented in veterinary patients; other serious adverse effects, including hypertension, lactic acidosis, seizures, and serotonin syndrome, have been reported in humans.
- Displays weak monoamine oxidase inhibitory effects; many drug interactions are possible

Uses/Indications

Linezolid is an antibacterial that should only be used for the treatment of gram-positive infections (with documented resistance to other antibiotics and susceptibility to linezolid) including methicillin-resistant *Staphylococcus aureus* (MRSA), methicillin-resistant *S pseudintermedius* (MRSP), and multidrug-resistant *Enterococcus* spp (including vancomycin-resistant *Enterococcus* [VRE]).

It is important to note there is little published information regarding safe and effective use of linezolid in veterinary patients. Because this drug is used for multidrug-resistant infections in humans, its use in veterinary medicine should be reserved for <u>documented</u> infections where cultures and susceptibilities suggest that the infection is resistant to all other options and is considered treatable, and where consultation with an infectious disease expert has concluded linezolid is a viable and reasonable treatment.[1]

The World Health Organization (WHO) classifies linezolid as a Critically Important, High Priority antibiotic for human use.[2]

Pharmacology/Actions

Linezolid binds to the bacterial 23S ribosomal RNA of the 50S subunit resulting in inhibition of bacterial protein synthesis. Linezolid prevents the formation of the 70S initiation complex needed for the bacterial translation process. It is bacteriostatic against enterococci and staphylococci and bactericidal against most streptococci strains. It is less active against gram-negative bacteria and anaerobes. Linezolid's effects are time dependent.

Resistance patterns have been shown to be linked to a mutation of the 23S rRNA.[3]

Linezolid also has weak, nonselective monoamine oxidase inhibitory effects.

Pharmacokinetics

In dogs, the bioavailability of linezolid after oral administration is more than 95% and it exhibits a pharmacokinetic profile similar to IV use. Linezolid is widely distributed throughout the body with low protein binding (less than 35%) and a volume of distribution nearly equal to total body water. Peak concentrations are reached quickly (T_{max} = 0.78 to 0.95 hours; C_{max} = 26.8 to 28.2 µg/mL).[4] In humans, time to peak concentration was slightly delayed by administration with a high-fat food (T_{max} increased from 1.5 hours to 2.2 hours); C_{max} was decreased by 17%, but overall AUC remained stable.[5] In humans, renal impairment does not alter the serum concentration of linezolid [5]; however, the concentration of linezolid metabolites, which are renally eliminated, are 2 to 3 times higher in patients with renal impairment.[6]

Linezolid is metabolized by oxidation into 2 metabolites with no significant antibacterial efficacy.

Linezolid undergoes renal tubular reabsorption but is primarily excreted via the kidneys unchanged (30%) or as metabolites (50%).[4] Approximately 15% is excreted in bile almost entirely as metabolites. The elimination half-life in dogs following IV and PO administration was 3.91 hours and 3.6 hours, respectively, with no measurable concentrations after 24 to 48 hours.[4] In dogs after IV administration, clearance was measured as 1.99 mL/minute/kg.

Pharmacokinetic studies in rats and mice resulted in pharmacokinetic profiles similar to that of dogs.[4]

Contraindications/Precautions/Warnings

Linezolid is contraindicated in patients with a history of hypersensitivity to oxazolidinone antibiotics or in patients that have received monoamine oxidase inhibitors (MAOIs) within the past 14 days.[5]

In humans, lactic acidosis, myelosuppression, peripheral and optic neuropathy, serotonin syndrome, and superinfection have been reported, with most cases associated with a treatment duration greater than 2 weeks.[5] The risk for thrombocytopenia appears to be increased in patients with impaired renal function.[7-10] Additionally, linezolid should be used with caution in patients with diabetes, uncontrolled hypertension, uncontrolled hyperthyroidism, pheochromocytoma, and seizure disorders.

In humans, it has been recommended to avoid consuming foods high in tyramine (eg, aged cheeses, and cured or processed meats) while taking linezolid, as this combination has caused unexpected and significant increases in blood pressure[5]; significance in veterinary medicine is unknown.

Do not confuse the trade names *Zyvox*® (linezolid) with *Zosyn*® (piperacillin/tazobactam).

Adverse Effects

In a case report of a dog that received 23 weeks of linezolid 20 mg/kg PO every 12 hours to treat methicillin-resistant *S pseudintermedius* (MRSP) bacteremia and discospondylitis, mild anemia and thrombocytopenia were observed at treatment weeks 4 and 7; a compensated lactic acidosis was observed at week 7.[11] All adverse effects resolved by treatment week 14. Vomiting, lethargy, and anorexia were noted in 2 dogs receiving 13 – 14 mg/kg every 12 hours; the adverse effects resolved with ≈50% dosage reduction.[12] A macrocytic, hypochromic, regenerative anemia occurring in a dog after 105 days of linezolid treatment resolved after the drug was discontinued. Reversible myelosuppression (eg, neutropenia, thrombocytopenia, anemia) also has been documented in a cat.[13]

In humans, commonly reported adverse effects (more than 10%) include diarrhea, nausea, and vomiting.[5] Other adverse effects include headache, rash, and dizziness. Myelosuppression, including leukopenia, thrombocytopenia, and anemia, has also been reported in humans, and was reversible after treatment discontinuation. Serotonin syndrome was reported in humans using linezolid alone or in combination with other medication, although the overall incidence was low.[14] Rare but serious adverse effects include lactic acidosis and peripheral and optic neuropathy.[5] Treatment duration exceeding 14 days increases the incidence of myelosuppression and neurologic adverse effects[5]; additionally, impaired renal function appears to increase the risk for thrombocytopenia.[7-10]

Reproductive/Nursing Safety

Linezolid was not teratogenic in animal models, but embryo and fetal toxicities were documented concurrently with maternal toxicities including decreased neonatal survival and decreased birth weights.[5] As linezolid should be reserved for use in serious infections only, the potential benefits of treatment likely outweigh the risks.

Linezolid is excreted into milk, reaching concentrations similar to maternal plasma, and caution should be used when administered to nursing patients.[5]

Overdose/Acute Toxicity

In dogs receiving a single oral dose of 2000 mg/kg/day, reported signs of toxicity were vomiting and tremors, but there were no deaths.[15] In dogs receiving repeated IV and oral doses of 40 mg/kg/day over 30 days, adverse effects noted were anemia, leukopenia, thrombocytopenia, and bone marrow hypoplasia.[4] In rats receiving oral doses up to 3000 mg/kg/day, decreased activity and ataxia were seen.[5] The minimum lethal dose was more than 5000 mg/kg in rats and more than 2000 mg/kg in dogs.[16] The reported LD_{50} in rabbits was 100 mg/kg following oral administration.

In the event of an overdose, supportive care is recommended. Approximately 30% of linezolid is removed via dialysis.[5] For patients that have experienced or are suspected to have experienced an overdose, consultation with a 24-hour poison consultation center specializing in providing veterinary-specific information is recommended. For general information related to overdose and toxin exposures, as well as contact information for poison control centers, refer to ***Appendix***.

Drug Interactions

The following drug interactions have either been reported or are theoretical in humans or animals receiving linezolid and may be of significance in veterinary patients. Unless otherwise noted, use together is not necessarily contraindicated but the potential risks must be weighed and additional monitoring performed when appropriate.

- Blood Glucose Lowering Agents (eg, **insulin, sulfonylureas** [eg, **glipizide**]): Linezolid may exacerbate hypoglycemic effects of blood glucose lowering agents.
- Carbamazepine: May worsen the adverse effects of monoamine oxidase inhibitors (MAOIs). Avoid combination within 14 days of treatment.
- Chloramphenicol: Potential for additive myelosuppression

- **Dipyrone**: Potential for additive myelosuppression
- **Food, Tyramine Containing** (eg, **aged cheese, cured meats, sauerkraut**): Food high in tyramine has caused unexpected and serious increases in blood pressure in humans taking MAOIs.
- **monoamine oxidase Inhibitors** (MAOIs; eg, **amitraz, selegiline**): Additive MAO inhibition may worsen serotonergic effect, resulting in serotonin syndrome. Avoid combination within 14 days of MAOI treatment.
- **Opioids** (eg, **buprenorphine, fentanyl, hydrocodone, tramadol**): Concurrent use may worsen serotonergic effects and may worsen adverse effects of MAOIs. Consider therapy modification.
- **Reserpine**: Use of MAOIs may worsen the adverse effects of reserpine. Addition of reserpine to linezolid therapy may cause paradoxical effects (eg, excitation, hypertension). Consider therapy modification.
- **Rifampin**: Reduced peak linezolid concentration and AUC may occur.
- **Selective Serotonin Reuptake Inhibitors** (SSRIs; eg, **fluoxetine, sertraline**): Concurrent use may increase risk for serotonin syndrome. Avoid combination.
- **Serotonergic Agents** (eg, **buspirone, dextromethorphan, metoclopramide, mirtazapine, ondansetron, trazodone**): Additive serotonergic effects increase the risk for serotonin syndrome. Avoid combination.
- **Sympathomimetics** (eg, **albuterol, dopamine, epinephrine, phenylephrine, phenylpropanolamine**): May worsen hypertensive effect. Reduce initial doses of sympathomimetics and monitor blood pressure closely.
- **Tricyclic Antidepressants** (eg, **amitriptyline, clomipramine**): Concurrent use may increase risk for serotonin syndrome. Avoid combination.

Laboratory Considerations

- None

Dosages

DOGS/CATS

NOTE: Based on pharmacokinetic information in dogs,[4] linezolid could be given by the IV route at these same dosages.

Multidrug-resistant bacterial infections (extra-label): 10 mg/kg PO every 8 to 12 hours[11-13,17]

Nocardiosis unresponsive to standard therapies (extra-label): 8 – 20 mg/kg PO every 12 hours[18]

Monitoring

- Culture and susceptibility documenting resistance to other antimicrobials and susceptibility to linezolid
- Baseline and periodic CBC if treatment duration will exceed 14 days
- Clinical efficacy
- Neurologic examination as needed
- Venous blood gas, serum lactate

Client Information

- It is important to give this medication exactly as prescribed and to complete the full course of therapy, even if your animal seems better. Missing doses or stopping treatment early may result in treatment failure.
- The most common side effects are gastrointestinal upset (eg, excessive drooling, vomiting, diarrhea, poor appetite).
- Linezolid can be given with or without food, but if your animal experiences nausea or vomiting after administration, try giving the medication with food. If side effects persist, contact your veterinarian.
- While your animal is being treated with linezolid, talk with your veterinarian before making changes to diet (including treats), additional medications, and flea/tick treatments (eg, collars, spot-on treatments).

Chemistry/Synonyms

Linezolid is an oxazolidinone antibacterial that occurs as a white to off-white crystalline powder. It has a pK_a of 1.8 and is slightly soluble in ethanol and water.

Linezolid may also be known as linezolide, U-100766, *Zyvox*®, and many other trade names internationally.

Storage/Stability

Linezolid tablets and powder for reconstitution should be stored at 25°C (77°F) and protected from light and moisture.[5] Following reconstitution, linezolid oral suspension should be stored at room temperature and discarded after 21 days.

Store unopened IV bags at 25°C (77°F) in the protective overwrap to protect from light and freezing. The solution may develop a yellow color over time but there is no effect on potency. The IV bags are intended for single use only.

Compatibility/Compounding Considerations

Linezolid IV solution is **compatible** with 0.9% sodium chloride injection, 5% dextrose injection, and lactated Ringer's injection.[5] The manufacturer recommends linezolid be administered separately from other medication and the IV line should be flushed before and after linezolid administration.

Dosage Forms/Regulatory Status

VETERINARY-LABELED PRODUCTS: NONE

HUMAN-LABELED PRODUCTS:

Linezolid Tablets: 600 mg; *Zyvox*®, generic; (Rx)

Linezolid Powder for Oral Suspension: 20 mg/mL after reconstitution in 150 mL bottles; *Zyvox*®, generic; (Rx)

Linezolid IV Solution: 2 mg/mL in 300 mL IV bag; generic; (Rx)

Linezolid IV Solution (preservative free): 2 mg/mL in 100 mL and 300 mL IV bag; *Zyvox*®, generic; (Rx)

References

For the complete list of references, see **wiley.com/go/budde/plumb**

Liothyronine

Triiodothyronine

(lye-oh-***thye***-roe-neen) *Cytomel*®, *Triostat*®

Thyroid Hormone

Prescriber Highlights

- Form of T_3 (active thyroid hormone) primarily used in cats as part of the T_3 suppression test for diagnosing hyperthyroidism
- Occasionally used for treatment of hypothyroidism, but only recommended when patients are unresponsive to levothyroxine; generally, it is not recommended in dogs
- Shorter duration of effect than levothyroxine
- Contraindications include in patients with severe cardiac disease, heart failure, thyrotoxicosis, or untreated adrenal insufficiency.
- Use with caution in patients with cardiac disease, in those being treated for adrenal insufficiency or diabetes mellitus, and in elderly patients.
- Do not confuse with levothyroxine or desiccated thyroid.

Uses/Indications

In cats, liothyronine is used to perform a T_3 suppression test as part of the diagnosis of hyperthyroidism.

Liothyronine is not recommended for initial therapy of hypothyroidism because only serum T_3 concentrations are normalized, whereas T_4 concentrations remain low. Because serum T_4 concentrations are important in the feedback regulation of the hypothalamic-pituitary-thyroid axis, dogs receiving T_3 supplementation may be more susceptible to iatrogenic thyrotoxicosis. Occasionally, animals not responding to levothyroxine due to inadequate GI absorption will respond to liothyronine; however, it is generally not recommended in dogs due to its shorter duration of effect that requires 3 times daily administration and its likelihood to cause iatrogenic hyperthyroidism. Combination products that contain both T_3 and T_4 should also be avoided for similar reasons.[1]

Pharmacology/Actions

Liothyronine is a synthetic form of triiodothyronine (T_3). In humans, T_3 is the primary hormone responsible for activity. Approximately 80% of T_3 found in the peripheral tissues is derived from thyroxine (T), which is the principal hormone released by the thyroid gland. Thyroid hormones affect the rate of many physiologic processes including fat, protein, and carbohydrate metabolism. Thyroid hormones increase protein synthesis, increase gluconeogenesis, and promote mobilization and utilization of glycogen stores. Thyroid hormones also increase oxygen consumption, body temperature, heart rate and cardiac output, blood volume, enzyme system activity, and growth and maturity. Thyroid hormones are particularly important for adequate development of the central nervous system.

Pharmacokinetics

In dogs, peak plasma concentrations of liothyronine occur 2 to 5 hours after oral dosing. The plasma half-life is ≈5 to 6 hours. In contrast to levothyroxine, it is believed that liothyronine is nearly completely absorbed by dogs and absorption is not as affected by stomach contents or intestinal flora changes.

Contraindications/Precautions/Warnings

Liothyronine and other thyroid replacement hormones are contraindicated in patients with severe cardiac disease, heart failure, thyrotoxicosis, or untreated adrenal insufficiency. Liothyronine should be used with caution and at a lower initial dose in patients with adrenal insufficiency, cardiac disease, or diabetes mellitus, and in elderly patients.

Adverse Effects

When liothyronine is administered at an appropriate dose to patients requiring thyroid hormone replacement, adverse effects are uncommon.

In humans, the most common adverse effects are clinical signs of hyperthyroidism including arrhythmias, irritability, insomnia, tremors, muscle weakness, increased appetite, weight loss, diarrhea, and skin rashes.[2]

Reproductive/Nursing Safety

Minimal amounts of thyroid hormones are excreted in milk and should not adversely affect nursing offspring.

Because safety has not been established in animals, this drug should only be used when the maternal benefits outweigh the potential risks to offspring.

Overdose/Acute Toxicity

Chronic overdoses will produce signs of hyperthyroidism, including tachycardia, polyphagia, polyuria, polydipsia, excitability, nervousness, and excessive panting. The dose should be reduced and/or temporarily withheld until signs subside. Some cats may exhibit signs of apathetic hyperthyroidism (eg, listlessness, anorexia).

Acute, massive overdoses can produce signs resembling a thyroid storm, such as fever, CNS effects (eg, agitation, seizures), GI and hepatic dysfunction (eg, vomiting, jaundice), and cardiovascular effects (eg, sinus tachycardia, atrial fibrillation, ventricular tachycardia, heart failure). After oral ingestion, treatment to reduce absorption of the drug should be accomplished using standard protocols (eg, emetics or gastric lavage, cathartics, charcoal) unless contraindicated by the patient's condition. Treatment is supportive and based on clinical signs. Oxygen, artificial ventilation, cardiac glycosides, beta-blockers (eg, propranolol), fluids, dextrose, and antipyretic agents have all been suggested for use if necessary.

For patients that have experienced or are suspected to have experienced an overdose, consultation with a 24-hour poison consultation center specializing in providing veterinary-specific information is recommended. For general information related to overdose and toxin exposures, as well as contact information for poison control centers, refer to ***Appendix***.

Drug Interactions

The following drug interactions have either been reported or are theoretical in humans or animals receiving liothyronine and may be of significance in veterinary patients. Unless otherwise noted, use together is not necessarily contraindicated, but weigh the potential risks and perform additional monitoring when appropriate.

- Antidepressants, Tricyclic/Tetracyclic (eg, **amitriptyline**, **clomipramine**): Increased risk for CNS stimulation and cardiac arrhythmias
- Antidiabetic Agents (eg, **glipizide**, **insulin**): May increase requirements for insulin or oral agents.
- Cholestyramine: May reduce liothyronine absorption; separate doses by 4 hours
- Digoxin: Potential for reduced digoxin concentrations
- Ketamine: May cause tachycardia and hypertension
- Sympathomimetics (eg, **epinephrine**, **norepinephrine**): May potentiate the sympathomimetic effects
- Warfarin: Thyroid hormones increase the catabolism of vitamin K-dependent clotting factors that may increase the anticoagulation effects in patients on warfarin.

Laboratory Considerations

- **Renal function tests**: Hypothyroid dogs can have decreased GFR (creatinine clearance); restoration to a euthyroid state can increase GFR and reduce serum creatinine concentrations.

The following drugs may have effects on thyroid function tests; evaluate results accordingly:

- **Effects on serum T_4**: aminoglutethimide, anabolic steroids/androgens, antithyroid drugs (eg, propylthiouracil [PTU], methimazole), asparaginase, barbiturates, corticosteroids, danazol, diazepam, estrogens, fluorouracil, heparin, insulin, lithium carbonate, mitotane (o,p-DDD), nitroprusside, phenylbutazone, phenytoin, propranolol, salicylates (large doses), sulfonamides, and sulfonylureas
- **Effects on serum T_3**: antithyroid drugs (eg, PTU, methimazole), barbiturates, corticosteroids, estrogens, fluorouracil, heparin, lithium carbonate, phenytoin, propranolol, salicylates (large doses), sulfonamides, and thiazides
- **Effects on T_3 uptake resin**: anabolic steroids/androgens, antithyroid drugs (eg, PTU, methimazole), asparaginase, corticosteroids, danazol, estrogens, fluorouracil, heparin, lithium carbonate, phenylbutazone, and salicylates (large doses)
- **Effects on serum TSH**: aminoglutethimide, antithyroid drugs (eg, PTU, methimazole), corticosteroids, danazol, lithium carbonate, and sulfonamides
- **Effects on free thyroxine index (FTI)**: antithyroid drugs (eg, PTU, methimazole), barbiturates, corticosteroids, heparin, lithium carbonate, and phenylbutazone

Dosages

DOGS:

Hypothyroidism (extra-label): Initially, 4 – 6 µg/kg PO every 8 hours.[1] Dose should be adjusted based on postdose serum T_3 concentrations. Once clinical control is achieved, the dosing frequency may be decreased to twice daily; if clinical signs recur, then frequency should be increased back to every 8 hours.

CATS:

T_3 suppression test to diagnose hyperthyroidism (extra-label): Measure baseline T_3 and T_4 concentrations, then administer liothyronine 25 µg/cat (NOT µg/kg) PO every 8 hours for 7 doses. Measure T_3 and T_4 concentrations again 2 to 4 hours after the last dose.[3] In euthyroid cats, the second T_4 concentration should be either less than 1.5 µg/dL (20 nmol/L) or at least 50% lower than the baseline T_4 concentration. Cats with hyperthyroidism fail to suppress. The measurement of T_3 concentrations before and after liothyronine administration helps to confirm that all doses were given and that the drug was adequately absorbed.[4]

Hypothyroidism (extra-label): Initially, 4.4 µg /kg PO 2 to 3 times daily.[5] Dose should be adjusted based on postdose serum T_3 concentrations. Once clinical control is achieved, the dosing frequency may be decreased to twice daily; if clinical signs recur, then frequency should be increased back to every 8 hours

Monitoring

- Clinical response: The goal of therapy is resolution of clinical signs of hypothyroidism.
- Serum total T_3: Draw serum just prior to dosing (trough) and again 2 to 4 hours after administering the drug.
- Serum total T_4: Unlike levothyroxine, T_4 concentrations will remain low with liothyronine treatment.
- Serum TSH: May be useful if TSH was abnormal prior to therapy

Client Information

- It is important to give this medication exactly as your veterinarian has prescribed. Missing doses or stopping treatment early may result in treatment failure.
- The most common side effects of this medicine are signs of too much thyroid hormone, such as increased hunger or thirst, excitability, or excessive panting. Contact your veterinarian if any of these signs occur.

Chemistry/Synonyms

Liothyronine is a synthetically prepared sodium salt of the naturally occurring hormone T_3 and occurs as an odorless, light tan crystalline powder. It is very slightly soluble in water and slightly soluble in alcohol. Each 25 µg of liothyronine is equivalent to ≈60 to 65 mg (1 grain) of thyroglobulin or desiccated thyroid and 100 µg or less of levothyroxine.

Liothyronine sodium may also be known as T_3, T_3 thyronine sodium, L-triiodothyronine, sodium L-triiodothyronine, liothyroninum natricum, sodium liothyronine, l-tri-iodothyronine sodium, 3,5,3'-Tri-iodo-L-thyronine sodium, or *Cytomel*®.

Storage/Stability

Liothyronine tablets should be stored at room temperature (15°C-30°C [59°F-86°F]) in tight containers.

The injection should be stored refrigerated (2°C-8°C [36°F-46°F]).

Compatibility/Compounding Considerations

No specific information was noted.

Dosage Forms/Regulatory Status

VETERINARY-LABELED PRODUCTS: NONE

HUMAN-LABELED PRODUCTS:

Liothyronine Sodium Tablets: 5 µg, 25 µg, and 50 µg; *Cytomel*®, generic; (Rx)

Liothyronine Sodium Injection Solution: 10 µg/mL in 1 mL vials; *Triostat*®, generic; (Rx)

References

For the complete list of references, see **wiley.com/go/budde/plumb**

Lipid Emulsion, Intravenous (ILE)

Fat Emulsion, Intravenous

Parenteral Nutritional Agent; Antidote *Intralipid*®

Prescriber Highlights

- Parenteral calorie and fatty acid source
- Can be useful in overdoses and poisonings to reduce free-drug blood concentrations of lipid-soluble toxins or drugs. Not a substitute for standard supportive measures in intoxicated patients. Only 20% lipid emulsion IV infusions should be used when treating toxicoses.
- The use of IV lipid emulsion (ILE) in toxicoses primarily consists of case reports and case series; the ideal dosages and protocols are still to be determined.
- Potentially serious adverse effects can occur (eg, hypersensitivity, lipemia, lipid overload).

Uses/Indications

IV lipid emulsions (ILEs), with or without dextrose and amino acids, can be used as a source of calories or essential fatty acids when parenteral feeding is required.

ILE may also be used as a rescue treatment for intoxications caused by lipid-soluble drugs and toxins when traditional treatments are not effective.[1,2] As certain treatments available for humans (eg, hemoperfusion, hemodialysis, long-term ventilator, or intensive care) are either widely unavailable or cost-prohibitive in veterinary medicine, early intervention with ILE for lipid-soluble (ie, lipophilic) toxin or drug toxicosis in patients with severe clinical signs may be a relatively low cost and safe intervention. A drug or toxin is considered lipophilic, and hence potentially amenable to ILE rescue treatment, when its oil:water partition coefficient ("log *P*") exceeds 2 (the greater the log *P* value, the more lipophilic the substance is).[1] Log *P* values can usually be found at the PubChem website. Note that lipophilicity/log *P* is not the only determinant to whether a toxicosis will respond to ILE treatment and contacting a 24-hour poison consultation center specializing in providing veterinary-specific information is recommended.

Most veterinary cases of lipid infusion in the management of toxicoses involve dogs and cats but it has been used in other species, including goats, a pony,[3] and a lion.[4]

Evidence exists that ILE could be useful for reducing free-drug concentrations for drugs or drug classes such as local anesthetics (eg, bupivacaine, mepivacaine, ropivacaine, lidocaine), macrocyclic lactones (eg, ivermectin, moxidectin), calcium channel blockers (eg, diltiazem, verapamil, amlodipine), beta-blockers (eg, propranolol, carvedilol), antidepressants (eg, bupropion, doxepin, sertraline, clomipramine), antipsychotics (eg, chlorpromazine, quetiapine), antiepileptics (eg, carbamazepine, lamotrigine[5-7]), cannabis and synthetic cannabinoids, and muscle relaxants (eg, baclofen, cyclobenzaprine).[8-10]

It has also been used in the management of poisoning with permethrin, grayanotoxins, loperamide, NSAIDs, cocaine, metaldehyde, bromethalin,[11] minoxidil, carbamate,[12] methamphetamine,[12] dextroamphetamine sulfate,[12] and tremorgenic mycotoxins.[13] A case report describes successful use of ILE to resuscitate a foal after IV lidocaine-induced cardiovascular collapse.[14] Another case report describes the use of low dose ILE in 2 goats with ivermectin overdose.

Pharmacology/Actions

IV lipid emulsion (ILE) administration is an efficient method of providing calories (1 mL of a 20% emulsion provides ≈2 kcal) and serves as a source of essential fatty acids. In addition, ILE can have immunosuppressive effects, increase pro-inflammatory cytokines, and affect pulmonary function.

When used for toxicologic indications, ILE's exact mechanism of action is unknown, but it may serve as a lipid sink or shuttle for lipid-soluble compounds, reducing the amount of free drug in the circulation, thereby reducing the drug's toxic effects. Other hypotheses include improving cardiac performance and function by increasing intracellular calcium and/or providing an energy substrate for myocytes, and increasing the pool of fatty acids, thus overcoming the inhibition of mitochondrial fatty acid metabolism by drugs such as bupivacaine. In experimental studies, cardiac output has been shown to improve with lipid therapy due to decreased tissue toxin concentrations, increased liver metabolism, and accelerated unbinding of toxin from ion channels.[15]

Pharmacokinetics

IV lipid emulsion (ILE) appears to be removed from the blood stream about as rapidly as chylomicrons, but the rate of removal requires prior lipolysis of ILE into free fatty acids and seems to be increased with heparin-activated lipoprotein. In humans, elimination half-life is ≈30 minutes, with clearance from the bloodstream in 5 to 6 hours.

Contraindications/Precautions/Warnings

IV lipid emulsions (ILEs) are contraindicated in patients with severe egg yolk allergies, abnormal lipid metabolism, hyperlipemia, increased bleeding tendency, hypokalemia, or hypophosphatemia. In humans, ILEs are used with caution in premature and low birth weight infants (black box warning; lipemia), patients with blood coagulation disorders, pulmonary disease, renal impairment, severe liver damage, and those at risk for lipid emboli.[16]

The volume of lipid administered over a short period can result in fluid overload. If this is a concern, temporarily stop or reduce the administration rate of other fluids.[16]

Strict aseptic technique and good IV catheter care are imperative when using ILE with or without amino acids and dextrose. When used alone, ILE may be administered via a peripheral line but when combined with amino acids and dextrose as central parenteral nutrition (CPN), a dedicated central line is required due to the solution's hypertonicity.

Use with caution in neonates, as an increased risk for lipid emboli has been reported in premature human infants.[16]

When managing poisoned patients, ILE is not a substitute for standard supportive care. Delayed toxicity is a potential risk, as the toxin diffuses out of the lipid or as the lipid is metabolized; therefore, animals must be monitored.

Although there are no studies specifically addressing the role or safety of lipids in critically ill animals, human data suggest that lipid administration may be associated with significant immunosuppression, exacerbation of pre-existing pulmonary pathology, and increased infection rates. Data also suggest that withholding lipids for moderate periods of time is not associated with an increase in morbidity or mortality.[17]

Adverse Effects

Although IV lipid emulsion's (ILE's) adverse effect profile and incidence rates in veterinary patients have not been thoroughly reported, they are likely similar to those seen in human patients. Adverse effects reported in veterinary cases include pancreatitis, hyperlipemia, unilateral facial pruritus, extravasation with pain and local swelling, prolonged gross lipemia (lasting more than 48 hours), hemolysis, and suspected corneal lipidosis.[10,18-22] Because of the high volume given over a short period, volume overload can be a concern.[2] One case report described suspected acute respiratory distress syndrome (ARDS) in a dog treated with ILE.[23]

In humans, adverse effects associated with ILE are infrequent and usually associated with ILE used for nutritional support. The most commonly reported adverse effects are sepsis or thrombophlebitis secondary to IV administration, but these can occur whether or not IV lipids are used in parenteral nutrition therapy. Lipid overload syndrome (hyperlipemia, hepatomegaly, icterus, splenomegaly, lipid embolism, thrombocytopenia, hemolysis, and prolonged clotting times) can occur, particularly if doses are too high or administration is too fast. More rarely (in less than 1% of cases), ILE can cause pulmonary toxicity, GI effects, somnolence, headache, flushing, lipid emboli, hyperlipemia, pancreatitis, hypercoagulability, and hypersensitivity. ILE effects on pulmonary function and oxygenation are temporary and resolve after discontinuation.

Reproductive/Nursing Safety

IV lipid emulsion (ILE) has been used in the management of poisonings and as parenteral nutrition in pregnant humans. When used in situations where it is clearly needed, the benefits of using ILE during pregnancy would likely outweigh the risks.

No data regarding the safe use of ILE during lactation are available, and although ILE is likely safe, nursing may not be appropriate for mothers that require ILE.

Because safety has not been established in animals, this drug should only be used when the maternal benefits outweigh the potential risks to offspring.

Overdose/Acute Toxicity

In the case of an inadvertent overdose, stop the infusion until the lipid has cleared. This can be evaluated in a gross manner by visually inspecting the plasma (hematocrit tubes), or by laboratory methods (eg, triglyceride concentrations, plasma light-scattering activity by nephelometry).

When using IV lipid emulsion (ILE) for drug toxicity and in cases where severe hyperlipemia is present, heparin therapy 75 – 250 units/kg SC every 6 hours can be considered. Heparin may increase lipid clearance (not proven) and the use of heparin may potentially affect the mechanism of action of ILE for lipid-soluble toxicosis. Some advocate using heparin when hyperlipemia occurs in dog breeds susceptible to pancreatitis (eg, Shetland sheepdog, miniature schnauzer, Yorkshire terrier, obese animals), although there is no direct proof that hyperlipemia secondary to ILE increases the risk for pancreatitis. Otherwise, heparin therapy is not recommended unless clinical signs or advanced diagnostics indicate otherwise. Monitor partial thromboplastin time (PTT) prior to use of heparin to ensure the patient is not already coagulopathic. If PTT exceeds 2 to 2.5 times the normal dose, the dose of heparin should either be reduced to 75 units/kg SC every 6 to 8 hours or discontinued.[24]

For patients that have experienced or are suspected to have experienced an overdose, consultation with a 24-hour poison consultation center specializing in providing veterinary-specific information is recommended. For general information related to overdose and toxin exposures, as well as contact information for poison control centers, refer to ***Appendix.***

Drug Interactions

The following drug interaction has either been reported or is theoretical in humans or animals receiving IV lipid emulsion (ILE) and may be of significance in veterinary patients. Unless otherwise noted, use together is not necessarily contraindicated, but weigh the potential risks and perform additional monitoring when appropriate.

- **Lipid-Soluble Drugs**: IV lipid emulsion (ILE) may affect the pharmacokinetics of lipid-soluble drugs by serving as a lipid sink or shuttle for free drug in circulation. At present, clinical significance is not clear; however, when ILE is used as a nutritional agent, concurrently with a lipid-soluble drug, be aware of possible decreased drug efficacy.

Laboratory Considerations

Blood samples for diagnostics should be collected prior to administration of IV lipid emulsion (ILE) to minimize effects from hyperlipemia.[25] This interference can be physical or chemical, particularly for electrophoretic testing methods, nonspecific interference in immunoassays, and most commonly interference in spectrophotometric testing methods, as lipid particles can absorb light.

- Falsely high **potassium, hemoglobin, MCH,** and **MCHC** values can occur if samples are drawn during or shortly after ILE infusion.
- Some analyzers (eg, *Hemocue®*) may report falsely high **blood glucose** values.
- **Serum bilirubin, phosphate, creatinine, oxygen saturation, AST,** and **lactate dehydrogenase** values may be affected by ILE.

Dosages

Nutritional agent for parenteral nutrition (extra-label): **NOTE**: If using IV lipid emulsion (ILE) for parenteral nutrition, it is recommended to consult with a veterinary nutritionist and refer to more detailed references.[26,27] The following are examples:

a) Most recommendations are to consider IV lipids as energy substrates, and to administer them at 30% to 40% of total calories. In veterinary medicine, lipid administration ranges from 25% to 60% of calories administered.[17] Traditionally, ILE administration is not recommended at more than 2 g/kg/day for parenteral nutrition therapy.[28]

b) There are 2 strategies employed by nutritionists to supply calories. One approach is to provide daily resting energy requirements (RER) with a mixture of all 3 nutrients (protein, dextrose, lipids) starting with a provision of adequate protein (4 – 6 g/100 kcal). Another approach is to supply the daily RER in dextrose and lipids and add protein "on top." This approach asserts that proteins not catabolized for energy can be used to maintain protein synthesis.

   Hyperalimentation may occur more frequently with the second approach. Generally, either approach can be used for central parenteral nutrition, but with peripheral parenteral nutrition, care should be taken with the second approach to keep the solution below 600 mOsm/L. Some nutritionists supplement lipids alone at RER for up to 3 days. For example, in a 10 kg (22 lb) dog with RER of 370 kcal/day, *Intralipid®* 20% solution (2 kcal/mL) could supply RER peripherally at 8 mL/hour. The lipid component of parenteral nutrition is controversial, and some nutritionists do not include lipids in parenteral nutrition for critically ill patients because of concerns of increased complications due to infection, immunosuppression, free radical generation, and inflammation. Use caution when using imbalanced strategies.[29]

Rescue agent for fat-soluble drug toxicoses and other toxicoses (extra-label): **NOTE**: For additional guidance, it is highly recommended to contact an animal poison center. See ***Appendix*** for contact information. The dosages listed below are for the use of ILE 20%, which is recommended for all suggested treatment protocols in small animal medicine. Additional information on using ILE for this purpose has been published.[19,20,30] Many treatment protocols exist; the following are examples:

a) 1.5 – 4 mL/kg over 1 minute, followed by 0.25 mL/kg/minute IV CRI over 30 to 60 minutes in dogs. In animals nonresponsive after this traditional dosing protocol, additional individual bolus doses can be administered slowly at up to 7 mL/kg IV. Authors have recommended intermittent IV boluses of 1.5 mL/kg every 4 to 6 hours for the initial 24 hours with anecdotal success.[1] In addition, it is likely safe to assume that follow-up IV CRI doses of 0.05 mL/kg/hour can be continued until clinical signs improve (not to exceed 24 hours). That said, there have been no safety studies evaluating the use of ILE in the clinically poisoned veterinary patient, and careful monitoring and risk assessment is important.

b) 1.5 mL/kg IV over 5 to 15 minutes, followed by 0.25 mL/kg per minute IV CRI over 1 to 2 hours. This dose can be repeated in several hours if clinical signs of toxicosis return. Prior to repeating the dose, a peripheral blood sample should be evaluated for evidence of lipemia; additional doses should not be given if serum is lipemic.[31]

c) 2.25 mL/kg IV initial loading dose of ILE 20%, followed by 0.025 mL/kg/minute IV CRI for up to 6.5 hours. This regimen aims to produce a modestly elevated plasma lipid concentration and is derived from pharmacokinetic and pharmacodynamics modeling.[25]

d) **For severe, protracted neurotoxicity caused by lipophilic substances (eg, permethrin, ivermectin, and other macro-lactones)**[2]: Initially, administer 1.5 mL/kg IV slowly over 1 to 2 minutes then begin 0.25 mL/kg/minute IV CRI for 30 to 60 minutes. If there is a risk for volume overload, consider a reduced rate of 0.07 mL/kg/minute for 4 hours. Evaluate patient 4 to 6 hours after stopping ILE administration. If insufficient or no clinical improvement, repeat dose once or twice as soon as the plasma/serum is no longer lipemic and there are no signs of hemolysis. Maximum total dose of ILE is 16.5 mL/kg in 60 minutes.

e) **For severe, potentially life-threatening cardiotoxicity induced by IV administered lipophilic substances**[2]: Initially, administer 1.5 mL/kg IV slowly over 1 minute then immediately begin 0.25 mL/kg/minute IV CRI. Evaluate patient after 5 minutes. If necessary, a second ILE bolus of 1.5 mL/kg IV over 1 minute can be administered. A final IV bolus may be given 5 minutes later, for a maximum of 3 total boluses. Alternatively, the CRI can be increased to 0.5 mL/kg/minute. As soon as heart function and circulation are restored, the CRI can be continued for a minimum of 10 minutes or until a maximum dose time of 30 minutes has been reached. Maximum total dose of ILE is 10 – 12 mL/kg in 30 minutes.

f) **Ivermectin overdose in 2 goats**: Initially, 2 mL/kg IV slowly over 15 minutes, followed by 0.008 mL/kg/minute IV CRI for 24 to 48 hours[32]

Monitoring

- When used for toxicity indications:
  - Drug concentrations (serum or plasma) to evaluate response to IV lipid emulsion (ILE) therapy. This information will aid in data collection for future retrospective study analysis. Although blood sampling times should be based on the pharmacokinetics of the drug, general recommendations for sampling times are time 0 (at the time of presentation), then 30 minutes, 1 hour, 6 hours, 12 hours, and 24 hours after administration of ILE.[24]
  - Monitor serum every 2 hours and consider additional infusions if the patient is still showing signs and the serum is clear of lipemia. Do not repeat ILE if the serum is very orange or yellow. If no improvement is noted after 3 doses (bolus and IV CRI), discontinue ILE therapy.[19]
  - Ensure tissue perfusion and oxygenation are maximized prior to administration of lipids. Animal studies suggest an adverse outcome of resuscitation and lipid infusion in the presence of hypoxia, possibly due to changes in the binding capacity of the lipid.

- Patients should be monitored for volume overload or allergic reactions during the infusion.[33] If there is concern for volume overload, either stop the infusion or decrease to 0.07 mL/kg/minute.

- When used for nutritional support, monitoring can be complicated and may include blood glucose, serum triglycerides, presence of lipemia, PCV, total protein, IV catheter patency and site status, hydration status, vital signs (eg, temperature, respiration rate, heart rate), serum electrolytes (including phosphorous), renal parameters (eg, BUN, creatinine) and hepatic enzyme monitoring (eg, ALT, AST, ALP), and CBC. It is recommended to consult with a veterinary nutritionist and refer to a veterinary nutrition reference for detailed information.

Client Information

- IV lipid emulsion (ILE) products should only be used by professionals in a setting where adequate patient monitoring is available.

Chemistry/Synonyms

IV lipid emulsion (ILE) products are emulsified soybean (*Intralipid*®; *Nutrilipid*®), or soybean and fish oils (*SMOFlipid*®) that provide the fatty acids linoleic, stearic, linolenic, oleic, and palmitic acids. Egg yolk phospholipids serve as the primary emulsifying agent and glycerol is used to adjust tonicity. Osmolarity varies with product, but ranges from 200 to 293 mOsm/L. The pH of ILE is between 6 and 9. Initially the pH is ≈9, but secondary to hydrolysis of triglycerides into free fatty acids (FFA), the pH decreases to 6 at the end of the product's shelf-life.

ILE may also be known as intravenous fat emulsion (IVFE), IVLE, and IFE.

Storage/Stability

Unopened IV lipid emulsion (ILE) products should be stored at room temperature (not above 25°C [77°F]) and not allowed to freeze.[16] If accidentally frozen, product should be discarded. If a partial amount of a bag or bottle is used, the remaining product should be stored protected in the refrigerator (2°C-8°C [36°F-46°F]) and discarded 24 hours after opening. A new bag or vial must be used within 24 hours.

Compatibility/Compounding Considerations

Compatibility is dependent on factors such as pH, concentration, temperature, and diluent used; specialized references or a hospital pharmacist should be consulted for more specific information.

IV lipid emulsion (ILE) is **compatible** when mixed with the usual components used in parenteral nutrition (dextrose, amino acids, parenteral multivitamins, and trace elements), but as concentrations and mixing order can affect compatibility, it is advisable to contact a hospital pharmacist or refer to a drug compatibility reference for more information. This is particularly important as the opaque nature of ILE makes detection of precipitates very difficult.

Admixtures must be prepared with strict aseptic technique. Do not add additives directly to ILE, and in no case, add lipid emulsion to the total parenteral nutrition container first. The correct order of mixing is as follows: 1) transfer dextrose to the admixture container; 2) transfer amino acid solution; then 3) transfer lipid emulsion. Alternatively, amino acids, dextrose, and lipid emulsion may be simultaneously transferred to the admixture container; gently agitate the mixture. Use these admixtures promptly; store under refrigeration (2°C-8°C [36°F-46°F]) for 24 hours or less and use within 24 hours after removal from refrigeration.

Dosage Forms/Regulatory Status

VETERINARY-LABELED PRODUCTS: NONE

HUMAN-LABELED PRODUCTS:

Fat Emulsion (plant-based; soybean), IV 10%, 20%, and 30%; depending on product, in 100 mL, 250 mL, 500 mL, and 1000 mL bottles or bags; *Intralipid*®, *Nutrilipid*®; (Rx)

Fat Emulsion (fish oil and plant-based), IV 20% depending on product, in 100 mL, 250 mL, and 500 mL bags; *SMOFlipid*®; (Rx)

References

For the complete list of references, see **wiley.com/go/budde/plumb**

Lisinopril

(lye-***sin***-oh-pril) *Prinivil*®, *Zestril*®

Angiotensin-Converting Enzyme (ACE) Inhibitor

Prescriber Highlights

- ► ACE inhibitor that may be useful as a vasodilator in the treatment of heart failure or hypertension; it may also be of benefit in the treatment of chronic renal failure or protein-losing nephropathies.
- ► May be less expensive than other ACE inhibitors and possibly can be dosed once daily. When compared to enalapril and benazepril, limited information or clinical experience for use in dogs or cats is available.
- ► Use caution in patients with renal insufficiency (doses may need to be reduced), hyponatremia, coronary or cerebrovascular insufficiency, or hepatic disease.
- ► Adverse effects may include GI distress (anorexia, vomiting, diarrhea), weakness, hypotension, renal dysfunction, and hyperkalemia.

Uses/Indications

The principal uses of lisinopril in veterinary medicine at present are as a vasodilator in the treatment of heart failure or hypertension. Studies have demonstrated that ACE inhibitors, particularly when used in conjunction with furosemide, improve the quality of life in dogs with heart failure. It is not clear, however, whether it has any significant effect on survival times. Lisinopril may also be of benefit in treating the effects associated with valvular heart disease (mitral regurgitation) and left to right shunts.[1] Lisinopril is being explored as adjunctive treatment in chronic renal failure and protein-losing nephropathies.[2]

Lisinopril may have advantages over other ACE inhibitors in that it may be dosed once daily but there is little published information on its use (efficacy, safety, dosing) in veterinary species.

Pharmacology/Actions

Unlike enalapril, lisinopril does not need to be converted in the liver to an active metabolite. Lisinopril prevents the formation of angiotensin-II (a potent vasoconstrictor) by competing with angiotensin-I for the enzyme angiotensin-converting enzyme (ACE). ACE has a much higher affinity for lisinopril than for angiotensin-I. Because angiotensin-II concentrations are decreased, aldosterone secretion is reduced, and plasma renin activity is increased. Lisinopril has a higher affinity for ACE than either enalapril or captopril.

The cardiovascular effects of lisinopril in patients with CHF include decreased total peripheral resistance, pulmonary vascular resistance, mean arterial and right atrial pressures, and pulmonary capillary wedge pressure, no change or decrease in heart rate, and increased cardiac index and output, stroke volume, and exercise tolerance. Renal blood flow can be increased with little change in hepatic blood flow. In animals with glomerular disease, ACE inhibitors probably decrease proteinuria and help to preserve renal function.

Pharmacokinetics

In dogs, lisinopril's bioavailability ranges from 25% to 50%, with peak concentrations occurring ≈4 hours after dosing. Lisinopril is distributed poorly into the CNS. It is unknown if it is distributed into maternal milk, but it does cross the placenta. Half-lives are increased in patients with renal failure or severe CHF. Duration of action in dogs has been described as being 24 hours, but effects tend to drop off with time.

No information was located for cats.

Contraindications/Precautions/Warnings

Lisinopril is contraindicated in patients that have demonstrated hypersensitivity to the ACE inhibitors. It should be used with caution and close supervision in patients with renal insufficiency, and doses may need to be reduced.

Lisinopril should be used with caution in patients with hyponatremia or sodium depletion, coronary or cerebrovascular insufficiency, or hepatic failure. Patients with severe CHF should be monitored closely upon initiation of therapy.

Adverse Effects

Lisinopril's adverse effect profile in dogs is reportedly similar to other ACE inhibitors, principally GI distress (anorexia, vomiting, diarrhea). Potentially, weakness, hypotension, renal dysfunction, and hyperkalemia could occur.

Reproductive/Nursing Safety

Lisinopril crosses the placenta. High doses in rodents have caused decreased fetal weights and increases in fetal and maternal death rates; teratogenic effects have not been reported. Current recommendations for humans are to discontinue ACE inhibitors as soon as pregnancy is detected.

It is not known whether lisinopril is excreted in the milk; use with caution.

Because safety has not been established in animals, this drug should only be used when the maternal benefits outweigh the potential risks to offspring.

Overdose/Acute Toxicity

The ASPCA Animal Poison Control Center (APCC) has over 3500 lisinopril exposure cases in its files, mostly involving dogs, but some birds and cats. The lowest dosage documented to cause hypotension in dogs is 27 mg/kg. Generally, dosages below 20 mg/kg cause mild signs only, most commonly vomiting and lethargy. Higher dosages warrant decontamination. Only a single cat out of 218 cats developed hypotension at a dosage of 4.9 mg/kg. In birds, only mild somnolence occurred at 41 mg/kg.

There were 1882 single-agent exposures to lisinopril reported to the ASPCA Animal Poison Control Center (APCC) from 2009 to 2013. There were 1781 dogs exposed and 156 that became symptomatic. The most common clinical signs included lethargy (24%), tachycardia (18%), vomiting (14%), and hypotension (13%). Of the 98 cats, 7 were symptomatic, with 29% hypertensive, 29% tachycardic, and 29% vomiting.

In overdose situations, the primary concern is hypotension; supportive treatment with volume expansion with normal saline is recommended to correct blood pressure. Because of the drug's long duration of action, prolonged monitoring and treatment may be required. Recent overdoses should be managed using gut-emptying protocols when warranted.

For patients that have experienced or are suspected of having experienced an overdose, consultation with a 24-hour poison consultation center specializing in providing veterinary-specific information is recommended. For general information related to overdose and toxin exposures, as well as contact information for poison control centers, refer to ***Appendix.***

Drug Interactions

The following drug interactions have either been reported or are theoretical in humans or animals receiving lisinopril and may be of significance in veterinary patients. Unless otherwise noted, use together is not necessarily contraindicated, but weigh the potential risks and perform additional monitoring when appropriate.

- **Anesthetics**: Concurrent use may increase the risk for hypotension.
- **Angiotensin Receptor Blockers** (eg, **telmisartan**): Concurrent use of an ACE inhibitor with an angiotensin II receptor antagonist may cause additive effects on the renin-angiotensin system causing hyperkalemia, hypotension, syncope, and acute kidney injury
- **Antacids, Aluminum-, Calcium-, or Magnesium-Containing**: Reduced oral absorption of lisinopril may occur if given concomitantly with antacids; it is suggested to separate dosing by at least 2 hours.
- **Antihypertensive Agents and Vasodilators** (eg, **amlodipine, hydralazine, nitrates, prazosin, sildenafil**): Concurrent use may increase the risk for hypotension and other adverse effects; doses should be titrated carefully.
- **Buspirone**: Concurrent use may increase the risk for hypotension.
- **Cabergoline**: Concurrent use may lead to additive hypotension.
- **Corticosteroids** (eg, **dexamethasone, fludrocortisone, predniso(lo)ne**): May decrease the antihypertensive effects of ACE inhibitors
- **Darbepoetin, Epoetin**: ACE inhibitors may interfere with erythropoietin.
- **Digoxin**: Levels may increase 15% to 30% when an ACE inhibitor is added, automatic reduction in dosage is not recommended, but monitoring of serum digoxin levels should be performed.
- **Diphenhydramine**: Concurrent use may increase the risk for hypotension.
- **Disopyramide**: Hypoglycemic effects may be enhanced.
- **Diuretics** (eg, **furosemide**): Concomitant diuretics may cause hypotension if used with lisinopril; titrate dosages carefully.
- **Doxepin**: Concurrent use may increase the risk for hypotension.
- **Glycerin, Oral**: Concurrent use may increase the risk for hypotension.
- **Heparin, Low Molecular Weight Heparins** (eg, **dalteparin, enoxaparin**): Concurrent use may increase the risk for hyperkalemia.
- **Lanthanum**: Reduced oral absorption of lisinopril may occur if given concomitantly; it is suggested to separate dosing by at least 2 hours.
- **Nonsteroidal Anti-inflammatory Agents** (**NSAIDs**; eg, **carprofen, meloxicam, robenacoxib**): May reduce the clinical efficacy of lisinopril when it is being used as an antihypertensive agent; combination may result in decreased renal function
- **Opioids** (eg, **butorphanol, hydrocodone, morphine**): Concurrent use may increase the risk for hypotension.
- **Potassium or Potassium Sparing Diuretics** (eg, **spironolactone**): Hyperkalemia may develop.

Laboratory Considerations

- ACE inhibitors may cause a reversible decrease in localization and excretion of **iodohippurate sodium** I^{123}/I^{134}, or **Technetium** Tc^{99} pentetate renal imaging in the affected kidney in patients with renal artery stenosis, that may lead to confusion in test interpretation.

Dosages

DOGS:

Adjunctive treatment of heart failure or for other uses when an ACE inhibitor is indicated: Anecdotally, 0.5 mg/kg PO once or twice daily. In a single-dose pharmacokinetic study, lisinopril

0.5 mg/kg PO reduced ACE activity to a similar degree as enalapril 0.5 mg/kg PO.

CATS:

Adjunctive treatment of heart failure or for other uses when an ACE inhibitor is indicated (extra-label): 2.5 mg total PO once daily in combination with a low sodium diet decreased arterial blood pressure.[3] Anecdotally: 0.25 – 0.5 mg/kg PO once daily.

Monitoring

- Clinical signs of CHF
- Serum electrolytes, creatinine, BUN, urine protein:creatinine ratio
- CBC with differential, periodic
- Blood pressure (if treating hypertension or signs associated with hypotension arise)

Client Information

- Lisinopril is used to treat heart failure, high blood pressure, and some forms of kidney disease in dogs and cats.
- This medicine is usually well tolerated but vomiting and diarrhea can occur. Give this medicine with food if vomiting or lack of appetite becomes a problem. If a rash or signs of infection occur (eg, fever), contact your veterinarian immediately.
- Very important to give lisinopril as prescribed. Do not stop or reduce the dosage without your veterinarian's guidance.
- Your animal will likely need to have blood pressure and lab tests performed while receiving lisinopril.

Chemistry/Synonyms

An oral angiotensin-converting enzyme inhibitor (ACE inhibitor), lisinopril is directly active and not a prodrug like enalapril. It occurs as a white crystalline powder. One milligram is soluble in 10 mL of water, 70 mL of methanol. It is practically insoluble in alcohol, chloroform, or ether.

Lisinopril may also be known as L-154826, lisinoprilum, and MK-521; many trade names are available.

Storage/Stability

Store lisinopril tablets at room temperature in tight containers unless otherwise directed by the manufacturer.

Compatibility/Compounding Considerations

Compounded preparation stability: Lisinopril oral suspension, compounded from the commercially available tablets, has been published.[4] Triturating ten (10) lisinopril 10 mg tablets with 50 mL of *Ora Plus*® and qs ad to 100 mL with *Ora Sweet*® yields a 1 mg/mL lisinopril oral suspension that retains greater than 95% potency for 91 days when stored at 4°C (39.2°F) and protected from light.

Dosage Forms/Regulatory Status

VETERINARY-LABELED PRODUCTS: NONE

The ARCI (Racing Commissioners International) has designated this drug as a class 3 substance. See the ***Appendix*** for more information.

HUMAN-LABELED PRODUCTS:

Lisinopril Oral Tablets: 2.5 mg, 5 mg, 10 mg, 20 mg, 30 mg, and 40 mg; *Prinivil*®, *Zestril*®; (Rx).

Lisinopril Oral Solution: 1 mg/mL; *Qbrelis*®; (Rx).

Also available are fixed-dose combinations of lisinopril with hydrochlorothiazide.

References

For the complete list of references, see **wiley.com/go/budde/plumb**

Lokivetmab

Canine Atopic Dermatitis Immunotherapeutic (CADI)

(loe-ki-***vet***-mab) *Cytopoint*®

Antipruritic, Monoclonal Antibody

Prescriber Highlights

- ► Used to treat clinical signs associated with allergic and atopic dermatitis in dogs only
- ► Reduced pruritus seen within 1 to 3 days in most dogs and lasts for 4 to 8 weeks; maximum effect achieved after the second dose
- ► Appears safe, well tolerated, and effective in reducing pruritus

Uses/Indications

Lokivetmab is indicated for the treatment of pruritus associated with allergic and atopic dermatitis in dogs of any age.[1,2] Lokivetmab provides dose-related relief of pruritus within 24 to 72 hours[3,4] that lasts for 4 to 8 weeks.[4,5] In studies, the majority of dogs with atopic dermatitis achieve significant reduction of pruritus after the first dose; however, maximum effect is achieved after the second dose.[5,6] Treatment with monthly lokivetmab injections was deemed noninferior to cyclosporine in controlling signs of atopic dermatitis over a 12-week study period.[7] The mean clinical scores of the cyclosporine and lokivetmab groups did not differ significantly at any time point. Lokivetmab efficacy may be improved with concurrent administration of topical treatments intended to repair the skin barrier.[8]

In a retrospective study in dogs with allergic dermatitis that received lokivetmab, 88% of dogs were determined to achieve treatment success defined as a 20 mm decrease in pruritus visual analogue scale (PVAS) scores and 77% of dogs attained a more than 50% improvement in pruritus scores.[3] A history of positive response to other anti-allergy treatment (eg, glucocorticoids, cyclosporine, allergen-specific immunotherapy) was predictive of a better response to lokivetmab. In addition, 71% of dogs with an inadequate response to oclacitinib responded to lokivetmab. In another study, significant reduction in clinical pruritus scores and skin lesions were also observed in lokivetmab treated dogs.[7]

Lokivetmab effectively treated pruritus in a dog with widespread cutaneous mastocytosis[9]; the skin lesions improved but did not resolve.

Pharmacology/Actions

Lokivetmab is a caninized monoclonal antibody that neutralizes interleukin-31 (IL-31). IL-31 is produced by cutaneous activated T helper cells in dogs with atopic dermatitis; it binds to receptors in the spinal cord that then send signals to the brain to stimulate peripheral nerves to cause pruritus. By neutralizing the action of IL-31, lokivetmab disrupts this itch signal that is activated in dogs with allergic and atopic dermatitis; this action may delay disease flares when used in advance of predictable allergen exposure.[10] Lokivetmab has also been shown to reduce transepidermal water loss (an indicator of skin barrier function) in dogs with atopic dermatitis.[11]

The degree and duration of response to lokivetmab vary in individual dogs.[5] In a retrospective study, a response occurred within 24 hours in ≈56% of dogs, between 1 to 3 days in another ≈40%, and after more than 3 days in 4%.[3] Duration of response was variable; the administration interval was less than 4 weeks in ≈20% of dogs, 4 weeks in ≈46%, and greater than 4 weeks in ≈34% of dogs. In a study conducted in a canine model of IL-31 induced pruritus, a single SC dose of lokivetmab (2 mg/kg) produced a significant reduction in pruritus starting at 3 hours postinjection and it was maintained for 42 days.[4]

Pharmacokinetics

Lokivetmab remains in the circulation for several weeks and has an onset of efficacy within 1 to 3 days of administration and a duration of activity for at least 1 month after a single dose.[2] Efficacy may persist for up to 2 months in some patients. Elimination is via protein-degradation pathways.

Contraindications/Precautions/Warnings

Lokivetmab is approved for use in dogs only and should not be used in any other species.

The US label lists no contraindications, precautions, or warnings; however, in other countries, lokivetmab is labeled as contraindicated in dogs hypersensitive to it.[12,13]

When giving lokivetmab concurrently with vaccinations, administer at separate injection sites.[13]

Adverse Effects

In the primary field safety study, pruritus as an adverse effect was reported less frequently in the lokivetmab-treated group versus placebo[14]; otitis and dermatitis occurred at a similar frequency between treatment groups and may be attributed to lokivetmab's mechanism of action (ie, reduces pruritus but does not affect inflammation related to allergic and atopic dermatitis). Adverse effects are more likely to occur during the first few days postinjection and include vomiting (7% to 15.5%), diarrhea (3.7% to 13.4%), lethargy (6% to 9.9%), pain at injection site (5.1%), anorexia (4.9%), and lameness (2.1%).[3,7,14]

Hypersensitivity-related effects (eg, anaphylaxis, facial edema, urticaria) may occur rarely; when they occur, they may cause temporary or persistent formation of antibodies to lokivetmab.[15] In studies, treatment-induced immunogenicity was found in up to 2.5% of treated dogs; antibodies to lokivetmab may reduce its efficacy in some dogs.[7,14,16]

Reproductive/Nursing Safety

Lokivetmab has not been tested in pregnant, lactating, or breeding animals.[2] Because safety has not been established in animals, this drug should only be used when the maternal benefits outweigh the potential risks to offspring.

Overdose/Acute Toxicity

In a long-term safety study, lokivetmab was administered at up to 10 mg/kg SC once monthly for 7 consecutive doses without adverse effects.[16]

For patients that have experienced or are suspected to have experienced an overdose, consultation with a 24-hour poison consultation center specializing in providing veterinary-specific information is recommended. For general information related to overdose and toxin exposures, as well as contact information for poison control centers, refer to ***Appendix***.

Drug Interactions

- No specific drug interactions have been reported and would not be expected to occur based on lokivetmab's mechanism of action as a monoclonal antibody biologic immunotherapy drug. A wide variety of concomitant medications were safely used in field safety studies, including parasiticides, antibiotics, antifungals, antidepressants, antiemetics, corticosteroids, NSAIDs, vaccines, immunotherapy, antihistamines, and other antipruritics (eg, oclacitinib, cyclosporine).[2]

Laboratory Interactions

- **Intradermal allergy testing (IDT):** One injection of lokivetmab did not interfere with circulating immunoglobulin E (IgE) concentrations in a model of *Dermatophagoides farinae*-sensitized beagles 2 weeks postinjection.[17]

Dosages

DOGS:

Allergic and atopic dermatitis (label dosage; USDA-approved): Administer SC at a minimum dose of 2 mg/kg (0.9 mg/lb) of body weight according to the table below.[2] Repeat administration every 4 to 8 weeks as needed for individual patients. Before administration, collect the number of vials indicated under each presentation according to the dog's body weight.

a) **Dogs weighing less than 2.3 kg (less than 5 lb):** Aseptically withdraw 0.2 mL/kg (0.09 mL/lb) from a single 10 mg (Sky) vial and administer SC. Discard any remaining product.

b) **Dogs weighing 2.3 kg to 18.1 kg (5 to 40 lb):** Aseptically withdraw the full volume of the appropriate vial according to the table below and administer SC.

c) **Dogs weighing greater than 18.1 kg (greater than 40 lb):** A single dose requires a combination of vials, as outlined in the table below. Aseptically draw the full volume from each vial into 1 syringe and administer SC as a single injection.

Body weight in kg (lb)	10 mg/vial (Sky)	20 mg/vial (Plum)	30 mg/vial (Blush)	40 mg/vial (Navy)
less than 2.3 (5)	less than 1 vial (0.2 mL/kg)			
2.3 to 4.5 (5-10)	1 vial			
4.6 to 9.1 (10.1-20)		1 vial		
9.2 to 13.6 (20.1-30)			1 vial	
13.7 to 18.1 (30.1-40)				1 vial
18.2 to 22.7 (40.1-50)	1 vial +			1 vial
22.8 to 27.2 (50.1-60)		1 vial +		1 vial
27.3 to 31.7 (60.1-70)			1 vial +	1 vial
31.8 to 36.3 (70.1-80)				2 vials
36.4 to 40.8 (80.1-90)	1 vial +			2 vials
40.9 to 45.4 (90.1-100)		1 vial +		2 vials
45.5 to 49.9 (100.1-110)			1 vial +	2 vials
50 to 54.4 (110.1-120)				3 vials
54.5 to 59 (120.1-130)	1 vial +			3 vials
59.1 to 63.5 (130.1-140)		1 vial +		3 vials
63.6 to 68 (140.1-150)			1 vial +	3 vials

Body weight in kg (lb)	10 mg/vial (Sky)	20 mg/vial (Plum)	30 mg/vial (Blush)	40 mg/vial (Navy)
68.1 to 72.6 (150.1-160)				4 vials
72.7 to 77.1 (160.1-170)	1 vial +			4 vials
77.2 to 81.6 (170.1-180)		1 vial +		4 vials
81.7 to 86.2 (180.1-190)			1 vial +	4 vials
86.3 to 90.7 (190.1-200)				5 vials

Atopic dermatitis (extra-label): 1 mg/kg SC once a month, as the recommended minimum dosage[4,13]

Monitoring

- Efficacy manifests as lessening of pruritus
- Regular monitoring of treated dogs is recommended.
- Any adverse effects suspected to be associated with lokivetmab should be reported to the manufacturer and the USDA. Refer to the important contact information in the ***Appendix*** for further information related to reporting adverse effects.

Client Information

- This product does not cure the underlying allergic condition but should help to relieve itching caused by it.
- This drug is safe for most dogs but very rarely may cause an allergic reaction. Contact your veterinarian immediately if you see signs of excessive lethargy, weakness, collapse, difficulty breathing, sudden onset of noisy breathing, vomiting, or facial swelling.
- Your veterinarian will need to monitor your dog's condition while receiving this medicine to help identify the needed frequency of injections. Do not miss these important follow-up visits.

Chemistry/Synonyms

Lokivetmab (ATCvet code QD11AH) may also be known as Canine Atopic Dermatitis Immunotherapeutic, CADI, ZTS-00103289, Immunoglobulin G2, anti-(*Canis familiaris* interleukin 31) (*Canis familiaris*-Mus musculus monoclonal PF-06443537 gamma2-chain), disulfide with *Canis familiaris*-Mus musculus monoclonal PF-06443537 kappa-chain, dimer, and *Cytopoint*®.

Storage/Stability

Store vials upright in original packaging between 2°C and 8°C (36°F-46°F). Do not freeze. Prolonged exposure to higher temperatures and/or direct sunlight may adversely affect potency. Product contains no preservatives. Vials are single-use only; discard vials after puncture.[2]

Compatibility/Compounding Considerations

No information noted

Dosage Forms/Regulatory Status

VETERINARY-LABELED PRODUCTS:

Lokivetmab Solution: 10 mg, 20 mg, 30 mg, and 40 mg in 1 mL vials; *Cytopoint*®; USDA Veterinary License No. 190; (Rx)

HUMAN-LABELED PRODUCTS: NONE

References

For the complete list of references, see **wiley.com/go/budde/plumb**

Lomustine

CCNU

(loe-mus-teen) *Gleostine*®, *CeeNu*®

Oral Antineoplastic

Prescriber Highlights

- ► Oral antineoplastic usually used for treatment of CNS neoplasms, mast cell tumors, and histiocytic sarcomas or as a rescue agent for lymphoma protocols
- ► Caution is advised in patients with anemia, myelosuppression, pulmonary function impairment, current infection, impaired renal or hepatic function, or a sensitivity to lomustine.Significant adverse effects include myelosuppression (eg, anemia, refractory thrombocytopenia, leukopenia) with nadirs in dogs occuring ≈1 to 3 weeks after treatment, idiosyncratic hepatocellular injury (dogs), corneal de-epithelization, renal toxicity, and pulmonary infiltrates or fibrosis. Additional adverse effects include anorexia, vomiting, diarrhea, stomatitis, and alopecia.
- ► Teratogenic
- ► The National Institute for Occupational Safety and Health (NIOSH) classifies lomustine as a hazardous drug; use appropriate precautions when handling.

Uses/Indications

Lomustine may be useful in the adjunctive treatment of CNS neoplasms, lymphomas, mast cell tumors, and sarcomas (histiocytic sarcoma [dogs], fibrosarcoma [cats]) in dogs and cats.[1-5] Lomustine is usually dosed in a pulse fashion (ie, higher dose every 2 to 6 weeks depending on the protocol), but metronomic dosing (ie, low dose, daily) could potentially be useful in dogs that do not have other standard-care treatment options.[6,7]

Pharmacology/Actions

Lomustine's mechanism of action is not totally understood, but it is cell cycle-phase nonspecific. Lomustine is believed to inhibit DNA, RNA, and protein synthesis through alkylation and carbamoylation.

Cross-resistance has occurred between lomustine and carmustine.

Pharmacokinetics

In humans, lomustine is absorbed rapidly and extensively from the GI tract, and some absorption occurs after topical administration. Lomustine and its active metabolites are widely distributed in the body, including across the blood–brain barrier. Lomustine is metabolized extensively in the liver to both active and inactive metabolites that are eliminated primarily in the urine. Lomustine half-life in humans is very short (≈15 minutes), but its biologic activity is significantly longer because of the longer elimination times of active metabolites (16 to 48 hours).

Contraindications/Precautions/Warnings

Lomustine is contraindicated in patients hypersensitive to it. Lomustine should be used only when its potential benefits outweigh its risks with the following conditions: anemia, myelosuppression, pulmonary function impairment, current infection, and impaired renal or hepatic function.

Fatalities have resulted from inadvertent daily administration of high-dose pulse therapy[8]; consider only administering high-dose pulse therapy in the clinic.

The National Institute for Occupational Safety and Health (NIOSH) classifies lomustine as a hazardous drug; personal protective equipment (PPE) should be used accordingly to minimize the risk for exposure.[9]

Adverse Effects

Lomustine can cause fatal adverse effects, particularly when used at higher dosages and for prolonged treatment periods. The most serious adverse effects are myelosuppression (eg, anemia, thrombocytopenia, leukopenia) and idiosyncratic hepatotoxicity. CBC nadirs in dogs generally occur ≈1 to 3 weeks after treatment is given but can range from 1 to 6 weeks. Neutropenia in cats (nadir is variable; usually 1 to 4 weeks but can range from 1 to 6 weeks) is usually the dose-limiting factor, but there is significant interpatient variation for dosage tolerance in cats. Neutropenia is common dogs and cats, although secondary infections or sepsis are relatively uncommon.

Lomustine may cause hepatotoxicity in dogs[10,11]; hepatotoxicity is reportedly less common in cats.[12] Because some studies in rats have shown that alpha-lipoic acid may reduce the incidence/severity of hepatotoxicity associated with some chemotherapeutic agents, alpha-lipoic acid (5 mg/kg PO every 12 hours) has been used in some canine treatment protocols using lomustine[13]; alpha-lipoic acid is generally not recommended for use in cats because of toxicity concerns.[14-16] S-adenosyl-methionine (SAMe) plus silymarin (*Denamarin*®) has also been used in dogs for the same purpose.[17,18]

Other potential adverse effects include GI effects (eg, anorexia, vomiting, diarrhea [more commonly seen in dogs]), stomatitis, alopecia, corneal de-epithelization and, rarely, renal toxicity, and pulmonary infiltrates or fibrosis.

A retrospective study of 185 dogs receiving lomustine reported the following adverse effects: neutropenia (57%), increased ALT (49%), GI toxicosis (38%; ≈the majority of which were because of vomiting), anemia (34%), thrombocytopenia (14%), azotemia (12%), and hepatic failure (1.2%).[11] The authors concluded that lomustine-induced toxicity is common in dogs but usually is not life-threatening.

Reproductive/Nursing Safety

Lomustine is a teratogen in laboratory animals. Use only during pregnancy when the benefits to the mother outweigh the risks to the offspring. Lomustine can suppress gonadal function.

Lomustine and its metabolites have been detected in maternal milk. Nursing neonates should be given a milk replacer when the dam is receiving lomustine.

Overdose/Acute Toxicity

The lowest reported fatal dose in a dog following IV and oral administration of lomustine was 5 mg/kg and 10 mg/kg, respectively.[19] Because lomustine can be toxic, overdoses should be treated aggressively, with gastric decontamination protocols employed when possible.

For patients that have experienced or are suspected to have experienced an overdose, it is strongly encouraged to consult with one of the 24-hour poison consultation centers that specialize in providing information specific for veterinary patients. For general information related to overdose and toxin exposures, as well as contact information for poison control centers, refer to ***Appendix.***

Drug Interactions

The following drug interactions have either been reported or are theoretical in humans or animals receiving lomustine and may be of significance in veterinary patients. Unless otherwise noted, use together is not necessarily contraindicated, but weigh the potential risks and perform additional monitoring when appropriate.

- **Myelosuppressive Agents** (eg, **antineoplastics, immunosuppressants, iron chelators**): Concurrent use with other bone marrow depressant medications may result in additive myelosuppression; avoid combination when possible.
- **Vaccines** (live and inactivated): Lomustine may diminish vaccine efficacy and enhance adverse effects of vaccines.

Dosages

NOTE: Because of the potential toxicity of this drug to patients, veterinary staff, and pet owners and because chemotherapy indications, treatment protocols, monitoring, and safety guidelines often change, the following are usual dosage ranges for this drug and should be used only as a general guide. Consultation with a veterinary oncologist and referral to current veterinary oncology references[20-24] are strongly recommended.

DOGS:

Chemotherapy indications (extra-label): 50 – 90 mg/m² (NOT mg/kg) PO every 2 to 6 weeks, depending on the indication and protocol

Metronomic chemotherapy for primary or metastatic tumors (extra-label): 1.8 – 3.8 mg/m² (median=2.84 mg/m²; NOT mg/kg) PO once daily[6]

CATS:

Chemotherapy indications (extra-label):

1) 40 – 60 mg/m² (NOT mg/kg) PO every 3 to 6 weeks depending on the indication and protocol[25]
2) 10 mg/cat (NOT mg/kg) PO every 3 weeks depending on the indication and protocol[26]

Monitoring

- Baseline CBC with platelet count, serum chemistry profile, and urinalysis
- CBC with platelet count 1 week after dosing and prior to next dose; as a general rule, if platelets are less than 50,000/μL, stop therapy until thrombocytopenia is resolved.[27]
- Serum chemistry profiles before each treatment (especially in dogs)

Client Information

- Lomustine is a chemotherapy (anticancer) drug. The drug and its byproducts can be hazardous to other animals and humans. On the day your animal receives the drug and for a few days after, all bodily waste (eg, urine, feces, litter), blood, or vomit should be handled only while wearing disposable gloves. Seal the waste in a plastic bag, then place both the bag and gloves in the regular trash.
- Bone marrow suppression can occur. The greatest effects on bone marrow are usually within a few weeks after treatment. Your veterinarian will do blood tests to watch for this. Do not miss these important follow-up visits.
- If you see bleeding, bruising, or fever (indicating an infection) or if your animal becomes very tired easily, contact your veterinarian right away.
- Lomustine can cause damage to the liver, kidney, and lungs. It is important to understand the need to immediately report any signs associated with toxicity (eg, abnormal bleeding, bruising, urination, depression, infection, shortness of breath, yellowing of whites of the eyes, skin, or gums).
- Ensure dosing regimen is completely understood if dispensing for owners to administer at home.

Chemistry/Synonyms

Lomustine, a nitrosourea derivative alkylating agent, occurs as a yellow powder that is practically insoluble in water and soluble in alcohol.

Lomustine may also be known as CCNU, lomustinum, NSC-79037, RB-1509, WR-139017, *CeeNu*®, and *Gleostine*®.

Storage/Stability

Store capsules in a well-closed container at room temperature between 20°C and 25°C (68°F-77°F). Avoid exposure to temperatures above 40°C (104°F).[28]

Compatibility/Compounding Considerations

Precautions (eg, use of a biological safety cabinet) must be taken to avoid exposure from capsule contents when compounding dosage forms from commercially available capsules. Recent studies suggest many of the compounded formulations do not contain the expected active drug content, and use of the FDA-approved product is recommended whenever possible.[29,30]

Dosage Forms/Regulatory Status

VETERINARY-LABELED PRODUCTS: NONE

HUMAN-LABELED PRODUCTS:

Lomustine Capsules: 5 mg, 10 mg, 40 mg, and 100 mg with mannitol; *Gleostine*®; (Rx)

References

For the complete list of references, see **wiley.com/go/budde/plumb**

Loperamide

(loe-***pair***-a-mide) *Imodium*®

Opioid Antidiarrheal

Prescriber Highlights

- ► Opioid GI motility modifier used primarily in dogs for treatment of noninfectious, intractable diarrhea
- ► Contraindications include dogs with *MDR1* genetic mutation (also known as *ABCB1-1*delta) or unknown *MDR1* status, known hypersensitivity to narcotic analgesics, or diarrhea caused by infectious etiologies or toxin ingestion.
- ► Use with caution in patients with respiratory disease, hepatic encephalopathy, hypothyroidism, hypoadrenocorticism (Addison's disease), head injury, increased intracranial pressure, acute abdominal conditions (eg, bowel obstruction), and in severely debilitated patients.
- ► Adverse effects in dogs include constipation, bloat, and sedation; potential for paralytic ileus, toxic megacolon, pancreatitis, and CNS effects.
- ► Use in cats may result in excitatory behavior.
- ► Calculate doses carefully in small dogs and cats to avoid overdose.

Uses/Indications

Loperamide is used as a GI motility modifier in small animal species (primarily dogs) with noninfectious, intractable diarrhea. Some have found that loperamide is useful for treating or helping to reduce chemotherapy-induced (eg, toceranib) diarrhea in dogs.[1,2] In combination with maropitant, loperamide may be useful in preventing paclitaxel-induced GI adverse effects in dogs.[3]

Anecdotally, loperamide has been used for short-term management of diarrhea in cats, although adverse effects (eg, excitatory behavior, constipation) may limit therapy.

Pharmacology/Actions

Loperamide acts on the circular and longitudinal muscles by binding to mu-opioid receptors in the GI tract to decrease GI motility and excessive GI propulsion. Loperamide also decreases intestinal secretion induced by the cholera toxin, prostaglandin E_2, and diarrhea caused by factors in which calcium is the second messenger (non-cyclic AMP/GMP mediated). Opioids may also enhance mucosal absorption and increase anal sphincter tone. It has no analgesic activity.

Pharmacokinetics

By altering GI motility, loperamide may alter its own absorption. In a small study of 2 wild-type *MDR1* homozygotes (*MDR1* normal/normal) and 3 *MDR1* mutant (also known as *ABCB1-1*delta) homozygotes (*MDR1* mutant/mutant) dogs, oral bioavailability was 46 and 67%, respectively, peak concentration occurred at 1 and 3.6 hours after administration, and half-life was ≈10 and ≈12 hours.[4]

In humans, peak concentrations are reached 2.5 to 5 hours after administration. Loperamide is metabolized in the liver by CYP450 and exhibits an extensive first-pass metabolism; it has a half-life of ≈11 hours and is eliminated in the feces via biliary excretion.

Contraindications/Precautions/Warnings

Loperamide is contraindicated in patients with known hypersensitivity to it. Loperamide is a P-glycoprotein substrate that is contraindicated in dogs that are homozygous (*MDR1* mutant/mutant) for the *MDR1* genetic mutation (also known as *ABCB-1*delta) due to loss of P-glycoprotein function needed to excrete loperamide from the CNS. Alternative antidiarrheals should be considered in untested dogs of high-risk breeds (eg, herding breeds: collies, Shetland sheepdogs, Australian shepherds) that may have the gene mutation. Dogs that are heterozygous for the mutation (*MDR1* mutant/normal) should receive loperamide at reduced dosages if no alternative therapies are available.

Opioid GI motility modifiers should be avoided if diarrhea is due to an infectious etiology or an ingested toxin. All opioids should be used with caution in patients with hypothyroidism, hypoadrenocorticism (Addison's disease), or in severely debilitated patients.

Opioid antidiarrheals should be used with caution in patients with head injuries or increased intracranial pressure and acute abdominal conditions (eg, bowel obstruction), as it may obscure the diagnosis or negatively impact clinical resolution. Loperamide should be used with extreme caution in patients suffering from respiratory disease or from acute respiratory dysfunction (eg, pulmonary edema). Opioid antidiarrheals should be used with extreme caution in patients with hepatic encephalopathy; hepatic coma may result. Loperamide should be used cautiously in patients with hepatic impairment as first-pass metabolism may be reduced.

Adverse Effects

In dogs, salivation, constipation, bloat, and sedation are the most likely adverse effects encountered when recommended dosages are used. Potentially, paralytic ileus, toxic megacolon, pancreatitis, and CNS effects (eg, sedation, ataxia) could be seen. Dogs with the *MDR1* genetic mutation (also known as *ABCB-1*delta; *MDR1* mutant/mutant) can develop severe CNS depression, ataxia, mydriasis and salivation after receiving a single 0.1 mg/kg PO dose of loperamide.[5] Naloxone may reverse CNS effects.[6] See ***Overdose/Acute Toxicity***.

Loperamide use in cats may cause excitatory behavior and constipation.

In humans, cardiotoxicity has been seen in patients receiving higher dosages.[7]

Reproductive/Nursing Safety

Rats experienced significant impairment of fertility at dosages of 20 – 40 mg/kg/day; this effect was not observed at 10 mg/kg/day. Loperamide is excreted in human maternal milk in small amounts; use with caution during lactation.

Because safety has not been established in animals, this drug should only be used when the maternal benefits outweigh the potential risks to offspring.

Overdose/Acute Toxicity

In dog toxicity studies, dosages of 1.25 – 5 mg/kg/day produced vomiting, depression, severe salivation, and weight loss. Breeds with either homozygous (*MDR1* mutant/mutant) or heterozygous (*MDR 1* mutant/normal) *MDR1* gene mutations (also known as *ABCB*-1delta) are more sensitive to CNS depression with loperamide than other breeds.[8]

Adverse effects seen in dogs with loperamide overdose include vomiting, lethargy, diarrhea, hypersalivation, hypothermia, bradycardia, vocalization, depression, sedation, circling, ataxia, limb weakness, non-reactive pupils and disorientation.[8-10]; in cats, vomiting, lethargy, and mydriasis are the most common.

Treatment should follow standard decontamination protocols,[11] although the use of emetics (eg, apomorphine, ropinirole) should be avoided because they may have additive CNS and/or respiratory depressant effects. Naloxone may be used to treat severe CNS or respiratory depression[8,9,11,12]; repeated doses of naloxone may be required. Intravenous lipid emulsion (ILE) rescue may be useful.[13]

For patients that have experienced or are suspected to have experienced an overdose, consultation with a 24-hour poison consultation center specializing in providing veterinary-specific information is recommended. For general information related to overdose and toxin exposures, as well as contact information for poison control centers, refer to ***Appendix***.

Drug Interactions

Loperamide is a substrate of P-glycoprotein and human CYP2C8 and 3A4 isoenzymes. The following drug interactions have either been reported or are theoretical in humans or animals receiving loperamide and may be of significance in veterinary patients. Unless otherwise noted, use together is not necessarily contraindicated, but weigh the potential risks and perform additional monitoring when appropriate.

- **Amiodarone**: By inhibiting P-glycoprotein, amiodarone may increase loperamide plasma concentrations.
- **Carvedilol**: By inhibiting P-glycoprotein, carvedilol may increase loperamide plasma concentrations.
- **CYP2B11 Substrates** (eg, **ketamine, midazolam, progesterone, propofol**): Loperamide can inhibit metabolism of this isoenzyme in dogs and potentially increase blood concentrations of substrates.
- **CYP2D15 Substrates** (eg, **imipramine, metoprolol, propranolol**): Loperamide can inhibit metabolism of this isoenzyme in dogs and potentially increase blood concentrations of substrates.
- **CYP3A12 Substrates** (eg, **cyclosporine, erythromycin, medetomidine, tacrolimus**): Loperamide can inhibit metabolism of this isoenzyme in dogs and potentially increase blood concentrations of substrates.
- **Desmopressin**: Loperamide may increase serum desmopressin concentrations.
- **Erythromycin**: By inhibiting P-glycoprotein, erythromycin may increase loperamide plasma concentrations.
- **Gemfibrozil**: Increased loperamide plasma concentrations
- **Ketoconazole, Itraconazole**: By inhibiting P-glycoprotein, these drugs may increase loperamide plasma concentrations.
- **Moxidectin**: Loperamide reduced moxidectin clearance and increased moxidectin plasma concentration and AUC.[14]
- **Quinidine**: By inhibiting P-glycoprotein, quinidine may increase loperamide plasma concentrations.
- **QT-Prolongation Agents**: Loperamide may enhance the QT-prolonging effect.
- **Sulfamethoxazole/Trimethoprim**: Increased loperamide plasma concentrations due to inhibition of first-pass metabolism
- **Verapamil**: By inhibiting P-glycoprotein, verapamil may increase loperamide plasma concentrations.

Laboratory Considerations

- Plasma **amylase** and **lipase** values may be increased for up to 24 hours following administration of opioids.

Dosages

DOGS:

NOTE: Avoid use in dogs with the *MDR1* genetic mutation as they are more sensitive to loperamide; there is no published evidence of a safe dosage for these patients. See ***Contraindications/Precautions/Warnings***.

Antidiarrheal agent (label dosage, not FDA-approved): Dosed based on body weight: 4.5 kg – 11.4 kg, 1 mg/dog (NOT mg/kg); 11.8 kg – 18.2 kg, 2 mg/dog (NOT mg/kg); 18.6 kg – 27.3 kg, 4 mg/dog (NOT mg/kg). Administer 1 dose every 8 hours as needed for the temporary relief of diarrhea; do not exceed 3 doses per 24 hours, or 3 days of treatment.[15]

Antidiarrheal (extra-label): Anecdotal dosage range from 0.08 – 0.1 mg/kg PO 3 times daily as needed, but dosages as high as 0.2 mg/kg PO 3 to 4 times daily have been noted.

CATS:

NOTE: Use is controversial; cats may react with excitatory behavior.

Antidiarrheal (extra-label): Anecdotal dosages ranging from 0.04 – 0.16 mg/kg PO every 12 hours have been noted. Practically, ¼ or ½ of a 2 mg tablet may be used, although the oral liquid dosage form is necessary to dose accurately.

RABBITS, RODENTS, SMALL MAMMALS:

Antidiarrheal agent (extra-label):

1. **Rabbits**: 0.1 mg/kg in 1 mL of water PO every 8 hours for 3 days, then once daily for 2 days[16]
2. **Mice, Rats, Gerbils, Hamsters, Guinea pigs, Chinchillas**: 0.1 mg/kg PO every 8 hours for 3 days, then once daily for 2 days; give in 1 mL of water.[17]

Monitoring

- Clinical efficacy
- Hydration and serum electrolytes especially in cases of severe diarrhea
- Adverse CNS effects (eg, sedation, depression, disorientation, ataxia, mydriasis, non-reactive pupils)

Client Information

- This medicine is used to treat diarrhea.
- Loperamide is generally well tolerated with few side effects. Loperamide can be toxic in dogs with a certain genetic mutation (MDR1; also known as *ABCB*-1delta) most commonly found in "white feet" breeds (eg, collies, Shetland sheepdogs, Australian shepherds).
- If diarrhea continues or if your animal appears listless or develops a high fever, contact your veterinarian immediately.
- Loperamide is available OTC (over the counter; without a prescription). Do not give loperamide (or any other OTC medication) to your animal without first consulting your veterinarian.

Chemistry/Synonyms

A synthetic piperidine-derivative antidiarrheal, loperamide occurs as a white to faintly yellow powder with a pK_a of 8.6. It is soluble in alcohol and slightly soluble in water.

Loperamide may also be known as PJ 185, or R 18553; a common trade name is *Imodium*®.

Storage/Stability

Loperamide capsules or oral solution should be stored at room temperature (20°C-25°C; 68°F-77°F), in well-closed containers protected from light. It is recommended that the oral solution not be diluted with other solvents.

Compatibility/Compounding Considerations

No specific information noted

Dosage Forms/Regulatory Status

VETERINARY-LABELED PRODUCTS:

The Association of Racing Commissioners International (ARCI) has designated this drug as a class 2 substance. Use of this drug may not be allowed in certain animal competitions. Check rules and regulations before entering in a competition while this medication is being administered. Contact local racing authorities for further guidance. See ***Appendix*** for more information.

Loperamide HCl Oral Liquid: 2 mg/mL in 10 mL; generic; (OTC). Not approved by the FDA.

Loperamide HCl Tablets: 2 mg; *Difixin*®; (OTC)

HUMAN-LABELED PRODUCTS:

Loperamide HCl Oral Liquid: 1 mg/5 mL (0.2 mg/mL) and 1 mg/7.5 mL (0.13 mg/mL) in 60 mL, 90 mL, 118 mL, and 120 mL solution or suspension; *Imodium® A-D*, generic; (OTC)

Loperamide HCl Capsules and Tablets: 2 mg; *Imodium® A-D*; other proprietary named products are available as well as generics; (OTC and Rx)

References

For the complete list of references, see **wiley.com/go/budde/plumb**

Loratadine

(lor-***at***-eh-deen) *Claritin®, Alavert®*

Antihistamine, Second-Generation

Prescriber Highlights

- Oral nonsedating antihistamine
- Limited experience in dogs or cats; efficacy (if any) has not been determined.

Uses/Indications

Loratadine is a nonsedating second-generation antihistamine. Although loratadine could be useful in treating histamine-mediated conditions in dogs and cats, there is no evidence documenting its efficacy. A double-blind, placebo-controlled, randomized clinical trial evaluating the efficacy of loratadine for the treatment of canine atopic dermatitis did not show sustained relief of pruritus in any of the dogs.[1] Guidelines for atopic dermatitis treatment in dogs state that antihistamines have modest efficacy in some dogs; loratadine should be given continuously (ie, daily) as preventive therapy before an acute flare.[2] Antihistamines may also be used as steroid-sparing agents and with essential fatty acids to improve potential efficacy.[3]

Pharmacology/Actions

Loratadine is a long-acting oral second-generation antihistamine from the piperidine class. It blocks peripheral histamine (H_1) receptors. Unlike some antihistamines, loratadine is not an alpha-1 antagonist, and at therapeutic dosages it does not have significant antimuscarinic activity.

Pharmacokinetics

No information was located for dogs or cats.

In humans, loratadine is rapidly absorbed from the GI tract; peak plasma concentrations occur in ≈1 hour. Food has variable effects on time to peak, but overall bioavailability is increased. It is extensively metabolized in the liver and its primary metabolite (desloratadine) is active. Loratadine is highly bound to plasma proteins (98%); plasma protein binding for desloratadine is lower. Minimal amounts of the drug enter the CNS at therapeutic dosages. Severe renal impairment does not appreciably alter blood concentrations of the drug or its active metabolite. Elimination half-life is ≈ 9 hours (loratadine) and 28 hours (desloratadine). Elimination occurs mostly as metabolites via urine and feces.

Contraindications/Precautions/Warnings

Loratadine is contraindicated in patients that are hypersensitive to it or desloratadine. Use with caution in dogs with keratoconjunctivitis (KCS), as loratadine has been shown to decrease tear production in humans. Lower dosages are recommended in humans with significant renal or hepatic impairment.

Adverse Effects

Adverse effects are not well-documented for loratadine in small animal species. At higher dosages in humans, it could have adverse CNS effects (eg, sedation, lethargy, paradoxical excitement), have GI effects (eg, vomiting), and/or cause tachycardia. Dry mouth and decreased tear production are possible.

Reproductive/Nursing Safety

Loratadine did not alter fertility of mice at 40 mg/kg and rats at 25 mg/kg; there is no evidence of teratogenicity in rats or rabbits given oral doses up to 96 mg/kg.[4] Loratadine and its metabolite are found in breast milk at concentrations roughly equivalent to maternal plasma, but the American Academy of Pediatrics has listed loratadine as compatible with breastfeeding in humans.[5]

Because safety has not been established in animals, this drug should only be used when the maternal benefits outweigh the potential risks to offspring.

Overdose/Acute Toxicity

Mild overdoses of loratadine are generally not serious, but moderate to severe overdoses can cause cardiac (eg, tachycardia) and CNS (eg, sedation) effects. Clinical signs usually occur within 30 minutes to 7 hours postingestion and can persist for 12 to 24 hours or more. Clinical signs in dogs have been noted at doses as low as 0.25 mg/kg, but doses as high as 72 mg/kg have been tolerated without serious effects or death.[6]

Common clinical signs associated with loratadine overdose in dogs include tachycardia, lethargy, and vomiting. Consider GI decontamination for patients that have ingested larger quantities of loratadine. Treatment is supportive; hemodialysis does not appear to be effective in removing loratadine or desloratadine from the body.

For patients that have experienced or are suspected to have experienced an overdose, consultation with a 24-hour poison consultation center specializing in providing veterinary-specific information is recommended. For general information related to overdose and toxin exposures, as well as contact information for poison control centers, refer to ***Appendix***.

Drug Interactions

The following drug interactions have either been reported or are theoretical in humans or animals receiving loratadine and may be of significance in veterinary patients. Unless otherwise noted, use together is not necessarily contraindicated, but weigh the potential risks and perform additional monitoring when appropriate.

- AMIODARONE: In humans, QT-interval prolongation and torsades de pointes have been reported[7]; clinical monitoring has been recommended.
- CIMETIDINE: May increase loratadine (and desloratadine) concentrations; no clinical effects noted in humans
- MACROLIDE ANTIBIOTICS (eg, **clarithromycin, erythromycin**): May increase loratadine (and desloratadine) concentrations
- KETOCONAZOLE: May increase loratadine (and desloratadine) concentrations; no clinical effects noted in humans

Laboratory Considerations

- **Intradermal allergy testing (IDT)**: Antihistamines may suppress IDT results. It is recommended to discontinue loratadine at least 7 days prior to testing in dogs.[2]

Dosages

NOTE: No published evidence was located that supports efficacy and safety for pruritus or atopic dermatitis.

DOGS:

Antihistamine (extra-label): Anecdotal dosages range from 0.25 – 1.1 mg/kg PO once daily or divided twice daily.[8-10]

Practically it could be dosed as follows:
- Small dogs: 5 mg/dog (NOT mg/kg) PO once daily
- Medium dogs: 10 mg/dog (NOT mg/kg) PO once daily
- Large dogs: 10 mg/dog (NOT mg/kg) PO twice daily

CATS:

Antihistamine (extra-label): Anecdotal dosages of 0.5 mg/kg PO once daily[11,12] or 2.5 – 5 mg/cat (NOT mg/kg) PO once daily[13,14] have been noted.

Monitoring

- No specific monitoring is required beyond clinical efficacy and adverse effects.

Client Information

- Use only products that contain loratadine as a single active ingredient. Decongestants found in human-label combination products can be toxic to animals.
- Antihistamines should be used on a regular, ongoing basis in animals that respond to them. They work better if used before exposure to an allergen (eg, pollens).
- This medicine may be given with or without food. If your animal vomits or acts sick after receiving the medication on an empty stomach, try giving the next dose with food or a small treat. If vomiting continues, contact your veterinarian.
- Causes less sleepiness than some other antihistamines, but sleepiness can still occur. Not used commonly in veterinary medicine so possible side effects are not well known.

Chemistry/Synonyms

Loratadine is a piperidine derivative related structurally to azatadine. It is a white to off-white powder that is insoluble in water but very soluble in acetone, chloroform, methyl alcohol, and toluene.

Loratadine may also be known as SCh-29851, loratadiini, loratadin, loratadinum, or loratadyna.

Storage/Stability

Loratadine products should be stored between 20°C to 25°C (68°F-77°F). Loratadine syrup or tablets should be stored in tight, light-resistant containers. The orally dispersing tablets should be protected from humidity.

Compatibility/Compounding Considerations

- No specific information is noted.

Dosage Forms/Regulatory Status

VETERINARY-LABELED PRODUCTS: NONE

The Association of Racing Commissioners International (ARCI) has designated this drug as a class 4 substance. Use of this drug may not be allowed in certain animal competitions. Check rules and regulations before entering in a competition while this medication is being administered. Contact local racing authorities for further guidance. See *Appendix* for more information.

HUMAN-LABELED PRODUCTS:

Loratadine Tablets, Oral Disintegrating Tablets, Chewable Tablets, and Gelcaps: 5 mg and 10 mg; generic; (OTC). Many proprietary brands are available; 2 common ones are *Claritin*® and *Alavert*®. NOTE: Oral dispersible tablets may contain xylitol (unknown quantity); avoid use in dogs. Chewable tablets may contain flavorings such as grape, citrus, or mint.

Loratadine Oral Solution/Syrup: 1 mg/mL (labeled as 5 mg/5 mL); generic; (OTC). Many proprietary brands are available; 2 common ones are *Claritin*® and *Alavert*®. May be flavored with grape or bubble gum. Do not use products containing propylene glycol in cats.

NOTE: *Do not use formulations containing pseudoephedrine, such as Claritin-D, to treat dogs and cats due to potential unpredictable adverse effects.*

References

For the complete list of references, see **wiley.com/go/budde/plumb**

Lorazepam

(lor-***ayz***-eh-pam) *Ativan*®

Benzodiazepine

Prescriber Highlights

- ▶ Benzodiazepine used as an anxiolytic in dogs and cats and as an alternative to diazepam for treating status epilepticus
- ▶ Can be administered IV for status epilepticus, or intranasally if IV access is difficult or delayed
- ▶ Most common adverse effects include activity or behavior changes (sedation, lethargy, hyperactivity, aggression) and increased appetite
- ▶ DEA Schedule IV (C-IV) controlled substance

Uses/Indications

Lorazepam is used to treat seizures and status epilepticus in dogs and for adjunctive treatment of behavior disorders (eg, fears, phobias, anxiety) in dogs and cats. As compared with diazepam, there are limited data using lorazepam in small animal medicine, but lorazepam has some advantages such as safer use in patients with liver dysfunction and in obese or geriatric patients. It appears to be as effective as diazepam, and may have a longer anticonvulsant duration of action.[1] Rectal administration of lorazepam is not recommended for status epilepticus.[2]

In human medicine, lorazepam is often used in place of diazepam for treating status epilepticus and anxiolytic indications. It is also used to treat chemotherapy-induced nausea and emesis, alcohol withdrawal, and akathisia secondary to antipsychotic drugs.

Pharmacology/Actions

Lorazepam is considered a long-acting benzodiazepine in humans, but it has a much shorter half-life in dogs. Lorazepam and other benzodiazepines depress CNS subcortical levels (primarily limbic, thalamic, and hypothalamic), thereby producing anxiolytic, sedative, skeletal muscle relaxation, and anticonvulsant effects. Lorazepam binds to gamma-aminobutyric acid type A (GABAA) receptors and increases the affinity of the receptor for GABA, which results in increased chloride conductance and hyperpolarization of the postsynaptic cell membrane. Other postulated mechanisms include antagonism of serotonin, increased release of GABA, and diminished release or turnover of acetylcholine in the CNS. Benzodiazepine-specific receptors have been located in the mammalian brain, kidney, liver, lung, and heart; receptors are lacking in the white matter of all species studied.

Pharmacokinetics

In dogs, lorazepam 0.2 mg/kg IV reached peak concentrations of ≈165 ng/mL, which remained above 30 ng/mL (considered necessary for anticonvulsant activity in humans) for 60 minutes.[3] Intranasal administration of lorazepam at 0.2 mg/kg in dogs reached peak concentrations of ≈106 ng/mL; in 3 out of 6 dogs studied, concentrations remained above 30 ng/mL for 60 minutes. Concentrations reached 30 ng/mL between 3 to 9 minutes after intranasal administration.[3] Although elimination half-life has been reported as ≈1 hour in dogs, concentrations in the brain may persist longer than in the serum, as lorazepam has a high affinity for benzodiazepine receptors in the CNS. Rectal administration of lorazepam in dogs does not appear to yield serum concentrations high enough for efficacious treatment of status epilepticus due to a high first-pass effect.[2] Lorazepam is converted into inactive glucuronide metabolites in the liver in most species.[4] The primary elimination route is via urine in dogs.

In cats, lorazepam is efficiently glucuronidated[4, 5]; elimination is ≈50% in the urine (primarily as the glucuronide) and 50% in the feces.[5]

In humans, absolute bioavailability is ≈90% after oral administration and, unlike diazepam, lorazepam is relatively rapidly and completely absorbed after IM dosing. Sublingual administration has similar bioavailability as oral dosing, but serum concentrations peak sooner. Elimination half-life appears to be much longer in humans (12 hours) than in dogs (≈1 hour).

Contraindications/Precautions/Warnings

Lorazepam is contraindicated in patients with known hypersensitivity to benzodiazepines, patients with acute narrow-angle glaucoma, and patients with severe respiratory insufficiency (unless they are being mechanically ventilated).

Lorazepam should be used with caution, if at all, in patients that have a history of aggression, as behavioral disinhibition may occur.

When using lorazepam to treat unwanted behaviors, behavior disorders, or with long-term administration, withdraw it gradually at the end of the treatment to prevent a possible rebound effect. Physical dependency has been induced in dogs, although it appears to be less intense than with diazepam.[6]

Injectable lorazepam must not be given intra-arterially; arteriospasm may occur, resulting in necrosis.[7] Use repeated high doses or CRIs with caution as the injection contains propylene glycol and benzyl alcohol.

Do not confuse LORazepam with other sound-alike/look-alike drugs (eg, CLONazepam, ALPRAZolam). Consider writing part of the drug's name in uppercase letters (tall-man designations) on prescriptions/orders to reduce the risk for errors.

Adverse Effects

In small animals, benzodiazepines can cause increased appetite, aggression, paradoxical increased activity/excitement/anxiety/agitation, and vocalization. Sedation, muscle relaxation, ataxia, somnolence, and lethargy can occur with initiation of therapy, with dosage increases, or at higher doses.

Lorazepam injection contains both propylene glycol 400 (0.18 mL/mL of injection) and 2% benzyl alcohol. Repeated high doses or CRIs may have toxic effects in dogs and cats.

Reproductive/Nursing Safety

Lorazepam crosses the placenta. Congenital anomalies, fetal resorption, and increased fetal loss have been observed in laboratory animals. In humans, the use of benzodiazepines during pregnancy resulted in premature births and low birth weights. "Floppy infant" syndrome has been seen in human neonates whose mothers receive high doses immediately prior to delivery.[8, 9]

Lorazepam is distributed into milk. Sedation and inability to suckle have occurred in human neonates of lactating mothers taking benzodiazepines.[9]

Because safety has not been established in animals, this drug should only be used when the maternal benefits outweigh the potential risks to offspring.

Overdose/Acute Toxicity

Overdose effects of lorazepam are generally limited to CNS depression. The most common clinical signs observed in dogs are sedation, lethargy, hyperactivity, ataxia, and vomiting. In cats, the most common clinical signs are ataxia, lethargy, vocalization, and agitation. Large overdoses can cause hypotension, coma, and death (rare). Repeated high doses or CRIs of the injectable formulation may cause propylene glycol or benzyl alcohol toxicity.

Treatment of acute orally ingested lorazepam toxicity consists of standard protocols for GI decontamination and supportive systemic measures. In patients with normal renal function, diuresis with IV fluids/electrolytes and mannitol may enhance excretion of lorazepam. The use of analeptic agents (CNS stimulants such as caffeine) is generally not recommended. Flumazenil may be considered for adjunctive treatment of severe overdoses of benzodiazepines, but its use does not replace proper supportive therapy. Flumazenil is not recommended in patients with seizure disorders as it may induce seizures.[7, 9]

For patients that have experienced or are suspected to have experienced an overdose, consultation with a 24-hour poison consultation center specializing in providing veterinary-specific information is recommended. For general information related to overdose and toxin exposures, as well as contact information for poison control centers, refer to ***Appendix***.

Drug Interactions

The following drug interactions have either been reported or are theoretical in humans or animals receiving lorazepam and may be of significance in veterinary patients. Unless otherwise noted, use together is not necessarily contraindicated, but weigh the potential risks and perform additional monitoring when appropriate.

- **Amiodarone**: Concurrent use may increase bioavailability and pharmacologic effects of benzodiazepines.
- **Anesthetic Agents** (eg, **alfaxalone, ketamine, propofol**): Combination may increase the risk for CNS and/or respiratory depression.
- **Antacids, Calcium- or Magnesium-Containing**: May slow the rate, but not the extent of oral absorption; administer 2 hours apart to avoid this potential interaction.
- **Antihypertensive Agents** (eg, **atenolol, lisinopril**): Concurrent use may increase risk for hypotension and orthostasis. Monitor blood pressure.
- **Carbonic Anhydrase Inhibitors** (CAIs; eg, **dichlorphenamide, methazolamide**): Benzodiazepines may interfere with the beneficial effects of CAIs by inhibiting respiratory responses to hypoxia. Avoid combination.
- **Cannabidiol**: Increased risk for CNS depression
- **Digoxin**: Serum levels may be increased; monitor serum digoxin concentrations and clinical signs of toxicity.
- **Fluoxetine, Fluvoxamine**: Concurrent use may increase lorazepam concentrations and lead to an increased risk for CNS and respiratory depression.
- **Hepatic Enzyme Inducers** (eg, **betamethasone, carbamazepine, rifampin**): Concurrent use may decrease benzodiazepine levels.
- **Hepatic Enzyme Inhibitors** (eg, **cimetidine, erythromycin, isoniazid, ketoconazole, itraconazole**): Metabolism of lorazepam may be decreased, and excessive sedation may occur.
- **Ifosfamide**: Concurrent use may increase the risk for ifosfamide-induced neurotoxic effects. Carefully monitor for adverse effects; discontinue both drugs if signs of encephalopathy occur.
- **Nondepolarizing Neuromuscular Blockers** (eg, **atracurium, pancuronium**): Concurrent use may potentiate, attenuate, or have no neuromuscular blocking effect.
- **Opioids** (eg, **buprenorphine, morphine**): Combination may increase the risk for CNS and/or respiratory depression.
- **Phenobarbital**: Combination may increase the risk for CNS and/or respiratory depression.
- **Phenothiazines** (eg, **acepromazine**): Combination may increase the risk for CNS and/or respiratory depression.
- **Theophylline/Aminophylline**: Concurrent use may de-

crease the levels and effectiveness of benzodiazepines. Withdrawing theophylline from a stable patient may increase the risk for benzodiazepine toxicity. Monitor and adjust doses accordingly.

- **Tricyclic Antidepressants** (TCAs; eg, **amitriptyline, clomipramine**): Lorazepam may increase concentrations of these drugs; clinical significance is not known. However, concurrent use may increase the risk for CNS and/or respiratory depression. Anticholinergic effects may be additive.
- **Yohimbine**: Limited data indicate that yohimbine may decrease therapeutic effects of anxiolytic drugs.

Laboratory Considerations

- Benzodiazepines may decrease the thyroidal uptake of I^{123} or I^{131}.

Dosages

DOGS:

Status epilepticus (extra-label): 0.2 mg/kg IV.[1] In humans, IV doses should be administered no faster than 2 mg/minute.[7] If IV access cannot be readily achieved (or for at-home use by pet owners), the IV dose can be administered intranasally; however, the delay in onset (3 to 9 minutes; see ***Pharmacokinetics***) may negate its practical use and midazolam IN may be more advantageous. Do not administer rectally.[2]

Behavior indications (eg, fears, anxieties, phobias, night waking; extra-label): No published evidence supporting any one dosage over the other was located. It is suggested to start therapy at the lower end of the dose range, choosing a practical dose for the patient based on available tablet sizes; adjust dose to desired effect. If used on an as-needed basis to treat episodic or situational anxiety, oral lorazepam may be most efficacious when administered prior to the triggering event, as the time to onset may be highly variable.

a) 0.02 – 0.2 mg/kg PO 1 to 3 times daily or on an as-needed basis

b) 0.02 – 0.5 mg/kg PO every 8 to 24 hours[10]

CATS:

Behavior indications (eg, fears, anxieties, phobias, night waking; extra-label): No published evidence supports any one dosage over the other. It is suggested to start therapy at the lower end of the dose range, choosing a practical dose for the patient based on available tablet sizes; adjust dose to desired effect. If used on an as-needed basis to treat episodic or situational anxiety, oral lorazepam may be most efficacious when administered prior to the triggering event, as the time to onset may be highly variable.

a) 0.025 – 0.08 mg/kg PO 1 to 2 times daily[10] or on an as-needed basis

b) 0.125 – 0.25 mg/cat (NOT mg/kg) PO every 12 to 24 hours[11]

Monitoring

- No specific monitoring is required beyond clinical efficacy and adverse effects.

Client Information

- When using lorazepam for thunderstorm phobias or other triggers that upset your animal (eg, owner separation anxiety), try to give this medicine about an hour before the event or trigger.
- Common side effects include drowsiness, sedation, and increased appetite. However, the drug can change your animal's behavior or work in the opposite way from what is expected.
- Tablets are relatively tasteless and readily dissolve in saliva. If administering the pill is difficult, place it inside your animal's cheek and follow up after about a minute with a small treat to facilitate swallowing of the medicine.
- If the whites of your animal's eyes, skin, or gums have a yellowish tint, or if your animal stops eating or seems depressed, contact your veterinarian immediately.
- Lorazepam is a controlled drug by the federal Drug Enforcement Agency (DEA). Use of this medication in animals or humans other than those for whom they are prescribed is illegal.

Chemistry/Synonyms

Lorazepam occurs as a white or practically white, practically odorless powder. It is insoluble in water and sparingly soluble in alcohol. Each mL of lorazepam for injection contains 0.18 mL of polyethylene glycol 400 and 2% benzyl alcohol in propylene glycol.

Lorazepam may also be known as BRN-07599084, CB-8133, Ro-7-8408, Wy-4036, lorazapamum, anxiedin, azurogen, bonatranquan, delormetazepam, lorazin, lorazon, lorenin, norlormetazepam, novhepar, novolorazem, o-Chloroxazepam, sinestron, *Ativan*®, and *Lorazepam Intensol*®; many international trade names are available.

Storage/Stability

Lorazepam tablets should be stored in airtight containers at room temperature (20°C-25°C [68°F-77°F]). The oral solution and injection should be stored refrigerated (2°C-8°C [36°F-46°F]) and protected from light.

The injection must be further diluted immediately prior to IV injection with an equal volume of D_5W, normal saline, or sterile water for injection. Do not shake the syringe vigorously; instead, gently invert it repeatedly until the injection is diluted and completely mixed in solution. Do not use if the solution is discolored or a precipitate forms. IV injections should be administered slowly (2 mg/minute).[7]

Lorazepam is a DEA Schedule IV (C-IV) controlled substance that should be stored in an area that is substantially constructed and securely locked. Follow applicable local, state, and federal rules regarding disposal of unused or wasted controlled drugs.

Compatibility/Compounding Considerations

Compatibility is dependent on factors such as pH, concentration, temperature, and diluent used; specialized references or a hospital pharmacist should be consulted for more specific information.

Lorazepam can be further diluted in D_5W or normal saline for IV infusion. (**NOTE**: This is not stated in the label information.) When used in this manner, lorazepam injection is most soluble in final concentrations of 0.1 to 0.2 mg/mL. For example, if the 2 mg/mL injection is used, further dilution with 9 mL or 19 mL of D_5W or normal saline would yield a final concentration of 0.2 or 0.1 mg/mL. The injection is very viscous; mix well before use. Because precipitation/crystallization can occur, observe the solution before and during the infusion. D_5W may be less prone to crystallization formation than is normal saline. Solutions for infusion mixed in this manner should be used within 12 hours of preparation.

Drugs reported to be **compatible** with lorazepam injection include (partial listing):

- **Syringe**: Hydromorphone, dimenhydrinate
- **Y-Site**: Albumin, amikacin, amphotericin B cholesteryl, atracurium, cefotaxime, ciprofloxacin, cisplatin, dexamethasone, diltiazem, diphenhydramine, dobutamine, doxorubicin, famotidine, fentanyl, fosphenytoin, furosemide, gentamicin, heparin, hydroxyethyl starches, hydromorphone, levetiracetam, methadone, metronidazole, morphine, piperacillin-tazobactam, propofol, ranitidine, vancomycin, and vecuronium

Drugs reported to be **incompatible** with lorazepam include (partial listing):

- **Syringe**: Buprenorphine and pantoprazole
- **Y-Site**: Aztreonam, gallium nitrate, imipenem-cilastatin, omeprazole, and ondansetron

Dosage Forms/Regulatory Status

Lorazepam is a DEA Schedule II controlled substance; report prescribing and/or dispensing to state monitoring programs where required

VETERINARY-LABELED PRODUCTS: NONE

The Association of Racing Commissioners International (ARCI) has designated this drug as a class 2 substance. See ***Appendix*** for more information. Use of this drug may not be allowed in certain animal competitions. Check rules and regulations before entering in a competition while this medication is being administered. Contact local racing authorities for further guidance.

HUMAN-LABELED PRODUCTS:

Lorazepam Tablets: 0.5 mg, 1 mg, and 2 mg; *Ativan*®, generic; (Rx; C-IV)

Lorazepam Concentrated Oral Solution: 2 mg/mL in 10 mL and 30 mL with dropper; *Lorazepam Intensol*®; (Rx; C-IV)

Lorazepam Injection: 2 mg/mL and 4 mg/mL in 1 mL prefilled syringes, 1 mL single use vials and 10 mL multidose vials; *Ativan*®, generic; (Rx; C-IV)

References

For the complete list of references, see **wiley.com/go/budde/plumb**

Losartan

(loe-***sar***-tan) *Cozaar*®

Angiotensin II Receptor Blocker (ARB)

Prescriber Highlights

- May be useful in dogs for the adjunctive treatment of proteinuria
- Limited data and experience in veterinary medicine to support clinical use in dogs or cats. Telmisartan is preferred in dogs and cats, as there is more research and clinical experience.
- Contraindications include volume and/or electrolyte depletion, hypotension, and hypersensitivity to losartan and possibly other angiotensin II receptor blockers (ARBs).
- Use caution in patients with hepatic impairment
- Not safe during pregnancy

Uses/Indications

Losartan may be useful for the adjunctive treatment of proteinuria in dogs,[1] but there is limited information on its safety and efficacy for veterinary species.

Any potential clinical usefulness of losartan in cats is in question, as one study in 6 cats with experimentally induced (angiotensin I given IV) hypertension did not show that losartan had any significant or consistent effect on blood pressure or pressor response.[2] Telmisartan is FDA-approved for use in cats, and its use would be preferred over losartan.

In dogs, potential clinical usefulness is tempered with the concern that dogs do not metabolize much losartan into an active metabolite (E-3174; EXP-3174)[3] that in humans is thought to produce much of the drug's therapeutic effect and allow once-daily dosing. A study measuring hemodynamic functions in dogs with experimental tachycardia-induced heart failure demonstrated that losartan was ≈3 times less potent than E-3174 in improving some measured functions (eg, reduced pulmonary artery pressure, mean arterial pressure, pulmonary capillary wedge pressure and peripheral resistance, and increased stroke volume).[4]

Additional studies are necessary to determine where losartan fits into the veterinary drug armamentarium.

Pharmacology/Actions

Losartan is an angiotensin II receptor blocker (ARB). By selectively blocking the AT1 receptor, aldosterone synthesis and secretion is reduced, resulting in vasodilation, decreased potassium excretion, and increased sodium excretion. Although plasma concentrations of renin and angiotensin II are increased, this does not counteract the blood pressure lowering effects of losartan. Losartan does not interfere with substance P or bradykinin responses.

In humans, losartan is converted in the liver, likely via P-450 2C9, into the active metabolite (E-3174). E-3174 is a reversible, noncompetitive inhibitor of the AT1 receptor and is more potent than losartan. Dogs do not appear to produce much of the active metabolite,[3] which, as compared with human patients, may considerably alter the dosing strategy, adverse effects, and efficacy of the drug.

Pharmacokinetics

In dogs, losartan, given as single oral doses, was rapidly absorbed with peak concentrations occurring within one hour and a bioavailability of 23% to 33%. Volume of distribution was 0.3 L/kg. Plasma protein binding was ≈97% with free drug between 2% and 3%. Elimination half-life was between 2 and 3 hours. It is thought that the majority of drug is eliminated in the bile/feces, but significant enterohepatic recirculation occurs.[3]

No losartan pharmacokinetic data were located for cats.

In humans, the pharmacokinetics of losartan differ markedly from what is seen in dogs. After oral dosing, absorption is rapid with a bioavailability of the parent compound of ≈33%. Presence of food can slow absorption but does not affect the extent. Significant first-pass metabolism converts much of the absorbed drug into a carboxylic metabolite (E-3174), which is responsible for much of the drug's therapeutic efficacy. Bioavailability of E-3174 is ≈14% of the administered dose. Peak concentrations of losartan and E-3174 occur at ≈1 and 4 hours, respectively. Free fractions of losartan/E-3174 are 1.3%/0.2%. Terminal half-lives are ≈2 hours for losartan and 8 hours for E-3174. Area under the curve for E-3174 is ≈4 times that of the parent compound. Approximately 10% of the drug and active metabolite are excreted unchanged in the urine with the remainder excreted primarily via bile and feces and as other metabolites in the urine.

Contraindications/Precautions/Warnings

Losartan is contraindicated in patients that are hypersensitive to it. It is not known if cross-reactivity occurs between other angiotensin II receptor blockers (ARBs) and losartan. Hypotensive patients should not receive this drug. Patients that are volume- or electrolyte-depleted should not receive this drug until they are rehydrated, and their electrolytes have been replenished and corrected.

Losartan should be used with caution in patients with hepatic impairment; dosage reduction may be warranted.

Adverse Effects

The adverse effect profile for losartan is not known when it is used clinically in veterinary species. In humans, adverse effects are not common. Adverse effects reported include dry cough, orthostatic dizziness, hypotension, nasal congestion, and back pain.[5] Changes in renal function and hyperkalemia are possible. Very rarely in humans, hypersensitivity and hepatopathy with increased liver enzymes have been reported.

Reproductive/Nursing Safety

Losartan is not considered safe to use during pregnancy. Studies in pregnant rats given high doses of angiotensin II receptor blockers (ARBs) demonstrated a variety of fetal abnormalities (eg, renal pelvic cavitation, hydroureter, absence of renal papilla). Smaller doses in rabbits caused increased maternal death and spontaneous abortion. In humans, the drug is considered teratogenic, particularly during the second and third trimesters. If pregnancy is detected in patients receiving losartan, the drug should be discontinued as soon as possible.

Because losartan and its active metabolite have been detected in substantial quantities in rat milk, there is significant concern about the safety of the drug during nursing.

Because safety has not been established in animals, this drug should only be used when the maternal benefits outweigh the potential risks to offspring.

Overdose/Acute Toxicity

Significant lethality was observed in mice and rats after oral administration of 1 g/kg. Hemodialysis is not effective in removing losartan or its active metabolites.

For patients that have experienced or are suspected to have experienced an overdose, consultation with a 24-hour poison consultation center specializing in providing veterinary-specific information is recommended. For general information related to overdose and toxin exposures, as well as contact information for poison control centers, refer to ***Appendix.***

Drug Interactions

The following drug interactions have either been reported or are theoretical in humans or animals receiving losartan and may be of significance in veterinary patients. Unless otherwise noted, use together is not necessarily contraindicated, but weigh the potential risks and perform additional monitoring when appropriate.

- **ACE INHIBITORS** (eg, **benazepril, enalapril**): Increased risk for adverse effects (eg, hypotension, hyperkalemia, renal function changes); increased monitoring may be warranted
- **ASPIRIN**: Possible reduced antihypertensive effects of losartan and increased risk for renal impairment; increased monitoring may be warranted
- **BACLOFEN**: Concurrent use may have additive blood pressure lowering effects.
- **BENZODIAZEPINES** (eg, **diazepam, lorazepam**): Concurrent use may increase risk for hypotension.
- **BUSPIRONE**: Concurrent use may increase risk for hypotension.
- **CABERGOLINE**: Concurrent use may increase risk for hypotension.
- **CLARITHROMYCIN**: Concurrent use may increase the risk for increased losartan concentrations.
- **CORTICOSTEROIDS** (eg, **betamethasone, dexamethasone**): May decrease the antihypertensive effects of angiotensin II receptor blockers (ARBs)
- **DEXMEDETOMIDINE**: Concurrent use may result in additive effects on blood pressure and heart rate.
- **DIAZOXIDE**: Concurrent use may increase risk for hypotension.
- **DICHLORPHENAMIDE**: Concurrent use may increase risk for hypotension.
- **DIGOXIN**: Concurrent use may increase digoxin concentration. Closely monitor digoxin concentration and therapeutic effects.
- **DIPHENHYDRAMINE**: Concurrent use may increase risk for hypotension.
- **DOXEPIN**: Concurrent use may increase risk for hypotension.
- **INSULIN**: Concurrent use may increase risk for hypoglycemia.
- **LOW MOLECULAR WEIGHT HEPARINS** (eg, **dalteparin, enoxaparin**): Concurrent use may increase risk for hyperkalemia.
- **NONSTEROIDAL ANTI-INFLAMMATORY DRUGS (NSAIDs**; eg, **carprofen, meloxicam**): Possible reduced antihypertensive effects of losartan and increased risk for renal impairment; increased monitoring may be warranted.
- **OPIOIDS** (eg, **buprenorphine, butorphanol**): Concurrent use may increase risk for hypotension.
- **POTASSIUM PREPARATIONS, POTASSIUM-SPARING DIURETICS** (eg, **spironolactone**): Increased risk for hyperkalemia; increased monitoring of serum potassium may be warranted.
- **YOHIMBINE**: Concurrent use may decrease the efficacy of ARBs.

Laboratory Considerations

None were noted.

Dosages

DOGS:

NOTE: There is little clinical experience using this drug in veterinary patients and very limited data published on its clinical usage. Losartan use at this time is experimental and use in clinically ill dogs and cats should be approached with caution. Given the differences in metabolization and lower concentrations of active metabolites noted in dogs, dosages and/or medication frequency may need to be adjusted to provide clinical effectiveness.

Adjunctive treatment of proteinuria in dogs with glomerular disease (extra-label): The International Renal Interest Society (IRIS) has published their consensus-recommended dosages: Azotemic dogs: Initial dose of 0.125 mg/kg PO per day and an escalating dose of 0.25 mg/kg per day. Nonazotemic dogs: 0.5 mg/kg per day and an escalating dose of 1 mg/kg per day. Concurrent administration of an ACE inhibitor is generally recommended.[1]

Monitoring

- Patients treated with losartan should be monitored for response to therapy as well as side effects.[1]
- Monitoring is recommended 1 to 2 weeks after starting losartan therapy and 1 to 2 weeks after increasing losartan dose or dose frequency.[1]
- Monitoring after starting or changing dosages should include UPC, serum creatinine, serum potassium, and blood pressure to verify the desired therapeutic effect was achieved.[1]
- In all dogs receiving losartan, UPC, urinalysis, systemic arterial blood pressure, serum albumin, creatinine, and potassium concentrations should be monitored at least quarterly.[1]

Client Information

- This medication may be given with or without food.
- Because this medication has not been used often in dogs or cats, side effects are not well known; watch carefully for any side effects and report them to your veterinarian. Possible side effects could include diarrhea, vomiting, lack of appetite, fatigue (tiredness), and low blood pressure (eg, fainting, weakness, intolerance to exercise).
- This drug has caused birth defects and should not be used in pregnant animals. If humans in the household are pregnant, they should be very careful not to ingest these tablets, wear disposable gloves when administering doses, and wash their hands after touching these tablets.

Chemistry/Synonyms

Losartan potassium [CAS Registry: 114798-26-4 (losartan); 124750-99-8 (losartan potassium); ATC: C09CA01] occurs as a white to off-white, hygroscopic crystalline powder. It is freely soluble in water and methyl alcohol; soluble in isopropyl alcohol and slightly soluble in acetonitrile.

Losartan potassium may also be known as DuP-753, E-3340, or MK-0954. A common trade name is *Cozaar®*.

Storage/Stability

Store losartan tablets at room temperature (up to 30°C [86°F]) and protect from light.

Compatibility/Compounding Considerations

Compatibility is dependent on factors such as pH, concentration, temperature, and diluent used; specialized references or a hospital pharmacist should be consulted for more specific information.

The manufacturer of the human-labeled tablets (Merck & Co)

describes a method to prepare an extemporaneous suspension containing losartan potassium 2.5 mg/mL: Add 10 mL of purified water to a 240 mL polyethylene terephthalate (PET) bottle containing ten 50 mg tablets of losartan potassium; shake contents for more than 2 minutes.[5] Allow concentrated suspension to stand for 60 minutes following reconstitution, then shake for an additional minute. Prepare a mixture containing equal parts (by volume) of syrup (*Ora-Sweet*®) and suspending vehicle (*Ora-Plus*®) separately. Dilute the concentrated suspension of losartan potassium with 190 mL of the *Ora-Sweet*® and *Ora-Plus*® mixture; shake the container an additional minute to disperse ingredients. Shake suspension before dispensing each dose. Store in the refrigerator (2°C-8°C [36°F-46°F]) for up to 30 days.

Dosage Forms/Regulatory Status

VETERINARY-LABELED PRODUCTS: NONE

HUMAN-LABELED PRODUCTS:

Oral Tablets: 25 mg, 50 mg, and 100 mg; *Cozaar*®, generic; (Rx)

References

For the complete list of references, see **wiley.com/go/budde/plumb**

Lotilaner

(loh-teh-***lan***-er) *Credelio*®

Isoxazoline Ectoparasiticide

Prescriber Highlights

- ► Chewable oral tablet for treatment and prevention of flea infestation in dogs and cats; treatment and control of American dog tick, black-legged tick, lone star tick, and brown dog tick infestation in dogs; and treatment and control of black-legged tick infestation in cats
- ► Must be administered with food
- ► Treatment can begin at any time of the year.
- ► Appears to be well tolerated when administered at the label dosage
- ► The FDA has warned that drugs in the isoxazoline class have the potential for causing neurologic adverse effects (eg, including muscle tremors, ataxia, and seizures) in dogs and cats.

Uses/Indications

Lotilaner is FDA-approved for the treatment and prevention of flea infestations (*Ctenocephalides felis*) and the treatment and control of infestations of American dog tick (*Dermacentor variabilis*, wood tick), black-legged tick (*Ixodes scapularis*, deer tick), lone star tick (*Amblyomma americanum*), and brown dog tick (*Rhipicephalus sanguineus*) for 1 month in dogs and puppies 8 weeks of age and older with a body weight of 2 kg (4.4 lb) or more.[1] Lotilaner may be used as part of a treatment strategy to control flea allergy dermatitis.[2]

In cats, lotilaner is FDA-approved for treatment and prevention of flea infestations (*Ctenocephalides felis*) for 1 month in cats and kittens 8 weeks of age and older weighing 2 pounds or more, as well as for the treatment and control of *Ixodes scapularis* (black-legged tick) infestations for 1 month in cats and kittens 6 months of age or older and weighing 2 pounds or more.[3]

Lotilaner is used extra-label to treat generalized demodicosis and sarcoptic mange in dogs.[4,5] When dogs with sarcoptic mange were treated with monthly label-recommended doses, pruritus ceased within 2 weeks, skin scrapings were negative in 1 month and active lesions in all dogs were absent at 2 months.[5] In dogs, lotilaner has demonstrated efficacy against *Ambylomma cajennense* (sensu lato),[6] *Ixodes holocyclus*,[7] and *Haemaphysalis longicornis*.[8]

In the European Union (EU), lotilaner is indicated for immediate and persistent killing activity for 1 month for fleas (*C felis* and *C canis*) and ticks (*R sanguineus, Ixodes ricinus* [castor bean tick], *I hexagonus* [hedgehog tick], and *Dermacentor reticulatus* [ornate cow/dog tick]) in dogs.[9] In cats, lotilaner has EU approval for the treatment of flea and tick infestations in cats 8 weeks of age and older and weighing 0.5 kg (1.1 lb) or more,[5] and can improve signs of flea allergy dermatitis.[9,10]

Pharmacology/Actions

Lotilaner is an isoxazoline insecticide and acaracide. Lotilaner inhibits gamma-aminobutyric acid (GABA)-gated chloride channels in insect and acarine peripheral and central nervous systems,[11] blocking transfer of chloride ions across cell membranes. The resulting neuronal hyperexcitation results in rapid death of susceptible insects and acarines. A difference between insect and acarine GABA receptor sensitivity to lotilaner in comparison to mammals is believed the reason for differential toxicity.[12] Lotilaner kills adult fleas and ticks only after they have bitten and fed.

In dogs, lotilaner begins killing fleas within 2 to 4 hours of infestation or administration,[1,13] with ≈99.8% of fleas killed within 8 hours[13,14] and 100% of fleas killed within 12 hours.[1,14] This speed of kill (ie, ≈99.8% of fleas killed within 8 hours, 100% of fleas killed within 12 hours) is maintained for 35 days after administration.[14] Fleas are killed before laying eggs.

In cats, lotilaner begins killing fleas within 8 hours of administration.[15] Efficacy was >99% against *I ricinus* in lotilaner-treated cats for up to 35 days, with >90% killing noted within 12 hours for the first 7 days following administration and within 18 hours for days 8 to 35.[16]

Lotilaner is 97% to 100% effective against the 4 major ticks when administered 48 hours after infestation, with ≈70% reduction in the number of live ticks observed on treated dogs at 4 hours after lotilaner administration. Effectiveness is maintained for 30 to 35 days after administration.[1,16-18]

Pharmacokinetics

In dogs, lotilaner peak levels occur 2 hours after oral administration.[13] Food increases absorption. Lotilaner is highly protein bound.[11] Biliary excretion is the major route of elimination.[9] Average elimination half-life is 9.6 days in beagles 2 months of age versus 28 days in beagles 10 months of age[19] and 30.7 days in adult beagles.[11]

In cats, peak lotilaner levels occur 4 hours after oral administration. Bioavailability approaches 100% when given with food but is only 8.4% when fasting. Maximum lotilaner concentration was ≈9 times higher when given with food versus fasting. Volume of distribution at steady state was 5.37 L/kg. Clearance was 0.13 L/kg/day, and the terminal half-life was 28.7 days after IV administration, and 33.6 days following oral administration.[20]

Contraindications/Precautions/Warnings

Lotilaner is contraindicated in patients with a known hypersensitivity to it.[1,3] In the United States, lotilaner is not approved for use in puppies or kittens less than 8 weeks of age, in kittens that weigh less than 0.9 kg (2 lb) or in dogs that weigh less than 2 kg (4.4 lb). Use lotilaner with caution in dogs or cats with a history of seizures or epilepsy.

Adverse Effects

In preapproval field studies (284 dogs over 90 days), no serious adverse effects were noted. The most common adverse effects in dogs included weight loss (1.5%), elevated BUN, polyuria, and diarrhea (1% each). Additionally, 1 dog experienced head tremors, and 1 dog with a history of seizures experienced seizure activity 6 days after lotilaner administration. Vomiting also has been reported.[1]

Field studies in cats did not result in significant adverse events. Adverse effects may include weight loss (2.2%), tachypnea (1.3%), vomiting (1.3%), diarrhea (0.9%), anorexia (0.9%), and elevated BUN (0.9%).[3]

The FDA has warned that in dogs and cats treated with drugs in the isoxazoline class have the potential for causing neurologic adverse effects, including muscle tremors, ataxia, and seizures.[21]

Reproductive/Nursing Safety

The label states that safe use in breeding, pregnant, or lactating dogs[1] and cats[3] has not been evaluated. No evidence[10] of reproductive or teratogenic effects was noted in laboratory studies of rats.[9]

Because safety has not been established in animals, this drug should only be used when the maternal benefits outweigh the potential risks to offspring.

Overdose/Acute Toxicity

No clinically relevant, treatment-related effects were observed when lotilaner was administered to beagles[1] or kittens[22] 8 weeks of age at 3 and 5 times the label dose every 28 days for 8 doses.[1]

For patients that have experienced or are suspected to have experienced an overdose, consultation with a 24-hour poison consultation center specializing in providing veterinary-specific information is recommended. For general information related to overdose and toxin exposures, as well as contact information for poison control centers, refer to ***Appendix***.

Drug Interactions

In a field study, lotilaner was administered with other medications (eg, vaccines, antibiotics, NSAIDs, anthelmintics, anesthetics) with no observed adverse effects.[1]

Laboratory Considerations

- None noted

Dosages

DOGS:

For labeled indications; treatment and prevention of flea infestations *(Ctenocephalides felis)*, and the treatment and control of black-legged tick *(Ixodes scapularis)*, American dog tick *(Dermacentor variabilis)*, lone star tick *(Amblyomma americanum)*, and **brown dog tick *(Rhipicephalus sanguineus)* infestations for 1 month in dogs and puppies 8 weeks of age and older weighing 2 kg (4.4 lb) of body weight or more** (label dosage; FDA-approved): Minimum dosage is 20 mg/kg PO once per month with food[1]

Patient weight	Tablet size (mg)	Number of tablets
2 kg to 2.7 kg (4.4 lb to 6 lb)	56.25	1
>2.8 kg to 5.5 kg (6.1 lb to 12 lb)	112.5	1
>5.5 kg to 11.4 kg (12.1 lb to 25 lb)	225	1
>11.5 kg to 22.7 kg (25.1 lb to 50 lb)	450	1
>22.8 kg to 45.5 kg (50.1 lb to 100 lb)	900	1

For dogs weighing more than 100 lb (45.5 kg), administer the appropriate combination of chewable tablets.

Generalized demodicosis (extra-label): Minimum dosage 20 mg/kg PO once every 4 weeks for 3 treatments was effective in reducing and eliminating live mite counts in dogs with naturally occurring *Demodex* spp infestation.[4]

Sarcoptic mange (extra-label): Treat according to manufacturer's label recommendations PO once every 4 weeks for 3 treatments (see table above for label dosages).[5]

CATS:

Treatment and prevention of flea infestations (*Ctenocephalides felis*) for 1 month in cats and kittens 8 weeks of age and older weighing 0.9 kg (2 lb) or greater (6 mg/kg), as well as the treatment and control of black-legged tick (*Ixodes scapularis*) infestations for 1 month in cats and kittens 6 months of age or older and weighing 0.9 kg (2 lb) or more (label dosage; FDA-approved): Minimum dose of 6 mg/kg orally once a month[3]

Patient weight	Tablet size (mg)	Number of tablets
0.9 kg to 1.8 kg (2 lb to 4 lb)	12	1
1.9 kg to 7.7 kg (4.1 lb to 17 lb)	48	1
Over 7.7 kg (17 lb)	Appropriate combination of tablets	

Treatment of flea and tick infestations in cats 8 weeks of age and older and weighing 0.5 kg (1.1 lb) or more (extra-label): 6 – 24 mg/kg PO once per month with food[22]

Patient weight	Tablet size (mg)	Number of tablets
0.5 kg to 2 kg (1.1 lb to 4.4 lb)	12	1
>2 kg to 8 kg (4.4 lb to 17.6 lb)	48	1
>8 kg (17.6 lb)	Appropriate combination of tablets	

Monitoring

- Efficacy of parasiticide activity
- Adverse effects (eg, muscle tremors, ataxia, seizures)

Client Information

- This medicine must be given with food or within 30 minutes before or after feeding.
- Be sure your animal consumes the full dose each time. Watch your animal for a few minutes after giving the medicine to be sure they do not spit out any part of the dose.
- If your dog or cat vomits within 2 hours of dosing, give another full dose. If a dose is missed, give it when you remember and start a new monthly dosing schedule.
- Treatment may start at any time of the year. In areas where fleas are common year-round, monthly treatment should continue the entire year without stopping.
- To minimize the likelihood of flea reinfestation, treat all animals in a household with an approved flea control product.
- Lotilaner kills adult fleas and ticks only after they have bitten your animal but before the fleas or ticks can lay eggs or transmit disease. Existing flea eggs will hatch and must feed in order to be killed.
- Wash hands after handling tablets.
- Contact your veterinarian if you see any side effects including neurologic problems such as tremors, difficulty walking, or seizures.

Chemistry/Synonyms

Lotilaner is a member of the isoxazoline family. It has a molecular weight of 596.8. Chewable tablets contain only the active S-enantiomer. Its ATCvet code is QP53BE04.

Lotilaner may also be known as *Credelio®*.

Storage/Stability

Chewable tablets should be stored at 15°C to 25°C (59°F-77°F); excursions are permitted between 5°C and 40°C (41°F-104°F). Keep out of reach of children.

Compatibility/Compounding Considerations

No specific information noted

Dosage Forms/Regulatory Status

VETERINARY-LABELED PRODUCTS:

Lotilaner Chewable (beef-flavored) Tablets: 56.25 mg, 112.5 mg, 225 mg, 450 mg, and 900 mg; *Credelio*®; (Rx). FDA-approved for use in dogs. NADA# 141-494

Lotilaner Chewable (vanilla and yeast-flavored) Tablets: 12mg and 48 mg; *Credelio*® CAT; (Rx). FDA-approved for use in cats. NADA# 141-528

HUMAN-LABELED PRODUCTS: NONE

References

For the complete list of references, see **wiley.com/go/budde/plumb**

Lufenuron/Lufenuron Combination Products

(loo-**fen**-yur-on) *Program®, Sentinel®, Sentinel® Spectrum®*

Chitin Synthesis Inhibitor; Insect Growth Regulator

*For information on the combination products, see **Milbemycin Oxime** and **Praziquantel/Praziquantel Combinations Products.***

Prescriber Highlights

- Used as a single agent for flea control in dogs and cats
- Also found in some antiparasitic products in combination with milbemycin oxime ± praziquantel
- Adverse effects are rarely seen at recommended oral doses; injectable lufenuron product can cause a local tissue reaction in cats.

Uses/Indications

Lufenuron is FDA-approved for oral use in dogs and cats for the control of flea populations[1,2]; however, the oral products with lufenuron as a single agent are no longer marketed. The 6-month injectable (*Program*®) is indicated for flea control in cats.[3] The lufenuron/milbemycin oxime combination product (*Sentinel*®) is labeled for prevention and control of flea populations, prevention of heartworm disease, control of adult hookworms, and the removal and control of adult roundworms and whipworms.[4] The oral chewable lufenuron/milbemycin oxime/praziquantel combination tablet (*Sentinel*® *Spectrum*®) extends the antiparasitic spectrum to also include treatment and control of tapeworms.[5]

Lufenuron has also been used in aquatic species (eg, salmonids,[6] stingrays,[7] loggerhead sea turtles[8]) for treatment of fish lice and copepods; however, no products are approved in the US for use in aquatics or for food species.

Lufenuron showed initial promise as a treatment for cutaneous fungal infections[9] (eg, dermatophytosis) but the early enthusiasm has dampened considerably as efficacy appears limited.[10,11]

Pharmacology/Actions

Lufenuron inhibits chitin synthesis, polymerization, and deposition in fleas, thereby preventing eggs from developing into adults. After biting a lufenuron-treated dog or cat, lufenuron is deposited in a female flea's eggs. These eggs are prevented from hatching, thereby breaking the flea life cycle. Lufenuron does not kill adult fleas. Therefore, pre-existing flea populations may continue to develop after treatment and noticeable control may not be observed for several weeks without additional flea control products.

It is believed that lufenuron's nonspecific effect on chitin synthesis is related to serine protease inhibition. Lufenuron's effect on chitin synthesis is specific to insects; lufenuron does not inhibit chitin synthesis in fungi.[12] However, a study in *Microsporum canis* infected cats found that pre-treatment with oral lufenuron prior to enilconazole or griseofulvin potentially had an immunomodulatory effect and could be of benefit in long-lasting infections that have been unsuccessfully treated with conventional drugs.[13]

Pharmacokinetics

Approximately 40% of an oral dose is absorbed with the remainder eliminated in the feces. To maximize oral absorption, the manufacturer recommends administering in conjunction with or immediately after (within 30 minutes) a full meal. The drug is absorbed in the small intestine and stored in adipose tissue that acts as a depot reservoir to slowly redistribute the drug back into the circulation. In dogs administered oral lufenuron, the drug was detected in the SC layer of the skin, not on the skin surface.[14]

After cats receive the lufenuron injectable product, 2 to 3 weeks are required before blood lufenuron concentrations are high enough to be effective. Cats require a substantially higher oral dose per kg than do dogs for equivalent efficacy. The drug is apparently not metabolized; it is excreted unchanged into the bile and eliminated in the feces.

Contraindications/Precautions/Warnings

Lufenuron injection should only be given SC; do NOT inject IM.[3] The feline-labeled injectable product should not be used in dogs as severe local reactions are possible.

Oral lufenuron (*Program*® *Flavor Tabs*) is indicated for use in dogs and cats 4 weeks of age and older[2] (oral suspension and *Program*® *Cat Flavor Tabs* are 6 weeks of age and older[2,15]); the feline injectable lufenuron (ie, *Program*® *6 Month for Cats*) is indicated for use in cats 6 weeks of age and older.[3] The lufenuron/milbemycin oxime combination product (ie, *Sentinel*®) is indicated for use in dogs and puppies 4 weeks and older and weighing at least 2 pounds.[4] The lufenuron/milbemycin oxime/praziquantel combination product (ie, *Sentinel*® *Spectrum*®) is indicated for use in dogs and puppies 6 weeks and older and weighing at least 2 pounds.[5]

For lufenuron combination products containing milbemycin oxime, dogs should be tested for pre-existing heartworm infections because some dogs with a high number of circulating heartworm microfilariae will develop a transient, shock-like syndrome after receiving milbemycin oxime. Infected dogs should be treated for heartworm infection to remove adult heartworms and microfilariae prior to initiating milbemycin oxime treatment.

Adverse Effects

Adverse effects reported in dogs and cats after oral lufenuron include vomiting, diarrhea, anorexia, lethargy/depression, pruritus/urticaria, erythema, and dyspnea.[1,2,15]

Adverse effects following lufenuron injection in cats include pain on injection, injection site lumps/granulomas, vomiting, listlessness/lethargy, and anorexia.[3] After receiving the injectable product, a small lump or tissue reaction at the injection site has been noted in some cats. A few weeks may be required for this to dissipate. There is one published case report of a cat that developed an injection-site sarcoma post lufenuron injection[16]; the FDA's adverse drug experience (ADE) database noted that "injection site neoplasm" had been reported 13 times between 1987 and April 30, 2013.

Reproductive/Nursing Safety

The oral lufenuron products appear to be safe to use in pregnant, breeding, or lactating animals[4]; safety of the injectable product in reproducing cats has not been formally established.[3] In dogs, lufenuron concentrates in the milk at concentrations greater than 60 times the concentrations found in blood; nursing puppies from treated dams may have blood lufenuron concentrations 8 to 9 times greater than the dam.[4,17]

Overdose/Acute Toxicity

Growing puppies were dosed at levels up to 30 times for 10 months without overt effect on growth or viability noted. Cats receiving oral dosages of up to 17 times apparently were unaffected. Kittens receiving a single dose of 266 mg/kg PO had no apparent adverse effects.[9]

Acute toxicity of lufenuron injection was evaluated in cats receiving 10 times the labeled dose, and cumulative toxicity was evaluated over a 2-month period in cats receiving 3 times the recommended dose. No clinical signs of toxicity were observed other than injection site reactions.[3]

Drug Interactions

Limited data are available; the manufacturer states that when used with a variety of adulticides, vaccines, antibiotics, anthelmintics, and steroids, no adverse effects or interactions were noted in either dogs or cats.

Laboratory Considerations

None

Dosages

DOGS:

Lufenuron as a single agent (*Program*®) for prevention and control of flea populations (label dosage; FDA-approved): lufenuron 10 mg/kg (minimum) PO once monthly given with or immediately after a meal. Dosed by body weight range: up to 4.5 kg (10 lb), 45 mg; 5 to 9.1 kg (11 to 20 lb), 90 mg; 9.5 to 20.5 kg (21 to 45 lb), 204.9 mg; 20.9 to 40.9 kg (46 to 90 lb), 409.8 mg; over 40.9 kg (90 lb), provide the appropriate combination of tablets based on body weight.[2] **NOTE**: This product remains listed in the FDA's Green Book but may no longer be marketed.

Lufenuron/milbemycin oxime combination product (*Sentinel*®) for heartworm prevention, control of fleas and hookworms, and control and removal of ascarids and whipworms (label dosage; FDA-approved): lufenuron 10 mg/kg (minimum) in combination with milbemycin oxime 0.5 mg/kg (minimum) PO once monthly given with or immediately after a meal.[4] Dosed by body weight range (see table below):

Body weight in kg (lb)	Lufenuron mg/tablet	Milbemycin oxime mg/tablet	Number of tablets to administer
0.9 to 4.5 (2-10)	46	2.3	1
5 to 11.4 (11-25)	115	5.75	1
11.8 to 22.7 (26-50)	230	11.5	1
23.2 to 45.5 (51-100)	460	23	1
Greater than 45.5 (100)	--	--	Appropriate combination of tablets

Lufenuron/milbemycin oxime/praziquantel combination product (*Sentinel*® *Spectrum*®) for heartworm prevention, prevention and control of fleas, treatment and control of roundworms, hookworms, whipworms, and tapeworms (label dosage; FDA-approved): lufenuron 10 mg/kg (minimum) in combination with milbemycin oxime 0.5 mg/kg (minimum), and praziquantel 5 mg/kg (minimum) PO once monthly with or immediately after a meal.[5] Dosed by body weight range (see table below):

Body weight in kg (lb)	Lufenuron mg/tablet	Milbemycin oxime mg/tablet	Praziquantel mg/tablet	Number of tablets to administer
0.9 to 3.6 (2-8)	46	2.3	22.8	1
3.7 to 11.4 (8.1-25)	115	5.75	57	1
11.4 to 22.7 (25.1-50)	230	11.5	114	1
22.8 to 45.5 (50.1-100)	460	23	228	1
Greater than 45.5 (100)	--	--	--	Appropriate combination of tablets

Lufenuron/nitenpyram (*Program*® *and Capstar*® *Flea Management System*®) to kill adult fleas and prevent flea eggs from hatching (label dosage; FDA-approved): lufenuron 10 mg/kg (minimum) PO once monthly used concurrently with nitenpyram 11.4 mg (dogs weighing less than 11.3 kg [25 lb]) OR nitenpyram 57 mg (dogs weighing more than 11.3 kg [25 lb]) PO once or twice weekly.[18] **NOTE**: This product remains listed in the FDA's Green Book but may no longer be marketed.

Lufenuron/milbemycin oxime/nitenpyram (*Sentinel*® *and Capstar*® *Flea Management System*®) to prevent heartworm disease, prevent and control of flea populations, control of hookworms, and the removal and control of roundworm and whipworm infections (label dosage; FDA-approved): lufenuron 10 mg/kg (minimum) in combination with milbemycin oxime 0.5 mg/kg PO once monthly used concurrently with nitenpyram 11.4 mg (dogs weighing less than 11.3 kg [25 lb]) OR nitenpyram 57 mg (dogs weighing more than 11.3 kg [25 lb]) PO once or twice weekly.[19] **NOTE**: This product remains listed in the FDA's Green Book but may no longer be marketed.

Adjunctive therapy for dermatophytosis using lufenuron as a single agent (extra-label): While efficacy is questionable, the following dosages have been suggested:

a) 65 – 100 mg/kg PO once every 2 weeks for 2 treatments.[11] If significant improvement is not seen, a different antifungal agent should be selected. If improvement is seen, re-treat monthly thereafter until at least 2 negative fungal cultures are obtained.

b) 54.2 – 68.3 mg/kg PO once[9]

CATS:

Lufenuron as a single agent (*Program*®) for control of flea populations (label dosage; FDA-approved):

- **Injectable**: 10 mg/kg (recommended minimum dose) SC once every 6 months. Shake well before administration.[3] Dosed by body weight range (see table below):

Body weight in kg (lb)	Syringe size (mL)	Lufenuron dose (mg)
Up to 4 kg (8.8)	0.4 (small)	40
4.1 to 8 kg (8.9-17.6)	0.8 (large)	80

- **Oral** (label dosage; FDA-approved): lufenuron 30 mg/kg (minimum) PO once monthly given with or immediately after a meal. **NOTE**: These products remain listed in the FDA's Green Book but may no longer be marketed.

a) *Suspension* dosed by body weight: up to 4.5 kg (10 lb), 135 mg; 4.6 to 9 kg (11 to 20 lb), 270 mg; over 10 kg (20 lb), provide the appropriate combination of packs based on body weight.[1]

b) *Tablets* dosed by body weight: up to 4.5 kg (10 lb), 135 mg; 5 to 9.1 kg (11 to 20 lb), 270 mg; over 9.1 kg (20 lb), provide the appropriate combination of tablets.[2,15]

Lufenuron with nitenpyram (*Program*® *and Capstar*® *Flea Management System*®) to kill adult fleas and prevent flea eggs from hatching (label dosage; FDA-approved): lufenuron 30 mg/kg (minimum) PO once monthly used concurrently with nitenpyram 11.4 mg/cat (NOT mg/kg) PO once or twice weekly. **NOTE**: This product remains listed in the FDA's Green Book but may no longer be marketed.[18]

Adjunctive treatment of dermatophytosis (extra-label): While efficacy is questionable, the following dosages have been suggested; re-treat after 14 days and monthly thereafter until at least 2 negative fungal cultures are obtained.

a) 80 mg/kg PO for house cats[11,20]

b) 100 mg/kg PO for cats housed in catteries

RABBITS/RODENTS/SMALL MAMMALS:

For control of flea populations in rabbits: 30 mg/kg PO once monthly[21]

For control of flea populations in ferrets: 30 mg/kg PO once monthly[22]

Monitoring

- Efficacy. It may take longer to see effect in colder geographic areas due to prolonged flea cycle in colder temperatures.
- Adverse effects (eg, vomiting, diarrhea, anorexia, lethargy/depression, pruritus/urticaria, erythema, dyspnea; pain on injection and injection site lumps/granulomas [injectable only]).

Client Information

- This medicine helps to control fleas by preventing development of flea eggs. It does not kill adult fleas.
- Give this medication with food.
- Oral products must be used every 30 days to work well.
- All animals in a household need to be treated for this treatment to work.
- Side effects are rare when given by mouth but vomiting after a dose is the most common side effect. If your animal vomits within 2 hours after dosing, the drug should be given again.
- If a dose is missed, give the medicine and then resume monthly treatments.
- Do not split tablets unless instructed to do so.

Chemistry/Synonyms

A benzoylphenylurea derivative, lufenuron is classified as an insect development inhibitor. The drug is lipophilic.

Lufenuron may also be known as CGA-184699, *Program*®, and *Sentinel*®.

Storage/Stability

The commercially available tablets and suspension and lufenuron injection suspension should be stored at room temperature between 15°C and 30°C (59°F-86°F). Lufenuron combinations with milbemycin oxime (+/- praziquantel) should be stored at controlled room temperature between 15°C and 25°C (59°F-77°F).

Compatibility/Compounding Considerations

- No specific information noted

Dosage Forms/Regulatory Status

VETERINARY-LABELED PRODUCTS:

Lufenuron Oral Suspension: 135 mg and 270 mg in 6-tube packs; *Program*® *Suspension*; (OTC). FDA-approved for use in cats and kittens 6 weeks of age or older. NADA #141-026. **NOTE**: This product remains listed in the FDA's Green Book but may no longer be marketed.

Lufenuron 6-Month Injectable for Cats: 100 mg/mL in 10 prefilled syringe packages; *Program*® *6 Month for Cats*; (Rx). FDA-approved for use in cats and kittens 6 weeks of age or older. NADA #141-105

Lufenuron Flavor Tabs for Dogs and Cats: 45 mg, 90 mg, 204.9 mg, and 409.8 mg; *Program Flavor Tabs* (OTC). FDA-approved for use dogs, puppies, cats, and kittens 4 weeks of age or older. NADA #141-035. **NOTE**: This product remains listed in the FDA's Green Book but may no longer be marketed.

Lufenuron Flavor Tabs for Cats: 135 mg and 270 mg; *Program*® *Cat Flavor Tabs*; (OTC). FDA-approved for use cats and kittens 6 weeks of age or older. NADA #141-062. **NOTE**: This product remains listed in the FDA's Green Book but may no longer be marketed.

Lufenuron Flavor Tabs used concurrently with Nitenpyram Oral Tablets: lufenuron 45 mg, 90 mg, 204.9 mg, and 409.8 mg; used concurrently with nitenpyram 11.4 mg or 57 mg; *Program*® *Flavor Tabs* and *Capstar*® *Flea Management System;* (OTC). FDA-approved for use in dogs, puppies, cats, and kittens 4 weeks of age or older. NADA #141-205. **NOTE**: This product remains listed in the FDA's Green Book but may no longer be marketed.

Lufenuron/Milbemycin oxime Oral Tablets for Dogs: lufenuron 46 mg/milbemycin oxime 2.3 mg; lufenuron 115 mg/milbemycin oxime 5.75 mg; lufenuron 230 mg/milbemycin oxime 11.5 mg; lufenuron 460 mg/milbemycin oxime 23 mg; *Sentinel*® *Flavor Tabs*; (Rx). FDA-approved for use in dogs and puppies 4 weeks of age or older and weighing at least 0.9 kg (2 lb). NADA #141-084. **NOTE**: This product remains listed in the FDA's Green Book but may no longer be marketed.

Lufenuron/Milbemycin oxime Oral Tablets used concurrently with Nitenpyram Flavored Tablets: lufenuron 46 mg/milbemycin oxime 2.3 mg, lufenuron 115 mg/milbemycin oxime 5.75 mg, lufenuron 230 mg/milbemycin oxime 11.5 mg; lufenuron 460 mg/milbemycin oxime 23 mg; used concurrently with nitenpyram 11.4 mg or 57 mg; *Sentinel*® *Flavor Tabs* and *Capstar*® *Flea Management System;* (Rx). FDA-approved for use in dogs and puppies 4 weeks of age or older. NADA #141-204. **NOTE**: This product remains listed in the FDA's Green Book but may no longer be marketed.

Lufenuron/Milbemycin oxime/Praziquantel Chewable Oral Tablets: lufenuron 46 mg/milbemycin oxime 2.3 mg/praziquantel 22.8 mg; lufenuron 115 mg/milbemycin oxime 5.75 mg/praziquantel 57 mg; lufenuron 230 mg/milbemycin oxime 11.5 mg/praziquantel 114 mg; lufenuron 460 mg/milbemycin oxime 23 mg/praziquantel 228 mg; *Sentinel*® *Spectrum*®; (Rx). FDA-approved for use in dogs and puppies 6 weeks of age or older and weighing at least 0.9 kg (2 lb). NADA #141-333

HUMAN-APPROVED PRODUCTS: NONE

References

For the complete list of references, see **wiley.com/go/budde/plumb**

Lysine

L-lysine

(*lye*-seen)

Nutritional Amino Acid; Anti-Feline Herpes Virus

Prescriber Highlights

- ► Amino acid that has questionable efficacy to suppress the shedding and reduce the severity of clinical signs associated with FHV-1 infections in cats
- ► Long-term treatment may be required.
- ► Usually well tolerated
- ► Most effective when administered as a bolus

Uses/Indications

Lysine has demonstrated efficacy for cats under experimental conditions to suppress shedding[1] and reduce the severity of conjunctivitis caused by feline herpesvirus-1 (FHV-1) infections.[2] Published studies, however, have not shown lysine to be effective to prevent or reduce the recurrence of FHV-1 upper respiratory tract infections in shelter cats,[3] and may even paradoxically exacerbate clinical disease or viral shedding.[4,5] Because of lysine's overall safety, and lack of studies in client-owned cats, lysine may be considered in that population to lessen viral shedding in latent infections and severity of clinical signs in cats undergoing primary virus exposure.[3,6-8]

Pharmacology/Actions

Lysine is an amino acid that is thought to compete with arginine for incorporation into many herpesviruses. As it is believed that arginine is required for producing infective viral particles, when lysine is incorporated, the virus becomes less infective.[9] Physiologic data from cats question this proposed mechanism.[10]

Pharmacokinetics

No specific information was located.

Contraindications/Precautions/Warnings

There are no specific contraindications.

The stress associated with lysine administration to shelter cats may negate beneficial effects in this population.[6] Lysine-enriched dry diets fed to shelter cats failed to control upper respiratory[7,8] and ocular[7] disease.

Adverse Effects

Adverse effects were not observed in clinical trials in cats.

Human patients taking lysine have occasionally complained of abdominal pain and diarrhea.

Reproductive/Nursing Safety

Lysine showed no teratogenic effects when given to pregnant rats, but reduced fetal weight and increased fetal mortality have been documented.[11] In humans, lysine crosses the placenta and is naturally found in breast milk; significance in veterinary medicine is unknown.[11]

Because safety has not been established in animals, this treatment should only be used when the maternal benefits outweigh the potential risks to offspring.

Overdose/Acute Toxicity

Significant toxicity is unlikely. GI effects (eg, nausea, vomiting, diarrhea) may occur. Reports of nephrotoxicity have been reported in humans as well as in canines receiving 4500 mg/kg/day IV over 3 days.[12]

For patients that have experienced or are suspected to have experienced an overdose, consultation with a 24-hour poison consultation center specializing in providing veterinary-specific information is recommended. For general information related to overdose and toxin exposures, as well as contact information for poison control centers, refer to ***Appendix.***

Drug Interactions

The following drug interactions have either been reported or are theoretical in humans or animals receiving lysine and may be of significance in veterinary patients. Unless otherwise noted, use together is not necessarily contraindicated, but weigh the potential risks and perform additional monitoring when appropriate.

- **ARGININE**: Arginine may negate the anti-herpesvirus effects of lysine. It is unlikely that the concentration of arginine found in feline diets would be significant.
- **CALCIUM, ORAL**: Concomitant use of lysine with calcium supplements may increase calcium absorption from the gut and decrease calcium loss in the urine.

Laboratory Considerations

- None noted

Dosages

CATS:

Preventing or reducing recurrent feline herpesvirus infections (extra-label): Although efficacy is not proven for any dosage, many clinicians recommend its use for household cats. It is recommended to administer lysine mixed in a very small amount of food to be eaten all at once and not simply applied over the food bowl to be eaten throughout the day. Of note, the stress of bolus administration (ie, "pilling" or squirting the medication directly into the cat's mouth) may negate any beneficial effects obtained from lysine.[13]

- **Kittens**: 250 mg/kitten (NOT mg/kg) PO once daily OR 125 – 250 mg/kitten (NOT mg/kg) PO twice daily[3]
- **Adult cats**:
  a) 250 – 500 mg/cat (NOT mg/kg) PO every 12 to 24 hours[3,13]
  b) 400 mg PO every 24 hours[1,14]

Reducing the severity of conjunctivitis caused by FHV-1 infection (extra-label): 500 mg/cat (NOT mg/kg) PO twice daily[2]

Monitoring

- Efficacy based on lack of or diminished clinical signs caused by feline herpesvirus upper respiratory infection

Client Information

- This medicine is a nutritional supplement that may lessen the signs related to herpesvirus infections in cats. This medicine will not cure the infection.
- If unable to administer this medicine all at once, it can be mixed with a small (treat-sized) amount of soft, moist food. Ensure the cat ingests the entire lysine-food mixture and receives the full dose.
- Side effects are not likely.
- Treatment, if helpful, may need to be long-term to control clinical signs related to feline herpesvirus infections.

Chemistry/Synonyms

An aliphatic amino acid, lysine has the chemical name L-2,6-diaminohexanoic acid and has a molecular weight of 146.2. It occurs as an odorless, white or almost white crystalline powder, or as colorless crystals, and is freely soluble in water and very slightly soluble in alcohol. It may be commercially available as the acetate or hydrochloride salts, or as the base.

Lysine may also be known as L-lysine. Many trade names are available.

Storage/Stability

Unless otherwise specified on the label, lysine should be stored at room temperature in tight containers.

Compatibility/Compounding Considerations

- No specific information noted

Dosage Forms/Regulatory Status

VETERINARY-LABELED PRODUCTS:

NOTE: There are many products containing lysine as one of many ingredients. No lysine products were located in FDA's Green Book of approved animal drugs. The following products were located with veterinary labeling where lysine is the sole active ingredient:

L-lysine Gel: 250 mg per 1.25 mL: *Viralys® Gel, Enisyl®* Paste, generic; (OTC). Labeled for use in cats and kittens.

L-lysine Powder: (in a palatable base) ≈250 mg per rounded scoop: *Viralys® Powder, Felisyl®*, generic; (OTC). Labeled for use in cats and kittens.

L-lysine chews: 500 mg per soft chewable treat; *Optixcare®*; (OTC). Other brands may have varying amounts of lysine per chewable treat/tablet.

L-Lysine Powder Feed Additive: in 16 oz jars and 5 lb pails; L-*Lysine Powder-Pure®*; (OTC) Labeled for use in horses.

HUMAN-LABELED PRODUCTS:

L-Lysine Tablets and Capsules: 312 mg, 334 mg, 500 mg, and 1000 mg; *Enisyl®*, generic; (OTC)

Lysine is considered a nutrient in the US; therefore, it is exempt from FDA drug approval requirements. There are many products available including tablets and capsules that usually range in strengths from 250 mg to 1000 mg. Combination products are also available.

References

For the complete list of references, see **wiley.com/go/budde/plumb**

Magnesium Hydroxide
Milk of Magnesia

(mag-***nee***-zee-um hye-***droks***-ide)

Antacid, Laxative

Prescriber Highlights

- ► May be used as an antacid or a laxative in small and large animal species
- ► In ruminants, the powder formulation is much more effective than the boluses.
- ► Magnesium hydroxide is contraindicated in patients with renal disease and should be used cautiously in patients with electrolyte restrictions or gastric outlet obstruction.
- ► In cattle, rumen pH should be determined before use, as oral magnesium hydroxide should only be used with documented rumen acidosis.
- ► Most common adverse effect is diarrhea
- ► Long-term use may lead to electrolyte abnormalities.
- ► Many potential drug interactions with orally administered drugs

Uses/Indications

Magnesium hydroxide alone, or in combination with aluminum salts, has been used for the adjunctive treatment of esophagitis, gastric hyperacidity, peptic ulcers, and gastritis. In foals and small animal species, because of difficulty in administration, frequency of dosing required, and availability of histamine-2 blocking agents (eg, ranitidine), proton pump inhibitors (eg, omeprazole), and sucralfate, antacids have largely been relegated to adjunctive roles for these indications.

Magnesium hydroxide alone may be used as an oral laxative in small animal species.

In ruminants, magnesium hydroxide is used to increase rumen pH and as a laxative in the treatment of rumen overload syndrome (ie, acute rumen engorgement, rumen acidosis, grain overload, engorgement toxemia, rumen impaction).

Pharmacology/Actions

Oral antacids used in veterinary medicine are generally relatively non-absorbable salts of aluminum, calcium, or magnesium. Up to 20% of an oral dose of magnesium can be absorbed. Antacids decrease HCl concentrations in the GI tract. One gram of these compounds generally neutralizes 20 to 35 mEq of acid (in vitro). Antacids will rarely bring the gastric fluid pH to near-neutral conditions; however, at a pH of 3.3, 99% of all gastric acid is neutralized, thereby reducing gastric acid back-diffusion through the gastric mucosa and thus, reducing the amount of acid presented to the duodenum. Pepsin proteolytic activity is reduced by raising the pH and can be minimized if the pH of the gastric contents can be increased to greater than 4.

In cattle, orally administered magnesium hydroxide can act as a rumen alkalinizing agent and decrease rumen antimicrobial activity.

Contraindications/Precautions/Warnings

Magnesium-containing antacids are contraindicated in patients with renal disease. Some products have significant quantities of sodium or potassium and should be used cautiously in patients who should have these electrolytes restricted in their diet. Aluminum-containing antacids may inhibit gastric emptying; use cautiously in patients with gastric outlet obstruction.

Oral magnesium hydroxide should only be used clinically in ruminants with documented rumen acidosis and should not be used for treatment of other suspected rumen disorders or hypomagnesemia.[1]

Adverse Effects

In monogastric animals, the most common side effects of magnesium-containing antacid therapy are diarrhea or frequent loose stools. Many products also contain aluminum and calcium salts, which can cause constipation and may balance the laxative actions of magnesium.

Magnesium-containing antacids can cause hypermagnesemia in patients with severe chronic kidney disease (CKD). Hypophosphatemia can develop in patients being fed a low phosphate diet with chronic use of magnesium antacids that also contain aluminum.

In ruminants, alkalinization of the rumen may enhance the absorption of ammonia, histamine, or other basic compounds.

Reproductive/Nursing Safety

In humans, magnesium crosses the placenta and is found in milk. Because safety has not been established in animals, this drug should only be used when the maternal benefits outweigh the potential risks to offspring.

Overdose/Acute Toxicity

Clinical signs associated with an overdose of magnesium salts are an extension of the adverse effects profile. See ***Adverse Effects***. Adverse GI effects and electrolyte imbalances should be treated as necessary based on clinical presentation.

Drug Interactions

The following drug interactions have either been reported or are theoretical in humans or animals receiving oral magnesium salts and may be of significance in veterinary patients. Unless otherwise noted, use together is not necessarily contraindicated, but weigh the potential risks and perform additional monitoring when appropriate.

- AMINOGLYCOSIDES (eg, **amikacin, gentamicin**): May result in neuromuscular weakness

- **Quinidine**: Increased absorption or pharmacologic effect of quinidine may occur.
- **Sodium Polystyrene Sulfonate** (*Kayexalate®*): Antacids may decrease the potassium lowering effectiveness of the sodium polystyrene sulfonate and may cause metabolic alkalosis in patients with renal failure.
- **Sustained- or Extended-Release Medications**: When magnesium hydroxide is used at laxative dosages, it may alter the absorption of these drugs by altering GI transit times.
- **Sympathomimetic Agents**: Increased absorption or pharmacologic effect of the sympathomimetic agent may occur.
- **Tacrolimus**: Concurrent use may result in increased tacrolimus exposure.

Oral magnesium salts can **decrease** the amount absorbed or the pharmacologic effect of the drugs listed below; separate oral doses of oral magnesium salts and these drugs by 2 hours to help reduce this interaction.

- **Allopurinol**
- **Aspirin**
- **Azole antifungals** (eg, **ketoconazole, itraconazole**)
- **Beta-blockers** (eg, **atenolol**)
- **Cefpodoxime**
- **Corticosteroids** (eg, **dexamethasone, prednisone**)
- **Digoxin**
- **Ethambutol**
- **Fluoroquinolones** (eg, **ciprofloxacin, enrofloxacin, marbofloxacin**)
- **Gabapentin**
- **H_2 Antagonists** (eg, **famotidine, ranitidine**)
- **Iron Salts**
- **Isoniazid**
- **Levothyroxine**
- **Macrolides** (eg, **azithromycin**)
- **Misoprostol**
- **Mycophenolate mofetil**
- **Penicillamine**
- **Phenothiazines**
- **Phenytoin**
- **Rifampin**
- **Tetracyclines** (eg, **doxycycline, minocycline**)

Dosages

DOGS:

Adjunctive treatment of hypomagnesemia in dogs with GI disease and severe hypocalcemia (extra-label): 5 – 15 mL/dog (NOT mL/kg) PO once daily[2]

CATS:

Antacid (extra-label): 5 – 15 mL/cat (NOT mL/kg) PO 1 to 2 times daily[3]

CATTLE:

NOTE: In ruminants, the powder formulation is more effective than the boluses.

Rumen overload syndrome (extra-label):

a) Adult animals: Up to 1 g/kg of magnesium hydroxide mixed in 2 to 3 gallons of warm water and given PO by tube. May repeat (use smaller doses) at 6- to 12-hour intervals. If the rumen has been evacuated, do not exceed a total dose of 225 g initially. Dehydration and systemic acidosis must be concomitantly corrected.

b) Calves: As above but use 1/8 – 1/4 the amount.[5]

SHEEP/GOATS:

NOTE: In ruminants, the powder formulation is more effective than the boluses.

Rumen overload syndrome (extra-label): As above for cattle but use 1/8 – 1/4 the amount.[5]

Monitoring

- Monitoring parameters are dependent upon the indication for the product. Patients receiving high-dose or long-term therapy should be monitored for electrolyte imbalances (eg, sodium, potassium, phosphorous, magnesium) and acid-base status.

Client Information

- Oral magnesium hydroxide products are available over the counter (OTC), without prescription; do not give on a regular basis without veterinary supervision.
- Generally well tolerated; constipation or diarrhea can occur.

Compatibility/Compounding Considerations

- No specific information noted

Dosage Forms/Regulatory Status

VETERINARY-LABELED PRODUCTS:

NOTE: No magnesium hydroxide or magnesium oxide products are FDA-approved.

Magnesium Hydroxide Oral Bolus: 17.9 – 27 g (**NOTE**: products may also contain ginger, capsicum, and methyl salicylate). The following may be available: *Magnalax®, Carmilax®, Polymag®, Rumen Bolus®, Instamag®, Polyox®II, Laxade®*; (OTC)

Magnesium Hydroxide Oral Powder: 350 – 361 g/lb (**NOTE**: products may also contain ginger, capsicum, and methyl salicylate). The following may be available: *Carmilax Powder®, Magnalax®, Polyox®, Laxade®*; (OTC)

Magnesium Hydroxide 80 mg/mL, 1 gallon jug; generic; (OTC). See also ***Saline Cathartics***.

HUMAN-LABELED PRODUCTS:

The following is a list of some magnesium hydroxide products available; it is not meant to be all-inclusive.

Magnesium Hydroxide

Chewable Tablets: 400 mg; *Pedia-Lax®*; (OTC)

Oral Liquid (Milk of Magnesia): 400 mg/5 mL in 129 mL, 355 mL, 360 mL, and 780 mL, pint, gallon, and UD 15 mL and 30 mL; liquid concentrate: 800 mg/5 mL (160 mg/mL) in 240 mL and 1200 mg/5 mL (240 mg/mL) in 400 mL; generic; (OTC). See also ***Saline Cathartics***.

Aluminum Hydroxide and Magnesium Hydroxide

Suspension (**NOTE**: Many products and concentrations exist; an example of a representative product is *Maalox®* Suspension, which contains aluminum hydroxide 200 mg and magnesium hydroxide 200 mg/5 mL.)

Other dosage forms that are available commercially include: tablets, chewable tablets, and aerosol foam suspension.

References

For the complete list of references, see **wiley.com/go/budde/plumb**

Magnesium, IV

Magnesium Chloride, Magnesium Sulfate

(mag-***nee***-zee-um)

Parenteral Electrolyte

See also ***Magnesium Hydroxide*** *and* ***Saline Cathartics***

Prescriber Highlights

- ► Used for treatment of hypomagnesemia in many species and for adjunctive therapy of malignant hyperthermia in swine
- ► Contraindications include significant myocardial damage or atrioventricular block; use with caution in patients with impaired renal function.
- ► Adverse effects are usually a result of overdose and can include drowsiness or other CNS depressant effects, muscular weakness, bradycardia, hypotension, respiratory depression, and prolonged QT intervals on ECG. Very high levels may cause neuromuscular blocking activity and, eventually, cardiac arrest.
- ► Monitor serum magnesium levels to avoid hypermagnesemia.
- ► Do not confuse mEq/mL and mg/mL concentrations or mEq/kg and mg/kg dosages.

Uses/Indications

Magnesium is used parenterally in many species for treatment of hypomagnesemia and to resolve clinical signs associated with hypomagnesemia (eg, seizures, refractory arrhythmias). It is also used in swine for adjunctive therapy of malignant hyperthermia. A case report of administering magnesium IV to a dog with generalized tetanus has been published.[1] In dogs and cats, routine use of magnesium during CPR is not recommended for cardiac arrhythmias; however, it may be considered as treatment for torsades de pointes.[2] A quick reference on magnesium in dogs and cats, including its role, deficit, clinical signs, and supplementation, has been published.[3]

In humans, IV magnesium has been used as a treatment of hypertensive crisis in patients with pheochromocytoma.

Pharmacology/Actions

Magnesium is used as a cofactor in a variety of enzyme systems and is involved in muscular excitement and neurochemical transmission.

Pharmacokinetics

In humans, IV magnesium results in immediate effects. Onset after IM administration is ≈1 hour. Magnesium is ≈30% to 35% bound to proteins, and the remainder exists as free ions. Duration of effect is ≈30 minutes after IV administration and 3 to 4 hours after IM administration. It is excreted by the kidneys at a rate proportional to the serum concentration and glomerular filtration rate.[4]

Contraindications/Precautions/Warnings

Parenteral magnesium is contraindicated in patients with myocardial damage or atrioventricular block. Because magnesium is renally cleared, it should be used with caution in patients with impaired renal function, as hypermagnesemia and magnesium intoxication can result.[4] Consider reducing the dose for patients with renal insufficiency.

When administering magnesium IV for treatment of hypomagnesemia, consider reducing potassium supplementation as hyperkalemia may result. Some magnesium products contain aluminum, which may accumulate with prolonged administration in patients with impaired renal function.[4] Patients receiving parenteral magnesium, especially in those with reduced renal function, should be observed and monitored carefully to avoid hypermagnesemia. See ***Monitoring***.

SC administration can cause necrosis of the skin. Only solutions containing a combination of calcium and magnesium should be given SC.

Magnesium sulfate for injection is considered a high-risk medication; additional dose determination and dose preparation safety checks should be employed.

Adverse Effects

Adverse effects of parenteral magnesium are generally the result of magnesium overdose and may include nausea, vomiting, drowsiness or other CNS depressant effects, muscular weakness, bradycardia, hypotension, hypocalcemia, respiratory depression, and prolonged QT intervals on ECG. Very high magnesium levels may cause neuromuscular blocking activity and eventually cardiac arrest.

Reproductive/Nursing Safety

In humans, continuous use of magnesium in pregnant women longer than 5 to 7 days has resulted in bone abnormalities in their offspring, including skeletal demineralization and osteopenia.[5] Magnesium should only be used when maternal benefits outweigh the risks to the fetus.

Magnesium is excreted in milk and should only be used when the benefits outweigh the risks.

Overdose/Acute Toxicity

Clinical signs of an overdose of magnesium are an extension of its adverse effects. See ***Adverse Effects***. Treatment of hypermagnesemia is dependent on the serum magnesium level and any associated clinical effects. Ventilatory support and administration of calcium 10 – 50 mg/kg IV[6] may be required for severe hypermagnesemia. Magnesium is dialyzable.

For patients that have experienced or are suspected to have experienced an overdose, consultation with a 24-hour poison consultation center specializing in providing veterinary-specific information is recommended. For general information related to overdose and toxin exposures, as well as contact information for poison control centers, refer to ***Appendix***.

Drug Interactions

The following drug interactions have either been reported or are theoretical in humans or animals receiving parenteral magnesium and may be of significance in veterinary patients. Unless otherwise noted, use together is not necessarily contraindicated, but weigh the potential risks and perform additional monitoring when appropriate.

- Aminoglycosides (eg, **amikacin, gentamicin**): Concurrent use may result in neuromuscular weakness.
- Calcium: Concurrent use of calcium salts may negate the effects of parenteral magnesium.
- CNS Depressant Drugs (eg, **barbiturates, general anesthetics**): Additive CNS depression may occur.
- Digoxin: Because serious conduction disturbances can occur, parenteral magnesium should be used with extreme caution with digitalis cardiac glycosides.
- Neuromuscular Blocking Agents (eg, **atracurium**): Excessive neuromuscular blockade is possible.

Dosages

NOTES:

1. Do not confuse magnesium dosages, which can be represented in mEq, mmol, and mg. Check dosages and concentrations carefully.
2. One gram of magnesium sulfate hexahydrate contains 8.1 mEq of magnesium. One gram of magnesium chloride contains 9.85 mEq of magnesium. Do not confuse dosages.
3. In adult humans, the maximum infusion rate for IV administration of magnesium sulfate is 150 mg/minute (with the exception of seizures during eclampsia). This is ≈2 mg/kg per minute for an average adult human. If this recommendation is extrapolated to animals, the maximum rate would be

≈0.016 mEq/kg/minute (0.027 mg/kg/minute of magnesium sulfate). Magnesium sulfate is diluted in 5% dextrose or 0.9% sodium chloride to a concentration of 200 mg/mL (20%) or less for IV administration.

DOGS/CATS:

Hypomagnesemia (extra-label):

Supplemental magnesium for animals with refractory hypokalemia, endocrine diseases (eg, DKA), or for critically ill animals (extra-label): 0.75 mEq/kg/day IV in combination with potassium supplementation[7]

Suspected or confirmed severe hypomagnesemia (extra-label): Dosage recommendations vary; most clinicians recommend a loading dose of magnesium sulfate of 0.15 – 0.3 mEq/kg (18.5 – 37 mg/kg) IV slowly over 10 to 20 minutes, followed by 0.75 – 1 mEq/kg/day (92 –123 mg/kg/day) given over 12 to 24 hours as an IV CRI. Some clinicians suggest reducing total daily dose after the first day.

Refractory ventricular arrhythmias (extra-label): 0.15 – 0.3 mEq/kg IV administered over 5 to 15 minutes.[8] Not recommended for routine use during CPR[2]

HORSES:

Hypomagnesemia (extra-label): Magnesium sulfate 25 – 150 mg/kg/day IV CRI diluted in 0.9% sodium chloride, 5% dextrose, or polyionic isotonic solutions for adult horses. Magnesium sulfate 100 – 150 mg/kg/day IV CRI should meet the daily requirements of foals and adult horses. **NOTE**: 100 mg/kg of magnesium *sulfate* provides 9.9 mg/kg of magnesium, whereas 100 mg/kg of magnesium *chloride* provides 12 mg/kg of magnesium. This distinction is critical as overdosing can be fatal.

Ventricular arrhythmias from quinidine intoxication (torsades de pointes) or refractory ileus and synchronous diaphragmatic flutter (extra-label): 50 – 100 mg/kg IV diluted in 0.9% sodium chloride over 30 minutes are considered safe.

Foals with ischemic encephalopathy (extra-label): Magnesium sulfate 50 mg/kg/hour IV CRI for the first hour, followed by 25 mg/kg/hour IV CRI has been proposed. This regimen can be continued for several days, adjusting the dose based on serum magnesium concentrations.[8]

Hypomagnesemia under general anesthesia during colic surgery (extra-label): Magnesium sulfate 25 mg/kg IV over 120 minutes[9]

Adjunctive treatment of perinatal asphyxia syndrome in foals (extra-label): Magnesium sulfate 50 mg/kg diluted to 10 mg/mL (1%) in 0.9% sodium chloride or 5% dextrose and given IV over 1 hour, then 25 mg/kg/hour IV CRI for 24 hours[10] or for 1 to 3 days

CATTLE:

Hypomagnesemia (grass and other magnesium-related tetanies) (extra-label):

a) A typical treatment for an adult beef cow has been slow IV administration (over at least 5 minutes) of 100 mL of the 25% Epsom salt solution. This solution provides 2.5 g of magnesium (0.025 g of magnesium/mL of solution). This solution is highly hypertonic (ie, 2028 mOsm/L). Hypomagnesemia is most commonly treated using commercially available combined calcium, magnesium, and phosphorous solutions; 500 mL of these solutions typically contain 1.6 to 2.7 g of magnesium in the form of a borogluconate, chloride, or hypophosphite salt (the phosphorous in hypophosphite salt form is unavailable to ruminants and therefore worthless). Combined calcium and magnesium solutions are preferred for IV administration to 25% Epsom salt solution because ruminants with hypomagnesemia frequently have hypocalcemia, and hypercalcemia provides some protection against the toxic effects of hypermagnesemia. The maximum safe rate of administration of magnesium in cattle is 0.04 mL of 25% Epsom salt solution/kg per minute. For a 500 kg beef cow with hypomagnesemia, this corresponds to a maximum safe rate of administration of 20 mL/minute. **NOTE**: In a seizing, hypomagnesemic beef cow, rectal administration may be the only safe and practical way to administer magnesium. After evacuating the rectal contents, an enema containing 60 g of Epsom salts (magnesium sulfate heptahydrate) or magnesium chloride in 200 mL of water can be placed in the descending colon (NOT the rectum) and the tail held down for 5 minutes. This treatment regimen increases plasma magnesium concentrations within 10 minutes. If enema solutions are prematurely evacuated, the chance for therapeutic success is eliminated; some degree of colonic mucosal injury is expected due to the high osmolarity of 30% solutions (≈2400 mOsm/L).[11]

b) 350 mL (250 mL of 25% calcium borogluconate and 100 mL of 10% magnesium sulfate) slow IV.[12] If not a proprietary mixture, give calcium first. Relapses occur frequently after IV therapy, and 350 mL SC of magnesium sulfate 20% may give more sustained magnesium levels. Alternating calcium and magnesium may prevent adverse effects. Continue control measures for 4 to 7 days to prevent relapse.

SHEEP/GOATS:

Hypomagnesemia (extra-label): 50 – 100 mL IV of calcium/magnesium solution[12]

SWINE:

Adjunctive therapy of malignant hyperthermia syndrome (extra-label): Using magnesium sulfate 50%, incremental doses of 1 g injected IV slowly, until heart rate and muscle tone are reduced. Use calcium if magnesium-related cardiac arrest occurs.[13]

Monitoring

- Serum magnesium: Total serum magnesium (tMg) measures magnesium in the serum in its 3 forms (ie, ionized, bound, and complexed). Unfortunately, it does not correlate well with total body magnesium but may be useful, especially when suspecting hypermagnesemia. Ionized magnesium (iMg) is preferred by some clinicians but alone may not be clinically useful due to methodology concerns and the low percentages of total body magnesium it represents. The iMg/tMg ratio may be more useful. In patients with normal renal function, pre-magnesium levels (iMg/tMg) are compared with levels after an IV loading dose. If the ratio is elevated, it suggests that a larger portion of stored body magnesium is being mobilized in response to a decrease in whole-body magnesium content. Alternatively, after an IV load, a 24-hour urine magnesium collection can be obtained. Retention of greater than 20% of the magnesium loading dose is considered suggestive of cellular magnesium depletion, and greater than 50% retention is considered diagnostic.[14]
- Clinical signs associated with hypomagnesemia (eg, tetany, seizures, ECG changes [eg, prolonged PR interval and/or QRS complexes]) or hypermagnesemia (eg, loss of deep tendon reflexes, hypotension, respiratory paralysis)[4]
- Serum calcium, potassium if indicated

Client Information

Only your veterinarian can give injectable magnesium.

Chemistry/Synonyms

Magnesium sulfate occurs as small, usually needle-like, colorless crystals with a cool, saline, bitter taste. It is freely soluble in water and sparingly soluble in alcohol. Magnesium sulfate injection has a pH of 5.5 to 7. One gram of magnesium sulfate hexahydrate contains 8.1 mEq of magnesium. Magnesium chloride contains 9.25 mEq of magnesium per gram.

When using commercially available magnesium sulfate injections:

- Magnesium sulfate 4% (40 mg/mL) injection contains 0.325 mEq/mL of elemental magnesium
- Magnesium sulfate 8% (80 mg/mL) injection contains 0.65 mEq/mL of elemental magnesium
- Magnesium sulfate 50% (500 mg/mL) injection contains 4 mEq/mL of elemental magnesium
- Magnesium sulfate 1% in dextrose 5% injection contains 0.081 mEq/mL elemental magnesium
- Magnesium sulfate 2% in dextrose 5% injection contains 0.162 mEq/mL elemental magnesium
- Magnesium chloride 200 mg/mL injection contains 1.97 mEq/mL of elemental magnesium

Magnesium sulfate may also be known as 518, Epsom salts, magnesii sulfas, magnesium sulfuricum heptahydricum, magnesium sulphate, sal amarum, sel anglais, and sel de sedlitz; many trade names are available.

Storage/Stability

Store magnesium sulfate and magnesium chloride for injection at room temperature (15°C to 30°C [59°F-86°F]); avoid freezing. Refrigeration may result in precipitation or crystallization.

Compatibility/Compounding Considerations

Compatibility is dependent upon factors such as pH, concentration, temperature, and diluent used; consult specialized references or a hospital pharmacist for more specific information.

Magnesium sulfate 50% must be diluted to 20% or less before administration. Dextrose 5% injection and sodium chloride 0.9% injection are commonly used as diluents.

Magnesium sulfate is reportedly physically **compatible** with the following IV solutions: dextrose 5%, lactated Ringer's solution, and sodium chloride 0.9%. It is also **compatible** with chloramphenicol sodium succinate, cisplatin, hydrocortisone sodium succinate, isoproterenol HCl, metoclopramide HCl (in syringes), norepinephrine bitartrate, penicillin G potassium, potassium phosphate, and verapamil HCl. Additionally, magnesium is **compatible at Y-sites** with sodium, amikacin sulfate, ampicillin sodium, cefazolin sodium, cefotaxime sodium, cefoxitin sodium, clindamycin phosphate, doxycycline phosphate, erythromycin lactobionate, esmolol HCl, gentamicin sulfate, heparin sodium, labetalol HCl, metronidazole (RTU), oxacillin sodium, piperacillin sodium, potassium chloride, tetracycline HCl, tobramycin sulfate, trimethoprim/sulfamethoxazole, vancomycin HCl, and vitamin B complex with C.

Magnesium sulfate has some concentration-dependent compatibility with calcium gluconate; low concentrations of both magnesium and calcium may be **compatible**. Contact a hospital pharmacist for specific information.

Magnesium sulfate is reportedly physically **incompatible** with alkali hydroxides, alkali carbonates, salicylates, and many metals. It is **incompatible** with 10% lipids, dobutamine HCl, polymyxin B sulfate, procaine HCl, and sodium bicarbonate solutions.

Dosage Forms/Regulatory Status

VETERINARY-LABELED PRODUCTS:

There are no parenteral magnesium-only products FDA-approved for veterinary medicine. There are, however, several proprietary magnesium-containing products available that may also include calcium, phosphorus, potassium, and/or dextrose; refer to the individual product's labeling for specific dosage information. Trade names for these products include *Norcalciphos®*, *Cal-Dextro® Special*, and *#2* and *CMPK®*, and *Cal-Phos® #2;* (Rx).

HUMAN-LABELED PRODUCTS:

Magnesium Sulfate in 5% Dextrose, Injection: 1% (10 mg/mL; 0.081 mEq/mL) in single-dose containers; 2% (20 mg/mL; 0.162 mEq/mL) in 500 mL and 1000 mL single-dose containers; generic; (Rx)

Magnesium Sulfate Injection, solution: 4% (40 mg/mL; 0.325 mEq/mL) in 50 mL, 100 mL, 500 mL, and 1000 mL; 8% (80 mg/mL; 0.65 mEq/mL) in 50 mL; 50% (500 mg/mL; 4 mEq/mL) in 2 mL, 10 mL, 20 mL, and 50 mL vials; generic; (Rx)

Magnesium Chloride Injection: 20% (200 mg/mL; 1.97 mEq/mL) in 50 mL multi-dose vials; generic; (Rx)

References

For the complete list of references, see **wiley.com/go/budde/plumb**

Mannitol

(***man***-i-tole) *Osmitrol®*

Osmotic Diuretic

Prescriber Highlights

- ▶ Used for acute oliguric renal failure, to reduce intraocular, treat cerebral edema, to enhance urinary excretion of some toxins, and, with other diuretics, to rapidly reduce edema
- ▶ Contraindications include anuria, hypovolemia, severe dehydration, severe pulmonary congestion, and pulmonary edema.
- ▶ Stop treatment if patient develops signs of heart failure, pulmonary congestion, or acute kidney injury.
- ▶ Adverse effects include fluid and electrolyte imbalances, GI (eg, nausea, vomiting), cardiovascular (eg, pulmonary edema, congestive heart failure, tachycardia), and CNS effects (eg, lethargy, coma).
- ▶ Fluid, electrolyte, and acid-base imbalances must be corrected prior to administration. Adequate monitoring of urine output, fluid, electrolyte, and neurologic status is mandatory.
- ▶ Ensure crystals are dissolved in solution before administering; warming the solution prior to administration and use of an in-line IV filter (5 micron) is recommended.

Uses/Indications

Mannitol is used in many species to promote diuresis in oliguric acute kidney injury, reduce intraocular pressure, treat cerebral edema, enhance urinary excretion of some toxins (eg, aspirin, some barbiturates, bromides, ethylene glycol), and, in conjunction with other diuretics, to rapidly reduce edema when appropriate (see ***Contraindications/Precautions/Warnings***). In stable cats with minimal renal compromise, mannitol has been used for IV fluid diuresis in an attempt to expel calcium oxalate uroliths.[1] In humans, it is also used as an irrigating solution during transurethral prostatic resections.

Mannitol may be used as emergency osmotic therapy for acute glaucoma in animals that are refractory to topical medications (eg, prostaglandin analogues, carbonic anhydrase inhibitors, beta-blockers, miotic agents).

Pharmacology/Actions

After IV administration, mannitol is freely filtered at the glomerulus and poorly reabsorbed in the tubule. The increased osmotic pressure prevents water from being reabsorbed at the tubule. To be effective, there must be sufficient renal blood flow and filtration for mannitol to reach the tubules. Although water is proportionately excreted at a higher rate, the excretion of sodium, chloride, bicarbonate ions, uric acid, and urea is also enhanced. Diuresis typically occurs within 1 to 3 hours.

Mannitol produces immediate reduction of cerebral edema (and thus, intracranial pressure) through its diuretic effects. The reduction in cerebral edema allows for improved cerebral blood flow and oxygenation of cerebral tissues. Mannitol also has free radical scavenging effects to help diminish tissue injury caused by cerebral hypoxia.

Mannitol may have a nephroprotective effect by preventing the accumulation of nephrotoxins in the tubular fluid. Additionally, it may minimize renal tubular swelling via its osmotic properties, and it may increase renal blood flow and glomerular filtration by causing renal arteriole dilatation, decreased vascular resistance, and decreased blood viscosity.

Pharmacokinetics

Mannitol is poorly absorbed from the GI tract. After IV dosing, mannitol is distributed to the extracellular compartment. It does not cross the blood–aqueous barrier or the blood–brain barrier unless the patient has received very high doses, is acidotic, or there is loss of integrity of the barrier.

Only 7% to 10% of mannitol is metabolized, with the remainder excreted unchanged in the urine. The elimination half-life of mannitol is ≈100 minutes in adult humans but may be prolonged by renal impairment. Half-lives in cattle and sheep are reported to be between 40 and 60 minutes.

Contraindications/Precautions/Warnings

Mannitol is contraindicated in patients that are hypersensitive to it, anuric, severely hypovolemic, or that have severe pulmonary congestion/edema. Only administer mannitol after correcting fluid, electrolyte, and acid-base imbalances. In humans, mannitol is also labeled as contraindicated in patients with intracranial bleeding; however, there is conflicting clinical evidence to support this contraindication as mannitol has been safely used in these patients without untoward effects (ie, worsening intracranial hemorrhage).

Use extreme caution when administering mannitol in hypovolemic patients, as the diuretic effect of mannitol can exacerbate hypovolemia. Patients treated with mannitol should be treated concurrently with isotonic crystalloid fluids and/or colloids to minimize the risk for hypovolemia. Hypertonic saline may be a better choice to treat elevated intracranial pressure and to increase intravascular volume in these patients. Adequate fluid replacement must be administered to dehydrated animals before mannitol therapy is started.

Use mannitol with caution when treating cerebral edema. Intermittent boluses of mannitol are preferred as CRIs will cause the blood-brain barrier to become more permeable and worsen cerebral edema. Similarly, mannitol should be used with caution when treating elevated intraocular pressure caused by secondary glaucoma (eg, uveitis, neoplasia), as the resulting inflammation may increase the permeability of the blood–aqueous barrier and cause an increase in intraocular pressure (IOP).

Mannitol should also be used with caution when treating ethylene glycol toxicity or other hyperosmolar states (eg, hyperosmolar hyperglycemia), as it can exacerbate intravascular hyperosmolarity. See ***Laboratory Considerations***.

Mannitol therapy should be discontinued if heart failure, pulmonary congestion, azotemia, or oliguria/anuria develop during therapy.

Crystals may form in mannitol solutions. To prevent inadvertent administration of crystals, warming of mannitol solutions (see ***Storage/Stability***) and using an in-line IV filter (5 micron) is recommended.

Adverse Effects

Mannitol therapy may cause imbalances of fluids (eg, volume depletion, volume overload in oliguric patients), electrolytes (eg, hypernatremia, hypokalemia, pseudohyponatremia), and acid-base status (eg, metabolic acidosis).

Mannitol affects canine whole blood coagulation and platelet function in vitro. Clinical significance is uncertain.

Other adverse effects include GI (nausea, vomiting), cardiovascular (pulmonary edema, congestive heart failure, tachycardia), acute kidney injury (if osmolality is more than 320 mOsm/L), and CNS effects (lethargy, coma). Mannitol is a vesicant, and the solutions are hyperosmotic; injection site reactions may occur.

Risks of mannitol therapy include the development of acute kidney injury, rebound cerebral edema, and blood–brain and blood–aqueous barrier disruption with repeated or high doses.

Reproductive/Nursing Safety

Mannitol crosses the placenta but has not demonstrated adverse embryo or fetal effects. It is not known whether this drug is excreted in milk, but it is unlikely that it would pose significant risk to nursing offspring.

Because safety has not been established in animals, this drug should only be used when the maternal benefits outweigh the potential risks to offspring.

Overdose/Acute Toxicity

Inadvertent overdoses can cause excessive excretion of sodium, potassium, and chloride. If urine output is inadequate, water intoxication, acute kidney injury, neurotoxicity,[2] or pulmonary edema may occur. Treat overdoses by discontinuing mannitol administration; monitor and correct electrolyte and fluid imbalances. Hemodialysis is effective in clearing mannitol.

For patients that have experienced or are suspected to have experienced an overdose, consultation with a 24-hour poison consultation center specializing in providing veterinary-specific information is recommended. For general information related to overdose and toxin exposures, as well as contact information for poison control centers, refer to ***Appendix.***

Drug Interactions

The following drug interactions have either been reported or are theoretical in humans or animals receiving mannitol and may be of significance in veterinary patients. Unless otherwise noted, use together is not necessarily contraindicated, but weigh the potential risks and perform additional monitoring when appropriate.

- Aminoglycosides (eg, **amikacin, gentamicin**): Mannitol may increase the nephrotoxic effect of aminoglycosides.
- **Blood Products**: Concurrent administration of mannitol with blood products through the same administration set may result in pseudoagglutination or hemolysis. See ***Compatibility/Compounding Considerations***.
- **Bromides:** Mannitol may enhance urinary bromide excretion.
- **Cyclosporine**: Concurrent use of cyclosporine with mannitol may increase the risk for nephrotoxicity.
- **Desmopressin:** Concurrent use may increase the risk for hyponatremia.
- **Diuretics** (eg, **furosemide**): Concurrent use of mannitol with diuretics may increase the risk for nephrotoxicity.
- **Hypotensive Agents** (eg, **amlodipine, enalapril, sildenafil, telmisartan**): Concurrent use may increase risk for hypotension.
- **Sotalol:** Mannitol's effects on potassium and magnesium may increase the risk for QT prolongation if it is administered with sotalol.

Laboratory Considerations

- Mannitol can interfere with **blood inorganic phosphorus** concentrations.
- Mannitol can give a false positive **ethylene glycol test**.

Dosages

NOTES:

1. Crystals may form in mannitol solutions. To prevent inadver-

tent administration of crystals, warming of mannitol solutions (see ***Storage/Stability***) and using an in-line IV filter (5 micron) is recommended.

2. Administer mannitol only after correcting fluid, electrolyte, and acid-base imbalances and determining that the patient is not anuric.

DOGS/CATS:

Osmotic diuresis (label dosage; not FDA-approved): 1.5 – 2 g/kg IV over 30 minutes[3]

Oliguric acute kidney injury (extra-label): Most clinicians recommend mannitol 0.25 – 0.5 g/kg as a slow IV bolus over 10 to 20 minutes. Recommendations range from 0.25 – 1 g/kg IV over 10 to 40 minutes, but no evidence was located that supports one recommendation over the other. If substantial diuresis occurs, can either start mannitol 60 – 120 mg/kg/hour IV CRI or give as intermittent repeated boluses of 0.25 – 0.5 g/kg IV every 4 to 6 hours.[4] Some clinicians recommend that total daily dose should not exceed 2 g/kg per day.

Adjunctive treatment of acute glaucoma refractory to topical agents (extra-label): Most clinicians recommend mannitol 0.5 – 1 g/kg as a slow IV bolus over 10 to 20 minutes. Recommendations range from 0.5 – 2 g/kg IV over 20 to 30 minutes, but no evidence was located that supports one recommendation over the other. Withholding water for 1 to 4 hours postdose is often recommended.[5]

Adjunctive treatment of increased intracranial pressure caused by cerebral edema (extra-label): 0.5 – 1 g/kg IV, IO over 15 to 20 minutes. If required, repeat boluses (usually ever 6 to 8 hours) may be administered; mannitol CRIs are not recommended for this indication.[6,7]

HORSES:

Oliguric acute kidney injury refractory to volume replacement (extra-label): 0.25 – 1 g/kg IV administered as a 20% solution over 15 to 20 minutes[8]

Increased intracranial pressure from traumatic brain injury (extra-label): 0.25 – 1 g/kg IV every 4 to 6 hours.[9] These effects are best accomplished with rapid mannitol bolus administration rather than continuous administration. The efficacy of mannitol wanes with repeated administration.[10]

Adjunctive treatment of hypoxic ischemic encephalopathy in foals (extra-label): 0.25 – 1 g/kg IV every 6 to 12 hours[11]

CATTLE, SWINE, SHEEP, GOATS:

Adjunctive treatment of cerebral edema (extra-label): 1 – 3 g/kg IV[12]

Diuretic for oliguric acute kidney injury (extra-label): 0.25 - 2 g/kg IV over 15 to 20 minutes[13]

FERRETS:

Increased intracranial pressure (extra-label): 0.5 – 1 g/kg IV administered over 20 minutes[14,15]

RABBITS/GUINEA PIGS/CHINCHILLAS:

Increased intracranial pressure (extra-label): 0.25 – 1 g/kg IV administered over 15 minutes[14,16]

Monitoring

- Serum electrolytes (especially sodium), serum osmolality (especially if multiple doses or CRIs are administered), acid-base status
- Serum BUN and creatinine
- Urine output
- Hydration status
- Blood pressure
- Central venous pressure, if possible
- Thoracic auscultation, respiratory rate and effort
- Neurologic status (eg, mentation, pupillary light reflex, pupil size and symmetry, Cushing reflex)

Client Information

- Mannitol should only be administered by professional staff in a setting where adequate monitoring can occur.

Chemistry/Synonyms

An osmotic diuretic, mannitol occurs as an odorless, sweet, white, crystalline powder with a melting range of 165°C to 168°C (329°F-334°F) and a pK_a of 3.4. One gram is soluble in ≈5.5 mL of water (at 25°C [77°F]); it is very slightly soluble in alcohol. The commercially available injectable products have a pH of ≈4.5 to 7.

Mannitol may also be known as cordycepic acid, E421, manita, manitol, manna sugar, mannite, mannitolum, or Eufusol M.

Storage/Stability

Mannitol solutions are recommended to be stored between 15°C and 30°C (59°F-86°F); avoid freezing.

Crystallization may occur at low temperatures in concentrations more than 15%. If crystals form, the solution can be gently heated to 60°C (140°F) to dissolve. Cool to body temperature before administering. If unsuccessful in dissolving the precipitate, discard. An in-line IV filter is recommended when administering concentrated mannitol solutions.

Compatibility/Compounding Considerations

Compatibility is dependent on factors such as pH, concentration, temperature, and diluent used; specialized references or a hospital pharmacist should be consulted for more specific information. It is not recommended to mix mannitol with any other drugs. Use of PVC, other plastics, or rough glass may potentiate crystallization.

Drugs reported to be physically **compatible** with mannitol include amikacin sulfate, cefoxitin sodium, cimetidine HCl, dopamine HCl, gentamicin sulfate, metoclopramide HCl, tobramycin sulfate, and verapamil HCl.

Mannitol should NOT be added to whole blood products to be used for transfusion. If administration of mannitol via a separate line or at different times from the blood products cannot be avoided, pseudoagglutination can be prevented by adding at least 20 mEq/L of sodium chloride to mannitol prior to administering it with the whole blood product. Sodium or potassium chloride can cause mannitol to precipitate out of solution when mannitol concentrations are 20% or greater. Mannitol may be physically **incompatible** when mixed with strongly acidic or alkaline solutions.

Dosage Forms/Regulatory Status

VETERINARY-LABELED PRODUCTS:

Mannitol Injection: 20% (200 mg/mL; 1100 mOsm/L) in 100 mL single-dose vials; generic; (Rx). Labeled for use as an osmotic diuretic in dogs; products have not been FDA-approved.

HUMAN-LABELED PRODUCTS:

Mannitol Injection: 5% (50 mg/mL; 275 mOsm/L) in 1000 mL; *Osmitrol*®; (Rx)

Mannitol Injection: 10% (100 mg/mL; 550 mOsm/L) in 500 mL and 1000 mL; *Osmitrol*®; (Rx)

Mannitol Injection: 15% (150 mg/mL; 825 mOsm/L) in 500 mL; *Osmitrol*®, generic; (Rx)

Mannitol Injection: 20% (200 mg/mL; 1100 mOsm/L) in 250 mL and 500 mL; *Osmitrol*®, generic; (Rx)

Mannitol Injection: 25% (250 mg/mL; 1375 mOsm/L) in 50 mL single use vials (12.5 g/vial); generic; (Rx)

References

For the complete list of references, see **wiley.com/go/budde/plumb**

Marbofloxacin

(mar-boe-***flox***-a-sin) *Zeniquin®*

Fluoroquinolone Antibiotic

Prescriber Highlights

- ▶ Veterinary oral fluoroquinolone antibiotic effective against a variety of bacterial pathogens
- ▶ Contraindications include hypersensitivity to fluoroquinolones, cats younger than 12 months, and immature dogs during the rapid growth phase.
- ▶ May produce erosions of cartilage in weight-bearing joints and other signs of arthropathy in immature animals of various species
- ▶ Use with caution in patients with hepatic or renal insufficiency or dehydration, in those that are prone to seizures, and in immature dogs and cats during the rapid growth phase.
- ▶ Adverse effects include GI distress; marbofloxacin has not been proven to cause ocular toxicity in cats or predispose to *Streptococcus canis* necrotizing fasciitis.
- ▶ Many drug interactions
- ▶ Prohibited for extra-label use in food animals in the United States

Uses/Indications

Marbofloxacin is labeled for treatment of susceptible bacterial infections in dogs and cats. It is recommended that marbofloxacin be reserved for cases of bacterial cystitis with documented resistance to first-line agents (eg, amoxicillin, amoxicillin/clavulanic acid); however, it is a good first-line choice for pyelonephritis or prostatic infections.[1] Fluoroquinolones are considered second-tier drugs for treatment of bacterial folliculitis.[2] In dogs, marbofloxacin appears to have some efficacy for treating the clinical signs associated with canine leishmaniasis.[3] Broad-spectrum antibacterial coverage can be achieved by combining marbofloxacin with an antibiotic with gram-positive and anaerobic activity (eg, clindamycin, ampicillin/amoxicillin).

The World Health Organization (WHO) has designated fluoroquinolones as Critically Important, Highest Priority antimicrobials for human medicine.[4] The Office International des Epizooties (OIE) has designated second-generation quinolones as Veterinary Critically Important Antimicrobial (VCIA) Agents in avian, bovine, equine, lagomorph, and swine species.[5]

Pharmacology/Actions

Marbofloxacin is a third-generation, concentration-dependent, bactericidal fluoroquinolone. It acts by inhibiting bacterial DNA-gyrase (type-II topoisomerase), thus preventing DNA supercoiling and DNA synthesis, with susceptible bacteria cell death occurring within 20 to 30 minutes of exposure. Like other fluoroquinolones, marbofloxacin has demonstrated a significant postantibiotic effect for both gram-negative and gram-positive bacteria and is active in both stationary and growth phases of bacterial replication. Clinical efficacy is associated with achieving a peak marbofloxacin concentration 10 times greater than bacterial MIC.[6,7]

Marbofloxacin has a similar spectrum of activity as the other veterinary commercially available fluoroquinolones, although marbofloxacin is considered more active against *Pseudomonas aeruginosa* as compared with enrofloxacin.[8] Fluoroquinolone agents have good activity against many gram-negative bacilli and cocci, including most species and strains of *Pseudomonas aeruginosa, Klebsiella* spp, *Escherichia coli, Enterobacter* spp, *Campylobacter* spp, *Shigella* spp, *Salmonella* spp, *Aeromonas* spp, *Haemophilus* spp, *Pasteurella* spp, *Proteus* spp, *Yersinia* spp, *Serratia* spp, and *Vibrio* spp. Other organisms that are generally susceptible include *Brucella* spp, *Chlamydia trachomatis, Staphylococcus* spp (including penicillinase-producing and methicillin-resistant strains), *Mycoplasma* spp, and some *Mycobacterium* spp. *Bordetella bronchiseptica* was susceptible, and a significant postantibiotic effect was demonstrated ex vivo.[9]

Fluoroquinolones have variable activity against most streptococci and are not usually recommended to treat these infections. Marbofloxacin is ineffective in treating anaerobic infections. Fluoroquinolones are ineffective against viral, protozoal, or fungal infections.

Resistance can occur by mutation, particularly with *Pseudomonas aeruginosa, Klebsiella pneumoniae, Acinetobacter* spp, *Staphylococcus* spp, and enterococci, but plasmid-mediated resistance is thought to occur only rarely.

Marbofloxacin's leishmanicidal activity is via the TNF-alpha and nitric oxide synthase pathways.[3]

Pharmacokinetics

In dogs, marbofloxacin is rapidly absorbed after oral administration and has a bioavailability of 94%.[10] Mean peak plasma concentrations in dogs given 2.75 mg/kg or 5.5 mg/kg PO were 2 µg/mL and 4.2 µg/mL, respectively. Peak concentrations occur in ≈1.5 hours. Protein binding is low, and the apparent volume of distribution is 1.2 to 1.9 L/kg. Marbofloxacin is widely distributed in canine tissues, and relatively high concentrations can be found in prostatic fluid. Elimination half-life averages 9 to 12 hours.[11,12] The drug is eliminated unchanged in the urine (40%) and bile/feces.[11] Only ≈15% of a dose is metabolized in the liver. Mild to moderate renal impairment does not significantly alter dose requirements in dogs.[13]

In cats, absorption after oral administration is nearly complete and peak serum concentrations occur ≈1 to 2 hours post-administration.[10,14] Mean peak plasma concentrations in cats given 5.5 mg/kg PO were 4.8 µg/mL. Terminal elimination half-life is ≈13 hours, with ≈70% of a dose excreted in the urine mostly as unchanged drug.

In rabbits, 5 mg/kg PO every 24 hours produced a peak plasma concentration of 1.7 µg/mL 24 hours after the first administration and 2.6 µg/mL after the tenth daily dose. Elimination half-life was 4 to 8 hours.[15]

Contraindications/Precautions/Warnings

Marbofloxacin is contraindicated in patients hypersensitive to it or other fluoroquinolones. Fluoroquinolones may cause cartilage erosions in weight-bearing joints in immature animals; dogs appear to be more susceptible to this effect.[10] To avoid cartilage damage, marbofloxacin is contraindicated in immature dogs during the rapid growth phase (small- and medium-breed dogs up to 8 months of age, large breeds to 12 months of age, and giant breeds to 18 months of age). It is also contraindicated in cats younger than 12 months.

Marbofloxacin can (rarely) cause CNS stimulation and should be used with caution in patients with seizure disorders. Patients with severe renal or hepatic impairment may require dosage adjustments (eg, increased dosing interval) to prevent drug accumulation.

Fluoroquinolones may cause photosensitization, and prolonged exposure of bare skin (eg, nose) or thinly haired skin to direct sunlight should be avoided.[10]

The FDA has prohibited the extra-label use of this drug in food-producing animals.

Adverse Effects

With the exception of potential cartilage abnormalities in young animals (see ***Contraindications/Precautions/Warnings***), the adverse effect profile of marbofloxacin is usually limited to GI distress (eg, vomiting, anorexia, diarrhea) and decreased activity.

Other fluoroquinolones have, in rare incidences, caused elevated hepatic enzymes, ataxia, seizures, depression, lethargy, and nervousness in dogs. Hypersensitivity reactions or crystalluria could occur.

Although unlikely to occur, the FDA's Adverse Drug Reaction database has received some reports of blindness associated with marbofloxacin. Unlike enrofloxacin, causal effect of ocular toxicity has not yet been proven with marbofloxacin, but higher dosages should be used carefully.

Induction of *Streptococcus canis* necrotizing fasciitis, which can be seen with enrofloxacin, does not appear to be a problem with marbofloxacin.

Reproductive/Nursing Safety

The safety of marbofloxacin in pregnant or lactating animals or those used for breeding purposes has not been demonstrated.[10] Fluoroquinolones should be used cautiously in pregnant animals due to their adverse effects on cartilage.

In cattle, marbofloxacin distributes into milk, attaining milk concentration similar to that of plasma.[16]

Because safety has not been established in animals, this drug should only be used when the maternal benefits outweigh the potential risks to offspring.

Overdose/Acute Toxicity

It is unlikely that an acute overdose of marbofloxacin would result in signs more serious than either anorexia or vomiting, but the adverse effects noted previously could occur. Dogs receiving 55 mg/kg per day PO for 12 days have developed anorexia, vomiting, dehydration, tremors, red skin, facial swelling, lethargy, and weight loss.[10] All large-breed, 3- to 4-month-old puppies given 11 mg/kg/day developed marked lameness due to articular cartilage lesions. Increased salivation, vomiting, and redness of the pinnae occurred in cats given 27.5 – 55 mg/kg/day.[10] Macroscopic and microscopic cartilage changes were noted but without accompanying lameness.

Acute bilateral blindness occurred in a dog following an accidental overdose of 35 mg/kg/day for 3 days.[17]

For patients that have experienced or are suspected to have experienced an overdose, consultation with a 24-hour poison consultation center specializing in providing veterinary-specific information is recommended. For general information related to overdose and toxin exposures, as well as contact information for poison control centers, refer to ***Appendix***.

Drug Interactions

The following drug interactions have either been reported or are theoretical in humans or animals receiving marbofloxacin or related fluoroquinolones and may be of significance in veterinary patients. Unless otherwise noted, use together is not necessarily contraindicated, but the potential risks should be weighed and additional monitoring performed when appropriate.

- Aluminum-, Calcium-, and Magnesium-Containing Oral Products: May bind to marbofloxacin and prevent its absorption; separate doses of by at least 2 hours.
- Antibiotics, Other (eg, **aminoglycosides, third-generation cephalosporins, penicillins—extended-spectrum**): Synergism may occur but is not predictable against some bacteria (particularly *Pseudomonas aeruginosa*) with these compounds. Although marbofloxacin has minimal activity against anaerobes, in vitro synergy has been reported when it was used with clindamycin against strains of *Peptostreptococcus* spp, *Lactobacillus* spp, and *Bacteroides fragilis*.
- Corticosteroids (eg, **dexamethasone, prednis(ol)one**): Concomitant use with fluoroquinolones may increase the risk for tendonitis and tendon rupture.
- Cyclosporine (**systemic**): Fluoroquinolones may exacerbate the nephrotoxicity and reduce the metabolism of cyclosporine when used systemically.
- Nonsteroidal Anti-Inflammatory Drugs (NSAIDs, eg, **flunixin**): Flunixin has been shown in dogs to increase the AUC and elimination half-life of enrofloxacin, and enrofloxacin increases the AUC and elimination half-life of flunixin; it is unknown if marbofloxacin also causes this effect, if other NSAIDs interact with marbofloxacin, or if this interaction applies to other species.
- Iron (**oral**): May decrease marbofloxacin absorption; doses should be separated by at least 2 hours after marbofloxacin.
- Methotrexate (MTX): May increase MTX concentrations and risk for MTX toxicity
- Nitrofurantoin: May antagonize the antimicrobial activity of the fluoroquinolones; concomitant use is not recommended
- Probenecid: May block tubular secretion of ciprofloxacin; may increase the blood concentration and half-life of marbofloxacin
- QT-Prolonging Agents (eg, **cisapride, sotalol, quinidine, erythromycin, ondansetron**): In humans, fluoroquinolones may enhance the QT-prolonging effect of other drugs.
- Sucralfate: May inhibit absorption of marbofloxacin; administration of these drugs should be separated by at least 2 hours after marbofloxacin.
- Theophylline, Aminophylline: Marbofloxacin may increase theophylline blood concentrations; this interaction is more likely to occur with enrofloxacin than with marbofloxacin.[18]
- Urine Acidifiers (eg, **ammonium chloride, methionine**): Low urinary pH could have an inhibitory effect on the activity of marbofloxacin.
- Warfarin: Potential for increased warfarin effects; monitor prothrombin time (PT)
- Zinc (**oral**): May decrease marbofloxacin absorption; doses should be separated by at least 2 hours after marbofloxacin.

Laboratory Considerations

- In some humans, fluoroquinolones have caused increases in **liver enzymes, BUN**, and **creatinine** and decreases in **hematocrit**. The clinical relevance of these mild changes in veterinary medicine is not known.

Dosages

DOGS:

Skin and soft tissue infections:

- **Label dosage; FDA-approved:** 2.75 – 5.5 mg/kg PO once daily.[10] Give for 2 to 3 days beyond cessation of clinical signs to a maximum duration of 30 days.
- **Extra-label dosage:** 5.5 mg/kg PO once daily[19]

UTIs:

- **Label dosage; FDA-approved:** 2.75 – 5.5 mg/kg PO once daily for at least 10 days to a maximum duration of 30 days. **NOTE:** A shorter treatment duration (ie, 3 to 5 days) is adequate for most cases of bacterial cystitis.[1]
- **Extra-label dosage for sporadic bacterial cystitis:** 2.75 – 5.5 mg/kg PO once daily for 3 to 5 days.[1] **NOTE:** When treating *Pseudomonas* spp infections, most clinicians recommend using the higher end of the dose range.

Leishmaniasis (extra-label): 2 mg/kg PO once daily for 28 days. At the one-year follow-up, marbofloxacin has shown some efficacy in 70% of treated dogs. At 3 months, there was a 61% decrease in the sum of clinical scores. Though clinically improved, dogs remained parasitologically positive.[3,20,21]

CATS:

Skin and soft tissue infections:

- **Label dosage; FDA-approved:** 2.75 – 5.5 mg/kg PO once daily.[10] Give for 2 to 3 days beyond cessation of clinical signs to a maximum duration of 30 days.

- **Extra-label dosage**: 5.5 mg/kg PO once daily[19]

UTIs:

- **Label dosage; FDA-approved**: 2.75 – 5.5 mg/kg PO once daily for at least 10 days to a maximum duration of 30 days. **NOTE**: a shorter treatment duration (ie, 3 to 5 days) is adequate for most cases of bacterial cystitis.[1]
- **Extra-label dosage for sporadic bacterial cystitis**: 2.75 – 5.5 mg/kg PO once daily for 3 to 5 days.[1] **NOTE**: When treating *Pseudomonas* spp infections, most clinicians recommend using the higher end of the dose range.

First-line treatment of feline mycobacterial infections (extra-label): If decision is made to treat localized cutaneous nontuberculous mycobacteria (NTM) infections; 2 mg/kg PO once daily in combination with rifampin and *either* azithromycin or clarithromycin for the initial 2 months, then continue with a combination of rifampin with either marbofloxacin or a macrolide for at least 4 months, with treatment continuing for at least 3 months beyond resolution of lesions and clinical signs.[22] Marbofloxacin is not effective against *M avium* complex (MAC) infection.

Hemotropic mycoplasma infections (extra-label): 2.75 mg/kg PO once daily for 14 to 28 days. Treatment up to 8 weeks with a goal to achieve a negative PCR has been suggested.[23,24] One protocol uses doxycycline 5 mg/kg PO twice daily for 28 days, and cats that remained PCR-positive or became positive again were treated with marbofloxacin 2 mg/kg PO once daily for 14 days.[25]

BIRDS:

Macaws (extra-label): From a single-dose pharmacokinetic study, 2.5 mg/kg PO every 24 hours may be considered.[26]

Mallard ducks (extra-label): 2 – 2.5 mg/kg PO or IV every 24 hours.[27,28] **NOTE**: Parenteral formulation is not available in the United States.

RABBITS:

Susceptible infections (extra-label): 5 mg/kg PO every 24 hours. 2 mg/kg IV, IM, or SC every 24 hours.[15,28,29] **NOTE**: Parenteral formulation is not available in the United States.

REPTILES:

Ball pythons (*Python regius*) (extra-label): 10 mg/kg PO at least every 48 hours. Dosage is based on a pharmacokinetic study; further studies are required to determine effective dosages and toxicity.[30]

Monitoring

- Fluoroquinolone use should be based on culture and susceptibility results.
- Clinical efficacy
- Adverse effects

Client Information

- Give this medicine to your animal as prescribed by your veterinarian. Do not stop the treatment even if your animal appears well.
- This medicine is best given without food on an empty stomach, but if your animal vomits or acts sick after receiving it, give it with food or small treat (no dairy products, antacids, or iron supplements). If vomiting continues, contact your veterinarian.
- Be sure to tell your veterinarian what medications (including vitamins, supplements, herbal therapies, and treats) you are giving your animal, including the amount and schedule of each. This medicine should not be given at the same time as some medications (eg, sucralfate) or vitamins that contain calcium, iron, or aluminum, as these can interfere with how well the medicine works.
- This medicine may cause bone and joint abnormalities if used in young animals or animals that are pregnant or nursing.
- The most common side effects are vomiting, nausea, or soft stool/diarrhea.
- For animals with thin hair coats, there may be a risk for sun sensitivity within a few hours of receiving fluoroquinolones.
- Your veterinarian will need to monitor your animal while it is taking this medicine. Do not miss important follow-up visits.

Chemistry/Synonyms

Marbofloxacin is a synthetic fluoroquinolone antibiotic that occurs as a light yellow, crystalline powder. It is soluble in water, but solubility decreases as pH increases.

Marbofloxacin may also be known as Ro 9-1168, *Aristos®*, *Boflox®*, *Efex®*, *Forcyl®*, *Kelacyl®*, *Marbocyl®*, *Marbocare®*, *Marbonor®*, *Marboquin®*, *Marbox®*, *Marfloquin®*, *Quiflor®*, or *Zeniquin®*.

Storage/Stability

Marbofloxacin tablets should be stored below 30°C (86°F).

Compatibility/Compounding Considerations

A marbofloxacin 20 mg/mL oral suspension was prepared by grinding twenty 100 mg tablets in a mortar with a pestle. The ground tablets were passed through a sieve to separate the powder from the tablet coating and returned to the mortar. The powder was wet with a small amount of glycerin. Equal amounts of *OraPlus®* and *OraSweet®* were added to form a smooth paste, and the liquid was transferred to an amber prescription liquid bottle and brought to 100 mL final volume with additional vehicle. Stability studies supported a beyond-use date (BUD) of 60 days when stored at controlled room temperature. The suspension should be shaken well prior to measuring a dose. **NOTE**: Use of *OraBlend®* resulted in a gritty suspension and a shorter BUD; *OraPlus®* and *OraSweet®* should be used separately.[31]

Dosage Forms/Regulatory Status

VETERINARY-LABELED PRODUCTS:

Marbofloxacin Oral Tablets: 25 mg, 50 mg, 100 mg, and 200 mg; *Zeniquin®*, *Marboquin®*; (Rx). FDA-approved for use in dogs and cats.

Extra-label use of fluoroquinolones is illegal in food animals in the United States.

HUMAN-LABELED PRODUCTS: NONE

References

For the complete list of references, see **wiley.com/go/budde/plumb**

Maropitant

(ma-**rahp**-it-ent) *Cerenia®*

Neurokinin-1 (NK-1) Receptor Antagonist, Antiemetic

Prescriber Highlights

- ▶ FDA-approved in dogs for the treatment of acute vomiting (SC injection), and for the prevention of acute vomiting (SC injection, oral tablets) and the prevention of vomiting due to motion sickness (tablets)
- ▶ The SC injection is also FDA-approved for the treatment of vomiting in cats.
- ▶ In animals that are actively vomiting, the injectable formulation is preferred to ensure the full dose is received.
- ▶ Because maropitant acts at the emetic center, it is effective for the treatment of emesis mediated via either peripheral or central mechanisms.
- ▶ SC injections may cause pain and swelling at the injection site. Refrigerating the injection may reduce pain.
- ▶ The PO dose is higher than the SC dose in dogs because of the decreased bioavailability of the oral tablet.
- ▶ Not for use in patients with suspected toxin ingestion

Uses/Indications

Maropitant tablets are indicated for the prevention of acute vomiting in dogs 2 months and older and vomiting due to motion sickness in dogs 4 months and older.[1]

Maropitant injectable solution is indicated for the prevention and treatment of acute vomiting in dogs 2 months and older and for the prevention of vomiting caused by emetogenic medication and chemotherapeutic agents in dogs 4 months and older.[2] Maropitant injectable solution also is approved for treatment of vomiting in cats 4 months or older.[2]

Maropitant has been effective for controlling vomiting secondary to a variety of stimuli, including xylazine (cats), hydromorphone (dogs),[3-6] morphine (dogs),[7-9] morphine with dexmedetomidine (cats),[10,11] cisplatin (dogs),[12-14] copper sulfate, apomorphine (dogs), brimonidine ophthalmic solution (cats),[15] tranexamic acid (dogs),[16] and parvovirus.[17-19] Maropitant demonstrated modest efficacy for controlling chemotherapy-induced nausea and ondansetron appeared to have a better effect.[14] In dogs hospitalized with parvoviral enteritis, maropitant was equally as effective as ondansetron in controlling clinical signs.[20] Maropitant reduced both nausea and vomiting when administered 2 hours before preoperative administration of hydromorphone, acepromazine, and glycopyrrolate[21]; however, preoperative maropitant does not appear to reduce perioperative gastroesophageal reflux.[22,23]

Maropitant appears to enhance the antinociceptive effect of other analgesic in dogs and cats[19,24-27] and has demonstrated a minimum alveolar concentration (MAC)-sparing effect (≈15% to 25% reduction) in dogs and cats maintained on inhalant anesthesia.[19,24,28-30]

Maropitant failed to improve clinical signs, airway hyperresponsiveness, or eosinophilia in experimental models of acute and chronic feline asthma.[31,32]

A 4-week treatment with oral maropitant seemed to be an effective, well-tolerated therapeutic option to control pruritus in cats with feline atopic skin condition.[33]

Pharmacology/Actions

Maropitant is a neurokinin-1 (NK-1) receptor antagonist that acts in the CNS by inhibiting the binding of substance P, which is the key neurotransmitter involved in vomiting. Maropitant can suppress both peripheral and centrally mediated emesis. Maropitant has been shown to reduce the MAC requirements of sevoflurane and to reduce visceral pain in dogs, as NK-1 receptors are stimulated by substance P.[28,30] Maropitant does not affect gastric emptying times or intestinal transit times, but it can decrease small intestine contraction pressure patterns.[34] Maropitant has been shown to possess anti-inflammatory activity in a mouse model of pancreatitis.[35]

Pharmacokinetics

In dogs, maropitant is rapidly absorbed after PO and SC administration. Peak plasma concentrations (C_{max}) are reached in less than 1 hour following 1 mg/kg SC administration and less than 2 hours following 2 or 8 mg/kg PO administration; C_{max} after IV administration is ≈3 times higher than the same dose given SC (297 ng/mL vs 103 ng/mL, respectively) and is ≈4 times higher than 2 mg/kg PO (81 ng/mL). After PO administration, bioavailability is 24% (2 mg/kg) and 37% (8 mg/kg), which suggests first-pass metabolism becomes saturated at the higher dose. Feeding status does not affect bioavailability. Bioavailability is 91% following SC administration of 1 mg/kg. An accumulation ratio of 1.5 occurs after use of maropitant every 24 hours for 5 consecutive days at 1 mg/kg SC or 2 mg/kg PO. Accumulation ratio is 2.18 after 2 consecutive days at 8 mg/kg PO daily. Accumulation ratios after 2 mg/kg and 8 mg/kg PO once daily for 14 days were 2.46 and 4.81 based on AUC, respectively, and 2.03 and 2.77 based on C_{max}.[36] However, no accumulation was demonstrated after administration of 2 mg/kg/day for 28 days.[37]

Maropitant is eliminated primarily by the liver. Hepatic metabolism of maropitant involves 2 cytochrome P450 enzymes: CYP2D15 (low capacity, high affinity) and CYP3A12 (high capacity, low affinity). The nonlinear kinetics at oral doses of 2 – 16 mg/kg may be due to saturation of the low-capacity enzyme and increased involvement of CYP3A12 at higher doses. Twenty-one metabolites have been identified and the major pharmacologically active metabolite is a product of hydroxylation. Plasma protein binding of maropitant is high (99.5%). Large interpatient PK variations have been observed. In dogs, the half-life is 8.8 hours (range: 6.07 to 17.7 hours) for 1 mg/kg SC, 6.9 hours for 1 mg/kg IV, and 4.03 hours (range: 2.58 to 7.09 hours) for 2 mg/kg PO. Urinary recovery of maropitant and its major metabolite is minimal (less than 1%).

In cats, bioavailability is ≈50% (PO) and 91% (SC). Protein plasma binding is high (99%). Maropitant displays linear kinetics when administered SC within the 0.25 – 3 mg/kg dose range. Terminal elimination half-life in cats is ≈15 hours. Feline isoforms of CYP1A and CYP3A enzymes are involved in the hepatic biotransformation of maropitant in cats. Less than 1% of a dose is excreted unchanged in urine or feces.[38,39]

There appears to be an age-related effect on pharmacokinetics, as puppies (10 weeks of age) and kittens (16 weeks of age) appear to have a faster clearance of maropitant than adults.[2]

Contraindications/Precautions/Warnings

Maropitant is most effective in preventing vomiting associated with chemotherapy if it is administered before the chemotherapeutic agent.[1,2] Safe use has not been evaluated in dogs or cats that have GI obstructions or ingested toxins. If vomiting persists despite treatment, reevaluation is needed to determine the cause.

Maropitant can cause prolongation of the QT interval because of cardiac potassium channel blockade. Safe use of maropitant has not been reported in patients with underlying cardiac disease when administered in combination with cardiac antiarrhythmic drugs.[40]

Caution is advised in patients with hepatic dysfunction, as maropitant is hepatically metabolized; the dose may need to be reduced by 50% if used in these patients.

Caution is also advised when administering the higher dose of maropitant to prevent vomiting due to motion sickness in puppies younger than 11 weeks. A higher frequency and greater severity of histologic evidence of bone marrow hypoplasia was seen in puppies treated with the higher dose of maropitant as compared with control puppies. In puppies 16 weeks or older, bone marrow hypocellularity was not observed.[1,2]

In humans, topical exposure may elicit allergic skin reactions in some individuals. In the event of accidental skin exposure, skin should be washed with soap and water. In the event of accidental eye exposure, eyes should be flushed with water for 15 minutes and medical attention should be sought.[1,2]

Adverse Effects

Maropitant appears to be well tolerated in dogs and cats. Allergic reactions are possible but rare and typically resolve with supportive treatment within 48 hours after the drug is discontinued.

In dogs given the higher oral dose required for prevention of motion sickness, the 2 most common adverse effects are pretravel vomiting and hypersalivation. Swelling or pain at the injection site has been reported following SC administration of this drug. A study found that dogs had less pain at the injection site when the injection was refrigerated and immediately injected,[41] and a formulation preserved with benzyl alcohol was less painful than the metacresol-containing product that is currently available in the US.[42] Other adverse effects include depression and lethargy, anorexia, diarrhea, anaphylaxis/anaphylactoid reactions (including swelling of the head and face), ataxia, tremors, fever, dyspnea, collapse/loss of consciousness, sedation, and convulsions.[1,2]

In healthy dogs, IV maropitant further decreased arterial blood pressure caused by isoflurane anesthesia, and clinically significant hypotension occurred in dogs premedicated with acepromazine.[43]

In cats, adverse effects include depression and lethargy, anorexia, injection site pain, hypersalivation, dyspnea, ataxia, fever, recumbency, vomiting, panting, convulsion, and muscle tremors.[2]

Reproductive/Nursing Safety

Safe use of maropitant in dogs or cats used for breeding or in pregnant or lactating bitches or queens has not been evaluated.[1,2] Because safety has not been established in animals, this drug should only be used when the maternal benefits outweigh the potential risks to offspring.

Overdose/Acute Toxicity

Single-dose toxicity was studied in mice and rats after PO and IV administration.[44] No adverse effects were reported after PO administration of up to 30 mg/kg (mice) and 100 mg/kg (rats) and after IV administration of 6.5 mg/kg (mice) and 2.5 mg/kg (rats). Clinical signs of overdose in mice and rats included decreased activity, irregular or labored respiration, ataxia, and tremors. Excretion of reddish urine was observed in some mice and rats following IV administration.

In dogs, no serious adverse effects were noted when oral doses up to 24 mg/kg (3 times the highest recommended dose) were administered 3 times longer than the proposed maximum duration of treatment.

Oral toxicokinetic studies with the primary metabolite were conducted in mice, rats, rabbits, and dogs; it was demonstrated that the metabolite was well tolerated.[44]

For patients that have experienced or are suspected to have experienced an overdose, consultation with a 24-hour poison consultation center specializing in providing veterinary-specific information is recommended. For general information related to overdose and toxin exposures, as well as contact information for poison control centers, refer to ***Appendix.***

Drug Interactions

During field safety and efficacy studies, a number of medications were used concomitantly with maropitant. The most common concomitant medication was metronidazole. Other commonly used concomitant medications included dextrose/Ringer's solution IV, sodium chloride IV, amoxicillin, ampicillin, cefazolin, cephalexin, enrofloxacin, sulfamethoxazole/trimethoprim, famotidine, sucralfate, cimetidine, dexamethasone, ivermectin, ivermectin/pyrantel, pyrantel, lufenuron/milbemycin, milbemycin, moxidectin, vitamin B, and vaccines. No problems were observed with any of these drugs when used in conjunction with maropitant.

Drug interactions with maropitant have not been thoroughly investigated. Maropitant may be susceptible to interactions because it is biotransformed in the liver by CYP3A12 and CYP2D15 in dogs and by CYP1A- and CYP3A-related enzymes in cats and is highly bound to plasma proteins. The following drug interactions are theoretical in animals receiving maropitant and may be of significance in veterinary patients. Unless otherwise noted, use together is not necessarily contraindicated, but the potential risks must be weighed and additional monitoring performed when appropriate.

- **CALCIUM CHANNEL BLOCKERS** (eg, **amlodipine, diltiazem, verapamil**): The UK label states maropitant *Should not be used concomitantly with Ca-channel antagonists as maropitant has affinity to Ca-channels.*[45]
- **CYP3A INHIBITORS** (eg, **amiodarone, diltiazem, cimetidine, erythromycin, ketoconazole, itraconazole**): May reduce maropitant metabolism
- **CYP2D INHIBITORS** (eg, **cimetidine, fluoxetine, terbinafine**): May reduce maropitant metabolism
- **HIGHLY PROTEIN BOUND DRUGS** (eg, **valproic acid, oral anticoagulants [rivaroxaban, warfarin], NSAIDs, salicylates, sulfonamides, sulfonylurea antidiabetic agents**): Because maropitant is highly bound to plasma proteins (99.5%), it could theoretically displace other highly bound drugs, causing a transient increase in serum concentrations of each drug. These interactions are unlikely to be of clinical concern because free drug concentrations will equilibrate through increased clearance. Monitor for adverse effects of each drug when using this combination.
- **QT PROLONGING AGENTS** (eg, **cisapride, domperidone, quinidine, sotalol**): Concurrent use may increase risk for QT prolongation and should be avoided.

Laboratory Considerations

- No specific concerns have been noted.

Dosages

NOTE: Refrigerating the injectable product may reduce the pain response associated with SC administration.

DOGS:

Label dosages (FDA-approved)[1,2]:

Indication	Dosage form	Minimum age for use	Dosage	Duration of therapy
Prevention and treatment of acute vomiting	Injection	2 months	1 mg/kg SC once daily	Up to 5 consecutive days
Prevention and treatment of acute vomiting	Injection	4 months	1 mg/kg SC or IV (over 1 to 2 minutes) once daily	Up to 5 consecutive days
Prevention of vomiting caused by emetogenic medications or chemotherapeutic agents	Injection	4 months	1 mg/kg SC or IV (over 1 to 2 minutes) once, 45 to 60 minutes prior to emetogenic medications or chemotherapeutic agents	Single injection

Indication	Dosage form	Minimum age for use	Dosage	Duration of therapy
Prevention of acute vomiting	Tablets	2 months	2 mg/kg PO once daily	5 days for dogs 2 to 7 months of age; until vomiting ceases in dogs older than 7 months
Prevention of vomiting due to motion sickness	Tablets	4 months	8 mg/kg PO once daily on an empty stomach or with a small amount of food; do not feed full meal prior to travel	Up to 2 consecutive days

Extra-label dosages:

Prevention of perioperative vomiting and improvement in recovery from general anesthesia after morphine use: 1 mg/kg SC or IV once daily more than 1 hour in advance of morphine administration; may be used for up to 5 consecutive days

Prevention and treatment of vomiting in dogs undergoing multiagent chemotherapy: 2 mg/kg PO once daily for 28 days[37]

Antitussive as part of a multimodal approach in dogs with airway disease: 2 mg/kg PO every 48 hours may be useful as an antitussive to break the cough cycle associated with tracheal collapse. A study showed that although cough was decreased in patients with chronic bronchitis, this dosage did not decrease airway inflammation.[46]

Analgesia/MAC-sparing effect during ovariohysterectomy:

a) 1 mg/kg SC at time of premedication. Maropitant also reduced postoperative nausea and vomiting and improved time to food intake.[9,24,29]
b) Intraoperatively, administration of 1 mg/kg IV followed by 0.03 mg/kg/hour CRI demonstrated an anesthetic sparing effect during visceral noxious stimulation of the ovarian ligament.[47] Higher doses (5 mg/kg IV followed by 0.15 mg/kg per hour CRI) have yielded marginally better results.[47,48] Doses involving continuous infusions do not appear to have superior MAC-sparing effects as compared with SC doses. Differences in study design make a direct comparison difficult.

CATS:

Treatment of vomiting in cats 4 months and older (label dosage; FDA-approved): 1 mg/kg SC or IV (over 1 to 2 minutes) once daily for up to 5 consecutive days[2]

Prevention of vomiting, including from motion sickness (extra-label): 1 mg/kg SC or PO.[45,49] A study reported that 8 mg/cat (NOT mg/kg) PO was effective in reducing emesis when administered as early as 18 hours before emetic medications.[11,50]

Prevention of vomiting associated with chronic kidney disease (CKD) (extra-label): 4 mg/cat (NOT mg/kg) PO every 24 hours for 2 weeks palliated vomiting associated with CKD.[51]

Analgesia/MAC-sparing effect during ovariohysterectomy (extra-label): In a proof-of-concept study, 1 mg/kg IV intraoperatively demonstrated an anesthetic sparing effect during visceral noxious stimulation of the ovarian ligament.[30] Alternatively, maropitant 1 mg/kg IV bolus followed maropitant 100 µg/kg/hour IV CRI experienced a lower heartrate and blood pressure during the procedure and required less analgesic rescue during the postoperative period compared to control cats.[52]

Feline atopic skin syndrome (extra-label): 2 mg/kg PO every 24 hours for 4 weeks seemed to be effective and well-tolerated.[33] **NOTE**: This dosage is from an open label, uncontrolled study, and further research to validate efficacy is warranted.

Monitoring

- Clinical efficacy as indicated by decreased episodes of vomiting
- Adverse effects

Client Information

- When using to prevent motion sickness, administer maropitant 2 hours before traveling with a small amount of food (not a full meal).
- Some dogs may vomit after taking this medication. Giving the drug with a small amount of food can help prevent vomiting.
- Do not wrap these pills tightly in food snacks, as this can prevent the drug from being released into the stomach.
- If giving your animal fractions (ie, half, quarter) of a tablet, wrap the remaining portion of the split tablet tightly in foil and store away from children and other animals.
- Do not give this medicine to puppies younger than 8 weeks, as bone marrow problems can occur.
- Side effects are uncommon. Contact your veterinarian if your animal experiences drooling, lethargy (ie, lack of energy), drowsiness/sleepiness, lack of appetite, or diarrhea.
- In humans, topical exposure may elicit allergic skin reactions in some individuals. In the event of accidental skin exposure, wash skin with soap and water. In the event of accidental eye exposure, flush the eye with water for 15 minutes and seek medical attention.

Chemistry/Synonyms

Commercial formulations containing maropitant citrate are classified as substituted quinuclidines and have a molecular weight of 678.81. Commercial formulations express drug potency or strength as milligrams of maropitant. The injection is a clear solution that may be colorless to light yellow and contains metacresol as a preservative.

Maropitant may also be known as CJ-11,972, *Cerenia*®, and *Prevomax*®.

Storage/Stability

The maropitant injectable solution contains a preservative and is designed for multidose use. The product label states the injectable solution should be stored at a controlled room temperature between 20°C and 25°C (68°F-77°F) with excursions between 15°C and 30°C (59°F-86°F) permitted. After the first vial puncture, the drug should be stored at a refrigerated temperature between 2°C and 8°C (36°F-46°F) and should be used within 90 days (56 days per UK label). The stopper may be punctured a maximum of 25 times.

Store maropitant tablets at room temperature 20°C to 25°C (68°F to 77°F) with excursions between 15°C to 30°C (59°F to 86°F). Maropitant tablets are packaged in foil to protect them from moisture uptake, which was observed in less protective packaging. A European stability study indicated that tablets removed from the blister pack and halved showed no loss of potency during the 48-hour testing period.

Compatibility/Compounding Considerations

Precipitation has been reported when maropitant and pantoprazole are coadministered in the same IV line. Given lack of compatibility information, consideration should be given to administering maropitant injections alone. The UK product label states that the maropitant injection *must not be mixed with other veterinary medicinal products in the same syringe*.[45] One study diluted maropitant in lactated Ringer's solution for use as an IV CRI, but the potency and stability of the admixture were not evaluated.[52]

Dosage Forms/Regulatory Status

VETERINARY-LABELED PRODUCTS:

Maropitant Citrate Injectable Solution: 10 mg/mL in 20 mL multi-dose vials; *Cerenia*®; (Rx). FDA-approved for use in dogs and cats. Licensed for use in other countries and available in a variety of vial sizes

Maropitant Citrate Oral Tablets: 16 mg, 24 mg, 60 mg, and 160 mg in blister packs (4 tablets per pack; carton of 10); *Cerenia*®; (Rx). Labeled for use in dogs

HUMAN-LABELED PRODUCTS: NONE

References

For the complete list of references, see **wiley.com/go/budde/plumb**

Mavacoxib

(mav-ah-***cox***-ib) *Trocoxil*®

Long-Acting NSAID

Prescriber Highlights

- Very long-acting NSAID for dogs; half-life averages 16 to 17 days. Not licensed/approved in the United States
- First 2 doses are given 14 days apart, then at 1 MONTH intervals for a maximum of 7 doses.
- Contraindications include pre-existing GI disorders, coagulopathies, impaired renal or hepatic function, cardiac insufficiency, or hypersensitivity to mavacoxib or sulfonamides.
- Adverse effect profile expected to be similar to other canine-approved NSAIDs: vomiting, diarrhea, loss of appetite, melena, and impairment of renal function.
- Primary benefit appears to be for patients whose owners have difficulty adhering to a daily oral dosing regimen.
- Although efficacy is long-lasting, adverse effects may persist and washout times to give other NSAIDs or glucocorticoids are prolonged.

Uses/Indications

Mavacoxib is a very long-acting oral NSAID licensed for use in dogs in the UK, Europe, and elsewhere. In the UK, it is labeled *for the treatment of pain and inflammation associated with degenerative joint disease in dogs aged 12 months or more in cases where continuous treatment exceeding 1 month is indicated.* Mavacoxib may be beneficial in cases in which long-term NSAID administration is indicated, but owners have difficulty adhering to a daily oral dosing regimen. However, because of its long half-life and duration of action, adverse effects could also persist for many weeks after the drug was last given.

In a study comparing the safety and efficacy of mavacoxib with carprofen in 124 dogs, the 2 were statistically equivalent, and each had a similar rate and profile of adverse effects.[1]

Pharmacology/Actions

In dogs, mavacoxib is a relatively selective inhibitor of cyclooxygenase-2 (COX-2) versus COX-1. At therapeutic dosages, this effect would inhibit the production of the prostaglandins that contribute to pain and inflammation (COX-2) and spare those that maintain normal GI and renal function (COX-1). However, COX-1 and COX-2 inhibition studies are done in vitro and do not necessarily correlate with clinical effects seen in patients.

Pharmacokinetics

Pharmacokinetic values for mavacoxib in dogs are widely patient variable. Average bioavailability after oral dosing is ≈46% when fasted but nearly doubles (87%) when given with food. Peak concentrations occur in ≈11 hours but range widely. In most dogs, blood concentrations are thought to be therapeutic, occurring ≈1 hour after dosing when given with food. The apparent volume of distribution at steady-state averaged 1.6 L/kg, and the drug is highly bound to canine plasma proteins (98%). Total body clearance was very low, 2.7 mL/hour/kg, and it is primarily cleared by biliary excretion. The average terminal half-life was 16.6 days (range: 8 to 39 days).[2] A population pharmacokinetic study in osteoarthritic dogs reported a typical elimination half-life of 44 days, but ≈5% of patients had Bayesian estimates greater than 80 days.[3]

Contraindications/Precautions/Warnings

Mavacoxib is contraindicated in dogs less than 12 months of age and/or less than 5 kg (11 lb) body weight, with GI disorders, including ulceration and bleeding, evidence of a hemorrhagic disorder, impaired renal or hepatic function, cardiac insufficiency, or with a history of hypersensitivity to the active substance, any of the excipients, or to sulfonamides.

Do not use concomitantly with glucocorticoids or other NSAIDs. Do not administer other NSAIDs within 1 month of the last administration of mavacoxib (washout period).

Avoid use in any dehydrated, hypovolemic, or hypotensive animal, as there is a potential risk for increased renal toxicity. Concurrent administration of potentially nephrotoxic medicinal products should be avoided.[4] Do not allow treated dogs to become dehydrated when receiving this or other NSAIDs.

Adverse Effects

Common adverse effects include vomiting and diarrhea, similar to other NSAIDs. Less common adverse effects include loss of appetite, hemorrhagic diarrhea, melena, and impaired renal function. GI ulceration can occur.

GI protectants and parenteral fluids may be required for dogs with GI or renal adverse effects.

Reproductive/Nursing Safety

The safety of mavacoxib has not been established during pregnancy and lactation. Per the UK label, do not use mavacoxib in pregnant, breeding, or lactating animals. Studies in pregnant rabbits receiving another coxib-class NSAID (eg, firocoxib) at dosages approximating those given to dogs demonstrated maternotoxic and fetotoxic effects.

Because safety has not been established in animals, this drug should only be used when the maternal benefits outweigh the potential risks to offspring.

Overdose/Acute Toxicity

In overdose safety studies performed in dogs, repeated doses (at the labeled frequency) of 5 mg/kg and 10 mg/kg did not demonstrate adverse effects, abnormal clinical chemistry, or significant histological abnormalities. At 15 mg/kg, vomiting, softened/mucoid feces, and increases in clinical chemistry parameters reflecting decreased renal function were noted. Doses of 25 mg/kg cause GI ulceration. In 1 study, a dog died from GI perforation and peritonitis at the 25 mg/kg dose.[5]

Oral acute overdoses of mavacoxib should be managed as with other NSAIDs toxicity, but because of the drug's long duration of effect, prolonged monitoring and treatment may be required; consulting a veterinary poison control center or the drug sponsor's hotline seems prudent until more experience has been gained with this agent.

As with any NSAID, overdoses can lead to GI and renal effects. The ASPCA Animal Poison Control Center (APCC) has not yet set a dosage level of concern for renal damage for dogs or cats. Decontamination with emetics and/or activated charcoal is appropriate. For doses at which GI effects are expected, the use of GI protectants is warranted. If renal effects are also expected, fluid diuresis is warranted.

For patients that have experienced or are suspected of having experienced an overdose, consultation with a 24-hour poison consultation center specializing in providing veterinary-specific information is recommended. For general information related to overdose and toxin exposures, as well as contact information for poison control centers, refer to ***Appendix.***

Drug Interactions

At the time of writing, no drug interactions have been reported with mavacoxib, but the manufacturer warns that use in conjunction with other **NSAIDs** or **corticosteroids** is contraindicated. It is also possible that mavacoxib could cause increased renal dysfunction if used with other drugs that can cause or contribute to **renal dysfunction** (eg, **diuretics, aminoglycosides**), but the clinical significance of this potential interaction is unclear. The following drug interactions are either expected or are theoretical in dogs receiving mavacoxib and may be of clinical significance:

- **ACE Inhibitors** (eg, **enalapril, benazepril**): Some NSAIDs can reduce effects on blood pressure. Because ACE inhibitors potentially can reduce renal blood flow, use with NSAIDs could increase the risk for renal injury. However, 1 study on dogs receiving tepoxalin did not show any adverse effects. It is unknown what effects, if any, occur if other NSAIDs and ACE inhibitors are used together in dogs.
- **Anticoagulants** (eg, **heparins, rivaroxaban, warfarin**): May increase the risk for bleeding
- **Aspirin**: May increase the risk for GI toxicity (eg, ulceration, bleeding, vomiting, diarrhea). Washout periods several weeks long are probably warranted when switching from mavacoxib to aspirin therapy in dogs.
- **Bisphosphonates** (eg, **alendronate**): May increase the risk for GI ulceration
- **Clopidogrel**: May increase the risk for bleeding
- **Glucocorticoids** (eg, **predniso(lo)ne**): May increase the risk for GI toxicity (eg, ulceration, bleeding, vomiting, diarrhea)
- **Digoxin**: NSAIDs may increase serum levels.
- **Fluconazole**: Administration has increased plasma concentrations of celecoxib in humans and potentially could also affect mavacoxib concentrations in dogs.
- **Furosemide**: NSAIDs may reduce saluretic and diuretic effects.
- **Methotrexate**: Serious toxicity has occurred when NSAIDs have been used concomitantly with methotrexate; use together with extreme caution.
- **Nephrotoxic Drugs** (eg, **furosemide, aminoglycosides, amphotericin B**): May enhance the risk for nephrotoxicity development
- **NSAIDs, Other** (eg, **carprofen, meloxicam**): May increase the risk for GI toxicity (eg, ulceration, bleeding, vomiting, diarrhea). The UK label states: *Should another NSAID be administered after Trocoxil® treatment, a treatment-free period of at least 1 MONTH should be ensured to avoid adverse effects.* Because of its long half-life (up to 39 days in 1 study dog),[6] however, mavacoxib may have a conservative washout time of 195 days.[7]

Laboratory Considerations

- None were identified.

Dosages

DOGS:

<u>UK Label:</u> **Treatment of pain and inflammation associated with degenerative joint disease in dogs aged 12 months or more in cases where continuous treatment exceeding 1 month is indicated** (extra-label in the United States): 2 mg/kg PO given immediately before or with the dog's main meal.[4] Care should be taken to ensure that the tablet is ingested. The treatment should be repeated 14 days later; thereafter, the dosing interval is 1 MONTH. A treatment cycle should not exceed 7 consecutive doses (6.5 months). **THIS IS NOT A DAILY NSAID.**

Monitoring

- Baseline and periodic CBC and serum chemistry (including BUN, serum creatinine, and liver function assessment)
- Baseline history and physical; repeat exam recommended 1 month after starting treatment with mavacoxib and prior to administering a third dose[4]
- Efficacy of therapy
- Adverse effects

Client Information

- Give doses exactly as directed by your veterinarian. Do not give extra doses or increase the dose without your veterinarian's guidance. Do NOT give this drug every day. After giving the first 2 doses 2 weeks apart, give this drug once a month for up to 5 doses, then an extra month off the drug is needed if you need to start the drug again.
- Do not administer steroids or other NSAIDs within 1 month of the last dose of mavacoxib (eg, carprofen, deracoxib, meloxicam).
- Give the medication with the dog's largest meal of the day. The drug is much better absorbed from the stomach if given with food.
- Contact your veterinarian if any of the following side effects persist or are severe: loss of appetite, vomiting, change in bowel movements (eg, stool color), change in behavior, or decrease in water consumption or urination; these could potentially occur many weeks after giving the last dose. Immediately report to your veterinarian if any of the following side effects occur: bloody stool/diarrhea, bloody vomiting, or allergic reaction (facial swelling, hives, red, itchy skin).
- Do not allow the dog to become dehydrated while receiving this drug. Ensure ready access to drinking water. Contact your veterinarian if your dog's fluid intake is reduced, or if your dog is losing bodily fluids (eg, vomiting, diarrhea).
- Dogs may find the chewable tablets' taste desirable; store the drug out of reach of animals and children.

Chemistry/Synonyms

Mavacoxib is structurally related to the human NSAID celecoxib and is a diaryl substituted pyrazole member of the sulphonamide group of coxibs. Mavacoxib's solubility in water is relatively low (0.006 mg/mL).

Mavacoxib may also be known as mavacoxibum; PHA 739,521; or UNII-YFT7X7SR77. A common trade name is *Trocoxil®*.

Storage/Stability

Store in the original packaging at room temperature, out of reach of pets and children.

Compatibility/Compounding Considerations

No specific information was noted.

Dosage Forms/Regulatory Status

VETERINARY-LABELED PRODUCTS:

None in the United States. In the UK and Europe: Mavacoxib Oral Chewable Tablets: 6 mg, 20 mg, 30 mg, 75 mg, and 95 mg; *Trocoxil®*; (Rx/POM-V)

HUMAN-LABELED PRODUCTS: NONE

References

For the complete list of references, see **wiley.com/go/budde/plumb**

Mechlorethamine

(me-klor-*eth*-a-meen) *Mustargen®*
Antineoplastic

Prescriber Highlights

- ► Highly toxic agent; handle with extreme caution.
- ► Antineoplastic for lymphoreticular neoplasms
- ► Contraindications include pre-existing myelosuppression or infection, and hypersensitivity to mechlorethamine.
- ► Adverse effects include myelosuppression, GI effects (vomiting, nausea), ototoxicity (high dosages); potentially alopecia, hyperuricemia, hepatotoxicity, peripheral neuropathy, GI ulcers.
- ► Avoid extravasation; vesicant injuries may be severe.
- ► Carcinogenic, mutagenic, and teratogenic
- ► The National Institute for Occupational Safety and Health (NIOSH) classifies mechlorethamine as a hazardous drug; use appropriate precautions when handling.

Uses/Indications

Mechlorethamine is used in dogs and cats as part of MOPP (mechlorethamine, vincristine, procarbazine, prednisone),[1,2] MPP (mechlorethamine, procarbazine, prednisone),[3] and MOMP (mechlorethamine, vincristine, melphalan, prednisone)[4] protocols to treat both naïve and relapse cases of lymphoma.

Pharmacology/Actions

Mechlorethamine is an alkylating agent, thereby interfering with DNA replication, RNA transcription, and protein synthesis. It is cell cycle–phase nonspecific.

Pharmacokinetics

Mechlorethamine is irritating to tissues and must be given IV for systemic use. It is incompletely absorbed after intracavitary administration. After injection, mechlorethamine combines with water and undergoes a rapid chemical transformation, resulting in no active drug within minutes of administration.

Contraindications/Precautions/Warnings

Mechlorethamine is contraindicated in patients with a known hypersensitivity to it or with known infections.

The risk versus benefits of therapy must be carefully considered in patients with pre-existing myelosuppression. Additive bone marrow depression may occur in patients undergoing concomitant radiation therapy. Therapy with mechlorethamine may increase the risk for a second malignant tumor, especially when combined with other antineoplastic agents or radiation therapy.[5] In humans, mechlorethamine can contribute to the rapid development of amyloidosis.

Only veterinarians with the experience and resources to monitor the toxicity of this agent should administer this drug.

Mechlorethamine is a severe vesicant; extravasation must be avoided. Mechlorethamine is highly toxic and must be handled with extreme caution in both powdered and liquid forms. Mechlorethamine is corrosive to skin and eyes, and is highly toxic by oral route. The drug is a respiratory tract irritant, and exposure to mechlorethamine dust or vapors must be avoided. It is carcinogenic, mutagenic, and teratogenic.

The National Institute for Occupational Safety and Health (NIOSH) classifies mechlorethamine as a hazardous drug; personal protective equipment (PPE, including respirators) and environmental controls should be used accordingly to minimize the risk for exposure. Clothing contaminated with mechlorethamine should be discarded.

Adverse Effects

Myelosuppression (leukopenia, thrombocytopenia) and GI effects (vomiting, nausea) are common and can be serious enough to halt therapy; pretreatment with antiemetics can be beneficial. In humans, it is preferred to administer at night if sedation for adverse effects is required; while this timing does not directly apply to veterinary patients, the severity of adverse effects should be closely monitored. Neutrophil and platelet nadir is ≈7 days.

Ototoxicity may occur with either high dosage. Hypersensitivity reactions have been reported in humans, including anaphylaxis.

Other potential effects include alopecia, hyperuricemia, hepatotoxicity, peripheral neuropathy, and GI ulcers.

Because it is often used in combination with other chemotherapy agents, myelosuppression and GI effects (hemorrhagic gastritis) may be enhanced.

Many dogs receiving chemotherapy will have minor hair coat changes (eg, shagginess, increased shedding, poor regrowth in shaved areas). Breeds with continuously growing hair coats (eg, poodles, terriers, Afghan hounds, or old English sheepdogs) are more likely to experience significant alopecia.

Mechlorethamine is a moderate to severe vesicant, and perivascular extravasation may lead to tissue damage and sloughing. If extravasation occurs, sodium thiosulfate may be administered (IV and SC around the extravasation site) to reduce vesicant damage. Ice compresses should be applied for 15 minutes every 6 hours for 48 hours. Other reported supportive therapies include local application of DMSO and/or perivascular infusion of corticosteroids, sodium chloride, and hyaluronidase.

Reproductive/Nursing Safety

Mechlorethamine is a teratogen in lab animals and fetal malformations have been documented. Use only during pregnancy when the benefits to the mother outweigh the risks to the offspring. Mechlorethamine can suppress gonadal function.

For sexually intact patients, verify pregnancy status prior to administration.

Although it is not known whether mechlorethamine enters maternal milk, nursing puppies or kittens should receive milk replacer when the dam is receiving mechlorethamine.

Overdose/Acute Toxicity

Because of the great toxic potential of this agent, determine dosages carefully. The LD_{50} in mice and rats following IV administration is 2 mg/kg and 1.6 mg/kg, respectively.[2] The drug is not dialyzable, and treatment is supportive.

In humans, overdoses may lead to severe leukopenia, anemia, and thrombocytopenia that can result in delayed bleeding and ultimately death. The only treatment is repeated blood transfusions, antibiotic therapy, and supportive care.[5]

For patients that have experienced or are suspected to have experienced an overdose, consultation with a 24-hour poison consultation center specializing in providing veterinary-specific information is recommended. For general information related to overdose and toxin exposures, as well as contact information for poison control centers, refer to ***Appendix***.

Drug Interactions

The following drug interactions have either been reported or are theoretical in humans or animals receiving mechlorethamine and may be of significance in veterinary patients. Unless otherwise noted, use together is not necessarily contraindicated, but weigh the potential risks and perform additional monitoring when appropriate.

- **Myelosuppressive Agents** (eg, **antineoplastics, immunosuppressants, iron chelators**): Concurrent use with other bone marrow depressant medications may result in additive myelosuppression.

- Vaccines (live and inactivated): Mechlorethamine may diminish vaccine efficacy and enhance adverse effects of vaccines.

Laboratory Considerations

- Mechlorethamine may raise **serum uric acid** levels. Drugs such as allopurinol may be required to control hyperuricemia.

Dosages

NOTE: Because of the potential toxicity of this drug to patients, veterinary personnel, and clients, and since chemotherapy indications, treatment protocols, and monitoring and safety guidelines often change, the following dosages should be used only as a general guide. Consultation with a veterinary oncologist and referral to current veterinary oncology references[6-10] are strongly recommended.

DOGS:

Lymphoma, first-line (T-cell) or rescue (extra-label): When mechlorethamine is used, it is given as part of a protocol in combination with other antineoplastic agents (MOPP, MPP, MOMP protocols) and usually given at a dose of 3 mg/m^2 (**NOT** mg/kg) IV given on Days 1 and 7 of a 21- to 28-day protocol.[1-4]

CATS:

Lymphoma, rescue (extra-label): When mechlorethamine is used, it is given as part of a protocol in combination with other antineoplastic agents (MOPP protocol, MOMP rescue protocol[11]) and usually given at a dose of 3 mg/m^2 (**NOT** mg/kg) IV given on Days 1 and 7 of a 21- to 28-day protocol.

Monitoring

- Baseline and weekly CBC
- Hepatic enzymes; initially before starting treatment and then every 3 to 4 months
- Renal function
- Injection site for signs of extravasation

Client Information

- This medication is considered to be a hazardous drug as defined by the National Institute for Occupational Safety and Health (NIOSH) because it may affect the reproductive ability of males or females actively trying to conceive, women who are pregnant or may become pregnant, and women who are breastfeeding. It is recommended that you wear gloves when administering this medication to your pet and wash your hands thoroughly afterwards. If you have questions about this medication's hazards, please speak with your veterinarian or pharmacist.
- On the day your animal gets the drug and then for ≈72 hours afterward, handle all bodily waste (urine, feces, litter), blood, or vomit only while wearing disposable gloves. Seal the waste in a plastic bag and then place both the bag and gloves in with the regular trash.
- Bone marrow suppression can occur. The greatest effects on bone marrow usually occur about 1 week after treatment. Your veterinarian will do blood tests to watch for this, but if you see bleeding, bruising, fever (indicating an infection), or if your animal becomes tired easily, contact your veterinarian right away.
- Immediately report any signs associated with toxicity (eg, vomiting, GI upset, abnormal bleeding, bruising, urination, depression, infection, shortness of breath).
- While your animal is taking this medication, it is important to return to your veterinarian for laboratory work. Do not miss these important follow-up visits.

Chemistry/Synonyms

Mechlorethamine, a bifunctional alkylating agent, occurs as a hygroscopic, light-yellow brown, crystalline powder that is very soluble in water. After reconstitution with sterile water or sterile saline, the resultant solution is clear and has a pH of 3 to 5.

Mechlorethamine may also be known as nitrogen mustard, mustine, HN2, chlormethine hydrochloride, chlorethazine hydrochloride, HN2 (mustine [chlormethine]), mechlorethamine hydrochloride, mustine hydrochloride, nitrogen mustard (mustine [chlormethine]), NSC-762, WR-147650, *Caryolysine®*, *Mustargen®*, and *Onco-Cloramin®*.

Storage/Stability

Store the powder for injection between 15°C and 30°C (59°F and 86°F), protected from light and humidity.[5] Mechlorethamine solution are highly unstable and decompose upon standing; administer the drug immediately after preparation.

Compatibility/Compounding Considerations

Compatibility is dependent on factors such as pH, concentration, temperature, and diluent used; specialized references or a hospital pharmacist should be consulted for more specific information.

When reconstituted, the solution should be clear and colorless. Do NOT use if the solution is discolored or if droplets of water are visible within the vial prior to reconstitution.[5] It is **NOT** recommended to mix mechlorethamine with any other medication or to dilute further beyond what is described in the package insert.

Drugs that have been reported to be **compatible** with mechlorethamine when given via an IV Y-site include aztreonam, filgrastim, granisetron, melphalan, and ondansetron.

Unused portions of the reconstituted drug must be neutralized; neutralization can be accomplished by mixing with equal volumes of 5% sodium thiosulfate and 5% sodium bicarbonate. Allow this solution to stand for 45 minutes and then discard appropriately. Empty mechlorethamine vials should be neutralized in this same manner.

Dosage Forms/Regulatory Status

VETERINARY-LABELED PRODUCTS: NONE

HUMAN-LABELED PRODUCTS:

Mechlorethamine Powder for Injection: 10 mg; *Mustargen®*; (Rx)

A Topical gel (*Valchlor®*) is also available.

References

For the complete list of references, see **wiley.com/go/budde/plumb**

Meclizine

(***mek***-li-zeen) *Antivert®*

Antihistamine, Antiemetic

Prescriber Highlights

- ► Antihistamine with sedative and antiemetic effects used primarily for motion sickness and vestibular disease
- ► Caution is advised in animals with prostatic hypertrophy, bladder neck obstruction, angle-closure glaucoma, or GI obstruction.
- ► Adverse effects include sedation; less frequently, anticholinergic effects (eg, dry mucous membranes, dry eyes, tachycardia) may be noted. Paradoxical CNS stimulation is possible.

Uses/Indications

Meclizine is principally used in small animal species as an antiemetic primarily for the treatment and prevention of motion sickness.

Pharmacology/Actions

Meclizine is an H_1 receptor blocking antihistamine agent with anticholinergic properties. This drug has antiemetic, CNS depressant, antispasmodic, and local anesthetic effects. The exact mechanisms of action for the antiemetic and anti-motion–sickness effects are not completely understood, but it is thought that they are at least partially a result of the drug's central anticholinergic and CNS depressant activity. The antiemetic effect is likely mediated through the chemoreceptor trigger zone. In humans, meclizine is considered less sedating than dimenhydrinate.

Pharmacokinetics

Little information is available. In humans, meclizine is absorbed following oral administration. The drug is metabolized in the liver predominantly via CYP2D6 and has a serum half-life of ≈6 hours.[1]

Contraindications/Precautions/Warnings

Meclizine is contraindicated in animals hypersensitive to it. It should be used with caution in animals with prostatic hypertrophy, bladder neck obstruction, and other forms of urinary retention, angle-closure glaucoma, asthma, or GI obstruction. Theoretically, renal or hepatic impairment can lead to drug accumulation and increased risk for adverse effects.

Adverse Effects

The typical adverse effect noted is sedation; less frequently, anticholinergic effects (eg, dry mucous membranes, dry eyes, tachycardia) may be seen. Paradoxical CNS stimulation has also been reported. Cats may develop inappetence while receiving this medication.[2]

Reproductive/Nursing Safety

Meclizine is considered teratogenic at high doses in laboratory animals, and cleft palates have been noted in rats given oral doses as low as 25 mg/kg (≈2 to 4 times the maximum human dose based on body surface area). However, in humans, it has been suggested that meclizine possesses low risk for teratogenicity for antiemetic drugs and can be used to treat nausea and vomiting associated with pregnancy.

It is unknown if meclizine enters milk; its anticholinergic activity may inhibit lactation.

Because safety has not been established in animals, this drug should only be used when the maternal benefits outweigh the potential risks to offspring.

Overdose/Acute Toxicity

Moderate overdose may result in drowsiness alternating with hyperexcitability; tachycardia and vomiting may also be seen. Massive overdose may result in profound CNS depression, hallucinations, seizures, and other anticholinergic effects (eg, tachycardia, urine retention).

Treatment is supportive and based on clinical signs. Consider gastric decontamination when animals are presented soon after ingestion. Avoid respiratory depressant medications.

For patients that have experienced or are suspected to have experienced an overdose, consultation with a 24-hour poison consultation center specializing in providing veterinary-specific information is recommended. For general information related to overdose and toxin exposures, as well as contact information for poison control centers, refer to ***Appendix***.

Drug Interactions

The following drug interactions have either been reported or are theoretical in humans or animals receiving meclizine and may be of significance in veterinary patients. Unless otherwise noted, use together is not necessarily contraindicated, but weigh the potential risks and perform additional monitoring when appropriate.

- **Anticholinergic Drugs** (eg, **atropine, glycopyrrolate, oxybutynin**): Other anticholinergic drugs may cause additive anticholinergic effects.
- **CNS Depressants** (eg, **benzodiazepines, gabapentin, trazodone**): Use with other CNS depressants may cause additive sedation.
- **Digoxin**: Meclizine may increase digoxin absorption by slowing GI motility.
- **Fluoxetine**: May increase meclizine concentrations and effects by inhibiting metabolism
- **Opioids** (eg, **hydrocodone, morphine**): May have additive CNS depression and anticholinergic effects (eg, constipation, urinary retention)
- **Potassium Salts, Oral/Solid**: Solid dose oral forms of potassium salts can cause focal upper GI injury, which can be worsened by drugs that may slow GI motility.
- **Prokinetic Agents** (eg, **cisapride, metoclopramide**): Meclizine may diminish the efficacy of prokinetic agents by decreasing GI motility.
- **Tricyclic Antidepressants** (eg, **amitriptyline, clomipramine**): Other anticholinergic drugs may cause additive anticholinergic effects.

Laboratory Considerations

- **Intradermal allergy testing (IDT)**: As an antihistamine, meclizine may suppress IDT results. Discontinue meclizine 2 (minimum) to 7 days (preferred) before IDT.[3]

Dosages

DOGS:

Vestibular disease; prevention of motion sickness and vomiting (extra-label): No controlled studies supporting any dosage regimen were found. Anecdotally: 4 mg/kg PO once daily. Practically: 12.5 mg – 50 mg/dog (NOT mg/kg) PO once daily[4]

CATS:

Vestibular disease; prevention of motion sickness and vomiting (extra-label): No controlled studies supporting any dosage regimen were found. Anecdotally: 6.25 – 12.5 mg/cat (NOT mg/kg) PO once daily

RABBITS, RODENTS, SMALL MAMMALS:

Rabbits: rolling, torticollis, motion sickness, head tilt (extra-label):

a) 2 – 12 mg/kg PO once daily[5,6]

b) 12.5 mg/rabbit (NOT mg/kg) PO every 12 to 24 hours[7]

Monitoring

- Efficacy
- Adverse effects

Client Information

- This medicine may be given with or without food. Giving this medicine with a small amount of food or a treat may help prevent vomiting.
- When using this medication for motion sickness prevention, give it 30 to 60 minutes before travel.
- The most common side effect is sedation (ie, drowsiness, sleepiness).

Chemistry/Synonyms

Meclizine HCl is a piperazine derivative antiemetic antihistamine that is structurally similar to hydroxyzine. It occurs as a white or yellowish-white crystalline powder. It is slightly soluble in water and soluble in alcohol. Meclizine is hygroscopic.

Meclizine may also be known as meclizinium, meclozine, or parachloramine. *Antivert®* and *Bonine®* are common trade names.

Storage/Stability

Meclizine products should be stored in well-closed, light-resistant containers at room temperature 20°C to 25°C (68°F-77°F); excursions are permitted between 15°C to 30°C (59°F-86°F).

Compatibility/Compounding Considerations

No specific information was noted.

Dosage Forms/Regulatory Status

VETERINARY-LABELED PRODUCTS: NONE

The Association of Racing Commissioners International (ARCI) has designated this drug as a class 4 substance. Use of this drug may not be allowed in certain animal competitions. Check rules and regulations before entering in a competition while this medication is being administered. Contact local racing authorities for further guidance. See ***Appendix*** for more information.

HUMAN-LABELED PRODUCTS:

Meclizine HCl Oral Tablets: 12.5 mg, 25 mg (plain and chewable), and 50 mg; *Antivert®*, *Dramamine® Less Drowsy Formula*, *Bonine®*, *Travel-Ease®*, generic; (Rx and OTC)

References

For the complete list of references, see **wiley.com/go/budde/plumb**

Medetomidine

(mee-de-***toe***-mi-deen) *Domitor®*

Alpha-2-Adrenergic Agonist

Prescriber Highlights

- Reversible sedative analgesic used primarily in dogs, cats, small mammals, and exotic species
- Contraindications include most forms of cardiac disease, respiratory disorders, shock, severe debilitation, or animals stressed due to heat, cold, or fatigue. Also contraindicated in liver or kidney disease, although some anesthesiologists consider those contraindications to be relative because medetomidine effects can be reversed.
- Use with caution in geriatric and pediatric animals.
- Adverse effects include bradycardia, occasional AV block, decreased respiratory rate, hypothermia, urination, vomiting, and hyperglycemia. Rarely, prolonged sedation, hypersensitivity, apnea, and death from circulatory failure may occur.
- Systemic and central effects may be reversed with atipamezole; however, analgesia will also be reversed, and additional analgesic agents may be required for adequate pain control.
- Do **NOT** confuse medetomidine with detomidine or dexmedetomidine.

Uses/Indications

Medetomidine is an alpha-2 agonist used as a sedative, premedication/anesthesia adjunct, and analgesic in dogs, cats, other small animal species, and in a wide variety of large animal species (eg, horses, cattle, camelids, small ruminants). Medetomidine is commonly used in combination with an opioid and/or ketamine to extend the depth and duration of action to minimize the need for redosing.

Pharmacology/Actions

An alpha-2 adrenergic receptor, medetomidine has an alpha-2:alpha-1 selectivity factor of 1620:1 and, as compared with xylazine, is reportedly 10 times more specific for alpha-2 receptors versus alpha-1 receptors. The pharmacologic effects of medetomidine include depression of CNS (sedation, anxiolysis), GI (nausea/vomiting, decreased secretions, varying effects on intestinal muscle tone), and endocrine functions; peripheral and cardiac vasoconstriction; bradycardia; respiratory depression; diuresis; hypothermia; analgesia (somatic and visceral); muscle relaxation; and blanched or cyanotic mucous membranes. Effects on blood pressure are variable, but medetomidine can cause hypertension for longer periods as compared with xylazine. Medetomidine also induces sedation for a longer period as compared with xylazine. Sedative effects persist longer than analgesic effects.

Pharmacokinetics

After IV or IM injection, onset of effect is rapid (5 minutes for IV; 10 to 15 minutes for IM). The drug is absorbed via the oral mucosa when administered sublingually in dogs, but efficacy at a given dose may be less than with IM dosing.

Contraindications/Precautions/Warnings

The label states that medetomidine is contraindicated in dogs having the following conditions: cardiac disease, respiratory disorders, liver or kidney disease, shock, severe debilitation, or dogs stressed due to heat, cold, or fatigue. However, not all forms of cardiac disease create a contraindication, for instance, medetomidine administered to cats with left ventricular outflow obstruction improved cardiac function secondary to slowed heart rate with subsequent increased ventricular filling.[1] Because medetomidine's effects are reversible, some anesthesiologists consider medetomidine contraindications to be relative, particularly in patients with hepatic or renal disease. Of note, reversal with atipamezole will counteract sedation, physiologic effects, and analgesia; additional analgesic agents may be required for adequate pain control.

Medetomidine should only be used in situations in which sufficient monitoring and patient-support capabilities (eg, intubation, ventilation) are available.

Dogs that are extremely agitated or excited may have a decreased response to medetomidine; the manufacturer suggests allowing these dogs to rest quietly before administration of the drug. Dogs not responding to medetomidine should not be redosed according to the label. Clinically, redose is common if a low dose was used initially and was not effective; however, the most effective process would be to combine medetomidine with an opioid and/or an anesthetic such as ketamine rather than to redose. Use medetomidine in pediatric or geriatric dogs should be done with caution.

Medetomidine reduces tear flow in dogs and cats.[2,3] Ophthalmic ointment should be used to protect eyes when using this drug.[4,5]

Do not confuse medetomidine with detomidine or dexmedetomidine. Do not interchange dexmedetomidine with medetomidine dosages. On a <u>**mg**</u>/kg basis, dexmedetomidine doses are ≈½ of the medetomidine dose since dexmedetomidine is more potent; however, dexmedetomidine is ½ the concentration of medetomidine so the doses are the same on a <u>**mL**</u>/kg basis.

Adverse Effects

The adverse effects reported with medetomidine are essentially extensions of its pharmacologic effects including bradycardia, occasional AV blocks, decreased respiratory rate, hypothermia, urination (particularly during recovery, 90 to 120 minutes following administration), vomiting, and hyperglycemia. Rare effects have also been reported, including prolonged sedation, paradoxical excitation[6] (particularly when combined with midazolam[7]), hypersensitivity, apnea, and death from circulatory failure.

Vomiting is common in cats and appears to be proportional to dose administered.[8-10]

Reduced tear flow has been documented in dogs[2] and cats.[3] However, in dogs, administration of medetomidine at 5, 10, 20, 40, and 80 µg/kg IM did not affect intraocular pressure except at the 80 µg/kg dose, which caused a decrease in intraocular pressure hours after ad ministration.[11] In cats, even high doses (100 µg/kg) of medetomidine do not affect intraocular pressure.[12]

Reproductive/Nursing Safety

Medetomidine is not recommended for use in pregnant dogs or dogs used for breeding[6]; medetomidine induces maternal uterine contractions in pregnant dogs.[13] Medetomidine 0.007 mg/kg IV has been used with propofol and sevoflurane for cesarean sections in dogs with resultant safety for the bitch and high puppy vigor scores and survival rate.[14]

Medetomidine crosses the placenta of pregnant goats and ewes, with equivalent fetal and maternal medetomidine concentrations.[15,16] In sheep, medetomidine induced maternal uterine contractions[15]; decreases in fetal heart rate and increases in fetal blood pressure were also noted.

Information on medetomidine use in lactating animals was not located.

Because safety has not been established in animals, this drug should only be used in pregnant or nursing animals when the maternal benefits outweigh the potential risks to offspring.

Overdose/Acute Toxicity

Single doses of medetomidine up to 5 times (IV) and 10 times (IM) the recommended dose were tolerated in dogs, but adverse effects can occur (see ***Adverse Effects***). Repeated doses may cause profound sedation, bradycardia, and reduced respiratory rate.[6] A single IV administration of 10 times the label dose may result in a prolonged anesthesia-like episode with muscle twitching. Death has occurred rarely in dogs (1 in 40,000) receiving 2 times the label dose.

Because of the potential of additional adverse effects occurring (heart block, PVCs, or tachycardia), treatment of medetomidine-induced bradycardia with anticholinergic agents (atropine or glycopyrrolate) is usually not recommended (see ***Drug Interactions***). Atipamezole is a safer choice to treat any medetomidine-induced effect provided reversal of analgesia or sedation is not contraindicated.

Drug Interactions

The following drug interactions have either been reported or are theoretical in humans or animals receiving medetomidine and may be of significance in veterinary patients. Unless otherwise noted, use together is not necessarily contraindicated, but weigh the potential risks and perform additional monitoring when appropriate. **NOTE**: Before attempting combination therapy with medetomidine, it is strongly advised to consult veterinary anesthesia references or veterinary anesthesiologists familiar with the use of this drug.

- ALFAXALONE: When alfaxalone is used after medetomidine, hypoxemia may occur secondary to respiratory depression. Oxygen delivery during induction or as soon as intubated is recommended. Dosages of alfaxalone should be adjusted based on the patient's level of sedation, ie, dose to effect.
- ANTICHOLINERGIC AGENTS (eg, **atropine, butylscopolamine, glycopyrrolate**): The use of atropine or glycopyrrolate to prevent or treat medetomidine-caused bradycardia is controversial as tachycardia and hypertension may result. This is more important when using higher doses of medetomidine (more than 20 µg/kg) and concomitant use is discouraged. However, in anesthetized patients that received medetomidine as premedication and that become hypotensive, anticholinergic use is often recommended to increase heart rate and improve blood pressure without reversing the sedation. Reversal of sedation can cause sudden arousal of the patient. One study showed tachycardia and hypertension developed when butylscopolamine was administered IV or IM before medetomidine in horses.[17]
- OPIOIDS (eg, **butorphanol, morphine**): Enhancement of sedation and analgesia occurs when medetomidine is used concurrently with all opioids; however, adverse effects (eg, bradycardia, hypoventilation) may be pronounced. Combination therapy of medetomidine with opioids is recommended for enhanced sedation and analgesia but reduced dosages (low end of the standard dosing range) of both drugs should be used and the patient should be observed for excessive sedation, bradyarrhythmias, and hypotension.
- PROPOFOL: When propofol is used after medetomidine, hypoxemia may occur secondary to respiratory depression. Oxygen delivery during induction or as soon as intubated is recommended. Dosages of propofol should be adjusted based on the patient's level of sedation, ie, dose to effect.
- SYMPATHOMIMETICS (eg, **dopamine, epinephrine**): Concurrent use contraindicated.[18] However, dopamine is often used in anesthetized patients that received medetomidine as premedication and that become hypotensive in spite of anticholinergic administration to normalize heart rate. Epinephrine is generally reserved for emergencies and is not contraindicated in a cardiovascular emergency.
- YOHIMBINE: May reverse the effects of medetomidine; but atipamezole is preferred for clinical use to reverse the drug's effects because atipamezole is more selective for the alpha receptors and is unlikely to cause hypotension, which is common following administration of yohimbine

Laboratory Considerations

- Medetomidine can inhibit ADP-induced **platelet aggregation** in cats, but this does not appear to be clinically significant.

Dosages

NOTES:

1. Medetomidine dosages depend on the combination of drugs used and the dosage(s) of the other drug(s). Dosage adjustments will also need to be made to account for the degree of desired sedation; type, duration, and pain level of the procedure, and patient temperament and body weight/size.
2. Dosing based on body surface area (BSA; or allometric scaling) is not common in clinical practice but decreases the variability in drug response between giant/large and small/toy breed dogs. See the United States label[1] for dosing based on BSA where, as an example, a 4 kg (8.8 lb) dog would receive ≈50 µg/kg IV versus a 40 kg (88 lb) dog would receive ≈20 µg/kg IV.
3. Premedication with medetomidine will significantly reduce the dose of the induction agent required and will reduce volatile anesthetic requirements for maintenance anesthesia. All anesthetic agents used for induction or maintenance of anesthesia should be administered to effect.
4. For all dosages, the low end of the dose range is generally appropriate for IV administration, whereas the mid-upper range is most appropriate for IM or SC administration. Higher dosages will provide more profound sedation and analgesia.
5. When SC administration is used, the speed of sedation is slower, and the level of sedation is lighter and inconsistent. For more predictable sedation, IM or IV administration is recommended.
6. The effects of medetomidine can be reversed with atipamezole. It is most often dosed by volume at ½ or same volume of medetomidine that was administered and given IM. See ***Atipamezole***.

DOGS:

Sedation/analgesia (label dosage; FDA-approved): 750 µg/m^2 (0.75 mg/m^2) IV or 1000 µg/m^2 (1 mg/m^2) IM.[6] For use in dogs over 12 weeks of age

Sedation/analgesia when medetomidine is used as sole agent (extra-label): Dosage ranges commonly used to achieve general sedation levels include:

a) **Light sedation (often also used for pre-anesthesia)**: 5 – 20 µg/kg IM, IV, SC[18]
b) **Moderate sedation (may be used for pre-anesthesia if deeper sedation is desired or the patient has a high energy or anxiety level)**: 20 – 40 µg/kg IM, IV, SC
c) **Deep sedation**: 30 – 80 µg/kg IM, IV, or SC[18]; repeat dose if necessary or consider using a combination protocol because these high doses can be dangerous.

Other routes of administration

a) Medetomidine can be administered oral transmucosally (OTM) but published papers are sparse. Based on the dexmedetomidine dose to sedate aggressive dogs by this route,[19] an average of ≈64 μg/kg OTM is suggested.

b) 40 μg/kg via nasal atomization produced sedation similar to IM administration; IN onset 7.2 minutes versus 6.3 minutes with IM.[20]

Sedation/analgesia when used in combination with other drugs (extra-label): More predictable sedation is obtained when medetomidine is administered in combination with other analgesic or sedative drugs. Use of medetomidine in combination with other sedatives allows for a reduced dose of medetomidine, which improves safety and, when used in combination with other analgesic agents, it enhances analgesia. Medetomidine has been combined with different opioids (eg, morphine, methadone, hydromorphone, buprenorphine, butorphanol, fentanyl) and induction agents (eg, propofol, alfaxalone, ketamine) to produce sedation/analgesia and decrease the amount of anesthesia maintenance drugs in healthy dogs with minimal adverse effects.[21-25] When combining medetomidine with other drugs, the low-mid range of the medetomidine dosage based on the desired level of sedation is generally adequate.

Examples of combinations used in clinical practice

a) Medetomidine 5 μg/kg combined with butorphanol 0.3 mg/kg and given IM followed by 1 – 2.5 mg/kg alfaxalone IM provided anesthesia with minimal to no cardiorespiratory depression.[26]

b) Medetomidine 24 μg/kg combined with butorphanol 0.24 mg/kg and given IM allowed for lower sevoflurane requirements to maintain general anesthesia.[27]

c) Medetomidine 20 μg/kg combined with butorphanol 0.3 mg/kg and given IM provided adequate clinical sedation.[28]

d) Medetomidine 2.5 μg/kg combined with either morphine 0.3 mg/kg or methadone 0.3 mg/kg and given IV prior to anesthesia induction with propofol and maintained with isoflurane.[21] Isoflurane-sparing effect and enhanced analgesia are noted.

e) Medetomidine 2.5 μg/kg combined with alfaxalone 2.5 mg/kg and butorphanol 0.25 mg/kg and given IM produced lateral recumbency and allowed intubation in dogs, without causing severe cardiopulmonary depression.[22]

f) Medetomidine 2.5 μg/kg combined with butorphanol 0.4 mg/kg or methadone 0.4 mg/kg in the same syringe and given IM.[23] Maximum sedation occurred at 20 to 30 minutes postinjection; heart rate decreased in both groups.

Refractory seizures (extra-label): Medetomidine 0.016 μg/kg per minute IV CRI was used to treat refractory seizures in a dog following portosystemic shunt ligation.[29]

CATS:

Sedation/analgesia when medetomidine is used as a sole agent (extra-label): Dosage ranges commonly used to achieve general sedation levels include:

a) **Light sedation (often also used for pre-anesthesia)**: 5 – 30 μg/kg IV, IM, or SC

b) **Moderate sedation (may be used for pre-anesthesia if deeper sedation is desired or the patient has a high energy or anxiety level)**: 30 – 50 μg/kg IV, IM or SC

c) **Deep sedation**: 50 – 80 μg/kg IV, IM,[8,9] SC. Doses up to 100 μg/kg have been used and up to 150 μg/kg are listed on the label of some countries[18] but an upper dose of 80 μg/kg is generally sufficient for most cats. Doses this high (ie, 100 to 150 μg/kg) are often dangerous and a combination protocol should be considered.

Sedation/analgesia when used in combination with other drugs (extra-label): Medetomidine has been combined with different opioids (eg, morphine, methadone, hydromorphone, buprenorphine, butorphanol, fentanyl) and induction agents (eg, propofol, alfaxalone, ketamine) to produce sedation/analgesia and decrease the amount of maintenance drugs in healthy cats with minimal adverse effects. When combining with other drugs, the low-mid range of the dose for the desired level of sedation is generally adequate. For many of these protocols, the drugs are combined in the same syringe and administered IM.

Examples of combinations used in clinical practice for *light* sedation

a) Medetomidine 20 μg/kg combined in the same syringe with butorphanol 0.4 mg/kg IM prior to induction[30]

b) Medetomidine 20 μg/kg combined with methadone 0.5 mg/kg and given IM prior to induction[30]

c) Medetomidine 20 μg/kg combined with buprenorphine 20 μg/kg and given IM prior to induction[30]

Other routes of administration

a) Medetomidine can be administered oral transmucosally (OTM) but published papers are sparse. Based on the dexmedetomidine dose to sedate cats by this route, a recommended dosage is medetomidine 20 μg/kg combined with buprenorphine 20 μg/kg and administered oral transmucosally (OTM) to provide sedation, although the degree of sedation is lower and less predictable as compared with IM administration of the same drugs at the same doses.[31]

Example of combination used in clinical practice for *moderate* sedation

a) Medetomidine 50 μg/kg combined in the same syringe with butorphanol 0.4 mg/kg IM prior to induction[18]

Examples of combinations used in clinical practice for *heavy* sedation/anesthesia (extra-label):

a) Medetomidine 60 μg/kg combined in the same syringe with ketamine 10 mg/kg IM[32]

b) Medetomidine 60 μg/kg combined in the same syringe with ketamine 10 mg/kg and morphine 0.2 mg/kg IM[32]

c) Medetomidine 60 μg/kg combined in the same syringe with ketamine 10 mg/kg and tramadol 2 mg/kg IM (injectable tramadol is not available in the US)[32]

General anesthesia when used in combination with ketamine (extra-label): Medetomidine 80 μg/kg combined in the same syringe with ketamine 2.5 – 7.5 mg/kg and given IM or SC; anesthesia occurs within 3 to 4 minutes and persists for 20 to 50 minutes.[18]

General anesthesia when used in combination with ketamine and butorphanol or buprenorphine | "Kitty Magic" (extra-label):

a) Medetomidine 20 – 40 μg/kg with ketamine 2 – 4 mg/kg and *either* butorphanol 0.2 – 0.4 mg/kg or buprenorphine 0.006 (generally considered too low for adequate analgesia) to 0.012 mg/kg combined in one syringe and given IM.[33] **NOTE**: This combination can also be calculated by drug *volume* when using drug concentrations of medetomidine 1 mg/mL, ketamine 100 mg/mL, butorphanol 10 mg/mL, buprenorphine 0.3 mg/mL: use 0.02 - 0.04 mL/kg of each drug combined in one syringe and given IM. The low end of the volume provides deep sedation whereas the high end provides anesthesia.

b) Medetomidine 70 – 80 μg/kg combined with ketamine 5 mg/kg and butorphanol 0.4 mg/kg OR buprenorphine 0.02 mg/kg in the same syringe and given IM[34]

General anesthesia when used in combination with alfaxalone (extra-label):

a) Medetomidine 40 µg/kg IM or SC followed 15 to 20 minutes later by alfaxalone 2.5 – 5 mg/kg IV

b) Medetomidine 20 µg/kg combined in the same syringe with butorphanol 0.2 mg/kg and alfaxalone 5 mg/kg and given IM; minimal cardiopulmonary effects expected but the cardiovascular effects of medetomidine are present. The mean time from induction to extubation was 114 minutes, from induction to standing 125 minutes (clinically prolonged), and analgesia lasted 55 minutes.[35] This protocol is limited to small patients due to the volume of injectate required. If 10 mg/mL butorphanol is used in this combination, the total volume of injectate at these dosages is a little over 2 mL IM.

HORSES:

Sedation/analgesia prior to general anesthesia or for short duration standing procedures (extra-label):

a) Medetomidine 5 – 7 µg/kg IV alone or in combination with butorphanol 0.02 mg/kg IV

b) Medetomidine 5 µg/kg IV bolus followed by medetomidine 1.25 – 3.5 µg/kg/hour IV CRI[36,37]

Total intravenous anesthesia (extra-label):

1. Premedication with medetomidine 7 µg/kg IV followed by anesthesia induction with ketamine 2.2 mg/kg IV and maintained by medetomidine 5 µg/kg/hour, ketamine 3 mg/kg per hour, and midazolam 0.1 mg/kg/hour IV CRI.[38]
2. Premedication with medetomidine 5 µg/kg combined with butorphanol 0.02 mg/kg IV; induce general anesthesia with guaifenesin 10 mg/kg IV, followed by either propofol 2 mg/kg IV or alfaxalone 1 mg/kg IV; anesthesia was maintained with IV CRI of either propofol 3 mg/kg/hour or alfaxalone 1.5 mg/kg/hour IV CRI in combination with medetomidine 3 µg/kg/hour and guaifenesin 80 mg/kg/hour IV CRI.[39]

CATTLE:

Sedation (extra-label): Calves were given medetomidine 8, 10, or 12 µg/kg IV. Onset of sedation was rapid and dose dependent. Duration of sedation ranged from 73 to 117 minutes with the longer duration seen at the higher dose.[40]

SHEEP/GOATS:

Analgesia (extra-label):

1. In sheep, medetomidine 2 µg/kg IV can provide analgesia for ≈20 minutes during surgery.[41]
2. In goats, medetomidine 10 µg/kg via lumbosacral subarachnoid administration produced mild sedation and moderate analgesia of the hind quarter, perineum, and flank for 158 minutes.[42]
3. In goats, medetomidine 20 µg/kg via lumbosacral epidural administration produced sedation and surgical analgesia; mean duration of lateral recumbency was 136 minutes.[43]

Sedation (extra-label):

1. In sheep, medetomidine 30 µg/kg IM[44]
2. In goats, medetomidine 20 µg/kg IV. Recumbency was observed 90 seconds after administration.[45] Doses as low as 4 – 6 µg/kg IV also resulted in sedation and analgesia.[46]
3. In goats, medetomidine 40 µg/kg IM. Recumbency lasted for 90 minutes.[47]

Heavy sedation/anesthesia (extra-label):

1. In sheep, medetomidine 10 µg/kg IV will produce recumbency.[48]
2. In sheep, medetomidine 2 µg/kg IV in combination with alfaxalone 2 mg/kg IV. Sheep showed minor excitatory effects, but those did not impact induction.[49]
3. In goats, medetomidine 15 µg/kg IM in combination with ketamine 5 mg/kg IM; surgical anesthesia was induced within ≈11 minutes and lasted ≈47 minutes with complete recovery at 121 minutes.[50]

CAMELIDS:

Sedation (extra-label): Medetomidine 10 µg/kg IM can produce standing sedation without analgesia.[48]

Heavy sedation (extra-label): Medetomidine 30 µg/kg IM; onset ≈7 minutes, duration ≈90 minutes[51]

BIRDS:

Sedation/analgesia (extra-label):

1. Medetomidine 75 – 100 µg/kg IM with ketamine 3 – 7 mg/kg IM[52]
2. Medetomidine 60 – 85 µg/kg IM with ketamine 1.5 – 2 mg/kg IM[53]

Anesthesia (extra-label): Medetomidine 50 - 200 µg/kg IM in combination with ketamine 3 – 10 mg/kg IM[54]

RABBITS:

Heavy sedation/ anesthesia (extra-label):

1. Medetomidine 250 µg/kg IM with atropine 0.5 mg/kg IM, midazolam 0.5 mg/kg IM followed 5 minutes later by propofol 2 mg/kg IV resulted in analgesia for 25 minutes; time from extubation to sternal recumbency was ≈27 minutes.[55]
2. Medetomidine 350 µg/kg IM followed by ketamine 5 mg/kg IV produced anesthesia of ≈19 minutes duration; medetomidine 350 µg/kg IM combined with propofol 3 mg/kg IV produced anesthesia for ≈11 minutes.[56]
3. Medetomidine 250 µg/kg with ketamine 15 mg/kg IM, SC.[57-59] Equivalent anesthetic effects were noted with either route of administration. **NOTE**: in one study all animals required supplemental oxygen.[58] SC administration appears to be better tolerated, but induction of anesthesia is faster with IM administration.[59,60] Another study determined that medetomidine 500 µg/kg and ketamine 25 mg/kg given SC offered reliable anesthesia and excellent muscle relaxation, but respiratory depression was noted.[61]
4. Medetomidine 250 µg/kg IM followed 5 minutes later by ketamine 60 mg/kg IM[62]
5. Medetomidine 200 µg/kg with ketamine 10 mg/kg administered intranasally to rabbits in sternal recumbency. 50% of the dose was repeated if swallowing occurred during intubation.[63]
6. Medetomidine 500 µg /kg IM, ketamine 35 mg/kg IM, and buprenorphine 0.03 mg/kg IM.[64] Another study administered buprenorphine 0.03 mg/kg SC one hour prior to medetomidine 250 µg/kg and ketamine 15 mg/kg SC, which prolonged the duration of analgesia and anesthesia.[65]
7. Medetomidine 200 µg/kg IM with morphine 1 – 2 mg/kg IM, followed by alfaxalone 10 mg/kg IV; anesthesia was suitable, but profound respiratory depression occurred.[66]

FERRETS:

Sedation/analgesia prior to general anesthesia (extra-label): 15 minutes prior to medetomidine, give atropine 0.05 mg/kg or glycopyrrolate 0.01 mg/kg IM or SC followed by medetomidine

60 – 80 µg/kg IM or SC.[8] Sedation lasts up to 3 hours. May be reversed with atipamezole 400 µg/kg IM

General anesthesia (extra-label):

1. Medetomidine 40 – 80 µg/kg in combination with butorphanol 0.1 – 0.4 mg/kg and ketamine 5 – 10 mg/kg and given IM[67]; may need to supplement with isoflurane 0.5% to 1.5% to maintain general anesthesia for abdominal surgery.
2. Medetomidine 20 µg/kg IM followed by alfaxalone 2.5 mg/kg IV provided anesthesia lasting ≈80 minutes.[68] **NOTE**: Alfaxalone used alone in the ferret produced unsatisfactory anesthetic results.

REPTILES:

Sedation/analgesia (extra-label): **NOTE**: Reversal of all dosages with atipamezole is 4 to 5 times the medetomidine dose.[69]

- **Medium to small land tortoises**: Medetomidine 100 to 150 µg/kg combined with ketamine 5 – 10 mg/kg and given IV or IM
- **Freshwater turtles**: Medetomidine 150 – 300 µg/kg combined with ketamine 10 – 20 mg/kg and given IV or IM
- **Giant land tortoises** (200 kg [440.9 lb] Aldabra tortoise): Medetomidine 40 µg/kg combined with ketamine 4 mg/kg and given IV or IM
- **Smaller Aldabra tortoises**: Medetomidine 40 – 80 µg/kg combined with ketamine 4 – 8 mg/kg and given IV or IM. Wait 30 to 40 minutes for peak effect.
- **Iguanas**: Medetomidine 100 – 150 µg/kg combined with ketamine 5 – 10 mg/kg and given IV or IM

Monitoring

- Level of sedation and analgesia; body temperature
- Heart rate and rhythm, blood pressure, respiratory depth and rate, $ETCO_2$, pulse oximetry, and body temperature should be considered in all patients, and mandatory in higher risk patients.

Client Information

- When given by injection (in the veterinary clinic), medetomidine should be used in a professionally supervised setting by individuals familiar with its properties.
- Withhold feed and water until the sedative effects of me detomidine have subsided.

Chemistry/Synonyms

An alpha-2-adrenergic agonist, medetomidine occurs as a white or off-white crystalline substance. It is soluble in water. Although the compound exists as 2 stereoisomers, only the D-isomer is active. 1 mg of medetomidine HCl is equivalent to 0.85 mg of medetomidine base. Dosages are expressed as medetomidine HCl.

Medetomidine HCl may also be known as MPV-785, *Domitor*®, *Dorbene*®, *Dormilan*®, and *Sedanorm*®.

Storage/Stability

The commercially available injection should be stored at room temperature (15°C-30°C [59°F-86°F]) and protected from freezing. Use within 28 days of first vial puncture.

Compatibility/Compounding Considerations

Compatibility is dependent on factors such as pH, concentration, temperature, and diluent used; specialized references or a hospital pharmacist should be consulted for more specific information.

See ***Dosage*** section for acceptable combinations; more information may also be found in the ***Dexmedetomidine*** monograph.

Dosage Forms/Regulatory Status

VETERINARY-LABELED PRODUCTS:

The Association of Racing Commissioners International (ARCI) has designated this drug as a class 3 substance. Use of this drug may not be allowed in certain animal competitions. Check rules and regulations before entering in a competition while this medication is being administered. Contact local racing authorities for further guidance. See the ***Appendix*** for more information.

Medetomidine HCl for Injection: 1 mg/mL in 10 mL multidose vials; *Domitor*®, generic; (Rx). FDA-approved for use in dogs over 12 weeks of age.

HUMAN-LABELED PRODUCTS: NONE

References

For the complete list of references, see **wiley.com/go/budde/plumb**

Medetomidine/Vatinoxan

(mee-de-***toe***-mi-deen/va-te-***nox***-an) *Zenalpha*®

Alpha-2-Adrenergic Agonist/Peripheral Antagonist Combination

Prescriber Highlights

- Reversible sedative-analgesic combination product approved for use in dogs to facilitate examinations, clinical procedures, or minor surgical procedures; the addition of vatinoxan reduces the risk for medetomidine's negative cardiovascular effects.
- Duration of sedation from the combination is typically shorter than that achieved by use of an equivalent dose of alpha-2 agonist alone
- Contraindicated in patients hypersensitive to either agent, and in dogs with cardiac disease, respiratory disorders, shock, or severe debilitation; that have or are at risk for developing hypoglycemia; and dogs stressed due to heat, cold, or fatigue. Additionally, do not administer to dogs with pre-existing hypotension, hypoxia (hypoxemia), or bradycardia.
- Use with caution in diabetic, geriatric, and pediatric dogs, and in dogs with renal or hepatic disease.
- Significant hypotension has been observed in cats and horses.
- Adverse effects include diarrhea, muscle tremors, and colitis; hypothermia, bradycardia, and arrhythmias are possible.
- Sedation and cardiac effects can be reversed with atipamezole.

Uses/Indications

Medetomidine/vatinoxan is indicated for use in clinically healthy dogs as a sedative and analgesic to facilitate clinical examinations or minor procedures. In field studies, the onset and duration of sedation after IM administration were ≈14 minutes and 38 minutes, respectively. In healthy dogs, medetomidine/vatinoxan has been safely used in combination with butorphanol[1,2] and as a premedication prior to propofol induction and isoflurane anesthesia,[3] and during isoflurane anesthesia.[4]

Pharmacology/Actions

An alpha-2-adrenergic receptor agonist, medetomidine is ≈10 times more specific for alpha-2 receptors versus alpha-1 receptors as compared with xylazine. The desirable pharmacologic effects of medetomidine include CNS depression (sedation, anxiolysis) and somatic and visceral analgesia. Other effects include GI (eg, nausea/vomiting, decreased secretions, varying effects on intestinal muscle tone), and endocrine (hyperglycemia) functions; peripheral vasoconstriction and hypertension with subsequent baroreflex-mediated bradycardia and decreased cardiac output; respiratory depression; diuresis; hypothermia; muscle relaxation; and blanched or cyanotic mucous membranes. The sedative effects of medetomidine generally persist longer than the analgesic effects.

Vatinoxan is a peripherally acting alpha-2-adrenergic antagonist. Vatinoxan attenuates the hemodynamic effects of alpha-2-adrenergic receptor agonists that occur outside the CNS in dogs when a plasma medetomidine:vatinoxan concentration ratio of 1:18 is reached or exceeded.[4] In dogs, the combination of medetomidine/vatinoxan resulted in higher heart rate and cardiac index, and lower mean arterial pressure and systemic vascular resistance as compared to medetomidine alone.[5,6] One study in dogs documented that IM vatinoxan did not prevent the initial hemodynamic changes (bradycardia, hypertension) caused by IM medetomidine, but vatinoxan resulted in the cardiovascular effects disappearing more rapidly.[7] Vatinoxan also prevented or abolished metabolic changes (eg, hyperglycemia, hypoinsulinemia, hyperlactatemia) induced by dexmedetomidine,[8] and mitigated the hypothermic effects of medetomidine and butorphanol combination.[9] Medetomidine/vatinoxan may decrease serum glucose in healthy dogs.[10]

Unlike atipamezole (a centrally and peripherally acting antagonist), vatinoxan appears to only minimally decrease the degree or depth of sedation caused by the alpha-2 agonist, and the difference does not appear to be clinically significant.[5,11-13] In dogs, the duration of sedation produced by medetomidine/vatinoxan is equivalent to its duration of analgesia; however, the duration of sedation from the combination is shorter than that achieved by medetomidine alone.[10,14] Vatinoxan did not diminish the visceral antinociceptive effects of medetomidine in healthy dogs, but vatinoxan's effect on somatic antinociception was variable.[15] Vatinoxan demonstrated a dose-related attenuation of the dexmedetomidine reduction of sevoflurane MAC in healthy dogs.[16] In horses, vatinoxan appeared to mitigate the reduced intestinal activity[17,18] and GI microperfusion[19] caused by alpha-2 agonists.

Pharmacokinetics

As a single agent, medetomidine is ≈90% bound to plasma proteins. In healthy dogs, its volume of distribution was 1.3 L/kg, clearance was 1.3 L/kg/hour, and terminal half-life was ≈1 hour.[20] Medetomidine is primarily oxidized in the liver and excreted renally.

Vatinoxan is ≈70% protein bound in canine plasma, and protein binding is not altered by the presence of medetomidine.[21] Vatinoxan only minimally distributes into the CNS; after IV administration, the CNS:plasma vatinoxan concentration ratio was ≈1:50.[22] Preliminary evidence suggests vatinoxan is not a substrate of P-gp.[23] Vatinoxan elimination has not been fully described, but less than 5% is excreted in the urine.

When a medetomidine and vatinoxan combination was administered IM to dogs as a 1:30 ratio (**NOTE**: The commercially available product contains a 1:20 ratio), peak plasma concentrations of dexmedetomidine (the active medetomidine isomer) and vatinoxan occurred ≈13 and 18 minutes after IM administration, respectively.[10] Vatinoxan decreased the apparent volume of distribution of dexmedetomidine,[24] and increased (more than doubled) the clearance of medetomidine and dexmedetomidine in dogs.[14] Vatinoxan reduced plasma concentrations of medetomidine and dexmedetomidine in dogs[14] but had variable effects in horses[25,26] and sheep.[27,28]

Contraindications/Precautions/Warnings

Medetomidine/vatinoxan is contraindicated in dogs that are hypersensitive to medetomidine or vatinoxan; dogs with cardiac disease, respiratory disorders, shock, or severe debilitation; that have or are at risk for developing hypoglycemia; and dogs that are stressed due to heat, cold, or fatigue.[10] Do not administer medetomidine/vatinoxan to patients with pre-existing hypotension, hypoxia (hypoxemia), or bradycardia. Use medetomidine/vatinoxan with caution in dogs with hepatic or renal disease, as the safe use in these conditions has not been evaluated.[10] Medetomidine/vatinoxan has not been evaluated in dogs younger than 4.5 months old. Because medetomidine's effects are reversible, some anesthesiologists consider these precautions to be relative, particularly in patients with hepatic or renal disease.

Medetomidine/vatinoxan should only be used in situations in which sufficient monitoring and patient-support capabilities (eg, intubation, oxygen administration, breathing support) are available.

Dogs that are extremely agitated, nervous, or excited may have a delayed or decreased response to medetomidine; the manufacturer suggests allowing these dogs to rest quietly for 10 to 15 minutes after administration of the drug. Repeat dosing of medetomidine/vatinoxan has not been evaluated by the manufacturer, but in one study, dogs that required additional sedation received a lower dose of medetomidine alone (ie, without vatinoxan).[2]

It is recommended that dogs fast for 4 to 6 hours prior to receiving medetomidine/vatinoxan.[29]

Medetomidine/vatinoxan use in cats[30-32] and horses[33] has been associated with significant hypotension, and the manufacturer states that medetomidine/vatinoxan is not intended for use in cats.[10]

Humans with cardiovascular disease and pregnant women should exercise caution when handling medetomidine/vatinoxan to avoid accidental exposure, as alpha-2 agonists cause changes to uterine contractility and blood flow which may result in fetal hypoxia and/or bradycardia.[10]

Do not confuse medetomidine/vatinoxan combination with medetomidine as a single agent, or with detomidine or dexmedetomidine.

Adverse Effects

Diarrhea, muscle tremors, and colitis were the most commonly reported adverse effects observed following IM use of medetomidine/vatinoxan during field studies, occurring in 2% to 4% of dogs.[10] Although decreased body temperature (ie, 99°F [37°C] or less) is common (52% of medetomidine/vatinoxan treated dogs), clinical hypothermia occurred only rarely and was of shorter duration and much less common in dogs receiving medetomidine/vatinoxan (0.9%) as compared with dogs receiving dexmedetomidine (11.5%); hypothermia may persist longer than sedation. Tachycardia occurring after recovery from sedation occurred rarely,[10] and may continue for up to 6 hours after administration.[29]

Medetomidine/vatinoxan use in cats has resulted in hypotension.[10]

Reproductive/Nursing Safety

Safe use of medetomidine/vatinoxan in dogs intended for breeding or pregnant or lactating bitches has not been established.[10] Extrapolating information from other alpha-2-adrenergic receptor agonists, medetomidine can induce uterine contractions in pregnant animals, and fetal bradycardia and hypoxia are possible.[34-36] Medetomidine crosses the placenta, with equivalent fetal and maternal medetomidine concentrations.[36,37]

Because safety has not been established in animals, this drug should only be used when the maternal benefits outweigh the potential risks to offspring.

Overdose/Acute Toxicity

Medetomidine/vatinoxan administered IV at doses 3 and 5 times the label IM dose resulted in sedation (4-to 8-hour duration), hypotension, hypothermia and an initial bradycardia followed later by sinus tachycardia during recovery.[10] Hypoglycemia occurred in 2 dogs receiving 5 times the label IM dose. Clinical signs included stool changes (eg, mucoid, soft, or watery), salivation, tremors, vocalization, defecation, vomiting, injected sclera, struggling after dosing, and skin that was cool to touch. Dogs returned to baseline physiologic state within 8 hours of administration.[10]

Atipamezole IM may be used to treat any medetomidine-induced effect provided reversal of analgesia or sedation is not contraindicated; reversal of sedation occurs within 5 to 10 minutes.[10]

For patients that have experienced or are suspected of having experienced an overdose, it is strongly encouraged to consult with one of the 24-hour poison consultation centers that specialize in providing information specific for veterinary patients. For general information related to overdose and toxin exposures, as well as contact information for poison control centers, refer to ***Appendix.***

Drug Interactions

The following drug interactions either have been reported or are theoretical in humans or animals receiving medetomidine and/or vatinoxan and may be of significance in veterinary patients. Unless otherwise noted, use together is not necessarily contraindicated, but weigh the potential risks and perform additional monitoring when appropriate. **NOTE**: Before attempting combination therapy with medetomidine, it is strongly advised to consult veterinary anesthesia references or veterinary anesthesiologists familiar with the use of this drug.

- ANALGESICS, SEDATIVES, TRANQUILIZERS, AND/OR ANESTHETIC AGENTS, OTHER (eg, **acepromazine, anesthetic agents** [**alfaxalone, isoflurane, ketamine, propofol**], **benzodiazepines** [eg, **midazolam**], **opioids** [eg, **fentanyl, morphine**]): When used in combination, lower dosages of medetomidine and/or other anesthetic or analgesic agents may be required. Additionally:
  a) Vatinoxan accelerated the time to peak midazolam concentration after IM administration.[38]
  b) Vatinoxan blocked the decrease in alfaxalone clearance caused by medetomidine.[39]
  c) Significant hypotension has been observed in studies using medetomidine/vatinoxan in combination with other anesthetic or analgesic drugs.[33,40]
- ANTICHOLINERGIC AGENTS (eg, **atropine, butylscopolamine, glycopyrrolate**): Vatinoxan minimizes the risk for medetomidine-induced bradycardia, and the concurrent administration of glycopyrrolate appeared to provide no benefit in dogs that received medetomidine/vatinoxan.[6]
- ANTIHYPERTENSIVE AGENTS/VASODILATORS (eg, **amlodipine, enalapril, hydralazine, telmisartan**): Concurrent use may increase the risk for hypotension.
- ATIPAMEZOLE: Atipamezole may be used to reverse the central effects of medetomidine when used in combination with vatinoxan[41]; reversal of sedation occurs within 5 to 10 minutes of IM atipamezole administration.[10]
- HYPOGLYCEMIC AGENTS (eg, **glipizide, insulin, metformin**): Medetomidine/vatinoxan may decrease serum glucose in healthy dogs.[10] Potentiation of hypoglycemic effect by medetomidine/vatinoxan was not observed in healthy dogs, but the study authors suggest using the combination cautiously in dogs at risk for hypoglycemia.[42]
- SYMPATHOMIMETICS (eg, **dopamine, epinephrine**): Concurrent use with medetomidine is contraindicated[43]; however, dopamine is often used in anesthetized patients that received medetomidine as premedication and that become hypotensive in spite of anticholinergic administration to normalize heart rate. Epinephrine is generally reserved for emergencies and is not contraindicated in a cardiovascular emergency.

Laboratory Considerations

- Medetomidine can inhibit ADP-induced **platelet aggregation** in cats, but this does not appear to be clinically significant.

Dosages

NOTE: Watch units closely when calculating doses. Do not confuse mg/m² with mg/kg, µg/m², or µg/kg.

DOGS:

Sedation and analgesia to facilitate examinations, clinical procedures, or minor surgical procedures in dogs (label dosage, FDA-approved): Calculate the dose based on medetomidine 1 mg/m² (NOT mg/kg) IM [which provides vatinoxan 20 mg/m² (NOT mg/kg)], or use the dosing table found in the United States product label and replicated below. Note that the mg/kg dosage decreases as body weight increases. Allow the dog to rest quietly until evidence of sedation has occurred (5 to 15 minutes).

Body weight – kg (lb)	Dose volume (mL)
2-3 (4.4-7)	0.3
3.1- 4 (7.1-9)	0.4
4.1-5 (9.1-11)	0.6
5.1-10 (11.1-22)	0.8
10.1-13 (22.1-29)	1
13.1-15 (29.1-33)	1.2
15.1-20 (33.1-44)	1.4
20.1-25 (44.1-55)	1.6
25.1-30 (55.1-66)	1.8
30.1-33 (66.1-73)	2
33.1-37 (73.1-81)	2.2
37.1-45 (81.1-99)	2.4
45.1-50 (99.1-110)	2.6
50.1-55 (110.1-121)	2.8
55.1-60 (121.1-132)	3
60.1-65 (132.1-143)	3.2
65.1-70 (143.1-154)	3.4
70.1-80 (154.1-176)	3.6
Greater than 80 (176)	3.8

Sedation and analgesia to facilitate diagnostic imaging of dogs (extra-label): Medetomidine 0.5 mg/m² (NOT mg/kg) in combination with vatinoxan 10 mg/m² (NOT mg/kg) IM and butorphanol 0.1 mg/kg IM. Medetomidine (as a single agent) 0.25 mg/m² (NOT mg/kg) IM was administered when additional sedation was needed.[2]

HORSES:

Multimodal sedation protocol (extra-label): Medetomidine 7 µg/kg in combination with vatinoxan 140 µg/kg IV prior to medetomidine (as a single agent) 3.5 µg/kg/hour IV CRI[25]

SHEEP:

Multimodal sedation protocol (extra-label): Medetomidine 30 µg/kg in combination with vatinoxan 600 µg/kg IM and ketamine 1 mg/kg IM[27]

Monitoring

- Quality of sedation and analgesia
- Heart rate and rhythm
- Blood pressure
- Respiratory rate, tidal volume or size of breath, $ETCO_2$, pulse oximetry, and body temperature

Client Information

- Medetomidine/vatinoxan should be used in a professionally supervised setting by individuals familiar with its properties and equipped with sufficient monitoring and patient-support capabilities.

Chemistry/Synonyms

An alpha-2-adrenergic agonist, medetomidine hydrochloride occurs as a white or off-white crystalline substance. It is soluble in water.

Although the compound exists as 2 stereoisomers, only the d-isomer (dexmedetomidine) is active. Medetomidine may also be known as MPV-785.

Vatinoxan hydrochloride occurs as a white to pale-yellow crystalline substance that is sparingly soluble in water. Vatinoxan may also be known as MK-467 and L-659066.

Medetomidine/vatinoxan may also be known as *Zenalpha*®.

Storage/Stability

Store medetomidine/vatinoxan below 25°C (77°F), protected from light and freezing. Discard in-use vials after 3 months.[10]

Compatibility/Compounding Considerations

Do not mix medetomidine/vatinoxan with other agents, as compatibility studies have not been performed.[29]

Dosage Forms/Regulatory Status

VETERINARY-LABELED PRODUCTS:

Medetomidine and Vatinoxan Injection: medetomidine 0.5 mg/mL and vatinoxan 10 mg/mL in 10 mL vials; *Zenalpha*®; (Rx). FDA-approved for use in dogs. NADA# 141-551

The Association of Racing Commissioners International (ARCI) has designated medetomidine as a class 3 substance. Use of this drug may not be allowed in certain animal competitions. Check rules and regulations before entering in a competition while this medication is being administered. Contact local racing authorities for further guidance. See the ***Appendix*** for more information.

HUMAN-LABELED PRODUCTS: NONE

References

For the complete list of references, see **wiley.com/go/budde/plumb**

Medium Chain Triglycerides; (MCT) Oil

Nutritional

Prescriber Highlights

- ► Lipid sometimes used to provide calories and fatty acids to dogs with restricted fat intake from chronic infiltrative diseases of the small intestine or fat malabsorption syndromes; may have benefit in canine epilepsy
- ► Most clinicians use dietary therapy instead of MCT oil.
- ► Use with caution in animals with significant hepatic disease (eg, portacaval shunts, cirrhosis).
- ► Adverse effects include unpalatability (dogs), bloating, flatulence, and diarrhea; may be associated with hepatic lipidosis in cats.

Uses/Indications

Medium chain triglycerides (MCT) oil, as a separate compound (not as an ingredient in commercial foods), can offset caloric reduction when dietary long chain triglycerides are restricted. Fat-restricted disease states include chronic infiltrative diseases of the small intestine or fat malabsorption of any cause. Many clinicians bypass MCT oil due to expense and unpalatability to dogs. Commercially made prescription diets, that are highly digestible with low fat content, can be used. Alternatively, a veterinary nutritionist can prepare a recipe for clients to make a homemade, complete, and balanced diet for their animals.

MCT oil may be useful as a base-vehicle to administer drugs to cats. A study evaluating the acceptance of low-dose (0.1 mL/kg) MCT oil, gelatin capsules, or thin-film dissolving strips found that owner-perceived acceptability by cats of MCT oil and thin-film strips was significantly higher than that of gelatin capsules.[1]

Diets with MCT may play a supporting role in prevention or treating cognitive dysfunction syndromes in dogs and cats.[2]

When added to standard antiepileptic treatment, supplementation with MCT decreased seizure frequency and number of days with seizure activity in dogs with idiopathic epilepsy.[3–5]

Pharmacology/Actions

Medium chain triglycerides (MCT) are more readily hydrolyzed than conventional food fat. MCT can pass through intestinal membranes into venous blood circulation. Bile acids or pancreatic lipase are not required for their absorption into portal circulation. MCT are not a source for essential fatty acids.

MCT oil supplementation (as coconut oil) to the diet of cats did not cause food aversion or significant effects on lipid metabolism.[6]

In epileptic brains, decreased metabolism of glucose and increased energy requirements from increased electrical activity creates an energy deficit. MCTs release octranoic and decanoic acids, which are hepatically converted into ketone bodies that can be used for fuel in the brain.[7]

Pharmacokinetics

No specific information located; see ***Pharmacology/Actions***.

Contraindications/Precautions/Warnings

Use medium chain triglycerides (MCT) oil with caution in patients with significant hepatic disease (eg, portacaval shunts, cirrhosis). MCTs are rapidly absorbed via the portal vein and if hepatic clearance is impaired, significantly high systemic blood and cerebral spinal fluid levels of medium chain fatty acids can occur. This may precipitate or exacerbate hepatic coma.

Patients experiencing diabetic ketoacidosis (DKA) should avoid MCT until the DKA has resolved.

Adverse Effects

Adverse effects seen with medium chain triglycerides (MCT) oil in small animals include unpalatability, bloating, flatulence, and diarrhea. In cats, higher dosages of MCT oil may induce hepatic lipidosis. Adverse effects may be transient and minimized by starting with low doses and gradually increasing the dose. Fat-soluble vitamin supplementation (vitamins A, D, E, and K) using a commercial feline or canine vitamin-mineral supplement has been recommended.

Reproductive/Nursing Safety

No reproductive or nursing safety data were located. Although medium chain triglycerides (MCT) use is unlikely to cause problems in pregnant or nursing animals, because safety has not been established in animals, this drug should only be used when the maternal benefits outweigh the potential risks to offspring.

Overdose/Acute Toxicity

Overdose would likely exacerbate the GI adverse effects noted (see ***Adverse Effects***). Treat severe diarrhea supportively if necessary.

For patients that have experienced or are suspected to have experienced an overdose, consultation with a 24-hour poison consultation center specializing in providing veterinary-specific information is recommended. For general information related to overdose and toxin exposures, as well as contact information for poison control centers, refer to ***Appendix.***

Drug Interactions

- None listed. Medium chain triglycerides (MCT) oil could theoretically affect absorption of drugs that are dependent on fat for oral absorption (eg, griseofulvin, fat-soluble vitamins).

Dosages

DOGS:

Offset caloric reduction when dietary long chain triglycerides are restricted (extra-label): Most clinicians prefer to use dietary therapy with foods containing additional medium chain triglycerides (MCT) in their formulation; but 0.5 – 2 mL/kg/day added to food is appropriate.

Adjunct to standard epilepsy treatment (extra-label): 6.5% – 9% of total caloric intake daily[3-5]

Monitoring

- Adverse effects (mostly GI-related)
- Efficacy (weight gain, improved seizure control)

Client Information

- Because of the unpalatability of the oil, it should be mixed with small quantities of food before offering to the animal.
- Contact your veterinarian if you notice side effects, including diarrhea or flatulence, or any other new problems.

Chemistry/Synonyms

Medium chain triglycerides (MCT) oil is a lipid fraction of coconut oil consisting principally of the triglycerides C8 (≈67%) and C10 (≈23%) saturated fatty acids. Each 15 mL contains 115 kCal (7.67 kCal/mL).

Medium chain triglycerides may also be known as triglycerida saturata media.

Storage/Stability

Unless otherwise noted by the manufacturer, store this product at room temperature in glass bottles, protected from light.

Compatibility/Compounding Considerations

No specific information noted

Dosage Forms/Regulatory Status

VETERINARY-LABELED PRODUCTS: NONE

HUMAN-LABELED PRODUCTS:

Medium Chain Triglycerides Oil: in quart bottles (946 mL); *MCT®*; (OTC).

References

For the complete list of references, see **wiley.com/go/budde/plumb**

Medroxyprogesterone

Medroxyprogesterone Acetate

(me-***drox***-ee-proe-***jess***-te-rone) *Provera®*

Progestin

Prescriber Highlights

- Used primarily to treat cats for sexually dimorphic behavior problems such as roaming, inter-male aggressive behaviors, spraying, and mounting; sometimes used to treat alopecia X in dogs
- Because of its serious adverse effect profile, particularly in small animal species, consider safer alternatives first.
- Contraindications include pre-pubescent dogs or cats, diabetes mellitus, pseudopregnancy in bitches, female patients in diestrus or with prolonged heat, and uterine hemorrhage or discharge.
- Adverse effects include increased thirst, increased appetite, weight gain, depression, lethargy, personality changes, adrenocortical depression, mammary changes (including enlargement, milk production, and neoplasms), diabetes mellitus, pyometra, and temporary inhibition of spermatogenesis.
- SC injection may cause permanent local alopecia or atrophy, and depigmentation may occur.
- The National Institute for Occupational Safety and Health (NIOSH) classifies medroxyprogesterone as a hazardous drug; use appropriate precautions when handling.

Uses/Indications

In cats, medroxyprogesterone has been used to treat sexually dimorphic behavior problems such as roaming, inter-male aggressive behaviors, spraying, and mounting when castration is either ineffective or undesirable.[1]

In dogs, medroxyprogesterone has been used to treat progestin-responsive dermatitis, aggressive behaviors,[1,2] long-term reproductive control, treatment of young German shepherd dwarfs, short-term treatment of benign prostatic hypertrophy, and luteal insufficiency. An open study in 8 Pomeranian dogs with alopecia X found that medroxyprogesterone administration resulted in partial hair regrowth in 3 and complete hair regrowth in 1 of the dogs treated.[3]

Progesterones have been used in horses for many purposes, including management of the spring transition period, prevention of estrus behavior, induction of estrous cycle synchrony, pregnancy maintenance, and modification of stallion behavior.[4] However, medroxyprogesterone does not appear to effectively suppress estrous behavior or follicular activity in normal cycling mares.[5]

In humans, parenteral medroxyprogesterone has been used as a long-acting contraceptive in women and as an antineoplastic agent for some carcinomas (see ***Pharmacology/Actions***). Oral medroxyprogesterone is used in women to treat secondary amenorrhea or abnormal uterine bleeding secondary to hormone imbalances.

Pharmacology/Actions

Progestins are primarily produced endogenously by the corpus luteum. They transform proliferative endometrium to secretory endometrium, enhance myometrium hypertrophy, and inhibit spontaneous uterine contraction. Progestins have a dose-dependent inhibitory effect on the secretion of pituitary gonadotropins and can have an anti-insulin effect. Medroxyprogesterone has exhibited a pronounced adrenocorticoid effect in animals (species not listed) and can suppress ACTH and cortisol release. Medroxyprogesterone is anti-estrogenic and will also decrease plasma testosterone levels in male humans and dogs.

Medroxyprogesterone has antineoplastic activity against endometrial carcinoma and renal carcinoma (efficacy in doubt) in humans.

Pharmacokinetics

No specific pharmacokinetic parameters in veterinary species were located for this drug. It has been reported that injectable MPA has an approximate duration of action of 30 days when used to treat behavior disorders in cats.[6] When administered IM to women, medroxyprogesterone has contraceptive activity for at least 3 months.[7] Single-dose half-life following oral administration in humans was ≈12 hours.[8]

Contraindications/Precautions/Warnings

When medroxyprogesterone is used for reproductive control, patients should 1) undergo a thorough reproductive history to rule out occurrence of estrus within the last 1 to 2 months (female patient in diestrus); 2) a complete physical examination; 3) palpation of mammary glands to rule out neoplasia; and 4) a vaginal cytology to rule out presence of estrus.[9]

This agent should not be used to treat bitches with pseudopregnancy. Female patients should not be treated during diestrus or if they have a uterine hemorrhage. Do not use medroxyprogesterone in female patients with prolonged heat unless cystic ovarian disease is confirmed and surgery, GNRH, or hCG are not viable options. Animals with diabetes mellitus should not receive medroxyprogesterone.

Do not use medroxyprogesterone prior to puberty in cats, as chronic, severe, mammary hypertrophy may result. Use in dogs before puberty may precipitate subclinical uterine or endocrine conditions (eg, cystic endometrial hyperplasia, pyometra, diabetes mellitus).

Because this drug can suppress adrenal function, exogenous steroids may need to be administered if the patient is stressed (eg, surgery, trauma).

In humans, medroxyprogesterone is contraindicated in patients that are hypersensitive to it and in patients with liver dysfunction.[10] Progestogen therapy can cause serious adverse effects (eg, thromboembolic disease), and safer alternative treatments should be considered when possible. Weigh the potential risks versus benefits before instituting therapy. Many clinicians believe that progestogens are grossly overused.

The National Institute for Occupational Safety and Health (NIOSH) classifies medroxyprogesterone as a hazardous drug; personal protective equipment (PPE) should be used accordingly to minimize the risk for exposure.

Adverse Effects

Adverse reactions that are possible in dogs and cats include increased appetite with weight gain, polyuria, polydipsia, depression, lethargy, personality changes, adrenocortical depression, mammary changes (including enlargement, milk production, and neoplasms), diabetes mellitus, hypothyroidism, pyometra, and temporary inhibition of spermatogenesis. In dogs, acromegaly and increased growth hormone levels have been seen when used in patients with diabetes mellitus.

SC administration may result in permanent local alopecia or atrophy, and depigmentation may occur. If injecting SC, it is recommended to use the inguinal area to avoid these manifestations.

Reproductive/Nursing Safety

In humans, progestins have caused congenital heart defects, limb reduction deformities, hypospadias in male fetuses, and mild virilization of the external genitalia of female fetuses, especially when administered to women during the first 4 months of pregnancy. Medroxyprogesterone is considered contraindicated in pregnant women. In general, medroxyprogesterone should be avoided in pregnant animals with some exceptions (eg, luteal deficiency); facial deformities were reported in 1 of 4 pups in a litter from a bitch treated with medroxyprogesterone for hypoluteoidism. In most instances, the potential benefits of progesterone treatment for hypoluteoidism during the second half of pregnancy outweigh the maternal and fetal risks.[11,12]

Medroxyprogesterone can be detected in maternal milk. Although no adverse effects have been noted in nursing infants, infant risk cannot be ruled out. Weigh the potential risks and benefits before using in nursing animals.

Overdose/Acute Toxicity

No reports or information were located on inadvertent overdoses with this agent. See ***Adverse Effects***.

For patients that have experienced or are suspected to have experienced an overdose, consultation with a 24-hour poison consultation center specializing in providing veterinary-specific information is recommended. For general information related to overdose and toxin exposures, as well as contact information for poison control centers, refer to ***Appendix***.

Drug Interactions

The following drug interactions have either been reported or are theoretical in humans or animals receiving medroxyprogesterone and may be of significance in veterinary patients. Unless otherwise noted, use together is not necessarily contraindicated, but weigh the potential risks and perform additional monitoring when appropriate.

- **Corticosteroids**: May result in an increased risk for corticosteroid adverse effects
- **Cyclosporine**: May increase risk for cyclosporine toxicity
- **Felbamate**: May increase medroxyprogesterone metabolism
- **Rifampin**: A potential interaction exists with rifampin, which may decrease progestin activity if administered concomitantly. This is presumably due to microsomal enzyme induction with resultant increase in progestin metabolism. The clinical significance of this potential interaction is unknown.
- **Selegiline**: May result in an increase in selegiline oral bioavailability and an increased risk for selegiline adverse reactions
- **Theophylline**: May result in theophylline toxicity

Laboratory Considerations

- In humans, progestins, in combination with estrogens (eg, oral contraceptives), have been demonstrated to increase thyroxine-binding globulin (TBG) with resultant increases in total circulating thyroid hormone. Decreased T_3 resin uptake also occurs, but free T_4 concentrations are unaltered. Liver function tests may also be altered.
- The manufacturer recommends notifying the pathologist of patient medroxyprogesterone exposure when submitting relevant specimens.

Dosages

DOGS:

Luteal insufficiency in pregnant bitches (extra-label): 0.1 mg/kg PO once daily.[11,12] Treatment is discontinued several days prior to the expected due date to avoid prolonged gestation. See ***Reproductive/Nursing Safety***.

Long-term reproductive control (extra-label): 2.5 – 3 mg/kg IM every 5 months[9,13,14]

Alopecia X (extra-label): A study done in Pomeranians found that 5 or 10 mg/kg SC every 4 weeks for 4 treatments resulted in partial hair regrowth in 3 and complete hair regrowth in 1 of 8 dogs treated.[3] The authors concluded that prolonged treatment could result in improved success with careful monitoring for adverse effects.

CATS:

Behavioral disorders (eg, to reduce marking in neutered male cats when all other drugs have been unsuccessful; extra-label): 5 – 20 mg/kg SC or IM 3 to 4 times yearly[15]

Long-term reproductive control (extra-label): 2 mg/kg IM every 5 months[9,13,14]

HORSES:

Management of the spring transition period, prevention of estrus behavior, induction of estrous cycle synchrony, pregnancy maintenance, or modification of stallion behavior (extra-label): ≈500 – 800 mg IM. The interval between doses varies between horses. Most injections last 2 to 3 months. Medroxyprogesterone will not prevent pregnancy loss and does not stop cyclicity,[4] and it does not appear to effectively suppress estrous behavior or follicular activity in normal cycling mares.[5]

Monitoring

- Body weight
- Baseline and periodic blood glucose
- Mammary gland palpation and examination to detect development of neoplasia
- Adrenocortical function (ie, ACTH stimulation test) as indicated by clinical situation
- Efficacy

Client Information

- Give this medicine as directed by your veterinarian.
- Side effects in dogs and cats can include loss of hair/fur at the site of injection, increased appetite with weight gain, increased thirst, depression and lethargy, changes in behavior, mammary changes (including enlargement, milk production, and tumors), diabetes

mellitus, low thyroid hormone (*hypothyroidism*), uterine infection (females), and temporary inhibition of sperm production (males).

- Your veterinarian will need to monitor your animal while it is receiving this medicine. Do not miss these important follow-up visits.
- This medication is considered to be a hazardous drug as defined by the National Institute for Occupational Safety and Health (NIOSH). Talk with your veterinarian or pharmacist about the use of personal protective equipment when handling this medicine.

Chemistry/Synonyms

A synthetic progestin, medroxyprogesterone acetate occurs as an odorless, white to off-white, crystalline powder. It is insoluble in water and sparingly soluble in alcohol. It has a melting range of 200°C to 210°C (392°F-410°F).

Medroxyprogesterone acetate may also be known as MPA, MAP, acetoxymethylprogesterone, medroxyprogesteroni acetas, methylacetoxyprogesterone, metipregnone, and NSC-26386; many trade names are available.

Storage/Stability

Medroxyprogesterone acetate suspensions for injection should be stored at room temperature (15°C-30°C [59°F-86°F]); avoid freezing and temperatures above 40°C (104°F). Tablets should be stored in well-closed containers at room temperature.

Compatibility/Compounding Considerations

No specific information is noted.

Dosage Forms/Regulatory Status

VETERINARY-LABELED PRODUCTS: NONE

HUMAN-LABELED PRODUCTS:

Medroxyprogesterone Acetate Tablets (scored): 2.5 mg, 5 mg, and 10 mg; *Provera*®, generic; (Rx)

Medroxyprogesterone Acetate Injection: 104 mg (160 mg/mL) in 0.65 mL prefilled syringes; 150 mg/mL in 1 mL vials; 400 mg/mL in 2.5 mL and 10 mL vials and 1 mL *U-ject*; *Depo-SubQ Provera 104*®, *Depo-Provera*®, generic; (Rx)

References

For the complete list of references, see **wiley.com/go/budde/plumb**

Megestrol

Megestrol Acetate

(me-***jess***-trole) *Ovaban*®, *Megace*®

Progestin

Prescriber Highlights

- Used in female dogs for postponement of estrus, in male dogs for benign prostatic hypertrophy, and in cats for many dermatologic and behavior-related conditions
- Contraindications include pregnant animals; animals with uterine disease, diabetes mellitus, or mammary neoplasias; and in female patients during diestrus or with uterine hemorrhage.
- Use with caution in patients with thrombophlebitis and pseudopregnancy; although indicated for alleviation of pseudopregnancy, it is no longer recommended for this indication.
- Adverse effects in dogs include increased appetite, weight gain, lethargy, change in behavior or hair color, mucometra, endometritis, cystic endometrial hyperplasia, mammary gland enlargement and neoplasia, acromegaly, adrenocortical suppression, or lactation (rare).
- Adverse effects in cats include profound adrenocortical suppression, adrenal atrophy, transient diabetes mellitus, polydipsia/polyuria, personality changes, weight gain, endometritis, cystic endometrial hyperplasia, mammary hypertrophy, neoplasias, and hepatotoxicity.
- The National Institute for Occupational Safety and Health (NIOSH) classifies megestrol as a hazardous drug; use appropriate precautions when handling.

Uses/Indications

Megestrol is FDA-approved for use in dogs for the postponement of estrus and the alleviation of pseudopregnancy; however, it has fallen out of favor for treatment of pseudopregnancy due to recurrence rates after drug withdrawal, adverse effects associated with its use, and availability of safer options (eg, cabergoline). In male dogs, it has also been used for benign prostatic hypertrophy. Megestrol has also been used clinically for many dermatologic and behavior-related conditions, primarily in cats. Low-dose megestrol may be an alternative to surgery for contraception in free-roaming cats, but safety, efficacy, regulatory pathways, and ethics remain questionable.[1]

Megestrol is indicated in humans for the palliative treatment of advanced carcinoma of the breast or endometrium.

Pharmacology/Actions

Megestrol possesses the pharmacologic actions expected of other progestational drugs (eg, medroxyprogesterone acetate). It has significant antiestrogen and glucocorticoid activity (with resultant adrenal suppression). It does not have anabolic or masculinizing effects on the developing fetus.

Pharmacokinetics

Megestrol is well absorbed from the GI tract and appears to be metabolized completely in the liver to conjugates and free steroids.

The half-life of megestrol acetate is reported to be 8 days in the dog.

Contraindications/Precautions/Warnings

Megestrol is contraindicated in pregnant animals or in animals with uterine disease, diabetes mellitus, or mammary neoplasias. Megestrol is not recommended in dogs prior to their first estrous cycle or for anestrus therapy in dogs with abnormal cycles. Prevent mating if estrus occurs within 30 days of cessation of megestrol therapy.[2]

Megestrol should not be used during pregnancy; it is no longer recommended to treat bitches with pseudopregnancy despite its labeled indication for this use. Female patients with uterine hemorrhage or those in diestrus should not be treated. Do not use megestrol in female patients with prolonged estrus unless cystic ovarian disease is confirmed and surgery, GNRH, or hCG are not viable options.

For estrus control, the drug must be given for the full treatment regimen to be effective.[2] It should not be given for more than 2 consecutive treatments, but the reasons for this are unclear; some theriogenologists question the need for this precaution. When megestrol is used for reproductive control, it has been recommended that patients undergo a thorough reproductive history (to rule out occurrence of estrus within the last 1 to 2 months), a complete physical examination, palpation of mammary glands (to rule out mammary nodules), and a vaginal cytology (to rule out the presence of estrus).[3,4]

Because this drug can suppress adrenal function, exogenous steroids may need to be administered if the patient is stressed (eg, surgery, trauma).

In humans, megestrol should be used with caution in patients with thrombophlebitis.[5]

The National Institute for Occupational Safety and Health (NIOSH) classifies megestrol as a hazardous drug; personal protective equipment (PPE) should be used accordingly to minimize the risk for exposure.

Adverse Effects

Adverse effects in dogs include increased appetite, weight gain, lethargy, change in behavior, change in hair color, mucometra, endometritis, pyometra, cystic endometrial hyperplasia, mammary enlargement and neoplasia, acromegaly, adrenocortical suppression, and, rarely, lactation. One dog reportedly developed diabetes mellitus after use.[6]

Adverse effects in cats include profound adrenocortical suppression and adrenal atrophy. Iatrogenic Addison syndrome can develop at standard dosages (2.5 – 5 mg every other day) within 1 to 2 weeks. After discontinuation, serum cortisol levels (both resting and ACTH-stimulated) will return to normal levels within a few weeks. Clinical signs of adrenocortical insufficiency (eg, vomiting, lethargy) are uncommon, but exogenous glucocorticoid support should be considered if the animal is stressed (eg, surgery, trauma). Cats may develop transient diabetes mellitus while receiving megestrol. Polydipsia/polyuria, personality changes, weight gain, endometritis, cystic endometrial hyperplasia, mammary hypertrophy, and neoplasias may also occur; however, increased appetite and weight gain are not consistently seen. Rarely, megestrol can cause hepatotoxicity in cats. Megestrol potentially can exacerbate latent viral infections (eg, FHV-1).

Limited clinical studies have suggested that megestrol may cause less cystic endometrial hyperplasia than other progestational agents, but cautious use and vigilant monitoring are still warranted.

Reproductive/Nursing Safety

No effects were noted in either the bitch or litter when pregnant dogs received megestrol 0.25 mg/kg PO daily for 32 days during the first half of pregnancy; however, reduced litter sizes and puppy survival were detected when the dose was given during the last half of pregnancy. Fetal hypospadias is possible if progestational agents are administered during pregnancy.

Detectable amounts of progestins enter the milk of mothers receiving these agents. Effects on nursing infants have not been established.

Because safety has not been established in animals, this drug should only be used when the maternal benefits outweigh the potential risks to offspring.

Overdose/Acute Toxicity

No information was located regarding acute megestrol overdoses. In humans, dosages of megestrol of up to 1600 mg/day caused no observable adverse reactions.[5]

Toxicity studies performed in dogs at dosages of 0.1 to 0.25 mg/kg/day PO for 36 months yielded no gross abnormalities in the study population. Histologically, cystic endometrial hyperplasia was noted at 36 months but resolved when therapy was discontinued. At dosages of 0.5 mg/kg/day PO for 5 months, reversible uterine hyperplasia was seen in treated dogs. Dosages of 2 mg/kg/day demonstrated early cystic endometritis in biopsies done on dogs at 64 days.

For patients that have experienced or are suspected to have experienced an overdose, consultation with a 24-hour poison consultation center specializing in providing veterinary-specific information is recommended. For general information related to overdose and toxin exposures, as well as contact information for poison control centers, refer to ***Appendix.***

Drug Interactions

- **Corticosteroids**: Megestrol used with corticosteroids (long-term) may exacerbate adrenocortical suppression and diabetes mellitus.
- **Rifampin**: May decrease progestin activity if administered concomitantly, presumably due to microsomal enzyme induction with a resultant increase in progestin metabolism. The clinical significance of this potential interaction is unknown.

Dosages

DOGS:

Postponement of estrus (label dosage; FDA-approved):

a) **During proestrus**: 2.2 mg/kg PO daily for 8 days during the first 3 days of proestrus[2]

b) **During anestrus**: 0.55 mg/kg PO daily for 32 days[2]

NOTE: If used properly during proestrus, physical manifestations of proestrus and estrus and breeding behavior will subside within days, and the bitch will not ovulate on that cycle. If used properly during anestrus, return to subsequent proestrus will be postponed for ≈3 months.[6]

Alleviation of clinical signs associated with false pregnancy (pseudopregnancy) (label dosage; FDA-approved): 2.2 mg/kg PO daily for 8 days.[2] **NOTE**: Despite this indication being listed on the label, the use of megestrol for alleviating clinical signs associated with pseudopregnancy are no longer recommended.[7]

Benign prostatic hypertrophy to maintain breeding potential for a short time prior to castration (extra-label): 0.1 – 0.5 mg/kg PO daily for 3 to 8 weeks[8]

Subinvolution of placental sites (SIPS) (extra-label): From a small non-blinded study in 9 dogs, 0.1 mg/kg PO once daily for the first week, then 0.05 mg/kg PO once daily for the second week.[9] Vaginal discharge ceased in all treated dogs within the treatment period, and 5 of 6 that were subsequently mated became pregnant.

CATS:

Postponement of estrus (extra-label):

a) **During proestrus**: 5 mg/cat (NOT mg/kg) PO daily for 4 days, then 5 mg/cat (NOT mg/kg) PO every 2 weeks[4,10]

b) **During anestrus**: 5 mg/cat (NOT mg/kg) PO every 2 weeks OR 2.5 mg/cat (NOT mg/kg) PO weekly, ideally divided into 2 doses given every 3.5 days

Alternative for treating feline atopy when standard treatments fail (extra-label): 2.5 – 5 mg/cat (NOT mg/kg) PO every 48 hours for 1 to 3 weeks may induce remission of clinical signs. Frequency can then be decreased to once weekly.[11]

Reduce marking in neutered male cats when all other drugs have been unsuccessful (extra-label): 2.5 – 10 mg/cat (NOT mg/kg) PO once daily for one week, then reduce to once or twice weekly[12]

Eosinophilic keratitis (extra-label): A compounded aqueous ophthalmic preparation of megestrol acetate 0.5% administered every 8 to 12 hours showed efficacy in one study, with 15 of 17 cats responding to treatment.[13]

Monitoring

- Body weight
- Baseline and periodic blood glucose
- Mammary gland development and appearance
- Adrenocortical function (ie, ACTH stimulation) with long-term treatment
- Liver enzymes if long-term treatment
- Efficacy

Client Information

- This medicine may be given with food or on an empty stomach but giving with food may help prevent vomiting.
- Megestrol can have many side effects; some of them are serious. Watch your animal for changes to the mammary glands/nipples or for any vaginal discharge.
- If you are pregnant, use caution when handling this medicine. Be sure to wear gloves and wash hands after handling any medication.
- This medication is considered to be a hazardous drug as defined by the National Institute for Occupational Safety and Health (NIOSH). Talk with your veterinarian or pharmacist about the use of personal protective equipment when handling this medicine.

Chemistry/Synonyms

Megestrol acetate is a synthetic progestin that occurs as an essentially odorless, tasteless, white to creamy white, crystalline powder that is insoluble in water, sparingly soluble in alcohol, and slightly soluble in fixed oils. It has a melting range of 213°C to 219°C (415°F-426°F) over a 3° range and a specific rotation of +8° to +12°.

Megestrol acetate may also be known as BDH-1298, compound 5071, megestroli acetas, NSC-71423, SC-10363. *Megace®* and *Ovaban®* are common trade names.

Storage/Stability

Store megestrol tablets in well-closed containers at a temperature of less than 40°C (104°F). Tablets may be crushed and administered with food; however, appropriate precautions are needed due to hazardous properties. The veterinary manufacturer recommends storing the tablets from 2°C to 30°C (36°F-86°F).

Compatibility/Compounding Considerations

Those who compound with this drug should wear appropriate PPE, as megestrol is classified as a hazardous drug.

Dosage Forms/Regulatory Status

VETERINARY-LABELED PRODUCTS:

Megestrol Acetate Oral Tablets: 20 mg; *Ovaban®*; (Rx). FDA-approved for use in dogs only. **NOTE**: This product is still listed in the FDA's Green Book of approved animal drugs but may no longer be marketed in the United States.

HUMAN-LABELED PRODUCTS:

Megestrol Acetate Tablets: 20 and 40 mg; *Megace®*, generic; (Rx)

Megestrol Acetate Oral Suspension: 40 mg/mL and 125 mg/mL; *Megace®*, *Megace ES®*, generic (40 mg/mL); (Rx)

References

For the complete list of references, see **wiley.com/go/budde/plumb**

Meglumine Antimoniate

(***meg***-loo-meen an-tih-***mohne***-ee-ate) *Glucantime®*

Antiprotozoal

Prescriber Highlights

- ► Used for treating leishmaniasis (with or without allopurinol) in dogs
- ► Not available in the United States
- ► Extreme caution (relatively contraindicated) in patients with cardiac, hepatic, or renal insufficiency
- ► Primary adverse effects noted in dogs with meglumine antimoniate are injection site reactions, lethargy, and GI effects (eg, inappetence, vomiting).
- ► Resistance to treatment has been reported.
- ► Treatment is prolonged, and the cost may be substantial.

Uses/Indications

Meglumine antimoniate is used to treat leishmaniasis in dogs, and combination therapy with allopurinol appears to be the treatment of choice for dogs with confirmed infection. It is available commercially in some Mediterranean and South American countries but not in the United States. The combination of meglumine antimoniate with allopurinol appears to have better clinical efficacy than a miltefosine/allopurinol combination.[1]

Meglumine antimoniate may be useful for treating feline leishmaniasis, but more evidence for safety and efficacy is needed before suggesting its use.

Liposomal formulations of meglumine antimoniate has been an active area of research,[2-4] but commercial dosage forms are not yet available.

Pharmacology/Actions

Pentavalent antimony compounds, such as meglumine antimoniate and sodium stibogluconate, selectively inhibit the leishmanial enzymes required for glycolytic and fatty acid oxidation. Pentavalent antimony compounds rarely are successful in completely eradicating *Leishmania* spp organisms in infected dogs. When used with allopurinol, synergy for treating leishmaniasis and reduced risk for antimonial drug-resistance development can occur.

Pharmacokinetics

After SC or IM injections in dogs, systemic bioavailability is ≈92%; the highest tissue concentrations are found in the liver, spleen, and skin. The elimination half-life is relatively short (≈2 hours when given SC). Within 9 hours of dosing, 80% of the antimony is excreted in the urine. Reduced renal function can cause increased antimoniate half-lives.

Contraindications/Precautions/Warnings

Hypersensitivity reactions have been reported in people, and any patient with the previous hypersensitivity to meglumine antimoniate or sulfites should not receive the drug.

Patients with renal, hepatic, or cardiac failure are more likely to develop serious adverse effects with this agent; weigh the potential risks vs benefits carefully before treating. Decreased renal function, in particular, may lead to drug accumulation and an increased risk for toxicity. In dogs with severe renal failure (IRIS stages III-IV), the correction of fluid and acid-base imbalances prior to treatment with allopurinol alone has been recommended.[5]

In humans, a protein-rich diet is required during treatment, and it is recommended to correct iron deficiencies prior to treatment.[6]

Adverse Effects

Primary adverse effects noted in dogs are injection site reactions (cutaneous abscesses/cellulitis), lethargy, and GI effects (inappetence, vomiting). Transient increases in liver enzymes have been reported.[7]

Potentially, the drug may be nephrotoxic in dogs, but this is difficult to evaluate in clinically infected dogs as renal dysfunction is one of the likely consequences of the infection. A study done in healthy dogs showed diffuse proximal tubule cell vacuolization and multifocal areas with coagulative necrosis under light microscopy. Electron microscopy showed reduced organellar content, loss or attenuation of brush border, cellular detachment from the basement membrane, apical blebbing, and individual cell necrosis. The authors concluded that meglumine antimoniate caused severe tubular damage.[8] A small study in dogs with leishmaniosis found that meglumine antimoniate 50 mg/kg SC every 12 hours for 28 days had no effects on glomerular filtration rate or urine specific gravity; urine protein to creatinine ratio was reduced following treatment.[9]

In a study in 28 dogs with clinical disease treated with meglumine antimoniate (75 mg/kg every 12 hours for 60 days), when compared pre-treatment and posttreatment (day 60), significant changes in serum cardiac troponin I concentrations or corrected QT intervals were not found.[10]

Drug resistance may occur. After several courses of treatment, decreased sensitivity of *Leishmania infantum* to meglumine antimoniate or antimonials has been reported.[11]

In humans, increased serum lipase, amylase, creatinine, urea nitrogen, and increased QT interval on ECG have been reported. Occasionally, decreases in white blood cell counts and hemoglobin have been reported in humans. Other adverse effects in humans include dyspnea, skin rash, facial edema, abdominal pain, elevated liver enzymes, and, rarely, pancreatitis.

Reproductive/Nursing Safety

There is limited information available. Pregnant rats given up to 300 mg/kg on days 6 to 15 of gestation caused increased fetal resorptions and increased rates of abnormalities of the atlas bone. A case report of a bitch that received meglumine antimoniate during pregnancy has been published.[12] Pregnancy and delivery were deemed normal. Three puppies died within 2 days of delivery, but the 2 surviving puppies were followed clinically, serologically, and with real-time PCR until 1 year of age. Neither puppy had clinical or serological evidence of *L. infantum* despite *L. infantum* DNA evidence being found in the uterine tissue of the bitch. The authors concluded that meglumine antimoniate may have prevented vertical transmission of leishmaniasis.

It is unknown if the drug enters maternal milk.

Because safety has not been established in animals, this drug should only be used when the maternal benefits outweigh the potential risks to offspring.

Overdose/Acute Toxicity

No specific overdose information was located. Depending on the dosage, a single overdose could potentially cause renal, hepatic, pancreatic, and hematologic effects, but GI effects (vomiting) and lethargy would be the most likely outcomes. It is recommended to observe the patient and contact an animal poison control center for further guidance with an overdose situation.

For patients that have experienced or are suspected of having experienced an overdose, consultation with a 24-hour poison consultation center specializing in providing veterinary-specific information is recommended. For general information related to overdose and toxin exposures, as well as contact information for poison control centers, refer to ***Appendix.***

Drug Interactions

The following drug interactions have either been reported or are theoretical in humans or animals receiving meglumine antimoniate and may be of significance in veterinary patients (dogs):

- **Agents That Can Prolong QT Interval** (eg, **tricyclic antidepressants, disopyramide, quinidine, procainamide**): Meglumine antimoniate may prolong QT interval further with increased risk for arrhythmias.
- **Other Potentially Nephrotoxic Drugs** (eg, **amphotericin B, aminoglycosides**): Avoid or use with caution in dogs with clinical leishmaniasis and kidney disease being treated with meglumine antimoniate.[13]

Laboratory Considerations

- No specific laboratory interactions or considerations were noted.

Dosages

DOGS:

Leishmaniasis (extra-label): 100 mg/kg SC once daily for 4 weeks[14-16] is the most commonly reported treatment regimen. However, because of the short half-life, giving meglumine antimoniate 50 – 75 mg/kg SC twice daily[10,16,17] for 4 to 8 weeks could be more effective. Combining it with allopurinol (10 mg/kg PO twice daily for at least 6 months) may yield a longer period of clinical remission than if treated with either drug alone.[1,10,18,19] The addition of deslorelin 4.7 mg SC implant to a combination of meglumine antimoniate 50 mg/kg SC twice daily for 28 days and allopurinol 10 mg/kg PO twice daily improved clinical signs and antibody levels beyond that observed ion dogs that only received meglumine antimoniate and allopurinol.[20]

Monitoring

- CBC (baseline and periodic)[14]
- Serum chemistry profile, including giver enzymes; renal function tests (serum creatinine, BUN); serum lipase and amylase (baseline and periodic)[14]
- Urinalysis (baseline and periodic), including urine protein:creatinine ratio[14]
- Antibody titer (controversial)

Client Information

- Clients should understand that treatment with this drug can be prolonged and expensive and that a cure (complete eradication) is unlikely.

Chemistry/Synonyms

Meglumine antimoniate is 1-Deoxy-1-methylamino-D-glucitol antimoniate. It has a molecular weight of 366. One gram contains ≈272 mg of antimony.

Meglumine antimoniate may also be known as meglumine antimonate, N-methylglucamine antimoniate, RP-2168, antimony meglumine, Protostib, 1-Deoxy-1-methylamino-D-glucitol antimoniate, *Glucantime*®, and *Glucantim*®. The chemical symbol for antimony is Sb.

Storage/Stability

Unless otherwise specified by the manufacturer, store commercially available ampules below 40°C (104°F), preferably between 15°C and 30°C (59°F and 86°F); protect from freezing. Check the solution for particles before use. If small particles are present, shake the vial well before use. If particles persist after shaking, do not use the product. Meglumine antimoniate may deteriorate with prolonged storage. Must be used immediately after opening.

Compatibility/Compounding Considerations

No specific information was noted.

Dosage Forms/Regulatory Status

VETERINARY-LABELED PRODUCTS:

None in the United States. May be available via the CDC, see: http://www.cdc.gov/laboratory/drug-service.html

HUMAN-LABELED PRODUCTS: NONE IN THE UNITED STATES

Meglumine antimoniate may be available in several countries, including Brazil, Venezuela, and Europe; trade names include *Glucantime*® and *Glucantim*®. Commercially, it is available as a solution containing 1.5 g of meglumine antimoniate (425 mg pentavalent antimony) per 5 mL.

References

For the complete list of references, see **wiley.com/go/budde/plumb**

Melarsomine

(mee-***lar***-soe-meen) *Diroban*®, *Immiticide*®

Arsenical Antiparasitic

Prescriber Highlights

- Organic arsenical adulticide for heartworm disease in dogs. American Heartworm Society recommends a 3-dose protocol (except for dogs with caval syndrome) that includes prior treatment with doxycycline and a macrocyclic lactone.
- Contraindications include caval syndrome; weigh risk versus benefits in pregnant, lactating, or breeding dogs. Reportedly toxic in cats; melarsomine is not currently recommended for use in this species.
- Many adverse effects are possible. The most common adverse effects are injection site reactions, coughing, gagging, depression/lethargy, anorexia/inappetence, excessive salivation, fever, lung congestion, vomiting, and pulmonary thromboembolism.
- Calculate dosages very carefully. Correct IM injection technique and site are required. Do not give IV or SC.
- Strict cage rest after treatment is essential.

Uses/Indications

Melarsomine is indicated for the treatment of stabilized class 1 (mild), class 2 (moderate), and class 3 (severe) heartworm disease caused by immature (4-month-old juvenile adults) to mature adult infections of *Dirofilaria immitis* in dogs.

The American Heartworm Society recommends that a 3-dose melarsomine protocol should be used. Prior to melarsomine treatment, it is recommended to administer doxycycline for 4 weeks concomitantly with a monthly macrocyclic lactone (at heartworm preventive doses) for 2 months. Doxycycline helps to reduce subsequent microfilaremia by eliminating *Wolbachia pipientis*, a bacterium associated with embryogenesis in *D immitis*.[1] The macrocyclic lactone prevents new infections and eliminates existing susceptible larvae.[2]

Although not optimal, if unexpected delays in melarsomine treatment occur, melarsomine injections should begin within 1 year after doxycycline therapy.[1] A heartworm preventive should be continued until melarsomine injections can begin. A delay of up to 6 months between the first and second melarsomine injection is considered acceptable as long as a heartworm preventive is continued; however, the second and third melarsomine injections ***must*** still be given within the recommended 24-hour timeframe.

Melarsomine is not recommended for use in cats.[3,4] Melarsomine may be useful for treating ferrets with adult heartworm infections.[5]

Pharmacology/Actions

Although melarsomine is an arsenical compound, its exact mechanism of action is not known. Both laboratory and field studies have demonstrated that melarsomine is 90% to 99% effective in killing adult and L_5 larvae of *Dirofilaria immitis* in dogs at recommended dosages. The 2-dose method kills only ≈90% of adult worms whereas the 3-dose method kills 98%.[2,6]

Pharmacokinetics

Melarsomine is reportedly rapidly absorbed after IM injection in dogs; time to peak plasma concentration is ≈11 minutes. The apparent volume of distribution is ≈0.7 L/kg. Terminal half-life is ≈3 hours.

Contraindications/Precautions/Warnings

Melarsomine is contraindicated in dogs with class 4 (caval syndrome) heartworm disease. Caval syndrome is when adult heartworms are present in the venae cavae and right atrium. Do **NOT** give melarsomine IV or SC as significant toxicity or tissue damage may occur.[6] Administer only by deep IM injection into the lumbar (L3-L5) epaxial muscles; do not administer at any other site. Dogs older than 8 years may be more susceptible to adverse effects than younger dogs.[6] Although all dogs with heartworm disease are at risk for posttreatment pulmonary thromboembolism, those with severe pulmonary artery disease are at increased risk for posttreatment morbidity and mortality.

It is imperative to strictly adhere to the manufacturer's instructions for administration. Exercise restriction during the recovery period is <u>essential</u> for minimizing cardiopulmonary complications.[2] Cage rest is recommended, beginning at the time of the first injection and continuing for 6 to 8 weeks after the last injection (10 to 12 weeks total).[2] The cage rest should occur where the animal can be observed and kept calm (eg, veterinary clinic, at home). If cage rest and observation are not possible, owners should be advised that, unless the patient's exercise is restricted, thromboembolic events are more likely and can be fatal.

Melarsomine is reportedly very toxic to cats; it is currently not recommended in this species.[4]

Because of the seriousness of heartworm infection and the potential for morbidity and mortality associated with treatment, consider requiring clients to give informed consent before electing to treat the patient.

Avoid drug contact with animal's eyes; if exposed, wash with copious amounts of water. Avoid human exposure. Wash hands after use or wear gloves when administering the drug. If human exposure occurs, contact a physician.[6]

Adverse Effects

Approximately ⅓ of dogs show signs of injection site reactions (pain, swelling, tenderness, reluctance to move) after receiving melarsomine, typically occurring within the first week after injection. This can be minimized by ensuring the injection is deposited deep into the belly of the epaxial musculature, with a needle newly changed after the drug is drawn into the syringe and that is an appropriate length and gauge for the size of dog and body condition. Most injection site signs resolve within weeks, but, rarely, severe injection reactions can occur. Firm nodules at the injection site could persist indefinitely.[6] The most severe local reactions are usually seen if the drug leaks back from the injection site into subcutaneous tissues. Applying firm pressure to the injection site for 1 to 2 minutes after administration may reduce the risk for this problem.

Creatine kinase (CK) elevations, up to 25-fold, and AST, up to 7-fold, were noted to be related to muscle damage at sites of injection; 2-fold elevations in ALT were also seen.[6] In a separate study, elevations of CK and AST of the same magnitude were observed within 8 hours of injection. These values approached pretest measurements by 72 hours and diminished to within the normal range by 1 month postinjection.[6]

Other reactions reported in 5% or more of treated dogs included coughing/gagging (22%), depression/lethargy (15%), anorexia/inappetence (13%), fever (7%), lung congestion (6%), and vomiting (5%). There is significant interpatient variance in both the date of onset and duration for the above effects. Dogs may also exhibit excessive salivation after dosing. Coughing may be exacerbated by the lack of exercise restriction.[7]

There are many other adverse effects in dogs with reported incidences less than 3%, including paresis and paralysis. Refer to the product label for further details.[6]

Animals not exhibiting adverse effects after the first dose or course may demonstrate them after the second dose or course.

Reproductive/Nursing Safety

Safety has not been established for use in pregnant, lactating, or breeding dogs. Because safety has not been established in animals, this drug should only be used when the maternal benefits outweigh the potential risks to offspring.

Overdose/Acute Toxicity

There is a low margin of safety with melarsomine dosages. At 7.5 mg/kg (3 times the recommended dose) in healthy dogs, melarsomine has demonstrated respiratory inflammation and distress, excessive salivation, restlessness, panting, vomiting, edema, tremors, lethargy, ataxia, cyanosis, stupor, and death. Signs of diarrhea, excessive salivation, restlessness, panting, vomiting, and fever have been noted in infected dogs that have received inadvertent overdoses (2 times the recommended dose).

Treatment with dimercaprol (BAL in Oil) may be considered to treat melarsomine overdoses; however, clinical efficacy of melarsomine may be reduced.[6]

For patients that have experienced or are suspected to have experienced an overdose, consultation with a 24-hour poison consultation center specializing in providing veterinary-specific information is recommended. For general information related to overdose and toxin exposures, as well as contact information for poison control centers, refer to ***Appendix***.

Drug Interactions

The manufacturer reports that during clinical field trials, melarsomine was given to dogs receiving anti-inflammatory agents, antibiotics, insecticides, heartworm prophylactic medications, and various other drugs commonly used to stabilize and support dogs with heartworm disease and that no adverse drug interactions were noted.

- **Aspirin**: Has been shown not to reduce adverse effects and may complicate therapy; use is not recommended.
- **CNS Depressant Drugs**: Drugs that have similar adverse effects (eg, depression caused by CNS depressant) may cause additive adverse effects or increase their incidence when used with melarsomine.

Laboratory Considerations

None noted

Dosages

CAUTION: Because of the low margin of safety, calculate dosages very carefully.

DOGS:

Refer to the most recent guidelines published by the American Heartworm Society at **www.heartwormsociety.org** for more information.

Treatment of heartworm disease (label dosage; FDA-approved): After diagnosis, determine the class (stage) of the disease. **NOTE**: The manufacturer provides worksheets that assist in determining the classification and treatment regimen. It is highly recommended to use these treatment records to avoid confusion and to document therapy. Recommended needle size for dogs 10 kg (22 lb) or less = 23 gauge x 1 inch; 10 kg (22 lb) or more = 22 gauge x 1.5 inch.

a) *Class 1 and 2*: melarsomine 2.5 mg/kg deep IM in the lumbar (L3-L5) epaxial muscles twice, 24 hours apart.[6] Use alternating sides with each administration. Based on response, the regimen may be repeated 4 months following the first treatment (2-dose protocol). **NOTE**: The 2-dose protocol is not recommended by the American Heartworm Society.
b) *Class 3 using the alternate dosing regimen*: In stabilized dogs, melarsomine 2.5 mg/kg deep IM once in the lumbar (L3-L5) epaxial muscles. One month later, give 2.5 mg/kg deep IM deep IM in the lumbar (L3-L5) epaxial muscles twice, 24 hours apart (3-dose protocol).[6]

Treatment of heartworm disease in both clinical (not caval syndrome) and subclinical dogs using the 3-dose protocol (extra-label): The American Heartworm Society (AHS) has a detailed management program table (including diagnostic, nursing, and monitoring guidelines) that can be accessed at **www.heartwormsociety.org**; the following is a summary.

1. Prior to melarsomine use, administer a macrocyclic lactone (eg, ivermectin, milbemycin, moxidectin, selamectin) at heartworm preventive doses for 2 months prior to melarsomine treatment (ie, Days 1, 30, 60) and doxycycline 10 mg/kg PO twice daily for 4 weeks (Days 1 to 28).[2] **NOTE**: Minocycline may be substituted for doxycycline, at the same dosage, but doxycycline is the antibiotic of choice.
   a) Dogs with clinical signs associated with the infection should begin treatment (Day 0) with oral prednisone 0.5 mg/kg twice daily for the first week, then 0.5 mg/kg once daily for the second week, followed by 0.5 mg/kg every other day for the third and fourth weeks.
   b) Dogs with microfilariae detected during the initial work-up, should be treated (Day 1) with an antihistamine and a glucocorticoid (if not already on prednisone) to reduce the risk for anaphylaxis from macrocyclic lactone treatment.
2. Melarsomine 2.5 mg/kg deep IM in the lumbar (L3-L5) epaxial muscles on Day 61, followed by 2 doses of melarsomine 2.5 mg/kg deep IM in the lumbar (L3-L5) epaxial muscles administered 24 hours apart on Days 90 and 91.
3. To reduce the risk for thromboembolism after melarsomine treatment is started, a glucocorticoid should be used in dogs that are in highly endemic areas for heartworm, where they are more likely to have significant worm burdens. On days 61 and 90, begin oral prednisone 0.5 mg/kg twice daily for the first week, then 0.5 mg/kg once daily for the second week, followed by 0.5 mg/kg every other day for the third and fourth weeks.
4. Strict cage rest/confinement is required at the time of the first melarsomine injection and continuing for 6 to 8 weeks after the last melarsomine injection (10 to 12 weeks total).[2]

Abbreviated treatment of heartworm disease in clinical (not caval syndrome) and subclinical dogs (extra-label): On Day 0, ivermectin 6 µg/kg PO every 30 days ongoing, and doxycycline 10 mg/kg PO twice daily for 30 days. Melarsomine 2.5 mg/kg IM was administered on Days 30, 60, and 61. On Days 90 and 240, all dogs ($n = 76$) were confirmed to be free of microfilaria, and circulating antigen was not detected.[8] **NOTE**: This study was performed in a geographic region where *Dirofilaria immitis* is hyperendemic; protocol is not recommended by the American Heartworm Society, but current data about the susceptibility gap[9] support this shortened protocol.

Monitoring

- Adverse effects including signs of thromboembolism (eg, low-grade fever, cough, hemoptysis, exacerbation of right-sided heart failure)
- Cardiac biomarkers (cardiac troponin I, MB isoenzyme of creatine kinase, myoglobin) may be useful to monitor the effects of worms and adulticide treatment on the heart, but additional research is necessary to confirm utility and application.[10,11]
- Clinical efficacy

- Microfilaria testing: Test 30 days after last melarsomine dose (Day 120 of the American Heartworm Society 3-dose protocol)
- Antigen test: Test 9 months after last melarsomine dose (Day 365 of the American Heartworm Society 3-dose protocol)

Client Information

- Strict exercise restriction after dosing with melarsomine is required. Follow your veterinarian's instructions closely.
- Your veterinarian will need to monitor your dog closely before, during, and after treatment. Do not miss these important follow-up visits.

Chemistry/Synonyms

An organic trivalent arsenical compound, melarsomine dihydrochloride has a molecular weight of 501 and is freely soluble in water.

Melarsomine may also be known as Cymelarsan, *Diroban*®, or *Immiticide*®. Its CAS registry is 128470-15-5.

Storage/Stability

The powder should be stored upright at room temperature (15°C-25°C [59°F-77°F]). Once reconstituted, the solution should be kept in the original container and kept protected from light and refrigerated for up to 24 hours. Do not freeze. Do not mix with any other drug.

Compatibility/Compounding Considerations

Reconstitute with 2 mL of the diluent provided (sterile water for injection) with a resultant concentration of 25 mg/mL.

Dosage Forms/Regulatory Status

VETERINARY-LABELED PRODUCTS:

Melarsomine Dihydrochloride Powder for Injection: 50 mg/vial; *Immiticide*®, *Diroban*®; (Rx). FDA-approved for use in dogs

HUMAN-LABELED PRODUCTS: NONE

References

For the complete list of references, see **wiley.com/go/budde/plumb**

Melatonin

(mel-ah-***tone***-in) *PrimeX*®, *Regulin*®

Hormone, Nutraceutical

Prescriber Highlights

- Oral and implantable pineal gland hormone
- FDA-approved to accelerate the fur priming cycle in mink. Other potential uses include as a reversible estrus suppression agent in cats; treatment of nonpruritic alopecia in dogs; treatment of sleep and behavior disorders in cats and dogs; adjusting seasonally controlled fertility in horses, sheep, and goats; and as adjunctive treatment for adrenal disease in ferrets.
- Adverse effects appear to be minimal; however, there are few data available for its use in veterinary medicine.
- Potential contraindications include pregnancy and liver dysfunction.

Uses/Indications

The only FDA-approved indication for melatonin is for SC implants in healthy male and female kits and adult female mink (*Mustela vison*) to accelerate the fur priming cycle. Although published evidence is weak to support clinical use of melatonin in animals, it has been proposed for many purposes. Many clinicians will use melatonin on a trial basis because the potential for adverse effects is very low.

In dogs, melatonin has been used anecdotally to treat alopecia-X in Nordic breeds (eg, Norwegian elkhound), canine pattern baldness, or canine recurrent flank alopecia, postclipping alopecia, and various follicular disorders such as follicular dysplasia.[1] The efficacy of melatonin on hair regrowth in dogs is variable and no published studies demonstrating efficacy were located; therefore, every effort to identify the underlying cause of alopecia should be made before starting therapy.[1] Melatonin has also been used for the treatment of sleep cycle disorders, cognitive dysfunction syndrome, idiopathic vacuolar hepatopathy,[2] phobias, and anxiety. Melatonin may have possible usefulness in reduction of anesthetic requirements[3] and postoperative phacoemulsification complications[4], promotion of sleep in hospitalized patients,[5] and for adjunctive treatment of canine mammary tumors,[6] hyperadrenocorticism,[7] and immune-mediated hemolytic anemia,[8] although clinical trials demonstrating efficacy for these indications are lacking.

In cats, melatonin has been used for the treatment of sleep cycle disorders. In queens, melatonin implants prolong the interestrus period by ≈60 to 120 days when they are placed during anovulatory interestrus.[9] In male cats, a melatonin implant reversibly reduced (but did not eliminate) sperm quantity and quality in male domestic cats for ≈120 days; spermatogenesis returned to baseline ≈140 days after implant.[10] The clinical utility of this finding in male cats is unclear.

Melatonin has been suggested for treating seasonal headshaking syndrome in horses.[11,12]

Supplementation of melatonin to the diets fed to late-gestation Holstein heifers resulted in calves with increased body weight and height at 8 weeks compared with the control group.[13]

In sheep and goats (and potentially in horses), melatonin implants are used to improve early breeding and ovulation rates.[14,15] Melatonin implants improved cashmere production and quality in adult goats.[16]

In ferrets, melatonin is widely used and appears to be effective in alleviating clinical signs associated with adrenal neoplasia, including alopecia, aggressive behavior, vulvar swelling, and prostatomegaly; however, it does not appear to alter tumor growth.[17]

Pharmacology/Actions

Melatonin is a tryptophan derivative. It is involved with the neuroendocrine control of photoperiod-dependent molting, hair growth, and pelage color. Melatonin stimulates winter coat growth and spring shedding occurs when melatonin decreases. The mechanism of how melatonin induces these effects is not well understood; however, it may be related to modulation of sex hormone concentrations, interference with cortisol production, blockage of estrogen receptors at the hair follicle concentration, or deficiency of melatonin. Melatonin may have direct effects on the hair follicle or alter the secretion of prolactin and/or melanocyte-stimulating hormone. In addition, melatonin's antiestrogenic properties seem to play an important role in tumor growth inhibition by reducing the mitogenic response in estrogen-dependent tumor cells.[6] Melatonin also increases serum prolactin concentrations, growth hormone, and the response to growth hormone-releasing hormone. Long-term use of melatonin may decrease luteinizing hormone concentrations. Melatonin is also ostensibly a free radical scavenger.

Pharmacokinetics

In cats, the calculated circulating shelf-life of orally administered melatonin was 45 minutes.[18]

In humans, melatonin has a short half-life (20-50 minutes); plasma concentrations return to baseline within 24 hours of a dose even after long-term dosing of less than 10 mg/day.

Contraindications/Precautions/Warnings

Melatonin is contraindicated in patients that are hypersensitive to it. Use melatonin implants cautiously in sexually immature animals. There are very specific times for melatonin administration, depending on indication for use, latitude, hemisphere, species, and breed. Animals that are pregnant or nursing may not benefit from implant therapy.[15]

In humans, melatonin is considered contraindicated in patients with hepatic insufficiency as it is cleared by the liver and should be used with caution in patients with renal impairment. Because of its CNS depressant qualities, caution is advised when using melatonin in patients with a history of cerebrovascular disease, depression, or neurologic disorders.

Adverse Effects

Melatonin appears to be quite safe in dogs and cats. Adverse effects in dogs are rare when melatonin is administered orally; it may cause sedation and affect sex hormone secretion and fertility. SC implants in dogs have been associated with sterile abscesses.

Adverse effects in ferrets are not commonly reported. Weight gain and/or lethargy could occur.

Adverse effects reported in humans include altered sleep patterns, hypothermia, sedation, tachycardia, confusion, headache, and pruritus. Increased blood glucose concentration has been reported, but the veterinary significance of this finding is unknown.[19]

Reproductive/Nursing Safety

Melatonin appears to cross the placenta. There are conflicting data from studies in rats: one study reported an inhibitory effect on the neuroendocrine reproductive axis in the offspring of pregnant rats that received 2.5 mg/kg SC daily throughout pregnancy, whereas another study using doses up to 200 mg/kg/day observed no maternal or fetal toxicity.[20] The melatonin implant labeled for mink states not to use it in breeding stock.[21]

Melatonin is excreted in breast milk; effects on nursing offspring are unknown. Melatonin implants in lactating cashmere goats had no impact on hair follicle development in the kids.[16]

Because safety has not been established in animals, this drug should only be used when the maternal benefits outweigh the potential risks to offspring.

Overdose/Acute Toxicity

Little information is available; however, melatonin is unlikely to cause significant morbidity after a single oral overdose.

For patients that have experienced or are suspected to have experienced an overdose, consultation with a 24-hour poison consultation center specializing in providing veterinary-specific information is recommended. For general information related to overdose and toxin exposures, as well as contact information for poison control centers, refer to ***Appendix.***

Drug Interactions

The following drug interactions have either been reported or are theoretical in humans or animals receiving melatonin and may be of significance in veterinary patients. Unless otherwise noted, use together is not necessarily contraindicated, but weigh the potential risks and perform additional monitoring when appropriate.

- **BENZODIAZEPINES**: Melatonin may potentiate the effects of benzodiazepines.
- **CIMETIDINE**: May increase melatonin concentration
- **SUCCINYLCHOLINE**: Melatonin may potentiate the effects of succinylcholine.
- **WARFARIN**: May increase risk for bleeding

Laboratory Considerations

- Melatonin can reduce **cortisol, progesterone,** and **estradiol** concentrations.[22]
- Melatonin can decrease total T_3 and total T_4 concentrations in dogs; free T_3 and free T_4 are not affected.[23]

Dosages

DOGS:

Dermatologic conditions such as alopecia-X in Nordic breeds, canine pattern baldness, postclipping alopecia, various follicular disorders such as follicular dysplasia, color dilution alopecia, recurrent or seasonal flank alopecia (extra-label):

- Oral formulations: Treat for at least 2 months for canine seasonal flank alopecia and 4 months for alopecia X to evaluate for maximal response.[1]
  a) 3 – 12 mg/dog (NOT mg/kg) PO 2 to 3 times daily, depending on the dog's size[1,24]
  b) Alternatively, 1 mg/kg/day PO *divided* into 2 or 3 doses
- SC Implant doses are based on dog's size according to the table below.[1] Re-treatment may be necessary 1 to 2 times a year.

Body weight in kg (lb)	Amount of melatonin (mg)/implant	Number of implants to insert
Less than 9 (19.8)	8	1
9-18 (19.8-39.9)	12	1
More than 18 (39.9)	18	1

Sleep disorders (eg, **nocturnal activity**), **phobias** (extra-label): 0.1 mg/kg PO 1 to 3 times daily initially.[5] Practically, round dose up to the nearest 1 mg/dog (NOT mg/kg). A single dose from 1 – 9 mg/dog (NOT mg/kg), depending on dog's size ≈30 minutes before bedtime may be sufficient to help with night waking.

Stressful situations (extra-label):

a. **Pre appointment calming**: Administered by body weight according to table below. As part of the "chill" protocol, give at least 2 hours prior to stressful event and use in combination with buccal (OTM) acepromazine and oral gabapentin ± trazodone.

Body weight in kg	Amount of melatonin to administer (mg/dog [NOT mg/kg])
Less than 5	1
5-15	1.5
15-50	3
More than 50	5

b. **Preoperative calming**: 5 mg/kg PO 2 hours prior to surgery. In dogs subjectively considered "trustful," melatonin reduced propofol requirements for anesthesia induction and endotracheal tube placement.[3]

Idiopathic vacuolar hepatopathy (extra-label): 3 mg/dog (NOT mg/kg) PO every 12 hours. Dogs over 15 kg (33.1 lb) may require a higher dose.[2]

CATS:

Sleep disorders | nocturnal activity (extra-label): Practically, 1.5 – 6 mg/cat (NOT mg/kg) PO before bedtime. Alternatively, 3 – 12 mg/cat (NOT mg/kg) PO every 12 to 24 hours[5]

Suppression of estrus (extra-label): 18 mg/cat (NOT mg/kg) implant administered SC suppressed estrus for 2 to 4 months.[9,25] Alternatively, 4 – 30 mg/cat (NOT mg/kg) PO once daily[9,18,26]

HORSES

Headshaking syndrome for seasonal headshakers that begin in spring and stop in late fall or winter (extra-label): Starting November 1 (Northern hemisphere), give 12 – 15 mg/horse (NOT mg/kg) PO once daily between 5 and 6 PM (1700 to 1800).[27,28] Administer this dose all year round; horse may not shed and may need body clipping.

SHEEP:

Stimulate early onset of reproductive activity in sexually mature ewes (extra-label): 18 mg/sheep (NOT mg/kg) implant administered SC near the base of ear 30 to 40 days prior to the selected joining date.[15] Follow label instructions for breed-based time of year to administer and guidance on separating ewes and rams.

GOATS:

Stimulate testosterone secretion in bucks during nonbreeding season (extra-label): Following 2.5 months of long days, two 18 mg implants (36 mg total dose) administered SC near the base of ears resulted in higher peak testosterone concentrations, which occurred 2 months earlier than in the control group.[29]

FERRETS:

Adjunctive treatment of adrenal disease to help control clinical signs (extra-label):

a) Oral formulations: Anecdotally, 0.5 – 1 mg/ferret (NOT mg/kg) PO once daily 7 to 9 hours after sunrise[17,30]
b) Implant dosages: 2.7 mg/ferret (NOT mg/kg [under 600 g body weight]) or 5.4 mg/ferret (NOT mg/kg [over 600 g body weight]) SC every 3 to 4 months

MINK:

Accelerate fur priming cycle (label dosage; FDA-approved): 2.7 mg/mink (NOT mg/kg) implanted SC[21]

Monitoring

- Clinical efficacy (eg, depending on indication: hair regrowth, estrus suppression, improvement in sleep/unwanted behaviors)
- Adverse effects (eg, sedation, lethargy, weight gain, sterile abscesses [implants only])

Client Information

- For treatment of hair loss, efficacy of melatonin varies. A 4-month trial is necessary to see if the treatment is beneficial.
- The oral medicine may be given with or without food.
- This medicine is usually well tolerated; sleepiness may occur.

Chemistry/Synonyms

Melatonin is a naturally occurring hormone produced in the pineal gland. It occurs as a white to pale yellow, crystalline solid that is slightly soluble in water and has a molecular weight of 232. It can be derived from natural sources or by synthetic means.

Melatonin may also be known as n-acetyl-5-methoxytryptamine, MEL, MLT, or pineal hormone.

Storage/Stability

Unless otherwise labeled, store at room temperature in tight containers.

Dosage Forms/Regulatory Status

VETERINARY-LABELED PRODUCTS:

Melatonin implant 2.7 mg; *PrimeX*®; (OTC). FDA-approved for use in mink. NADA# 140-846. Although this product is still listed in FDA's Green Book of approved animal drugs, marketing status is uncertain.

The following products are marketed for ferret and dog use. Their FDA approval status is not known, and they are not listed in FDA's Green Book of approved animal drugs.

Melatonin Implant 2.7 mg and 5.4 mg; *Ferretonin*®; (OTC); marketed for ferrets

Melatonin Implant 8 mg, 12 mg, 18 mg, and 24 mg; *Dermatonin*®; (OTC); marketed for dogs, cats, sheep, goats, skunk, cattle, and horses.

An 18 mg implant for sustained SC release is available in a variety of countries. One trade name is *Regulin*®. It is labeled for use in sheep (UK and AUS/NZ) and goats (AUS/NZ) to improve early breeding and ovulation rates.

HUMAN-LABELED PRODUCTS:

Melatonin Capsules, Tablets, Chewable Tablets, Disintegrating Oral Tablets, Gummies, Extended-Release Tablets, Sublingual Tablets: 0.2 – 20 mg, although 1 – 10 mg are most common; (OTC). Because melatonin is considered a "nutraceutical," there is no official labeling or central quality control systems for it in the US. Purchase from reputable sources.

Melatonin Oral Solution: 0.25 mg/mL, 0.33 mg/mL, and 1 mg/mL; generic; (OTC)

References

For the complete list of references, see **wiley.com/go/budde/plumb**

Meloxicam

(mel-***ox***-i-kam) *Metacam*®

Nonsteroidal Anti-Inflammatory Drug (NSAID)

Prescriber Highlights

- ► COX-2–preferential NSAID used in many species
- ► Long-term use in cats is controversial.
- ► Available as both injectable and oral products
- ► Primary adverse effects are GI- and renal-related, but idiosyncratic hepatotoxicity has occurred in dogs (rare).

Uses/Indications

Meloxicam is FDA-approved for the treatment of pain, inflammation, and osteoarthritis in dogs.[1,2] Short-term use (eg, single-dose injectable, administered before surgery) of meloxicam is also FDA-approved in the United States in cats to control postoperative pain and inflammation associated with orthopedic surgery, ovariohysterectomy, and castration.[3] Meloxicam is licensed in several countries for long-term use (at lower doses) in cats.

Oral meloxicam may be a cost-effective agent for use during painful procedures such as castration or dehorning in calves[4]; however, meloxicam administration in calves prior to transportation did not affect movement or feeding or drinking behaviors[5] and did not mitigate leukocyte function or inflammatory markers.[6]

Metronomic cyclophosphamide and meloxicam successfully managed oral squamous cell carcinoma in a horse.[7]

Pharmacology/Actions

Like other NSAIDs, meloxicam exhibits analgesic, anti-inflammatory, and antipyretic activity, most likely through its inhibition of cyclooxygenase (COX) and prostaglandin synthesis. Meloxicam is considered COX-2 preferential (not COX-2 specific) because at higher doses, its COX-2 specificity is diminished.

Pharmacokinetics

In dogs, meloxicam is almost completely absorbed after PO and SC administration. The oral transmucosal spray product (not currently marketed in the United States) is bioequivalent to the canine-approved oral suspension.[8] Peak blood concentrations occur ≈4 to 8 hours after oral administration and 2.5 hours after SC administration.[1,3,9,10] The volume of distribution in dogs is 0.3 L/kg and ≈97% is bound to plasma proteins. Meloxicam is extensively biotransformed to several different metabolites in the liver; none of these appear to have pharmacologic activity. The majority of these metabolites (and unchanged drug) are eliminated in the feces. A significant amount of enterohepatic recirculation occurs. Elimination half-life is species-specific. The elimination half-life in dogs averages 24 hours (range, 12 to 36 hours).

In cats, SC injection is nearly completely absorbed. Peak concentrations occur ≈1.5 hours after injection. Meloxicam is relatively highly bound to feline plasma proteins (97%), and volume of distribution is ≈0.27 L/kg. After a single dose, total systemic clearance is

≈130 mL/hour/kg, and elimination half-life is ≈15 hours. The major pathway for biotransformation is oxidation, and the major elimination route is fecal.

In horses, oral meloxicam tablets appear to be well absorbed, regardless of feeding status.[11] Elimination half-life in horses given 0.6 mg/kg IV toward the end of laparotomy for colic syndrome was 6.9 hours[12] and 5 hours in horses given 0.6 mg/kg PO once daily for 14 days.[13] Absorption was similar in foals younger than 6 weeks of age, but elimination half-life was 2.5 hours.[14]

In ruminant calves (≈3 months of age), meloxicam 1 mg/kg PO was well absorbed and had an elimination half-life of ≈24 hours.[4] Half-life was 25.7 hours in 4- to 6-month-old beef calves given 0.5 mg/kg PO every 24 hours for 4 days, and meloxicam tissue concentrations were below the concentration of quantification 15 days after treatment.[15] In 6-month-old Holstein steers given 1 mg/kg PO, the terminal half-life was 16.7 hours, and mean residence time (MRT) was 34 hours.[16] In adult cows given a single 1 mg/kg PO dose, elimination half-life was 10 to 13 hours.[15,17] MRT was 30.3 hours in postpartum cows as compared with 22.3 hours in mid-lactation cows. Meloxicam was detected in the milk of postpartum cows up to 144 hours after administration, as compared with 96 hours in mid-lactation cows, and the authors suggest that a 96-hour milk withdrawal period may be insufficient in postpartum cows to avoid a violative residue.[10]

In lactating goats, meloxicam 0.5 mg/kg IM was completely absorbed, and elimination half-life was 10.8 hours.[19] Administration once every 24 hours was predicted to provide an analgesic plasma concentration. Meloxicam was quantifiable in milk up to 48 hours after IM administration.

Elimination half-life was 15.4 hours in healthy sheep given 0.5 mg/kg IV or 1 mg/kg PO; oral bioavailability was 72%, and time to peak concentration was 19 hours.[20]

Meloxicam was well absorbed (bioavailability, ≈90%) in mature swine given 0.5 mg/kg IV and PO, and elimination half-life was ≈6 hours.[21]

In African gray parrots given 1 mg/kg IV, IM, and PO as a single dose, peak drug concentrations were reached 30 minutes and 13 hours after IM and PO administration, respectively. Bioavailability was 78% (IM) and 38% (PO) as compared with IV administration. Elimination half-life with IV administration was 31 hours.[22] Plasma accumulation ratios of 2 (IM) and 2.4 (PO) were noted with meloxicam dosages of 1 mg/kg PO or IM every 24 hours for 7 (IM) or 12 (PO) days.[23] In Hispaniolan parrots, peak meloxicam concentration occurred at 15 minutes, with 100% bioavailability after IM administration, while peak concentrations occurred 6 hours after oral administration with 50% to 75% bioavailability. Elimination half-life was ≈15 hours regardless of the route of administration.[24]

In healthy white leghorn hens, a single dose of meloxicam 1 mg/kg PO produced peak concentrations after 2 hours, and the plasma elimination half-life was 2.8 hours. Meloxicam was not detected after 4 days in egg whites and after 8 days in egg yolks.[25]

Contraindications/Precautions/Warnings

Meloxicam is contraindicated in animals that are hypersensitive to it. The European and United Kingdom labels state that safe use has not been evaluated in dogs younger than 6 weeks of age[9,10]; the United States FDA label states that safe use has not been established in dogs younger than 6 months of age.[1] The drug should not be used or should be used with extreme caution in dogs with active GI ulceration or bleeding or in dogs receiving glucocorticoids.[10,26] To avoid accidental overdosing, dogs weighing less than 4.5 kg (10 lb) should have meloxicam doses carefully measured and applied on food only, never directly into the mouth.[2]

Meloxicam, like all NSAIDs, should be used with caution in animals with impaired hepatic, cardiac, or renal function and animals with hemorrhagic disorders. Hypotension, high doses, hypovolemia, sodium depletion, and inhalant anesthesia all appear to increase risk for NSAID renal toxicity.[27]

Concurrent use with other anti-inflammatory drugs may result in additional or increased adverse effects; therefore, a treatment-free period from all other anti-inflammatories should be observed for at least 24 hours before beginning treatment with meloxicam. The treatment-free period, however, should take into account the pharmacokinetic properties of the products used previously. Use meloxicam under strict veterinary monitoring in animals with a risk for GI ulcers, or if the animal previously displayed intolerance to other NSAIDs.

The manufacturer warns that additional doses of meloxicam or other NSAIDs are contraindicated in cats, as no safe dose for repeated NSAID administration has been established, and the United States product labels contain a boxed warning stating that repeated use of meloxicam in cats has been associated with acute renal failure and death.[3] Safe use in cats younger than 4 months of age has not been established. Preoperative use in cats undergoing major surgery, in which hypotensive episodes are possible, may result in a higher risk for renal damage.

The human label states that no dose adjustment is necessary in patients with mild to moderate hepatic or renal impairment.

The veterinary oral suspension comes with a dosing syringe that is marked in pounds. If providing dosing directions in mL, make sure to supply an appropriately marked dosing syringe.

Adverse Effects

Experience in Europe and Canada has demonstrated a relatively safe adverse effect profile for meloxicam at labeled doses in healthy dogs.[26] GI distress is the most commonly reported adverse effect, and in United States field trials, vomiting, soft stools, diarrhea, and inappetence were the most common adverse effects. Renal toxicity appears to be quite low in animals with normal renal blood flow. Adverse effects reported postapproval have included GI effects (eg, vomiting, anorexia, diarrhea, melena, ulceration), elevated liver enzymes/hepatotoxicity, pruritus, azotemia, elevated creatinine, and renal failure. When NSAIDs are used long term in dogs, gastroprotectant drugs (eg, proton pump inhibitors [PPIs], H_2 blockers, misoprostol) have been used in an attempt to prevent or limit GI adverse effects, but the benefits of these drugs have not been proven.[28]

Like other COX-2 NSAIDs, meloxicam may have effects on platelet function, although no effect was demonstrated in healthy dogs in a small study.[29] A case report of a dog developing vasculitis with ulcers, vesicles, and erosions has been published.[30] In cats, single doses of meloxicam appear relatively safe. In field trials, some cats developed elevated BUN, posttreatment anemia, and residual pain at the injection site (rare). In other studies, meloxicam has caused GI effects (eg, vomiting, diarrhea, inappetence), behavior changes, and lethargy. Repeated use of meloxicam in cats is controversial, as repeated doses have been associated with renal failure and death. The FDA warns against repeated doses in cats; however, low-dose long-term use is licensed in some countries, and guidelines for long-term NSAID use in cats suggest the benefits of treatment often outweigh the risks.[31]

Acute dosing studies in dogs have not demonstrated any hepatic toxicity.[1,3] Administration to piglets for ≈2 months demonstrated no adverse effects on trabecular bone or growth plates.[32]

Meloxicam is relatively safe in other species (eg, horses, cattle, camelids, swine, rabbits, small ruminants) when used at recommended doses.

Reproductive/Nursing Safety

Safe use has not been established in dogs or cats used for breeding or in pregnant or lactating animals. Meloxicam had a positive effect on pregnancy rates after embryo transfer in heifers.[33,34] Meloxicam reduced deslorelin-induced ovulation and induced intrafollicular hemorrhage and luteinization of anovulatory follicles in mares.[35]

Most NSAIDs are excreted in milk. Because safety has not been established, this drug should only be used when the maternal benefits outweigh the potential fetal risks.

Overdose/Acute Toxicity

GI effects (eg, vomiting, diarrhea) and renomegaly with minimal degeneration and necrosis were noted in dogs given 3 and 5 times the label dosage during 6-week safety studies. Overdoses should be treated supportively based on clinical signs. Therapeutic plasma exchange was successful in the overdose management of one dog.[36]

For patients that have experienced or are suspected to have experienced an overdose, consultation with a 24-hour poison consultation center that specializes in providing veterinary-specific information is recommended. For general information related to overdose and toxin exposures, as well as contact information for poison control centers, refer to ***Appendix***.

Drug Interactions

In humans, meloxicam is a CYP2C9 substrate. The following drug interactions have either been reported or are theoretical in humans or animals receiving meloxicam and may be of significance in veterinary patients. Unless otherwise noted, use together is not necessarily contraindicated, but weigh the potential risks and perform additional monitoring when appropriate.

- **Angiotensin Converting Enzyme Inhibitors** (ACEIs; eg, **benazepril, enalapril**): NSAIDs can reduce effects on blood pressure.
- **Amiodarone**: May increase meloxicam concentrations
- **Amlodipine**: Some NSAIDs can reduce effects on blood pressure.
- **Anesthetics, Inhalant** (eg, **isoflurane, sevoflurane**): May increase risk for renal hypotension and NSAID renal toxicity
- **Angiotensin-II Receptor Blockers** (ARBs; eg, **telmisartan**): Some NSAIDs can reduce effects on blood pressure.
- **Anticoagulants** (eg, **heparins, rivaroxaban, warfarin**): Increased chance for bleeding
- **Bisphosphonates** (eg, **alendronate**): May increase risk for GI ulceration
- **Clopidogrel**: Increased chance for bleeding
- **Corticosteroids** (eg, **dexamethasone, prednis(ol)one**): May increase risk for GI toxicity (eg, ulceration, bleeding, vomiting, diarrhea); avoid use with NSAIDs
- **Cyclosporine** (**systemic**): Concurrent use may result in increased risk for cyclosporine nephrotoxicity.
- **Digoxin**: NSAIDs may increase serum concentrations.
- **Diuretics** (eg, **furosemide, hydrochlorothiazide**): Concurrent use may result in reduced diuretic efficacy and possible nephrotoxicity.
- **Fluconazole**: Administration has increased plasma concentrations of celecoxib in humans and could also affect meloxicam concentrations in dogs.
- **Fluoroquinolones** (eg, **enrofloxacin, marbofloxacin**): Meloxicam may increase fluoroquinolone concentrations, increasing risk for CNS toxicity.
- **Leflunomide**: May increase meloxicam exposure; risk for leflunomide hepatotoxicity may be increased
- **Methotrexate**: Concomitant NSAID use with methotrexate may increase risk for myelosuppression, nephropathy, hepatotoxicity, and GI toxicity; use together with extreme caution.
- **Nephrotoxic Drugs** (eg, **aminoglycosides, amphotericin B, furosemide**): May enhance risk for nephrotoxicity
- **NSAIDs** (eg, **carprofen**): May increase risk for GI toxicity (eg, ulceration, bleeding, vomiting, diarrhea)
- **Pentoxifylline**: May increase risk for bleeding
- **Salicylates** (eg, **aspirin, bismuth subsalicylate**): Concurrent use may increase risk for GI toxicity and bleeding.
- **Selective Serotonin Reuptake Inhibitors** (SSRIs; eg, **fluoxetine**): Concurrent use may result in an increased risk for bleeding.
- **Sulfonamides** (eg, **sulfamethoxazole**): May inhibit meloxicam metabolism, increasing meloxicam exposure and risk for toxicity
- **Tricyclic Antidepressants** (eg, **amitriptyline, clomipramine**): Concurrent use may increase risk for bleeding.

Dosages

When doses are listed in drops, use with caution; drug concentration per drop may be different in products marketed in different countries.

DOGS:

Control of pain and inflammation associated with osteoarthritis (label dosage; FDA-approved): 0.2 mg/kg PO, IV, or SC on the first day of treatment; subsequent doses of 0.1 mg/kg PO every 24 hours.[1-3] For dogs weighing less than 4.5 kg (10 lb), administer drops on food only, never directly into the mouth; for dogs weighing more than 4.5 kg (10 lb), drops can be placed in food or directly into the mouth. Consult product labels for additional oral dosing instructions for dogs weighing less than 2.3 kg (5 lb).[2] Use the lowest effective dose for the shortest duration consistent with individual response.

CATS:

Control of postoperative pain and inflammation associated with orthopedic surgery, ovariohysterectomy, and castration (label dosage; FDA-approved): 0.3 mg/kg SC once; should not be followed by additional doses of meloxicam or other NSAIDs.[3]

NOTE: The following dosages for cats are extra-label in the United States, and in 2010, the drug sponsor and the FDA issued the following: *WARNING: Repeated use of meloxicam in cats has been associated with acute renal failure and death. Do not administer additional doses of injectable or oral meloxicam to cats.*[1] See ***Contraindications/Precautions/Warnings***. However, the ISFM and AAFP Consensus Guidelines: Long-Term Use of NSAIDs in Cats include the following statements:

It is only recently that NSAIDs have become licensed for long-term use in cats in some countries. The panel believe that these drugs have a major role to play in the management of chronic pain in cats, but at present only limited feline-specific data are available. To date published studies of the medium- to long-term use of the COX-1 sparing drug meloxicam in older cats and cats with chronic kidney disease provide encouraging data that these drugs can be used safely and should be used to relieve pain when needed. While further data are needed and would undoubtedly lead to refinement of the guidelines presented here, the panel hope that these recommendations will encourage rational and safe long-term use of NSAIDs in cats, thereby improving patients' quality of life in the face of painful disease conditions.[31]

Prevention of mild to moderate postoperative pain and inflammation following surgical procedures: 0.2 mg/kg SC once before surgery. To continue treatment for up to 5 days, the initial dose may be followed 24 hours later by administration of oral suspension at 0.05 mg/kg PO every 24 hours for a total of up to 4 oral doses. For cats not receiving additional oral doses, a single injection of meloxicam 0.3 mg/kg SC has also been shown to be safe and effective.[37]

Alleviation of pain and inflammation associated with acute or chronic musculoskeletal disorders: On the first day of treatment, 0.1 – 0.2 mg/kg PO once for acute disorders or 0.1 mg/kg PO once for chronic disorders.[38–40] Thereafter, maintenance treatment should be 0.05 mg/kg PO every 24 hours. A clinical response is normally seen within 7 days. Treatment should be discontinued after 14 days if no clinical improvement is apparent.[38,41] Many cats may experience pain relief at even lower doses given every 2 to 3 days. Titrating to the lowest effective dose may help avoid adverse effects.[42,43]

HORSES:

Inflammation and pain associated with musculoskeletal disorders or colic pain (extra-label):

a) **IV**: 0.6 mg/kg IV once; oral dose may be given after 24 hours.
b) **Oral**: 0.6 mg/kg PO either mixed with food or given directly in the mouth every 24 hours, for up to 14 days. When administering this product with food, add to a small quantity of feed to be fed before providing full meal.[44,45]

Pain and inflammation (extra-label):

a) **Foals**: In a pharmacokinetic study in healthy foals, the authors concluded 0.6 mg/kg PO every 12 hours would likely be therapeutic in foals younger than 7 weeks of age.[14]
b) **Adults**: 0.6 mg/kg PO every 24 hours was effective in a lipopolysaccharide-induced synovitis model of pain.[46]

CATTLE:

Acute respiratory infection with appropriate antibiotic therapy to reduce clinical signs in cattle; diarrhea, in combination with oral rehydration therapy, to reduce clinical signs in calves older than 1 week of age and young nonlactating cattle; as adjunctive therapy in the treatment of acute mastitis, in combination with antibiotic therapy (extra-label): 0.5 mg/kg SC, IV, or IM once[47]

Analgesia for surgical pain (extra-label):

a) **Oral**: 0.5 – 1 mg/kg PO every 24 to 48 hours.[48] Single doses appear effective for dehorning.[16]
b) **Buccal**: 0.5 mg/kg buccal meloxicam gel reduced pain and inflammation related to castration[49] and dehorning[50] in unweaned beef calves.

Lameness (extra-label): 0.5 mg/kg PO once daily for 4 days alone or in combination with gabapentin (15 mg/kg PO once daily) was effective in experimentally induced lameness in 4- to 6-month-old beef calves.[51]

SMALL RUMINANTS:

Pain and inflammation (extra-label):

a) **Sheep**: 0.5 mg/kg IV every 12 hours. 2 mg/kg PO on first day and then 1 mg/kg PO every 24 hours. A single 1 mg/kg SC injection provided analgesia in an experimental pain model.[52,53]
b) **Goats**: 0.5 mg/kg IV every 8 hours; 0.5 mg/kg IM or PO every 24 hours.[54] 1 mg/kg of buccal meloxicam was shown to be effective when given to lambs immediately before marking[55] or surgical mulesing and hot-knife tail docking.[56]

CAMELIDS:

Pain and inflammation (extra-label): 0.5 mg/kg IV; 1 mg/kg PO every third day[54]

SWINE:

Noninfectious locomotor disorders to reduce the clinical signs of lameness and inflammation; for adjunctive therapy in the treatment of puerperal septicemia and toxemia (mastitis-metritis-agalactia syndrome) with appropriate antibiotic therapy (extra-label): 0.4 mg/kg IM once. If required, a second administration of meloxicam can be given after 24 hours.

BIRDS:

Analgesic (extra-label): 0.5 mg/kg IM once is also commonly used in birds and may be the safest of the NSAID analgesics for avian species. Because the adverse effects of all analgesics have not been studied in birds, these drugs should be used carefully in avian patients.[57] Another source states, *Injectable forms of meloxicam and carprofen will cause myositis/muscle necrosis and therefore oral formulations are recommended . . . however oral bioavailability of NSAIDs varies greatly between avian species. Therefore, it is critical to monitor response to dosage and frequency of NSAID treatment for each avian patient.*[58]

FERRETS:

Anti-inflammatory/analgesic for postsurgical pain (extra-label): 0.2 mg/kg PO or SC once[59,60]

SMALL MAMMALS:

Pain and inflammation (extra-label):

a) **Rabbits**: Pharmacokinetic studies in healthy rabbits receiving 1 mg/kg PO every 24 hours for 5 to 29 days concluded that meloxicam at this dose and treatment duration may be safe and effective.[61,62]
b) **Rats**: 1 mg/kg PO or SC every 12 to 24 hours[63]
c) **Guinea pigs**:
   i. 0.2 mg/kg PO as a single presurgical dose, followed by 0.1 mg/kg PO every 24 hours for postoperative days 2 and 3. Dose may be titrated up to 0.5 mg/kg in individual cases; do not exceed 0.6 mg/kg per dose.[38]
   ii. 0.1 – 0.3 mg/kg PO or SC every 24 hours has also been recommended.[63]

REPTILES:

Pain and inflammation (extra-label): 0.2 mg/kg PO every 24 hours for 5 days. Subsequent administration should be 0.2 mg/kg every 48 hours. A study in ball pythons failed to demonstrate analgesic effects when meloxicam was used at 0.3 mg/kg.[64]

Monitoring

- Clinical efficacy
- Adverse effects, especially GI effects in dogs
- Baseline and periodic serum renal and hepatic chemistry panels when used chronically. One recommendation is to perform baseline renal and hepatic panels; repeat within the first 2 weeks and periodically thereafter.[27] When liver enzymes are elevated and concern for liver function is present, liver function tests (eg, serum bile acids) should be performed.[65]

Client Information

- If using the oral liquid, shake the bottle well before using, and carefully measure the dose. Do not confuse the markings on the syringe (provided by the manufacturer). Give with food. For dogs weighing less than 4.5 kg (10 lb), it is safest to carefully measure the amount of medicine to give and apply it directly to a small amount of food. Do not give this medicine directly in the mouth.
- Most animals tolerate meloxicam well, but ulcers or serious kidney and liver problems can develop (rare), especially in cats. Contact your veterinarian if your animal develops side effects such as eating less than normal, vomiting, changes in bowel movements, changes in behavior or activity (ie, more or less active than normal), weakness (eg, stumbling, clumsiness), seizures (ie, convulsions), aggression (ie, threatening behavior/actions), changes in drinking habits (ie, frequency, amount consumed), changes in urination habits (ie, frequency, color, or smell), and/or yellowing of gums, skin, or whites of the eyes (ie, jaundice).

- Store this medicine well out of reach of animals and children, especially the honey-flavored oral liquid.
- Periodic laboratory tests to check for liver and kidney side effects are required.

Chemistry/Synonyms

Meloxicam is a COX-2–preferential NSAID that occurs as a pale-yellow powder. It is in the oxicam class, related to piroxicam.

Meloxicam may also be known as UH-AC-62 and/or UH-AC-62XX; many trade names are available, including *Alloxate®, Inflacam®, Loxicom®, M-eloxyn®, Meloxadin®, Meloxidolor®, Meloxidyl®, Meloximed®, Metacam®, Ostilox® Recocam®, Rheumocam®, and Zeleris®.*

Storage/Stability

Unless otherwise labeled, store the injection and oral liquid at controlled room temperature (20°C to 25°C [68°F-77°F]), with excursions permitted between 15°C to 30°C (59°F-86°F) for the oral suspension. The oral suspension labeled for use in the United Kingdom has a 6-month shelf life after the immediate package is first opened.

Dosage Forms/Regulatory Status

VETERINARY-LABELED PRODUCTS:

Meloxicam Oral Suspension: 0.5 mg/mL (0.02 mg/drop) and 1.5 mg/mL (0.05 mg/drop) in a honey-flavored base: 10 mL, 32 mL, 100 mL, and 180 mL dropper bottles with measuring syringe (marked in 5-lb body weight increments); *Metacam®*, generic; (Rx). FDA-approved for use in dogs. NADA# 141-213

Meloxicam 5 mg/mL for Injection: 10 mL vial; *Metacam®*, generic; (Rx). FDA-approved for use in dogs and cats. NADA# 141-219

The Association of Racing Commissioners International (ARCI) has designated this drug as a class 3 substance. Use of this drug may not be allowed in certain animal competitions. Check rules and regulations before entering in a competition while this medication is being administered. Contact local racing authorities for further guidance. See ***Appendix*** for more information.

Suggested withdrawal periods for extra-label use; always consult with local regulatory agencies prior to prescribing:

Horses: meat/offal, 5 days[44,45]

Cattle: Conservative 21- to 30-day meat withdrawal and 5-day milk withdrawal times have been recommended.[66,67] United Kingdom withdrawal periods: 15-day meat withdrawal; milk: 120 hours[47]

Swine: meat/offal, 5 days[45]

Sheep and goats: 15-day meat withdrawal time has been recommended.[67]

HUMAN-LABELED PRODUCTS:

Meloxicam Tablets: 7.5 mg and 15 mg; *Mobic®*, generic; (Rx)

Meloxicam Capsules: 5 mg and 10 mg; *Vivlodex®*; (Rx)

Meloxicam Oral Suspension: 7.5 mg/5 mL in 100 mL bottle; *Mobic®*, generic; (Rx)

References

For the complete list of references, see **wiley.com/go/budde/plumb**

Melphalan

(***mel***-fa-lan) *Alkeran®, Evomela®*

Antineoplastic

Prescriber Highlights

- ► Alkylating antineoplastic agent primarily used for multiple myeloma, resistant leukemia or lymphoma, and various other neoplasms
- ► Use with caution in patients with anemia, leukopenia, thrombocytopenia, previous chemotherapy or radiotherapy, impaired hepatic or renal function, or in those for whom immunosuppression may be dangerous (eg, infection).
- ► Adverse effects include chronic bone marrow suppression (eg, anemia, thrombocytopenia, leukopenia), GI effects (eg, anorexia, vomiting, diarrhea), and pulmonary infiltrates or fibrosis.
- ► Potentially teratogenic and fetotoxic
- ► The National Institute for Occupational Safety and Health (NIOSH) classifies melphalan as a hazardous drug; use appropriate precautions when handling it.

Uses/Indications

Melphalan may be useful in the treatment of a variety of neoplastic diseases, including lymphoreticular neoplasms particularly of plasma cell neoplasms, osteosarcoma, and mammary or pulmonary neoplasms. When combined with prednisone, it is considered the drug of choice for treating multiple myeloma. Melphalan can be used for treating primary (essential) thrombocythemia in dogs or cats. It has been used with some success in a variety of rescue protocols, including dexamethasone, melphalan, dactinomycin, and cytarabine (DMAC) for relapsed multicentric lymphoma in dogs and cats,[1-4] and mechlorethamine, vincristine, melphalan, and prednisolone (MOMP) for relapsed canine lymphoma[5] and resistant feline lymphoma.[6] Melphalan has been used successfully in combination with prednisone for canine cutaneous plasmacytosis.[7]

Pharmacology/Actions

Melphalan is a bifunctional alkylating agent and interferes with RNA transcription and DNA replication, thereby disrupting nucleic acid function. Because it is bifunctional, it has effects on both dividing and resting cells. Melphalan does not require activation by the liver (unlike cyclophosphamide).

Pharmacokinetics

Melphalan absorption is variable and often incomplete. It is distributed throughout the body water, but it is unknown whether it crosses the placenta, blood–brain barrier, or enters maternal milk. Melphalan is eliminated principally by hydrolysis. In humans, protein binding varies from 50% to 92%, and terminal half-lives are ≈75 minutes following IV administration.

Contraindications/Precautions/Warnings

Melphalan should not be used in patients with a history of hypersensitivity and should be used with caution in the following conditions: anemia, bone marrow depression, current infection, impaired hepatic or renal function, tumor cell infiltration of bone marrow, or patients that have received previous chemotherapy or radiotherapy. Severe bone marrow suppression resulting in infection or bleeding can occur in humans. Melphalan is considered an irritant, and care should be taken to avoid extravasation.

In humans with impaired renal function receiving IV melphalan, a 50% dose reduction is suggested.[8]

The National Institute for Occupational Safety and Health (NIOSH) classifies melphalan as a hazardous drug; personal protective equipment (PPE) should be used accordingly to minimize the risk for exposure.

Melphalan hydrochloride for injection is available in 2 formulations, which have different storage and preparation instructions. Melphalan flufenamide is a prodrug of melphalan and should not be interchanged with melphalan hydrochloride.

Adverse Effects

The most serious adverse effect likely with melphalan is bone marrow depression (eg, anemia, thrombocytopenia, leukopenia); the onset of, and recovery from, leukopenia can be delayed. Other potential adverse effects include GI effects (eg, anorexia, vomiting, diarrhea), pulmonary infiltrates or fibrosis, or neurotoxic effects. Prophylactic antiemetics are recommended in humans. Hepatotoxicity, secondary malignancies, and skin hypersensitivity reactions[9] have also been reported in humans.

Many dogs receiving chemotherapy will have minor hair coat changes (eg, shagginess, loss of luster). Breeds with continuously growing hair coats (eg, poodles, terriers, Afghan hounds, or old English sheepdogs) are more likely to experience significant alopecia.

Reproductive/Nursing Safety

Safe use of melphalan during pregnancy has not been established. Other alkylating agents are known teratogens, and melphalan is considered potentially mutagenic in humans. Melphalan should only be used during pregnancy when the benefits to the mother outweigh the risks to the offspring. Melphalan can suppress gonadal function. For sexually intact patients, verify pregnancy status prior to administration.

Although it is unknown whether melphalan enters maternal milk, nursing is generally not recommended when dams are receiving the drug.

Because safety has not been established in animals, this drug should only be used when the maternal benefits outweigh the potential risks to offspring.

Overdose/Acute Toxicity

Because of the toxic potential of this agent, overdoses must be avoided. Determine dosages carefully. The reported lowest lethal dose (LD_{Lo}) following IV administration in a dog is 3 mg/kg, with the dog exhibiting diarrhea, somnolence, and anemia. The drug is not considered dialyzable, and the recommended treatment is supportive.

For patients that have experienced or are suspected of having experienced an overdose, consultation with a 24-hour poison consultation center specializing in providing veterinary-specific information is recommended. For general information related to overdose and toxin exposures, as well as contact information for poison control centers, refer to ***Appendix***.

Drug Interactions

The following drug interactions have either been reported or are theoretical in humans or animals receiving melphalan and may be of significance in veterinary patients. Unless otherwise noted, use together is not necessarily contraindicated, but weigh the potential risks and perform additional monitoring when appropriate.

- **Cyclosporine**: There are anecdotal reports of melphalan causing increased nephrotoxicity associated with systemic cyclosporine use in humans.
- **Immunosuppressants** (eg, **cyclosporine, leflunomide, tacrolimus**): May increase the immunosuppressive effect and decrease cyclosporine concentration
- **Myelosuppressive Agents** (eg, **azathioprine, chloramphenicol**): May increase the risk for neutropenia or other hematologic effects
- **Vaccines, Live**: Melphalan may diminish vaccine efficacy.

Laboratory Considerations

- Melphalan may raise serum **uric acid** levels. Drugs such as allopurinol may be required to control hyperuricemia.

Dosages

NOTE: Because of the potential toxicity of this drug to patients, veterinary personnel, and clients, and since chemotherapy indications, treatment protocols, and monitoring and safety guidelines often change, the following dosages should be used only as a general guide. Consultation with a veterinary oncologist and referral to current veterinary oncology references[10-14] are strongly recommended.

DOGS:

Melphalan dosages for dogs vary depending on the source, the disease treated, and the protocol being used. As a general guide, it is usually dosed from 1.5 – 2 mg/m² (NOT mg/kg) or 0.1 – 0.2 mg/kg in dogs, but higher dosages have been used.[8,9] Dosage frequencies range from daily to every other day to pulse dosing (eg, daily for 5 days, then 16 days off). The following are examples:

Multiple myeloma (extra-label): Several dosing schedules have been developed to treat canine multiple myeloma with melphalan. One recommended dosing regimen is 0.1 mg/kg PO every 24 hours for 10 days, followed by 0.05 mg/kg PO every 48 hours thereafter. Another source recommends 0.25 mg/kg/day PO for 4 days and 2 – 4 mg/day PO maintenance. Pulse therapy is another reported option: 7 mg/m² (NOT mg/kg) PO every 24 hours for 5 days every 21 days.[15] One retrospective study reported similar efficacy and adverse effect profiles for daily and pulse dosing protocols, although pulse dosing allows for fewer days of handling chemotherapy and reduces hazardous waste exposure.

Anecdotally, the human dosage 16 mg/m² (NOT mg/kg) IV every 2 weeks has been used in dogs. A 50% dose reduction is recommended for animals with pre-existing renal insufficiency. Clinical response can be assessed by improved clinical signs and reduced serum immunoglobulin. Melphalan should be administered indefinitely until clinical relapse, which may involve worsened bone pain, recurrence of bleeding diathesis, funduscopic changes, or elevated serum immunoglobulins.[16] **NOTE**: Melphalan flufenamide (*Pepaxto®*) is not interchangeable with melphalan hydrochloride.

Rescue protocol (DMAC) to treat relapsed multicentric lymphoma (extra-label): Dactinomycin 0.75 mg/m² (NOT mg/kg) IV with cytarabine 300 mg/m² (NOT mg/kg) IV over 4 hours or SC and dexamethasone 1 mg/kg PO on Day 0, then melphalan 20 mg/m² (NOT mg/kg) PO and dexamethasone (1 mg/kg PO) on Day 7. The cycle was repeated continuously every 2 weeks as long as a complete or partial remission is achieved. After 4 cycles, chlorambucil was substituted for melphalan at the same dose. If complete remission was achieved, the protocol was discontinued after 5 to 8 cycles, and maintenance therapy with the LMP (chlorambucil, methotrexate, prednisone) or lomustine/prednisone protocols was instituted. If dogs developed grades 3 or 4 toxicosis, DMAC was discontinued, and maintenance protocol was started.[1,17]

CATS:

Melphalan dosages for cats vary depending on the source, the disease treated, and the protocol being used. As a general guide, it is usually dosed from 1.5 – 2 mg/m² (NOT mg/kg) or 0.5 mg/cat (NOT mg/kg) PO. Dosage frequencies range from daily to every other day to pulse dosing (eg, daily for 7 to 10 days, then 3 weeks off). The following listed indication and dosage is an example:

Chronic lymphocytic leukemia (extra-label): 2 mg/m² (NOT mg/kg) PO every other day with or without prednisone at 20 mg/m² (NOT mg/kg) PO every other day[18]

Monitoring

- CBC with platelets at least every week for 2 weeks and then monthly thereafter. Significant myelosuppression requires an alteration in dose or frequency of administration.

Client Information

- Wear gloves when handling the medication and give it with food.
- Melphalan is a chemotherapy (cancer) drug. The drug and its by-products can be hazardous to other animals and people that come in contact with it. On the day your animal gets the drug and then for a few days afterward, handle all bodily waste (ie, urine, feces, litter), blood, or vomit only while wearing disposable gloves. Seal the waste in a plastic bag, then place both the bag and gloves in with the regular trash.
- Bone marrow suppression can occur. The greatest effects on bone marrow usually occur within a few weeks after treatment. Your veterinarian will do blood tests to watch for this, but if you see bleeding, bruising, fever (indicating an infection), or if your animal becomes tired easily, contact your veterinarian right away.
- Give melphalan as your veterinarian has directed; immediately report any signs associated with toxicity (eg, abnormal bleeding, bruising, urination, depression, infection, shortness of breath).
- This medication is considered to be a hazardous drug as defined by the National Institute for Occupational Safety and Health (NIOSH). Talk with your veterinarian or pharmacist about the use of personal protective equipment when handling this medicine.

Chemistry/Synonyms

Melphalan is a nitrogen mustard derivative that occurs as an off-white to buff-colored powder that is practically insoluble in water.

Melphalan may also be known as CB-3025, NSC-8806, PAM, L-PAM, L-phenylalanine mustard, phenylalanine mustard, phenylalanine nitrogen mustard, L-sarcolysine, WR-19813, *Alkeran*®, or *Alkerana*®.

Storage/Stability

Store melphalan tablets in well-closed, light-resistant glass containers in the refrigerator (2°C-8°C [36°F-46°F]).

Store intact powder vials between 15°C and 30°C (59°F-86°F), protected from light. Complete administration within 60 minutes of reconstitution. Once reconstituted, the injectable product should not be refrigerated, or a precipitate may form. For IV administration of *Alkeran*® and the generic, the reconstituted solution should be further diluted with sterile 0.9% sodium chloride to a concentration of not more than 0.45 mg/mL.[15] Further dilution or refrigeration of the solution increases the stability of certain products; check package insert of the specific product used.

Compatibility/Compounding Considerations

Compatibility is dependent on factors such as pH, concentration, temperature, and diluent used; specialized references or a hospital pharmacist should be consulted for more specific information.

Melphalan has **variable compatibility** with 0.9% sodium chloride; concentration should not exceed 0.45 mg/mL.

Melphalan is **incompatible** with 5% dextrose in water and lactated Ringer's solution.

Melphalan is also **incompatible** with amphotericin B, chlorpromazine, and pantoprazole for Y-site administration.

Compounded oral formulations have been shown to have variable stability and potency.[19] The risks vs benefits of using a compounded formulation should be carefully considered.

Dosage Forms/Regulatory Status

VETERINARY-LABELED PRODUCTS: NONE

HUMAN-LABELED PRODUCTS:

Melphalan Oral Tablets: 2 mg; *Alkeran*®; (Rx)

Melphalan Powder for Injection (lyophilized): 50 mg in single-use vials; *Alkeran*®, *Evomela*®, generic; (Rx). Melphalan flufenamide (*Pepaxto*®) is not interchangeable with melphalan hydrochloride.

References

For the complete list of references, see **wiley.com/go/budde/plumb**

Meperidine

Pethidine

(me-***per***-i-deen) *Demerol*®

Opioid Agonist

Prescriber Highlights

- ► Infrequently used due to short duration of analgesia and potential for more adverse effects than other commonly used injectable opioids
- ► Contraindicated in patients hypersensitive to it, patients with diarrhea caused by a toxic ingestion, and patients taking MAOIs
- ► Use with extreme caution in patients with head injuries, respiratory disease, acute respiratory dysfunction, or acute abdominal conditions (eg, colic).
- ► Use with caution in patients with hypothyroidism, adrenocortical insufficiency, seizures, renal/hepatic impairment, or in geriatric or severely debilitated patients.
- ► Adverse effects include respiratory depression, histamine release, bronchoconstriction, central nervous system (CNS) depression, and GI effects (eg, nausea, vomiting, decreased intestinal peristalsis). Mydriasis can be seen in dogs, and salivation can occur, especially in cats. Horses may also experience tachycardia with premature or polymorphic ventricular contractions (PVCs), profuse sweating, or hyperpnea. Meperidine may potentiate intestinal obstruction secondary to reduced intestinal motility.
- ► Must be administered slowly if given IV; may be irritating when given SC
- ► Overdoses can cause CNS excitatory effects (eg, agitation, seizures); naloxone may enhance rather than reverse these effects.
- ► DEA Schedule II (C-II) controlled substance

Uses/Indications

Meperidine has been used as a sedative/analgesic in small animal species for both postoperative pain and medical conditions, such as acute pancreatitis and thermal burns; however, other opioids are usually preferred as meperidine has a short analgesic duration and can cause significant histamine release. Meperidine is occasionally used in horses and other large animal species for pain control; however, when meperidine is used a single agent, it does not provide much restraint in large animal species.

Pharmacology/Actions

Meperidine is an opioid agonist with activity at the mu-OP_3 receptor. It has ≈20% to 25% the potency of morphine. Receptors for opioid analgesics are found in high concentrations in the limbic system, spinal cord, thalamus, hypothalamus, striatum, and midbrain. The GI tract, urinary tract, and other smooth muscle tissues also contain opioid receptors.

The morphine-like agonists (morphine, meperidine, oxymorphone, hydromorphone, fentanyl) have primary activity at the mu-opioid receptors. The primary pharmacologic effects of these agents include analgesia, antitussive activity, respiratory depression, sedation, emesis, physical dependence, and intestinal effects (constipation/defecation). Secondary pharmacologic effects include effects on the central nervous system (euphoria and confusion), cardiovascular system (bradycardia due to central vagal stimulation, depressed alpha-adrenergic receptors resulting in peripheral vasodilation, decreased peripheral resistance, and baroreceptor inhibition, possible orthostatic hypotension and syncope), and urinary effects (increased bladder sphincter tone and resulting urinary retention).

Meperidine produces equivalent respiratory depression at equianalgesic doses as morphine. Like morphine, it can cause histamine release. Meperidine does not have antitussive activity at doses lower than those causing analgesia. Meperidine is the only used opioid that has vagolytic (can cause tachycardia) and negative inotropic properties at clinically used doses. One study in ponies demonstrated changes in jejunal activity after meperidine administration, but no effects on transit time or colonic electrical activity were noted.

Pharmacokinetics

Although meperidine is generally well absorbed after oral administration, a marked first-pass effect limits oral effectiveness. Therefore, meperidine is rarely used orally in the clinical setting. Oral bioavailability in dogs (beagles; $n = 3$) ranged from 3% to 25%. After IM or SC injection, peak analgesic effects occur between 30 and 60 minutes, with the IM route having a slightly faster onset. Duration of action is variable, with effects generally lasting from 1 to 6 hours in most species. In dogs and cats, analgesic duration is less than 2 hours and often less than 1 hour at clinically used doses. The drug is metabolized primarily in the liver (mostly hydrolysis with some conjugation), and ≈5% is excreted unchanged in the urine. One metabolite is normeperidine, which is active with ≈50% of the analgesic effects of the parent compound. Accumulation of normeperidine is associated with central nervous system excitatory effects that appear to be mediated by other than mu-opioid receptors and are not amenable to reversal by naloxone or other mu antagonists.

In horses, IM and SC administration resulted in low plasma concentrations.[1]

Contraindications/Precautions/Warnings

Meperidine is contraindicated in patients that are hypersensitive to narcotic analgesics and in patients currently receiving or that have received monoamine oxidase inhibitors (MAOIs) within 14 days. Avoid use in patients with diarrhea caused by toxic ingestion until the toxin is eliminated from the gastric tract.

Use meperidine with extreme caution in patients with head injuries, increased intracranial pressure, and acute abdominal conditions (eg, colic) as it may obscure the diagnosis or clinical course of these conditions. Use with extreme caution in patients suffering from respiratory disease or acute respiratory dysfunction (eg, pulmonary edema secondary to smoke inhalation). In humans, meperidine is contraindicated in patients with acute or severe bronchial asthma.[2]

Meperidine should be used with caution in patients with hypothyroidism, hypoadrenocorticism (Addison's disease), prostatic hypertrophy, urethral stricture, and geriatric or severely debilitated patients. Use with caution in patients with renal or hepatic impairment, as meperidine and its active metabolite, normeperidine, may accumulate.[2] Use caution in patients with biliary tract impairment, including pancreatitis, as Sphincter of Oddi constriction may occur. Consider using an alternate analgesic in patients with seizure disorders, as normeperidine can cause central nervous system excitement and precipitate anxiety, tremors, and seizures. Hypotension may occur with meperidine. Use caution in patients with cardiovascular disease and in those that are hypovolemic. Use caution in patients with tachycardia due to potential increased ventricular response rate.

Use meperidine with caution in cats. Some recommend avoiding meperidine use in feline patients.

Many clinicians recommend meperidine not be administered IV. If meperidine must be given IV, it must be given very slowly to prevent severe hypotension. In humans, it should only be given IV when necessary and should preferably be administered in a diluted solution, as rapid injection can increase incidence of adverse effects.[2]

Although naloxone will reverse respiratory depression associated with meperidine overdoses, it will not reverse CNS excitement mediated by normeperidine and may exacerbate CNS excitement and seizures.[3]

Opioid analgesics are contraindicated in patients that have been stung by the scorpion species *Centruroides sculpturatus Ewing* and *Centruroides gertschi Stahnke* as opioids may potentiate their venoms. Meperidine should not be used for pain secondary to envenomations from Gila monsters or Mexican beaded lizards.[4]

In humans, the American Pain Society and Institute for Safe Medication Practices do not recommend meperidine use due to neurotoxicity related to meperidine's metabolite, normeperidine. If using meperidine, it is generally not recommended to use it for longer than 48 hours.

Adverse Effects

Meperidine may be irritating when administered SC. Severe hypotension can occur with rapid IV administration. Meperidine can cause pronounced histamine release, particularly with IV administration. At usual doses, the primary concern is the effect meperidine has on respiratory function. Decreased tidal volume, depressed cough reflex, and the drying of respiratory secretions may all have a detrimental effect on susceptible patients. Bronchoconstriction following IV doses has been noted in dogs. GI effects may include nausea, vomiting, and decreased intestinal peristalsis. In dogs, meperidine causes mydriasis (unlike morphine). If given orally, meperidine may be irritating to the buccal mucosa and cause salivation; this is of particular concern in cats. Chronic administration can lead to physical dependence.

In horses undergoing general anesthesia, meperidine has been associated with a reaction that manifests as tachycardia with premature ventricular contractions, profuse sweating, and hyperpnea. Urticaria induced by IV meperidine is presumably due to histamine release.

Cutaneous eruptions and localized sweating have been reported after SC administration in horses.[5] Meperidine can reduce colonic activity and increase the risk for postanesthetic colic. Doses greater than 2 mg/kg may induce locomotor activity; 5 mg/kg initially causes incoordination, shaking, and immobility, followed by a substantial locomotor response.[6]

Reproductive/Nursing Safety

Meperidine is more lipophilic than several other opioids (eg, morphine, hydromorphone) and can more readily cross the placenta. Meperidine is generally not recommended for use in pregnant animals.

Most opioids are excreted into milk. Meperidine enters human breast milk. Central nervous system and respiratory depression may occur in nursing human infants. Use in breastfeeding humans is not recommended, and either breastfeeding or meperidine should be discontinued.

Because safety has not been established in animals, this drug should only be used when the maternal benefits outweigh the potential risks to offspring.

Overdose/Acute Toxicity

Overdoses may produce profound respiratory and/or central nervous system (CNS) depression in most species. Other effects include cardiovascular collapse, hypothermia, and skeletal muscle hypotonia. A metabolite of meperidine, normeperidine, can have CNS excitatory effects (eg, agitation, hyperreflexia, seizures), and these effects can predominate in meperidine overdoses. While naloxone (at low doses) can be used for treating profound respiratory depression when ventilator support is unavailable, it is not recommended when treating suspected normeperidine-induced CNS excitotoxicity.[7] Benzodiazepines or barbiturates may be considered if treatment of CNS excitement is needed. Use caution as additive respiratory depression can occur.

For patients that have experienced or are suspected to have experienced an overdose, consultation with a 24-hour poison consultation center specializing in providing veterinary-specific information is recommended. For general information related to overdose and toxin exposures, as well as contact information for poison control centers, refer to ***Appendix***.

Drug Interactions

The following drug interactions have either been reported or are theoretical in humans or animals receiving meperidine and may be of significance in veterinary patients. Unless otherwise noted, use together is not necessarily contraindicated, but weigh the potential risks and perform additional monitoring when appropriate.

- **ACYCLOVIR**: May increase plasma concentrations of meperidine and normeperidine[2]
- **ANTICHOLINERGIC AGENTS**: Medications with anticholinergic properties may increase the risk for urinary retention and constipation when combined with opioids.
- **ANTIHYPERTENSIVE AGENTS/VASODILATORS** (eg, **amlodipine, enalapril, hydralazine, prazosin, sildenafil**): Concurrent use may increase the risk for hypotension and other adverse effects.
- **BUTORPHANOL, NALBUPHINE, NALTREXONE, NALOXONE**: Opioid antagonists and partial agonists may contribute to central nervous system (CNS) excitatory effects of normeperidine (see ***Overdose/Acute Toxicity***). In cases where normeperidine excitotoxicity is suspected, avoid the use of naloxone or butorphanol unless severe respiratory depression is present without a method of ventilatory support.[7]
- **CENTRAL NERVOUS SYSTEM DEPRESSANTS, OTHER** (eg, **anesthetic agents, antihistamines, barbiturates, benzodiazepines,[2] ethanol, phenothiazines**): May cause increased central nervous system or respiratory depression when used with meperidine
- **CIMETIDINE**: Serum concentrations of meperidine may be increased when given concurrently.
- **DESMOPRESSIN**: Opioids may increase the risk for water intoxication or hyponatremia when combined with desmopressin.
- **GASTROINTESTINAL AGENTS, PROKINETIC** (eg, **metoclopramide, cisapride**): Opioids may antagonize the GI motility effects of these agents.
- **DIURETICS**: Opioids may decrease efficacy in congestive heart failure patients.
- **IOHEXOL**: Meperidine may lower the seizure threshold, increasing the risk for seizure and potential adverse/toxic effects from iohexol. Discontinue meperidine 2 days prior to iohexol use and wait 24 hours after iohexol administration to restart meperidine.
- **ISONIAZID**: Meperidine may enhance isoniazid's adverse effects.
- **MINOCYCLINE**: IV minocycline therapy may enhance the central nervous system depressant effects of meperidine.
- **MONOAMINE OXIDASE INHIBITORS** (MAOIs; eg, **amitraz, linezolid, methylene blue,** possibly **selegiline**): Meperidine is contraindicated in patients receiving MAOIs and for at least 14 days after receiving MAOIs in humans. Some human patients have exhibited signs of opioid overdose after receiving therapeutic doses of meperidine while taking MAO inhibitors.
- **MUSCLE RELAXANTS, SKELETAL**: Meperidine may enhance neuromuscular blockade, and additive CNS depression may be seen.
- **SUCCINYLCHOLINE**: Opioids, combined with succinylcholine, may enhance the bradycardic effects of opioids.
- **SEROTONIN MODULATORS** (eg, **metoclopramide, mirtazapine, ondansetron, SSRIs [eg, fluoxetine], trazodone**): Opioids may enhance the serotonergic effect of other serotonin modulators, potentially causing serotonin syndrome.
- **TRICYCLIC ANTIDEPRESSANTS** (TCAs; eg, **amitriptyline, clomipramine**): Meperidine may exacerbate the effects of tricyclic antidepressants.
- **WARFARIN**: Opioids may potentiate anticoagulant activity.

Laboratory Considerations

- Opioids may increase biliary tract pressure, resulting in increased **plasma amylase** and **lipase** values up to 24 hours following opioid administration.
- Increased **bromosulfophthalein (BSP)** retention.
- Increased **creatine kinase (CK)** with IM injections.

Dosages

DOGS:

Analgesic (extra-label): Dosage recommendations vary but generally are 3 – 5 mg/kg (up to 11 mg/kg has been noted) IM or SC. Analgesic duration in dogs usually lasts 30 minutes to 2 hours.

Analgesic for anesthetic premedication (extra-label):

a) One study recommended atropine 0.04 mg/kg IM 20 minutes before administering meperidine 2 mg/kg IM with propofol to effect until loss of pedal reflexes.[8]

b) 3 – 4 mg/kg IM have been used to pre-medicate dogs undergoing pacemaker placement due to the potential positive chronotropic effects of meperidine.[9]

c) 2 mg/kg administered as premedication reduced the dose of propofol required to induce general anesthesia, but muscle twitching and defecation were noted.

CATS:

NOTE: Meperidine is generally not recommended for use in cats.

Analgesic for perioperative pain (extra-label): Dosage recommendations vary but generally are 2 – 5 mg/kg IM or SC. Analgesic duration of in cats lasts 30 minutes to greater than 1 hour. A premedication dose of meperidine 6 mg/kg IM was reported to be inferior to tramadol 2 – 4 mg/kg IM to control postoperative pain in cats undergoing ovariohysterectomy.[10]

HORSES:

Analgesic (extra-label): 1 – 2 mg/kg IM or 0.3 – 0.6 mg/kg slow IV. A study comparing meperidine 1 mg/kg IM vs placebo for treating pain associated with experimental laminitis found meperidine was more effective, but analgesic effects only lasted 2 to 3.7 hours. The authors concluded that it could be used as an alternative analgesic for acute foot pain, with efficacy lasting 2 to 3 hours.[11] **NOTE**: Meperidine may cause central nervous system excitement or ataxia in horses. Some clinicians recommend pretreatment with acepromazine 0.02 – 0.04 mg/kg IV or xylazine 0.3 – 0.5 mg/kg IV to reduce drug-induced behavioral changes. **WARNING**: Narcotic analgesics can mask behavioral and cardiovascular signs associated with mild colic.

CATTLE:

Perioperative analgesic (extra-label): 3.3 – 4.4 mg/kg IM or SC[12]

FERRETS:

Analgesic (extra-label): 5 – 10 mg/kg IM or SC every 2 to 3 hours[13]

RABBITS:

Analgesic for moderate pain (extra-label): 5 – 10 mg/kg IM or SC every 2 to 3 hours. Use banana flavored oral syrup: 0.2 mg/mL in drinking water[14]

SMALL MAMMALS (RODENTS):

Analgesic (extra-label): 5 – 10 mg/kg IM, IV, or SC every 2 to 4 hours[13]

Monitoring

- Respiratory rate and depth; $ETCO_2$; pulse oximetry (SpO_2)
- Heart rate
- CNS level of depression/excitation

- Blood pressure (especially with IV use)
- Analgesic efficacy
- Body temperature

Client Information

- Give this medicine to your animal as directed by your veterinarian.
- Oral formulations of this medicine may cause mouth irritation.
- Meperidine is classified as a Schedule II controlled drug by the federal Drug Enforcement Agency (DEA) and requires a new written prescription for every refill. The use of this medication in animals or humans without a prescription is illegal.

Chemistry/Synonyms

Meperidine HCl, a synthetic opioid analgesic, is a fine, white, crystalline, odorless powder that is very soluble in water, sparingly soluble in ether, and soluble in alcohol. Meperidine has a pK_a of 7.7 to 8.15 and a melting range of 186°C to 189°C (367°F-372°F). The pH of the commercially available injectable preparation is between 3.5 and 6.

Meperidine HCl may also be known as pethidine HCl, isonipecaine, meperidine hydrochloride, pethidini hydrochloridum, or *Demerol*®.

Storage/Stability

Meperidine is a DEA Schedule II controlled substance. It should be stored in an area that is substantially constructed and securely locked. Follow applicable local, state, and federal rules regarding the disposal of unused or wasted controlled drugs.

Meperidine is stable at room temperature. Avoid freezing the injectable solution and protect from light during storage. Meperidine has not exhibited significant adsorption to polyvinyl chloride (PVC) IV bags or tubing in studies to date.

Compatibility/Compounding Considerations

Compatibility is dependent on factors such as pH, concentration, temperature, and diluent used; specialized references or a hospital pharmacist should be consulted for more specific information.

Meperidine is reported to be physically **compatible** with the following fluids and drugs: 0.45% and 0.9% sodium chloride; Ringer's injection; lactated Ringer's; 2.5%, 5%, and 10% dextrose for injection; dextrose/sodium chloride combinations; dextrose/lactated Ringer's solutions; atropine, butorphanol, chlorpromazine, dimenhydrinate, diphenhydramine HCl, dobutamine, fentanyl citrate, glycopyrrolate, metoclopramide, pentazocine lactate, promazine HCl, succinylcholine, verapamil HCl as well as other drugs. Consult a specialized reference for additional information.

Meperidine is reported to have **variable compatibility** when admixed with sodium bicarbonate and when mixed in a syringe with atropine and promethazine. Meperidine is reported to have **variable compatibility at Y-sites** with the following agents: acyclovir, ampicillin, ampicillin-sulbactam, cefotetan, chloramphenicol, dexamethasone, doxorubicin, furosemide, haloperidol, heparin, hydralazine, hydrocortisone sodium succinate, imipenem, magnesium sulfate, methylprednisolone sodium succinate, minocycline, oxacillin, and sulfamethoxazoletrimethoprim.

Meperidine is reported to be **incompatible** when admixed with the following agents: aminophylline, heparin sodium, morphine sulfate, pentobarbital sodium, phenobarbital sodium, phenytoin sodium, and thiopental. It is reported to be **incompatible** when mixed in a syringe with the following agents: heparin sodium, morphine sulfate, pantoprazole, pentobarbital sodium, and thiopental. Meperidine is reported to be **incompatible at Y-sites** with the following agents: allopurinol, amphotericin B, azathioprine, cefepime, cefoperazone, dantrolene, diazepam, diazoxide, idarubicin, lorazepam, pantoprazole, pentobarbital, phenobarbital, phenytoin, sodium bicarbonate, and thiopental.

Dosage Forms/Regulatory Status

VETERINARY-LABELED PRODUCTS: NONE

HUMAN-LABELED PRODUCTS:

Meperidine HCl Injection: 10 mg/mL (30 mL), 25 mg/0.5 mL (0.5 mL), 25 mg/mL (1 mL), 50 mg/mL (1 mL, 30 mL), 75 mg/1.5 mL (1.5 mL), 75 mg/mL (1 mL), and 100 mg/mL (1 mL, 20 mL); *Demerol*®, generic; (Rx, C-II)

Meperidine HCl Tablets: 50 mg and 100 mg; *Demerol*®, generic; (Rx, C-II)

Meperidine HCl Syrup/Oral Solution: 50 mg/5 mL (500 mL); generic; (Rx, C-II)

NOTE: Report dispensing to state monitoring programs where required.

References

For the complete list of references, see **wiley.com/go/budde/plumb**

Mepivacaine

(me-***piv***-a-kane) *Carbocaine®-V, Isocaine®*

Local Anesthetic

Prescriber Highlights

- ▶ Amide type local anesthetic with a quick onset (5 to 10 minutes) and intermediate duration of action (2 to 3 hours) compared with others in its class
- ▶ FDA-approved for infiltration, nerve block, intra-articular, and epidural anesthesia in horses
- ▶ Local anesthetics are absorbed from the site of administration and may have systemic effects.
- ▶ Adverse effects are usually minimal when used correctly, but local anesthetic systemic toxicity, including cardiac and CNS effects, may occur.
- ▶ Use should be limited to clinicians experienced in the diagnosis and management of local anesthetic systemic toxicity; resources for treating acute emergencies must be readily available.

Uses/Indications

Mepivacaine is indicated for infiltration, nerve block, intra-articular and epidural anesthesia, and anesthesia of the laryngeal mucosa prior to ventriculectomy for horses. Perineural analgesic duration during lameness evaluations may be shorter than observed for soft-tissue analgesia.[1] Adding mepivacaine to an IV regional limb perfusion with amikacin provided analgesia without altering amikacin's antimicrobial activity under experimental conditions.[2] Combination with triamcinolone acetonide for intra-articular injection into the metacarpophalangeal joints of horses did not alter the potency or duration of triamcinolone's action.[3] Topical ocular administration decreased corneal sensitivity immediately, and this persisted for 35 minutes.[4] When used in dogs intra-articularly before elbow arthroscopy, mepivacaine blunts the hemodynamic response and reduces interventional analgesia requirement.[5] Similarly, intra-articular mepivacaine prior to carpal arthroscopy in horses resulted in fewer detectable reactions to surgical stimulation, with similar recovery scores and blood pressure support requirements.[6]

The duration of analgesia from local anesthetics can be extended when combined with opioids. Mepivacaine can have a MAC-sparing effect on general anesthesia in dogs and horses,[7,8] and leads to better postoperative recovery.[9]

Intra-articular mepivacaine facilitated diagnostic evaluations of canine elbows, although false negative results were observed.[10] Intra-articular mepivacaine combined with iohexol was determined to be safe and reliable when used in a diagnostic test for identifying and confirming the source of pain in dogs with shoulder joint lameness.[11]

Mepivacaine has been used to provide local or epidural anesthesia in a variety of other species, including cattle, small ruminants, and swine.

Pharmacology/Actions

Local anesthetics block sodium ion channels on the nerve cell membrane, thereby altering electrical excitability, depolarization, and action potential propagation. They block the generation and conduction of impulses in motor, sensory, and autonomic nerve fibers around the site of application. Nerve fiber diameter, conduction velocity, and myelination determine loss of nerve function. Clinically, the progressive loss of nerve function occurs in the following order: pain, temperature, touch, proprioception, and skeletal muscle tone. Anesthetic effect is lost in reverse order.

Mepivacaine produces analgesia typically within 3 to 20 minutes of administration, and this persists for 2 to 2.5 hours. Mepivacaine has a slower onset of analgesia than lidocaine but is more rapid than bupivacaine. Its duration of action is longer than lidocaine but shorter than bupivacaine. However, after palmar digital nerve block in horses, desensitization of the skin was observed for ≈107 minutes as compared with only 25 and 53 minutes with lidocaine and bupivacaine, respectively.[12] The duration of action after IV regional perfusion is ≈150 minutes.[13]

Pharmacokinetics

Local anesthetics are absorbed from their site of administration into systemic circulation. The rate and extent of systemic absorption increases with the dose and volume given, repeated administration, administration in the head and neck region, and administration into highly vascularized sites.

Mepivacaine may diffuse into surrounding tissue after intrasynovial[14-17] and perineural[18,19] administration. The extent of tissue diffusion may be dependent on administration volume and injection approach.[20]

Pharmacokinetic information was not found for veterinary species. In humans, peak concentrations occur ≈3 to 20 minutes after administration. Systemically absorbed drug distributes into all tissues, including the CNS, placenta, and into breast milk. Protein binding is ≈75%. Mepivacaine is hepatically metabolized and undergoes enterohepatic recirculation but is predominantly excreted in the urine as metabolites. Elimination half-life in humans is ≈2 to 3 hours in adults and ≈9 hours in neonates.

Epinephrine (at a very low concentration) may be added to mepivacaine products to cause vasoconstriction at the site of administration, thereby reducing the rate of systemic absorption. Epinephrine prolongs the duration of action at the site of administration, as well as minimizes systemic mepivacaine toxicity. Dexmedetomidine also prolongs the duration of mepivacaine anesthesia at the palmar digital nerves of horses.[21]

Contraindications/Precautions/Warnings

Mepivacaine is contraindicated in patients with a known hypersensitivity to it or to other amide-type local anesthetic agents. Injections should be administered aseptically, aspirating frequently and relocating the needle if blood is aspirated. Ensure adequacy of local anesthesia prior to starting painful procedures. Care should be taken when administering epidural anesthesia to avoid injecting the local anesthetic into the subarachnoid space. Local anesthetics with preservatives should not be used for epidural or intrathecal anesthesia. Epidural injections should be administered incrementally, with aspiration prior to each dose to avoid intravascular injection.

To reduce potential toxicoses, high doses should be used with caution in patients with hepatic or renal disease or impaired cardiovascular function. Chondrolysis has occurred in humans receiving intra-articular infusions. Mepivacaine maintained equine chondrocyte viability to a greater extent than lidocaine or bupivacaine, and mepivacaine was less toxic to equine chondrocytes than bupivacaine in in vitro studies.[22,23]

Mepivacaine products that contain epinephrine should be used with caution, or not at all, in patients with hypertension, if the integrity of the nerve is compromised (it might cause nerve ischemic injury), or to block extremities without collateral circulation (eg, digits, ears, nose, or penis), as it may cause tissue necrosis.

Adverse Effects

Local anesthetics are generally well tolerated when administered correctly. Adverse effects (ie, local anesthetic systemic toxicity) are related to high plasma concentrations, which may result from the dosage or mepivacaine concentration used, rapid absorption from the injection site, and unintentional intravascular or subarachnoid injection.

Adverse cardiovascular effects include bradycardia, AV block, and decreased cardiac output; hypotension may occur but is less likely with mepivacaine than other amide-class anesthetics. Either CNS excitation (eg, restlessness, tremors) or depression (eg, drowsiness, loss of consciousness) may occur. Nausea and vomiting may occur in species with the ability to vomit. Other local anesthetics have caused methemoglobinemia, but this has not been reported with mepivacaine.

Reproductive/Nursing Safety

Local anesthetics readily cross the placenta; however, animal reproductive studies have not been conducted with mepivacaine. Use during labor and delivery may cause fetal and neonatal toxicity, including cardiovascular and CNS effects.

The extent to which mepivacaine is excreted in milk is unknown; use with caution during lactation.

Because safety has not been established in animals, this drug should only be used when the maternal benefits outweigh the potential risks to offspring.

Overdose/Acute Toxicity

Toxic blood concentrations are most likely to occur after unintended intravascular administration. Toxic effects may occur rapidly and simultaneously. Cardiac conduction and excitability are depressed, which may lead to AV block, ventricular arrhythmias, and cardiac arrest; arrhythmias may be refractory to treatment. In addition, myocardial contractility is depressed, and peripheral vasodilation occurs, leading to decreased cardiac output and arterial blood pressure. CNS stimulation (eg, restlessness, tremors, and shivering progressing to convulsions) may precede CNS depression, coma, and respiratory arrest. The mean dosage that induced seizures in rhesus monkeys was 18.8 mg/kg. The LD_{50} in mice was 23 to 35 mg/kg IV.

Management must begin with delivery of oxygen via a patent airway. Benzodiazepines or barbiturates can be used for seizure management but may cause further CNS depression. Cardiovascular support should be provided and may include IV fluids and vasopressor drugs (eg, epinephrine); use of lidocaine, calcium channel blockers, and beta blockers should generally be avoided. Prolonged resuscitative efforts may be required. IV lipid emulsion therapy may be beneficial.

For patients that have experienced or are suspected to have experienced an overdose, consultation with a 24-hour poison consultation center specializing in providing veterinary-specific information is recommended. For general information related to overdose and toxin exposures, as well as contact information for poison control centers, refer to ***Appendix***.

Drug Interactions

The following drug interactions have either been reported or are theoretical in humans or animals receiving mepivacaine and may be of significance in veterinary patients. Unless otherwise noted, use

together is not necessarily contraindicated, but weigh the potential risks and perform additional monitoring when appropriate.

- **Propranolol**: May increase mepivacaine concentration and risk for toxicity

Severe, prolonged hypertension may result when using mepivacaine/epinephrine combination products with the following:

- **Ergot Alkaloids**
- **Monoamine Oxidase Inhibitors** (eg, **selegiline, linezolid, amitraz)**
- **Tricyclic Antidepressants** (eg, **amitriptyline, clomipramine)**
- **Vasopressors** (eg, **dobutamine, norepinephrine)**

Laboratory Considerations

- Mepivacaine may increase **(99m) Technetium hydroxymethylene diphosphonate** tissue uptake following peroneal nerve block in horses.[24]

Dosages

NOTE: Mepivacaine product concentration, administration volume, site of administration, administration technique, and underlying patient condition(s) are important interrelated factors that determine mepivacaine's safe and effective use. Local anesthetics should only be used by clinicians well versed in correct administration technique, diagnosis, and management of local anesthetic toxicity, and who have completed resuscitative resources immediately available. All dosages are for a 2% solution unless otherwise stated.

DOGS:

Local analgesia (extra-label): 1 – 5 mg/kg [25,26]

Epidural analgesia and anesthesia (extra-label): 3 – 4.5 mg/kg[27]

CATS:

Local analgesia (extra-label): 0.5 – 2.5 mg/kg[25]

Epidural analgesia and anesthesia (extra-label): 1 – 1.5 mg/kg[27]

HORSES:

The following FDA-approved dosages are a general guide[28]:

Nerve block (diagnosis of lameness, firing, pain relief in osteoarthritis, navicular disease): 3 – 15 mL total dose (NOT mg/kg)

Epidural anesthesia (animal standing): 5 – 20 mL total dose (NOT mg/kg)

Intra-articular anesthesia (removal of fracture chips, bone and bog spavin, arthritis): 10 – 15 mL total dose (NOT mg/kg)

Infiltration (alone or in combination with nerve block or intra-articular anesthesia): As required

Anesthesia of the laryngeal mucosa prior to ventriculectomy: Administer topically, or by infiltration, or by a combination of the 2. For topical application, a total of 25 – 40 mL applied by spray (3 mL per application) is usually adequate. For infiltration, 20 to 50 mL will suffice.

Diagnostic analgesia of the foot (extra-label): The following doses use a mepivacaine 2% solution.[29]

a) **Palmar/plantar digital nerve**: 1.5 mL over each nerve
b) **Abaxial sesamoid nerve**: 2.5 mL over each nerve; a larger volume may anesthetize the fetlock.
c) **DIP joint**: 5 – 6 mL administered into the joint will also anesthetize the navicular apparatus. 10 mL may anesthetize the entire sole.

Retrobulbar block (extra-label): 10 – 12 mL total dose (NOT mg/kg) injected into the retrobulbar space[30]

Stifle joint anesthesia and analgesia (extra-label): 20 mL total dose (NOT mg/kg) injected into each stifle joint synovial compartment.[31]

Local block (extra-label): Less than 4 mg/kg[8]

Epidural analgesia and anesthesia for urogenital surgery (extra-label): 5 – 7 mL total dose (NOT mg/kg) alone or in combination with 0.1 mg/kg morphine[32]

IV regional limb perfusion (extra-label): Mepivacaine 500 mg was added to 1 gallon amikacin, diluted with saline to 60 mL final volume, and administered by cephalic vein for 30-minute duration.[2]

CATTLE:

Local analgesia (extra-label): 5 mg/kg[33]

SHEEP/GOATS:

Local analgesia (extra-label): 6 mg/kg. Dilute to 1% solution when administering to lambs or kids.[33]

Caudal epidural analgesia and anesthesia (extra-label): 2 – 4 mL total dose (NOT mg/kg) in the sacrocaudal or the first intercoccygeal space should anesthetize the perineum and vagina without interfering with motor function.[34]

SWINE:

Analgesia during castration (extra-label): 0.5 mL total dose (NOT mg/kg) injected intratesticularly and 0.5 mL total dose (NOT mg/kg) injected subscrotally[35]

Monitoring

- Adequacy of analgesia and anesthesia
- Cardiovascular and respiratory function as well as state of consciousness, after each injection

Client Information

- This drug should only be used by professionals familiar with its use and in a setting where adequate patient monitoring can be performed.
- This medication causes temporary loss of feeling. The area where it was injected may not have usual function for several hours.

Chemistry/Synonyms

Mepivacaine hydrochloride is an amide-class local anesthetic. It occurs as a white, odorless crystalline powder and is freely soluble in water and alcohol.

Mepivacaine hydrochloride is also known as mepivacaini hydrochloridum, *Carbocaine*®, and *Isocaine*®.

Storage/Stability

Mepivacaine should be stored at controlled room temperatures of 20°C to 25°C (68°F-77°F). Mepivacaine stored under field conditions for equine use was found to maintain pH and potency without microbial contamination in a variety of storage conditions and with repeated vial use over 12 months.[36]

Compatibility/Compounding Considerations

Compatibility is dependent on factors such as pH, concentration, temperature, and diluent used; specialized references or a hospital pharmacist should be consulted for more specific information.

Mepivacaine HCl is **compatible** with 0.9% sodium chloride solutions, epinephrine, and gentamicin. Mepivacaine HCl is reported to be **variably compatible** with sodium bicarbonate, and to be **incompatible** with bupivacaine. Mepivacaine solutions to which sodium bicarbonate have been added (to reduce pain on infiltration) should be used immediately and promptly discarded.

The recommended final concentration of epinephrine for combined use with mepivacaine is 5 µg/mL. To reach this concentration, add 0.1 mL of epinephrine 1 mg/mL to 20 mL of local anesthetic.

Dosage Forms/Regulatory Status

VETERINARY-LABELED PRODUCTS:

Mepivacaine Hydrochloride Injection: 2% (20 mg/mL) in 50 mL

multidose vials; *Carbocaine®-V*; (Rx). FDA-approved for use in horses not intended for human consumption. NADA# 100-703

The Association of Racing Commissioners International (ARCI) has designated this drug as a class 2 substance. Use of this drug may not be allowed in certain animal competitions. Check rules and regulations before entering in a competition while this medication is being administered. Contact local racing authorities for further guidance. See the ***Appendix*** for more information.

HUMAN -LABELED PRODUCTS:

Mepivacaine Hydrochloride Injection: 1%, 1.5%, and 2% in 20 mL or 30 mL single-dose vials, and 50 mL multidose vials; *Carbocaine®*, *Isocaine®*, generic; (Rx)

References

For the complete list of references, see **wiley.com/go/budde/plumb**

Meropenem

(mare-oh-***pen***-ehm) *Merrem IV®*

Carbapenem Antibiotic

Prescriber Highlights

- Broad-spectrum parenteral antibiotic
- Can be administered more rapidly and with less volume than imipenem
- Adverse effects are uncommon; drug is usually well tolerated
- Use in veterinary medicine is controversial because of the drug's importance in human medicine. Veterinary infectious disease specialists should be consulted prior to treatment. Use should be reserved for infections with confirmed susceptibility that are resistant to lower-tier options.

Uses/Indications

Meropenem is a carbapenem that is used to provide broad coverage for both gram-positive and gram-negative infections, but it is especially useful in infections caused by extended-spectrum beta-lactamase–producing Enterobacterales or *Pseudomonas aeruginosa.*[1] Because this antibiotic is used for multidrug-resistant infections in humans, its use in veterinary medicine should be reserved for confirmed infections where culture and susceptibility testing demonstrates resistance to all other options, the infection is considered treatable, and consultation with an infectious disease expert has concluded that meropenem is a viable and reasonable treatment.[1-3]

Parenteral administration of meropenem is required. Meropenem can be used judiciously for outpatient treatment of stable patients, as it is amenable for SC administration; however, it is not intended for home management of critical patients (eg, sepsis).

The World Health Organization (WHO) classifies meropenem as a Critically Important, High Priority antibiotic for human use.[4]

Pharmacology/Actions

Meropenem has a broad antibacterial spectrum similar to that of imipenem, but meropenem is more active against Enterobacterales and less so against gram-positive bacteria. Synergy against *Pseudomonas aeruginosa* could occur when meropenem is used with aminoglycosides. Meropenem resistance is currently rare in dogs and cats, but carbapenemase-producing bacteria are a serious and increasing problem in humans and sporadic carbapenem-resistant infections in animals have been reported.[5-7] Methicillin-resistant *Staphylococcus* spp are resistant to carbapenems. Meropenem has demonstrated in vitro or in vivo activity against the following bacteria: *Enterococcus faecalis, Staphylococcus aureus, Staphylococcus epidermidis* (methicillin-susceptible isolates only), *Streptococcus* spp, *Escherichia coli, Haemophilus influenzae, Klebsiella pneumoniae, Klebsiella oxytoca, Neisseria meningitides, Pseudomonas aeruginosa, Proteus mirabilis, Aeromonas hydrophila, Campylobacter jejuni, Citrobacter koseri, Citrobacter freundii, Enterobacter cloacae, Hafnia alvei, Moraxella catarrhalis, Morganella morganii, Pasteurella multocida, Proteus vulgaris, Bacteroides* spp, *Peptostreptococcus* spp, *Clostridium difficile, Clostridium perfringens, Eubacterium lentum, Fusobacterium* spp, *Prevotella* spp, and *Porphyromonas asaccharolytica.*

Because meropenem is more resistant to renal dehydropeptidase-I than imipenem is, meropenem does not require the addition of cilastatin to inhibit that enzyme.

Pharmacokinetics

Meropenem is a time-dependent antibacterial that must be administered parenterally.

After SC injection in dogs, bioavailability is 84%.[8] After IV injection in dogs, the volume of distribution is ≈0.37 L/kg, protein binding is ≈12%, half-life is ≈40 minutes, and clearance is ≈6.5 mL/minute/kg. Concentrations of total and unbound drug in tissue or interstitial fluid and plasma are similar.[8,9] In dogs receiving intermittent hemodialysis, the extraction ratio was 0.46 and dialysis clearance was 71 mL/hour/kg.[10]

After IV injection in cats, peak concentration was 101 µg/mL, volume of distribution was 0.21 L/kg, and the drug was minimally protein bound (1.54% to 9.38%).[11] Half-life was ≈1.35 hours and clearance was ≈0.11 L/hour/kg. Following SC and IM administration in cats, bioavailability was 96.5% and 99.6%, respectively. Absorption was significantly faster after IM administration compared with SC (0.5 vs 1.7 hours). Half-life was ≈2.2 hours following either SC or IM administration.

Following a single IV injection in horses, peak concentration (77 µg/mL) was reached in ≈1 hour, the volume of distribution was 136 mL/kg, and protein binding was 7% to 11%.[2] Half-life was 0.8 hours and clearance was 165 mL/hour/kg. Meropenem penetrated into synovial fluid, reaching peak concentration of 7.5 µg/mL 1 hour after IV administration, and the half-life in synovial fluid was 2.4 hours. Following IV regional limb perfusion, the concentration of meropenem in synovial fluid remained above 1 µg/mL for 3 hours.[12]

In ewes, after IM injection meropenem was rapidly absorbed and had a bioavailability equal to that of IV dosing.[13] Volume of distribution at steady state was 0.06 L/kg and protein binding was ≈43%; elimination half-life was ≈43 minutes. After IM injection, 91% of the drug was recovered in the urine over 24 hours.

Pharmacokinetic data for humans include wide distribution in body tissues and fluids, including into the CSF and bile and very low protein binding.[3] In patients with normal renal function, elimination half-life is ≈1 hour. One inactive metabolite has been identified, but the majority of the drug is eliminated via renal mechanisms (tubular secretions and glomerular filtration) and 70% of a dose is recovered unchanged in the urine over 12 hours.

Contraindications/Precautions/Warnings

Meropenem is contraindicated in patients that are hypersensitive to it or other carbapenems and in patients that have developed anaphylaxis after receiving any beta-lactam antibiotic.[3]

In humans, carbapenems have been associated with CNS toxicities, including seizures.[3] Meropenem has less associated seizure risk than other carbapenems,[14-16] but it should be used cautiously in patients with a history of seizure disorders or with renal impairment, as accumulation may increase risk for CNS toxicity.[3]

Adverse Effects

Meropenem is usually well tolerated. Anecdotally, animals receiving the drug SC may show changes in fur color or slight fur loss over injection sites. In human patients receiving meropenem, GI effects (nausea, vomiting, diarrhea, constipation), headache, and skin rashes have been reported to occur in more than 1% of patients.[3] Meropenem use in humans is associated with a low risk of seizures, but the risk of meropenem-induced seizures in clinically ill veterinary patients has not been described.[15]

Reproductive/Nursing Safety

Meropenem has not demonstrated fetal toxicity or malformations in laboratory animals.[3,17]

Meropenem is found in the breast milk of humans,[3] but as meropenem is not orally absorbed, it is likely safe to use during lactation. Because safety has not been established in animals, this drug should only be used when the maternal benefits outweigh the potential risks to offspring. As meropenem is used for serious infections only, the potential benefits of treatment likely outweigh the risks.

Overdose/Acute Toxicity

Overdoses of meropenem are unlikely to occur in patients that have normal renal function. In mice and rats, large IV doses of meropenem (2200 mg/kg – 4000 mg/kg) have been associated with ataxia, dyspnea, convulsions, and mortalities.[3] In human trials, doses of 2 g every 8 hours failed to demonstrate any significant adversity. If an overdose occurs, the drug can be discontinued, or the next dose could be delayed by a few hours. Meropenem can be removed via hemodialysis when necessary.

For patients that have experienced or are suspected to have experienced an overdose, consultation with a 24-hour poison consultation center specializing in providing veterinary-specific information is recommended. For general information related to overdose and toxin exposures, as well as contact information for poison control centers, refer to ***Appendix.***

Drug Interactions

The following drug interactions have either been reported or are theoretical in humans or animals receiving meropenem and may be of significance in veterinary patients. Unless otherwise noted, use together is not necessarily contraindicated, but weigh the potential risks and perform additional monitoring when appropriate.

- **Aminoglycosides**: The combination of aminoglycosides and meropenem can be synergistic against some isolates of *Pseudomonas aeruginosa.*
- **Probenecid**: May increase serum concentrations and elimination half-life of meropenem

Laboratory Considerations

- No specific laboratory interactions noted

Dosages

NOTES:

1. Meropenem susceptibility and resistance to first-line antibacterial drugs should be confirmed prior to using the drug.
2. Consultation with a veterinary infectious disease specialist or veterinary pharmacologist prior to use is recommended.[1]
3. Concurrent aminoglycoside therapy is indicated for infections caused by *Pseudomonas aeruginosa*.
4. De-escalate therapy to a lower-tier antibiotic class if culture and susceptibility results indicate an antibacterial agent with a narrower spectrum would be effective.
5. Usually administered IV over 15 to 30 minutes, although low volumes can be given over 3 to 5 minutes

DOGS:

Documented multidrug-resistant UTIs, particularly those caused by multidrug-resistant Enterobacterales *or P aeruginosa* (extra-label): 8.5 mg/kg SC every 12 hours or slowly IV every 8 hours[1]

Documented multidrug-resistant systemic or soft tissue infections caused by Enterobacterales (extra-label): 8.5 mg/kg SC every 12 hours or 24 mg/kg IV every 12 hours[8,18]

Documented multidrug-resistant systemic or soft tissue infections caused by *P aeruginosa* or other similar organisms with MIC values near 1 μg/mL (extra-label): 12 mg/kg SC every 8 hours or 25 mg/kg IV every 8 hours.[8,19] A pharmacokinetic study has determined that a loading dose of 0.37 mg/kg IV bolus followed by 0.38 mg/kg/hour IV CRI could maintain plasma meropenem concentration of 1 μg/mL.[9]

***Escherichia coli*-associated granulomatous colitis** (extra-label): 10 mg/kg SC every 12 hours for at least 6 weeks[20]

CATS:

Documented multidrug-resistant UTIs, particularly those caused by multidrug-resistant Enterobacteriaceae *or P aeruginosa* (extra-label): 10 mg/kg IV, SC, or IM every 12 hours[1]

Documented multidrug-resistant systemic or soft tissue infections, specifically caused by Enterobacteriaceae (extra-label): 10 mg/kg SC, IM, or IV every 12 hours[19]

HORSES:

Documented multidrug-resistant systemic or soft tissue infections (extra-label): Based on a pharmacokinetic study, 5 mg/kg IV every 8 hours or 0.5 mg/kg/hour as a CRI should maintain meropenem concentration above the MIC target of 1 μg/mL for an adequate time.[2]

Monitoring

- Clinical efficacy: resolution of clinical signs associated with UTI or other systemic infection[1]
- Recheck urinalysis (for UTI) and aerobic bacterial culture and susceptibility 5 to 7 days after cessation of antimicrobials[1]

Client Information

- Meropenem must be injected in the vein or under the skin of your animal; it does not work if given by mouth.
- Your animal's fur may become thinner or change color over the injection site.
- It is important to give this medication exactly as prescribed, to complete the full course of therapy, and to follow up with your veterinarian as instructed, even if your animal seems better. Missing doses, stopping treatment early, or failing to perform recommended recheck testing may result in treatment failure.
- Your veterinarian will need to monitor your animal closely during treatment. Do not miss these important follow-up appointments.

Chemistry/Synonyms

Meropenem is a synthetic carbapenem antibiotic that occurs as a clear to white to pale yellow powder or crystals. It is very slightly soluble in water or hydrated alcohol and practically insoluble in acetone or ether. When the commercially available injection is reconstituted, the resulting pH is between 7.3 and 8.3.

Meropenem may also be known as ICI-194660, SM-7338, *Meronem®*, *Meropen®*, *Merrem®*, *Optinem®*, or *Zeropenem®*.

Storage/Stability

The powder for injection should be stored at controlled room temperature (20°C-25°C [69°F-77°F]). When the commercially available powder for injection is reconstituted with sterile water for injection (up to a concentration of 50 mg/mL), it is labeled as stable (per the manufacturer) for up to 3 hours at room temperature and up to 13 hours when refrigerated. When reconstituted with normal saline in concentrations ranging from 1 to 20 mg/mL, it is stable per the manufacturer for up to 1 hour at temperatures up to 25°C (77°F) and up to 15 hours at temperatures up to 5°C (41°F). When reconstituted with dextrose injection 5%, the solution should be used immediately.

When the dry meropenem powder is reconstituted with sterile water and further diluted to a concentration of 20 mg/mL with sodium chloride 0.9%, the solution is stable for up to 5 days if kept refrigerated

(5°C [41°F]) and protected from light.[21] Once the refrigerated solution is brought back to room temperature, it should be used within 1 hour.[17]

Meropenem and sodium chloride injection solution in DUPLEX containers should be stored at controlled room temperature (20°C-25°C [69°F-77°F]). Reconstituted solution should be used within 1 hour but may be stored under refrigeration for up to 15 hours. Administer only if solution is clear and free from particulates.

The manufacturer recommends that solutions of meropenem should not be frozen.[17] Additionally, one study noted the formation of a precipitate after thawing of a frozen meropenem solution.[22]

Compatibility/Compounding Considerations

Compatibility is dependent on factors such as pH, concentration, temperature, and diluent used; specialized references or a hospital pharmacist should be consulted for more specific information.

Meropenem has been reported **compatible** with vancomycin, ranitidine, morphine sulfate, metoclopramide, heparin, gentamicin, furosemide, dopamine, dobutamine, dexamethasone sodium phosphate, atropine, and aminophylline.

Additives should not be added to meropenem and sodium chloride injection solution in DUPLEX containers.

Dosage Forms/Regulatory Status

VETERINARY-LABELED PRODUCTS: NONE

HUMAN-LABELED PRODUCTS:

Meropenem Powder for solution for Injection: 500 mg and 1 g in 20 mL, and 30 mL vials; *Merrem® IV*, generic; (Rx)

Meropenem and Sodium Chloride Injection Solution: 500 mg and 1 g in DUPLEX containers with 50 mL 0.9% NaCl; generic; (Rx)

References

For the complete list of references, see **wiley.com/go/budde/plumb**

Metergoline

(meh-***tir***-goe-leen) *Contralac®, Liserdol®*

Serotonin Antagonist; Prolactin Inhibitor

Prescriber Highlights

- ▶ Serotonin antagonist prolactin inhibitor used primarily for pseudopregnancy in dogs
- ▶ Primary adverse effects are GI (especially vomiting) and behavior related
- ▶ Not commercially available in the United States
- ▶ Metergoline should be handled as a hazardous drug; use appropriate precautions when handling.

Uses/Indications

Metergoline is used to treat pseudopregnancy in dogs. It is available as a veterinary product in several European and South American countries. Metergoline has been investigated as an abortifacient in dogs at high doses (0.4 – 0.6 mg/kg); however, similar to other ergot prolactin inhibitors, it can only be used reliably for this effect during the last 3 weeks of gestation.[1] Metergoline could potentially be used to induce estrus or treat pyometra in bitches.

In humans, metergoline has been used for hyperprolactinemia, prolactinomas, and migraine prophylaxis.

Pharmacology/Actions

Metergoline reduces prolactin primarily via its serotonin antagonism effects. It differs from cabergoline and bromocriptine in that it has both strong central and peripheral antiserotonin effects, and only weak direct dopamine-2-agonist effects. Like those drugs, it also is an antagonist at dopamine-1 receptors. Potentially, metergoline could be used to induce estrus or treat pyometra in bitches.

Pharmacokinetics

Limited pharmacokinetic information is available for dogs. The half-life of metergoline is reportedly short (≈4 hours), and twice-daily dosing is required.

In humans, metergoline oral bioavailability is ≈25% and volume of distribution is 0.8 L/kg. It is metabolized in the liver to at least 1 active metabolite (1-desmethylmetergoline), which attains plasma concentrations higher than that of the parent drug. Elimination half-life is ≈50 minutes for the parent drug and 80 to 100 minutes for 1-desmethylmetergoline.

Contraindications/Precautions/Warnings

Metergoline is contraindicated in dogs and cats that are pregnant unless abortion is desired. It should not be used in patients who are hypersensitive to ergot derivatives. Patients that do not tolerate cabergoline or bromocriptine may or may not tolerate metergoline. Use metergoline with caution in patients with significantly impaired liver function; lower doses may be required.

The National Institute for Occupational Safety and Health (NIOSH) classifies cabergoline, a related drug, as a hazardous drug; personal protective equipment (PPE) should be used accordingly to minimize the risk for exposure. Women who are pregnant or of child-bearing age should avoid contact with or wear disposable gloves when administering metergoline.

Adverse Effects

Reported adverse effects for metergoline in dogs include behavior-related effects (eg, anxiety, aggressiveness, depression, hyperexcitation, whining, escaping) and GI effects (eg, anorexia, vomiting, nausea).[2]

Reproductive/Nursing Safety

Metergoline is contraindicated in dogs and cats that are pregnant unless abortion is desired. Because it suppresses prolactin, metergoline should not be used in nursing mothers.

Overdose/Acute Toxicity

Limited information is available. Vomiting is the most likely effect after an overdose of metergoline.

For patients that have experienced or are suspected to have experienced an overdose, consultation with a 24-hour poison consultation center specializing in providing veterinary-specific information is recommended. For general information related to overdose and toxin exposures, as well as contact information for poison control centers, refer to ***Appendix.***

Drug Interactions

The following drug interactions have either been reported or are theoretical in humans or animals receiving metergoline and may be of significance in veterinary patients. Unless otherwise noted, use together is not necessarily contraindicated, but weigh the potential risks and perform additional monitoring when appropriate.

- **Bromocriptine, Cabergoline**: May cause additive effects if used with metergoline
- **Cyproheptadine**: May cause additive effects if used with metergoline
- **Metoclopramide**: May reduce the efficacy of both drugs and should be avoided.
- **Selective Serotonergic Receptor Inhibitors** (**SSRIs**; eg, **fluoxetine, paroxetine, sertraline**): May reduce the efficacy of each drug

Laboratory Considerations

- No particular laboratory interactions or considerations were located for this drug.

Dosages

DOGS:

Pseudopregnancy or to halt lactation (extra-label): 0.5 mg/kg PO twice daily for 4 to 5 days is effective for the treatment of most bitches. Treatment failures can be managed by repeating the treatment protocol and extending the duration to 8 to 10 days, or by using joint protocols of cabergoline plus metergoline or cabergoline plus bromocriptine.[2]

Pregnancy termination (extra-label): 0.4 – 0.5 mg/kg PO once daily for 5 days[3]

Induce estrus (extra-label): Cabergoline and bromocriptine have consistently given positive results, while metergoline's results have been more variable depending on dosage. Using low dose metergoline 0.1 mg/kg PO twice a day, the commercial oral formulation (administered from 100 days after ovulation until the following proestrus) caused the interestrus interval to be significantly shortened.[4]

CATS:

Pseudopregnancy or to halt lactation (extra-label): 0.125 mg/kg PO twice a day for 4 to 8 days[5]

Monitoring

- Efficacy
- Adverse effects

Client Information

- Give this medicine with food. Contact your veterinarian if your animal has vomiting that does not stop.
- Keep this medication and all other medications away from animals.
- This medication is considered to be a hazardous drug as defined by the National Institute for Occupational Safety and Health (NIOSH). Talk with your veterinarian or pharmacist about the use of personal protective equipment when handling this medicine.

Chemistry/Synonyms

Metergoline is an ergot derivative and has the chemical name benzyl (8S,10S)-(1,6-dimethylergolin-8-ylmethyl)carbamate.

Metergoline may also be known as FI-6337, MCE, Metergoliini, Metergolin, Metergolina, Métergoline, Metergolinum, or Methergoline. Common trade names are *Contralac®* (veterinary) and *Liserdol®* (human).

Storage/Stability

Metergoline tablets should be stored at room temperature and protected from light.

Compatibility/Compounding Considerations

No specific information was noted.

Dosage Forms/Regulatory Status

VETERINARY-LABELED PRODUCTS:

None in the United States. Metergoline 0.5 mg and 2 mg oral tablets are available in some European and South American countries; *Contralac®*

HUMAN-LABELED PRODUCTS:

None in the United States. Metergoline 4 mg tablets are available in some countries.

References

For the complete list of references, see **wiley.com/go/budde/plumb**

Metformin

(met-***fore***-min) *Glucophage®*

Antihyperglycemic

Prescriber Highlights

- ► Oral anti-hyperglycemic agent that could be useful in the adjunctive treatment of noninsulin-dependent diabetes (NIDDM) in dogs and cats or in equine metabolic syndrome; however, its use is controversial
- ► Contraindications include patients hypersensitive to it, patients with renal dysfunction or metabolic acidosis, or temporarily when iodinated contrast agents are required.
- ► Adverse effects may include lethargy, inappetence, vomiting, and weight loss.
- ► Potentially significant drug interactions
- ► Human dosage forms may be difficult to accurately dose in cats; compounded formulations may be required.

Uses/Indications

Metformin may be useful in the adjunctive treatment of noninsulin-dependent diabetes mellitus (NIDDM) in cats. Limited trials of the drug have been performed in cats, with only limited success when the drug is used alone. Currently, metformin should only be used in cats with functional beta cells known to have type 2 diabetes mellitus.[1] Studies comparing its safety and efficacy with other oral antihyperglycemics (eg, glipizide or insulin) were not located.

Metformin may also be useful in dogs with NIDDM; however, evidence is limited, and incidence of NIDDM is rare in canines.[2]

There has been some research evaluating metformin for treating insulin resistance associated with equine metabolic syndrome in horses, but data conflict regarding its efficacy.[3,4] Because of the drug's low cost and low adverse effect profile, further investigation of its clinical usefulness is warranted.

Pharmacology/Actions

Metformin's actions are multifaceted. At usual dosages, it increases insulin's ability to transport glucose across cell membranes in skeletal muscle without increasing lactate production and inhibits the formation of advanced glycosylation end-products. Metformin decreases hepatic glucose production and may decrease intestinal absorption of glucose. It does not stimulate insulin production or release from the pancreas and therefore does not cause hypoglycemia.

In horses, metformin has poor oral bioavailability (around 5%) and is not likely to act systemically; however, there is some indication that metformin may act locally and limit gut glucose uptake. A recently published study in 7 normal horses found that metformin at 30 mg/kg via NG tube 1 hour prior to an oral glucose challenge test (dextrose powder 0.5 g/kg PO in feed) reduced glycemic and insulinemic responses. Further work is required to determine whether these effects may translate into clinical benefits in horses with equine metabolic syndrome and hyperinsulinemia.[4]

In a study evaluating the whole blood of 4 horses, metformin displayed anti-inflammatory properties by reducing TNF-alpha production. Further studies are warranted to determine whether or not these properties have a role in the treatment of equine endotoxemia or other infections.[5]

Pharmacokinetics

A pharmacokinetic study done in cats showed that metformin is variably absorbed (35% to 67%) after oral administration.[6] In cats, the steady-state volume of distribution was 0.55 L/kg, the elimination half-life was ≈12 hours, and total clearance was 0.15 L/hour/kg. Metformin is primarily eliminated via the kidneys. The authors concluded that the drug's pharmacokinetics are similar to those seen in humans, and that a dosage of 2 mg/kg twice daily would give plasma concentrations known to be effective in humans.

In a small (4 subjects) pharmacokinetic study in horses, metformin demonstrated very low oral bioavailability (4% fed, 7% fasted).[7] Maximum blood concentrations were around 0.4 µg/mL. The elimination half-life after IV dosing was ≈25 minutes.

Contraindications/Precautions/Warnings

In humans (and presumably cats), metformin is contraindicated in patients that are hypersensitive to it, patients with severe renal dysfunction, and patients with metabolic acidosis. It is also temporarily contraindicated when iodinated contrast agents are to be used (see ***Drug Interactions***).

In humans, metformin rarely can cause lactic acidosis that may lead to death. The onset can be subtle with nonspecific symptoms, including malaise, myalgia, respiratory distress, somnolence, and abdominal pain.[8] Risk factors for lactic acidosis include renal impairment, old age, hypoxic states (eg, acute congestive heart failure), and hepatic impairment.

In a study evaluating metformin in 5 diabetic cats, 1 cat died unexpectedly 11 days after receiving metformin.[9] As the cause of death was undetermined, metformin could not be ruled out as a causative factor.

Adverse Effects

Metformin caused adverse GI effects (eg, diarrhea, inappetence, vomiting) in ≈40% of dogs, which were managed with dose reduction and weekly dose increases.

In cats, metformin may cause lethargy, inappetence, vomiting, and weight loss. Hypoglycemia would not be an expected adverse effect when metformin is used as a single agent.

Reproductive/Nursing Safety

Metformin is excreted in maternal milk in levels equivalent to those found in plasma. Although adverse effects in nursing kittens would be unlikely, use with caution in lactating queens.

Because safety has not been established in animals, this drug should only be used when the maternal benefits outweigh the potential risks to offspring.

Overdose/Acute Toxicity

In small animals, hypoglycemia is not commonly seen in overdoses with metformin alone, but it has a narrow margin of safety regarding GI upset. Vomiting commonly occurs with ingestion of metformin in small animals. Another common clinical sign associated with overdose is lethargy.

Massive overdoses in humans (100 g) caused hypoglycemia only 10% of the time, but lactic acidosis has occurred. Lactic acidosis has been seen in human overdoses of 7 and 20 g (total dose). It is unknown at what dose acidosis may occur in domestic animals. Ingestion of up to 1700 mg by children is not usually associated with significant toxicity. Enhancement of metformin elimination may be amenable to dialysis.

In 2 case reports in dogs, lactic acidosis and hypoglycemia were reported after ingestion of 198 to 291 mg/kg of metformin.[10,11] Treatment included fluids, dextrose, and sodium bicarbonate, and clinical signs resolved within 24 to 34 hours.

For patients that have experienced or are suspected of having experienced an overdose, consultation with a 24-hour poison consultation center specializing in providing veterinary-specific information is recommended. For general information related to overdose and toxin exposures, as well as contact information for poison control centers, refer to ***Appendix.***

Drug Interactions

The following drug interactions have either been reported or are theoretical in humans or animals receiving metformin and may be of significance in veterinary patients. Unless otherwise noted, use together is not necessarily contraindicated, but weigh the potential risks and perform additional monitoring when appropriate.

- **ACE Inhibitors**: May increase the risk for hypoglycemia
- **Carbonic acid inhibitors** (eg, **acetazolamide, zonisamide**): May increase the risk for lactic acidosis, as carbonic acid inhibitors frequently cause decreased serum bicarbonate.
- **Cimetidine**: In humans, cimetidine can cause a 60% increase in peak metformin plasma levels and a 40% increase in AUC.
- **Corticosteroids** (eg, **dexamethasone, predniso(lo)ne**): May reduce metformin efficacy
- **Diuretics, Thiazide**: May reduce hypoglycemic efficacy
- **Fluoroquinolones** (eg, **enrofloxacin**): May increase the risk for hyperglycemia or hypoglycemia. If the combination is necessary, monitor blood glucose closely.
- **Furosemide**: Can increase the AUC and plasma levels of metformin by 22% in humans; metformin can decrease the peak plasma concentrations and AUC of furosemide.
- **Iodinated Contrast Agents, Parenteral**: May cause acute renal failure and lactic acidosis if used within 48 hours of a metformin dose
- **Isoniazid**: May reduce hypoglycemic efficacy
- **Sympathomimetic Agents** (eg, **phenylpropanolamine**): May reduce hypoglycemic efficacy

Laboratory Considerations

- No specific laboratory interactions or considerations were noted.

Dosages

CATS:

Noninsulin-dependent diabetes mellitus (patients with detectable concentrations of insulin) (extra-label): 2 mg/kg PO twice daily,[6] which generally equals 25 – 50 mg/cat (NOT mg/kg) PO twice daily.[1] If using tablets, must be compounded. No information on the use of the oral liquid (100 mg/mL) or extended-release tablets for use in cats was noted. One 14-day study found the maximum tolerated dose in cats to be 10 mg/kg.[12]

HORSES:

Adjunctive treatment of equine metabolic syndrome (extra-label): NOTE: Use is controversial, and evidence for efficacy conflicts. Reserve metformin treatment for horses and ponies with markedly increased oral sugar test (OST; corn syrup-based) insulin concentrations, even after the loss of body fat mass and dietary management. Current recommendations are metformin 30 mg/kg PO every 8 to 12 hours, preferably 30 to 60 minutes before the horse is fed.[4,13]

Monitoring

- Efficacy: Standard methods of monitoring efficacy for diabetes treatment should be followed (eg, blood glucose, appetite, attitude, body condition, PU/PD resolution, and perhaps serum fructosamine and/or glycosylated hemoglobin levels).
- Renal function (baseline and annually)
- Adverse effects

Client Information

- Monitor your animal for vomiting, decrease in appetite, diarrhea, lethargy, or any other new problems and report them to your veterinarian.
- While your animal is taking this medication, it is important to return to your veterinarian for physical examinations and laboratory work. Do not miss these important follow-up visits.

Chemistry/Synonyms

Metformin HCl is a biguanide oral anti-hyperglycemic agent that occurs as white to off-white crystals that are slightly soluble in alcohol and freely soluble in water. It is a weak base—a 1% aqueous solution of metformin HCl has a pK_a of 6.68, and a metformin base has a pK_a of 12.4.

Metformin HCl may also be known as dimethylbiguanide HCl or metforimini hydrochloridium. There are many proprietary names outside of the United States for this drug.

Storage/Stability

Store metformin HCl oral products (tablets, sustained-release tablets) protected from light at a controlled room temperature of 20°C to 25°C (68°F-77°F). Excursions permitted to 15°C to 30°C (59°F-86°F).

Compatibility/Compounding Considerations

No specific information was noted.

Dosage Forms/Regulatory Status

VETERINARY-LABELED PRODUCTS: NONE

HUMAN-LABELED PRODUCTS:

Metformin HCl Oral Tablets: 500 mg, 850 mg, and 1000 mg; *Glucophage®*, generic; (Rx)

Metformin HCl Extended-Release Oral Tablets: 500 mg, 750 mg, and 1000 mg; *Glucophage XR®*, *Glumetza®*, *Fortamet®*, generic; (Rx)

Metformin HCl Oral Solution: 500 mg/5 mL (100 mg/mL) in 118 mL and 473 mL; *Riomet®*; (Rx)

There are also fixed-dose oral tablet combination products available containing metformin and glyburide or glipizide.

References

For the complete list of references, see **wiley.com/go/budde/plumb**

Methadone

(***meth***-a-done) *Dolophine®, Methadose®*

Opioid Agonist

Prescriber Highlights

- Opioid mu-receptor agonist with NMDA blocking properties used in dogs, cats, and horses
- Can be used for sedation, as premedication before anesthesia, and for analgesia
- Adverse effects include panting, vomiting, vocalization, defecation postinjection, bradycardia, and respiratory depression.
- Many possible drug interactions
- DEA Schedule II (C-II) controlled substance in the United States
- Effects can be reversed with naloxone.

Uses/Indications

Methadone may be used as an opioid sedative, preanesthetic, or analgesic agent. Methadone use as a premedication reduces MAC requirements.[1] Methadone has demonstrated an analgesic effect after epidural use in horses.[2] Poor bioavailability precludes oral administration in dogs.[3]

Pharmacology/Actions

In small animal species, methadone acts similarly to morphine with regard to its degree of analgesia and duration of action. Methadone is a synthetic mu-receptor agonist that is supplied as a racemic mixture; the L-isomer is up to 50 times more potent as a µ-agonist than the D-isomer. Agonism of the mu-opioid receptor (a g-protein coupled receptor) on both pre- and postsynaptic neurons results in decreased transmission and modulation of pain. Presynaptically, binding of the mu-opioid receptor results in closure of calcium ion channels and reduction of neurotransmitter release. Postsynaptically, agonism will open potassium channels, resulting in hyperpolarization and inhibition of postsynaptic neurons.[4] Both methadone isomers are noncompetitive inhibitors of NMDA (N-methyl-D-aspartate) receptors[5] and can reduce reuptake of norepinephrine,[6] which may also contribute to its analgesic effects, especially in patients tolerant to other opioids[7,8]; however, the therapeutic application of this is unknown.

Methadone's depression of the medullary respiratory center results in respiratory depression, and stimulation at the vagal center can cause bradycardia. Methadone is more lipid-soluble than morphine and is therefore more potent due to having more favorable pharmacokinetics. IV administration of methadone has potential for histamine release, but studies have shown no resulting hemodynamic instability[9]; histamine release following administration of methadone by other routes is unknown but possible.

Pharmacokinetics

In dogs, methadone has poor oral bioavailability due to extensive first-pass metabolism.[3,10] Coadministration of multiple CYP450 inhibitors (eg, ketoconazole, fluconazole, fluoxetine, trimethoprim, chloramphenicol) presumably affects different isoenzymes in dogs and has been shown to significantly increase oral absorption, area under the curve (AUC), and plasma concentrations of methadone.[3,11] Methadone absorption after oral transmucosal administration is slower and reduced as compared with methadone given IM.[12] SC administration has a bioavailability of ≈80%, with peak concentrations occurring ≈1 hour after administration. Bioavailability is ≈90% after IM administration,[6] with peak concentrations occurring within 5 to 15 minutes. Vd_{SS} is ≈5 to 6 L/kg, and protein binding is 60% to 90%.[6] Terminal elimination half-life after IV administration is ≈1.75 to 4 hours; clearance is ≈25 to 50 mL/kg/minute.[13,14] After SC and IM administration, half-life is ≈11 hours and ≈1 to 2 hours, respectively; however, there is wide interpatient variation.[6,14]

In cats, bioavailability of buccal (ie, oral transmucosal [OTM]) methadone is 44%.[15] After administration of methadone 0.3 mg/kg IV or 0.6 mg/kg via OTM administration, peak concentrations occurred at 10 minutes (IV) and 2 hours (OTM).[16] A 0.6 mg/kg IM dose provides 4 hours of analgesia and reaches plasma concentration between 40 to 124 ng/mL. T_{max} and clearance were 20 minutes and 9.1 mL/kg/minute, respectively.[17]

In horses, methadone given PO appears to be well absorbed, but bioavailability is ≈3 times lower when administered intragastrically. P-glycoprotein may play a role in the poor intestinal absorption of methadone in vivo. Elimination half-life is ≈1 to 2 hours, and clearance is 5 to 8 mL/kg/minute.[18,19]

In goats, methadone has a high bioavailability and volume of distribution (7 L/kg) after SC administration, with a half-life of ≈3.6 hours. IV administration resulted in a terminal half-life of ≈1.5 hours.[20] Elimination half-life after IM administration was ≈1.4 hours.[21]

In humans, methadone is well absorbed from the GI tract via PO administration and after parenteral injection (SC or IM). Methadone is widely distributed and extensively bound to plasma proteins (60% to 90%, principally $alpha_1$-acid glycoprotein). Methadone is metabolized in the liver to inactive metabolites primarily by the CYPP450, CYP3A, and CYP2B6 isoenzymes, but other isoenzymes also play metabolic roles. Methadone's half-life in humans is widely variable (15 to 60 hours). Elimination half-lives of methadone may be extended if giving multiple doses.

Contraindications/Precautions/Warnings

Methadone is contraindicated in animals hypersensitive to narcotic analgesics and in animals with any condition associated with respiratory depression, acute respiratory dysfunction, advanced respiratory failure, and severe hepatic or renal dysfunction, as well as during parturition.[6,22,23]

Use methadone with extreme caution in patients with head injuries, increased intracranial pressure, or acute abdominal conditions (eg, colic), as it may obscure the diagnosis or clinical course of these conditions.

Use opioids with caution in patients with hypothyroidism and hypoadrenocorticism (ie, Addison's disease), as well as geriatric and severely debilitated patients. Neonatal, debilitated, and geriatric patients or patients with severe hepatic disease may be more susceptible to the effects of methadone, may require lower doses, and should be monitored closely. Greyhounds may require higher doses than other breeds.[24]

Methadone can cause bradycardia and therefore should be used cautiously in patients with pre-existing bradyarrhythmia. Hypotension may occur and result in decreased cardiac output and blood pressure.

Because vomiting may occur, methadone as a preanesthetic in animals with suspected gastric dilatation-volvulus or intestinal obstruction is usually not recommended.

Opioid analgesics are contraindicated in patients stung by scorpions (eg, *Centruroides* spp) as it may potentiate venom effects.[25]

Some dosage forms may contain benzylalcohol as a preservative. In human newborns, benzylalcohol and derivatives can potentially displace bilirubin from protein binding sites; caution in human neonates is advised. There is an FDA black-box warning regarding the risk for misuse and abuse, respiratory depression, QT prolongation, neonatal withdrawal syndrome, accidental ingestion, and addiction treatment when prescribing methadone for humans. QT intervals may be prolonged in patients taking methadone, which can result in life-threatening arrhythmia. Use caution in patients with prolonged QT intervals or those receiving medications that can further prolong QT intervals. See ***Drug Interactions***.

Extreme care should be taken when administering methadone; spillage onto the skin can result in respiratory depression. If methadone comes in contact with skin, wash the area thoroughly and seek medical advice.

Adverse Effects

In dogs, adverse effects can include panting,[26] whining/vocalization,[14] dysphoria, sedation, anorexia,[27] emesis, urination and/or defecation (shortly after injection), constipation or paralytic ileus, reduced body temperature,[3] bradycardia, and respiratory depression or apnea. Systemic vascular resistance may increase.[28,29] Adverse effects appear to be dose-related.[1,30] Methadone tends to cause less sedation or vomiting than morphine.[31] Methadone has a greater cardiodepressant effect than morphine.[32]

In cats, methadone appears to cause less excitation (eg, lip licking, salivation, tremors, urination, vocalization) and vomiting than some other mu-agonists, but these effects can occur. Pupil dilation persists after analgesia in cats.[6] Hyperalgesia has also been reported in cats.

In horses, methadone 0.1 mg/kg IV or greater has caused pronounced CNS excitement. Gut sounds may be diminished.[33] Mean arterial pressure may be increased when administered in combination with detomidine.[34]

In sheep, methadone 0.5 mg/kg IV may result in drooling, bruxism, mydriasis, nystagmus, vocalization, and tremors. Rumination was inhibited in goats receiving SC methadone.[20]

Reproductive/Nursing Safety

Effects on the hypothalamic–pituitary–gonadal axis may cause testicular regression, decreased testosterone concentrations, and reduced sexual activity in males. Administration to animals from the time of organogenesis through lactation has resulted in increased neonate mortality, decreased litter size, neural tube defects, and lifelong behavior alterations.[35]

In humans, methadone is relatively safe to use at low doses for short periods during the first 2 trimesters of pregnancy; methadone administered late in term has caused significant respiratory depression and increased stillbirths.

Epidural administration results in lower umbilical cord methadone concentration than IV methadone.[36] Some veterinary-approved product labels outside of the United States state that methadone is contraindicated for use in animals during parturition.[23]

Methadone has been found in breast milk and there are subsequently low plasma concentrations in nursing human infants.

Although methadone enters maternal milk, it is considered compatible with breastfeeding in women.[37]

Overdose/Acute Toxicity

Overdose may produce profound respiratory and/or CNS depression in most species. Newborn animals may be more susceptible to these effects than adults. In dogs, a lethal dose of 50% (LD_{50}) is reported to be 29 mg/kg.[38] A dose of 4 mg/kg can be fatal in cats.[6] Other toxic effects can include cardiovascular collapse, hypothermia, and skeletal muscle hypotonia. Seizures may occur at very high doses (ie, 10 times the therapeutic dose).[22,23]

Naloxone, an opioid antagonist, is the agent of choice in treating respiratory depression. Naloxone may need to be readministered in cases of larger overdoses. Patients given naloxone must be observed closely because naloxone's effects may diminish before subtoxic concentrations of methadone are reached. Mechanical respiratory support should be considered in cases of severe respiratory depression. Dialysis, charcoal hemoperfusion, and forced diuresis do not appear to be beneficial in treating methadone overdose.

For patients that have experienced or are suspected to have experienced an overdose, consultation with a 24-hour poison consultation center specializing in providing veterinary-specific information is recommended. For general information related to overdose and toxin exposures, as well as contact information for poison control centers, refer to ***Appendix***.

Drug Interactions

The following drug interactions have either been reported or are theoretical in humans or animals receiving methadone and may be of significance in veterinary patients. Unless otherwise noted, use together is not necessarily contraindicated, but weigh the potential risks and perform additional monitoring when appropriate. In humans, the FDA-approved product has a black-box warning regarding the risk for fatal respiratory depression when methadone is administered with other CYP inhibitors.

- **ALPHA$_2$-RECEPTOR AGONISTS** (eg, **detomidine, dexmedetomidine, xylazine**): Although methadone combinations with alpha$_2$-receptoragonists are generally safe and effective,[39] severe hypoxemia was seen in dogs breathing room air in one study using methadone/medetomidine combination.[40] Detomidine may reduce methadone clearance in horses[41]
- **ANTIARRHYTHMICS, CLASS I AND III** (eg, **amiodarone, lidocaine, procainamide, quinidine**): Use with methadone may increase the risk for arrhythmia, including QT prolongation.
- **ANTICHOLINERGIC AGENTS** (eg, **atropine, clomipramine, diphenhydramine, hyoscyamine, procainamide**): Medications with anticholinergic properties may increase the risk for urinary retention and constipation when combined with opioids.
- **AZOLE ANTIFUNGALS** (eg, **fluconazole, itraconazole, ketoconazole**): May increase methadone plasma concentrations. Methadone is contraindicated with ketoconazole in humans. In dogs, ketoconazole did not appreciably increase methadone absorption following oral administration in one study[10] but appeared to increase oral methadone absorption, peak methadone concentration, and total drug exposure (AUC) in another study.[3] Fluconazole appears to increase oral methadone absorption, peak

methadone concentration, and exposure in dogs.[11]

- **Benzodiazepines** (eg, **alprazolam, diazepam, midazolam**): May potentiate the CNS and respiratory depressant effects of methadone
- **Calcium Channel Blockers**: Use with methadone may increase the risk for arrhythmias.
- **Central Nervous System Depressants, Other** (eg, **anesthetic agents, antihistamines, , ethanol, methocarbamol, phenothiazines**): May cause increased CNS or respiratory depression when used with methadone
- **Chloramphenicol**: May increase methadone concentrations. Chloramphenicol given to greyhounds that had also received methadone resulted in increased peak drug concentrations, total drug exposure (AUC), and persistence of drug concentrations. Coadministration of chloramphenicol with methadone may result in exaggerated and prolonged effects of methadone if methadone doses are not adjusted.[26]
- **Cimetidine**: May reduce methadone metabolism
- **Corticosteroids With Mineralocorticoid Activity** (eg, **desoxycorticosterone pivalate [DOCP], fludrocortisone**): Use with methadone may increase potential for electrolyte abnormalities.
- **Desmopressin**: Opioids may increase the risk for water intoxication or hyponatremia when combined with desmopressin.
- **Diuretics** (eg, **furosemide**): Opioids may decrease diuretic efficacy in patients with congestive heart failure and increase the adverse effects of diuretics.
- **Interferon Alfa**: May increase methadone concentrations
- **Macrolide Antibiotics** (eg, **clarithromycin, erythromycin**): May inhibit metabolism of methadone and increase methadone concentrations
- **Magnesium Sulfate**: The CNS effects of methadone may be increased; this is more likely with higher magnesium doses or IV magnesium therapy.
- **Minocycline**: IV minocycline therapy may enhance the CNS depressant effects of methadone.
- **Monoamine Oxidase Inhibitors** (MAOIs; eg, **amitraz, linezolid, selegiline**): Methadone may enhance the serotonergic effect of MAOIs and lead to possible serotonin syndrome; avoid concurrent use.
- **Naloxone**: Used clinically to reverse opioid CNS and respiratory depression.
- **Opioid Agonist/Antagonist** (eg, **buprenorphine, butorphanol, nalbuphine**): Combined use could antagonize opioid effects.
- **Phenobarbital, Primidone**: May decrease methadone concentrations; additive CNS or respiratory depression is possible
- **QT Prolongation** (eg, **cisapride, fluoxetine, metronidazole, ondansetron**): Methadone may prolong QT intervals in humans; this effect may be increased with agents that also prolong QT intervals. In dogs, methadone does not appear to prolong the QT interval.[30] Use with caution with other QT-prolonging agents.
- **Rifampin**: May decrease methadone concentrations, but potentially not in dogs
- **Selective Serotonin Reuptake Inhibitors** (SSRIs; eg, **fluoxetine, sertraline**): Concurrent fluoxetine increases oral methadone absorption, peak methadone concentration, and exposure in dogs.[3] May have additive serotonergic effects. Monitor for serotonin syndrome.
- **Serotonin Modulators** (eg, **metoclopramide, mirtazapine, ondansetron, tramadol, trazodone**): Serotonin effects may be enhanced when serotonin modulators are given concomitantly with methadone. Monitor for serotonin syndrome.
- **St John's Wort**: May decrease methadone concentrations
- **Succinylcholine**: Opioids combined with succinylcholine may enhance the bradycardic effects of opioids.
- **Tricyclic Antidepressants** (eg, **amitriptyline, clomipramine**): Methadone may exacerbate the CNS depressant effects of tricyclic antidepressants; serotonin effects may be enhanced.
- **Trimethoprim**: Concurrent use appears to increase oral methadone absorption, peak methadone concentration, and exposure in dogs.[3]
- **Zidovudine**: Methadone may increase zidovudine concentrations.

Laboratory Considerations

- Opioids may increase biliary tract pressure, resulting in increased plasma **amylase** and **lipase** values up to 24 hours following their administration.
- The following drugs can reportedly cause false positive results on **urine screening tests for methadone**: chlorpromazine, clomipramine, diphenhydramine, doxylamine, quetiapine, quinolones, thioridazine, and verapamil.

Dosages

NOTE: All listed dosages are based on the methadone HCl salt formulation (10 mg methadone HCl is equivalent to ≈8.9 mg of methadone). Most products are labeled with methadone HCl strength but check before administering to patients.

DOGS:

Perioperative pain control (extra-label):

IM: Methadone 0.5 mg/kg IM and acepromazine 0.03 mg/kg IM as a premedication prior to orthopedic surgery and meloxicam 0.2 mg/kg at induction produced superior analgesia to buprenorphine for 8 hours postoperatively.[42] Methadone 0.3 mg/kg combined with acepromazine 0.05 mg/kg or medetomidine 10 µg/kg and given IM as premedication for ovariohysterectomy produced superior analgesia to buprenorphine for 8 hours postoperatively.[43]

IV: Methadone 0.2 mg/kg IV; dexmedetomidine 1 µg/kg IV preceded[44]

Epidural: Methadone 0.1 mg/kg at induction; may combine this dose with ropivacaine 1.65 mg/kg.[45] Methadone 0.5 mg/kg lumbosacrally has also been used[46]; isoflurane MAC can be reduced by up to 30% with this higher methadone dose.

Analgesia (extra-label):

Continuous rate infusion (CRI): Methadone 0.1 – 0.2 mg/kg IV as a loading dose followed by methadone 0.12 mg/kg/hour IV CRI. Practically, add methadone 60 mg (6 mL of the 10 mg/mL injection) to 500 mL IV fluid (eg, 0.9% NaCl, Ringer's, 5% dextrose) at 1 mL/kg/hour. May be combined with ketamine and/or lidocaine[47]

Intermittent dosing:

1. Dosage recommendations vary but range from methadone 0.1 – 1 mg/kg IV,[45] SC, or IM every 4 to 8 hours.[6,22]
2. Methadone 0.2 mg/kg IV every 4 hours provided analgesia equivalent to fentanyl CRI following spinal surgery.[48]
3. Methadone 0.7 mg/kg IM provides sedation and analgesia as a premedication prior to orthopedic surgery.[49]
4. Methadone 0.5 mg/kg combined with acepromazine 0.02 mg/kg and given IM decreases isoflurane MAC.[50]
5. Methadone 0.3 mg/kg IV after medetomidine 2.5 µg/kg IV enhances sedation and provides postoperative analgesia.[51]

Premedication to general anesthesia (extra-label):

IM:

1. Methadone 0.2 – 0.3 mg/kg IM[52]

2. Methadone 0.2 mg/kg combined with acepromazine 0.02 mg/kg and given IM[53]
3. Methadone 0.2 mg/kg combined with dexmedetomidine 2 μg/kg and given IM prior to brachycephalic obstructive airway syndrome surgery[54]
4. Methadone 0.2 – 0.3 mg/kg combined with dexmedetomidine 5 μg/kg and given IM[55]
5. Methadone 0.2 – 0.3 mg/kg combined with dexmedetomidine 5 μg/kg and midazolam 0.3 mg/kg and given IM[56]
6. Methadone 0.2 – 0.3 mg/kg combined with medetomidine 20 μg/kg and given IM[57]

IV:

1. Methadone 0.2 mg/kg IV was used as a premedication, followed by isoflurane for anesthesia in a study of 32 dogs undergoing orthopedic surgery.[55]
2. Methadone 0.2 – 0.3 mg/kg IV with acepromazine 0.05 mg/kg IV[58]

SC: Methadone 1.1 mg/kg SC[22]

Extradural: Methadone 0.3 mg/kg diluted with saline to 0.2 mL/kg; acepromazine 0.05 mg/kg IV was used as a preanesthetic agent[58]

Sedative combinations (extra-label):

IM:

1. Methadone 0.25 – 0.75 mg/kg combined with acepromazine 0.05 mg/kg and given IM. For shorter sedation requirements (30 to 90 minutes), use methadone 0.25 mg/kg; for longer sedation requirements (up to 120 minutes), use methadone 0.5 – 0.75 mg/kg IM. Peak effect is achieved within 30 minutes.[39,59]
2. Methadone 0.5 mg/kg IM; can be combined with dexmedetomidine 10 μg/kg[60] or xylazine 0.5 mg/kg and given IM[39]
3. Methadone 0.4 mg/kg combined with medetomidine 2.5 μg/kg and given IM enhances sedation; bradycardia and panting may occur.[61]

IV: Methadone 0.2 mg/kg IV with dexmedetomidine 2 μg/kg IV[62]

CATS:

Perioperative pain control (extra-label):

IM combinations:

1. Methadone 0.5 mg/kg IM combined with medetomidine 20 μg/kg IM[63] or acepromazine 0.05 mg/kg IM[64]
2. Methadone 0.3 mg/kg IM, dexmedetomidine 15 μg/kg IM, and either alfaxalone 3 mg/kg IM or ketamine 3 mg/kg IM provided adequate analgesia and anesthesia and smooth recoveries for cats undergoing ovariectomy.[65]
3. **QUAD protocol**: methadone 5 mg/m^2 (NOT mg/kg), medetomidine 600 μg/m^2 (NOT μg/kg), ketamine 60 mg/m^2 (NOT mg/kg), midazolam 3 mg/m^2 (NOT mg/kg) mixed in the same syringe and given IM 10 minutes prior to anesthesia[66]

SC: Methadone 0.6 mg/kg with acepromazine 0.02 mg/kg SC as preoperative combination provided effective analgesia for 6 hours following ovariohysterectomy in most cats.[67]

Epidural:

1. In cats undergoing ovariohysterectomy, lumbosacral epidural combination of lidocaine 2% 4 mg/kg with methadone 0.3 mg/kg resulted in adequate surgical analgesia and prolonged (ie, greater than 18 hours) postoperative analgesia.[68]
2. Under maintenance anesthesia, methadone 0.2 mg/kg epidural reduced and delayed the need for postoperative rescue analgesia.[69]

Analgesia (extra-label):

Continuous rate infusion (CRI): Loading dose of 0.1 – 0.2 mg/kg IV; followed by 0.12 mg/kg/hour IV CRI. Practically, add methadone HCl 60 mg (6 mL of the 10 mg/mL injection) to 500 mL IV fluid and run at 1 mL/kg/hour IV CRI. May combine with ketamine and/or lidocaine[47]

Intermittent dosing:

1. Dosage recommendations vary but range from methadone 0.05 – 0.5 mg/kg IV, SC, or IM every 4 to 6 hours.
2. Methadone 0.2 – 0.6 mg/kg SC[17,70-72]; may repeat at 3 time points at 5 hour intervals.[22]
3. Methadone 0.5 mg/kg IM with ketamine 0.3 mg/kg IM 20 minutes before induction of anesthesia[73]
4. Methadone 0.75 mg/kg oral transmucosal provided transient antinociception under experimental conditions.[72]

Anesthesia premedication (extra-label): Methadone 0.1 – 0.6 mg/kg IV, IM, or SC[70,74]

IM combinations:

1. Methadone 0.2 mg/kg combined with acepromazine 0.05 mg/kg and given IM[75]
2. Methadone 0.2 mg/kg combined with dexmedetomidine 5 μg/kg and given IM[76]
3. Methadone 0.2 mg/kg combined with tiletamine/zolazepam 3 mg/kg and given IM[77]
4. Methadone 0.3 mg/kg combined with dexmedetomidine 3 – 4 μg/kg and given IM[78,79]

HORSES:

Analgesia (extra-label): 0.22 mg/kg IM or SC[23]

IV combination: Methadone 0.2 – 0.5 mg/kg IV. Can be combined with detomidine 10 μg/kg IV or acepromazine 0.05 mg/kg IV and given IV.[80-82] In one study, more pronounced antinociception occurred with the methadone/detomidine combination as compared with methadone/acepromazine.[81] Use of methadone 0.5 mg/kg IV provided better analgesia but more adverse effects.[80]

Continuous rate infusion (CRI):

1. Methadone 0.2 mg/kg combined with detomidine 5 μg/kg and given IV as a loading dose followed by methadone 0.05 mg/kg per hour and detomidine 12.5 μg/kg/hour IV CRI.[83,84] Decreased gut sounds occurred.

Epidural (extra-label): Methadone 0.1 mg/kg in the first intercoccygeal space (ie, Co1-Co2) diluted with sterile 0.9% sodium chloride solution to a total volume of 20 mL and administered at a rate of 1 mL/second; analgesia was attained 15 minutes after administration and lasted 5 hours.[2]

Restraint (extra-label): Methadone 0.11 mg/kg combined with acepromazine 0.055 mg/kg and given IV[23]

Premedication (extra-label): Methadone 0.1 mg/kg combined with romifidine 80 μg/kg and given IV; combination administered 30 to 120 minutes after acepromazine 0.02 mg/kg IM[85]

SHEEP:

Sedation (extra-label): Methadone 0.5 mg/kg IV combined with *either* xylazine 0.1 mg/kg *or* acepromazine 0.05 mg/kg IV[87,88]

Lumbosacral epidural (extra-label):

1. Methadone 0.15 – 0.3 mg/kg combined with bupivacaine 0.25 – 0.5 mg/kg[89,90,68]

Monitoring

- Analgesic or preanesthetic effect
- Respiratory depression at higher doses

Client Information

- Methadone should only be used in the clinic or with direct professional supervision when given as an injection.
- Methadone is a C-II controlled drug and requires a new written prescription for refills. Use of this medication in animals or humans other than those for whom they are prescribed is illegal.

Chemistry/Synonyms

Methadone HCl, a synthetic diphenylheptane-derivative narcotic agonist, occurs as an odorless, white crystalline powder. Methadone is freely soluble in water, chloroform, and alcohol and practically insoluble in ether or glycerol. The pH of a 1% solution in water is between 4.5 to 6.5. The commercially available injection has a pH from 3 to 6.5. Methadone is typically supplied as methadone hydrochloride (HCl) salt and doses are based on the concentration of the salt formulation (ie, 10 mg methadone HCl is equivalent to 8.9 mg methadone). The dispersible tablet formulation (ie, *Diskets*®) contains insoluble ingredients that deter their use for injection. Methadone injectable products and oral suspensions should be protected from light.[6]

Methadone may also be known as amidine HCl, amidone HCl, methadoni hydrochloridum, Phenadone, *Adolan*®, *Biodone*®, *Cloro Nona*®, *Comfortan*®, *Dolmed*®, *Eptadone*®, *Gobbidona*®, *Heptadon*®, *Ketalgine*®, *Metadol*®, *Metasedin*®, *Methaddict*®, *Methadose*®, *Methatabs*®, *Methex*®, *Methodyne*®, *Methone*®, *Pallidone*®, *Phymet*®, *Physeptone*®, *Pinadone*®, *Sedo*®, *Symoron*®, *Synastone*®, or *Synthadon*®.

Storage/Stability

Methadone injection should be stored at room temperature of 20°C to 25°C (68°F-77°F) and protected from light. Store vials in the manufacturer's carton until ready for use.

Methadone is a schedule II (C-II) controlled substance. In accordance with DEA regulations, it must be stored in an area that is substantially constructed and securely locked. Follow applicable local, state, and federal rules regarding disposal of unused or wasted controlled drugs.

Compatibility/Compounding Considerations

Compatibility is dependent on factors such as pH, concentration, temperature, and diluent used; consult specialized references or a hospital pharmacist for more specific information.

Methadone injection is reportedly stable when mixed in a syringe with acepromazine and compatible with propofol and alfaxalone.

Methadone is **compatible** in solution with 0.9% sodium chloride, and appears **Y-site compatible** with the following drugs (partial list): ampicillin/sulbactam, calcium chloride/gluconate, cefazolin, dexamethasone sodium phosphate, dexmedetomidine, diazepam, dobutamine, dopamine, esmolol, esomeprazole, famotidine, hydrocortisone sodium succinate, magnesium sulfate, methylprednisolone sodium succinate, metoclopramide, midazolam, pantoprazole, phenobarbital, potassium chloride, and sodium bicarbonate.

Methadone injection is reportedly **incompatible** at Y-sites with acyclovir, allopurinol, amphotericin B conventional, dantrolene, fluorouracil, meloxicam, methohexital, pentobarbital, piperacillin-tazobactam, sulfamethoxazole-trimethoprim, and thiopental.

Methadone has reported **variable compatibility** at Y-sites with furosemide.

Dosage Forms/Regulatory Status

VETERINARY-LABELED PRODUCTS: NONE IN THE UNITED STATES

Methadone HCl Injection: (10 mg/mL) is approved for veterinary use in some countries (ie, United Kingdom, Australia).

The Association of Racing Commissioners International (ARCI) has designated this drug as a Class 1 substance. Use of this drug may not be allowed in certain animal competitions. Check rules and regulations before entering in a competition while this medication is being administered. Contact local racing authorities for further guidance. See ***Appendix*** for more information.

HUMAN-LABELED PRODUCTS:

Methadone HCl Injection: 10 mg/mL in 20 mL multidose vials; generic; (Rx, C-II)

Methadone HCl Oral Tablets: 5 and 10 mg; *Dolophine*®; generic; (Rx, C-II)

Methadone HCl Dispersible Tablet: 40 mg; *Methadose*®; generic; (Rx, C-II)

Methadone HCl Oral Solution: 1 mg/mL and 2 mg/mL in 500 mL bottles; *Methadose*®; generic; (Rx, C-II)

Methadone HCl Oral Liquid Concentrate: 10 mg/mL in 30 mL (with calibrated dropper) and 1000 mL bottles; *Methadose*®, *Intensol*®; generic; (Rx, C-II)

Report dispensing to state monitoring programs where required.

References

For the complete list of references, see **wiley.com/go/budde/plumb**

Methazolamide

(meth-a-***zoe***-la-mide) *Neptazane*®

Carbonic Anhydrase Inhibitor

Prescriber Highlights

- ► Oral carbonic anhydrase inhibitor used primarily for open angle glaucoma; reportedly is becoming difficult to obtain at an affordable cost
- ► Contraindications include patients with significant hepatic, renal, or pulmonary disease, hyponatremia, hypokalemia, hypoadrenocorticism, hyperchloremic acidosis, or electrolyte imbalance.
- ► Primary adverse effects include GI (eg, vomiting, diarrhea, inappetence), hypokalemia, and metabolic acidosis. Cats may be more susceptible to developing adverse effects.
- ► Give oral doses with food if GI adverse effects occur.
- ► Monitor with tonometry for glaucoma; check electrolytes

Uses/Indications

Orally administered methazolamide is used for the medical treatment of glaucoma. Topical carbonic anhydrase inhibitors (eg, dorzolamide) are more commonly used today, as they can lower intraocular pressure as effectively as systemic drugs and have fewer adverse effects.

Pharmacology/Actions

The carbonic anhydrase inhibitors are noncompetitive, reversible inhibitors of carbonic anhydrase. Inhibition of carbonic anhydrase results in a reduction of the formation of hydrogen and bicarbonate ions from carbon dioxide and decreases the availability of these ions for active transport into body secretions.

Pharmacologic effects of the carbonic anhydrase inhibitors include decreased formation of aqueous humor, thereby reducing intraocular pressure; increased renal tubular secretion of sodium and potassium and, to a greater extent, bicarbonate, leading to increased urine alkalinity and volume; and anticonvulsant activity, which is independent of its diuretic effects (mechanism not fully understood, but may be due to carbonic anhydrase or a metabolic acidosis effect).

Pharmacokinetics

Little information is available. Methazolamide is absorbed from the GI tract, albeit more slowly than acetazolamide. It is distributed throughout the body, including the CSF and aqueous humor. Methazolamide is at least partially metabolized in the liver.

Contraindications/Precautions/Warnings

Carbonic anhydrase inhibitors are contraindicated in patients with significant hepatic disease (may precipitate hepatic coma), renal or adrenocortical insufficiency, hyponatremia, hypokalemia, hyperchloremic acidosis, or electrolyte imbalance. They should not be used in patients with severe pulmonary obstruction unable to increase alveolar ventilation (may precipitate acidosis) or in those that are hypersensitive to them. Long-term use of carbonic anhydrase inhibitors is contraindicated in patients with chronic, noncongestive, angle-closure glaucoma, as angle closure may occur, and the drug may mask the condition by lowering intraocular pressure.

Methazolamide is a sulfonamide derivative and has the potential to cause severe reactions. Stevens-Johnson syndrome, toxic epidermal necrolysis, and aplastic anemia have been reported in humans.[1]

Do not confuse methaZOLAMIDE with methIMAZOLE, or methENAMINE.

Adverse Effects

Adverse effects may include GI disturbances (eg, vomiting, diarrhea, inappetence), metabolic acidosis (with heavy panting), CNS effects (eg, sedation, depression, disorientation, excitement), hypokalemia, hematologic effects (eg, bone marrow depression, thrombocytopenia), renal effects (eg, crystalluria, dysuria, renal colic, polyuria, polydipsia), hyperglycemia, hyponatremia, hyperuricemia, hepatic insufficiency, dermatologic effects (eg, rash), and hypersensitivity reactions. Electrolyte imbalances may manifest as weakness or cardiac arrhythmias.

Cats may be more prone to developing adverse effects than are dogs.

Combining methazolamide (oral dosing) with topical (ophthalmic) dorzolamide does not apparently yield additive reductions in intraocular pressure and may cause increased adverse effects.

Reproductive/Nursing Safety

Methazolamide is teratogenic in rats at high doses. Safety for use of methazolamide during nursing has not been established, but a related compound, acetazolamide, is excreted in milk in concentrations that are unlikely to have pharmacologic effect.

Because safety has not been established in animals, this drug should only be used when the maternal benefits outweigh the potential risks to offspring.

Overdose/Acute Toxicity

Information regarding overdoses of this drug is not readily available. It is suggested to monitor serum electrolytes, blood gases, volume status, and CNS status during an acute overdose. Treat overdoses symptomatically and supportively.

For patients that have experienced or are suspected of having experienced an overdose, consultation with a 24-hour poison consultation center specializing in providing veterinary-specific information is recommended. For general information related to overdose and toxin exposures, as well as contact information for poison control centers, refer to ***Appendix***.

Drug Interactions

The following drug interactions have either been reported or are theoretical in humans or animals receiving methazolamide and may be of significance in veterinary patients. Unless otherwise noted, use together is not necessarily contraindicated, but weigh the potential risks and perform additional monitoring when appropriate.

- **Antidepressants, Tricyclic**: Alkaline urine caused by methazolamide may decrease excretion.
- **Aspirin (or Other Salicylates)**: Increased risk for methazolamide accumulation and toxicity and metabolic acidosis; methazolamide increases salicylate excretion.
- **Digoxin**: As methazolamide may cause hypokalemia, there is increased risk for toxicity.
- **Insulin**: Rarely, carbonic anhydrase inhibitors interfere with the hypoglycemic effects of insulin.
- **Metformin**: Increased risk for lactic acidosis
- **Methenamine Compounds**: Methazolamide may negate effects in the urine.
- **Potassium And Drugs Affecting Potassium** (eg, **corticosteroids, amphotericin B, corticotropin, or other diuretics**): Concomitant use may exacerbate potassium depletion.
- **Phenobarbital, Primidone**: May increase urinary excretion and reduce phenobarbital levels
- **Quinidine**: Alkaline urine caused by methazolamide may decrease excretion.

Laboratory Considerations

- By alkalinizing the urine, carbonic anhydrase inhibitors may cause false positive results in determining **urine protein** using bromphenol blue reagent (*Albustix*®, *Albutest*®, *Labstix*®), sulfosalicylic acid (*Bumintest*®, *Exton's*® *Test Reagent*), nitric acid ring test, or heat and acetic acid test methods.
- Carbonic anhydrase inhibitors may **decrease iodine uptake** by the thyroid gland in hyperthyroid or euthyroid patients.

Dosages

DOGS:

Open-angle glaucoma (extra-label): Dosages usually range from 2 – 5 mg/kg PO 2 to 3 times a day.

CATS:

Open-angle glaucoma (extra-label): Dosages usually range from 1 – 4 mg/kg PO 2 to 3 times a day.

Monitoring

- Intraocular pressure/tonometry
- Serum electrolytes; pH. May need to supplement potassium.
- Baseline CBC with differential and periodic retests if using long term
- Adverse effects including GI disturbances, altered CNS status, and dermatologic abnormalities

Client Information

- This medicine must be given 2 to 3 times a day.
- If gastrointestinal upset (eg, vomiting, lack of appetite) occurs, give the medicine with food.
- Notify your veterinarian if abnormal bleeding or bruising occurs, or if your animal develops tremors or a rash.
- While your animal is taking this medication, it is important to return to your veterinarian for physical examinations and laboratory work. Do not miss these important follow-up visits.

Chemistry/Synonyms

A carbonic anhydrase inhibitor similar to dichlorphenamide, methazolamide occurs as a white to slightly yellow crystalline powder. It is very slightly soluble in water.

Methazolamide may also be known as *GlaucTabs*®, *Glaumetax*®, *MZM*®, and *Neptazane*®.

Storage/Stability

Methazolamide tablets should be stored in tightly closed containers at room temperature (20°C-25°C [68°F-77°F]), with excursions permitted to 15°C to 30°C (59°F-86°F).

Compatibility/Compounding Considerations

No specific information is noted.

Dosage Forms/Regulatory Status

VETERINARY-LABELED PRODUCTS: NONE

The American Racing Commissioners International (ARCI) has designated this drug as a class 4 substance. Use of this drug may not be allowed in certain animal competitions. Check rules and regulations before entering in a competition while this medication is being administered. Contact local racing authorities for further guidance. See ***Appendix*** for more information.

HUMAN-LABELED PRODUCTS:

Methazolamide Tablets: 25 and 50 mg; *Neptazane®*; generic; (Rx)

References

For the complete list of references, see **wiley.com/go/budde/plumb**

Methenamine

(meth-***en***-a-meen) *Hiprex®, Urex®*

Urinary Antiseptic

Prescriber Highlights

- ► Urinary antiseptic used for recurrent UTIs in dogs and cats, but efficacy is questionable and no evidence supports its use
- ► Contraindications include metabolic acidosis, hypersensitivity to methenamine, concurrent treatment with sulfonamides, renal insufficiency, severe hepatic impairment (due to ammonia production), or severe dehydration
- ► Adverse effects include GI irritation; dysuria is possible if used long term.
- ► Urine pH must be less than or equal to 6 (ideally less than 5.5) to be effective.

Uses/Indications

Methenamine is used as an antimicrobial agent for prophylaxis of recurrent UTIs. It is not commonly used in veterinary medicine and little good evidence is available to confirm its efficacy in dogs or cats.[1]

Pharmacology/Actions

In an acidic urinary environment (pH less than 6.5), methenamine is converted to formaldehyde. Formaldehyde is a nonspecific antibacterial agent that exerts a bactericidal effect. It can have activity against a variety of bacteria, including both gram-positive (*Staphylococcus aureus, Staphylococcus epidermidis, Enterococcus* spp) and gram-negative organisms (*Escherichia coli, Enterobacter* spp, *Klebsiella* spp, *Proteus* spp, and *Pseudomonas aeruginosa*), but may be less effective against those bacteria that produce urease (and increase urine pH). Reportedly, methenamine has activity against fungal UTIs.

Hippuric acid or mandelic acid is added primarily to help acidify the urine, but it also has some nonspecific antibacterial activity. Bacterial resistance to formaldehyde or hippuric acid does not usually occur.

Pharmacokinetics

Human data: Although methenamine and its salts are well absorbed from the GI tract, up to 30% of a dose may be hydrolyzed by gastric acid to ammonia and formaldehyde. With enteric-coated tablets, the amount hydrolyzed in the gut is reduced. While absorbed, plasma concentrations of both formaldehyde and methenamine are very low and have negligible systemic antibacterial activity. Methenamine does cross the placenta and is distributed into milk.

Within 24 hours, 70% to 90% of a dose is excreted unchanged into the urine.[2] In acidic urine, conversion to ammonia and formaldehyde takes place. Peak formaldehyde concentrations occur in the urine at ≈2 hours postdose (3 to 8 hours with enteric-coated tablets).

Contraindications/Precautions/Warnings

Methenamine and its salts are contraindicated in patients with known hypersensitivity to it, renal insufficiency, metabolic acidosis, severe hepatic impairment (due to ammonia production), or severe dehydration.

Because methenamine requires acidic urine to be beneficial, urine pH should ideally be kept at or below 5.5. Some urea-splitting bacteria (eg, *Proteus* spp and some strains of staphylococci, *Enterobacter* spp, and *Pseudomonas* spp) may increase urine pH. Addition of a urinary acidification program may be required using dietary modification and acidifying drugs (eg, ascorbic acid, methionine, sodium biphosphate, ammonium chloride).

Do not confuse meTHENAMine with meTHIOnine.

Adverse Effects

The most likely adverse effect noted is GI upset, with nausea, vomiting, and anorexia predominant. Some patients may develop dysuria, likely secondary to irritation due to high formaldehyde concentrations. Cats reportedly do not tolerate methenamine as well as dogs. Potentially, systemic acidosis could occur.

In humans, increased liver enzymes, pruritus, and rashes have rarely been reported, and large doses have caused bladder irritation, albuminuria, and hematuria. Lipoid pneumonitis has been reported in some humans that receive prolonged therapy with the suspension.

Reproductive/Nursing Safety

Methenamine crosses the placenta. Although laboratory animal studies have not demonstrated any teratogenic effects, it should be used with caution during pregnancy. Administration to pregnant dogs has been reported to cause a slight increase in stillborn rate and slight impairment of weight gain and survival in offspring.[2]

Methenamine enters milk; in humans, it is recommended to discontinue nursing or discontinue methenamine.[2]

Because safety has not been established in animals, this drug should only be used when the maternal benefits outweigh the potential risks to offspring.

Overdose/Acute Toxicity

Dogs have received single IV dosages of up to 600 mg/kg of methenamine hippurate without overt toxic effects. Large oral overdoses should be handled using established GI decontamination protocols, maintaining hydration status, and supportive care as required.

For patients that have experienced or are suspected to have experienced an overdose, consultation with a 24-hour poison consultation center specializing in providing veterinary-specific information is recommended. For general information related to overdose and toxin exposures, as well as contact information for poison control centers, refer to ***Appendix***.

Drug Interactions

The following drug interactions have either been reported or are theoretical in humans or animals receiving methenamine and may be of significance in veterinary patients. Unless otherwise noted, use together is not necessarily contraindicated, but weigh the potential risks and perform additional monitoring when appropriate.

- Carbonic Anhydrase Inhibitors (eg, **acetazolamide, methazolamide**): Use of drugs that alkalinize the urine may reduce the efficacy of the methenamine.
- Salicylates (eg, **aspirin, bismuth subsalicylate**): Acidified urine may reduce salicylate excretion and increase salicylate concentrations.
- Sulfonamides (eg, **sulfa-/trimethoprim, zonisamide**): Use of methenamine with sulfonamides is not recommended. An insoluble precipitate may form in urine.
- Thiazide Diuretics (eg, **hydrochlorothiazide**): Use of drugs that alkalinize the urine may reduce the efficacy of the methenamine.
- Urine Alkalinizing Drugs (eg, **calcium or magnesium containing antacids, citrates, sodium bicarbonate**): Use of urinary

alkalinizing drugs may reduce the efficacy of the methenamine.

Laboratory Considerations

- Urinary values of the following compounds may be falsely elevated: **catecholamines, vanillylmandelic acid** (**VMA**), and **17-hydrocorticosteroid.**
- Falsely decreased urinary values of **estriol** or **5-HIAA** may occur.
- Methenamine may cause false-positive **urine glucose determinations** when using cupric sulfate solution (Benedict's Solution, *Clinitest*®) and false-negative tests utilizing the glucose oxidase (*Tes-Tape*®, *Clinistix*®) method.

Dosages

DOGS/CATS:

Recurrent UTI (extra-label): No prospective studies supporting any dosage protocol were noted, and there is little evidence to support clinical use, but it theoretically could be effective. Recommended anecdotal dosages usually range from 10 – 20 mg/kg PO every 8 to 12 hours or 500 mg/dog (NOT mg/kg) every 12 hours or 250 mg/cat (NOT mg/kg) every 12 hours.[3] Practically, this is rounded off to the nearest 250 mg (as usually only available in 1 gram tablets). Requires acidic urine (pH less than or equal to 6; optimally less than 5.5) for efficacy and an acidifying diet and/or urinary acidifiers may be required. It reportedly is not tolerated well in cats.

Monitoring

- Urine pH
- Liver function tests periodically in patients with hepatic impairment[2]
- Efficacy (decreased frequency of UTI; monitor for clinical symptoms of UTI and urine culture periodically)

Client Information

- Give this medication with food to prevent stomach upset. Tablets are large but can be split.
- Vomiting, nausea (acting "sick"), and reduced appetite are common. Cats may not tolerate the drug as well as dogs.
- Requires urine to be acidic to work properly. Your veterinarian may recommend other drugs (eg, vitamin C, methionine) or dietary changes to increase urine acidity.
- While your animal is taking this medication, it is important to return to your veterinarian for physical examinations and laboratory work. Do not miss these important follow-up visits.

Chemistry/Synonyms

Methenamine is chemically unrelated to other anti-infective agents. It is commercially available as methenamine hippurate or methenamine mandelate. Methenamine mandelate occurs as a white crystalline powder and contains ≈48% methenamine and 52% mandelic acid. It is very soluble in water. Methenamine hippurate occurs as a white crystalline powder with a sour taste and contains ≈44% methenamine and 56% hippuric acid. It is freely soluble in water.

Methenamine may also be known as hexamine amygdalate, hexamine mandelate, mandelato de metenamina, *Aci-Steril*®, *Mandelamine*®, *Hiprex*®, *Reflux*®, *Urocedulamin*®, and *Urex*®.

Storage/Stability

Commercially available methenamine products should be stored at 15°C to 30°C (59°F-86°F). Because acids hydrolyze methenamine to formaldehyde and ammonia, do not mix with acidic vehicles before administering.

Compatibility/Compounding Considerations

Methenamine is physically **incompatible** when mixed with most alkaloids and metallic salts (eg, ferric, mercuric, or silver salts). Ammonium salts or alkalis will darken methenamine.

Dosage Forms/Regulatory Status

VETERINARY-LABELED PRODUCTS: NONE

HUMAN-LABELED PRODUCTS:

Methenamine Hippurate Oral Tablets: 1 g; generic; (Rx)

Methenamine Mandelate Tablets: 0.5 g and 1 g; generic; (Rx). These products are available but are not listed as an FDA-approved drug.

References

For the complete list of references, see **wiley.com/go/budde/plumb**

Methimazole

Thiamazole

(meth-***im***-a-zole) *Felimazole*®, *Tapazole*®

Antithyroid

Prescriber Highlights

- ▶ FDA-approved for treatment of feline hyperthyroidism
- ▶ The sugar coating on the veterinary-approved product masks the bitter taste that is noticed with uncoated human products.
- ▶ Transdermal methimazole gels can be considered in cats that do not tolerate oral administration.
- ▶ Review ***Contraindications/Precautions/Warnings*** before prescribing.
- ▶ Adverse GI effects occur most commonly in the first 3 months of therapy and are usually transient. Adverse hematologic or hepatic effects and facial excoriations may require discontinuation of therapy.
- ▶ Nursing should not be allowed for queens receiving methimazole; kittens should be placed on a milk replacer.
- ▶ Blood samples for monitoring thyroid hormone concentrations can be collected at any time of the day.
- ▶ The National Institute for Occupational Safety and Health (NIOSH) classifies methimazole as a hazardous drug; use appropriate precautions when handling.

Uses/Indications

Methimazole is considered by most clinicians in North America to be the drug of choice to treat feline hyperthyroidism. More than 90% of cats that tolerate methimazole respond to the drug.[1] In a retrospective case series, iodine 131 was more effective than methimazole in the treatment of hyperthyroid cats, and cats treated with iodine 131 had a survival time of 4 years as compared with 2 years for those treated with methimazole and 5.3 years in those that received methimazole followed by radioiodine.[2]

Transdermal methimazole (in pluronic lecithin organogel [PLO]) has been used with some therapeutic success in cats that cannot tolerate oral administration.[3-5] Four or more weeks of therapy may be required for the drug to reach efficacy. Orally administered methimazole is more effective than transdermal methimazole.[4]

Pharmacology/Actions

Methimazole inhibits thyroid peroxidase and interferes with iodine incorporation into tyrosyl residues of thyroglobulin, thereby inhibiting thyroid hormone synthesis. It also inhibits iodinated tyrosyl residues from coupling to form iodothyronine. Methimazole has no effect on the release or activity of thyroid hormones already formed or in general circulation. Significant reductions in serum thyroxine (T_4) usually occur within 2 to 3 weeks of therapy.[1,6]

Pharmacokinetics

In a study of healthy cats, peak drug concentration occurred 30 to 60 minutes after oral administration.[7-9] Average oral bioavailability was 80%, and elimination half-life was 5.1 to 6.6 hours, with wide interpatient variability (≈2 to 15 hours).[8,9] Administration in a fasted state increases absorption.[6] Protein binding is minimal. Absorption and steady-state volume of distribution (1.1 L/kg) are similar in normal and hyperthyroid cats, but elimination half-life is shorter (2.5 hours) in hyperthyroid cats.[9] The drug is renally eliminated.[10]

Drug absorption using compounded (pluronic lecithin organogel [PLO]-base) transdermal methimazole can be highly variable; in a study, methimazole was detectable in only 2 of 6 cats given a 5 mg dose.[11] However, in another study[12] in cats receiving methimazole PLO (either 2.5 mg/cat [NOT mg/kg] twice daily or 5 mg/cat [NOT mg/kg] once daily), at 1 and 3 weeks after starting treatment, all cats showed sustained suppression of T_4 concentration 10 hours after administration. In both groups, T_4 concentrations measured immediately before the next methimazole treatment were not significantly different as compared with measurements at any time point after application.[12] An alternative non-PLO–based transdermal methimazole formulation applied to the pinnae of healthy cats demonstrated more reliable absorption after a 10 mg/cat (NOT mg/kg) dose as compared with a 5 mg/cat (NOT mg/kg) dose.[13]

In dogs, methimazole has a serum half-life of 8 to 9 hours. Methimazole apparently concentrates in canine thyroid tissue.

Contraindications/Precautions/Warnings

Methimazole is contraindicated in patients that are hypersensitive to it, carbimazole, or the excipient, polyethylene glycol. The US veterinary label states that methimazole is contraindicated in cats with autoimmune disease, primary liver disease, renal failure, or hematologic disorders (ie, anemia, neutropenia, lymphopenia, thrombocytopenia) or coagulopathies[6]; the UK veterinary label also states, *Do not use in cats suffering from systemic disease such as primary liver disease or diabetes mellitus.*[10] Cats with liver disease can potentially receive the drug at lower doses with dose titration and liver function tests intensely monitored.

Treatment of hyperthyroid cats with methimazole can unmask underlying renal disease because lowering thyroid hormone concentrations decreases glomerular filtration rates.[14] An estimated 40% of hyperthyroid cats also have chronic kidney disease.[15] As such, the cat's renal parameters should be monitored closely during treatment (see ***Monitoring***). A significant reduction in serum creatinine was noted after restoration of euthyroidism in cats with iatrogenic hypothyroidism caused by methimazole or carbimazole.[16] Appropriate dose adjustments to avoid iatrogenic hypothyroidism are important, as cats with iatrogenic hypothyroidism are at an increased risk for azotemia.

An increasing prevalence of moderate-to-severe thyroid disease (eg, large thyroid tumors, multifocal disease, intrathoracic thyroid masses) was associated with an increased duration of methimazole treatment, which the study authors speculated may indicate a progressive nature of feline hyperthyroidism that is not stopped by maintaining euthyroidism with methimazole.[17]

Methimazole has antivitamin K activity, which may increase risk for bleeding.[6]

The National Institute for Occupational Safety and Health (NIOSH) classifies methimazole as a hazardous drug representing an occupational hazard to healthcare workers; wash hands after handling and use personal protective equipment (PPE) accordingly to minimize the risk for exposure.[18]

MethIMAzole should not be confused with meTAMizole (dipyrone), methazolamide, or metOLazone.

Adverse Effects

Most adverse effects associated with methimazole use in cats occur within the first 3 months of therapy, with vomiting, anorexia, depression/lethargy, and abnormal vocalization occurring most frequently.[6,19] GI effects occur in ≈10% of treated cats and may be related to the drug's bitter taste or direct gastric irritation and are usually transient. Cats that cannot tolerate GI adverse effects may tolerate transdermal methimazole. Other systemic adverse effects occur at similar rates when comparing oral with transdermal methimazole, although skin reactions (eg, erythema) may occur at the transdermal application site.[3]

Eosinophilia, leukopenia, thrombocytopenia, and lymphocytosis may be noted in ≈15% of cats in the first 8 weeks of therapy[19]; these hematologic effects usually resolve within a week of drug withdrawal.[1] Blood dyscrasias (eg, severe thrombocytopenia, bleeding, neutropenia, agranulocytosis) can occur in ≈4% of cats and typically occurs within the first 1 to 2 months of treatment.[19] Methimazole use should be discontinued in these patients, and prophylactic antibiotic therapy and other supportive measures can be considered.[10] Methimazole rechallenge can cause recurrence of adverse effects.[20]

Methimazole-treated cats can develop pruritus and facial excoriations. Incidence of these effects has been reported to be 2% to 3%, with most cases occurring within the first 3 weeks of treatment,[20] although an incidence rate of up to 15% has been reported.[21] Discontinuation of methimazole is warranted in these cases.

Increased ALT may occur early in therapy and normalize with continued therapy. Other serious but rare adverse effects include hepatopathy (1.5% of cases) and a positive direct antiglobulin test result (1.9% of cases).[19] Methimazole and carbimazole are thought to be potential triggers for immune-mediated hemolytic anemia and/or immune-mediated thrombocytopenia in cats[22]; in such cases, drug withdrawal is generally required. If methimazole must be discontinued due to adverse effects, alternative therapies (eg, radioiodine, antithyroid diet) should be considered.

Up to 20% of cats receiving methimazole chronically (longer than 6 months) will develop a dose-dependent positive antinuclear antibody result and require dose reduction.[6,19]

Rarely, cats can develop an acquired myasthenia gravis that requires drug withdrawal or concomitant glucocorticoid therapy. Pyogranulomatous mural folliculitis[23] and lymphadenomegaly[24] have been reported.

Reproductive/Nursing Safety

Delayed testes maturation was noted in a 12-week safety study.[6] High concentrations of methimazole cross the placenta and may induce hypothyroidism in kittens born of queens receiving the drug. The drug is contraindicated in pregnant or lactating queens, as laboratory studies in mice and rats have shown evidence of teratogenic and embryotoxic effects.

Methimazole concentrations higher than those found in plasma have been detected in human breast milk, so it has been suggested that queens not allow kittens to nurse; kittens should be placed on a milk replacer after receiving colostrum from a queen on methimazole.

Overdose/Acute Toxicity

Signs of acute toxicity that may be seen with overdoses include those listed in ***Adverse Effects***. Agranulocytosis, hepatopathy, immune-mediated hemolytic anemia, and thrombocytopenia are likely the most serious effects that may be seen. Treatment of overdose/toxicity consists of following standard protocols for handling an oral ingestion (eg, empty stomach, administer charcoal if not contraindicated) and treat supportively and based on clinical signs.

For patients that have experienced or are suspected to have experienced an overdose, it is strongly encouraged to consult with one of the 24-hour poison consultation centers that specialize in providing information specific for veterinary patients. For general information related to overdose and toxin exposures, as well as contact information for poison control centers, refer to ***Appendix***.

Drug Interactions

Hyperthyroidism increases glomerular filtration rate (GFR). Methimazole restores euthyroidism, thereby reducing GFR,[14] which may alter the pharmacokinetics of drugs that rely on GFR for elimination from the body. The following drug interactions have either been reported or are theoretical in humans or animals receiving methimazole and may be of significance in veterinary patients. Unless otherwise noted, use together is not necessarily contraindicated, but the potential risks should be weighed and additional monitoring performed when appropriate.

- **ANTICOAGULANTS** (eg, **heparin, rivaroxaban**): Methimazole may potentiate anticoagulant activity.
- **BENZIMIDAZOLE ANTIPARASITICS** (eg, **albendazole, fenbendazole, thiabendazole**): Concurrent methimazole use can reduce hepatic oxidation of benzimidazoles and increase blood concentrations of the parent drug or its metabolites.[6,25-27]
- **BETA-BLOCKERS** (eg, **atenolol, propranolol**): Reduction in the beta-blocker dose may be needed when the patient becomes euthyroid.[6]
- **CHLORAMPHENICOL**: Combination may increase the risk for myelosuppression.
- **DIGOXIN**: Correction to euthyroidism reduces digoxin clearance, resulting in increased digoxin exposure and risk for toxicity. A reduction in the digoxin dose may be needed when the patient becomes euthyroid.[6]
- **DIPYRONE**: Combination may increase the risk for myelosuppression.
- **IODINE 131**: Methimazole does not appear to have a significant impact on radioiodine efficacy and discontinuing methimazole prior to radioiodine does not appear necessary.[1]
- **PHENOBARBITAL**: Concurrent use of phenobarbital may reduce the clinical effectiveness of methimazole.[6]
- **PREDNIS(OL)ONE**: A reduction in dose may be needed when the patient becomes euthyroid.
- **TECHNETIUM-99M PERTECHNETATE**: Thyroid scintigraphy has not been shown to be significantly altered by methimazole in hyperthyroid cats.[28]
- **THEOPHYLLINE**: A reduction in the theophylline dose may be needed when the patient becomes euthyroid.[6]
- **WARFARIN**: In humans with hyperthyroidism, the metabolism of vitamin K clotting factors is increased, resulting in increased sensitivity to oral anticoagulants. By reducing the effects of hyperthyroidism, methimazole may decrease clotting factor metabolism, thus reducing the effects of warfarin. However, patients that are euthyroid on methimazole and receiving warfarin may develop hypoprothrombinemia if methimazole is stopped and they become thyrotoxic again. Methimazole also has antivitamin K activity, and the veterinary label states that anticoagulants may be potentiated by methimazole.[6] Recommendation: If methimazole and warfarin are used together, increased monitoring of anticoagulant effect is warranted.

Laboratory Considerations

None were noted.

Dosages

CATS:

Hyperthyroidism (label dosage; FDA-approved): Starting dose is 2.5 mg/cat (NOT mg/kg) PO every 12 hours.[6] After 3 weeks of treatment, the dose should be titrated to effect based on individual serum total T_4 (TT_4) concentrations and clinical response. Dose adjustments should be made in 2.5 mg increments. The maximum total dose is 20 mg per day divided, not to exceed 10 mg as a single administration. In an extended-use field study, the average maintenance dose was 2.5 mg/cat (NOT mg/kg) twice daily, with a range of 2.5 – 15 mg/cat (NOT mg/kg) per day.

Hyperthyroidism (extra-label):

Oral: An initial methimazole dose of 1.25 – 2.5 mg/cat (NOT mg/kg) PO twice a day; in cases of extremely elevated TT_4, an initial dose of 5 mg/cat (NOT mg/kg) PO twice a day can be used. TT_4 should be evaluated 2 to 3 weeks after starting therapy or after any treatment adjustment(s) until euthyroidism is achieved; most cats will become euthyroid after this time. Doses are titrated in 2.5 mg/day increments to obtain and maintain circulating TT_4 concentrations in the lower half of the reference interval. Once euthyroidism is achieved, once-daily dosing can be considered.[1,15,29]

Transdermal: Methimazole (50 mg/mL; 5 mg/0.1 mL) in pluronic lecithin organogel (PLO) for transdermal administration: 2.5 – 5 mg/cat (NOT mg/kg) to inner pinna every 12 hours; alternate ear with each application.[3,4,12] See ***Compatibility/Compounding Considerations***. Gloves or finger cots should be worn when applying the medication. Convenience of administration must be weighed against somewhat lower efficacy than the oral form (67% vs 82% euthyroid at 4 weeks).[4] Lower incidence of GI effects with transdermal as compared with the oral form (4% vs 24%). No difference in facial excoriation, neutropenia, hepatotoxicity, or thrombocytopenia between the transdermal and oral form has been reported. Drawbacks of transdermal administration include erythema at the application site (alternating application site location helps prevent this), increased cost, and stability of compounded medication (guaranteed stable for 2 weeks).[30] Considering these drawbacks, topical preparations are a good alternative in cats intolerant of administration of oral dose forms.[29]

SMALL MAMMALS:

Hyperthyroidism in guinea pigs (from a case report of 3 animals treated medically[31]): Initial dose was methimazole 1 – 1.4 mg/kg PO once daily. Maintenance dosages were 2 – 3 mg/kg PO once daily for 2 animals, and 2.5 mg/kg PO every 8 hours in the third animal. All 3 animals showed improvement of clinical signs during therapy but not until the dose or frequency of administration was increased. Therefore, regular monitoring of circulating TT_4 concentrations may be required to determine appropriate dosage.[31]

Monitoring

Published guidelines recommend the following[20]:

- Owners should be counseled to monitor for lethargy, vomiting, inappetence, jaundice, or pruritus.
- The drug should be stopped at the first potential sign of adverse effects.
- The cat should be evaluated as soon as possible by performing a physical examination for skin excoriations, ruling out blood dyscrasia (CBC), ruling out hepatotoxicity (ALT, bilirubin, ALP) and comparing values with pretreatment liver enzymes (often reversibly increased in hyperthyroid cats), evaluating for renal decompensation (BUN, creatinine), and checking serum TT_4.
- If simple GI upset (ie, blood work is normal): A dose reduction should be initiated or the animal switched to transdermal methimazole, which has a lower incidence of GI upset than oral methimazole.

During the first 3 months of therapy (baseline values and after 3 and 6 weeks of treatment)[6]:

NOTE: Cats receiving daily doses that exceed 10 mg should be monitored more frequently.

- CBC with platelet count
- Serum chemistry profile

- Serum TT_4: Blood samples can be collected at any time and do not need to be collected at a prescribed time after methimazole treatment.
- Antinuclear antibody (ANA) testing, if indicated by clinical signs

After stabilization (at least 3 months of therapy)[6]:

- TT_4 at 3- to 6-month intervals
- Other diagnostic tests as indicated by adverse effects

Client Information

- Although this medicine decreases excessive thyroid hormones, it does not cure the condition. Give this medicine as directed by your veterinarian. It may take several weeks before your cat shows clinical improvement.
- Most side effects, including vomiting, decreased appetite, or lethargy (eg, tiredness, lack of energy), occur in the first 3 months of therapy.
- This medicine is available in different dosage forms, including a compounded topical gel that can be applied to your animal's skin.
- Wear gloves when the transdermal/topical formulation is applied to your animal's skin. Wash hands with soap and water after handling the medicine (even if gloves are worn) and when cleaning waste from the litter box.
- Pregnant women, women who may become pregnant, and nursing mothers should wear gloves when handling this medicine, litter, or bodily fluids of treated cats.
- Do not use the transdermal gel if it appears visibly separated (ie, not uniform in appearance).
- Crusted material that forms on your cat's ear can be removed with moistened gauze or cotton ball prior to the next dose. Alternate ears with each application.
- This medication is considered to be a hazardous drug as defined by the National Institute for Occupational Safety and Health (NIOSH). Talk with your veterinarian or pharmacist about the use of personal protective equipment when handling this medicine.

Chemistry/Synonyms

Methimazole, a thioimidazole-derivative (thioureylene) antithyroid drug, occurs as a white to pale-buff crystalline powder and has a faint characteristic odor and a melting point of 144°C to 147°C (291.2°F-296.6°F). It is freely soluble (1 gram in 5 mL) in water or alcohol.

Methimazole may also be known as thiamazole, mercazolylum, methylmercaptoimidazole, thiamazolum, tiamazol, *Felimazole*®, and *Tapazole*®.

Storage/Stability

Methimazole tablets should be stored in well-closed, light-resistant containers at room temperature 25°C (77°F) with excursions between 15°C and 30°C (59°F-86°F) permitted; protect from moisture.

Compatibility/Compounding Considerations

Compounded transdermal formulations of methimazole in a pluronic lecithin organogel (PLO) vehicle have been investigated,[3,4,11,12] and, although another proprietary formulation has been reported,[13,32] studies validating other common compounding vehicles (eg, *Lipoderm*®) were not located.

Dosage Forms/Regulatory Status

VETERINARY-LABELED PRODUCTS:

Methimazole Tablets (sugar-coated): 2.5 mg and 5 mg; *Felimazole*®; (Rx). FDA-approved for use in cats. NADA #141-292. 1.25 mg tablets are available in the UK, in addition to 2.5 mg and 5 mg (POM-V).

HUMAN-LABELED PRODUCTS:

Methimazole Tablets (plain and scored): 5 mg and 10 mg; *Tapazole*®, generic; (Rx)

References

For the complete list of references, see **wiley.com/go/budde/plumb**

Methionine

DL-Methionine

Racemethionine

(me-***thye***-oh-neen) *Methio-Form*®

Urinary Acidifier, Nutritional

Prescriber Highlights

- Used primarily as a urinary acidifier; may be useful in managing struvite urolithiasis
- Contraindications include renal failure, pancreatic disease, hepatic insufficiency, pre-existing acidosis, and oxalate or urate calculi. Not recommended for kittens
- Adverse effects include GI distress (food may alleviate) and Heinz-body hemolytic anemia (cats).

Uses/Indications

In small animal species, methionine has been used primarily for its urine acidification effect in the treatment and prevention of certain types of urolith formation (eg, struvite) and to reduce ammoniacal urine odor. Use of methionine is generally not recommended unless urine pH is more than 6.5. Feeding of acidifying commercial feline diets can successfully minimize or dissolve struvite urolith formation,[1,2] and methionine can be considered for cats for which these diets are contraindicated or that cannot be fed.

In food animal species, methionine has been used as a nutritional supplement in swine and poultry feed and in the treatment of ketosis in cattle. It has been suggested as a treatment for laminitis in horses and cattle (purportedly provides a disulfide bond substrate to maintain the hoof-pedal bone bond), but definitive studies demonstrating its effectiveness for this indication are lacking. A small study in male goats (wethers) concluded that methionine may be a more palatable alternative for urine acidification in small ruminants.[3]

Pharmacology/Actions

Methionine has several pharmacologic effects. It is an essential amino acid (l-form) and nutrient, a lipotrope (prevents or corrects fatty liver in choline deficiency), and a urine acidifier. Two molecules of methionine can be converted to one molecule of cysteine. Methionine supplies both sulfhydryl and methyl groups to the liver for metabolic processes. Choline is formed when methionine supplies a methyl group to ethanolamine. After methionine is metabolized, sulfate is excreted in the urine as sulfuric acid, thereby acidifying the urine.

Pharmacokinetics

No information is available on the pharmacokinetics of this agent in veterinary species or humans.

Contraindications/Precautions/Warnings

Methionine (at pharmacologic doses) is contraindicated in patients with severe renal or pancreatic disease.[4] If used in patients with severe hepatic disease, methionine can cause increased production of mercaptan-like compounds and intensify the signs of hepatic encephalopathy or coma. Methionine should not be given to animals with pre-existing acidosis (eg, diabetic ketoacidosis) or with oxalate or urate calculi. It is not recommended for use in kittens, as excess dietary methionine has been shown to alter growth.[5]

Use of methionine in combination with a urinary acidifying diet is not recommended.

Do not confuse methionine with methenamine or S-adenosyl-L-methionine (SAMe).

Adverse Effects

At recommended dosages, GI distress can occur; give with food or divide into multiple meals to alleviate this effect.[4] Methionine may cause Heinz-body hemolytic anemia in cats. See ***Overdose/Acute Toxicity*** (below) for other potential adverse effects.

Unmonitored use of methionine with an acidifying diet may increase the risk for adverse effects or acute toxicity.

Reproductive/Nursing Safety

No specific information was located. Methionine administration to the dam could cause fetal acidosis.

Because safety has not been established in animals, this drug should only be used when the maternal benefits outweigh the potential risks to offspring.

Overdose/Acute Toxicity

Vomiting and ataxia are the most common clinical signs of overdose in dogs. Vomiting may occur at doses as low as 22.5 mg/kg. At higher doses (300 mg/kg), vocalization, tremors, hypermetria, tremors, and disorientation may occur. Methionine may be toxic to kittens that consume food in which methionine has been added. When methionine was administered at a dose of 2 g/kg PO daily to mature cats, anorexia, methemoglobinemia, Heinz-body formation (with resultant hemolytic anemia), ataxia, and cyanosis were noted. An ingestion of 20 grams/cat (NOT mg/kg) is likely to be fatal without treatment.[1] Metabolic acidosis may occur with overdoses in any species, particularly in combination with an acidifying diet.

Treatment can include GI decontamination (if the ingestion occurred within 2 to 4 hours prior to presentation), supportive therapy, and correction of acid/base abnormalities. Clinical signs generally resolve within 24 to 48 hours.[6]

For patients that have experienced or are suspected to have experienced an overdose, consultation with a 24-hour poison consultation center specializing in providing veterinary-specific information is recommended. For general information related to overdose and toxin exposures, as well as contact information for poison control centers, refer to ***Appendix***.

Drug Interactions

The following drug interactions have either been reported or are theoretical in humans or animals receiving methionine and may be of significance in veterinary patients. Unless otherwise noted, use together is not necessarily contraindicated, but weigh the potential risks and perform additional monitoring when appropriate.

- **Aminoglycosides** (eg, **amikacin, gentamicin**): Aminoglycosides are more effective in an alkaline medium; urine acidification may diminish the effectiveness of these drugs in treating bacterial UTIs.
- **Antiarrhythmic Agents (lidocaine, mexiletine, procainamide, quinidine)**: Urine acidification may increase excretion of these antiarrhythmic agents, potentially reducing their efficacy.
- **Carbonic Anhydrase Inhibitors** (eg, **acetazolamide, methazolamide**): May negate the effect of each drug on urine pH. Avoid combination.
- **Citrate, Potassium**: May negate the effect of each drug on urine pH. Avoid combination.
- **Colchicine**: Urine acidification may increase colchicine excretion, potentially reducing its efficacy.
- **Ephedrine**: Urine acidification may increase ephedrine excretion, potentially reducing its efficacy.
- **Erythromycin**: Erythromycin is more effective in an alkaline medium; urine acidification may diminish the effectiveness of erythromycin in treating bacterial UTIs.
- **Phenylpropanolamine (PPA)**: Urine acidification may increase PPA excretion, potentially reducing its efficacy.
- **Salicylates** (eg, **aspirin, bismuth subsalicylate**): Urine acidification may decrease salicylate excretion and increase plasma salicylate concentration.
- **Zonisamide**: May reduce the ability of methionine to acidify the urine.

Laboratory Considerations

- No known laboratory considerations

Dosages

DOGS:

Urine acidification (label dosage; not FDA-approved): 150 – 300 mg (2 – 4 mEq)/kg PO daily.[3] Practically, small breeds (less than 7 kg [15 lb]): ½ – 4 tablets PO daily; medium breeds (7 to 15 kg [15 to 33 lb]): 2 – 7 tablets PO daily; large breeds (15 to 30 kg [33 to 66 lb]): 4 – 13 tablets PO daily. Once-daily dosing is appropriate, but daily dose may be administered in 2 or 3 divided doses. **NOTE**: Tablets can be crushed and sprinkled over the food.

Urine acidification; infection-induced struvite dissolution (extra-label): 75 – 100 mg/kg PO every 12 hours in combination with an appropriate antibiotic microbial agent and without using a struvite dissolution diet. Continue antibiotic until urolith is dissolved. Reconsider diagnosis and/or choice of antibiotic if uroliths have not decreased in size by 50% within one month of treatment initiation.[7]

CATS:

Urine acidification (label dosage; not FDA-approved): 188 – 375 mg (2.5 – 5 mEq)/kg PO daily.[3] Practically, ½ – 1 tablet/1 to 1.5 kg (2.5 to 3 lb) body weight; average-sized cats typically receive 1-½ – 3 tablets (10 – 20 mEq) PO daily. Once-daily dosing is appropriate, but daily dose may be administered in 2 or 3 divided doses. **NOTE**: Tablets can be crushed and sprinkled over the food.

Urine acidification (extra-label): 1000 – 1500 mg/cat (NOT mg/kg) PO daily given in the food once daily[8] if diet and antimicrobials do not reduce urine pH.[9]

SMALL RUMINANTS:

Urine acidification (extra-label): 200 mg/kg PO daily in feed.

Monitoring

- Urine pH (urine pH of less than or equal to 6.5 has been recommended as goal of therapy)
- Blood pH if signs of toxicity are present
- CBC in cats exhibiting signs of toxicity
- If attempting medical dissolution of struvite uroliths, monthly monitoring of abdominal radiographs and/or ultrasonography monthly until calculi are no longer visible

Client Information

- Give with meals or mixed in food, unless otherwise instructed by your veterinarian.
- Do not use in combination with a urinary acidifying diet unless directed to do so by a veterinarian.
- Discontinue use and contact your veterinarian if your animal starts vomiting, has difficulty walking, or develops any new signs.
- While your animal is taking this medication, it is important to return to your veterinarian for urine and other testing. Do not miss these important follow-up visits.

Chemistry/Synonyms

A sulfur-containing amino acid, methionine occurs as a white, crystalline powder with a characteristic odor. One gram is soluble in ≈30 mL of water and it is very slightly soluble in alcohol. 74.6 mg is equivalent to 1 mEq of methionine.

Methionine may also be known as dl-methionine, racemethionine, M, s-methionine, l-methionine, methioninum, *Ammonil®*, *Methigel®*, *Methio-Form®*, *Pedameth®*, and *Uracid®*.

Storage/Stability

Methionine should be stored at room temperature.

Compatibility/Compounding Considerations

No specific information noted

Dosage Forms/Regulatory Status

VETERINARY-LABELED PRODUCTS:

Methionine is labeled for use in dogs, cats, and horses in pharmaceutical dosage forms; however, there are no methionine products listed in the FDA's Green Book of approved products. Products labeled as nutritional supplements may be approved for use in other species. Depending on the product, methionine may be available without prescription. Methionine is an ingredient found in many other nutritional products.

Methionine Tablets: 200 mg and 500 mg; *Ammonil® Tablets*, generic; (Rx). Labeled for use in cats and dogs

Methionine Tablets Chewable: 500 mg; *Methio-Form®*; (Rx). Labeled for use in cats and dogs

Methionine Powder (concentration varies with product); may also be called d-l-Methionine Powder. Labeled for use in dogs and cats

Methionine Gel: 480 mg/6 g (8%) in 120.5 g tubes; *Methigel®*; (OTC). Labeled for use in cats and dogs

HUMAN-LABELED PRODUCTS:

Methionine Capsules: 200 mg and 500 mg; (OTC, Rx)

Methionine Tablets: 500 mg; generic; (OTC, Rx)

Methionine Oral Powder 100 mg/packet; generic; (OTC)

Topical ointments, cream, lotion, pads, and powder available

References

For the complete list of references, see **wiley.com/go/budde/plumb**

Methocarbamol

(meth-oh-***kar***-ba-mole) *Robaxin®*

Muscle Relaxant

Prescriber Highlights

- Oral and injectable centrally acting muscle relaxant; appears useful in treating muscle tremors associated with toxic agents
- Contraindications include food animals, animals with renal disease (injectable only), and animals with a hypersensitivity to methocarbamol.
- Adverse effects include sedation, salivation, emesis, lethargy, weakness, and ataxia.
- IV administration should be slow, not to exceed 2 mL/minute in dogs and cats. Avoid extravasation. May be given IM but not SC
- Use caution when using with other CNS depressant drugs, as additive CNS and respiratory depression can occur.

Uses/Indications

Methocarbamol is FDA-approved for oral and IV use in dogs and cats as an adjunctive treatment for acute inflammatory and traumatic conditions of skeletal muscle and for reduction of muscular spasms.[1] Methocarbamol has been effective in treating skeletal muscle hyperactivity due to intervertebral disc syndrome, myelitis, spinal cord injury (where cord remains intact), sprains and strains, and myositis/bursitis/synovitis. It has also been used for muscular spasms prior to or following surgical procedures and to maintain muscle relaxation in tetanus. Methocarbamol has also been found useful in treating tremors and muscle fasciculations associated with various toxicities (eg, metaldehyde, pyrethroids, strychnine, CNS stimulants [eg, caffeine, amphetamines, guarana], SSRIs, tremorgenic mycotoxins, compost ingestions) in dogs and cats. One retrospective study in cats found that after permethrin toxicity, cats that received methocarbamol had a shorter duration of hospitalization compared with cats that did not receive methocarbamol.[2]

In horses, methocarbamol is FDA-approved for IV use as an adjunctive therapy for acute inflammatory and traumatic conditions of the skeletal muscle to reduce muscular spasms and affect striated muscle relaxation.[1] Efficacy has been demonstrated for sprains and strains, myositis/fibrositis/bursitis/synovitis, and tying-up syndrome. It has also been used for muscular spasms prior to or following surgical procedures and to maintain muscle relaxation in tetanus.

Pharmacology/Actions

Methocarbamol is a central nervous system depressant with sedative and musculoskeletal relaxant properties.[3] The exact mechanism for causing skeletal muscle relaxation is uncertain, but it is thought to work centrally on the internuncial neurons. Its prolonged blocking effect on polysynaptic neurons reduces skeletal muscle hyperactivity. Methocarbamol has no direct relaxant effects on striated muscle, nerve fibers, or the motor endplate.[4] It will not directly relax contracted skeletal muscles. The drug has a secondary sedative effect at higher doses.

Pharmacokinetics

Methocarbamol is readily absorbed orally in dogs, with peak concentrations at 2 hours and a dose-dependent half-life of 0.6 to 2 hours. Methocarbamol and its metabolites are extensively conjugated before excretion in urine. There is limited excretion (ie, 2%) in feces, and most methocarbamol is eliminated within 24 hours.[5]

In horses, oral paste bioavailability is ≈50%[6]; the volume of distribution is 1.6 L/kg, clearance is 6 to 9 mL/kg/minute, and elimination halflife is 3 to 4 hours.[7] In a study,[7] the elimination half-life for single 5 g and 15 g oral (paste) doses were 32 and 3.7 hours, respectively, and there was no significant difference between the single dose of 15 g and multiple doses of 15 g (4.1 hours). The majority of horses given a single oral dose or multiple oral doses of 15 g were above the regulatory threshold set by the Association of Racing Commissioners International (ARCI) at the recommended withdrawal time. The study concluded that, because of the similarities between absorption and elimination half-lives, the difference in the time above the regulatory threshold with a 15 g oral dose (as compared with a 5 g dose) is likely due to higher drug exposure rather than lower clearance.

In humans, methocarbamol has an onset of action ≈30 minutes after oral administration. Peak concentrations occur ≈2 hours after administration, and plasma protein binding is ≈50%. The serum half-life is ≈1 to 2 hours. The drug is metabolized, and the inactive metabolites are excreted into the urine and the feces (small amounts).

Guaifenesin is a minor metabolite of methocarbamol and was quantifiable after oral administration, which may have regulatory ramifications in racing; however, it probably has little clinical effect.

Contraindications/Precautions/Warnings

Methocarbamol should not be used in patients that are hypersensitive to it or in food animals.

Methocarbamol should not be administered SC, and extravasation should be avoided, as the injection is hypertonic; IV administration should not exceed 2 mL/minute in dogs and cats.[4]

Because the injectable product contains polyethylene glycol (PEG) 300, the manufacturer lists known or suspected renal pathology as a contraindication to injectable methocarbamol therapy.[3] PEG 300 has been noted to increase pre-existing acidosis and urea retention in humans with renal impairment. In addition, drug clearance is reduced with severe renal impairment or severe hepatic impairment; dosage reduction may be necessary. Use methocarbamol with caution in patients with known or suspected seizure disorders. In humans, IV administration rate should not exceed 3 mL/minute due to the risk for bradycardia and hypotension attributable to PEG 300.[3]

Adverse Effects

Adverse effects can include sedation, salivation, emesis, lethargy, weakness, loss of righting reflex, and ataxia in dogs and cats. These effects appear to be related to dose and rate of injection. Sedation and ataxia are possible in horses. Because of its CNS depressant effects, methocarbamol may impair the abilities of working animals.

In humans, serious adverse effects include anaphylactic reactions and seizures.[3] Onset of convulsive seizures during IV administration of methocarbamol has been reported in patients with seizure disorders.

Reproductive/Nursing Safety

It is unknown whether methocarbamol crosses the placenta and what the effects are, if any, on the developing fetus. It should be used with caution during pregnancy, as studies demonstrating its safety during pregnancy are lacking.

Methocarbamol or its metabolites are excreted in the milk in dogs.[8] In humans, the Briggs breastfeeding recommendation states that methocarbamol is likely compatible with breastfeeding. Caution should be used in nursing dams.[9]

Because safety has not been established in animals, this drug should only be used when the maternal benefits outweigh the potential risks to offspring.

Overdose/Acute Toxicity

The reported oral LD_{50} in rats and dogs is 1.32 g/kg and 2 g/kg, respectively.[10] Overdose is generally characterized by CNS depressant effects (eg, loss of righting reflex, prostration). In dogs and cats, excessive doses may cause emesis, salivation, weakness, and ataxia.

GI decontamination protocols may be indicated if the patient presents within 2 to 3 hours of a toxic ingestion. Emesis should not be induced if the patient's continued consciousness cannot be assured. Severe clinical signs should be treated supportively, including maintenance of an adequate airway and administration of IV fluids if necessary.

For patients that have experienced or are suspected of having experienced an overdose, consultation with a 24-hour poison consultation center specializing in providing veterinary-specific information is recommended. For general information related to overdose and toxin exposures, as well as contact information for poison control centers, refer to ***Appendix***.

Drug Interactions

The following drug interactions have either been reported or are theoretical in humans or animals receiving methocarbamol and may be of significance in veterinary patients. Unless otherwise noted, use together is not necessarily contraindicated, but weigh the potential risks and perform additional monitoring when appropriate.

- **Antihistamines** (eg, **diphenhydramine**): Increased risk for CNS depression
- **Benzodiazepines** (eg, **diazepam, midazolam**): Increased risk for CNS depression
- **Buprenorphine**: Methocarbamol may enhance the CNS depressant effect of buprenorphine.
- **CNS Depressants** (eg, **acepromazine, baclofen, dexmedetomidine, trazodone**): Additive depression may occur when methocarbamol is given with other CNS depressant agents.
- **Gabapentin**: Concurrent use may result in respiratory depression.
- **Metoclopramide**: Increased risk for CNS depression
- **Mirtazapine**: Methocarbamol may enhance the CNS depressant effect of mirtazapine.
- **Opioids** (eg, **buprenorphine, morphine, tramadol**): Increased risk for CNS depression
- **Phenobarbital**: May result in additive respiratory depression
- **Pyridostigmine**: Methocarbamol may diminish the therapeutic effect of pyridostigmine.
- **Selective Serotonin Reuptake Inhibitors (SSRIs; eg, fluoxetine, paroxetine)**: Methocarbamol may enhance the adverse/toxic effects of SSRIs.

Laboratory Considerations

- Methocarbamol may cause color interference in certain screening tests for **5-hydroxyindoleacetic acid** using nitrosonaphthol reagent and in screening tests for urinary **vanillylmandelic acid** using the Gitlow method.

Dosages

DOGS/CATS:

Reducing muscle spasms from acute inflammatory and traumatic conditions of the skeletal muscle (label dosage; FDA-approved):

a) **Injectable:**

i. For relief of moderate conditions: 44 mg/kg IV initial dose[4]

ii. For controlling severe effects of strychnine and tetanus: 55 – 220 mg/kg IV initial dose.[4] Rapidly administer 1/2 of the total dosage, allow muscle relaxation to occur, then administer the remainder of the dosage. Additional doses may be needed to relieve residual effects or prevent a recurrence. The total cumulative dose should not exceed 330 mg/kg.[4] Administer IV at a rate no faster than 2 mL/minute.

b) **Oral (tablets)**: 132 mg/kg PO on Day 1 in 2 or 3 equally divided doses (ie, every 8 to 12 hours), then 66 – 132 mg/kg/day PO divided every 8 to 12 hours.[11] Discontinue therapy if there is no response within 5 days.[12]

Adjunctive treatment of toxicities associated with muscle tremors (extra-label): Although there are no controlled studies documenting efficacy in animals, consider using an initial IV bolus, followed by a CRI or multiple (if required) IV boluses. Initially, 40 – 50 mg/kg IV slowly over 3 to 5 minutes to clinical effect (ie, resolution or near-resolution of clinical signs). Repeat as necessary or follow with a CRI at an initial rate of 10 mg/kg/hour IV. Titrate the bolus dose/frequency or CRI administration rate to clinical effect. There are 3 case reports of this method being used successfully for pyrethroid intoxication, and IV CRI rates of 8.8, 11.6, and 12.2 mg/kg/hour were used.[13] The labeled maximum dose of 330 mg/kg/day can be exceeded if necessary, but the patient must be monitored for profound CNS depression, seizures, and hypotension.[14] The IV CRI can be administered with a syringe pump or with the drug added to a fluid bag (eg, 0.9% NaCl). If the parenteral product is not available and the oral route is not appropriate, tablets can be crushed and given rectally.

Muscle relaxant for the adjunctive treatment of intervertebral disk disease in dogs (extra-label): Anecdotal dosages of 15 – 20 mg/kg PO every 8 hours are usually noted.

HORSES:

Reducing muscle spasms from acute inflammatory and traumatic conditions of the skeletal muscle (label dosage; FDA-approved):

a) For moderate conditions: 4.4 – 22 mg/kg IV to effect[1]

b) For severe conditions (tetanus): 22 – 55 mg/kg IV[1]

Monitoring

- Level of muscle relaxation/sedation
- Adverse effects (eg, salivation, emesis, ataxia, CNS depression)

Client Information

- May be given with or without food
- Drowsiness/sedation is the most common side effect.
- May cause dark or blue–green urine, but this is not clinically significant

Chemistry/Synonyms

Methocarbamol, a centrally acting muscle relaxant related structurally to guaifenesin, occurs as a fine white powder with a characteristic odor. In water, it has a solubility of 25 mg/mL. The commercial injection is hypertonic, and the pH is ≈3.5 to 6.

Methocarbamol may also be known as guaiphenesin carbamate, *Robinax*®, and *Robaxin*®.

Storage/Stability

Store methocarbamol tablets at 20°C to 25°C (68°F-77°F), protected from light and moisture. Store the injection at 20°C to 25°C (68°F-77°F), with excursions permitted to 15°C to 30°C (59°F-86°F); do not freeze. Do not refrigerate solutions prepared for IV infusion, as a precipitate may form. Because a haze or precipitate may form, physically inspect all diluted IV solutions before administration.

Compatibility/Compounding Considerations

Methocarbamol solutions diluted to 4 mg/mL in 5% dextrose or 0.9% sodium chloride are stable for 6 days at room temperature.

Dosage Forms/Regulatory Status

VETERINARY-LABELED PRODUCTS:

NOTE: Although these products are still listed in the FDA Green Book of approved animal drugs, they may no longer be commercially available in the United States.

The Association of Racing Commissioners International (ARCI) has designated this drug as a class 4 substance. Use of this drug may not be allowed in certain animal competitions. Check rules and regulations before entering a competition while this medication is being administered. Contact local racing authorities for further guidance. See ***Appendix*** for more information.

Methocarbamol Tablets: 500 mg; *Robaxin*®*-V*; (Rx). FDA-approved for use in dogs and cats. NADA# 045-715

Methocarbamol Injection: 100 mg/mL in vials of 20 mL and 100 mL; *Robaxin*®*-V*; (Rx). FDA-approved for use in dogs, cats, and horses not intended for food. NADA 038-838

HUMAN-LABELED PRODUCTS:

Methocarbamol Tablets: 500 mg and 750 mg; *Robaxin*®, *Robaxin*®*-750*, generic; (Rx)

Methocarbamol Injection: 100 mg/mL in 10 mL vials; *Robaxin*®; (Rx)

References

For the complete list of references, see **wiley.com/go/budde/plumb**

Methotrexate

Methotrexate Sodium

(meth-oh-***trex***-ate)

Antineoplastic, Immunosuppressive

Prescriber Highlights

- ▶ Used primarily for lymphoma in dogs and cats
- ▶ Contraindications include pre-existing myelosuppression, severe hepatic or renal insufficiency, or known hypersensitivity to methotrexate.
- ▶ Common adverse effects include inappetence, vomiting, and diarrhea.
- ▶ Many potential drug interactions
- ▶ Teratogenic; may affect spermatogenesis. The National Institute for Occupational Safety and Health (NIOSH) classifies methotrexate as a hazardous drug; use appropriate precautions when handling it.

Uses/Indications

Methotrexate was used in original multiagent protocols for the treatment of lymphoproliferative diseases in dogs and cats; however, as less toxic and more potent agents became available, methotrexate has fallen out of favor and is now rarely used in veterinary oncology protocols. Methotrexate has been suggested as part of a possible rescue therapy combination with lomustine and cytarabine for relapsed feline lymphoma, failing more standardized multiagent protocols (COP and CHOP), but strong evidence of efficacy is lacking.[1]

Although there is little clinical experience with methotrexate as an immunomodulating drug in animals, low-dose methotrexate has been used as an alternate immunosuppressive agent when other drugs (eg, prednisone, azathioprine) have not been effective, or as an add-on drug to enhance efficacy and/or allow dosage reductions of other drugs.

Pharmacology/Actions

Methotrexate is an S-phase specific antimetabolite antineoplastic agent that competitively inhibits folic acid reductase, preventing the reduction of dihydrofolate to tetrahydrofolate and affecting the production of purines and pyrimidines. Rapidly proliferating cells (eg, neoplasms, bone marrow, GI tract epithelium, fetal cells) are most sensitive to the drug's effects.

Dihydrofolate reductase has a much greater affinity for methotrexate than either folic acid or dihydrofolic acid, and coadministration of folic acid will not reduce methotrexate's effects. Leucovorin calcium (a derivative of tetrahydrofolic acid) can block the effects of methotrexate.

Methotrexate also has immunosuppressive activity, possibly due to its effects on lymphocyte replication. Neoplastic cells have been noted to develop resistance to methotrexate, possibly due to decreased cellular uptake of the drug. One study demonstrated that the 50% inhibitory concentration for methotrexate was higher in histiocytic sarcoma lines than in lymphoma.[2]

Pharmacokinetics

In a pharmacokinetic study in dogs, the oral bioavailability of low-dose methotrexate (≈0.5 mg/kg) was 30%, but inter-individual variability was high. SC bioavailability was much higher at ≈93% and was more consistent. The half-life was ≈2 to 3 hours.[3]

In one pharmacokinetic study in horses, oral bioavailability was less than 1%, but SC bioavailability was 73%. The half-life was ≈2 to 2.5 hours.[4]

In humans, oral absorption is dose-dependent, and the absorption rate appears to decrease with the increasing dose. After oral administration of dosages less than 30 mg/m^2, the average bioavailability of methotrexate was ≈60%. Peak concentrations occur within 4 hours after oral dosing and between 30 minutes and 2 hours after IM injection.

Methotrexate is widely distributed in the body and is actively transported across cell membranes. The highest concentrations are found in the kidneys, spleen, gallbladder, liver, and skin. When given orally or parenterally, methotrexate does not reach therapeutic concentrations in the CSF. When given intrathecally, methotrexate attains therapeutic concentrations in the CSF and also passes into the systemic circulation. In humans, methotrexate is ≈50% bound to plasma proteins and crosses the placenta. Methotrexate is excreted almost entirely by the kidneys via both glomerular filtration and active transport. Serum half-life is between 3 and 10 hours.

Contraindications/Precautions/Warnings

Methotrexate is contraindicated in patients with pre-existing bone marrow depression, severe hepatic or renal insufficiency, or hypersensitivity to the drug. It should be used with caution in patients that are susceptible to or have pre-existing clinical signs associated with the adverse reactions associated with this drug (see ***Adverse Effects***).

Unexpected and severe myelosuppression has been reported in humans. Respiratory clinical signs, especially coughing, may indicate a severe methotrexate-induced interstitial pneumonitis and should prompt further investigation. Diarrhea and stomatitis require interruption of therapy in humans, as there is a risk for fatal hemorrhagic enteritis and intestinal perforation. Severe skin reactions have been reported in humans. Hepatotoxicity is possible but typically only after prolonged use. Although acute increases in liver enzymes are often seen, they are usually transient. Methotrexate may cause renal damage that can lead to acute renal failure. Potentially fatal opportunistic infections are possible. Elimination is reduced in patients with ascites or pleural effusion.[5]

In human medicine, methotrexate is considered a high-alert medication (medications that require special safeguards to reduce the risk for errors). Consider instituting practices such as redundant drug dosage and volume checking and special alert labels.

Some formulations contain benzyl alcohol.

The National Institute for Occupational Safety and Health (NIOSH) classifies methotrexate as a hazardous drug; personal protective equipment (PPE) should be used accordingly to minimize the risk for exposure.

Adverse Effects

In dogs and cats, GI adverse effects are most prevalent, including diarrhea, nausea, inappetence (especially cats), and vomiting (especially dogs). Leukopenia, thrombocytopenia, temporary alopecia, depigmentation, or oral lesions can occur but are uncommon. Transient elevations in liver enzymes are possible, including with low dosages in dogs and horses.[3,4] Higher doses may lead to nephrotoxicity due to the precipitation of the drug in the renal tubules. CNS toxicity (encephalopathy) may be noted if methotrexate is given intrathecally; however, a retrospective evaluation of 112 dogs and 8 cats receiving cytosine arabinoside alone or in combination with methotrexate found that only 1 patient developed generalized tonic-clonic seizure activity after intrathecal administration of this drug combination.[6] From this evaluation, it was concluded that intrathecal administration of cytosine arabinoside alone or in combination with methotrexate is a safe procedure in dogs and cats. Anaphylaxis has rarely been seen. One case of granulomatous mural folliculitis has been reported in a dog receiving cyclosporine and methotrexate.[7]

Reproductive/Nursing Safety

Methotrexate is teratogenic, embryotoxic, and may affect spermatogenesis in male animals.

For sexually intact patients, verify pregnancy status prior to administration.

Methotrexate is contraindicated in nursing mothers. It is excreted in breast milk in low concentrations with a milk:plasma ratio of 0.08:1. Nursing offspring should be switched to milk replacer if the dam requires methotrexate.

Because safety has not been established in animals, this drug should only be used when the maternal benefits outweigh the potential risks to offspring.

Overdose/Acute Toxicity

The oral LD_{50} for single doses of methotrexate in mice and rats is 146 mg/kg and 135 mg/kg, respectively. The LD_{50} for single IV doses in mice and rats is 65 mg/kg and 14 mg/kg, respectively. Acute overdoses in dogs are associated with exacerbations of the adverse effects outlined above, particularly myelosuppression and acute renal failure. Acute tubular necrosis is secondary to drug precipitation in the tubules. In dogs, the maximum tolerated dose is reported to be 0.12 mg/kg once daily for 5 days; 10 mg/kg is considered a lethal dose if leucovorin rescue is not performed.

Treatment of acute oral overdoses includes GI decontamination and prevention of drug absorption using standard protocols if the ingestion is recent. Additionally, oral neomycin has been suggested to help prevent the absorption of methotrexate from the GI tract. In order to minimize renal damage, forced alkaline diuresis should be considered. Urine pH should be maintained between 7.5 and 8 by the addition of sodium bicarbonate 0.5 – 1 mEq/kg per 500 mL of IV fluid. One case of successful serial use of charcoal hemoperfusion and hemodialysis following a methotrexate overdose in a dog has been reported.[8]

Leucovorin calcium is specific therapy for methotrexate overdoses. It should be given as soon as possible, preferably within the first hour and within 48 hours. Doses of leucovorin required are dependent on the methotrexate serum concentration. See ***Leucovorin***.

For patients that have experienced or are suspected of having experienced an overdose, consultation with a 24-hour poison consultation center specializing in providing veterinary-specific information is recommended. For general information related to overdose and toxin exposures, as well as contact information for poison control centers, refer to ***Appendix.***

Drug Interactions

Methotrexate has been shown to be a substrate of the drug transporter ABCG-2, and there are potentially many interactions with other drugs that may be clinically significant. The following drug interactions have either been reported or are theoretical in humans or animals receiving methotrexate and may be of significance in veterinary patients. Unless otherwise noted, use together is not necessarily contraindicated, but weigh the potential risks and perform additional monitoring when appropriate.

- **Amiodarone**: May increase the risk for methotrexate toxicity
- **Asparaginase**: May decrease the antineoplastic activity of methotrexate, as asparaginase inhibits cell replication that is required for methotrexate activity
- **Chloramphenicol**: May decrease methotrexate efficacy
- **Ciprofloxacin**: May increase methotrexate concentrations
- **Cyclosporine**: May increase methotrexate levels; consider therapy modification.
- **Doxycycline**: May increase the risk for methotrexate toxicity
- **Hepatotoxic Drugs** (eg, **halothane, ketoconazole, valproic acid, phenobarbital, primidone**): Methotrexate should be used cautiously with other drugs that can cause hepatotoxicity.
- **Hydrochlorothiazide**: May increase methotrexate exposure and increase the risk for myelosuppression
- **Immunosuppressive Drugs** (eg, **azathioprine, cyclophosphamide, corticosteroids**): Use with other immunosuppressant drugs may increase the risk for infection.

- **Leflunomide**: May result in increased methotrexate exposure and increased risk for hepatotoxicity and bone marrow toxicity
- **Levetiracetam**: May increase methotrexate exposure and toxicity
- **Loop Diuretics** (eg, **furosemide**): Methotrexate may decrease the efficacy of loop diuretics; consider therapy modification.
- **Myelosuppressive Agents** (eg, **antineoplastics, immunosuppressants, iron chelators**): Concurrent use with other bone marrow depressant medications may result in additive myelosuppression; avoid combination when possible.
- **Neomycin (oral)**: Oral neomycin may decrease the absorption of oral methotrexate if given concomitantly.
- **Nonsteroidal Anti-Inflammatory Drugs (NSAIDs), Salicylates**: In humans, severe hematologic and GI toxicity has resulted in patients receiving both methotrexate and NSAIDs; avoid or use very cautiously in dogs on methotrexate.
- **Proton Pump Inhibitors** (eg, **omeprazole, pantoprazole**): May increase concentrations of methotrexate and its metabolite; increased risk for methotrexate toxicity
- **Penicillins**: Penicillins may interfere with the excretion of methotrexate and increase the risk for methotrexate toxicity. Avoid concurrent use. If the combination cannot be avoided, consider decreasing the methotrexate dose and monitoring closely for adverse effects.
- **Probenecid**: May inhibit the tubular secretion of methotrexate and increase its half-life
- **Sulfonamides** (eg, **sulfadimethoxine, sulfamethoxazole**): May displace methotrexate from plasma proteins, increasing the risk for toxicity
- **Theophylline**: May increase theophylline exposure
- **Vaccines** (live and inactivated): Methotrexate may diminish vaccine efficacy and enhance adverse effects of vaccines.
- **Warfarin**: May cause prolonged bleeding times and increased risk for bleeding

Laboratory Considerations

- Methotrexate may cause invalid **vitamin B_{12}** results.
- Methotrexate may interfere with the microbiologic assay for **folic acid**.

Dosages

NOTE: Dosages and dosage forms of methotrexate sodium are expressed in terms of methotrexate. Because of the potential toxicity of methotrexate, when used at antineoplastic dosages, to patients, veterinary personnel, and clients, and since chemotherapy indications, treatment protocols, monitoring, and safety guidelines often change, the following dosages should be used only as a general guide. Consultation with a veterinary oncologist and referral to current veterinary oncology references[9-13] are strongly recommended. It is not recommended to crush, split, or formulate oral tablets into liquid, as this practice increases the risk for environmental contamination, and personal and/or occupational exposure to chemotherapy. Dosages are commonly listed as mg/m^2. Do not confuse with mg/kg dosages.

DOGS:

Susceptible neoplastic diseases (usually as part of a multi-drug protocol) (extra-label):

a) As part of the LMP protocol for maintenance of canine lymphoma: Chlorambucil 20 mg/m^2 (NOT mg/kg) PO every 15 days; methotrexate 2.5 – 5 mg/m^2 (NOT mg/kg) PO twice a week; prednisone 20 mg/m^2 (NOT mg/kg) PO every other day. Vincristine can be added to this protocol at a dosage of 0.5 – 0.7 mg/m2 (NOT mg/kg) IV given every 15 days, alternating weeks with chlorambucil.[14]

b) Combining with other antineoplastics (per protocol): methotrexate 5 mg/m^2 (NOT mg/kg) PO twice weekly or 0.8 mg/kg IV every 21 days; alternatively, 2.5 mg/m^2 (NOT mg/kg) PO daily[15]

As an immunosuppressive agent (extra-label): There is not much experience using methotrexate as an immunosuppressant agent in animals. Anecdotal dosages noted include 2.5 mg/m^2 (NOT mg/kg) PO every 24 hours.

CATS:

Susceptible neoplastic diseases (usually as part of a multi-drug protocol); (extra-label): 2.5 mg/m^2 (NOT mg/kg) PO 2 to 3 times weekly; 0.3 – 0.8 mg/m^2 (NOT mg/kg) IV every 7 days.[16] A study evaluating the combination of alternating lomustine, cytarabine, and methotrexate used a target methotrexate dosage of 0.5 – 0.6 mg/m^2 (NOT mg/kg) IV.[1]

Immunosuppressive agent (extra-label): One dosage recommendation for treating rheumatoid arthritis with leflunomide is: Initially, 10 mg of leflunomide per cat (NOT mg/kg) PO once daily with 2.5 mg of methotrexate per cat (NOT mg/kg) PO 3 times on 1 day per week (ie, 7.5 mg of methotrexate per cat [NOT mg/kg] is divided and given as 3 separate 2.5 mg doses over a single day). When significant improvement occurs, reduce doses to 10 mg of leflunomide per cat (NOT mg/kg) PO twice weekly and 2.5 mg of methotrexate (NOT mg/kg) PO once weekly.[17,18]

HORSES:

Immunomodulatory agent (extra-label): 0.2 mg/kg SC weekly was suggested based on a pharmacokinetic study, further studies are warranted to verify efficacy and safety.[4]

Monitoring

- Efficacy: serial lymph node measurements by physical caliper measurements and/or radiologic methods (thoracic and abdominal radiographs and ultrasound)
- Baseline CBC, serum chemistry profile, and urinalysis:
  - CBCs should be performed weekly early in therapy and eventually every 4 to 6 weeks when stabilized. If absolute neutrophil count is less than 2500/µL or platelet count is less than 75,000/µL, therapy should be delayed until these values return to normal. The chemistry panel should be evaluated monthly while on therapy or more frequently if abnormalities are noted at baseline.
  - Frequency of CBC and serum chemistry profile monitoring depends on the protocol employed. Consultation with a veterinary oncologist is recommended.
- Monitor for clinical signs of toxicity, including vomiting, diarrhea, inappetence, and fever.

Client Information

- It is important to follow your veterinarian's directions when giving this medication to your animal to minimize the risks for side effects.
- Methotrexate is a chemotherapy (anticancer) drug. It can be hazardous to other animals and humans that come in contact with it.
- Wear gloves when handling this medication. On the day your animal gets the drug and then for a few days afterward, handle all bodily waste (ie, urine, feces, litter), blood, or vomit only while wearing disposable gloves. Seal the waste in a plastic bag, then place both the bag and gloves in with the regular trash.
- Give this medicine with food.
- This medicine can affect your animal's ability to fight infection (bone marrow suppression). The greatest effects on bone marrow usually occur within a few weeks after treatment.

- Methotrexate can be toxic to the gastrointestinal tract and cause vomiting and gastrointestinal upset.
- Contact your veterinarian immediately if you see bleeding, bruising, shortness of breath, vomiting, diarrhea, lack of an appetite, fever (indicating an infection), or if your animal becomes very tired easily.
- While your animal is taking this medication, it is important to return to your veterinarian for physical examinations and laboratory work. Do not miss these important follow-up visits.
- This medication is considered to be a hazardous drug as defined by the National Institute for Occupational Safety and Health (NIOSH). Talk with your veterinarian or pharmacist about the use of personal protective equipment when handling this medicine.

Chemistry/Synonyms

Methotrexate is a folic acid antagonist that is available commercially as sodium salt. It occurs as a yellow powder that is soluble in water. Methotrexate sodium injection has a pH of 7.5 to 9.

Methotrexate and methotrexate sodium may also be known as MTX, amethopterin, 4-Amino-4-deoxy-10-methylpteroyl-L-glutamic acid, 4-Amino-10-methylfolic acid, CL-14377, alpha-methopterin, methotrexatum, metotrexato, NSC-740, WR-19039; there are many trade names available.

Storage/Stability

Store methotrexate tablets and injectables between 20°C and 25°C (68°F-77°F) in well-closed containers and protect from light.

Store methotrexate oral solution in the original container with tightly closed lid and refrigerated (2°C-8°C [36°F-46°F]); may store at room temperature for up to 60 days. Avoid freezing and excessive heat.

Compatibility/Compounding Considerations

Compatibility is dependent on factors such as pH, concentration, temperature, and diluent used; specialized references or a hospital pharmacist should be consulted for more specific information.

Methotrexate sodium is reportedly physically **compatible** with the following IV solutions and drugs: Amino acids 4.25%/dextrose 25%, D_5W, sodium bicarbonate 0.05 M, cytarabine, mercaptopurine sodium, sodium bicarbonate, and vincristine sulfate. In syringes, methotrexate is physically **compatible** with bleomycin sulfate, cyclophosphamide, doxorubicin HCl, fluorouracil, furosemide, leucovorin calcium, mitomycin, vinblastine sulfate, and vincristine sulfate.

Methotrexate sodium **compatibility information conflicts** or is dependent on diluent or concentration factors with the following drugs or solutions: heparin sodium and metoclopramide HCl.

Methotrexate sodium is reportedly physically **incompatible** when mixed with the following solutions or drugs: bleomycin sulfate (as an IV additive only; **compatible** in syringes and Y-lines), fluorouracil (as an IV additive only; **compatible** in syringes and Y-lines), prednisolone sodium phosphate, and ranitidine HCl.

Dosage Forms/Regulatory Status

VETERINARY-LABELED PRODUCTS: NONE

The Association of Racing Commissioners International (ARCI) has designated this drug as a class 4 substance. Use of this drug may not be allowed in certain animal competitions. Check rules and regulations before entering a competition while this medication is being administered. Contact local racing authorities for further guidance. See ***Appendix*** for more information.

HUMAN-LABELED PRODUCTS:

Methotrexate Tablets: 2.5 mg, 5 mg, 7.5 mg, 10 mg, and 15 mg; *Trexall*®, generic (2.5 mg only); (Rx)

Methotrexate Oral Solution: 2.5 mg/mL in 120 mL bottles; *Xatmep*®; (Rx)

Methotrexate Injection for SC use; available in numerous strengths and configurations:

- 7.5 mg, 10 mg, 12.5 mg, 15 mg, 17.5 mg, 20 mg, 22.5 mg, and 25 mg in 0.4 mL auto-injectors (concentration varies); *Otrexup*®; (Rx)
- 7.5 mg, 10 mg, 12.5 mg, 15 mg, 17.5 mg, 20 mg, 22.5 mg, 25 mg, 27.5 mg, and 30 mg auto-injectors as 50 mg/mL solution (injection volume varies); *Rasuvo*®(Rx)
- 7.5 mg, 10 mg, 12.5 mg, 15 mg, 17.5 mg, 20 mg, 22.5 mg, and 25 mg pre-filled syringes as a 25 mg/mL solution (injection volume varies); *Reditrex*®; (Rx)

Methotrexate Sodium Injection: 25 mg/mL preservative-free in 2 mL, 10 mL, 20 mL, and 40 mL singleuse vials; generic; (Rx)

Methotrexate Powder for Injection, lyophilized: 1 g preservative-free in single-use vials; generic; (Rx)

References

For the complete list of references, see **wiley.com/go/budde/plumb**

Methylene Blue

(***meth***-i-leen ***bloo***) *ProvayBlue*®

Antidote

Prescriber Highlights

- ► Thiazine dye primarily used to treat methemoglobinemia in ruminants; can be used in dogs and horses, but considered relatively ineffective in horses
- ► Contraindications include lactating dairy animals, renal insufficiency, and hypersensitivity to methylene blue. It is generally considered contraindicated for use in cats. Not for intrathecal use.
- ► Adverse effects include Heinz body anemia or other red cell morphological changes, methemoglobinemia, and decreased red cell life spans; cats are particularly sensitive to these effects.

Uses/Indications

Methylene blue is used primarily in ruminants for treating methemoglobinemia secondary to oxidative agents[1] (eg, nitrates, nitrites, chlorates) and occasionally as an adjunctive or alternative therapy for cyanide toxicity.

In dogs, methylene blue may be considered for treating methemoglobinemia secondary to drugs or toxins (eg, phenol, mothballs, hydroxyurea, phenazopyridine[2]). It can also be used intra-operatively to preferentially stain islet-cell tumors of the pancreas in order to aid in their surgical removal or in determining the prognosis[3]; however, IV methylene blue is rarely used for this purpose due to its adverse effects and delayed effect of colorizing pancreatic cells.

Although it has been used for treatment of methemoglobinemia in horses caused by chlorate toxicity, methylene blue is considered relatively ineffective for this purpose.

In humans, methylene blue has been used to treat histamine-induced vasodilation. It may be an option in the future to treat anaphylactic shock in animals; however, further studies are needed.[4]

Pharmacology/Actions

Methylene blue is rapidly converted to leucomethylene blue in tissues. This compound serves as a reducing agent that helps to convert methemoglobin (Fe^{+++}) to hemoglobin (Fe^{++}). Methylene blue is an oxidating agent and may actually cause methemoglobinemia if high doses are administered (species-dependent).

Methylene blue also has antimicrobial activity. Methylene blue is a potent guanylyl cyclase inhibitor and blocks the release of cyclic guanosine monophosphate (cGMP), thereby preventing vascular smooth muscle relaxation. It is used in human medicine to improve hypotension associated with various clinical states (eg, vasoplegic shock, septic shock).

Pharmacokinetics

Oral absorption of methylene blue is species dependent. It is well absorbed from the GI tract of humans but poorly absorbed when given orally to dogs.[5] Therefore, it is usually administered parenterally in veterinary medicine. Methylene blue is excreted in the urine and bile, primarily in the colorless form, but some unchanged drug may be also excreted.

Contraindications/Precautions/Warnings

Methylene blue is contraindicated in patients with renal insufficiency and in patients that are hypersensitive to it. It cannot be given as an intrathecal injection.

Methylene blue is generally considered contraindicated in cats, as it can result in Heinz body anemia and methemoglobinemia. Although the number of cells with Heinz bodies increased after two doses of methylene blue, no increase was seen after a single dose.[6]

Methylene blue has the potential to cause severe serotonin syndrome when used in combination with other serotonergic drugs.

Adverse Effects

The greatest concerns with methylene blue therapy are the development of Heinz body anemia or other erythrocyte morphological changes, methemoglobinemia, and decreased erythrocyte life spans. Cats tend to be very sensitive to these effects and it is generally considered contraindicated in feline patients; however, dogs and horses can also develop hematologic adverse effects at relatively low doses.

Necrotic abscesses may develop if injected SC or extravasation occurs during IV administration.

Adverse effects in humans include pain in extremity, discoloration of skin, nausea, and dizziness.[7]

Reproductive/Nursing Safety

Safe use of this agent during pregnancy has not been demonstrated. Human data suggest risk to the fetus when administered to women in the second and third trimesters.[7,8]

No information on lactation safety in animals was found. In humans, it is recommended to discontinue nursing during treatment and for up to 8 days after.[7]

Because safety has not been established in animals, this drug should only be used when the maternal benefits outweigh the potential risks to offspring.

Overdose/Acute Toxicity

In sheep, the IV LD_{50} for 3% methylene blue is ≈42.3 mg/kg.[9]

For patients that have experienced or are suspected to have experienced an overdose, consultation with a 24-hour poison consultation center specializing in providing veterinary-specific information is recommended. For general information related to overdose and toxin exposures, as well as contact information for poison control centers, refer to ***Appendix.***

Drug Interactions

The following drug interactions have either been reported or are theoretical in humans or animals receiving methylene blue and may be of significance in veterinary patients. Unless otherwise noted, use together is not necessarily contraindicated, but weigh the potential risks and perform additional monitoring when appropriate.

- SEROTONERGIC DRUGS (eg, **linezolid, monoamine oxidase inhibitors** [eg, **selegiline**], **selective serotonin reuptake inhibitors** [eg, **fluoxetine, paroxetine**], **tricyclic antidepressants** [eg, **amitriptyline, clomipramine**], **tramadol**): Methylene blue used in combination with drugs that increase serotonin levels may increase the risk for severe serotonin syndrome; combination is considered contraindicated in humans.

Laboratory Considerations

- Methylene blue can cause a green-blue color in urine and may affect the accuracy of **urinalysis.**
- **Pulse oximetry**. Methemoglobinemia optically interferes with the accuracy of pulse oximeters.

Dosages

DOGS:

Preferential staining of islet-cell tumors of the pancreas (extra-label): 3 mg/kg diluted in a total fluid volume of 250 mL and administered IV over 30 to 40 minutes intraoperatively.[3] **NOTE:** Dextrose 5% is recommended for dilution as sodium-chloride may reduce the solubility of methylene blue. Initial tumor staining occurs ≈20 minutes after infusion initiation and is maximal at ≈25 to 35 minutes after start of infusion. Tumors generally appear to be reddish-violet in color as opposed to the dusky blue color of the background staining.

Severe methemoglobinemia secondary to toxic exposures (eg, **phenol, mothballs, hydroxyurea**; extra-label): Using a 1% solution, 1 – 1.5 mg/kg given IV slowly over several minutes. A dramatic response should occur during the first 30 minutes after treatment. Dose may be repeated if necessary, but should be done cautiously as Heinz body anemia can result. Measure hematocrit for 3 days after treatment.[10]

Severe methemoglobinemia due to toxic phenazopyridine exposure (extra-label): 4 mg/kg IV was used in one case report.[2]

CATS:

NOTE: Use methylene blue with extreme caution in cats. Methylene blue is often considered contraindicated; however, single doses have been tolerated.[6]

Severe methemoglobinemia (extra-label): A single dose of 1 – 1.5 mg/kg IV infused slowly over several minutes

HORSES:

Methemoglobinemia secondary to chlorate toxicity (extra-label): Although generally considered ineffective, using a 1% solution, 4.4 mg/kg IV has been used; dose may be repeated after 15 to 30 minutes if clinical response is not obtained.[11]

RUMINANTS:

Methemoglobinemia due to toxins (eg, **nitrites, nitrates, chlorates**; extra-label): Using a 1% solution, 4 – 15 mg/kg IV every 6 hours.[1] See ***Dosage Forms/Regulatory Status.***

Monitoring

- Methemoglobinemia using co-oximetry or multi-wavelength pulse oximetry; pulse oximetry is not reliable
- Erythrocyte morphology, indices (eg, MCV, MCHC), hematocrit, hemoglobin

Client Information

- Because of the potential toxicity of this agent and the seriousness of methemoglobin-related intoxications, this medicine should be used with close professional supervision only.
- Methylene blue will stain clothing and skin. Removal may be accomplished using hypochlorite solutions (bleach).

Chemistry/Synonyms

A thiazine dye, methylene blue occurs as hygroscopic, dark-green crystals or crystalline powder that has a bronze-like luster. It may have a slight odor and is soluble in water and sparingly soluble in alcohol. When dissolved, a dark blue solution results. Commercially available methylene blue injection (human-labeled) has a pH from 3 to 4.5.

Methylene blue may also be known as methylthioninium chloride, azul de metileno, blu di metilene, CI basic blue 9, colour index no. 52015, methylenii caeruleum, methylthioninii chloridum, schultz no. 1038, tetramethylthionine chloride trihydrate, *Azul Metile®*, *Collubleu®*, *Desmoidpillen®*, *Vitableu®*, *Urolene Blue®* and *Zumetil®*.

Storage/Stability

Unless otherwise instructed by the manufacturer, store methylene blue at room temperature.

Compatibility/Compounding Considerations

Methylene blue is reportedly physically **incompatible** when mixed with caustic alkalis, dichromates, iodides, and oxidizing or reducing agents.

ProvayBlue® may be diluted with 50 mL of dextrose 5% in water. Do NOT dilute with sodium chloride 0.9% due to a decrease in solubility of the methylene blue.[7]

Dosage Forms/Regulatory Status

VETERINARY-LABELED PRODUCTS:

No FDA-approved products as pharmaceuticals for internal use. A non-sterile 1% (10 mg/mL) methylene blue solution is labeled for animal use as a dye, laboratory indicator, and reagent. It is available in pint and gallon bottles. Methylene Blue, USP powder may be available from chemical supply houses.

The recommended minimum milk withdrawal is 4 days and minimum meat withdrawal is an extremely conservative 180 days due to carcinogenicity concerns; however, available data suggest that a much shorter withdrawal time of 14 days may be sufficient.[12]

HUMAN-LABELED PRODUCTS:

Methylene Blue Injection: 1% (10 mg/mL) in 1 mL and 10 mL vials; generic; (Rx; not FDA-approved)[13]

Methylene Blue Injection: 5 mg/mL in 10 mL amp; *ProvayBlue®*; (Rx)

References

For the complete list of references, see **wiley.com/go/budde/plumb**

Methylphenidate

(meth-ill-***fen***-i-date) *Concerta®, Ritalin®*

CNS Stimulant

Prescriber Highlights

- Amphetamine-like drug that may be useful for treating cataplexy/narcolepsy or hyperkinesis/hyperactivity in dogs
- Contraindicated in patients receiving monoamine oxidase inhibitors or within 14 days after their discontinuation
- Use with caution in dogs with seizure disorders, cardiac disease, hypertension, or in aggressive animals.
- Adverse effects are primarily related to CNS stimulation.
- DEA Schedule II (C-II) controlled substance

Uses/Indications

Methylphenidate may be useful for diagnosing and treating cataplexy/narcolepsy or hyperactivity in dogs.

Pharmacology/Actions

Methylphenidate has stimulating effects on the central nervous and respiratory systems similar to that of amphetamine. It also has weak sympathomimetic activity and, at normal dosages, has little effect on peripheral circulation.

Pharmacokinetics

There is limited pharmacokinetic information available for methylphenidate in dogs. Single PO doses of immediate-release 20 mg tablets to 7 to 19 kg (15 to 42 lb) beagles resulted in peak concentrations of ≈60 µg/mL in ≈15 minutes after dosing. Clearance was ≈0.27 L/hour and elimination half-life was ≈1 hour. Interpatient variability was much higher with 20 mg sustained-release tablets; serum concentrations peaked ≈30 minutes after dosing, and peak concentrations were much lower than immediate-release tablets at 19 µg/mL. Clearance was ≈0.97 L/hour and elimination half-life was ≈40 minutes. Therapeutic plasma concentrations of methylphenidate are thought to be between 1 and 10 µg/mL.[1]

In humans, methylphenidate immediate-release tablets are rapidly and well absorbed from the GI tract. Food in the GI tract may increase the rate but not the extent of drug absorbed. Peak concentrations occur ≈2 hours postdose. Methylphenidate undergoes extensive first-pass metabolism; protein binding is low. Terminal elimination half-life is ≈3 hours; less than 1% is excreted unchanged in the urine.

Contraindications/Precautions/Warnings

Methylphenidate is contraindicated in patients receiving monoamine oxidase inhibitors or within 14 days of discontinuing them.[2] The risks associated with methylphenidate should be carefully considered before using this drug in dogs with seizure disorders, cardiac disease, hypertension, or aggressive behaviors.

Hypersensitivity reactions including angioedema and anaphylaxis have been reported in humans.[2]

Be alert for drug-seeking individuals as methylphenidate is a DEA Schedule II controlled drug in the United States. A written prescription (typically limited to a maximum of a 30-day supply) is required each time the drug is dispensed by a pharmacy.

Adverse Effects

The most likely adverse effects of methylphenidate are increased heart and respiratory rates, anorexia, tremors, and hyperthermia, particularly exercise-induced hyperthermia. CNS stimulation can occur (see ***Overdose/Acute Toxicity***).

Reproductive/Nursing Safety

Methylphenidate was associated with teratogenic effects in rabbits at massive dosages (200 mg/kg/day; ≈40 times the maximum recommended human dose).[2]

It is unknown if methylphenidate enters maternal milk.

Because safety has not been established in animals, this drug should only be used when the maternal benefits outweigh the potential risks to offspring.

Overdose/Acute Toxicity

In dogs, even relatively low doses can cause serious toxicosis. Methylphenidate doses of 1 mg/kg or less have caused toxic reactions. One fatality has been reported after a dog ingested 3.1 mg/kg[3]; however, research dogs have survived doses of 20 mg/kg/day for 90 days. Expected signs associated with an overdose in dogs are generally CNS overstimulation and excessive sympathomimetic effects, including hyperactivity, salivation, diarrhea, head bobbing, agitation, tachycardia, hypertension, tremors, seizures, and hyperthermia. Consider the dosage form (extended-release vs regular tablets) when considering treatment options and expected onset and duration of effects; extended-release formulations are associated with more severe clinical signs.

In one cat, given methylphenidate 5 mg PO developed tremors, agitation, mydriasis, tachycardia, tachypnea, and hypertension; signs resolved 25 hours postingestion with supportive care (eg, dark cage, diazepam, fluids).[4]

Typical GI decontamination protocols can be considered, but

emetics should be used with caution as CNS signs can occur rapidly. Treatment is supportive and aimed at controlling signs associated with toxicity. Phenothiazines (eg, acepromazine, chlorpromazine) may be useful in controlling agitation. Benzodiazepines (eg, diazepam) potentially could increase the severity of agitation and are typically avoided. Seizures may be controlled with propofol, followed by barbiturates if necessary. Additional treatments that may be considered include injectable methocarbamol for tremors; beta-blockers for tachycardia; prazosin, amlodipine, nitroprusside, or hydralazine for hypertension; external cooling for hyperthermia; and cyproheptadine to help prevent serotonin syndrome.

For patients that have experienced or are suspected to have experienced an overdose, consultation with a 24-hour poison consultation center specializing in providing veterinary-specific information is recommended. For general information related to overdose and toxin exposures, as well as contact information for poison control centers, refer to ***Appendix.***

Drug Interactions

The following drug interactions have either been reported or are theoretical in humans or animals receiving methylphenidate and may be of significance in veterinary patients. Unless otherwise noted, use together is not necessarily contraindicated, but weigh the potential risks and perform additional monitoring when appropriate.

- **ANTICONVULSANTS** (eg, **phenobarbital, primidone**): Methylphenidate may increase anticonvulsant serum concentrations.
- **ANTIHYPERTENSIVE DRUGS**: Methylphenidate may reduce effects.
- **CLONIDINE**: Methylphenidate may enhance toxic effects of clonidine. Historically, serious adverse events including death were reported with combination use in humans; however, more recent safety studies have found no evidence of adverse events from this combination.[5,6]
- **INHALANT ANESTHETIC AGENTS** (eg, **isoflurane, sevoflurane**): Concurrent use with methylphenidate may increase risk for interoperative hypertension, tachycardia, and arrhythmias; it is recommended to withhold methylphenidate on day of surgery.
- **MONOAMINE OXIDASE INHIBITORS** (MAOIs; eg, **amitraz, linezolid, selegiline**): Concurrent therapy may lead to hypertensive crisis; combination is contraindicated.
- **SELECTIVE SEROTONIN REUPTAKE INHIBITORS** (SSRIs; eg, **fluoxetine, sertraline**): Methylphenidate may inhibit metabolism and increase SSRI concentrations.
- **TRICYCLIC ANTIDEPRESSANTS** (TCAs; eg, **amitriptyline, clomipramine**): Methylphenidate may inhibit metabolism and increase TCA concentrations.
- **WARFARIN**: Methylphenidate may inhibit warfarin metabolism and prolong coagulation times.

Laboratory Considerations

- No specific laboratory interactions were noted for this drug.

Dosages

DOGS:

NOTES:

1. It is assumed that the following dosages are for the use of the immediate-release formulation of methylphenidate; dosages may not apply to extended-release formulations.
2. **Dosages listed below are anecdotal and widely variable.** It is recommended to start with the low end of the dosing range and titrate up as the patient's condition requires for clinical control.

Adjunctive treatment of narcolepsy/cataplexy (extra-label): 0.25 – 0.5 mg/kg PO or 5 – 10 mg/dog (NOT mg/kg) PO every 12 to 24 hours[7]

Diagnosis and treatment of hyperkinesis/hyperactivity (extra-label):

a) For diagnosis, doses of 5 – 20 mg/dog (NOT mg/kg), depending on the size of the dog, are given PO every 8 to 12 hours for 3 days, and the patient is assessed for improvement of target behaviors (anxiety, overactivity, learning ability).[8,9] If effective, treatment can be started at a lower dose given 1 to 2 times daily, then increased if necessary. Treatment is accompanied by training and behavior modification therapy. Breaks from therapy (drug holidays) can occur on days when the dog's behavior is less important.[8,10]

b) 0.25 – 4 mg/kg PO every 24 hours[11]

Monitoring

- Clinical efficacy
- Baseline and periodic physical exam to monitor vital signs and body weight (especially in young, growing puppies)
- Baseline and periodic blood pressure

Client Information

- A common side effect of this medicine is a decreased appetite.
- Be sure to let your veterinarian know if your animal has worn a flea or tick collar in the past 2 weeks. Do not use one of these collars on your animal while it is taking this medicine without first talking to your veterinarian.
- Contact your veterinarian immediately if your animal has a seizure while taking this medicine.
- Methylphenidate has significant potential for abuse by humans and should be kept secure.
- If using an extended-release product, do not crush the tablet or capsule.
- The Federal Drug Enforcement Agency (DEA) classifies methylphenidate as a schedule II (C-II) controlled drug, and it requires a new written prescription for refills. The use of this medication in animals or humans other than those for whom they are prescribed is illegal.

Chemistry/Synonyms

Methylphenidate HCl is a CNS stimulant related to amphetamine and occurs as a fine white odorless, crystalline powder. It is freely soluble in water and soluble in alcohol.

Methylphenidate may also be known as *Attenta®*, *Daytrana®*, *Equasym®*, *Focalin®*, *Metadate ER®*, *Methylin®*, *Rilatine®*, *Riphenidate®*, *Ritalina®*, *Ritalin®*, *Ritaphen®*, *Rubifen®*, or *Tranquilyn®*.

Storage/Stability

Unless otherwise noted on the label, store methylphenidate tablets and extended-release tablets and capsules in tight, light-resistant containers at room temperature.

Methylphenidate is a DEA schedule II (C-II) controlled substance. Store it in a substantially constructed and securely locked area. Follow applicable local, state, and federal rules regarding the disposal of unused or wasted controlled drugs.

Compatibility/Compounding Considerations

No specific information was noted.

Dosage Forms/Regulatory Status

VETERINARY-LABELED PRODUCTS: NONE

The American Racing Commissioners International (ARCI) has designated this drug as a class 1 substance. Use of this drug may not be allowed in certain animal competitions. Check rules and regulations before entering in a competition while this medication is being administered. Contact local racing authorities for further guidance. See ***Appendix*** for more information.

HUMAN-LABELED PRODUCTS:

Methylphenidate Oral Tablets (immediate release): 5 mg, 10 mg, and 20 mg; *Ritalin*®, generic; (Rx; C-II).

Methylphenidate Oral Chewable Tablets (immediate release): 2.5 mg, 5 mg, and 10 mg; *Methylin*®, generic; (Rx; C-II).

A wide variety of extended-release tablets, suspensions and transdermal formulations are also available; do not confuse these formulations.

References

For the complete list of references, see **wiley.com/go/budde/plumb**

Methylprednisolone
Methylprednisolone Acetate
Methylprednisolone Sodium Succinate

(meth-ill-pred-***niss***-oh-lone)

Medrol®, *Depo-Medrol*®, *Solu-Medrol*®

Glucocorticoid

For more information, see ***Glucocorticoid Agents, General Information***

Prescriber Highlights

- Oral and parenteral glucocorticoid that is 4 to 5 times more potent than hydrocortisone; no appreciable mineralocorticoid activity
- Relatively contraindicated with systemic fungal infections
- Use with caution in animals with active bacterial or viral infections, peptic ulcer, corneal ulcer, hyperadrenocorticism, diabetes mellitus, osteoporosis, predisposition to thrombophlebitis, hypertension, CHF, and renal insufficiency.
- Acetate form can cause marked HPA axis suppression. In cats, extracellular hyperglycemia can cause volume expansion and may predispose cats to diabetes mellitus and congestive heart failure. IM administration is generally reserved for when owners cannot adhere to oral treatment regimens.
- Goal of therapy should be to use the lowest dose possible for the least amount of time to treat and control patient's condition.
- Primary adverse effects are related to iatrogenic hyperadrenocorticism with sustained use.
- Many potential drug and laboratory interactions

Uses/Indications

Methylprednisolone is similar to prednisone or prednisolone but is slightly more potent. Methylprednisolone is effective in dogs with atopic dermatitis[1-3] and cats with allergies[4] or hypersensitivity dermatitis.[5] The drug did not show benefit in dogs with thoracolumbar intervertebral disk herniation.[6-8]

Although glucocorticoids have been used to treat many conditions in humans and animals, methylprednisolone has 4 primary uses with accompanying dosage ranges: 1) replacement or supplementation for glucocorticoid deficiency secondary to hypoadrenocorticism or relative adrenal insufficiency (eg, septic shock) for glucocorticoid deficiency secondary to hypoadrenocorticism, 2) anti-inflammatory agent, 3) immunosuppressive, and 4) antineoplastic agent. High-dose use is not supported for hemorrhagic or hypovolemic shock, head trauma, spinal cord trauma,[9] or sepsis. In general, when administering glucocorticoids, the following principles should be followed:

- A specific diagnosis is needed before glucocorticoids are administered, as they can mask disease.
- A course of treatment should be determined prior to treatment.
- A therapeutic endpoint should be determined prior to treatment.
- The least potent glucocorticoid should be used at the lowest dose for a minimal amount of time.
- It is important to understand when glucocorticoid use is inappropriate (eg, acute infection, diabetes mellitus).[10]

See ***Glucocorticoid Agents, General Information***

Pharmacology/Actions

Methylprednisolone may be administered orally or parenterally (sodium succinate, IV and IM; acetate, IM only). Its relative anti-inflammatory potency is ≈5 times that of cortisol. It has negligible to very slight mineralocorticoid activity. Once in the systemic circulation, it has an approximate duration of activity of 12 to 36 hours.

For further information, see ***Glucocorticoid Agents, General Information***

Pharmacokinetics

Methylprednisolone administered orally is relatively well absorbed and extensively distributed. The liver is the primary site for metabolism (oxidation); most of the drug is excreted renally as metabolites. The pharmacokinetics of methylprednisolone do not translate into pharmacologic effect, and duration of activity is independent of elimination half-life. Methylprednisolone is an intermediate-acting corticosteroid with a biologic half-life of ≈12 to 36 hours.

Methylprednisolone sodium succinate IV injection is water soluble and considered fast acting.

Methylprednisolone acetate IM injection is absorbed slowly and can have a duration of effect of weeks to months. Intra-articular (IA) or intrasynovial injection of methylprednisolone acetate in horses results in systemic methylprednisolone exposure.[11-16] In horses receiving methylprednisolone acetate 100 mg or 200 mg IA, the last quantifiable plasma concentration was measured at 7 days (100 mg) and 18 days (200 mg).[14]

Contraindications/Precautions/Warnings

Methylprednisolone acetate is contraindicated for IM administration in animals with arrested tuberculosis, peptic ulcer, and hyperadrenocorticism. Use with caution in patients with diabetes mellitus, osteoporosis, predisposition to thrombophlebitis, hypertension, CHF, renal insufficiency, and active tuberculosis.[17,18] Epidural use of glucocorticoids is associated with severe adverse CNS reactions (eg, blindness, paralysis, seizures).

Do not administer methylprednisolone acetate IV. When injected locally (eg, intrasynovially, intratendinously), methylprednisolone acetate is contraindicated in the presence of acute infections. If pain or further loss of joint mobility occurs with fever following intrasynovial or intratendon injection, immediate appropriate antibiotic therapy is warranted, as sepsis may be present.

Systemic glucocorticoids suppress adrenal function. Unless very short-term burst therapy is used, patients that have received systemic glucocorticoids systemically should be tapered off the drug. Tapering should be gradual if the patient has been receiving a glucocorticoid chronically, as endogenous ACTH and corticosteroid function may return slowly. Should the animal undergo a stressful event (eg, surgery, trauma, illness) during the tapering process and/or until normal adrenal and pituitary functions resume, additional glucocorticoids should be administered.

Corticosteroids may mask signs of infection and delay wound healing. Systemic use of glucocorticoids is generally considered contraindicated in patients with ocular herpetic or systemic fungal infections (unless used for replacement therapy in Addison's disease), when administered IM in patients with idiopathic thrombocytopenia, and in patients with hypersensitivities to glucocorticoids. Animals, particularly cats, at risk for diabetes mellitus or with concurrent cardiovascular disease should receive glucocorticoids with caution because of the potent hyperglycemic effect of these agents.

Sustained-release injectable glucocorticoids are contraindicated for chronic corticosteroid therapy of systemic diseases because of their long duration of action and the increased risks for adverse effects. Most clinicians do not recommend use of methylprednisolone acetate IM when alternate day oral glucocorticoid therapy could be used. In difficult-to-pill cats, however, it may be a viable alternative to oral glucocorticoids. A study in cats ($n = 8$) with feline herpesvirus 1 (FHV-1) administered 5 mg/kg methylprednisolone acetate IM on day 0 and day 21 reported that clinical signs of activated FHV-1 occurred in some cats, but in most it was mild and self-limited.[19]

Do not confuse methylPREDNISolone with medroxyPROGESTERone or methylTESTOSTERone.

Adverse Effects

Adverse effects are generally associated with long-term administration of these drugs, especially if the drugs are administered at high doses or not on an alternate-day regimen. Effects typically manifest as clinical signs of hyperadrenocorticism. A complete listing of potential effects is outlined in ***Glucocorticoid Agents, General Information***.

In dogs, polyuria (PU), polydipsia (PD), and polyphagia (PP) may occur during short-term burst therapy and on days when the drug is administered during alternate-day maintenance therapy. Adverse effects in dogs can include dull/dry coat, bilaterally asymmetrical alopecia, weight gain, panting, vomiting, diarrhea, elevated liver enzymes, pancreatitis, GI ulceration (especially with high parenteral or oral doses); hypercoagulability; hyperlipidemia, activation or worsening of diabetes mellitus, muscle wasting, and/or behavior changes (eg, depression, lethargy, aggression). Glucocorticoids have been known to delay growth in young animals. Discontinuation of the drug may be necessary; changing to an alternate steroid may also alleviate adverse effects. Adverse effects associated with anti-inflammatory therapy are relatively uncommon, with the exception of PU, PD, and PP. Adverse effects associated with immunosuppressive dosages are more common and potentially more severe.

Cats generally require higher glucocorticoid doses than dogs for clinical effect but tend to develop fewer adverse effects. Occasionally, PD, PU, PP with weight gain, diarrhea, or depression can be seen. Long-term high-dose therapy can lead to effects related to hyperadrenocorticism. A study in 12 cats receiving the long-acting acetate salt demonstrated that methylprednisolone causes extracellular hyperglycemia leading to volume expansion and may predispose patients to diabetes mellitus and congestive heart failure.[20]

Rapid IV administration of methylprednisolone sodium succinate may cause vomiting; high doses may also reduce blood pressure.

Experimental data in sheep support the osteoporosis-inducing effects of glucocorticoids in animals.[21]

In humans, corticosteroid-related diabetes mellitus may be related to increased urinary excretion of chromium and potentially could respond to chromium supplementation.[22-25] Significance in animals is unknown.

Reproductive/Nursing Safety

Excessive glucocorticoid doses early in pregnancy may lead to teratogenic effects. When administered in the latter stages of pregnancy, exogenous steroid administration may induce parturition, including premature parturition followed by dystocia, fetal death retained placenta and metritis. Cleft palate, foreleg deformities, phocomelia, and anasarca have occurred in offspring of dogs that received corticosteroids during pregnancy.[18]

Use with caution in nursing animals. Glucocorticoids unbound to plasma proteins will enter milk. High doses or prolonged administration to mothers may inhibit growth, interfere with endogenous corticosteroid production, or cause other unwanted effects in nursing offspring. However, in humans, several studies suggest that amounts excreted in breast milk are negligible when methylprednisolone doses are less than or equal to 8 mg/day. Larger doses for short periods may not harm the infant.

Overdose/Acute Toxicity

The oral LD_{50} for methylprednisolone in mice is 450 mg/kg and in rats is greater than 4 g/kg.[26] Overdoses of glucocorticoids used alone are unlikely to cause harmful effects; GI effects (eg, vomiting, diarrhea), that are sometimes severe, can be seen in dogs. One incidence of a dog developing acute CNS effects after accidental ingestion of glucocorticoids has been reported. Consider GI decontamination for recent oral ingestion. If clinical signs occur, use supportive treatment if required.

For patients that have experienced or are suspected to have experienced an overdose, consultation with a 24-hour poison consultation center specializing in providing veterinary-specific information is recommended. For general information related to overdose and toxin exposures, as well as contact information for poison control centers, refer to ***Appendix***.

Drug Interactions

The following drug interactions have been reported or are theoretical in humans or animals receiving methylprednisolone and may be of significance in veterinary patients. Unless otherwise noted, use together is not necessarily contraindicated, but weigh the potential risks and perform additional monitoring when appropriate.

- **AMPHOTERICIN B**: Concomitant administration with glucocorticoids may cause hypokalemia; in humans, CHF and cardiomegaly have been reported after methylprednisolone was used to treat amphotericin B adverse effects.
- **ANALGESICS, OPIOIDS and/or LOCAL ANESTHETICS (EPIDURAL)**: Combination with glucocorticoids in epidural injections has caused serious CNS injuries and death; use only very small intrathecal test doses of these agents with glucocorticoids.
- **ANTICHOLINESTERASE AGENTS** (eg, **pyridostigmine, neostigmine**): In patients with myasthenia gravis, concomitant glucocorticoid and anticholinesterase agent administration may lead to profound muscle weakness. If possible, discontinue anticholinesterase medication at least 24 hours prior to corticosteroid administration.
- **ANTIDIABETIC AGENTS, ORAL** (eg, **glimepiride, glipizide, glyburide, metformin**): Glucocorticoids may worsen glycemic control.
- **ASPIRIN**: Glucocorticoids may reduce salicylate blood concentrations. Combination may increase risk for GI ulceration.
- **AZOLE ANTIFUNGALS** (eg, **itraconazole, ketoconazole**): May decrease the metabolism of glucocorticoids and increase methylprednisolone blood concentrations; ketoconazole may induce adrenal insufficiency when glucocorticoids are withdrawn by inhibiting adrenal corticosteroid synthesis.
- **CHOLESTYRAMINE**: May reduce methylprednisolone absorption
- **CYCLOPHOSPHAMIDE**: Glucocorticoids may inhibit the hepatic metabolism of cyclophosphamide; dosage adjustments may be required.
- **CYCLOSPORINE**: Concomitant administration of glucocorticoids and cyclosporine may increase the blood concentration of each drug by mutually inhibiting each drug's hepatic metabolism; the clinical significance of this interaction is not clear.
- **DESMOPRESSIN (DDAVP)**: Concomitant administration of DDAVP and glucocorticoids may increase the risk for hyponatremia.
- **DIGOXIN**: When glucocorticoids are used concurrently with digitalis glycosides, an increased chance of digitalis toxicity may oc-

cur should hypokalemia develop; diligent monitoring of potassium and digitalis glycoside concentrations is recommended.

- **Diltiazem**: Concurrent use may increase plasma concentrations of methylprednisolone.
- **Diuretics, Potassium-Depleting** (eg, **furosemide, thiazides**): Concurrent use increases the risk for hypokalemia.
- **Ephedrine**: May reduce methylprednisolone blood concentrations
- **Estrogens**: The effects of methylprednisolone, and possibly other glucocorticoids may be potentiated by concomitant administration with estrogens.
- **Fluoroquinolones** (eg, **ciprofloxacin, enrofloxacin**): Concurrent use may increase risk for tendinitis and tendon rupture.
- **Immunosuppressive Agents** (eg, **azathioprine, hydroxychloroquine, mycophenolate**): Additive immunosuppressive effects possible.
- **Insulin**: Insulin requirements may increase in patients receiving glucocorticoids.
- **Leflunomide**: Increased risk for pancytopenia, agranulocytosis, thrombocytopenia, and infection
- **Macrolide Antibiotics** (eg, **erythromycin, clarithromycin**): May decrease the metabolism of glucocorticoids and increase methylprednisolone blood concentrations
- **Mitotane**: May alter the metabolism of steroids; higher than usual doses of steroids may be necessary to treat mitotane-induced adrenal insufficiency.
- **Nonsteroidal Anti-Inflammatory Drugs** (eg, **carprofen, flunixin, meloxicam**): Administration of ulcerogenic drugs with glucocorticoids may increase the risk for GI ulceration.
- **Phenobarbital**: May increase the metabolism of glucocorticoids and decrease methylprednisolone blood concentrations
- **Rifampin**: May increase the metabolism of glucocorticoids and decrease methylprednisolone blood concentrations
- **Theophylline, Aminophylline**: Concomitant use can alter the pharmacologic effects of both drugs.
- **Vaccines**: Patients receiving corticosteroids at immunosuppressive dosages should generally not receive live attenuated-virus vaccines, as virus replication may be augmented; a diminished immune response may occur after vaccine, toxoid, or bacterin administration in patients receiving glucocorticoids.
- **Warfarin**: Methylprednisolone may affect clotting times; monitor prothrombin times.

Laboratory Considerations

- Methylprednisolone can cross-react with cortisol when measuring cortisol for adrenal function testing with a **cortisol assay**, and spurious results can occur. Dexamethasone does not interfere with the assay for cortisol.
- Reactions to **intradermal allergy skin tests** may be suppressed by glucocorticoids. Suggested methylprednisolone withdrawal time prior to testing is 3 to 4 weeks for oral formulations and 8 weeks for IM methylprednisolone acetate.
- False-negative results of the **nitroblue tetrazolium** test for systemic bacterial infections may be induced by glucocorticoids.
- Glucocorticoids may increase **serum cholesterol.**
- Glucocorticoids may increase **serum and urine glucose**.
- Glucocorticoids may decrease **serum potassium.**
- Glucocorticoids can suppress the release of thyroid stimulating hormone (TSH) and reduce **total T_3** and **total T_4** values. Thyroid gland atrophy has been reported after chronic glucocorticoid administration. Uptake of **I^{131}** by the thyroid may be decreased by glucocorticoids.
- Glucocorticoids may cause **neutrophilia** within 4 to 8 hours after dosing and return to baseline within 24 to 48 hours after drug discontinuation.
- In dogs, glucocorticoids can cause **lymphopenia** that can persist for weeks after drug discontinuation.

Dosages

NOTES:

1) If using methylprednisolone tablets orally or methylprednisolone sodium succinate for IV injection, refer to the ***Prednisolone/Prednisone Dosages*** section to determine an appropriate dose for the condition treated. A near equivalent dose for methylprednisolone can be determined by dividing the dose of prednis(ol)one by 1.25 (eg, if the prednis(ol)one dose is 5 mg, the methylprednisolone dose is 4 mg).
2) If given daily, therapy for longer than 1 to 2 weeks will suppress the hypothalamic-pituitary-adrenal (HPA) axis, and recovery will take longer than 1 week. Therefore, if corticosteroids are used for longer than a few days, the dosage must be tapered using alternate-day therapy. Many glucocorticoid responsive diseases can be managed with chronic alternate-day therapy. If possible, it is suggested to avoid giving doses greater than 1 mg/kg (prednisolone equivalent) every other day; larger doses saturate a dog's ability to fully metabolize the last dose before the next dose is given and can negate the benefits of alternate-day therapy. However, to induce remission of clinical signs or manage their recurrence initially requires daily therapy at an appropriate dose to control clinical signs, then tapering the drug to reach a minimum daily dose that will control clinical signs, followed by alternate-day therapy to manage the disease. Animals vary greatly in their response to the therapeutic and adverse effects of glucocorticoids, and qualitative differences may exist between the effects of different glucocorticoids in the same animal.[27]

DOGS:

Label indications (FDA-approved):

NOTE: Label dosages are listed as mg/dog (NOT mg/kg).

1. Oral: Dogs weighing 2.3 to 6.8 kg (5-15 lb): 2 mg/dog (NOT mg/kg); dogs weighing 6.8 to 18.1 kg (15-40 lb): 2 – 4 mg/dog (NOT mg/kg); dogs weighing 18.1 to 36.3 kg (40-80 lb): 4 – 8 mg/dog (NOT mg/kg); these are average total daily doses, which should be divided into 2 equal doses and given 6 to 10 hours apart. Once clinical response has been obtained, gradually reduce dosage until treatment is terminated or the lowest effective dose has been achieved.[18]
2. IM (methylprednisolone *acetate*): 2 – 120 mg/dog (NOT mg/kg) IM (average 20 mg/dog; NOT mg/kg); depending on breed (ie, 2 mg/dog [NOT mg/kg] in miniature breeds; 40 mg/dog [NOT mg/kg] in medium breed; as high as 120 mg/dog [NOT mg/kg] in extremely large breeds or dogs with severe involvement), severity of condition, and response. May repeat at weekly intervals or in accordance with the severity of the condition and the response.[17] The manufacturer has specific directions for use of the drug intrasynovially.

Adjunctive treatment of canine atopic dermatitis (extra-label): Initial dosage of ≈0.4 – 0.8 mg/kg PO once to twice daily to be tapered as needed.[28,29]

Adjunctive treatment of anaphylaxis (extra-label): Methylprednisolone *sodium succinate* (NOT acetate) 2 – 6 mg/kg IV, not a substitute for epinephrine. Pre-treatment does NOT prevent anaphylaxis.[30] Infuse at no faster than 1 – 2 mg/kg/minute.[31]

CATS:

Label indications (FDA-approved):

NOTE: Labeled dosages are listed as mg/cat (NOT mg/kg.)

1. Oral: Cats weighing 2.3 to 6.8 kg (5-15 lb): 2 mg/cat (NOT mg/kg); Cats weighing more than 6.8 kg (15 lb): 2 – 4 mg/cat (NOT mg/kg). These are average total daily doses which should be divided into 2 equal doses and given 6 to 10 hours apart. Once clinical response has been obtained, gradually reduce the dose until treatment is terminated or the lowest effective dose has been achieved.[18]
2. Intramuscularly (methylprednisolone acetate): The average dose is 10 mg/cat (NOT mg/kg) IM with a range up to 20 mg/cat (NOT mg/kg); depending on breed (size), severity of condition, and response. May repeat at weekly intervals or in accordance with the severity of the condition and the response.[17]

Adjunctive treatment for allergic cats (extra-label):

a) Pruritus: Initial induction dosage was 4 mg/cat (NOT mg/kg) PO once daily for cats weighing less than or equal to 5 kg (11 lb), and 6 mg/cat (NOT mg/kg) PO once daily for cats more than 5 kg (11 lb). Cats that did not achieve remission by day 7 had their once daily induction dose doubled for the next 7 days. Mean dose required for induction of remission was 1.41 mg/kg (range 0.8 – 2.2 mg/kg) PO once daily, and 88% of treated cats achieved remission by the end of the second week. Dosages used to achieve remission were then given every other day and tapered (from 100% to 25% of induction dose in 25% increments) to the lowest every other day dosage that maintained remission. Sixty-seven percent of cats that achieved remission were maintained at 25% of the induction dose given every other day.[4]
b) Feline atopic dermatitis, as part of a multimodal treatment protocol: 1 – 2 mg/kg PO once daily for 7 days and then taper to the lowest effective dose.[32]

Adjunctive treatment of anaphylaxis (extra-label): Methylprednisolone *sodium succinate* (NOT acetate) 2 – 6 mg/kg IV. Not a substitute for epinephrine. Pre-treatment does NOT prevent anaphylaxis.[30] Infuse no faster than 1 – 2 mg/kg/minute.[31]

HORSES:

Anti-inflammatory (glucocorticoid effects); (label dosage; FDA-approved): Methylprednisolone acetate 200 mg IM repeated as necessary.[17] The manufacturer has specific directions for use of the drug intrasynovially.

Intra-articular use (extra-label): Methylprednisolone acetate 100 mg IA[33]

Monitoring

Monitoring of glucocorticoid therapy is dependent on the reason for use, dosage used, agent used (amount of mineralocorticoid activity), duration of therapy, and animal's age and condition. The following list may not be appropriate or complete for all animals; use clinical assessment and judgment should adverse effects be noted:

- Weight, appetite, signs of edema
- Serum and/or urine electrolytes
- Total plasma proteins, albumin
- Blood glucose
- Growth and development in young animals
- ACTH stimulation test if necessary (**NOTE**: Methylprednisolone can interfere with cortisol assay.)

Client Information

- Give oral products with food.
- Goal is to find the lowest dose possible and use for the shortest period.
- Many side effects are possible, especially when the medication is used long term. Most common side effects are increased panting, appetite, thirst, and need to urinate.
- In dogs, stomach or intestinal ulcers, perforation, or bleeding can occur. If your animal stops eating, or you notice a high fever, black tarry stools, or bloody vomit, contact your veterinarian right away.
- Do not stop therapy abruptly without a veterinarian's guidance as serious side effects could occur.

Chemistry/Synonyms

Methylprednisolone is a synthetically produced glucocorticoid. Both the free alcohol and the acetate ester occur as an odorless, white or practically white, crystalline powder. The powder is practically insoluble in water and sparingly soluble in alcohol.

Methylprednisolone sodium succinate occurs as an odorless, white or nearly white, hygroscopic, amorphous solid. It is very soluble in both water and alcohol. Methylprednisolone sodium succinate has equivalent biologic activity as methylprednisolone.

Methylprednisolone may also be known as 6α-methylprednisolone, methylprednisolonum, NSC-19987, *A-Methapred®*, *Depo-Medrol®*, *Medrol®* or *Solu-Medrol®*, *Medrone® V*, *Solu-Medrone® V*, and *Depo-Medrone® V*.

Storage/Stability

Commercially available products of methylprednisolone should be stored at room temperature (20°C to 25°C [68°F-77°F]); avoid freezing the acetate injection. Vial contents should be used within 12 weeks of first vial puncture or discarded. After reconstituting the sodium succinate injection, store at room temperature and use within 48 hours; only use solutions that are clear.

Compatibility/Compounding Considerations

Compatibility is dependent upon factors such as pH, concentration, temperature, and diluent used; consult specialized references or a hospital pharmacist for more specific information.

Methylprednisolone sodium succinate injection is reportedly **Y-site compatible** with the following fluids and drugs: amino acids 4.25%/dextrose 25%, amphotericin B (limited amounts), butorphanol, cefazolin, chloramphenicol sodium succinate, cimetidine, clindamycin phosphate, dobutamine, dopamine, epinephrine, furosemide, heparin sodium, lactated Ringer's solution, metoclopramide, morphine, norepinephrine, parenteral nutrition (3-in-1 and 2-in-1), penicillin G potassium, piperacillin/tazobactam, polymyxin B, and verapamil.

The following drugs and fluids have been reported to be physically **incompatible** when mixed with methylprednisolone sodium succinate, compatible dependent upon concentration, or the data are conflicting: dextrose 5%/sodium chloride 0.45%, dextrose 5%/sodium chloride 0.9% (80 mg/L reported compatible), dextrose 5% (up to 5 g/L reported compatible), lactated Ringer's (up to 80 mg/L reported compatible), sodium chloride 0.9% (some reports of up to 60 g/L compatible), ampicillin, calcium gluconate, diazepam, famotidine, glycopyrrolate, insulin, pantoprazole, potassium chloride, and tetracycline HCl.

Dosage Forms/Regulatory Status

VETERINARY-LABELED PRODUCTS:

Methylprednisolone Tablets: 1 mg, 2 mg, and 4 mg tablets, *Medrol®*, generic; (Rx). FDA-approved for use in dogs and cats. NADA# 011-403

Methylprednisolone Acetate Injection: 20 mg/mL in 20 mL vials and 40 mg/mL in 5 mL vials; *Depo-Medrol®*, generic; (Rx). FDA-approved for IM injection in dogs, cats, and horses; intrasynovial injection in dogs and horses. The veterinary label states that the drug is not to be used in horses intended for human consumption. NADA# 012-204

The Association of Racing Commissioners International (ARCI) has designated this drug as a class 4 substance. See ***Appendix*** for more information. Use of this drug may not be allowed in certain animal competitions. Check rules and regulations before entering in a competition while this medication is being administered. Contact local racing authorities for further guidance.

HUMAN-LABELED PRODUCTS:

Methylprednisolone Oral Tablets: 2 mg, 4 mg, 8 mg, 16 mg, and 32 mg; *Medrol®*, generic; (Rx)

Methylprednisolone Acetate Injection: 20 mg/mL, 40 mg/mL, and 80 mg/mL suspension in 1 mL (40 and 80 mg only), 5 mL, and 10 mL vials; *Depo-Medrol®*, generic; (Rx)

Methylprednisolone Sodium Succinate Powder for Injection: 40 mg, 125 mg, 500 mg, 1 gram, and 2 gram vials for reconstitution; *Solu-Medrol®*, *A-Methapred®*, generic; (Rx)

References

For the complete list of references, see **wiley.com/go/budde/plumb**

Metoclopramide

(met-oh-***kloe***-pra-mide) *Reglan®, Emeprid®*

GI Prokinetic Agent; Antiemetic

Prescriber Highlights

- Stimulates upper GI motility and has antiemetic properties
- In dogs, it is more potent as an antiemetic than a prokinetic agent; may be a poor antiemetic in cats
- May work best when used as an IV CRI
- Contraindications include GI hemorrhage, obstruction, perforation, and hypersensitivity. Relative contraindications include seizure disorders and pheochromocytoma.
- In dogs, adverse effects include changes in mentation and behavior and constipation. In cats, adverse effects include signs of frenzied behavior or disorientation, and constipation. When given IV in horses, adverse effects include severe CNS effects, behavior changes, and abdominal pain; adverse effects are less common in foals.
- Several potentially serious drug interactions

Uses/Indications

Metoclopramide has been used in animals for both its GI prokinetic and antiemetic properties. It has been used clinically for gastric stasis disorders, gastroesophageal reflux, intubation of the small intestine, and as an antiemetic for parvoviral enteritis, bilious vomiting syndrome, uremic gastritis, and to prevent or treat chemotherapy-induced vomiting. Although metoclopramide is widely accepted as an antiemetic in dogs, other drugs (eg, maropitant, ondansetron) are more effective and appear to be better tolerated.[1-4]

Distinct differences between antiemetic and prokinetic effects can be seen in different species. Antiemetic effects appear more pronounced in dogs than in cats; distal esophageal motility effects are greater in cats. Metoclopramide has gastric prokinetic effects in both species; however, in dogs, metoclopramide did not facilitate duodenal passage of a flexible endoscope[5,6] or promote gastric emptying following gastric dilatation and volvulus.[7] Breed and dose may influence prokinetic response.[8]

Pharmacology/Actions

The primary pharmacologic effects of metoclopramide are associated with the GI tract and the CNS. Metoclopramide stimulates motility of the upper GI tract without stimulating gastric, pancreatic, or biliary secretions. Although the exact mechanisms for these actions are unknown, it appears that metoclopramide sensitizes upper GI smooth muscle to the effects of acetylcholine. Intact vagal innervation is not necessary for enhanced motility, but anticholinergic drugs negate metoclopramide's effects. GI effects seen after metoclopramide administration include increased tone and amplitude of gastric contractions, relaxed pyloric sphincter, and increased duodenal and jejunal peristalsis. Gastric emptying and intestinal transit times can be significantly reduced. There is little or no effect on colon motility. In addition, metoclopramide may increase lower esophageal sphincter (LES) pressure and reduce gastroesophageal reflux; however, one study showed no significant change in LES pressure after metoclopramide administration in dogs.[9] The drug did not reduce gastroesophageal reflux in dogs undergoing anesthesia with acepromazine, propofol, and isoflurane[10] or the incidence of aspiration pneumonia in dogs with idiopathic laryngeal paralysis undergoing unilateral arytenoid lateralization.[11,12] A protocol involving metoclopramide and famotidine in brachycephalic dogs undergoing airway surgery was associated with a decreased incidence of postoperative regurgitation.[13] The drug ameliorated delayed gastric emptying caused by endotoxin administration in horses.[14]

The stimulatory effect of metoclopramide on distal esophageal peristalsis is species specific, with more effect seen in humans, cats, and guinea pigs and less effect seen in dogs.

In the CNS, metoclopramide apparently antagonizes dopamine (D_2) at receptor sites. It is also a weak inhibitor of serotonin 5-HT_3 receptors and an agonist for serotonin 5-HT_4 receptors. These actions help explain its sedative, central antiemetic, extrapyramidal, and prolactin secretion stimulation effects.

Antiemetic effects of metoclopramide are secondary to both central and peripheral (local) effects. Cats reportedly have few CNS dopamine receptors; therefore, metoclopramide may be a poor antiemetic choice in this species.[15] Nevertheless, metoclopramide delayed time to onset of vomiting and reduced the number of vomiting episodes following xylazine administration in cats by 50% to 88%.[16,17] Metoclopramide 0.5 mg/kg IV every 8 hours decreased the severity and frequency of vomiting in dogs hospitalized with parvoviral enteritis.[18] Another study showed that metoclopramide given at 0.5 mg/kg SC 45 minutes before morphine administration decreased incidence of emesis in dogs by 53%, and animals had a lower incidence of injection site pain as compared with maropitant.[4]

In humans, metoclopramide can induce transient increases in aldosterone concentrations, which increase sodium and fluid retention[19]; this effect was not found to occur in dogs or rabbits.[20] In cats and horses, there are no data pertaining to the effects of metoclopramide on aldosterone secretion.

In a study in horses comparing the effects of certain prokinetic drugs (eg, metoclopramide, cisapride, mosapride) on gastric emptying and small intestinal and cecal motility, metoclopramide promoted jejunal motility but did not significantly affect gastric emptying or cecal motility.[21] In a different study in healthy Arabian horses comparing the effects of neostigmine and metoclopramide on GI motility via ultrasound evaluation, metoclopramide improved cecal and colonic contractions compared to control, but not duodenal contractions.[22]

Pharmacokinetics

In dogs and cats, metoclopramide is almost completely absorbed; it is metabolized in the liver and 65% of the dose is eliminated in the urine. The elimination half-life is ≈0.9 hours.[3] Metoclopramide formulated for and used as a nasal spray has been shown to have a higher bioavailability and shorter T_{MAX} as compared to oral tablets.[23]

In goats given metoclopramide IV, volume of distribution was 1.34 L/kg and elimination half-life was 0.6 hours; the drug was undetectable in serum 120 minutes after administration. With IM administration, biologic half-life was 1 hour.[24]

In rabbits, bioavailability of metoclopramide was shown in a study to be 96% and 112% when administered at 2 mg/kg IM and SC, respectively; bioavailability was poor when administered per rectum (13% at a dose of 4 mg/kg). Terminal half-lives were 0.81 hours (IM), 0.89 hours (SC), and 1.68 hours (per rectum). Peak drug concentration occurred at ≈0.2 hours when given IM and SC.[25]

In humans, metoclopramide is well absorbed after oral administration, but a significant first-pass effect in some patients may reduce systemic bioavailability to 30%. Apparently, there is a great deal of interpatient variation with this effect. Bioavailability after IM administration is 74% to 96%. After oral administration, peak plasma concentrations generally occur within 2 hours. Metoclopramide is well distributed throughout the body and enters the CNS. Up to 30% of the drug is protein-bound.[19,26]

In humans, metoclopramide is primarily excreted in urine, and ≈20% to 25% of the drug is excreted unchanged. The remaining drug is primarily metabolized to glucuronidated or sulfated conjugate forms and then excreted in the urine. Approximately 5% is excreted in the feces. Elimination half-life is 5 to 6 hours.

Contraindications/Precautions/Warnings

Metoclopramide is contraindicated in animals with GI hemorrhage, obstruction, or perforation and in animals hypersensitive to it. It is relatively (some say absolutely) contraindicated in animals with seizure disorders. Catecholamine release may occur following IV injection, and the drug is contraindicated in animals with pheochromocytoma, as it may induce a hypertensive crisis. In humans, it is recommended to use metoclopramide with caution in patients with hypertension.[27]

Metoclopramide has a black box warning regarding the risk for development of tardive dyskinesia in humans; it is recommended that the drug not be used for longer than 12 weeks. Use should be avoided in animals with tardive dyskinesia or a history of dystonic reactions.

Metoclopramide has been associated with cases of neuroleptic malignant syndrome in humans.

Because of its effects on aldosterone in humans, metoclopramide should be used with caution in animals with congestive heart failure.[19]

A dose adjustment may be required when metoclopramide is used as a CRI in animals with renal failure. Anecdotal experience in a study suggests reducing the CRI to 25% to 50% of the standard dose.[28] Dose reduction should also be considered in animals with moderate to severe hepatic impairment.

Adverse Effects

In dogs, the most common (although infrequent) adverse effects are changes in mentation and behavior (eg, motor restlessness, involuntary spasms, aggression, vocalization, hyperactivity, drowsiness, depression). Metoclopramide can increase detrusor muscle contractility and reduce bladder capacity. Tremors may occur, particularly in dogs with renal insufficiency.[29] Extrapyramidal signs (head tremors, dystonia of the dorsal back and lateral thorax muscles) were observed in a dog after it received metoclopramide via IV bolus.[30]

Cats may exhibit signs of frenzied behavior or disorientation. Cats and dogs can develop constipation.

In adult horses, IV metoclopramide administration has been associated with the development of severe CNS effects.[31] Alternating periods of sedation and excitement, behavior changes, and abdominal pain have been noted. These effects appear to be less common in foals.

Other adverse effects that have been reported in humans and are plausible in animals include extrapyramidal effects (eg, dyskinesia, dystonia, akathisia), nausea, diarrhea, transient hypertension, and elevated prolactin concentrations.

Reproductive/Nursing Safety

Studies in laboratory animals have not produced any evidence of teratogenic or fetotoxic effects. Metoclopramide may elevate prolactin concentrations, which may lead to galactorrhea, gynecomastia, impotence, and anestrus; use should be avoided in dogs with pseudopregnancy.[32]

Metoclopramide is excreted into milk and may concentrate at approximately twice the plasma concentration; breastfed infants exposed to metoclopramide in milk have experienced adverse GI effects. Metoclopramide-induced hyperprolactinemia stimulated milk production in postpartum healthy bitches, but the effect on their offspring was not assessed.[33] Caution is advised when using in nursing animals.

Overdose/Acute Toxicity

The oral LD_{50} doses of metoclopramide in mice, rats, and rabbits are 465 mg/kg, 760 mg/kg, and 870 mg/kg, respectively. Because of the high doses required for lethality, it is unlikely an oral overdose will cause death in a veterinary patient. Clinical signs of an overdose include sedation, ataxia, agitation, extrapyramidal effects, nausea, vomiting, and constipation. Serotonin syndrome is possible.

There is no specific antidotal therapy for metoclopramide intoxication. If an oral ingestion was recent, standard GI decontamination protocols can be employed. Metoclopramide may reduce the efficacy of emetics (eg, ropinirole, apomorphine). Anticholinergic agents (eg, diphenhydramine, 2.2 mg/kg IV) that enter the CNS may be helpful in controlling extrapyramidal effects. Peritoneal dialysis or hemodialysis is not thought to be effective in removal of this drug.

For patients that have experienced or are suspected to have experienced an overdose, consultation with a 24-hour poison consultation center specializing in providing veterinary-specific information is recommended. For general information related to overdose and toxin exposures, as well as contact information for poison control centers, refer to ***Appendix***.

Drug Interactions

The following drug interactions have either been reported or are theoretical in humans or animals receiving oral metoclopramide and may be of significance in veterinary patients. Unless otherwise noted, use together is not necessarily contraindicated, but the potential risks must be weighed and additional monitoring performed when appropriate.

- **Acetaminophen**: In overdose situations in humans, metoclopramide has enhanced absorption of these agents.
- **Alpha-2 Adrenergic Receptor Agonists** (eg, **dexmedetomidine, xylazine**): In cats, metoclopramide may reduce the emetic effects of alpha-2 agonists.[34]
- **Anesthetics**: Acute hypotension has been reported when metoclopramide is used concurrently IV.
- **Anticholinergic agents** (eg, **atropine, dimenhydrinate, diphenhydramine, glycopyrrolate, meclizine, oxybutynin**): May antagonize the GI motility effects of metoclopramide
- **Apomorphine**: Metoclopramide may negate the emetic effects of apomorphine.
- **Aspirin**: In overdose situations in humans, metoclopramide has enhanced absorption of these agents.
- **Butyrophenones** (eg, **azaperone, droperidol**): May potentiate the extrapyramidal effects of metoclopramide[35,36]
- **Cephalexin**: In dogs, oral metoclopramide was shown to increase cephalexin peak plasma concentrations and area under the curve (AUC). No dosage adjustments are required.[37]
- **Cholinergic Drugs** (eg, **bethanechol**): May enhance metoclopramide's GI effects

- **CNS Depressants** (eg, **anesthetic agents, antihistamines, anxiolytics, barbiturates, phenothiazines, sedatives, tranquilizers**): Metoclopramide may enhance CNS depressant effects.
- **Cyclosporine**: Metoclopramide can potentially increase the rate and extent of GI absorption of cyclosporine; however, this does not appear to be an issue in dogs.[38]
- **Dopamine and Dopaminergic Drugs** (eg, **bromocriptine, cabergoline**): Metoclopramide could theoretically antagonize dopamine or dopaminergic drugs, and vice versa, but clinical significance has not been established.
- **Monoamine Oxidase Inhibitors** (**MAOIs**; eg, **amitraz, linezolid, selegiline**): May cause hypertension
- **Mirtazapine**: Increased risk for extrapyramidal adverse effects; use together is contraindicated in humans
- **Opioid Analgesics** (eg, **fentanyl, hydromorphone, morphine**): May antagonize the GI motility effects of metoclopramide and enhance metoclopramide's CNS depressant effects; combination may also reduce the emetic effects of hydromorphone.
- **Phenothiazines** (eg, **acepromazine, chlorpromazine**): May potentiate the extrapyramidal effects of metoclopramide[35,36]
- **Posaconazole**: May reduce posaconazole concentrations
- **Propofol**: In humans, metoclopramide reduces induction requirements of propofol by 20% to 25%.
- **Quinidine**: May inhibit metoclopramide metabolism
- **Ropinirole**: Metoclopramide may negate the emetic effects of ropinirole.
- **Selective Serotonin Reuptake Inhibitors** (**SSRIs**; eg, **fluoxetine, paroxetine, sertraline,**): Potential for enhanced extrapyramidal effects or neuroleptic malignant syndrome. In addition, SSRIs may inhibit metoclopramide metabolism and increase the risk for toxicity.
- **Tetracyclines**: Metoclopramide can increase the rate and extent of GI absorption.
- **Tramadol**: Use together may increase risk for seizures
- **Tricyclic Antidepressants** (eg, **amitriptyline, clomipramine**): Potential for enhanced extrapyramidal effects or neuroleptic malignant syndrome

Laboratory Considerations

- Metoclopramide may induce secretion of **vasopressin** and alter fluid and electrolyte values.
- Metoclopramide may induce secretion of **prolactin**.

Dosages

DOGS:

Antiemetic and gastric prokinetic (extra-label):

Intermittent doses: Most published studies used a dose of 0.5 mg/kg IV or SC; historically, 0.2 – 0.5 mg/kg every 6 to 8 hours PO, SC, IV, or IM has been used.[39] When used as a prokinetic, administer 30 to 60 minutes before a meal. A higher dose (eg, 1 mg/kg SC, IM) may be required when used as an antiemetic for chemotherapy-induced emesis.

Constant rate infusion (CRI): 0.04 – 0.09 mg/kg/hour (1 – 2 mg/kg/day) IV[39]

Reduction of morphine-induced nausea and vomiting: 0.2 – 0.5 mg/kg SC 30 to 45 minutes prior to morphine administration[4,40]

Reduction of reflux or aspiration associated with surgery for laryngeal paralysis (extra-label): 1 mg/kg IV loading dose followed by 1 mg/kg/hour IV CRI during surgery. Postoperatively, rate was reduced to 0.083 mg/kg/hour IV CRI for a total treatment duration of 24 hours.[11]

Treatment for vomiting and reduced GI motility associated with gastritis, pyloric spasm, chronic nephritis, and digestive intolerance to some drugs (extra-label): 0.25 – 0.5 mg/kg twice daily or 0.17 – 0.33 mg/kg three times daily PO, IV, IM, or SC. Doses may be given up to every 6 hours.[35,36]

Induction of milk letdown reflex for secondary agalactia (extra-label): Oxytocin 0.25 – 1 unit (total dose; NOT units/kg) SC every 2 hours. Neonates are removed for 30 minutes postinjection and then encouraged to suckle or gentle stripping of the glands is performed. Metoclopramide 0.1 – 0.2 mg/kg SC every 12 hours can be used to promote milk production. Therapy is usually successful within 24 hours.[41]

Reduction of regurgitation and respiratory complications in brachycephalic dogs undergoing airway surgery (extra-label): 0.5 mg/kg SC in combination with famotidine 1 mg/kg IV or SC given either shortly before or as part of premedication.[13] In patients with no history of regurgitation or vomiting, this protocol was followed with no additional medications preoperatively. For non-emergent procedures in patients with a history of regurgitation or vomiting, patients were treated with oral metoclopramide and a proton pump inhibitor for one week prior to surgery, and the injectable protocol followed as described above. Implementation of this protocol decreased the incidence of postoperative regurgitation in brachycephalic dogs undergoing anesthesia.

CATS:

Antiemetic (extra-label): Other antiemetics (eg, ondansetron, maropitant) and prokinetic agents (eg, cisapride) are typically used, but metoclopramide dosages in dogs can be tried. 0.2 – 1 mg/kg IM delayed or reduced xylazine-induced emesis[16,17]

Gastric prokinetic (extra-label): 0.5 mg/kg SC every 8 hours[42]

Treatment for vomiting and reduced GI motility associated with gastritis, pyloric spasm, chronic nephritis, and digestive intolerance to some drugs (extra-label): 0.25 – 0.5 mg/kg twice daily or 0.17 – 0.33 mg/kg three times daily PO, IV, IM, or SC. Doses may be given up to every 6 hours.[35,36]

HORSES:

GI prokinetic (extra label):

a) 0.2 mg/kg SC improved jejunal motility[21]

b) 0.04 mg/kg/hour IV CRI reduced ileus following small intestinal resection and anastamosis[43]

c) 0.25 mg/kg IM improved cecal and colonic contractions, but not duodenal contractions, when evaluated by ultrasound in healthy Arabian horses[22]

RABBITS/RODENTS/SMALL MAMMALS:

a) Anecdotal dosages of 0.2 – 1 mg/kg PO, IM, or SC every 8 to 24 hours have been noted.

b) In a pharmacokinetic study, single doses of 2 mg/kg were used intra-arterial, IM, and SC in rabbits with no apparent adverse effects.[25]

c) **Gastric dilation in rabbits** (extra-label): 0.5 mg/kg SC three times daily[44]

Monitoring

- Clinical efficacy
- Adverse effects, including monitoring for tremors

Client Information

- When administering this medicine orally, it may be given ≈15 to 30 minutes before feeding or on an empty stomach. If your animal vomits or acts sick after receiving this medicine on an empty stomach, try giving the next dose with food or a small treat. If vomiting continues, contact your veterinarian.

- If vomiting occurs after giving your animal the oral liquid solution, do not repeat the dose. Give the next dose at the next scheduled time and continue the regular schedule of administration.
- This medicine may be injected under the skin, especially when vomiting in small animals is being treated or prevented. Your veterinarian will instruct you on how to give the injections. Do not give the oral liquid as an injection.
- There are no specific precautions required when handling this medication unless you are allergic to it.
- This medicine is typically well tolerated in dogs and cats. Contact your veterinarian if your animal develops severe restlessness, hyperactivity, rigid posture, spasms, aggression, or severe drowsiness/depression. Your animal may need to urinate more often while taking this medicine.
- Cats may show signs of frenzied behavior or disorientation.
- Dogs and cats can become constipated when taking this medicine.

Chemistry/Synonyms

Metoclopramide HCl, a derivative of para-aminobenzoic acid, occurs as an odorless, white, crystalline powder with pK_as of 0.6 and 9.3. One gram is soluble in ≈0.7 mL of water or ≈3 mL of alcohol. The injectable product has a pH of 2.5 to 6.5. Dosage form potency is expressed in mg of metoclopramide base.

Metoclopramide HCl may also be known as AHR-3070-C, DEL-1267, metoclopramidi hydrochloridum, and MK-745; many trade names are available.

Storage/Stability

Metoclopramide is photosensitive and must be stored in light-resistant containers at room temperatures of 20°C to 25°C (68°F-77°F), with excursions permitted between 15°C to 30°C (59°F-86°F) for the injectable solution. Metoclopramide tablets should be kept in tight containers.

The injectable solution is reportedly stable in solutions with a pH range between 2 and 9 and with the following IV solutions: 5% dextrose, 0.9% sodium chloride, 5% dextrose/0.45% sodium chloride, Ringer's, and lactated Ringer's injection.

Compatibility/Compounding Considerations

Compatibility is dependent on factors such as pH, concentration, temperature, and diluent used; specialized references or a hospital pharmacist should be consulted for more specific information.

The following drugs have been stated to be physically **compatible** with metoclopramide for at least 24 hours: aminophylline, ascorbic acid, atropine sulfate, chlorpromazine HCl, cimetidine HCl, clindamycin phosphate, cyclophosphamide, cytarabine, dexamethasone sodium phosphate, dimenhydrinate, diphenhydramine HCl, doxorubicin HCl, fentanyl citrate, heparin sodium, hydrocortisone sodium phosphate, hydroxyzine HCl, insulin (regular), lidocaine HCl, magnesium sulfate, mannitol, meperidine HCl, methylprednisolone sodium succinate, morphine sulfate, multivitamin infusion (MVI), pentazocine lactate, potassium acetate/chloride/phosphate, prochlorperazine edisylate, ranitidine, TPN solution (25% dextrose with 4.25% *Travasol*®, with or without electrolytes), verapamil, and vitamin B complex with vitamin C.

Metoclopramide is reported to be physically **incompatible** when mixed with the following drugs: ampicillin sodium, calcium gluconate, chloramphenicol sodium succinate, cisplatin, erythromycin lactobionate, methotrexate sodium, penicillin G potassium, sodium bicarbonate, and tetracycline.

Dosage Forms/Regulatory Status

VETERINARY-LABELED PRODUCTS: NONE IN THE UNITED STATES

The Association or Racing Commissioners International (ARCI) has designated this drug as a class 4 substance. Use of this drug may not be allowed in certain animal competitions. Check rules and regulations before entering in a competition while this medication is being administered. Contact local racing authorities for further guidance. See ***Appendix*** for more information.

HUMAN-LABELED PRODUCTS:

All are expressed in terms of metoclopramide monohydrate:

Metoclopramide HCl Oral Tablets: 5 mg and 10 mg; *Reglan*®, generic; (Rx)

Metoclopramide Oral Dispersible Tablets (ODT): 5 mg; *Metozolv*®, generic; (Rx)

Metoclopramide HCl Oral Syrup: 1 mg/mL in 473 mL bottles; generic; (Rx)

Metoclopramide HCl Injection Solution: 5 mg/mL in 2, 10, and 30 mL single-use vials; generic; (Rx)

References

For the complete list of references, see **wiley.com/go/budde/plumb**

Metoprolol
Metoprolol Succinate
Metoprolol Tartrate

(me-***toe***-pro-lole) *Lopressor*®, *Toprol XL*®

Beta-Adrenergic Blocker

Prescriber Highlights

- Used in dogs for supraventricular tachyarrhythmias, premature ventricular contractions (PVCs), and systemic hypertension, and in cats for treatment of hypertrophic cardiomyopathy
- Due to its selectivity for beta-1 over beta-2, metoprolol is likely safer than propranolol in animals with bronchoconstrictive disease.
- Contraindications include overt or unstable heart failure, hypersensitivity to any beta-blocker, atrioventricular block greater than first-degree, and sinus bradycardia.
- Use with caution in animals with significant hepatic insufficiency, bronchospastic lung disease, stable CHF, pheochromocytoma, hyperthyroidism, diabetes mellitus, and sinus node dysfunction.
- Adverse effects include bradycardia, lethargy and depression, impaired AV conduction, worsening of heart failure, hypotension, hypoglycemia, bronchoconstriction, syncope, and diarrhea.
- Adverse effects are more likely in geriatric animals or animals with acute decompensating heart disease.
- Metoprolol should be gradually tapered when discontinuing after chronic use.

Uses/Indications

Metoprolol may be effective in treating dogs with supraventricular tachyarrhythmias, premature ventricular contractions (PVCs), and systemic hypertension. It may also be effective for treating cats with hypertrophic cardiomyopathy. Because metoprolol is relatively safe to use in animals with bronchospastic disease, it is often chosen over propranolol.

One retrospective study showed increased survival times when dogs were given metoprolol; however, no prospective studies documenting increased survival with beta-blockers in dogs with heart failure have been reported. Beta-blockers are generally not recommended for treatment of congestive heart failure (CHF) associated with myxomatous mitral valve disease (MMVD) except as potential adjunct treatment for heart rate control in atrial fibrillation.[1,2] Beta-blockers should be used cautiously due to negative inotropic effects and should not be used in dogs with active signs of CHF.

Pharmacology/Actions

Metoprolol is a relatively selective beta-1-blocker and is sometimes characterized as a second-generation beta-blocker. At higher doses, nonselective beta-1 and beta-2-blockade can occur. Metoprolol does not possess any intrinsic sympathomimetic activity like pindolol, nor does it possess membrane-stabilizing activity like pindolol or propranolol. Metoprolol has negative inotropic and chronotropic actions, resulting in a decreased sinus heart rate, slowed AV conduction, diminished cardiac output at rest and during exercise, decreased myocardial oxygen demand, and reduced blood pressure.

Pharmacokinetics

No information on the pharmacokinetics of metoprolol succinate was located for dogs or cats. When a sustained-release tablet containing metoprolol 50 mg and felodipine 5 mg was administered orally to beagle dogs, the maximum plasma concentration of metoprolol was 532 µg/mL and occurred after 3.8 hours. The plasma half-life, clearance, and volume of distribution were 9.1 hours, 1.2 L/hour/kg, and 16.4 L/kg, respectively.[3]

In humans, metoprolol tartrate is rapidly and completely absorbed from the GI tract; however, bioavailability is only ≈50% due to high first-pass metabolism.[4] Metoprolol is only ≈5% to 15% bound to plasma proteins and is distributed well into most tissues. It crosses the blood-brain barrier, and CSF concentrations are ≈78% of those found in the plasma. It also crosses the placenta, and concentrations in milk are 3 to 4 times higher than those found in plasma. Metoprolol is extensively metabolized in the liver, and both unchanged drug and metabolites are excreted in the urine. The half-life in humans varies depending on CYP2D6 polymorphisms, and ranges from 3 to 4 hours in extensive metabolizers to 7 to 9 hours in poor metabolizers. Reported half-life of metoprolol tartrate in dogs is 1.7 hours; reported half-life in cats is 1.3 hours.

Contraindications/Precautions/Warnings

Metoprolol is contraindicated in patients with overt or unstable heart failure, hypersensitivity to any beta-blocker, atrioventricular block greater than firstdegree, or sinus bradycardia. In humans, metoprolol is contraindicated in patients with severe peripheral arterial circulatory disorders and pheochromocytoma. Nonselective beta-blockers are contraindicated in patients with bronchospastic lung disease; however, because metoprolol is relatively selective for beta-2 receptors, it can be used with extreme caution in patients with bronchospastic disease.

Metoprolol should be used cautiously in patients with history of cardiac failure as beta-blockade depresses myocardial contractility and can lead to failure over time.[4] It should also be used with caution in patients with significant hepatic insufficiency or sinus node dysfunction. At high doses, metoprolol can mask the clinical signs associated with hypoglycemia. It can also cause hypoglycemia or hyperglycemia and, therefore, should be used cautiously in labile diabetic patients. Metoprolol can also mask some clinical signs associated with thyrotoxicosis, but it may be used clinically to treat the clinical signs associated with this condition (eg, tachycardia, hypertension).

When discontinuing metoprolol after chronic administration, the dose should be gradually tapered.[4]

Do not confuse metoprolol succinate (extended-release) with metoprolol tartrate (immediate-release).

Adverse Effects

Adverse effects of metoprolol include bradycardia, lethargy, weakness, depression, impaired AV-node conduction, CHF or worsening of heart failure, hypotension, and hypoglycemia. Bronchoconstriction is possible, but less likely with beta-1 selective drugs like metoprolol. Syncope and diarrhea have also been reported in canine patients with beta-blockers. Cats with hypertrophic cardiomyopathy may be at an increased risk for pulmonary edema. It is reported that adverse effects most commonly occur in geriatric animals or those that have acute decompensating heart disease.

Exacerbation of clinical signs has been reported following abrupt cessation of beta-blockers in humans. Gradual discontinuation of therapy is recommended in patients that have been receiving metoprolol chronically.

Reproductive/Nursing Safety

Metoprolol crosses the placenta. No teratogenic effects have been reported, but safe use during pregnancy has not been established.

Metoprolol is excreted in milk in very small quantities. Use with caution in nursing animals and monitor offspring for adverse effects.

Because safety has not been established in animals, this drug should only be used when the maternal benefits outweigh the potential risks to offspring.

Overdose/Acute Toxicity

There is limited information available on metoprolol overdoses. The predominant clinical signs of an overdose of other beta-blockers (eg, propranolol) include hypotension and bradycardia. Other possible effects include CNS (eg, depressed consciousness, seizures), bronchospasm, hypoglycemia, hyperkalemia, respiratory depression, pulmonary edema, other arrhythmias (especially AV block), and asystole.

If overdose is secondary to recent oral ingestion, GI decontamination protocols may be considered; however, use caution inducing emesis as coma and seizures may develop rapidly. Monitor ECG, blood glucose, potassium, and blood pressure. Treatment of the cardiovascular effects is based on clinical signs; fluids and pressor agents can be used to treat hypotension, and bradycardia may be treated with atropine. If atropine fails, isoproterenol, given cautiously, has been recommended. Use of a transvenous pacemaker may be necessary. Heart failure can be treated with digitalis glycosides, diuretics, and oxygen. Glucagon 5 – 10 mg IV may increase heart rate and blood pressure and reduce the cardiodepressant effects of metoprolol. Intravenous lipid emulsion (ILE) infusions are likely not beneficial for metoprolol intoxication.

Humans have reportedly survived doses of up to 5 g.

For patients that have experienced or are suspected to have experienced an overdose, consultation with a 24-hour poison consultation center specializing in providing veterinary-specific information is recommended. For general information related to overdose and toxin exposures, as well as contact information for poison control centers, refer to ***Appendix.***

Drug Interactions

The following drug interactions have either been reported or are theoretical in humans or animals receiving metoprolol and may be of significance in veterinary patients. Unless otherwise noted, use together is not necessarily contraindicated, but weigh the potential risks and perform additional monitoring when appropriate.

- **Anesthetics Agents, Inhalant** (eg, **halothane**): Increased risk for heart failure and hypotension
- **Antidiabetic Agents** (eg, **glipizide, insulin**): May result in hypoglycemia or hyperglycemia; metoprolol may mask signs of hypoglycemia
- **Calcium Channel Blockers** (eg, **amlodipine, diltiazem, verapamil**): Increased risk for hypotension, bradycardia, and AV node disturbances. Concurrent use of beta-blockers with calcium channel blockers (or other negative inotropics) should be done with caution, particularly in patients with pre-existing cardiomyopathy or CHF.

- **Digoxin**: May increase negative effects on SA or AV node conduction
- **Diuretics** (eg, **furosemide, thiazides**): May increase hypotensive effect of metoprolol
- **Hydralazine**: May increase the risks for pulmonary hypertension in uremic patients
- **Lidocaine, Systemic**: May result in lidocaine toxicity including myocardial depression and cardiac arrest
- **Methimazole**: Change from hyperthyroid to euthyroid state may alter metoprolol metabolism; metoprolol dose adjustment may be required
- **Nonsteroidal Anti-Inflammatory Drugs** (**NSAIDs**; eg, **carprofen, meloxicam, robenacoxib**): May result in increased blood pressure
- **Phenobarbital**: May reduce metoprolol efficacy
- **Quinidine**: May increase metoprolol plasma concentrations
- **Reserpine**: Potential for additive hypotension and bradycardia
- **Rifampin**: May reduce metoprolol efficacy
- **Selective Serotonin Receptor Inhibitors** (**SSRIs**; eg, **fluoxetine, paroxetine, sertraline**): May increase metoprolol plasma concentrations
- **Sympathomimetics** (eg, **epinephrine, phenylpropanolamine, terbutaline**): Use together may reduce the efficacy of both agents
- **Terbinafine**: May increase metoprolol plasma concentrations

Dosages

DOGS:

Adjunctive treatment for heart rate control in atrial fibrillation (extra-label): Using metoprolol tartrate (immediate-release tablets), doses are typically started low at ≈0.2 mg/kg PO every 12 hours and slowly titrated upwards every 2 to 3 weeks as tolerated. Practically, 6.25 mg (1/4 of a 25 mg tablet) is the minimum dose using commercial tablets. Commonly, dosages of 0.4 – 1 mg/kg PO every 8 to 12 hours are used, but dosages as high as 6.6 mg/kg PO 3 times daily have been noted; however, many dogs will not tolerate upward dose titration. Extended-release metoprolol succinate tablets could be considered, but pharmacokinetic data supporting their use in dogs are not available.

CATS:

Beta-blockade (extra-label): Anecdotal dosages of 2 – 15 mg/cat (NOT mg/kg) PO every 8 hours have been noted. Compounded products may be necessary for small doses.

Monitoring

- Baseline and periodic physical exam, including heart rate, pulse, and pulse quality
- Baseline and periodic ECG as necessary
- Baseline and periodic blood pressure
- Echocardiography as clinically indicated
- Signs of toxicity (see ***Adverse Effects*** and ***Overdose/Acute Toxicity***)

Client Information

- This medicine may be given with or without food.
- The most common side effects are related to drops in heart rate and blood pressure and may include tiredness, lack of energy, and weakness. Contact your veterinarian if these signs occur.
- Notify your veterinarian if your animal becomes exercise intolerant, has shortness of breath or cough, or develops a change in behavior or attitude.
- When starting this medicine, your veterinarian may start with a low dose and gradually increase it over time to see how your animal reacts to it. Do not administer more than your veterinarian prescribes at one time.
- Your veterinarian will need to monitor your animal closely while it is taking this medicine. Do not miss these important follow-up visits.
- It is very important to not suddenly stop giving this medicine without your veterinarian's guidance.

Chemistry/Synonyms

Metoprolol tartrate, a beta-1 selective adrenergic blocker, occurs as a white, crystalline powder having a bitter taste. It is very soluble in water. Metoprolol succinate occurs as a white, crystalline powder and is freely soluble in water.

Metoprolol may also be known as CGP-2175E, H-93/26, and metoprolol; many trade names are available.

Storage/Stability

Protect metoprolol products from light. Store tablets in tight, light-resistant containers at room temperature. Avoid freezing the injection.

Compatibility/Compounding Considerations

The injection is **compatible** with D_5W and normal saline and at Y-sites with morphine sulfate.

Compounded preparation stability: Metoprolol oral suspension compounded from the commercially available tablets has been published.[5] Triturating twelve (12) metoprolol tartrate 100 mg tablets with 60 mL of *Ora-Plus*® and *qs ad* to 120 mL with *Ora-Sweet*® or *Ora-Sweet SF*® yields a 10 mg/mL metoprolol tartrate oral suspension that retains greater than 95% potency for 60 days when stored at both 4°C (39°F) and 25°C (77°F) and protected from light.

Dosage Forms/Regulatory Status

VETERINARY-LABELED PRODUCTS: NONE

The Association of Racing Commissioners International (ARCI) has designated this drug as a class 3 substance. Use of this drug may not be allowed in certain animal competitions. Check rules and regulations before entering in a competition while this medication is being administered. Contact local racing authorities for further guidance. See the ***Appendix*** for more information.

HUMAN-LABELED PRODUCTS:

Metoprolol Tartrate Oral Tablets: 25 mg, 37.5 mg, 50 mg, 75 mg, and 100 mg; *Lopressor*®, generic; (Rx)

Metoprolol Succinate Extended-Release Tablets: 25 mg, 50 mg, 100 mg, and 200 mg; *Toprol XL*®, generic; (Rx)

Metoprolol Tartrate Injection: 1 mg/mL; *Lopressor*®, generic; (Rx)

References

For the complete list of references, see **wiley.com/go/budde/plumb**

Metronidazole

(me-troe-***ni***-da-zole) *Flagyl®*

Antibiotic, Antiparasitic

Prescriber Highlights

- Injectable and oral antibacterial (anaerobes) and antiprotozoal agent
- Prohibited by the FDA for use in food animals
- Contraindications include hypersensitivity to it or other nitroimidazole derivatives.
- Use with extreme caution in patients that are severely debilitated, pregnant, nursing, or that have hepatic dysfunction. Metronidazole may be a teratogen, especially in early pregnancy.
- Adverse effects include neurologic disorders, lethargy, weakness, neutropenia, hepatotoxicity, hematuria, anorexia, nausea, vomiting, and diarrhea.
- Very bitter taste; metronidazole benzoate may be more palatable when compounded.

Uses/Indications

Metronidazole has been used extensively in the treatment of *Giardia* spp in both dogs and cats, although it is not the drug of choice. It is also used clinically in small animal species for the treatment of other parasites (*Trichomonas* spp and *Balantidium coli*), as well as for treating both enteric and systemic anaerobic infections. It is sometimes used as a perioperative surgical prophylaxis antibiotic where anaerobes are likely (eg, colorectal surgery).

Although metronidazole is frequently used for acute nonspecific diarrhea in dogs, there is little evidence to support this use. One small study found that metronidazole shortened the duration of acute nonspecific diarrhea by ≈1.5 days compared with placebo.[1] Another study found no statistically significant difference in time to acceptable fecal consistency between metronidazole, probiotics, or placebo.[2] Metronidazole should not be used indiscriminately, as its use may have a significant and potentially sustained impact on the GI microbiota.[3,4]

In the United Kingdom, metronidazole is approved in dogs and cats for the treatment of GI tract infections caused by *Giardia* spp and *Clostridium* spp and for the treatment of infections of the urogenital tract, oral cavity, throat, and skin caused by obligate anaerobic bacteria susceptible to metronidazole.[5]

In horses, metronidazole has been used clinically for the treatment of systemic and enteric anaerobic infections.

The World Health Organization (WHO) has designated metronidazole as an Important antimicrobial for human medicine.[6]

Pharmacology/Actions

Metronidazole is a concentration-dependent bactericidal agent against susceptible bacteria. Metronidazole diffuses across the cell membranes of anaerobic bacteria where it interacts with DNA to cause strand breaks, resulting in inhibition of protein synthesis and cell death. Metronidazole has activity against most obligate anaerobes, including *Bacteroides* spp (including *Bacteroides fragilis*), *Eubacterium* spp, *Fusobacterium* spp, *Veillonella* spp, *Clostridium* spp, *Peptococcus* spp, *Peptostreptococcus* spp, and *Prevotella* spp. Resistance to metronidazole appears to be rare, although *Actinomyces* spp are frequently resistant.

Metronidazole is also trichomonacidal and amoebicidal. The mechanism of action for its antiprotozoal activity is not understood. It has therapeutic activity against *Entamoeba histolytica*, *Trichomonas* spp, *Giardia* spp, and *Balantidium coli*. It acts primarily against the trophozoite forms of Entamoeba rather than encysted forms.

Metronidazole has some inhibitive actions on cell-mediated immunity that may play a role in its use for treating inflammatory bowel disease; however, the clinical relevance of these properties is unclear.

Pharmacokinetics

Metronidazole is well absorbed after oral administration. It is lipophilic and is rapidly and widely distributed to most body tissues and fluids, including bone, abscesses, CSF, and seminal fluid. Metronidazole is less than 20% bound to plasma proteins in humans. Metronidazole is primarily metabolized in the liver via several pathways. Both the metabolites and unchanged drug are eliminated in the urine and feces.

The oral bioavailability of metronidazole in dogs is high, but there is interpatient variability, with ranges from 50% to 100% reported. If the drug is given with food, absorption is enhanced in dogs but delayed in humans. Peak concentrations occur ≈1 hour after oral administration.

In a single-dose study in cats, the oral bioavailability of metronidazole benzoate was variable but averaged ≈65%.[7] Peak concentrations after oral administration appear to be highly variable in cats (ranging from 1 to 8 hours), and peak serum concentrations are somewhat lower in cats than in dogs or humans. Mean systemic clearance is slower in cats than in dogs (cats, 1.53 mL/kg/minute; dogs, 2.49 mL/kg/minute). Despite the concern that glucuronidation is a metabolic pathway for metronidazole, terminal elimination half-life is only slightly (not significantly) longer (5 to 6 hours) in cats.

The oral bioavailability of the drug in horses averages ≈80% (range, 57% to 100%). In neonatal foals (1 to 2.5 days of age), volume of distribution (Vd) was 0.87 L/kg and elimination half-life (t½) was 11.8 hours; in the same foals at 10 to 12 days of age, t½ was 9 hours and Vd was unchanged. Oral bioavailability was 100%.[8] In adult horses, food does not appreciably alter oral absorption.[9] Metronidazole accumulation in pleural fluid after oral administration may be sufficient for targeting *Bacteroides* spp pneumonia or pleuropneumonia.[10] If the drug is administered rectally to horses, bioavailability is decreased by ≈50%. Manually evacuating the rectal contents prior to rectal administration improves metronidazole absorption only slightly and appears unnecessary.[11] Elimination half-life in horses is ≈2.9 to 4.3 hours. After IV regional limb perfusion (IVRLP) with metronidazole in standing horses, concentrations in the distal interphalangeal joint of the thoracic limb were high but rapidly declined below the MIC of target pathogens.[12] Studies are needed to determine if IVRLP with metronidazole is a plausible treatment for synovial anaerobic infections.

Contraindications/Precautions/Warnings

Metronidazole is prohibited for use in food animals by the FDA.

Metronidazole is contraindicated in animals that are hypersensitive to it or nitroimidazole derivatives. Metronidazole should be used with caution in animals with hepatic dysfunction. If the drug must be used in animals with significant liver impairment, the total daily dose should be reduced to ⅓ of the standard anti-anaerobe dose and administered once daily.[13] Hepatic disorders are listed as a contraindication in the United Kingdom product label.[5]

Neurotoxicity is a concern, particularly at high doses. In dogs, total daily doses of metronidazole should not exceed 60 mg/kg.[14] However, the median dosage identified in a more recent retrospective study of 26 dogs with metronidazole neurotoxicity was 21 mg/kg every 12 hours.[15] The primary clinical signs were cerebellovestibular ataxia (85%) and pathologic nystagmus (50%), and the median time to resolution was 3 days after metronidazole discontinuation. In a separate case report, neurologic status improved rapidly within 72 hours after discontinuation of high-dose (65 mg/kg/day) oral metronidazole.[16]

Metronidazole use (25 mg/kg PO twice daily) resulted in degradation in the ability to detect odors in 50% of explosives detection dogs.

Further studies are required to determine if a lower metronidazole dosage would have the same effect.[17]

Metronidazole tablets have a sharp, metallic taste that animals find unpleasant. Placing in capsules, using compounded oral suspensions, or hiding in pungent food may help alleviate avoidance.

Do not confuse metronidazole with metformin, mebendazole, or metoclopramide.

Adverse Effects

Adverse effects reported in dogs include neurologic disorders, lethargy, weakness, neutropenia, hepatotoxicity, hematuria, anorexia, nausea, vomiting, and diarrhea. Rare cases of cutaneous vasculitis associated with metronidazole have been reported. Neurologic toxicity in dogs may occur after acute high dosages or, more likely, with long-term moderate to high-dose therapy. See ***Overdose/Acute Toxicity***.

In cats, vomiting, inappetence, hepatotoxicity, and, rarely, CNS toxicity can occur with metronidazole therapy.[18] Genotoxicity was detected in peripheral blood mononuclear cells collected from cats after 7 days of oral metronidazole but resolved within 6 days of discontinuation of the drug. Clinical significance, particularly with long-term therapy, is yet to be determined.[7]

In horses, metronidazole may occasionally cause anorexia, ataxia, and depression, particularly when used at higher dosages. There have been reported cases of *Clostridium difficile* and *Clostridium perfringens* diarrhea and death after use of metronidazole.

In humans, convulsive seizures and peripheral neuropathy have been reported.[19]

Reproductive/Nursing Safety

Metronidazole has not demonstrated impairment of fertility or reproductive performance in mice or rats. Metronidazole's potential for teratogenicity is somewhat controversial; some references state that it has been teratogenic in some laboratory animal studies,[20,21] but others state that it has not. However, unless the benefits to the mother outweigh the risks for the fetus(es), it should not be used during pregnancy, particularly during the first 3 weeks of gestation. In humans, metronidazole is contraindicated in the first trimester of pregnancy.[14]

Metronidazole is present in human milk at concentrations similar to maternal serum concentrations. According to the American Academy of Pediatrics, metronidazole has unknown effects and may be of concern during breastfeeding. Because of the potential for tumorigenicity, using an alternative therapy or switching to milk replacer for nursing patients should be considered.

Overdose/Acute Toxicity

Signs of intoxication associated with metronidazole in dogs and cats include anorexia and/or vomiting, depression, mydriasis, nystagmus, ataxia, head tilt, deficits of proprioception, joint knuckling, disorientation, tremors, seizures, bradycardia, rigidity, and stiffness. These effects may be seen with acute overdoses, doses in dogs above 60 mg/kg per day, or in some animals on long-term therapy when using older recommended dosages (eg, 30 mg/kg/day).

In dogs, common signs of metronidazole toxicity include generalized ataxia with a rapid positional nystagmus. Most often, dogs have neurologic deficits localized to the central vestibular system and/or cerebellum. Dogs with mild to moderate clinical signs usually improve rapidly within 1 to 2 days, once metronidazole has been discontinued.[22]

Diazepam has been used successfully to decrease the CNS effects associated with metronidazole toxicity, but it has not been evaluated in a controlled manner.[15,23] See ***Diazepam*** for more information.

Acute overdoses should be handled by attempting to limit the absorption of the drug using standard protocols. Extreme caution should be used before attempting to induce vomiting in patients demonstrating CNS effects or aspiration may result. If acute toxicity is seen after long-term therapy, the drug should be discontinued. Neurologic clinical signs may require several days before showing signs of resolving. Patient management should consist of treatment of clinical signs and supportive therapy.

For patients that have experienced or are suspected to have experienced an overdose, consultation with a 24-hour poison consultation center specializing in providing veterinary-specific information is recommended. For general information related to overdose and toxin exposures, as well as contact information for poison control centers, refer to ***Appendix***.

Drug Interactions

The following drug interactions have either been reported or are theoretical in humans or animals receiving metronidazole and may be of significance in veterinary patients. Unless otherwise noted, use together is not necessarily contraindicated, but the potential risks should be weighed and additional monitoring performed when appropriate.

- **BUSULFAN**: May result in increased busulfan concentrations and toxicity
- **CIMETIDINE**: May decrease the metabolism of metronidazole and increase the likelihood of dose-related adverse effects
- **CYCLOSPORINE**: Use with metronidazole may increase cyclosporine concentrations.
- **ETHANOL**: May induce a disulfiram-like reaction (eg, nausea, vomiting, cramps) when given with metronidazole
- **FLUOROURACIL (5-FU)**: May result in increased fluorouracil levels and toxicity
- **MYCOPHENOLATE**: Metronidazole may reduce formation of the active mycophenolate metabolite.
- **PHENOBARBITAL, PRIMIDONE**: May increase the metabolism of metronidazole, thereby decreasing blood concentrations
- **QT PROLONGATION DRUGS** (eg, **amiodarone, cisapride, procainamide, quinidine, sotalol**): May increase risk for QT prolongation
- **WARFARIN**: Metronidazole may prolong PT in patients receiving warfarin or other coumarin anticoagulants. Concurrent use should be avoided if possible; otherwise, monitoring with prothrombin times should be intensified.

Laboratory Considerations

- Metronidazole can cause falsely decreased readings of **AST** and **ALT** when determined using methods measuring decreases in ultraviolet absorbance when NADH is reduced to NAD.
- Metronidazole can interfere with measurement of serum **triglycerides**.

Dosages

NOTES:

1. Dosages are for metronidazole base unless otherwise noted. If metronidazole benzoate is being used, dosages should be adjusted unless provided by pharmacy as "mg/mL of the base." One mg of metronidazole base = 1.6 mg of metronidazole benzoate. For example, if the calculated metronidazole dose is 200 mg (of the base), the corresponding dose using metronidazole benzoate would be 320 mg (metronidazole benzoate).
2. Because of the drug's extreme bitterness, using a flavored, compounded metronidazole benzoate or putting quartered tablets in an empty gelatin capsule may be considered.

DOGS:

Giardiasis (extra-label):

a) 25 mg/kg PO twice daily in combination with fenbendazole 50 mg/kg PO once daily for 5 days.[24] **NOTE**: The Companion

Animal Parasite Council (CAPC) recommends monotherapy with fenbendazole 50 mg/kg PO once daily for 5 days as its first choice, but combination therapy may result in better resolution of clinical disease and cyst shedding. If treatment, combined with bathing, does not eliminate infection, as evidenced by testing feces for persistence of cysts, treatment with either fenbendazole alone or in combination with metronidazole may be extended for another 10 days. All dogs in the household should be treated. Repeated courses of treatment are not indicated in dogs without clinical signs.

b) 50 mg/kg PO once daily for 5 to 7 days; dose may be divided equally for twice-daily administration[5]

Other protozoal infections (eg, *Entamoeba histolytica* or *Pentatrichomonas hominis*) (extra-label): 25 mg/kg PO every 12 hours for 8 days[25]

Perioperative surgical prophylaxis (eg, colorectal surgery) (extra-label): There is no consensus for dosages in veterinary medicine, but anecdotally, metronidazole 15 mg/kg IV over 30 to 60 minutes and completed ≈1 hour before surgery may be considered. Usually used in conjunction with cefazolin.

Anaerobic infections (extra-label):

a) For less severe anaerobic infections: 10 – 15 mg/kg PO every 8 to 12 hours
b) Severe infections (ie, sepsis): 15 mg/kg IV every 12 hours

Clostridial enteritis (extra-label):

a) 10 – 15 mg/kg PO every 8 to 12 hours for 5 days.
b) 15 mg/kg IV every 12 hours for 5 days can be used if PO is not an option
c) 50 mg/kg PO every 24 hours for 5 to 7 days; dose may be divided equally for twice-daily administration[5]

Adjunctive therapy of inflammatory GI conditions (IBD) (extra-label): 10 – 15 mg/kg PO twice daily. Dosage can be reduced to 7.5 – 10 mg/kg PO twice daily in patients with concomitant hepatic disease. Long-term therapy has potential risks for neurotoxicosis and hepatotoxicosis.

Confirmed *Helicobacter* spp gastritis infections in dogs showing clinical signs (extra-label):

a) Metronidazole 15.4 mg/kg PO every 8 hours in combination with amoxicillin 11 mg/kg PO every 8 hours and bismuth subsalicylate (original *Pepto-Bismol*®) 0.22 mL/kg PO every 4 to 6 hours for 3 weeks[26]
b) Metronidazole 10 mg/kg PO every 12 hours in combination with amoxicillin 15 mg/kg PO every 12 hours and bismuth subsalicylate 262 mg tablets given based on body weight (less than 5 kg [11 lb] = 0.25 tablet; 5 to 9.9 kg [11 to 21.8 lb] = 0.5 tablet; 10 to 24.9 kg [22 to 54.8 lb] = 1 tablet; greater than 25 kg [55 lb] = 2 tablets) PO every 12 hours for 2 weeks.[27]
c) Metronidazole 11 – 15 mg/kg PO every 12 hours in combination with amoxicillin 22 mg/kg PO every 12 hours and bismuth subsalicylate suspension 0.22 mL/kg (3.85 mg/kg) PO every 6 to 8 hours for 3 weeks[28]

Alternative treatment for *Babesia gibsoni* after atovaquone and azithromycin failed to eliminate infection on PCR test: Metronidazole 15 mg/kg PO twice daily in combination with clindamycin 25 mg/kg PO twice daily and doxycycline 5 mg/kg PO once daily for 30 to 90 days[29]

Hepatic encephalopathy (extra-label): 7.5 mg/kg PO every 8 to 12 hours[30]

CATS:

Giardiasis (extra-label):

a) 25 mg/kg PO twice daily for 5 days.[31] The CAPC states: Data on treatment of cats with Giardia are lacking. However, cats may be treated with either fenbendazole 50 mg/kg PO once daily for 5 days or metronidazole 25 mg/kg PO twice daily for 5 days, or a combination of the two as described for dogs. There is anecdotal evidence that metronidazole benzoate is tolerated better in cats than metronidazole (USP). If other pets live with an infected dog or cat, all those of the same species may also be treated with a single course of antigiardial therapy. Repeated courses of treatment are not indicated in dogs or cats without clinical signs.[24]
b) 50 mg/kg/day for 5 to 7 days; dose may be divided equally for twice-daily administration[5]

Trichomoniasis (*Tritrichomonas foetus*, most prevalent; *Pentatrichomonas hominis*); (extra-label): 30 – 50 mg/kg PO twice daily for 3 to 14 days has been used in the past for *T foetus*, but clearance of infections appears less common than when ronidazole is used.[32]

Perioperative surgical prophylaxis (colorectal surgery) (extra-label): There is no consensus for dosages in veterinary medicine, but metronidazole 15 mg/kg IV over 30 to 60 minutes and completed ≈1 hour before surgery may be considered. Usually used in conjunction with cefazolin.

Confirmed *Helicobacter* spp gastritis infections in cats showing clinical signs (extra-label):

a) Metronidazole 10 – 15 mg/kg PO twice daily in combination with clarithromycin 7.5 mg/kg PO twice daily and amoxicillin 20 mg/kg PO twice daily for 14 days[33]
b) Metronidazole 11 – 15.4 mg/kg PO every 8 – 12 hours in combination with amoxicillin 11 – 22 mg/kg PO every 8 hours and bismuth subsalicylate suspension (original *Pepto-Bismol*®) 0.22 mL/kg (3.85 mg/kg) PO every 4 to 8 hours and for 3 weeks[28,34]
c) Metronidazole 10 mg/kg PO twice daily in combination with amoxicillin 10 – 20 mg/kg PO 3 times daily and bismuth subsalicylate (262 mg tablets; *Pepto-Bismol*®) ¼ tablet/cat (total dose) PO twice daily, ± H_2 blocker (eg, famotidine) or omeprazole for 2 weeks.[27]

Anaerobic infections (extra-label):

a) For less severe anaerobic infections: 10 – 15 mg/kg PO every 12 hours or 15 – 25 mg/kg PO once daily can be considered. Practically, ¼ of a 250 mg tablet (62.5 mg) per cat is often chosen for a PO dose.
b) Severe infections (ie, sepsis): 15 mg/kg IV every 12 hours

Clostridial enteritis (extra-label):

a) 62.5 mg/cat (NOT mg/kg) PO every 12 hours for 5 days
b) 50 mg/kg PO daily for 5 to 7 days; dose may be divided equally for twice-daily administration[5]

Adjunctive therapy of inflammatory GI conditions (IBD) (extra-label): 10 – 15 mg/kg PO twice daily. Long-term therapy has potential risks for neurotoxicity and hepatotoxicity.[35] Practically, ¼ of a 250 mg tablet (62.5 mg) per cat is often chosen for a PO dose.

Hepatic encephalopathy (extra-label): 7.5 mg/kg PO every 8 to 12 hours[30]

HORSES:

Clostridial enterocolitis (extra-label): Dosage recommendations vary, but 15 mg/kg PO every 8 to 12 hours appears reasonable. IV route can be used if PO is not possible. Consider lower dosages (ie, 10 mg/kg IV every 12 hours) in newborn (ie, less than 5 days old) foals.

Metritis secondary to *Bacteroides fragilis* (extra-label): 15 – 25 mg/kg PO every 12 hours[36]

Periodontal disease (extra-label): Metronidazole tablets were cut into 1 to 2 mm pieces and filled into mandibular periodontal pockets to the level of the gingiva.[37]

BIRDS:

Susceptible infections (anaerobes; *Giardia* spp) (extra-label): 10 – 50 mg/kg PO every 12 hours[38]

FERRETS:

***Helicobacter mustelae* gastritis infections** (extra-label): Metronidazole 20 mg/kg PO every 8 hours in combination with *either* amoxicillin 30 mg/kg PO every 8 hours OR clarithromycin 12.5 mg/kg PO every 12 hours for 21 to 28 days; the addition of bismuth subsalicylate 7.5 mg/kg PO every 8 hours to the combination is optional.[39,40]

Anaerobic infections (extra-label): 10 – 30 mg/kg PO 1 to 2 times daily

Inflammatory bowel disease (extra-label): 50 mg/kg PO once daily[39]

RABBITS, RODENTS, SMALL MAMMALS:

Anaerobic infections (extra-label):

a) **Rabbits:**
   i. 20 mg/kg PO every 12 hours for 3 to 5 days[41]
   ii. 40 mg/kg PO once daily[41]
   iii. 5 mg/kg slow IV every 12 hours[41]
b) **Mice:**
   i 3.5 mg/mL in water for 5 days[42]
   ii. ***Spironucleus muris:*** 10 – 40 mg/kg PO twice, 5 days apart[43]
c) **Rats**: 10 – 40 mg/rat (NOT mg/kg) PO once daily[42]
d) **Chinchillas, guinea pigs**: 10 – 40 mg/kg PO once daily[42]
e) **Gerbils, hamsters**: 7.5 mg/70 to 90 g body weight PO every 8 hours[42]

REPTILES/AMPHIBIANS:

Treatment of amoebae, flagellates, and ciliates in reptiles and amphibians (extra-label): Typically, metronidazole 100 mg/kg PO repeated in 2 weeks or 50 mg/kg PO once daily for 3 to 5 days; repeat treatment as needed.[44]

Anaerobic respiratory infections in reptiles (extra-label): 20 mg/kg PO every 48 hours[45]

Monitoring

- Clinical efficacy
- Adverse effects; clients should report any neurologic signs

Client Information

- Give this medication with food.
- This medicine can cause nervous system side effects, especially when administered at higher doses. Tell your veterinarian about any changes in your animal's behavior or coordination.
- Do not give this medicine to pregnant or nursing animals.
- Metronidazole is banned for use in animals that are used for food (including egg-laying chickens and dairy animals).
- Pregnant women and people who are allergic to this drug should be very careful not to accidentally take it.

Chemistry/Synonyms

Metronidazole is a synthetic, nitroimidazole antibacterial and antiprotozoal agent. It occurs as white to pale-yellow crystalline powder or crystals with a pK_a of 2.6. It is sparingly soluble in water or alcohol. Metronidazole base is commercially available as tablets or solution for IV injection. The hydrochloride is very soluble in water.

Metronidazole benzoate is the benzoic ester of metronidazole. It occurs as a white to slightly yellow crystalline powder that is practically insoluble in water, slightly soluble in alcohol, and soluble in acetone. Because it is less soluble in aqueous solutions as compared with the base, it does not taste as bad. Based on the molecular weights of metronidazole (171.1 g/mol) and metronidazole benzoate (275.3 g/mol), 1.6 mg metronidazole benzoate contains 1 mg metronidazole.

Metronidazole may also be known as Bayer-5360, metronidazolum, SC-32642, NSC-50364, RP-8823, and SC-10295; many trade names are available.

Storage/Stability

Metronidazole tablets and solution for injection should be stored at temperatures less than 30°C (86°F) and protected from light. The shelf life of divided tablets is 3 days.[5]

Compatibility/Compounding Considerations

Compatibility is dependent on factors such as pH, concentration, temperature, and diluent used; specialized references or a hospital pharmacist should be consulted for more specific information.

The manufacturer states that metronidazole should not be mixed with other drugs, and other IV infusions should be discontinued, when possible, while metronidazole is being infused. The following drugs and solutions are reportedly physically **Y-site compatible** with metronidazole ready-to-use solutions for injection: amikacin sulfate, aminophylline, ampicillin, cefazolin sodium, cefotaxime sodium, cefoxitin sodium, cefuroxime sodium, chloramphenicol sodium succinate, clindamycin phosphate, dexamethasone sodium phosphate, gentamicin sulfate, heparin sodium, hydrocortisone sodium succinate, hydromorphone HCl, ketamine, magnesium sulfate, metoclopramide, morphine sulfate, multi-electrolyte concentrate, multivitamins, penicillin G sodium, and tobramycin sulfate.

The following drugs and solutions are reportedly physically **incompatible** (or compatibility data conflict) with metronidazole ready-to-use solutions for injection: amphotericin B (all formulations), aztreonam, cefamandole naftate, diazepam, dopamine HCl, pantoprazole, and propofol.

Metronidazole hydrochloride is bitter tasting and, even with taste-masking or flavoring agents, is universally unpalatable to veterinary patients. Although not commercially available in the United States, the metronidazole ester of benzoic acid, metronidazole benzoate, is relatively palatable to animal patients and is often used in extemporaneously compounded suspensions, particularly in cats to reduce the drug's bitterness. If metronidazole benzoate is being used, dosages should be adjusted from those used for the base unless provided by the pharmacy as "mg/mL of the base." One mg of metronidazole base = ≈1.6 mg of metronidazole benzoate. Crystallization and sedimentation can occur in aqueous metronidazole benzoate suspensions when conversion from the anhydrous to the monohydrate form occurs.

Compounded preparation stability: One method for compounding a metronidazole benzoate suspension (80 mg/mL; equivalent to 50 mg/mL metronidazole hydrochloride) that is stable (when protected from light and kept at an ambient temperature) for at least a year has been published.[46] To make 750 mL of an 80 mg/mL suspension: 60 grams metronidazole benzoate powder is placed in a suitable mortar then triturated with 1.25 grams of Propylene Glycol, NF, to a smooth paste; increasing amounts of *SyrSpend® SF* are then added until the suspension is pourable. The liquid suspension is then transferred to a suitable graduated container and the mortar rinsed with 3 small aliquots of *SyrSpend® SF*, which are added to the suspension. Additional *SyrSpend® SF* is added to bring the suspension to the final volume of 750 mL. The suspension should be stored in light-resistant containers and kept refrigerated or at room temperature.

Another published method is to triturate 9.6 g (9600 mg) of metronidazole benzoate powder with 60 mL of *Ora-Plus®* and *qs ad* to 120 mL with *Ora-Sweet®* or *Ora-Sweet® SF®* to yield a 80 mg/mL metronidazole benzoate oral suspension (equivalent to 50 mg/mL metronidazole hydrochloride) that retains greater than 90% potency for 90 days when stored at both 4°C (39.2°F) and 25°C (77°F) and protected from light.[47]

Dosage Forms/Regulatory Status

VETERINARY-LABELED PRODUCTS: NONE IN THE UNITED STATES. VETERINARY TABLETS AND ORAL SUSPENSIONS ARE AVAILABLE IN OTHER COUNTRIES FOR DOGS AND CATS.

Metronidazole is prohibited for use in food animals by the FDA.

HUMAN-LABELED PRODUCTS:

Metronidazole Oral Tablets: 250 mg and 500 mg; *Flagyl®*, generic; (Rx)

Metronidazole Oral Capsules: 375 mg; *Flagyl 375®*, generic; (Rx)

Metronidazole Oral Suspension: 50 mg/mL in 150 mL (grape); generic; (Rx)

Metronidazole Injection 500 mg pre-mixed in 100 mL sodium chloride; generic; (Rx)

Metronidazole is available in combination with other medications (eg, bismuth, tetracycline) for treatment of *H pylori*. Lotions, gels, creams, and vaginal products are also available.

References

For the complete list of references, see **wiley.com/go/budde/plumb**

Metyrapone

(me-***teer***-a-pone) *Metopirone®*

Adrenal Steroid Inhibitor

Prescriber Highlights

- Primarily used in cats with hyperadrenocorticism; may be most useful for short-term treatment to stabilize patient before adrenalectomy
- Well tolerated in cats at recommended dosages
- May alter insulin requirements; monitor blood glucose closely.
- Inconsistent availability

Uses/Indications

Metyrapone may be useful to treat cats with hyperadrenocorticism, though it is not considered a first-line therapy. Effectiveness appears variable and may be transient, so it may be best used short-term in an attempt to stabilize the patient prior to adrenalectomy.[1,2] Metyrapone may potentially be useful in treating hyperadrenocorticism in ferrets and small mammals (eg, hamsters), but there is little, if any, information available on its use in these species.[2]

In humans, an overnight metyrapone test may be used in conjunction with other dynamic tests in the diagnosis of specific hypothalamic/pituitary/adrenal disorders.

Pharmacology/Actions

Metyrapone reduces cortisol and corticosterone production by inhibiting 11-beta-hydroxlase; this converts 11-deoxycortisol to cortisol within the adrenal cortex. ACTH production can subsequently increase as negative feedback is lost. With time, this effect may override the effects of metyrapone on the adrenal gland. Metyrapone can also suppress synthesis of aldosterone and cause a mild natriuresis. Mineralocorticoid deficiency does not usually occur with long-term metyrapone therapy because inhibition of the 11-beta-hydroxylation reaction increases production of 11-desoxycorticosterone; this has a mineralocorticoid effect and has been associated with hypertension in patients receiving long-term metyrapone therapy.

Pharmacokinetics

No information on the pharmacokinetics of metyrapone is available for cats. In humans, metyrapone is well absorbed after oral administration. Peak concentrations occur in ≈ 1 hour; however, pharmacological response to metyrapone does not occur immediately. It is rapidly cleared from the plasma and has an average elimination half-life of around 2 hours. Metyrapone's major metabolite, metyrapol, is active and formed via reduction; its half-life is about twice as long as that of metyrapone. Both metyrapol and metyrapone are conjugated with glucuronide in humans. As cats are unable to effectively glucuronidate, it is unclear what metabolic path(s) metyrapone takes in this species.

Contraindications/Precautions/Warnings

Metyrapone should not be used in animals that are hypersensitive to it or have adrenal cortical insufficiency. Metyrapone may induce acute adrenal insufficiency in patients that have reduced adrenal secretory capacity.[3]

Use cautiously in cats with concurrent diabetes mellitus; monitor blood glucose closely in these patients, as insulin requirements in may decrease.[1]

Adverse Effects

Metyrapone appears to be relatively well-tolerated in cats. Dosages ranging from 195 – 500 mg/cat/day (divided) have been used in cats with hyperadrenocorticism without observed toxicity.[4] Some cats may experience vomiting and anorexia.[5]

In humans, reported adverse effects include headache, dizziness, sedation, allergic rash, nausea, vomiting, and abdominal pain.[3] Rarely, metyrapone can cause myelosuppression.

Reproductive/Nursing Safety

Animal reproduction studies have not been conducted with metyrapone. In humans, metyrapone has been shown to cross the placenta.[6] In women given the drug in the 2nd and 3rd trimesters, evidence of fetal pituitary response to the enzymatic block was detected; a subnormal response to metyrapone may also occur during pregnancy.[3]

Metyrapone's safety in lactating animals and their offspring is not known. Because safety has not been established in animals, this drug should only be used when the maternal benefits outweigh the potential risks to offspring.

Overdose/Acute Toxicity

The oral LD_{50} in rats (mg/kg) was 521 mg/kg. Metyrapone overdoses likely would cause GI effects and, possibly, acute adrenocortical insufficiency. Other effects that may be seen include hypoglycemia, hyponatremia, hypochloremia, hyperkalemia, cardiac arrhythmias, hypotension, dehydration, and impairment of consciousness. There is no specific antidote. Standard decontamination protocols should be considered with IV hydrocortisone, saline, and glucose. Monitoring and support for several days may be required.

For patients that have experienced or are suspected to have experienced an overdose, consultation with a 24-hour poison consultation center specializing in providing veterinary-specific information is recommended. For general information related to overdose and toxin exposures, as well as contact information for poison control centers, refer to ***Appendix.***

Drug Interactions

The following drug interactions have either been reported or are theoretical in humans or animals receiving metyrapone and may be of significance in veterinary patients. Unless otherwise noted, use together is not necessarily contraindicated, but weigh the potential risks and perform additional monitoring when appropriate.

- **Acetaminophen (do NOT use in cats)**: In humans, there is an increased risk for acetaminophen toxicity.
- **Corticosteroids**: Decrease the efficacy of metyrapone

Laboratory Considerations

- In humans, the following drugs have been reported to interfere with the results of the metyrapone test: antidepressants (eg, amitriptyline), antithyroid drugs, phenothiazines, barbiturates, corticosteroids, cyproheptadine, and hormones such as estrogens and progesterone.
- The metyrapone test may not be reliable in humans with hyper- or hypothyroidism.

Dosages

CATS:

Hyperadrenocorticism (extra-label): Metyrapone has been used to successfully treat hyperadrenocorticism in the cat, but results are variable:

a) 30 – 70 mg/kg PO twice daily. Begin with the lower end of the range for the first 2 to 4 weeks.[1,7] Increase dose in small increments as indicated by clinical signs and ACTH stimulation testing.

b) 250 – 500 mg/cat (NOT mg/kg) PO daily.[4] If effective, results are generally noted within 5 days.

Monitoring

- Blood glucose should be closely monitored in cats with diabetes mellitus, as insulin requirements may change.
- Clinical signs associated with hyperadrenocorticism or hypoadrenocorticism should prompt dose adjustment.
- Adrenocorticotropic hormone (ACTH) stimulation tests may be used to assess adrenal function.

Client Information

- Do not stop giving this medicine to your animal unless instructed to do so by your veterinarian. Serious side effects can occur if the medicine is stopped suddenly.
- This medicine may be given with or without food but giving with food may reduce the likelihood of vomiting.
- This medicine is usually well tolerated. Side effects (eg, increased panting, appetite, thirst, and need to urinate) are possible, especially when the medicine is used long-term.
- Cats with diabetes will need their blood glucose monitored carefully while receiving this medicine. Do not miss these important follow-up visits.

Chemistry/Synonyms

Metyrapone occurs as a white to light amber, fine, crystalline powder, with a characteristic odor. It is sparingly soluble in water, soluble in chloroform and methyl alcohol.

Metyrapone may also be known as SU-4885, metirapon, metirapona, or metyraponum. A common trade name is *Metopirone*®.

Storage/Stability

Store metyrapone at room temperature (15°C-25°C [59°F-77°F]) in a well-closed, light-resistant container.[3] Protect from moisture.

Compatibility/Compounding Considerations

No specific information noted

Dosage Forms/Regulatory Status

VETERINARY-LABELED PRODUCTS: NONE

HUMAN-LABELED PRODUCTS:

Metyrapone Oral Capsules: 250 mg; *Metopirone*®; (Rx)

References

For the complete list of references, see **wiley.com/go/budde/plumb**

Mexiletine

(mex-***ill***-i-teen) *Mexitil*®

Oral Antiarrhythmic

Prescriber Highlights

- ► Oral antiarrhythmic with similar effects to lidocaine
- ► Used for ventricular tachycardia, premature ventricular contractions (PVCs)
- ► Strict dosing frequency (every 8 hours) may be a barrier to clinical use; may be used in combination with sotalol to allow for less frequent dosing.
- ► Use with extreme caution in patients with pre-existing second- or third-degree AV block (without pacemaker) or in patients with cardiogenic shock.
- ► Use with caution in patients with severe congestive heart failure or acute myocardial infarction, hepatic function impairment, hypotension, sinus node dysfunction, seizure disorder, or sensitivity to the drug.
- ► Adverse effects include GI distress (eg, vomiting, inappetence); give with meals to alleviate.

Uses/Indications

Mexiletine is used to treat some ventricular arrhythmias, including premature ventricular contractions (PVCs) and ventricular tachycardia in dogs. Ventricular tachycardias that have responded to lidocaine may respond to mexiletine. There is some evidence for efficacy for arrhythmogenic right ventricular cardiomyopathy in boxers,[1,2] and other breeds,[3] as well as for inherited ventricular arrhythmias in German shepherd dogs but the drug's dosing frequency may be challenging. See ***Pharmacokinetics***.

Mexiletine may be useful for treating certain myopathies in dogs such as myotonia congenita (most studied in miniature schnauzers[4] and chow chows) and myokymia in Jack Russell terriers.[5-7]

Pharmacology/Actions

Mexiletine is considered a class IB antiarrhythmic agent and is similar to lidocaine in its mechanism of antiarrhythmic activity. It inhibits the inward sodium current (fast sodium channel), thereby reducing the rate of rise of the action potential, Phase 0. In cardiomyocytes, automaticity is decreased and action potential duration is shortened; however, the effective refractory period is minimally affected. Usually conduction is unaffected but may be slowed in patients with pre-existing conduction abnormalities. No effect on sinus automaticity has been noted clinically.

Pharmacokinetics

There is limited information available for dogs. Mexiletine is relatively well absorbed from the GI tract and has a low first-pass effect. A preliminary report of a study in 6 healthy dogs (4 beagles, 2 hounds) reported that sotalol 2.5 mg/kg PO twice daily, combined with mexiletine 8 to 10 mg/kg PO twice daily for 10 days, resulted in mexiletine serum concentrations within the described therapeutic range (for humans) for the 12 hour postdose period in the 3 dogs weighing more than 10 kg (22 lb).[8] There are no published studies evaluating the pharmacokinetics of mexiletine in cats.

In humans, mexiletine is moderately bound to plasma proteins (60% to 75%) and is metabolized in the liver to inactive metabolites with an elimination half-life of ≈10 to 12 hours. Half-lives may be significantly increased in patients with moderate to severe hepatic disease,[9] or in those having severely reduced cardiac output. Half-lives may be slightly prolonged in patients with severe renal disease or after acute myocardial infarction.

Contraindications/Precautions/Warnings

Mexiletine should be used with extreme caution, if at all, in patients with pre-existing second- or third-degree AV block (without pacemaker), or with cardiogenic shock.[9] It should only be used when the benefits of therapy outweigh the risks when the following medical conditions exist: severe congestive heart failure or acute myocardial infarction, hepatic function impairment, hypotension, intraventricular conduction abnormalities, sinus node function impairment, seizure disorder, or sensitivity to the drug.

A single case report of a collie with the *MDR1* genetic mutation (also known as *ABCB1-1delta*) was reported to have developed mexiletine toxicity with a standard dosage.[10,11] Although mexiletine is not known to be a P-glycoprotein substrate, consider testing for the mutation in susceptible breeds before treatment or if toxicity develops.

It is anecdotally reported that cats are more sensitive than dogs to mexiletine's adverse effects.

Do not confuse mexiletine with meclizine.

Adverse Effects

The most likely adverse effect noted in animals is GI distress, including vomiting and inappetence; giving with meals may alleviate GI effects.[9] Cats administered a wide range of dosages for 24 hours were noted to have anorexia, tremors, and incoordination with these signs most evident at 20 mg/kg and 40 mg/kg.[12] Trembling, dizziness, depression, chest pain, and, rarely, seizures and severe liver injury have been reported in humans.[9] In some humans (1% to 3%), AST values increased by as much as 3 times or more above the upper limit of normal. AST elevations were reportedly transient with no elevations in bilirubin; patients were asymptomatic and did not require discontinuation of therapy.[9]

Reproductive/Nursing Safety

Laboratory animal studies have not demonstrated teratogenicity.[9] Because mexiletine is secreted into maternal milk, it has been recommended to use milk replacer if the dam is receiving this drug. Because safety has not been established in animals, this drug should only be used when the maternal benefits outweigh the potential risks to offspring.

Overdose/Acute Toxicity

Toxicity associated with a mexiletine overdose may be significant. A small series of healthy cats receiving doses of 4 – 40 mg/kg developed neurologic and GI signs, most commonly at a dose over 20 mg/kg.[12] Case reports in humans have noted that CNS signs always preceded cardiovascular signs. Treatment should consist of GI decontamination protocols when indicated, acidification of the urine to enhance urinary excretion, and supportive therapy. Atropine or pressor agents may be useful if bradycardia or hypotension occur.[9]

For patients that have experienced or are suspected to have experienced an overdose, consultation with a 24-hour poison consultation center specializing in providing veterinary-specific information is recommended. For general information related to overdose and toxin exposures, as well as contact information for poison control centers, refer to ***Appendix.***

Drug Interactions

The following drug interactions have either been reported or are theoretical in humans or animals receiving mexiletine and may be of significance in veterinary patients. Unless otherwise noted, use together is not necessarily contraindicated, but weigh the potential risks and perform additional monitoring when appropriate.

- **Amiodarone**: Concurrent use may increase mexiletine blood concentrations.
- **Antacids, Aluminum-Magnesium**: May slow the absorption of mexiletine
- **Atropine**: May reduce the rate of oral absorption
- **Bupropion**: Concurrent use may increase mexiletine blood concentrations.
- **Cimetidine**: May increase or decrease mexiletine blood concentrations
- **Clozapine**: Concurrent use may increase clozapine exposure and risk for adverse effects.
- **Griseofulvin**: May accelerate the metabolism of mexiletine
- **Lidocaine**: May cause additive adverse effects
- **Metoclopramide**: May accelerate the absorption of mexiletine
- **Opioids**: May slow the absorption of mexiletine
- **Paroxetine**: Concurrent use may increase mexiletine blood concentrations.
- **Phenobarbital, Primidone, Phenytoin**: May accelerate the metabolism of mexiletine
- **Propranolol**: Concurrent use may result in increased propranolol blood concentrations.
- **Quinidine**: Concurrent use may increase mexiletine bioavailability and risk for cardiotoxicity.
- **Rifampin**: May accelerate the metabolism of mexiletine
- **Sotalol**: May increase mexiletine plasma concentrations.[13] This may be used for therapeutic effect but could also increase potential for adverse effects.
- **Theophylline, Aminophylline**: Metabolism may be reduced by mexiletine, thereby leading to theophylline toxicity
- **Urinary Acidifying Drugs** (eg, **ammonium chloride, methionine, potassium phosphate, sodium phosphate**): May accelerate the renal excretion of mexiletine
- **Urinary Alkalinizing Drugs** (eg, **bicarb, carbonic anhydrase inhibitors, citrates**): May reduce the urinary excretion of mexiletine

Laboratory Considerations

- None noted

Dosages

DOGS:

Ventricular arrhythmias (extra-label): 4 – 6 mg/kg PO every 8 hours.[14,15] Higher dosages of 5 – 8 mg/kg PO every 8 hours have also been described.[1,13] Twice-daily dosing at 8 – 10 mg/kg PO every 12 hours has been described as yielding therapeutic concentrations of mexiletine when sotalol was concomitantly administered at 2.5 mg/kg PO every 12 hours,[8] though this dosage is not commonly administered in practice.

Myotonia congenita in chow chows and miniature schnauzers (extra-label): 8.3 mg/kg PO every 8 hours[16]

Myokymia in Jack Russell terriers (extra-label): 4 mg/kg PO every 12 hours has been suggested to decrease frequency of attacks.[5-7]

CATS:

Ventricular arrhythmias (extra-label): Anecdotal reports describe use of mexiletine in cats at similar dosages to that used in dogs, 4 – 6 mg/kg PO every 8 hours.[12]

Monitoring

- In humans, therapeutic plasma concentrations are 0.5 – 2 µg/mL; toxicity may be noted at therapeutic concentrations.
- ECG and 24-hour Holter monitoring
- Adverse effects (eg, vomiting, inappetence)

Client Information

- This medicine needs to be given 3 times a day (every 8 hours; even through the night) in order to work.
- Give with food to reduce the risk for vomiting or nausea.
- Vomiting is the most likely side effect; contact your veterinarian if it worsens or does not stop.

Chemistry/Synonyms

A class IB antiarrhythmic, mexiletine HCl occurs as a white or almost white, odorless, crystalline powder. It is freely soluble in water.

Mexiletine may also be known as Ko-1173, mexiletini hydrochloridum, *Mexilen*®, *Mexitil*®, *Mexitilen*®, *Myovek*®, and *Ritalmex*®.

Storage/Stability

Mexiletine capsules should be stored at controlled room temperature (20°C-25°C [68°F-77°F]) in a tight, light-resistant container with a child-resistant closure (as required).[9]

Compatibility/Compounding Considerations

No specific information noted

Dosage Forms/Regulatory Status

VETERINARY-LABELED PRODUCTS: NONE

The Association of Racing Commissioners International (ARCI) has designated this drug as a class 4 substance. Use of this drug may not be allowed in certain animal competitions. Check rules and regulations before entering in a competition while this medication is being administered. Contact local racing authorities for further guidance. See ***Appendix*** for more information.

HUMAN-LABELED PRODUCTS:

Mexiletine Oral Capsules: 150 mg, 200 mg, and 250 mg; generic; (Rx)

References

For the complete list of references, see **wiley.com/go/budde/plumb**

Midazolam

(mih-***day***-zoe-lam) *Versed*®

Benzodiazepine

Prescriber Highlights

- Injectable benzodiazepine used primarily as a preoperative and co-induction medication and, unlike diazepam, may be given IM and can be used intranasally for seizures
- Contraindications include hypersensitivity to benzodiazepines and acute narrow-angle glaucoma.
- Caution is advised with hepatic or renal disease, open-angle glaucoma, debilitated or geriatric animals, significant respiratory depression, and animals in a coma or shock.
- The adverse effect of most concern is the potential for respiratory depression. Cats may develop excited behaviors; this drug should be used with sedatives/tranquilizers in this species.
- DEA Schedule IV (C-IV) controlled substance
- Effects are reversible with flumazenil.

Uses/Indications

Midazolam is principally used for its sedative, anxiolytic, and muscle relaxant properties as a premedication and co-induction agent (combined with other drugs) prior to induction of general anesthesia. When midazolam is used alone, sedation may be adequate in ruminants, camelids, swine, rabbits, ferrets, and some birds; it does not appear to provide predictable sedation in dogs, cats, or horses, as they may become sedated or dysphoric and excited. Cats may be more prone to developing an excited effect/disinhibition as compared with dogs. When used in combination with other drugs (eg, opioids, ketamine, acepromazine, dexmedetomidine), midazolam provides more reliable sedation.

Midazolam IV, IM, or intranasal (but not per rectum) may be used to treat status epilepticus. Midazolam given intranasally controlled status epilepticus in ≈70% to 75% of dogs, was more effective than rectal diazepam, and controlled seizures faster than midazolam IV.[1,2]

Pharmacology/Actions

Midazolam exhibits similar pharmacologic actions as other benzodiazepines; subcortical levels (primarily limbic, thalamic, and hypothalamic) of the CNS are depressed, which produces anxiolytic, sedative, skeletal muscle relaxant, and anticonvulsant effects. The exact mechanism of action is unknown, but postulated mechanisms include antagonism of serotonin, increased release of and/or facilitation of gamma-aminobutyric acid (GABA) activity, and diminished release or turnover of acetylcholine in the CNS.

Benzodiazepine-specific receptors have been located in the mammalian brain, kidney, liver, lungs, and heart. In all species studied, receptors are lacking in white matter.

Midazolam has unique solubility characteristics (eg, water-soluble injection formulation but lipid-soluble at pH greater than 4) that provide a rapid onset of action after injection. As compared with diazepam, midazolam has ≈2 times the affinity for benzodiazepine receptors, is nearly 3 times as potent, and has a faster onset of action and a shorter duration of effect.

Pharmacokinetics

After IM administration in healthy dogs, bioavailability was ≈47%, and peak plasma concentrations occurred ≈7 to 8 minutes postinjection.[3] The authors concluded that midazolam IM may be useful in treating seizures in dogs when venous access is unavailable but higher doses may be necessary. In dogs, midazolam is absorbed when the commercially available injection is administered intranasally, and peak plasma concentrations following intranasal administration are higher than when the drug is administered rectally. In dogs, a 50 mg/mL compounded gel (0.2% hydroxypropyl methylcellulose) demonstrated significantly higher peak plasma concentrations after intranasal administration as compared with the injectable formulation administered rectally or intranasally.[4] Buccal administration of midazolam 0.6 mg/kg using a 20 mg/mL hydroxypropyl methylcellulose gel resulted in a peak plasma concentration of 187 ng/mL.[5] The average midazolam elimination halflife is 77 minutes in dogs. Midazolam is metabolized in the liver via the cytochrome P450 enzyme 3A12, 3A26 (minor), and 2B11 isoenzymes[6]; this is in contrast to humans, in which CYP3A4 and CYP3A5 are largely responsible for the metabolism of midazolam.

In horses given midazolam 0.05 or 0.1 mg/kg IV, total clearance was ≈10.5 mL/minute/kg (median), volume of distribution (V_d) at steady state was 2 to 3 L/kg, and terminal half-life varied widely and ranged from 120 to 924 minutes (medians, 216 minutes after 0.05 mg/kg, 408 minutes after 0.1 mg/kg). Cardiorespiratory parameters and sedation scores did not change; however, agitation, postural sway, and weakness were noted, and a horse became recumbent after receiving a 0.1 mg/kg dose.[7]

In alpacas given midazolam 0.05 mg/kg IM or IV, IM bioavailability was 92%, and peak plasma concentrations were ≈3 times lower than after IV administration. Mean elimination half-lives were 98 minutes (IV) and 234 minutes (IM). The authors concluded that midazolam appears to provide a short duration of action with moderate levels of sedation and minimal cardiovascular or behavioral adverse effects in alpacas.[8]

In sheep receiving midazolam 0.5 mg IV, V_d was 0.84 L/kg, and the elimination half-life was 0.79 hours. After IM administration at 0.5 mg/kg, the total drug exposure as calculated by the area under the curve (AUC) was 3.3 times higher than with IV administration.[9] Time to peak plasma concentration following IM injection was ≈28 minutes.

In humans, the onset of action following IV administration is rapid due to the high lipophilicity of the agent, and loss of the lash reflex or counting occurs within 30 to 97 seconds after administration. Following IM injection, midazolam is rapidly and almost completely

(91%) absorbed. The drug is well absorbed after oral administration, but bioavailability suffers (≈36% in pediatric animals) because of a rapid first-pass effect.

Midazolam is highly protein-bound (ie, 94% to 97%) and rapidly crosses the blood–brain barrier. Changes in plasma protein concentrations and resultant protein binding may significantly alter the response to a given dose because only unbound drugs cross into the CNS. The serum halflife and duration of activity of midazolam in humans are shorter than diazepam. Midazolam is eliminated almost entirely by renal mechanisms as conjugates of hydroxylated metabolites. Elimination half-life in humans is ≈2 hours (diazepam is ≈30 hours) and is almost doubled in patients with significant hepatic impairment. The active metabolite alpha-hydroxymidazolam has a pharmacologic activity that contributes to midazolam's clinical effects. Alpha-hydroxymidazolam has a half-life of ≈1 to 1.5 hours, which is prolonged in patients with renal impairment.

Contraindications/Precautions/Warnings

In humans, hypersensitivity to benzodiazepines and acute narrow-angle glaucoma are contraindications. Intracarotid or other intra-arterial injections should also be avoided.

Caution should be used in animals with hepatic or renal disease and debilitated or geriatric animals. Animals with congestive heart failure or hepatic dysfunction may eliminate the drug more slowly, and prolonged effects can occur. This drug should be administered cautiously in animals in a coma or in shock and in animals with significant respiratory depression or open-angle glaucoma (contraindicated if untreated).

When used alone, midazolam does not possess significant effects on cardiorespiratory function; however, cardiorespiratory effects may be noted when it is used in combination with other agents. Increased heart rate and blood pressure may be noted when this drug is used with ketamine. Effects may be diminished if this combination is used after an opioid has been administered.

Midazolam given in combination with opioids can cause less cardiovascular depression but greater respiratory depression as compared with acepromazine given in combination with opioids. Midazolam in combination with butorphanol may cause anxiousness, aggressiveness, and restraint difficulties in some cats and is best reserved for geriatric or very ill cats.[10]

Midazolam given with etomidate should be used with caution in dogs undergoing ocular surgery. A study found this combination caused clinically relevant miosis; significantly increased intraocular pressure; and commonly induced ptyalism, gagging, and abdominal heaving. Midazolam given with propofol caused only a minor decrease in pupil diameter.[11]

Adverse Effects

At usual doses, midazolam is well tolerated in veterinary patients. Midazolam IV CRIs may cause thrombophlebitis less often than diazepam CRIs.

In dogs, after morphine and acepromazine are given prior to surgery, midazolam given 0.2 mg/kg IV prior to propofol anesthesia caused excitement in some dogs.[12,13] Hypothermia was noted in dogs premedicated with buprenorphine 0.02 mg/kg and acepromazine 0.05 mg/kg IM prior to induction with midazolam or diazepam 0.25 mg/kg IV combined with either ketamine 5 mg/kg IV or propofol 4 mg/kg IV and maintained on isoflurane for ovariohysterectomy. All dogs became hypothermic within 5 minutes of induction. Dogs receiving a combination of benzodiazepine and propofol had a greater temperature decrease and longer interval to the restoration of normothermia.[14] A combination of midazolam and medetomidine premedication resulted in a high incidence of paradoxical behavior in healthy dogs; the authors did not recommend this combination.[15] In healthy dogs undergoing ovariohysterectomy or castration following a combination of acepromazine and meperidine prior to surgery, midazolam 0.25 mg/kg administered IV prior to propofol anesthesia resulted in a significantly longer time to standing, an increased incidence of hypotension, and an overall negative effect on recovery as compared with dogs that did not receive midazolam. Pigmenturia occurred in dogs premedicated with hydromorphone and induced with midazolam followed by etomidate.[16]

In horses, midazolam administered as a sole agent at 0.05 and 0.1 mg/kg IV produces agitation and ataxia but not sedation.[7]

In humans receiving midazolam, effects on respiratory rate, heart rate, and blood pressure have been most frequently reported.[17] Respiratory depression has been reported in patients receiving narcotics or that have chronic obstructive pulmonary disease (COPD). Between 1% and 5% of patients receiving midazolam had pain on injection, local irritation, headache, nausea, vomiting, and/or hiccups. Midazolam impairs memory recall for several hours after administration; it is unclear whether this occurs in veterinary patients.

Reproductive/Nursing Safety

Although midazolam has not been demonstrated to cause fetal abnormalities, in humans, other benzodiazepines have been implicated in causing congenital abnormalities when administered during the first trimester of pregnancy. Anesthetic agents administered to animals during the third trimester of pregnancy (and during other periods of rapid brain growth) may adversely affect the developing brain. Infants born to mothers given large doses of benzodiazepines shortly before delivery have been reported to suffer from apnea, impaired metabolic response to cold stress, difficulty feeding, hyperbilirubinemia, and hypotonia. Signs of withdrawal have occurred in infants whose mothers chronically took benzodiazepines during pregnancy. The veterinary significance of these effects is unclear, but these agents should only be used during the first trimester of pregnancy when the benefits clearly outweigh the risks associated with their use.

Midazolam and alpha-hydroxymidazolam are excreted in milk and may cause CNS effects in nursing neonates. Caution should be used when administering this drug to a nursing mother.

Overdose/Acute Toxicity

The IV LD_{50} has been reported to be 50 mg/kg in mice and 75 mg/kg in rats.[18] It is suggested that accidental overdoses should be managed with supportive therapy (eg, cardiopulmonary support, IV fluids). In addition, flumazenil can be used to antagonize midazolam effects; however, supportive therapy may be more suitable in all but the largest overdoses because midazolam has a short duration of effect.

For patients that have experienced or are suspected of having experienced an overdose, consultation with a 24-hour poison consultation center specializing in providing veterinary-specific information is recommended. For general information related to overdose and toxin exposures, as well as contact information for poison control centers, refer to ***Appendix***.

Drug Interactions

Although midazolam is a CYP3A4 substrate in humans, it is a CYP3A12 and CYP2B11 substrate in dogs. Caution should be used when extrapolating midazolam human drug interactions to veterinary species. The following drug interactions have either been reported or are theoretical in humans or animals receiving midazolam and may be of significance in veterinary patients. Unless otherwise noted, use together is not necessarily contraindicated, but weigh the potential risks and perform additional monitoring when appropriate.

- Anesthetic Agents (eg, **alfaxolone,**[19,20] **etomidate,**[21] **isoflurane,**[22] **propofol**[13,20,23]): Midazolam reduces anesthetic requirements.
- Antihypertensive Agents (eg, **amlodipine, enalapril, telmisartan**): Concurrent use may increase the risk for hypotension

and orthostasis. Blood pressure should be monitored.

- **Azole Antifungals** (eg, **itraconazole, ketoconazole, voriconazole**): May increase midazolam concentration; excessive sedation may occur. In healthy dogs given oral fluconazole, clearance of IV midazolam and ketamine was ≈50% slower, and the duration of the sedative effect was increased.[24]
- **Carbonic Anhydrase Inhibitors** (CAIs; eg, **dichlorphenamide, methazolamide**): Benzodiazepines may interfere with the beneficial effects of CAIs by inhibiting respiratory responses to hypoxia; this combination should be avoided.
- **CNS Depressant Agents** (eg, **buspirone, cannabidiol, gabapentin, methocarbamol, trazodone**): Combination may increase the risk for CNS depression; monitoring and adjustment of doses are needed.
- **Hepatic Enzyme Inhibitors** (eg, **cimetidine, erythromycin, isoniazid**): Metabolism of midazolam may be decreased, and excessive sedation may occur.
- **Ifosfamide**: Concurrent use may increase the risk for ifosfamide-induced neurotoxic effects. Careful monitoring is needed, and discontinuation of both drugs may be necessary if signs of encephalopathy occur.
- **Nondepolarizing Neuromuscular Blockers** (eg, **atracurium, rocuronium**): Concurrent use may potentiate, attenuate, or have no effect; respiratory status should be monitored.
- **Opioids** (eg, **butorphanol, fentanyl, hydromorphone**): Combination may increase the risk for CNS and/or respiratory depression.
- **Phenobarbital, Primidone**: May induce hepatic microsomal enzymes and decrease the pharmacologic effects of benzodiazepines; additive CNS depression is possible.
- **Rifampin**: May induce hepatic microsomal enzymes and decrease the pharmacologic effects of benzodiazepines
- **Theophylline, Aminophylline**: Concurrent use may decrease the levels and effectiveness of benzodiazepines. Withdrawing theophylline from a stable patient may increase the risk for benzodiazepine toxicity.
- **Tricyclic Antidepressants** (eg, **amitriptyline, clomipramine, imipramine**): Midazolam may increase the levels of these drugs; clinical significance is not known. Concurrent use may increase the risk for CNS and/or respiratory depression.
- **Yohimbine**: May decrease therapeutic effects of anxiolytic drugs

Laboratory Considerations

- Benzodiazepines may decrease the thyroidal uptake of $\mathbf{I^{123}}$ or $\mathbf{I^{131}}$.

Dosages

NOTE: There are many potential combinations that have been suggested; the following are examples and not inclusive. For additional information, refer to other anesthesia-specific references.[25]

DOGS:

Preoperative agent (extra-label): Used in combination with other premedications or co-induction agents (eg, ketamine, acepromazine, opioids, alpha-2 agonists), 0.1 – 0.3 mg/kg SC, IM, IV

a) Dogs were premedicated with acepromazine 0.02 mg/kg and morphine 0.4 mg/kg IM and induced with midazolam 0.25 mg/kg IV followed by propofol 1 mg/kg IV or induced first with propofol 1 mg/kg IV followed by midazolam 0.25 mg/kg IV.[26] If intubation was not possible, propofol was titrated to effect until intubation was achieved. Dogs given midazolam before propofol had mild to moderate excitement. The total dose of propofol for intubation was decreased with the use of midazolam.

b) Dogs were sedated with fentanyl 7 µg/kg IV and induced with either propofol or alfaxalone with or without midazolam 0.3 mg/kg IV.[20] The addition of midazolam reduced the induction doses of both propofol and alfaxalone.

c) Dogs premedicated with acepromazine 0.025 mg/kg and morphine 0.25 mg/kg IM were induced with midazolam 0.2 mg/kg IV followed by propofol IV titrated until intubation was possible.[13] After midazolam administration, some dogs had excitement (eg, paddling, myoclonic twitching) that resolved after induction. Midazolam significantly decreased the amount of propofol needed for induction.

d) Dogs can be premedicated with midazolam 0.5 mg/kg and morphine 0.5 mg/kg IM, or they can be premedicated with midazolam 0.5 mg/kg, morphine 0.5 mg/kg, and acepromazine 0.05 mg/kg mixed in the same syringe and given IM.[27]

e) Dogs receiving butorphanol 0.2 mg/kg combined with midazolam 0.2 mg/kg IV followed by alfaxalone 2 mg/kg IV had an excellent quality of induction and recovery.[28] Premedication with acepromazine 0.02 mg/kg and hydromorphone 0.1 mg/kg mixed in the same syringe and administered IM with midazolam 0.3 mg/kg IV significantly reduced the alfaxalone dose required for intubation.[29]

f) Dogs were premedicated with buprenorphine 0.02 mg/kg and acepromazine 0.05 mg/kg IM prior to induction with midazolam or diazepam 0.25 mg/kg IV combined with either ketamine 5 mg/kg IV or propofol 4 mg/kg IV and maintained on isoflurane for ovariohysterectomy.[14] All dogs became hypothermic within 5 minutes of induction. Dogs receiving a combination of benzodiazepine and propofol had a greater temperature decrease and longer interval to the restoration of normothermia.

g) Dogs can be premedicated with a combination of alfaxalone 5 mg/kg, morphine 0.4 mg/kg, and midazolam 1 mg/kg IM prior to induction with alfaxalone IV and maintenance on sevoflurane.[30]

h) Midazolam 0.1 mg/kg IV with butorphanol 0.2 mg/kg IV did not cause significant influence on duodenal contrast-enhanced ultrasonography parameters in dogs.[31]

i) Following premedication with acepromazine 0.02 mg/kg and methadone 0.3 mg/kg IM, the addition of midazolam 0.4 mg/kg to induction protocol significantly reduced the total alfaxalone dose required for intubation (ie, 0.65 mg/kg vs 0.94 mg/kg) with no significant changes to heart rate or blood pressure; however, the incidence of apnea was increased.[32]

Status epilepticus (extra-label): Dose recommendations vary, and there is no evidence that supports a specific dosing protocol is better than others.

IV or IM: Most clinicians recommend 0.1 – 0.3 mg/kg, but doses can range from 0.07 – 0.5 mg/kg IM or IV; IM doses may need to be higher than IV doses. Doses up to 0.5 mg/kg may be repeated twice if no response is noted. If seizures recur, rebolus and consider a CRI.

Intranasal: 0.2 mg/kg intranasal; readminister dose as above. Midazolam was delivered via a nasal adaptor attached to the end of a syringe. In a study, the median time to seizure cessation was 33 to 47 seconds, and seizures were controlled in 70% to 75% of dogs.[1,2]

Continuous rate IV infusion: 0.25 – 0.4 mg/kg/hour IV CRI (range 0.1 – 2.5 mg/kg/hour); seizures were controlled in 77% of dogs.[33] In general, the dose should be started at the low end, and the rate should be increased until seizures are controlled.

CATS:

Preoperative agent (extra-label): Used in combination with other premedications (eg, ketamine, acepromazine, opioids, alpha-2 agonists); 0.1 – 0.3 mg/kg SC, IM, IV. **NOTE**: Midazolam in combination with butorphanol may cause anxiousness, aggressiveness, and restraint difficulties in some cats and is best reserved for geriatric or very ill cats.[10]

a) Cats were premedicated with acepromazine 0.01 mg/kg and methadone 0.2 mg/kg IV. Induction was achieved with propofol 2 mg/kg IV followed by midazolam at 0.2 mg/kg, 0.3 mg/kg, 0.4 mg/kg, and 0.5 mg/kg IV; additional propofol was given as needed for intubation.[34] All doses of midazolam decreased the amount of propofol needed for induction.
b) Cats were sedated with dexmedetomidine 3 μg/kg and methadone 0.3 mg/kg IM.[35] Optimal induction was achieved with alfaxalone 0.25 mg/kg IV over 60 seconds followed 1 minute later by midazolam 0.08 mg/kg IV.
c) Cats were given ketamine 14 mg/kg and midazolam 0.5 mg/kg IM or intranasally by dropping the solution into both nostrils.[36] This drug combination was diluted with saline to a volume of 1 mL. Cats vocalized with the IM administration and sneezed or snorted with the intranasal administration. With both techniques, the onset was 3 minutes, and the duration of sedation was 23 (nasal) to 33 (IM) minutes.
d) Cats can be sedated with medetomidine 0.05 mg/kg and midazolam 0.5 mg/kg combined and given IM followed by ketamine 10 mg/kg IM.[37] This drug combination can cause hyperglycemia and decreases in epinephrine, norepinephrine, cortisol, and nonesterified fatty acids. These effects can be reversed with atipamezole 0.2 mg/kg IV.

Opioid-free injectable protocol for cats undergoing ovariohysterectomy (extra-label): Midazolam 0.25 mg/kg IM in combination with ketamine 5 – 7 mg/kg IM, dexmedetomidine 40 μg/kg IM, bupivacaine 2 mg/kg intraperitoneal, and meloxicam 0.2 mg/kg SC postoperatively.[38] Most adult cats in the study required an opioid for postoperative pain relief.

Placement of IV catheter (extra-label): Midazolam 0.2 mg/kg combined in the same syringe with alfaxalone 1.5 mg/kg and hydromorphone 0.1 mg/kg and administered IM in the epaxial muscles.[39] Combination may be beneficial when prolonged sedation is required.

EQUINE:

Preoperative agent/total IV anesthesia (TIVA) (extra-label): Midazolam may be used or substituted for diazepam in protocols in combination with ketamine ± xylazine. See ***Ketamine*** and ***Diazepam*** for more information.

a) Medetomidine 6 μg/kg and midazolam 20 μg/kg IV in the same syringe prior to induction[40]
b) **Castration in the field** can be done in ponies with premedication of xylazine 1.1 mg/kg IM or detomidine 20 – 30 μg/kg IV, along with or followed by either midazolam or diazepam 0.05 – 0.06 mg/kg in combination with ketamine 2.2 mg/kg IV in the same syringe.[41,42]
c) **TIVA for field castration**: Premedicate with acepromazine 0.01 – 0.02 mg/kg IV, medetomidine 7 μg/kg IV, and methadone 0.1 mg/kg IV; induce anesthesia with ketamine 2.2 mg/kg IV and midazolam 0.06 mg/kg IV; maintain anesthesia with IV infusion of ketamine 3 mg/kg/hour, medetomidine 5 μg/kg/hour, and midazolam 0.1 mg/kg/hour.[43]
d) Ponies can be premedicated with romifidine 80 μg/kg IV and induced with midazolam 0.06 mg/kg and ketamine 2.5 mg/kg IV.[44] General anesthesia was maintained with romifidine 120 μg/kg/hour, midazolam 0.09 mg/kg/hour, and ketamine 3.3 mg/kg/hour given IV as a CRI. Oxygen supplementation is recommended. Recovery was uneventful.
e) Premedicate with acepromazine 0.03 mg/kg IM followed 15 minutes later by either xylazine 0.5 mg/kg IV or dexmedetomidine 3.5 μg/kg IV and induced with ketamine 2.2 mg/kg and midazolam 0.05 mg/kg IV.[45] The TIVA protocol included ketamine 3 – 5 mg/kg/hour, midazolam 0.1 mg/kg/hour, and either xylazine 1 mg/kg/hour or dexmedetomidine 7 μg/kg/hour IV. TIVA was discontinued after 120 minutes; 20 minutes later, flumazenil 0.01 mg/kg IV was given, and recovery was good to excellent.
f) **Horses**: Midazolam 25 mg, ketamine 650 mg, and xylazine 325 mg were admixed into a 500 mL bag of 0.9% sodium chloride.[46] The average IV infusion rate was 0.04 mL/kg/minute, which provided midazolam 0.002 mg/kg/minute, ketamine 0.048 mg/kg/minute, and xylazine 0.024 mg/kg/minute. Premedication included the use of an alpha-2 agonist alone or with an additional agent (eg, butorphanol, acepromazine). Anesthesia induction was achieved with midazolam 0.05 mg/kg and ketamine 2.2 mg/kg IV. Times to extubation and standing were 18 and 33 minutes, respectively. A combination of ketamine, midazolam, and medetomidine also produced adequate anesthesia but better recovery than a combination of ketamine, medetomidine, and guaifenesin.[47] A combination of ketamine, midazolam, and xylazine was inferior to a combination of ketamine, xylazine, and propofol.[48]
g) Thoroughbreds received medetomidine 6 μg/kg and midazolam 0.02 mg/kg (the route was not specified, but IV is assumed) premedication prior to anesthesia with alfaxalone, ketamine, or thiopental. All horses were well sedated prior to induction.[40]
h) **Dental extractions**: an initial bolus of romifidine 0.03 mg/kg combined with midazolam 0.02 mg/kg IV followed by romifidine 0.05 mg/kg/hour with midazolam 0.06 mg/kg/hour IV CRI had improved sedation and surgical condition as compared with horses that received only romifidine.[49]
i) **Donkeys** that were premedicated with xylazine 0.5 mg/kg IM followed 3 minutes later by midazolam 0.05 mg/kg IV and either alfaxalone 1 mg/kg IV or ketamine 2.2 mg/kg IV had a smooth anesthesia induction and average recumbency of ≈1 hour (alfaxalone) or ≈0.5 hours (ketamine).[50] Time to recumbency was somewhat shorter with alfaxalone (29 seconds) than with ketamine (51 seconds).

Seizure control in foals (extra-label): 2 – 5 mg (NOT mg/kg) for a 50 kg (110 lb) foal IV, IM.[51,52] Rapid IV administration may result in apnea and hypotension. Repeat as necessary. An IV CRI may be used at 1 – 3 mg/hour (NOT mg/kg/hour) for a 50 kg (110 lb) foal.

RUMINANTS:

a) **Calves** (extra-label): Induced general anesthesia with xylazine 0.05 mg/kg IV followed by ketamine 2 mg/kg and midazolam 0.1 mg/kg IV, which allows endotracheal intubation.[53]
b) **Goats** (extra-label): Premedicate with midazolam 0.3 mg/kg IM or midazolam 0.3 mg/kg and butorphanol 0.1 mg/kg IM.[54] This premedication decreases the induction dose of alfaxalone.

BIRDS:

Intranasal sedative/restraining agent (extra-label):

a) A study in Hispaniolan Amazon parrots given midazolam 2 mg/kg intranasally (IN) 15 minutes prior to manual restraint; sedation occurred within 3 minutes of administration, and vocalization, flight, and defense responses were significantly reduced.[55] Flumazenil antagonized the effects of midazolam within 10 minutes. A study in pigeons found that midazolam 5 mg/kg IN with dexmedetomidine 80 μg/kg IN was effective.[56] In cockatiels, midazolam 3 mg/kg IN with butorphanol 3 mg/kg IN provided sedation within ≈90 seconds.[57]
b) **Intranasal** midazolam 5 mg/kg mixed with dexmedetomidine 80 μg/kg slowly dripped into the nares provided short-term immobilization of 20 to 30 minutes in pigeons.[56] Atipa-

mezole 250 µg/kg dripped into the nares resulted in decreased sedation but not full responsiveness. Intranasal midazolam 3 mg/kg used alone or with butorphanol 3 mg/kg provided safe and effective sedation in cockatiels.[57]

Parenteral sedative/restraining agent (extra-label): In budgerigars, midazolam 3 mg/kg IM in combination with dexmedetomidine 10 – 40 µg/kg IM.[58] Reverse with atipamezole and flumazenil.

Premedication for anxious or easily stressed birds (eg, macaws, African greys, raptors, wild birds) (extra-label): 1 mg/kg IM.[59] This causes mild sedation and relaxation. Doses as high as 6 mg/kg have been reported to result in considerable sedation.

Part of an injectable anesthetic regimen (extra-label): Injectable anesthetics are only occasionally used in birds for short procedures or in situations where inhalant anesthetics are not available.[59] Ketamine 10 – 30 mg/kg and midazolam 2 – 6 mg/kg can be used. Midazolam can be reversed with flumazenil 0.1 mg/kg if necessary. Butorphanol 1 – 2 mg/kg can be added for analgesia.

Psittacid species (extra-label): Midazolam 0.5 mg/kg in combination with butorphanol 1 mg/kg and given IM in the pectoral muscle provided good anesthetic premedication prior to isoflurane.[60] This combination improved the quality and time of induction without adverse effects on cardiorespiratory parameters.

RABBITS, RODENTS, SMALL MAMMALS:

Hamsters, Gerbils, Mice, Rats, Guinea pigs, Chinchillas (extra-label): 1 – 2 mg/kg IM

a) **Preanesthetic agent for rodents** (extra-label): 3 – 5 mg/kg IM or IV; often beneficial to minimize stress and anxiety. If needed, reversal is possible with flumazenil 0.1 mg/kg IV, but it may precipitate seizures.[61]
b) **Rodents** (extra-label): Midazolam 5 mg/kg in combination with ketamine 100 mg/kg and buprenorphine 0.05 mg/kg intraperitoneal
c) **Rats** (extra-label): Midazolam 2.5 mg/kg in combination with butorphanol 2 mg/kg intraperitoneal prior to isoflurane anesthesia can provide smooth induction and can attenuate the respiratory depression of isoflurane.[62]

Rabbits:

Preanesthetic agent (extra-label): 0.5 – 5 mg/kg IM or IV

Combination Dosages:

a) Midazolam 2 mg/kg in combination with dexmedetomidine 0.1 mg/kg and butorphanol 0.4 mg/kg mixed in the same syringe and delivered via transnasal catheter to the nasopharyngeal mucosa. Loss of righting reflex, sedation, and analgesia occurred within 1 to 2 minutes with a duration of 45 minutes.[63] Blood pressure decreased, and hypoventilation with hypoxemia occurred; close monitoring and oxygen supplementation are recommended.
b) Midazolam 0.2 mg/kg in combination with ketamine 30 mg/kg IM OR midazolam 0.2 mg/kg in combination with dexmedetomidine 25 µg/kg IM. Deeper sedation occurred with the combination of dexmedetomidine and midazolam.[64]

Induction agent:

a) Midazolam 0.05 – 0.5 mg/kg IV (typically via a marginal ear vein). The low end of the dose range is usually given and topped up as necessary. In nonsedated animals, prior preparation of the area with topical local anesthetics may be useful. Midazolam IV leads to further sedation of the animal, which is sufficient to allow intubation but may also induce apnea. This, together with fentanyl's respiratory depression, can potentially compound the possibility of hypoxia. It is therefore important that midazolam is given to effect and that preoxygenation is performed. Intubation is considered essential when using this protocol. **NOTE**: Not all animals require midazolam induction for purposes of intubation.[65] An assessment of the animal can be made in the first 10 minutes after premedication delivery. Some rabbits may be sufficiently sedated to allow intubation at this point.
b) A combination of midazolam 3 mg/kg and ketamine 25 mg/kg IM followed by isoflurane was superior to using midazolam alone or a combination of midazolam and ketamine.[66]

Injectable anesthesia: Premedication with medetomidine 0.1 mg/kg SC, sufentanil 2.5 µg/mL, and midazolam 0.45 mg/mL administered at 0.3 mL/kg/hour IV CRI for induction with 0.1 mL of the mixture given every 20 seconds until the righting reflex was lost.[67] Following endotracheal intubation, the infusion rate was adjusted to suppress the pedal withdrawal reflex. Although induction and recovery were smooth, this drug combination caused marked hypotension and respiratory depression that required intubation and ventilation.

Monitoring

- Signs of sedation or paradoxical excitement
- Baseline and periodic blood pressure
- Respiratory rate, $ETCO_2$, and pulse oximetry
- Horses should be observed carefully for ataxia.
- Clinical response to treatment

Client Information

- Do not give this medicine as an injection at home, as it requires special medical monitoring for safe use.
- If giving this medicine into the nose to stop a seizure in dogs, follow your veterinarian's instructions exactly and contact your veterinarian immediately for further instruction.

Chemistry/Synonyms

Midazolam HCl is a benzodiazepine that occurs as a white or yellowish crystalline powder. It is soluble in alcohol, but solubility in water is dependent on pH. At a pH of 3.4 (≈ the pH of the commercial injection and syrup), 10.3 mg are soluble in 1 mL of water.

Midazolam HCl may also be known as Ro-21-3981/003 or *Versed*®.

Storage/Stability

Store midazolam injection at room temperature (15°C-30°C [59°F-86°F]) and protected from light. After being frozen for 3 days and allowed to thaw at room temperature, the injectable product is physically stable. Midazolam is stable at a pH range of 3 to 3.6.

Midazolam is a DEA Schedule IV (C-IV) controlled substance. Store it in an area that is substantially constructed and securely locked. Follow applicable local, state, and federal rules regarding the disposal of unused or wasted controlled drugs.

Compatibility/Compounding Considerations

Compatibility is dependent on factors such as pH, concentration, temperature, and diluent used; specialized references or a hospital pharmacist should be consulted for more specific information.

Midazolam is reportedly physically **compatible** when mixed with the following products: D_5W, normal saline, lactated Ringer's, atracurium, atropine sulfate, buprenorphine, butorphanol, calcium chloride/gluconate, cefazolin, cefuroxime, chlorpromazine, ciprofloxacin, fentanyl citrate, gentamicin, glycopyrrolate, fluconazole, hydromorphone, hydroxyzine, ketamine, lidocaine, mannitol, meperidine, metoclopramide, morphine sulfate (not in a syringe; compatibility appears to be concentration-dependent), nalbuphine, ondansetron, penicillin G potassium/sodium, promethazine HCl, potassium chloride, sufentanil citrate, and scopolamine HBr.

Midazolam is physically **incompatible** with amphotericin B, ampicillin sodium, ceftazidime, dexamethasone sodium phosphate, dimenhydrinate, esomeprazole, furosemide, heparin, hydrocortisone sodium succinate, pantoprazole, pentobarbital, phenobarbital, piperacillin/tazobactam, ranitidine, and sodium bicarbonate.

A midazolam hydrochloride oral suspension compounded from the commercially available injectable solution has been published.[68] Diluting midazolam 5 mg/mL injection in a 1:1 ratio with *Syrpalta*® yields a 2.5 mg/mL midazolam hydrochloride oral solution that retains more than 90% potency for 56 days when stored at 7°C (44.6°F), 20°C (68°F), or 40°C (104°F) and protected from light.

Dosage Forms/Regulatory Status

VETERINARY-LABELED PRODUCTS: NONE

The Association of Racing Commissioners International (ARCI) has designated this drug as a class 2 substance. Use of this drug may not be allowed in certain animal competitions. Check rules and regulations before entering a competition while this medication is being administered. Contact local racing authorities for further guidance. See ***Appendix*** for more information.

HUMAN-LABELED PRODUCTS:

Midazolam HCl Injection: 1 mg (as HCl)/mL; 5 mg (as HCl)/mL; generic; (Rx, C-IV)

Midazolam HCl Syrup: 2 mg/mL; generic; (Rx, C-IV)

Midazolam HCl Nasal Spray: packaged in 5 mg units, 2 units per box; *Nayzilam*®; (Rx)

Report dispensing to state monitoring programs where required.

References

For the complete list of references, see **wiley.com/go/budde/plumb**

Milbemycin Oxime

(mil-beh-***my***-sin) *Interceptor*®

Macrolide Antiparasitic

For information on the combination products with lufenuron, see ***Lufenuron***. For information on the combination product with spinosad, see ***Spinosad***. For information on the combination product with praziquantel, see ***Praziquantel/Praziquantel Combination Products***

Prescriber Highlights

- Used as a heartworm preventive and for the removal and/or control of hookworms, roundworms, and whipworms in dogs and puppies
- Available in combination with other anthelmintics or insecticides
- Prevents heartworm disease and removes adult roundworms and hookworms in cats and kittens
- No absolute contraindications
- Animals with a high number of circulating microfilariae may develop a transient shock-like syndrome.
- Adverse effects appear unlikely at labeled dosages; at higher doses, neurologic signs become more likely.

Uses/Indications

Milbemycin tablets for dogs and puppies are labeled as a monthly heartworm preventive (*Dirofilaria immitis*), for hookworm control (*Ancylostoma caninum*), and for control and removal of adult roundworms (*Toxocara canis, Toxascaris leonina*) and whipworms (*Trichuris vulpis*).[1] It can also be used extra-label for treatment of infestations of *Demodex canis, Demodex injai*, and *Sarcoptes scabiei* var. *canis*. In a systematic review of published clinical trials, the optimal determined treatments for demodicosis were daily oral milbemycin and weekly[2,3] or monthly[4-6] topical moxidectin (± imidacloprid); however, isoxazolines (eg, fluralaner, sarolaner) are as effective as the moxidectin/imidacloprid combination and have supplanted macrolide antiparasitics for the treatment of demodicosis.[3-5]

In cats, milbemycin tablets are labeled as a monthly heartworm preventive (*D. immitis*) and for removal of adult hookworms (*Ancylostoma tubaeforme*) and roundworms (*Toxocara cati*).

Pharmacology/Actions

The primary mode of action of milbemycins is binding to glutamate-gated chloride ion channels in the nervous system of nematodes and arthropods. Cell membrane permeability to chloride ions is increased, inhibiting the electrical activity of nerve cells in nematodes and muscle cells in arthropods and causing paralysis and death of the parasites.

Milbemycins also enhance the release of Gamma-aminobutyric acid (GABA) at presynaptic neurons. GABA acts as an inhibitory neurotransmitter and blocks postsynaptic stimulation of the adjacent neuron in nematodes or the muscle fiber in arthropods.

Milbemycins are generally not toxic to mammals, as mammals do not have glutamate-gated chloride channels and because these compounds do not readily cross the blood–brain barrier and therefore cannot reach the mammalian GABA receptors.

Pharmacokinetics

No specific information was located. At labeled doses, milbemycin is considered effective for at least 45 days after infection by *D immitis* larvae.

Contraindications/Precautions/Warnings

Manufacturers do not list any absolute contraindications to milbemycin use. Because some dogs with a high number of circulating microfilariae will develop a transient, shock-like syndrome after receiving milbemycin, the manufacturer recommends testing for pre-existing heartworm infections and treating infected dogs to remove adult heartworms and microfilariae prior to initiating milbemycin.

If using milbemycin at doses greater than labeled in breeds susceptible to the *MDR1* gene mutation (also known as *ABCB1*-1delta), genetic testing is recommended before initiating milbemycin.

The manufacturer states to only use the product (*Interceptor*®) in dogs 4 weeks of age or older and weighing at least 0.9 kg (2 lb) and in cats and kittens 6 weeks of age and older and weighing at least 0.7 kg (1.5 lb). Age and weight restrictions vary slightly for combination products labelled for use in dogs and puppies; consult specific product labels for further information.

Adverse Effects

At label dosages, adverse effects appear to be infrequent in microfilaria-free dogs, including breeds susceptible to neurologic toxicity (see ***Overdose/Acute Toxicity***). Lethargy, vomiting, ataxia, anorexia, diarrhea, convulsions, and weakness have been reported in dogs.

In a study of dog breeds susceptible to the *MDR1* mutation, milbemycin was given at dosages of 1 – 2.2 mg/kg PO daily for the treatment of demodicosis. All *MDR1* mutant/mutant dogs exhibited signs of CNS toxicity, whereas no *MDR1* wild-type/wild-type or *MDR1* mutant/wild-type dogs exhibited signs of toxicity.[7]

Reproductive/Nursing Safety

Studies in pregnant dogs at daily doses 3 times those labeled showed no adverse effects to offspring or bitch.[1] In cats, safety in breeding, pregnant, and lactating queens and breeding toms has not been established.

Milbemycin enters maternal milk. At labeled doses, no adverse effects have been noted in nursing puppies.

Because safety has not been established in animals, this drug should only be used when the maternal benefits outweigh the potential risks to offspring.

Overdose/Acute Toxicity

Eight-week-old puppies receiving 2.5 mg/kg (5 times the label dose) for 3 consecutive days showed no clinical signs after the first day, but after the second or third consecutive dose, showed some ataxia and trembling.

Beagles have tolerated a single oral dose of 200 mg/kg (400 times the label dose). Rough-coated collies have tolerated doses of 10 mg/kg (20 times the label dose) without adversity (label information; *Interceptor*®). Avermectin-sensitive collies tolerated 10 mg/kg milbemycin when combined with 300 mg/kg spinosad.[8] Toxic doses can cause mydriasis, ptyalism, lethargy, ataxia, pyrexia, seizures, coma, and death. Intravenous lipid emulsion (ILE) has been recommended for management of macrocyclic lactone toxicity,[9] and ILE was used to manage milbemycin toxicity in one dog[10] and one cat.[11] Supportive therapy is recommended.

Safety studies were conducted in young cats and kittens and doses of 1, 3, and 5 times the minimum recommended dose of 2 mg/kg demonstrated no drug-related effects. Tolerability studies at 10 times the label dose also demonstrated no drug-related adverse effects in kittens and young adult cats.

For patients that have experienced or are suspected to have experienced an overdose, consultation with a 24-hour poison consultation center specializing in providing veterinary-specific information is recommended. For general information related to overdose and toxin exposures, as well as contact information for poison control centers, refer to ***Appendix.***

Drug Interactions

The manufacturer states that milbemycin was used safely during testing in dogs and cats receiving other frequently used veterinary products, including vaccines, anthelmintics, antibiotics, steroids, flea collars, shampoos, and dips. The following drug interactions have either been reported or are theoretical in humans or animals receiving GABA agonists and may be of significance in veterinary patients. Unless otherwise noted, use together is not necessarily contraindicated, but weigh the potential risks and perform additional monitoring when appropriate.

- BENZODIAZEPINES: Effects may be potentiated by milbemycin; use together not advised in humans

Caution is advised if using milbemycin with other drugs that can inhibit **p-glycoprotein**, particularly in those dogs at risk for *MDR1* genetic mutation (collies, Australian shepherds, shelties, long-haired whippet, "white feet" breeds), unless tested normal. Drugs and drug classes involved include:

- AMIODARONE
- CARVEDILOL
- CLARITHROMYCIN
- CYCLOSPORINE
- DILTIAZEM
- ERYTHROMYCIN
- ITRACONAZOLE
- KETOCONAZOLE
- QUINIDINE
- SPIRONOLACTONE
- VERAPAMIL

Laboratory Considerations

None noted

Dosages

DOGS:

Parasiticide for labeled indications using milbemycin as a single agent (label dosages; FDA-approved): Appropriate dose is based on body weight and given orally, once a month, at the recommended minimum dosage of 0.5 mg/kg (0.23 mg/lb body weight).

Recommended Dosage Schedule for Dogs

Body weight	INTERCEPTOR® Flavor Tabs
0.9-4.5 kg (2-10 lb)	One tablet (2.3 mg)
5-11.3 kg (11-25 lb)	One tablet (5.75 mg)
11.8-22.7 kg (26-50 lb)	One tablet (11.5 mg)
23.2-45.5kg (51-100 lb)	One tablet (23.0 mg)

Dogs over 45.5 kg (100 lb) are provided the appropriate combination of tablets (Label information; *Interceptor*®)

Treatment of canine demodicosis (extra-label):

a) 0.5 – 1.6 mg/kg/day (mean dose 0.75 mg/kg/d) PO for 1 to 6 months and/or until skin scrape is negative. Cure more likely with juvenile-onset patients[12]

b) 1 – 2 mg/kg/day PO[13,14]

Treatment of canine sarcoptic mange (extra-label):

a) 0.75 mg/kg/day PO for 30 days[15]

b) 2 mg/kg PO once weekly for 3 treatments[16]

Prevention of *Angiostrongylus vasorum* infection (extra-label): milbemycin oxime/spinosad combination tablet at 0.75 – 1 mg/kg and 45 – 60 mg/kg PO, respectively. From a laboratory study, monthly doses would be expected to be effective.[17]

CATS:

Parasiticide for labeled indications using milbemycin as a single agent (label dosages; FDA-approved): Appropriate dose is based on body weight and given orally, once a month, at the recommended minimum dosage of 2 mg/kg (0.9 mg/lb body weight).

Recommended Dosage Schedule for Cats

Body weight	INTERCEPTOR® Flavor Tabs
0.7-2.7 kg (1.5-6 lb)	One tablet (5.75 mg)
2.8-5.5 kg (6.1-12 lb)	One tablet (11.5 mg)
5.4-11.4 kg (12.1-25 lb)	One tablet (23.0 mg)

Cats over 11.4 kg (25 lb) are provided the appropriate combination of tablets. (Label information; *Interceptor*®)

Treatment of Lungworm infections (extra-label): milbemycin 2 mg/kg with praziquantel 5 mg/kg PO every 15 days for 3 doses[18]

Monitoring

- Efficacy based on clinical signs and diagnostic testing (eg, fecal flotation, heartworm antigen testing, external parasite elimination)
- For demodicosis, clinical signs and monthly skin scraping; continue treatment for 4 weeks beyond 2 negative monthly skin scrapings.[14]
- Adverse effects

Client Information

- Used monthly in dogs to control heartworm and hookworms and to control and remove roundworms and whipworms.
- Used monthly in cats to control heartworm and to control and remove hookworms.
- Appears very safe when used at recommended dosages for prevention of heartworm, even in dogs with the *MDR1* genetic mutation.
- Store flavored tablets out of reach of children and animals. This medicine may be toxic to wildlife so dispose of unused tablets responsibly.

- When using milbemycin for heartworm prevention it is important to administer each monthly dose on schedule, as a late or missed dose may allow a heartworm infection to become established. Be certain that your pet fully consumes each dose.
- It is recommended to administer heartworm preventives year-round. If being administered seasonally, the first dose should be given within one month of the first mosquito exposure and continued monthly thereafter until the end of the mosquito season.

Chemistry/Synonyms

Milbemycin oxime consists of ≈80% of the A_4 derivatives and 20% of the A_3 derivatives of 5-didehydromilbemycin. Milbemycin is considered to be a macrolide antibiotic structurally. Milbemycin oxime occurs as a white to yellow powder.

Milbemycin may also be known as CGA-179246, *Interceptor*®, *Milbeguard*®, and *Milbehart*®.

Storage/Stability

Store milbemycin oxime tablets at room temperature between 15°C and 25°C (59°F-77°F).

Compatibility/Compounding Considerations

An analysis of aqueous milbemycin suspensions compounded by two national compounding pharmacies found that potency varied from 67.5% to 135% of labeled strength, and that potency decreased by ≈20% over the 3-week study period.[19]

Dosage Forms/Regulatory Status

VETERINARY-LABELED PRODUCTS:

Milbemycin Oxime Oral Tablets for dogs: 0.9 to 4.5 kg (2 to 10 lb): 2.3 mg; 5 to 11.4 kg (11 to 25 lb): 5.75 mg; 11.8 to 22.7 kg (26 to 50 lb): 11.5 mg; 23.2 to 45.5 kg (51 to 100 lb): 23 mg; dogs more than 45.5 kg (100 lb) are provided the appropriate combination of tablets; *Interceptor*® *Flavor Tabs*, generic (Rx). FDA-approved for use in dogs and puppies older than 4 weeks of age and at least 0.9 kg (2 lb).

Milbemycin Oxime Oral Tablets for cats: 0.7 to 2.7 kg (1.5 to 6 lb): 5.75 mg; 2.8 to 5.5 kg (6.1 to 12 lb): 11.5 mg; 5.5 to 11.4 kg (12.1 to 25 lb): 23 mg; *Interceptor*® *Flavor Tabs*, generic; (Rx). FDA-approved for cats and kittens older than 6 weeks of age and at least 0.7 kg (1.5 lb).

Milbemycin/Lufenuron Oral Tablets for dogs: 0.9 to 4.5 kg (2 to 10 lb): 2.3 mg/46 mg; 5 to 11.4 kg (11 to 25 lb): 5.75 mg/115 mg; 11.8 to 22.7 kg (26 to 50 lb): 11.5 mg/230 mg; 23.2 to 45.5 kg (51 to 100 lb): 23 mg/460 mg milbemycin/lufenuron; *Sentinel*® *Flavor Tabs*; (Rx). FDA-approved for use in dogs and puppies older than 4 weeks of age and at least 0.9 kg (2 lb). Also available with nitenpyram (*Capstar*®).

Milbemycin/Praziquantel Chewable Oral Tablets for dogs: 0.9 to 3.6 kg (2 to 8 lb): 2.3 mg/22.8 mg; 3.7 to 11.4 kg (8.1 to 25 lb): 5.75 mg/57 mg; 11.4 to 22.7 kg (25.1 to 50 lb): 11.5 mg/114 mg; 22.7 to 45.5 kg (50.1 to 100 lb): 23 mg/228 mg; *Interceptor*® *Plus* (Rx). FDA-approved for use in dogs and puppies 6 weeks of age or older and at least 0.9 kg (2 lb).

Milbemycin/Lufenuron/Praziquantel Chewable Oral Tablets for dogs: 0.9 to 3.6 kg (2 to 8 lb): 2.3 mg/46 mg/22.8 mg; 3.7 to 11.4 kg (8.1 to 25 lb): 5.75 mg/115 mg/57 mg; 11.4 to 22.7 kg (25.1 to 50 lb): 11.5 mg/230 mg/114 mg; 22.7 to 45.5 kg (50.1 to 100 lb): 23 mg/460 mg/228 mg; *Sentinel*® *Spectrum*®; (Rx). FDA-approved for use in dogs and puppies older than 6 weeks of age and at least 0.9 kg (2 lb).

Milbemycin/Spinosad Chewable Oral Tablets for dogs: 2.3 to 4.5 kg (5 to 10 lb): 2.3 mg/140 mg; 4.5 to 9.1 kg (10.1 to 20 lb): 4.5 mg/270 mg; 9.1 to 18.2 kg (20.1 to 40 lb): 9.3 mg/560 mg; 18.2 to 27.3 kg (40.1 to 60 lb): 13.5 mg/810 mg; 27.3 to 54.5 kg (60.1 to 120 lb): 27 mg/1620 mg; *Trifexis*®, *Comboguard*®; (Rx). FDA-approved for use in dogs and puppies 8 weeks of age or older and at least 2.2 kg (5 lb).

Milbemycin 0.1% otic solution (*Milbemite*®) available for treatment of ear mite (*Otodectes cynotis*) infestations in cats and kittens 4 weeks of age and older.

HUMAN-LABELED PRODUCTS: NONE

References

For the complete list of references, see **wiley.com/go/budde/plumb**

Miltefosine

(mil-***tef***-oh-seen) *Milteforan*®, *Impavido*®

Antileishmanial

Prescriber Highlights

- Oral treatment for canine leishmaniasis; improves clinical status but is unlikely to fully clear the organism
- Appears to be more effective when used with allopurinol
- Contraindicated in patients hypersensitive to it, in pregnant or lactating animals, and in breeding animals
- Use caution in animals with hepatic dysfunction or cardiac insufficiency.
- Adverse effects include vomiting and diarrhea.
- The National Institute for Occupational Safety and Health (NIOSH) classifies miltefosine as a hazardous drug; use appropriate precautions when handling and do not handle if pregnant.

Uses/Indications

Originally developed as an antineoplastic agent, miltefosine can be used alone or with allopurinol to treat canine leishmaniasis. Like other drugs, it does not completely clear the organism in dogs, but can substantially reduce the parasitic load.[1,2] Clinical efficacy is improved when used with allopurinol.[1] Clinical signs decrease substantially immediately after beginning treatment and are significantly reduced after 2 weeks.[3] The combination of meglumine antimoniate with allopurinol appears to have better clinical efficacy than a miltefosine-allopurinol combination.[4]

One case report demonstrates efficacy of miltefosin and allopurinol combination therapy for leishmaniasis in a ferret.[5]

Pharmacology/Actions

Although the exact mechanism of action for miltefosine against *Leishmania infantum* is not understood, it is thought that it inhibits the penetration of the organism into macrophages by interacting with glycosomes and glycosylphosphatidyl-inositol anchors that are essential for the survival of *Leishmania* organisms intracellularly. Also, by inhibiting phospholipase, miltefosine disrupts *Leishmania* membrane signal transduction. Other possible mechanisms include inhibition of mitochondrial function and cell death from an apoptosis-like effect. Miltefosine has antineoplastic, immunomodulatory, anti-amebic, and antiviral activity.

Pharmacokinetics

After oral administration in dogs, miltefosine has a bioavailability of 94% with peak plasma concentrations occurring around 5 hours postdose. The drug is distributed throughout the major organs, including the brain. Intravascularly, it is nearly evenly distributed between plasma and erythrocytes. Miltefosine undergoes phospholipase D-like cleavage in the liver; it is mainly eliminated via the feces, with ≈10% of a dose eliminated unchanged. Renal elimination appears negligible. Miltefosine has a long half-life of around 6.5 days.

Contraindications/Precautions/Warnings

Miltefosine is labeled as contraindicated in patients hypersensitive to it and in pregnant, lactating, or breeding animals.

Use with caution in patients with severe hepatic dysfunction or cardiac impairment. Do not underdose as it may increase the risk for drug resistance to occur.

The National Institute for Occupational Safety and Health (NIOSH) classifies miltefosine as a hazardous drug; personal protective equipment (PPE) should be used accordingly to minimize the risk for exposure.

Adverse Effects

Clinical signs of GI distress (eg, vomiting, diarrhea, inappetence) are the most common adverse effects seen in dogs.[6] In clinical studies, these adverse effects occurred on average within 5 to 7 days of starting treatment and lasted for 1 to 2 days, but may last longer in some animals. Giving with food may reduce GI signs.[3] Miltefosine potentially may cause nephrotoxicity and/or hepatotoxicity, but as leishmaniasis can cause kidney and liver damage, it is difficult to ascribe any specific risk for these potential adverse effects in dogs. One study in healthy beagles found that miltefosine 2 mg/kg/day PO in 8 dogs did not cause renal tubular damage, but meglumine antimoniate 100 mg/kg/day SC caused severe tubular damage (cell necrosis and apoptosis).[7]

In humans, the most common (>10%) adverse effects are abdominal pain, nausea, vomiting, diarrhea, reduced appetite, and an increase in liver enzymes.[8] Nephrotoxicity and thrombocytopenia have also been reported in humans.

Reproductive/Nursing Safety

Miltefosine is contraindicated during pregnancy in humans[8] and should be considered contraindicated in pregnant, lactating, and breeding animals. When pregnant rats were dosed at 1.2 mg/kg/day and higher during the early embryonic development (up to day 7 of pregnancy), an increased risk for embryotoxic, fetotoxic, and teratogenic effects was determined. In pregnant rabbits given 2.4 mg/kg/day and higher during the organogenesis phase, embryotoxic and fetotoxic effects were also seen.

Male rats given miltefosine 8.25 mg/kg daily showed testicular atrophy and impaired fertility; this was at least partially reversible within 10 weeks.

It is not known if miltefosine is excreted into milk. The canine and human labels state that it should not be used in nursing mothers.

Because safety has not been established in animals, this drug should only be used when the maternal benefits outweigh the potential risks to offspring.

Overdose/Acute Toxicity

Overdoses can result in uncontrollable vomiting.[3] Potentially, hepatic, renal, and retinal toxicity are possible in large overdoses. A specific antidote for miltefosine overdose is not known.

For patients that have experienced or are suspected to have experienced an overdose, consultation with a 24-hour poison consultation center specializing in providing veterinary-specific information is recommended. For general information related to overdose and toxin exposures, as well as contact information for poison control centers, refer to ***Appendix.***

Drug Interactions

No drug interactions have been reported for miltefosine.

Laboratory Considerations

- No specific concerns noted

Dosages

DOGS:

Canine leishmaniasis (extra-label):

a) 2 mg/kg PO, poured onto food, with a full or partial meal once a day for 28 days[2,3,9]

b) As an alternative treatment to meglumine antimoniate and allopurinol: miltefosine 2 mg/kg PO once daily for 28 days with allopurinol 5 – 20 mg/kg PO every 12 hours, for at least 6 months[1,10–12]

c) Miltefosine 1.5 mg/kg PO once daily for 5 days, then 2.5 mg/kg PO once daily for 25 days; used in combination with allopurinol 10 mg/kg PO twice daily, for at least 6 months[4,9]

FERRETS:

Leishmaniosis (extra-label): From a case report: miltefosine 2 mg/kg PO once daily for 28 days with allopurinol 10 mg/kg PO every 12 hours[5]

Monitoring

- Baseline and periodic renal function and hepatic enzymes
- Adverse effects (especially vomiting)
- Body weight

Client Information

- Give with food to help reduce the chance for vomiting.
- If vomiting or severe diarrhea occurs, contact your veterinarian.
- Because this drug has caused birth defects, it should not be handled by pregnant women.
- Do not allow treated dogs to lick persons immediately after intake of the veterinary liquid form of the medication.
- If using a veterinary oral solution (imported), wear disposable gloves when administering this product as it has caused skin reactions.
- To avoid foaming, do not shake the vial of the veterinary oral solution (imported).
- This medication is considered to be a hazardous drug as defined by the National Institute for Occupational Safety and Health (NIOSH). Talk with your veterinarian or pharmacist about the use of personal protective equipment when handling this medicine.

Chemistry/Synonyms

Miltefosine is a phospholipid derivative (alkylphosphocholine) that is structurally related to the phospholipid components of cell membranes. It occurs as a white powder freely soluble in water or ethanol. The commercially available canine product (*Milteforan®*) is a clear, colorless, viscous solution containing 20 mg/mL of miltefosine. Excipients in the solution include hydroxypropylcellulose, propylene glycol, and water.

Miltefosine may also be known as D-18506, HDPC, hexadecilfosfocolina, hexadecylphosphocholine, miltefosiini, miltefosina, miltéfosine, or miltefosinum. Trade names include *Milteforan®*, *Miltex®*, and *Impavido®*.

Storage/Stability

Miltefosine capsules should be protected from moisture and stored at 20°C to 25°C (68°F-77°F); excursions permitted from 15°C to 30°C (59°F-86°F). Avoid freezing. Veterinary liquid should be discarded 1 month after first opening the container.

Compatibility/Compounding Considerations

No specific information noted

Dosage Forms/Regulatory Status

VETERINARY-LABELED PRODUCTS:

None in the United States. Elsewhere, a canine licensed product may be available. Miltefosine Oral Solution: 20 mg/mL in 30 mL, 60 mL, and 90 mL vials; *Milteforan®*; (Rx)

HUMAN-LABELED PRODUCTS:

Miltefosine capsules: 50 mg; *Impavido®*; (Rx). Approved as an orphan drug by FDA. For availability, see www.impavido.com

References

For the complete list of references, see **wiley.com/go/budde/plumb**

Mineral Oil

Liquid Paraffin

Lubricant Laxative

Prescriber Highlights

- ► Laxative used mainly in horses to treat constipation and fecal impaction
- ► Use with caution in debilitated or pregnant patients, patients with hiatal hernia, dysphagia, or esophageal or gastric retention.
- ► Use caution when administering by tube to avoid aspiration.
- ► Adverse effects include lipid pneumonitis if aspirated, granulomatous reactions in liver if significant amounts are absorbed from gut, and oil leakage from the anus.
- ► Long-term use may lead to decreased absorption of fat-soluble vitamins (A, D, E, K).

Uses/Indications

Mineral oil is commonly used in horses to treat constipation and fecal impactions. Mineral oil has also been administered after ingestion of lipid-soluble toxins (eg, kerosene, metaldehyde) to delay the absorption of these toxins through its laxative and solubility properties.

Mineral oil products containing petrolatum (eg, *Laxatone*®) may be used in dogs and cats as a laxative or to prevent and reduce hairballs in cats. Mineral oil has been used with some success to treat gastric impaction in certain raptor species.[1]

Pharmacology/Actions

Mineral oil acts as a laxative by lubricating fecal material and the intestinal mucosa. It also reduces reabsorption of water from the GI tract, thereby increasing fecal bulk and decreasing intestinal transit time.

Pharmacokinetics

It has been reported that after oral administration, emulsions of mineral oil may be up to 60% absorbed, but most reports state that mineral oil preparations are only minimally absorbed from the gut.

Contraindications/Precautions/Warnings

No specific contraindications were noted with regard to veterinary patients. In humans, orally administered mineral oil is considered contraindicated in patients less than 6 years of age; debilitated or pregnant patients; and patients with hiatal hernia, dysphagia, or esophageal or gastric retention.

Use caution when administering mineral oil by nasogastric tube to avoid aspiration, especially in debilitated or recalcitrant animals. To avoid aspiration in small animal species, oral administration of mineral oil should not be attempted when there is a pre-existing difficulty with swallowing or if there is an increased risk for vomiting or regurgitation. Many clinicians believe that mineral oil should not be administered orally to small animal species due to the risk for aspiration and should be administered rectally when used as a laxative.

In horses, administration of mineral oil is contraindicated to remove an esophageal blockage, as aspiration can occur.

Adverse Effects

When used on a short-term basis and at recommended doses, mineral oil should cause minimal adverse effects. The most serious effect that could be encountered is aspiration of the oil with resultant lipid pneumonitis. This effect can be prevented by using mineral oil only in appropriate cases when the risk for aspiration is minimal and by ensuring that the tube is in the stomach when administering via tube, and by administering the oil at a reasonable rate.

Granulomatous reactions have occurred in the liver, spleen, and mesenteric lymph nodes when significant quantities of mineral oil are absorbed from the gut. Oil leakage from the anus may occur and be of concern in animals with rectal lesions or house pets. Long-term administration of mineral oil may lead to decreased absorption of fat-soluble vitamins (A, D, E, K). No reports were found documenting clinically significant hypovitaminosis in cats receiving long-term petrolatum therapy, however.

Reproductive/Nursing Safety

Oral mineral oil should be safe to use during nursing.

Because safety has not been established in animals, this drug should only be used when the maternal benefits outweigh the potential risks to offspring.

Overdose/Acute Toxicity

No specific information was located regarding overdoses of mineral oil; but it would be expected that with the exception of aspiration, the effects would be self-limiting. See ***Adverse Effects*** for more information.

For patients that have experienced or are suspected to have experienced an overdose, consultation with a 24-hour poison consultation center specializing in providing veterinary-specific information is recommended. For general information related to overdose and toxin exposures, as well as contact information for poison control centers, refer to ***Appendix.***

Drug Interactions

The following drug interactions have either been reported or are theoretical in humans or animals receiving mineral oil and may be of significance in veterinary patients. Unless otherwise noted, use together is not necessarily contraindicated, but weigh the potential risks and perform additional monitoring when appropriate.

- **Docusate**: Theoretically, mineral oil should not be given with docusate (DSS), as enhanced absorption of the mineral oil could occur; however, this does not appear to be of significant clinical concern with large animal species.
- **Vitamins A, D, E, K**: Long-term administration of mineral oil may affect absorption of fat-soluble vitamins (A, D, E, K). It has been recommended to administer mineral oil products between meals to minimize this problem.

Dosages

DOGS/CATS:

Lubricant laxative (extra-label): Because of the risk for aspiration, liquid mineral oil is rarely recommended for oral administration. Occasionally, some clinicians administer liquid mineral oil rectally at 5 – 30 mL/dog (NOT mL/kg) and 5 – 10 mL/cat (NOT mL/kg). Cat laxative (petrolatum-based) products are sometimes recommended at 1 – 5 mL/cat (NOT mL/kg) PO daily.

Preventing hairballs (label dosage; NOT FDA-approved): ½ – 1 teaspoonful PO daily for 2 to 3 days, then ¼ – ½ teaspoonful 2 to 3 times per week.[2]

HORSES:

Laxative (extra-label):

a) **Large colon impactions**:
   i. Adults: 2 – 4 liters/horse via nasogastric (NG) tube; may be repeated every 12 hours
   ii. Foals: 60 – 240 mL/foal (NOT mL/kg). Not recommended for foals less than 24 hours old

b) **Sand colic**: In one experimental study, 0.5 kg psyllium was mixed with 1 liter of mash and given twice daily. Two liters of mineral oil via NG tube were administered once daily. This combination was more effective (measured ash content of feces) than giving mineral oil alone.[3]

CATTLE:

Laxative (extra-label):

a) Adults: 0.5 – 4 liters/animal via stomach tube

b) Calves: 60 – 120 mL (NOT mL/kg) via stomach tube

SHEEP & GOATS:

Laxative (extra-label): 100 – 500 mL/animal (NOT mL/kg) via stomach tube[4]

SWINE:

Laxative (extra-label): 50 – 100 mL/animal (NOT mL/kg) via stomach tube[4]

BIRDS:

Laxative and to aid in the removal of lead from the gizzard (extra-label): 1 – 3 drops/30 grams of body weight or 5 mL/kg PO once. Repeat as necessary. Give via tube or give slowly to avoid aspiration.[5]

RABBITS, RODENTS, SMALL MAMMALS:

Laxative or to remove hairballs in rabbits (extra-label): Using a feline laxative product: 1 – 2 mL/rabbit (NOT mL/kg) PO per day for 3 to 5 days[6]

Monitoring

- Clinical efficacy (eg, stool consistency and frequency)
- If aspiration is suspected, auscultate and perform thoracic radiographs.

Client Information

- Follow your veterinarian's instructions or label directions for cat laxative products.
- Do not increase the amount you are giving your animal or prolong treatment beyond your veterinarian's recommendations.

Chemistry/Synonyms

Mineral oil, also known as liquid petrolatum, liquid paraffin, or white mineral oil, occurs as a tasteless, odorless (when cold), transparent, colorless, oily liquid that is insoluble in both water and alcohol. It is a mixture of complex hydrocarbons and is derived from crude petroleum. For pharmaceutical purposes, heavy mineral oil is recommended over light mineral oil, as it is believed to have a lesser tendency to be absorbed in the gut or aspirated after oral administration.

White petrolatum, also known as white petroleum jelly or white soft paraffin, occurs as a white or faintly yellow unctuous mass. It is insoluble in water and almost insoluble in alcohol. White petrolatum differs from petrolatum only in that it is further refined to remove more of the yellow color.

Mineral oil may also be known as liquid paraffin, 905 (mineral hydrocarbons), dickflussiges paraffin, heavy liquid petrolatum, huile de vaseline epaisse, liquid petrolatum, oleum petrolei, oleum vaselini, paraffinum liquidum, paraffin oil, paraffinum subliquidum, vaselinol, vaselinum liquidum, and white mineral oil; many trade names are available.

Storage/Stability

Mineral oil products should be stored at room temperature between 10°C and 30°C (50°F-86°F).

Compatibility/Compounding Considerations

No specific information was noted.

Dosage Forms/Regulatory Status

VETERINARY-LABELED PRODUCTS:

Mineral oil products have not been formally FDA-approved for use in animals. These products and preparations are available without a prescription (OTC).

Mineral Oil Oral Preparations:

Liquid Mineral Oil: Available in gallons or 55 gallon drums

Cat Laxative Products: Products may vary in actual composition; some contain liquid petrolatum in place of white petrolatum and may have various flavors (eg, tuna, caviar, malt). There are many proprietary products marketed.

HUMAN-LABELED PRODUCTS:

Mineral Oil Liquid: in 180 mL and 473 mL; generic; (OTC)

Mineral Oil Emulsions: There are several products available that are emulsions of mineral oil and may be more palatable for oral administration. Trade names include: *Kondremul® Plain*; (OTC). Various generic products are available.

References

For the complete list of references, see **wiley.com/go/budde/plumb**

Minocycline

(mi-noe-***sye***-kleen) *Minocin®, Solodyn®*

Tetracycline Antibiotic

Prescriber Highlights

- ► Oral and parenteral tetracycline antibiotic; potential alternative to doxycycline
- ► Less likely to cause bone and teeth abnormalities than other tetracyclines, but use in pregnant and/or young animals should be avoided when possible
- ► May be used in patients with mild to moderate renal insufficiency without dosage adjustment
- ► Administration on an empty stomach is preferred.
- ► Adverse effects are most commonly GI-related (eg, nausea, vomiting).

Uses/Indications

Minocycline is a tetracycline-derived antibiotic used for the treatment of a variety of bacterial infections, particularly when doxycycline is unavailable. It can be effective against some doxycycline-resistant staphylococci.[1] Minocycline is not recommended for the treatment of bacterial cystitis or prostatitis,[2] as it does not reach adequate concentrations in these sites.[3,4] Minocycline may be used instead of doxycycline as part of the American Heartworm Society's recommended canine heartworm treatment protocol.[5]

Minocycline is effective in the treatment of periodontitis in dogs when applied locally after scaling and root planing were performed.[6,7] Minocycline purportedly has antiangiogenic effects but was ineffective as adjuvant therapy when given to dogs with hemangiosarcoma treated with standard chemotherapy[8]; however, concerns have been expressed about the use of antimicrobials for nonantimicrobial effects.[9]

Minocycline has been suggested as a potential alternative to doxycycline in the treatment of Lyme disease (ie, *Borrelia burgdorferi* infection) in horses, although minocycline may not attain MIC concentrations.[10,11] Minocycline is a preferred choice for the treament of Lyme borreliosis in dogs.[12]

The World Health Organization (WHO) has designated minocycline as a Highly Important antimicrobial in human medicine.[13] The World Organization for Animal Health (OIE) has designated tetracyclines as a Veterinary Critically Important Antimicrobial Agent.[14]

Pharmacology/Actions

Tetracyclines are time-dependent, bacteriostatic antibiotics. In susceptible organisms, tetracyclines inhibit bacterial protein synthesis by reversibly binding to the bacterial 30S ribosomal subunits, thus preventing aminoacyl tRNA attachment to the ribosome. Tetracyclines also alter cytoplasmic membrane permeability in susceptible organisms. At high concentrations, tetracyclines inhibit protein synthesis in mammalian cells.

A study in 6 beagles reported a mean oral bioavailability of ≈50%, but bioavailability ranged from 28% to 74%. This study concluded that minocycline at a dosage of 5 mg/kg PO twice daily is sufficient for inhibiting *Staphylococcus pseudintermedius* isolates with MICs less than or equal to 0.25 µg/mL.[15] A small pharmacokinetic/drug interaction study in 5 healthy greyhounds found that a dose of 7.5 mg/kg PO every 12 hours achieved the pharmacodynamic index for a bacterial MIC of 0.25 µg/mL (AUC:MIC greater than or equal to 33.9), but the authors cautioned that this was not an efficacy study and that further studies are required.[16] Staphylococcal resistance to tetracyclines occurs via the *tet*(K) and *tet*(M) genes. *tet*(K) confers resistance to tetracycline but not doxycycline or minocycline, whereas *tet*(M) confers resistance to all 3. These findings indicate that minocycline can be a useful second-tier drug in the treatment of canine infections caused by some strains of MRSP (eg, ST71) and other multidrug- and doxycycline-resistant strains harboring the tetracycline-resistance gene *tet*(K).[15] Minocycline susceptibility testing should be performed to determine whether minocycline is a valid choice in the treatment of MRSP.

Although doxycycline and minocycline are sometimes considered interchangeable, they have differences in pharmacokinetics and antibacterial activity. Human interpretive breakpoints may overreport minocycline susceptibility, potentially leading to treatment failure; thus, a lower canine-specific breakpoint (ie, susceptibility less than or equal to 0.25 µg/mL as compared with the human breakpoint of 4 µg/mL) has been recommended.[17] A retrospective review of MRSP found that of the 107 isolates tested, 36% were susceptible to tetracycline, 38% to doxycycline, and 65% to minocycline.[1] In the treatment of MRSP, minocycline susceptibility testing should be performed if doxycycline resistance is reported. Resistance to minocycline is indicative of presence of the *tet*(M) gene, whereas susceptibility to minocycline but resistance to doxycycline can occur with presence of the *tet*(K) gene.[18] Therefore, some doxycycline-resistant staphylococci will be susceptible to minocycline. A small prospective study determined that minocycline is an acceptable alternative to doxycycline in the treatment of *Ehrlichia canis* infection in dogs.[19]

As a class, tetracyclines have activity against most *Mycoplasma* spp, spirochetes (including *Borrelia burgdorferi*), *Chlamydia* spp, and *Rickettsia* spp. Against gram-positive bacteria, tetracyclines have inherent activity against staphylococci and streptococci, but resistance in these organisms to tetracyclines is increasing.[1] Gram-positive bacteria usually covered by tetracyclines include *Actinomyces* spp, *Bacillus anthracis, Clostridium perfringens, Clostridium tetani, Listeria monocytogenes*, and *Nocardia* spp. Among gram-negative bacteria, tetracyclines usually have in vitro and in vivo activity against *Bordetella* spp, *Brucella* spp, *Bartonella* spp, *Haemophilus* spp, *Pasteurella multocida, Shigella* spp, and *Yersinia pestis*. Many or most strains of *Escherichia coli, Klebsiella* spp, *Bacteroides* spp, *Enterobacter* spp, *Proteus* spp, and *Pseudomonas aeruginosa* are resistant to tetracyclines.[20]

Minocycline and doxycycline have significant inhibitory properties against the activity of matrix metalloproteinases (eg, collagenase, gelatinase) and can act as a disease-modifying agent for osteoarthritis. The clinical benefits of this approach are unclear, and concern has been expressed about the use of antimicrobials for nonantimicrobial properties.[21]

Pharmacokinetics

Minocycline is highly lipid-soluble and distributed widely throughout the body. In dogs, minocycline appears to be cleared more rapidly than doxycycline. Therapeutic concentrations can be found in CSF (whether meninges are inflamed or not), saliva, and eyes. Minocycline is extensively metabolized in the liver and excreted primarily as inactive metabolites in the feces and urine. Less than 20% is excreted unchanged in the urine. The half-life in dogs after an oral dose is ≈4 hours.[15] In dogs, administration without food has been recommended due to the impact of food on drug pharmacokinetics. In a study, administration of minocycline with a meal to hounds reduced the peak concentration as compared with fasted dogs, with the overall extent of absorption reduced but not considered significant.[22]

In cats, a dose of minocycline at 5 mg/kg IV resulted in a mean volume of distribution at steady-state (Vdss) of 1.5 L/kg. Plasma protein binding was 60%, total body clearance was 2.9 mL/kg/minute, and elimination half-life was 6.7 hours. An oral dose of minocycline at 50 mg/cat (NOT mg/kg) (mean, 13.9 mg/kg) resulted in a mean oral bioavailability of 62%, and elimination half-life was 6.3 hours.[23]

In a study of adult horses given a single dose of minocycline (2.2 mg/kg IV), mean Vdss was 1.53 L/kg, total body clearance was 0.16 L/hour/kg, and elimination half-life was ≈8 hours. Plasma protein-binding was 68%, and concentration of free minocycline was 0.12 µg/mL at 12 hours.[24] In studies of healthy horses given minocycline at 4 mg/kg PO every 12 hours, time to maximum concentration was 1 to 1.3 hours, maximum serum concentration was 1.6 to 2.3 µg/mL, and steady-state elimination half-life was 8.6 to 12 hours.[25-27] Oral bioavailability was more than doubled (39% vs 16%) when horses underwent a 12 hour fast prior to drug administration and access to hay was delayed for 2 hours after administration.[28] Minocycline pharmacokinetics in foals are similar to pharmacokinetics in adult horses, except oral bioavailability in foals was ≈58%.[27] Minocycline has been detected 1 to 3 hours after administration in pulmonary epithelial lining fluid,[27] brain tissue,[24] CSF,[24,25] tear fluid,[29] synovial fluid, and aqueous humor.[25] Minocycline concentrations in plasma, CSF, and synovial fluid exceeded MIC_{90} for many gram-positive equine pathogens.[25] However, tear fluid levels were inconsistent and oral administration may not be effective in the treatment of ocular infections.[29]

Contraindications/Precautions/Warnings

Minocycline is contraindicated in patients that are hypersensitive to tetracyclines and should be used with caution in patients that are pregnant, nursing, or younger than 6 months due to the potential for enamel hypoplasia or permanent discoloration of the teeth.[30,31] Minocycline is much less likely to cause dental abnormalities than other more water-soluble tetracyclines (eg, oxytetracycline, tetracycline). Unlike either oxytetracycline or tetracycline, minocycline can be used in patients with moderate renal insufficiency without dosage adjustment; however, patients with oliguric renal failure may require dosage adjustment or use of an alternative antibiotic.

Because urine concentrations are low, minocycline is not recommended in the treatment of bacterial cystitis.

For oral use of minocycline, the doxycycline recommendations for administration should be followed to reduce the risk for oroesophageal erosions, particularly in cats. In the use of oral tablets or capsules, pilling should be followed by a bolus of water or food (at least 6 mL for cats).[32] Dry pilling should not be performed.

Adverse Effects

The most commonly reported adverse effects of oral minocycline in dogs and cats are nausea and vomiting. To alleviate these effects, the drug could be given with food although this may impair drug absorption. Dental or bone staining can occur when minocycline exposure occurs in utero or early in life. More rarely, increases in hepatic enzymes and/or ototoxicity are possible. Two research cats (50%) became lethargic and tachypneic after IV administration, and vomiting occurred in 3 (≈30%) cats.[23]

Similar to doxycycline, oral minocycline can cause esophagitis and esophageal strictures, particularly in cats. See ***Contraindications/Precautions/Warnings*** for more information.

IV injections of minocycline in dogs have caused urticaria, shivering, hypotension, dyspnea, cardiac arrhythmias, and shock when given rapidly[15]; IV administration should be done slowly over a minimum of 10 minutes,[33,34] although 60 minutes is recommended for humans.[31]

Tetracycline therapy—especially long-term—may result in overgrowth (eg, superinfections) of nonsusceptible bacteria or fungi.[30,31]

In humans, minocycline (or other tetracyclines) has also been associated with photosensitivity reactions and, rarely, hepatotoxicity or blood dyscrasias. CNS effects (eg, dizziness, lightheadedness) are commonly reported in humans taking minocycline. A blue-gray pigmentation of skin and mucous membranes may occur.[30,31] Erythema multiforme and Stevens-Johnson syndrome have also been reported in humans; significance in veterinary medicine is unknown.[30,31]

Reproductive/Nursing Safety

Because tetracyclines can delay fetal skeletal development and discolor deciduous teeth, they should only be used in the last half of pregnancy when the benefits outweigh the fetal risks. Minocycline is much less likely to cause these abnormalities than other more water-soluble tetracyclines (eg, oxytetracycline, tetracycline). Minocycline has been shown to impair fertility in male rats.[30,31]

Tetracyclines are excreted in milk. Milk:plasma ratios vary between 0.25 and 1.5. In humans, minocycline may alter milk production or composition. Although minocycline probably has less effect on teeth and bones than other tetracyclines, its use should be avoided during nursing.

Because safety has not been established in animals, this drug should only be used when the maternal benefits outweigh the potential risks to offspring.

Overdose/Acute Toxicity

Oral overdoses of minocycline would most likely be associated with GI disturbances (eg, vomiting, anorexia, diarrhea). Although this drug is less vulnerable to chelation with cations than other tetracyclines, oral administration of divalent or trivalent cation antacids may bind some of the drug and reduce GI distress. Treatment is supportive based on clinical signs. If patients develop severe emesis or diarrhea, hydration and electrolytes should be monitored and corrected if necessary.

For patients that have experienced or are suspected to have experienced an overdose, consultation with a 24-hour poison consultation center specializing in providing veterinary-specific information is recommended. For general information related to overdose and toxin exposures, as well as contact information for poison control centers, refer to ***Appendix.***

Drug Interactions

The following drug interactions have either been reported or are theoretical in humans or animals receiving minocycline and may be of significance in veterinary patients. Unless otherwise noted, use together is not necessarily contraindicated, but the potential risks should be weighed and additional monitoring performed when appropriate.

- **ANTACIDS, ALUMINUM-, CALCIUM-, AND MAGNESIUM CONTAINING**: When orally administered, tetracyclines can chelate divalent or trivalent cations and decrease the absorption of the tetracycline or another drug if it contains these cations. Minocycline has a relatively low affinity for divalent or trivalent cations, but it is recommended that all oral tetracyclines be given at least 1 to 2 hours before or after the cation-containing product.
- **BISMUTH SUBSALICYLATE, KAOLIN, PECTIN**: May reduce absorption of minocycline
- **DIGOXIN**: Concurrent use with minocycline may cause digoxin toxicity. These effects may persist for months after discontinuation of the tetracycline.
- **IRON, ORAL**: Oral iron products are associated with decreased tetracycline absorption, and iron salts should preferably be given 3 hours before or 2 hours after the tetracycline dose.
- **KAOLIN/PECTIN**: Decreased minocycline absorption is possible; administer oral tetracyclines at least 1 to 2 hours before or after kaolin/pectin.
- **PENICILLINS**: Bacteriostatic drugs (eg, tetracyclines including minocycline) may interfere with the bactericidal activity of penicillins, cephalosporins, and aminoglycosides; however, there is a fair amount of controversy regarding the actual clinical significance of this interaction.
- **RIFAMPIN**: Synergistic activity against *Rhodococcus equi* in foals may occur.
- **SEVOFLURANE**: In a study of rats, minocycline reduced sevoflurane MAC requirement by 23%.[35]
- **SUCRALFATE**: Significantly decreases the oral bioavailability of minocycline in healthy dogs. Administration 2 hours after minocycline did not have a significant impact on absorption of minocycline.[16]
- **VITAMIN A**: May result in an increased risk for pseudotumor cerebri
- **WARFARIN**: Tetracyclines may depress plasma prothrombin activity; patients on anticoagulant therapy may need dosage adjustment.
- **ZINC, ORAL**: Decreased minocycline absorption is possible; administer oral tetracyclines at least 1 to 2 hours before or after oral zinc preparations.

Laboratory Considerations

- Tetracyclines can reportedly cause false-positive **urine glucose** results if the cupric sulfate method of determination (eg, Benedict's reagent, *Clinitest*®) is used, but this may be the result of ascorbic acid that is found in some parenteral formulations of tetracyclines.
- Tetracyclines have reportedly caused false-negative results in determining **urine glucose** when the glucose oxidase method (eg, *Clinistix*®, *Tes-Tape*®) is used.
- Minocycline may interfere with the fluorescence test for **urinary catecholamines**, causing falsely elevated values.

Dosages

NOTE: No clinical studies using IV minocycline were located. Considering minocycline's bioavailability, use of IV dosages at the lower end of the oral range appears to be reasonable. Doses administered IV should be given over at least 10 minutes.[33,34] Immediate-release formulations are used for oral dosages.

DOGS:

Susceptible infections (extra-label): Dosage information is derived from pharmacokinetic studies rather than clinical trials.[15,16,22,36] 5 – 10 mg/kg PO every 12 hours without food has been suggested. Practically, doses are rounded to the nearest 25 mg if using commercially available, solid, immediate-release dosage forms. 5 mg/kg PO every 12 hours has been recommended for dogs with respiratory disease.[37]

***E canis* infection** (extra-label): 5 – 10 mg/kg PO twice daily for 28 days[19,38]

Adjunctive treatment of canine heartworm disease (extra-label): If doxycycline is unavailable, use minocycline 10 mg/kg PO twice daily for 4 weeks (days 1 through 28 of the American Heartworm Society protocol) along with an approved heartworm preventive.[5,39]

Lyme borreliosis (extra-label): 10 mg/kg IV or PO once or twice daily for 30 days[12]

CATS:

Susceptible infections including respiratory tract infections (extra-label): Based on a pharmacokinetic study and typical bacterial MIC, 8.8 mg/kg PO every 24 hours.[23,37] Anecdotal dosing recommendations range from 5 – 25 mg/kg PO twice daily, whereas 5 – 12.5 mg/kg PO twice daily is commonly noted. Practically, 50 mg/cat (NOT mg/kg) PO every 24 hours is recommended.

HORSES:

Susceptible (MIC less than or equal to 0.25 µg/mL) nonocular infections (extra-label): Based on pharmacokinetic data, 4 mg/kg PO every 12 hours.[25,40] Oral absorption is improved if hay is withheld for 2 hours after administration.[28]

Monitoring

- Clinical efficacy: resolving signs of infection; culture and susceptibility testing if indicated
- Adverse effects (eg, nausea, vomiting)

Client Information

- Oral minocycline works best when given without food. If your animal vomits or acts sick after receiving the medicine on an empty stomach, try giving the next dose with a small amount of food or a treat.
- Do not give as a dry pill. Give this medicine with a moist treat or small amount of liquid to be sure it reaches the stomach. This is especially important in cats as minocycline may cause ulcers in the throat and esophagus if the pill gets stuck there before it reaches the stomach. If your animal has trouble swallowing or eating, contact your veterinarian immediately.
- Do not give antacids, including sucralfate, oral iron, and antidiarrheal medicine, within 2 hours before or after giving minocycline. These other medications will reduce the effectiveness of this antibiotic.
- This drug may make your animal's skin more sensitive to sunlight and increase the risk for sunburn on hairless areas (eg, nose, abdomen, around the eyelids and ears). Tell your veterinarian if you notice any reddening/sunburn on the skin while your animal is on this medication.
- For this medication to work, give it exactly as your veterinarian has prescribed. Always check the prescription label to be sure you are giving the drug correctly. Avoid missing doses and give the full course of medication as directed by your veterinarian even if your animal seems to be back to normal.
- Your veterinarian will need to monitor your animal while it is taking this medicine. Do not miss these important follow-up visits.

Chemistry/Synonyms

Minocycline HCl is a semisynthetic tetracycline that occurs as a yellow crystalline powder. It is soluble in water and slightly soluble in alcohol. Commercial minocycline dosage forms contain minocycline hydrochloride.

Minocycline may also be known as minocyclini hydrochloridum, *Arestin*®, *Minocin*®, or *Solodyn*®; many other trade names are available.

Storage/Stability

Store oral preparations at room temperature in tight containers. Do not freeze oral suspensions. The injectable should be stored at room temperature (20°C-25°C [68°F-77°F]) and protected from light, moisture, and excessive heat. After reconstitution with sterile water for injection, solutions with a concentration of 20 mg/mL are stable for 4 hours at room temperature or for 24 hours if refrigerated.

Compatibility/Compounding Considerations

Compatibility is dependent on factors such as pH, concentration, temperature, and diluent used; specialized references or a hospital pharmacist should be consulted for more specific information.

Minocycline lyophilized powder for injection should be reconstituted with 5 mL sterile water for injection and immediately further diluted with sodium chloride injection USP, dextrose injection USP, dextrose and sodium chloride injection USP, Ringer's injection USP, or lactated Ringer's injection USP. Minocycline is **incompatible** with most medications. If the same IV line is being used for sequential drug administration, the line should be flushed with saline before and after minocycline infusion.

Dosage Forms/Regulatory Status

VETERINARY-LABELED PRODUCTS: NONE

HUMAN-LABELED PRODUCTS:

Minocycline HCl Oral Tablets: 50 mg, 75 mg, and 100 mg; generic; (Rx)

Minocycline Extended-Release Tablets: 45 mg, 55 mg, 65 mg, 80 mg, 90 mg, 105 mg, 115 mg, and 135 mg; *Solodyn*®, generic; (Rx)

Minocycline HCl Oral Capsules: 50 mg, 75 mg, and 100 mg; generic; (Rx)

Minocycline HCl Pellet-Filled Oral Capsules: 50 mg and 100 mg; *Minocin*®; (Rx)

Minocycline HCl Powder for Injection: 100 mg in vials; *Minocin*®; (Rx)

Minocycline HCl Powdered Microspheres, Extended-Release, Dental: 1 mg; *Arestin*®; (Rx)

References

For the complete list of references, see **wiley.com/go/budde/plumb**

Mirtazapine

(mir-***taz***-ah-peen) *Remeron*®, *Mirataz*®

Tetracyclic Antidepressant; 5-HT_3 Antagonist

Prescriber Highlights

- Transdermal formulation is labeled for management of weight loss in cats. Also used in tablet form as an appetite stimulant and antiemetic in dogs and cats with chronic kidney disease (CKD).
- It can be used in conjunction with other antiemetics.
- Primary adverse effect is sedation. In cats, vocalization and increased affection can be noted. Serotonin syndrome is possible; check for drug interactions when administering with other medications.
- The lowest effective dose should be used to reduce sedative properties. Doses should not exceed 30 mg/day in dogs when using it for appetite stimulation.
- Gloves should be worn when handling transdermal mirtazapine. Humans and other animals in the household should avoid contact with the treated cat for at least 2 hours after transdermal administration.

Uses/Indications

Transdermal mirtazapine is indicated in the management of weight loss in cats[1]; the average weight gain in cats was 3.9% of body weight after a 2-week course of therapy.[2] Mirtazapine is an effective appetite stimulant and has antiemetic activity in cats with CKD.[3] Cats receiving mirtazapine tablets ingested significantly more food as compared with placebo. Food ingestion did not correlate with mirtazapine dose, but high doses (ie, 3.75 mg/cat [NOT mg/kg]) of mirtazapine were associated with noticeable behavior changes.[4] In cats with stage 2 or 3 chronic kidney disease, administration of compounded transdermal mirtazapine demonstrated an increased appetite and weight gain; this formulation may benefit cats in countries where the commercial product is not available.[5]

In a study of healthy dogs, mirtazapine accelerated gastric emptying and colonic transit without having an effect on small intestine transit.[6] Mirtazapine can also be used for the treatment of chemotherapy-induced nausea and vomiting.[7]

Pharmacology/Actions

The antidepressant activity of mirtazapine appears to be mediated by antagonism at central presynaptic alpha-2 receptors, which normally act as a negative feedback mechanism, inhibiting further norepinephrine (NE) release. By blocking these receptors, mirtazapine overcomes the negative feedback loop and causes a net increase in NE. This mechanism may also contribute to the appetitestimulating effects of the medication, as NE acts at other α receptors to increase appetite. In addition, mirtazapine antagonizes several serotonin (5-HT) receptor subtypes. The drug is a potent inhibitor of the 5-HT_2, 5-HT_3, and histamine (H_1) receptors. Antagonism at 5-HT_3 receptors accounts for the antinausea and antiemetic effects of the drug, and its action at H_1 receptors produces prominent sedative effects. It is a moderate peripheral α_1-adrenergic antagonist, a property that may explain the occasional orthostatic hypotension associated with its use; it is also a moderate antagonist of muscarinic receptors, which may explain the relatively low incidence of anticholinergic effects.

Pharmacokinetics

In a pilot study in healthy beagles, the mean clearance of mirtazapine was 1193 mL/kg/hour and the mean half-life was 6.17 hours after 20 mg/dog PO.[8]

After administration of oral mirtazapine at either 1.88 mg (low dose [LD]) or 3.75 mg (high dose [HD]) in a study of healthy cats, median elimination half-lives were 9.2 hours and 15.9 hours, respectively. Mean clearance was 10.5 mL/kg/minute (LD) and 18 mL/kg/minute (HD). A single LD of mirtazapine was well tolerated, and the half-life (9 hours) was compatible with 24-hour dose intervals in healthy cats. Mirtazapine does not appear to have linear kinetics in cats.[4] A study in cats with CKD (n = 6) found that the mean half-life was 15.2 hours and the mean oral clearance was 0.6 L/hour/kg.[9] The authors concluded that the results were compatible with administration every 48 hours in cats with CKD.[9] Liver disease delays time to peak concentration (4 hours vs 1 hour) and prolongs elimination half-life (14 hours vs 7 hours) in cats.[10]

Transdermal mirtazapine bioavailability in cats is ≈65%, and peak drug concentration is reached ≈16 hours after administration of a single dose and ≈2 hours after repeated administration.[11] Half-life is 21 to 27 hours,[11] although a shorter half-life (10 to 11 hours) may reflect both topical and oral (ie, grooming) exposure. In healthy cats, transdermal mirtazapine has been shown to reach a steady-state within 14 days. Transdermal time to maximum concentration is 6 hours, with a peak plasma concentration (C_{max}) of 32.1 ng/mL.

After a single PO dose of mirtazapine 2 mg/kg (fasted or fed) in horses, peak concentrations occurred at 2.2 hours (fasted) and 1.3 hours (fed) after administration. The mean residence time of mirtazapine was 6 to 7 hours, and elimination half-life was ≈4 to 5 hours. The authors concluded that mirtazapine might be amenable for long-term oral administration but obtaining additional information concerning safety and efficacy before it is used clinically is critical.[12]

Following oral administration in humans, mirtazapine is rapidly and completely absorbed, but oral bioavailability is ≈50%. C_{max} is reached within ≈2 hours after oral administration. Food has minimal effects on both the rate and extent of absorption and does not require dose adjustment. Plasma protein binding (PPB) for mirtazapine appears to be ≈70% to 72% in mice, rats, and dogs, whereas in humans and rabbits, it is ≈85%. Despite the interspecies differences in PPB, no displacement interactions or dose adjustments for mirtazapine are expected because of its large therapeutic window and nonspecific, relatively low affinity for plasma proteins. Mirtazapine is metabolized via multiple pathways and varies by species. In all species tested (ie, humans and laboratory animals), the drug is metabolized via the following mechanisms: 8-hydroxylation followed by conjugation, *N*-oxidation, and demethylation followed by conjugation. Humans and guinea pigs also produce metabolites via N^+-glucuronidation, whereas mice are the only species that have been found to use demethylation followed by CO_2 addition and conjugation and 13-hydroxylation followed by conjugation as methods of mirtazapine breakdown. These processes are conducted primarily by CYP2D6, CYP1A2, and CYP3A4, but mirtazapine exerts minimal inhibition on these cytochromes. Several metabolic pathways of mirtazapine involve conjugation with glucuronide (glucuronidation). Because cats have a limited capacity for glucuronidation, mirtazapine is cleared less rapidly from the system; therefore, extended dosing intervals may be required.

In humans, elimination occurs via urine (75%) and feces (15%). Renal impairment may reduce elimination by 30% to 50% as compared with normal subjects, and hepatic impairment may reduce clearance by up to 30%. The elimination half-life of mirtazapine ranges from 20 to 40 hours across age and gender subgroups, so dose increases should occur no more frequently than every 7 to 14 days. Females (both human and animal) of all ages exhibit significantly longer elimination half-lives than males (in humans, mean half-life of 37 hours for females versus 26 hours for males).

Contraindications/Precautions/Warnings

Mirtazapine is contraindicated in patients hypersensitive to it and in those that have received monoamine oxidase inhibitors (eg, selegiline) in the past 14 days. Transdermal mirtazapine should not be administered orally or in the eye.

Mirtazapine has been associated with orthostatic hypotension in humans and should, therefore, be used with caution in patients with known cardiac disease or cerebrovascular disease that could be exacerbated by hypotension. Patients with renal impairment, renal failure, or hepatic disease may require lower doses of mirtazapine and should be closely monitored while receiving mirtazapine. Mirtazapine has rarely been associated with hyponatremia in humans; caution should be used in patients receiving a diuretic or other medication that could decrease sodium levels.

In humans, abrupt discontinuation of mirtazapine after long-term administration has resulted in withdrawal symptoms, (eg, nausea, headache, malaise). In general, antidepressants may affect blood glucose concentrations because of their indirect effects on the endocrine system; caution should be used in patients with diabetes mellitus.

Mirtazapine exhibits very weak anticholinergic activity; consequently, vigilance should be used in patients that might be more susceptible to these effects (eg, those with urinary retention; prostatic hypertrophy; acute, untreated closed-angle glaucoma, or increased intraocular pressure; GI obstruction or ileus). Effects of mirtazapine may also be additive to anticholinergic medications.

Extra care should be taken in active animals, as mirtazapine may impair concentration and alertness. Although extremely rare, mirtazapine has been associated with blood dyscrasias in humans and should be used cautiously in patients with the pre-existing hematologic disease, especially leukopenia, neutropenia, and/or thrombocytopenia. Prolongation of the QT interval has been reported, and risk may increase with other QT-prolonging drugs.

Adverse Effects

Mirtazapine appears to be well tolerated in both dogs and cats at the appropriately prescribed dosages. In a study evaluating the adverse effects of mirtazapine in cats, the 10 most common adverse effects seen (listed from most frequent to least frequent) were vocalization (56%), agitation (31%), vomiting (26.2%), abnormal gait/ataxia (16.7%), restlessness (14.3%), tremors/trembling (14.3%), hypersalivation (13%), tachypnea (11.9%), tachycardia (10.7%), and lethargy (10.7%).[13] Only 1 cat that received a dose of 1.88 mg/cat (NOT mg/kg) dose had adverse effects, whereas 25 cats that received a dose of 3.75 mg/cat (NOT mg/kg) displayed adverse effects. Other adverse effects reported during the study included anorexia, disorientation, dyspnea, hypothermia, mouth breathing/panting, mydriasis, behavior changes, depression/sedation, fasciculations, hyperactivity, hypertension, pacing, dysphoria, inappropriate elimination, polyphagia, circling, discomfort, hiding, inappetence, seizures, and weakness.[13] Increases in liver enzymes have been reported in some cats receiving mirtazapine. Cats experienced more behavioral effects (vocalization, interactions) with 3.75 mg doses as compared with 1.88 mg doses.

Transdermal mirtazapine may cause application site reactions (eg, erythema, crusting/scabbing, residue) in ≈10% of cats.

Reproductive/Nursing Safety

Reproductive studies in rats, rabbits, and dogs have shown no evidence of teratogenicity. Additional studies in hamsters, rabbits, and rats have shown no evidence of fetal genetic mutation or reduction in parental fertility, although there were increases in postimplantation losses and pup deaths, as well as decreases in birth weight.

Mirtazapine is distributed in human breast milk and can be detected in the serum of breastfed infants; caution should be used in nursing dams.

Overdose/Acute Toxicity

Clinical signs associated with mirtazapine overdose include agitation, lethargy, vocalization, panting, and tremors; cats may also develop tachycardia and ataxia.

In humans, mirtazapine ingestion upwards of 10 times the therapeutic dose exhibits minimal toxicity, requiring no acute intervention and only 6 hours of observation. Similar effects were seen in patients receiving up to 30 times the recommended dose. However, serotonin syndrome is possible, and the package insert for mirtazapine recommends that activated charcoal be administered in addition to other standard monitoring activities in an overdose situation.

For patients that have experienced or are suspected of having experienced an overdose, consultation with a 24-hour poison consultation center specializing in providing veterinary-specific information is recommended. For general information related to overdose and toxin exposures, as well as contact information for poison control centers, refer to *Appendix.*

Drug Interactions

Mirtazapine is a substrate for several hepatic cytochrome P450 isoenzymes, including 2D6, 1A2, and 3A4. The following drug interactions have either been reported or are theoretical in humans or animals receiving mirtazapine and may be of significance in veterinary patients. Unless otherwise noted, use together is not necessarily contraindicated, but weigh the potential risks and perform additional monitoring when appropriate.

- BENZODIAZEPINES (eg, **diazepam, midazolam**): Concurrent use has minimal effects on mirtazapine blood levels, but use together may cause additive impairment of motor skills.
- BUPRENORPHINE: Concurrent use with mirtazapine may increase the risk for serotonin syndrome.
- BUTORPHANOL: Concurrent use with mirtazapine may increase the risk for serotonin syndrome.
- CIMETIDINE: May increase mirtazapine exposure
- CLONIDINE: Concurrent use with mirtazapine may cause increases in blood pressure.
- CNS DEPRESSANTS (eg, **acepromazine, antihistamines, gabapentin**): Concurrent use with mirtazapine may increase the risk for sedation and CNS depression.
- CYPROHEPTADINE: May negate the effects of mirtazapine
- DIURETICS (eg, **furosemide**): May increase the risk for hyponatremia
- ERYTHROMYCIN: May increase mirtazapine exposure
- KETOCONAZOLE: May increase mirtazapine exposure
- MONOAMINE OXIDASE INHIBITORS (MAOIs; eg, **amitraz, linezolid, methylene blue, selegiline**): Increased risk for serotonin syndrome when used concurrently with mirtazapine. Concurrent use or use within 14 days is contraindicated.
- OPIOIDS (eg, **morphine**): May increase the risk for hyponatremia, sedation, and CNS depression
- SEROTONERGIC AGENTS, MISCELLANEOUS (eg, **buspirone, metoclopramide, ondansetron, trazodone**): Concurrent use with mirtazapine increases the risk for serotonin syndrome.
- SELECTIVE SEROTONIN REUPTAKE INHIBITORS (SSRIs; eg, **fluoxetine, fluvoxamine**): Concurrent use with mirtazapine increases the risk for serotonin syndrome.
- TRICYCLIC ANTIDEPRESSANTS (eg, **amitriptyline, clomipramine**): Concurrent use with mirtazapine increases the risk for serotonin syndrome.
- TRAMADOL: Increased risk for serotonin syndrome when used concurrently with mirtazapine
- WARFARIN: May prolong prothrombin time (PT) when used concurrently with mirtazapine

Laboratory Considerations

- No specific concerns were noted.

Dosages

DOGS:

Appetite stimulant and/or antiemetic (extra-label): There is little data on mirtazapine pharmacokinetics or efficacy in dogs. Anecdotal dosages ranging from 3.75 – 30 mg/dog (depending on dog size; NOT mg/kg) PO every 24 hours have been suggested. Alternatively, 1.1 – 1.3 mg/kg PO every 24 hours.[14] Doses should not exceed 30 mg/dog (NOT mg/kg) PO once daily.

Chemotherapy-induced anorexia: 0.5 mg/kg PO every 24 hours[7]

CATS:

Management of weight loss (label dosage; FDA-approved): Using the transdermal formulation, apply 1.5-inch ribbon (≈2 mg/cat) to the inner pinna of the cat's ear every 24 hours for 14 days.[1] The person applying medication should wear gloves. Alternate application of ointment between the left and right inner pinnae of the ears.

Appetite stimulant and/or antiemetic (extra-label): **NOTE:** Higher initial doses are not more effective and have more adverse effects.

a) **Healthy cats**: 1.88 mg/cat (NOT mg/kg) PO every 24 hours.[4] Practically, ¼ of a 7.5 mg tablet or ⅛ of a 15 mg tablet PO every 24 hours

b) **Cats with chronic kidney or hepatic disease**: 1.88 mg/cat (NOT mg/kg) PO every 48 hours.[3,10] Practically, ¼ of a 7.5 mg tablet or ⅛ of a 15 mg tablet PO every 48 hours

Chemotherapy-induced anorexia: 0.5 mg/kg PO every 24 to 72 hours[7]

Monitoring

- Clinical efficacy measured by the following parameters: increased appetite, decreased episodes of vomiting, and weight gain
- Liver enzymes in cats
- Adverse effects (eg, behavior, sedation) and signs of serotonin

syndrome (eg, sedation, GI signs, vocalization, agitation, tremors, difficulty breathing, hyperactivity, hyperthermia)

Client Information

- This medicine may be given with or without food. If your animal vomits after receiving the medication on an empty stomach, give it with food or a small treat. If vomiting continues, contact your veterinarian.
- Mirtazapine is usually tolerated well in dogs. Contact your veterinarian if your cat develops side effects as the dose may need to be adjusted. Common side effects include vocalization, behavior changes, and tremors/shaking. Report excessive drowsiness or vocalization to your veterinarian.
- If your animal is receiving orally disintegrating tablets, make sure your hands are dry before handling the tablet. Place the tablet under the animal's tongue and hold the animal's mouth closed for several seconds to allow it to dissolve (should occur quickly). After the tablet has melted, offer the animal water.
- You should wear gloves when handling the transdermal formulation and dispose of them afterward in the regular trash. Be sure you understand how to give this medicine to your animal. Apply the medicine to the inner side of the ear flap and not into the ear canal. After applying the medication, wash your hands with soap and water. Caregivers should avoid contact with the treated area for 2 hours after administration, as the medicine can be absorbed through the skin.

Chemistry/Synonyms

Mirtazapine, a member of the piperazinoazepine group of compounds, is classified as an atypical tetracyclic antidepressant and is not chemically related to other antidepressants. Mirtazapine occurs as a white to creamy white crystalline powder that is slightly soluble in water.

Mirtazapine may also be known as 6-azamianserin, Org-3770, mepirzapine, and *Remeron*®; many trade names for international products are available.

Storage/Stability

Store mirtazapine transdermal ointment at 25°C (77°F) and use it within 30 days after opening.

Store the coated tablets and orally disintegrating tablets between 20°C and 25°C (68°F and 77°F), with excursions permitted between 15°C and 30°C (59°F and 86°F). Protect from light and moisture. The orally disintegrating tablets must be used immediately upon removal from the tablet blister and cannot be stored.

Compatibility/Compounding Considerations

Compounded preparation stability: Mirtazapine 10 mg/mL oral suspension can be compounded from commercially available tablets. Triturate 10 mirtazapine 30 mg tablets with 15 mL of *Ora-Plus*® and qs ad to 30 mL with *Ora-Sweet*®. The resulting suspension retains 90% potency for 90 days stored at both 5°C (41°F) and 25°C (77°F). Compounded mirtazapine suspensions should be protected from light and shaken well before use.[15]

Mirtazapine powder compounded into a transdermal *Lipoderm*® gel at concentrations of 1.88 mg/0.1 mL and 3.75 mg/0.1 mL did not reliably meet compendial standards for potency, as mirtazapine concentration within the gel varied by greater than 10% of target despite concerted efforts of the compounding staff.[5] Transdermal mirtazapine gel prepared by commercial compounding pharmacies have also demonstrated significant variation from the intended product concentration.[16]

Dosage Forms/Regulatory Status

VETERINARY-LABELED PRODUCTS:

Mirtazapine Transdermal Ointment: 100 mg/tube in 5 g tube (20 mg/1 g); *Mirataz*®, (Rx)

HUMAN-LABELED PRODUCTS:

Mirtazapine Oral Tablets: 7.5 mg, 15 mg, 30 mg, and 45 mg; *Remeron*®, generic; (Rx)

Mirtazapine Orally Disintegrating Tablets (ODT): 15 mg, 30 mg, and 45 mg; *Remeron SolTab*®, generic; (Rx). **NOTE**: Some generic ODTs may contain xylitol (unknown quantity).

References

For the complete list of references, see **wiley.com/go/budde/plumb**

Misoprostol

(mye-soe-***prost***-ole) *Cytotec*®

Prostaglandin Analogue

Prescriber Highlights

- ▶ Prostaglandin E1 analogue for treatment or prevention of GI lesions, especially those associated with aspirin therapy; may also be useful for reproductive purposes. Appears ineffective in prevention of glucocorticoid-induced lesions
- ▶ Contraindications include pregnant animals (but has been used in horses mid-gestation and intravaginally for cervical ripening) and nursing dams (diarrhea in the nursing offspring).
- ▶ Caution is advised in patients sensitive to prostaglandins or prostaglandin analogues.
- ▶ Adverse effects include GI distress (eg, diarrhea, abdominal pain, vomiting, flatulence) and potentially uterine contractions and vaginal bleeding in female dogs.
- ▶ The National Institute for Occupational Safety and Health (NIOSH) classifies misoprostol as a hazardous drug; use appropriate precautions when handling.

Uses/Indications

Misoprostol may be useful as primary or adjunctive therapy in *preventing* gastroduodenal ulceration in dogs, especially when caused or aggravated by NSAIDs.[1] Although misoprostol can be used for *treatment* of gastric ulcers, other drugs may be equally effective and better tolerated; it does not appear to be effective in reduction of gastric ulceration secondary to glucocorticoid therapy.[2-6] Misoprostol reduces basal gastric acid secretion in horses.[7]

There is limited evidence of efficacy for misoprostol in the treatment of atopic dermatitis in dogs.[8]

Misoprostol's effects on uterine contractility and cervical ripening make it effective as an adjunct treatment for reproductive indications (eg, abortifacient, pyometra) in multiple species.

Pharmacology/Actions

Misoprostol is a synthetic prostaglandin E_1 analogue. It has 2 main pharmacologic effects that make it a potentially useful agent in prevention of upper GI ulceration. It acts via direct action on parietal cells to inhibit basal and nocturnal gastric acid secretion as well as gastric acid secretions stimulated by food, pentagastrin, or histamine—pepsin secretion is decreased under basal conditions, but not when stimulated by histamine. Misoprostol also has a cytoprotective effect on gastric mucosa, likely by increasing production of gastric mucosa and bicarbonate and increasing turnover and blood supply of gastric mucosal cells. Misoprostol enhances mucosal defense mechanisms and healing in response to acid-related injuries.

Other pharmacologic effects include increased amplitude and frequency of uterine contractions, cervical thinning and relaxation, stimulation of uterine bleeding, and total or partial expulsion of uterine contents in pregnant animals.

Pharmacokinetics

Approximately 88% of an oral dose of misoprostol is rapidly absorbed from the GI tract in humans, but a significant amount is metabolized via the first-pass effect. The presence of food and antacids will delay the absorption of the drug. Misoprostol is rapidly de-esterified to misoprostol acid, which is the primary active metabolite. Misoprostol and misoprostol acid are equal in their effects on gastric mucosa.[9] Plasma protein binding of both misoprostol and the acid metabolite is between 81% and 89%.[10]

Misoprostol acid is further biotransformed via oxidative mechanisms to pharmacologically inactive metabolites. These metabolites, free acid, and small amounts of unchanged drug are principally excreted into the urine. In humans, the serum half-life of misoprostol is ≈30 minutes and its duration of pharmacologic effects is ≈3 to 6 hours.

Contraindications/Precautions/Warnings

Misoprostol is contraindicated in patients hypersensitive to it and during pregnancy. The misoprostol product label has a black-box warning against administration in pregnant women due to risk for abortion, premature birth, uterine rupture, or birth defects[11]; this drug should be used with caution in female veterinary patients with reproductive potential that may become pregnant.

Do not confuse miSOPROstol with miFEPRIStone.

The National Institute for Occupational Safety and Health (NIOSH) classifies misoprostol as a hazardous drug; personal protective equipment (PPE) should be used accordingly to minimize the risk for exposure.[12]

Adverse Effects

In humans, the most prevalent adverse effect seen with misoprostol is GI distress, which usually manifests as diarrhea, abdominal pain, vomiting, and flatulence.[11] Adverse effects are often transient and resolve over several days or may be minimized by dosage adjustment or giving doses with food. Potentially, uterine contractions and vaginal bleeding could occur in female dogs. See ***Contraindications/ Precautions/Warnings*** and ***Reproductive/Nursing Safety***.

Reproductive/Nursing Safety

Misoprostol may cause abortion, premature birth, uterine rupture, or birth defects (eg, skull and limb defects, facial malformations) and is contraindicated during pregnancy. However, in humans, it is used intravaginally for cervical ripening to induce labor when spontaneous labor and vaginal delivery is indicated. Misoprostol may impair fertility as pre- and postimplantation losses, and a significant decrease in the number of live pups were noted when high doses were given to male and female breeding rats.

In horses, a study[13] in midgestational pregnant mares given a 5-day course of oral misoprostol 5 µg/kg PO twice daily as a GI mucosal cytoprotectant during colic found that pregnancy was not disrupted and no adverse effects were noted. Cervical tone, ultrasonographic characteristics of the uterus, cervix and conceptus, and progesterone and estrone sulfate concentrations were similar before misoprostol treatment. The authors concluded that additional investigation of treatment at earlier and later stages of gestation, for longer term treatment, and evaluating neonates for developmental disturbances would add further information on safety of misoprostol during gestation.

Misoprostol acid is excreted in milk. Misoprostol is not recommended for lactating dams, as it could potentially cause significant diarrhea in nursing offspring.

Overdose/Acute Toxicity

There is limited information available. Overdoses in laboratory animals have produced diarrhea, GI lesions, emesis, tremors, focal cardiac, hepatic, or renal tubular necrosis, dyspnea, abdominal pain, sedation, tremors, fever, seizures, bradycardia, and hypotension.[11] GI distress (eg, vomiting, diarrhea, abdominal pain) is the most common clinical sign seen in dogs.

Overdoses should be treated seriously, and standard GI decontamination techniques should be employed when applicable. Resultant toxicity should be treated supportively and based on clinical signs.

For patients that have experienced or are suspected to have experienced an overdose, consultation with a 24-hour poison consultation center specializing in providing veterinary-specific information is recommended. For general information related to overdose and toxin exposures, as well as contact information for poison control centers, refer to ***Appendix.***

Drug Interactions

The following drug interactions have either been reported or are theoretical in humans or animals receiving misoprostol and may be of significance in veterinary patients. Unless otherwise noted, use together is not necessarily contraindicated, but weigh the potential risks and perform additional monitoring when appropriate.

- **Antacids, Magnesium-Containing**: Magnesium-containing antacids may aggravate misoprostol-induced diarrhea. If an antacid is required, an aluminum-only antacid may be a better choice. Antacids and food reduce the rate of misoprostol absorption and may reduce the systemic availability, but these probably do not affect therapeutic efficacy.
- **Oxytocin**: Misoprostol may enhance effects.
- **Phenylbutazone**: Concurrent use may result in neurosensory effects (eg, dizziness, ataxia).

Dosages

DOGS:

Prevention of aspirin-induced gastric injury (extra-label): 3 µg/kg PO every 8 to 12 hours. Efficacy appears similar with dosing intervals of every 8 hours and every 12 hours.[14,15]

Prevention of gastric injury caused by other NSAIDs (extra-label): No controlled studies documenting safety and efficacy were located and no clear evidence currently is available that supports any dosage in dogs.[5] Anecdotal dosage recommendations usually range from 2 – 5 µg/kg PO every 8 to 12 hours, although some have suggested that longer times between doses may be effective and that dosages above 3 µg/kg may be associated with more GI adverse effects.

Adjunctive therapy as an abortifacient (extra-label):

a) Aglepristone 10 mg/kg SC every 24 hours on 2 consecutive days and misoprostol 200 µg/bitch (NOT µg/kg) for bitches weighing less than or equal to 20 kg (44 lb) or 400 µg/bitch (NOT µg/kg) for bitches weighing more than 20 kg (44 lb) intravaginally once daily until completion of abortion. In a study, all bitches in the treatment group aborted within 6 days.[16]
b) Misoprostol 1 – 3 µg/kg administered as a vaginal suppository once daily to promote cervical dilation. This allows for a reduced dinoprost (PGF2alpha) dose of 0.1 mg/kg SC every 8 hours for 2 days, then 0.2 mg/kg SC every 8 hours to effect. Abortion usually occurs after 5 days.[17]

Pyometra and metritis (extra-label): Give aglepristone 10 mg/kg SC on days 1, 2, 8, 15, and 29. Give misoprostol 10 µg/kg PO twice daily on days 3 through 12. Approximately 75% of cases showed significant clinical improvement without developing the adverse effects associated with the prostaglandins (PGF2alpha, cloprostenol).[18]

Adjunctive therapy for atopic dermatitis (extra-label): Target dosage of 5 µg/kg PO 3 times daily. Modest improvement in clinical signs.[19] **NOTE**: This is not recommended as a first-choice therapy, and efficacy is questionable.

CATS:

GI adverse effects associated with NSAID use (extra-label): No controlled studies documenting safety or efficacy in cats were located. When adverse GI effects are observed in cats receiving NSAIDs, NSAID therapy should be withheld and appropriate supportive therapy introduced until any mucosal lesions have healed.[20] If NSAID therapy is reinstituted, it should be done so at the lowest effective dose, with consideration given to the concomitant use of misoprostol 5 µg/kg PO every 8 hours or omeprazole 0.7 – 1 mg/kg PO once daily and/or a different NSAID where licensing/approval permits.[20]

Adjunctive therapy as an abortifacient (extra-label): Aglepristone 10 mg/kg SC every 24 hours on 2 consecutive days and misoprostol 200 µg/queen (NOT mg/kg) PO every 12 hours until the start of abortion. In a study, treatments began on the same day; abortion began within ≈3 to 6 days of beginning treatment and were completed within ≈5 to 7 days of beginning treatment.[21] Misoprostol as a single agent was ineffective as an abortifacient.

HORSES:

GI mucosal cytoprotectant (extra-label): 5 µg/kg PO every 8 to 12 hours[7,13]

Equine glandular disease (extra-label): 5 µg/kg PO every 12 hours, 1 hour prior to feeding[22]

Inducing cervical relaxation (extra-label): From a case report of postbreeding endometritis in a maiden mare in which the cervix remained closed during estrus and acted as a barrier to uterine clearance[23]: After uterus was lavaged and catheter removed, misoprostol 1000 µg/mare (NOT µg/kg) as a compounded cream was applied to the caudal os and lumen of the cervix. Oxytocin 20 Units/mare (NOT µg/kg) IM was administered immediately following lavage and again every 6 hours until the following morning. Separately, a study using misoprostol 1000 µg/mare (NOT µg/kg) in 1.5 g of a compounded cream applied to the external cervical os failed to induce a measurable degree of cervical relaxation.[24]

Unexplained infertility (extra-label): 200 µg (total amount; NOT µg/kg) diluted in 3 mL sterile water and applied deep in the uterine horn, as close as possible to the papilla of the uterine tube; perform in each horn[25]

COWS:

Induction of parturition (extra-label): 200 – 400 µg/cow (NOT µg/kg) intravaginally every 6 hours to a maximum of 6 doses. Misoprostol tablets were moistened with drops of water prior to insertion.[26]

SHEEP:

Cervical relaxation (extra-label): May improve depth of cervical penetration when nonsurgical access to the uterus is needed.

a) 200 µg/ewe (NOT µg/kg) diluted in 1.5 mL 0.9% NaCl and applied directly to the cervix 5 hours prior to the procedure (eg, artificial insemination, embryo collection/transfer). NOTE: Ewes were also given cloprostenol 37.5 µg/ewe (NOT µg/kg) IM 12 hours prior to the procedure. Degree of cervical dilation improved when treatment was also combined with a compounded formulation of estradiol benzoate 100 µg/ewe (NOT µg/kg; diluted with 2.5 mL 0.9% NaCl and 2.5 mL ethanol) IV 12 hours prior and oxytocin 100 Units/ewe (NOT Units/kg) IV 15 minutes prior to cervical transposition.[27]
b) Misoprostol 1000 µg/ewe (NOT µg/kg) and terbutaline 5 mg/ewe (NOT mg/kg) combined and dissolved in 4 mL glycerol. The resulting mixture was filtered and applied vaginally near the cervix 6 hours prior to artificial insemination.[28]

Monitoring

- Efficacy based on indication for use
- Adverse effects (eg, vomiting, diarrhea, flatulence)
- Absence of pregnancy prior to initiating misoprostol therapy when it is being used for non-abortifacient indications.

Client Information

- Give this medicine with food if stomach upset occurs or to prevent stomach upset.
- Common side effects include diarrhea, abdominal/stomach pain, vomiting, and flatulence (ie, gas). These effects may only last a few days, and giving the drug with food may help, but if any of these effects are severe, get worse, or continue to be a problem, contact your veterinarian.
- This medicine is considered to be a hazardous drug because it may affect the reproductive ability of males or females actively trying to conceive, women who are pregnant or may become pregnant, as it can cause miscarriage, and women who are breastfeeding. It is recommended that you wear gloves when administering this medicine to your animal and wash your hands thoroughly afterwards. If you have questions about this medicine's hazards, please speak with your veterinarian or pharmacist.

Chemistry/Synonyms

Misoprostol, a synthetic prostaglandin E_1 analogue, occurs as a yellow, viscous liquid with a musty odor.

Misoprostol may also be known as SC-29333, *Arthrotec®*, or *Cytotec®*.

Storage/Stability

Misoprostol tablets should be stored in well-closed containers at room temperature of 25°C (77°F) or less.

Compatibility/Compounding Considerations

Misoprostol has been compounded into a variety of vehicles (eg, sterile water,[25] sterile saline solution,[27] glycerol,[28] gum acacia[29]) for inducing cervical relaxation. As stability and potency were not validated, these formulations should be prepared at the time of administration for 'immediate-use' only.

Dosage Forms/Regulatory Status

VETERINARY-LABELED PRODUCTS: NONE

The Association of Racing Commissioners International (ARCI) has designated this drug as a class 5 substance. See ***Appendix*** for more information. Use of this drug may not be allowed in certain animal competitions. Check rules and regulations before entering in a competition while this medication is being administered. Contact local racing authorities for further guidance.

HUMAN-LABELED PRODUCTS:

Misoprostol Tablets: 100 and 200 µg; *Cytotec®*, generic; (Rx)

References

For the complete list of references, see **wiley.com/go/budde/plumb**

Mitotane

(*mye*-toe-tane) *Lysodren®, o,p'-DDD*
Antineoplastic

Prescriber Highlights

- ▶ Adrenal cytotoxic agent used for medical treatment of pituitary-dependent hyperadrenocorticism in dogs and ferrets
- ▶ Caution with pregnancy, diabetes mellitus, and pre-existing renal or hepatic disease
- ▶ Adverse effects include lethargy, ataxia, weakness, anorexia, vomiting, and/or diarrhea; liver changes possible
- ▶ Relapses are not uncommon.
- ▶ All dogs receiving mitotane therapy should receive additional glucocorticoid supplementation if undergoing stress (eg, surgery, trauma, acute illness).
- ▶ Monitoring is mandatory.
- ▶ The National Institute for Occupational Safety and Health (NIOSH) classifies mitotane as a hazardous drug; use appropriate precautions when handling.

Uses/Indications

In veterinary medicine, mitotane is used primarily for the medical treatment of pituitary-dependent hyperadrenocorticism (PDH) when there are clinical signs present (eg, polyuria, polydipsia, polyphagia) that are consistent with this condition. Mitotane has also been used for the palliative treatment of adrenal carcinoma in humans and dogs.[1]

Approximately 80% of dogs with PDH respond to mitotane treatment.[1] However, trilostane is the preferred treatment of PDH, as retrospective studies[2-4] found no qualitative or statistical difference in survival times in dogs treated with mitotane or trilostane, and mitotane typically causes more adverse effects than trilostane.

In cats, mitotane is not recommended, as it is ineffective and may be poorly tolerated.[5]

Pharmacology/Actions

Although mitotane is considered an adrenal cytotoxic agent, it apparently can also inhibit adrenocortical function without causing cell destruction. The exact mechanisms of action for these effects are not clearly understood. Mitotane also inhibits several enzymes responsible for corticosteroid production.

In dogs with PDH, mitotane has been demonstrated to cause severe, progressive necrosis of the zona fasciculata and zona reticularis. These effects occur quite rapidly (usually within 5-10 days of starting therapy). It has been stated that mitotane spares the zona glomerulosa and therefore aldosterone synthesis is unaffected; however, this is only partially true as the zona glomerulosa may also be affected by mitotane therapy although it is uncommon for clinically significant effects on aldosterone production to be noted with therapy. Additionally, dogs with PDH that are treated with mitotane demonstrate decreased aldosterone secretion 30 and 60 minutes after ACTH stimulation compared to healthy controls.[6]

Pharmacokinetics

In dogs, the systemic bioavailability of mitotane is poor. Oral absorption can be enhanced by giving the drug with food (especially food high in oil/fat). In humans, ≈40% of an oral dose of mitotane is absorbed after dosing, with peak serum concentrations occurring ≈3 to 5 hours after a single dose. Distribution of the drug occurs to virtually all tissues in the body. The drug is stored in the fat and does not accumulate in the adrenal glands. A small amount may enter the CSF.

Mitotane has a very long plasma half-life in humans, ranging from 18 to 159 days. Serum half-lives may increase in a given patient with continued dosing, perhaps due to a depot effect from adipose tissue releasing the drug. The drug is metabolized in the liver and is excreted as metabolites in the urine and bile. Within 24 hours of dosing, ≈15% of an oral dose is excreted in the bile and 10% in the urine.

Contraindications/Precautions/Warnings

Mitotane is contraindicated in patients known to be hypersensitive to it. Mitotane should only be used to treat patients that have clinical signs *and* laboratory testing consistent with hyperadrenocorticism; it should never be administered to sick patients (eg, lethargy, inappetence).

Hepatic impairment may interfere with mitotane metabolism. Dogs with pre-existing renal or hepatic disease should receive the drug with caution and with more intense monitoring.

Patients with concurrent diabetes mellitus may have rapidly changing insulin requirements during the initial treatment period; closely monitor insulin requirements to avoid insulin overdose until effects of hyperadrenocorticism are controlled.

Some clinicians recommend giving prednis(ol)one at 0.2 mg/kg/day (0.4 mg/kg/day to diabetic dogs) PO during the induction treatment period to reduce the potential for adverse effects from acute endogenous steroid withdrawal.[7] Other clinicians have argued that routinely administering glucocorticoids masks the clinical markers that signify when the endpoint of therapy has been reached and that steroids must be withdrawn 2 to 3 days before ACTH stimulation tests can be done. The benefits of routine glucocorticoid administration may not be warranted because, in adequately observed patients, adverse effects requiring glucocorticoid therapy may only be necessary in 5% of patients.

When mitotane is prescribed, owners should always be provided a small supply of predniso(lo)ne or dexamethasone tablets so that they can initiate emergency treatment for Addisonian crisis if this occurs. Dexamethasone is the preferred corticosteroid for treatment, as it will not interfere with the ACTH stimulation test. If prednisone or prednisolone are used, an ACTH stimulation test cannot be accurately performed for at least 24 hours after administration because of cross reactivity of these drugs in cortisol assays.

The National Institute for Occupational Safety and Health (NIOSH) classifies mitotane as a hazardous drug; personal protective equipment (PPE) should be used accordingly to minimize the risk for exposure.[8]

Adverse Effects

The most common adverse effects seen with initial therapy in dogs include lethargy, ataxia, weakness, anorexia, vomiting, and/or diarrhea. Neurologic signs can be seen but are not common. Adverse effects are commonly associated with plasma cortisol concentrations of less than 1 µg/dL or a too rapid decrease of plasma cortisol concentrations into the normal range. Adverse effects may also be more commonly seen in dogs weighing less than 5 kg, which may be due to the inability to accurately dose mitotane because of limited tablet size availability. The incidence of one or more of these effects is ≈25%, and they are usually mild. If mild adverse effects are noted, it is recommended to halt mitotane therapy. If moderate to severe signs are noted (especially GI in nature; moderate to severe vomiting, and/or diarrhea), halt mitotane therapy and supplement with glucocorticoid therapy.

Mitotane decreases aldosterone secretory reserve.[9] Rarely, an Addisonian crisis can occur during therapy. Owners should be warned about this life-threatening complication and counseled on the clinical signs of an Addisonian crisis. If such signs occur, owners need to discontinue mitotane therapy, administer glucocorticoid replacement therapy, and seek veterinary care immediately.

Liver changes (congestion, centrilobular atrophy, and moderate to severe fatty degeneration) have been noted in dogs given mitotane.

Although not commonly associated with clinical signs, these effects may be more pronounced with long-term therapy or in dogs with pre-existing liver disease.

In ≈5% of dogs treated, long-term glucocorticoid and sometimes mineralocorticoid replacement therapy may be required. All dogs receiving mitotane therapy should receive additional glucocorticoid supplementation if undergoing a stressful event (eg, surgery, trauma, acute illness).

Relapses are not uncommon in dogs receiving mitotane for hyperadrenocorticism.

Reasons for treatment failure include misdiagnosis, adrenal tumors unresponsive to mitotane, loss of drug potency, administration of drugs that interfere with mitotane metabolism (eg, phenobarbital), or inadequate mitotane dose for that particular patient.

Reproductive/Nursing Safety

Mitotane crosses the placenta and is known to have caused preterm births and early pregnancy loss in humans.

Mitotane is excreted in human maternal milk and nursing is not recommended during mitotane therapy.

Overdose/Acute Toxicity

There are no specific recommendations regarding overdoses of mitotane. Because of the drug's toxicity and long half-life, emptying the stomach and administering charcoal and a cathartic should be considered after a recent ingestion. It is recommended that the patient be closely monitored; clinical signs associated with hypoadrenocorticism may require treatment with corticosteroids, mineralocorticoids, and IV fluids.

For patients that have experienced or are suspected to have experienced an overdose, it is strongly encouraged to consult with one of the 24-hour poison consultation centers that specialize in providing information specific for veterinary patients. For general information related to overdose and toxin exposures, as well as contact information for poison control centers, refer to ***Appendix.***

Drug Interactions

In humans, mitotane induces the CYP3A4 enzyme and may increase the metabolism of other drugs that are substrates of this cytochrome P450 enzyme system. The following drug interactions have either been reported or are theoretical in humans or animals receiving mitotane and may be of significance in veterinary patients. Unless otherwise noted, use together is not necessarily contraindicated, but weigh the potential risks and perform additional monitoring when appropriate.

- **CNS Depressant Drugs** (eg, **acepromazine, methocarbamol**): If mitotane is used concomitantly with drugs that cause CNS depression, additive depressant effects may be seen.
- **Dexamethasone**: Mitotane may reduce dexamethasone concentration.
- **Estrogens** (eg, **diethylstilbestrol [DES], estriol**): Mitotane may reduce estrogen concentration.
- **Fentanyl**: Mitotane may increase fentanyl metabolism.
- **Insulin**: Diabetic dogs receiving insulin may have decreased insulin requirements after starting mitotane therapy.
- **Itraconazole**: Mitotane may reduce itraconazole concentration; it is recommended to avoid this combination in humans.
- **Midazolam**: Mitotane may increase midazolam metabolism.
- **Phenobarbital**: Phenobarbital can induce enzymes and reduce the efficacy of mitotane; conversely mitotane can induce hepatic microsomal enzymes and increase the metabolism of phenobarbital.
- **Praziquantel**: Mitotane may reduce praziquantel concentration; it is recommended to avoid this combination in humans.
- **Rivaroxaban**: Mitotane may reduce rivaroxaban concentration; it is recommended to avoid this combination in humans.
- **Selegiline**: Mitotane may increase selegiline metabolism and result in loss of efficacy.
- **Spironolactone**: In dogs, spironolactone has been demonstrated to block the action of mitotane; it is recommended to use an alternate diuretic if possible.
- **Warfarin**: Mitotane may increase warfarin metabolism.

Laboratory Considerations

- Mitotane will bind competitively to thyroxine-binding globulin and decreases the amount of serum protein-bound iodine. Serum **total thyroxine (tT_4)** concentrations may be unchanged or slightly decreased, but free thyroxine (fT_4) concentrations remain in the normal range. Mitotane does not affect the results of the resin triiodothyronine uptake test.
- Mitotane can reduce the amount of measurable **17-OHCS** in the urine, which may or may not reflect a decrease in serum cortisol levels or adrenal secretion.

Dosages

DOGS:

Medical treatment of pituitary-dependent hyperadrenocorticism (bilateral adrenal hyperplasia) (extra-label): **NOTE**: Treatment with mitotane can be very complex and potentially serious adverse effects can occur. Use requires vigilance by the veterinarian and pet owner for monitoring therapy. The reader is advised to refer to the original references for more detail or to the review by Reine.[1] The following are synopses of published dosing protocols; choose one ONLY:

a) Induction phase: Mitotane 30 – 50 mg/kg/day PO with a meal once daily or divided every 12 hours for 7 to 10 days. If adverse effects (lethargy, vomiting, weakness, diarrhea) occur, discontinue mitotane and give glucocorticoids (prednis(ol)one at 0.15 – 0.25 mg/kg/day) until dog can be evaluated. If decreased appetite occurs, discontinue mitotane and evaluate with an ACTH stimulation test. Perform ACTH stimulation test at end of 10-day period or sooner if adverse effects occur. Goal is to have basal and post-ACTH cortisol between 1 and 5 µg/dL (normal basal level for most labs). If basal and post-ACTH cortisol falls below 1 µg/dL, temporarily suspend mitotane and supplement with glucocorticoids until circulating cortisol normalizes (usually 2 to 4 weeks, but may take several weeks to months). If basal or post-ACTH cortisol is above normal, continue daily mitotane and recheck ACTH stimulation tests at 5 to 10 days intervals until serum cortisol falls within normal resting range. Begin maintenance dose when desired cortisol concentrations are documented by ACTH stimulation testing. Mitotane given initially at 35 – 50 mg/kg per week in 2 to 3 divided doses. If adverse effects occur, discontinue mitotane and supplement with glucocorticoids until dog can be evaluated by serum electrolytes and ACTH stimulation test. If ACTH stimulation tests are above desired range, the maintenance dose can be cautiously increased. If dose increase fails to normalize clinical signs and cortisol levels, induction can be repeated.[10]

b) Initial dose: Mitotane 50 mg/kg divided every 12 hours. Glucocorticoids are not usually administered concurrently, but a small supply of prednis(ol)one should be made available to the owner for emergencies. Continue until water consumption decreases to less than 100 mL/kg/day, or until a decreased appetite, depression, diarrhea, or vomiting are observed. The time for clinical response is quite variable but most dogs respond within 3 to 7 days. At this point the dog should be re-evaluated and an ACTH stimulation test performed. Prednis(ol) one treatment (0.2 mg/kg/day) should be initiated in patients that are showing clinical signs of hypocortisolemia, until the results of the ACTH stimulation test are known. In patients that are not polydipsic prior to therapy, where water consumption cannot be monitored, and whose polydipsia is due to another cause (eg, diabetes mellitus), mitotane should be administered for a maximum of 5 to 7 days prior to ACTH stimulation testing. The goal of treatment is to have both the pre- and post-cortisol measurement in the normal resting range (2 - 6 µg/dL). Maintenance therapy: Mitotane 50 mg/kg every 7 to 10 days divided over multiple days is started once the ACTH stimulation test shows adequate suppression and prednis(ol)one therapy (if necessary) has been discontinued. Failure to use maintenance therapy will result in regrowth of the adrenal cortex and recurrence of clinical signs. Efficacy of maintenance therapy is monitored by an ACTH stimulation test after 1 month of maintenance treatment and then every 3 months. The dose of mitotane required for long-term maintenance is variable: 26 – 330 mg/kg/week.[11]

c) Intentionally causing complete destruction of the adrenal cortex as an alternative to the traditional mitotane treatment: Mitotane 75 – 100 mg/kg/day for 25 consecutive days, given in 3 to 4 doses per day with food. Lifelong prednisone at 0.1 – 0.5 mg/kg PO twice daily initially and mineralocorticoid therapy is begun at the start of mitotane therapy. Prednisone dose is tapered after completion of the 25 day protocol. Relapse is common and periodic ACTH stimulation testing is necessary. May be considerably more expensive than traditional therapy because of the expense associated with treating Addisonian dogs.[12]

d) Total adrenal ablation for management of Cushing's disease: Mitotane 100 mg/kg/day divided twice daily for 30 days. Supplemental cortisone acetate 2 mg/kg/day divided twice daily and fludrocortisone acetate 0.1 mg/4.5 kg (10 lb) of body weight PO once daily are begun on day 1 of mitotane therapy. Diet is supplemented with 1 – 5 g of sodium chloride per day. One week after induction phase with mitotane, cortisone acetate is reduced to 1 mg/kg/day. Electrolytes and ACTH stimulation test are performed at end of induction, every 6 months thereafter, and at any time the patient demonstrates signs of either hypo- or hyperadrenocorticism. This form of management requires close patient monitoring and lifelong daily therapy. Close attention during stress and nonadrenal illnesses required.[13]

Palliative medical treatment of adrenal carcinomas or medical treatment of adrenal adenomas (extra-label):

a) Mitotane 50 – 75 mg/kg PO in daily divided doses for 5 days then every other day for over 40 days. Smaller dog breeds may require up to 100 mg/kg/day. Beginning on the third day of treatment, supplement with predniso(lo)ne 0.4 mg/kg/day, fludrocortisone 0.0125 mg/kg/day, and salt 0.1 g/kg/day. If adverse effects occur, stop mitotane (but not supplemental corticosteroids) therapy and evaluate dog. After day 45, assess treatment by withholding the evening doses of prednis(ol)one and fludrocortisone and the re-evaluate the following morning. After initial therapy, continue mitotane 50 – 75 mg/kg PO once per week and predniso(lo)ne 0.1 – 0.2 mg/kg/day, fludrocortisone 0.0125 mg/kg/day, and salt for at least 6 months.[14]

b) Initially, mitotane 50 – 75 mg/kg PO in daily divided doses for 10 to 14 days.[15,16] May supplement with predniso(lo)ne 0.2 mg/kg/day. Stop therapy and evaluate dog if adverse effects occur. After initial therapy, run ACTH stimulation test (do not give prednis(ol)one the morning of the test). If basal or post-ACTH serum cortisol values are decreased, but still above the therapeutic end-point (less than 1 µg/dL), repeat therapy for an additional 7 to 14 days and repeat testing. If post-ACTH serum cortisol values remain greatly elevated or unchanged, increase mitotane to 100 mg/kg/day and repeat ACTH stimulation test at 7- to 14-day intervals. If ACTH continues to remain elevated, increase dosage by 50 mg/kg/day every 7 to 14 days until response occurs or drug intolerance ensues. Adjust dosage as necessary as patient tolerates or ACTH-responsive dictates. Once undetectable or low-normal post-ACTH cortisol levels are attained, continue mitotane 100 – 200 mg/kg/week in divided doses with glucocorticoid supplementation (predniso(lo)ne 0.2 mg/kg/day). Repeat ACTH stimulation test in 1 to 2 months. Continue at present dose if cortisol remains below 1 µg/dL. If cortisol increases to 1 – 4 µg/dL, increase maintenance dose by 50%. If basal or post-ACTH cortisol goes above 4 µg/dL, restart daily treatment of mitotane 50 to 100 mg/kg/day as outlined above. Once patient is stabilized, repeat ACTH stimulation tests at 3 to 6 month intervals.[17]

FERRETS:

Medical treatment of hyperadrenocorticism where surgery has not been performed or tumor has not been fully resected (extra-label): 50 mg per ferret (NOT mg/kg) PO once daily for 1 week, then 50 mg per ferret (NOT mg/kg) PO 2 to 3 times per week. Have a compounding pharmacy make 50 mg capsules. Capsules can be easily administered if coated with a substance such as *Nutrical*.[18,19] This treatment may no longer be recommended.

Monitoring

Initially and as needed (see ***Dosages***):

- Physical examination and history (including water and food consumption, weight)
- Reduction of clinical signs related to hyperadrenocorticism
- Adverse effects. A life-threatening adverse effect of mitotane therapy can be an Addisonian crisis (eg, vomiting, diarrhea, collapse, shock). Monitor closely during therapy for this potential complication; daily communication with the pet owner during the induction period of mitotane therapy (ie, the first 7 to 10 days) is recommended.
- ACTH stimulation testing: See ***Dosages*** for monitoring during induction phase of treatment. Once maintenance therapy is started, perform ACTH stimulation test after 1, 3, and 6 months; repeat every 3 months to monitor level of control (sooner if dog develops clinical signs). See ***Cosyntropin***.
- Periodic CBC and serum chemistry profile with electrolytes
- Blood pressure

Client Information

- Mitotane treatment requires intensive monitoring and close supervision by your veterinarian. Keep in close contact with your veterinarian while your animal is on this medication and report any concerns you may have as soon as possible. **Contact your veterinarian immediately if you notice any vomiting, diarrhea, poor appetite, low energy level, weakness, or stumbling.**
- The drug should be given with food.
- You will usually see positive effects (ie, animal eats, drinks, and urinates less) in 5 to 14 days after starting this medicine. Contact your veterinarian when this occurs so that your animal can be tested for completion of the initial phase of treatment.
- Your animal will need to be monitored closely while on this medication. Do not miss important follow-up visits.
- If your animal requires surgery or has been injured, be sure to tell your veterinarian that your animal has been taking this medication. Mitotane can decrease the body's ability to handle stress,

and medications such as prednisone may be needed during these times.

- Pregnant women should not handle this drug; others should wear disposable gloves whenever handling the drug.
- This medication is considered to be a hazardous drug as defined by the National Institute for Occupational Safety and Health (NIOSH). Talk with your veterinarian or pharmacist about the use of personal protective equipment when handling this medicine.

Chemistry/Synonyms

Mitotane, also commonly known in veterinary medicine as o,p'-DDD, is structurally related to the infamous insecticide, chlorophenothane (DDT). It occurs as a white, crystalline powder with a slightly aromatic odor. It is practically insoluble in water and soluble in alcohol.

Mitotane may also be known as CB-313, o,p'DDD, NSC-38721, WR-13045, *Lysodren*®, or *Lisodren*®.

Storage/Stability

Mitotane tablets should be stored at room temperature (15°C-30°C [59°F-86°F]) in tight, light-resistant containers.

Compatibility/Compounding Considerations

No specific information noted

Dosage Forms/Regulatory Status

VETERINARY-LABELED PRODUCTS: NONE

HUMAN-LABELED PRODUCTS:

Mitotane Tablets (scored): 500 mg; *Lysodren*®; (Rx)

References

For the complete list of references, see **wiley.com/go/budde/plumb**

Mitoxantrone

(mye-toe-***zan***-trone) *Novantrone*®

Antineoplastic

Prescriber Highlights

- Used to treat a variety of neoplastic diseases in dogs and cats
- Less risk for nephrotoxicity and less cardiotoxic than doxorubicin, but more myelosuppressive than doxorubicin
- Contraindications include hypersensitivity to the drug.
- Use with caution in patients with myelosuppression, concurrent infection, hyperuricemia or hyperuricuria, hepatic dysfunction, and in patients that have received prior cytotoxic drug or radiation exposure.
- Adverse effects include dose-dependent GI distress (eg, vomiting, diarrhea, anorexia), myelosuppression (primarily neutropenia), lethargy, and seizures (in cats).
- The National Institute for Occupational Safety and Health (NIOSH) classifies mitoxantrone as a hazardous drug; use appropriate precautions when handling.

Uses/Indications

Mitoxantrone may be used in the treatment of several neoplastic diseases in dogs and cats, including lymphoma, mammary adenocarcinoma, squamous cell carcinoma, renal adenocarcinoma, fibrosarcoma, thyroid or prostate carcinoma, anal sac adenocarcinoma, and hemangiopericytoma. When used with piroxicam, mitoxantrone has shown efficacy for treating transitional cell bladder carcinoma in dogs.[1-3] Mitoxantrone is commonly used in veterinary medicine as an alternative to doxorubicin in the presence of cardiac dysfunction, and may be a reasonable substitution in a CHOP protocol.[4,5] In dogs, mitoxantrone has limited value when used as a single agent for treatment of the first relapse of lymphoma[6]; however, it may be useful as part of a rescue protocol when combined with dacarbazine for resistant lymphoma.[7]

Mitoxantrone is less nephrotoxic than doxorubicin and may be a safer option in cats with renal insufficiency.

Pharmacology/Actions

Mitoxantrone is a DNA-reactive agent that binds in between DNA base pairs, causing crosslinks and strand breaks. Mitoxantrone also interferes with RNA synthesis and is a potent topoisomerase II inhibitor. Mitoxantrone is not cell cycle phase-specific but appears to be most active during the S phase.

Pharmacokinetics

Mitoxantrone is rapidly and extensively distributed after IV infusion. The highest concentrations of the drug are found in the liver, heart, thyroid, and red blood cells. Penetration into the CNS is low. In humans, it is ≈78% bound to plasma proteins. Mitoxantrone metabolism is poorly understood, but the drug's clearance is reduced in patients with hepatic impairment. Roughly 10% of the drug is excreted in the urine, and ≈25% in the feces. In humans, half-life is based on a 3-compartment model, and the drug can be detected for ≈5 days following administration secondary to the drug being taken up, bound, and then slowly released by tissues.

Contraindications/Precautions/Warnings

Mitoxantrone is contraindicated in patients with a history of hypersensitivity and should be used with caution in patients with myelosuppression, concurrent infection, hyperuricemia or hyperuricuria, or those that have received prior cytotoxic drug or radiation exposure. Use mitoxantrone with caution in patients with hepatic impairment and dose adjustment may be required.

One study in dogs receiving their first dose of mitoxantrone 5 mg/m^2 found that dogs weighing 10 kg (22 lb) or less were significantly more likely to develop grade 3 or grade 4 neutropenia than dogs over 10 kg (22 lb); a reduction of the initial dose can be considered for dogs weighing less than 10 kg (22 lb).[8]

Mitoxantrone is not for intrathecal use; severe injury can occur. In humans, congestive heart failure can occur during or long after therapy with mitoxantrone; cardiotoxicity risk increases with increasing cumulative dose.[9]

Mitoxantrone is considered an irritant (rarely, a vesicant) and care should be taken to avoid extravasation.[9]

The National Institute for Occupational Safety and Health (NIOSH) classifies mitoxantrone HCl as a hazardous drug; personal protective equipment (PPE) should be used accordingly to minimize the risk for exposure.

Mitoxantrone is considered a high-alert medication (medications that require special safeguards to reduce the risk for errors). Consider instituting practices such as redundant drug dosage and volume checking, and special alert labels.

Adverse Effects

In dogs and cats, adverse effects include dose-dependent GI distress (eg, nausea, vomiting, anorexia, diarrhea) and myelosuppression, which can lead to infection and sepsis. Neutropenia has been established as the dose-limiting toxicity in dogs.[8,10,11] Nonregenerative anemias may be detected, and white cell nadirs generally occur on day 7 to 10. Some evidence exists that by giving recombinant granulocyte-colony stimulating factor, myelosuppression severity and duration may be reduced.[12] Lethargy may also be noticed. Some cats receiving this drug have developed seizures. Many dogs receiving chemotherapy will have minor hair coat changes (eg, shagginess, loss of luster). Breeds with continuously growing hair coats (eg, poodles, terriers, Afghan hounds, or Old English sheepdogs) are more likely to experience significant alopecia.

Unlike doxorubicin, cardiotoxicity has not yet been reported in dogs and rarely occurs in humans. Other adverse effects less frequently or rarely noted in humans and possible in dogs include conjunctivitis, jaundice, renal failure, seizures, allergic reactions, cough or dyspnea, thrombocytopenia, bleeding or bruising, and irritation or phlebitis at the injection site. Tissue necrosis associated with extravasation has only been reported in a few human cases.

Reproductive/Nursing Safety

In humans, mitoxantrone is excreted in maternal milk and significant concentrations (18 ng/mL) have been reported for 28 days after the last administration.[9] Because of the potential for serious adverse effects in offspring, it is recommended to use milk replacer if mitoxantrone is administered. For sexually intact patients, verify pregnancy status prior to administration.

Because safety has not been established in animals, this drug should only be used when the maternal benefits outweigh the potential risks to offspring.

Overdose/Acute Toxicity

The LD_{50} following IV administration to mice is 66 mg/kg. Because of the potential serious toxicity associated with this agent, dosage determinations must be made carefully. No specific antidote is known; treatment is supportive. Reported effects after an overdose in dogs include neutropenia, thrombocytopenia, anemia, diarrhea, anorexia, vomiting, lethargy, nausea, and death.[13]

For patients that have experienced or are suspected to have experienced an overdose, consultation with a 24-hour poison consultation center specializing in providing veterinary-specific information is recommended. For general information related to overdose and toxin exposures, as well as contact information for poison control centers, refer to ***Appendix***.

Drug Interactions

Mitoxantrone is a substrate for ABCB1 (P-glycoprotein) and ABCG2 and it is likely that there are other interacting drugs yet to be identified. The following drug interactions have either been reported or are theoretical in humans or animals receiving mitoxantrone and may be of significance in veterinary patients. Unless otherwise noted, use together is not necessarily contraindicated, but weigh the potential risks and perform additional monitoring when appropriate.

- **Cyclosporine**: May increase mitoxantrone's toxic effects
- **Doxorubicin**, **Daunorubicin**, or **Radiation Therapy**: Cardiotoxicity risks may be enhanced in patients that have previously received doxorubicin, daunorubicin, or radiation therapy to the mediastinum.
- **Immunosuppressive Drugs** (eg, **azathioprine, cyclophosphamide, corticosteroids**): Use with other immunosuppressant drugs may increase the risk for infection.
- **Myelosuppressive Agents** (eg, **antineoplastics, immunosuppressants, iron chelators**): Concurrent use with other myelosuppressive drugs may result in additive myelosuppression; avoid combination when possible.
- **Vaccines** (live and inactivated): Mitoxantrone may diminish vaccine efficacy and enhance adverse effects of vaccines.

Laboratory Considerations

- Mitoxantrone may raise serum **uric acid** concentrations. Drugs such as allopurinol may be required to control hyperuricemia.
- **Liver function tests** may become abnormal, indicating hepatotoxicity.
- Mitoxantrone may discolor **urine** to a green-blue color.

Dosages

NOTE: Because of the potential toxicity of this drug to patients, veterinary personnel, and clients, and because chemotherapy indications, treatment protocols, monitoring and safety guidelines often change, the following dosages should be used only as a general guide. Consultation with a veterinary oncologist and referral to current veterinary oncology references[14-18] are strongly recommended.

DOGS:

Treatment of susceptible neoplastic diseases (extra-label): Used in chemotherapy protocols with other chemotherapeutic agents; commonly dosed at 5 – 6 mg/m^2 (NOT mg/kg) IV once every 21 days.[4-7,19-21] Must be diluted in 0.9% sodium chloride or 5% dextrose prior to administration and should be infused over a minimum of 5 minutes. Consider using a lower first dose for dogs weighing 10 kg (22 lb) or less due to increased risk for severe neutropenia.[8]

CATS:

Treatment of neoplastic diseases (extra-label): 5.5 – 6.5 mg/m^2 (NOT mg/kg) IV once every 21 days.[22] Must be diluted in 0.9% sodium chloride or 5% dextrose prior to administration, and should be infused over a minimum of 5 minutes

Monitoring

- Efficacy: tumor or lymph node measurements, thoracic or abdominal imaging
- Baseline and periodic CBC, serum chemistry profile, and urinalysis:
  - CBCs should be performed weekly early in therapy and eventually every 4 to 6 weeks when stabilized.
  - Frequency of CBC and serum chemistry profile monitoring depends on protocol employed. Consultation with a veterinary oncologist is recommended.
  - Consider serum uric acid concentrations for susceptible patients
- Monitor for clinical signs of toxicity (eg, vomiting, diarrhea, inappetence, fever)

Client Information

- Mitoxantrone is a chemotherapy (anticancer) medicine. It can be harmful to other animals and people that come in contact with it. This medicine may be detected in urine up to 6 days, and in feces up to 7 days after your animal receives it. On the day your animal gets the medicine and then for a few days afterward, all bodily waste (ie, urine, feces, litter), blood, or vomit should only be handled while wearing disposable gloves. Seal the waste in a plastic bag, then place both the bag and gloves in with the regular trash.
- A blue-green color urine or a bluish color to the whites of the eyes can be seen but is not a problem.
- This medicine can affect your animal's ability to fight infection (bone marrow suppression). The greatest effects on the bone marrow usually occur within a few weeks after treatment. Your veterinarian will need to do blood tests on your animal while it is taking this medicine. Do not miss these important follow-up visits.
- Mitoxantrone can be toxic to the gastrointestinal tract and cause vomiting and gastrointestinal upset. Contact your veterinarian immediately if your animal has any bleeding, bruising, shortness of breath, vomiting, diarrhea, lack of an appetite, fever (indicating an infection), or if your animal becomes very tired easily.
- This medicine is considered to be a hazardous drug as defined by the National Institute for Occupational Safety and Health (NIOSH). Talk with your veterinarian or pharmacist about the safe handling of this medicine.

Chemistry/Synonyms

Mitoxantrone HCl is a synthetic anthracenedione antineoplastic. It occurs as a dark-blue powder that is sparingly soluble in water, practically insoluble in acetone, acetonitrile, and chloroform, and slightly soluble in methyl alcohol.

Mitoxantrone may also be known as: L-232315, DHAD, dihydroxyanthracenedione dihydrochloride, mitoxantroni hydrochloridum, NSC-301739, or *Novantrone*®.

Storage/Stability

Mitoxantrone HCl should be stored between 20°C and 25°C (68°F-77°F). Store multidose vials no longer than 7 days at room temperature and no longer than 14 days under refrigeration.[9] Although the manufacturer recommends not to freeze this drug, one study demonstrated that the drug maintained its cytotoxic effects when frozen and thawed at various intervals over a 12-month period.[23] Do not mix or use the same IV line with heparin infusions (precipitate may form). It is not recommended to mix this drug with other IV drugs.

Compatibility/Compounding Considerations

Compatibility is dependent on factors such as pH, concentration, temperature, and diluent used; specialized references or a hospital pharmacist should be consulted for more specific information.

Compatible for dilution with 0.9% sodium chloride or 5% dextrose. Do not mix or use the same IV line with heparin infusions (precipitate may form). It is recommended to not mix with other IV drugs.

Dosage Forms/Regulatory Status

VETERINARY-LABELED PRODUCTS: NONE

HUMAN-LABELED PRODUCTS:

Mitoxantrone HCl for Injection Solution Concentrate: 2 mg/mL, preservative-free in 10 mL, 12.5 mL, and 15 mL multi-dose vials; generic; (Rx)

References

For the complete list of references, see **wiley.com/go/budde/plumb**

Molybdates
Ammonium Molybdate
Ammonium Tetrathiomolybdate
Choline Tetrathiomolybdate
Sodium Molybdate

(moe-***lib***-dates) Molypen®

Copper Toxicosis Treatment

Prescriber Highlights

- Used primarily to treat copper toxicosis in food animals (especially sheep)
- May be useful in the treatment of copper-associated chronic hepatopathy in dogs
- Consider contacting FDA Center for Veterinary Medicine (CVM) for guidance in treating food animals

Uses/Indications

Molybdates are used for the investigational or compassionate treatment of copper toxicosis in food animals, primarily sheep.[1,2] A 12-week study demonstrated that oral administration of ammonium tetrathiomolybdate (TTM) to dogs with copper-associated chronic hepatopathy can effectively lower hepatic copper concentrations[3]; however, further investigation is needed to determine the long-term safety and efficacy of this treatment as compared with established therapies (eg, d-penicillamine).

Pharmacology/Actions

Molybdates are chelating agents that irreversibly bind and promote the excretion of copper. They also prevent intestinal copper absorption by binding copper in the GI tract.[4]

Pharmacokinetics

A study on ammonium tetrathiomolybdate (TTM) reported the following pharmacokinetic information after single IV and oral dosing of 1 mg/kg in dogs: oral bioavailability was 21 ± 22%, Vdss was 1 L/kg, and half-life was ≈27 hours.[5] TTM has high affinity for hepatocytes in other species and a high first-pass effect may be responsible for the low relative drug exposures in the study. Elimination characteristics described in the study suggested that a long dosing interval may be appropriate. The study also found that pretreatment with maropitant to dogs that had a history of vomiting with TTM treatment might have resulted in an increase in the bioavailability of TTM and could prove useful in preventing emesis and improving TTM efficacy. Both maropitant and TTM are highly protein-bound substances and are hepatically metabolized and eliminated. The study authors concluded that the increased serum copper concentrations observed in response to TTM were suggestive of mobilization of tissue copper stores, but more investigation is needed.

One study of TTM in sheep found a volume of distribution of 0.8 L/kg and serum elimination half-life of ≈7 hours.[6]

Adverse Effects

After apparent successful treatment for copper toxicosis with ammonium tetrathiomolybdate (TTM), a flock of sheep became infertile and progressively unthrifty and died 2 to 3 years later. The authors concluded the TTM was retained in the CNS, pituitary glands, and adrenal glands and caused a toxic endocrinopathy.[7] Increased AST was observed in dairy goats with copper toxicosis that were treated with ammonium molybdate, penicillamine, and sodium thiosulfate.[8]

Molybates are usually well tolerated by dogs; vomiting is the most common adverse effect seen.[5] One dog developed anorexia, lethargy, and presumed immune-mediated hemolytic anemia (IMHA) and thrombocytopenia during the 11th week of TTM treatment, but it remains undetermined whether IMHA was a direct result of TTM use.[3] Substantial hepatic molybdenum accumulation occurs with treatment in dogs, although the clinical significance of this finding is unknown.[3]

Reproductive/Nursing Safety

Ammonium molybdate is secreted in the breast milk in substantial amounts in humans.[9] Because safety has not been established in animals, this drug should only be used when the maternal benefits outweigh the potential risks to offspring.

Dosages

DOGS:

Copper-associated chronic hepatopathy (extra-label):

Ammonium <u>tetrathiomolybdate</u> (TTM): ≈0.5 mg/kg PO 4 times daily; from a 12-week safety and efficacy study, the administered dose was between 0.4 – 0.7 mg/kg.[3]

FOOD ANIMALS:

Copper toxicosis (extra-label):

Ammonium <u>molybdate</u>:

a) 50 – 500 mg/animal (NOT mg/kg) PO once daily in combination with sodium thiosulfate 300 – 1000 mg/animal (NOT mg/kg) PO once daily for 3 weeks[10,11]
b) 500 mg/animal (NOT mg/kg) PO once daily in combination with sodium thiosulfate 1000 mg/animal (NOT mg/kg) PO once daily for 5 days[12]
c) 200 mg/animal (NOT mg/kg) PO once daily for 3 weeks[13]

Ammonium <u>tetrathiomolybdate</u> (TTM):

a) 235 mg/calf (≈1 mg/kg) in 7 mL 0.9% sodium chloride SC every other day for 3 doses[14]
b) 2 – 15 mg/kg IV every 24 hours for 3 to 6 days.[15] **NOTE**: Until more is known about the significance of TTM cuproenzyme

inhibition, it is recommended that it be used conservatively (eg, 1 mg/kg IV once). Dose could be repeated if there is recurrence of prehemolytic copper toxicosis. Reduction in available copper in dietary supply is necessary. Zinc 150 mg/kg (route not stated) may be useful along with the antagonists, molybdate, and sulfate.[16]

Sodium molybdate: 200 mg/animal (NOT mg/kg) per day PO in combination with removal of copper-containing supplements[17]

SHEEP:

Copper toxicosis (extra-label):

Ammonium molybdate: 3.4 mg/kg SC every other day (ie, every 48 hours) for 3 doses[1]

Ammonium tetrathiomolybdate (TTM): 1.7 – 3.4 mg/kg SC every other day (ie, every 48 hours) for 3 doses[16]

GOATS:

Copper toxicosis (extra-label):

Ammonium molybdate: 300 mg/animal (NOT mg/kg) PO every 24 hours in combination with penicillamine 50 mg/kg and sodium thiosulfate 300 mg/animal (NOT mg/kg) PO every 24 hours[8]

Monitoring

- Baseline and periodic liver enzymes
- Copper concentration: serum, hepatic (requires biopsy)

Chemistry/Synonyms

Ammonium molybdate is an inorganic salt that occurs as odorless white crystals. Ammonium tetrathiomolybdate (TTM) occurs as a red crystalline powder. Specific solubility information was not located, but anecdotally, ammonium molybdate is more water-soluble than is TTM.

Ammonium molybdate may also be known as *Molybdene®* or *Molypen®*. Ammonium tetrathiomolybdate may also be known as TTM and tiomolibdate diammonium.

Dosage Forms/Regulatory Status

VETERINARY-LABELED PRODUCTS: NONE

HUMAN-LABELED PRODUCTS: NONE

NOTE: Ammonium molybdate or ammonium tetrathiomolybdate (TTM) can be obtained from various chemical supply houses. There are no FDA-approved products, but the FDA has historically used discretion in enforcement when molybdate is used for copper toxicosis in animals. It is recommended to contact the FDA Center for Veterinary Medicine (CVM) before treating for guidance.

In food animals, FARAD recommends a minimum 10-day preslaughter withdrawal time and a minimum 5-day milk withholding interval.[18]

References

For the complete list of references, see **wiley.com/go/budde/plumb**

Montelukast

(mon-teh-***loo***-kast) *Singulair®*

Leukotriene Antagonist

Prescriber Highlights

- Potentially useful in cats for feline asthma, IBD, upper respiratory disease, and heartworm-associated respiratory disease syndrome; however, there is limited evidence to support use in this species and limited clinical experience in veterinary species
- No significant adverse effects reported in cats

Uses/Indications

In veterinary medicine, montelukast has been used primarily in cats. Potential indications include feline asthma, atopy, upper respiratory disease, inflammatory bowel disease, and heartworm disease. Its use in treating feline asthma has been disappointing, and few clinicians recommend it for this purpose. At the time of writing, there was only anecdotal evidence for efficacy of this class of drugs in cats. A small trial in horses with recurrent airway obstruction (RAO) did not show efficacy.[1]

In humans, montelukast is FDA-approved for allergic rhinitis and asthma. It is used off-label in humans for atopic dermatitis, urticaria (chronic and NSAID-induced), and eosinophilic esophagitis.

Pharmacology/Actions

Montelukast is a leukotriene antagonist that inhibits at the cysteinyl leukotriene (CysLT1) receptor. The cysteinyl leukotrienes (ie, LTC4, LTD4, LTE4) are proinflammatory products of arachidonic acid metabolism released from certain cells, including mast cells and eosinophils.

Pharmacokinetics

No pharmacokinetic information for montelukast in cats was located.

In humans, oral bioavailability is 64% and peak concentrations occur 3 to 4 hours after dosing.[2] The presence of food does not affect bioavailability. Montelukast is highly bound (99%+) to human plasma proteins. It is extensively metabolized in the liver via cytochrome P450 isoenzymes CYP3A4, CYP2A6, and CYP2C9. Based on in vitro studies in human liver microsomes, therapeutic plasma concentrations of montelukast do not inhibit CYP450 isoenzymes 3A4, 2C9, 1A2, 2A6, 2C19, or 2D6. Metabolites are excreted primarily in the bile and eliminated in the feces. In healthy young adults, plasma half-life is ≈4 hours.

Contraindications/Precautions/Warnings

Montelukast is contraindicated in patients that are hypersensitive to it. Humans are warned not to use it to attempt to reverse acute bronchospasm.[2]

Adverse Effects

No adverse effects were noted for montelukast in cats, but the drug has not been extensively studied or used in cats.

In humans, the drug is usually well tolerated with minimal adverse effects reported. Rarely, behavioral effects (eg, aggression, suicidal thoughts), palpitations, cholestatic hepatitis, and allergic granulomatous angiitis have been reported.[2]

Reproductive/Nursing Safety

Montelukast appears safe to use during pregnancy. No teratogenicity was observed in rats at oral dosages up to 100 times the recommended human dose, or in rabbits at 110 times the recommended human dose.[2]

Although studies in rats have shown that montelukast is excreted in milk, data from breastfeeding women suggest the drug is safe to use during nursing.[2]

Because safety has not been established in animals, this drug should only be used when the maternal benefits outweigh the potential risks to offspring.

Overdose/Acute Toxicity

Montelukast is relatively safe in overdose situations. Rats and mice survived oral doses of ≈230 times and 335 times the recommended human adult dose, respectively. Cases of human adults and children receiving doses as high as 1000 mg have been reported and the majority of overdoses had no adverse effects. The most frequent adverse effects observed in humans are headache, vomiting, psychomotor hyperactivity, thirst, somnolence, mydriasis, hyperkinesia, and abdominal pain. Treatment is supportive.

For patients that have experienced or are suspected to have expe-

rienced an overdose, consultation with a 24-hour poison consultation center specializing in providing veterinary-specific information is recommended. For general information related to overdose and toxin exposures, as well as contact information for poison control centers, refer to ***Appendix***.

Drug Interactions

The following drug interactions have either been reported or are theoretical in humans receiving montelukast and may be of significance in veterinary patients. Unless otherwise noted, use together is not necessarily contraindicated, but weigh the potential risks and perform additional monitoring when appropriate.

- **CYP450 Enzyme Inducers** (eg, **phenobarbital, rifampin**): May reduce the montelukast plasma concentrations and efficacy
- **Gemfibrozil**: May increase montelukast concentration

Laboratory Considerations

- None were noted.

Dosages

CATS:

Adjunctive treatment of feline asthma, allergic rhinitis, mild cases of IBD, atopy, or feline heartworm (extra-label): There is no clear evidence that montelukast is effective for any of these indications. Anecdotal dosages are 0.25 – 1 mg/kg PO once daily. Practically, this would be ⅛ to ¼ of a 10 mg tablet per cat PO once daily.

Monitoring

- Clinical efficacy

Client Information

- This medicine may be given with or without food. Food may help if the animal vomits or acts sick after getting the drug. If vomiting continues, contact your veterinarian.
- Montelukast does not reverse an active asthma attack and it is not useful for immediate treatment of asthma.
- No significant side effects were reported when montelukast was used in cats, but the drug has not been used in many cats. Contact your veterinarian if any new problems or side effects occur after starting this medication.

Chemistry/Synonyms

Montelukast is a cyclopropaneacetic acid derivative leukotriene inhibitor. It is freely soluble in ethanol, methanol, and water.

Montelukast may also be known as MK-476, L-706631, or montelukastum.

Storage/Stability

Store tablets or granules at room temperature; excursions are permitted between 15°C and 30°C (59°F-86°F). Protect from moisture and light.

Compatibility/Compounding Considerations

No specific information was noted.

Dosage Forms/Regulatory Status

VETERINARY-LABELED PRODUCTS: NONE

The Association of Racing Commissioners International (ARCI) Uniform Classification Guidelines for Foreign Substances (UCGFS) Class 4 Drug. Use of this drug may not be allowed in certain animal competitions. Check rules and regulations before entering in a competition while this medication is being administered. Contact local racing authorities for further guidance. See ***Appendix*** for more information.

HUMAN-LABELED PRODUCTS:

Montelukast Sodium Oral Tablets: 4 mg (chewable), 5 mg (chewable), and 10 mg; *Singulair®*, generic; (Rx)

Montelukast Sodium Oral Granules: 4 mg/packet; *Singulair®*, generic; (Rx)

References

For the complete list of references, see **wiley.com/go/budde/plumb**

Morantel

(mor-***an***-tel) *Rumatel®*

Antiparasitic Agent

Prescriber Highlights

- ▶ Infrequently used anthelmintic that is available as a medicated feed for cattle and goats
- ▶ Use with caution in severely debilitated animals.
- ▶ Adverse effects are uncommon.
- ▶ Clinical signs of overdose include increased respiratory rate, profuse sweating, ataxia, or other cholinergic effects.

Uses/Indications

Morantel is an FDA-approved Type A medicated feed that is labeled for the removal and control of mature forms of *Haemonchus* spp, *Ostertagia* spp, *Trichostrongylus* spp, *Nematodirus* spp, *Cooperia* spp, and *Oesophagostomum radiatum* in cattle. In goats, it is indicated for the removal and control of mature *Haemonchus contortus, Ostertagia (Teladorsagia) circumcincta*, and *Trichostrongylus axei*.

Pharmacology/Actions

Morantel is a depolarizing neuromuscular blocking agent that paralyzes susceptible parasites, similar to pyrantel. It possesses nicotine-like properties and acts similarly to acetylcholine. Morantel also inhibits fumarate reductase in *Haemonchus* spp.

Morantel has a slower onset of action than pyrantel but is ≈100 times as potent.

Pharmacokinetics

After oral administration, morantel is absorbed rapidly from the upper abomasum and small intestine. Peak concentrations occur ≈4 to 6 hours after dosing. The drug is promptly metabolized in the liver. Within 96 hours of administration, 17% of the drug is excreted in the urine, with the remainder in the feces.

Contraindications/Precautions/Warnings

There are no absolute contraindications for use.

Morantel should be used with caution in severely debilitated animals.[1] Do not underdose morantel, as underdosing can result in ineffective treatment and lead to development of parasite resistance.

Adverse Effects

At recommended dosages, adverse effects are uncommon.

Reproductive/Nursing Safety

Morantel is generally considered safe to use during pregnancy.

Overdose/Acute Toxicity

Morantel tartrate has a large safety margin. In cattle, doses of up to 200 mg/kg (20 times the recommended dose) resulted in no toxic reactions. The LD_{50} in mice is 5 g/kg. Clinical signs of toxicity that might possibly be seen include increased respiratory rates, profuse sweating (in species with sweat glands), ataxia, or other cholinergic effects.

Chronic toxicity studies have been conducted in cattle and sheep. Four times the recommended dose of morantel was given to sheep with no detectable deleterious effects. Cattle receiving 2.5 times the recommended dose for 2 weeks showed no toxic signs.

For patients that have experienced or are suspected to have experienced an overdose, consultation with a 24-hour poison consultation center specializing in providing veterinary-specific information

is recommended. For general information related to overdose and toxin exposures, as well as contact information for poison control centers, refer to ***Appendix***.

Drug Interactions

The following drug interactions have either been reported or are theoretical in animals receiving morantel and may be of significance. Unless otherwise noted, use together is not necessarily contraindicated, but weigh the potential risks and perform additional monitoring when appropriate.

- **Bentonite**: Do not add morantel to feeds containing bentonite.
- **Levamisole, Pyrantel**: Because of similar mechanisms of action (and toxicity), morantel is not recommended for use concurrently with pyrantel or levamisole.
- **Organophosphates, Diethylcarbamazine**: Increased risk for adverse effects; additional monitoring may be required
- **Piperazine**: Piperazine and morantel have antagonistic mechanisms of action; do not use together.

Dosages

CATTLE:

Susceptible parasites (label dosage; FDA-approved): Feed at a rate of morantel tartrate 0.44 g/45.36 kg (100 lb) of body weight as a single treatment, which results in a 10 mg/kg morantel dose.[1] Medicated feed should be consumed within 6 hours of mixing. It can be fed as the sole ration, mixed with 1 to 2 parts of complete feed, or used as a top dress. When used as a top dress, the medication (as well as the underlying feed) should be evenly distributed. Animals should be grouped by size for optimum efficacy. Fresh water should be available at all times. Resume normal feeding once all medicated feed is consumed. Conditions of constant parasite exposure may require repeat treatment within 2 to 4 weeks.

GOATS:

Susceptible parasites (label dosage; FDA-approved): Feed at a rate of morantel tartrate 0.44 g/45.36 kg (100 lb) of body weight as a single treatment, which results in a 10 mg/kg morantel dose. Medicated feed should be consumed within 6 hours of mixing. Fresh water should be available at all times. Conditions of constant parasite exposure may require retreatment in 2 to 4 weeks.[1]

SHEEP:

Susceptible parasites (extra-label): Feed at a rate of morantel tartrate 0.44 g/45.36 kg (100 lb) of body weight as a single treatment, which results in a 10 mg/kg morantel dose. Medicated feed should be consumed within 6 hours of mixing. Fresh water should be available at all times. Conditions of constant parasite exposure may require retreatment in 2 to 4 weeks.[2]

Client Information

- Follow all label directions and withdrawal times.
- Contact your veterinarian before using this medicine in sick animals.

Chemistry/Synonyms

A tetrahydropyrimidine anthelmintic, morantel tartrate occurs as a practically odorless, off-white to pale-yellow crystalline solid that is soluble in water. It has a melting range of 167°C to 171°C (332.6°F-339.8°F). The tartrate salt is equivalent to 59.5% of base activity.

Morantel tartrate may also be known as CP-12009-18, moranteli hydrogenotartras, UK-2964-18, *Goat Care-2X*®, or *Rumatel*®.

Storage/Stability

Morantel tartrate products should be stored at or below 25°C (77°F) and protected from light unless otherwise instructed by the manufacturer. Excursions are permitted up to 40°C (104°F).

Compatibility/Compounding Considerations

No specific information is noted.

Dosage Forms/Regulatory Status

VETERINARY-LABELED PRODUCTS:

Morantel Tartrate Medicated Pellets: 0.194% (880 mg/lb) in 3 lb bags (treats 12 to 50 lb goats) and 10 lb bags (treats 40 to 50 lb goats). *Goat Care-2X*®; (OTC, Type C medicated feed); 30-day slaughter withdrawal. Do not mix this product in feeds containing bentonite.

Morantel Tartrate Medicated Premix: 19.4% (morantel tartrate 88 g/lb) in 25 lb bags. *Rumatel*®*-88*; (OTC, Type A medicated article). FDA-approved for use in beef or dairy cattle and goats. Do not mix this product in feeds containing bentonite. No milk withdrawal at label dosages; 14-day meat withdrawal in cattle and 30-day meat withdrawal in goats at label dosages

HUMAN-LABELED PRODUCTS: NONE

References

For the complete list of references, see **wiley.com/go/budde/plumb**

Morphine

(***mor***-feen)

Opioid Agonist

Prescriber Highlights

- Classic opioid analgesic that can be reversed with naloxone
- Response varies by species
- Contraindications include hypersensitivity to morphine; recent treatment with monoamine oxidase inhibitors; diarrhea caused by a toxic ingestion; ileus or GI obstruction; and scorpion or coral snake envenomation.
- Use with extreme caution in patients with severe respiratory disease or acute respiratory dysfunction, or with head injuries or increased intracranial pressure (particularly in cases of impaired consciousness or coma); ventilatory monitoring and support are warranted in these cases.
- Use with caution in patients with hypothyroidism, severe renal insufficiency (acute azotemia), severe hepatic disease, or adrenocortical insufficiency; severely hypotensive or hypovolemic patients; geriatric or severely debilitated patients; brachycephalic patients; and patients with acute abdominal conditions (eg, colic). Morphine may obscure clinical signs of acute abdominal conditions during diagnosis.
- Adverse effects include histamine release/vasodilation (with rapid IV injection), CNS system depression or excitation (varies by species), hyperthermia (cats, horses, cattle, goats, and camelids), hypothermia, GI effects (may include nausea, vomiting, and decreased intestinal peristalsis), defecation or micturition, respiratory depression, and bronchoconstriction.
- Dogs can develop physical dependence with chronic use; dose needs to be tapered to minimize clinical signs associated with withdrawal.
- DEA Schedule II (C-II) controlled substance

Uses/Indications

Morphine is used to treat acute pain in dogs, cats, horses, swine, sheep, and goats. Morphine is used as a preanesthetic in several species. For sedation and analgesia in critically ill small animals, a combination of a sedative agent (eg, midazolam) and a mu-opioid (eg, morphine, hydromorphone) is often preferred because of its minimal effect on cardiac output, systemic blood pressure, and oxygen delivery. Additionally, sedative effects from opioids can be reversed with naloxone if necessary.

Morphine is typically administered by parenteral (ie, IV, IM, SC) routes. Oral morphine is not recommended in dogs because of poor oral bioavailability.[1] Epidural administration is used to provide analgesia primarily in the hindlimbs and, to a lesser extent, in the forelimbs and perineal region in small and large animals species. Intra-articular morphine administration as part of a balanced analgesic protocol may be beneficial in horses for synovitis or after joint surgery.[2,3] Morphine has been used for IV limb perfusion in standing sedated horses.[4]

Pharmacology/Actions

The morphine-like agonists (eg, morphine, meperidine, hydromorphone) have primary activity at mu-opioid receptors, with some activity at delta- and kappa-opioid receptors. The primary pharmacologic effects of these agents are species-specific but can include analgesia, antitussive activity, respiratory depression, sedation, emesis, physical dependence, and intestinal effects (defecation followed by constipation). Secondary pharmacologic effects include CNS (euphoria, sedation, and confusion), cardiovascular (bradycardia due to central vagal stimulation, depressed alpha-adrenergic receptors resulting in peripheral vasodilation, decreased peripheral resistance, and baroreceptor inhibition [orthostatic hypotension and syncope may occur]), and urinary (increased bladder sphincter tone can induce urinary retention).

When morphine was administered intra-articularly (0.05 mg/kg) in horses with experimentally induced synovitis, it demonstrated anti-inflammatory effects such as reducing swelling, synovial total protein, serum amyloid, and white blood cell counts.[3] In a study where morphine (120 mg) was injected into the talocrural joint of horses 1 hour after inducing synovitis, significant decreases were found in synovial white blood cell count, prostaglandin E_2, and bradykinin levels, and there was improvement in clinical lameness of kinematic and behavioral parameters as compared with placebo.[2]

Morphine's CNS effects are irregular and are species-specific. Generally, cats, horses, cattle, sheep, goats, and swine may exhibit stimulatory effects after morphine injection. Dogs, humans, and other primates exhibit CNS depression. Dogs and cats are sensitive to the emetic effects of morphine. Significantly higher morphine doses are required in cats before vomiting occurs from direct stimulation of the chemoreceptor trigger zone (CRTZ). Other species (horses, ruminants, and swine) do not respond to the emetic effects of morphine.

Morphine is an effective centrally acting antitussive in dogs. Morphine can cause miosis in humans and rabbits. A study in healthy dogs following IV morphine (dose not specified) showed no significant effect on pupil size or intraocular pressure.[5]

Morphine is a respiratory depressant. In dogs, morphine can cause alterations to the thermoregulatory center, leading to an initial increase in respiratory rate with a decrease in tidal volume (panting). The overall effect on minute ventilation is minimal. As CNS depression progresses, respirations may become depressed. Morphine at moderate to high doses can also cause bronchoconstriction in dogs.

The cardiovascular effects of morphine in dogs are minimal when recommended doses are used and if slow IV administration is performed. Like meperidine, morphine can affect the release of histamine from mast cells. When administered at 0.5 – 1 mg/kg IV or 0.3 – 0.6 mg/kg followed by 0.17 – 0.34 mg/kg/hour IV CRI, histamine release is present with no cardiovascular effects at the lower doses and minimal cardiovascular depression at the higher doses.[6,7] In contrast, when high doses (3 mg/kg IV) of morphine were used in dogs that were anesthetized with pentobarbital, profound hypotension was noted.[8] However, when the same dose is used in awake dogs, minimal system effects on hemodynamics were observed.[9]

The effects of morphine on the GI tract consist primarily of decreased motility and secretions. Horses that received morphine doses as low as 0.05 mg/kg IM had decreased GI motility 1 to 2 hours later.[10] Dogs may defecate following morphine injection then exhibit signs of decreased intestinal motility and can cause constipation. Biliary, pancreatic, and gastric secretions (including hydrochloric acid) are reduced following morphine administration.[11]

Initially, morphine can induce micturition. Higher morphine doses (greater than 2.4 mg/kg IV) may substantially reduce urine production by an increase in antidiuretic hormone (ADH) release. Morphine may cause bladder hypertonia, which can lead to increased urinary difficulties.[3]

Refer to ***Appendix: Pharmacology of Narcotic (Opioid) Agonist Analgesics*** for more information.

Pharmacokinetics

Morphine is absorbed after IM, SC, buccal (oral transmucosal, OTM), and rectal administration. Although absorbed after PO administration, bioavailability is reduced, likely from the high first-pass effect. Morphine's very low oral bioavailability (less than 20%) and erratic absorption of the oral extended-release formulation limit oral usefulness in canines.[12-14] Morphine concentrates in the kidneys, liver, and lungs; lower concentrations are found in the CNS. Most free morphine is found in skeletal muscle, with lower concentrations found in parenchymatous tissue.

The majority of morphine is eliminated via hepatic metabolism, primarily by glucuronidation. Cats are deficient in this metabolic pathway and morphine's half-life in cats is prolonged compared with other species (reported to be ≈3 hours). The glucuronidated metabolite M6G (active) is renally excreted.

After administration of morphine 0.5 mg/kg IV in dogs, morphine had a half-life of 1.2 hours, a volume of distribution of ≈4.6 L/kg, and a clearance of ≈62.5 mL/minute/kg.[14]

In horses, morphine's serum half-life is reported to be 1.5 hours after a dose of 0.1 mg/kg IV or IM.[15] At this dose, morphine was detectable in serum for 48 hours and urine for 6 days. Epidurally administered morphine in horses caused rapid, short-lasting serum concentrations and delayed, long-lasting CSF concentrations (elimination half-life ≈8 hours). Isoflurane anesthesia did not significantly alter values.[16]

Contraindications/Precautions/Warnings

Morphine is contraindicated in patients that are hypersensitive to narcotic analgesics, are receiving or are within 14 days of receiving monoamine oxidase inhibitors (MAOIs), have diarrhea caused by a toxic ingestion until the toxin is eliminated from the GI tract, or have GI tract obstruction or paralytic ileus. Avoid morphine in envenomation situations, as clinical signs associated with histamine release can be confused with anaphylaxis. Respiratory depressants, including morphine, should not be used in coral snake envenomation in dogs or cats.[17] Opioid analgesics are contraindicated in patients that are stung by scorpions (eg, *Centruroides* spp), as they may potentiate venom effects.[18]

Use extreme caution with morphine in patients with brain tumors, head injuries, or increased intracerebral pressure and avoid use in patients with impaired consciousness or coma as morphine may increase intracerebral pressure secondary to cerebral vasodilation caused by increased $PaCO_2$ stemming from respiratory depression. Also use extreme caution in patients that are suffering from severe respiratory disease or acute respiratory dysfunction (eg, pulmonary edema secondary to smoke inhalation). Ventilatory monitoring and support are warranted in these cases.

Use opioids with caution in patients with hypothyroidism, hypoadrenocorticism, severe hypotension or hypovolemia, or in severely debilitated patients.[19] Caution is warranted in acute abdominal conditions (eg, colic), as morphine may obscure the diagnosis or clinical course of these conditions. Because of the drug's effects on vasopressin (ADH), morphine should be used cautiously in patients that are suffering from acute azotemia or severe renal insufficiency. Urine flow is reported to decrease as much as 90% in dogs following large morphine doses. If administering the drug IV, give morphine slowly or significant hypotension can result. Hypotension may result in decreased cardiac output and blood pressure. Biliary tract impairment may be worsened, and caution is recommended. Morphine may constrict the sphincter of Oddi, decreasing pancreatic and biliary secretions. Patients with severe hepatic disease may have prolonged duration of action of the drug.

Neonatal, debilitated, or geriatric patients may be more susceptible to the effects of morphine and require lower dosages. Anecdotally, some clinicians have suggested that animals with brachycephalic airway syndrome are potentially sensitive to morphine's adverse effects, but no scientific documentation for this was located.

Intrathecal administration is contraindicated in patients with upper airway obstruction. Intrathecal and epidural administration are both contraindicated by presence of infection at injection site, anticoagulant therapy, or uncontrolled bleeding.

Some dosage forms may contain benzyl alcohol as a preservative. In human newborns, benzyl alcohol and its derivatives can potentially displace bilirubin from protein-binding sites and caution for use in human neonates is advised. Some dosage forms may contain sulfites, which could cause allergic reactions in susceptible patients. The significance of these cautions for veterinary patients is unclear.

Morphine has significant potential for drug abuse and drug diversion in humans; caution is advised when prescribing this drug.

Sedative drugs such as morphine should only be used in situations in which sufficient monitoring and patient-support capabilities (eg, intubation, ventilation) are available.

Adverse Effects

At recommended dosages, opioids have limited respiratory depressant effects in veterinary species compared to humans. Decreased tidal volume, depressed cough reflex, and drying of respiratory secretions may have a detrimental effect on susceptible patients (eg, patients with brachycephalic airway syndrome, aspiration, or pneumonia). Bronchoconstriction following IV morphine doses may be noted in dogs[20]; significant hypotension results if morphine is administered rapidly IV. Panting and bradycardia may be seen in dogs after morphine administration.[21]

GI effects may include nausea, vomiting, and decreased intestinal peristalsis. Maropitant can significantly decrease the incidence of morphine-induced vomiting in dogs[22,23] and cats.[24] Dogs may defecate after an initial dose of morphine, but this is uncommon when used postoperatively. Horses exhibiting signs of mild colic may have their clinical signs masked by narcotic analgesics. Horses may be prone to developing colic, constipation, and ileus, particularly when an opioid-alpha-2 agonist combination is used.[20] In ferrets, morphine can induce nausea and vomiting and is often avoided in this species.[25]

CNS excitation is typically only seen after rapid IV administration, or with doses that are higher than those used clinically. Dose-related excitatory changes appear more likely in cats, horses, ruminants, and camelids, and may include dysphoria, vocalization, thrashing, increased locomotor activity (eg, pacing), restlessness, ataxia, and convulsions at very high doses. Morphine-induced CNS depression may hinder the abilities of working animals. Long-term administration may lead to physical dependence in dogs.[26,27]

Morphine initially may induce micturition which may be followed by substantially reduced urine production and/or urethral sphincter hypertonia, which can lead to urine retention.[19]

Body temperature changes, including hypothermia, may be seen. Panting is often seen in dogs after morphine administration and contributes to the development of hypothermia. Cats, horses, cattle, and goats may develop hyperthermia.

Sheep may exhibit drooling, bruxism, facial tremors, vocalization, and mydriasis.[28]

In one case report of a Holstein calf epidural of morphine 0.1 mg/kg with a fentanyl patch, adverse effects included altered consciousness, mydriasis, nystagmus, increased locomotion, vocalization, tail myoclonus, hyper-responsiveness, hyperthermia, tachycardia, and tachypnea.[29]

Reproductive/Nursing Safety

Placental transfer of opioids is rapid, but morphine appears safe to use during pregnancy when given at recommended dosages. Administration during late stages of pregnancy may result in respiratory depression of the offspring.[30]

Morphine appears in maternal milk, but the effects on offspring may not be significant when used for short periods.

Because safety has not been established in animals, this drug should only be used when the maternal benefits outweigh the potential risks to offspring.

Overdose/Acute Toxicity

Overdoses may produce profound respiratory and/or CNS depression in most species. Newborns may be more susceptible to these effects than adult animals. Parenteral doses greater than 100 mg/kg are thought to be fatal in dogs. Other toxic effects can include cardiovascular collapse, hypothermia/hyperthermia, and skeletal muscle hypotonia. Some species such as cats, horses, cattle, and swine may demonstrate CNS excitability (hyperreflexia, tremors) and seizures at high doses of morphine, or if it is administered rapidly IV.

Naloxone is the reversal agent for morphine. In cases of massive overdoses, naloxone doses may be repeated. Observe animals closely as naloxone's effects might diminish before attaining subtoxic morphine levels. Consider mechanical respiratory support in cases of severe respiratory depression.

Pentobarbital has been suggested as a treatment for CNS excitement and seizures in cats. Extreme caution should be used in administering this treatment, as barbiturates and narcotics can have additive effects on respiratory depression.

For patients that have experienced or are suspected to have experienced an overdose, consultation with a 24-hour poison consultation center specializing in providing veterinary-specific information is recommended. For general information related to overdose and toxin exposures, as well as contact information for poison control centers, refer to ***Appendix***.

Drug Interactions

The following drug interactions have either been reported or are theoretical in humans or animals receiving morphine and may be of significance in veterinary patients. Unless otherwise noted, use together is not necessarily contraindicated, but weigh the potential risks and perform additional monitoring when appropriate.

- **Anticholinergic Agents** (eg, **atropine, glycopyrrolate, oxybutynin**): Medications with anticholinergic properties may increase the risk for urinary retention and constipation when combined with opioids.
- **Clopidogrel**: Morphine may diminish clopidogrel's antiplatelet effect and serum concentration.
- **Blood Pressure Lowering Agents** (eg, **amlodipine, enalapril, telmisartan**): Agents that lower blood pressure may have additive hypotensive effects when used with morphine.
- **CNS Depressants, Other** (eg, **anesthetic agents, antihistamines, barbiturates, phenothiazines**): May cause increased CNS or respiratory depression when used with morphine
- **Desmopressin**: Opioids may increase the risk for water intoxi-

cation or hyponatremia when combined with desmopressin.

- **Diuretics**: Opioids may decrease diuretic efficacy in congestive heart failure patients.
- **Esmolol**: Serum concentrations of esmolol may be increased with concomitant morphine use.
- **GI Prokinetic Agents** (eg, **cisapride, metoclopramide**): Opioids may decrease the effectiveness of GI prokinetic agents.
- **Magnesium Sulfate**: The CNS depressant effects of morphine may be increased, more likely with higher magnesium doses or IV magnesium therapy.
- **Minocycline**: IV minocycline therapy may enhance the CNS depressant effects of morphine.
- **Mixed Opioid Agonist/Antagonist** (eg, **butorphanol, nalbuphine**): Combined use with morphine could antagonize opioid effects.
- **Monoamine Oxidase Inhibitors** (MAOIs; eg, **amitraz, linezolid, selegiline**): Morphine may enhance the serotonergic effect of MAOIs and lead to possible serotonin syndrome; avoid concurrent use or use of morphine within 14 days of stopping MAOIs.
- **Muscle Relaxants, Skeletal** (eg, **atracurium**): Morphine may enhance neuromuscular blockade.
- **Naloxone**: Antagonizes opioid effects. NOTE: This action is an expected outcome when naloxone is used as a reversal agent.
- **P-Glycoprotein Modulators** (eg, **ketoconazole**): Medication that induces, inhibits, or is a substrate of P-glycoproteins may affect morphine bioavailability and serum concentration.
- **Rifampin**: May induce morphine metabolism and decrease morphine serum concentration
- **Serotonin Modulators** (eg, **SSRIs, linezolid, methylene blue, metoclopramide**): Serotonin levels may be enhanced when serotonin modulators are given concomitantly with morphine. Monitor for serotonin syndrome.
- **Succinylcholine**: Opioids combined with succinylcholine may enhance the bradycardic effects of opioids.
- **Tricyclic Antidepressants** (eg, **clomipramine, amitriptyline**): Morphine may exacerbate the effects of tricyclic antidepressants.
- **Warfarin**: Opioids may potentiate anticoagulant activity.

Laboratory Considerations

- Opioids may increase biliary tract pressure, resulting in increased plasma **amylase** and **lipase** values up to 24 hours following their administration.
- Quinolones may cause false positive results on urine screening tests for morphine.

Dosages

NOTES:

1. Preservative-free morphine formulations should be used for epidural administration.
2. Do not confuse CRI dosages listed as mg/kg/hour with those listed as µg/kg/minute.
3. For additional dosages/protocols for using morphine in combination with other drugs (eg, ketamine, lidocaine, dexmedetomidine) for pain/sedation in dogs or cats, see the dosages and their accompanying references in the ***Dexmedetomidine***, ***Ketamine***, and ***Lidocaine*** monographs.

DOGS:

Analgesia (extra-label):

a) **Intermittent dosing**: 0.5 – 1 mg/kg IM, SC, or IV (slowly). Lower doses may be necessary in severely debilitated animals, and higher doses may be required for treatment of extreme pain. Duration of effect can vary, and re-dosing is often needed after 2 hours.

b) **CRI dosing**: Initial loading dose of 0.3 – 0.5 mg/kg IM, IV (slowly), followed by 0.1 – 1 mg/kg/<u>hour</u> IV CRI.[31,32] Adjust dosage based on clinical analgesic response and/or adverse effects, which may be pronounced at higher infusion rates or with prolonged duration of use.

c) **Epidural**: Using preservative-free morphine, 0.1 mg/kg diluted with saline to a volume of 0.3 mL/kg (maximum 6 mL). Opioids provide analgesia without loss of hindlimb function or muscle tone. Extended analgesia can be maintained with an epidural catheter (although catheter placement and maintenance may be difficult). One advantage of epidural morphine is that analgesia will migrate cranially and be effective up to 18 hours.[33]

In combination as a preanesthetic agent or perioperative sedative analgesic (extra-label): Many combinations can be used. Morphine is usually dosed between 0.1 – 0.5 mg/kg IM in combination with drugs such as acepromazine, midazolam, dexmedetomidine, and/or ketamine. Lower morphine doses (eg, 0.05 mg/kg) may be necessary in debilitated or critically ill animals.

Morphine/Lidocaine/Ketamine (MLK) low-dose CRI: Morphine 3.3 **µg**/kg/*<u>minute</u>* in combination with lidocaine 50 **µg**/kg/*<u>minute</u>* and ketamine 10 **µg**/kg/*<u>minute</u>* IV CRI decreases isoflurane minimum alveolar concentration (MAC) in dogs and is not associated with adverse hemodynamic effects.[34,35]

Dexmedetomidine/morphine/lidocaine/ketamine (DMLK): Dexmedetomidine 0.5 µg/kg/<u>hour</u> in combination with morphine 0.2 mg/kg/<u>hour</u>, lidocaine 3 mg/kg/<u>hour</u>, and ketamine 0.6 mg/kg per <u>hour</u> admixed in IV fluids and administered IV as CRI.[36]

CATS:

Analgesia (extra-label):

a) **Intermittent dosing**: 0.1 – 0.25 mg/kg IV, IM, or SC every 2 to 4 hours as needed.[31] Duration of effect can vary, and often re-dosing is needed after 3 hours.

b) **CRI dosing**: 0.05 – 0.1 mg/kg/<u>hour</u> IV CRI[31]

c) **Epidural analgesia** (extra-label): In one study, using preservative-free morphine 0.1 mg/kg diluted with saline to a volume of 0.22 mL/kg was administered over 1 minute.[37] Morphine provided analgesia for 12 hours postadministration. In another study of 24 cats undergoing ovariohysterectomy, morphine 0.1 mg/kg with 2% lidocaine 4 mg/kg was administered as an epidural and provided adequate analgesia for the procedure.[38]

HORSES:

NOTE: Some clinicians recommend pretreatment with acepromazine, detomidine, or xylazine to reduce drug-induced behavioral changes caused by morphine.

Analgesia (extra-label):

a) **Intermittent dosing**:
   i. 0.1 mg/kg IM every 4 hours; this dose reduces morphine's impact on GI motility.[39]
   ii. 0.012 – 0.66 mg/kg IV in combination with alpha-2 agonists[40]

b) **CRI dosing**: Initial loading dose of 0.12 – 0.15 mg/kg IV (slowly) or IM, followed by 0.05 – 0.1 mg/kg/hour IV CRI[41,42]

c) **Epidural analgesia**: **NOTE**: Use preservative-free morphine for epidural administration.
   i. In one study, 6 hours after inducing carpal synovitis in ponies, morphine 0.1 mg/kg (diluted in a 0.9% saline solution to a final volume of 0.15 mL/kg) was administered epidurally at a rate of 1 mL per 10 seconds.[43] The authors conclud-

ed that epidural morphine produced analgesia that lasted more than 12 hours without adverse effects and would be an analgesic option to alleviate joint pain in ponies' fore-limbs.[43]

ii. Morphine 0.1 – 0.2 mg/kg diluted in 10 to 20 mL of 0.9% saline solution (total volume of 0.04 mL/kg body weight) epidurally alone or in combination with detomidine 0.015 – 0.03 mg/kg epidurally to provide effective analgesia of the caudal half of the body.[40,44,45] Analgesic effects are seen within 20 to 30 minutes and may last 8 to 24 hours without adverse effects on motor function.

iii. Adult horses: Preservative-free morphine 0.1 – 0.2 mg/kg; dilute with saline to a total volume of 0.04 mL/kg or 20 mL/450 kg (992 lb) and administer epidurally[31]

iv. Foals: Preservative-free morphine 0.1 mg/kg epidurally. Use of preservative-containing morphine is not recommended, but if unavoidable then dilute to a volume of 0.2 mL/kg.

d) **Intraregional limb perfusion**: Morphine 0.1 mg/kg IV has been used for IV limb perfusion in standing sedated horses. Measurable levels were detected in the synovial fluid and this technique did not cause adverse effects.[4]

e) **Intra-articular injection for acute inflammatory joint pain** (extra-label): Two single-dose experimental studies suggest that intra-articular morphine has anti-inflammatory effects for acute synovitis. One study used morphine 0.05 mg/kg IA (radiocarpal joint) and another used 120 mg diluted in 20 mL saline (talocrural joint).[2,3]

CAMELIDS:

Epidural (extra-label): 0.1 – 0.3 mg/kg of preservative-free morphine diluted to 12 mL and administered epidurally[46]

SHEEP:

Sedation (extra-label):

a) In a study of 6 Santa Inês sheep, dexmedetomidine 0.005 mg/kg combined with morphine 0.5 mg/kg and given IV resulted in similar sedation scores and cardiopulmonary effects compared with dexmedetomidine alone.[47]

b) In another study of 6 Santa Inês sheep administered xylazine 0.1 mg/kg combined with morphine 0.5 mg/kg and given IV, the combination produced superior sedation for 30 minutes compared with xylazine alone.[28]

RABBITS, RODENTS, SMALL MAMMALS:

Analgesic/sedative (extra-label):
Rats: 2.5 mg/kg SC every 4 hours
Mice: 2.5 mg/kg SC every 2 to 4 hours
Guinea pigs: 2 – 5 mg/kg SC or IM every 4 hours[48]
Rabbits: 2 – 5 mg/kg IM or SC every 2 to 4 hours; epidurally at 0.1 mg/kg[49]

Monitoring

- Respiratory rate and depth; $ETCO_2$; pulse oximetry (SpO_2)
- Heart rate
- CNS level of depression/excitation
- Blood pressure (especially with IV use)
- Analgesic efficacy
- Body temperature

Client Information

- Morphine is a pain reliever for dogs or cats that is not suitable for use at home.
- Use of morphine may lead to nausea, vomiting, and constipation. Contact your veterinarian if these effects do not resolve within a few days.

Chemistry/Synonyms

The sulfate salt of a naturally occurring (derived from opium) opioid analgesic, morphine sulfate occurs as white, odorless crystals. One gram of morphine is soluble in 16 mL of water (62.5 mg/mL) or 570 mL of alcohol (1.75 mg/mL). Morphine is insoluble in chloroform or ether. Morphine sulfate injection pH ranges from 2.5 to 6.

Morphine sulfate may also be known as morphini sulfas, *Astramorph PF®*, *Avinza®*, *DepoDur®*, *Infumorph®*, *Kadian®*, *MSIR®*, *MS Contin®*, *Oramorph SR*, *RMS®*, and *Roxanol®*.

Storage/Stability

Morphine is a DEA schedule II (C-II) controlled substance that should be stored in an area that is substantially constructed and securely locked. Follow applicable local, state, and federal rules regarding disposal of unused or wasted controlled drugs.

Morphine injection should be stored at room temperature (20°C-25°F [68°F-77°F]), protected from light; do not freeze.[19] Morphine gradually darkens in color when exposed to light. Morphine does not appear to adsorb to plastic or polyvinyl chloride (PVC) syringes, tubing, or bags.

Compatibility/Compounding Considerations

Compatibility is dependent on factors such as pH, concentration, temperature, and diluent used; consult specialized references or a hospital pharmacist for more specific information.

Morphine sulfate has been shown to be physically **compatible** at a concentration of 16.2 mg/L with the following IV fluids: dextrose 2.5%, 5%, and 10% in water; Ringer's injection and lactated Ringer's injection; and sodium chloride 0.45% and 0.9% for injection.[50] Morphine sulfate has been demonstrated to be generally physically **compatible** when mixed at Y-sites with a wide variety of agents.

The following drugs have been shown to be physically **incompatible** when mixed at Y-sites with morphine sulfate: amphotericin B, azathioprine, cloxacillin, dantrolene, diazoxide, doxorubicin, folic acid, inamrinone, pentobarbital sodium, and phenytoin sodium.

The following drugs have been shown to have **variable** compatibility and should be used cautiously when mixed at Y-sites with morphine sulfate: acyclovir, ampicillin ± sulbactam, azithromycin, cefepime, cefoperazone, cisplatin, diazepam, furosemide, gallium nitrate, hydralazine, regular insulin, levofloxacin, minocycline, nutrient admixtures, pantoprazole, propofol, sulfamethoxazole-trimethoprim, and thiopental sodium.

Morphine sulfate has been shown to physically **incompatible** when admixed with the following: aminophylline, chlorothiazide sodium, fluorouracil, heparin sodium, meperidine HCl, phenobarbital sodium, phenytoin sodium, sodium bicarbonate, and thiopental sodium.

Morphine sulfate has been shown to have **variable** compatibility and should be used cautiously when admixed with alteplase.

Dosage Forms/Regulatory Status

VETERINARY-LABELED PRODUCTS: NONE

The Association of Racing Commissioners International (ARCI) has designated this drug as a class 1 substance. Use of this drug may not be allowed in certain animal competitions. Check rules and regulations before entering in a competition while this medication is being administered. Contact local racing authorities for further guidance. See ***Appendix*** for more information.

HUMAN-LABELED PRODUCTS:

NOTE: Accurate record keeping is required regarding use and disposition of stock. Report dispensing to state monitoring programs where required.

Morphine Sulfate for Injection: 1 mg/mL, 2 mg/mL, 4 mg/mL, 5 mg/mL, 8 mg/mL, 10 mg/mL, and 50 mg/mL in ampules, vials, syringes, and prefilled IV bags in sizes that range from 1 mL to 250 mL depending on manufacturer and concentration; generic; (Rx; C-II)

Morphine Sulfate for Injection (preservative-free): 0.5 mg/mL: 10 mL ampules; 1 mg/mL: 10 mL ampules and vials, 30 mL vials and syringes; 2 mg/mL: 1 mL syringes; 4 mg/mL: 1 mL syringes and vials; 5 mg/mL: 30 mL vials; 8 mg/mL: 1 mL syringes and vials; 10 mg/mL: 1 mL syringes and vials, 20 mL ampules; 25 mg/mL: 20 mL ampules and vials; *Duramorph®*, *Infumorph®*, *Astramorph PF®*, generic; (Rx, C-II)

References

For the complete list of references, see **wiley.com/go/budde/plumb**

Moxidectin/Moxidectin Combination Products

(mox-i-**dek**-tin) *Cydectin®, ProHeart®, Quest®; Advantage Multi®, Bravecto® Plus, Simparica Trio®*

Macrocyclic Lactone Antiparasitic

Prescriber Highlights

- ▶ Milbemycin-class antiparasitic that is FDA-approved for use in cattle, dogs, cats, ferrets, sheep, and horses
- ▶ Contraindications include hypersensitivity to the drug, or in female dairy cattle of breeding age, veal calves, and horses intended for food purposes or foals younger than 4 months of age. Use with extreme caution in sick, debilitated, or underweight animals.
- ▶ Adverse effects with oral and topical formulations in dogs potentially include lethargy, vomiting, ataxia, anorexia, diarrhea, nervousness, weakness, increased thirst, and itching. Adverse effects are minimal in cattle and appear to be minimal in horses at labeled doses. Adverse effects with the injection formulation include swelling and slight edema at the injection site.
- ▶ Current data indicate moxidectin at labeled doses is safe to use in dogs with the *MDR1* mutation (also known as *ABCB1*-1delta); higher doses may cause neurotoxicity in these dogs.

Uses/Indications

For dogs, an extended-release injectable moxidectin product is FDA-approved for the prevention of heartworm disease caused by *D immitis* and for the treatment of existing larval and adult hookworm (*A caninum, U stenocephala*) infections. A 6-month injectable product (*ProHeart® 6*)[1] is approved for dogs aged 6 months and older, and a 12-month injectable product (*ProHeart® 12*)[2] is approved for dogs aged 12 months and older.

Moxidectin/fluralaner topical solution (*Bravecto® Plus*) is labeled for the prevention of heartworm disease caused by *D immitis*, treatment of intestinal roundworms (*T cati*) and hookworms (*A tubaeforme*), treatment and prevention of flea infestations (*C felis*), and treatment and control of tick infestations (*Ixodes scapularis* [black-legged tick] and *Dermacentor variabilis* [American dog tick]) for 2 months duration in cats 6 months of age and older and weighing 1.2 kg (2.6 lb) or more.[3] In infected cats, a single dose of topical moxidectin/fluralaner was 100% effective at eliminating *Capillaria* spp, hookworm, and *Toxascaris* spp ova and was 99% effective in clearing *T cati* infection.[4]

In dogs and cats, moxidectin/imidacloprid (*Advantage Multi®*)[5,6] is labeled for use as a once-monthly topical solution for the prevention of heartworm disease caused by *D immitis*, as a flea (*Ctenocephalides felis*) adulticide, and for the treatment and control of hookworms (*A caninum, U stenocephala)* and roundworms (*T cati, Toxascaris leonina*). In cats, this combination drug is also approved for the treatment of ear mites. In dogs, it is also approved for the treatment of whipworms (*T vulpis*), sarcoptic mange (*Sarcoptes scabiei* var *canis*), and circulating heartworm microfilariae, as well as having been shown to be effective for extra-label treatment of fox lungworm (*Crenosoma vulpis*) in dogs after a single treatment.[7] The moxidectin/imidacloprid combined product is approved for use in cats and kittens 9 weeks of age and older and that weigh at least 2 lb and in dogs and puppies 7 weeks of age and older and weighing 3 to 9 lb.

In ferrets, moxidectin/imidacloprid (*Advantage Multi® for Cats*) is labeled for the treatment and control of adult fleas and flea infestations (*Ctenocephalides felis*) and the prevention of heartworm disease caused by *D immitis*.[5]

Moxidectin/pyrantel/sarolaner (*Simparica Trio®*) is labeled as a monthly oral treatment for the prevention of heartworm disease caused by *D immitis*; treatment and prevention of flea infestations (*C felis*); treatment and control of tick infestations with *A americanum* (lone star tick), *A maculatum* (Gulf Coast tick), *D variabilis* (American dog tick), *I scapularis* (black-legged tick), and *Rhipicephalus sanguineus* (brown dog tick); and treatment and control of roundworms (*T canis, T leonina*) and hookworms (*A caninum, U stenocephala*) in dogs 8 weeks of age and older and weighing 1.3 kg (2.8 lb) or more.[8]

The use of moxidectin in slow-kill protocols for treatment of heartworm infection is no longer recommended and is considered a salvage procedure only for dogs in which melarsomine therapy is not possible or is contraindicated.[9] An accelerated dosage protocol that combined oral doxycycline for 7 to 14 days with topical moxidectin/imidacloprid every 10 to 15 days for 50 to 90 days, followed by monthly administration, was found to eradicate microfilariae and adult heartworms within 3 and 7 months, respectively.[10] Similar results have been noted with monthly topical moxidectin/imidacloprid administration when combined with doxycycline at 10 mg/kg every 12 hours for the first 30 days.[11,12]

Generalized demodicosis in dogs has been treated with extra-label oral moxidectin and increased frequency of administration of the canine topical product. In a systematic review of published clinical trials, the optimal determined treatments for demodicosis were daily oral milbemycin and weekly[13,14] or monthly[15-17] topical moxidectin (± imidacloprid); however, isoxazolines (eg, fluralaner, sarolaner) are as effective as the moxidectin/imidacloprid combination, and have supplanted macrocyclic lactones for the treatment of demodicosis.[14-16,18]

In horses and ponies 6 months of age and older, moxidectin is indicated for the treatment and control of the following stages of GI parasites:

- **Large strongyles**: *Strongylus vulgaris* (adults and L4, L5 arterial stages), *S edentatus* (adults and tissue stages), *Triodontophorus brevicauda* (adults), *T serratus* (adults)
- **Small strongyles** (adults and undifferentiated luminal larvae): *Cyathostomum* spp; *Cylicocyclus* spp; *Cylicostephanus* spp; *Coronocyclus* spp, *Gyalocephalus capitatus* (adults); *Petrovinema poculatus* (adults); undifferentiated lumenal larvae
- **Encysted cyathostomes**: Late L3 and L4 mucosal cyathostome larvae
- **Ascarids**: *Parascaris equorum* (adults and L4 larval stages)
- **Pin worms**: *Oxyuris equi* (adults and L4 larval stages)
- **Hair worms**: *T axei* (adults)
- **Large-mouth stomach worms**: *Habronema muscae* (adults)
- **Horse stomach bots**: *Gasterophilus intestinalis* (second and third instars) and *G nasalis* (third instars)

Resistance to antiparasitic agents is an ongoing problem in horses. Moxidectin has demonstrated efficacy against fenbendazole-resistant adult and encysted cyathostomins and continues to be a foundation for control of strongyle parasites.[19,20] Strongyle egg production is suppressed for 84 days after a single labeled dose of moxidectin. When moxidectin is combined with praziquantel (*Quest® Plus*), additional coverage against *Anoplocephala* spp occurs.

In cattle, moxidectin (topical and injection) is indicated for the treatment and control of the following internal (ie, adult and fourth stage larvae [L4]) and external parasites:

GI roundworms: *Ostertagia ostertagi* (adult and L4, including inhibited larvae), *Haemonchus placei* (adult), *Trichostrongylus axei* (adult and L4), *Trichostrongylus colubriformis* (adult and L4), *Cooperia oncophora* (adult), *C pectinata* (adult), *C punctata* (adult and L4), *C spatulata* (adult), *C surnabada* (adult and L4), *Bunostomum phlebotomum* (adult), *Oesophagostomum radiatum* (adult and L4), *Nematodirus helvetianus* (adult), *Trichuris* spp (adult)

Lungworm: *Dictyocaulus viviparus* (adult and L4)

Cattle grubs: *Hypoderma bovis, H lineatum*

Mites: *Chorioptes bovis, Psoroptes ovis* (*Psoroptes communis* var *bovis*)

Lice: *Linognathus vituli, Haematopinus eurysternus, Solenopotes capillatus, Bovicola (Damalinia) bovis*

Horn flies: *Haematobia irritans*

Moxidectin for injection (or pour-on, as indicated) is also used to control infections and protect from reinfection of *Haemonchus placei* for 35 days (14 days for pour-on) after treatment, 42 days (28 days for pour-on) after treatment for *Oesophagostomum radiatum*, 14 days (28 days for pour-on) after treatment for *Ostertagia ostertagi*, 14 days after injectable treatment for *Trichostrongylus axei*, and 42 days after treatment for *Dictyocaulus viviparous*. Moxidectin demonstrated efficacy in the treatment of feedlot cattle that were infected with ivermectin-resistant GI nematodes.[21]

In sheep, oral moxidectin is indicated for the treatment and control of adult and L4 stages of *Haemonchus contortus*; *Teladorsagia circumcincta* and *T trifurcate*; *Trichostrongylus colubriformis, T axei*, and *T vitrinius*; *Cooperia curticei* and *C oncophora*; *Oesophagostomum columbianum* and *O venolosum*; and *Nematodirus battus, N filicollis*, and *N spathiger*.

Pharmacology/Actions

The primary mode of action of milbemycin drugs is to affect chloride ion channel activity in the nervous system of nematodes and arthropods. The drug binds to receptors that increase membrane permeability to chloride ions, inhibiting the electrical activity of nerve cells in nematodes and muscle cells in arthropods and causing paralysis and death of the parasites.

Milbemycins also enhance the release of gamma-aminobutyric acid (GABA) at presynaptic neurons. GABA acts as an inhibitory neurotransmitter and blocks postsynaptic stimulation of the adjacent neuron in nematodes or the muscle fiber in arthropods.

Milbemycins are generally not toxic to mammals, as they do not have glutamate-gated chloride channels and because these compounds do not readily cross the blood–brain barrier in which mammalian GABA receptors occur.

Pharmacokinetics

Moxidectin's metabolism is unknown in small animal species.

Peak moxidectin blood concentrations occur ≈7 to 14 days after administration of either the 6- month or 12-month injection.[1,2] The half-life is 50 days; residual drug concentrations are negligible at the end of the treatment intervals (ie, 6 months for *ProHeart® 6* and 12 months for *ProHeart® 12*).

After topical application in cats, peak moxidectin concentration occurred between 1 to 5 days after administration, and elimination half-life was 20 to 30 days.

In large animal species, moxidectin is metabolized by the liver and excreted in the bile.

In horses, moxidectin may have a duration of action of up to 12 weeks.

In cattle, the drug apparently has a long duration (ie, 14 to 15 days) of plasma residence. A pharmacokinetic study of SC administration in feedlot calves showed a time to peak concentration (T_{max}) of 9.6 hours and elimination half-life of 11 days.[21]

In sheep, elimination half-life is ≈18 days and mean residence time is ≈27 days; pregnancy reduced these values to ≈12 and ≈21 days, respectively.[22]

In alpacas, elimination half-life was ≈12 days after SC administration. Oral bioavailability was 11% relative to SC administration.[23]

In swine, V_d was 89.6 L/kg after IV administration, elimination half-life was ≈10 days after IV administration and 6.2 days after pour-on administration. T_{max} was 1.7 days after pour-on administration.[24]

Because moxidectin is lipophilic (100 times that of ivermectin), the volume of distribution (V_d) is likely to be very high. Animals with very low body fat (eg, neonates, cachectic animals) could potentially have serum concentrations much higher than patients with normal body condition.

Contraindications/Precautions/Warnings

Do not use moxidectin in animals hypersensitive to it, or in sick, debilitated, or underweight animals. Animals with poor body condition (eg, neonates, cachectic animals) may be more prone to adverse effects.

DOGS:

Labeled heartworm preventive doses for the oral (up to 3 µg/kg per month) and topical (2500 µg/kg/month) formulations are safe for all dogs with the *MDR1* mutation (also known as *ABCB1*-1delta; see ***Appendix***).[25] High-dose treatment can be neurotoxic in all dogs, particularly dogs with the *MDR1* mutation.

Moxidectin as a sole agent:

Injectable products (*ProHeart® 6, ProHeart® 12*): Use with caution in dogs with pre-existing allergic disease, including food allergy, atopy, and flea allergy dermatitis. Use with caution when administering the drug concurrently with vaccinations; adverse effects, including anaphylaxis, have been reported following concomitant use of *ProHeart® 6* and vaccinations.[1] Dogs should be tested for existing heartworm infections before this drug is administered; caution should be used if it is administered to heartworm positive dogs. The safety and effectiveness of *ProHeart® 6* have not been evaluated in dogs younger than 6 months of age. *ProHeart® 12* is approved for use in dogs 12 months of age and older.[2] Do not provide an overdose to growing puppies in anticipation of their expected adult weight.

Combination products:

Moxidectin/imidacloprid (*Advantage Multi®*): For the first 30 minutes after application, ensure that dogs cannot lick the product from application sites on themselves or other treated dogs, and separate all treated dogs and other household pets to reduce the risk for accidental ingestion. Ingestion of this product by dogs may cause serious adverse effects, including depression, salivation, dilated pupils, incoordination, panting, and generalized muscle tremors. In dogs sensitive to milbemycin, signs may be more severe and can include coma and death. **Do not use canine products on cats.**[6]

Moxidectin/pyrantel/sarolaner (*Simparica Trio®*): This product contains sarolaner, which is an isoxazoline. This class of drugs has been associated with neurologic adverse effects (eg, muscle tremors, ataxia, seizures), even in dogs with no known history of neurologic problems. Use with caution in dogs with a history of seizures or neurologic disorder. Dogs should test negative for heartworm infection before being treated with this product, which is not effective against adult *D immitis* infection. This combination product should not be used in dogs younger than 8 weeks of age or weighing less than 1.3 kg (2.8 lb).[8]

CATS:

Moxidectin/imidacloprid (*Advantage Multi® for Cats*): Not indicated for use in cats weighing less than 0.91 kg (2 lb) or in kittens younger than 9 weeks of age. **Do not use canine products on cats.**[5]

Moxidectin/fluralaner (*Bravecto® Plus*): Not indicated for use in kittens younger than 6 months of age and/or weighing less than 1.2 kg (2.6 lb)[3]

FERRETS:

Moxidectin/imidacloprid (*Advantage Multi® for Cats*): Not indicated for use in ferrets weighing less than 0.91 kg (2 lb)[5]

HORSES:

Moxidectin is not for use in horses intended for food purposes and is not labeled for use in foals younger than 6 months of age.[26,27] Extreme caution should be used when administering this product to foals and young and miniature horses, as overdose may result in serious adverse effects.

CATTLE:

Moxidectin injection is not for use in female dairy cattle of breeding age or in calves younger than 8 weeks of age.[28]

SHEEP:

The sheep product should not be used in other animal species, as severe adverse effects, including fatalities in dogs, may result.[29]

Adverse Effects

DOGS:

<u>Moxidectin as a sole agent:</u>

Injectable products (*ProHeart® 6, ProHeart® 12*): Previously, the injectable product (*ProHeart® 6*) was implicated in serious adverse effects. In 2004, at the request of the FDA, the manufacturer instituted a voluntary recall of *ProHeart® 6* after reports of serious adverse effects (including anaphylaxis, liver disease, autoimmune hemolytic disease, convulsions, and death) were discovered to have been caused by contamination from residual solvent. The product reentered the market in 2013 after data analysis and label revision. In 2019, the 12-month injectable product (*ProHeart® 12*) was approved with a restricted distribution program that allows only clinicians to order and administer the product after the clinician and pet owner complete a Risk Mitigation Action Plan (RiskMAP) program. <u>Anaphylaxis</u>, vomiting, diarrhea, listlessness, weight loss, seizures, injection site reactions, and elevated body temperature have been reported. Coughing and dyspnea may occur in heartworm-positive dogs. Elevated BUN, elevated creatinine, elevated liver enzymes, hypoproteinemia, hyperbilirubinemia, and hepatopathy were reported as rare adverse effects; for this reason, the drug should be used cautiously in dogs with renal or hepatic dysfunction.[1,2]

<u>Combination products:</u>

Moxidectin/imidacloprid (*Advantage Multi®*): In heartworm-negative dogs, field studies report pruritus, mild erythema, and a dry residue at the site of application.[6] Some dogs had GI signs (eg, vomiting, diarrhea, anorexia), lethargy, coughing, nasal discharge, or ocular discharge; these signs were postulated to have been caused by drug administration or underlying worm burdens.

Moxidectin/pyrantel/sarolaner (*Simparica Trio®*): This product contains sarolaner, which is an isoxazoline. This class of drug has been associated with neurologic adverse effects (eg, muscle tremors, ataxia, seizures), even in dogs with no known history of neurologic problems. Use with caution in dogs with a history of seizures or neurologic disorder. Adverse effects reported in field safety studies in dogs receiving this oral combination product include vomiting (14.3%), diarrhea (13.2%), and lethargy (8.5%).[8]

CATS:

Moxidectin/imidacloprid (*Advantage Multi® for Cats*): In field studies, behavioral changes (eg, agitation, excessive grooming, hiding, pacing, spinning), discomfort (eg, scratching, rubbing, headshaking), lethargy, hypersalivation, polydipsia, and coughing or gagging were noted. Cats may experience hypersalivation, tremors, vomiting, and decreased appetite if the topical solution is ingested. Postapproval adverse effect reports include pyrexia, tachypnea, hypersalivation, depression/lethargy, application site reactions (eg, alopecia, pruritus, lesions, erythema), decreased appetite, vomiting, bloody stool, hyperactivity, ataxia, trembling, and behavior changes.[5]

Moxidectin/fluralaner (*Bravecto® Plus*): Fluralaner, an isooxazoline, has been associated with neurologic adverse effects (eg, muscle tremors, ataxia, seizures), even in cats with no known history of neurologic problems. Use this product with caution in cats with a history of neurologic disease.[3]

FERRETS:

Moxidectin/imidacloprid (*Advantage Multi® for Cats*): Ferrets may experience lethargy, pruritus/scratching, scabbing, redness, wounds, and/or inflammation at the treatment site, and they may emit a chemical odor.[5]

HORSES:

Adverse effects appear to be nonexistent or minimal in horses given a label-recommended dose of moxidectin.[26,27] A case report in which 4 foals developed CNS depression and coma after receiving high doses has been reported.[30]

CATTLE:

Adverse effects appear to be nonexistent or minimal in cattle given a label-recommended dose of moxidectin.[28,31]

Reproductive/Nursing Safety

DOGS/CATS/FERRETS:

Reproductive studies have demonstrated no evidence of adverse effects on fertility, reproductive performance, or offspring of dogs given moxidectin as a single agent.[1,2]

Safe use of moxidectin combination products has not been evaluated in dogs, cats, and ferrets used for breeding and those that are pregnant or lactating.[3,5,6,8]

CATTLE/HORSES:

Reproductive studies have not demonstrated evidence of adverse effects on fertility, reproductive performance, or offspring in male or female cattle or horses.[26-28,31] After SC injection, ≈5% of a dose given to the cow can be passed to suckling calves. Calves as young as 8 weeks of age showed no signs of toxicity when treated with up to 3 times the recommended dose while nursing from cows being concurrently treated with the label-recommended injection dose of moxidectin.[28]

Overdose/Acute Toxicity

DOGS:

<u>Moxidectin as a sole agent</u>:

Injectable products (*ProHeart® 6, ProHeart® 12*): In safety studies, no clinical signs of moxidectin toxicity were observed in dogs receiving 3 or 5 times the recommended dose.[1,2]

<u>Combination products:</u>

Moxidectin/imidacloprid (*Advantage Multi®*): In safety studies, loose stools, diarrhea, reduced appetite, and vomiting were noted in puppies 7 weeks of age given up to 5 times the labeled dose every 2 weeks. After oral administration of the topical solution, vomiting, nervousness, and neurologic signs (eg, circling, ataxia, tremors) were noted.[6] Topical exposure of up to 5 times the labeled dose did not cause clinical abnormalities in ivermectin-sensitive collies, but neurologic signs (eg, depression, ataxia, mydriasis, salivation) occurred after oral administration of 40% of the label-recommended dose.

Moxidectin/pyrantel/sarolaner (*Simparica Trio®*): Puppies 8 weeks of age receiving 5 times the maximum recommended dose did not have clinically relevant adverse effects.[8] Collies with the *MDR1* mutation (also known as *ABCB1*-1delta) demonstrated signs of avermectin sensitivity (eg, ataxia, muscle fasciculations, mydriasis) after receiving 5 times the label-recommended dose.

CATS:

Combination products:

Moxidectin/imidacloprid (*Advantage Multi® for Cats*): Topical overdoses as low as 3 times the label-recommended dose caused lethargy, ataxia, and disorientation in a healthy 9-week-old kitten. Oral ingestion of the topical solution (at the maximum labeled dose) caused vomiting, inappetence, tremor, cough, and/or hypersalivation.[5]

Moxidectin/fluralaner (*Bravecto® Plus*): No clinically relevant effects were noted in kittens after topical administration of up to 5 times the labeled dose. Oral administration of the topical solution to kittens and adult cats at the labeled dose caused hypersalivation, vomiting, and transient reduction in food consumption; coughing after administration was also noted in adult cats.

HORSES:

In one report, 5 horses (4 of which were foals) showed clinical signs (eg, coma, dyspnea, depression, ataxia, tremors, seizures, weakness) after receiving an oral moxidectin overdose greater than 1.7 mg/kg (≈4 times the label-recommended dose). Four other horses received an oral overdose of 0.9 – 1.7 mg/kg and did not show clinical signs.[30]

CATTLE:

In studies on cattle, application of the pour-on moxidectin solution at 5 times the label-recommended dose for 5 consecutive days, 10 times for 2 consecutive days, and 25 times for 1 day did not produce any significant adverse clinical or pathological effects.[31] No signs of toxicity were seen in growing cattle that were given up to 5 times the labeled dose of moxidectin injection or in calves as young as 8 weeks of age given 3 times the recommended dose. Mild, transient ataxia occurred in growing cattle given 10 times the recommended injection dose.

For patients that have experienced or are suspected to have experienced an overdose, consultation with a 24-hour poison consultation center specializing in providing veterinary-specific information is recommended. For general information related to overdose and toxin exposures, as well as contact information for poison control centers, refer to ***Appendix***.

Drug Interactions

Use caution when administering injectable moxidectin (*ProHeart® 6 or ProHeart® 12*) in conjunction with vaccinations, as there is an increased potential for anaphylaxis and other immune-mediated reactions.[1,2]

Although no other specific drug interactions for moxidectin have been reported, the following drug interactions have either been reported or are theoretical in humans or animals receiving ivermectin (a related compound) and may be of significance in veterinary patients. Unless otherwise noted, use together is not necessarily contraindicated, but weigh the potential risks and perform additional monitoring when appropriate.

- **BENZODIAZEPINES**: Effects may be potentiated by moxidectin; use together not advised in humans
- **P-GLYCOPROTEIN INHIBITORS**: Caution is advised if using moxidectin with other p-glycoprotein inhibitors. Those dogs at risk for the *MDR1* mutation (also known as *ABCB1*-1delta; eg, collies, Australian shepherds, shelties, long-haired whippets, "white feet" breeds) should probably not be given moxidectin with the following drugs (unless determined to be unaffected):
  - **AMIODARONE**
  - **CARVEDILOL**
  - **CLARITHROMYCIN**
  - **CYCLOSPORINE**
  - **DILTIAZEM**
  - **ERYTHROMYCIN**
  - **ITRACONAZOLE**
  - **KETOCONAZOLE**
  - **QUINIDINE**
  - **SPINOSAD**
  - **SPIRONOLACTONE**
  - **TAMOXIFEN**
  - **VERAPAMIL**

Laboratory Considerations

- When performing a **fecal egg count reduction (FECR) test** in horses, it is preferable to wait at least 12 weeks after the previous moxidectin administration before collecting another pretreatment sample.[32]

Dosages

DOGS:

Moxidectin 10% (*ProHeart® 6 or ProHeart® 12*) labeled indications (label dosage; FDA-approved): 0.05 mL of the constituted suspension/kg SC (delivers moxidectin at 0.17 mg/kg for *ProHeart® 6* and 0.5 mg/kg for *ProHeart® 12*).[1,2] Alternate injection sites (either right or left of the dorsum of the neck cranial to the scapula) with subsequent administrations. Calculate the dose based on the dog's weight at the time of treatment; a dose chart in the package insert can be used as a guide. **NOTE**: Clinicians must complete the RiskMAP training and certification program before administering *ProHeart®*. Dogs should be monitored for 30 minutes after injection. Educational materials should be provided to the owners, and the dog should be carefully observed at home for 24 hours following administration.

Frequency of treatment: *ProHeart® 6* and *ProHeart® 12* prevent infection by *Dirofilaria immitis* for 6 months and 12 months, respectively.[1,2] *ProHeart®* should be administered within 1 month of the dog's first exposure to mosquitoes. Follow-up treatments can be given every 6 months for *ProHeart® 6* or 12 months for *ProHeart® 12* if the dog has continued exposure to mosquitoes and continues to be healthy without weight loss. When switching from a different heartworm preventive product, *ProHeart®* should be given within 1 month of the last dose of the former medication.[1]

Moxidectin 2.5%/imidacloprid 10% (*Advantage Multi®*) label indications (label dosage; FDA-approved): The recommended minimum dose is imidacloprid 10 mg/kg with moxidectin 2.5 mg/kg once a month by topical administration (**NOTE**: See package insert for specific instructions on application and safety).[6] For dogs 1.4 to 4 kg (3 to 9 lb) = 0.4 mL, 4.1 to 9 kg (9.1 to 20 lb) = 1 mL, 9.1 to 24.9 kg (20.1 to 55 lb) = 2.5 mL, 25 to 39.9 kg (55.1 to 88 lb) = 4 mL, 40 to 49.9 kg (88.1 to 110 lb) = 5 mL; dogs weighing more than 49.9 kg (110 lb) should be treated with an appropriate combination for their weight. For prevention of heartworm disease, moxidectin should be administered at 1-month intervals. For treatment and control of intestinal nematode infections, moxidectin should be administered once.

Moxidectin/pyrantel/sarolaner (*Simparica Trio*®) (label dosage; FDA-approved): Chewable tablets are available in sizes for dogs weighing 1.3 to 59.9 kg (2.8 to 132 lb). Each tablet size is formulated to provide minimum dosages of moxidectin 24 µg/kg (0.011 mg/lb), sarolaner 1.2 mg/kg (0.54 mg/lb), and pyrantel pamoate 5 mg/kg (2.27 mg/lb) PO with or without food once monthly.[8]

Canine demodicosis (extra-label): **NOTE**: Isoxazolines (eg, fluralaner, sarolaner) have supplanted avermectins for ectoparasite management.

1. Moxidectin 0.2 – 0.5 mg/kg PO daily (oral dosage forms not available in the US).[33] **WARNING**: Because these doses can cause serious neurotoxicity in dogs with the *MDR1* mutation (also known as *ABCB1*-1delta), it is highly recommended that this mutation be tested for before milbemycins (eg, moxidectin) are used to treat demodicosis in dogs. Because a negative *MDR1* test (normal/normal) does not ensure tolerance to this medication, it is recommended to begin with a test dose of moxidectin 50 µg/kg PO on the first day with gradual daily dose increases of 50 µg/kg until the desired dose is achieved without adverse effects.[34]
2. **Moxidectin 2.5 %/imidacloprid 10% (*Advantage Multi*® *for Dogs*)**: Apply product based on body weight recommendations found on product label once weekly for dogs with juvenile-onset and mild cases of demodicosis.[35] If clinical improvement is not seen in the first few weeks, other therapy (eg, isoxazolines[15]) should be considered.

Ocular *Thelazia callipaeda* (eyeworm) (extra-label): moxidectin 2.5%/imidacloprid 10% (*Advantage Multi*®) applied topically according to product weight-range dose recommendations for label indications; repeat dose 28 days after initial treatment[36]

CATS:

Moxidectin 1%/imidacloprid 10% (*Advantage Multi*® *for Cats*) label indications (label dosage; FDA-approved): The recommended minimum dose is imidacloprid 10 mg/kg with moxidectin 1 mg/kg once a month by topical administration (**NOTE**: See package insert for specific instructions on application and safety).[5] For cats 0.9 to 2.2 kg (2 to 5 lb) = 0.23 mL; 2.3 to 4 kg (5.1 to 9 lb) = 0.4 mL; 4.1 to 8.2 kg (9.1 to 18 lb) = 0.8 mL; cats weighing more than 8.2 kg (18 lb) should be treated with an appropriate combination for their weight. For prevention of heartworm disease, moxidectin should be administered at 1-month intervals. For the treatment and control of intestinal nematode infections, moxidectin should be administered once.

Moxidectin/fluralaner (*Bravecto*® *Plus*) labeled indications (label dosage; FDA-approved): Based on body weight, each applicator contains moxidectin 2 mg/kg and fluralaner 40 mg/kg applied topically as a single dose every 2 months. For cats 1.2 to 2.8 kg (2.6 to 6.2 lb) = 0.4 mL; more than 2.8 to 6.3 kg (6.2 to 13.8 lb) = 0.9 mL; more than 6.3 to 12.5 kg (13.8 to 27.5 lb) = 1.8 mL.[3] Cats weighing more than 12.5 kg (27.5 lb) should be administered the appropriate combination of tubes for their weight. The drug may be administered year-round or, at a minimum, should be administered at 2-month intervals beginning with the cat's first seasonal exposure to mosquitoes.

Feline aelurostrongylosis (*Aelurostrongylus abstrusus*) (extra-label): 1 to 3 topical applications of moxidectin 1% with imidacloprid 10% (*Advantage Multi*® *for Cats*) according to product weight range and applied every two weeks appeared to be effective in the treatment of cats infected with *A abstrusus*.[37,38] Monthly applications also appear to be effective.[39]

Notoedric mange (feline scabies) (extra-label): Moxidectin 1% / imidacloprid 10% (*Advantage Multi*® *for Cats*) according to product label-recommended dosing according to body weight[40]

FERRETS:

Moxidectin 1%/imidacloprid 10% (*Advantage Multi*® *for Cats*) labeled indications (label dosage; FDA-approved): The recommended minimum dose is imidacloprid 20 mg/kg (9 mg/lb) and moxidectin 2 mg/kg (0.9 mg/lb) once a month by topical administration.[5] Only the 0.4 mL applicator tube volume should be used on ferrets; the 0.23 mL applicator tube volume can result in an underdose, and the 0.8 mL size can result in an overdose.

HORSES:

Combination oral gel with or without praziquantel (*Quest*®, *Quest*® *Plus*) label indications (label dosage; FDA-approved): Moxidectin 0.4 mg/kg PO.[26,27] Dial in the weight of the animal on the syringe. Administer gel by inserting the syringe applicator into the animal's mouth through the interdental space and depositing the gel in the back of the mouth near the base of the tongue. After the syringe is removed, the animal's head should be raised to ensure proper swallowing of the gel. Horses weighing more than 680 kg (1500 lb) require additional gel from a second syringe.

CATTLE:

Pour-on label indications (label dosage; FDA-approved): Moxidectin 1 mL (5 mg)/10 kg (22 lb) body weight applied slowly in a narrow strip directly to the hair and skin along the top of the back from the withers to the base of the tail.[31] Application should be made to healthy skin and avoiding mange scabs, skin lesions, or extraneous foreign matter. Varying weather conditions do not affect pour-on efficacy.

Injection label indications (label dosage; FDA-approved): Moxidectin 0.2 mg/kg (1 mL for each 50 kg [110 lb] of body weight) SC under the loose skin in front of or behind the shoulder.[28] Needles ½ to ¾ inch in length and 16 to 18 gauge are recommended. Do not give this product by any other route.

Injection (extra-label): Moxidectin 1 mg/kg SC was more effective against helminths than the labeled dose in feedlot calves, but the authors expressed caution regarding the potential for moxidectin resistance with this dose.[41]

SHEEP/GOATS:

Label indications for sheep (label dosage; FDA-approved): Moxidectin 0.2 mg/kg (1 mL per 5 kg [11 lb] body weight) PO (drench)[42]

Goats (extra-label): Moxidectin dosing in goats should be used at 2 times the oral dose for sheep.[43] In countries in which the injection is licensed for use in sheep, 1.5 times the injectable sheep dose can be given to goats.[44]

NEW WORLD CAMELIDS:

Antiparasitic agent (extra-label): Moxidectin 0.2 mg/kg PO for GI helminths[45]

Monitoring

- Efficacy based on clinical signs and diagnostic testing (eg, FECR testing, fecal flotation, heartworm antigen testing, external parasite elimination)
- For demodicosis, clinical signs and monthly skin scrapings; continue treatment for 4 weeks beyond 2 negative monthly skin scrapings[33]
- Adverse effects
- Fecal egg count reduction testing (FECR testing) for horses and ruminants[49]

Client Information

- If your animal is receiving *ProHeart®* injection, your veterinarian will provide guidance according to the FDA-required RiskMAP program.
- Do not apply topical products to irritated skin.
- Children should not come into contact with the topical small animal products for 30 minutes (*Advantage® Multi for Cats)* to 2 hours (*Bravecto® Plus, Advantage® Multi for Dogs*) after application. For the first 30 minutes after application of *Advantage® Multi* products, ensure that dogs and cats cannot lick the product from application sites on themselves or other treated pets, and separate all treated animals and other pets to reduce the risk for accidental ingestion. Ingestion of this product by dogs or cats may cause serious side effects, including depression, salivation, dilated pupils, incoordination, panting, and generalized muscle tremors. In dogs and cats sensitive to milbemycins, the side effects may be more severe and can include coma and death.
- When using topical products on dogs, cats, and ferrets, part the animal's hair and apply the product directly to the skin at the base of the head (cats and ferrets) or between the shoulder blades (dogs). For dogs weighing more than 9.1 kg (20 lb), apply the solution in 3 or 4 spots that cannot be licked. Do not apply to irritated skin. Pink skin, damp hair, or a powdery residue may be seen temporarily.
- Wash your hands well after application. Contact a physician if any skin irritation occurs in humans.
- Treated cattle can be easily identified by a characteristic purple color of the topical pour-on, which remains for a short period after application. To avoid inadvertent residue, untreated animals should be housed separately from treated animals for the duration of the withdrawal period.
- In horses, oral gels are safe to use when used as directed.
- Moxidectin is toxic to aquatic organisms, including fish. Do not contaminate water by direct application or improper disposal of drug containers. Dispose of containers in an approved landfill site.
- The topical products are flammable; keep away from open flames, heat, sparks, or other sources of ignition.

Chemistry/Synonyms

Moxidectin, a milbemycin-class antiparasitic agent, is a semisynthetic, methoxime derivative of nemadectin. Moxidectin is a white or pale-yellow, amorphous powder that is practically insoluble in water and very soluble in alcohol.

Moxidectin may also be known as CL-301423, *Advantage® Multi, Advocate®, Barrier®, Bravecto® Plus, ComboCare®, Coraxis®, Cydectin®, Imoxi®, Midamox®, Parasedge® Multi, Quest®*, or *Simparica Trio®*.

Storage/Stability

Store the unconstituted sustained-release injection product at or below 25°C (77°F). Do not expose to light for extended periods of time. After constitution, *ProHeart® 6* is stable for 4 weeks when refrigerated at 2°C to 8°C (36°F-46°F).[1] *ProHeart® 12* is stable for 8 weeks when refrigerated at 2°C to 8°C (36°F-46°F).[2]

The topical solution for small animal species should be stored between 4°C and 25°C (39°F-77°F); avoid excess heat or cold.[5,6] Only open the outer pouch immediately before administration.

The oral gel for horses should be stored at or near room temperature (15°C-30°C [59°F-86°F]); avoid freezing.[26,27] If the product freezes, thaw completely before using. Partially used syringes should have the cap tightly secured.

The topical solution for cattle should be stored at or below room temperature.[31] Do not allow prolonged exposure to temperatures above 25°C (77°F). If the product becomes frozen, thaw completely and shake well before using.

The commercially available injection and the oral drench for sheep should be stored at or below 25°C (77°F) and protected from light.[28,42] The moxidectin solution for injection for sheep should be used within 12 months of first puncture.

Compatibility/Compounding Considerations

When constituting the sustained-release injectable product (*ProHeart®6* or *ProHeart® 12*), the provided diluent must be used and there are very specific directions for proper preparation. Refer to the package insert for more information.[1,2]

Do not mix moxidectin oral drench for sheep with any other product.[42]

Dosage Forms/Regulatory Status

VETERINARY-LABELED PRODUCTS:

Single Agent Products:

Moxidectin 2.5% Topical Solution; *Coraxis®*; (Rx). FDA-approved for use in dogs NADA# 141-417. While this product is still listed in FDA's Green Book of approved animal drugs, it may no longer be commercially available in the United States.

Moxidectin 10% Sustained-Release (microspheres) Injectable: 598 mg/vial with 17 mL diluent vial; *ProHeart® 6*; (Rx).[1] FDA-approved for use in dogs 6 months of age or older. NADA# 141-189

Moxidectin 10% Sustained-Release (microspheres) Injectable: 889 mg/vial with 8 mL diluent vial, and 4444 mg/vial with 40 mL diluent vial; *ProHeart® 12*; (Rx). FDA-approved for use in dogs 12 months of age or older. NADA# 141-519

Moxidectin 0.5% (5 mg/mL) Pour-On for Cattle in 500 mL and 1 L squeeze-measure pour bottles, and 2.5 L, 5 L, and 10 L containers for use with commercial applicators; *Cydectin®*; (OTC). FDA-approved for use in cattle; not to be used in veal calves. No meat or milk withdrawal times required, but the FDA has established tolerances of 50 ppb and 200 ppb for parent moxidectin in muscle and liver, respectively, in cattle. NADA# 141-099

Moxidectin 10 mg/mL Injectable Solution in 200 mL and 500 mL; *Cydectin® Injectable Solution*; (OTC). FDA-approved for use in cattle. Not to be used in female dairy cattle 20 months of age or older, veal calves, or calves younger than 8 weeks of age. Meat withdrawal is 21 days. NADA# 141-220

Moxidectin 1 mg/mL Oral Drench Solution in 1 L and 4 L; *Cydectin® Oral Drench for Sheep*; (OTC).[29] FDA-approved for use in sheep. Not to be used in female sheep providing milk for human consumption. Meat withdrawal is 7 days. NADA# 141-247

Moxidectin Oral Gel containing 20 mg/mL in 14.4 g syringes (sufficient to treat one 680 kg [1500 lb] horse); *Quest®*; (OTC).[26] FDA-approved for use in horses or ponies 6 months of age and older and not intended for food purposes. NADA# 141-087

Combination Products:

Moxidectin 1.4% (14 mg/mL) and Fluralaner 28% (280 mg/mL) Topical Solution in 0.4 mL, 0.9 mL, and 1.8 mL tubes; *Bravecto® Plus*; (Rx).[3] FDA-approved for use in cats and kittens 6 months of age and older. NADA# 141-518

Moxidectin 1% (10 mg/mL) and Imidacloprid 10% (100 mg/mL) Topical Solution in three 0.23 mL tubes, six 0.4 mL tubes, and six 0.8 mL tubes; *Advantage Multi® for Cats*, generic; (Rx).[46] FDA-approved for use in cats 9 weeks of age or older and weighing 0.9 kg (2 lb) or more. FDA-approved (0.4 mL only) for ferrets weighing 0.9 kg (2 lb) or more. NADA# 141-254

Moxidectin 2.5% (25 mg/mL) and Imidacloprid 10% (100 mg/mL) Topical Solution in six 0.4 mL tubes, six 1 mL tubes, six 2.5 mL tubes, six 4 mL tubes, and six 5 mL tubes; *Advantage Multi® for Dogs*; generic; (Rx).[47] FDA-approved for use on dogs 7 weeks of age or older and weighing more than 1.4 kg (3 lb). This product may be known as *Advocate®* in some countries. Do not use canine product on cats. NADA# 141-251

Moxidectin 20 mg/mL and Praziquantel 125 mg/mL Oral Gel in 14 g syringes (sufficient to treat one 680 kg [1500 lb] horse); *Quest Plus®*; (OTC). FDA-approved for use in horses or ponies 6 months of age and older and not intended for food purposes. NADA# 141-216

Moxidectin with Pyrantel Pamoate and Sarolaner Chewable (flavored) Tablets for dogs: 1.3 to 2.4 kg (2.8 to 5.5 lb): moxidectin 0.06 mg, pyrantel pamoate 12.5 mg, and sarolaner 3 mg; 2.5 to 4.9 kg (5.6 to 11 lb): moxidectin 0.12 mg, pyrantel pamoate 25 mg, and sarolaner 6 mg; 5 to 9.9 kg (11.1 to 22 lb): moxidectin 0.24 mg, pyrantel pamoate 50 mg, and sarolaner 12 mg; 10 to 19.9 kg (22.1 to 44 lb): moxidectin 0.48 mg, pyrantel pamoate 100 mg, and sarolaner 24 mg; 20 to 39.9 kg (44.1 to 88 lb): moxidectin 0.96 mg, pyrantel pamoate 200 mg, and sarolaner 48 mg; 40 to 60 kg (88.1 to 132 lb): moxidectin 1.44 mg, pyrantel pamoate 300 mg, and sarolaner 72 mg; *Simparica Trio®* (Rx). FDA-approved for use in dogs 8 weeks of age and older and weighing 1.3 kg (2.8 lb) or more. NADA# 141-521

In the United Kingdom and other countries, moxidectin is available in combination with triclabendazole (*Cydectin® TriclaMox*) as topical pour-on solutions for use in sheep and cattle.

HUMAN-LABELED PRODUCTS: NONE

References

For the complete list of references, see **wiley.com/go/budde/plumb**

Mycobacterial Cell Wall Fraction Immunomodulator

(my-koe-bak-***tear***-ee-al)

Immunostimulant

Prescriber Highlights

- ► Biologic agent labeled for treatment of mixed mammary tumors and mammary adenocarcinomas in dogs, treatment of sarcoids, equine respiratory disease complex (ERDC), or endometritis in horses, and the reduction of mortality and clinical signs associated with scours in calves.
- ► Contraindications include hypersensitivity and mycobacterial infection.
- ► Use with caution in patients with hyperimmune disease and discontinue use if clinical signs such as urticaria, lymphadenitis, cellulitis, or abscessation develop.
- ► Patients receiving corticosteroids or immunosuppressants may not respond to therapy.
- ► Adverse effects include transient fever, depression, decreased appetite, and localized pain. Hypersensitivity and systemic inflammatory reactions are also possible.

Uses/Indications

Mycobacterial cell wall fraction (MCWF) immunomodulator is USDA-approved for use in dogs, horses, and cattle for a variety of indications. The canine product is approved for the treatment of mixed mammary tumors and mammary adenocarcinomas.[1]

There are multiple equine products with different indications, including treatment of sarcoids, equine respiratory disease complex (ERDC), and treatment of equine endometritis caused by *Streptococcus zooepidemicus*.[2]

Although these are not labeled indications, *Equimune®* has also been used anecdotally in horses as an adjuvant immunostimulant for equine protozoal myeloencephalitis (EPM) treatment and as an adjuvant for herpesvirus vaccines when injected IM at a separate site from the vaccine.

The bovine product is labeled for treatment of neonatal calves 1 to 5 days of age to reduce mortality and clinical signs associated with calf scours caused by enterotoxigenic *Escherichia coli* K99.[3]

Pharmacology/Actions

Mycobacteriaceae have been known for many years to have antitumor activity. Mycobacterial cell wall fractionated compounds are an emulsion of mycobacterial cell wall fractions derived from *Mycobacterium phlei* that have been modified to reduce their toxic and allergic effects but retain their antitumor activity.[1]

Mycobacterial cell wall fractionated compounds require a functional immune system for efficacy.[1] They stimulate the activation of macrophages and thymic lymphocytes which indirectly kill tumor cells through antitumor cytokines. Interleukin-1 release from macrophages is thought to be the primary mediator for their actions.

Pharmacokinetics

No information was located.

Contraindications/Precautions/Warnings

Mycobacterial fractionated compounds should not be used in patients with prior hypersensitivity to them or those with mycobacterial infections. They should be used with caution in animals with a history of hyperimmune diseases. Discontinue use of mycobacterial fractionated compounds in animals that develop clinical signs such as urticaria, lymphadenitis, cellulitis, or abscessation.[1-4]

The inflammatory response can occasionally be severe after initial treatment, leading to edema and malaise. Discontinue treatment until clinical signs have resolved.[1]

Patients receiving corticosteroids or immunosuppressants may not respond to treatment.[1,2,4]

Adverse Effects

Adverse effects may occur for 1 to 2 days following and can include fever, drowsiness, and decreased appetite. Local inflammation commonly occurs and can cause pain and tenderness at the injection site. Necrosis and draining may occur in regressing tumors, which can last for several weeks. Anaphylaxis or hypersensitivity reactions are possible[1-4]; severe respiratory inflammatory reactions have also been reported in horses.

Reproductive/Nursing Safety

Some equine products are safe to use in pregnant mares[2,4]; refer to specific labels for detailed information prior to administration. No other information was located. Because safety has not been established in animals, this drug should only be used when the maternal benefits outweigh the potential risks to offspring.

Overdose/Acute Toxicity

For patients that have experienced or are suspected to have experienced an overdose, consultation with a 24-hour poison consultation center specializing in providing veterinary-specific information is recommended. For general information related to overdose and toxin exposures, as well as contact information for poison control centers, refer to ***Appendix***.

Drug Interactions

The following drug interactions have either been reported or are theoretical in animals receiving mycobacterial cell wall fraction (MCWF) immunomodulator and may be of significance in veterinary patients. Unless otherwise noted, use together is not necessarily contraindicated, but weigh the potential risks and perform additional monitoring when appropriate.

- **CORTICOSTEROIDS** (eg, **dexamethasone, prednis(ol)one**): May reduce the effectiveness of MCWF immunostimulants

- **Corticotropin (ACTH), Cosyntropin**: May reduce the effectiveness of MCWF immunostimulants
- **Immunosuppressive Drugs** (eg, **cyclosporine**): May reduce the effectiveness of MCWF immunostimulants

Laboratory Considerations

- None identified

Dosages

DOGS:

Immunotherapy for mixed mammary tumor and mammary adenocarcinoma (label dosage; USDA-approved): Administer by intratumoral injection only. Using no larger than a 20-gauge needle, infiltrate entire tumor and a small region of adjacent and underlying tissue. Dose varies with tumor size, but 1 mL should be considered a minimum dose. Administer as a single dose 2 to 4 weeks prior to surgery or repeat treatment every 1 to 3 weeks as an alternative to surgery. Discontinue therapy if there is no response after 4 treatments.[1] Mix the emulsion thoroughly prior to administration; inject shortly after mixing, as the emulsion can separate rapidly. As pain may occur from injection, additional anesthetics or analgesics may be used.

HORSES:

NOTE: Various equine products exist. Ensure the correct product is being used for the intended indication via the labeled route. See ***Dosage Forms/Regulatory Status.***

Immunotherapy for sarcoids (label-dosage; USDA-approved): Administer by intratumoral injection only. Using no larger than a 20-gauge needle, infiltrate entire tumor and a small region of adjacent and underlying tissue. Dose varies with tumor size, but 1 mL should be considered a minimum dose. Repeat treatment every 1 to 3 weeks. Discontinue therapy if no response after 4 treatments.[4] Mix the emulsion thoroughly prior to administration; inject shortly after mixing, as the emulsion can separate rapidly. Large pedunculated sarcoids should be debulked by partial excision prior to treatment. As pain may occur from injection, additional anesthetics or analgesics may be used.

Immunotherapeutic agent for the treatment of equine respiratory disease complex (ERDC) (label dosage; USDA-approved): 1.5 mL IV into the jugular vein; may repeat dose in 1 to 3 weeks[2]

Treatment of equine metritis caused by *Streptococcus zooepidemicus* (label dosage; USDA-approved):

a) IV administration: 1.5 mL IV into the jugular vein during the early estrus period[5]

b) Intrauterine instillation: 1.5 mL mL diluted in sterile LRS, 0.9% sodium chloride, water for injection, or semen extender to a total volume of 25 – 50 mL and aseptically instilled into the uterus using a sterile catheter[5]

CATTLE:

Immunotherapeutic treatment for calves 1 to 5 days of age to reduce mortality and clinical signs associated with calf scours caused by enterotoxigenic *Escherichia coli* K99 (label dosage; USDA-approved): 1 mL IV once[3]

Monitoring

- Clinical efficacy: tumor size, metritis improvement, or respiratory infection improvement
- Adverse effects: fever, local reactions, anaphylaxis, appetite suppression

Client Information

- Your animal may be painful around the tumor injection site. As the medicine begins to work, tumors may ooze and drain. If this occurs and is bothersome, contact your veterinarian for further instructions on management.
- Treated animals may have a low-energy level, develop fever, or have a reduced appetite for a few days after treatment. If these signs persist, or are severe, contact your veterinarian.

Chemistry/Synonyms

Mycobacterial cell wall fraction (MCWF) compounds are oil-in-water emulsions containing purified cell wall fractions obtained from *Mycobacterium phlei* that are modified to reduce their toxic and allergic effect.[1] MCWF may also be known as mycobacterial cell wall extract; bacillus Calmette-Guerin, or BCG; *Amplimune®*; *Equimune®*; *Immunocidin®*; *Immunocidin® Equine;* and *Settle®*.

Storage/Stability

These products should be stored refrigerated (2°C-8°C [36°F-46°F]). Do not freeze. Unused product from vials not labeled for multi-dose use should be discarded after use. The emulsion breaks upon standing and the product must be re-emulsified prior to administration. To re-emulsify to a milky appearance, shake vial or roll syringe between hands.

Compatibility/Compounding Considerations

No specific information noted

Dosage Forms/Regulatory Status

VETERINARY-LABELED PRODUCTS:

NOTE: These products are USDA-licensed biologics, not FDA-approved products.

Mycobacterial Cell Wall Fraction (MCWF) Immunomodulator products:

Immunocidin®: **Intratumoral injection** for mixed mammary tumors and adenocarcinomas in **dogs**; 1 mg/mL of MCWF in a 2.5 mL vial. Contains gentamicin as a preservative

Immunocidin® Equine: **Intratumoral injection** for sarcoid tumors in **horses**; 5 mL vial. Contains gentamicin as a preservative. Do not administer within 21 days of slaughter.

Equimune®: **IV administration** for Equine Respiratory Disease Complex (ERDC) in **horses**; 1.5 mL single-dose vial. Contains gentamicin as a preservative. Do not administer within 21 days of slaughter.

Settle®: **IV or intrauterine administration** for endometritis in **horses**; 1.5 mL single-dose vial. Contains gentamicin as a preservative. Do not administer within 21 days of slaughter.

Amplimune®: **IV administration** for scours in **calves** 1 to 5 days of age; 5 mL, 20 mL, and 100 mL vials. Contains gentamicin as a preservative. Do not administer within 21 days of slaughter.

HUMAN-LABELED PRODUCTS: NONE

References

For the complete list of references, see **wiley.com/go/budde/plumb**

Mycophenolate

Mycophenolate Mofetil (MMF)

(mye-koe-***fen***-oh-late) *Cellcept*®

Immunosuppressant

Prescriber Highlights

- ► Immunosuppressive drug that may be useful for treating dogs with IMHA, IMTP, glomerulonephritis, myasthenia gravis, or meningoencephalomyelitis of unknown etiology in dogs; potentially useful in cats, but there is little information available on safety or efficacy.
- ► Limited experience in veterinary medicine, especially in cats or with long-term use
- ► Adverse effects include GI signs (eg, diarrhea, vomiting, anorexia) most commonly are dose-limiting and can be severe.
- ► Can be administered PO or IV. Compounding into appropriate oral dosage forms may be needed.
- ► Teratogenic in humans
- ► The National Institute for Occupational Safety and Health (NIOSH) classifies mycophenolate as a hazardous drug; use appropriate precautions when handling.

Uses/Indications

Although clinical experience using mycophenolate in veterinary medicine has been limited and no large well-controlled studies were located, mycophenolate appears useful in the treatment of a variety of autoimmune diseases, including immune-mediated hemolytic anemia (IMHA),[1-4] immune-mediated thrombocytopenia (IMTP),[5,6] myasthenia gravis,[7,8] meningoencephalomyelitis,[9,10] glomerulonephritis,[11] and pemphigus foliaceous.[12] Mycophenolate has been suggested for use in treating inflammatory bowel disease in dogs; however, the drug's primary adverse effects in dogs are gastritis, diarrhea, and intestinal inflammation. Mycophenolate is also used in anti-rejection protocols for organ transplants in animals. Mycophenolate is often used as part of a combination immunosuppressive therapy protocol in a patient, although it has also been used alone as monotherapy. The drug was ineffective for the treatment of sudden acquired retinal degeneration syndrome (SARDS) in dogs.[13]

In humans, although this drug is used off-label for a variety of autoimmune disease indications, it is labeled only for use in preventing transplant rejection.

Pharmacology/Actions

Mycophenolate mofetil (MMF) is a prodrug that must be hydrolyzed in vivo to mycophenolic acid (MPA) to be pharmacologically active. Mycophenolic acid noncompetitively, but reversibly, inhibits inosine monophosphate dehydrogenase (IMPDH). Two distinct forms of IMPDH exist in the body, including type 1 found in most cells and type 2 existing in activated lymphocytes. Mycophenolic acid has a 5-fold greater affinity for the type 2 IMPDH isoform. Inosine monophosphate dehydrogenase is the rate-limiting enzyme in de novo synthesis of guanosine nucleotides. As T cells and B cells are dependent on de novo synthesis of purines (eg, guanosine) and, unlike other cells, cannot use salvage pathways, proliferative responses of T cells and B cells are inhibited, and suppression of B cell antibody formation occurs, thus inhibiting both cell-mediated and humoral immune responses. These effects enable MPA to inhibit leukocyte recruitment to inflammatory sites and allotransplant tissues.

In a study in juvenile dachshunds, MMF administration did not inhibit proliferating CD5+ T lymphocytes at any time point.[14] In healthy cats, MMF administration resulted in little change in peripheral blood mononuclear cell counts or CD4+/CD8+:T-cell ratios.[15]

Pharmacokinetics

Mycophenolate mofetil is absorbed after oral administration, but limited bioavailability studies in dogs have shown both a wide interpatient and interdose variation. A study performed in a single dog showed bioavailabilities of 54%, 65%, and 87% after administration of 10, 15, and 20 mg/kg of MMF, respectively.[16]

A study in dogs compared the pharmacokinetic parameters of mycophenolic acid (MPA) with its pharmacodynamic effects on inosine monophosphate dehydrogenase (IMPDH) activity in lymphocytes[17]; volume of distribution at steady-state was ≈5 L/kg, but inter-patient variability (±4.5) was wide. Elimination half-life for MPA was ≈8 hours (±4 hours). In a study performed in juvenile dachshunds receiving 13 mg/kg PO, peak MPA concentration occurred within 1 hour of administration, and half-life was 5.5 minutes.[14] Mycophenolic acid is primarily excreted in the urine, both unchanged (≈5%) and as the glucuronide metabolite (≈90%). In this study, the authors concluded that the pharmacokinetic/pharmacodynamic profile of MMF in dogs suggests that an every 8-hour dosing schedule would be required for optimization of immunosuppressive efficacy. However, dosing every 8 hours can be clinically challenging because of the severity of adverse effects, and thus has not entered common clinical usage (see ***Adverse Effects***).

In a study in healthy cats, administration of 20 mg/kg MMF IV as a CRI over 2 hours resulted in all cats forming the active MPA metabolite. Disposition of plasma MPA was highly variable and unpredictable. The major metabolite was a glucoside product, and a glucuronide product was found in only 3 of 6 cats.[18] An in vitro study similarly demonstrated a relative deficiency of MPA glucuronidation in cats.[19]

In humans, oral bioavailability averages 94%; food reduces peak MPA concentrations by 40%.[20] After absorption, MMF is rapidly and completely hydrolyzed to mycophenolic acid. Peak blood concentrations are seen ≈1 to 2 hours after oral administration. Mycophenolic acid 97% protein (albumin) bound and undergoes extensive hepatic metabolism, primarily via glucuronidation. Mycophenolic acid undergoes extensive enterohepatic recirculation, and reactivation to MPA within the gut may result in a second peak blood concentration 4 to 12 hours after administration. Elimination half-life of MPA is ≈17 hours. Metabolites are eliminated primarily via the kidneys.

Contraindications/Precautions/Warnings

Do not use mycophenolate in patients with documented hypersensitivity reactions to mycophenolate. Patients with severe renal dysfunction may require dosage adjustment. Because MMF can cause diarrhea, use with caution in patients with inflammatory bowel disease.

IV mycophenolate must be administered over at least 2 hours; do not give it as an IV bolus or via rapid IV infusion.

In humans, the active metabolite, MPA, is primarily excreted as the MPA-glucuronide metabolite. Mycophenolate should be used with caution in cats because of deficient MPA glucuronidation in this species.

For humans, mycophenolate has a black box warning regarding potential increased risk for lymphoma and serious infection associated with its use. Severe neutropenia has occurred in human transplant patients receiving mycophenolate.

The National Institute for Occupational Safety and Health (NIOSH) classifies mycophenolate as a group II hazardous drug (non-antineoplastic agent representing an occupational hazard to healthcare workers); personal protective equipment (PPE) should be used accordingly to minimize the risk of exposure.[21]

Do not confuse mycophenolate mofetil with mycophenolic acid. A study comparing adverse effects in dogs with MMF capsules and mycophenolate sodium (the sodium salt of mycophenolic acid) enteric-coated tablets demonstrated significantly greater occurrences and severity of diarrhea, weight loss, and decreased activity in dogs that received the sodium salt enteric-coated tablets.[22]

Adverse Effects

Because of limited experience with mycophenolate in veterinary patients, the adverse effect profile is not well established. At usual doses (10 mg/kg PO twice daily), mycophenolate is usually well tolerated in dogs. Dose-dependent diarrhea appears to be the most common adverse effect, but vomiting, anorexia, lethargy/reduced activity, lymphopenia, papillomatosis, and increased rates of dermal infections can be seen. In a study evaluating MMF in dogs for the treatment of IMHA at a dosage of 10 to 15 mg/kg PO every 8 hours, the authors concluded that the level of GI toxicity observed could not justify the use of MMF with this dosing regimen, despite the fact that 4 of 5 dogs achieved disease remission.[1] Ulcerative colitis may develop.[4] Mild hypersensitivity reactions after IV administration are possible. Because of the drug's immunosuppressive actions, increased systemic infection and malignancy rates are possible, especially with long-term use.

Diarrhea was the most common adverse effect in healthy cats enrolled in mycophenolate pharmacokinetic studies. Diarrhea was less frequent after IV administration and appeared dose related with oral use. Hyporexia was noted in 1 cat. Decreases in PCV and platelet counts have been noted, but the reduced values remained within the reference range.[15,18,23] Hepatopathy and pancreatitis were reported in one cat after receiving MMF for treatment of IMHA.[24]

In humans, the most common adverse effects include constipation, diarrhea, nausea, vomiting, and headache. Hypertension and peripheral edema occur in ≈30% of patients. Leukopenia has been reported in 25% to 45% of patients taking the medication. Other effects that occur more rarely include GI bleeding, severe neutropenia, cough, confusion, tremor, fatal neurologic disease, infection, and malignant lymphoma (0.4% to 1%).

Reproductive/Nursing Safety

Mycophenolate should be avoided, if at all possible, during pregnancy. Mycophenolate is a known teratogen in humans, causing congenital malformations and first trimester pregnancy loss. At doses significantly lower than those used in humans, increased resorptions and malformations were noted in rabbits and rats.

Mycophenolic acid is distributed in rat milk. It is unknown if mycophenolate is safe to use during nursing and it should be considered contraindicated.[25]

Overdose/Acute Toxicity

In acute toxicity studies performed in mice and monkeys, no deaths occurred in oral doses of mycophenolate up to 4000 mg/kg and 1000 mg/kg, respectively. In small animals, acute GI disturbances or neutropenia are possible. Treat supportively, if required. Cholestyramine may increase mycophenolate excretion.

For patients that have experienced or are suspected to have experienced an overdose, consultation with a 24-hour poison consultation center specializing in providing veterinary-specific information is recommended. For general information related to overdose and toxin exposures, as well as contact information for poison control centers, refer to ***Appendix.***

Drug Interactions

The following drug interactions have either been reported or are theoretical in humans or animals receiving mycophenolate and may be of significance in veterinary patients. Unless otherwise noted, use together is not necessarily contraindicated, but weigh the potential risks and perform additional monitoring when appropriate.

- **Acyclovir and Valacyclovir**: Increased serum concentrations of acyclovir and the phenolic glucuronide of mycophenolic acid
- **Aminoglycosides** (eg, **amikacin, gentamicin**): In rats, use together induced greater nephrotoxicity.
- **Antacids, Oral (Aluminum-, Calcium-, or Magnesium-Containing)**: Decreased absorption of mycophenolate; separate dosing by at least 2 hours.
- **Azathioprine**: Increased risk for myelosuppression; concurrent use is not recommended.
- **Cholestyramine**: May inhibit enterohepatic recycling of mycophenolate, reducing serum concentrations
- **Immunosuppressive Agents** (eg, **corticosteroids** [eg, **dexamethasone, predniso(lo)ne**], **leflunomide**): Additive immunosuppressant effects could occur
- **Iron (oral)**: Decreased absorption of mycophenolate; separate dosing by at least 2 hours.
- **Lanthanum Carbonate**: May decrease mycophenolate plasma concentrations
- **Probenecid**: Potentially increased serum concentrations of mycophenolic acid and the phenolic glucuronide of mycophenolic acid
- **Proton Pump Inhibitors (PPIs;** eg, **omeprazole, pantoprazole)**: May reduce mycophenolate absorption, decreasing MPA exposure (AUC)
- **Salicylates** (eg, **aspirin, bismuth subsalicylate**): Potentially increased concentrations of free mycophenolic acid
- **Sevelamer**: Decreased absorption of mycophenolate; administer MMF at least 2 hours prior to sevelamer.
- **Telmisartan**: May decrease mycophenolate exposure (AUC)
- **Vaccines, Modified Live**: Vaccines may be less effective; administer vaccines prior to initiating mycophenolate therapy and avoid concurrent use.

The following drugs or drug classes may reduce MPA exposure by inhibiting the enterohepatic recycling of the mycophenolate glucuronide metabolite:

- **Cephalosporins** (eg, **cephalexin, cefpodoxime**)
- **Clindamycin**
- **Cyclosporine**: additive immunosuppressant effects also possible
- **Fluoroquinolones** (eg, **ciprofloxacin, enrofloxacin**)
- **Metronidazole**
- **Rifampin**
- **Penicillins** (eg, **amoxicillin/clavulanate**)
- **Sulfonamides, Potentiated** (eg, **sulfa-/trimethoprim**)

Laboratory Considerations

- No issues noted

Dosages

DOGS:

Immune-mediated hemolytic anemia (extra-label): 8 – 12 mg/kg PO or IV every 12 hours in combination with predniso(lo)ne 2 – 3 mg/kg/day PO (50 – 60 mg/m2/day [NOT mg/kg/day] for dogs greater than 25 kg)[2,4]

Immune-mediated thrombocytopenia (IMTP) (extra-label): 7 – 9 mg/kg PO every 12 hours in combination with predniso(lo)ne (≈2 mg/kg/day)[5,6]

Meningoencephalomyelitis of unknown etiology (extra-label): 10 – 20 mg/kg PO or IV every 12 hours in conjunction with corticosteroids.[9,10] One study described administering MMF IV over 20 minutes using a syringe pump.[10]

Adjunctive immunosuppressive treatment of glomerular disease based on established pathology (extra-label): The International Renal Interest Society (IRIS) consensus statement recommends mycophenolate alone or in combination with prednisolone for peracute and/or rapidly progressive glomerular disease: mycophenolate 10 mg/kg PO every 12 hours. For stable or slowly progressive glomerular diseases, IRIS recommends mycophenolate alone. In the absence of overt adverse effects, therapy should continue for at least 8 weeks before altering or discontinuing the drug. Therapy should be continued in dogs demonstrating a complete or partial response to initial treatment for a minimum of 12 to 16 weeks. Thereafter, consideration should be given to tapering the treatment to a dose/schedule that maintains the response without worsening the proteinuria, azotemia, or clinical signs.[11]

Myasthenia gravis (extra-label): 15 – 20 mg/kg diluted and given IV over 2 to 4 hours every 24 hours until able to swallow, then 10 – 20 mg/kg PO every 12 hours.[7] One retrospective study found that when compared to using pyridostigmine alone, MMF with pyridostigmine did not significantly affect remission rate, time to remission, or survival time.[8]

Aplastic anemia (extra-label): From a case report in a single dog: mycophenolate 10 mg/kg PO every 12 hours. The first effects (improvements in hematocrit) were observed 2 weeks later, and complete remission of all blood cell counts were obtained in ≈3 weeks.[26]

Immune-mediated skin disease (extra-label): Dosages varied, but 10 – 20 mg/kg PO twice daily was typical. Adverse GI effects were noted with higher dosages.[12,27] In one study, dogs that achieved remission still required glucocorticoids.[12]

CATS:

Adjunctive treatment of IMHA (extra-label): From a case report of 2 cats: mycophenolate 10 mg/kg PO every 12 hours.[28] Use for immune-mediated disorders in cats is not recommended by some based on pharmacokinetic and pharmacodynamic data.[15]

Monitoring

- Efficacy
- Baseline and periodic CBCs every 2 to 3 weeks for the first month, then every 2 to 3 months during treatment.[4]
- Baseline and periodic serum chemistry profile, urinalysis, and urine culture
- Signs associated with infection (eg, fever, malaise, inappetence)
- GI effects (eg, inappetence, vomiting, diarrhea)

Client Information

- Preferably give on an empty stomach; if vomiting or lack of appetite occurs, try giving with food.
- Limited experience in veterinary medicine, especially in cats or for long-term use
- Diarrhea, vomiting, and anorexia are the most likely adverse effects and can be severe. If any of these signs persist or are severe, contact your veterinarian.
- Because of concerns that this drug can suppress the immune system and cause birth defects, pregnant women should wear gloves when handling this drug and avoid inhaling dust from capsules or split or crushed tablets. The manufacturer recommends that tablets or capsules not be crushed, split, or opened.
- This medicine is considered to be a hazardous drug as defined by the National Institute for Occupational Safety and Health (NIOSH) because it may affect the reproductive ability of males or females actively trying to conceive, women who are pregnant or may become pregnant, and women who are breastfeeding. It is recommended to wear gloves when administering this medication to your animal, and wash hands thoroughly afterwards. If you have any concerns about the risks associated with exposure to this medicine, speak with your veterinarian or health care provider.

Chemistry/Synonyms

Mycophenolate mofetil occurs as a white or almost white, crystalline powder. It is sparingly soluble in alcohol and practically insoluble in water at neutral pH; aqueous solubility increases as pH decreases. The pH of mycophenolate for injection after reconstitution is 2.2 to 4.1.

Mycophenolic acid is derived from *Penicillium stoloniferum*.

Mycophenolate mofetil may also be known as RS-61443 or MMF. International trade names include *CellCept*®, *Cellmune*®, *Imuxgen*®, *Munotras*®, *Mycept*®, *Myfortic*®, and *Refrat*®.

Storage/Compatibility

Mycophenolate mofetil tablets and capsules should be stored between 20°C and 25°C (68°F-77°F) and protected from light. Mycophenolate mofetil powder for oral suspension should be stored between 15°C and 30°C (59°F-86°F), preferably at 25°C (77°F). Once reconstituted with 94 mL of water, the solution may be stored at room temperature or in the refrigerator; do not freeze. The unused drug should be discarded after 60 days. Refer to the product label of generic formulations for specific reconstitution recommendations.

The injectable product should be stored between 15°C and 30°C (59°F-86°F); preferably at 25°C (77°F). Each vial should be reconstituted with 14 mL of 5% dextrose injection; the final volume is ≈15 mL. Gently agitate to dissolve the powder. Mycophenolate injection should not be mixed or given with any other medication or diluent. Administer mycophenolate within 6 hours of dilution. The drug must be administered over at least 2 hours and is not to be given as an IV bolus or via rapid IV infusion. For human use, the manufacturer recommends further diluting with dextrose 5% to a concentration of 6 mg/mL for IV administration. Mycophenolate diluted in dextrose 5% to a final concentration between 1 – 10 mg/mL in PVC bags was stable for seven days when stored under refrigeration or at room temperature.[29]

Compatibility/Compounding Considerations

The manufacturer states that mycophenolate injection should not be mixed or given with any other medication or diluent. The drug appears **Y-site compatible** with buprenorphine, butorphanol, calcium chloride, dexmedetomidine, dobutamine, dopamine, hydromorphone, magnesium sulfate, metoclopramide, metronidazole, ondansetron, potassium chloride, and ranitidine. The drug appears **Y-site incompatible** with amphotericin B, calcium gluconate, cefazolin, dexamethasone sodium phosphate, furosemide, heparin, meropenem, pantoprazole, phenobarbital, and sodium bicarbonate.

Compatibility is dependent on factors such as pH, concentration, temperature, and diluent used; consult specialized references or a hospital pharmacist for more specific information.

Dosage Forms/Regulatory Status

VETERINARY-LABELED PRODUCTS: NONE

HUMAN-LABELED PRODUCTS:

Mycophenolate Mofetil Oral Capsules: 250 mg; *CellCept*®, generic; (Rx)

Mycophenolate Mofetil Oral Tablets: 500 mg; *CellCept*®, generic; (Rx)

Mycophenolate Mofetil Powder for Oral Suspension: 200 mg/mL (reconstituted) in 225 mL bottles; *CellCept*®; (Rx)

Mycophenolate Mofetil Lyophilized Powder for Injection: 500 mg in 20 mL vials; *CellCept*®; (Rx)

Mycophenolate is also available as the sodium salt of mycophenolic acid in oral, delayed-release tablets; however, this dosage form cannot be used interchangeably with mycophenolate mofetils.[22]

References

For the complete list of references, see **wiley.com/go/budde/plumb**

Nalbuphine

(*nal*-byoo-feen) *Nubain®*

Opioid Partial Agonist

See also ***Nalbuphine Ophthalmic***

Prescriber Highlights

- Injectable opioid mixed agonist/antagonist used in combination as a premedication prior to general anesthesia in small animal species
- May also be used for mild-to-moderate pain relief or to reverse effects of full mu-opioid agonists without complete elimination of analgesic effects
- Has a relatively short duration of action in dogs and cats
- Use cautiously in patients with hepatic or renal impairment, bradyarrhythmias, or head trauma.
- Limited information about its use in veterinary medicine, but appears to be relatively safe and effective in small animal species
- Not a controlled substance in the United States

Uses/Indications

Nalbuphine may be used as premedication prior to general anesthesia. It could theoretically be used for analgesia, but it is only effective for relief of mild-to-moderate pain and has a relatively short duration of effect. Nalbuphine may be used to reverse the adverse effects (eg, respiratory depression) of mu-agonists (eg, morphine) while retaining some analgesic effects.

Nalbuphine has been used in dogs epidurally to decrease the MAC of isoflurane and to provide postoperative analgesia for ovariohysterectomy.[1] In calves undergoing surgical castration, nalbuphine reduces some pain-related behaviors but does not eliminate physiological signs of distress.[2]

When compared with other mixed agonist/antagonists (eg, butorphanol, buprenorphine), the potential benefit of nalbuphine is that it is not a controlled substance in the United States; however, there is considerably less clinical experience and published information about its use in animals.

Pharmacology/Actions

Nalbuphine is a synthetic opioid-receptor agonist-antagonist of the phenanthrene series. Nalbuphine binds to kappa-, mu-, and delta-opioid receptors. Its primary analgesic pharmacologic activity is due to its agonist activity at kappa receptors. Nalbuphine can cause respiratory depression, but above a certain dose (30 mg in adult humans), further respiratory depression does not occur.[3]

Nalbuphine does not increase plasma histamine in dogs.[4]

Pharmacokinetics

Nalbuphine has a similar pharmacokinetic profile as morphine.[5] Nalbuphine must be administered parenterally as it has very low oral bioavailability secondary to GI mucosal metabolism and a high first-pass effect. In humans, the onset of action is usually within 3 minutes after IV administration and 15 minutes after SC or IM doses. In humans, plasma half-life is ≈5 hours. Analgesic effects usually last from 3 to 6 hours after a dose. Analgesic duration of action in dogs and cats has anecdotally been reported as significantly shorter than in humans.

In calves, after 0.4 mg/kg IV, half-life, volume of distribution, and clearance were 0.68 hours, 6.8 L/kg, and 114 mL/minute/kg, respectively. Plasma concentrations were only detectable 3 hours after the injection.[2]

In Hispaniolan Amazon parrots, IM dosages of nalbuphine HCl had complete bioavailability. After IV administration, the measured volume of distribution was 2 L/kg and clearance was ≈70 mL per minute/kg. Terminal half-life was ≈20 minutes for both IV and IM doses.[6] A follow-up study using a sustained-release IM form (nalbuphine decanoate 37.5 mg/kg IM) showed a mean terminal half-life of 20.4 hours. Plasma concentrations that could be associated with antinociception (20 ng/mL) were maintained for 24 hours after injection.[7]

Contraindications/Precautions/Warnings

Nalbuphine is contraindicated in patients hypersensitive to it. Severe pain should be treated with other analgesics (eg, mu-opioid agonists). Use nalbuphine cautiously in patients with hepatic or renal impairment, bradyarrhythmias, or head trauma.

When used alone, nalbuphine rarely causes clinically significant respiratory depression, but it should be used with caution in patients with impaired respiratory function or when used concomitantly with other CNS- or respiratory-depressant agents; respiratory depression can be severe in these patients—adequate monitoring is required. Naloxone can reverse nalbuphine-induced respiratory depression.

In humans, nalbuphine is contraindicated in patients with significant respiratory depression, acute or severe asthma, and known or suspected GI obstruction.[3]

Nalbuphine can precipitate withdrawal signs in patients that are physically dependent on opioid drugs. While the potential for abuse of nalbuphine by humans is less than with other opioids (especially mu-receptor agonist agents), there have been reports of diversion, abuse, and dependence. Although there are no special recordkeeping or storage requirements, veterinarians should be alert to this potential.

Adverse Effects

Respiratory depression is unlikely but can occur. Other adverse effects that can be seen with nalbuphine include excitement (high doses), dysphoria, vomiting, and bradycardia.

Reproductive/Nursing Safety

Safe use of nalbuphine during pregnancy has not been established.

Very little drug is excreted into milk, and nalbuphine is considered relatively safe in humans to use while nursing; however, offspring exposed to nalbuphine should be monitored for excess sedation or respiratory depression.[3]

Because safety has not been established in animals, this drug should only be used when the maternal benefits outweigh the potential risks to offspring.

Overdose/Acute Toxicity

Overdoses of nalbuphine are rarely serious, particularly when used on an inpatient basis and with adequate monitoring when used with other CNS and respiratory depressant drugs. Respiratory depression can be reversed with naloxone.[3] In humans, single doses of nalbuphine 72 mg SC administered to healthy subjects caused sedation, sleepiness, and mild dysphoria. Oral ingestions are not serious as the drug has low oral bioavailability.

For patients that have experienced or are suspected to have experienced an overdose, consultation with a 24-hour poison consultation center specializing in providing veterinary-specific information is recommended. For general information related to overdose and toxin exposures, as well as contact information for poison control centers, refer to ***Appendix.***

Drug Interactions

The following drug interactions have either been reported or are theoretical in humans or animals receiving nalbuphine and may be of significance in veterinary patients. Unless otherwise noted, use together is not necessarily contraindicated, but weigh the potential risks and perform additional monitoring when appropriate.

- **Cimetidine**: Increased nalbuphine effects possible
- **CNS or Respiratory Depressants**: Additive CNS and/or respiratory depression can occur.

- **Mu-Opioid Agonists** (eg, **fentanyl, morphine**): Administration of nalbuphine with or following a mu agonist may result in a reduced analgesic effect.

Laboratory Considerations

- Opioid **screening tests.** Nalbuphine may interfere with enzymatic tests.

Dosages

DOGS/CATS:

In combination as a preanesthetic adjunct (extra-label): 0.2 – 0.4 mg/kg IV, IM, or SC in combination with other preanesthetic agents (eg, midazolam, acepromazine, alpha-2 agonists)

Sole agent for mild-to-moderate pain (extra-label): 0.25 – 1 mg/kg IV, IM, or SC.[8] Up to 2 mg/kg IV or IM has been suggested for use in dogs.

CALVES:

Pain relief after surgical castration (extra-label): 0.4 mg/kg IV reduced some pain-related behaviors but did not significantly eliminate signs of distress in calves.[2]

SMALL MAMMALS:

Analgesic (extra-label):
Rabbits, Ferrets: 0.5 – 1.5 mg/kg IV, IM every 4 hours
Guinea Pigs: 1 – 4 mg/kg IM, SC every 3 hours
Gerbils, Mice, Rats, Hamsters: 1 – 2 mg/kg IM, SC every 2 to 4 hours (dosages have been recommended up to 8 mg/kg IM)

Monitoring

- Level of sedation and analgesia
- Respiratory depth and rate especially when used in combination with other respiratory depressant drugs

Client Information

- Nalbuphine is only used in an inpatient setting.

Chemistry/Synonyms

Nalbuphine HCl is a synthetic opioid agonist/antagonist in the phenanthrene series and is structurally related to both naloxone (opioid antagonist) and oxymorphone (opioid agonist). Nalbuphine HCl is soluble in water and ethanol; insoluble in chloroform and ether.

The commercially available injection in 10 mL vials also contains sodium citrate hydrous 0.94%, citric acid anhydrous 1.26%, methyl- and propylparabens 0.2%, and hydrochloric acid to adjust pH to 3.5 to 3.7.

Nalbuphine HCl may also be known as EN-2234A, Nubian (street name), and *Nubain®*.

Storage/Stability

Store intact vials and ampules at 15°C to 30°C (59°F-86°F) and protect from light.

Compatibility/Compounding Considerations

Compatibility is dependent on factors such as pH, concentration, temperature, and diluent used; specialized references or a hospital pharmacist should be consulted for more specific information.

Nalbuphine HCl injection has been found **compatible** with the following IV solutions: dextrose 5% in sodium chloride 0.9%; dextrose 10%; lactated Ringer's solution (LRS); sodium chloride 0.9%.[9]

At usual concentrations, nalbuphine has been found **compatible** with the following drugs (partial listing) when mixed in syringes: atropine sulfate, diphenhydramine, glycopyrrolate, hydroxyzine, lidocaine, midazolam, and ranitidine. Diazepam, ketorolac, and pentobarbital are **incompatible**. Propofol is **compatible** at a 1:1 ratio at Y-site.[9] There are anecdotal reports of syringe mixtures successfully combining nalbuphine with acepromazine, dexmedetomidine, or medetomidine, although published stability data were not located.

Dosage Forms/Regulatory Status

VETERINARY-LABELED PRODUCTS: NONE

HUMAN-LABELED PRODUCTS:

Nalbuphine HCl Injectable Solution: 10 mg/mL and 20 mg/mL in 1 mL ampules and 10 mL multi-dose vials; generic; (Rx)

References

For the complete list of references, see **wiley.com/go/budde/plumb**

Naloxone

(nal-***ox***-one) *Narcan®*
Antidote; Opioid Antagonist

Prescriber Highlights

- Most effective at reversing pure mu-opioid receptor agonists (eg, fentanyl, morphine); less effective reversal agent for partial opioid agonists (eg, buprenorphine)
- Use with caution in animals with pre-existing cardiac abnormalities or patients that are opioid dependent. At reversal dosages, can negate opioid analgesic effects.
- Reversal effect may last for a shorter time than opioid effect; monitor and re-dose as needed.

Uses/Indications

Naloxone is used almost exclusively for its opioid reversal effects, but the drug has been investigated for treating other conditions (eg, septic, hypovolemic, or cardiogenic shock). Frequent administration of low-dose naloxone is advocated by some to reverse opioid effects while minimizing consequences of opioid withdrawal. Some have found low-dose naloxone useful in treating postanesthetic dysphoria associated with perioperative opioids,[1] but this practice is somewhat controversial due to the difficulty in distinguishing pain from dysphoria in animal patients. Naloxone has been employed as a test drug to see if endogenous opioid blockade will result in diminished tail chasing or other self-mutilating behaviors.[2]

Pharmacology/Actions

Naloxone is considered a pure opioid antagonist and has no analgesic activity at usual dosages. The drug acts as a competitive antagonist by binding to the mu, kappa, and delta opioid receptor sites, and has its highest affinity for the mu receptor. It also has some GABA antagonistic effects, which can elicit convulsions, although this is usually not clinically relevant.

Naloxone reverses the majority of effects associated with high-dose opioid administration (eg, respiratory and CNS depression). In dogs, naloxone does not reverse the emetic or hypotensive actions of apomorphine.[3]

At higher doses, naloxone has other pharmacologic activity including effects on dopaminergic mechanisms (increases dopamine levels) and GABA antagonism.

Pharmacokinetics

Naloxone is only minimally absorbed when given orally due to an extensive first-pass metabolism. Much higher doses are required if using this route of administration for any pharmacologic effect. When given IV, naloxone has a rapid onset of action (usually 1 to 2 minutes). If given IM, the drug generally has an onset of action within 5 minutes of administration. The duration of action usually persists from 45 to 90 minutes but may have an effect for up to 3 hours.

Naloxone is distributed rapidly throughout the body with high concentrations found in the brain, kidneys, spleen, skeletal muscle, lung, and heart. Naloxone is metabolized in the liver, principally via glucuronidative conjugation, with metabolites excreted into the urine. In humans, the serum half-life is ≈60 minutes, but ≈3 hours in neonates.[4]

Contraindications/Precautions/Warnings

Naloxone is contraindicated in patients hypersensitive to it.[4] It should be used cautiously in animals that have preexisting cardiac abnormalities or that may be opioid dependent. Excessive naloxone doses or abrupt reversal following surgery may result in vomiting, tachycardia, blood pressure changes, ventricular arrhythmias, pulmonary edema, and seizures.[4] The drug should be used cautiously (and in smaller doses) in animals who have received exceedingly large doses of narcotics as it may produce an acute withdrawal syndrome.

Naloxone is reportedly not effective for reversing meperidine-induced seizures. In a case of a dog that received an overdose of meperidine at ten times the labeled dosage, naloxone administration elicited CNS excitement. The authors recommend that naloxone (and butorphanol) should be avoided when normeperidine (active metabolite of meperidine) excitotoxicity is suspected, unless severe respiratory depression is present without a method of ventilatory support available.[5]

Naloxone has not been shown to be an effective therapy to reverse apnea of newborns and its routine use is not recommended. However, if the dam received opioids during parturition, it may reverse opioid-induced respiratory depression.

Large doses of naloxone may be required to reverse the effects of buprenorphine because buprenorphine has a long duration of action due to its slow rate of binding and subsequent slow dissociation from the opioid receptor.[4] Doses 100 times the label dosage have been required to reverse buprenorphine effects in a normal dog.

When used to reduce postoperative dysphoria associated with perioperative opioids, naloxone dose and administration rate must be carefully titrated or hyperalgesia can occur.

Do not confuse nalOXone with nalTREXone.

Adverse Effects

At recommended dosages, naloxone is relatively free of adverse effects in non-opioid dependent patients; however, when used to reverse opioid effects, it can also reverse any analgesic effects of the opioid (see ***Contraindications/Precautions/Warnings***). Because the duration of action of naloxone may be shorter than that of the narcotic being reversed, animals that are being treated for opioid intoxication or with clinical signs of respiratory depression should be closely monitored, as additional doses of naloxone and/or ventilatory support may be required.

Rare cases of noncardiogenic pulmonary edema have been reported following IV administration of naloxone at standard dosages in dogs and humans.[4,6]

Reproductive/Nursing Safety

Naloxone readily crosses the placenta.[4] No embryotoxic or teratogenic effects were observed in mice and rats treated with naloxone hydrochloride during the period of organogenesis. Opioid withdrawal may occur in the fetuses of dams that have received opioids during the course of pregnancy or in those that are or may be opioid-dependent.

It is not known whether the drug is excreted in maternal milk. Although oral absorption of naloxone by the offspring would be unlikely, use with caution when administering to nursing patients. Because safety has not been established in animals, this drug should only be used when the maternal benefits outweigh the potential risks to offspring.

Overdose/Acute Toxicity

Naloxone is considered a safe agent with a wide margin of safety, but very high doses have initiated seizures (possibly secondary to GABA antagonism) in a few patients. Abdominal distress (eg, rapid-onset diarrhea, abdominal checking), restlessness, tachycardia and tachypnea, and diaphoresis were noted in horses given naloxone 0.75 mg/kg IV.[7]

For patients that have experienced or are suspected to have experienced an overdose, consultation with a 24-hour poison consultation center specializing in providing veterinary-specific information is recommended. For general information related to overdose and toxin exposures, as well as contact information for poison control centers, refer to ***Appendix***.

Drug Interactions

The following drug interactions either have been reported or are theoretical in humans or animals receiving naloxone and may be of significance in veterinary patients. Unless otherwise noted, use together is not necessarily contraindicated, but weigh the potential risks and perform additional monitoring when appropriate.

- **APOMORPHINE**: Emetic effect may be prolonged.[8] Naloxone can reverse the respiratory depressant effects but not the emetic or cardiovascular effects of apomorphine.
- **CLONIDINE**: Naloxone may reduce the hypotensive and bradycardic effects of clonidine; potentially useful for clonidine overdoses.
- **MEPERIDINE** (overdose): Naloxone may contribute to CNS excitatory effects of normeperidine (meperidine metabolite). In cases where normeperidine excitotoxicity is suspected, avoid use of naloxone (or butorphanol), unless severe respiratory depression is present without a method of ventilatory support.[5]
- **OPIOID AGONIST-ANTAGONISTS** (eg, **butorphanol**, **pentazocine**, **nalbuphine**): Naloxone may also antagonize the effects of these agents (respiratory depression, analgesia).
- **OPIOID PARTIAL-AGONISTS** (eg, **buprenorphine**): Naloxone may also antagonize the effects of these agents (respiratory depression, analgesia), although higher naloxone doses maybe needed. It should not be relied upon to treat respiratory depression caused by buprenorphine.
- **YOHIMBINE**: Naloxone may increase the CNS effects of yohimbine (eg, anxiety, tremors, nausea, palpitations) and increase plasma cortisol levels.

Laboratory Considerations

None noted

Dosages

DOGS & CATS:

Opioid reversal (extra-label):

a) 0.001 – 0.04 mg/kg IV, IM, SC; the IO route has also been used.[9,10] Dosages up to 0.1 – 0.2 mg/kg have been suggested depending on severity of the patient.[11] IV doses may be repeated every 2 to 3 minutes as necessary for re-narcotization. If given IM or SC, effects may be delayed up to 5 minutes.

b) **As a constant rate infusion (CRI)**: 0.001 – 0.004 mg/kg per minute (1 – 4 µg/kg/minute) IV CRI[12]

c) **Respiratory depression in newborns when opioids given to dam:**
   i. 0.1 mg/kg IV, SC, or IM; repeat as necessary[13]
   ii. **Transmucosal**: Using the 0.4 mg/mL injection, 1 – 2 drops given under tongue or intranasally (approximately 0.2 mg/kg)[14]; repeat as necessary.

d) **During CPR in cases of opioid toxicity or if recent opioids were administered:** 0.04 mg/kg IV; IO may be considered[15]

e) **Postoperative dysphoria**: If the patient is clearly dysphoric or returns to a whining state shortly after opioid administration or if suspicion exists related to the use of high doses of opioid during surgery, a slow titration of IV naloxone can be given to effect. Depending on the size of the patient, either dilute 0.1 mL of the 0.4 mg/mL injection (0.04 mg; 40 µg) into 5 mL sterile saline (to make an 8 µg/mL solution) OR 0.25 mL of the 0.4 mg/mL injection (0.1 mg; 100 µg) into 10 mL sterile saline (to make a 10 μg/mL). Give 1 mL of the diluted solution IV over 30 to 60 seconds at the Y-site injection port nearest to the patient. Observe patient carefully during infusion. Infusion can be stopped once patient calms or sleeps. Most patients do not require the full 1 mL. Overdosing can induce hyperalgesia. If dysphoria recurs, may need to repeat.[16,17]

f) **Postepidural urinary retention**: 0.01 - 0.04 mg/kg IV can be used to reverse urinary retention that follows epidural morphine.[10]

g) **Adjunctive treatment of postanesthesia hyperthermia in cats** (extra-label): Postanesthesia hyperthermia (ie, exceeding 41.1°C [106°F]) has been treated with naloxone at 0.01 – 0.02 mg/kg IV, IM or SC. Temperatures have returned to normal under 30 minutes.[18]

HORSES:

Opioid reversal (extra-label): 0.01 – 0.05 mg/kg IV; low end of dosing range can limit opioid-induced locomotor activity; upper end may stimulate colonic propulsion. Duration of effect can be very short (under 30 minutes).

RABBITS, RODENTS, SMALL MAMMALS:

Opioid reversal (extra-label): Wide range of anecdotal dosages noted naloxone 0.005 – 0.1 mg/kg; consider an initial dose of 0.01 – 0.02 mg/kg IV, IM, SC, or IP, repeat as necessary

REPTILES:

Opioid reversal (extra-label): for significant respiratory depression, 0.04 – 0.2 mg/kg SC[19]

Monitoring

- Because the duration of action of naloxone may be shorter than that of the narcotic being reversed, animals that are being treated for opioid intoxication or that have clinical signs of respiratory depression should be closely monitored for re-narcotization, as additional doses of naloxone and/or ventilatory support may be required.
- Respiratory rate/depth
- CNS function
- Pain associated with opioid reversal

Client Information

- Should be used with direct veterinary professional supervision only

Chemistry/Synonyms

An opioid antagonist, naloxone HCl is structurally related to oxymorphone. It occurs as a white to slightly off-white powder with a pK_a of 7.94. Naloxone is soluble in water and slightly soluble in alcohol. The pH ranges of commercially available injectable solutions are from 3 to 4.5.

Naloxone HCl may also be known as N-allylnoroxymorphone, naloxona, EN-15304, naloxoni and by the trade name, *Narcan*®.

Storage/Stability

Naloxone HCl for injection should be stored at room temperature (15 to 30°C) and protected from light.

When given as an IV infusion, dilute naloxone in either dextrose 5% or sodium chloride 0.9%.[4] Sterile water for injection may be used to dilute naloxone injection prior to SC, IM or bolus IV injection.

Compatibility/Compounding Considerations

Naloxone HCl injection **should not** be mixed with solutions containing sulfites, bisulfites, long-chain or high molecular weight anions or any solutions at alkaline pH. Naloxone HCl is reportedly **Y-site compatible** with the following IV solutions and drugs (partial list): D_5W, 0.9% NaCl, lactated Ringer's solution, acetylcysteine, aminocaproic acid, amiodarone HCl, atropine sulfate, calcium salts, dexamethasone sodium phosphate, dexmedetomidine, dobutamine HCl, epinephrine HCl, esmolol, famotidine, heparin sodium, hydrocortisone sodium succinate, lidocaine HCl, mannitol, methylprednisolone sodium succinate, midazolam HCl, ondansetron, potassium chloride, propofol, and sodium bicarbonate.

Naloxone HCl is reportedly **incompatible** or compatibility varies with the following: cefazolin, diazepam, magnesium sulfate, and pantoprazole sodium. Compatibility is dependent upon factors such as pH, concentration, temperature, and diluent used; consult specialized references or a hospital pharmacist for more specific information.

Dosage Forms/Regulatory Status

VETERINARY-LABELED PRODUCTS: NONE

There were approved products in the past, but these have been discontinued. The Association of Racing Commissioners International (ARCI) has designated this drug as a class 3 substance. Use of this drug may not be allowed in certain animal competitions. Check rules and regulations before entering in a competition while this medication is being administered. Contact local racing authorities for further guidance. See the ***Appendix*** for more information.

HUMAN-LABELED PRODUCTS:

Naloxone HCl Injection: 0.4 mg/mL (400 μg/mL) and 1 mg/mL; generic; (Rx)

Naloxone HCl Auto-Injector: 0.4 mg/0.4 mL and 2 mg/0.4 mL; *Evzio*®; (Rx)

Naloxone Nasal Spray: 2 mg and 4 mg in 0.1 mL single-dose applicators; *Narcan*®; (Rx)

References

For the complete list of references, see **wiley.com/go/budde/plumb**

Naltrexone

(nal-trex-ohne) *ReVia*®

Opioid Antagonist

Prescriber Highlights

- ► Oral opioid antagonist that may be useful in determining if adverse behaviors have a significant endorphin component and for short-term treatment of adverse behaviors. Compounded injection may be an alternative to naloxone for reversing opioid effects.
- ► Contraindications include patients that are physically dependent on opioid drugs, are in hepatic failure, or have acute hepatitis.
- ► Use with caution in patients with hepatic dysfunction or patients with a history of allergic reaction to naltrexone or naloxone.
- ► Relatively free of adverse effects. Potential adverse effects include abdominal cramping, nausea, vomiting, nervousness, joint or muscle pain, skin rashes, and pruritus. Dose-dependent hepatotoxicity is also possible.
- ► May cause clinical signs of withdrawal in physically dependent patients
- ► Oral treatment can be expensive.

Uses/Indications

Naltrexone may be useful in determining if adverse behaviors (eg, self-mutilating or tail-chasing) in dogs or cats have a significant endorphin component. Naltrexone has largely been supplanted for treatment of behavior disorders by other more accepted treatments. Compounded injectable naltrexone may be an acceptable replacement for reversing opioids when commercial naloxone injection is not available. A study in cats found that hourly naltrexone 600 µg/kg IV antagonized the dysphoric and antinociceptive effects of high doses of remifentanil.[1]

Adjunctive use of low-dose oral naltrexone in female dogs with surgically resected mammary carcinoma reduced the incidence of chemotherapy-related adverse effects and improved quality of life.[2]

Due to its long duration of action (approximately twice that of naloxone), naltrexone is preferred in wildlife and zoo animals when potent opioids, such as etorphine and thiafentanil, are used. These potent opioids are long-acting, and the use of naltrexone minimizes the potential of renarcotization, especially when redosing of antagonists is not possible for personnel safety reasons.

Pharmacology/Actions

Naltrexone is an orally available narcotic antagonist. It competitively binds to opioid receptors in the CNS, thereby preventing both endogenous opioids (eg, endorphins) and exogenously administered opioid agonists or agonist/antagonists from occupying the site. Naltrexone may be more effective in blocking the euphoric aspects of the opioids and less effective at blocking the respiratory depressive or miotic effects.

Naltrexone may also increase plasma concentrations of luteinizing hormone (LH), cortisol, and ACTH. In dogs with experimentally induced hypovolemic shock, naltrexone (like naloxone) given IV in high doses increased mean arterial pressure, cardiac output, stroke volume, and left ventricular contractility.[3]

Pharmacokinetics

In humans, naltrexone is rapidly and nearly completely absorbed, but it undergoes a significant first-pass effect as only 5% to 12% of a dose reaches systemic circulation. Naltrexone circulates throughout the body and CSF concentrations are ≈30% of those found in plasma. Approximately 20% to 30% is bound to plasma proteins. Naltrexone is metabolized in the liver primarily to 6-beta-naltrexol, which has some opioid-blocking activity. The metabolites are eliminated primarily via the kidney. In humans, the serum half-life of naltrexone is ≈4 hours and ≈13 hours for 6-beta-naltrexol.[4]

Contraindications/Precautions/Warnings

Naltrexone is contraindicated in patients physically dependent on opioid drugs, in hepatic failure, or acute hepatitis. The benefits of the drug versus its risks should be weighed in patients with hepatic dysfunction or with a history of allergic reaction to naltrexone or naloxone.

Do not confuse NALTREXone with NALOxone.

Adverse Effects

At recommended dosages, naltrexone is relatively free of adverse effects in non-opioid–dependent patients.[4] Some human patients have developed abdominal cramping, nausea and vomiting, nervousness, insomnia, joint or muscle pain, skin rashes, and pruritus. Dose-dependent hepatotoxicity has been described in humans on occasion.[4]

Naltrexone will block the analgesic, antidiarrheal, and antitussive effects of opioid agonist or agonist/antagonist agents. Withdrawal clinical signs may be precipitated in physically dependent patients.

Reproductive/Nursing Safety

In humans, naltrexone crosses the placenta.[4] It is unknown whether it enters human milk; however, animal studies have shown that naltrexone and its metabolite, 6-beta-naltrexol are excreted in the milk of rats dosed orally with naltrexone. Very high doses (5 times the recommended label dose based on body surface area) have caused increased embryotoxicity in some laboratory animals.[4]

Because safety has not been established in animals, this drug should only be used when the maternal benefits outweigh the potential risks to offspring.

Overdose/Acute Toxicity

Naltrexone appears to be relatively safe even after very large doses. The LD_{50} in dogs after SC injection has been reported to be 200 mg/kg. Oral LD_{50} in species tested ranged from 1.1 g/kg in mice to 3 g/kg in monkeys (dogs and cats not tested). Deaths at these doses were a result of respiratory depression and/or tonic-clonic seizures. Massive overdoses should be treated using GI decontamination protocols when warranted and supportive treatment.

For patients that have experienced or are suspected to have experienced an overdose, consultation with a 24-hour poison consultation center specializing in providing veterinary-specific information is recommended. For general information related to overdose and toxin exposures, as well as contact information for poison control centers, refer to ***Appendix.***

Drug Interactions

The following drug interactions have either been reported or are theoretical in humans or animals receiving naltrexone and may be of significance in veterinary patients. Unless otherwise noted, use together is not necessarily contraindicated, but weigh the potential risks and perform additional monitoring when appropriate.

- **Opiods** (eg, **etorphine, fentanyl, thiafentanil**): May result in decreased opioid effectiveness; naltrexone can be used clinically to reverse adverse opioid effects (eg, CNS or respiratory depression).
- **Yohimbine**: Naltrexone may increase the CNS effects of yohimbine (anxiety, tremors, nausea, palpitations) and increase plasma cortisol concentrations.

Laboratory Considerations

Naltrexone reportedly does not interfere with TLC, GLC, or HPLC methods of determining **urinary opioids** or **quinine**, but can interfere with some enzymatic assays.

Dosages

DOGS:

Adjunctive therapy in behavior disorders (eg, stereotypy); (extra-label): 1.1 – 2.2 mg/kg PO every 8 to 12 hours. Dosage recommendations vary but naltrexone 2 – 5 mg/kg PO once daily[5] or divided every 12 hours have been noted. If using commercially available tablets (50 mg), dose is typically rounded to nearest 25 mg. Tablets can be bitter. **NOTE**: Limited evidence to support use

Adjunctive treatment of surgically resected canine mammary carcinoma (extra-label): 0.1 mg/kg PO every 24 hours for 24 weeks, in addition to chemotherapy with carboplatin[2]

CATS:

Adjunctive therapy in behavior disorders (eg, stereotypy); (extra-label): 25 – 50 mg/cat (NOT mg/kg) PO every 24 hours[6]

Monitoring

- Efficacy
- Liver enzymes if using high doses with prolonged therapy

Client Information

Give this medicine as directed by your veterinarian.

Additional behavior modification techniques may be required to improve undesired behavior and clinical signs. Follow your veterinarian's recommendations.

Chemistry/Synonyms

A synthetic opioid antagonist, naltrexone HCl occurs as white crystals having a bitter taste. 100 mg are soluble in 1 mL of water.

Naltrexone may also be known as EN-1639A, *ReVia*®, and *Vivitrol*®.

Storage/Stability

Naltrexone tablets should be stored at controlled room temperature (15°C-30°C [59°F-86°F]) in well-closed containers.

Compatibility/Compounding Considerations

No specific information noted

Dosage Forms/Regulatory Status

VETERINARY-LABELED PRODUCTS: NONE

The Association of Racing Commissioners International (ARCI) has designated this drug as a class 3 substance. Use of this drug may not be allowed in certain animal competitions. Check rules and regulations before entering in a competition while this medication is being administered. Contact local racing authorities for further guidance. See ***Appendix*** for more information.

Compounded naltrexone for injection may be available for use as an opioid reversal agent.

HUMAN-LABELED PRODUCTS:

Naltrexone HCl Oral Tablets: 50 mg; *ReVia®*, generic; (Rx).

References

For the complete list of references, see **wiley.com/go/budde/plumb**

Neomycin

(nee-o-**mye**-sin) *Biosol®, Neomix®*

Aminoglycoside Antibiotic

NOTE:** For topical formulations of neomycin, refer to **Neomycin Ophthalmic, Triple Antibiotic Ophthalmic, Corticosteroid/Antimicrobial Otic Preparations

Prescriber Highlights

- ▶ Orally administered aminoglycoside antibiotic used to treat enteric infections; it is also used for adjunctive treatment of hepatic encephalopathy.
- ▶ Contraindications include hypersensitivity to aminoglycosides, intestinal obstruction, and use in hindgut fermenters (eg, rabbits, horses).
- ▶ Adverse effects include ototoxicity, nephrotoxicity, severe diarrhea, and intestinal malabsorption. Long-term use can lead to GI superinfections.
- ▶ Minimal amounts absorbed via GI tract

Uses/Indications

Orally administered neomycin is indicated to treat enteric infections in cattle, sheep, goats, and swine; it may also be administered orally or as an enema to reduce ammonia-producing bacteria as adjunctive treatment of hepatic encephalopathy. In humans, neomycin is no longer considered a first-line choice for the treatment of hepatic encephalopathy due to lack of evidentiary support and increased risk for nephrotoxicity and ototoxicity compared with other treatment options.[1] Unlike other aminoglycoside antibiotics (eg, amikacin, gentamicin), neomycin is not used for treatment of systemic infections because of poor oral absorption and adverse effect profile.

The World Health Organization (WHO) has designated aminoglycosides as Critically Important (High Priority) antimicrobials for human medicine.[2] The Office International des Epizooties (OIE) has designated aminoglycosides as Veterinary Critically Important Antimicrobial Agents (VCIA) in bee, avian, bovine, caprine, equine, lagomorph, ovine, and swine species.[3]

Pharmacology/Actions

Neomycin has a mechanism of action and spectrum of activity (primarily gram-negative aerobes) similar to the other aminoglycosides, but in comparison with either gentamicin or amikacin, it is significantly less effective against several species of gram-negative organisms, including strains of *Klebsiella* spp, *Escherichia coli*, and *Pseudomonas* spp. Neomycin-resistant bacteria often remain susceptible to amikacin.

More detailed information on the aminoglycoside mechanism of action and spectrum of activity is outlined in the ***Amikacin*** monograph. Neomycin has been shown to decrease the production of ammonia and reduce glutamine activity.[4]

Pharmacokinetics

Approximately 3% of a dose of neomycin is absorbed after oral or rectal (retention enema) administration, but this can be increased if gut motility is slowed or if the bowel wall is damaged. Therapeutic levels are not attained in systemic circulation after oral administration. In humans, growth of gut bacteria is rapidly suppressed following oral administration and persists for 48 to 72 hours. Orally administered neomycin is nearly all excreted unchanged in the feces.

After IM administration, therapeutic levels can be attained with peak levels occurring within 1 hour of dosing. Neomycin apparently distributes to tissues and is eliminated like the other aminoglycosides (see ***Amikacin***). It is minimally protein bound.

Contraindications/Precautions/Warnings

Oral neomycin is contraindicated in the presence of intestinal obstruction or if the patient is hypersensitive to aminoglycosides.

In neonates, orally administered neomycin can yield high systemic levels and corresponding toxic effects; it should be avoided in neonatal patients.

Aminoglycosides are generally considered contraindicated in rabbits and hares, as this class of drugs adversely affects the GI microbiota in these animals. Oral neomycin has been associated with antibiotic-associated diarrhea (enterocolitis) in horses and should not be used in this species.

Long-term use of oral aminoglycosides may result in bacterial or fungal superinfections.

The human product contains a black box warning stating that neurotoxicity, irreversible ototoxicity, and nephrotoxicity can occur after oral administration. The risk for these toxicities is increased with higher neomycin doses and in patients with decreased renal function, advanced age, and dehydration. Neomycin should be avoided in patients that are azotemic or who have any evidence of intestinal bleeding or ulcerations. See package insert for the full warning.[5]

Adverse Effects

Antibiotic-associated diarrhea can occur, and some species may be more susceptible, particularly hindgut fermenters (eg, rabbits, horses). Rarely, oral neomycin may cause ototoxicity, nephrotoxicity, severe diarrhea, and intestinal malabsorption.

Reproductive/Nursing Safety

Aminoglycosides cross the placenta and have very rarely been associated with congenital deafness in humans.[5] The safety of neomycin has not been established in pregnant animals.

Neomycin is excreted in cow's milk following a single IM injection.[5] If used orally, neomycin may negatively alter gut flora and cause diarrhea in nursing offspring; the risk for more serious adverse effects (eg, otoxicity) is unknown.

Because safety has not been established in animals, this drug should only be used when the maternal benefits outweigh the potential risks to offspring.

Overdose/Acute Toxicity

An acute overdose of oral neomycin is not expected to result in significant systemic toxicity due to poor oral absorption.[5] Ototoxicity, nephrotoxicity, and severe diarrhea are possible, particularly with prolonged exposure or in patients with underlying renal impairment, advanced age, or dehydration.

For patients that have or are suspected of having experienced an overdose, consultation with a 24-hour poison center specializing in providing veterinary-specific information is recommended. For general information related to overdose and toxin exposures, as well as contact information for poison control centers, refer to ***Appendix.***

Drug Interactions

The following drug interactions have either been reported or are theoretical in humans or animals receiving oral neomycin and may be of significance in veterinary patients. Unless otherwise noted, use together is not necessarily contraindicated, but weigh the potential risks and perform additional monitoring when appropriate.

- **Cephalosporins** (eg, **ceftiofur, cephalexin**): Concurrent use may enhance the nephrotoxic effect of neomycin.
- **Cyclosporine**: Neomycin may increase the nephrotoxic potential of cyclosporine.
- **Digoxin**: Oral neomycin may decrease oral digoxin absorption. Separating the doses of the 2 medications may not alleviate this effect. Some human patients (less than 10%) metabolize digoxin in the GI tract, and neomycin may increase serum digoxin levels in these patients. It is recommended that therapeutic drug monitoring be performed if oral neomycin is added or withdrawn from the drug regimen of a patient stabilized on a digitalis glycoside.
- **Mannitol**: Concurrent use should be avoided as it may enhance the nephrotoxic effect of neomycin.
- **Methotrexate**: Absorption may be reduced by oral neomycin but is increased by oral kanamycin (another aminoglycoside).
- **Neuromuscular-Blocking Agents** (eg, **atracurium, pancuronium**): Concomitant use with neuromuscular-blocking agents could potentiate neuromuscular blockade.[6]
- **Ototoxic, Nephrotoxic Drugs**: Although only minimal amounts of neomycin are absorbed after oral or rectal administration, the concurrent use of other ototoxic or nephrotoxic drugs with neomycin should be done with caution. Topical use for the treatment of otitis should be avoided if an intact tympanic membrane has not been confirmed.
- **Penicillin V Potassium (oral)**: Oral neomycin should not be given concurrently with oral penicillin V potassium, as malabsorption of the penicillin may occur.
- **Vancomycin**: May enhance the nephrotoxic effect of neomycin
- **Vitamin K Antagonists** (eg, **warfarin**): Oral neomycin may decrease the amount of vitamin K absorbed from the gut; this may have ramifications for patients receiving oral anticoagulants.

Laboratory Considerations

- No specific concerns were noted.

Dosages

DOGS/CATS:

Adjunctive treatment of hepatic encephalopathy (extra-label): 20 mg/kg PO every 8 to 12 hours[7]

CATTLE:

Oral administration to treat and control colibacillosis (bacterial enteritis) caused by *Escherichia coli* (label dosage; FDA-approved): 22 mg/kg PO daily[8]; administer to individual animals as a drench in divided doses or mix in drinking water that will be consumed in 12 to 24 hours. Treat for a maximum of 14 days. NOTE: One reference states, *Published studies do not support the oral administration of potentiated sulfonamides, tetracyclines or neomycin in the treatment of calf scours.*[9]

SHEEP & GOATS:

Oral administration to treat and control colibacillosis (bacterial enteritis) caused by *E coli* (label dosage; FDA-approved): 22 mg/kg PO daily[8]; administer to individual animals as a drench in divided doses or mix in drinking water that will be consumed in 12 to 24 hours. Treat for a maximum of 14 days.

SWINE:

Oral administration to treat and control colibacillosis (bacterial enteritis) caused by *E coli* (label dosage; FDA-approved): 22 mg/kg PO daily[8]; administer to individual animals as a drench in divided doses or mix in drinking water that will be consumed in 12 to 24 hours. Treat for a maximum of 14 days.

FERRETS:

Susceptible enteric infections (extra-label): 10 – 20 mg/kg PO 2 to 4 times daily[10]

TURKEYS:

Oral administration for control of mortality associated with *E coli* (label dosage; FDA-approved): 22 mg/kg PO daily for 5 days[8]; administer to individual animals as a drench in divided doses or mix in drinking water that will be consumed in 12 to 24 hours.

Monitoring

- Clinical efficacy
- Systemic and GI adverse effects with prolonged use

Client Information

- This medication should **not** be given to horses, hamsters, or rabbits.
- This medicine may be given by mouth with or without food. If your animal vomits or acts sick after receiving the medicine on an empty stomach, give with food or a small treat to see if this helps. If vomiting continues, contact your veterinarian.
- When neomycin is given by mouth for short periods, it is usually tolerated well. Contact your veterinarian if your animal develops diarrhea while taking this medicine.
- Rarely, this medicine can cause hearing loss and damage to the kidneys and nerves when used for long periods of time. Contact your veterinarian if your animal develops hearing loss, a head tilt, weakness, changes in appetite, or with drinking and urination habits.

Chemistry/Synonyms

An aminoglycoside antibiotic obtained from *Streptomyces fradiae*, neomycin is a complex of 3 separate compounds: neomycin A (neamine; inactive), neomycin C, and neomycin B (framycetin). The commercially available product almost entirely consists of the sulfate salt of neomycin B. It occurs as an odorless or almost odorless, white to slightly yellow, hygroscopic powder or cryodessicated solid. It is freely soluble in water and very slightly soluble in alcohol. One mg of pure neomycin sulfate is equivalent to not less than 650 units.

Neomycin sulfate may also be known as fradiomycin sulfate, neomycin sulphate, or neomycini sulfas, *Neo-325®*, *Neo-fradin®*, *Neo-Sol 50®*, *Neomix® 325*, and *Neovet®*.

Storage/Stability

Neomycin sulfate oral solution should be stored at room temperature (15°C-30°C [59°F-86°F]) in airtight, light-resistant containers. Unless otherwise instructed by the manufacturer, oral tablets/boluses should be stored in airtight containers at room temperature.

In the dry state, neomycin is stable for at least 2 years at room temperature.

Compatibility/Compounding Considerations

No specific information is noted.

Dosage Forms/Regulatory Status

VETERINARY-LABELED PRODUCTS:

Neomycin Sulfate; Oral Liquid: 200 mg/mL (140 mg neomycin base/mL); generic. Depending on labeling, FDA-approved for use in cattle, swine, sheep, goats, turkeys, laying hens, and broilers.

Neomycin Sulfate Soluble Powder: 325 g/lb: *Neo-325® Soluble Powder*, *Neovet® 325/100*, and *NeoVet® 325 AG Grade* (includes turkey label), *Neo-Sol 50®*; (Rx). FDA-approved for use in cattle (not veal calves), swine, sheep, goats, and turkeys (some products).

Check labels for slaughter withdrawals; may vary with product. General withdrawal times (when used as labeled): Cattle = 1 day; sheep = 2 days; and swine and goats = 3 days. Withdrawal period has not been established in pre-ruminating calves. Do not use in calves to be processed for veal. A milk discard period has not been established in lactating dairy cattle. Do not use in female dairy cattle 20 months of age or older.

HUMAN-LABELED PRODUCTS:
Neomycin Sulfate Tablets: 500 mg; generic; (Rx)

References

For the complete list of references, see **wiley.com/go/budde/plumb**

Neostigmine

(nee-oh-***stig***-meen) *Bloxiverz®*
Parasympathomimetic (Cholinergic)

Prescriber Highlights

- ▶ Parasympathomimetic used to initiate peristalsis, empty the bladder, and stimulate skeletal muscle contractions. Also used for diagnosis and treatment of myasthenia gravis and to reverse or treat overdoses of nondepolarizing neuromuscular blocking agents (eg, curare-type).
- ▶ Contraindications include peritonitis, mechanical intestinal or urinary tract obstructions, late stages of pregnancy, hypersensitivity to this class of compounds, or treatment with other cholinesterase inhibitors.
- ▶ Adverse effects are cholinergic in nature and dose related and include nausea, vomiting, diarrhea, excessive salivation and drooling, sweating, miosis, lacrimation, increased bronchial secretions, bradycardia or tachycardia, cardiac arrhythmias, bronchospasm, hypotension, muscle cramps, extreme weakness, agitation, restlessness, or paralysis.
- ▶ Do not confuse cholinergic crisis with myasthenic crisis.
- ▶ Use may be cost-prohibitive due to significant expense.

Uses/Indications

Neostigmine is labeled for treatment of rumen atony, initiating peristalsis, urinary bladder emptying, and skeletal muscle contraction stimulation in horses, cattle, sheep, and swine.[1] It has also been used in dogs for the diagnosis and treatment of myasthenia gravis and to reverse or treat overdoses of nondepolarizing neuromuscular blocking agents (eg, curare-type).[2] Under experimental conditions in beagles, edrophonium demonstrated better reversal of neuromuscular blocking agents and thus may be preferred over neostigmine for this use[3]; however, the lack of commercial availability of edrophonium may limit its use.

In horses, it has been reported that neostigmine decreases jejunal activity and delays gastric emptying; however, a study in horses given neostigmine 0.008 mg/kg/hour IV CRI reported increased fecal production and urination frequency and no decrease in gastric emptying.[5] The study also found that neostigmine stimulated contractile activity of jejunum and pelvic flexure smooth muscle strips in vitro. Neostigmine's use for treating colon impactions and postoperative ileus is controversial and more studies are necessary to determine its clinical usefulness for these indications in horses.

Pharmacology/Actions

Neostigmine competes with acetylcholine for binding of acetylcholinesterase, which forms a carbamyl-ester complex. The neostigmine-acetylcholinesterase complex is hydrolyzed at a slower rate than that of an acetylcholine-acetylcholinesterase complex, resulting in acetylcholine accumulation with a resultant exaggeration and prolongation of its effects. These effects can include increased tone of intestinal and skeletal musculature, stimulation of salivary and sweat glands, bronchoconstriction, ureter constriction, miosis, and bradycardia. Of note, the effects of the neostigmine-acetylcholinesterase complex last longer compared to edrophonium. Neostigmine also has a direct cholinomimetic effect on skeletal muscle. Neostigmine effects may be diminished in patients with metabolic acidosis.[4]

Pharmacokinetics

After IV administration in dogs, neostigmine is rapidly removed from the circulation. The apparent volume of distribution and clearance are ≈150 mL/kg and ≈6.9 mL/minute/kg, respectively.[6]

In humans, neostigmine effects on peristaltic activity begin within 10 to 30 minutes after parenteral administration and can persist for up to 4 hours. It is ≈15% to 25% bound to plasma proteins, and the half-life is ≈1 hour. Neostigmine is metabolized in the liver and hydrolyzed by cholinesterases to 3-OH PTM, which is weakly active. When administered parenterally, ≈80% of the drug is excreted in the urine within 24 hours, with 50% excreted unchanged.

Contraindications/Precautions/Warnings

Neostigmine is contraindicated in patients with peritonitis, with mechanical obstruction of the intestinal or urinary tract, in animals hypersensitive to this class of compounds, or in animals treated with other cholinesterase inhibitors. Neostigmine is contraindicated in lactating animals.[1]

Use with extreme caution in patients with recent urinary bladder or intestinal surgery. Use with caution in patients with epilepsy, peptic ulcer disease, bronchial asthma, cardiac arrhythmias, hyperthyroidism, vagotonia, or megacolon. In humans, neostigmine has been associated with bradycardia.[7]

Adverse Effects

Adverse effects of neostigmine are dose-related and cholinergic in nature. Postoperative diarrhea may occur in humans that have had neuromuscular blockade reversal.[8] A case report of a dog developing a cholinergic crisis after receiving a dose of neostigmine 0.05 mg/kg SC has been published.[9] For more information on cholinergic signs, see ***Overdose/Acute Toxicity***. Rapid administration to horses increases likelihood of bradycardia and hypotension.[4]

In humans, common adverse effects include hypotension, nausea, and vomiting.[7]

Reproductive/Nursing Safety

No adverse effects on organogenesis were noted in rats or rabbits. In humans, acetylcholinesterase inhibitors given IV to pregnant patients near term may lead to premature labor.[7]

Neostigmine has not been detected in human milk and would not be expected to cross the placenta when given at recommended doses due to its ionization at physiologic pH; however, it is not labeled for use in lactating animals due to risk of milk contamination.[1]

Because safety has not been established in animals, this drug should only be used when the maternal benefits outweigh the potential risks to offspring.

Overdose/Acute Toxicity

Overdoses of neostigmine can induce a cholinergic crisis. Clinical signs may include nausea, vomiting, diarrhea, excessive salivation and drooling, sweating (in animals with sweat glands), miosis, lacrimation, increased bronchial secretions, bradycardia or tachycardia, cardiac arrhythmias, bronchospasm, hypotension, muscle cramps and extreme weakness, agitation, restlessness, or paralysis. Death may occur secondary to respiratory paralysis. In patients with myasthenia gravis, it may be difficult to distinguish between a cholinergic crisis and myasthenic crisis.

Treat a cholinergic crisis by temporarily ceasing neostigmine therapy and instituting treatment with atropine. Maintain adequate ventilation using mechanical assistance if necessary.

For patients that have experienced or are suspected to have experienced an overdose, consultation with a 24-hour poison consultation center specializing in providing veterinary-specific information is recommended. For general information related to overdose and toxin exposures, as well as contact information for poison control centers, refer to ***Appendix.***

Drug Interactions

The following drug interactions have either been reported or are theoretical in humans or animals receiving neostigmine and may be of significance in veterinary patients. Unless otherwise noted, use together is not necessarily contraindicated, but weigh the potential risks and perform additional monitoring when appropriate.

- **ATROPINE**: Atropine will antagonize the muscarinic effects of neostigmine and some clinicians routinely use the two together, but concurrent use should be done cautiously as atropine can mask the early clinical signs of a cholinergic crisis.
- **BETA-BLOCKERS** (eg, **atenolol, propranolol**): May increase risk for bradycardia or hypotension caused by beta-blockers. Beta-blockers may worsen clinical signs of myasthenia gravis and reduce efficacy of neostigmine.
- **CORTICOSTEROIDS** (eg, **dexamethasone, prednis(ol)one**): May decrease the anticholinesterase activity of neostigmine; after stopping corticosteroid therapy, neostigmine may cause increased anticholinesterase activity
- **DEXPANTHENOL**: Theoretically, dexpanthenol may have additive effects when used with neostigmine.
- **MAGNESIUM**: Anticholinesterase therapy may be antagonized by administration of parenteral magnesium therapy, as it can have a direct depressant effect on skeletal muscle.
- **MUSCLE RELAXANTS**: Neostigmine may prolong the Phase I block of depolarizing muscle relaxants (eg, **succinylcholine, decamethonium**) and neostigmine antagonizes the actions of nondepolarizing neuromuscular blocking agents (eg, **pancuronium, tubocurarine, gallamine, vecuronium, atracurium**). Effect may be seen with certain antibiotics that also possess mild nondepolarizing blocking effects (eg, **aminoglycosides, clindamycin**).
- **TETRACYCLINES, LINCOMYCIN, and CLINDAMYCIN**: These drugs can enhance the blockade of neuromuscular blocking agents. This blockade is difficult to reverse with neostigmine in the presence of these antibiotics.[10]

Laboratory Considerations

- No specific concerns noted

Dosages

DOGS/CATS:

Diagnosis of myasthenia gravis (extra-label): From a retrospective study, 0.01 – 0.05 mg/kg SC, IM, IV[2]; IV administration should be over 1 minute. Some pretreat with atropine, but this must be done with caution as it can mask the early signs associated with a cholinergic crisis. If clinical improvement occurs in 15 to 30 minutes, it is suggestive of a diagnosis.

Treatment of myasthenia gravis when administration of oral pyridostigmine is not possible (extra-label): If pyridostigmine is not available or oral medication cannot be given in actively regurgitating animals: neostigmine 0.04 mg/kg IM, SC every 6 hours.[2] (**NOTE**: Currently available human products are only labeled for IV use, to be given over 1 minute.)

Adjuvant epidural analgesia for orthopedic surgery in dogs (extra-label): neostigmine 5 µg/kg epidurally with morphine 0.1 mg/kg administered at the end of surgery resulted in improved pain scores and fewer doses of rescue analgesia.[11]

Reversal agent for neuromuscular blockade in dogs (extra-label): **NOTE**: use for this indication should be limited to individuals familiar with neuromuscular blockade and Train of Four (TOF) monitoring.

a) Neostigmine 0.01 – 0.1 mg/kg IV (over 1 minute) in combination with atropine 0.02 mg/kg IV or glycopyrrolate 0.01 mg/kg IV[4]

b) Neostigmine 0.02 – 0.07 mg/kg IV in combination with atropine 0.03 mg/kg IV. Reversal time was 5 to 10 minutes and was faster when higher doses of neostigmine were used.[12]

HORSES:

Initiating peristalsis to cause evacuation of the bowel; emptying the urinary bladder; and stimulating skeletal muscle contractions (label dosage; FDA-approved): 1 mg/45.3 kg (100 lb) of body weight SC; repeat as indicated[1]

Reversal agent for neuromuscular blockade (extra-label): 0.007 mg/kg IV over 1 to 2 minutes is recommended. Reversal should not be attempted until some degree of spontaneous recovery has been established and ECG monitoring is in use; atropine should be readily available.[4,13-15] Edrophonium is preferred to neostigmine due to its shorter duration of action and milder muscarinic effect, which may reduce the need for administration of anticholinergic drugs; however, the lack of commercially available edrophonium may limit its use.

Decrease clinical signs associated with botulism A toxin (extra-label): From a case report, neostigmine 0.025 mg/kg SC 3 times daily improved palpebral reflexes and tongue and tail tone. Although the horse regained limited ability to stand and defecate, neostigmine did not restore chewing and swallowing function.[16]

Adjuvant for epidural injection (extra-label): 1 µg/kg combined with 2% lidocaine 0.2 mg/kg epidurally provided analgesia for ≈2.5 hours with moderate ataxia.[17,18]

CATTLE:

Rumen atony; initiating peristalsis to cause evacuation of the bowel; emptying the urinary bladder; and stimulating skeletal muscle contractions (label dosage; FDA-approved): 1 mg/45.3 kg (100 lb) of body weight SC; repeat as indicated[1]

SWINE:

Initiating peristalsis to cause evacuation of the bowel; emptying the urinary bladder; and stimulating skeletal muscle contractions (label dosage; FDA-approved): 2 – 3 mg/45.3 kg (100 lb) of body weight IM; repeat as indicated[1]

SHEEP:

Rumen atony; initiating peristalsis that causes evacuation of the bowel; emptying the urinary bladder; and stimulating skeletal muscle contractions (label dosage; FDA-approved): 1 – 1.5 mg/45.3 kg (100 lb) of body weight SC; repeat as indicated[1]

Monitoring

Dependent on reason for use:

- Adverse effects
- Clinical efficacy

Client Information

- Neostigmine should only be administered by a veterinary professional under close monitoring.

Chemistry/Synonyms

Synthetic quaternary ammonium parasympathomimetic agents, neostigmine bromide and neostigmine methylsulfate both occur as odorless, bitter, white, crystalline powders that are very soluble in water and soluble in alcohol. The melting point of neostigmine methylsulfate is 144°C-149°C (291.2°F-300.2°F). The pH of the commercially available neostigmine methylsulfate injection is from 5 to 6.5.

Neostigmine methylsulfate may also be known as neostigmine metilsulfate, neostigmine methylsulphate, neostigmini metilsulfas, proserinum, *Bloxiverz®*, *Prostigmin®*, *Prostigmina®, or Stiglyn®*.

Storage/Stability

Neostigmine methylsulfate injection should be stored at room temperature (20°C-25°C; 68°F-77°F) with excursions permitted between 15°C and 30°C (59°F-86°F). Protect from light; avoid freezing.

Compatibility/Compounding Considerations

Compatibility is dependent on factors such as pH, concentration, temperature, and diluent used; specialized references or a hospital pharmacist should be consulted for more specific information.

Neostigmine methylsulfate injection is reportedly physically **Y-site compatible** with the following IV replacement solutions and drugs: 0.9% sodium chloride, heparin sodium, hydrocortisone sodium succinate, and potassium chloride.

Dosage Forms/Regulatory Status

VETERINARY-LABELED PRODUCTS: NONE

Historically, there was an approved injectable product (*Stiglyn®* 1:500), but although still listed in FDA's Green Book, it does not appear to be marketed.

The Association of Racing Commissioners International (ARCI) has designated this drug as a class 3 substance. Use of this drug may not be allowed in certain animal competitions. Check rules and regulations before entering in a competition while this medication is being administered. Contact local racing authorities for further guidance. See ***Appendix*** for more information.

HUMAN-LABELED PRODUCTS:

Neostigmine Methylsulfate Injection: 0.5 mg/mL and 1 mg/mL in 10 mL vials; *Bloxiverz®*, *Prostigmin®*, generic; (Rx)

References

For the complete list of references, see **wiley.com/go/budde/plumb**

Niacinamide

Nicotinamide

(nye-a-***sin***-a-mide)

Immunomodulator; Nutritional; Vitamin

Prescriber Highlights

- Used in combination with a tetracycline for a variety of sterile inflammatory and autoimmune conditions in dogs
- Possible contraindications include seizures, liver disease, active peptic ulcers, or hypersensitivity to the drug.
- Adverse effects include anorexia, vomiting, and lethargy; rarely increases in liver enzymes.
- Clinical response may be gradual and take at least 6 to 8 weeks.
- Nicacinamide is inexpensive, but 3 times daily dosing may be problematic for some owners.

Uses/Indications

Niacinamide is used in conjunction with a tetracycline antibiotic (eg, tetracycline, doxycycline) in controlling a variety of sterile inflammatory or autoimmune conditions in dogs. Some examples of indications include localized and generalized discoid lupus erythematosus (DLE),[1,2] cutaneous vesicular lupus erythematosus,[3] sterile granulomatous/pyogranulomatous syndrome, sterile nodular panniculitis,[4] cutaneous reactive histiocytosis,[5] pemphigus complex,[6] mucous membrane pemphigoid,[7,8] idiopathic symmetrical (lupoid) onychodystrophy/onychitis,[9] metatarsal fistulae, vasculitis, arteritis of the nasal philtrum,[10] sebaceous adenitis, dermatomyositis,[11] nodular granulomatous conjunctivitis,[12] and chronic ulcerative paradental stomatitis (CUPS).[13]

Controlled prospective studies demonstrating clear efficacy are lacking, but niacinamide appears effective in some patients, including 70% of dogs treated for DLE in one study.[2] It is often used in conjunction with other immunomodulating drugs such as glucocorticoids[1] or omega-3 fatty acids, especially in the initial treatment phase. Niacinamide may be particularly efficacious for milder disease forms or as a steroid-sparing agent. It may take 6 to 8 weeks of using niacinamide (with a tetracycline) before efficacy is noted.

Pharmacology/Actions

Niacinamide is an essential nutrient in humans; it is necessary for lipid metabolism, tissue respiration, and glycogenolysis. Its primary pharmacologic use (in combination with a tetracycline) for autoimmune disorders in dogs is secondary to its ability to block IgE-induced histamine release and degranulation of mast cells. When niacinamide is used with a tetracycline, it may suppress leukocyte chemotaxis secondary to complement activation by antibody antigen complexes. It also inhibits phosphodiesterases and decreases the release of proteases.

Niacinamide is a product of niacin metabolism. Although niacinamide and niacin act identically as vitamins, at higher (pharmacologic) doses, they exert different effects. For example, niacinamide does not affect blood lipid levels or the cardiovascular system.

Pharmacokinetics

Niacinamide is absorbed well after oral administration and widely distributed to body tissues. Niacinamide is metabolized in the liver to several metabolites that are excreted into the urine. At physiologic doses, only a small amount of niacinamide is excreted into the urine unchanged, but as dosages increase, larger quantities are excreted unchanged.

Contraindications/Precautions/Warnings

In humans, niacinamide therapy is contraindicated in patients with liver disease, active peptic ulcers, or hypersensitivity to the drug.

Use niacinamide/tetracycline drug combination with caution, or avoid use, in dogs with a seizure history.

Do not confuse niacinamide with niacin (see ***Pharmacology/Actions***).

Adverse Effects

Adverse effects of niacinamide in dogs are uncommon, but may include anorexia, vomiting, diarrhea, and lethargy. Administration of niacinamide with food may help alleviate adverse GI effects. Occasionally, increases in liver enzymes may be noted; loss of glycemic control is possible in diabetic patients, although documentation of this adverse effect was not located. There have been some anecdotal reports of increased seizure frequencies in dogs.[5] Because niacinamide is used clinically in combination with a tetracycline, adverse effects noted may be due to niacinamide and/or the tetracycline.

Reproductive/Nursing Safety

Although niacinamide alone should be safe to use in pregnant and lactating animals, its use in combination with a tetracycline may not be safe.

Because safety has not been established in animals, this drug should only be used when the maternal benefits outweigh the potential risks to offspring.

Overdose/Acute Toxicity

Niacinamide overdoses are unlikely to cause adverse effects other than acute GI distress.

For patients that have experienced or are suspected to have experienced an overdose, consultation with a 24-hour poison consultation center specializing in providing veterinary-specific information is recommended. For general information related to overdose and toxin exposures, as well as contact information for poison control centers, refer to ***Appendix***.

Drug Interactions

Niacinamide and tetracycline treatment does not interfere with antibody production associated with routine vaccinations in dogs.[14] Also see ***Tetracycline, Doxycycline,*** *or* ***Minocycline*** monographs for additional drug interactions if using combination therapy.

The following drug interactions have either been reported or are theoretical in humans or animals receiving niacinamide and may be of significance in veterinary patients. Unless otherwise noted, use together is not necessarily contraindicated, but weigh the potential risks and perform additional monitoring when appropriate.

- INSULIN/ORAL ANTIDIABETIC AGENTS (eg, **glipizide, metformin**): In diabetic humans, dosage increases for insulin or oral antidiabetic agents have sometimes been necessary after initiating niacinamide therapy; significance in veterinary patients is unknown.

Laboratory Considerations

- Potentially could interfere with intradermal or serum **allergy testing**; withdraw the drug 1 to 2 weeks before testing.

Dosages

DOGS:

Adjunctive treatment of sterile inflammatory or autoimmune diseases (extra-label): Niacinamide is typically used in combination with a tetracycline. Recommended dosages are empirical and vary.

- **Dogs 10 kg (22 lb) or less:** Niacinamide 250 mg/dog (NOT mg/kg) PO 3 times daily in combination with tetracycline 250 mg/dog (NOT mg/kg) PO 3 times daily[5]
- **Dogs more than 10 kg (22 lb):** Niacinamide 500 mg/dog (NOT mg/kg) PO 3 times daily in combination with tetracycline 500 mg/dog (NOT mg/kg) PO 3 times daily[5]

NOTES:

1. If efficacious, may reduce niacinamide dose to twice-daily administration and then taper further over time when possible.
2. Tetracycline may be replaced with doxycycline 5 – 10 mg/kg PO every 12 hours OR minocycline 5 – 10 mg/kg PO every 12 hours.[15]
3. Some clinicians have used 15 kg (33.1 lb) as the weight cutoff (ie, dogs 15 kg [33.1 lb] or less receive 250 mg/dog [NOT mg/kg]; dogs more than 15 kg [33.1 lb] receive 500 mg/dog [NOT mg/kg]).[9] Other clinicians have suggested niacinamide 45 mg/kg PO every 8 hours in combination with tetracycline 45 mg/kg PO every 8 hours.[1]

Monitoring

- Efficacy: Clinical response may be gradual and take up to 6 to 8 weeks.
- Adverse effects (baseline and occasional monitoring of liver enzymes is suggested), particularly when combined with other drugs that may increase liver enzymes such as doxycycline or minocycline

Client Information

- Niacinamide is used in dogs in combination with a tetracycline for treatment of a variety of serious skin conditions and other autoimmune diseases.
- Give as directed to your animal; usually 3 times daily at first. Improvement may be gradual and may take up to 6 to 8 weeks.
- Side effects from niacinamide are rare. Vomiting, diarrhea, and reduced appetite (eating less than normal) are the most common side effects. When niacinamide is used in combination with a tetracycline, the risk for side effects is greater and includes lethargy (tiredness or lack of energy) and, rarely, liver problems.
- Be careful to purchase the correct product; niacinamide is not the same as niacin (which is more readily available).
- Your veterinarian will need to monitor your animal with recheck examinations while it is receiving this medicine. Do not miss these important follow-up visits.

Chemistry/Synonyms

Niacinamide, also commonly known as nicotinamide, occurs as a white crystalline powder. It is odorless or nearly odorless and has a bitter taste. It is freely soluble in water or alcohol.

Niacinamide may also be known as nicotinamide, nicotinamidum, nicotinic acid amide, nicotylamide, vitamin B (3), or vitamin PP.

Storage/Stability

Store niacinamide tablets in tight containers at room temperature unless otherwise labeled. Niacinamide is **incompatible** with alkalis or strong acids.

Compatibility/Compounding Considerations

No specific information noted

Dosage Forms/Regulatory Status

VETERINARY-LABELED PRODUCTS: NONE

HUMAN-LABELED PRODUCTS:

Niacinamide Tablets and Capsules: 100 and 500 mg; generic; (OTC)

References

For the complete list of references, see **wiley.com/go/budde/plumb**

Nitazoxanide

(nye-tah-***zox***-ah-nide)

Antiparasitic Agent

Prescriber Highlights

- ► Drug that has activity against a variety of protozoa, nematodes, bacteria, and trematodes, including *Sarcocystis neurona*, *Giardia* spp, *Cryptosporidia* spp, and *Helicobacter pylori*
- ► Historically approved for use in horses for equine protozoal myeloencephalitis (EPM), but veterinary paste no longer marketed
- ► Interest in using in other companion animals (eg, dogs, cats), but data are lacking to support use
- ► Adverse effects in dogs include GI (eg, hypersalivation, vomiting, diarrhea), which may be therapy limiting.

Uses/Indications

Nitazoxanide may be useful as an alternative treatment for cryptosporidiosis in cats. A single nitazoxanide dose reduces shedding of *Giardia* spp cysts and *Cryptosporidium* spp oocysts in dogs.[1] Because of the drug's spectrum of activity and apparent safety, there is potential for using it in a variety of companion animal species, but data are lacking for specific indications and dosages.

Nitazoxanide oral paste was approved for the treatment of horses with equine protozoal myeloencephalitis (EPM) caused by *Sarcocystis neurona*, but the product is no longer marketed in the United States.

In humans, nitazoxanide is FDA-approved to treat diarrhea caused by *Cryptosporidium parvum* and *Giardia lamblia.*

Pharmacology

Although the precise mechanism of action of nitazoxanide is unknown, its active metabolites (tizoxanide and tizoxanide glucuronide) are thought to inhibit the pyruvate ferredoxin oxidoreductase (PFOR) enzyme-dependent electron transfer reactions essential to anaerobic energy metabolism. Nitazoxanide has activity against a variety of protozoa, nematodes, bacteria, and trematodes, including *Sarcocystis neurona, Giardia* spp, *Cryptosporidia* spp, and *Helicobacter pylori.*

Pharmacokinetics

Following oral administration in horses, nitazoxanide is absorbed and rapidly converted to its active metabolite (tizoxanide [desacetyl-nitazoxanide]). Peak concentrations of tizoxanide are attained between 2 to 3 hours and are not detectable by 24 hours postadministration. In humans, nitazoxanide is not detectable in plasma, but peak concentrations of tizoxanide and tizoxanide glucuronide occur ≈3 to 4 hours postadministration. More than 99% of tizoxanide is bound to plasma proteins. Tizoxanide is excreted in the urine, bile, and feces; the glucuronide metabolite is secreted in the urine and bile.

Contraindications/Precautions/Warnings

Nitazoxanide is contraindicated in patients that are hypersensitive to it. Safety for use in animals with compromised renal or hepatic function has not been established; use with caution.

Do not confuse niTAZOXanide with niZATidine.

Adverse Effects

In cats, GI irritation can occur.

In a study using nitazoxanide in 9 dogs with naturally occurring *Giardia* spp infections, 5 of the dogs developed excessive salivation, vomiting, or diarrhea that resulted in removal from the study.[2]

In humans, nitazoxanide appears to be well tolerated and adverse effect rates are similar to placebo. Rarely, sclera may turn yellow secondary to drug disposition (not jaundice) but return to normal after drug discontinuation.

Reproductive/Nursing Safety

Reproduction studies have been performed using dosages of up to 3200 mg/kg/day PO in rats (≈48 times the clinical dose adjusted for body surface area) and 100 mg/kg/day PO in rabbits (≈3 times the clinical dose adjusted for body surface area) and have revealed no evidence of impaired fertility or harm to the fetus due to nitazoxanide.[3] It is unknown if nitazoxanide is excreted into milk. Because safety has not been established in animals, this drug should only be used when the maternal benefits outweigh the potential risks to offspring.

Overdose/Acute Toxicity

There is limited information available on the acute toxicity of nitazoxanide. It has been reported that overdoses of 2.5 times in horses have been associated with fatalities. The oral LD_{50} for dogs and cats is greater than 10 g/kg. Repeated doses of 450 mg/kg in rats caused intense salivation and increased liver and spleen weights. In a study of horses given ≈5 times the label-recommended dose, all of the horses developed anorexia, diarrhea, and lethargy, and testing was halted after 4 days of study. Human volunteers have taken doses of up to 4 g without significant adverse effects occurring.

For patients that have experienced or are suspected of having experienced an overdose, consultation with a 24-hour poison consultation center specializing in providing veterinary-specific information is recommended. For general information related to overdose and toxin exposures, as well as contact information for poison control centers, refer to ***Appendix.***

Drug Interactions

The following drug interactions have either been reported or are theoretical in humans or animals receiving nitazoxanide and may be of significance in veterinary patients. Unless otherwise noted, use together is not necessarily contraindicated, but weigh the potential risks and perform additional monitoring when appropriate.

- **Highly Protein Bound Drugs** (eg, **NSAIDs [eg, meloxicam], salicylates, sulfonamides** [eg, **sulfadimethoxine**], **warfarin**): Because nitazoxanide is highly protein bound, it could theoretically displace other highly bound drugs, causing a transient increase in serum concentrations of each drug. These interactions are unlikely to be of clinical concern because increased free drug concentrations will equilibrate through increased clearance. Monitor for adverse effects of each drug when using this combination.

Laboratory Considerations

- No specific laboratory interactions or considerations were noted.

Dosages

DOGS:

***Giardia* spp associated diarrhea** (extra-label): 75 – 150 mg/kg PO once[1]

***Cryptosporidia* spp associated diarrhea** (extra-label): 75 – 150 mg/kg PO once[1]

CATS:

***Cryptosporidia* spp associated diarrhea** (extra-label): 10 – 25 mg/kg PO every 12 to 24 hours for up to 28 days[4,5]

HORSES:

Equine protozoal myeloencephalitis (EPM) caused by *Sarcocystis neurona*: For a 28-day course of therapy, 25 mg/kg PO once daily on days 1 through 5 followed by 50 mg/kg PO once daily on days 6 through 28[6]

Monitoring

- Clinical efficacy
- Weekly body weight
- Adverse effects

Client Information

- This medicine has not been commonly used in dogs or cats, and adverse effects such as excessive salivation, vomiting, or diarrhea may occur.

Chemistry/Synonyms

A nitrothiazolyl-salicylamide derivative antiparasitic agent, nitazoxanide occurs as a light-yellow powder. It is slightly soluble in ethanol and practically insoluble in water.

Nitazoxanide may also be known as PH-5776, *Alinia*®, *Daxon*®, *Heliton*®, and *Navigator*®.

Storage/Stability

The human-approved powder for oral suspension should be stored at 25°C (77°F); excursions permitted to 15°C to 30°C (59°F-86°F). Once suspended with tap water, the oral suspension should be kept in tightly closed containers at room temperature and discarded after 7 days.

Compatibility/Compounding Considerations

No specific information was noted.

Dosage Forms/Regulatory Status

VETERINARY-LABELED PRODUCTS: NONE

Nitazoxanide oral paste (32%) *Navigator*® was FDA-approved in the United States for use in horses. Although this product is still listed in FDA's Green Book of approved animal drugs, it is no longer commercially available in the United States.

HUMAN-LABELED PRODUCTS:

Nitazoxanide Oral Tablets: 500 mg; *Alinia*®, generic; (Rx)

Nitazoxanide Powder for Oral Suspension: 20 mg/mL in 60 mL; *Alinia*®; (Rx)

References

For the complete list of references, see **wiley.com/go/budde/plumb**

Nitenpyram

(nye-ten-***pye***-rum) *Capstar*®

Oral Insecticide

Prescriber Highlights

- Oral insecticide used primarily as a flea (*Ctenocephalides felis*) adulticide in dogs and cats; may also be used for the treatment of myiasis
- Fast onset of action: fleas begin to die within 30 minutes of administration
- Not effective for killing flea eggs or other immature forms when used as a single agent
- Safe and well tolerated, including in pregnant and lactating dogs and cats
- Available over the counter (OTC)

Uses/Indications

Nitenpyram is indicated as a flea (*Ctenocephalides felis*) adulticide in dogs and cats that are at least 0.9 kg (2 lb) in weight and 4 weeks old.[1] It does not repel fleas or ticks and does not reliably kill ticks or fleas in other life stages (ie, eggs, larvae, or immature fleas). Nitenpyram tablets begin working within 30 minutes of administration and kill 90% of fleas within 4 hours in dogs and 6 hours in cats.[1,2] It has been anecdotally reported that rectal administration is effective when PO administration is not possible.

Nitenpyram is also effective for treating myiasis (ie, fly larvae/maggot infestation) in dogs due to various species, including *Cochliomyia hominivorax* and *Chrysomya bezziana*.[3,4]

Pharmacology/Actions

Nitenpyram is in the class of neonicotinoid insecticides. It enters the systemic circulation of the adult flea after consuming a blood meal from a treated animal. It binds to nicotinic acetylcholine receptors in the postsynaptic membranes and blocks acetylcholine-mediated neuronal transmission, causing paralysis and death of the flea. Nitenpyram is 3500 times more selective for insect alpha-4 beta-2 nicotinic receptors than vertebrate receptors. It does not inhibit acetylcholinesterase. Efficacy appears to be greater than 98% (kill rate) in dogs or cats within 6 hours of treatment.[2] When combined with an insect growth regulator (eg, lufenuron), immature stages of fleas may also be controlled.

Pharmacokinetics

Nitenpyram is rapidly and almost completely absorbed after oral administration. Tablets begin working within 30 minutes, with peak levels occurring ≈80 minutes after dosing in dogs and ≈40 minutes in cats.[1] Elimination half-life is ≈3 hours in dogs and 8 hours in cats. Nitenpyram is excreted primarily as conjugated metabolites in the urine, and excretion is complete within 48 hours of dosing. In dogs and cats, ≈3% and ≈5% of doses are excreted in the feces, respectively.

Contraindications/Precautions/Warnings

Nitenpyram is not to be used in animals under 0.9 kg (2 lb) of body weight or 4 weeks of age. Use it with caution in animals under 8 weeks old.

Adverse Effects

Nitenpyram is usually well tolerated.[5]

Based on postapproval adverse drug experience reporting, the following adverse effects (listed in decreasing order of frequency) have been reported:

Cats: Hyperactivity, panting, lethargy, itching, vocalization, vomiting, fever, decreased appetite, nervousness, diarrhea, difficulty breathing, salivation, incoordination, seizures, pupil dilation, increased heart rate, and trembling[1]

Dogs: Lethargy/depression, vomiting, itching, decreased appetite, diarrhea, hyperactivity, incoordination, trembling, seizures, panting, allergic reactions including hives, vocalization, salivation, fever, and nervousness[1]

Reported clinical signs are generally associated with flea die-off and are not related to the medication. Clinical signs are usually self-limiting and resolve without any treatment.

The frequency of severe signs, including neurologic signs and death, was higher in animals under 0.9 kg (2 lb) of body weight, less than 8 weeks of age, and/or reported to be in poor body condition.[1]

Reproductive/Nursing Safety

Nitenpyram is considered safe to use in pregnant or lactating dogs and cats.[1] In some instances, birth defects and fetal/neonatal loss were reported after treatment of pregnant and/or lactating animals.

Because safety has not been established in animals, this drug should only be used in breeding animals when the maternal benefits outweigh the potential risks to offspring.

Overdose/Acute Toxicity

Nitenpyram is relatively safe in high doses to mammals. The oral LD_{50} in rats is ≈1.6 g/kg.[5] Adult dogs and cats were dosed up to 10 times a therapeutic dose daily for 14 days without adverse effects.[2] Cats receiving 125 mg/kg (125 times the therapeutic dose) exhibited hypersalivation, lethargy, vomiting, and tachypnea.[6] These clinical signs typically occurred within 2 hours of treatment and resolved within 24 hours.

For patients that have experienced or are suspected of having experienced an overdose, consultation with a 24-hour poison consultation center specializing in providing veterinary-specific information is recommended. For general information on overdose and toxin exposures, as well as for poison control centers' contact information, refer to ***Appendix.***

Drug Interactions

- No specific drug interactions were located. Nitenpyram has reportedly been used safely with a variety of other medications and other flea products.

Laboratory Considerations

- No specific laboratory interactions or considerations were noted.

Dosages

DOGS/CATS:

Flea infestations (label dosage; FDA-approved): Appropriate dose is given orally based on body weight according to the table below. If reinfestation occurs, the dose may be safely repeated as often as once daily. Tablets may be administered with or without food.

Recommended Dosing Schedule[1]

Species	Body weight (kg [lb])	Dose	Nitenpyram per tablet
Dog or Cat	0.9 -11.4 (2-25)	1 tablet	11.4 mg
Dog	11.4-56.8 (25.1-125)	1 tablet	57 mg

Canine screwworm myiasis (extra-label): Using the label dosage for fleas, administer one dose by mouth once, or one dose followed by a second dose 6 hours later.[3,4] Medication targets the screwworm larvae. Spontaneous expulsion of larvae combined with mechanical removal of dead larvae resulted in 100% efficacy within 18 hours.[7]

REPTILES:

Myiasis (extra-label): Crush one 11.4 mg tablet into powder and administer once orally, as an enema, or on the wound.[8]

Monitoring

- Efficacy (ie, reduction in number of adult fleas)

Client Information

- This medicine is used primarily to kill adult fleas on dogs and cats.
- When used alone, this medicine does not kill flea eggs or other immature forms. Your veterinarian will discuss any additional treatments needed to control the flea problem. All animals in the household must be treated.
- Give this medicine as directed by your veterinarian.
- This medicine is usually tolerated well in dogs and cats. Serious side effects are rare and occur most often in animals that weigh less than 0.9 kg (2 lb), are less than 8 weeks old, or are in poor health.
- Keep this medicine out of reach of children.

Chemistry/Synonyms

Nitenpyram, a neonicotinoid insecticide, occurs as a pale-yellow crystalline powder and is very soluble in water (840 mg/mL).

Nitenpyram may also be known as TI-304, (E)-Nitenpyram, *Bestguard*®, and *Capstar*®.

Storage/Stability

Store commercially available nitenpyram tablets at room temperature (15°C to 25°C [59°F-77°F]).

Compatibility/Compounding Considerations

No specific information was noted.

Dosage Forms/Regulatory Status

VETERINARY-LABELED PRODUCTS:

Nitenpyram Oral Tablets: 11.4 mg and 57 mg in boxes containing blister packs of 6 tablets; *Capstar*®, generic; (OTC); FDA-approved for use in dogs and cats

Combination products:

Nitenpyram with Lufenuron [*Program*® *Flavor Tabs* and *Capstar*® *Flea Management System for Dogs* and *Program*® *Flavor Tabs* (OTC); *Capstar*® *Flea Management System for Cats* (OTC)]. Refer to the ***Lufenuron*** monograph for details. Although this combination product is listed in the FDA Green Book, it does not appear to be commercially available.

Nitenpyram with milbemycin and lufenuron (*Sentinel*® *Flavor Tabs* and *Capstar*® *Flea Management System for Dogs* [Rx]). Refer to ***Lufenuron*** and ***Milbemycin*** monographs for details. Although this combination product is listed in the FDA Green Book, it does not appear to be commercially available

HUMAN-LABELED PRODUCTS: NONE

References

For the complete list of references, see **wiley.com/go/budde/plumb**

Nitrofurantoin

(nye-troe-fyoor-***an***-toyn) *Macrodantin*®, *Macrobid*®

Urinary Antimicrobial

Prescriber Highlights

- Antibacterial that is useful for the treatment of some cases of bacterial cystitis that are resistant to first-line drugs
- Only achieves therapeutic concentrations in urine, so this drug should only be used for bacterial cystitis (not pyelonephritis or other infections)
- Contraindications include food-producing species, renal impairment, and hypersensitivity to nitrofurantoin.
- Adverse effects include GI disturbances, peripheral neuropathy, and hepatopathy.

Uses/Indications

Nitrofurantoin is used primarily in small animal species as a potential treatment for bacterial cystitis in cases where resistance to first-line antibiotics (eg, amoxicillin ± clavunate, sulfa-/trimethoprim) is present.[1-4] It is recommended as a second-line option for sporadic bacterial cystitis.[3] Because nitrofurantoin only reaches therapeutic concentrations in urine, it is not an appropriate choice for the treatment of infections that require tissue drug concentrations (eg, pyelonephritis).

The World Health Organization (WHO) has designated nitrofurantoin as an Important antimicrobial in human medicine.[5]

Pharmacology/Actions

Nitrofurantoin usually acts as a bacteriostatic antimicrobial, but it may be bactericidal depending on the concentration of the drug and the susceptibility of the organism. Although the exact mechanism of action of nitrofurantoin has not been fully elucidated, the drug apparently inhibits various bacterial enzyme systems, including synthesis of DNA, RNA, and proteins, acetyl coenzyme A, as well as energy metabolism and cell wall synthesis. Nitrofurantoin has greater antibacterial activity in acidic environments. Bacterial resistance to nitrofurantoin has remained inconsequential.

Nitrofurantoin has activity against several gram-negative and some gram-positive organisms, including many strains of *Escherichia coli, Klebsiella* spp, *Enterobacter* spp, *Enterococcus* spp, *Streptococcus* spp, *Staphylococcus* spp, *Enterobacter* spp, *Citrobacter* spp, *Salmonella* spp, *Shigella* spp, and *Corynebacterium* spp. It has little or no activity against most strains of *Proteus* spp, *Serratia* spp, or *Acinetobacter* spp and has no activity against *Pseudomonas* and *Corynebacterium* spp.

Pharmacokinetics

There are 3 commercial (human label) oral forms of nitrofurantoin (regular nitrofurantoin in an oral suspension, macrocrystalline capsules, and monohydrate/macrocrystals capsules). No pharmacokinetic studies comparing these different forms in dogs or cats were located. In humans, nitrofurantoin is rapidly absorbed from the GI tract; the presence of food may enhance the absorption of the drug. Macrocrystalline (eg, *Macrodantin*®) capsules are more slowly absorbed, but they are still dosed 3 to 4 times daily for treating UTIs in humans. Monohydrate/macrocrystalline forms of the drug (eg, *Macrobid*®) are absorbed even more slowly, with less GI upset. Because of the monohydrate/macrocrystalline form's slower absorption, urine concentrations of the drug may be prolonged with the monohydrate macrocrystalline form and so it is dosed twice daily in humans.

In dogs, absorption was widely variable (38% to 120%) following oral administration, although absorption half-lives were higher with solid dosage forms versus suspension.[6] Elimination half-lives after oral administration ranged from 19 to 87 minutes.

Therapeutic concentrations in the systemic circulation are not maintained because of the rapid elimination of the drug. Approximately 20% to 60% of the drug is bound to serum proteins. Administration of the macrocrystalline form results in therapeutic peak urine concentrations occurring within 30 minutes of dosing.

Approximately 40% to 50% of the drug is eliminated into the urine unchanged. Some of the drug is metabolized, primarily in the liver. The elimination half-lives in humans with normal renal function average 20 minutes.

Contraindications/Precautions/Warnings

Nitrofurantoin is contraindicated in patients that have renal impairment as the drug is much less efficacious, and the development of neurotoxicity is much more likely. The drug is also contraindicated in patients that are hypersensitive to it.

Use nitrofurantoin with caution in patients with pre-existing hepatic dysfunction. Although rare, significant hepatic reactions (eg, jaundice, hepatitis, hepatitis necrosis) have been documented in humans with its use.

In humans, pulmonary reactions have also been reported rarely in patients receiving treatment for greater than 6 months. Treatment should be immediately discontinued in the event of pulmonary toxicity.

Rats can develop neurotoxicity when they are given nitrofurantoin; avoid using the drug in this species.

Adverse Effects

In dogs and cats, GI disturbances (primarily vomiting and diarrhea), peripheral neuropathies (reversible), pulmonary hypersensitivity reactions, and hepatopathy can occur. Chronic active hepatitis, hemolytic anemia, and pneumonitis have been described in humans. These effects are believed to occur very rarely in animals with nitrofurantoin's use.

Reproductive/Nursing Safety

Nitrofurantoin crosses the placenta. In humans, nitrofurantoin is contraindicated in pregnant patients at term and neonates, as hemolytic anemia can occur secondary to immature enzyme systems. Safe use of the drug during earlier stages of pregnancy has not been determined in animals. Nitrofurantoin has been implicated in decreasing spermatogenesis in rats and humans, as well as in causing infertility in male dogs.

Nitrofurantoin is excreted into maternal milk in very low concentrations. Safety for use in the nursing mother or offspring has not been established. In humans, nitrofurantoin is considered compatible with breastfeeding in healthy, full-term infants over 1 month old.[7,8]

Because safety has not been established in animals, this drug should only be used when the maternal benefits outweigh the potential risks to offspring.

Overdose/Acute Toxicity

No specific information was located. Because the drug is rapidly absorbed and excreted, patients with normal renal function should require little therapy when mild overdoses occur. A high fluid intake should be maintained to promote urinary excretion of the drug. Nitrofurantoin is dialyzable. If the ingestion was relatively recent, massive overdoses should be handled with standard GI decontamination protocols; the patient should then be monitored for adverse effects (see ***Adverse Effects***).

For patients that have experienced or are suspected to have experienced an overdose, consultation with a 24-hour poison consultation center specializing in providing veterinary-specific information is recommended. For general information related to overdose and toxin exposures, as well as contact information for poison control centers, refer to ***Appendix***.

Drug Interactions

The following drug interactions have either been reported or are theoretical in humans or animals receiving nitrofurantoin and may be of significance in veterinary patients. Unless otherwise noted, use together is not necessarily contraindicated, but weigh the potential risks and perform additional monitoring when appropriate.

- **ANTICHOLINERGIC DRUGS** (eg, **atropine, glycopyrrolate**): May increase the oral bioavailability of nitrofurantoin
- **FLUCONAZOLE**: Increased risk for hepatic and pulmonary toxicity.
- **FLUOROQUINOLONES** (eg, **ciprofloxacin, enrofloxacin**): Nitrofurantoin may antagonize the antimicrobial activity of the fluoroquinolones. Concomitant use is best avoided.
- **LOCAL ANESTHETICS** (eg, **bupivacaine, lidocaine**): In humans, nitrofurantoin may increase the risk for methemoglobinemia when used with local anesthetics. The significance in veterinary medicine is unknown.
- **PROBENECID**: May inhibit the renal excretion of nitrofurantoin, potentially increasing its toxicity and reducing its effectiveness in UTIs
- **PSYLLIUM**: Psyllium may bind and reduce nitrofurantoin absorption if given at the same time; if possible, separate doses by 3 or more hours.
- **SPIRONOLACTONE**: Nitrofurantoin may increase hyperkalemic effects.

Laboratory Considerations

- Nitrofurantoin may cause false-positive **urine glucose** determinations if using cupric-sulfate solutions (Benedict's reagent, *Clinitest*®). Tests using glucose oxidase methods (*Tes-Tape*®, *Clinistix*®) are not affected by nitrofurantoin.
- Nitrofurantoin may cause decreases in **blood glucose** and increases in **serum creatinine, bilirubin,** and ALP.

Dosages

DOGS/CATS:

NOTE: Neither reference below states which form is being used (macrocrystalline [eg, *Macrodantin*®] or monohydrate/macrocrystals [eg, *Macrobid*®]).

As a second-line antimicrobial for sporadic bacterial cystitis, particularly when multidrug-resistant pathogens are involved (extra-label): 4.4 – 5 mg/kg PO every 8 hours for 5 days.[3] Longer treatment courses (eg, 7 to 14 days may be reasonable for persistent, recurrent, or relapsing infections). Amoxicillin (+/- clavulanic acid) and sulfa-/trimethoprim are considered first-line agents.

HORSES:

Sporadic bacterial cystitis, particularly when multidrug-resistant pathogens are involved (extra-label): 4.5 mg/kg PO for the first dose, then 2.25 mg/kg PO every 8 hours for 7 days

Monitoring

- Clinical efficacy
- Adverse effects
- Culture and susceptibility for recurrent or persistent infections[3]
- Baseline and periodic hepatic enzymes should be considered with chronic therapy

Client Information

- Give this medicine with food.
- Your animal may develop brownish-colored urine while taking this medicine.
- Stomach upset (acting sick) and vomiting are the most common side effects, but muscle weakness may indicate nerve toxicity (se-

rious). Contact your veterinarian if any of these signs occur.

- Be sure your animal always has access to fresh water while receiving this medication.

Chemistry/Synonyms

Nitrofurantoin is a synthetic and nitrofuran antibacterial, which occurs as a bitter-tasting, lemon-yellow, crystalline powder with a pK_a of 7.2. It is very slightly soluble in water or alcohol.

Nitrofurantoin may also be known as furadoninum or nitrofurantoinum, *Furadantin*®, *Macrobid*®, and *Macrodantin*®.

Storage/Stability

Nitrofurantoin preparations should be stored in tight containers at room temperature and protected from light. The oral suspension should not be frozen. Nitrofurantoin will decompose if it comes into contact with metals other than aluminum or stainless steel.

Compatibility/Compounding Considerations

No specific information was noted.

Dosage Forms/Regulatory Status

VETERINARY-LABELED PRODUCTS: NONE

Nitrofurantoin use in food-producing animals is strictly prohibited.

HUMAN-LABELED PRODUCTS:

Nitrofurantoin Macrocrystalline Oral Capsules: 25 mg, 50 mg, and 100 mg; *Macrodantin*®, generic; (Rx)

Nitrofurantoin Monohydrate/Macrocrystals Oral Capsules: 100 mg; *Macrobid*®, generic; (Rx)

Nitrofurantoin Oral Suspension: 5 mg/mL (25 mg/5 mL) in 230 mL and 240 mL bottles; *Furadantin*®, generic; (Rx)

References

For the complete list of references, see **wiley.com/go/budde/plumb**

Nitroglycerin, Transdermal

(nye-troe-***gli***-ser-in) *NTG, Nitro-bid*®

Venodilator; Afterload Reducer

Prescriber Highlights

- Transdermal, oral, and injectable venodilator; occasionally used topically in veterinary medicine for congestive heart failure (CHF) or hypertension
- Continuous use results in tolerance after 48 to 72 hours.
- Contraindications include severe anemia and hypersensitivity.
- Use cautiously (if at all) in patients with cerebral hemorrhage, head trauma, diuretic-induced hypovolemia, or other hypotensive conditions.
- Adverse effects include rashes at the application sites; hypotension is possible. Transient headaches (common in humans); may be a problem for some animals.
- Rotate application sites.
- Wear gloves when applying; avoid human skin contact.

Uses/Indications

Transdermal nitroglycerin (NTG) in small animal medicine is used primarily as an adjunctive vasodilator in heart failure and cardiogenic edema. Because of questionable efficacy and rapid development of tolerance, topical nitroglycerin is not commonly used in veterinary medicine today. In humans, NTG is also used as an anti-anginal agent, antihypertensive (acute), and topically to treat Raynaud's disease.

For horses, topical nitroglycerin is ineffective in increasing digital blood flow in laminitis.[1,2]

Pharmacology/Actions

Nitroglycerin relaxes vascular smooth muscle primarily on the venous side, but a dose-related effect on arterioles is possible. Preload (left end-diastolic pressure) is reduced from the peripheral pooling of blood and decreased venous return to the heart. Because of its arteriolar effects, depending on the dose, afterload may also be reduced. Myocardial oxygen demand and workload are reduced, and coronary circulation can be improved.

Pharmacokinetics

Nitroglycerin transdermal ointment is absorbed through the skin, with an onset of action usually within 1 hour and duration of action of 2 to 12 hours. It is generally dosed in dogs and cats every 6 to 8 hours (3 to 4 times a day). The transdermal patches have a wide inter-patient bioavailability. Reportedly, the topical paste can be absorbed when rubbed on the gums of dogs and cats. Nitroglycerin has a very short half-life (1 to 4 minutes in humans) and is metabolized in the liver. At least 2 metabolites have some vasodilator activity and have longer half-lives than NTG.

Contraindications/Precautions/Warnings

Nitrates are contraindicated in patients with severe anemia or those hypersensitive to them. They should be used with caution (if at all) in patients with cerebral hemorrhage, head trauma, diuretic-induced hypovolemia, or other hypotensive conditions.

Continuous use (48 to 72 hours) of nitroglycerin results in the rapid development of tolerance to the effects of the drug.

Do not confuse nitroGLYCERIN with nitroPRUSSIDE or nitrofurantoin.

Adverse Effects

Most common adverse effect seen is a rash at the application site. If hypotension is a problem, reduce dosage. Transient headaches are a common adverse effect seen in humans and may be a problem for some animals.

Reproductive/Nursing Safety

No toxic effects were observed in pregnant rats or rabbits receiving doses up to 80 mg/kg/day and 240 mg/kg/day, respectively.[3] It is not known whether nitrates are excreted in maternal milk; use with caution in nursing animals.

Because safety has not been established in animals, this drug should only be used when the maternal benefits outweigh the potential risks to offspring.

Overdose/Acute Toxicity

If severe hypotension results after topical administration, wash the site of application to prevent any more absorption of ointment. Fluids may be administered if necessary. Epinephrine is contraindicated as it is ineffective and may complicate the animal's condition.

For patients that have experienced or are suspected to have experienced an overdose, consultation with a 24-hour poison consultation center specializing in providing veterinary-specific information is recommended. For general information related to overdose and toxin exposures, as well as contact information for poison control centers, refer to ***Appendix.***

Drug Interactions

The following drug interactions have either been reported or are theoretical in humans or animals receiving nitroglycerin and may be of significance in veterinary patients. Unless otherwise noted, use together is not necessarily contraindicated, but weigh the potential risks and perform additional monitoring when appropriate.

- **ACETYLCYSTEINE**: Concurrent use may result in enhanced hypotension.
- **ANTIHYPERTENSIVE DRUGS, OTHER** (eg, **amlodipine**, **enalapril**, **telmisartan**): Use of nitroglycerin with other antihypertensive drugs may cause additive hypotensive effects.
- **ASPIRIN**: Concurrent use may result in increased nitroglycerin

concentrations and additive platelet function depression.

- PHENOTHIAZINES (eg, **acepromazine**): May increase hypotensive effects
- SILDENAFIL (and other **PDE inhibitors**): May profoundly increase risk for hypotension. Concurrent use is contraindicated in humans.

Dosages

NOTE: Transdermal nitroglycerin is not used alone for the treatment of acute heart failure. It must be used with a loop diuretic (eg, furosemide). There is very limited evidence of efficacy of topical nitroglycerin in dogs and cats, but it is unlikely to cause harm.

DOGS/CATS:

Adjunctive treatment of acute heart failure using the transdermal ointment (*Nitro-bid®*) (extra-label): Dosed semi-quantitatively based on animal size. Cats: 1/8 – 1/4 inch; small dogs: 1/4 – 1/2 inch; medium dogs: 1/2 – 1 inch; large dogs: 1 – 2 inches every 6 to 12 hours for first 24 to 48 hours. Applied with a gloved finger to the inner ear pinna, groin, or axilla. Some clinicians have suggested that it can be applied to oral mucous membranes and is absorbed and tolerated well. Alternatively for dogs: 0.5 inch per 10 kg[4]

FERRETS:

Adjunctive therapy for heart failure (extra-label): 1/8 inch strip applied to inside of pinna every 12 hours for the first 24 hours of therapy[5]

Monitoring

- Clinical efficacy
- Sites of application for signs of rash
- Blood pressure, particularly if hypotensive effects are seen

Client Information

- Dosage is measured in inches of ointment; use papers supplied with product to measure appropriate dose.
- Wear gloves (nonpermeable) when applying the medicine.
- Do not pet animal where ointment has been applied.
- Rotate application sites. Recommended application sites include groin, inside the ears, and axilla (arm pits). Rub ointment into skin well. If rash develops, do not use on that site again until it has cleared. Sometimes, veterinarians will have you rub it onto the gums of your animal.
- Contact your veterinarian if rash persists or if your animal's condition deteriorates.
- There is no danger of explosion or fire with the use of this product.
- While your animal is taking this medication, it is important to return to your veterinarian for blood pressure checks. Do not miss these important follow-up visits.

Chemistry/Synonyms

Famous as an explosive, nitroglycerin (NTG) occurs undiluted as a thick, volatile, white-pale yellow flammable, explosive liquid with a sweet, burning taste. The undiluted drug is soluble in alcohol and slightly soluble in water. Because of obvious safety reasons, nitroglycerin is diluted with lactose, dextrose, propylene glycol, and so on when used for pharmaceutical purposes.

Nitroglycerin may also be known as glyceryl trinitrate, glonoine, GTN, nitroglycerol, NTG, trinitrin, or trinitroglycerin, *Nitro-bid®*, and *Nitro-Dur®*.

Storage/Stability

The topical ointment should be stored at room temperature and the cap firmly attached. For storage/stability and compatibility for dosage forms other than the topical ointment, see specialized references or the package inserts for each product.

Compatibility/Compounding Considerations

No specific information noted

Dosage Forms/Regulatory Status

VETERINARY-LABELED PRODUCTS: NONE

The Association of Racing Commissioners International (ARCI) has designated this drug as a class 2 substance. Use of this drug may not be allowed in certain animal competitions. Check rules and regulations before entering in a competition while this medication is being administered. Contact local racing authorities for further guidance. See ***Appendix*** for more information.

HUMAN-LABELED PRODUCTS:

NOTE: Many dosage forms of nitroglycerin are available for human use, including sublingual or buccal tablets and powders, lingual spray, extended-release oral capsules and tablets, and parenteral solutions for IV infusion. Because the use of nitroglycerin in small animal medicine has been limited to the use of topical ointment or transdermal patches, those other dosage forms are not listed here.

Nitroglycerin Topical Ointment: 2% in a lanolin-white petrolatum base in 30 gram and 60 gram tubes and 1 gram unit-dose foil packets; *Nitro-bid®*; (Rx)

Nitroglycerin Transdermal Systems (patches): 0.1 mg/hour, 0.2 mg/hour, 0.3 mg/hour, 0.4 mg/hour, 0.6 mg/hour, and 0.8 mg/hour; *Nitro-Dur®*, generic; (Rx) **NOTE**: Various products contain differing quantities of nitroglycerin and patch surface area size, but release rates of drug are identical for a given mg/hr.

References

For the complete list of references, see **wiley.com/go/budde/plumb**

Nitroprusside

(nye-troe-***pruss***-ide) *Nitropress®*

Vasodilator

Prescriber Highlights

- ► Vascular, smooth muscle relaxant used for acute/severe hypertension; acute heart failure secondary to mitral regurgitation and in combination with dobutamine for refractory congestive heart failure (CHF). Use only in an ICU setting; monitoring essential, including continuous measurement of direct or, less ideally, indirect arterial blood pressure.
- ► Drug of choice in animals under general anesthesia to treat severe hypertension caused by manipulation of pheochromocytomas.
- ► Contraindications include compensatory hypertension, inadequate cerebral circulation, or during emergency surgery in patients near death. Use caution in geriatric patients, hepatic insufficiency, severe renal impairment, hyponatremia, cobalamin deficiency, or hypothyroidism.
- ► Adverse effects include hypotensive effects; potentially: nausea, retching, restlessness, apprehension, muscle twitching, dizziness.
- ► Solution for infusion (but not the IV tubing) must be protected from light.
- ► Continued use at high dosages may lead to potential thiocyanate and cyanide toxicity.

Uses/Indications

Nitroprusside is used for adjunctive treatment of severe, acute heart failure, and hypertensive crisis when blood pressure must be reduced relatively rapidly. Its use in veterinary medicine is generally reserved for the treatment of critically ill patients only when constant blood pressure monitoring can be performed. In patients with dilated cardiomyopathy, administering dobutamine first to improve contractility and increase cardiac output can offset the hypotensive effects of sodium nitroprusside.[1] Due to its potency, rapid onset, and duration of action, it is considered the drug of choice in anesthetized animals undergoing adrenalectomy to treat acute and severe hypertension due to manipulation of pheochromocytomas.[2]

Pharmacology/Actions

Sodium nitroprusside provides intracellular nitric oxide, which activates guanylate cyclase. This effect produces an increase in intracellular cyclic-GMP, which inhibits vascular smooth muscle contraction. Nitroprusside is an immediate acting IV hypotensive agent that directly causes peripheral vasodilation (arterial and venous) independent of autonomic innervation. It produces a lowering of blood pressure, an increase in heart rate, a mild decrease in cardiac output, and a significant reduction in total peripheral resistance. Preload, afterload, and left ventricular end-diastolic pressures are reduced. Unlike the organic nitrates, tolerance does not develop to nitroprusside.

Pharmacokinetics

After starting an IV infusion of nitroprusside, reduction in blood pressure and other pharmacologic effects begin almost immediately. Blood pressure will return to pretreatment concentrations within 1 to 10 minutes following cessation of therapy.

Nitroprusside is metabolized nonenzymatically in the blood and tissues to cyanogen (cyanide radical). Cyanogen is converted in the liver to thiocyanate, then eliminated in the urine, feces, and exhaled air. The half-life of cyanogen is 2.7 to 7 days if renal function is normal, but prolonged in patients with impaired renal function or with hyponatremia.

Contraindications/Precautions/Warnings

Nitroprusside is contraindicated in patients with compensatory hypertension (eg, arteriovenous shunts or coarctation of the aorta; Cushing's reflex), inadequate cerebral circulation, or during emergency surgery in patients near death.

Nitroprusside must be used with caution in patients with hepatic insufficiency, severe renal impairment, hyponatremia, cobalamin deficiency, or hypothyroidism. When nitroprusside is used for controlled hypotension during surgery, patients may have less tolerance to hypovolemia, anemia, or blood loss. Geriatric patients may be more sensitive to the hypotensive effects of nitroprusside.

Do **NOT** flush IV line or severe hypotension can result secondary to acute overdose.

The FDA label (human use)[3] includes a black box warning that includes the following: *Nitroprusside is not suitable for direct injection. The solution must be further diluted in dextrose 5% injection before infusion. Nitroprusside can cause precipitous decreases in blood pressure. In patients not properly monitored, these decreases can lead to irreversible ischemic injuries or death. Use only when available equipment and personnel allow blood pressure to be continuously monitored. Except when used briefly or at low (less than 2 µg/kg/minute) infusion rates, nitroprusside injection gives rise to important quantities of cyanide ion, which can reach toxic and potentially lethal levels. The usual dose rate is 0.5 to 10 µg/kg/minute, but infusion at the maximum dose rates should never last more than 10 minutes. If blood pressure has not been adequately controlled after 10 minutes of infusion at the maximum rate, terminate administration immediately. Although acid-base balance and venous oxygen concentration should be monitored and may indicate cyanide toxicity, these laboratory tests provide imperfect guidance.*

Nitroprusside is considered a high alert medication (medications that require special safeguards to reduce the risk of errors). Consider instituting practices such as redundant drug dosage and volume checking, and special alert labels.

Do not confuse nitroPRUSSIDE with nitroGLYCERIN or nitroFURANTOIN.

Adverse Effects

Most adverse reactions from nitroprusside are associated with its hypotensive effects, particularly if blood pressure is reduced too rapidly. Clinical signs such as nausea, retching, restlessness, apprehension, muscle twitching, and dizziness have been reported in humans. These effects disappear when the infusion rate is reduced or stopped. Nitroprusside may be irritating at the infusion site; avoid extravasation.

Continued use may lead to potential thiocyanate and cyanide toxicity (see ***Overdose/Acute Toxicity*** section). Cats may be more susceptible to nitroprusside-induced oxidative damage; use minimum dosage required for efficacy.

Reproductive/Nursing Safety

Nitroprusside crosses the placenta, and fetal cyanide concentration is dose-related to maternal nitroprusside concentration, and lethal cyanide concentrations have been detected in fetal sheep.[3] It is not known whether nitroprusside and its metabolites are excreted in maternal milk.

Because safety has not been established in animals, this drug should only be used when the maternal benefits outweigh the potential risks to offspring.

Overdose/Acute Toxicity

Acute overdoses are characterized by profound hypotension, tachycardia, hyperventilation, metabolic acidosis, and seizures. Treat by reducing or stopping the infusion and giving IV fluids. Monitor blood pressure constantly.

Excessive doses, prolonged therapy, a depleted hepatic thiosulfate (sulfur) supply, or severe hepatic or renal insufficiency may lead to profound hypotension, and cyanogen or thiocyanate toxicity. Acid-base status should be monitored to evaluate therapy and to detect metabolic acidosis (early sign of cyanogen toxicity). Tolerance to therapy is also an early sign of nitroprusside toxicity. Hydroxocobalamin (vitamin B_{12a}) may prevent cyanogen toxicity and sodium thiosulfate may be used to treat cyanogen or thiocyanate toxicity. Thiocyanate toxicity may be exhibited as delirium in dogs. Serum thiocyanate concentration may need to be monitored in patients on prolonged therapy, especially in those patients with concurrent renal dysfunction. Serum thiocyanate concentration greater than 100 µg/mL are considered toxic.

For patients that have experienced or are suspected of having experienced an overdose, consultation with a 24-hour poison consultation center specializing in providing veterinary-specific information is recommended. For general information related to overdose and toxin exposures, as well as contact information for poison control centers, refer to ***Appendix.***

Drug Interactions

The following drug interactions have either been reported or are theoretical in humans or animals receiving nitroprusside and may be of significance in veterinary patients. Unless otherwise noted, use together is not necessarily contraindicated, but weigh the potential risks and perform additional monitoring when appropriate.

- **ANESTHETICS, INHALANT** (eg, **isoflurane**): Concurrent use may potentiate hypotensive effects.
- **DOBUTAMINE**: Synergistic effects (increased cardiac output and reduced wedge pressure) may result if dobutamine is used with nitroprusside.
- **HYPOTENSIVE AGENTS, OTHER** (eg, **amlodipine, enalapril, telmisartan**): Patients receiving other hypotensive agents may be more sensitive to the hypotensive effects of nitroprusside.

- **Negative Inotropic Agents** (eg, **propranolol, verapamil**): Concurrent use may potentiate hypotensive effects.
- **Phenothiazines** (eg, **acepromazine**): May increase hypotensive effects
- **Sildenafil**: Concurrent use may potentiate hypotensive effects. Combination is contraindicated in humans.

Dosages

NOTE: Must be diluted before use. See ***Compatibility/Compounding Considerations*** for information on preparing the infusion and protecting the solution from light.

DOGS/CATS:

Hypertensive crisis (systolic arterial blood pressure greater than 180 mm Hg with accompanying target organ damage) (extra-label): 0.5 – 3.5 µg/kg/minute IV CRI. Begin infusion at 0.5 µg/kg per minute[4] and titrate upwards every 5 minutes until target blood pressure is attained. Reduce blood pressure 25% over 4-hour period.

Adjunctive treatment of acute heart failure (cardiogenic shock; fulminant pulmonary edema; acute treatment for myxomatous mitral valve disease stage C and D) (extra-label): Initially, infuse 0.5 – 1 µg/kg/minute IV CRI. Titrate dosage upwards to effect in 0.5 – 1 µg/kg/minute increments every 10 to 30 minutes. Maximum CRI rate is 10 – 15 µg/kg/minute IV, although most animals are improved at 2 – 3 µg/kg/minute IV CRI. May use for 12 to 48 hours. Dobutamine can be used to treat or prevent hypotension if severe heart failure is confirmed by echocardiogram.[5,6]

Monitoring

- Blood pressure must be constantly monitored. Direct arterial blood pressure monitoring is recommended; however, if an arterial catheter cannot be placed (eg, smaller dogs and cats), continuous indirect blood pressures (eg, Doppler) can be used.
- Respiratory rate
- Acid-base balance and venous oxygen concentration, as acidemia and hypoxemia are early signs of cyanide toxicity
- Electrolytes (especially Na^+)

Client Information

- Must only be used by professionals in a setting where precise IV infusion and constant blood pressure monitoring can be performed.

Chemistry/Synonyms

A vascular smooth muscle relaxant, nitroprusside sodium occurs as practically odorless, reddish-brown crystals or powder. It is freely soluble in water and slightly soluble in alcohol. After reconstitution in D_5W, solution may have a brownish, straw, or light orange color and have a pH of 3.5 to 6.

Nitroprusside sodium may also be known as natrii nitroprussias, sodium nitroferricyanide dihydrate, sodium nitroprusside, SNP, or sodium nitroprussiate, and *Nitropress®*.

Storage/Stability

Nitroprusside sodium for injection should be stored protected from light and moisture and kept at room temperature (15°C-30°C [59°F-86°F)]. Nitroprusside solutions exposed to light will cause a reduction of the ferric ion to the ferrous ion with a resultant loss in potency and a change from a brownish color to a blue color. Degradation is enhanced with nitroprusside solutions in *Viaflex®* (Baxter) plastic bags exposed to fluorescent light. After dilution, protect immediately by covering infusion bag with aluminum foil or other opaque material. Discard solutions that turn to a blue, dark red, or green color. IV infusion tubing does not need to be protected from light while the infusion is running. It is not recommended to use IV infusion solutions other than 5% dextrose or to add any other medications to the infusion solution.

Compatibility/Compounding Considerations

Compatibility is dependent on factors such as pH, concentration, temperature, and diluent used; specialized references or a hospital pharmacist should be consulted for more specific information.

It is not recommended to use IV infusion solutions other than 5% dextrose or to add any other medications to the prepared infusion solution. However, nitroprusside is considered **compatible at Y-sites** with the following drugs: atracurium, dexmedetomidine, diltiazem, dopamine, enalaprilat, esmolol, furosemide, heparin, lidocaine, midazolam, morphine, norepinephrine, potassium chloride, propofol, and vecuronium. ***Dobutamine Y-site compatibility with nitroprusside is variable*** depending on drug concentration. Nitroprusside solutions with concentrations up to 1.2 mg/mL were compatible with dobutamine 12.5 mg/mL solutions for 48 hours in one study.[7]

Directions for preparation of infusion: Add 2 – 3 mL 5% dextrose to 50 mg vial to dissolve powder. Add dissolved solution to 1000 mL of 5% dextrose and promptly protect solution from light (using aluminum foil or other opaque covering). Resultant solution contains 50 µg/mL of nitroprusside. Different concentrations may be necessary for precise administration and/or restricting IV fluids. The administration set (IV line) does not need to be protected from light. Solution may have a slight brownish tint, but discard solutions that turn to a blue, dark red or green color. Solution is stable for 24 hours after reconstitution. Do not add any other medications to IV running nitroprusside. Avoid extravasation at IV site. Use an accurate flow control device (infusion pump, controller) for administration. If a mini-drip IV set must be used: 60 drops ≈1 mL; 1 drop contains ≈0.83 µg of nitroprusside.

Dosage Forms/Regulatory Status

VETERINARY-LABELED PRODUCTS: NONE

HUMAN-LABELED PRODUCTS:

Nitroprusside Sodium for Injection: 25 mg/mL in 2 mL single-dose vials; *Nitropress®*, generic; (Rx)

Nitroprusside Sodium Injection in 0.9% Sodium Chloride: 0.2 mg/mL in 50 mL and 100 mL vials, and 0.5 mg/mL in 100 mL vials; *Nipride® RTU*; (Rx)

References

For the complete list of references, see **wiley.com/go/budde/plumb**

Nizatidine

(ni-***za***-ti-dine) *Axid®*

H_2-Receptor Antagonist; Prokinetic

Prescriber Highlights

- H_2-receptor antagonist similar to ranitidine; reduces gastric acid and has prokinetic activity
- Use with caution in geriatric patients and those with hepatic or renal insufficiency.
- Adverse effects are rare.

Uses/Indications

Although nizatidine acts similarly to cimetidine and ranitidine as an H_2 blocker to reduce gastric acid secretion in the stomach,[1,2] in small animal medicine its use has been primarily for its prokinetic effects. It may be useful to treat delayed gastric emptying, pseudo-obstruction of the intestine, and constipation.[3]

Pharmacology/Actions

At the H_2 receptors of the parietal cells, nizatidine competitively inhibits histamine, thereby reducing gastric acid output both during basal conditions and when stimulated by food, amino acids, pentagastrin, histamine, or insulin.

Nizatidine stimulates gastric emptying and intestinal motility by inhibiting acetylcholinesterase (thereby increasing acetylcholine at muscarinic receptors).[1,4-6] It may also have direct agonist effects on M3 muscarinic receptors. Lower esophageal sphincter pressures may be increased by nizatidine. By decreasing the amount of gastric juice produced, nizatidine decreases the amount of pepsin secreted.

Pharmacokinetics

In dogs, oral absorption is rapid and nearly complete with minimal first pass effect.[7] Food can enhance the absorption of nizatidine, but this is not considered clinically important. The drug is only marginally bound to plasma proteins. It is unknown if it enters the CNS. Nizatidine is metabolized in the liver to several metabolites, including at least one that has some activity.[7] Elimination half-life is 1 to 2 hours.[2] In animals with normal renal function over half the drug is excreted in the urine unchanged.

Contraindications/Precautions/Warnings

Nizatidine is contraindicated in patients who are hypersensitive to it. It should be used cautiously and, possibly, at reduced dosage in patients with diminished renal function. Nizatidine has caused increased serum ALT levels in humans receiving high IV doses for longer than 5 days. The manufacturer recommends that with high dose, chronic therapy, serum ALT values be monitored.

Do not confuse niZATidine with niTAZOXanide.

Adverse Effects

Nizatidine was reportedly well tolerated in animal studies.[2]

In humans, nizatidine appears to be well tolerated. Rarely, anemia has been reported. CNS effects have been noted (headache, dizziness) but incidence is similar to those taking placebo. Rash and pruritus have also been reported in a few humans taking nizatidine.

Reproductive/Nursing Safety

Doses of nizatidine up to 275 mg/kg per day in pregnant rabbits did not reveal any teratogenic or fetotoxic effects. Nizatidine is excreted in maternal milk in a concentration of 0.1% of the oral dose in proportion to plasma concentrations.

Because safety has not been established in animals, this drug should only be used when the maternal benefits outweigh the potential risks to offspring.

Overdose/Acute Toxicity

Single nizatidine doses of 75 mg/kg IV and single or daily (up to 3 months) doses of 800 mg/kg PO were not lethal in dogs.[8] Adverse effects could include cholinergic effects (lacrimation, salivation, emesis, miosis and diarrhea); suggest treating supportively based on clinical presentation.

For patients that have experienced or are suspected of having experienced an overdose, consultation with a 24-hour poison consultation center specializing in providing veterinary-specific information is recommended. For general information related to overdose and toxin exposures, as well as contact information for poison control centers, refer to ***Appendix***.

Drug Interactions

The following drug interactions have either been reported or are theoretical in humans or animals receiving nizatidine and may be of significance in veterinary patients. Unless otherwise noted, use together is not necessarily contraindicated, but weigh the potential risks and perform additional monitoring when appropriate.

- ANTICHOLINERGIC AGENTS (eg, **atropine, propantheline**): May negate the prokinetic effects of nizatidine
- ANTACIDS, ALUMINUM-, CALCIUM- OR MAGNESIUM-CONTAINING (high doses): May decrease the absorption of nizatidine; give at separate times (2 hours apart) if used concurrently.
- ANTIHISTAMINES, FIRST GENERATION (eg, **diphenhydramine, meclizine**): Anticholinergic effects may negate the prokinetic effects of nizatidine.
- AZOLE ANTIFUNGALS (eg, **ketoconazole, itraconazole**): By raising gastric pH, nizatidine may decrease the absorption of these agents; if both drugs are required, administer the azole antifungal one hour prior to nizatidine.
- CEFPODOXIME, CEFUROXIME: Nizatidine may decrease the absorption of these cephalosporins; giving with food may alleviate this effect.
- IRON SALTS (**oral**): Nizatidine may decrease the absorption of oral iron; administer iron at least one hour prior to nizatidine.
- PHENOTHIAZINES (eg, **acepromazine**): Anticholinergic effects may negate the prokinetic effects of nizatidine.
- SALICYLATES (eg, **aspirin, bismuth subsalicylate**): Nizatidine may increase salicylate concentrations in patients receiving high salicylate doses.
- TRICYCLIC ANTIDEPRESSANTS (TCAs; eg, **amitriptyline, clomipramine**): Anticholinergic effects may negate the prokinetic effects of nizatidine.

Laboratory Considerations

- False positive tests for **urobilinogen** may occur with patients receiving nizatidine.

Dosages

DOGS/CATS:

Prokinetic agent, reduce gastric acid production (extra-label): 2.5 – 5 mg/kg PO once daily[3,9]

Monitoring

- Clinical efficacy (dependent on reason for use) monitored by decrease in clinical signs, endoscopic examination, and blood in feces.

Client Information

- This medicine is used to treat or prevent stomach ulcers or to stimulate the movement of food through the stomach and intestines.
- If this medicine is given once each day, it works best if given before the first meal of the day.
- Nizatidine is available over the counter (OTC), without a prescription, but only give it to your animal if your veterinarian recommends it.

Chemistry/Synonyms

Nizatidine occurs as an off-white to buff-colored crystalline powder. It has a bitter taste and a slight sulfur-like odor. Nizatidine is sparingly soluble in water.

Nizatidine may also be known as LY-139037, nizatidinum, and *Axid®*.

Storage/Stability

Nizatidine products should be stored in tight, light-resistant containers at room temperature (20°C-25°C [68°F-77°F]); for the oral solution, excursions permitted between 15°C to 30°C (59°F-86°F).

Compatibility/Compounding Considerations

No specific information noted

Dosage Forms/Regulatory Status

VETERINARY-LABELED PRODUCTS: NONE

The Association of Racing Commissioners International (ARCI) has designated this drug as a class 5 substance. Use of this drug may not be allowed in certain animal competitions. Check rules and regulations before entering a competition while this medication is being administered. Contact local racing authorities for further guidance.

See *Appendix* for more information.

HUMAN-LABELED PRODUCTS:
Nizatidine Tablets: 75 mg; *Axid® AR;* (OTC)

Nizatidine Capsules: 150 mg & 300 mg; *Axid®*, generic; (Rx)

Nizatidine Oral Solution: 15 mg/mL in 480 mL; *Axid®*, generic; (Rx) Peppermint flavor

References

For the complete list of references, see **wiley.com/go/budde/plumb**

Norepinephrine

Noradrenaline

(nor-eh-pih-***nef***-rin) *Levophed®*

Alpha- and Beta- Adrenergic Pressor Agent

Prescriber Highlights

- ▶ Vasopressor agent for persistent, profound shock (after fluid deficits replaced)
- ▶ Specifically indicated for hypotension associated with septic shock; may also be useful for isoflurane-induced hypotension
- ▶ Administration requires IV constant rate infusion (CRI) and continuous monitoring.
- ▶ Extravasation injuries possible
- ▶ Norepinephrine is considered a high alert medication (medication that requires special safeguards to reduce the risk for errors). Consider instituting practices such as redundant drug dosage and volume checks and special alert labels.

Uses/Indications

Norepinephrine (NE) is a direct-acting sympathomimetic vasopressor and cardiac inotrope used for treatment of profound hypotension in small and large animal species. NE is the first choice vasopressor for septic shock in volume-replete animals, and it can be used to raise blood pressure and as a cardiac stimulant in these patients.[1] In humans, NE is a first-line agent for hypotension associated with post-resuscitation shock[2,3]; these established guidelines have been extrapolated into use for dogs and cats although further research is warranted.[1,4] NE has been shown to correct hypotension secondary to isoflurane anesthesia in a variety of species. In humans, NE may also be useful when administered intragastrically or intraperitoneally for treatment of upper GI bleeding.[5,6]

Pharmacology/Actions

Norepinephrine (NE) is a strong alpha-1- and alpha-2-adrenergic receptor agonist, and a moderate beta-1 agonist.

NE acts as a peripheral vasoconstrictor (alpha-adrenergic), inotropic cardiostimulant, and coronary artery dilator (beta-adrenergic). Total peripheral resistance is increased, resulting in increased systolic and diastolic blood pressure. Perfusion to vital organs, skin, and skeletal muscle can be reduced, especially at higher dosages.

Pharmacokinetics

When administered IV, norepinephrine's (NE) onset of action occurs within 1 to 2 minutes and persists for an additional 1 to 2 minutes. Due to its vasoconstrictive effects, it can cause tissue damage and is poorly absorbed when given SC. After oral administration, NE is destroyed in the GI tract and not absorbed. After uptake by sympathetic nerve endings, it is rapidly metabolized via catechol-*O*-methyltransferase (COMT) and monoamine oxidase (MAO) to inactive metabolites.

Contraindications/Precautions/Warnings

In life-threatening situations, there are no absolute contraindications to norepinephrine (NE) use. Vasopressors are not a substitute for adequate blood, fluid, or electrolyte replacement. NE should not be given to patients that are hypotensive from hypovolemia,[7] except as an emergency measure to maintain coronary and cerebral artery perfusion until volume replacement therapy can be completed. If used in the absence of volume replacement, severe peripheral and visceral vasoconstriction, decreased renal perfusion and urine output, and poor systemic blood flow can occur despite normal blood pressures.[7] NE should not be used if severe peripheral vasoconstriction exists because it may be ineffective and may cause further reductions in blood flow to vital organs. Because it increases myocardial oxygen demand, risks for use during cardiac events (eg, arrhythmias) may outweigh the drug's benefits.

NE is a drug used in the critical care setting. Animals must be observed and infusion rates titrated. See ***Monitoring***. Avoid abrupt withdrawal of the infusion.[7]

In humans, it is recommended that NE be administered through a central venous catheter, if possible, to minimize risks for tissue ischemia from extravasation that can occur with a peripheral catheter. If a peripheral catheter must be used, it should be placed in a large vein[7] with the largest gauge catheter possible, and a slow infusion rate is advised. NE should not be used in patients with pre-existing vascular thrombosis, as this may increase ischemia.[7]

Do **NOT** confuse NOR-EPInephrine with EPInephrine. NE is considered a high alert medication (medication that requires special safeguards to reduce the risk for errors).[8] Consider instituting practices such as redundant drug dosage and volume checking and special alert labels.

Adverse Effects

If used in the absence of blood volume replacement, the following may occur: severe peripheral and visceral vasoconstriction, decreased renal perfusion and urine output, and poor systemic blood flow despite normal blood pressures.[7] Higher doses can cause arrhythmias.[7] Cats may be more susceptible to these adverse effects. In humans, reported adverse effects for norepinephrine (NE) include headache, weakness, dizziness, anxiety, pallor, respiratory difficulty, and pulmonary edema.[7]

The human label has a black box warning regarding extravasation injuries from NE.[7] To prevent sloughing and necrosis in areas where extravasation has taken place, the area should be infiltrated as soon as possible with 10 – 15 mL 0.9% sodium chloride solution containing 5 to 10 mg of phentolamine,[7] an adrenergic-receptor blocking agent (this product may need to be obtained from a human hospital pharmacy). A syringe with a fine hypodermic needle should be used to administer the saline solution, with the solution being infiltrated liberally throughout the area, which is easily identified by its cold, hard, and pallid appearance. Sympathetic blockade with phentolamine causes immediate and conspicuous local hyperemic changes if the area is infiltrated within 12 hours. Therefore, phentolamine should be given as soon as possible after the extravasation is noted.

Reproductive/Nursing Safety

Placental blood flow was diminished in pregnant sheep receiving high dose norepinephrine (NE) (40 µg/minute [NOT µg/kg/minute] IV).[7] It is not known if NE enters maternal milk.

Because safety has not been established in animals, this drug should only be used when the maternal benefits outweigh the potential risks to offspring.

Overdose/Acute Toxicity

Overdose with norepinephrine (NE) can result in severe hypertension, arrhythmias, reflex bradycardia, cardiac ischemia, increase in peripheral resistance with resulting decreased perfusion to vital organs, digital or other satellite tissue necrosis, and decreased cardiac output. If any of these signs occur, discontinue administration of the drug. Immediate toxic effects from NE should resolve within 1 to 2 minutes, but ischemic lesions may not become evident for hours to days later. Propranolol may be used to treat NE-induced cardiac arrhythmias.

For patients that have experienced or are suspected to have experienced an overdose, consultation with a 24-hour poison consultation center specializing in providing veterinary-specific information is recommended. For general information related to overdose and toxin exposures, as well as contact information for poison control centers, refer to ***Appendix.***

Drug Interactions

The following drug interactions have either been reported or are theoretical in humans or animals receiving norepinephrine (NE) and may be of significance in veterinary patients. Unless otherwise noted, use together is not necessarily contraindicated, but weigh the potential risks and perform additional monitoring when appropriate.

- **ALPHA-2-ADRENERGIC AGONISTS** (eg, **detomidine, dexmedetomidine, medetomidine, xylazine**): NE possesses alpha-agonist effects; thus, it should **NOT** be used to treat cardiac effects caused by alpha-2-adrenergic agonists.
- **ALPHA-ADRENERGIC ANTAGONISTS** (eg, **phenoxybenzamine, phentolamine, prazosin**): May reverse the pressor effects of NE due to alpha-1 blockade
- **ANTIHISTAMINES**: Certain antihistamines (eg, **chlorpheniramine, diphenhydramine**) may potentiate the effects of NE.
- **ATROPINE**: May block the reflex bradycardia caused by NE and enhance the pressor response
- **BETA-ADRENERGIC ANTAGONISTS** (eg, **atenolol, esmolol, propranolol**): May result in higher blood pressures secondary to antagonizing beta-2 receptors to cause arteriole dilation. Can antagonize cardiac stimulating effects; propranolol may be used to treat NE-induced cardiac arrhythmias.
- **DIGOXIN**: Increased risk for arrhythmias
- **DIURETICS** (eg, **furosemide**): May decrease arterial responsiveness to NE
- **MONOAMINE OXIDASE INHIBITORS** (MAOIs; eg, **amitraz, linezolid, selegiline**): Hypertension can result.
- **NITRATES** (eg, **nitroglycerin**): May reverse the pressor effects of NE
- **OXYTOCIN**: Hypertension may result if NE is used with oxytocic agents.
- **PHENOTHIAZINES** (eg, **acepromazine**): May reverse the pressor effects of NE due to alpha-1 blockade
- **TRICYCLIC ANTIDEPRESSANTS** (eg, **amitriptyline, clomipramine**): Hypertension, cardiac arrhythmias, and tachycardia can result.

Laboratory Considerations

None noted

Dosages

NOTE: Dosages and drug concentrations are listed as norepinephrine base; injectable product concentration is labeled as norepinephrine base.

DOGS/CATS:

Persistent, profound hypotension after adequate fluid volume replacement (extra-label): Initial dosage: 0.05 – 0.1 µg/kg per <u>minute</u> IV CRI then titrated up to desired effect[9,10]; most recommend a maximum rate of 1 – 2 µg/kg/<u>minute</u> IV CRI. Can be used in combination with dopamine, dobutamine, or vasopressin.

Isoflurane-induced hypotension (extra-label): In a study comparing 12 healthy beagles, the average effective dose was 0.44 µg/kg/<u>minute</u> IV CRI.[11] Dosages ranged from 0.1 – 2 µg/kg per <u>minute</u> IV CRI.

HORSES:

Hypotension in critically ill foals (extra-label): Initial dosage: 0.1 µg/kg/<u>minute</u> IV CRI then titrated up to desired effect.[10] Upper end of dosage range is ≈1.5 µg/kg/<u>minute</u> IV CRI.[12] Use with dobutamine could be considered.[13]

Isoflurane-induced hypotension (extra-label):

a) **Neonatal foals**: 0.3 – 1 µg/kg/<u>minute</u> IV CRI. Norepinephrine improved cardiac index and O_2 delivery; high dosage significantly increased blood pressure.[14]

b) **Adult horses**: 0.1 – 0.5 µg/kg/<u>minute</u> IV CRI[15]

Acepromazine-induced hypotension (extra-label): The hypotensive effect of acepromazine in the awake horse was treated by a norepinephrine infusion of 1 µg/kg/<u>minute</u> IV CRI for 15 minutes. When these horses received the norepinephrine infusion without prior acepromazine, second degree AV block developed.[16]

ALPACAS:

Isoflurane-induced hypotension (extra-label): 0.3 – 1 µg/kg per <u>minute</u> IV CRI. It is recommended to titrate the dose starting at the lowest dose to avoid excessive vasoconstriction.[17]

SHEEP:

Hypotension after adequate fluid volume replacement during septic shock (extra-label): 0.4 – 1 µg/kg/<u>minute</u> IV CRI has been safely used in experimentally induced sepsis in sheep.[12,18] Norepinephrine in combination with dobutamine may be more effective than norepinephrine alone.[19]

Monitoring

Norepinephrine is a drug used in the intensive care unit (ICU) for critical patients. Animals must be observed, and dosage rates titrated. Avoid abrupt withdrawal of the infusion.

- Blood pressure. Preferably including central venous pressure or pulmonary arterial diastolic pressure; maintain mean arterial pressure at more than 65 mm Hg
- Continuous ECG
- Urine output

Client Information

- Must only be used by veterinary professionals in a hospital critical care setting.

Chemistry/Synonyms

Norepinephrine bitartrate (noradrenaline acid tartrate) occurs as a white or grey-white, odorless, crystalline powder that slowly darkens on exposure to air and light. One part is soluble in 2.5 parts water. Solutions in water have a pH of ≈3.5. The bitartrate injection contains sulfites.

Norepinephrine may also be known as levarterenol, noradrenaline, or L-arterenol. A commonly known trade name is *Levophed®*.

Storage/Stability

Store at room temperature (25°C [77°F]). Excursions are permitted to 15°C to 30°C (59°F-86°F). Protect from light.

Compatibility/Compounding Considerations

Compatibility is dependent on factors such as pH, concentration, temperature, and diluent used; consult specialized references or a hospital pharmacist for more specific information.

The following drugs are listed as **compatible** with norepinephrine infusions: amikacin sulfate, calcium chloride/gluconate, ciprofloxacin, dimenhydrinate, dobutamine HCl, heparin sodium, hydrocortisone sodium succinate, magnesium sulfate, meropenem, methylprednisolone sodium succinate, multivitamins, potassium chloride, succinylcholine chloride, and verapamil HCl.

Avoid contact with iron salts, alkalis, or oxidizing agents. Norepinephrine is **incompatible** with aminophylline, sodium bicarbonate, ranitidine, or pantoprazole. Administer whole blood or plasma separately (via a Ytube and individual containers if given simultaneously).

Dilute norepinephrine in dextrose 5% or dextrose 5% with 0.9% sodium chloride. Administration in 0.9% sodium chloride alone is not recommended as significant loss of potency can occur due to oxidation. Dextrose-containing fluids can help prevent oxidation. A 4 mL vial (4 mg) is added to a 250 mL, 500 mL, or 1 L bag of a dextrose 5%-containing IV solution. Each mL of this dilution then contains either 16 µg/mL (250 mL bag), 8 µg/mL (500 mL bag), or 4 µg/mL (1 L bag) of norepinephrine bitartrate base. Do not use if solution color is pinkish, darker than slightly yellow, or if it contains a precipitate.

Dosage Forms/Regulatory Status

VETERINARY-LABELED PRODUCTS: NONE

The Association of Racing Commissioners International (ARCI) has designated norepinephrine as a class 2 substance. Use of this drug may not be allowed in certain animal competitions. Check rules and regulations before entering in a competition while this medication is being administered. Contact local racing authorities for further guidance. See the ***Appendix*** for more information.

HUMAN-LABELED PRODUCTS:

Norepinephrine bitartrate for injection (must be diluted before use): 1 mg/mL in 4 mL vials; *Levophed*®, generic; (Rx). Concentrations are listed as norepinephrine base.

References

For the complete list of references, see **wiley.com/go/budde/plumb**

Novobiocin

(noe-ve-***bye***-oh-sin) *Albadry Plus*®

Antibiotic

Prescriber Highlights

- ► Used as an intramammary treatment of subclinical mastitis in dry cows caused by susceptible strains of *Staphylococcus aureus* and *Streptococcus agalactiae*
- ► Primarily effective against some gram-positive cocci but is uncommonly used clinically
- ► Oral formulations no longer available

Uses/Indications

Novobiocin is FDA-approved in combination with penicillin G for use in dry dairy cattle for the treatment of subclinical mastitis caused by susceptible strains of *Staphylococcus aureus* and *Streptococcus agalactiae*.

The Office International des Epizooties (OIE) has designated novobiocin as a Veterinary Important Antimicrobial (VIA) Agent in veterinary species.[1]

Pharmacology/Actions

Novobiocin is believed to act in a bactericidal manner. It inhibits bacterial DNA gyrase, interfering with protein and nucleic acid synthesis, and also interferes with bacterial cell wall synthesis. Activity of the drug is enhanced in an alkaline medium.

The spectrum of activity of novobiocin includes some gram-positive cocci (staphylococci, *Streptococcus pneumoniae,* and some group A streptococci). Novobiocin resistance is not associated with methicillin resistance and some methicillin-resistant staphylococci are susceptible.[2] Activity is variable against other streptococci and weak against the enterococci. Most gram-negative organisms are resistant to the drug, but some *Haemophilus* spp, *Neisseria* spp, and *Proteus* spp may be susceptible.

Pharmacokinetics

After oral administration, novobiocin is well absorbed from the GI tract. Peak concentrations occur within 1 to 4 hours. The presence of food can decrease peak concentrations of the drug.

Novobiocin is only poorly distributed to body fluids with concentrations in synovial, pleural, and ascitic fluids less than those found in plasma. Only minimal quantities of the drug cross the blood-brain barrier, even when meninges are inflamed. Highest concentrations of novobiocin are found in the small intestine and liver. The drug is ≈90% protein bound and is distributed into milk.

Novobiocin is primarily eliminated in the bile and feces. Approximately 3% is excreted into the urine; urine concentrations are usually less than those found in serum.

Contraindications/Precautions/Warnings

Novobiocin is contraindicated in patients hypersensitive to it. Additionally, systemic use of the drug should be undertaken with extreme caution in patients with preexisting hepatic or hematopoietic dysfunction.

Adverse Effects

Adverse effects reported with the systemic use of this drug include fever, GI disturbances (eg, nausea, vomiting, diarrhea), rashes, and blood dyscrasias. In humans, occurrences of hypersensitivity reactions, hepatotoxicity, and blood dyscrasias have significantly limited the use of this drug. A novobiocin degradation product may cause a yellow skin discoloration.

Reproductive/Nursing Safety

Intramammary novobiocin infusions are safe to administer to pregnant cattle when used as a dry cow treatment; however, they are not intended for use in lactating cows.

Overdose/Acute Toxicity

Little information is available regarding overdoses of novobiocin. It is suggested that large oral overdoses be handled by emptying the gut following standard protocols; monitor and treat adverse effects symptomatically if necessary.

For patients that have experienced or are suspected of having experienced an overdose, consultation with a 24-hour poison consultation center specializing in providing veterinary-specific information is recommended. For general information related to overdose and toxin exposures, as well as contact information for poison control centers, refer to ***Appendix.***

Drug Interactions

The following drug interactions have either been reported or are theoretical in humans or animals receiving novobiocin and may be of significance in veterinary patients. Unless otherwise noted, use together is not necessarily contraindicated, but weigh the potential risks and perform additional monitoring when appropriate.

- Beta-Lactam Antibiotics: Novobiocin may block the renal tubular transport of drugs (similar to probenecid). Although the clinical significance of this action is unclear, the elimination rates of drugs excreted in this manner (eg, **cephalosporins, penicillins**) could be decreased and half-lives prolonged.

Laboratory Considerations

- Novobiocin can be metabolized into a yellow-colored product that can interfere with **serum bilirubin** determinations.
- Novobiocin may interfere with the determination of **BSP** (bromosulfophthalein, sulfobromophthalein) uptake tests by altering BSP uptake or biliary excretion.

Dosages

CATTLE:

Subclinical mastitis in dry cows (label dosage; FDA-approved): Infuse the entire contents of one syringe into each quarter at the time of drying off, but not less than 30 days prior to calving.[3] Warm to body temperature and shake well before using.

Monitoring

- Clinical efficacy
- Adverse effects

Client Information

- Be sure you understand how to give this medicine to your cow. Shake the medicine tubes well before placing into each quarter.
- Only give this medicine as directed by your veterinarian. Do not give more medicine or treat for longer than is recommended by your veterinarian.

Chemistry/Synonyms

An antibiotic obtained from *Streptomyces niveus* (*S spheroids*), novobiocin sodium occurs as white to light yellow, crystalline powder and is very soluble in water.

Novobiocin or novobiocin sodium may also be known as crystallinic acid, PA-93, streptonivicin, U-6591, novobiocinum natricum, sodium novobiocin, *Albadry Plus*®, *Albamycin*®, *Biodry*®, and *Delta Albaplex*®.

Storage/Stability

Novobiocin should be stored at room temperature, 20°C to 25°C (68°F-77°F).

Compatibility/Compounding Considerations

No specific information noted

Dosage Forms/Regulatory Status

VETERINARY-LABELED PRODUCTS:

Novobiocin Combination Products:

Novobiocin sodium 400 mg and Penicillin G Procaine 200,000 units per 10 mL *Plastet*® Syringe; *Albadry Plus*®; (OTC). FDA-approved for use in dry cows only. Do not use 30 days prior to calving. Milk must not be used for food for 72 hours after calving. Slaughter withdrawal at label dosages is 30 days.

Historically, novobiocins have been available as single-agent intramammary infusions for lactating and dry cows, and in combination with tetracycline with or without prednisolone for oral use in dogs. These products are still listed in FDA's Green Book but are no longer marketed in the United States.

HUMAN-LABELED PRODUCTS: NONE

References

For the complete list of references, see **wiley.com/go/budde/plumb**

Nystatin

(nye-***stat***-in)

Antifungal

See also ***Nystatin/Nystatin Combinations, Topical***

Prescriber Highlights

- ▶ Oral antifungal used for treatment of oral and GI *Candida* spp infections
- ▶ Do not use for treatment of systemic infections, as nystatin is not absorbed systemically after PO administration.
- ▶ Adverse effects include GI signs at high doses or hypersensitivity.
- ▶ Dosed in units; calculate doses carefully.

Uses/Indications

Orally administered nystatin is used primarily for the treatment of oral or GI *Candida* spp infections or overgrowth in dogs, cats, and birds. It has been used less commonly in other species for the same indications.

Pharmacology/Actions

Nystatin is a polyene antifungal and has a mechanism of action similar to that of amphotericin B. It binds to sterols in the membrane of the fungal cell, altering the permeability of the membrane and thus allowing intracellular potassium and other cellular constituents to leak out. Nystatin must come into contact with the target organism to be effective.

Nystatin is fungistatic and fungicidal against yeasts and yeast-like fungi, particularly *Candida* spp.[1] It has no activity against bacteria, protozoa, or viruses.

Pharmacokinetics

Nystatin is not measurably absorbed after oral administration and is almost entirely excreted unchanged in the feces. The drug is not used parenterally because it is reportedly extremely toxic to internal tissues.

Contraindications/Precautions/Warnings

Nystatin is contraindicated in patients with known hypersensitivity to it. Do not use for treatment of systemic mycoses.[1]

Do not confuse nystatin with HMG-CoA reductase inhibitors (ie, statin drugs such as simvastatin).

Adverse Effects

Occasionally, high dosages of nystatin may cause oral irritation or GI upset (anorexia, vomiting, diarrhea). Hypersensitivity reactions have rarely been reported in humans.

Reproductive/Nursing Safety

Effects of nystatin on fertility have not been studied. Although the safety of the drug during pregnancy has not been firmly established, the lack of appreciable absorption appears to make it safe to use.

It is not known whether nystatin is excreted in maternal milk; however, milk concentrations are likely insignificant due to its lack of systemic absorption.

Because safety has not been established in animals, this drug should only be used when the maternal benefits outweigh the potential risks to offspring.

Overdose/Acute Toxicity

Because the drug is not absorbed after oral administration, acute toxicity after an oral overdose is extremely unlikely, but transient GI distress may result.

For patients that have experienced or are suspected to have experienced an overdose, consultation with a 24-hour poison consultation center specializing in providing veterinary-specific information is recommended. For general information related to overdose and toxin exposures, as well as contact information for poison control centers, refer to ***Appendix.***

Drug Interactions

- No significant interactions reported for oral nystatin

Laboratory Considerations

- No significant laboratory considerations noted

Dosages

DOGS/CATS:

Oral candidiasis (extra-label): Dosages are not well established. Anecdotal dosages of nystatin range from 100,000 – 150,000 units/dog or units/cat (NOT units/kg) PO 3 to 4 times daily.

HORSES:

Intrauterine infusion for *Candida* spp overgrowth (extra-label): 250,000 – 1,000,000 units mixed with sterile water; precipitates in saline. Limited evidence is available for a recommended dose, volume infused, frequency, or diluent. Most intrauterine treatments are performed every day or every other day for 3 to 7 days.[2]

BIRDS:

Enteric yeast (*Candida* spp) infections (extra-label):

a) 200,000 – 300,000 units/kg PO every 8 to 12 hours. **NOTE**: Oral lesions may be missed if bird is tubed.[3]

b) **Neonates on antibiotic therapy**: Crush one fluconazole 100 mg tablet and mix with 20 mL of nystatin 100,000 units/mL oral suspension. Then dose the solution at 0.5 mL/kg (2.2 lb) of body weight PO twice daily for duration of antibiotic therapy.[4]

c) **Candidiasis after antibiotic or in conjunction with antibiotics**: Using the nystatin 100,000 units/mL suspension, 1 mL/300 grams (0.66 lb) body weight PO 1 to 3 times daily for 7 to 14 days. If treating mouth lesions, do not give by gavage. Hand-fed baby birds should receive antifungal therapy if being treated with antibiotics.[5]

REPTILES:

Candidiasis (extra-label):

a) **Turtles with enteric yeast infections**: 100,000 units/kg PO once daily for 10 days[6]

b) **All reptiles**: 100,000 units/kg PO once daily[7]

Monitoring

- Clinical efficacy

Client Information

- Shake suspension well before administering

Chemistry/Synonyms

A polyene antifungal antibiotic produced by *Streptomyces noursei*, nystatin occurs as a yellow to light tan, hygroscopic powder having a cereal-like odor. It is very slightly soluble in water and slightly to sparingly soluble in alcohol. One mg of nystatin contains not less than 4400 units of activity. According to the USP, nystatin used in the preparation of oral suspensions should not contain less than 5000 units per mg.

Nystatin may also be known as fungicidin, nistatina, nystatinum, *Mycostatin*®, and *Nilstat*®.

Storage/Stability

Nystatin tablets and oral suspension should be stored at room temperature (15°C-30°C [59°F-86°F]) in airtight, light-resistant containers. Avoid freezing the oral suspension or exposing to temperatures above 40°C (104°F).

Nystatin deteriorates when exposed to heat, light, air, or moisture.

Compatibility/Compounding Considerations

No specific information noted

Dosage Forms/Regulatory Status

VETERINARY-LABELED PRODUCTS:

None for oral use

HUMAN-LABELED PRODUCTS:

Nystatin Oral Suspension: 100,000 units/mL in 5 mL, 60 mL, 473 mL, and 480 mL; generic; (Rx)

Nystatin Oral Tablets: 500,000 units; generic; (Rx)

Also available in topical creams, powders, and ointments

References

For the complete list of references, see **wiley.com/go/budde/plumb**

Oclacitinib

(***ok***-la-***sit***-ih-nib) *Apoquel*®

Janus Kinase (JAK) Inhibitor, Antipruritic, Anti-Inflammatory

Prescriber Highlights

- FDA-approved for treating allergic skin diseases in dogs
- Studies have demonstrated short-term effectiveness and safety in cats with feline atopic skin syndrome. Pruritus relief in dogs starts within 4 hours of administration of the first dose, with significant itch relief by 24 hours.
- Oclacitinib may increase susceptibility to infections. Avoid use in dogs with serious infection, and use with caution in dogs with history of recurrent infection.
- Patients should be monitored for the development of any new (or exacerbations of existing) neoplastic conditions, including cutaneous or subcutaneous masses.
- Extra-label use may be considered in cats, but safety data are limited.

Uses/Indications

Oclacitinib is FDA-approved in dogs at least 12 months of age for controlling pruritus associated with allergic dermatitis, including flea allergies and atopic dermatitis.[1] Oclacitinib is suitable for the treatment of both acute flares and long-term management of atopic dermatitis.[2,3] Studies in dogs with atopic dermatitis indicate an efficacy rate comparable to glucocorticoids and cyclosporine except that oclacitinib has a faster onset of action (within 24 hours) for control of pruritus.[4,5] Oclacitinib appears to reduce antimicrobial usage in dogs with allergic dermatitis.[6]

Based on case reports in dogs, oclacitinib has also been shown to be effective for treatment of ischemic dermatopathy,[7-9] hyperkeratotic erythema multiforme,[10] autoimmune subepidermal blistering dermatosis,[11] ear tip ulcerative dermatitis,[12] cutaneous epitheliotropic T-cell lymphoma (partial remission),[13] and as a temporary treatment to relieve pruritus associated with sarcoptic mange.[14] Anecdotal reports also suggest that oclacitinib may be beneficial for the treatment of canine lupus and pemphigus.

Oclacitinib is not approved for use in cats; however, cats with feline atopic skin syndrome (FASS) showed improvement in clinical signs and pruritus when they were treated with oclacitinib.[15-18] Oclacitinib appeared to be as effective as methylprednisolone. Cats that responded to treatment did so within one month. Successful reports for oclacitinib use in cats also exist for cutaneous mastocytosis,[19] asthma,[20] head and neck pruritus,[17,21] idiopathic ulcerative dermatitis,[22] and pemphigus foliaceus.[23] Long-term studies with a larger number of cats are needed to investigate the true efficacy and safety of oclacitinib in cats and identify the proper dose range.

Pharmacology/Actions

Oclacitinib is a nonselective JAK inhibitor. It inhibits cytokines that are dependent on the JAK enzyme, inhibiting mostly JAK1 enzyme activity with some inhibition of JAK2 and JAK3. Specifically, oclacitinib inhibits IL-31, an important pruritogenic cytokine in atopic dogs, as well as pro-inflammatory cytokines such as IL-2, IL-4, IL-6, and IL-13 that also play an important role in canine atopic dermatitis. At the approved regimen, oclacitinib appears to have no effect on hematologic parameters, but at higher extra-label doses or frequencies, inhibition of hematopoiesis might occur in some dogs. Oclacitinib is not an antihistamine or glucocorticoid.[1]

Under experimental conditions, oclacitinib delayed the development of dermatitis at the site of cutaneous antigen exposure in atopic beagles.[24] In a study of client-owned dogs with allergic dermatitis, pruritus scores were reduced by 31% within 4 hours of the first dose and by 67% at 14 days.[4] Anecdotally, a subset of dogs that responded favorably to oclacitinib every 12 hours experienced partial loss of clinical sign control when administration frequency was reduced to every 24 hours. Chronic administration of the initial dose every 12 hours is extra-label use, as it may increase the risk for immunosuppression and is not recommended.

A study in mice showed a significant rebound phenomenon in pruritus after abrupt withdrawal of oclacitinib, which correlated with increased concentrations of pruritogenic cytokines that cause scratching; this has been reported anecdotally in dogs as well.[25] Further studies in allergic dogs are needed to corroborate these findings.

Pharmacokinetics

After oral administration in dogs, oclacitinib maleate had a bioavailability of 89%, and peak plasma concentrations occurred in less than 1 hour.[1] The feeding state did not affect pharmacokinetics. Oclacitinib was not significantly bound to plasma proteins in dogs (66% to 69%). The apparent volume of distribution (steady-state) was 942 mL/kg, and total body plasma clearance was 5.3 mL/minute/kg. The terminal half-life was 3.5 hours (IV) and 4.1 hours (PO). Oclacitinib was metabolized to several metabolites, with an oxidative form being the major metabolite. Less than 4% of the drug was excreted unchanged in the urine within 24 hours of administration.[26,27]

After oral administration in cats, oclacitinib bioavailability was 87%, T_{max} was 35 minutes, and the elimination half-life was 2.3 hours.[28] Volume of distribution (steady state) was 0.67 L/kg and clearance was calculated as 4.45 mL/minute/kg following IV administration). In cats with feline atopic skin syndrome (FASS), control of clinical signs did not correlate with plasma oclacitinib concentration.[18]

Contraindications/Precautions/Warnings

Oclacitinib should not be used in dogs younger than 12 months, dogs with serious infections, breeding dogs, or pregnant or lactating bitches.[1] At label dosages, there is increased potential for susceptibility to infections, demodicosis, and exacerbation or development of neoplastic conditions.[1] Clinicians should avoid or carefully consider the use of oclacitinib in animals with pre-existing disorders, such as demodicosis, severe infections (eg, pneumonia), and neoplastic diseases. Cats should be screened for FIV or FeLV prior to treatment with oclacitinib.[15]

Adverse Effects

Oclacitinib appears to be well tolerated in dogs, with an incidence of adverse effects similar to placebo. One study in allergic dogs showed that chronic use of oclacitinib for up to 630 days is generally safe.[5] Most commonly, GI effects (eg, vomiting, diarrhea, anorexia) or lethargy have been noted; in most cases these effects are transient and resolve spontaneously.[1,5] Polydipsia, lymphadenopathy, polyphagia, aggression, and weight loss were noted in less than 1.5% of treated dogs.

In dogs, oclacitinib may increase susceptibility to infections (eg, pneumonia, demodicosis, pododermatitis, pyoderma, otitis).[2,5] Proteinuria, hematuria, hyposthenuria, and microalbuminemia have also been reported.[5]

The rate of UTI/cystitis was reported as 11.3% in one long-term study,[5] whereas a small prospective study in healthy dogs without a prior history of UTI concluded that oclacitinib did not increase the risk for bacterial UTI over the average 6-month study.[29] Caution may be warranted when treating dogs with prior history of or predisposing factors for UTI, as the risk of UTI with oclacitinib administration in this population has not been determined.

New (or exacerbations of existing) benign and malignant neoplastic conditions have been observed in dogs treated with oclacitinib.[1] Unspecified benign cutaneous and subcutaneous masses, histiocytomas, and papillomas have also been reported in dogs.[2,5] A retrospective cohort study (660 client-owned dogs followed for a mean of 36 months) indicated that long-term treatment with oclacitinib did not increase the risk for malignancy as compared to an age- and breed-matched control group that was treated with other systemic atopic dermatitis medications (eg, cyclosporine, glucocorticoids).[30] Reductions of leukocyte (neutrophil, eosinophil, monocyte) counts, transient increased lymphocyte counts, and decreased serum globulin have occurred; however, study population mean values remained within normal ranges.[1]

In small, short-term studies of up to 28 days in cats, oclacitinib seems to be well tolerated; adverse effects appear more frequently at higher doses. In a placebo-controlled safety study, healthy cats were administered oclacitinib 1 or 2 mg/kg PO every 12 hours for 28 days.[31] In the 2 mg/kg dose group, adverse GI effects (vomiting, soft stools) were noted. There were no differences in CBC parameters and serum chemistry profiles between the 2 treatment groups and placebo. A different study (oclacitinib 0.7 – 1.2 mg/kg PO every 12 hours) showed that 4 of 14 cats had mild increases in BUN and creatinine.[15] In a study of cats with experimental asthma, no adverse effects were noted when cats were administered oclacitinib 0.5 or 1 mg/kg PO twice daily for 28 days[20]; however, a case report described fatal toxoplasmosis in a feline immunodeficiency virus-positive domestic short hair cat with feline atopic skin syndrome after treatment with oclacitinib for 5 months.[32] Until more studies with a larger number of cats, longer duration of monitoring, and more extensive safety data are available, oclacitinib should only be used in cats when other medications with known safety data in cats cannot be used or are not effective.[33]

Reproductive/Nursing Safety

Safe use of oclacitinib during pregnancy, breeding, or nursing has not been established; it should not be used in breeding dogs or pregnant or lactating bitches.[1]

Overdose/Acute Toxicity

Limited information is available on acute toxicity. In rats, the oral LD_{50} is 310 mg/kg.[34] In preapproval margin of safety studies in beagles receiving 5 times the label dosages (3 mg/kg PO every 12 hours for 6 weeks, then every 24 hours for 20 weeks), clinically observed adverse effects attributable to the drug included vomiting, diarrhea, interdigital furunculosis/dermatitis, papillomas, microscopic evidence of mild interstitial pneumonia, and lymphoid hyperplasia and chronic active inflammation in lymph nodes draining feet affected by interdigital furunculosis. No deaths or serious effects were reported.[1]

For patients that have experienced or are suspected to have experienced an overdose, consultation with a 24-hour poison consultation center specializing in providing veterinary-specific information is recommended. For general information related to overdose and toxin exposures, as well as contact information for poison control centers, refer to ***Appendix***.

Drug Interactions

Oclacitinib causes minimal inhibition of canine cytochrome P450, and no significant drug interactions have been reported to date. It has been reported to be safely used in conjunction with other common medications, including **vaccines, NSAIDs, antibiotics, parasiticides, anticonvulsants**, and **allergen immunotherapy**.[4,5,35,36] Oclacitinib at label dosages was shown to be well tolerated when given in combination with **carboplatin** or **doxorubicin** in a small pilot study.[37]

- **Cyclosporine**: Although concurrent administration of oclacitinib and cyclosporine appears safe when administered for up to 3 weeks,[38] the combination of cyclosporine and oclacitinib is relatively contraindicated for long-term use, especially in cases in which infection is present, because of the theoretical increased risk for immunosuppression.[3]
- **Immunosuppressive Agents** (eg, **azathioprine, glucocor-**

Severe esophagitis: 1 – 1.5 mg/kg PO every 12 hours, often in combination with a prokinetic (cisapride) and sucralfate.[40] Some have recommended giving omeprazole up to 2 mg/kg every 12 hours.[41]

Prevention of exercise-induced gastritis (extra-label): In a study, racing Alaskan sled dogs were administered omeprazole at ≈0.85 mg/kg (one 20 mg tablet) every 24 hours, 30 minutes before being fed. The administration began ≈48 hours before exercise.[1]

***Helicobacter* spp infection/gastritis** (extra-label): Omeprazole 0.5 – 1 mg/kg PO every 24 hours in combination with amoxicillin 20 mg/kg PO every 12 hours and clarithromycin 7.5 mg/kg PO every 24 hours for 21 days.[6] Diarrhea can be an adverse effect of this treatment protocol.

Decrease CSF production: 0.5 – 1 mg/kg PO every 24 hours.[7,10] In 1 study, omeprazole was evaluated in 12 dogs with hydrocephalus at a dose of 10 mg/kg PO every 24 hours and showed medical improvement in all dogs and reduced ventricular size in most dogs.[11]

CATS:

GI ulcer management/prevention (extra-label): 1.1 – 1.3 mg/kg PO every 12 hours.[12] Enteric-coated tablets may be split.[42]

HORSES:

Gastric ulcers (label dosage; FDA-approved):

a) **Treatment of gastric ulcers**: 4 mg/kg PO every 24 hours for 4 weeks[30]

b) **Prevention of gastric ulcers**:

   i. 2 mg/kg PO every 24 hours for at least another 4 weeks[30]

   ii. 1 mg/kg minimum dose PO every 24 hours[25]

Treatment of squamous ulceration (extra-label): Dosages as low as 1 mg/kg PO once daily were effective when administered following a brief fast and prior to exercise.[43]

Prevention of gastric ulcers (extra-label): One study found that dosages as low as 0.5 mg/kg PO every 24 hours were as effective as the higher, label dosage.[21]

Treatment or prophylaxis of gastric ulcers in foals (extra-label):

a) **Treatment**: 4 mg/kg PO every 24 hours[44]

b) **Prophylaxis**: 1 – 2 mg/kg PO every 24 hours for prophylaxis[44]

SWINE:

Ulcer management (extra-label): 40 mg PO every 24 hours for 2 days; fasted for 48 hours[45]

FERRETS:

Short-term treatment of gastroenteritis (extra-label): 0.7 mg/kg PO every 24 hours[46]

Monitoring

- Efficacy
- Adverse effects

Client Information

- This medicine is used to treat or prevent stomach ulcers and usually only used short-term.
- This medicine works best if given before the first meal of the day.
- Before giving the oral paste to your horse, set the lock ring so that the side nearest the barrel is at the intended dose. Syringes are marked either for body weight or in precalibrated individual doses. Make sure there is no feed in the horse's mouth then deposit the dose on the back of the tongue or deep in the cheek pouch. Redose if any of the doses are lost or rejected.

Chemistry/Synonyms

Omeprazole, a substituted benzimidazole proton pump inhibitor, has a molecular weight of 345.4 and pK_as of 4 and 8.8. Omeprazole occurs as a white to off-white crystalline powder that is slightly soluble in water and soluble in ethanol. The equine oral paste is in a paraffin-based vehicle.

Omeprazole may also be known as H-168/68, omeprazolum, *GastroGard*®, *Peptizole*®, *Prilosec*®, *UlcerGard*®, and *Zegerid*®.

Storage/Stability

Store omeprazole oral paste between 20°C and 25°C (68°F and 77°F); excursions between 15°C and 30°C (59°F and 86°F) are permitted; discard tube 28 days after first opening.[47] Store omeprazole tablets at room temperature in tight, light-resistant containers. Omeprazole pellets found in the capsules should not be crushed.

Compatibility/Compounding Considerations

Caution should be used when administering compounded omeprazole products; bioequivalence has been an issue with some compounded preparations. Omeprazole capsules or tablets should not be crushed or chewed. A study in cats found that fractionated enteric-coated omeprazole tablets were effective in suppressing gastric acid.[42] If the dose of the commercially available capsules is being reduced, the capsule contents should be reinserted into a gelatin capsule so they cannot be chewed.

Compounded preparation stability: A formula for an omeprazole oral suspension compounded from the commercially available powder packets has been published.[48] Dissolving one (1) omeprazole 20 mg powder packet qs ad to 10 mL of sterile water yields 2 mg/mL omeprazole oral suspension that retains more than 98% potency for 45 days when stored at 4°C (39.2°F); however, the resulting low concentration and strawberry flavoring may not be suitable for administration to veterinary patients. Information on the efficacy of omeprazole 40 mg/mL oral suspension compounded by diluting commercially available equine paste 1:9 with sesame oil for use in dogs has been published.[3] Although the long-term stability of this preparation has not yet been assayed, it meets the default beyonduse date criteria of 180 days for nonaqueous oral suspensions.

Dosage Forms/Regulatory Status

VETERINARY-LABELED PRODUCTS:

Omeprazole Oral Paste, 2.28 g per syringe; *GastroGard*®, (Rx); *UlcerGard*®; (OTC). Contains 370 mg omeprazole per gram of paste.

The Association of Racing Commissioners International (ARCI) Uniform Classification Guidelines for Foreign Substances (UCGFS) has designated this drug as a class 5 substance. Use of this drug may not be allowed in certain animal competitions. Check rules and regulations before entering a competition while this medication is being administered. Contact local racing authorities for further guidance. See ***Appendix*** for more information.

Use of this drug may not be allowed in certain animal competitions. Check rules and regulations before entering a competition while this medication is being administered. Contact local racing authorities for further guidance.

HUMAN-LABELED PRODUCTS:

Omeprazole Delayed-Release Capsules: 10 mg, 20 mg, and 40 mg; *Prilosec*® (*Losec*® in Canada), generic; (Rx)

Omeprazole Delayed-Release Tablets: 20 mg; *Prilosec*® *OTC*, generic; (OTC)

Omeprazole Delayed-Release Oral Suspension: 2.5 mg and 10 mg packets; *Prilosec*®; (Rx). Packet contents are reconstituted with water.

Omeprazole Suspension: 2 mg/mL; *First*®*-Omeprazole, Omeprazole+Syrspend*® *SF Alka*; (Rx)

Omeprazole/Sodium Bicarbonate Capsules (Immediate Release):

20 mg omeprazole/1100 mg sodium bicarbonate and 40 mg omeprazole/1100 mg sodium bicarbonate; *Zegerid*®, *Zegerid*® OTC; (Rx and OTC)

Omeprazole/Sodium Bicarbonate Powder for Suspension: 20 mg omeprazole/1680 sodium bicarbonate and 40 mg omeprazole/1680 sodium bicarbonate in 30 unit-dose packets; *Zegerid*®; (Rx)

References

For the complete list of references, see **wiley.com/go/budde/plumb**

Ondansetron

(on-***dan***-sah-tron) *Zofran*®

5-HT_3 Receptor Antagonist

Prescriber Highlights

- Oral and injectable agent used for prevention and treatment of vomiting and nausea
- Can be used in combination with other antiemetics
- Use with caution when administering it with other drugs that increase serotonin in order to avoid serotonin syndrome.
- Appears to be well tolerated

Uses/Indications

Ondansetron is an antiemetic that may be used to treat nausea and vomiting in dogs and cats. Ondansetron, metoclopramide, and maropitant can be equally effective in reducing the frequency of vomiting in dogs with parvoviral enteritis.[1,2] Ondansetron is effective for treating chemotherapy-associated nausea and vomiting[3-5]; in preventing the incidence of emesis and nausea in healthy dogs premedicated with hydromorphone, acepromazine, and glycopyrrolate[6]; and in treating nausea in dogs with vestibular syndrome.[7] As an antiemetic and antinausea agent, ondansetron is as effective or more effective than metoclopramide[1,4,8]; however, maropitant appears to be as effective or more effective than ondansetron.[1-4,8,9] Ondansetron has shown promise in the management of obstructive sleep apnea.[10,11]

A study in cats found that ondansetron 0.22 mg/kg IM administered with dexmedetomidine and buprenorphine (in the same syringe) reduced the incidence (≈33%) and severity of nausea and vomiting as compared with ondansetron given 30 minutes before dexmedetomidine and buprenorphine (67%) or when ondansetron was not given (76%).[12]

In donkeys, IV ondansetron decreased duodenal, jejunal, and cecal contractility, as well as small and large intestinal motility.[13] Six out of 30 donkeys experienced a cardiac arrhythmia that began 30 minutes postinfusion and lasted up to 180 minutes.

In humans, ondansetron is approved for the prevention and treatment of nausea and vomiting due to chemotherapy, radiation, and surgery. It may be used in combination with other antiemetics.[14]

Pharmacology/Actions

Ondansetron is a 5-HT_3 receptor antagonist. 5-HT_3 receptors are found peripherally on vagal nerve terminals and centrally in the chemoreceptor trigger zone (CRTZ). Ondansetron's effects appear to be mediated by the antagonism of these receptors both centrally and peripherally. At typical dosages, ondansetron does not have an effect on GI motility or transit time.

Pharmacokinetics

In cats, ondansetron's oral bioavailability is ≈32%, but bioavailability is 75% when the drug is injected SC. Elimination half-life is ≈2 hours (IV), 1.2 hours (PO), and 3.2 hours (SC).[15] Administration of ondansetron 2 mg SC to geriatric cats and cats with renal and hepatic disease revealed reductions in clearance, which were greatest in cats with hepatic disease.[16] Application of ondansetron in *Lipoderm*® transdermal gel to the inner ear pinnae of healthy cats resulted in no measurable serum ondansetron concentrations.[17]

After a single 8 mg oral dose was given to healthy beagles, peak concentrations were reached at 1.1 hours, and the elimination half-life was ≈1.3 hours.[18]

In humans, ondansetron is well absorbed from the GI tract but exhibits some first-pass hepatic metabolism. Oral bioavailability is ≈50% to 60%; bioavailability is ≈75% after IM administration. Oral dosage forms are bioequivalent. Protein binding is ≈75%. Peak plasma concentrations occur ≈2 hours after oral administration. Ondansetron is extensively metabolized in the liver by several cytochrome P450 enzymes, primarily via CYP3A4. Elimination half-lives are ≈3 to 4 hours but are prolonged in elderly patients and pediatric patients 1 to 4 months of age, whereas half-life is reduced in pediatric patients younger than 4 months.

Contraindications/Precautions/Warnings

Ondansetron is contraindicated in patients hypersensitive to it or other agents in this class. Ondansetron may mask ileus or gastric distention; it should not be used in place of nasogastric suction or appropriate diagnostic assessment. Ondansetron should be used with caution in patients with hepatic dysfunction, as absorption may be increased because of reduced first-pass metabolism and halflife may be prolonged; dosage adjustment may be warranted in severe hepatic impairment.

In humans, ondansetron is pumped by P-glycoprotein (the protein encoded by the *MDR1* gene, also known as *ABCB1*-1delta gene), but there are currently no data stating whether it is pumped by canine P-glycoprotein. It is suggested to use caution when administering ondansetron to dogs with the MDR1 gene mutation.[19]

Dose-related prolongation of the QT interval and cases of torsades de pointes have been reported in humans. Patients that have electrolyte abnormalities, have underlying cardiac conditions, or take other QT-prolonging drugs can be at greater risk. Ondansetron caused QT prolongation in healthy dogs,[20] but QT prolongation in sick dogs was identified by only 1 of the 2 methods used to calculate the QT interval.[21]

Serotonin syndrome has occurred in humans receiving ondansetron.[22]

Adverse Effects

Ondansetron appears to be well tolerated. GI effects (ie, constipation, diarrhea), sedation, extrapyramidal clinical signs (eg, head shaking), increased liver enzymes, arrhythmias, and hypotension can be possible (incidence in humans is less than 10%). Headaches occur in 10% to 25% of humans; relevance for veterinary patients is unknown. Transient vision changes, including blindness, during IV administration, have been reported rarely in humans.

Reproductive/Nursing Safety

Safety in pregnancy is not clearly established, but high-dose studies in rodents did not demonstrate overt fetal toxicity or teratogenicity. A review of ondansetron use in women during pregnancy and the risk for birth defects noted a small increase in the incidence of cardiac abnormalities, and the authors concluded that ondansetron should be avoided during the first trimester if possible.[23]

Ondansetron is excreted in the maternal milk of rats.[22] Caution should be used when 5-HT_3 antagonists are administered to nursing patients.

Overdose/Acute Toxicity

Overdoses of up to 10 times the label dosage did not cause significant morbidity in humans. If an overdose occurs, it should be treated supportively.

For patients that have experienced or are suspected of having experienced an overdose, consultation with a 24-hour poison consulta-

tion center specializing in providing veterinary-specific information is recommended. For general information related to overdose and toxin exposures, as well as contact information for poison control centers, refer to ***Appendix.***

Drug Interactions/Laboratory Considerations

In humans, ondansetron is a substrate of P-glycoprotein and CYP 3A4, although other CYP isoenzymes (eg, 2D6, 1A2) are involved in the drug's metabolism to a lesser extent. The following drug interactions have either been reported or are theoretical in humans or animals receiving ondansetron and may be of significance in veterinary patients. Unless otherwise noted, use together is not necessarily contraindicated, but weigh the potential risks and perform additional monitoring when appropriate.

- **Apomorphine**: Ondansetron may reduce the emetic effect of apomorphine. A human patient that received ondansetron and apomorphine developed severe hypotension and loss of consciousness. In humans, use together is contraindicated.
- **Azole Antifungals** (eg, **itraconazole, posaconazole**): May inhibit ondansetron metabolism, and concurrent use may increase prolong QTc interval.
- **Cisplatin**: Plasma cisplatin concentrations may be decreased.
- **Cyclophosphamide**: Plasma cyclophosphamide concentrations may be decreased.
- **Drugs Affecting QTc Interval** (eg, **amiodarone, cisapride, procainamide, quinidine, sotalol**): Theoretically, ondansetron may have additive effects on QTc interval; possible serious arrhythmias may result.[21]
- **Monoamine Oxidase Inhibitors** (**MAOIs;** eg, **amitraz, methylene blue, selegiline**): Increased risk for serotonin syndrome has been reported in humans.
- **Metformin**: Ondansetron may increase the serum concentration of metformin.
- **P-glycoprotein Inhibitors** (eg, **amiodarone, cyclosporine, diltiazem, quinidine**): In humans, these drugs may increase serum concentrations of ondansetron. It is unclear if ondansetron is a P-glycoprotein substrate in veterinary patients.
- **Ropinirole**: Ondansetron may reduce the emetic effect of ropinirole.
- **Serotonergic Drugs** (eg, **clomipramine, fluoxetine, mirtazapine, trazodone**): Increased risk for serotonin syndrome has been reported in humans.
- **Tramadol**: In humans, use together may reduce the efficacy of both drugs. Veterinary significance is not known.

Dosages

NOTE: In humans, it is recommended that IV administration of ondansetron occur over at least 30 seconds, and preferably over 2 to 5 minutes.[24]

DOGS:

Antiemetic (extra-label): 0.5 – 1 mg/kg PO or IV (slowly) every 8 to 12 hours is commonly used, although studies supporting these dosages are limited; however, doses of 0.1 – 0.2 mg/kg IV have been noted and are closer to human pediatric recommendations.

Chemotherapy-induced nausea and vomiting (extra-label): 0.3 – 0.5 mg/kg IV (slowly) 30 minutes before chemotherapy administration[3,5,8,25]; may repeat every 8 to 12 hours

Parvovirus-induced nausea and vomiting (extra-label): 0.5 mg/kg IV (slowly) every 8 hours[1,2]

Obstructive Sleep Apnea (extra-label): 1 – 2 mg/kg PO twice daily[10,11]

Vestibular syndrome-associated nausea (extra-label): 0.5 mg/kg IV (slowly) as a single dose[7]

CATS:

Acute vomiting (extra-label): Dosage recommendations vary somewhat; 0.1 – 1 mg/kg IV (slowly), SC, IM, or PO every 6 to 12 hours. Based on a pharmacokinetic study,[15] oral dosages may need to be toward the high end and given more frequently than IV or SC. If using before chemotherapy, give IV (slowly) 30 minutes before treatment; may repeat every 6 to 12 hours.

Vomiting associated with chronic kidney disease (extra-label):

a) IRIS Stage 1 or 2: 0.1 – 0.2 mg/kg slow IV, SC, PO every 6 to 12 hours[26]

b) IRIS Stage 3: 0.05 – 0.1 mg/kg slow IV, SC, PO every 6 to 12 hours[26]

c) IRIS Stage 4: 0.025 – 0.05 mg/kg slow IV, SC, or PO every 6 to 12 hours[26]

Reducing the incidence and severity of vomiting associated with dexmedetomidine/buprenorphine premedication (extra-label): Ondansetron 0.22 mg/kg IM administered with dexmedetomidine and buprenorphine (in the same syringe)[12]

Monitoring

- Clinical efficacy

Client Information

- This medicine is used to treat or prevent severe vomiting. The oral medication may be given with or without food.
- This medicine is usually tolerated well.
- If using orally disintegrating tablets, protect the tablets from moisture, and be sure hands are dry when handling them. Place the tablet on top of the animal's tongue after removing it from the package.

Chemistry/Synonyms

Ondansetron HCl dihydrate is a selective inhibitor of the 5-HT_3 receptor. It occurs as a white to off-white powder that is sparingly soluble in water and alcohol. Solutions for injections have a pH of 3.3 to 4. The potency of commercial dosage forms is expressed as an ondansetron base; 1 mg ondansetron is equivalent to 1.25 mg ondansetron HCl dihydrate.

Ondansetron HCl may also be known as GR-38032F or ondansetroni hydrochloridum, and *Zofran*®.

Storage/Stability

Unless otherwise labeled, store oral products in tight, light-resistant containers between 20°C and 25°C (68°F-77°F); temperature excursions of 15°C to 30°C (59°F-86°F) are permitted for the oral solution. Store orally disintegrating tablets in the original foil blisters and administer immediately upon opening; discard opened/unused tablets or tablet remnants. Store the injection between 2°C and 25°C (36°F-77°F) and protected from light. Solutions diluted for IV infusion retain potency for 48 hours at room temperature, but the manufacturer recommends discarding them 24 hours after dilution.

Compatibility/Compounding Considerations

Compatibility is dependent on factors such as pH, concentration, temperature, and diluent used; specialized references or a hospital pharmacist may be consulted for more specific information.

An ondansetron 0.8 mg/mL oral suspension can be compounded by crushing oral tablets to a fine powder, suspending with *Ora-Plus*®, and diluting with an equal amount of *Ora-Sweet*® (regular or sugar-free), *Syrpalta*®, or Cherry syrup USP[27]; the resulting product is stable for 6 weeks when refrigerated. Alternatively, using the suspending vehicle, *SyrSpend*® *SF* pH 4 results in a 90-day beyond-use date when refrigerated or stored at room temperature.[28]

Drugs reported to be **compatible** with ondansetron when combined in a syringe and administered via a Y-site include alfentanil, atropine, fentanyl, glycopyrrolate, metoclopramide, midazolam, morphine, naloxone, neostigmine, and propofol. Ondansetron is also reported to be **compatible** with dextrose, saline, and lactated Ringer's solutions, as well as with the following drugs when administered via a **Y-site**: amikacin, aminocaproic acid, amiodarone, azithromycin, bleomycin, butorphanol, carboplatin, carmustine, cefazolin, cefotaxime, cefuroxime, cisplatin, clindamycin, cyclophosphamide, cyclosporine, cytarabine, dacarbazine, dactinomycin, daunorubicin, dexamethasone sodium phosphate, dexmedetomidine, dexrazoxane, digoxin, diphenhydramine, dopamine, doxorubicin HCL (also liposome form), doxycycline, famotidine, filgrastim, fluconazole, gemcitabine, gentamicin, heparin, hydromorphone, hydroxyzine, ifosfamide, lidocaine, mannitol, methotrexate, mitoxantrone, norepinephrine, pamidronate, piperacillin-tazobactam, potassium chloride, procainamide, prochlorperazine, promethazine, ranitidine, vancomycin, vinblastine, vincristine, zidovudine, and zoledronic acid.

A precipitate may form when mixed with alkaline solutions. Ondansetron is reportedly **incompatible** with amphotericin B (conventional and lipid-based forms), ampicillin/sulbactam, furosemide, pantoprazole, and phenobarbital sodium.

Dosage Forms/Regulatory Status

VETERINARY-LABELED PRODUCTS: NONE

HUMAN-LABELED PRODUCTS:

Ondansetron HCl Tablets: 4 mg and 8 mg; *Zofran®*, generic; (Rx)

Ondansetron Orally Disintegrating Tablets or Oral Film: 4 mg and 8 mg (as base); *Zofran® ODT, Zuplenz®*, generic; (Rx)

Ondansetron HCl Oral Solution: 0.8 mg/mL (4 mg/5 mL) in 50 mL; *Zofran®*, generic; (Rx)

Ondansetron HCl Injection: 2 mg/mL in 2 mL single-dose syringes and 20 mL single- or multi-dose vials; *Zofran®*, generic; (Rx)

References

For the complete list of references, see **wiley.com/go/budde/plumb**

Orbifloxacin

(or-bi-***flox***-a-sin) *Orbax®*

Fluoroquinolone Antibiotic

Prescriber Highlights

- Fluoroquinolone antibiotic labeled for treating skin and soft tissue infections in dogs and cats and for treating bacterial urinary infections in dogs.
- Contraindications: Immature dogs during the rapid growth phase; known hypersensitivity to this class of drugs. Caution: Known or suspected CNS disorders
- Adverse effects: GI effects most likely
- In cats, tablet and suspension formulations are not bioequivalent.
- Many potential drug interactions
- Federal law prohibits extra-label use in food-producing animals.

Uses/Indications

Orbifloxacin is indicated for treatment of susceptible skin and soft tissue bacterial infections in dogs and cats. In dogs, it is also indicated for treatment of UTIs. It is recommended that orbifloxacin be reserved for documented resistant UTIs, but it is a good first-line choice for pyelonephritis or infections that involve the prostate.[1] In addition, fluoroquinolones are recommended as second-tier drugs for treatment of bacterial folliculitis.[2]

Orbifloxacin may also be of benefit in treating susceptible gram-negative infections in horses, although clinical data are lacking and an equine formulation is not available.

The World Health Organization has designated orbifloxacin as a Critically Important (Highest Priority) antimicrobial for human medicine.[3] The Office International des Epizooties (OIE) has designated quinolones as Veterinary Critically Important Antimicrobial (VCIA) Agents in veterinary species.[4]

Pharmacology/Actions

Orbifloxacin is a concentration-dependent bactericidal agent. It acts by inhibiting bacterial DNA-gyrase (a type II topoisomerase), thereby preventing DNA supercoiling and DNA synthesis. The net result is disruption of bacterial cell replication. Like other fluoroquinolones, orbifloxacin has demonstrated a significant postantibiotic effect for both gram-negative and gram-positive bacteria. Clinical efficacy is associated with achieving a peak orbifloxacin concentration 10 times greater than bacterial MIC,[5,6] resulting in infrequent (once-daily) administration of high doses.

Like other fluoroquinolones, orbifloxacin has excellent activity against many gram-negative bacteria and many gram-positive bacteria. This includes most species and strains of *Klebsiella* spp, *Staphylococcus pseudintermedius* or *S aureus, E coli, Enterobacter* spp, *Campylobacter* spp, *Bartonella* spp, *Shigella* spp, *Proteus* spp, and *Pasteurella* spp. Some strains of *Pseudomonas aeruginosa* and other *Pseudomonas* spp are resistant to orbifloxacin and most *Enterococcus* spp are resistant. Like other fluoroquinolones, orbifloxacin has weak activity against most anaerobes and is not a good choice when treating known or suspected anaerobic infections. Acquired resistance can occur in virtually any bacterial species but is most commonly encountered in Enterobacteriaceae (*E coli* and related species) and staphylococci.

Pharmacokinetics

After oral administration in dogs or cats, orbifloxacin is apparently nearly completely absorbed, although the suspension formulation results in lower and more variable plasma levels in cats as compared with tablets.[7] Dogs receiving 7.5 mg/kg PO had an average peak orbifloxacin concentration of ≈6 µg/mL 2 hours after administration. Cats receiving orbifloxacin tablets 7.5 mg/kg PO had peak plasma level of 6 µg/mL as compared with 3 µg/mL in cats receiving an equivalent dose of orbifloxacin suspension. The drug is distributed well (V_d=1.2 L/kg in dogs; 1.3 L/kg in cats) and only slightly bound to plasma proteins (8% dogs; 15% cats). Orbifloxacin is eliminated primarily via the kidneys. Approximately 50% of the drug is excreted unchanged. Serum half-life after oral dosing is ≈5.5 hours in dogs and 4.5 to 7.5 hours in cats. Urine levels remain well above MICs for susceptible organisms for at least 24 hours after dosing.

In horses, orbifloxacin is well absorbed after oral administration (bioavailability is ≈70%) and distributes in many body fluids and endometrial tissue. Protein binding is relatively low (≈20%). Elimination half-life is ≈3.5 to 9 hours.[8,9]

Rabbits receiving 20 mg/kg PO reached a peak concentration of 3 µg/mL at 2 hours after administration. Volume of distribution was 1.3 L/kg, and terminal half-life was 8.6 hours.[10]

Contraindications/Precautions/Warnings

Some fluoroquinolones can cause arthropathies in immature, growing animals, and the risk posed by orbifloxacin is unclear. Because dogs appear to be more sensitive to this effect, the manufacturer states that the drug is contraindicated in immature dogs during the rapid growth phase (age 2 to 8 months in small- and medium-sized breeds and up to 18 months in large and giant breeds). The drug is also contraindicated in dogs and cats known to be hypersensitive to orbifloxacin or other drugs in its class (quinolones). Orbifloxacin use is contraindicated in patients receiving cyclosporine.

The manufacturer states that orbifloxacin should be used with caution in animals with known or suspected hepatic and CNS disorders (eg, seizure disorders) as, rarely, drugs in this class have been associated with CNS stimulation. Because fluoroquinolones, including orbifloxacin, are known to adversely affect the retina in cats, the manufacturer cautions to not exceed doses of 7.5 mg/kg per day in cats.[7]

Adverse Effects

Although the manufacturer states that no adverse effects were reported during clinical studies (at 2.5 mg/kg dosing) in adult animals, GI effects (eg, anorexia, vomiting, hypersalivation), depression/lethargy, and convulsions have been reported.[7]

Blindness has been reported in cats receiving orbifloxacin.[7]

Induction of *Streptococcus canis* necrotizing fasciitis, which can be seen with enrofloxacin, does not appear to be a problem with orbifloxacin.

Reproductive/Nursing Safety

Safety in breeding or pregnant dogs or cats has not been established. Other fluoroquinolones are known to cross the placenta.

It is not known whether orbifloxacin enters maternal milk. Other fluoroquinolones are known to be excreted in milk.

Because safety has not been established in animals, this drug should only be used when the maternal benefits outweigh the potential fetal risks.

Overdose/Acute Toxicity

Dogs and cats receiving up to 5 times (37.5 mg/kg) the label dose for 30 days did not exhibit any significant adverse effects. At 75 mg/kg, dogs experienced adverse GI effects, including anorexia, vomiting, diarrhea, and mild weight loss. Glucosuria was also noted. Cats receiving the higher doses exhibited emesis, salivation, lacrimation, soft feces, and decreased food consumption. Ophthalmic changes were apparent in cats receiving 45 and 75 mg/kg/day, including retinal degeneration.

For patients that have experienced or are suspected to have experienced an overdose, it is strongly encouraged to consult with one of the 24-hour poison consultation centers that specialize in providing information specific for veterinary patients. For general information related to overdose and toxin exposures, as well as contact information for poison control centers, refer to ***Appendix***.

Drug Interactions

The following drug interactions have either been reported or are theoretical in humans or animals receiving orbifloxacin or related fluoroquinolones and may be of significance in veterinary patients. Orbifloxacin has been shown to inhibit CYP1A activity in dogs.[11] Unless otherwise noted, use together is not necessarily contraindicated, but weigh the potential risks and perform additional monitoring when appropriate.

- **Antacids/Dairy Products** (containing cations Mg^{++}, Al^{+++}, Ca^{++}): May bind to orbifloxacin and prevent its absorption; separate doses of these products by at least 2 hours.
- **Antibiotics, Other** (eg, **aminoglycosides, 3rd-generation cephalosporins, penicillins—extended-spectrum**): Synergism may occur, but is not predictable, against some bacteria (particularly *Pseudomonas aeruginosa*) with these compounds. Although orbifloxacin has minimal activity against anaerobes, in vitro synergy has been reported when the drug is used with **clindamycin** against strains of *Peptostreptococcus* spp, *Lactobacillus* spp, and *Bacteroides fragilis*.
- **Cimetidine**: May impair fluoroquinolone metabolism
- **Cyclosporine**: Fluoroquinolones may exacerbate the nephrotoxicity and reduce the metabolism of systemically administered cyclosporine. The manufacturer states concurrent orbifloxacin use with cyclosporine is contraindicated.
- **Flunixin**: Has been shown in dogs to increase the AUC and elimination half-life of enrofloxacin, and enrofloxacin increases the AUC and elimination half-life of flunixin; it is unknown whether orbifloxacin also causes this effect or other NSAIDs interact with orbifloxacin in dogs.
- **Glyburide**: Severe hypoglycemia possible
- **Iron, Zinc (oral)**: Decreased orbifloxacin absorption; separate doses by at least 2 hours.
- **Methotrexate**: Increased methotrexate levels possible with resultant toxicity
- **Nitrofurantoin**: May antagonize the antimicrobial activity of the fluoroquinolones, and their concomitant use is not recommended.
- **Phenytoin**: Orbifloxacin may alter phenytoin levels.
- **Probenecid**: Blocks tubular secretion of ciprofloxacin and may also increase the blood level and half-life of orbifloxacin
- **Sucralfate**: May inhibit absorption of orbifloxacin; separate doses of these drugs by at least 2 hours.
- **Theophylline**: Orbifloxacin may increase theophylline blood levels.
- **Warfarin**: Potential for increased warfarin effects

Dosages

DOGS/CATS:

Susceptible infections (label dose; FDA-approved):

Tablets: *Dogs and cats,* **For the treatment of susceptible bacterial infections***:* 2.5– 7.5 mg/kg PO once daily. Treatment duration is 10 days for UTI, and treatment for other infections should continue for 2 to 3 days past resolution of clinical signs to a maximum of 30 days. Do not exceed 7.5 mg/kg/day in cats.[7] **NOTE**: Higher doses may be preferable for any situation because of the concentration-dependent nature of the drug.

Suspension:

Dogs: **For the treatment of UTIs and skin and soft tissue infections** (wounds and abscesses) caused by susceptible bacteria: 2.5 – 7.5 mg/kg PO once daily. Treatment duration is 10 days for UTI; treatment for other infections should continue for 2 to 3 days past resolution of clinical signs to a maximum of 30 days. **NOTE**: Higher doses may be preferable for any situation because of the concentration-dependent nature of the drug.

Cats: **For the treatment of skin infections (wounds and abscesses) caused by susceptible strains of *S aureus, E coli,* and *P multocida***: 7.5 mg/kg PO once daily. Treatment should continue for 2 to 3 days past resolution of clinical signs. Do not exceed 7.5 mg/kg/day in cats.[7]

Sporadic cystitis for which amoxicillin (±clavulanic acid) and trimethoprim-sulfonamide are not appropriate based on culture and susceptibility or patient factors (extra-label): 2.5 – 7.5 mg/kg PO once daily (7.5 mg/kg/day PO in cats treated with oral suspension) for 3 to 5 days.[1]

HORSES:

Susceptible infections (extra-label): Little documentation exists for clinical use of orbifloxacin in horses. Two PK studies suggested 5 mg/kg PO once daily[12] and 7.5 mg/kg PO once daily.[13]

BIRDS:

Japanese Quail (extra-label): From a PK/PD study: Authors concluded that 20 mg/kg PO once daily would be a rational dose to treat susceptible infections in Japanese quail not intended for food; for more susceptible organisms, 15 mg/kg PO may also be effective.[14]

RABBITS:

Susceptible infections (extra-label): 20 mg/kg PO once daily[10]

Monitoring
- Efficacy
- Adverse effects

Client Information
- This drug is best given without food on an empty stomach, but if your animal vomits or acts sick after receiving it, give with small amount of food or a small treat (**no** dairy products, antacids, or anything containing iron). If vomiting continues, contact your veterinarian.
- Do not give at the same time with other drugs or vitamins that contain calcium, iron, or aluminum, as these can reduce the amount of drug absorbed.
- Most common side effects are vomiting, nausea (animal acts sick), or diarrhea. May discolor feces
- The suspension form does not require refrigeration but must be shaken well before use; the oral dosing syringe should be rinsed after use.
- Give the medicine for as long as your veterinarian has prescribed it for, even if your animal appears well.

Chemistry/Synonyms
A 4-fluoroquinolone antibiotic, orbifloxacin occurs as a white to pale yellow, odorless crystalline powder. It is slightly soluble in water at neutral pH. Solubility increases in either an acidic or basic medium.

Orbifloxacin may also be known as marufloxacin, orbifloxacine, orbifloxacinum, or *Orbax*®.

Storage/Stability
The commercially available tablets should be stored between 2°C to 30°C (36°F-86°F) and protected from excessive moisture.

The oral suspension should be stored between 2°C to 25°C (36°F-77°F). It does not require refrigeration. Store upright. Shake well before use.

Compatibility/Compounding Considerations
An orbifloxacin 22.7 mg tablet crushed and mixed with molasses, dark corn syrup, water from canned tuna, Kame fish sauce, *Ora-Plus*®, *Syrplata*®, or simple syrup was relatively stable (greater than 85% expected value) for up to 7 days when stored unrefrigerated but protected from light. Mixing with oral supplements that contain calcium or magnesium (eg, *Lixotinic*®) showed significant inactivation of orbifloxacin after 4 days.[15]

Dosage Forms/Regulatory Status
VETERINARY-LABELED PRODUCTS:

Orbifloxacin Oral Tablets: 22.7 mg (green) and 68 mg (blue) E-Z Break tablets; *Orbax*®[7]; (Rx). FDA-approved for use in dogs and cats. Federal law prohibits the use of the drug in food-producing animals. NADA# 141-081

Orbifloxacin Oral Suspension: 30 mg/mL malt-flavored in 20 mL bottles; *Orbax® Suspension*[16]; (Rx). FDA-approved for use in dogs and cats. Federal law prohibits the use of the drug in food-producing animals. NADA# 141-305

An otic suspension containing orbifloxacin, mometasone furoate monohydrate, and posaconazole is also available; *Posatex® Otic Suspension* (Rx). For otic use in dogs only. See ***Corticosteroid/Antimicrobial Preparations***.

HUMAN-LABELED PRODUCTS: NONE

References
For the complete list of references, see **wiley.com/go/budde/plumb**

Osaterone

(oh-***sat***-eh-rone) *Ypozane*®

Antiandrogenic; Progestational

Prescriber Highlights
- ► Approved in other countries for benign prostatic hypertrophy (BPH) in intact male dogs. Not commercially available in the United States
- ► Labeled as a 7-day treatment course; efficacy persists for several months
- ► Contraindications include in female dogs and patients that are hypersensitive to it.
- ► Most common adverse effects include transient appetite stimulation and behavioral changes.
- ► May decrease cortisol levels and affect ACTH stimulation tests
- ► Women of child-bearing age should avoid contact with, or wear disposable gloves when administering, osaterone.

Uses/Indications
Osaterone is used in male dogs to treat benign prostatic hypertrophy (BPH). It is also being investigated as a treatment for alopecia X in dogs.[1]

Osaterone is not available in the United States but is available in other countries.

Pharmacology/Actions
Osaterone acetate is structurally related to progesterone and has anti-androgenic effects. It is thought to act primarily by decreasing testosterone transport into the prostate, inhibiting 5-alpha reductase, competitively inhibiting binding to prostate androgen receptors, and decreasing androgen nuclear receptors.[2] The 15-beta hydroxylated metabolite (PB-4) also has anti-androgenic activity. Although osaterone has weak affinity for glucocorticoid receptors, PB-4 can cause some adrenosuppression. Osaterone has some progestational activity but does not have mineralocorticoid activity.

Pharmacokinetics
In dogs, osaterone is rapidly absorbed after oral administration and peak concentrations occur ≈2 hours after dosing. Plasma protein binding of osaterone is ≈90% and ≈80% for its active metabolite (PB-4). Osaterone is primarily metabolized via hydroxylation to PB-4.[3] Elimination half-life is ≈80 hours. It is eliminated primarily in feces via biliary excretion and, to a lesser extent, in urine. After a single dose, osaterone and its metabolites can be detected in urine and feces for up to 14 days.

Contraindications/Precautions/Warnings
Osaterone is contraindicated in female animals and animals that are hypersensitive to it. Use osaterone cautiously in animals with hepatic dysfunction.

Wash hands after handling osaterone.[4] Women of child-bearing age should avoid contact with, or wear disposable gloves when administering, osaterone.

Adverse Effects
The most common adverse effect reported in dogs is a temporary increase in appetite. Transient behavioral changes are common, including changes in activity level and sociability. Polyuria, polydipsia, mammary gland hyperplasia (rare), hair coat changes (rare), and GI effects (eg, vomiting, diarrhea) have been reported. Decreased cortisol plasma levels occur commonly early in treatment and can persist for several weeks. In dogs with hypoadrenocorticism or that are under physiological stress (eg, postsurgery, posttrauma), consider additional monitoring and glucocorticoid support, if required.

Reproductive/Nursing Safety

Osaterone should not be used in female animals.[4] In laboratory animals, it has caused serious adverse effects on reproductive functions. Women of child-bearing age should wear gloves and avoid handling osaterone when possible.

No adverse effects on semen quality have been reported[4,5]; however, an early study in beagles reported transient abnormalities in semen quality likely secondary to decreased testosterone effects on the epididymis.[6]

Overdose/Acute Toxicity

Limited information is available for clinical overdoses of osaterone. Doses greater than 10 mg/kg may cause ataxia and tremors. Dogs given 1.25 mg/kg (2.5 times the label dose) for 10 days only showed decreased plasma cortisol levels.[4] A single 40 mg dose in human males resulted in sporadic decreases of LH, FSH, and testosterone levels, but no associated clinical signs.

For patients that have experienced or are suspected to have experienced an overdose, consultation with a 24-hour poison consultation center specializing in providing veterinary-specific information is recommended. For general information related to overdose and toxin exposures, as well as contact information for poison control centers, refer to ***Appendix.***

Drug Interactions

There are no known interactions.[4] Osaterone may be administered concurrently with antimicrobials.

Laboratory Considerations

- Plasma cortisol levels may decrease after starting treatment and persist for several weeks. ACTH stimulation tests may be suppressed.[4]

Dosages

DOGS:

Benign prostatic hypertrophy (BPH) in male dogs (extra-label): 0.25 – 0.5 mg/kg PO once daily for 7 days.[4] Re-evaluate 5 months after treatment or earlier if clinical signs recur. The decision to retreat should be based on examination findings as well as the risks and benefits of treatment.

Monitoring

- Clinical efficacy (reduced prostate size, improvement in constipation, ease of urination)
- Liver enzymes (ALT, ALP) in dogs with a history or signs of hepatic dysfunction
- Monitor for the development of clinical signs related to hypoadrenocorticism

Client Information

- This medicine can be given with or without food.
- Osaterone is usually given for 7 days and then stopped. Improvement is usually seen within 2 weeks and can last for 5 months or more. Your veterinarian will need to evaluate your dog 5 months after treatment or sooner if the effects of the medicine wear off.
- Side effects include increased appetite or changes in activity level and sociability but are usually temporary.
- Wash hands after administration. In the case of accidental human ingestion, seek medical advice immediately and show the product label to the physician. Women of childbearing age should avoid handling this medication when possible, or they should wear disposable gloves when handling.

Chemistry/Synonyms

Osaterone acetate is structurally related to progesterone and is a derivative of chlormadinone. The commercially available tablets also contain pre-gelatinized starch, carmellose calcium, corn (maize) starch, talc, and magnesium stearate as excipients.

Osaterone acetate may also be known as TZP-4238, 17alpha-acetoxy-6-chloro-2-oxa-4, 6-pregnadiene-3, or 20-dione. The trade name is *Ypozane®*.

Storage/Stability

Osaterone tablets should be stored at room temperature (15°C-30°C [59°F-86°F]). Expiration dates of 3 years postmanufacture are assigned.

Compatibility/Compounding Considerations

No specific information is noted.

Dosage Forms/Regulatory Status

VETERINARY-LABELED PRODUCTS: NONE IN THE UNITED STATES

Oral Tablets: 1.875 mg, 3.75 mg, 7.5 mg, and 15 mg; *Ypozane®*; (Rx). Approved for use in dogs in countries other than the United States

HUMAN-LABELED PRODUCTS: NONE

References

For the complete list of references, see **wiley.com/go/budde/plumb**

Oseltamivir

(oh-sell-***tam***-ih-vir) *Tamiflu®*

Antiviral; Neuraminidase Inhibitor

Prescriber Highlights

- Neuraminidase inhibitor that has been suggested as a treatment for canine parvovirus infections or other mixed bacterial/viral infections; evidence supporting its use is lacking
- Treatment must begin as early as possible for it to be effective.
- Limited information on efficacy and safety in animals
- Use in veterinary medicine is controversial due to public health concerns.
- Expense may be an issue, especially when treating horses.

Uses/Indications

Oseltamivir has been suggested as a treatment for canine parvovirus infections. In a small, prospective, randomized, blinded, placebo-controlled clinical trial of 35 dogs with parvovirus, 19 were treated with oseltamivir.[1] Although the oseltamivir group showed statistically significant differences in weight gain and maintenance of white blood cell count compared with untreated dogs, no significant decreases in hospitalization time, treatments needed, clinical scores, morbidity, or mortality were seen. Another study in 50 dogs also found no significant reduction in mortality or morbidity.[2]

Oseltamivir may be beneficial for adjunctive treatment of other viral infections, particularly those with associated secondary bacterial components, but evidence and experience are lacking. One small study in horses experimentally infected with equine influenza A (H3N8) documented some efficacy in the attenuation of pyrexia, viral shedding, and secondary bacterial pneumonia.[3] Oseltamivir given to swine prior to H1N2 exposure prevented clinical signs and significantly reduced virus shedding.[4]

Because oseltamivir is the primary antiviral agent proposed for treatment or prophylaxis for influenza in humans, its use in veterinary patients is controversial. Concerns include adequate drug supply for the human population and the potential for the development of viral resistance. Extra-label use of oseltamivir and other influenza antivirals in chickens, turkeys, and ducks is prohibited by the FDA.[5]

Pharmacology/Actions

Oseltamivir phosphate is a prodrug that is hydrolyzed after absorption into its active form, oseltamivir carboxylate. Oseltamivir carboxylate competitively inhibits influenza virus neuraminidase, an enzyme that is required for viral replication, release of virus from infected cells, and the prevention of formation of viral aggregates after release from cells. Resistance to oseltamivir has been induced in the laboratory and from posttreatment isolates from infected humans.

It has been postulated that oseltamivir may limit the ability of canine parvovirus to pass through the intestinal mucosa and infect intestinal crypt cells. There is some evidence that oseltamivir has this effect (increased mucous inactivation) on influenza viruses in the respiratory tract of humans. It may also reduce GI bacteria colonization, translocation, and toxin production.

Pharmacokinetics

No information was located for the pharmacokinetic profiles of oseltamivir in dogs or cats.

The pharmacokinetics of oseltamivir and the active metabolite (oseltamivir carboxylate) were evaluated in horses.[6] After NG administration of a 2 mg/kg dose, the drug was rapidly absorbed with peak concentrations attained between 1 and 2 hours postdose. The elimination half-life was ≈2 hours for oseltamivir and 2.5 hours for oseltamivir carboxylate. At 2 mg/kg, it was concluded that the dosing interval should be less than 10 hours to maintain concentrations above the inhibitory concentrations of equine influenza A viruses.

In humans, oseltamivir phosphate is readily absorbed and converted into the active carboxylate metabolite predominantly via liver esterases. The bioavailability of oseltamivir carboxylate is ≈75%, and it is minimally bound to plasma proteins. Elimination of oseltamivir carboxylate is primarily via renal mechanisms, including both glomerular filtration and tubular secretion. The elimination half-life is ≈6 to 10 hours in patients with normal renal function. Up to 20% of a dose may be eliminated in the feces.

Neither oseltamivir nor oseltamivir carboxylate act as substrates or inhibitors for any CYP-450 isoenzymes.

Contraindications/Precautions/Warnings

Oseltamivir is contraindicated in patients with documented hypersensitivity to it.[7] Treatment must begin as early as possible for it to be effective; delay in treatment beyond 40 hours after the onset of clinical signs in humans with influenza is associated with minimal efficacy. Dosage adjustments may be needed in patients with impaired renal function.

In humans, anaphylaxis and skin reactions have been reported.[7]

Extra-label use of oseltamivir and other influenza antivirals in chickens, turkeys, and ducks is prohibited by the FDA.[5]

Oseltamivir is not recommended for the treatment of canine influenza at this time, as it represents a primary line of defense against a human influenza pandemic.

Adverse Effects

The adverse effect profile in animals is not known. In small canine and equine studies, no major adverse effects were noted in the treatment groups.[1,3]

In humans, the most common adverse effects are nausea and vomiting. GI effects are usually transient and may be alleviated by giving the medication with food. Serious skin reactions (eg, erythema multiforme, toxic epidermal necrolysis) have also been reported.

Reproductive/Nursing Safety

Oseltamivir has not been shown to increase the risk for adverse outcomes during pregnancy. In humans, it is the preferred agent during pregnancy because it has the most evidence to suggest safety and benefit. Oseltamivir and oseltamivir carboxylate have been detected in milk, but adverse events have not been reported in breastfed infants.

Because safety has not been established in animals, this drug should only be used when the maternal benefits outweigh the potential risks to offspring.

Overdose/Acute Toxicity

Oseltamivir has relatively low toxic potential. In humans, overdoses of up to 1000 mg have caused only nausea and vomiting.

In studies where neonatal rats were administered oseltamivir 1 g/kg, concentrations of the prodrug in the brain were 1500 times greater, and the active metabolite was 3 times higher than those found in adult rats. Potentially, newborn puppies could exhibit similar findings; neurotoxicity is a possibility.

For patients that have experienced or are suspected to have experienced an overdose, consultation with a 24-hour poison consultation center specializing in providing veterinary-specific information is recommended. For general information related to overdose and toxin exposures, as well as contact information for poison control centers, refer to ***Appendix***.

Drug Interactions

The following drug interactions have either been reported or are theoretical in humans or animals receiving oseltamivir and may be of significance in veterinary patients. Unless otherwise noted, use together is not necessarily contraindicated, but weigh the potential risks and perform additional monitoring when appropriate.

- **PROBENECID**: May increase 2-fold the exposure to the active metabolite, oseltamivir carboxylate, by reducing tubular secretion. This could potentially be useful in reducing drug doses or dosing frequency or increasing serum concentrations at the usual dosage; however, supporting data are not readily available.
- **VACCINES, INFLUENZA (live)**: Oseltamivir may potentially reduce the immune response to live influenza virus vaccines. There does not appear to be any effect on inactivated (killed) vaccines.
- **WARFARIN**: May increase risk for bleeding

Laboratory Considerations

- None noted

Dosages

DOGS:

Adjunctive treatment of canine parvovirus enteritis (extra-label): 2 mg/kg PO every 12 hours for 5 days was used in one small study but did not significantly reduce morbidity or mortality.[1]

HORSES:

Treatment of equine influenza A (extra-label): 2 mg/kg PO twice daily for 5 days was used in a small experimental study based on human pediatric dosages, not equine pharmacokinetic or pharmacodynamic data.[3]

Prophylaxis of equine influenza A (extra-label): 2 mg/kg PO once daily for 5 days was experimentally studied; however, it was concluded that a different dose or longer administration may provide better prophylaxis.[3]

Monitoring

- Efficacy

Client Information

- This medicine has not been commonly used in animals. It is not known how well this medicine works and how safe it is to use in animals. Contact your veterinarian if your animal has any side effects of concern.

Chemistry/Synonyms

Oseltamivir phosphate occurs as a white crystalline solid that is freely soluble in water, soluble in propylene glycol, and slightly soluble in alcohol.

Oseltamivir phosphate may also be known as GS-4104/002, or Ro-64-0796/002 and *Tamiflu*®.

Storage/Stability

Store oseltamivir capsules at 25°C (77°F), with excursions permitted from 15°C to 30°C (59°F-86°F). Store the oral powder for reconstitution between 15°C and 30°C (59°F-86°F). Once reconstituted with

55 mL of water, it may be stored at room temperature (15°C-30°C [59°F-86°F]) for 10 days or in the refrigerator (2°C-8°C [36°F-46°F]) for 17 days. Protect this product from freezing.

Compatibility/Compounding Considerations

An extemporaneously compounded oral suspension (6 mg/mL) may be made using the commercially available capsules with cherry syrup, simple syrup, or *OraSweet® SF* when the commercially available oral suspension product is in short supply.[7] The compounded suspension is stable for 5 days at room temperature, and for 5 weeks if refrigerated.

Dosage Forms/Regulatory Status

VETERINARY-LABELED PRODUCTS: NONE

Extra-label use of oseltamivir and other influenza antivirals in chickens, turkeys, and ducks is prohibited by the FDA.[5]

HUMAN-LABELED PRODUCTS:

Oseltamivir Phosphate Oral Capsules: 30 mg, 45 mg, and 75 mg; *Tamiflu®*; (Rx)

Oseltamivir Phosphate Powder for Oral Suspension: 6 mg/mL after reconstitution in 60 mL bottles; *Tamiflu®*; (Rx)

References

For the complete list of references, see **wiley.com/go/budde/plumb**

Oxacillin

(ox-a-***sill***-in) *Bactocill®*

Anti-Staphylococcal Penicillin

Prescriber Highlights

- Penicillinase-resistant penicillin that is rarely used therapeutically; only parenteral dosage forms are available in the United States.
- Oxacillin resistance is a marker for methicillin-resistance in staphylococci.
- Predominant adverse effects are GI in nature.

Uses/Indications

Oxacillin has been primarily used in veterinary medicine for the treatment of bone, skin, and other soft tissue infections in small animal species when penicillinase-producing *Staphylococcus* spp have been isolated. It is rarely used due to frequency of dosing and lack of oral dosage forms.

Pharmacology/Actions

Oxacillin, cloxacillin, and dicloxacillin are penicillinase-resistant penicillins. They have a nearly identical spectrum of activity and can be considered therapeutically equivalent when comparing in vitro activity. Penicillinase-resistant penicillins have a narrower overall spectrum of activity than the natural penicillins (penicillin G, penicillin V); however, unlike the natural penicillins, they are effective against penicillinase-producing bacteria. Their antimicrobial efficacy is aimed directly against penicillinase-producing strains of gram-positive cocci, particularly staphylococcal species, and they are sometimes referred to as anti-staphylococcal penicillins.

Oxacillin resistance is a marker for methicillin resistance in staphylococci. Although this class of penicillins does have activity against some other gram-positive and gram-negative aerobes and anaerobes, other antibiotics are usually better choices. Oxacillin is inactive against rickettsial organisms, mycobacteria, fungi, *Mycoplasma* spp, and viruses.

Pharmacokinetics

Although oxacillin sodium is resistant to acid inactivation in the gut, it is only partially absorbed after oral administration. The bioavailability after oral administration in humans has been reported to range from 30% to 35%. Both the rate and extent of absorption are decreased when given with food. In humans, oxacillin is rapidly absorbed after IM administration and peak concentrations generally occur within 30 minutes.[1]

Oxacillin is distributed to the lungs, kidneys, bone, bile, pleural fluid, synovial fluid, and ascitic fluid. The volume of distribution is reportedly 0.3 L/kg in dogs and 0.4 L/kg in humans. As with other penicillins, CSF penetration is limited but increased with meningeal inflammation. In humans, ≈89% to 94% of the drug is bound to plasma proteins.[1]

Oxacillin is partially metabolized to both active and inactive metabolites. These metabolites and the parent compound are rapidly excreted in the urine via both glomerular filtration and tubular secretion mechanisms. A small amount of the drug is also excreted in the feces via biliary elimination. The serum half-life in humans with normal renal function ranges from ≈18 to 48 minutes. In dogs, the reported elimination half-life is 20 to 30 minutes.

Contraindications/Precautions/Warnings

Penicillins are contraindicated in patients with a history of hypersensitivity to them. Because cross-reactivity is possible, use with caution in patients that have documented hypersensitivity to other beta-lactam antibiotics (eg, cephalosporins, carbapenems).

Adverse Effects

Adverse effects of penicillins are generally mild. Hypersensitivity reactions are possible, including rash, fever, eosinophilia, neutropenia, agranulocytosis, thrombocytopenia, leukopenia, anemias, lymphadenopathy, or anaphylaxis. In humans, it is estimated that 1% to 15% of patients hypersensitive to cephalosporins will also be hypersensitive to penicillins. The incidence of cross-reactivity in veterinary patients is unknown.

After oral administration, penicillins may cause GI effects (eg, anorexia, vomiting, diarrhea). Because the penicillins may also alter gut flora, antibiotic-associated diarrhea can occur and allow the proliferation of resistant bacteria in the colon (superinfections).

Neurotoxicity (eg, ataxia in dogs) has been associated with high doses or prolonged use. Although the penicillins are not considered hepatotoxic, elevated liver enzymes have been reported. Other effects reported in dogs include tachypnea, dyspnea, edema, and tachycardia.

Reproductive/Nursing Safety

Reproduction studies in mice, rats, and rabbits using penicillinase-resistant penicillins have not revealed evidence of impaired fertility or teratogenic effects; however, penicillins have been shown to cross the placenta and safe use during pregnancy has not been firmly established.[1]

Penicillins are excreted in maternal milk in low concentrations; use may cause diarrhea, candidiasis, or allergic response in nursing offspring.

Because safety has not been established in animals, this drug should only be used when the maternal benefits outweigh the potential risks to offspring.

Overdose/Acute Toxicity

Acute oral penicillin overdoses are unlikely to cause significant effects other than GI distress, but other effects are possible (see ***Adverse Effects***). In humans, high doses of parenteral penicillins have resulted in CNS effects, especially in patients with renal disease.[1]

For patients that have experienced or are suspected to have experienced an overdose, consultation with a 24-hour poison consultation center specializing in providing veterinary-specific information is recommended. For general information related to overdose and

toxin exposures, as well as contact information for poison control centers, refer to ***Appendix.***

Drug Interactions

The following drug interactions have either been reported or are theoretical in humans or animals receiving oxacillin and may be of significance in veterinary patients. Unless otherwise noted, use together is not necessarily contraindicated, but weigh the potential risks and perform additional monitoring when appropriate.

- **Aminoglycosides**: In vitro evidence of synergism with oxacillin against staphylococci
- **Probenecid**: May increase oxacillin concentrations by competitively inhibiting the tubular secretion of oxacillin
- **Tetracyclines**: Theoretical antagonism; use together typically not recommended
- **Warfarin**: Oxacillin may cause decreased warfarin efficacy.

Laboratory Considerations

Penicillinase-resistant penicillins may interfere with or cause false-positive results in a variety of test methods used to determine urinary or serum proteins.

Dosages

NOTE: Oxacillin is rarely used due to availability of other licensed and/or proven therapies. It is only available commercially in the US as a parenteral injection. Dicloxacillin capsules may be substituted for oxacillin for oral therapy.

DOGS/CATS:

Susceptible infections (extra-label): 22 – 40 mg/kg SC, IM, or IV every 8 hours[2]

HORSES:

Susceptible infections in foals (extra-label): 20 – 30 mg/kg IV every 6 to 8 hours (Dose extrapolated from adult horse data; use lower dose or longer interval in premature foals or those less than 7 days old)[3,4]

Monitoring

- Clinical efficacy
- Adverse effects (eg, GI signs, hypersensitivity reactions)

Client Information

- This medication is only available as an injection. Be sure you understand how to give this medicine to your animal.
- The most common side effects of this medicine are mild in nature but may include a decrease in appetite, vomiting, and diarrhea. Contact your veterinarian if you have any concerns about your animal.

Chemistry/Synonyms

Oxacillin sodium is a semi-synthetic, penicillinase-resistant, isoxazolyl-penicillin. It is available commercially as the monohydrate sodium salt, which occurs as a fine, white, crystalline powder that is odorless or has a slight odor. It is freely soluble in water and has a pK_a of ≈2.8. One milligram of oxacillin sodium contains not less than 815 to 950 µg of oxacillin. Each gram of the commercially available powder for injection contains 2.8 to 3.1 mEq of sodium.

Oxacillin sodium may also be known as sodium oxacillin, methylphenyl isoxazolyl penicillin, (5-methyl-3-phenyl-4-isoxazolyl) penicillin sodium, oxacillinum natricum, oxacillinum natrium, P-12, SQ-16423, or *Bactocill®*.

Storage/Stability

Store oxacillin sodium powder for injection at room temperature (15°C-30°C [59°F-86°F]).

Powder for injection reconstituted with sterile water to 167 mg/mL for IM injection is stable for 3 days at room temperature or 7 days if refrigerated.[1] Quantity of diluent depends on route of administration; stability of IV solutions depends on the diluent used, storage temperature, and final concentration; refer to the package insert for specific instructions.

Compatibility/Compounding Considerations

Compatibility is dependent on factors such as pH, concentration, temperature, and diluent used; specialized references or a hospital pharmacist should be consulted for more specific information.

Oxacillin sodium injection is reportedly physically **compatible** with the following fluids/drugs: 5% and 10% dextrose in water, 5% and 10% dextrose in 0.9% sodium chloride 0.9%, lactated Ringer's injection, cefazolin, chloramphenicol sodium succinate, dopamine HCl, famotidine, metoclopramide, midazolam, and potassium chloride.

Oxacillin sodium injection is reportedly physically **incompatible** with the following fluids/drugs: calcium salts, oxytetracycline HCl, and tetracycline HCl. As penicillins can inactivate aminoglycosides *in vitro*, they should never be mixed together in the same syringe or administration set.

Dosage Forms/Regulatory Status

VETERINARY-LABELED PRODUCTS: NONE

HUMAN-LABELED PRODUCTS:

Oxacillin Sodium Powder for Injection: 1 g, 2 g, and 10 g; generic; (Rx)

References

For the complete list of references, see **wiley.com/go/budde/plumb**

Oxazepam

(ox-***a***-ze-pam) *Serax®*

Benzodiazepine

Prescriber Highlights

- Benzodiazepine used primarily as an appetite stimulant in cats, but may also be useful to treat behavior problems in dogs and cats
- Contraindications include known benzodiazepine hypersensitivity and acute narrow-angle glaucoma.
- Use with caution in animals with myasthenia gravis, hepatic dysfunction, or seizure disorders.
- Sedation is the primary adverse effect; ataxia is occasionally seen.
- DEA Schedule IV (C-IV) controlled substance

Uses/Indications

Oxazepam is used most frequently in small animal medicine as an appetite stimulant in cats. It may also be useful as an oral anxiolytic agent for adjunctive therapy of behavior-related disorders for both dogs and cats. Like lorazepam, it does not have any active metabolites so it may be a good choice for treating geriatric patients and those with liver dysfunction. However, use in feline patients is controversial, as fulminant hepatic failure has been anecdotally reported.

Pharmacology/Actions

Oxazepam is classified as an intermediate acting benzodiazepine. The subcortical levels (primarily limbic, thalamic, and hypothalamic) of the CNS are depressed by oxazepam and other benzodiazepines, thus producing the anxiolytic, sedative, skeletal muscle relaxant and anticonvulsant effects seen. The exact mechanism of action is unknown, but postulated mechanisms include antagonism of serotonin, increased release of gamma-aminobutyric acid (GABA) and/or facilitation of GABA activity, and diminished release or turnover of acetylcholine in the CNS. Benzodiazepine-specific receptors have been located in the mammalian brain, kidney, liver, lung, and heart. In all species studied, receptors were lacking in the white matter.

Pharmacokinetics

Oxazepam is absorbed from the GI tract, but it is one of the more slowly absorbed oral benzodiazepines. Oxazepam, like other benzodiazepines, is widely distributed and is highly bound to plasma proteins (97% in humans). Although not confirmed, oxazepam may cross the placenta and enter maternal milk. Oxazepam is principally conjugated in the liver via glucuronidation to an inactive metabolite. Serum half-life in humans ranges from 3 to 21 hours.

Contraindications/Precautions/Warnings

Oxazepam is contraindicated in patients that are hypersensitive to it or other benzodiazepines and in those with acute narrow-angle glaucoma. Caution is advised when using oxazepam in animals that have hepatic or renal disease; that are comatose or in shock; that have respiratory depression; or that are debilitated, obese, or geriatric. Although oxazepam is less susceptible to accumulation than many other benzodiazepines in patients with hepatic dysfunction, it should still be used with caution.

Use of oxazepam in feline patients is controversial, as anecdotal fulminant hepatic failure in cats has rarely been reported.

Adverse Effects

The most common adverse effect seen with oxazepam in small animal species is sedation. Ataxia is also seen occasionally. Adverse effects may be transient, and dosage adjustment may be required to alleviate them. Paradoxical effects such as excitability, vocalization, or aggression are possible. When oxazepam is used to treat negative behaviors, a rebound effect can occur, particularly if the drug is not withdrawn slowly.

Reproductive/Nursing Safety

Safe use of oxazepam during pregnancy has not been established; teratogenic effects of similar benzodiazepines have been noted in rabbits and rats. In humans, mild tranquilizers have been associated with increased risk for congenital malformations when used in the first trimester.[1]

Benzodiazepines are excreted in maternal milk. Neonates metabolize benzodiazepines more slowly than adults do, and accumulation of toxic levels of the drug and its metabolites is possible. Long-term diazepam use in nursing mothers has reportedly caused lethargy and weight loss in human infants; avoid the use of benzodiazepines in nursing patients.

Because safety has not been established in animals, this drug should only be used when the maternal benefits outweigh the potential risks to offspring.

Overdose/Acute Toxicity

When oxazepam is used alone, overdoses are generally limited to significant CNS depression (eg, confusion, coma, decreased reflexes). Treatment of significant oral oxazepam overdoses consists of standard GI decontamination protocols and supportive therapy based on clinical presentation. CNS stimulants such as caffeine or amphetamines are generally not recommended. Flumazenil could potentially be used in life-threatening overdoses.

For patients that have experienced or are suspected to have experienced an overdose, consultation with a 24-hour poison consultation center specializing in providing veterinary-specific information is recommended. For general information related to overdose and toxin exposures, as well as contact information for poison control centers, refer to ***Appendix.***

Drug Interactions

The following drug interactions have either been reported or are theoretical in humans or animals receiving oxazepam and may be of significance in veterinary patients. Unless otherwise noted, use together is not necessarily contraindicated, but weigh the potential risks and perform additional monitoring when appropriate.

- CNS DEPRESSANTS (eg, **anesthetics, barbiturates, opioids**): Additive CNS depressant effects may occur.
- METOCLOPRAMIDE: May increase risk for CNS depression
- MIRTAZAPINE: May increase risk for somnolence
- PROBENECID: May impair glucuronide conjugation in dogs and prolong effects
- RIFAMPIN: May induce hepatic microsomal enzymes and decrease the pharmacologic effects of benzodiazepines
- ST. JOHN'S WORT: May decrease oxazepam effectiveness
- THEOPHYLLINE, AMINOPHYLLINE: May decrease oxazepam effectiveness

Laboratory Considerations

- Benzodiazepines may decrease the thyroidal uptake of I^{123} or I^{131}.

Dosages

NOTE: Because 10 mg capsules are the smallest dosage form available, compounded dosage forms may be required for cats and smaller dogs.

DOGS:

Fears and phobias (extra-label): Anecdotally, 0.2 – 1 mg/kg PO every 12 to 24 hours. Dosage recommendations vary and no published evidence supporting one dose over the other was located.

CATS:

Appetite stimulation or behavior-related conditions (extra-label): Anecdotally, 0.2 – 0.5 mg/kg PO every 12 to 24 hours. Dosage recommendations vary and no published evidence supporting one dose over the other was located.

Monitoring

- Efficacy
- Adverse effects
- Consider baseline and period serum liver chemistry panels with long-term administration

Client Information

- When using this medicine for thunderstorm phobias or other triggers (eg, separation anxiety), try to give it about an hour before the event or trigger.
- If you see yellowing of the whites of the eyes, gums, or skin, contact your veterinarian immediately.
- Sleepiness is the most common side effect, but sometimes this medicine can change behavior or cause unexpected excitement.
- This medicine may increase appetite, especially in cats.
- Contact your veterinarian immediately if your animal stops eating or has a low-energy level.
- Oxazepam is classified as a Schedule IV (C-IV) controlled drug by the federal Drug Enforcement Agency (DEA). Use of this medication in animals or humans other than those for whom it is prescribed is illegal.

Chemistry/Synonyms

Oxazepam is a benzodiazepine that occurs as a creamy white to pale-yellow powder. It is practically insoluble in water.

Oxazepam may also be known as oxazepamum, Wy-3498, or *Serax®*.

Storage/Stability

Store oxazepam capsules and tablets at room temperature, 20°C to 25°C (68°F-77°F), in well-closed containers.

Oxazepam is a DEA Schedule IV (C-IV) controlled substance that should be stored in an area that is substantially constructed and securely locked. Follow applicable local, state, and federal rules regarding disposal of unused or wasted controlled drugs.

Dosage Forms/Regulatory Status

VETERINARY-LABELED PRODUCTS: NONE

The Association of Racing Commissioners International (ARCI) has designated this drug as a class 2 substance. Use of this drug may not be allowed in certain animal competitions. Check rules and regulations before entering in a competition while this medication is being administered. Contact local racing authorities for further guidance. See ***Appendix*** for more information.

HUMAN-LABELED PRODUCTS:

Oxazepam Capsules: 10 mg, 15 mg, and 30 mg; generic; (Rx; C-IV). Report dispensing to state monitoring programs where required.

References

For the complete list of references, see **wiley.com/go/budde/plumb**

Oxfendazole

(ox-***fen***-da-zole) *Synanthic*®

Antiparasitic Agent (Anthelmintic)

Prescriber Highlights

- ▶ Benzimidazole anthelmintic used primarily in cattle
- ▶ Contraindicated for use in female dairy cattle of breeding age
- ▶ Use caution in debilitated or sick horses
- ▶ Adverse effects appear unlikely; hypersensitivity possible

Uses/Indications

Oxfendazole (*Synanthic*®) is indicated in cattle for the removal and control of lungworms, stomach worms, intestinal worms (including inhibited forms of *Ostertagia ostertagi*), and tapeworms. See product label for specific parasite species covered for the indication.

In swine, oxfendazole has demonstrated activity against nematodes (*Ascaris suum, Oesophagostomum* spp, *Trichuris suis, Metastrongylus* spp) and liver flukes (*Fasciola hepatica*).

Oxfendazole, marketed as *Benzelmin*®, was indicated (no longer marketed in the US) for the removal of the following parasites in horses: large roundworms (*Parascaris equorum*), large strongyles (*Strongylus edentatus, Strongylus equinus, Strongylus vulgaris*), small strongyles, and pinworms (*Oxyuris equi*).

Oxfendazole has shown efficacy in sheep and goats[1] and is approved for use in sheep in the UK.[2]

Pharmacology/Actions

Benzimidazole antiparasitic agents have a broad spectrum of activity against a variety of pathogenic internal parasites. In susceptible parasites, their mechanism of action is believed to be due to disrupting intracellular microtubular transport systems by binding selectively and damaging tubulin, preventing tubulin polymerization, and inhibiting microtubule formation. Benzimidazoles also act at higher concentrations to disrupt metabolic pathways within the helminth and inhibit metabolic enzymes, including malate dehydrogenase and fumarate reductase.

Pharmacokinetics

Limited information is available regarding this compound's pharmacokinetics. Unlike most of the other benzimidazole compounds, oxfendazole is absorbed more readily from the GI tract. The elimination half-life has been reported to be ≈7.5 hours in sheep and 5.25 hours in goats. Absorbed oxfendazole is metabolized to oxfendazole sulfone (inactive).

After a single oral dose of 50 mg/kg to dogs, oxfendazole levels peaked at 8 hours. The elimination half-lives for the parent compound and the sulfoxide metabolite (active) were both ≈5.5 hours. In dogs, oxfendazole plasma concentrations were significantly higher and resident times longer than that of either fenbendazole or albendazole following single oral administration at the same dose (50 mg/kg).[3]

Contraindications/Precautions/Warnings

Oxfendazole is not for use in female dairy cattle of breeding age.

There are no contraindications to using this drug in horses, but it is recommended to use oxfendazole cautiously in debilitated or sick horses.

Adverse Effects

When used as labeled, it is unlikely that any adverse effects will be noted. Hypersensitivity reactions secondary to antigen release by dying parasites are theoretically possible, particularly at high dosages.

Reproductive/Nursing Safety

Oxfendazole may be safely used in pregnant mares and foals. It is not labeled for use in female dairy cattle of breeding age.

Overdose/Acute Toxicity

Doses of 10 times the recommended dose elicited no adverse reactions in horses tested. It is unlikely that this compound would cause serious toxicity when given alone.

For patients that have experienced or are suspected of having experienced an overdose, consultation with a 24-hour poison consultation center specializing in providing veterinary-specific information is recommended. For general information related to overdose and toxin exposures, as well as contact information for poison control centers, refer to ***Appendix***.

Drug Interactions

The following drug interactions have either been reported or are theoretical in humans or animals receiving oxfendazole and may be of significance in veterinary patients. Unless otherwise noted, use together is not necessarily contraindicated, but weigh the potential risks and perform additional monitoring when appropriate.

- **Bromsalan Flukicides** (eg, **dibromsalan**, **tribromsalan**): Oxfendazole should not be given concurrently with these agents; abortions in cattle and death in sheep have been reported after using these compounds together.

Dosages

NOTE: Ensure animals receive a complete dose based on a current and accurate estimate of weight. Underdosing may result in ineffective treatment and promote parasite resistance.

HORSES:

Susceptible parasites: 10 mg/kg PO.[4] **NOTE**: No longer marketed

CATTLE:

Removal and control of lungworms, roundworms (including inhibited forms of *Ostertagia ostertagi*), and tapeworms. See product label for the specific parasite species covered for the indication (label dose; FDA-approved): 4.5 mg/kg PO. May repeat in 4 to 6 weeks.[5]

SWINE:

Adult stages of *Ascaris suum, Oesophagostomum* spp, *Trichuris suis, Metastrongylus* spp, and ***Fasciola hepatica*** (extra-label): 30 mg/kg PO once[6,7]

SHEEP/GOATS:

GI nematodes (extra-label): 5 mg/kg PO once [1,2]

Monitoring

- Efficacy, including fecal examination/FECRT

Client Information

- Do not use in horses intended for food purposes.
- Shake suspension well immediately before use.
- Administer oxfendazole oral suspension using an accurate dose syringe.

- Slaughter withdrawal in cattle is 7 days; not FDA-approved for lactating dairy cattle.

Chemistry/Synonyms

Oxfendazole, a benzimidazole anthelmintic, occurs as white or almost white powder possessing a characteristic odor. It is practically insoluble in water. Oxfendazole is the active sulfoxide metabolite of fenbendazole.

Oxfendazole may also be known as RS 8858; there are many international trade names.

Storage/Stability

Store this product at or below 25°C (77°F). Brief excursions up to 30°C (86°F) are permitted. Do not freeze.

Dosage Forms/Regulatory Status

VETERINARY-LABELED PRODUCTS:

Oxfendazole Oral Suspension: 9.06% in 1 L and 4 L; *Synanthic®*; (OTC). FDA-approved for use in beef cattle and female dairy cattle not of breeding age. Because a withdrawal time in milk has not been established, do not use in female dairy cattle of breeding age. At recommended dosages, slaughter withdrawal is 7 days.

Oxfendazole Oral Suspension: 22.5% in 500 mL and 1 L; *Synanthic®*; (OTC). FDA-approved for use in beef cattle and female dairy cattle not of breeding age. Because a withdrawal time in milk has not been established, do not use in female dairy cattle of breeding age. At recommended dosages, slaughter withdrawal is 7 days.

HUMAN-LABELED PRODUCTS: NONE

References

For the complete list of references, see **wiley.com/go/budde/plumb**

Oxibendazole

(ox-i-**ben**-da-zole) *Anthelcide EQ®*

Antiparasitic Agent

Prescriber Highlights

- ► Benzimidazole anthelmintic used primarily in horses
- ► Resistance development is an ongoing concern.
- ► Contraindications include severely debilitated horses or horses suffering from colic, toxemia, or infectious disease.
- ► Adverse effects are uncommon; hypersensitivity is possible.

Uses/Indications

Oxibendazole is FDA-approved in horses for the removal and control of large roundworms (*Parascaris equorum*), large strongyles (*Strongylus edentatus, S equinus, S vulgaris*), small strongyles (various genera), threadworms, and pinworms (*Oxyuris equi*). Resistance to antiparasitic agents is an ongoing concern. Fecal egg count reduction testing (FECRT) is recommended for strongyle nematodes. A value of less than 90% in 5 to 10 horses is the suggested cut-off for determining resistance on a given farm.[1] One study in horses found that the combination of oxibendazole and pyrantel pamoate demonstrated additive effects in reducing fecal egg counts compared to either drug alone.[2]

Oxibendazole has also been used in rabbits for adjunctive treatment of *Encephalitozoon cuniculi*.

Pharmacology/Actions

Benzimidazole antiparasitic agents have a broad spectrum of activity against a variety of pathogenic internal parasites. In susceptible parasites, their mechanism of action disrupts intracellular microtubular transport systems by binding tubulin, preventing tubulin polymerization, and inhibiting microtubule formation. Benzimidazoles are also believed to act at higher concentrations to disrupt metabolic pathways within the helminth, and inhibit metabolic enzymes, including malate dehydrogenase and fumarate reductase.

Pharmacokinetics

No information was located.

Contraindications/Precautions/Warnings

Oxibendazole is contraindicated in severely debilitated horses and horses suffering from colic, toxemia, or infectious disease.[3]

Treatment with oxibendazole should be in conjunction with parasite management practices to help prevent parasite resistance.[3] Do not underdose, as underdosing can result in ineffective treatment and encourage development of resistance.

Do not use in horses intended for human consumption.

Adverse Effects

At recommended doses, adverse effects in horses are uncommon. Hypersensitivity reactions are theoretically possible secondary to antigen release by dying parasites, particularly at high doses.

Oxibendazole in combination with diethylcarbamazine (*Filaribits Plus®*) was implicated in causing periportal hepatitis in dogs when it was marketed (1980s).

Myelosuppression has been reported in rabbits.[4]

Reproductive/Nursing Safety

Oxibendazole is considered safe to use in pregnant mares.

Overdose/Acute Toxicity

Doses of 60 times those recommended on the product label elicited no adverse reactions in horses tested. Serious toxicity from overdose of oxibendazole alone is unlikely in horses.

For patients that have experienced or are suspected to have experienced an overdose, consultation with a 24-hour poison consultation center specializing in providing veterinary-specific information is recommended. For general information related to overdose and toxin exposures, as well as contact information for poison control centers, refer to ***Appendix.***

Drug Interactions

- No significant interactions have been reported.

Dosages

HORSES:

Removal and control of susceptible parasites other than threadworms (label dosage; FDA-approved): 10 mg/kg PO once.[3] Re-treat in 6 to 8 weeks if reinfection is likely.

Removal and control of *Strongyloides westeri* (threadworms; label dosage; FDA-approved): 15 mg/kg PO once.[3] Re-treat in 6 to 8 weeks if reinfection is likely.

RABBITS:

Adjunctive treatment of *E cuniculi* (extra-label): Published evidence is limited; suggested dosage is 30 mg/kg PO once daily for 7 to 14 days, then 15 mg/kg once daily for 30 to 60 days. For palliative treatment of larval migrans, 60 mg/kg PO once daily indefinitely has been suggested.[5]

Monitoring

- Efficacy (eg, fecal egg count reduction test)
- For rabbits, consider baseline CBC prior to treatment and 14 days later.

Client Information

- Protect suspension from freezing.
- Not for use in horses intended for food.
- Side effects are uncommon.

Chemistry/Synonyms

Oxibendazole is a benzimidazole anthelmintic that occurs as a white powder and is practically insoluble in water.

Oxibendazole may also be known as SKF-30310 and *Anthelcide EQ®* and in the UK by the proprietary names: *Dio®*, *Equidin®*, *Equitac®* or *Loditac®*.

Storage/Stability

Oxibendazole oral paste should be stored at controlled room temperature 15°–30°C (59°–86°F) and protected from freezing.

Dosage Forms/Regulatory Status

VETERINARY-LABELED PRODUCTS:

Oxibendazole Oral Paste: 227 mg/g (22.7%) in 24-g syringes. *Anthelcide EQ® Paste*; (OTC). FDA-approved for use in horses not intended for food. NADA# 121-042

HUMAN-LABELED PRODUCTS: NONE

References

For the complete list of references, see **wiley.com/go/budde/plumb**

Oxybutynin

(ox-i-***byoo***-tin-in) *Ditropan®, Oxytrol®*

Genitourinary Smooth Muscle Relaxant

Prescriber Highlights

- ► Urinary antispasmodic potentially useful in dogs or cats
- ► Use with caution (risk vs benefit) in animals with obstructive GI tract disease, gastric retention or conditions that decrease intestinal motility, gastroesophageal reflux, angle closure glaucoma, hiatal hernia, cardiac disease (particularly associated with mitral stenosis, associated arrhythmias, tachycardia, CHF), myasthenia gravis, hyperthyroidism, prostatic hypertrophy, severe ulcerative colitis, urinary retention, or other obstructive uropathies.
- ► Adverse effects include diarrhea, constipation, urinary retention, dry mouth, hypersalivation, and sedation.

Uses/Indications

Oxybutynin may be useful for the adjunctive therapy of detrusor hyperreflexia in dogs and in cats with FeLV-associated detrusor instability.

Pharmacology/Actions

Considered a urinary antispasmodic, oxybutynin has direct antimuscarinic (atropine-like) and spasmolytic (papaverine-like) effects on smooth muscle. Spasmolytic effects appear to be most predominant on the detrusor muscle of the bladder and small and large intestine. It does not have appreciable effects on vascular smooth muscle. In humans with neurogenic bladders, oxybutynin increases bladder capacity, reduces the frequency of uninhibited contractions of the detrusor muscle, and delays the initial desire to void.[1] Effects were more pronounced in patients with uninhibited neurogenic bladders than in patients with reflex neurogenic bladders. Other effects noted in laboratory animal studies include moderate antihistaminic, local anesthetic, mild analgesic, very low mydriatic, and antisialagogue effects.

Pharmacokinetics

Oxybutynin is rapidly and well absorbed from the GI tract. Studies done in rats show the drug is distributed into the brain, lungs, kidneys, and liver. Although elimination characteristics have not been well documented, oxybutynin apparently is metabolized in the liver and excreted in the urine. In humans, the duration of action is from 6 to 10 hours after a dose.

Contraindications/Precautions/Warnings

Oxybutynin is contraindicated in patients that are hypersensitive to the drug substance or other components of the product.

Because of the drug's pharmacologic actions, oxybutynin should only be used when its benefits outweigh its risks if the following conditions are present: obstructive GI tract disease, gastric retention or conditions that decrease intestinal motility, gastroesophageal reflux, hiatal hernia, severe ulcerative colitis, angle closure glaucoma, cardiac disease (particularly associated with mitral stenosis, associated arrhythmias, tachycardia, CHF), myasthenia gravis, hyperthyroidism, prostatic hypertrophy, or urinary retention or other obstructive uropathies. Use with caution in patients with hepatic impairment.

Adverse Effects

Although use of oxybutynin in small animals is limited, diarrhea, constipation, urinary retention, hypersalivation, and sedation have been reported. Other adverse effects reported in humans, and potentially seen in animals, primarily result from the drug's pharmacologic effects, including dry mouth or eyes, tachycardia, anorexia, vomiting, weakness, or mydriasis.

Reproductive/Nursing Safety

Although safety during pregnancy has not been firmly established, studies in a variety of laboratory animals have demonstrated no teratogenic effect associated with the drug.

It is not known whether this drug is excreted in maternal milk. Although oxybutynin may inhibit lactation, no documented problems associated with its use in nursing offspring have been noted.

Because safety has not been established in animals, this drug should only be used when the maternal benefits outweigh the potential risks to offspring.

Overdose/Acute Toxicity

Overdoses may cause CNS effects (eg, restlessness, excitement, seizures), cardiovascular effects (eg, hyper- or hypotension, tachycardia, circulatory failure), fever, nausea, or vomiting. Massive overdoses may lead to paralysis, coma, respiratory failure, and death. Treatment of overdoses should consist of general techniques to limit absorption of the drug from the GI tract and supportive care as required; IV physostigmine may be useful. See the ***Atropine*** monograph (***Overdoses/Acute Toxicity***) for more information on the use of physostigmine. Oxybutynin is highly protein bound; excessive overdose leading to paralysis or coma would require therapeutic plasma exchange to rapidly remove the drug from the patient.

For patients that have experienced or are suspected of having experienced an overdose, consultation with a 24-hour poison consultation center specializing in providing veterinary-specific information is recommended. For general information related to overdose and toxin exposures, as well as contact information for poison control centers, refer to ***Appendix.***

Drug Interactions

The following drug interactions have either been reported or are theoretical in humans or animals receiving oxybutynin and may be of significance in veterinary patients. Unless otherwise noted, use together is not necessarily contraindicated, but weigh the potential risks and perform additional monitoring when appropriate.

- AMANTADINE: May increase anticholinergic adverse effects of oxybutynin
- ANTICHOLINERGIC AGENTS (eg, **atropine, propantheline, scopolamine, isopropamide, glycopyrrolate, hyoscyamine, tricyclic antidepressants, disopyramide, procainamide, antihistamines**): May intensify oxybutynin's anticholinergic effects
- AZOLE ANTIFUNGALS (eg, **ketoconazole**): May increase oxybutynin concentration
- BENZODIAZEPINES (eg, **diazepam, midazolam**): May exacerbate the sedating effects of oxybutynin
- BETA-RECEPTOR ANTAGONISTS (eg, **atenolol**): Oxybutynin may increase the bioavailability of atenolol.

- **CNS Depressants** (eg, **methocarbamol, trazodone**): Other sedating drugs may exacerbate the sedating effects of oxybutynin.
- **Macrolide Antibiotics** (eg, **erythromycin, clarithromycin**): May increase oxybutynin concentration
- **Opioids** (eg, **buprenorphine, hydrocodone, morphine**): May exacerbate the anticholinergic and sedating effects of oxybutynin

Dosages

NOTE: All dosages are for using regular 5 mg oxybutynin tablets or oral syrup unless otherwise noted. There are also sustained-release tablets for humans and transdermal gels/patches commercially available. No dosages for these products for dogs or cats were found.

DOGS:

Refractory incontinence (detrusor hyperreflexia) (extra-label): 0.2 – 0.3 mg/kg PO every 8 to 12 hours; practically, most dogs are dosed at 1.25 – 5 mg per dog (NOT mg/kg) PO every 8 to 12 hours (¼ to 1 tablet)

CATS:

Refractory incontinence (detrusor hyperreflexia) (extra-label): 0.5 – 1.25 mg per cat (NOT mg/kg) every 8 to 12 hours ≈⅛ to ¼ of a 5 mg tablet)

Monitoring

- Efficacy (eg, frequency of urination)
- Adverse effects (eg, drowsiness/sleepiness, dry mouth, and constipation)

Client Information

- In dogs and cats, oxybutynin is used to help stop bladder spasms that cause leaking of urine.
- Side effects include constipation, urinary retention (ie, trouble urinating), dry mouth, and sedation/drowsiness.
- The most common side effects are drowsiness/sleepiness, dry mouth, and constipation. Diarrhea and hypersalivation are also possible. Be sure your animal has access to fresh water at all times.

Chemistry/Synonyms

Oxybutynin chloride is a synthetic tertiary amine that occurs as white to off-white crystals. It is freely soluble in water.

Oxybutynin chloride may also be known as oxybutinyn HCl, 5058, MJ-4309-1, oxybutynini hydrochloridum, *Ditropan®* and *Oxytrol®*.

Storage/Stability

Tablets and oral solution should be stored in tight, light-resistant containers at room temperature 20°C to 25°C (68°F-77°F); excursions permitted within 15°C to 30°C (59°F-86°F).

Dosage Forms/Regulatory Status

VETERINARY-LABELED PRODUCTS: NONE

HUMAN-LABELED PRODUCTS:

Oxybutynin Chloride Oral Tablets: 5 mg; generic; (Rx)

Oxybutynin Chloride Oral Syrup: 1 mg/mL in 473 mL; generic; (Rx)

Oxybutynin extended-release tablets (*Ditropan® XL*), transdermal system (*Oxytrol®*), and topical gel (*Gelnique®*) also are available.

References

For the complete list of references, see **wiley.com/go/budde/plumb**

Oxymorphone

(ox-ee-***mor***-fone) *Numorphan®*

Opioid Agonist

Prescriber Highlights

- ► Injectable opioid used as a sedative/premedication and analgesic agent
- ► Injectable oxymorphone was discontinued in 2017; ***hydromorphone*** is a commonly used alternative.
- ► DEA Schedule II (C-II) controlled substance

Uses/Indications

Oxymorphone is used in dogs and cats as a sedative and analgesic agent. It is occasionally used in horses as an analgesic and as an induction agent for anesthesia. In swine, oxymorphone is used as an adjunctive analgesic with ketamine and xylazine for anesthesia. Oxymorphone is used in small rodents as an analgesic and anesthetic agent for minor surgical procedures.

Oxymorphone is effective for moderate to severe pain and has minimal effects on the cardiovascular system. Oxymorphone causes less histamine release than morphine.

One study in dogs found that oxymorphone was comparable to hydromorphone in potency and efficacy for pain control and caused less vomiting than hydromorphone.[1]

Pharmacology/Actions

Oxymorphone is a mu-opiate receptor agonist and is ≈10 times more potent than morphine. Opioid receptors are in high concentrations in the limbic system, spinal cord, thalamus, hypothalamus, striatum, and midbrain. The GI tract, urinary tract, and other smooth muscle tissues also contain opioid receptors.

Oxymorphone primarily has activity at mu-opioid receptors and potentially some activity at delta-receptors. Primary pharmacologic effects include analgesia and sedation. In dogs at usual doses, oxymorphone alone has good sedative qualities. Respiratory depression is another primary effect of oxymorphone. Like morphine, oxymorphone initially increases respiratory rates (eg, panting in dogs); however, actual oxygenation may be decreased, and blood CO_2 levels may increase by 10 mm Hg or more. In dogs, oxymorphone may cause more panting and has less antitussive activity than morphine. GI effects include emesis, constipation, defecation, and decreased gut motility with resultant delayed gastric emptying time.

Oxymorphone has many secondary pharmacologic effects. Central nervous system effects include euphoria, sedation, and confusion. Cardiovascular effects include bradycardia due to central vagal stimulation, peripheral vasodilation due to depressed alpha-adrenergic receptors, decreased peripheral resistance, baroreceptor inhibition, orthostatic hypotension, syncope, and slight decreases in cardiac contractility and/or blood pressure. Urinary effects can also occur, including urinary retention due to increased bladder sphincter tone.

Contradictory effects are possible from mu-opioid agonists, including oxymorphone. Morphine administration in dogs may cause defecation rather than the expected effect of constipation. Dogs and humans may develop miosis, whereas cats and some other species may develop mydriasis. Horses, cattle, swine, and cats may develop excitement after morphine administration rather than sedation. However, unlike morphine or meperidine, oxymorphone does not appear to cause histamine release when administered IV and may cause less excitement.

Pharmacokinetics

Oxymorphone is bioavailable after IM, SC, and rectal administration. In humans, oral, bioavailability is ≈10%. After IV administration, analgesic efficacy usually occurs within 3 to 5 minutes.

After oxymorphone 0.1 mg/kg IM administration to dogs, onset of action is ≈15 minutes and duration of effect is 2 to 4 hours.

In cats, oxymorphone exhibits a moderate steady state volume of distribution (≈2.5 L/kg), clearance of ≈26 mL/minute/kg, and a short elimination half-life of ≈1.6 hours.[2] After buccal administration to cats, bioavailability is ≈17%.[3]

Like morphine, oxymorphone concentrates in the kidneys, liver, and lungs with lower concentrations found in the CNS. Oxymorphone crosses the placenta and narcotized newborns can result if mothers are given the drug before giving birth. Effects can be rapidly reversed with naloxone.

The drug is metabolized in the liver primarily by glucuronidation and is excreted by the kidneys.

Contraindications/Precautions/Warnings

Oxymorphone is contraindicated in patients hypersensitive to narcotic analgesics and patients with diarrhea caused by a toxic ingestion (until the toxin is eliminated from the GI tract). Additionally, oxymorphone is considered contraindicated in humans with GI tract obstruction and paralytic ileus. Patients with severe hepatic disease may have prolonged duration of drug action; moderate to severe hepatic impairment is a contraindication in humans.

Because oxymorphone may cause vomiting, use as a preanesthetic medication is generally considered contraindicated in animals with suspected gastric dilation-volvulus, intestinal obstruction, or increased intracerebral and intraocular pressure. Pretreatment with maropitant may help prevent vomiting in dogs medicated with hydromorphone and presumably oxymorphone.[4-7]

Use extreme caution in patients with head injuries, increased intracranial or intraocular pressure, and acute abdominal conditions (eg, colic) as oxymorphone may obscure the diagnosis or clinical course of these conditions. In horses, opioids can mask behavioral and cardiovascular clinical signs associated with mild colic. Use oxymorphone with extreme caution in patients suffering from respiratory disease or acute respiratory dysfunction (eg, pulmonary edema secondary to smoke inhalation).

Use opioids with caution in patients with hypothyroidism, severe renal insufficiency, and hypoadrenocorticism. Use cautiously in geriatric or severely debilitated patients. Neonatal, debilitated, or geriatric patients may be more susceptible to the effects of oxymorphone, including respiratory depression, and may require lower doses. Use cautiously in patients with seizures as oxymorphone, may induce or aggravate seizures. Hypotension following oxymorphone administration may result in decreased cardiac output and blood pressure. Use with caution in hypotensive patients or those in circulatory shock. Oxymorphone can cause bradycardia and should be used cautiously in patients with pre-existing bradyarrhythmias. Use with caution in patients with biliary tract impairment, including acute pancreatitis, as oxymorphone may cause sphincter of Oddi spasm.

At high doses in cats, concurrent administration with a tranquilizing agent is typically recommended with any mu-opioid agonist, as unpredictable behavioral changes may occur.

Opioid analgesics are contraindicated in patients stung by the scorpion species *Centruroides sculpturatus Ewing* and *C gertschi Stahnke* as oxymorphone may potentiate the effect of the venom.[8]

There is an FDA black box warning to call attention to the risk for abuse, respiratory depression, neonatal withdrawal syndrome, and accidental ingestion in humans.

Adverse Effects

In general, oxymorphone has a similar adverse effect profile to hydromorphone or morphine in dogs and cats. Dose-related respiratory depression is possible and is more likely during general anesthesia. Panting can occur but may be less than with hydromorphone, and cough suppression may occur. Secondary to enhanced vagal tone, oxymorphone can cause bradycardia. Although oxymorphone may cause histamine release, it is significantly less than histamine release from morphine and is usually clinically insignificant; however, it may be significant in critically ill animals. Constipation is possible with chronic oxymorphone dosing.

In dogs, adverse effects include vomiting, sedation, panting, whining/vocalization, and defecation. Vomiting, nausea, and defecation reportedly occurs more frequently after SC administration than IV administration. CNS depression may be greater than desired, particularly when treating moderate to severe pain. In dogs, IV constant rate infusions greater than 0.05 mg/kg/hour administered for more than 12 hours may cause sedation and adverse effects severe enough to require rate reduction.[9]

In cats, high doses of oxymorphone may cause ataxia, hyperesthesia, and behavioral changes such as hyperexcitability or aggression. Behavioral changes can be unpredictable, and concomitant tranquilization is recommended.

In horses, opioids may cause CNS excitement and pretreatment (eg, xylazine) is usually administered to reduce CNS behavioral changes.

Humans have an increased tendency to experience nausea and vomiting with oxymorphone than with morphine.

Reproductive/Nursing Safety

Opioids cross the placenta. In humans, there is a boxed warning that prolonged use of oxymorphone during pregnancy can result in potentially life-threatening neonatal opioid withdrawal syndrome.[10]

Most opioids appear in maternal milk. In humans, withdrawal signs have occurred in breastfeeding infants after stopping maternal administration of an opioid-analgesic.[10]

Because safety has not been established in animals, this drug should only be used when the maternal benefits outweigh the potential risks to offspring.

Overdose/Acute Toxicity

Massive overdoses of oxymorphone may produce profound respiratory and/or CNS depression. Other effects may include cardiovascular collapse, hypothermia, and skeletal muscle hypotonia. Naloxone is the agent of choice to treat respiratory depression. Animals should be closely monitored after naloxone administration as effects may diminish before subtoxic concentrations of oxymorphone are attained, and naloxone doses may need to be repeated. Consider mechanical respiratory support in cases of severe respiratory depression.

For patients that have experienced or are suspected to have experienced an overdose, consultation with a 24-hour poison consultation center specializing in providing veterinary-specific information is recommended. For general information related to overdose and toxin exposures, as well as contact information for poison control centers, refer to ***Appendix***.

Drug Interactions

The following drug interactions have either been reported or are theoretical in humans or animals receiving oxymorphone and may be of significance in veterinary patients. Unless otherwise noted, use together is not necessarily contraindicated, but weigh the potential risks and perform additional monitoring when appropriate.

- **Anticholinergic Agents**: Medications with anticholinergic properties may increase risk for urinary retention and constipation when combined with opioids.
- **Butorphanol, Buprenorphine, Nalbuphine**: May antagonize opioid effects
- **Clopidogrel**: Opioids may decrease metabolism of clopidogrel to its active metabolite and thus decrease clopidogrel's antiplatelet effect.
- **Central Nervous System (CNS) Depressants** (eg, **anesthetic agents, antihistamines, barbiturates, ethanol, gabapen-**

tin, phenothiazines, tranquilizers): May increase risk for CNS or respiratory depression

- **Desmopressin**: Opioids may increase the risk for water intoxication or hyponatremia when combined with desmopressin.
- **Diuretics**: Opioids may decrease efficacy in congestive heart failure patients.
- **Gastrointestinal (GI) Prokinetic Agents** (eg, **cisapride, metoclopramide**): Opioids may decrease the effectiveness of GI prokinetic agents.
- **Magnesium Sulfate**: The CNS depressant effects of oxymorphone may be increased; more likely with higher magnesium doses or IV magnesium therapy.
- **Minocycline**: IV minocycline therapy may enhance the CNS depressant effects of oxymorphone.
- **Opioid Antagonists** (eg, **naloxone, naltrexone**): Combined use negates opioid effects.
- **Monoamine Oxidase Inhibitors** (**MAOIs**; eg, **amitraz, linezolid, selegiline**): Use MAOIs with oxymorphone with extreme caution as meperidine (a related opioid) is contraindicated in human patients receiving MAOIs and for at least 14 days after receiving MAOIs. Some human patients have exhibited signs of opioid overdose after receiving therapeutic doses of meperidine while taking MAOIs.
- **Muscle Relaxants, Skeletal**: Oxymorphone may enhance effects.
- **Phenothiazines** (eg, **acepromazine, chlorpromazine**): Some phenothiazines may antagonize analgesic effects and increase risk for hypotension.
- **Rufinamide**: The CNS effects of oxymorphone may be increased when used concurrently, specifically dizziness and sleepiness.
- **Serotonin Modulators** (eg, **linezolid, methylene blue, metoclopramide, SSRIs, trazodone**): Serotonin concentrations may be enhanced when serotonin modulators are given concomitantly with oxymorphone. Monitor for serotonin syndrome.
- **Succinylcholine**: Opioids combined with succinylcholine may enhance the bradycardic effects of opioids.
- **Tricyclic Antidepressants** (eg, **amitriptyline, clomipramine**): Oxymorphone may exacerbate the effects of tricyclic antidepressants.
- **Warfarin**: Opioids may potentiate the anticoagulant activity of warfarin.

Laboratory Considerations

- As they may increase biliary tract pressure, opioids can increase plasma **amylase** and **lipase** values up to 24 hours following their administration.
- Quinolones may cause false positive results on urine screening tests for oxymorphone.[11]

Dosages

DOGS/CATS:

Analgesia for acute pain, sedation, premedication agent (extra-label):

a) 0.05 – 0.2 mg/kg IV, IM, or SC every 1 to 6 hours as needed. May be given in combination with a sedative.

b) Epidural administration: 0.05 – 0.1 mg/kg diluted in 0.3 mL/kg of 0.9% sodium chloride.[12] Some recommend a maximum of 6 mL. Use of preservative-free product is recommended.[13]

HORSES:

Analgesia (extra-label): 0.01 – 0.03 mg/kg IV or IM. NOTE: Oxymorphone may cause CNS excitement in horses. Pretreatment with acepromazine or xylazine is recommended to reduce the severity of this effect.

SHEEP:

Premedication (extra-label): 0.05 mg/kg IV once[14]

BIRDS:

Premedication (in most species; extra-label): 0.05 – 0.2 mg/kg IV, IM, or SC once

FERRETS:

Analgesia (extra-label): 0.05 – 0.2 mg/kg IV, IM, or SC every 6 to 12 hours as needed

SMALL MAMMALS:

Analgesia (extra-label):

Rabbits: 0.1 – 0.3 mg/kg IV, IM, or SC every 2 to 4 hours as needed

Hamsters, Gerbils, Mice, Rats, Guinea pigs, Chinchillas: 0.2 – 0.5 mg/kg SC every 6 to 12 hours as needed

Monitoring

- Respiratory rate and depth
- Level of central nervous system depression or excitation
- Blood pressure (especially with IV use)
- Analgesia
- Cardiac rate

Client Information

- This medication is normally given intramuscularly, intravenously, subcutaneously, or rectally. This drug is normally only used in the veterinary clinic or under direct professional supervision.
- Oxymorphone is classified as a schedule II (C-II) controlled drug by the federal Drug Enforcement Agency (DEA) and requires a new written prescription for refills. Use of this medication in animals or humans other than that for which it is prescribed is illegal.

Chemistry/Synonyms

A semi-synthetic phenanthrene narcotic agonist, oxymorphone HCl occurs as odorless white crystals or a white to off-white powder. Oxymorphone will darken with prolonged exposure to light. One gram of oxymorphone HCl is soluble in 4 mL of water and sparingly soluble in alcohol or ether. Commercially available oxymorphone injection has a pH of 2.7 to 4.5.

Oxymorphone HCl may also be known as 7,8-Dihydro-14-hydroxymorphinone hydrochloride, oximorphone hydrochloride, *Numorphan®*, and *Opana®*.

Storage/Stability

Store vials protected from light at room temperature 15°C to 30°C (59°F-86°F) and avoid freezing. Store commercially available suppositories at 2°C to 15°C (35.6°F-59°F). Store commercially available oral products at 25°C (77°F) with excursions permitted from 15°C to 30°C (59°F-86°F).

Compatibility/Compounding Considerations

Oxymorphone is reported to be physically **compatible** when mixed with acepromazine, atropine, glycopyrrolate, and ranitidine.

Oxymorphone is physically **incompatible** when mixed with barbiturates or diazepam.

Dosage Forms/Regulatory Status

VETERINARY-LABELED PRODUCTS: NONE

The Association of Racing Commissioners International (ARCI) has designated this drug a Class 1 substance. Use of this drug may not be allowed in certain animal competitions. Check rules and regulations before entering in a competition while this medication is being administered. Contact local racing authorities for further guidance.

See ***Appendix*** for more information.

HUMAN-LABELED PRODUCTS:

Oxymorphone HCl for Injection: 1 mg/mL in 1 mL ampules; *Opa-*

na®; (Rx, C-II). **NOTE**: manufacturing of the injection was stopped in 2017.

Oxymorphone oral tablets (*Opana*®) and extended-release tablets (*Opana ER*®) are also available.

NOTE: Oxymorphone is a DEA schedule-II (C-II) controlled substance. Report dispensing to state monitoring programs where required.

References

For the complete list of references, see **wiley.com/go/budde/plumb**

Oxytetracycline

(ox-ee-tet-ra-***sye***-kleen) *Terramycin*®, *Pennox*®, *LA-200*®

Tetracycline Antibiotic

For ophthalmic use, refer to ***Oxytetracycline/Polymyxin B Ophthalmic***

Prescriber Highlights

- Although many bacteria are now resistant, oxytetracycline is still used to treat *Mycoplasma* spp, *Rickettsia* spp, spirochetes, and *Chlamydia* spp.
- When used in food animals, refer to product labels for indications, restrictions, dosages, and withdrawal times.
- Contraindications include hypersensitivity to tetracyclines.
- Use with extreme caution in pregnancy due to risk for impaired fetal skeletal development and discoloration of deciduous teeth.
- Use with caution in liver or renal insufficiency
- Adverse effects include GI distress (diarrhea, alteration of microbiota, ruminoreticular stasis); staining and impaired development of teeth and bones in young, growing animals; superinfections; and photosensitivity. Long-term use may cause uroliths.
- Avoid rapid IV administration of undiluted propylene glycol-based products due to risk for intravascular hemolysis and cardiodepressant effects. Local reactions, yellow staining, and necrosis may be seen at IM injection sites.

Uses/Indications

Certain oxytetracycline products are FDA-approved for use in dogs and cats (no known products are currently being marketed), calves, nonlactating dairy cattle, preruminating calves, beef cattle, sheep, swine, fish, honeybees, and poultry.

In dogs and cats, oxytetracycline has been used to treat susceptible infections including for the treatment of infections caused by *Neorickettsia helminthoeca* (salmon poisoning disease)[1] and antibiotic-responsive diarrhea.[2] Oxytetracycline also has been used to address tear staining that may develop near the medial canthus[3] ; however, the use of an antimicrobial for non-antimicrobial effects is under increasing scrutiny.

For cattle, there are several injectable oxytetracycline products, concentrations, and formulations. Depending on the product, they may be indicated for infectious diseases such as bovine respiratory disease (BRD), diphtheria, foot rot, infectious bovine keratoconjunctivitis (pink eye), bacterial enteritis (scours), wooden tongue, leptospirosis, wound infections, and acute metritis. Concentrated formulations (200 mg/mL and 300 mg/mL) have been used for the control of respiratory infections in cattle at high risk for BRD. Historical overuse has limited the efficacy of oxytetracycline for conditions such as BRD in many areas.[4–6]

For swine, oxytetracycline is FDA-approved for the treatment of pneumonia caused by *Pasteurella multocida*, bacterial enteritis caused by *Escherichia coli*, leptospirosis caused by *Leptospira pomona*, and for use in farrowing sows to control bacterial enteritis in suckling piglets caused by *E coli*.

The World Health Organization (WHO) has designated oxytetracycline as a Highly Important antimicrobial for human medicine.[7] The Office International des Epizooties (OIE) has designated tetracyclines as Veterinary Critically Important Antimicrobial (VCIA) Agents in avian, bovine, camelids, caprine, equine, lagomorph, ovine, and swine species.[8]

Pharmacology/Actions

Tetracyclines are time-dependent bacteriostatic antibiotics that inhibit protein synthesis by reversibly binding to 30S ribosomal subunits of susceptible organisms, thereby preventing aminoacyl transfer-RNA binding to those ribosomes. Tetracyclines are alter cytoplasmic membrane permeability in susceptible organisms. In high concentrations, tetracyclines can also inhibit protein synthesis by mammalian cells.

As a class, the tetracyclines have activity against most *Mycoplasma* spp, spirochetes (including *Borrelia burgdorferi*), *Chlamydia* spp, and *Rickettsia* spp. For gram-positive bacteria, tetracyclines have activity against some strains of staphylococci and streptococci, but resistance of these organisms is increasing. Gram-positive bacteria that are usually susceptible to tetracyclines include *Actinomyces* spp, *Bacillus anthracis, Clostridium perfringens, Clostridium tetani, Listeria monocytogenes*, and *Nocardia* spp. Tetracyclines usually have in vivo and in vitro activity against some gram-negative bacteria, including *Bordetella* spp, *Brucella* spp, *Bartonella* spp, *Haemophilus* spp, *Pasteurella multocida, Shigella* spp, and *Yersinia pestis*. Many or most strains of *Escherichia coli, Klebsiella* spp, *Bacteroides* spp, *Enterobacter* spp, *Proteus* spp, and *Pseudomonas aeruginosa* are resistant to tetracyclines. Although most strains of *Pseudomonas aeruginosa* show in vitro resistance to tetracyclines, tetracycline and oxytetracycline attain high levels in urine and have been associated with clinical cures in dogs with UTI caused by *P aeruginosa*.

Oxytetracycline and tetracycline share nearly identical spectrums of activity and patterns of cross-resistance. A tetracycline susceptibility disk is usually used for in vitro testing for oxytetracycline susceptibility. Tetracycline susceptibility indicates oxytetracycline susceptibility.

Oxytetracycline appears to have immunomodulatory effects that may contribute to its clinical efficacy. In horses, oxytetracycline appears to be a potent inhibitor of matrix metalloproteinase-9 and a modest inhibitor of matrix metalloproteinase-2[9]; however, the clinical relevance of this is unclear.

Pharmacokinetics

Both oxytetracycline and tetracycline are readily absorbed after oral administration to fasting animals. Bioavailability ranges from ≈60% to 80%. The presence of food, and especially dairy products, can reduce the amount of tetracycline absorbed by as much as 50% or more. After IM administration of oxytetracycline (short-acting), peak levels may occur in 30 minutes to several hours, depending on the volume and site of injection. The long-acting product (*LA-200*®) has significantly slower absorption after IM injection. Pharmacokinetic data for 200 mg/mL single injection oxytetracycline products administered IM as per the label single injection regimen of 20 mg/kg suggest that plasma concentrations are ≈1, 0.2, and 0.1 mg/mL at 48, 72, and 96 hours, respectively.[10]

Tetracyclines are widely distributed in the body, including to the heart, kidney, lungs, muscle, pleural fluid, bronchial secretions, sputum, bile, saliva, urine, synovial fluid, ascitic fluid, and aqueous and vitreous humor. Only small quantities of tetracycline and oxytetracycline are distributed to the CSF and therapeutic levels may not be attainable. Although all tetracyclines distribute to the prostate and eye, doxycycline or minocycline penetrate better into these and most other tissues. Tetracyclines cross the placenta, enter fetal circulation, and are distributed into milk. The volume of distribution of oxytetracycline is ≈2.1 L/kg in small animals, 1.4 L/kg in horses, and 0.8 L/kg in cattle. The amount of plasma protein binding is ≈10% to 40% for oxytetracycline. Oxytetracycline tissue concentrations are higher in diseased lung than in healthy lung and concentrations in milk are higher than serum when mammary glands are inflamed.

Both oxytetracycline and tetracycline are eliminated unchanged, primarily via glomerular filtration. Patients with impaired renal function can have prolonged elimination half-lives and may accumulate the drug with repeated dosing. These drugs are apparently not metabolized but are excreted into the GI tract via both biliary and nonbiliary routes and may become inactive after chelation with fecal material. The elimination half-life of oxytetracycline is ≈4 to 6 hours in dogs and cats, 4.3 to 9.7 hours in cattle, 10.5 hours in horses, 6.7 hours in swine, and 3.6 hours in sheep.

In broilers, oxytetracycline absorption was significantly slower in chickens that were treated with the long-acting formulation compared with those administered short-acting formulation. However, a therapeutic plasma concentration (greater than 1 µg/mL) was maintained for 72 hours following a single long-acting injection.[11] Oxytetracycline soluble powder is poorly absorbed from the GI tract following oral administration, even in the absence of food and with the use of deionized water. The oxytetracycline injectable products, given SC and IM, are rapidly absorbed to a similar extent, irrespective of the administration route.[12]

Contraindications/Precautions/Warnings

Oxytetracycline is contraindicated in patients that are hypersensitive to it or other tetracyclines. Because tetracyclines can impair fetal skeletal development, discolor deciduous teeth, and lead to enamel hypoplasia, they should only be used in the last half of pregnancy when the benefits outweigh the fetal risks. Oxytetracycline and tetracycline are considered more likely to cause these abnormalities than doxycycline or minocycline.

In patients with renal insufficiency or hepatic impairment, oxytetracycline and tetracycline must be used cautiously. In these situations, lower than usual doses are recommended, with enhanced monitoring of renal and hepatic function if an alternative antibiotic is unavailable. Avoid concurrent administration of other nephrotoxic or hepatotoxic drugs with tetracyclines. Monitoring of serum levels should be considered if long-term treatment is required.

Oral administration of tetracycline, chlortetracycline, or oxytetracycline appears safe in mice and rats, but little appears to be absorbed, which limits efficacy. Oral tetracyclines are known to be toxic to guinea pigs, and may be toxic to hamsters, gerbils, and rabbits.[13]

Adverse Effects

Oxytetracycline and tetracycline given to young animals can cause a yellow, brown, or gray discoloration of bones and teeth. High doses or long-term administration may delay bone growth and healing. In humans, tetracyclines in high concentrations have been shown to exert an antianabolic effect, which can cause an increase in BUN and/or hepatotoxicity, particularly in patients with pre-existing renal dysfunction.[14] As renal function deteriorates secondary to drug accumulation, this effect may be exacerbated. Veterinary significance is unclear.

In small animal species, tetracyclines can cause nausea, vomiting, anorexia, and diarrhea. Cats do not tolerate oral tetracycline or oxytetracycline well, and may present with GI distress, fever, hair loss, and depression. There are reports that long-term tetracycline use may cause urolith formation in dogs, but this is thought to occur very rarely.

Diarrhea in horses is possible. Acute kidney injury has been observed in foals receiving high-dose oxytetracycline treatment for flexural limb deformities.[15,16]

In ruminants, high oral doses can cause ruminal microflora depression and ruminoreticular stasis. Rapid IV injection of undiluted propylene glycol-based products can cause intravascular hemolysis with resultant hemoglobinuria. Perivascular injection or leakage from an IV injection may cause severe swelling at the injection site. Propylene glycol-based products have also caused cardiodepressant effects when administered to calves. When the drug is administered IM, local reactions, yellow staining, and necrosis may be seen at the injection site. Reports of adverse effects associated with oxytetracycline administration in cattle include injection site swelling; restlessness; ataxia; trembling; swelling of eyelids, ears, muzzle, anus, vulva (or scrotum and sheath in males); respiratory abnormalities (labored breathing); frothing at the mouth; collapse; and death. Some of these reactions may be attributed to anaphylaxis or to cardiovascular collapse of unknown cause.

Tetracycline therapy (especially long-term) may result in overgrowth (superinfections) of nonsusceptible bacteria or fungi.

Tetracyclines have also been associated with photosensitivity reactions and, rarely, hepatotoxicity or blood dyscrasias.

Reproductive/Nursing Safety

Tetracyclines cross the placenta; they are embryotoxic when used early in pregnancy and can retard fetal skeletal growth and permanently discolor teeth.

Tetracyclines are excreted in maternal milk. Milk to plasma ratios vary between 0.25 and 1.5. Because safety has not been established in animals, this drug should only be used when the maternal benefits outweigh the potential risks to offspring.

Overdose/Acute Toxicity

Tetracyclines are generally well tolerated after acute overdoses. Dogs given more than 400 mg/kg/day PO or 100 mg/kg/day IM of oxytetracycline did not demonstrate any toxicity. Oral overdoses would most likely be associated with GI disturbances (vomiting, anorexia, and/or diarrhea). If the patient develops severe emesis or diarrhea, fluids and electrolytes should be monitored and replaced if necessary. Chronic overdoses may lead to drug accumulation and nephrotoxicity.

High oral doses given to ruminants can cause ruminal microflora depression and ruminoreticular stasis. Rapid IV administration of undiluted propylene glycol-based products can cause intravascular hemolysis with resultant hemoglobinuria.

Rapid IV injection of tetracyclines has induced transient collapse and cardiac arrhythmias in several species, presumably due to chelation with intravascular calcium ions and/or the cardiodepressant effects of the propylene glycol vehicle. If the drug must be given rapidly IV (in less than 5 minutes), some clinicians recommend pretreating the animal with IV calcium gluconate.

For patients that have experienced or are suspected to have experienced an overdose, consultation with a 24-hour poison consultation center specializing in providing veterinary-specific information is recommended. For general information related to overdose and toxin exposures, as well as contact information for poison control centers, refer to ***Appendix.***

Drug Interactions

The following drug interactions have either been reported or are theoretical in humans or animals receiving oxytetracycline and may be of significance in veterinary patients. Unless otherwise noted, use together is not necessarily contraindicated, but weigh the potential risks and perform additional monitoring when appropriate.

- **Atovaquone**: Tetracyclines have caused decreased atovaquone concentrations.
- **Beta-Lactam** or **Aminoglycoside Antibiotics**: Bacteriostatic drugs, such as the tetracyclines, may interfere with bacte-

ricidal activity of the penicillins, cephalosporins, and aminoglycosides; actual clinical significance of this interaction is in doubt.

- **Cholestyramine**: May decrease oxytetracycline absorption
- **Digoxin**: Tetracyclines may increase the bioavailability of digoxin in a small percentage of human patients and lead to digoxin toxicity. These effects may persist for months after discontinuation of the tetracycline.
- **Divalent or Trivalent Cations** (eg, **oral antacids, saline cathartics or other orally administered products containing aluminum** [eg, **sucralfate**], **bismuth, calcium, iron, magnesium, or zinc cations**): When administered orally, tetracyclines can chelate divalent or trivalent cations that can decrease the absorption of the tetracycline or the other drug if it contains these cations. It is recommended that all oral tetracyclines be given at least 1 to 2 hours before or after the cation-containing product.
- **Furosemide**: Increased risk for acute kidney injury and renal failure
- **Lanthanum**: May decrease oxytetracycline absorption
- **Retinoid Acids** (eg, **acitretin, isotretinoin**): May increase the potential for the occurrence of intracranial hypertension. Combination is contraindicated.
- **Warfarin**: Tetracyclines may depress plasma prothrombin activity, and patients on anticoagulant therapy may need dosage adjustment.

Laboratory Considerations

- Tetracyclines (except minocycline) may cause falsely elevated values of **urine catecholamines** when using fluorometric methods of determination.
- Tetracyclines can reportedly cause false positive **urine glucose** results if the cupric sulfate method of determination (Benedict's reagent, *Clinitest*®) is used, but this effect may be the result of ascorbic acid, which is found in some parenteral formulations of tetracyclines. Tetracyclines have also reportedly caused false negative results in determining urine glucose when the glucose oxidase method (*Clinistix*®, *Tes-Tape*®) is used.

Dosages

DOGS/CATS:

Susceptible systemic infections (extra-label):

a) 10 mg/kg IV every 12 hours
b) 20 mg/kg PO every 8 to 12 hours

Adjunctive treatment of *Neorickettsia helminthoeca* | Salmon poisoning (extra-label): 7 mg/kg IV every 8 hours for 3 to 5 days[1]

HORSES:

Susceptible infections (extra-label): Dosage recommendations can vary considerably. For short-acting oxytetracycline injection, 6.6 – 10 mg/kg IV once daily is commonly used. Some clinicians use oxytetracycline 5 – 6.6 mg/kg IV every 12 hours. The following are representative indications and dosages:

a) **Foals**: 5 – 10 mg/kg IV every 12 hours diluted and given slowly, or 10 – 20 mg/kg IV once daily, diluted and given slowly. Monitor creatinine and UA.[17]
b) **Equine monocytic or granulocytic ehrlichiosis**: 6.6 – 7 mg/kg IV once daily for 5 to 7 days; to safeguard against adverse effects (muscle tremors, agitation, or acute collapse), dilute in a 1:1 ratio (at least) and give IV slowly, or deliver it as an infusion in 500 mL or 1 L of fluids.[17,18]
c) **Lyme disease**: 5 – 6.6 mg/kg every 12 to 24 hours IV for 1 month[19]
d) **Potomac horse fever (*Neorickettsia risticii*) early in the clinical course of the disease**: 6.6 mg/kg IV twice a day. Usually no more than 5 days treatment is necessary.[18]
e) **Proliferative enteropathy (*Lawsonia intracellularis*) in foals**: Oxytetracycline 6.6 mg/kg IV (slowly) once daily; typically administered for 2 to 4 weeks.[20] Alternatively, oxytetracycline 5 – 6.6. mg/kg IV every 12 hours for 3 to 7 days followed by doxycycline 10 mg/kg PO every 12 hours for 7 to 17 days[21]
f) **Intrauterine infusion**: 1 – 5 g/horse (NOT g/kg); use povidone-based products only. There is limited information available for recommending doses, volume infused, frequency, and diluents. Most intrauterine treatments are commonly performed every day or every other day for 3 to 7 days.[22]

Adjunctive treatment of flexural limb deformities in foals: 44 – 70 mg/kg (3 g for a 50 kg [110 lb] foal) diluted in 250 to 500 mL of normal saline and given IV.[23,24] May repeat once daily for 2 to 3 days

CATTLE:

Susceptible infections in beef cattle, dairy cattle, and calves, including preruminating (veal) calves (label dosages; FDA-approved):

a) Using the short-acting (100 mg/mL) product:
Treatment of pneumonia and shipping fever complex associated with *Pasteurella* spp; bacterial enteritis (scours) caused by *Escherichia coli*; foot rot and calf diphtheria caused by *Fusobacterium necrophorum;* wooden tongue caused by *Actinobacillus lignieresi*; wound infections, metritis, and traumatic injury caused by sensitive strains of *Staphylococcus* spp and *Streptococcus* spp: 6.6 – 11 mg/kg (3 – 5 mg/lb) IV (*slowly* over a period of at least 5 minutes) once daily; use of the higher end of the dosage range (11 mg/kg) is recommended for severe forms of indicated diseases. Treatment should continue for 24 to 48 hours following remission of clinical signs related to infection and should not exceed a total of 4 consecutive days.[25]
b) Using the *Liquamycin LA-200*® product: **NOTE**: Do not exceed 10 mL per SC or IM injection site.
Treatment of pneumonia and shipping fever complex caused by *Pasteurella* spp and *Haemophilus* spp and infectious bovine keratoconjunctivitis (pink eye) caused by *Moraxella bovis* in calves and yearlings where re-treatment is impractical because of husbandry conditions, such as cattle on range, or where their repeated restraint is inadvisable or for infectious bovine keratoconjunctivitis (pink eye) caused by *Moraxella bovis*: 20 mg/kg (9 mg/lb) IM or SC once[26]
Treatment of pneumonia and shipping fever complex caused by *Pasteurella* spp and *Haemophilus* spp; foot rot and diphtheria caused by *Fusobacterium;* wooden tongue caused by *Actinobacillus lignieresii;* leptospirosis caused by *Leptospira pomona*; and wound infections and acute metritis caused by sensitive strains of *Staphylococcus* spp and *Streptococcus* spp: 6.6 – 11 mg/kg (3 – 5 mg/lb) IM, SC, or IV (*slowly* over a period of at least 5 minutes) once daily; use of the higher end of the dosage range (11 mg/kg SC or IV slow) is recommended when used to treat severe foot rot and other advanced cases of other indicated diseases.[26] Treatment should continue for 24 to 48 hours following resolution of clinical signs related to infection and should not exceed a total of 4 consecutive days.
c) Using *300 PRO LA*®: **NOTE**: Do not exceed 10 mL per SC or IM injection site.
Control of respiratory disease in cattle at high risk for developing bovine respiratory disease (BRD) associated with *Mannheimia (Pasteurella) haemolytica*: 30 mg/kg (13.6 mg/lb) IM or SC once
Treatment of pneumonia and shipping fever complex caused by *Pasteurella* spp (shipping fever) in calves and yearlings

where re-treatment is impractical due to husbandry conditions, such as cattle on range, or where their repeated restraint is inadvisable; or infectious bovine keratoconjunctivitis (pink eye) caused by *Moraxella bovis*: 20 – 30 mg/kg (9 – 13.6 mg/lb) IM or SC once[27]

Treatment of pneumonia and shipping fever complex caused by *Pasteurella* spp and *Histophilus* spp; foot rot and diphtheria caused by *Fusobacterium necrophorum*; bacterial enteritis (scours) caused by *E coli*; or wooden tongue caused by *Actinobacillus lignieresii*; leptospirosis caused by *Leptospira pomona*; and wound infections and acute metritis caused by sensitive strains of *Staphylococcus* spp and *Streptococcus* spp: 6.6 – 11 mg/kg (3 – 5 mg/lb) IM, SC, or IV (IV *slowly* over a period of at least 5 minutes) once daily[27]; use of the higher end of the dosage range (11 mg/kg SC or IV slow) is recommended when used to treat severe foot rot and other advanced cases of other indicated diseases. Treatment should continue for 24 to 48 hours following resolution of clinical signs related to infection and should not exceed a total of 4 consecutive days.

d) Using the combination product with flunixin (*Hexasol*®): **NOTE**: Do not exceed 10 mL per SC or IM injection site.

Treatment of pneumonia associated with *Pasteurella* spp and for the control of associated pyrexia in beef and non-lactating dairy cattle: oxytetracycline 30 mg/kg (13.6 mg/lb) and flunixin 2 mg/kg (0.9 mg/lb) IM or SC once.[28] Do not administer more than 10 mL per injection site (1 to 2 mL per site in small calves). Recommended where re-treatment of calves and yearlings is impractical because of husbandry conditions, such as cattle on range, or where their repeated restraint is inadvisable.

Listeria monocytogenes (extra-label): 10 mg/kg IV (*slowly* over a period of at least 5 minutes) every 12 hours for at least 5 days.[29]

SHEEP & GOATS:

Enteritis caused by *E coli* and for pneumonia caused by *Pasteurella multocida* (extra-label): oxytetracycline (for use in water) 22 mg/kg PO in water daily for 7 to 14 days[21]

***Chlamydophila abortus* in pregnant ewes** (extra-label): Long-acting oxytetracycline 20 mg/kg IM.[30] In the face of an outbreak, all pregnant ewes should be treated.

***Coxiella burnetii* | Q fever** (extra-label): Aborting ewes or does and other females in late pregnancy were given 2 doses of oxytetracycline 20 mg/kg IM during the last month of gestation; injections were typically separated by 7 to 27 days (mean = 16 days). Treatment does not totally suppress abortions and shedding of *C burnetii* at lambing.[31]

Foot rot in sheep *(Dichelobacter nodosus or Fusobacterium necrophorum)*: 20 mg/kg IM, once[32]

SWINE:

Susceptible infections (label dosages, FDA-approved):

a) Using the *Liquamycin*® *100* product[33]:

Treatment of sows as an aid in the control infectious enteritis (baby pig scours, colibacillosis) in suckling piglets caused by *E coli*: 6.6 mg/kg (3 mg/lb) IM once ≈8 hours before farrowing or immediately after completion of farrowing

b) Using the *Liquamycin*® *LA-200*® product: **NOTE**: Do not exceed 5 mL per SC or IM injection site. For pigs weighing less than 11.3 kg (25 lb), see product label for specific administration instructions.

Treatment of bacterial enteritis (scours, colibacillosis) caused by *E coli*, pneumonia caused by *P multocida*, and leptospirosis caused by *Leptospira pomona* where retreatment is impractical due to husbandry conditions or where repeated restraint is inadvisable: 20 mg/kg (9 mg/lb) IM, once in the neck region[34]

Treatment of bacterial enteritis (scours, colibacillosis) caused by *E coli*, pneumonia caused by *P multocida*, and leptospirosis caused by *Leptospira pomona*: 6.6 – 11 mg/kg (3 – 5 mg/lb) IM daily.[34] Treatment should continue for 24 to 48 hours following resolution of clinical signs related to infection and should not exceed a total of 4 consecutive days.

Treatment of sows as an aid in the control infectious enteritis (baby pig scours, colibacillosis) in suckling piglets caused by *E coli*: 6.6 mg/kg (3 mg/lb) IM once ≈8 hours before farrowing or immediately after completion of farrowing[34]

c) Using the *300 PRO LA*® product: **NOTE**: Do not exceed 5 mL per injection site. For pigs weighing less than 11.3 kg (25 lb), see product label for specific administration instructions.

Treatment of pneumonia caused by *P multocida* where re-treatment is impractical because of husbandry conditions or where repeated restraint is inadvisable: 20 mg/kg (9 mg/lb) IM once[27]

Treatment of bacterial enteritis (scours, colibacillosis) caused by *E coli*; pneumonia caused by *P multocida*; and leptospirosis caused by *Leptospira pomona*: 6.6 – 11 mg/kg (3 – 5 mg/lb) IM once daily.[27] Treatment should be continued for 24 to 48 hours following resolution of clinical signs related in infection and should not exceed a total of 4 consecutive days.

Treatment of sows as an aid in the control of infectious enteritis (baby pig scours, colibacillosis) in suckling piglets caused by *E coli*: 6.6.mg/kg (3 mg/lb) IM once ≈8 hours before farrowing or immediately after completion of farrowing[27]

Susceptible infections (extra-label): 2 - 10 mg/kg IM, SC every 12 to 24 hours[35]

BIRDS:

Chlamydiosis (psittacosis) (extra-label): Using 200 mg/mL product (*Liquamycin*® *LA-200*®*)*: 50 mg/kg IM once every 3 to 5 days in birds suspected or confirmed of having disease. Using 300 mg/mL product: single dose 20 mg/kg IM in broilers.[11] **NOTE**: IM injections may cause severe local tissue reactions.[36]

REPTILES:

Susceptible infections in turtle and tortoises (extra-label): 10 mg/kg PO once daily for 7 days (useful to treat ulcerative stomatitis caused by *Vibrio* spp)[37]

Monitoring

- Adverse effects (eg, GI distress, staining of teeth, overgrowth (superinfections) of nonsusceptible bacteria or fungi infections)
- Clinical efficacy (ie, improvement in clinical signs of disease being treated)
- Long-term use or in susceptible patients: periodic CBC and serum biochemistry profiles as indicated by clinical condition

Client Information

- When this medicine is given orally, oxytetracycline should be administered on an empty stomach 1 to 2 hours before or after consumption of food, milk, other dairy products, and minerals such as calcium or iron. If your animal vomits or acts sick after receiving the medicine on an empty stomach, give it with a small amount of food to see if this helps. If vomiting continues, contact your veterinarian.
- Oxytetracycline may permanently stain teeth and interfere with developing bones in young animals.

- Darkening of your animal's urine may occur. In some cases, this change may occur shortly after the first dose. Contact your veterinarian if this effect persists, or if you notice blood in the urine.
- This medicine may make your animal's skin more sensitive to sunlight and increase the risk for sunburn on hairless areas such as the nose and around the eyelids and ears. Keep treated animals out of the sun or apply a veterinary-approved sunblock product to protect the skin. Tell your veterinarian if you notice any reddening/sunburn on the skin while your animal is on this medication.
- Administration of injectable forms of this medicine drug may be painful and cause staining of the skin around the injection and result in trim losses. Be sure you understand how to give the medications.

Chemistry/Synonyms

A tetracycline derivative obtained from *Streptomyces rimosus*, oxytetracycline base occurs as a pale yellow to tan crystalline powder that is very slightly soluble in water and sparingly soluble in alcohol. Oxytetracycline HCl occurs as a bitter, hygroscopic, yellow crystalline powder that is freely soluble in water and sparingly soluble in alcohol. Commercially available 50 mg/mL and 100 mg/mL oxytetracycline HCl injections are usually available in either propylene glycol- or povidone-based products.

Oxytetracycline may also be known as glomycin, hydroxytetracycline, oxytetracyclinum, riomitsin, terrafungine, *Agrimycin®*, *Biomycin®*, *Liquamycin®*, *Medamycin®*, *Oxybiotic®*, *Oxytet®*, *Terramycin®*, and *Vetrimycin®*.

Storage/Stability

Unless otherwise directed by the manufacturer, oxytetracycline HCl and oxytetracycline products should be stored in airtight, light-resistant containers at temperatures of less than 40°C (104°F) and preferably at room temperature (15°C-30°C [59°F-86°F]); avoid freezing. Products do not require refrigeration. Because storage requirements and discard specifications vary slightly by manufacturer and by product, refer to product label for specific information.

Some products state to discard vial after a defined number of stopper punctures or days after first use.

Compatibility/Compounding Considerations

The following information pertains to short-acting (not long-acting) forms of oxytetracycline HCl. It is generally considered to be physically **compatible** with most commonly used IV infusion solutions, including D_5W, sodium chloride 0.9%, and lactated Ringer's, but can become relatively unstable in solutions with a pH more than 6, particularly in those containing calcium. This is apparently more of a problem with the veterinary injections that are propylene glycol-based rather than those that are povidone-based. Other drugs that are reported to be physically **compatible** with oxytetracycline for injection include: corticotropin, dimenhydrinate, insulin (regular), isoproterenol HCl, norepinephrine bitartrate, potassium chloride, tetracycline HCl, and vitamin B complex with C.

Drugs that are reportedly physically **incompatible** with oxytetracycline, data conflict, or compatibility is concentration/time dependent include: amikacin sulfate, aminophylline, amphotericin B, calcium chloride/gluconate, chloramphenicol sodium succinate, erythromycin gluceptate, heparin sodium, hydrocortisone sodium succinate, iron dextran, methohexital sodium, oxacillin sodium, penicillin G potassium/sodium, pentobarbital sodium, phenobarbital sodium, and sodium bicarbonate.

Compatibility is dependent upon factors such as pH, concentration, temperature, and diluent used; consult specialized references or a hospital pharmacist for more specific information.

Dosage Forms/Regulatory Status

VETERINARY-LABELED PRODUCTS:

Oxytetracycline HCl 100 mg/mL Injection: There are many FDA-approved oxytetracycline products marketed in these concentrations. Some trade names for these products include: *Terramycin®*, *Liquamycin® 100*, *Biomycin®*, *Duramycin®*, *Oxybiotic®*, and *Oxytet®*. Some are labeled for Rx (prescription) use only, whereas some are OTC. Depending on the product, this drug may be FDA-approved for use in cattle, beef cattle, swine, chickens, or turkeys. Products may also be labeled for IV, IM, or SC use. Withdrawal times vary with regard to individual products; when used as labeled, slaughter withdrawal times vary in cattle from 15 to 22 days, swine 20 to 26 days, and 5 days for chickens and turkeys. Refer to the labeled information for the product used for more information.

Oxytetracycline base 200 mg/mL Injection in 100 mL, 250 mL, and 500 mL bottles; *Liquamycin® LA-200®*, *Vetrimycin®* 200, *Biomycin®-200* generic; (OTC). FDA-approved for use in swine and cattle. When used as labeled, slaughter withdrawal = 28 days for swine and cattle; milk withdrawal = 96 hours.

Oxytetracycline base 300 mg/mL Injection in 100 mL, 250 mL, and 500 mL vials; *Noromycin® 300*-LA (OTC), *300 Pro® LA*; (Rx). FDA-approved for use in beef cattle, nonlactating dairy cattle, calves, including preruminating (veal) calves, and swine. When used as labeled, slaughter withdrawal = 28 days.

Oxytetracycline Oral Tablets (Boluses) 250 mg and 500 mg tablets; *Calf Scour Bolus®*, *Oxy 500 Calf Bolus, Terramycin® Scours Tablets*; (OTC). FDA-approved for use in nonlactating dairy and beef cattle. Withdrawal periods may vary; refer to the product label.

Combination Products:

Oxytetracycline 300 mg/mL and Flunixin (as flunixin meglumine) 20 mg/mL in 100 mL, 250 mL, and 500 mL; *Hexasol®*; (Rx). When used as labeled, slaughter withdrawal = 21 days. Restricted drug in California. Do not use in female dairy cattle 20 months of age or older. A withdrawal period has not been established for this product in preruminating calves. Do not use in calves to be processed for veal.

Water Soluble, VFD, and Milk Replacer Products:

Water soluble oxytetracycline products transitioned from OTC to Rx status on January 1, 2017. Some trade names include *Pennox 343®*, *Tetroxy® 25*, *Tetroxy 343®*; *Tetroxy HCA®*; (Rx)

Feed additive products transitioned from OTC to VFD status on January 1, 2017. Some trade names for these products include *Neo-Oxy®*, *Neo-Terramycin®*, *NT Concentrate®*, *Pennox®*, *Terramycin®*; (VFD)

Milk replacer products available for use in calves. Some trade names include *Sav-A-Caf®*, *Scour-Ease®* (OTC), *Calf Solutions®* (VFD)

Oxytetracycline is also available as an ophthalmic ointment for use in beef and dairy cattle for the treatment of eye infections; *Terramycin Ophthalmic Ointment®*; (OTC). See ***Oxytetracycline/Polymyxin B Ophthalmic***.

HUMAN-LABELED PRODUCTS: NONE

References

For the complete list of references, see **wiley.com/go/budde/plumb**

Oxytocin

(ox-ee-***toe***-sin) *Pitocin®*
Hormone

Prescriber Highlights

- Hypothalamic hormone used for induction or enhancement of uterine contractions during parturition, postpartum retained placenta and metritis, uterine involution after manual correction of prolapsed uterus in dogs, and agalactia. It is also used for stimulation of milk letdown in dairy animals.
- Contraindications include a known hypersensitivity and dystocia due to abnormal maternal anatomy and/or presentation of fetus(es) unless correction is made. When used prepartum, oxytocin should be used only when the cervix is relaxed naturally or by prior administration of estrogens.
- Correct hypocalcemia before using oxytocin.
- Adverse effects usually occur only when used at a dosage that is too high.
- The National Institute for Occupational Safety and Health (NIOSH) classifies oxytocin as a hazardous drug; use appropriate precautions when handling.

Uses/Indications

Oxytocin has been used in veterinary medicine for induction or enhancement of uterine contractions at parturition, postpartum evacuation of uterine debris or control of uterine bleeding, uterine involution after manual correction of prolapsed uterus in dogs, and treatment of agalactia.

Pharmacology/Actions

Oxytocin stimulates uterine contractions by increasing the sodium permeability of uterine myofibrils. The threshold for oxytocin-induced uterine contraction is reduced with pregnancy duration, in the presence of high estrogen levels, and in patients already in labor.

Oxytocin can facilitate milk ejection, but it does not have any galactopoietic properties. Oxytocin has weak antidiuretic properties.

Pharmacokinetics

Oxytocin must be administered parenterally because it is destroyed in the GI tract. Uterine response occurs almost immediately after IV administration. Following IM administration, the uterus generally responds within 3 to 5 minutes. The duration of effect in dogs after IV or IM/SC administration has been reported to be 13 minutes and 20 minutes, respectively. Although oxytocin can be administered intranasally, absorption can be erratic. Oxytocin is distributed throughout the extracellular fluid. It is believed that small quantities of the drug cross the placenta and enter the fetal circulation.

In most mammals, the plasma half-life of oxytocin is ≈1 to 6 minutes. In goats, this value has been reported to be ≈22 minutes. Oxytocin is metabolized rapidly in the liver and kidneys; oxytocinase, a circulating enzyme, can also destroy the hormone. Very small amounts of oxytocin are excreted unchanged in the urine.

Contraindications/Precautions/Warnings

Oxytocin is considered contraindicated in animals hypersensitive to it or with obstructive dystocia due to abnormal presentation of fetus(es) unless correction is made. It is also contraindicated when female anatomy does not allow vaginal birth. When used prepartum, oxytocin should be used only when the cervix is fully relaxed, either naturally or by prior administration of estrogens. (**NOTE**: Most clinicians avoid the use of estrogens, as natural relaxation is a better indicator of when to induce contractions.)

Oxytocin is ineffective for treatment of primary uterine inertia (uterine muscles do not contract normally at parturition). Correcting hypocalcemia may improve the effectiveness of oxytocin in stimulating uterine contractions.[1]

In humans, oxytocin is contraindicated in patients with significant cephalopelvic disproportion, with unfavorable fetal positions, in obstetrical emergencies when surgical intervention is warranted, with grand multiparity, with uterine hypertonia or severe toxemia, or in which vaginal delivery is contraindicated. This drug should be used with caution in patients with uterine overdistention, previous major cervical or uterine surgery, or cervical carcinoma. Nasally administered oxytocin is contraindicated in pregnancy.

In human medicine, IV oxytocin is considered to be a high-alert medication (ie, medication that requires special safeguards to reduce the risk for errors). Consider instituting practices such as redundant drug dosages, volume checking, and using special alert labels. The National Institute for Occupational Safety and Health (NIOSH) classifies oxytocin as a hazardous drug; personal protective equipment (PPE) should be used accordingly to minimize the risk of exposure.[2]

Adverse Effects

Oxytocin used appropriately at reasonable doses rarely causes significant adverse effects. Most adverse effects are a result of the drug being used at dosages that are too high (see ***Overdose/Acute Toxicity***) or in patients that should not receive oxytocin (see ***Contraindications/Precautions/Warnings***); adequate physical examination and monitoring of the patient are essential. Most older (ie, higher) dosage recommendations for dogs and cats are obsolete, as mini-doses have been found to improve the frequency of uterine contractility and are less hazardous to the bitch (ie, uterine rupture) and fetus(es) (ie, placental compromise).[1] Hypersensitivity reactions are a possibility with products derived from animal sources. Repeat bolus injections of oxytocin may cause uterine cramping and discomfort.

The human product lists QT interval prolongation and cardiac arrhythmias as possible adverse effects. Water intoxication can occur if the drug is administered too quickly IV and/or if excessively large volumes of electrolyte-free IV fluids are co-administered.

Overdose/Acute Toxicity

Effects of overdose on the uterus depend on the stage of parturition and position of the fetus(es). Hypertonic or tetanic contractions can occur, leading to tumultuous labor, uterine rupture, and/or fetal injury or death.

Water intoxication can occur if large doses of oxytocin are infused for a long period of time, especially if there is free access to drinking water or large volumes of electrolyte-free IV fluids are concomitantly administered. Clinical signs can range from listlessness and/or depression to coma, seizures, and eventual death. Treatment includes stopping oxytocin therapy and restricting water access until signs are resolved. Severe intoxication may require the use of osmotic diuretics (eg, mannitol, urea, dextrose) with or without furosemide

For patients that have experienced or are suspected to have experienced an overdose, consultation with a 24-hour poison consultation center specializing in providing veterinary-specific information is recommended. For general information related to overdose and toxin exposures, as well as contact information for poison control centers, refer to ***Appendix.***

Reproductive/Nursing Safety

Oxytocin is contraindicated in humans with significant cephalopelvic disproportion, with unfavorable fetal positions, in obstetrical emergencies in which surgical intervention is warranted, with severe toxemia, or when vaginal delivery is contraindicated. Nasally administered oxytocin is contraindicated in pregnancy.

There are no known indications for use of oxytocin in the first trimester other than in relation to spontaneous or induced abortion. When used as indicated, oxytocin is not expected to present a risk for fetal abnormalities.

Oxytocin may be found in small quantities in maternal milk but is unlikely to have significant effects. Oxytocin may alter milk flow.

Drug Interactions

The following drug interactions have either been reported or are theoretical in humans or animals receiving oxytocin and may be of significance in veterinary patients. Unless otherwise noted, use together is not necessarily contraindicated, but weigh the potential risks and perform additional monitoring when appropriate.

- **Beta-Adrenergic Agonists** (eg, **albuterol, clenbuterol**): May reduce effects of oxytocin and delay labor
- **Dinoprost**: May enhance effects of oxytocin
- **Misoprostol**: May enhance effects of oxytocin
- **Nonsteroidal anti-inflammatory drugs (NSAIDs**; eg, **flunixin**): Attenuation of oxytocic effects has been demonstrated in postpartum cows.[3]
- **Vasoconstrictors** (eg, **ephedrine, epinephrine**): Concurrent use with sympathomimetic agents or other vasoconstrictors increases the risk for hypertension.

Dosages

NOTE: Unless otherwise indicated, all dosages are extra-label.

DOGS/CATS:

Uterine inertia: In most cases, calcium is given *before* oxytocin to improve contraction strength. See ***Calcium IV (-Borogluconate, -Chloride, -Gluconate)*** for further information.

a) Initial oxytocin doses of 0.1 units/kg IM; repeat doses every 30 to 40 minutes, and increase doses incrementally to a maximum of 2 units/kg (maximum of 20 units/kg).[4]

b) Oxytocin 2 units (total dose, NOT units/kg) IV, repeated in 30 to 60 minutes[5]

c) Oxytocin 0.25 units per bitch or queen (NOT units/kg) SC or IM to a maximum dose of 4 units per bitch or queen (NOT units/kg). The frequency of oxytocin administration is dictated by the labor pattern; oxytocin should generally not be given more frequently than hourly.[6]

Secondary agalactia: Oxytocin 0.25 – 1 unit per bitch or queen (NOT units/kg) SC every 2 hours. Neonates are removed for 30 minutes postinjection and encouraged to suckle, or gentle stripping of the glands is performed. Metoclopramide (dopamine antagonist) 0.1 – 0.2 mg/kg SC every 12 hours can also be given to promote milk production. Therapy is usually rewarding within 24 hours.[7]

Adjunctive treatment of acute metritis: Start broad-spectrum antibiotic therapy with good tissue penetration into the reproductive tract (eg, clindamycin plus gentamicin, ampicillin/sulbactam, amoxicillin/clavulanate, second generation cephalosporin), while waiting for culture and susceptibility results. Institute fluid therapy if the patient is dehydrated or in shock. Oxytocin 0.5 – 5 units per bitch or queen (NOT units/kg) IM may be used if birth has occurred less than 24 hours prior, or dinoprost (prostaglandin [PGF2-alpha] analogue) 0.25 mg/kg SC may be used at any time to promote evacuation of the uterus.[8]

Promotion of uterine involution after uterine prolapse manual reduction:

a) Digital manipulation to replace the uterus can be attempted using general and/or epidural anesthesia. If the tissue is very swollen, hyperosmotic fluids (eg, 50% dextrose, mannitol) may be used to assist in replacement. In some cases, an episiotomy is required to successfully reduce the prolapse. Following reduction, oxytocin 0.5 – 5 units per bitch or queen (NOT units/kg) IM will promote uterine involution.

b) Anesthetize the patient and apply sterile lubricant liberally to the exposed tissue. The uterine horn is flushed with sterile saline under pressure. Mannitol or hypertonic saline can be used to reduce edema, if necessary, before attempting reduction. Once the uterus is replaced, give oxytocin 5 – 10 units per bitch or queen (NOT units/kg) IM to cause uterine involution.

HORSES:

Augmentation or initiation of uterine contractions during parturition in properly evaluated mares: Ideally, colostrum should be present in the udder prior to induction, the cervix should be soft and dilating, and the mare should be as close to her normal due date as possible. The optimal dose and route of administration for induction remains controversial. Three protocols have been suggested: (1) low-dose oxytocin 2.5 – 5 units (total dose; NOT units/kg) IV every 15 to 30 minutes; (2) oxytocin 1 unit (total dose; NOT units/kg)/minute IV CRI; or (3) multiple smaller doses of oxytocin 15 units (total dose; NOT units/kg) IM every 15 to 20 minutes.[9]

Prevention of luteolysis:

a) Oxytocin 60 units (total dose; NOT units/kg) IM once daily can be given from day 7 to day 14 postovulation to prolong corpus luteum lifespan. With this protocol, mares have remained out of heat for up to 45 to 60 days; however, ovulation must be documented (or estimated closely) when oxytocin is used this manner.[10]

b) A similar protocol (ie, oxytocin 60 units IM from days 8 to 17) prolonged luteal maintenance past 30 days in most mares.[11]

Evacuation of uterine fluid: 10 – 20 units (total dose; NOT units/kg) IV or IM every 4 to 8 hours[12]

Assistance in removal of retained fetal membranes: 20 units (total dose; NOT units/kg) IV or IM given every hour beginning 2 to 3 hours after foaling; repeat as needed.[12] Alternatively, 20 units IV or IM every 15 min for one 2-hour block in the morning and one 2-hour block in the evening.[13]

Treatment of esophageal obstruction ("choke"): Butylscopolamine 0.3 mg/kg IV once and oxytocin 0.11 – 0.22 units/kg IV once. Oxytocin use should be avoided in mares, or the dose should be significantly reduced. Do not use in pregnant mares.

CATTLE:

Milk letdown (label dosage; FDA-approved): 10 – 20 units IV; may be repeated as necessary[14]

Obstetrical use in cows (label dosage; FDA-approved): 100 units IV, IM, or SC; may be repeated as necessary.[14] **NOTE**: Many clinicians believe this dosage to be higher than necessary.

Retained fetal membranes: 20 – 30 units (total dose; NOT units/kg) IM immediately following calving, repeated 2 to 4 hours later[15–17]

Mild to moderate cases of acute postpartum metritis: 20 units (total dose; NOT units/kg) IM 3 to 4 times daily for 2 to 3 days[15]

Augmentation of uterine contractions during parturition: 30 units (total dose; NOT units/kg) IM; repeat no sooner than 30 minutes, if necessary[18]

SHEEP/GOATS:

Obstetrical use in ewes (label dosage; FDA-approved): 30 – 50 units (total dose; NOT units/kg) IV, IM, or SC; may be repeated as necessary[14]

Retained placenta in patients with uterine atony: 10 – 20 units (total dose; NOT units/kg) IM; this drug is of limited value 48 hours postpartum, as uterine sensitivity is reduced. Treat with antibiotics if signs of metritis develop.[19]

Mild to moderate cases of acute postpartum metritis: 5 – 10 units (total dose; NOT units/kg) IM 3 to 4 times daily for

2 to 3 days[15]

Control of postextraction cervical and uterine bleeding in goats after internal manipulations (eg, fetotomy): 10 – 20 units (total dose; NOT units/kg) IV; may repeat SC in 2 hours[20]

Nonsurgical embryo recovery: Oxytocin 50 units (total dose; NOT units/kg) IV or intravaginally given 20 minutes before embryo flushing. Cloprostenol 37.5 **µg (total dose, NOT mg/kg)** via latero-vulvar injection and estradiol benzoate 1 mg (total dose, NOT mg/kg) by either IM or intravaginal route were administered 16 hours before embryo flushing.[21,22]

NEW WORLD CAMELIDS:

Retained placenta: 5 – 30 units (total dose; NOT units/kg) IM may be given at 10-minute intervals, with or without gentle traction. Strenuous traction may induce uterine prolapse.[23,24]

Agalactia: 20 units (total dose; NOT units/kg) IM up to every 2 hours[24]

SWINE:

Milk letdown in sows (label dosage): 5 – 20 units (total dose; NOT units/kg) IV; may be repeated as necessary[14]

Augmentation of uterine contractions during parturition:

a) **Obstetrical use in sows** (label dosage; FDA-approved): 30 – 50 units (total dose; NOT units/kg) IV, IM, or SC; may be repeated as necessary[14]
b) 10 units (total dose; NOT units/kg) IM; repeat no sooner than 30 minutes, if necessary[18]

Mild to moderate cases of acute postpartum metritis: 5 units (total dose; NOT units/kg) IM; may need to be repeated, as effect may be as short as 30 minutes[25]

Adjunctive treatment for mastitis, metritis, agalactia (MMA) syndrome: 20 – 50 units (total dose; NOT units/kg) IM or 5 – 10 units IV[26]

Retained placenta in patients with uterine atony: 20 – 30 units (total dose; NOT units/kg) every 2 to 3 hours as necessary in conjunction with antimicrobial therapy [19] 5 – 10 units (total dose; NOT units/kg) around the time of expulsion of first placental part (route not specified, assume IM; editors).[27]

BIRDS:

Egg binding (nonobstructive): 0.2 – 2 units per hen (total dose; NOT unit/kg) IM once. Adequate calcium must be present. In general, prostaglandins are considered superior to oxytocin because they can increase uterine contraction and relax the vaginal sphincter.[28] Oxytocin 0.5 – 10 units/kg have been reported, up to 30 units/bird, often repeated in 30 to 60 minutes. Oxytocin should be used in conjunction with other therapeutics (eg, PGE2, PGF2alpha, calcium gluconate).[24]

RABBITS, RODENTS, SMALL MAMMALS:

Dystocia:

Mice, Rats, Gerbils, Hamsters, Guinea pigs, Chinchillas: 0.2 – 3 units/kg IV, IM, or SC[29]

Rabbits: Calcium glubionate 10%, 5 – 10 mL PO 30 minutes before giving oxytocin 1 – 3 units (total dose; not units/kg) IM[24]

Ferrets: 5 – 10 units per ferret (NOT units/kg) IM[30]

REPTILES:

Egg binding (nonobstructive): Depending on the species, oxytocin 1 – 40 units/kg have been effective, especially in chelonians. A second dose is generally given anywhere from 20 minutes to 12 hours after the first dose has been administered. Keep reptiles near their optimal body temperature, as temperature likely influences the effect of oxytocin on the oviduct. For best results, use with a therapy protocol that includes environmental optimization, rehydration, and calcium supplementation.

Snakes: 5 – 20 units/kg IM[24]

Lizards: 5 – 30 units/kg IM or intracoelomically[24]

Chelonians: Generally, 1 – 3 units/kg IM, IV, or by intraosseous infusion; 50% to 100% of the initial dose can be repeated IV or IM 1 to 12 hours later.[24,31]

Monitoring

- Uterine contractions, status of cervix
- Fetal monitoring if available and indicated

Client Information

- Do not use during obstructed labor, if cervix is not ready/relaxed, or if vaginal birth is not possible or recommended.
- Oxytocin should only be used in animals that can be adequately monitored for its effects.
- Use this medication only in close communication with your veterinarian.
- Oxytocin is administered by injection. Be sure you understand the instructions from your veterinarian about how and when to give this medication.
- Place used needles and syringes in a sharps disposal container immediately after use.
- Contact your veterinarian immediately if the fetus fails to be delivered within the expected timeframe or if your animal develops a fever, vomiting, or seizures.
- Those trying to conceive, and women who are pregnant or breastfeeding, should handle oxytocin carefully.
- This medication is considered to be a hazardous drug as defined by the National Institute for Occupational Safety and Health (NIOSH). Talk with your veterinarian or pharmacist about the use of personal protective equipment when handling this medicine.

Chemistry/Synonyms

Oxytocin, a nonapeptide hypothalamic hormone stored in the posterior pituitary (in mammals), occurs as a white powder that is soluble in water. The commercially available preparations are highly purified and have virtually no antidiuretic or vasopressor activity when administered at usual doses. Oxytocin potency is standardized according to its vasopressor activity in chickens and is expressed in USP Posterior Pituitary Units. One unit is equivalent to ≈2 – 2.2 µg of pure hormone.

Commercial preparations of oxytocin injection have the pH adjusted with acetic acid to 2.5 to 4.5, and multidose vials generally contain chlorobutanol 0.5% as a preservative.

Oxytocin may also be known as alpha-hypophamine, oxytocinum, or *Pitocin®*.

Storage/Stability

Oxytocin injection should be stored at temperatures of less than 25°C (77°F) but not frozen. Some manufacturers recommend storing the product under refrigeration (2°C-8°C [36°F-46°F]), but some products have been demonstrated to be stable for up to 5 years when stored at less than 26°C (78.8°F).

Compatibility/Compounding Considerations

Oxytocin is reportedly physically **compatible** with most commonly used IV fluids and amikacin, buprenorphine, butorphanol, calcium salts (eg, chloride, gluconate), cefazolin, clindamycin, dexamethasone sodium phosphate, famotidine, ketamine, lidocaine, metoclopramide, metronidazole, midazolam, ondansetron, penicillin G potassium/sodium, sodium bicarbonate, and verapamil.

Oxytocin is reportedly physically **incompatible** with ampicillin sodium, diazepam, pantoprazole, and sulfamethoxazole/trimethoprim.

Compatibility is dependent on factors such as pH, concentration, temperature, and diluent used; consult specialized references or a hospital pharmacist for more specific information.

Dosage Forms/Regulatory Status

VETERINARY-LABELED PRODUCTS:

Oxytocin for Injection: 20 USP units/mL in 100 mL vials; generic; (Rx). Oxytocin products are labeled for several species, including horses, dairy cattle, beef cattle, sheep, swine, cats, and dogs. There are no milk or meat withdrawal times specified for oxytocin. Other strengths may be available in some countries.

HUMAN-LABELED PRODUCTS:

Oxytocin Solution for Injection: 10 units/mL in 1 mL single-dose vials, and 10 mL and 30 mL multiple-dose vials; *Pitocin*®, generic; (Rx)

References

For the complete list of references, see **wiley.com/go/budde/plumb**

Pamidronate

(pah-***mih***-dro-nate) *Aredia*®

Bisphosphonate

Prescriber Highlights

- IV bisphosphonate used for the treatment of hypercalcemia and for the palliative treatment of bone cancer
- Must be given IV in saline over several hours
- Use with caution in patients with renal insufficiency as pamidronate can cause renal toxicity.
- Adverse effects include electrolyte abnormalities and anemia.
- The National Institute for Occupational Safety and Health (NIOSH) classifies pamidronate as a hazardous drug; use appropriate precautions when handling.

Uses/Indications

In companion animals, pamidronate has been used to treat refractory idiopathic hypercalcemia, hypercalcemia associated with malignancy, or vitamin D–related toxicosis. Pamidronate is also utilized in the adjunctive treatment of pain associated with osteolytic bone tumors.

Pamidronate administered to horses with osteoarthritis had a beneficial effect on clinical scores and reduced inflammatory biomarkers of disease.[1]

Pharmacology/Actions

Bisphosphonates, at therapeutic concentrations, inhibit bone resorption and do not inhibit bone mineralization via binding to hydroxyapatite crystals. They impede osteoclast activity and induce osteoclast apoptosis. Pamidronate has ≈100 times greater relative antiresorptive potency when compared to etidronate.

Bisphosphonates in vitro have direct cytotoxic or cytostatic effects on human osteosarcoma cell lines. They may also have antiangiogenic effects and inhibit cell migration in certain cancers.

Pharmacokinetics

After IV infusion in rats, 50% to 60% of the dose is rapidly absorbed by bone.[2] Bone uptake is highest in areas of rapid bone turnover. Pamidronate is not metabolized, and the kidneys very slowly eliminate the drug. Terminal half-life is on the order of 300 days in rats. When used for hypercalcemia, pamidronate's onset of action is in 24 to 48 hours, and its duration of effect ranges from 2 to 4 weeks.

Contraindications/Precautions/Warnings

Pamidronate is contraindicated in patients hypersensitive to it or any of the bisphosphonate drugs or mannitol (many commercial pamidronate products also contain mannitol—see ***Dosage Forms/Regulatory Status***). Use with caution in juvenile animals in which skeletal development is still occurring and in those animals healing from a bone fracture.

Pamidronate should be used with caution in patients with impaired renal function as it has been associated with renal toxicity. Pamidronate potentially causes renal toxicity in dogs; infuse over at least 2 hours. In humans, infusions are administered over 2 to 24 hours, and infusions longer than 2 hours may reduce the risk for renal toxicity, particularly in patients with pre-existing renal impairment. In humans, it has not been tested in patients with serum creatinine levels greater than 5 mg/dL.

The National Institute for Occupational Safety and Health (NIOSH) classifies pamidronate as a hazardous drug[3]; personal protective equipment (PPE) should be used accordingly to minimize the risk for exposure.

Adverse Effects

Electrolyte abnormalities (g, calcium, phosphorus, potassium, magnesium) may occur with pamidronate therapy. One case of a dog developing hypomagnesemia and arrhythmias after pamidronate has been reported.[4] In dogs, injection site reactions in association with pamidronate extravasation have been described.[5] In humans, fever, dose-related injection site reactions, ocular inflammation, transient musculoskeletal pain, electrolyte disturbances, osteonecrosis of the jaw, atypical fractures, anemia, thrombocytopenia, and leukopenia have been reported.[2] One case of medication-related osteonecrosis of the jaw (MRONJ) has been reported in a cat that had received long-term pamidronate therapy.[6]

Reproductive/Nursing Safety

Pamidronate has produced both maternal and embryo/fetal toxicity in laboratory animals when given at dosages therapeutically used in humans.[2] If it is used in pregnant veterinary patients, informed consent by the owner accepting the risks to both dam and offspring is recommended. It is unknown if pamidronate is excreted into milk. Use it with caution in nursing mothers. Because safety has not been established in animals, this drug should only be used when the maternal benefits outweigh the potential risks to offspring.

Overdose/Acute Toxicity

Overdoses of pamidronate may cause hypocalcemia, including tetany. If this occurs, treat with short-term IV calcium. For patients that have experienced or are suspected of having experienced an overdose, consultation with a 24-hour poison consultation center specializing in providing veterinary-specific information is recommended. For general information related to overdose and toxin exposures, as well as contact information for poison control centers, refer to ***Appendix.***

Drug Interactions

The following drug interactions have either been reported or are theoretical in humans or animals receiving pamidronate and may be of significance in veterinary patients. Unless otherwise noted, use together is not necessarily contraindicated, but weigh the potential risks and perform additional monitoring when appropriate.

- **AMINOGLYCOSIDES**: May enhance hypocalcemic effects of pamidronate; monitor
- **CORTICOSTEROIDS** (eg, **dexamethasone, fludrocortisone, prednis(ol)one**): Pamidronate must be used carefully (with monitoring) when used in conjunction with other drugs that can affect calcium.
- **LOOP DIURETICS** (eg, **furosemide**): Loop diuretics promote calcium excretion and may result in additive effects on calcium concentrations.
- **NEPHROTOXIC DRUGS** (eg, **aminoglycosides, amphotericin B, cisplatin**): Use with caution; potential for increased risk for nephrotoxicity
- **NONSTEROIDAL ANTI-INFLAMMATORY DRUGS** (**NSAIDs**; eg,

carprofen, flunixin, meloxicam): Use with caution; potential for increased risk for nephrotoxicity

- THIAZIDE DIURETICS (eg, **hydrochlorothiazide**): Thiazide diuretics promote calcium retention and may impair the hypocalcemic effects of pamidronate.

Laboratory Considerations

- No specific laboratory interactions or considerations were noted.

Dosages

DOGS/CATS

Refractory hypercalcemia (extra-label): 1.3 – 2.3 mg/kg diluted in 150 to 250 mL of 0.9% sodium chloride and administered IV as a CRI over 2 to 4 hours.[7,8] May be repeated every 21 to 28 days

Treatment of vitamin D (cholecalciferol, calcipotriene, and related compounds) induced hypercalcemia: 1.3 – 2 mg/kg diluted into 250 mL of 0.9% sodium chloride and administered IV as a CRI over 2 hours; may repeat dose after 3 days. In most cases, a single dose will lower calcium levels back to normal. Recommended monitoring calcium levels daily for at least 10 days after they have returned to normal, and some patients may need to be retreated in 5 to 7 days.[9,10]

Palliative adjunctive analgesia for osteosarcoma bone pain (extra-label): 1 – 2 mg/kg; diluted into 250 mL of 0.9% sodium chloride and administered IV as a CRI over 2 hours every 28 days.[11-16] **NOTE**: Some sources anecdotally recommend giving as frequently as once per week.

HORSES:

Osteoarthritis (extra-label): 90 mg (0.4 – 0.8 mg/kg) IV with a second dose repeated 9 days later resulted in improved clinical scores and reduced proinflammatory markers.[1]

Monitoring

- Baseline and periodic (prior to each dose) serum renal chemistry panel
- Hydration status
- Baseline and periodic serum calcium, phosphate, magnesium, potassium
- Baseline and periodic CBC
- Baseline and periodic urinalysis
- Injection site should be checked periodically during infusion

Client Information

- This medicine must only be given at the veterinary hospital.
- Owners should understand the costs for the medication, care, and monitoring associated with its use.

Chemistry/Synonyms

Pamidronate disodium, a bisphosphonate inhibitor of bone resorption, occurs as a white, crystalline powder that is soluble in water and practically insoluble in organic solvents.

Pamidronate may also be known as ADP sodium, AHPrBP sodium, GCP-23339A, *Aminomux®*, *Aredia®*, *Aredronet®*, *Ostepam®*, or *Pamidran®*.

Storage/Stability

Store at room temperature, 20°C to 25°C (68°F-77°F).

Once the lyophilized powder for injection is reconstituted (10 mL) with sterile water for injection, it may be stored in the refrigerator for 24 hours. Be sure drug is completely dissolved before withdrawing into syringe.

Compatibility/Compounding Considerations

Compatibility is dependent upon factors, such as pH, concentration, temperature, and diluent used; consult specialized references or a hospital pharmacist for more specific information.

Do **NOT** mix pamidronate with any IV fluid containing calcium (eg, lactated Ringer's solution [LRS]). It is recommended to use a dedicated IV solution (0.45% or 0.9% sodium chloride or 5% dextrose) and line.

Pamidronate disodium is reported **compatible** with dextrose and saline solutions and the following drugs when administered via a **Y-site**: aminocaproic acid, ampicillin/sulbactam, azithromycin, bleomycin, butorphanol, carboplatin, carmustine, cefazolin, cefotaxime, ceftazidime, cisplatin, clindamycin, cyclophosphamide, cytarabine, dacarbazine, daunorubicin (liposomal), dexamethasone sodium phosphate, dexmedetomidine, dexrazoxane, diphenhydramine, dopamine, doxorubicin HCL (also liposome form), doxycycline, erythromycin lactobionate, famotidine, fentanyl citrate, fluconazole, fluorouracil, gemcitabine, heparin, hydromorphone, hydroxyzine, ifosfamide, imipenem-cilastatin, mannitol, mesna, methotrexate, metoclopramide, methylprednisolone sodium succinate, mitoxantrone, morphine, ondansetron, piperacillin-tazobactam, potassium chloride, prochlorperazine, promethazine, ranitidine, vinblastine, and vincristine.

Dosage Forms/Regulatory Status

VETERINARY-LABELED PRODUCTS: NONE

HUMAN-LABELED PRODUCTS:

Pamidronate Disodium Lyophilized Powder for Injection: 30 mg, 60 mg, and 90 mg vials; generic; (Rx). Also contains mannitol 375 mg, 400 mg, or 470 mg per vial, respectively.

Pamidronate Disodium Injection: 3 mg/mL, 6 mg/mL, and 9 mg/mL (may contain mannitol) in 10 mL vials; generic; (Rx).

References

For the complete list of references, see **wiley.com/go/budde/plumb**

Pancrelipase

(pan-kree-***lih***-pase) *Viokase®*

Pancreatic Enzymes

Prescriber Highlights

- ▶ Used to treat exocrine pancreatic insufficiency
- ▶ Contraindications include hypersensitivity to pork products.
- ▶ Adverse effects include GI effects (eg, diarrhea, cramping, nausea), and oral or esophageal irritation are possible.
- ▶ Most human products are enteric-coated delayed-release formulations; veterinary products are not coated.
- ▶ Respiratory irritant: avoid inhalation of powder; may cause skin irritation: wash hands after handling

Uses/Indications

Pancrelipase is used to treat patients with exocrine pancreatic enzyme insufficiency (EPI).

Dogs may have EPI and not respond to pancreatic enzyme replacement because a) the enzyme product is poorly effective, b) the diet is too high in fat, and/or c) the dog has concurrent antibiotic responsive enteropathy. About 15% of dogs with EPI simply will not respond to therapy and have a bad prognosis.[1]

Pharmacology/Actions

Pancrelipase is a combination of porcine lipase, proteases, and amylase, which help to digest and absorb fats, proteins, and carbohydrates. It catalyzes the hydrolysis of fats to glycerol and fatty acids, degrades protein into amino acids, and converts starch into dextrin and sugars. In humans, the enteric-coated form is preferred as it is more stable in gastric acid; however, it is not recommended in patients with rapid gastrojejunal transit.[2] This may indicate that non-enteric-coated formulations would be more effective in dogs, and most GI experts advocate for powdered non–enteric-coated formulations.[3] However, one study revealed a positive treatment response to an enteric-coated pancreatic supplementation product.[4] Another study found no difference between the 2 formulations, although it was too underpowered to determine clinical significance.[5]

Pharmacokinetics

Pancrelipase is inactivated by gastric acid. The enteric coating of delayed-release products prevents destruction and inactivation in gastric acid. In humans, non–enteric-coated products are recommended to be given with proton pump inhibitors to help prevent their breakdown in the stomach.[6] Pancrelipase is not absorbed from the GI tract and is not systemically active.

Contraindications/Precautions/Warnings

Pancrelipase products are contraindicated in animals that are hypersensitive to pork proteins. Use pancrelipase with caution in patients with gout, renal impairment, or hyperuricemia, as pancrelipase has been shown to increase blood uric acid concentrations in humans.[7] Because pancrelipase is a porcine product, human products contain a warning that there is a theoretical risk for transmission of viral diseases.

Do not crush capsule contents of delayed-release capsules or mix with foods with a pH greater than 4, as this disrupts the protective coating.[7] In humans, non–enteric-coated tablets are intended to be swallowed whole and should not be crushed or chewed.[7] One veterinary product specifies that tablets are intended to be administered prior to being fed and they are not intended for being mixed directly with food[8]; other products do not specify. However, crushing tablets should be avoided when possible due to risks associated with the inhalation of powders.

Do not inhale the powder, as it may cause respiratory irritation, including coughing, chest tightness, allergies, or asthma clinical signs.[9] Avoid contact with mucous membranes or skin; wash hands after handling.

Adverse Effects

The most common adverse effects are GI-related (eg, diarrhea, cramping, nausea). Pancreatic enzymes can cause oral or esophageal irritation or ulcers; follow dosing with food or water. Oral bleeding has been reported in dogs after receiving pancrelipase.[10] Dose reduction and moistening the food-pancreatic powder mix may also decrease the incidence of this adverse effect.

Reproductive/Nursing Safety

These enzymes are unlikely to be excreted in maternal milk or pose a risk for offspring.

Because safety has not been established in animals, this drug should only be used when the maternal benefits outweigh the potential risks to offspring.

Overdose/Acute Toxicity

Overdoses may cause diarrhea or other intestinal upset. The effects should be temporary and may be treated by reducing the dose and providing supportive care if diarrhea is severe.

For patients that have experienced or are suspected of having experienced an overdose, consultation with a 24-hour poison consultation center specializing in providing veterinary-specific information is recommended. For general information related to overdose and toxin exposures, as well as contact information for poison control centers, refer to ***Appendix.***

Drug Interactions

The following drug interactions have either been reported or are theoretical in humans or animals receiving pancrelipase and may be of significance in veterinary patients. Unless otherwise noted, use together is not necessarily contraindicated, but weigh the potential risks and perform additional monitoring when appropriate.

- **ANTACIDS** (magnesium hydroxide, calcium carbonate): May diminish the effectiveness of pancrelipase[11]
- **CIMETIDINE** (or other H2 Antagonists): May increase the amount of pancrelipase that reaches the duodenum

Laboratory Considerations

None noted

Dosages

DOGS:

Exocrine pancreatic insufficiency (extra-label):

a) Initially, 1 teaspoon/10 kg (22 lb; NOT mg/kg) body weight per meal. Mix with food immediately prior to feeding. When clinical signs have resolved, the amount of pancreatic enzymes given can be gradually decreased to the lowest effective dose, which may vary from patient to patient and from batch to batch of the pancreatic supplement.[12,13]

b) 1 – 2 teaspoons of powder to each of 2 meals of balanced canine ration. Tailor regimen to maintain optimal body weight.[14]

CATS:

Exocrine pancreatic insufficiency (extra-label): **NOTE:** Cats reportedly dislike the taste of the powder but may accept the powder if mixed with fish/tuna oil and then thoroughly mixed with canned food. If using solid dosage forms (enteric-coated tablets or compounded capsules made from powder or crushed tablets), be certain that immediately after dosing, water or food is consumed to reduce the risk for esophageal damage.

a) 1 teaspoon of powder to each of 2 meals of balanced feline ration. Cats that refuse to eat food treated with powder may be dosed with capsules filled with powder. Tailor regimen to maintain optimal body weight.[14]

b) Initially, 1 teaspoon/cat (NOT teaspoon/kg) with each meal. When clinical signs have resolved, the amount of pancreatic enzymes given can be gradually decreased to the lowest effective dose, which may vary from patient to patient and from batch to batch of the pancreatic supplement.[12]

c) 0.5 – 1 teaspoon/cat (NOT teaspoon/kg) with each meal. Mix within the food immediately prior to feeding. Enteric-coated tablets, granules, and capsules are not recommended due to their variable efficacy.[15]

BIRDS:

Exocrine pancreatic insufficiency (extra-label): ⅛ teaspoon/kg mixed with moistened feed or administer by gavage. Incubate with food for 15 minutes prior to gavage.[17] Used in birds that are polyphagic "going light", passing whole seeds, and slow in emptying crops

RABBITS, RODENTS, SMALL MAMMALS:

Gastric trichobezoars in rabbits (extra-label): 1 teaspoon pancrelipase powder plus 3 teaspoons (15 mL) of yogurt; let stand for 15 minutes, then give 2 – 3 mL PO every 12 hours. Questionable efficacy for removing hairballs, but might help dissolve the protein matrix surrounding hair[16]

Monitoring

- Animal's weight
- Stool consistency, frequency

Client Information

- Pancrelipase powder is usually mixed in the food and left to stand for 15 to 20 minutes before feeding. Your veterinarian may instruct you to mix it into food and offer it to your animal without waiting.
- Cats often dislike the taste of the powder and pancrelipase may be more easily given using tablets or specially compounded capsules.

Some cats will eat food mixed with one brand of veterinary powder and refuse another.

- If using capsules or tablets, be certain that your animal gets plenty of water or food right after dosing to reduce the risk for esophageal damage.
- Use caution to avoid inhaling powder, as it can cause lung irritation and asthma. If your skin comes into contact with the powder, wash it off immediately.

Chemistry/Synonyms

Pancrelipase contains pancreatic enzymes, primarily lipase but also amylase and protease, and is obtained from the pancreas of hogs. Each milligram of pancrelipase contains not less than 24 USP units of lipase activity, not less than 100 USP units of protease activity, and not less than 100 USP units of amylase activity. When compared on a per weight basis, pancrelipase has at least 4 times the trypsin and amylase content of pancreatin, and at least 12 times the lipolytic activity of pancreatin.

Pancrelipase may also be known as pancrelipasa, *Epizyme®*, *Panakare®*, *Pancrepowder Plus®*, *Pancreved®*, *Pancrezyme®*, and *Viokase®*.

Storage/Stability

Unless otherwise recommended by the manufacturer, store this product at room temperature (20°C-25°C [68°F-77°F]) in a dry place in tight containers. When present in quantities greater than trace amounts, acids will inactivate pancrelipase.

Dosage Forms/Regulatory Status

NOTE: There are several dosage forms (both human and veterinary-label) available containing pancrelipase, including oral capsules, oral delayed-release capsules, tablets, and delayed-released tablets. Most small animal practitioners believe the oral powder is most effective in dogs.

VETERINARY-LABELED PRODUCTS: (**NOTE**: NONE OF THE VETERINARY PRODUCTS ARE FDA-APPROVED.)

Pancrelipase Powder containing ≈2.8 g per teaspoonful: 71,400 units lipase; 388,000 units protease; 460,000 units amylase; in 8 oz bottle; *Viokase®-V Powder, Pancrezyme® Powder, Pancrepowder Plus®, Pancreved® Powder, Epizyme® Powder, Panakare® Plus Powder*; (Rx). Labeled for use in dogs and cats

Pancreatic enzyme concentrate plus fat-soluble vitamins in tablet form: each tablet contains a minimum of 9000 USP units of lipase; 57,000 units of protease; 64,000 USP units of amylase; and is fortified with vitamins A, D_3, and E; *Panakare® Plus Tablets, Pancreplus® Tablets, Pancreved®* Tablets. Labeled for use in dogs and cats

HUMAN-LABELED PRODUCTS:

There are capsules, tablets, and powders available containing lipase, protease, and amylase in varying units available for human consumption from many distributors. Most formulations are enteric-coated/delayed-release. Human formulations are not directly interchangeable.

References

For the complete list of references, see **wiley.com/go/budde/plumb**

Pantoprazole

(pan-***toe***-prah-zohl) *Protonix®, Pantoloc®*
Proton Pump Inhibitor

Prescriber Highlights

- ► Used for the treatment of gastric acid-related pathologies in dogs, cats, foals, camelids, and ruminants; more effective than histamine-2 receptor antagonists (eg, famotidine)
- ► Administer every 12 hours for optimal efficacy; available in IV dosage form
- ► Appears to be well tolerated
- ► Tapering dose after long-term (ie, 3 to 4 weeks) use is recommended.

Uses/Indications

Pantoprazole may be useful in the treatment of gastric acid-related pathologies in dogs, cats, foals, camelids, and ruminants, particularly when the IV route is required.

Based on studies conducted in healthy dogs,[1,2] IV pantoprazole significantly increased gastric pH and the percentage of time gastric pH was greater than 3 or 4.[1,2] Under these experimental conditions, twice-daily esomeprazole IV or omeprazole PO and famotidine CRI were the only treatments that attained intragastric pH goals (ie, pH greater than 3 for 75% of the day, and greater than 4 for 67% of the day) established for treatment of humans with duodenal ulcers and/or gastroesophageal reflux.[1,2] There were no significant differences in intragastric pH in dogs given combination pantoprazole with famotidine as compared with dogs given pantoprazole alone,[3] and combining a histamine-2 receptor antagonist with a proton pump inhibitor is not recommended.[4] If pantoprazole has been used for 3 weeks or longer, it is recommended to taper the dose by decreasing to once-daily administration for 7 days before discontinuing to minimize the risk for developing rebound gastric acid hypersecretion.[4,5]

Pantoprazole use has been described in case reports for ruminant species.[6-8] One retrospective study found that pantoprazole may be a safe adjunct therapy in cattle, sheep, and goats[9]; however, further studies are needed to assess safety and toxicity.

Pantoprazole is used in some *Helicobacter pylori* treatment protocols for humans; however, there is no evidence that acid suppression is indicated for the treatment of *Helicobacter* spp infections in dogs and cats.[4]

Pharmacology/Actions

Pantoprazole is a substituted benzimidazole proton pump inhibitor. At the secretory surface of gastric parietal cells, pantoprazole forms a covalent bond at 2 sites of active H^+/K^+ ATPase (proton pump), inhibiting the transport of hydrogen ions into the stomach. Pantoprazole reduces acid secretion during both basal and stimulated conditions. Inactivation of the proton pump is permanent, which contributes to the durability of pantoprazole's acid suppressing effect.[10] Steady state acid suppression is reached after 2 to 4 days, as some proton pumps are dormant.[11,12]

In alpacas, pantoprazole has been shown to increase the pH of the third compartment.[13]

Pharmacokinetics

No specific information was located for pantoprazole pharmacokinetics in dogs or cats.

In neonatal foals, intragastric (IG) administered pantoprazole bioavailability was 41%, and the drug was detected in plasma within 5 minutes of administration.[14] Gastric pH was significantly increased 2 hours after administration by either IV or IG routes, and mean hourly gastric pH remained elevated for the remainder of the 24-hour study-period.[14]

In neonatal calves given 1 mg/kg IV, plasma clearance was ≈4.5 mL/kg/minute, elimination half-life was ≈2.8 hours, and volume of distribution was ≈0.3 L/kg.[15]

In goats given 1 mg/kg IV, plasma clearance was ≈0.3 mL/kg/minute, elimination half-life was ≈0.7 hours, and volume of distribution was ≈0.9 L/kg.[16]

In alpacas, pantoprazole has a high SC bioavailability (ie, greater than 100% in some animals). A dose of 2 mg/kg SC produced significantly higher area under the curve (AUC) and longer half-life than when given IV, but the half-life remained short (mean, 0.58 hours).[13]

In humans, the drug is rapidly absorbed after oral administration, with an oral bioavailability of 77%. Food can reduce the rate of absorption but does not appear to affect the extent of absorption. On average, 51% of gastric acid secretion is inhibited 2.5 hours after a single dose and 85% is inhibited after 7 days of daily administration. Protein binding is 98%, primarily to albumin. The drug is metabolized in the liver, primarily by CYP2C19 isoenzymes. CYP3A4, 2D6, 2C9, and 1A2 are minor components of pantoprazole biotransformation; pantoprazole does not appear to clinically affect (ie, induce or inhibit) the metabolism of other drugs using these isoenzymes for biotransformation. Metabolites of pantoprazole do not appear to have pharmacologic activity. The elimination half-life for both PO and IV administration is ≈1 hour, but the drug's pharmacologic action can last 24 hours or longer, presumably due to irreversible binding at the receptor site. Approximately 71% of a dose is excreted as metabolites in the urine, with the remainder in the feces as metabolites and unabsorbed drug.

Contraindications/Precautions/Warnings

Pantoprazole is contraindicated in those known to be hypersensitive to it or other proton pump inhibitors.

In humans, pantoprazole is not for SC or IM use due to the pH of the reconstituted solution.[17] Anecdotally, SC dosing in camelids and ruminants appears to be tolerated. When given IV, the reconstituted injection (4 mg/mL) must be administered over at least 2 minutes. Hypomagnesemia has been reported in humans, typically after long-term use.[17]

Adverse Effects

Pantoprazole appears to be well tolerated.

In a retrospective study of 36 cattle receiving pantoprazole, edema was reported in 7 (16%) cattle.[9] Safe duration of use has not been established in ruminants; increasing abomasal pH for extended periods may lead to growth of enteropathogenic bacteria.[6]

In humans, the most commonly reported adverse effects are diarrhea and headache.[17] Hyperglycemia has been reported in ≈1% of patients. Proton pump inhibitors have been associated with an increased risk for developing community-acquired pneumonia in humans. Injection site reactions (eg, thrombophlebitis, abscess) have occurred with IV administration.

Reproductive/Nursing Safety

Daily administration of pantoprazole 20 mg/kg IV to rats and 15mg/kg IV to rabbits during organogenesis had no effects on fertility, and no teratogenic effects were noted; however, daily pantoprazole 5 – 30 mg/kg given to pregnant rats from the sixth gestational day through the twenty-first day of lactation resulted in changes in bone morphology in rat pups.[17]

Pantoprazole and its metabolites are excreted in milk. Use pantoprazole with caution during lactation.

Because safety has not been established in animals, this drug should only be used when the maternal benefits outweigh the potential fetal risks.

Overdose/Acute Toxicity

Limited information is available. A single dose of 266 mg/kg IV or 887 mg/kg PO was lethal in dogs. Acute toxic signs included ataxia, hypoactivity, and tremors. In humans, single overdoses of up to 600 mg (total dose) PO have been reported without adverse effects. In the event of a large overdose, it is recommended to contact an animal poison control center for guidance.

For patients that have experienced or are suspected to have experienced an overdose, consultation with a 24-hour poison consultation center specializing in providing veterinary-specific information is recommended. For general information related to overdose and toxin exposures, as well as contact information for poison control centers, refer to ***Appendix***.

Drug Interactions

The following drug interactions have either been reported or are theoretical in humans or animals receiving pantoprazole and may be of significance in veterinary patients. Unless otherwise noted, use together is not necessarily contraindicated, but weigh the potential risks and perform additional monitoring when appropriate.

- **Bisphosphonate Derivatives** (eg, **alendronate, etidronate**): Pantoprazole may diminish therapeutic effects.
- **Drugs Requiring Decreased Gastric pH for Optimal Absorption** (eg, **ampicillin esters, iron, itraconazole, ketoconazole**): Pantoprazole may decrease drug absorption.
- **Levothyroxine**: Concurrent use may result in increased TSH concentrations.
- **Mycophenolate mofetil**: May result in decreased exposure to the active metabolite of mycophenolate
- **Sucralfate**: Concurrent use may decrease bioavailability of orally administered pantoprazole.
- **Warfarin**: Pantoprazole may increase the anticoagulant effect.

Laboratory Considerations

- Although not likely to be important for veterinary patients, pantoprazole may cause false-positive results for urine screening tests for THC (tetrahydrocannabinol).[17]

Dosages

DOGS/CATS:

Gastric acid suppression (extra-label): 0.7 – 1 mg/kg IV over 15 minutes every 12 hours[1,3]

HORSES:

Gastric acid suppression in neonatal foals (extra-label): 1.5 mg/kg IV once daily. **NOTE**: From an experimental study evaluating the pharmacokinetics and pharmacodynamics in normal neonatal foals.[14] Further studies are required to investigate the use of this drug in critically ill patients.

CATTLE:

Prevention of abomasal ulceration (extra-label): 1 mg/kg IV once daily, or 2 mg/kg SC once daily[9]

SHEEP/GOATS:

Prevention of abomasal ulceration (extra-label): 1 mg/kg IV once daily, or 2 mg/kg SC once daily[9]

NEW WORLD CAMELIDS:

Gastric acid suppression(extra-label): 1 mg/kg IV or 2 mg/kg SC every 24 hours for 3 days (from a pharmacokinetic and efficacy study in alpacas)[13]

Monitoring

- Efficacy
- Adverse effects (eg, vomiting, diarrhea, injection site reactions)

Client Information

- This medicine is used on a short-term basis to treat stomach or intestinal ulcers.
- This medicine works best if it is given before the first meal of the day.
- Do not break or cut tablets.

Chemistry/Synonyms

Pantoprazole sodium sesquihydrate occurs as a white to off-white crystalline powder and is racemic. It is freely soluble in water and very slightly soluble in phosphate buffer at a pH of 7.4. Stability of aqueous solutions is pH dependent. At room temperature, solutions are stable for ≈3 hours at a pH of 5 and 220 hours at a pH of 7.8.

Pantoprazole may also be known as BY-1023 or SKF-96022. International trade names include *Controloc®*, *Pantoloc®*, *Pantop®*, *Pantozol®*, *Protium®*, *Protonix®*, *Somac-MA®*, and *Zurcal®*.

Storage/Stability

Delayed-release tablets should be stored at between 15°C and 30°C (59°F-86°F).

The powder for injection should be stored protected from light at 20°C to 25°C (68°F-77°F); excursions are permitted between 15°C and 30°C (59°F-86°F).

Reconstituted solutions (10 mL) are stable for up to 6 hours at room temperature prior to further dilution. If the reconstituted solution is further diluted (according to the label 15-minute infusion protocol), the solution is stable at room temperature for up to 24 hours from the time of initial reconstitution.[17] Reconstituted and admixed solutions do not require protection from light. Do not freeze. Do not use any of the IV solutions if discoloration or precipitates are seen; stop infusion immediately if these are observed during the infusion. A study demonstrated that pantoprazole 4 mg/mL was stable (at least 90% of initial concentration) for 3 days when stored in glass vials at 20°C to 25°C (68°F-77°F) or for 28 days when stored in polypropylene syringes at 2°C to 8°C (36°F-46°F).[18] Pantoprazole 0.4 mg/mL diluted in 5% dextrose and stored in PVC mini-bags was stable for 2 days at 20°C to 25°C (68°F-77°F) or for 14 days at 2°C to 8°C (36°F-46°F). At 0.8 mg/mL, pantoprazole in 5% dextrose was stable for 3 days at 20°C to 25°C (68°F-77°F) or 28 days at 2°C to 8°C (36°F-46°F). Pantoprazole diluted to either 0.4 or 0.8 mg/mL in 0.9% sodium chloride and stored in PVC mini-bags was stable for 3 days at 20°C to 25°C (68°F-77°F) or 28 days at 2°C to 8°C (36°F-46°F).

Compatibility/Compounding Considerations

Compatibility is dependent on factors such as pH, concentration, temperature, and diluent used; specialized references or a hospital pharmacist should be consulted for more specific information.

Precipitation has been reported in cases in which maropitant and pantoprazole are coadministered in the same IV line.

At Y-sites, pantoprazole injection is **incompatible** with dobutamine, esmolol, mannitol, midazolam, and multivitamins and may not be compatible with solutions containing zinc. It is reportedly **compatible** (at Y-sites) with ampicillin, cefazolin, ceftriaxone, dimenhydrinate, dopamine, epinephrine, furosemide, morphine, nitroglycerin, potassium chloride, and vasopressin.

For a 2-minute IV infusion, reconstitute with 10 mL of 0.9% sodium chloride injection. To prepare the injection for a 15-minute IV infusion, reconstitute with 10 mL of 0.9% sodium chloride injection, then dilute further with 100 mL of 5% dextrose, 0.9% sodium chloride, or lactated Ringer's injection to a final concentration of ≈0.4 mg/mL.

Dosage Forms/Regulatory Status

VETERINARY-LABELED PRODUCTS: NONE

The Association of Racing Commissioners International (ARCI) has designated this drug as a class 5 substance. Use of this drug may not be allowed in certain animal competitions. Check rules and regulations before entering in a competition while this medication is being administered. Contact local racing authorities for further guidance. See ***Appendix*** for more information.

HUMAN-LABELED PRODUCTS:

Pantoprazole Sodium Delayed-Release Tablets: 20 mg (as base) and 40 mg (as base); *Protonix®*, generic; (Rx)

Pantoprazole Lyophilized Powder for Injection Solution: 40 mg (as base) in vials; *Protonix I.V.®*, generic; (Rx)

Pantoprazole Sodium Delayed-Release Granules for Suspension: 40 mg; *Protonix®*; (Rx)

References

For the complete list of references, see **wiley.com/go/budde/plumb**

Parapox Ovis Virus Immunomodulator

(pair-ah-***poks oh***-vis) *Zylexis®*

Immunostimulant

Prescriber Highlights

- Biologic immunostimulant that may be used as an aid in reducing upper respiratory disease caused by equine herpesvirus types 1 and 4 in healthy horses 4 months of age and older
- 3-dose regimen; important to give all doses
- Limited published information available on safety and clinical efficacy
- Contraindicated in patients with prior hypersensitivity to it or in patients that have chronic conditions with unclear causality
- Rare adverse effects include hypersensitivity reactions, hyperthermia, general malaise, and musculoskeletal signs.

Uses/Indications

Parapox ovis virus immunomodulator (inactivated *Parapoxvirus ovis*, iPPVO) is labeled as an aid in reducing upper respiratory disease caused by equine herpesvirus types 1 and 4 in healthy horses 4 months of age and older.

There is conflicting evidence regarding the clinical efficacy of iPPVO for reducing the incidence of equine respiratory disease complex (ERDC). A placebo-controlled study in foals 24 to 48 hours old (n = 59) on a farm with endemic *Rhodococcus equi* infections found no significant difference in the pneumonia incidence between foals treated with iPPVO versus placebo.[1] One review concluded that although immunomodulators such as iPPVO provide non-specific stimulation of an innate immune response, they may not provide protection against direct infection or transmission of respiratory pathogens associated with ERDC. They may, however, contribute to the reduction of the disease severity and reduce the frequency of complications, and improve the rate of recovery.[2]

Parapoxvirus products may also be available in other countries for use in small animal species.

Pharmacology/Actions

Parapox ovis virus immunomodulator stimulates non-specific immune mechanisms[3] and is believed to prevent viral infection by infecting host cells with a non-replicating virus, which interferes with pathogenic virus infection. Postulated mechanisms of action include induction of interferons, cytokines and colony-stimulating factors, and activation of natural killer cells.

Parapoxvirus ovis is the DNA virus responsible for orf, a contagious pustular dermatitis in sheep.

Pharmacokinetics

Effects on the immune system are reported to occur 4 to 6 hours after administration and persist for 1 to 2 weeks.

Contraindications/Precautions/Warnings

Parapox ovis virus immunomodulator is contraindicated in patients with prior hypersensitivity to it. If anaphylaxis occurs, administer epinephrine or equivalent. Do not use in animals that have chronic diseases with unclear causality.[3]

The first dose of *Parapox ovis* virus immunomodulator should be administered shortly before or up to the day of crowding or exposure to other stressful conditions to ensure efficacy.[3]

Reproductive/Nursing Safety

No information was located. Because safety has not been established in animals, this biologic agent should only be used when the maternal benefits outweigh the potential risks to offspring.

Adverse Effects

Hypersensitivity or anaphylactic reactions are possible. Hyperthermia, general malaise, and musculoskeletal signs (eg, stiffness, abnormal posture) have rarely been reported.[3]

Overdose/Acute Toxicity

No systemic or local reactions were seen in horses given double the recommended dose.[3]

For patients that have experienced or are suspected to have experienced an overdose, consultation with a 24-hour poison consultation center specializing in providing veterinary-specific information is recommended. For general information related to overdose and toxin exposures, as well as contact information for poison control centers, refer to ***Appendix.***

Drug Interactions

- None noted

Laboratory Considerations

- None identified

Dosages

HORSES:

Aid in reducing upper airway disease caused by herpesvirus types 1 and 4 (label dosage): Reconstitute with the provided sterile diluent and administer 2 mL/horse (NOT mL/kg) IM (day 0). Repeat dose on day 2 and day 9. Retreatment is recommended during subsequent disease episodes or prior to stress inducing situations.

Monitoring

- Clinical efficacy (respiratory infection improvement)

Chemistry/Synonyms

Parapox ovis virus immunomodulator is provided commercially as a freeze-dried inactivated (killed) virus component with separate 2 mL vial of sterile diluent.

Parapox ovis virus immunomodulator may also be known as iPPVO, PPOV, PIND-ORF, *Baypamun*®, and *Zylexis*®.

Storage/Stability

Parapox ovis virus immunomodulator should be stored refrigerated (2°C-8°C [36°F-46°F]), but not be frozen. After reconstituting, entire contents of vial should be used.

Dosage Forms/Regulatory Status

VETERINARY-LABELED PRODUCTS:

NOTE: This product was a USDA-licensed biologic but is no longer listed on the USDA-licensed veterinary biologics product summary and appears to no longer be marketed in the US.

Parapox Ovis Virus Immunomodulator Injection in boxes of 5 single dose vials for reconstitution with 5-2mL vials of sterile diluent; *Zylexis*®. Labeled for use in horses. Refer to specific product label and local regulations for potential withdrawal times.

HUMAN-LABELED PRODUCTS: NONE

References

For the complete list of references, see **wiley.com/go/budde/plumb**

Paromomycin

(pair-oh-moe-***my***-sin) *Humatin*®

Oral Aminoglycoside Antiparasitic

Prescriber Highlights

- ▶ Oral aminoglycoside used primarily as a treatment of cryptosporidiosis in small animal species
- ▶ Not appreciably absorbed when given orally if the gut is intact
- ▶ Adverse effects are usually limited to GI effects (nausea, vomiting, diarrhea); cats may be susceptible to renal and ophthalmic toxicity and some clinicians consider it contraindicated in cats because of toxicity.
- ▶ Use it with caution in patients with intestinal ulceration.

Uses/Indications

Paromomycin may be useful as a treatment for cryptosporidiosis in dogs and cats. Although some clinicians consider paromomycin to be the second-line treatment for dogs and should be avoided in cats, others recommended it as a first choice.[1]

In dogs, paromomycin is also used topically to treat cutaneous leishmaniasis. Subcutaneously administered paromomycin (no dosage forms available in the United States) in combination with meglumine antimoniate is used in some protocols for treating systemic leishmaniasis, but serious adverse effects limit usefulness.[2-4]

Paromomycin has been used successfully to treat cryptosporidiosis in cattle,[5] goats, lambs,[6] and reptiles.[7]

In humans, paromomycin has been used as an alternative oral treatment for intestinal amebiasis and for management of hepatic coma.[8]

The World Health Organization has designated aminoglycosides as Critically Important, High Priority antimicrobial agents for human medicine.[9] The Office International des Epizooties (OIE) has designated paromomycin as a Veterinary Critically Important Antimicrobial (VCIA) Agent in avian, bovine, caprine, ovine, rabbit, and swine species.[10]

Pharmacology/Actions

Like other aminoglycoside antibiotics, paromomycin irreversibly binds bacterial 30S ribosomal subunits, thereby inhibiting protein synthesis. It is considered a bactericidal, concentration-dependent antibiotic. Paromomycin has an antimicrobial spectrum of activity similar to neomycin, including aerobic gram-positive and gram-negative bacteria, but its primary therapeutic uses are for the treatment of intestinal protozoa, including *Leishmania* spp, *Entamoeba histolytica*, and *Cryptosporidium* spp. It also has activity against a variety of tapeworms, but there are better choices available for clinical use.

Pharmacokinetics

Like neomycin, paromomycin is poorly absorbed when given orally. It is excreted unchanged in the feces.

Contraindications/Precautions/Warnings

Paromomycin is contraindicated in patients with known hypersensitivity to the drug or with ileus or intestinal obstruction. Patients should be well-hydrated prior to treatment to minimize risk for nephrotoxicity. The foreign label for paromomycin solution cautions against using it in animals with impaired renal or hepatic function.[11] It should be used with caution in patients with GI ulceration or blood in feces, which increases the likelihood of systemic absorption with resultant toxic effects. Use with caution in newborn animals as paromomycin has increased GI absorption in neonates.[11]

Use with caution in cats; because of potential toxicity, some clinicians consider paromomycin contraindicated in cats due to this risk.

Do not confuse *Humatin*® (paromomycin trade name) with *Humulin*® (insulin trade name).

Adverse Effects

GI effects (eg, nausea, inappetence, vomiting, diarrhea) are the most likely adverse effects to be noted with therapy.[8] Because paromomycin can affect the gut flora, nonsusceptible bacterial or fungal overgrowths are a possibility. In patients with significant gut ulceration or degradation of GI mucosal barriers, paromomycin may be absorbed systemically with resultant nephrotoxicity, ototoxicity, or pancreatitis. Use in cats has been associated with renal dysfunction, ototoxicity, and blindness.

Reproductive/Nursing Safety

Because minimal amounts are absorbed when administered orally, paromomycin should be safe to use during pregnancy.[12] It should not be used parenterally during pregnancy. When used orally, paromomycin should be safe to use during lactation. Because safety has not been established in animals, this drug should only be used when the maternal benefits outweigh the potential risks to offspring.

Overdose/Acute Toxicity

Because paromomycin is not appreciably absorbed after oral administration, acute overdose adverse effects should be limited to GI distress in patients with an intact GI system. Chronic overdoses may lead to systemic toxicity.

For patients that have experienced or are suspected of having experienced an overdose, consultation with a 24-hour poison consultation center specializing in providing veterinary-specific information is recommended. For general information related to overdose and toxin exposures, as well as contact information for poison control centers, refer to ***Appendix.***

Drug Interactions

The following drug interactions have either been reported or are theoretical in humans or animals receiving paromomycin and may be of significance in veterinary patients. Unless otherwise noted, use together is not necessarily contraindicated, but weigh the potential risks and perform additional monitoring when appropriate.

- Digoxin: Paromomycin may reduce digoxin absorption.
- Methotrexate: Paromomycin may reduce methotrexate absorption.

Laboratory Considerations

- None were noted.

Dosages

DOGS:

Cryptosporidiosis (extra-label): 125 – 165 mg/kg PO twice daily for 5 days has been suggested[13]; commonly, 150 mg/kg PO once daily for 5 days is recommended.[14]

CATS:

Cryptosporidiosis (extra-label): **NOTE**: Higher doses of paromomycin have caused renal or otic toxicity and/or blindness in some treated cats. Consider using an alternative treatment first (eg, azithromycin) or paromomycin at an initially reduced dose.

a) 150 mg/kg PO every 12 to 24 hours.[15] If the cat is responding to the first 7 days of therapy and toxicity has not been noted, continue treatment for 1 week past clinical resolution of diarrhea.

b) 150 mg/kg PO once daily for 5 days[14]

CATTLE:

Cryptosporidiosis (extra-label): 25 mg/kg PO daily for 5 days[5]

Reduction of diarrhea due to *Cryptosporidium parvum* in pre-ruminating calves (extra-label): 35 mg/kg PO daily for 7 consecutive days[16]

NEW WORLD CAMELIDS:

Cryptosporidiosis in crias (extra-label): 50 mg/kg PO (*dosing interval not specified, assume once per day—Plumb*) for 5 to 10 days[17,18]

Clinical endoparasitism (extra-label): 25 – 100 mg/kg PO every 12 hours[19]; however, this has **not** been studied for safety or efficacy, and extreme caution is recommended.

SHEEP:

***Giardia duodenalis* in lambs** (extra-label): 100 mg/kg PO once daily for 3 days resulted in no cysts shed in feces 6 days after treatment.[20]

***Cryptosporidium parvum* in lambs** (extra-label): 100 mg/kg/day for 3 consecutive days significantly decreased oocyst shedding and improved clinical signs.[6] 200 mg/kg/day for 2 consecutive days did not improve efficacy and appeared to stunt weight gain; further studies are needed to determine the optimal dose and duration of treatment.

Reduction of diarrhea due to *Cryptosporidium parvum* in pre-ruminating lambs (extra-label): 35 mg/kg PO daily for 7 consecutive days[21]

GOATS:

Reduction of diarrhea due to *Cryptosporidium parvum* in pre-ruminating kids (extra-label): 35 mg/kg PO daily for 7 consecutive days[21]

REPTILES:

Cryptosporidiosis (extra-label):

General: 300 – 800 mg/kg PO every 24 to 48 hours for 7 to 14 days or as needed[7]

Bearded dragons: 100 mg/kg once daily for 7 days, then 100 mg/kg twice per week for 6 weeks, then 360 mg/kg every 48 hours for 10 days[22] (*route not specified, assume PO- Plumb*)

Leopard geckos: 100 mg/kg PO once daily for 7 days, then once weekly thereafter. Clinical signs and shedding in stool 6 weeks after drug discontinuation[23]

King cobra: 360 mg/kg PO twice weekly for 6 weeks was successful in 1 case report.[24]

Monitoring

- Serial fecal examinations
- GI adverse effects
- If used in cats, monitor renal function.

Client Information

- Unless otherwise instructed, give this medicine with food.
- When paromomycin is given by mouth for short periods, it is usually tolerated well. Contact your veterinarian if your animal develops diarrhea while taking this medicine.
- Rarely, this medicine can cause hearing loss and damage to the kidneys and nerves when used for long periods of time. Contact your veterinarian if your animal develops hearing loss, a head tilt, weakness, changes in appetite, or with drinking and urination habits.

Chemistry/Synonyms

Paromomycin sulfate, an aminoglycoside antibiotic, occurs as an odorless, creamy white to light yellow, hygroscopic, amorphous powder having a saline taste. Paromomycin is very soluble in water (greater than 1 g/mL).

Paromomycin may also be known as aminosidin sulphate, aminosidine sulphate, catenulin sulphate, crestomycin sulphate, estomycin sulphate, hydroxymycin sulphate, monomycin A sulphate, neomycin E sulphate, paucimycin sulphate, and *Humatin*®.

Storage/Stability

Store paromomycin capsules at room temperature (15°C-30°C [59°F-86°F]) in tight containers protected from moisture.

Dosage Forms/Regulatory Status

VETERINARY-LABELED PRODUCTS: None in the United States. In some countries, it is available as:

Paromomycin solution: 140 mg/mL in 125 mL, 250 mL, 500 mL, or 1 L; for use in drinking water, milk, or milk replacer in pre-ruminant cattle (20-day withdrawal) and pigs (3-day withdrawal); *Gabbrovet*®

Paromomycin powder: 70,000 IU/g in a 25 g package; for use in drinking water, milk, or milk replacer in pre-ruminant cattle (20-day withdrawal) and pigs (3-day withdrawal); *Parofor*®

Paromomycin oral solution: 140 mg/mL in 125 mL, 250 mL, 500 mL, or 1 L; for use in pre-ruminating cattle (62-day withdrawal); *Parofor crypto*

Paromomycin oral solution: 140 mg/mL in 125 mL, 250 mL, 500 mL, or 1 L; for use in pre-ruminating lambs and pre-ruminating kids (24-day withdrawal); *Parofor crypto*

HUMAN-LABELED PRODUCTS:

Paromomycin Sulfate Oral Capsules: 250 mg; generic; (Rx).

References

For the complete list of references, see **wiley.com/go/budde/plumb**

Paroxetine

(pah-***rox***-a-teen) *Paxil*®

Selective Serotonin Reuptake Inhibitor (SSRI)

Prescriber Highlights

- ► Selective serotonin reuptake inhibitor (SSRI) used extra-label in dogs and cats to treat a variety of behavior disorders
- ► Contraindications include patients with known hypersensitivity or receiving monoamine oxidase inhibitors. Caution in patients with severe cardiac, renal, or hepatic disease. Dosages may need to be reduced in patients with severe renal or hepatic impairment.
- ► If patient is on the drug for an extended period, gradual withdrawal is recommended.
- ► Potential adverse effects in dogs: anorexia, lethargy, GI effects, anxiety, irritability, insomnia, hyperactivity, panting, or aggression; in cats: behavior changes (anxiety, aggression, sleep disturbances), anorexia, constipation, or changes in elimination patterns
- ► The National Institute for Occupational Safety and Health (NIOSH) classifies paroxetine as a hazardous drug; use appropriate precautions when handling.

Uses/Indications

Paroxetine may be beneficial for the treatment of canine aggression, anxiety, and stereotypic or other obsessive-compulsive behaviors. It has been used occasionally in cats for urine marking, aggression, and feline hyperesthesia syndrome.

Pharmacology/Actions

Paroxetine is a highly selective inhibitor of the reuptake of serotonin (SSRI) in the CNS, thus potentiating the pharmacologic activity of serotonin. Paroxetine has a very weak effect on dopamine and norepinephrine reuptake and little affinity for other neurotransmitter (eg, histamine) receptors; it also has mild anticholinergic effects.[1,2]

Pharmacokinetics

No data for cats or dogs were located.

In Grey parrots, paroxetine HCl dissolved in water given PO was slowly absorbed and had a bioavailability (mean) of 31%, but there was significant interpatient variation.[3] Repeated administration increased bioavailability. Terminal elimination half-life was ≈5 hours.

In humans, paroxetine is slowly and nearly completely absorbed from the GI tract. Because of a relatively high first-pass effect, relatively small amounts reach the systemic circulation unchanged. Food does not impair absorption.

The drug is ≈95% bound to plasma proteins. Paroxetine is extensively metabolized, probably in the liver. Half-life in humans ranges from 7 to 65 hours and averages ≈24 hours.

Contraindications/Precautions/Warnings

Paroxetine is contraindicated in patients with known hypersensitivity to it; it should also not be used in combination with monoamine oxidase inhibitors (MAOIs) or other serotonergic drugs (eg, mirtazapine, ondansetron) due to the risk for developing serotonin syndrome (see ***Drug Interactions***). Use with caution in patients with seizure disorders or severe cardiac, hepatic, or renal disease; dosages may need to be reduced in patients with severe hepatic or renal impairment.

If paroxetine is discontinued and the patient has been receiving the drug for an extended period, a gradual withdrawal over several weeks is recommended to minimize withdrawal reactions (eg, nausea, behavior changes [eg, agitation, anxiety, dysphoria], tremors).

Do not confuse paroxetine with fluoxetine or piroxicam. Do not confuse paroxetine *hydrochloride* with paroxetine *mesylate* (*Brisdelle*®, *Pexeva*®). Do not confuse PAXil with PLAVix or PACLitaxel.

The National Institute for Occupational Safety and Health (NIOSH) classifies paroxetine as a hazardous drug; personal protective equipment (PPE) should be used accordingly to minimize the risk for exposure.[4]

Adverse Effects

In dogs, paroxetine can cause lethargy, salivation, GI effects, anxiety, irritability, insomnia, hyperactivity, or panting. Anorexia is a common adverse effect in dogs (usually transient and may be negated by temporarily increasing the palatability of food and/or hand feeding). Some dogs have persistent anorexia that precludes further use of paroxetine.

There seems to be less incidence of anorexia in paroxetine than in fluoxetine. Aggressive behavior in previously unaggressive dogs has been reported. Selective serotonin reuptake inhibitors (SSRIs) may also cause changes in blood glucose levels and potentially reduce seizure threshold.

Paroxetine in cats can cause behavior changes (eg, anxiety, irritability, sleep disturbances), anorexia, constipation, or changes in elimination patterns.

Paroxetine has mild anticholinergic effects; anticholinergic adverse effects are possible, including constipation, urinary retention, and arrhythmias. Serotonergic effects may reduce platelet aggregation and increase the risk of bleeding. Hyponatremia has been reported in humans.

Reproductive/Nursing Safety

Paroxetine crosses the placenta. Paroxetine's safety during pregnancy in veterinary medicine has not been established. No teratogenic effects were noted in laboratory animals receiving paroxetine during periods of organogenesis, but increased pup deaths were observed in rats given the drug during the third trimester and through lactation.[5] Use of paroxetine during human pregnancies, particularly in the first trimester, is associated with increased risk of congenital malformations, including cardiac defects.

The drug is excreted into milk but at low levels; caution is advised in nursing patients.

Because safety has not been established in animals, this drug should only be used when the maternal benefits outweigh the potential risks to offspring.

Overdose/Acute Toxicity

Although paroxetine is not as toxic as the tricyclic antidepressants, fatalities and significant morbidity have occurred after paroxetine overdoses. In one retrospective study in dogs, a median dose of 7.7 mg/kg (range: 0.3 – 25.9 mg/kg; $n = 5$) was associated with clinical signs of overdoses, but no clinical significance could be differentiated from doses that did not cause clinical signs.[6] Another retrospective review in dogs found the following overdoses and associated clinical signs: 1 – 3 mg/kg: vomiting, drooling, and lethargy; greater than 3 mg/kg: agitation and seizures; greater than 4 mg/kg (sustained-release product): sedation, drooling, and vomiting; greater than 4.5 mg/kg (sustained-release product): agitation—no seizures reported from the sustained-release product.[7]

There were 222 single-agent exposures to paroxetine reported to the ASPCA Animal Poison Control Center (APCC) from 2009 to 2013. Of the 194 dogs, 33 showed clinical signs with lethargy (36%) and vomiting (18%) being the most common. Of the 30 cats, 9 showed clinical signs, with 56% having behavior changes and 44% being mydriatic.

When ingestion amounts are associated with significant morbidity or when the ingested amount is unknown, consider GI decontamination (if not contraindicated). Activated charcoal can be very effective in binding paroxetine; induction of emesis is not recommended. Treat supportively based on clinical signs at the time of presentation. For overdoses in patients that are subclinical, the animal should be monitored for the first 12 hours for development of clinical signs.

For patients that have experienced or are suspected to have experienced an overdose, it is strongly encouraged to consult with one of the 24-hour poison consultation centers that specialize in providing information specific for veterinary patients. For general information related to overdose and toxin exposures, as well as contact information for poison control centers, refer to ***Appendix***.

Drug Interactions

Paroxetine is both a substrate and an inhibitor of CYP2D6 in humans. The following drug interactions have either been reported or are theoretical in humans or animals receiving paroxetine and may be of significance in veterinary patients. Unless otherwise noted, use together is not necessarily contraindicated, but weigh the potential risks and perform additional monitoring when appropriate.

- **Anticoagulants** (eg, **heparin, rivaroxaban, warfarin**): Paroxetine may increase the risk for bleeding.
- **Antiplatelet Agents** (eg, **aspirin, clopidogrel**): Paroxetine may increase the risk for bleeding.
- **Beta-Adrenergic Blocking Agents** (eg, **atenolol, propranolol, sotalol**): Selective serotonin reuptake inhibitors (SSRIs) may increase serum concentrations of beta-blockers and the combination may increase risk for arrhythmias due to prolongation of the QT interval. Atenolol may be safer to use if paroxetine is required.
- **Buspirone**: Increased risk for serotonin syndrome
- **Codeine**: Paroxetine may reduce codeine's conversion into morphine.
- **Cyproheptadine**: May decrease or reverse the effects of SSRIs
- **Diuretics** (eg, **furosemide, hydrochlorothiazide**): Increased risk for hyponatremia
- **Doxorubicin**: Paroxetine may increase doxorubicin concentration.
- **Insulin**: May alter insulin requirements
- **Isoniazid**: Increased risk for serotonin syndrome
- **MAO Inhibitors** (amitraz, linezolid, selegiline): High risk for serotonin syndrome; use contraindicated; in humans, a 5-week washout period is required after discontinuing paroxetine and a 2-week washout period if first discontinuing the MAO inhibitor.
- **Methylene Blue**: Increased risk for serotonin syndrome; avoid concomitant use.
- **Metoclopramide**: May enhance adverse/toxic effects of SSRIs and increase risk for serotonin syndrome
- **Mexiletine**: SSRIs may decrease the metabolism of mexiletine.
- **Mirtazapine**: Increased risk for serotonin syndrome
- **Nonsteroidal Anti-Inflammatory Drugs** (NSAIDs; eg, aspirin, carprofen, meloxicam): SSRIs may increase the risk for bleeding and GI ulceration.
- **Ondansetron**: Increased risk for serotonin syndrome
- **Opioids** (eg, fentanyl, methadone): Increased risk for serotonin syndrome
- **Pentazocine**: Serotonin syndrome-like adverse effects are possible.
- **Phenobarbital**: May reduce paroxetine concentration and exposure
- **Phenytoin**: Increased plasma levels of phenytoin are possible.
- **St John's Wort**: Increased risk for serotonin syndrome.
- **Tramadol**: SSRIs can inhibit the metabolism of tramadol to its active metabolites, decreasing its efficacy and increasing the risk for toxicity (serotonin syndrome, seizures).
- **Tricyclic antidepressants** (eg, clomipramine, amitriptyline): Paroxetine may increase TCA blood levels and the risk for serotonin syndrome.
- **Trazodone**: Increased plasma levels of trazodone possible. Increased risk for serotonin syndrome

Dosages

DOGS:

Selective serotonin reuptake inhibitor (SSRI)-responsive behavior problems (extra-label): Using regular (not extended-release) tablets: 0.5 – 2 mg/kg PO once daily. Used in conjunction with behavior modification. Usually start at the low end of the dosing range and treat for ≈2 months; evaluate and adjust dosage if necessary.

CATS:

SSRI-responsive behavior problems (extra-label): Using regular (not extended release) tablets: 0.25 – 1 mg/kg once to twice daily; practically, 1.25 – 5 mg (⅛ – ½ of a regular 10 mg tablet) per cat (NOT mg/kg) once or twice daily. Usually start at the low end of the dosing range and treat for ≈2 months; evaluate and adjust dosage if necessary.

BIRDS:

Stress- or anxiety-related behavior disorders (eg, feather picking; extra-label): From a pharmacokinetic study in Grey parrots: Paroxetine HCl dissolved in water (human oral suspension was not consistently absorbed) and given at 4 mg/kg PO twice daily was sufficient to reach plasma concentrations reported to be effective in humans.[3]

Monitoring

- Efficacy
- Adverse effects; including appetite (weight)
- Baseline CBC, serum chemistry profile, urinalysis, and thyroid testing. Repeat yearly during treatment; consider twice-yearly testing in senior animals.

Client Information

- May take up to 6 weeks to determine if the drug is effective.
- Most common side effects are drowsiness, sleepiness, and reduced appetite.
- Rare side effects that can be serious (contact veterinarian immediately) include seizures, aggression (threatening behavior and actions).
- Overdoses can be very serious; keep out of the reach of animals and children.
- If your animal wore a flea and tick collar 2 weeks prior to starting

this drug, let your veterinarian know. Do not use one of these collars on your animal while it's receiving this medicine without first talking to your veterinarian.

- Do not abruptly discontinue this medication without speaking with a veterinarian. A gradual withdrawal is usually recommended if your animal has been on this medication for an extended period.
- This medication is considered to be a hazardous drug as defined by the National Institute for Occupational Safety and Health (NIOSH). Talk with your veterinarian or pharmacist about the use of personal protective equipment when handling this medicine.

Chemistry/Synonyms

Paroxetine HCl is a selective serotonin reuptake inhibitor (SSRI) antidepressant that occurs as an off-white, odorless powder. Its solubility in water is 5.4 mg/mL and pK_a is 9.9.

Paroxetine may also be known as BRL-29060, FG-7051, and *Paxil®*.

Storage/Stability

Paroxetine oral tablets should be stored at 15°C to 30°C (59°F-86°F). The oral suspension should be stored below 25°C (77°F).

Dosage Forms/Regulatory Status

VETERINARY-LABELED PRODUCTS: NONE

The Association of Racing Commissioners International (ARCI) has designated this drug as a class 2 substance. See the ***Appendix*** for more information. Use of this drug may not be allowed in certain animal competitions. Check rules and regulations before entering in a competition while this medication is being administered. Contact local racing authorities for further guidance.

HUMAN-LABELED PRODUCTS:

Paroxetine HCl Oral Tablets: 10 mg, 20 mg, 30 mg, and 40 mg; *Paxil®*, generic; (Rx)

Paroxetine HCl Oral Tablets Controlled-Release: 12.5 mg, 25 mg, and 37.5 mg; *Paxil® CR*, generic; (Rx)

Paroxetine HCl Oral Suspension: 2 mg/mL in 250 mL; *Paxil®*, generic; (Rx)

References

For the complete list of references, see **wiley.com/go/budde/plumb**

Penicillamine

(pen-i-***sill***-a-meen) *Depen®, Cuprimine®*

Antidote; Chelating Agent

Prescriber Highlights

- ► Chelating agent used primarily for copper-storage hepatopathies in dogs. Can be considered for lead poisoning or cystine urolithiasis, but other therapies are preferred
- ► Contraindications: history of penicillamine-related blood dyscrasias, lead present in GI tract
- ► Potentially teratogenic
- ► Adverse effects: nausea, vomiting, and hyporexia. Can reduce GI dietary mineral absorption (zinc, iron, copper, and calcium) and cause deficiencies; Rarely: fever, lymphadenopathy, skin hypersensitivity reactions, or immune-complex glomerulonephropathy
- ► Pyridoxine deficiency may occur; consider supplementation.
- ► Food significantly reduces oral bioavailability. Give on an empty stomach (if it can be tolerated).

Uses/Indications

Penicillamine is used primarily for its chelating ability in veterinary medicine. It is the drug of choice for copper-associated hepatopathies in dogs[1]; clinical improvement may require weeks to months of treatment. It can also be used for the long-term oral treatment of lead or mercury poisoning or in cystine urolithiasis. It was effective in treating zinc toxicosis in a dog.[2]

Because it has antifibrotic effects,[1] penicillamine may be of benefit in chronic hepatitis, but doses necessary for effective treatment are likely too high to be tolerated.

Pharmacology/Actions

Penicillamine chelates a variety of metals, including copper, lead, iron, and mercury, forming stable water-soluble complexes that are excreted by the kidneys. Urinary copper excretion does not correlate with baseline hepatic copper concentration.[3] Penicillamine combines chemically with cystine to form a stable, soluble complex that can be readily excreted.

Penicillamine has antirheumatic activity; however, the exact mechanisms for this action are not understood. Penicillamine has been shown to improve lymphocyte function, depress T-cell activity, and decrease IgM rheumatoid factor and immune complex formation in serum and synovial fluid.

Penicillamine possesses antifibrotic activity via inhibition of collagen crosslinking, thereby causing collagen to be more susceptible to degradation.

Although penicillamine is a degradation product of penicillins, it has no antimicrobial activity.

Pharmacokinetics

In dogs, giving penicillamine with food reduces bioavailability, peak concentration, and area under the curve (AUC) (24 hours) by ≈70%, as compared with the fasted state.[4]

In humans, penicillamine is 40% to 70% absorbed after oral administration and peak serum concentrations occur ≈1 hour after dosing. It is ≈80% bound to plasma proteins. The drug apparently crosses the placenta, but little information is known about its distribution. Penicillamine that is not complexed with either a metal or cystine is thought to be metabolized by the liver and excreted in the urine and feces.

Contraindications/Precautions/Warnings

Penicillamine is contraindicated in patients with a history of penicillin hypersensitivity or penicillamine-related blood dyscrasias and should be avoided in patients with renal insufficiency. Penicillamine can potentially enhance absorption of lead from the GI tract. If lead is still present in the gut, penicillamine should not be administered.

Adverse Effects

In dogs, the most common adverse effects associated with penicillamine includes nausea, vomiting, and hyporexia. Although penicillamine should be given on an empty stomach (at least 30 minutes before feeding), if the animal develops problems with vomiting or anorexia, consider one or more of the following suggestions:

1) Give the same total daily dose but divide into smaller individual doses and give more frequently.
2) Temporarily reduce the daily dose and gradually increase to recommended dosage.
3) Give a long-acting antiemetic 1 hour before dosing.
4) Give with a small amount of food (eg, small piece of meat[1]) if one of the above does not alleviate vomiting.

Rare adverse effects in dogs include proteinuria, fever, lymphadenopathy, skin hypersensitivity reactions, or immune-complex glomerulonephropathy. A case of hemolytic anemia in a cat has been reported.[5]

In humans, other rare side effects include oral ulcerations, rashes, hepatic failure, pancreatitis, and adverse hematologic effects (eg, leukopenia, thrombocytopenia; see ***Contraindications/Precautions/Warnings***).

Penicillamine can reduce GI dietary mineral absorption (zinc, iron, copper, and calcium) and cause deficiencies with long-term use. Pyridoxine-deficient states may occur; supplementation advised. Interference with collagen and elastin production may lead to increased skin friability and impaired wound healing.

Reproductive/Nursing Safety

Penicillamine has been associated with the development of birth defects in offspring of rats given 6 times the recommended dose.[6,7] There are also some reports of human teratogenicity, including skin and collagen defects. Penicillamine is relatively contraindicated during human pregnancy.

The manufacturer warns that mothers taking penicillamine should not nurse offspring.[6,7]

Because safety has not been established in animals, this drug should only be used when the maternal benefits outweigh the potential risks to offspring.

Overdose/Acute Toxicity

No specific acute toxic dose has been established for penicillamine and toxic effects generally occur in patients taking the drug chronically. Any relationship of toxicity to dose is unclear; patients on small doses may also develop toxicity.

For patients that have experienced or are suspected of having experienced an overdose, consultation with a 24-hour poison consultation center specializing in providing veterinary-specific information is recommended. For general information related to overdose and toxin exposures, as well as contact information for poison control centers, refer to ***Appendix***.

Drug Interactions

The following drug interactions have either been reported or are theoretical in humans or animals receiving penicillamine and may be of significance in veterinary patients. Unless otherwise noted, use together is not necessarily contraindicated, but weigh the potential risks and perform additional monitoring when appropriate.

- 4-AMINOQUINOLINE DRUGS (eg, **chloroquine, quinacrine**): Concomitant administration with these agents may increase the risks for severe dermatologic adverse effects.
- CATIONS, ORAL INCLUDING ZINC, IRON, CALCIUM, & MAGNESIUM: May decrease the effectiveness of penicillamine if given orally together. Long-term use of penicillamine may induce deficient states.
- FOOD: The amount of penicillamine absorbed from the GI tract may be significantly reduced by the concurrent administration of food or antacids.
- GOLD COMPOUNDS (eg, **auranofin**): May increase the risk for hematologic and/or renal adverse reactions
- IMMUNOSUPPRESSANT DRUGS (eg, **cyclophosphamide, azathioprine**, but not corticosteroids): May increase the risk for hematologic and/or renal adverse effects
- PHENYLBUTAZONE: May increase the risk for hematologic and/or renal adverse effects
- PYRIDOXINE: Penicillamine may induce deficient states. Supplementation is advised in human patients.

Laboratory Considerations

- When using technetium Tc 99m gluceptate to visualize the kidneys, penicillamine may chelate this agent and form a compound that is excreted via the hepatobiliary system resulting in gallbladder visualization that could confuse the results.
- In humans, penicillamine may cause a positive ANA test.

Dosages

DOGS:

Copper-associated hepatopathy (extra-label): The standard recommended dosage is 10 – 15 mg/kg PO twice daily on an empty stomach (at least 20 to 30 minutes before feeding). However, in a pharmacokinetic study, the authors suggest that a lower dosage (7 mg/kg PO twice daily on an empty stomach) might be efficacious and also reduce drug cost and the incidence of vomiting. Alternatively, a long-acting antiemetic could be administered 1 hour before dosing in dogs that have a proclivity to vomit.[4,8]

Copper-associated chronic hepatitis (extra-label): 10 – 15 mg/kg PO every 12 hours, 30 minutes before or 2 hours after a meal. Treatment duration is based on hepatic copper quantification. Some dogs need maintenance with chronic intermittent low-dose (5 – 10 mg/kg PO) administration 2 to 3 times weekly; however, this has not been studied.[1]

Cystine urolithiasis (extra-label): 15 mg/kg PO twice daily with food.[9]

Subclinical hepatitis in Doberman pinschers (extra-label): 6.7 mg/kg PO twice daily 30 minutes prior to feeding for 4 months improved liver appearance on histopathology.[10]

Lead poisoning (extra-label): As an alternative or adjunct to CaEDTA: penicillamine 110 mg/kg/day divided every 6 to 8 hours PO 30 minutes before feeding for 1 to 2 weeks. If vomiting is a problem, may premedicate with dimenhydrinate 2 – 4 mg/kg PO. Alternatively, may give penicillamine 33 – 55 mg/kg/day divided as above. Dissolving medication in juice may facilitate administration.[11,12]

CATS:

Primary copper hepatopathy (extra-label): From a retrospective study where 5 cats received penicillamine: 10 – 15 mg/kg PO every 12 hours. One cat developed hemolytic anemia.[5]

Lead toxicosis (extra-label): 125 mg/cat (NOT mg/kg) PO every 12 hours for 5 days. Do not administer if any lead remains in the GI tract, as it will increase systemic lead absorption.

RUMINANTS:

NOTE: When used in food animals, FARAD recommends a minimum milk withdrawal time of 3 days after the last treatment and a 21-day preslaughter withdrawal.[13]

Copper toxicity in small ruminants (extra-label): 26 – 52 mg/kg PO once daily for 6 days[14,15]

Lead or mercury toxicity (extra-label): 110 mg/kg PO for 1 to 3 weeks. To prevent continued metal absorption, must clear GI tract of toxic metal before treatment.[16]

BIRDS:

Adjunctive treatment of lead poisoning (extra-label): 55 mg/kg PO every 12 hours for 1 to 2 weeks. It has been recommended to combine CaEDTA and penicillamine for several days until clinical signs dissipate, followed by a 3- to 6-week treatment with penicillamine.[17]

Monitoring

- NOTE: The manufacturer cautions that penicillamine can produce severe toxic reactions, and that patients receiving the drug should be continuously monitored for adverse effects.
- Monitoring for efficacy is dependent on the reason for its use (eg, liver copper concentrations, blood lead concentrations)
- CBC (including platelets) and renal function (including urinalysis) should be routinely monitored.
- Adverse effects

Client Information

- Used to remove excess metals (eg, copper, lead, mercury) from the body
- Can cause nausea (acting sick) and vomiting
- Should be given on an empty stomach, at least 30 minutes before feeding
- Does not have any antibiotic activity

Chemistry/Synonyms

A monothiol chelating agent that is a degradation product of penicillins, penicillamine occurs as a white or practically white, crystalline powder with a characteristic odor. Penicillamine is freely soluble in water and slightly soluble in alcohol with pK_a values of 1.83, 8.03, and 10.83.

Penicillamine may also be known as D-Penicillamine; beta,beta-Dimethylcysteine; D-3-Mercaptovaline; penicillaminum; *Depen*®; and *Cuprimine*®.

Storage/Stability

Penicillamine should be stored at room temperature, 20°C to 25°C (68°F-77°F), protected from moisture, and in tight containers.

Dosage Forms/Regulatory Status

VETERINARY-LABELED PRODUCTS: NONE

HUMAN-LABELED PRODUCTS:

Penicillamine Titratable Oral Tablets: 250 mg (scored); *Depen*®; (Rx)

Penicillamine Oral Capsules: 250 mg; *Cuprimine*®; (Rx)

References

For the complete list of references, see **wiley.com/go/budde/plumb**

Penicillin G

(pen-i-***sill***-in ***jee***)

Penicillin Antibiotic

Prescriber Highlights

- Prototypical penicillin agent used parenterally for treatment of susceptible infections
- Contraindications include known hypersensitivity.
- Adverse effects may include hypersensitivity. Very high doses or IV injection of procaine-containing products may cause adverse CNS effects.
- Label dosages may be too low.
- Benzathine penicillin only effective against extremely susceptible agents and has limited clinical use

Uses/Indications

Penicillin G is FDA-approved for systemic use in horses, cattle, and sheep for respiratory infections, and in swine for treatment of erysipelas. Natural penicillins (G and V) remain the drugs of choice for a variety of bacteria, including group A beta-hemolytic streptococci, many gram-positive anaerobes, spirochetes, and some gram-negative aerobic bacilli and cocci. Generally, if bacteria remain susceptible to a natural penicillin, either penicillin G or V is preferred for treating that infection as long as adequate penetration of the drug to the site of the infection occurs and the patient is not hypersensitive to penicillins. The high prevalence of penicillinase production by clinically relevant bacteria has limited the use of natural penicillins.

The World Health Organization (WHO) has designated penicillin G as a Critically Important, High Priority antimicrobial for human medicine.[1] The Office International des Epizooties (OIE) has designated natural penicillins as Veterinary Critically Important Antimicrobial (VCIA) Agents in avian, bovine, camelids, caprine, equine, lagomorph, ovine, and swine species.[2]

Pharmacology/Actions

Penicillins are usually bactericidal against susceptible bacteria and act by inhibiting mucopeptide synthesis in the cell wall, resulting in a defective barrier and an osmotically unstable spheroplast. The exact mechanism for this effect has not been definitively determined, but beta-lactam antibiotics have been shown to bind to several enzymes (carboxypeptidases, transpeptidases, and endopeptidases) within the bacterial cytoplasmic membrane that are involved with cell wall synthesis. The different affinities that various beta-lactam antibiotics have for these enzymes (also known as penicillin-binding proteins [PBPs]) help explain the differences in spectrums of activity the drugs have that are not explained by the influence of beta-lactamases. Like other beta-lactam antibiotics, penicillins are generally considered more effective against actively growing bacteria. Penicillins are considered time-dependent antibiotics, as efficacy depends on the length of time that plasma (or tissue) concentrations exceed the MIC of pathogens.

The natural penicillins (G and V) have similar spectrums of activity, but penicillin G is slightly more active in vitro on a per weight basis against many organisms. The natural penicillins are narrow in spectrum and have in vitro activity against most spirochetes and gram-positive and gram-negative aerobic cocci, but not penicillinase-producing strains. They have activity against some aerobic and anaerobic gram-positive bacilli such as *Bacillus anthracis*, *Clostridium* spp, *Fusobacterium* spp, and *Arcanobacterium* spp. The natural penicillins are inactive against most gram-negative aerobic and anaerobic bacilli, and all *Rickettsia* spp, mycobacteria, fungi, *Mycoplasma* spp, and viruses. Natural penicillins are consistently inactive against *Pseudomonas* spp, most Enterobacteriaceae, and penicillinase-producing *Staphylococcus* spp.

Pharmacokinetics

Penicillin G potassium is poorly absorbed orally because of rapid acid-catalyzed hydrolysis. When penicillin G is administered on an empty (fasted) stomach, oral bioavailability is ≈15% to 30%. If penicillin G is given with food, absorption rate and extent will be decreased.

Penicillin G potassium and sodium salts are rapidly absorbed after IM injections and yield high peak concentrations usually within 20 minutes of administration. In horses, equivalent doses given either IV or IM demonstrated that IM dosing will provide serum concentrations above 0.5 µg/mL for approximately twice as long as IV administration (≈3 to 4 hours [IV] vs 6 to 7 hours [IM]). Penicillin G potassium administered IM to rabbits yielded peak concentration at 30 minutes, with a half-life of 2 hours.[3]

Penicillin G procaine is slowly hydrolyzed to penicillin G after IM injection. Peak levels are much lower than with parenterally administered aqueous penicillin G sodium or potassium, but serum concentrations are more prolonged.

Penicillin G benzathine is also very slowly absorbed after IM injection after being hydrolyzed to the parent compound. Serum concentrations can be very prolonged, but concentrations attained generally only exceed MICs for the most susceptible streptococci, and the use of penicillin G benzathine should be limited to these infections when other penicillin use is impractical.

After absorption, penicillin G is widely distributed throughout the body with the exception of the CSF, joints, and milk. In lactating dairy cattle, the milk to plasma ratio is ≈0.2. CSF concentrations are generally 10% or less of that found in the serum when meninges are not inflamed. Concentrations in the CSF may be greater in patients with inflamed meninges or if probenecid is given concurrently. Binding to plasma proteins is ≈50% in most species.

Penicillin G is principally excreted unchanged in the urine through renal mechanisms via both glomerular filtration and tubular secretion. Elimination half-lives are rapid and are usually 1 hour or less in most species (if normal renal function exists).

Contraindications/Precautions/Warnings

Penicillins are contraindicated in patients with a history of hypersensitivity to them.[4] Because there may be cross-reactivity, use penicillins cautiously in patients documented as hypersensitive to other beta-lactam antibiotics (eg, cephalosporins, cefamycins, carbapenems).

High doses of penicillin G sodium or potassium, particularly in small animal species with a pre-existing electrolyte abnormality, renal disease, or congestive heart failure, may cause electrolyte imbalances.[5] Certain species (eg, snakes, birds, turtles) are reportedly sensitive to penicillin G procaine.

A retrospective observational study in horses found an association between perioperative penicillin G sodium administration and postanesthetic colic.[6] The authors concluded an alternative to penicillin G sodium should be investigated to reduce the incidence of postanesthetic colic.

Accidental IV injection of procaine- or benzathine-containing penicillin products to humans may lead to immediate excitatory CNS toxicity (procaine) or cardiovascular arrest and death (benzathine).[4,7] Injections near major peripheral nerves or blood vessels may lead to tissue damage, necrosis, or permanent neurologic damage.

Adverse Effects

Adverse effects from the penicillins in animals are usually not severe and have a relatively low frequency of occurrence.

Hypersensitivity reactions, unrelated to dose, can occur with these agents and manifest as rashes, fever, eosinophilia, neutropenia, agranulocytosis, thrombocytopenia, leukopenia, anemia, lymphadenopathy, or anaphylaxis. In humans, it is estimated that up to 15% of patients that are hypersensitive to cephalosporins will also be hypersensitive to penicillins.[8] The incidence of cross-reactivity in veterinary patients is unknown.

Neurotoxicity (eg, ataxia in dogs) has been associated with very high doses or prolonged use. Although the penicillins are not considered hepatotoxic, elevated liver enzymes have been reported. Other effects noted in dogs include tachypnea, dyspnea, edema, and tachycardia.

Procaine toxicity can occur when procaine penicillin is administered at high doses or is inadvertently administered IV. These reactions are poorly characterized in animals but rapid onset behavioral, locomotor, neurologic, and vascular reactions have been reported in multiple animal species.[9-12] Some cases have resulted in death.

Reproductive/Nursing Safety

Penicillins have been shown to cross the placenta and safe use of them during pregnancy has not been firmly established, but there have not been any documented teratogenic problems associated with these drugs.

Penicillins are excreted in maternal milk in low concentrations; use could potentially cause diarrhea, candidiasis, or allergic responses in nursing offspring. Milk replacer could be considered.

Because safety has not been established in animals, this drug should only be used when the maternal benefits outweigh the potential risks to offspring.

Overdose/Acute Toxicity

Acute oral penicillin overdoses are unlikely to cause significant problems other than GI distress, but other effects are possible (see ***Adverse Effects***). In humans (especially those with renal disease), very high doses of parenteral penicillins have induced CNS effects. Rapid-onset behavioral, locomotor, neurologic, and vascular reactions have been reported in dogs, cats, horses, and sows, particularly when penicillin procaine has been administered IV or at high doses. Some cases have resulted in death.[9-13] Treatment, if required, should be supportive and include anticonvulsants, centrally acting muscle relaxants, and sedation as indicated.

For patients that have experienced or are suspected to have experienced an overdose, consultation with a 24-hour poison consultation center specializing in providing veterinary-specific information is recommended. For general information related to overdose and toxin exposures, as well as contact information for poison control centers, refer to ***Appendix.***

Drug Interactions

The following drug interactions have either been reported or are theoretical in humans or animals receiving penicillin G and may be of significance in veterinary patients. Unless otherwise noted, use together is not necessarily contraindicated, but weigh the potential risks and perform additional monitoring when appropriate.

- **Aminoglycosides or Cephalosporins**: In vitro studies have demonstrated that penicillins can have synergistic or additive activity against certain bacteria when used with aminoglycosides or cephalosporins.
- **Bacteriostatic Antibiotics** (eg, **chloramphenicol, erythromycin, tetracyclines**): Use with penicillins is generally not recommended, particularly in acute infections where the organism is proliferating rapidly as penicillins tend to perform better on actively growing bacteria. However, clinical significance is unknown.
- **Methotrexate**: Penicillins may decrease renal elimination of methotrexate.
- **Probenecid**: Competitively blocks the tubular secretion of most penicillins, thereby increasing serum concentrations and serum half-lives

Laboratory Considerations

- As penicillins and other beta-lactams can inactivate **aminoglycosides** in vitro (and in vivo in patients in renal failure), serum concentrations of aminoglycosides may be falsely decreased if the patient is also receiving beta-lactam antibiotics and the serum is stored prior to analysis. It is recommended that if the assay is delayed, samples be frozen and, if possible, drawn at times when the beta-lactam antibiotic is at a trough.
- Penicillin G can cause falsely elevated **serum uric acid** values if the copper-chelate method is used; phosphotungstate and uricase methods are not affected.
- Penicillins may cause false positive **urine glucose** determinations when using cupric-sulfate solution (Benedict's Solution, *Clinitest*®). Tests utilizing glucose oxidase (*Tes-Tape*®, *Clinistix*®) are not affected by penicillin.

Dosages

NOTE: Label dosages of penicillin have been unchanged for decades and may result in marked underdosing based on current understanding of antibiotic therapy. Although consideration of the label recommendations is required, present-day recommended dosing regimens should be used.

DOGS/CATS:

Susceptible infections (extra-label):

Penicillin G procaine: 20,000 – 40,000 units/kg IM or SC every 12 to 24 hours

Penicillin G sodium or potassium: 20,000 – 40,000 units/kg IV or IM every 4 to 8 hours

Leptospirosis (extra-label): Penicillin G sodium or potassium 25,000 – 40,000 units/kg IV every 12 hours initially, followed by doxycycline 5 mg/kg PO every 12 hours or 10 mg/kg PO every 24 hours for 2 weeks, starting once the patient can tolerate PO administration[14]

HORSES:

Strangles caused by *Streptococcus equi* (label dosage; FDA-approved): Penicillin G procaine: 3000 units per 0.45 kg (1 lb) of body weight (1 mL per 45.3 kg [100 lb] body weight) IM daily. **NOTE**: According to modern principles of antibiotic therapy the labeled dosage is understood to be too low and the dosing interval too infrequent to effectively treat infections.

Susceptible infections caused by gram-positive aerobes (extra-label):

Penicillin G procaine: 22,000 – 44,000 units/kg IM every 12 hours

Penicillin G potassium or sodium: 20,000 units/kg IV or IM every 6 hours

Serious gram-positive infections (eg, tetanus, clostridial myonecrosis): Penicillin G sodium or potassium: 22,000 – 44,000 units/kg IV every 6 hours[15]

Carriers with *Streptococcus equi* infections of the guttural pouches (extra-label): Administration of both systemic and topical penicillin G may improve treatment success rate. Before topical therapy, remove all visible inflammatory material from guttural pouch. To make a gelatin-penicillin G mix of 50 mL for guttural pouch instillation:

1) Measure 2 g gelatin (Sigma G-6650 or household) and add 40 mL of sterile water.
2) Heat or microwave to dissolve. Cool to 45°C to 50°C (113°F-133°F).
3) Add 10 mL sterile water to a vial of 10 million units penicillin G sodium for injection and mix with the cooled gelatin to a total volume of 50 mL.
4) Dispense into syringes and leave overnight in the refrigerator.
5) Instillation is easiest through a catheter inserted up the nose and endoscopically guided into the pouch opening, with the last inch bent at an angle to aid entry under the pouch flap. Elevate horse's head for 20 minutes after instillation.[16]

Foals (extra-label):

Penicillin G procaine: 22,000 units/kg every 12 hours IM (painful, lower blood concentrations than penicillin G potassium)[17]

Penicillin G potassium: 22,000 units/kg every 6 hours IV or IM[17]

CATTLE (AND OTHER RUMINANTS UNLESS SPECIFIED):

NOTE: When penicillin G procaine is administered in an extra-label manner, the dose, dosage frequency, treatment duration, injection site, and injection route (IM vs SC) can all affect drug residues.[18] Veterinarians seeking information for determination of a withdrawal interval following extra-label drug use should contact the Food Animal Residue Avoidance Databank (FARAD) for assistance.

Susceptible infections in beef cattle (label dosage; FDA-approved): Penicillin G benzathine and Penicillin G procaine: 2 mL per 68 kg (150 lb) body weight, SC only. Repeat in 48 hours. **NOTE**: According to modern principles of antibiotic therapy the labeled dosage is understood to be too low and the dosing interval too infrequent to effectively treat infections.

Bacterial pneumonia (shipping fever) caused by *Pasteurella multocida* in cattle and sheep (label dosage; FDA-approved): Penicillin G procaine: 3000 units per 0.45 kg (1 lb) of body weight (1 mL per 45.3 kg [100 lb] body weight) IM daily. Treatment duration varies by manufacturer; follow the directions found on product label. **NOTE**: According to modern principles of antibiotic therapy the labeled dose is understood to be too low and the dosing interval too infrequent to effectively treat infections.

Susceptible infections (extra-label): Penicillin G procaine: 24,000 – 66,000 units/kg IM once per day[19]

Clostridial abomasitis and enteritis in calves (extra-label): Penicillin G procaine: 22,000 units/kg PO every 24 hours for 3 to 5 days. Oral penicillin is preferred over systemic as oral penicillin is poorly absorbed from the GI tract and will provide activity in the intestinal lumen where the target bacteria reside.[20]

SWINE:

NOTE: When penicillin G procaine is administered in an extra-label manner, the dose, dosage frequency, treatment duration, injection site, and injection route (IM vs SC) can all affect drug residues.[21] Veterinarians seeking information for determination of a withdrawal interval following extra-label drug use should contact the Food Animal Residue Avoidance Databank (FARAD) for assistance.

Erysipelas caused by *Erysipelothrix rhusiopathiae* (label dosage; FDA-approved): Penicillin G procaine: 3000 units per 0.45 kg (1 lb) of body weight (1 mL per 45.3 kg [100 lb] body weight) IM daily. Treatment duration varies by product; consult label for specific information. **NOTE**: According to modern principles of antibiotic therapy the labeled dose is understood to be too low and the dosing interval too infrequent to effectively treat infections.

Susceptible infections (extra-label):

Penicillin G procaine: 40,000 units/kg IM once daily[22]

Penicillin G procaine/penicillin G benzathine combination: 40,000 units/kg IM once[23]

BIRDS:

Susceptible infections in turkeys (extra-label): Penicillin G procaine/penicillin G benzathine combination: 200 mg/kg IM once daily.[24,25] Use cautiously in small birds as it may cause procaine toxicity[26]

FERRETS:

Susceptible infections (extra-label): Penicillin G procaine: 20,000 – 40,000 units/kg IM once or twice daily[27]

RABBITS, RODENTS, SMALL MAMMALS:

Rabbits (extra-label): Penicillin G procaine: 20,000 – 84,000 units/kg SC or IM every 24 hours for 5 to 7 days for venereal spirochetosis.[28] **NOTE**: Parenteral administration of penicillin, unlike the oral route, appears to be tolerated by rabbits and other hindgut fermenters.

Hedgehogs (extra-label): Penicillin G procaine: 40,000 units/kg IM once daily[29]

Monitoring

- Because penicillins usually have minimal toxicity associated with their use, monitoring for efficacy is usually all that is required unless toxic signs develop. Serum concentrations and therapeutic drug monitoring are not routinely done with these agents.

Client Information

- This medicine is not usually given orally.
- Penicillin G procaine and/or Penicillin G benzathine should not be administered in the vein. Inadvertent administration into a vein (IV) may result in serious toxicity and death. Be sure you understand the proper injection technique.
- Injectable solutions may cause stinging when injected under the skin (subcutaneously).
- Side effects to penicillin G are uncommon. Contact your veterinarian if you have any concerns about your animal's condition.

Chemistry/Synonyms

Penicillin G is a natural penicillin obtained from cultures of *Penicillium chrysogenum* and is available in several different salt forms. Penicillin G potassium (also known as benzylpenicillin potassium, aqueous or crystalline penicillin) occurs as colorless or white crystals, or white crystalline powder. It is very soluble in water and sparingly soluble in alcohol. The potency of penicillin G potassium is generally expressed in terms of units. One mg of penicillin G potassium is equivalent to 1440 to 1680 USP units (1355 to 1595 USP units for the powder for injection). After reconstitution, penicillin G potassium powder for injection has a pH of 6 to 8.5 and contains 1.7 mEq of potassium per 1 million units.

Penicillin G sodium (also known as benzylpenicillin sodium, aqueous or crystalline penicillin) occurs as colorless or white crystals, or white to slightly yellow, crystalline powder. Approximately 25 mg are soluble in 1 mL of water. The potency of penicillin G sodium is generally expressed in terms of units. One mg of penicillin G sodium is equivalent to 1500 to 1750 USP units (1420 to 1667 USP units for the powder for injection). After reconstitution, penicillin G sodium powder for injection has a pH of 6 to 7.5 and contains 2 mEq of sodium per 1 million units.

Penicillin G procaine (also known as procaine penicillin G, aqueous procaine penicillin G, APPG, benzylpenicillin procaine, procaine benzylpenicillin) is the procaine monohydrate salt of penicillin G. In vivo it is hydrolyzed to penicillin G and acts as a depot or repository form of penicillin G. It occurs as white crystals or a very fine, white crystalline powder. Approximately 4 to 4.5 mg is soluble in 1 mL of water and 3.3 mg is soluble in 1 mL of alcohol. The potency of penicillin G procaine is generally expressed in terms of units. One mg of penicillin G procaine is equivalent to 900 to 1050 USP units. The commercially available suspension for injection is buffered with sodium citrate and has a pH of 5 to 7.5. It is preserved with methylparaben and propylparaben.

Penicillin G benzathine (also known as benzathine benzylpenicillin, benzathine penicillin G, benzylpenicillin benzathine, dibenzylethylenediamine benzylpenicillin) is the benzathine tetrahydrate salt of penicillin G. It is hydrolyzed in vivo to penicillin G and acts as a long-acting form of penicillin G. It occurs as an odorless, white, crystalline powder. Solubility ranges from 0.2 to 0.3 mg/mL in water and 15 mg/mL in alcohol. One mg of penicillin G benzathine is equivalent to 1090 to 1272 USP units. The commercially available suspension for injection is buffered with sodium citrate and has a pH of 5 to 7.5. It is preserved with methylparaben and propylparaben.

Penicillin G may also be known as benzylpenicillin, crystalline penicillin G, pen G, penicillin, *Bicillin C-R*®, and *Pfizerpen*®.

Storage/Stability

Penicillin G procaine should be stored at 2°C to 8°C (36°F-46°F); avoid freezing. Penicillin G benzathine should be stored at 2°C to 8°C (36°F-46°F).

Penicillin G sodium and potassium powder for injection can be stored at room temperature (15°C-30°C [59°F-86°F]). After reconstituting, the injectable solution is stable for 7 days when kept refrigerated (2°C-8°C [36°F-46°F]) and for 24 hours at room temperature.

Compatibility/Compounding Considerations

All commonly used IV fluids (some Dextran products are physically **incompatible**) and the following drugs are reportedly physically **compatible** with penicillin G potassium: ascorbic acid injection, calcium chloride/gluconate, chloramphenicol sodium succinate, cimetidine HCl, clindamycin phosphate, corticotropin, dexamethasone sodium phosphate, diphenhydramine HCl, ephedrine sulfate, famotidine, gentamicin, hydrocortisone sodium succinate, ketamine hydrochloride, lidocaine HCl, methicillin sodium, methylprednisolone sodium succinate, metronidazole with sodium bicarbonate, nitroprusside sodium, potassium chloride, prednisolone sodium phosphate, procaine HCl, prochlorperazine edisylate, sodium iodide, and verapamil HCl.

The following drugs/solutions are either physically **incompatible** or the data conflict regarding compatibility with penicillin G potassium injection: amikacin sulfate, aminophylline, chlorpromazine HCl, dopamine HCl, erythromycin lactobionate, heparin sodium, hydroxyzine HCl, metoclopramide HCl, oxytetracycline HCl, pentobarbital sodium, prochlorperazine mesylate, promazine HCl, promethazine HCl, sodium bicarbonate, tetracycline HCl, and vitamin B complex with C.

The following drugs/solutions are reportedly physically **compatible** with penicillin G sodium injection: Dextran 40 10%, dextrose 5% (some degradation may occur if stored for 24 hours), sodium chloride 0.9% (some degradation may occur if stored for 24 hours), calcium chloride/gluconate, chloramphenicol sodium succinate, cimetidine HCl, clindamycin phosphate, dexamethasone sodium phosphate, diphenhydramine HCl, famotidine, gentamicin sulfate, hydrocortisone sodium succinate, ketamine hydrochloride, prednisolone sodium phosphate, procaine HCl, verapamil HCl, and vitamin B complex with C.

The following drugs/solutions are either physically **incompatible** or the data conflict regarding compatibility with penicillin G sodium injection: amphotericin B, bleomycin sulfate, chlorpromazine HCl, dobutamine hydrochloride, erythromycin lactobionate, heparin sodium, hydroxyzine HCl, methylprednisolone sodium succinate, oxytetracycline HCl, polymyxin B sulfate, potassium chloride, prochlorperazine mesylate, promethazine HCl, and tetracycline HCl.

Compatibility is dependent on factors such as pH, concentration, temperature, and diluent used; consult specialized references or a hospital pharmacist for more specific information.

Dosage Forms/Regulatory Status

VETERINARY-LABELED PRODUCTS:

NOTE: Withdrawal times are for labeled dosages only. Contact Food Animal Residue Avoidance Databank (FARAD) when used in an extra-label manner for assistance in determining a withdrawal interval.

Penicillin G Procaine Injection 300,000 units/mL in 100 mL, 250 mL, and 500 mL vials: Variety of trade names available (OTC). Depending on product, FDA-approved for use in horses, cattle, sheep, and swine. Not intended for use in horses used for food. Withdrawal times vary depending on the product and are for the labeled dosage of 6600 units/kg once daily (rarely used today). Milk withdrawal times (at labeled doses) = 48 hours. Slaughter withdrawal: Calves (nonruminating) = 7 days; cattle = 4 to 14 days; sheep = 8 to 9 days; swine = 6 to 7 days; refer to label for more information.

Penicillin G benzathine 150,000 units/mL with Penicillin G procaine Injection 150,000 units/mL for Injection in 100 mL, 250 mL, and 500 mL vials: Variety of trade names available (Rx). FDA-approved (most products) in horses and beef cattle. Not FDA-approved for horses intended for food. Slaughter withdrawal: cattle = 30 days (at labeled doses). Actual species approvals and withdrawal times vary with the product; refer to the product label.

Penicillin G is also available in syringes for intramammary administration and as a powder for use in poultry drinking water systems.

The Association of Racing Commissioners International (ARCI) has designated procaine (including penicillin G procaine) as a class 3 substance. Use of this drug may not be allowed in certain animal competitions. Check rules and regulations before entering in a competition while this medication is being administered. Contact local racing authorities for further guidance. See the ***Appendix*** for more information.

HUMAN-LABELED PRODUCTS:

Penicillin G (aqueous) sodium powder for injection: 5 million units/vial; generic; (Rx)

Penicillin G (aqueous) premixed injectable solution: 1, 2, or 3 million units/50 mL (Rx)

Penicillin G (aqueous) potassium powder for injection: 5 million, and 20 million units; *Pfizerpen-G®*, generic; (Rx)

Penicillin G procaine injection: 600,000 units/vial in 1 mL *Tubex* and 1.2 million units/vial in 2 mL *Tubex*; generic; (Rx)

Penicillin G benzathine injection: 600,000 units/dose in 1 mL *Tubex*; 1.2 million units/dose in 2 mL; 2.4 million units/dose in 4 mL prefilled syringes; *Bicillin L-A®*; (Rx)

Penicillin G Benzathine 600,000 units/mL with Penicillin G Procaine Injection 600,000 units/mL for Injection: in 2 mL syringes; *Bicillin C-R®*; (Rx)

Penicillin G Benzathine 900,000 units/mL with Penicillin G Procaine Injection 300,000 units/mL for Injection: in 2 mL syringes; *Bicillin CR 900/300®*; (Rx)

References

For the complete list of references, see **wiley.com/go/budde/plumb**

Penicillin V

Phenoxymethylpenicillin

(pen-i-***sill***-in ***vee***)

Oral Penicillin Antibiotic

Prescriber Highlights

- Requires frequent administration on an empty stomach, which limits its utility in veterinary medicine
- Contraindications include known hypersensitivity, and hindgut fermenters.
- Adverse effects include anorexia, vomiting, and diarrhea.

Uses/Indications

Penicillin V is a natural penicillin that is active against many streptococci. It is rarely used today in veterinary medicine because it requires frequent administration on an empty stomach and has no significant advantages over other available related drugs.

The World Health Organization (WHO) has designated penicillin V as a Critically Important, High Priority antimicrobial for human medicine.[1] The Office International des Epizooties (OIE) has designated natural penicillins as Veterinary Critically Important Antimicrobial (VCIA) Agents in avian and swine species.[2]

Pharmacology/Actions

Penicillins are usually bactericidal against susceptible bacteria and act by inhibiting mucopeptide synthesis in the cell wall, resulting in a defective barrier and an osmotically unstable spheroplast. The exact mechanism for this effect has not been definitively determined, but beta-lactam antibiotics have been shown to bind to several enzymes (carboxypeptidases, transpeptidases, and endopeptidases) within the bacterial cytoplasmic membrane that are involved with cell wall synthesis. The different affinities that various beta-lactam antibiotics have for these enzymes (also known as penicillin-binding proteins [PBPs]) help explain the differences in spectrums of activity the drugs have that are not explained by the influence of beta-lactamases. Like other beta-lactam antibiotics, penicillins are generally considered more effective against actively growing bacteria. Penicillin V is considered a time-dependent antibiotic as its efficacy depends on the length of time that plasma (or tissue) concentrations exceed the MIC of pathogens.

The natural penicillins (G and V) have similar spectrums of activity, but penicillin G is slightly more active in vitro on a per weight basis against many organisms. The natural penicillins are narrow in spectrum and have in vitro activity against most spirochetes and gram-positive and gram-negative aerobic cocci, but not penicillinase-producing strains. They have activity against some aerobic and anaerobic gram-positive bacilli such as *Bacillus anthracis*, *Clostridium* spp, *Fusobacterium* spp, and *Arcanobacterium* spp. The natural penicillins are inactive against most gram-negative aerobic and anaerobic bacilli, and all *Rickettsia* spp, mycobacteria, fungi, *Mycoplasma* spp, and viruses. Natural penicillins are consistently inactive against *Pseudomonas* spp, most Enterobacteriaceae, and penicillinase-producing *Staphylococcus* spp. Although penicillin V may be slightly less active than penicillin G against organisms that are susceptible to the natural penicillins, its superior absorptive characteristics after oral administration make it a better choice against mild to moderately severe infections in monogastric animals when oral administration is desired.

Pharmacokinetics

The pharmacokinetics of penicillin V are very similar to penicillin G with the exception of oral bioavailability and the percentage of the drug that is bound to plasma proteins. Penicillin V is significantly more resistant to acid-catalyzed inactivation in the gut and bioavailability after oral administration in humans is ≈60% to 73%. Bioavailability in calves is only 30%, but studies performed in horses and dogs demonstrated that therapeutic serum concentrations can be achieved after oral administration. In dogs, food will decrease the rate and extent of absorption.[3]

Distribution of penicillin V follows that of penicillin G but, in humans, the drug is bound to a larger extent to plasma proteins (≈80% with penicillin V vs 50% with penicillin G).

Like penicillin G, penicillin V is excreted rapidly in the urine via the kidney. Elimination half-lives are generally less than 1 hour in animals with normal renal function. An elimination half-life of 3.7 hours has been reported after oral dosing in horses.[4]

Contraindications/Precautions/Warnings

Penicillins are contraindicated in patients with a history of hypersensitivity to them. Because there may be cross-reactivity, use penicillins cautiously in patients documented as hypersensitive to other beta-lactam antibiotics (eg, cephalosporins, cefamycins, carbapenems).[5]

Oral penicillins should be avoided in hindgut fermenters (eg, horses, rabbits, guinea pigs, hamsters, gerbils, chinchillas) because of potential for *Clostridium* spp bacterial overgrowth.

Do not administer systemic antibiotics orally in patients with septicemia, shock, or other grave illnesses as absorption of the medication from the GI tract may be significantly delayed or diminished.

Adverse Effects

Adverse effects from the penicillins are usually not severe and have a relatively low frequency of occurrence.

Hypersensitivity reactions, unrelated to dose, can occur with these agents and manifest in humans as rashes, fever, eosinophilia, neutropenia, agranulocytosis, thrombocytopenia, leukopenia, anemia, or anaphylaxis.[6] In humans, it is estimated that up to 15% of patients that are hypersensitive to cephalosporins will also be hypersensitive to penicillins.[7] The incidence of hypersensitivity and cross-reactivity in veterinary patients is unknown.

When penicillins are given orally, they may cause GI effects (eg, anorexia, vomiting, diarrhea). Because the penicillins may also alter gut flora, antibiotic-associated diarrhea can occur and can allow for the proliferation of resistant bacteria in the colon (superinfections).[5]

Neurotoxicity (eg, ataxia in dogs) has been associated with very high doses or prolonged use. Although the penicillins are not considered hepatotoxic, elevated liver enzymes have been reported. Other effects reported in dogs include tachypnea, dyspnea, edema, and tachycardia.

Reproductive/Nursing Safety

Penicillins have been shown to cross the placenta and safe use of them during pregnancy has not been firmly established, but there have not been any documented teratogenic problems associated with these drugs. Despite this, use penicillins only when the potential benefits outweigh the risks.

Penicillins are excreted in maternal milk in low concentrations. Use of penicillins in the dam could potentially cause diarrhea, candidiasis, or allergic response in nursing offspring; consider using a milk replacer if treatment is necessary.

Overdose/Acute Toxicity

Acute oral penicillin overdoses are unlikely to cause significant problems other than GI distress, but other effects are possible (see ***Adverse Effects***). In humans (especially in patients with renal disease), very high doses of parenteral penicillins have induced CNS effects.

For patients that have experienced or are suspected to have experienced an overdose, consultation with a 24-hour poison consultation center specializing in providing veterinary-specific information is recommended. For general information related to overdose and toxin exposures, as well as contact information for poison control centers, refer to ***Appendix.***

Drug Interactions

The following drug interactions have either been reported or are theoretical in humans or animals receiving penicillin V and may be of significance in veterinary patients. Unless otherwise noted, use together is not necessarily contraindicated, but weigh the potential risks and perform additional monitoring when appropriate.

- **Aminoglycosides or Cephalosporins**: In vitro studies have demonstrated that penicillins can have synergistic or additive activity against certain bacteria when used with aminoglycosides or cephalosporins.
- **Bacteriostatic Antibiotics** (eg, **chloramphenicol, erythromycin, tetracyclines**): Use of bacteriostatic antibiotics with penicillins is generally not recommended, particularly in acute infections where the organism is proliferating rapidly, as penicillins tend to perform better on actively growing bacteria. The clinical significance of this interaction is unknown.
- **Methotrexate**: Penicillins may decrease renal elimination of methotrexate.
- **Probenecid**: Competitively blocks the tubular secretion of most penicillins, thereby increasing serum concentrations and serum half-lives.

Laboratory Considerations

- As penicillins and other beta-lactams can inactivate **aminoglycosides** in vitro (and in vivo in patients in renal failure), serum concentrations of aminoglycosides may be falsely decreased if the patient is also receiving beta-lactam antibiotics and the serum is stored prior to analysis. It is recommended that if the assay is delayed, samples be frozen and, if possible, drawn at times when the beta-lactam antibiotic is at a trough.
- Penicillin V can cause falsely elevated **serum uric acid** values if the copper-chelate method is used; phosphotungstate and uricase methods are not affected.
- Penicillins may cause false positive **urine glucose** determinations when using cupric-sulfate solution (Benedict's Solution, *Clinitest*®). Tests utilizing glucose oxidase (*Tes-Tape*®, *Clinistix*®) are not affected by penicillin.

Dosages

DOGS/CATS:

Susceptible infections (extra-label): 10 mg/kg PO every 8 hours for 7 days[8]

Monitoring

- Because penicillins usually have minimal toxicity associated with their use, monitoring for efficacy is usually all that is required unless toxic signs develop. Serum concentrations and therapeutic drug monitoring are not routinely done with these agents.

Client Information

- Penicillin V should not be given to horses, rabbits, guinea pigs, gerbils, hamsters, and chinchillas, as life-threatening diarrhea may occur.
- Penicillin V is best given without food, but if your animal vomits or acts sick after receiving this medicine on an empty stomach, try giving the next dose with food or a small treat. If vomiting continues, contact your veterinarian.
- Liquid forms of this medication must be measured carefully and should be stored in the refrigerator. Your veterinarian or pharmacist can help by providing special measuring spoons or syringes. Liquid forms of this medication should be discarded 14 days after mixing.
- This medication can be given for various lengths of time. Be sure you understand how long your veterinarian wants you to continue giving this medication. Prescription refills may be necessary before the therapy will be complete. Before stopping this medication, talk to your veterinarian, as there may be important reasons to continue its use.
- It is uncommon for side effects to occur in animals treated with penicillin V. The most common side effects are loss of appetite, vomiting, and diarrhea. It is important to contact your veterinarian if you have any concerns.
- Allergic reactions to penicillin V are rare but can be severe with signs including rashes, fever, collapse, or difficulty breathing. In the event of such signs, contact your veterinarian immediately.

Chemistry/Synonyms

A natural penicillin, penicillin V is produced from *Penicillium chrysogenum* and is commercially available as the potassium salt. Penicillin V potassium occurs as an odorless, white, crystalline powder that is very slightly soluble in water and slightly soluble in alcohol. The potency of penicillin V potassium is usually expressed in terms of weight (in mg) of penicillin V, but penicillin V units may also be used. One mg of penicillin V potassium is equivalent to 1380 to 1610 USP units. Manufacturers generally state that 125 mg of penicillin V potassium is ≈200,000 USP units. Each 5 mL of reconstituted penicillin V potassium oral solution (250 mg/5 mL) contains contain 0.85 mEq (32.8 mg) of potassium; each 250 mg tablet contains 0.71 mEq (27.9 mg) of potassium.

Penicillin V may also be known as phenoxymethylpenicillin, fenoximetilpenicilina, penicillin, phenoxymethyl phenomycilline, phenoxymethyl penicillin, phenoxymethylpenicillinum, and *Veetids*®.

Storage/Stability

Penicillin V potassium tablets and powder for oral solution should be stored in tight containers at room temperature (20°C-25°C [68°F-77°F]). Refer to each product label for specific storage temperature recommendations as they may vary by manufacturer. The powder for oral solution should be reconstituted by adding water in 2 portions; the solutions should be shaken vigorously after each addition. After reconstitution, the oral solution should be stored in the refrigerator at 2°C to 8°C (36°F-46°F) and any unused portion discarded after 14 days.

Dosage Forms/Regulatory Status

VETERINARY-LABELED PRODUCTS: NONE

HUMAN-LABELED PRODUCTS:

Penicillin V Potassium Tablets: 250 and 500 mg; generic; (Rx)

Penicillin V Potassium Powder for Oral Solution: 25 mg/mL (labeled as 125 mg/5 mL) and 50 mg/mL (labeled as 250 mg/5 mL) in 100 mL and 200 mL; generic; (Rx)

References

For the complete list of references, see **wiley.com/go/budde/plumb**

Pentobarbital

(pen-toe-***bar***-bi-tal) *Nembutal®*
Barbiturate

NOTE: *For information related to pentobarbital and pentobarbital combinations for euthanasia, see* ***Euthanasia Agents****.*

Prescriber Highlights

- ► Used therapeutically as a sedative/anesthetic and for treating intractable seizures; also used for euthanasia
- ► Contraindications include in patients with known hypersensitivity and porphyria.
- ► Use with caution in patients with liver dysfunction, renal dysfunction, severe respiratory depression, hypovolemia, anemia, borderline hypoadrenal function, or with cardiac or respiratory disease.
- ► Must have ventilatory support available if using for anesthesia
- ► Adverse effects include respiratory depression, hypothermia, or excitement postanesthesia (dogs).
- ► Extravasation or SC administration can cause local tissue damage or necrosis; do not give intra-arterially.
- ► IV administration must be done slowly; during induction of anesthesia, administer ⅓ to ½ of the calculated dose as a bolus and wait to see effects, then give the rest SLOWLY to effect.
- ► Numerous drug interactions
- ► DEA Schedule II (C-II) controlled substance

Uses/Indications

Pentobarbital is used therapeutically as a sedative/restraining agent in patients being mechanically ventilated and has been used as a sedative and anesthetic agent in horses, cattle, swine, sheep, and goats. It is also commonly used as an anesthetic for rodents in laboratory situations. Although pentobarbital was once the principal agent used for general anesthesia in small animal species, it has been largely supplanted by the use of inhalant and other injectable anesthetic agents.

Pentobarbital can also be used for treating intractable seizures secondary to convulsant agents (eg, strychnine) or secondary to CNS toxins (eg, tetanus). It should not be used to treat seizures caused by lidocaine intoxication. Pentobarbital may be used for refractory status epilepticus that is not controlled with diazepam and phenobarbital; however, propofol or inhalant anesthetics are generally preferred.

Pentobarbital is a major active ingredient in several euthanasia solutions; see ***Euthanasia Agents.***

Pharmacology/Actions

Although barbiturates are generally considered CNS depressants, they can invoke all levels of CNS mood alteration from paradoxical excitement to deep coma and death. Barbiturates have been shown to inhibit the release of acetylcholine, norepinephrine, and glutamate. They also have effects on GABA receptors; pentobarbital has been shown to be GABA-mimetic. Pentobarbital may have neuroprotective effects via decreasing cerebral metabolic rate and oxygen consumption, scavenging of free radicals, and stabilization of endothelial and glial membranes. At high anesthetic doses, barbiturates have been demonstrated to inhibit the uptake of calcium at nerve endings.

The degree of depression produced by pentobarbital is dependent on the dose, route of administration, and species treated. Additionally, effects may be altered by patient age, physical condition, or concurrent use of other drugs. The barbiturates depress the sensory cortex, lessen motor activity, and produce sedation at low dosages. Barbiturates have no true intrinsic analgesic activity.

Although barbiturates cause dose-dependent respiratory depression in most species, they can also cause slight respiratory stimulation in some species. At lower sedative/hypnotic doses, respiratory depression is similar to that during normal physiologic sleep. As doses increase, the medullary respiratory center is progressively depressed with resultant decreases in rate, depth, and volume. Respiratory arrest may occur at doses 4 times lower than those that cause cardiac arrest.

Cardiovascular effects of pentobarbital in dogs include tachycardia, decreased myocardial contractility and stroke volume, and decreased mean arterial pressure and total peripheral resistance. At high doses, pentobarbital has cardiac arresting effects.

Barbiturates cause reduced tone and motility of the intestinal musculature, likely secondary to its central depressant action. Thiobarbiturates (thiamylal, thiopental) may, after initial depression, cause an increase in both tone and motility of the intestinal musculature; however, these effects do not appear to have much clinical significance. Administration of barbiturates reduces the sensitivity of the motor endplate to acetylcholine, thereby slightly relaxing skeletal muscle. Because the musculature is not completely relaxed, other skeletal muscle relaxants may be necessary for surgical procedures.

Barbiturates have no direct effect on the kidney, but overdoses may cause severe renal impairment secondary to hypotensive effects. Liver function is not directly affected with short-term use, but hepatic microsomal enzyme induction is well documented with extended barbiturate administration, especially pentobarbital. Although barbiturates reduce oxygen consumption of all tissues, no change in metabolic rate is measurable at sedative doses; however, at anesthetic doses, basal metabolic rates may be reduced with resultant decreases in body temperature.

Pharmacokinetics

In humans, pentobarbital is rapidly absorbed from the GI tract after oral and rectal administration.[1] Peak plasma concentrations occur between 30 and 60 minutes after oral dosing. The onset of action usually occurs within 15 to 60 minutes after oral dosing and within 1 minute after IV administration.

Pentobarbital, like all barbiturates, distributes rapidly to all body tissues, with the highest concentrations found in the liver, brain, and kidneys.[1] It is 35% to 45% bound to plasma proteins in humans. Although less lipophilic than the ultra-short-acting barbiturates (eg, thiopental), pentobarbital is highly lipid soluble, and the amount of adipose tissue may alter the distribution of the drug.

Pentobarbital is metabolized in the liver principally by oxidation. Ruminants, especially sheep and goats, metabolize pentobarbital at a rapid rate. Reported elimination half-life in goats is ≈0.9 hours. Conversely, the half-life in dogs is ≈8 hours. In humans, half-life ranges from 15 to 50 hours.[1]

Contraindications/Precautions/Warnings

Barbiturates are contraindicated in patients that have demonstrated previous hypersensitivity reactions to them and in patients with porphyria.[1] Large doses are contraindicated in patients with nephritis or severe respiratory dysfunction. Use of barbiturates for cesarean section is not recommended because of fetal respiratory depression.

Use pentobarbital with caution in patients with renal or hepatic dysfunction; dose reduction is required. Use pentobarbital cautiously in patients that are hypovolemic, anemic, have borderline hypoadrenal function, or cardiac or respiratory disease. Doses should be reduced in geriatric and debilitated patients, as significant excitement and/or depression may occur. Use this medicine with caution in neonates, as pentobarbital concentrations in the CNS may be substantially higher than in adults; exposure to sedatives or anesthetics may have detrimental effects on fetal/neonatal brain development. Female cats appear to be more susceptible to the effects of pentobarbital than male cats.

If pentobarbital is administered IV too rapidly, respiratory depression, apnea, laryngospasm, or vasodilation and subsequent blood pressure decrease may occur. It is recommended to administer ⅓ to ½ of the calculated dose initially as a bolus, then administer the remainder slowly after the initial effects are ascertained. Concurrent IV fluids are recommended during administration of the bolus to decrease pain on injection. Pentobarbital is highly alkaline and can cause local tissue damage or necrosis if extravasated or administered SC. Do not administer pentobarbital intra-arterially.

Do not confuse PENTObarbital with PHENObarbital. Consider writing orders and prescriptions using tall man letters to reduce the risk of errors.

Adverse Effects

Pentobarbital causes respiratory depression; respiratory activity must be closely monitored, and ventilatory support must be readily available. Hypotension can occur at high doses. Pentobarbital may cause excitement in dogs during recovery from anesthetic doses; this can be confused with seizure activity. Hypothermia may develop in animals receiving pentobarbital if exposed to temperatures below 27°C (80.6°F).

Reproductive/Nursing Safety

All barbiturates cross the placenta and enter milk at concentrations far below those of plasma. In neonates, pentobarbital may cross into the CNS at concentrations up to 6 times those in adult animals.

Barbiturates can cause fetal damage when administered to pregnant patients. Studies have suggested a connection between maternal barbiturate administration and fetal abnormalities.[1]

Exercise caution when administering pentobarbital to nursing mothers, as small amounts are excreted in maternal milk. Drowsiness in nursing offspring has been reported.

Overdose/Acute Toxicity

In dogs, the reported oral LD_{50} is 85 mg/kg and IV LD_{50} is 40 – 60 mg/kg. Fatalities from ingestion of meat from animals euthanized by pentobarbital have been reported in dogs. Treatment of pentobarbital overdose consists of GI decontamination protocols if appropriate and offering ventilatory and cardiovascular support.

For patients that have experienced or are suspected to have experienced an overdose, consultation with a 24-hour poison consultation center specializing in providing veterinary-specific information is recommended. For general information related to overdose and toxin exposures, as well as contact information for poison control centers, refer to ***Appendix.***

Drug Interactions

The following drug interactions with pentobarbital have either been reported or are theoretical in humans or animals and may be of significance in veterinary patients. Unless otherwise noted, use together is not necessarily contraindicated, but the potential risks must be weighed, and additional monitoring performed when appropriate.

- **Acetaminophen**: Increased risk for hepatotoxicity, particularly with large doses or long-term administration of barbiturates
- **Lidocaine**: Fatalities have been reported when dogs suffering from lidocaine-induced seizures were treated with pentobarbital. Until this interaction is further clarified, diazepam is recommended for initial treatment of lidocaine-induced seizures in dogs.
- **Rifampin**: May induce enzymes that increase the metabolism of barbiturates

The following drugs may increase the effect of pentobarbital:

- **Antihistamines**
- **Benzodiazepines**
- **Chloramphenicol**
- **Opioids**
- **Phenothiazines**
- **Valproic Acid**

Pentobarbital (particularly after chronic therapy) may decrease the effect of the following drugs/drug classes by lowering their serum concentrations:

- **Anticoagulants, Oral (Warfarin)**
- **Beta-Blockers**
- **Chloramphenicol**
- **Clarithromycin**
- **Clonazepam**
- **Corticosteroids**
- **Cyclosporine**
- **Doxorubicin**
- **Doxycycline** (may persist for weeks after barbiturate discontinued)
- **Estrogens**
- **Griseofulvin**
- **Methadone**
- **Metronidazole**
- **Paroxetine**
- **Phenothiazines**
- **Progestins**
- **Quinidine**
- **Selegiline**
- **Theophylline**
- **Tricyclic Antidepressants**
- **Verapamil**

Laboratory Considerations

- Barbiturates may cause increased retention of **bromosulfophthalein** (BSP; sulfobromophthalein) and give falsely elevated results. It is recommended that barbiturates not be administered within the 24 hours before BSP retention tests.

Dosages

NOTES:

1. To avoid confusion, doses used for euthanasia are listed separately under the monograph for ***Euthanasia Agents***.
2. Due to the potential lethal nature of this drug, it is highly recommended to review ***Contraindications/Precautions/Warnings*** and ***Adverse Effects*** prior to administration.

DOGS/CATS:

Maintenance of chemical restraint in patients being mechanically ventilated (extra-label): 1 – 3 mg/kg/hour IV CRI. Switching to a shorter-acting agent such as propofol ≈12 hours prior to weaning from the ventilator will allow the pentobarbital concentrations to decrease and will help attenuate any seizure-like activity.[2]

Intractable seizures refractory to benzodiazepine boluses (extra-label): 3 – 15 mg/kg IV slowly to effect; may require several minutes for full therapeutic effect. Once seizures are controlled, consider 0.5 – 5 mg/kg/hour IV CRI. After seizures have been controlled for at least 6 hours, patient may be slowly weaned from the CRI while standard anticonvulsant therapy is initiated. NOTE: Patients may require intubation.

HORSES:

NOTE: Pentobarbital is generally not considered an ideal agent for use in adult horses due to possible development of excitement and injury when the animal is being induced for anesthesia.

Sedative/anesthetic (extra-label): Doses of 3 – 18 mg/kg IV have been noted.

SMALL MAMMALS/RODENTS:

Chemical restraint (extra-label):

a) **Mice**: 30 – 80 mg/kg IP
b) **Rats**: 40 – 60 mg/kg IP
c) **Hamsters/Gerbils**: 70 – 80 mg/kg IP
d) **Guinea pigs**:
  i) 15 – 40 mg/kg IP
  ii) 30 mg/kg IV
e) **Rabbits**: 20 – 60 mg/kg IV[3]

Monitoring

- Levels of consciousness and/or seizure control. EEG monitoring may be helpful in patients with intractable seizures.
- Protect and maintain airway patency.
- Heart and respiratory rate; $ETCO_2$, SpO_2
- Blood pressure
- Body temperature
- Hydration status; body weight

Client Information

- This medicine is used in an inpatient setting with close professional supervision.

Chemistry/Synonyms

Pentobarbital sodium occurs as a white, odorless, slightly bitter, crystalline powder or granules. It is very soluble in water and freely soluble in alcohol. The pK_a of the drug has been reported to range from 7.85 to 8.03 and the pH of the injection is from 9 to 10.5.

Alcohol or propylene glycol may be added to enhance the stability of the injectable product.

Pentobarbital may also be known as aethaminalum, mebubarbital, mebumal, pentobarbitalum, or pentobarbitone.

Storage/Stability

The injectable product should be stored at room temperature. The aqueous solution is not stable and should not be used if it contains a precipitate. Because precipitates may occur, pentobarbital sodium should not be added to acidic solutions.

Pentobarbital is a DEA Schedule II (C-II) controlled substance that should be stored in an area that is substantially constructed and securely locked. Follow applicable local, state, and federal rules regarding disposal of unused or wasted controlled drugs.

Compatibility/Compounding Considerations

Compatibility is dependent on factors such as pH, concentration, temperature, and diluent used; specialized references or a hospital pharmacist should be consulted for more specific information.

The following solutions and drugs have been reported to be physically **compatible** with pentobarbital sodium: dextrose IV solutions, Ringer's injection, lactated Ringer's injection, saline IV solutions, dextrose-saline combinations, dextrose-Ringer's combinations, dextrose-Ringer's lactate combinations, amikacin sulfate, aminophylline, atropine sulfate (for at least 15 minutes, not 24 hours), calcium chloride, cephapirin sodium, chloramphenicol sodium succinate, hyaluronidase, hydromorphone HCl, lidocaine HCl, neostigmine methylsulfate, scopolamine HBr, sodium bicarbonate, sodium iodide, thiopental sodium, and verapamil HCl.

The following drugs have been reported to be physically **incompatible** with pentobarbital sodium: butorphanol tartrate, chlorpromazine HCl, cimetidine HCl, chlorpheniramine maleate, codeine phosphate, diphenhydramine HCl, droperidol, fentanyl citrate, glycopyrrolate, hydrocortisone sodium succinate, hydroxyzine HCl, insulin (regular), meperidine HCl, nalbuphine HCl, norepinephrine bitartrate, oxytetracycline HCl, penicillin G potassium, pentazocine lactate, phenytoin sodium, prochlorperazine edisylate, promazine HCl, and promethazine HCl.

Dosage Forms/Regulatory Status

VETERINARY-LABELED PRODUCTS:

NOTE: The Association of Racing Commissioners International (ARCI) has designated this drug as a class 2 substance. Use of this drug may not be allowed in certain animal competitions. Check rules and regulations before entering in a competition while this medication is being administered. Contact local racing authorities for further guidance. See ***Appendix*** for more information.

Pentobarbital sodium injection: 64.8 mg/mL; *Somnopentyl®* Injection; (Rx, C-II). Approved for use in dogs, cats, and horses as a general anesthetic; although still listed in FDA's Green Book of approved animal drugs, it is no longer commercially available. NADA # 004-536.

HUMAN-LABELED PRODUCTS:

Pentobarbital Sodium Injection: 50 mg/mL in 2 mL *Tubex*; *Nembutal®*, generic; (Rx, C-II). Report prescribing and/or dispensing to state monitoring programs where required.

References

For the complete list of references, see **wiley.com/go/budde/plumb**

Pentosan Polysulfate (PPS)

Sodium Pentosan Polysulfate

(***pen***-toe-san) *Cartrophen-Vet®, Elmiron®*

Anti-inflammatory, Osteoarthritis Disease-Modifier

Prescriber Highlights

- ► Injectable pentosan polysulfate (PPS) may be beneficial in treating osteoarthritis in dogs, cats, and horses.
- ► Contraindications include hypersensitivity to PPS, advanced kidney or liver impairment, infection, active bleeding or bleeding disorders, impending surgical procedures, skeletal immaturity, and periparturient animals.
- ► Use with caution when combining with other drugs affecting coagulation.
- ► Adverse effects are uncommon but may include bleeding and GI effects (eg, vomiting, anorexia).

Uses/Indications

Pentosan polysulfate (PPS) may be beneficial for treating osteoarthritis in dogs, cats, and horses. No products are approved for use in animals in the United States; however, an injectable product is licensed in the UK (dogs), Canada (dogs), and Australia (dogs, horses).

Strong evidence of PPS efficacy for the treatment of osteoarthritis in dogs is lacking.[1,2]

It has been suggested that orally, intravesically, and parenterally administered PPS may benefit cats with lower urinary tract disease as an adjunctive treatment; however, studies have shown no significant difference between PPS treatment and placebo.[3,4]

In a small study, horses with experimentally induced osteoarthritis experienced significantly reduced articular cartilage fibrillation and an increase in chondroitin sulfate concentration in the joints of PPS treated horses. The study authors concluded that PPS may be considered a therapeutic option for treatment of osteoarthritis in horses.[5]

Pharmacology/Actions

Pentosan polysufate (PPS) has disease-modifying effects on osteoarthritic joints similar to polysulfated glycosoaminoglycans.[6,7] Proposed mechanisms of action include modulation of cytokine action, preservation of proteoglycan content, and stimulation of hyaluronic acid synthesis. PPS has anti-inflammatory, hypolipidemic, anticoagulant (considerably weaker than heparin—1/15th), and fibrinolytic properties. These effects may increase synovial blood flow and reduce joint inflammation. Proposed modes of action for PPS's efficacy include increasing proteoglycan synthesis, reducing matrix metalloproteinase activity, inducing synoviocyte biosynthesis of high molecular weight hyaluronan, and increasing subchondral blood flow via thrombolytic activity.

PPS has a mild analgesic effect when used for interstitial cystitis. The mechanism for its action in treating interstitial cystitis is not known. However, it is postulated that it may adhere to bladder wall mucosal membranes and act as a buffer to prevent irritating compounds in urine from reaching bladder cells.

Pharmacokinetics

In rats, 10% to 20% of the calcium derivative (pentosan polysulfate calcium) is absorbed after oral dosing. In humans, only ≈3% of an oral dose of pentosan polysulfate sodium is absorbed. It distributes primarily to the uroepithelium of the genitourinary tract. Smaller concentrations are found in the liver, spleen, lung skin, bone marrow, and periosteum. About 2/3 of the absorbed drug is desulfated in the liver and spleen within one hour; ≈3.5% of the absorbed drug is excreted into the urine.

In dogs, peak plasma concentrations were reached within 15 minutes following subcutaneous administration. The volume of distribution was 0.43 L, with higher concentrations in the liver, kidneys, and reticuloendothelial system. Low levels were found in the connective tissue and muscle. The elimination half-life was ≈3 hours.

Contraindications/Precautions/Warnings

Contraindications to the use of pentosan polysulfate include septic arthritis, advanced kidney or liver impairment, infection, active bleeding or bleeding disorders, malignancy (especially hemangiosarcoma), peri-operative or peri-parturient animals, skeletally immature animals, and in animals that are hypersensitive to it. Use this drug with caution when combining with other drugs that affect coagulation.

No more than 3 courses of 4 injections should be administered in 12 months.

Adverse Effects

Parenterally administered pentosan polysulfate (PPS) is usually well tolerated, and adverse effects in veterinary species appear mild and transitory. In dogs, vomiting, anorexia, lethargy, or mild depression are possible. Because PPS has some anticoagulant effects, bleeding is possible in any species, perhaps more likely in animals receiving other drugs that affect coagulation (eg, aspirin, anticoagulants) or during stressful exercise. PPS can cause dose-dependent increases in activated partial thromboplastin time (aPTT) up to 24 hours postdose.[8]

When used orally in cats, PPS seems to be well tolerated.

In a small percentage (less than 2%) of humans taking PPS, transient increases in liver enzymes have been reported. There is also some evidence that chronic use of PPS can cause ocular changes in humans[9]; this has not been documented in veterinary species.

Reproductive/Nursing Safety

Safe use of pentosan polysulfate (PPS) in animals intended for breeding or during pregnancy has not been demonstrated. PPS should not be used at the time of parturition due to its anticoagulant effects. Embryotoxic effects resulted when PPS was administered to rabbits at 2.5 times the recommended dose.[8]

Because safety has not been established in animals, this drug should only be used when the maternal benefits outweigh the potential risks to offspring.

Overdose/Acute Toxicity

Information regarding overdoses is not readily available. Potentially, overdoses could cause bleeding, thrombocytopenia, GI distress, and increased liver enzyme (ALT) elevations. At present, treatment recommendations are supportive. If an oral overdose occurs, consider GI decontamination. In healthy dogs receiving repeated daily doses 5 times or more than the recommended dose, increases in aPTT and thrombin time (TT) persisted for over 1 week.[8]

For patients that have experienced or are suspected of having experienced an overdose, consultation with a 24-hour poison consultation center specializing in providing veterinary-specific information is recommended. For general information on overdose and toxin exposures, as well as poison control centers' contact information, refer to ***Appendix***.

Drug Interactions

The following drug interactions have either been reported or are theoretical in humans or animals receiving pentosan polysulfate and may be of significance in veterinary patients. Unless otherwise noted, use together is not necessarily contraindicated, but weigh the potential risks and perform additional monitoring when appropriate.

- **Anticoagulants** (eg, **rivoroxaban, warfarin**): Concurrent use may increase the risk for bleeding.
- **Antiplatelet Agents** (eg, **aspirin, clopidogrel**): Concurrent use may increase the risk for bleeding.
- **Corticosteroids** (eg, **dexamethasone, prednis(ol)one, triamcinolone**): Glucocorticoids could mask the clinical signs associated with septic joints.
- **Heparin, Low Molecular Weight Heparins** (eg, **dalteparin, enoxaparin**): Concurrent use may increase the risk for bleeding.
- **NSAIDs** (eg, **carprofen, phenylbutazone**): NSAIDs could mask the clinical signs associated with septic joints and increase the risk for bleeding.

Laboratory Considerations

- No laboratory interactions or considerations were noted.

Dosages

DOGS:

Treatment of lameness and pain of degenerative joint disease/osteoarthritis (noninfectious arthrosis) in the skeletally mature dog (extra-label): 3 mg/kg SC on 4 occasions with an interval of 5 to 7 days between injections.[7,8] **NOTE**: Other products, with an interval of 5 to 7 days between injections, may be labeled in some markets for IM or SC use.

CATS:

Chondroprotective agent for osteoarthritis (extra-label): 3 mg/kg SC or IM once weekly for 4 weeks has been used anecdotally in cats.[10]

HORSES:

Aid in the treatment of noninfectious, inflammatory joint disease (extra-label): Intramuscular administration: 3 mg/kg IM on 4 occasions with an interval of 5 to 7 days between injections.[7] Intra-articular injection: 1 mL (250 mg) IA. It may be repeated at weekly intervals for 3 to 4 treatments.[11] More than one joint may be treated at one time. The horse should be rested for 2 weeks after the final injection, followed by a further 2 weeks of graded walking exercise before returning to work. (**NOTE**: See the label for specific directions on injection technique.)

Monitoring

- Clinical efficacy (eg, decrease in pain and inflammation in arthritic joints, improved mobility)

- Baseline and periodic packed cell volume (PCV), capillary refill time
- Signs of blood loss. When administered into joints, animals should be assessed for intra-articular bleeding.
- Consider coagulation testing before surgical procedures for patients that have recently received this medication.

Client Information

- If giving this medicine to your animal at home, be sure you understand how to give it.
- Monitor for side effects, including vomiting, decreased appetite, low energy level, and bleeding.
- Pentosan polysulfate is typically administered more than once. Follow the treatment recommendations of your veterinarian. Do not miss important follow up visits.

Chemistry/Synonyms

Pentosan polysulfate sodium, a heparin-like compound, is a mixture of linear polymers of beta-1->4-linked xylose, which is usually sulfated at the 2- and 3- positions. The average molecular weight is between 4000 and 6000. It is not derived from animal sources but Beechwood hemicellulose.

Pentosan may also be known as pentosan polysulphate sodium; PPS; PZ-68; sodium pentosan polysulphate; NaPPS; sodium xylanpolysulphate; SP-54, *Arthropen Vet® 250; Cartrophen-Vet®, AU-PEN5000®, Zydax®*, and *Elmiron®*.

Storage/Stability

Unless otherwise labeled, store oral pentosan products at controlled room temperature (15°C-30°C [59°F-86°F]) and injectable pentosan products under refrigeration (2°C-8°C [36°F-46°F]) and protected from light.

Compatibility/Compounding Considerations

No specific information was noted.

Dosage Forms/Regulatory Status

VETERINARY-LABELED PRODUCTS:

No products are currently FDA-approved in the United States.

Injectable pentosan polysulfate sodium 100 mg/mL (*Cartrophen-Vet®* Injection) labeled for use in dogs and pentosan polysulfate sodium 250 mg/mL products (eg, *Arthropen Vet® 250, Cartrophen-Vet Forte®* Injection) labeled for use in horses are available in several other countries. Be sure to check local regulations for withdrawal times when used in animals intended for human consumption.

HUMAN-LABELED PRODUCTS:

Pentosan Polysulfate Sodium Oral Capsules: 100 mg; *Elmiron®*; (Rx)

References

For the complete list of references, see **wiley.com/go/budde/plumb**

Pentoxifylline

(pen-tox-***ih***-fi-leen) *Trental®*

Hemorrheologic, Immunomodulatory Agent

Prescriber Highlights

- ► Increases erythrocyte flexibility, reduces blood viscosity, and reduces inflammation; used for the treatment of numerous immune-mediated, inflammatory, and ischemic conditions, and may be beneficial for other conditions in which improved microcirculation would be helpful
- ► Contraindications include retinal or cerebral hemorrhage and intolerance or hypersensitivity to pentoxifylline or other xanthines (eg, theophylline).
- ► Use with caution in patients that are at risk for hemorrhage and avoid or dose-reduce in patients with severe hepatic or renal impairment.
- ► Adverse effects are infrequent and when present, typically affect the GI tract (eg, vomiting, inappetence); adverse CNS or cardiovascular effects could also occur.

Uses/Indications

Pentoxifylline is used to treat immune-mediated dermatologic conditions, enhance tissue healing, reduce inflammation, and to improve microcirculation in ischemic conditions and vasculitis.

Reported indications in dogs include[1,2] exfoliative cutaneous lupus erythematosus, idiopathic sterile nodular and vaccine-associated panniculitis,[3] sterile nodular pyogranulomatous/granulomatous syndrome, erythema multiforme,[4] interdigital furunculosis, pemphigus foliaceus,[5] symmetrical lupoid onychodystrophy,[6] proliferative arteritis of the nasal philtrum,[7] antivenom-associated serum sickness,[8] cutaneous and renal vasculopathy of greyhounds,[9] and vasculitis.[10] It is also used for ischemic dermatopathies[11] including familial canine dermatomyositis,[12] ischemic reactions to vaccines,[13] ear tip ulcerative dermatitis/necrosis,[14] and thermal necrosis.[15] There is some evidence for efficacy for pentoxifylline in the treatment of IgE-mediated allergic reactions,[16] contact dermatitis,[17] and as an adjunctive treatment for canine atopic dermatitis.[18]

Limited experience exists for use of pentoxifylline in cats with reported indications including inflammatory dermatologic conditions[19] and cutaneous vasculitis[20] similar to dogs. Pentoxifylline has been used in cats to decrease vasculitis associated with FIP but has failed to demonstrate benefit.[21]

In horses, pentoxifylline has been used as adjunctive therapy for cutaneous vasculitis, placentitis,[22] and atopic dermatitis, and has demonstrated benefit in experimental models of endotoxemia.[23,24] Additionally, the results of one study suggested a potential use for pentoxifylline in treating horses with recurrent airway obstruction, as it effectively reduced reactive oxygen and nitrogen species in pulmonary tissues of affected horses.[25]

Pharmacology/Actions

The mechanisms for pentoxifylline's actions to improve microcirculatory blood flow are not fully understood. The drug increases flexibility of newly formed erythrocytes probably by inhibiting erythrocyte phosphodiesterase and altering erythrocyte electrolyte concentrations. It decreases blood viscosity possibly by stimulating prostacyclin synthesis and release, reducing plasma fibrinogen, decreasing collagen synthesis, and increasing fibrinolytic activity. Pentoxifylline increases leukocyte deformability (flexibility), inhibits neutrophil adhesion and activation and inhibits tumor necrosis factor alpha (TNF-alpha),[26] a cytokine implicated in the pathogenesis of many microvascular disease states. Pentoxifylline is postulated to reduce negative endotoxic effects of cytokine mediators via its phosphodiesterase inhibition.

In healthy dogs, pentoxifylline was also shown to inhibit mast cell degranulation and to significantly decrease the total numbers of cutaneous inflammatory cells, especially eosinophils, impairing late phase reactions but not immediate reactions at site of intradermal injection of IgE-specific antibodies.[27] Several weeks of treatment may be required before beneficial effects are realized.

In horses, pentoxifylline appears to be a potent inhibitor of matrix metalloproteinase-9 and a modest inhibitor of matrix metalloproteinase-2.[28]

Pharmacokinetics

In dogs, pentoxifylline reportedly has a bioavailability of ≈50% with peak concentrations occurring ≈1 to 3 hours after dosing.[29] Serum half-life is ≈6 to 7 hours for the parent compound, 36 hours for active metabolite 1, and 8 hours for active metabolite 2.

In horses, after PO administration of crushed, sustained-release tablets, pentoxifylline is rapidly absorbed with a wide interpatient variation of bioavailability that averages around 68%. Bioavailability may decrease with continued administration over several days. The authors concluded that 10 mg/kg every 12 hours PO yields serum concentrations equivalent to those observed after administration of therapeutic doses to humans and horses.[30]

In humans, pentoxifylline absorption from the GI tract is rapid and almost complete but a significant first-pass effect occurs. Food affects the rate, but not the extent, of absorption. Pentoxifylline is metabolized both in the liver and erythrocytes; all identified metabolites appear to be active. Elimination half-life of drug and metabolites is ≈1 to 2 hours. Metabolites are eliminated in the urine.

Contraindications/Precautions/Warnings

Pentoxifylline should be considered contraindicated in patients that have been intolerant to the drug or xanthines (eg, theophylline, caffeine, theobromine) in the past and those with cerebral hemorrhage or retinal hemorrhage.[31] It should be used cautiously in patients with hepatic or renal impairment.[31]

Adverse Effects

Pentoxifylline is generally well-tolerated in dogs. Most commonly reported adverse effects involve the GI tract (eg, vomiting, inappetence, loose stools) or CNS (eg, excitement, nervousness) in dogs[29,32] and cats.

In horses, IV administration may be associated with transient leukocytosis, muscle fasciculations, sweating on shoulders and flanks, and mild increases in heart rate.[30] Oral dosing at 10 mg/kg or less appears to be well tolerated.

There are reports of dizziness and headache occurring in a small percentage of humans receiving the drug. Other adverse effects, primarily GI, CNS, and cardiovascular related, have been reported in humans but are considered to occur rarely; dosage reduction is recommended in such cases, and the drug should be discontinued if the adverse effects persist.[31] Veterinary experience is limited with pentoxifylline, and animal adverse effects may differ.

Reproductive/Nursing Safety

Pentoxifylline may be teratogenic at high doses. In dogs, high concentration of pentoxifylline was shown to induce capacitation and acrosome reaction and improve quality of motility in ejaculated spermatozoa.[33] Pentoxifylline showed no deleterious effect on sperm motility, viability, and capacitation of cryopreserved stallion epididymal sperm.

Studies in rats and rabbits revealed no evidence of fetal malformation but increased resorption was noted in rats receiving 25 times the maximum labeled dose.

In humans, pentoxifylline and its metabolites are excreted in maternal milk. Because of the potential for tumorigenicity (seen in rats), use cautiously in nursing patients.

Because safety has not been established in animals, this drug should only be used when the maternal benefits outweigh the potential risks to offspring.

Overdose/Acute Toxicity

Humans overdosed with pentoxifylline have demonstrated signs of flushing, seizures, hypotension, unconsciousness, agitation, fever, somnolence, GI distress, and ECG changes. One human patient who ingested 80 mg/kg recovered completely. Symptoms appear dose-related, and typically persist for ≈12 hours. Overdoses should be treated using appropriate GI decontamination and supportive therapies.

For patients that have experienced or are suspected to have experienced an overdose, consultation with a 24-hour poison consultation center specializing in providing veterinary-specific information is recommended. For general information related to overdose and toxin exposures, as well as contact information for poison control centers, refer to ***Appendix***.

Drug Interactions

The following drug interactions have either been reported or are theoretical in humans or animals receiving pentoxifylline and may be of significance in veterinary patients. Unless otherwise noted, use together is not necessarily contraindicated, but weigh the potential risks and perform additional monitoring when appropriate.

- **Anticoagulants** (eg, **rivaroxaban**, **warfarin**): When pentoxifylline is used with anticoagulants, increased risk for bleeding may result; use together with enhanced monitoring and caution.
- **Antihypertensive Drugs** (eg, **amlodipine, enalapril, telmisartan**): Pentoxifylline may increase hypotensive effect.
- **Cimetidine**: May increase pentoxifylline concentration
- **Fluoroquinolones** (eg, **ciprofloxacin**): May increase pentoxifylline concentration
- **Insulin**: May increase risk of hypoglycemia
- **Macrolides** (eg, **clarithromycin, erythromycin** [not azithromycin]): May increase pentoxifylline concentration
- **Nonsteroidal Anti-Inflammatory Drugs (NSAIDs**; eg, **carprofen, meloxicam, phenylbutazone**): Concurrent use may increase risk for bleeding. In horses, use of NSAIDs with pentoxifylline is controversial. Some sources state that when used for endotoxemia in horses, pentoxifylline's beneficial effects are negated by NSAIDs, but one study showed superior efficacy when flunixin and pentoxifylline were used together, compared with either used alone.
- **Platelet-Aggregation Inhibitors** (eg, **aspirin, clopidogrel**): Increased risk for bleeding
- **Theophylline**: Theophylline serum concentration may be increased when used concurrently with pentoxifylline.

Laboratory Considerations

- Pentoxifylline could potentially alter **intradermal allergen testing** results. It is advised to discontinue treatment at least one week prior to testing.

Dosages

NOTE: The commercially available pentoxifylline product is a 400 mg extended-release tablet. Cutting or crushing the tablets may negate the extended-release characteristics and alter pharmacokinetics but splitting tablets may be necessary to administer or accurately dose. Avoid crushing tablets for small animal use.

DOGS:

Inflammatory/autoimmune dermatologic conditions (extra-label): 10 – 30 mg/kg PO every 8 to 12 hours. Typically, 15 – 20 mg/kg PO every 8 to 12 hours[34]

Symmetric lupoid onychitis (extra-label): 15 - 25 mg/kg PO every 12 hours[35]

Ischemic dermatopathies (extra-label): 15 mg/kg PO every 8 hours to 30 mg/kg PO every 12 hours.[11] One open label study used 25 mg/kg PO every 12 hours.[36]

Vasculitis (extra-label): 10 – 15 mg/kg PO every 12 hours[37]

CATS:

Inflammatory dermatologic conditions (extra-label): 100 mg/cat (NOT mg/kg) PO every 12 hours[19]

Cutaneous vasculitis (extra-label): 10 – 15 mg/kg PO every 12 hours[37]

HORSES:

Cutaneous vasculitis (extra-label): From a pharmacokinetic study, 10 mg/kg PO every 12 hours yields serum concentrations equivalent to those observed after administration of therapeutic doses to humans and horses. Sustained-release tablets may be crushed and mixed with molasses. If efficacy wanes with time, consider increasing the dosage to 15 mg/kg PO twice daily or 10 mg/kg PO 3 times a day. In the experience of the authors, 10 mg/kg PO twice daily for 30 days results in clinical response in horses with cutaneous vasculitis.[38]

Inflammatory/autoimmune dermatologic conditions (extra-label): 8 – 10 mg/kg PO every 8 to 12 hours[39]

Placentitis (extra-label): From a study in pony mares with experimentally induced equine placentitis. Treated group was given trimethoprim/sulfamethoxazole 30 mg/kg PO every 12 hours, pentoxifylline 8.5 mg/kg PO every 12 hours, and altrenogest 0.088 mg/kg PO every 24 hours from the onset of clinical signs to delivery of a live foal or abortion. 83% of treated mares delivered viable foals.[40]

Monitoring

- Efficacy
- Adverse effects (eg, hyporexia, vomiting, diarrhea, hyperexcitability)
- Consider more intensive monitoring for evidence of hemorrhage (eg, PCV) in patients with increased risk of bleeding, such as recent surgery or GI ulceration.

Client Information

- Give this medicine with food.
- Side effects are not common in dogs but may include loss of appetite, vomiting, and nervousness or excitement. This medicine is usually well tolerated in horses.
- This medicine may cause an increased risk for bleeding, particularly in animals that may be predisposed to this problem.
- This medicine can take 1 to 2 weeks (or longer) to see its full effect.
- Extended-release tablets can be split if necessary to give the appropriate dose. Crushing the tablets may increase the risk for side effects and should be avoided when possible.

Chemistry/Synonyms

A synthetic xanthine derivative structurally related to caffeine and theophylline, pentoxifylline occurs as a white, odorless, bitter-tasting, crystalline powder that is soluble in water and sparingly soluble in alcohol.

Pentoxifylline may also be known as BL-191, oxpentifylline, pentoxifyllinum, *Pentoxil*®, PTX, and *Trental*®.

Storage/Stability

The commercially available tablets should be stored in well-closed containers, protected from light at 20°C to 25°C (68°F -77°F).

Compatibility/Compounding Considerations

The commercially available product in the United States is a 400 mg extended-release tablet (labeled for human use). Cutting or crushing tablets may negate the sustained-release characteristics and alter pharmacokinetics[41]; however, splitting tablets may be necessary to administer or accurately dose. Avoid use of crushed tablets in dogs or cats as adverse effects (hyperexcitability, diarrhea) may occur; crushing tablets may be required for horses.

Dosage Forms/Regulatory Status

VETERINARY-LABELED PRODUCTS: NONE

The Association of Racing Commissioners International (ARCI) has designated this drug as a class 4 substance. Use of this drug may not be allowed in certain animal competitions. Check rules and regulations before entering in a competition while this medication is being administered. Contact local racing authorities for further guidance. See ***Appendix*** for more information.

HUMAN-LABELED PRODUCTS:

Pentoxifylline Controlled-/Extended-Release Tablets: 400 mg; generic; (Rx). See ***Compatibility/Compounding Considerations***.

References

For the complete list of references, see **wiley.com/go/budde/plumb**

Pergolide

(***per***-go-lide) *Prascend*®

Dopamine Agonist

Prescriber Highlights

- ► Used in horses to control clinical signs associated with pituitary pars intermedia dysfunction (PPID)
- ► Contraindications include in patients that are hypersensitive to ergot derivatives.
- ► Well tolerated in horses; anorexia may occur

Uses/Indications

Pergolide is FDA-approved for use in horses for the control of clinical signs associated with pituitary pars intermedia dysfunction (PPID).

Pharmacology/Actions

Pergolide is a potent agonist at dopamine (D_1 and D_2) receptors and is 10 to 1000 times more potent than bromocriptine.[1] It is thought that pituitary pars intermedia dysfunction (PPID) in horses is a degenerative disease associated with loss of dopaminergic control of the melanotropes of the pars intermedia, with a subsequent overproduction of proopiomelanocortin (POMC) and POMC-derived peptides. These POMC-derived peptides are implicated in causing the signs associated with PPID. In horses with PPID, pergolide is believed to exert its therapeutic effect by stimulating dopamine receptors and has been shown to decrease the plasma levels of adrenocorticotropic hormone (ACTH), alpha-melanocyte-stimulating hormone (MSH), and other POMC-derived peptides. Additionally, pergolide inhibits the release of prolactin, which suggests that it may interfere with lactation.

Pharmacokinetics

Pharmacokinetic studies of pergolide in horses are limited and provide varying information. In horses, pergolide is reportedly 90% plasma protein-bound.[2] Pharmacokinetic information in horses is based on a study using single oral doses of 10 µg/kg in 6 healthy mares between 3 and 17 years of age. Pergolide was rapidly absorbed with an average maximum concentration (C_{max}) of ≈4 ng/mL and a median time to maximum concentration (T_{max}) of ≈0.4 hours. The area under the curve (AUC) was ≈14 hours ng/mL. The mean half-life was ≈5.9 hours; mean apparent oral clearance (CL/F) was 1204 mL/kg/hour; and mean apparent volume of distribution (V/F) was ≈3082 mL/kg. Below are summaries of each study.

In horses (6 in the study), pergolide was rapidly absorbed following oral administration (0.01 mg/kg), with plasma concentrations reaching maximum concentrations within 1 hour of dosing.[3] Maximum plasma concentrations ranged from 1.07 to 3.38 ng/mL. Pergolide appears to be rapidly and widely distributed. Elimination half-life averaged 27 hours, but there was high interpatient variation.

In a study evaluating 6 aged (18 to 28 years old) horses with PPID, 2 mg (≈0.004 mg/kg) of pergolide was dissolved in water and immediately given in the feed each day over a period of 6 months.[4] Pharmacokinetic parameters were measured after the last dose. Maximum plasma concentrations were reached on average within 1 hour of dosing at concentrations ranging from 0 to 1.38 ng/mL. The average elimination half-life was determined to be 19.7 hours.

In a study evaluating 8 healthy, young horses, pergolide 0.02 mg/kg IV was given.[5] The mean C_{max} was found to be 15.62 ng/mL, with a mean terminal elimination half-life of 5.64 hours.

In humans, the drug is orally absorbed (estimated 60% bioavailable) and 90% bound to plasma proteins. At least 10 different metabolites have been identified, some of which are active. The principal route of elimination is via the kidneys.

Contraindications/Precautions

Pergolide is contraindicated in patients that are hypersensitive to it or other ergot derivatives. Treatment with pergolide may cause inappetence.[2]

In humans, caution is recommended in patients that are prone to cardiac arrhythmias.[1]

Pergolide should not be handled by anyone who has experienced adverse reactions to ergotamine or ergot derivatives (eg, bromocriptine). Pergolide has been reported to cause eye irritation, an irritating smell, or headache when tablets are split or crushed[2]; therefore, tablets should not be crushed, and care should be taken to minimize exposure when tablets are split. Wear gloves when handling this product if pregnant or nursing.[2]

Adverse Effects

Pergolide appears to be well tolerated in horses. Decreased appetite is seen during the first week of therapy[2]; temporary dose reduction is often beneficial in alleviating this effect. Lethargy, colic, diarrhea, and weight loss have been reported to occur more rarely.

In post-approval reports, additional adverse effects included dermatologic effects such as alopecia, hyperhidrosis, and dermatitis; musculoskeletal effects such as laminitis and muscle stiffness/soreness; and neurologic effects such as ataxia, seizures, and muscle tremors.[2] Behavioral aggression was also reported.

In humans, common adverse effects reported include CNS effects (eg, dyskinesia, hallucinations, somnolence, insomnia), GI effects (eg, nausea, vomiting, diarrhea, constipation), transient hypotension, and rhinitis.[1]

Reproductive/Nursing Safety

In pregnant mice and rabbits given pergolide, no evidence of fetal harm was seen[1]; however, the safety of pergolide in pregnant horses has not been established.[2] It is not known if pergolide enters maternal milk; however, like other ergot-derivative dopamine agonists, it may interfere with lactation.

Because safety has not been established in animals, this drug should only be used when the maternal benefits outweigh the potential risks to offspring.

Overdose/Acute Toxicity

There is limited information available on pergolide overdoses. Potential effects include GI disturbances, CNS effects, seizures, and hypotension. One pony that was given a single 110-fold overdose of pergolide demonstrated transient tachycardia, a decreased appetite, and anxiety.[6]

Clinical signs associated with a pergolide overdose in dogs include vomiting, lethargy, and trembling. In cats, hyperthermia, mydriasis, and elevation of the third eyelids may be seen.

Treatment is supportive based on clinical presentation. Activated charcoal may help prevent absorption; phenothiazines may decrease CNS stimulation effects.

For patients that have experienced or are suspected to have experienced an overdose, consultation with a 24-hour poison consultation center specializing in providing veterinary-specific information is recommended. For general information related to overdose and toxin exposures, as well as contact information for poison control centers, refer to ***Appendix.***

Drug Interactions

The following drug interactions have either been reported or are theoretical in humans or animals receiving pergolide and may be of significance in veterinary patients. Unless otherwise noted, use together is not necessarily contraindicated, but weigh the potential risks and perform additional monitoring when appropriate.

- **Dopamine Antagonists** (eg, **phenothiazines**): May decrease the effects of pergolide
- **Metoclopramide**: May decrease the effects of pergolide

Laboratory Considerations

- None noted

Dosages

HORSES:

Control of clinical signs associated with pituitary pars intermedia dysfunction (PPID; label dosage; FDA approved): Starting dosage of 2 µg/kg PO once daily, then adjust to effect.[2] Dose titration is based on individual response to therapy, including improvement in clinical signs associated with PPID and/or improvement or normalization of endocrine tests. Titrate to achieve the lowest effective dose. Tablets are scored and dose should be rounded to the nearest half-tablet increment, not to exceed 4 µg/kg daily. If signs of dose intolerance develop, decrease the dose by 50% for 3 to 5 days, then titrate back up in 2 µg/kg increments every 2 weeks until the desired effect is achieved.[2] **NOTE**: Although early studies noted maximum daily doses of 10 µg/kg, the currently recommended daily maximum dose is 4 µg/kg. Doses higher than 4 µg/kg should be only used in extenuating circumstances where no effect is achieved with doses between 2 and 4 µg/kg.[5]

Monitoring

- Baseline and periodic endogenous adrenocorticotropic hormone (ACTH). Periodic testing should begin 1 to 3 months after starting treatment or changing the dose. Once clinical signs are controlled, testing can be done every 6 to 12 months.[7] **NOTE**: The results of this testing should take seasonal variation into account. A TRH stimulation test may be necessary for those horses with equivocal ACTH levels.
- Clinical signs (improvements in quality of hair coat, body weight, PU/PD)

Client Information

- Pergolide does not cure your horse's condition. This medicine is intended to help control the signs associated with it. This medicine may take several weeks to months to see positive effects.
- It is important to not crush tablets to avoid exposure to the medicine.
- People who have had adverse reactions to ergotamine or other ergot derivatives should not administer pergolide.
- Pregnant or nursing women should wear gloves when handling this medicine.
- Keep pergolide tablets in a secure location out of reach of children and animals to prevent accidental ingestion or overdose. Animals

may get sick if they eat horse feed mixed with this medicine.

- Decreased appetite is the most common side effect seen with this medicine.
- Watch for unpredictable behavior and colic while your horse is taking this medicine. Contact your veterinarian if you have any concerns.
- Your veterinarian will need to monitor your horse while it is taking this medicine. Do not miss these important follow-up visits.

Chemistry/Synonyms

Pergolide is an ergot derivative that occurs as white to off-white powder and is slightly soluble in water, dehydrated alcohol, or chloroform. It is very slightly soluble in acetone, practically insoluble in ether, and sparingly soluble in methyl alcohol.

Pergolide mesylate may also be known as LY-127809, pergolide mesilate, pergolidi mesilas, *Prascend®*, *Celance®*, *Nopar®*, *Parkotil®*, *Parlide®*, or *Pharken®*.

Storage/Stability

Store pergolide tablets in tight containers at room temperature (25°C [77°F]); excursions permitted to 15°C to 30°C (59°F-86°F).

Compatibility/Compounding Considerations

FDA-approved products should be the first choice when prescribing pergolide for pituitary pars intermedia dysfunction (PPID). Compounded products are available; however, because of concerns regarding stability, the use of this product is questionable when the approved product is accessible.

A 1 mg/mL oral suspension of pergolide mesylate was prepared using bulk powder obtained from a commercial supplier. 20 mg of pergolide mesylate was added to the plunger of a 35 mL Luer-lock syringe containing 10 mL of *Ora-Plus®* suspending liquid. The 35 mL syringe was connected to an empty 35 mL Luer-lock syringe using a fluid-dispensing connector. Using the plunger of the original 35 mL syringe, the suspension was mixed by depressing the plungers back and forth for a total of 50 depressions (or until uniformly mixed). 10 mL of *OraSweet®* was added to the suspension and mixed in a similar manner for a final suspension volume of 20 mL. The suspension was found to be stable for 30 days when protected from light and stored under refrigeration (2°C-8°C [36°F-46°F]). Formulations that have undergone a color change should be considered unstable and discarded. **NOTE**: The use of a mortar and pestle to prepare this suspension is not recommended, as it has resulted in a loss of suspending vehicle that caused a 20% increase in final concentration. Proper precautions to prevent eye and skin irritation from exposure to free powder should be taken.[8]

Dosage Forms/Regulatory Status

VETERINARY-LABELED PRODUCTS:

Pergolide Mesylate Tablets: 1 mg; *Prascend®*; (Rx) FDA-approved for use in horses. NADA# 141-331. Do not use this product in horses intended for human consumption.

HUMAN-LABELED PRODUCTS: NONE

Because of an increased potential for heart valve damage associated with pergolide use in humans, all dosage forms were withdrawn from the United States market in the spring of 2007.

References

For the complete list of references, see **wiley.com/go/budde/plumb**

Phenobarbital

Phenobarbitone

(fee-noe-***bar***-bi-tal)

Barbiturate

Prescriber Highlights

- ► Used primarily as an antiseizure medication
- ► Contraindicated in patients with known hypersensitivity, severe liver disease, severe respiratory distress, or nephritis (with large doses). Phenobarbital should be used with caution in patients with hypovolemia, anemia, borderline hypoadrenal function, or severe cardiac or respiratory disease.
- ► Cats are more sensitive to respiratory depression when receiving phenobarbital at high doses.
- ► Adverse effects in dogs include anxiety/agitation or lethargy (when treatment is initiated); profound depression is possible even at low doses. Sedation, ataxia, polyuria/polydipsia, and polyphagia can be seen at moderate to high serum phenobarbital concentrations. An increase in liver enzymes (ALP more so than ALT) is common; however, overt hepatotoxicity is not. Anemia, thrombocytopenia, and neutropenia are rarely seen.
- ► Adverse effects in cats include ataxia, lethargy, facial pruritus, polyphagia with weight gain, and polyuria/polydipsia. Immunemediated reactions and bone marrow hypoplasia are rare. Hepatotoxicity has not been reported in cats.
- ► Should be given slowly when administered IV; should not be administered SC or perivascularly, as it can cause severe irritation
- ► Drug and drug–laboratory test interactions are possible.
- ► When therapy is discontinued, phenobarbital doses should be tapered over several weeks (see ***Dosages***).
- ► DEA Schedule IV (C-IV) controlled substance

Uses/Indications

Based on its efficacy, relative safety, and reasonable dose frequency (every 12 hours), phenobarbital is considered a first-line treatment for epilepsy in dogs and cats.[1,2] Phenobarbital has a slower onset of action than benzodiazepines, which should be used first to manage status epilepticus. Phenobarbital is generally used for long-term control to prevent seizure recurrence in dogs, cats, and horses. In a study, more dogs receiving phenobarbital were seizure-free as compared with those receiving potassium bromide (85% vs 52%); phenobarbital reduced seizure duration more than potassium bromide.[3]

Phenobarbital may also be useful in controlling excessive drooling (ie, sialadenosis) in horses[4] and dogs.[5-9] Phenobarbital improves clinical signs in dogs with orthostatic tremor; however, most responses were partial rather than complete.[10]

In cattle, it has been suggested that the microsomal–enzyme-stimulating properties of phenobarbital increase the detoxification process of organochlorine (ie, chlorinated hydrocarbon) insecticide poisoning.

Phenobarbital has also been used in the treatment and prevention of neonatal hyperbilirubinemia in human infants. It is unknown if phenobarbital effectively treats hyperbilirubinemia in veterinary patients.

Pharmacology/Actions

Although barbiturates are nonselective CNS depressants, they can invoke all levels of CNS mood alteration, from paradoxical excitement to deep coma and death. The exact mechanisms of the CNS effects caused by barbiturates are unknown. Barbiturates have been shown to inhibit the release of acetylcholine, norepinephrine, and glutamate; they also have effects on gamma-aminobutyric acid

(GABA). At high anesthetic doses, barbiturates have been demonstrated to inhibit the uptake of calcium at nerve endings. The seizure threshold is raised, and the spread of seizures is limited. In humans, selective anticonvulsant activity of phenobarbital is independent of the degree of sedation produced.

The degree of CNS depression produced is dependent on the dose, route of administration, the pharmacokinetics of the drug, and species treated. In addition, patient age, physical condition, and/or concurrent use of other drugs can alter drug effects. Barbiturates may depress the sensory cortex, lessen motor activity, and produce sedation at low doses. In humans, barbiturates have been shown to reduce the rapid eye movement (REM) stage of sleep. Barbiturates have no true intrinsic analgesic activity.

In most species, barbiturates can cause dose-dependent respiratory depression and, in some species, can cause slight respiratory stimulation. At sedative/hypnotic doses, respiratory depression is similar to that during normal physiologic sleep. As doses increase, the medullary respiratory center is progressively depressed, with resultant decreases in rate, depth, and volume. Respiratory arrest can occur at doses 4 times lower than those that can cause cardiac arrest. Barbiturates must be used very cautiously in cats, as cats are particularly sensitive to their respiratory depressant effects.

Barbiturates can cause reduced tone and motility of the intestinal, uterine, ureteral, and bladder musculature, likely secondary to their central depressant action. Barbiturates can reduce the sensitivity of the motor endplate to acetylcholine, thereby slightly relaxing the skeletal muscle.

Liver function is not directly affected when barbiturates are used short-term, but hepatic microsomal enzyme induction is well documented with extended barbiturate administration,[11-14] particularly with phenobarbital, and may persist for up to 4 weeks after discontinuation.[11] Although barbiturates reduce oxygen consumption in all tissue, no change in metabolic rate is measurable when barbiturates are administered at sedative doses; however, basal metabolic rates may be reduced with resultant decreases in body temperature when barbiturates are administered at anesthetic doses.

Pharmacokinetics

Phenobarbital is slowly absorbed from the GI tract. Bioavailability ranges from 70% to 90% in humans and ≈90% in dogs.[15,16] Absorption is practically complete in cats[17] and adult horses.[18] Peak concentrations occur 4 to 8 hours after oral administration in dogs[19] and 8 to 12 hours in humans. One study in cats showed that phenobarbital compounded in PLO gel and applied transdermally to the pinna twice daily achieved steady-state serum concentrations within the therapeutic range in some cats; more individual variation was seen when *Lipoderm ActiveMax*® was used instead of PLO.[20]

Phenobarbital is widely distributed throughout the body, but because of its lower lipid solubility, it does not distribute as rapidly into the CNS as compared with most other barbiturates. In humans, peak drug concentration in the CNS may be delayed up to 15 minutes after IV administration. In humans, the amount of phenobarbital bound to plasma proteins has been reported to be 40% to 60%. The reported apparent volumes of distribution are ≈0.8 to 1 L/kg in horses,[21,22] ≈0.86 L/kg in foals, ≈0.7 L/kg in cats,[23] and ≈0.75 L/kg in dogs.[24]

The drug is metabolized in the liver primarily by hydroxylated oxidation to p-hydroxyphenobarbital; sulfate and glucuronide conjugates are also formed. In humans, elimination half-life ranges from 2 to 6 days compared to 12 to 125 hours (average of ≈2 days) in dogs.[16,19,24] Elimination half-life in dogs fed protein- or fat-restricted diets appears to be shorter (26 and 24 hours, respectively).[25] Because of phenobarbital's ability to induce the hepatic enzymes used to metabolize itself and other drugs, elimination half-life may decrease with time, along with concomitant reductions in serum concentrations. The half-life of phenobarbital may be less than 24 hours in some dogs that may require 3 times daily administration for maximal control.[26] An elimination half-life of 34 to 43 hours has been reported in cats.[23] Elimination half-life in horses is considerably shorter, with reported values of ≈13 hours in foals and 10 to 12 hours in adult horses with chronic administration.[21,22] Approximately 25% of a dose is excreted unchanged by the kidney; alkalinizing urine and/or substantially increasing urine flow increases phenobarbital excretion rates. The remaining 75% of a dose is renally excreted as metabolites. Anuric or oliguric patients may accumulate the unmetabolized drug; dose adjustments may be required.

In dogs, changes in diet, body weight, and body composition may alter the pharmacokinetics of phenobarbital and necessitate dosage adjustment.

In goats given phenobarbital 10 mg/kg IV and PO, bioavailability was ≈25%, and half-life was ≈4 hours for both routes.[27]

Contraindications/Precautions/Warnings

Barbiturates are contraindicated in patients that have severe liver disease, severe respiratory distress, or those that have demonstrated previous hypersensitivity reactions to these drugs.[28] Large doses are contraindicated in patients with nephritis.[29] Barbiturates should be used cautiously in patients with hypovolemia, anemia, borderline hypoadrenal function, and/or cardiac or respiratory disease. Dose reductions may be necessary in patients with significant renal impairment.

The drug should be given slowly (not more than 1 – 2 mg/kg per minute) when administered IV; IV administration that is too rapid can cause respiratory depression. Commercially available injectable preparations are very alkaline and must not be administered SC, intraarterially, or perivascularly, as significant pain, tissue irritation, and possible necrosis can result.[29] Extreme care should be taken to avoid extravasation. Applications of moist heat and local infiltration of 0.5% procaine solution have been recommended to treat extravasation reactions.

In humans, IM injection is limited to a total volume of 5 mL and injected into a large muscle to avoid tissue irritation.[29]

PHENobarbital should not be confused with PENTobarbital.

Adverse Effects

Dogs may exhibit increased clinical signs of anxiety/agitation or lethargy when therapy is initiated. These effects are generally transitory in nature. Occasionally, dogs will exhibit profound depression at lower doses (and plasma concentrations). Decreased physical activity levels have been observed in dogs receiving phenobarbital-containing antiepileptic drug combinations.[30]

Polydipsia, polyuria, and polyphagia are also commonly observed; these signs usually begin 2 to 3 weeks after initiating phenobarbital therapy. Sedation and/or ataxia often become significant concerns as serum phenobarbital concentrations reach the higher ends of the therapeutic range. Anemia, thrombocytopenia, and/or neutropenia occur rarely and are reversible if detected early.[31-33] Increased triglycerides[34] and pancreatic lipase activity[35,36] have been reported in dogs.

Increases in liver enzymes with phenobarbital in dogs are well described[37-39] and are not necessarily indicative of liver dysfunction but should raise concern if serum ALT or ALP is more than 4 to 5 times the upper limit of normal or if any elevation in gamma-glutamyltransferase (GGT) is noted. Of note, in a study, serum ALP was higher in dogs receiving phenobarbital and fed protein- or fat-restricted diets as compared with dogs receiving a maintenance diet.[25] Phenobarbital should generally be discontinued if any increases in serum bilirubin, total serum bile acids, or hypoalbuminemia are detected. If phenobarbital needs to be discontinued yet antiepileptic medication is required, alternative antiepileptic therapy (eg, potassium bromide, levetiracetam) should be started immediately. Frank hepatic failure is uncommon and is usually associated with higher serum phenobarbital levels (greater than 30 to 40 µg/mL).[39] In a study, hematologic abnormalities occurred within the first 3 months of therapy in 4.2% of dogs treated with standard doses.[40]

In dogs, phenobarbital rarely causes superficial necrolytic dermatitis (SND) associated with changes in hepatocytes (ie, severe parenchymal collapse with glycogen-laden hepatocytes and moderate fibrosis sharply demarcated by nodules of normal hepatic parenchyma)[41] distinct from that seen with phenobarbital hepatotoxicity (ie, chronic hepatic fibrosis with nodular regeneration [cirrhosis]).[39] A presumed case of Stevens-Johnson syndrome in a dog has also been reported.[42]

Phenobarbital may increase the metabolism of cortisol and has been implicated in contributing to relative adrenal insufficiency,[43] including a case of Addisonian crisis in an Irish setter.[44] Pseudolymphoma has been documented or suspected in at least 1 dog[45] and 2 cats.[46,47]

Cats may develop ataxia, persistent sedation and/or lethargy, facial pruritus, polyphagia/weight gain, and/or polydipsia/polyuria. Rarely, immune-mediated reactions and bone marrow hypoplasia (eg, thrombocytopenia, neutropenia) may be seen.[48] A presumed case of phenobarbital-induced fever has been reported in a cat.[49] Phenobarbital-induced anticonvulsant hypersensitivity syndrome has also been reported. In 1 cat, tachypnea, hyperthermia, high serum amyloid A, and abdominal lymph node enlargement were seen 8 days after initiation of phenobarbital.[50] Another cat presented immune-mediated anemia 2 weeks after starting phenobarbital.[51]

Cats, unlike dogs, do not develop increased liver enzymes; increases in liver enzymes in cats on phenobarbital should prompt further investigation. High doses (ie, 10 – 40 mg/kg/day) have caused coagulopathies in cats.[52,53]

Although there is much less information regarding phenobarbital use in horses (and foals in particular), cattle, goats, and ferrets, it would generally be expected for adverse effects to mirror those seen in other species.

In humans, phenobarbital can cause rare, possibly fatal, hypersensitivity reactions, including exfoliative dermatitis and Stevens-Johnson syndrome.[28] It is recommended to discontinue use whenever dermatologic reactions occur.

Reproductive/Nursing Safety

Barbiturates readily cross the placenta.[28,29] Phenobarbital has been associated with rare congenital defects and bleeding problems in newborns but may be safer than other anticonvulsants. Clinical signs related to withdrawal can occur in offspring born to dams receiving phenobarbital.

Caution should be used when administering to a nursing dam, as small amounts are excreted in maternal milk. Drowsiness in nursing offspring has been reported. A foal born to a mare receiving phenobarbital reportedly had a serum phenobarbital concentration of 12.2 µg/mL, and the concentration in the mare's milk was 7.5 µg/mL.[54]

Because safety has not been established in animals, this drug should only be used when the maternal benefits outweigh the potential risks to offspring.

Overdose/Acute Toxicity

Clinical signs caused by overdoses of phenobarbital are an extension of its adverse effect profile. Animals may present with ataxia, lethargy/sedation, hypothermia, recumbency, and mydriasis (cats).

Barbiturates have no direct effect on the kidneys, but severe renal impairment can occur secondary to hypotensive effects in overdose situations.

Treatment of phenobarbital overdose consists of GI decontamination, if appropriate, and respiratory and cardiovascular support. Activated charcoal has been shown to be of considerable benefit in enhancing the clearance of phenobarbital even when the drug was administered parenterally. Charcoal acts as a sink for the drug to diffuse from the vasculature back into the gut. Forced alkaline diuresis can also be of substantial benefit in augmenting the elimination of phenobarbital in patients with normal renal function. Peritoneal dialysis or hemodialysis can be helpful in severe intoxications or anuric patients.[55]

For patients that have experienced or are suspected of having experienced an overdose, consultation with a 24-hour poison consultation center specializing in providing veterinary-specific information is recommended. For general information related to overdose and toxin exposures, as well as contact information for poison control centers, refer to ***Appendix***.

Drug Interactions

In humans, phenobarbital induces CYP 3A strongly and most other CYP isoenzymes to a lesser degree; it is a substrate of CYP 2C19. The following drug interactions have either been reported or are theoretical in humans or animals receiving phenobarbital and may be of significance in veterinary patients. Unless otherwise noted, use together is not necessarily contraindicated, but weigh the potential risks and perform additional monitoring when appropriate.

- **ACETAMINOPHEN**: Increased risk for hepatotoxicity, particularly when large or chronic doses of barbiturates are administered
- **ALPHA-2 AGONISTS** (eg, **dexmedetomidine, xylazine**): Concurrent use may result in additive respiratory depression.
- **ANTIHISTAMINES** (eg, **diphenhydramine**): May increase the effects of phenobarbital
- **BENZODIAZEPINES** (eg, **diazepam, midazolam**): Concurrent use may result in additive respiratory depression.
- **BROMIDES**: Synergistic efficacy and toxicity
- **CARPROFEN**: There may be an increased risk for hepatotoxicity secondary to carprofen metabolites. One source states that patients should not receive phenobarbital or other hepatic drug-metabolizing enzyme inducers when receiving carprofen.[56]
- **CHLORAMPHENICOL**: May increase the effects of phenobarbital
- **CHOLESTYRAMINE**: May reduce phenobarbital absorption and/or levels. Should be administered separately
- **CNS DEPRESSANTS** (eg, **methocarbamol, mirtazapine, trazodone**): Concurrent use may result in additive respiratory and CNS depression.
- **FELBAMATE**: May increase the effects of phenobarbital
- **MONOAMINE OXIDASE INHIBITORS** (MAOIs; eg, **amitraz, selegiline**): May prolong phenobarbital effects
- **OPIOIDS** (eg, **buprenorphine, hydrocodone, morphine, tramadol**): Concurrent use may result in additive respiratory and CNS depression.
- **PHENOTHIAZINES** (eg, **acepromazine**): May increase the effects of phenobarbital
- **RIFAMPIN**: May induce enzymes that increase the metabolism of barbiturates
- **URINARY ACIDIFIERS** (eg, **ammonium chloride**): Unchanged phenobarbital elimination in urine may be decreased and cause an increase in serum half-life.[57]

Phenobarbital (particularly after chronic therapy) may <u>decrease the effects</u> of the following drugs/drug classes by lowering their serum concentrations; effects may persist for several weeks after phenobarbital is discontinued[11]; these drugs may require initial or maintenance doses that are at or above the higher end of the dosing range, and doses of these drugs may need to be reduced when phenobarbital is being discontinued:

- **Azole Antifungals** (eg, **itraconazole, ketoconazole, voriconazole**): Phenobarbital levels may be increased, and antifungal levels may be decreased. Concurrent use is contraindicated in humans.
- **Benzimidazoles** (eg, **albendazole, fenbendazole**): May reduce active metabolite concentration
- **Benzodiazepines** (eg, **clorazepate, diazepam**)[58]
- **Buspirone**
- **Chloramphenicol**: Concurrent use also may increase the risk for phenobarbital toxicity.
- **Clarithromycin**
- **Clindamycin**
- **Corticosteroids** (eg, **dexamethasone, methylprednisolone, prednis[ol]one**)
- **Cyclosporine**[59]
- **Digoxin**[60]
- **Doxorubicin**
- **Doxycycline**
- **Estrogens** (eg, **diethylstilbestrol [DES], estriol**)
- **Felbamate**: Phenobarbital concentrations may increase, and felbamate concentrations may decrease.
- **Griseofulvin**
- **Ivermectin**
- **Levetiracetam**: Levetiracetam dosage requirements are increased by phenobarbital. In dogs receiving immediate-release levetiracetam, phenobarbital therapy reduced levetiracetam elimination half-life by ≈35% to 50%.[61] In dogs receiving extended-release levetiracetam, phenobarbital reduced levetiracetam peak concentration and increased clearance, although half-life appeared to be unaffected.[62]
- **Levothyroxine**
- **Methadone**
- **Metoprolol**
- **Metronidazole**
- **Quinidine**
- **Paroxetine**
- **Phenothiazines** (eg, **acepromazine**)
- **Praziquantel**
- **Progestins** (eg, **medroxyprogesterone**)
- **Sulfonamides**[14]
- **Tacrolimus**
- **Theophylline, Aminophylline**
- **Topiramate**
- **Tricyclic Antidepressants**
- **Urinary Alkalinizers** (eg, **potassium citrate**): Unchanged phenobarbital elimination in urine may be increased and cause a decrease in serum half-life.[57]
- **Verapamil**
- **Vincristine**
- **Vitamin D**
- **Warfarin**
- **Zonisamide**[63]

Laboratory Considerations

- Barbiturates may cause increased retention of **bromosulfophthalein** (BSP; sulfobromophthalein) and give falsely elevated results. It is recommended that barbiturates not be administered within the 24 hours before a BSP retention test is performed or, if they must be administered (eg, for seizure control), the results be interpreted accordingly.[64,65]
- Phenobarbital can alter the results of **thyroid** testing. Decreased total and free thyroxine (T_4), normal triiodothyronine (T_3), and either normal or increased thyroid-stimulating hormone (TSH) have been reported. It has been suggested to wait at least 4 weeks after discontinuing phenobarbital to perform thyroid testing.[38,66]
- In some dogs, phenobarbital may cause a false-positive **low dose dexamethasone suppression test** by increasing the clearance of dexamethasone. Phenobarbital apparently has no effect either on adrenocorticotropic hormone (ACTH) stimulation tests or on the hormonal equilibrium of the adrenal axis. Because phenobarbital can potentially increase the metabolism of cortisol, it has been implicated in contributing to relative adrenal insufficiency.

Dosages

DOGS:

Idiopathic epilepsy (extra-label): Initially, 2.5 – 3 mg/kg PO every 12 hours is commonly recommended, although starting dosages may vary. To achieve therapeutic phenobarbital concentrations sooner in phenobarbital-naïve dogs, some clinicians suggest an initial loading dose of 12 – 20 mg/kg (total dose); this dose can be administered as a single, slow (over at least 5 minutes) IV injection but may cause profound sedation and respiratory depression.[67] To minimize these effects, the total dose can be divided into increments of 3 – 4 mg/kg IV every 1 to 4 hours; the degree of sedation and respiratory depression during administration should be monitored, and subsequent doses should be adjusted accordingly. Doses should be adjusted based on phenobarbital concentrations, efficacy, and adverse effects. Administration of 3 – 5.6 mg/kg PO every 8 hours in dogs with a shorter phenobarbital elimination half-life appeared safe and improved seizure management in some patients.[26] Combination with other anticonvulsants is common.

Adjunctive treatment of status epilepticus (extra-label): After use of benzodiazepines (eg, diazepam, midazolam), phenobarbital 4 – 8 mg/kg IV slow (over at least 5 minutes) can be administered. If seizure activity continues, additional increments of phenobarbital can be administered at 4 mg/kg IV every 20 to 30 minutes with a maximum total phenobarbital dose of 20 – 24 mg/kg IV.[67,68] Once seizure activity has diminished and the patient is alert, the patient can be transitioned to oral phenobarbital, as noted above.

Sialadenosis (extra-label): In case reports, 1 mg/kg PO every 12 hours appears to be most common, although dosages up to 2.5 mg/kg PO twice daily have been noted.[69] In one case,[5] 6 mg/kg IM every 12 hours was initially prescribed. In several but not all cases, dogs were slowly weaned off phenobarbital without relapse.[5,6,9,70]

Discontinuing phenobarbital therapy (taper guidelines): Tapering guidelines may vary and are anecdotal. In general, for patients stabilized on another anticonvulsant, a typical tapering schedule involves reducing the phenobarbital dose by 25% every 2 weeks. Smaller dose decreases (eg, 10% to 20%) or longer intervals between reductions (eg, every 3 to 4 weeks) can be considered. Available tablet size may dictate actual dose decrease. Reductions can be made more rapidly (eg, every 7 days) if necessary (eg, fulminant phenobarbital hepatotoxicity); because seizure activity may increase during a rapid taper, concurrently initiating another anticonvulsant is recommended. Doses of other anticonvulsants may need to be reduced as phenobarbital's effects on CYP enzyme induction wane, which may take several weeks after discontinuation.

CATS:

Idiopathic epilepsy (extra-label): Initially, 1 – 3 mg/kg PO every 12 hours is commonly recommended, although starting dosages may vary. Cats receiving phenobarbital 2.5 – 8.6 mg/kg/day PO had a therapeutic serum phenobarbital concentration between 15 and 45 μg/mL; seizure control can be achieved in most cats in this range regardless of the cause of the seizures.[71] Practically, ½ to one 15 mg tablet/cat (NOT mg/kg) PO every 12 hours is used. To achieve therapeutic phenobarbital concentrations sooner in phenobarbital-naïve cats, some suggest an initial phenobarbital loading dose of 12 – 24 mg/kg IV given in increments of 3 to 4 mg/kg IV every 2 to 6 hours. The dose should be adjusted based on phenobarbital concentrations, efficacy, and adverse effects.

Transdermal phenobarbital compounded in PLO (extra-label): 9 mg/kg applied to the inside of the pinna every 12 hours (18 mg/kg/day). Therapeutic concentrations may be achieved in some cats, and consistent monitoring is recommended.[20,72] Further study is warranted to prove this route effectively controls seizures.

Adjunctive treatment of status epilepticus (extra-label): After use of benzodiazepines (eg, diazepam, midazolam), phenobarbital 3 mg/kg IV can be administered. Phenobarbital can be repeated every 20 minutes up to 24 mg/kg in a 24-hour period or given as loading of 10 mg/kg IV bolus.[67,68,73]

Discontinuing phenobarbital therapy (taper guidelines): In patients stabilized on another anticonvulsant, a typical tapering schedule involves reducing the phenobarbital dose by 25% every 2 weeks. Smaller dose decreases (eg, 10% to 20%) or longer intervals between reductions (eg, every 3 to 4 weeks) can be considered. Available tablet size may dictate actual dose decrease. Reductions can be made more rapidly (eg, every 7 days) if necessary; because seizure activity may increase during a rapid taper, concurrently initiating another anticonvulsant is recommended. Doses of other anticonvulsants may need to be reduced as phenobarbital's effects on CYP enzyme induction wane, which may take several weeks after discontinuation.

HORSES:

Seizure control (extra-label):

a) Adult horses: Loading dose of 16 – 20 mg/kg IV once; maintenance dose of 1 – 5 mg/kg PO every 12 hours
b) Foals: Loading dose of 16 – 20 mg/kg IV once; maintenance dose of 100 – 500 mg/foal (NOT mg/kg) PO every 12 hours[74,75]

CATTLE:

Enzyme induction in organochlorine toxicity (extra-label): 5 g/animal (NOT mg/kg) PO for 3 to 4 weeks, off 3 to 4 weeks, then repeat for 3 to 4 more weeks[76]

FERRETS:

Seizure control (extra-label): Loading dose of 16 – 20 mg/kg IV once; maintenance dose of 1 – 2 mg/kg PO every 8 to 12 hours[74,75]

Monitoring

- Anticonvulsant efficacy
- Adverse effects (eg, CNS related, polyuria/polydipsia, weight gain)
- Serum phenobarbital concentration:
  - After initiation of therapy or dosage change:
    - If a loading dose of phenobarbital was not administered, at least 5 to 6 half-lives (dogs, ≈12 to 14 days; cats, 9 to 10 days) should be allowed to pass before measuring serum phenobarbital concentrations to confirm that therapeutic levels have been reached; on the day of sampling, the time between drug administration sampling does not appear to be significant.[77,78]
    - Re-measure at 6 weeks postinitiation of phenobarbital to determine the patient's steady-state concentration and the extent of autoinduction of phenobarbital metabolism.[2]
  - Once steady-state is achieved and the patient's clinical condition is controlled with a maintenance dose: measure serum phenobarbital concentrations every 6 months in dogs and cats. Rechecking concentration more often should be considered when efficacy is reduced or adverse effects are suspected.
  - Dogs: Serum phenobarbital concentrations of 15 to 35 μg/mL (86 to 150 mmol/L) have been recommended, with the high end of the range reflecting suggested changes to minimize the potential for hepatotoxicity.[2] Approximately ⅓ of dogs receiving phenobarbital with bromides may require lower phenobarbital doses and serum concentrations that are ≈33% less for seizure control.[79]
  - Cats: In a retrospective study of 30 cats, 93% of cats had seizures controlled with serum phenobarbital concentrations between 15 and 45 μg/mL.[71] Optimum therapeutic levels of 23 to 30 μg/mL (100 to 130 mmol/L) have been recommended in cats in an attempt to maximize seizure control with the lowest potential for adverse effects.[80] Cats being treated with a transdermal formulation will require more frequent monitoring.
- If phenobarbital is used long term, routine CBC and comprehensive serum chemistry profile are recommended at least every 6 months.
- If results of routine serum chemistry profile suggest possible hepatotoxicity, bile acids and abdominal ultrasonography should be considered for further evaluation.

Client Information

- This medicine may be given with or without food. If your animal vomits or acts sick after getting it on an empty stomach, give it with food or a small treat. If vomiting continues, contact your veterinarian.
- Do not skip doses. Try to give doses at the same time each day. Do not suddenly stop giving this medicine to your animal.
- Do not change the amount you are giving your animal without first talking with your veterinarian.
- Sleepiness, lack of energy, greater thirst, appetite, and increased need to urinate commonly occur when starting therapy.
- Liver problems can occur in dogs. Contact your veterinarians if your animal has any vomiting, diarrhea, lethargy, loss of appetite, or swollen abdomen. Your veterinarian will need to perform examinations and blood work on your dog while it is taking this medicine. Do not miss these important follow-up visits.
- Phenobarbital is classified as a schedule-IV controlled drug by the federal Drug Enforcement Agency (DEA). The use of this medication in animals or humans other than those for whom they are prescribed is illegal.

Chemistry/Synonyms

Phenobarbital, a barbiturate, occurs as glistening, odorless, small, white crystals or a white crystalline powder with a melting point of 174°C to 178°C (345.2°F-352.4°F) and a pK_a of 7.41. One gram is slightly soluble in ≈1000 mL of water and freely soluble in 10 mL of alcohol. Compared with other barbiturates, it has a low lipid solubility.

Phenobarbital sodium occurs as bitter-tasting, odorless, flaky, white crystals, crystalline granules, or powder. It is very soluble in water, soluble in alcohol, and freely soluble in propylene glycol. The injectable product has a pH of 8.5 to 10.5.

SI units (mmol/L) are multiplied by 0.232 to convert phenobarbital levels to conventional units (μg/mL); conversely, conventional units are multiplied by 4.31 to obtain SI units.

Phenobarbital may also be known as fenobarbital, phenemalum, phenobarbitalum, phenobarbitone, phenylethylbarbituric acid, phenylethylmalonylurea, *Luminal Sodium*®, or *Solfoton*®.

Storage/Stability

Store phenobarbital tablets in tight, light-resistant containers at room temperature 20°C to 25°C (68°F-77°F); protect from moisture.

Store phenobarbital elixir in tight containers at room temperature (15°C-30°C [59°F-86°F]).

Store phenobarbital sodium injection at room temperature (15°C-30°C [59°F-86°F]). Do not add solutions of phenobarbital sodium to acidic solutions or use them if they contain a precipitate or are grossly discolored.

Aqueous solutions of phenobarbital are not very stable. Propylene glycol is often used in injectable products to help stabilize the solution.

Phenobarbital is a DEA Schedule-IV controlled substance (C-IV) that should be stored in an area that is substantially constructed and securely locked. Follow applicable local, state, and federal rules regarding the disposal of unused or wasted controlled drugs.

Compatibility/Compounding Considerations

Compatibility is dependent on factors such as pH, concentration, temperature, and diluent used; specialized references or a hospital pharmacist should be consulted for more specific information.

The following solutions and drugs have been reported to be physically **compatible** with phenobarbital sodium: dextrose IV solutions, Ringer's injection, lactated Ringer's injection, sodium chloride IV solutions, dextrose-sodium chloride combinations, dextrose Ringer's combinations, dextrose-Ringer's lactate combinations, amikacin sulfate, aminophylline, atropine sulfate (stable for at least 15 minutes but not 24 hours), calcium chloride and gluconate, dexmedetomidine, dimenhydrinate, glycopyrrolate, heparin sodium, methylprednisolone sodium succinate, piperacillin-tazobactam, polymyxin B sulfate, ranitidine, sodium bicarbonate, and verapamil.

The following drugs have been reported to be physically **incompatible** with phenobarbital sodium: buprenorphine, chlorpromazine, codeine phosphate, cyclosporine, diazepam, diphenhydramine, dobutamine, ephedrine sulfate, fentanyl citrate, glycopyrrolate, hydralazine, hydrocortisone sodium succinate, hydroxyzine, insulin (regular), ketamine, meperidine, midazolam, morphine sulfate, nalbuphine, norepinephrine bitartrate, oxytetracycline, pentazocine lactate, procaine, prochlorperazine, promazine, and promethazine.

Phenobarbital 10 mg/mL oral suspension can be made by crushing the appropriate number of tablets and suspending in *ORA-Blend*® (regular or sugar-free). In a study, potency was maintained over the 115-day study period when stored at room temperature in amber plastic bottles.[81]

Dosage Forms/Regulatory Status

VETERINARY-LABELED PRODUCTS: NONE

The Association of Racing Commissioners International [ARCI] Uniform Classification Guidelines for Foreign Substances [UCGFS] has designated this drug as a class 2 substance. Use of this drug may not be allowed in certain animal competitions. Check rules and regulations before entering a competition while this medication is being administered. Contact local racing authorities for further guidance. See ***Appendix*** for more information.

HUMAN-LABELED PRODUCTS:

Phenobarbital Tablets: 15 mg, 16.2 mg, 30 mg, 32.4 mg, 60 mg, 64.8 mg, 97.2 mg, and 100 mg; *Solfoton*®, generic; (Rx; C-IV). **NOTE**: Phenobarbital strengths previously were expressed in grains, whose abbreviation ("gr") can easily be confused with gram (g). To prevent medication errors, using grains to express strength should be avoided when prescribing phenobarbital.

Phenobarbital Elixir/Oral Solution: 20 mg/5 mL (4 mg/mL); generic; (Rx, C-IV). Contains 15% ethanol

Phenobarbital Sodium Injection: 65 mg/mL and 130 mg/mL; *Luminal Sodium*®, generic; (Rx; C-IV). Contains benzyl alcohol

References

For the complete list of references, see **wiley.com/go/budde/plumb**

Phenoxybenzamine

(fen-ox-ee-***ben***-za-meen) *Dibenzyline*®

Alpha-adrenergic Antagonist (nonselective), Vasodilator

Prescriber Highlights

- An alpha-adrenergic antagonist used primarily in small animals for urethral hypertonus and urethral obstruction and to control hypertension in cases of pheochromocytoma
- May be contraindicated in patients with hypotension, glaucoma, or diabetes mellitus and in horses with colic
- Use with caution in patients with congestive heart failure or other heart disease, renal impairment, or cerebral/coronary arteriosclerosis.
- Adverse effects include hypotension, rebound hypertension, miosis, increased intraocular pressure, tachycardia, inhibition of ejaculation, nasal congestion, weakness, ataxia, and GI effects (eg, nausea, vomiting). Constipation may occur in horses.
- Availability and cost can be problematic; product may need to be obtained from compounding pharmacy.
- The National Institute for Occupational Safety and Health (NIOSH) classifies phenoxybenzamine as a hazardous drug; use appropriate precautions when handling.

Uses/Indications

Phenoxybenzamine is used primarily for its effect in reducing internal urethral sphincter tone when urethral sphincter hypertonus is present. It can also be used to treat hypertension associated with pheochromocytoma before surgery. It was used in the management of tachycardia resulting from phenylpropanolamine overdose in a dog.[1] In cats with recurrence of urethral obstruction, prazosin appears to be more effective to prevent the incidence of reobstruction as compared with phenoxybenzamine.[2,3]

Phenoxybenzamine has been anecdotally reported to increase acupuncture effectiveness.[4]

In horses, phenoxybenzamine has been used to decrease urethral sphincter tone with bladder paresis. It has also been historically tried for preventing or treating laminitis in early stages[5-7] and treating secretory diarrhea.[8,9]

Pharmacology/Actions

Phenoxybenzamine noncompetitively blocks the alpha-adrenergic response to circulating epinephrine or norepinephrine; it is considered a nonselective alpha-adrenergic antagonist, with greater affinity for alpha-1 receptors than alpha-2 receptors. The effect of phenoxybenzamine has been described as a chemical sympathectomy. Phenoxybenzamine has no effects on beta-adrenergic receptors or on the parasympathetic nervous system.

Phenoxybenzamine increases cutaneous blood flow, but little effect is noted on skeletal muscle or cerebral blood flow.

Phenoxybenzamine can also block pupillary dilation, lid retraction, and nictitating membrane contraction. Prevention of epinephrine inhibitory action on insulin secretion is noted. Both standing and supine systolic blood pressures are decreased when this drug is used in humans.

Pharmacokinetics

No information was located on the pharmacokinetics of this agent in veterinary species. In humans, phenoxybenzamine is variably absorbed from the GI tract and has a bioavailability of 20% to 30%.

Onset of action is slow (several hours) and increases over several days after regular dosing. Effects persist for 3 to 4 days after discontinuation.

Phenoxybenzamine is highly lipid soluble and may accumulate in body fat. The serum half-life is ≈24 hours in humans. It is metabolized (dealkylated) and excreted in both urine and bile.

Contraindications/Precautions/Warnings

Phenoxybenzamine is contraindicated in patients hypersensitive to it, in horses with clinical signs of colic, and in patients in which hypotension would be deleterious (eg, those with renal impairment or shock) unless blood pressure can be adequately monitored and maintained. One source[10] lists glaucoma and diabetes mellitus as contraindications to the use of phenoxybenzamine in dogs.

Phenoxybenzamine should be used with caution in patients with congestive heart failure or other heart disease due to drug-induced tachycardia. It should also be used cautiously in patients with renal impairment or cerebral/coronary arteriosclerosis. Adrenergic blockade may worsen signs of respiratory infections.

Phenoxybenzamine is not recommended for long-term use in humans because it has been shown to be mutagenic and carcinogenic in mice, rats, and humans.

The National Institute for Occupational Safety and Health (NIOSH) classifies phenoxybenzamine as a hazardous drug; personal protective equipment (PPE) should be used accordingly to minimize the risk for exposure.[11]

Adverse Effects

Adverse effects associated with alpha-adrenergic blockade include hypotension, weakness/dizziness, GI effects (eg, nausea, vomiting), miosis, increased intraocular pressure, tachycardia, sodium retention, inhibition of ejaculation, and nasal congestion.

When used in dogs for controlling hypertension before surgery for pheochromocytoma, phenoxybenzamine can cause prolonged postoperative hypotension; volume expansion may be required. Increased preoperative sodium intake has been suggested in human medicine.

Phenoxybenzamine can cause constipation in horses.

Reproductive/Nursing Safety

It is unknown if phenoxybenzamine crosses the placenta. Phenoxybenzamine has been shown to cause abnormalities in the closure of the patent ductus in guinea pigs. Long-term phenoxybenzamine is mutagenic and carcinogenic to humans.

Whether phenoxybenzamine is excreted into milk is also unknown, but this activity could be expected.[12] Because safety has not been established in animals, this drug should only be used when the maternal benefits outweigh the potential risks to offspring.

Overdose/Acute Toxicity

Overdoses of phenoxybenzamine may yield signs of hypotension (eg, ataxia, syncope), tachycardia, vomiting, lethargy, shock.

Treatment should consist of GI decontamination if the ingestion was recent, and there are no contraindications to those procedures. Hypotension can be treated with fluid support. Epinephrine is contraindicated (see ***Drug Interactions***), and most vasopressor drugs are ineffective in reversing the effects of alpha-blockade. IV norepinephrine (ie, levarterenol) may be beneficial, however, if clinical signs are severe.

For patients that have experienced or are suspected to have experienced an overdose, it is strongly encouraged to consult with one of the 24-hour poison consultation centers that specialize in providing information specific for veterinary patients. For general information related to overdose and toxin exposures, as well as contact information for poison control centers, refer to ***Appendix.***

Drug Interactions

The following drug interactions have either been reported or are theoretical in humans or animals receiving phenoxybenzamine and may be of significance in veterinary patients. Unless otherwise noted, use together is not necessarily contraindicated, but weigh the potential risks and perform additional monitoring when appropriate.

- **ANTIHYPERTENSIVE AGENTS** (eg, **amlodipine**): Concurrent use may result in hypotension.
- **BETA-BLOCKERS** (eg, **atenolol**): May enhance hypotensive effects
- **EPINEPHRINE**: Use in combination with drugs that have both alpha- and beta-adrenergic effects may result in increased hypotension, vasodilation or tachycardia.
- **PHENYLEPHRINE**: Phenoxybenzamine will antagonize the effects of alpha-adrenergic agonists.
- **RESERPINE**: Phenoxybenzamine can antagonize the hypothermic effects of reserpine.
- **SILDENAFIL**: May enhance hypotensive effects

Dosages

DOGS:

Functional urethral obstruction caused by increased sympathetic urethral tone (extra-label): A common dosage recommendation is 0.25 mg/kg PO every 12 hours, or practically 5 – 20 mg/dog (NOT mg/kg) PO every 12 hours.

Hypertension associated with pheochromocytoma (extra-label): Initially 0.25 – 0.5 mg/kg PO every 12 hours. Dosage is gradually increased to a maximum of 2.5 mg/kg PO every 12 hours or until clinical signs of hypotension (eg, lethargy, weakness, syncope), or adverse effects (eg, vomiting) occur. Median dosage in one study was 0.6 mg/kg PO every 12 hours.[6] Continue until surgery; close monitoring during the perioperative period is critical for a successful outcome.

CATS:

Functional urethral obstruction caused by increased sympathetic urethral tone (extra-label): 2 – 4 mg/cat (NOT mg/kg) every 12 hours[2,13] If using in combination with bethanechol, it is recommended that phenoxybenzamine be started 2-3 days prior to bethanechol (1.25 mg – 7.5 mg per cat [NOT mg/kg] PO every 8 to 12 hours).

HORSES:

Decreasing urethral sphincter tone in horses with bladder paresis (extra-label): 0.7 mg/kg PO 4 times a day (in combination with bethanechol at 0.25 – 0.75 mg/kg PO 2 to 4 times a day)[14]

Diarrhea unresponsive to other intervention (extra-label): 1 – 1.5 mg/kg IV infusion with a second dose given 12 to 24 hours later; total cumulative dose is 2 mg/kg[8,9]

Monitoring

- Clinical efficacy (eg, adequate urination, controlled blood pressure)
- Efficacy for urinary problems may take a week or longer, and the drug should be given for several weeks before it is determined to be ineffective.
- Baseline and periodic blood pressure

Client Information

- May be given with or without food
- Efficacy for urinary problems may take a week or longer, and the drug should be given for several weeks before it is determined to be ineffective.
- Can cause GI effects (eg, vomiting and diarrhea in small animals, constipation in horses), rapid heartbeat, small pupils, and runny nose

- If the animal collapses while receiving this medication, contact your veterinarian immediately.

Chemistry/Synonyms

An alpha-adrenergic–blocking agent, phenoxybenzamine HCl is an odorless, white crystalline powder with a melting range of 136°C to 141°C (277°F-304°F) and a pK_a of 4.4. Approximately 40 mg are soluble in 1 mL of water, and 167 mg are soluble in 1 mL of alcohol.

Phenoxybenzamine may also be known as SKF-688A, *Dibenyline®*, *Dibenzyran®*, or *Fenoxene®*.

Storage/Stability

Phenoxybenzamine capsules should be stored at room temperature (20°C-25°C [68°F-77°F]) in well-sealed containers.

Dosage Forms/Regulatory Status

VETERINARY-LABELED PRODUCTS: NONE

The Association of Racing Commissioners International (ARCI) has designated phenoxybenzamine as a class 3 substance. See ***Appendix*** for more information. Use of this drug may not be allowed in certain animal competitions. Check rules and regulations before entering in a competition while this medication is being administered. Contact local racing authorities for further guidance.

HUMAN-LABELED PRODUCTS:

Phenoxybenzamine HCl capsules: 10 mg; *Dibenzyline®*; generic; (Rx)

References

For the complete list of references, see **wiley.com/go/budde/plumb**

Phenylbutazone

(fen-ill-***byoo***-ta-zone) *Butazolidin®, Bute*

Non-Steroidal Anti-inflammatory Drug (NSAID)

Prescriber Highlights

- NSAID used primarily in horses
- Contraindications include known hypersensitivity, history of or pre-existing hematologic or bone marrow abnormalities, pre-existing GI ulcers; use in horses and dairy cattle intended for food is prohibited.
- Use with caution in foals or ponies, and in patients with pre-existing renal disease or CHF.
- Adverse effects in horses include oral and GI erosions and ulcers, hypoalbuminemia, diarrhea, anorexia, azotemia, and renal papillary necrosis.
- Parenteral injections should be administered only by the IV route.

Uses/Indications

Phenylbutazone is used primarily for treating pain and inflammation in horses. It has been used in other species (eg, dogs, cattle, swine), but generally other NSAIDs are preferred.

Pharmacology/Actions

Phenylbutazone is an NSAID with analgesic, anti-inflammatory, antipyretic, and mild uricosuric properties. The proposed mechanism of action is by the inhibition of cyclooxygenase, thereby reducing prostaglandin synthesis. Additional pharmacologic actions include reduced renal blood flow, decreased glomerular filtration rate, decreased platelet aggregation, and gastric mucosal damage.

Pharmacokinetics

Following oral administration, phenylbutazone is absorbed from both the stomach and small intestine. The drug is distributed throughout the body with highest concentrations attained in the liver, heart, lungs, kidneys, and blood. Plasma protein binding in horses exceeds 99%.

The serum half-life in horses ranges from 3.5 to 6 hours and, like aspirin, it is dose dependent. Therapeutic efficacy, however, may last for more than 24 hours, likely due to the irreversible binding of phenylbutazone to cyclooxygenase. In horses and other species, phenylbutazone is nearly completely metabolized, primarily to oxyphenbutazone (active) and gamma-hydroxyphenylbutazone. Oxyphenbutazone has been detected in horse urine up to 48 hours after a single dose. Phenylbutazone is more rapidly excreted into alkaline than acidic urine. One study suggests equine CYP 3A97 is responsible for in vitro conversion of phenylbutazone to oxyphenbutazone.[1] Another study in 17 horses showed the following pharmacokinetic parameters: volume of distribution at steady state was 0.194 L/kg; systemic clearance was 23.9 mL/hour/kg; terminal half-life following IV administration was 10.9 hours; terminal half-life after PO administration with paste was 13.4 hours; and terminal half-life after PO administration with tablets was 15.1 hours.[2] Complete elimination of phenylbutazone in horses may take 2 months and phenylbutazone can be detected in the urine for at least 7 days following administration.

Serum half-lives reported for other animals are as follows: dogs ≈2 to 6 hours, cattle ≈42 to 55 hours, swine ≈2 to 6 hours, and rabbits ≈2 hours.[3]

Contraindications/Precautions/Warnings

Phenylbutazone is contraindicated in patients that are hypersensitive to it or have a history of or pre-existing hematologic or bone marrow abnormalities. Avoid use of phenylbutazone in horses with known or suspected equine gastric ulcer syndrome (EGUS); single doses of phenylbutazone will likely not result in catastrophic consequences, but repeated doses can exacerbate gastric ulcers.[4] Phenylbutazone may cause decreased renal blood flow and sodium and water retention; use cautiously in animals with pre-existing renal disease or CHF. Use with caution in patients who have a history of drug allergy.

Cautious use in both foals and ponies is recommended because of increased incidences of hypoproteinemia and GI ulceration. Foals with a heavy parasite burden or that are undernourished may be more susceptible to developing adverse effects.

Therapeutic response to phenylbutazone typically occurs within 24 hours.[5,6] Re-evaluate diagnosis and treatment if patient's condition does not improve after 5 days.

Because phenylbutazone may mask clinical signs of lameness in horses for several days following therapy, it may be used to mask lameness prior to soundness examinations.

Parenteral phenylbutazone should only be administered IV; do not administer phenylbutazone IM or SC, as it may cause local tissue swelling, necrosis, and sloughing. Intracarotid injections may cause CNS stimulation and seizures.

Phenylbutazone is labeled for use in horses that are not intended to be used for food. A thorough evaluation of phenylbutazone residues and toxicology in humans and horses concluded that the illegal and erratic presence of trace amount residues of phenylbutazone in horse meat is not a public health issue.[3]

Adverse Effects

Adverse effects that have been reported in horses include oral and GI erosions and ulcers, hypoalbuminemia, diarrhea, right dorsal colitis, anorexia, azotemia, and renal papillary necrosis. Unlike in humans, it does not appear that phenylbutazone causes much sodium and water retention in horses at labeled dosages, but edema has been reported. In dogs, however, phenylbutazone may cause sodium and water retention and diminished renal blood flow. Phenylbutazone-induced blood dyscrasias and hepatotoxicity have also been reported in dogs. Therapy should be halted at first signs of anorexia, oral lesions, depression, reduced plasma proteins, increased serum creatinine or BUN, leukopenia, or anemias.

Although gastric ulceration is frequently observed in adult horses and foals, evidence of an association between this disease and administration of NSAIDs such as phenylbutazone or flunixin at recommended dosages is lacking. On the basis of the current evidence, prophylactic anti-ulcer medications for horses receiving therapeutic doses of NSAIDs are likely unnecessary in patients that are otherwise at low risk for gastric ulceration.[7] Use of sucralfate or H_2 blockers (eg, ranitidine, famotidine) has been suggested to treat the adverse GI effects. Misoprostol, a prostaglandin E analogue, may also be useful in reducing the GI effects of phenylbutazone.

IM or SC injection can cause swelling, necrosis, and sloughing. Intracarotid injections may cause CNS stimulation and seizures.

The primary concerns with phenylbutazone therapy in humans include its bone marrow effects (agranulocytosis, aplastic anemia), renal and cardiovascular effects (fluid retention to acute renal failure), and GI effects (dyspepsia to perforated ulcers). Other serious concerns with phenylbutazone include hypersensitivity reactions, neurologic, dermatologic, and hepatic toxicities.

Reproductive/Nursing Safety

Both phenylbutazone and oxyphenbutazone (active metabolite) cross the placenta and are excreted into milk. Although phenylbutazone has shown no direct teratogenic effects, rodent studies have demonstrated reduced litter sizes, increased neonatal mortality, and increased stillbirth rates. Phenylbutazone should, therefore, be used in pregnancy only when the potential benefits of therapy outweigh the risks associated with it.

The safety of phenylbutazone during nursing has not been determined. Because safety has not been established in animals, this drug should only be used when the maternal benefits outweigh the potential risks to offspring.

Overdose/Acute Toxicity

In humans, manifestations of an acute phenylbutazone overdose include a prompt respiratory or metabolic acidosis with compensatory hyperventilation, renal failure (oliguric, with proteinuria and hematuria), liver injury (hepatomegaly and jaundice), bone marrow depression, ulceration (and perforation) of the GI tract, seizures, coma, and acute hypotensive crisis. Other symptoms reported in humans include nausea, vomiting, abdominal pain, diaphoresis, neurologic and psychiatric symptoms, edema, hypertension, respiratory depression, and cyanosis.

The most common clinical signs in dogs with a phenylbutazone toxicity (per unpublished ASPCA Animal Poison Control Center [APCC] data) include tremors, seizures, ataxia, vomiting, tachypnea, and tachycardia. Oral LD_{50} in dogs is 332 mg/kg.[3] In horses, the most common clinical signs (per unpublished APCC data) are colic, anorexia, and ataxia. Horses receiving 30 mg/kg/day PO for up to 2 weeks became anorectic and depressed; reduced neutrophils count, decreasing serum calcium, and increased serum BUN and creatinine were noted.[8] In the same study, all horses given 15 or 30 mg/kg/day IV died within 4 to 7 days. Pathology findings included GI ulcerations, renal papillary necrosis, and vascular thromboses.

Standard overdose procedures should be followed (eg, GI decontamination, IV fluid diuresis). Benzodiazepines IV may be used to help control seizures. Monitor for fluid overload as phenylbutazone may cause fluid retention.

For patients that have experienced or are suspected to have experienced an overdose, consultation with a 24-hour poison control center specializing in providing veterinary-specific information is recommended. For general information related to overdose and toxin exposures, as well as contact information for poison control centers, refer to ***Appendix.***

Drug Interactions

The following drug interactions either have been reported or are theoretical in humans or animals receiving phenylbutazone and may be of significance in veterinary patients. Unless otherwise noted, use together is not necessarily contraindicated, but weigh the potential risks and perform additional monitoring when appropriate.

- **Angiotensin Converting Enzyme Inhibitors (ACEIs; benazepril, enalapril)**: Combined use with phenylbutazone may increase the risk for renal dysfunction and/or may decrease the efficacy of the ACEI.
- **Anticoagulants** (eg, **enoxaparin, heparin, rivaroxaban, warfarin**): May increase risk for bleeding. Avoid combination
- **Corticosteroids** (eg, **dexamethasone, prednis(ol)one**): May increase the risk for GI ulceration or bleeding and risk for hepatotoxicity
- **Cyclosporine**: May increase risk for renal dysfunction
- **Digoxin**: Phenylbutazone may increase serum digoxin concentrations, prolong digoxin half-life, and thus increase the risk for adverse effects related to digoxin toxicity (eg, arrhythmias, GI adverse effects).
- **Diuretics, Loop** (eg, **furosemide, torsemide**): May increase risk for renal toxicity
- **Diuretics, Potassium-Sparing** (eg, **spironolactone**): May decrease diuretic and antihypertensive efficacy; increased risk for hyperkalemia and nephrotoxicity
- **Hepatotoxic Drugs** (eg, **acetaminophen, chlorpromazine, isoniazid**): May increase risk for hepatotoxicity
- **Methotrexate**: May increase risk for methotrexate toxicity, especially with higher methotrexate doses. Avoid combination
- **Misoprostol**: May result in CNS adverse effects (eg, **ataxia**)
- **Nonsteroidal Anti-Inflammatory Drugs (NSAIDs**; eg, **firocoxib, flunixin**): May increase the potential for GI ulceration and renal toxicity
- **Penicillamine**: May increase the risk for hematologic and/or renal adverse reactions
- **Penicillin G**: Phenylbutazone may increase plasma half-life of penicillin G.
- **Pentoxifylline**: May increase risk for bleeding
- **Phenobarbital**: May result in decreased phenylbutazone half-life and increased risk for hepatotoxicity
- **Selective Serotonin Reuptake Inhibitors** (**SSRIs**; eg, **fluoxetine, paroxetine**): May increase risk for bleeding
- **Sulfonamides** (eg, **sulfa-/trimethoprim, sulfadimethoxine**): Phenylbutazone could potentially displace sulfonamides from plasma proteins, increasing the risk for adverse effects.[9]
- **Tricyclic Antidepressants** (**TCAs**; eg, **amitriptyline, clomipramine**): May increase risk for bleeding

Laboratory Considerations

- Phenylbutazone and oxyphenbutazone may interfere with thyroid function tests by competing with thyroxine at protein-binding sites or by inhibiting thyroid iodine uptake.

Dosages

DOGS:

Anti-inflammatory for musculoskeletal conditions (label dosage; FDA-approved): 14.7 mg/kg PO 3 times daily initially (maximum of 800 mg/dog [NOT mg/kg] daily regardless of weight); titrate to lowest effective dose.[10] **NOTE**: The lack of suitable tablet sizes and the ready availability of safer NSAIDs precludes use of phenylbutazone in dogs.

HORSES:

Anti-inflammatory for musculoskeletal conditions (label dosage; FDA-approved):

a) 1 – 2 g/454 kg (1000 lb) horse (NOT mg/kg) IV slowly once daily.[6] Limit IV administration to no more than 5 successive days of therapy. Follow with oral forms if treatment needs to be continued.

b) 2 – 4 g/454 kg (1000 lb) horse (NOT per kg) PO once daily.[5] Do not exceed 4 g/day. Use high end of dose range for the first 48 hours, then titrate to lowest effective dose.

Extra-label dosage: 2 – 4.4 mg/kg PO, IV every 12 to 24 hours[11,12]

RUMINANTS:

NOTE: The FDA has issued an order prohibiting the extra-label use of phenylbutazone in female dairy cattle 20 months of age or older. In the United States, there is zero tolerance for phenylbutazone residues in any edible tissue from any animal and many believe that phenylbutazone use in any food animal should be banned.[13]

Analgesia for surgical pain (extra-label):

a) 5 mg/kg PO every 24 to 48 hours or 10 mg/kg PO every 48 to 72 hours[14]

b) 4 mg/kg IV every 24 hours[11]

Monitoring

- Analgesic/anti-inflammatory/antipyretic effect
- Baseline and periodic CBCs with chronic therapy (especially if used in dogs); consider weekly CBCs early in therapy and every other week with long-term therapy.
- Baseline and periodic urinalysis and renal chemistry profile (including albumin, total protein) with long-term therapy

Client Information

- This medicine works best when given to your animal with food.
- Injections must only be administered in the vein (IV).
- Side effects can include mouth/stomach ulcers, kidney damage, loss of appetite, and swelling of the limbs.

Chemistry/Synonyms

A synthetic pyrazolone derivative related chemically to aminopyrine, phenylbutazone occurs as a white to off-white, odorless crystalline powder that has a pK_a of 4.5. It is very slightly soluble in water and 1 g will dissolve in 28 mL of alcohol. It is tasteless at first but has a slightly bitter aftertaste.

Phenylbutazone may also be known as butadiene, fenilbutazona, bute, phenylbutazonum, or phenylbute.

Storage/Stability

Oral products should be stored at 15°C to 30°C (59°-86°F) in tight, child-resistant containers if possible. The injectable product should be refrigerated 2°C to 8°C (36°F-46°F).

Dosage Forms/Regulatory Status

VETERINARY-LABELED PRODUCTS:

The extra-label use of phenylbutazone in female dairy cattle 20 months of age or older is prohibited.[15] Not to be used in animals used for food. Some products are listed in the Green Book but appear to no longer be marketed. Except where otherwise noted, the following are labeled for use in horses. Different racing jurisdictions and equine disciplines have different standards regarding the use of phenylbutazone in racing and nonracing performance animals.

Phenylbutazone Tablets: 100 mg, 200 mg, and 1 g; many tradename and generic products available; (Rx). FDA-approved for use in dogs (only 100 mg and 200 mg size) and horses (all strengths).

Phenylbutazone Oral Powder: 1 g in 10 g of powder to be mixed into feed. *generic*; (Rx)

Phenylbutazone Paste Oral Syringes: Contains 6 g, 12 g, or 20 g/syringe; many tradename and generic products available; (Rx)

Phenylbutazone Granules: Contains 8 g of phenylbutazone per package. *Butazolidin®* Granules; (Rx)

Phenylbutazone Injection: 100 mg/mL (approved for use in dogs) and 200 mg/mL in 100 mL vials; many tradename and generic products available; (Rx)

HUMAN APPROVED PRODUCTS: NONE

References

For the complete list of references, see **wiley.com/go/budde/plumb**

Phenylephrine

(fen-ill-***ef***-rin) *Neo-Synephrine®*

Alpha-adrenergic Agonist

For ophthalmic use, see ***Phenylephrine, Ophthalmic***

Prescriber Highlights

- Used parenterally to treat hypotension without overt cardiostimulation
- Contraindicated in patients with severe hypertension, ventricular tachycardia, or that are hypersensitive to it
- Use with extreme caution in geriatric patients, patients with hyperthyroidism, bradycardia, partial heart block, or other heart disease.
- Not a replacement for adequate volume therapy in patients with shock
- Adverse effects include reflex bradycardia, CNS effects (eg, excitement, restlessness), and rarely, arrhythmias. Hemorrhage is possible in horses.
- Blood pressure must be monitored.
- Extravasation injuries with phenylephrine can be very serious.

Uses/Indications

Phenylephrine has been used to treat hypotension and shock after adequate volume replacement in dogs, cats, horses, and sheep. Phenylephrine is rarely used in dogs but may be useful when profound vasodilation occurs, such as with septic shock. In cats, it may be useful in patients with pronounced systemic vasodilation (eg, visceral inflammation) or to increase blood pressure when increasing myocardial contractility may be disadvantageous (eg, hypertrophic cardiomyopathy).

Phenylephrine is sometimes recommended to treat hypotension secondary to general anesthesia, drug overdoses, or idiosyncratic hypotensive reactions to drugs such as phenothiazines, adrenergic blocking agents, and ganglionic blockers. Its use to treat hypotension resulting from barbiturate or other CNS depressant agents is controversial.

In horses, phenylephrine has been used as adjunctive treatment of ascending colon displacement[1]; however, one case series found that pretreatment with phenylephrine did not affect efficacy of the rolling technique or surgery for nephrosplenic entrapment of the colon,[2] and a retrospective study found that rolling was more effective than phenylephrine and exercise.[3]

Ophthalmic uses of phenylephrine include diagnostic eye examinations, reducing posterior synechiae formation, and relieving pain associated with complicated uveitis. In horses, it has also been applied intranasally in an attempt to reduce nasal congestion by reducing nasal mucous membrane thickness and upper airway resistance.

In humans, phenylephrine has been used to treat hypotension and prolong the effects of spinal anesthesia.[4,5]

Pharmacology/Actions

Phenylephrine is an alpha-1-adrenergic agonist that has predominantly postsynaptic alpha effects at therapeutic doses. Beta-adrenergic effects are typically negligible but can occur at high doses.

After IV administration, the primary effects of phenylephrine include peripheral vasoconstriction with resultant increases in diastolic and systolic blood pressure, small decreases in cardiac output, and an increase in circulation time. As mean arterial pressure increases, vagal activity also increases which can result in reflex bradycardia. Renal splanchnic, pulmonary, and cutaneous vascular beds are constricted, but coronary blood flow is increased. Its alpha effects can cause contraction of the uterus during pregnancy and constriction of uterine blood vessels.[6]

Pharmacokinetics

In humans, bioavailability after oral administration is ≈1.3%. Phenylephrine is rapidly metabolized in the GI tract, and cardiovascular effects are generally unattainable when administered orally. Following IV administration, pressor effects begin almost immediately and will persist for up to 20 minutes.

Phenylephrine is metabolized by the liver, and the effects of the drug are also terminated by uptake into tissues.

Contraindications/Precautions/Warnings

Phenylephrine is contraindicated in patients with severe hypertension, ventricular tachycardia, or those that are hypersensitive to it. It should be used with extreme caution in geriatric patients (especially horses), patients with hyperthyroidism, bradycardia, partial heart block, or other heart disease. Phenylephrine is not a replacement for adequate volume therapy in patients with shock.

Extravasation injuries with phenylephrine can be serious and result in necrosis and sloughing of surrounding tissue.[6] Monitor infusion site routinely for signs of extravasation. If extravasation occurs, infiltrate ischemic areas with a solution of phentolamine 5 – 10 mg in 10 to 15 mL of normal saline. A syringe with a fine needle should be used to infiltrate the site with many injections.

Some products contain sodium metabisulfite which can cause anaphylactic in humans.[6] Phenylephrine can cause excessive peripheral and visceral vasoconstriction and ischemia to vital organs. In humans, renal function should be monitored during use. Phenylephrine can also exacerbate underlying heart failure and increase pulmonary arterial pressure.

Adverse Effects

At recommended doses, adverse effects reported in humans include reflex bradycardia and CNS effects such as excitement and restlessness; arrhythmias have rarely been reported. Blood pressure must be monitored to prevent hypertension. Hemorrhage is possible in horses, with the highest risk in aged horses.[7]

In humans, arrythmias, decreased cardiac output, hypertensive crisis, ischemia, severe bradycardia, headache, nausea, vomiting, tremors, dyspnea, and increased pulmonary arterial pressure have been reported.[6]

Reproductive/Nursing Safety

In humans, phenylephrine crosses the placenta at term. It is unknown whether phenylephrine is excreted in maternal milk.[6]

Because safety has not been established in animals, this drug should only be used when the maternal benefits outweigh the potential risks to offspring.

Overdose/Acute Toxicity

Overdoses of phenylephrine can cause hypertension, seizures, vomiting, paresthesias, ventricular extrasystoles/tachycardia, lethargy, depression, hyperactivity, reflex bradycardia, hypertension, and cerebral hemorrhage; however, the margin of safety with phenylephrine overdose is fairly wide, especially after oral administration. Vomiting is commonly seen with overdoses. Overdose can also cause CNS stimulation including agitation, hyperactivity, and muscle tremors. Cardiovascular changes often respond well to fluids. Beta-blockers or nitroprusside may be indicated when cardiovascular signs are refractory to fluids.

For patients that have experienced or are suspected to have experienced an overdose, consultation with a 24-hour poison consultation center specializing in providing veterinary-specific information is recommended. For general information related to overdose and toxin exposures, as well as contact information for poison control centers, refer to ***Appendix.***

Drug Interactions

The following drug interactions have either been reported or are theoretical in humans or animals receiving phenylephrine systemically and may be of significance in veterinary patients. Unless otherwise noted, use together is not necessarily contraindicated, but weigh the potential risks and perform additional monitoring when appropriate.

- **Alpha-Adrenergic Receptor Antagonists** (eg, **phenothiazines, phenoxybenzamine, phentolamine**): Higher doses of phenylephrine may be required to attain a pressor effect if these agents have been used prior to therapy.
- **Anesthetics, General/Halogenated** (eg, **halothane**): Phenylephrine may potentially induce cardiac arrhythmias when used with halothane anesthesia.
- **Anticholinergics** (eg, **atropine**): Block reflex bradycardia caused by phenylephrine and can precipitate cardiac arrhythmias
- **Beta-Adrenergic Receptor Antagonists** (eg, **propranolol**): The cardiostimulatory effects of phenylephrine can be blocked.
- **Digoxin**: Use with phenylephrine may cause increased myocardial sensitization and increase risk for arrhythmias.
- **Insulins** : May decrease blood glucose lowering effect of insulin
- **Monoamine Oxidase Inhibitors** (MAOIs; eg, **amitraz, linezolid, methylene blue, selegiline**): MAOIs should not be used with phenylephrine because of a pronounced pressor effect; combination is considered contraindicated in humans.
- **Oxytocin**: When used concurrently with oxytocic agents, pressor effects may be enhanced; severe, persistent hypertension can occur.
- **Pergolide**: May enhance hypertensive effect of phenylephrine
- **Sympathomimetic Agents** (eg, **epinephrine**): Tachycardia and serious arrhythmias are possible.

Laboratory Considerations

None noted

Dosages

DOGS:

Hypotension (extra-label): 1 – 3 µg/kg/minute IV CRI; doses up to 10 µg/kg/minute IV CRI have been used.[8]

CATS:

Hypotension (extra-label): 1 – 2 µg/kg/minute IV CRI. Infusions of 1 µg/kg/minute IV CRI significantly increased mean arterial pressure without a change in cardiac output; however, at 2 µg/kg/minute, cardiac index also was increased with an increase in stroke volume index.[9]

HORSES:

Adjunctive medical treatment of ascending (large) colon displacement (extra-label): 3 µg/kg/minute IV CRI for 15 minutes; repeat every 12 hours if horse does not respond.[1]

Decrease postanesthesia intranasal airway obstruction and edema (extra-label): Dilute phenylephrine 15 mg with 0.9% sodium chloride to a final volume of 10 mL, then administer 5 mL into each nostril.[10]

Hypotension during general anesthesia (extra-label): 0.5 – 2 µg/kg/minute IV CRI. Increased blood pressure and systemic vascular resistance are seen at these doses; however, cardiac output and oxygen delivery are decreased. Phenylephrine should not be used routinely, and its use is recommended only when other treatments have failed to reverse hypotension.[11,12]

SHEEP

Hypotension due to sepsis (extra-label): 1 – 2 µg/kg/minute IV CRI resulted in increased mean arterial blood pressure and decreased heart rate in septic sheep with hypotension. Stroke volume increased but cardiac output decreased, and renal blood flow also increased.[13]

Monitoring

- Heart rate and rhythm
- Blood pressure
- Blood gases if possible
- Infusion site

Client Information

- Parenteral phenylephrine should only be used by professionals in a setting where adequate monitoring is possible.

Chemistry/Synonyms

Phenylephrine is an alpha-adrenergic sympathomimetic amine that occurs as bitter, odorless, white to off-white crystals with a melting point of 145°C to 146°C (293°F-294°F). It is freely soluble in water and alcohol. The pH of the commercially available injection is 3 to 6.5.

Phenylephrine may also be known as fenilefrina, phenylephrinum, m-synephrine, or *Neo-Synephrine®*.

Storage/Stability

The injectable product should be stored protected from light. Do not use solutions if they are brown or contain a precipitate. Oxidation of the drug can occur without a color change. To protect against oxidation, the air in commercially available ampules for injection is replaced with nitrogen and a sulfite added.

Compatibility/Compounding Considerations

Compatibility is dependent on factors such as pH, concentration, temperature, and diluent used; specialized references or a hospital pharmacist should be consulted for more specific information.

Phenylephrine is reported to be physically **compatible** with all commonly used IV solutions and the following drugs: chloramphenicol sodium succinate, dobutamine HCl, lidocaine HCl, potassium chloride, and sodium bicarbonate. Although stated to be physically **incompatible** with alkalis, it is stable with sodium bicarbonate solutions. Phenylephrine is reported to be **incompatible** with ferric salts, oxidizing agents, and metals.

Dosage Forms/Regulatory Status

VETERINARY-LABELED PRODUCTS:

The Association of Racing Commissioners International (ARCI) has designated this drug as a class 3 substance. Use of this drug may not be allowed in certain animal competitions. Check rules and regulations before entering in a competition while this medication is being administered. Contact local racing authorities for further guidance. See ***Appendix*** for more information.

HUMAN-LABELED PRODUCTS:

Phenylephrine HCl Injection: 1% (10 mg/mL); generic; (Rx)

Phenylephrine is also available in oral tablets (eg, *Sudafed PE®*), oral solutions, ophthalmic solutions, and intranasal dosage forms. It is also available in combination with antihistamines, analgesics, and decongestants for oral administration.

References

For the complete list of references, see **wiley.com/go/budde/plumb**

Phenylpropanolamine

(fen-ill-proe-pa-***nole***-a-meen) *Proin®*

Sympathomimetic

Prescriber Highlights

- Sympathomimetic used primarily to treat acquired urethral sphincter hypotonus in spayed dogs
- Should be used with caution in animals with glaucoma, prostatic hypertrophy, hyperthyroidism, diabetes mellitus, cardiovascular disorders, liver disease, hypertension or conditions that predispose to hypertension, or renal insufficiency
- Adverse effects include vomiting, hypertension, anorexia, weight loss, proteinuria, restlessness, and irritability.
- Those prescribing this drug should be aware of human abuse potential as it is a precursor to methamphetamine.

Uses/Indications

Phenylpropanolamine is FDA-approved for the control of urinary incontinence caused by urethral sphincter hypotonus in dogs.[1]

Pharmacology/Actions

It is believed that phenylpropanolamine indirectly stimulates both alpha- and, to a lesser degree, beta-adrenergic receptors of smooth muscle by causing the release of norepinephrine and inhibition of reuptake at the synaptic junction. Phenylpropanolamine's alpha-adrenergic stimulation increases urethral sphincter tone[2-6] and produces closure of the bladder neck. Prolonged use or excessive dosing frequency can deplete norepinephrine from storage sites and tachyphylaxis can occur, although this has not been documented in dogs or cats when used to treat urethral sphincter hypotonus.

Other pharmacologic effects of phenylpropanolamine include increased vasoconstriction, heart rate (although bradycardia may also occur), coronary blood flow, and blood pressure; mild CNS stimulation; and decreased nasal congestion and appetite.

Pharmacokinetics

In a study of 4 female beagles given phenylpropanolamine chewable tablets, peak concentration was reached 2 hours after administration and elimination half-life was 4 hours.[7] Extended-release phenylpropanolamine tablets result in a lower peak concentration and overall drug exposure as compared with chewable tablets.

Contraindications/Precautions/Warnings

Phenylpropanolamine is contraindicated in animals hypersensitive to it.

Because it is a sympathomimetic agent, phenylpropanolamine should be used with caution in animals with cardiovascular disease. It should also be used with caution in patients with glaucoma, prostatic hypertrophy, hyperthyroidism, diabetes mellitus, hyperadrenocorticism, liver disease, hypertension or conditions that predispose to hypertension, or renal insufficiency.[1] Phenylpropanolamine does not treat incontinence caused by UTI, anatomical abnormalities, behavioral disorders, or neurologic disease. In female dogs younger than 1 year of age, anatomical abnormalities should be ruled out prior to treatment with phenylpropanolamine.

Animals should have access to plenty of fresh water while receiving phenylpropanolamine, as it can cause increased thirst.[1]

Overdose has been associated with dogs chewing through closed bottles; store bottles securely out of reach.[1]

Human use of phenylpropanolamine has been withdrawn in the United States and Canada due to increased risk for stroke in women; it is not clear if this is applicable to veterinary patients.

Adverse Effects

Most adverse effects are dose related. Typical adverse effects include hypertension, arrhythmias, weight loss, vomiting, proteinuria, anorexia, restlessness, anxiety, irritability, increased thirst, urine retention, tachycardia or bradycardia, panting, diarrhea, and mydriasis.[1,8,9] Severe left and mild right ventricular hypertrophy have been reported in a dog receiving phenylpropanolamine long-term.[10] Effects of phenylpropanolamine on blood pressure can be seen within 2 hours of administration.[11] Hypersensitivity has been reported in rare cases.[9]

Reproductive/Nursing Safety

Drug labels in some countries outside of the United States state that phenylpropanolamine is contraindicated during pregnancy.[9] Phenylpropanolamine may cause decreased ovum implantation; however, uncontrolled clinical experience has not demonstrated any untoward effects during pregnancy.

Safe use during lactation has not been studied. Drug labels in other countries state that it should not be administered to pregnant or lactating dogs.[1,9]

Because safety has not been established in animals, this drug should only be used when the maternal benefits outweigh the potential risks to offspring.

Overdose/Acute Toxicity

Clinical signs of overdose may consist of an exacerbation of the adverse effects listed above. In the case of a very large overdose, severe cardiovascular effects (ie, hypertension to rebound hypotension, bradycardias to tachycardias, cardiovascular collapse) or CNS effects (ie, stimulation to coma) may occur.

In a case report of a dog ingesting phenylpropanolamine 56 – 69 mg/kg, clinical signs included anxiety, piloerection, mucosal ulceration, mydriasis, hyphema, and retinal detachment.[8] Laboratory findings included elevated creatine kinase (CK) and AST, proteinuria, and pigmenturia; cardiac arrhythmia (eg, ventricular tachycardia) and severe systemic hypertension were also noted. Ventricular tachycardia and hypertension were successfully treated with phenoxybenzamine, sotalol, esmolol, and nitroprusside.

Survival rate in a 2011 retrospective case study of phenylpropanolamine overdose in dogs was 99.4%, with one death out of 170 dogs studied.[12] Adverse effects were dose dependent. Thirty-nine percent of dogs studied experienced no clinical signs, and the median dose ingested for dogs that experienced no clinical signs was 18 mg/kg. Median dose for dogs that experienced adverse effects was 37.3 mg/kg. For the dogs that developed clinical signs, most developed signs within 8 hours of ingestion. Common signs included agitation, vomiting, lethargy, tremor or twitching, adverse cardiac effects, and erythema. Most dogs did well with decontamination and supportive care. The dog that died had ingested multiple medications from the trash; the exact amount of phenylpropanolamine ingested was not known but could have been as much as 145 mg/kg.[12]

If the overdose was within 2 to 3 hours before presentation, the stomach should be emptied using the usual precautions and activated charcoal with a cathartic administered. Clinical signs should be treated supportively as they occur. Propranolol, a nonspecific beta-blocker, should *not* be used to treat hypertension in bradycardic patients, and atropine should *not* be used to treat bradycardia. Use of alpha-adrenergic blockers (eg, acepromazine [low dose such as 0.02 mg/kg IV or IM]) may be appropriate in cases of hypertension caused by a severe overdose.[9] If phenothiazines do not normalize blood pressure, a nitroprusside IV CRI can be considered.

For patients that have experienced or are suspected to have experienced an overdose, consultation with a 24-hour poison consultation center specializing in providing veterinary-specific information is recommended. For general information related to overdose and toxin exposures, as well as contact information for poison control centers, refer to ***Appendix***.

Drug Interactions

The following drug interactions have either been reported or are theoretical in humans or animals receiving phenylpropanolamine and may be of significance in veterinary patients. Unless otherwise noted, use together is not necessarily contraindicated, but the potential risks should be weighed and additional monitoring performed when appropriate.

- **Aspirin**: Phenylpropanolamine may potentiate decreased platelet aggregation.[1]
- **Estriol**: In a study of female dogs receiving estriol, the addition of phenylpropanolamine did not result in further increases of urethral resistance.[13]
- **Isoflurane, Desflurane, and Sevoflurane**: Phenylpropanolamine may increase potential for cardiac arrhythmias; use combination with caution.
- **Monoamine Oxidase Inhibitors** (MAOIs; eg, **amitraz, linezolid, selegiline**): Phenylpropanolamine should not be given within 2 weeks of a patient receiving MAO inhibitors, as concurrent use may result in severe hypertension. Combination is contraindicated in humans.[1,9] NOTE: In one small study, selegiline and phenylpropanolamine were used together in healthy dogs without noticeable adverse effects.[14]
- **Reserpine**: Phenylpropanolamine may reduce the antihypertensive effect of reserpine.
- **Sympathomimetic Agents, Other** (eg, **ephedrine**): Phenylpropanolamine should not be administered with other sympathomimetic agents, as increased toxicity may result.
- **Tricyclic Antidepressants** (eg, **amitriptyline, clomipramine**): Concurrent use increases the risk for hypertension and arrhythmias.

Laboratory Considerations

None noted

Dosages

DOGS:

Control of urinary incontinence due to urethral sphincter hypotonus (label dosage, FDA-approved):

Immediate-release formulation: 2 mg/kg PO twice daily. The dose should be calculated in half-tablet increments.[1]

Extended-release formulation: 2 – 4 mg/kg PO once daily with food.[15] Dogs weighing less than 4.5 kg (10 lb) cannot be safely dosed with available tablet sizes. Dogs weighing more than 56.8 kg (125 lb) should receive the appropriate combination of tablets. Tablets should not be split or crushed.

Control of urinary incontinence due to urethral sphincter hypotonus (extra-label): 1.5 mg/kg twice daily.[16-18] Some dogs may require administration every 8 hours (eg, 0.8 mg/kg PO 3 times daily[9]), and some may respond adequately to once-daily administration[19]

Retrograde ejaculation (extra-label): 3 – 4 mg/kg PO twice daily may be tried.[20]

CATS:

Control of urinary incontinence due to urethral sphincter hypotonus (extra-label): From a case report, 1.5 mg/kg PO once daily.[21] Anecdotally, 1 – 2.2 mg/kg PO 2 to 3 times daily; practically, 12.5 mg/cat (NOT mg/kg) PO 2 to 3 times a daily

Monitoring

- Clinical effectiveness
- Adverse effects
- Baseline blood pressure (BP) and soon after initiating therapy or increasing the dose. BP should be monitored twice a year in animals that are predisposed to hypertension or have comorbid conditions that may be impacted by hypertension.[22]

Client Information

- Improvement in incontinence may not be apparent until several days after beginning treatment.
- If your pet is incontinent at night, give the largest dose at night before sleeping.
- May be given with or without food; however, giving it with food may help if your animal vomits or acts sick after getting the drug on an empty stomach.
- If you miss a dose, give it as soon as you remember. If it is close to the time for the next dose, skip the dose you missed and give it at the next scheduled time. After that, return to the regular dosing schedule. Do not give 2 doses at once or give extra doses.
- May cause increased thirst; provide ample fresh water.
- Tablets are liver flavored, so keep out of reach of animals and children. Instances of dogs chewing through closed bottles and ingesting the contents have been reported. Contact your veterinarian immediately if your dog ingests more than the prescribed dose.

Chemistry/Synonyms

Phenylpropanolamine HCl, a sympathomimetic amine analogue, occurs as a white crystalline powder with a slightly aromatic odor. It has a melting range between 191°C and 194°C (375.8°F-381.2°F) and a pK_a of 9.4. One gram is soluble in ≈1.1 mL of water or 7 mL of alcohol.

Phenylpropanolamine may also be known as (±)-norephedrine, dl-norephedrine, PPA, *Cystolamine*®, *Proin*®, *Propalin*®, *Uricon*®, *Urilin*®, and *Uriflex-PT*®.

Storage/Stability

Store phenylpropanolamine products in light-resistant, tight containers at controlled room temperature (20°C-25°C [68°F-77°F]). Excursions between 15°C and 40°C (59°F-104°F) are permitted. Phenylpropanolamine syrup (available outside the United States) should be discarded 3 months after first use.

Dosage Forms/Regulatory Status

VETERINARY-LABELED PRODUCTS:

Phenylpropanolamine Chewable Tablets: 25 mg, 50 mg, and 75 mg; *Proin*®; (Rx). FDA-approved for use in dogs. NADA# 141-324

Phenylpropanolamine Extended-Release Tablets: 18 mg, 38 mg, 74 mg, and 145 mg; *Proin ER*®; (Rx). FDA-approved for use in dogs. NADA# 141-517

Phenylpropanolamine Oral Liquid: 50 mg/mL; *Propalin*®; (Rx). Approved in Australia, Canada, and the United Kingdom for use in dogs. Not available in the United States

The Association of Racing Commissioners International (ARCI) has designated this drug as a class 3 substance. Use of this drug may not be allowed in certain animal competitions. Check rules and regulations before entering in a competition while this medication is being administered. Contact local racing authorities for further guidance. See ***Appendix*** for more information.

In the United States, phenylpropanolamine is classified as a list 1 chemical (drugs that can be used as precursors to manufacture methamphetamine), and in some states, it may be a controlled substance or have other restrictions placed on its sale. Those prescribing this medication should be alert to persons desiring to purchase this medication.

HUMAN-LABELED PRODUCTS:

NOTE: Because of potential adverse effects in humans, phenylpropanolamine has been removed from the United States market for human use.

References

For the complete list of references, see **wiley.com/go/budde/plumb**

Pheromones

(***fer***-i-mones) *Feliway*®, *D.A.P.*®, *Adaptil*®, *Comfort Zone*®
Pheromone Behavior Modifier

Prescriber Highlights

- ► May be useful in cats, dogs, and horses for a variety of behavioral concerns
- ► May need adjunctive therapy such as behavior modification or drug therapy for treating unwanted behaviors
- ► Dog and cat products are administered environmentally; the equine product is administered at the base of the nostrils.

Uses/Indications

Pheromones may be useful as adjunct therapy for a variety of behavioral concerns in dogs, cats, and horses. Behavioral modification and/or concomitant drug therapy may be required.

In dogs, pheromone products may be useful for treating behaviors associated with fear or stress (eg, separation anxiety, destruction, excessive barking, house soiling, licking, phobias) or calming animals in new environments or situations.

In cats, feline facial pheromones may be useful for treating urine marking or spraying, vertical scratching, avoidance of social contact, loss of appetite, stressful situations, or inter-cat aggression; it may also be useful for reducing tension or conflict between cats in the same household.

In horses, pheromones may be useful for reducing stress in situations such as transport, shoeing, clipping, new environments, or training.

Pharmacology/Actions

Appeasing pheromones are thought to be produced during nursing by all mammals. They are detected by the Jacobson's organ or vomero-nasal organ (VNO). The VNO is more sensitive in young animals but is believed to continue to function in older animals as well. It is not well understood what neurotransmitters or neurochemical processes are involved for pheromones to exhibit their effects. In most animals, pheromones have a general calming effect. In cats, the F3 facial pheromone is thought to inhibit urine marking, encourage feeding, and enhance exploratory behaviors in unfamiliar situations. The F4 pheromone is an allomarking pheromone that calms and familiarizes the cat with its surroundings.

Pharmacokinetics

No information was located.

Contraindications/Precautions/Warnings

Do not touch diffusers with wet hands or metal objects while plugged in. Do not touch diffuser with uncovered hands during or immediately after use. Never use diffusers with extension cords or adaptors.

Do not spray products directly onto animals.[1,2]

Reproductive Safety

No risks are expected following inhalation of pheromone products.

Adverse Effects

No adverse effects have been reported.

Overdose/Acute Toxicity

No specific animal toxicity data were located. Do **not** induce vomiting if ingested.[2,3] Although pheromone products are considered non-toxic, humans that are accidentally exposed and experiencing adverse reactions should report to a physician or poison control center.

For patients that have experienced or are suspected to have experienced an overdose, consultation with a 24-hour poison consultation center specializing in providing veterinary-specific information is recommended. For general information related to overdose and

toxin exposures, as well as contact information for poison control centers, refer to ***Appendix***.

Drug Interactions

- Effects may be reduced or negated by concurrent administration of drugs that cause CNS stimulation.

Laboratory Considerations

- No information was located.

Dosages

DOGS:

Provide calming and comfort during stressful situations (label use; not FDA-approved): Using a canine appeasing pheromone product:

a) Diffuser: Plug diffuser into electric outlet in the room where dogs spend the most time.[4] Ensure airflow from the diffuser is not covered or obstructed. Diffuser vial lasts ≈4 weeks and covers 700 sq ft. Effects are not immediate as diffuser may require up to 72 hours to saturate area.

b) Collar: Apply collar with enough room for 2 fingers between the collar and the neck.[5] Collar should be worn continuously and lasts ≈30 days.

Provide comfort during travel (label use; not FDA-approved): Using a canine appeasing pheromone product.

Spray: Spray 8 pumps per treatment area 10 minutes before travel.[1] May spray in car and kennels or on collars, leashes, bandanas, and blankets; wait 10 minutes after application before introducing dogs to treated items or environment. Application lasts ≈4 to 5 hours.

CATS:

Provide calming and comfort to reduce unwanted behaviors (label use; not FDA-approved): Using a feline facial pheromone (F3) product:

Diffuser: Plug diffuser into electric outlet in an area where cats spend the most time or where spraying behavior occurs.[3] Ensure airflow from the diffuser is not covered or obstructed. Diffuser vial lasts ≈4 weeks and covers 700 sq ft. Effects are not immediate as diffuser may require up to 72 hours to saturate the area.

Spray: Spray 5 to 8 pumps per treatment area 15 minutes prior to introducing cat into the treated environment.[2,6] May be applied to bedding, carriers, or areas of the home that are affected by spraying or scratching behaviors. Spray lasts ≈4 to 5 hours and may be re-applied as needed. For urine spraying behaviors, area should be sprayed at least once daily. If cat is observed rubbing its own facial pheromones onto a spot, treatment is no longer necessary at that location.

Reduce tension and conflict between cats (label use; not FDA-approved): Using a feline facial pheromone (F3) product:

Diffuser: Plug diffuser into an electric outlet in an area where cats spend the most time, ensuring airflow from the diffuser is not covered or obstructed.[7] One diffuser covers 700 sq ft and contents last ≈30 days. Diffusers should be replaced after 6 months. Inter-cat aggression problems may also require behavior modification and concomitant drug therapy.

HORSES:

Reduce or prevent situational stress (label use; not FDA-approved): Apply gel from 1 packet to the base of the nostril 30 minutes before anticipated stressful situation.[8] Takes effect in 30 minutes and lasts 2.5 hours; may be re-applied as needed.

Monitoring

- Clinical efficacy

Client Information

- This product may be useful in treating behaviors associated with stress and anxiety.
- Administered to dogs and cats by sprays, diffusers, and collars.
- Administered to horses via gel at the base of the nostrils.
- No known side effects.

Chemistry

Mammalian pheromones are fatty acids. Canine appeasing pheromone is a synthetic derivative of bitch intermammary pheromone. Feline pheromone is a synthetic analog of feline cheek gland secretions (feline facial pheromone; FFP). The commercially available product available in the US is an analog of the F3 fraction of the pheromone. Equine appeasing pheromone (EAP) is derived from maternal pheromones found in the "wax area" close to the mammae of nursing mares.

Storage/Stability

Unless otherwise labeled, store at room temperature and do not mix with other ingredients or substances. Keep products out of reach of children.

Compatibility/Compounding Considerations

No specific information was noted.

Dosage Forms/Regulatory Status

VETERINARY-LABELED PRODUCTS:

NOTE: These products have not been evaluated for safety or efficacy by the FDA.

Canine products

Canine Appeasing Pheromone Diffuser: Canine Appeasing Pheromone 2% in 48 mL vials; *Adaptil® Calm Diffuser*; (OTC)

Canine Appeasing Pheromone (DAP) Spray: Canine Appeasing Pheromone 2% in 60 mL bottles; *Adpatil® Travel Spray*; (OTC)

Caine Appeasing Pheromone Collar: Canine Appeasing Pheromone 5% in 3 collar sizes; *Adaptil® Calm Collar*; (OTC)

Feline products

Feline Facial Pheromone (FFP-F3 fraction) Diffuser: FFP 2% in 48 mL vials; *Feliway® Classic Diffuser*; (OTC)

Feline Facial Pheromone (FFP-F3 fraction) Spray: 10% in 60 mL bottles; *Feliway® Classic Spray*; (OTC)

Cat Appeasing Pheromone (CAP) Diffuser: CAP 2% in a 48 mL vial; *Feliway®* MultiCat Diffuser; (OTC)

Feline Pheromone (unspecified) Diffuser: 5% in 48 mL vials; *Comfort Zone® Calming Diffuser*; *Comfort Zone® Multi-Cat Diffuser*; (OTC)

Feline Pheromone (unspecified) Spray: 15% in 60 mL and 120 mL bottles; *Comfort Zone® Spray and Scratch Control*; (OTC)

Equine products

Equine Appeasing Pheromone (EAP) Gel: 1% gel 5 mL packets, *Confidence EQ®*; (OTC)

HUMAN-LABELED PRODUCTS: NONE

References

For the complete list of references, see **wiley.com/go/budde/plumb**

Phosphate (Potassium-, Sodium-), IV

(*fos*-fayt)

Electrolyte

Prescriber Highlights

- ▶ Used for treatment or prevention of acute, severe hypophosphatemia
- ▶ Available as either sodium or potassium salts
- ▶ Contraindications include hyperphosphatemia, hypocalcemia, oliguric renal failure, and tissue necrosis.
- ▶ Hyperkalemia is a contraindication for *potassium* phosphate; hypernatremia is a contraindication for *sodium* phosphate.
- ▶ Use with caution in animals with cardiac (especially if receiving digoxin) or renal disease.
- ▶ Adverse effects include hyperphosphatemia, hypocalcemia, hypotension, renal failure, or soft tissue mineralization; hyperkalemia or hypernatremia are possible.
- ▶ Must be diluted prior to administration

Uses/Indications

Parenteral phosphate is used to correct or prevent hypophosphatemia when adequate oral phosphorous intake is not possible. Parenteral phosphate is typically recommended when serum phosphorous is less than 1.5 mg/dL or less than 2 mg/dL if concurrent clinical signs (eg, hemolysis, ileus, rhabdomyolysis, decreased contractility, platelet dysfunction) are present. Acute, severe hypophosphatemia can cause hemolytic anemia, thrombocytopenia, neuromuscular and CNS disorders, bone and joint pain, and decompensation in patients with cirrhotic liver disease.

Pharmacology/Actions

Phosphorous is involved in several functions in the body, including calcium metabolism, acid-base buffering, B-vitamin utilization, bone deposition, and several enzyme systems.

Pharmacokinetics

Phosphate administered IV is eliminated by the kidneys. It is glomerularly filtered, but up to 80% is reabsorbed by the tubules.[1]

Contraindications/Precautions/Warnings

Potassium and sodium phosphates are contraindicated in patients with hyperphosphatemia, hypercalcemia or significant hypocalcemia, oliguric renal failure, and patients with tissue necrosis. Potassium phosphate is contraindicated in patients with hyperkalemia[2]; sodium phosphate is contraindicated in patients with hypernatremia.[3]

Sodium and potassium phosphates should be used with caution in patients with cardiac or renal disease. Use potassium phosphate with extreme caution in patients receiving digoxin, as life-threatening hyperkalemia may result.

In humans, undiluted or rapid IV administration has resulted in seizures, cardiac arrhythmias, cardiac arrest, and death.[2]

Adverse Effects

Oversupplementation with parenteral phosphate can result in hypocalcemia, hypotension, renal failure, or soft tissue mineralization. Either hyperkalemia or hypernatremia may occur in susceptible patients.

Reproductive/Nursing Safety

Safety has not been established in animals; this drug should only be used when the maternal benefits outweigh the potential risks to offspring.

Overdose/Acute Toxicity

Phosphorous intoxication may result in hypocalcemia that manifests as hypocalcemic tetany.[2,3] Stop phosphate infusion in patients that are developing hyperphosphatemia secondary to parenteral phosphate therapy and administer appropriate parenteral calcium therapy to restore serum calcium levels. Monitor serum potassium and treat if required.

For patients that have experienced or are suspected to have experienced an overdose, consultation with a 24-hour poison consultation center specializing in providing veterinary-specific information is recommended. For general information related to overdose and toxin exposures, as well as contact information for poison control centers, refer to ***Appendix***.

Drug Interactions

The following drug interactions have either been reported or are theoretical in humans or animals receiving phosphate and may be of significance in veterinary patients. Unless otherwise noted, use together is not necessarily contraindicated, but weigh the potential risks and perform additional monitoring when appropriate.

- **Angiotensin Converting Enzyme Inhibitors (ACEIs;** eg, **benazepril, enalapril**): May result in hyperkalemia when used with potassium phosphate
- **Digoxin**: Potassium phosphate must be used with extreme caution in patients taking digoxin, as life-threatening hyperkalemia can result; do not use in digitalized patients with heart block.
- **Potassium Sparing Diuretics** (eg, **spironolactone**): May result in hyperkalemia when used with potassium phosphate

Dosages

NOTE: Sodium and potassium phosphate injections **must be diluted** before IV administration. Dilute in a calcium-free IV fluid such as 0.9% sodium chloride or 5% dextrose (ie, **NOT** lactated Ringer's solution [LRS]).

DOGS/CATS:

Hypophosphatemia (extra-label): Sodium or potassium phosphate 0.01 – 0.03 mmol/kg/hour IV CRI is typically suggested.[4] For diabetic ketoacidosis (DKA), dosages ranging up to 0.12 mmol/kg/hour have been noted.[5] When treating DKA, it is sometimes recommended to provide ⅓ to ½ of the supplemented phosphate as potassium phosphate due to the concurrent need for potassium supplementation in these patients.[6] **NOTE**: When using this protocol, it is important to account for all sources of potassium being administered to the patient in the overall fluid therapy plan to minimize the risk for hyperkalemia. Monitor serum phosphorous levels every 4 to 6 hours initially and adjust infusion rate to maintain serum phosphorous above 2 mg/dL. Use caution not to induce hyperphosphatemia. Correct the underlying cause for hypophosphatemia if possible. Once patient is stabilized and phosphorous levels are maintained above 2 to 2.5 mg/dL, consider transitioning to oral phosphate if continued supplementation is needed.

Monitoring

- Serum inorganic phosphorous
- Serum electrolytes, including calcium, potassium, and sodium

Chemistry

Potassium phosphate injection is a combination of 224 mg of monobasic potassium phosphate and 236 mg of dibasic potassium phosphate. The pH of the injection is 6.5 to 7.5 and has an osmolarity of ≈7700 mOsm/L.[2]

Sodium phosphate injection is a combination of 276 mg of monobasic sodium phosphate and 142 mg of dibasic sodium phosphate. The pH of the injection is 5.5 and has an osmolarity of ≈7000 mOsm/L.[3]

Because commercial preparations are a combination of monobasic and dibasic forms, dosages are calculated in mmol of phosphate.

Storage/Stability

Potassium and sodium phosphate injections should be stored at room temperature and protected from freezing.

Compatibility/Compounding Considerations

Compatibility is dependent on factors such as pH, concentration, temperature, and diluent used; specialized references or a hospital pharmacist should be consulted for more specific information.

Potassium phosphate injection is reportedly physically **compatible** with the following IV solutions and drugs: 4% amino acids/25% dextrose, 2.5% to 10% dextrose injection, 0.45% to 0.9% sodium chloride, magnesium sulfate, metoclopramide HCl, and verapamil HCl.

Phosphates may be physically **incompatible** with metals such as calcium and magnesium.

Potassium phosphate injection is reportedly physically **incompatible** with the following solutions or drugs: 2.5% dextrose in half-strength lactated Ringer's solution (LRS), 5% dextrose in Ringer's, 10% dextrose in 0.9% sodium chloride, Ringer's injection, LRS, and dobutamine HCl.

Dosage Forms/Regulatory Status

VETERINARY-LABELED PRODUCTS: NONE

There are no FDA-approved parenteral phosphate products for veterinary use and no veterinary phosphate-only injectable products. There are several proprietary phosphate-containing products labeled for large animal species that may also include calcium, magnesium, potassium, and/or dextrose; refer to the individual product labeling for specific dosage information. Trade names for these products include *Magnadex*®, *Norcalciphos*®, *Cal-Dextro*® *Special* and *#2*, *CMPK*®, and *Cal-Phos*® *#2*; (Rx)

HUMAN-LABELED PRODUCTS:

Potassium Phosphates (monobasic/dibasic) Injection: Each mL contains monobasic potassium phosphate 175 mg and dibasic potassium phosphate 300 mg and provides phosphorous 3 mmol (93 mg) and potassium 4.7 mEq (184 mg); available in 15 mL vials; generic; (Rx)

Potassium Phosphates (monobasic/dibasic) Injection: Each mL contains monobasic potassium phosphate 224 mg and dibasic potassium phosphate 236 mg and provides phosphorous 3 mmol (93 mg) and potassium 4.4 mEq (172 mg); available in 15 mL vials; generic; (Rx)

Sodium Phosphate Injection: Each mL contains monobasic sodium phosphate monohydrate 276 mg and dibasic sodium phosphate, anhydrous, 142 mg, and provides phosphorous 3 mmol (93 mg) and sodium 4 mEq (92 mg); available in 5 mL, 15 mL, and 50 mL vials; generic; (Rx)

References

For the complete list of references, see **wiley.com/go/budde/plumb**

Physostigmine

(fye-zoh-***stig***-meen) *Antilirium*®

Cholinesterase Inhibitor

Prescriber Highlights

- ▶ May be used as a diagnostic aid for ivermectin toxicity in dogs and narcolepsy in dogs and horses. May be useful to improve recovery after isoflurane anesthesia in horses and to treat tall larkspur poisoning in cattle
- ▶ Enters the CNS and is therefore effective for treating central anticholinergic toxicity; however, it is not recommended for use as an antidote due to availability of safer alternatives
- ▶ Contraindications include hypersensitivity reactions, asthma, gangrene, diabetes mellitus, cardiovascular disease, mechanical obstruction of the GI or urinary tract, and vagotonic states.
- ▶ Adverse effects are cholinergic in nature; diarrhea and colic are possible in horses. Cholinergic crisis can occur with high doses; must be administered with direct patient supervision as adverse effects can be serious

Uses/Indications

Physostigmine has been used as a diagnostic aid for ivermectin toxicity in dogs and narcolepsy in dogs[1] and horses.[2,3] It has been used to treat experimentally induced anticholinergic toxicity in dogs[4] and to antagonize CNS depressant effects of benzodiazepines in humans; however, use as an antidote in animals is not recommended due to potential serious adverse effects and availability of safer alternatives, such as neostigmine and pyridostigmine.

One small study in horses demonstrated that physostigmine, but not neostigmine, may be useful for improving recovery and reducing emergence delirium after general anesthesia with isoflurane.[5]

Physostigmine has been used in cattle to treat tall larkspur (*Delphinium barbeyi*) poisoning.[6,7]

Pharmacology/Actions

Physostigmine reversibly inhibits the breakdown of acetylcholine by acetylcholinesterase, thereby prolonging the effect of acetylcholine at receptor sites. Physostigmine is a tertiary amine that crosses the blood–brain barrier and therefore inhibits acetylcholinesterase both centrally and peripherally. This distinguishes physostigmine from quaternary amine cholinesterase inhibitors (eg, neostigmine, pyridostigmine) that cannot cross the blood–brain barrier.

Pharmacologic effects of physostigmine include miosis, bronchial constriction, hypersalivation, muscle weakness, and sweating (in species with sweat glands). At higher doses, a cholinergic crisis can occur. See ***Adverse Effects***.

Pharmacokinetics

Physostigmine is rapidly absorbed from subcutaneous tissue and mucous membranes. After parenteral administration, physostigmine readily crosses the blood–brain barrier into the CNS. Peak effects occur within 5 minutes after IV administration and ≈25 minutes after IM administration. The mean elimination half-life in dogs is ≈30 minutes. The majority of the administered drug is rapidly metabolized via hydrolysis by cholinesterases. Very small amounts can be eliminated unchanged into the urine. The duration of pharmacologic effect can range from 30 minutes to 5 hours with an average duration of 30 to 60 minutes. After administration of 0.1 mg/kg IV to beagles, maximal inhibition of cholinesterase (78%) in plasma occurred at 2 minutes; cholinesterase activity in plasma was still 60% inhibited at 45 minutes.[8]

Contraindications/Precautions/Warnings

Physostigmine is contraindicated in patients with prior hypersensitivity reactions to it or sulfites, bronchoconstrictive disease (asthma), gangrene, diabetes mellitus, cardiovascular disease, mechanical obstruction of the GI or urinary tract, and patients in vagotonic states.

Use of physostigmine in the absence of anticholinergic toxicity or for treatment of tricyclic or tetracyclic antidepressant overdoses increases risk for a cholinergic crisis. Rapid IV administration increases the potential for bradycardia, hypersalivation, and seizures. In humans, it should be given IV at a slow, controlled rate not exceeding 1 mg/minute in adults or 0.5 mg/minute in children.[9]

Because of the risks for toxicity, atropine should be readily available (see ***Overdose/Acute Toxicity***).

Physostigmine injection contains benzyl alcohol that may be toxic in neonatal animals.

Do not confuse PHYSOstigmine with PYRIDOstigmine or phytosophingosine. Consider writing part of the drug's name in uppercase letters (tall man designations) on prescriptions/orders to reduce the risk of errors.

Adverse Effects

Adverse effects of physostigmine include hypersensitivity and cholinergic effects. Cholinergic effects are dose-related and include miosis, bronchial constriction, hypersalivation, muscle weakness, and sweating (in species with sweat glands). In horses, diarrhea or colic are also possible.[10]

At higher doses, a cholinergic crisis can occur with clinical signs such as seizures, bradycardia, tachycardia, hypotension, asystole, nausea, vomiting, diarrhea, depolarizing neuromuscular block, pulmonary edema, and respiratory paralysis.

In humans, bradycardia and convulsions can occur if IV administration is too rapid.[9]

Reproductive/Nursing Safety

Limited information is available, but physostigmine would be expected to cross the placenta. Behavioral, biochemical, and metabolic teratogenic effects have been observed in mice studies. It is unknown if physostigmine enters milk. Because safety has not been established in animals, this drug should only be used when the maternal benefits outweigh the potential risks to offspring.

Overdose/Acute Toxicity

The IV LD_{50} in cats is 0.66 mg/kg.[11] Overdoses or acute toxicity can result in a cholinergic crisis, which can be life-threatening (see ***Adverse Effects***); however, because of the short duration of effect, supportive care may be sufficient. Treatment of serious acute toxicity includes mechanical ventilation, repeated bronchial aspiration, and administration of IV atropine. See ***Atropine***. Readministration of atropine may be required. Pralidoxime (2-PAM) may be useful to reverse the ganglionic and skeletal muscle effects of physostigmine. See ***Pralidoxime***.

For patients that have experienced or are suspected to have experienced an overdose, consultation with a 24-hour poison consultation center specializing in providing veterinary-specific information is recommended. For general information related to overdose and toxin exposures, as well as contact information for poison control centers, refer to ***Appendix***.

Drug Interactions

The following drug interactions have either been reported or are theoretical in humans or animals receiving physostigmine and may be of significance in veterinary patients. Unless otherwise noted, use together is not necessarily contraindicated, but weigh the potential risks and perform additional monitoring when appropriate.

- **ANTICHOLINERGICS** (eg, **atropine, glycopyrrolate**): Concurrent use may diminish the effects of physostigmine and the anticholinergic agent.
- **ANTIDEPRESSANTS, TRICYCLIC, TETRACYCLIC** (eg, **clomipramine, mirtazapine**): Concurrent use may diminish the effects of physostigmine and the anticholinergic agent.
- **CHOLINE ESTERS** (eg, **bethanechol, carbachol, methacholine**): Concurrent use may cause additive adverse effects; monitor for signs of toxicity.
- **INHALATION ANESTHETICS**: The efficacy of anticholinesterases in reversing neuromuscular blockade may be impaired by inhalation anesthetics.
- **ORGANOPHOSPHATES**: May cause additive adverse effects.
- **SUCCINYLCHOLINE**: May increase succinylcholine concentrations and prolong neuromuscular blockade; avoid concurrent use

Laboratory Considerations

- None noted

Dosages

DOGS:

Temporarily reverse the CNS effects of ivermectin toxicosis to support the diagnosis (extra-label): 1 mg/dog (NOT mg/kg) IV once[12]

Provocative test for narcolepsy/cataplexy (extra-label): 0.025 – 0.1 mg/kg IV increases the chance of cataplexy occurring within 15 minutes for mild cases.[13] Starting at the low end of the range is recommended.

HORSES:

Provocative test to diagnose cataplexy or narcolepsy (extra-label): 0.05 – 0.1 mg/kg IV slowly will precipitate a cataplectic attack within 3 to 10 minutes after administration in affected horses.[10,14] A lack of positive response does not rule out the diagnosis of narcolepsy as the response may be variable, even with repeated doses in the same animal.

Improve recovery after isoflurane anesthesia (extra-label): 0.04 mg/kg IV over 8 to 10 minutes during the anesthetic weaning process prior to moving to the recovery stall[1]

CATTLE:

Reversal of clinical effects caused by tall larkspur (*Delphinium barbeyi*) poisoning (extra-label): 0.04 – 0.08 mg/kg IV reversal lasts ≈2 hours and multiple doses may be necessary.[6,7]

Monitoring

- Adverse effects such as miosis, bronchial constriction, hypersalivation, muscle weakness, and sweating (in species with sweat glands); colic and diarrhea in horses
- Heart rate and rhythm
- Blood pressure

Client Information

- This medication is administered in a hospital setting with close monitoring.

Chemistry/Synonyms

Physostigmine salicylate is made from an extract of *Physostigma venenosum* (Calabar bean) seeds. It occurs as white, shiny, odorless crystals or crystalline powder. Degradation occurs upon exposure to heat, light, air, or exposure to traces of metals for a long period, causing a red tint to develop. Solutions for injection use should not be used if more than slightly discolored. One gram is soluble in 75 mL of water or 16 mL of alcohol. The injection has a pH of 3.5 to 5.

Physostigmine salicylate may also be known as eserine salicylate, physostigmine monosalicylate, and *Anticholium*®.

Storage/Stability

Store the injection (ampules) below 40°C (104°F); preferably between 15°C and 30°C (59°F-86°F). Protect this product from light and freezing.

Compatibility/Compounding Considerations

Physostigmine is administered undiluted in humans. It may be given

IV via a Y-site or stopcock port on IV sets but should **not** be added to IV solutions.

Dosage Forms/Regulatory Status

VETERINARY-LABELED PRODUCTS: NONE

The Association of Racing Commissioners International (ARCI) has designated this drug as a class 3 substance. Use of this drug may not be allowed in certain animal competitions. Check rules and regulations before entering a competition while this medication is being administered. Contact local racing authorities for further guidance. See ***Appendix*** for more information.

HUMAN-LABELED PRODUCTS:

Physostigmine Salicylate Injection: 1 mg/mL (contains benzyl alcohol 2% and 0.1% sodium metabisulfite) in 1 mL ampules; generic; (Rx; not FDA-approved)

References

For the complete list of references, see **wiley.com/go/budde/plumb**

Phytonadione

Vitamin K_1

(fye-toe-na-***dye***-ohne) *Mephyton®*

Antidote, Fat Soluble Vitamin

Prescriber Highlights

- ► Used for the treatment of anticoagulant rodenticide toxicity, dicumarol toxicity associated with sweet clover ingestion in ruminants, sulfaquinoxaline toxicity, and bleeding disorders associated with faulty formation of vitamin K-dependent coagulation factors
- ► Contraindicated in patients with hypersensitivity; does not correct hypoprothrombinemia due to hepatocellular damage
- ► Adverse effects include severe reactions that resemble hypersensitivity reactions after IV administration; IM use may result in acute bleeding at the injection site during the early stages of treatment. SC injections or PO doses may be slowly or poorly absorbed in hypovolemic animals.
- ► May require 6 to 12 hours for effect. When dosing orally, absorption is significantly enhanced when given with a meal.
- ► Small-gauge needles are recommended for use when injecting SC or IM.

Uses/Indications

The principal use of exogenously administered phytonadione (ie, vitamin K_1) is in the treatment of anticoagulant rodenticide toxicity. Phytonadione is also used for treatment of dicumarol toxicity associated with sweet clover ingestion in ruminants, sulfaquinoxaline toxicity, and bleeding disorders associated with faulty formation of vitamin K-dependent coagulation factors (eg, liver failure). Disorders of fat absorption can lead to decreased vitamin K absorption, including inflammatory bowel disease, exocrine pancreatic insufficiency, and bile duct obstruction. In cases of anticoagulant rodenticide ingestion, GI decontamination within 6 hours of oral ingestion may reduce the need for phytonadione therapy.[1]

Pharmacology/Actions

Vitamin K is a cofactor in hepatic activation of blood coagulation factors II (ie, prothrombin), VII, IX, and X, as well as anticoagulant proteins C and S. Without vitamin K, these coagulation proteins remain inactivated and thus nonfunctional. Intestinal microorganisms produce small amounts of endogenous vitamin K.[2,3] Exogenous phytonadione appears to have a pharmacologic effect only in vitamin K-deficient patients; it appears to have no effect in normal, healthy patients.[4] In humans, vitamin K storage is much less than that of other fat-soluble vitamins, and reserves may be rapidly depleted.[4]

Increases in clotting factors may not occur until 6 to 12 hours after oral administration but may be detected within 1 to 2 hours after parenteral administration.[4,5]

Vitamin K also appears to be necessary for bone mineralization and cell growth regulation[6] and possibly for CNS sphingolipid metabolism.[7]

Pharmacokinetics

Phytonadione is absorbed from the GI tract in monogastric animals via the intestinal lymphatics in the jejunum and ileum, only in the presence of bile salts. Oral absorption of phytonadione may be significantly enhanced by giving the drug with food. The relative oral bioavailability of vitamin K is increased 4 to 5 times when given to dogs with canned food. Phytonadione is readily absorbed after IM administration.[4]

In humans, oral administration may be more rapidly absorbed than SC administration.

Phytonadione may concentrate in the liver for a short period but is not appreciably stored in the liver or other tissue; its elimination is not well understood.

Contraindications/Precautions/Warnings

Phytonadione is labeled as contraindicated in patients hypersensitive to it or any component of its formulation.

After oral phytonadione administration, new clotting factors can take up to 6 to 12 hours to be synthesized; therefore, in an emergency, clotting factors must be provided by giving blood products (ie, whole blood, fresh plasma, fresh frozen plasma).[8,9]

Intravenous use of phytonadione preparations may cause severe reactions that resemble hypersensitivity reactions or anaphylaxis (eg, cardiac arrest, death)[4]; the trigger appears to be excipients (emulsifier of the injection's castor oil solution) versus phytonadione itself.[10,11] In human medicine, IV phytonadione using a slow infusion rate (ie, no faster than 1 mg/minute[4]) is cautiously recommended for severe bleeding associated with prolonged clotting times. In small animals, oral treatment is preferred unless the oral route is contraindicated (eg, vomiting, recently received activated charcoal).

Use caution when giving phytonadione to correct hypoprothrombinemia caused by anticoagulant therapy, as overzealous phytonadione dosing may restore conditions that caused thromboembolic events. It is important to note that phytonadione does not counteract anticoagulant effects of heparin or direct-acting anticoagulants (eg, rivaroxaban) or correct hypoprothrombinemia caused by hepatocellular damage. Absorption after oral or SC administration may be delayed in animals that are hypovolemic, and oral absorption may be impaired in patients with bile acid deficiency (eg, biliary obstruction) and malabsorptive conditions (eg, inflammatory bowel disease, GI neoplasia).

Other forms of vitamin K (eg, vitamin K_3 [ie, menadione]) are not recommended as alternatives for phytonadione.

Adverse Effects

Severe hypersensitivity-like reactions have been reported following IV administration of phytonadione (see ***Contraindications/Precautions/Warnings***) and are also possible when injecting IM and SC.[10] These reactions are due to the emulsifier in phytonadione products and are more common with older formulations.[12] Rarely, venous irritation or phlebitis have been reported in association with IV administration. IM or SC administration may cause injection site reactions, as well as acute bleeding from the injection site during the early stages of treatment. Use small-gauge needles (eg, 25-gauge) when injecting SC or IM and administer into large-muscle groups.

Reproductive/Nursing Safety

Phytonadione crosses the placenta only in small amounts, but its safety has not been documented in pregnant animals. It has been used without apparent adverse effects in pregnant dogs with anticoagulant rodenticide poisoning.[13] Pregnancy in animals with anticoagulant rodenticide poisoning are high risk; neonates are at risk for hemorrhage even if there are no toxic signs in the dam.[14] Phytonadione is considered compatible with pregnancy in humans.[15]

Vitamin K is excreted in maternal milk but is unlikely to have negative effects in nursing offspring. In humans, phytonadione is considered compatible with breastfeeding.[15]

Overdose/Acute Toxicity

Phytonadione is relatively nontoxic. It is unlikely that toxic clinical signs would result after a single overdose; however, refer to ***Adverse Effects*** for more information.

For patients that have experienced or are suspected to have experienced an overdose, it is strongly encouraged that a 24-hour poison consultation center that specializes in providing information specific for veterinary patients be consulted. For general information related to overdose and toxin exposures, as well as contact information for poison control centers, refer to ***Appendix***.

Drug Interactions

There are many drugs that may prolong or enhance the effects of coumarin anticoagulants (including ingested coumarin rodenticides) and thus impede some of the therapeutic effects of phytonadione. See ***Warfarin*** for more details.

The following drug interactions have either been reported or are theoretical in humans or animals receiving phytonadione and may be of significance in veterinary patients. Unless otherwise noted, use together is not necessarily contraindicated, but weigh the potential risks and perform additional monitoring when appropriate.

- **ANTIBIOTICS, ORAL**: Although chronic antibiotic therapy should have no significant effect on the absorption of phytonadione, these drugs may decrease the numbers of vitamin K-producing bacteria in the colon.
- **CHOLESTYRAMINE**: May reduce oral absorption of phytonadione
- **MINERAL OIL**: Concomitant oral administration of mineral oil may reduce the absorption of oral vitamin K.
- **WARFARIN**: Phytonadione antagonizes the anticoagulant effects of coumarin and indanedione agents.

Dosages

DOGS/CATS:

Acute hypoprothrombinemia (with hemorrhage) and nonacute hypoprothrombinemia (label dosage; NOT FDA-approved): 0.25 – 5 mg/kg SC or IM. Use higher end of dosing range for second generation rodenticides.[16]

Adjunctive treatment of anticoagulant rodenticide toxicity (extra-label): **NOTE**: For short-acting anticoagulant rodenticides (eg, warfarin, pindone), the minimum duration of treatment with phytonadione is 14 days, bromadiolone is 21 days, and other second-generation anticoagulant rodenticides (eg, brodifacoum, difethialone, difenacoum) is 28 days. More than 4 weeks of treatment with phytonadione may be necessary if PT remains prolonged due to ingestion of a large anticoagulant dose.

a) **Subclinical patients**: After gastric decontamination (if appropriate) either begin prophylactic phytonadione 1.5 – 2.5 mg/kg PO (with a fatty meal) twice daily without monitoring prothrombin time (PT) OR monitor PT and give phytonadione only if PT becomes elevated.[1] If PT is to be monitored, perform baseline test (to determine if any prior exposure occurred) and repeat the test 48 and 72 hours after exposure.[17] Phytonadione treatment is not needed if PT remains normal after 48 to 72 hours; however, a full course of treatment with phytonadione is needed if any PT prolongation occurs.

b) **Bleeding patients**:
   - i. 2.5 mg/kg PO twice daily with a fatty meal; duration of treatment depends on type of anticoagulant exposure.
   - ii. 5 mg/kg once daily, preferably with a meal, PO or slow IV injection, depending on the clinical condition. If IV administration is required, switch to oral administration as soon as practicable. Alternatively, a second injection can be given after 12 to 18 hours if oral treatment is not immediately possible.[16]
   - iii. Initial dose of 2.5 – 5 mg/kg PO or SC followed by 5 mg/kg per day PO in 2 or 3 divided doses.[18] Most dogs also received fresh whole blood or plasma. Phytonadione treatment continued for 14 days in dogs exposed to warfarin and 21 to 42 days in dogs exposed to second-generation anticoagulants.

Excessive bleeding secondary to hepatic disease (extra-label):

a) Prior to venipuncture, hepatic biopsy, feeding tube placement: 0.5 – 1.5 mg/kg SC every 12 hours for 2 or 3 doses. Initiating treatment early in disease course allows earlier use of invasive procedures. PT normalizes within 1 to 2 days. Weekly doses can be continued if hepatic disease progresses or persists.[19-22]

b) From a case series in 7 cats, phytonadione 3.7 – 5 mg/kg SC or PO initially, then continued at 1 – 2 mg/kg PO twice daily for 31 to 61 days.[23] Five cats received fresh whole blood transfusions on day 0.

Adjunctive treatment of hepatic failure due to blue-green algae (*Microcystis* spp) exposure (extra-label): From a case report in a dog, 5 mg/kg SC initially, then 4 mg/kg SC every 8 hours for 2 days, followed by 4 mg/kg PO every 8 hours for an additional 9 days.[24] Treatment also included whole blood transfusion on the third hospital day.

HORSES:

NOTE: Label dosages and route and rate of administration vary by manufacturer; refer to specific product label.

Acute or nonacute hypoprothrombinemia, anticoagulant rodenticide toxicity, or moldy/spoiled sweet clover ingestion (label dosage; NOT FDA approved): 0.5 – 2.5 mg/kg IM or SC once daily.[16] For acute cases (with hemorrhage) that may require IV administration, recommended administration rates vary from 1 mg/minute up to but not exceeding 10 mg/minute (5 mg/minute in newborn and very young animals). Treatment duration depends on anticoagulant. See ***Dogs/Cats*** for estimated treatment times.

Moldy sweet clover (dicumarol) toxicosis (extra-label): 1.5 mg/kg SC or IM twice daily for up to 3 days

Vitamin K deficiency in foals (extra-label): From a case report of a 4-week-old colt: 2 mg/kg SC every 12 hours for 2 days, then 0.5 mg/kg PO every 12 hours for 17 days normalized clotting factors and terminated spontaneous bleeding.[25]

CATTLE, SHEEP, GOATS, SWINE:

NOTE: Label dosages and route and rate of administration vary by manufacturer; refer to specific product label.

Acute hypoprothrombinemia, anticoagulant rodenticide toxicity, or moldy/spoiled sweet clover ingestion (label dosage; NOT FDA approved): 0.5 – 2.5 mg/kg IM or SC once daily.[16] For acute cases (with hemorrhage) that may require IV administration, recommended administration rates vary from 1 mg/minute[5] up to but not exceeding 10 mg/minute (5 mg/minute in newborn and very young animals).[16] Treatment duration may require several weeks. See ***Dogs/Cats*** for estimated treatment times.

Sweet clover (*Melilotus* spp) or lespedeza (*Lespedeza* spp) toxic-

ity (extra-label): 1 – 1.5 mg/kg SC once daily for several days. Remove the animal from the source and avoid stress and/or injury.[26]

BIRDS:

Anticoagulant rodenticide toxicity (extra-label): 0.2 – 2.2 mg/kg IM every 4 to 8 hours until stable, then daily.[27,28] See ***Dogs/Cats*** for estimated treatment times.

Secondary brodifacoum toxicity (extra-label): From a case report in a red-tailed hawk,[29] 2.5 mg/kg SC every 12 hours for 4 days, followed by 2.5 mg/kg PO in food every 24 hours for 4 weeks

Vitamin K-related hemorrhagic disorders (extra-label): 0.2 – 2.5 mg/kg IM as needed; usually only 1 to 2 injections are required[30]

RABBITS, GUINEA PIGS:

Anticoagulant rodenticide toxicity (extra-label): 3 – 5 mg/kg PO every 12 hours.[31,32] See ***Dogs/Cats*** for estimated treatment times.

Monitoring

- Clinical efficacy (lack of hemorrhage)
- Prothrombin time (PT)
- A study in dogs with GI decontamination performed within 6 hours of anticoagulant rodenticide ingestion1 suggests that phytonadione therapy could be delayed until a follow-up PT check is performed 48 to 72 hours later and found to be prolonged.
- For anticoagulant poisoning treatment regimens, PT should be checked 48 to 72 hours after the last phytonadione dose is administered. If PT is still elevated, continue phytonadione therapy for an additional week, then repeat PT 48 to 72 hours after the last dose was given.[17,33-35]

Client Information

- Oral phytonadione is best given with food that is high in fat content.
- This vitamin is considered very safe when given by mouth for treatment of anticoagulant rodenticide poisoning (ie, mouse/rat poison).
- Do not skip doses, or your animal may start to bleed. If you miss a dose, give it as soon as possible. If it is time for the next dose, give both doses at that time.
- Your animal will need to have clotting times checked at the end of treatment. Do not miss these important follow-up visits.

Chemistry/Synonyms

Phytonadione, a naphthoquinone derivative identical to naturally occurring vitamin K_1, occurs as an odorless, clear, yellow to amber, viscous liquid. It is insoluble in water, slightly soluble in alcohol, and soluble in lipids.

Phytonadione may also be known as methylphytylnaphthochinonum, phylloquinone, phytomenadione, phytomenadionum, vitamin K_1, *Aqua-Mephyton*®, K_1®, *K-Caps*®, *Konakion*®, or *Mephyton*®.

Storage/Stability

Phytonadione is resistant to heat and moisture but is oxygen sensitive and subject to photodegradation; protect from light at all times. If used as an IV infusion, the container should be wrapped with an opaque material. All phytonadione products should be stored protected from light at room temperature between 15°C to 30°C (59°F-86°F). Tablets and capsules should be stored in well-closed containers.

Compatibility/Compounding Considerations

Most sources state that phytonadione is contraindicated for IV use; consult specialized references or a hospital pharmacist for more specific information on compatibility of phytonadione with other agents.

Injectable phytonadione may be administered orally, directly into the mouth.

Dosage Forms/Regulatory Status

VETERINARY-LABELED PRODUCTS:

NOTE: The following veterinary products may not be FDA approved, as no phytonadione products were located in the FDA-Approved Animal Drug Products (Green Book).

Phytonadione Oral Capsules: 25 mg and 50 mg; generic; (Rx). Labeled for use in dogs and cats

Phytonadione Oral Tablets, Chewable: 25 mg and 50 mg; *Vitamin K_1 Chewable*®, generic; (Rx). Labeled for use in dogs and cats

Phytonadione Aqueous Colloidal Solution for Injection: 10 mg/mL in 100 mL vials; *Vitamin K_1*, generic; (Rx). May be labeled for use in dogs, cats, cattle, calves, horses, swine, sheep, or goats. Product labels do not list withdrawal times. Food Animal Residue Avoidance Databank (FARAD) currently lists a 0 day milk and slaughter withdrawal interval in all indicated species; it is recommended to check withdrawal times with FARAD prior to administration.

HUMAN-LABELED PRODUCTS:

Phytonadione Oral Tablets: 5 mg; *Mephyton*®; (Rx)

Phytonadione Oral Tablets and Gelcaps: 0.1 mg (100 μg); generic; (OTC)

Phytonadione Injection, Emulsion: 2 mg/mL and 10 mg/mL in 0.5 mL and 1 mL amps; generic; (Rx)

References

For the complete list of references, see **wiley.com/go/budde/plumb**

Pimobendan

(pi-moe-***ben***-den) *Vetmedin*®

Inodilator

Prescriber Highlights

- ▶ Used for treatment of heart disease in dogs (FDA-approved) and cats (extra-label)
- ▶ Effects of food on drug absorption are unknown; should be given consistently (with or without food)
- ▶ May increase the risk for arrhythmias

Uses/Indications

Pimobendan is FDA-approved for congestive heart failure (CHF) in dogs secondary to dilated cardiomyopathy (DCM) or chronic myxomatous/degenerative atrioventricular valve insufficiency (AVVI). Two studies reported that, in dogs with AVVI and CHF, administration of pimobendan and furosemide can improve survival times and quality of life when compared with standard treatment (ie, ACE inhibitor and furosemide).[1,2] The QUEST study also concluded that although dogs given pimobendan or benazepril had a similar quality of life during the study, patients treated with pimobendan had increased time before CHF treatment intensified, which resulted in the patient having a smaller heart size and higher body temperature as well as less retention of free water.[3]

In other countries, pimobendan also has a labeled indication to delay the onset of clinical signs of heart failure, to reduce heart size, and to increase survival time in dogs with evidence of increased heart size secondary to asymptomatic (preclinical) AVVI. A large international multicenter trial (known as the EPIC trial) of dogs in stage B2 AVVI (meaning substantial cardiomegaly but no CHF) showed a delay of over 15 months to reach a composite endpoint of CHF, cardiac-related death, or euthanasia in dogs receiving pimobendan as compared with dogs receiving placebo.[4] In the ACVIM consensus guidelines for the diagnosis and treatment of myxomatous mitral valve disease in dogs, the panel recommended incorporation of pimobendan in the treatment of dogs in stage B2 preclinical disease. The guidelines also recommend pimobendan in the acute and chronic treatment of dogs in stage C (current or historical signs of CHF) heart failure.[5] An abstract has suggested administration of pimobendan at an escalated total daily dose for dogs in stage D (end stage, refractory) heart failure.[6]

Some countries have a labeled indication for pimobendan in large breed dogs with DCM to prolong the time to the onset of CHF or sudden death. A study performed in Doberman pinschers concluded that pimobendan should be used as first-line therapy for the treatment of CHF caused by DCM.[7] In addition, the PROTECT trial concluded that administration of pimobendan to Doberman pinschers with preclinical DCM can prolong the onset of clinical signs and extend survival time compared to placebo.[8]

Pimobendan has been suggested as an adjunctive treatment option for dogs with pulmonary arterial hypertension secondary to AAVI.[9]

Pimobendan is not FDA-approved for use in cats. A prospective, double-blind, randomized, non-pivotal, exploratory field study in 83 cats with hypertrophic cardiomyopathy and CHF found no benefit at 180 days for pimobendan as compared to placebo.[10] However, in the cats without obstructive disease, treatment with pimobendan was associated with a tendency toward benefit while cats with dynamic outflow tract obstruction had an increased likelihood of early removal from the study or an increase of furosemide dose if treated with pimobendan.[10] Retrospective studies have previously suggested that pimobendan is tolerated in cats and may have potential benefits.[11-13] A case-control study of cats with hypertrophic cardiomyopathy and CHF suggested that pimobendan prolonged survival time as compared with cats not receiving pimobendan.[14]

Pharmacology/Actions

Pimobendan is an inodilator, with both positive inotropic and vasodilatory effects. Pimobendan typically (indirectly) decreases heart rate (negative chronotrope) in animals with CHF. Pimobendan's inotropic effects occur via inhibition of phosphodiesterase III (PDE-III) and by increasing intracellular calcium sensitivity in the cardiac contractile apparatus. Cardiac contractility is enhanced without an increase in myocardial oxygen consumption, as pimobendan does not increase intracellular calcium levels. Commercially available pimobendan is a 50:50 mixture of *l*- and *d*-isomers. In dogs, the *l*-isomer of pimobendan has ≈1.5 times greater inotropic activity than the *d*-isomer. Pimobendan's vasodilator effects are via vascular PDE-III inhibition, and both arterial and venous dilation occur. In dogs, pimobendan administered at high dosages (0.6 mg/kg PO every 12 hours for 10 days) with furosemide 2 mg/kg PO every 12 hours did not substantially affect the renin–angiotensin–aldosterone system.[15] Pimobendan also possesses some antithrombotic activity, but at clinically used doses pimobendan does not have an effect on platelet function in dogs.[16] Pimobendan is occasionally used as adjunct therapy for pulmonary arterial hypertension, with experimental data suggesting it may have some activity against phosphodiesterase V and may result in an increase in cyclic guanosine monophosphate (cGMP), although this has not been confirmed in vivo.[17]

One study noted that pimobendan administered IV has positive chronotropic and inotropic effects for healthy mature horses when administered at 0.25 mg/kg slowly over 15 minutes. Additional studies are needed to determine clinical applications.[18]

Pharmacokinetics

Peak concentrations of the parent compound and the active metabolite were observed 1 to 4 hours after administration (mean, 2 and 3 hours, respectively) of a single dose of pimobendan 0.25 mg/kg PO to dogs. Food decreased the bioavailability of an aqueous solution of pimobendan, but the effect of food on absorption of pimobendan from chewable tablets is unknown. The steady-state volume of distribution of pimobendan is 2.6 L/kg in dogs. Protein binding of pimobendan and the active metabolite in dog plasma is greater than 90%. Pimobendan is oxidatively demethylated to a pharmacologically active metabolite that is then conjugated with sulfate or glucuronic acid and excreted mainly via feces. Clearance of pimobendan is ≈90 mL/min/kg, and the terminal elimination half-lives of pimobendan and the active metabolite are ≈0.5 hours and 2 hours, respectively. After oral administration, plasma concentrations of pimobendan and the active metabolite were below quantifiable concentrations by 4 and 8 hours, respectively.

In healthy cats, the pharmacokinetics of pimobendan after a single oral dose (≈0.28 mg/kg) were determined; peak concentrations of the parent compound occurred at 0.9 hours, apparent volume of distribution was high, and mean elimination half-life was 1.3 hours.[19] In another study of oral pimobendan pharmacokinetics in cats that evaluated low-dose (0.625 mg per cat; ≈0.14 mg/kg) and high-dose (1.25 mg per cat; ≈0.28 mg/kg) administration, both the compound and the active metabolite (*O*-desmethylpimobendan) rapidly reached peak plasma concentration, with a volume of distribution of ≈3 L/kg, a clearance of 42.9 – 51.1 mL/min/kg, and an elimination half-life of 0.7 to 0.8 hours.[20]

The pharmacokinetics of pimobendan after single PO doses were determined in healthy Hispaniolan Amazon parrots. A suspension prepared using commercially available tablets and stored for no more than 1 hour was administered at 10 mg/kg and reached a C_{max} of 8.26 ng/mL at 3 hours with a half-life of 2.1 hours; when pimobendan was administered with a suspension prepared using bulk pimobendan powder, the C_{max} was 1.28 ng/mL at 12 hours and half-life was 2.3 hours.[21]

Pimobendan is rapidly absorbed in humans with heart failure, with peak concentrations occurring less than 1 hour after an oral dose. The volume of distribution is ≈3.2 L/kg and clearance is ≈25 mL/min/kg. The terminal half-life is slightly less than 3 hours.

Contraindications/Precautions/Warnings

Pimobendan is contraindicated in animals hypersensitive to it and relatively contraindicated in animals with semilunar valve stenosis or any condition in which an augmentation of cardiac output is inappropriate for functional or anatomic reasons. Pimobendan should be used with caution in patients with uncontrolled cardiac arrhythmias.

The label states pimobendan has not been evaluated for use in dogs younger than 6 months; or dogs with congenital heart defects, diabetes mellitus, or other serious metabolic diseases.

Adverse Effects

GI effects (eg, decreased appetite, vomiting, diarrhea) and lethargy are the primary adverse effects noted in dogs.

There is variable evidence that pimobendan may increase the development of arrhythmias. Atrial fibrillation or increased ventricular ectopic beats have been reported in dogs receiving pimobendan, but a causative effect has not been established because the underlying heart disease can cause arrhythmias. A small (n = 8) prospective study in small-breed dogs with AVVI and CHF did not find evidence of increased incidence of cardiac arrhythmias as compared with dogs given a placebo over a 2-week evaluation period.[22] A trial of pimobendan demonstrated an increased patient mortality rate when administered to humans with heart failure. In a US field trial (56 days duration) performed on dogs with heart disease, the adverse effect incidence (at least 1 occurrence reported per dog) included poor appetite (38%), lethargy (33%), diarrhea (30%), dyspnea (29%), azotemia (14%), weakness and ataxia (13%), pleural effusion (10%), syncope (9%), cough (7%), sudden death (6%), ascites (6%), and heart murmur (3%).[23] In the EPIC study of 360 dogs with preclinical AVVI, 12 of 178 dogs (6.7%) receiving pimobendan experienced sudden cardiac death as compared with 5 of 176 dogs (2.8%) receiving a placebo[4]; these rates were not statistically different. The primary endpoint of time to CHF or cardiac death was strongly favorable for the group receiving pimobendan.

In a study comparing the cardiac adverse effects of pimobendan versus benazepril,[24] dogs with mitral valve regurgitation that were given pimobendan had increases in systolic function and developed worsening mitral valve disease and specific mitral valve lesions (eg, acute hemorrhages, endocardial papilliform hyperplasia on the dorsal surfaces of the leaflets, infiltration of chordae tendinae by glycosaminoglycans) not seen in the group receiving benazepril.

A retrospective study concluded that cats (n = 27) with systolic anterior motion of the mitral valve may develop systemic hypotension when treated with pimobendan.[13] However, a prospective crossover study of 13 cats with hypertrophic cardiomyopathy found no increase in left ventricular outflow tract obstruction in cats receiving pimobendan as compared with cats receiving a placebo, whereas pimobendan improved left atrial function.[25] As noted above, in the exploratory field study of pimobendan compared to placebo in cats with CHF those with left ventricular outflow tract obstruction had a tendency to do worse when receiving pimobendan as compared to those cats with no obstruction.[10]

Reproductive/Nursing Safety

The product label states pimobendan has not been evaluated in dogs used for breeding or for pregnant or lactating bitches. Increased fetal resorptions occurred when pimobendan was administered at high doses (300 mg/kg) to pregnant laboratory animals. Rabbits receiving pimobendan 100 mg/kg showed no adverse effects on fetuses.

No information on the safety of pimobendan during nursing was noted.

Because safety has not been established in animals, this drug should only be used when the maternal benefits outweigh the potential risks to offspring.

Overdose/Acute Toxicity

In nonclinical dogs, prompt decontamination, including emesis induction and administration of activated charcoal (once the patient has stopped vomiting), is advised. For patients exhibiting clinical signs associated with toxicity, supportive care is recommended. Hypotension should be treated as needed with IV fluid therapy and vasopressors; monitoring of heart rate, blood pressure, and an electrocardiogram is advised.[26] In the event of any potential overdose, clinicians are encouraged to contact a poison control center for patient decontamination and management advice.

In a 4-week study of dogs, dose-dependent increases in heart rate were seen after administration of pimobendan 2 and 8 mg/kg IV. In a 6-month toxicity study of dogs, mild heart murmurs developed in one dog at 3 times (1.5 mg/kg) the labeled dosage and in 2 dogs at 5 times (2.5 mg/kg) the labeled dosage; the murmurs were nonclinical.

There were 468 single-agent exposures to pimobendan reported to the ASPCA Animal Poison Control Center (APCC) from 2009 to 2013. Of the 427 reported dogs, 111 showed clinical signs, with tachycardia (48%), vomiting (24%), hypertension (12%), lethargy (12%), and hypotension (9%) being the most common. Of the 41 cats reported, only 6 showed clinical signs, with 33% experiencing vomiting.

A review of the Pet Poison Helpline database from November 2004 to April 2010 identified 98 cases of pimobendan toxicosis.[26] Of those, 7 dogs that ingested between 2.6 to 21.3 mg/kg of pimobendan were selected for further evaluation. Clinical signs of cardiovascular abnormalities, including severe tachycardia in 4 out of 7 dogs, hypotension in 2 of 7 dogs, and hypertension in 2 of 7 dogs, were noted. No clinical signs were seen in 2 dogs.

For patients that have experienced or are suspected to have experienced an overdose, consultation with a 24-hour poison consultation control center specializing in providing veterinary-specific information is recommended. For general information related to overdose and toxin exposures, as well as contact information for poison control centers, refer to ***Appendix.***

Drug Interactions

In field studies pimobendan was safely used with furosemide, digoxin, enalapril, atenolol, nitroglycerin, hydralazine, diltiazem, antiparasitic products (including heartworm preventative), antibiotics, famotidine, theophylline, levothyroxine, diphenhydramine, hydrocodone, metoclopramide, and butorphanol.[27] The following drug interactions have either been reported or are theoretical in animals receiving pimobendan and may be of significance in veterinary patients. Unless otherwise noted, use together is not necessarily contraindicated, but weigh the potential risks and perform additional monitoring when appropriate.

- **Beta-Adrenergic Blocking Agents** (eg, **propranolol**): The positive inotropic effect of pimobendan may be reduced.[28]
- **Calcium Channel Blockers** (eg, **diltiazem, verapamil**): The positive inotropic effect of pimobendan may be reduced.[28]

Laboratory Considerations

- No laboratory interactions or special considerations were located.

Dosages

DOGS:

Management of the signs of mild, moderate, or severe congestive heart failure due to AV valve insufficiency or dilated cardiomyopathy (label dosage; FDA-approved): 0.5 mg/kg PO total daily dose divided into 2 portions that are not necessarily equal (using whole or half tablets) and should be administered ≈12 hours apart. Calculated dose should be rounded to the nearest half-tablet increment.[27]

Adjunctive treatment of preclinical dilated cardiomyopathy (extra-label): Same as the labeled dosage. In the PROTECT study, all dogs that weighed more than 35.1 kg (77.4 lb) received pimobendan 10 mg PO twice daily.[8] All dogs that weighed less than 35 kg (77 lb) received 5 mg pimobendan PO twice daily.

Adjunctive treatment of stage B2 and stage C atrioventricular valve insufficiency (AVVI) (extra-label): 0.25 – 0.3 mg/kg PO every 12 hours.[5] In the EPIC study, all dogs received 0.4 – 0.6 mg/kg/day divided into 2 doses.[4] It is important to note that dogs were required to have relevant cardiac remodeling, including both radiographic and echocardiographic evidence of cardiomegaly. Administration of pimobendan to dogs with AVVI before CHF is not advised unless criteria for cardiac enlargement, as established by the EPIC study, are met.

Adjunctive treatment of acute or chronic stage D heart failure (extra-label): 0.3 mg/kg PO 3 times (every 8 hours) daily.[5,6]

CATS:

Heart failure with left ventricular systolic dysfunction, pleural effusion, renal insufficiency, or severe refractory pulmonary edema (extra-label): 0.25 mg/kg PO twice daily; practically, one 1.25 mg tablet/cat (NOT per kg) twice daily. Generally used in combination with an ACE inhibitor and furosemide[14]

Monitoring

Cardiovascular parameters used to monitor heart function including:

- Resting respiratory rate
- Heart rate and rhythm (ECG)
- Blood pressure
- Thoracic auscultation and radiographs
- Echocardiography

Client Information

- Give this medicine as directed by your veterinarian. Do not stop giving this medicine to your pet without discussing with your veterinarian.
- This medicine works best when given on an empty stomach.
- Gastrointestinal effects (eg, poor appetite, vomiting, diarrhea) are the most likely side effects. Contact your veterinarian if these signs persist, worsen, or if your pet is having other signs that are of concern.
- Your veterinarian will need to monitor your pet closely while it is taking this medicine. Do not miss these important follow-up visits.

Chemistry/Synonyms

Pimobendan, a benzimidazole-derivative phosphodiesterase inhibitor, occurs as a white or slightly yellowish, hygroscopic powder. Pimobendan is practically insoluble in water and slightly soluble in acetone or methyl alcohol. Pimobendan's chemical name is 4,5-Dihydro-6-[2-(p-methyoxyphenyl)-5-benzimidazolyl]-5-methyl-3(2H) pyridazinone. Pimobendan has a molecular weight of 334.4.

Pimobendan may also be known as UDCG-115, *Acardi*®, *Vetmedin*®, or *Zelys*®.

Storage/Stability

Unless otherwise labeled, store pimobendan chewable tablets or capsules at room temperature below 25°C (77°F) in a dry place. Store commercial pimobendan oral solution at 25°C (77°F) and protected from light. Pimobendan injection has no storage requirement; use single-dose vials immediately after opening and discard any unused drug.

Compatibility/Compounding Considerations

Compounded suspensions may not be stable[29]; use should be avoided unless stability data are available.

Dosage Forms/Regulatory Status

VETERINARY-LABELED PRODUCTS:

Pimobendan Chewable Tablets (artificial beef-flavored): 1.25 mg, 2.5 mg, 5 mg, and 10 mg; *Vetmedin*®; (Rx). NADA# 141-273. FDA-approved for use in dogs. Pimobendan capsules and chews may be available in other countries.

Pimobendan 0.75 mg/mL Injectable Solution: 5 mL and 10 mL single dose vials; *Vetmedin*® Injectable Solution for Dogs; (Rx). Approved in some countries (not the United States) for use in dogs

Pimobendan 3.5 mg/mL Oral Solution for Dogs is available in Australia in 21 mL, 42 mL, and 168 mL bottles; *Vetmedin*®; (Rx)

HUMAN-LABELED PRODUCTS: NONE

References

For the complete list of references, see **wiley.com/go/budde/plumb**

Piperacillin/Tazobactam

(***pype***-er-ah-sill-in; tay-zoh-***bak***-tam) *Zosyn*®

Extended Spectrum Penicillin/Beta-Lactamase Inhibitor Combination

Prescriber Highlights

- Parenteral penicillin and beta-lactamase inhibitor combination
- Broad-spectrum agent; covers many gram-positive, gram-negative, and anaerobic pathogens including *Pseudomonas* and *Enterobacter* spp
- Limited experience and research in veterinary medicine

Uses/Indications

Although veterinary experience is limited with piperacillin/tazobactam, it has broad-spectrum activity against many bacteria and may be used to treat bacterial infections based on culture and susceptibility data, or for surgical prophylaxis when gram-negative or mixed aerobic/anaerobic infections are concerns.

Pharmacology/Actions

Piperacillin is a bactericidal, extended-action acylaminopenicillin that inhibits septum formation and cell wall synthesis in susceptible bacteria. It has a wide spectrum of activity against many aerobic and anaerobic gram-positive (including some enterococci eg, *E faecalis*) and gram-negative bacteria. It has a similar spectrum of activity as the aminopenicillins, but with additional activity against several gram-negative organisms of the family Enterobacteriaceae, including *Enterobacter* spp and many strains of *Pseudomonas aeruginosa*. *Klebsiella* spp are often resistant. Alone, it is susceptible to inactivation by beta-lactamases; the addition of tazobactam increases piperacillin's spectrum of activity against many strains of bacteria that produce beta-lactamase.

Tazobactam is a beta-lactamase inhibitor that irreversibly binds to beta-lactamases. It has minimal antibacterial activity when used alone, but when combined with piperacillin, it protects the beta-lactam ring of piperacillin from hydrolysis. This extends piperacillin's spectrum of activity to those bacteria that produce beta-lactamases of Richmond-Sykes types II-V that would otherwise render it ineffective. It has slightly more activity than either clavulanate or sulbactam against some Type I beta-lactamases. Unlike clavulanic acid, tazobactam does not induce chromosomal beta-lactamases at the serum concentrations achieved.

Pharmacokinetics

Limited information is available for veterinary species. In mares, piperacillin has an elimination half-life of ≈7 hours.[1] IM bioavailability is 86% and protein binding is ≈19%.

In humans, piperacillin is not appreciably absorbed from the gut so it must be administered parenterally. After IM administration, peak concentrations occur in ≈30 minutes. The drug exhibits low protein binding and has a volume of distribution of 0.1 L/kg. It is widely distributed into many tissues and fluids including lung, gallbladder, intestinal mucosa, uterus, bile, and interstitial fluid. With inflamed meninges, piperacillin concentrations in the CSF are ≈30% those in serum. If meninges are normal, CSF concentrations are only ≈6% of serum concentrations. Piperacillin crosses the placenta and is distributed into milk in low concentrations. Piperacillin is partly metabolized in the liver to a desethyl metabolite that only has minimal antibacterial activity. Piperacillin is primarily (68%) eliminated unchanged in the urine via active tubular secretion and glomerular filtration; it is also excreted in the bile. Elimination half-life in humans is ≈1 hour.

Tazobactam's pharmacokinetics generally mirror that of piperacillin. In dogs, piperacillin reduced the renal clearance of tazobactam, presumably due to competition for tubular secretion.[2]

Contraindications/Precautions/Warnings

Piperacillin/tazobactam should not be used in patients with documented hypersensitivity reactions to penicillins, cepholosporins, or beta-lactamase inhibitors.

Because of the sodium content, high doses of piperacillin/tazobactam may adversely affect patients with cardiac failure or hypernatremic conditions.

Dosage adjustment (ie, reduced dosing frequency) may be required in patients with significantly decreased renal function.

Penicillins, cephalosporins, and macrolides should not be administered to rabbits, guinea pigs, chinchillas, or hamsters as serious enteritis and clostridial enterotoxemia may occur.

Adverse Effects

Piperacillin/tazobactam is generally well tolerated. Hypersensitivity reactions and GI effects (eg, nausea, vomiting, diarrhea, constipation) are possible. Local effects (eg, thrombophlebitis) associated with IV injection may occur. Alterations in gut microbiota may lead to antibiotic-associated diarrhea.

In humans, bleeding has been reported in patients receiving some beta-lactams, including piperacillin. Very high doses may cause neurotoxicity (seizures). These effects are more likely in patients with diminished renal function. Dermatologic effects have been reported in humans, including rash and pruritus.[3] Superinfections with *Clostridium difficile* have been reported (rare).

Reproductive/Nursing Safety

Piperacillin/tazobactam is relatively safe to use during pregnancy. No teratogenic effects have been attributed to either drug in humans or laboratory animals.

Piperacillin is distributed in milk in low concentrations. It is not known if tazobactam enters milk. This drug combination is likely safe to use during nursing.

Because safety has not been established in animals, this drug should only be used when the maternal benefits outweigh the potential risks to offspring.

Overdose/Acute Toxicity

One-time overdoses are unlikely to pose much risk although very large overdoses may cause vomiting, diarrhea, or neurotoxicity. Dogs receiving up to 800 mg/kg/day of piperacillin/tazobactam for 6 months demonstrated no serious toxic effects. Doses of 400 mg/kg/day or more caused some transient effects to the liver (glycogen granules in the cytoplasm and increases in smooth endoplasmic reticulum in hepatocytes) that were mostly reversed after discontinuing the drug for one month.[4] Treatment for overdoses, if required, is supportive.

For patients that have experienced or are suspected to have experienced an overdose, consultation with a 24-hour poison consultation center specializing in providing veterinary-specific information is recommended. For general information related to overdose and toxin exposures, as well as contact information for poison control centers, refer to ***Appendix.***

Drug Interactions

The following drug interactions have either been reported or are theoretical in humans or animals receiving piperacillin/tazobactam and may be of significance in veterinary patients. Unless otherwise noted, use together is not necessarily contraindicated, but weigh the potential risks and perform additional monitoring when appropriate.

- **Aminoglycosides** (eg, **amikacin, gentamicin, tobramycin**): In vitro studies have demonstrated that penicillins can have synergistic or additive activity against certain bacteria when used with aminoglycosides. However, beta-lactam antibiotics can inactivate aminoglycosides in vitro and in vivo in patients in renal failure or when penicillins are used in massive dosages. Amikacin is considered the most resistant aminoglycoside to this inactivation.
- **Anticoagulants**: Because piperacillin may rarely affect platelets, increased monitoring of coagulation parameters is suggested for patients on heparin or warfarin.
- **Methotrexate**: Piperacillin may increase methotrexate serum concentrations.
- **Probenecid**: Can reduce the renal tubular secretion of both piperacillin and tazobactam, thereby maintaining higher systemic concentrations for a longer period; this potential beneficial interaction requires further investigation before dosing recommendations can be made for veterinary patients.
- **Vancomycin**: Increased risk for acute kidney injury
- **Vecuronium**: Piperacillin may prolong neuromuscular blockade.

Laboratory Considerations

- Urine glucose determinations when using cupric sulfate solution (Benedict's solution, *Clinitest®*): Piperacillin may cause false positive results. Tests using glucose oxidase (*Tes-Tape®*, *Clinistix®*) are not affected by piperacillin.
- Aminoglycoside serum quantitative analysis: As penicillins and other beta-lactams can inactivate aminoglycosides in vitro (and in vivo in patients in renal failure or when penicillins are used in massive dosages), serum concentrations of aminoglycosides may be falsely decreased if the patient is also receiving beta-lactam antibiotics and the serum is stored prior to analysis. It is recommended that if the aminoglycoside assay is delayed, samples be frozen and, if possible, drawn at times when the beta-lactam antibiotic is at a trough.
- Aspergillus galactomannan antigen assay: False positive results may occur.
- Direct antiglobulin (Coombs) tests: False positive results may occur.
- Urine protein: Piperacillin may produce false positive urine protein results with the sulfosalicylic acid and boiling test, nitric acid test, or the acetic acid test. Strips using bromophenol blue reagent (eg, *Multi-Stix®*) do not appear to be affected by high concentrations of penicillins in the urine.

Dosages

DOGS/CATS:

Bacterial sepsis (extra-label):

a) 40 – 50 mg/kg IV over 30 minutes every 6 hours have been suggested.[5-7]

b) 3 mg/kg IV loading dose, followed by 3.2 mg/kg/hour IV CRI[7]

BIRDS:

Susceptible infections (extra-label): Reconstitute to 200 mg/mL and administer 100 mg/kg IM every 8 to 12 hours; <u>for severe polymicrobic bacteremia:</u> give 100 mg/kg IV every 6 hours; <u>for preoperative orthopedic or coelomic surgery</u>: 100 mg/kg IM every 12 hours[8]

REPTILES:

Susceptible respiratory tract infections (extra-label): 100 – 200 mg/kg IM every 24 hours. 10 mg/mL in saline and nebulized every 4 to 6 hours.[9] **NOTE**: This reference was for using piperacillin alone; if using piperacillin/tazobactam, calculate dose per the piperacillin component.

Monitoring

- Clinical signs of infection
- CBC
- Electrolytes

Client Information

- Piperacillin/tazobactam is an antibiotic that is reserved for serious infections and must be given by infusion into the vein. It should only be used in a setting where adequate patient monitoring is available.

Chemistry/Synonyms

Piperacillin sodium/tazobactam sodium occurs as a white to off-white, cryodessicated powder. Tazobactam is structurally related to sulbactam and a penicillanic acid sulfone derivative. The commercially available piperacillin/tazobactam injection contains 2.79 mEq of sodium and 0.25 mg of EDTA per gram of piperacillin.

Tazobactam may also be known as CL 298741 or YTR 830H. Piperacillin may also be known as piperacillinum, BL-P 1908, Cl 867, CL 227193, T 12220, and TA 058. International trade names for piperacillin/tazobactam include *Tazobac®*, *Tazocin®*, *Zosyn®*, and others.

Storage/Stability

Piperacillin/tazobactam injection vials and *ADD-Vantage* vials should be stored at controlled room temperature (20°C-25°C [68°F-77°F]). Piperacillin/tazobactam pre-mixed solution for injection must be frozen at -20°C (-4°F) and thawed only under refrigeration (2°C-8°C [36°F-46°F]) or at room temperature (20°C to 25°C [68°F-77°F]); never force thawing with a hot water bath or microwave. Thawed solutions are stable at room temperature for 24 hours, or 14 days when refrigerated.

Conventional vials should be reconstituted with 5 mL of diluent per gram of piperacillin. Suitable diluents include 0.9% sodium chloride, sterile water for injection, and bacteriostatic saline or water for injection. Once reconstituted, further dilute for intravenous infusion with 50 to 150 mL of 0.9% sodium chloride, lactated Ringer's solution (reformulated product only; see below) or 5% dextrose. IV infusion should be over at least 30 minutes.

Once reconstituted, vials should be used immediately. It is recommended to discard after 24 hours if kept at room temperature or 48 hours if stored in the refrigerator. The manufacturer recommends not freezing reconstituted vials. IV bags (50 to 150 mL) containing further diluted product are stable for up to 24 hours at room temperature and one week if refrigerated. As no preservatives are used, sterility is not assured in stored reconstituted products.

Compatibility/Compounding Considerations

Compatibility is dependent on factors such as pH, concentration, temperature, and diluent used; specialized references or a hospital pharmacist can be consulted for more specific information.

Zosyn® (piperacillin/tazobactam) injection underwent a formulation change in 2006. Sodium citrate (buffer) and EDTA (metal chelator) were added, which made it **compatible** with lactated Ringer's injection and via simultaneous Y-site administration at specific concentrations of gentamicin and amikacin (but not tobramycin). This reformulated product has a yellow background behind the *Zosyn*® name on the label. The manufacturer states that other medications should **not** be added to piperacillin/tazobactam solutions, or mixed within the same syringe. Consult specialized references or a hospital pharmacist for more specific information.

Dosage Forms/Regulatory Status

VETERINARY-LABELED PRODUCTS: NONE

HUMAN-LABELED PRODUCTS:

Piperacillin Sodium and Tazobactam Injection (powder for solution); 2.25 g (piperacillin 2 g; tazobactam 0.25 g), 3.375 g (piperacillin 3 g; tazobactam 0.375 g), 4.5 g (piperacillin 4 g; tazobactam 0.5 g), and 40.5 g (piperacillin 36 g; tazobactam 4.5 g); *Zosyn*®, generic; (Rx)

Piperacillin Sodium and Tazobactam Injection (solution in D_5W); 2.25 g/50 mL (piperacillin 2 g; tazobactam 0.25 g), 3.375 g/50 mL (piperacillin 3 g; tazobactam 0.375 g), and 4.5 g/100 mL (piperacillin 4 g; tazobactam 0.5 g); *Zosyn*® in Galaxy container; (Rx). Must be kept frozen.

References

For the complete list of references, see **wiley.com/go/budde/plumb**

Piperazine

(pi-per-a-***zeen***)

Antiparasitic

Prescriber Highlights

- Anthelmintic for ascarids in a variety of species. Limited efficacy. Rarely recommended today
- Adverse effects are unlikely, but diarrhea, emesis, or ataxia are possible.

Uses/Indications

Piperazine may be used for the treatment of ascarids, but its use is rarely recommended, as more effective treatments are preferred. Piperazine is considered safe to use in animals with concurrent gastroenteritis.

Pharmacology/Actions

Piperazine is thought to paralyze susceptible nematodes. The neuromuscular blocking effect is believed to be caused by stimulation of GABA-gated chloride ion channels.[1] In ascarids, succinic acid production is also inhibited.

Pharmacokinetics

Piperazine and its salts are reportedly readily absorbed from the proximal sections of the GI tract, and the drug is metabolized and excreted by the kidneys. Absorptive, distribution, and elimination kinetics on individual species were not located.

Contraindications/Precautions/Warnings

Piperazine is contraindicated in patients with chronic liver or kidney disease and with GI hypomotility. Do not use piperazine in puppies or kittens less than 6 weeks old. It should not be used in sick, feverish, underweight, or physically weak animals.[2,3] There is some evidence in humans that high-dose piperazine may provoke seizures in patients with a seizure history or renal disease.

If piperazine is used in horses with heavy infestations of *Parascarus equorum*, rupture or blockage of intestines is possible due to the rapid death and detachment of the parasite.

Adverse Effects

Adverse effects are uncommon at recommended dosages, but diarrhea, emesis, and ataxia may be noted in dogs or cats. Horses and foals generally tolerate the drug quite well, even at high doses, but transient soft stools may be seen.

Reproductive/Nursing Safety

Piperazine is considered safe to use during pregnancy. No information was located on use during nursing, but it appears to be safe to use.

Overdose/Acute Toxicity

Piperazine is considered to have a wide margin of safety; however, acute massive overdoses can lead to paralysis and death. The oral LD_{50} of piperazine adipate in mice is 11.4 g/kg.

In cats, adverse effects occur within 24 hours after a toxic dose is ingested. Emesis; weakness; dyspnea; muscular fasciculations of ears, whiskers, tail, and eyes; rear limb ataxia, hypersalivation, depression, dehydration, head-pressing, positional nystagmus, and slowed pupillary responses have all been described after toxic ingestions. Many of these effects may also be seen in dogs after toxic piperazine ingestions.

Treatment is supportive and based on clinical presentation. If ingestion was recent, use of activated charcoal with a cathartic has been suggested. IV fluid therapy and keeping the animal in a quiet, dark place is recommended. Recovery generally takes place within 3 to 4 days.

For patients that have experienced or are suspected to have experienced an overdose, consultation with a 24-hour poison consultation center specializing in providing veterinary-specific information is recommended. For general information related to overdose and toxin exposures, as well as contact information for poison control centers, refer to ***Appendix.***

Drug Interactions

The following drug interactions have either been reported or are theoretical in humans or animals receiving piperazine and may be of significance in veterinary patients. Unless otherwise noted, use together is not necessarily contraindicated, but weigh the potential risks and perform additional monitoring when appropriate.

- **Chlorpromazine**: Although data conflict, piperazine and chlorpromazine may precipitate seizures if used concomitantly.
- **Laxatives**: The use of purgatives (laxatives) with piperazine is not recommended, as the drug may be eliminated before its full efficacy is established.
- **Pyrantel/Morantel**: Piperazine and pyrantel/morantel have antagonistic modes of action and should generally not be used together.

Laboratory Considerations

- Piperazine can have an effect on uric acid blood levels, but references conflict with regard to the effect. Both falsely high and low values have been reported; interpret results cautiously.

Dosages

CAUTION: Piperazine is available in several salts that contain varying amounts of piperazine base (see ***Chemistry/Synonyms*** below). Refer to specific label information for the product being used.

DOGS/CATS:

NOTE: Rarely recommended today

Ascarids (label dosage; NOT FDA-approved): 50 – 55 mg/kg (as base) PO once; repeat in 10 days[4,5] then every 30 days to prevent reinfestation[5]

Ascarids (extra-label): 100 – 110 mg/kg PO once; repeat in 21 days[6]

SWINE:

Large roundworms (*Ascaris suum*) and nodular worms (label dosage): 112 mg/kg of piperazine base in sole source drinking water for 24 hours.[2,3] May repeat dosing every 30 days. Refer to specific product label for instructions on how to prepare medicated water.

BIRDS:

***Ascaridia galli* in poultry** (extra-label): 32 mg/kg (as base) (≈0.3 grams for each adult) given in each of 2 successive feedings or for 2 days in drinking water. Citrate or adipate salts are usually used in feed and the hexahydrate in drinking water.[7]

RABBITS, RODENTS, SMALL MAMMALS:

a) **Mice, rats, hamsters, gerbils, and rabbits for pinworms** (extra-label): Piperazine citrate in drinking water at 3 g/liter for 2 weeks[8]

b) **Rabbits for pinworms** (extra-label): Piperazine citrate 100 mg/kg PO once a day for 2 days. Piperazine adipate: Adults: 200 – 500 mg/kg PO once a day for 2 days. **Young rabbits**: 750 mg/kg PO once daily for 2 days. Wash the perianal area[9]

c) **Mice, rats, hamsters, gerbils, guinea pigs, and chinchillas for pinworms/tapeworms** (extra-label): Using piperazine citrate: 2 – 5 mg/mL drinking water for 7 days, off 7 days and repeat[10]

REPTILES:

Nematodes (extra-label): 40 – 60 mg/kg PO. Repeat in 2 weeks, followed by fecal examination 14 days after the second dose. If positive for parasites, a third dose is given, and the cycle continues until the parasites are cleared from the animal.[11]

Monitoring

- Clinical efficacy (eg, serial fecal flotations)
- Adverse effects

Client Information

- This medicine is used to rid your animal of roundworm infections only. It does not work for treatment of many other intestinal parasites.
- Side effects are unlikely, but diarrhea, vomiting, and incoordination/weakness (eg, stumbling, clumsiness) are possible in dogs and cats.

Chemistry/Synonyms

Piperazine occurs as a white, crystalline powder that may have a slight odor. It is soluble in water and alcohol.

Piperazine is available commercially in a variety of salts, including citrate, adipate, phosphate, hexahydrate, monohydrochloride, and dihydrochloride. Each salt contains a variable amount of piperazine (base): adipate (37%), chloride (48%), citrate (35%), dihydrochloride (50% to 53%), hexahydrate (44%), phosphate (42%), and sulfate (46%).

Piperazine may also be known as diethylendiamin, dispermin, hexahydropropyrazin, piperazinum, and *Pipa-Tabs*®.

Storage/Stability

Unless otherwise specified by the manufacturer, piperazine products should be stored at room temperature (15°C-30°C [59°F-86°F]).

Dosage Forms/Regulatory Status

VETERINARY-LABELED PRODUCTS:

OTC products may be available under a variety of trade names labeled for use in dogs, cats, chickens, turkeys, or swine. Read and carefully follow all label instructions. Meat withdrawal is 14 days for poultry and 21 days for swine.[2,3]

HUMAN-LABELED PRODUCTS: NONE

References

For the complete list of references, see **wiley.com/go/budde/plumb**

Pirlimycin

(per-li-***mye***-sin) *Pirsue*®

Lincosamide Antibiotic

Prescriber Highlights

- ▶ For intramammary use in lactating dairy cattle
- ▶ Repeated infusion with pirlimycin may increase the potential for intramammary infections and subsequent clinical mastitis.
- ▶ Be sure to observe longer withdrawal times when using extended therapy.

Uses/Indications

Pirlimycin is FDA-approved for the treatment of clinical and subclinical mastitis in lactating dairy cattle associated with *Staphylococcus* spp and *Streptococcus* spp.

The World Health Organization (WHO) has designated pirlimycin as a Highly Important antimicrobial agent for human medicine.[1] The Office International des Epizooties (OIE) Antimicrobial Classification has designated pirlimycin as a Veterinary Highly Important Antimicrobial agent.[2]

Pharmacology/Actions

Like other lincosamides, pirlimycin acts by binding to the 50S ribosomal subunit of susceptible bacterial RNA, thus interfering with bacterial protein synthesis. It is primarily active against gram-positive bacteria, including a variety of *Staphylococcus* spp (eg, *S aureus, S epidermidis, S chromogenes, S hyicus, S xylosus*), *Streptococcus* spp (eg, *S agalactiae, S dysgalactiae, S uberis, S bovis*) and *Enterococcus faecalis*. It is not active against gram-negative bacteria.

Pharmacokinetics

Systemic absorption after intramammary (IMM) administration is ≈50%. Pirlimycin is lipophilic and diffuses readily across tissue membranes. After systemic absorption, it is secreted into the milk of all four quarters. Tissue pirlimycin concentrations in treated quarters are ≈2-3 times those found in the extracellular fluid. It is eliminated primarily as parent drug when administered via IMM; however, 4% of the dose is oxidized by the liver to pirlimycin sulfoxide.

Contraindications/Precautions/Warnings

Repeated infusion for extended-duration therapy regimens (ie, infusion longer than twice in a 24-hour interval, up to 8 days) can result in elevated somatic cell counts or clinical mastitis, which can be fatal.[3] Failure to thoroughly clean quarters or use aseptic infusion technique may increase this risk. Discontinue use if acute clinical mastitis or other signs of illness develop during extended-duration therapy.

Milk from untreated quarters must be disposed of during withdrawal time as residues may be detected from untreated quarters.

Adverse Effects

Repeated infusion with pirlimycin may increase the potential for intramammary infections and subsequent clinical mastitis (see ***Contraindications/Precautions/Warnings***).[3]

Reproductive/Nursing Safety

No information was noted. Because safety has not been established in animals, this drug should only be used when the maternal benefits outweigh the potential risks to offspring.

Overdose/Acute Toxicity

No data were located. For patients that have experienced or are suspected to have experienced an overdose, consultation with a 24-hour poison consultation center specializing in providing veterinary-specific information is recommended. For general information related to overdose and toxin exposures, as well as contact information for poison control centers, refer to ***Appendix.***

Drug Interactions

- Because erythromycin and clindamycin have shown antagonism in vitro, antagonism may also occur with pirlimycin.

Laboratory Considerations

- The established tolerance of pirlimycin in milk is 0.4 ppm.

Dosages

CATTLE:

Clinical and subclinical mastitis caused by susceptible organisms in lactating dairy cattle (label dosage; FDA-approved): Using proper teat end preparation, sanitation, and intramammary infusion technique, infuse contents of one syringe (50 mg/10 mL) into each affected quarter.[3] Repeat treatment after 24 hours. For extended therapy, treatment may be repeated at 24-hour intervals for up to 8 consecutive days. **NOTE**: US withdrawal times are extended when used daily for longer than 2 consecutive days. See ***Dosage Forms/Regulatory Status.***

Monitoring

- Efficacy: resolution of clinical signs related to mastitis

Client Information

- It is important to follow and understand your veterinarian's recommendations for how to give this medicine to your cow.
- Be sure you understand how long to treat your cow. Repeated infusion during extended duration therapy regimens, even with adequate teat end preparation and sanitation, can result in serious illness, including death of the animal.
- Carefully follow your veterinarian's instructions for appropriate milk and meat withdrawal times.
- Milk from untreated quarters must also be disposed of during withdrawal time as residues may be detected from untreated quarters.

Chemistry/Synonyms

Pirlimycin HCl is a lincosamide antibiotic. It has a molecular weight of 465.4.

Pirlimycin HCl may also be known as U-57930E and *Pirsue*®.

Storage/Stability

Store syringes at or below 25°C (77°F); protect from freezing.

Dosage Forms/Regulatory Status

VETERINARY-LABELED PRODUCTS:

Pirlimycin HCl Sterile Solution: pirlimycin base 50 mg in a 10 mL disposable teat syringe; *Pirsue*®; (Rx). FDA-approved for use in lactating dairy cattle. At United States label dosages, milk withdrawal is 36 hours. Meat withdrawal is 9 days if 2 infusions 24 hours apart are used; however, if administering *any* extended duration of therapy (ie, more than 2 daily infusions, up to 8 consecutive days), meat withdrawal is 21 days.

HUMAN-LABELED PRODUCTS: NONE

References

For the complete list of references, see **wiley.com/go/budde/plumb**

Piroxicam

(peer-**ox**-i-kam) *Feldene*®

Nonsteroidal Anti-Inflammatory Drug (NSAID), Anti-Tumor

Prescriber Highlights

- NSAID primarily used for its antitumor (indirect) activity. Safer FDA approved NSAIDs are available for treatment of pain and inflammation in dogs and cats.
- Contraindications include hypersensitivity or animals with allergic-type reactions to aspirin or other NSAIDs.
- Extreme caution is advised in animals with active or history of GI ulcer disease or bleeding disorders. Caution should be used in those with severely compromised cardiac function.
- Adverse effects include GI ulceration and bleeding, GI distress (eg, vomiting, anorexia, diarrhea), elevated liver enzymes, and, rarely, renal papillary necrosis.

Uses/Indications

In dogs and cats, piroxicam is primarily indicated for adjunctive treatment of bladder transitional cell carcinoma.[1-4] This drug may also be beneficial in the treatment of squamous cell carcinoma,[5,6] inflammatory mammary carcinoma,[7] soft tissue sarcoma,[8] primary lung carcinoma,[9] and transmissible venereal tumor (TVT).[2] Piroxicam may be beneficial in reducing the pain and inflammation associated with degenerative joint disease; however, FDA-approved, safer alternatives are available. When used in combination with oral alkylator therapy, piroxicam also has anti-angiogenic effects, thereby delaying tumor recurrence and/or metastases in dogs.[10]

Piroxicam has shown benefits in treating cats with transitional cell carcinoma[11,12] and cats with oral squamous cell carcinoma.[13-15]

Piroxicam administered after surgical debulking successfully treated transitional cell carcinoma in a horse.[16] Other case reports for adjunctive treatment of squamous cell carcinoma in horses have been published.[17,18]

Pharmacology/Actions

Like other NSAIDs, piroxicam has anti-inflammatory, analgesic, and antipyretic activity. The drug's anti-inflammatory activity is thought to be primarily due to its inhibition of prostaglandin synthesis, but additional mechanisms (eg, superoxide formation inhibition) may also be important. As with other NSAIDs, piroxicam can affect renal function, cause GI mucosal damage, and inhibit platelet aggregation.

Piroxicam's antitumor effects are believed to be due to its action on the immune system[2] and its antiangiogenic effect[19] rather than direct effects on tumor cells. Piroxicam has been shown to enhance the activity of vinblastine in dogs with transitional cell carcinoma.[20]

Pharmacokinetics

After oral administration, piroxicam is well absorbed from the GI tract. Although the presence of food decreases the rate of absorption, the amount absorbed is not decreased. It is not believed that antacids significantly affect absorption.

In dogs, piroxicam has a high oral bioavailability of 100%, with peak plasma levels reached ≈3 hours after administration. Volume of distribution is ≈0.3 L/kg; total body clearance is 0.066 L/hour, and elimination half-life is ≈40 hours.[21]

In cats given single oral doses, piroxicam is well absorbed with an oral bioavailability of ≈80%. Peak levels occur in ≈3 hours. Elimination half-life after IV or PO administration is ≈12 to 13 hours.[22]

Piroxicam is highly bound to plasma proteins. In humans, synovial levels are ≈40% of those found in plasma. Maternal milk concentrations are only ≈1% of plasma levels.

In humans, piroxicam has a long plasma half-life (ie, ≈50 hours). The drug is principally excreted as metabolites in the urine after hepatic (CYP2C9) biotransformation.

Contraindications/Precautions/Warnings

Piroxicam is contraindicated in patients hypersensitive to it or in those with allergic-type reactions to aspirin or other NSAIDs. This drug should be used only when its potential benefits outweigh the risks in patients with active or history of GI ulcer disease or bleeding disorders. Because peripheral edema has been noted in some human patients, piroxicam should be used with caution in patients with severely compromised cardiac function. Antipyretic effects may mask signs of infection (eg, fever).

Do not confuse PIRoxicam with PARoxetine.

Adverse Effects

Like other NSAIDs used in dogs, piroxicam has the potential for causing significant GI ulceration and bleeding. The therapeutic window for the drug is narrow, as doses as low as 1 mg/kg given daily have caused significant GI ulceration and peritonitis. Other adverse effects reported in humans that are possible in dogs include CNS effects (eg, headache, dizziness), otic effects (eg, tinnitus), elevations in hepatic enzymes, pruritus and rash, reduced renal function, hyperkalemia, heart failure, and peripheral edema. Renal papillary necrosis has been seen in dogs postmortem but, apparently, clinical effects have not been noted with these occurrences.[2,23] In dogs, advanced age increases the likelihood of adverse effects.[24]

Cats may have GI effects (eg, vomiting, anorexia, diarrhea), particularly early in therapy[13]; vomiting is the most common clinical sign, affecting ≈15% to 20% of cats treated with piroxicam. Gastric erosions[25] and elevated liver enzymes[13] have been documented. There are anecdotal reports of piroxicam decreasing hematocrits in cats given a daily regimen for 7 to 14 days. Renal toxicity is possible if used for prolonged periods.

Reproductive/Nursing Safety

Studies in animals have not demonstrated any teratogenic effects associated with piroxicam. Postimplantation losses occurred in rats, but not rabbits, given piroxicam during organogenesis. Premature closure of fetal ductus arteriosus has occurred in human pregnancies, and the drug should be avoided starting at gestational week 30. NSAIDs inhibit prostaglandin synthesis, which may delay parturition and increase the risk for stillbirth.

The drug is excreted into maternal milk in very low concentrations (ie, ≈1% found in maternal plasma). Use with caution in nursing patients.

Overdose/Acute Toxicity

Limited information is available, but dogs may be more sensitive to piroxicam's ulcerative effects than are humans.

Common clinical signs associated with overdose include vomiting and bloody vomitus.

As with any NSAID, overdoses can lead to GI and renal effects. In monogastric animals, acute toxicity can also result in neurologic effects. Decontamination with emetics and/or activated charcoal is appropriate. For doses with expected GI effects, the use of GI protectants is warranted. If renal effects are also expected, fluid diuresis should be considered. Patients with significant overdose should be monitored carefully and treated supportively.

For patients that have experienced or are suspected to have experienced an overdose, it is strongly encouraged that a 24-hour poison consultation center that specializes in providing information specific for veterinary patients be consulted. For general information related to overdose and toxin exposures, as well as contact information for poison control centers, refer to ***Appendix***.

Drug Interactions

The following drug interactions have either been reported or are theoretical in humans or animals receiving piroxicam and may be of significance in veterinary patients. Unless otherwise noted, use together is not necessarily contraindicated, but weigh the potential risks and perform additional monitoring when appropriate.

- ACE INHIBITORS (eg, **benazepril, enalapril**): Concurrent piroxicam use may reduce ACE inhibitor efficacy.
- AMINOGLYCOSIDES (eg, **amikacin, gentamicin**): Increased risk for nephrotoxicity
- ANGIOTENSIN RECEPTOR BLOCKERS (ARB; eg, **telmisartan**): Concurrent piroxicam use may reduce ACE inhibitor efficacy.
- ANTICOAGULANTS (eg, **enoxaparin, heparin, rivaroxaban, warfarin**): Increased risk for bleeding is possible.
- ASPIRIN: Increased risk for bleeding. When aspirin is used concurrently with piroxicam, plasma levels of piroxicam could decrease, and there may be an increased likelihood of GI adverse effects (eg, blood loss). Concomitant administration of aspirin with piroxicam is not recommended.
- BISPHOSPHONATES, ORAL (eg, **alendronate**): May increase the risk for GI ulceration
- CISPLATIN: Piroxicam may potentiate the renal toxicity of cisplatin when used in combination.
- CLOPIDOGREL: Increased risk for bleeding
- CORTICOSTEROIDS (eg, **dexamethasone, predniso(lo)ne**): Concomitant administration with NSAIDs may significantly increase the risk for GI adverse effects.
- CYCLOSPORINE: Concurrent use may result in increased risk for cyclosporine nephrotoxicity.
- DIGOXIN: Concurrent use may result in increased serum concentration of digoxin and prolonged digoxin half-life.
- DIURETICS (eg, **furosemide**): Concurrent use may result in reduced diuretic efficacy and possible nephrotoxicity.
- HIGHLY PROTEIN BOUND DRUGS (eg, oral anticoagulants, other anti-inflammatory agents, phenytoin, salicylates, sulfonamides, sulfonylurea antidiabetic agents [eg, **glipizide, glyburide**]): Because piroxicam is highly bound to plasma proteins (99%), it could theoretically displace other highly bound drugs; a temporary increase serum levels may occur. These interactions have not been shown to be of clinical concern.
- METHOTREXATE: Serious toxicity (eg, bone marrow suppression, nephrotoxicity) has occurred when NSAIDs were used concomitantly with methotrexate; use together with extreme caution.
- SSRIs (eg, **fluoxetine, paroxetine, sertraline**): Concurrent use may result in an increased risk for bleeding.

- **Tacrolimus**: Concurrent use may result in acute renal failure.
- **Tricyclic Antidepressants** (eg, **amitriptyline, clomipramine**): Concurrent use may result in increased risk for bleeding.

Laboratory Considerations

- Piroxicam may cause falsely elevated **blood glucose** values when using the glucose oxidase and peroxidase method, with ABTS as a chromogen.

Dosages

DOGS:

Adjunctive therapy for neoplastic diseases (extra-label): 0.3 mg/kg PO with food once daily (preferred, if tolerated) or once every other day (every 48 hours).[2] Adding misoprostol may be considered in dogs that do not tolerate GI effects of NSAIDs.

Adjunctive treatment for idiopathic lymphoplasmacytic rhinitis (LPR; extra-label): Piroxicam 0.3 mg/kg PO once a day is recommended. Long-term administration of antibiotics with immunomodulatory effects (eg, doxycycline 3 – 5 mg/kg PO every 12 hours or azithromycin 5 mg/kg PO once a day) combined with NSAIDs can be helpful in some dogs. If clinical improvement is observed within 2 weeks, daily piroxicam therapy should be continued but the frequency of administration of doxycycline should be reduced to once daily or azithromycin to twice weekly. Therapy will likely be required for a minimum of 6 months, if not indefinitely.[26]

CATS:

Adjunctive therapy for transitional cell carcinomas (extra-label): 0.3 mg/kg PO every 48 hours (every other day)[11]

Adjunctive treatment for other neoplasias (eg, oral squamous cell carcinoma (OSCC), solid tumors) (extra-label): 0.13 – 0.41 mg/kg PO daily.[13,14] 0.3 mg/kg PO every 48 hours has also been used in cats with OSCC.[15]

Anti-inflammatory/analgesic (extra-label): 1 mg/cat (NOT mg/kg) PO once a day for a maximum of 7 days[27,28]

Idiopathic chronic rhinosinusitis (extra-label): 0.3 mg/kg PO once daily or every other day may reduce clinical signs in some cats[26]

HORSES:

Neoplastic diseases (extra-label):

a) From a case report treating mucocutaneous squamous cell carcinoma[17]: 80 mg/horse (NOT mg/kg) PO once daily; lip lesion resolved completely over 3 months, but the patient developed signs of colic twice. The dose was eventually reduced to every other day or every third day.

b) From a case report treating a squamous cell carcinoma of the third eyelid after surgical excision[18]: 80 mg/horse (NOT mg/kg) PO once daily

c) From a case report treating bladder TCC after surgical debulking[16]: 0.2 mg/kg PO once daily, started 10 days postoperatively and continued for 4 months, then reduced to 0.1 mg/kg PO once daily

RABBITS, RODENTS, SMALL MAMMALS:

Fracture with associated limb swelling in rabbits (extra-label): 0.1 – 0.2 mg/kg PO every 8 hours for 3 weeks[29]

Monitoring

- Adverse effects (eg, inappetence, vomiting, diarrhea, melena)
- Liver enzymes and renal function tests should be monitored occasionally with chronic use, especially in cats.

Client Information

- This drug is best given with food to reduce the chance for stomach upset.
- Gastrointestinal (stomach) ulcers and bleeding and kidney problems (especially in cats) are possible.

Chemistry/Synonyms

Piroxicam, an oxicam derivative NSAID, occurs as a white crystalline solid. It is sparingly soluble in water. Piroxicam is not structurally related to other NSAIDs.

Piroxicam may also be known as CP-16171, piroxicamum, or PIRO; many trade names are available.

Storage/Stability

Capsules should be stored at temperatures less than 30°C (86°F) in tight, light-resistant containers. When stored as recommended, capsules have an expiration date of 36 months after manufacture.

Dosage Forms/Regulatory Status

VETERINARY-LABELED PRODUCTS: NONE

The Association of Racing Commissioners International (ARCI) has designated this drug as a class 4 substance. See ***Appendix*** for more information. Use of this drug may not be allowed in certain animal competitions. Check rules and regulations before entering in a competition while this medication is being administered. Contact local racing authorities for further guidance.

HUMAN-LABELED PRODUCTS:

Piroxicam Oral Capsules: 10 and 20 mg; *Feldene*®, generic; (Rx)

References

For the complete list of references, see **wiley.com/go/budde/plumb**

Polyethylene Glycol 3350 (PEG 3350)

(pah-lee-**eth**-il-een **gly**-kol) *MiraLAX*®, *CoLyte*®, *GoLYTELY*®

Laxative, Hyperosmotic

NOTE: Within this monograph, "PEG 3350 with electrolytes" refers to polyethylene glycol 3350 products that also contain electrolytes (eg, GoLYTELY®) while PEG 3350 refers to polyethylene glycol 3350 as a single agent (ie, no electrolytes; eg, *Miralax*®).

Prescriber Highlights

- Indications include constipation, bowel cleansing in preparation for colonoscopy, or to increase elimination of GI toxins
- For enteral use only.
- Contraindicated in patients hypersensitive to it. When used for bowel cleansing, contraindications include patients with GI obstruction, gastric retention, bowel perforation, toxic colitis, or megacolon.
- Adverse effects may include cramping and nausea; electrolyte disturbances may occur with repeated use.

Uses/Indications

Polyethylene glycol 3350 (PEG 3350) is an osmotic laxative agent and is used as an adjunct therapy for feline constipation. When balanced electrolytes are added (PEG 3350 with electrolytes; eg, *CoLyte*®, *GoLYTELY*®), it is used as a bowel cleansing solution. It could also be used to reduce intestinal transit time to reduce the absorption of orally ingested toxicants and poisons, but usually sorbitol is chosen for this indication. It is without odor, taste, or texture, allowing it to easily be added to food or fluids.

Pharmacology/Actions

Polyethylene glycol 3350 is a non-absorbable compound that acts as an osmotic laxative agent that does not alter nutrient, glucose, or electrolyte absorption. PEG 3350 with electrolytes is used as a bowel cleansing solution (eg, *CoLyte*®, *GoLYTELY*®), and the additional electrolytes are added to help prevent electrolyte imbalance. Sodium sulfate is the primary sodium source, so sodium absorption is minimized. Other electrolytes (bicarbonate, potassium, chloride) are also added so that no net change occurs with either absorption or secretion of electrolytes or water in the gut.

Pharmacokinetics

PEG 3350 is not absorbed after oral administration. Depending on formulation, dose and additional fluid consumed, PEG 3350 can have a laxative effect within one hour of dosing.

Contraindications/Precautions/Warnings

In humans, all PEG 3350 solutions are contraindicated in patients that are hypersensitive to it. PEG 3350 with electrolytes also is contraindicated in patients with GI obstruction, gastric retention, bowel perforation, toxic colitis, or megacolon. PEG 3350 solutions with electrolytes should be used with caution in patients with inflammatory bowel disease and in patients already receiving laxatives, as fluid or electrolyte imbalances may occur. Patients should have electrolyte imbalances corrected and be adequately hydrated prior to using PEG 3350 with electrolytes. Enteral infusions of large volumes may increase the risk of aspiration.

Do not confuse PEG 3350 without electrolytes (eg, *Miralax*®) with PEG 3350 containing electrolytes (eg, *GoLYTELY*®).

Adverse Effects

Vomiting, nausea, and cramping are possible. Vomiting occurring during acute administration of PEG 3350 with electrolytes may be managed with metoclopramide or by reducing the flow rate by 50% for one hour, then resuming the original rate.[1] Long-term use could potentially cause hyponatremia, dehydration, or hyperkalemia. If PEG 3350 is absorbed systemically, oxidative injury to red blood cells could occur in cats, but this has not been documented to date.

In one small study ($n = 6$) in cats where PEG 3350 with electrolytes (powder in food and dose titrated to produce soft, but formed stools) was given for 4 weeks, 1 cat sporadically vomited after dosing, mild erythrocytosis was noted in 1 cat, and 3 cats developed mild hyperkalemia. The authors concluded that PEG 3350 was a safe and palatable oral laxative in cats for long-term use; potential side effects include hyperkalemia and subclinical dehydration.[2]

In humans, PEG 3350 has rarely caused hyponatremia secondary to syndrome of inappropriate vasopressin release (SIADH). Contact dermatitis has also been reported in humans. Neither of these adverse effects have been reported in veterinary patients.

Reproductive/Nursing Safety

Minimal amounts are systemically absorbed, and it is therefore likely that these products are safe to use in pregnant or lactating animals at recommended dosages.

Because safety has not been established in animals, this drug should only be used when the maternal benefits outweigh the potential risks to offspring.

Overdose/Acute Toxicity

A single oral overdose event could cause diarrhea and fluid or electrolyte abnormalities.

Toxicity may occur when there is aspiration of the PEG 3350 solution or administration through an unintended route. A case report describes the successful use of bronchoscopy to lavage the lungs of a dog that aspirated PEG 3350 solution.[3] The authors recommend early intervention with cases of aspiration due to the rapid progression of the pulmonary edema that occurs.

Another case report describes inadvertent 6 g/kg IV administration of PEG 3350 to a cat which resulted in severe hypernatremia (Na = 203 mmol/L), encephalopathy (initially laterally recumbent with diminished cranial nerve reflexes, with head pressing and vocalization on day 4 of hospitalization), transient hemolysis, and azotemia (Cr = 3.1 mg/dL).[4] Treatment with supportive care (including appropriate IV and oral fluid therapy) allowed for correction of the hypernatremia and azotemia, as well as improved clinical signs. One month after discharge, there was complete resolution of clinical signs.

For patients that have experienced or are suspected to have experienced an overdose, consultation with a 24-hour poison consultation center specializing in providing veterinary-specific information is recommended. For general information related to overdose and toxin exposures, as well as contact information for poison control centers, refer to ***Appendix.***

Drug Interactions

The following drug interactions with PEG 3350 (single agent, or with electrolytes) either have been reported or are theoretical in humans or animals and may be of significance in veterinary patients. Unless otherwise noted, use together is not necessarily contraindicated, but the potential risks should be weighed and additional monitoring should be performed when appropriate.

- **Anticholinergic Agents** (eg, **atropine**): May decrease GI motility and reduce laxative effect
- **Diuretics** (eg, **furosemide**): May increase risk for dehydration
- **Laxatives, Other** (eg, **bisacodyl, lactulose**): May have additive effects on GI motility and increase risk for adverse effects. Stimulant laxatives may increase the risk for GI mucosal ulceration.
- **Opioids** (eg, **morphine**): May decrease GI motility and reduce laxative effect
- **Other Drugs, Oral**: Reduced absorption of other oral drugs (especially extended-release) could occur if given concomitantly. Administer any necessary oral medications at least 1 hour prior to PEG 3350 administration to ensure adequate absorption.
- **Tricyclic Antidepressants (TCAs**, eg, **amitriptyline, clomipramine**): May decrease GI motility and reduce laxative effect

Dosages

DOGS:

Polyethylene Glycol 3350-Electrolyte Solution (eg, *CoLyte*®, *GoLYTELY*®):

Colonic cleansing prior to colonoscopy (extra-label): Several slightly different protocols have been suggested. The following is an example: Keep animal from food for a minimum of 24 to 36 hours. On the evening prior to a morning colonoscopy (or the morning for an afternoon colonoscopy), give 60 mL/kg *GoLYTELY*® via orogastric tube. Repeat in 2 hours. A warm water enema should follow each dose and a third enema given prior to anesthesia.[5-7]

Enterogastric lavage for decontamination (extra-label): 25 mL/kg/hour delivered via NG tube. Do not exceed 175 mL/kg total.[1] Alternatively, 500 mL/hour (NOT mL/kg/hour) via NG tube. Administer until fecal effluent runs clear, which may take several hours.

CATS:

Laxative (extra-label): Using the polyethylene 3350 powder (eg, *MiraLax*®), ⅛ to ¼ teaspoon/cat (NOT teaspoon/kg) twice daily in food.

Polyethylene Glycol 3350-Electrolyte Solution (eg, *CoLyte*®, *GoLYTELY*®):

Adjunctive treatment of obstipation/constipation (extra-label): From an observational study in 9 cats, *CoLyte*® was administered via naso-esophageal tube at rates between 6 – 10 mL/kg/hr. The median total dose given was 80 mL/kg (range 40 – 156 mL/kg). Median time to significant defecation was 8 hours (range 5 to 24 hours). Side effects were limited to vomiting in 1 cat (was vomiting prior to admission).[8]

Colonic cleansing prior to colonoscopy (extra-label): Keep animal from food for 24 to 36 hours. On the evening prior to a morning colonoscopy, give 30 mL/kg *GoLYTELY*® via nasogastric tube. Repeat in 2 hours. A warm water enema should follow each dose and a third enema given prior to anesthesia.[6,7] **NOTE**: An antiemetic may be given before the first *GoLYTELY*® dose is given to reduce vomiting.

Monitoring

- Fluid and electrolyte status; in particular, if using high doses or with long-term use
- Clinical efficacy (eg, production of feces)
- Adverse effects, especially vomiting and aspiration when a large volume is administered

Client Information

- This medicine is used to treat constipation, for bowel cleansing before procedures (eg, colonoscopy), or to help remove toxins from the gastrointestinal tract.
- Polyethylene glycol 3350 (PEG 3350) powders are mixed into canned food or dissolved in liquid before using. Follow your veterinarian's or pharmacist's measuring instructions carefully.
- PEG 3350 is available OTC (over-the-counter; without a prescription). Do not give PEG 3350 (or any other OTC medications) to your animal without first consulting your veterinarian.
- Contact your veterinarian if your animal begins vomiting or develops any new signs after starting this medication.
- While your animal is taking this medication, it is important to return to your veterinarian for periodic examinations and bloodwork monitoring. Do not miss these important follow-up visits.

Chemistry/Synonyms

Polyethylene glycol 3350 is a non-absorbable compound that acts as an osmotic agent. It occurs as white or almost white solid with a waxy appearance and is very soluble in water and very slightly soluble in alcohol. One common trade name is *Miralax*®.

Storage/Stability

Store powder at 25°C (77°F); excursions are permitted from 15°C-30°C (59°F-86°F). Reconstituted PEG 3350 solutions (from powder by the pharmacy, client, clinic) should be kept refrigerated and used within 24 hours.

Dosage Forms/Regulatory Status

VETERINARY-LABELED PRODUCTS: NONE

The Association of Racing Commissioners International (ARCI) has designated this drug as a class 5 substance. Use of this drug may not be allowed in certain animal competitions. Check rules and regulations before entering in a competition while this medication is being administered. Contact local racing authorities for further guidance. See ***Appendix*** for more information.

HUMAN-LABELED PRODUCTS:

Polyethylene Glycol 3350 Powder for solution: *MiraLax*®, *GlycoLax*®, *ClearLax*®, *Gavilax*®, *Dulcolax Balance*®, generic; (OTC). Available in either pre-measured 17 g packets or bulk powder

Polyethylene Glycol 3350 and Electrolyte Solutions (Rx): There are a variety of products available. The following are representative:

CoLyte®; (Rx); 1 gallon of Powder for Oral Solution in bottles: 227.1 g PEG 3350, 5.53 g sodium chloride (NaCl), 6.36 g sodium bicarbonate, 21.5 g sodium sulfate, 2.82 g potassium chloride (KCl); 4 L of solution: 240 g PEG 3350, 22.72 g sodium sulfate, 6.72 g sodium bicarbonate, 5.84 g NaCl, 2.98 g KCl

GoLYTELY®; (Rx); Powder for Oral Solution in jugs: 5.86 g NaCl, 6.74 g sodium bicarbonate, 22.74 g sodium sulfate, 2.97 g KCl, 236 g PEG 3350; Packets: 227.1 g PEG 3350, 21.5 g sodium sulfate, 6.36 g sodium bicarbonate, 5.53 g NaCl, 2.82 g KCl

NuLytely®, *TriLyte*®, (Rx); Powder for Reconstitution in 4 L jugs: 420 g PEG 3350, 5.72 g sodium bicarbonate, 11.2 g NaCl, 1.48 g KCl

MoviPrep®; (Rx); Powder for Reconstitution in pouches (amount per 1 L): 100 g PEG 3350, 7.5 g sodium sulfate, 2.691 g NaCl, 1.015 g KCl

References

For the complete list of references, see **wiley.com/go/budde/plumb**

Polymyxin B, Systemic

(***pol***-lee-***mix***-in ***B***)

Polymyxin Antibiotic

For specific information related to topical use of polymyxin B, see ***Corticosteroid/Antimicrobial Preparations, Otic; Oxytetracycline/Polymyxin B Ophthalmic, Triple Antibiotic Ophthalmic.***

Prescriber Highlights

- Concentration-dependent polypeptide bactericidal antibiotic effective against most gram-negative bacilli
- Primarily used at subantimicrobial dosages to treat endotoxemia in equine patients
- Rarely given at antimicrobial doses because of dose-related adverse effects, including nephrotoxicity and neurotoxicity
- Thrombophlebitis at the administration site is possible.

Uses/Indications

Polymyxin B is primarily used in equine patients at subantimicrobial dosages to treat endotoxemia. No studies have been performed in naturally occurring cases of endotoxemia. Polymyxin B administration to healthy foals or horses given lipopolysaccharide (LPS) under experimental conditions resulted in dose-dependent decreases in rectal temperature, decreases in respiratory and heart rates, improved attitude, reduced incidence of hypoglycemia, and decreased concentrations of blood lactate, tumor necrosis factor-alpha, thromboxane B_2, and IL-6.[1-5] The beneficial effects of polymyxin B for endotoxemia appear to be both time- and dose-dependent, with early administration of higher doses proving more beneficial than delayed treatment or lower doses. Similar beneficial results for experimentally induced endotoxemia were found in cats,[6,7] sheep,[8] and dwarf goats.[9] IV regional limb perfusions of polymyxin B may be used as an alternative treatment of horses with induced gram-negative bacteria synovial infections.[10]

In humans, polymyxin B is used to treat sepsis, bacteremia, and serious urinary or respiratory tract infections caused by susceptible bacteria, when safer antibiotics cannot be used.

The World Health Organization has designated polymyxin B as a Critically Important, Highest Priority antimicrobial for human medicine.[11]

Pharmacology/Actions

As an antibacterial agent, polymyxin B binds to phospholipids in bacterial cytoplastic membranes, increasing permeability and causing loss of intracellular components and cell death. It has concentration-dependent bactericidal activity against most gram-negative bacilli, including *Escherichia coli*, *Enterobacter* spp, *Klebsiella* spp, *Haemophilus* spp, and *Pseudomonas* spp, but not *Proteus* spp. Polymyxin B may have synergistic antibacterial effects against *Pseudomonas* spp, *Klebsiella* spp, and *Acinetobacter* spp when combined with imipenem, rifampin, and/or azithromycin. Pus and cellular debris reduce effectiveness. Polymyxin B is ineffective against gram-positive bacteria, gram-negative cocci, or obligate anaerobes. It lacks activity against viral, fungal, or parasitic pathogens.

When administered at subantimicrobial dosages to equine patients with endotoxemia, polymyxin B binds to and inactivates the lipopolysaccharide (LPS) component of endotoxin. Polymyxin B inhibited TNF-alpha production in an equine ex vivo study.[12]

Pharmacokinetics

In horses receiving 6000 units/kg polymyxin B sulfate as an IV infusion over 15 minutes, elimination half-life averaged ≈3.3 hours. Administration of 6000 units/kg every 8 hours for 5 treatments was determined to maintain an effective anti-lipopolysaccharide (LPS) polymyxin B concentration.[13]

In humans, polymyxin B is not orally bioavailable. After parenteral administration, polymyxin B distributes poorly into tissues and does not cross the blood–brain barrier. Approximately 50% is bound to cell membrane phospholipids. It is renally excreted. Half-life is 6 hours, which may increase to 48 to 72 hours in anuric patients.

Contraindications/Precautions/Warnings

Polymyxin B is contraindicated in patients that are hypersensitive to it or other polymyxins. It should be used with caution in patients with, or at risk for, renal impairment or respiratory paralysis; it should only be used in hospitalized patients being monitored for these conditions. Fluid support should be provided to maintain renal perfusion; dose reduction may be required in patients with significant renal dysfunction. Overgrowth infections caused by fungi or nonsusceptible bacteria, including *Clostridia* spp, may occur during or after treatment with polymyxin B.

Adverse Effects

Few veterinary data are available. One dog developed pemphigus vulgaris after 1 week of otic polymyxin B application.[14] Transient ataxia during administration was observed in healthy horses.[15]

In humans, most adverse effects are dose related. Polymyxin B may cause renal tubule damage, and hyponatremia, hypokalemia, hypochloremia, and hypocalcemia have been noted. Thrombophlebitis is possible at administration sites. Additional adverse effects may include fever, rash and other skin reactions, and eosinophilia. Neurotoxicity (eg, irritability, weakness, lethargy, ataxia) may occur but is rare; patients with renal impairment that receive high-dose polymyxin B therapy are at increased risk. Rapid IV injection or infusion increases the risk for neuromuscular blockade. IM administration is not advised due to significant pain at the injection site.

Reproductive/Nursing Safety

Although polymyxin B does not cross the placenta and is not absorbed orally, safe use in pregnant or lactating women has not been established; thus, the drug should be used with caution in pregnant or nursing veterinary patients.

Because safety has not been established in animals, this drug should only be used when the maternal benefits outweigh the potential risks to offspring.

Overdosage/Acute Toxicity

Polymyxin B may cause renal tubule damage, which may reduce its elimination and prolong its half-life. Respiratory paralysis and other signs of neuromuscular blockade are possible.

Dialysis may remove only 5% to 13% of polymyxin B and is considered ineffective. Neither neostigmine nor calcium administration reverse neuromuscular blockade. Supportive treatment is recommended, including mechanical ventilation when required.

For patients that have experienced or are suspected to have experienced an overdose, consultation with a 24-hour poison consultation center specializing in providing veterinary-specific information is recommended. For general information related to overdose and toxin exposures, as well as contact information for poison control centers, refer to ***Appendix***.

Drug Interactions

The following drug interactions have either been reported or are theoretical in humans or animals receiving polymyxin B and may be of significance in veterinary patients. Unless otherwise noted, use together is not necessarily contraindicated, but the potential risks should be weighed and additional monitoring performed when appropriate.

- **Aminoglycosides** (eg, **amikacin, gentamicin**): Combination may increase risk for nephropathy.[15]
- **Bisphosphonates** (eg, **clodronate, pamidronate, zoledronic acid**): Combination may increase risk for nephropathy.
- **Loop Diuretics** (eg, **furosemide**): Combination may increase risk for nephropathy.
- **Nephrotoxic Drugs, Other** (eg, **amphotericin B, carboplatin, cyclosporine, iohexol**): Combination may increase risk for nephropathy.
- **Neuromuscular Blockers** (eg, **atracurium, pancuronium, succinylcholine**): Combination may enhance or prolong neuromuscular blockade and increase risk for respiratory paralysis.
- **Nonsteroidal Anti-inflammatory Drugs (NSAIDs**; eg, **flunixin, meloxicam**): Combination may increase risk for nephropathy.
- **Polymyxins, Other** (eg, **colistin – polymyxin E**): Combination may increase risk for toxicity.
- **Sodium Citrate**: Combination may increase risk for respiratory depression.

Laboratory Considerations

None noted

Dosages

NOTE: All dosages are for polymyxin B *sulfate* unless otherwise noted.

CATS:

Reduce clinical signs related to endotoxemia (extra-label): 6000 units/kg IV infusion administered over 30 minutes as a single dose under experimental conditions.[7] Further clinical study is warranted to validate the safety and efficacy of this dosage.

HORSES:

Reduce clinical signs related to endotoxemia (extra-label): 6000 units/kg IV bolus every 8 to 12 hours is most commonly recommended, but an effective dosage range of 1000 – 10,000 units/kg has been supported in experimental studies. Polymyxin B doses were typically further diluted with 0.9% NaCl to a total volume of 12 to 50 mL and administered as an IV bolus.[1,3-5] No cases of nephrotoxicity were observed at these doses in the study patients (healthy foals or horses). Administration early in the disease course is believed to improve outcomes.

Synovial infections (extra-label): From a pharmacokinetic study: 250,000 units (NOT units/kg) via IV regional limb perfusion (IV-RLP) achieved therapeutic concentration in synovial fluid.[10] Further clinical study is warranted to validate the safety and efficacy of this dosage.

SHEEP/GOATS:

Reduce clinical signs related to endotoxemia (extra-label):

a) In sheep, under experimental conditions: 6000 units/kg IV infusion along with 2.5 L of isotonic fluids at 20 mL/kg/hour[8]

b) In dwarf goats, under experimental conditions: 3 mg/kg IV infusion administered over 30 minutes (0.1 mg/kg/minute).[9] Study methods do not state whether polymyxin B or polymyxin B sulfate was used.

Monitoring

- Resolution of clinical signs related to endotoxemia (eg, vital signs, CBC)

- Baseline and periodic renal chemistry panel with electrolytes, urinalysis (check for proteinuria), and urine output. In humans, decreased urine output and increasing BUN are indications to discontinue treatment.
- Clinical signs related to neurotoxicity (eg, irritability, weakness, lethargy, ataxia) and respiratory depression or paralysis
- Culture and susceptibility testing prior to treatment when this drug is used for its antimicrobial properties (rare); this testing is not indicated when polymyxin B is used to treat endotoxemia.

Client Information

- Polymyxin B is an antibiotic administered only in the clinic to severely ill patients.
- Polymyxin B use may result in antibiotic-related diarrhea, which may persist for up to 2 months after treatment. Inform your veterinarian if diarrhea develops.

Chemistry/Synonyms

Polymyxin B is a polypeptide antibiotic derived from *Bacillus polymyxa* (*B aerosporous*) that contains Polymyxin B_1 and B_2. Parenteral formulations contain polymyxin B sulfate, which occurs as a white or almost-white, hygroscopic powder and is freely soluble in water and slightly soluble in alcohol. Available formulations of polymyxin B sulfate for injection contain no less than 6000 units polymyxin B per 1 mg. 1 mg pure polymyxin B base is equal to 10,000 units polymyxin B.

Storage/Stability

Prior to reconstitution, polymyxin B sulfate should be stored at controlled room temperature (20°C to 25°C [68°F-77°F]) and protected from light. Reconstituted polymyxin B sulfate solution must be refrigerated (2°C to 8°C [36°F-46°F]); the manufacturer recommends discarding any unused portion after 72 hours. Polymyxin B should not be mixed or stored in strongly acidic or alkaline solutions.

Compatibility/Compounding Considerations

Polymyxin B sulfate for injection requires reconstitution with 2 mL sterile water for injection, 0.9% sodium chloride for injection, or 5% dextrose for injection. In humans, further dilution with 5% dextrose to a final concentration of 1000 to 1667 units/mL is recommended. IV infusions should be administered over 30 to 90 minutes. In studies conducted in healthy foals or horses, polymyxin B doses were diluted with 0.9% NaCl to a total volume of 12 to 50 mL and safely administered as an IV bolus.[4,5]

Polymyxin B is reportedly **compatible** with 5% dextrose and 0.9% sodium chloride solutions. Polymyxin B is reportedly **incompatible** with IV solutions containing calcium or magnesium and is **incompatible** with amphotericin B, ampicillin, calcium salts, cefazolin, cefoxitin, chloramphenicol sodium succinate, diazepam, heparin sodium, insulin, magnesium salts, pantoprazole, and piperacillin-tazobactam.

Compatibility is dependent on factors such as pH, concentration, temperature, and diluent used. Specialized references or a hospital pharmacist should be consulted for more specific information.

Dosage Forms/Regulatory Status

VETERINARY-LABELED PRODUCTS: NONE

HUMAN-LABELED PRODUCTS:

Polymyxin B Sulfate for Injection: Each vial of lyophilized powder contains the equivalent of 500,000 polymyxin B units; generic; (Rx)

Polymyxin B may be found in a multitude of otic, ophthalmic, and topical products.

References

For the complete list of references, see **wiley.com/go/budde/plumb**

Polysulfated Glycosaminoglycan

(***pol***-ee-***sulf***-ayte-ed glye-***kose***-a-meen-ohe-***glye***-kan) *Adequan®*

Proteolytic Enzyme Inhibitor; Chondroprotectant

Prescriber Highlights

- ▶ FDA-approved for the treatment of noninfectious degenerative and/or traumatic arthritis/joint dysfunction in dogs (IM) and horses (IM or IA)
- ▶ Contraindications include hypersensitivity to polysulfated glycosaminoglycan (PSGAG) or known or suspected bleeding disorders. Should not be used in place of other treatments when infection suspected or present or in place of necessary surgical repair or joint immobilization
- ▶ Use it with caution in patients that have hepatic or renal impairment.
- ▶ Adverse effects are unlikely after IM injection. IA use in horses may result in postinjection inflammation; discontinue therapy if inflammation is excessive.

Uses/Indications

Polysulfated glycosaminoglycan (PSGAG) is FDA-approved in dogs for the control of signs associated with noninfectious degenerative and/or traumatic arthritis of synovial joints.[1] PSGAG had a beneficial and steroid-sparing effect in 3 dogs with pemphigus foliaceus.[2]

PSGAG is indicated in horses for the treatment of noninfectious degenerative and/or traumatic joint dysfunction and associated lameness of the carpal and hock joints.[3,4] The intra-articular product is labeled only for use in the carpal joint. PSGAG can be characterized as a disease-modifying agent in horses with osteoarthritis.[5] Additionally, the drug has demonstrated a positive effect on tendon healing under experimental conditions in horses.[6] PSGAG reduced the lameness score in horses with moderate to severe lameness caused by traumatic arthritis.[7]

Pharmacology/Actions

In joint tissue, polysulfated glycosaminoglycan (PSGAG) inhibits catabolic and proteolytic enzymes (eg, serine proteases, elastase, metalloproteases, hyaluronidases) that can degrade proteoglycans (including naturally occurring glycosaminoglycans), collagen, and hyaluronic acid, all of which increase connective tissue flexibility, resistance to compression, and resiliency. PSGAG also inhibits the synthesis of prostaglandin E_2, which is released in response to joint injury and is associated with the loss of proteoglycan from cartilage. By acting as a precursor, PSGAG increases the synthesis of proteoglycans[8] and hyaluronate in the joint to reduce inflammation and restore synovial fluid viscosity.

Pharmacokinetics

After IM injection, polysulfated glycosaminoglycan (PSGAG) is widely distributed throughout the body. Studies in rabbits and dogs showed peak serum concentrations ≈20 to 40 minutes after IM injection,[1] and peak joint concentrations are reached in 48 hours and persist for up to 96 hours. The drug passively diffuses from the synovial fluid into cartilage. PSGAG is deposited in all layers of articular cartilage and is preferentially taken up by osteoarthritic cartilage. When administered IM, articular concentrations will, over time, exceed those found in the serum.

In rabbits, metabolism occurs in the liver, spleen, bone marrow, and possibly the kidneys. The unchanged drug is primarily renally excreted.[1]

Pharmacokinetic information for horses was not located.

In humans, PSGAG was found to be 30% to 40% bound to plasma proteins.

Contraindications/Precautions/Warnings

Polysulfated glycosaminoglycan (PSGAG) is contraindicated in patients hypersensitive to it. Use is contraindicated in dogs with known or suspected bleeding disorders.[1] Use it with caution in patients with hepatic or renal impairment. PSGAG should not be used in place of other therapies in cases where the infection is present or suspected or in place of necessary surgical repair or joint immobilization.

In horses, concomitant use of PSGAG and NSAIDs or steroids may mask the clinical signs associated with joint sepsis.[3]

Products formulated for intramuscular use must not be injected intra-articularly.[1,3,4]

Adverse Effects

In dogs, adverse effects include pain at the injection site, transient diarrhea or vomiting, and abnormal bleeding.[1] Adverse effects are uncommon and are typically self-limiting without requiring treatment modification. Dose-related inhibition of hemostasis has been described.

In horses, intra-articular administration may cause inflammatory joint reactions, including joint pain, effusion, swelling, and associated lameness.[3] Joint reactions may be due to sensitivity or may be secondary to traumatic injection technique, overdose, or the number or frequency of the injections. Treatment consists of anti-inflammatory drugs, cold hydrotherapy, and rest. Discontinue therapy if excessive inflammation develops. Although uncommon, intra-articular administration can result in septic arthritis[3]; strict aseptic technique should be employed to minimize this occurrence. Amikacin 125 mg has been added to polysulfated glycosaminoglycan (PSGAG) solution (extra-label) when the intra-articular route is used in horses.[5] Nonseptic arthritis, hemathrosis, and cellulitis at the injection site have also rarely been reported.[3]

A case series reported fatal coagulopathies in avian species.[9] Another study in chickens found that thrombin-clotting times were significantly prolonged at 5 and 10 mg/kg doses, but at 1 mg/kg, there was no significant difference compared to control.[10] The results suggested that lower doses could potentially be safely used in avian species, but more research is needed to confirm safety and efficacy.

Reproductive/Nursing Safety

Safe use of polysulfated glycosaminoglycan (PSGAG) in animals intended for breeding or during pregnancy has not been demonstrated. It is not known whether glycosaminoglycans are excreted in maternal milk, but because PSGAG is not orally absorbed,[11] this effect is unlikely to be of clinical significance to the nursing offspring.

Because safety has not been established in animals, this drug should only be used when the maternal benefits outweigh the potential risks to offspring.

Overdose/Acute Toxicity

In dogs, dose-related intramuscular inflammation, hemorrhage, and degeneration have been noted. Dogs that received 3 times the recommended dose for 3 times the recommended duration were found to have increased cholesterol and microscopic lesions in the liver, kidneys, and lymph nodes. Dogs administered 10 times the recommended dose for 3 times the recommended duration also showed increased prothrombin time, reduced platelet count, increased ALT, and 1 large hematoma, which necessitated euthanasia.[1]

Horses that received 5 times (2.5 g) the recommended dose IM twice weekly for 6 weeks exhibited no untoward effects. ≈2% of horses receiving overdoses (up to 1250 mg) intra-articularly showed transient clinical signs associated with joint inflammation; dose-related increased partial thromboplastin time was noted. Hematoma, increased prothrombin time, and reduced platelet count occurred in dogs receiving 50 mg/kg IM twice weekly for 13 weeks (10 times the labeled dose and triple the labeled duration).

For patients that have experienced or are suspected of having experienced an overdose, consultation with a 24-hour poison consultation center specializing in providing veterinary-specific information is recommended. For general information related to overdose and toxin exposures, as well as contact information for poison control centers, refer to ***Appendix***.

Drug Interactions

The following drug interactions have either been reported or are theoretical in humans or animals receiving polysulfated glycosaminoglycan (PSGAG) and may be of significance in veterinary patients. Unless otherwise noted, use together is not necessarily contraindicated, but weigh the potential risks and perform additional monitoring when appropriate.

- **Anticoagulants** (eg, **rivoroxaban, warfarin**): Concurrent use may increase the risk for bleeding.
- **Antiplatelet Agents** (eg, **aspirin, clopidogrel**): Concurrent use may increase the risk for bleeding.
- **Corticosteroids** (eg, **dexamethasone, prednis(ol)one, triamcinolone**): Glucocorticoids could mask the clinical signs associated with septic joints.
- **Heparin, Low Molecular Weight Heparins** (eg, **dalteparin, enoxaparin**): Concurrent use may increase the risk for bleeding.

Dosages

DOGS:

Noninfectious degenerative and/or traumatic arthritis (label dosage; FDA-approved): 4.4 mg/kg IM twice weekly for up to 4 weeks (maximum of 8 injections)[1]

Noninfectious degenerative and/or traumatic arthritis (extra-label): 4.4 mg/kg SC twice weekly. Only anecdotal evidence supports the use via a nonapproved route and/or for a longer duration of treatment.

Pemphigus foliaceus (extra-label): Only case studies exist, which suggest a dosage of 4.4 – 4.6 mg/kg SC every 4 days for 4 weeks, then once weekly, in addition to standard treatment.[2]

CATS:

Chondroprotectant agent (extra-label): 2 mg/kg IM every 3 to 5 days for 4 treatments; only anecdotal experience in cats.[12] Many protocols exist for administering polysulfated glycosaminoglycan (PSGAG) to cats, such as 5 mg/kg SC twice weekly for 4 weeks, then once weekly for 4 weeks, then once monthly. No long-term data exist for cats.[13]

HORSES:

Noninfectious and/or traumatic joint dysfunction and associated lameness (label dosage; FDA-approved):

IM administration: 500 mg/horse (NOT mg/kg) IM every 4 days for 28 days[4]

IA administration in the carpal joint (IA-labeled product only): 250 mg total dose (NOT mg/kg) intra-articularly once a week for 5 weeks. The joint area must be shaved, cleansed, and sterilized as in a surgical procedure prior to injecting.[3]

RABBITS, RODENTS, SMALL MAMMALS:

Rabbits for arthritis (extra-label): 2.2 mg/kg SC or IM every 3 days for 21 to 28 days, then once every 2 weeks[14]

Monitoring

- Efficacy
- Joint inflammation and/or signs of infection if administered intra-articularly

Client Information

- Only veterinary professionals should administer the intra-articular product. If using the product used for intramuscular injections, be sure you understand how to give the injections properly.

- This medicine must be given as an injection as it is not effective when given by mouth.
- It may take up to 4 weeks of treatment to see if the medicine is helping.
- Side effects from this medicine are unlikely.

Chemistry/Synonyms

Polysulfated glycosaminoglycan (PSGAG) is chemically similar to natural mucopolysaccharides found in cartilaginous tissues. It contains repeating disaccharide units primarily composed of chondroitin with 3 or 4 sulfate esters per disaccharide unit and has a molecular weight between 3000 and 150,000. Solutions for injection are clear and colorless to slightly yellow. Multidose vials are preserved with benzyl alcohol. PSGAG is reportedly an analog of heparin.

Polysulfated glycosaminoglycan is also known as PSGAG and *Adequan®*.

Storage/Stability

Store polysulfated glycosaminoglycan (PSGAG) products (canine or equine) at 20°C to 25°C (68°F to 77°F). Products intended for IM use may tolerate excursions of 15°C to 30°C (59°F to 86°F). Avoid prolonged exposure to temperatures greater than 40°C (104°F).

Use multidose containers within 28 days of the first puncture and puncture a maximum of 10 times. When using single-dose vials, discard any unused portions.

The manufacturer does not recommend mixing with any other drug or solvent.[1,3,4]

Compatibility/Compounding Considerations

The manufacturer states that polysulfated glycosaminoglycan (PSGAG) should not be mixed with other drugs or solvents,[1,3,4] although amikacin has been added to PSGAG solution (extra-label) for intra-articular administration to horses.[5]

Dosage Forms/Regulatory Status

VETERINARY-LABELED PRODUCTS:

Polysulfated Glycosaminoglycan for IM Injection: 100 mg/mL in 5 mL vials.; *Adequan® Canine*; (Rx). FDA-approved for use in dogs. NADA #141038

Polysulfated Glycosaminoglycan for Intra-Articular Injection: 250 mg/mL in 1 mL single-use vials, boxes of 6; *Adequan® I.A.*; (Rx). FDA-approved for use in horses (not in those intended for food). NADA# 136-383

Polysulfated Glycosaminoglycan for Intramuscular Injection: 100 mg/mL in 5 mL single-dose vials and 50 mL multidose vials; *Adequan® I.M.*; (Rx). FDA-approved for use in horses (not in those intended for food). NADA# 140-901

HUMAN-LABELED PRODUCTS: NONE

References

For the complete list of references, see **wiley.com/go/budde/plumb**

Ponazuril

Toltrazuril Sulfone

(poe-***naz***-yoor-ill) *Marquis®*

Antiprotozoal

Prescriber Highlights

- ► Triazine approved to treat equine protozoal myeloencephalitis (EPM) caused by *Sarcocystis neurona*
- ► May also be used to treat other protozoal infections in various species, including coccidiosis in shelter dogs and cats
- ► Usually well tolerated; in equine field trials, rashes, hives, blisters, and GI signs were noted.

Uses/Indications

Ponazuril is indicated for the treatment of equine protozoal myeloencephalitis (EPM) caused by *Sarcocystis neurona*.[1] Clinical improvement was noted in 60% to 75% of horses that were treated with ponazuril.

One study of shelter dogs and cats with coccidiosis reported ≈90% clearance of infection after a 3-day treatment with ponazuril; animals with low oocyst burdens appeared to respond better than those with high counts.[2]

Pharmacology/Actions

Ponazuril (also known as toltrazuril sulfone) is a metabolite of toltrazuril. The triazine class of antiprotozoals is believed to target the plastid body, an organelle found in the members of the Apicomplexa phylum, including *Sarcocystis neurona*.[3] Ponazuril is coccidiocidal; in vitro concentrations required to kill *Sarcocystis neurona* range from 0.1 to 1 µg/mL. Ponazuril also has activity against several genera of the Apicomplexa phylum and may also be useful in treating *Neospora caninum, Toxoplasma* spp, and other protozoal infections (eg, *Isospora* spp, *Cryptosporidium* spp) in other species (eg, dogs, cats, birds, reptiles, ruminants).

Pharmacokinetics

When ponazuril is administered orally to horses in water, it has a bioavailability of ≈30% and elimination half-life of 80 hours.[4] After daily (5 mg/kg) oral administration to horses, ponazuril reaches its peak serum concentrations in ≈18 days and peak CSF concentrations in ≈15 days. Peak CSF concentrations are 1/20th (0.21 µg/mL) of those found in the serum.[5] Because ponazuril has a long terminal half-life, it takes ≈8 days to reach steady state serum/CSF concentrations in horses dosed at 5 mg/kg once daily.[6] Therefore, a single loading dose of 15 mg/kg is recommended to achieve steady state concentrations more quickly, in ≈1 to 2 days. Elimination half-life from serum averages ≈4.5 days.[1]

Ponazuril dissolved in DMSO and administered orally significantly enhanced bioavailability and peak plasma concentration.[7] Ponazuril administered orally with corn oil increased steady state serum and CSF concentrations by ≈30%.[8]

In cattle, oral doses of ponazuril 5 mg/kg are relatively well absorbed and have an approximate elimination half-life of 58 hours.[4]

Piglets receiving a single 5 mg/kg PO dose had peak plasma concentrations of 5.8 µg/mL at 42 hours, and a terminal half-life of 135 hours.[9]

In goats, a single 10 mg/kg oral dose reached peak plasma levels of 9 µg/mL in 36 hours, with an average half-life of 129 hours.[10]

In healthy llamas given a single 20 mg/kg PO dose, a peak serum concentration of 24 µg/mL was reached at 84 hours, and the elimination half-life was 136 hours.[11]

In tortoises, absorption appears to be prolonged and variable compared with mammals. A 20 mg/kg dose failed to reach serum concentrations that are considered therapeutic in mammals.[12]

Contraindications/Precautions/Warnings

No contraindications were noted. Before treating horses for EPM, other conditions that can cause ataxia should be ruled out. Neurologic deficits may worsen early in the treatment period. Successful treatment may not resolve all the clinical signs associated with equine protozoal myeloencephalitis (EPM).[1]

Adverse Effects

Ponazuril appears to be well tolerated in most species. Equine field trials showed some animals developing blisters on the nose and mouth or a rash/hives.[1] Individual horses developed diarrhea, mild colic, or seizures.[1]

Reproductive/Nursing Safety

Safety during pregnancy has not been evaluated in lactating mares, or horses used for breeding purposes. Because safety has not been established in animals, this drug should only be used when the maternal benefits outweigh the potential risks to offspring.

Overdose/Acute Toxicity

Daily doses of up to 30 mg/kg (2 times the loading dose and 6 times the maintenance dose) of ponazuril primarily caused loose feces. Moderate edema of the uterine epithelium was also noted on histopathology for female horses at this higher dose.

For patients that have experienced or are suspected to have experienced an overdose, consultation with a 24-hour poison consultation center specializing in providing veterinary-specific information is recommended. For general information related to overdose and toxin exposures, as well as contact information for poison control centers, refer to ***Appendix.***

Drug Interactions/Laboratory Considerations

- None noted

Dosages

NOTE: The commercially available paste (*Marquis*®) is too concentrated to be given to very small animals and should be diluted before being administered. See ***Compatibility/Compounding Considerations.***

DOGS/CATS:

Coccidiosis (extra-label):

a) 20 mg/kg PO once daily for 3 days[13]

b) 50 mg/kg PO once daily for 3 days; extended courses (two 3-day courses) are sometimes necessary for fecal flotation results to become negative in dogs and cats with coccidiosis[2]

c) 30 mg/kg PO given on days 0 and 7 (2 doses total)

Neosporosis or toxoplasmosis (extra-label): 7.5 – 15 mg/kg PO once daily for 28 days. Dosage extrapolated between known dosages for horses and mice.[14]

Canine hepatozoonosis (extra-label): 10 mg/kg PO every 12 hours for 14 days followed by long-term treatment with decoquinate[15,16]

HORSES:

Equine protozoal myeloencephalitis (EPM) caused by *Sarcocystis neurona* (label dosage; FDA-approved): 15 mg/kg PO as a loading dose on the first day of treatment, followed by 5 mg/kg PO once daily for 27 days[11]

EPM caused by *S neurona* or *Neospora hughesi* (extra-label): 5 mg/kg PO once daily for 28 days.[5] Treatment may continue for 6 to 8 weeks (or longer) if clinical signs continue to improve.[17,18]

Prevention of EPM (extra-label): Therapy minimized, but did not eliminate, infection in horses experimentally infected with *S neurona.*[17]

a) 2.5 – 5 mg/kg PO every 24 hours for 30 to 60 days[19]

b) 20 mg/kg PO every 7 days for 28 days

NEW WORLD CAMELIDS:

Eimeria macusaniensis (extra-label): 20 mg/kg PO once daily for 3 days. Because *E macusaniensis* can cause clinical disease or even death before oocysts are present in feces, prophylactic treatment should be considered in camelids that have unexplained weight loss with concurrent hypoproteinemia and without severe anemia.[11,20]

GOATS:

Coccidiosis (extra-label): 10 mg/kg PO once resulted in decreased oocyst counts. Goats receiving amprolium appeared to respond more favorably than goats that received ponazuril.[21]

BIRDS:

***Cryptosporidium* spp respiratory disease in falcons** (extra-label): From a case report of 2 patients, 20 mg/kg PO (as a compounded suspension) once daily for 7 days[22]

SMALL MAMMALS:

Adjunctive treatment of *Eimeria* spp in rabbits (extra-label): 20 mg/kg PO once a day for 7 days[16]

REPTILES:

Coccidiosis in bearded dragons (extra-label): Anecdotal dosage recommendations vary considerably. Daily spot cleaning of the environment with weekly deep cleaning and disinfection is essential to prevent reinfection.

a) 30 mg/kg PO twice 48 hours apart[23]

b) 30 – 45 mg/kg PO once daily for 28 days[24]

Testudine intranuclear coccidiosis (TINC) in tortoises (extra-label): 20 mg/kg PO every other day for 3 months.[25] Long-term subclinical infection may be possible after treatment despite resolution of clinical signs.[26]

Monitoring

- Clinical efficacy (ie, improvement in neurologic signs such as ataxia and muscle weakness)
- Adverse effects (eg, diarrhea, colic, skin rash, and blisters on the nose and mouth)

Client Information

- It is very important to not miss any doses of this medicine or it may not be effective.
- Ponazuril can be given with or without food.
- Contact your veterinarian if your animal develops a rash, hives, blisters, poor appetite, diarrhea, or redness or discharge from the eyes.

Chemistry/Synonyms

Related to other antiprotozoals such as toltrazuril, ponazuril is a triazine antiprotozoal (anticoccidial) agent. The commercially available oral paste is white to off-white in color and odorless; pH is 5.7 to 6. Solubility of ponazuril in DMSO is 250 mg/mL.

Ponazuril may also be known as toltrazolone sulfone, toltrazuril sulfone, ICI-128436, *Marquis*®, and *Ponalrestat*®.

Storage/Stability

Store the paste at room temperature, 20°C to 25°C (68-77°F), with excursions permitted between 15°C to 30°C (59°F-86°F).

Compatibility/Compounding Considerations

For use in small animal species, particularly in shelter situations, various dilutions of the equine paste can be made. One recommendation is to dilute the paste to 100 mg/mL by weighing out 40 g of ponazuril paste, adding sufficient distilled water to reach a total weight of 60 g, and mixing well. The paste is water-soluble and can be easily syringed into the animal.[11,20]

For practical purposes, 1 g of paste is roughly equivalent to 1 mL of paste and contains ≈150 mg of ponazuril. No specific stability data were located for these dilutions.

Dosage Forms/Regulatory Status

VETERINARY-LABELED PRODUCTS:

Ponazuril Oral Paste (15% w/w): 127 g tubes; each gram of paste contains 150 mg of ponazuril; each syringe is enough to treat a 1200-lb horse for 7 days. *Marquis*®; (Rx). Do not use in horses intended for food.

HUMAN-LABELED PRODUCTS: NONE

References

For the complete list of references, see **wiley.com/go/budde/plumb**

Posaconazole

(**poe**-sa-**kon**-a-zole) *Noxafil*®

Azole Antifungal

Prescriber Highlights

- Second-generation triazole antifungal with a wide spectrum of activity, but little information on clinical efficacy and safety has been published in veterinary medicine
- Currently cost-prohibitive for most clients. May be cost-effective in cats and small dogs for itraconazole- or fluconazole-resistant infections
- Full adverse effect profile for animals is not known. GI effects and increases in liver enzymes have been reported.
- Treatment may be required for months, and infection may not be fully cleared.
- Many potential drug interactions

Uses/Indications

Posaconazole has demonstrated efficacy (eg, improved clinical signs, clinical remission) against severe refractory or resistant systemic fungal infections in dogs and cats, including aspergillosis[1-4] and coccidioidomycosis,[5] and may be useful for treating blastomycosis, histoplasmosis, sporotrichosis, and zygomycosis.

In humans, posaconazole is labeled for prophylaxis (in at-risk patients) or treatment of candidiasis or aspergillosis. It is also used in an extra-label manner for the treatment of other fungal infections.

The currently available dosage forms are expensive and may prohibit posaconazole's clinical use for many animals.

Pharmacology/Actions

Posaconazole is structurally related to itraconazole but has a wider spectrum of activity and, at present, significantly less potential for fungal resistance. Like other triazoles, posaconazole inhibits a fungal cytochrome P450-dependent demethylation enzyme that produces ergosterol in the cell membrane. The resultant intracellular accumulation of methylated sterols weakens the cellular membranes of susceptible fungi, increasing membrane permeability, allowing leakage of cellular contents, and impairing uptake of purine and pyrimidine precursors.

Posaconazole's spectrum of activity includes a variety of organisms, including many species of *Blastomyces*, *Coccidioides*, *Cryptococcus*, *Histoplasma*, *Aspergillus*, *Fusarium*, *Candida*, *Mucor*, and zygomycetes. Fungi that are resistant to posaconazole may also be resistant to other azole antifungals (eg, fluconazole, itraconazole).

Pharmacokinetics

In dogs, the oral bioavailability of 2 different posaconazole oral suspension formulations was 43% to 59%; food increased bioavailability (peak concentration and area under the curve) ≈4 times. The terminal half-life was 15 hours (after IV dosing). Multiple-day dosing caused some accumulation of the drug. Based on the kinetics results and minimum fungicidal concentrations for most organisms, the authors concluded that a dosage of 10 mg/kg/day should be effective.[5]

Another study in dogs compared commercially available oral suspension, delayed-release tablet (DRT), and IV formulations. DRTs resulted in markedly greater absorption compared with oral suspension. Peak concentrations of 0.42 µg/mL (oral suspension) and 1.8 µg/mL (DRT) occurred 7.5 to 9.5 hours after administration (with a meal). Terminal half-lives were 24 hours (oral suspension) and 42 hours (DRT).[6]

In cats that received the oral suspension after a small meal, a peak concentration of 1.2 µg/mL was reached roughly 18 hours after administration. The volume of distribution was 1.9 L/kg, with a terminal half-life of 38 hours.[7]

In humans, DRTs result in greater posaconazole bioavailability compared with oral suspension. Therefore, the 2 dosage forms are not interchangeable at equal doses. Peak concentration after oral suspension administration occurs in 3 to 6 hours. Bioavailability is significantly increased if posaconazole is given with food. Maximum concentration and total exposure were 3 times higher when administered with food compared with fasting and 4 times higher than fasting when given with a high-fat meal. It is widely distributed in tissues, and protein binding is greater than 98%. Posaconazole is metabolized primarily via glucuronidation. ≈71% of a dose is eliminated in feces, primarily as an unchanged drug. About 13% of a dose is eliminated in the urine as metabolites. The average elimination half-life is 35 hours.

Contraindications/Precautions/Warnings

Posaconazole is contraindicated in patients with hypersensitivity to the drug or any component in the suspension. In humans, posaconazole use is contraindicated with concomitant use with HMG-CoA reductase inhibitors (eg, atorvastatin, simvastatin), sirolimus, ergot alkaloids, or CYP3A4 substrates that can prolong QT interval (eg, pimozide, quinidine). Dosage adjustment for patients with decreased renal function is not required when using oral formulations of posaconazole; however, the parenteral formulation contains an inactive ingredient that could accumulate in patients with impaired renal function. Additionally, patients with severe renal impairment should be monitored closely for breakthrough infections, as variable exposure was shown in humans with severe renal insufficiency.

No dose adjustment is needed for patients with hepatic impairment, but caution is recommended. Patients experiencing severe vomiting or diarrhea should be closely monitored for breakthrough infections.

Adverse Effects

There is limited information on the adverse effect profile for posaconazole in dogs or cats. The only adverse effect possibly associated with a 16-week posaconazole treatment in a cat with orbital aspergillosis was facial and ear pruritus with erythema. In a retrospective study of cats with sino-nasal and sino-orbital aspergillosis that had received posaconazole, 2 out of 10 cats developed transient 1.1 to 2 times elevations in ALT activity, but it was otherwise well tolerated.[8]

In 10 dogs with disseminated aspergillosis treated with posaconazole for an average of 7.5 months, adverse effects included vomiting, inappetence, diarrhea, polyuria/polydipsia, and mild increases in ALT.[2] One dog experienced mild thrombocytopenia, and 1 experienced leukopenia/neutropenia. No discontinuation or alteration of dosage was required.[2]

The most commonly reported adverse effects in humans are GI-related and include nausea, vomiting, abdominal pain, and diarrhea. Rare but serious adverse effects include liver failure and cholestasis (associated with high dosages), prolonged QT interval/torsade des pointes, and hypokalemia. Other adverse effects reported include skin rash, headache, tremors, hypertension, anorexia, and weakness.

Mild to moderate increases in liver enzymes and bilirubin can be seen but are usually reversible with therapy discontinuation; monitor for the development of more severe hepatic injury. Consider discontinuing the drug if clinical signs of liver disease occur.

Reproductive/Nursing Safety

Safe use of posaconazole during pregnancy or nursing has not been established. In rats, skeletal malformations were seen in some offspring of mothers given posaconazole while pregnant. Other azole antifungal drugs are associated with teratogenic effects or early embryonic loss and are not recommended for use in pregnancy except in life-threatening maternal diseases without therapeutic alternatives.[9,10]

Posaconazole is excreted into rat milk, and safe use during nursing is not known.

Because safety has not been established in animals, this drug should only be used when the maternal benefits outweigh the potential risks to offspring.

Overdose/Acute Toxicity

Acute toxicity due to a posaconazole overdose is unlikely. Humans have tolerated up to 1600 mg/day in clinical studies, and 1 patient that ingested 1200 mg twice daily for 3 days did not develop adverse effects. In dogs, single oral doses of 240 mg/kg (females) and 480 mg/kg (males) were tolerated with no observable adverse effects; the nonlethal oral dose in dogs was 2000 mg/kg. Repeated dose safety studies with 30 mg/kg/day orally in dogs for up to 1 year showed minimal clinical adverse effects but mild histopathologic changes consistent with other azole antifungal drugs.[11]

Hemodialysis does not remove posaconazole.

For patients that have experienced or are suspected of having experienced an overdose, consultation with a 24-hour poison consultation center specializing in providing veterinary-specific information is recommended. For general information related to overdose and toxin exposures, as well as contact information for poison control centers, refer to ***Appendix.***

Drug Interactions

Posaconazole can inhibit CYP3A4 and can potentially cause increased plasma concentrations of drugs that are metabolized by CYP3A4. Posaconazole is also a substrate of the P-glycoprotein transport system and can potentially interact with other drugs that inhibit or induce this system.

The following drug interactions (partial list) have either been reported or are theoretical in humans or animals receiving posaconazole and may be of significance in veterinary patients. Unless otherwise noted, use together is not necessarily contraindicated, but weigh the potential risks and perform additional monitoring when appropriate.

- BENZODIAZEPINES (eg, **alprazolam, midazolam**): Increased benzodiazepine concentration (up to 5-fold) possible
- CIMETIDINE: Decreased concentration of posaconazole possible; avoid use together. No interactions reported with other H2 blockers (eg, **famotidine**)
- CISAPRIDE: Possible prolonged QT interval. In humans, the use of cisapride and posaconazole together is contraindicated, but any clinical relevance for animal patients is unknown.
- CYCLOSPORINE: Increased cyclosporine concentration possible; in humans, it is recommended to decrease cyclosporine dose by 25% when starting posaconazole in patients that are already receiving cyclosporine.
- DIGOXIN: Possibility for increased digoxin concentration
- DILTIAZEM: May increase diltiazem concentration
- METOCLOPRAMIDE: Decreased absorption of posaconazole oral suspension is possible; there is no effect on the absorption of posaconazole delayed-release tablets (DRTs)
- PROTON PUMP INHIBITORS (eg, **omeprazole**): Decreased absorption of posaconazole oral suspension only; there is no effect on the absorption of posaconazole DRTs.
- QUINIDINE: Increased quinidine concentration, possible prolonged QT interval
- RIFAMPIN: Decreased posaconazole concentration
- VINCA ALKALOIDS (eg, **vincristine, vinblastine**): Increased risk for vinca alkaloid toxicity possible
- WARFARIN: Increased bleeding risk

Laboratory Considerations

No laboratory test interactions were noted.

Dosages

NOTES:

1. The dosing regimens for the oral suspension and the delayed-release tablets (DRTs) are different; do not interchange dosage forms on a mg per mg basis.
2. Oral doses should be administered with food, preferably right after a high-fat meal.[9] Several months of treatment may be required.

DOGS:

Susceptible fungal infections (extra-label):

a) **Suspension:** 5 – 10 mg/kg PO every 12 to 24 hours. A preclinical study suggested that a dosage of 10 mg/kg/day PO should be effective.[2,5]

b) **DRTs**: Based on the results of a pharmacokinetic study, a dosage of 5 mg/kg PO every 48 hours may be considered.[6]

CATS:

Susceptible fungal infections (extra-label):

a) 30 mg/kg PO loading dose followed by 15 mg/kg PO every 48 hours or 15 mg/kg PO loading dose followed by 7.5 mg/kg every 24 hours[3,7]

b) 5 – 7.5 mg/kg PO every 24 hours or divided into 2 doses per day[4,12]

Monitoring

- Efficacy and adverse effects
- Liver enzymes and serum electrolytes; baseline and periodically during treatment
- Patients with severe renal impairment should be monitored closely for breakthrough fungal infections.

Client Information

- When using the oral suspension, shake the bottle well before measuring the dose.
- Delayed-release tablets must be swallowed whole and not chewed or crushed.
- Give this medicine after food; a full meal if possible.
- This medicine may be dosed once per day, but if your animal vomits or acts sick after a dose, your veterinarian may have you give ½ of the daily dose twice per day.
- Treatment for many months may be required.
- There is not much experience with this medication in animals, so if you see any side effects, contact your veterinarian.

Chemistry/Synonyms

Posaconazole is a triazole antifungal that occurs as a white powder that is insoluble in water. The commercially available oral suspension is a white, cherry-flavored immediate-release oral suspension that contains polysorbate 80, simethicone, sodium benzoate, sodium citrate dihydrate, citric acid monohydrate, glycerin, xanthan gum, glucose, titanium dioxide, artificial cherry flavor, and purified water.

Posaconazole may also be known as Sch-56592. Trade names include *Noxafil®* and *Spriafil®*.

Storage/Stability

Store the commercially available oral products at room temperature 25°C (77°F), with excursions permitted to 15°C to 30°C (59°F-86°F); do not freeze. Store the formulation for injection refrigerated 2°C to 8°C (36°F-46°F).

Compatibility/Compounding Considerations

Compatibility is dependent on factors such as pH, concentration, temperature, and diluent used; specialized references or a hospital pharmacist should be consulted for more specific information.

Posaconazole injection must be further diluted to a final concentration between 1 and 2 mg/mL using a saline or saline/dextrose IV solution. The manufacturer cautions to inspect for particulates prior to administration. Posaconazole should be administered over 90 minutes through a central line with an in-line 0.22-micron filter. The manufacturer states posaconazole for injection is **Y-site compatible** with (partial list) amikacin sulfate, ciprofloxacin, dobutamine HCl, famotidine, gentamicin sulfate, hydromorphone HCl, meropenem, morphine sulfate, and potassium chloride. Posaconazole for injection is **incompatible** with lactated Ringer's solution.

Dosage Forms/Regulatory Status

VETERINARY-LABELED PRODUCTS: No systemic products are labeled in the United States.

An otic suspension containing posaconazole 0.1%, orbifloxacin 1%, and mometasone 0.1% is available (for use in dogs with otitis externa); *Posatex®*; (Rx). Refer to ***Corticosteroid/Antimicrobial Preparations, Otic***.

HUMAN-LABELED PRODUCTS:

Posaconazole Oral Suspension: 40 mg/mL in 105 mL bottles; *Noxafil®*; (Rx)

Posaconazole Delayed-Release Tablets: 100 mg; *Noxafil®*; generic; (Rx)

Posaconazole Injection: 300 mg in 16.7 mL vials (18 mg/mL); *Noxafil®*; (Rx)

It is also available as a veterinary otic preparation (*Posatex®*) containing orbifloxacin, posaconazole, and mometasone.

References

For the complete list of references, see **wiley.com/go/budde/plumb**

Potassium (-Acetate, -Chloride, -Gluconate)

(po-***tass***-ee-um)

Electrolyte

See also ***Bromides; Iodide (Potassium-, Sodium-);*** and ***Citrate, Potassium***

Prescriber Highlights

- Parenteral and oral electrolyte used for treatment or prevention of hypokalemia
- Contraindications include hyperkalemia, renal failure or severe renal impairment, severe hemolysis, untreated hypoadrenocorticism, acute dehydration, and GI motility impairment (solid oral dosage forms).
- Use with caution in patients receiving digoxin.
- Adverse effects include hyperkalemia. Specific adverse effects with oral therapy include GI distress and, with IV therapy, phlebitis.
- ***Rapid IV potassium supplementation can cause cardiac arrest and death; potassium salts must be diluted before administering IV slowly.***
- Serum potassium and acid-base and hydration status must be monitored during therapy.

Uses/Indications

Potassium supplementation is used to prevent or treat potassium deficits associated with a variety of conditions (eg, vomiting, diarrhea, diabetic ketoacidosis, feline hyperaldosteronism, chronic kidney disease[1]). When it is feasible and appropriate, oral or nutritional supplementation is generally preferred over parenteral potassium administration because oral and nutritional routes carry fewer risks for adverse effects such as cardiac arrest.

Potassium chloride injection can be used for euthanasia of unconscious or fully anesthetized animals (ie, a surgical plane of anesthesia is required *before* using), although its use is generally reserved for situations when other euthanasia methods are unavailable, or when predators or scavengers may consume the euthanized remains.[2]

Pharmacology/Actions

Potassium is the principal intracellular cation in the body. It is essential in maintaining cellular tonicity; nerve impulse transmission; smooth, skeletal, and cardiac muscle contraction; and maintenance of normal renal function. Potassium is also used in carbohydrate metabolism and protein synthesis. Magnesium is a cofactor for potassium regulation, and correction of potassium imbalance may also require addressing serum magnesium.

Potassium requirements in mature dogs are ≈3.7 mEq/kg/day and ≈1.5 mEq/kg/day in mature cats. Puppies and kittens have higher dietary potassium requirements than do mature animals.

Pharmacokinetics

Approximately 98% of total body potassium is found in the intracellular fluid space, with only 2% found in the extracellular fluid space. Plasma pH can alter potassium distribution. Acidosis can shift potassium out of the intracellular space and, conversely, alkalosis shifts potassium into the intracellular space. Insulin shifts potassium to the intracellular space; glucose may also accomplish this effect by stimulating insulin release. Potassium is primarily (80% to 90%) excreted via the kidneys, with the majority of the remainder excreted in the feces. Potassium concentration in GI secretions exceeds that of plasma. Small amounts of potassium may be excreted in perspiration (in animals with sweat glands).

Contraindications/Precautions/Warnings

Potassium salts are contraindicated in patients with hyperkalemia.

Potassium supplementation should be administered with extreme caution when administered IV in patients with renal failure or severe renal impairment, severe hemolysis, extensive tissue damage, untreated hypoadrenocorticism, or acute dehydration. IV potassium salts must be diluted and thoroughly mixed before being administered[3] (see ***Overdose/Acute Toxicity***), then given slowly (see ***Dosages***). ***Rapid IV potassium supplementation can cause cardiac arrest and death***; infusion rate must not exceed 0.5 mEq/kg/hour.

Use oral potassium supplementation with caution in patients with renal failure or severe renal impairment, severe hemolysis, extensive tissue damage, untreated hypoadrenocorticism, GI motility impairment, or acute dehydration.

Potassium salts of any formulation should be used with caution in patients that are receiving digoxin (see ***Drug Interactions***) and in horses with hyperkalemic periodic paralysis (HYPP).

Because potassium is primarily an intracellular electrolyte, serum measurements may not adequately reflect the total body stores of potassium. Acid-base balance may also impact potassium measurements. Patients with systemic acidosis conditions may appear to have hyperkalemia when, in fact, they may be significantly low in total body potassium. Conversely, alkalosis may cause a falsely low serum potassium value. Assess renal and cardiac function prior to potassium therapy and closely monitor serum potassium levels. IV potassium supplementation should generally occur over 3 to 5 days to allow equilibration to occur between extracellular and intracellular fluids. Some clinicians believe that if acidosis is present or a concern, potassium acetate, citrate, gluconate, or sodium bicarbonate should be used. If alkalosis is present, potassium chloride should be used.

Adverse Effects

The biggest risk associated with potassium supplementation is the development of hyperkalemia, which may be more serious than hypokalemia. Clinical signs associated with hyperkalemia can range from muscular weakness and/or GI disturbances to cardiac conduction disturbances and cardiac arrest.[4] In dogs and cats, ECG changes seen in critical patients with hyperkalemia may be affected by concurrent metabolic derangements (eg, metabolic acidosis, hypermagnesemia, hyponatremia, hypocalcemia) and thus may not typify the expected ECG changes (eg, bradyarrhythmias, loss of P wave, wide QRS complexes, peaked T waves) commonly described for hyperkalemia.[5] In humans, treatment for hyperkalemia is recommended when serum potassium is greater than 5.5 mEq/L if there are ECG changes, or when serum potassium is greater than 6 mEq/L, regardless of ECG findings.[6]

Oral potassium therapy can cause GI distress, including ulceration and GI bleeding, and IV therapy may cause phlebitis.

Reproductive/Nursing Safety

Monitored potassium supplementation is unlikely to have negative effects during pregnancy or lactation. Potassium supplementation that results in hyperkalemia in the dam may also have adverse effects on the fetus or lactating offspring.

Overdose/Acute Toxicity

Fatal hyperkalemia may develop if potassium salts are administered too rapidly IV or if potassium renal excretory mechanisms are impaired (eg, urethral obstruction). Clinical signs associated with hyperkalemia are noted in ***Adverse Effects***. Treatment of hyperkalemia is dependent on the cause and/or severity of the condition and can consist of discontinuation of the drug with ECG, acid-base and electrolyte monitoring, dextrose/insulin infusions, sodium bicarbonate, calcium therapy, polystyrene sulfonate resin, and dialysis.

For patients that have experienced or are suspected to have experienced an overdose, consultation with a 24-hour poison consultation center specializing in providing veterinary-specific information is recommended. For general information related to overdose and toxin exposures, as well as contact information for poison control centers, refer to ***Appendix***.

Drug Interactions

The following drug interactions have either been reported or are theoretical in humans or animals receiving potassium and may be of significance in veterinary patients. Unless otherwise noted, use together is not necessarily contraindicated, but weigh the potential risks and perform additional monitoring when appropriate.

- **Angiotensin Converting Enzyme Inhibitors** (**ACEIs**; eg, **benazepril, enalapril**): Potassium retention may occur; increased risk for hyperkalemia
- **Angiotensin-Receptor Blockers** (**ARBs**; eg, **irbesartan, telmisartan**): Potassium retention may occur; increased risk for hyperkalemia
- **Antimuscarinic Agents** (eg, **atropine, opioids**): Delay GI transit, increasing risk for adverse GI effects from tablet or capsule formulations
- **Digoxin**: In patients with severe or complete heart block that are receiving digitalis therapy, potassium salts are generally not recommended.
- **Diuretics, Potassium-Sparing** (eg, **spironolactone**): Potassium retention may occur; increased risk for hyperkalemia. Avoid concomitant use.
- **Nonsteroidal Anti-inflammatory Drugs** (**NSAIDs**; eg, **carprofen, meloxicam, robenacoxib**): Oral potassium administered with NSAIDs may increase the risk for GI adverse effects.

Dosages

DOGS/CATS:

NOTE: There are no exact formulas for calculating the total body potassium depletion or the requirement for supplementation needed to restore normokalemia. Guidelines should always be modified based on patient response. Patients with hypokalemia and osmotic diuresis will have a much higher requirement for potassium than patients with normal urine output. Hypokalemia associated with diabetic ketoacidosis and postobstructive diuresis requires additional monitoring and treatment; refer to specific references for additional information.

Chronic mild hypokalemia (3.0 – 3.5 mEq/L):

a) **Potassium gluconate** (label dosage; not FDA-approved): 2 mEq/4.5 kg (10 lb) PO with food twice daily; adjust dosage as necessary based on periodic serum potassium measurements.

b) **Potassium chloride** (extra-label): 0.5 – 1 mEq/kg PO mixed in food once or twice daily; adjust dosage as necessary based on periodic serum potassium measurements.

Moderate to severe (less than 3.0 mEq/L) hypokalemia | acute hypokalemia with or without metabolic alkalosis:

a) The <u>rate</u> of IV administration of KCl is more critical than the total amount administered. Under most circumstances, the rate should not exceed 0.5 mEq/kg/hour. Under the most dire circumstances (serum potassium less than 2.0 mEq/L), the rate of potassium administration can be increased to 1.5 mEq/kg per hour along with close, continuous ECG monitoring.[7] **NOTE**: Administering more than 10 mEq/hour of KCl to a small animal (less than 10 kg [22 lb] body weight) can be potentially life-threatening because of the effects of a more concentrated solution on the wall of the right ventricle if the solution is given through a central IV line.[4] Although potassium administration should be determined by how much potassium to administer to the patient (not by how much KCl to add to a bag of fluid), see table below for suggested guidelines:

Measured serum K+ (mEq/L or mmol/L)	mEq KCl/1000 mL IV fluid*
Less than 2	60 – 80
2 – 2.5	40 – 60
2.5 – 3	30 – 40
3 – 3.5	20 – 30

*Be sure to take into consideration the amount of potassium already present in polyionic crystalloids (eg, LRS contains 4 mEq potassium/1000 mL of fluid) when deciding how much potassium to add to the fluid bag.

b) For patients less than 10 kg that are not able to be hospitalized and require outpatient treatment, isotonic fluids such as lactated Ringer's or 0.9% saline with added 30 – 35 mEq KCL/L can be given at a dose of 150 mL SC every 12 hours.[8]

HORSES:

Hypokalemia (extra-label): To counteract potassium depletion in a completely anorectic adult horse, IV fluids should be supplemented to deliver at least 50 mEq KCl/hour. Hypertonic oral KCl pastes can be administered to horses with diarrhea.[9] **NOTE**: IV administration rate should not exceed 0.5 mEq/kg/hour.

Euthanasia of unconscious or fully anesthetized animals (extra-label): 1 – 2 mEq/kg rapid IV or intracardiac.[2] Animal ***must*** be fully unconscious prior to administration. Administered volume may be quite large (eg, 250 mL – 500 mL of KCl 2 mEq/mL solution for a 500 kg [1102.3 lb] horse).

RUMINANTS:

Severe hypokalemia (less than 2.3 mEq/L) with severe muscle weakness or recumbency (extra-label): Isotonic potassium chloride 11.5 g/1 L of sterile water at a rate of 4 mL/kg/hour IV CRI in combination with large doses of oral potassium salts (ie, KCl 200 g/day).[10]

Hypokalemia (less than 3.5 mEq/L): Potassium chloride 100 – 120 g PO dissolved in water every 12 hours; doses exceeding 0.4 g/kg/day PO are not recommended, except in cattle with profound hypokalemia.[11,12]

Euthanasia of unconscious or fully anesthetized animals (extra-label): 1 – 2 mEq/kg rapid IV or intracardiac.[2] Animal ***must*** be fully unconscious prior to administration. Administered volume may be quite large (eg, 350 to 700 mL of 2 mEq/mL solution for a 700 kg cow).

Monitoring

The degree and frequency of monitoring associated with potassium therapy is dependent on the cause and/or severity of hypokalemia, the route of potassium administration, acid-base abnormalities, renal function, concomitant drugs administered, and disease states and can include:

- Serum potassium; other electrolytes; frequent monitoring of serum potassium is strongly recommended when potassium supplementation ia administered by the IV route
- Acid-base status
- Glucose
- ECG; continuous ECG monitoring is strongly recommended when correcting moderate to severe hypokalemia with aggressive potassium supplementation and/or when other metabolic derangements (eg, metabolic acidosis) are encountered with critical patients.[13]
- CBC
- Urinalysis

Client Information

- Oral potassium is best administered with food to help prevent stomach upset.
- Overdoses (both one time and over a period of time) of potassium can be life-threatening. Contact your veterinarian immediately if you suspect an overdose.

Chemistry/Synonyms

Potassium acetate occurs as a white crystalline powder or as flakes. It is odorless or has a slight acetic odor and is freely soluble in water. The 2 mEq/mL commercial solution has a pH of 6.2 (5.5 to 8). One gram of potassium acetate contains 10 mEq of potassium.

Potassium acetate may also be known as E262, hocura-diureticum, kalii acetas, kaliumacetat, *Onixol*®, and Trikates oral solution.

Potassium chloride occurs as either a white, granular powder or as colorless, elongated, prismatic, or cubical crystals. It is odorless and has a saline taste. One gram is soluble in ≈3 mL of water and is insoluble in alcohol. The pH of the injection ranges from 4 to 8. One gram of potassium chloride contains 13.4 mEq of potassium. A 2 mEq/mL solution has an osmolarity of 4000 mOsm/L.

Potassium chloride may also be known as cloreto de potassio, E508, kalii chloridum, kalium chloratum, *Kaochlor*®, KCl, *K-Dur 20*®, *K-lor*®, *Klorvess*®, *K-lyte*®, potash muriate, and potassium muriate.

Potassium gluconate occurs as a white to yellow-white, crystalline powder or as granules. It is odorless, has a slightly bitter taste, and is freely soluble in water. One gram of potassium gluconate contains 4.3 mEq of potassium.

Potassium gluconate may also be known as E577, *K-G Elixir*®, *Kaon*®, *Kaylixir*®, *Potasoral*®, *Potassiject*®, *Potassium-Rougier*®, *Renakare*®, *Sopa-K*®, *Tumil-K*®, and *Ultra-K*®.

Storage/Stability

Potassium acetate injection should be stored at controlled room temperature (20°C-25°C [68°F-77°F]).

Unless otherwise directed by the manufacturer, potassium chloride products should be stored in tight containers at room temperature (15°C-30°C [59°F-86°F]); protect from freezing.

Potassium gluconate oral products should be stored in tight, light-resistant containers at room temperature (15°C-30°C [59°F-86°F]), unless otherwise instructed by the manufacturer.

Compatibility/Compounding Considerations

Compatibility is dependent on factors such as pH, concentration, temperature, and diluent used; specialized references or a hospital pharmacist should be consulted for more specific information.

Adequate mixing of IV solutions to which potassium has been added must occur prior to administration; multiple inversions of the bag are recommended.[3]

Potassium chloride for injection is reportedly physically **compatible** with the following IV solutions and drugs (as an additive): all commonly used IV replacement fluids (not 10% fat emulsion), aminocaproic acid, aminophylline, amiodarone HCl, ampicillin, calcium gluconate, cefazolin, chloramphenicol sodium succinate, cimetidine HCl, clindamycin phosphate, corticotropin (ACTH), cytarabine, diphenhydramine, dopamine HCl, erythromycin gluceptate/lactobionate, famotidine, fentanyl citrate, fluconazole, gentamicin, heparin sodium, hydrocortisone sodium succinate, isoproterenol HCl, lidocaine HCl, magnesium sulfate, metoclopramide HCl, morphine sulfate, norepinephrine bitartrate, oxacillin sodium, oxytetracycline HCl, penicillin G potassium, phenylephrine HCl, ranitidine, tetracycline HCl, vancomycin HCl, verapamil HCl, and vitamin B-complex with C.

Potassium chloride for injection **compatibility information con-**

flicts or is dependent on diluent or concentration factors with the following drugs or solutions: fat emulsion 10%, amikacin sulfate, dobutamine HCl, mannitol, methylprednisolone sodium succinate **(at Y-site)**, ondansetron, penicillin G sodium, promethazine HCl (**at Y-site**), and sodium bicarbonate.

Potassium chloride for injection is reportedly physically **incompatible** with the following solutions or drugs: amphotericin B, diazepam **(at Y-site),** and phenytoin sodium **(at Y-site).**

Dosage Forms/Regulatory Status

VETERINARY-LABELED PRODUCTS:

Parenteral Products: There are several products for parenteral use that contain potassium; refer to ***Appendix*** tables or individual proprietary veterinary products for additional information.

Oral Products: These products are not found in the FDA Green Book; approval status is uncertain.

Potassium Gluconate Tablets: 2 mEq (468 mg); *Tumil-K®*, *Renakare®*, generic; (Rx). Labeled for use in cats and dogs

Potassium Gluconate Oral Powder: Each 0.65 g (¼ teaspoon) contains 2 mEq of potassium in 4 oz containers; *Renakare®*, *Tumil-K®*; (Rx). Labeled for use in dogs and cats

Potassium Gluconate Gel: Each 2.34 g (½ teaspoon) contains 2 mEq of potassium in 5 oz tubes; *Tumil-K® Gel*, *Renakare®*; (Rx). Labeled for use in dogs and cats

HUMAN-LABELED PRODUCTS (NOT A COMPLETE LIST):

Parenteral Products:

Potassium Chloride for Injection Concentrate: 2 mEq/mL in single-dose and multi-dose vials and ***must be diluted before administering***; generic; (Rx)

Potassium Chloride for Injection, Highly Concentrated: 10 mEq and 20 mEq in 50 mL or 100 mL bags, and 40 mEq/100 mL bags; generic; (Rx). Ready-to-use solution for fluid-restricted patients; requires administration through a central line via calibrated infusion device.

There are also premixed IV bags of saline and dextrose (both separately and in various combinations) that contain potassium 10 mEq/L, 20 mEq/L, 30 mEq/L, or 40 mEq/L.

Potassium Acetate for Injection Concentrate: 2 mEq/mL and 4 mEq/mL and ***must be diluted before administering***; (Rx)

Potassium Phosphate for Injection (see ***Phosphate, Intravenous***) is also available.

Oral Products: There are many human-labeled potassium salts for oral use available in several dosage forms; refer to human drug references for more information on these products. Tablets, controlled/sustained release tablets and capsules, effervescent tablets, liquids, and powder in varying strengths available; (OTC, Rx)

References

For the complete list of references, see **wiley.com/go/budde/plumb**

Pradofloxacin

(pra-doe-***flox***-a-sin) *Veraflox®*

Fluoroquinolone Antibiotic

Prescriber Highlights

- FDA-approved for use in cats; approved for dogs in some countries
- Enhanced aerobic gram-positive activity and activity against anaerobes; its gram-negative activity is similar to other fluoroquinolones.
- Contraindications include hypersensitivity to fluoroquinolones; do not administer to pregnant or lactating animals, or kittens less than 12 weeks of age, as safety has not been determined.
- May produce erosions of cartilage of weight-bearing joints and other signs of arthropathy in immature animals of various species
- Use with caution in patients with renal insufficiency, pre-existing CNS disorders (eg, epilepsy), or underlying conditions that predispose to arrhythmias (eg, electrolyte imbalances, cardiac disease); use with caution in immunocompromised cats (ie, infected with feline leukemia and/or feline immunodeficiency virus), as safety has not been determined.
- Adverse effects may include GI distress, photosensitivity, myelosuppression, and arrhythmias (dogs only).
- Many potential drug interactions
- FDA prohibits extra-label use in food animals. Should not be used in humans

Uses/Indications

In cats, pradofloxacin oral suspension is FDA-approved for the treatment of skin infections (wounds and abscesses) caused by susceptible strains of *Pasteurella multocida, Streptococcus canis, Staphylococcus aureus, Staphylococcus felis,* and *Staphylococcus pseudintermedius.* Pradofloxacin has also been used clinically in cats for the treatment of bacterial UTIs, *Bartonella* spp,[1] *Mycoplasma haemofelis* upper respiratory infections, and in combination with other antimycobacterial drugs for feline leprosy syndromes. One study showed pradofloxacin to be equivalent to amoxicillin for treatment of bacterial upper respiratory infections.[2]

Pradofloxacin is not FDA-approved for use in dogs (see ***Contraindications/Precautions/Warnings***). In other countries, pradofloxacin is labeled for the treatment of wound infections, superficial and deep pyoderma caused by susceptible strains of the *S pseudintermedius* group (including *S pseudintermedius*); acute UTIs caused by susceptible strains of *Escherichia coli* and the *S pseudintermedius* group (including *S pseudintermedius*); and as adjunctive treatment to mechanical or surgical periodontal therapy in the treatment of severe infections of the gingiva and periodontal tissues caused by susceptible strains of anaerobic organisms (eg, *Porphyromonas* spp and *Prevotella* spp).

The World Health Organization (WHO) has designated fluoroquinolones as Critically Important (Highest Priority) antimicrobials for human medicine.[3] The Office International des Epizooties (OIE) has designated fluoroquinolones as Veterinary Critically Important Antimicrobial (VCIA) Agents for veterinary species.[4]

Pharmacology/Actions

Pradofloxacin is a broad-spectrum third-generation bactericidal fluoroquinolone antibiotic. The bactericidal activity of pradofloxacin is concentration dependent, so its antibacterial activity is dependent on high peak concentrations. Its antibacterial action is via inhibition of DNA gyrase and topoisomerase IV, thereby preventing DNA supercoiling and DNA synthesis.

Pradofloxacin is unique among veterinary fluoroquinolones in that it has enhanced aerobic gram-positive activity and activity against anaerobes; its gram-negative activity is similar to other fluoroquinolones. This spectrum of activity is similar to the human fluoroquinolone, moxifloxacin. Pradofloxacin, compared with other veterinary fluoroquinolones, also has enhanced activity against *Mycoplasma* spp. It is the only antibiotic shown to date that can eliminate *Mycoplasma haemofelis* from the blood of experimentally inoculated cats.[5] Methicillin-resistant staphylococci (MRSP) isolates are usually resistant to all fluoroquinolones, including pradofloxacin.[6] Proposed ALCS breakpoints during the FDA approval process of less than 1 µg/mL were considered susceptible and breakpoints greater than 2 µg/mL were considered resistant.

Pradofloxacin has weak activity against streptococci and enterococci and is not recommended in the treatment of these infections.

Unlike enrofloxacin, pradofloxacin does not cause retinal toxicity in cats.[7] It has also not been linked to *Streptococcus canis*-associated necrotizing fasciitis.

Pharmacokinetics

In dogs, after oral administration, pradofloxacin is rapidly absorbed with peak plasma concentrations occurring ≈2 hours after a dose.[8] Bioavailability is reported to be high and not affected by tablet size or the dose administered. Repeated doses do not impact pharmacokinetics. Volume of distribution is more than 2 L/kg, and only ≈35% of the drug is bound to plasma proteins. Peak drug concentrations are slightly higher in serum than in interstitial fluid but persist at concentrations higher than in plasma for most of the 24-hour dosing period. Pradofloxacin at 3 mg/kg PO resulted in 5 times as high PK-PD values in leukocytes compared with plasma, with the lowest values in CSF, synovial fluid, and aqueous humor.[9] Highest tissue concentrations were found in cartilage, liver, and kidneys and measured 1 to 1.5 hours after a dose. Clearance was 0.24 L/hour/kg, and plasma elimination half-life was ≈8 hours. Pradofloxacin is primarily metabolized via glucuronidation and sulfation; ≈40% of a dose is excreted in the urine. Approximately 85% of a dose is excreted into the urine within 24 hours—40% is excreted unchanged and the rest is excreted primarily as glucuronide metabolites.[10-13]

In cats, pradofloxacin is rapidly absorbed with peak plasma concentrations occurring within 1 to 2 hours.[8,14] Oral bioavailability is ≈60% with oral suspension and ≈70% with oral tablets. Repeat doses do not significantly alter the pharmacokinetics. A 5 mg/kg PO dose produced a peak concentration of 2.1 µg /mL when given to fasted cats; administration with food reduces peak concentrations by 50% and total absorption by ≈25%. Volume of distribution is relatively high, and only ≈30% of the drug is bound to plasma proteins. Like in dogs, glucuronidation is the major metabolic pathway for cats; 70% of a dose is excreted into the urine within 24 hours, but only ≈10% of it is excreted as unchanged drug. Clearance is 0.27 L/hour/kg, and terminal plasma elimination half-life has been variably reported from 3 to 8 hours.[11,12,15] Clinical efficacy is associated with achieving a peak pradofloxacin concentration 10 times greater than bacterial MIC.[16,17]

Contraindications/Precautions/Warnings

Pradofloxacin is contraindicated in animals that are hypersensitive to it or other quinolones. It should not be used in kittens younger than 12 weeks of age[18] (younger than 6 weeks on United Kingdom label[14]), as safety has not been evaluated. Pradofloxacin has been shown to produce erosions of cartilage of weight-bearing joints and other signs of arthropathy in immature animals of various species.[18] Pradofloxacin should not be used in dogs and cats with pre-existing articular cartilage lesions.[8,14] Additionally, pradofloxacin administration to healthy cats for longer than 7 days resulted in reversible leukopenia, neutropenia, and lymphopenia.[18]

Although pradofloxacin is approved for use in dogs in other countries (eg, United Kingdom, Europe), it is not FDA-approved in the United States due to myelosuppression (thrombocytopenia and leukopenia) observed in canine safety studies at daily oral pradofloxacin doses of 27 mg/kg (6 times the maximum recommended dose) and above, but not at lower, recommended doses.[12,18] Additional contraindications for dogs include use in dogs less than 12 months of age (most breeds), in giant breeds less than 18 months old due to effects on articular cartilage, and with CNS disorders (eg, epilepsy).[19]

Use with caution in animals with impaired renal function or severely impaired hepatic function. It should also be used with caution in dogs predisposed to arrhythmias and in cats with pre-existing CNS disorders[18] (eg, epilepsy, a contraindication on the United Kingdom label[8,14]). The safety of pradofloxacin in immune-compromised cats (eg, cats infected with feline leukemia virus and/or feline immunodeficiency virus) has not been evaluated.[18]

Fluoroquinolones may cause photosensitization, and prolonged exposure of bare (eg, nose) or thinly haired skin to direct sunlight should be avoided.

The artificial beef flavor used in the tablets originates from irradiated (to inactivate any viruses or micro-organisms) pig livers. Dogs that are hypersensitive to pork products could potentially react to these proteins.

Extra-label use of fluoroquinolones is prohibited in food animals.

Adverse Effects

In dogs and cats, pradofloxacin at recommended dosages appears to be well tolerated with diarrhea/loose stools occasionally reported. Articular cartilage abnormalities have been noted in young, rapidly growing animals given fluoroquinolones (see ***Contraindications/ Precautions/Warnings***).[8,14,18]

Myelosuppression (thrombocytopenia, neutropenia, lymphopenia) is possible in dogs and cats (when used for longer than 7 days).[18] Therapy should be discontinued if this occurs. See ***Contraindications/Precautions/Warnings***

In dogs, QT interval can be increased and pradofloxacin potentially could have proarrhythmic effects, especially in patients with coexisting risk factors (eg, hypothyroidism, bradycardia, electrolyte disturbances, heart failure, or liver or kidney disease).[20]

Reproductive/Nursing Safety

Pradofloxacin is labeled as contraindicated for use during pregnancy or lactation.[8,14] The drug does not pose additional risk when used in breeding animals.[8]

Because safety has not been established in animals, this drug should only be used when the maternal benefits outweigh the potential risks to offspring.

Overdose/Acute Toxicity

Pradofloxacin appears to be quite safe in acute overdose situations, with vomiting and diarrhea possible. The approximate LD_{50} after a single intraperitoneal application in rats was more than 50 mg/kg, and single oral doses of 100 mg/kg were tolerated well in young cats, and in dogs; however, in one dog there was temporary overloading of renal excretory capacity.[12]

Acute overdoses should be managed supportively. Consider performing baseline white blood cell counts in dogs with overdoses.

For patients that have experienced or are suspected to have experienced an overdose, consultation with a 24-hour poison consultation center specializing in providing veterinary-specific information is recommended. For general information related to overdose and toxin exposures, as well as contact information for poison control centers, refer to ***Appendix***.

Drug Interactions

The following drug interactions either have been reported or are theoretical in humans or animals receiving pradofloxacin or other fluoroquinolones and may be of significance in veterinary patients. Unless otherwise noted, use together is not necessarily contraindicated, but weigh the potential risks and perform additional monitoring when appropriate.

- **Antacids, Aluminum-, Calcium- or Magnesium-Containing**: May bind to pradofloxacin and prevent its absorption; separate doses of these products by at least 2 hours.
- **Cimetidine**: Cimetidine has been shown to interfere with the metabolism of quinolones and should be used with care when used concurrently.[18]
- **Corticosteroids** (eg, **dexamethasone, prednisone**): May enhance the toxic effect of quinolones, specifically the risk for tendonitis and tendon rupture
- **Cyclosporine**: Fluoroquinolones may exacerbate the nephrotoxicity and reduce the metabolism of cyclosporine. Concurrent use of pradofloxacin with oral cyclosporine should be avoided.[18]
- **Dairy Products**: May bind to pradofloxacin and prevent its absorption; do not administer pradofloxacin with dairy products.
- **Digoxin**: Concurrent use of pradofloxacin with digoxin should be avoided, as it may increase the oral bioavailability of digoxin.
- **NonSteroidal Anti-Inflammatory Drugs** (**NSAIDs**; eg, **flunixin**): Flunixin has been shown in dogs to increase the AUC and elimination half-life of enrofloxacin, and enrofloxacin increases the AUC and elimination half-life of flunixin; it is unknown if pradofloxacin also causes this effect or if other NSAIDs interact with pradofloxacin in dogs. Fluoroquinolones should not be used in combination with NSAIDs in animals with a history of seizures due to potential pharmacodynamic interactions in the CNS.[8,14]
- **Glyburide**: Severe hypoglycemia is possible with concurrent use of glyburide with pradofloxacin.
- **Iron, Zinc** (oral): Decreased pradofloxacin absorption; separate doses by at least 2 hours.
- **Lanthanum**: May decrease pradofloxacin absorption
- **Methotrexate**: When used concurrently with pradofloxacin, increased methotrexate levels possible with resultant toxicity
- **Nitrofurantoin**: May antagonize the antimicrobial activity of fluoroquinolones, and concomitant use of nitrofurantoin with pradofloxacin is not recommended.
- **Probenecid**: Blocks tubular secretion of ciprofloxacin and may also increase the blood level and half-life of pradofloxacin
- **QT-Prolonging Agents** (eg, **cisapride, sotalol, quinidine, erythromycin, ondansetron**): May enhance the QT-prolonging effect of pradofloxacin
- **Sevelamer**: May decrease pradofloxacin absorption
- **Sucralfate**: May inhibit absorption of pradofloxacin; separate doses of these drugs by at least 2 hours.
- **Theophylline**: Pradofloxacin may increase theophylline blood concentration. The United States label states, The dosage of theophylline should be reduced when used concurrently with quinolones.[18] The United Kingdom labels state, The combination of fluoroquinolones with theophylline could increase the plasma levels of theophylline by altering its metabolism and thus should be avoided.[8,14]

Laboratory Considerations

No specific concerns noted.

Dosages

DOGS:

Wound infections, superficial and deep pyoderma caused by susceptible strains of the *Staphylococcus pseudintermedius* group (including *S pseudintermedius*); acute UTIs caused by susceptible strains of *Escherichia coli* and the *Staphylococcus pseudintermedius* group (including *S pseudintermedius*); and as adjunctive treatment to mechanical or surgical periodontal therapy in the treatment of severe infections of the gingiva and periodontal tissues caused by susceptible strains of anaerobic organisms (extra-label):
3 – 4.5 mg/kg PO once daily.[8] As with other fluoroquinolones, the upper end of the dosing range may be preferable. The duration of the treatment depends on the nature and severity of the infection and on the response to treatment.

CATS:

Skin infections (wounds and abscesses) caused by susceptible strains of *Pasteurella multocida, Streptococcus canis, Staphylococcus aureus, Staphylococcus felis,* and *Staphylococcus pseudintermedius* (label dosage; FDA-approved): 7.5 mg/kg (3.4 mg/lb) PO once daily for 7 consecutive days. If acceptable response to treatment is not observed, or if no improvement is seen within 3 to 4 days, then the diagnosis should be re-evaluated and appropriate alternative therapy considered.[18]

Bartonellosis (extra-label): 5 – 10 mg/kg PO once or twice daily for 28 to 42 days.[1,21] (**NOTE**: larger, once-daily dosages of fluoroquinolones are preferred over twice-daily administration.) Elimination of infection often requires use of more than one class of antibiotic. For cats that are reasonably stable (eg, when treating *Bartonella* spp-linked polyarthritis), one recommendation is to start with one antibiotic (eg, doxycycline 5 mg/kg PO every 12 hours), then add the second antibiotic (eg, pradofloxacin) 5 to 7 days later. Initiation of both antibiotics simultaneously has been associated with a Jarisch-Herxheimer-like reaction, which can be confused with an adverse drug reaction.[1,21]

Mycoplasma haemofelis (extra-label): 5 – 10 mg/kg PO once daily for 14 days[5]

Acute infections of the upper respiratory tract caused by susceptible strains of *Pasteurella multocida, E coli,* and the *Staphylococcus intermedius* group (including *S pseudintermedius*) (extra-label): Oral suspension, 5 – 7.5 mg/kg PO once daily[14]; oral tablets, 3 – 4.5 mg/kg PO once daily.[8] The duration of the treatment depends on the nature and severity of the infection and on the response to treatment. For most infections the following treatment courses will be sufficient: wound infections and abscesses, 7 days; acute infections of the upper respiratory tract, 5 days.

BIRDS:

Infections caused by susceptible strains of *Staphylococcus* spp and *Streptococcus* spp species (extra-label): 15 mg/kg PO every 24 hours[22]

Monitoring

- Clinical efficacy, including culture and susceptibility when indicated
- Consider performing baseline and periodic white blood cell counts. Discontinue therapy if an unexplained drop in leukocyte, neutrophil, and/or lymphocyte counts is noted.[18]

Client Information

- This medicine is an antibiotic used to treat bacterial infections. Be sure to give your animal this medicine exactly as prescribed by your veterinarian.
- If using the liquid form, shake the container well before measuring each dose. Use the syringe provided to ensure accurate dosing. Rinse syringe between doses.
- This medicine is best given without food on an empty stomach,

but if your animal vomits or acts sick afterwards, give it with food or a small treat (no dairy products, antacids, or anything containing iron). If vomiting continues, contact your veterinarian.

- Be sure to finish the entire course of treatment even if your animal appears to feel better.
- Pradofloxacin may stunt bone growth or cause joint abnormalities if used in young animals, or during pregnancy or while nursing.
- The most common side effects are vomiting, nausea (acting sick), or diarrhea.
- For animals with thin hair coats, there may be a risk of sun sensitivity within a few hours after receiving this type of antibiotic.
- Your veterinarian will need to monitor your animal while it is taking this medicine. Do not miss these important follow-up visits.

Chemistry/Synonyms

Pradofloxacin (CAS Registry 0195532-12-8; ATCvet: QJ01MA97, QJ01MA) is an 8-cyano fluoroquinolone antibiotic structurally similar to moxifloxacin. It occurs as a brownish, light yellow to yellow, fine crystalline powder. Pradofloxacin has 4 enantiomeric forms, but secondary to its high antimicrobial potency, the S,S-isomer is used in the pharmaceutical products.

The oral suspension contains 2 mg/mL sorbic acid (E200) as a preservative.

Pradofloxacin may also be known as UNII-6O0T5E048I. Its trade name is *Veraflox*®.

Storage/Stability

The oral suspension should be stored below 30°C (86°F) in the original container and kept tightly closed; after opening, it is stable for 60 days[18] (3 months on United Kingdom label[19]). Oral tablets require no special storage conditions, but once the container is opened, they should be protected from light and moisture.

Compatibility/Compounding Considerations

No information has been located.

Dosage Forms/Regulatory Status

VETERINARY-LABELED PRODUCTS:

Pradofloxacin Oral Suspension: 25 mg/mL in 15 mL and 30 mL bottles; *Veraflox*®; (Rx). Approved for use in cats. NADA 141-344#

Pradofloxacin Oral Tablets: 15 mg, 60 mg, and 120 mg. Approved in United Kingdom and Europe for cats (15 mg only) and dogs (15 mg, 60 mg, 120 mg); POM-V; *Veraflox*®; (Rx)

HUMAN-LABELED PRODUCTS: NONE

References

For the complete list of references, see **wiley.com/go/budde/plumb**

Pralidoxime (2-PAM)

(pra-li-***dox***-eem) *Protopam Chloride*®

Antidote; Cholinesterase Reactivator

Prescriber Highlights

- Cholinesterase reactivator used for adjunctive treatment of organophosphate poisoning
- Contraindications include hypersensitivity; generally not recommended for carbamate poisoning.
- Use with caution in animals with renal impairment and patients receiving anticholinesterase agents for the treatment of myasthenia gravis.
- Adverse effects appear to be uncommon; rapid IV injection may cause tachycardia, muscle rigidity, transient neuromuscular blockade, or laryngospasm.
- Most effective if given within 24 hours of exposure
- Available dosage forms and significant cost may be a limiting factor.

Uses/Indications

Pralidoxime is used in the treatment of organophosphate poisoning, in conjunction with atropine and supportive therapy.

Pralidoxime must generally be given within 24 hours of exposure to be effective, but some benefits may occur, particularly in large exposures, if given within 36 to 48 hours.

Pralidoxime has been shown to have vasoconstrictive properties. When pralidoxime is administered during CPR in pig models, it has been shown to increase coronary perfusion pressure leading to higher rates of restoration of spontaneous circulation[1-3]; however, clinical significance is not yet determined.

Pharmacology/Actions

Pralidoxime reactivates cholinesterase that has been inactivated by phosphorylation secondary to certain organophosphates. Via nucleophilic attack, the drug removes and binds the offending phosphoryl group attached to the enzyme, which is then excreted. Pralidoxime may have protective effects on cholinesterase and may directly detoxify some organophosphates. It has greater activity at nicotinic sites. Its effects occur primarily at the neuromuscular junction of respiratory and skeletal muscle. Because it acts in the periphery, atropine is needed to block the effect of accumulated acetylcholine in the respiratory center.

Pharmacokinetics

Pralidoxime is only marginally absorbed after oral dosing, and oral dosage forms are no longer available in the United States. It is rapidly distributed, primarily throughout the extracellular fluid. Because of its quaternary ammonium structure, it has limited CNS penetration.

Pralidoxime is thought to be metabolized by the liver and rapidly excreted as both metabolite(s) and unchanged drug in the urine. Elimination half-life in humans is ≈75 minutes. The half-life in ruminants is ≈2 to 5 hours.[4]

Contraindications/Precautions/Warnings

Pralidoxime is contraindicated in patients that are hypersensitive to it. Pralidoxime is generally not recommended for use in instances of carbamate poisoning because cholinesterase inhibition by carbamates is rapidly reversible, but there is some controversy regarding this issue. One case report has demonstrated efficacy in a dog with carbamate toxicity using a lower, more frequent dosing regimen.[5]

Pralidoxime should be used with caution in patients receiving anticholinesterase agents for the treatment of myasthenia gravis, as it may precipitate a myasthenic crisis. It should also be used cautiously and at a reduced dose in patients with renal impairment. Temporary worsening of cholinergic signs can occur if pralidoxime is administered IV too rapidly.

Adverse Effects

At usual doses, pralidoxime generally is safe and free of significant adverse effects. Transient increases in liver enzymes and creatine phosphokinase may occur. Rapid IV injection may cause tachycardia, muscle rigidity, transient neuromuscular blockade, and laryngospasm.

In humans, pain at injection site has been reported after IM administration.

Reproductive/Nursing Safety

It is not known whether this drug causes fetal harm or is excreted in maternal milk.

Because safety has not been established in animals, this drug should only be used when the maternal benefits outweigh the potential risks to offspring.

Overdose/Acute Toxicity

The acute LD_{50} of pralidoxime in dogs is 190 mg/kg. Signs of overdose may include dizziness, nausea, or increased heart rate; however, it may be difficult to distinguish these signs from effects of the poisoning being treated.

For patients that have experienced or are suspected of having experienced an overdose, consultation with a 24-hour poison consultation center specializing in providing veterinary-specific information is recommended. For general information related to overdose and toxin exposures, as well as contact information for poison control centers, refer to ***Appendix.***

Drug Interactions

The following drug interactions have either been reported or are theoretical in humans or animals receiving pralidoxime and may be of significance in veterinary patients. Unless otherwise noted, use together is not necessarily contraindicated, but weigh the potential risks and perform additional monitoring when appropriate.

- **ATROPINE**: Effects of atropine occur more rapidly with concomitant use.
- **BARBITURATES**: Anticholinesterases can potentiate the action of barbiturates; use with caution.
- **BENZODIAZEPINES** (eg, **diazepam, midazolam**): Respiratory depressants should be avoided in patients with organophosphate toxicity.
- **CIMETIDINE**: Use should be avoided in patients with organophosphate toxicity.
- **RESERPINE**: Use should be avoided in patients with organophosphate toxicity
- **OPIOIDS** (eg, **morphine**): Respiratory depressants should be avoided in patients with organophosphate toxicity.
- **SUCCINYLCHOLINE**: Use should be avoided in patients with organophosphate toxicity.
- **THEOPHYLLINE**: Use should be avoided in patients with organophosphate toxicity.

Dosages

NOTES:

1) Usually used in conjunction with ***Atropine***; refer to that monograph and/or the references below for more information.
2) Treatment may vary depending on patient factors such as type of poisoning, amount ingested, and time since ingestion.

DOGS/CATS:

Organophosphate poisoning (extra-label):

a) 25 mg/kg IM; repeat in 1 hour if muscle weakness has not been resolved
b) Cats: 20 – 25 mg/kg IM every 12 hours[6]
c) Initial dose of 20 mg/kg IV, IM, or SC. IV administration is preferred; dilute in saline and administer over at least 5 minutes (see ***Compatibility/Compounding Considerations*** below). Subsequent doses of 20 mg/kg IM, SC, or IV (slowly) every 6 to 12 hours can be administered until nicotinic signs (eg, tachycardia, hypertension, muscle fasciculations, respiratory depression) are present. Discontinue after 3 to 4 treatments if no response or if nicotinic signs are aggravated.
   i. Alternatively, 50 mg/kg/day IV CRI may be used[7]
   ii. Kittens: 50 mg/kg initial dose followed by a 20 mg/kg dose the next day in a kitten[8]
   iii. Dogs: 66 mg/kg given IV over 12 hours in a dog[9]

HORSES:

Organophosphate poisoning (extra-label): 20 mg/kg (may require up to 35 mg/kg) IV and repeat every 4 to 6 hours[10]

RUMINANTS:

Organophosphate poisoning in cattle (extra-label): 30 mg/kg IM every 8 hours[11]

CAMELIDS:

Organophosphate poisoning (extra-label): 20 mg/kg (route not specified)[12]

BIRDS:

Organophosphate poisoning (extra-label):

a) 10 – 20 mg/kg every 8 to 12 hours (route not specified) with atropine 0.2 – 0.5 mg/kg IM every 3 to 4 hours.[13] Use lower dose when given with atropine[14]
b) 10 – 100 mg/kg IM every 24 to 48 hours or repeat once in 6 hours[15]

Monitoring

- Pralidoxime therapy is monitored via improvement in the clinical signs associated with organophosphate poisoning (eg, salivation, lacrimation, urination, defecation/diaphoresis, gastrointestinal upset, emesis [SLUDGE]). For more information, refer to one of the references outlined in the dosage section.

Client Information

- This agent should only be used with close professional supervision.

Chemistry/Synonyms

A quaternary ammonium oxime cholinesterase reactivator, pralidoxime chloride occurs as a white to pale yellow, crystalline powder with a pK_a of 7.8 to 8. It is freely soluble in water. The commercially available injection has a pH of 3.5 to 4.5 after reconstitution.

Pralidoxime chloride may also be known as 2-Formyl-1-methylpyridinium chloride oxime, 2-PAM, 2-PAM chloride, 2-PAMCl, 2-pyridine aldoxime methochloride and *Protopam*®.

Storage/Stability

Unless otherwise instructed by the manufacturer, pralidoxime chloride powder for injection should be stored at room temperature, with excursions permitted to 15° to 30°C (59°F-86°F). After reconstituting with sterile water (preservative-free) for injection, the solution should be used immediately. Do not use sterile water with preservatives to reconstitute the powder for injection.

Compatibility/Compounding Considerations

Reconstitute with 20 mL of sterile water for injection to yield 50 mg/mL. For IV infusion, a concentration of 10 – 20 mg/mL in sodium chloride 0.9% is recommended. For IM injection when IV administration is not feasible, reconstitute each vial with 3.3 mL of sterile water for injection (with no preservatives added) to yield 300 mg/mL.

Dosage Forms/Regulatory Status

VETERINARY-LABELED PRODUCTS: NONE

NOTE: When used in food animals, FARAD recommends a 28-day meat and a 6-day milk withdrawal time.[16]

HUMAN-LABELED PRODUCTS:

Pralidoxime Chloride Powder for Injection: 1 g in 20 mL single-use vials; *Protopam® Chloride*; (Rx)

Also available in 600 mg/2 mL IM auto-injectors as single agent, or in combination with atropine sulfate 2.1 mg/0.7 mL.

References

For the complete list of references, see **wiley.com/go/budde/plumb**

Praziquantel/Praziquantel Combination Products

(pra-zi-***kwon***-tel) *Droncit®, Drontal®, Drontal Plus®*

Anticestodal Antiparasitic

For information on other combination products that contain praziquantel, see ***Emodepside/Praziquantel, Eprinomectin/ Praziquantel, Ivermectin, Lufenuron, Milbemycin Oxime, Moxidectin/Moxidectin Combination Products,*** *and* ***Pyrantel.***

Prescriber Highlights

- Anthelmintic approved for treatment of cestodes (tapeworms) in dogs and cats. It may also be useful for some trematodes.
- Many combination products exist with different anthelmintic spectrums of activity.
- Contraindications include puppies younger than 4 weeks, kittens younger than 6 weeks, and hypersensitivity to the drug.
- Use with caution in patients with hepatic impairment.
- Adverse effects are uncommon after oral use but may include GI upset or lethargy. Adverse effects appear more common after injection and include pain at the injection site, anorexia, salivation, vomiting, lethargy, weakness, or diarrhea.

Uses/Indications

Praziquantel is FDA-approved in dogs for the treatment of *Dipylidium caninum, Taenia pisiformis, Echinococcus granulosus* and treatment and control of *E multilocularis*. In cats, it is FDA-approved for the treatment of *D caninum* and *T taeniaeformis*. A single dose is usually effective, but measures should be taken to prevent reinfection (eg, flea control), particularly against *D caninum*.

Praziquantel can also be used extra-label to treat trematodes (eg, *Alaria* spp, *Paragonimus kellicoti, Heterobilharzia americana*) and other cestodes (eg, *Diphyllobothrium* spp, *Spirometra* spp) in dogs and cats.

Praziquantel has been used in birds and other animals, including horses and small ruminants; however, use in large animal species (ie, cattle, horses, small ruminants) is usually not economically feasible.

Combination products with praziquantel can control a wide spectrum of internal parasites in a variety of species. The combination products containing pyrantel pamoate have additional activity against hookworms and roundworms; adding febantel broadens the spectrum of activity to include whipworms.

Pharmacology/Actions

The mechanism of action of praziquantel against cestodes is thought to be the result of the drug interacting with phospholipids in the parasite integument, causing ion fluxes of sodium, potassium, and calcium. At low concentrations in vitro, the drug appears to paralyze the worm's sucker function and stimulate worm motility. At higher concentrations in vitro, praziquantel contracts and paralyzes (irreversibly at very high concentrations) the worm's strobilla (ie, chain of proglottids). In addition, praziquantel causes irreversible focal vacuolization, with subsequent cestodal disintegration at specific sites of the cestodal integument. The parasite ultimately becomes susceptible to digestion.

In schistosomes and trematodes, praziquantel directly kills the parasite, possibly by increasing calcium ion flux in the worm. This is followed by focal vacuolization of the integument, and the parasite is phagocytized by the host.

Details related to additional components of combination products can be found in the respective drug monographs. Febantel is an anthelmintic with activity against nematode parasites, including whipworms, and is partially metabolized into the active metabolites fenbendazole and oxibendazole. For more information, refer to ***Fenbendazole*** and ***Oxibendazole***. Pyrantel pamoate is active against hookworms and roundworms. It acts on the cholinergic receptors of the nematode, resulting in spastic paralysis. For more information, refer to ***Pyrantel***.

Pharmacokinetics

Praziquantel is nearly completely absorbed after oral administration, but there is a significant first-pass effect. Peak serum concentrations are achieved between 30 to 120 minutes in dogs.[1] It is distributed throughout the body. It crosses the intestinal wall and blood–brain barrier into the CNS. Protein binding is ≈80%.[1]

Praziquantel is metabolized in the liver via CYP3A enzymes to metabolites of unknown activity. It is excreted primarily in the urine; elimination half-life is 1 hour in cats[2] and ≈3 hours in dogs[1] (a half-life of 7.4 hours has been reported in greyhounds[3]). Elimination half-life after administration of a topical combination product containing praziquantel was 347 hours in dogs and 152 hours in cats.[3] In dogs, orally administered grapefruit juice can increase drug exposure (area under the curve; AUC) by 150% to 200%.[4] Hepatic impairment may result in prolonged, higher praziquantel concentration; elimination half-life was 1.5 to 3 times longer in humans with moderate to severe hepatic impairment.[5]

Praziquantel pharmacokinetics in parasites have not been described, but drug uptake appears to occur readily.

Contraindications/Precautions/Warnings

Praziquantel is contraindicated in patients that have previously shown hypersensitivity to it or any excipients. The manufacturer recommends not using praziquantel in puppies younger than 4 weeks or kittens younger than 6 weeks.

In humans, praziquantel is contraindicated in patients with ocular parasitism and should be used with caution in patients with moderate to severe liver dysfunction or a history of epilepsy.[6]

Adverse Effects

In dogs, oral administration of praziquantel can cause anorexia, vomiting, lethargy, or diarrhea; the incidence of these effects is less than 5%.[7] In cats, salivation and diarrhea were reported after oral administration; in field trials, the incidence of adverse effects was less than 2%.[7]

A greater incidence of adverse effects has been reported after use of the injectable product. In dogs, pain at the injection site was the most frequent adverse effect, with vomiting, drowsiness, and/or a staggering gait also reported.[8] Approximately 9.4% of cats showed clinical signs of diarrhea, weakness, vomiting, salivation, sleepiness, transient anorexia, and/or pain at the injection site.

Reproductive/Nursing Safety

Praziquantel is considered safe for use in pregnant dogs or cats. Praziquantel (up to 300 mg/kg/day) did not impair fertility or reproductive performance in rats and was not harmful to rabbit or rat fetuses.[6] However, the label for the combination product containing praziquantel, pyrantel pamoate, and febantel states to not use in pregnant animals, as doses 3 times the label dosage increased the incidence of abortion and fetal abnormalities in dogs.[9]

Praziquantel appears in maternal milk at a concentration of ≈25% of that in maternal serum but appears safe for use in nursing patients.

Overdose/Acute Toxicity

Praziquantel has a wide margin of safety. In rats and mice, oral LD_{50} is at least 2 g/kg. Praziquantel at 25 – 50 mg/kg IM or SC every 14 days did not cause clinical toxicity in dogs as young as 4 weeks or cats as young as 5.5 weeks. Vomiting, salivation, and depression occurred in dogs given praziquantel at 150 – 200 mg/kg. Parenteral doses of 100 – 200 mg/kg in cats caused vomiting, muscle tremors, transient ataxia, and depression; death occurred in ≈80% of cats. In dogs homozygous for the *ABCB1* (*MDR-1*) gene mutation, tremors, ataxia, salivation, agitation, panting, and seizures followed administration of a topical praziquantel/emodepside combination.[10,11]

For patients that have experienced or are suspected of having experienced an overdose, consultation with a 24-hour poison consultation center specializing in providing veterinary-specific information is recommended. For general information related to overdose and toxin exposures, as well as contact information for poison control centers, refer to ***Appendix***.

Drug Interactions

Praziquantel is metabolized by the CYP3A enzyme.[12] The following drug interactions have either been reported or are theoretical in humans or animals receiving praziquantel and may be of significance in veterinary patients. Unless otherwise noted, use together is not necessarily contraindicated, but weigh the potential risks and perform additional monitoring when appropriate.

- ALBENDAZOLE: May increase albendazole sulfoxide concentration
- CIMETIDINE: May increase the serum concentration of praziquantel
- CYP3A4 INDUCERS (eg, **dexamethasone, phenobarbital, rifampin**): May decrease praziquantel concentrations.[12,13] In humans, it is recommended to discontinue rifampin 4 weeks before administering praziquantel.
- GRAPEFRUIT JUICE: Can significantly increase praziquantel serum concentrations[4]
- ITRACONAZOLE, KETOCONAZOLE: May increase praziquantel concentrations

Laboratory Considerations

None noted

Dosages

NOTE: For dosages of other combination products that contain praziquantel, *see* ***Emodepside/Praziquantel, Eprinomectin/Praziquantel, Ivermectin, Lufenuron, Milbemycin Oxime, Moxidectin/Moxidectin Combination Products,*** *and* ***Pyrantel.***

DOGS:

<u>Praziquantel as a single agent</u>:

Removal of tapeworms (eg, *Dipylidium caninum, Taenia pisiformis, Echinococcus granulosus*) and removal and control of *E multilocularis* (label dosage; FDA-approved): For use in dogs and puppies 4 weeks of age and older

Injectable: IM or SC dose using the 56.8 mg/mL injectable product is determined by body weight. In dogs, IM may be preferred, as it appears less painful than SC administration.

Droncit® Injectable

Body weight	Dose
Up to 2.3 kg (5 lb)	17 mg (0.3 mL)
2.7-4.5 kg (6-10 lb)	28.4 mg (0.5 mL)
5-11.4 kg (11-25 lb)	56.8 mg (1 mL)
Over 11.4 kg (25 lb)	5 mg/kg (0.2 mL per 5 lb); maximum of 3 mL

Oral: Using the 34 mg canine tablet in dogs 4 weeks of age and older[8]:

Droncit® Tablets for Puppies and Adult Dogs

Body weight	Number of tablets
2.3 kg (5 lb) and under	0.5
2.7-4.5 kg (6-10 lb)	1
5-6.8 kg (11-15 lb)	1.5
7.2-13.6 kg (16-30 lb)	2
14.1-20.5 kg (31-45 lb)	3
20.9-27.3 kg (46-60 lb)	4
Over 27.3 kg (60 lb)	5 (maximum)

<u>Praziquantel combination products:</u>

Praziquantel/Febantel/Pyrantel Pamoate (*Drontal® Plus*):

Removal of tapeworms (eg, *Dipylidium caninum, Taenia pisiformis, Echinococcus granulosus*), hookworms (eg, *Ancylostoma caninum, Uncinaria stenocephala*), ascarids (eg, *Toxocara canis, Toxascaris leonina*), and whipworms (*Trichuris vulpis*) and removal and control of *Echinococcus multilocularis* (label dosage; FDA-approved): Three tablet sizes are available: Puppies and small dogs, 0.9 to 11.3 kg (2 to 25 lb); medium-sized dogs, 11.8 to 27.2 kg (26 to 60 lb); large dogs, more than 20.4 kg (45 lb). See table below to determine the correct tablet size and dose. **NOTE**: Dogs from 45 to 60 lb can be dosed with either 2 medium tablets or 1 large tablet. Ensure correct dose is given for tablet size used. Not for use in puppies younger than 3 weeks of age or dogs weighing less than 0.9 kg (2 lb).[9]

Drontal® Plus Tablets and Taste Tabs® for Puppies and Small Dogs (0.9 to 11.3 kg [2 to 25 lb])

Body weight	Number of tablets
0.9-1.8 kg (2-4 lb)	0.5
2.3-3.2 kg (5-7 lb)	1
3.6-5.5 kg (8-12 lb)	1.5
5.9-8.2 kg (13-18 lb)	2
8.6-11.4 kg (19-25 lb)	2.5

Drontal® Plus Tablets and Taste Tabs® for Medium-Sized Dogs (11.8 to 27.2 kg [26 to 60 lb])

Body weight	Number of tablets
11.8-13.6 kg (26-30 lb)	1
14.1-20 kg (31-44 lb)	1.5
20.5-27.3 kg (45-60 lb)	2

Drontal® Plus Tablets and Taste Tabs® for Large Dogs (20.4 kg [45 lb] and greater)

Body weight	Number of tablets
20.5-27.3 kg (45-60 lb)	1
27.7-40.9 kg (61-90 lb)	1.5
41.4-54.5 kg (91-120 lb)	2

Praziquantel as a single agent (extra-label):

a) ***Taenia* spp, *Echinococcus* spp, *Dipylidium caninum*, *Mesocestoides* spp (adult)**: 5 mg/kg PO or SC[14]
b) ***Diphyllobothrium* spp**: 7.5 mg/kg PO once daily for 2 days.[14] Alternatively, 25 mg/kg PO daily for 2 consecutive days[15]
c) ***Sparganum proliferum* (adult)**: 7.5 mg/kg or 25 mg/kg PO or SC daily for 2 days[14]
d) ***Spirometra mansonoides* or *Diphyllobothrium erinacei***: 7.5 mg/kg PO once daily for 2 days[16]
e) **Paragonimiasis (*Paragonimus kellicotti*)**: 23 – 25 mg/kg PO every 8 hours for 3 days[17,18]
f) **Liver flukes (*Platynosomum* spp or Opisthorchiidae families)**: 20 – 40 mg/kg PO once daily for 3 to 10 days.[19] Alternatively, 20 mg/kg PO as a single dose appeared effective in an infected kennel of huskies.[20]
g) ***Alaria* spp**: 20 mg/kg PO once[21] or once daily for 2 to 10 days[22]
h) **Adjunctive treatment of flukes (*Nanophyetus salmincola*) associated with Salmon poisoning**: 10 – 30 mg/kg PO or SC once[23]
i) ***Heterobilharzia americana***: From a case report, 25 mg/kg PO every 8 hours for 2 days; the dog had previously received 3 courses of fenbendazole[24]
j) **Peritoneal larval cestodiasis*:*** From a case report, 5 mg/kg SC; the dog was previously treated with a 10-day course of fenbendazole 50 mg/kg PO every 12 hours[25]

Praziquantel combination products (extra-label):

a) **Giardiasis using *Drontal® Plus***: Use the label dosage according to weight-based dosing tables on the product label once daily PO for 3 days[26]
b) **Persistent *Ancylostoma caninum*:** Label dosages according to weight-based dosing tables on the product labels for topical moxidectin combination products or oral praziquantel/febantel/pyrantel pamoate administered once monthly were effective in 8 greyhounds with persistent *Ancylostoma caninum*, as measured by monthly fecal ova testing.[27]

CATS:

Praziquantel as a single agent:

Removal of *Dipylidium caninum* and *Taenia taeniaeformis* (label dosage; FDA-approved): For use in cats 6 weeks of age and older

Injectable: IM or SC dose using the 56.8 mg/mL injectable product as a single dose:

Droncit® Injectable

Body weight	Dose
Less than 2.3 kg (5 lb)	11.4 mg (0.2 mL)
2.3-4.5 kg (5-10 lb)	22.7 mg (0.4 mL)
5 kg (11 lb) and over	34.1 mg (0.6 mL); maximum dose

Oral: Using the 23 mg feline tab as a single dose:[8]

Droncit® Tablets for Cats and Kittens

Body weight	Number of tablets
1.8 kg (4 lb) and under[39]	0.5
2.3-5 kg (5-11 lb)	1
Over 5 kg (11 lb)	1.5

Praziquantel combination products:

Praziquantel/Pyrantel Pamoate *(Drontal®)*:

Removal of tapeworms (*Dipylidium caninum*, *Taenia pisiformis*), hookworms (*Ancylostoma tubaeforme*), and ascarids (*Toxocara cati*) (label dosage; FDA-approved): In cats and kittens at least 2 months of age and weighing 0.9 kg (2 lb) or more.[28]

Drontal® Tablets for Cats

Body weight	Number of tablets
0.9-1.4 kg (2-3 lb)	0.5
1.8-3.6 kg (4-8 lb)	1
4.1-5.4 kg (9-12 lb)	1.5
5.9-7.3 (13-16 lb)	2

Praziquantel as a single agent (extra-label):

a) **Paragonimiasis (*Paragonimus kellicotti*)**: 23 – 25 mg/kg PO every 8 hours for 3 days[17,18]
b) ***Diphyllobothrium* spp (adult)**: 25 mg/kg PO daily for 2 consecutive days or 35 mg/kg PO once has been recommended[14,15]
c) ***Sparganum proliferum* (adult)**: 7.5 mg/kg or 25 mg/kg PO or SC daily for 2 days[14]
d) ***Alaria* spp**: 20 mg/kg PO once[21] or once daily for 2 to 10 days[22]
e) ***Taenia* spp, *Echinococcus* spp, *Dipylidium caninum*, *Mesocestoides* spp (adult)**: 5 mg/kg PO or SC once[14]
f) ***Spirometra mansonoides***: 30 – 35 mg/kg PO once[29] or once daily for 2 days[30]
g) ***Platynosomum* spp*:*** 30 mg/kg PO every 24 hours for 5 to 10 days[31]

Praziquantel combination products (extra-label):

a) ***Aelurostrongylus abstrusus* (adult) using praziquantel/emodepside (*Profender®*)*:*** Emodepside 3 mg/kg and praziquantel 12 mg/kg, applied topically; repeat dose 14 days after initial treatment[32]
b) ***Giardia* spp infections using praziquantel/febantel/pyrantel (*Drontal®* Plus)**: Give 2 small dog tablets (praziquantel, 22.7 mg; febantel, 113.4 mg; pyrantel, 22.7 mg) PO once daily for 5 days[33]

HORSES:

Susceptible parasites (label dosage; FDA-approved): 1 – 2.5 mg/kg PO using combination products containing praziquantel with ivermectin or moxidectin[34,35]

Anoplocephala perfoliata (extra-label): 1.5 – 2 mg/kg PO was 100% effective in treated horses; 1 mg/kg PO was 99.7% effective[36]

NEW WORLD CAMELIDS:

Dicrocoelium dendriticum (extra-label): 50 mg/kg PO once (**NOTE**: concentrated [250 mg/mL] galenic paste formulation[37])

SHEEP, GOATS:

a) ***Moniezia* spp, *Stilesia* spp, or *Avitellina* spp** (extra-label): 10 – 15 mg/kg PO[16]
b) **Cestodes** (extra-label): 10 – 15 mg/kg PO once[38]
c) ***Dicrocoelium dendriticum*** (extra-label): 50 mg/kg PO once was 95.9% effective[39]
d) ***Schistosoma bovis* in goats** (extra-label): 60 mg/kg PO once[40]

BIRDS:

Susceptible parasites (tapeworms) (extra-label):

a) ¼ of one 23 mg tablet/kg PO, repeated after 10 to 14 days. Add to feed or give by gavage. Injectable form is toxic to finches.[41]

b) **Common tapeworms in chickens**: 10 mg/kg PO[16]

c) **Cestodes and some trematodes**: Direct dose: 5 – 10 mg/kg PO or IM once or 12 mg of crushed tablets baked into a 9 × 2-inch cake. Finches should have their regular food withheld and be pre-exposed to a non-medicated cake.[42]

RABBITS, RODENTS, SMALL MAMMALS:

NOTE: All dosages are extra-label.

a) **Chinchillas**: 6 – 10 mg/kg PO[43]

b) **Cestodes in chinchillas, rats, mice, hamsters, gerbils, and guinea pigs**: 6 – 10 mg/kg PO or SC once[44]

c) **Ferrets**: 5 mg/kg PO once[45]; alternatively, 5 – 10 mg/kg PO, repeated after 10 to 14 days[44]

d) **Trematodes in ferrets**: 25 mg/kg PO once daily for 3 days (depending on type of trematode)[45]

e) **Cestodes and trematodes in rabbits**: 5 – 10 mg/kg PO once[46]; may be repeated after 10 days[44]

f) ***Schistosoma bovis* in rabbits**: 40 mg/kg PO

REPTILES/AMPHIBIANS:

NOTE: All dosages are extra-label.

a) **Reptiles**: Cestodes and some trematodes in most species: 7.5 mg/kg PO once, repeated after 2 weeks PO[47]

b) **Removal of common tapeworms in snakes**: 3.5 – 7 mg/kg[16]

c) **Cestodes and trematodes in reptiles and amphibians**: 7 – 8 mg/kg PO, IM, SC[48]

d) **Removal of susceptible cestodes in tortoises**: 8 mg/kg SC, repeated after 14 days[49]

Monitoring

- Clinical efficacy: Confirm presence of parasites with fecal laboratory examination

Client Information

- This medicine can be given with or without food. The tablets may be crushed or mixed with food. Your animal does not need to have food withheld prior to treatment.
- When this medicine is given by mouth, side effects are rare, but this medicine can cause loss of appetite, salivation or drooling (in cats), vomiting, lethargy/tiredness/lack of energy, and/or diarrhea. Persistent vomiting, bloody stool, or profuse/watery diarrhea should be reported to your veterinarian.
- Dead tapeworms are not usually seen in the feces after treatment.
- Praziquantel removes tapeworms but does not prevent re-infestation, which may occur as early as 1 month after treatment. It is important to discuss parasite control with your veterinarian.

Chemistry/Synonyms

Praziquantel, a prazinoisoquinoline derivative anthelmintic, occurs as a white to practically white, hygroscopic, bitter, crystalline powder, either odorless or having a faint odor. It is very slightly soluble in water and freely soluble in alcohol.

Praziquantel may also be known as EMBAY-8440, praziquantelum, *Anthelmin*®, *Biltricide*®, *Bio-Cest*®, *Cazitel*®, *Cercon*®, *Cesol*®, *Cestox*®, *Cisticid*®, *ComboCare*®, *Cysticide*®, *Doplac*®, *Droncit*®, *Dronspot*®, *Drontal*®, *Ehliten*®, *Endogard*®, *Equimax*®, *Eqvalan*®, *Extiser*® *Q*®, *Mycotricide*®, *Opticide*®, *Praquantel*®, *Prasikon*®, *Prazite*®, *Prozitel*®, *Quest*® *Plus*, *Sincerck*®, *Teniken*®, *Veloxa*®, *Virbantel*®, *Waycital*®, *Zifartel*®, or *Zimecterin Gold Paste*®.

Storage/Stability

Unless otherwise instructed by the manufacturer, praziquantel tablets should be stored in tight containers at room temperature (25°C [77°F]). Protect from light. Praziquantel injection should be stored at or below 25°C (77°F) and not allowed to freeze. Vials of praziquantel injection should be used within 6 months of first vial puncture and discarded after a maximum number of punctures (10 mL vial, 25 times; 50 mL vial, 90 times).

Dosage Forms/Regulatory Status

VETERINARY-LABELED PRODUCTS:

Praziquantel Tablets: 23 mg (feline); 34 mg (canine); *Droncit*® *Canine Tablets*, *Droncit*® *Feline Tablets*, generic; (Rx; OTC). FDA-approved for use in cats and dogs

Praziquantel Injection: 56.8 mg/mL in 10 mL and 50 mL vials; *Droncit*® *Injection*, generic; (Rx). FDA-approved for use in cats and dogs

Combination Products:

Praziquantel/Emodepside: Praziquantel 7.94% w/w (85.8 mg/mL) and emodepside 1.98% w/w (21.4 mg/mL) topical solution for cats in 0.35 mL (2.2-5.5 lb), 0.7 mL (5.5-11 lb) and 1.12 mL (over 11-17.6 lb) tubes; *Profender*®; (Rx). FDA-approved for use on cats 8 weeks of age and older and weighing at least 1 kg (2.2 lb).

Praziquantel/Eprinomectin: Praziquantel (83 mg/mL) and eprinomectin (4 mg/mL) topical solution for cats in 0.3 mL (1.8-5.5 lb) and 0.9 mL (5.6-16.5 lb); *Centragard*®; (Rx). FDA-approved for use on cats 7 weeks of age and older and weighing at least 1.8 lb.

Praziquantel/Febantel/Pyrantel Oral Tablets and Chewable Tablets: 22.7 mg/113.4 mg/22.7 mg (puppies and small dogs 2-25 lb); 68 mg/340.2 mg/68 mg (Medium-Sized Dogs 26-60 lb); 136 mg/680.4 mg/136 mg (Large Dogs more than 45 lb); *Drontal*® Plus Tablets and *Taste Tabs*®, generic; (Rx). FDA-approved for use in dogs 3 weeks of age and older.

Praziquantel/Ivermectin Oral Paste: 14.03% praziquantel and 1.87% ivermectin in oral syringes (sufficient to treat a 1320 lb horse); *Equimax*®, generic; (OTC). FDA-approved for use in horses or ponies not intended for food purposes.

Praziquantel/Ivermectin Oral Paste: 7.75% praziquantel and 1.55% ivermectin in oral syringes; *Zimecterin Gold*®; (OTC). FDA-approved for use in horses or ponies not intended for food purposes

Praziquantel/Milbemycin Chewable Oral Tablets for Dogs: 22.8 mg/2.3 mg (2-8 lb); 57 mg/5.75 mg (8.1-25 lb); 114 mg/11.5 mg (25.1-50 lb); 228 mg/23 mg (50.1-100 lb); *Interceptor*® *Plus* (Rx). FDA-approved for use in dogs and puppies 6 weeks of age or older and weighing 0.9 kg (2 lb) or greater

Praziquantel/Milbemycin/Lufenuron Chewable Oral Tablets for dogs: 2.3 mg/46 mg/22.8 mg (2-8 lb); 5.75 mg/115 mg/57 mg (8.1-25 lb); 11.5 mg/230 mg/114 mg (25.1-50 lb); 23 mg/460 mg/228 mg (50.1-100 lb); *Sentinel*® *Spectrum*® (Rx). FDA-approved for use in dogs and puppies 6 weeks of age or older

Praziquantel/Moxidectin: Praziquantel 125 mg/mL and moxidectin 20 mg/mL oral gel in 11.6 g syringes (sufficient to treat one 1250 lb horse); *Quest Plus*®; (OTC). FDA-approved for use in horses or ponies 6 months of age and older and not intended for food purposes

Praziquantel/Pyrantel Tablets: Praziquantel 18.2 mg/pyrantel base 72.6 mg (as pamoate); *Drontal*® *Tablets*; (OTC). FDA-approved for use in cats and kittens that are 2 months of age or older and weighing 0.9 kg (2 lb) or greater

Praziquantel/Pyrantel Chewable Tablets: Praziquantel 30 mg/pyrantel pamoate 30 mg; Praziquantel 114 mg/pyrantel pamoate 114 mg chewable tablets; *Virbantel*® Flavored *Chewables*, generic; (OTC). FDA-approved for use in dogs

Praziquantel/Pyrantel/Ivermectin Chewable Tablets: 28.5 mg/28.5 mg/34 µg (6-12 lb), 57 mg/57 mg/68 µg (12.1-25 lb); 114 mg/114 mg/136 µg (25.1-50 lb); 228 mg/228 mg/272 µg (50.1-100 lb); *Iverhart® Max, Quadriguard®*; (Rx). FDA-approved for use in dogs 8 weeks of age and older

HUMAN-LABELED PRODUCTS:

Praziquantel Oral Tablets (film-coated): 600 mg; *Biltricide®*; (Rx)

References

For the complete list of references, see **wiley.com/go/budde/plumb**

Prazosin

(pra-zoe-***sin***) *Minipress®*

Alpha-1-Adrenergic Blocker

Prescriber Highlights

- Alpha-1-adrenergic blocker that may be useful to treat functional urethral obstruction in dogs and cats
- May also be used as adjunctive treatment for congestive heart failure (CHF) or systemic hypertension in dogs; however, prazosin is not considered a first-line choice
- Should be used with caution in patients that have chronic kidney disease (CKD) or pre-existing hypotensive conditions
- Adverse effects include hypotension and CNS (lethargy, dizziness) and GI effects.

Uses/Indications

Prazosin may be useful in the treatment of functional urethral obstruction (eg, vesicourethral reflex dyssynergia [VURD]) in dogs. It has been successfully used to manage dysuria in dogs with prostatic carcinoma.[1] Its usefulness for this purpose in male cats is somewhat controversial,[2] and its efficacy is unknown. In a study of cats with recurrent urethral obstruction, prazosin appeared to be more effective in preventing reobstruction as compared with phenoxybenzamine[3]; however, subsequent placebo-controlled studies have demonstrated that prazosin does not lessen the severity or prevent the recurrence of urethral obstruction in male cats[4,5] and may increase the likelihood of recurrent urethral obstruction.[6]

Prazosin could be considered for adjunctive treatment of CHF, but its use for this indication has fallen out of favor as other medications are more effective. Prazosin may also be used for the treatment of systemic hypertension in dogs but is not typically a first-line drug for this indication.[7]

Pharmacology/Actions

Prazosin's effects are a result of its selective, competitive inhibition of postsynaptic alpha-1-adrenergic receptors. It directly relaxes vascular smooth muscle, which reduces blood pressure and peripheral vascular resistance. Prazosin has dilatory effects on the arterial and venous side.

Prazosin reduces systemic arterial and venous blood pressure and right atrial pressure in patients with CHF, resulting in increased cardiac output and reduced pulmonary and systemic vascular resistance. Heart rates can be moderately decreased or unchanged. Glomerular filtration rate and renal blood flow are unchanged or may be increased. Unlike hydralazine, prazosin does not seem to increase renin release.

Prazosin has not been shown to antagonize medetomidine-[8] or xylazine-induced[9] diuresis in cats.

Laminar microcirculation has not been shown to change in healthy horses given IV prazosin.[10]

Pharmacokinetics

The pharmacokinetic parameters for this agent were not located for veterinary species.

In humans, prazosin is variably absorbed after oral administration. Peak concentrations occur 2 to 3 hours after administration. Prazosin is widely distributed throughout the body and is ≈97% bound to plasma proteins. Prazosin is metabolized in the liver, and some metabolites have activity. Elimination half-life is ≈3 hours. Metabolites, some of which are active, and some unchanged drug (5%-10%) are primarily eliminated in feces via bile.

Contraindications/Precautions/Warnings

Prazosin is contraindicated in patients hypersensitive to it or other quinazolines (eg, tamsulosin). The drug should be used with caution in patients with CKD or pre-existing hypotensive conditions.

There are some anecdotal reports that dogs with the multidrug sensitivity gene (*MDR1* gene, also known as *ABCB1* gene) mutation may be overly sensitive to the effects of prazosin; it should be used with caution in breeds known to be susceptible to this mutation. Alternative drugs should be considered for dogs that have tested positive for the *MDR1* mutation until more information becomes available; if this is not possible, reducing the dose and increased monitoring, particularly blood pressure, should be considered.

Adverse Effects

In an experimental study of dogs receiving prazosin, 0.025 mg/kg IV caused significant decreases in systolic, diastolic, and mean arterial blood pressures.[11] Whether this is a clinical concern when using prazosin orally to decrease urethral resistance is unclear. Other reported adverse effects include CNS effects (lethargy, dizziness [usually transient]), GI effects (nausea, vomiting, diarrhea, constipation), and nictitans elevation. Drug tolerance has been reported in humans, but dose adjustment, temporarily withdrawing the drug, and/or adding an aldosterone antagonist (eg, spironolactone) usually corrects this effect.

Syncope secondary to orthostatic hypotension has been reported in humans after the first dose of the drug. This effect may persist if the dose is too high for the patient.

Reproductive/Nursing Safety

In a study, testicular atrophy and necrosis occurred in dogs and rats receiving 25 mg/kg daily for one year, and decreased fertility was noted in male rats receiving 75 mg/kg/day.[12] Decreased litter size occurred in rats receiving very high dosages, but no fetal abnormalities were observed in rats or rabbits.[12]

Prazosin is excreted into maternal milk in small amounts.[12]

Because safety has not been established in animals, this drug should only be used when the maternal benefits outweigh the potential risks to offspring.

Overdose/Acute Toxicity

Clinical signs associated with a prazosin overdose in dogs include ataxia, lethargy, trembling; hypotension is the most common clinical finding in cats.

GI decontamination with activated charcoal using standard precautionary measures should be considered if the ingestion was recent, the animal is conscious with control of its airway, and the animal is hemodynamically stable. Heart rate and blood pressure should be monitored. Shock should be treated using volume expanders and, if necessary, pressor agents. Renal function should be monitored and supported. Prazosin is not removed by dialysis.

For patients that have experienced or are suspected of having experienced an overdose, consultation with a 24-hour poison consultation center specializing in providing veterinary-specific information is recommended. For general information related to overdose and toxin exposures, as well as contact information for poison control centers, refer to ***Appendix***.

Drug Interactions

The following drug interactions have either been reported or are theoretical in humans or animals receiving prazosin and may be of significance in veterinary patients. Unless otherwise noted, use together is not necessarily contraindicated, but the potential risks should be weighed and additional monitoring performed when appropriate.

- **Angiotensin-Converting Enzyme Inhibitors** (**ACEIs;** eg, benazepril, enalapril): May increase risk for hypotension
- **Amlodipine**: May increase risk for hypotension
- **Beta-Blocking Agents** (eg, propranolol): May enhance the postural hypotensive effects seen after the first dose of prazosin
- **Clonidine**: May decrease prazosin antihypertensive effects
- **Pentoxifylline**: May increase risk for hypotension
- **Phosphodiesterase Inhibitors** (eg, sildenafil): May increase risk for hypotension
- **Telmisartan**: May increase risk for hypotension
- **Vasopressors** (eg, dopamine, norepinephrine): Prazosin may reduce dopamine pressor effect.
- **Verapamil**: May cause synergistic hypotensive effects when used concomitantly with prazosin

Laboratory Considerations

None noted

Dosages

DOGS:

Decrease urethral resistance in idiopathic vesico-urethral reflex dyssynergia (VURD; extra-label):

a) 0.5 mg/kg PO twice daily. If adverse effects develop, decrease the dose by 50%. Moderate to good effect was noted in 60% of the dogs treated.[13]

b) Anecdotally, 1 mg/15 kg (33 lb) PO 2 to 3 times daily

Dysuria in patients with prostatic carcinoma (extra-label): From a case report, 0.1 – 0.4 mg/kg PO daily was helpful in managing dysuria associated with prostatic carcinoma.[1]

Systemic hypertension (extra-label):

a) Weight-based dosage: 0.5 – 2 mg/kg PO every 8 to 12 hours[7]

b) Dosage per dog: 0.5 – 2 mg/dog (NOT mg/kg) PO every 8 to 12 hours[14,15]

Adjunctive treatment of heart failure (extra-label): 1 mg/dog (NOT mg/kg) PO 3 times daily for dogs weighing less than 15 kg (33 lb); 2 mg/dog (NOT mg/kg) 3 times daily PO for dogs weighing more than 15 kg (33 lb)[16,17]

CATS:

Decreasing urethral resistance with functional urethral obstruction (extra-label): Use is controversial, and efficacy has been questioned.[2,6] Several dosages have been suggested, but most commonly 0.25 – 1 mg/cat (NOT mg/kg) PO every 12 hours for 1 to 2 weeks[4-6]

Hypertension (extra-label): 0.25 – 0.5 mg/cat (NOT mg/kg) PO once daily[7]

Monitoring

- Clinical efficacy
- Baseline and periodic blood pressure
- Mucous membrane color, capillary refill time (CRT), pulse oximetry

Client Information

- This medicine may be given with or without food. If your animal vomits, stops eating, or acts sick after getting prazosin on an empty stomach, give the medicine with food or a small treat to see if this helps. If vomiting continues, contact your veterinarian.
- The most common side effect with this medicine is lethargy (tiredness/lack of energy).

Chemistry/Synonyms

Prazosin HCl, a quinazoline-derivative postsynaptic alpha-1-adrenergic blocker, occurs as a white to tan powder. It is slightly soluble in water and very slightly soluble in alcohol. Dosage forms contain prazosin HCl, but potency and dosage are expressed (and calculated) as prazosin base.

Prazosin may also be known as CP-12299-1, furazosin hydrochloride, prazosini hydrochloridum; many trade names are available.

Storage/Stability

Prazosin capsules should be stored in well-closed containers and protected from light and moisture at room temperature (20°C-25°C [68°F-77°F]).

Dosage Forms/Regulatory Status

VETERINARY-LABELED PRODUCTS: NONE

The Association of Racing Commissioners International (ARCI) has designated this drug as a class 3 substance. Use of this drug may not be allowed in certain animal competitions. Check rules and regulations before entering in a competition while this medication is being administered. Contact local racing authorities for further guidance. See ***Appendix*** for more information.

HUMAN-LABELED PRODUCTS:

Prazosin Capsules: 1 mg, 2 mg, and 5 mg (as base); *Minipress*®, generic; (Rx)

References

For the complete list of references, see **wiley.com/go/budde/plumb**

PrednisoLONE/Prednisone/ PrednisoLONE Sodium Succinate

(pred-***niss***-oh-lone; ***pred***-ni-zone)

Glucocorticoid

For more information, see ***Glucocorticoid Agents, General Information*** *and* ***Trimeprazine/Prednisolone***

NOTE: *Prednisone and prednisoLONE are distinct drugs. This monograph uses TALL man letters to differentiate prednisoLONE from prednisone. They are often considered bioequivalent as most species rapidly convert prednisone to its active form, prednisolone, in the liver; however, horses, cats, and animals that have severe hepatic failure may not efficiently absorb or convert prednisone to prednisoLONE. PrednisoLONE or an alternative glucocorticoid should be used for these animals when possible.*

Prescriber Highlights

- ► Used to treat many conditions in a variety of species.
- ► Prednisone's anti-inflammatory activity is 4 times more potent than hydrocortisone and it has some mineralocorticoid activity.
- ► Contraindications (relative) include systemic fungal infections. Increased risk of GI ulceration when used concurrently with NSAIDS or aspirin.
- ► Caution is advised for use in animals with an active bacterial infection, corneal ulcer, hyperadrenocorticism, diabetes mellitus, osteoporosis, chronic psychotic reactions, predisposition to thrombophlebitis, hypertension, congestive heart failure, and renal insufficiency.
- ► Goal of therapy should be to use the lowest dose possible for the least amount of time to treat and control patient's condition.
- ► PrednisoLONE is recommended for use in cats and horses because of the poor bioavailability of prednisone.
- ► Primary adverse effects are related to iatrogenic hyperadrenocorticism with sustained use.
- ► Many potential drug and laboratory interactions

Uses/Indications

Although glucocorticoids have been used to treat many conditions in humans and animals, prednisoLONE and prednisone have 4 primary uses with accompanying dosage ranges: 1) replacement or supplementation (eg, relative adrenal insufficiency associated with septic shock) for glucocorticoid deficiency secondary to hypoadrenocorticism, 2) anti-inflammatory agent, 3) immunosuppression, and 4) antineoplastic agent.

Glucocorticoids are used in the treatment of endocrine conditions (eg, adrenal insufficiency), autoimmune and immune-mediated diseases (eg, rheumatoid arthritis, systemic lupus, masticatory myositis), severe allergic conditions, anaphylaxis, envenomation, respiratory diseases (eg, asthma), dermatologic diseases (eg, pemphigus, allergic dermatoses), hematologic disorders (eg, thrombocytopenia, autoimmune hemolytic anemia), neoplasias, nervous system disorders (eg, increased CSF pressure), GI diseases (eg, ulcerative colitis exacerbations, inflammatory bowel disease), renal diseases (eg, nephrotic syndrome), and induction of fetal maturation. Some glucocorticoids are used topically on the eye and skin or are injected intra-articularly or intralesionally. This list is not exhaustive. High-dose use is not supported for hemorrhagic or hypovolemic shock, head trauma, spinal cord trauma,[1] or sepsis.

In general, when administering glucocorticoids, the following principles should be followed:

- A specific diagnosis is ideally obtained before glucocorticoids are administered as they can mask disease.
- A course of treatment should be determined prior to treatment.
- A therapeutic endpoint should be determined prior to treatment.
- The least potent glucocorticoid should be used at the lowest dose for a minimal amount of time.
- It is important to understand when glucocorticoid use is inappropriate (eg, acute infection, diabetes).[2]

Pharmacology/Actions

PrednisoLONE and prednisone are intermediate-acting corticosteroids with biologic half-lives of 12 to 36 hours. Glucocorticoids have effects on almost every cell type and system in mammals.

Cardiovascular system: Glucocorticoids can reduce capillary permeability and enhance vasoconstriction. A clinically insignificant positive inotropic effect can occur after glucocorticoid administration. This drug's vasoconstrictive properties and increased blood volume can result in increased blood pressure.

Cells: Glucocorticoids can inhibit fibroblast proliferation, macrophage response to migration inhibiting factor, sensitization of lymphocytes, and the cellular response to mediators of inflammation; they can also stabilize lysosomal membranes.

CNS/autonomic nervous system: Glucocorticoids can lower the seizure threshold, alter mood and behavior, diminish response to pyrogens, stimulate appetite, and maintain alpha rhythm. Glucocorticoids are necessary for normal adrenergic receptor sensitivity.

Endocrine system: When an animal is not stressed, glucocorticoids suppress the release of corticotropin (adrenocorticotropic hormone [ACTH]) from the anterior pituitary, which reduces or prevents the release of endogenous corticosteroids. Stress factors (eg, renal disease, liver disease, diabetes) may occasionally nullify the suppressing aspects of exogenously administered steroids. The release of thyroid-stimulating hormone (TSH), follicle-stimulating hormone (FSH), prolactin, and luteinizing hormone may be reduced when glucocorticoids are administered at pharmacologic doses. Conversion of thyroxine (T_4) to triiodothyronine (T_3) may be reduced by glucocorticoids, and plasma levels of parathyroid hormone may be increased. Glucocorticoids may inhibit osteoblast function. Vasopressin (antidiuretic hormone [ADH]) activity is reduced at the renal tubules and diuresis may occur. Glucocorticoids inhibit insulin binding to insulin-receptors and the post-receptor effects of insulin.

Fluid and electrolyte balance: Glucocorticoids can increase renal potassium and calcium excretion, sodium and chloride reabsorption, and extracellular fluid volume. Hypokalemia and/or hypocalcemia rarely occur. Diuresis may develop following glucocorticoid administration.

GI tract and hepatic system: Glucocorticoids increase the secretion of gastric acid, pepsin, and trypsin. They alter the structure of mucin and decrease mucosal cell proliferation. Iron salts and calcium absorption are decreased, whereas fat absorption is increased. Hepatic changes can include increased fat and glycogen deposits in hepatocytes and increased serum levels of ALT and gamma-glutamyl transpeptidase (GGT). Significant increases can be seen in serum ALP levels. Glucocorticoids can cause minor increases in bromosulfophthalein (BSP) retention time.

Hematopoietic system: Glucocorticoids can increase the number of circulating platelets, neutrophils, and RBCs, but platelet aggregation is inhibited. Decreased amounts of lymphocytes (peripheral), monocytes, and eosinophils are seen because glucocorticoids can sequester these cells into the lungs and spleen and can prompt decreased release from bone marrow; removal of old RBCs becomes diminished. Glucocorticoids can cause involution of lymphoid tissue.

Immune system (also see ***Cells*** and ***Hematopoietic system***): Glucocorticoids can decrease circulating levels of T-lymphocytes; inhibit lymphokines; inhibit neutrophil, macrophage, and monocyte migration; reduce production of interferon; and inhibit phagocytosis, chemotaxis, antigen processing, and intracellular killing. Specific acquired immunity is affected less than nonspecific immune responses. Glucocorticoids can also antagonize the complement cascade and mask the clinical signs of infection. Mast cells are decreased in number and histamine synthesis is suppressed. Many of these effects only occur at high doses and species have different responses.

Metabolic effects: Glucocorticoids stimulate gluconeogenesis. Lipogenesis is enhanced in certain areas of the body (eg, abdomen), and adipose tissue can be redistributed away from the extremities to the trunk. Fatty acids are mobilized from tissues and their oxidation is increased. Plasma levels of triglycerides, cholesterol, and glycerol are increased. Protein is mobilized from most areas of the body (not the liver).

Musculoskeletal: Glucocorticoids may cause muscular weakness, atrophy, and osteoporosis. Bone growth can be inhibited via growth hormone and somatomedin inhibition, increased calcium excretion, and inhibition of vitamin D activation. Resorption of bone can be enhanced. Fibrocartilage growth is also inhibited.

Ophthalmic: Prolonged corticosteroid use (both systemic or topically to the eye) can cause increased intraocular pressure and glaucoma, cataracts, and exophthalmos.

Skin: Thinning of dermal tissue and skin atrophy can be seen with glucocorticoid therapy. Hair follicles can become distended and alopecia may occur.

Pharmacokinetics

Prednisone is a prodrug and requires hepatic bioactivation.

In cats, prednisoLONE has a higher bioavailability when administered orally as compared with prednisone.[3] Reported bioavailabilities (of active prednisoLONE) are 100% and 21%, respectively. Although it is not clear if this is due to decreased GI absorption or decreased hepatic conversion of prednisone to prednisoLONE, oral prednisoLONE is the superior choice in cats.[3,4] In a study, overconditioned cats had significantly higher plasma prednisoLONE concentrations (2 times) as compared with normal-conditioned cats.[5]

In horses, oral prednisone has been shown to have poor oral bioavailability and minimal conversion to prednisoLONE, and therefore prednisoLONE is recommended over prednisone in horses.[6]

In humans, prednisoLONE is hepatically conjugated and metabolites are primarily excreted in the urine. Plasma half-life is not meaningful from a therapy standpoint when evaluating systemic corticosteroids. PrednisoLONE and prednisone are intermediate-acting corticosteroids with biologic half-lives of 12 to 36 hours in humans.

Contraindications/Precautions/Warnings

Systemic use of glucocorticoids is considered contraindicated in systemic fungal infections (unless it is being used as replacement therapy for Addison's disease), when administered IM in animals with idiopathic thrombocytopenia and in those hypersensitive to a particular compound. Sustained-released injectable glucocorticoids are considered contraindicated for chronic corticosteroid therapy for systemic diseases.

The veterinary injectable product label states: *Contraindicated in animals with tuberculosis, Cushingoid syndrome, and peptic ulcer. Existence of congestive heart failure, diabetes, chronic nephritis, and osteoporosis are relative contraindications. In the presence of infection, appropriate antibacterial agents should also be administered and should be continued for at least 3 days after discontinuance of the glucocorticoid and disappearance of all signs of infection. Do not use in viral infections.*[7]

Caution is advised when using predis(ol)one in animals with concomitant renal disease, as they may be at increased risk for adverse GI effects. Animals with hepatic dysfunction may have impaired ability to metabolize prednisone to prednisoLONE.

Systemic glucocorticoids can suppress adrenal function. Animals that have received these drugs chronically should be tapered off slowly, as endogenous ACTH release and corticosteroid function may return slowly. Additional glucocorticoids should be administered if the animal undergoes a stressor (eg, surgery, trauma, illness) during the tapering process or until normal adrenal and pituitary functions resume.

Animals, particularly cats, at risk for diabetes mellitus should be administered glucocorticoids with caution because of the potent hyperglycemic effects of these agents. Patients with cardiovascular disease should be monitored closely, as glucocorticoids can cause fluid retention, which may cause the patient's condition to decompensate. Glucocorticoids are immunosuppressive at higher doses (greater than or equal to 2 mg/kg/day) and may increase the risk for infection. In humans, long-term glucocorticoids may increase intraocular pressure and may increase the risk for cataracts and/or osteoporosis.

Do not confuse prednisoLONE with predniSONE, particularly in cats and horses.

Adverse Effects

Adverse effects are generally associated with long-term administration of these drugs, especially if the drugs are administered at high doses or not on an alternate-day regimen. Effects typically manifest as clinical signs of hyperadrenocorticism. Glucocorticoids can delay growth when administered to young, growing animals. A listing of potential effects are outlined in ***Glucocorticoid Agents, General Information***.

In dogs, polydipsia (PD), polyphagia (PP), and polyuria (PU) may occur during short-term burst therapy and on days when the drug is administered during alternate-day maintenance therapy. Adverse effects in dogs can include dull/dry coat, weight gain, panting, vomiting, diarrhea, elevated liver enzymes, GI ulceration (especially with high parenteral or oral doses); hypercoagulability; hyperlipidemia, activation or worsening of diabetes mellitus, muscle wasting, and/or behavior changes (eg, depression, lethargy, aggression). Glucocorticoids have been known to delay growth in young animals. Discontinuation of the drug may be necessary; changing to an alternate steroid may also alleviate adverse effects. Adverse effects associated with anti-inflammatory therapy are relatively uncommon, with the exception of PU, PD, and PP. Adverse effects associated with immunosuppressive dosages are more common and potentially more severe. In healthy dogs, immunosuppressive dosages of prednis(ol)one 2 – 4 mg/kg/day PO for 1 to 3 weeks did not enhance platelet function or coagulation[8] or produce clinical or histologic evidence of pancreatitis.[9] PrednisoLONE reduced gallbladder emptying in healthy beagles.[10] Bone mineral density, as assessed by quantitative CT, was reduced ≈15% from baseline after a 9-week tapered prednisoLONE dose, which recovered to near baseline 30 months after prednisoLONE was discontinued.[11]

Cats generally require higher doses than dogs for clinical effects but typically develop fewer adverse effects. Glucocorticoids appear to have a greater hyperglycemic effect in cats than other species. Occasionally, PU, PD, and PP with weight gain, diarrhea, and/or depression will be present. Long-term, high-dose therapy can lead to Cushingoid effects. Systemic steroid administration may increase the chance for development of acute bullous keratopathy.[12]

Reproductive/Nursing Safety

Corticosteroid therapy may induce parturition in large animal species during the latter stages of pregnancy. The veterinary label states: *Clinical and experimental data have demonstrated that corticosteroids administered orally or by injection to animals may induce the first stage or parturition is used during the last trimester of pregnancy and may precipitate premature parturition followed by dystocia, fetal death, retained placenta, and metritis. Additionally, corticosteroids administered to dogs, rabbits, and rodents during pregnancy have resulted in cleft palate in offspring. Corticosteroids administered to dogs during pregnancy have also resulted in other congenital anomalies, including deformed forelegs, phocomelia, and anasarca.* Multiple midline defects were noted in a litter of golden retriever puppies with gestation exposure to doxycycline and prednisone.[13] In humans, maternal glucocorticoid use may lead to hypoadrenalism in newborns.[12]

Caution is advised when using in nursing dams; glucocorticoids unbound to plasma proteins can enter milk. High doses or prolonged administration to nursing dams may potentially inhibit growth, interfere with endogenous corticosteroid production, or cause other unwanted effects in nursing offspring. In humans, several studies suggest that amounts excreted in milk are negligible when the prednisone or prednisoLONE dose given to the mother is less than or equal to 20 mg/day or when the methylprednisoLONE dose is less than or equal to 8 mg/day. Larger doses given for short periods may not harm the infant.

Overdose/Acute Toxicity

Overdoses of glucocorticoids used alone are unlikely to cause harmful effects, but GI effects that are sometimes severe can be seen in dogs. Supportive treatment may be required if clinical signs occur. Other clinical signs associated with an overdose in dogs include polyuria and polydipsia.

For patients that have experienced or are suspected to have experienced an overdose, consultation with a 24-hour poison consultation center specializing in providing veterinary-specific information is recommended. For general information related to overdose and toxin exposures, as well as contact information for poison control centers, refer to ***Appendix***.

Drug Interactions

The following drug interactions have either been reported or are theoretical in humans or animals receiving oral prednisoLONE/prednisone and may be of significance in veterinary patients. Unless otherwise noted, use together is not necessarily contraindicated, but the potential risks must be weighed and additional monitoring performed when appropriate.

- **Amphotericin B**: May cause hypokalemia when administered concomitantly with glucocorticoids
- **Anticholinesterase Agents** (eg, **neostigmine, pyridostigmine**): In animals with myasthenia gravis, concomitant glucocorticoid use with these agents may lead to profound muscle weakness. If possible, anticholinesterase medication should be discontinued at least 24 hours before corticosteroid administration.
- **Aspirin** (salicylates): Glucocorticoids may reduce salicylate blood levels. Combination may increase the risk for GI ulcers or erosions. In dogs, prednisone given with ultra-low–dose aspirin (0.5 mg/kg/day is often used in the treatment of immune-mediated hemolytic anemia (IMHA) does not increase the severity of GI lesions as compared with prednisone alone but may increase incidence of diarrhea.[14]
- **Barbiturates**: May increase the metabolism of glucocorticoids
- **Cholestyramine**: May reduce prednis(ol)one absorption
- **Cyclophosphamide**: Glucocorticoids may also inhibit the hepatic metabolism of cyclophosphamide; dosage adjustments may be required.
- **Cyclosporine**: Concomitant administration with glucocorticoids may increase the blood levels of each by mutually inhibiting the hepatic metabolism of the other; clinical significance of this interaction is not clear.
- **Digoxin**: Secondary to hypokalemia, increased risk for arrhythmias
- **Diuretics, Potassium-Depleting** (eg, **furosemide, thiazides**): May cause hypokalemia when administered concomitantly with glucocorticoids
- **Ephedrine**: May increase metabolism of glucocorticoids
- **Estrogens**: Effects of hydrocortisone, and possibly other glucocorticoids, may be potentiated by concomitant administration with estrogens.
- **Fluoroquinolones**: Concurrent use may increase risk for tendinitis and tendon rupture.
- **Insulin**: Insulin requirements may increase in animals receiving glucocorticoids.
- **Ketoconazole**: May decrease the metabolism of glucocorticoids
- **Macrolide Antibiotics** (eg, **clarithromycin, erythromycin**): May decrease the metabolism of glucocorticoids
- **Mitotane**: May alter the metabolism of steroids; higher than usual doses of steroids may be necessary to treat mitotane-induced adrenal insufficiency.
- **Mycophenolate**: PrednisoLONE increased the in vitro unbound (active) fraction of mycophenolic acid in dogs but not in cats.[15]
- **Nonsteroidal Anti-Inflammatory Drugs** (**NSAIDs**; eg, **carprofen, meloxicam, phenylbutazone, robenacoxib**): Administration of other ulcerogenic drugs with glucocorticoids may increase risk for GI ulceration.
- **Phenobarbital, Primidone**: May increase the metabolism of glucocorticoids
- **Rifampin**: May increase the metabolism of glucocorticoids
- **Vaccines**: Animals receiving corticosteroids at immunosuppressive dosages should generally not receive live attenuated-virus vaccines, as virus replication may be augmented; a diminished immune response may occur after vaccine, toxoid, or bacterin administration in animals receiving glucocorticoids.
- **Warfarin**: Glucocorticoids may affect clotting times; monitoring is advised.

Laboratory Considerations

- Glucocorticoids may increase serum cholesterol and urine glucose levels.
- Glucocorticoids may decrease serum potassium.
- In cats, increases in ALP are not attributable to glucocorticoid administration due to lack of a steroid-induced ALP isoenzyme.
- Glucocorticoids can suppress the release of TSH and reduce T_3 and T_4 values. Thyroid gland atrophy has been reported after chronic glucocorticoid administration. Uptake of I^{131} by the thyroid may be decreased by glucocorticoids.
- Reactions to allergen intradermal skin tests may be suppressed by glucocorticoids.[16,17] A 2-week (14-day) withdrawal time before intradermal skin testing is recommended for dogs and cats[18,19]; no withdrawal time is required before serum IgE testing to identify sensitizing allergens in cats.[19]
- False-negative results of the nitroblue tetrazolium test for systemic bacterial infections may be induced by glucocorticoids.
- High-dose prednisone increases serum cystatin C in dogs.[20]
- Bovine urinary prednisoLONE:cortisol ratio of greater than or equal to 0.26 may discriminate between endogenous and exogenous prednisoLONE.[21]

Dosages

NOTE: Currently, there are no injectable prednisone/prednisoLONE products available for use in animals in the United States.

Unless cited by a veterinary-approved product, all dosages should be considered extra-label.

DOGS/CATS:

NOTES:

1. PrednisoLONE should be used in place of prednisone in cats whenever possible, as cats do not absorb or convert prednisone to prednisoLONE as well as dogs.[3]
2. If given daily, therapy for longer than 1 to 2 weeks will suppress the hypothalamic-pituitary-adrenal (HPA) axis and recovery will take longer than 1 week. Therefore, if corticosteroids are used for longer than a few days, dosage must be tapered off using alternate-day therapy. Many glucocorticoid responsive diseases can be managed with chronic alternate-day therapy. If possible, it is suggested to avoid giving doses greater than 1 mg/kg (prednisoLONE equivalent) every other day; larger doses saturate a dog's ability to fully metabolize the last dose before the next dose is given and can negate the benefits of alternate-day therapy. However, to induce remission of clinical signs or manage their recurrence initially requires daily therapy at an appropriate dose to control clinical signs, then tapering the drug to reach a minimum daily dose that will control clinical signs, followed by alternate-day therapy to manage the disease. Animals vary greatly in their response to the therapeutic and adverse effects of glucocorticoids, and there may be qualitative differences between the effects of different glucocorticoids in the same animal.[22]

Anti-inflammatory agent:

Dogs: 0.5 – 1 mg/kg PO once daily; not to exceed 40 mg/dog (NOT mg/kg) in large breed dogs.[23] Dose can be given once daily, or the total dose can be divided and given twice daily.[4,24]

Cats: prednisoLONE 1 – 2 mg/kg PO once daily[4,24]

Immunosuppressive agent:

Dogs: Initial dose of 2 – 4 mg/kg PO once daily.[4,24] 50 – 60 mg/m^2 once daily for dogs over 25 kg (55 lb) can be considered an initial dosage to provide immunosuppression and minimize adverse effects in larger dogs.[25] Many suggest beginning with 2 mg/kg PO once daily and dividing the total dose and giving it twice daily. Administration of a dose at the upper end of the range may not provide additional immune suppression but may cause more pronounced adverse effects. Many internists believe that the prednisone total daily dose should not exceed 60 – 80 mg, regardless of a dog's weight.[23] A sample prednisone immunosuppressive protocol for dogs is (dosages should be tailored to the ongoing requirements of the individual animal): 2.2 mg/kg daily (daily dose not to exceed 60 – 80 total) for 3 weeks, then 1 mg/kg daily for 3 weeks, then 0.5 mg/kg daily for 3 weeks, then 0.5 mg/kg every other day, provided disease remission is maintained.

Cats: Initial dose of prednisolone 2 – 8 mg/kg PO once daily.[4,24,26] Many start with 4 mg/kg PO daily then dividing the total dose and giving it twice daily.[4]

Antineoplastic/cytotoxic agent: When prednis(ol)one is used as an antineoplastic agent, alone or in a multidrug chemotherapy protocol, the following dosages should be used only as a general guide. Consultations with a veterinary oncologist and referral to current veterinary oncology references are strongly recommended.

Dogs: 2 mg/kg PO daily. Omission of prednisone from the L-CHOP protocol did not improve progression-free survival in dogs with peripheral nodal lymphoma.[27]

Cats: PrednisoLONE should be used. Cats are relatively steroid resistant and require higher doses than dogs. Doses can typically be safely doubled as compared with dogs. See above note for additional information.[22] **NOTE**: When used with other cytotoxic agents in chemotherapy protocols, prednisoLONE doses may be reduced.

Adjunctive treatment for hypoadrenocorticism:

Acute treatment using prednisoLONE sodium succinate: 1 – 2 mg/kg IV after second blood draw for cortisol measurement (ACTH stimulation test).[28] Injectable glucocorticoid therapy (eg, prednisoLONE sodium succinate 0.5 mg/kg IV every 6 hours) should be continued until the animal can be safely switched to oral glucocorticoid therapy.[29] Alternatively, injectable dexamethasone sodium phosphate can be used in the acute management of hypoadrenocorticism.

Oral glucocorticoid replacement (ongoing, with a mineralocorticoid): Oral glucocorticoid therapy can begin after a confirmed diagnosis of hypoadrenocorticism has been made and parenteral therapy has achieved a positive clinical response. Prednisone can be given initially at 0.1 – 0.22 mg/kg PO once daily, then tapered to the lowest dose to control clinical signs.[28] An increase in dose is often needed in times of stress (eg, surgery, illness). It is common for dogs to require no more than 0.1 mg/kg once per day of prednis(ol)one and less may be sufficient to prevent recurrence of signs of glucocorticoid insufficiency. When using fludrocortisone for mineralocorticoid replacement therapy, up to 50% of dogs will not require any additional prednisone, as there is enough glucocorticoid activity in fludrocortisone for those dogs. One study reported 11 out of 13 dogs receiving fludrocortisone 0.022 mg/kg PO daily required a mean prednisoLONE dosage of 0.06 mg/kg daily and suggested that most dogs receiving fludrocortisone may benefit from the addition of a small prednisoLONE dose.[30] All dogs receiving desoxycorticosterone pivalate (DOCP) will also require prednis(ol)one, as it only has mineralocorticoid activity.[4] In one study, dogs receiving DOCP initially received prednisoLONE 0.22 mg/kg PO daily, but it was possible to reduce the dosage to 0.13 mg/kg PO daily.[31]

HORSES:

NOTE: Prednisone does not appear to be absorbed well after oral administration; prednisoLONE or another oral steroid should be used.

Glucocorticoid effects (label dosage; FDA-approved): prednisoLONE sodium succinate 50 – 100 mg/horse (NOT mg/kg) as an initial dose, IV or IM over a period of 30 seconds to 1 minute. Dose may be repeated in inflammatory, allergic, or other stress conditions at intervals of 12, 24, or 48 hours based on the size of the animal, the severity of the condition, and the response to treatment.[7]

Adjunctive therapy of severe equine asthma (SEA):

a) **Short-term treatment with environmental control**: In the study, dexamethasone sodium phosphate was given 0.1 mg/kg IM once daily for 4 days, 0.075 mg/kg IM once daily for 4 days, and 0.05 mg/kg IM for 4 days or oral prednisoLONE was given 1 mg/kg PO for 4 days, 0.75 mg/kg for 4 days, and 0.5 mg/kg PO for 4 days. Except for bronchoalveolar lavage cytology, PO prednisoLONE was as effective as IM dexamethasone.[32]
b) In horses under continuous antigen exposure, dexamethasone was given 0.05 mg/kg PO once daily for 7 days or prednisoLONE was given 2 mg/kg PO once daily for 7 days. Although both were effective, dexamethasone was more so.[33]

Pruritus: Topical therapy is preferred, but for more severe cases, oral prednisoLONE can be considered. Induction dose of 2 mg/kg PO once daily for 3 to 10 days. Dose can be tapered to 0.5 mg/kg PO every 48 hours once pruritus is controlled.[34]

Adjunctive therapy of neoplasia responsive to glucocorticoid therapy: Typical dose is prednisoLONE 1 mg/kg PO every other day.[35]

CATTLE:

Glucocorticoid activity: PrednisoLONE sodium succinate 0.2 – 1 mg/kg IV or IM[36]

NEW WORLD CAMELIDS:

Steroid-responsive pruritic dermatoses secondary to allergic origins: 0.5 – 1 mg/kg PO initially; can be gradually reduced to lowest effective dose given every 48 hours.[37]

BIRDS:

Anti-inflammatory: 0.2 mg/30 g (1 oz) body weight, or one 5-mg tablet can be dissolved in 2.5 mL of water and 2 drops administered orally, twice daily. Administration schedule should be tapered if using long-term.[38]

Shock: PrednisoLONE sodium succinate (10 mg/mL) 0.1 – 0.2 mL/100 g (3.5 oz) body weight repeated every 15 minutes to effect. Dose may be decreased by half in large birds.[38]

RABBITS/RODENTS/SMALL MAMMALS:

Rabbits: Rarely indicated. As an anti-inflammatory agent: 0.5 – 2 mg/kg PO

Mice, rats, gerbils, hamsters, guinea pigs, chinchillas: 0.5 – 2.2 mg/kg IM or SC

REPTILES:

Shock in most species: PrednisoLONE sodium succinate 5 – 10 mg/kg IV[39,40]

Monitoring

Monitoring of glucocorticoid therapy is dependent on reason for use, dosage, agent used (amount of mineralocorticoid activity), dose schedule (daily vs alternate-day therapy), duration of therapy, and the animal's age and condition. The following list may not be appropriate or complete for all animals; clinical assessment and judgment should be used if adverse effects are noted.

- Response to therapy
- Weight, appetite, and/or signs of fluid retention
- Serum and/or urine electrolytes
- Total plasma proteins and albumin
- Blood glucose
- Urine culture
- Growth and development in young animals

Client Information

- Follow your veterinarian's instructions on how to give this medicine. Give this medicine with food.
- The goal of treatment is to find the lowest dose possible and use it for the shortest period of time. Do not change the amount of medicine you give your animal without talking to your veterinarian first.
- Many side effects are possible, especially when used long-term or when given in higher doses. The most common side effects are increased appetite, thirst, and need to urinate.
- In dogs, stomach or intestinal ulcers, perforation, or bleeding can occur while taking this medicine. Contact your veterinarian right away if your animal stops eating or if you notice a high fever, black tarry stools, or bloody vomit (looks like coffee grounds).
- Do not suddenly stop giving this medicine to your animal without talking to your veterinarian first, as serious side effects could occur.
- Be sure to tell your veterinarian what other medications (including vitamins, supplements, or herbal therapies) you give your animal.

Chemistry/Synonyms

PrednisoLONE and prednisone are synthetic glucocorticoids. PrednisoLONE and prednisoLONE acetate occur as odorless, white to practically white crystalline powders. PrednisoLONE is very slightly soluble in water and slightly soluble in alcohol. The acetate ester is practically insoluble in water and slightly soluble in alcohol. The sodium succinate ester is highly water-soluble. The sodium phosphate ester occurs as a slightly yellow or white powder or as granules, is odorless or may have a slight odor, and is freely soluble in water and soluble in methanol.

Prednisone occurs as an odorless, white to practically white crystalline powder. Prednisone is very slightly soluble in water and slightly soluble in alcohol.

PrednisoLONE is also known as deltahydrocortisone or metacortandralone.

Prednisone may also be known as delta(1)-cortisone, 1,2-dehydrocortisone, deltacortisone, deltadehydrocortisone, metacortandracin, NSC-10023, prednisonum; many trade names are available.

Storage/Stability

Store prednisoLONE and prednisone tablets in tightly closed containers below 40°C (104°F), ideally between 15°C to 30°C (59°F-86°F). PrednisoLONE oral solution storage requirements vary by product and manufacturer; refer to product label for specific information. Avoid freezing all liquid prednisoLONE products. Do not autoclave. Store oral liquid preparations of prednisone in tightly closed containers.

PrednisoLONE sodium succinate should be stored at room temperature and protected from light (stored in a carton). After reconstitution, the product is recommended for immediate use and should not be stored for later use. If the solution becomes cloudy after reconstituting, it should not be used IV.

Compatibility/Compounding Considerations

Compatibility is dependent on factors such as pH, concentration, temperature, and diluent used; specialized references or a hospital pharmacist should be consulted for more specific information.

Few data appear to be available regarding the compatibility of prednisoLONE sodium succinate injection (*Solu-Delta Cortef*®) with other products. A related compound, prednisoLONE sodium phosphate is reportedly physically **compatible** with the following drugs/solutions: ascorbic acid injection, cytarabine, erythromycin lactobionate, fluorouracil, heparin sodium, penicillin G potassium/sodium, tetracycline HCl, and vitamin B-complex with C. It is reportedly physically **incompatible** with calcium gluconate/gluceptate, dimenhydrinate, metaraminol bitartrate, methotrexate sodium, prochlorperazine edisylate, polymyxin B sulfate, promazine HCl, and promethazine.

Dosage Forms/Regulatory Status

VETERINARY-LABELED PRODUCTS:

A zero-tolerance residue in milk for these compounds has been established for dairy cattle. All of these agents require a prescription (Rx). Known FDA-approved veterinary products for systemic use are indicated below; not all products may be marketed.

The Association of Racing Commissioners International (ARCI) has designated this drug as a class 4 substance. Use of this drug may not be allowed in certain animal competitions. Check rules and regulations before entering in a competition while this medication is being administered. Contact local racing authorities for further guidance. See ***Appendix*** for more information.

PrednisoLONE Tablets: 5 mg and 20 mg: *Prednis-Tab*® (various), generic; (Rx). FDA-approved for use in dogs

PrednisoLONE Acetate Injection: 25 mg/mL; *Meticortelone Acetate*®; (Rx). FDA-approved for use in dogs, cats, and horses

PrednisoLONE Sodium Succinate for Injection *act-o-vial*® System 100 mg (equivalent to 10 mg prednisoLONE) and 500 mg (equivalent to 50 mg prednisoLONE) per 10-mL vial; *Solu-Delta-Cortef*®; (Rx). FDA-approved for use in dogs, cats, and horses. May be unavailable in some countries.

PrednisoLONE Sodium Succinate Powder for Injection: 10 mg/mL, 20 mg/mL, and 50 mg/mL of prednisoLONE; *Solu-Delta Cortef*® Sterile Powder; (Rx). FDA-approved for use in dogs, cats, and horses. May be unavailable in some countries.

PrednisoLONE Tertiary Butylacetate Injection: 20 mg/mL; *Hydeltrone-TBA*® *Suspension*; (Rx). FDA-approved for use in cats, dogs, and horses

Prednisone Injection: 10 mg/mL and 40 mg/mL; *Meticorten*®; (Rx). FDA-approved for use in dogs, cats, and horses

PrednisoLONE and Trimeprazine Tartrate Tablets: Each tablet contains trimeprazine 5 mg and prednisoLONE 2 mg; *Temaril-P*®; (Rx). FDA-approved for use in dogs

HUMAN-LABELED PRODUCTS:

PrednisoLONE Oral Tablets: 5 mg; *Millipred*®, generic; (Rx).

PrednisoLONE Sodium Phosphate Orally Disintegrating Tablets: 10 mg, 15 mg, and 30 mg (as base); *Orapred ODT*®; (Rx)

PrednisoLONE Syrup/Oral Liquid or Solution: 5 mg/5 mL (1 mg/mL), 10 mg/5 mL (2 mg/mL), 15 mg/5 mL (3 mg/mL), 20 mg/5 mL (4 mg/mL), and 25 mg/5 mL (5 mg/mL); *Pediapred*®, *Millipred*®, *Orapred*®, *Flo-Pred*®, *Veripred*® 20, generic; (Rx)

Prednisone Tablets: 1 mg, 2.5 mg, 5 mg, 10 mg, 20 mg, and 50 mg; *Deltasone*®, generic; (Rx)

Prednisone Oral Tablet (Delayed Release): 1 mg, 2 mg, and 5 mg; *Rayos*®; (Rx)

Prednisone Oral Solution/Syrup: 5 mg/5 mL (1 mg/mL); *Prednisone* and *Prednisone Intensol*® *Concentrate*; (Rx)

Ophthalmic solutions/suspensions are available.

References

For the complete list of references, see **wiley.com/go/budde/plumb**

Pregabalin

(pre-***gab***-ah-lin) *Lyrica®*

Anticonvulsant; Neuropathic Pain Agent

Prescriber Highlights

- ▶ Similar to gabapentin; may be useful as an anticonvulsant or to treat tremors and neuropathic pain
- ▶ Little information is available on safety and efficacy in dogs or cats.
- ▶ The most common adverse effects are sedation and ataxia.
- ▶ May be cost prohibitive
- ▶ DEA Schedule V (C-V) controlled substance

Uses/Indications

Like gabapentin, pregabalin may be useful as adjunctive therapy for refractory or complex partial seizures,[1] and treating chronic pain, particularly neuropathic pain in small animal species. In an open-label, noncomparative study in epileptic dogs that were not controlled with phenobarbital and/or bromides, pregabalin reduced seizures by ~60% in 7 out of 9 dogs.[1] When pregabalin is administered pre- and postoperatively in combination with opioids after surgical treatment of intervertebral disc herniation in dogs, it reduces pain more than opioids alone.[2] Pregabalin has been successfully used to reduce clinical signs related to central neuropathic pain associated with syringomyelia in dogs.[3,4] Other potential uses include treatment of orthostatic tremors in dogs[5] and as a pre-transportation anxiolytic for cats.[6]

In humans, pregabalin is used to treat pain associated with diabetic peripheral neuropathy, partial-onset seizures, postherpetic neuralgia, and fibromyalgia. Extra-label uses include treatment of generalized anxiety, possible reduction of opioid demand for postsurgical analgesia, and to decrease postoperative nausea and vomiting.

Pharmacology/Actions

Pregabalin has antiepileptic, analgesic, and anxiolytic activity. Like gabapentin, pregabalin is a structural analogue of the inhibitory neurotransmitter gamma-aminobutyric acid (GABA). The mechanism of action of pregabalin, for either its anticonvulsant or analgesic actions, is not fully understood, but it appears to bind to CaVa2-d (alpha2-delta subunit of the voltage-gated calcium channels). By decreasing calcium influx, release of excitatory neurotransmitters (eg, substance P, glutamate, norepinephrine) is inhibited. It is ≈5 times as potent as gabapentin.[7,8]

Pharmacokinetics

After a single oral pregabalin dose of 4 mg/kg in 6 dogs, median parameters included the following: T_{max} = 1.5 hours; C_{max} = 7.15 µg /mL; elimination half-life = 6.9 hours.[9]

In 6 cats receiving a single oral dose (4 mg/kg using pregabalin capsules), pregabalin median parameters included the following: T_{max} = 2.9 hours; C_{max} = 8.3 µg /mL; elimination half-life = 10.4 hours.[10]

After a single dose of 4 mg/kg administered via nasogastric tube in 5 horses, pregabalin median parameters included the following: T_{max} = 1 hour; C_{max} = 5 µg/mL; and elimination half-life = 8 hours.[11] After IV administration of 4 mg/kg the initial concentration was 22.2 µg/mL and elimination half-life was 7.74 hours. Bioavailability was 97.7%. Signs of mild, transient colic and behavioral abnormalities were observed after IV administration.

In humans, oral bioavailability is ≈90%.[12] Presence of food can delay the rate, but not the amount absorbed, and it can be administered regardless of feeding status. Pregabalin is not bound to plasma proteins, and it has an apparent volume of distribution of ≈500 mL/kg. Hepatic metabolism is negligible, and it does not appear to affect hepatic enzymes. The drug is almost exclusively cleared unchanged by renal routes with a renal clearance of 67 to 81 mL/minute in young, healthy subjects. Elimination half-life is ≈6 hours. Dosage adjustment may be required in patients with diminished renal function.

Contraindications/Precautions/Warnings

Pregabalin is contraindicated in patients that are hypersensitive to it. Use with caution in patients with renal insufficiency; if required, dosage adjustment should be considered. In humans, pregabalin doses are adjusted based on creatinine clearance. Pregabalin is used with caution in human patients with heart failure or underlying respiratory impairment.

In humans, abrupt discontinuation may lead to increased seizure frequency, diarrhea, headache, insomnia, or nausea.[12]

Adverse Effects

The most common adverse effects reported include sedation and ataxia. Because use to date is limited in animals, the adverse effect profile may evolve with additional clinical experience. Superficial dermatitis lesions on the face were reported in 1 cat that was receiving pregabalin.[13] Transient sedation, ataxia, tremor, and salivation were observed in cats receiving a single oral dose.[6,10]

In humans, the most commonly reported adverse effects include somnolence, dizziness, ataxia, difficulty with concentration/attention/memory, blurred vision, dry mouth, peripheral edema, constipation, and weight gain.[12] Syncope and congestive heart failure have been reported less frequently. Rarely, renal failure (reversible) and rhabdomyolysis have been reported.

Hypersensitivity reactions have included angioedema, rash, blisters, and wheezing. Pregabalin therapy has been associated with decreased platelet production or increased creatine kinase levels in some human patients.[12]

Reproductive/Nursing Safety

Very high doses of pregabalin have caused skeletal malformations in offspring when administered to pregnant rats and rabbits.[12] Pregabalin is excreted into milk, and safety during nursing has not been established.

Because safety has not been established in animals, this drug should only be used when the maternal benefits outweigh the potential risks to offspring.

Overdose/Acute Toxicity

Clinical signs most commonly seen in dogs and cats with a pregabalin overdose include ataxia and lethargy. There is no specific antidote for overdose with pregabalin. Standard GI decontamination protocols with supportive care based on clinical presentation can be employed if indicated.

For patients that have experienced or are suspected to have experienced an overdose, consultation with a 24-hour poison control center specializing in providing veterinary-specific information is recommended. For general information related to overdose and toxin exposures, as well as contact information for poison control centers, refer to ***Appendix***.

Drug Interactions

The following drug interactions either have been reported or are theoretical in humans or animals receiving pregabalin and may be of significance in veterinary patients. Unless otherwise noted, use together is not necessarily contraindicated, but weigh the potential risks and perform additional monitoring when appropriate.

- ANGIOTENSIN-CONVERTING ENZYME INHIBITORS (eg, **benazepril, enalapril**): In humans, co-administration with pregabalin may increase risks for edema and hives.
- BENZODIAZEPINES (eg, **alprazolam, diazepam, midazolam**):

Pregabalin may cause additive CNS and respiratory depression.

- **Central Nervous System (CNS) Depressants** (eg, **acepromazine, dexmedetomidine, phenobarbital**): Pregabalin may cause additive CNS and respiratory depression.
- **Nonsteroidal Anti-Inflammatory Drugs (NSAIDs)**: In humans, ketorolac and naproxen have been cited as possibly reducing anticonvulsant effectiveness. Substantive evidence is weak, however.
- **Opioids** (eg, **morphine**): Pregabalin may cause additive CNS and respiratory depression.

Laboratory Considerations

- None noted

Dosages

DOGS:

Seizure disorders (extra-label): 3 – 4 mg/kg PO every 8 hours.[1] Generally used when seizure control cannot be obtained with a combination of phenobarbital and bromides. In a small single-dose pharmacokinetic study, the authors concluded that 4 mg/kg PO twice daily would produce plasma concentrations within the therapeutic range extrapolated from humans[9]; further studies evaluating its safety and efficacy for the treatment of seizures in dogs are warranted. To reduce sedation, consider starting at 2 mg/kg PO every 12 hours and titrating dosage upwards in 1 mg/kg increments per week to 3 – 4 mg/kg PO every 8 to 12 hours.

Neuropathic pain (extra-label): 2 – 5 mg/kg PO every 8 to 12 hours.[4,14] In another study in King Charles Cavalier spaniels, 150 mg/dog (NOT mg/kg) PO once daily for 2 days, then 150 mg/dog (NOT mg/kg) PO twice daily was used.[3] This latter dosage equated to ≈13 – 19 mg/kg PO twice daily.

Control of perioperative pain (extra-label): 4 mg/kg PO 1 hour before anesthesia, followed by postoperative treatment of 4 mg/kg PO 3 times daily for 5 days[2]

Orthostatic tremor (extra-label): 3.5 mg/kg PO every 8 to 12 hours[5]

CATS:

Seizure disorders (extra-label): Anecdotally, 1 – 2 mg/kg PO every 12 hours is most commonly mentioned.[15] Based on their single-dose pharmacokinetic study in 6 cats, the authors theorize that a dose of 1 – 2 mg/kg PO twice daily would be a reasonable starting dosage. Further clinical trials are warranted based on a favorable pharmacokinetic profile.[16]

Neuropathic pain (extra-label):

a) 1 mg/kg PO every 8 to 12 hours[15,17]

b) 3 mg/kg PO every 12 hours from a case report[18]

Anxiolytic for carrier transportation (extra-label): 5 – 10 mg/kg PO 90 minutes prior to transportation.[6] The study used pregabalin oral solution; anxiolysis in association with veterinary visits was not assessed.

HORSES:

Neuropathic pain, seizures (extra-label): 4 mg/kg PO every 8 hours; based on single-dose pharmacokinetic study.[11] Efficacy and safety of this dosage requires validation.

Monitoring

- Efficacy/adverse effects
- At present, pregabalin plasma concentrations are not routinely monitored in human medicine. In humans, plasma pregabalin concentrations greater than 2.8 mg/mL have been suggested as being therapeutic.

Client Information

- This medicine may be given with or without food. If your animal vomits or acts sick after getting it on an empty stomach, try giving the medicine with food or a small treat to see if this helps. If vomiting continues, contact your veterinarian.
- Sleepiness and loss of coordination (eg, stumbling) and weakness are the most likely side effects. Pregabalin is a controlled drug in the US. It is against federal law to use, give away, or sell this medication to others than for whom it was prescribed.
- When it is used for seizure control, do not suddenly stop giving this medicine.

Chemistry/Synonyms

Pregabalin is (S)-3-(aminomethyl)-5-methylhexanoic acid. It is freely soluble in water and in both basic and acidic aqueous solutions.

Pregabalin may also be known as CI-1008, PD-144723, pregabalina, prégabaline, or pregabalinum. A common trade name is *Lyrica*®.

Storage/Stability

Store capsules and oral solution at room temperature (25°C [77°F]); excursions permitted between 15°C to 30°C (59°F-86°F).

Dosage Forms/Regulatory Status

VETERINARY-LABELED PRODUCTS: NONE

HUMAN-LABELED PRODUCTS:

Pregabalin Oral Capsules: 25 mg, 50 mg, 75 mg, 100 mg, 150 mg, 200 mg, 225 mg, and 300 mg; *Lyrica*®, generic; (Rx; C-V controlled substance)

Pregabalin Oral Solution: 20 mg/mL; *Lyrica*®, generic; (Rx; C-V controlled substance)

References

For the complete list of references, see **wiley.com/go/budde/plumb**

Primaquine

(***prim***-ah-kwin)

Antiprotozoal Agent

Prescriber Highlights

- ► Considered the drug of choice for treating *Babesia felis* in cats. May not eliminate infection, and repeated courses of therapy may be necessary.
- ► Most common adverse effect in cats is vomiting; give with food.
- ► Very narrow therapeutic index; use extreme caution when determining a dose, particularly considering the large difference between primaquine base and salt (phosphate) doses. In cats, doses of primaquine phosphate greater than 1 mg/kg can be lethal.
- ► Compounded formulations may be necessary for accurate dosing.
- ► Monitor CBC weekly during treatment

Uses/Indications

Primaquine is considered the drug of choice for treating *Babesia felis* in cats. Primaquine typically resolves anemia and clinical signs of disease; however, it often does not eliminate the infection and repeated courses of therapy may be necessary.[1,2] Relapse rates of 20% to 80% have been reported but these are lower than other therapy protocols.[1] Primaquine may be useful in treating *Hepatazoon* spp infection in dogs and cats, or *Plasmodium* spp in birds.

In humans, primaquine is used in the treatment and prophylaxis for malaria and treating *Pneumocystis* spp pneumonia.[3]

Pharmacology/Actions

The antiprotozoal mechanism of primaquine is not well understood; it may be related to the drug binding and altering protozoal DNA. When used for *Babesia felis* in cats, decreased parasitemia and improvement in clinical signs is usually seen within 1-3 days.

Pharmacokinetics

No pharmacokinetic information was located for small animal species.

In humans, primaquine is rapidly absorbed with ≈96% systemic bioavailability.[4] It is extensively distributed and rapidly metabolized in the liver to carboxyprimaquine. Antiprotozoal activity of the metabolite is unknown. Elimination half-life is ≈6 hours for primaquine and ≈24 hours for carboxyprimaquine.

Contraindications/Precautions/Warnings

Primaquine is contraindicated in patients with known hypersensitivity to it. In humans, it is contraindicated in patients receiving other myelosuppressive medications or patients susceptible to granulocytopenia (eg, lupus, rheumatoid arthritis). Primaquine is also contraindicated in humans with glucose-6-phosphate dehydrogenase (G6PD) deficiency, as there is increased risk for hemolytic anemia when exposed to drugs that cause oxidative stress, such as primaquine.[5]

Safety margin is particularly narrow with this drug in cats (see ***Overdose/Acute Toxicity***).

Adverse Effects

The most common adverse effect associated with primaquine in cats is vomiting[1,2]; administration with food may decrease GI upset. Other potential adverse effects include myelosuppression, methemoglobinemia, and hemolysis.

Reproductive/Nursing Safety

In humans, primaquine is considered contraindicated during pregnancy as it can cause hemolytic anemia in G6PD deficient fetuses. Chloroquine should be used instead. Primaquine may be used during lactation if infants have normal G6PD activity.[3] Although significance for veterinary patients is unclear, primaquine should be avoided during pregnancy and lactation.

Overdose/Acute Toxicity

In cats, the lethal dose of primaquine phosphate has been reported as greater than 1 mg/kg.[2] Overdoses should initially be handled aggressively using standardized GI decontamination protocols.

For patients that have experienced or are suspected to have experienced an overdose, consultation with a 24-hour poison consultation center specializing in providing veterinary-specific information is recommended. For general information related to overdose and toxin exposures, as well as contact information for poison control centers, refer to ***Appendix***.

Drug Interactions

The following drug interactions have either been reported or are theoretical in humans or animals receiving primaquine and may be of significance in veterinary patients. Unless otherwise noted, use together is not necessarily contraindicated, but weigh the potential risks and perform additional monitoring when appropriate.

- GRAPEFRUIT JUICE: May increase primaquine concentrations
- HEMOLYSIS-INDUCING DRUGS (eg, **acetohydroxamic acid, quinidine, sulfonamides, sulfonylureas**): Use with primaquine may cause increased risk for toxicity.
- MYELOSUPPRESSIVE DRUGS (eg, **amphotericin B, antineoplastic drugs, azathioprine, chloramphenicol**): Use with primaquine may cause increased risk for myelotoxicity.
- QUINACRINE: May potentiate the toxicity of one another; use of primaquine within 3 months of quinacrine is not recommended.
- QT PROLONGING AGENTS (eg, **cisapride, domperidone, erythromycin, sotalol**): Concurrent use may increase the risk for QT prolongation and should be avoided.[5]
- RABIES VACCINE: In humans, primaquine can decrease the immune response to rabies vaccine.[6] Significance to veterinary patients is unknown.

Laboratory Considerations

- No specific concerns noted

Dosages

CATS:

NOTES:

1. Primaquine has an extremely narrow therapeutic index in cats.
2. Primaquine dosing for humans is typically described in terms of primaquine ***base***; however, dosages for cats may not distinguish between primaquine base or phosphate. ***Primaquine phosphate 26.3 mg tablets contain 15 mg of primaquine base.*** Due to the large difference between doses of phosphate and base and the narrow therapeutic index, it is important to have a clear understanding of the desired amount of primaquine to be given per dose.
3. The strength of the commercially available tablet is typically too high to be accurately dosed in cats; compounded formulations may be required. See ***Compounding: How to Find a Quality-Assured Pharmacy***.

Babesia felis (extra-label):

a) Primaquine ***base*** 0.5 – 1 mg/kg (as base) PO once or administered daily on 3 consecutive days. Duration of therapy should be based on hematologic variables and clinical signs rather than parasitemia. Do not exceed dosages of 1 mg/kg/day as fatalities have occurred.[2]

b) Primaquine ***phosphate*** 1 mg/cat (NOT mg/kg) PO every 36 hours for 4 doses followed by 1 mg/cat (NOT mg/kg) every 7 days for 4 additional doses[7,8]

Monitoring

- Baseline and weekly CBC during treatment
- Improvement of clinical signs (increased appetite and body weight, improvement in anemia)

Client Information

- This medicine can be very toxic to cats if they are given too much. Be sure to follow your veterinarian's instructions closely.
- In case of a missed dose, do not double-up the next dose.
- Give with food to decrease vomiting and upset stomach.
- Your veterinarian will need to monitor your cat closely while it is taking this medicine. Do not miss these important follow-up visits.

Chemistry/Synonyms

Primaquine phosphate is an 8-amino-quinoline compound that occurs as an orange-red, odorless, bitter-tasting, crystalline powder. It is soluble (1 gram in 15 mL) in water and practically insoluble in alcohol. 1 mg of primaquine phosphate contains 0.57 mg of primaquine base.

Primaquine may also be known as primachina, primachinum, primaquina or SN 13272.

Storage/Stability

Primaquine phosphate tablets should be stored in a tight, light resistant container below 40°C (104°F), preferably between 15 and 30°C (59 to 86°F).

Dosage Forms/Regulatory Status

VETERINARY-LABELED PRODUCTS: NONE

HUMAN-LABELED PRODUCTS:

Primaquine Phosphate Oral Tablets: 26.3 mg (equivalent to 15 mg primaquine base); generic; (Rx)

References

For the complete list of references, see **wiley.com/go/budde/plumb**

Probenecid

(proh-***ben***-eh-sid)

Uricosuric; Renal Tubular Secretion Inhibitor

Prescriber Highlights

- ► Uricosuric and renal tubular secretion inhibitor that may be useful for treating gout (particularly in reptiles)
- ► Probenecid is associated with many drug interactions as it inhibits the renal tubular secretion of numerous drugs, including several beta-lactam antibiotics; some interactions may be beneficial, whereas others may increase potential for toxicity.
- ► Little experience using this drug in mammals other than humans

Uses/Indications

Although there has been limited clinical use or research on probenecid in veterinary medicine, it may be useful in treating gout (hyperuricemia), particularly in reptiles.

Probenecid's effect in inhibiting renal tubular secretion of certain beta-lactam antibiotics and other weak organic acids is of interest for increasing serum concentrations or reducing doses and dosing frequency of these drugs. This effect may allow greater efficacy and reduce the cost or dosing frequency of expensive human drugs. Probenecid has a significantly long elimination half-life in dogs (≈18 hours), which may make it particularly useful in this species; however, at present there is little research supporting this in veterinary patients.

Pharmacology/Actions

Probenecid reduces serum uric acid concentrations by enhancing uric acid excretion into the urine by competitively inhibiting urate reabsorption at the proximal renal tubules.

Probenecid competitively inhibits tubular secretion of weak organic acids (eg, penicillins, some cephalosporins, sulbactam, tazobactam, oseltamivir).

Pharmacokinetics

There is limited information available for veterinary species. In dogs, after IV administration of probenecid, the distribution half-life was 2.3 hours and apparent volume of distribution at steady state was 0.46 L/kg.[1] Probenecid exhibits biphasic concentration-dependent plasma protein binding characteristics; probenecid plasma protein binding appeared to be less than that occurring in humans. Plasma clearance was 0.343 mL/minute/kg and elimination half-life was 17.7 hours, which is considerably longer than in humans (6.5 hours) or sheep (1.55 hours).[1]

After administration to mares (10 mg/kg), probenecid had an oral bioavailability of ≈90%.[2] The drug was highly bound (99.9%) to equine plasma proteins. Elimination half-life was ≈90 to 120 minutes.

In humans, absorption after oral administration is rapid and complete. The drug is converted in the liver to glucuronidated, carboxylated, and hydroxylated compounds that have uricosuric and renal tubular secretion inhibition activity. Elimination half-life is dose dependent and large doses (greater than 500 mg) have longer half-lives.

Contraindications/Precautions/Warnings

Probenecid is contraindicated in patients with a history of hypersensitivity to it, and should not be used in patients with, or that are susceptible to, uric acid renal or bladder calculus formation or urate nephropathy (eg, receiving chemotherapy with rapidly cytolytic agents). Probenecid requires sufficient renal function to be effective; efficacy decreases with increasing renal function impairment. The drug may not be effective in human patients with a creatinine clearance of less than 30 mL/minute.[3]

Probenecid is not usually recommended for treating gout in birds, as it can exacerbate the condition.

Adverse Effects

An accurate adverse effect profile for probenecid has not been determined for animal patients. In humans, probenecid occasionally causes headaches, GI effects (eg, inappetence, nausea, mild vomiting), or rashes. When probenecid is used for gout, it can initially cause an increased rate of gouty attacks unless prophylaxis with colchicine is used concurrently. Rarely, hypersensitivity, bone marrow suppression, hepatotoxicity, or nephrotic syndrome have been reported in humans.

Reproductive/Nursing Safety

Probenecid apparently crosses the placenta, but adverse effects to fetuses have not been reported.

It is unknown if probenecid enters milk.

Because safety has not been established in animals, this drug should only be used when the maternal benefits outweigh the potential risks to offspring.

Overdose/Acute Toxicity

Limited information is available. One massive (ie, greater than 45 g) overdose in a human patient caused CNS stimulation, seizures, protracted vomiting, and respiratory failure. The reported LD_{50} in a dog following IV administration was 230 mg/kg.[4]

Generally, probenecid overdoses should initially be handled using standardized protocols for removal of drug from the gut to prevent absorption. Treat supportively but use caution co-administrating drugs that may compete with probenecid for tubular secretion.

For patients that have experienced or are suspected to have experienced an overdose, consultation with a 24-hour poison consultation center specializing in providing veterinary-specific information is recommended. For general information related to overdose and toxin exposures, as well as contact information for poison control centers, refer to ***Appendix***.

Drug Interactions

The following drug interactions have either been reported or are theoretical in humans or animals receiving probenecid and may be of significance in veterinary patients. Unless otherwise noted, use together is not necessarily contraindicated, but weigh the potential risks and perform additional monitoring when appropriate.

- ANTINEOPLASTICS (rapidly cytolytic): Increased chance of uric acid nephropathy
- ASPIRIN (and other salicylates): Salicylates antagonize the uricosuric effects of probenecid.
- BENZODIAZEPINES (eg, **lorazepam, oxazepam**): Probenecid may prolong action or reduce time for onset of action.
- BETA-LACTAM ANTIBIOTICS (eg, **penicillins**, some **cephalosporins**): Probenecid may increase serum concentrations by reducing renal excretion.
- BETA-LACTAMASE INHIBITORS (eg, **sulbactam, tazobactam**, but not **clavulanic acid**): Probenecid may increase serum concentrations by reducing renal excretion.
- CIPROFLOXACIN/ENROFLOXACIN: Probenecid reduces renal tubular secretion of ciprofloxacin by ≈50%. In goats, probenecid significantly reduced renal excretion of enrofloxacin.[5,6]
- DAPSONE: Possible accumulation of dapsone or its active metabolites

- **Furosemide**: Increased serum furosemide concentrations are possible.
- **Heparin**: Probenecid may increase and prolong heparin's effects.
- **Methotrexate**: Probenecid may increase methotrexate concentrations and increase the risk for toxicity.
- **Nonsteroidal Anti-Inflammatory Drugs** (eg, **carprofen, ketoprofen**): Probenecid may increase plasma NSAID concentrations and increase the risk for toxicity.
- **Nitrofurantoin**: Reduced urine nitrofurantoin concentrations causing an increased risk for therapeutic failure and systemic toxicity
- **Penicillamine**: May reduce penicillamine efficacy
- **Oseltamivir**: May increase serum oseltamivir concentrations by reducing renal excretion
- **Ranitidine**: May increase serum ranitidine concentrations by reducing renal excretion
- **Rifampin**: May reduce hepatic uptake of rifampin and serum concentrations can be increased; use together is not recommended, as effect is inconsistent and can lead to toxicity.
- **Sulfonamides**: Probenecid decreases renal elimination of sulfonamides; however, as free serum concentrations of sulfonamides are not increased, this interaction is not therapeutically beneficial and may increase risks for sulfonamide toxicity.

Laboratory Considerations

- Urine glucose determinations: When using cupric sulfate solution (Benedict's Solution, *Clinitest*®): Probenecid may cause false-positive results. Tests utilizing glucose oxidase (*Tes-Tape*®, *Clinistix*®) are not affected.
- Theophylline concentrations: Serum theophylline concentrations may be falsely elevated (Schack and Waxtler technique).
- 17-ketosteroid concentrations in urine: May be decreased
- Phosphorus: Probenecid may increase phosphorus reabsorption in hypoparathyroid patients.
- Aminohippuric acid (PAH) or phenolsulphonphthalein (PSP) clearance studies: Probenecid decreases renal clearance.
- Renal function studies using iodohippurate sodium I 123 or I 131, or technetium TC 99: Decreased kidney uptake
- Homovanillic acid (HVA) or 5-hydroxyindoleacetic acid (5-HIAA): Probenecid inhibits transport from CSF into blood.

Dosages

HORSES:

Adjunct to increase antibiotic serum concentration and/or increase dosing interval (extra-label): Limited data are available. Probenecid administered 75 mg/kg PO one hour prior to an IV ampicillin bolus increased AUC and prolonged elimination half-life. The authors concluded that with this protocol, ampicillin administration may be extended to every 12 hours.[7]

REPTILES:

NOTE: Dosages are not well defined for reptiles.

Gout (extra-label):

a) 250 mg/reptile (NOT mg/kg) PO every 12 hours; can be increased as needed. Suggested dosage based upon human data, as dose is not established for reptiles[8]

b) 40 mg/kg PO every 12 hours[9,10]

Monitoring

- Serum and urine uric acid; if concomitant urine alkalinization is used, consider monitoring acid-base balance.

Client Information

- This medicine may be used to treat reptiles with a joint disease caused by excess uric acid (gout).
- This medicine has many drug interactions. Be sure to tell your veterinarian and pharmacist what medications (including vitamins, supplements, or herbal therapies) you give your animal, including the amount and time you give each. Some interactions may be helpful while others may increase risk for side effects.
- Side effects caused by probenecid in small animals (eg, dogs, cats) are not well known. Be sure to contact your veterinarian if you have concerns about your animal.

Chemistry/Synonyms

Probenecid is a sulfonamide derivative that occurs as a white to practically white, practically odorless, fine, crystalline powder. It is practically insoluble in water and soluble in alcohol.

Probenecid may also be known as probenecidas, probenecidum, *Benemid*®, and *Benuryl*®.

Storage/Stability

Probenecid tablets should be stored at room temperature (15°C-30°C [59°F-86°F]) in well-closed containers protected from light. Expiration dates are generally 3 to 5 years after manufacture.

Dosage Forms/Regulatory Status

VETERINARY-LABELED PRODUCTS: NONE

The Association of Racing Commissioners International (ARCI) has designated probenecid as a class 4 substance. Use of this drug may not be allowed in certain animal competitions. Check rules and regulations before entering in a competition while this medication is being administered. Contact local racing authorities for further guidance. See ***Appendix*** for more information. The International Federation for Equestrian Sports (FEI) lists this drug as a "prohibited substance – banned."

HUMAN-LABELED PRODUCTS:

Probenecid Tablets: 500 mg; generic; (Rx)

References

For the complete list of references, see **wiley.com/go/budde/plumb**

Procainamide

(proe-kane-***a***-mide) *Procanbid*®, *Pronestyl*®

Antiarrhythmic

Prescriber Highlights

- ► Used primarily for treatment of atrial fibrillation, premature ventricular complexes (PVC), and ventricular tachycardia
- ► Contraindications include myasthenia gravis; hypersensitivity to drug, procaine, or other chemically related drugs; torsade de pointes; second- or third-degree AV block (unless artificially paced)
- ► Use with extreme caution in patients with cardiac glycoside intoxication or systemic lupus.
- ► Use with caution in patients with significant hepatic and/or renal disease or congestive heart failure; consider dose reduction in these patients and in those that are critically ill.
- ► Adverse effects are related to serum drug concentrations and include GI effects, weakness, hypotension, negative inotropism, widened QRS complex and QT intervals, AV block, and multiform ventricular tachycardias. Fever and leukopenia are also possible.
- ► Profound hypotension can occur if injected too rapidly IV.
- ► Oral products are no longer commercially marketed and must be compounded.
- ► Many potential drug interactions

Uses/Indications

Procainamide may be used to treat premature ventricular complexes (PVC), ventricular tachycardia, or supraventricular tachycardias (SVTs). For a wide complex tachycardia that is present on ECG and that cannot be definitively identified as supraventricular or ventricular in origin, procainamide is an ideal first-line IV therapeutic agent because of its broad spectrum of activity for atrial and ventricular arrhythmias.[1]

In an open-label human study comparing IV procainamide and IV amiodarone for acute termination of stable wide QRS complex tachycardia (likely ventricular tachycardia), procainamide was more effective at terminating the tachycardic episode within 40 minutes. In the following 24 hours, procainamide was also associated with fewer major cardiac adverse events.[2]

Pharmacology/Actions

A class 1A antiarrhythmic agent, procainamide binds and inhibits fast sodium channels. It exhibits cardiac action similar to that of quinidine. It is considered both a supraventricular and ventricular antidysrhythmic. Procainamide prolongs the refractory times in both the atria and ventricles, decreases myocardial excitability, and depresses automaticity and conduction velocity. It has anticholinergic properties that may contribute to its effects. Procainamide's effects on heart rate are unpredictable, but it usually causes only slight increases or no change. It may exhibit negative inotropic actions on the heart, although cardiac outputs are generally not affected. One ex vivo study using rat hearts found that procainamide did not negatively affect contractility, cardiac output, or diastolic function.[3]

On ECG, QRS widening and prolonged PR and QT intervals can be seen. The QRS complex and T wave may occasionally show some slight decreases in voltage.

Pharmacokinetics

After IM or IV administration, the onset of action is practically immediate. After oral administration in humans, ≈75% to 95% of a dose is absorbed in the intestine, but some patients absorb less than 50% of a dose. Food, delayed gastric emptying, or decreased stomach pH may delay oral absorption. In dogs, it has been reported that the oral bioavailability is ≈85% and the absorption half-life is 0.5 hours[4]; however, there is an apparent large degree of variability in both bioavailability and half-life of absorption.

FDA-approved oral procainamide products are no longer available, but a small (n = 6) pharmacokinetic study was performed in healthy dogs using a compounded delayed-release formulation.[5] After dosing at 30 mg/kg PO, the average time that procainamide serum concentrations were above 4 µg/mL was 9.65 hours. The authors concluded: *Although specific dosing recommendations cannot be made from this data due to individual animal variability, it appears that twice daily administration of delayed-release procainamide could be efficacious in dogs. Due to individual patient variability, evaluation of serum trough concentrations should be considered to confirm concentrations within the reported therapeutic range.*

Distribution of procainamide is highest into the CSF, liver, spleen, kidneys, lungs, heart, and muscles. The volume of distribution in dogs is ≈1.4 to 3 L/kg.[4] It is only ≈20% protein-bound in humans and 15% in dogs. The elimination half-life in dogs has been reported to be variable; most studies report values between 2 and 3 hours.[4] In humans, procainamide is metabolized to N-acetyl-procainamide (NAPA), an active metabolite. Dogs do not form appreciable amounts of NAPA from procainamide, as they are unable to appreciably acetylate aromatic and hydrazine amino groups.[2,4] In dogs, ≈90% (50% to 70% unchanged) of an IV dose is excreted in the urine as procainamide and metabolites within 24 hours of dosing.

Contraindications/Precautions/Warnings

Procainamide may be contraindicated in patients with myasthenia gravis, as it may worsen clinical signs (see ***Drug Interactions***). Procainamide is contraindicated in patients hypersensitive to it, procaine, or other local anesthetic esters. In humans, procainamide is contraindicated in patients with systemic lupus erythematosus (SLE), but it is unknown if it adversely affects dogs with this condition. Procainamide should not be used in patients with torsade de pointes, or with second- or third-degree heart block (unless artificially paced).

Procainamide should be used with extreme caution, if at all, in patients with cardiac glycoside (eg, digitalis, digoxin) intoxication. It should be used with caution in patients with significant hepatic or renal disease or with congestive heart failure. Dosages should usually be reduced in patients with renal failure, congestive heart failure, or those that are critically ill.

It has been recommended to not use procainamide in Doberman pinschers and boxers with dilated cardiomyopathy or dogs with subaortic stenosis; the drug may be proarrhythmic in certain patients susceptible to tachyarrhythmic-induced sudden death.[6]

Adverse Effects

In dogs, adverse effects are generally related to dose and serum drug concentrations. GI effects may include anorexia, vomiting, or diarrhea. Effects related to the cardiovascular system can include weakness, hypotension, negative inotropism, widened QRS complex and QT intervals, AV block, and multiform ventricular tachycardias. Fevers and leukopenias are a possibility. Profound hypotension can occur if injected too rapidly IV. In humans, an SLE syndrome can occur, but its incidence has not been established in dogs.

Agranulocytosis, neutropenia, bone marrow suppression, hypoplastic anemia, and thrombocytopenia have been rarely reported in humans (≈0.5%).

Reproductive/Nursing Safety

Procainamide can cross the placenta. Both procainamide and NAPA are excreted in maternal milk and absorbed in nursing offspring. It should be used with caution in nursing patients; consider using milk replacer if the drug is to be continued.

Because safety has not been established in animals, this drug should only be used when the maternal benefits outweigh the potential risks to offspring.

Overdose/Acute Toxicity

Clinical signs of overdose can include hypotension, lethargy, confusion, nausea, vomiting, and oliguria. Cardiac signs may include widening of the QRS complex, junctional tachycardia, ventricular fibrillation, or intraventricular conduction delays.

If the overdose is from an oral ingestion, GI decontamination and charcoal administration may be beneficial to remove any unabsorbed drug. IV fluids, plus dopamine, phenylephrine, or norepinephrine could be considered to treat hypotensive effects. A $^1/_6$ molar IV infusion of sodium lactate may be used in an attempt to reduce the cardiotoxic effects of procainamide. Forced diuresis using fluids and diuretics along with reduction of urinary pH can enhance the renal excretion of the drug. Temporary cardiac pacing may be necessary should severe AV block occur.

For patients that have experienced or are suspected to have experienced an overdose, consultation with a 24-hour poison consultation center specializing in providing veterinary-specific information is recommended. For general information related to overdose and toxin exposures, as well as contact information for poison control centers, refer to ***Appendix***.

Drug Interactions

The following drug interactions have either been reported or are theoretical in humans or animals receiving procainamide and may be of significance in veterinary patients. Unless otherwise noted, use together is not necessarily contraindicated, but weigh the potential risks and perform additional monitoring when appropriate.

Use with caution with other antidysrhythmic agents, as additive cardiotoxic or other toxic effects may result.

- **Anticholinesterase Agents** (eg, **neostigmine, pyridostigmine**): Procainamide may antagonize effects in patients with myasthenia gravis.
- **H2 Antagonists** (eg, **cimetidine, ranitidine**): May increase procainamide concentrations
- **Hypotensive Drugs** (eg, **amlodipine, enalapril**): Procainamide may enhance effect.
- **Neuromuscular Blocking Agents** (eg, **atracurium, succinylcholine**): Procainamide may potentiate or prolong the neuromuscular blocking activity.
- **Trimethoprim**: May increase procainamide concentrations

Concurrent use with the following drugs may increase risk for cardiotoxicity, including QT prolongation, torsades de pointes, or cardiac arrest:

- **Amiodarone**: May increase procainamide concentrations, procainamide dose may need to be reduced
- **Amitriptyline**
- **Azithromycin**
- **Azole Antifungals** (eg, itraconazole, fluconazole)
- **Buprenorphine**
- **Cisapride**
- **Clomipramine**
- **Erythromycin**
- **Fluoroquinolones** (eg, ciprofloxacin)
- **Fluoxetine**
- **Hydroxychloroquine**
- **Hydroxyzine**
- **Isoflurane**
- **Lidocaine**: Toxic effects may be additive, and cardiac effects are unpredictable. Cardiotoxicity may include decreases in cardiac output, total peripheral resistance, and mean arterial pressure.
- **Methadone**
- **Metronidazole**
- **Mirtazapine**
- **Ondansetron**
- **Quinidine**
- **Sevoflurane**
- **Sodium Phosphate**
- **Sotalol**: Discontinue use of procainamide for at least 3 half-lives before dosing sotalol.
- **Tacrolimus**
- **Trazodone**

Laboratory Considerations

- Propranolol and very high concentrations of lidocaine can affect fluorescent tests for procainamide or NAPA.

Dosages

DOGS:

Severe or clinical ventricular tachycardia (extra-label): Lidocaine is usually the drug of first choice, but procainamide can be considered when lidocaine is ineffective and serum potassium and magnesium concentrations are adequate. Dosage recommendations vary. Consider procainamide slow IV boluses (over 2 to 5 minutes) of 2 – 4 mg/kg to a maximum of 20 mg/kg. If successful, follow with 20 – 50 µg/kg/minute IV CRI. If a CRI is not feasible, 7 – 10 mg/kg IM every 6 to 8 hours.

Compounded oral delayed-release procainamide may be useful for maintenance therapy but documentation of efficacy is lacking. One pharmacokinetic study[5] using a compounded product at 30 mg/kg PO every 12 hours concluded that dosing every 12 hours could be efficacious, but evaluation of serum drug concentrations should be considered.

Acute management of supraventricular tachycardias (SVTs) (extra-label): After drugs have been used to slow AV nodal conduction (eg, diltiazem), procainamide 6 – 8 mg/kg IV over 3 minutes or 6 – 20 mg/kg IM may terminate atrial tachyarrhythmias.[7]

CATS:

Acute, clinical ventricular tachycardia or SVTs (extra-label): 1 – 2 mg/kg IV slowly over 20 minutes.[8] For maintenance therapy, 3 – 8 mg/kg PO every 6 to 8 hours.[9] Rarely used, but could be considered in refractory arrhythmia

HORSES:

Atrial fibrillation (extra-label): 1 – 2 mg/kg/minute IV CRI, not to exceed 20 mg/kg (10 to 20 minutes) total dose. Alternatively, administer 25 – 35 mg/kg PO every 8 hours.[10] Not as effective as quinidine

Ventricular tachycardia (extra-label): 1 – 2 mg/kg/minute IV CRI up to a total dose of 20 mg/kg (10 to 20 minutes) has been suggested.[10,11]

Monitoring

- Cardiovascular parameters: ECG (continuous with IV administration); blood pressure; heart rate
- Adverse effects (eg, vomiting, diarrhea)
- Therapeutic drug monitoring: Because of the variability in pharmacokinetics reported in the dog, it is recommended to monitor therapy using serum drug concentrations. Because dogs do not form the active metabolite NAPA in appreciable quantities, the therapeutic range for procainamide is controversial. Therapeutic ranges from 3 – 8 µg/mL to 8 – 20 µg/mL have been suggested. Due to the lack of conversion to NAPA (which contributes to the antiarrhythmic effects of procainamide) in dogs, a higher procainamide concentration may be required. This author (Plumb) would suggest using the lower range as a guideline to initiate therapy, but not to hesitate increasing doses to attain higher concentrations if efficacy is not achieved and toxicity is not a problem. Digitalis-induced ventricular arrhythmias may require substantially higher blood concentrations for control. Trough drug concentrations are usually specified when monitoring oral therapy. Because NAPA is routinely monitored with procainamide in human medicine, it may be necessary to tell the laboratory that NAPA values need not be automatically run for canine patients.
- In horses, therapeutic levels have been suggested as 4 – 10 µg/mL for procainamide and 10 – 30 µg/dL as procainamide and NAPA together.[10]
- Because of serious and potentially fatal blood dyscrasias seen in humans, it is recommended to perform a CBC at weekly intervals for the first 3 months of therapy, and periodically thereafter.[12]

Client Information

- Procainamide oral medicine should be administered at evenly spaced intervals throughout the day/night. Unless otherwise directed, give the medication on an empty stomach, at least 1 hour before feeding or 2 hours after.
- Notify your veterinarian if your animal's condition gets worse or clinical signs of toxicity (eg, vomiting, diarrhea, weakness) occur.

- While your animal is taking this medication, it is important to return to your veterinarian for laboratory work, physical examination, and testing of heart rate and rhythm. Do not miss these important follow-up visits.

Chemistry/Synonyms

Structurally related to procaine, procainamide is used as an antiarrhythmic agent. Procainamide HCl differs from procaine by the substitution of an amide group for the ester group found on procaine. It occurs as an odorless, white to tan, hygroscopic, crystalline powder with a pK_a of 9.23 and a melting range from 165°C to 169°C (329°F-336°F). It is very soluble in water and soluble in alcohol. The pH of the injectable product ranges from 4 to 6.

Procainamide may also be known as novocainamidum, procainamidi chloridum, procainamidi hydrochloridum, *Biocoryl®*, *Procan®*, *Procanbid®*, or *Pronestyl®*.

Storage/Stability

The solution may be used if the color is no darker than light amber. Refrigeration may delay the development of oxidation, but the solution may be stored at room temperature.

Compatibility/Compounding Considerations

Compatibility is dependent on factors such as pH, concentration, temperature, and diluent used; specialized references or a hospital pharmacist should be consulted for more specific information.

The injectable product is reportedly physically **compatible** with sodium chloride 0.9% injection, and water for injection. Procainamide is also physically **compatible** with dobutamine HCl, lidocaine HCl, and verapamil HCl.

Dosage Forms/Regulatory Status

VETERINARY-LABELED PRODUCTS: NONE

The Association of Racing Commissioners International (ARCI) has designated this drug as a class 4 substance. Use of this drug may not be allowed in certain animal competitions. Check rules and regulations before entering in a competition while this medication is being administered. Contact local racing authorities for further guidance. See ***Appendix*** for more information.

HUMAN-LABELED PRODUCTS:

Procainamide HCl Injection Solution: 100 mg/mL in 10 mL vials and 500 mg/mL in 2 mL vials; generic; (Rx)

Procainamide HCl Immediate Release Capsules in 250 mg, 375 mg, and 500 mg, and Extended-Release Tablets in 250 mg, 500 mg, and 750 mg are available in Canada; generic; (Rx)

References

For the complete list of references, see **wiley.com/go/budde/plumb**

Procarbazine

(proe-***kar***-ba-zeen) *Matulane®*

Antineoplastic

Prescriber Highlights

- ► Atypical alkylating agent that is used in multiagent lymphoma protocols for dogs/cats and for granulomatous meningoencephalitis (GME) in dogs; enters CNS
- ► Contraindicated in patients that are hypersensitive to the drug and have myelosuppression
- ► Use with caution in patients with hepatic and renal impairment and when used with other CNS depressant drugs.
- ► Adverse effects include GI (eg, vomiting, diarrhea, acute hemorrhagic diarrhea syndrome), myelosuppression, and hepatotoxicity.
- ► Potentially teratogenic and embryotoxic. The National Institute for Occupational Safety and Health (NIOSH) classifies procarbazine as a hazardous drug; use appropriate precautions when handling it.

Uses/Indications

Procarbazine is used as part of MOPP (mechlorethamine, vincristine, procarbazine, prednisone),[1-4] MPP (mechlorethamine, procarbazine, prednisone),[5] LOPP (lomustine, vincristine, procarbazine, prednisone),[6-9] LPP (modified LOPP; lomustine, procarbazine, prednisone),[10] and BOPP (bendamustine, vincristine, procarbazine, prednisone)[7] protocols to treat both naïve and relapsed/refractory lymphoma in dogs and cats.

It may be of benefit in treating granulomatous meningoencephalitis (GME) in dogs.[11]

Pharmacology/Actions

Procarbazine's precise mode of action is not well understood, but it is considered to be an alkylating agent, and it appears to inhibit protein, RNA, and DNA synthesis. Procarbazine is auto-oxidized into hydrogen peroxide, which may also directly damage DNA.

Pharmacokinetics

No data specific for dogs or cats are available. In humans, procarbazine is completely absorbed after oral administration and rapidly equilibrates between the CSF and plasma.[12] Peak concentrations in plasma occur in ≈1 hour; in the CSF, ≈30 to 90 minutes after dosing. Procarbazine is almost entirely metabolized in the liver and kidney. Metabolic products are cytotoxic, and nearly 70% are excreted in the urine within 24 hours.

Contraindications/Precautions/Warnings

Procarbazine is contraindicated in patients known to be hypersensitive to the drug. The risk vs benefits of therapy must be carefully considered in patients with pre-existing myelosuppression or concurrent infections. Additive myelosuppression may occur in patients undergoing concomitant radiation therapy. Because procarbazine can cause CNS depression, use it with extreme caution with other CNS depressant drugs. Use procarbazine with caution in patients with impaired renal or hepatic function.

Only veterinarians with the experience and resources to monitor the toxicity of this agent should administer procarbazine.

Significant treatment-related toxicities in humans include the long-term risk for secondary cancers, infertility, neuropathy, and monoamine oxidase (MAO) inhibition.[12]

The National Institute for Occupational Safety and Health (NIOSH) classifies procarbazine as a hazardous drug; personal protective equipment (PPE) should be used accordingly to minimize the risk for exposure.[13]

Adverse Effects

When dosed as recommended for dogs and cats, procarbazine is relatively well tolerated. GI effects (eg, nausea, vomiting), hepatotoxicity, and myelosuppression (eg, thrombocytopenia, leukopenia) can be seen. Platelet nadir usually occurs at ≈3 to 4 weeks.

Many dogs receiving chemotherapy will have minor hair coat changes (eg, shagginess, loss of luster). Breeds with continuously growing hair coats (eg, poodles, terriers, Afghan hounds, or old English sheepdogs) are more likely to experience significant alopecia.

Because it is often used in combination with other chemotherapy agents, myelosuppression, and GI effects (hemorrhagic gastritis) may be enhanced. Alternate-day dosing or concurrent administration of antiemetics and appetite stimulants may alleviate severe anorexia in cats.

In humans, CNS effects may be noted and include sedation or agitation. Peripheral neuropathy can occur and includes loss of tendon reflexes, paresthesias, and myalgia.[12] Other reported adverse effects in humans include thrombosis, stomatitis, pancreatitis, ataxia, convulsions, cardiotoxicity, retinal hemorrhage, pulmonary toxicity, dermatitis, pruritus, nervousness, confusion, and hearing loss.[14]

In humans, it is recommended to discontinue or withhold therapy if any of the following occur: CNS signs, leukopenia (WBC less than 4000/μL), thrombocytopenia (platelets less than 100,000/μL), hypersensitivity, stomatitis (at the sign of first ulceration), diarrhea, and hemorrhage or bleeding. Resume therapy at a lower dose only if adverse effects resolve.

Reproductive/Nursing Safety

Procarbazine is potential teratogen. For sexually intact patients, verify pregnancy status prior to administration. It is unknown if procarbazine enters the milk. It is recommended to use milk replacer if the dam requires procarbazine. Because safety has not been established in animals, this drug should only be used when the maternal benefits outweigh the potential risks to offspring.

Overdose/Acute Toxicity

The LD_{50} for laboratory animals ranges from 150 mg/kg (rabbits) to 1.3 g/kg (mice).[15] There is no known antidote, and treatment is supportive. If the overdose was within a few hours, it is recommended to treat aggressively to remove the drug from the gut. Anticipated adverse effects would be extensions of the drug's adverse effect profile (eg, GI, myelosuppression, CNS effects).

For patients that have experienced or are suspected to have experienced an overdose, consultation with a 24-hour poison consultation center specializing in providing veterinary-specific information is recommended. For general information related to overdose and toxin exposures, as well as contact information for poison control centers, refer to ***Appendix.***

Drug Interactions

The following drug interactions have either been reported or are theoretical in humans or animals receiving procarbazine and may be of significance in veterinary patients. Unless otherwise noted, use together is not necessarily contraindicated, but weigh the potential risks and perform additional monitoring when appropriate.

- **Antidepressants** (eg, **amitriptyline, clomipramine, fluoxetine**): Procarbazine exhibits some monoamine oxidase inhibitory (MAOI) activity. Do not use concurrently with antidepressant drugs.
- **CNS Depressant Drugs** (eg, **barbiturates, opiates, antihistamines, phenothiazines**): Because procarbazine can cause CNS depression, use with extreme caution with other CNS depressant drugs. Coma and death have been reported when procarbazine has been used with opiates.
- **Ethanol**: May cause severe nausea and vomiting
- **Foods and Supplements With High Tyramine Content** (eg, aged cheese, yogurt, pepperoni/salami/summer sausage, ginseng): Procarbazine exhibits some MAOI activity; serious hypertension may result.
- **Myelosuppressive Agents** (eg, antineoplastics, immunosuppressants, iron chelators): Concurrent use with other bone marrow depressant medications may result in additive myelosuppression; avoid combination when possible.
- **Sympathomimetics** (eg, **phenylpropanolamine**): Procarbazine exhibits some MAOI activity; serious hypertension may result.
- **Vaccines** (live and inactivated): Procarbazine may diminish vaccine efficacy and enhance adverse effects of vaccines.

Laboratory Considerations

- None were noted.

Dosages

NOTES:

- Because of the potential toxicity of this drug to patients, veterinary staff, and pet owners, and because chemotherapy indications, treatment protocols, monitoring, and safety guidelines often change, the following dosages should be used only as a general guide. Consultation with a veterinary oncologist and referral to current veterinary oncology references[16-20] are strongly recommended.
- Dose calculations should be checked thoroughly to avoid overdosing because of the potential for serious toxicity associated with this agent.

DOGS:

Lymphoma, first-line (T-cell), or rescue (extra-label): When procarbazine is used, it is as part of a protocol in combination with other antineoplastic agents (MOPP, MPP, LOPP, LPP, BOPP protocols) and is usually given for the first 14 days of the treatment cycle.[1,2,5-7] The usual dose for dogs is 50 mg/m² (NOT mg/kg) PO daily.

Granulomatous meningoencephalitis (GME) (extra-label): 25 – 50 mg/m² (NOT mg/kg) PO once daily, initially with prednisone treatment. After the first month of therapy, attempt to reduce the procarbazine dose to every other day.

CATS:

Lymphoma, rescue (extra-label): When procarbazine is used, it is as part of a protocol in combination with other antineoplastic agents (MOPP protocol) and is usually given for the first 14 days of the treatment cycle. Usual doses for cats are 50 mg/m² (NOT mg/kg) PO daily or every other day; 10 mg/cat (NOT mg/m² or mg/kg) PO once daily has also been reported.[4]

Monitoring

- Baseline and weekly CBC, particularly platelet count. When giving the drug long term as part of treatment for granulomatous meningoencephalitis (GME), monitor CBC weekly for the first month and then monthly thereafter.
- Baseline and periodic serum liver and renal chemistry panels

Client Information

- Procarbazine is a chemotherapy (anticancer) medicine. It can be hazardous to other animals and humans that come in contact with them. Wear gloves when handling and administering procarbazine. On the day your animal gets the medicine, and then for ≈72 hours afterward, handle all bodily waste (ie, urine, feces, litter), blood, or vomit while wearing disposable gloves. Seal the waste in a plastic bag and then place both the bag and gloves in with the regular trash.
- Gastrointestinal toxicity (eg, ulcers, diarrhea) can occur. If diarrhea is severe or continues, contact your veterinarian.

- Bone marrow suppression can occur and make your animal at risk for developing infections. The greatest effects on bone marrow usually occur within a few weeks after treatment. Your veterinarian will do blood tests to watch for this problem. Do not miss these important follow-up visits.
- Contact your veterinarian right away if you see bleeding, bruising, or fever (indicating an infection) or if your animal becomes tired easily.
- Procarbazine can also be toxic to the nerves and cause numbness, tingling, or lameness. Contact your veterinarian if you have any concerns that your animal is having these side effects.
- This medication is considered to be a hazardous drug as defined by the National Institute for Occupational Safety and Health (NIOSH). Talk with your veterinarian or pharmacist about the use of personal protective equipment when handling this medicine.

Chemistry/Synonyms

Procarbazine HCl, a derivative of hydrazine, occurs as a white to a pale-yellow crystalline powder having a slight odor. It is soluble but unstable in water or aqueous solutions.

Procarbazine may also be known as ibenzemethyzin, NSC-77213, Ro-4-6467/1, MIH, N-Methylhydrazine, *Matulane*®, *Natulan*®, and *Natulanar*®.

Storage/Stability

Store procarbazine capsules in airtight containers, protected from light at temperatures between 20°C and 25°C (68°F-77°F).

Compatibility/Compounding Considerations

Procarbazine is a hazardous drug and should only be compounded by trained personnel with adequate hazardous drug facilities and precautions. Precautions (eg, use of a biological safety cabinet) must be taken to avoid exposure from capsule contents when compounding dosage forms from commercially available capsules.

Dosage Forms/Regulatory Status

VETERINARY-LABELED PRODUCTS: NONE

HUMAN-LABELED PRODUCTS:

Procarbazine HCl Capsules: 50 mg; *Matulane*®; (Rx)

References

For the complete list of references, see **wiley.com/go/budde/plumb**

Prochlorperazine

(proe-klor-***per***-a-zeen) *Compazine*®, *Compro*®

Phenothiazine Antiemetic

Prescriber Highlights

- ► Used as an antiemetic in dogs and cats
- ► Relatively contraindicated in patients that are hypovolemic, dehydrated, or in shock, and in patients with tetanus or strychnine intoxication
- ► Use with caution in patients with hepatic dysfunction, cardiac disease, general debilitation, and in very young animals.
- ► Adverse effects include sedation and hypotension.

Uses/Indications

Prochlorperazine is used in dogs and cats as an antiemetic. It has a mild sedative effect that may be advantageous in an inpatient setting. There is limited published information to support clinical use in dogs or cats.

Prochlorperazine was FDA-approved in combination with isopropamide, with or without neomycin, for vomiting, nonspecific gastroenteritis, drug-induced diarrhea, infectious diarrhea, spastic colitis, and motion sickness in dogs and cats; however, these products are no longer marketed in the United States.

Pharmacology/Actions

Prochlorperazine is a phenothiazine derivative. It has multiple mechanisms of action, including antagonism of dopamine, histamine type-1, alpha-2-adrenergic, and muscarinic receptors. The antiemetic activity of prochlorperazine is due to its effects primarily in the brain's emetic center and chemoreceptor trigger zone, but it also has some peripheral activity. Prochlorperazine has weak anticholinergic effects, strong extrapyramidal effects, and moderate sedative effects.

Pharmacokinetics

Limited information is available regarding the pharmacokinetics of prochlorperazine in animals, although it likely follows the general pattern of other phenothiazine agents in absorption, distribution, and elimination.

In humans, the onset of action is 10 to 20 minutes after IM administration with a duration of 3 to 4 hours. IV administration is generally avoided due to the increased risk for hypotension; SC administration is avoided due to local irritation.

Contraindications/Precautions/Warnings

Prochlorperazine is contraindicated in patients with a known hypersensitivity to it or other phenothiazines and in patients in comatose states due to large amounts of CNS depressants. Phenothiazines are relatively contraindicated in patients with hypovolemia, dehydration, or shock due to their hypotensive effects. Do not use prochlorperazine for tetanus or strychnine intoxication due to its effects on the extrapyramidal system.

Use prochlorperazine with caution in animals with hepatic dysfunction, cardiac disease, or general debilitation; smaller doses are recommended. Phenothiazines may exacerbate CNS depression. Use prochlorperazine with caution in very young or debilitated animals. Animals may require lower doses of general anesthetics following phenothiazines.

Some dosage forms contain large amounts of benzyl alcohol.

Avoid skin contact with the injectable solution during dose preparation and administration, as contact dermatitis has occurred. Do not confuse prochlorPERAZINE with chlorproMAZINE.

Adverse Effects

The most frequent adverse effects of prochlorperazine are sedation and hypotension. Muscle fasciculations, tremors, and prolactin release have been reported in small animal species.

In humans, the most common adverse effects include drowsiness, dizziness, skin reactions, and hypotension.

Reproductive/Nursing Safety

It is unknown if prochlorperazine is excreted in milk; however, other phenothiazines have been detected in maternal milk. Because safety has not been established in animals, this drug should only be used when the maternal benefits outweigh the potential risks to offspring.

Overdose/Acute Toxicity

The reported LD_{50} in dogs following PO and IV administration was 102 and 100 mg/kg, respectively.[1] Acute extrapyramidal clinical signs such as torticollis, tremor, and salivation have been successfully treated with injectable diphenhydramine in humans. Treatment is supportive as there is no known antidote, and prochlorperazine is unlikely to be removed via dialysis. Refer to ***Overdose/Acute Toxicity*** in ***Acepromazine*** for further information.

For patients that have experienced or are suspected to have experienced an overdose, consultation with a 24-hour poison consultation center specializing in providing veterinary-specific information is recommended. For general information related to overdose and

toxin exposures, as well as contact information for poison control centers, refer to ***Appendix***.

Drug Interactions

The following drug interactions have either been reported or are theoretical in humans or animals receiving prochlorperazine or other phenothiazines and may be of significance in veterinary patients. Unless otherwise noted, use together is not necessarily contraindicated, but weigh the potential risks and perform additional monitoring when appropriate.

- Anticholinergic Agents (eg, **atropine, glycopyrrolate, hyoscyamine**): Increased risk for anticholinergic effects (eg, dry mucous membranes, constipation, urinary retention)
- Beta-Adrenergic Receptor Antagonists: May increase risk for hypotension
- CNS Depressant Agents (eg, anesthetics, barbiturates): May cause additive CNS depression
- Dopamine: Phenothiazines may decrease pressor effects.
- Emetics (eg, **apomorphine, ropinirole**): Prochlorperazine may decrease the effectiveness of emetics and increase risk for sedation and hypotension
- Epinephrine: Contraindicated in the treatment of acute hypotension produced by prochlorperazine or other phenothiazines, as further depression of blood pressure can occur (also referred to as epinephrine reversal)
- Metoclopramide: Phenothiazines may potentiate the extrapyramidal effects of metoclopramide.
- Opioids (eg, **buprenorphine, morphine, tramadol**): May enhance the hypotensive effects of the phenothiazines; dosages of prochlorperazine may need to be reduced when used with an opioid.
- Organophosphate Agents: Phenothiazines should not be given within 1 month of deworming with organophosphates, as organophosphate toxicity may be potentiated.
- Paraquat: Toxicity of the herbicide paraquat may be increased by prochlorperazine.
- Physostigmine: Toxicity may be enhanced by prochlorperazine.
- Procaine: Activity may be enhanced by phenothiazines.
- QT Prolonging Agents (eg, **cisapride, fluoroquinolones, sotalol, selective serotonin reuptake inhibitors** [**SSRIs**]): Increased risk for QT prolongation and torsade de pointes

Dosages

DOGS/CATS:

Antiemetic (extra-label): 0.1 – 0.5 mg/kg SC every 6 to 8 hours; ensure adequate hydration

Monitoring

- Heart rate, rhythm, and blood pressure if indicated
- Antiemetic/antispasmodic efficacy
- Periodic chemistry and hydration status as indicated by clinical presentation
- Body temperature (especially if the ambient temperature is very hot or cold)

Client Information

- Observe animals for at least 1 hour following dosing. Keep treated animal in a quiet environment at a comfortable temperature.
- This medicine may cause your animal's urine color to change to a pink or red-brown color. This change does not cause any harm.
- Vomiting and diarrhea that does not improve or worsens can be a serious problem. Contact your veterinarian if this occurs.
- Contact your veterinarian if you notice abnormal behavior, rigidity, or other abnormal body movements.

Chemistry/Synonyms

Prochlorperazine is a piperazine phenothiazine derivative that is available commercially as the base in rectal formulations, the edisylate salt in injectable and oral solutions, and as the maleate salt in oral tablets and capsules. Each 8 mg of the maleate salt and 7.5 mg of the edisylate salt are ≈5 mg of prochlorperazine base.

The base occurs as a clear to pale-yellow, viscous liquid that is very slightly soluble in water and freely soluble in alcohol. The edisylate salt occurs as white to very light yellow, odorless, crystalline powder. Five hundred milligrams are soluble in 1 mL of water or 750 mL of alcohol. The maleate salt occurs as a white or pale-yellow, practically odorless, crystalline powder. It is practically insoluble in water or alcohol.

The commercial injection is a solution of the edisylate salt in sterile water. It has a pH of 4.2 to 6.2.

Prochlorperazine may also be known as chlormeprazine, prochlorpemazine, *Compazine*®, *Compro*®, *Prochlor*®, *Prorazin*®, *Stemetil*®, or *Tementil*®.

Storage/Stability

Store intact vials and tablets between 20°C and 25°C (68°F-77°F); avoid freezing. Protect from light. Slight yellowing of oral or injectable solutions does not affect potency or efficacy. Do not use if precipitate forms or if the solution is substantially discolored.

Compatibility/Compounding Considerations

Compatibility is dependent on factors such as pH, concentration, temperature, and diluent used; specialized references or a hospital pharmacist should be consulted for more specific information.

The following products have been reported to be physically **compatible** when mixed with prochlorperazine edisylate injection: all usual IV fluids, ascorbic acid injection, atropine sulfate, butorphanol tartrate, chlorpromazine HCl, dexamethasone sodium phosphate, fentanyl citrate, glycopyrrolate, hydroxyzine HCl, lidocaine HCl, meperidine HCl, metoclopramide, morphine sulfate, nalbuphine HCl, pentazocine lactate, perphenazine, promazine HCl, promethazine, scopolamine HBr, sodium bicarbonate, and vitamin B complex with C.

The following drugs have been reported to be physically **incompatible** when mixed with prochlorperazine edisylate: aminophylline, amphotericin B, ampicillin sodium, calcium gluceptate, chloramphenicol sodium succinate, dimenhydrinate, hydrocortisone sodium succinate, methohexital sodium, penicillin G sodium, phenobarbital sodium, pentobarbital sodium, and thiopental sodium. Do not mix with other drugs/diluents having parabens as preservatives.

Dosage Forms/Regulatory Status

VETERINARY-LABELED PRODUCTS:

None; *Darbazine*® is no longer available.

The Association of Racing Commissioners International (ARCI) has designated this drug as a class 2 substance. Use of this drug may not be allowed in certain animal competitions. Check rules and regulations before entering in a competition while this medication is being administered. Contact local racing authorities for further guidance. See ***Appendix*** for more information. The FEI (International Federation for Equestrian Sports) lists this drug as a "prohibited substance – banned."[2]

HUMAN-LABELED PRODUCTS:

Prochlorperazine for Injection: 5 mg/mL in 2 mL vials (as edisylate); generic; (Rx)

Prochlorperazine Tablets: 5 mg and 10 mg (as maleate); generic; (Rx)

Prochlorperazine Suppositories: 25 mg (as base); *Compro*®, generic; (Rx)

References

For the complete list of references, see **wiley.com/go/budde/plumb**

Promethazine

(proe-***meth***-a-zeen) *Phenergan®*

Phenothiazine

Prescriber Highlights

- Used as an antiemetic and antihistamine in small animal species
- In horses, may cause less sedation and peripheral vasodilation than acepromazine
- Limited experience with promethazine in veterinary medicine
- Contraindications include hypersensitivity, hypovolemia, and shock. Do not inject IA or SC.
- Use with caution in patients with hepatic dysfunction, patients with cardiac disease, very young patients, and debilitated patients.
- Adverse effects include sedation and anticholinergic effects.

Uses/Indications

Promethazine has been used in dogs and cats as an antiemetic. A small study in cats found that IM doses of 2 and 4 mg/kg given 1 hour prior to xylazine administration significantly reduced the frequency of emesis.[1] Despite its antihistamine actions, efficacy for treatment of pruritus in atopic dogs has been poor. Oral H_1 antihistamines may provide limited benefit in some dogs with atopic dermatitis for preventing pruritus when given before a flare but are of little to no benefit for long-term treatment.[2]

A study in standing horses compared the sedative and hemodynamic effects of acepromazine 0.1 mg/kg IV with those of promethazine 0.1, 0.2, and 0.3 mg/kg IV. At the doses used, promethazine appeared to have less sedative and peripheral vasodilator effects than acepromazine.[3] Promethazine may be safer than acepromazine in horses at risk for hypotension[3] and may be of benefit in horses suffering from shock or cardiovascular depression if anti-inflammatory and antioxidative properties are confirmed in vivo.[4]

Pharmacology/Actions

Promethazine is similar to other phenothiazines with multiple mechanisms of action, including antagonism of H_1, alpha$_2$-adrenergic, and muscarinic receptors; it also antagonizes dopamine but to a lesser extent than other phenothiazines. Antiemetic activity of promethazine is primarily due to its effects in the brain's emetic center and chemoreceptor trigger zone, but it also has some peripheral activity.

Pharmacokinetics

Limited pharmacokinetic information is available in animals. Oral bioavailability in dogs is very low at ≈10%.[5]

In humans, promethazine is well absorbed following oral, rectal, and IM administration. Sedative effects occur within minutes of IV administration and persist for several hours. Promethazine is widely distributed. It is metabolized in the liver and metabolites are eliminated primarily in the urine.[6] Elimination half-life in humans is ≈10 hours.

Contraindications/Precautions/Warnings

Promethazine is contraindicated in patients that are hypersensitive to it or other phenothiazines. In humans, promethazine is contraindicated in children less than 2 years old due to risk for fatal respiratory depression.[6,7] Phenothiazines are relatively contraindicated in patients with hypovolemia or shock due to their hypotensive effects. Do not use in patients with tetanus or strychnine intoxication due to effects on the extrapyramidal system.

Promethazine is absolutely contraindicated for intra-arterial injection due to the likelihood of arteriospasm, which could lead to gangrene. It should not be given SC as chemical irritation and necrotic lesions are possible.[7]

Use with caution in patients with hepatic dysfunction, or cardiac disease; smaller doses may be required. Use cautiously in very young or debilitated animals. Drugs with anticholinergic properties such as promethazine should be used with caution in patients with narrow-angle glaucoma, prostatic hypertrophy, stenosing peptic ulcer, pyloroduodenal obstruction, or bladder-neck obstruction.

Animals may require lower doses of general anesthetics following phenothiazine administration. Promethazine discolors blood on contact, making it difficult to assess needle placement upon drawback.

Adverse Effects

Limited information is available in animals but sedation and anticholinergic effects such as dry mucous membranes, constipation, and urinary retention occur with other phenothiazines. Promethazine can cause paradoxical CNS stimulation leading to hyperexcitability, tremors, abnormal muscle movements, or convulsions. Promethazine may lower seizure threshold. Injection-site reactions are also possible.

Reproductive/Nursing Safety

Whether promethazine is distributed in milk is unknown; however, a related compound, chlorpromazine, has been detected in maternal milk. In humans, it is recommended to either discontinue promethazine or discontinue nursing due to the risk for serious adverse effects in nursing infants.[6,7]

Because safety has not been established in pregnant animals, this drug should only be used when the maternal benefits outweigh the potential risks to offspring.

Overdose/Acute Toxicity

Acute extrapyramidal clinical signs of overdose such as torticollis, tremor, and salivation have been treated successfully with injectable diphenhydramine in humans. See ***Acepromazine*** for more information.

For patients that have experienced or are suspected to have experienced an overdose, consultation with a 24-hour poison consultation center specializing in providing veterinary-specific information is recommended. For general information related to overdose and toxin exposures, as well as contact information for poison control centers, refer to ***Appendix.***

Drug Interactions

The following drug interactions have either been reported or are theoretical in humans or animals receiving promethazine or other phenothiazines and may be of significance in veterinary patients. Unless otherwise noted, use together is not necessarily contraindicated, but weigh the potential risks and perform additional monitoring when appropriate.

- ANTACIDS: May reduce GI absorption of oral phenothiazines
- ANTIDIARRHEAL MIXTURES (eg, **kaolin/pectin, bismuth subsalicylate**): May reduce GI absorption of oral phenothiazines
- ANTICHOLINERGIC AGENTS (eg, **atropine, glycopyrrolate, hyoscyamine**): May have additive effects when used with promethazine
- CNS DEPRESSANT AGENTS (eg, **anesthetics, barbiturates, narcotics, sedatives**): May cause additive CNS depression if used with phenothiazines
- EMETICS (eg, **apomorphine, ropinirole**): Prochlorperazine may decrease the effectiveness of emetics and increase risk for sedation and hypotension
- EPINEPHRINE: Phenothiazines may reduce or reverse pressor effects of epinephrine.
- METOCLOPRAMIDE: Phenothiazines may potentiate the extrapyramidal effects of metoclopramide.

- **Monoamine Oxidase Inhibitors** (MAOIs; eg, **amitraz, linezolid, selegeline**): May potentiate extrapyramidal effects
- **Myelosuppressants**: Promethazine may potentiate the myelosuppressive effects.
- **Opioids** (eg, **buprenorphine, morphine, tramadol**): May enhance the hypotensive effects of the phenothiazines; dosages of promethazine may need to be reduced when used with an opioid.
- **Organophosphate Agents**: Phenothiazines should not be given within 1 month of deworming with organophosphates as their effects may be potentiated.
- **QT Prolonging Agents** (eg, **cisapride, fluoroquinolones, sotalol, SSRIs**): Increased risk for QT prolongation and torsade de pointes; concurrent administration of cisapride and promethazine is contraindicated in humans.

Laboratory Considerations

- Promethazine can cause false-positive results for salicylates in urine.
- Promethazine can cause false-positive or false-negative results for chorionic gonadotropin in urine.

Dosages

NOTE: Do not administer intra-arterially or SC (see *Contraindications/Precautions/Warnings*). IM is the preferred parenteral route.

DOGS:

Antiemetic | Prevention of motion sickness (extra-label): 0.2 – 0.5 mg/kg PO every 6 to 8 hours; oral bioavailability is low so efficacy may be limited.[8]

CATS:

Antiemetic (extra-label): 2 mg/kg IM given 1 hour prior to xylazine administration has been shown to significantly reduce the frequency of emesis.[1]

HORSES:

Alternative to acepromazine in horses at risk for hypotension (extra-label): 0.1 – 0.2 mg/kg IV based on one small study[3]

Monitoring

- Efficacy (eg, signs of nausea, vomiting)

Client Information

- This medicine may cause dry mouth. Applying small amounts of water to the animal's tongue for 10 to 15 minutes may provide relief.
- Promethazine may cause sedation or behavior changes. Contact your veterinarian if these are a concern.
- Vomiting or diarrhea that does not resolve can be serious. Contact your veterinarian if these signs worsen or do not stop.
- Contact your veterinarian if your animal develops abnormal movements, tremors, or becomes rigid.

Chemistry/Synonyms

Promethazine HCl occurs as a white to faint yellow, practically odorless, crystalline powder. It slowly oxidizes and acquires a blue color on prolonged exposure to air. Promethazine HCl is freely soluble in water, hot dehydrated alcohol, or chloroform, but practically insoluble in acetone, ether, or ethyl acetate. The pH of a 5% solution in water is between 4 and 5.

Promethazine may also be known as Lilly 01516, PM 284, RP 3277, diprazinum, prometazina, or *Phenergan*®. There are many other branded products available.

Storage/Stability

Store tablets at room temperature (20°C-25°C [68°F-77°F]) in tight, light-resistant containers. Store the syrup at 15°C-25°C (59°F-77°F) and protect it from light and freezing.

Store the injection at room temperature (20°C-25°C [68°F-77°F]) and protect it from light. Keep in covered carton until time of use. Do not use if a precipitate forms or the solution is discolored. Promethazine can be adsorbed to plastic IV bags and tubing.

Store promethazine suppositories in the refrigerator (2°C-8°C [36°F-46°F]).

Compatibility/Compounding Considerations

Compatibility is dependent on factors such as pH, concentration, temperature, and diluent used; consult specialized references or a hospital pharmacist for more specific information.

The following products have been reported to be physically **compatible** when mixed with promethazine injection: all commonly used IV fluids, amikacin, ascorbic acid, buprenorphine, butorphanol, calcium salts, cimetidine, diphenhydramine, fentanyl, fluconazole, gentamicin sulfate, glycopyrrolate, hydromorphone, hydroxyzine, ketamine, lidocaine, meperidine, metoclopramide, midazolam, ondansetron, pancuronium, pentazocine, procainamide, and ranitidine.

Solutions of promethazine hydrochloride are **incompatible** with alkaline substances, which can precipitate promethazine base.

The following drugs have been reported to be physically **incompatible** when mixed with promethazine HCl: aminophylline, amphotericin B (all forms), ampicillin, barbiturates, benzylpenicillin salts, most cephalosporins, chloramphenicol sodium succinate, dexamethasone sodium phosphate, diazepam, dimenhydrinate, doxorubicin (in a liposomal formulation), furosemide, heparin sodium, hydrocortisone sodium succinate, morphine sulfate, nalbuphine HCl, and pantoprazole.

Dosage Forms/Regulatory Status

VETERINARY-LABELED PRODUCTS: NONE

The Association of Racing Commissioners International (ARCI) has designated this drug as a class 3 substance. Use of this drug may not be allowed in certain animal competitions. Check rules and regulations before entering in a competition while this medication is being administered. Contact local racing authorities for further guidance. See ***Appendix*** for more information.

HUMAN-LABELED PRODUCTS:

Promethazine HCl for Injection: 25 mg/mL and 50 mg/mL in 1 mL ampules; generic; (Rx)

Promethazine HCl Oral Syrup: 1.25 mg/mL in 118 mL and 473 mL; generic; (Rx)

Promethazine HCl Oral Tablets: 12.5 mg, 25 mg, and 50 mg; generic; (Rx)

Promethazine HCl Rectal Suppositories: 12.5 mg, 25 mg, and 50 mg; *Phenadoz*®, *Promethegan*®, generic; (Rx)

References

For the complete list of references, see **wiley.com/go/budde/plumb**

Propantheline

(proe-***pan***-the-leen) *Pro-Banthine®*
Quaternary Antimuscarinic

Prescriber Highlights

- ► Quaternary antimuscarinic agent used for its antispasmodic/antisecretory effects for the treatment of diarrhea, detrusor hyperreflexia or urge incontinence, and anticholinergic responsive bradycardias. In horses, it is used IV to reduce colonic peristalsis and relax the rectum to allow easier examination and surgery.
- ► Contraindications include hypersensitivity to anticholinergics, tachycardia secondary to thyrotoxicosis or cardiac insufficiency, myocardial ischemia, unstable cardiac status during acute hemorrhage, GI obstructive disease, paralytic ileus, severe ulcerative colitis, obstructive uropathy, or myasthenia gravis (unless used to reverse adverse muscarinic effects secondary to therapy).
- ► Use with extreme caution in patients that have known or suspected GI infections or autonomic neuropathy.
- ► Use with caution in patients that have hepatic or renal disease, hyperthyroidism, hypertension, CHF, tachyarrhythmias, prostatic hypertrophy, or esophageal reflux, and in geriatric or pediatric patients.
- ► Adverse effects are similar to atropine (eg, dry mouth, dry eyes, urinary hesitancy, tachycardia, constipation), but there are fewer effects on the eye or CNS. Cats may exhibit vomiting and hypersalivation. High doses may cause ileus.

Uses/Indications

In small animal medicine, propantheline has been used for its antispasmodic/antisecretory effects in the treatment of diarrhea. It is also employed in the treatment of detrusor hyperreflexia or urge incontinence, and as an oral treatment for anticholinergic responsive bradycardias.

In horses, propantheline has been used IV to reduce colonic peristalsis and for relaxing the rectum to allow easier rectal examination and surgery.

Pharmacology/Actions

Propantheline, an antimuscarinic with similar actions as atropine, is a quaternary ammonium compound and does not cross appreciably into the CNS. It should not exhibit the same extent of CNS adverse effects that atropine possesses. After a 100 mg IV injection to horses, propantheline reduced GI tract sounds for 2-plus hours and elevated heart rate relative to the control. Maximum heart rates were noted between 60 and 90 minutes postinjection.[1]

Pharmacokinetics

Quaternary anticholinergic agents are not completely absorbed after oral administration because they are completely ionized. In humans, peak concentrations occur 1 to 2 hours after oral administration. Propantheline's half-life in humans is 1.6 hours. Food apparently decreases the amount of drug absorbed. Propantheline is reportedly variably absorbed in dogs; dosages should be adjusted for each patient.

The distribution of propantheline has not been extensively studied, but, like other quaternary antimuscarinics, propantheline is poorly lipid-soluble and does not extensively penetrate into the CNS or eye.

Propantheline is believed to be primarily metabolized in the GI tract and/or liver; its primary pathway in humans is by hydrolysis to inactive metabolites. Less than 5% of an oral dose is excreted unchanged in the urine.

Contraindications/Precautions/Warnings

The equine product (Australia) is labeled as contraindicated in cases of tympanic colic. Do not use propantheline in cases of dry choke where saliva is deficient, as the anticholinergic properties will further inhibit the secretion of saliva. Propantheline should be considered contraindicated if the patient has a history of hypersensitivity to anticholinergic drugs, tachycardia secondary to thyrotoxicosis or cardiac insufficiency, myocardial ischemia, unstable cardiac status during acute hemorrhage, GI obstructive disease, paralytic ileus, severe ulcerative colitis, obstructive uropathy, glaucoma, or myasthenia gravis (unless used to reverse adverse muscarinic effects secondary to therapy).

Propantheline should be used with extreme caution in patients with known or suspected GI infections, as it can decrease GI motility and prolong retention of the causative agent(s) or toxin(s), resulting in prolonged clinical signs. Antimuscarinic agents must also be used with extreme caution in patients with autonomic neuropathy.

Antimuscarinic agents should be used with caution in patients with hepatic disease, renal disease, hyperthyroidism, hypertension, CHF, tachyarrhythmias, prostatic hypertrophy, esophageal reflux, and in geriatric or pediatric patients. The human product contains a warning for heat prostration; use caution in the presence of high environmental heat.

Adverse Effects

With the exception of fewer effects on the eye and the CNS, propantheline can be assumed to have a similar adverse reaction profile as atropine (eg, dry mouth, dry eyes, urinary hesitancy, tachycardia, constipation). Vomiting and hypersalivation have also been reported in cats. High doses may lead to the development of ileus with resultant bacterial overgrowth in susceptible animals. For more information, refer to the ***Atropine*** monograph.

Reproductive/Nursing Safety

Although anticholinergics (especially atropine) may be excreted in milk and cause toxicity and reduce milk production, it is unknown if propantheline enters maternal milk. Use propantheline with caution in nursing patients.

Because safety has not been established in animals, this drug should only be used when the maternal benefits outweigh the potential risks to offspring.

Overdose/Acute Toxicity

Because of propantheline's quaternary structure, it would be expected that minimal CNS effects would occur after an overdose when compared to atropine. See the information listed in the ***Atropine*** monograph for more information on the clinical signs that may be seen following an overdose.

In case of recent oral ingestion, GI decontamination and administration of activated charcoal and saline cathartics may be warranted. Treat clinical signs supportively and symptomatically. Do not use phenothiazines, as they may contribute to anticholinergic effects. Fluid therapy and standard treatments for shock may be instituted. The oral LD_{50} of propantheline bromide is 780 mg/kg in a mouse and 370 mg/kg in a rat.

The use of physostigmine is controversial and should likely be reserved for cases where the patient exhibits either extreme agitation and is at risk for injuring themselves or others, or where supraventricular tachycardias and sinus tachycardias are severe or life-threatening. The usual human dose for physostigmine is 2 mg IV slowly (for an average-sized adult); if there is no response, it may be repeated every 20 minutes until reversal of toxic antimuscarinic effects or cholinergic effects takes place. The human pediatric physostigmine dose is 0.02 mg/kg slow IV (repeat every 10 minutes as above) and may be a reasonable choice for the treatment of small animals. Physostigmine adverse effects (eg, bronchoconstriction, bradycardia, seizures) may be treated with small doses of atropine IV.

For patients that have experienced or are suspected of having experienced an overdose, consultation with a 24-hour poison consultation center specializing in providing veterinary-specific information is recommended. For general information related to overdose and toxin exposures, as well as contact information for poison control centers, refer to ***Appendix***.

Drug Interactions

The following drug interactions have either been reported or are theoretical in humans or animals receiving propantheline and may be of significance in veterinary patients. Unless otherwise noted, use together is not necessarily contraindicated, but weigh the potential risks and perform additional monitoring when appropriate.

- **Antihistamines, first generation** (eg, **diphenhydramine**): May enhance the activity of propantheline
- **Antiarrhythmics, Type 1** (eg, **procainamide, quinidine**): May enhance the activity of propantheline
- **Benzodiazepines** (eg, **diazepam**): May enhance the activity of propantheline
- **Cimetidine**: Propantheline may decrease the absorption of cimetidine.
- **Corticosteroids** (eg, **dexamethasone, predniso(lo)ne**): May increase intraocular pressure (IOP) with long-term use
- **Digoxin**: May cause increased serum digoxin levels
- **Nitrates** (eg, **nitroglycerine, nitroprusside**): May potentiate the adverse effects of propantheline
- **Nitrofurantoin**: Propantheline may enhance actions.
- **Opioids** (eg, **buprenorphine, hydrocodone, meperidine, morphine**): May have additive anticholinergic effects
- **Phenothiazines** (eg, **acepromazine**): May enhance the activity of propantheline
- **Prokinetic Agents** (eg, **cisapride, metoclopramide**): Propantheline may decrease prokinetic effects.
- **Sympathomimetics** (eg, **phenylpropanolamine**): Propantheline may enhance actions.
- **Ranitidine**: Propantheline delays the absorption but increases the peak serum level of ranitidine; the relative bioavailability of ranitidine may be increased by 23% when propantheline is administered concomitantly with ranitidine.
- **Thiazide Diuretics** (eg, **hydrochlorothiazide**): Propantheline may enhance actions.

Dosages

DOGS/CATS:

Detrusor hyperreflexia, urge incontinence (extra-label): Dogs: 7.5 – 30 mg/dog (NOT mg/kg) PO every 8 to 24 hours. Cats: Suggested dosages vary significantly, ranging from 5 – 7.5 mg/cat (NOT mg/kg) PO every 8 hours to 7.5 mg/cat (NOT mg/kg) PO every 3 days. Use the lowest dose that will control clinical signs.

Chronic diarrhea (noninfectious) (extra-label): Dogs: 2.5 mg/kg PO 2 to 3 times per day[2]

Antiemetic (extra-label): 0.25 mg/kg PO 2 to 3 times per day has been suggested. However, propantheline is a poor antiemetic when compared with other options and has the negative effect of altering GI motility.[2]

Short-term treatment of sinus bradycardia, incomplete AV block (extra-label): Dogs: 7.5 – 30 mg/dog (NOT mg/kg) PO every 8 to 12 hours. Cats: 7.5 mg/cat (NOT mg/kg) PO every 8 to 12 hours. Improvement is usually partial and often temporary.[3]

HORSES:

Parasympatholytic (extra-label): **For rectal palpation**: 50 – 100 mg/horse (NOT mg/kg) IV. **Acute spasmodic colic**: 100 – 300 mg/horse (NOT mg/kg) IV. **Rectal tears**: If rectal tears are suspected, use immediately at a dose of 50 – 100 mg/horse (NOT mg/kg) IV. Rectal relaxation will usually follow within 1 minute.[4]

Monitoring

- Clinical efficacy
- Heart rate and rhythm, if indicated
- Adverse effects

Client Information

- It is best to give this medicine on an empty stomach, but if the animal vomits after getting a dose, give with a small amount of food or treat to see if this helps. If vomiting continues, contact your veterinarian.
- Side effects can include dry mouth, dry eyes, trouble urinating or defecating, fast heartbeat, vomiting (in cats), and drooling/hypersalivation (in cats).
- Dry mouth may be relieved by applying small amounts of water to the animal's tongue for 10 to 15 minutes.
- Severe constipation can be serious. If your animal has not passed any stool for several days, contact your veterinarian right away.

Chemistry/Synonyms

Propantheline bromide, a quaternary ammonium antimuscarinic agent, occurs as bitter-tasting, odorless, white or practically white crystals, with a melting range of 156°C to 162°C (313°F-324°F; with decomposition). It is very soluble in both water and alcohol.

Propantheline bromide may also be known as bromuro de propantelina, propanthelini bromidum, *Propan B*®, or *Pro-Banthine*®.

Storage/Stability

Store propantheline bromide tablets at room temperature 20° to 25°C (68°F-77°F) in tight, light-resistant containers.

Store the dry powder for reconstitution (*Propan B*®) below 25°C (77°F). Protect this product from light. Use prepared solution within 10 days.

Compatibility/Compounding Considerations

Reconstitute the powder for injection with 10 mL of sterile water for injection. As there is no commercially available injectable product available in the United States, if preparation is made from oral tablets, it should be freshly prepared and filtered through a 0.22-micron filter before administering. Use this product with caution. If using a compounded product, reconstitute as directed.

Dosage Forms/Regulatory Status

VETERINARY-LABELED PRODUCTS:

None in the United States. In Australia: Propantheline Bromide 300 mg sterile powder for reconstitution (for IV use) in 10 mL vials; *Propan B*®; S4 By Veterinary Prescription (APVMA 51275). The meat withholding period for horses is 28 days.

HUMAN-LABELED PRODUCTS:

None. Propantheline Bromide Tablets: 15 mg; generic; (Rx) have been discontinued.

References

For the complete list of references, see **wiley.com/go/budde/plumb**

Propionibacterium Acnes Injection

(**proe**-pee-nuh-ohe-bak-**ter**-ee-um **ak**-nees) *ImmunoRegulin®, EqStim®*

Immunostimulant

Prescriber Highlights

- ► Indicated as adjunct treatment for canine pyoderma and equine respiratory disease complex; anecdotally used for canine viral papillomatosis, FeLV, and feline herpes infections
- ► Contraindications include hypersensitivity, cardiac dysfunction, and canine lymphoma or leukemia with CNS involvement.
- ► Adverse effects include lethargy, hyperthermia, chills, and anorexia. Anaphylactic reactions are possible.
- ► Extravasation may cause local tissue inflammation.

Uses/Indications

Propionibacterium acnes is a USDA-licensed immunostimulant indicated in dogs as adjunct treatment for controlling and reducing lesions of chronic recurring pyoderma.[1] In horses, it is indicated for adjunctive treatment of equine respiratory disease complex (ERDC).[2]

Anecdotally, *P acnes* may be of benefit as a treatment for canine papillomatosis.[3] It has also been used anecdotally in the adjunctive treatment of canine oral melanoma and mastocytoma. *P acnes* injection has been used as an immunostimulant for the adjunctive treatment of feline rhinotracheitis (feline herpesvirus-1) and feline leukemia virus-induced disease. Controlled studies documenting efficacy for these potential indications were not located.

A study in neonatal foals less than 30 days old did not demonstrate any effect from *P acnes* injection on interferon-gamma production.[4] Another study in neonatal foals exposed ex vivo to *Rhodococcus equi* had similar negative effects on interferon-gamma, but treated foals did have significantly less intracellular proliferation of *R equi* within monocyte-derived macrophages on day 12 compared to control foals.[5] Another study showed that *P acnes* administration had no effect on the incidences of nasal shedding of respiratory pathogens or other clinical parameters in 21 weaning pony foals; however, it did appear to modulate rises in cortisol after weaning and possibly enhance innate immunity.[6]

Pharmacology/Actions

Propionibacterium acnes products are nonspecific immunostimulants derived from nonviable *P acnes*, a gram-positive anaerobic bacterium currently known as *Cutibacterium acnes*. They induce macrophage activation and lymphokine production, increase natural killer cell activity, enhance cell-mediated immunity, and display oncolytic properties. They may not provide protection against direct infection or transmission of respiratory pathogens, but they may contribute to the reduction of the disease severity, subsequently reducing the frequency of complications and improving the rate of recovery.[7]

Pharmacokinetics

No information was noted.

Contraindications/Precautions/Warnings

Propionibacterium acnes injection is contraindicated in patients that are hypersensitive to it and should not be used in patients with cardiac conditions.[1] It should not be used in dogs that have lymphoma or leukemia with CNS involvement. Glucocorticoids should be discontinued at least 7 days prior to starting *P acnes* treatment.[1,2]

Anaphylactic reactions can occur and should be treated with epinephrine.[1]

Adverse Effects

Adverse effects include lethargy, increased body temperature, chills, and anorexia, which can occur within hours after injection.[1,2] Anaphylactic reactions have also been reported. Injection extravasation may cause local tissue inflammation. Pain at the injection site is possible, particularly with larger volumes and repeated administration. In these cases, administration may be divided into different muscle sites.

Long-term toxicity studies have demonstrated vomiting, anorexia, malaise, fever, acidosis, increased water consumption, and hepatitis.

Reproductive/Nursing Safety

Propionibacterium acnes immunostimulant is not recommended for use during pregnancy or when pregnancy is suspected.[1,2]

Overdose/Acute Toxicity

No overdose information was noted.

For patients that have experienced or are suspected to have experienced an overdose, consultation with a 24-hour poison consultation center specializing in providing veterinary-specific information is recommended. For general information related to overdose and toxin exposures, as well as contact information for poison control centers, refer to ***Appendix***.

Drug Interactions

The following drug interactions have either been reported or are theoretical in humans or animals receiving *Propionibacterium acnes* and may be of significance in veterinary patients. Unless otherwise noted, use together is not necessarily contraindicated, but weigh the potential risks and perform additional monitoring when appropriate.

- **Glucocorticoids** (eg, **dexamethasone, prednis(ol)one**): Immunostimulant effects may be compromised if given concomitantly; discontinue glucocorticoid therapy at least 7 days prior to starting P acnes treatment.[1,2]
- **Immunosuppressants** (eg, **azathioprine, cyclosporine, mycophenolate**): Immunostimulant effects may be compromised if given concomitantly.

Dosages

DOGS:

Adjunct treatment for chronic recurring pyoderma (label dosage; USDA-approved): Administer IV according to body weight twice weekly for the first 2 weeks, then once weekly until week 12, then once monthly until clinical signs abate or stabilize.[1] Shake well before use.

***ImmunoRegulin*® Recommended Dosage**

Body weight in kg (lb)	IV dose/dog (NOT mL/kg [lb])
Up to 6.8 (15)	0.25 mL
6.8-20.4 (15-45)	0.5 mL
20.4-34 (45-75)	1 mL
34 (75) or greater	2 mL

Adjunctive treatment for severe cases of oral and cutaneous viral papillomatosis (extra-label): 2 mg/dog (NOT mg/kg) as a deep IM injection every 5 to 7 days. Repeat until regression of lesions occurs; may take 6 doses for complete resolution. Dose may be divided into different muscle sites if pain at the injection site is noted.[3]

CATS:

Immunostimulant for adjunctive treatment of FeLV and feline herpesvirus infections (extra-label):

a) **For a 2.3 kg (5 lb) cat**: Anecdotally, give 0.25 mL/cat (NOT mL/kg) IV or IP twice weekly for 2 weeks, then once weekly until remission, then once monthly to maintain clinical improvement.

b) **For a 4.5 kg (10 lb) cat**: Anecdotally, give 0.5 mL/cat (NOT mL/kg) IV or IP twice weekly for 2 weeks, then once weekly for

3 weeks, then once monthly for 2 months to maintain clinical improvement for a total of 9 injections. Some protocols suggest follow-up with injections once weekly for 20 weeks or longer as needed. Other clinicians suggest once-weekly dosing until clinical remission, then once-monthly administration. It has also been suggested to discontinue treatment after 12 weeks if no improvement is seen.

HORSES:

Immunostimulant for adjunctive therapy of equine respiratory disease complex (ERDC) (label dosage; USDA-approved):

a) **Foals**: 1 mL/foal (NOT mL/kg) IV; repeat dose on day 3 or 4, day 7, and weekly as needed[2]

b) **Adult horses**: 1 mL/114 kg (250 lb; NOT mL/kg) IV; repeat dose on day 3 or 4, day 7, and weekly as needed[2]

Adjunctive treatment to improve fertility in mares with endometritis (extra-label): 1 mL/114 kg (250 lb) IV on days 0, 2, and 6. Best results occur in mares bred 2 days before to 8 days after initial administration.[8,9]

Monitoring

- Efficacy
- Adverse effects (eg, lethargy, chills, fever, anorexia)

Chemistry/Synonyms

Propionibacterium acnes injection is an immunostimulant agent that contains nonviable *P acnes* suspended in 12.5% ethanol in saline.

P acnes may also be known as *Corynebacterium parvum* and *Cutibacterium acnes*; NSC-220537, *Arthrokehlan A*®, *Coparvax*®, *Corymunun*®, *EqStim*®, *Imunoparvum*®, and *ImmunoRegulin*®.

Storage/Stability

Store this product refrigerated; do not freeze. Shake well before using.

Dosage Forms/Regulatory Status

VETERINARY-LABELED PRODUCTS:

Propionibacterium acnes (nonviable) IV: 0.4 mg/mL in 5 mL vials; *ImmunoRegulin*®; (Rx). USDA-licensed biologic labeled for use in dogs

Propionibacterium acnes (nonviable) IV: 0.4 mg/mL in 5 mL and 50 mL vials; *EqStim*®; (Rx). USDA-licensed biologic labeled for use in horses

HUMAN-LABELED PRODUCTS: NONE

References

For the complete list of references, see **wiley.com/go/budde/plumb**

Propofol

(***proe***-poe-fol) *PropoFlo*®, *Diprivan*®, *Rapanofal*®

Injectable Anesthetic

Prescriber Highlights

- Injectable (IV) sedative-hypnotic anesthetic agent labeled for dogs and cats, extra-label in other species
- Rapid onset of action; titrated to effect
- Short duration of action so additional doses may be needed in unpremedicated patients transitioning to inhalants
- Rapid, smooth recoveries. Repeated doses in greyhounds and cats may cause prolonged anesthetic recovery; however, this is generally clinically insignificant.
- Adverse effects include transient respiratory depression, which is common but usually clinically tolerable, and vasodilation, which can be significant. Apnea is also possible, especially if given too rapidly.
- Debilitated patients generally require lower doses of propofol and may experience exaggerated cardiovascular and respiratory depression.
- No analgesia is provided.
- Lower doses are needed when premedications (eg, alpha-2 agonists, opioids) and/or co-induction agents (eg midazolam, ketamine) are used.
- Continuous monitoring is required; respiratory and cardiovascular support must be readily available.

Uses/Indications

In dogs and cats, propofol's labeled indications are for use as a single injection to provide general anesthesia for short procedures; induction and maintenance of anesthesia, using incremental doses to effect, for short periods of up to 20 minutes; or induction of general anesthesia in which maintenance is provided by inhalant anesthetics.

In both dogs and cats, the dose to achieve induction of general anesthesia can be significantly reduced when used in combination with premedications, such as an opioid and/or alpha-2 agonists and acepromazine.[1] Co-administration with a benzodiazepine or ketamine also decreases the propofol dose.

For relatively short procedures, propofol can be used as a CRI for total intravenous anesthesia (TIVA) beyond 20 minutes, especially when inhalants may be contraindicated to maintain general anesthesia; however, it is important to note that propofol does not provide analgesia. The dose required to maintain dogs under general anesthesia and propofol minimum infusion rate (MIR) can be reduced when midazolam or ketamine, but not systemic lidocaine, are added to the induction protocol.[2,3] Propofol combined with ketamine for induction and TIVA in dogs increases heart rate and blood pressure, causes respiratory depression, and has no difference in recovery quality as compared with propofol given alone.[4]

Propofol is also used to treat refractory status epilepticus, as it tends to cause less cardiovascular depression and respiratory depression as compared with barbiturates, and recovery can be smoother and shorter than with pentobarbital; however, apnea is possible and supplemental oxygen and ventilatory support should be readily available.

Propofol may be safely used in animals with liver or renal disease and mild to moderate cardiac disease.

Propofol administered to dogs prior to chemical euthanasia with pentobarbital/phenytoin did not require a change in the euthanasia dose or reduce the incidence of adverse events, other than a significant decrease in perimortem muscle activity, related to euthanasia.[5] However, injection of propofol prior to administration of euthanasia solution is clinically perceived to decrease perimortem muscle activity (eg, paddling, involuntary movement and fasciculations) and agonal breathing and is a commonly used technique in both dogs and cats. Sedation or anesthesia is recommended prior to euthanasia.[6]

Pharmacology/Actions

Propofol is a short-acting sedative-hypnotic injectable anesthetic unrelated to other general anesthetic agents. The mechanism of action is similar to barbiturates. Propofol potentiates the effects of gamma-aminobutyric acid (GABA; an inhibitory neurotransmitter) by decreasing the rate of dissociation of GABA from its receptors. This prolonged binding results in an influx of chloride, causing hyperpolarization of the postsynaptic cell membrane. Propofol may also have activity at the glycine and *N*-methyl-D-aspartate (NMDA) receptors, but this is unclear.

In dogs and cats, propofol produces rapid, smooth, and excitement-free anesthesia induction in 20 to 60 seconds when administered IV slowly (ie, over 60 to 90 seconds) with a duration of ≈10 minutes following a single injection. Time to unconsciousness may be longer (up to 2 minutes) in patients with low cardiac output states and the drug should be slowly titrated to effect. Subanesthetic doses produce sedation, restraint, and an unawareness of surroundings. Anesthetic dosages produce unconsciousness and muscle relaxation.

During induction of general anesthesia, propofol can cause a dose-dependent decrease in systemic vascular resistance without increased heart rate, which causes transient vasodilatory hypotension; decreased cardiac output is possible (especially in combination with opioid premedications). Propofol does not appear to be arrhythmogenic at clinical doses, but it can enhance the ability of epinephrine to induce arrhythmias.[7] Propofol causes significant respiratory depression, particularly with rapid administration or high doses. The drug does not precipitate malignant hyperthermia.

Propofol decreases cerebral oxygen consumption, intracranial pressure, and cerebral perfusion pressure.[8] This is an advantage when used to treat patients with intracranial disease, including seizures, tumors, hydrocephalus, and traumatic brain injury.

In dogs, propofol can cause an initial increase in intraocular pressure (IOP),[9] which decreases below baseline values 5 minutes after induction[10]; muscle-relaxing premedication[11] or gabapentin[12] may blunt propofol-induced increases in IOP. IOP did not change in dogs with glaucoma that received propofol for anesthetic induction.[11] The drug minimally (8%) increased IOP in horses[13] but does not appear to increase IOP in sheep.[14]

Recoveries are smooth. Recoveries are documented to be longer in greyhounds (effects in other sighthounds are unknown) and cats as compared with dogs.[15,16]

Pharmacokinetics

After IV administration, propofol rapidly crosses the blood–brain barrier and has an onset of action usually within 1 to 2 minutes. Speed of induction depends on drug dose, delivery rate, and patient cardiac output. Propofol is preferentially distributed into highly perfused tissues and is highly bound to plasma proteins (95% to 99%). In dogs, the steady state volume of distribution is greater than 3 L/kg.[17]

In dogs, the duration of action after a single IV induction dose lasts ≈5 to 7 minutes and ≈2 to 6 minutes following maintenance doses. In cats, the duration of action after induction and maintenance doses is 5 to 12 minutes and 5 to 7 minutes, respectively. Propofol's short duration of action is principally due to its rapid redistribution from the CNS to other tissue. The drug is rapidly and almost completely biotransformed in the liver via glucuronide conjugation (predominantly) and hydroxylation to inactive metabolites, which are then excreted primarily by the kidneys. In dogs, the elimination half-life is ≈1.4 hours, and clearance is ≈50 mL/kg/minute.[17] Canine CYP2B11 may be the isoenzyme responsible for propofol metabolism in dogs. Plasma clearance exceeds hepatic blood flow, suggesting extrahepatic metabolism.[18] In humans, propofol may accumulate in tissue during prolonged infusion (ie, over several days), with slower clearance and elimination half-life.

The addition of 2% benzyl alcohol (as found in *PropoFlo® 28*) does not appear to significantly alter propofol pharmacokinetics or pharmacodynamics (single-dose induction) in cats.[19]

Contraindications/Precautions/Warnings

Propofol is contraindicated in animals hypersensitive to it or any component of the product, including eggs and soybeans, and it should not be used in animals in which general anesthesia or sedation is contraindicated.

Propofol does not provide analgesia; peri-, intra-, and postoperative analgesics should be considered.

Theoretically, recoveries from propofol could be slower in cats as the drug is metabolized in part by glucuronidation and cats have a lower glucuronidation capacity; however, slow recovery times have only been reported after propofol infusions of longer than 30 minutes, leading to the recommendation that infusions be of short duration in cats.[15] A benzyl alcohol-containing formulation of propofol (ie, *PropoFlo® 28*) is only labeled for use in dogs in the US but has been shown to be safe in cats.[20] In addition, the benzyl alcohol-containing propofol formulation available in the EU/UK is approved for anesthetic induction or short-duration use in both species.[21]

As with all anesthetics, continuous monitoring and readily available respiratory and cardiovascular support are recommended.

Patients that are debilitated will generally require lower doses of propofol and may experience exaggerated cardiovascular and respiratory depression.

Propofol may have both anticonvulsant and seizure-causing properties. Theoretically it should be used with caution in animals with a history of or active seizure disorders; however, propofol-induced seizures are rare and propofol is commonly used to treat seizures[22] and as an anesthetic to study dogs with seizures.[23] Thus, propofol is often a component of the anesthetic protocol in patients with a history of seizures.

Propofol should be used with caution in patients with pre-existing cardiac arrhythmias,[24,25] as propofol has demonstrated both proarrhythmic and antiarrhythmic effects.[26] Anecdotally, it has been safely used in dogs with pre-existing arrhythmias.

A decrease in the dose of ≈40% to 60% (from the single-agent dose) should be anticipated in cases in which propofol is used in combination with other CNS depressants (eg, acepromazine, opioids, diazepam), especially in debilitated or critically ill animals or those with moderate to severe cardiac disease. A reduction in dose should also be anticipated in animals with poor body condition due to a potential for decreased volume of distribution. Induction of general anesthesia with propofol in overweight dogs may occur at lower doses than in normal weight dogs.[27]

A study in dogs found that propofol administered before midazolam resulted in less benzodiazepine-induced excitation and a greater reduction of total propofol requirements than when midazolam was administered before propofol.[28] With this technique, ≈1 mg/kg of propofol is administered slowly followed by the total dose of midazolam or diazepam. Once the patient is relaxed (1 to 2 minutes), the remainder of the propofol is slowly titrated until the patient is anesthetized to a depth that allows smooth intubation.

Greyhounds metabolize propofol more slowly than beagles or crossbreed dogs, potentially resulting in prolonged recovery; however, prolonged recovery is more likely with multiple repeat doses or infusions and generally does not occur with 1 to 2 propofol boluses for anesthesia induction, especially if followed by inhalants as the propofol has time to undergo metabolism. Slow metabolism of propofol in greyhounds is due to decreased cytochrome P450 (CYP) 2B11 gene expression.[29,30] Interestingly, American Kennel Club greyhounds have greater deficiency compared to racing greyhounds.[29] In addition, caution should be used when extrapolating greyhound information to other breeds as not all sighthounds had a deficiency whereas some other breeds of dogs were deficient.

Theoretically, as propofol is highly bound to plasma proteins, animals with hypoproteinemia may be susceptible to adverse effects; this interaction has not been shown to be of clinical concern.

Theoretically the benefits of propofol should be weighed against risks in animals with a history of hyperlipidemia; however, use of propofol did not increase morbidity or fatalities in cats with primary hepatic lipidosis undergoing anesthesia for placement of feeding tubes.[31]

Adverse Effects

Transient respiratory depression is common but usually clinically tolerable. However, because there is a relatively high incidence of apnea with occasional cyanosis if propofol is given rapidly, the drug should be given slowly. Treatment of apnea is endotracheal intubation and assisted ventilation until spontaneous ventilation resumes. The incidence of hypoxemia can increase when combined with opioids (eg, alfentanil).[32] One study in cats premedicated with medetomidine showed that alfaxalone had less adverse influence on respiration as compared with propofol[33]; however, most studies report that propofol and alfaxalone have similar cardiovascular and respiratory effects. There were no differences in cardiopulmonary parameters or apnea in dogs induced with propofol, alfaxalone, or ketamine/diazepam.[34] Respiratory depression following induction is more common when either drug is administered rapidly IV.[35] Following premedication with dexmedetomidine and methadone, propofol administered at 4 mg/kg/minute caused apnea in 100% of dogs, whereas propofol at 1 mg/kg/minute caused apnea in 25%.[36] In addition, slow administration also resulted in a lower induction dose needed to achieve endotracheal intubation.[37]

Propofol can cause histamine release in some animals and anaphylactoid reactions, although rare, have been noted.[38] Propofol can cause direct myocardial depression, arrhythmias, and hypotension. In dogs, the number of interventions needed to deepen the plane of anesthesia or treat hemodynamic depression is significantly lower with propofol as compared with inhalant anesthesia (eg, isoflurane).[39] A study in dogs premedicated with methadone and acepromazine showed a drop in arterial pressure in cases in which propofol was used for induction, but cardiac output was maintained by compensatory chronotropic response.[40]

Propofol combined with a benzodiazepine can cause hypothermia and longer time to return to preanesthetic temperature than in animals induced with ketamine combined with a benzodiazepine.[41]

Dogs may occasionally exhibit seizure-like clinical signs (eg, paddling, opisthotonus, myoclonic twitching) during induction that, if persistent, may be treated with a benzodiazepine (eg, diazepam, midazolam), low-dose ketamine, or paralytic agent (eg, atracurium); the mechanism of action is unknown and it occurs in ≈1.2% of dogs.[42] Sneezing and paddling during recovery has also been observed in dogs and cats.

A potentially clinically significant increase in IOP may occur in dogs following induction with propofol.[10,11,43] Increased IOP appears to be transient and may be mitigated with muscle-relaxing premedication (eg, midazolam[11]) or gabapentin.[12]

In cats, increased Heinz body production, prolonged recovery, anorexia, lethargy, malaise, and diarrhea have been noted (but do not occur commonly) in cases in which propofol has been used repeatedly or as a prolonged CRI.[44] Consecutive use in dogs appears to be safe.

Pain on injection has been reported in humans; dogs and cats very occasionally react to an IV propofol injection, but this does not appear to be a clinically significant problem in dogs or cats.[45] Extravasation of propofol injection is not irritating nor does it cause tissue sloughing.

Propofol infusion syndrome is a very rare complication reported in humans receiving prolonged administration of propofol. Neonates and sick patients appear to be at higher risk, and clinical signs include metabolic acidosis, rhabdomyolysis, hyperlipidemia, cardiac arrhythmia, and cardiac and renal failure.[46,47] A case of propofol infusion-like syndrome in a dog has been published.[48]

Reproductive/Nursing Safety

Propofol crosses the placenta, and its safe use during pregnancy has not been established. Fetal toxicity was not observed in studies with pregnant laboratory animals given propofol at clinical doses. In humans, brain development may be negatively affected by prolonged or repeated use of anesthetic or sedative drugs. The significance in dogs and cats has not been determined. Puppies delivered via C-section from bitches that received propofol generally had high Apgar scores, with the lowest Apgar scores occurring in cases in which extra propofol doses were required.[49] Apgar scores were higher when an alpha-2 agonist was used as a premedicant before propofol administration[49,50] or when an opioid epidural was used as part of the intraoperative analgesia.[51]

In humans, propofol is not recommended for use in nursing mothers because propofol is excreted in maternal milk, and the effects of oral absorption of small amounts of propofol are not known.[52] Should potentially be used with caution in nursing animals, however propofol is a common induction drug for dogs and cats undergoing cesarean sections with no clinical reports of adverse effects.

Overdose/Acute Toxicity

The LD_{50} in mice and rats given propofol IV is 53 mg/kg and 42 mg/kg, respectively.[53] Single doses of 19.5 mg/kg IV did not cause harm in dogs. A cumulative dose of 19.5 mg/kg IV in cats was tolerated, but 38.6 mg/kg produced prolonged recovery in all treated cats and paraesthesia in 1 cat.[54] Overdoses are likely to cause significant respiratory and cardiovascular depression.

Treatment should consist of discontinuation of propofol, artificial ventilation with oxygen after endotracheal intubation, and supportive care measures for cardiovascular depression (eg, IV fluids, vasopressors, anticholinergics) if necessary.

Drug Interactions

Propofol is a substrate of CYP2B6 in humans and CYP2B11 in dogs. Propofol has been used in association with anticholinergics, phenothiazines, alpha-2 agonists, opioids, and benzodiazepines, as well as inhalant anesthetics.[24,25] The following drug interactions have either been reported or are theoretical in humans or animals receiving propofol and may be of significance in veterinary patients. Unless otherwise noted, use together is not necessarily contraindicated, but weigh the potential risks and perform additional monitoring when appropriate.

- **Alpha-2-Adrenergic Receptor Agonists** (eg, **clonidine, dexmedetomidine, medetomidine**): Propofol given after medetomidine or dexmedetomidine may result in hypoxemia; a reduction in the propofol dose should be anticipated and respiratory monitoring and support available. Premedication with dexmedetomidine caused a dose-dependent decrease in the induction dose of propofol or barbiturates in dogs (30% to 61% reduction) and propofol in cats (48.9% reduction).[55]
- **Anesthetics, Inhalation** (eg, **isoflurane**): Propofol serum concentrations may be increased.
- **Anesthetics, Local** (eg, **bupivacaine, lidocaine**): Use of local anesthetics can reduce propofol dose requirements for sedation.

- **Benzodiazepines** (eg, **diazepam, midazolam**): Concurrent use has been shown to increase the risk for hypothermia in dogs.[41] Midazolam may have synergistic effects with propofol, and midazolam plasma concentrations may be increased up to 20%.
- **Drugs That Inhibit The Hepatic P-450 Enzyme System** (eg, **chloramphenicol,**[56] **cimetidine, ketoconazole**): May potentially prolong the recovery times associated with propofol; clinical significance is unclear
- **Epinephrine**: Propofol enhances epinephrine-induced arrhythmia in a dose-dependent manner in dogs.[7]
- **Melatonin**: Administration 2 hours prior to induction may modestly reduce the propofol dose required for intubation and anesthetic induction.[57]
- **Metoclopramide**: In humans, metoclopramide reduced the propofol dose required for induction by 20% to 25%.
- **Opioids** (eg, **fentanyl, hydromorphone, meperidine, morphine, remifentanil**): May increase the serum concentrations of the opioid and propofol if used together. Propofol dose requirements may be reduced. In dogs, fentanyl causes a small reduction in heart rate,[58] and remifentanil decreased heart rate, cardiac index, and stroke volume and increased systemic vascular resistance index, central venous pressure, and pulmonary artery occlusion pressure.[59]
- **Phenothiazines** (eg, **acepromazine**): Increased sedation and cardiorespiratory depression are possible.
- **St. John's Wort**: Concurrent use may result in an increased risk for cardiovascular collapse and/or delayed emergence from anesthesia.

Laboratory Considerations

None noted

Dosages

DOGS:

Label dosages

NOTES:

1. Product labels state clearly that all dosages are provided *for guidance only* and that individual animal response should dictate the dose used.
2. Because the label dosage is different for each of the veterinary products, the details listed below in the tables compile dosages from 3 veterinary-labeled propofol products.[24,25,60]
3. Use of premedications reduces propofol dose requirements.
   a) **Induction of general anesthesia** (label dosage; FDA approved): IV dosing should be titrated against the response of the animal over 30 to 60 seconds or until clinical signs show the onset of anesthesia. Rapid injection of propofol (ie, less than 5 seconds) may be associated with an increased incidence of apnea. An inadequate plane of anesthesia may occur if injected too slowly; additional propofol may need to be administered if this occurs. The average propofol induction dose rates for healthy dogs given propofol alone, or in cases in which propofol is preceded by a premedication, are indicated in the table, which should be used for guidance only.

   NOTE: Premedications reduce propofol requirements by 40% to 60%. As with other sedative-hypnotic agents, the amount of opioid and/or alpha-2 agonist premedication influences the animal's response to an induction dose of propofol. With premedications, the propofol dose may also need to be reduced with increasing age of the animal. During induction, additional low doses of propofol, similar to those used for maintenance with propofol, may be administered to facilitate intubation or the transition to inhalant maintenance anesthesia.

Induction Dosage Guidelines for *Dogs*[24,25,60]

Preanesthetic agent(s)	Propofol INDUCTION dose (mg/kg)	Propofol rate of administration (seconds)
None#†‡	5.5 – 7.6	40-90
Acepromazine#†	4 – 4.4† 3.7#	60-90 30-50
Xylazine†	2.2 – 3.3	60-90
Medetomidine†	2.2 – 2.8	60-90
Benzodiazepine + opioid‡	4.7	60-90
Acepromazine + opioid‡	4‡ 2.6#	60-90 30-50
Alpha-2 agonist + opioid‡	3.2	60-90

#*Propoflo*®, †*Rapanofal*®, ‡*Propoflo*® *28*

   b) **Maintenance of general anesthesia by intermittent IV propofol injection** (label dosage; FDA-approved): Anesthesia can be maintained by administering propofol in intermittent IV injections. The clinical response will be determined by the amount and frequency of maintenance injections. The following table is provided for guidance.

NOTE: Maintenance dose sparing was ≈48% with benzodiazepine and opioid preanesthesia and 37% in dogs preanesthetized with phenothiazine and an opioid.[25] Repeated maintenance doses of propofol do not result in increased recovery times or administration intervals, indicating the anesthetic effects of propofol are not cumulative.

Maintenance Dosage Guidelines Using Intermittent IV Propofol Injection for *Dogs*[24,25,60]

Preanesthetic agent(s)	Intermittent propofol MAINTENANCE dose (mg/kg)	Propofol rate of administration (seconds)
None	1.1 – 3.2	10 - 60
Acepromazine#†	1.1	30 - 60
Xylazine†	1.1	30 – 60
Medetomidine†	1.1	30 – 60
Benzodiazepine + opioid‡	1.7	60
Acepromazine + opioid#‡	2	30 – 60

#*Propofol*®,†*Rapanofal*®, ‡*Propoflo*® *28*

   c) **Maintenance by inhalant anesthetics** (label dosage; FDA approved): Because of the rapid metabolism of propofol, additional low doses of propofol (similar to those used for maintenance with propofol) may be required to complete the transition to inhalant maintenance anesthesia.[24,25] Because of the rapid recovery from propofol, clinical trials using propofol have shown higher initial concentrations of the inhalant anesthetic halothane may be needed than is usually required following induction using barbiturate anesthetics.[57]

Extra-label dosages

NOTE: There are many extra-label drug combinations for induction and maintenance of anesthesia using propofol. The following are representative, but not necessarily inclusive; it is suggested to refer to a recent anesthesia reference.[61,62]

Anesthetic induction (extra-label): 30 minutes after IM premedication (ie, methadone/acepromazine or methadone/dexmedetomidine), propofol 1 – 1.3 mg/kg/minute IV infusion safely and effectively replaced propofol bolus 4 mg/kg IV to facilitate intubation and reduced overall propofol requirements in healthy dogs.[37,63]

Total intravenous anesthesia (TIVA) maintenance (extra-label):

a) Propofol for induction is dosed to effect. Most clinicians recommend between 2 – 8 mg/kg IV slowly (over ≈60 seconds) to effect. Preanesthetic medications can reduce propofol requirements for induction by 25% or more. Using propofol to maintain general anesthesia: 0.1 – 0.5 mg/kg/minute IV CRI.
b) A study in healthy dogs undergoing ovariohysterectomy (OHE) compared propofol with alfaxalone.[64] Dogs received acepromazine 0.01 mg/kg and morphine 0.4 mg/kg SC ≈30 minutes prior to general anesthesia. Induction was performed with propofol ≈6 mg/kg IV over ≈40 seconds to effect. Using propofol to maintain general anesthesia: 0.3 – 0.5 mg/kg/minute IV CRI.
c) Propofol for induction (dosed to effect) 6.5 mg/kg IV slowly; premedication that includes an alpha-2 agonist may reduce the propofol dose by as much as 85%. Using propofol to maintain general anesthesia (dosed to effect): 0.25 – 0.5 mg/kg/minute IV[62]

Refractory status epilepticus (extra-label): 2 – 8 mg/kg IV bolus, followed by 0.1 – 0.25 mg/kg/minute IV CRI.[22] The propofol dose should be kept as low, and duration of treatment kept as short, as possible. Infusion should be maintained for 6 to 12 hours and then gradually decreased. The maximum duration of propofol CRI is ≈48 hours.

CATS:

__Label dosages__

a) **Induction of general anesthesia** (label dosage; FDA-approved): The average propofol induction dose ranges and rates for healthy cats given propofol alone, or in cases in which propofol is preceded by a premedication, are indicated in the table, which should be used for guidance only. The dose and rate should be based on animal response. Preanesthetic agent and dose influences the animal's response to an induction dose of propofol. The induction dose will also be influenced by the interval between the administration of premedication and induction and by the rate of administration of propofol.

NOTE: Many clinicians consider the labeled propofol dosages to be higher than necessary. Expect larger dose reductions than are indicated in this table when premedicants are used.

Induction Dosage Guidelines for *Cats*[60]

Preanesthetic agent(s)	Propofol INDUCTION dose (mg/kg)	Propofol rate of administration (seconds)
None	8 – 13.2	60-90
Acepromazine	8 – 13.2	60-90
Butorphanol	8 – 13.2	60-90
Oxymorphone	8 – 13.2	60-90
Xylazine	7 – 12	60-90

b) **Maintenance of general anesthesia by __intermittent__ IV propofol injection for *cats*** (label dosage; FDA-approved): Anesthesia can be maintained by administering propofol in intermittent IV injections. The clinical response will be determined by the amount, rate of administration, and frequency of maintenance injections. The following table is provided for guidance.

NOTE: Repeated maintenance doses of propofol do not result in increased recovery times or administration intervals, indicating that the anesthetic effects of propofol are not cumulative in cats.[60]

Maintenance of General Anesthesia by __Intermittent__ IV Propofol Injection for *Cats*[60]:

Preanesthetic agent(s)	__Intermittent__ propofol MAINTENANCE dose (mg/kg)	Propofol rate of administration (seconds)
None	1.1 – 4.4	30-60
Acepromazine	1.1 – 4.4	30-60
Butorphanol	1.1 – 4.4	30-60
Oxymorphone	1.1 – 4.4	30-60
Xylazine	1.1 – 2.2	30-60
Acepromazine + butorphanol	1.1 – 3.3	30-60
Acepromazine + opioid	1.1 – 3.3	30-60

c) **Maintenance by inhalant anesthetics** (label dosage; FDA-approved): Because of the rapid recovery from propofol injections, clinical trials using propofol have shown higher initial concentrations of the inhalant anesthetic may be needed than is usually required following induction using barbiturate anesthetics.[60]

__Extra-label dosages:__

Anesthetic induction and total intravenous anesthesia maintenance:

a) Propofol for induction is dosed to effect. Most recommend a dose between 2 – 8 mg/kg IV slowly (over ≈60 seconds) to effect.[65-67] Induction doses as high as 11.7 mg/kg have been used.[33] Preanesthetic medications can reduce propofol requirements for induction by 25% (or more). General anesthesia can be maintained with 0.1 – 0.5 mg/kg/minute IV CRI.[33] **NOTE:** Cats may be susceptible to long recoveries when propofol is used alone as a CRI, or with continuous, prolonged exposure.
b) 30 minutes after IM premedication, propofol 1 mg/kg/minute IV infusion facilitated intubation and resulted in a lower propofol induction dose (≈5.3 mg/kg IV) and slower anesthetic induction (≈5.5 minutes) as compared with a rapid propofol bolus (induction dose ≈8 mg/kg IV, induction time ≈2.3 minutes) in healthy female cats undergoing OHE.[68]
c) **Propofol/Ketamine TIVA**: In cats undergoing OHE, anesthesia was induced with a combination of propofol 2 mg/kg and ketamine 2 mg/kg administered IV ± dexmedetomidine 3 µg/kg IV.[69] Anesthesia was maintained with propofol 10 mg/kg/hour IV CRI and ketamine 10 mg/kg/hour IV CRI. Short-term infusions produced smooth recovery and adequate analgesia during the postoperative period. The number of RBCs with Heinz bodies was not increased. **NOTE**: Although both ketamine and dexmedetomidine provide analgesia, a more potent analgesic (eg, opioid, local anesthetic) is recommended as an addition to this protocol for clinical use.[70]

Refractory status epilepticus (extra-label): 2 – 8 mg/kg IV initial bolus, followed by 0.1 – 0.25 mg/kg/minute IV CRI.[22] The propofol dose should be kept as low, and duration of treatment as short as possible. Infusion should be maintained for 6 to 12 hours and then gradually decreased.

HORSES:

NOTE: Use of propofol as a single agent (ie, without premedication or co-induction agent) for anesthesia induction typically results in poor induction quality.[71]

Induction of general anesthesia using ketamine and propofol after xylazine sedation (extra-label): In a retrospective study (n = 100), all horses were sedated with xylazine 0.99 ± 0.2 mg/kg IV; some horses also received IV butorphanol.[72] After visually apparent sedation, a combination of propofol 0.4 ± 0.1 mg/kg and ketamine 2.8 ± 0.3 mg/kg were given via IV bolus. The order of administration was not standardized, and in some cases, the 2 drugs were mixed together before administration. Following induction, 6 horses required a one-time administration of additional ketamine 0.7 ± 0.4 mg/kg. Anesthesia was maintained with GKX (ie, guaifenesin/ketamine/xylazine) in 34 horses and isoflurane in oxygen in 66 horses. Anesthetic recoveries were satisfactory.

Maintenance of general anesthesia (extra-label):

a) Propofol 0.5 mg/kg IV loading dose, followed by propofol 0.2 mg/kg/minute with ketamine 1 mg/kg/hour and medetomidine 1.25 µg/kg/hour IV CRI provided satisfactory quality and control of anesthesia with minimal cardiovascular depression for ≈175 minutes.[73]

b) **Arthroscopic surgery**: propofol 8 mg/kg/hour with dexmedetomidine 1.5 µg/kg/hour and ketamine 1 mg/kg/hour IV[74]

c) **Adjuvant during inhalant anesthesia** (extra-label): propofol 3 mg/kg/hour with medetomidine 1.25 – 3 µg/kg/hour IV CRI significantly decreases the amount of isoflurane[75] or sevoflurane[76] required for general anesthesia, improves stability of blood pressure, and provides good quality of recovery.

d) **Alternative to GKX** (extra-label): Following sedation with xylazine and induction with ketamine, propofol 0.05 to 0.1 mg/kg/minute IV CRI with xylazine 0.016 mg/kg/minute IV CRI and ketamine 0.03 mg/kg/minute IV CRI[77]

DONKEYS:

Maintenance of general anesthesia (extra-label):

a) After premedication with xylazine 1 mg/kg IV and induction with ketamine 1.5 mg/kg and propofol 0.5 mg/kg IV, giving propofol 0.15 mg/kg/minute with ketamine 0.05 mg/kg/minute IV CRI produced a stable plane of anesthesia. Hypoxemia was noted during the study, but no other cardiorespiratory complications were recorded.[78]

b) After premedication with acepromazine 0.04 mg/kg IV and induction with propofol 2 mg/kg IV, donkeys were maintained with propofol 0.2 mg/kg/minute IV CRI. This protocol provided good cardiovascular stability.[79]

SHEEP, GOATS:

General anesthesia (goats) (extra-label): Induction dose 3 – 7 mg/kg IV is smooth and rapid, but myoclonic activity of the face or limbs may occur; anesthesia lasts 5 to 10 minutes and is suitable for endotracheal intubation. Anesthesia can be maintained with 0.3 – 0.6 mg/kg/minute IV CRI.[80]

ALPACAS:

Induction of general anesthesia (extra-label): 3.3 mg/kg IV was sufficient to achieve an adequate plane of anesthesia to allow tracheal intubation.[81]

RABBITS, RODENTS, SMALL MAMMALS:

Rabbits:

a) 5 – 14 mg/kg IV slow to effect or 20 mg/kg/minute IV CRI; not recommended as the sole agent for maintenance

b) **Maintenance of anesthesia**: propofol 0.6 – 0.8 mg/kg/minute alone[82,83] or combined with sufentanil 0.033 mg/kg/minute IV.[84] The sufentanil combination resulted in a significant drop in blood pressure.

c) Propofol 5 mg/kg IV admixed in same syringe with ketamine 5 mg/kg produced a smooth anesthetic induction; hypoxemia, respiratory depression, and apnea were observed[85]

Mice: 26 mg/kg IV

Rats: 10 mg/kg IV

REPTILES:

Sedation/Anesthesia (extra-label):

Chelonians: *Sedation*: 2 – 5 mg/kg IV (also provides light anesthesia)[86]; *Anesthesia*: 2 – 10 mg/kg IV[86-88]

Lizards: *Sedation*: 3 – 5 mg/kg IV or IO[86,87]; *Anesthesia*: 5 to 10 mg/kg IV, IO[87,89]

Snakes: *Sedation*: 3 – 5 mg/kg IV [90]; *Anesthesia*: 3-10 mg/kg IV, IC[86]

Anesthesia induction (extra-label): 5 – 15 mg/kg IV or IO; in snakes, intracardiac route is usually used[91]

Monitoring

- Depth of anesthesia and CNS effects (eg, excitement, paddling, myoclonus)
- Respiratory effects (eg, respiratory rate, pulse oximetry (SpO_2), end-tidal CO_2 ($ETCO_2$)
- Cardiovascular effects (eg, heart rate and rhythm; blood pressure)
- Cats: CBC to check for Heinz body anemia with repeated exposure

Chemistry/Synonyms

Propofol is an alkylphenol derivative (2,6-diisopropylphenol). Commercially available 1% injections are isotonic, milky white macroemulsions, containing soybean oil, glycerol, and egg lecithin.

Propofol products are not identical; some contain oleic acid. *Propoflo® 28* is preserved with benzyl alcohol. Disodium edetate is the antimicrobial agent in *Diprivan®*, but human generic products use either sodium metabisulfite or benzyl alcohol. *Propoflo® 28, Diprivan®*, and the generic human propofol with benzyl alcohol have a pH range of 7 to 8.5. In products that use sodium metabisulfite, pH is adjusted to ≈4.5 to 6.5.

Propofol may also be known as disoprofol, ICI-35868, propofolum, *Ansiven®*, *Bioprofol®*, *Cryotol®*, *Diprivan®*, *Diprofol®*, *PropoFlo®*, *Propoflo® Plus*, *Propothesia®*, *Propovan®*, *Provive®*, *Rapinovet®*, or *Recofol®*.

Storage/Stability

NOTE: Storage varies by manufacturer and product. Consult the product label to ensure proper storage. Do *not* confuse storage of PropoFlo® with that of PropoFlo® 28. For all products, store protected from light; do not freeze. Shake the vial thoroughly before opening. Do not use if there is evidence of excessive creaming or aggregation, if large droplets are visible, or if there are other forms of phase separation indicating the stability of the product has been compromised. Slight creaming, which should disappear after shaking, may be visible after prolonged standing. Do not use if particulate matter and discoloration are present. Do not use if contamination is suspected.

PropoFlo® 28: Store at room temperature. Open vials should be placed in a covered container, stored at room temperature, and discarded after 28 days.[25]

Other veterinary-labeled products: Store between 4°C to 25°C (40°F-77°F) but not below 4°C (40°F). Unused product should be discarded within 6 hours of opening.

Human-labeled products: Store below 22°C (72°F) but not below 4°C (40°F). The manufacturer recommends discarding any unused portion at the end of the anesthetic procedure or after 12 hours of opening, whichever occurs first. If using inline filters, do not use sizes less than 5 µm.

Compatibility/Compounding Considerations

Propofol labels state: *The emulsion should not be mixed with other therapeutic agents or into infusion fluids prior to administration.*

Propofol (macroemulsion; *Diprivan*® human-label product): If dilution is necessary, only dilute with dextrose 5% injection, and do not dilute to a concentration of less than 2 mg/mL. In diluted form, the drug is more stable when in contact with glass than with plastic (95% potency after 2 hours of running infusion in plastics).

Propofol macroemulsion (human-label) is physically **compatible** with the commonly used IV solutions (eg, lactated Ringer's solution (LRS), D_5W) when injected into a running IV line.

Drugs that are reported to be **compatible** with propofol (macroemulsion) at Y-site administration include (partial listing): alfentanil, ampicillin, butorphanol, calcium gluconate, cefazolin, cefoxitin, clindamycin, dexamethasone sodium phosphate, dexmedetomidine, diphenhydramine, esmolol, fentanyl, furosemide, glycopyrrolate, heparin sodium, insulin, isoproterenol, ketamine, lorazepam, magnesium sulfate, mannitol, midazolam, morphine sulfate, naloxone, nitroprusside sodium, norepinephrine, ondansetron, pentobarbital, phenobarbital, potassium chloride, propranolol, sodium bicarbonate, succinylcholine, thiopental, and vecuronium.

Drugs known to be **incompatible** with propofol at Y-site administration include amphotericin B, atracurium, calcium chloride, ceftazidime, diazepam, gentamicin, lidocaine (concentration dependent), methylprednisolone sodium succinate, metoclopramide, tobramycin, and verapamil. Refer to specialized references or a veterinary pharmacist for more information.

Dosage Forms/Regulatory Status

VETERINARY-LABELED PRODUCTS:

Propofol Injection: 10 mg/mL in 20 mL (single use) vials; *PropoFlo*®; (Rx). FDA-approved for use in dogs. NADA# 141-098

Propofol Injection: 10 mg/mL in 20 and 50 mL (multi-dose) vials; *Propoflo® 28*; (Rx). FDA-approved for use in dogs. NADA# 141-098

Propofol Injection: 10 mg/mL in 20 mL vials; *Rapanofal*®; *Propothesia*®; (Rx). FDA-approved for use in dogs and cats. NADA# 141-070

The Association of Racing Commissioners International (ARCI) has designated this drug as a class 2 substance. Use of this drug may not be allowed in certain animal competitions. Check rules and regulations before entering in a competition while this medication is being administered. Contact local racing authorities for further guidance. See ***Appendix*** for more information.

HUMAN-LABELED PRODUCTS:

Propofol Injectable Emulsion: 10 mg/mL in 20 mL amps and vials, 10 mL, 50 mL, and 100 mL vials; 50 mL and 100 mL infusion vials; and 50 mL prefilled single-use syringes; *Diprivan*®; generic; (Rx)

The Drug Enforcement Agency does not list propofol as a federally controlled substance, but it is regulated as a controlled drug in some states. Report dispensing to state monitoring programs where required.

References

For the complete list of references, see **wiley.com/go/budde/plumb**

Propranolol

(proe-***pran***-oh-lole) *Inderal*®

Beta-Adrenergic Antagonist

Prescriber Highlights

- Nonspecific beta-adrenergic antagonist primarily used in veterinary medicine as an antiarrhythmic agent. Sometimes used for short-term treatment of clinical signs associated with thyrotoxicosis or pheochromocytoma
- Contraindications include congestive heart failure (unless secondary to a tachyarrhythmia responsive to beta-adrenergic antagonist therapy), hypersensitivity to this class of agents, sinus bradycardia, second- or third-degree atrioventricular block, or bronchospastic lung disease.
- Use with caution in labile diabetic patients, digitalized or digitalis intoxicated patients, with significant renal or hepatic insufficiency, with first-degree heart block, or with sinus node dysfunction.
- Adverse effects include bradycardia, lethargy and depression, impaired AV conduction, CHF or worsening of heart failure, hypotension, syncope, diarrhea, hypoglycemia, and bronchoconstriction.
- If discontinuing drug, consider gradual withdrawal if it has been used chronically.
- Many potential drug interactions

Uses/Indications

In veterinary medicine, propranolol is used in small animal species and horses primarily for tachyarrhythmias or when a beta-blocker is indicated in a patient with a right-to-left shunt (eg, tetralogy of Fallot).

Propranolol has also been used for the short-term treatment of systemic hypertension and clinical signs associated with thyrotoxicosis and pheochromocytoma in small animal species,[1] although a cardioselective beta-1-adrenergic antagonist (eg, atenolol, esmolol) may be preferred if the effects of beta-2 blockade are not desired. Propranolol may also be useful in the management of beta-2-agonist (eg, albuterol, terbutaline) toxicity.[2,3] It has also been used in ferrets as adjunctive treatment of hypertrophic cardiomyopathy to prolong cardiac filling and decrease myocardial ischemia.[4]

Other beta-adrenergic antagonists have largely supplanted propranolol's use due to propranolol's poor oral bioavailability, short half-life, and nonspecificity.

Pharmacology/Actions

Propranolol blocks both beta-1- and beta-2-adrenergic receptors in the myocardium, bronchi, and vascular smooth muscle. Propranolol does not have any intrinsic sympathomimetic activity (ISA). Additionally, propranolol possesses membrane-stabilizing effects (quinidine-like) affecting the cardiac action potential and direct myocardial depressant effects. Cardiovascular effects secondary to propranolol include decreased sinus node rate, depressed conduction through the atrioventricular node, diminished cardiac output at rest and during exercise, decreased myocardial oxygen demand, decreased hepatic and renal blood flow, reduced systemic blood pressure, and inhibition of isoproterenol-induced tachycardia. Electrophysiologic effects on the heart include decreased automaticity, increased or no effect on effective refractory period, and no effect on conduction velocity.

The nonselective effects of propranolol may be beneficial in the setting of a right-to-left shunting ventricular septal defect (eg, tetralogy of Fallot) as blocking the beta-1-adrenergic receptor may limit hypercontraction of the right ventricle while the beta-2-adrenergic receptor blockade may limit peripheral vasodilation.[5]

Additional pharmacologic effects of propranolol include increased airway resistance (especially in patients with bronchoconstrictive disease), prevention of migraine headaches, increased uterine activity (more so in the nonpregnant uterus), decreased platelet aggregability, inhibited glycogenolysis in cardiac and skeletal muscle, and increased numbers of circulating eosinophils.

Propranolol has been proposed as adjunctive therapy for hyperthyroidism in cats due to its ability to inhibit the conversion of thyroxine (T_4) to triiodothyronine (T_3).[6]

Pharmacokinetics

Propranolol is well absorbed after oral administration, but a rapid first-pass effect through the liver reduces systemic bioavailability to ≈2% to 27% in dogs, thereby explaining the significant difference between PO and IV dosages. These values reportedly increase with chronic dosing. Hyperthyroid cats may have increased bioavailability of propranolol when compared with healthy cats.[7]

Propranolol is highly lipid soluble and readily crosses the blood-brain barrier. The apparent volume of distribution has been reported to be 3.3 to 11 L/kg in the dog. In horses receiving 1 mg/kg IV bolus, peak concentration, volume of distribution at steady state, and elimination half-life were 628 ng/mL, 3070 mL/kg, and 180 minutes, respectively.[8] In humans, propranolol is ≈90% bound to plasma proteins.

Propranolol is metabolized principally by the liver and the CYP2D15 isoenzyme is responsible for a significant percentage of its metabolism in dogs. An active metabolite, 4-hydroxypropranolol, has been identified after oral administration in humans. Less than 1% of a dose is excreted unchanged into the urine. The half-life has been reported to range from 0.77 to 2 hours in dogs, and less than 2 hours in horses. Hyperthyroid cats may have a decreased clearance of propranolol when compared with healthy cats.[7]

Contraindications/Precautions/Warnings

Propranolol is contraindicated in patients with hypersensitivity to this class of agents, second- or third-degree atrioventricular heart block, sick sinus syndrome, or sinus bradycardia. Nonspecific beta-blockers are also generally contraindicated in patients with CHF unless secondary to a tachyarrhythmia responsive to beta-blocker therapy. They are also contraindicated in patients with bronchospastic lung disease.

Propranolol should be used cautiously in patients with significant renal or hepatic insufficiency. In humans, it has been suggested to reduce dosage by 50% (or more) in patients with impaired renal or hepatic function. Patients with sinus node dysfunction, first degree atrioventricular block, or conduction disorders may be at increased risk for bradycardia (including sinus pause, heart block, and cardiac arrest).[9]

Propranolol given by the IV route is considered a high alert medication (medication that requires special safeguards to reduce the risk for errors). Consider instituting practices such as redundant drug dosage and volume checking and special alert labels.

Propranolol can mask tachycardia associated with hypoglycemia. It can also cause hypoglycemia or hyperglycemia and, therefore, should be used cautiously in labile diabetic patients.

Propranolol can mask the clinical signs associated with thyrotoxicosis.

Use propranolol cautiously with digoxin or in digoxin-intoxicated patients; severe bradycardia may result.

Adverse Effects

Clinically relevant adverse effects include bradycardia, lethargy and depression, impaired AV conduction, negative inotropy, CHF or worsening of heart failure, hypotension, hypoglycemia, and bronchoconstriction. Syncope and diarrhea have also been reported in canine patients. Adverse effects may be more likely in geriatric animals or those that have acute decompensating heart disease.

Exacerbations of clinical signs (eg, rebound hypertension, thyrotoxicosis) have been reported following abrupt cessation of beta-blockers in humans. Significance in veterinary patients is unclear but it is recommended to withdraw therapy gradually in patients that have been receiving the drug chronically.

Reproductive/Nursing Safety

Propranolol crosses the placenta and enters milk at very low concentrations. Because safety has not been established in animals, this drug should only be used when the maternal benefits outweigh the potential risks to offspring.

Overdose/Acute Toxicity

The predominant clinical signs of an overdose include hypotension and bradycardia. Other possible effects include CNS (eg, depressed consciousness, seizures), bronchospasm, hypoglycemia, hyperkalemia, respiratory depression, pulmonary edema, other arrhythmias (especially AV block), and asystole. Seizures are reported in humans but have not been reported in animals.

If overdose is secondary to a recent oral ingestion, GI decontamination and charcoal administration may be considered. Monitor patient's ECG, blood glucose, potassium, and blood pressure; treatment of cardiovascular and CNS effects are based on clinical presentation. Use IV fluids and/or vasopressor agents to treat hypotension. Bradycardia may be treated with atropine or isoproterenol; a transvenous pacemaker may be necessary. Glucagon 5 – 10 mg/hour IV (human dose) may increase heart rate and blood pressure and reduce the cardiodepressant effects of propranolol. Branchospasm may be treated with aminophylline or isoproterenol. Seizures will generally respond to diazepam IV. Intravenous lipid emulsion therapy may be beneficial.[10,11]

For patients that have experienced or are suspected to have experienced an overdose, consultation with a 24-hour poison consultation center specializing in providing veterinary-specific information is recommended. For general information related to overdose and toxin exposures, as well as contact information for poison control centers, refer to ***Appendix.***

Drug Interactions

The following drug interactions have either been reported or are theoretical in humans or animals receiving propranolol and may be of significance in veterinary patients. Unless otherwise noted, use together is not necessarily contraindicated, but weigh the potential risks and perform additional monitoring when appropriate.

- **Alpha-2-Adrenergic Agonists** (eg, **clonidine, dexmedetomidine, romifidine**): Concurrent administration may increase the degree of sedation but may also cause severe bradycardia. Concurrent use is not recommended.[8]
- **Amiodarone**: Concurrent use may increase risk for bradycardia, hypotension, sinus arrest, and AV block.
- **Anesthetic Agents, General**: Additive myocardial depression may occur with the concurrent use of propranolol and myocardial depressant anesthetic agents.
- **Anticholinergics** (eg, **atropine**): May negate bradycardic effects of beta-blockers
- **Beta-2-Adrenergic Agonists** (eg, **albuterol, terbutaline**): At higher doses, atenolol may impair bronchodilation.
- **Calcium Channel Blockers** (eg, **amlodipine,diltiazem, verapamil**): May increase risk of hypotension and bradycardia, and may precipitate heart failure in patients with pre-existing cardiac conditions
- **Cimetidine**: May decrease the metabolism of propranolol and increase propranolol blood concentrations
- **Digoxin**: Concurrent use may increase risk for bradycardia and digitalis toxicity.

- **Epinephrine, Norepinephrine**: Unopposed alpha-adrenergic agonist effects of epinephrine may lead to a rapid increase in blood pressure and decrease in heart rate.
- **Fluoxetine**: May decrease propranolol metabolism
- **Furosemide**: Concurrent use may increase risk for hypotension and bradycardia.
- **Hydrochlorothiazide**: Concurrent use may increase risk for hypotension, hyperglycemia, and hypertriglyceridemia.
- **Hypotensive Agents** (eg, **enalapril, telmisartan**): Concurrent use may increase the risk for hypotension.
- **Insulin** and other **Antidiabetic Drugs**: Propranolol may prolong the hypoglycemic effects of insulin therapy.
- **Local Anesthetics** (eg, **bupivacaine, lidocaine**): Clearance may be impaired by propranolol.
- **Methimazole**: Propranolol dosages may need to be decreased when initiating therapy.
- **Nonsteroidal Anti-Inflammatory Drugs** (eg, **carprofen, meloxicam, robenacoxib**): Concurrent use may decrease antihypertensive effect.
- **Phenobarbital**: May increase the metabolism of propranolol
- **Phenothiazines** (eg, **acepromazine, chlorpromazine**): May increase risk for hypotension
- **Quinidine**: Concurrent use may increase risk for hypotension, bradycardia, arrhythmias, and heart failure.
- **Reserpine**: May have additive effects with propranolol
- **Succinylcholine, Tubocurarine**: Effects may be enhanced with propranolol therapy
- **Sympathomimetics** (eg, **phenylpropanolamine**): May have their actions blocked by propranolol
- **Theophylline/Aminophylline**: Bronchodilatory effects may be blocked by propranolol.
- **Thyroid Hormones** (eg, **levothyroxine**): May decrease the effects of beta-blocking agents
- **Tricyclic Antidepressants** (eg, **amitriptyline, clomipramine**): Concurrent use may increase risk for postural hypotension. Amitriptyline may increase propranolol exposure.

Laboratory Considerations

None noted

Dosages

NOTE: Because of a high first-pass effect after oral dosing, IV dosages are ≈10% of oral dosages. Do not confuse the dosages.

DOGS:

Susceptible cardiac arrhythmias (extra-label):

a) IV dosage: 0.02 mg/kg IV slowly over 2 to 3 minutes, titrate dosage up to effect (to a maximum of 0.1 mg/kg). Can be repeated every 8 hours

b) Oral dosage: 0.1 – 0.2 mg/kg PO initially (practically 2.5 – 10 mg/dog [NOT mg/kg] PO) every 8 hours, titrated to effect up to a maximum of 1.5 mg/kg every 8 hours (practically 10 – 80 mg/dog [NOT mg/kg] PO every 8 hours)

Tetralogy of Fallot (extra-label): Initially 0.25 mg/kg PO every 8 hours, increase gradually to 1 mg/kg PO every 8 hours over 4 weeks[12]

Antihypertensive agent (extra-label): 0.2 – 1 mg/kg PO every 8 hours[1]

CATS:

Susceptible cardiac arrhythmias (extra-label):

a) IV dosage: 0.02 mg/kg IV slowly over 2 to 3 minutes, titrate dosage up to effect (to a maximum of 0.1 mg/kg). Can be repeated every 8 hours

b) Oral dosage: 2.5 – 10 mg/cat (NOT mg/kg) PO every 8 to 12 hours. Start at the low end of the dosage range and titrate to effect.

Tetralogy of Fallot (extra-label): Initially 0.25 mg/kg PO every 8 hours, increase gradually to 1 mg/kg PO every 8 hours over 4 weeks[12]

Antihypertensive agent (extra-label): 2.5 – 5 mg/cat (NOT mg/kg) PO every 8 hours[1]

Adjunctive treatment of severe thyrotoxicosis (extra-label):

a) IV dosage: 0.02 mg/kg IV slowly over 1 minute

b) Oral dosage: 2.5 – 5 mg/cat (NOT mg/kg) PO every 8 hours[5,13]

HORSES:

Refractory ventricular tachycardia and management of rapid ventricular response rate during quinidine therapy for atrial fibrillation (extra-label): 0.03 – 0.16 mg/kg IV or 0.38 – 0.78 mg/kg PO every 8 hours. Considered not as effective as lidocaine; decreases ventricular rate even if it does not restore sinus rhythm[14]

FERRETS:

Hypertrophic cardiomyopathy (extra-label): 0.5 – 2 mg/kg PO or SC once a day to twice a day

Monitoring

- Adverse effects (eg, CNS changes, bronchospasm, respiratory depression)
- Electrocardiogram to monitor heart rate and rhythm
- Blood pressure

Client Information

- Give this medicine as prescribed by your veterinarian.
- This medicine can be given with or without food.
- The most common side effects include tiredness/lack of energy and weakness. Contact your veterinarian if your animal becomes exercise-intolerant, has difficulty breathing, develops a cough, or has a change in behavior or attitude.
- When starting this medicine, your veterinarian may start with a low dose and gradually increase it over time to see how your animal reacts to it. Do not administer more than your veterinarian prescribes.
- Do not suddenly stop giving propranolol to your animal as it can make your animal's condition worse.
- Your veterinarian will need to monitor your animal closely while it is receiving this medicine. Do not miss these important follow-up visits.

Chemistry/Synonyms

A nonspecific beta-adrenergic blocking agent, propranolol HCl occurs as a bitter tasting, odorless, white to off-white powder with a pK_a of 9.45 and a melting point of ≈161°C (321°F). One gram of propranolol is soluble in ≈20 mL of water or alcohol. At a pH from 4 to 5, solutions of propranolol will fluoresce. The commercially available injectable solutions are adjusted with citric acid to a pH 2.8 to 3.5.

Propranolol may also be known as AY-64043, ICI-45520, NSC-91523, propranololi hydrochloridum; many trade names are available.

Storage/Stability

All propranolol preparations should be stored at room temperature (15°C-30°C [59°F-86°F]) and protected from light. Propranolol solutions will decompose rapidly at alkaline pH.

Compatibility/Compounding Considerations

Compatibility is dependent on factors such as pH, concentration, temperature, and diluent used; specialized references or a hospital pharmacist should be consulted for more specific information.

Propranolol injection is reported to be physically **compatible** with 5% dextrose, 0.9% sodium chloride, or lactated Ringer's injection. It is also physically **compatible** with dobutamine HCl and verapamil HCl.

Dosage Forms/Regulatory Status

VETERINARY-LABELED PRODUCTS: NONE

The Association of Racing Commissioners International (ARCI) has designated this drug as a class 3 substance. Use of this drug may not be allowed in certain animal competitions. Check rules and regulations before entering in a competition while this medication is being administered. Contact local racing authorities for further guidance. See ***Appendix*** for more information.

HUMAN-LABELED PRODUCTS:

Propranolol HCl Oral Tablets: 10 mg, 20 mg, 40 mg, 60 mg, and 80 mg; generic; (Rx)

Propranolol HCl Extended/Sustained-Release Capsules: 60 mg, 80 mg, 120 mg, and 160 mg; *Inderal® LA, Inderal XL®, InnoPran® XL*, generic; (Rx)

Propranolol for Injection: 1 mg/mL in 1 mL ampules or vials; *Inderal®*, generic; (Rx)

Propranolol Oral Solution: 4 mg/mL and 8 mg/mL in 500 mL; generic; (Rx)

References

For the complete list of references, see **wiley.com/go/budde/plumb**

Pseudoephedrine

(soo-doe-e-***fed***-rin) *Equiphed®, Sudafed®*

Sympathomimetic

Prescriber Highlights

- ► Oral sympathomimetic primarily used for urethral sphincter hypotonus. Therapeutic index is narrow in dogs; use is controversial.
- ► Contraindications include hypersensitivity and severe hypertension.
- ► Use with caution in patients with glaucoma, prostatic hypertrophy, hyperthyroidism, diabetes mellitus, cardiovascular disorders, or hypertension.
- ► Adverse effects include restlessness, irritability, hypertension, and anorexia.
- ► Restricted drug in the United States; has been used to manufacture methamphetamine

Uses/Indications

Pseudoephedrine is primarily used as a substitute for phenylpropanolamine for the treatment of urinary incontinence in dogs; however, it has a narrow therapeutic index and can result in severe toxicity (see ***Overdose/Acute Toxicity***). One study in dogs with urinary incontinence found that it was not as effective as phenylpropanolamine (PPA) and had more adverse effects.[1] Pseudoephedrine is typically not recommended due to the availability of alternative FDA-approved agents.

Pseudoephedrine could be useful as a decongestant or for treating retrograde ejaculation; however, efficacy and safety is lacking.

Pharmacology/Actions

The exact mechanism of actions for pseudoephedrine are unknown. It is thought that it indirectly stimulates both alpha- and, to a lesser degree, beta-adrenergic receptors by causing the release of norepinephrine.

Pharmacologic effects of pseudoephedrine include vasoconstriction, increased heart rate, increase coronary blood flow, increased blood pressure, mild CNS stimulation, decreased nasal congestion, and decreased appetite. Pseudoephedrine can also increase urethral sphincter tone and produce closure of the bladder neck.[2]

Pharmacokinetics

Pseudoephedrine is rapidly and nearly completely absorbed from the GI tract. Food may delay the absorption of pseudoephedrine but not the extent. In children, the apparent volume of distribution is ≈2.5 L/kg. Pseudoephedrine is only partially metabolized, and the bulk is excreted unchanged in the urine. Urine pH can affect excretion rates. Alkaline urine (ie, pH ≈ 8) can prolong half-life while acidic urine (ie, pH ≈ 5) can decrease it.

Contraindications/Precautions/Warnings

Pseudoephedrine is contraindicated in patients that are hypersensitive to it or in patients with severe hypertension. It should be used with caution in patients with glaucoma, prostatic hypertrophy, hyperthyroidism, diabetes mellitus, cardiovascular disorders, or hypertension.

Because it may be used to manufacture methamphetamine, pseudoephedrine is a restricted drug and regulations may vary by state. Use caution when prescribing pseudoephedrine and be alert for drug seeking behavior.

Adverse Effects

Adverse effects are dose-related and adrenergic in nature. Panting, decreased appetite, lethargy, and rapid heart rate are the most likely adverse effects at typical doses; however, CNS excitement, restlessness, insomnia, and other behavioral changes are possible. Increases in blood pressure and arrhythmias can occur in susceptible individuals, particularly at high doses.

Reproductive/Nursing Safety

Safe use has not been established during pregnancy. In humans, pseudoephedrine enters maternal milk. Because safety has not been established in animals, this drug should only be used when the maternal benefits outweigh the potential risks to offspring.

Overdose/Acute Toxicity

Overdoses of pseudoephedrine can cause hyperactivity/agitation, hyperthermia, mydriasis, tachycardia, hypertension, vomiting, disorientation, and seizures. In small animal species, adverse reactions may develop at doses of 5 – 6 mg/kg. Fatalities have occurred at doses greater than 10 – 12 mg/kg.

Large overdoses should be treated with GI decontamination protocols when indicated. Treatment is otherwise supportive and based on clinical signs. Carvedilol (0.5 mg/kg PO twice daily) was successfully used in a dog to treat tachycardia from a pseudoephedrine overdose.[3] Phenothiazines are preferred to treat hyperactivity, agitation, and tremors; benzodiazepines are not recommended, as they may worsen dysphoria.

For patients that have experienced or are suspected to have experienced an overdose, consultation with a 24-hour poison consultation center specializing in providing veterinary-specific information is recommended. For general information related to overdose and toxin exposures, as well as contact information for poison control centers, refer to ***Appendix.***

Drug Interactions

The following drug interactions have either been reported or are theoretical in humans or animals receiving pseudoephedrine and may be of significance in veterinary patients. Unless otherwise noted, use together is not necessarily contraindicated, but weigh the potential risks and perform additional monitoring when appropriate.

- **MONOAMINE OXIDASE INHIBITORS (MAOIs, eg, amitraz, selegiline)**: Pseudoephedrine should not be given within 2 weeks of MAOI administration.

- **Reserpine**: Increased risk for hypertension if given concomitantly
- **Sympathomimetic Agents, Other** (eg, **phenylpropanolamine**): Increased risk for toxicity
- **Tricyclic Antidepressants** (eg, **clomipramine, amitriptyline**): Increased risk for hypertension if given concomitantly

Dosages

DOGS:

Increase urethral tone (extra-label): 1.5 mg/kg PO 2 to 3 times daily. Nighttime incontinence may be effectively managed with once-daily dosing at night.

Retrograde ejaculation (extra-label): **NOTE**: Doses at or above 5 mg/kg have been associated with significant toxic effects (see ***Overdose/Acute Toxicity***).

a) 4 – 5 mg/kg PO 3 times daily

b) 4 – 5 mg/kg PO 1 to 3 hours before semen collection or attempted breeding

CATS:

Decongestant (extra-label): 1 mg/kg PO every 8 hours[4]

Monitoring

- Efficacy
- Adverse effects including tachycardia, CNS stimulation, and increased appetite

Client Information

- Side effects of this medicine include lack of appetite, restlessness (unable to settle down), reduced energy, and rapid heartbeat.
- Overdoses can be serious. Only give this medicine as directed by your veterinarian.
- Store this medicine out of reach of other animals and children.

Chemistry/Synonyms

A sympathomimetic, pseudoephedrine HCl is the stereoisomer of ephedrine. It occurs as a fine, white to off-white powder or crystals. Approximately 2 grams are soluble in 1 mL of water.

Pseudoephedrine may also be known as pseudoephedrini, pseudoephedrina, or *Sudafed*®.

Storage/Stability

Oral pseudoephedrine products should be stored at room temperature in tight containers. Oral liquid preparations should be protected from light and freezing.

Dosage Forms/Regulatory Status

Pseudoephedrine is classified as a DEA List I chemical, as it can be used as a precursor to manufacture methamphetamine. Regulations vary by state; it may be a controlled substance in some states or have other restrictions placed upon its sale. Pseudoephedrine products are available without a prescription, but sales are restricted to behind-the-counter status; purchase quantities are limited, and purchases are tracked.

VETERINARY-LABELED PRODUCTS: NONE

The Association of Racing Commissioners International (ARCI) has designated this drug as a class 3 substance. Use of this drug may not be allowed in certain animal competitions. Check rules and regulations before entering in a competition while this medication is being administered. Contact local racing authorities for further guidance. See ***Appendix*** for more information.

HUMAN-LABELED PRODUCTS:

Pseudoephedrine HCl Tablets: 30 mg and 60 mg; *Sudafed*®, generic; (OTC, restricted)

Pseudoephedrine HCl Capsules: 30 mg; *Zephrex D*®; (OTC, restricted)

Pseudoephedrine HCl Extended-Release Tablets: 120 mg and 240 mg; *Sudafed*®, *Contac*®, generic; (OTC, restricted)

Pseudoephedrine Liquid: 3 mg/mL and 6 mg/mL; *Sudafed*®, generic; (OTC, restricted)

NOTE: Pseudoephedrine is also available in a wide variety of cold and allergy combination products; use caution when selecting and recommending products.

References

For the complete list of references, see **wiley.com/go/budde/plumb**

Psyllium

(***sill***-i-yum) *Metamucil*®

Bulk-Forming GI Laxative/Antidiarrheal

Prescriber Highlights

- ► Bulk-forming agent used for the treatment and prevention of sand colic in horses, as a laxative, and to increase stool consistency in patients with chronic, large-bowel diarrhea
- ► Contraindications include use in rabbits, situations when prompt intestinal evacuation is required, and situations when a fecal impaction or intestinal obstruction is present.
- ► Adverse effects include flatulence; if insufficient fluids are given, there is increased risk for esophageal or bowel obstruction.

Uses/Indications

Bulk-forming laxatives may be used in patients with constipation resulting from a lack of dietary fibers or when straining to defecate may be deleterious.

Psyllium is considered the laxative of choice in the treatment and prevention of sand colic in horses. The combination of psyllium with magnesium sulfate or mineral oil was more effective than any of the products given alone.[1,2]

Psyllium has also been used to increase stool consistency in patients with chronic, large-bowel diarrhea.[3,4]

Psyllium added to the diet may help to control metabolic syndrome in horses.

Pharmacology/Actions

Psyllium is a soluble, slowly fermenting fiber. By swelling into a gel after absorbing water, psyllium increases bulk in the intestine and is believed to induce peristalsis and decrease intestinal transit time. The total amount of water in the stool remains unchanged. In the treatment of sand colic in horses, psyllium is thought to help collect sand and lubricate its passage through the GI tract.

In normal, non-obese, unexercised horses, psyllium fed for 60 days reduced postprandial blood glucose (at 90, 180, and 270 g/day) and insulin levels (at 270 g/day).[5]

Pharmacokinetics

Psyllium is not absorbed when administered orally. Laxative action may take up to 72 hours to occur and is likely highly dependent on species being treated.

Contraindications/Precautions/Warnings

Bulk-forming laxatives should not be used where prompt intestinal evacuation is required or when fecal impaction (no feces being passed) or intestinal obstruction is present. Psyllium products are not recommended for rabbits as they may damage intestinal mucosa and cause bowel obstruction.

In dogs and cats, initiating treatment at ¼ – ½ of the recommended dosage and gradually increasing the dosage may facilitate adaptation to the effects of psyllium fermentation in the GI tract.

Do not confuse teaspoon dosages with tablespoon dosages.

Adverse Effects

With the exception of increased flatulence, psyllium very rarely produces any adverse reactions if adequate water is given or is available to the patient. If insufficient fluids are given, there is increased risk for esophageal or bowel obstruction.

Reproductive/Nursing Safety

Because there is no appreciable systemic absorption of psyllium from the GI tract, it should be safe to use in pregnant and lactating animals.

Overdose/Acute Toxicity

If psyllium is administered with sufficient liquid, overdose should cause only an increased amount of soft or loose stools. A horse receiving 4 times the recommended dosage of a pelleted psyllium product experienced a gastric rupture caused by 2 psyllium bezoars (1 in the pylorus and 1 in the proximal duodenum).[6]

For patients that have experienced or are suspected to have experienced an overdose, consultation with a 24-hour poison consultation center specializing in providing veterinary-specific information is recommended. For general information related to overdose and toxin exposures, as well as contact information for poison control centers, refer to ***Appendix.***

Drug Interactions

The following drug interactions have either been reported or are theoretical in humans or animals receiving psyllium and may be of significance in veterinary patients. Unless otherwise noted, use together is not necessarily contraindicated, but weigh the potential risks and perform additional monitoring when appropriate.

- **Antidiabetic Agents**: Concurrent use may result in an increased risk for hypoglycemia
- **Aspirin** (and other **Salicylates**): Potential exists for psyllium to bind and reduce absorption if given with aspirin; if possible, separate doses by 3 or more hours.
- **Digoxin**: Potential exists for psyllium to bind and reduce absorption if given with digoxin; if possible, separate doses by 3 or more hours.
- **Lithium**: Concurrent use may result in decreased plasma levels and effectiveness of lithium
- **Nitrofurantoin**: Potential exists for psyllium to bind and reduce absorption if given at the same time; if possible, separate doses by 3 or more hours

Dosages

DOGS:

Adjunctive treatment of idiopathic large bowel diarrhea (extra-label): Median dose is 2 tablespoons (30 cc) daily (1.33 g of psyllium/kg/day; range: 0.31 – 4.9 g/kg/day) added to a highly digestible diet.[3] It is recommended to start with ¼ – ½ of this dosage and gradually titrate upward to effect. Four tablespoons (60 cc) added to the diet daily improved stool frequency and consistency in police working dogs.[4]

Adjunct for treatment of hepatic encephalopathy (extra-label): 1 – 3 teaspoons (5 to 15 cc) daily as a source of soluble fiber[7]

CATS:

Chronic constipation (extra-label): 1 – 4 teaspoons (5 to 20 cc) per meal added to canned cat food. It is recommended to start with ¼ – ½ of this dosage and gradually titrate upwards to effect. Be sure the cat is properly hydrated.[8]

HORSES:

Adjunctive treatment of sand colic (extra-label):

a) 1 g/kg twice daily. Mix ≈0.45 kg (1 lb) of psyllium (in powdered form) with water and administer immediately via NG tube; delayed administration will cause the mixture to thicken. If giving this mixture orally to foals, esophageal obstruction can occur. Give small amounts of the mixture at a time, and confirm the foal swallows after each bolus. A liquid-like mixture (versus a paste-like one) can also help. Pelleted psyllium is also available, and most horses find this form more palatable than if the powdered form is mixed with dry or moistened feed. If the horse refuses the pelleted form, experimentation with different flavors and smells produced by different suppliers of psyllium pellets may be helpful. Another option is to blend the psyllium pellets with the horse's favorite treat or grain source to improve intake.[9]
b) 1 g/kg twice daily in combination with magnesium sulfate 1 g/kg via NG tube once daily for 4 days cleared sand accumulation in horses presented without clinical signs of colic.[10]
c) In this experimental study, 0.5 kg psyllium was mixed with 1 L of mash and given twice daily, and 2 L of mineral oil via NG tube was administered once daily. This combination was more effective (measured ash content of feces) than giving mineral oil alone.[2]

Monitoring

- Stool consistency, frequency

Client Information

- Be sure your animal always has plenty of clean water to drink while taking psyllium.
- Psyllium is available OTC (over-the-counter; without a prescription). Do not give psyllium (or any other OTC medications) to your animal without consulting your veterinarian.
- Psyllium products are not recommended for use in rabbits.

Chemistry/Synonyms

Psyllium is obtained from the ripe seeds of varieties of *Plantago* species. The seed coating is high in the content of hemicellulose mucilage that absorbs and swells in the presence of water.

Psyllium is also known as *Metamucil*®; many other trade names are available.

Storage/Stability

Store psyllium products in tightly closed containers; protect from excess moisture or humidity.

Dosage Forms/Regulatory Status

VETERINARY-LABELED PRODUCTS: There are numerous psyllium products sold for use in animals, however, none have been evaluated or approved by the FDA for safety and efficacy in animals.

Equine Enteric Colloid®, *Equi-Phar*® *Sweet Psyllium* (not for horses intended for food), *Sandclear*®, *Anipsyll*® *Powder* (AHC), *Purepsyll*® *Powder*, *Vita-Flex Sand Relief*®, *Equa Aid Psyllium*®; (OTC). Products may be available in 28 oz, 56 oz, 1 lb, 10 lb, and 30 lb pails and are labeled for use in horses.

Vetasyl Fiber Tablets for Cats® 500 mg and 1000 mg tablets in bottles of 60 and 180; (OTC); Labeled for use in cats. Contains barley malt extract powder, acacia, and thiamine.

HUMAN-LABELED PRODUCTS:

There are many human-approved products containing psyllium; most products have ≈3.4 g of psyllium per rounded teaspoonful. Dosages of sugar-free products may be different from those containing sugar. Many products on the human market are orange flavored, but unflavored products are available and may be more palatable for veterinary patients.

References

For the complete list of references, see **wiley.com/go/budde/plumb**

Pyrantel

(pie-***ran***-tel) *Strongid T®, Nemex®*
Antiparasitic

Prescriber Highlights

- ▶ Pyrimidine anthelmintic FDA-approved in dogs and horses and used in a variety of species primarily for treatment of ascarids
- ▶ Due to poor absorption, pyrantel is only useful for GI parasites.
- ▶ Use is contraindicated in severely debilitated animals.
- ▶ Adverse effects are uncommon, but emesis and diarrhea are possible in small animal species.

Uses/Indications

Pyrantel is FDA-approved for removal of ascarids (eg, *Toxocara canis, Toxascaris leonina*) and hookworms (eg, *Ancylostoma caninum, Uncinaria stenocephala*) in dogs.[1] *A caninum* resistance to pyrantel has been reported.[2,3] In greyhounds naturally infected with *T canis*, fenbendazole had a slightly greater reduction in fecal egg count reduction (FECR) than pyrantel.[4]

Pyrantel is not FDA-approved as a single entity for use in cats; however, its use is considered safe to address similar internal parasites as described for dogs.

Pyrantel is FDA-approved in horses for the removal of *Strongylus vulgaris, S equinus*, and *Parasacaris equorum*.[5] It has variable activity against *Oxyuris equi, S edentatus*, and small strongyles. Pyrantel at twice the recommended dose is active against ileocecal tapeworms (eg, *Anoplocephala perfoliata*); however, resistance has been reported. Resistance to pyrantel is an ongoing concern,[6] particularly for large strongyles[7] and cyathostomins.[8] It is recommended to perform fecal egg count reduction (FECR) testing for strongyle nematodes. A value of greater than 90% in treated horses is the suggested cutoff for determining pyrantel efficacy in an individual horse and on a given farm; FECR testing values less than 90% indicate resistance.[9]

Although no pyrantel products are FDA-approved for use in cattle, sheep, or goats, the pyrantel tartrate is effective for the removal of *Haemonchus* spp, *Ostertagia* spp, *Trichostrongylus* spp, *Nematodirus* spp, *Chabertia* spp, *Cooperia* spp, and *Oesophagostomum* spp.[10,11]

In swine, pyrantel tartrate medicated feed is indicated for the prevention or removal and control of large roundworms (ie, *Ascaris suum*) and nodular worms (ie, *Oesophagostomum* spp). The drug also has activity against the swine stomach worm (ie, *Hyostrongylus rubidus*).

Pyrantel has also been used in birds and llamas, although use is not FDA-approved. See ***Dosages*** for more information.

Pyrantel resistance is a growing concern for canine hookworms.[3,12]

Pharmacology/Actions

Pyrantel is a cholinergic agonist that binds to the nicotinic receptors of susceptible parasites to cause depolarization and acts as a neuromuscular-blocking agent to paralyze the organism. It also inhibits cholinesterase.

Pharmacokinetics

Because pyrantel pamoate is poorly absorbed from the GI tract, its antiparasitic effects remain active in the lower GI tract of dogs, cats, and horses. Pyrantel tartrate is absorbed more readily than the pamoate salt. In swine and dogs, pyrantel tartrate reaches peak plasma concentrations 2 to 3 hours after administration. Peak plasma concentrations occur at highly variable times in ruminants. In horses given pyrantel embonate (not available in the United States), peak concentration was reached 7.5 hours after administration.[13]

The absorbed drug is rapidly metabolized and excreted into urine and feces. Elimination half-life is 1.4 hours in cats and 13.4 hours in horses.[14] The maximum pyrantel concentration in equine feces is ≈11 times higher than that reached in plasma.[13]

Contraindications/Precautions/Warnings

Pyrantel is contraindicated in patients that are hypersensitive to it. Use with caution in severely debilitated animals.

In humans, it is recommended to use with caution in patients with hepatic disease.[15]

Adverse Effects

Adverse effects are unlikely when pyrantel is administered at recommended doses. Emesis, diarrhea, or inappetence can occur in small animal species receiving pyrantel pamoate and may be related to expulsion of parasites.

In humans, abdominal cramps, nausea, vomiting, diarrhea, and dizziness have been reported.[15]

Reproductive/Nursing Safety

Pyrantel does not appear to impact the reproductive performance of pregnant mares or stud horses.[5] There has been no evidence of impaired fertility in rats.

Pyrantel is considered safe for use in nursing animals. Several over the counter (OTC) products labeled for dogs contain dosing information for lactating bitches.

Overdose/Acute Toxicity

Pyrantel has a moderate margin of safety. Doses up to ≈7 times the label dose generally do not result in toxic reactions. In horses, doses of 20 times the label dose yielded no adverse effects. The LD_{50} for pyrantel tartrate is 170 mg/kg in mice and rats, and the LD_{50} for pyrantel *base* is more than 690 mg/kg in dogs.[1] Oral dosages of ≈200 mg/kg/day for up to 90 days did not cause morphologic abnormalities in dogs.[1]

In dogs, chronic administration of pyrantel pamoate at 50 mg/kg/day, but not at 20 mg/kg/day over 3 months, resulted in clinical signs of toxicity (eg, increased respiratory rate, profuse sweating [in species with sweat glands], ataxia, other cholinergic effects).

For patients that have experienced or are suspected to have experienced an overdose, it is strongly encouraged to consult with a 24-hour poison consultation center that specialize in providing information specific for veterinary patients. For general information related to overdose and toxin exposures, as well as contact information for poison control centers, refer to ***Appendix.***

Drug Interactions

The following drug interactions have either been reported or are theoretical in humans or animals receiving pyrantel and may be of significance in veterinary patients. Unless otherwise noted, use together is not necessarily contraindicated, but weigh the potential risks and perform additional monitoring when appropriate.

- **LEVAMISOLE**: Because of similar mechanisms of action (and toxicity), do not use concurrently with pyrantel.
- **MORANTEL**: Because of similar mechanisms of action (and toxicity), do not use concurrently with pyrantel.
- **ORGANOPHOSPHATES**: Increased risk for adverse effects
- **PIPERAZINE**: Pyrantel and piperazine have antagonistic mechanisms of action; do not use together.

Dosages

NOTE: Listed dosages specify whether dose is based on the salt (ie, pyrantel pamoate) or pyrantel base; always check the product label to determine the appropriate dose for the specific product being prescribed. For additional information on using this drug in dogs and cats, see the Companion Animal Parasite Council recommendations at capcvet.org.

DOGS:

Pyrantel as a single agent:

Susceptible parasites (label-dosage; FDA-approved): Using pyrantel base, for dogs weighing less than 2.3 kg (5 lb), 10 mg/kg PO; for dogs weighing more than 2.3 kg (5 lb), 5 mg/kg PO. Treat puppies at 2, 3, 4, 6, 8, and 10 weeks of age. Treat lactating bitches 2 to 3 weeks after whelping; perform follow-up fecal examinations 2 to 4 weeks after treating to determine need for retreatment. Adult dogs kept in a heavily contaminated environment may need to be treated at monthly intervals.[1]

Susceptible parasites (extra-label):

a) **Hookworms or roundworms**: Pyrantel pamoate 5 mg/kg PO once after a meal; repeat after 7 to 10 days[16]
b) **Puppies**: To prevent environmental contamination, all puppies should be routinely treated with pyrantel pamoate (10 mg/kg for dogs weighing less than 2.3 kg [5 lb]; 5 mg/kg for dogs weighing more than 2.3 kg [5 lb]) at 2, 4, 6, and 8 weeks of age and then placed on a monthly heartworm preventative with efficacy against *Toxocara* spp.[17]
c) ***Physaloptera* spp nematodes**:
   i. Pyrantel pamoate 5 mg/kg PO once[18]
   ii. Pyrantel pamoate 20 mg/kg PO every 2 weeks for at least 3 treatments[19]

Combination Products:

Pyrantel/Praziquantel/Febantel (*Drontal*® Plus) label indications (FDA-approved): Available in several weight-based sizes that provide minimum dosages of 5 mg/kg pyrantel pamoate, 5 mg/kg praziquantel and 25 mg/kg febantel. See ***Praziquantel/Praziquantel Combination Products.***

Pyrantel/Moxidectin/Sarolaner (*Simparica Trio*®) label indications (FDA-approved): Available in several weight-based sizes that provide minimum dosages of 5 mg/kg pyrantel pamoate, 1.2 mg/kg sarolaner, and 24 µg/kg moxidectin PO once monthly. See ***Sarolaner*** and ***Moxidectin/Moxidectin Combination Products.***

Pyrantel/Ivermectin (*Heartgard Plus*®, *Tri-Heart Plus*®, *Iverhart Plus*®) label indications (FDA-approved): Available in several weight-based sizes that provide minimum dosages of 5 mg/kg pyrantel pamoate and 6 µg/kg ivermectin PO once monthly. See ***Ivermectin.***

CATS:

Pyrantel as a single agent:

Susceptible parasites (extra-label):

a) Pyrantel pamoate 20 mg/kg PO; repeat when necessary[20]
b) **Kittens**: Can be treated as early as 2 to 3 weeks of age at 5 – 10 mg/kg PO; dose can be repeated every 2 to 3 weeks until kittens are at least 12 weeks of age.[21]
c) ***Physaloptera* spp nematodes**: 20 mg/kg PO every 2 weeks for at least 3 treatments[19]

Combination Products:

Pyrantel/Praziquantel (*Drontal*®) label indications (FDA-approved): The tablet provides a minimum dosage of 20 mg/kg pyrantel pamoate and 5 mg/kg praziquantel. See ***Praziquantel/Praziquantel Combination Products.***[22]

HORSES:

Removal and control of mature infections of large strongyles (*Strongylus vulgaris, S edentatus, S equinus*), small strongyles, pinworms (*Oxyuris equi*), and large roundworms (*Parascaris equorum*) in horses and ponies (label dosage; FDA-approved): Pyrantel pamoate 6.6 mg/kg PO. It is recommended that foals (2 to 8 months of age) be given a dose every 4 weeks. Treat mares 1 month before the anticipated foaling date and give retreatment 10 days to 2 weeks after birth in order to minimize any potential source of infection the mare may pose to the foal. Horses and ponies over 8 months of age should be routinely treated every 6 weeks.[5,23]

Control of mature infections of adult large strongyles, adult and larval stages of small strongyles, pinworms, and ascarids in horses (label dosage; FDA-approved): pyrantel tartrate 2.64 mg/kg PO administered on a continuous basis either as a top dress or mixed in the daily grain.[24]

Removal and control of mature infections of large strongyles, small strongyles, pinworms, and large roundworms (extra-label): Pyrantel pamoate 13.2 mg/kg PO (two times the label dosage) may be effective in herds with documented pyrantel resistance.[25]

Control of cestodes (extra-label): 13.2 mg/kg PO (two times the labeled dose)[26]

Combination treatment with oxibendazole (extra-label): Pyrantel pamoate 6.6 mg/kg PO combined with oxibendazole 10 mg/kg PO achieved a more than 90% FECR for cyathostomins on all studied farms, including farms in which FECR was less than <90% for the agents given individually.[27]

DONKEYS

Removal of GI nematodes in donkeys (extra-label): Pyrantel pamoate 20 mg/kg PO using equine oral paste[28,29]

LLAMAS:

Susceptible parasites (extra-label): 18 mg/kg PO once[30,31]

BIRDS:

Intestinal nematodes (extra-label):

a) ***Ascaridia* spp in psittacines**: In endemic areas, outdoor breeding birds and their offspring should be routinely dewormed for ascarids: pyrantel pamoate 25 mg/kg PO every 2 weeks.[32]
b) 7 mg/kg PO; repeat after 14 days[33]
c) 100 mg/kg PO once in psittacines and passerines[34]

RABBITS, RODENTS, SMALL MAMMALS:

Rabbits (extra-label): 5 – 10 mg/kg PO, repeat after 2 to 3 weeks[35]

Monitoring

- Efficacy (eg, fecal float, fecal egg count reduction test)

Client Information

- This medicine may be given with or without food; can be mixed into food.
- Usually no side effects. Rarely, some small animal species may vomit after receiving the drug; give with food if this happens.
- In small animal species, dose is usually repeated at various weekly intervals; follow your veterinarian's recommendation for best control of parasites.
- If using a liquid suspension, shake the container thoroughly before each use; protect from sunlight.
- Most intestinal parasites are digested after treatment; it is uncommon to see parasites passed in the stool.

Chemistry/Synonyms

Pyrantel pamoate, a pyrimidine-derivative anthelmintic, occurs as yellow to tan solid and is practically insoluble in water and alcohol. Each gram of pyrantel pamoate is ≈347 mg (34.7%) of the base.

Pyrantel may also be known as CP-10423-16, pyrantel embonate, pirantel pamoate, *Anthel*®, *Antiminth*®, *Ascarical*®, *Aut*®, *Bantel*®, *Cobantril*®, *Combantrin*®, *Early Bird*®, *Helmex*®, *Helmintox*®, *Jaa Pyral*®, *Lombriareu*®, *Nemex*®, *Nemocid*®, *Pin-X*®, *Pirantrim*®, *Pyrantin*®, *Pyrantrin*®, *Pyrapam*®, *Reese's*® *Pinworm*, *Strongid*®, *Trilombrin*®, or *Vertel*®.

Storage/Stability

Pyrantel pamoate products should be stored in tight, light-resistant containers at room temperature (15°C-30°C [59°F-86°F]) unless otherwise directed by the manufacturer. Do not expose pyrantel products to direct sunlight.

Dosage Forms/Regulatory Status

VETERINARY-LABELED PRODUCTS:

NOTE: Many products are available; a partial listing of products follows:

Pyrantel Pamoate Tablets: 22.7 mg (of base), 113.5 mg (of base); (OTC). FDA-approved for use in dogs. A commonly known product is *Nemex® Tabs.*

Pyrantel Pamoate Oral Suspension: 2.27 mg/mL and 4.54 mg/mL (as base) (for dogs only); in 60 mL, 120 mL, 280 mL, and 473 mL bottles. Many products are available; a commonly known trade name is *Nemex-2®*; (OTC).

Pyrantel Pamoate Oral Suspension: 50 mg/mL (of base). Many products are available; a commonly known trade name *is Strongid®* T; (OTC). FDA-approved for use in horses and foals 2 months of age and older and not intended for food purposes

Pyrantel Pamoate Oral Paste: 43.9% w/w pyrantel base in 23.6 g paste (171 to 180 mg pyrantel base/mL); *Strongid®* Paste, Exodus® Paste, generic; (OTC). FDA-approved for use in horses and foals 2 months of age and older and not intended for food purposes

Pyrantel Tartrate 1.06% (4.8 g/lb) Top Dress: in 25 lb pails: *Strongid®* C; (OTC). Labeled for use in horses not intended for food purposes.

Pyrantel Tartrate 2.12% (9.6 g/lb) Top Dress: in 10 lb, 25 lb, and 50 lb pails: *Strongid®* C 2X; (OTC). Labeled for use in horses not intended for food purposes.

Pyrantel embonate is available in countries outside the United States. Dose requirements differ from that of pyrantel pamoate and pyrantel tartrate; consult the product label.

Combination Products:

With Febantel and Praziquantel: Tablets and Taste Tabs: For Puppies and Small Dogs (0.9 to 11.3 kg [2 to 25 lb]): praziquantel, 22.7 mg/pyrantel pamoate, 22.7 mg/febantel, 113.4 mg; For Medium-Sized Dogs (11.8 to 27.2 kg [26 to 60 lb]): praziquantel, 68 mg/pyrantel pamoate, 68 mg/febantel, 340.2 mg; For Large Dogs (more than 20.4 kg [45 lb]): praziquantel, 136 mg/pyrantel pamoate, 136 mg/febantel, 680.4 mg; *Drontal®* Plus (Rx, OTC). Approved for use in dogs 3 weeks of age and older. See ***Fenbendazole*** and ***Praziquantel/Praziquantel Combination Products*** for more information.

With Ivermectin: Chewable Tablets: For dogs up to 11.3 kg (25 lb): ivermectin 68 µg/pyrantel pamoate 57 mg; For dogs 11.8 to 22.7 kg (26 to 50 lb): ivermectin 136 µg/pyrantel pamoate 114 mg; For dogs 23.1 to 45.4 kg (51 to 100 lb): ivermectin 272 µg/pyrantel pamoate 227 mg; *Heartgard®* Plus Chewables, generic; (Rx). FDA-approved for use in dogs 6 weeks of age and older. See ***Ivermectin*** for more information.

With Ivermectin and Praziquantel: Ivermectin/Pyrantel Pamoate/Praziquantel Oral Chewable Tablets: For dogs 2.7 to 5.4 kg (6 to 12 lb): 34 µg/28.5 mg/28.5 mg; For dogs 5.5 to 11.3 kg (12.1 to 25 lb): 68 µg/57 mg/57 mg; For dogs 11.4 to 22.7 kg (25.1 to 50 lb): 136 µg/114 mg/114 mg; For dogs 22.7 to 45.4 kg (50.1 to 100 lb): 272 µg/228 mg/228 mg; *Iverhart®* Max; (Rx). FDA-approved for use in dogs 6 weeks of age and older. See ***Ivermectin*** and ***Praziquantel/Praziquantel Combination Products*** for more information.

With Moxidectin and Sarolaner: Chewable (flavored) Tablets: For dogs, 1.3 to 2.5 kg (2.8 to 5.5 lb): moxidectin 0.06 mg, pyrantel pamoate 12.5 mg, and sarolaner 3 mg; For Dogs, 2.5 to 5 kg (5.6 to 11 lb): moxidectin 0.12 mg, pyrantel pamoate 25 mg, and sarolaner 6 mg; For dogs, 5 – 10 kg (11.1 to 22 lb): moxidectin 0.24 mg, pyrantel pamoate 50 mg, and sarolaner 12 mg; For Dogs, 10 to 20 kg (22.1 to 44 lb): moxidectin 0.48 mg, pyrantel pamoate 100 mg, and sarolaner 24 mg; For dogs, 20 to 40 kg (44.1 to 88 lb): moxidectin 0.96 mg, pyrantel pamoate 200 mg, and sarolaner 48 mg; For dogs, 40 to 60 kg (88.1 to 132 lb): moxidectin 1.44 mg, pyrantel pamoate 300 mg, and sarolaner 72 mg; *Simparica Trio®* (Rx). Approved for use in dogs 8 weeks of age and older and weighing 1.3 kg (2.8 lb) or greater. NADA# 141-521. See ***Moxidectin*** and ***Sarolaner*** for more information.

With Praziquantel: Tablets: 18.2 mg praziquantel/72.6 mg pyrantel pamoate (of base); *Drontal®* Tablets; some sizes may be available as generics or under various trade names (OTC). FDA-approved for use in cats and kittens older than 2 months of age and weighing more than 0.9 kg (2 lb). See ***Praziquantel/Praziquantel Combination Products*** for more information.

With Praziquantel: Chewable Tablets: Praziquantel 30 mg/pyrantel pamoate 30 mg and praziquantel 114 mg/pyrantel pamoate 114 mg; *Virbantel®*; generic; (OTC). FDA-approved for use in dogs 12 weeks of age and older. See ***Praziquantel/Praziquantel Combination Products*** for more information.

HUMAN-LABELED PRODUCTS:

Pyrantel Pamoate Oral Suspension: 144 mg/mL (equivalent to 50 mg/mL pyrantel base); generic; (OTC)

Pyrantel Pamoate Chewable Oral Tablets: 180 mg and 720.5 mg (equivalent to 62.5 mg and 250 mg pyrantel base, respectively); *Pin-X®*, *Vermisol®*; generic; (OTC)

References

For the complete list of references, see **wiley.com/go/budde/plumb**

Pyridostigmine

(peer-id-oh-***stig***-meen) *Mestinon®*

Anticholinesterase Agent

Prescriber Highlights

- ▶ Anticholinesterase inhibitor used for treatment of myasthenia gravis
- ▶ Contraindications include hypersensitivity to this class of compounds or bromides, as well as patients with mechanical (physical) obstructions of the urinary or GI tract.
- ▶ Use with caution in patients with bronchospastic disease, epilepsy, hyperthyroidism, bradycardia or other arrhythmias, vagotonia, or GI ulcer diseases.
- ▶ Adverse effects are usually dose-related cholinergic signs, including GI effects (nausea, vomiting, diarrhea, salivation), respiratory effects (increased bronchial secretions, bronchospasm, pulmonary edema, respiratory paralysis), ophthalmic effects (miosis, blurred vision, lacrimation), cardiovascular effects (bradycardia or tachycardia, cardiospasm, hypotension, cardiac arrest), muscle cramps, sweating, and weakness.

Uses/Indications

Pyridostigmine is used in the treatment of myasthenia gravis (MG) in dogs and, rarely, in cats. It is considered to be much more effective in treating acquired MG than congenital MG.

Pharmacology/Actions

Pyridostigmine inhibits the hydrolysis of acetylcholine by directly competing with acetylcholine for attachment to acetylcholinesterase.

Because the pyridostigmine-acetylcholinesterase complex is hydrolyzed at a much slower rate than the acetylcholine-acetylcholinesterase complex, acetylcholine tends to accumulate at cholinergic synapses with resultant cholinergic activity. Compared with neostigmine, pyridostigmine is ≈4.4 times less potent, has a slower onset and longer duration of action, and has fewer adverse GI effects.

At usual doses, pyridostigmine does not cross into the CNS (quaternary ammonium structure), but overdoses can cause CNS effects.

Pharmacokinetics

Pyridostigmine is only marginally absorbed from the GI tract (≈10% to 20%). Absorption may be delayed by food and be more erratic with the extended-release tablets than the regular tablets. In humans, oral dosage is ≈30 times greater than IV dosage. The onset of action after oral dosing is generally within 1 hour.

At recommended dosages, pyridostigmine is apparently distributed to most tissues except the brain, intestinal wall, fat, or thymus.

Pyridostigmine is both hydrolyzed by cholinesterases and metabolized by the liver (≈25% of the dose administered) but is largely excreted unchanged in the urine. Elimination half-life is ≈1.5 to 3 hours in humans. Patients with renal failure will have prolonged elimination.

The extended-release tablet is intended to have an immediate effect equivalent to a 60 mg tablet, and the effect is then sustained over time.

Contraindications/Precautions/Warnings

Pyridostigmine is contraindicated in patients that are hypersensitive to this class of compounds or bromides, or in those that have mechanical (physical) obstructions of the urinary or GI tract.

The drug should be used with caution in patients with bronchospastic disease, epilepsy, hyperthyroidism, bradycardia or other arrhythmias, vagotonia, or GI ulcer diseases. Lower doses may be needed in patients with renal impairment. Atropine sulfate should be readily available to block excessive cholinergic effects.

Do not confuse PYRIDostigmine with PHYSostigmine.

Adverse Effects

Adverse effects are generally dose-related and cholinergic in nature such as increased GI motility, salivation, urination, abdominal pain, diarrhea, bradycardia, and increased lacrimation. These effects are usually mild and easily treatable with dosage reduction, but severe adverse effects are possible (see ***Overdose/Acute Toxicity***).

Reproductive/Nursing Safety

Pyridostigmine crosses the placenta and is excreted in maternal milk.

Because safety has not been established in animals, this drug should only be used when the maternal benefits outweigh the potential risks to offspring.

Overdose/Acute Toxicity

Overdoses of pyridostigmine may induce a cholinergic crisis. Clinical signs of cholinergic toxicity can include GI effects (eg, nausea, vomiting, diarrhea, salivation), respiratory effects (eg, increased bronchial secretions, bronchospasm, pulmonary edema, respiratory paralysis), ophthalmic effects (eg, miosis, blurred vision, lacrimation), cardiovascular effects (eg, bradycardia or tachycardia, cardiospasm, hypotension, cardiac arrest), sweating (ie, species with sweat glands), muscle cramps, and weakness.

Overdoses in myasthenic patients can be difficult to distinguish from the effects associated with a myasthenic crisis. The time of onset of clinical signs or an edrophonium challenge may help to distinguish between the two.

Treatment of pyridostigmine overdose consists of both respiratory and cardiac supportive therapy and administration of atropine, if necessary. Refer to the ***Atropine*** monograph for more information on its use for cholinergic toxicity.

For patients that have experienced or are suspected to have experienced an overdose, consultation with a 24-hour poison consultation center specializing in providing veterinary-specific information is recommended. For general information related to overdose and toxin exposures, as well as contact information for poison control centers, refer to ***Appendix.***

Drug Interactions

The following drug interactions have either been reported or are theoretical in humans or animals receiving pyridostigmine and may be of significance in veterinary patients. Unless otherwise noted, use together is not necessarily contraindicated, but weigh the potential risks and perform additional monitoring when appropriate.

- **Anticholinergic Agents** (eg, **atropine, diphenhydramine**): Concurrent use may reduce efficacy of both agents.
- **Beta-Blockers** (eg, **atenolol, propranolol**): May result in adverse effects in heart rate or blood pressure
- **Bethanechol**: Additive cholinergic effects (eg, salivation, diarrhea, micturition) are possible.
- **Corticosteroids** (eg, **dexamethasone, prednis(ol)one**): May decrease the anticholinesterase activity of pyridostigmine. After stopping corticosteroid therapy, drugs like pyridostigmine may cause increased anticholinesterase activity.
- **Dexpanthenol**: Theoretically, dexpanthenol may have additive effects when used with pyridostigmine.
- **Drugs With Neuromuscular Blocking Ability** (eg, **aminoglycoside antibiotics**): May necessitate increased dosages of pyridostigmine in treating or diagnosing myasthenic patients
- **Magnesium**: Parenteral magnesium can have a depressant effect on skeletal muscle, necessitating increased dosages of pyridostigmine.
- **Neuromuscular Blocking Agents, Depolarizing** (eg, **succinylcholine, decamethonium**): Pyridostigmine may prolong the phase I block of depolarizing muscle relaxants.
- **Neuromuscular Blocking Agents, NonDepolarizing** (eg, **pancuronium, tubocurarine, gallamine, vecuronium, atracurium**): Pyridostigmine antagonizes the actions of nondepolarizing neuromuscular blocking agents.
- **Quinidine**: Recurrent paralysis may occur when quinidine is administered during recovery from use of nondepolarizing neuromuscular blocking agents, necessitating increased dosages of pyridostigmine.

Laboratory Considerations

- None known

Dosages

DOGS:

Adjunctive treatment of myasthenia gravis (extra-label):

a) 0.2 – 2 mg/kg PO every 8 to 12 hours with food once able to swallow.[1] Practically, either round dose to nearest ¼ of a regular 60 mg tablet or use the oral liquid for more precise dosing. Dose should start low and be carefully titrated to effect to minimize adverse effects and maximize muscle strength.

b) 0.01 – 0.03 mg/kg/hour IV CRI for patients unable to swallow, especially in critically ill animals[1,2]

CATS:

Myasthenia gravis (extra-label): Rarely used but can be dosed similarly as dogs[3-7]

FERRETS:

Myasthenia gravis (extra-label): 1 mg/kg PO every 12 hours in combination with prednisolone[8]

Monitoring

- Animals should be routinely monitored for clinical signs of cholinergic toxicity (see ***Overdose/Acute Toxicity***) and efficacy of the therapy.

Client Information

- Give this medicine as directed by your veterinarian. It may be given with or without food but give the same way each time.
- Dosage adjustments may occur frequently early in the course of treatment, and periodically thereafter. Always follow your veterinarian's instructions. Do not change the amount you give your animal without speaking to your veterinarian first.
- Giving a dose too early or too late should be avoided. Discuss with your veterinarian if you are having difficulty giving the medication at the prescribed dosing interval.
- Contact your veterinarian if your animal has side effects such as excessive salivation, gastrointestinal disturbances (nausea, vomiting, diarrhea), weakness, or difficulty breathing.
- Overdoses can be very serious. Be sure to measure liquid doses very carefully.
- Keep this medicine out of reach of children and animals.

Chemistry/Synonyms

An anticholinesterase agent, pyridostigmine bromide is a synthetic quaternary ammonium compound that occurs as an agreeable smelling, bitter tasting, hydroscopic, white or practically white, crystalline powder. It is freely soluble in water and alcohol. The pH of the commercially available injection is ≈5.

Pyridostigmine bromide may also be known as pyridostigmini bromidum, *Distinon*®, *Gravitor*®, *Kalymin*®, *Mestinon*®, or *Regonol*®.

Storage/Stability

Unless otherwise instructed by the manufacturer, store pyridostigmine products at room temperature. The oral solution and injection should be protected from light and freezing. Pyridostigmine tablets should be kept in tight containers.

The extended-release tablets may become mottled with time, but this does not affect their potency.

Pyridostigmine injection is unstable in alkaline solutions. It contains 1% benzyl alcohol.

Compatibility/Compounding Considerations

Compatibility is dependent upon factors such as pH, concentration, temperature, and diluent used; consult specialized references or a hospital pharmacist for more specific information.

Pyridostigmine injection is reportedly physically **compatible** with glycopyrrolate, heparin sodium, hydrocortisone sodium succinate, potassium chloride, and vitamin B complex with C.

Dosage Forms/Regulatory Status

VETERINARY-LABELED PRODUCTS: NONE

The Association of Racing Commissioners International (ARCI) has designated this drug as a class 3 substance. Use of this drug may not be allowed in certain animal competitions. Check rules and regulations before entering in a competition while this medication is being administered. Contact local racing authorities for further guidance. See ***Appendix*** for more information.

HUMAN-LABELED PRODUCTS:

Pyridostigmine Bromide Tablets: 60 mg; *Mestinon*®, generic, (Rx)

Pyridostigmine Bromide Extended-Release Tablets: 180 mg; *Mestinon*®, generic; (Rx)

Pyridostigmine Bromide Syrup: 12 mg/mL (labeled as 60 mg/5 mL) in 480 mL; *Mestinon*®; (Rx)

Pyridostigmine Bromide Injection: 5 mg/mL in 2 mL ampules; *Regonol*®; (Rx)

References

For the complete list of references, see **wiley.com/go/budde/plumb**

Pyridoxine

Vitamin B_6

(peer-ih-***dox***-een)

Nutritional B Vitamin; Antidote

Prescriber Highlights

- ▶ Pyridoxine may be beneficial in the treatment of isoniazid, crimidine, or hydrazine mushroom toxicity, delaying cutaneous toxicity of *Doxil*® (liposomal doxorubicin), or to supplement while patients are receiving penicillamine.
- ▶ Use caution when using in patients with renal insufficiency or are hypersensitive to pyridoxine.
- ▶ Overdoses may cause peripheral neuropathy.

Uses/Indications

Pyridoxine use in veterinary medicine is relatively infrequent. It may be of benefit in the treatment of isoniazid (INH) or crimidine (an older rodenticide) toxicity. Pyridoxine deficiency is extremely rare in dogs or cats that are able to ingest food. Cats with severe intestinal disease may have a greater requirement for pyridoxine in their diet. Experimentally, pyridoxine has been successfully used in dogs to reduce the cutaneous toxicity associated with doxorubicin containing pegylated liposomes (*Doxil*®). Pyridoxine has been demonstrated to suppress the growth of feline mammary tumors (cell line FRM) in vitro.

In humans, labeled uses for pyridoxine include pyridoxine deficiency and intractable neonatal seizures secondary to pyridoxine dependency syndrome.[1] Pyridoxine has also been used in humans for sideroblastic anemia associated with elevated serum iron levels. Unlabeled uses include premenstrual syndrome (PMS); carpal tunnel syndrome; tardive dyskinesia secondary to antipsychotic drugs; nausea and vomiting in pregnancy; hyperoxaluria type 1 and oxalate kidney stones; and for the treatment of INH, cycloserine, hydrazine, or *Gyromitra* mushroom poisonings.

Pharmacology/Actions

In erythrocytes, pyridoxine is converted to pyridoxal phosphate and, to a lesser extent, pyridoxamine, which serve as coenzymes for amino acid metabolism, as well as lipid and carbohydrate utilization. Pyridoxine is necessary for tryptophan conversion to serotonin or niacin, glycogen breakdown, heme synthesis, synthesis of GABA in the CNS, and oxalate conversion to glycine. Pyridoxine can act as an antidote by enhancing the excretion of cycloserine or isoniazid.

Pyridoxine requirements increase as protein ingestion increases, with carnivores having higher pyridoxine requirements than omnivores.

Pharmacokinetics

Pyridoxine is absorbed from the GI tract, primarily in the jejunum. Malabsorption syndromes can significantly impair pyridoxine absorption. Pyridoxine is not bound to plasma proteins, but pyridoxal phosphate is completely bound to plasma proteins. Pyridoxine is stored primarily in the liver, with smaller amounts stored in the brain and muscle. It is biotransformed in the liver and various other tissues and excreted almost entirely as metabolites into the urine. Elimination half-life in humans is ≈15 to 20 days.[1]

Contraindications/Precautions/Warnings

Weigh potential risks versus benefits in patients with documented sensitivity to pyridoxine. Parenteral pyridoxine solutions contain aluminum and prolonged use should be undertaken with caution in patients with renal impairment.

Adverse Effects

Pyridoxine is generally well tolerated unless doses are large (see ***Overdose/Acute Toxicity***). In humans, nausea and vomiting, headache, paresthesia, and somnolence have been reported with long-term use at high doses. Reduced serum folic acid levels have occurred. Worsening of metabolic acidosis has occurred following rapid infusion of large doses of pyridoxine injection, which has a pH of 2 to 3.8.

Reproductive/Nursing Safety

Pyridoxine crosses the placenta reaching concentrations 5 times higher in the fetus than in maternal plasma concentrations. Although pyridoxine is a nutritional agent and very safe at recommended doses during pregnancy, large doses during pregnancy can cause a pyridoxine dependency syndrome in neonates. Pyridoxine requirements increase during pregnancy.

Pyridoxine is excreted in breast milk. Pyridoxine administration at low dosages should be safe during nursing. Pyridoxine requirements of the dam may be increased during nursing.

Because safety has not been established in animals, this drug should only be used when the maternal benefits outweigh the potential risks to offspring.

Overdose/Acute Toxicity

Single overdoses are not considered overly problematic unless they are massive. Single doses of up to 1 g/kg are tolerated by dogs, rats, and rabbits. A dose of 1 g/kg caused ataxia in dogs, with recovery within 1 week. Laboratory animals given 3 – 4 g/kg developed seizures and died. Chronic excessive doses of pyridoxine have been associated with severe peripheral neuropathy. Beagles given 50 mg/kg/day developed no signs, although there was a bilateral loss of myelin in the dorsal nerve roots; 150 mg/kg/day caused ataxia, muscle weakness, and loss of balance after 40 to 75 days.[2,3] Beagles repeatedly given 3 g oral daily doses developed uncoordinated gait and neurologic signs. Neuronal lesions were noted in sensory, dorsal root ganglia, and trigeminal ganglia. Signs generally resolved over a 2-month drug-free period.[4,5]

For patients that have experienced or are suspected of having experienced an overdose, consultation with a 24-hour poison consultation center specializing in providing veterinary-specific information is recommended. For general information related to overdose and toxin exposures, as well as contact information for poison control centers, refer to ***Appendix.***

Drug Interactions

The following drug interactions have either been reported or are theoretical in humans or animals receiving pyridoxine and may be of significance in veterinary patients. Unless otherwise noted, use together is not necessarily contraindicated, but weigh the potential risks and perform additional monitoring when appropriate.

- **CHLORAMPHENICOL**: May cause increased pyridoxine requirements
- **ESTROGENS**: May cause increased pyridoxine requirements
- **HYDRALAZINE**: May cause increased pyridoxine requirements
- **IMMUNOSUPPRESSANTS** (eg, **azathioprine, chlorambucil, cyclophosphamide, corticosteroids**): May cause increased pyridoxine requirements
- **ISONIAZID**: May cause increased pyridoxine requirements
- **PENICILLAMINE**: May cause increased pyridoxine requirements
- **PHENOBARBITAL, PRIMIDONE**: High-dose pyridoxine may decrease phenobarbital serum concentration.

Laboratory Considerations

- Urobilinogen in the spot test using Ehrlich reagent: Pyridoxine may cause false-positive results.
- AST: Excessive dosages of pyridoxine may elevate AST.

Dosages

DOGS/CATS:

Isoniazid (INH) toxicity in dogs (extra-label): If the quantity of INH ingested is known, give pyridoxine on an mg-for-mg (1:1) basis. If it is not known, give pyridoxine initially at 71 mg/kg as a 5% to 10% IV infusion over 30 to 60 minutes. (Some sources say it can be given as an IV bolus.) Pyridoxine injection can usually be obtained from human hospital pharmacies. Do not use injectable B-complex vitamins.[6-8]

Provide cofactors for the metabolism of toxic compounds, including ethylene glycol (extra-label): 1 – 2 mg/kg IV every 6 hours[9]

Replace pyridoxine antagonized by crimidine ingestion (extra-label): 20 mg/kg IV[10]

Adjunctive treatment (acute seizures) of hydrazine mushroom (*Gyromitra* spp) poisoning (extra-label): 75 – 150 mg/kg IV[11]

Supplementation while on penicillamine (extra-label): 25 mg/animal (NOT mg/kg) per day PO given concurrently with d-penicillamine to prevent pyridoxine depletion [10]

To delay the development of cutaneous toxicity (palmar-plantar erythrodysesthesia) associated with doxorubicin containing pegylated liposomes *(Doxil®)* in dogs (extra-label): 50 mg/animal (NOT mg/kg) PO 3 times daily during chemotherapy protocol period[12]

Interruption of lactation during pseudopregnancy in dogs (extra-label): 50 mg/kg PO once daily[13]

Monitoring

- Other than evaluating efficacy for its intended use, no significant monitoring is required.

Client Information

- Very safe; usually no side effects
- Do not give more medicine than your veterinarian has ordered.

Chemistry/Synonyms

Pyridoxine (vitamin B_6) is a water-soluble vitamin that is present in many foods (eg, liver, meat, eggs, cereals, legumes, and vegetables). The commercially available form (pyridoxine HCl) found in medications is obtained synthetically. Pyridoxine HCl occurs as white or practically white crystals or crystalline powder with a slightly bitter, salty taste. It is freely soluble in water and slightly soluble in alcohol.

Pyridoxine or vitamin B_6 may also be known by the following synonyms or analogues: adermine, pyridoxal, pyridoxal-5-phosphate, pyridoxamine, pirodoxamina, piridossima, piridoxolum, piridossina, *Aminoxin®*, and *Vitelle Nestrex®*.

Storage/Stability

Unless otherwise specified by the manufacturer, store pyridoxine tablets below 40°C (104°F), preferably between 15°C and 30°C (59°F-86°F), in well-closed containers protected from light.

Store pyridoxine HCl injection at 20°C to 25°C (68°F-77°F), protected from light and freezing.

Compatibility/Compounding Considerations

Compatibility is dependent on factors such as pH, concentration, temperature, and diluent used; specialized references or a hospital pharmacist should be consulted for more specific information.

Pyridoxine HCl injection can be administered undiluted or added to commonly used IV solutions. It is reportedly **compatible** with ascorbic acid, atropine sulfate, buprenorphine, butorphanol, calcium salts, dexamethasone sodium phosphate, diphenhydramine, dobutamine, famotidine, glycopyrrolate, heparin sodium, lidocaine, magnesium sulfate, metoclopramide, midazolam, ondansetron, potassium chloride, and thiamine HCl.

It is reportedly **incompatible** with alkaline or oxidizing solutions, iron salts, and the following drugs (partial list): cefazolin, diazepam, furosemide, hydrocortisone sodium succinate, and methylprednisolone sodium succinate.

Dosage Forms/Regulatory Status

VETERINARY-LABELED PRODUCTS:

No single ingredient pyridoxine products were located. There is a multitude of veterinary-labeled products that contain pyridoxine as one of several ingredients.

HUMAN-LABELED PRODUCTS:

Pyridoxine Tablets: 25 mg, 50 mg, 100 mg; generic; (OTC)

Pyridoxine HCl Injection: 100 mg/mL in 1 mL vials; generic; (Rx)

Pyridoxine is also an ingredient in many combination products (eg, B-Complex, multivitamins).

References

For the complete list of references, see **wiley.com/go/budde/plumb**

Pyrilamine

(pye-***ril***-a-meen) *Histall®*

Antihistamine

Prescriber Highlights

- ► Used for allergic conditions in horses
- ► Use with caution in patients with narrow-angle glaucoma, prostatic hypertrophy, pyloroduodenal or bladder neck obstruction, or asthma.
- ► Adverse effects in horses include CNS stimulation (eg, nervousness, insomnia, convulsions, tremors, ataxia) or CNS depression (eg, sedation), palpitation, GI disturbances, muscle weakness, inappetence, and lassitude.

Uses/Indications

Pyrilamine is a first-generation antihistamine that may provide an alternative to glucocorticoids in managing allergic conditions in horses.

Pharmacology/Actions

Antihistamines competitively inhibit histamine at H_1 receptor sites. They do not inactivate or prevent the release of histamine but can prevent histamine's action on the cell. H_1 receptor antagonists also have varying degrees of anticholinergic activity and CNS effects such as sedation. Pyrilamine is considered to be less potent, cause less sedation, and have fewer anticholinergic effects than most other first-generation antihistamines.

Pharmacokinetics

The pharmacokinetics of this agent have not been extensively studied in cattle, dogs, or cats. In horses, pyrilamine is poorly bioavailable (18%) after oral administration. After IV administration, elimination half-life was ≈1.7 hours. After a single dose, the principal metabolite, *O*-desmethylpyrilamine (O-DMP), can be detected in urine for at least two days, and possibly up to one week after administration.[1]

Contraindications/Precautions/Warnings

Although there are no specific contraindications or precautions listed for pyrilamine, first-generation antihistamines should be used with caution in patients with narrow-angle glaucoma, prostatic hypertrophy, pyloroduodenal or bladder neck obstruction, and asthma due to their anticholinergic activity.

Adverse Effects

Adverse effects in horses can include CNS stimulation (eg, nervousness, insomnia, convulsions, tremors, ataxia), palpitation, temporary anhidrosis, GI disturbances, CNS depression (eg, sedation), muscular weakness, inappetence, and lassitude.

Reproductive/Nursing Safety

Rats and mice treated with 10 to 20 times the human dose had an increased frequency of embryonic, fetal, or perinatal death, but a study in pregnant women showed no increase in teratogenic or fetocidal rates. It is unknown if pyrilamine enters milk. Because safety has not been established in animals, this drug should only be used when the maternal benefits outweigh the potential risks to offspring.

Overdose/Acute Toxicity

Treatment of overdoses is supportive and based on clinical signs. For patients that have experienced or are suspected to have experienced an overdose, consultation with a 24-hour poison consultation center specializing in providing veterinary-specific information is recommended. For general information related to overdose and toxin exposures, as well as contact information for poison control centers, refer to ***Appendix***.

Drug Interactions

The following drug interactions have either been reported or are theoretical in humans or animals receiving pyrilamine and may be of significance in veterinary patients. Unless otherwise noted, use together is not necessarily contraindicated, but weigh the potential risks and perform additional monitoring when appropriate.

- Anticoagulants (eg, **heparin, warfarin**): Antihistamines may partially counteract the anticoagulation effects of heparin or warfarin.
- CNS Depressants (eg, **benzodiazepines, detomidine, methocarbamol**): Increased sedation can occur if pyrilamine is combined with other CNS depressant drugs.
- Epinephrine: Pyrilamine may enhance the effects of epinephrine.

Laboratory Considerations

- Antihistamines can decrease the wheal and flare response to antigen skin testing. In humans, it is suggested that antihistamines be discontinued at least 4 days before testing. In dogs, it is recommended to discontinue antihistamines a minimum of 2 days before testing, with 7 days being optimal.[2]

Dosages

HORSES:

Treatment of conditions in which antihistaminic therapy will alleviate clinical signs (label dosage; FDA-approved):

a) **Foals**: 0.44 mg/kg IV slowly every 6 to 12 hours as needed[3]

b) **Adult horses**: 0.88 – 1.3 mg/kg IV slowly every 6 to 12 hours as needed[3]

Antihistamine (label dosage; not FDA-approved): 0.66 mg/kg PO every 12 hours as needed.[4]

Monitoring

- Clinical efficacy
- Adverse effects

Chemistry/Synonyms

An ethylenediamine antihistamine, pyrilamine maleate occurs as a white, crystalline powder with a melting range of 99°C to 103°C (210°F-217.4°F). One gram is soluble in ≈0.5 mL of water or 3 mL of alcohol.

Pyrilamine maleate may also be known as pyranisamine hydrochloride, pyrilamine hydrochloride, mepyramine hydrochloride, mepyramini maleas, myranisamine maleate, myrilamine maleate, mepyramine maleate, *Anihist*®, *Alergitanil*®, *Antemesyl*®, *Anthisan*®, *Anthisan*®, *Equi-Phar*® *Equi-Hist*®, *Equiphed*®, *Fluidasa*®, *Histall*®, *Histagranules*®, *Histamed*®, *Mepyraderm*®, *Mepyrimal*, *Pyramine*®, *Pyripea*®, *Relaxa-Tabs*®, and *Tri-Hist*®.

Storage/Stability

Keep lid tightly closed and store in a dry place below 30°C (86°F).

Dosage Forms/Regulatory Status

VETERINARY-LABELED PRODUCTS:

NOTE: The marketing status of pyrilamine products changes frequently. Marketed products may not be FDA-approved for safe and effective use.

The Association of Racing Commissioners International (ARCI) has designated this drug as a class 3 substance. Use of this drug may not be allowed in certain animal competitions. Check rules and regulations before entering a competition while this medication is being administered. Contact local racing authorities for further guidance. See ***Appendix*** for more information.

Pyrilamine Maleate Solution for Injection: 20 mg/mL; (Rx). This product is still listed in the FDA Green Book of approved animal drugs but is no longer commercially available.

Pyrilamine Granules: 600 mg/oz in 20 oz containers; *Histall*® (OTC). Labeled for use in horses

Pyrilamine is also available in combination with guaifenesin or pseudoephedrine:

Pyrilamine Maleate 600 mg/oz and Pseudoephedrine HCl 600 mg/oz Granules: 20 oz, 5 lb and 10 lb containers; *Tri-Hist*® *Granules* (Rx). Labeled for use in horses. Not for use in horses intended for food. **NOTE**: Pseudoephedrine regulations may vary by state. See ***Pseudoephedrine*** for more information.

Pyrilamine 600 mg/oz and Guaifenesin 2400 mg/oz Granules: 20 oz and 5 lb containers; *Anihist*®; (OTC). Labeled for use in horses

HUMAN-LABELED PRODUCTS:

Pyrilamine is available in OTC combination products marketed for allergies, cough, and colds.

References

For the complete list of references, see **wiley.com/go/budde/plumb**

Pyrimethamine

(pye-ri-***meth***-a-meen) *Daraprim*®

Antiprotozoal

NOTE: Also see the ***Pyrimethamine/Sulfadiazine*** and ***Sulfadiazine/Trimethoprim*** monographs

Prescriber Highlights

- Folic acid inhibitor used primarily in combination with a sulfonamide for toxoplasmosis, *Hepatozoon americanum*, neosporosis, and equine protozoal encephalomyelitis
- Contraindications include hypersensitivity to pyrimethamine, and hematologic disorders caused by folate deficiency.
- Adverse effects in small animals, which may be more severe in cats, include anorexia, malaise, vomiting, depression, and bone marrow depression (eg, anemia, thrombocytopenia, leukopenia); adverse effects in horses include leukopenias, thrombocytopenia, and anemias.
- Potentially teratogenic; avoid use in pregnancy
- Dosage form (25 mg tab only) may be inconvenient for accurate dosing; unpalatable to cats

Uses/Indications

Pyrimethamine is used to treat *Hepatozoon americanum* infections, canine neosporosis, and toxoplasmosis in small animals (often in combination with sulfonamides). In horses, it is approved, in combination with sulfadiazine, to treat equine protozoal myeloencephalitis.

In humans, pyrimethamine is used for the treatment of toxoplasmosis when used in combination with a sulfonamide[1]; drug resistance has rendered it ineffective as an anti-malarial agent.

Pharmacology/Actions

Pyrimethamine is a folic acid antagonist similar to trimethoprim. It acts by inhibiting dihydrofolate reductase, which catalyzes the conversion of dihydrofolic acid to tetrahydrofolic acid. It more readily binds to protozoal dihydrofolate reductase than the mammalian enzyme. The resulting depletion of folic acid impairs protozoal production of proteins and nucleic acids. Pyrimethamine has in vitro activity against *Toxoplasma gondii*; adding sulfadiazine can synergistically enhance activity.

Pharmacokinetics

Pyrimethamine administered to adult horses at 1 mg/kg IV or PO for 1 dose and 1 mg/kg PO once daily for 10 days resulted in oral bioavailability ≈55%. Food, including alfalfa hay, may reduce pyrimethamine absorption by up to 50%. Steady-state plasma concentrations were reached within 5 days, with CSF concentrations 25% to 50% of plasma values. The steady-state volume of distribution was ≈1.5 L/kg, and the elimination half-life was 12 hours.[2,3]

In humans, pyrimethamine is well absorbed from the gut after oral administration. It is distributed primarily to the kidneys, liver, spleen, and lungs but does cross the blood–brain barrier. It has a volume of distribution of ≈3 L/kg and is 80% bound to plasma proteins. Pyrimethamine enters milk in concentrations greater than those found in serum and can be detected in milk up to 48 hours after dosing. In humans, plasma half-life is ≈3 to 5 days. It is metabolized at least in part by the liver, and metabolites are found in the urine.

Contraindications/Precautions/Warnings

Pyrimethamine is contraindicated in patients that are hypersensitive to it and in patients with pre-existing hematologic disorders caused by folate deficiency. Pyrimethamine has a narrow therapeutic window; reduce the dose or discontinue if signs of folate deficiency develop. Use pyrimethamine with caution in patients with pre-existing folate deficiency or that have hepatic or renal impairment.[1] Some clinicians recommend avoiding pyrimethamine in cats because of its adverse effect profile.

In humans with seizure disorders, it is recommended to initiate therapy at a lower dose to avoid potential CNS toxicity.

Adverse Effects

In small animals, anorexia, malaise, vomiting, depression, and bone marrow depression (eg, anemia, thrombocytopenia, leukopenia) have been seen. Adverse effects may be more prominent in cats and noted 4 to 6 days after starting combination therapy. Some clinicians recommend avoiding its use in this species. Hematologic effects can develop rapidly, and frequent monitoring is recommended, particularly if therapy persists longer than 2 weeks. Administration of folinic acid (leucovorin) has been suggested to alleviate adverse hematologic effects.

The drug is unpalatable to cats when mixed with food, and the 25 mg tablet dosage size makes accurate dosing a challenge.

In horses, pyrimethamine has caused leukopenias, thrombocytopenia, and anemias when used in combination with sulfonamides.

In humans, hypersensitivity reactions have been reported, including Stevens-Johnson syndrome and toxic epidermal necrolysis. Other reported adverse effects in humans include megaloblastic anemia, thrombocytopenia, neutropenia, hematuria, and cardiac rhythm disorders.[1]

Reproductive/Nursing Safety

In stallions, pyrimethamine did not affect semen quality or sperm production, but physical performance (eg, mounting, thrusting, ejaculatory force) was adversely impacted.[4] Pyrimethamine has been demonstrated to be teratogenic in rats. Fetal abnormalities have been seen in foals after mares have been treated; however, it has been used in treating women with toxoplasmosis during pregnancy. Clearly, the risks associated with therapy must be weighed against the potential for toxicity, the severity of the disease, and any alternative therapies available (eg, clindamycin in small animals). Concomitant administration of folinic acid has been recommended (strongly recommended for humans) if the drug is to be used during pregnancy by some clinicians, but others state that pregnant mares should not receive folic acid during therapy, as it may exacerbate fetal abnormalities or mortality.[5]

Pyrimethamine is excreted in maternal milk; consider using milk replacer.

Because safety has not been established in animals, this drug should only be used when the maternal benefits outweigh the potential risks to offspring.

Overdose/Acute Toxicity

Reports of acute overdose of pyrimethamine in animals were not located. In humans, vomiting, nausea, anorexia, CNS stimulation (including seizures), and hematologic effects can be seen. Neurologic effects may occur within a few hours. Recommendations for treatment include GI decontamination, parenteral benzodiazepines (eg, midazolam) for seizures, folinic acid for hematologic effects, and long-term monitoring (at least 1 month) of renal and hematopoietic systems.

For patients that have experienced or are suspected of having experienced an overdose, consultation with a 24-hour poison consultation center specializing in providing veterinary-specific information is recommended. For general information related to overdose and toxin exposures, as well as contact information for poison control centers, refer to ***Appendix.***

Drug Interactions

The following drug interactions have either been reported or are theoretical in humans or animals receiving pyrimethamine and may be of significance in veterinary patients. Unless otherwise noted, use together is not necessarily contraindicated, but weigh the potential risks and perform additional monitoring when appropriate.

- **DAPSONE**: May increase the risk for myelosuppression
- **FOLIC ACID**: May reduce pyrimethamine efficacy
- **METHOTREXATE**: Antifolate effects may be additive, increasing the risk of myelosuppression
- **SULFONAMIDES** (eg, **sulfadiazine, sulfadimethoxine**): Pyrimethamine is synergistic with sulfonamides in activity against toxoplasmosis (and malaria).
- **TRIMETHOPRIM**: Use with pyrimethamine/sulfa is not recommended in humans, as adverse effects may be additive. Although this combination has been used clinically in horses, it is currently not recommended as trimethoprim competitively inhibits pyrimethamine, thus decreasing the efficacy of the more effective dihydrofolate reductase inhibitor.[6]
- **ZIDOVUDINE**: May reduce pyrimethamine efficacy; also may increase the risk for myelosuppression

Laboratory Considerations

- Pyrimethamine may cause inaccurate results for vitamin B_{12} and folic acid blood assays.

Dosages

DOGS:

Toxoplasmosis (extra-label): Pyrimethamine 0.25 – 0.5 mg/kg twice daily plus a sulfonamide 30 mg/kg twice daily for 2 to 4 weeks to treat disseminated toxoplasmosis and to reduce oocyst shedding[7]

Hepatazoon americanum (extra-label): Pyrimethamine 0.25 mg/kg PO every 24 hours in combination with trimethoprim/sulfadiazine 15 mg/kg PO every 12 hours and clindamycin 10 mg/kg every 8 hours. Once remission is attained, decoquinate 15 mg/kg mixed in food every 12 hours for 2 years can maintain a disease-free interval.[8,9]

Canine neosporosis (extra-label): Pyrimethamine 1 mg/kg PO every 24 hours for 4 weeks in combination with trimethoprim/sulfadiazine 15 – 20 mg/kg PO every 12 hours for 4 weeks. If observable clinical improvement is slow, treatment should be extended beyond the recommended 4 weeks until 2 weeks after clinical signs have plateaued. All littermates of affected puppies should be treated regardless of clinical signs.

CATS:

NOTE: See ***Contraindications/Precautions/Warnings*** above.

Toxoplasmosis (extra-label):

a) For disseminated toxoplasmosis, pyrimethamine 0.25 – 0.5 mg/kg PO twice daily with a sulfonamide 30 mg/kg PO twice daily for 2 to 4 weeks can be used to treat disseminated toxoplasmosis and to reduce oocyst shedding.[7]

b) In critical cases of pulmonary toxoplasmosis, pyrimethamine 0.25 – 0.5 mg/kg PO every 12 hours in combination with clindamycin 12.5 mg/kg PO once daily (follow with food or water) may be a better option than using clindamycin alone, especially in cats immunosuppressed with cyclosporine.[11]

HORSES:

See ***Pyrimethamine/Sulfadiazine.***

BIRDS:

Coccidian organisms in raptors (extra-label): 0.5 mg/kg PO twice daily for 14 to 28 days (especially effective against toxoplasmosis, atoxoplasmosis, and sarcocystis)[12]

Monitoring

- CBC with platelet count
- Adverse effects (eg, GI signs, malaise, depression)
- Clinical efficacy

Client Information

- For dogs, cats, and birds, this medicine can be given with or without food. It is unpleasant tasting if mixed into food.

- Cats may be more likely to develop side effects while on this drug; use with caution.
- Side effects include vomiting, lack of appetite, depression/malaise (tiredness/lack of energy), and bone marrow depression. If bleeding, extreme tiredness/lack of energy, infection, or fever are seen, contact veterinarian right away.
- Pregnant women should handle this drug very carefully.
- While your animal is taking this medication, it is important to return to your veterinarian for blood tests. Do not miss these important follow-up visits.

Chemistry/Synonyms

Pyrimethamine, an aminopyrimidine agent structurally related to trimethoprim, occurs as an odorless, white, or almost white crystalline powder or crystals. It is practically insoluble in water and slightly soluble in alcohol.

Pyrimethamine may also be known as BW-50-63, pirimetamina, pyrimethaminum, RP-4753, *Daraprim*®, *Malocide*®, or *Pirimecidan*®.

Storage/Stability

Store pyrimethamine tablets at 15°C to 25°C (59°F-77°F) in tight, light-resistant containers.

Compatibility/Compounding Considerations

Pyrimethamine tablets may be crushed to make oral suspensions of the drug. Although stable in an aqueous solution, sugars tend to adversely affect the stability of pyrimethamine. If cherry syrup, corn syrup, or sucrose-containing liquids are used in the preparation of the suspension, it is recommended to store the suspension at room temperature and discard it after 7 days.

Dosage Forms/Regulatory Status

VETERINARY-LABELED PRODUCTS: NONE

HUMAN-LABELED PRODUCTS:

Pyrimethamine Tablets: 25 mg; *Daraprim*®; (Rx)

References

For the complete list of references, see **wiley.com/go/budde/plumb**

Pyrimethamine/Sulfadiazine

(pye-ri-***meth***-a-meen/sul-fa-***dye***-a-zeen) *ReBalance*®

Antiprotozoal

Prescriber Highlights

- ► Combination antiprotozoal labeled for the treatment of horses with equine protozoal myeloencephalitis (EPM) caused by *Sarcocystis neurona*.
- ► Use with caution in patients with pre-existing hematologic abnormalities, renal or hepatic dysfunction, or patients with folate deficiency.
- ► Adverse effects include myelosuppression, GI effects, and worsening of neurologic signs after beginning therapy (treatment crisis).
- ► Daily treatment may be required for 3 to 9 months.

Uses/Indications

Pyrimethamine/sulfadiazine is FDA-approved in horses for the treatment of equine protozoal myeloencephalitis (EPM) caused by *Sarcocystis neurona*. Anecdotally, some combine pyrimethamine/sulfadiazine with ponazuril or diclazuril when treating relapsing EPM.

Although not labeled for use in small animal species, it potentially could be used for treating protozoal infections, such as toxoplasmosis, in cats or neosporosis in dogs.

Pharmacology/Actions

Pyrimethamine is a dihydrofolate reductase inhibitor that blocks the conversion of dihydrofolic acid (DFA) to tetrahydrofolic acid by inhibiting dihydrofolate reductase. Sulfonamides inhibit the conversion of para-aminobenzoic acid (PABA) to DFA by competing with PABA for dihydropteroate synthase binding sites. Sulfonamides and dihydrofolate reductase inhibitors are synergistic when used together. Although trimethoprim is more active than pyrimethamine against bacterial dihydrofolate reductase, pyrimethamine is more active against protozoal dihydrofolate reductase.

When used as labeled for EPM in horses, the estimated success rate is 60% to 70%, with a 10% estimated relapse rate.[1]

Pharmacokinetics

No specific pharmacokinetic information was located for this drug combination and dosage form (oral suspension) in horses. Previous reports in horses using other dosage forms reported pyrimethamine oral bioavailability as ≈56% and elimination half-life of ≈12 hours. Food, including alfalfa hay, may reduce pyrimethamine absorption by up to 50%. CNS concentrations are ≈25% to 50% of those found in plasma.[2,3]

Sulfadiazine is well absorbed after oral administration to horses. It has a volume of distribution of ≈0.58 L/kg and distributes into the CSF. Sulfonamides are metabolized via acetylation and other pathways and are primarily removed via the kidneys, with an elimination half-life of ≈3 to 4 hours.

Contraindications/Precautions/Warnings

Pyrimethamine/sulfadiazine is contraindicated in horses that are hypersensitive to either drug. Do not use in horses intended for human consumption.[4]

Use with caution in horses with pre-existing hematologic abnormalities due to the potential for myelosuppression. Use cautiously in patients with renal or hepatic impairment, or those with folate deficiency. EPM should be distinguished from other ataxic conditions prior to beginning treatment with pyrimethamine/sulfadiazine.[4]

Adverse Effects

Adverse effects reported in horses include reversible myelosuppression (eg, anemia, leukopenia, neutropenia, thrombocytopenia), reduced appetite or anorexia, loose stools/diarrhea, and urticaria.[4] CNS effects such as seizures and depression are also possible but are more likely signs of EPM.

Baker's yeast or folinic acid have been suggested to antagonize the drug combination's myelosuppressive effects, but evidence of efficacy is lacking.

Neurologic signs may worsen (treatment crisis) during the first few days of treatment and may persist up to 5 weeks.[4] This may be the result of an inflammatory reaction secondary to dying parasites in the central nervous system.

Reproductive/Nursing Safety

The safe use of pyrimethamine/sulfadiazine combination in horses for breeding purposes, during pregnancy, or in lactating mares has not been evaluated.[4]

Pyrimethamine has been demonstrated to be teratogenic in rats,[5] and fetal abnormalities have been seen in foals following treatment of pregnant mares[6]; however, it has been used to treat pregnant women with toxoplasmosis when the benefits outweigh the risks.[5] Similarly, in horses, risks associated with therapy must be weighed against the potential for toxicity, the severity of the disease, and any alternative therapies available. Some clinicians have recommended concomitant administration of folinic acid if pyrimethamine is to be used during pregnancy, but others state that pregnant mares should not receive folic acid during therapy as it may exacerbate fetal abnormalities or mortality.[7] Additionally, pyrimethamine may adversely impact the physical performance (eg, mounting, thrusting, ejaculatory force) of stallions.[8]

Sulfonamides cross the placenta and fetal serum concentrations may be up to 50% of that found in maternal serum. Teratogenicity has been reported in some laboratory animals when given at high doses. Sulfonamides should be used in pregnant animals only when the benefits clearly outweigh the risks of therapy.

Pyrimethamine and sulfonamides are distributed into milk. Safety for nursing offspring has not been established[4]; consider using milk replacer.

Overdose/Acute Toxicity

Acute overdose information for pyrimethamine/sulfadiazine in horses was not located. At 2 times the label dose for 92 days in 49 horses, signs included loose stools, slight increases in ALP in some horses, declines in RBC, HCT, Hgb, and PCV, and decreased appetite.[4]

For patients that have experienced or are suspected to have experienced an overdose, consultation with a 24-hour poison consultation center specializing in providing veterinary-specific information is recommended. For general information related to overdose and toxin exposures, as well as contact information for poison control centers, refer to ***Appendix***.

Drug Interactions

The safety of pyrimethamine/sulfadiazine has not been evaluated with concomitant therapies in horses. In humans, the following drug interactions with pyrimethamine and/or sulfonamides have been reported or are theoretical and may be of significance in veterinary patients. Unless otherwise noted, use together is not necessarily contraindicated, but weigh the potential risks and perform additional monitoring when appropriate.

- **ANTACIDS**: May decrease the bioavailability of sulfonamides if administered concurrently
- **CYCLOSPORINE**: May decrease cyclosporine effectiveness
- **HIGHLY PROTEIN-BOUND DRUGS** (eg, **methotrexate, phenylbutazone, thiazide diuretics, salicylates, probenecid, phenytoin, warfarin**): Because sulfonamides are highly bound to plasma proteins, they could theoretically displace other highly bound drugs causing a transient increase in serum concentrations of each drug. These interactions are unlikely to be of clinical concern because increased free drug concentrations will equilibrate through increased clearance. Monitor for adverse effects of each drug when using this combination.
- **PARA-AMINOBENZOIC ACID (PABA)**: PABA is reportedly antagonistic towards the activity of pyrimethamine; the clinical significance is unclear.
- **TRIMETHOPRIM**: Use with pyrimethamine/sulfadiazine is not recommended as adverse effects may be additive. Although this combination has been used clinically in horses, it is not recommended as trimethoprim competitively inhibits pyrimethamine, thus decreasing the efficacy of the more effective dihydrofolate reductase inhibitor.[1]
- **WARFARIN**: Sulfonamides may potentiate the effects of warfarin.

Laboratory Considerations

The following laboratory alterations have been reported in humans taking sulfonamides or pyrimethamine and may be of significance in veterinary patients.

- Urine glucose: Sulfonamides may give false-positive results when using Benedict's method.
- Vitamin B_{12} and folic acid: Pyrimethamine may cause inaccurate results for blood assays.

Dosages

HORSES:

Equine protozoal myeloencephalitis (EPM) (label dosage; FDA-approved): Pyrimethamine 1 mg/kg and sulfadiazine 20 mg/kg PO once daily, at least 1 hour before feeding with hay or grain.[4] Treatment duration is based upon clinical response but typically ranges from 90 to 270 days.

Monitoring

- Baseline and monthly CBC with platelets
- GI adverse effects
- Clinical efficacy, including improvement in neurologic signs and negative CSF Western Blot test

Client Information

- Shake this medicine well before each use.
- Give this medicine at least 1 hour before feeding with hay or grain.
- Use an oral dosing syringe to give this medicine to your horse. Place the tip of the syringe in the interdental space (entering side of the mouth behind front teeth) and apply the dose on the back of the tongue.
- During the first few days of treatment, neurologic signs (eg, weakness, trouble walking) may get worse and may last up to 5 weeks. These signs may be due to inflammation caused by dying parasites.
- Side effects include loose stools, diarrhea, reduced appetite, and itching.
- This medicine can put your horse at risk for developing infections. Contact your veterinarian immediately if you notice bleeding, extreme tiredness or lack of energy, fever, or other signs of infection.

Chemistry/Synonyms

Pyrimethamine is an aminopyrimidine agent structurally related to trimethoprim. It occurs as an odorless, white, or almost white crystalline powder or crystals. It is practically insoluble in water and slightly soluble in alcohol.

Sulfadiazine occurs as an odorless or nearly odorless, white to slightly yellow powder. It is practically insoluble in water and sparingly soluble in alcohol.

Sulfadiazine and Pyrimethamine may also be known as *ReBalance*®. Sulfadoxine and pyrimethamine may also be known as *Fansidar*®.

Storage/Stability

Store suspension at controlled room temperature (20°C-25°C [68°F-77°F]), with excursions permitted between 15°C and 30°C (59°F- 86°F) and protected from light and freezing.[4]

Dosage Forms/Regulatory Status

VETERINARY-LABELED PRODUCTS:

Pyrimethamine 12.5 mg/mL and Sulfadiazine (as the sodium salt) 250 mg/mL Oral Suspension in 946.4 mL bottles; *ReBalance*®; (Rx) FDA-approved for use in horses; not for use in horses intended for human consumption

HUMAN-LABELED PRODUCTS:

None

References

For the complete list of references, see **wiley.com/go/budde/plumb**

Quinacrine

(*qwin*-a-krin)

Antiprotozoal

Prescriber Highlights

- ► May be used for treatment of a variety of protozoans and helminths
- ► Use should be avoided in patients with hepatic dysfunction.
- ► Adverse effects include benign yellowing of skin and urine, GI effects (eg, anorexia, nausea, vomiting, diarrhea), abnormal behaviors (eg, fly biting, agitation), lethargy, pruritus, and fever.
- ► Give with meals; ensure plenty of water is available.
- ► Not commercially available in the United States

Uses/Indications

Quinacrine has activity against a variety of protozoans and helminths; however, it is no longer available in the United States. Newer, safer, or more effective agents have largely replaced its use in small animal species, except as an alternative treatment for *Giardia* spp or *Trichomonas* spp.

In humans, quinacrine is an antimalarial drug that has been used for treatment of mild to moderate discoid lupus erythematosus.

Pharmacology/Actions

Quinacrine's mechanism of action for its antiprotozoal activity against *Giardia* spp is not understood; however, it is known that it binds to DNA by intercalation to adjacent base pairs, thereby inhibiting RNA transcription and translocation. Additionally, quinacrine interferes with electron transport and inhibits succinate oxidation and cholinesterase. Quinacrine binds to nucleoproteins that, in humans, can suppress lupus erythematosus cell factor.

Pharmacokinetics

Quinacrine is absorbed well from the GI tract or after intrapleural administration. It is distributed throughout the body, but CSF concentrations are only 1% to 5% of those found in plasma. Quinacrine is concentrated in the liver, spleen, lungs, and adrenals. It is relatively highly bound to plasma proteins in humans (80% to 90%).

Quinacrine is metabolized slowly and eliminated slowly, primarily by the kidneys. Its half-life in humans ranges from 5 to 14 days. Acidifying the urine may increase renal excretion. Significant amounts may be detected in urine up to 2 months after drug discontinuation.

Contraindications/Precautions/Warnings

Use quinacrine with extreme caution in patients with hepatic dysfunction. In humans, quinacrine is relatively contraindicated in patients with psychotic disorders, psoriasis, or porphyria, as it may exacerbate these conditions; relevance for veterinary patients is unknown.

Do not confuse quinaCRINE with quiniDINE. Consider writing part of the drug's name in uppercase letters (tall-man designations) on prescriptions/orders to reduce the risk for errors.

Adverse Effects

In small animal species, a benign yellowing of skin and urine color can occur; yellowing does not indicate jaundice. GI disturbances (eg, anorexia, nausea, vomiting, diarrhea), abnormal behaviors (eg, fly biting, agitation), lethargy, pruritus, and fever have also been noted.

In humans, hypersensitivity reactions, hepatopathy, aplastic anemia, corneal edema, and retinopathy have rarely been reported, primarily with high-dose, long-term use.

Reproductive/Nursing Safety

Quinacrine crosses the placenta and has been implicated in causing a case of renal agenesis and hydrocephalus in a human infant. In high doses, it has caused increased fetal death rates in rats. Quinacrine enters maternal milk in only small amounts. Because safety has not been established in animals, this drug should only be used when the maternal benefits outweigh the potential risks to offspring.

Overdose/Acute Toxicity

Severity of overdose is dose dependent. In humans, a dose as low as 6.8 g administered intraduodenally was fatal. Clinical signs associated with acute toxicity include CNS excitation (including seizures), GI disturbances, vascular collapse, and cardiac arrhythmias. Treatment consists of GI decontamination protocol, and supportive and symptomatic therapies. Urinary acidification with ammonium chloride and forced diuresis with adequate fluid therapy may enhance urinary excretion of the drug.

For patients that have experienced or are suspected to have experienced an overdose, consultation with a 24-hour poison consultation center specializing in providing veterinary-specific information is recommended. For general information related to overdose and toxin exposures, as well as contact information for poison control centers, refer to ***Appendix.***

Drug Interactions

The following drug interactions have either been reported or are theoretical in humans or animals receiving quinacrine and may be of significance in veterinary patients. Unless otherwise noted, use together is not necessarily contraindicated, but weigh the potential risks and perform additional monitoring when appropriate.

- ETHANOL: Quinacrine may cause a disulfiram-reaction if used with alcohol.
- HEPATOTOXIC DRUGS (eg, **androgens, azole antifungals, estrogens, NSAIDs**): Quinacrine concentrates in the liver and should be used cautiously with other hepatotoxic drugs.
- PRIMAQUINE: Quinacrine increases the toxicity of primaquine; use together is contraindicated.

Laboratory Considerations

- Quinacrine may cause acidic urine to turn a deep yellow color.
- Quinacrine can cause falsely elevated values of plasma and urine cortisol values by causing an interfering fluorescence.

Dosages

DOGS:

Last-line drug for treatment of *Giardia* spp or other susceptible protozoa (extra-label): 6.6 mg/kg PO every 12 hours for 5 days[1,2]

CATS:

Last-line drug for treatment of *Giardia* spp (extra-label): 9 mg/kg PO once daily for 6 days[1,2]

Last-line drug for treatment of *Coccidia* spp (extra-label): 10 mg/kg PO once daily for 5 days[1,2]

REPTILES:

Hemoprotozoal infections (extra-label): 19 – 100 mg/kg PO every 48 hours for 2 to 3 weeks[3]

Monitoring

- Fecal examinations
- Efficacy: resolution of clinical signs associated with infection being treated
- Adverse effects

Client Information

- Give this medicine after meals with access to plenty of fresh water to drink.
- Watch for signs of adverse effects, including vomiting, diarrhea, decreased appetite, abnormal behaviors, low-energy level, itching, or fever.
- Yellowing of skin or urine is due to the dye characteristics of quin-

acrine and is not serious. However, you should contact your veterinarian if yellowing of the eyes occurs.

Chemistry/Synonyms

Quinacrine is a synthetic acridine derivative anthelmintic that occurs as a bright-yellow, odorless, crystalline powder and has a bitter taste. It is sparingly soluble in water.

Quinacrine HCl may also be known as mepacrine HCl, acrichinum, or acrinamine.

Storage/Stability

Tablets should be stored in tight, light-resistant containers at room temperature. Quinacrine is not stable in solution for any length of time; however, it may be crushed and mixed with foods to mask its very bitter taste.

Compatibility/Compounding Considerations

No specific information noted

Dosage Forms/Regulatory Status

VETERINARY-LABELED PRODUCTS: NONE

HUMAN-LABELED PRODUCTS: NONE

There currently are no quinacrine products being marketed in the United States. It may be available from compounding pharmacies.

References

For the complete list of references, see **wiley.com/go/budde/plumb**

Quinidine

(***qwin***-i-deen)

Antiarrhythmic (Systemic Drug)

Prescriber Highlights

- ▶ Antiarrhythmic agent used in horses and, less commonly, in small animals
- ▶ Contraindications include hypersensitivity, myasthenia gravis, complete AV block with an AV junctional or idioventricular pacemaker, intraventricular conduction defects, digitalis intoxication with associated arrhythmias or AV conduction disorders, aberrant ectopic impulses, and abnormal rhythms secondary to escape mechanisms.
- ▶ Use extreme caution with any form of AV block or any clinical signs of digoxin toxicity.
- ▶ Use caution with uncorrected hypokalemia, hypoxia, or acid-base imbalances; hepatic or renal insufficiency; congestive heart failure.
- ▶ Adverse effects in dogs include GI effects, weakness, hypotension (especially with too rapid IV administration), negative inotropism, widened QRS complex and QT intervals, AV block, and multiform ventricular tachycardias and hypotension.
- ▶ Adverse effects in horses include inappetence, depression, swelling of the nasal mucosa, ataxia, diarrhea, colic, hypotension, and, rarely, laminitis, paraphimosis, and the development of urticarial wheals; cardiac arrhythmias including AV block, circulatory collapse, and sudden death.
- ▶ Consider monitoring blood concentrations.
- ▶ Administer at evenly spaced intervals throughout the day and night.
- ▶ Many possible drug interactions, including some with significant risk for patient harm

Uses/Indications

Quinidine is used in equine medicine for medical cardioconversion of atrial fibrillation. In small animals it is used for the treatment of ventricular arrhythmias (PVCs, ventricular tachycardia), refractory supraventricular tachycardias, and supraventricular arrhythmias associated with anomalous conduction in Wolff-Parkinson-White (WPW) syndrome. Long-term use of quinidine for controlling ventricular arrhythmias and supraventricular tachycardia in dogs has diminished over the years as other drugs appear to be more effective. It is still used in dogs and horses to convert atrial fibrillation to sinus rhythm. One retrospective study in horses found quinidine to be more effective than flecainide at achieving cardioversion in horses with naturally occurring, recent-onset atrial fibrillation.[1] Oral therapy is generally not used in cats.

Pharmacology/Actions

Quinidine is a class IA antiarrhythmic, which has effects similar to that of procainamide. It blocks the fast sodium channels during the depolarization of the action potential (phase 0). It depresses myocardial excitability, conduction velocity, and contractility. Quinidine prolongs the duration of the action potential and the effective refractory period, which prevents the reentry phenomenon and increases conduction times. Quinidine also possesses anticholinergic activity, which decreases vagal tone and may facilitate AV conduction.

Pharmacokinetics

After oral administration, quinidine salts are nearly completely absorbed from the GI tract; however, the amount that reaches systemic circulation is reduced due to the hepatic first-pass effect. The extended-release formulations of quinidine sulfate and gluconate, as well as the polygalacturonate tablets, are more slowly absorbed than the conventional tablets or capsules.

Quinidine is distributed rapidly to all body tissues except the brain. Protein binding varies from 82% to 92%. The reported volumes of distribution in various species are as follows: dogs, ≈2.9 L/kg; cats, ≈2.2 L/kg; horses, ≈15.1 L/kg; and cattle, ≈3.8 L/kg. Quinidine is distributed into milk and crosses the placenta.

Quinidine is metabolized in the liver, primarily by hydroxylation. Approximately 20% of a dose may be excreted unchanged in the urine within 24 hours of dosing. Serum half-lives reported in various species are as follows: dogs, ≈5.6 hours; cats, ≈1.9 hours; horses, ≈8.1 hours; cattle, ≈2.3 hours; swine, ≈5.5 hours; and goats, ≈0.9 hours. Acidic urine (pH less than 6) can increase renal excretion of quinidine and decrease its serum half-life.

Contraindications/Precautions/Warnings

Quinidine is generally contraindicated in patients that have demonstrated previous hypersensitivity reactions to it, or in patients with myasthenia gravis, complete AV block with an AV junctional or an idioventricular pacemaker, intraventricular conduction defects (especially with pronounced QRS widening), digitalis intoxication with associated arrhythmias or AV conduction disorders, aberrant ectopic impulses, or abnormal rhythms secondary to escape mechanisms. It should be used with extreme caution, if at all, in any form of AV block or if any clinical signs of digitalis toxicity are exhibited. In humans, mortality associated with the use of quinidine was 3 times higher than placebo when quinidine was used to prevent recurrence of atrial flutter/fibrillation. Mortality associated with quinidine was also higher than other antiarrhythmics when used for various non-life–threatening ventricular arrhythmias.[2,3] The significance of these findings for veterinary patients is unclear.

Quinidine should be used with caution in patients with uncorrected hypokalemia, hypoxia, and acid-base imbalances. Quinidine and other class IA antiarrhythmics prolong the QT interval, which can potentially lead to torsades de pointes. In humans, this risk is increased in patients with hypokalemia, hypomagnesemia, or high quinidine concentrations. In humans with sick sinus syndrome, sinus node depression and bradycardia can occur. Use quinidine cautiously in patients with hepatic or renal insufficiency, as accumulation of the drug and subsequent toxicity may result. Use quinidine with caution in patients with congestive heart failure, as apparent volume of distribution is reduced, which can lead to quinidine toxicity. Consider dose reduction.[2,3]

Quinidine has many significant drug interactions; see ***Drug Interactions***.

When using quinidine to cardiovert horses with atrial fibrillation, monitor the ECG throughout treatment. Indicators to discontinue medication include heart rates above 80 bpm, a widening of QRS beyond 125% of baseline, and abnormal complexes.[4]

Adverse Effects

In dogs, GI effects may include anorexia, vomiting, or diarrhea. Effects related to the cardiovascular system can include weakness, hypotension (especially with too rapid IV administration), negative inotropism, widened QRS complex and QT intervals, AV block, and multiform ventricular tachycardias.

In horses, inappetence and depression are commonly seen after quinidine therapy, but this does not necessarily indicate toxicity. Signs of toxicity can include swelling of the nasal mucosa; ataxia; diarrhea; colic; ventricular rate exceeding 120 bpm; QRS broadening by 25% of baseline or more; hypotension; and, rarely, laminitis, paraphimosis, and the development of urticarial wheals. Urticaria or upper respiratory tract obstruction can be treated, if required, by discontinuing the drug and administering corticosteroids. If obstruction persists, nasotracheal tube placement or tracheostomy may be required. Horses may develop cardiac arrhythmias including AV block, circulatory collapse, and sudden death.

Patients exhibiting signs of toxicity or lack of response may be candidates for therapeutic serum monitoring. The therapeutic range is thought to be 2.5 to 5 µg/mL in dogs. Quinidine concentrations above 5 µg/mL are associated with adverse effects.[5]

Reproductive/Nursing Safety

No animal data were located. In humans, quinidine crosses the placenta; maternal and fetal quinidine concentrations are roughly equivalent.[6]

Quinidine is excreted into maternal milk with a milk to serum ratio of ≈0.71. Use caution when quinidine is administered to nursing patients. The American Academy of Pediatrics considers quinidine compatible with breastfeeding.

Because safety has not been established in animals, this drug should only be used when the maternal benefits outweigh the potential risks to offspring.

Overdose/Acute Toxicity

Clinical signs of overdose can include depression, hypotension, lethargy, confusion, seizures, vomiting, diarrhea, and oliguria. Cardiac signs may include depressed automaticity and conduction, or tachyarrhythmias. The CNS effects are often delayed after the onset of cardiovascular effects but may persist after the cardiovascular effects have begun to resolve.

If the overdose was from a recent oral ingestion, GI decontamination may be beneficial to remove any unabsorbed drug. IV fluids, plus metaraminol or norepinephrine, can be considered to treat hypotensive effects. Digoxin has been recommended for treating quinidine-induced profound hypotension or supraventricular tachycardia (more than 200 bpm) in horses.[7] A 1/6 molar IV infusion of sodium lactate may be used in an attempt to reduce the cardiotoxic effects of quinidine. Forced diuresis using fluids and diuretics along with urinary acidification may enhance the renal excretion of the drug. Temporary cardiac pacing may be necessary should severe AV block occur. Hemodialysis will effectively remove quinidine, but peritoneal dialysis will not.

For patients that have experienced or are suspected to have experienced an overdose, consultation with a 24-hour poison consultation center specializing in providing veterinary-specific information is recommended. For general information related to overdose and toxin exposures, as well as contact information for poison control centers, refer to ***Appendix***.

Drug Interactions

The following drug interactions have either been reported or are theoretical in humans or animals receiving quinidine and may be of significance in veterinary patients. Unless otherwise noted, use together is not necessarily contraindicated, but weigh the potential risks and perform additional monitoring when appropriate.

- ACETAZOLAMIDE: May reduce quinidine clearance
- AMIODARONE: May significantly increase quinidine concentrations and risk for cardiotoxicity
- ANTACIDS, ALUMINUM-, CALCIUM-, OR MAGNESIUM-CONTAINING: May delay oral absorption; separate dosages
- ANTICHOLINESTERASES (eg, **pyridostigmine, neostigmine**): Quinidine may antagonize the effects of anticholinesterases in patients with myasthenia gravis.
- ANTIHYPERTENSIVE AGENTS (eg, **amlodipine, enalapril, sildenafil, telmisartan**): Quinidine may potentiate hypotensive effects.
- AUROTHIOGLUCOSE: Increased risk for blood dyscrasias
- AZOLE ANTIFUNGALS (eg, **fluconazole, itraconazole, ketoconazole**): Increased risk for cardiotoxicity. Combination contraindicated in humans
- CIMETIDINE: Cimetidine may increase the concentrations of quinidine by inhibiting hepatic microsomal enzymes.
- CISAPRIDE: Increased risk for QTc interval prolongation
- COLCHICINE: Quinidine may increase colchicine concentrations.
- DEXAMETHASONE: In dogs, dexamethasone increased quinidine volume of distribution (49% to 78%) and elimination half-life (1.5 to 2.3 times).[8]
- DIGOXIN: Digoxin concentrations may increase considerably in patients stabilized on digoxin that receive quinidine. Some cardiologists recommend decreasing the digoxin dose by ½ when adding quinidine. Therapeutic drug monitoring of both quinidine and digoxin may be warranted in these cases. Digoxin has been recommended for treating quinidine-induced profound hypotension or supraventricular tachycardia (more than 200 bpm) in horses.[7]
- DILTIAZEM: Possible decreased clearance; increased elimination half-life of quinidine. Diltiazem has been recommended for treating quinidine-induced profound hypotension or supraventricular tachycardia (more than 200 bpm) in horses.[7]
- DOXORUBICIN: Concurrent use may increase doxorubicin exposure.
- HYDROXYZINE: Concurrent use may increase the risk for QT interval prolongation.
- FLUOROQUINOLONE ANTIBIOTICS (eg, **ciprofloxacin, enrofloxacin**): Increased risk for cardiotoxicity
- LIDOCAINE, MEXILETINE: Concurrent use may increase risk for cardiotoxicity.
- MACROLIDE ANTIBIOTICS (eg, **clarithromycin, erythromycin**): Concurrent use may increase risk for cardiotoxicity.
- METHADONE: Concurrent use may increase risk for QT interval prolongation.
- METRONIDAZOLE: Concurrent use may increase risk for QT interval prolongation.
- MORPHINE: Concurrent use may increase morphine exposure.
- NEUROMUSCULAR BLOCKING AGENTS (eg, **succinylcholine, tubocurarine, atracurium**): Quinidine may increase the neuromuscular blocking effects of these drugs.
- ONDANSETRON: Concurrent use may increase risk for QT interval prolongation.

- **Paroxetine**: Concurrent use may increase paroxetine plasma concentrations and risk for paroxetine toxicity.
- **Phenobarbital, Primidone**: May induce hepatic enzymes that metabolize quinidine, thus reducing quinidine serum half-life by 50%
- **Phenothiazines** (eg, **acepromazine**): Additive cardiac depressant effects may be seen.
- **Procainamide**: Concurrent use may increase risk for cardiotoxicity.
- **Rifampin**: May induce hepatic enzymes that metabolize quinidine, thus reducing quinidine serum half-life by 50%
- **Sotalol**: Concurrent use may increase risk for QT interval prolongation.
- **Trazodone**: Concurrent use may increase risk for QT interval prolongation.
- **Tricyclic Antidepressants** (eg, **amitriptyline, clomipramine, doxepin, imipramine**): Increased risk for QTc interval prolongation and tricyclic adverse effects
- **Urinary Acidifiers** (eg, **methionine, ammonium chloride**): Drugs that acidify the urine may increase the excretion of quinidine and decrease serum concentration.
- **Urinary Alkalinizers** (eg, **carbonic anhydrase inhibitors, thiazide diuretics, sodium bicarbonate, antacids**): Drugs that alkalinize the urine may decrease the excretion of quinidine, prolonging its half-life.
- **Verapamil**: Possible decreased clearance; increased elimination half-life of quinidine; increased risk for hypotension
- **Vincristine**: Concurrent use may increase vincristine plasma concentrations.
- **Warfarin**: Coumarin anticoagulants with quinidine may increase the likelihood of bleeding problems.

Laboratory Considerations

- None noted

Dosages

DOGS:

PVCs or ventricular tachycardia (extra-label): immediate-release products, 6 – 16 mg/kg PO every 6 hours; extended-release products, 6 – 16 mg/kg PO every 8 hours[9]

Conversion of atrial fibrillation to sinus rhythm in dogs without underlying heart disease (extra-label): Initially attempted with quinidine gluconate 6 – 11 mg/kg IM every 6 hours. Some dogs will convert in the first 24 hours of therapy. If rapid ventricular response occurs, may give either digoxin or a beta-blocker to slow rate of conduction across AV node.[10,11]

HORSES:

Atrial fibrillation in a horse without heart failure (extra-label): Quinidine sulfate 22 mg/kg via nasogastric (NG) tube every 2 hours until cardioversion occurs, toxic effects are noted, or 6 doses have been given (4 doses if quinidine plasma concentrations cannot be monitored).[5,12] If atrial fibrillation remains, continue quinidine 22 mg/kg via NG tube every 6 hours until cardioversion or adverse effects. Check ECG prior to administering each dose. Do not administer directly into the mouth, as quinidine is a mucosal irritant.[12] Alternate IV dosing: 0.5 – 2.2 mg/kg IV bolus every 5 to 10 minutes to effect or until adverse effects seen. Maximum IV dose is 12 mg/kg. Conversion of ventricular tachycardia has occurred with a single 0.5 mg/kg dose.

Sustained narrow-QRS tachycardia (extra-label): From a case report: 22 mg/kg via NG tube every 2 hours for 3 doses. The rate of the tachycardia slowed gradually from 150 bpm to ≈100 bpm. Approximately 1 hour after the third dose, the cardiac rhythm abruptly converted to sinus tachycardia at a rate of 80 bpm.[13]

Monitoring

- ECG, continuous if possible
- Blood pressure, during IV administration
- Clinical signs of toxicity (see ***Overdose/Acute Toxicity*** and ***Adverse Effects***)
- Serum quinidine concentrations. Therapeutic serum concentrations are believed to range from 2 to 7 µg/mL in dogs and 2 to 5 µg/mL in horses. Concentrations more than 10 µg/mL are considered toxic.
- Atrial fibrillatory rate (AFR); one study found that a lower AFR may be associated with successful quinidine cardioversion[14]
- When using quinidine to cardiovert horses with atrial fibrillation, monitor the ECG throughout treatment. Indicators to discontinue medication include heart rates above 80 bpm, a widening of QRS beyond 125% of baseline, and abnormal complexes, or signs of toxicity (eg, nasal edema, diarrhea or colic, neurologic signs; see ***Adverse Effects***).[4]

Client Information

- Oral products should be administered at evenly spaced intervals throughout the day and night. Gastrointestinal upset (eg, anorexia, vomiting, or diarrhea) may be decreased if administered with food.
- Do not allow your animal to chew or crush sustained-release oral dosage forms.
- Notify your veterinarian if your animal's condition deteriorates or signs of toxicity (eg, vomiting, diarrhea, weakness) occur.

Chemistry/Synonyms

Used as an antiarrhythmic agent, quinidine is an alkaloid obtained from cinchona or related plants, or prepared from quinine. It is available commercially in two salts: gluconate and sulfate. Quinidine polygalacturonate is no longer commercially available.

Quinidine gluconate occurs as a very bitter tasting, odorless, white powder. It is freely soluble in water and slightly soluble in alcohol. The injectable form has a pH of 5.5 to 7. Quinidine gluconate contains 62% anhydrous quinidine alkaloid. Quinidine sulfate occurs as very bitter tasting, odorless, fine, needle-like, white crystals that may cohere in masses. One gram is soluble in ≈100 mL of water or 10 mL of alcohol. Quinidine sulfate contains 83% anhydrous quinidine alkaloid.

Quinidine gluconate may also be known as quinidinium gluconate, *Duraquin®*, *Quinaglute®*, *Quinalan®*, and *Quinate®*.

Quinidine sulfate may also be known as chinidini sulfas, chinidinsulfate, chinidinum sulfuricum, or quinidini sulfas; many trade names are available.

Storage/Stability

All quinidine salts darken on exposure to light (acquire a brownish tint) and should be stored in light-resistant, well-closed containers. Use only colorless, clear solutions of quinidine gluconate for injection.

Compatibility/Compounding Considerations

Compatibility is dependent on factors such as pH, concentration, temperature, and diluent used; specialized references or a hospital pharmacist should be consulted for more specific information.

Quinidine gluconate is reported to be physically **compatible** with bretylium tosylate, cimetidine HCl, and verapamil HCl. It is reportedly physically **incompatible** with alkalis and iodides.

Quinidine gluconate injection is usually administered IM but may be given very slowly (1 mL/minute) IV. It may be diluted by adding 10 to 40 mL of 5% dextrose.

Dosage Forms/Regulatory Status

VETERINARY-LABELED PRODUCTS: NONE

The Association of Racing Commissioners International (ARCI) has designated this drug as a class 4 substance. Use of this drug may not be allowed in certain animal competitions. Check rules and regulations before entering in a competition while this medication is being administered. Contact local racing authorities for further guidance. See ***Appendix*** for more information.

HUMAN-LABELED PRODUCTS:

Quinidine Sulfate (83% anhydrous quinidine alkaloid) Tablets: 200 and 300 mg; generic; (Rx)

Quinidine Gluconate (62% anhydrous quinidine alkaloid) Sustained-Release Tablets: 324 mg; generic; (Rx)

Quinidine Gluconate Injection has been discontinued.

References

For the complete list of references, see **wiley.com/go/budde/plumb**

Rabacfosadine

(***ra***-bak-***fos***-a-deen) *Tanovea®*

Antineoplastic

Prescriber Highlights

- Guanine nucleotide analogue that is FDA-approved for the treatment of lymphoma in dogs
- Narrow therapeutic index; calculate dosages carefully
- Most common adverse effects include diarrhea, vomiting, decreased/loss of appetite, neutropenia, lethargy, and cumulative dermatopathy (dermatitis, hyperpigmentation, alopecia, pruritus, and otitis).
- More serious adverse effects can occur, requiring treatment delay or dose reduction.
- Administration can be associated with life-threatening or fatal pulmonary fibrosis in a small percentage of patients (less than 5%). Contraindicated in dogs with or susceptible to pulmonary fibrosis, including West Highland white terriers
- Careful monitoring is essential, including CBC, renal function, and liver enzymes.
- Precautions required for handling waste for 5 days following administration

Uses/Indications

Rabacfosadine is indicated for the treatment of lymphoma in dogs. The drug appears to show promise for combined chemotherapy of naïve canine lymphoma[1] as well as relapsed or refractory lymphoma,[2] and as a single agent for the treatment of canine cutaneous Tcell lymphoma[3] and multiple myeloma.[4]

In 2 pilot field studies, the overall response rate (ORR) in 22 dogs with B-cell or T-cell lymphoma receiving rabacfosadine once every 21 days was 77% (46% complete response; 32% partial response). The ORR was 100% (8 of 8 dogs) in naïve dogs and 64% (9 of 14 dogs) in pretreated dogs. The overall median progression-free survival time in the 17 dogs experiencing response was 134 days.[5]

In a study of 60 treatment-naïve dogs, the ORR was 87%. The ORR in dogs with B-cell lymphoma was 97% compared to an ORR of 50% in dogs with T-cell lymphoma.[6] Considering these results, the novel mechanism of action, and the unique toxicities that do not overlap with other chemotherapeutics, the authors concluded that rabacfosadine could potentially be combined with other agents or incorporated into standard first-line protocols.

In a multicenter, randomized, double-blinded, placebo-controlled study, dogs with both naïve and relapsed lymphoma treated with rabacfosadine had a statistically significant improvement in progression-free survival (PFS) compared to placebo.[7] ORR was calculated for a given study visit and ranged from 48.2% to 63.4%. One month after the last treatment, 33% of rabacfosadine-treated dogs were progression-free compared to 0% of placebo dogs. Similar to previous studies, PFS was longer in dogs with B-cell lymphoma compared to those with T-cell lymphoma.

In an open-label, single-arm study, the combination of rabacfosadine and L-asparaginase appeared to be effective in dogs with lymphoma that had relapsed after previous treatment with a doxorubicin protocol.[2]

Pharmacology/Actions

Rabacfosadine is a guanine nucleotide analogue. Intracellularly, the prodrug is sequentially hydrolyzed, deaminated, and then undergoes 2 separate phosphorylation reactions. Its active form, 9-[2-(phosphonomethoxy)ethyl] guanine diphosphate (PMEGpp), is a potent, chain-terminating inhibitor of the major deoxyribonucleic acid (DNA) polymerases. In vitro studies have demonstrated the drug to inhibit DNA synthesis, resulting in S phase arrest and induction of apoptosis.[8] It also inhibits the proliferation of mitogen-stimulated lymphocytes and lymphoma/leukemia cell lines.[9]

Resistance may be mediated by mutations in the deamination gene[10] and by the acquisition of point mutations in the enzyme guanidylate kinase, impairing PMEG phosphorylation to PMEGpp.[11]

Pharmacokinetics

Rabacfosadine is not orally absorbed. Following a 30-minute IV infusion, the mean peak plasma concentrations for rabacfosadine and an interim metabolite occurred at ≈30 minutes (T_{max}) and 1 to 2 hours, respectively.[9] After administration, the drug and metabolites are widely distributed throughout the body. Some of the highest rabacfosadine concentrations are found in lymphoid tissue, and the drug preferentially accumulates in peripheral blood mononuclear cells (PBMCs). It is not known if rabacfosadine or metabolites cross the placenta or enter the milk; it does not penetrate the CNS. In dogs with lymphoma, rabacfosadine and the interim metabolite had a plasma half-life of less than 0.5 and 6 hours, respectively. In lymphoid cells, high concentrations of the active metabolite PMEGpp accumulate and persist for more than 24 hours. In PBMCs, the active metabolite PMEGpp showed a terminal half-life of 68.7 hours. Overall elimination of [^{14}C]-rabacfosadine after IV dosing was 80% over 120 hours. It undergoes both fecal and renal elimination.[9]

Contraindications/Precautions/Warnings

The drug is contraindicated in dogs with pulmonary fibrosis, a history of chronic pulmonary disease that could lead to fibrosis, and in West Highland white terriers or other breeds with a genetic predisposition for the development of pulmonary fibrosis.[9] Rabacfosadine was associated with life-threatening or fatal pulmonary fibrosis in a small percentage of patients in the field studies (less than 5%). Pulmonary fibrosis may be an idiosyncratic toxicity. This adverse effect generally occurs several months after treatment has been discontinued and can range from clinically normal to life-threatening. While pulmonary fibrosis is a rare adverse toxicity, baseline thoracic radiographs can be recommended prior to and during treatment with rabacfosadine.

Rabacfosadine can cause severe toxicity. It should only be used where adequate monitoring and support can be administered. It should be used with caution in patients with pre-existing myleosuppression or infection. Safety and effectiveness in conjunction with other chemotherapeutic agents or other treatment modalities have not been evaluated.

There is increasing evidence that chronic exposure by health care givers to antineoplastic drugs increases the mutagenic, teratogenic, and carcinogenic risks associated with these agents. Proper training and precautions in the handling, preparation, administration, and disposal of these drugs and supplies associated with their use are strongly recommended. Use caution when handling this medication. See the product's package insert and client information sheet for more details.

Adverse Effects

The most common acute adverse effects observed with rabacfosadine in dogs include diarrhea, vomiting, decreased/loss of appetite, weight loss, lethargy, and neutropenia.[9] Leukopenia nadirs were observed between Days 6 and 9 following administration, with recovery by Day 12. Other adverse effects include hematochezia, tachypnea, dyspnea, tachycardia, thrombocytopenia, anemia, hypokalemia, hypophosphatemia, otitis media, and dermal changes (eg, alopecia, dermatitis, pyoderma). A cumulative dermatopathy can be observed, consisting of erythema and alopecia, which can progress to crusting and exudate; the ears/periauricular region, the dorsum, the axillae, and inguinal regions are most commonly affected and generally appear following 2 to 4 treatments. GI toxicity and dermatopathy have been reported as dose-limiting toxicities.[2] Most adverse effects are Veterinary Cooperative Oncology Group grade 1 or 2 and resolve with supportive therapy and/or dose reduction/delay.

Rabacfosadine was associated with suspected or confirmed pulmonary fibrosis in a small percentage of patients in the field studies (less than 5%).

Similar to other cytotoxic agents, sequential dose reductions and/or delays can be utilized to reduce the severity of adverse effects. Treatment with antiemetics (eg, maropitant, ondansetron), antidiarrheals (eg, metronidazole, loperamide, tylosin), topical or systemic anti-inflammatories (eg, NSAIDs, corticosteroids), and/or antibiotics may mitigate adverse effects and are not in violation of the FDA label.

Rabacfosadine may cause pain and tissue damage at the site of injection; avoid extravasation injuries.[9] If signs of extravasation occur, it is recommended to stop the infusion immediately and, if possible, withdraw 3 mL to 5 mL of blood to remove some of the drug, and try to aspirate additional fluids from any swelling through separate percutaneous aspirations using a 25-gauge needle. Remove the infusion catheter. Delineate the infiltrated area on the patient's skin with a felt tip marker. Consider cold packing the affected area for 48 to 72 hours. Avoid pressure or friction; do not rub the area. Observe for signs of increased erythema, pain, or skin necrosis. Ensure that no medication is given distal to the extravasation site. After 48 hours, encourage the patient to use the extremity normally to promote a full range of motion. The use of an Elizabethan collar may prevent self-trauma.

Reproductive/Nursing Safety

Rabacfosadine is contraindicated in dogs that are pregnant, lactating, or intended for breeding.[9] It is a likely teratogen. For sexually intact patients, verify pregnancy status prior to administration. Its effects on male fertility have not been studied.

It is not known if rabacfosadine or metabolites cross the placenta or enter the milk. Because of possible risks to nursing offspring, consider using milk replacer if the dam is receiving rabacfosadine.

Overdose/Acute Toxicity

Dogs receiving single IV doses of 2.5 mg/kg (2.5 times the label dose) developed moderate to severe GI signs (eg, diarrhea, vomiting, hyporexia, weight loss) starting on Day 4 and resolving by Day 10.[9] Moderate to severe neutropenia and leukopenia were observed, with the nadir occurring between Days 6 and 9 and recovery occurring by Day 12. Dogs receiving doses of 8.2 mg/kg IV (8.2 times the label dose) developed severe neutropenia, GI signs, salivation, fever, tremors, and weakness, resulting in a moribund state, and were either preterminally found dead or were euthanized by Day 7. For sequential dosing, dogs receiving up to 0.82 mg/kg IV every 24 hours for 5 days experienced dose-related neutropenia, dehydration, anorexia, vomiting, abnormal feces, fever, and decreased activity. When administered at doses up to 1 mg/kg IV every 7 days, dose-related neutropenia, anorexia, and weight loss were noted. Pathology changes across all dosage groups included dosedependent atrophy and/or necrosis in lymphoid tissue, GI tract, pancreas, mandibular salivary gland, kidneys, adrenal cortex, and the male reproductive tract.[9]

In case of accidental overdose, aggressive supportive care measures (eg, IV fluids, antiemetics, antidiarrheals, antibiotics, ± granulocyte colony-stimulating factor) are indicated.

Because of the narrow therapeutic index of this agent, iatrogenic overdoses must be avoided. Recheck dosage calculations carefully.

For patients that have experienced or are suspected of having experienced an overdose, consultation with a 24-hour poison consultation center specializing in providing veterinary-specific information is recommended. For general information related to overdose and toxin exposures, as well as contact information for poison control centers, refer to ***Appendix.***

Drug Interactions

The following drug interactions are theoretical in animals receiving rabacfosadine and may be of significance in veterinary patients. Unless otherwise noted, use together is not necessarily contraindicated, but weigh the potential risks and perform additional monitoring when appropriate. The use of concomitant medications with rabacfosadine has not been evaluated by the FDA for safety or efficacy.

- Other Cytotoxic Antineoplastic Agents (eg, **other antineoplastics, immunosuppressives, chloramphenicol, flucytosine, colchicine**): May cause additive myelosuppression and/or GI toxicity when used with rabacfosadine. Safety and effectiveness with other chemotherapy drugs or treatment agents have not been evaluated. The effect of concomitant medications on the metabolism of rabacfosadine has also not been evaluated.[9]
- Radiation Therapy: Rabacfosadine is a potent inhibitor of DNA repair.[12] There is the potential for enhancement of radiation-associated acute effects when coadministered with rabacfosadine.

Laboratory Considerations

- None were noted.

Dosages

NOTE: There is a significant amount of ongoing research evaluating rabacfosadine for use with other drugs, other species, and for extra-label indications. Because of the potential toxicity of this drug to patients, veterinary staff, and pet owners and because chemotherapy indications, treatment protocols, monitoring, and safety guidelines often change, the following dosages should be used only as a general guide. Consultation with a veterinary oncologist and referral to current veterinary oncology references are strongly recommended.[13-16]

DOGS:

Treatment of lymphoma (label dosage; FDA-approved): 1 mg/kg administered as a 30-minute IV infusion, once every 3 weeks for up to 5 doses.[9] For dogs intolerant of 1 mg/kg dosing, noninferior clinical activity can be achieved with 0.82 mg/kg dosing. Stepwise dose reductions to 0.8 mg/kg and 0.66 mg/kg or dose delays may be used to manage adverse reactions. After adding 2 mL 0.9% sodium chloride for injection to the vial, gently invert the vial several times until the drug has completely dissolved and the solution is particle free. Do not use the solution if particulates are observed. The reconstituted solution contains 8.2 mg/mL. Add the calculated volume of reconstituted drug to

0.9% sodium chloride in a polyvinyl chloride (PVC) infusion bag or polypropylene infusion syringe to yield a total infusion volume of 2 mL/kg body weight. See the product label for an example dosage and administration chart.

Monitoring

- Baseline complete blood count, serum biochemistry profile, urinalysis, and thoracic radiographs
- CBC 7 days after the first treatment and immediately before each subsequent treatment
- Baseline and periodic (eg, every 2 to 3 treatments) serum biochemistry profile, including renal and hepatic parameters
- Monitoring for signs of pulmonary dysfunction consistent with pulmonary fibrosis, including serial monitoring of thoracic radiographs every 2 to 3 months, is recommended, or if clinical signs support respiratory compromise (tachypnea, coughing, exercise intolerance)
- Antitumor efficacy
- Monitor infusion site for signs of extravasation.

Client Information

- Always provide Client Information Sheet with prescription. In addition, it is highly recommended to verbally reiterate key points found on the sheet. Specifically, those sections related to when the veterinarian should be contacted and how to minimize exposure to the drug.
- Rabacfosadine is a cytotoxic (anti-cancer) medicine. The medicine can be hazardous to other animals and people that come in contact with it. On the day that your animal gets the medicine and then for 5 days afterward, handle all bodily waste (eg, urine, feces, litter), blood, or vomit only while wearing chemotherapy-resistant gloves. Place all waste materials in a plastic bag and seal before disposal in the regular trash. Those who are pregnant, attempting to conceive, or nursing should not clean up the animal's waste.
- Do not wash any items soiled with waste, vomit, or saliva from your dog with other laundry. Take precautions in handling the dog's toys, food bowl, and water bowl. All items should be washed separately from other household items.
- Your veterinarian will need to perform regular monitoring, including blood tests and/or radiographs, to be sure this drug is not causing toxic effects to your animal. Do not miss these important follow up visits.
- Observe your dog for lack of appetite, vomiting, or diarrhea. If these signs are severe, or if you notice your dog having difficulty breathing or signs of infection (eg, fever, lack of energy), contact your veterinarian immediately.

Chemistry/Synonyms

Rabacfosadine is an acyclic nucleotide phosphonate with a molecular weight of 526.5 g/mole. It is supplied as a sterile white to off-white lyophilized powder in the form of a cake contained in a 3 mL amber glass vial. Each single-use vial contains 16.4 mg of rabacfosadine, present as the succinate salt, along with 20 mg of mannitol and 1.6 mg of citrate as excipients. Once reconstituted with 0.9% sodium chloride injection, USP, the resulting solution contains 8.2 mg rabacfosadine per mL.

Rabacfosadine may also be known as GS-9219, VDC-1101, and *Tanovea*®.

Storage/Stability

Refrigerate the vials at 2°C to 8°C (36°F-46°F). Retain in the original package to protect from light. After reconstitution, dilute the solution further within 4 hours. Discard the unused infusion solution within 24 hours of admixture and within 4 hours of attachment to an IV administration set. Dispose of any unused product or waste materials in accordance with proper procedures for cytotoxic drugs.

Compatibility/Compounding Considerations

None were noted.

Dosage Forms/Regulatory Status

VETERINARY-LABELED PRODUCTS:

Rabacfosadine Injection: 16.4 mg vial for reconstitution; *Tanovea*®; (Rx). NADA # 141-475

HUMAN-LABELED PRODUCTS: NONE

References

For the complete list of references, see **wiley.com/go/budde/plumb**

Ramipril

(***ram***-ih-prill) *Altace*®, *Vasotop*®

Angiotensin-Converting Enzyme (ACE) Inhibitor

Prescriber Highlights

- ► Used primarily as a vasodilator in the treatment of heart failure or systemic hypertension; may be of benefit in the treatment of chronic kidney disease or protein-losing nephropathies
- ► Not as much information or experience available as some other angiotensin-converting enzyme (ACE) inhibitors (eg, enalapril, benazepril) in dogs or cats
- ► Contraindications include in animals that are hypersensitive it or to other ACE inhibitors.
- ► Use with caution during pregnancy, in patients with vascular stenosis or obstructive hypertrophic cardiomyopathy, in patients taking potassium-sparing diuretics, and in hypovolemic patients
- ► Appears well-tolerated in both dogs and cats. Adverse effects may include GI distress (eg, anorexia, vomiting, diarrhea), and, less commonly, weakness, hypotension, and hyperkalemia.

Uses/Indications

Ramipril is a long-acting angiotensin-converting enzyme (ACE) inhibitor that may be useful in treating heart failure or systemic hypertension in dogs or cats. It is an approved product in the UK for treating heart failure in dogs. However, in dogs in heart failure due to MMVD, ramipril was less effective than pimobendan[1], and the addition of ramipril to the combination of pimobendan plus furosemide did not improve survival.[2] In cats, ramipril has been used for treating arterial hypertension. A study did not show any significant benefit in using ramipril in treating Maine coon cats with hypertrophic cardiomyopathy without heart failure.[3]

Like other ACE inhibitors, ramipril may be useful as adjunctive treatment in chronic kidney disease and protein-losing nephropathies. In dogs with moderate renal impairment (such as might be found with heart failure), there is apparently no need to adjust the ramipril dose.[4]

In healthy horses, oral benazepril was found to be more effective than ramipril (0.3 or 0.1 mg/kg) at inhibiting serum ACE activity.[5] When ramipril 0.2 mg/kg PO was administered to healthy horses before exercise, the exercise-induced increase in systolic blood pressure was reduced by 26.6%, and the diastolic blood pressure was reduced by 16.6%. Mean maximum serum ACE inhibition 2 hours after ramipril administration was 55%.[6]

Pharmacology/Actions

Ramipril is a prodrug that has little pharmacologic activity until it is converted into ramiprilat. Ramiprilat prevents the formation of angiotensin-II (a potent vasoconstrictor) by competing with angiotensin-I for the enzyme angiotensin-converting enzyme (ACE). ACE has a much higher affinity for ramiprilat than for angiotensin-I. Because angiotensin-II concentrations are decreased, aldosterone secretion is reduced, and plasma renin activity is increased.

The cardiovascular effects of ramiprilat in patients with CHF include decreased total peripheral resistance, pulmonary vascular resistance, mean arterial and right atrial pressures, and pulmonary capillary wedge pressure with no change or decrease in heart rate. Increased cardiac index and output, stroke volume, and exercise tolerance also occur. Renal blood flow can be increased with little change in hepatic blood flow. In animals with glomerular disease, ACE inhibitors likely decrease proteinuria and help to preserve renal function.

Pharmacokinetics

After oral administration to dogs, ramipril is rapidly converted via de-esterification into ramiprilat. The bioavailability of ramiprilat after a dose of 0.25 mg/kg per day of ramipril is ≈6.7%. At this dose, angiotensin-converting enzyme (ACE) activity never exceeded 60% in either healthy dogs or those with experimentally induced renal dysfunction (GFR reduced to 58%).[4]

After oral administration to cats with ramipril doses ranging from 0.125 mg/kg to 1 mg/kg once daily for 9 days, ramipril peak concentrations occurred in ≈0.5 hours. Absorption was not significantly affected by food. Ramipril is rapidly converted into its active metabolite ramiprilat, which peaks at 1 to 1.5 hours postadministration. Half-life was ≈20 hours and excretion occurred primarily in the feces. Repeated doses of ramipril 0.125 mg/kg inhibited serum ACE activity by 94% at maximum and 55% inhibited 24 hours postdose. At a dose of 1 mg/kg, ACE activity was 97% inhibited at maximum, and it was 83% inhibited 24 hours postdose.[7,8]

When cats were administered radiolabeled ramipril PO, 85% to 89% of the radioactivity was recovered in the feces. It is unclear how much of this represents the unabsorbed drug or absorbed parent compound/metabolites eliminated in the feces. Approximately 10% of the administered drug was recovered in the urine. Excretion of radiolabeled compounds was complete by 168 hours after dosing.

In horses, after ramipril 0.05 mg/kg IV and 0.05, 0.1, 0.2, 0.4, and 0.8 mg/kg PO, the serum ACE activity was only suppressed by 84.27% at the 0.8 mg/kg dose and by 98.88% with the IV dose. The PO availability of ramipril at doses ranging from 0.05 to 0.8 mg/kg was low. It is unknown if 80% suppression would be sufficient to counteract vasoconstriction in pathological conditions.[9]

Contraindications/Precautions/Warnings

Ramipril is contraindicated in patients that are hypersensitive to it or to any other ACE inhibitor. The labeling for the UK product approved for dogs states that it should not be used in clinical cases of obstructive heart disease (eg, aortic/subaortic stenosis and hypertrophic obstructive cardiomyopathy), or with potassium-sparing diuretics (see ***Drug Interactions***).[10] In humans, dosage reduction may be recommended in cases of hepatic or renal impairment.

The use of ACE inhibitors in dehydrated patients can lead to acute hypotension. In patients at risk for hypovolemia, starting at a ½ dose and gradually increasing over 1 week is recommended.

Ramipril is a prodrug that is converted to the active form in the liver. This conversion may be reduced in patients with hepatic dysfunction.

Pregnant women should exercise caution to avoid exposure and wash their hands after handling.

Adverse Effects

Although information is limited, ramipril appears to be well tolerated in dogs and cats. GI effects are probably the most likely adverse effects to be noted. Weakness, hypotension, or hyperkalemia are possible. The UK product label states that if clinical signs of hypotension occur (apathy or ataxia), treatment should be suspended until signs resolve, then continued at 50% of the original dose.

In humans, bradykinin accumulation caused by angiotensin-converting enzyme (ACE) inhibitors can lead to angioedema and cough. These effects appear to be rare but possible in dogs. ACE inhibitors can rarely cause cholestatic jaundice in humans that may progress fulminant hepatic necrosis.

Reproductive/Nursing Safety

No studies have been carried out to assess the use of ramipril in pregnant bitches.[10] Doses of ramipril up to 500 mg/kg/day did not impair fertility in rats. Although no teratogenic effects have been detected with ramipril in studies performed in mice, rats, rabbits, and cynomolgus monkeys, there is increased fetal risk for humans.

If used in humans during the second and third trimesters, increased rates of fetal death, neonatal hypotension, skull hypoplasia, anuria, renal failure, oligohydramnios leading to fetal limb contractures, craniofacial deformation, and hypoplastic lung development were noted. In humans, ramipril has a black box warning regarding its use in pregnancy, which states, *When used in pregnancy during the second and third trimesters, angiotensin-converting enzyme (ACE) inhibitors can cause injury and even death to the developing fetus. When pregnancy is detected, ramipril should be discontinued as soon as possible.*

No studies have been carried out to assess the use of ramipril in lactating bitches. The human (US) label recommends not using the drug during nursing.

Because safety has not been established in animals, this drug should only be used when the maternal benefits outweigh the potential risks to offspring.

Overdose/Acute Toxicity

In dogs, ramipril appears quite safe; dosages as high as 1 g/kg induced only mild GI distress. Lethal doses in rats and mice were noted at 10 to 11 g/kg. No information was located on overdoses in cats. In overdose situations, the primary concern is hypotension; supportive treatment with volume expansion with normal saline is recommended to correct blood pressure. Because of the drug's long duration of action, prolonged monitoring and treatment may be required.

For patients that have experienced or are suspected of having experienced an overdose, consultation with a 24-hour poison consultation center specializing in providing veterinary-specific information is recommended. For general information related to overdose and toxin exposures, as well as contact information for poison control centers, refer to ***Appendix***.

Drug Interactions

The following drug interactions have either been reported or are theoretical in humans or animals receiving ramipril and may be of significance in veterinary patients. Unless otherwise noted, use together is not necessarily contraindicated, but weigh the potential risks and perform additional monitoring when appropriate.

- ANESTHETICS: Concurrent use may increase the risk for hypotension.
- ANGIOTENSIN RECEPTOR BLOCKERS (eg, **losartan, telmisartan**): In humans, dual blockade of the RAAS system with angiotensin-converting enzyme (ACE) inhibitors and ARBs is associated with an increased risk for hypotension, hyperkalemia, and changes in renal function. The ONTARGET trial in humans found no benefit with dual therapy compared to ACE or ARB therapy alone but found an increased incidence of renal dysfunction.[11]
- ANTACIDS, ALUMINUM-, CALCIUM-, AND MAGNESIUM-CONTAINING: Reduced oral absorption of ramipril may occur if given concomitantly with antacids; it is suggested to separate dosing by at least 2 hours.
- ANTIHYPERTENSIVE AGENTS/VASODILATORS (eg, **amlodipine,**

hydralazine, prazosin, sildenafil): Concurrent use may increase the risk for hypotension and other adverse effects.

- **Baclofen**: Concurrent administration may increase the risk for hypotension.
- **Buspirone**: Concurrent use may increase the risk for hypotension.
- **Cabergoline**: Concurrent use may lead to additive hypotension.
- **Cimetidine**: Use with ACE inhibitors has caused neurologic dysfunction in 2 human patients
- **Corticosteroids** (eg, **dexamethasone, fludrocortisone, predniso(lo)ne**): May decrease the antihypertensive effects of ACE inhibitors
- **Darbepoetin Alfa**: ACE inhibitors may interfere with erythropoietin.
- **Digoxin**: Concentration may increase 15% to 30% when ACE inhibitors are added; automatic reduction in dosage is not recommended but monitoring of serum digoxin concentration should be performed.
- **Diphenhydramine**: Concurrent use may increase the risk for hypotension.
- **Disopyramide**: Hypoglycemic effects may be enhanced.
- **Diuretics** (eg, **furosemide**): Concomitant diuretics may cause hypotension if used with ramipril; titrate dosages carefully.
- **Doxepin**: Concurrent use may increase the risk for hypotension.
- **Glycerin, Oral**: Concurrent use may increase the risk for hypotension.
- **Heparin, Low Molecular Weight Heparins** (eg, **dalteparin, enoxaparin**): Concurrent use may increase the risk for hyperkalemia.
- **Nonsteroidal Anti-inflammatory Agents (NSAIDs**; eg, **carprofen, meloxicam**): May reduce the clinical efficacy of ramipril when it is being used as an antihypertensive agent
- **Opioids** (eg, **buprenorphine, hydrocodone, morphine**): Concurrent use may increase the risk for hypotension.
- **Potassium** or **Potassium Sparing Diuretics** (eg, **spironolactone**): Hyperkalemia may develop.
- **Probenecid**: Can decrease renal excretion of ramipril and possibly enhance the clinical and toxic effects of the drug

Laboratory Considerations

- Angiotensin-converting enzyme (ACE) inhibitors may cause a reversible decrease in localization and excretion of iodohippurate sodium I123/I134 or Technetium Tc99 pententate renal imaging in the affected kidney in patients with renal artery stenosis, which could lead to confusion in test interpretation.

Dosages

DOGS:

Heart failure (extra-label): Initially, 0.125 mg/kg PO once daily; depending on the severity of pulmonary congestion, the dose may be increased to 0.25 mg/kg PO once daily[10]

CATS:

Systemic hypertension (extra-label): Initially, 0.125 mg/kg PO once daily. In cats where systemic blood pressure (SBP) was still above 160 mm Hg on Day 14, the dose was increased to 0.25 mg/kg PO once daily up to the end of the trial (Day 63). A total of 62% had a decrease in SBP of 20 mm Hg or more; of these cats, 69% had had a final SBP below 160 mm Hg.[12]

Monitoring

- Clinical signs
- Renal function; baseline and 7 days after initiation or alteration in the dose of ramipril or concurrently administered diuretics[10]
- Serum electrolytes, liver enzymes, creatinine, BUN, urine protein:creatinine ratio
- CBC with differential, periodic
- Blood pressure (if treating hypertension or clinical signs associated with hypotension arise)

Client Information

- Ramipril is used to treat heart failure, high blood pressure, and some forms of kidney disease in dogs and cats.
- This medicine is usually well tolerated but vomiting and diarrhea can occur. Give this medicine with food if vomiting or lack of appetite becomes a problem. If a rash or signs of infection occur (eg, fever), contact your veterinarian immediately.
- It is important to give this medicine exactly as prescribed. Do not stop or reduce the dosage without first talking with your veterinarian.
- While your animal is taking this medication, it is important to return to your veterinarian for blood pressure and laboratory tests. Do not miss these important follow-up visits.

Chemistry/Synonyms

Ramipril occurs as a white to almost white, crystalline powder that is sparingly soluble in water and freely soluble in methyl alcohol.

Ramipril may also be known as Hoe-498, ramiprilis, or ramiprilium. There are many international trade names, including *Altace®*, *Cardase®*, *Delix®*, *Ramase®*, *Triatec®*, and *Vasotop®*.

Storage/Stability

Store capsules at room temperature (15°C-30°C [59°F-86°F]) protected from light in tight containers.

Compatibility/Compounding Considerations

No specific information was noted.

Dosage Forms/Regulatory Status

VETERINARY-LABELED PRODUCTS:

None in the United States. In some countries, ramipril is available in 1.25 mg, 2.5 mg, and 5 mg tablets.

HUMAN-LABELED PRODUCTS:

Ramipril Oral Capsules: 1.25 mg, 2.5 mg, 5 mg, and 10 mg; *Altace®*, generic; (Rx)

References

For the complete list of references, see **wiley.com/go/budde/plumb**

Ranitidine

(rah-***nih***-tih-deen) *Zantac®*

H_2 Receptor Antagonist; Prokinetic

Prescriber Highlights

- Used to reduce acid output in the stomach, to prevent and/or treat esophageal reflux, esophagitis, gastritis, and GI ulcers; also has prokinetic activity
- Contraindications include hypersensitivity. Use caution in geriatric patients and in patients with hepatic or renal insufficiency
- Adverse effects are rare. IV boluses may cause vomiting. Pain at the injection site after IM administration. Potentially: agranulocytosis, and transient cardiac arrhythmias (too rapid IV injection)
- Product may not be commercially available due to an FDA total market recall announced April 2020.

Uses/Indications

In veterinary medicine, ranitidine has been used to decrease gastric acid production for the treatment and/or prophylaxis of gastric, abomasal, and duodenal ulcers; uremic gastritis; stress-related or drug-induced erosive gastritis; esophagitis; and duodenogastric and esophageal reflux. One study did not demonstrate any reduction in the incidence of gastroesophageal reflux in anesthetized dogs from either ranitidine or metoclopramide.[1] Ranitidine has also been employed to treat hypersecretory conditions associated with gastrinomas and systemic mastocytosis. Because of its effects on gastric motility, ranitidine may be useful in increasing gastric emptying, particularly when delayed gastric emptying is associated with gastric ulcer disease. Ranitidine may also be useful for stimulating colonic activity in cats via its prokinetic effects. Ranitidine had no effect on gastric emptying in healthy foals.[2]

Increased intragastric pH has been reported to diminish after twice-daily famotidine administration to dogs,[3] cats,[4] and cattle[5]; however, this effect did not occur with ranitidine.[6]

Pharmacology/Actions

At the H_2 receptors of the parietal cells, ranitidine competitively inhibits histamine, thereby reducing gastric acid output both during basal conditions and when stimulated by food, amino acids, pentagastrin, histamine, or insulin. Ranitidine is 3 to 13 times more potent (on a molar basis) than cimetidine.

Ranitidine may stimulate GI motility, especially in the stomach, by inhibiting acetylcholinesterase (thereby increasing acetylcholine at muscarinic receptors). Lower esophageal sphincter pressures may be increased by ranitidine. By decreasing the amount of gastric juice produced, ranitidine decreases the amount of pepsin secreted.

Ranitidine, unlike cimetidine, does not appear to have any appreciable effect on serum prolactin levels, although it may inhibit the release of vasopressin.

Pharmacokinetics

In dogs, the oral bioavailability is ≈81%, serum half-life is 2.2 hours, and volume of distribution is 2.6 L/kg.

In horses, oral ranitidine has a bioavailability of ≈27% in adults and 38% in foals. Peak levels after oral dosing occur in ≈100 minutes in adults and 60 minutes in foals. Apparent volume of distribution is ≈1.1 L/kg and 1.5 L/kg in adults and foals, respectively. Clearance in adults is ≈10 mL/minute/kg and 13.3 mL/minute/kg in foals. A recent study reported that the terminal half-life in performance horses after 8 mg/kg PO twice daily (7 doses total) was 7.4 hours, which is higher than previous reports (1.5 hours). Since the use of this drug is regulated in racing horses (class 5 foreign substance by the Association of Racing Commissioners International), an extended withdrawal time may be necessary prior to competition.[7]

In humans, ranitidine is absorbed rapidly after oral administration, but undergoes extensive first-pass metabolism with a net systemic bioavailability of ≈50%. Peak levels occur at ≈2 to 3 hours after oral dosing. Food does not appreciably alter the extent of absorption or the peak serum levels attained.

Ranitidine is distributed widely throughout the body and is only 10% to 19% bound to plasma proteins. Ranitidine is distributed into human milk at levels 25% to 100% of those found in plasma.

Ranitidine is excreted in the urine by the kidneys (via glomerular filtration and tubular secretion) and metabolized in the liver to inactive metabolites; accumulation of the drug can occur in patients with renal insufficiency. The serum half-life of ranitidine in humans averages 2 to 3 hours. The duration of action at usual doses is 8 to 12 hours.

Contraindications/Precautions/Warnings

Ranitidine is contraindicated in patients who are hypersensitive to it. It should be used cautiously and possibly at a reduced dose in patients with diminished renal function. Use with caution in patients with impaired hepatic function. Ranitidine has caused increased serum ALT levels in humans receiving high IV doses for longer than 5 days. The manufacturer recommends that with high-dose chronic therapy, serum ALT values be considered for monitoring.

Acid-suppressing therapy has been associated with increased risk for pneumonia in humans.[8]

Do not confuse raNITIdine with riMANTAdine, or amantadine, or *Zantac*® with *Zyrtec*® or *Zofran*®.

Adverse Effects

Adverse effects appear to be uncommon in animals at clinical dosages. Potential adverse effects in humans include mental confusion and headache; relevance to animals is unknown. Rarely, agranulocytosis may develop and, if given rapidly IV, transient cardiac arrhythmias may be seen. Pain at the injection site may be noted after IM administration. IV boluses have been associated with vomiting in small animals and transient hypotension in cats.

Reproductive/Nursing Safety

Studies in laboratory animals have revealed no evidence of fetal toxicity.

Ranitidine is excreted in human breast milk with milk:plasma ratios of ≈5:1 to 12:1. Use with caution in nursing veterinary patients.

Overdose/Acute Toxicity

Clinical experience with ranitidine overdose is limited. In laboratory animals, very high dosages (225 mg/kg/day) have been associated with muscular tremors, vomiting, and rapid respiration. Single doses of 1 g/kg PO in rodents did not cause death.

Treatment of overdoses in animals should be handled using standard protocols for oral ingestions of drugs; clinical signs may be treated symptomatically and supportively if necessary. Hemodialysis and peritoneal dialysis have been noted to remove ranitidine from the body.

For patients that have experienced or are suspected to have experienced an overdose, it is strongly encouraged to consult with one of the 24-hour poison consultation centers that specialize in providing information specific for veterinary patients. For general information related to overdose and toxin exposures, as well as contact information for poison control centers, refer to ***Appendix.***

Drug Interactions

Unlike cimetidine, ranitidine appears to have much less effect on the hepatic metabolism of drugs and is unlikely to cause clinically relevant drug interactions via this mechanism. The following drug interactions have either been reported or are theoretical in humans or animals receiving ranitidine and may be of significance in veterinary patients. Unless otherwise noted, use together is not necessarily contraindicated, but weigh the potential risks and perform additional monitoring when appropriate.

- Acetaminophen: Ranitidine (dose-dependent) may inhibit acetaminophen metabolism.
- Antacids (high doses) (eg, **calcium carbonate, magnesium/aluminum combinations**): May decrease the oral absorption of ranitidine; give at separate times (2 hours apart) if used concurrently.
- Azole Antifungals (eg, **ketoconazole, itraconazole, fluconazole**): By raising gastric pH, ranitidine may decrease the absorption of these agents; if both drugs are required, administer the azole 1 hour prior to ranitidine.
- Cefpodoxime, Cefuroxime: Ranitidine may decrease the absorption of these cephalosporins; giving with food may alleviate this effect.
- Iron Salts (oral): Ranitidine may decrease the absorption of oral iron; administer iron at least 1 hour prior to ranitidine.
- Metoprolol: Ranitidine may increase metoprolol half-life and peak levels.

- **Probenecid**: May reduce the excretion of ranitidine
- **Procainamide**: Concurrent use may result in increased serum concentrations of procainamide.
- **Propantheline**: Delays the absorption but increases the peak serum level of ranitidine; relative bioavailability of ranitidine may be increased by 23% when propantheline is administered concomitantly with ranitidine.
- **Vitamin B12**: Long-term ranitidine use may reduce oral absorption of B12.

Laboratory Considerations

- Ranitidine may cause a false-positive urine protein reading when using *Multistix*®. The sulfosalicylic acid reagent is recommended for determining urine protein when the patient is concomitantly receiving ranitidine.
- Gastric acid secretion testing: H_2 blockers may antagonize the effects of histamine and pentagastrin in the evaluation of gastric acid secretion; it is recommended that H_2 blockers be discontinued at least 24 hours before performing this test.
- Intradermal allergy testing: H_2 antagonists may inhibit histamine responses[9]; consider discontinuation at least 24 hours before performing this test.

Dosages

NOTE: In humans, the manufacturer recommends dilution of ranitidine when administering IV; doses must be diluted to a concentration of 2.5 mg/mL using dextrose 5%, 0.9% NaCl, or another suitable IV solution and be administered at a 10 – 25 mg/minute. Significance in animals is not known, but precautions should be considered.

DOGS:

Esophagitis, ulcer disease, gastritis, or gastric prokinetic (extra-label): Common anecdotal dosages generally range from 1 – 2 mg/kg PO, SC, IM, or slow IV (max = 25 mg/minute) every 8 to 12 hours,[10] but one study found that ranitidine at 2 mg/kg IV every 12 hours did not significantly increase gastric pH as compared with saline.[6] One source states *Therefore, current dose recommendations (0.5 – 2 mg/kg every 8 to 12 hours) seem to be too low to be of any effect.*[11] *Currently, clinical studies on the effect of ranitidine on gastric disorders in dogs and cats are lacking.*

CATS:

Esophagitis, ulcer disease, or as a prokinetic agent to stimulate colonic motility (extra-label): Based on pharmacokinetic data: 2.5 mg/kg slow IV twice daily or 3.5 mg/kg PO twice daily.[12] One study found that 1.4 – 2.3 mg/kg PO every 12 hours did not significantly suppress gastric acid.[13]

FERRETS:

Helicobacter mustelae (extra-label): Ranitidine bismuth citrate (**NOTE**: Not available commercially in US; must be compounded) 24 mg/kg PO every 8 to 12 hours and clarithromycin 12.5 mg/kg PO every 8-12 hours for 14 days[14]

HORSES:

Gastroprotectant/reduce stomach acid (extra-label): 1.5 – 2 mg/kg IV every 8 hours or 6.6 – 10 mg/kg PO every 8 hours

SMALL MAMMALS:

Rabbits: Prokinetic: 0.5 mg/kg IV every 24 hours with cisapride (0.5 mg/kg PO every 8 hours)[15]

Suspected gastric ulceration: 2 – 5 mg/kg PO twice daily[16]

Monitoring

- Clinical efficacy (dependent on reason for use); monitored by decrease in clinical signs, endoscopic examination, and blood in feces.

Client Information

- Used to treat or prevent stomach ulcers
- Usually well tolerated; side effects are uncommon.
- Works best if given before the first meal of the day
- Ranitidine is available OTC (over the counter; without a prescription), but only give it to your animal if recommended by your veterinarian.

Chemistry/Synonyms

An H_2-receptor antagonist, ranitidine HCl occurs as a white to pale yellow granular substance with a bitter taste and a sulfur-like odor. The drug has pK_as of 8.2 and 2.7. One gram is soluble in ≈1.5 mL of water or 6 mL of alcohol. The commercially available injection has a pH of 6.7 to 7.3.

Ranitidine HCl may also be known as AH-19065, ranitidini hydrochloridum. Many trade names are available; a common trade name is *Zantac*®.

Storage/Stability

Ranitidine tablets and syrup/solution should be stored in tight, light-resistant containers at room temperature 20°C to 25°C (68°F-77°F). The injectable product should be stored protected from light and at a temperature less than 30°C (86°F). A slight darkening of the injectable solution does not affect the potency of the drug.

Compatibility/Compounding Considerations

Ranitidine injection is reportedly stable for up to 48 hours when mixed with commonly used IV solutions (including 5% sodium bicarbonate).

Dosage Forms/Regulatory Status

VETERINARY-LABELED PRODUCTS: NONE

The Association of Racing Commissioners International (ARCI) has designated this drug as a class 5 substance. See ***Appendix*** for more information.

HUMAN-LABELED PRODUCTS:

NOTE: Product may not be commercially available due to an FDA total market recall announced April 2020.

Ranitidine HCl Oral Tablets: 75 mg, 150 mg, & 300 mg; *Zantac*®, generic; (Rx or OTC)

Ranitidine HCl Oral Capsules: 150 and 300 mg (traditional and liquid filled); generic; (Rx or OTC)

Ranitidine HCl Oral Solution/Oral Syrup: 15 mg/mL in 473 mL and 480 mL; generic; (Rx) May contain alcohol or sorbitol

Ranitidine HCl Injection: 25 mg/mL in 2 mL, 6 mL, and 40 mL vials; *Zantac*®, generic; (Rx)

References

For the complete list of references, see **wiley.com/go/budde/plumb**

Remifentanil

(rem-i-***fen***-ta-nil) *Ultiva®*
Ultrashort-Acting Opioid Analgesic

Prescriber Highlights

- ► Opioid similar to fentanyl with an even shorter duration of action, which may reduce recovery times; used primarily as an anesthesia adjunct.
- ► Degraded by esterases in plasma, red blood cells, and tissues; can be used for prolonged procedures in patients with renal or hepatic dysfunction
- ► Currently much more expensive than fentanyl
- ► DEA Schedule II (C-II) controlled substance

Uses/Indications

Remifentanil is a mu-opioid that is structurally related to fentanyl. Because remifentanil is primarily metabolized by plasma, tissue, and red blood cell esterases, it can safely be used in patients with either hepatic or renal impairment, and patients with hepatic dysfunction (eg, hepatic shunts) still have a constant and predictable excretion of this drug.[1] Its short duration of action is also beneficial, because if adverse effects occur (eg, respiratory depression, bradycardia), reversal with naloxone should rarely be required. One possible advantage of using remifentanil instead of fentanyl as an anesthesia adjunct is that recovery times may be faster with remifentanil.

Pharmacology/Actions

Remifentanil is a mu-opioid agonist that is structurally related to fentanyl with a rapid onset of analgesic action and peak effect and short duration of action. Mu receptors are found primarily in the pain-regulating areas of the brain. They are thought to contribute to the analgesia, euphoria, respiratory depression, physical dependence, miosis, and hypothermic actions of opioids. Receptors for opioid analgesics are found in high concentrations in the limbic system, spinal cord, thalamus, hypothalamus, striatum, and midbrain. They are also found in tissues such as the GI tract, urinary tract, and other smooth muscles. The pharmacology of the opioid agonists is discussed in more detail in ***Opioids, General Information***.

Unlike other opioids, remifentanil is rapidly metabolized by hydrolysis of the propanoic acid-methyl ester linkage by nonspecific blood and tissue esterases. Remifentanil is not appreciably metabolized by the liver or plasma cholinesterase (pseudocholinesterase). Adverse effects (eg, bradycardia, respiratory depression, hypotension) are dose-dependent and similar to other mu-opioids. When used as an anesthesia adjunct, remifentanil, like other opioids, has a ceiling effect (ie, increased doses do not enhance analgesia).

Antagonists such as naloxone antagonize the opioid activity of remifentanil. Hourly dosages of naltrexone (600 µg/kg IV) antagonized the behavioral and antinociceptive effects of a high dose of remifentanil in cats.[2]

In dogs, remifentanil is equally efficacious but about half as potent as fentanyl; recovery from remifentanil anesthesia is much more rapid, especially after continuous infusions maintained for 6-plus hours.[3] Remifentanil reduced sevoflurane MAC similarly to fentanyl in dogs but allowed shorter recovery times.[4] In another dog study, remifentanil given as an IV CRI reduced the dosage requirements of propofol for maintaining target-controlled infusion system-based anesthesia.[5] A dose of 0.3 µg/kg/minute IV CRI resulted in nearly maximal isoflurane-sparing effects; a ceiling effect was observed at higher infusion rates.[6] Remifentanil infusions of 0.25 – 0.5 µg/kg/minute IV CRI combined with propofol 0.2 mg/kg per minute IV CRI produced minimal effects on arterial blood pressure and led to a good recovery, and analgesia was sufficient to control the nociceptive response applied by electrical stimulation.[7] Another study showed a significant decrease in heart rate and cardiac index and no difference in mean arterial pressure when anesthesia was maintained with remifentanil 0.3 µg/kg/minute IV CRI combined with a target-controlled infusion of propofol compared to propofol alone.[8] The principal carboxylic acid metabolite of remifentanil (GR90291) has been shown to be at least 4000 times less potent in dogs as the parent drug.[9]

In cats, remifentanil reduced isoflurane MAC similarly (≈25% reduction) at the 3 doses studied[10]; however, in another cat study, remifentanil did not alter the MAC value of isoflurane but did produce analgesia, reflected by increased thermal thresholds.[11]

In horses anesthetized with isoflurane and receiving dexmedetomidine 1 µg/kg/hour IV CRI with remifentanil 6 µg/kg/hour, a decreased heart rate and increased systemic vascular resistance were seen during the anesthetic event (60 minutes). Remifentanil was not associated with adverse effects during anesthesia and did not affect recovery time or recovery score.[12]

Pharmacokinetics

In dogs, remifentanil is rapidly distributed into the CNS with a blood–brain equilibration half-life of 2.3 to 5.2 minutes. It has a terminal elimination half-life of 6 minutes.[9] On termination of an IV infusion, dogs recover in 5 to 20 minutes regardless of the infusion duration.

In cats, remifentanil has a moderately high volume of distribution (7.6 L/kg), a high clearance (766 mL/minute/kg), and a short terminal elimination half-life (17.4 minutes). In anesthetized (isoflurane) cats, the volume of distribution of remifentanil is decreased (1.65 L/kg), but elimination half-life is not significantly altered.[13]

In horses, after remifentanil IV infusions of 6 µg/kg/hour for a minimum of 60 minutes while anesthesia was maintained with isoflurane, the mean peak remifentanil concentration was 7.14 ng/mL at 50 minutes postinfusion start, mean Vd was 268 ± 40 mL/kg, and mean half-life was 12.8 minutes. Blood concentration decreased to 1 ng/mL 27 minutes after the infusion was terminated.[14]

In humans after IV doses, remifentanil is rapidly distributed into the CNS and has a peak effect 1 to 3 minutes after administration. Remifentanil is ≈70% bound to plasma proteins with the majority bound to alpha-1-acid-glycoprotein. Remifentanil has an effective biological half-life of 3 to 10 minutes in human patients. The pharmacokinetics of remifentanil are not appreciably altered in patients with renal or hepatic failure.

Contraindications/Precautions/Warnings

Remifentanil is contraindicated in patients that are hypersensitive to it or other fentanyl analogues.[15] As the injection contains glycine, it is contraindicated for epidural or intrathecal administration.

Because of the possibility of significant respiratory depression or bradycardia, it should only be administered in a monitored anesthesia care setting. Continuous infusions should only be administered with an infusion device.

In morbidly obese patients, the drug dose should be based on ideal body weight.

Opioid analgesics are contraindicated in patients stung by scorpions (eg, *Centruroides* spp), as they may potentiate venom effects.[16]

Adverse Effects

Remifentanil has an adverse effect profile similar to other mu-opioids. Respiratory depression, including apnea, bradyarrhythmias, and hypotension, is possible. Increased body temperatures in cats may be noted. Anaphylaxis is rare, but possible.

In cats, doses higher than 1 µg/kg/minute IV CRI may be associated with dysphoria and frenetic locomotor activity.[11]

Reproductive/Nursing Safety

Remifentanil appears to be relatively safe to use during pregnancy. No teratogenic effects were observed after administration of remifentanil at doses up to 5 mg/kg in rats and 0.8 mg/kg in rabbits. It is unknown if remifentanil is excreted into milk, but clinical effects in offspring seem unlikely.

Because safety has not been established in animals, this drug should only be used when the maternal benefits outweigh the potential risks to offspring.

Overdose/Acute Toxicity

As with all potent opioid analgesics, overdoses manifest as enhancement of the drug's nonanalgesic pharmacological effects. Clinical signs may include apnea, chest-wall rigidity, seizures, hypoxemia, hypotension, and bradycardia.

If an overdose occurs, discontinue drug administration and give supportive therapy including mechanical ventilation and oxygen administration. Often, this is all that is required because the drug is cleared rapidly. Additional supportive therapy can include IV fluids and glycopyrrolate or atropine for bradycardia or hypotension. Naloxone may also be used to reverse the drug's mu-activity but can lead to acute pain and sympathetic hyperactivity.

For patients that have experienced or are suspected to have experienced an overdose, consultation with a 24-hour poison consultation center specializing in providing veterinary-specific information is recommended. For general information related to overdose and toxin exposures, as well as contact information for poison control centers, refer to ***Appendix.***

Drug Interactions

Remifentanil clearance is not altered by concomitant administration of thiopental, isoflurane, or propofol.

The following drug interactions with remifentanil and fentanyl have either been reported or are theoretical in humans or animals and may be of significance in veterinary patients. Unless otherwise noted, use together is not necessarily contraindicated, but weigh the potential risks and perform additional monitoring when appropriate.

- **Alpha-2 Agonists** (eg, **dexmedetomidine, xylazine**): Concurrent use may increase the risk for CNS and/or respiratory depression.
- **Anesthetic Agents** (eg, **alfaxalone, isoflurane, ketamine, propofol**): Concurrent use may increase the risk for CNS and/or respiratory depression.
- **Anticholinergic Agents** (eg, **acepromazine, atropine, disopyramide**): Concurrent use may increase the risk for urinary retention, constipation, and CNS and respiratory depression.
- **Antihypertensive Agents** (eg, **atenolol, lisinopril, spironolactone**): Concurrent use may increase the risk for bradycardia, hypotension, and orthostasis. Use cautiously and monitor blood pressure and heart rate. Opioids may decrease therapeutic effects of diuretics.
- **Benzodiazepines** (eg, **diazepam, midazolam**): Concurrent use may increase the risk for CNS and/or respiratory depression.
- **Bethanechol**: Concurrent use may antagonize the beneficial effects of bethanechol on GI motility. Avoid combination.
- **CNS Depressants** (eg, **methocarbamol, phenobarbital**): Concurrent use may increase the risk for CNS and/or respiratory depression. Monitor and adjust doses accordingly.
- **Desmopressin**: Concurrent use may increase concentrations of oral desmopressin and increase the risk for water intoxication and/or hyponatremia, which can progress to seizures, coma, respiratory arrest, and death. Monitor electrolytes and renal function.
- **Domperidone**: Concurrent use may antagonize the GI effects of domperidone.
- **Drugs That Inhibit Hepatic Isoenzymes** (eg, **cimetidine, diltiazem, erythromycin, fluconazole, itraconazole, ketoconazole**): May increase the half-life and decrease the clearance of fentanyl, leading to prolonged effects and an increased risk for respiratory depression. However, a study in dogs showed that ketoconazole did not significantly alter the elimination of fentanyl.[17] Monitor and considering adjusting doses accordingly.
- **Drugs That Induce Hepatic Isoenzymes** (eg, **griseofulvin, mitotane, phenobarbital**): Current use may decrease concentrations of fentanyl. Monitor clinical response and adjust doses accordingly.
- **Drugs That Depress Cardiac Function Or Reduce Vagal Tone** (eg, **beta-blockers** or **other anesthetic agents**): May produce bradycardia or hypotension if used concurrently with fentanyl
- **Ifosfamide**: Concurrent use may increase risk for neurotoxicity including somnolence, confusion, hallucinations, blurred vision, urinary incontinence, seizures, and coma. Use cautiously and monitor
- **Iohexol**: Concurrent use of opioids with intrathecal iohexol may increase risk for seizures. Opioids should be withheld for 48 hours before and 24 hours after intrathecal administration of iohexol.
- **Loperamide**: Concurrent use may increase risk for constipation.
- **Monoamine Oxidase Inhibitors** (MAOIs; eg, **amitraz, selegiline**): Concurrent use may increase the risk for anxiety, confusion, hypotension, respiratory depression, cyanosis, and coma. MAOIs should be withheld for 14 days prior to administration of opioids. Avoid combination.
- **Metoclopramide**: Concurrent use may antagonize the prokinetic effects of metoclopramide.
- **Neuromuscular Blocking Agents** (eg, **atracurium, pancuronium**): Concurrent use may increase the risk for tachycardia, bradycardia, and/or hypotension. Use cautiously and monitor.
- **Propofol**: Concurrent use has been shown to decrease heart rate, cardiac index, and stroke volume. Systemic vascular resistance index, central venous pressure, and pulmonary artery occlusion pressure increased in dogs.[18]
- **Serotonin Receptor Antagonists** (eg, **dolasetron, fluoxetine**): Concurrent use may increase the risk for serotonin syndrome. Avoid combination.
- **Tramadol**: Concurrent use may increase risk for seizures, serotonin syndrome, urinary retention, and constipation. Risk for CNS and respiratory depression may be additive.
- **Tricyclic Antidepressants** (TCAs; eg, **amitriptyline, clomipramine**): Concurrent use may increase the risk for urinary retention, constipation, and CNS and respiratory depression.

Laboratory Considerations

- Because opioids can increase biliary tract pressure and raise serum amylase and lipase values, these values may be unreliable for 24 hours after sufentanil is administered.

Dosages

NOTE: Do not confuse CRI dosages listed as µg/kg/*HOUR* with those listed as µg/kg/*MINUTE.*

DOGS:

Analgesic adjunct to general anesthesia (extra-label): 1 µg/kg bolus IV, followed by 0.1 – 0.3 µg/kg/*MINUTE* IV CRI.[5,19-24] IV boluses prior to CRI administration are generally avoided due to potential severe bradycardia. Because of the drug's short duration of activity, consider additional analgesia on termination of remifentanil if painful condition persists.

CATS:

Analgesic adjunct to general anesthesia (extra-label): 2.5 µg/kg IV bolus followed by 0.2 – 0.4 µg/kg/*MINUTE* IV CRI.[25-27] IV boluses prior to CRI administration are generally avoided due to potential severe bradycardia.

HORSES:

Adjunct for general anesthesia (extra-label): Remifentanil 3 µg/kg/*HOUR* IV CRI in combination with dexmedetomidine 1 µg/kg/*HOUR* IV CRI ± alfaxalone 6 µg/kg/*HOUR* IV CRI[28,29]

Standing sedation (extra-label): Remifentanil 6 µg/kg/*HOUR* IV CRI in combination with xylazine 0.65 µg/kg/*HOUR*.[30] Prior to administration of remifentanil/xylazine IV CRI, horses were premedicated with xylazine 0.8 mg/kg IV.

Monitoring

- Anesthetic and/or analgesic efficacy
- Cardiac and respiratory rate
- Pulse oximetry or other methods to measure blood oxygenation when used for anesthesia
- Blood pressure

Client Information

- Remifentanil is a very potent opioid that should only be used by professionals in a setting where adequate animal monitoring is available.

Chemistry/Synonyms

Remifentanil hydrochloride has a pK_a of 7.07 and partition coefficient n-octanol:water of 17.9 at pH 7.3. The commercially available injection has a pH of 2.5 to 3.5.

Remifentanil may also be known as GI-87084B, remifentanilo, rémifentanil, or remifentanili. Trade names include *Ultiva®* and *Remicit®*.

Storage/Stability

Prior to reconstitution, store lyophilized powder for solution between 2°C and 25°C (36°F-77°F). It is stable for 24 hours at room temperature after reconstitution and further dilution to concentrations of 20 – 250 µg/mL with the following IV fluids: sterile water for injection, 5% dextrose, 5% dextrose and 0.9% sodium chloride, 0.9% sodium chloride, 0.45% sodium chloride, and 5% dextrose in lactated Ringer's injection. It is stable for 4 hours at room temperature after reconstitution and further dilution to concentrations of 20 – 250 µg/mL with lactated Ringer's injection. The UK licensed product information states that it should **NOT** be mixed with lactated Ringer's injection with or without 5% glucose.

Remifentanil is a DEA Schedule II (C-II) controlled substance that should be stored in an area that is substantially constructed and securely locked. Follow applicable local, state, and federal rules regarding disposal of unused or wasted controlled drugs.

Compatibility/Compounding Considerations

To reconstitute solution, add 1 mL of diluent per mg of remifentanil. Shake well to dissolve. When reconstituted as directed, the solution contains ≈1 mg of remifentanil activity per mL. It should then be further diluted to a final concentration of 20, 25, 50, or 250 µg/mL prior to administration. Do not administer remifentanil without dilution.

Dosage Forms/Regulatory Status

VETERINARY-LABELED PRODUCTS: NONE

The Association of Racing Commissioners International (ARCI) has designated this drug as a class 1 substance. Use of this drug may not be allowed in certain animal competitions. Check rules and regulations before entering in a competition while this medication is being administered. Contact local racing authorities for further guidance. See the *Appendix* for more information.

HUMAN-LABELED PRODUCTS:

Remifentanil HCl Powder for reconstitution (IV use only): 1 mg (3 mL vial), 2 mg (5 mL vial), and 5 mg (10 mL vial); *Ultiva®*; (Rx, C-II controlled substance)

References

For the complete list of references, see **wiley.com/go/budde/plumb**

Reserpine

(re-***ser***-peen)

Rauwolfia Alkaloid

Prescriber Highlights

- Used as a long-term tranquilizer to sedate excitable or difficult horses or horses on forced stall rest
- Reserpine is contraindicated in patients that are hypersensitive to it.
- Horses may experience a prolonged hypotensive effect. Use this medicine with extreme caution in patients with hypotension or bradycardia. Concurrent or subsequent administration of sedative agents that can lower BP (eg, xylazine) must also be undertaken with caution.
- Relatively narrow therapeutic index–dose carefully
- Not commercially available in the United States

Uses/Indications

Reserpine is a long-acting central monoamine-depleting agent used for long-term sedation in horses.[1] It may be beneficial in managing difficult horses or horses on forced stall rest. Reserpine has historically been used as a treatment for agalactia in mares with fescue toxicosis; however, this use has mainly been replaced by domperidone.

Reserpine was used in humans for the treatment of hypertension and schizophrenia but has been replaced with safer, more effective therapies.

Pharmacology/Actions

Reserpine irreversibly blocks the transport of norepinephrine, serotonin, and dopamine into storage vesicles. Without storage, the neurotransmitters are metabolized in the cytoplasm of presynaptic nerve terminals by monoamine oxidase and catechol-O-methyltransferase. Depletion of brain amines and serotonin causes sedation and behavior changes, and long-term use may induce extrapyramidal effects (eg, dystonia, dyskinesia, akinesia). The actions of reserpine are long-lasting, as it can take days to weeks for the body to replenish the depleted neurotransmitters.

Reserpine's use in fescue toxicosis is related to the depletion of dopamine, which counteracts the effects of the dopaminergic alkaloids found in tall fescue. Dopamine itself decreases prolactin production and, therefore, milk production. In one study, reserpine was ineffective in treating prepartum agalactia and prolonged gestation from fescue toxicosis but did resolve postpartum agalactia.[1]

Pharmacokinetics

Reserpine is highly lipid-soluble and can penetrate the blood–brain barrier, resulting in further prolonged duration of action. After a single 2.5 mg IM administration of reserpine (0.0045 – 0.005 mg/kg) in horses, peak plasma concentrations occurred at 6 hours, and the drug was detectable for 28 to 56 hours.[2] Following oral administration of the same dose, concentrations similarly peaked at 6 hours, but concentrations were low (C_{max} 0.2 ng/mL) and more variable than with IM dosing; half-life was ≈24 hours.[3] Maximum effects of reserpine have been seen 5 days after repeated dosing. After administration of reserpine, serotonin uptake was decreased for 3 days and returned to normal after 7 days.[4] Reserpine is widely distributed in the brain, liver, kidneys, and adipose tissue.

In humans, the oral bioavailability of reserpine is ≈50%, with peak concentrations achieved ≈2 hours after administration. Reserpine undergoes hepatic metabolism in humans and is excreted predominantly in feces (30% to 60%) and urine (10%).

Contraindications/Precautions/Warnings

Reserpine is contraindicated in patients that are hypersensitive to it or its inactive ingredients. Use reserpine with extreme caution in patients with low blood pressure or low heart rate.

Reserpine is considered a prohibited substance in most sanctioned competitions and can be detected through high-performance liquid chromatography.

Reserpine was withdrawn from the human market because of risks for serious adverse effects, such as severe depression, seizures, and drug-induced Parkinson disease, and the availability of safer alternatives.

Adverse Effects

Adverse effects of reserpine in horses are associated with decreased sympathetic tone and adrenergic inhibition. Common adverse effects reported in horses include diarrhea with or without signs of abdominal pain or colic (eg, pawing, getting up and down, pacing, restlessness, rolling, kicking or biting at the side, stretching out/straining, shifting weight), muscle tremors/fasciculations, bradycardia, and hypotension.[5,6] There are anecdotal reports of severe, prolonged, and sometimes fatal hypotension, and many clinicians recommend waiting 3 to 4 weeks after discontinuation of reserpine before elective anesthetic procedures. Transient or permanent penile prolapse, paralysis, and paraphimosis may occur in male horses.[7] Increases in dose or IM dosing of reserpine may increase the severity of adverse effects, although the individual patient response is variable. In vitro, equine platelets exposed to reserpine demonstrated increased aggregation and adhesion,[3] although bleeding has not been reported.

Reproductive/Nursing Safety

Reserpine crosses the placenta, resulting in potential teratogenic effects. Nasal discharge, lethargy, and anorexia have been reported in newborns exposed to reserpine in the third trimester.[8] Reserpine is excreted into breast milk, although no adverse effects have been reported.

A possible adverse effect is a penile paralysis in stallions, resulting in paraphimosis and penile edema.[7]

Because safety has not been established in animals, this drug should only be used when the maternal benefits outweigh the potential risks to offspring.

Overdose/Acute Toxicity

Limited information is available. Reports have shown that 10 mg (total dose) of reserpine IV in horses causes generalized sweating and flatulence within 3 hours.[9] Pupillary miosis, upper eyelid ptosis, and marked depression may last for 48 hours. Doses of 5 – 10 mg (total dose) have caused colic, sweating, flatulence, miosis, and depression. Dose-dependent increases in the frequency and severity of adverse effects have been noted.

Methamphetamine is considered an antidote in cases of severe hypotension caused by reserpine overdose[6,9]; presumably other (legal) amphetamines (eg, dextroamphetamine) may be used, although no data were located. Other treatments include supportive care and supplemental vitamin C and vitamin E.[10]

For patients that have experienced or are suspected of having experienced an overdose, consultation with a 24-hour poison consultation center specializing in providing veterinary-specific information is recommended. For general information related to overdose and toxin exposures, as well as contact information for poison control centers, refer to ***Appendix.***

Drug Interactions

The following drug interactions (partial listing) have either been reported or are theoretical in humans or animals receiving reserpine and may be of significance in veterinary patients. Unless otherwise noted, use together is not necessarily contraindicated, but weigh the potential risks and perform additional monitoring when appropriate.

- **Anesthetic Agents, General** (eg, **isoflurane, propofol**): Reserpine may potentiate hypotensive effects.
- **Antihypertensive Agents**: Reserpine may potentiate the hypotensive effects of these agents.
- **Alpha-2 agonists** (eg, **detomidine, xylazine**): Reserpine may potentiate the hypotensive effects of these agents.
- **CNS Depressants**: Reserpine may enhance CNS depressant effects.
- **Digoxin**: Coadministration may result in additive bradycardia.
- **Insulin And Other Diabetic Agents**: Reserpine may mask clinical signs associated with hypoglycemia.
- **Monoamine Oxidase Inhibitors** (**MAOIs**; eg, **furazolidone, methylene blue**): Initially may increase the risk for hypertensive crisis. Concurrent long-term use may increase the risk for hypotension. The combination is contraindicated.
- **Pentoxifylline**: May increase the risk for hypotension
- **Quinidine**: May increase the risk for hypotension, orthostasis, and cardiac depression and/or arrhythmias
- **St. John's Wort**: Antagonizes the effects of reserpine
- **Sympathomimetics** (eg, **epinephrine, norepinephrine, pseudoephedrine**): Increased risk for hypertension and arrhythmias

Laboratory Considerations

- Reserpine may increase serum prolactin levels.
- Urinary catecholamine excretion may initially increase but is reduced with long-term use.
- May interfere with colorimetric assays for 17-hydroxycorticosteroids and 17-ketosteroids

Dosages

HORSES:

Tranquilizer (extra-label): 0.002 – 0.008 mg/kg (1 – 4 mg/500 kg [1102 lb] horse) PO once daily.[11] Dosages are not well established and should be adjusted to the individual horse based on response. A similar IM dose is recommended; however, the administration is every 48 hours to once weekly, or even less often, based on response.[12,13]

Fescue toxicosis (extra-label): 0.01 mg/kg by mouth every 24 hours[1]

Monitoring

- Clinical efficacy, signs of sedation
- Heart rate, blood pressure, mucous membrane color, capillary refill time
- Adverse effects: signs of hypotension (eg, pale mucous membranes, mental dullness, cold extremities, weakness), colic, and diarrhea

Client Information

- A veterinary professional must administer this medication. Consult with your veterinarian before using reserpine.
- Monitor for signs of side effects (eg, diarrhea, decrease in blood pressure, colic).
- Reserpine may cause male horses to drop their penises.
- Reserpine is a prohibited substance in most sanctioned competitions.

Chemistry/Synonyms

Reserpine is a natural indole alkaloid purified from the *Rauwolfia serpentine* shrub. Reserpine is available as a white to slightly yellow crystalline powder, with a pK_a of 6.6. It is odorless with a slightly bitter taste.

Reserpine may also be known as NSC-757309, raunervil, raupasil, rausedil, and *Serpasil*®.

Storage/Stability

Store powder at controlled room temperature between 20°C and 25°C (68°F-77°F) and protect from light. Compounded products should be stored according to the product label.

Compatibility/Compounding Considerations

It is suggested to consult specialized references or a veterinary compounding pharmacist for more specific information.

Dosage Forms/Regulatory Status

VETERINARY-LABELED PRODUCTS:

None. Products may be available from compounding pharmacies.

The Association of Racing Commissioners International (ARCI) has designated this drug as a class 2 substance. Use of this drug may not be allowed in certain animal competitions. Check rules and regulations before entering a competition while this medication is being administered. Contact local racing authorities for further guidance. See ***Appendix.***

HUMAN-LABELED PRODUCTS:

None. The product has been discontinued in the United States.

References

For the complete list of references, see **wiley.com/go/budde/plumb**

Rifampin

Rifampicin

(***rif***-am-pin) *Rifadin*®

Antimicrobial

Prescriber Highlights

- Antimicrobial with activity against a variety of microbes (*Rhodococcus* spp, mycobacteria, staphylococci)
- Contraindications include hypersensitivity to it or other rifamycins.
- Use with caution in pre-existing hepatic dysfunction; dogs may be more susceptible to hepatotoxic effects.
- Adverse effects include increases in liver enzymes (especially in dogs). Uncommon adverse effects include rashes, GI distress, and hepatitis.
- Preferable to give this drug on an empty stomach
- May cause red/orange urine, tears, and sweat (harmless, but can stain fabrics)
- Many drug interactions are possible.

Uses/Indications

Rifampin is primarily used to treat *Rhodococcus equi* infections in young horses. A combination of rifampin with a macrolide (eg, erythromycin, azithromycin, or clarithromycin) is the recommended treatment for infection caused by *R equi*[1]; however, a controlled, randomized, double-blinded clinical trial found no difference in efficacy between foals with mild pneumonia associated with *R equi* that received azithromycin/rifampin and those that received azithromycin alone.[2] Studies suggest a macrolide/tetracycline combination (eg, azithromycin or clarithromycin with doxycycline or minocycline) can be used for treatment of *R equi* in foals.[3,4] Rifampin may also be useful to treat proliferative enteropathy caused by *Lawsonia intracellularis* in foals.[5-8]

In dogs, rifampin may be a useful adjunctive antibiotic for treating methicillin-resistant *Staphylococcus pseudintermedius* pyoderma or as an alternative treatment of *Ehrlichia canis;* however, resistance emerges rapidly when rifampin is used alone, so combination therapy with another effective antimicrobial is recommended. When canine brucellosis treatment is attempted (not recommended[9,10]), rifampin may be used in combination with doxycycline and gentamicin. In small animals, rifampin is sometimes combined with other antimycobacterial drugs to treat nontubercular mycobacterial infections or with other antifungal agents (amphotericin B and flucytosine) in the treatment of histoplasmosis or aspergillosis with CNS involvement.

The World Health Organization (WHO) has designated rifampin as a Critically Important (High Priority) Antimicrobial for human medicine.[11] The Office International des Epizooties (OIE) has designated rifampin as a Veterinary Highly Important Antimicrobial (VHIA) Agent in equine species.[12]

Pharmacology/Actions

Rifampin may act as either a bactericidal or bacteriostatic antimicrobial depending on the susceptibility of the organism and the concentration of the drug. For *Rhodococcus equi,* it is considered a time-dependent antibiotic. Rifampin inhibits bacterial, but not mammalian, DNA-dependent RNA polymerase, thereby suppressing the initiation of chain formation for RNA transcription in susceptible organisms. Rifampin is most active against susceptible bacteria undergoing cell division. Rifampin is active against a variety of mycobacterium species and gram-positive bacteria such as staphylococci, *Neisseria* spp, and *Haemophilus* spp.

Although the prevalence of equine *R equi* isolates that are resistant to rifampin is relatively low, tolerance by *R equi* with increasing MICs appears to be growing. Rifampin is used in combination with another active antibiotic in an attempt to reduce the potential for resistance development.[13] Resistance is thought to occur via mutation with resistant strains spreading clonally.

Rifampin has some antifungal activity when combined with other antifungal agents.

Pharmacokinetics

After oral administration, rifampin is relatively well absorbed from the GI tract. Oral bioavailability is reportedly ≈40% to 70% in horses and 37% in adult sheep. If food is given concurrently, peak plasma concentrations may be delayed and slightly reduced.

Rifampin is very lipophilic and readily penetrates into, and achieves effective concentrations in, most body tissues (including bone and prostate), cells, and fluids (including CSF). It also penetrates abscesses and caseous material. Rifampin is 70% to 90% bound to serum proteins, is distributed into milk, and crosses the placenta. Mean volume of distribution is ≈0.9 L/kg in horses, and 1.3 L/kg in sheep.

Rifampin is metabolized in the liver to a deacetylated form that also has antibacterial activity. Both this metabolite and unchanged drug are excreted primarily in the bile, but up to 30% may be excreted in the urine. The parent drug is substantially reabsorbed in the gut but the metabolite is not. Reported elimination half-lives for various species are 6 to 8 hours in horses, 8 hours in dogs, and 3 to 5 hours in sheep. Because rifampin can induce hepatic microsomal enzymes, elimination rates may increase with time.

Contraindications/Precautions/Warnings

Rifampin is contraindicated in patients that are hypersensitive to it or other rifamycins. It should be used with caution in patients with pre-existing hepatic dysfunction. Small animal species should be closely monitored for signs of hepatopathy; dogs may be more susceptible to hepatotoxicity than some other species.[13] To reduce chances for hepatopathy, some clinicians have suggested that PO doses should not exceed 10 mg/kg/day in dogs.

Adverse Effects

Rifampin can cause red/orange colored urine, tears, sweat, and saliva. There are no harmful consequences from this effect. A retrospective study in dogs found that at dosages from 2.9 – 16 mg/kg per day, 16% of treated dogs showed adverse effects, including vomiting (7%), anorexia (6%), and lethargy (4%).[14] Commonly used dosages can cause increased liver enzymes (ALT) in ≈25% of treated dogs.[1] Hepatitis has been reported in some treated dogs.

If rifampin is used in cats for mycobacterial infections, signs of liver dysfunction, including inappetence, vomiting, or jaundice, may occur. Hepatopathy can be fatal.

In some species (eg, humans), rashes, GI distress, and increases in liver enzymes may occur, particularly with long-term use.

Oral dosage forms may be unpalatable.

Adverse effects in horses are apparently rare, but when rifampin is combined with erythromycin, mild diarrhea (self-limiting) to severe enterocolitis in foals and mares, hyperthermia, and acute respiratory distress can occur. When it is used in combination with doxycycline, rifampin can result in hemolytic anemia and elevated liver enzymes.[15] Although not commercially available, IV rifampin has caused CNS depression, sweating, hemolysis, and anorexia in horses.

Reproductive/Nursing Safety

Rodents given high doses of rifampin (150 – 250 mg/kg/day) showed some congenital malformations in their offspring, but the drug has been used in pregnant women with no reported increases in teratogenicity.[16]

Rifampin is excreted in maternal milk; use with caution in nursing patients.

Because safety has not been established in animals, this drug should only be used when the maternal benefits outweigh the potential risks to offspring.

Overdose/Acute Toxicity

Clinical signs associated with oral rifampin overdose are generally extensions of the adverse effects outlined in the ***Adverse Effects*** section (GI, red/orange coloring of fluids and skin), but massive overdoses may cause hepatotoxicity.

Should a massive oral overdose occur, standard GI decontamination protocols should be followed. Liver enzymes should be monitored, and supportive treatment should be initiated if necessary.

For patients that have experienced or are suspected to have experienced an overdose, consultation with a 24-hour poison consultation center specializing in providing veterinary-specific information is recommended. For general information related to overdose and toxin exposures, as well as contact information for poison control centers, refer to ***Appendix***.

Drug Interactions

There are a multitude of potential drug interactions with rifampin. The following drug interactions (partial listing) have either been reported or are theoretical in humans or animals receiving rifampin and may be of significance in veterinary patients. Unless otherwise noted, use together is not necessarily contraindicated, but weigh the potential risks and perform additional monitoring when appropriate.

- **ACETAMINOPHEN**: Rifampin may increase acetaminophen toxicity.
- **ATOVAQUONE**: Rifampin may decrease serum concentrations of atovaquone.
- **CLARITHROMYCIN**: Rifampin may reduce clarithromycin concentrations and oral bioavailability may be significantly decreased in foals[17-19]; however, effective clarithromycin concentrations against *Rhodococcus equi* are still achieved.[18,20]
- **CLOPIDOGREL**: Rifampin may increase the risk for bleeding by increasing formation of clopidogrel's active metabolite.
- **CYCLOPHOSPHAMIDE**: Rifampin may increase concentrations of active metabolites of cyclophosphamide.
- **ISONIAZID**: Increased risk for hepatotoxicity
- **FLUOROQUINOLONES** (eg, **enrofloxacin**): Rifampin may reduce fluoroquinolone concentrations. In vitro antagonism also has been reported when rifampin is used concurrently with fluoroquinolone antibiotics, and concurrent use should be avoided.
- **IFOSFAMIDE**: Rifampin may increase the risk for nephrotoxicity and neurotoxicity by increasing formation of the ifosfamide-active metabolite.
- **LEFLUNOMIDE**: Rifampin may increase the risk for hepatotoxicity by increasing the formation of the active leflunomide metabolite.
- **PROPOFOL**: Rifampin may enhance the hypotensive effect of propofol.

Because rifampin has been documented to induce hepatic microsomal enzymes, drugs that are metabolized by these enzymes, such as cytochrome P450, may have their elimination half-lives shortened and serum levels decreased. This effect may persist for up to one month after rifampin is discontinued. Examples of drugs/classes that may be affected include:

- **AMIODARONE**
- **AZOLE ANTIFUNGALS** (eg, **fluconazole, itraconazole, ketoconazole, voriconazole**)
- **BENZODIAZEPINES** (eg, **diazepam, midazolam**)
- **BETA BLOCKERS** (eg, **carvedilol, propranolol**)
- **BUSPIRONE**
- **CALCITRIOL**
- **CANNABIDIOL**
- **CHLORAMPHENICOL**
- **CORTICOSTEROIDS** (eg, **dexamethasone, prednisone/prednisolone**)
- **CYCLOSPORINE**
- **DAPSONE**
- **DIGOXIN**
- **DILTIAZEM**
- **DOXORUBICIN**
- **DOXYCYCLINE**
- **ENALAPRIL**
- **ESTROGENS**
- **GLIPIZIDE**
- **KETAMINE**
- **LIDOCAINE, MEXILETINE**
- **MYCOPHENOLATE**
- **ONDANSETRON**
- **OPIOIDS** (eg, **fentanyl, hydrocodone, morphine, tramadol**)
- **PHENOBARBITAL**
- **PRAZIQUANTEL** (combination is contraindicated in humans)
- **PROGESTINS**
- **PROTON PUMP INHIBITORS** (eg, **omeprazole, pantoprazole**)
- **QUINIDINE**
- **RIVAROXABAN**
- **SERTRALINE**
- **SULFA-/TRIMETHOPRIM**
- **THEOPHYLLINE**
- **VINCRISTINE**
- **WARFARIN**

Laboratory Considerations

- Microbiologic methods of assaying serum folate and vitamin B12 are interfered with by rifampin.

- Rifampin can cause false positive BSP (bromosulfophthalein, sulfobromophthalein) test results by inhibiting the hepatic uptake of the drug.

Dosages

DOGS:

Superficial bacterial folliculitis (extra-label):

a) 5 – 10 mg/kg PO twice daily when empirical selection of a first-tier systemic antimicrobial agent (eg, cephalexin, amoxicillin/clavulanate, clindamycin) and topical therapy are not appropriate and when cultures indicate susceptibility.[21] Use in combination with another antimicrobial agent is recommended to reduce development of resistance; consultation with a specialist is recommended prior to using this treatment.

b) **Methicillin-resistant *Staphylococcus* spp pyoderma**: 5 mg/kg PO twice daily in combination with topical antimicrobials for 4 to 5 weeks[22]; consultation with a specialist is recommended prior to using this treatment.

Canine leproid granuloma (extra-label): 10 – 15 mg/kg (maximum of 600 mg total) PO once daily in combination with antimicrobial agents known to be effective against slow-growing nontuberculous mycobacteria (eg, clofazimine, clarithromycin, pradofloxacin) may facilitate disease resolution.[23] A combination of rifampin 10 – 15 mg/kg PO once daily and clarithromycin 7.5 – 12.5 mg/kg PO 2 to 3 times a day is recommended for treating severe or refractory canine leproid granuloma in concert with topical silver sulfasalazine.[24]

Canine brucellosis (extra-label): Antibiotic therapy is not encouraged except in select cases due to the zoonotic risk and because there is no known cure.[9,10] If therapy is attempted, infected dogs must be isolated from other dogs and breeding animals. Use combination therapy of rifampin 5 mg/kg PO once daily with doxycycline 10 mg/kg PO every 12 hours and gentamicin 5 mg/kg SC once daily for 3 months. After this antibiotic trial, retest and repeat treatment until the patient has a negative test. After reaching a negative serology test, continue to test every 4 to 6 months and repeat treatment as necessary.[25]

CATS:

Feline leprosy syndromes (extra-label): 10 – 15 mg/kg PO once daily in combination with antimicrobial agents known to be effective against slow-growing nontuberculous mycobacteria (eg, clofazimine, clarithromycin, pradofloxacin) may facilitate disease resolution.[24]

HORSES:

***Rhodococcus equi* infections in foals** (extra-label): There does not appear to be a clear consensus on the treatment of choice for *R equi* in foals. Commonly, rifampin 5 mg/kg PO twice daily is used in combination with either clarithromycin 7.5 mg/kg PO every 12 hours OR azithromycin 10 mg/kg PO once a day for 5 days, then every 48 hours (every other day).[1] Treatment may be required for 4 to 9 weeks but can be reduced with early diagnosis and treatment.

Proliferative enteropathy caused by *Lawsonia intracellularis* in foals (extra-label): Primary treatment consists of a macrolide antibiotic; rifampin 10 mg/kg PO once daily can be added as adjunctive therapy; treat for a minimum of 21 days.[5-8]

Monitoring

- Clinical efficacy
- For monitoring *Rhodococcus equi* infections in foals and response to rifampin/macrolide: Chest radiographs and plasma fibrinogen levels have been suggested as prognostic indicators when performed after 1 week of treatment.
- Adverse effects (especially clinical signs for hepatopathy in small animal species)
- Liver function monitoring (especially in dogs or cats): baseline liver enzymes with rechecks at 10 to 14 days, then at least monthly with long-term therapy

Client Information

- This medicine is best given on an empty stomach. If it causes stomach upset or vomiting, give the medicine with food to see if this helps.
- Rifampin causes red/orange urine, tears, and saliva (and sweat in horses). This effect is not harmful but can stain fabrics.
- Rifampin can have a bitter taste, especially for horses, and may cause your animal to avoid food and develop a decreased appetite during treatment.
- Other medications can interact with rifampin, so be sure to tell your veterinarian and pharmacist what medications (including vitamins, supplements, or herbal therapies) you give your animal, including the amount and time you give each.
- This medicine may cause liver damage, which may be worse in older animals. Your veterinarian will do periodic blood tests to monitor for this problem. Do not miss these important follow-up visits.

Chemistry/Synonyms

A semi-synthetic zwitterion derivative of rifamycin B, rifampin occurs as a red-brown, crystalline powder with a pK_a of 7.9. It is very slightly soluble in water and slightly soluble in alcohol.

Rifampin may also be known as rifampicin, Ba-41166/E, L-5103, NSC-113926, rifaldazine, rifampicinum, or rifamycin AMP; many trade names are available.

Storage/Stability

Rifampin capsules should be stored in tight, light-resistant containers, preferably at room temperature (15°C-30°C [59°F-86°F]).

Compatibility/Compounding Considerations

Compatibility is dependent on factors such as pH, concentration, temperature, and diluent used; specialized references or a hospital pharmacist should be consulted for more specific information.

Rifampin for injection is reported as wholly or variably **incompatible** with typical IV solutions as well as other drugs for injection. It is suggested to consult specialized references or a hospital pharmacist for more specific information. If used, rifampin for injection must be administered only by IV infusion over at least 30 minutes in 5% dextrose solution within 4 hours of preparation. Extravasation must be avoided, and never administer rifampin by IM or SC routes.

Dosage Forms/Regulatory Status

VETERINARY-LABELED PRODUCTS: NONE

HUMAN-LABELED PRODUCTS:

Rifampin Oral Capsules: 150 mg and 300 mg; *Rifadin®*, generic; (Rx)

Rifampin Lyophilized Powder for Injection Solution: 600 mg; *Rifadin®*, generic; (Rx)

References

For the complete list of references, see **wiley.com/go/budde/plumb**

Rifaximin

(rif-**ax**-i-min) *Xifaxan®*

Antimicrobial

Prescriber Highlights

- Nonsystemic antibiotic used to treat hepatic encephalopathy and diarrhea in humans
- Has induced remission in dogs with chronic enteropathy but is rarely used clinically
- Drug interactions are limited and likely clinically insignificant.
- Significantly more expensive than metronidazole or lactulose

Uses/Indications

Rifaximin can be used orally to modify the gut microbiota, as a treatment for chronic diarrhea, or in an attempt to ameliorate hepatic encephalopathy in dogs. In a study with dogs, rifaximin induced complete (86%) or partial (14%) remission of chronic enteropathy; it was shown to be as effective as metronidazole.[1] Rifaximin may have utility in treating or preventing recurrence of hepatic encephalopathy in veterinary patients, but use is limited, as it is prohibitively more expensive than current, accepted treatments.

Rifaximin is used in humans to treat uncomplicated traveler's diarrhea caused by *Escherichia coli* and diarrhea due to irritable bowel syndrome and to treat and reduce the risk for hepatic encephalopathy.

The World Health Organization has designated rifaximin as a Critically Important antimicrobial for human medicine.[2]

Pharmacology/Actions

Rifaximin inhibits bacterial protein synthesis by binding the beta-subunit of bacterial DNA-dependent RNA polymerase. In humans, it is effective against *Escherichia coli* but is ineffective against *Campylobacter jejuni*; efficacy for other causes of infectious diarrhea (eg, *Salmonella* spp, *Shigella* spp) has not been established. Rifaximin may also be active against some protozoa (eg, *Blastocystis hominis*, *Cryptosporidium parvum*).[3]

Pharmacokinetics

In a study of dogs receiving rifaximin at either 25 mg/kg PO as a single dose or at 10 mg/kg PO per day for 8 days, serum rifaximin was not detectable.[4]

Systemic exposure to rifaximin is limited after oral administration. In patients with hepatic impairment, systemic exposure increases 10- to 25-fold after oral administration, although dosage adjustment is usually not necessary.[5] Administration with food increases systemic exposure, but this effect is clinically insignificant. Over 95% of the drug is excreted unchanged in the feces. Of the limited drug that is absorbed, ≈65% is protein-bound, and extensive hepatic metabolism occurs via CYP 3A4. The elimination half-life is ≈6 hours.

Contraindications/Precautions/Warnings

Rifaximin is contraindicated in patients with a known hypersensitivity to it or other rifamycin antimicrobials.[5] The effectiveness of rifaximin in humans with infectious diarrhea caused by pathogens other than *Escherichia coli* has not been demonstrated. Rifaximin use has been associated with the development of *Clostridium difficile* infection in humans. Severe hepatic impairment may lead to increased systemic exposure and may be substantially increased with concurrent use of rifaximin with P-glycoprotein inhibitors (eg, verapamil). Hypersensitivity reactions, including exfoliative dermatitis, rash, angioneurotic edema, urticaria, flushing, pruritus, and anaphylaxis, have occurred as early as within 15 minutes of drug administration. It is not appropriate for use in patients with bloody diarrhea or with diarrhea and fever.

Do not confuse rifaXIMin with rifaMPin.

Adverse Effects

Rifaximin appears to be well tolerated. Adverse effects reported in humans include peripheral edema, dizziness, fatigue, pruritus, anemia, and nausea.

Reproductive/Nursing Safety

Rifaximin was teratogenic when given to rats at 150 – 300 mg/kg and in rabbits receiving 62.5 – 1000 mg/kg.[5] Data about the safe use of rifaximin in pregnant women are lacking. It is unknown if rifaximin is excreted into milk.

Because safety has not been established in animals, this drug should only be used when the maternal benefits outweigh the potential risks to offspring.

Overdosage/Acute Toxicity

Because rifaximin is not systemically absorbed, clinical signs from overdoses are unlikely. Gut decontamination is not considered necessary. Provide supportive care and monitor the patient closely. Consultation with a veterinary poison center can be considered.

For patients that have experienced or are suspected of having experienced an overdose, consultation with a 24-hour poison consultation center specializing in providing veterinary-specific information is recommended. For general information related to overdose and toxin exposures, as well as contact information for poison control centers, refer to ***Appendix.***

Drug Interactions

Induction of hepatic enzymes by rifaximin is not expected in humans receiving recommended rifaximin doses. Rifaximin is a substrate of CYP 3A4 in humans, as well as a substrate and possible inhibitor of P-glycoprotein and several organic-anion-transporting polypeptides (OATPs). Clinically significant alteration of rifaximin by other drugs is unlikely because of the limited bioavailability of rifaximin. The following drug interactions have either been reported or are theoretical in humans or animals receiving rifaximin and may be of significance in veterinary patients. Unless otherwise noted, use together is not necessarily contraindicated, but weigh the potential risks and perform additional monitoring when appropriate.

- **CYCLOSPORINE**: May increase rifaximin exposure
- **CYP 3A4 INHIBITORS** (eg, **clarithromycin, fluoxetine, ketoconazole, verapamil**): May increase rifaximin exposure
- **P-GLYCOPROTEIN INHIBITORS** (eg, **amiodarone, clarithromycin, itraconazole, verapamil**): May increase rifaximin exposure
- **VACCINES (LIVE, ORAL)**: Antibiotics may reduce immunologic response to the live vaccines.
- **WARFARIN**: Prothrombin time (PT) and anticoagulant effect may be reduced.

Laboratory Considerations

- None were noted.

Dosages

DOGS:

Chronic enteropathy (extra-label): 25 mg/kg PO every 12 hours for 21 days was as effective as metronidazole.[1] All dogs concurrently received metoclopramide and ranitidine for the first 15 days, a weekly cyanocobalamin injection, and were fed a limited diet of boiled chicken and rice; the study lacked a control group to account for the possible therapeutic role of these interventions.

Monitoring

- Clinical efficacy
- Development of antibiotic-related diarrhea

Client Information

- This medicine may be given with or without food.
- Report bloody diarrhea to your veterinarian immediately.

Chemistry/Synonyms

Rifaximin is a semi-synthetic derivative of rifamycin SV and is structurally related to rifampin. It occurs as a red-orange crystalline powder that is insoluble in water and soluble in acetone and methanol.

Rifaximin is also known as L/105, rifaxidin, rifaximinum, and *Xifaxin*®.

Storage/Stability

Store rifaximin protected from light at controlled room temperature 20°C to 25°C (68°F-77°F); excursions are permitted to 15°C to 30°C (59°F-86°F).[5]

Compatibility/Compounding Considerations

No information was noted.

Dosage Forms/Regulatory Status

VETERINARY-LABELED PRODUCTS: NONE

HUMAN-LABELED PRODUCTS:

Rifaximin Tablets: 200 mg and 550 mg tablets; *Xifaxin*®; (Rx)

References

For the complete list of references, see **wiley.com/go/budde/plumb**

Rivaroxaban

(riv-a-**rox**-a-ban) *Xarelto*®

Factor Xa Inhibitor

Prescriber Highlights

- ► Oral anticoagulant used to prevent or treat thrombosis in high-risk patients, with prompt and predictable anticoagulant effect
- ► Contraindicated in patients with uncontrolled pathologic bleeding, severe hepatic disease, hepatic disease associated with coagulopathy, or with significant renal impairment.
- ► Appears to be well tolerated but use in veterinary patients is limited. Minor bleeding is possible.
- ► Specific guidelines for monitoring therapy in clinical patients are lacking.
- ► Cost may be a limiting factor.

Uses/Indications

Rivaroxaban has been used to treat thromboembolic disease in dogs[1-7] and cats.[8] Rivaroxaban may be preferred over unfractionated heparin in dogs due to evidence of equivalent efficacy, as well as reliable pharmacokinetics and the ease of oral administration. Direct Xa inhibitors can be considered in cats based on reliable pharmacokinetics and favorable safety profile.[9]

In humans, it is used to treat deep-vein thrombosis (DVT) and pulmonary embolism (PE) for the prevention of DVT following orthopedic surgery or before DVT/PE, and for stroke and systemic embolism prevention in patients with atrial fibrillation. Rivaroxaban has not been proven to be either safer or more effective than other available anticoagulants.

Pharmacology/Actions

Rivaroxaban is an inhibitor of activated clotting factor X (FXa) and prothrombinase activity. Unlike heparins, its anticoagulant effect does not require a cofactor. It indirectly inhibits platelet aggregation induced by thrombin.

In vitro data suggest FXa in dogs has a lower affinity for rivaroxaban than in humans; a concentration of ≈0.4 µg/mL was required to inhibit 50% thrombin generation.[10] Peak anti-FXa activity occurred 2 to 4 hours after administration to dogs,[11] and 2 to 3 hours after administration to cats.[12]

Pharmacokinetics

In healthy dogs given a single dose of rivaroxaban 1 mg/kg PO, the drug was rapidly absorbed, with 60% to 85% bioavailability.[13] Food does not appear to have a clinically relevant effect on rivaroxaban aborption.[11] Peak concentrations were 1.28 µg/mL and occurred 30 minutes after administration. The elimination half-life was ≈1 hour.[13]

In healthy cats, a single 2.5 mg/cat (NOT mg/kg) rivaroxaban dose PO resulted in peak concentrations of 0.27 µg/mL attained 2.5 hours after administration. The elimination half-life was 7.5 hours.[12]

In humans, rivaroxaban is 66% to 100% bioavailable after oral administration, although absorption decreases with increasing doses. Peak concentrations occur within 2 to 4 hours after dosing. Food increases the extent of the drug's absorption while delaying the time to peak concentration, but this effect only occurs at higher doses. Absorption is greatest when rivaroxaban is administered into the stomach and diminishes when it is administered directly into the intestinal tract. It is ≈95% protein-bound to albumin. Rivaroxaban is hepatically metabolized, including cytochrome P450 3A4 isozyme (CYP3A4). It is also a P-glycoprotein substrate. The drug and metabolites are renally eliminated, with an elimination half-life between 5 and 9 hours. Half-life is prolonged in elderly patients (11 to 13 hours) and in patients with renal (8 to 10 hours) or hepatic (10 hours) dysfunction.

Contraindications/Precautions/Warnings

Rivaroxaban is contraindicated in patients that are allergic to it or have uncontrolled pathologic bleeding. The drug should be avoided in patients with severe hepatic disease, a hepatic disease associated with coagulopathy, or with significant renal impairment. It may be used with caution in patients with moderate hepatic impairment; a lower dose is recommended in patients with moderate renal impairment. Use rivaroxaban with caution in patients with minor bleeding and in patients with bleeding disorders or coagulopathies. Patients undergoing neuraxial anesthesia or spinal puncture are at increased risk for epidural or spinal hematoma.

Thrombotic events have been observed in humans following discontinuation of rivaroxban.[14] The significance for veterinary patients is unclear, but it has been suggested to taper rivaroxaban before discontining.[15]

In humans with atrial fibrillation, a rebound risk for stroke has been noted after discontinuing rivaroxaban; alternative anticoagulant coverage may be needed during that time. Rivaroxaban should be stopped at least 24 hours before surgery or high-risk procedures; resume rivaroxaban once hemostasis has been established.[16] Consult the product label for guidance when transitioning to and from rivaroxaban with other anticoagulants to ensure continuous anticoagulation while minimizing the risk for bleeding.

Adverse Effects

The most common adverse effect in humans is bleeding.[16] Nausea, vomiting, diarrhea, and an increase in liver enzymes can also occur. Pruritus and rash have been noted but are uncommon.

Rivaroxaban is generally safe and well tolerated in dogs and cats, although the number of animals that have received rivaroxaban is small. Reported adverse effects include minor bleeding (eg, epistaxis, hematemesis, hematuria, hematochezia, and anemia) and vomiting.[8,17-19]

Reproductive/Nursing Safety

Rivaroxaban crosses the placenta of rats and rabbits.[16] Pronounced maternal hemorrhagic complications have occurred in rats, and decreased fetal weights occurred in pregnant rats receiving 120 mg/kg (14 times the human exposure). Postimplantation pregnancy losses have occurred in rabbits, as has fetal toxicity (eg, decreases in fetal weights, live fetuses, increased resorption) in rabbits receiving 10 mg/kg (4 times the human exposure) or more during organogenesis. In animal studies, during labor and delivery, increased maternal bleeding and death and increased fetal death occurred in animals receiving 40 mg/kg.[16]

Rivaroxaban is excreted into the breast milk of rats[16]; use with caution in lactating animals.

Because safety has not been established in animals, this drug should only be used when the maternal benefits outweigh the potential risks to offspring.

Overdose/Acute Toxicity

Overdoses are expected to increase the risk for hemorrhage, but overdoses in humans have not been universally associated with significant bleeding. Treatment is supportive and based on clinical signs; monitoring with prothrombin time (PT), international normalized ratio (INR), activated partial thromboplastin time (aPTT), thromboelastography, and thrombin generation tests may also be helpful. GI decontamination can be considered for recent ingestions. Hemorrhagic complications may be treated with appropriate blood products. It is not dialyzable. An antidote to FXa anticoagulants (andexanet alfa [recombinant coagulation factor Xa, inactivated zhzo])[20] is available and may be considered, but its use in animals is limited.

For patients that have experienced or are suspected of having experienced an overdose, consultation with a 24-hour poison consultation center specializing in providing veterinary-specific information is recommended. For general information related to overdose and toxin exposures, as well as contact information for poison control centers, refer to ***Appendix***.

Drug Interactions

In humans, rivaroxaban is a substrate of CYP3A4 and P-glycoprotein. Drugs that inhibit both enzyme pathways may increase rivaroxaban exposure and the risk for bleeding. The following drug interactions have either been reported or are theoretical in humans or animals receiving rivaroxaban and may be of significance in veterinary patients. Unless otherwise noted, use together is not necessarily contraindicated, but weigh the potential risks and perform additional monitoring when appropriate.

- **Azole Antifungals** (eg, **itraconazole, ketoconazole, voriconazole**): May substantially increase rivaroxaban exposure and increase the risk for bleeding
- **Anticoagulants, Other** (eg, **heparins, warfarin**): May increase the risk for bleeding
- **Antiplatelet Agents** (eg, **aspirin, clopidogrel**): May increase the risk for bleeding
- **CYP3A4 Inducers** (eg, **rifampin, phenobarbital**): May increase rivaroxaban metabolism and increase the risk for a thrombotic event
- **Fluoxetine**: May increase the risk for bleeding
- **Macrolide Antibiotics** (eg, **clarithromycin, erythromycin**): May substantially increase rivaroxaban exposure and increase the risk for bleeding
- **Nonsteroidal Anti-Inflammatory Drugs** (**NSAIDs**; eg, **carprofen, deracoxib, firocoxib, meloxicam, robenacoxib**): May increase the risk for bleeding

Laboratory Interactions

- Rivaroxaban may result in a decreased factor VIII: C serum level because of assay interference.
- Falsely elevated INR has been noted.

Dosages

NOTE: Thrombotic events have been observed in humans following discontinuation of rivaroxaban. The significance for veterinary patients is unclear, but it has been suggested to taper rivaroxaban before discontinuing.[15]

DOGS:

Antithrombotic agent (extra-label):

a) 0.5 –1 mg/kg PO every 24 hours.[2-7] Based on in vivo coagulation assessments, administration every 12 hours may be more appropriate.[21]

b) 1 – 2 mg/kg PO every 24 hours[22,23]

CATS:

Antithrombotic agent (extra-label):

a) 1.25 mg/cat (NOT mg/kg) PO every 24 hours provided less than 12 hours of anti-FXa activity in healthy cats. Further studies of higher doses are warranted.[12]

b) 0.5 – 1 mg/kg PO every 12 to 24 hours[12,23]; practically, 2.5 – 5 mg/cat (NOT mg/kg) PO every 24 hours

c) 2.5 mg/cat (NOT mg/kg) PO every 24 hours in combination with clopidogrel 18.75 mg/cat (NOT mg/kg) PO every 24 hours[8]

Monitoring

- Routine coagulation monitoring is not required[17]; however, prothrombin time (PT) and thromboelastography can be considered.[24,25]
- CBC with platelets
- Renal and hepatic function
- Clinical efficacy
- Signs of bleeding (eg, lethargy, dyspnea, collapse)

Client Information

- Give this medicine as directed by your veterinarian.
- Your animal may bruise or bleed more easily while taking this medication. Contact your veterinarian immediately if you notice bleeding or suspect your animal may be experiencing internal bleeding.
- If you miss a dose, give it as soon as you remember then restart the regular schedule.
- Give this medicine with or without food and at the same time each day.
- Do not stop giving this medicine to your animal without discussing with your veterinarian.

Chemistry/Synonyms

Rivaroxaban occurs as an odorless white to yellowish powder that is practically insoluble in water and only slightly soluble in organic solvents. The commercial tablets contain pure (*S*)-enantiomer.

Rivaroxaban is also known as Bay-59-7939, rivaroxabana, rivaroxabanum, and *Xarelto*®.

Storage/Stability

Store rivaroxaban at room temperature (ie, 25°C [77°F]); excursions to 15°C to 30°C (59°F-86°F) are permitted. Store out of reach of pets and children.

Compatibility/Compounding Considerations

Rivaroxaban may be crushed and mixed with applesauce immediately before oral administration. It may also be crushed and suspended in 50 mL of water for administration via nasogastric or gastric feeding tube. The drug is stable for up to 4 hours when crushed and mixed in water or applesauce.[16]

Dosage Forms/Regulatory Status

VETERINARY-LABELED PRODUCTS: NONE

HUMAN-LABELED PRODUCTS:

Rivaroxaban Tablets: 2.5 mg, 10 mg, 15 mg, and 20 mg tablets; *Xarelto*®; (Rx)

References

For the complete list of references, see **wiley.com/go/budde/plumb**

Robenacoxib

(roe-ben-ah-***cox***-ib) *Onsior®*

Nonsteroidal Anti-inflammatory Drug (NSAID)

Prescriber Highlights

- COX-2–selective NSAID for use in dogs and cats to control postoperative pain for up to 3 days
- Only NSAID approved for multiple doses in cats in the United States
- In cats, the oral dose is different than the injection dose.
- Contraindications include hypersensitivity, known NSAID intolerance, and GI ulceration.
- Use with caution in patients with impaired renal and hepatic function, that are dehydrated, hypovolemic, or hypotensive, and in patients with a risk for GI ulceration.
- GI effects are the most common adverse effect.

Uses/Indications

Robenacoxib is a cyclooxygenase-2 (COX-2)–selective NSAID that is FDA-approved for use in dogs and cats 4 months of age and older, weighing 2.5 kg (5.5 lb) or more. In the United States, it is indicated for use in cats for the control of postoperative pain and inflammation associated with orthopedic surgery, ovariohysterectomy, and castration for a maximum of 3 days.[1,2] In dogs, robenacoxib is indicated for the control of postoperative pain and inflammation associated with soft tissue surgery for a maximum of 3 days.[1,3]

In other countries, the oral tablets are labeled for the treatment of pain and inflammation associated with chronic osteoarthritis in dogs and for the treatment of acute pain and inflammation associated with musculoskeletal disorders in cats. The injection is labeled for the treatment of pain and inflammation associated with orthopedic or soft tissue surgery in dogs and for the treatment of pain and inflammation associated with soft tissue surgery in cats.[4]

In cats, robenacoxib had equivalent (noninferior) efficacy and tolerability as compared with ketoprofen tablets,[5,6] meloxicam injection,[7] and tolfenamic acid injection.[8] Robenacoxib given SC prior to hysterectomy provided analgesia for up to 24 hours and was more effective than a single dose of buprenorphine (0.02 mg/kg SC) for the first 8 hours after surgery.[9] Robenacoxib did not change the extent of blood–aqueous barrier breakdown in cats undergoing anterior chamber paracentesis.[10] The tablets and injection can safely be interchanged in cats, although the dose is different for each formulation.[11]

In an acute synovitis model in dogs, robenacoxib had equivalent analgesic and anti-inflammatory efficacy as meloxicam.[12] In a multicenter, prospective, randomized, blinded field trial, robenacoxib provided efficacy and tolerability similar to that of meloxicam for the management of perioperative pain and inflammation in dogs undergoing orthopedic surgery[13] and to carprofen in dogs with arthritis.[14,15] Meloxicam appeared more effective than robenacoxib in dogs undergoing combined laparoscopic ovariectomy and laparoscopic-assisted gastropexy.[16] Robenacoxib tablets appear safe when given daily for up to 6 months in dogs.[17] The tablets and injection can safely and effectively be interchanged in dogs without interruption of daily therapy.[18]

Pharmacology/Actions

Robenacoxib is a selective inhibitor of cyclooxygenase-2 (COX-2) in cats[19,20] and dogs.[21,22] It is ≈130 times more selective for COX-2 than COX-1 in dogs[21] and ≈500 times more selective in cats[19] when using an in vitro whole blood assay. COX-2 is the inducible form of the enzyme and is primarily responsible for the production of mediators (eg, prostaglandin E) that can induce pain, inflammation, and fever.

In dogs, robenacoxib 2 mg/kg given SC 1 hour before administration of sevoflurane decreased the sevoflurane minimum alveolar concentration (MAC) for blunting the adrenergic response (BAR) by ≈16%.[23]

Creatinine clearance in cats was not altered when determined immediately after a single dose (2 mg/kg SC) of robenacoxib or ketoprofen.[24]

Pharmacokinetics

In dogs, peak blood concentrations occur ≈30 minutes after oral administration. Oral bioavailability is 62% when robenacoxib is given with food and 84% when it is given without food; SC bioavailability is 67% to 100%.[1,25] Peak concentration occurred 90 minutes after SC administration in conscious dogs but 120 minutes in sevoflurane-anesthetized mechanically ventilated dogs.[26] The volume of distribution (steady state) is 0.24 L/kg.[25] It is highly bound to plasma proteins (greater than 98%). Robenacoxib is metabolized by the liver. Terminal half-life in blood is ≈0.9 to 1.2 hours after oral administration and 1 to 4 hours when given SC. Robenacoxib persists longer and at higher concentrations at sites of inflammation than in blood.[27] Excretion is primarily via the biliary route (≈65%); the remainder is excreted renally.[28] Robenacoxib does not appear to induce hepatic enzymes in dogs.

In cats, bioavailability is ≈69% after SC administration. After PO administration, peak blood concentrations of robenacoxib occur at ≈30 minutes, and, although the presence of a small amount of food does not significantly affect bioavailability, full rations may significantly reduce oral bioavailability (49% fasted vs 10% full ration).[29] The volume of distribution is 0.19 L/kg, and robenacoxib is 99% bound to plasma proteins. It is extensively metabolized by the liver, with ≈25% converted into a gamma-lactam metabolite. Terminal elimination half-life is ≈1.1 hours after SC injection and 1.7 hours after oral administration. Elimination is 60% biliary and 17% renal. Robenacoxib crossed the blood-aqueous barrier in 5 of 6 cats.[10]

Contraindications/Precautions/Warnings

Robenacoxib is contraindicated in patients with hypersensitivity to robenacoxib or known intolerance to NSAIDs or with GI ulcers.[4] Robenacoxib injection contains sodium metabisulfite and should not be used in patients with sulfite hypersensitivity.[4] Robenacoxib should not be used concurrently with corticosteroids or other NSAIDs.[1-3]

Use robenacoxib with caution in patients with impaired renal function, patients that are dehydrated, hypovolemic, or hypotensive, and in patients with a risk for GI ulceration. Use with caution in dogs and cats with hepatic dysfunction[1-3]; on some foreign labels, hepatic dysfunction is listed as being a contraindication.[30] Robenacoxib has been shown to prolong the QT interval and should be used with caution in patients with cardiac disease. Use with other QT prolonging agents is not recommended.[1,2] If use cannot be avoided in these cases, careful monitoring is required.

Stop administration in patients that develop hyporexia or patients that become lethargic. Use has not been evaluated in cats or dogs less than 4 months of age, weighing less than 2.5 kg (5.5 lb), that are used for breeding, or are pregnant or lactating.[1-3]

Concurrent use with other anti-inflammatory drugs may result in additional or increased adverse effects; therefore, a treatment-free period from all other anti-inflammatories should be observed for at least 24 hours before beginning treatment with robenacoxib.[4,31] The treatment-free period, however, should take into account the pharmacokinetic properties of the products used previously. Use robenacoxib under strict veterinary monitoring in dogs or cats with a risk for GI ulcers, or if the animal previously displayed intolerance to other NSAIDs.

Robenacoxib should be used cautiously with other drugs that may affect renal blood flow (eg, diuretics, ACE inhibitors), and additional clinical monitoring is recommended. Avoid use with other potentially nephrotoxic drugs, as this may increase risk for renal toxicity. When NSAIDs are used, fluid therapy during surgery is recommended to decrease potential renal complications.[1,2]

Adverse Effects

Adverse effects commonly reported in dogs include GI effects (eg, decreased appetite, vomiting, soft feces, diarrhea)[1,3] and pain on injection and are usually mild and self-limiting.[1,31] Blood in the feces was seen in some patients. Increased liver enzymes were common in dogs given robenacoxib for longer than 2 weeks. No significant adverse cardiovascular effects were noted in healthy dogs.[32] Injection site reactions (eg, swelling, necrosis, and abscesses) have been reported.[1]

Robenacoxib administered IV to healthy adult beagles did not alter ECG readings, arterial blood pressure, clinical chemistry, coagulation or hematologic parameters, or mucosal bleeding time for up to 8 hours after administration.[32] Another study in healthy adult beagles demonstrated no decrease in GFR when robenacoxib was given orally alone or with benazepril; however, different effects may occur in dogs with cardiovascular or renal disaease.[33]

Adverse effects reported in cats include infections, dehiscence, and increased bleeding at *incision* sites.[1,2] Decreased appetite, vomiting, lethargy, and pain at the *injection* site may also occur. Patients at greatest risk for adverse effects are those that are dehydrated, on concomitant diuretic therapy, or with existing renal, cardiovascular, and/or hepatic dysfunction. Acute kidney injury and death have been reported.

Administration of the labeled dose for 28 days was well-tolerated in cats with osteoarthritis.[34] Administration of the label-recommended dose to cats with chronic musculoskeletal disease for 4 to 12 weeks was not associated with an increased risk for adverse effects compared to placebo.[35]

Reproductive/Nursing Safety

Because the safety of robenacoxib has not been established during pregnancy or lactation in dogs or cats used for breeding, this drug should only be used when the maternal benefits outweigh the potential risks to offspring.

Overdose/Acute Toxicity

No acute toxicity data were located. Acute overdoses may potentially cause GI, kidney, or liver toxicity.

In chronic toxicity studies in healthy young (ie, 6 to 7 months old) beagles, robenacoxib up to 10 mg/kg/day for 6 months did not produce any signs of toxicity.[22] In preclinical safety studies, dosages in beagles of up to 20 times the label dose (40 mg/kg) PO for 1 month and 5 times the label dose (10 mg/kg) for 6 months did not cause significant clinical adverse effects, hematologic and clinical chemistry variables, or macroscopic or microscopic lesions at necropsy.[22] Oral robenacoxib administered daily for 21 days to healthy beagles resulted in microscopic mucosal lesions in the descending colon of 4 of 7 dogs.[36] The clinical relevance of this finding is uncertain.

In healthy young cats (ie, 10 months of age), dosages of 4 mg/kg (2 times label dose) SC every 24 hours for 2 days and 10 mg/kg (5 times label dose) SC for 3 consecutive days did not produce any signs of toxicity. Safety trials in healthy young cats receiving up to 10 mg/kg (≈5 times label dose) PO every 24 hours for 28 days or PO every 12 hours for 42 days showed that robenacoxib, as compared with placebo, did not cause toxicologically significant effects on general observations of health, hematologic and clinical chemistry variables, urinalyses, or postmortem organ weight, gross pathology, or histopathology assessment.[37]

Supportive therapy based on clinical presentation, including administration of GI protective agents and forced diuresis, may be appropriate.

For patients that have experienced or are suspected to have experienced an overdose, it is strongly encouraged to consult with one of the 24-hour poison consultation centers that specialize in providing information specific for veterinary patients. For general information related to overdose and toxin exposures, as well as contact information for poison control centers, refer to ***Appendix.***

Drug Interactions

See the ***Contraindications/Precautions/Warnings*** section for the manufacturer's warnings regarding use of robenacoxib with other medications. In addition, the following drug interactions have either been reported or are theoretical in humans or animals receiving NSAIDs and may be of significance in animals receiving robenacoxib. Unless otherwise noted, use of these drugs with robenacoxib is not necessarily contraindicated, but the potential risks should be weighed and additional monitoring performed when appropriate.

- ANGIOTENSIN-CONVERTING ENZYME INHIBITORS (ACEIs; eg, **benazepril, enalapril**): NSAIDs can reduce effects on blood pressure.
- ANESTHETIC AGENTS (eg, **alfaxalone, propofol, sevoflurane**): Anesthetic use may reduce renal perfusion, which may alter robenacoxib pharmacokinetics[26] and possibly increase the risk for renal complications. Robenacoxib has a minimum alveolar concentration (MAC)-sparing effect in dogs.[23]
- ASPIRIN: May increase the risk for GI toxicity (eg, ulceration, bleeding, vomiting, diarrhea)
- CORTICOSTEROIDS (eg, **dexamethasone, prednis(ol)one**): May increase the risk for GI toxicity (eg, ulceration, bleeding, vomiting, diarrhea); use together is contraindicated.
- DIGOXIN: NSAIDs may increase serum digoxin concentrations.
- FLUCONAZOLE: Administration has increased plasma concentrations of celecoxib in humans and could potentially affect robenacoxib concentrations in dogs.
- FUROSEMIDE: NSAIDs may reduce the saluretic and diuretic effects.
- HIGHLY PROTEIN BOUND DRUGS (eg, **anticoagulants [oral], phenytoin, other anti-inflammatory agents, salicylates, sulfonamides, sulfonylurea antidiabetic agents, valproic acid**): Because robenacoxib is highly bound to plasma proteins (more than 99%) in dogs and cats, it could theoretically displace other highly bound drugs. These interactions are unlikely to be of clinical concern because increased free drug concentrations will equilibrate through increased clearance. Monitor for adverse effects of each drug when using this combination.
- METHOTREXATE: Serious toxicity has occurred when NSAIDs have been used concomitantly with methotrexate; use together with extreme caution.
- NEPHROTOXIC DRUGS (eg, **aminoglycosides, amphotericin B, furosemide**): May enhance the risk for nephrotoxicity
- NONSTEROIDAL ANTI-INFLAMMATORY DRUGS (NSAIDs; eg, **carprofen, deracoxib, meloxicam**): Concurrent use with robenacoxib duplicates therapy and is contraindicated.
- QT PROLONGATION DRUGS (eg, **cisapride, quinidine, sotalol**): Robenacoxib prolongs the QT interval; use with other QT prolonging drugs is not recommended.[1,2]

Laboratory Considerations

- None noted

Dosages

DOGS:

Control of postoperative pain and inflammation associated

with soft tissue surgery (label dosage; FDA-approved): 2 mg/kg SC, PO once daily for a maximum of 3 days. The first dose should be administered ≈45 minutes before surgery, at the same time as preanesthetic agents. Subsequent doses can be given as SC injections (rotate injection sites) or using oral tablets. Use the lowest effective dose for the shortest duration consistent with individual response. Giving without food increases bioavailability; however, it may also be given with food. Tablets are not scored and should not be broken.[1]

Pain and inflammation associated with chronic osteoarthritis (extra-label): 1 mg/kg with a range of 1 – 2 mg/kg PO every 24 hours (at the same time every day). A clinical response is normally seen within a week; discontinue and reassess diagnosis if no clinical improvement is seen after 10 days. For long-term treatment, dose can be adjusted to lowest effective dose for the patient.[4]

CATS:

Control of postoperative pain and inflammation associated with orthopedic surgery, ovariohysterectomy, and castration (label dosage; FDA-approved): **NOTE**: In cats, the dosages of robenacoxib tablets and injection are different.[1,2]

a) SC: 2 mg/kg SC once daily for a maximum of 3 days.[1] The first dose should be administered ≈30 minutes prior to surgery, at the same time as preanesthetic agents. Subsequent doses can be given as SC injection (rotate injection sites) or using oral tablets.

b) PO: 1 mg/kg with a range of 1 – 2.4 mg/kg PO once daily; dosed based on body weight according to table below.[2] The first dose should be administered ≈30 minutes prior to surgery, at the same time as preanesthetic agents. May be given with or without food. Tablets are not scored and should not be broken.

Robenacoxib Tablet Dosing Chart for Cats

Body weight in kg (lb)	Number of robenacoxib 6 mg tablets PO daily
2.5-6 (5.5-13.2)	1
6.1-12 (13.3-26.4)	2

Acute or chronic pain and inflammation associated with musculoskeletal disorders (extra-label): 1 mg/kg; with a range of 1 – 2.4 mg/kg PO once daily (at the same time each day) for up to 6 days for acute pain. This equates to 1 tablet for cats weighing 2.5 kg (5.5 lb) to less than 6 kg (13.2 lb) and 2 tablets for cats weighing 6 to 12 kg (13.2 to 26.4 lb). Giving without food increases bioavailability; however, it may also be given with food. Tablets are not scored and should not be broken. Duration of treatment for chronic musculoskeletal disorders should be decided on an individual basis.[38]

Osteoarthritis (extra-label): 1 – 2.4 mg/kg PO every 24 hours for 28 days was well tolerated in cats with osteoarthritis, including cats with evidence of concurrent CKD. After 28 days of administration, there was no clinical indication of damage to the GI tract, kidneys, or liver.[34]

Monitoring

- Baseline and periodic physical examination, including clinical efficacy and adverse effect queries
- GI adverse effects; appetite in cats
- Baseline and periodic CBC
- With long-term therapy, baseline and periodic serum liver chemistry profile (eg, 2, 4, and 8 weeks after beginning treatment, then every 3 to 6 months); discontinue treatment if liver enzyme activity increases markedly or increases in liver enzymes are accompanied by clinical signs (eg, anorexia, lethargy, vomiting)[30]
- Baseline and periodic serum renal chemistry profile with electrolytes and urinalysis

Client Information

- NSAID that is approved for short-term treatment (up to 3 days) of postoperative pain and inflammation in dogs and cats.
- For dogs, give this medicine at the same time each day about 30 minutes before letting the dog eat; however, if the dog vomits shortly after being given the drug, try giving another dose with food to see if this helps. If vomiting continues, contact your veterinarian. Most dogs tolerate the drug well, but in rare cases some dogs can develop ulcers or serious kidney and liver problems.
- Contact your veterinarian if your animal has any decreased or increased appetite; vomiting; change in bowel movements; change in behavior or activity (eg, more or less active than normal); incoordination/weakness (eg, stumbling, clumsiness); seizures (convulsions); aggression (threatening behavior/actions); yellowing of gums, skin, or whites of the eyes (jaundice); and changes in drinking (eg, frequency, amount consumed) or urination habits (eg, frequency, color, or smell).
- If your animal is taking this medicine long term, your veterinarian will need to monitor your animal closely for side effects by doing examinations and blood tests. Do not miss these important follow-up visits.
- Do not divide or break tablets. Store chewable tablets out of reach of animals and children.
- Wash hands after handling tablets. Pregnant women who are near term should wear gloves when handling this medicine.

Chemistry/Synonyms

A coxib-class NSAID, robenacoxib is a diclofenac analogue. The commercially available injection is a clear, colorless to slightly pink solution. A lactam degradation product is formed over time with normal storage.[1]

Robenacoxib may also be known as robenacoxibum or robénacoxib. Its trade name is *Onsior*®.

Storage/Stability

Store tablets at controlled room temperature of 15°C to 25°C (59°F-77°F). The injection should be stored in the refrigerator at 2°C to 8°C (36°F-46°F) in its original outer carton.

Compatibility/Compounding Considerations

Robenacoxib must not be mixed with other drugs as compatibility studies have not been done.[31]

Dosage Forms/Regulatory Status

VETERINARY-LABELED PRODUCTS:

Robenacoxib-Flavored (yeast) Tablets: 6 mg; *Onsior*®; (Rx). FDA-approved for use in cats. NADA# 141-320. Tablets are not scored and should not be split. The *Information for Cat Owners* sheet should be included whenever tablets are dispensed for administration by clients at home.

Robenacoxib-Flavored (yeast, pork liver) Oral Tablets: 10 mg, 20 mg, and 40 mg; *Onsior*®; (Rx). FDA-approved for use in dogs. NADA# 141-463. Tablets are not scored and should not be split. The *Information for Dog Owners* sheet should be included whenever tablets are dispensed for administration by clients at home.

Robenacoxib Solution for Injection: 20 mg/mL in 20 mL multi-dose vials; *Onsior*®; (Rx). FDA-approved for dogs and cats. NADA# 141-443

HUMAN-LABELED PRODUCTS: NONE

References

For the complete list of references, see **wiley.com/go/budde/plumb**

Rocuronium

(roe-kyoo-***roe***-nee-um) *Zemuron®*

Nondepolarizing Neuromuscular Blocker

Prescriber Highlights

- Nondepolarizing neuromuscular blocking agent with a rapid to intermediate onset and intermediate duration of action
- Faster onset of action than vecuronium and atracurium and fewer adverse effects than succinylcholine
- Use with caution in patients with renal or hepatic dysfunction or myasthenia gravis.
- Adverse effects may include changes in heart rate and blood pressure.
- Not for use as a sole agent; no analgesic or sedative actions
- Must only be used under close monitoring with intubation and mechanical ventilation
- High alert medication; consider extra dosage checks and warning labels

Uses/Indications

Clinical experience with rocuronium in veterinary patients is relatively limited, but it potentially can be used in dogs, cats, and horses for muscle relaxation during surgery. Rocuronium can be used under general anesthesia during ophthalmic procedures to achieve a central position of the eye.

In cats, it has been shown that recovery of the train-of-four (TOF) ratio of 0.9 does not reliably exclude residual block, and it is prudent to reverse rocuronium and other neuromuscular blocking agents even when no fade can be detected by objective means.[1]

Pharmacology/Actions

Rocuronium is an aminosteroidal competitive, nondepolarizing neuromuscular blocking agent structurally similar to vecuronium. It has a dose-dependent rapid to intermediate onset and intermediate duration of action. Rocuronium onset is nearly as rapid onset as succinylcholine and is 2 to 3 times faster than vercuronium. Its duration is similar to vercuronium and atracurium. It antagonizes acetylcholine by competitively binding cholinergic receptor sites on the motor end plate, resulting in paralysis of striated muscles. Rocuronium does not appear to induce malignant hyperthermia (MH) as it did not cause hyperthermia in MH-susceptible swine. Rocuronium is mildly vagolytic, and a slight, transient tachycardia is occasionally seen in humans.

Pharmacokinetics

In dogs, rocuronium 0.4 mg/kg IV produces complete neuromuscular blockade in ≈2 to 3 minutes.[2] Complete neuromuscular blockade was observed in 90% of cats receiving 0.6 mg/kg IV within 30 to 60 seconds without significant effects on HR. At doses of 0.6 mg/kg, the duration of action of rocuronium is 20 minutes in dogs, 13 minutes in cats, and 55 minutes in horses.[3,4]

It has been reported that rocuronium is eliminated primarily by the liver in dogs and cats. The principal metabolite, 17-desacetyl-rocuronium, has ≈1/20 the neuromuscular blocking potency of rocuronium in cats.

In humans, rocuronium is ≈30% bound to plasma proteins.[5] The half-life ranges from 66 to 144 minutes; ≈26% of the drug is excreted by the kidneys, and the remainder is excreted in the bile (31%). Patients with hepatic impairment or cirrhosis exhibited prolonged plasma half-lives and 2.5 times longer recovery periods compared to patients with normal function.

Contraindications/Precautions/Warnings

Rocuronium is contraindicated in patients hypersensitive to it or other neuromuscular blocking agents. In humans, severe anaphylactic reactions have been reported.

Rocuronium should only be used in patients that are adequately anesthetized and mechanically ventilated. It should only be used in settings where patients can be fully monitored and where oxygen therapy and antagonist drugs are immediately available. Rocuronium has no analgesic or sedative/anesthetic actions.

Atracurium may be preferred in patients with renal or hepatic impairments as there are conflicting reports on whether rocuronium should be used in these patients. Use with caution in patients with myasthenia gravis as small doses of nondepolarizing neuromuscular blocking agents may have profound effects.[5] Extravasation may result in local irritation.

Rocuronium is considered a high alert medication, meaning it requires special safeguards to reduce the risk for errors. Consider instituting practices, such as redundant drug dosage and volume checking or special alert labels.

Adverse Effects

Rocuronium has fewer adverse effects than succinylcholine, as it has minimal cardiovascular and histamine-releasing effects. Other than the effects associated with pharmacologic neuromuscular blockade, rocuronium appears to be well tolerated. Changes in heart rate and blood pressure may be noted.

In humans, the most common adverse reactions are hypotension or hypertension which are reported in ≈2% of patients.[5] These effects are transient and typically mild. Severe anaphylaxis has also been reported. Although rocuronium has minimal histamine-releasing effects, histaminoid reactions have been reported. Rocuronium can cause severe burning pain at the injection site; giving only after a deep stage of anesthesia has been achieved has been recommended.

Reproductive/Nursing Safety

In pregnant laboratory animals, rocuronium did not demonstrate teratogenic effects; however, rate of embryonic death was increased likely due to oxygen deficiency. The molecular weight of rocuronium is low enough for excretion into milk, but because the drug is ionized at physiologic pH, clinical effect in offspring would likely be minimal. Because safety has not been established in animals, this drug should only be used when the maternal benefits outweigh the potential risks to offspring.

Overdose/Acute Toxicity

Overdoses with neuromuscular blocking agents may result in a prolonged neuromuscular blockade. The primary treatment is the maintenance of the patient's airway, mechanical ventilation and oxygenation, and adequate sedation until recovery of normal neuromuscular function is assured.[5] Only after evidence of recovery is seen should the administration of an acetylcholinesterase inhibitor (eg, neostigmine) with an anticholinergic agent (eg, atropine) be considered. Sugammadex is the specific reversal agent for rocuronium.[6] Blood pressure and heart rate should be monitored during an overdose, with any necessary supportive treatment performed.

For patients that have experienced or are suspected to have experienced an overdose, consultation with a 24-hour poison consultation center specializing in providing veterinary-specific information is recommended. For general information related to overdose and toxin exposures, as well as contact information for poison control centers, refer to ***Appendix***.

Drug Interactions

The following drug interactions have either been reported or are theoretical in humans or animals receiving rocuronium and may be of significance in veterinary patients. Unless otherwise noted, use together is not necessarily contraindicated, but weigh the potential risks and perform additional monitoring when appropriate.

- **Acetylcholinesterase Inhibitors** (eg, **neostigmine, pyridostigmine**): Antagonize the effects of rocuronium

- **Anesthetics, General**: In humans, rocuronium use with general anesthetics can prolong the QT interval.
- **Corticosteroids** (eg, **dexamethasone, prednis(ol)one**): May decrease rocuronium effectiveness, prolong muscle weakness, and result in myopathy
- **Nondepolarizing Muscle Relaxant Drugs, Other**: Some nondepolaring muscle relaxant drugs may have a synergistic effect if used with rocuronium
- **Succinylcholine**: May speed the onset of action and enhance the neuromuscular blocking actions of rocuronium; do not give rocuronium until succinylcholine effects have subsided.
- **Sugammadex**: Antagonizes the effects of rocuronium

The following agents may enhance or prolong the neuromuscular blocking activity of rocuronium:

- **Aminoglycoside Antibiotics** (eg, **gentamicin**)
- **Anesthetics, Inhalation** (eg, **halothane, isoflurane**)
- **Antiarrhythmic Agents** (eg, **procainamide, quinidine**)
- **Bacitracin or Polymyxin B, Systemic**: Consider therapy modification.
- **Calcium Channel Blockers** (eg, **amlodipine, diltiazem**)
- **Cyclosporine, Systemic**
- **Lincosamide Antibiotics** (eg, **clindamycin**)
- **Lithium**
- **Magnesium Salts**
- **Polymyxin B**
- **Quinine**: Avoid combination
- **Tetracyclines** (eg, **doxycycline, minocycline**)
- **Vancomycin**

Laboratory Considerations

- None were noted.

Dosages

DOGS:

Neuromuscular blocker (extra-label): 0.5 mg/kg IV followed by 0.2 mg/kg/hour IV CRI. The authors concluded that rocuronium administered in this way was effective in dogs and easily applicable to clinical practice, but that further work is required on infusion titration.[7]

To achieve a central position of the eye for ophthalmic procedures: 0.03 – 0.05 mg/kg IV in combination with isoflurane may be useful for short ophthalmic procedures.[8]

CATS:

Neuromuscular blocker (extra-label): 0.3 – 0.6 mg/kg IV[1,3,9]

HORSES:

Neuromuscular blocker (extra-label): Although a formal dose-finding study for rocuronium has not yet been reported, doses ranging between 0.2 and 0.6 mg/kg have been used extensively in horses under inhalational anesthesia; doses of 0.2 mg/kg provide ≈90% twitch depression and 0.4 – 0.6 mg/kg produces full blockade. Block lasts less than 20 minutes at 0.2 mg/kg and as long as 1 hour at 0.6 mg/kg.[4,10,11]

Monitoring

- When nondepolarizing neuromuscular blocking agents are administered, the paralysis should be monitored via acceleromyography (train-of-four or TOF) or electromyography. A recent study in dogs showed that, after rocuronium administration, the laryngeal neuromuscular function recovered 36% slower than the pelvic limb. Monitoring the recovery from paralysis induced by rocuronium at the pelvic limb site might not exclude residual block at the larynx.[12]
- Heart rate and blood pressure

Client Information

- This drug should only be used by professionals familiar with using neuromuscular blocking agents in a supervised setting with adequate ventilatory support.

Chemistry/Synonyms

Rocuronium bromide is an aminosteroidal competitive, nondepolarizing neuromuscular blocking agent. It occurs as an almost white or pale yellow, slightly hygroscopic powder. It is freely soluble in water or dehydrated alcohol. A 1% solution (in water) has a pH of 8.9 to 9.5. The commercially available injection is a sterile, nonpyrogenic, isotonic solution that is clear, colorless to yellow/orange. Each mL contains 10 mg rocuronium bromide and 2 mg sodium acetate and is adjusted to isotonicity with sodium chloride. The pH is adjusted to 4 with acetic acid and/or sodium hydroxide.

Rocuronium may also be known as ORG-9426, rocuronii, rocuronio, rokuroniowy, or rokuronyum. Rocuronium may also be known by the trade names *Zemuron*® or *Esmeron*®.

Storage/Stability

Store intact rocuronium vials at 2°C to 8°C (36°F-46°F) and protect against freezing. When removed from refrigeration to room temperature storage conditions (25°C [77°F]), use within 60 days. Use opened vials of rocuronium within 30 days. Infusion solutions are stable for 24 hours at room temperature at dilutions up to 5 mg/mL. Discard unused portions of infusion solutions.

Compatibility/Compounding Considerations

Compatibility is dependent on factors such as pH, concentration, temperature, and diluent used; specialized references or a hospital pharmacist should be consulted for more specific information.

Unlike both vecuronium and atracurium, rocuronium is stable in aqueous solutions.

Rocuronium is **compatible** with 0.9% sodium chloride, 5% dextrose in water, 5% dextrose in 0.9% sodium chloride, and lactated Ringer's for dilution.

Rocuronium is physically **incompatible** when mixed with amphotericin B, hydrocortisone sodium succinate, amoxicillin, insulin, azathioprine, lipid emulsion (*Intralipid*®), cefazolin, ketorolac, cloxacillin, lorazepam, dexamethasone, methohexital, diazepam, methylprednisolone, erythromycin, thiopental, famotidine, trimethoprim, furosemide, or vancomycin.

Dosage Forms/Regulatory Status

VETERINARY-LABELED PRODUCTS: NONE.

The Association of Racing Commissioners International (ARCI) has designated this drug as a class 2 substance. Use of this drug may not be allowed in certain animal competitions. Check rules and regulations before entering a competition while this medication is being administered. Contact local racing authorities for further guidance. See ***Appendix*** for more information.

HUMAN-LABELED PRODUCTS:

Rocuronium Bromide for Injection: 10 mg/mL in 5 mL and 10 mL multi-dose vials; generic; (Rx)

References

For the complete list of references, see **wiley.com/go/budde/plumb**

Romifidine

(roe-***mif***-ih-deen) *Sedivet®*

Alpha-2 Agonist Sedative Analgesic

Prescriber Highlights

- ► Indicated for use in adult horses as a sedative and analgesic to facilitate handling, clinical examinations, procedures, and minor surgical procedures and as a preanesthetic agent prior to the induction of general anesthesia
- ► Contraindicated in patients hypersensitive to it. Do not use in horses with respiratory, hepatic, or renal disease, dehydration, or other systemic conditions of compromised health.
- ► Adverse effects in horses may include profound bradycardia, first- and second-degree atrioventricular heart block, dose-dependent sinus arrhythmias, hypertension followed by hypotension, ataxia, sweating, piloerection, salivation, muscle tremors, penile-relaxation, urination, stridor, decreased GI motility, flatulence, and mild colic; passive congestion and swelling of the face, lips, and upper airways can also be seen due to head lowering
- ► Anaphylactic reactions are possible.
- ► Decrease dose of concurrent anesthetics as romifidine has anesthetic sparing effects.

Uses/Indications

Romifidine is FDA-approved for use as a sedative and analgesic in adult horses to facilitate handling, clinical examinations, clinical procedures, and minor surgical procedures and for use as a preanesthetic prior to the induction of general anesthesia.

Romifidine has been used extra-label in cattle and foals.

Pharmacology/Actions

Romifidine is a potent alpha-2-adrenergic agonist with sedative, analgesic, and muscle relaxant properties. Alpha-2-adrenergic receptors are found in the CNS and several tissues peripherally both presynaptically and postsynaptically. In the CNS, the primary action is feedback inhibition of norepinephrine release. Opioids and alpha-2 agonists may have synergistic analgesic effects.

Pharmacologic effects of romifidine include sedation, analgesia, muscle relaxation, and reduced catecholamine release from the CNS. Thermoregulatory mechanisms may be altered. Peripherally, an initial vasoconstrictive response occurs with increases in blood pressure. Within 45 to 60 minutes, a hypotensive phase may occur. Heart rate can significantly decrease secondary to a vagal response to hypertension. A second-degree atrioventricular block may also occur. Antimuscarinic agents can prevent bradycardia, but their use is controversial as they can potentially cause hypertension, increase myocardial oxygen demand, and reduce GI motility. Alpha-2-receptor agonists can transiently slow duodenal motility and increase micturition in horses and can inhibit insulin release from pancreatic islet cells, resulting in hyperglycemia. Other effects seen in horses include sweating, mydriasis, decreases in hematocrit, and increased uterine pressure in nonpregnant mares.

In horses, romifidine may cause less ataxia and postural sway than xylazine or detomidine.[1,2] Romifidine may decrease reactivity to visual and acoustic stimulation at sedative doses compared to xylazine.[3] Romifidine has the longest duration of sedation.[1-3] For these reasons, romifidine may be preferred to other alpha-2 agonists for standing procedures and during recovery after inhalant anesthesia. The duration of analgesia is shorter than the duration of sedation, which may last up to 2 hours. Romifidine has a ceiling effect whereby increasing the dose beyond a certain amount can increase the duration of sedation but not sedation intensity. Romifidine has been shown to decrease intraocular pressure in healthy horses.[4,5]

Pharmacokinetics

In horses, the onset of action of romifidine is 30 seconds to 5 minutes and the effect gradually decreases over 2 to 4 hours. Romifidine 80 µg/kg IV has a volume of distribution of ≈2 L/kg, a clearance of ≈32 mL/minute/kg, and an elimination half-life of ≈135 minutes.[6]

In dogs and cats, bioavailability after IM administration is 86% and 95%, respectively. Bioavailability after SC injection in dogs is 92%. Peak levels after IM injection occur in ≈50 minutes in dogs and 25 minutes in cats. After IV injection, volumes of distribution are ≈3 L/kg in dogs and 6 L/kg in cats. Romifidine is biotransformed in the liver. In dogs, ≈80% of an administered dose is eliminated in the urine, 20% in the feces. Elimination half-lives are ≈2 hours for dogs and 6 hours for cats.

Contraindications/Precautions/Warnings

Romifidine is contraindicated in patients that are hypersensitive to it. Do not use in combination with IV potentiated sulfonamides. Do not use in horses with respiratory, hepatic, or renal disease, dehydration, or other systemic conditions of compromised health.

Romifidine has not been evaluated in horses with colic or in foals. Use with caution in horses with pre-existing cardiac conditions due to the effects on heart rhythm and blood pressure. Romifidine should only be used in situations in which sufficient monitoring and patient-support capabilities (eg, intubation, ventilation) are available. Although animals may appear to be deeply sedated, some may respond (eg, kick) to external stimuli; use appropriate caution. Raising the horse's head can help prevent sudden kicking. Anesthetic doses should be reduced to prevent overdose as romifidine has anesthetic sparing effects.

This medication can be absorbed through the skin and via oral routes; handle with caution to avoid accidental exposure.

Do not use in horses intended for human consumption.

Adverse Effects

In horses, romifidine may cause profound bradycardia, first- and second-degree atrioventricular heart block, and dose-dependent sinus arrhythmias. Initially, hypertension may occur, followed by hypotension. Other adverse effects can include ataxia, sweating, piloerection, salivation, muscle tremors, penile relaxation, urination (occurs ≈1 hour after dose), stridor, decreased GI motility, flatulence, and mild colic. Passive congestion and swelling of the face, lips, and upper airways can also be seen due to head lowering. When used alone as a premedication agent, romifidine can cause twitching. Paradoxical excitation is also possible. Anaphylactic reactions to alpha-2 agonists have rarely been reported in horses.

Reproductive/Nursing Safety

Romifidine is contraindicated for use in pregnant mares.[7]

Overdose/Acute Toxicity

Horses that received romifidine up to 600 µg/kg (5 times the maximum recommended dose) exhibited sinus bradycardia, second-degree heart block, occasional apnea and mild respiratory stridor, deep sedation, severe ataxia, frequent urination, and sweating. No clinically significant alterations in blood gases, acid-base, or hematological or chemical parameters were noted. If necessary, a reversal agent (eg, atipamezole, yohimbine) may be used to reduce the duration and extent of adverse effects associated with acute toxicity.

For patients that have experienced or are suspected to have experienced an overdose, consultation with a 24-hour poison consultation center specializing in providing veterinary-specific information is recommended. For general information related to overdose and toxin exposures, as well as contact information for poison control centers, refer to ***Appendix***.

Drug Interactions

The following drug interactions have either been reported or are theoretical in humans or animals receiving romifidine and may be of significance in veterinary patients. Unless otherwise noted, use together is not necessarily contraindicated, but weigh the potential risks and perform additional monitoring when appropriate.

- **Anesthetics, Opioids, Sedative/Hypnotics**: Effects may be additive; dosage reduction of 1 or both agents may be required; potential for increased risk for arrhythmias when used in combination with thiopental, ketamine, or halothane
- **Epinephrine**: May potentiate adverse effects of alpha-2 agonists
- **Other Alpha-2 Agonists** (eg, **clonidine, detomidine, medetomidine, xylazine**): May potentiate adverse effects of romifidine; concurrent use not recommended
- **Phenothiazines** (eg, **acepromazine**): Severe hypotension can result.
- **Potentiated Sulfonamides, Intravenous** (eg, **trimethoprim/sulfa**): Use with IV potentiated sulfonamides may result in fatal dysrhythmias; combination is contraindicated.

Laboratory Considerations

- ADP-induced platelet aggregation: Can be inhibited in cats by medetomidine (a related alpha-2 agonist); not known if romifidine can have this effect in horses.
- PCV and TS: Clinically significant transient changes have been observed in horses.[8]

Dosages

HORSES:

Sedation and analgesia (label dosage; FDA-approved): 40 – 120 µg/kg IV slowly once.[9] The degree of sedation and analgesia is dose- and time-dependent. The duration of analgesia is shorter than the duration of sedation.

Preanesthetic agent (label dosage; FDA-approved): 100 µg/kg as a single, slow IV injection.[9] Induce anesthesia after maximal sedation is achieved. Anesthetic dose should be decreased to prevent overdose as romifidine has anesthesia-sparing effects.

Part of a 'GKR triple drip' total intravenous anesthesia (TIVA) protocol (extra-label): Add romifidine 40 mg (total; NOT mg/kg) and ketamine 3.3 g (total; NOT mg/kg) to 500 mL of 5% guaifenesin. Resultant solution contains guaifenesin 50 mg/mL, ketamine 6.6 mg/mL, and romifidine 80 µg/mL. Infuse at a rate of 1 mL/kg/hour.[10]

Part of a ketamine/romifidine partial intravenous anesthesia (PIVA) protocol (extra-label): After induction of general anesthesia, a surgical plane of anesthesia can be maintained with a combination of isoflurane and romifidine 18 – 24 µg/kg/hour and ketamine 1.8 – 2.4 mg/kg/hour IV CRI.[11]

Postanesthesia sedation (extra-label): 20 µg/kg IV administered once the breathing circuit is disconnected and the patient is spontaneously breathing.[12]

Standing sedation (extra-label):

a) **Single injection in ponies**: 50 µg/kg IV in combination with tramadol 3 mg/kg provides sedation and antinociceptive effects for up to 120 minutes. Slight ataxia was noted without excitatory behavioral adverse effects.[13]

b) **Constant rate infusion in horses**: 46 µg/kg IV loading dose, followed by 126 µg/kg/hour IV CRI[1]

CATTLE:

Epidural anesthesia for paralumbar analgesia or laparotomy: Romifidine 50 µg/kg in combination with morphine 0.1 mg/kg administered epidurally. The duration of analgesia is 12 hours maximum.[14] Doses of 30, 40, and 50 µg/kg diluted in sterile saline to a total volume 25 mL were administered epidurally to dairy cows. Antinociceptive effects were dosedependent and covered the tail, anus, perineum, vulva, and inguinal area and extended to the pelvic limb and thoracic area. Moderate sedation was observed at 30 and 40 µg/kg and deep sedation at 50 µg/kg.[15]

Monitoring

- Level of sedation and analgesia
- Heart rate and rhythm, blood pressure, pulse oximetry
- Respiratory depth and rate, $ETCO_2$
- Body temperature

Client Information

- This medication is only to be administered by veterinary professionals.
- After receiving romifidine, your horse may look fully sedated but may still respond defensively (eg, kick) when stimulated.

Chemistry/Synonyms

Romifidine HCl is an alpha-2-adrenoreceptor agonist that is structurally related to clonidine. It has a molecular weight of 258.1 and occurs as a crystalline, white, odorless substance that is soluble in water.

Romifidine may also be known as STH-2130, romifidini, romifidin, romifidina, romifidinum, *Romidys®*, *Sedivet®*, and *Sedivan®*.

Storage/Stability

Store romifidine HCl injection at controlled room temperature (15°C to 30°C [59°F-86°F]).

Compatibility/Compounding Considerations

No specific information was noted.

Dosage Forms/Regulatory Status

VETERINARY-LABELED PRODUCTS:

The Association of Racing Commissioners International (ARCI) has designated this drug as a class 3 substance. Use of this drug may not be allowed in certain animal competitions. Check rules and regulations before entering a competition while this medication is being administered. Contact local racing authorities for further guidance. See ***Appendix*** for more information.

Romifidine HCl 1% (10 mg/mL) Injection; *Sedivet®*; (Rx). FDA-approved for use in horses not intended for human consumption. Although this product is still listed in FDA's Green Book of approved animal drugs, it may no longer be commercially available in the US. In the UK, slaughter withdrawal is 6 days for horses.

HUMAN-LABELED PRODUCTS: NONE

References

For the complete list of references, see **wiley.com/go/budde/plumb**

Ronidazole

(roe-***nid***-ah-zole)

Antiprotozoal

Prescriber Highlights

- ▶ Nitroimidazole antibiotic/antiparasitic drug for treating *Tritrichomonas* foetus infections in cats; also used to treat *Trichomonas* spp infections in birds not intended for consumption. Potentially useful as an alternative treatment for giardiasis.
- ▶ Prohibited by the FDA for use in food animals
- ▶ Contraindications include hypersensitivity to it or other nitroimidazole derivatives.
- ▶ Potentially carcinogenic; avoid human exposure
- ▶ Adverse effects include reversible neurotoxicity (more likely at higher doses but can occur at lower dosages) and GI effects.
- ▶ Many potential drug interactions
- ▶ Must be compounded from bulk powder and, ideally, put in gelatin capsules

Uses/Indications

Ronidazole is a nitroimidazole antibiotic/antiparasitic drug that is considered the treatment of choice for *Tritrichomonas foetus* infections,[1-3] with resolution of diarrhea occurring in 60% to 70% of cats.[4,5] Formulations that delay ronidazole release until arrival of the drug in the large intestine may limit neurotoxicity while maintaining efficacy.[6,7] Ronidazole is also used for treating *Trichomonas* spp infections in birds not intended for consumption. Ronidazole is prohibited in food animals and belongs to a class of antibiotics important for human medicine. It should only be used for *Tritrichomonas* when infection has been confirmed.

Ronidazole may also be a viable alternative treatment for giardiasis in dogs and cats.[8]

The drug is not commercially available in the United States and must be compounded from bulk powder by a compounding pharmacy. To improve palatability, compounded capsules are recommended over flavored liquids.

The World Health Organization (WHO) has designated ronidazole as a Critically Important, Highest Priority antimicrobial for human medicine.[9] The Office International des Epizooties (OIE) Antimicrobial Classification has designated ronidazole as a Veterinary Critically Important antimicrobial.[10]

Pharmacology/Actions

Ronidazole, like other 5-nitroimidazoles such as metronidazole, is converted by hydrogenosomes (an organelle found in trichomonads) into polar autotoxic anion radicals. *T foetus* infections in cats have been resistant to treatment by metronidazole, and ronidazole appears to have greater activity against the organism, but ronidazole resistance has been documented.[11]

Pharmacokinetics

In cats, ronidazole is completely absorbed and bioavailable after oral dosing. Volume of distribution (steady-state) is ≈0.7 L/kg and clearance is ≈0.8 mL/kg/minute. Elimination half-life is ≈10 hours.[12]

A guar gum-coated colon-targeted delayed-release tablet formulation had negligible release until 6 hours after administration. Peak plasma concentrations occurred at ≈14.5 hours, coinciding with colonic arrival. Repeated dosing did not appreciably affect bioavailability or other pharmacokinetic parameters.[7]

Contraindications/Precautions/Warnings

Ronidazole should not be used in patients hypersensitive to it or other 5-nitroimidazoles (eg, metronidazole).

The compound has been demonstrated to be carcinogenic in mice but not rats. Although humans should avoid contact with this compound or animal waste from treated patients, it can be safely compounded using a biological safety cabinet.

The FDA prohibits the use of this drug in food animals.

Adverse Effects

Reversible neurotoxicity similar to that reported with metronidazole has been reported with ronidazole in cats. Initial signs may include tremors, lethargy, anorexia, ataxia, nystagmus, seizures, or behavior changes (agitation). If neurotoxicity is diagnosed, discontinue ronidazole, treat supportively, and, if necessary, consider administering a benzodiazepine such as diazepam to competitively inhibit GABA receptors in the CNS. The incidence of neurotoxicity appears to be higher with a 50 mg/kg twice-daily dosage, but may occur at lower doses as well. Potentially, GI effects can occur (anorexia, vomiting). Ronidazole is very bitter and should be administered to cats in capsule form.

Ronidazole has been shown to increase the risk for benign mammary tumors in rats, and benign and malignant pulmonary tumors in mice at dosages more than or equal to 20 mg/kg/day.

Dogs given 30 mg/kg per day for 2 years (40 mg/kg/day the first month) showed some testicular toxicity (type not specified), but no tumors.

Reproductive/Nursing Safety

Safety of this compound during pregnancy has not been established. Teratology studies have been performed in mice, rats, and rabbits. In rabbits given 30 mg/kg/day, no embryotoxicity occurred, but fetal weights were significantly decreased. Mice demonstrated no teratogenic effects at dosages up to 200 mg/kg/day. Rats given up to 150 mg/kg/day demonstrated no embryotoxic effects, but at dosages of 200 mg/kg/day, both maternal and fetal weights were decreased.

It is not known if ronidazole is distributed into milk and safety cannot be assured. Consider using milk replacer if treating nursing queens.

Because safety has not been established in animals, this drug should only be used when the maternal benefits outweigh the potential risks to offspring.

Overdose/Acute Toxicity

No specific information was located. Cats receiving doses of 50 mg/kg twice daily appear to have greater incidences of neurotoxicity (see ***Adverse Effects***). A case report of an overdose causing neurotoxicity, hemorrhage, and death in society finches after consuming ronidazole in drinking water has been published.[13] If overdoses cause neurotoxicity, discontinue further therapy and treat supportively. Consider administering a GABA inhibitor such as diazepam to competitively inhibit GABA receptors in the CNS.

For patients that have experienced or are suspected to have experienced an overdose, consultation with a 24-hour poison consultation center specializing in providing veterinary-specific information is recommended. For general information related to overdose and toxin exposures, as well as contact information for poison control centers, refer to ***Appendix.***

Drug Interactions

In humans, the following drug interactions with metronidazole, a compound similar to ronidazole, have been reported or are theoretical and may be of significance in veterinary patients in patients receiving ronidazole. Unless otherwise noted, use together is not necessarily contraindicated, but weigh the potential risks and perform additional monitoring when appropriate.

- ALCOHOL: May induce a disulfiram-like (nausea, vomiting, cramps) reaction
- CIMETIDINE, KETOCONAZOLE: May decrease the metabolism of ronidazole and increase the likelihood of dose-related adverse effects

- **Cyclosporine, Tacrolimus** (systemic): Ronidazole may increase the serum concentrations of cyclosporine or tacrolimus.
- **Fluorouracil** (systemic): Ronidazole may increase the serum concentrations of fluorouracil and risk for toxicity.
- **Lithium**: Ronidazole may increase lithium serum concentrations and risk for lithium toxicity.
- **Oxytetracycline**: May antagonize the therapeutic effects of metronidazole (and presumably ronidazole)
- **Phenobarbital, Rifampin, or Phenytoin**: May increase the metabolism of ronidazole thereby decreasing blood concentrations
- **Warfarin**: Metronidazole (and potentially ronidazole) may prolong INR/PT in patients taking coumarin anticoagulants; avoid concurrent use if possible; otherwise intensify monitoring.

Laboratory Considerations

- AST, ALT, LDH (lactic dehydrogenase), triglycerides, hexokinase glucose: A related compound, metronidazole can cause falsely decreased readings when determined using methods measuring decreases in ultraviolet absorbance when NADH is reduced to NAD. It is not known if ronidazole also causes falsely decreased values.

Dosages

DOGS:

Giardia **spp** (extra-label). Study was in a kennel setting and combined strict hygiene control/disinfection, chlorhexidine shampoos, and ronidazole 30 – 50 mg/kg PO twice daily for 7 days. Authors concluded this "*was highly effective in reducing Giardia cyst excretion and may therefore constitute an alternative control strategy for canine giardiasis.*"[8]

CATS:

T foetus **infections** (extra-label): 30 mg/kg PO every 24 hours for 14 days[5,6,14]

Monitoring

- Clinical efficacy (diarrhea improvement)
- Adverse effects (neurotoxicity, vomiting, anorexia)
- PCR testing can be used to confirm infection, but negative results after treatment do not conclusively prove that infection has been eradicated.

Client Information

- Keep medicine stored in the freezer.
- Give with food to avoid stomach or intestinal problems.
- Side effects in cats can include fever, loss of appetite, ataxia (eg, trouble keeping balance, trouble walking or climbing stairs), muscle twitching or weakness, seizures, lethargy (tiredness/lack of energy), nystagmus (eyes uncontrollably moving back and forth). Contact your veterinarian immediately if any of these signs are seen.
- This drug has caused cancer at high doses in laboratory animals. Do not open or crush capsules; administer whole. Wear disposable gloves when handling and wash your hands afterwards.
- After treatment has started, wear disposable gloves when cleaning the litter box, double-bag feces, and throw both gloves and feces in trash. Do not flush feces down toilet.
- Must not be used in any animals that will be consumed by humans.

Chemistry/Synonyms

Ronidazole is a 5-nitroimidazole compound that occurs as a white to yellowish-brown, odorless or almost odorless, bitter powder. It is very slightly soluble in water or alcohol.

Ronidazole may also be known as ronidazol, ronidazolum, *Belga*®, *Ridsol-S*®, *Ronida*®, *Ronivet*®, *Ronizol*®, *Turbosol*®, *Tricho Plus*®, *Trichocure*®, or *Trichorex*®.

Storage/Stability

Compounded capsules should be stored in child-resistant, airtight containers protected from light. Until further stability studies can be performed, capsules should be stored in the freezer.

Aqueous solutions are reportedly not very stable. It is recommended that fresh solutions using the 10% powder for addition to drinking water (used for pigeons) be freshly prepared every day.

Compatibility/Compounding Considerations

No specific information noted. See additional information in ***Dosage Forms/Regulatory Status*** section.

Dosage Forms/Regulatory Status

VETERINARY-LABELED PRODUCTS:

None in the United States; a 10% ronidazole powder to be added to drinking water for treating *Trichomonas* infections in pigeons is available in some countries, but these products are unsuitable for use in cats due to the dosage required and the unpalatability (bitter taste) of the powder and solution. Capsules prepared from 100% bulk powder for individual feline patient should be obtained from a compounding pharmacy that can prepare the capsules in a bio-safety hood that will protect the compounder from drug exposure.

The FDA prohibits the use of this drug in food animals.

HUMAN-LABELED PRODUCTS: NONE.

References

For the complete list of references, see **wiley.com/go/budde/plumb**

Ropinirole

(roe-***pin***-i-role) *Clevor*®

Emetic

Prescriber Highlights

- ► Ophthalmic formulation FDA-approved to induce vomiting in dogs 4.5 months of age and older and weighing at least 1.8 kg (4 lb)
- ► On average, the onset of vomiting is ≈12 minutes, the dog vomits 4 to 5 times, and vomiting typically subsides within 25 minutes after administration.
- ► Most dogs (95%) vomit within 30 minutes of application. A second dose can be administered 20 minutes after the first dose if the dog has not vomited.
- ► Contraindications include dogs with hypersensitivity, lack of laryngeal reflexes, neurological impairment or conditions that increase the risk for aspiration, or corneal ulceration or ocular injury/irritation, as well as when vomiting is contraindicated (eg, shock, seizures, ingestion of sharp foreign objects, corrosive agents). Use cautiously in cases in which stimulating vomiting may be detrimental (eg, history of aspiration pneumonia, CNS stimulant ingestion). Do not use in species that cannot vomit.
- ► Adverse effects include tremors, lethargy, hypotension, tachycardia, and hypotension. Ocular effects (eg, redness, discharge, blepharospasm, ptosis, ulceration) may occur.
- ► Metoclopramide can be used to halt protracted vomiting and relieve other dopaminergic signs. Maropitant may be used to ameliorate protracted vomiting but must be administered via the IV route and has no effects on other dopaminergic signs.
- ► Wear gloves when handling, as absorption across human skin can occur with resultant potential for human exposure. Those who are pregnant, breastfeeding, or attempting to become pregnant should avoid contact with the product.

Uses/Indications

In situations in which vomiting is appropriate, ropinirole is FDA-approved to induce vomiting in dogs. In a study, 50% of dogs vomited within 10 minutes of administration (range, 3 to 37 minutes), 87% vomited within 20 minutes, and 95% vomited within 30 minutes.[1] The number of vomiting episodes was 4 to 5 per dog (range, 1 to 13), and the duration of vomiting was 16 to 25 minutes (maximum, 108 minutes).[1,2] In European approval studies, vomiting occurred within 5 to 7 minutes of administration and lasted ≈20 to 25 minutes with 6 to 10 vomiting episodes.[3]

Ropinirole is a dopaminergic agent indicated for the treatment of Parkinson's disease and restless leg syndrome in humans.

Pharmacology/Actions

Dopamine receptor subtypes belong to 2 families of dopamine receptors: D1 (including the D_1 and D_5 subtypes) and D2 (including D_2, D_3, and D_4 receptor subtypes).[4] Ropinirole is a dopamine agonist that preferentially targets the D2 family receptors, specifically the D_2 and D_3 receptor subtypes.[4] Ropinirole stimulates emesis via activity on both the peripheral and central dopamine receptors but primarily via the D_2 receptor in the chemoreceptor trigger zone. Unlike other available emetics, ropinirole is more selective for dopamine receptors and is expected to have less off-target effects due to binding of other receptors (eg, serotonergic, adrenergic).

Ropinirole's dopaminergic effects may blunt norepinephrine action, resulting in hypotension and tachycardia. In beagles receiving ropinirole IV, mean arterial pressure decreased by 16 mm Hg, heart rate increased by 29 bpm, and (on ECG) PR interval shortened by 13 milliseconds and QTc length increased by 33 milliseconds.[5] Peak ropinirole concentration was 5.9 ng/mL, which is ≈¼ that achieved after ophthalmic administration. Studies performed in canine myocytes suggest ropinirole may carry a proarrhythmic risk in patients with inherited or acquired long QT syndrome.[6]

As a dopamine agonist specific for the D_2 receptor subtype, ropinirole suppresses prolactin.

Pharmacokinetics

Bioavailability is 18% to 28% after ocular administration to dogs.[2,7] The drug is rapidly absorbed into systemic circulation, with peak concentration (C_{max}) of 26 ng/mL occurring ≈15 minutes after application; however, vomiting may occur before C_{max} is reached.[2,7] Volume of distribution is 5.6 L/kg, and protein binding is ≈40%.[2] Terminal half-life is 4 to 6 hours.[2,3] Metabolism occurs by dealkylation, hydroxylation, and subsequent conjugation with glucuronic acid or oxidation to carboxylic acid. Excretion occurs mainly as metabolites in the urine.[2] Although duration of vomiting does not appear to correlate with plasma ropinirole concentration, vomiting occurred earlier in dogs receiving doses at the higher end of the dosage range.[7]

In humans, bioavailability of the immediate-release tablet is ≈50%.[8] Peak concentration occurs 1 to 2 hours after oral administration but taking the drug along with a high-fat meal can delay peak concentration to 2.5 hours. Protein binding is 40%, apparent volume of distribution is 7.5 L/kg, and half-life is ≈6 hours. Ropinirole is extensively metabolized, predominantly via N-despropylation and hydroxylation pathways with subsequent conjugation, forming inactive metabolites. CYP1A2 is the major cytochrome P450 isoenzyme involved in phase I metabolism. The drug is eliminated in the urine, principally as metabolites.

Contraindications/Precautions/Warnings

Emetics can be an important aspect in the treatment of orally ingested toxins, but they must be used judiciously. Most emetics cause emesis when administered within 2 hours of foreign material or toxin ingestion[9]; however, induction of emesis should be performed as soon as possible, especially for cases of toxin ingestion. Emetics should not be used in rodents or rabbits because these patients are either unable to vomit or do not have stomach walls strong enough to tolerate emesis. Emetics are also contraindicated in patients that are hypoxic, have evidence of cardiovascular shock or respiratory distress, are actively having seizures, and/or lack normal pharyngeal reflexes (ie, laryngeal paralysis). The risks and benefits of administering an emetic should also be considered for animals with a recurrent history of aspiration pneumonia, seizures, coma, severe CNS depression or deteriorating CNS function, or extreme physical weakness. Emetics should also be withheld in patients that have previously vomited repeatedly. Because of the risk for additional esophageal or gastric injury with emesis, emetics are contraindicated in patients that have ingested a sharp object, strong acids, alkalis, or other caustic agents. Because of the risk for aspiration, emetics are usually contraindicated after petroleum distillate ingestion but may be employed when the risk for toxicity of the compound is greater than the risk for aspiration. Use of emetics after ingestion of strychnine or other CNS stimulants may precipitate seizures.

Ropinirole is contraindicated in patients hypersensitive to it. Do not use ropinirole in dogs with CNS depression or seizures, ocular irritation or injury, or corneal ulceration, or in dogs that have ingested sharp foreign objects, corrosive agents (eg, acids, alkalis), volatile substances, or organic solvents.[2,7] Use cautiously in patients with conditions that may increase the risk for aspiration pneumonia. Safety has not been studied in dogs that have ingested foreign material or in dogs with GI disease, cardiac disease or cardiovascular compromise, hepatic impairment, younger than 4.5 months old, or weighing less than 1.8 kg (4 lb).[3,7] Dogs that weigh less than 1.8 kg (4 lb) cannot be accurately dosed; 1 drop in one eye would deliver a higher dose than the target dose range.

In an effectiveness study, 99 dogs were given ropinirole.[10] Three dogs did not vomit (even after multiple administrations). Two dogs required a second dose when no vomiting occurred after 20 minutes—vomiting then occurred between 30 to 40 minutes after the first administration. Repeating administration of medication(s) prescribed for chronic conditions may be necessary if they were impacted by emesis.

Ropinirole may be absorbed across intact skin. Exposure to humans handling ropinirole, particularly when opening the unit-dose container, may cause adverse effects (eg, headache, nausea, vomiting, dizziness, orthostatic hypotension, sleepiness). This product should be handled with caution. Use of personal protective equipment (eg, gloves, eye protection) is recommended. In cases of accidental exposure, rinse the affected area immediately with plenty of fresh water, and seek medical attention if symptoms occur. Ropinirole ophthalmic solution should not be administered those who are pregnant, breastfeeding, or attempting to become pregnant.[2,7]

Do not confuse rOPINIRole with reserpine, risperiDONE, or *Rocaltrol®*.

Adverse Effects

The most common systemic adverse effect with ropinirole use in dogs is lethargy (41%). Other adverse effects (less than 5%) include diarrhea, salivation, and CNS signs (eg, ataxia, tremors).[2,3] Elevated ALT (3%) has also been reported.[2] CNS adverse effects resolved within 8 hours after administration.[10]

Prolonged emesis (ie, more than 60 minutes) occurred in 8% of dogs.[10] Metoclopramide (0.5 mg/kg IV or SC) terminates protracted vomiting and may reverse other ropinirole adverse effects (eg, lethargy, muscle tremors).[2,3] Maropitant given by the IV route (not SC) stops protracted vomiting but has no effect on other dopaminergic signs. See ***Overdose/Acute Toxicity***.

Tachycardia was noted in 14% of dogs after ophthalmic administration.[3] The average heart rate increased ≈55 bpm within 10 minutes of administration; however, this resolved within 4 hours after administration.

Moderate eye irritation (eg, conjunctival hyperemia [51%], third eyelid protrusion [38%], conjunctival discharge [30%], blepharospasm [19%]) may occur but typically improves within 2 hours after administration and is usually completely resolved within 8 to 24 hours.[2,3]

Reproductive/Nursing Safety

The manufacturer does not recommend ropinirole use during pregnancy or lactation.[2,7]

Implantation was disrupted in rats given ropinirole 20 mg/kg/day PO. In rats, developmental effects occurred at clinically used doses, and teratogenicity and embryo lethality occurred at 120 mg/kg/day PO. No developmental toxicity was noted in rabbits receiving 20 mg/kg/day PO.[3]

Ropinirole reduces serum prolactin concentration due to its activity at D_2 receptor subtypes, and prolonged use would be expected to reduce lactation. Ropinirole is excreted in maternal milk, but effects on offspring are unknown. Use with caution in nursing patients or consider a milk replacer.

Safe use of ropinirole during pregnancy has not been established; thus, this drug should only be used when the maternal benefits outweigh the potential fetal risks.

Overdose/Acute Toxicity

Oral LD_{50} in rats is 400 – 500 mg/kg.[3] Clinical signs in dogs receiving up to ≈50 – 59 mg/m²/day (up to 5 times the labeled dose) mirrored the drugs clinical and adverse effects, including vomiting, retching, hunched posture, salivation, hypotension, tachycardia, lethargy, and tremors.[2,3] At these doses, vomiting lasted up to 2 hours, and other clinical signs returned to normal 6 hours after administration.[2]

The effects of ropinirole overdose are mild to moderate and transient; therefore, supportive therapy is likely sufficient. Ophthalmic irrigation is likely of limited value, as ropinirole reaches peak concentration (C_{max}) within 12 minutes of administration, and vomiting may occur prior reaching C_{max}. Metoclopramide (0.5 mg/kg SC or IV) ameliorates clinical signs (eg, protracted vomiting, lethargy, tremors) caused by ropinirole in 100% of dogs.[2,7] Maropitant must be administered via the IV route to stop protracted vomiting; however, it is important to note that maropitant does not relieve ropinirole's other dopaminergic signs (eg, lethargy, tremors).[2,7,10]

For patients that have experienced or are suspected of having experienced an overdose, it is strongly encouraged to consult with one of the 24-hour poison consultation centers that specialize in providing information specific for veterinary patients. For general information related to overdose and toxin exposures, as well as contact information for poison control centers, refer to ***Appendix***.

Laboratory Considerations

- None

Drug Interactions

The following drug interactions have either been reported or are theoretical in humans or animals receiving ropinirole and may be of significance in veterinary patients. Unless otherwise noted, use together is not necessarily contraindicated, but the potential risks should be weighed and additional monitoring performed when appropriate.

- **Antiemetics** (eg, **maropitant, ondansetron**): May reduce emetogenic effects of ropinirole[7,10]
- **Antihistamines, First Generation** (eg, **dimenhydrinate, meclizine**): Antihistamines with antiemetic effects may reduce emetogenic effects of ropinirole.
- **Antihypertensive Agents** (eg, **amlodipine, enalapril, sildenafil, telmisartan**): Additive hypotensive effects may occur.
- **CNS Depressants** (eg, **phenobarbital**): Additive CNS depressant effects (eg, lethargy, ataxia) may occur.
- **Dopamine Antagonists** (eg, **domperidone, metoclopramide**): May antagonize ropinirole action at dopaminergic receptors and block its emetogenic effect. May be used to treat or reverse adverse ropinirole effects—see ***Overdose/Acute Toxicity***
- **Phenothiazines** (eg, **acepromazine, promethazine**): May reduce emetogenic effects of ropinirole

In humans, ropinirole is metabolized by CYP1A2, and inhibitors of this enzyme increase ropinirole concentration and AUC. Veterinary significance of this interaction is unclear, but, theoretically, prolonged vomiting may occur when ropinirole is combined with the following CYP1A2 inhibitors:

- **Amiodarone**
- **Ciprofloxacin**: In humans, coadministration of ciprofloxacin with immediate-release ropinirole tablets increased ropinirole AUC by 84% and C_{max} by 60%.[8]
- **Erythromycin**
- **Mexiletine**

Dosages

DOGS:

Induction of vomiting (labeled dose, FDA-approved): Administer the appropriate number of drops to deliver a target dose of 3.75 mg/m² (NOT mg/kg; dose range 2.7 – 5.4 mg/m² [NOT mg/kg]) according to the table below.* A second dose of the same number of drops may be administered if the dog does not vomit within 20 minutes of receiving the first dose.[2]

Ropinirole Dose Administration

Body weight (kg)	Body weight (lb)	Total number of eye drops	Example administration
1.8-5	4-11.1	1	1 drop in one eye (either left **OR** right)
5.1-10	11.2-22.1	2	1 drop in each eye
10.1-20	22.2-44.1	3	2 drops in one eye, and 1 drop in the other eye
20.1-35	44.2-77.2	4	2 drops in each eye
35.1-60	77.3-132.3	6	An initial dose of 2 drops in each eye, followed 2 minutes later by 1 drop in each eye
60.1-100	132.4-220.5	8	An initial dose of 2 drops in each eye, followed 2 minutes later by 2 drops in each eye

*Table adapted from *CLEVOR®* ropinirole ophthalmic solution US product label, 2020[2]

Monitoring

- Clinical efficacy
- Blood pressure and heart rate
- Signs of ocular irritation (eg, conjunctival hyperemia, blepharospasm, protrusion of the third eyelid)
- Adverse effects (eg, protracted vomiting, aspiration of vomitus)

Client Information

- Ropinirole ophthalmic solution should be administered only under the supervision of your veterinarian to induce vomiting when it is appropriate and safe to do so.
- Visibility of the third eyelid and eye irritation (eg, redness, discharge, squinting) may occur after administration but should resolve within 24 hours.

- Your dog may appear sleepy, have difficulty walking, or have a reduced appetite for a short period of time after administration. Contact your veterinarian if your dog's appetite has not returned to normal within 1 to 2 days.

Chemistry/Synonyms

Ropinirole is a nonergoline indoline that occurs as white or cream-colored crystalline powder that is freely soluble in water. The log-P n-octanol:water coefficient is 2.7. The commercial solution (*Clevor*®) is a clear, slightly yellow, sterile aqueous solution that contains citric acid monohydrate, sodium citrate, and sodium chloride.

Ropinirole may also be known as ORM-145704, SKF 101468, *Clevor*®, or *Requip*®.

Storage/Stability

Store ropinirole solution at room temperature between 20°C to 25°C (68°F-77°F) and protected from light. Opened droppers may be stored upright inside the manufacturer's pouch for up to 30 minutes after opening; discard any unused portion.

Compatibility/Compounding Considerations

None noted

Dosage Forms/Regulatory Status

VETERINARY-LABELED PRODUCTS:

Ropinirole Ophthalmic Solution: 3% in 0.3 mL prefilled single dose dropper (contains 9 mg ropinirole; each mL contains 30 mg of ropinirole [equivalent to 34.2 mg of ropinirole hydrochloride]) packaged in an opaque foil pouch in cartons of 1 or 5 droppers. Each drop delivers 27 µL (810 µg). *Clevor*®; (Rx). NADA# 141-534.

HUMAN-LABELED PRODUCTS:

Ropinirole Tablets: 0.25 mg, 0.5 mg, 1 mg, 2 mg, 3 mg, 4 mg, and 5 mg tablets; *Requip*®, generic; (Rx). An extended-release tablet (*Requip XL*®) is also available.

References

For the complete list of references, see **wiley.com/go/budde/plumb**

Ropivacaine

(roe-***piv***-a-kane) *Naropin*®

Local Anesthetic

Prescriber Highlights

- Local anesthetic with delayed onset (20 minutes) and intermediate duration of action (3 to 5 hours) compared to others in its class
- Local anesthetics are absorbed from the site of administration and may have systemic effects.
- Adverse effects are usually minimal when ropivacaine is used correctly, but cardiac and CNS toxicity may occur.
- Use should be limited to clinicians experienced in the diagnosis and management of local anesthetic toxicity; resources for treating acute emergencies must be readily available.

Uses/Indications

Ropivacaine is used to produce local or regional analgesia or anesthesia for surgery and diagnostic or therapeutic procedures. The local block can have a MAC-sparing effect on general anesthesia and results in better postoperative recovery. The duration of analgesia can be extended by combining ropivacaine with opioids or alpha-2 agonists, and the accuracy of the block can be increased with use of a nerve stimulator[1] or with ultrasound-guided administration. Ropivacaine can be used for epidural and spinal anesthesia, and, when combined with magnesium sulfate for intrathecal administration, it increases the intensity and duration of analgesia, but prolonged motor block may be a limiting factor.[2] Ropivacaine also provides corneal anesthesia when applied topically to the eye.[3]

In dogs, epinephrine does not appear to alter the onset ropivacaine effect but may slightly prolong its duration of action.[4]

Pharmacology/Actions

Local anesthetics block sodium ion channels on the nerve cell membrane, thereby altering electrical excitability, depolarization, and action potential propagation. They block the generation and conduction of impulses in motor, sensory, and autonomic nerve fibers around the site of application. Nerve fiber diameter, conduction velocity, and myelination determine the loss of nerve function. Clinically, the progressive loss of nerve function occurs in the following order: pain, temperature, touch, proprioception, and skeletal muscle tone. The anesthetic effect is lost in reverse order. Ropivacaine produces less motor block than bupivacaine.[4,5]

After epidural administration, ropivacaine produces analgesia typically within 3 to 15 minutes, and the analgesic effect persists for 3 to 5 hours. Compared to lidocaine, ropivacaine has a slower onset but longer duration of action. When ropivacaine is used as a peripheral nerve block, analgesia onset occurs after ≈10 minutes, and the analgesic effect lasts ≈3.5 hours but varies with nerve block location and technique.

Pharmacokinetics

Local anesthetics are absorbed from their site of administration into the systemic circulation. The rate and extent of systemic absorption increase with the dose and volume given, repeated administration, administration in the head and neck region, and administration into highly vascularized sites.

In dogs, peak arterial concentrations occurred 5 to 10 minutes after epidural administration of ≈1.5 mg/kg, and the elimination half-life and clearance were ≈200 minutes and ≈25 mL/minute/kg, respectively. The elimination half-life and clearance after IV administration were ≈26 minutes and 41 mL/minute/kg, respectively.[6]

In humans, peak concentrations occur ≈35 to 45 minutes after epidural block and ≈1 hour after brachial plexus block. Systemically absorbed drug distributes into all tissues, including the CNS. Protein binding is ≈95% to alpha-1-acid glycoprotein, which may limit but not prevent ropivacaine from crossing the placenta and being excreted in milk. It is metabolized in the liver by cytochrome P450 1A2 isozyme and is excreted in the urine principally as metabolites. Elimination half-life after IV administration is ≈1.8 hours in adults and ≈8 hours in neonates; with epidural use, the half-life is ≈4 hours.

Contraindications/Precautions/Warnings

Ropivacaine is contraindicated in patients with a known hypersensitivity to it or to another amide-type local anesthetic agent. It is not recommended for obstetrical paracervical block, spinal anesthesia, or IV regional anesthesia (Bier block). Epidural injections should be administered incrementally, with aspiration before each dose. Local anesthetics with preservatives should not be used for epidural or intrathecal anesthesia.

Use it with caution in patients with hepatic or renal disease or impaired cardiovascular function.

Ropivacaine products in which epinephrine has been added should be used with caution, or not at all, in patients with hypertension or for anesthesia of extremities without collateral circulation, such as digits, ears, nose, or penis, as it may cause tissue necrosis.

Ropivacaine should only be used in situations in which sufficient monitoring and patient-support capabilities (eg, intubation, ventilation) are available.

Adverse Effects

Local anesthetics are generally well tolerated when administered correctly. Adverse effects are related to high plasma concentrations, which may result from the dosage or ropivacaine concentration used, rapid absorption from the injection site, and unintentional intravascular or subarachnoid injection.

Cardiovascular effects include hypotension, bradycardia, AV block, and decreased cardiac output; severe hypotension caused by epidural ropivacaine was deemed responsible for the death of a healthy beagle enrolled in an experimental study.[7] It has greater cardiac toxicity (eg, hypotension, QRS widening) than lidocaine but less than bupivacaine.[8] It slows respiratory rate, but the rate typically remains within normal parameters. CNS excitation (eg, restlessness, tremors), depression (eg, drowsiness, loss of consciousness), or both may occur. Other noted adverse effects include nausea, vomiting, fever, urinary retention, and transient Horner's syndrome. Ataxia may occur with epidural administration.[9,10]

Chondrolysis has occurred with an intra-articular infusion of local anesthetics.

Reproductive/Nursing Safety

Local anesthetics readily cross the placenta. Animal reproductive studies with ropivacaine in rats and rabbits have not revealed adverse effects on fetal development, viability, or mortality.

Approximately 4% of the maternal dose is estimated to reach the nursing pup in breast milk; use with caution during lactation.

Overdose/Acute Toxicity

Toxic blood levels are most likely to occur after unintended intravascular ropivacaine administration. Toxic effects may occur rapidly and simultaneously. Cardiac conduction and excitability are depressed and may lead to AV block, ventricular arrhythmias, and cardiac arrest; arrhythmias may be refractory to treatment. In addition, myocardial contractility is depressed, and peripheral vasodilation occurs, leading to decreased cardiac output and arterial blood pressure. CNS stimulation (eg, restlessness, tremors, and shivering progressing to convulsions) may precede CNS depression, coma, and respiratory arrest. The mean dose that induced seizures in dogs and sheep was 4.9 mg/kg and 6.1 mg/kg, respectively.

Management must begin with the delivery of oxygen via a patent airway. Benzodiazepines or barbiturates can be used for seizure management but may cause further CNS depression. Cardiovascular support should be provided and may include IV fluids and vasopressor drugs. Prolonged resuscitative efforts may be required. Lipid emulsion therapy may be beneficial.

For patients that have experienced or are suspected to have experienced an overdose, consultation with a 24-hour poison consultation center specializing in providing veterinary-specific information is recommended. For general information related to overdose and toxin exposures, as well as contact information for poison control centers, refer to ***Appendix.***

Drug Interactions

The following drug interactions have either been reported or are theoretical in humans or animals receiving ropivacaine and may be of significance in veterinary patients. Unless otherwise noted, use together is not necessarily contraindicated, but weigh the potential risks and perform additional monitoring when appropriate.

- **AMIODARONE**: May increase the risk for cardiac toxicity
- **ANGIOTENSIN-CONVERTING ENZYME INHIBITORS** (ACEIs; eg, **benazepril, enalapril**): Increased risk for bradycardia and hypotension
- **BETA-ADRENERGIC ANTAGONISTS**: (eg, **atenolol, esmolol, propranolol, sotalol**): May increase serum bupivacaine concentrations by reducing bupivacaine clearance
- **CIPROFLOXACIN/ENROFLOXACIN**: May impair ropivacaine metabolism
- **THEOPHYLLINE**: May impair ropivacaine metabolism

Severe, prolonged hypertension may result when using ropivacaine/epinephrine combination products with the following:

- **ANTIDEPRESSANTS, TRICYCLIC** (eg, **amitriptyline, clomipramine**): Use in combination with epinephrine-containing ropivacaine products may produce severe, prolonged hypertension.
- **ERGOT ALKALOIDS** (eg, **bromocriptine, pergolide**)
- **MONOAMINE OXIDASE INHIBITORS** (eg, **selegiline, linezolid, amitraz**)
- **VASOPRESSORS** (eg, **dobutamine, norepinephrine**)

Laboratory Considerations

- None were noted.

Dosages

NOTE: Ropivacaine product concentration, administration volume, site of administration, administration technique, and underlying patient condition(s) are important interrelated factors that determine ropivacaine's safe and effective use. Local anesthetics should be used only by clinicians well versed in correct administration technique, diagnosis, and management of local anesthetic toxicity and who have complete resuscitative resources immediately available.

DOGS:

Local analgesia (extra-label):

a) 2 mg/kg is a generally recommended dosage for local block.

b) Using ropivacaine 0.75% solution, give 0.75 mg/kg perineurally. **NOTE:** The combination with dexmedetomidine 0.1 µg/kg provided analgesia similar to ropivacaine alone.[11]

c) **Peribulbar injection**: Using ropivacaine 1% solution, administer 3 mg/kg (0.3 mL/kg). Ultrasound-guided injection resulted in lower postinjection intraocular pressure, faster restoration of conjugate eye movement, and lower risk for a subconjunctival hemorrhage.[12] Another separate study found satisfactory results using ropivacaine 0.75% solution.[13]

d) **Tumescent local anesthesia**: Ropivacaine 0.05% and 0.1% solutions (diluted in lactated Ringer's solution) at temperatures between 8°C and 12°C (46°F and 54°F) infused through a multi-hole needle at 15 mL/kg over 10 minutes provided analgesia for 7 hours following mastectomy.[14]

e) **Intraperitoneal administration during ovariohysterectomy**:
   - 3 mg/kg using 1% ropivacaine diluted in saline solution 0.9% to a final volume of 1.2 mL/kg (final concentration of ropivacaine 0.25%) administered after the abdomen had been surgically opened and before ligation of the ovarian pedicles and uterus.[15]
   - 3 mg/kg ropivacaine using 0.75% solution diluted with sterile water to 0.5% and administered just prior to closure.[16]

Epidural analgesia and anesthesia (extra-label): 0.2 – 1.65 mg/kg alone or in combination with an opioid (eg, methadone, morphine), alpha-2 agonist (xylazine) or both (ie, ropivacaine + opioid + xylazine).[17–24]

a) Using ropivacaine 1% solution, give 0.2 mg/kg with preservative-free morphine 0.2 mg/kg epidurally at L7-S1; total volume delivered is 1 mL/4.5 kg (10 lb) of body weight to a maximum of 10 mL.[21]

b) Using ropivacaine 0.75% solution, give 1.65 mg/kg with methadone 0.1 mg/kg. This dosage reduced intraoperative isoflurane and fentanyl requirements and prolonged postoperative analgesia; time to standing was also delayed.[17,18]

c) Using butorphanol 0.1 mg/kg with ropivacaine 0.75% solution

2.175 mg/kg to make a final total volume (butorphanol + ropivacaine) of 0.3 mL/kg allowed ovariosalpingohysterectomy without the need for anesthesia in 12 of 16 bitches.[20]

d) In a study comparing 1 mg/kg ropivacaine to 0.5 mg/kg ropivacaine alone or in combination with sufentanil or sufentanil-epinephrine: the combination of ropivacaine-sufentanil-epinephrine resulted in no rescue analgesia and the lowest postoperative pain scores. The 1 mg/kg ropivacaine group had a significantly greater motor block.[19]

e) Ropivacaine 0.75 mg/kg with morphine 0.1 mg/kg ± xylazine 0.1 mg/kg[22]

CATS:

Local analgesia (extra-label): 1.5 – 2 mg/kg is a generally recommended dose for local block.

Epidural analgesia and anesthesia (extra-label): Using ropivacaine 1% solution, administer 2 mg/kg in the L7-S1 epidural space.[25] Morphine can be added to ropivacaine. In another study, ropivacaine 1.95 mg/kg with morphine 0.1 mg/kg decreased postoperative analgesic requirement.[26]

HORSES:

Local analgesia (extra-label): Palmar digital nerve block: Using ropivacaine 0.75% solution, inject 1.5 mL SC just palmar to the medial and lateral neurovascular bundles and just proximal to the collateral cartilages of the foot.[27]

Intra-articular analgesia (extra-label): Using ropivacaine 1% solution, 20 mg (NOT mg/kg) combined with morphine 20 mg (NOT mg/kg) administered into the radio-carpal joint produced a strong analgesic effect for 24 hours under experimental conditions. Ropivacaine alone (40 mg total dose) produced analgesia for ≈2.5 to 3.5 hours.

Epidural analgesia and anesthesia (extra-label):

a) **Lumbosacral epidural**: 0.15 mg/kg administered between the first and second coccygeal vertebrae. The study used 0.3% ropivacaine in saline solution.[9]

b) **Caudal epidural**: Using ropivacaine 0.5% solution, 0.08 mg/kg with fentanyl citrate 100 µg (total dose, NOT µg/kg) produced perineal analgesia within an average of ≈7 minutes, and the analgesic effect lasted ≈3.6 hours. Ropivacaine alone (0.1 mg/kg) had a slower onset (≈12 minutes) and shorter duration (≈3 hours) with inferior quality of surgical analgesia.[28]

CATTLE:

Caudal epidural analgesia and anesthesia (extra-label): Using ropivacaine 0.75% solution, 0.11 mg/kg induced perineal analgesia within 15 minutes and lasted for 6 hours. Mild ataxia occurred in 50% of patients.[10]

SWINE:

Epidural analgesia and anesthesia (extra-label): Using ropivacaine 0.75% solution, 1.5 mg/kg reduced isoflurane requirement while improving blood pressure and heart rate in pigs undergoing abdominal and nonabdominal surgery.[29]

SHEEP/GOATS:

Local analgesia (extra-label): Using ropivacaine 0.5% solution, 12 mL (1.3 mg/kg) for thoracolumbar paravertebral nerve block for ruminal fistulation provided ≈9 to 10 hours of analgesia.[30]

Epidural analgesia and anesthesia (extra-label): 0.6 mg/kg administered lumbosacrally provided complete analgesia of the tail, perineum, thighs, and inguinal region of healthy goats.[31]

Monitoring

- Adequacy of analgesia and anesthesia
- Cardiovascular and respiratory function as well as state of consciousness after each injection
- ECG for patients taking class III antiarrhythmics (eg, sotalol, amiodarone) and for patients with a history of arrhythmias

Client Information

- This drug should only be used systemically by professionals familiar with its use and in a setting in which adequate patient monitoring can be performed.
- This medication causes temporary loss of feeling. The injected area may not have the usual function for several hours.

Chemistry/Synonyms

Ropivacaine hydrochloride is an amide-class local anesthetic. It occurs as a white crystalline powder that is soluble in water and alcohol. Commercial solutions contain only the S-enantiomer. Solubility is limited at pH above 6.

Ropivacaine hydrochloride is also known as AL-281, ropivacaini hydrochloridum, and *Naropin*®.

Storage/Stability

Store ropivacaine at controlled room temperature between 20°C and 25°C (68°F and 77°F); excursions are permitted to 15°C to 30°C (59°F-86°F).

Compatibility/Compounding Considerations

Ropivacaine HCl is **compatible** with 0.9% sodium chloride solutions and the following drugs (partial list): ketamine, methylprednisolone acetate, and morphine sulfate. Ropivacaine HCl is reported to be **variably compatible** with fentanyl citrate.

Dosage Forms/Regulatory Status

VETERINARY-LABELED PRODUCTS: NONE.

The Association of Racing Commissioners International (ARCI) has designated this drug as a class 2 substance. See ***Appendix*** for more information.

Use of this drug may not be allowed in certain animal competitions. Check rules and regulations before entering a competition while this medication is being administered. Contact local racing authorities for further guidance.

HUMAN-LABELED PRODUCTS:

Ropivacaine Hydrochloride Injection: 0.2%, 0.5%, 0.75%, and 1% solution in 10 mL, 20 mL, 30 mL, and 100 mL single-dose ampules, bottles, or vials; *Naropin*®, generic; (Rx)

References

For the complete list of references, see **wiley.com/go/budde/plumb**

S-Adenosyl-Methionine (SAMe)

(***ess***-ah-***den***-oh-seel meth-***ie***-oh-neen) *Denosyl*®

Hepatoprotectant

See also ***S-Adenosyl-Methionine (SAMe)/Silybin*** and ***Silymarin***

Prescriber Highlights

- Nutraceutical that has been used in small animals as an adjunctive treatment for acute and chronic liver disease (hepatitis) including hepatotoxicity and for cognitive dysfunction
- Evidence is scant supporting clinical efficacy, but it is well tolerated.
- Should be administered on an empty stomach but may be hidden in a small amount of food if necessary
- Not a regulated drug; choose products carefully

Uses/Indications

S-adenosyl-methionine (SAMe) is most commonly used in small animal species as an adjunctive treatment for liver disease[1] (chronic hepatitis, hepatic lipidosis, cholangiohepatitis), feline triaditis, gallbladder leiomyoma[2] or mucocele,[3] and blue-green algae ingestion.[4]

It potentially could be of benefit for age-related cognitive dysfunction,[5,6] treatment of acute hepatotoxin-induced liver toxicity (eg, acetaminophen,[7,8] xylitol,[9] amatoxin), and in at-risk patients on long-term therapy using drugs with hepatotoxic potential. The authors in a 2013 review assessing the evidence for nutraceuticals for treating canine liver disease state: *Despite the lack of data supporting the use of SAMe as a hepatoprotectant, the compound is frequently recommended for dogs with hepatobiliary disease. Before veterinarians recommend use of SAMe, they should ensure that owners understand (informed consent) that data on its efficacy is lacking.*[10]

Although a benefit has been reported for in vitro use of SAMe combined with glucosamine in preserving the integrity of bovine articular cartilage, a double-blinded, placebo-controlled clinical trial (6 weeks) evaluating SAMe efficacy for the treatment of clinically inferred osteoarthritis (OA) did not find that it was an effective standalone treatment for reducing clinical signs of OA in dogs.[11]

Pharmacology/Actions

S-adenosyl-methionine (SAMe) is an endogenous molecule synthesized by cells throughout the body. It is formed from the amino acid methionine and ATP, in conjunction with SAMe synthetase enzyme (an enzyme manufactured in the liver; a rate-limiting step in the presence of liver compromise). SAMe is an essential part of three major biochemical pathways: transmethylation, transsulfuration, and aminopropylation. Normal function of these pathways is especially vital to the liver as many metabolic and detoxifying reactions occur there.

In the transmethylation pathway, SAMe serves as a methyl donor (necessary for many substances and drugs to be activated and/or eliminated). Transmethylation is essential in phospholipid synthesis important to cell membrane structure, fluidity, and function. In aminopropylation, SAMe donates aminopropyl groups and is a source of polyamines. Aminopropylation is important in producing substances that have anti-inflammatory effects, protein and DNA synthesis, and promoting cell replication and liver mass regeneration.

In transsulfuration, SAMe generates sulfur-containing compounds important for conjugation reactions used in detoxification and as a precursor to glutathione (GSH). Glutathione is important in many metabolic processes and cell detoxification. The conversion of SAMe to glutathione requires the presence of folate, cyanocobalamin (B_{12}), and pyridoxine (B_6). Normally, the liver produces ample SAMe, but in liver disease or in the presence of hepatotoxic substances, endogenous conversion to glutathione may be deficient. Exogenous SAMe has been shown to increase liver and red blood cell glutathione levels and/or prevent its depletion. SAMe inhibits apoptosis secondary to alcohol or bile acids in hepatocytes.

In humans, the mechanism for its antidepressant effects is not well understood, but it apparently increases serotonin turnover and increases dopamine and norepinephrine levels. Neuro-imaging studies in humans show that SAMe affects the brain similarly to other antidepressant medications.

Pharmacokinetics

Oral bioavailability is dependent on the salt used to stabilize SAMe. Oral bioavailability of the tosylate salt is reportedly 1% whereas the 1,4-butanedisulfonate form has a bioavailability of 5%. Regardless of oral dosage form administered, presence of food in the gut can substantially reduce the amount of drug absorbed. Peak concentrations occur in 1 to 6 hours after oral dosing with the enteric-coated tablets. Once absorbed, SAMe enters the portal circulation and is primarily metabolized in the liver. In humans, 17% of a dose of radiolabeled SAMe was recovered in the urine within 48 hours of dosing and 27% in the feces; veterinary significance is unclear.

In dogs, a chewable non-hygroscopic formulation of SAMe yielded similar areas under-the-curve when compared with the enteric-coated tablets, but peak levels occurred sooner with the chewable tablets.[12]

Contraindications/Precautions/Warnings

There are no apparent contraindications to the use of SAMe.

An analysis comparing the measured amount of SAMe present in commercial dosage forms compared with the amount stated on product labels found a greater than 3-fold variance.[13]

Adverse Effects

Adverse effects appear to be minimal or nonexistent in treated animals. Most studies in humans have shown adverse effects similar to that of placebo.

Reproductive/Nursing Safety

The safety of exogenous SAMe has not been proven in pregnancy; use with caution. Limited studies in laboratory animals and pregnant women with liver disease have not demonstrated any ill effects to mother or fetus.

It is unknown if SAMe enters maternal milk.

Because safety has not been established in animals, this drug should only be used when the maternal benefits outweigh the potential risks to offspring.

Overdose/Acute Toxicity

SAMe appears to be quite safe. LD_{50} in rodents exceeds 4.65 g/kg, and toxicity studies in dogs and cats at the usual prescribed doses demonstrated no deleterious effects.[14] In the case of an overdose, GI effects may be observed, but are unlikely to require treatment.

For patients that have experienced or are suspected to have experienced an overdose, consultation with a 24-hour poison consultation center specializing in providing veterinary-specific information is recommended. For general information related to overdose and toxin exposures, as well as contact information for poison control centers, refer to ***Appendix.***

Drug Interactions

No drug interactions have been documented with SAMe; however, theoretically, some drug interactions in humans may be of significance in veterinary patients. Unless otherwise noted, use together is not necessarily contraindicated, but the potential risks must be weighed and additional monitoring performed when appropriate.

- CHOLESTYRAMINE: Decreased efficacy of SAMe possible

The following drugs can theoretically cause additive serotonergic effects:

- **DEXTROMETHORPHAN**
- **MEPERIDINE**
- **MIRTAZAPINE**
- **MONOAMINE OXIDASE INHIBITORS (MAOIs; eg, selegiline)**
- **PENTAZOCINE**
- **SELECTIVE SEROTONIN REUPTAKE INHIBITORS (SSRIs; eg, fluoxetine)**
- **TRAMADOL**
- **TRAZODONE**
- **TRICYCLIC ANTIDEPRESSANTS (TCAs; eg, amitriptyline, clomipramine)**

Laboratory Considerations

- No specific laboratory interactions or considerations noted

Dosages

NOTE: None of these dosages are FDA-approved and should be treated as extra-label. Use a product from a reputable manufacturer and with proven bioavailability.[13,15] See ***Contraindications/ Precautions/Warnings.***

DOGS:

Increase hepatic glutathione levels (product insert dosage; not FDA-approved): Administer the appropriate number of tablets according to body weight using the dosing table below. The daily dosage may also be calculated based on 20 mg/kg of body weight and rounded to the closest tablet size or combination of sizes.[16] Product should be given on an empty stomach, at least one hour before feeding. The daily dose can be gradually increased or decreased based on the dog's needs. Many dogs are maintained long-term using every-other-day or every-third-day dosing. If giving more than one tablet, may divide total daily dose and give twice daily.

Body weight	Tablet size (mg)	Number of tablets daily
Up to 5.5 kg (12 lb)	90	1
6 to 15.5 kg (13-34 lb)	225	1
16 to 29.5 kg (35-65 lb)	425	1
30 to 54.5 kg (66-120 lb)	425	2
Over 54.5 kg (120 lb)	425	3

Adjunctive treatment of necro-inflammatory/cholestatic liver disease, vacuolar hepatopathy: 20 mg/kg PO once daily on an empty stomach[15]

CATS:

Increase hepatic glutathione levels (product insert dosage; not FDA-approved): Administer the appropriate number of tablets according to body weight using the dosing table below. The daily dosage may also be calculated based on 20 mg/kg of body weight and rounded to the closest tablet size or combination of sizes.[16] Product should be given on an empty stomach, at least one hour before feeding. Because tablets can become lodged in the esophagus, administer 3 to 6 mL of water immediately after SAMe. The daily dose can be gradually increased or decreased based on the cat's needs. Many cats are maintained long-term using every-other-day or every-third-day dosing. If giving more than one tablet, may divide total daily dose and give twice daily.

Body weight	Tablet size (mg)	Number of tablets daily
Up to 5.5 kg (12 lb)	90	1
Over 5.5 kg (12 lb)	90	2

Adjunctive treatment of necro-inflammatory/cholestatic liver disease, vacuolar hepatopathy, or feline hepatic lipidosis: 20 mg/kg PO once daily on an empty stomach[17]

Monitoring

- Clinical signs (appetite, activity, attitude)
- Liver enzymes, bilirubin, bile acids; may require 1 to 4 months before any changes in lab values are noted

Client Information

- Keep tablets in original packaging until administration. Do not crush or split enteric-coated tablets.
- Very well tolerated, usually with no side effects
- Give on an empty stomach, at least an hour before or 2 hours after feeding. Total daily dosage may be given as 1 dose or divided and given as 2 doses.
- For cats: follow all oral tablets with 3 to 6 mL of water to make sure tablets pass into the stomach.
- SAMe is considered a nutritional supplement by the FDA, not a medication. Product quality (and thus effectiveness) may vary between manufacturers. Use only the medication prescribed by your veterinarian.
- While your animal is taking this medication, it is important to return to your veterinarian for any recommended bloodwork or physical exam rechecks. Do not miss these important follow-up visits.

Chemistry/Synonyms

S-adenosyl-methionine (SAMe) is a naturally occurring molecule found throughout the body. Because pure SAMe is highly reactive and unstable, commercially available forms of SAMe are salt forms; sulfate, sulfate-p-toluenesulfonate (also known as tosylate), and butanedisulfonate salts can all be procured.

SAMe may also be known as S-adenosyl-L-methionine, S-adenosylmethionine, SAM, SAM-e, ademetionine, adenosylmethionine, Sammy, or methioninyl adenylate. Many trade names are available.

Storage/Stability

Unless otherwise labeled, SAMe tablets should be stored at room temperature. Avoid conditions of high temperature or humidity. SAMe is inherently unstable in acidic or aqueous environments; store in tightly sealed, moisture-resistant containers.

Compatibility/Compounding Considerations

No specific information noted. SAMe is inherently unstable in acidic or aqueous environments.

Dosage Forms/Regulatory Status

VETERINARY-LABELED PRODUCTS:

None as a pharmaceutical. The FDA considers SAMe a nutritional supplement. No standards have been accepted for potency, purity, safety, or efficacy by regulatory bodies. Supplements are available from a wide variety of sources and dosage forms include tablets in a variety of strengths.

There are specific products marketed for use in animals, including:

Enteric-coated tablets: *Denosyl® for cats and small dogs* (SAMe 90 mg), *Denosyl® for medium dogs* (SAMe 225 mg), and *Denosyl® for large dogs* (SAMe 425 mg); (OTC)

Chewable tablets: SAMe 225 mg; *Denosyl®*; (OTC)

A combination product *Denamarin®*, containing SAMe and silybin (silymarin), is also labeled for use in dogs and cats.

HUMAN-LABELED PRODUCTS:

Many OTC products available.

References

For the complete list of references, see **wiley.com/go/budde/plumb**

S-Adenosyl-Methionine (SAMe)/ Silybin

(***ess***-ah-***den***-oh-seel meth-***ie***-oh-neen/***sill***-eh-bin) *Denamarin®*

Hepatoprotectant

See also ***S-Adenosyl-Methionine***.

Prescriber Highlights

- Nutraceutical combination used in small animal species as adjunctive treatment for acute and chronic liver disease (eg, chronic hepatitis), including hepatotoxicity
- Evidence supporting clinical efficacy is scant, but the combination is well tolerated; GI effects are possible.
- Should be administered on an empty stomach but may be hidden in a small amount of food if necessary
- Products are not regulated and should be chosen carefully.
- Some drug interactions may be possible.

Uses/Indications

The FDA considers S-adenosyl-methionine (SAMe)/silybin to be a combination nutritional supplement (not a medication); thus, no standards for potency, purity, safety, or efficacy have been accepted by regulatory bodies. An analysis comparing the measured amount of SAMe present in commercial dosage forms compared with the amount stated on product labels found a greater than 3-fold variance.[1]

In small animal medicine, SAMe (ie, ademetionine) combined with silybin is most commonly used as an adjunctive treatment for liver disease (eg, chronic hepatitis, hepatic lipidosis, cholangiohepatitis, feline triad disease). This combination may potentially be beneficial for treatment of acute hepatotoxin-induced liver toxicity (eg, acetaminophen, xylitol toxicity, amatoxins) and for at-risk animals receiving long-term therapy involving drugs with hepatotoxic potential.

Silymarin (silybin) is used to treat a variety of liver diseases in humans and domestic companion animals (eg, dogs, cats, horses, birds, rabbits), although controlled clinical studies demonstrating the efficacy for a standardized form and concentration are lacking. Silymarin (silybin) is most commonly used for treatment of chronic and acute liver disease and cirrhosis and as a hepatoprotective agent when hepatotoxic agents (eg, *Amanita phalloides*; death cap mushroom) are ingested. A study in cats found that silymarin had some hepatoprotective effects on hepatotoxicity induced by acetaminophen and tetracycline.[2,3] Silymarin appears to attenuate gentamicin-induced nephrotoxicity in dogs.[4]

The proprietary combination of silybin and SAMe (ie, *Denamarin*®) minimized liver enzyme elevations in dogs receiving lomustine (ie, CCNU) chemotherapy, which increased the likelihood that dogs could complete the prescribed lomustine therapy course.[5] However, according to a later review, the original study had several weaknesses, including a low number of dogs undergoing additional liver testing with bile acids, abdominal ultrasonography examination, and liver biopsies; low incidence of dogs with severe liver disease; lack of placebo in the control group; the study was nonblinded; some dogs had pre-existing occult liver disease; use of a fixed combination of 2 distinct agents; and potential author conflicts of interest.[6] In a small study in dogs with experimentally induced endotoxemia, the proprietary combination of silybin and SAMe protected the dog's hepatorenal function and had beneficial effects on coagulation.[7]

Pharmacology/Actions

SAMe, an endogenous molecule synthesized by cells throughout the body, is formed from the amino acid methionine and adenosine triphosphate (ATP) in conjunction with the SAMe synthetase enzyme (an enzyme manufactured in the liver; a rate-limiting step in the presence of liver compromise). SAMe is an essential part of 3 major biochemical pathways: transmethylation, transsulfuration, and aminopropylation. Normal functioning of these pathways is particularly vital to the liver, as the liver is where many metabolic and detoxifying reactions occur.

In the transmethylation pathway, SAMe serves as a methyl donor, which is necessary for the activation and/or elimination of many substances and drugs. Transmethylation is essential to phospholipid synthesis that is important to cell membrane structure, fluidity, and function.

In the aminopropylation pathway, SAMe donates aminopropyl groups and is a source of polyamines. Aminopropylation is important in producing substances that have anti-inflammatory effects, for protein and DNA synthesis, and in promoting cell replication and liver mass regeneration.

In the transsulfuration pathway, SAMe generates sulfur-containing compounds important for conjugation reactions used in detoxification and as a precursor to glutathione (GSH). GSH is important in many metabolic processes and cell detoxification. The conversion of SAMe to GSH requires the presence of folate, cyanocobalamin (vitamin B_{12}), and pyridoxine (vitamin B_6). The liver typically produces ample SAMe, but endogenous conversion to GSH may be deficient in animals with liver disease or in the presence of hepatotoxic substances. Exogenous SAMe has been shown to increase liver and erythrocyte GSH levels and/or prevent GSH depletion. SAMe inhibits apoptosis secondary to alcohol or bile acids in hepatocytes.

Silybin, which is the major active constituent of silymarin, has a variety of pharmacologic actions that may contribute to its apparent treatment for liver disease. Silymarin inhibits lipid peroxidase and beta-glucoronidase and acts as an antioxidant and free radical scavenger. Silymarin also inhibits the cytotoxic, inflammatory, and apoptotic effects of tumor necrosis factor (TNF); apparently silymarin can alter outer hepatocyte cell membranes that can prevent toxin penetration. Silymarin is thought to reduce hepatic collagen formation and increase hepatic GSH concentrations.

Pharmacokinetics

Oral bioavailability is dependent on the salt used to stabilize SAMe. Oral bioavailability of the tosylate salt is reportedly 1%, whereas the 1,4-butanedisulfonate form has a bioavailability of 5%. The presence of food in the gut can substantially reduce the amount of drug absorbed, regardless of the oral dose administered. Peak concentrations occur 1 to 6 hours after oral administration of enteric-coated tablets. After SAMe is absorbed, it enters the portal circulation and is primarily metabolized in the liver. In humans, 17% of a dose of radiolabeled SAMe was recovered in urine within 48 hours of administration; 27% of a dose was recovered in feces.

Few pharmacokinetic data exist regarding silymarin use in animals. Oral silybin absorption is increased in dogs, cats, and horses when the drug is administered as a phosphatidylcholine complex.[8–10] Oral bioavailability of silybin phosphatidylcholine complex was 7% in cats and 2.9% in horses.[9,10]

In humans, silymarin has an oral bioavailability of less than 50% and peak concentrations occur 2 to 4 hours after administration. Oral absorption can increase when silybin (ie, silibinin, sylibin) is complexed with phosphatidylcholine. The drug undergoes extensive enterohepatic circulation and has significantly higher concentrations in liver cells and bile than in plasma. The elimination half-life in humans averages 6 hours. The majority of the drug is eliminated unchanged in feces, but 20% to 40% is converted into glucuronide and sulfate conjugates, which are eliminated in feces; only about 8% of the drug is excreted in urine.

Contraindications/Precautions/Warnings

None

Adverse Effects

Adverse effects appear to be minimal or nonexistent in treated animals. Most studies in humans have shown adverse effects similar to that of placebo treatment; there have been reports of vomiting, anorexia, and anxiety immediately after administration. Oral SAMe in humans may cause anorexia, nausea, vomiting, diarrhea, flatulence, constipation, dry mouth, insomnia/nervousness, headache, sweating, and dizziness.

Reproductive/Nursing Safety

Exogenous SAMe/silybin should be used with caution during pregnancy, as it has not been proven to be safe during pregnancy. Limited studies in laboratory animals and pregnant women with liver disease did not demonstrate any adverse effects.

It is unknown whether SAMe/silybin enters maternal milk.

Because safety has not been established in animals, this drug should only be used when the maternal benefits outweigh the potential risks to offspring.

Overdose/Acute Toxicity

SAMe appears to be safe. LD_{50} in rodents exceeds 4.65 g/kg, and toxicity studies in dogs and cats demonstrated no adverse effects at the usual prescribed doses. Overdoses are unlikely to cause significant morbidity. GI effects may be noted and treated as necessary in a supportive manner.

For patients that have experienced or are suspected to have experienced an overdose, consultation with a 24-hour poison consultation center specializing in providing veterinary-specific information is recommended. For general information related to overdose and toxin exposures, as well as contact information for poison control centers, refer to ***Appendix.***

Drug Interactions

No drug interactions have been documented with SAMe/silybin; however, theoretically, some drug interactions in humans may be of significance in veterinary patients. Unless otherwise noted, use together is not necessarily contraindicated, but the potential risks must be weighed and additional monitoring performed when appropriate.

The following drugs can theoretically cause additive serotonergic effects:

- **Dextromethorphan**
- **Meperidine**
- **Mirtazapine**
- **Monoamine Oxidase Inhibitors** (MAOIs; eg, **amitraz, linezolid, selegiline**)
- **Pentazocine**
- **Selective Serotonin Reuptake Inhibitors** (SSRIs; eg, **fluoxetine**)
- **Tramadol**
- **Trazodone**
- **Tricyclic Antidepressants** (eg, **amitriptyline, clomipramine**)

Other potential drug interactions include:

- **Antiviral Drugs**: Decreased efficacy possible
- **Cholestyramine**: Decreased SAMe absorption
- **Drugs Affected By Cytochrome P450 Inhibition** (eg, **amitriptyline, NSAIDs, verapamil, warfarin**): Silybin may inhibit CYP2C9. Drugs with narrow therapeutic indexes that are metabolized by this isoenzyme should be used with caution.
- **Drugs Cleared Via Hepatic Glucuronidation** (eg, **acetaminophen, diazepam, metronidazole**[11], **morphine**): Silybin may increase the clearance of drugs that undergo hepatic glucuronidation (interaction does not apply to cats).

Laboratory Considerations

- No specific laboratory interactions or considerations are noted.

Dosages

DOGS/CATS: NOTE: Dosing is different for regular and chewable tablet formulations; chewable formulations are only available for dogs.

Adjunctive treatment in animals with acute hepatopathies or hepatic fibrosis: Recommended dosages are often significantly higher than what is listed on the label. Anecdotally, SAMe 20 – 40 mg/kg PO daily has been suggested for dogs and 200 – 400 mg/cat (NOT mg/kg) PO daily for cats. For chronic hepatitis or other acute hepatopathies, silybin (ie, silymarin) 7 – 15 mg/kg PO daily has been suggested. To attempt to reduce fibrosis, silybin 20 – 50 mg/kg PO daily has been suggested.

- Tablets should be given on an empty stomach at least 1 hour before feeding, as food decreases absorption of SAMe.
- Enteric-coated tablets may be hidden in a small amount of food if there is difficulty in pilling.
- Dry-pilling cats is not recommended; 3 – 6 mL of water can be given immediately after pilling to facilitate passage to the stomach.
- The number of tablets given can be gradually reduced or increased at any time depending on the animal's needs.
- Many animals can be maintained long-term with every-other-day or every-third-day administration.

***Denamarin*® Tablets**[12]

Species	Body weight*	Tablet size (SAMe/ Silybin)	Number of tablets	Frequency of administration
Dogs, cats	Less than 5.5 kg (12 lb)	90 mg/ 9 mg	1	Once daily
Dogs, cats	More than 5.5 kg (12 lb)	90 mg/ 9 mg	1	Twice daily
Dogs	6-15.5 kg (13-34 lb)	225 mg/ 24 mg	1	Once daily
Dogs	16-29.5 kg (35-65 lb)	425 mg/ 35 mg	1	Once daily
Dogs	30-54.5 kg (66-120 lb)	425 mg/ 35 mg	2	Once daily or 1 tablet twice daily
Dogs	More than 54.5 kg (120 lb)	425 mg/ 35 mg	3	Once daily or divided and given twice daily

*Manufacturer lists dosages per lb, not per kg.

***Denamarin*® *Advanced* Tablets**[13]

Species	Body weight*	Tablet size (SAMe/ Silybin)	Number of tablets	Frequency of administration
Cats	All sizes	30 mg/9 mg	1	Once daily
Dogs	Less than 5.5 kg (12 lb)	30 mg/9 mg	1	Once daily
Dogs	5.5-15.5 kg (12-34 lb)	82 mg/24 mg	1	Once daily
Dogs	16-29.5 kg (35-65 lb)	172 mg/35 mg	1	Once daily
Dogs	30-54.5 kg (66-120 lb)	172 mg/35 mg	2	Once daily
Dogs	More than 54.5 kg (120 lb)	172 mg/35 mg	3	Once daily

*Manufacturer lists dosages per lb, not per kg.

***Denamarin*® Chewable Tablets**[14]

Species	Body weight*	Tablet size (SAMe/ Silybin)	Number of tablets	Frequency of administration
Dogs	Less than 2.7 kg (6 lb)	225 mg/ 24 mg	0.25	Once daily
Dogs	3.2-6.8 kg (7-15 lb)	225 mg/ 24 mg	0.5	Once daily
Dogs	7.3-13.6 kg (16-30 lb)	225 mg/ 24 mg	1	Once daily
Dogs	14.1-20.4 kg (31-45 lb)	225 mg/ 24 mg	1.5	Once daily

Species	Body weight*	Tablet size (SAMe/ Silybin)	Number of tablets	Frequency of administration
Dogs	20.4 kg-27.2 kg (46-60 lb)	225 mg/ 24 mg	2	Once daily
Dogs	27.7-34 kg (61-75 lb)	225 mg/ 24 mg	2.5	Once daily
Dogs	34.5-40.8 kg (76-90 lb)	225 mg/ 24 mg	3	Once daily
Dogs	41.3-47.6 kg (91-105 lb)	225 mg/ 24 mg	3.5	Once daily
Dogs	More than 47.6 kg (105 lb)	225 mg/ 24 mg	4	Once daily

*Manufacturer lists dosages per lb, not per kg.

Denamarin® Advanced Chewable Tablets[15]

Species	Body weight*	Tablet size (SAMe/ Silybin)	Number of tablets	Frequency of administration
Dogs	3.2-6.4 kg (7-14 lb)	120 mg/ 35 mg	0.25	Once daily
Dogs	6.8-11.3 kg (15-25 lb)	120 mg/ 35 mg	0.5	Once daily
Dogs	11.8-22.7 kg (26-50 lb)	120 mg/ 35 mg	1	Once daily
Dogs	23.1-38.6 kg (51-85 lb)	215 mg/ 70 mg	1	Once daily
Dogs	39-58.9 kg (86-130 lb)	215 mg/ 70 mg	1.5	Once daily
Dogs	More than 58.9 kg (130 lb)	215 mg/ 70 mg	2	Once daily

*Manufacturer lists dosages per lb, not per kg.

Monitoring

- Clinical signs (eg, changes in appetite, activity, temperament)
- Liver enzymes, bilirubin, liver function testing (eg, serum bile acids or ammonia); may require 1 to 4 months before any changes in laboratory values are noted

Client Information

- Keep tablets in original packaging until used. Do not crush or split enteric-coated tablets.
- SAMe/silybin is well tolerated in animals and typically does not have side effects.
- Give this medicine on an empty stomach, at least an hour before or 2 hours after feeding. Total daily dose may be given as a single dose or divided and given as 2 separate doses.
- For cats, follow all oral tablets with 3 to 6 mL of water to ensure tablets pass into the stomach.
- SAMe/silybin is considered a combination nutritional supplement by the FDA (not a medication). Use only the medication prescribed by your veterinarian.
- Your veterinarian will need to monitor your animal while it is taking this medication. Do not miss these important follow-up visits.

Chemistry / Synonyms

S-adenosyl-methionine (SAMe) is a naturally occurring molecule found throughout the body. Because pure SAMe is highly reactive and unstable, commercially available forms of SAMe are salt forms (eg, sulfate, sulfate *p*-toluenesulfonate [also known as tosylate], 1,4-butanedisulfonate).

Silybin (ie, silibinin, sylibin, silibide) is a flavolignan and is the most biologically active component found in silymarin, which is the medicinal extract from the seeds of milk thistle (*Silybum marianum*).

Silymarin is reportedly fairly insoluble in water but is soluble in organic solvents (eg, ethanol, dimethylsulfoxide [DMSO]).

Storage / Stability

Unless otherwise labeled, store in a cool dry place not to exceed 30°C (86°F). Keep tablets in original bottle or blister pack until used; do not discard the desiccant that comes in the bottle.

Tablets are sensitive to moisture and extreme heat and should not be split or crumbled.

Compatibility / Compounding Considerations

No specific information was noted.

Dosage Forms / Regulatory Status

VETERINARY-LABELED PRODUCTS:

The FDA considers SAMe and silymarin (silybin) to be nutritional supplements. No standards for potency, purity, safety, or efficacy have been accepted by regulatory bodies.

Specific products are marketed for use in animals, including *Denamarin®*, which is a patented product labeled for use in dogs and cats.

Enteric-Coated Tablets: *Denamarin® for Cats and Small Dogs* (SAMe 90 mg/silybin 9 mg); *Denamarin® for Medium Dogs* (SAMe 225 mg/silybin 24 mg); *Denamarin® for Large Dogs* (SAMe 425 mg/silybin 35 mg). Silybin provided as phosphatidylcholine complex.

Hard Tablets: *Denamarin® Advanced Hard Tablets for Cats and Small Dogs* (SAMe 30 mg, Silybin 9 mg); *Denamarin® Advanced Hard Tablets Medium Dogs* (SAMe 82 mg, Silybin 24 mg); *Denamarin® Advanced Hard Tablets for Cats and Small Dogs* (SAMe 172 mg, Silybin 35 mg). SAMe provided as a proprietary formulation; silybin provided as phosphatidylcholine complex

Chewable Tablets:

Denamarin® Chewable Tablets for Dogs (SAMe 225 mg/silybin 24 mg);

Denamarin® Advanced Chewable Tablets for Small to Medium Dogs (SAMe 120 mg/Silybin 35 mg); *Denamarin® Advanced Chewable Tablets for Large Dogs* (SAMe 215 mg/Silybin 70 mg). SAMe provided as a proprietary formulation; silybin provided as phosphatidylcholine complex

HUMAN-LABELED PRODUCTS: None as an FDA-approved pharmaceutical

References

For the complete list of references, see **wiley.com/go/budde/plumb**

Saline Cathartics

Magnesium Citrate, Magnesium Hydroxide, Magnesium Oxide, Magnesium Sulfate, Sodium Sulfate

Laxative/Cathartic

See also ***Magnesium Hydroxide***.

Prescriber Highlights

- Hyperosmotic agents used for constipation or to increase elimination of GI toxins
- Contraindications include dehydration and long-term use. Sodium sulfate is also contraindicated in patients with CHF or congenital megacolon.
- Use with extreme caution in patients with renal insufficiency, pre-existing water imbalance, electrolyte abnormalities, or cardiac disease.
- Adverse effects include cramping and nausea. Electrolyte disturbances are possible, particularly with repeated use. Hypermagnesemia (muscle weakness, ECG changes, and CNS effects) can occur with chronic use of magnesium salts.
- Many drug interactions are possible.

Uses/Indications

Saline cathartics (laxatives) include oral magnesium sulfate (Epsom salts), magnesium hydroxide (milk of magnesia), magnesium citrate, and sodium sulfate (Glauber's salt). Saline cathartics can be used to relieve constipation or shorten intestinal transit time to reduce the absorption of orally ingested toxicants. In small animal species, saline cathartics are rarely recommended for treating constipation or obstipation but can be used with or without activated charcoal to enhance toxin removal. Sodium sulfate is typically preferred to magnesium sulfate in small animal species.

Pharmacology/Actions

It is thought that the hyperosmotic effect of poorly absorbed magnesium cations causes water retention, stimulates stretch receptors, and enhances peristalsis in the small intestine and colon. Magnesium ions may also directly shorten transit times and increase cholecystokinin release.

Pharmacokinetics

Up to 30% of an orally administered dose of magnesium salts can be absorbed.

The onset of action of saline cathartics (characterized by a loose, watery stool) typically occurs in 3 to 12 hours after administration in monogastric animals and within 18 hours in ruminants.

Contraindications/Precautions/Warnings

Saline cathartics are contraindicated in dehydrated patients. Saline cathartics are not for long-term use. Sodium-containing laxatives are contraindicated in patients with congestive heart failure or congenital megacolon.

Saline cathartics should be used with extreme caution in patients with significant diarrhea, renal insufficiency, pre-existing water imbalance, electrolyte abnormalities, or cardiac disease, and in severely depressed animals. Routine use as a sole treatment is not recommended due to risk for volume depletion, hypotension, and electrolyte disturbances.

Adverse Effects

Adverse effects are uncommon in healthy patients but may include cramping and nausea. Electrolyte disturbances (eg, hypernatremia, hypermagnesemia) are possible but typically only occur with chronic use or overdoses. Hypermagnesemia may manifest as muscle weakness, ECG changes, or CNS depression.

Reproductive/Nursing Safety

Magnesium emulsions administered orally did not affect the stools of nursing infants, although magnesium content in breast milk was slightly elevated compared with untreated patients. In veterinary patients, magnesium-containing cathartics should be safe to use during nursing if used infrequently. Because safety has not been established in animals, this drug should only be used when the maternal benefits outweigh the potential risks to offspring.

Overdose/Acute Toxicity

An overdose of saline cathartics can result in electrolyte disturbances such as hypernatremia or hypermagnesemia. Hypermagnesemia may result in muscle weakness, ECG changes, and CNS depression. Treatment consists of monitoring and correcting fluid imbalances with parenteral fluid therapy. Concurrent furosemide may be used to enhance the renal excretion of excess magnesium. Calcium has been suggested to help antagonize the CNS effects of magnesium.

For patients that have experienced or are suspected to have experienced an overdose, consultation with a 24-hour poison consultation center specializing in providing veterinary-specific information is recommended. For general information related to overdose and toxin exposures, as well as contact information for poison control centers, refer to ***Appendix.***

Drug Interactions

All orally administered saline cathartics may alter the rate and extent of absorption of other *orally* administered drugs by shortening intestinal transit times; however, the extent of these effects has not been well characterized for individual drugs. The following drug interactions have either been reported or are theoretical in humans or animals receiving magnesium-containing oral products and may be of significance in veterinary patients receiving saline cathartics. Unless otherwise noted, use together is not necessarily contraindicated, but weigh the potential risks and perform additional monitoring when appropriate.

- **Quinidine**: Increased risk for quinidine toxicity
- **Sodium Polystyrene Sulfonate**: Increased risk for metabolic acidosis

The following drugs or drug classes may have reduced oral bioavailability if administered with magnesium-containing cathartics; separate dosages by at least 2 hours:

- **Allopurinol**
- **Captopril**
- **Digoxin**
- **Fexofenadine**
- **Fluoroquinolones** (eg, **ciprofloxacin, enrofloxacin, marbofloxacin**)
- **Gabapentin**
- **Iron**
- **Ketoconazole, Itraconazole**
- **Levothyroxine**[1]
- **Misoprostol**
- **Mycophenolate**
- **Penicillamine**
- **Quinidine**
- **Sotalol**
- **Sucralfate**
- **Tacrolimus**
- **Tetracyclines** (eg, **doxycycline, minocycline**)

Laboratory Considerations

- No specific information was noted.

Dosages

DOGS/CATS:

Cathartic to enhance toxin removal from the GI tract (extra-label):

a) **Magnesium hydroxide (milk of magnesia)**: Rarely used in small animals as a laxative but has been recommended as a cathartic for zinc phosphide ingestions at 5 – 15 mL/dog or cat PO[1]

b) **Magnesium sulfate or sodium sulfate** (extra-label): 250 mg/kg administered as a suspension in water up to a concentration of 20%. Activated charcoal (AC) 1 – 4 g/kg may also be combined with the cathartic as a suspension in water (10 times water). In cases where repeated doses of AC are indicated and magnesium sulfate is used, the cathartic should *only* be given with the initial dose of AC.[1]

HORSES:

Cathartic for plant intoxications using magnesium sulfate or sodium sulfate (extra-label): 250 – ≈500 mg/kg mixed with an activated charcoal (AC) slurry dosed at 1 – 5 g/kg (≈1 g of AC/5 mL of water). There is little need to administer a cathartic if significant diarrhea is already present.[2]

Cecal impactions using magnesium sulfate (extra-label): 1 g/kg dissolved in water and given via NG tube concomitantly with a balanced electrolyte solution IV.[3]

RUMINANTS:

Cathartic in cattle using sodium sulfate (extra-label): 500 – 750 g PO as a 6% solution via stomach tube[4]

Cathartic for plant intoxications using magnesium sulfate or sodium sulfate (extra-label): 250 – 500 mg/kg mixed in an activated charcoal (AC) slurry dosed at 1 – 5 g/kg (≈1 g of AC/5 mL water). There is little need to administer a cathartic if significant diarrhea is already present.[2]

Monitoring

- Clinical efficacy
- Hydration status
- Baseline and periodic serum electrolytes in susceptible patients, especially with high or repeated doses

Client Information

- Give this medicine as directed by your veterinarian.
- Contact your veterinarian if your animal begins vomiting.

Chemistry/Synonyms

Magnesium cation containing solutions of magnesium citrate, magnesium hydroxide, magnesium oxide, and magnesium sulfate act as saline laxatives. Magnesium citrate solutions contain magnesium 4.71 mEq/5 mL. Magnesium hydroxide contains magnesium 34.3 mEq /g and milk of magnesia contains magnesium 13.66 mEq/5 mL. One gram of magnesium sulfate (Epsom salt) contains ≈8.1 mEq of magnesium.

Sodium sulfate (hexahydrate form) occurs as large, colorless, odorless crystals or as white crystalline powder. It will effloresce in dry air and partially dissolve in its own water of crystallization at about 33°C (91°F). One gram is soluble in ≈2.5 mL of water. Sodium sulfate may also be known as E514, Glauber's Salt, natrii sulphas, natrio sulfata, or natrium sulfuricum.

Storage/Stability

Store milk of magnesia at temperatures less than 35°C (95°F), but do not freeze.

Compatibility/Compounding Considerations

No specific information was noted.

Dosage Forms/Regulatory Status

VETERINARY-LABELED PRODUCTS:

Saline cathartic products are not FDA-approved for use in veterinary species. They are available without a prescription (OTC).

HUMAN-LABELED PRODUCTS:

Saline Laxatives: **NOTE**: Many commercial products exist; below is a representative list and is not all-inclusive.

Magnesium Hydroxide Suspension (Milk of Magnesia): 400 mg/5 mL (80 mg/mL); generic; (OTC)

Magnesium Hydroxide Suspension concentrated (Milk of Magnesia concentrated): 800 mg/5 mL (160 mg/mL); generic; (OTC)

Magnesium Sulfate (Epsom Salt) Granules: 120 g, 0.5 kg (1 lb), and 2 kg (4 lb) bags; generic; (OTC)

Magnesium Citrate Solution: 1.75 g/30 mL in 296 mL bottles; generic; (OTC)

Sodium sulfate (hexahydrate) is available from chemical supply houses. **NOTE**: A 24-hour meat withdrawal is recommended as sodium sulfate is rapidly excreted.[5]

References

For the complete list of references, see **wiley.com/go/budde/plumb**

Sarolaner

(***sar***-oh-***lan***-er) *Simparica®, Simparica TRIO®*

Isoxazoline Ectoparasiticide

*See also **Selamectin/Sarolaner, Moxidectin/Moxidectin Combination Products.***

Prescriber Highlights

- ▶ Monthly chewable ectoparasiticide (insecticide/acaricide) for use in dogs and puppies 6 months of age and older weighing more than or equal to 1.3 kg (2.8 lb)
- ▶ Indicated for treatment and prevention of flea infestations and treatment and control of tick infestations
- ▶ Combination product with moxidectin and pyrantel is used in dogs as a monthly heartworm preventive that also kills adult fleas, treats and prevents flea infestation, and treats and controls tick infestation, roundworms, and intestinal hookworms.
- ▶ Extra-label use of the single-agent product for treatment of generalized demodicosis, scabies, and ear mites.
- ▶ FDA has warned that drugs in the isoxazoline class have the potential for causing neurologic adverse effects (eg, muscle tremors, ataxia, and seizures) in dogs and cats.

Uses/Indications

Sarolaner is FDA-approved for use in dogs for the treatment and prevention of flea infestations (*Ctenocephalides felis*) and for treatment and control of tick infestations (*Amblyomma americanum* [lone star tick], *Amblyomma maculatum* [Gulf Coast tick], *Dermacentor variabilis* [American dog tick], *Ixodes scapularis* [black-legged tick, also called deer tick], and *Rhipicephalus sanguineus* [brown dog tick]) for 1 month in dogs 6 months of age or older and weighing 1.3 kg (2.8 lb) or more.[1]

Sarolaner effectively treats (extra-label) dogs naturally infested with the mite species *Demodex canis*,[2] *Sarcoptes scabiei*,[3] and *Otodectes cynotis*.[4]

In dogs exposed to ticks under experimental conditions, sarolaner at label dosages prevented transmission of *Babesia canis*,[5] *Borrelia burgdorferi*, and *Anaplasma phagocytophilum*.[6] At 35 days after administration, sarolaner was 99.6% effective against *Amblyomma cajennense* nymphs (Cayenne tick),[7] 100% effective against adult *Haemaphysalis elliptica* (African yellow dog tick),[8] and more than 97% effective against *Haemaphysalis longicornis* nymphs (New Zealand cattle tick, Asian long-horned bush tick).[9] It demonstrated 100% larvicidal effect in dogs 24 hours after a single dose for *Cochliomyia hominivorax* (New World screwworm).[10]

In experimental, comparative speed-of-kill studies, sarolaner-treated dogs had significantly lower mean tick counts than afoxolaner at 8 and/or 12 hours post-treatment against *Rhipicephalus sanguineus sensu lato*[11] and *Ixodes* spp.[12,13] Similarly, sarolaner-treated dogs had lower flea counts at 8 hours after administration compared with the combination milbemycin/spinosad[14] or afoxolaner.[15] In all studies, equivalent efficacy was demonstrated at 24 hours after administration of all drugs. Sarolaner appeared to have equivalent speed-of-kill times as fluralaner against *R sanguineus sensu lato*[16,17] and *Ctenocephalides felis*.[18]

In dogs, the European label indicates sarolaner for the treatment of infestations of the tick species *Dermacentor reticulatus* (ornate cow tick), *Ixodes hexagonus* (hedgehog tick), *Ixodes ricinus* (castor bean tick), and *R sanguineus*; flea species *C felis* and *Ctenocephalides canis*; as well as *Sarcoptes scabiei* (sarcoptic mange) and *Otodectes cynotis* (ear mites).[19]

Sarolaner/selamectin is available as a topical spot-on solution for cats (8 weeks of age and older and weighing more than 1.3 kg [2.8 lb]) to treat and prevent parasitic infestations by ticks, fleas, lice, mites, and GI nematodes, and for prevention of heartworm infection. See also ***Selamectin/Sarolaner***.

Sarolaner/moxidectin/pyrantel is labeled for dogs 8 weeks of age and older and weighing 1.3 kg (2.8 lb) or more as a monthly oral treatment for prevention of heartworm disease caused by *Dirofilaria immitis*, treatment and prevention of flea infestations (*C felis*), treatment and control of tick infestations of *A americanum*, *A maculatum*, *D variabilis*, *Ixodes scapularis*, and *R sanguineus*, and for the treatment and control of roundworms (*Toxocara canis*, *Toxascaris leonina*) and hookworms (*A caninum*, *Uncinaria stenocephala*).[20]

Pharmacology/Actions

Sarolaner is an isoxazoline acaricide/insecticide that inhibits gamma-aminobutyric acid (GABA) and glutamate receptors at the neuromuscular junction in insects or acarines, resulting in uncontrolled neuromuscular activity leading to death of the parasite. Sarolaner does not interact with known insecticidal binding sites of nicotinic or other GABAergic insecticides (eg, neonicotinoids, fiproles, milbemycins, avermectins, cyclodienes).[19] Sarolaner kills adult fleas and ticks only after they have bitten and fed.

Controlled laboratory studies have demonstrated that fleas start dying 3 hours after the dose is administered. Live fleas are reduced by 96.2% or more within 8 hours. A 100% effectiveness within 24 hours of treatment has been reported, with 100% effectiveness maintained against weekly reinfestations for 35 days.[11,13] For 35 days after administration, sarolaner kills fleas before they can lay eggs.[1]

For indicated tick species, sarolaner demonstrated 99% or more effectiveness against initial infestation 48 hours after administration and maintained more than 96% effectiveness 48 hours after reinfestation for 30 days.[1]

Pharmacokinetics

After oral administration, absorption of sarolaner is extensive and rapid; mean oral bioavailability is 86% and 107% in fasted and fed dogs, respectively. Sarolaner has wide distribution with a mean volume of distribution (steady-state) of 2.81 L/kg (after IV dose of 2 mg/kg). Sarolaner is highly bound to canine plasma proteins (more than or equal to 99.9%). Clearance is low (0.12 mL/minute/kg) and the mean half-life after oral administration is 10 to 12 days. Primary route of drug elimination is thought to occur via biliary excretion of unchanged drug into the feces. Metabolism appears to be minimal.[1,19]

Contraindications/Precautions/Warnings

There are no known contraindications for the use of sarolaner; however, it is not labeled for use in dogs weighing less than 1.3 kg (2.8 lb) or less than 6 months of age, or as a single agent for oral use in cats.[1] Sarolaner may cause abnormal neurologic signs (eg, tremors, decreased conscious proprioception, ataxia, decreased or absent menace, seizures).[1] The FDA has warned that drugs in the isoxazoline class have the potential for causing neurologic adverse effects in dogs and cats, including muscle tremors, ataxia, and seizures.[21]

No adverse effects were noted after 3 times the label doses were administered to collies homozygous for the *MDR1* genetic mutation (also known as *ABCB1*-1delta).[22]

Sarolaner/moxidectin/pyrantel should be used with caution in dogs with a history of seizures or neurologic disorders. Dogs should return a negative result for heartworm infection prior to being treated with this product. This product is not an effective treatment for adult *Dirofilaria immitis* infections. Not to be used in dogs less than 8 weeks of age or weighing less than 1.3 kg (2.8 lb).[20]

Adverse Effects

Sarolaner appears to be well tolerated in the majority of dogs. In a 3-month field study in dogs, vomiting, diarrhea, inappetence, and lethargy were the most commonly reported adverse effects. Isoxazolines, including sarolaner, have been associated with neurologic adverse effects (eg, muscle tremors, ataxia, seizures) even in dogs with no known history of neurologic problems.[1,20]

Field safety studies in dogs receiving sarolaner/moxidectin/pyrantel reported vomiting (14.3%), diarrhea (13.2%), and lethargy (8.5%).[20]

Reproductive/Nursing Safety

The safety of sarolaner has not been established during pregnancy or lactation or in animals intended for breeding. Studies performed in rats and rabbits have not produced evidence of teratogenic effects.[19]

Safe use of the combination product sarolaner/moxidectin/pyrantel has not been evaluated in dogs used for breeding and those that are pregnant or lactating.[20]

Because safety has not been established in animals, this drug should only be used when the maternal benefits outweigh the potential risks to offspring.

Overdose/Acute Toxicity

In rats, the oral (acute) LD_{50} is 783 mg/kg and dermal (acute) LD_{50} is greater than 2020 mg/kg.[19] In one study, 8-week-old beagle puppies were given up to 5 times (20 mg/kg) doses PO at 28-day intervals for 10 doses. Some animals in the 3 times and 5 times groups showed transient and self-limiting neurologic signs: ataxia, lethargy, disorientation, hypersalivation, absent menace, and tremors at 3 times the labeled dose; and convulsions, tremors, and abnormal head coordination at 5 times the labeled dose. All dogs recovered without treatment.[1]

Following single oral administration at 5 times the recommended dose, sarolaner as a single agent is reportedly well tolerated in collies with the *MDR1* gene mutation (also known as *ABCB1*-1delta). No treatment-related clinical signs were observed.[1]

Eight-week-old puppies receiving 5 times the maximum recommended dose of sarolaner/moxidectin/pyrantel (*Simparica TRIO*®) did not have any clinically relevant adverse effects.[20] Collies with the *MDR1* mutation demonstrated signs of avermectin sensitivity (eg, ataxia, muscle fasciculations, mydriasis) after receiving 5 times the recommended dose of the combination product.

For patients that have experienced or are suspected to have experienced an overdose, it is strongly encouraged to consult with one of the 24-hour poison consultation centers that specialize in providing information specific for veterinary patients. For general information related to overdose and toxin exposures, as well as contact information for poison control centers, refer to ***Appendix.***

Drug Interactions

No clinically significant drug interactions have been reported to date with sarolaner or sarolaner/selamectin when used at label dosages. See also ***Moxidectin/Moxidectin Combination Products*** and ***Pyrantel*** for potential drug interactions for the sarolaner combination product containing moxidectin and pyrantel.

In one field study, 1 dog developed lethargy, ataxia while posturing to eliminate, elevated third eyelids, and inappetence 1 day after receiving sarolaner concurrently with ivermectin and pyrantel pamoate combination. Clinical signs resolved 1 day later.[1] No causation of a drug interaction should be inferred from this single case.

Dosages

DOGS:

Single-agent Product:

Label indications (label dosage; FDA-approved): Administer orally once a month at the recommended minimum dose of 2 mg/kg (0.91 mg/lb).[1]

Body weight in kg (lb)	Sarolaner (mg) per tablet	Number of tablets administered
1.3-2.5 (2.8-5.5)	5	1
2.5-5 (5.6-11)	10	1
5-10 (11.1-22)	20	1
10-20 (22.1-44)	40	1
20-40 (44.1-88)	80	1
40-60 (88.1-132)	120	1
Greater than 60 (132.1)	Administer appropriate combination of tablets	

Susceptible ectoparasites (extra-label): 2 – 4 mg/kg PO has effectively treated the following:

1. Mites:
   a. *Otodectes cynotis*: 1 or 2 doses administered 30 days apart[4,23]
   b. Generalized demodicosis: 3 to 5 monthly doses achieved parasitological cure in client-owed dogs.[2] Cure was achieved after 2 doses in an experimental (induced) infection.[23]
   c. *Sarcoptes scabiei*: 2 doses administered 30 days apart achieved parasitological cure in 100% of dogs.[3]
2. Ticks: Naturally occurring infestations with *Ixodes ricinus, Ixodes hexagonus, Rhipicephalus sanguineus,* and *Dermacentor reticulatus*: 3 monthly (as per label) doses resulted in 97% to 100% reduction of all tick species 14 days after the first dose, and 100% of dogs becoming tick-free after 90 days.[24] Experimentally induced infestation with adult *R sanguineus,*[11,16,17] *Haemaphysalis elliptica,*[8] *Amblyomma cajennense,*[7] and *Haemaphysalis longicornis* nymphs[9] also showed effectiveness with sarolaner at labeled dosages.
3. Myiasis caused by *Cochliomyia hominivorax* (New World screwworm) larvae: A single dose of sarolaner 2 mg/kg had a 100% larvicidal effect after 24 hours.[10]

Prevention of tick-borne disease (extra-label): 2 – 4 mg/kg PO in single doses under laboratory conditions prevented transmission of *Babesia canis*[5], as well as *Borrelia burgdorferi* and *Anaplasma phagocytophilum.*[6]

Combination Products:

Sarolaner/Moxidectin/Pyrantel (label dosage; FDA-approved): Each tablet is formulated to provide minimum dosages of 1.2 mg/kg (0.54 mg/lb) sarolaner, 24 µg/kg (0.011 mg/lb) moxidectin, and 5 mg/kg (2.27 mg/lb) pyrantel (as pamoate salt) PO with or without food once monthly.[20]

Body weight in kg (lb)	Sarolaner (mg) per tablet	Moxidectin (mg) per tablet	Pyrantel (mg) per tablet	Number of tablets administered
1.3-2.5 (2.8-5.5)	3	0.06	12.5	1
2.5-5 (5.6 -11)	6	0.12	25	1
5-10 (11.1-22)	12	0.24	50	1
10-20 (22.1-44)	24	0.48	100	1
20-40 (44.1-88)	48	0.96	200	1
40 -60 (88.1-132)	72	1.44	300	1
Greater than 60 (132.1)	Administer appropriate combination of tablets			

CATS:

See ***Selamectin/Sarolaner***

Monitoring

- Efficacy of parasiticide activity
- Adverse effects (eg, muscle tremors, ataxia, seizures)

Client Information

- Treatment may start at any time of the year. In areas where fleas and ticks are common year-round, monthly treatment should continue for the entire year without stopping.
- Prior to being treated with the combination product sarolaner/moxidectin/pyrantel, dogs should return a negative test for heartworm infection.
- Tablets are chewable, palatable, and readily consumed by dogs. If the dog does not take the tablet voluntarily, the tablet can also be given with food.
- Be sure your dog consumes the complete dose. Watch your dog for a few minutes after giving the dose to be sure it does not spit out any part of the dose.
- Sarolaner kills adult fleas and ticks only after they have bitten your animal but before the fleas or ticks can lay eggs or transmit disease. Existing flea eggs will hatch and must feed in order to be killed. Keep this medicine out of the reach of other animals and children. Keep the tablets in the original packaging until you are ready to give the medicine to your animal.
- Report any side effects, including tremors, difficulty walking, or seizures, to your veterinarian as soon as possible.

Chemistry/Synonyms

Sarolaner is in the isoxazoline class of parasiticides. Its chemical name is 1-(5'-((5S)-5-(3,5-Dichloro-4-fluorophenyl)-5-(trifluoromethyl)-4,5-dihydroisoxazol-3-yl)-3'-Hspiro(azetidine-3,1'-(2)benzofuran)-1-yl)-2-(methylsulfonyl)ethanone. The commercially available product is the *S*-enantiomer. The CAS registry number is 1398609-39-6 and ATC vet code is QP53BX06.

The commercially available chewable tablets also contain the excipients hydrolyzed soy protein, corn starch, sucrose, wheat germ, anhydrous dibasic calcium phosphate, corn syrup, and gelatin.[1,19]

Sarolaner may also be known by its trade names, which also include the following combination products: *Revolution® Plus*, *Simparica®*, *Simparica TRIO®*.

Storage/Stability

Store at or below 30°C (86°F) with excursions permitted up to 40°C (104°F).

Compatibility/Compounding Considerations

No known incompatibilities.

Dosage Forms/Regulatory Status

VETERINARY-LABELED PRODUCTS:

Single-agent Products:

Sarolaner Chewable (flavored) Tablets: 5 mg, 10 mg, 20 mg, 40 mg, 80 mg, and 120 mg. Each tablet size is available in packages of 1, 3, or 6 tablets. *Simparica®* (NADA 141-452; approved by FDA); (Rx)

Combination Products:

Sarolaner with Moxidectin and Pyrantel Pamoate Chewable (flavored) Tablets for dogs: 1.3 to 2.5 kg (2.8 to 5.5 lb): moxidectin 0.06 mg, pyrantel pamoate 12.5 mg, and sarolaner 3 mg; 2.5 to 5 kg (5.6 to 11 lb): moxidectin 0.12 mg, pyrantel pamoate 25 mg, and sarolaner 6 mg; 5 to 10 kg (11.1 to 22 lb): moxidectin 0.24 mg, pyrantel pamoate 50 mg, and sarolaner 12 mg; 10 to 20 kg (22.1 to 44 lb): moxidectin 0.48 mg, pyrantel pamoate 100 mg, and sarolaner 24 mg; 20 to 40 kg (44.1 to 88 lb): moxidectin 0.96 mg, pyrantel pamoate 200 mg, and sarolaner 48 mg; 40 to 60 kg (88.1 to 132 lb): moxidectin 1.44 mg, pyrantel pamoate 300 mg, and sarolaner 72 mg. Each tablet size is available in packages of 1, 3, or 6 tablets; *Simparica TRIO®* (Rx). Approved for use in dogs 8 weeks of age and older that weigh 1.3 kg (2.8 lb) or greater. NADA 141-521

Sarolaner and Selamectin Topical Solution: 60 mg/mL selamectin and 10 mg/mL sarolaner in 0.25 mL, 0.5 mL, and 1 mL tubes, available in boxes of 1, 3, or 6 single-dose tubes; *Revolution® Plus*; (Rx). Each tube provides a minimum of 6 mg/kg selamectin and 1 mg/kg sarolaner. For use on cats and kittens 8 weeks of age or older weighing at least 1.3 kg (2.8 lb). NADA# 141-502. See ***Selamectin/Sarolaner***.

HUMAN-LABELED PRODUCTS: NONE

References

For the complete list of references, see **wiley.com/go/budde/plumb**

Selamectin

(sell-a-***mek***-tin) *Revolution®*

Avermectin (Topical) Antiparasitic

See also ***Selamectin/Sarolaner***.

Prescriber Highlights

- FDA-approved as a monthly endo- and ectoparasiticide for use in dogs and cats
- Some extra-label indications only require one-time dosing while more frequent dosing may be necessary for others.
- Adverse effect profile appears minimal when used as labeled. Oral exposure should be avoided.

Uses/Indications

Topical selamectin is indicated for the prevention and control of flea infestations (*Ctenocephalides felis*), prevention of heartworm disease (*Dirofilaria immitis*), and the treatment and control of ear mites (*Otodectes cynotis*) in dogs 6 weeks of age or older and cats 8 weeks of age or older.[1] Additionally, in dogs, it is indicated for treatment and control of sarcoptic mange (*Sarcoptes scabiei*) and control of tick infestations (*Dermacentor variabilis*). In cats, it is indicated for treatment and control of hookworms (*Ancylostoma tubaeforme*) and roundworms (*Toxocara cati*). A systematic review of treatments for ear mites in cats found fair evidence for recommending topical selamectin.[2]

Selamectin is labeled as not effective against adult heartworms or for clearing circulating microfilariae, but it has some efficacy with prolonged, continuous administration.[3]

Topical selamectin has been successfully used extra label to treat a variety of ectoparasites in small animal species, including notoedric mange (*Notoedres cati*); nasal mites in dogs (*Pneumonyssoides caninum*); cheyletiellosis in dogs, cats, and rabbits; and cordylobiolosis (cutaneous myiasis, *Cordylobia anthropophaga*) in dogs.

Selamectin has not been successful for treating generalized demodicosis; other treatments (eg, isoxazolines) are preferred.

Pharmacology/Actions

Like other compounds in its class, selamectin is believed to act by enhancing chloride permeability or enhancing the release of gamma amino butyric acid (GABA) at presynaptic neurons. GABA acts as an inhibitory neurotransmitter and blocks the postsynaptic stimulation of the adjacent neuron in nematodes or the muscle fiber in arthropods. By stimulating the release of GABA, selamectin causes paralysis and eventual death of the parasite. As liver flukes and tapeworms do not use GABA as a peripheral nerve transmitter, selamectin is unlikely to be effective against these parasites.

Pharmacokinetics

After topical administration to dogs, ≈5% of the drug is bioavailable and peak plasma concentrations occur ≈3 days later.[4] Selamectin bioavailability may be higher in female dogs.[5] Elimination half-life after topical administration is ≈11 days.

After topical administration to cats, ≈75% of the drug is bioavailable and peak plasma concentration occur ≈15 hours later.[4] Peak concentrations may be 64 times those in dogs. Elimination half-life after topical administration is ≈8 days.

In rabbits given topical selamectin at doses of 10 or 20 mg/kg, mean terminal half-life was slightly less than 1 day. Maximum plasma concentrations of selamectin were 91.7 ng/mL (10 mg/kg) and 304.2 ng/mL (20 mg/kg).[6]

The persistence of selamectin in the body is believed to be due to the drug forming reservoirs in skin sebaceous glands. It is secreted into the intestine to kill susceptible endoparasites in cats.

Contraindications/Precautions/Warnings

The manufacturer recommends caution when using in sick, underweight, or debilitated dogs or cats. At labeled doses of selamectin, dogs positive for the *MDR1* mutation (also known as *ABCB1*-1delta; eg, collies, Australian shepherds, shelties, long-haired whippets) should tolerate the medication, but use cautiously. Higher doses may cause neurological toxicity in these dogs.

Adverse Effects

In field trials (limited numbers of animals), adverse effects were rare. Approximately 1% of cats showed a transient, localized alopecia at the area of administration. Other effects reported (less than or equal to 0.5% incidence) include diarrhea, vomiting, muscle tremors, anorexia, pruritus/urticaria, erythema, lethargy, salivation, and tachypnea. Rarely, seizures and ataxia have been reported in dogs. Adverse effects are more likely after oral exposure to selamectin.

Reproductive/Nursing Safety

Selamectin appears to be safe to use in pregnant or lactating dogs or cats.[1] However, because safety has not been established in animals, this drug should only be used when the maternal benefits outweigh the potential risks to offspring.

Overdose/Acute Toxicity

Dogs: Oral overdoses of the topical product up to 15 mg/kg did not cause adverse effects except for transient ataxia in 1 avermectin-sensitive collie after receiving a 5 mg/kg oral dose[1] ; hypersalivation and polydipsia have been observed. Topical overdoses (10 times the label dosage) to puppies caused no adverse effects; topical overdoses to avermectin-sensitive collies caused salivation. Selamectin was also administered at 3 times the recommended dose to heartworm-infected dogs, and no adverse effects were observed.

Cats: Oral ingestion of the topical product may cause hypersalivation and vomiting[1] ; anorexia and lethargy may also be observed. Topical overdoses of up to 10 times the label dosage caused no observable adverse effects in 6-week-old kittens.

For patients that have experienced or are suspected to have experienced an overdose, consultation with a 24-hour poison control center specializing in providing veterinary-specific information is recommended. For general information related to overdose and toxin exposures, as well as contact information for poison control centers, refer to ***Appendix.***

Drug Interactions

No drug interactions have been documented. In controlled clinical studies, selamectin was used safely in animals receiving other frequently used veterinary products such as vaccines, anthelmintics, antiparasitics, antibiotics, steroids, collars, shampoos, and dips.

Caution is advised if using other drugs that can inhibit p-glycoprotein. Those dogs at risk for the *MDR1* mutation (also known as *ABCB1*-1delta; eg, collies, Australian shepherds, shelties, long-haired whippets, "white feet" breeds) should probably not receive selamectin with the following drugs and drug classes, unless confirmed to not possess the mutation:

- **Amiodarone**
- **Carvedilol**
- **Clarithromycin**
- **Cyclosporine**
- **Diltiazem**
- **Erythromycin**
- **Itraconazole**
- **Ketoconazole**
- **Quinidine**
- **Spironolactone**
- **Tamoxifen**
- **Verapamil**

Laboratory Considerations

- None were reported.

Doses

DOGS:

Labeled indications (label dosage; FDA-approved): For prophylaxis of dirofilariasis, it is suggested to review the guidelines published by the American Heartworm Society at www.heartwormsociety.org for more information. The recommended minimum topical dose is 6 mg/kg[1]; dosed based on body weight (see table below). **NOTE**: Dogs weighing greater than 59.1 kg (130 lb) should receive the appropriate combinations of tubes. Dosing frequency: Heartworm prevention, flea control = monthly; *Dermacentor variabilis* ticks = monthly (if heavy infestations, may repeat 2 weeks after the first dose); ear mites, *Sarcoptes* spp = once, repeat in one month if necessary. See package for specific instructions on administration technique.

Body weight in kg (lb)	mg selamectin/ tube	mg/mL	Volume (mL)
Up 2.3 (up to 5)	15	60	0.25
2.3-4.5 (5.1-10)	30	120	0.25
4.6-9.1 (10.1-20)	60	120	0.5
9.1-18.2 (20.1-40)	120	120	1
18.2-38.6 (40.1-85)	240	120	2
38.7-59.1 (85.1-130)	360	120	3

Sarcoptic mange (extra-label): 6 – 13 mg/kg topically every 2 weeks for 4 to 6 treatments[7]

Nasal mites in dogs (*Pneumonyssoides caninum*) (extra-label): 6 – 24 mg/kg topically for 3 times at 2-week intervals[8]

Cheyletiellosis (extra-label): 6 – 12 mg/kg topically every other week for a total of 4 treatments[9]

Biting lice (extra-label): 6 mg/kg topically once[10]

***Cordylobia* spp** (extra-label): 6 mg/kg topically once, repeat monthly for control[11]

CATS:

Labeled indications (label dosage; FDA-approved): The recommended minimum topical dose is 6 mg/kg[1], dosed based on body weight (see table below). **NOTE**: Cats weighing greater than 10 kg (22 lb) should receive the appropriate combinations of tubes. Dosing frequency: Heartworm prevention, flea control = monthly; ear mites = once, repeat in one month if necessary; hookworms, roundworms = once. See package for specific instructions on administration technique.

Body weight in kg (lb)	mg selamectin/ tube	mg/mL	Volume (mL)
Up to 2.3 (up to 5)	15	60	0.25
4.5-6.8 (5.1-15)	45	60	0.75
6.9-10 (15.1-22)	60	60	1

Ancylostoma ceylanicum (extra-label): 6 – 12 mg/kg topically once[12]

Cheyletiellosis (extra-label): 6 – 12 mg/kg topically once monthly for a total of 3 treatments[7]

Notoedric (face/head) mange (*Notoedres cati*) (extra-label): 6 mg/kg topically once[13]

Biting lice (extra-label): 6 mg/kg topically once[10]

FERRETS:

Heartworm prevention (extra-label): 18 mg/kg topically every 30 days[14]

Ear mites (*Otodectes* ***cynotis***) (extra-label): 45 mg/ferret (NOT mg/kg) topically every 30 days

Sarcoptes scabiei (extra-label): 15 mg/kg topically[15]

SMALL MAMMALS:

Rabbits; ear mites (*Psoroptes cuniculi*) (extra-label): 6 – 18 mg/kg topically[16]

Rabbits; psoroptic mange, sarcoptic mange, *Cheyletiella* spp (extra-label): 6 – 18 mg/kg topically every 30 days. *Cheyletiella* spp may require treatment as high as 20 mg/kg repeated every 2 to 4 weeks[17–19]

Rabbits; fleas (*Ctenocephalides felis, Ctenocephalides canis*) (extra-label): Results of a safety, efficacy and pharmacokinetic study suggested that topical administration at 20 mg/kg every 7 days is efficacious; further studies are needed to assess long-term safety in rabbits following repeated applications.[6]

Guinea pigs; *Trixacarus caviae* mange (extra-label): Results from the study suggested that a single topical application of selamectin 15 mg/kg can eliminate *T caviae* mites from guinea pigs within 30 days.[20]

Guinea pigs; ear mites (extra-label): 6 – 10 mg/kg topically[21]

Monitoring

- Clinical efficacy
- Owner compliance with treatment regimen

Client Information

- Follow label directions for administration technique. Part hair and apply directly to skin; do not massage into skin, and do not apply if hair coat is wet. Because the product contains alcohol, do not apply to broken skin.
- Ensure entire contents of the tube are applied.
- Stiff or clumped hair, discoloration of hair, or a powdery residue may be seen after administration. This is temporary and does not affect the safety or efficacy of the product.
- Wait 2 hours or more after applying to bathe the animal (or allow to go swimming).
- Avoid contact with animal while the application site is wet.
- Avoid getting the product on human skin; if contact occurs, wash off immediately. If eye contact occurs, flush eyes with copious amounts of water. If ingestion occurs, contact a physician immediately.
- Dispose of empty tubes in regular household refuse.
- Do not expose to flame, as the product is flammable.

Chemistry/Synonyms

A semi-synthetic avermectin, selamectin occurs as a white hygroscopic powder. It is practically insoluble in water, soluble in acetone and freely soluble in isopropyl alcohol. Selamectin is commercially available as a colorless to yellow solution (flammable).

Selamectin may also be known as UK-124114, *Revolution*®, *Paradyne*® or *Stronghold*®, *Revolt*®, *Selarid*®, *Selaspot*®, or *Senergy*®.

Storage/Stability

The commercially available solution should be stored below 30°C (86°F). Keep away from flame or other igniters.

Compatibility/Compounding Considerations

No specific information was noted.

Dosage Forms/Regulatory Status

VETERINARY-LABELED PRODUCTS:

Selamectin Topical Solution for Cats; *Revolution*®, generic; (Rx). For use in cats 8 weeks of age and older. For cats over 10 kg (22 lb) use the appropriate combination of tubes. NADA 141-152.

Up to 2.3 kg (5 lb), Pkg. Color: mauve. 15 mg/tube. Tube volume: 0.25 mL

4.5 to 6.8 kg (5.1 to 15 lb), Pkg. Color: blue. 45 mg/tube. Tube volume: 0.75 mL

6.9 to 10 kg (15.1 to 22 lb), Pkg. Color: taupe. 60 mg/tube. Tube volume: 1 mL

Selamectin Topical Solution for Dogs; *Revolution*®, generic; (Rx). For use in dogs 6 weeks of age and older. For dogs over 59.1 kg (131 lb), use the appropriate combination of tubes. NADA 141-152.

Up to 2.3 kg (5 lb), Pkg. Color: mauve. 15 mg/tube. Tube volume: 0.25 mL

2.3 to 4.5 kg (5.1 to 10 lb), Pkg. Color: purple. 30 mg/tube. Tube volume: 0.25 mL

4.6 to 9.1 kg (10.1 to 20 lb), Pkg. Color: brown. 60 mg/tube. Tube volume: 0.5 mL

9.1 to 18.2 kg (20.1 to 40 lb), Pkg. Color: red. 120 mg/tube. Tube volume: 1 mL

18.2 to 38.6 kg (40.1 to 85 lb), Pkg. Color: teal. 240 mg/tube. Tube volume: 2 mL

38.7 to 59.1 kg (85.1 to 130 lb), Pkg. Color: plum. 360 mg/tube. Total volume: 3 mL

HUMAN-LABELED PRODUCTS: NONE

References

For the complete list of references, see **wiley.com/go/budde/plumb**

Selamectin/Sarolaner

(sell-a-***mek***-tin; ***sar***-oh-***lan***-er) *Revolution® Plus*

Avermectin Antiparasitic and Isoxazoline Ectoparasiticide (Topical)

See also ***Selamectin*** and ***Sarolaner***

Prescriber Highlights

- ▶ Topical combination antiparasitic agent FDA-approved for use in cats and kittens 8 weeks of age and older, and weighing 1.3 kg (2.8 lb) or more
- ▶ Monthly heartworm preventive that also kills adult fleas; treats and prevents flea infestation; and treats and controls tick infestation, ear mites, roundworms, and intestinal hookworms
- ▶ Use with caution on cats that are debilitated and underweight for their size and age.
- ▶ Use with caution in cats with a history of neurologic disease.
- ▶ FDA has warned that drugs in the isoxazoline class have the potential to cause neurologic adverse effects (eg, muscle tremors, ataxia, seizures) in dogs and cats.
- ▶ Adverse effects may include lethargy, anorexia, alopecia, administration site reactions, and other skin changes.

Uses/Indications

The combination selamectin/sarolaner topical solution is FDA-approved for monthly use in cats and kittens 8 weeks of age and older and weighing 1.3 kg (2.8 lb) or more.[1] This combination is indicated for the prevention of heartworm disease (*Dirofilaria immitis*), treatment and prevention of flea infestations (*Ctenocephalides felis*), and the treatment and control of ear mite (*Otodectes cynotis*) infestations, roundworm (*Toxocara cati*) and intestinal hookworm (*Ancylostoma tubaeforme*) infections, and tick infestations with *Ixodes scapularis* (black-legged tick), *Amblyomma maculatum* (Gulf Coast tick), and *Dermacentor variabilis* (American dog tick) for one month. Selamectin/sarolaner topical solution prevented transmission of the parasite *Cytauxzoon felis* from lone star ticks under experimental conditions.[2] Monthly selamectin/sarolaner application was more consistently effective against *Ixodes ricinus* than a single application of fluralaner topical solution when assessed at 8 and 12 weeks after fluralaner application.[3] The combination of selamectin/sarolaner has been shown to be effective at eradicating natural flea infestations in a heavy flea-challenged environment[4] and under a range of geological conditions, including tropical and subtropical environments.[5] In one case report, once monthly administration of selamectin/sarolaner applied topically to the back of the neck was effective at treating otodemodicosis caused by *Demodex cati*. Complete resolution was seen after 4 doses.[6]

An experimental combination of selamectin 6 mg/kg and sarolaner 2 mg/kg (double the sarolaner dose of approved products) was effective at preventing the development of a macrocyclic lactone resistant strain of *D immitis*. In 10 cats that were infected with L3 larvae and then given monthly selamectin/sarolaner for 3 consecutive doses, no adult heartworms were found in any cat at study conclusion; however, selamectin alone was also highly effective. It is also uncertain whether macrocyclic lactone resistance can be reversible, as the strain of *D immitis* used had not been exposed to any macrocyclic lactones for ≈2.5 years prior to this study.[7]

In other countries, the selamectin/sarolaner combination products are also indicated for the treatment of biting lice infestations (*Felicola subrostratus*).[8–10]

Pharmacology/Actions

Selamectin is thought to enhance chloride permeability or the release of gamma-aminobutyric acid (GABA) at presynaptic neurons. GABA acts as an inhibitory neurotransmitter and blocks postsynaptic stimulation of the adjacent neuron in nematodes or the muscle fiber in arthropods. Stimulating the release of GABA causes paralysis and eventual death of the parasite. Selamectin is likely ineffective against liver flukes and tapeworms, as they do not use GABA as a peripheral nerve transmitter.

Sarolaner is an isoxazoline acaricide/insecticide that inhibits GABA and glutamate receptors at the neuromuscular junction in insects and acarines, which results in uncontrolled neuromuscular activity leading to death. Sarolaner does not interact with known insecticidal binding sites of nicotinic or other GABAergic insecticides (eg, neonicotinoids, fiproles, milbemycins, avermectins, cyclodienes).[11]

Under experimental conditions, a single application of selamectin and sarolaner topical solution starts killing adult fleas within 6 to 12 hours for up to 5 weeks.[12] Adult fleas are killed before eggs can be laid. Most ticks (90% to 95%) are killed within 24 to 72 hours post-infestation for up to one month after application.[13]

Labels in other countries state that the selamectin and sarolaner topical combination solution has ovicidal and larvicidal action against fleas.[8–10]

Pharmacokinetics

Bioavailability is ≈40% for selamectin (elimination half-life, ≈12.5 days) and 58% for sarolaner (elimination half-life, 41.5 days) after topical administration.[1] When administered monthly, drug accumulation will plateau after the third selamectin and sixth sarolaner dose. Elimination occurs primarily via hepatobiliary excretion, and ≈50% of the dose is excreted in the feces.

Contraindications/Precautions/Warnings

There are no known contraindications for the use of selamectin/sarolaner[1]; however, the UK label lists contraindications for cats with concomitant disease, hypersensitivity, and that are debilitated and underweight for their age and size.[9] Use product with caution when treating cats with a history of neurologic disease.[1] The FDA has warned that drugs in the isoxazoline class have the potential to cause neurologic adverse effects in dogs and cats, such as muscle tremors, ataxia, and seizures, including in animals that do not have a history of neurologic disease.[14]

Do not apply when the cat's hair coat is wet. Do not apply directly to the ear canal. The product is highly flammable, so it is important to keep treated animals away from heat, sparks, open flames, or other sources of ignition for at least 30 minutes after application or until the site of application is dry.[15]

In humans, reactions including redness, hives, and itching have rarely been reported following accidental dermal exposure; children should not be allowed to play with treated cats for 4 hours after application.[9]

Adverse Effects

Adverse effects were uncommon in field trials using a limited number of animals. In a field study that evaluated the safety and efficacy of selamectin and sarolaner topical solution in treating fleas, the following adverse effects were reported: lethargy (4.3%), nonapplication site skin lesions (3.5%), anorexia (3.2%), pruritus (2.5%), conjunctivitis (2.5%), and application site skin changes or alopecia (2.5%).[16] Adverse effects reported in other field studies included emesis, diarrhea, ataxia, seizures, and tremors.[1]

Reproductive/Nursing Safety

Safe use of selamectin and sarolaner topical solution has not been evaluated in breeding, pregnant, or lactating cats; however, selamectin is considered safe for use in breeding, pregnant, or lactating cats.[1,8–10,15] Laboratory studies of sarolaner in rats and rabbits have not shown evidence of teratogenic effects, but safety in cats has not been established.

Because safety has not been established in animals, this drug should only be used when the maternal benefits outweigh the potential risks to offspring.

Overdose/Acute Toxicity

The death of a single cat exposed to 3.75 times the label dose under experimental conditions was determined to be caused by thrombocytopenia and internal hemorrhage.[1] The role of selamectin and sarolaner in the cat's death was undetermined and no other significant changes were noted in other subjects that received up to 5 times the labeled dose. Oral ingestion of the highest recommended topical dose of selamectin and sarolaner topical solution may cause vomiting, soft stools, reduced food intake, mild tremors, and salivation.

Topical overdoses up to 10 times the label dose of selamectin (without sarolaner) caused no observable adverse effects in kittens 6 weeks of age.[17] Commonly reported findings in cats with an overdose recorded in decreasing frequency included hypersalivation, licking lips, vomiting, anorexia, depression, and lethargy.

In rats, the oral (acute) LD_{50} for sarolaner is 783 mg/kg and dermal (acute) LD_{50} is greater than 2020 mg/kg.[11]

For patients that have experienced or are suspected of having experienced an overdose, consultation with a 24-hour poison consultation center specializing in providing veterinary-specific information is recommended. For general information related to overdose and toxin exposures, as well as contact information for poison control centers, refer to ***Appendix.***

Drug Interactions

No drug interactions have been documented. In controlled field studies, selamectin and sarolaner topical solution, as well as selamectin and sarolaner individually, were used safely on animals receiving other frequently used veterinary products (eg, vaccines, cestocide anthelmintics, antibiotics, sedatives, anesthetics, opioids, corticosteroids, NSAIDs).[1]

Laboratory Considerations

- None reported

Dosages

CATS:

Label indications (FDA-approved): The recommended minimum topical dose is selamectin 6 mg/kg and sarolaner 1 mg/kg[1]; dosed based on body weight according to table below. Administer monthly for heartworm prevention, flea control, and ticks. Administer once as a single dose for ear mite, hookworms, and roundworms. Cats weighing over 10 kg (22 lb) should be treated with the appropriate combination of tubes. See package for specific instructions on administration technique.

Body weight in kg (lb)	Tube cap color	Tube volume (mL)	Selamectin (mg/tube)	Sarolaner (mg/tube)
1.3-2.5 (2.8-5.5)	Gold	0.25	15	2.5
2.6-5 (5.6-11)	Orange	0.5	30	5
5.1-10 (11.1-22)	Green	1	60	10
Over 10 (22)	Use the appropriate combination of tubes			

Treatment of chewing lice (extra-label): Apply topically based on body weight dosage listed on the product label, corresponding to a minimum of selamectin 6 mg/kg and sarolaner 1 mg/kg) once as a single dose.[15]

Monitoring

- Clinical efficacy (eg, heartworm antigen testing, fecal float, FECR testing)
- Owner compliance with treatment regimen

Client Information

- Treatment may be started any time of the year and should continue year-round. If not administered year-round, monthly treatment should begin at least 1 month before fleas and/or ticks become active and within 1 month of the first exposure to mosquitos. Monthly treatment should continue until the end of the mosquito season, with the final dose given within 1 month of the last exposure to mosquitos.
- Fleas and ticks need to start feeding on the animal before they will die.
- Read label directions for full administration technique. Part the cat's hair and apply directly to the skin in one spot at the base of the neck, in front of the shoulder blades.
- Clumping or spiking of the hair, greasiness, and dry white deposits may occur; these are normal and do not affect the medication's safety or efficacy.
- Do not massage medication into the skin
- Do not apply to wet hair or coat, to broken skin, or inside the ear canal.
- Do not bathe the cat for at least 24 hours after application.
- Avoid contact with human skin and avoid contact with the animal while the application site is wet. If contact occurs, wash the affected area immediately.
- This product is flammable and should not be exposed to flames. Empty tubes may be disposed in regular household refuse.
- Report any side effects, including nerve-related effects (eg, tremors, difficulty walking, seizures), to your veterinarian.

Chemistry/Synonyms

A semi-synthetic avermectin, selamectin occurs as a white hygroscopic powder. It is practically insoluble in water, soluble in acetone, and freely soluble in isopropyl alcohol. Selamectin is commercially available as a flammable, colorless to yellow solution.

Selamectin may also be known as UK-124114, *Revolution®*, *Paradyne®*, or *Stronghold®*.

Sarolaner is an isoxazoline class of parasiticides. Sarolaner may also be known as *Simparica®*.

Storage/Stability

The commercially available solution should be stored at or below 30°C (86°F) and should be kept away from flames or other igniters.

Compatibility/Compounding Considerations

No specific information noted.

Dosage Forms/Regulatory Status

VETERINARY-LABELED PRODUCTS:

Selamectin and Sarolaner Topical Solution: 60 mg/mL selamectin and 10 mg/mL sarolaner in 0.25 mL, 0.5 mL, and 1 mL tubes; *Revolution® Plus*; (Rx). NADA# 141-502

HUMAN-LABELED PRODUCTS: NONE

References

For the complete list of references, see **wiley.com/go/budde/plumb**

Selegiline

L-deprenyl

(se-*le*-ji-leen) *Anipryl®, Eldepryl®*

Monoamine Oxidase Inhibitor (MAOI)

Prescriber Highlights

- May be useful for cognitive dysfunction syndrome (CDS) in dogs or cats, or for canine hyperadrenocorticism (efficacy in doubt for hyperadrenocorticism)
- May require 2 to 6 weeks of administration to show clinical improvement for CDS
- Adverse effects include vomiting and diarrhea; CNS effects manifested by restlessness, repetitive movements, or lethargy; salivation and anorexia. Diminished hearing/deafness, pruritus, licking, shivers/trembles/shakes are possible.
- Many serious drug interactions are possible.

Uses/Indications

Selegiline is FDA-approved for use in dogs to control the clinical signs associated with canine cognitive dysfunction syndrome (CDS; "old dog dementia") as well as the clinical signs associated with uncomplicated canine pituitary-dependent hyperadrenocorticism (PDH). Although selegiline is FDA-approved, its use for PDH is controversial, as clinical studies evaluating its efficacy have shown disappointing results.[1,2] Selegiline may have a role in treating dogs with chronic anxiety, particularly those that have high prolactin levels.[3] Combined with a benzodiazepine and a beta-blocker such as propranolol, selegiline may be particularly useful in treating social or noise phobias.

Selegiline may be of use in feline cognitive dysfunction syndrome.[4]

In humans, selegiline's primary indication is for the adjunctive treatment of Parkinson disease.[5]

Pharmacology/Actions

Selegiline's mechanism of action for treatment of pituitary-dependent hyperadrenocorticism (PDH) is complex; a somewhat simplified explanation follows: In the hypothalamus, corticotropin-releasing hormone (CRH) acts to stimulate the production of ACTH in the pituitary, and dopamine acts to inhibit the release of ACTH. As dogs age, there is a tendency for a decrease in dopamine production that can contribute to the development of PDH.

As dopamine is metabolized by monoamine oxidase-B (MAO-B) and selegiline irreversibly inhibits MAO-B, dopamine concentrations can be increased at receptor sites after selegiline administration.[5] In theory, this allows the concentration of dopamine and CRH to be in balance in the hypothalamus, thereby reducing the amount of ACTH produced and, ultimately, cortisol.

Although selegiline is labeled as a MAO-B inhibitor, at higher-than-label dosages, the drug loses its MAO-B specificity and also inhibits MAO-A. Two of the 3 metabolites of selegiline are amphetamine and methamphetamine. These metabolites may contribute to both the efficacy and the adverse effects of the drug.

Pharmacokinetics

There is only limited information on the pharmacokinetics of selegiline in dogs. A study done in 4 dogs showed that selegiline was absorbed rapidly and had an absolute bioavailability of ≈10%.[6] The volume of distribution of the central compartment was measured at ≈7 L/kg. Terminal half-life was ≈1 hour.

In humans, selegiline pharmacokinetics have wide interpatient variability. The drug has a high first pass effect where extensive metabolism to N-desmethylselegiline, L-methamphetamine, and L-amphetamine occurs.[5] Each of these metabolites is active. N-desmethylselegiline inhibits monoamine oxidase-B (MAO-B). The other 2 metabolites are CNS stimulants and do not inhibit MAO-B. The drug is excreted in the urine, primarily as conjugated and unconjugated metabolites.

Contraindications/Precautions/Warnings

Selegiline is contraindicated in patients that are known to be hypersensitive to it. In humans, severe CNS toxicity has resulted from concurrent use of selegiline with certain medications (eg, antidepressants, meperidine, tramadol), and some combinations are considered contraindicated. See ***Drug Interactions.***

Selegiline should only be used to treat hyperadrenocorticism that is of pituitary origin.[7] Be sure to confirm the diagnosis before starting therapy.

During clinical trials, 3 dogs showed an increase in aggression while on selegiline[7]; therefore, it is not recommended for the treatment of aggression or other behavioral problems aside from those associated with canine cognitive dysfunction.

Selegiline has not been tested for safety in animals with debilitating diseases other than hyperadrenocorticism[7]; use with caution.

Do not confuse selegiline with sertraline.

Adverse Effects

Adverse effects reported in dogs include vomiting, diarrhea, CNS effects manifested by restlessness, disorientation, aggression, repetitive movements or lethargy, salivation, and anorexia. Should GI effects be a problem, discontinue the drug for a few days and then restart it at a lower dose. Diminished hearing/deafness, pruritus, licking, and shivers/trembles/shakes have also been reported. The manufacturer advises to observe animals carefully for atypical responses.

Adverse effects that have been reported in humans include nausea (10%), hallucinations, confusion, depression, loss of balance, insomnia, and hypersexuality.[5] These effects are noted because of their subjective nature and if they occur, they could help explain untoward behavioral changes in canine patients.

Because selegiline could potentially be abused by humans, veterinarians should be alert for the potential for drug diversion.

Reproductive/Nursing Safety

Safety of selegiline in pregnant, breeding, or lactating animals has not been established. Rat studies have not demonstrated overt teratogenicity.

It is not known whether selegiline is excreted in maternal milk.

Because safety has not been established in animals, this drug should only be used when the maternal benefits outweigh the potential risks to offspring.

Overdose/Acute Toxicity

Oral LD_{50} in laboratory animals was ≈200 – 445 mg/kg.[8,9] In limited data, dogs that received 3 times the labeled doses showed signs of decreased weight, salivation, decreased pupillary response, panting, stereotypic behaviors, and decreased skin elasticity (dehydration).[7] Overdoses, if severe, should be treated with appropriate GI decontamination and supportive treatments.

For patients that have experienced or are suspected to have experienced an overdose, consultation with a 24-hour poison consultation center specializing in providing veterinary-specific information is recommended. For general information related to overdose and toxin exposures, as well as contact information for poison control centers, refer to ***Appendix.***

Drug Interactions

Evaluating the potential for drug interactions for selegiline in dogs and cats is problematic. There is a plethora of significant interactions with monoamine oxidase inhibitors in humans for selegiline, but because there are significant species differences in quantities and locations of monoamine oxidase-A and monoamine oxidase-B (MOA-A and MOA-B), and the effect of selegiline at various dosages on these enzymes, may not apply to dogs and cats. However, the following are some of the more significant interactions reported (or theoretical) in humans or animals; caution is advised, particularly if using selegiline at higher than label dosages:

- **Alpha-2 Agonists** (eg, **medetomidine**): Concurrent use in humans has resulted in extreme blood pressure fluctuations; however, concurrent administration of selegiline with medetomidine to healthy dogs did not affect cardiopulmonary parameters (eg, heart rate, blood pressure, mean arterial pressure, systemic vascular resistance, cardiac output) beyond those caused by medetomidine alone.[10]
- **Atropine**: Increased risk for hypertension and hypertensive crisis
- **Buspirone**: Increased risk for hypertension
- **CNS Stimulants** (eg, **doxapram, methylphenidate**): Increased risk for hypertension
- **Dextromethorphan**: Increased risk for serotonin syndrome; avoid combination
- **Diphenoxylate**: Increased risk for hypertension; avoid combination
- **Meperidine/Opioids**: In humans, severe agitation, hallucinations, serotonin syndrome, and death have occurred in some patients receiving meperidine and a monoamine oxidase inhibitor (MAOI).[5] Until the data can be clarified, it is recommended not to use selegiline and meperidine together. A separation of 2 weeks has been recommended. Other opioids (eg, **morphine**) should be safer, but use with extreme caution, if at all.[10]
- **Monoamine oxidase inhibitors** (MAOIs; eg, **amitraz, linezolid, methylene blue**): Concurrent use can contribute to serotonin syndrome. The manufacturer recommends not using selegiline concurrently with amitraz (*Mitaban®*) in dogs. Avoid combination
- **Metoclopramide**: Concurrent use may result in increased risk for hypertensive crisis and loss of selegiline efficacy.
- **Mirtazapine**: Potential for serotonin syndrome with concurrent use
- **Phenylpropanolamine (PPA), Pseudoephedrine**: Possibility for increased risk for hypertension and hyperpyrexia; however, adverse effects were not observed when selegiline was given with PPA to healthy dogs.[11]
- **Serotonin 5-HT3 receptor Antagonists** (eg, **ondansetron**): Increased risk for hypertension
- **Selective Serotonin Reuptake Inhibitors (SSRIs**; eg, **fluoxetine**): Potential for serotonin syndrome could occur if selegiline is used concurrently with SSRIs; several sources recommend a 5-week washout before administering selegiline to dogs after fluoxetine is discontinued, and to wait 2 weeks if switching from selegiline to an SSRI.

- **Sympathomimetic Agents** (eg, **dopamine, ephedrine, epinephrine, norepinephrine, phenylephrine**): Concurrent selegiline use may enhance hypertensive effects.
- **Tramadol**: Use together is contraindicated in humans due to the potential for serotonin syndrome or cardiovascular collapse.
- **Trazodone**: Concurrent use may increase risk for serotonin syndrome.
- **Tricyclic Antidepressants** (eg, **clomipramine, amitriptyline**): Potential for serotonin syndrome to occur if selegiline is used concurrently with these agents, and use together is not advised at this time; a 2-week separation between these compounds and selegiline is recommended.

Dosages

DOGS:

Canine pituitary-dependent hyperadrenocorticism (label dosage; FDA-approved): 1 mg/kg PO in the AM (with food as needed). Reevaluate clinically over the next 2 months[7]; if no improvement, may increase to 2 mg/kg once daily; if no improvement or signs increase after 1 month at the higher dose, reevaluate diagnosis or consider alternate treatment. Dogs should be monitored closely for possible adverse effects associated with any increase in dose.

Canine cognitive dysfunction (label dosage; FDA-approved): 0.5 – 1 mg/kg, PO once daily, preferably in the AM.[7] Initially, dose to the nearest whole tablet; adjustments should then be made based upon response and tolerance to the drug.

CATS:

Feline cognitive dysfunction syndrome (extra-label): 0.25 – 1 mg/kg PO once daily[4,12,13]

Monitoring

- Clinical efficacy
- Adverse effects: There is no correlation between low-dose dexamethasone suppression test results and clinical efficacy of the drug. The manufacturer recommends physical examination and history as the primary methods to measure response to therapy.

Client Information

- This medicine may be given with or without food. Dogs usually get the daily dose in the morning and cats in the evening.
- It may take several weeks to see if this medicine is working.
- Talk with your veterinarian before making changes to your animal's diet, medications, and flea/tick treatments (eg, collars, spot-ons) before giving selegiline to your animal.
- Side effects include gastrointestinal problems (eg, vomiting, diarrhea, lack of appetite, drooling) and behavioral changes.

Chemistry/Synonyms

Selegiline HCl, also commonly called L-deprenyl, occurs as a white to off-white crystalline powder that is freely soluble in water. It has a pK_a of 7.5.

Selegiline HCl may also be known as deprenyl, l-deprenyl, selegilini hydrochloridum; many trade names are available including *Anipryl*® and *Selgian*®.

Storage/Stability

Commercially available veterinary tablets should be stored at controlled room temperature 20°C to 25°C (68°F-77°F).

Compatibility/Compounding Considerations

No specific information was noted.

Dosage Forms/Regulatory Status

VETERINARY-LABELED PRODUCTS:

Selegiline HCl Oral Tablets: 2 mg, 5 mg, 10 mg, 15 mg, and 30 mg in blister-packs of 30 tablets; *Anipryl*®; (Rx). FDA-approved for use in dogs. NADA #141-080

The Association of Racing Commissioners International (ARCI) has designated this drug as a class 2 substance. Use of this drug may not be allowed in certain animal competitions. Check rules and regulations before entering in a competition while this medication is being administered. Contact local racing authorities for further guidance. See the ***Appendix*** for more information.

HUMAN-LABELED PRODUCTS:

Selegiline HCl Tablets and Capsules 5 mg; *Eldepryl*®, generic; (Rx)

Selegiline Orally Disintegrating Tablets 1.25 mg; *Zelapar*®; (Rx)

Selegiline HCl Transdermal Patch: 6 mg/24 hours (20 mg/20 cm²); 9 mg/24 hours (30 mg/30 cm²), and 12 mg/24 hours (40 mg/40 cm²); *Emsam*®; (Rx)

References

For the complete list of references, see **wiley.com/go/budde/plumb**

Sertraline

(***sir***-trah-leen) *Zoloft*®

Selective Serotonin Reuptake Inhibitor (SSRI)

Prescriber Highlights

- May be useful in treating a variety of behavior-related diagnoses in dogs and cats, including aggression, anxiety-related behaviors, and other obsessive-compulsive behaviors
- Use with caution in diabetic or geriatric patients or those with severe hepatic disease.
- Adverse effect profile is not well established for this drug. In dogs, sertraline can potentially cause anorexia, lethargy, GI effects, anxiety, irritability, insomnia/hyperactivity, or panting. In cats, sedation, decreased appetite/anorexia, vomiting, diarrhea, and behavior changes (eg, anxiety, irritability, sleep disturbances) could occur.
- Many potential drug interactions

Uses/Indications

Sertraline may be considered for use in treating a variety of behavior-related diagnoses in dogs and cats, including aggression and anxiety-related or other obsessive-compulsive behaviors,[1] as well as inappropriate elimination in cats.

Pharmacology/Actions

Sertraline is a highly selective inhibitor of the reuptake of serotonin (5-hydroxytryptamine, 5-HT) in the CNS, thus potentiating its pharmacologic activity. Sertraline apparently has little effect on dopamine or norepinephrine, and no effect on other neurotransmitters.

Pharmacokinetics

In dogs, sertraline's volume of distribution is 25 L/kg, and it is 97% bound to plasma proteins.[2] High first-pass metabolism occurs; clearance is greater than 35 mL/minute/kg. Bile appears to be the major route of excretion.

In humans, sertraline peak concentrations occur ≈4.5 to 8 hours after oral dosing.[3] It is 98% bound to plasma proteins. Sertraline appears to be highly metabolized primarily to N-desmethylsertraline, which is active. Elimination half-lives for sertraline and desmethylsertraline average 26 and 80 hours, respectively.

Contraindications/Precautions/Warnings

Sertraline is contraindicated in patients that are hypersensitive to it or any selective serotonin reuptake inhibitor (SSRI), or are receiving a monoamine oxidase inhibitor (MAOI). Use with caution in geriatric patients and in those with hepatic impairment; doses may need to be decreased, or dosing interval may need to be increased. Sertraline may alter blood glucose and should be used with caution in diabetic patients.

Do not confuse sertraline with selegiline or cetirizine.

Adverse Effects

Because there has been limited use of sertraline in dogs or cats, it is difficult to compare its adverse effect profile with other selective serotonin reuptake inhibitors (SSRIs; eg, fluoxetine, paroxetine, fluvoxamine). In dogs, SSRIs can cause lethargy, GI effects, anxiety, irritability, insomnia/hyperactivity, or panting. Anorexia is a common adverse effect in dogs (this effect is usually transient and may be negated by temporarily increasing the palatability of food and/or hand feeding). SSRIs in cats can cause sedation, decreased appetite/anorexia, vomiting, diarrhea, behavior changes (eg, anxiety, irritability, sleep disturbances), and changes in elimination patterns.

In humans, sertraline use may precipitate serotonin syndrome, which is a potentially life-threatening condition with symptoms that may include CNS (eg, agitation, seizures), GI (eg, vomiting, diarrhea), autonomic (eg, blood pressure changes, tachycardia, hyperthermia), and neuromuscular (eg, tremor, rigidity, myoclonus) changes. Other adverse effects noted in humans include hyponatremia, QTc prolongation, and torsade de pointes, as well as increased risks for bleeding and angle-closure glaucoma attacks.

Reproductive/Nursing Safety

Delayed fetal ossification occurred when sertraline, at doses used clinically, was administered to pregnant rats and rabbits during the period of organogenesis.[3] Increased stillbirths and neonatal pup death occurred after sertraline use during the third trimester.

Sertraline enters maternal milk at low levels.

Because safety has not been established in animals, this drug should only be used when the maternal benefits outweigh the potential risks to offspring.

Overdose/Acute Toxicity

An overdose of a selective serotonin reuptake inhibitor (SSRI) can cause vomiting, diarrhea, hypersalivation, and lethargy. Serotonin syndrome may occur with clinical signs that include muscle tremors, rigidity, agitation, hyperthermia, vocalization, hypertension or hypotension, tachycardia, seizures, coma, and death. Most exposures below 20 mg/kg in dogs are not serious. The reported median lethal dosage for dogs following a single ingestion is 80 mg/kg of body weight.[4]

A retrospective review of sertraline ingestions reported to Pet Poison Helpline found ≈⅓ of reports of ingestions in dogs had clinical signs, including CNS depression (60%), CNS stimulation (24%), cardiovascular signs (8%), respiratory signs (12%), GI signs (16%), and hyperthermia (8%).[5] The median dose for causing clinical signs was 11.6 mg/kg, but the range was very wide (0.4 – 264 mg/kg). More severe signs such as tremoring and hyperthermia were not seen until the dose reached between 8 – 10 mg/kg of sertraline, and seizure activity was not noted until the dose exceeded 25 mg/kg. No deaths were reported.

Management of sertraline overdoses should be handled aggressively with supportive therapy based on clinical presentation.

For patients that have experienced or are suspected to have experienced an overdose, consultation with a 24-hour poison consultation center specializing in providing veterinary-specific information is recommended. For general information related to overdose and toxin exposures, as well as contact information for poison control centers, refer to ***Appendix.***

Drug Interactions

The following drug interactions either have been reported or are theoretical in humans or animals receiving sertraline and may be of significance in veterinary patients. Unless otherwise noted, use together is not necessarily contraindicated, but weigh the potential risks and perform additional monitoring when appropriate.

- **ANTICOAGULANTS** (eg, **heparins, rivaroxaban, warfarin**): Increased risk for bleeding has been reported in humans.
- **ANTIPLATELET AGENTS** (eg, **aspirin, clopidogrel**): Increased risk for bleeding has been reported in humans.
- **BUSPIRONE**: Increased risk for serotonin syndrome
- **CYP3A INHIBITORS** (eg, **clarithromycin, ketoconazole**): May decrease sertraline metabolism and increase risk for adverse effects
- **CYP3A INDUCERS** (eg, **phenobarbital, rifampin**): May increase sertraline metabolism; higher dosage may be required to achieve clinical response
- **CYPROHEPTADINE**: May decrease or reverse the effects of selective serotonin reuptake inhibitors (SSRIs)
- **DIAZEPAM**: Sertraline may decrease diazepam clearance.
- **ISONIAZID**: Increased risk for serotonin syndrome
- **METOCLOPRAMIDE**: May enhance adverse/toxic effects of SSRIs and increase the risk for serotonin syndrome
- **MEXILETINE**: SSRIs may decrease the metabolism of mexiletine.
- **MONOAMINE OXIDASE INHIBITORS** (MAOIs; eg, **amitraz, linezolid, selegiline**): High risk for serotonin syndrome; use is contraindicated. In humans, a 5-week washout period is required after discontinuing sertraline, and a 2-week washout period is required if first discontinuing the MAO inhibitor.
- **NONSTEROIDAL ANTI-INFLAMMATORY DRUGS** (**NSAIDs**; eg, **carprofen, meloxicam, robenacoxib**): Increased risk for bleeding
- **OPIOIDS** (eg, **fentanyl, meperidine**): Serotonin syndrome-like adverse effects possible
- **PENTAZOCINE**: Serotonin syndrome-like adverse effects possible
- **QT PROLONGING AGENTS** (eg, **amiodarone, ciprofloxacin, cisapride, erythromycin, ondansetron, quinidine**): Increased risk of QT prolongation and arrhythmias
- **SEROTONERGIC AGENTS, OTHER** (eg, **dextromethorphan, mirtazapine, trazodone**): Increased risk for serotonin syndrome
- **ST JOHN'S WORT**: Increased risk for serotonin syndrome. Avoid use if possible.
- **TRAMADOL**: SSRIs can inhibit the metabolism of tramadol to the active metabolites, decreasing its efficacy and increasing the risk for toxicity (serotonin syndrome, seizures).
- **TRICYCLIC ANTIDEPRESSANTS** (eg, **clomipramine, amitriptyline**): Sertraline may increase TCA blood levels and the risk for serotonin syndrome.
- **WARFARIN**: Sertraline may increase the risk for bleeding.

Laboratory Considerations

- False-positive benzodiazepine urine immunoassay screening tests[3]

Dosages

DOGS:

Adjunctive treatment (with behavior modification) of behavior disorders (eg, **obsessive/compulsive disorders, anxiety**) (extra-label): Anecdotal dosage recommendations range from 0.5 – 4 mg/kg PO every 24 hours.[1] Most clinicians recommend starting at the low end of the dosing range in combination with behavioral therapy. No specific studies supporting any one dosage were located. Anecdotally, dosing every 12 hours has also been used. A minimum of a 6- to 8-week trial is usually recommended before assessing efficacy. If discontinuing treatment, wean off over at least 2 to 3 weeks (or longer).

CATS:

Adjunctive treatment (with behavior modification) of behavior disorders (eg, **obsessive/compulsive disorders, anxiety, spraying**) (extra-label): Anecdotal dosage recommendations range from 0.5 – 1.5 mg/kg PO every 24 hours.[1] Most clinicians recommend starting at the low end of the dosing range. No specific studies supporting any one dosage were located. Anecdotally, dosing every 12 hours has also been used. A minimum of a 6- to 8-week trial is usually recommended before assessing efficacy. If discontinuing treatment, wean off over at least 2 to 3 weeks (or longer).

Monitoring

- Efficacy
- Adverse effects (eg, lethargy, hyporexia)
- Baseline and periodic serum liver enzymes and ECG

Client Information

- This medicine may take several days or weeks to see how well it works.
- The most common side effects with this medicine are drowsiness/sleepiness and a decreased appetite.
- Rare side effects that can be serious include seizures and aggression (threatening behavior/actions). Contact your veterinarian immediately if your pet experiences any of these side effects.
- Let your veterinarian know if your animal has worn a flea/tick collar in the past 2 weeks as some of these collars may make your animal sick if worn while taking this medicine.
- Do not stop giving this medicine to your animal without speaking with your veterinarian. A gradual withdrawal of the medicine is usually recommended if your animal has been taking this medicine for an extended period of time.

Chemistry/Synonyms

A selective serotonin reuptake inhibitor (SSRI), sertraline hydrochloride is a white crystalline powder that is slightly soluble in water and isopropyl alcohol; it is sparingly soluble in ethanol. The commercially available oral solution contains 12% ethanol and has a menthol scent.

Sertraline may also be known as CP-51974-01; *Altruline*®, *Anilar*®, *Aremis*®, *Atenix*®, *Besitran*®, *Bicromil*®, *Gladem*®, *Insertec*®, *Irradial*®, *Lustral*®, *Novativ*®, *Sealdin*®, *Serad*®, *Sercerin*®, *Serlain*®, *Serta*®, *Tatig*®, *Tolrest*®, *Tresleen*®, or *Zoloft*®.

Storage/Stability

Store commercially available sertraline tablets and oral solution at controlled room temperature (25°C [77°F]); excursions permitted to 15°C to 30°C (59°F-86°F).

Compatibility/Compounding Considerations

The manufacturer states to dilute the oral solution before administration, and to dilute only in the following liquids: water, orange juice, ginger ale, lemonade, or lemon-lime soda; use immediately after dilution.

Dosage Forms/Regulatory Status

VETERINARY-LABELED PRODUCTS: NONE

The Association of Racing Commissioners International (ARCI) has designated this drug as a class 2 substance. Use of this drug may not be allowed in certain animal competitions. Check rules and regulations before entering in a competition while this medication is being administered. Contact local racing authorities for further guidance. See ***Appendix*** for more information.

HUMAN-LABELED PRODUCTS:

Sertraline HCl Tablets: 25 mg, 50 mg, and 100 mg (as base); *Zoloft*®, generic; (Rx)

Sertraline HCl Oral Solution Concentrate: 20 mg/mL in 60 mL; *Zoloft*®, generic; (Rx)

References

For the complete list of references, see **wiley.com/go/budde/plumb**

Sevelamer

(se-***vel***-a-mer) *Renagel*®, *Renvela*®

Phosphorus-Binding Agent

Prescriber Highlights

- ► Orally administered phosphorus-binding agent used to treat hyperphosphatemia associated with chronic kidney disease
- ► May be useful when aluminum- or calcium-containing phosphate binders cannot be used
- ► Expensive when compared to aluminum hydroxide or calcium carbonate products
- ► Caution of drug–drug interactions including nutrients

Uses/Indications

Sevelamer may be useful for treating hyperphosphatemia associated with chronic kidney disease, particularly when dietary phosphorus restriction fails and aluminum- or calcium-containing phosphorus-binding agents are not tolerated.

Pharmacology/Actions

Sevelamer binds phosphorus in the gut; when combined with decreased phosphorus in the diet it can substantially reduce serum phosphorus levels. Sevelamer also binds bile acids, which interferes with fat and fat-soluble vitamin absorption. It also reduces serum low-density lipoproteins and total cholesterol.

Pharmacokinetics

Sevelamer is administered orally but is not absorbed systemically.

Contraindications/Precautions/Warnings

Sevelamer is contraindicated in patients with hypophosphatemia or bowel obstruction and in patients that are hypersensitive to it. Safety of sevelamer products has not been established in patients with dysmotility, dysphagia, or history of major GI surgery; use with caution in these patients. Worsening of metabolic acidosis has been reported in humans that take the hydrochloride salt (ie, *Renagel*®).

Adverse Effects

Adverse effects in humans include nausea, vomiting, diarrhea, dyspepsia, constipation, and abdominal pain.[1] Esophageal tablet retention and ileus have also been reported. Absorption of certain vitamins (eg, A, D, E, K) may be reduced by sevelamer; consider vitamin supplementation during therapy. In theory, sevelamer HCl could exacerbate metabolic acidosis; this would not be expected with sevelamer carbonate.

Reproductive/Nursing Safety

Safety of sevelamer during pregnancy is not established; because of the potential for binding vitamins, additional vitamins (both fat- and water-soluble) may be necessary. There are no adequate and well-controlled studies in nursing mothers, but as sevelamer is not absorbed, safe use during nursing would be expected.[1]

Because safety has not been established in animals, this drug should only be used when the maternal benefits outweigh the potential risks to offspring.

Overdose/Acute Toxicity

As sevelamer is not absorbed, acute toxicity potential appears to be negligible,[1] but chronic overdoses may affect serum electrolytes and nutrient absorption.

For patients that have experienced or are suspected to have experienced an overdose, consultation with a 24-hour poison consultation center specializing in providing veterinary-specific information is recommended. For general information related to overdose and toxin exposures, as well as contact information for poison control centers, refer to ***Appendix***.

Drug Interactions

The following drug interactions have either been reported or are theoretical in humans or animals receiving sevelamer and may be of significance in veterinary patients. Unless otherwise noted, use together is not necessarily contraindicated, but weigh the potential risks and perform additional monitoring when appropriate.

- FLUOROQUINOLONES: Concurrent administration with sevelamer may decrease absorption by 50%; administer oral fluoroquinolones at least 1 hour before or 3 hours after sevelamer.
- MYCOPHENOLATE: Sevelamer may reduce absorption; administer 2 hours after mycophenolate.
- ORAL MEDICATIONS: There are only a few medications that have documented reductions in oral absorption when administered with sevelamer; consider dosing other oral drugs separately, particularly for drugs with narrow therapeutic indexes.
- THYROID HORMONES: Sevelamer may reduce absorption; separate administering the 2 drugs by at least 4 hours.
- VITAMINS: Sevelamer may reduce vitamin absorption from food; consider administering vitamin supplements separately from sevelamer dose.
- WARFARIN: Single-dose studies demonstrated no drug interaction between warfarin and sevelamer, but reduced vitamin K absorption with long-term use may alter warfarin requirements.

Dosages

DOGS/CATS:

Adjunctive treatment of hyperphosphatemia in animals with chronic kidney disease (extra-label): No specific studies were noted that support any dosage. 30 – 150 mg/kg PO daily, divided into 2 or 3 doses and given with meals.[2-4] Practically, cats and small dogs would receive 200 – 400 mg/dose (NOT mg/kg) PO every 8 to 12 hours with meals. Medium to large dogs would receive 400 – 1600 mg/dose (NOT mg/kg) PO every 8 to 12 hours with meals. Adjust dose based on serum electrolytes and phosphorous. **NOTE**: When switching between carbonate and hydrochloride forms, it is recommended in humans to use an equivalent dose and then titrate if needed.

Monitoring

- Baseline and periodic serum phosphorus and other electrolytes (eg, calcium, bicarbonate, chloride)
- Consider a baseline coagulation-screening test before and after sevelamer therapy implementation as vitamin K absorption may be impacted.
- After beginning therapy, check serum phosphorus (after a 12-hour fast) every 4 to 6 weeks until target phosphorous levels are attained. Once phosphorous levels are stable, check phosphorous levels at the time of renal chemistry rechecks (eg, every 12 weeks). For chronic kidney disease (CKD), the International Renal Interest Society (IRIS) recommends a target phosphorous range for dogs and cats at each stage5,6:
  - Stage 2 CKD target phosphorous levels: greater than 2.7 and less than 4.6 mg/dL (0.9 – less than 1.5 mmol/L)
  - Stage 3 CKD target phosphorous levels: greater than 2.7 and less than 5 mg/dL (0.9 – less than 1.6 mmol/L)
  - Stage 4 CKD target phosphorous levels: greater than 2.7 and less than 6 mg/dL (0.9 – less than 1.9 mmol/L)

Client Information

- Give this medicine with meals.
- Sevelamer powder may be mixed with water or into a small amount of food. Do not add this medicine to hot foods or liquids or heat the powder.
- Give this medicine separately (at least an hour apart) from other oral medicines or vitamins.
- Sevelamer is well tolerated, but may cause reduced appetite, vomiting, constipation, or diarrhea.
- Follow-up blood tests to measure phosphorus and other electrolytes are necessary. Do not miss these important follow-up visits.

Chemistry/Synonyms

A phosphorus-binding agent, sevelamer HCl is a complex chemical that is hydrophilic but insoluble in water. Sevelamer carbonate is also insoluble in water but is hygroscopic.

Sevelamer may also be known as GT16-026A, sevelamerum, *Renagel®*, or *Renvela®*.

Storage/Stability

Sevelamer capsules should be stored at room temperature 25°C (77°F), with excursions permitted to 15°C to 30°C (59°F-86°F).[1] Protect from moisture.

Compatibility/Compounding Considerations

No specific information was noted.

Dosage Forms/Regulatory Status

VETERINARY-LABELED PRODUCTS: NONE

HUMAN-LABELED PRODUCTS:

Sevelamer HCl Oral Tablets: 400 mg and 800 mg; *Renagel®*; (Rx)

Sevelamer Carbonate Oral Tablets: 800 mg; *Renvela®*; (Rx)

Sevelamer Carbonate Powder for Oral Suspension: 0.8 g/packet and 2.4 g/packet; *Renvela®*; (Rx)

References

For the complete list of references, see **wiley.com/go/budde/plumb**

Sevoflurane

(see-voe-***floo***-rane) *SevoFlo®, Ultane®*

General Anesthetic, Inhalant

Prescriber Highlights

- ► Inhalant general anesthetic similar to isoflurane, but with more rapid induction and recovery
- ► MAC is reduced by concurrent use of injectable premedicants and/or induction agents.
- ► Contraindicated in patients with a history or predisposition to malignant hyperthermia
- ► Use with caution in patients with elevated intracranial pressure or head injury, or renal insufficiency.
- ► Adverse effects (cardiovascular or respiratory depression, nausea, vomiting) are uncommon at maintenance doses providing surgical anesthesia but are more common when it is used for masked anesthetic induction.
- ► Currently more expensive than isoflurane

Uses/Indications

While only FDA-approved for use in dogs and humans, sevoflurane may be useful in a variety of species (including cats, horses, small mammals, and ruminants, birds, reptiles) when rapid induction and/or rapid recoveries are desired with an inhalant anesthetic. When mask inductions are necessary, sevoflurane is preferred over isoflurane because of the faster onset of action and over desflurane as it is better accepted and inductions are smoother. Sevoflurane may be of particularly useful in debilitated or geriatric patients as it is more easily dosed to effect than isoflurane because of lower blood solubility (blood–gas partition coefficient).

Pharmacology/Actions

While the precise mechanisms of how inhalant anesthetics produce their general anesthetic effects are not precisely known, they may interfere with the functioning of nerve cells in the brain by acting on the lipid matrix of the membrane. They alter the activity of neuronal ion channels, particularly the fast synaptic neurotransmitter receptors. Sevoflurane has low blood–gas partition coefficient (0.6), allowing very rapid anesthesia induction and recovery. Rapid mask induction is possible.

Pharmacologic effects of sevoflurane are similar to isoflurane when used at equipotent doses and include CNS depression, depression of body temperature regulating centers, increased cerebral blood flow, respiratory depression, hypotension, vasodilation, myocardial depression (less than with halothane), and muscular relaxation.

Approximate minimal alveolar concentration (MAC) in oxygen reported for sevoflurane in various species: Dog = 2.1% to 2.4%; Cat = 2.6% to 3.4%; Horse = 2.3% to 2.8%; Sheep = 1.9% to 2%; Swine = 2% to 2.7%; Human (adult) = 1.6% to 2.1%.[1,2] Several factors, including acid/base status, temperature, other CNS depressants or stimulants on board, age, ongoing acute disease, pregnancy, severe hypoxemia, and hypercarbia, may alter MAC.

Pharmacokinetics

At the labeled dose, surgical anesthesia is obtained in 3 to 14 minutes. Because of its low solubility in blood, only small concentrations of sevoflurane in the blood are required before alveolar partial pressures are in equilibrium with arterial partial pressures. This low solubility means that sevoflurane is rapidly removed from the lungs. It is unknown what percent sevoflurane is bound to plasma proteins. The majority of sevoflurane is excreted via the lungs, but ≈3% to 5% is metabolized in the liver via the cytochrome P450 2E1 isoenzyme.

Contraindications/Precautions/Warnings

Sevoflurane is contraindicated in patients with a history or predisposition toward malignant hyperthermia. It should be used with caution (benefits vs risks) in patients with elevated intracranial pressure or head injury, or renal insufficiency.

Because of its rapid action, use caution not to overdose during the induction phase. Because of the rapid recovery associated with sevoflurane, use caution (and appropriate sedation during the recovery phase), particularly with large animals.

Geriatric animals may require less inhalant anesthetic.

In rabbits and other small mammals, sevoflurane (and isoflurane) can cause breath-holding and struggling; premedication and close observation are required. Sevoflurane may have a low margin of safety in guinea pigs.[3]

Sevoflurane can react with carbon dioxide absorbents to produce compound A, which is nephrotoxic. After extensive clinical use in humans and dogs, nephrotoxicity has not been demonstrated to be of clinical concern. However, sevoflurane should be used with good maintenance of the carbon dioxide absorbent (ie, should be changed regularly to prevent exhaustion or excessive drying) and should not be used with extremely low oxygen flows (ie, less than 500 mL/minute).[4] Fluoride is another degradation product of sevoflurane, which has been associated with renal damage; however, it has not been shown to cause significant changes in renal function.[5]

Sevoflurane should be used in precision, agent-specific, out-of-circuit vaporizers. Sevoflurane should only be used in situations in which sufficient monitoring and patient-support capabilities (eg, intubation, ventilation) are available.

The National Institute for Occupational Safety and Health (NIOSH) has recommended that no worker should be exposed at ceiling concentrations greater than 2 ppm of any halogenated anesthetic agent over a sampling period not to exceed 1 hour.

Adverse Effects

Sevoflurane seems to be well-tolerated. Hypotension and respiratory depression may occur and are considered dose dependent. GI effects (nausea, vomiting, ileus) have been reported. Cardiodepression (ie, decreased heart rate and contractility) is possible but generally minimal at sevoflurane doses causing surgical planes of anesthesia. Chamber or facemask induction can significantly increase the risks for respiratory or cardiovascular depression because of the high percentage of inspired inhalant used during this phase.

Like other inhalant anesthetics, sevoflurane may rarely trigger malignant hyperthermia in predisposed patients.

A study in dogs found a decrease in gastric motility during sevoflurane anesthesia. While gastric motility returned to normal within 12 to 15 hours, gastric emptying was delayed for 30 to 40 hours, possibly increasing the risk for postoperative ileus.[6]

Sinus arrhythmias have been detected when used in birds.[7] Prolongation of the QT interval has been reported in humans.

In ferrets, sevoflurane (and isoflurane) can cause temporary decreases in erythrocyte and white blood cell counts and total protein. Within 45 minutes after discontinuation of sevoflurane, this effect begins to revert to normal and is reversed within 2 hours.

Volatile anesthetics contribute to the greenhouse effect. When scavenged to the atmosphere, sevoflurane rises to the troposphere and remains nondegraded for 1.1 years. This degradation time equates to a global warming potential of 130 years. However, sevoflurane does not react with the highly reactive ozone in the stratosphere and does not damage the earth's protective ozone barrier like isoflurane and nitrous oxide do. The shorter degradation time and the absence of reaction with the ozone in the stratosphere make sevoflurane the inhalant with the least negative impact on the environment.

Reproductive/Nursing Safety

No overt fetotoxicity or teratogenicity has been demonstrated in lab animal studies, but safety has not been definitively established for use during pregnancy.

The MAC of inhalation agents is 25% to 40% lower during pregnancy.[8]

Limited information is available regarding lactation. In humans, sevoflurane appears compatible with breastfeeding, and breastfeeding may resume after recovery from anesthesia.[9]

Because safety has not been established in animals, this drug should only be used when the maternal benefits outweigh the potential risks to offspring.

Overdose/Acute Toxicity

In the event of an overdose, discontinue sevoflurane, maintain a patent airway, and support respiratory and cardiac function as necessary.

For patients that have experienced or are suspected to have experienced an overdose, consultation with a 24-hour poison consultation center specializing in providing veterinary-specific information is recommended. For general information related to overdose and toxin exposures, as well as contact information for poison control centers, refer to ***Appendix.***

Drug Interactions

The following drug interactions have either been reported or are theoretical in humans or animals receiving sevoflurane and may be of significance in veterinary patients. Unless otherwise noted, use together is not necessarily contraindicated, but weigh the potential risks and perform additional monitoring when appropriate.

- **Aminoglycosides, Lincosamides**: May enhance neuromuscular blockade
- **Barbiturates** (eg, **phenobarbital, pentobarbital**): May increase concentrations of inorganic fluoride
- **Dexmedetomidine**: May potentiate sevoflurane effects; decrease MAC[10]
- **Isoniazid**: May increase concentrations of inorganic fluoride
- **Ketamine**: May decrease MAC requirements
- **Lidocaine**: IV lidocaine can significantly reduce MAC in horses[11] and dogs.[12]

- **Methimazole**: May decrease the metabolism of sevoflurane and prolong recovery
- **Midazolam**: May potentiate sevoflurane effects; decrease MAC
- **Nondepolarizing Neuromuscular Blocking Agents** (eg, **atracurium, pancuronium, vecuronium**): Additive neuromuscular blockade may occur.
- **Opioids**: May potentiate sevoflurane effects; decrease MAC
- **Propofol**: IV propofol CRI can significantly reduce MAC in dogs in a dose-dependent manner.[13]
- **QT Prolonging Agents** (eg, **amiodarone, cisapride, quinidine, sotalol**): May increase the risk for arrhythmias
- **Sildenafil**: May decrease the metabolism of sevoflurane and prolong recovery
- **St. John's Wort**: Increased risk for anesthetic complications; recommend discontinuing St. John's Wort 5 days in advance of surgery.
- **Succinylcholine**: Sevoflurane may enhance effects.
- **Sympathomimetics** (eg, **dopamine, epinephrine, norepinephrine, ephedrine, metaraminol**): While sevoflurane sensitizes the myocardium to the effects of sympathomimetics less than halothane, arrhythmias may still result; caution and monitoring are advised.
- **Tramadol**: May decrease MAC requirements
- **Verapamil**: May cause cardiovascular depression

Laboratory Considerations

- Inhalant anesthetics may cause transient increases in **liver enzymes, WBCs, and glucose.**

Dosages

Minimal alveolar concentration (MAC; %) in oxygen reported for sevoflurane in various species: dog = 2.1% to 2.4%; cat = 2.6% to 3.4%; horse = 2.3% to 2.8%; sheep = 1.9% to 2%; swine = 2% to 2.7%; human (adult) = 1.6% to 2.1%.[1,2]

NOTES:

1. Sevoflurane should be used with well-maintained anesthetic machines with proper scavenging equipment and in areas with adequate ventilation to prevent escape of gases that could result in exposure of veterinary personnel to anesthetic vapors.
2. General anesthesia using inhalants must be performed with adequate monitoring and support and cannot be dosed in a purely textbook fashion.
3. MAC is affected by many variables, including:
   a) type and location of stimulus,
   b) concurrent administration of MAC reducing drugs,
   c) type of ventilation, type of breathing system,
   d) age of the animal (younger animals may have higher MAC values), and
   e) patient variables (acid/base status, temperature, ongoing acute disease, pregnancy, severe hypoxemia, and hypercarbia)

DOGS/CATS:

General anesthesia (label dosage; FDA-approved): **Dogs:** Inspired Concentration: The delivered concentration of *SevoFlo*® (sevoflurane) should be known. Since the depth of anesthesia may be altered easily and rapidly, only vaporizers producing predictable percentage concentrations of sevoflurane should be used. Sevoflurane should be vaporized using a precision vaporizer specifically calibrated for sevoflurane. Sevoflurane contains no stabilizer. Nothing in the drug product alters the calibration or operation of these vaporizers. The administration of general anesthesia must be individualized based on the patient's response. **When using sevoflurane, patients should be continuously monitored, and facilities for maintenance of patient airway, artificial ventilation, and oxygen supplementation must be immediately available.**

Replacement of Desiccated CO_2 Absorbents: When a clinician suspects that the CO_2 absorbent may be desiccated, it should be replaced. An exothermic reaction occurs when sevoflurane is exposed to CO_2 absorbents. This reaction is increased when the CO_2 absorbent becomes desiccated.

Premedication: No specific premedication is either indicated or contraindicated with sevoflurane. The necessity for and choice of premedication is left to the discretion of the veterinarian. Preanesthetic doses for premedicants may be lower than the label directions for their use as a single medication.

Induction: For mask induction using sevoflurane, inspired concentrations of up to 7% sevoflurane with oxygen are employed to induce surgical anesthesia in the healthy dog. These concentrations can be expected to produce a deep plane of anesthesia in 3 to 14 minutes. **Because of the rapid and dose-dependent changes in anesthetic depth, care should be taken to prevent overdosing. Respiration must be monitored closely in the dog and supported when necessary with supplemental oxygen and/or assisted ventilation. If painful procedures are performed, analgesic drugs should be administered as sevoflurane has no analgesic effects.**

Maintenance: *SevoFlo*® may be used for maintenance of anesthesia following mask induction using sevoflurane or following injectable induction agents. The concentration of vapor necessary to maintain anesthesia is much less than that required to induce it. Surgical levels of anesthesia in the healthy dog may be maintained with inhaled concentrations of 3.7% to 4% sevoflurane in oxygen in the absence of premedication and 3.3% to 3.6% in the presence of premedication. The use of injectable induction agents without premedication has little effect on the concentrations of sevoflurane required for maintenance. Anesthetic regimens that include opioid, alpha-2-agonist benzodiazepine, or phenothiazine premedication will allow the use of lower sevoflurane maintenance concentrations.[14]

Extra-label doses:

a) **Dogs/Cats**: Where required, mask induction (particularly of cats) is achieved easily via a nonrebreathing system, usually starting at a concentration of around 4% to 4.5%. Maximum concentration (8%) is possible using the vaporizer can be used for fresh gas flow for chamber inductions as the concentrations in the box take time to reach high levels. However, concentrations administered must be reduced as soon as the animal loses consciousness (ie, take the animal out of the box). For maintenance, a vaporizer setting of 3% for a circle system is a reasonable initial concentration that can be adjusted based on the residual effects of injectable drugs and/or the patient's health status.[15]

b) **Cats**: From a retrospective review of studies reporting sevoflurane MAC. Average MAC for sevoflurane in cats was 3.08% ± 0.4% but ranged from 2.5% ± 0.2% to 3.95% ± 0.33%, reflecting a relatively wide range. Multiple variables and study methodology likely contributed to this wide range.[16]

SMALL MAMMALS:

General anesthesia: (extra-label): Induction: 4% to 6% sevoflurane to effect has been used in hedgehogs via induction chamber or facemask. Maintenance: 0.5% to 3% sevoflurane to effect with facemask has been used in hedgehogs.[17]

HORSES:

General anesthesia: (extra-label): Approximate MAC is 2.31% to 2.84%.

ALPACAS:

General anesthesia: (extra-label): Induction: sevoflurane 6% in oxygen delivered by face mask from a circle system attached to a small animal anesthetic machine. Maintenance: sevoflurane 2.3%. MAC is 1.9 to 2.3.[18]

SHEEP/GOATS:

General anesthesia (extra-label): Small animal anesthetic circuits can be used to deliver inhalational anesthetics in small ruminants. During maintenance, the vaporizer setting should be adjusted to 2.5% to 4%. The oxygen flow rate should be 2 to 4 L/minute during induction and reduced to 0.5 to 1 L/minute during maintenance.[19]

BIRDS:

General anesthesia (extra-label): Induction: 5% to 8% sevoflurane via a mask using a nonrebreathing (Bain) system.[20] Maintenance: 1% to 4% sevoflurane to effect via a mask or endotracheal tube.[17] Approximate MAC was found to be 3 in pigeons.[7] Birds should always be intubated during general anesthesia.

AMPHIBIANS:

General anesthesia (extra-label): A 38% sevoflurane jelly has been compounded for use in cane toads and applied at 37.5 µL/g of body weight for induction. (See ***Compatibility/Compounding Considerations***)

Monitoring

- Respiratory and ventilatory status
- Cardiac rate/rhythm; blood pressure (particularly with at-risk patients)
- Level of anesthesia

Client Information

- Sevoflurane is used for general anesthesia only by veterinarians.

Chemistry/Synonyms

Sevoflurane is an isopropyl ether inhalational anesthetic with a molecular weight of 200, a saturated vapor pressure of 20°C (68°F) of 160 mm Hg, and a boiling point of 58.5°C (137°F). It is reported to have a pleasant odor and is not irritating to the airways. It is nonflammable and nonexplosive. Sevoflurane is a clear, colorless liquid that is miscible with ethanol or ether and slightly soluble in water.

Sevoflurane may also be known as BAX-3084, MR-654, *Sevocris®*, *SevoFlo®*, *Sevorane®*, *Petrem®*, or *Ultane®*.

Storage/Stability

Store sevoflurane at room temperature. Sevoflurane does not react with metal but can react with Lewis acids to form hydrofluoric acid.

Compatibility/Compounding Considerations

A 38% sevoflurane jelly was compounded for use in amphibians, composed of 3 parts liquid sevoflurane, 3.5 parts aqueous nonspermacidal jelly, and 1.5 parts distilled water. Each component of the mixture was added to a catheter-tip 60 mL syringe, and the syringe was shaken vigorously while the end of the syringe was occluded with a finger. When mixed thoroughly, the mixture changed from colorless to an opaque, white jelly of uniform consistency. Attempts at higher concentrations of sevoflurane were unsuccessful as this caused separation. No stability analysis was performed. See cited study for more information.[21]

Dosage Forms/Regulatory Status

VETERINARY-LABELED PRODUCTS:

Sevoflurane in 250 mL bottles; *SevoFlo®*, *Petrem®*; (Rx). FDA-approved for use in dogs

HUMAN-LABELED PRODUCTS:

Sevoflurane in 250 mL bottles; *Ultane®*, *Sojourn®*, generic; (Rx)

References

For the complete list of references, see **wiley.com/go/budde/plumb**

Sildenafil

(sil-***den***-ah-fil) *Viagra®, Revatio®*

Vasodilator; Phosphodiesterase Type 5 Inhibitor

Prescriber Highlights

- Used in veterinary medicine for the treatment of pulmonary arterial hypertension or to improve clinical signs associated with congenital megaesophagus
- Contraindicated in patients receiving organic nitrates (eg, nitroglycerin)
- Adverse effects appear to be uncommon; inguinal flushing and possible GI effects have been reported.

Uses/Indications

Sildenafil may be of benefit in the adjunctive treatment of pulmonary hypertension of a variety of causes in small animals. Studies have demonstrated reduced estimates of pulmonary arterial pressure, lessened clinical signs, and improved exercise capacity and quality of life after sildenafil administration.[1-5] An open label study in 5 dogs with Eisenmenger's syndrome found that sildenafil improved clinical signs and secondary erythrocytosis.[6] Sildenafil has also been shown to resolve alveolar infiltrates in dogs with pulmonary arterial hypertension[5] and to slow the rate of cardiac remodeling in dogs with myxomatous mitral valve disease, as compared with dogs receiving no therapy.[7] Sildenafil and pimobendan administered to 4 dogs with heartworms entangled in the tricuspid apparatus resulted in worm migration to the pulmonary arteries.

In a study of puppies with congenital megaesophagus, sildenafil reduced the number of regurgitation episodes and improved weight gain.[8] Sildenafil also reduced basal tone and increased electrically induced relaxation of the lower esophageal sphincter (in vitro) in a dose-dependent manner, thus, suggesting that sildenafil may be useful as an alternative treatment for controlling signs related to congenital megaesophagus.

In cattle, an intrauterine sildenafil infusion increased intensity of blood flow in the uterine wall; this may be beneficial in conditions of reduced uterine blood flow (eg, endometritis) or help initiate luteolysis.[9]

In humans, sildenafil is indicated for erectile dysfunction or pulmonary arterial hypertension.

Pharmacology/Actions

Sildenafil inhibits cyclic guanosine monophosphate (cGMP) specific phosphodiesterase type-5 (PDE5) found in the smooth muscle of the pulmonary vasculature, corpus cavernosum, and elsewhere where PDE5 is responsible for degradation of cGMP. Sildenafil increases cGMP thereby, resulting in nitric oxide mediated vasodilation within pulmonary vascular smooth muscle cells.

In Thoroughbred horses, sildenafil 5 mg/kg PO did not alleviate pulmonary hemorrhage or enhance performance-related indices.[10]

Pharmacokinetics

The pharmacokinetics of sildenafil have been reported in dogs.[11-13] Oral bioavailability is ≈50% to 80% (approximately the same as in humans); giving the drug with food significantly reduces peak concentration. Volume of distribution is 4.5 to 6.5 L/kg (vs 1.2 L/kg in humans); elimination half-life is ≈3 to 6 hours (significant inter-patient variability; average human half-life is ≈4 hours). Humans metabolize sildenafil (mainly via CYP3A4) to an active metabolite, which has an elimination half-life of ≈4 hours.

Contraindications/Precautions/Warnings

Sildenafil should not be used concurrently with nitrates (see ***Drug Interactions***) or in patients documented as being hypersensitive to the drug.

Pulmonary arterial vasodilators may significantly worsen the cardiovascular status of patients with pulmonary veno-occlusive disease (PVOD). Sildenafil should be used cautiously in animals with pulmonary arterial hypertension from congenital cardiac shunts or left-sided heart disease because vascular reactivity or responsiveness to sildenafil can be hard to predict, and sildenafil may increase venous return to the left side of the heart, resulting in congestive heart failure in some cases.[4]

An in vitro study demonstrated that sildenafil at supratherapeutic concentrations possesses direct, positive inotropic and chronotropic effects together with coronary vasodilator action. Caution should be used when giving sildenafil to patients with ischemic heart disease, obstructive hypertrophic cardiomyopathy, or ventricular arrhythmias.[14]

Use with extreme caution in patients with resting hypotension, fluid depletion, severe left ventricular outflow obstruction, bleeding disorder, or autonomic dysfunction. One dose of sildenafil caused acute decompensation leading to euthanasia in a cat with a vasoproliferative disorder resembling pulmonary capillary hemangiomatosis.[15] Dosage reduction may be required in patients with significant hepatic or renal impairment.

Adverse Effects

Sildenafil appears to be well tolerated. Cutaneous flushing of the inguinal region has been reported,[1] and GI adverse effects (eg hyporexia, vomiting, diarrhea)[12,13,16] are possible. The magnitude of systolic blood pressure reduction (12 – 24 mm Hg) did not reach statistical significance in clinical reports.[1,3,17] In humans, hypotension, headache, visual disturbances (including retinal toxicity and vision loss), dyspepsia, epistaxis, nasal congestion, hearing loss, myalgia, priapism, dizziness, and back pain have been reported.

Reproductive/Nursing Safety

No evidence of teratogenicity, embryotoxicity, or fetotoxicity was observed in pregnant rats or rabbits given sildenafil 200 mg/kg/day during organogenesis. In a pre- and postnatal development study in rats given 30 mg/kg/day, there were no observed adverse effects. Sildenafil did not impair fertility in male or female rats.

Sildenafil and its metabolites are excreted into maternal milk.

Because safety has not been established in animals, this drug should only be used when the maternal benefits outweigh the potential risks to offspring.

Overdose/Acute Toxicity

Little information is available. An adult woman ingested 2000 mg and survived but developed tachycardia, nonspecific ST-T changes on ECG, headache, dizziness, and flushing.

It is expected that overdoses in animals would mirror the drug's adverse effect profile; treat supportively.

For patients that have experienced or are suspected to have experienced an overdose, it is strongly encouraged that a 24-hour poison consultation center that specializes in providing information specific for veterinary patients be consulted. For general information related to overdose and toxin exposures, as well as contact information for poison control centers, refer to ***Appendix.***

Drug Interactions

The following drug interactions have either been reported or are theoretical in humans or animals receiving sildenafil and may be of significance in veterinary patients. Unless otherwise noted, use together is not necessarily contraindicated, but weigh the potential risks and perform additional monitoring when appropriate.

- ACE INHIBITORS (eg, **benazepril, enalapril**): Potential to increase hypotensive effects
- ALPHA-1-ADRENERGIC RECEPTOR ANTAGONISTS (eg, **phenothiazines [eg, acepromazine], phenoxybenzamine, phentolamine, prazosin**): May increase hypotensive effects
- ALPHA-2-ADRENERGIC RECEPTOR AGONISTS (eg, **dexmedetomidine, xylazine**): Potential to increase hypotensive effects
- AMLODIPINE: Potential to increase hypotensive effects
- ANGIOTENSIN RECEPTOR BLOCKERS (ARBs, eg, **telmisartan**): Potential to increase hypotensive effects
- AZOLE ANTIFUNGALS (eg, **itraconazole, ketoconazole**): May reduce sildenafil metabolism and increase AUC; consider lower sildenafil dosages
- CIMETIDINE: May reduce sildenafil metabolism and increase AUC
- CIPROFLOXACIN: May reduce sildenafil metabolism and increase AUC
- CLARITHROMYCIN, ERYTHROMYCIN (not azithromycin): May reduce sildenafil metabolism and increase AUC; consider lower sildenafil dosages
- FUROSEMIDE: Concurrent use may increase the risk for hearing loss. May increase concentration of sildenafil active metabolite
- HEPARIN: May increase bleeding risks
- NITRATES (eg, **isosorbide, nitroglycerin**): Significant potentiation of vasodilatory effects; life-threatening hypotension is possible. Combination is contraindicated
- NITROPRUSSIDE SODIUM: Significant potentiation of vasodilatory effects; life-threatening hypotension is possible. May increase bleeding risks
- PACLITAXEL: May alter paclitaxel plasma concentrations
- PHENOBARBITAL: May decrease sildenafil concentrations
- PROPRANOLOL: May increase concentration of sildenafil active metabolite
- RIFAMPIN: May decrease sildenafil concentrations

Laboratory Considerations

- None noted

Dosages

DOGS:

Pulmonary hypertension (extra-label): Initially, 0.5 – 1 mg/kg PO every 8 hours, may increase to 3 mg/kg PO every 8 hours based on clinical signs[1-3,5,16,17]

Congenital idiopathic megaesophagus (extra-label): 1 mg/kg PO every 12 hours; from a prospective study[8]

Eisenmenger's syndrome (extra-label): 0.5 mg/kg PO twice daily improved clinical signs and secondary erythrocytosis[6]

Subclinical myxomatous mitral valve disease (extra-label): 1 – 3 mg/kg PO every 12 hours[7,18]

CATS:

Pulmonary hypertension (extra-label): A case report of a cat with atrial septal defect that developed pulmonary hypertension leading to Eisenmenger's syndrome (ie, right to left shunting) was treated with sildenafil 0.25 to 1.6 mg/kg PO every 12 hours for 10 months. There was improvement in clinical signs but increasing doses of sildenafil were required. After 10 months the cat deteriorated and was euthanized.[19]

Monitoring

- Clinical efficacy: improved exercise capacity, cough, respiratory effort, regurgitation frequency, or weight gain; fewer episodes of syncope
- Pulmonary arterial pressure, systemic blood pressure
- Adverse effects

Client Information

- Give this medicine on an empty stomach (ie, 1 hour before or 2 hours after feeding). If your animal vomits or acts sick after receiving this drug on an empty stomach, try giving the next dose with food or a small treat. If vomiting continues, contact your veterinarian.

- Be sure to give this medicine exactly as prescribed.
- This medicine may cause flushing (ie, redness) in the groin area; gastrointestinal side effects (eg, lack of appetite, vomiting, diarrhea) are also possible.

Chemistry/Synonyms

Sildenafil citrate occurs as a white to off-white crystalline powder with a solubility of 3.5 mg/mL in water and a molecular weight of 666.7.

Sildenafil may also be known as UK 92480, UK 92480-10, *Aphrodil®*, *Revatio®*, or *Viagra®*.

Storage/Stability

Sildenafil tablets and oral suspension should be stored at room temperature (25°C [77°F]); excursions are permitted to 15°C to 30°C (59°F-86°F). Oral suspension may be refrigerated at 2°C to 8°C (36°F-46°F) after reconstitution; do not freeze. Discard 60 days after reconstitution. Store sildenafil injection at room temperature of 20°C to 25°C (68°F-77°F).

Compatibility/Compounding Considerations

A stable 2.5 mg/mL sildenafil citrate oral suspension can be made with tablets and either a 1:1 mixture of methylcellulose 1% and simple syrup NF or a 1:1 mixture of *Ora-Sweet®* and *Ora-Plus®*. Crush 30 sildenafil 25 mg tablets in a mortar and reduce to a fine powder. Add small portions of the chosen vehicle and mix to a uniform paste. Continue to add the vehicle in incremental proportions to almost 300 mL and then transfer to a graduated cylinder, rinse mortar with vehicle, and add a quantity of the vehicle sufficient to make a total of 300 mL. Store in amber plastic bottles and label "shake well." The drug is stable for 90 days at room temperature or when refrigerated.[20]

Dosage Forms/Regulatory Status

VETERINARY-LABELED PRODUCTS: NONE

HUMAN-LABELED PRODUCTS:

Sildenafil Citrate Oral Tablets: 20 mg, 25 mg, 50 mg, and 100 mg (of sildenafil); *Revatio®* (20 mg only), *Viagra®*, generic; (Rx)

Sildenafil Citrate Oral Powder for Suspension: 10 mg/1 mL; *Revatio®*, generic; (Rx). Cost may be prohibitive.

Sildenafil Injection Solution: 10 mg/12.5 mL (dextrose 50.5 mg/mL) in 12.5 mL single-use vials; *Revatio®*, generic; (Rx)

References

For the complete list of references, see **wiley.com/go/budde/plumb**

Sodium Bicarbonate

(soe-***dee***-um bye-***kar***-boe-nate)

Alkalinizer

Prescriber Highlights

- ► Alkalinizing agent used to treat metabolic acidosis and to alkalinize urine; may also be used adjunctively for hypercalcemic or hyperkalemic crises. Not commonly used secondary to potential complications/adverse effects
- ► Contraindications include patients with metabolic or respiratory alkalosis, excessive chloride loss secondary to vomiting or GI suction, patients at risk for developing diuretic-induced hypochloremic alkalosis, and patients with hypocalcemia where alkalosis may induce tetany.
- ► Use with extreme caution in patients with hypocalcemia.
- ► Caution in patients with CHF, nephrotic syndrome, hypertension, oliguria, or volume overload
- ► Adverse effects, especially with parenteral administration or high doses, include metabolic alkalosis, hypokalemia, hypocalcemia, overshoot alkalosis, hypernatremia, volume overload, CHF, shifts in the oxygen dissociation curve causing decreased tissue oxygenation, and paradoxical CNS acidosis leading to respiratory arrest.
- ► If used during CPR, hypercapnia can occur if the patient is not well ventilated; patients may be predisposed to ventricular fibrillation.

Uses/Indications

Sodium bicarbonate may be used to treat severe metabolic acidosis. It is not a substitute for diagnosing and treating the underlying cause of the acid/base disturbance. In small animal species, acidotic conditions that may be amenable to bicarbonate therapy include those that occur as a result of cardiopulmonary arrest, renal failure, renal tubular acidosis, or toxin exposure. The use of bicarbonate for metabolic acidosis secondary to diabetic crises (eg, diabetic ketoacidosis) is controversial.

Sodium bicarbonate can also be used as adjunctive therapy for the treatment of hypercalcemia or hyperkalemia crises and to alkalinize the urine.

Pharmacology/Actions

The bicarbonate ion is the conjugate base component of bicarbonate:carbonic acid buffer, the principal extracellular buffer in the body.

Contraindications/Precautions/Warnings

Parenterally administered sodium bicarbonate is considered generally contraindicated in patients with metabolic or respiratory alkalosis, excessive chloride loss secondary to vomiting or GI suction, those at risk for development of diuretic-induced hypochloremic alkalosis, or with hypocalcemia where alkalosis may induce tetany. Patients that are unable to adequately ventilate are at risk for developing hypercapnia.

Use with extreme caution and give very slowly in patients with hypocalcemia. Ideally, low calcium or potassium serum concentrations should be corrected prior to administration. Bicarbonate therapy during a diabetic crisis (ie, diabetic ketoacidosis) is rarely indicated. Administering sodium bicarbonate before potassium replenishment can be detrimental and potentially life-threatening as it can exacerbate hypokalemia.

Because of the potential sodium load, use with caution in patients with CHF, renal insufficiency, nephrotic syndrome, hypertension, oliguria, or volume overload.

Rapid IV boluses of sodium bicarbonate should be avoided because of the production of carbon dioxide and its diffusion into the central nervous system, making CSF acidosis even worse. Other disadvantages of sodium bicarbonate administration include shifting of the oxygen/hemoglobin dissociation curve to the left and increasing osmolality.

Sodium bicarbonate is generally not effective for treating lactic acidosis, and fluid therapy remains the mainstay of treatment.

Adverse Effects

Sodium bicarbonate therapy (particularly high-dose parenteral use) can lead to metabolic alkalosis, hypokalemia, hypocalcemia, overshoot alkalosis, hypernatremia, volume overload, CHF, shifts in the oxygen dissociation curve causing decreased tissue oxygenation, and paradoxical CNS acidosis, leading to depression, stupor, coma, respiratory arrest, and death.

When sodium bicarbonate is used during cardiopulmonary resuscitation, hypercapnia may result if the patient is not well ventilated; patients may be predisposed to ventricular fibrillation.

Oral and parenteral bicarbonate (especially at higher doses) may contribute significant amounts of sodium and result in hypernatremia and volume overload; use with caution in patients with CHF or acute kidney injury. Inadvertent extravasation during IV administration of hypertonic sodium bicarbonate solutions has caused cellulitis, tissue necrosis, and sloughing at the infiltration site.

Reproductive/Nursing Safety

Because safety has not been established in animals, this drug should only be used when the maternal benefits outweigh the potential risks to offspring.

Overdose/Acute Toxicity

Sodium bicarbonate can cause severe alkalosis if overdosed or given too rapidly, with signs including irritability or tetany. Doses should be thoroughly checked prior to administration, and patients should be frequently monitored of electrolyte and acid/base status performed. Treatment of mild alkalosis may only require discontinuing bicarbonate or use of a rebreathing mask. Severe alkalosis may require IV calcium therapy. Sodium chloride or potassium chloride may be necessary if hypokalemia is present.

For patients that have experienced or are suspected to have experienced an overdose, consultation with a 24-hour poison consultation center specializing in providing veterinary-specific information is recommended. For general information related to overdose and toxin exposures, as well as contact information for poison control centers, refer to ***Appendix***.

Drug Interactions

The following drug interactions have either been reported or are theoretical in humans or animals receiving sodium bicarbonate and may be of significance in veterinary patients. Unless otherwise noted, use together is not necessarily contraindicated, but weigh the potential risks and perform additional monitoring when appropriate.

- Anticholinergic Agents (eg, **hyoscyamine, oxybutynin**): Concomitant oral sodium bicarbonate may reduce absorption of oral anticholinergic agents; administer separately.
- Azole Antifungals (eg, **ketoconazole, itraconazole**): Concomitant oral sodium bicarbonate may reduce absorption; administer separately.
- Ciprofloxacin; Enrofloxacin: The solubility of ciprofloxacin and enrofloxacin is decreased in an alkaline environment; patients with alkaline urine should be monitored for signs of crystalluria.
- Corticosteroids (eg, **dexamethasone, prednis(ol)one**): Patients receiving high dosages of sodium bicarbonate and ACTH or glucocorticoids may develop hypernatremia.
- Digoxin: Concomitant oral sodium bicarbonate may reduce digoxin concentrations.
- Diuretics (eg, **furosemide, thiazides**): Concurrent use of sodium bicarbonate in patients receiving potassium-wasting diuretics may cause hypochloremic alkalosis.
- Ephedrine: When urine is alkalinized by sodium bicarbonate, excretion may be decreased.
- Histamine Type 2 Receptor Antagonists (eg, **famotidine**): Concomitant oral sodium bicarbonate may reduce absorption; separate dosages by at least 2 hours.
- Iron Products: Concomitant oral sodium bicarbonate may reduce absorption; separate dosages by at least 2 hours.
- Methenamine: Methenamine efficacy may be decreased when urine is alkalinized by sodium bicarbonate.
- Oral Medications: Because oral sodium bicarbonate can either increase or reduce the rate and/or extent of absorption of many orally administered drugs, it is recommended to avoid giving other drugs within 1 to 2 hours of oral sodium bicarbonate.
- Quinidine: When urine is alkalinized by sodium bicarbonate, excretion may be decreased.
- Salicylates: (eg, **aspirin**): When urine is alkalinized by sodium bicarbonate, excretion of weakly acidic drugs may be increased.
- Sucralfate: Oral sodium bicarbonate may reduce the efficacy of sucralfate if administered concurrently; separate dosages by at least 2 hours.
- Tetracyclines (eg, **doxycycline**): Concomitant oral sodium bicarbonate may reduce absorption; separate dosages by at least 2 hours.

Dosages

NOTE: In most cases it is suggested to administer sodium bicarbonate IV infusions as an isotonic 1.4% sodium bicarbonate solution (≈150 mEq/L). See ***Compatibility/Compounding Considerations*** for preparation instructions.

DOGS/CATS:

Severe metabolic acidosis (extra-label): The main therapeutic goal should be to first eliminate the underlying cause of acidosis. If causes are not readily reversible, arterial pH is less than 7 to 7.2, and fluid therapy and ventilatory procedures have not reduced acidemia, bicarbonate therapy should be considered.

a) Sodium bicarbonate requirement (dose, in mEq) = 0.3 × body weight (kg) × (desired HCO_3^- - measured patient HCO_3^-). Administer ¼ to ⅓ of the calculated dose as a slow IV bolus, and the remaining amount via IV infusion over 4 to 6 hours.[1] To minimize the risk for alkalinization, recheck blood gases and assess the clinical status of the patient.

b) **Prolonged cardiac arrest (ie, greater than 10-15 minutes) or if blood gas measurement is not possible, and it is believed that the animal is severely acidotic**: 1 – 2 mEq/kg slow IV/IO.[2,3]

Adjunctive therapy for hyperkalemic crisis (extra-label): Must be used judiciously. Hyperkalemia associated with hypoadrenocorticism typically improves with fluid resuscitation alone.[4] Empirical dosage of 1 – 2 mEq/kg slow IV (over 10 to 20 minutes) can be used[5]; alternatively, bicarbonate dose in mEq can be calculated as 0.3 × body weight (kg) × (desired HCO_3^- - measured HCO_3^-).[6]

Alkalinizing the urine (extra-label): Rarely recommended. Initially, 650 mg – 5.85 g/animal (NOT mg or g/kg) PO daily, depending on the size of the patient and the pretreatment urine pH value. Dosage must be individualized to the patient, with the goal of maintaining a urine pH of ≈7 to 7.5.[7]

HORSES:

Metabolic acidosis associated with colic (extra-label): If pH is less than 7.3 and the base deficit is greater than 10 mEq/L, estimate the sodium bicarbonate requirement (dose in mEq) = base deficit (mEq/L) × body weight (kg) × 0.4 (use 0.6 for foals[8]). It is suggested to administer as an isotonic sodium bicarbonate 1.4% solution (150 mEq/L). Alternatively, may administer as a sodium bicarbonate 5% solution, which contains 600 mEq of bicarbonate/L (hypertonic) and should be administered IV but at a rate no faster than 1 – 2 L/hour.[9,10]

CATTLE:

Correction of acidosis in mature cattle (extra-label): Estimate the sodium bicarbonate requirement (dose in mEq) = base deficit (mEq/L) × body weight (kg) × 0.3. When laboratory data are unavailable, estimate a base deficit of 10 mEq/L.[11] Sodium bicarbonate may be administered IV as an isotonic (1.4%, 150 mEq/L) or hypertonic (8.4%) solution.

Severely dehydrated (10% to 16% dehydrated) acidotic calves (usually comatose) (extra-label): Using isotonic sodium bicarbonate (1.4%, 150 mEq/L), most calves require ≈2 L of this solution IV given over 1 to 2 hours, then change to isotonic saline and sodium bicarbonate or a balanced electrolyte solution.[12] Isotonic saline and sodium bicarbonate can be made by mixing 1 L of isotonic saline with 1 L of isotonic sodium bicarbonate.

Empiric correction of acidosis in calves dehydrated due to diarrhea (extra-label): For situations where prolonged IV fluid administration is difficult or impractical: using sodium bicarbonate 8.4% solution, administer 10 mL/kg IV over 10 to 20 minutes. Sodium bicarbonate may be given alone, followed by oral administration of isotonic electrolyte solutions or given concurrently with IV fluids.[13]

CAMELIDS:

Correction of acidosis in New World Camelids (extra-label): Determine the bicarbonate requirement and give up to ½ of the calculated dose IV over 2 to 4 hours, with adjustments made based on blood gases and patient status to avoid over alkalinization. Sodium bicarbonate may be administered as an isotonic (1.4%) or hypertonic (8.4%) solution. Calculate the bicarbonate requirement with the following formulas:

a) Neonates: mEq bicarbonate needed = base deficit × body weight (kg) × 0.6

b) Adults: mEq bicarbonate needed = base deficit × body weight (kg) × 0.3.

GOATS:

Floppy kid syndrome in goats (extra-label): Give 1 or 2 doses of 2.5 – 3 g/kid (NOT g/kg) PO mixed in water. For severe cases or cases where the kid is unable to swallow, determine the bicarbonate requirement and administer IV as an isotonic (1.4%, 150 mEq/L) sodium bicarbonate solution, giving up to ½ of the calculated dose over 2 to 4 hours, with adjustments made based on blood gases and patient status to avoid over alkalinization. Estimate the sodium bicarbonate requirement (dose in mEq) = base deficit (mEq/L) × body weight (kg) × 0.5.

BIRDS:

Metabolic acidosis (extra-label): 1 mEq/kg initially IV (then SC) for 15 to 30 minutes to a maximum of 4 mEq/kg[14]

Monitoring

- Acid/base status. Blood gas analysis should be performed ≈2 to 4 hours after initiating sodium bicarbonate treatment, and periodically as treatment continues.[2]
- Serum electrolytes
- IV infusion site for infiltration
- Urine pH (if being used to alkalinize urine)

Chemistry/Synonyms

Sodium bicarbonate is an alkalinizing agent that occurs as a white, crystalline powder and has a slightly saline or alkaline taste. It is soluble in water and insoluble in alcohol. One gram of sodium bicarbonate contains ≈12 mEq (mMol) each of sodium and bicarbonate; 84 mg of sodium bicarbonate contains 1 mEq each of sodium and bicarbonate. Instructions to prepare an isotonic sodium bicarbonate solution are found in ***Compatibility/Compounding Considerations***.

Sodium bicarbonate may also be known as baking soda, E500, monosodium carbonate, natrii bicarbonas, natrii hydrogenocarbonas, sal de vichy, sodium acid carbonate, $NaHCO_3$, sodium hydrogen carbonate; many trade names are available.

Storage/Stability

Store sodium bicarbonate tablets in tight containers at room temperature (15°C-30°C [59°F-86°F]). Store sodium bicarbonate injection at temperatures less than 40°C (104°F), preferably at room temperature; avoid freezing.

Sodium bicarbonate powder is stable in dry air but will slowly decompose upon exposure to moist air.

Compatibility/Compounding Considerations

Compatibility is dependent on factors such as pH, concentration, temperature, and diluent used; specialized references or a hospital pharmacist can be consulted for more specific information.

Sodium bicarbonate for injection is reportedly physically **compatible** with the following IV solutions and drugs: Dextrose in water, dextrose/sodium chloride combinations, sodium chloride injections, amikacin sulfate, aminophylline, atropine sulfate, cefazolin, ceftazidime, ceftriaxone sodium, chloramphenicol sodium succinate, clindamycin phosphate, cyclosporine, dexamethasone sodium phosphate, dexmedetomidine, erythromycin gluceptate/lactobionate, fentanyl citrate, fluconazole, furosemide, gentamicin sulfate, glycopyrrolate, heparin sodium, hyaluronidase, hydrocortisone sodium succinate, regular insulin, labetalol HCl, mannitol, naloxone HCl, oxytocin, pamidronate disodium, penicillin G potassium, phenobarbital sodium, phenylephrine HCl, phenytoin sodium, phytonadione, piperacillin/tazobactam, potassium chloride, propofol, ranitidine HCl, sodium iodide, vasopressin, vincristine, and zoledronic acid.

Sodium bicarbonate for injection **compatibility information conflicts** or is dependent on diluent or concentration factors with the following drugs or solutions: lactated Ringer's injection, Ringer's injection, sodium lactate 1/6 M, ampicillin sodium, bupivacaine HCl, doxorubicin, famotidine, hydralazine, methylprednisolone sodium succinate, pentobarbital sodium, promazine HCl, thiopental sodium, verapamil HCl, vitamin B-complex with C, and voriconazole.

Sodium bicarbonate for injection is reportedly physically **incompatible** with the following solutions or drugs: alcohol 5%/dextrose 5%, D5-lactated Ringer's, amiodarone HCl, amphotericin B (all formulations), ascorbic acid injection, atracurium besylate, buprenorphine HCl, butorphanol HCl, calcium chloride/gluconate, carboplatin, cefoxitin sodium, ciprofloxacin, codeine phosphate, corticotropin, diazepam, diphenhydramine HCl, dobutamine HCl, dolasetron HCl, dopamine HCl, epinephrine HCl, glycopyrrolate, hydromorphone HCl, imipenem-cilastatin, isoproterenol, lidocaine HCl, HCl, ketamine HCl, levorphanol bitartrate, magnesium sulfate, meperidine HCl, meropenem, metoclopramide HCl, midazolam, morphine sulfate, norepinephrine bitartrate, ondansetron HCl, oxytetracycline HCl, pantoprazole sodium, pentazocine lactate, and succinylcholine chloride.

A 1.4% solution of sodium bicarbonate (≈13 g sodium bicarbonate/L) is approximately isotonic. An 8.4% solution of sodium bicarbonate, with a calculated osmolarity of 2000 mOsm/L, can be made isotonic by diluting each mL with 4.6 mL of sterile water for injection; remove 150 mL from a 1 L bag of sterile water for injection (or other isotonic fluid) and add 150 mL of 8.4% sodium bicarbonate for injection. Practically, a slightly hypertonic solution can be prepared by adding 200 mL of sodium bicarbonate 8.4% solution to a 1000 mL bag of sterile water for injection or other isotonic solution; ***do not*** remove any fluid from the bag prior to adding sodium bicarbonate.

Because converting volume measurements into weights is not very accurate for powders, it is recommended to actually weigh powders when using them for pharmaceutical purposes. However, if this is not possible, one (1) level teaspoon (5 mL) of commercially available baking soda contains ≈4.8 to 5.9 g of sodium bicarbonate.

Dosage Forms/Regulatory Status

VETERINARY-LABELED PRODUCTS:

Sodium Bicarbonate Injection: 8.4% (1 mEq/mL) in 50 mL and 100 mL vials; generic; (Rx). Not FDA-approved

HUMAN-LABELED PRODUCTS:

Injectable Products:

Sodium Bicarbonate Neutralizing Additive Solution: 4% (0.48 mEq/mL) in 5 mL vials; 4.2% (0.5 mEq/mL) in 5 mL vials (2.5 mEq); *Neut®*, generic; (Rx).

Sodium Bicarbonate Injection: 4.2% (0.5 mEq/mL) in 10 mL syringes; generic; (Rx)

Sodium Bicarbonate Injection: 7.5% (0.9 mEq/mL) in 50 mL syringes; generic; (Rx)

Sodium Bicarbonate Injection: 8.4% (1 mEq/mL) in 10 mL syringes, 50 mL syringes, and 50 mL vials; generic; (Rx)

Oral Products:

Sodium Bicarbonate Tablets: 325 mg and 650 mg; generic; (OTC)

Sodium Bicarbonate Powder: 113 g, 120 g, and 0.5 kg (1 lb); generic; (OTC)

Omeprazole/Sodium Bicarbonate Capsules (immediate release): 20 mg or 40 mg omeprazole/1100 mg sodium bicarbonate; *Zegerid®*, generic; (Rx)

Omeprazole/Sodium Bicarbonate Powder for Oral Suspension: 20 mg or 40 mg omeprazole/1680 mg sodium bicarbonate in unit-dose packets; *Zegerid®*; (Rx)

References

For the complete list of references, see **wiley.com/go/budde/plumb**

Sodium Stibogluconate

(sti-boe-***gloo***-koe-nate) *Pentostam®*

Antileishmanial

Prescriber Highlights

- ► Antimony compound for treatment of leishmaniasis in dogs
- ► Not commercially available in the United States
- ► Contraindicated in patients with renal failure or pre-existing arrhythmias
- ► Many potential severe adverse effects are possible.

Uses/Indications

Sodium stibogluconate has been used for the treatment of leishmaniasis in dogs. Availability and adverse effects limit clinical use; therefore, meglumine antimoniate is typically the preferred antimony product.

Pharmacology/Actions

Sodium stibogluconate is a pentavalent antimonial. Its exact mechanism of action is unknown, but it is believed to reduce ATP and GTP synthesis in susceptible amistagotes.[1] It may also alter membrane permeability or active transport mechanisms.

Pharmacokinetics

In dogs, the steady-state volume of distribution of sodium stibogluconate was 0.25 L/kg, with a clearance of 1.71 L/kg/hr. Terminal half-life ranged from 0.6 to 1.5 hours.[2] The main route of excretion is via the kidneys; glomerular filtration rate determines excretion rate.

Contraindications/Precautions/Warnings

Sodium stibogluconate is contraindicated in patients with pre-existing cardiac arrhythmias or significantly impaired renal function. It should not be used in patients that have had a serious adverse reaction to a previous dose.

Adverse Effects

Dogs given stibogluconate 40 mg/kg developed increased AST levels.[2] Other reported adverse effects include pain on injection, musculoskeletal pain, hemolytic anemia, leukopenia, vomiting, diarrhea, pancreatitis, myocardial injury and arrhythmias, renal toxicity, shock, and sudden death. IV administration can cause thrombophlebitis. The incidence of adverse effects reportedly increases with duration of use longer than 2 months.

Reproductive/Nursing Safety

Sodium stibogluconate has not been shown to cause fetal harm, but it should be withheld during pregnancy unless the benefits outweigh the risks. Sodium stibogluconate use during nursing is controversial; it is usually compatible with nursing,[3] the manufacturer states that it should not be used in nursing mothers. Because safety has not been established in animals, this drug should only be used when the maternal benefits outweigh the potential risks to offspring.

Overdose/Acute Toxicity

Antimony can potentially be chelated with dimercaprol (BAL in oil), dimercaptosuccinic acid (DMSA) or d-penicillamine.

For patients that have experienced or are suspected to have experienced an overdose, consultation with a 24-hour poison consultation center specializing in providing veterinary-specific information is recommended. For general information related to overdose and toxin exposures, as well as contact information for poison control centers, refer to ***Appendix.***

Drug Interactions

- No specific drug interactions were noted. Stibogluconate has reportedly been used with allopurinol, paromomycin, or pentamidine without problems.

Laboratory Considerations

- No specific laboratory interactions or considerations noted.

Dosages

DOGS:

Cutaneous leishmaniasis (extra-label): 30 – 50 mg/kg IV or SC daily for 3 to 4 weeks. May be administered every other day for longer durations if adverse effects occur. If administered IV, give slowly over 5 minutes or longer using a fine needle or catheter to avoid thrombophlebitis. Concomitant allopurinol (10 mg/kg PO twice daily) is recommended.[4,5]

Monitoring

- Baseline and periodic (ie, 1 month after therapy begins then every 3 to 4 months) CBC, serum chemistry panel including amylase and lipase, urinalysis with urine:protein creatinine ratio[6]
- Baseline and periodic ECG
- Clinical efficacy; serology +/- PCR at least 6 months after the start of therapy then every 6 months[6]

Client Information

- Clients should understand the potential public health implications of this disease in dogs (dependent on country), the guarded prognosis (even with treatment), risks of treatment, and associated expenses.

Chemistry/Synonyms

Sodium stibogluconate is a pentavalent antimony compound that contains between 30% and 34% antimony. It is a colorless, odorless or almost odorless, amorphous powder. Sodium stibogluconate is very soluble in water and practically insoluble in alcohol or ether. The injection commercially available in other countries has a pH between 5 and 5.6.

Sodium stibogluconate may also be known as sodium antimony gluconate, *stiboglucat-natrium*, natriumstibogluconat-9-wasser, solusurmin, stibogluconat, *sodio stibogluconato*, and *natrii stibogluconas*.

Storage/Stability

Store the injection at temperatures below 25°C (76°F) and protect from freezing and exposure to light. After removing the first dose, the vial should not be used after one month. Use of a 5 micron filter during preparation is recommended to remove particulates that may be formed by an interaction between the vial stopper and the solution's preservative.

Compatibility/Compounding Considerations

No specific information noted

Dosage Forms/Regulatory Status

VETERINARY-LABELED PRODUCTS: NONE

HUMAN-LABELED PRODUCTS:

Sodium Stibogluconate for Injection: Sodium antimony gluconate 100 mg (of pentavalent antimony) per mL in 100 mL vials; *Pentostam®*. Not available in the United States. Check with the Centers for Disease Control and Prevention (CDC) for availability. https://www.cdc.gov/laboratory/drugservice/formulary.html

References

For the complete list of references, see **wiley.com/go/budde/plumb**

Sodium Thiosulfate

(soe-***dee***-um thye-oh-***sul***-fayte) *Sodium Hyposulfite*

Antidote (Arsenic, Cyanide)

Prescriber Highlights

- ▶ Used for cyanide, arsenic, or copper poisoning; localized treatment for chemotherapy extravasation injuries
- ▶ No known contraindications
- ▶ Adverse effects may include profuse diarrhea when large doses are given by mouth.
- ▶ Injectable forms should be given slowly IV.

Uses/Indications

Sodium thiosulfate is used in the treatment of cyanide toxicity, including poisoning from cyanogenic glycoside-containing plants. It has synergistic effects when used in sequence with sodium nitrate. It has been used in treating arsenic toxicosis in cattle,[1,2] and has been proposed for other heavy metal poisonings but its efficacy is in question for these purposes. When used in combination with sodium molybdate, sodium thiosulfate may be useful for the treatment of copper poisoning,[3] although penicillamine may be preferable but cost may be an issue.

In humans, sodium thiosulfate has been used to reduce cisplatin nephrotoxicity[4,5] and has been shown to reduce cisplatin related ototoxicity.[6] A 3% or 4% solution has been used to infiltrate the site of extravasations of cisplatin, carboplatin, or dactinomycin.[7,8] Sodium thiosulfate has been used in the management of mechlorethamine extravasation,[9,10] and, in combination with steroids, sodium thiosulfate may reduce the healing time associated with doxorubicin extravasation. It is also used in humans in the management of calciphylaxis in dialysis patients.

Pharmacology/Actions

Administration of thiosulfate provides an exogenous source of sulfur to the body, thereby hastening the detoxification of cyanide using the enzyme rhodanese. Rhodanese (*thiosulfate cyanide sulfurtransferase*) converts cyanide to the relatively nontoxic thiocyanate ion; thiocyanate is then excreted in the urine.

Sodium thiosulfate's topical antifungal activity is probably due to its slow release of colloidal sulfur.

Although sodium thiosulfate has been recommended for treating arsenic (and some other heavy metal) poisoning, the proposed mechanism of action is not known and its efficacy is in question. Presumably, the sulfate moiety may react with and chelate the metal allowing its removal.

Pharmacokinetics

Sodium thiosulfate is relatively poorly absorbed from the GI tract. When substantial doses are given PO, it acts as a saline cathartic. When administered IV, it is distributed in the extracellular fluid and then rapidly excreted via the urine. In dogs, a therapeutic IV dose is eliminated in urine within 90 minutes. In dogs with renal failure, metabolic clearance rate is reduced, and the plasma thiosulfate concentration is increased and remains elevated for at least 16 hours.[11]

Elimination half-life in humans is ≈1.5 hours.

Contraindications/Precautions/Warnings

Sodium thiosulfate may exacerbate hypertension or edema and should be used with caution in patients who may have these signs including those with congestive heart failure or renal impairment.

NOTE: With cyanide poisoning, sodium nitrite is given first, followed by sodium thiosulfate, except in cases involving smoke inhalation, as nitrite acts by converting hemoglobin to methemoglobin; however, in subjects with carbon monoxide inhalation (from smoke) increasing the concentration of methemoglobin would worsen oxygen carrying capacity already reduced by CO exposure. In cyanide poisoning the dose of sodium thiosulfate can be repeated if required, but only one dose of sodium nitrite should be given because of the risk of producing a high concentration of methemoglobinemia and exacerbating tissue hypoxia.

Adverse Effects

Sodium thiosulfate is relatively nontoxic. Large doses by mouth may cause profuse diarrhea. Hypernatremia and edema are possible. Injectable forms should be given slowly IV to minimize the risk of nausea, vomiting, and hypotension.

In humans, hypernatremia, hypotension, nausea and vomiting, diarrhea, diuresis, and metabolic acidosis have been reported and are thought to be due to both the intrinsic osmotic properties of sodium thiosulfate, and from thiocyanate formed when it is used to treat cyanide poisoning. Increased clotting times 1 to 3 days after dosing have also been reported. Sodium thiosulfate preparations may contain trace impurities of sodium sulfite; however, in an emergency sodium thiosulfate should not be withheld in subjects with sulfite hypersensitivity.

Reproductive/Nursing Safety

There were no teratogenic effects in the offspring of hamsters treated with sodium thiosulfate during pregnancy. Sodium thiosulfate reduces cyanide maternal toxicity in animal studies.[12,13] In addition sodium thiosulfate was not embryotoxic or teratogenic in rodents or rabbits at maternal doses of up to 580 mg/kg/day.

No lactation information was found; use when the maternal benefits outweigh the potential risks to offspring.

Overdose/Acute Toxicity

In dogs the LD_{50} of IV sodium thiosulfate is greater than 3000 mg/kg.

For patients that have experienced or are suspected of having experienced an overdose, consultation with a 24-hour poison consultation center specializing in providing veterinary-specific information is recommended. For general information related to overdose and toxin exposures, as well as contact information for poison control centers, refer to ***Appendix***.

Drug Interactions

No specific drug interactions were noted.

Laboratory Considerations

- Sodium thiosulfate may produce clinically significant falsely increased chloride measurements, depending on the analyzer used.[14,15]

Dosages

DOGS, CATS:

Cyanide toxicity (extra-label): First give sodium nitrite 3% solution 10 – 20 mg/kg IV followed by sodium thiosulfate 25% solution 150 – 500 mg/kg IV bolus or CRI.[16] In mild cases sodium thiosulfate alone may be sufficient.

Treating extravasation injuries secondary to doxorubicin, carboplatin, cisplatin, and mechlorethamine infusions (extra-label): Prepare a 0.17 Mol/L solution by mixing 4 mL sodium thiosulfate 10% w/v with 6 mL sterile water for injection. Inject into extravasation site. **NOTE**: These are recommendations for human patients.[8-10]

HORSES:

Cyanide toxicity (extra-label): First give sodium nitrite 20% solution 10 – 20 mg/kg IV followed by sodium thiosulfate 20% solution 30 – 40 mg/kg IV[17]

Arsenic toxicity (extra-label): Sodium thiosulfate 20 – 30 grams per horse (NOT mg/kg) in 300 mL of water orally with dimercaprol (BAL) 3 mg/kg IM every 4 hours[18]

RUMINANTS:

Note: When used in food animals, FARAD states that this salt is rapidly excreted and not considered a residue concern in animal tissues; therefore a 24-hour preslaughter withdrawal interval (WDI) would be sufficient.[19]

Copper poisoning in combination with sodium molybdate (extra-label): In conjunction with fluid replacement therapy, sodium thiosulfate 500 mg with ammonium or sodium molybdate 200 mg PO daily for up to 3 weeks will help decrease total body burden of copper[20]

Cyanide toxicity secondary to cyanogenic plants (extra-label): Sodium thiosulfate in a 30% solution 660 mg/kg IV given rapidly using a 12- or 14- gauge needle.[21]

Arsenic poisoning: (extra-label) In a meta-analysis, the most commonly administered antidote was sodium thiosulfate 20 – 40 mg/kg IV every 8 hours and 80 mg/kg PO once a day, but one study using 40 mg/kg IV every 8 hours and 80 mg/kg PO once a day reported better outcomes. Administration of oral or IV fluids was highly associated with survival.[1]

Monitoring

For cyanide poisoning, vital signs (eg, respiratory rate, heart rate, blood pressure, CNS) and acid-base status.

For heavy metal poisoning, blood and/or urinary concentrations of the metal.

Client Information

- This agent should only be used with close professional supervision.

Chemistry/Synonyms

Sodium thiosulfate occurs as large, colorless, odorless crystals or coarse, crystalline powder. It is very soluble in water, deliquescent in moist air and effloresces in dry air at temperatures greater than 33°C (91.4°F).

Sodium thiosulfate may also be known as natrii thiosulfas, natrium thiosulfuricum, sodium hyposulphite, sodium thiosulphate, *Consept Step 2®*, *Hiposul®*, *Hyposulfene®*, or *S-hydril®*.

Storage/Stability

Unless otherwise stated by the manufacturer, store at room temperature 20° to 25°C (68°F-77°F); excursions permitted from 15°C to 30°C (59°F-86°F). Crystals should be stored in tight containers.

Compatibility/Compounding Considerations

Compatibility is dependent on factors such as pH, concentration, temperature, and diluent used; specialized references or a hospital pharmacist should be consulted for more specific information.

Sodium thiosulfate is **compatible** with sodium nitrate and sodium nitroprusside and is **not compatible** mixed with hydroxocobalamin.

No chemical incompatibility has been reported between sodium thiosulfate and sodium nitrite, when administered sequentially through the same IV line.

Dosage Forms/Regulatory Status

VETERINARY-LABELED PRODUCTS: NONE

HUMAN-LABELED PRODUCTS:

Sodium Thiosulfate for Injection: 10% (100 mg/mL, as pentahydrate) and 25% (250 mg/mL as pentahydrate) preservative-free in 10 mL and 50 mL single-use vials; generic; (Rx)

Sodium thiosulfate crystals or powder may be available from chemical suppliers, and the use of pharmaceutical grade (USP- or NF- designation) is recommended.

References

For the complete list of references, see **wiley.com/go/budde/plumb**

Somatotropin

Growth Hormone

(soe-ma-toe-***troe***-pin) *Posilac®*

Hormone

Prescriber Highlights

- ▶ Used for treatment of canine hypopituitary dwarfism; it may also be used to increase milk production in cows.
- ▶ Hypersensitivity reactions are possible. May cause irreversible diabetes mellitus in dogs
- ▶ Products used for dogs may be expensive and difficult to obtain.

Uses/Indications

Somatotropin may be useful in treating hypopituitary dwarfism. Historically, it was used to treat alopecia X (also previously known as growth hormone-responsive dermatosis) in adult dogs; however, somatotropin is no longer recommended given the current understating of the disease etiology.

Bovine somatotropin is indicated for increasing production of marketable milk in healthy lactating dairy cattle.

Pharmacology/Actions

Somatotropin (growth hormone) is responsible for and contributes to musculoskeletal growth (linear growth and increased bone and muscle mass) as well as other cellular and organ growth. It is also a factor in protein, carbohydrate, lipid, connective tissue, and mineral metabolism, and it plays an important role in thymus development and T-cell function.

Pharmacokinetics

No canine-specific information was located. Somatotropin is a peptide, and elimination via the liver and kidneys would be expected.

Contraindications/Precautions/Warnings

Growth hormone is contraindicated in patients that are hypersensitive to it.

In humans, active malignancy is considered a contraindication for use of recombinant growth factor and increased risk for neoplasm is listed as a warning[1]; however, this is controversial.[2] The drug should not be used for growth promotion in pediatric patients with closed epiphyses.[1] Use somatotropin with caution in patients with impaired glucose tolerance or diabetes mellitus, and hypoadrenocorticism. Concurrent secondary adrenocortical insufficiency and hypothyroidism must be treated appropriately. Patients with hypothyroidism may experience a suboptimal response to somatotropin.

Lactating cows receiving bovine somatotropin may require diets that meet or exceed typical nutritional requirements.[3]

Adverse Effects

Growth hormone may cause diabetes mellitus in dogs and may be transient or permanent even after discontinuing treatment. Blood and urine glucose should be routinely monitored. Discontinue therapy if hyperglycemia occurs. Hypersensitivity reactions are possible, but less so if using products of porcine origin in dogs; porcine growth hormone appears to have little immunogenicity in dogs. Long-term treatment at high doses may cause acromegaly. Acromegaly in dogs can cause increased size of paws and head, increased skin folds around head and neck area, prognathism, and inspiratory stridor.

Cows receiving somatotropin may have increased body temperature and injection site reactions and are at increased risk for clinical mastitis.[3]

In humans receiving recombinant growth hormone, adverse effects include upper respiratory infections, fever, pharyngitis, otitis media, edema, arthralgia, paresthesia, myalgia, peripheral edema, hypothyroidism, pancreatitis, hyperglycemia, and impaired glucose tolerance.[1,4]

Reproductive/Nursing Safety

Because safety has not been established in small animal species, this drug should only be used when the maternal benefits outweigh the potential risks to offspring.

Overdose/Acute Toxicity

Acute overdoses could cause hypoglycemia initially and then hyperglycemia. Blood glucose should be monitored, and supportive treatment (eg, dextrose or insulin) should be provided.

For patients that have experienced or are suspected of having experienced an overdose, consultation with a 24-hour poison consultation center specializing in providing veterinary-specific information is recommended. For general information related to overdose and toxin exposures, as well as contact information for poison control centers, refer to ***Appendix***.

Drug Interactions

The following drug interactions have either been reported or are theoretical in humans or animals receiving somatotropin and may be of significance in veterinary patients. Unless otherwise noted, use together is not necessarily contraindicated, but weigh the potential risks and perform additional monitoring when appropriate.

- **Glucocorticoids** (eg, **dexamethasone, prednis(ol)one**): May inhibit the growth-promoting effect of somatotropin. If concurrent adrenal insufficiency is diagnosed, adjust glucocorticoid dose carefully to avoid negative effects on growth.
- **Insulin/Oral Hypoglycemic Agents** (eg, **glipizide, metformin**): Doses of hypoglycemic agents may require modification when somatotropin is initiated and/or discontinued.

Dosages

DOGS:

Hypopituitary dwarfism using porcine growth hormone (extra-label): 2 units/dog (NOT units/kg) SC every other day OR 0.1 unit/kg SC 3 times weekly for 4 to 6 weeks[5,6]; adjust dose based on clinical response and IGF-1 measurements. See ***Monitoring***. Improvement of skin and hair coat signs can be seen within 6 to 8 weeks. Because growth plates close rapidly, no significant change in stature (ie, minimal linear growth) is noted.

CATTLE:

Increasing production of marketable milk in lactating dairy cows: 500 mg (one syringe) SC every 14 days.[3] Start during the ninth or tenth week after calving and continue until the end of lactation. Recommended administration sites are the neck area, behind the shoulder, or in the depression on either side of the tailhead.

Monitoring

When used in dogs:

- Clinical efficacy
- Blood glucose (weekly)
- Urine glucose (daily)
- Baseline and periodic thyroid function and adrenal function

When used in lactating dairy cows:

- Milk output
- Mastitis

Client Information

- Clients should be instructed on the methods for SC injection and testing urine glucose.
- Be sure to understand the cost of this medicine, as it may be a barrier to treatment.
- Dogs treated with this medicine may develop diabetes mellitus that does not go away once the medicine is stopped.

Chemistry/Synonyms

Somatotropin may also be known as CB-311, hGH, human growth hormone, LY-137998, somatropinum; many trade names are available. The bovine somatotropin product is also known as sometribove zinc, BGH, rBGH. Synthetic recombinant human forms (rhGH) are known as somatropin.

Storage/Stability

Porcine growth hormone should be stored according to product label. Store the bovine somatotropin product under refrigeration (2°C-8°C [36°F-46°F]); do not freeze.[3] Avoid prolonged exposure to excessive heat or sunlight. Allow syringes to warm to room temperature (15°C-30°C [59°F-86°F]) before use.

Compatibility/Compounding Considerations

No specific information noted

Dosage Forms/Regulatory Status

VETERINARY-LABELED PRODUCTS:

The Association of Racing Commissioners International (ARCI) has designated this drug as a class 2 substance. Use of this drug may not be allowed in certain animal competitions. Check rules and regulations before entering in a competition while this medication is being administered. Contact local racing authorities for further guidance. See ***Appendix*** for more information.

No FDA-approved formulations of porcine growth hormone are commercially available.

Bovine somatotropin, prolonged-release injectable: 500 mg single-dose syringes in 25 or 100 count boxes; *Posilac*®; (OTC). Approved for use in lactating dairy cattle. Withdrawal intervals: slaughter, 2 weeks; milk, none. **NOTE**: This formulation is not suitable for canine use as it is a sustained release formulation and not easily diluted to smaller doses that are required for dogs.

HUMAN-LABELED PRODUCTS:

There are several manufacturers of human recombinant growth hormone (somatropin) products; however, these products are expensive, can cause immunogenicity reactions in dogs, and are not sold for veterinary use.

References

For the complete list of references, see **wiley.com/go/budde/plumb**

Sorbitol

(***sore***-bit-ahl)

Laxative/Cathartic

Prescriber Highlights

- Orally administered cathartic that is often used in combination with activated charcoal to accelerate expulsion of GI toxins or with sodium polystyrene sulfonate (SPS) for hyperkalemia
- Do not use as part of a retention enema due to risk for colonic necrosis.
- Adverse effects include loose stools, diarrhea, vomiting, and potential fluid and electrolyte disturbances (eg, hypernatremia).

Uses/Indications

Sorbitol is an osmotic laxative that can is typically used in combination with activated charcoal for GI decontamination or with sodium polystyrene sulfonate (SPS) for treating mild hyperkalemia. Sorbitol is also used as a sweetener (½ the sweetening power of sucrose).

Pharmacology/Actions

Sorbitol is a nonabsorbable sugar alcohol that acts as an osmotic laxative. Stool pH may be reduced in patients taking sorbitol, thus trapping ammonia in the stool, which may be useful in patients with hepatic encephalopathy.

Pharmacokinetics

Depending on dose and additional fluid consumed, sorbitol can have a laxative effect within 1 hour of dosing.

Contraindications/Precautions/Warnings

Do not use sorbitol mixed with sodium polystyrene sulfonate (SPS) as a retention enema. Retention enemas with sorbitol and SPS have been implicated in some human cases of colonic necrosis,[1] presumably secondary to sorbitol causing cellular dehydration.

When sorbitol is used in combination with activated charcoal, only the first dose should contain sorbitol, as multiple doses can increase the risks for hypernatremia and dehydration.

Adverse Effects

Products containing sorbitol may cause loose stools, diarrhea, and vomiting. Fluid and electrolyte imbalances are also possible.

There have been reports of hypernatremia occurring in small dogs and cats after activated charcoal and sorbitol administration, presumably due an osmotic effect pulling water into the GI tract. Administration of reduced-sodium IV fluids (eg, 5% dextrose, 0.45% sodium chloride with 2.5% dextrose) in conjunction with warm water enemas may be helpful to alleviate hypernatremia.

Reproductive/Nursing Safety

Safe use during nursing has not been established but it is unlikely to pose much risk to nursing offspring. Because safety has not been established in animals, this drug should only be used when the maternal benefits outweigh the potential risks to offspring.

Overdose/Acute Toxicity

Overdoses or multiple doses can cause fluid and electrolyte disorders including dehydration and hypernatremia.

For patients that have experienced or are suspected to have experienced an overdose, consultation with a 24-hour poison consultation center specializing in providing veterinary-specific information is recommended. For general information related to overdose and toxin exposures, as well as contact information for poison control centers, refer to ***Appendix.***

Drug Interactions

The following drug interactions have either been reported or are theoretical in humans or animals receiving sorbitol and may be of significance in veterinary patients. Unless otherwise noted, use together is not necessarily contraindicated, but weigh the potential risks and perform additional monitoring when appropriate.

- **Sodium Polystyrene Sulfonate (SPS)**: Although commonly used together for oral administration in veterinary patients, there is an increased risk for colon necrosis, especially if used as a retention enema.

Laboratory Considerations

- Sorbitol may cause false-positive ethylene glycol test results.

Dosages

DOGS/CATS:

Adjunctive treatment for toxin ingestion using sorbitol with activated charcoal (extra-label): Using activated charcoal containing sorbitol, 1 – 2 g/kg PO but doses up to 5 g/kg have been described. Charcoal with sorbitol is commonly employed (only with the first dose) to shorten GI transit time. For drugs and toxins that undergo enterohepatic recirculation (eg, caffeine, phenobarbital, theobromine, theophylline, bromethalin, pyrethrins, marijuana, NSAIDs, organophosphate insecticides, ivermectin, digoxin, antidepressants), multiple subsequent doses of activated charcoal WITHOUT sorbitol at 1 – 2 g/kg PO every 4 to 8 hours for 24 to 48 hours are recommended. Dogs and cats with no clinical signs may freely consume the charcoal suspension if administered via syringe. A small amount of food may be added to the solution to enhance palatability.[2] In animals exhibiting clinical signs, administration of activated charcoal suspensions may be done via a nasogastric tube, as it may be better accepted, easier to place (especially in cats), and offer a greater margin of safety; always ensure adequate airway protection.[3-6] There is little need to administer a cathartic if significant diarrhea is already present. See also ***Charcoal, Activated.***

Adjunctive treatment of hyperkalemia using sorbitol with sodium polystyrene sulfonate (SPS) (extra-label): SPS resin 2 g/kg mixed with 70% sorbitol PO, DIVIDED into 3 to 4 doses per day. Do not mix with potassium-rich foods (eg, bananas, potatoes).[7,8] See also ***Sodium Polystyrene Sulfonate.***

Shorten GI transit time, cathartic (extra-label): 0.5 – 2 mL/kg PO once daily, adjusted to effect[9]

HORSES:

Cathartic for plant intoxications using sorbitol with activated charcoal (extra-label): 70% sorbitol 3 mL/kg mixed with an activated charcoal slurry 1 – 5 g/kg (≈1 g of activated charcoal/5 mL of water). There is little need to administer a cathartic if significant diarrhea is already present.[10] See also ***Charcoal, Activated.***

Monitoring

- Monitoring for efficacy of charcoal is usually dependent on the toxin/drug's mechanism of action, extent of toxicity, and patient's clinical signs.

- When sorbitol is given with activated charcoal, repeated serum sodium measurements (eg, every 8 to 12 hours) are recommended to address potential hypernatremia before clinical signs (eg, tremors, ataxia, seizures) occur. Serum sodium increases can be seen 6 to 10 hours after cathartic administration.[11]
- Hydration status

Client Information

- This medicine may cause diarrhea, excess gas (flatulence), cramping, and vomiting.
- Although sorbitol is available without a prescription, do not give this medicine without first consulting your veterinarian.

Chemistry/Synonyms

Sorbitol is a sugar alcohol and occurs as a white, odorless, hygroscopic powder, granules, or crystalline masses having a sweet taste with a cold sensation. It is very soluble in water; it is sparingly soluble in alcohol and practically insoluble in solvent ether.

Sorbitol may also be known as D-glucitol, E420, D-sorbitol, sorbitoli, sorbitolis, sorbitolum, or szorbit.

Storage/Stability

Store the 70% oral solution at controlled room temperature (20°C-25°C [68°F-77°F]).

Compatibility/Compounding Considerations

No specific information noted

Dosage Forms/Regulatory Status

VETERINARY-LABELED PRODUCTS:

Only available in combination products.

Oral Suspension: Sorbitol 10%, activated charcoal 10%, and kaolin 6.25% in 240 mL bottles; *Toxiban® Suspension with Sorbitol*; (OTC)

Oral Granules: Sorbitol 20%, activated charcoal 47.5%, and kaolin 10% in 1 lb jars and 5 kg pails; *Toxiban® Granules*; (OTC)

HUMAN-LABELED PRODUCTS:

Sorbitol 70% Enema Solution: 16 oz; generic; (OTC)

In combination with activated charcoal:

Activated Charcoal Oral Suspension in Sorbitol Base: Sorbitol 26 g and activated charcoal 25 g in 120 mL; *Insta-Char®*; and Sorbitol 48 g and activated charcoal 25 g in 120 mL containers and sorbitol 96 g and activated charcoal 50 g in 240 mL containers; *ActiDose® with Sorbitol*; (OTC)

References

For the complete list of references, see **wiley.com/go/budde/plumb**

Sotalol

(***soh***-ta-lole) *Betapace®*

Beta-Adrenergic Antagonist

Prescriber Highlights

- ► Nonselective beta-adrenergic receptor antagonist and potassium channel blocker commonly used to control ventricular tachyarrhythmias, as well as some forms of supraventricular tachyarrhythmia in dogs, cats, and horses
- ► Contraindicated in patients hypersensitive to it, with asthma, sinus bradycardia, second- or third-degree AV block, sick sinus syndrome, hypokalemic bradycardia, long QT syndromes, cardiogenic shock, or uncontrolled congestive heart failure (CHF).
- ► Use with caution in patients with controlled CHF, decreased myocardial function, diabetes mellitus, or hyperthyroidism.
- ► Dose reduction or extended dosing intervals may be needed for patients with renal dysfunction.
- ► Most serious adverse effects include negative inotropic and pro-arrhythmic effects but dyspnea, bronchospasm, fatigue, and nausea or vomiting are also possible.

Uses/Indications

Sotalol can be useful in the long-term oral management of ventricular and supraventricular tachycardias in dogs, cats, and horses. It is used alone or as combination therapy (eg, mexiletine) in dogs with ventricular tachycardia that are refractory to IV antiarrhythmic therapy (eg, lidocaine, procainamide, amiodarone), in boxer dogs, and in other breeds with arrhythmogenic right ventricular cardiomyopathy (ARVC), and in German shepherd dogs with inherited arrhythmias.[1] Although research data support its efficacy to suppress ventricular ectopy, it is unknown if it significantly impacts survival, particularly when compared with other therapies.[2,3] Sotalol has been used for the treatment of supraventricular tachyarrhythmias such as in dogs with accessory pathway-mediated reciprocating tachycardia,[4] in a dog with atrial flutter,[5] and in a cat with supraventricular tachycardia.[6]

In horses, it has been used to treat both supraventricular and ventricular tachyarrhythmias.[7-9] Based on a small clinical trial,[10] sotalol may lower the cardioversion threshold for atrial fibrillation in horses and has been postulated to have potential for limiting recurrence of atrial fibrillation in that species.[11]

Pharmacology/Actions

Sotalol is a nonselective beta-blocker and class III antiarrhythmic agent (potassium channel blocker). The beta-blocking activity of sotalol is ≈30% that of propranolol. The pharmacologic action is believed to be caused by selectively inhibiting potassium channels. Like other class III drugs, it prolongs repolarization and refractoriness without affecting conduction. In animals with supraventricular tachycardias, sotalol may be more effective in preventing recurrence of the arrhythmia than in terminating it.

Pharmacokinetics

Unlike propranolol, sotalol does not have any appreciable first pass effect after oral administration. Food may reduce the bioavailability of sotalol by ≈20% in humans and, if given on an empty stomach, bioavailability is 90% to 100%. Peak plasma concentrations occur between 2 to 4 hours after a dose. The drug has relatively low lipid solubility and virtually no protein binding. Elimination is almost all via the kidney and most of the drug is excreted unchanged. In dogs, sotalol's elimination half-life is 5 hours; in humans, it is ≈12 hours.

In horses, after IV administration of 1 mg/kg, maximum plasma concentration, clearance, and elimination half-life were 1624 ng/mL, 0.15 L/hour/kg, and 8.7 hours, respectively. When the same dose was administered orally, maximum plasma concentration, time to reach maximum plasma concentration, clearance, elimination half-life, and bioavailability were 317 ng/mL, 0.9 hours, 0.15 L/hour/kg, 15.2 hours, and 47.8%, respectively.[12] In a follow-up study, mean steady-state plasma concentrations were 287 ng/mL (range 234 to 339), 409 ng/mL (359 to 458), and 543 ng/mL (439 to 646) for oral dosages of 2, 3, and 4 mg/kg (respectively) of sotalol given orally every 12 hours over 9 days.[13] Pharmacodynamic effects in the horse include a significant increase in QT interval and the effective refractory period after oral dosing.[13]

In dogs, sotalol administered at 1 – 2 mg/kg orally twice daily for 12 to 16 days resulted in a 5.8% mean reduction in ejection fraction by echocardiography and a reduction in maximum heart rate of 17 beats per minute on 24-hour Holter monitor, demonstrating mild negative inotropic and chronotropic effects in healthy dogs.[14]

Contraindications/Precautions/Warnings

Sotalol is contraindicated in patients hypersensitive to it and in patients with asthma, sinus bradycardia, second- or third-degree heart block (unless artificially paced), sick sinus syndrome, hypokalemia, long QT syndromes, cardiogenic shock, or uncontrolled congestive heart failure (CHF). Because of the potential for negative inotropic effects, use with caution in controlled CHF and in those with decreased myocardial function. Also, use sotalol with caution in patients with diabetes mellitus or hyperthyroidism, as it may mask clinical signs associated with both conditions. Use with caution in patients with renal dysfunction; dosages may need to be decreased or dosage intervals may need to be extended.

Adverse Effects

Primary concerns with sotalol in dogs are the potential for negative inotropic, chronotropic, and proarrhythmic effects. These effects generally are not clinically important if dosage is not excessive. Rarely, dogs receiving sotalol will demonstrate an increase in arrhythmia number or complexity on follow-up ambulatory ECG; it is not well studied how often this perceived proarrhythmic effect occurs nor is it known which patient factors may contribute. Other potential adverse effects include dyspnea, bronchospasm, fatigue/dizziness, nausea, and vomiting.[15] Sotalol's beta-blocking effects can worsen syncope or cause lethargy, particularly if the ventricular tachyarrhythmia coexists with intermittent bradycardia (eg, AV block).

Reproductive/Nursing Safety

Sotalol did not cause any fetotoxicity or teratogenicity when given to pregnant laboratory animals at high dosages, but clear safety in pregnancy has not been established.

Sotalol enters human breastmilk in concentrations ≈5 times those found in the serum and is not recommended for use in nursing humans.[15] Consider using a milk replacer in nursing animals.

Because safety has not been established in animals, this drug should only be used when the maternal benefits outweigh the potential risks to offspring.

Overdose/Acute Toxicity

Overdoses may result in panting, bradycardia, lethargy, vomiting, hypotension, CHF, bronchospasm, and hypoglycemia. Use GI decontamination (if not contraindicated) when significant risk of morbidity is possible. Treat adverse effects symptomatically and supportively.

For patients that have experienced or are suspected to have experienced an overdose, consultation with a 24-hour poison consultation center specializing in providing veterinary-specific information is recommended. For general information related to overdose and toxin exposures, as well as contact information for poison control centers, refer to ***Appendix***.

Drug Interactions

The following drug interactions have either been reported or are theoretical in humans or animals receiving sotalol and may be of significance in veterinary patients. Unless otherwise noted, use together is not necessarily contraindicated, but weigh the potential risks and perform additional monitoring when appropriate.

- **Amiodarone**: May prolong refractory periods; concurrent use not recommended in human patients
- **Anesthetics, General**: Additive myocardial depression may occur with the concurrent use of sotalol and myocardial depressant anesthetic agents.
- **Antacids, Aluminum- or Magnesium- Containing**: May reduce oral sotalol absorption; separate doses by at least 2 hours.
- **Antiarrhythmics, Class 1A** (eg, **disopyramide, procainamide, quinidine**): May prolong refractory periods; concurrent use not recommended in human patients; may also prolong QT interval
- **Antiarrhythmics, Class 1B, 1C** (eg, **lidocaine, mexiletine, phenytoin**): May prolong QT interval
- **Azithromycin**: May increase risk for cardiotoxicity
- **Beta-2-Adrenergic Agonists** (eg, **metaproterenol, terbutaline, albuterol**): May have their actions blocked by sotalol
- **Calcium Channel Blockers** (eg, **diltiazem, verapamil**): Potential to increase hypotensive effects; may have additive effects on AV conduction or ventricular function; use with caution, particularly in patients with pre-existing cardiomyopathy or CHF.
- **Cisapride**: May prolong QT interval
- **Clonidine**: If clonidine is discontinued after concomitant therapy with sotalol, there is an increased risk for rebound hypertension.
- **Digoxin**: Potential for increased risks for proarrhythmic events
- **Diuretics** (eg, **furosemide**): May increase risk for cardiotoxicity
- **Erythromycin; Clarithromycin**: May prolong QT interval
- **Fluoroquinolones**: May increase risk for QT interval prolongation
- **Fluoxetine**: May increase risk for cardiotoxicity
- **Lidocaine**: Clearance may be impaired by sotalol
- **Methimazole, Carbimazole**: May result in altered metabolism of sotalol
- **Nonsteroidal Anti-Inflammatory Drugs (NSAIDs**; May decrease antihypertensive effect of sotalol
- **Phenothiazines** (eg, **acepromazine**): May prolong QT interval
- **Reserpine**: May have additive effects (hypotension, bradycardia) with sotalol
- **Sympathomimetics** (eg, **phenylpropanolamine**): May have their actions blocked by sotalol
- **Tricyclic Antidepressants (TCAs**; eg, **amitriptyline, clomipramine**): May prolong QT interval

Laboratory Considerations

- Beta-adrenergic antagonists may potentiate hypoglycemia and interfere with **glucose** or insulin tolerance tests.
- Sotalol may falsely elevate urine **metanephrine** concentrations (pheochromocytoma screen) if using a fluorometric or photometric assay.

Dosages

DOGS/CATS:

Nonurgent control of ventricular tachyarrhythmias ± supraventricular tachycardia (extra-label): Anecdotal dosage range recommendations are 1 – 3.5 mg/kg (most clinicians advocate 2 – 2.5 mg/kg) PO every 12 hours. Often, patients are initially started at the low end of the dosing range and the dosage is escalated based on control of the arrhythmia. Patients with significant renal dysfunction may require reduced dosages or increased time between dosages.

Ventricular tachyarrhythmias associated with arrhythmogenic right ventricular cardiomyopathy (ARVC; eg in boxers) (extra-label):

a) **Single agent**: 1.5 – 3.5 mg/kg PO twice daily[2]
b) **In combination with mexiletine**: Sotalol 1.5 – 3 mg/kg PO twice daily in combination with mexiletine 5 – 7.5 mg/kg PO 3 times daily.[16,17] Evidence in normal dogs suggests that when mexiletine is used with sotalol in dogs weighing more than 10 kg, mexiletine could be dosed at 8 – 10 mg/kg PO every 12 hours, though confirmation in clinically affected dogs is needed.[18]

Ventricular arrhythmias in German shepherds with inherited arrhythmias (extra-label): Sotalol 2.5 mg/kg PO every 12 hours in combination with mexiletine 8 mg/kg PO every 8 hours were more effective than either drug alone in suppressing ventricular premature complexes. Mexiletine concentrations were also higher when sotalol was added.[1]

HORSES:

Lower cardioversion threshold and prevent recurrence of atrial fibrillation in horses (extra-label): Sotalol at 2 – 3 mg/kg PO twice daily used for 3 days before cardioversion and for a few weeks after has been proposed as a potential strategy to reduce the risk of recurrent atrial fibrillation though this has not been confirmed by clinical studies.[10,11]

Control of ventricular arrhythmias (extra-label): Sotalol 1 – 2 mg/kg PO twice daily for 1 day, followed by 2 – 3 mg/kg PO twice daily[9]

Monitoring

- Efficacy: ECG, heart rate, and pulse
- Resting respiratory rate
- Blood pressure
- Adverse effects (eg, dyspnea, bronchospasm, lethargy, syncope, nausea/vomiting, worsening of arrhythmias, and progression of heart failure)

Client Information

- Sotalol is best given on an empty stomach.
- Most common side effects include lack of energy and weakness, poor appetite, and vomiting. Contact your veterinarian if these signs persist or worsen.
- If your animal has trouble breathing or has episodes of collapse, call your veterinarian immediately.
- Your veterinarian may start with a low dose and gradually increase the dose. Do not administer more than your veterinarian prescribes.
- Your veterinarian will need to monitor your animal closely while it is taking this medication. Do not miss these important follow-up visits.

Chemistry/Synonyms

A non-selective beta-adrenergic antagonist and class III antiarrhythmic agent, sotalol HCl is a racemic mixture of the d- and l- forms. Both isomers exhibit antiarrhythmic (class II) activity, but only the levo- form has beta-adrenergic receptor antagonist activity. Sotalol HCl occurs as white, crystalline solid that is soluble in water.

Sotalol may also be known as MJ-1999, d,l-sotalol hydrochloride, or sotaloli hydrochloridum; many trade names are available.

Storage/Stability

Store tablets at room temperature.

Compatibility/Compounding Considerations

No specific information noted

Dosage Forms/Approval

VETERINARY-LABELED PRODUCTS: NONE

The Association of Racing Commissioners International (ARCI) has designated this drug as a class 3 substance. Use of this drug may not be allowed in certain animal competitions. Check rules and regulations before entering in a competition while this medication is being administered. Contact local racing authorities for further guidance. See ***Appendix*** for more information.

HUMAN-LABELED PRODUCTS:

Sotalol HCl Tablets: 80 mg, 120 mg, 160 mg, and 240 mg; *Betapace®*, *Sorine®*, generic; (Rx)

Sotalol HCl Oral Solution: 5 mg/mL; *Sotylize®*; (Rx)

References

For the complete list of references, see **wiley.com/go/budde/plumb**

Spectinomycin

(spek-ti-noe-***mye***-sin) *Spectogard®*

Aminocyclitol Antibiotic

Prescriber Highlights

- Aminocyclitol antibiotic used primarily in food-producing animals; relatively broad spectrum but minimal activity against anaerobes and most strains of *Pseudomonas* spp
- Contraindicated in patients hypersensitive to it
- Adverse effects appear to be minimal at labeled dosages; can cause neuromuscular blockade and swelling at SC injection sites

Uses/Indications

Spectinomycin is FDA-approved for infectious synovitis and *chronic respiratory disease* in chickens and for *bacterial enteritis* (scours) in swine. It is only rarely used in dogs, cats, and horses for susceptible infections, and there are no suitable dosage forms available for these species. There are FDA-approved uses in cattle and dogs but no currently available products. In addition, spectinomycin/lincomycin combination products are FDA-approved for *airsacculitis and chronic respiratory disease in chickens.*

The World Health Organization (WHO) has designated spectinomycin as an Important antimicrobial for human medicine.[1] The Office International des Epizooties (OIE) Antimicrobial Classification has designated spectinomycin as a Veterinary Critically Important antimicrobial.

Pharmacology/Actions

Spectinomycin is primarily a bacteriostatic antibiotic that inhibits protein synthesis in susceptible bacteria by binding to the 30S ribosomal subunit.

Spectinomycin has activity against a wide variety of gram-positive and gram-negative bacteria, including *Escherichia coli*, *Klebsiella* spp, *Proteus* spp, *Enterobacter* spp, *Salmonella* spp, *Streptococcus* spp, and *Staphylococcus* spp. It has minimal activity against anaerobes, most strains of *Pseudomonas* spp, *Chlamydia* spp, *Moraxella bovis*, or *Treponema* spp.

In human medicine, spectinomycin is used principally for its activity against *Neisseria gonorrhoeae*.

Pharmacokinetics

After oral administration, only ≈7% of the dose is absorbed, but the drug that remains in the GI tract is active. When injected SC or IM, the drug is reportedly absorbed well, with peak levels occurring in ≈1 hour.

Tissue levels of the absorbed drug are lower than those found in the serum. Spectinomycin does not appreciably enter the CSF or the eye and is not bound significantly to plasma proteins.

The absorbed drug is excreted via glomerular filtration into the urine, mostly unchanged. In cattle, the terminal half-life is ≈2 hours.

Contraindications/Precautions/Warnings

Spectinomycin is contraindicated in patients hypersensitive to it.

Adverse Effects

When used as labeled, adverse effects are unlikely with this drug. It is reported that parenteral use of this drug is much safer than with other aminocyclitol antibiotics, but little is known regarding its prolonged use. Hypersensitivity reactions and injection site reactions have been reported.[2] Spectinomycin could potentially cause neuromuscular blockade; parenteral calcium administration will generally reverse the blockade.

Adverse effects that have been reported in human patients receiving the drug in single or multidose studies include soreness at the injection site, rash, increases in BUN, alkaline phosphatase, and ALT, and decreases in hemoglobin, hematocrit, and creatinine clearance. Although increases in BUN and decreases in creatinine clearance and urine output have been noted, overt renal toxicity has not been demonstrated with this drug.

Cattle receiving the sulfate form subcutaneously have developed swelling at the injection site.

Reproductive/Nursing Safety

It is unknown whether spectinomycin crosses the placenta. Spectinomycin is excreted into milk.[3]

Because safety has not been established in animals, this drug should only be used when the maternal benefits outweigh the potential risks to offspring.

Overdose/Acute Toxicity

No specific information was located on oral overdoses, but because the drug is negligibly absorbed after oral administration, significant toxicity is unlikely via this route.

Cattle receiving 150 mg/kg/day SC for 5 days experienced injection site reactions.[2] Injected doses of 90 mg produced transient ataxia in turkey poults.

For patients that have experienced or are suspected of having experienced an overdose, consultation with a 24-hour poison consultation center specializing in providing veterinary-specific information is recommended. For general information related to overdose and toxin exposures, as well as contact information for poison control centers, refer to ***Appendix***.

Drug Interactions

The following drug interactions with spectinomycin have either been reported or are theoretical in humans or animals and may be of significance in veterinary patients. Unless otherwise noted, use together is not necessarily contraindicated, but weigh the potential risks and perform additional monitoring when appropriate.

- **CHLORAMPHENICOL**: Antagonism has been reported when used with spectinomycin.
- **TETRACYCLINE**: Antagonism has been reported when used with spectinomycin.

Dosages

SMALL MAMMALS:

Rabbits; susceptible infections (extra-label): 1 g/L in drinking water for 7 days in weanling rabbits; may cause diarrhea[4]

SWINE:

Bacterial enteritis (white scours) in piglets associated with *E coli* susceptible to spectinomycin (label dose; FDA-approved): Piglets weighing less than 4.5 kg (10 lb): 50 mg/piglet (NOT mg/kg) PO twice daily for 3 to 5 days; Piglets weighing more than 4.5 kg (10 lb): 100 mg/piglet (NOT mg/kg) PO twice daily for 3 to 5 days.[5]

BIRDS:

Prevention and control of chronic respiratory disease associated with *Mycoplasma gallisepticum* in broilers (label dose; FDA-approved): Add sufficient amount to drinking water to attain a final concentration of 2 g/gallon. (Label directions; *Spectam® Water-Soluble*)[6]

Infectious synovitis associated with *Mycoplasma synoviae* in broilers (label dose; FDA-approved): Add sufficient amount to drinking water to attain a final concentration of 1 g/gallon. (Label directions; *Spectam® Water-Soluble*)[6]

Monitoring

- Clinical efficacy

Chemistry/Synonyms

Spectinomycin, an aminocyclitol antibiotic obtained from *Streptomyces spectabilis*, is available as the dihydrochloride pentahydrate and hexahydrate sulfate salts. It occurs as a white to pale buff, crystalline powder with pK_a of 7 and 8.7. It is freely soluble in water and practically insoluble in alcohol.

Spectinomycin may also be known as M-141, actinospectacin, spectinomycini, U-18409AE, *Adspec®*, *Amtech Spectam®*, *Kempi®*, *Kirin®*, *Spectoguard Scour-Chek®*, *Stanilo®*, *Togamycin®*, *Trobicin®*, *Trobicine®*, or *Vabicin®*.

Storage/Stability

Unless otherwise instructed by the manufacturer, store spectinomycin products at room temperature (15°C to 30°C [59°F to 86°F]). Protect from freezing.

Compatibility/Compounding Considerations

No specific information was noted.

Dosage Forms/Regulatory Status

VETERINARY-LABELED PRODUCTS:

Spectinomycin Water Soluble Powder: 0.5 g of spectinomycin per gram in 1 kg containers. *Spectogard® Water Soluble Powder*; (Rx). FDA-approved for use in broiler chickens (not layers). Slaughter withdrawal (at labeled doses) = 5 days.

Spectinomycin Oral Solution: 50 mg/mL in 240 mL pump bottle, 1000 mL pump bottle, and 1-gallon refill without pump; *Spectogard Scour-Chek®*, (OTC). FDA-approved for use in swine (weighing less than 6.8 kg [15 lb] and not older than 4 weeks of age). Slaughter withdrawal (at labeled doses) = 21 days.

The following products are listed in FDA's Green Book of approved animal drugs but may no longer be commercially available in the US:

- Spectinomycin Dihydrochloride Oral Tablets: 100 mg; (Rx)
- Spectinomycin Dihydrochloride Injection: 100 mg/mL; (Rx)
- Spectinomycin Sulfate Injection: 100 mg/mL in 500 mL vials; *Adspec®*; (Rx). When used as labeled, slaughter withdrawal in cattle = 11 days; not to be used in veal calves or in dairy cattle 20 months of age or older
- Spectinomycin Dihydrochloride Pentahydrate Injection: 100 mg/mL, *Prospec®*; (OTC). For use in 1 to 3 days old chicks and poults
- Spectinomycin/Lincomycin in a 2:1 ratio; in 2.65 oz packets. Each packet contains lincomycin 16.7 g and spectinomycin 33.3 g; *LS 50 Water Soluble Powder®*, *SepcLinx-50®*, generic; (Rx). FDA-approved for use in chickens up to 7 days of age

HUMAN-LABELED PRODUCTS: NONE

References

For the complete list of references, see **wiley.com/go/budde/plumb**

Spinosad

(***spin***-oh-sad) *Comfortis®, Trifexis®*

Oral Flea Adulticide

Prescriber Highlights

- Oral flea adulticide for dogs and cats; labeled for one month prevention/treatment; not effective for flea eggs or other immature flea forms
- Combination product with milbemycin approved for dogs for heartworm prevention, prevention and treatment of flea infestations, and for the treatment and control of adult hookworms, roundworms, and whipworms.
- Fast onset of action; fleas begin to die within 30 minutes of administration
- Appears safe and well tolerated in dogs and cats.
- Give with food.
- Potentially serious drug interaction with extra-label doses of ivermectin (and possibly other drugs)

Uses/Indications

In dogs, oral spinosad is FDA-approved for the prevention and treatment of flea (*Ctenocephalides felis*) infestations for one month in dogs 14 weeks of age and older and weighing 2.2 kg (5 lb) or more.[1] Spinosad has also been shown to be effective in the prevention of *Pulex irritans* (human flea) infestation in dogs that live in close proximity to flea-infested sheep.[2]

In cats, oral spinosad is FDA-approved to kill fleas (*C felis*) and for the prevention and treatment of flea infestations (*C felis*) for one month in cats 14 weeks of age and older and weighing 1.8 kg (4.1 lb) or more.[1]

Spinosad is not labeled for use against ticks and it has been stated as not effective for this use; however, in a pilot study evaluating the efficacy of spinosad dosed at 50 mg/kg (1.7 times minimum flea dose) and 100 mg/kg (3.3 times minimum flea dose) against adult brown dog tick (*Rhipicephalus sanguineus*) infestations in dogs, ≈95% of ticks were killed within 24 hours of dosing. The results suggested that some posttreatment residual tick control persisted up to 1 month.[3]

The spinosad/milbemycin combination product is FDA-approved for the prevention of heartworm infection (*Dirofilaria immitis*), for the prevention and treatment of flea infestations (*C felis*), and for the treatment and control of adult hookworm (*Ancylostoma caninum*), adult roundworm (*Toxocara canis* and *Toxascaris leonina*) and adult whipworm (*Trichuris vulpis*) infections in dogs 8 weeks of age or older and weighing 2.2 kg (5 lb) or more.[4] Monthly treatments with spinosad/milbemycin may prevent *Angiostrongylus vasorum* (French heartworm) infection in dogs.[5]

Pharmacology/Actions

Spinosad is a macrocyclic lactone containing a combination of two naturally occurring macrocyclic lactones (spinosyn A and spinosyn D). Its primary mode of action in insects is as a nicotinic acetylcholine D-alpha receptor agonist causing involuntary muscle contractions and tremors secondary to motor neuron activation.[6] Prolonged exposure causes paralysis and flea death. Flea death is rapid, beginning within 30 minutes of dosing and is complete in 4 hours in dogs and 24 hours in cats.[1] In insects, spinosad also opens chloride channels similarly to other macrocyclic lactones.

Pharmacokinetics

After oral administration of spinosad (with food) to dogs, peak plasma concentrations for spinosyn A and spinosyn D occur in ≈2 and 3 hours, respectively. Spinosyn D concentrations are ≈5 times greater than those of spinosyn A. Spinosyn A and D are extensively bound (≈99%) to canine plasma proteins. Spinosad is hepatically biotransformed with glutathione conjugates and 70% to 90% is eliminated in the feces via the bile. The plasma elimination half-life is ≈10 days.

Contraindications/Precautions/Warnings

There are no labeled contraindications.

For treatment of flea infestations, it is recommended to combine treatment with an insect growth regulator or insect development inhibitor (eg, methoprene, lufenuron) as well as environmental control measures.

It has been recommended not to use spinosad in combination with high extra-label doses of ivermectin due to potential severe neurotoxicity.[7,8]

Use with caution in breeding females and dogs with pre-existing epilepsy at higher than label dosages as this may decrease seizure threshold.[1,4]

The chewable tablets are beef flavored and although they do not contain beef proteins, pork proteins and hydrolyzed soy are used. Dogs with pork or soy allergies may develop adverse effects.[9]

A study evaluating the safety of spinosad (doses up to 5 times the maximum label recommendation) with or without milbemycin (doses up to 10 times the maximum label recommendation) in collies homozygous and heterozygous for the *MDR1* mutation (also known as *ABCB1*-1delta) did not cause signs of neurotoxicosis.[10]

When using the spinosad/milbemycin combination product for dogs, ensure the patient has recently tested negative for heartworm; do not use in patients with heartworm infection.

Adverse Effects

Spinosad appears to be well tolerated in dogs and most animals will not show any adverse effects after dosing. In field studies, vomiting was the most frequent adverse effect, occurring in up to 12% of dogs.[6] The following additional adverse effects are possible and based on postapproval adverse drug event reporting (listed in decreasing order of frequency): depression/lethargy, anorexia, ataxia, diarrhea, pruritus, trembling, hypersalivation, and seizures.[1]

In cats, adverse effects are infrequent but vomiting (≈14%), lethargy, reduced appetite, weight loss, and diarrhea have been reported.[1]

Reproductive/Nursing Safety

Use spinosad and spinosad/milbemycin with caution in breeding bitches; however, the drug appears to be relatively safe to use during pregnancy and lactation.[1,4] In female beagles dosed at 1.3 times and 4.4 times the recommended dose every 28 days prior to mating, during gestation, and during a 6 week lactation period, no changes in dam conception rates or mortality, body temperature, necropsy, or histopathology were seen in dams or puppies.[6] Treated dams experienced more frequent vomiting, especially at 1 hour postdose, than control dams.[11] Puppies from dams treated at 1.3 times the recommended rate had lower body weights; those from the 4.4 times group experienced more lethargy, dehydration, weakness, and felt cold to the touch. Safe use in breeding males has not been evaluated.

Safe use in breeding, pregnant, or lactating cats has not been evaluated.[6]

In a pilot study in 3 dogs, spinosyns were excreted in milk at concentrations ≈2.5 times of that found in the plasma.[6] Puppy mortality and morbidity was highest in puppies from the dam with the highest spinosyn milk concentrations, but causal effect cannot be inferred due to the small sample size of the study.

Overdose/Acute Toxicity

Spinosad appears to be safe in mammals, with an oral LD_{50} in mice and rats of more than 5000 mg/kg.[12] Acute overdoses in dogs appear to be relatively harmless. Common adverse effects seen in dogs with a spinosad overdose include lethargy, vomiting, ataxia, and trembling; with vomiting the most common adverse effect in cats. In a dose tolerance study in adult beagles dosed orally up to 100 mg/kg PO once daily (16.7 times recommended dose) for 10 consecutive days, vomiting was routinely seen after the dose was administered.[6] No significant changes in hematology, blood coagulation, or urinalysis parameters were noted, but phospholipidosis (vacuolation) of the lymphoid tissue and mild elevations in ALT occurred in all dogs.

Vomiting and anorexia was noted in kittens receiving monthly oral doses as high as 500 mg/kg.[6] Phospholipidosis occurred in the liver, lung, and adrenal gland of dogs (4.4 times label dosage for 6 months) and cats (3 times label dosage for 6 months)[6]

For patients that have experienced or are suspected to have experienced an overdose, consultation with a 24-hour poison consultation center specializing in providing veterinary-specific information is recommended. For general information related to overdose and toxin exposures, as well as contact information for poison control centers, refer to ***Appendix***.

Drug Interactions

The following drug interactions have either been reported or are theoretical in humans or animals receiving spinosad and may be of significance in veterinary patients. Unless otherwise noted, use together is not necessarily contraindicated, but weigh the potential risks and perform additional monitoring when appropriate.

- **IVERMECTIN**: It has been recommended not to use spinosad with high extra-label doses of ivermectin,[7] as spinosad can increase the plasma concentrations of ivermectin in dogs with the area under curve (AUC) increasing 3.6-fold.[13] When used with heartworm preventives at their label dosages, spinosad appears safe to use. No signs of neurotoxicosis were seen in collies homozygous and heterozygous for the MDR1 genetic mutation receiving up to 5 times the recommended spinosad label dose with or without milbemycin (up to 10 times the recommended label dose).[10]
- **OTHER DRUGS AFFECTED BY P-GLYCOPROTEIN INHIBITORS**: Spinosad has been shown to be a substrate and potent inhibitor of canine p-glycoprotein, and other orally dosed drugs such as cyclosporine, verapamil, ketoconazole, or loperamide could potentially interact at the level of the intestinal tract. Because spinosad is so highly bound to plasma proteins, the risk for additional interactions at the blood-brain barrier appear to be limited.[14]

Laboratory Considerations

- No specific concerns noted.

Dosages

DOGS:

Spinosad as a single agent - prevention and treatment of flea infestations in dogs 14 weeks of age and older and weighing 2.2 kg (5 lb) or more (label dosage; FDA-approved): Given orally once a month with food at the minimum dosage of spinosad 30 mg/kg.[1] Dogs weighing more than 54.5 kg (120 lb) should be administered the appropriate combination of tablets. See weight-based dosage table below specifically for dogs. **NOTE**: Do not use the cat dosing table for dogs as overdoses could occur.

Body weight in kg (lb)	Spinosad per tablet (mg)	Number of tablets to administer
2.3-4.5 (5-10)	140	1
4.6-9.1 (10.1-20)	270	1
9.1-18.2 (20.1-40)	560	1
18.2-27.3 (40.1-60)	810	1
27.3-54.5 (60.1-120)	1620	1

Spinosad/Milbemycin - prevention of heartworm disease, prevention and treatment of flea infestations, and treatment and control of adult hookworm, adult roundworm, and adult whipworm infections in dogs 8 weeks of age or older and weighing 2.2 kg (5 lb) or more (label dosage; FDA-approved): Given orally once a month at the minimum dosage of spinosad 30 mg/kg with milbemycin oxime 0.5 mg/kg.[4] For heartworm prevention, give once monthly for at least 3 months after exposure to mosquitoes. Dogs weighing more than 54.5 kg (120 lb) should be administered the appropriate combination of tablets. See weight-based dosage table below.

Body weight in kg (lb)	Spinosad/Milbemycin per tablet (mg)	Number of tablets to administer
2.3-4.5 (5-10)	140/2.3	1
4.6-9.1 (10.1-20)	270/4.5	1
9.1-18.2 (20.1-40)	560/9.3	1
18.2-27.3 (40.1-60)	810/13.5	1
27.3-54.5 (60.1-120)	1620/27	1

CATS:

Prevention and treatment of flea infestations in cats 14 weeks of age and older and weighing 1.8 kg (4.1 lb) or more (label dosage; FDA-approved): Given orally once a month at the minimum dosage of spinosad 50 mg/kg just prior to or after feeding, once monthly.[1] Alternatively, it may be offered in food or administered like other tablet medications. For cats weighing more than 10.9 kg (24 lb), the appropriate combination of tablets should be administered. See weight-based dosage table below specifically for cats. **NOTE**: Do not use the dog dosing table for cats as underdosing could occur.

Body weight in kg (lb)	Spinosad per tablet (mg)	Number of tablets to administer
1.9-2.7 (4.1-6)	140	1
2.8-5.5 (6.1-12)	270	1
5.5-10.9 (12.1-24)	560	1

Monitoring

- Efficacy and adverse effects
- Heartworm status prior to administration of *Trifexis®* to dogs

Client Information

- Spinosad is an oral tablet given monthly that kills adult fleas on dogs and cats. It begins to kill fleas 30 minutes after dosing. When used alone, this medicine does not kill flea eggs or other immature flea forms. Your veterinarian will talk with you about a flea control program. This medicine does not kill ticks.
- The spinosad/milbemycin oral combination product is given monthly to kill adult fleas, prevent heartworm infection, and control hookworms, roundworms, and whipworms in dogs. This combination product does not kill ticks.
- Give this medicine with food or immediately after a meal.
- When used as directed on the label, this medication appears safe.
- Keep chewable tablets well out of reach of children and animals.

Chemistry/Synonyms

Spinosad is a spinosyn class insecticide and contains two major factors, spinosyn A and spinosyn D, that are both derived from the naturally occurring bacterium, *Saccharopolyspora spinosa*. Spinosad may also be known as spinosyn A and D, DE-105, or XDE-105. Trade names include *Comfortis®*, *Natroba®* (human topical), *Acuguard®*, or *Extinosad®*.

Storage/Stability

Chewable tablets should be stored at 20°C to 25°C (68°F-77°F). Excursions are permitted between 15°C to 30°C (59°F-86°F).

Compatibility/Compounding Considerations

No specific information noted.

Dosage Forms/Regulatory Status

VETERINARY-LABELED PRODUCTS:

Spinosad Chewable Tablets: 140 mg (dogs 2.3-4.5 kg [5-10 lb]), 270 mg (dogs 4.6-9.1 kg [10.1-20 lb]), 560 mg (dogs 9.1-18.2 kg [20.1-40 lb]), 810 mg (dogs 18.2-27.3 kg [40.1-60 lb]), 1620 mg (dogs 27.3-54.5 kg [60.1-120 lb]); *Comfortis*®; (Rx). FDA-approved for use in dogs. Dogs over 54.5 kg (120 lb) should be administered the appropriate combination of tablets.

Spinosad Chewable Tablets: 140 mg (cats 1.9-2.7 kg [4.1-6 lb]), 270 mg (cats 2.8-5.5 kg [6.1-12 lb]), 560 mg (cats 5.5-10.9 kg [12.1-24 lb]); *Comfortis® for Cats*; (Rx). FDA-approved for cats. Cats over 10.8 kg (24 lb) should be administered the appropriate combination of tablets.

Spinosad/Milbemycin Chewable Tablets: 140 mg/2.3 mg (dogs 2.3-4.5 kg [5-10 lb]); 270 mg/4.5 mg (dogs 4.6-9.1 kg [10.1-20 lb]); 560 mg/9.3 mg (dogs 9.1-18.2 kg [20.1-40 lb]); 810 mg/13.5 mg (dogs 18.2-27.3 kg [40.1-60 lb]); 1620 mg/27 mg (dogs 27.3-54.5 kg [60.1-120 lb]); *Trifexis*®; (Rx). FDA-approved for use in dogs. Dogs over 54.5 kg (120 lb) should be administered the appropriate combination of tablets.

NOTE: Tablets are beef flavored (but contain pork and soy proteins), and the sizes are color-coded and provided in packets of 6 or 12 tablets.

HUMAN-LABELED PRODUCTS:

None for systemic use

Spinosad 0.9% Topical Suspension (120 mL): *Natroba*®; (Rx)

References

For the complete list of references, see **wiley.com/go/budde/plumb**

Spironolactone

(speer-on-oh-***lak***-tone) *Aldactone*®

Aldosterone Antagonist

Prescriber Highlights

- Aldosterone antagonist used as a potassium-sparing diuretic and for adjunctive treatment for heart failure or ascites; should not be substituted for furosemide in patients with CHF
- Contraindications include hyperkalemia, Addison's disease, anuria, acute kidney injury, or significant renal impairment.
- Caution in patients with renal impairment or hepatic disease
- Adverse effects include facial dermatitis in cats. Hyperkalemia, hyponatremia, and dehydration possible; increased BUN and mild acidosis in patients with renal impairment. GI distress (eg, vomiting, anorexia), CNS effects (eg, lethargy, ataxia), and endocrine changes (eg, reduced testosterone, increased estrogen) possible.
- The National Institute of Occupational Safety and Health (NIOSH) classifies spironolactone as a hazardous drug; use appropriate precautions when handling.

Uses/Indications

Spironolactone may be used in patients with congestive heart failure (CHF) for its cardioprotective effects. It is also administered to patients that develop hypokalemia while receiving other diuretics and are unwilling or unable to supplement with exogenous potassium sources. In a study evaluating spironolactone's efficacy for improving survival in dogs with naturally occurring mitral regurgitation in myxomatous mitral valve disease (MMVD), the authors concluded that spironolactone added to conventional cardiac therapy decreased the risk for cardiac-related death, euthanasia, or severe worsening of the disease.[1] However, the clinical relevance of these findings has been questioned due to the study design, event rate, patient withdrawals, and patient categorization with regard to heart failure.[2] A prospective, randomized, single-blinded, placebo-controlled study evaluating the efficacy of spironolactone in combination with benazepril in dogs with preclinical MMVD failed to demonstrate a protective effect of the 2 drugs as compared with placebo.[3] Although efficacy remains in doubt, a randomized, double-blinded, prospective study found that spironolactone added to conventional treatment (ACE inhibitors, furosemide ± digoxin) did not increase risk for adverse effects, death caused by cardiac disease, renal disease, hyperkalemia, or azotemia.[4]

Spironolactone may also be effective in treating ascites, as it has less potential to increase ammonia concentrations than other diuretics.

Spironolactone may find a role in treating renal disease. In rats, it has been shown to decrease proteinuria and glomerulosclerosis in experimental models of renal disease, but clinical effectiveness in dogs has been disappointing. It has potential therapeutic benefit in feline chronic kidney disease,[5] but studies demonstrating efficacy are lacking.

Pharmacology/Actions

Spironolactone is also categorized as a potassium-sparing diuretic or a mineralocorticoid-receptor antagonist. Aldosterone is competitively inhibited by spironolactone in the distal renal tubules with resultant increased excretion of sodium, chloride, and water, and decreased excretion of potassium, ammonium, phosphate, and titratable acid. Spironolactone has no effect on carbonic anhydrase or renal transport mechanisms and has its greatest effect in patients with hyperaldosteronism. When used alone in healthy dogs, spironolactone does not appear to cause significant diuresis.[6] As a diuretic, spironolactone is not commonly used alone, as most sodium is reabsorbed at the proximal tubules. Combining it with a thiazide or loop diuretic maximizes its diuretic effect. Aldosterone also plays a role in the progression of myocardial fibrosis, vascular remodeling, and endothelial dysfunction in heart failure. In humans with heart failure, spironolactone has been shown to reduce remodeling, cardiac fibrosis, and the progression of left ventricular dysfunction.[7] Whether this occurs in veterinary patients with heart failure is controversial. One study in Maine Coon cats with hypertrophic cardiomyopathy but not heart failure showed that spironolactone did not cause significant changes in diastolic function or left ventricular mass after 4 months of treatment.[8]

Pharmacokinetics

Because spironolactone is unstable if frozen and thawed, pharmacokinetic studies in animals are not readily performed. In fasted dogs, oral bioavailability of spironolactone (measured via its main metabolites) is ≈50% but increases up to 90% when the drug is given with food. Approximately 70% of a dose is found in the feces and 18% in the urine. In a recent pharmacodynamic study in 15 beagles, the dose required to inhibit the action of aldosterone by 50% was estimated to be ≈1.1 mg/kg, and the authors suggest that the dose for spironolactone would be ≈2 mg/kg PO once daily to effectively inhibit the aldosterone concentrations associated with CHF in dogs.[9]

In humans, spironolactone is more than 90% bioavailable and peak concentrations are reached within 1 to 2 hours. The diuretic action of spironolactone when used alone is gradually attained and generally reaches its maximal effect on the third day of therapy. Spironolactone and its active metabolite, canrenone, are both ≈98% bound to plasma proteins. Both spironolactone and its metabolites may cross the placenta. Canrenone has been detected in breast milk.

Spironolactone is rapidly metabolized (half-life of 1 to 2 hours) to several metabolites, including canrenone, which has diuretic activity. Canrenone is more slowly eliminated, with an average half-life of ≈20 hours.

Contraindications/Precautions/Warnings

Spironolactone is contraindicated in patients hypersensitive to it and those with hyperkalemia, Addison's disease, anuria, or acute renal failure. It should be used cautiously in patients with significant renal impairment or hepatic disease but is often used to treat ascites.

The label for *Prilactone®Next* (the canine product licensed in the UK) states *Do not use in dogs suffering from hypoadrenocorticism, hyperkalemia, or hyponatremia. Do not administer spironolactone in conjunction with NSAIDs to dogs with renal insufficiency. As spironolactone has an antiandrogenic effect, it is not recommended to administer the product to growing dogs.*

The National Institute for Occupational Safety and Health (NIOSH) classifies spironolactone as a hazardous drug; personal protective equipment (PPE) should be used accordingly to minimize the risk of exposure.[10]

Adverse Effects

Adverse effects are usually considered mild and reversible upon discontinuation of the drug. The most likely adverse effects are GI effects (eg, anorexia, vomiting, diarrhea) and electrolyte (hyperkalemia, hyponatremia) and water balance (dehydration) abnormalities. In dogs, electrolytes do not appear to be significantly affected. After cats received spironolactone 2.7 mg/kg PO twice daily for 7 to 9 days, the following serum values significantly increased (on average): potassium 0.39 mEq/L, calcium 0.48 mg/dL, creatinine 0.22 mg/dL, phosphorus 0.63 mg/dL, and total protein 0.51 mg/dL.[12]

A study in dogs found that spironolactone added to conventional treatment (ACE inhibitors, furosemide ± digoxin) did not increase risk for adverse effects, death caused by cardiac disease, renal disease, hyperkalemia, or azotemia.[4] In the prospective study evaluating the efficacy of spironolactone in combination with benazepril in dogs with preclinical MMVD, there was no difference in adverse events between those dogs receiving active medication as compared with the placebo group.[3]

In cats, an interim report of a study using spironolactone 1.7 – 3.3 mg/kg PO once daily (n = 16) with benazepril and furosemide reported no severe adverse events except worsening of heart failure (death, euthanasia, aortic thromboembolism, and one case of severe anorexia). However, of the original 16 cats enrolled, 11 died or were euthanized, 2 were withdrawn, 1 completed 15 month follow-up ,and 2 cats remain in the study.[13] The final report from this study reported that 9 of 11 cats in the placebo group reached the primary endpoint of death due to cardiac causes as compared with 2 of 9 cats in the spironolactone group.[14] In the study in Maine Coon cats,[8] ≈⅓ of treated subjects developed severe facial dermatitis.

Transient increases in BUN and mild acidosis may occur in patients with renal impairment. Use of spironolactone in patients with severe renal impairment may lead to hyperkalemia.

Spironolactone reportedly inhibits the synthesis of testosterone and may increase the peripheral conversion of testosterone to estradiol; gynecomastia has been reported in human males. Long-term toxicity studies in rats have demonstrated that spironolactone is tumorigenic in that species.

Reproductive/Nursing Safety

Spironolactone or its metabolites may cross the placental barrier. Feminization occurs in male rat fetuses, and endocrine dysfunction in females with in utero spironolactone exposure.

Canrenone, a metabolite of spironolactone, appears in maternal milk. In humans, the estimated maximum dose to the infant is ≈0.2% of the mother's daily dose. Use with caution in nursing patients, but it is unlikely to have clinical significance in veterinary patients.

Overdose/Acute Toxicity

Information on spironolactone overdoses is limited. Dose-dependent adverse effects (see ***Adverse Effects***) were noted in healthy dogs after administration of up to 10 times the recommended dose. If an acute overdose occurs, it is suggested to follow the guidelines outlined in the ***Chlorothiazide*** and ***Furosemide*** monographs.

For patients that have experienced or are suspected to have experienced an overdose, it is strongly encouraged to consult with one of the 24-hour poison consultation centers that specialize in providing information specific for veterinary patients. For general information related to overdose and toxin exposures, as well as contact information for poison control centers, refer to ***Appendix***.

Drug Interactions

The following drug interactions have either been reported or are theoretical in humans or animals receiving spironolactone and may be of significance in veterinary patients. Unless otherwise noted, use together is not necessarily contraindicated, but weigh the potential risks and perform additional monitoring when appropriate.

- **ACE INHIBITORS** (eg, enalapril, lisinopril): Hyperkalemia is possible but unlikely and usually clinically irrelevant if it occurs.[4,11]
- **ANGIOTENSIN RECEPTOR BLOCKERS (ARBs)** (eg, **irbesartan, telmisartan**): Hyperkalemia is possible.
- **BETA-ADRENERGIC ANTAGONISTS** (eg, **atenolol, carvedilol, propranolol**): Hyperkalemia is possible.
- **CHOLESTYRAMINE**: Hyperkalemic metabolic acidosis is possible.
- **DEOXYCORTICOSTERONE PIVALATE (DOCP)**: May reduce diuretic and natriuretic effects of spironolactone
- **DIGOXIN**: Spironolactone may increase the half-life of digoxin; enhanced monitoring of digoxin serum concentrations and effects is warranted when spironolactone is used with these agents.
- **MITOTANE**: Spironolactone may mute the effects of mitotane if given concurrently, but very limited information is available on this potential interaction; monitor carefully.
- **NEUROMUSCULAR BLOCKERS, NON-DEPOLARIZING** (eg, **pancuronium, rocuronium, vecuronium**): Increase in neuromuscular blockade effects is possible
- **NONSTEROIDAL ANTI-INFLAMMATORY DRUGS (NSAIDs**; eg, **carprofen, robenacoxib**): NSAIDs may reduce diuretic and natriuretic effects of spironolactone. Ensure adequate hydration before using combination.[15]
- **POTASSIUM-SPARING DIURETICS, OTHER** (eg, **triamterene**): Hyperkalemia is possible.
- **POTASSIUM SUPPLEMENTS**: Hyperkalemia is possible.
- **SALICYLATES** (eg, **aspirin, bismuth subsalicylate**): Spironolactone's diuretic effects may be decreased if aspirin or other salicylates are administered concomitantly.

Laboratory Considerations

- Spironolactone may give falsely elevated **digoxin** values if using a radioimmunoassay (RIA) method.
- Fluorometric methods of determining plasma and urinary **17-hydroxycorticosteroids** (cortisol) may be interfered with by spironolactone.

Dosages

DOGS:

Preclinical myxomatous mitral valve disease (extra-label): 2 – 4 mg/kg PO once daily in combination with benazepril, although this study failed to demonstrate the drug combination could delay onset of heart failure compared to placebo.[3]

Compensated MMVD (extra-label): 2 mg/kg PO once daily in combination with ACE-inhibitor and furosemide. Pilot study suggestive of benefit from spironolactone, but further studies are warranted.[16]

Adjunctive treatment of congestive heart failure caused by MMVD (extra-label):

a) 2 mg/kg PO once daily with food[17,18]

b) 1 – 2 mg/kg PO every 12 to 24 hours[19]; dosing ranges of 0.5 – 4 mg/kg PO every 12 to 24 hours have been noted.

Ascites (extra-label): 1 – 2 mg/kg PO once daily. If no response observed within 7 to 10 days, titrate dose upward every 3 to 5 days to a maximum of 4 mg/kg/day.[20]

Adjunctive treatment of hypertension (extra-label): 1 – 2 mg/kg PO every 12 hours.[21] Not first-line therapy; effectiveness has been marginal when the drug is used as sole therapy for the management of hypertension.[22]

CATS:

Diuretic in heart failure (extra-label): No definitive studies documenting efficacy were located. Anecdotally, some may add spironolactone using dog dosages when furosemide and ACE inhibitors do not control fluid accumulation in refractory CHF.

Cardiomyopathy (extra-label): 1.7 – 3.3 mg/kg once daily.[14] This was a pilot study, and the authors suggest further study is warranted.

Adjunctive treatment of hypertension (extra-label): 1 – 2 mg/kg PO every 12 hours.[21] Not first-line therapy; effectiveness has been marginal when the drug is used as sole therapy for the management of hypertension, even in cats with hyperaldosteronism. Cutaneous drug reactions may also limit usefulness.[22]

Monitoring

- Serum electrolytes, BUN, creatinine. Initially, 5 to 14 days after starting therapy and every 2 months thereafter[23]
- Hydration status and body weight
- Respiratory rate and effort
- Blood pressure, if indicated
- Clinical signs of edema and ascites; serial girth measurements

Client Information

- When beginning this medicine, your animal may urinate more often than normal.
- Administer with a meal.
- Because this drug can change electrolytes (salts) in the blood, more frequent blood testing may be required. Do not miss these important follow-up visits.
- If your animal shows any of the following signs, contact your veterinarian immediately: sores or face scratching (cats), severe or continuing vomiting or diarrhea, acting extremely tired, trouble walking or keeping balance, or stopping eating, drinking, or urinating.

Chemistry/Synonyms

Spironolactone is a synthetically produced aldosterone antagonist that occurs as a cream to light tan, crystalline powder with a faint mercaptan-like odor. Spironolactone is practically insoluble in water and soluble in alcohol.

Spironolactone may also be known as espironolactona, SC-9420, spirolactone, and spironolactonum; many trade names are available.

Storage/Stability

Spironolactone tablets should be stored at room temperature in tight, light-resistant containers.

Compatibility/Compounding Considerations

An extemporaneously prepared oral suspension can be prepared by pulverizing commercially available tablets and adding cherry syrup, simple syrup, or a mixture of *Ora-Sweet*® and *Ora-Plus*®. This preparation is reportedly stable for 60 days.

Dosage Forms/Regulatory Status

VETERINARY-LABELED PRODUCTS:

No single-agent FDA-approved formulations in the United States; may be available in other countries

Spironolactone/Benazepril Tablets: 20 mg/2.5 mg, 40 mg/5 mg, and 80 mg/10 mg; *Cardalis*®;(Rx)

The Association of Racing Commissioners International (ARCI) has designated this drug as a class 4 substance. Use of this drug may not be allowed in certain animal competitions. Check rules and regulations before entering in a competition while this medication is being administered. Contact local racing authorities for further guidance. See ***Appendix*** for more information.

HUMAN-LABELED PRODUCTS:

Spironolactone Oral Tablets: 25 mg, 50 mg, and 100 mg; *Aldactone*®, generic; (Rx)

Spironolactone/Hydrochlorothiazide Oral Tablets: 25 mg/25 mg and 50 mg/50 mg; *Aldactazide*®, generic; (Rx)

References

For the complete list of references, see **wiley.com/go/budde/plumb**

Spironolactone/Benazepril

(speer-on-oh-***lak***-tone /ben-***a***-za-pril) *Cardalis*®

Aldosterone Antagonist/Angiotensin-Converting Enzyme (ACE) Inhibitor

Prescriber Highlights

- Indicated for the adjunctive management of clinical signs of mild, moderate, or severe congestive heart failure in dogs due to atrioventricular valvular insufficiency (AVVI)
- Contraindications include hypersensitivity, hypoadrenocorticism, hyperkalemia, hyponatremia, in cases of cardiac output failure due to aortic or pulmonary stenosis, pregnancy, or in growing dogs or dogs with renal impairment that are receiving NSAIDs.
- Use with caution in dogs with renal or hepatic impairment.
- Adverse effects include vomiting and elevations of serum magnesium and potassium.
- The National Institute of Occupational Safety and Health (NIOSH) classifies spironolactone as a hazardous drug; use appropriate precautions when handling.

Uses/Indications

The spironolactone/benazepril combination product is FDA-approved with concurrent therapy (eg, furosemide) for the management of clinical signs related to mild, moderate, or severe congestive heart failure in dogs due to atrioventricular valvular insufficiency (AVVI). In a field study,[1] all dogs received furosemide in addition to spironolactone/benazepril; digoxin or calcium channel blockers were used to control supraventricular arrhythmias.[1]

Spironolactone/benazepril delayed the onset of cardiac death, recurrent or worsening pulmonary edema, new cardiogenic ascites, or clinical signs of heart failure requiring high-dose furosemide, although treatment failure rates were high (81% for spironolactone/benazepril; 88% for benazepril alone).[2] In contrast, a prospective, randomized, single-blinded, placebo-controlled study evaluating the efficacy of the spironolactone/benazepril combination in dogs with *preclinical* MMVD failed to demonstrate a protective effect from the combination product compared with placebo.[3]

Pharmacology/Actions

Spironolactone is an aldosterone antagonist and a potassium-sparing diuretic; it also has an affinity for androgen and progesterone receptors. Aldosterone is competitively inhibited by spironolactone in the distal renal tubules with resultant increased excretion of sodium, chloride, and water, and decreased excretion of potassium, ammonium, phosphate, and titratable acid. In dogs, aldosterone also plays a role in the progression of myocardial fibrosis, vascular remodeling, and endothelial dysfunction in heart failure, and spironolactone has been shown to reduce these effects in dogs.[4] The addition of spironolactone to an ACE inhibitor treatment regimen helps prevent the unwanted effects of aldosterone synthesized from other (ie, non-ACE) pathways.

In a pharmacodynamic study in 15 beagles,[5] the spironolactone dose required to inhibit the action of aldosterone by 50% was estimated to be ≈1.1 mg/kg, and the authors suggest that the dose for spironolactone would be ≈2 mg/kg PO once daily to obtain concentrations effective at inhibiting the aldosterone levels associated with CHF in dogs. The spironolactone/benazepril combination inhibited plasma ACE activity by 95% at peak effect, and by over 80% over 24 hours.[6]

Benazepril is a prodrug and has little pharmacologic activity of its own. After being hydrolyzed in the liver to benazeprilat, the drug inhibits angiotensin converting enzyme (ACE), preventing the conversion of angiotensin-I to angiotensin-II. Angiotensin-II is a potent vasoconstrictor and stimulates production of aldosterone in the adrenal cortex. By blocking angiotensin-II formation, ACE inhibitors reduce blood pressure in hypertensive patients and vascular resistance in patients with congestive heart failure. Aldosterone breakthrough (ie, insufficient suppression of aldosterone secretion) has been documented with ACE inhibitor administration to healthy dogs.[7]

Pharmacokinetics

In fasted dogs, oral bioavailability of spironolactone (measured via its primary active metabolites: 7-alpha-thiomethyl-spironolactone and canrenone) is ≈50%, but increases up to 90% when given with food.[6] Metabolite half-lives are ≈7 to 10 hours.[2,6] Approximately 70% of a dose is found in the feces and 20% in the urine.[2,6]

After oral administration in healthy dogs, benazepril is rapidly absorbed and converted into the active metabolite benazeprilat, with peak concentrations of benazeprilat occurring 85 to 120 minutes after administration.[8-11] Protein binding is ≈85%. Benazeprilat half-life is 12 to 21 hours[9,11] and it is cleared via both renal (45%) and hepatic (55%) routes.[2] Renal impairment does not alter benazeprilat clearance.[8]

Contraindications/Precautions/Warnings

Spironolactone/benazepril is contraindicated in patients hypersensitive to either spironolactone or ACE inhibitors, and in patients with hypoadrenocorticism, hyperkalemia, or hyponatremia.[2,6] Do not use in cases of cardiac output failure due to aortic or pulmonary stenosis.[6] Pulmonary edema should be stabilized prior to use of the combination.[2] Use with caution in growing dogs due to antiandrogenic effects associated with spironolactone, and in patients with renal or hepatic impairment.[2,6]

Do not administer spironolactone/benazepril in conjunction with NSAIDs to dogs with renal insufficiency.[2,6] Adequate hydration should be ensured in all treated dogs to reduce the risk for renal toxicity.

The National Institute for Occupational Safety and Health (NIOSH) classifies spironolactone as a hazardous drug. Therefore, personal protective equipment (PPE) should be used to minimize the risk for exposure.[12]

Do not confuse *Cardalis*® with *Cialis*® or *Cardizem*®.

Adverse Effects

Adverse effects reported in FDA field studies included anorexia, vomiting, lethargy, diarrhea, renal insufficiency, collapse, hepatopathy, and urinary incontinence.[1] In one study,[3] adverse effects from the combination did not differ from dogs that received placebo. Renal insufficiency was seen more frequently in dogs treated with the spironolactone/benazepril combination; however, renal function values were not statistically different between the treatment groups. In dogs receiving spironolactone/benazepril, elevations of serum magnesium and potassium can be significantly higher than dogs receiving only benazepril. Reversible prostatic atrophy has been observed in male dogs.[6] Spironolactone inhibits the synthesis of testosterone and may increase the peripheral conversion of testosterone to estradiol. Adverse endocrine effects in humans include menstrual irregularities and gynecomastia; significance in veterinary patients is unclear.

Reproductive/Nursing Safety

Spironolactone/benazepril is contraindicated during pregnancy.[6] In rats, use of ACE inhibitors (eg, benazepril) at labeled dosages during the second and third trimesters is associated with fetal malformation and fetal and neonatal morbidity and mortality. Spironolactone or its metabolites may cross the placental barrier. Feminization occurs in male rat fetuses, and endocrine dysfunction in females with utero spironolactone exposure. Reversible prostatic atrophy has been observed in male dogs treated with spironolactone, and in dogs receiving 3 to 5 times the labeled dosage of the spironolactone/benazepril combination.[2,6]

Canrenone, a metabolite of spironolactone, appears in maternal milk. Benazepril is excreted in maternal milk. Use this combination product with caution in nursing patients.

Overdose/Acute Toxicity

Clinical signs associated with an overdose typically are extensions of the adverse effects of both drugs and may include hypotension and vomiting. Hyperkalemia and hyponatremia may occur. Compensatory hypertrophy of the zona glomerulosa occurred at doses 3 times or greater than the recommended dose.[2]

Supportive treatment including volume expansion with appropriate IV fluid therapy is recommended if hypotension is documented. Because of benazepril's long duration of action, prolonged monitoring and treatment may be required. The manufacturer recommends inducing vomiting, gastric lavage, and electrolyte monitoring as appropriate.

For patients that have experienced or are suspected to have experienced an overdose, it is strongly encouraged to consult with one of the 24-hour poison consultation centers that specialize in providing information specific for veterinary patients. For general information related to overdose and toxin exposures, as well as contact information for poison control centers, refer to ***Appendix.***

Drug Interactions

The following drug interactions have either been reported or are theoretical in humans or animals receiving spironolactone and/or benazepril and may be of significance in veterinary patients. Unless otherwise noted, use together is not necessarily contraindicated, but weigh the potential risks and perform additional monitoring when appropriate.

- **Allopurinol**: Concurrent use may cause severe hypersensitivity reactions, neutropenia, agranulocytosis, or serious infections.
- **Alpha-2-Adrenergic Agonists** (eg, **clonidine, dexmedetomidine**): Concurrent use may result in additive effects on blood pressure and heart rate.
- **Antidiabetic agents** (eg, **glipizide, insulin**): Possible increased risk for hypoglycemia; enhanced monitoring is recommended
- **Histamine H1 Receptor Antagonists** (eg, **diphenhydramine**): Concurrent use may result in additive hypotension.
- **Apomorphine**: Concurrent use may result in additive hypoten-

sion.

- **Angiotensin Receptor Blockers** (ARBs; eg, **candesartan, telmisartan**): Concurrent use may increase the risk for adverse effects such as hypotension, syncope, hyperkalemia, changes in renal function, or acute renal insufficiency.
- **Aspirin**: Aspirin may potentially negate the decrease in systemic vascular resistance induced by ACE inhibitors; however, one study in dogs using low-dose aspirin showed that the hemodynamic effects of enalaprilat (active metabolite of enalapril, a related drug) were not affected.[13]
- **Azathioprine**: Concurrent use may result in an increased risk for neutropenia or leukopenia.
- **Barbiturates** (eg, **phenobarbital**): Concurrent use may enhance the hypotensive effects of benazepril.
- **Benzodiazepines** (eg, **diazepam, midazolam**): Concurrent use may lead to low blood pressure.
- **Beta-Blockers** (eg, **atenolol, propranolol**): Concurrent use may result in additive hypotension or hyperkalemia.
- **Buspirone**: Concurrent use may increase risk for hypotension.
- **Cabergoline**: Concurrent use may lead to additive hypotension.
- **Calcium Channel Blockers** (eg, **amlodipine, diltiazem**): Concurrent use may result in hypotension.
- **Cholestyramine**: Concurrent use may increase risk for hyperkalemic metabolic acidosis due to spironolactone.
- **Corticosteroids** (eg, **dexamethasone, prednis(ol)one**): May decrease antihypertensive effects by causing fluid and sodium retention
- **Cyclosporine**: Concurrent administration may increase the risk for hyperkalemia or precipitate acute renal failure.
- **Dalteparin/Enoxaparin**: Concurrent use may increase risk for hyperkalemia.
- **Desoxycorticosterone Pivalate (DOCP)**: DOCP may cause moderate reduction in the natriuretic effect of spironolactone.6 Spironolactone may reduce the effect of DOCP.[2]
- **Diazoxide**: Concurrent use may lead to hypotension and orthostasis.
- **Digoxin**: Spironolactone may increase the half-life of digoxin; however, field studies supported that digoxin can be safely used with the spironolactone/benazepril combination.[1] Enhanced monitoring of digoxin serum levels and effects should be considered.
- **Diuretics** (eg, **furosemide, hydrochlorothiazide**): Potential for increased hypotensive effects. Field studies demonstrated that furosemide can be safely used with the spironolactone/benazepril combination.
- **Diuretics, Potassium-Sparing** (eg, **triamterene**): Concurrent use may increase hyperkalemic effects. Enhanced monitoring of serum potassium is recommended.
- **Fenoldopam**: Concurrent administration may theoretically increase the risk for severe hypotension.
- **Heparin**: Concurrent use may increase the risk for hyperkalemia.
- **Interferon Alfa**: Concurrent use may increase risk for granulocytopenia.
- **Iodinated Contrast Agents** (eg, **iohexol**): Concurrent use may increase risk for nephrotoxicity.
- **Iron**: Benazepril may increase severity and risk for systemic adverse effects associated with parenteral administration of iron.
- **Lanthanum**: In theory, lanthanum may bind with drugs in the GI tract and interfere with absorption. Lanthanum should be given 2 hours before or after benazepril.
- **Methotrexate**: Concurrent use may potentiate risk for liver injury.
- **Mirtazapine**: Concurrent administration may result in additive hypotension and orthostasis.
- **Mitotane**: Spironolactone may mute the effects of mitotane if given concurrently, but very limited information is available on this potential interaction; monitor carefully.
- **Muscle Relaxants** (eg, **baclofen, methocarbamol**): Concurrent use may have additive blood pressure lowering effects.
- **Naltrexone**: Concurrent administration may increase risk for hepatotoxicity.
- **Nitroglycerin**: Benazepril may enhance the vasodilatory and hypotensive effects.
- **Nonsteroidal Anti-Inflammatory Drugs** (NSAIDs; eg, **carprofen, meloxicam, robenacoxib**): Potentially could increase the risk for nephrotoxicity and/or reduce efficacy of the ACE inhibitor in animals with cardiac or renal disease. Combination is considered contraindicated in dogs with renal insufficiency.[2,6,14,15]
- **Opioids** (eg, **butorphanol, morphine**): Concurrent use may result in additive hypotension and orthostasis.
- **Pentoxifylline**: Concurrent use may increase risk for hypotension.
- **Phenothiazines** (eg, **acepromazine, chlorpromazine**): Concurrent administration may cause orthostatic hypotension and syncope associated with vasodilation.
- **Polyethylene Glycol 3350**: Concurrent use may increase risk for fluid and electrolyte imbalances leading to renal impairment, cardiac arrhythmias, or seizures.
- **Potassium Supplements**: Increased risk for hyperkalemia
- **Prazosin**: Concurrent use can cause additive hypotension.
- **Pregabalin**: Concurrent use may increase risk for angioedema.
- **QT Prolonging Agents** (eg, **amiodarone, cisapride, fluoroquinolones, ondansetron, sotalol**): Concurrent use may increase risk for QTc prolongation and arrhythmias.
- **Salicylates** (eg, **aspirin**): Spironolactone's diuretic effects may be decreased if aspirin or other salicylates are administered concomitantly.
- **Selegiline**: Concurrent use can cause additive hypotension and orthostasis.
- **Sildenafil**: Concurrent use may potentiate the blood pressure lowering effects of benazepril and cause orthostasis and hypotension.
- **Sulfa-/Trimethoprim**: Concurrent use may increase the risk for hyperkalemia.
- **Trazodone**: Concurrent use may result in additive hypotension and orthostasis.
- **Tricyclic Antidepressants** (TCAs; eg, **amitriptyline, clomipramine**): Concurrent use may result in additive hypotension and orthostasis.

Laboratory Considerations

- Spironolactone may give falsely elevated digoxin values, if using a radioimmunoassay (**RIA**) method.
- Fluorometric methods of determining plasma and urinary 17-hydroxycorticosteroids (cortisol) may be interfered with by spironolactone.

Dosages

DOGS:

Management of clinical signs of mild, moderate, or severe congestive heart failure due to AVVI (label dosage, FDA-approved): Spironolactone 2 mg/kg with benazepril 0.25 mg/kg PO once daily with food, using an appropriate combination of whole and/or half tablets.[1] Begin use once pulmonary edema is stabilized; use in conjunction with concomitant therapy (eg, furosemide).

Monitoring

- Clinical efficacy: respiratory rate and effort and other clinical signs of heart failure
- Hydration status and body weight
- Clinical signs of pulmonary edema and ascites; serial girth measurements
- Baseline and periodic serum electrolytes (particularly potassium and magnesium), BUN, and creatinine[2,16]
- Measure digoxin levels regularly if dog is receiving concomitant digoxin; spironolactone can decrease the elimination (and thus increase plasma concentrations) of digoxin and cause toxicity.
- Cardiovascular parameters: blood pressure, ECG, thoracic radiographs, echocardiogram

Client Information

- This medicine should be given with food, or within 30 minutes of feeding.
- Ensure that your dog always has access to fresh water
- It is important to give this medicine as prescribed. Do not stop or change the amount you are giving your dog without your veterinarian's guidance.
- Your dog will need to have periodic examinations, blood pressure measurements, and blood tests performed while taking this medicine. Do not miss these important follow-up visits.
- If your dog shows any of the following side effects, contact your veterinarian immediately: severe or continuing vomiting or diarrhea, acting extremely tired, panting or increased breathing rate, trouble walking or keeping balance, or stopping eating, drinking, or urinating.
- The National Institute for Occupational Safety and Health (NIOSH) classifies spironolactone as a hazardous drug; wearing gloves should be considered (especially if you are pregnant) when giving this medicine to your dog.

Chemistry/Synonyms

Spironolactone is a synthetically produced aldosterone antagonist that occurs as a cream to light tan crystalline powder with a faint mercaptan-like odor and is practically insoluble in water and soluble in alcohol. Benazepril HCl occurs as a white to off-white crystalline powder that is soluble in water and ethanol.

Storage/Stability

Store in the manufacturer's original container at room temperature 20°C to 25°C (68°F-77°F), with excursions permitted between 15°C to 30°C (59°F-86°F). Store securely out of reach of pets or children.

Compatibility/Compounding Considerations

No information noted.

Dosage Forms/Regulatory Status

VETERINARY-LABELED PRODUCTS:

Spironolactone and Benazepril HCl Chewable Tablets (scored; in a fixed 8:1 ratio of spironolactone to benazepril hydrochloride): 20 mg spironolactone + 2.5 mg benazepril, 40 mg spironolactone + 5 mg benazepril, and 80 mg spironolactone + 10 mg benazepril in 30-count bottles; *Cardalis*®; (Rx). NADA # 141-538. Contains meat flavoring.

HUMAN-LABELED PRODUCTS:

None, although separate formulations of spironolactone and benazepril as a sole agent are readily available and generic.

References

For the complete list of references, see **wiley.com/go/budde/plumb**

Stanozolol

(stah-***no***-zo-lahl) *Winstrol*®*-V*

Anabolic Steroid

Prescriber Highlights

- ► FDA-approved controlled substance that is no longer marketed in the United States. Potentially useful in dogs for medical treatment of tracheal collapse
- ► Contraindications include in pregnant animals, breeding stallions, and food animals.
- ► Use extreme caution if using in cats or animals with hepatic dysfunction, hypercalcemia, history of myocardial infarction, pituitary insufficiency, prostate carcinoma, mammary carcinoma, benign prostatic hypertrophy, or are in the nephrotic stage of nephritis.
- ► Use caution in animals with cardiac and renal dysfunction; perform enhanced fluid and electrolyte monitoring.
- ► Adverse effects include high incidence of hepatotoxicity in cats. Other possible effects include sodium, calcium, potassium, water, chloride, and phosphate retention; hepatotoxicity; behavioral (androgenic) changes; and reproductive abnormalities (oligospermia, estrus suppression).
- ► Drug interactions and laboratory interactions are possible.
- ► The National Institute for Occupational Safety and Health (NIOSH) classifies androgens as hazardous drugs; use appropriate precautions when handling.

Uses/Indications

The previously marketed veterinary stanozolol product *Winstrol*®*-V* was approved as an adjunct to other specific and supportive therapy, including nutritional therapy to improve appetite, promote weight gain, and increase strength and vitality in dogs, cats, and horses. In a review of the evidence supporting anabolic steroid use in horses, the authors conclude: *Level 1 evidence for the efficacy of anabolic steroids in horses for therapeutic uses is not found in the biomedical literature. Evidence in other species exists for the efficacy of anabolic steroids in treating anemia and increasing muscle mass after illness or injury, but that evidence is not unequivocal, and the applicability to horses has not been demonstrated. There is little evidence in other species for the efficacy of anabolic steroids for increasing appetite.*[1]

In sheep, a study that used an experimental model of osteoarthritis (OA) found intra-articular stanozolol reduced osteophytes formation and subchondral bone reaction and promoted articular cartilage regeneration.[2] Intra-articular administration once weekly to horses with both acute and chronic OA improved physical characteristics of synovial fluid as well as lameness scores.[3] Intra-articular bilateral stanozolol improved clinical signs in police dogs with OA, but was less effective than hyaluranate.[4]

Stanozolol has been used to treat anemia of chronic disease. Because stanozolol has been demonstrated to enhance fibrinolysis after parenteral injection, it may be efficacious in the treatment of feline aortic thromboembolism or thrombosis in nephrotic syndrome; however, clinical studies and/or experience are apparently lacking for this indication at present. In humans, stanozolol may also raise plasma antithrombin III and plasminogen levels.

A controlled study in dogs using stanozolol as a conservative treatment for collapsing trachea (without bronchitis) reported that at the end of the study (75 days), 93% of dogs in the stanozolol group had an improvement in the tracheal collapse grade. Eight of the 14 treated dogs were deemed cured.[5]

Pharmacology/Actions

Stanozolol possesses the actions of other anabolic agents, but it may be less androgenic than other anabolics used in veterinary medicine.

In the presence of adequate protein and calories, anabolic steroids promote body tissue-building processes and can reverse catabolism. As these agents are either derived from or are closely related to testosterone, the anabolics have varying degrees of androgenic effects. Endogenous testosterone release may be suppressed by inhibiting luteinizing hormone (LH). Large doses can impede spermatogenesis by negative feedback inhibition of follicle stimulating hormone (FSH).

Anabolic steroids can also stimulate erythropoiesis, possibly by stimulation of erythropoietic stimulating factor. Anabolics can cause nitrogen, sodium, potassium, and phosphorus retention and decrease the urinary excretion of calcium.

For medical treatment of tracheal collapse in dogs, it is postulated that stanozolol could increase tracheal wall strength via enhancing protein or collagen synthesis, increasing chondroitin sulfate content, increasing lean body mass, and decreasing inflammation.

Pharmacokinetics

In horses (n = 26), following a 0.55 mg/kg IM injection of compounded stanozolol suspension, peak levels occur at 7 days.[6] The median halflife was 3 to 4 days but ranged from 1.6 to 14.7 days.[6]

In horses (n = 10), following a 5 mg intra-articular injection into both tarsal joints, a maximum plasma concentration (1.7 ng/mL) was observed 6 hours postdose.[7] The elimination half-life was between 4 and 12 hours and was completed cleared from plasma within 36 hours after dosing.

In humans, stanozolol is extensively metabolized by the liver.

Contraindications/Precautions/Warnings

Stanozolol is contraindicated in pregnant animals and in breeding stallions and should not be administered to horses intended for food purposes.

Because of reported hepatotoxicity associated with stanozolol in cats, it should only be used in this species with extreme caution.

The manufacturer recommends using stanozolol cautiously in patients with cardiac and renal dysfunction with enhanced fluid and electrolyte monitoring.

In humans, anabolic agents are contraindicated in patients with hepatic dysfunction, hypercalcemia, patients with a history of myocardial infarction (can cause hypercholesterolemia), pituitary insufficiency, prostate carcinoma, benign prostatic hypertrophy, during the nephrotic stage of nephritis, and in selected patients with breast carcinoma. In children, anabolic agents should be used with caution because of hormonal effects and possible effects on bone growth.

The National Institute for Occupational Safety and Health (NIOSH) classifies androgens as hazardous drugs representing an occupational hazard to healthcare workers; personal protective equipment (PPE) should be used accordingly to minimize the risk for exposure.[8]

Adverse Effects

The manufacturer lists only *mild androgenic effects* in dogs, cats, and horses and then only when used with excessively high doses for a prolonged period.

One study in cats demonstrated a high incidence of hepatotoxicity associated with stanozolol use.

Transient postinjection swelling was observed after IA administration to horses.[3] A horse that received stanozolol monthly for 8 years developed adrenal insufficiency following abrupt discontinuation, which the authors attributed to stanozolol-induced adrenal suppression.[9]

Potentially (from human data), adverse reactions of the anabolic agents in dogs and cats could include sodium, calcium, potassium, water, chloride, and phosphate retention, hepatotoxicity, behavioral (androgenic) changes, and reproductive abnormalities (eg, oligospermia, estrus suppression).

Reproductive/Nursing Safety

Stanozolol is contraindicated in pregnant animals and in breeding stallions. It is not known whether anabolic steroids are excreted in maternal milk. Because of the potential for serious adverse reactions in nursing offspring, use it with extreme caution in patients that are nursing.

Overdose/Acute Toxicity

No information was located for this specific agent. In humans, sodium and water retention can occur after overdosage of anabolic steroids. It is suggested to treat supportively and monitor liver function should an inadvertent overdose be administered.

For patients that have experienced or are suspected of having experienced an overdose, consultation with a 24-hour poison consultation center specializing in providing veterinary-specific information is recommended. For general information related to overdose and toxin exposures, as well as contact information for poison control centers, refer to ***Appendix.***

Drug Interactions

The following drug interactions have either been reported or are theoretical in humans or animals receiving stanozolol and may be of significance in veterinary patients. Unless otherwise noted, use together is not necessarily contraindicated, but weigh the potential risks and perform additional monitoring when appropriate.

- **ANTICOAGULANTS** (eg, **heparin, warfarin**): Anabolic agents as a class may potentiate the effects of anticoagulants; monitor anticoagulation (eg, aPTT, PT) closely and adjust dosage if necessary.
- **CORTICOSTEROIDS** (eg, **dexamethasone, predniso(lo)ne**): Anabolics may enhance the edema that can be associated with ACTH or adrenal steroid therapy.
- **INSULIN**: Diabetic patients receiving insulin may need dosage adjustments if anabolic therapy is added or discontinued; anabolics may decrease blood glucose and decrease insulin requirements.

Laboratory Considerations

- Concentrations of protein-bound iodine (PBI) can be decreased in patients receiving androgen/anabolic therapy, but the clinical significance of this is probably not important. Androgen/anabolic agents can decrease amounts of thyroxine-binding globulin and decrease total T_4 concentrations and increase resin uptake of $\mathbf{T_3}$ **and** $\mathbf{T_4}$. Free thyroid hormones are unaltered, and there is no evidence of dysfunction.
- Both **creatinine** and **creatine** excretion can be decreased by anabolic steroids.
- Anabolic steroids can increase the urinary excretion of **17-ketosteroids**.
- Androgenic/anabolic steroids may alter **blood glucose** levels.
- Androgenic/anabolic steroids may suppress clotting factors II, V, VII, and X.
- Anabolic agents can affect **liver function tests** and **liver enzymes** (BSP retention, AST, ALT, bilirubin, and ALP).

Dosages

DOGS:

Anabolic agent (label dosage; FDA-approved): Small breeds: 1 – 2 mg/dog (NOT mg/kg) PO twice daily or 25 mg/dog (NOT mg/kg) deep IM, may repeat weekly. Large breeds: 2 – 4 mg/dog (NOT mg/kg) PO twice daily or 50 mg/dog (NOT mg/kg) deep IM, may repeat weekly. Treatment should continue for several weeks, depending on the response and condition of the animal.[10–12]

Tracheal collapse: (extra-label): In the study, dogs in the treatment group received 0.15 mg/kg PO twice daily for 2 months, then tapered for 15 days.[5]

Hip osteoarthritis (extra-label): 0.3 mg/kg via intra-articular injection into both hip joints[4]

CATS:

NOTE: See ***Contraindications/Precautions/Warnings*** regarding hepatotoxicity in cats. Most clinicians do not recommend using stanozolol in cats.

Anabolic agent (label dosage; FDA-approved): 1 – 2 mg/cat (NOT mg/kg) PO twice daily or 25 mg/cat (NOT mg/kg) deep IM; may repeat weekly. Treatment should continue for several weeks, depending on the response and condition of the animal.[11,12]

HORSES:

Anabolic agent per (former) labeled indications: 0.55 mg/kg (25 mg/45 kg [100 lb] of body weight) deep IM. May repeat weekly for not more than 4 weeks[11]

Acute or chronic osteoarthritis (OA) (extra-label): 5 mg/joint (NOT mg/kg) via intra-articular injection into affected joint, repeated weekly up to 4 times (acute OA) or 6 times (chronic OA)[3]

BIRDS:

Anabolic agent to promote weight gain and recovery from disease (extra-label): 0.5 – 1 mL/kg (25 – 50 mg/kg) IM once or twice weekly. Use with caution in birds with renal disease.[13]

FERRETS:

Anabolic agent (extra-label): 0.5 mg/kg PO or SC twice daily; use with caution in ferrets with hepatic disease.[14]

RABBITS, RODENTS, SMALL MAMMALS:

Rabbits; Appetite stimulant (extra-label): 0.5 – 2 mg/rabbit (NOT mg/kg) PO once[15]

REPTILES:

Most species postsurgically and in debilitated animals (extra-label): 5 mg/kg IM once weekly as needed[16]

Monitoring

- Androgenic adverse effects
- Fluid and electrolyte status, if indicated
- Liver enzymes, if indicated
- RBC count, indices, hemoglobin, if indicated
- Weight, appetite

Client Information

- This medicine may be given with or without food. If your animal vomits or acts sick after receiving the drug on an empty stomach, try giving the next dose with food or a small treat. If vomiting continues, contact your veterinarian.
- This medicine can cause behavior changes, including more sexual behaviors.
- Cats may be prone to developing liver problems while receiving this medication.
- Pregnant women should handle this medicine with caution.
- This medicine is a controlled substance in the United States. It is against federal law to use, give away, or sell this medication to others than for whom it was prescribed.

Chemistry/Synonyms

Stanozolol is an anabolic steroid that occurs as an odorless, nearly colorless, crystalline powder that can exist in 2 forms: prisms that melt at ≈235°C (455°F) and needles that melt at ≈155°C (311°F). It is sparingly soluble in alcohol and insoluble in water.

Stanozolol may also be known as androstanazole, estanozolol, methylstanazole, NSC-43193, stanozololum, win-14833, *Menabol*®, *Neurabol*®, *Stanol*®, *Stromba*®, *Strombaject*®, and *Winstrol*®.

Storage/Stability

Store stanozolol in light-resistant packaging, preferably at room temperature; store tablets in tight containers.

Compatibility/Compounding Considerations

No specific information was noted.

Dosage Forms/Regulatory Status

VETERINARY-LABELED PRODUCTS: NONE

Although *Winstrol*®*-V* tablets and injections still appear in the FDA's Green Book, they are no longer commercially marketed but may be available from reputable compounding pharmacies. See ***Compounding: How to Find a Quality Assured Pharmacy.***

The Association of Racing Commissioners International (ARCI) has designated this drug as a class 3 substance. Use of this drug may not be allowed in certain animal competitions. Check rules and regulations before entering a competition while this medication is being administered. Contact local racing authorities for further guidance. See ***Appendix*** for more information.

HUMAN-LABELED PRODUCTS: NONE

References

For the complete list of references, see **wiley.com/go/budde/plumb**

Staphylococcus Aureus Phage Lysate

(***staf***-ih-loe-***kok-us or***-ee-us fayj ***lie***-sayt) *Staphage Lysate*®

Immunostimulant

Prescriber Highlights

- Used to treat dogs with recurrent and idiopathic staphylococcal pyodermas
- Use with caution in highly allergic patients; desensitizing doses are required.
- May cause local or systemic hypersensitivity reactions, including redness, itching, swelling, and anaphylaxis

Uses/Indications

Staphylococcus aureus phage lysate (SPL) is USDA-licensed for treatment of canine pyoderma and related staphylococcal hypersensitivity or polymicrobial skin infections with a staphylococcal component. SPL, or similar *Staphylococcus aureus* bacterins, reduces pruritus and recurrence of superficial and deep pyodermas in dogs.[1-3] One small study in dogs showed a 77% reduction of recurrent canine pyoderma caused by *Staphylococcus pseudintermedius* when treated with antibiotics and SPL compared to antibiotics alone.[4]

Pharmacology/Actions

Staphylococcus aureus phage lysate (SPL) enhances cell-mediated immunity and increases the capability of macrophages to inactivate staphylococci. It stimulates production of tumor necrosis factor, interleukin-6, interleukin-gamma, and gamma-interferon.

Pharmacokinetics

No information was located.

Contraindications/Precautions/Warnings

In highly allergic patients, it is recommended to first perform a skin test to evaluate the patient's response to Staphylococcus aureus phage lysate (SPL); if the skin test indicates tolerance, then weekly doses should be gradually increased until the full weekly label dose is achieved.[5] Use SPL with extreme caution, if at all, in patients with prior systemic hypersensitivity reactions to SPL or documented hypersensitivity reactions to beef products, as the product contains ultrafiltered beef heart infusion broth.

Avoid administering subsequent doses at the same injection site.[5] The product contains no preservative so it must be handled aseptically.

Adverse Effects

Adverse effects reported for Staphylococcus aureus phage lysate (SPL) include vaccine-type reactions (eg, fever, malaise) and injection site reactions, including redness, itching, and swelling, that may occur within 2 to 3 hours after injection and persist up to 3 days.[5] Reduce dose by 50% if significant injection site reaction occurs.

Although thought to be rare, systemic hypersensitivity reactions are possible. Signs may include weakness, vomiting, diarrhea, severe itching, rapid breathing, and fatigue or lassitude. Should an anaphylactic-type reaction occur, treat the patient supportively (eg, epinephrine and atropine).

Reproductive/Nursing Safety

Studies performed in rats and rabbits demonstrated no impaired fertility or fetal harm.[5] No information was located on safety during nursing. Because safety has not been established, this drug should only be used when the maternal benefits outweigh the potential risks to offspring.

Overdose/Acute Toxicity

No specific information was located. Other than an increased risk for local or systemic hypersensitivity reactions, significant morbidity appears unlikely.

For patients that have experienced or are suspected to have experienced an overdose, consultation with a 24-hour poison consultation center specializing in providing veterinary-specific information is recommended. For general information related to overdose and toxin exposures, as well as contact information for poison control centers, refer to ***Appendix.***

Drug Interactions

The following drug interactions have either been reported or are theoretical in animals receiving SPL. Unless otherwise noted, use together is not necessarily contraindicated, but weigh the potential risks and perform additional monitoring when appropriate.

- **IMMUNOSUPPRESSANTS** (eg, **corticosteroids, cyclosporine**): May reduce the efficacy of Staphylococcus aureus phage lysate (SPL)

Laboratory Considerations

- No significant concerns noted

Dosages

DOGS:

Treatment of canine pyoderma and related staphylococcal hypersensitivity or treatment of polymicrobial skin infections with a staphylococcal component (label dosage; USDA-licensed): **NOTE:** It is recommended to administer this agent with concomitant topical and/or systemic antibiotic therapy according to current antimicrobial stewardship guidelines. Avoid administration in previous injection sites.

a) **Highly allergic patients**: Skin test with 0.05 – 0.1 mL intradermally. If no immediate reactions are seen within 1 hour and no delayed reactions are seen after 48 hours, initiate treatment at 0.2 mL SC. Incrementally increase by 0.2 mL once weekly to 1 mL (a total of 5 injections). Then continue at 1 mL SC weekly for ≈10 to 12 weeks.[5]

b) **Nonallergic patients**: 0.5 mL SC twice weekly for 10 to 12 weeks, then 0.5 – 1 mL SC every 1 to 2 weeks. Skin testing is not required prior to treatment.[5]

c) **All patients**: Dosage adjustments should be guided by infection severity and patient response to treatment.[5] The maximum dose should be decreased in small dogs and can be cautiously increased to 1.5 mL in large dogs if necessary. Continue this dosage regimen until clinical signs improve, then gradually lengthen dosing interval to the longest interval that maintains adequate clinical control.

Adjunctive treatment of chronic recurrent idiopathic pyoderma (extra-label):

a) 0.5 mL SC twice weekly, slowly reducing to 0.5 mL every 2 weeks[6]

b) 1 mL SC once weekly or 0.5 mL twice weekly for 4 to 6 months. If no significant recurrence of pyoderma, decrease administration to every 2 weeks, then every 3 weeks. SPL is best used to prevent pyoderma from recurring and should be used with antibiotics initially to induce remission.[7]

Recurrent staphylococcal infection in dogs with atopic dermatitis following treatment with antibiotics to resolve active pyoderma (extra-label): 0.5 mL SC twice weekly for 12 weeks, then 1 mL once weekly for 4 weeks, then 1 mL every 15 days for 2 doses, then 1 mL every 3 weeks for 2 doses[3]

Monitoring

- Clinical efficacy
- Local and systemic reactions which may occur within 2 to 3 hours after injection and persist up to 3 days

Client Information

- The first dose of this medication should be administered at a veterinary practice where suitable treatment can be given if a serious reaction to the medicine (eg, anaphylaxis) occurs.
- Report any side effects to your veterinarian, including injection site redness or irritation, itching, changes in behavior or activity level, difficulty breathing, unexplained rapid breathing, vomiting, or diarrhea.

Chemistry/Synonyms

Staphylococcus aureus phage lysate (SPL) is prepared by lysing cultures of *Staphylococcus aureus* (Cowan serologic types I and III; human strains) by a staphylococcal bacteriophage. Pre-lysed cell counts (120 to 180 CFU/mL) are used to standardize the product; ultrafiltration achieves bacteriologic sterility. The prepared solution contains *Staphylococcus aureus* components (protein A extracts), bacteriophage, and unfiltered beef heart infusion.

Storage/Stability

Staphylococcus aureus phage lysate (SPL) should be stored in the refrigerator at 2°C to 7°C (36°F-45°F); do not freeze.[5]

Unopened, properly stored vials and ampules have an average expiration date of one year past the shipment date. The product contains no preservative and must be handled aseptically. Do not use if contents are cloudy.

Compatibility/Compounding Considerations

Do not mix Staphylococcus aureus phage lysate (SPL) with other drugs or solutions prior to administration.

Dosage Forms/Regulatory Status

VETERINARY-LABELED PRODUCTS:

Staphylococcal Phage Lysate (serotypes I and III): in 1 mL ampules and 10 mL multi-dose vials; *Staphage Lysate (SPL)®*; (OTC); USDA license #339

HUMAN-LABELED PRODUCTS: NONE

References

For the complete list of references, see **wiley.com/go/budde/plumb**

Streptozocin

(strep-toe-***zoe***-sin) *Zanosar®*

Antineoplastic

Prescriber Highlights

- ► Used primarily for treating recurrent insulinoma in dogs
- ► Severe nephrotoxicity is known to occur with streptozocin; myelotoxicity and hepatotoxicity are also possible.
- ► Adverse effects include severe vomiting after treatment, transient hypoglycemia, or diabetes mellitus.
- ► Saline diuresis is required before, during, and after administration to reduce risk for nephrotoxicity.
- ► The National Institute for Occupational Safety and Health (NIOSH) classifies streptozocin as a hazardous drug; use appropriate precautions when handling.

Uses/Indications

The primary indication for streptozocin use in veterinary medicine is for treatment for insulinomas in dogs, particularly those with refractory hypoglycemia and when tumors are nonresectable or have metastasized. Its use has been limited by high rates of nephrotoxicity and other serious adverse effects. Streptozocin potentially could be used for other neoplastic conditions as well.

Pharmacology/Actions

Streptozocin is a nitrosourea antineoplastic. Although its antineoplastic activity is not well understood, streptozocin is considered an alkylating agent, and it inhibits DNA synthesis, likely by inhibiting precursor incorporation into DNA and cross-linking DNA strands. It is cell cycle–phase nonspecific.

Streptozocin also exhibits a diabetogenic effect by reducing nicotinamide adenine dinucleotide (NAD) concentration in pancreatic beta cells. This effect is usually irreversible in animals with a pre-existing normal beta cell function. Although streptozocin has activity against gram-positive and gram-negative bacteria, its cytotoxicity prevents it from clinical usefulness for this purpose.

Pharmacokinetics

Streptozocin must be administered IV. Its distribution characteristics are not well known, but the drug does distribute to most tissues; concentrations in the pancreas are higher than those found in plasma. Streptozocin is metabolized, probably in the liver and kidneys. Both the unchanged and metabolized drug are excreted in the urine.

Contraindications/Precautions/Warnings

Streptozocin should only be used for recurrent insulinoma in dogs that have undergone previous surgery in which complete tumor resection was not possible. A confirmed histologic diagnosis is mandatory.

Streptozocin must be used with extreme caution in patients with decreased renal, bone marrow, or hepatic function. Streptozocin is known to cause renal toxicity. In humans, nephrotoxicity is dose-related, cumulative, can be irreversible, and can be fatal.[1] Monitor renal function before and after each treatment. Streptozocin is a tissue irritant and may cause severe irritation or necrosis if extravasated.

Streptozocin is known to be carcinogenic and tumorigenic in lab rodents. The National Institute for Occupational Safety and Health (NIOSH) classifies streptozocin as a hazardous drug; personal protective equipment (PPE) should be used accordingly to minimize the risk for exposure.[2]

Adverse Effects

The primary concern with streptozocin is the potential for serious, permanent renal toxicity. In dogs, Fanconi syndrome and likely nephrogenic diabetes insipidus have been reported.[3] In humans, nephrotoxicity is dose-related, cumulative, can be irreversible, and can be fatal. Nephrotoxicity in humans can present as azotemia, anuria, hypophosphatemia, glycosuria, and renal tubular acidosis.[1] Adequate hydration during drug administration is strongly recommended in order to reduce the risk for nephrotoxicity.

GI effects (eg, nausea, vomiting) often occur and can be severe or protracted; increased liver enzymes (ALT) may also occur. Acute, transient hypoglycemia has been reported secondary to streptozocin-damaged tumor cells releasing intracellular insulin stores. Permanent diabetes mellitus has also been reported. Less commonly, hematologic changes such as mild myelosuppression can be seen. Injection site reactions (including severe necrosis) can occur if the drug extravasates.[1]

In one small study, adverse effects included GI signs (eg, nausea, anorexia, vomiting, regurgitation, diarrhea, colitis) diabetes mellitus, renal injury, increased ALT, and hypoglycemic collapse or seizure; no neutropenia or thrombocytopenia was observed.[3]

Many dogs receiving chemotherapy will have minor hair coat changes (eg, shagginess, loss of luster). Breeds with continuously growing hair coats (eg, poodles, terriers, Afghan hounds, or old English sheepdogs) are more likely to experience significant alopecia.

Reproductive/Nursing Safety

Streptozocin has been shown to be teratogenic in rats and abortifacient in rabbits. For sexually intact patients, verify pregnancy status prior to administration.

It is not known whether streptozocin is excreted in milk. Because of the potential for serious adverse reactions in nursing offspring, milk replacer should be used if treating nursing patients.

Because safety has not been established in animals, this drug should only be used when the maternal benefits outweigh the potential risks to offspring.

Overdose/Acute Toxicity

Severe toxicity may result if acutely overdosed (see ***Adverse Effects***); calculate dosages carefully.

For patients that have experienced or are suspected to have experienced an overdose, consultation with a 24-hour poison consultation center specializing in providing veterinary-specific information is recommended. For general information related to overdose and toxin exposures, as well as contact information for poison control centers, refer to ***Appendix.***

Drug Interactions

The following drug interactions have either been reported or are theoretical in humans or animals receiving streptozocin and may be of significance in veterinary patients. Unless otherwise noted, use together is not necessarily contraindicated, but weigh the potential risks and perform additional monitoring when appropriate.

- **Doxorubicin**: Streptozocin may prolong the half-life of doxorubicin; dosage adjustment may be required.[4]
- **Myelosuppressive Drugs, Other**: When streptozocin is used with other myelosuppressive drugs (eg, **lomustine**), additive or synergistic myelosuppression may occur.
- **Nephrotoxic Drugs, Other** (eg, **aminoglycosides, amphotericin B, cisplatin**): May cause additive nephrotoxicity when used with streptozocin
- **Niacinamide/Nicotinamide**: Can block the diabetogenic effects of streptozocin without altering its antineoplastic activity; this may be beneficial or detrimental depending on the reason for use.

Dosages

DOGS:

NOTE: Because of the potential toxicity of this drug to patients, veterinary personnel, and clients, and since chemotherapy indications, treatment protocols, monitoring, and safety guidelines often change, the following dosages should be used only as a general guide. Consultation with a veterinary oncologist and referral to current veterinary oncology references[5-9] are strongly recommended.

Insulinoma (extra-label):

a) Dilute 500 mg/m² (NOT mg/kg) in 36.6 mL/kg of 0.9% sodium chloride and administer IV over 2 hours every 2 weeks for a total of 5 doses. Administer 0.9% sodium chloride 18.3 mL/kg per hour IV CRI for 3 hours before streptozocin and continuing for 2 hours after streptozocin administration. Prophylactic antiemetics may be administered with each dose, and prednisone 0.5 – 1 mg/kg PO every 24 hours or divided every 12 hours may be used for patients with persistent hypoglycemia.[3]
b) 500 mg/m² (NOT mg/kg) IV over 2 hours. Prior to administration of streptozocin, administer 0.9% sodium chloride 18.3 mL/kg/hour IV CRI for 3 hours. Dilute the dose of streptozocin to the appropriate volume of IV fluids to be administered over 2 hours. Following the streptozocin infusion, continue 0.9% sodium chloride 18.3 mL/kg/hour IV CRI for an additional 2 hours. May repeat this protocol at 3week intervals until evidence of tumor progression, recurrence of hypoglycemia, or drug toxicity occurs. Give with antiemetics.[10]
c) 500 mg/m² (NOT mg/kg) IV over 2 hours every 3 weeks. Administer only with aggressive saline diuresis: 0.9% sodium chloride 18 to 20 mL/kg/hour IV CRI for 7 to 8 hours, starting 4 hours before streptozocin administration. Give maropitant at the beginning of the 0.9% sodium chloride infusion and continue daily for 3 to 4 days following streptozocin administration.[11]

Monitoring

- Blood glucose (efficacy)
- Baseline and periodic (eg, prior to each treatment) CBC, serum chemistry profile with electrolytes, and urinalysis; proteinuria is usually the first indicator of renal toxicity.
- Hydration status, especially for the first few days after treatment or if vomiting is persistent
- Baseline and periodic (eg, every 2 to 3 months) abdominal ultrasound or CT scan to assess tumor size during therapy

Client Information

- Streptozocin is a chemotherapy (anticancer) drug. This medicine can be hazardous to other animals and people that come in contact with it. On the day your animal gets the drug and then for a few days afterward, wear disposable gloves when handling all bodily waste (urine, feces, litter), blood, and vomit of the animal. Seal the waste in a plastic bag and then place both the bag and gloves in with the regular trash.
- Be sure that your animal has ready access to plenty of clean drinking water.

Chemistry/Synonyms

Streptozocin is a nitrosourea antineoplastic antibiotic produced by *Streptomyces achromogenes*, although the commercial product is prepared synthetically. It occurs as an ivory-colored, crystalline powder. It is very soluble in water and saline and has a pK_a of 1.35.

Streptozocin may also be known as NSC-85998, streptozotocin, U-9889, and *Zanosar*®.

Storage/Stability

Store the lyophilized powder for injection in the refrigerator at 2°C to 8°C (36°F-46°F) and protect it from light. It is stable for at least 3 years after manufacture when refrigerated. If stored at room temperature, it is stable for at least 1 year after manufacture.

After reconstitution, the lyophilized powder for injection has a pH of 3.5 to 4.5. Add citric acid to buffer the solution at a concentration of 22 mg/mL. The solution is stable for 48 hours at room temperature and 96 hours if refrigerated, but as there is no preservative, the manufacturer recommends using the drug within 12 hours of mixing.

Compatibility/Compounding Considerations

Compatibility is dependent upon factors such as pH, concentration, temperature, and diluent used; consult specialized references or a hospital pharmacist for more specific information.

Reconstitute the vial using 9.5 mL of either 5% dextrose or 0.9% sodium chloride, and it can be further diluted with either solution if desired. Streptozocin is reported to be **Y-site compatible** with the following drugs (partial list): dolasetron, hydromorphone, octreotide, and ondansetron. It is **incompatible** with amphotericin B (lipid complex), pantoprazole, and piperacillin-tazobactam.

Dosage Forms/Regulatory Status

VETERINARY-LABELED PRODUCTS: NONE

HUMAN-LABELED PRODUCTS:

Streptozocin Powder for Injection: 1 g (100 mg/mL) vials; *Zanosar*®; (Rx)

References

For the complete list of references, see **wiley.com/go/budde/plumb**

Succimer

(***sux***-i-mer) *Chemet*®

Antidote; Chelator

Prescriber Highlights

- ► Oral heavy metal chelator used for lead poisoning in dogs, cats, and birds
- ► Appears to be safe and effective despite limited experience
- ► Most common adverse effects noted are GI in nature; may also cause increased liver enzymes or rash.
- ► Unpleasant odor of capsules may cause odorous feces, urine, and saliva.
- ► May be cost prohibitive

Uses/Indications

Succimer may be useful for the oral treatment of lead poisoning in dogs, cats, and birds. It may also be beneficial for the treatment of other toxic heavy metals such as arsenic or mercury. Succimer is not nephrotoxic, does not increase lead absorption from the GI tract and does not significantly increase elimination of other essential minerals.

Pharmacology/Actions

Succimer physically chelates heavy metals such as lead, mercury, and arsenic. These water-soluble chelates are then excreted via the kidneys. Succimer-lead complexes are also eliminated in the feces and undergo enterohepatic recycling.

Pharmacokinetics

The absorption of oral succimer is less than or equal to 20% in monkeys and less than or equal to 32% in rabbits. In rats, oral succimer is rapidly absorbed and 95% is eliminated from the body by 24 hours. In experimental animals succimer is eliminated in feces and urine after oral administration. After IV administration, most is eliminated in the urine with only trace amounts in the feces.

In humans, the drug is rapidly but incompletely absorbed after oral ingestion. Absorbed drug is excreted primarily through the kidneys into the urine. Half-life in humans is ≈2 days.

Contraindications/Precautions/Warnings

Succimer is contraindicated in patients that are hypersensitive to it.[1] Chelation therapy should only be attempted after the source of lead is removed to prevent further exposure. Use with caution in patients with renal or hepatic impairment. In humans, treatment courses longer than 3 weeks have not been proven safe.

Adverse Effects

In humans, the most common adverse effects are GI related (eg, vomiting, diarrhea) or flu-like symptoms (eg, body aches, fatigue, rhinitis, cough).[1] Clinically insignificant increases in liver enzymes occur in up to 60% of patients. Rashes and allergic mucocutaneous reactions (which can be severe) may occur; skin reactions occur in ≈6% of patients. Mild to moderate neutropenia has also been reported. Adverse effects in humans are usually mild, self-limiting and do not require cessation of therapy. In humans succimer produces a small increase in urinary excretion of zinc and copper.

Reproductive/Nursing Safety

It is unknown if succimer is safe to use during pregnancy. At high doses, it was fetotoxic and teratogenic in mice and rats.[1] It is not known whether this drug is excreted in breast milk, but mothers are discouraged from nursing when taking succimer. Because safety has not been established in animals, this drug should only be used when the maternal benefits outweigh the potential risks to offspring.

Overdose/Acute Toxicity

Succimer is generally well tolerated in overdoses. In toxicology studies, there was no renal toxicity in dogs given 50 mg/kg/day orally for 14 days.[1] In a 28-day oral toxicity study dogs given 30 or 100 mg/kg/day had lower urine specific gravity and an increase in renal tubular regenerative hyperplasia. Doses of less than or equal to 200 mg/kg/day in dogs did not cause overt toxicity. Doses of 300 mg/day did cause fatalities in dogs; primarily kidney and GI tract lesions were seen. Doses of 80 mg/kg PO every 12 hours caused a significant number of fatalities in cockatiels (but 40 mg/kg every 12 hours did not). Doses up to 270 mg/kg twice daily for 15 days caused an initial increase in plasma uric acid concentration but did not cause significant adverse effects in pigeons with experimental lead-intoxication.[2]

If overdose occurs, standard GI decontamination protocols with subsequent activated charcoal may be used.

For patients that have experienced or are suspected to have experienced an overdose, consultation with a 24-hour poison consultation center specializing in providing veterinary-specific information is recommended. For general information related to overdose and toxin exposures, as well as contact information for poison control centers, refer to ***Appendix.***

Drug Interactions

The following drug interactions have either been reported or are theoretical in humans or animals receiving succimer and may be of significance in veterinary patients. Unless otherwise noted, use together is not necessarily contraindicated, but weigh the potential risks and perform additional monitoring when appropriate.

- **Chelating Agents, Other** (eg, **CaEDTA, dimercaprol, penicillamine, trientine**): Concomitant use with other chelating agents is not recommended in humans.1 Succimer may be used 4 weeks after CaEDTA treatment.

Laboratory Considerations

- False positive urine ketones can be reported when using nitroprusside reagents (eg, *Ketostix*®).
- Falsely low measurements of CPK or serum uric acid can be caused by succimer.

Dosages

DOGS/CATS:

Lead poisoning (extra-label): 10 mg/kg PO every 8 hours for 5 to 10 days. Blood lead concentrations should be rechecked a few days following the last dose of succimer; a second round of chelation therapy may be necessary to reduce the lead load.[3] The total length of treatment should be based on clinical improvement and blood lead concentrations.[4]

HORSES:

Lead poisoning (extra-label): Anecdotally, 30 mg/kg/day PO in divided doses

BIRDS:

Lead poisoning (extra-label): 20 – 40 mg/kg twice daily for a minimum of 7 days[5,6]

Monitoring

- Baseline and periodic complete blood count and measurement of blood lead concentration
- GI adverse effects
- Baseline and periodic liver enzymes (AST, ALT)

Client Information

- This medicine is used to remove excess metals, particularly lead, from the body
- Capsules can be opened and sprinkled on soft food. The capsules may have an unpleasant odor, which may increase the odor of saliva, urine, and feces.
- Animals should always have plenty of clean drinking water available while taking this medicine.
- This medicine may cause diarrhea and vomiting. Contact your veterinarian if you have any concerns.
- Your veterinarian will need to monitor your animal while it is taking this medicine. Do not miss these important follow-up visits.

Chemistry/Synonyms

A heavy metal chelating agent also known as meso-2,3 dimercaptosuccinic acid (DMSA), succimer is a water-soluble analog of dimercaprol. It occurs as a white crystalline powder with a sulfurous odor.

Succimer may also be known as meso-2,3 dimercaptosuccinic acid, dimercaptosuccinic acid, DIM-SA, DMSA, *Chemet*®, or *Succicaptal*®.

Storage/Stability

Unless otherwise labeled, store succimer capsules in tight containers at room temperature. Protect from light.

Compatibility/Compounding Considerations

No specific information noted

Dosage Forms/Regulatory Status

VETERINARY-LABELED PRODUCTS: NONE

HUMAN-LABELED PRODUCTS:

Succimer Capsules: 100 mg; *Chemet*®; (Rx)

Succimer 200 mg capsules may be available in some countries.

References

For the complete list of references, see **wiley.com/go/budde/plumb**

Succinylcholine

(***suks***-sin-nil-***koe***-leen) *Anectine*®

Neuromuscular Blocking Agent

Prescriber Highlights

- Used for short-term muscle relaxation during surgery, diagnostic procedures, or mechanical ventilation
- No analgesic or anesthetic effects
- Contraindications include severe liver disease, chronic anemia, malnourishment, glaucoma or penetrating eye injuries, predisposition to malignant hyperthermia, and increased CPK values with resultant myopathies.
- Use with extreme caution in patients with traumatic wounds or burns, patients receiving quinidine or digoxin therapy, and patients with hyperkalemia or other electrolyte imbalances.
- Use with caution in patients with pulmonary, renal, cardiovascular, metabolic, or hepatic dysfunction.
- Adverse effects include muscle soreness, malignant hyperthermia, excessive salivation, hyperkalemia, rash, myoglobinemia/myoglobinuria, and cardiovascular effects (eg, bradycardia, tachycardia, hypertension, hypotension, arrhythmias).
- High-alert drug; ensure appropriate respiratory support, reversal agents, and error-reducing safeguards are in place to minimize risk for patient harm.

Uses/Indications

Succinylcholine is indicated for short-term muscle relaxation needed during surgery, diagnostic procedures, and mechanical ventilation. Newer nondepolarizing agents with fewer adverse effects (eg, atracurium, vecuronium, rocuronium) have largely replaced succinylcholine.

In humans, succinylcholine can be used to facilitate endotracheal intubation.[1]

Pharmacology/Actions

Succinylcholine is an ultrashort-acting depolarizing skeletal muscle relaxant that binds to motor endplate nicotinic cholinergic receptors to produce depolarization (perceived as fasciculations). The neuromuscular block remains as long as sufficient quantities of succinylcholine remain and is characterized by flaccid paralysis.

Pharmacokinetics

After IV administration, the onset of action with complete muscle relaxation is usually within ≈60 seconds.[1] In humans, this effect lasts for 2 to 3 minutes and then gradually diminishes within 10 minutes. The very short duration of action after a single IV dose is thought to occur because the drug diffuses away from the motor endplate. If multiple injections or a continuous infusion are performed, the brief activity is a result of rapid hydrolysis by pseudocholinesterases at the site of action. After IM injection, the onset of action is generally within 2 to 3 minutes and may persist for 10 to 30 minutes. Dogs exhibit a prolonged duration of action of ≈20 minutes; this species appears unique in this idiosyncratic response.

Succinylcholine is metabolized by plasma pseudocholinesterases to succinylmonocholine and choline; 10% is excreted unchanged in the urine. Succinylmonocholine is partially excreted in the urine and may accumulate in patients with impaired renal function. Succinylmonocholine has ≈1/20 the neuromuscular blocking activity of succinylcholine, but if it accumulates, prolonged periods of apnea may result.

Contraindications/Precautions/Warnings

Succinylcholine is contraindicated in patients with severe liver disease, chronic anemia, chronic malnourishment, increased intracranial pressure, glaucoma or penetrating eye injuries, predisposition to malignant hyperthermia, and increased creatine phosphokinase (CPK) values with resultant myopathies. As succinylcholine can exacerbate the effects of hyperkalemia, it should be used with extreme caution in patients that have suffered traumatic wounds or burns, are receiving quinidine or digoxin therapy, or have pre-existing hyperkalemia or electrolyte imbalances, as arrhythmias or cardiac arrest may occur. Use succinylcholine with caution in patients with pulmonary, renal, cardiovascular, metabolic, or hepatic dysfunction.

Succinylcholine should only be used in patients that are adequately anesthetized as it has no analgesic or sedative/anesthetic actions. Respiratory support (eg, intubation, mechanical ventilation), neuromuscular blocker reversal agents, and staff experienced in the use of these agents must be readily available. Inadvertent administration of neuromuscular blocking agents to patients for which they were not intended may cause significant harm, including death. Neuromuscular blocking agents should be sequestered from other medications, and with access limited to those familiar with their use.[2] Prominent placement of warning labels (eg, *paralyzing agent- causes respiratory arrest, causes respiratory paralysis; patient must be ventilated*) on storage containers is highly recommended.

Ruminants are deficient in pseudocholinesterase, and succinylcholine is considered contraindicated these species.[3] The drug should be used with caution in horses due to the risk for malignant hyperthermia.[4-6]

Succinylcholine should not be used if organophosphate agents have been given or applied recently.[7]

Adverse Effects

Succinylcholine chloride can cause muscle soreness, malignant hyperthermia, excessive salivation, hyperkalemia, rash, and myoglobinemia/myoglobinuria. Cardiovascular effects can include bradycardia, tachycardia, hypertension, hypotension, or arrhythmias.

Reproductive/Nursing Safety

It is unknown if succinylcholine can cause fetal harm. The drug does cross the placenta in low concentrations, and a newly delivered neonate may show signs of neuromuscular blockade if the dam received high doses or prolonged administration of the drug prior to delivery. It is not known whether this drug is excreted into milk; exercise caution when succinylcholine is administered to a nursing patient. Because safety has not been established in animals, this drug should only be used when the maternal benefits outweigh the potential risks to offspring.

Overdose/Acute Toxicity

Inadvertent overdoses or standard doses in patients deficient in pseudocholinesterase may result in prolonged apnea. Mechanical ventilation with oxygen should be used until recovery.

Repeated or prolonged high doses may cause patients to convert from a phase I to a phase II block.

For patients that have experienced or are suspected to have experienced an overdose, consultation with a 24-hour poison consultation center specializing in providing veterinary-specific information is recommended. For general information related to overdose and toxin exposures, as well as contact information for poison control centers, refer to ***Appendix.***

Drug Interactions

The following drug interactions have either been reported or are theoretical in humans or animals receiving succinylcholine and may be of significance in veterinary patients. Unless otherwise noted, use together is not necessarily contraindicated, but weigh the potential risks and perform additional monitoring when appropriate.

- **Acetylcholinesterase Inhibitors** (eg, **neostigmine, pyridostigmine**): May prolong depolarizing phase I block but may antagonize phase II block

- **Amphotericin B**: May increase succinylcholine's effects by causing electrolyte imbalances
- **Digoxin**: Succinylcholine may cause a sudden outflux of potassium from muscle cells, thus causing arrhythmias in digitalized patients.
- **Opioids**: Potential for increased incidences of bradycardia and sinus arrest
- **Thiazide Diuretics** (eg, **hydrochlorothiazide**): May increase succinylcholine's effects by causing electrolyte imbalances

The following drugs/drug classes may increase or prolong neuromuscular blockade if used concurrently with succinylcholine:

- **Aminoglycosides**
- **Anesthetics, Inhalation** (eg, **desflurane, isoflurane**)
- **Antiarrhythmics** (eg, **quinidine, lidocaine, procainamide**)
- **Beta-Adrenergic Receptor Antagonists** (eg, **atenolol**)
- **Chloroquine**
- **Clindamycin**
- **Corticosteroids** (eg, **dexamethasone, prednis(ol)one**)
- **Cyclophosphamide**
- **Magnesium Salts**
- **Monoamine Oxidase Inhibitors**
- **Metoclopramide**
- **Organophosphates**
- **Oxytocin**
- **Pancuronium**
- **Phenothiazines** (eg, **acepromazine**)
- **Terbutaline**

Dosages

DOGS:

Neuromuscular blockade (extra-label): 0.3 – 0.4 mg/kg IV are recommended[8]; rarely used today

CATS:

Neuromuscular blockade (extra-label): 0.2 mg/kg IV1 mg/kg IV[8]; rarely used today

HORSES:

Neuromuscular blockade (extra-label): 0.12 – 0.15 mg/kg IV[8]

SWINE:

Intubation/abolish laryngospasm (extra-label): 1 – 2 mg/kg IV[9-11]

REPTILES:

Neuromuscular blockade in *Crocodilia* spp, chelonians, and lizards (extra-label): 0.4 – 1 mg/kg IM with time to onset of 5 to 30 minutes. The recovery period is based on the administered dose and the patient's metabolic activity; however, recovery generally occurs within 1 hour with doses in this range. Some large crocodiles require 2 – 5 mg/kg IM, which results in a recovery of 7 to 9 hours. Administration of an anxiolytic prior to induction is helpful. The clinician must have the means to ventilate the patient.[12]

Monitoring

- Level of neuromuscular blockade. It is strongly recommended to be familiar with techniques required to monitor the level of neuromuscular blockade (eg, acceleromyography, train-of-four twitch ratio) when using succinylcholine.[13] Visual or tactile assessments of the level of blockade are inaccurate and unreliable. Correct placement of electrodes is essential to minimize direct muscle stimulation and prevent misinterpretation of the degree of the blockade and minimize risk for overdose.
- Assess ventilation (eg, arterial blood gas, $ETCO_2$)
- Heart rate and rhythm
- Blood pressure

Client Information

- Only professionals familiar with the use of succinylcholine should use this drug.

Chemistry/Synonyms

Succinylcholine chloride is a depolarizing neuromuscular blocking agent that occurs as an odorless, white, crystalline powder. The dihydrate form melts at 190°C (374°F) and the anhydrous form at 160°C (320°F). Aqueous solutions are acidic, with a pH of ≈4. One gram is soluble in ≈1 mL of water and ≈350 mL of alcohol. Commercially available injections have a pH from 3 to 4.5.

Succinylcholine chloride may also be known as choline chloride succinate, succicurarium chloride, succinylcholine chloride, suxamethonii chloridum, suxametonklorid, suxamethonium chloride; many trade names are available.

Storage/Stability

Store commercial injectable solutions refrigerated (2°C-8°C [36°F-46°F]). One manufacturer states that multiple-dose vials are stable for up to 2 weeks at room temperature with no significant loss of potency.[14]

Compatibility/Compounding Considerations

Compatibility is dependent on factors such as pH, concentration, temperature, and diluent used; specialized references or a hospital pharmacist should be consulted for more specific information.

Succinylcholine chloride is physically **compatible** with all commonly used IV solutions, amikacin sulfate, isoproterenol HCl, meperidine HCl, norepinephrine bitartrate, and scopolamine HBr. It **may not be compatible** with pentobarbital sodium and is physically **incompatible** with sodium bicarbonate and thiopental sodium.

Dosage Forms/Regulatory Status

VETERINARY-LABELED PRODUCTS: NONE

The Association of Racing Commissioners International (ARCI) has designated this drug as a class 2 substance. Use of this drug may not be allowed in certain animal competitions. Check rules and regulations before entering a competition while this medication is being administered. Contact local racing authorities for further guidance. See ***Appendix*** for more information.

HUMAN-LABELED PRODUCTS:

Succinylcholine Chloride Injection: 20 mg/mL; *Anectine*®, *Quelicin*®; (Rx)

Succinylcholine Chloride Injection: 100 mg/mL; *Quelicin-1000*®; (Rx)

References

For the complete list of references, see **wiley.com/go/budde/plumb**

Sucralfate

(soo-***kral***-fate) *Carafate®*

GI-Mucosal Protectant

Prescriber Highlights

- ▶ Local-acting treatment for GI ulcers/esophagitis; may also protect somewhat against GI ulceration
- ▶ No contraindications have been identified; however, sucralfate should be used with caution when decreased GI transit times may be harmful.
- ▶ Adverse effects are unlikely, although constipation is possible. Vomiting has been reported in cats.
- ▶ Tablets should be dissolved in water before administration. Should be administered on an empty stomach, if possible
- ▶ To avoid possible drug interactions (eg, drug binding, decreased drug bioavailability), other medications should be administered 2 hours before sucralfate is administered.

Uses/Indications

Sucralfate has been used to treat oral, esophageal, gastric, and duodenal ulcers and to prevent drug (eg, aspirin)-induced gastric erosions. Despite sucralfate's theoretical benefits and widespread use, research has shown limited or no evidence to support the effectiveness of sucralfate for these indications.[1-3] A consensus panel has determined that evidence supporting sucralfate use in small animal species for the prevention or treatment of esophageal injury is weak[4]; however, sucralfate in combination with omeprazole is recommended for treating horses with equine glandular gastric disease.[5]

Sucralfate has been used in humans with hyperphosphatemia secondary to renal failure and could be useful for this indication in animals; however, in a study, sucralfate did not significantly change serum or urine phosphorus levels in healthy cats or normophosphatemic cats with CKD, and adverse effects (eg, vomiting, anorexia, constipation, worsening azotemia) may interfere with treatment.[6]

Pharmacology/Actions

Although the exact mechanism of action of sucralfate as an antiulcer agent is unknown, the drug appears to have a local effect rather than a systemic one. After oral administration, sucralfate may react with hydrochloric acid in the stomach to form a paste-like complex that preferentially binds to the proteinaceous exudates that are generally found at ulcer sites (eg, albumin, fibrinogen). This insoluble complex may form a barrier at the site and protect the ulcer from further damage caused by pepsin, acid, or bile. Sucralfate can bind bile acids and reduce pepsin activity. As an aluminum salt, sucralfate can bind to GI phosphorus.

Sucralfate may have some cytoprotective effects, possibly by stimulation of prostaglandins E_2 and I_2. It also has some antacid activity, although this may not be of clinical importance. Sucralfate may also bind to intact GI mucosa to form a protective layer.

Sucralfate does not significantly affect gastric acid output or trypsin or pancreatic amylase activity. It may slightly decrease the rate of gastric emptying but will not alter peristalsis.

Pharmacokinetics

By reacting with hydrochloric acid in the gut, most of the drug is converted to sucrose sulfate, which is excreted in the feces within 48 hours.[7] The duration of action (binding to ulcer site) may persist up to 6 hours after oral administration. A negligible amount of an oral dose is absorbed into the systemic circulation and excreted in the urine unchanged within 48 hours.[8]

Dissolving tablets in water before administration to dogs and cats is recommended to increase the dispersion of the drug, as tablet fractions have been observed in dog feces.[9]

Contraindications/Precautions/Warnings

Sucralfate is contraindicated in patients with known hypersensitivity to it. Because it may cause constipation, it should be used with caution in animals in which decreased GI transit times might be deleterious. Hyperglycemia has been reported rarely in diabetic humans receiving sucralfate suspension. Small amounts of aluminum may be absorbed following oral administration and may accumulate in patients with renal failure.

Concurrent use of sucralfate with proton pump inhibitors (eg, omeprazole) or histamine-H_2 receptor antagonists (eg, ranitidine) does not enhance the treatment of gastroduodenal injury in small animal species.[4]

Adverse Effects

Adverse effects are uncommon with sucralfate therapy. Constipation is the most prominent adverse effect reported in humans (2%) and dogs receiving the drug. Vomiting has been reported in cats. Sucralfate can have an unpalatable taste, and patient acceptance may be a problem.

Sucralfate administration to cats with CKD resulted in clinical decompensation (vomiting, anorexia, constipation, worsening azotemia) in 3 of the 5 studied cats.[6]

Reproductive/Nursing Safety

In rats, sucralfate doses up to 38 times those used in humans have not been shown to cause impaired fertility, and doses up to 50 times normal used in humans have not been shown to cause signs of teratogenicity.[7]

Sucralfate is most likely not excreted in breast milk because of minimal systemic absorption.

Overdose/Acute Toxicity

Overdoses are unlikely to cause significant problems. Laboratory animals receiving up to 12 g/kg PO have demonstrated no incidence of mortality.[7]

For patients that have experienced or are suspected of having experienced an overdose, consultation with a 24-hour poison consultation center specializing in providing veterinary-specific information is recommended. For general information related to overdose and toxin exposures, as well as contact information for poison control centers, refer to ***Appendix***.

Drug Interactions

The following drug interactions have either been reported or are theoretical in humans or animals receiving sucralfate and may be of significance in veterinary patients. Unless otherwise noted, use together is not necessarily contraindicated, but weigh the potential risks and perform additional monitoring when appropriate.

- **Antacids, Aluminum Containing**: Additive absorption of aluminum may occur, particularly in patients with renal insufficiency.

Sucralfate may impair the oral absorption of the following medications; administration should be separated by at least 2 hours to minimize this effect (with other medication being administered before sucralfate)[4]:

- **Alendronate**: Other oral bisphosphonates should be assumed to have the same effects.
- **Antacids, Aluminum Containing**: Can decrease sucralfate effectiveness; administration should be separated by 30 minutes. Additive absorption of aluminum may occur, particularly in patients with renal insufficiency.
- **Antacids, Calcium/Magnesium Containing**: Can decrease sucralfate effectiveness; administration should be separated by 30 minutes.
- **Ciprofloxacin**: Other oral fluoroquinolones, except enrofloxacin, should be assumed to be affected.[9,10]

- **Diclofenac**
- **Digoxin**
- **Feeding, Enteral**: Administration should be separated by an hour.
- **Ferrous Sulfate**
- **Furosemide**
- **Ketoconazole**
- **Lanthanum**
- **Levothyroxine**: Administration should be separated by 4 hours.
- **Macrolide Antibiotics** (eg, azithromycin, clarithromycin, erythromycin)
- **Penicillamine**
- **Tetracyclines** (eg, doxycycline, minocycline, tetracycline)[11,12]
- **Theophylline**
- **Vitamins, Fat Soluble**
- **Warfarin**

Dosages

DOGS/CATS:

GI-mucosal protectant for conditions such as esophagitis, gastric or duodenal ulcers, and uremic gastritis (extra-label): Empirically administered at ¼ to ½ of a 1 g tablet (250 – 500 mg)/animal (NOT g/kg) for toy-breed dogs and cats and 1 g/animal (NOT g/kg) PO 2 to 4 times daily for large-sized dogs. When using tablet formulations, it is recommended to crush the tablet then suspend it in a small amount of water prior to administration.

FERRETS:

GI-mucosal protectant (extra-label):

a) 75 mg/kg PO every 4 to 6 hours; should be administered 10 minutes prior to feeding[13]

b) 25 – 125 mg/kg PO every 8 to 12 hours[14]

HORSES:

GI-mucosal protectant (extra-label):

a) **Gastric glandular disease**: Sucralfate 12 – 20 mg/kg PO twice daily in combination with omeprazole 4 mg/kg PO once daily.[5,15,16]

b) **Prevention of stress-induced ulcers (used with acid-suppressive drugs) in foals**:
   i. 10 – 20 mg/kg PO every 6 to 8 hours[17]
   ii. 20 – 40 mg/kg PO every 6 hours[18]
   iii. 2 – 4 g/foal (NOT g/kg) PO every 6 hours[18]

c) **Right dorsal colitis | colonic ulcers**: 22 mg/kg PO every 6 to 8 hours[19,20]

REPTILES:

GI irritation in most species (extra-label): 500 – 1000 mg/kg PO every 6 to 8 hours[21]

BIRDS:

Upper GI mucosal hemorrhage (extra-label): 50 – 100 mg/kg PO every 12 hours[22]

Monitoring

- Clinical efficacy (dependent on the reason for use); may be monitored by a decrease in clinical signs, endoscopic examination, and fecal occult blood testing

Client Information

- This medicine is best given on an empty stomach and not at the same time as other medications. If you are giving your animal any other medication, be sure to give the other medications 2 hours before you give the sucralfate.
- Sucralfate be given several times a day to be most effective.
- Shake liquids well before using. If using tablets, it is best to dissolve the tablets in lukewarm water just before giving them.
- This medicine is usually tolerated well. Some animals may develop constipation. Some cats may vomit after receiving this medicine. Contact your veterinarian if you have concerns about your animal taking this medicine.

Chemistry/Synonyms

Sucralfate, a basic aluminum complex of sucrose sulfate, can occur as a white, amorphous powder. It is practically insoluble in alcohol or water. Each 1 g sucralfate tablet contains ≈207 mg of aluminum.

Sucralfate is structurally related to heparin but does not possess any appreciable anticoagulant activity. It is also structurally related to sucrose but is not utilized as sugar by the body.

Sucralfate is also known as basic aluminum sucrose sulfate and *Carafate*®, *Sulcrate*®, and *Cytogard*®.

Storage/Stability

Store sucralfate tablets in tight containers at room temperature (15°C-30°C [59°F-86°F]). Store sucralfate suspension at controlled room temperature (20°C-25°C [68°F-77°F]); do not freeze.

Compatibility/Compounding Considerations

A sucralfate 200 mg/mL suspension can be extemporaneously prepared. For a volume of 100 mL, twenty (20) sucralfate 1 g tablets should be crushed, and a sufficient quantity of distilled water added to bring the volume to 100 mL. Suspending agents (eg, acacia, tragacanth) should not be used, as they can bind to sucralfate and make it inactive. "Shake well" and "refrigerate" should be labeled on the compounded solution. When refrigerated, it is stable for 14 days.

Dosage Forms/Regulatory Status

VETERINARY-LABELED PRODUCTS: NONE

HUMAN-LABELED PRODUCTS:

Sucralfate Tablets: 1 g; *Carafate*®, generic; (Rx)

Sucralfate Suspension: 1 g/10 mL in 10 mL unit-dose cups and 415 mL bottles; *Carafate*®, generic; (Rx)

Formulations are available as oral mucosal coating agents and regulated by the FDA as medical devices.

References

For the complete list of references, see **wiley.com/go/budde/plumb**

Sufentanil

(soo-***fen***-ta-nil) *Sufenta*®

Opioid Agonist

Prescriber Highlights

- ► Injectable opioid that is 5 to 7 times more potent than fentanyl. May be useful for adjunctive anesthesia or epidural analgesia
- ► Dose-related respiratory and CNS depression most likely adverse effects
- ► DEA Schedule II (C-II) controlled substance

Uses/Indications

Sufentanil is an opioid analgesic that may be useful as an anesthesia adjunct or as an epidural analgesic. In humans, it has been used as the primary anesthetic in intubated patients with assisted ventilation and as a postoperative analgesic.

Pharmacology/Actions

Sufentanil is a potent mu opioid with the expected sedative, analgesic, and anesthetic properties. When comparing analgesic potencies when injecting IM, 0.01 to 0.04 mg of sufentanil is equivalent to

0.4 to 0.8 mg of alfentanil, 0.1 to 0.2 mg of fentanyl, and ≈10 mg of morphine. Like fentanyl, sufentanil appears to have less circulatory effects than morphine. Sufentanil has a rapid onset of action (1 to 3 minutes) and a faster recovery time than fentanyl.

Pharmacokinetics

In isoflurane-anesthetized cats, a sufentanil 1 µg/kg IV bolus had a volume of distribution (at steady-state) of ≈0.77 L/kg, a clearance of ≈17.6 mL/minute/kg, and a terminal half-life of ≈54 minutes. Elimination of sufentanil is expected to be more rapid than either fentanyl or alfentanil because of a small volume of distribution and moderate clearance.[1]

In humans, the drug has a rapid onset of action (1 to 3 minutes) after IV injection. The drug is highly lipid-soluble and has a volume of distribution in the central compartment of 0.1 L/kg. Approximately 93% is bound to plasma proteins. Plasma concentrations rapidly decline because of redistribution, and its terminal elimination half-life is ≈2.5 hours. Plasma clearance has been reported to be ≈12 mL/minute/kg. Sufentanil is metabolized primarily in the liver and small intestine via O-demethylation and N-dealkylation. The parent drug and these metabolites are excreted primarily in the urine. Although the manufacturer states to use sufentanil with caution in patients with impaired renal or hepatic function, limited pharmacokinetic studies in these patients rarely showed any drug accumulation.

Contraindications/Precautions/Warnings

Sufentanil is contraindicated in patients that are hypersensitive to it or other opioids.[2] It should be used with caution in debilitated or geriatric patients and those with severely diminished renal or hepatic function. Initial dose reduction may be required in geriatric or debilitated patients, particularly those with diminished cardiopulmonary function.

Because of the drug's potency, the use of a tuberculin syringe to measure doses less than 1 mL in addition to a double-check system for dose calculations and measurement is recommended. It should only be used in situations where patient vital signs can be continuously monitored.

Opioid analgesics are contraindicated in patients stung by scorpions (eg, *Centruroides* spp), as they may potentiate venom effects.[3]

Do not confuse SUfentanil with fentanyl or ALfentanil.

Adverse Effects

Adverse effects are generally dose-related and consistent with other opioid agonists. Respiratory depression and/or CNS depression are most likely to be encountered and can be exacerbated if sufentanil is given with other drugs that can cause those effects.

In humans, bradycardia may occur, but it is usually responsive to anticholinergic agents. Dose-related skeletal muscle rigidity has been reported, particularly with high doses and/or rapid IV administration and can be managed with concurrent use of neuromuscular blockers. Sufentanil has rarely been associated with asystole, hypercarbia, and hypersensitivity reactions.

Reproductive/Nursing Safety

Although sufentanil is indicated for epidural use (mixed with bupivacaine ± epinephrine) in women for labor/delivery, it should not be administered systemically to a dam close to giving birth, as offspring may show behavioral alterations (eg, hypotonia, depression) associated with opioid administration.

The effects of sufentanil on lactation and its safety for nursing offspring are not well defined, but sufentanil milk levels approximate those found in serum. This, coupled with its low oral bioavailability, makes it unlikely to cause significant effects in nursing offspring.

Overdose/Acute Toxicity

In dogs, the LD_{50} of IV sufentanil is 10.1 to 19.5 mg/kg. Severe IV overdoses may cause apnea, circulatory collapse, pulmonary edema, seizures, cardiac arrest, and death. Treatment is a combination of supportive therapy and administration of an opioid antagonist, such as naloxone. Although sufentanil has a fairly rapid half-life, multiple doses of naloxone may be necessary.

For patients that have experienced or are suspected of having experienced an overdose, consultation with a 24-hour poison consultation center specializing in providing veterinary-specific information is recommended. For general information related to overdose and toxin exposures, as well as contact information for poison control centers, refer to ***Appendix***.

Drug Interactions

The following drug interactions have either been reported or are theoretical in humans or animals receiving sufentanil and may be of significance in veterinary patients. Unless otherwise noted, use together is not necessarily contraindicated, but weigh the potential risks and perform additional monitoring when appropriate.

- Alpha-2 Receptor Agonists (eg, **dexmedetomidine, xylazine**): Concurrent use may increase the risk for CNS and/or respiratory depression.
- Anesthetic Agents (eg, **alfaxalone, isoflurane, ketamine, propofol**): Concurrent use may increase the risk for CNS and/or respiratory depression.
- Anticholinergic Agents (eg, **acepromazine, atropine, glycopyrrolate**): Concurrent use may increase the risk for urinary retention, constipation, and CNS and respiratory depression.
- Antihypertensive Agents (eg, **atenolol, lisinopril**): Concurrent use may increase the risk for bradycardia, hypotension, and orthostasis. Use cautiously and monitor blood pressure and heart rate. Opioids may decrease the therapeutic effects of diuretics.
- Benzodiazepines (eg, **diazepam, midazolam**): Concurrent use may increase the risk for CNS and/or respiratory depression.
- Bethanechol: Concurrent use may antagonize the beneficial effects of bethanechol on GI motility. Avoid combination.
- CNS Depressants (eg, **methocarbamol, phenobarbital**): Concurrent use may increase the risk for CNS and/or respiratory depression. Monitor and adjust dosages accordingly.
- Desmopressin: Concurrent use may increase levels of oral desmopressin and increase the risk for water intoxication and/or hyponatremia, which can progress to seizures, coma, respiratory arrest, and death. Monitor electrolytes and renal function.
- Domperidone: Concurrent use may antagonize the GI effects of domperidone.
- Drugs That Inhibit Hepatic Isoenzymes (eg, **cimetidine, diltiazem, erythromycin, fluconazole, itraconazole, ketoconazole**) May increase the half-life and decrease the clearance of sufentanil, leading to prolonged effects and an increased risk for respiratory depression. Consider adjusting doses accordingly.
- Drugs That Induce Hepatic Isoenzymes (eg, **griseofulvin, mitotane, phenobarbital**): Current use may decrease levels of sufentanil. Monitor clinical response and adjust doses accordingly.
- Drugs That Depress Cardiac Function Or Reduce Vagal Tone (eg, **beta-blockers or other anesthetic agents**): May produce bradycardia or hypotension if used concurrently with sufentanil
- Ifosfamide: Concurrent use may increase the risk for neurotoxicity, including somnolence, confusion, hallucinations, blurred vision, urinary incontinence, seizures, and coma. Use cautiously and monitor.
- Iohexol: Concurrent use of opioids with intrathecal iohexol may increase the risk for seizures. Opioids should be withheld for 48 hours before and 24 hours after intrathecal administration of iohexol.

- **Loperamide**: Concurrent use may increase the risk for constipation.
- **Monoamine Oxidase Inhibitors** (MAOIs; eg, **amitraz, selegiline**): Concurrent use may increase the risk for anxiety, confusion, hypotension, respiratory depression, cyanosis, and coma. MAOIs should be withheld for 14 days prior to administration of opioids. Avoid combination.
- **Metoclopramide**: Concurrent use may antagonize the prokinetic effects of metoclopramide.
- **Neuromuscular Blocking Agents** (eg, **atracurium**): Concurrent use may increase the risk for tachycardia, bradycardia, and/or hypotension. Use cautiously and monitor
- **Serotonin Receptor Antagonists** (eg, **dolasetron, fluoxetine**): Concurrent use may increase the risk for serotonin syndrome. Avoid combination.
- **Tramadol**: Concurrent use may increase the risk for seizures, serotonin syndrome, urinary retention, and constipation. The risk for CNS and respiratory depression may be additive.
- **Tricyclic Antidepressants** (TCAs; eg, **amitriptyline, clomipramine**): Concurrent use may increase risk for urinary retention, constipation, and CNS and respiratory depression.

Laboratory Considerations

- Because opioids can increase biliary tract pressure and raise serum amylase and lipase values, these values may be unreliable for 24 hours after sufentanil is administered.

Dosages

NOTE: In obese patients, calculate doses based on lean body weight.

DOGS/CATS:

Opioid analgesic (extra-label): 0.5 – 1 µg/kg slow IV followed by 0.5 – 1 µg/kg/*HOUR* IV CRI has been noted.[1,4-8] Dosage is titrated to effect. Dosages as high as 2.5 µg/kg slow IV followed by 2 – 4 µg/kg/*HOUR* IV CRI have been noted.[9]

Epidural analgesia in dogs (extra-label): 0.5 – 1 µg/kg diluted to a volume of 0.2 – 0.36 mL/kg with sterile saline. The onset of action is 10 to 15 minutes; duration 1 to 4 hours.[10-12]

RABBITS:

Anesthesia (extra-label): 0.5 µg/kg IV bolus, followed by 0.72 µg/kg/*HOUR* IV CRI[13]

Monitoring

- Anesthetic and/or analgesic efficacy
- Cardiac and respiratory rate
- Pulse oximetry or other methods to measure blood oxygenation when used for anesthesia
- Blood pressure

Client Information

- Sufentanil is a very potent opioid that should only be used by professionals in a setting where adequate patient monitoring is available.

Chemistry/Synonyms

Sufentanil citrate is a phenylpiperidine derivative opioid related to fentanyl. It occurs as a white or almost white powder that is soluble in water and sparingly soluble in alcohol, acetone, and chloroform. The commercially available injection has a pH (adjusted with citric acid) of 3.5 to 6.

Sufentanil citrate may also be known as R-33800, sufentanili citras, fentathienel citrate, sufentanyl citrate, sulfentanil citrate, *Fastfen*®, *Fentaientel*®, and *Sufenta*®.

Storage/Stability

Unless otherwise labeled, store sufentanil injection protected from light at room temperature 20°C to 25°C (68°F-77°F). Sufentanil citrate is hydrolyzable in acidic solutions.

Sufentanil citrate is a DEA Schedule II (C-II) controlled substance; store it in a substantially constructed and securely locked area. Follow applicable local, state, and federal rules regarding the disposal of unused or wasted controlled drugs.

Compatibility/Compounding Considerations

Sufentanil citrate is reportedly **compatible** with 5% dextrose and bupivacaine. Sufentanil is **Y-site compatible** with solutions containing atropine, dexamethasone sodium phosphate, diazepam, diphenhydramine, etomidate, metoclopramide, midazolam, phenobarbital, and propofol. It is **incompatible** with lorazepam, phenytoin, and thiopental.

Dosage Forms/Regulatory Status

VETERINARY-LABELED PRODUCTS: NONE.

The Association of Racing Commissioners International (ARCI) has designated this drug as a class 1 substance. Use of this drug may not be allowed in certain animal competitions. Check rules and regulations before entering in a competition while this medication is being administered. Contact local racing authorities for further guidance. See the *Appendix* for more information.

HUMAN-LABELED PRODUCTS:

Sufentanil Citrate Injection: 50 µg/mL (as base) in 1 mL, 2 mL, and 5 mL ampules; *Sufenta*® (preservative free), generic; (Rx, C-II)

References

For the complete list of references, see **wiley.com/go/budde/plumb**

Sulfa-/Trimethoprim
Sulfadiazine/Trimethoprim
Sulfamethoxazole/Trimethoprim

(sul-fa-***dye***-a-zeen; sul-fa-meth-***ox***-a-zole/trye-***meth***-ohe-prim)

Bactrim®, EquiSul-SDT®, Uniprim®

Potentiated Sulfonamide Antimicrobial

NOTE: In the United States, 2 FDA-approved combinations of sulfonamide with trimethoprim (ie, sulfa-/trimethoprim) are used clinically in animals: sulfadiazine/trimethoprim for parenteral and oral use in dogs, cats, and horses and sulfamethoxazole/trimethoprim for oral use in humans. In Canada, sulfadoxine is also available in combination with trimethoprim for veterinary use.

Prescriber Highlights

- ► Combination antimicrobial agent, often referred to as a potentiated sulfonamide, used to treat bacterial and protozoal infections
- ► Contraindications include hypersensitivity to sulfonamides and severe renal or hepatic impairment.
- ► Caution is advised in cases of diminished renal or hepatic function, urinary obstruction, urolithiasis, and in dog breeds predisposed to sulfonamide hypersensitivity (eg, Doberman pinschers).
- ► Adverse effects in dogs include keratoconjunctivitis sicca, hypersensitivity (type 1 or type 3), acute neutrophilic hepatitis with icterus, vomiting, anorexia, diarrhea, fever, hemolytic anemia, urticaria, polyarthritis, facial swelling, polydipsia, crystalluria, hematuria, polyuria, cholestasis, hypothyroidism, anemia, agranulocytosis, and idiosyncratic hepatic necrosis.
- ► Adverse effects in cats include anorexia, crystalluria, hematuria, leukopenia, and anemia.
- ► Adverse effects in horses include diarrhea, hypersensitivity reactions, and hematologic effects (eg, anemia, thrombocytopenia, leukopenia) when administered orally and transient pruritus after IV injection.
- ► Local injection adverse effects (eg, warmth, edema, pain) are possible.
- ► Sulfa-/trimethoprim is potentially teratogenic; weigh the risks versus the benefits before prescribing.
- ► In the United States, extra-label use of sulfonamides is prohibited in lactating dairy cattle.

Uses/Indications

Although sulfadiazine/trimethoprim is only FDA-approved for use in dogs and horses, this drug is used to treat infections caused by susceptible bacteria and parasitic organisms in various species.

Sulfadiazine/trimethoprim is commonly used in horses because it is 1 of a limited number of safe oral options. Although use in dogs is more limited because of concerns about adverse effects and availability of other antimicrobial options, this antibiotic is a potential choice for treatment of various infections (eg, cystitis, prostatitis) and is also sometimes used for treatment of atypical pathogens (eg, *Nocardia* spp). Prophylactic use of sulfadiazine/trimethoprim reduced morbidity in dogs receiving doxorubicin.[1]

The World Health Organization (WHO) has designated sulfamethoxazole/trimethoprim as a Highly Important antimicrobial for human medicine.[2] The Office International des Epizooties (OIE) Antimicrobial Classification has designated sulfadiazine/trimethoprim as a Veterinary Critically Important antimicrobial.[3]

Pharmacology/Actions

Sulfonamides are bacteriostatic agents while trimethoprim is bactericidal; both agents are time-dependent antibiotics. When used in combination, the resulting potentiated sulfonamides are bactericidal. Potentiated sulfonamides sequentially inhibit enzymes in the folic acid pathway, inhibiting bacterial thymidine synthesis. Sulfonamides compete with para-aminobenzoic acid (PABA) to reduce bacterial dihydrofolic acid (DFA) formation, and trimethoprim blocks the conversion of DFA to tetrahydrofolic acid by preferentially inhibiting bacterial dihydrofolate reductase. Infected tissue and cellular debris can inhibit the activity of sulfa-/trimethoprim by secreting PABA and thymidine. The effects of sulfa-/trimethoprim on the equine GI microbiome appear to be reversible.[4]

The in vitro optimal ratio for most susceptible bacteria is ≈1:20 (trimethoprim:sulfonamide), but synergistic activity can reportedly occur with ratios of 1:1 to 1:40. The serum concentration of the trimethoprim component is considered more important than the sulfonamide concentration.

Potentiated sulfonamides have a fairly broad spectrum of activity. Generally susceptible gram-positive bacteria include most streptococci and staphylococci and *Nocardia* spp. Many gram-negative organisms of the Enterobacteriaceae family are inherently susceptible to potentiated sulfonamides but acquired resistance can occur. Sulfa-/trimethoprim is ineffective against *Pseudomonas aeruginosa*; some protozoa (ie, *Pneumocystis jiroveci*, *Coccidia* spp, *Neospora* spp, *Toxoplasma* spp) are also inhibited. Potentiated sulfonamides appear to have little activity against most atypical bacteria and anaerobes; methicillin-resistant staphylococci are usually resistant. *Enterococcus* spp infections may appear to be susceptible to sulfonamide-containing antibiotics in vitro; however, they are intrinsically resistant, so sulfa-/trimethoprim should not be used for these bacteria.

Resistance development is thought to occur more slowly to the combination of drugs than to either drug alone. In gram-negative organisms, sulfamethoxazole resistance is usually plasmid mediated, although a point mutation for dihydropteroate synthase also may confer resistance.

Pharmacokinetics

Sulfa-/trimethoprim is relatively well absorbed after oral administration, with peak concentrations occurring ≈1 to 4 hours after administration; however, the drug is absorbed more slowly after SC absorption. Oral bioavailability in fed horses after a single dose of 30 mg/kg paste was 74% for sulfadiazine and 46% for trimethoprim.[5] Bioavailability was ≈84% in male goats.[6] Food has no apparent effect on the absorption of sulfadiazine, but trimethoprim absorption is decreased.

In calves 1 day and 1 week of age, trimethoprim and sulfadiazine were absorbed after oral administration, although serum trimethoprim concentration was diminished in the 1-week-old calves. In calves 6 weeks of age, peak sulfadiazine concentration was only 60% as compared with calves 1 day of age, and trimethoprim was undetectable.[7] In a separate study, sulfadiazine half-life was 8.5 to 10 hours in calves 6 weeks of age and ≈8 to 13 hours in calves 12 weeks of age.[8] In ruminants older than 8 weeks of age, trimethoprim is apparently trapped in the ruminoreticulum after oral administration and undergoes some degradation that limits its usefulness.

Sulfa-/trimethoprim is well distributed in the body; however, in horses, concentrations are lower in the pulmonary epithelial lining fluid than in plasma.[5] Both sulfadiazine and trimethoprim attain therapeutic concentrations in the equine endometrium.[9] In dogs, therapeutic concentrations of both agents are reached in the skin.[10] In patients with inflamed meninges, the drugs enter the CSF in concentrations ≈50% of those found in the serum. Sulfa-/trimethoprim is relatively well distributed into the prostate, and both drugs concentrate in the urine. The volume of distribution for trimethoprim is 1.49 L/kg in dogs; 0.59 to 1.51 L/kg in horses; and 2.7 L/kg in donkeys.[11] The volume of distribution for sulfadiazine is 1.02 L/kg in dogs and 0.6 L/kg in donkeys.[11] Sulfadiazine and trimethoprim are 20% and 35% bound to equine plasma proteins.[12]

Sulfa-/trimethoprim is both renally excreted unchanged via glomerular filtration and tubular secretion and metabolized by the liver. Sulfonamides are primarily acetylated (not in dogs) and conjugated with glucuronic acid, and trimethoprim is metabolized to oxide and hydroxylated metabolites. Trimethoprim may be more extensively metabolized in the liver of adult ruminants than in other species. The serum elimination half-life for trimethoprim is 2.5 hours in dogs, ≈2 to 3 hours in horses, 10.9 hours in goats,[6] and 1.5 hours in cattle. The serum elimination half-life for sulfadiazine is 9.84 hours in dogs, ≈4 to 8 hours in horses, and 2.5 hours in cattle. Sulfadiazine and trimethoprim clearances in donkeys were 1.7 and 4.4 mL/minute/kg, respectively.[11] Although trimethoprim is rapidly eliminated from the serum, the drug may persist for a longer period of time in tissue.

Because of the number of variables involved, it is extremely difficult to apply pharmacokinetic values in making dosage recommendations with these combinations. Each drug (ie, trimethoprim, sulfonamide) has different pharmacokinetic parameters (eg, absorption, distribution, elimination) in each species. Because different organisms have different MIC values and the optimal ratio of trimethoprim to sulfonamides differs from organism to organism, this problem is exacerbated.

Considerable controversy exists regarding the frequency of administration of these combinations. Sulfadiazine/trimethoprim is labeled for once daily administration in dogs and horses, but many clinicians believe that sulfa-/trimethoprim is more efficacious if given twice daily, regardless of the sulfonamide used.

Contraindications/Precautions/Warnings

The veterinary manufacturer states that sulfadiazine/trimethoprim should not be used in dogs or horses with marked liver parenchymal damage, impaired hepatic function, blood dyscrasias, or a history of sulfonamide or trimethoprim sensitivity. Sulfadiazine/trimethoprim is not for use in horses (or FDA-approved for other animals) intended for food. Sulfonamides are _not_ considered contraindicated in patients allergic to thiazide diuretics or sulfonylurea agents.[13]

Doberman pinschers, Samoyeds, and miniature schnauzers appear to be more susceptible to sulfonamide-induced polysystemic immune complex disease[14]; use sulfa-/trimethoprim with caution in these breeds.

Sulfa-/trimethoprim should be used with caution in patients with pre-existing hepatic or renal disease or folate deficiency. In animals with moderate to severe renal dysfunction, consider dosage reduction; avoid products containing sulfadiazine.

Sulfadiazine has potential for crystallization in the urine, so use should be avoided in dogs with uroliths, at increased risk for developing uroliths, with highly concentrated urine (from dehydration), or with acidic urine.

Horses receiving sulfadiazine/trimethoprim that are under conditions of stress may develop potentially fatal acute diarrhea.[15] Discontinue antimicrobial therapy if acute diarrhea or persistent changes in fecal consistency are observed and initiate appropriate treatment. Sulfadiazine/trimethoprim should not be administered to horses with drug-induced cardiac arrhythmias (eg, anesthetic and sedative agents) and it should not be given IV concurrently or with previous administration of CNS depressants (eg, anesthetic agents, phenothiazines).[16]

In humans, sulfamethoxazole/trimethoprim is contraindicated in patients younger than 2 months of age, with known hypersensitivity to either drug component, with marked hepatic or renal impairment, and with megaloblastic anemia due to folate deficiency.

Adverse Effects

Adverse effects noted in dogs include keratoconjunctivitis sicca (KCS; which may be irreversible), acute neutrophilic hepatitis with icterus, vomiting, anorexia, diarrhea, fever, hemolytic anemia, urticaria, polyarthritis, facial swelling, polydipsia, polyuria, and cholestasis. Potentiated sulfonamides may cause clinical hypothyroidism in dogs, particularly with extended therapy. Acute hypersensitivity reactions manifesting as type I (ie, anaphylaxis) or type III (ie, formation of antigen:antibody complexes) reactions can be seen. Hypersensitivity reactions appear to be more common in large-breed dogs. Doberman pinschers, Samoyeds, and miniature schnauzers may be more susceptible to hypersensitivity reactions than other breeds.[14] Other hematologic effects (eg, anemia, agranulocytosis) are possible but are rare, although the incidence may increase with prolonged use of high doses.[17] Sulfa-/trimethoprim has rarely caused an idiosyncratic, moderate to massive hepatic necrosis in dogs.[18] Use of sulfa-/trimethoprim may increase the risk for developing acute pancreatitis,[14] but cause and effect have not been definitively shown.

Adverse effects noted in cats may include anorexia, leukopenia, and anemia.

In horses, transient pruritus has been noted after IV injection. Oral therapy has resulted in dose-related diarrhea, but incidence is relatively low. Previous administration of potentiated sulfonamides has been implicated in increasing the mortality rate associated with severe diarrhea. If the 48% injectable product is administered IM or SC, or if it extravasates after IV administration, swelling, pain, and minor tissue damage may result. Hypersensitivity reactions, neurologic effects (eg, gait alterations, behavior changes), cutaneous vasculitis, and hematologic effects (eg, anemia, thrombocytopenia, leukopenia) may also be seen.[19] In experimental models, trimethoprim inhibited equine voltage-gated K+ channel K(v)11.1, suggesting that trimethoprim could induce repolarization disorders in horses[20,21]; validation with in vivo studies are needed. Neurologic adverse effects (agitation, erratic behavior, hypermetric gait) have been noted in horses being treated with typical doses of sulfa-/trimethoprim; all adverse effects resolved with discontinuation of the drug.[22]

Sulfonamides (and their metabolites) can precipitate in the urine, particularly when given at high dosages for prolonged periods. Acidic or highly concentrated urine may also contribute to increased risk for crystalluria, hematuria, and renal tubule obstruction.

Regurgitation may occur in birds.

Sulfamethoxazole/trimethoprim can markedly reduce tear production in rabbits,[23] but sulfadiazine/trimethoprim had no effect in horses.[24]

Reproductive/Nursing Safety

Trimethoprim and sulfonamides cross the placenta. Safety of sulfa-/trimethoprim has not been clearly established in pregnant animals. Reports of teratogenicity (eg, cleft palate, fetal loss) have been reported in rats and rabbits. Studies in male animals have not demonstrated reduced reproductive performance. First trimester exposure in humans has been associated with increased risk for congenital malformations.

Trimethoprim and sulfonamides are distributed into milk. Use sulfa-/trimethoprim products in nursing animals with caution. Sulfonamides are distributed into maternal milk, but in humans are considered compatible with breastfeeding in healthy, full-term infants.[25,26] Premature infants and infants with hyperbilirubinemia may be at risk for adverse effects.

Overdose/Acute Toxicity

Manifestations of an acute overdose can include clinical signs of GI distress (eg, nausea, vomiting, diarrhea), CNS toxicity (eg, depression,), facial swelling, bone marrow depression, and increased serum aminotransferase (ie, ALT, AST) activity. Oral overdoses can be treated by emptying the stomach (following typical protocols) and initiating supportive therapy based on clinical signs. Acidification of the urine may increase the renal elimination of trimethoprim but could also cause sulfonamide crystalluria, particularly with sulfadiazine-containing products. CBC and other laboratory parameters should be monitored as necessary. Severe bone marrow suppression associated with chronic overdoses can be treated with folinic acid (leucovorin). Peritoneal dialysis is not effective in removing trimethoprim or sulfonamides from circulation.

For patients that have experienced or are suspected of having experienced an overdose, consultation with a 24-hour poison consultation center specializing in providing veterinary-specific information is recommended. For general information related to overdose and toxin exposures, as well as contact information for poison control centers, refer to ***Appendix***.

Drug Interactions

In humans, trimethoprim may be a substrate of p-glycoprotein, sulfamethoxazole is a substrate of the CYP2C family, and both trimethoprim and sulfamethoxazole may inhibit CYP2C enzymes. The following drug interactions have either been reported or are theoretical in humans or animals receiving sulfa-/trimethoprim and may be of significance in veterinary patients. Unless otherwise noted, use together is not necessarily contraindicated, but weigh the potential risks and perform additional monitoring when appropriate.

- **Amantadine**: A human patient developed toxic delirium while receiving amantadine in conjunction with sulfamethoxazole/trimethoprim.[27]
- **Amiodarone**: May reduce sulfonamide metabolism and increase the risk for adverse effects.
- **Anesthetic Agents**: Concurrent IV administration is contraindicated. Ester-type local anesthetics (eg, **procaine, tetracaine**) may locally inhibit sulfonamide effects.[28,29]
- **Angiotensin II-Receptor Blockers** (ARBs; eg, **telmisartan**): May increase the risk for hyperkalemia when used with potassium-sparing drugs
- **Angiotensin-Converting Enzyme Inhibitors** (ACEIs; eg, **benazepril, enalapril**): May increase the risk for hyperkalemia when used with potassium-sparing drugs
- **Antacids**: Concurrent administration may decrease sulfonamide bioavailability.
- **Azathioprine, Mercaptopurine**: Increased risk for myelosuppression
- **Cyclosporine**: Sulfa-/trimethoprim may increase the risk for nephrotoxicity.
- **Detomidine**: Concurrent use has resulted in fatal arrhythmias in horses.[21]
- **Digoxin**: Sulfa-/trimethoprim may increase digoxin concentration.
- **Diuretics, Thiazide**: May increase the risk for thrombocytopenia
- **Hypoglycemic Agents, Oral** (eg, **glipizide, metformin**): Sulfa-/trimethoprim may potentiate hypoglycemic effects.
- **Leucovorin**: May reduce therapeutic effect of sulfa-/trimethoprim
- **Methenamine**: May form an insoluble precipitate in the urine
- **Methotrexate** (MTX): Sulfa-/trimethoprim may displace from plasma proteins and increase the risk for toxic effects; it can also interfere with MTX assays (competitive protein binding technique, but not when measured by radioimmunoassay).
- **Phenothiazines** (eg, **acepromazine, promethazine**): Concurrent administration is contraindicated.
- **Potassium Supplements**: Increased risk for hyperkalemia
- **Procainamide**: Sulfa-/trimethoprim may increase the concentration of procainamide and its active metabolite.
- **Pyrimethamine**: May increase the risk for megaloblastic anemia and myelosuppression
- **Rifampin**: May reduce serum concentrations of trimethoprim and sulfonamide
- **Spironolactone**: May increase the risk for hyperkalemia when used with potassium-sparing drugs
- **Tricyclic Antidepressants** (TCAs; eg, **amitriptyline, clomipramine**): Sulfa-/trimethoprim may decrease efficacy.
- **Warfarin**: Sulfa-/trimethoprim may prolong prothrombin time and INR.

Laboratory Considerations

- When using the Jaffe alkaline picrate reaction assay for **creatinine** determination, sulfa-/trimethoprim may cause an overestimation of ≈10%.
- Sulfonamides may give false-positive results for **urine glucose** determinations when using the Benedict's method.

Dosages

NOTE: There is significant controversy regarding the frequency of administration of these drugs. See ***Pharmacokinetics*** for more information. Unless otherwise noted, doses are for combined sulfa-/trimethoprim. See ***Monitoring*** if treatment is expected to be longer than 7 days.

DOGS:

For systemic antibacterial action against sensitive organisms, either alone or as an adjunct to surgery or debridement with associated infection; treatment of acute urinary tract infections, acute bacterial complications of distemper, acute respiratory tract infections, acute alimentary tract infections, wound infections, and abscesses (label dosage; FDA-approved): 30 mg/kg PO once daily. Alternatively, especially in severe infections, the initial dose may be followed by 15 mg/kg every 12 hours.[30]

Superficial bacterial folliculitis (extra-label): 15 – 30 mg/kg PO twice daily.[31] Potentiated sulfonamides (ie, sulfa-/trimethoprim, sulfadimethoxine/ormetoprim) are first-tier drugs only if regional susceptibility of *Staphylococcus pseudintermedius* is known.

Bacterial cystitis (extra-label): Potentiated sulfonamides (ie, sulfa-/trimethoprim, sulfadimethoxine/ormetoprim) are first-tier drugs only if regional pathogen susceptibility patterns are known.[32]

a) **Uncomplicated UTI**: 15 mg/kg PO every 12 hours. Treatment may be as short as 3 days.[32,33]
b) **Complicated UTI**: 15 – 30 mg/kg PO every 12 hours[32]

Parasitic diseases (extra-label):

Coccidiosis:

a) Body weight less than 4 kg (8.8 lb): 15 – 30 mg/kg PO every 12 to 24 hours[34]
b) Body weight greater than 4 kg (8.8 lb): 30 – 60 mg/kg PO every 24 hours[34]

Neosporosis: Sulfadiazine/trimethoprim 15 – 20 mg/kg PO every 12 hours for 4 weeks in combination with pyrimethamine 1 mg/kg PO once daily for 4 weeks. If observable clinical improvement is slow, treatment should be extended beyond the recommended 4 weeks until 2 weeks after clinical signs have plateaued. All littermates of affected puppies should be treated regardless of clinical signs. Alternative treatment is clindamycin 12.5 – 25 mg/kg PO or IM every 12 hours for 4 weeks.[35] **NOTE**: There is no approved or curative treatment for canine neosporosis. Arrestment of clinical disease is best achieved when treatment is initiated before the occurrence of contracture or paralysis.

Toxoplasmosis: Sulfa-/trimethoprim 15 mg/kg PO every 12 hours for 4 weeks can be used. Supportive care should be provided as needed.[35] There is no approved treatment for toxoplasmosis in dogs.

Pneumocystosis (*Pneumocystis jiroveci*): 15 mg/kg PO every 8 hours for 3 weeks or 30 mg/kg PO every 12 hours for 3 weeks

American canine hepatozoonosis (*Hepatozoon americanum*): Triple-combination therapy (TCP) consists of sulfadiazine/trimethoprim 15 mg/kg PO every 12 hours for 14 days, clindamycin 10 mg/kg PO every 8 hours for 14 days, and pyrimethamine 0.25 mg/kg PO every 24 hours for 14 days or ponazuril 10 mg/kg PO every 12 hours for 14 days. Prolonged therapy consists of decoquinate 10 – 20 mg/kg mixed in food twice daily; treatment is continued for 2 years. If relapse occurs, either ponazuril or TCP should be administered again for 14 days, followed by long-term decoquinate therapy.[36] **NOTE**: No treatment is effective in eliminating *H americanum* in infected dogs. Treatment can increase survival time, improve quality of life, and decrease the number and severity of clinical relapses. Supportive care can ensure hydration, and NSAIDs can assist with pain control.

CATS:

Bacterial cystitis (extra-label): Potentiated sulfonamides (ie, sulfa-/trimethoprim, sulfadimethoxine/ormetoprim) are first-tier drugs only if regional pathogen susceptibility patterns are known.[32]

a) **Uncomplicated UTI**: 15 mg/kg PO every 12 hours. Treatment may be as short as 3 days.[32,33]
b) **Complicated UTI**: 15 – 30 mg/kg PO every 12 hours.[32]

Parasitic diseases (extra-label):

Coccidiosis: 15 – 30 mg/kg PO every 12 to 24 hours[34]

Toxoplasmosis: 15 mg/kg PO every 12 hours for 4 weeks can be used. Supportive care should be provided as needed.[35]

HORSES:

Control of bacterial infections of horses during treatment of acute strangles, respiratory tract infections, acute urogenital infections, wound infections, and abscesses (label dosage; FDA-approved):

a) **Powder and paste formulations**: 75 mg/kg PO once daily; administer in a small amount of feed. Continue treatment for 2 to 3 days after clinical signs have subsided. Usual treatment course is 5 to 7 days.[37,38]
b) **IV injection formulation**: 21.3 mg/kg IV once daily[38]

Lower respiratory tract infections by susceptible strains of *Streptococcus equi* subsp *zooepidemicus* (label dosage; FDA-approved): 24 mg/kg (combined active ingredients) PO twice daily for 10 days[15]

Respiratory infections (extra-label): 30 mg/kg PO or IV twice daily.[5] **NOTE**: Potentiated sulfonamides for treatment of lower airway infections in horses should be restricted to treatment against highly susceptible pathogens.

***Pneumocystis jiroveci* (formerly *P carinii*) in foals** (extra-label): 30 mg/kg PO every 12 hours

Dermatologic infections (extra-label): 15 – 30 mg/kg PO every 12 hours, often in conjunction with topical antibacterial shampoo. Treatment for 3 weeks may be necessary.[39]

BIRDS:

Susceptible infections (extra-label):

a) **Respiratory and enteric infections in psittacines** using the 24% (240 mg/mL) injectable suspension: 0.22 mL/kg IM once to twice daily
b) **Respiratory and enteric infections in hand-fed baby psittacines**: Using the sulfamethoxazole/trimethoprim oral suspension 240 mg/5 mL (48 mg/mL): 0.22 mL/30 g 2 to 3 times daily for 5 to 7 days
c) **Coccidiosis in toucans and mynahs**: Using the sulfamethoxazole/trimethoprim oral suspension 240 mg/5 mL (48 mg/mL): 2.2 mL/kg once daily for 5 days; may be added to feed.
d) **Canaries, finches, and mynah birds**: Sulfadiazine/trimethoprim 100 mg/kg PO twice daily is recommended for treatment of avian coccidian parasitic diseases.[40] **NOTE**: *Atoxoplasma* spp treatment is difficult.
e) **GI protozoal infections in pigeons**: 25 – 50 mg/kg PO twice daily for 10 to 14 days[41]

FERRETS:

Susceptible infections (extra-label):

a) 30 mg/kg PO twice daily
b) **Coccidiosis**: 30 mg/kg PO once daily for 14 days

RABBITS, RODENTS, SMALL MAMMALS:

Susceptible infections (extra-label):

a) **Rabbits**:
   i. 15 – 30 mg/kg PO every 12 to 24 hours; 30 – 48 mg/kg SC every 12 hours. Sulfadiazine has a very short half-life (ie, ≈1 hour) in rabbits.[42]
   ii. **GI protozoal infections**: 25 – 30 mg/kg PO twice daily for 10 to 14 days[41]
b) **Chinchillas, Gerbils, Guinea Pigs, Hamsters, Mice, Rats**: 15 – 30 mg/kg PO every 12 hours
c) **Chinchillas, Hedgehogs**: 30 mg/kg PO or SC every 12 hours[43]

REPTILES:

Susceptible infections (extra-label):

a) **Most species**: 30 mg/kg IM (upper part of body) once daily for 2 treatments, then every other day for 5 to 12 treatments; may be useful for enteric infections.[44]
b) **All species**: 30 mg/kg IM, first 2 doses should be 24 hours apart, then every other day[45]
c) 15 – 25 mg/kg/day IM for 7 to 14 days[46]
d) **GI protozoal infections in bearded dragons**: 15 – 20 mg/kg PO once daily for 7 to 14 days; may consider giving dose every other day after the second dose.[41]

Monitoring

- Clinical efficacy
- Adverse effects
- Renal function (creatinine, BUN) and potassium
- If prolonged therapy (ie, greater than 7 days) is anticipated, the following is recommended:
- Baseline and periodic CBC and hepatic profile
- In dogs, baseline Schirmer tear testing, with periodic re-evaluation (eg, in 5 days, then every 2-3 weeks) and owner monitoring for ocular discharge
- Thyroid function tests should also be considered (baseline and ongoing) in dogs

Client Information

- Shake the oral suspension well before using. It does not need to be refrigerated.
- Give to horses on an empty stomach.
- Animals must be allowed free access to water and not become dehydrated while receiving this medication.
- If the animal's eyes are dry, develop a discharge, or become irritated, contact your veterinarian.
- In horses, discontinue treatment and contact your veterinarian immediately if there are changes in stool consistency or diarrhea.

Chemistry/Synonyms

Trimethoprim occurs as odorless, bitter-tasting, white to cream-colored crystals or crystalline powder. It is very slightly soluble in water and slightly soluble in alcohol.

Sulfadiazine occurs as an odorless or nearly odorless, white to slightly yellow powder. It is practically insoluble in water and sparingly soluble in alcohol.

Sulfamethoxazole occurs as a practically odorless and tasteless, white to off-white, crystalline powder. Approximately 0.29 mg is soluble in 1 mL of water, and 20 mg is soluble in 1 mL of alcohol.

In combination, sulfadiazine and trimethoprim may be known as co-trimazine, sulfadiazine/trimethoprim, trimethoprim/sulfadiazine, SDZ-TMP, TMP-SDZ, and various trade names.

In combination, sulfamethoxazole and trimethoprim may be known as co-trimoxazole, sulfamethoxazole/trimethoprim, trimethoprim/sulfamethoxazole, SMX-TMP, TMP-SMX, and various trade names.

Storage/Stability

Unless otherwise instructed by the manufacturer, sulfa-/trimethoprim products should be stored at room temperature of 20°C to 25°C (68°F-77°F) in tight containers and protected from freezing. Shake suspensions well before use.

Compatibility/Compounding Considerations

No specific information noted

Dosage Forms/Regulatory Status

VETERINARY-LABELED PRODUCTS:

Trimethoprim/Sulfadiazine Oral Suspension: Each gram contains 67 mg trimethoprim and 333 mg sulfadiazine (proprietary formulation) in 135 mL, 280 mL, 560 mL, and 900 mL bottles; *Equisul-SDT®*; (Rx). FDA-approved for use in horses not intended for food. NADA# 141-360

Trimethoprim/Sulfadiazine Powder: Each gram contains 67 mg trimethoprim and 333 mg sulfadiazine; *Uniprim® Powder* in 37.5 g and 1125 g packets; 200 g, 400 g, and 1200 g jars; 2000 g pails; and 12 kg box; (Rx). FDA-approved for use in horses not intended for food. NADA# 200-033

Trimethoprim/Sulfadiazine Oral Paste: Each gram contains 67 mg trimethoprim and 333 mg sulfadiazine. Available in 37.5 g (total weight) syringes; *Tribrissen® 400 Oral Paste*; (Rx). FDA-approved for use in horses not intended for food. **NOTE**: Not currently marketed in the United States; approved products are available in other countries.

Trimethoprim/Sulfadiazine Sterile Injection: 48% in 100 mL vials: *Di-Biotic® 48%, Tribrissen® 48% Injection*; (Rx). FDA-approved for use in horses not intended for food. **NOTE**: Not currently marketed in the United States; approved products are available in other countries under different trade names. A 24% solution may also be available.

In Canada, trimethoprim and sulfadoxine are available for use in cattle and swine (*Trimidox®*; *Borgal®*). Slaughter withdrawal = 10 days; milk withdrawal = 96 hours. (In the United States, extra-label use of sulfonamides is prohibited in lactating dairy cattle.)

In the United Kingdom, trimethoprim and sulfamethoxazole oral drops (*Sulfatrim®*) are available for use in rabbits, pigeons, and bearded dragons.

HUMAN-LABELED PRODUCTS:

Trimethoprim Tablets: 100 mg; generic; (Rx). A 50 mg/5 mL oral solution (trimethoprim HCl, *Primsol®*) is also available.

Trimethoprim and Sulfamethoxazole (Co-Trimoxazole; TMP-SMZ) Oral Tablets: 80 mg trimethoprim and 400 mg sulfamethoxazole; Double Strength Tablets: 160 mg trimethoprim and 800 mg sulfamethoxazole; *Bactrim®* and *Bactrim® DS*; generic; (Rx)

Trimethoprim 8 mg/mL and Sulfamethoxazole 40 mg/mL (labeled as 40 mg/5 mL and 200 mg/5mL) oral suspension; *Sulfatrim®*; generic; (Rx)

Trimethoprim and Sulfamethoxazole Injection: 80 mg sulfamethoxazole, 16 mg trimethoprim per mL in 5 mL single-use vials, 10 mL, or 30 mL multiple-dose vials; generic; (Rx). Contains benzyl alcohol, propylene glycol (40%); pH ≈10. **NOTE**: Refer to product label for administration guidelines.

References

For the complete list of references, see **wiley.com/go/budde/plumb**

Sulfadimethoxine

(sul-fa-***dye***-meth-***ox***-een) *Albon®*

Sulfonamide Antimicrobial

See also ***Sulfadimethoxine/Ormetoprim***

Prescriber Highlights

- Used to treat bacterial and protozoal infections
- Contraindications include hypersensitivity to sulfonamides and severe renal or hepatic impairment.
- Use with caution in breeds that are prone to sulfonamide hypersensitivity (ie, Doberman pinschers, Samoyeds, miniature schnauzers).
- Adverse effects include the possibility of the drug precipitating in the urine (particularly with high doses administered for prolonged periods, acidic urine, or highly concentrated urine). In dogs, keratoconjunctivitis sicca, hypersensitivity reactions (eg, rashes, fever, bone marrow suppression, dermatitis, nonseptic polyarthritis), focal retinitis, and vomiting are possible. Diminished renal or hepatic function or urinary obstruction may occur.
- Potentially teratogenic; potential risks versus benefits should be considered.
- In the United States, extra-label use of sulfonamides is prohibited in lactating dairy cattle.

Uses/Indications

Sulfadimethoxine injection and tablets are FDA-approved for use in dogs and cats for respiratory, genitourinary, enteric, and soft tissue infections caused by susceptible organisms. Efficacy is greater when treatment is initiated early in the course of disease. Sulfadimethoxine is also used to treat coccidial infections in small animals.

In horses, sulfadimethoxine injection is FDA-approved for the treatment of respiratory infections caused by *Streptococcus equi*.

In cattle, sulfadimethoxine is FDA-approved for treatment of shipping fever complex, calf diphtheria, bacterial pneumonia, and foot rot caused by susceptible organisms.

In poultry, sulfadimethoxine is added to drinking water to treat coccidiosis, fowl cholera, and infectious coryza.

Although sulfadimethoxine is not used in human medicine, the World Health Organization (WHO) has designated sulfonamides as highly important antimicrobials for human medicine.[1] The Office International des Epizooties (OIE) has designated sulfonamides as Veterinary Critically Important Antimicrobial (VCIA) Agents for veterinary species.[2]

Pharmacology/Actions

Sulfonamides are time-dependent, bacteriostatic agents when used alone, but are considered bactericidal when used in combination with dihydrofolate reductase inhibitors (eg, ormetoprim, trimethoprim). They are thought to prevent bacterial replication by competing with para-aminobenzoic acid (PABA) in the biosynthesis of tetrahydrofolic acid in the pathway to form folic acid. Only microorganisms that synthesize their own folic acid are affected by sulfonamides.

Microorganisms usually affected by sulfonamides include some gram-positive bacteria, including some strains of streptococci, staphylococcus, *Bacillus anthracis*, *Clostridium tetani*, *Clostridium perfringens*, and many strains of *Nocardia* spp. Sulfonamides also have in vitro activity against some gram-negative species, including some strains of *Shigella* spp, *Salmonella* spp, *Escherichia coli*, *Klebsiella* spp, *Enterobacter* spp, *Pasteurella* spp, and *Proteus* spp. Sulfonamides have activity against some protozoa (eg, *Toxoplasma* spp, *Coccidia* spp). Sulfonamides are inactive against atypical bacterial, viral, or fungal infections.

Sulfonamides are less efficacious in pus, necrotic tissue, or in areas with extensive cellular debris.

Pharmacokinetics

In dogs, cats, swine, and sheep, sulfadimethoxine is reportedly readily absorbed and well distributed. Relative volumes of distribution range from 0.17 L/kg in sheep to 0.35 L/kg in horses and cattle. Parameters in dogs include 33% bioavailability, 75% protein binding, and 13.1-hour elimination half-life.[3] Bioavailability was 52% in llamas and ≈100% in camels.[4,5]

In most species, sulfadimethoxine is acetylated in the liver to acetylsulfadimethoxine and excreted unchanged in the kidneys. In dogs, the drug is not appreciably metabolized by the liver; renal excretion is the major route of drug elimination as the unchanged drug. Sulfadimethoxine's long elimination half-lives are a result of its appreciable reabsorption in the renal tubules. Serum half-lives reported in various species are 9 to 10 hours in llamas, 11.7 hours in camels, 13 hours in swine, 15 hours in sheep, and 11.3 hours in horses.[4-6]

Contraindications/Precautions/Warnings

Sulfonamides are contraindicated in patients that are hypersensitive to them. They are also considered contraindicated in patients with severe renal or hepatic impairment. They should be used with caution in animals with diminished renal or hepatic function or urinary obstruction. Sulfonamides are _not_ considered contraindicated in patients that are allergic to thiazide diuretics or sulfonylurea agents.[7]

Doberman pinschers, Samoyeds, and miniature schnauzers appear to be highly susceptible to sulfonamide-induced polysystemic immune complex disease,[8-11] and these drugs should be used with caution in these breeds.

IV injection of sulfonamides given too rapidly can cause muscle weakness, blindness, ataxia, and collapse.

Adverse Effects

Sulfonamides (or their metabolites) can precipitate in the urine, particularly when given at high doses for prolonged periods. Acidic urine or highly concentrated urine may also contribute to increased risk for crystalluria, hematuria, and renal tubule obstruction. Different sulfonamides have different solubilities at various pH levels. Alkalinization of the urine using sodium bicarbonate may prevent crystalluria, but the amount available for tubular reabsorption decreases. Crystalluria can usually be avoided with most commercially available sulfonamides by maintaining an adequate urine flow. Normal urine pH in herbivores is usually 8 or more, so crystalluria is not frequently a problem. Sulfonamides can also cause various hypersensitivity reactions or diarrhea by altering the normal gut flora.

In dogs, keratoconjunctivitis sicca, hypersensitivity reactions (eg, rashes, dermatitis, fever, myelosuppression, nonseptic polyarthritis), focal retinitis, and vomiting have been reported with sulfonamides.[8] Dose-dependent hypothyroidism has been reported in dogs receiving sulfonamides.[12]

Oral sulfonamides can depress the normal cellulytic function of the ruminoreticulum, but this effect is generally temporary, and the animal typically adapts.

Because solutions of sulfonamides are usually alkaline, they can cause tissue irritation and necrosis if injected IM or SC.

Reproductive/Nursing Safety

Sulfonamides cross the placenta and may reach fetal concentrations of greater than or equal to 50% of those found in maternal serum; teratogenicity has been reported in some laboratory animals when sulfonamides are given at high doses.

Sulfonamides are distributed into maternal milk, but in humans, they are considered compatible with breastfeeding in healthy, full-term infants.[13,14] Premature infants and infants with hyperbilirubinemia may be at risk for adverse effects.

Overdose/Acute Toxicity

Acute toxicity secondary to overdoses apparently occurs only rarely in veterinary species. Dogs receiving single oral doses of 3.2 g/kg of body weight experienced only diarrhea. Dogs receiving 160 mg/kg PO daily for 13 weeks showed no signs of toxicity.[15] In addition to the adverse effects listed above, CNS stimulation and myelin degeneration have been noted after high doses are given.

For patients that have experienced or are suspected to have experienced an overdose, consultation with a 24-hour poison consultation center specializing in providing veterinary-specific information is recommended. For general information related to overdose and toxin exposures, as well as contact information for poison control centers, refer to ***Appendix***.

Drug Interactions

The following drug interactions have either been reported or are theoretical in humans or animals receiving sulfonamides and may be of significance in veterinary patients. Unless otherwise noted, use together is not necessarily contraindicated, but the potential risks must be weighed and additional monitoring performed when appropriate.

- **AMIODARONE**: May reduce sulfonamide metabolism and increase the risk for adverse effects
- **ANTACIDS, ALUMINUM-, CALCIUM- AND MAGNESIUM- CONTAINING**: May decrease oral bioavailability of sulfonamides if administered concurrently
- **AZATHIOPRINE, MERCAPTOPURINE**: Increased risk for myelosuppression
- **CYCLOSPORINE**: Increased risk for cyclosporine nephrotoxicity; decreased cyclosporine concentration is possible.
- **LEUCOVORIN**: May reduce therapeutic effect of sulfadimethoxine
- **METHOTREXATE**: Concurrent use of sulfonamides may potentiate methotrexate toxicity by interfering with plasma protein binding and/or renal clearance of methotrexate and its toxic metabolite.
- **PYRIMETHAMINE**: Concurrent use of sulfonamides with high doses of pyrimethamine may increase the risk for megaloblastic anemia and pancytopenia through additive antifolate effects.
- **WARFARIN**: Sulfonamides may prolong prothrombin time (PT).

Laboratory Considerations

- Sulfonamides may give false-positive results for **urine glucose** determinations when using the Benedict's method.

Dosages

DOGS/CATS:

Sulfadimethoxine-susceptible bacterial infections in dogs and cats and bacterial enteritis associated with coccidiosis in dogs (label dosage; FDA-approved): 55 mg/kg PO once on the first day, with subsequent daily doses of 27.5 mg/kg PO every 24 hours.[15] Length of treatment depends on the clinical response. Treatment should be continued until the animal shows no clinical signs for 48 hours. In most cases, treatment for 3 to 5 days is adequate.

Coccidiosis (extra-label): 50 – 60 mg/kg PO once daily for 5 to 20 days[16]

Coccidiosis in dogs (extra label): 25 mg/kg PO in combination with amprolium 150 mg/kg PO once daily for 14 days[17]

HORSES:

Susceptible infections (label dosage; FDA-approved): 55 mg/kg IV initially, then 27.5 mg/kg every 24 hours IV until free of clinical signs for 48 hours[18]

CATTLE:

Susceptible infections (label dosage; FDA-approved):

a) **Bolus tablets**: 55 mg/kg PO initially, then 27.5 mg/kg PO every 24 hours.[19] Length of treatment depends on the clinical response but should not exceed 5 days.

b) **Injection**: 55 mg/kg IV initially, then 27.5 mg/kg IV every 24 hours until free of clinical signs for 48 hours.[20] The injection should be made moderately slow, never rapidly.

NEW-WORLD CAMELIDS:

Coccidiosis (*Eimeria alpacae, Eimeria lamae, Eimeria punoensis, Eimeria peruviana*) (extra-label): 15 mg/kg PO twice daily for 5 days; monitor for signs of polioencephalomalacia[21]

***Eimeria* spp infection** (extra-label): Treatment is generally directed at clinically affected animals using sulfadimethoxine 110 mg/kg PO every 24 hours (or amprolium). Treatments are effective only against the immature stages and therefore may not have a significant impact on fecal oocyst count initially. *Eimeria macusaniensis* infections have a long prepatent period, treatment should last 10 to 15 days and should be directly administered to the animal rather than by medicating water supplies.[22]

FERRETS:

Coccidiosis (extra-label): 50 mg/kg PO once, then 25 mg/kg every 24 hours for 5 to 10 days. Alternatively, 25 mg/kg PO every 24 hours for 21 days.[23] Treatment may not clear the organism.

RABBITS/RODENTS/SMALL MAMMALS:

a) **Rabbits** (extra-label): 10 – 15 mg/kg PO every 12 hours[24]

b) **Coccidiosis in rabbits** (extra-label):

   i. 25 mg/kg PO once daily[25]

   ii. 50 mg/kg PO once, followed by inclusion in drinking water at 1 g/4 L for 9 days[26]

c) **Hedgehogs** (extra-label): 2 – 20 mg/kg/day IM, SC, or PO[27]

d) **Coccidiosis in mice, rats, gerbils, hamsters, guinea pigs, chinchillas** (extra-label): 50 mg/kg PO once, then 25 mg/kg PO once daily for 10 to 20 days or 75 mg/kg PO for 7 to 14 days

REPTILES:

***Coccidia* spp** (extra-label): 90 mg/kg PO once initially, followed by 45 mg/kg PO every 24 hours for 5 successive days; may also be given IM or IV. Maintain adequate hydration during treatment.[28]

***Isospora* spp** (extra-label): 50 mg/kg PO once daily for 21 days has been recommended for bearded dragons.[29]

Monitoring

- Clinical efficacy
- Adverse effects
- Baseline and periodic CBC and serum liver chemistry panel should be considered with long-term therapy.
- Baseline Schirmer tear testing is recommended in dogs if prolonged therapy (ie, more than 7 days) is anticipated or in dogs with a predisposition for KCS (eg, shih tzus, cocker spaniels). Dogs should be re-evaluated periodically (ie, within 5 days of starting therapy, then every 2 to 3 weeks during treatment). Owners should monitor dogs for red eye and ocular discharge.

Client Information

- If using the oral suspension, shake well before using. The oral suspension does not need to be refrigerated.
- It is important that your animal has access to plenty of fresh water while taking this medicine.
- Contact your veterinarian if the dog's eyes are dry, become red or irritated, or develops a discharge. You should also contact your veterinarian if your dog develops a rash or other skin lesions, low energy level, poor appetite, or has difficulty walking.

Chemistry/Synonyms

Sulfadimethoxine, a long-acting sulfonamide, occurs as an odorless or almost odorless, almost tasteless white powder. It is practically insoluble in water and slightly soluble in alcohol.

Sulfadimethoxine may also be known as solfadimetossina, solfadimetossipirimidina, sulphadimethoxine, *Albon®*, *Bactrovet®*, *Agribon®*, *Chemiosalfa®*, *Deltin®*, *Di-Methox®*, *Levosin®*, *Risulpir®*, *Ritarsulfa®*, *SDM®*, *Sulfadren®*, *Sulfastop®*, *Sulfasol®*, and *Sulfathox®*.

Storage/Stability

Unless otherwise instructed by the manufacturer, store sulfadimethoxine products protected from light at a room temperature of 15°C to 30°C (59°F-86°F). Solutions may discolor if exposed to direct sunlight. If crystals form due to exposure to cold temperatures, either gently warm the vial in a warm water bath or store at room temperature until crystals dissolve. Freezing and discoloration of liquid formulations do not alter potency.

Compatibility/Compounding Considerations

No specific information noted

Dosage Forms/Regulatory Status

VETERINARY-LABELED PRODUCTS:

Sulfadimethoxine Injection: 400 mg/mL (40%) in 250 mL vials; generic; (OTC). FDA-approved for use in cattle. Not to be used in calves to be processed for veal. Slaughter withdrawal (at labeled doses) is 5 days (cattle); milk withdrawal (at labeled doses) is 60 hours (5 milkings). A withdrawal period has not been established for preruminating calves.

Sulfadimethoxine Oral Tablets: 125 mg, 250 mg, and 500 mg; *Albon® Tablets*; (Rx). FDA-approved for use in dogs and cats

Sulfadimethoxine Oral Suspension: 50 mg/mL (5%) in 60- and 473-mL bottles; *Albon®*; (Rx). FDA-approved for use in dogs and cats

Sulfadimethoxine Oral Boluses: 2.5 g, 5 g, and 15 g; *Albon®*; (OTC). FDA-approved for use in cattle. Not to be used in calves to be processed for veal. No withdrawal period has been established for preruminating calves. Slaughter withdrawal (at labeled doses) is 7 days (cattle); milk withdrawal (at labeled doses) is 60 hours.

Sulfadimethoxine Soluble Powder: 94.6 g sulfadimethoxine/107 g packet (88.4% w/w) (for addition to drinking water); *Albon®*, generic; (OTC). FDA-approved for use in dairy calves, dairy heifers, beef cattle, broiler and replacement chickens only, and meat-producing turkeys. Slaughter withdrawal (at labeled doses) is 5 days in poultry (not for use in chickens older than 16 weeks or in turkeys older than 24 weeks) and 7 days in dairy calves, dairy heifers, and beef cattle only (withdrawal for preruminating calves has not been established; not to be used in calves to be processed for veal).

Sulfadimethoxine 12.5% Concentrated Solution: 3.8 L (1 gal) containers (for addition to drinking water): *Albon®*, generic; (OTC). FDA-approved for use in chickens, turkeys, and cattle. Slaughter withdrawal (at labeled doses) is 7 days in dairy calves, dairy heifers, and beef cattle only (withdrawal for preruminating calves has not been established; not to be used in calves to be processed for veal) and 5 days in poultry (not for use in chickens older than 16 weeks or in turkeys older than 24 weeks).

HUMAN-LABELED PRODUCTS: NONE

References

For the complete list of references, see **wiley.com/go/budde/plumb**

Sulfadimethoxine/Ormetoprim

(sul-fa-***dye***-meth-***ox***-een/or-meh-***toe***-prim) *Primor*®

Potentiated Sulfonamide Antimicrobial

Prescriber Highlights

- Potentiated sulfa similar to sulfa-/trimethoprim but may have fewer adverse effects and is labeled for once daily administration

NOTE: The following points apply to sulfa-/trimethoprim and may also apply to sulfadimethoxine/ormetoprim.

- Contraindications include hypersensitivity to sulfonamides, thiazides, or sulfonylurea agents; severe renal or hepatic impairment; and Doberman pinschers.
- Caution is advised in diminished renal or hepatic function, urinary obstruction, and urolithiasis.
- Adverse effects in dogs include keratoconjunctivitis sicca (KCS), hypersensitivity reactions (type 1 or type 3), acute neutrophilic hepatitis with icterus, vomiting, anorexia, diarrhea, fever, hemolytic anemia, urticaria, polyarthritis, facial swelling, polydipsia, crystalluria, hematuria, polyuria, cholestasis, hypothyroidism, anemia, agranulocytosis, and idiosyncratic hepatic necrosis.
- Sulfadimethoxine/ormetoprim is potentially teratogenic; weigh the risks versus the benefits before prescribing.
- In the United States, extra-label use of sulfonamides is prohibited in lactating dairy cattle.

Uses/Indications

In dogs, sulfadimethoxine/ormetoprim is FDA-approved for the treatment of skin and soft tissue infections caused by susceptible strains of *Staphylococcus aureus* and *Escherichia coli* and UTIs caused by *E coli*, *Staphylococcus* spp, and *Proteus mirabilis*. Sulfadimethoxine/ormetoprim effectively treats superficial pyoderma. Sulfadimethoxine/ormetoprim may have fewer adverse effects in dogs as compared with sulfa-/trimethoprim and can be given once daily.

Pharmacology/Actions

Sulfadimethoxine/ormetoprim shares mechanism of action and (probably) the bacterial spectrum of activity with sulfa-/trimethoprim. Sulfonamides are bacteriostatic agents. When used in combination with either ormetoprim or trimethoprim, the resulting potentiated sulfonamides are bactericidal. Combining sulfonamides and dihydrofolate reductase inhibitors (eg, ormetoprim, trimethoprim) results in synergistic antimicrobial effects.[1] Potentiated sulfonamides sequentially inhibit enzymes in the folic acid pathway, inhibiting bacterial thymidine synthesis. The sulfonamide competes with para-aminobenzoic acid (PABA) to reduce bacterial dihydrofolic acid (DFA) formation, and ormetoprim blocks the conversion of DFA to tetrahydrofolic acid by preferentially inhibiting bacterial dihydrofolate reductase.

Potentiated sulfonamides have a fairly broad spectrum of activity. Generally susceptible gram-positive bacteria include most streptococci, many strains of staphylococcus, and *Nocardia* spp. Although many gram-negative organisms of the Enterobacteriaceae family are susceptible to potentiated sulfonamides, this does not include *Pseudomonas aeruginosa*. Some protozoa (ie, *Pneumocystis jiroveci*, *Coccidia* spp, *Toxoplasma* spp, *Neospora* spp) are also inhibited by the combination. Potentiated sulfonamides appear to have little activity against most atypical bacteria and anaerobes; methicillin-resistant staphylococci are usually resistant. *Enterococcus* infections may appear to be susceptible to sulfonamide-containing antibiotics in vitro; however, they are intrinsically resistant, so sulfonamide-containing antibiotics should not be used for these bacteria.

Resistance development is thought to occur more slowly to the combination of drugs than to either drug alone.[1] In gram-negative organisms, sulfamethoxazole resistance is usually plasmid mediated, although a point mutation for dihydropteroate synthase also may confer resistance.

The Office International des Epizooties (OIE) Antimicrobial Classification is a Veterinary Critically Important antimicrobial.[2]

Pharmacokinetics

In dogs, cats, swine, and sheep, sulfadimethoxine is reportedly readily absorbed and well distributed. Relative volumes of distribution range from 0.17 L/kg in sheep to 0.35 L/kg in cattle and horses. Parameters in dogs include 33% bioavailability, 75% protein binding, and 13.1-hour elimination half-life.[3] Bioavailability was 52% in llamas and ≈100% in camels.[4,5]

In most species, sulfadimethoxine is acetylated in the liver to acetylsulfadimethoxine and excreted unchanged in the kidneys. In dogs, the drug is not appreciably metabolized by the liver; renal excretion is the major route of drug elimination. Sulfadimethoxine's long elimination half-lives are a result of its appreciable reabsorption in the renal tubules. Serum half-lives reported in various species are 9 to 10 hours in llamas, 11.7 hours in camels, 13 hours in swine, 15 hours in sheep, and 11.3 hours in horses.[4-6]

Pharmacokinetic data for ormetoprim are not currently available, but the manufacturer states that therapeutic levels are maintained over 24 hours at recommended doses.[7]

Contraindications/Precautions/Warnings

The manufacturer states that sulfadimethoxine/ormetoprim should not be used in dogs with marked liver parenchymal damage, blood dyscrasias, or history of sulfonamide sensitivity.

Avoid use of this antibiotic in dogs that may be sensitive to potential adverse effects (eg, keratoconjunctivitis sicca, hepatopathy, hypersensitivity, skin eruptions).[8]

Doberman pinschers, Samoyeds, and miniature schnauzers appear to be more susceptible to sulfonamide-induced polysystemic immune complex disease[9]; use sulfadimethoxine/ormetoprim with caution in these breeds.

Sulfonamides (and their metabolites) can precipitate in the urine, particularly when given at high dosages for prolonged periods. Sulfadimethoxine is less likely to cause formation of sulfonamide crystalluria because it has a relatively high solubility at the normal pH found in the kidney; however, acidic or highly concentrated urine may cause precipitation.

This drug combination should be used with caution in patients with pre-existing hepatic or thyroid disease.

Adverse Effects

In dogs, sulfadimethoxine/ormetoprim may have adverse effects similar to sulfa-/trimethoprim, including keratoconjunctivitis sicca (KCS; which may be irreversible), acute neutrophilic hepatitis with icterus, vomiting, anorexia, diarrhea, fever, hemolytic anemia, urticaria, polyarthritis, facial swelling, polydipsia, polyuria, and cholestasis.[7] Acute hypersensitivity reactions manifesting as type I (ie, immediate) or type III (ie, formation of antigen:antibody complexes) reactions can also be seen. Hypersensitivity reactions appear to be more common in large breed dogs.[9] Doberman pinschers may be more susceptible to this effect than other breeds. In humans, other hematologic effects (eg, anemia, agranulocytosis) are possible but are rare.[10]

Long-term therapy (ie, 8 weeks) at recommended doses of sulfadimethoxine/ormetoprim (27.5 mg/kg once daily) resulted in elevated serum cholesterol, thyroid and liver weights, mild follicular thyroid hyperplasia, and enlarged basophilic cells in the pituitary.

The manufacturer states that the principal treatment-related effect of extended or excessive use is hypothyroidism.

Reproductive/Nursing Safety

Sulfonamides cross the placenta and may reach fetal levels of greater than or equal to 50% of those found in maternal serum; teratogenicity (eg, cleft palate, fetal loss) has been reported in some laboratory animals given sulfonamides at high doses.

Sulfonamides are distributed into milk. This drug should be used in pregnant animals only when the benefits clearly outweigh the risks.

Overdose/Acute Toxicity

In experimental studies in dogs, doses greater than 80 mg/kg resulted in slight tremors and increased motor activity in some dogs.[11] Higher doses may result in depression, anorexia, or seizures.

It is suggested that very high oral overdoses be handled by gastric decontamination using standard precautions and protocols and by treating clinical signs supportively and symptomatically.

For patients that have experienced or are suspected to have experienced an overdose, consultation with a 24-hour poison consultation center specializing in providing veterinary-specific information is recommended. For general information related to overdose and toxin exposures, as well as contact information for poison control centers, refer to ***Appendix***.

Drug Interactions

None have been noted for sulfadimethoxine/ormetoprim, but the potential interactions for sulfa-/trimethoprim (listed below) may also apply to this drug combination; refer to ***Sulfa-/Trimethoprim*** for more information.

- AMANTADINE: A human patient developed toxic delirium when receiving amantadine with sulfamethoxazole/trimethoprim.[12]
- ANESTHETIC AGENTS: Concurrent IV administration is contraindicated. Ester-type local anesthetics (eg, **procaine, tetracaine**) may locally inhibit sulfonamide effects.[13,14]
- ANGIOTENSIN II-RECEPTOR BLOCKERS (ARBs; eg, **telmisartan**): May increase risk of hyperkalemia when used with potassium-sparing drugs
- ANGIOTENSIN-CONVERTING ENZYME INHIBITORS (ACEIs; eg, **benazepril, enalapril**): May increase risk of hyperkalemia when used with potassium-sparing drugs
- ANTACIDS: Concurrent administration may decrease sulfonamide bioavailability.
- AZATHIOPRINE: Increased risk for myelosuppression
- CYCLOSPORINE: May increase the risk for nephrotoxicity
- DETOMIDINE: Concurrent use has resulted in fatal arrhythmias in horses.[15]
- DIGOXIN: May increase digoxin levels
- DIURETICS, THIAZIDE: May increase risk for thrombocytopenia
- HYPOGLYCEMIC AGENTS, ORAL (eg, **glipizide, metformin**): May potentiate hypoglycemic effects
- METHENAMINE: May form an insoluble precipitate in the urine
- METHOTREXATE (MTX): May displace from plasma proteins and increase risk for toxic effects; can also interfere with MTX assays (competitive protein binding technique, but not when measured by radioimmunoassay)
- PHENOTHIAZINES (eg, **acepromazine, promethazine**): Concurrent administration contraindicated[13]
- PHENYTOIN: May increase half-life
- POTASSIUM SUPPLEMENTS: Increased risk of hyperkalemia
- PROCAINAMIDE: May increase levels of procainamide and its active metabolite
- PYRIMETHAMINE: May increase risk for megaloblastic anemia and myelosuppression
- RIFAMPIN: May reduce serum concentrations of both trimethoprim and sulfonamide
- SPIRONOLACTONE: May increase risk for hyperkalemia when used with potassium-sparing drugs
- TRICYCLIC ANTIDEPRESSANTS (TCAs; eg, **amitriptyline, clomipramine**): May decrease efficacy
- WARFARIN: May prolong prothrombin time and INR

Laboratory Considerations

NOTE: The following points apply to sulfa-/trimethoprim and may also apply to sulfadimethoxine/ormetoprim.

- When using the Jaffe alkaline picrate reaction assay for **creatinine** determination, sulfa-/trimethoprim may cause an overestimation of ≈10%.
- Sulfonamides may give false-positive results for **urine glucose** determinations when using the Benedict's method.

Dosages

DOGS:

NOTE: Unless otherwise noted, doses are for combined amounts of sulfadimethoxine and ormetoprim. See *Monitoring* if treatment is expected to be longer than 7 days.

Labeled indications (skin and soft tissue infections caused by susceptible strains of *Staphylococcus aureus* and *Escherichia coli*; UTIs caused by susceptible strains of *E coli, Staphylococcus* spp, and *Proteus mirabilis*) (FDA-approved): 55 mg/kg (combined drug) PO on the first day of therapy, then 27.5 mg/kg PO once daily, continuing for at least 2 days after remission of clinical signs. Not approved for treatment longer than 21 days.[7]

***Isospora* spp infections** (extra-label): 66 mg/kg (combined drug) PO once daily for 23 days[16]

Superficial bacterial folliculitis (extra-label): 55 mg/kg PO the first day, then 27.5 mg/kg PO once daily.[8] Potentiated sulfonamides (ie, sulfa-/trimethoprim, sulfadimethoxine/ormetoprim) are first-tier drugs only if regional susceptibility of *Staphylococcus pseudintermedius* is known.

Bacterial cystitis (extra-label): Potentiated sulfonamides (ie, sulfa-/trimethoprim, sulfadimethoxine/ormetoprim) are first-tier drugs only if regional pathogen susceptibility patterns are known.[17]

a) Uncomplicated UTI: 15 mg/kg PO every 12 hours. Treatment may be as short as 3 days.[17,18]
b) Complicated UTI: 15 – 30 mg/kg PO every 12 hours[17]

Monitoring

- Clinical efficacy
- Adverse effects
- Renal function (creatinine, BUN) and potassium
- If prolonged therapy (ie, greater than 7 days) is anticipated in dogs, the following is recommended:
- Baseline Schirmer tear testing, with periodic reevaluation (eg, in 5 days, then every 2 to 3 weeks) and owner monitoring for ocular discharge[8]
- Baseline and periodic CBC and hepatic profile
- Thyroid function tests should be considered (baseline and ongoing) particularly in dogs receiving long-term treatment.

Client Information

- Animals must be allowed free access to water and not become dehydrated while receiving this medication.
- If dog's eyes are dry, develop a discharge, or become irritated, contact your veterinarian.

Chemistry/Synonyms

Ormetoprim is a diaminopyrimidine structurally related to trimethoprim and occurs as a white, odorless, almost tasteless powder.

Sulfadimethoxine, a long-acting sulfonamide, occurs as an odorless or almost odorless, almost tasteless white powder. It is practically insoluble in water and slightly soluble in alcohol.

Sulfadimethoxine may also be known as solfadimetossina, solfadimetossipirimidina, sulphadimethoxine, *Albon®, Chemiosalfa®, Deltin®, Di-Methox®, Levosin®, Risulpir®, Ritarsulfa®, SDM®, Sulfadren®, Sulfasol®, Sulfastop®, and Sulfathox®.*

Ormetoprim may also be known as NSC-95072, ormetoprima, ormétoprime, ormetoprimum, or Ro-5-9754.

Storage/Stability

Unless otherwise instructed by the manufacturer, store tablets in tight, light-resistant containers at room temperature of 15°C to 30°C (59°F-86°F).

Compatibility/Compounding Considerations

No specific information noted

Dosage Forms/Regulatory Status

VETERINARY-LABELED PRODUCTS:

Sulfadimethoxine/Ormetoprim Tablets (scored)

120's: 100 mg Sulfadimethoxine, 20 mg Ormetoprim

240's: 200 mg Sulfadimethoxine, 40 mg Ormetoprim

600's: 500 mg Sulfadimethoxine, 100 mg Ormetoprim

1200's: 1000 mg Sulfadimethoxine, 200 mg Ormetoprim; *Primor®*; (Rx). FDA-approved for use in dogs. NADA# 100-929

HUMAN-LABELED PRODUCTS: NONE

References

For the complete list of references, see **wiley.com/go/budde/plumb**

Sulfasalazine

(sul-fa-***sal***-a-zeen) *Azulfidine®*

Sulfonamide/Salicylate Antibacterial/Immunosuppressive

Prescriber Highlights

- Sulfa-analogue that has GI antibacterial and anti-inflammatory activity used for inflammatory bowel disease; has also been used for vasculitis
- Contraindications include hypersensitivity to sulfasalazine, sulfas, or salicylates; intestinal or urinary obstructions; and Dobermans.
- Use with caution in cats and in patients that have liver, renal, or hematologic diseases.
- Adverse effects in dogs include keratoconjunctivitis sicca (KCS), anorexia, vomiting, cholestatic jaundice, hemolytic anemia, leukopenia, vomiting, decreased sperm counts, and allergic dermatitis.
- Adverse effects in cats include anorexia, vomiting, anemia.

Uses/Indications

Sulfasalazine may be used as adjunctive treatment of inflammatory large bowel (colonic) disease in dogs and cats. It has also been suggested for adjunctive use in treating vasculitis in dogs. It is not effective for small intestinal inflammation, as colonic bacteria are required to cleave the drug into sulfapyridine and 5-aminosalicylic acid (5-ASA, mesalamine). In humans, sulfasalazine is also used as adjunctive treatment for inflammatory arthropathies.

Pharmacology/Actions

Sulfasalazine is cleaved into sulfapyridine and 5-aminosalicylic acid (5-ASA, mesalamine) by colonic bacteria. Although the exact mechanism of action for its therapeutic effects in treating colitis in small animal species has not been determined, it is believed that mesalamine's local (not systemic) anti-inflammatory activity, including cyclooxygenase and lipoxygenase inhibition, provides the main therapeutic effect. Its antibacterial (sulfapyridine) and/or immunomodulatory activity may contribute to controlling clinical signs and course of the disease. In humans, concentrations of both metabolites in the colon are higher than by giving them orally as separate agents.

Pharmacokinetics

No pharmacokinetic data for dogs or cats were located.

In humans, only ≈10 to 33% of an orally administered dose of sulfasalazine is absorbed.[1] Of the absorbed drug, sulfasalazine is 99.3% bound to albumin, and sulfapyridine is 70% bound to albumin. Both sulfasalazine and sulfapyridine are widely distributed to the synovial fluid and connective tissue. Sulfasalazine reaches high concentrations in the intestinal wall. Some of the absorbed drug is then excreted unchanged in the bile and some is metabolized in the liver.

Unabsorbed and biliary excreted drug is cleaved into 5-ASA and sulfapyridine in the colon by bacterial flora. The sulfapyridine component is rapidly absorbed, but only a small percentage of the 5-ASA is absorbed. Absorbed sulfapyridine and 5-ASA are hepatically metabolized and then renally excreted. Unabsorbed sulfapyridine and 5-ASA is excreted in the feces. Elimination half-life is prolonged in elderly human patients, but clinical impact has yet to be established.

Contraindications/Precautions/Warnings

Sulfasalazine is contraindicated in animals hypersensitive to it, sulfonamides, or salicylates. Doberman pinschers, Samoyeds, and miniature schnauzers appear to be more susceptible to sulfonamide-induced polysystemic immune complex disease[2]; use sulfasalazine with caution in these breeds. Alternative medications should be considered in these dogs. It is also contraindicated in patients with intestinal or urinary obstructions.

Sulfasalazine should be used with caution in animals with pre-existing liver, renal, or hematologic diseases. Because cats can be sensitive to salicylates (see ***Aspirin***), use this drug cautiously in this species.

Do not confuse sulfaSALAzine with sulfaDIAzine.

Adverse Effects

Adverse effects occur relatively uncommonly in dogs and may include anorexia, vomiting, cholestatic jaundice, hemolytic anemia, leukopenia, hypersensitivity reactions, vomiting, decreased sperm counts, and allergic dermatitis. Yellow or orange discoloration of skin and body fluids may occur (harmless but may stain clothing). Keratoconjunctivitis sicca (KCS) has also been reported.[3-5] If decreased tear production is noted early, either reducing the dose or discontinuing the drug may prevent progression of KCS or increase tear production.

Cats can occasionally develop anorexia and vomiting, which may be alleviated by use of the enteric-coated tablets. Anemias secondary to sulfasalazine are also potentially possible in cats.

Adverse effects in humans are associated with serum sulfapyridine concentrations greater than 50 µg/mL. Blood dyscrasias (eg, agranulocytosis, aplastic anemia) and severe dermatologic reactions (eg, Stevens-Johnson reaction, drug reaction with eosinophilia and systemic symptoms [DRESS]) have been reported in humans receiving sulfasalazine or other sulfonamides.[1]

Reproductive/Nursing Safety

Sulfonamides cross the placenta. Although sulfasalazine has not been proven harmful to use during pregnancy and incidences of neonatal kernicterus in infants born to women taking sulfasalazine are low, it should only be used when it is clearly indicated. In laboratory animal studies (rats, rabbits), doses of 6 times the normal (human) amount caused impairment of fertility in male animals[1]; this effect is thought to be caused by the sulfapyridine component and was reversible upon discontinuation of the drug. Folic acid supplementation may be advised for women taking sulfasalazine during pregnancy.[1] Sulfasalazine has caused oligospermia in humans.

Sulfonamides, including sulfasalazine, are excreted in milk. In human newborns, they compete with bilirubin for binding sites on plasma proteins and may cause kernicterus. Use with caution in nursing patients.

Because safety has not been established in animals, this drug should only be used when the maternal benefits outweigh the potential risks to offspring.

Overdose/Acute Toxicity

Little specific information is available regarding overdoses with this agent, but because massive overdoses could cause significant salicylate and/or sulfonamide toxicity, standard decontamination protocols (empty stomach, cathartics) should be considered. Urine alkalinization and forced diuresis may also be beneficial in selected cases. Dialysis may remove sulfasalazine and its metabolites.

For patients that have experienced or are suspected to have experienced an overdose, consultation with a 24-hour poison control center specializing in providing veterinary-specific information is recommended. For general information related to overdose and toxin exposures, as well as contact information for poison control centers, refer to ***Appendix.***

Drug Interactions

Sulfasalazine and sulfapyridine are metabolized primarily by acetylation, along with glucuronidation and hydroxylation pathways. The following drug interactions either have been reported or are theoretical in humans or animals receiving sulfasalazine and may be of significance in veterinary patients. Unless otherwise noted, use together is not necessarily contraindicated, but weigh the potential risks and perform additional monitoring when appropriate.

- **Antibacterial Agents**: Reduction in GI flora caused by antibiotics may reduce bacterial cleavage of sulfasalazine and subsequent production of 5-ASA.
- **Cyclosporine**: Sulfadiazine has been reported to decrease cyclosporine concentrations in humans; interaction may apply to sulfasalazine. Monitor serum cyclosporine concentrations if using this combination.[6]
- **Digoxin**: Concomitant use may reduce absorption of digoxin.
- **Ferrous Sulfate** or **Other Iron Salts**: Concomitant use may decrease the blood concentrations of sulfasalazine; clinical significance is unknown.
- **Folic Acid**: Concomitant use may reduce oral absorption of folic acid.
- **Methenamine**: In humans, concurrent use may result in the formation of an insoluble precipitate in the urine, and the combination is considered contraindicated.
- **Nonsteroidal Anti-Inflammatory Drugs (NSAIDs**; eg, **carprofen, flunixin, meloxicam, robenacoxib)**: Concomitant use of NSAIDs may increase risk for bleeding.
- **Warfarin**: Concomitant use may potentiate the anticoagulant effects of warfarin.

Laboratory Interactions

- Sulfasalazine may cause false-positive urinary normetanephrine performed by liquid chromatography.
- Sulfasalazine may interfere with ALT, AST, ammonia, thyroxine, or glucose tests that use ultraviolet absorbance around wavelength 340 nm.[1]

Dosages

NOTE: Unless otherwise noted, assume the following dosages are for the standard-release tablets.

DOGS:

Inflammatory large bowel disease (extra-label):

a) Initial dosages range from 15 – 30 mg/kg PO every 8 to 12 hours, not to exceed a total daily dose of 6 g.[7] Anecdotal dosage recommendations vary considerably, and no definitive studies were located supporting any one dose. After 2 to 4 weeks (longer if at the low end of the dosing range) most taper off (reducing dosage every 2 weeks) until eventual drug discontinuation while maintaining dietary treatment. Some dogs may require long-term therapy.

b) As adjunct to dietary modification: 10 – 30 mg/kg (maximum dose of 1 g) PO with food every 8 hours for 4 to 6 weeks, then reduce dosing interval to every 12 hours.[8] If clinical signs remain controlled after 10 to 14 days, then decrease again to once-daily dosing.

Adjunctive treatment of vasculitis (extra-label): 20 – 40 mg/kg PO every 8 hours[9,10]

CATS:

Inflammatory large bowel disease (extra-label):

a) Use cautiously in cats because of their sensitivity to salicylates. Dosages range from 10 – 20 mg/kg PO 1 to 3 times a day (most clinicians recommend once daily). Anecdotal dosage recommendations vary somewhat, and no definitive studies were located supporting any one dose. Some clinicians state to treat no longer than 10 days and other clinicians advise to taper to the lowest effective dose.

b) As adjunct to dietary modification: 5 – 12.5 mg/kg PO with food every 8 hours for 2 to 3 weeks[8]

HORSES:

Chronic diarrhea (extra-label): Sulfasalazine (with dietary adjustment) 16 mg/kg PO once a day for 5 days, followed by 8 mg/kg PO once a day for 10 days.[13] **NOTE**: The product used in this case report (*Salazopyrin® EN*) was a delayed-release product.

FERRETS:

a) 10 – 20 mg/kg PO 2 to 3 times a day[11]
b) 25 mg (total dose) PO twice daily[12]

Monitoring

- Efficacy
- Baseline and periodic Schirmer tear tests, especially for breeds that are predisposed to developing keratoconjunctivitis sicca (KCS)
- Adverse effects
- Occasional CBC, liver enzymes are warranted with long-term therapy.

Client Information

- Give this medicine with food. Dose is often increased until diarrhea is controlled and then reduced to the lowest effective dose.
- Contact your veterinarian if your animal begins to have discharge from the eye(s) or the eyes become red.
- Cats may be sensitive to this medicine. Contact your veterinarian if you have any concerns about your cat.
- People allergic to sulfa drugs should handle this drug with caution.
- Skin or body fluids may become yellow-orange in color while your animal is taking this medicine. The fluids may cause staining.

Chemistry/Synonyms

Sulfasalazine is basically a molecule of sulfapyridine linked by a diazo bond to the diazonium salt of salicylic acid. It occurs as an odorless, bright yellow to brownish-yellow fine powder. Less than 0.1 mg is soluble in 1 mL of water and ≈0.34 mg is soluble in 1 mL of alcohol.

Sulfasalazine may also be known as salazosulfapyridine, salicylazosulfapyridine, sulfasalazinum, sulphasalazine, *Sulfazine®* and *Azulfidine®*.

Storage/Stability

Sulfasalazine tablets (either plain or enteric-coated) should be stored protected from light at temperatures less than 40°C (104°F) and preferably at room temperature 20°C to 25°C (68°F-77°F) in well-closed containers.

Compatibility/Compounding Considerations

No specific information is noted.

Dosage Forms/Regulatory Status

VETERINARY-LABELED PRODUCTS: NONE.

The Association of Racing Commissioners International (ARCI) has designated this drug as a class 4 substance. Use of this drug may not be allowed in certain animal competitions. Check rules and regulations before entering in a competition while this medication is being administered. Contact local racing authorities for further guidance. See ***Appendix*** for more information.

HUMAN-LABELED PRODUCTS:

Sulfasalazine Tablets: 500 mg; *Azulfidine®*, *Sulfazine®*, generic; (Rx)

Sulfasalazine Delayed-Release Tablets: 500 mg (enteric coated); *Azulfidine® EN-tabs®*, *Sulfazine EC®*, generic; (Rx)

References

For the complete list of references, see **wiley.com/go/budde/plumb**

Tadalafil

(ta-***dal***-a-fil) *Cialis®*

Phosphodiesterase Type 5 Inhibitor

Prescriber Highlights

- Used for treating pulmonary arterial hypertension and possibly benign prostatic hyperplasia in dogs
- Limited clinical experience or published data for use in dogs
- Appears to have a longer duration of action than sildenafil
- Contraindicated in patients receiving organic nitrates (eg, nitroglycerin, isosorbide)
- Adverse effects not well known for dogs; decreased appetite has been noted, as well as inguinal flushing and GI effects

Uses/Indications

Tadalafil is a phosphodiesterase-5 (PDE5) inhibitor, related to sildenafil, that is used to treat pulmonary arterial hypertension (PAH) in dogs.[1-3]

In dogs with PAH, tadalafil added to conventional heart failure therapy decreased diastolic pulmonary arterial pressure (PAP), mean PAP, and tricuspid regurgitation.[1] Both tadalafil and sildenafil improved quality of life and activity measures in dogs with moderate to severe pulmonary hypertension with various etiologies.[3] Because of its longer duration of action, tadalafil has some advantages over sildenafil. A study in humans has suggested that tadalafil may be tolerated in some patients experiencing sildenafil intolerance.[4]

Tadalafil reduced biochemical markers of benign prostatic hyperplasia (BPH) in dogs with experimentally induced BPH;[5] further research is needed to determine the drug's effect on clinical signs of BPH.

In humans, tadalafil is approved for use in treating pulmonary artery hypertension and erectile dysfunction. Offlabel uses include treating Raynaud's phenomenon.

Pharmacology/Actions

Tadalafil is a selective inhibitor of cyclic guanosine monophosphate (cGMP)-specific phosphodiesterase type 5 (PDE5). PDE5 is the enzyme responsible for the degradation of cGMP and is found (in humans) in the corpus cavernosum smooth muscle, pulmonary vascular and visceral smooth muscle, skeletal muscle, platelets, kidney, lung, cerebellum, and pancreas. In patients with PAH, vascular endothelium nitric oxide release is impaired with an associated reduction of cGMP. PDE5 is the primary phosphodiesterase in the pulmonary vasculature, and tadalafil's PDE5 inhibition increases cGMP, thereby relaxing pulmonary vascular smooth muscle with resultant vasodilation.

Pharmacokinetics

In healthy dogs, peak plasma concentration occurred ≈1.5 hours after oral administration, and half-life was 4.2 hours.[6] In the same study, tadalafil plasma concentration peaked ≈1.7 hours following intranasal administration, and half-life was 5.8 hours.

In humans, after oral administration, maximum plasma concentrations occur in ≈4 hours in patients with PAH. Food does not alter the rate or extent of absorption. Tadalafil is 94% bound to human plasma proteins. Tadalafil is metabolized by CYP3A4 to a catechol metabolite that then undergoes methylation and glucuronidation. These metabolites are not thought to be active. In PAH patients, the mean terminal half-life is 35 hours. Excretion is primarily of the drug's metabolites via fecal routes (61%), with the majority of the remainder in the urine (~36%).

Contraindications/Precautions/Warnings

Tadalafil is contraindicated in human patients using any form of organic nitrate (either regularly or intermittently) and in those with serious hypersensitivity to tadalafil. Dosage reductions may be required in patients with severe hepatic or renal impairment.

Adverse Effects

An adverse effect profile for dogs at suggested doses for PAH has not been determined. GI effects are possible, and decreased appetite has been noted.[3] In a 12-month tadalafil chronic toxicity study done in dogs, no disseminated arteritis was observed as was seen in rodent studies, but 2 dogs exhibited marked decreases in neutrophils and moderate decreases in platelets with inflammatory signs when dosed at ≈4 to 18 times the equivalent human dose. These effects were reversible within 2 weeks after discontinuing the drug. Cutaneous flushing of the inguinal region has been reported with sildenafil, a related drug, in dogs.

The most common adverse effects of tadalafil reported in humans with PAH include dyspepsia, nausea, back pain, myalgia, nasal congestion, flushing, and headache. Rare but serious adverse effects include optic neuropathy, seizures, hypersensitivity reactions (eg, Stevens-Johnson syndrome, exfoliative dermatitis), and deafness.

Reproductive/Nursing Safety

Tadalafil animal reproduction studies in rats and mice demonstrated no evidence of teratogenicity, embryotoxicity, or fetotoxicity when tadalafil was given to pregnant rats or mice at exposures of up to 11 times (human equivalent dose).

Tadalafil and/or its metabolites are secreted into the milk in lactating rats at concentrations ≈2.4-fold those found in the plasma. It is unlikely to pose much risk to nursing offspring.

Overdose/Acute Toxicity

Little information is available. Single doses of up to 500 mg have been given to healthy men, and multiple daily doses of up to 100 mg have been given to men with erectile dysfunction; adverse reactions were similar to those seen at lower doses.

It is expected that overdoses in animals would mirror the drug's adverse effect profile; treat supportively.

For patients that have experienced or are suspected of having experienced an overdose, consultation with a 24-hour poison consulta-

tion center specializing in providing veterinary-specific information is recommended. For general information related to overdose and toxin exposures, as well as contact information for poison control centers, refer to ***Appendix.***

Drug Interactions

The following drug interactions have either been reported or are theoretical in humans or animals receiving tadalafil and may be of significance in veterinary patients. Unless otherwise noted, use together is not necessarily contraindicated, but weigh the potential risks and perform additional monitoring when appropriate.

- **Alpha-Adrenergic Blockers** (eg, **tamsulosin, prazosin, phenothiazines** [eg, **acepromazine**], **phenoxybenzamine**): May increase hypotensive effects
- **Amlodipine**: Potential to increase hypotensive effects
- **Antihypertensive, Hypotensive Drugs**: Potentially could increase hypotensive effects
- **Azole Antifungals** (eg, **ketoconazole, itraconazole**): May reduce tadalafil metabolism and increase AUC
- **Cimetidine**: May reduce tadalafil metabolism and increase AUC
- **Clarithromycin/Erythromycin**: May increase tadalafil bioavailability, reduce tadalafil metabolism, and increase AUC
- **Nitrates** (eg, **nitroglycerin, isosorbide**): Significant potentiation of vasodilatory effects; life-threatening hypotension possible
- **Nitroprusside Sodium**: Significant potentiation of vasodilatory effects; life-threatening hypotension possible
- **Phenobarbital**: May decrease tadalafil concentrations
- **Rifampin**: May decrease tadalafil concentrations
- **Rivaroxaban**: Tadalafil decreased P-glycoprotein mediated efflux of rivaroxaban in an in vitro model; clinical significance remains unclear.[7]

Laboratory Considerations

- None was noted.

Dosages

DOGS:

Pulmonary arterial hypertension (extra-label):

a) 1-2 mg/kg PO once daily[3,8]

b) From a case report in a Yorkshire terrier: 1 mg/kg PO every 48 hours (every other day) was added to the background treatment (furosemide, spironolactone, benazepril, dexamethasone, and oxygen). The dog's condition rapidly improved (less than 24 hours), and a 7-day follow-up showed a decrease (up to 26 mm Hg) in systolic pulmonary arterial pressure and disappearance of all respiratory and cardiac signs of PAH (cyanosis, syncope, and tachypnea).[9]

Benign prostatic hyperplasia (extra-label): 5 mg/dog (NOT mg/kg) PO once daily[5]

Monitoring

- Clinical efficacy: improved exercise capacity, cough, respiratory effort; fewer episodes of syncope
- Pulmonary artery pressure, systemic blood pressure
- Adverse effects

Client Information

- May give this medicine with or without food. Be sure to give it exactly as prescribed.
- Tadalafil may cause flushing (redness) in the groin area. Lack of appetite, vomiting, and diarrhea are also possible.
- This medicine has not been used often in veterinary medicine, so it is important to report any other side effects to your veterinarian.
- Do not give with nitroglycerin or isosorbide, as it may cause severely low blood pressure.
- While your animal is taking this medication, it is important to return to your veterinarian for important tests. Do not miss these important follow-up visits.

Chemistry/Synonyms

Tadalafil has a molecular weight of 389.41. It is insoluble in water and slightly soluble in ethanol.

Tadalafil may also be known as GF-196960, IC-351, tadalafili, tadalafilo, or tadalafilum. *Cialis*® and *Adcirca*® are trade names for tadalafil.

Storage/Stability

Store tadalafil tablets at room temperature between 15°C and 30°C (59°F-86°F).

Compatibility/Compounding Considerations

A method of preparing a stable 5 mg/mL oral suspension from tablets has been published. Crush fifteen 20 mg tadalafil tablets to a fine powder in a glass mortar. Mix together 30 mL of *Ora-Sweet*® and 30 mL of *Ora-Plus*®; stir vigorously. Add 30 mL of this solution in geometric proportions to the powder and mix to form a smooth suspension. Transfer the mixture to a 2-ounce (60 mL) amber plastic prescription bottle. Rinse mortar with a quantity of the vehicle sufficient to make a final volume of 60 mL. Label "shake well." Suspension is stable for 91 days when stored at room temperature in an amber plastic prescription bottle.[10]

Dosage Forms/Regulatory Status

VETERINARY-LABELED PRODUCTS: NONE

HUMAN-LABELED PRODUCTS:

Tadalafil Oral Tablets: 2.5 mg, 5 mg, 10 mg, and 20 mg: *Cialis*®, *Adcirca*® (20 mg only); generic; (Rx)

References

For the complete list of references, see **wiley.com/go/budde/plumb**

Tamsulosin

(tam-suh-***low***-sin) *Flomax*®

Alpha-1 Adrenergic Antagonist

Prescriber Highlights

- ▶ Potentially useful as a lower urinary tract (ureteral/urethral) relaxant in dogs and cats; limited published clinical experience
- ▶ Contraindications include use in patients known to be hypersensitive to it.
- ▶ Higher doses could cause hypotension.
- ▶ Do not crush sustained-release pellets in capsules as rapid oral absorption may result in hypotension.

Uses/Indications

Tamsulosin is an alpha-1 adrenergic blocking agent that is similar to prazosin and phenoxybenzamine but longer-acting. Although evidence for efficacy in animals is limited, tamsulosin could be useful to facilitate passage of nephroliths and ureteroliths and for treating functional urinary obstruction, benign prostatic hypertrophy, or detrusor-urethral dyssynergia in dogs and cats, and postobstructive urethral spasm in cats.

In humans, tamsulosin is labeled for treatment of benign prostatic hyperplasia (BPH). It is also used for ureteral relaxation to facilitate passage of urinary calculi.

Pharmacology/Actions

Tamsulosin blocks sympathetic nervous stimulation of alpha-1 adrenoceptors. It is more selective for the 1A receptor subtype, which is the primary alpha-1 adrenoceptor found in the prostate, prostatic capsule, prostatic urethra, and bladder neck and is less common in vascular or other smooth muscle. Blockade of these adrenoceptors can cause smooth muscles in the bladder neck and prostate to relax resulting in improvement in urine flow rate and expulsion of urinary calculi. In conscious male dogs, tamsulosin caused a sustained inhibitory effect on phenylephrine-induced prostatic intraurethral pressure (IUP) response that was related to higher concentrations in the prostate and urethra, rather than in plasma and vascular tissues.[1]

Pharmacokinetics

Tamsulosin exhibits significant interspecies variation in its pharmacokinetics. After oral dosing of a nonsustained release formulation in dogs, tamsulosin bioavailability was ≈30% and peak plasma concentrations occurred ≈0.5 hours postdose. Volume of distribution Vd_{ss} was 1.74 L/kg; protein binding was 90%; clearance was 4 L/hour/kg (estimated unbound clearance: 31 to 41 L/hour/kg), and elimination half-life was ≈1.5 hours.[2] Tamsulosin concentrations are significantly higher and retained longer in prostatic and urethral tissues than in plasma. At 6 hours postdose (0.03 mg/kg), prostate/plasma and urethra/plasma ratios were 10.5 and 6.6 respectively.[1,3] Therefore despite a relatively fast plasma half-life, once or twice daily dosing may be possible in dogs, although pharmacokinetic/pharmacodynamic studies using the commercially available sustained-release formulation are required to determine appropriate dosages. In dogs, cytochrome CYP3A4 is responsible for metabolism of tamsulosin to the M1 and AM-1 metabolites.[4]

Pharmacokinetic data for cats were not located.

In humans, fasted state oral bioavailability is essentially complete (more than 90%). Tamsulosin exhibits linear kinetics following single and multiple dosing, with achievement of steady-state concentrations by the fifth day of once-a-day dosing. Plasma protein binding in humans is significant (98% to 99%). The terminal half-life of tamsulosin in humans is ≈6 to 15 hours.[2]

Contraindications/Precautions/Warnings

Tamsulosin is contraindicated in patients known to be hypersensitive to it. Some humans with sulfonamide drug allergies have reportedly experienced hypersensitivity reactions (skin rash, urticaria, pruritus, angioedema, and respiratory symptoms).[5] Priapism has been reported in humans; significance for veterinary patients is unknown.

Tamsulosin capsules are manufactured in a sustained-release (beads) presentation to avoid rapid absorption and associated hypotensive effects; therefore, they should not be crushed or compounded into an oral suspension.

Adverse Effects

The adverse effect profile in animals is not well documented, but hypotensive effects are possible. Hypotension may be more likely at high doses or in older dogs.[6] When tamsulosin was administered to anesthetized female beagles at doses from 0.003 – 0.01 mg/kg IV, urethral pressures were reduced in a dose-dependent fashion; almost no effect on mean arterial blood pressure was seen.[7]

In humans, reported adverse effects include headache, dizziness, blurred vision, rhinitis, muscle weakness, abnormal ejaculation, decreased libido, back pain, diarrhea, and nausea.[5] Intraoperative floppy iris syndrome and other postoperative ophthalmic adverse effects have also been reported in humans receiving tamsulosin undergoing cataract surgery; significance for veterinary patients is unknown. Administration on an empty stomach improves absorption, but also increases the risk for orthostasis.

Reproductive/Nursing Safety

Teratogenic effects or fetal harm were not observed when tamsulosin was administered to pregnant rats and rabbits. Tamsulosin may impair or alter ejaculation in humans and in rats[5]; it is presumed this effect may also occur in breeding males.

Tamsulosin is present in the milk of lactating rats.[5] Use with caution in nursing veterinary patients.

Because safety has not been established in animals, this drug should only be used when the maternal benefits outweigh the potential risks to offspring.

Overdose/Acute Toxicity

Moderate toxicity in humans generally occurs at 10 times recommended doses, but severe toxicity is uncommon. If hypotension occurs, it is usually responsive to IV fluid therapy; severe hypotension may require vasopressors. Dialysis is unlikely to be of benefit.

Adverse effects in dogs and cats with a tamsulosin overdose include lethargy/sedation, tachycardia, vomiting, and hypotension; older dogs may be at higher risk for hypotension.[6]

For patients that have experienced or are suspected to have experienced an overdose, consultation with a 24-hour poison consultation center specializing in providing veterinary-specific information is recommended. For general information related to overdose and toxin exposures, as well as contact information for poison control centers, refer to ***Appendix***.

Drug Interactions

In humans, tamsulosin is a substrate of CYP 2D and 3A enzyme families. The following drug interactions have either been reported or are theoretical in humans or animals receiving tamsulosin and may be of significance in veterinary patients. Unless otherwise noted, use together is not necessarily contraindicated, but weigh the potential risks and perform additional monitoring when appropriate.

- **Alpha-1 Adrenergic Receptor Agonists** (eg, **phenylephrine**): May decrease the effects of each other
- **Cimetidine**: May increase tamsulosin concentration
- **Clarithromycin & Erythromycin**: May increase plasma concentration of tamsulosin
- **Hypotensive Agents** (eg, **amlodipine, atenolol, enalapril, telmisartan**): May have additive hypotensive effects
- **Ketoconazole**: May increase plasma concentration of tamsulosin
- **Phosphodiesterase Type 5 (PDE5) Inhibitors** (eg, **sildenafil, tadalafil**): May have additive hypotensive effects
- **Terbinafine**: May increase plasma concentration of tamsulosin
- **Warfarin**: Drug interaction studies with tamsulosin are inconclusive; use together with caution.

Laboratory Considerations

- No laboratory test interactions reported

Dosages

DOGS:

Ureteral/urethral relaxant (extra-label): 0.01 – 0.2 mg/kg PO once daily.[8-10] Anecdotally, may increase frequency to every 12 hours if no effects are seen with once-daily dosing. Safety, efficacy, and dosages have not been determined; compounded capsules may be required for dosing.

CATS:

Ureteral/urethral relaxant (extra-label): An anecdotal dosage of 0.004 – 0.006 mg/kg PO once daily has been noted.[11] Safety, efficacy, and dosages have not been determined; compounded capsules are required.

Monitoring

- Clinical efficacy
- Baseline blood pressure; periodic blood pressure checks if adverse effects related to hypotension occur

Client Information

- Do not crush or allow animal to chew beads found inside capsule.
- This medicine may take several days to work at its peak effect.

Chemistry/Synonyms

Tamsulosin hydrochloride is a white or almost white crystalline powder that melts with decomposition at ≈230°C (446°F). It is slightly soluble in water or ethanol, sparingly soluble in methanol, and practically insoluble in ether.

Tamsulosin may also be known as LY253351, YM-12617-1, YM617, *Flomax*®, *Flowmaxtra*®, *Omexel*®, or *Omnic*®.

Storage/Stability

Do not store tablets above 25°C (77°F); protect from moisture.

Compatibility/Compounding Considerations

Tamsulosin capsules are manufactured in a sustained-release presentation to avoid rapid absorption and the associated hypotensive effects; therefore, they should not be crushed or compounded into an oral suspension. Capsule contents are small sustained-release beads that could be compounded into smaller sized capsules for use in dogs or cats.

Dosage Forms/Regulatory Status

VETERINARY-LABELED PRODUCTS: NONE

HUMAN-LABELED PRODUCTS:

Tamsulosin HCl Capsules: 0.4 mg; *Flomax*®, generic; (Rx)

References

For the complete list of references, see **wiley.com/go/budde/plumb**

Taurine

(***tor***-een)

Amino Acid Nutritional

Prescriber Highlights

- ► Used primarily for the treatment of taurine deficiency cardiomyopathies in dogs and cats
- ► Because of its low cost, low potential for toxicity, and the limitations of testing for taurine deficiency, routine taurine supplementation in cats with dilated cardiomyopathy (DCM) is advised.
- ► May also be useful for many other conditions (eg, seizures, hepatic lipidosis), but little or no supporting data available

Uses/Indications

Taurine has proven beneficial in preventing retinal degeneration and the prevention and adjunctive treatment of dilated cardiomyopathy (DCM) in cats caused by taurine deficiency. These conditions are rarely seen today when a modern, reputable commercial feline diet is fed. Supplementation with taurine (± carnitine) is also used in dogs with DCM in susceptible breeds (eg, American cocker spaniels, golden retrievers).[1] Studies have shown that taurine supplementation may be useful as adjunctive treatment for DCM in animals even if taurine deficiency is not present.[2] Because of taurine's low toxicity, some clinicians have also suggested it can be tried for a multitude of conditions (eg, seizures, hepatic lipidosis) in humans and animals; unfortunately, little scientific evidence exists for these other uses.

Pharmacology/Actions

Taurine is an important amino acid for bile acid conjugation, especially in dogs and cats. In vivo, taurine is synthesized from methionine. Cysteinesulfinic acid decarboxylase (CSAD) and vitamin B_6 are involved with this synthesis. Deficiencies of either will depress taurine synthesis. Cats are particularly susceptible to taurine deficiency, as they have low CSAD activity and use taurine almost exclusively for bile acid conjugation.

Additionally, taurine is important in the modulation of calcium flux, thereby reducing platelet aggregation, stabilizing neuronal membranes, and affecting cardiac function. Taurine's effects on cardiac function include positive inotropic activity without affecting resting potential and modulating ionic currents across the cell membrane. Taurine is important for normal development of the CNS, and it has a GABA-like effect that may make it useful for treating some seizure disorders.

Pharmacokinetics

No specific information was located. Excess taurine is rapidly excreted in the kidneys, but if a deficiency exists, urinary excretion is reduced via reabsorption.

Contraindications/Precautions/Warnings

Although taurine is safe, it should not be used as a substitute for adequate diagnosis.

Adverse Effects

Taurine appears to be well tolerated. Minor GI distress potentially could occur after oral dosing.

Overdose/Acute Toxicity

No specific information was located, but toxic potential appears to be low.

For patients that have experienced or are suspected to have experienced an overdose, consultation with a 24-hour poison consultation center specializing in providing veterinary-specific information is recommended. For general information related to overdose and toxin exposures, as well as contact information for poison control centers, refer to ***Appendix***.

Drug Interactions

- None noted

Laboratory Considerations

- To determine actual status of taurine in the body, whole blood taurine levels are preferred to plasma levels. Intracellular levels of taurine are much higher than in plasma, and hemolysis or collection of the buffy coat will negate the results. However, whole blood assays may also yield false-positive results in animals that are in a prolonged fasting state or anorectic; false-negative results may be obtained after postprandial sampling, a recent dietary change, or recent thromboembolism.[3]

Dosages

DOGS:

Dilated cardiomyopathy (DCM) (extra-label):

a) 500 – 1000 mg/dog (NOT mg/kg) PO every 8 to 12 hours for dogs weighing less than 25 kg (55.1 lb) and 1 – 2 g/dog (NOT g/kg) PO every 8 to 12 hours for dogs weighing more than 25 kg (55.1 lb)[4,5]

b) 30 – 100 mg/kg/day PO subjectively improved some echocardiographic left ventricular measurements in English cocker spaniels.[6]

Adjunctive antiepileptic (extra-label): 22 mg/kg PO twice daily may help decrease seizure activity.[7]

CATS:

Adjunctive therapy for DCM associated with taurine deficiency (extra-label): 250 mg/cat (NOT mg/kg) PO every 12 hours[8]

Adjunctive antiepileptic (extra-label): 100 – 400 mg/cat (NOT mg/kg) PO once daily[9]

Adjunctive treatment of hepatopathies (extra-label): Anecdotally, 250 – 500 mg/cat (NOT mg/kg) PO twice daily. No clinical studies document efficacy, but some in vitro data support use.

Monitoring

- Clinical efficacy. Clinical improvement in cats with taurine-responsive dilated cardiomyopathy (DCM) is usually seen within 2 weeks; significant echocardiographic improvement may take 4 weeks or more.[3]
- Taurine levels: whole blood levels preferable to plasma/serum

levels

Client Information

- This medicine is usually tolerated well but may cause vomiting. If your animal vomits or acts sick after receiving the medicine on an empty stomach, try giving the next dose with food or a small treat. If vomiting continues, contact your veterinarian.
- Your veterinarian will need to monitor your animal while it is taking this medicine. Do not miss these important follow-up visits.
- If using a powder form of this medicine, it can be mixed into your animal's food.

Chemistry/Synonyms

Taurine, an amino acid also known as 2-aminosulphonic acid, has a molecular weight of 125. Solubility in 100 mL of water at 20°C (68°F) is 8.8 grams.

Storage/Stability

Unless otherwise labeled, store taurine tablets or capsules at room temperature. Protect this product from light and moisture.

Compatibility/Compounding Considerations

No specific information was noted.

Dosage Forms/Regulatory Status

VETERINARY-LABELED PRODUCTS:

The following products are labeled (not FDA-approved drugs) for use in animals:

Taurine Tablets: 250 mg; *Formula V® Taurine Tablets*. Labeled for use in cats

Taurine Liquid: 375 mg/4 mL (one pump); *Dyna-Taurine®*. Labeled for use in dogs and cats

HUMAN-LABELED PRODUCTS:

There are several oral dosage form products available for taurine. Technically considered a nutrient they are all OTC and may need to be obtained from health food stores. Most dosage forms available range from 125 mg to 500 mg.

References

For the complete list of references, see **wiley.com/go/budde/plumb**

Telmisartan

(***tel***-mi-***sar***-tan) *Semintra®, Micardis®*
Angiotensin-II Receptor Blocker (ARB)

Prescriber Highlights

- Indicated in cats for control of systemic hypertension and for treatment of proteinuria associated with chronic kidney disease (CKD)
- May also be useful in dogs for the adjunctive treatment of proteinuria and systemic hypertension secondary to CKD
- GI effects (vomiting, diarrhea) and lethargy are the most commonly reported adverse effects in cats. Hypotension, increases in liver enzymes, and anemia are possible but uncommon.
- Not safe for use during pregnancy
- Dispense with Client Information Sheet

Uses/Indications

Telmisartan is used for the adjunctive treatment of systemic hypertension and proteinuria in both dogs and cats.

Telmisartan is approved for control of systemic hypertension in cats. In both a United States clinical trial[1] as well as a European clinical trial,[2] telmisartan significantly reduced mean systolic blood pressure compared to placebo in hypertensive cats. In the United States trial, systolic blood pressure at 28 days decreased on average by ≈24 mm Hg compared to ≈12 mm Hg in the placebo group and this decrease persisted over the 6 months of the trial.[1] In the European trial, telmisartan reduced mean baseline systolic blood pressure by ≈25 mm Hg compared to an ≈11 mm Hg decrease in the placebo group.[2] In the EU, the drug is approved for the reduction of proteinuria associated with chronic kidney disease (CKD) in cats.

An open-label study of telmisartan in 28 dogs with proteinuric chronic kidney disease found that telmisartan reduced the urine protein-to-creatinine ratio by 65% and the systolic blood pressure by 10% compared to placebo.[3] A prospective, randomized, double-masked clinical trial in 39 dogs found that telmisartan resulted in a greater decrease (-65%) in urine protein-to-creatinine ratio compared to enalapril (-35%).[4] Finally, in an observational study of 42 dogs, telmisartan in combination with an angiotensin-converting enzyme inhibitor significantly reduced systolic blood pressure and urine protein-to-creatinine ratio.[5]

Telmisartan is being investigated as an adjunctive antiepileptic drug in dogs with refractory idiopathic epilepsy.[6]

Pharmacology/Actions

Telmisartan is an angiotensin-II receptor blocker (ARB). By selectively blocking the AT1-receptor, aldosterone synthesis and secretion is reduced causing vasodilation and decreased potassium and increased sodium excretion. While plasma concentrations of renin and angiotensin-II are increased, this does not counteract the blood pressure lowering effects of telmisartan. Telmisartan does not interfere with substance P or bradykinin responses. The product label (UK) for cats states that, *...telmisartan does not affect potassium excretion, as shown in the clinical field trial in cats.*

A study in healthy cats ($n = 6$) found that telmisartan 3 mg/kg PO, when compared to benazepril 2.5 mg/cat PO, significantly better attenuated blood pressure increases secondary to angiotensin I administration at 90 minutes and 24 hours.[7]

Pharmacokinetics

In cats, telmisartan oral solution bioavailability is ≈33% and peak concentrations occur in ≈30 minutes. Food delays the magnitude of and time to peak concentration, and also reduces overall absorption.[8,9] Systemic exposure is ≈60% lower in female cats compared to male cats.[8] Distribution data for cats were not located, but the drug is highly lipophilic and, in other species (rats, dogs, humans), is highly bound (greater than 99.5%) to plasma proteins. Absorbed drug is primarily metabolized via glucuronidation; the cat genetic defect UGT1A6 does not affect glucuronidation.[10] The major metabolite is telmisartan-O-acylglucuronide, which is not active. Elimination half-life is ≈8 hours.[8,9]

In dogs, peak plasma concentrations occur 45 minutes after oral administration and the half-life is 5.4 hours.[11]

In humans, oral bioavailability of telmisartan is dose dependent and ranges from 42% (40 mg) to 58% (160 mg).[12] Food slightly reduces bioavailability. Absorbed drug is highly protein bound (greater than 99.5%) and volume of distribution ≈500 L. It is conjugated via glucuronidation to the pharmacologically inactive acylglucuronide. Elimination kinetics are bi-exponential and the terminal half-life is ≈1 day.

Contraindications/Precautions/Warnings

Telmisartan is contraindicated in patients that are hypersensitive to it. It is not known if cross-reactivity occurs between other ARBs and telmisartan. The drug has not been evaluated in patients with systolic blood pressure greater than 200 mmHg, with hepatic disease, or less than 6[13] to 9 months old.[8]

Hypotensive patients should not receive this drug. Patients that are volume or electrolyte depleted should not receive this drug until blood volume and electrolytes have been replenished and corrected.

This drug should not be used in pregnant animals. The human label has the following black box warning[12]: *Fetal toxicity: When pregnancy is detected, discontinue telmisartan as soon as possible. Drugs that act directly on the renin-angiotensin system can cause injury and even death to the developing fetus.* See ***Reproductive/Nursing Safety***.

Telmisartan should be used with caution in patients with moderate to severe hepatic impairment; dose reduction may be warranted.

Adverse Effects

In FDA field studies in cats, gastrointestinal distress (vomiting, diarrhea), lethargy, dehydration and weight loss were the most commonly reported side effects.[8,9] Hypotension, requiring dosage reduction, occurred in 16% to 24% of patients. Non-regenerative anemia occurred in 5% to 15% of patients.[9] Less commonly, increases in liver enzyme values, tachycardia, azotemia, and renal insufficiency or failure have been noted.[8,9]

Adverse effects in dogs are comparable, with adverse GI signs (eg, inappetence, vomiting, diarrhea) being the most common (11% of dogs in one study[5]).[4,5] A greater than 30% increase in serum creatinine has been reported in 5% to 25% of dogs.[4,5] Hyperkalemia at 6.2 mEq/L was noted in one of 42 dogs that was also receiving an angiotensin converting enzyme inhibitor in another study.[14]

Reproductive/Nursing Safety

Telmisartan is not considered safe to use during pregnancy. The EU label for the cat product reads: *Do not use during pregnancy or lactation. The safety of Semintra® has not been established in breeding, pregnant or lactating cats.*

Studies in pregnant rats given high doses of ARBs demonstrated a variety of fetal abnormalities (renal pelvic cavitation, hydroureter, absence of renal papilla). Smaller doses in rabbits caused increased maternal death and spontaneous abortion. In humans, the drug is considered teratogenic, particularly during the second and third trimesters. If pregnancy is detected in patients receiving telmisartan, the drug should be discontinued as soon as possible.

It is not known if telmisartan is excreted into cat or dog milk and it is recommended to either halt nursing and use milk replacer or discontinue the drug in nursing animals.

Because safety has not been established in animals, this drug should only be used when the maternal benefits outweigh the potential risks to offspring.

Overdose/Acute Toxicity

Limited information is available. Hypotension and tachycardia are possible; bradycardia could occur from parasympathetic (vagal) stimulation. Patients may present with lethargy, anorexia, trembling, and vomiting. Treat supportively. Telmisartan is not removed by hemodialysis.

In chronic toxicity studies done in cats of up to 5 mg/kg/day (5 times recommended dose) for 6 months, telmisartan did not cause lethality. Hypotension, decreased red blood cell and reticulocyte counts, and reduced food intake occurred[9]; increased BUN and gastrointestinal effects are possible.

For patients that have experienced or are suspected to have experienced an overdose, consultation with a 24-hour poison control center specializing in providing veterinary-specific information is recommended. For general information related to overdose and toxin exposures, as well as contact information for poison control centers, refer to ***Appendix***.

Drug Interactions

The following drug interactions either have been reported or are theoretical in humans or animals receiving telmisartan and may be of significance in veterinary patients. Unless otherwise noted, use together is not necessarily contraindicated, but weigh the potential risks and perform additional monitoring when appropriate.

- **Angiotensin Converting Enzyme Inhibitors** (ACEIs; eg, **benazepril, enalapril**): Increased risk for adverse effects (eg, hypotension, hyperkalemia, renal function changes); increased monitoring may be warranted.
- **Aspirin**: Possible reduced antihypertensive effect of telmisartan and increased risk for renal impairment; increased monitoring may be warranted.
- **Baclofen**: Concurrent use may have additive blood pressure lower effects.
- **Benzodiazepines** (eg, **diazepam, lorazepam**): Concurrent use may increase risk for hypotension.
- **Buspirone**: Concurrent use may increase risk for hypotension.
- **Cabergoline**: Concurrent use may increase risk for hypotension.
- **Corticosteroids** (eg, **betamethasone, dexamethasone**): May decrease the antihypertensive effects of ARBs
- **Dexmedetomidine**: Concurrent use may result in additive effects on blood pressure and heart rate.
- **Diazoxide**: Concurrent use may increase risk for hypotension.
- **Dichlorphenamide**: Concurrent use may increase risk for hypotension.
- **Digoxin**: Concurrent use may increase digoxin levels. Closely monitor digoxin levels and therapeutic effects.
- **Diphenhydramine**: Concurrent use may increase risk for hypotension.
- **Doxepin**: Concurrent use may increase risk for hypotension.
- **Insulin**: Concurrent use may increase risk for hypoglycemia.
- **Heparin, Low Molecular Weight Heparins** (eg, **dalteparin, enoxaparin**): Concurrent use may increase risk for hyperkalemia.
- **Nonsteroidal Anti-Inflammatory Drugs** (NSAIDs; eg, **carprofen, meloxicam**): Possible reduced antihypertensive effects of telmisartan and increased risk for renal impairment; increased monitoring may be warranted.
- **Opioids** (eg, **buprenorphine, butorphanol**): Concurrent use may increase risk for hypotension.
- **Potassium Preparations** (including potassium bromide): Increased risk for hyperkalemia; increased monitoring of serum potassium may be warranted.
- **Potassium-Sparing Diuretics** (eg, **spironolactone**): Increased risk for hyperkalemia; increased monitoring of serum potassium may be warranted.
- **Yohimbine**: Concurrent use may decrease the efficacy of ARBs.

Laboratory Considerations

No specific information noted.

Dosages

DOGS:

Reduction of proteinuria associated with chronic kidney disease | CKD (extra-label): 1 mg/kg PO once daily.[3-5] One study escalated the dosage to a maximum of 3 mg/kg PO once daily for cases with persistent proteinuria.[4]

Systemic hypertension (extra-label): 1 mg/kg PO once daily[15]

CATS:

Control of systemic hypertension (label dosage; FDA-approved): 1.5 mg/kg PO twice daily for the first 14 days, then 2 mg/kg PO once daily. Reduce dose in 0.5 mg/kg increments to manage hypotension; the minimum dose is 0.5 mg/kg PO once daily. May be administered either directly into the cat's mouth or on top of a small amount of food (do not mix into food). Cats that vomit within 30 minutes of administration may be redosed.[8]

Reduction of proteinuria associated with chronic kidney disease | CKD (extra-label): Using the oral solution: 1 mg/kg PO (directly into mouth or with a small amount of food) once daily.[16]

Monitoring

- Blood pressure, signs of target organ damage (eg, retinal lesions). In field studies in cats, dosage reduction for systolic BP less than 120 mm Hg was allowed.
- Depending on reason for use and patient's clinical condition: baseline and periodic serum chemistry panel (including renal values, liver enzymes, and electrolytes [especially potassium]), urine protein, UPC, volume/hydration status, and body weight
- Baseline and periodic CBC[17]
- Monitor for vomiting, diarrhea, or weight loss after initiating therapy.

Client Information

- Dispense with Client Information Sheet
- This medication is best absorbed when given on an empty stomach but may be given with or without food.
- The most common side effects are vomiting, diarrhea, lack of appetite, low energy level, anemia, dehydration, and low blood pressure (fainting, weakness, inability to exercise).
- This medicine has caused birth defects and should not be used in pregnant animals. If a human in the household is pregnant, they should be very careful not to ingest the medication and should avoid contact with telmisartan (ie, wear disposable gloves when administering doses and wash their hands after handling).

Chemistry/Synonyms

Telmisartan [CAS Registry: 144701-48-4; ATCvet code: QC09CA07] occurs as a white or slightly yellowish, crystalline powder. It is practically insoluble in water, slightly soluble in methyl alcohol, sparingly soluble in dichloromethane, and dissolves in 1M sodium hydroxide.

The feline product (*Semintra*®) is a clear, colorless to yellowish viscous oral solution; excipients include: hydroxyethylcellulose, manitol, and benzalkonium chloride.

Telmisartan may also be known as BIBR 277 SE. Trade names include *Micardis*® and *Semintra*®.

Storage/Stability

Telmisartan solution for cats may be stored at room temperature (at or below 25°C; 77°F) with excursions permitted up to 40°C (104°F) with the cap tightly closed. The label states that shelf life is 6 months after first opening the bottle. Telmisartan tablets should be stored at room temperature (up to 30°C; 86°F); do not remove from blisters until immediately before administration.

Compatibility/Compounding Considerations

The UK label for the cat product states: "In the absence of compatibility studies, this veterinary medicinal product must not be mixed with other veterinary products."

Dosage Forms/Regulatory Status

VETERINARY-LABELED PRODUCTS:

Telmisartan Oral Solution: 10 mg/mL in 35 mL bottle with oral measuring syringe; *Semintra*®; (Rx). NADA# 141-501.

Telmisartan Oral Solution: 4 mg/mL in 30 mL bottle with oral measuring syringe; *Semintra*®; (In the UK/EU and Canada: POM-V).

HUMAN-LABELED PRODUCTS:

Oral Tablets: 20 mg, 40 mg, and 80 mg; *Micardis*®, generic; (Rx)

References

For the complete list of references, see **wiley.com/go/budde/plumb**

Terbinafine

(***ter***-bih-nah-feen) *Lamisil*®

Antifungal

Prescriber Highlights

- ▶ Used primarily for dermatophytosis; may also be useful for systemic fungal infections
- ▶ Fewer drug interactions than azole antifungals
- ▶ Appears to be well tolerated; adverse effects are primarily GI related (eg, vomiting, diarrhea)
- ▶ Use with caution in patients with liver or renal disease.

Uses/Indications

Terbinafine may be useful for treating dermatophyte and systemic fungal infections (eg, blastomycosis, histoplasmosis, coccidioidomycosis, cryptococcosis, sporotrichosis) in dogs, cats, birds, and other species. Terbinafine may also be used for the treatment of *Malassezia* spp dermatitis, and *Aspergillus* spp and *Candida* spp infections.

Pharmacology/Actions

Terbinafine is an inhibitor of the synthesis of ergosterol, a component of fungal cell membranes. By blocking the enzyme squalene monooxygenase (ie, squalene 2,3-epoxidase), terbinafine inhibits the conversion of squalene to sterols (especially ergosterol) and causes accumulation of squalene. Both of these effects are thought to contribute to its antifungal action.

Terbinafine has far greater activity (1000 times or more) on fungal squalene monooxygenase as compared with the similar human enzyme. Unlike azole antifungals, terbinafine's mechanism for inhibiting ergosterol is not mediated via the cytochrome P450 enzyme system and therefore does not alter testosterone or cortisol production and has fewer drug interactions. However, terbinafine is a competitive inhibitor of CYP2D6 in humans.

Terbinafine primarily has clinical activity (fungicidal) against dermatophytes (eg, *Microsporum* spp, *Trichophyton* spp). It may only be fungistatic against the yeasts (eg, *Candida* spp). Terbinafine has activity against *Aspergillus* spp, *Blastomyces dermatitidis*, *Coccidioidomyces immitis*, *Histoplasma capsulatum*, *Sporothrix schenckii*, and *Cryptococcus neoformans*. When used by itself, terbinafine is not very effective for pythiosis, but it displays synergy when combined with other antifungals.[1] Terbinafine resistance in *Microsporum canis* has been documented in a cat.[2]

In an in vivo human experimental model, terbinafine was shown to possess anti-inflammatory properties, although the exact mechanism and veterinary clinical significance remains unclear.[3]

Pharmacokinetics

In dogs, a single-dose study of terbinafine (30 – 35 mg/kg with food) showed maximum serum concentrations of ≈3.5 µg/mL and average time to maximum concentration of ≈3.5 hours after administration.[4] In greyhounds, the same dose resulted in slightly higher maximum serum concentrations (≈4 µg/mL) and a shorter time to maximum concentration (≈2 hours). Terbinafine is widely distributed and highly protein bound (more than 99%).[5] A half-life of ≈8.6 hours was reported for greyhounds.[6] Following the 30 – 35 mg/kg PO dose, the time above MIC was maintained for ≈18 to 19 hours.[4] After 21 days of 30 mg/kg PO once-daily dosing, low skin and sebum concentrations were seen compared to serum. Maximum concentration in the stratum corneum and the sebum barely exceeded *Malassezia* spp MIC_{90}.[7]

In cats, after a single fasted oral dose of 30 mg/kg, peak concentrations (≈3.2 µg/mL) occurred ≈1.3 hours after dosing. Elimination half-life was ≈8 to 10 hours.[8] Although oral bioavailability was low at ≈30%, terbinafine appears to achieve high enough concentrations at the site of action; cats dosed at 34 – 46 mg/kg PO once daily for 14 days had terbinafine concentrations in hair that persisted above the MIC of most dermatophytes for several weeks.[9]

In horses, maximum plasma concentration after oral dosing was ≈0.3 µg/mL,[6,10] and time to maximum concentration was ≈1.5 hours. Half-life is ≈8 hours.[6,10] Volume of distribution (Vd/F) was ≈131 L/kg, and clearance was 187 mL/minute/kg. Because IV terbinafine was not administered, volume of distribution and clearance are reported as per fraction of drug available.[11] Rectal administration resulted in low plasma concentrations compared with oral administration.[10]

In humans, more than 70% of terbinafine given orally is absorbed; after first-pass metabolism, bioavailability is ≈40%. Food may increase absorption by up to 20%. Terbinafine is distributed into and attains high concentration in hair, nails, skin, and sebum. More than 99% of drug in plasma is bound to plasma proteins. Drug in the circulation is metabolized in the liver and the effective half-life is ≈36 hours. Approximately 70% of the drug is renally excreted as metabolites, and another 20% is excreted in the feces.[12] Terbinafine clearance is decreased ≈50% in patients with renal impairment or hepatic cirrhosis. The drug may persist in adipose tissue and skin for long periods of time.

Contraindications/Precautions/Warnings

Terbinafine is contraindicated in patients that are hypersensitive to it and in patients with active or chronic liver disease.[12] Use terbinafine with caution in patients with significantly impaired renal function. If terbinafine is to be used in veterinary patients with markedly impaired liver or renal function, do so with extreme caution; dosage adjustments should be considered. Liver failure leading to transplant or death has occurred in humans with and without pre-existing liver disease.

In humans, loss of taste and smell have been reported.[12] It is unknown if this effect occurs in animals; use terbinafine with caution in working dogs that rely on olfaction.

Do not confuse LamISIL with LaMICtal or LOMOtil, or terbINAafine with terBUTaline.

Adverse Effects

Because of limited use in veterinary patients, the adverse effect profile is not well defined. In general, terbinafine appears to be well tolerated. GI effects (eg, vomiting, inappetence, diarrhea) are possible. Reportedly, the oral tablets can have an unpleasant taste and may contribute to GI or behavioral adverse effects or dosing avoidance.

In dogs, excessive panting and elevated liver enzymes have been noted.[13] Ocular effects have also been reported in 2 dogs including periocular swelling, chemosis, and conjunctival erythema. Signs resolved within 24 to 36 hours of terbinafine administration, and ophthalmological examination after study completion was within normal limits. No recurrence of ocular effects was seen with follow-up administration.[4]

In a case report in 2 cats, 1 cat developed lethargy.[14] Facial pruritus in some treated cats has also been reported.[9]

In horses, signs of unpleasant taste or oral irritation (eg, lip curling, pawing at ground, opening/closing mouth, head shaking, excessive tongue movements, nostril flaring) were seen after PO administration.[6,10] Subclinical fever was reported in 1 horse.[10] Signs resolved spontaneously, but transient colic could not be ruled out.

Regurgitation was common in red-tailed hawks.[15]

In humans, photosensitivity has been reported with terbinafine use. Very rarely, liver failure, neutropenia, or serious skin reactions (eg, toxic epidermal necrolysis [TEN], Stevens-Johnson syndrome) have occurred after terbinafine use. Disturbances or loss of smell and taste have also been reported[12]; whether or how this may impact working animals is uncertain.

Reproductive/Nursing Safety

It is unknown if terbinafine crosses the placenta. High-dose studies in pregnant rabbits and rats have not demonstrated overt fetotoxicity or teratogenicity. Although risk appears low, use with caution in pregnant animals.

The drug enters maternal milk at concentrations 7 times that found in plasma; the manufacturer recommends that mothers do not nurse while taking this drug.

Because safety has not been established, this drug should only be used when the maternal benefits outweigh the potential fetal risks.

Overdose/Acute Toxicity

Limited information available; humans have taken doses up to 5 g (total dose) without serious effects. Clinical signs are expected to be extensions of the drug's adverse effects. See ***Adverse Effects***.

For patients that have experienced or are suspected of having experienced an overdose, it is strongly encouraged to consult with one of the 24-hour poison consultation centers that specialize in providing information specific for veterinary patients. For general information related to overdose and toxin exposures, as well as contact information for poison control centers, refer to ***Appendix***.

Drug Interactions

The following drug interactions have either been reported or are theoretical in humans or animals receiving terbinafine and may be of significance in veterinary patients. Unless otherwise noted, use together is not necessarily contraindicated, but weigh the potential risks and perform additional monitoring when appropriate.

- CIMETIDINE: Inhibits terbinafine metabolism and increases terbinafine absorption and exposure[10]
- CYCLOSPORINE: Terbinafine may increase the elimination of cyclosporine.
- FLUCONAZOLE: Inhibits terbinafine metabolism and increases terbinafine exposure
- RIFAMPIN: May increase terbinafine clearance

Because terbinafine is an inhibitor of CYP2D6 in humans, it could reduce the metabolism of:

- ANTIARRHYTHMICS (eg, **lidocaine, mexiletine, procainamide**)
- BETA-BLOCKERS (eg, **metoprolol, propranolol**)
- CODEINE (blocks the conversion to morphine)
- DEXTROMETHORPHAN
- DOXORUBICIN
- MONOAMINE OXIDASE INHIBITORS (MAOIs; eg, **amitraz, selegiline**)
- METHADONE
- METOCLOPRAMIDE
- ONDANESTRON
- SELECTIVE SEROTONIN RECEPTOR INHIBITORS (SSRIs; eg, **fluoxetine, sertraline**)
- TAMSULOSIN
- TRAMADOL
- TRAZODONE
- TRICYCLIC ANTIDEPRESSANTS (TCAs; eg, **amitriptyline, clomipramine, doxepin**)

Laboratory Considerations

- None

Dosages

DOGS:

Systemic mycoses | blastomycosis, coccidioidomycosis, cryptococcosis, histoplasmosis, sporotrichosis (extra-label): 30 mg/kg PO every 24 hours.[16-19] Based on a pharmacokinetic study, twice-daily dosing may be considered.[4] Use of terbinafine as a single agent is not recommended.[4]

Cryptococcosis (extra-label): From a case report, after primary therapy with amphotericin B and fluconazole had failed, a dog received terbinafine 30 mg/kg PO once daily. Insufficient data are currently available to recommend terbinafine as a first-line agent, but in cases where primary therapy has failed to yield a response, it may prove beneficial.[19]

Colonic pythiosis (extra-label): Terbinafine 6 – 12 mg/kg PO once daily in combination with itraconazole 5 – 10 mg/kg PO once daily.[20–24] This combination may be used in conjunction with mefenoxam 4 mg/kg PO every 12 hours[20–22] or prednisone.[23] Terbinafine as a single agent is not recommended for treatment of pythiosis.[4]

Refractory sinonasal aspergillosis (extra-label): For dogs that have not responded to conventional topical and systemic therapy for sinonasal aspergillosis, terbinafine 30 mg/kg PO every 12 hours in combination with posaconazole 5 mg/kg PO every 12 hours and doxycycline 5 mg/kg PO every 12 hours; treatment continued for 6 to 18 months. 70% of dogs achieved complete remission and 30% partial remission.[25]

Dermatophytosis (extra-label): 30 – 40 mg/kg PO every 24 hours[26]; treatment should continue until mycological cure (ie, 2 negative skin cultures taken 2 weeks apart).

***Malassezia* spp dermatitis** (extra-label): 30 mg/kg PO once daily.[7] **NOTE**: Terbinafine was only partially effective, and concentration achieved in the stratum corneum and sebum was only slightly higher than *Malassezia* spp MIC_{90}. Higher terbinafine doses or other drug therapy (eg, ketoconazole, itraconazole) may be required.

CATS:

Systemic mycoses:

Cryptococcal CNS infections (extra-label): 10 mg/kg PO once daily can rectify the clinical signs though cats with CNS cryptococcosis usually require lifelong treatment.[27]

Sporotrichosis (extra-label): 30 mg/cat (NOT mg/kg) PO once daily as an alternative for the treatment of cats that do not tolerate itraconazole, in cases that respond poorly, and/or if an azole resistance is suspected. May be used in combination with itraconazole 5 – 10 mg/kg PO every 24 hours[28,29] or posaconazole.[30]

Dermatophytosis (extra-label):

a) **Pulse therapy**: 20 mg/kg PO once daily for 7 days, then 21 days off, followed by 40 mg/kg PO daily for 7 days[31]
b) Using terbinafine 250 mg tablets, cats weighing less than 2.8 kg (6.1 lb) received ¼ of a tablet (62.5 mg) per dose, cats weighing 2.8 to 5.5 kg (6.1 to 12.1 lb) received ½ a tablet (125 mg) per dose, and cats weighing greater than 5.5 kg (12.1 lb) received 1 tablet (250 mg) per dose. Administered once daily with food for 21 days in combination with twice-weekly lime sulfur rinses[32]

Sinonasal aspergillosis (extra-label): 15 mg/kg PO every 12 hours.[33] Lower dosages 5 – 10 mg/kg PO every 12 to 24 hours also have been reported,[34–36] and are based primarily on author experience or case reports.

BIRDS:

Aspergillosis (extra-label):

a) Terbinafine 10 – 15 mg/kg PO every 12 to 24 hours in combination with itraconazole 5 – 10 mg/kg PO every 12 hours[37]
b) A single oral dose pharmacokinetic study in red-tailed hawks concluded that terbinafine 22 mg/kg PO once a day results in steady-state trough plasma concentrations above the MIC and is recommended as a potential treatment option for aspergillosis in raptors; however, additional research is required to determine both treatment efficacy and safety.[38]
c) **Nebulization therapy**: A pharmacokinetic study using nebulized terbinafine (1 mg/mL solution nebulized for 15 minutes) in Hispaniolan Amazon parrots concluded that higher concentrations of nebulization solutions, nebulization times greater than 15 minutes, or more frequent nebulization is likely needed to reach clinically relevant systemic terbinafine concentrations.[39] The relationship between plasma concentrations and lung or air sac concentrations after nebulization of terbinafine still needs to be determined and further studies are warranted to determine the optimal technique for dissolving terbinafine in solution, as well as to determine the best concentration of terbinafine and particle size to nebulize. Pharmacodynamic studies are also necessary to determine therapeutic plasma concentrations.

REPTILES:

Antifungal (extra-label):

a) **Nebulization therapy**: From a pharmacokinetic study, 18 mg/reptile (NOT mg/kg) delivered via 30-minute nebulization into a sealed 10-gallon aquarium achieved therapeutic plasma concentrations.[40] Terbinafine 2 mg/mL solution was prepared by dissolving terbinafine powder, USP in sterile saline. Efficacy would need to be confirmed with clinical studies.
b) From a case report in an Aldabra tortoise, 3.3 mg/kg PO once daily for 15 months was used to treat phaeohyphomycosis of the carapace.[41]

HEDGEHOGS:

Dermatophytosis (extra-label): 100 mg/kg PO twice daily for 28 days reduced clinical lesions and resulted in ≈99% mycological cure rate. The mycological cure rate was significantly better than with itraconazole.[42]

Monitoring

- Clinical efficacy
- Baseline liver enzymes; repeat periodically as needed (especially if treating long-term) based on clinical signs and development of adverse effects.
- Fungal cultures (eg, Dermatophyte Test Media [DTM]) for dermatophytosis

Client Information

- This medicine may be given with or without food.
- This medicine is usually tolerated well. The most common side effect is vomiting.
- If your animal vomits after receiving this medicine on an empty stomach, try giving it with food. Contact your veterinarian if your animal continues to vomit after receiving this medicine.
- Your veterinarian will need to monitor your animal while it is taking this medicine. Do not miss these important follow-up visits.

Chemistry/Synonyms

A synthetic allylamine antifungal, terbinafine HCl occurs as a white to off-white, fine, crystalline powder. It is slightly soluble in water and soluble in ethanol.

Terbinafine HCl may also be known as *Alamil®*, *Daskil®*, *Daskyl®*, *DesenexMax®*, *Finex®*, *Lamisil®*, *Micosil®*, *Terbinex®*, *Terbisil®*, or *Terekol®*.

Storage/Stability

Terbinafine tablets should be stored at room temperature (25°C [77°F]) in tight containers, with excursions permitted from 15°C to 30°C (59°F-86°F); protect from light.

Compatibility/Compounding Considerations

In a pharmacokinetic study for terbinafine nebulization in parrots, one 250 mg tablet was crushed and dissolved into 250 mL sterile water to make a 1 mg/mL solution. Before nebulization, the solution was agitated before being mixed with a stir bar for 12 hours. Terbinafine concentrations of solutions made with a crushed tablet were significantly lower than those made with raw powder, but plasma concentrations did not differ significantly.[43]

Dosage Forms/Regulatory Status

VETERINARY-LABELED PRODUCTS:

No oral products are FDA-approved. An otic solution containing terbinafine (1.48%), florfenicol (1.66%), and mometasone furoate (0.22%) is FDA-approved for treatment of otitis externa in dogs; *Claro*®; (Rx)

HUMAN-LABELED PRODUCTS:

Terbinafine HCl Oral Tablets: 250 mg; *Lamisil*®, generic; (Rx)

A topical cream and a spray (1%) are also available (OTC)

References

For the complete list of references, see **wiley.com/go/budde/plumb**

Terbutaline

(ter-***byoo***-ta-leen) *Brethine*®

Beta-2-Adrenergic Agonist, Tocolytic

Prescriber Highlights

- Used as a bronchodilator or tocolytic; sometimes used to treat bradyarrhythmia or hyperkalemia
- Oral administration is not practical in horses due to low bioavailability.
- May be used in horses to confirm and quantitate anhidrosis
- Caution should be used in patients with diabetes, hyperthyroidism, hypertension, seizure disorders, or cardiac disease (especially with concurrent arrhythmias).
- Adverse effects include increased heart rate, tremors, CNS excitement (eg, nervousness), and hypotension; after parenteral injection in horses, sweating and CNS excitation are possible.

Uses/Indications

Terbutaline is used as a bronchodilating agent in the adjunctive treatment of bronchospasm caused by pulmonary disease (including tracheobronchitis, collapsing trachea, chronic bronchitis, and asthma) in small animal species. Its use for airway collapse in dogs is controversial, as some sources state that terbutaline is not helpful for the treatment of airway collapse,[1,2] while others advocate that it may be helpful in certain patients.[1,3,4] Terbutaline is primarily used as adjunctive therapy in cats with asthma that are already receiving corticosteroid therapy. The drug may be used pre-emptively or intraoperatively for management of bronchospasm in cats undergoing transtracheal wash, bronchoscopy, and bronchoalveolar lavage.[5-9]

Terbutaline may also be beneficial in the treatment of bradyarrhythmias and hyperkalemia in dogs and cats.

In horses, terbutaline has occasionally been used for its bronchodilating effects, but adverse effects, short duration of activity after IV administration, and poor oral absorption have limited its use. Terbutaline can help diagnose anhidrosis in horses after intradermal injection.[10]

Oral and parenteral terbutaline has been used successfully as a tocolytic agent in humans, dogs, and cats for short-term inhibition of premature labor.

Pharmacology/Actions

Terbutaline is a sympathomimetic drug that preferentially stimulates beta-2-adrenergic receptors found primarily in vascular smooth muscle (including bronchial, GI, and uterine tissues) to cause relaxation of bronchial smooth muscle cells, reduced airway resistance, vasodilation, and tocolysis, as well as to inhibit release of bronchoconstrictive mediators from mast cells. At recommended doses, terbutaline spares the beta-1 receptor found primarily in the heart, thus lowering the likelihood for cardiac adverse events; terbutaline's specificity is not as precise at higher doses and some beta-1 activity may occur, resulting in tachycardia and increased myocardial contractility. Occasionally, tachycardia may develop at recommended doses and can be a result of either direct beta-1 stimulation or a reflex response secondary to peripheral vasodilation. Terbutaline also promotes intracellular shift of potassium through activation of Na^+ K^+ ATPase enzyme system.

Terbutaline has virtually no alpha-adrenergic activity.

Pharmacokinetics

Studies in dogs found that 16.9% to 46.6% of the IV dose was excreted within 2 to 4 hours and greater than 95% of doses administered IV, SC, or PO were excreted within 24 hours.[11,12] Peak serum concentrations of terbutaline administered SC in dogs occurred within ≈30 minutes; peak serum concentrations following PO administration occurred between 2 to 6 hours.[12]

In horses, terbutaline is poorly absorbed after oral administration and has a bioavailability less than 1%.[13] Mean residence time is ≈30 minutes in horses when the drug is given IV; administration via IV CRI appears to be necessary to maintain therapeutic serum concentrations.

In humans, only ≈33% to 50% of an oral dose is absorbed; peak bronchial effects occur within 2 to 3 hours and activity persists up to 8 hours.[14]

Terbutaline is well absorbed following SC administration in humans; onset of action occurs within 15 minutes, peak effects are at 30 to 60 minutes, and duration of activity is up to 4 hours. Although terbutaline is principally excreted unchanged in the urine (60%), it is also metabolized in the liver to an inactive sulfate conjugate.[15]

Contraindications/Precautions/Warnings

Terbutaline is contraindicated in patients hypersensitive to it and should be used with caution in patients with diabetes, hyperthyroidism, hypertension, seizure disorders, glaucoma, or cardiac disease (especially with concurrent arrhythmias).

Adverse Effects

Most adverse effects are dose-related and are similar to those of sympathomimetic agents, including increased heart rate, tremors, CNS excitement (eg, nervousness), and dizziness. These effects are generally transient, mild, and do not require discontinuation of therapy. Tachycardia, trembling, sweating, and CNS excitation were reported after IV injection in horses.[13] In horses under injectable general anesthesia, terbutaline at 2 µg/kg IV (once) did not improve PaO_2 and was associated with adverse cardiovascular effects (eg, increased heart rate, decreased blood pressure).[16]

Transient hypokalemia has been reported in humans receiving beta-adrenergic agents. Hyperglycemia, cardiac arrhythmias, and pulmonary edema have been reported in humans.

Reproductive/Nursing Safety

Terbutaline crosses the placenta. No teratogenic effects were noted in pregnant laboratory animals given terbutaline during embryofetal development, but alterations in neonatal behavior and brain development have been noted. Increased fetal heart rate and neonatal hypoglycemia may occur when terbutaline is administered in late pregnancy. Terbutaline has tocolytic effects, but it is recommended that use in humans for this effect be limited to 48 to 72 hours due to adverse maternal effects. In humans, use of this drug should be avoided or minimized during early pregnancy due to the risk for asthma and cardiac defects, and prolonged use should be avoided in the second and third trimesters.[17]

Although terbutaline is excreted in milk at concentrations similar to those found in maternal plasma, use is only recommended when the potential maternal benefit outweighs possible risks for offspring.[15,17]

Overdose/Acute Toxicity

Clinical signs of significant overdose after systemic administration may include arrhythmias (eg, bradycardia, tachycardia, heart block, extrasystoles), hypokalemia, hypertension, fever, muscle tremors, vomiting, mydriasis, and CNS stimulation resulting in seizures. Recent oral ingestion should be handled like other overdoses (eg, gastrointestinal decontamination) if the animal does not have significant cardiac or CNS effects. Treatment should be supportive and based on clinical presentation. Potassium supplementation may be required. If cardiac arrhythmias require treatment, a beta-blocking agent (eg, propranolol[18]) can be used but may precipitate bronchoconstriction.

For patients that have experienced or are suspected to have experienced an overdose, consultation with a 24-hour poison consultation centers that specialize in providing veterinary-specific information is recommended. For general information related to overdose and toxin exposures, as well as contact information for poison control centers, refer to ***Appendix***.

Drug Interactions

The following drug interactions have either been reported or are theoretical in humans or animals receiving terbutaline and may be of significance in veterinary patients. Unless otherwise noted, use together is not necessarily contraindicated, but weigh the potential risks and perform additional monitoring when appropriate.

- **Anesthetics, Inhalation** (eg, **isoflurane**): Use with inhalation anesthetics may predispose the patient to ventricular arrhythmias, particularly in patients with pre-existing cardiac disease—use cautiously.
- **Beta-Adrenergic Receptor Antagonists** (eg, **propranolol**): May antagonize the actions of terbutaline
- **Digoxin**: Use with digitalis glycosides may increase the risk for cardiac arrhythmias.
- **Diuretics** (eg, **furosemide, hydrochlorothiazide**): Beta-agonists may increase the risk for hypokalemia.
- **Monoamine Oxidase Inhibitors (MAOIs**; eg, **amitraz, linezolid, selegiline**): May potentiate the vascular effects of terbutaline
- **Succinylcholine**: Concurrent use may result in enhanced neuromuscular blockade.
- **Sympathomimetics, Other** (eg, **phenylpropanolamine**): Use of terbutaline with other sympathomimetic amines may increase the risk for developing adverse cardiovascular effects.
- **Theophylline**: May result in decreased theophylline concentrations. Combination may precipitate cardiac arrhythmias; sudden death has occurred in humans.
- **Tricyclic Antidepressants** (eg, **amitriptyline, clomipramine**): May potentiate the vascular effects of terbutaline

Laboratory Considerations

- **Macrolide Antibiotics** (eg, azithromycin, clarithromycin): Macrolides induce anhidrosis in foals and may interfere with quantitative intradermal terbutaline sweat test (QITST).[19]

Dosages

NOTES:

1. Do not confuse mg/kg dosages with mg/dog or mg/cat.
2. Terbutaline should not be administered as an IV bolus; administer slowly if IV use cannot be avoided.

DOGS:

Bradyarrhythmias (extra-label): 0.2 mg/kg PO every 8 to 12 hours; improvement is usually partial and often temporary.[20]

Hyperkalemia (extra-label): 0.01 mg/kg IV over 5 to 10 minutes[21,22]

Bronchodilator for small airway collapse/disease (extra-label): 0.625 - 5 mg/dog (NOT mg/kg) every 8 to 12 hours.[3,4,23] Efficacy is debatable for its use in airway collapse/disease in dogs; however, it may be useful in some cases.[1,3,4] If used, it is often instituted for a 1-to-2-week trial to determine its effectiveness in the individual patient, and continued use is based on efficacy as well development of unwanted side effects.

Premature labor as a tocolytic (extra-label): 0.03 mg/kg PO every 8 hours as an initial dose to suppress uterine contractility in bitches with historical loss of otherwise normal pregnancies preterm. The dose should ideally be titrated to effect using tocodynamometry. Terbutaline should be discontinued 48 hours prior to the calculated delivery date so normal labor and delivery can occur. Exogenous progesterone can be added if myometrial contractility cannot be controlled with tocolytics.[24]

Nonischemic priapism (extra-label): 1.25 – 5 mg/dog (NOT mg/kg) PO every 8 to 12 hours in combination with other conservative therapies (eg, lubrication, analgesia) may be beneficial.[24]

CATS:

Bronchodilator (extra-label):

a) **Status asthmaticus**: 0.01 mg/kg SC, IM, or slow IV. Can be considered for home management (SC or IM only) of acute asthma in cats that cannot or will not tolerate use of an albuterol metered-dose inhaler (see ***Albuterol***); positive response (ie, decrease of respiratory rate or effort by 50%) occurs in 15 to 30 minutes.[25,26]
b) **To minimize bronchospasm prior to tracheal wash or bronchoalveolar lavage (BAL)**: 0.625 mg/cat (NOT mg/kg) PO (alternatively, 0.01 mg/kg IM or SC if the cat is intolerant of oral administration) twice daily administered 12 to 24 hours prior to the procedure, with the last dose given 2 to 4 hours before anesthesia induction.[9]

Bradyarrhythmias (extra-label): 0.625 mg/cat (NOT mg/kg) PO every 8 to 12 hours; improvement is usually partial and often temporary.[20]

Hyperkalemia (extra-label): 0.01 mg/kg slow IV over 5 to 10 minutes[21,22]

Premature labor as a tocolytic (extra-label): 0.03 mg/kg PO every 8 hours as an initial dose to suppress uterine contractility in queens with historical loss of otherwise normal pregnancies preterm. The dose should ideally be titrated to effect using tocodynamometry. Terbutaline should be discontinued 48 hours prior to the calculated delivery date so normal labor and delivery can occur. Exogenous progesterone can be added if myometrial contractility cannot be controlled with tocolytics.[24]

HORSES:

Quantitative intradermal terbutaline sweat test (QITST) to identify anhidrosis (extra-label): Prepare eight 0.1 mL intradermal injections of serial 10-fold terbutaline dilutions (0 [control], 0.001, 0.01, 0.1, 1, 10, 100, and 1000 mg/L) using 0.9% sodium chloride; sequentially administer diluted solutions with a 25-gauge needle at ≈5 cm intervals. Apply preweighed absorbent padding over each injection site. After 30 minutes, remove and reweigh padding. Anhidrotic horses do not sweat, even at the highest concentrations. See ***Laboratory Considerations***.[10]

BIRDS:

Adjunctive treatment of respiratory distress (extra-label): Terbutaline 0.01 mg/kg IM every 6 to 8 hours in combination with butorphanol 1 – 2 mg/kg IM every 2 to 3 hours are usually given to birds in respiratory distress before placing them in an oxygen-enriched incubator. Treatment can be continued via nebulizer.[27]

REPTILES:

Bronchodilator (extra-label): 0.01 – 0.02 mg/kg IM[28]

Monitoring

- Improvement in clinical signs (eg, cough, respiratory rate and effort); thoracic auscultation
- Cardiac rate and rhythm (if indicated)
- Serum potassium, early in therapy if animal is susceptible to hypokalemia (eg, diuretic therapy)
- Adverse effects, including signs of CNS excitation

Client Information

- This medication can increase heart rate and cause excitement.
- Terbutaline can delay labor in pregnant animals.
- Contact your veterinarian if your animal's condition deteriorates or it becomes acutely ill.
- Overdoses can be serious. Keep this medication out of reach of children and animals.

Chemistry/Synonyms

Terbutaline sulfate, a synthetic sympathomimetic amine, occurs as a slightly bitter-tasting, white to gray-white crystalline powder that may have a faint odor of acetic acid. One gram is soluble in 1.5 mL of water or 250 mL of alcohol. The commercially available injection has its pH adjusted to 3 to 5 with hydrochloric acid.

Terbutaline may also be known as KWD-2019, terbutaline sulphate, or terbutalini sulfas; there are many trade names, including *Brethine®*.

Storage/Stability

Terbutaline should be stored in tight containers at room temperature of 20°C to 25°C (68°F-77°F) and protected from light. Discolored solutions should not be used. Unused portions of terbutaline injection should be discarded.

Compatibility/Compounding Considerations

Compatibility is dependent on factors such as pH, concentration, temperature, and diluent used; specialized references or a hospital pharmacist should be consulted for more specific information.

Terbutaline injection is physically **compatible** with sodium chloride solutions, 5% dextrose, aminophylline, doxapram, and regular insulin.

Dosage Forms/Regulatory Status

VETERINARY-LABELED PRODUCTS: NONE

The Association of Racing Commissioners International (ARCI) has designated this drug as a class 3 substance. Use of this drug may not be allowed in certain animal competitions. Check rules and regulations before entering in a competition while this medication is being administered. Contact local racing authorities for further guidance. See ***Appendix*** for more information.

HUMAN-LABELED PRODUCTS:

Terbutaline Tablets: 2.5 mg and 5 mg; generic; (Rx)

Terbutaline Injection: 1 mg/mL in 1 mL single-dose vials; generic; (Rx)

References

For the complete list of references, see **wiley.com/go/budde/plumb**

Testosterone

(tess-***toss***-ter-ohn)

Androgenic Hormone

Prescriber Highlights

- Principal endogenous androgen used primarily for the treatment of testosterone-responsive urinary incontinence in neutered male dogs and cats; in bovine medicine, it is used to produce an estrus-detector animal.
- Contraindications include known hypersensitivity to the drug, pregnancy, and prostate carcinoma.
- Use with caution in animals with renal, cardiac, or hepatic dysfunction.
- Adverse effects are uncommon in males; however, perianal adenomas, perineal hernias, prostatic disorders, and behavior changes possible. Masculinization and aggression may occur in females.
- The National Institute for Occupational Safety and Health (NIOSH) classifies testosterone as a hazardous drug; use appropriate precautions when handling.
- DEA Schedule III (C-III) controlled substance

Uses/Indications

The use of injectable esters of testosterone in veterinary medicine is primarily limited to its use in dogs (and perhaps cats) for the treatment of testosterone-responsive urinary incontinence in neutered males. Testosterone has been used to treat a rare form of dermatitis (exhibited by bilateral alopecia) in neutered male dogs. Testosterone products are also used in bovine medicine to produce an estrus-detector (teaser) animal in cull cows, heifers, and steers.

The effectiveness of testosterone to increase libido and treat hypogonadism, aspermia, and infertility in domestic animals has been disappointing and is generally not recommended.

Theoretically, topically applied human transdermal products could be effective in animals, but no information was located on their efficacy or safety.

Pharmacology/Actions

Testosterone, the principal endogenous androgenic steroid, is responsible for many secondary sex characteristics of the male, as well as the maturation and growth of the male reproductive organs and increasing libido.

Testosterone has anabolic activity with resultant increased protein anabolism and decreased protein catabolism. Testosterone causes nitrogen, sodium, potassium, and phosphorus retention and decreases the urinary excretion of calcium. Nitrogen balance is improved only when an adequate intake of both calories and protein occurs. By stimulating erythropoietic stimulating factors, testosterone can stimulate the production of red blood cells. Large doses of exogenous testosterone can inhibit spermatogenesis through a negative feedback mechanism, inhibiting luteinizing hormone (LH).

Testosterone may help maintain the normal urethral muscle tone and integrity of the urethral mucosa in male dogs. It may also be necessary to prevent some types of dermatoses.

Pharmacokinetics

Orally administered testosterone is rapidly metabolized by the GI mucosa and the liver (first-pass effect); very little reaches the systemic circulation. The esterified compounds, testosterone enanthate and cypionate, are less polar than testosterone and more slowly absorbed from lipid tissue after IM injection.[1] The duration of action of these compounds may persist for 2 to 4 weeks after IM injection. Because testosterone absorption is dependent upon several factors (volume injected, perfusion), the duration of action may be variable.

Testosterone is highly bound to a specific testosterone-estradiol globulin (98% in humans).[1] The quantity of this globulin determines the amount of drug that is in the free or bound form. The free form concentration determines the plasma half-life of the hormone.

Testosterone is metabolized in the liver and is, with its metabolites, excreted in the urine (≈90%) and feces (≈6%).[1] The plasma half-life of testosterone has been reported to be between 10 and 100 minutes in humans. The plasma half-life of testosterone cypionate has been reported to be 8 days.

Contraindications/Precautions/Warnings

Testosterone therapy is contraindicated during pregnancy and in patients with known hypersensitivity to the drug; it should not be used in males with prostate carcinoma.[1] It should be used with caution in patients with renal, cardiac, or hepatic dysfunction.

Testosterone depot formulations are formulated for deep IM injection and should not be given by the IV route.[1]

The National Institute for Occupational Safety and Health (NIOSH) classifies androgens as hazardous drugs representing an occupational hazard to healthcare workers; personal protective equipment (PPE) should be used accordingly to minimize the risk for exposure.[2]

Adverse Effects

Adverse effects are reportedly uncommon when injectable testosterone products are used in male dogs to treat hormone-responsive incontinence; however, perianal adenomas, perineal hernias, prostatic disorders, and behavior changes (aggression) are all possible. In bitches, testosterone can cause clitoral hypertrophy, masculinization, and aggression. In cats, behavioral changes have been reported. High doses or chronic use may result in priapism, oligospermia, or infertility in intact males.

Polycythemia, hepatitis, hepatocellular carcinoma, and reduced clotting factors have been reported in humans receiving high doses of testosterone.[1] Use in pediatric patients may result in early epiphyseal closure.

Reproductive/Nursing Safety

Testosterone use during pregnancy causes virilization of female fetuses. In humans, testosterone is contraindicated during pregnancy.[1] It is not known whether androgens are excreted in the milk; consider using milk replacer if using testosterone in nursing patients.

Because safety has not been established in animals, this drug should only be used when the maternal benefits outweigh the potential risks to offspring.

Overdose/Acute Toxicity

No specific information was located; refer to ***Adverse Effects*** for further information.

For patients that have experienced or are suspected of having experienced an overdose, consultation with a 24-hour poison consultation center specializing in providing veterinary-specific information is recommended. For general information related to overdose and toxin exposures, as well as contact information for poison control centers, refer to ***Appendix.***

Drug Interactions

The following drug interactions have either been reported or are theoretical in humans or animals receiving testosterone and may be of significance in veterinary patients. Unless otherwise noted, use together is not necessarily contraindicated, but weigh the potential risks and perform additional monitoring when appropriate.

- **CORTICOSTEROIDS** (eg, **dexamethasone, fludrocortisone, prednis(ol)one**): Androgens may enhance the edema that can be associated with ACTH or adrenal steroid therapy.
- **CYCLOSPORINE**: Increased risk for cyclosporine toxicity
- **INSULIN; ORAL ANTIDIABETIC AGENTS**: May decrease serum glucose levels
- **PROPRANOLOL**: Testosterone cypionate may increase propranolol clearance.
- **WARFARIN**: May increase anticoagulant effects

Laboratory Considerations

- Concentrations of **protein-bound iodine (PBI)** can be decreased in patients receiving testosterone therapy, but the clinical significance of this is probably not important. Androgen agents can decrease amounts of **thyroxine-binding globulin** and decrease **total T_4 concentrations** and increase resin uptake of T_3 **and** T_4. Free thyroid hormones are unaltered, and clinically, there is no evidence of dysfunction.
- Both **creatinine** and **creatine** excretion can be decreased by testosterone.
- Testosterone can increase the urinary excretion of **17-ketosteroids**.
- Androgenic/anabolic steroids may alter **blood glucose** levels.
- Androgenic/anabolic steroids may suppress **clotting factors II, V, VII, and X**.

Dosages

NOTE: Older references may list dosages using testosterone propionate (a shorter-acting injectable form), but commercially available products are no longer available in the United States.

DOGS:

Testosterone-responsive urinary incontinence (may be used with phenylpropanolamine) in males (extra-label): Testosterone cypionate 2.2 mg/kg IM once every 30 to 45 days[3]

Estrus control (extra-label): **NOTE**: Rarely recommended. Concerns have been expressed about adverse effects as well as the long-term suppression of estrous activity in bitches treated with testosterone. Research results disagree as to whether treatment with testosterone interferes with the subsequent ability to induce estrus in bitches.[4] Testosterone enanthate (or cypionate) 0.5 mg/kg IM once every 5 days.[5]

Reducing mammary gland enlargement seen in pseudopregnancy (extra-label): **NOTE**: Rarely recommended. Testosterone enanthate (or cypionate) 0.5 – 1 mg/kg IM once[5]

CATTLE:

Producing an estrus-detector (teaser) animal (cull cows, heifers, steers) (extra-label): Testosterone enanthate 0.5 g IM and 1.5 g SC (divided into 2 separate locations). After 4 days, attach the chin ball marker and put the animal in with the breeding herd. To maintain, give 0.5 – 0.75 g SC every 10 to 14 days[6]

Monitoring

- Efficacy
- Adverse effects
- Consider baseline and periodic CBC, serum chemistry profile with electrolytes especially with long-term administration or with high doses.

Chemistry/Synonyms

The esterified compounds, testosterone cypionate and enanthate, are available commercially as injectable (in oil) products.

Testosterone cypionate occurs as an odorless to having a faint odor, creamy white or white crystalline powder. It is insoluble in water, soluble in vegetable oils, and freely soluble in alcohol. Testosterone cypionate has a melting range of 98°C to 104°C (208°F-219°F). It may also be known as testosterone cyclopentyl propionate.

Testosterone enanthate occurs as an odorless to having a faint odor, creamy white or white crystalline powder. It is soluble in vegetable oils and insoluble in water and melts between 34°C and 39°C (93°F-102°F).

Storage/Stability

Store the commercially available injectable preparations of testosterone cypionate, enanthate, and propionate at room temperature (20°C-25°C [68°F-77°F]); avoid freezing or exposure to temperatures greater than 40°C (104°F). If exposed to low temperatures, a precipitate may form but should redissolve with shaking and rewarming. If a wet (aqueous) needle or syringe is used to draw up the parenteral solutions, cloudy solutions may result, but this will not affect the drug's potency.

Testosterone is a DEA Schedule III (C-III) controlled substance. Store it in a substantially constructed and securely locked area. Follow applicable local, state, and federal rules regarding the disposal of unused or wasted controlled drugs.

Compatibility/Compounding Considerations

No specific information was noted.

Dosage Forms/Regulatory Status

VETERINARY-LABELED PRODUCTS:

The Association of Racing Commissioners International (ARCI) has designated this drug as a class 4 substance. Use of this drug may not be allowed in certain animal competitions. Check rules and regulations before entering a competition while this medication is being administered. Contact local racing authorities for further guidance. See ***Appendix*** for more information.

No known testosterone products (with the exception of combinations with estradiol as growth promotant implants) that are FDA-approved for use in veterinary species were located. Testosterone propionate (200 mg) is available in combination with estradiol benzoate (20 mg) as a growth promotant. Trade names include *Component E-H*®; (OTC) and *Synovex-H*®; (OTC). For use in heifers weighing at least 181 kg (400 lb).

HUMAN-LABELED PRODUCTS:

Testosterone Cypionate (in oil) Injection: 100 mg/mL and 200 mg/mL in 1 mL and 10 mL vials; *Depo-Testosterone*® generic; (Rx, C-III)

Testosterone Enanthate (in oil) Injection: 50 mg, 75 mg, 100mg and 200 mg in 0.5 mL prefilled syringes, and 200 mg/mL in 5 mL multi-dose vials; generic; (Rx, C-III)

Testosterone Undecanoate solution for injection: 250 mg/ mL in 3 mL single-dose vials; *Aveed*®; (Rx; C-III)

Testosterone Pellets Implant for subcutaneous implantation: 75 mg in 1 pellet/vials; *Testopel*®; (Rx, C-III)

There are also testosterone transdermal patches, topical solutions and gels, and oral capsules available.

References

For the complete list of references, see **wiley.com/go/budde/plumb**

Tetracycline

(tet-ra-***sye***-kleen)

Tetracycline Antibiotic

Prescriber Highlights

- Prototype tetracycline antibiotic; many bacteria are now resistant, but may still be useful to treat *Mycoplasma* spp, *Rickettsia*, spirochetes, and *Chlamydia* spp. Used with niacinamide to help control sterile inflammatory skin conditions in dogs
- Doxycycline or minocycline are usually preferred antimicrobial indications in small animals due to more favorable dosing frequency and adverse effect profile.
- Extreme caution: pregnancy
- Caution: renal insufficiency
- Adverse effects: GI distress, staining of developing teeth and bones, photosensitivity; long-term use may cause uroliths. Cats: do not tolerate well. Horses: if stressed, diarrhea is possible (oral use). Ruminants: high oral doses can alter ruminal microbiota and cause ruminoreticular stasis

Uses/Indications

Although tetracycline is still used as an antimicrobial, its use has largely been supplanted by doxycycline or minocycline in dogs and cats, and oxytetracycline in most food animals. It is also used for non-antimicrobial effects in combination with niacinamide, which may be useful in controlling a variety of sterile inflammatory skin conditions in dogs including: discoid lupus erythematosus (DLE), sterile granulomatous/pyogranulomatous syndrome, sterile nodular panniculitis, cutaneous reactive histiocytosis, cutaneous vesicular lupus erythematosus, pemphigus erythematosus, pemphigus foliaceus, lupoid onychodystrophy/onychitis, German shepherd dog metatarsal fistulae, vasculitis, arteritis of the nasal philtrum, sebaceous adenitis, and dermatomyositis.[1] Controlled studies demonstrating clear efficacy are lacking, but anecdotally this combination appears effective in some patients, including up to ⅔ of dogs that are treated for DLE. Often used in conjunction with other immunomodulating drugs, especially in the initial treatment phase. Niacinamide/tetracycline may take 1 to 2 months before efficacy is noted.

Tetracycline soluble powder is labeled for treatment and control of bacterial enteritis and bacterial pneumonia in swine and calves; chronic respiratory disease, air sac disease, and infectious synovitis in chickens; and infectious synovitis and enteritis in turkeys that are caused by susceptible bacteria.[2] Tetracycline has also been used topically in an extra-label manner to treat digital dermatitis in cows.

The World Health Organization (WHO) has designated tetracycline as a Highly Important antimicrobial for human medicine.[3] The Office International des Epizooties (OIE) Antimicrobial Classification has designated tetracycline as a Veterinary Critically Important antimicrobial.[4]

Pharmacology/Actions

Tetracyclines generally act as time-dependent antibiotics and inhibit protein synthesis by reversibly binding to 30S ribosomal subunits of susceptible organisms, thereby preventing binding to those ribosomes of aminoacyl transfer-RNA. Tetracyclines are bacteriostatic antibiotics at usual doses and may be bactericidal at higher doses or against susceptible bacteria. Tetracyclines are believed to reversibly bind to 50S ribosomes and additionally alter cytoplasmic membrane permeability in susceptible organisms. At high concentrations, tetracyclines can inhibit protein synthesis by mammalian cells.

As a class, the tetracyclines have activity against most *Mycoplasma* spp, spirochetes (including *Borrelia burgdorferi*), *Chlamydia* spp, and rickettsia. Against gram-positive bacteria, the tetracyclines have activity against some strains of *Staphylococcus* spp and *Streptococcus* spp, but resistance of these organisms is increasing. Gram-positive bacteria that are usually susceptible to tetracyclines include *Bacillus anthracis*, *Clostridium perfringens* and *C tetani*, *Listeria monocytogenes*, and *Nocardia* spp. Gram-negative bacteria against which tetracyclines usually have in vitro and in vivo activity include *Bordetella* spp, *Brucella* spp, *Bartonella* spp, *Haemophilus* spp, *Pasteurella multocida*, *Shigella* spp, and *Yersinia pestis*. Many or most strains of *Escherichia coli*, *Klebsiella* spp, *Bacteroides* spp, *Enterobacter* spp, *Proteus* spp, and *Pseudomonas aeruginosa* are resistant to the tetracyclines. Hemoglobin at the site of the infection can reduce the antimicrobial activity of tetracycline.

Oxytetracycline and tetracycline share nearly identical spectrums of activity and patterns of cross-resistance and a tetracycline susceptibility disk is usually used for in vitro testing for oxytetracycline susceptibility.

Tetracyclines have anti-inflammatory and immunomodulating effects. They can suppress antibody production and chemotaxis of neutrophils; inhibit lipases, collagenases, prostaglandin synthesis; and inhibit activation of complement component 3. The clinical relevance of these is largely unknown.

Tetracycline susceptibility cannot be predicted by susceptibility to doxycycline or minocycline. If doxycycline or minocycline resistance is present, tetracycline resistance is also present. However, doxycycline or minocycline susceptibility can be present in some tetracycline-resistant bacteria.

Pharmacokinetics

Both oxytetracycline and tetracycline are readily absorbed after oral administration to fasting animals. Bioavailabilities are ≈60% to 80%. The presence of food or dairy products can significantly reduce the amount of tetracycline absorbed, with reductions of 50% or more possible. After IM administration, tetracycline is erratically and poorly absorbed with serum concentrations usually lower than those attainable with oral therapy.

Tetracyclines, as a class, are widely distributed to the heart, kidneys, lungs, muscles, pleural fluid, bronchial secretions, sputum, bile, saliva, urine, synovial fluid, ascitic fluid, and aqueous and vitreous humor. Only small quantities of tetracycline and oxytetracycline are distributed to the CSF, and therapeutic concentrations may not be achievable. Although all tetracyclines distribute to the prostate and eye, doxycycline or minocycline penetrate better into these and most other tissues. Tetracyclines cross the placenta, enter fetal circulation, and are distributed into milk. The volume of distribution of tetracycline is ≈1.2 to 1.3 L/kg in small animals. The amount of plasma protein binding is ≈20% to 67% for tetracycline. In cattle, the volume of distribution for oxytetracycline is between 1 and 2.5 L/kg. Milk to plasma ratios for oxytetracycline and tetracycline are 0.75 and 1.2 to 1.9, respectively.

Both oxytetracycline and tetracycline are eliminated unchanged primarily via glomerular filtration and in the feces. Patients with impaired renal function can have prolonged elimination half-lives and accumulate the drug with repeated dosing. These drugs are not metabolized but are excreted unchanged into the urine as well as into the GI tract via both biliary and nonbiliary routes. The elimination half-life of tetracycline is ≈5 to 6 hours in dogs and cats.

Contraindications/Precautions/Warnings

Tetracycline is contraindicated in patients hypersensitive to it or other tetracyclines.

Use with caution in patients with renal insufficiency, as tetracycline can accumulate and lead to liver toxicity.[5] Dose reduction is recommended. In humans, tetracycline can cause an increase in BUN. In patients with impaired renal function, this can lead to azotemia, hyperphosphatemia, and acidosis. Avoid concurrent administration with other nephrotoxic drugs. Monitoring of serum tetracycline concentrations should be considered if long-term therapy is required.

In humans, tetracyclines can cause increased photosensitivity that presents as severe sunburns.[5] Limit sun exposure for patients with thin or light-colored coats while taking tetracycline.

Adverse Effects

Oxytetracycline and tetracycline given to young animals can cause discoloration (yellow, brown, or gray color) of teeth. High doses or chronic administration may delay bone growth and healing.

In small animal species, tetracyclines can cause nausea, vomiting, anorexia, and diarrhea. Esophageal injuries (esophagitis, ulceration) have occurred with administration of capsule and tablet forms of tetracyclines; a water bolus after administering solid dosage forms is recommended.

Cats do not tolerate oral tetracycline well and may present with clinical signs of colic, fever, hair loss, and depression. There are reports that long-term tetracycline use may cause urolith formation in dogs. Tetracyclines have caused thyroid hyperpigmentation and induced thyroid hyperplasia in many small animal species. Horses that are stressed by surgery, anesthesia, or trauma, may develop severe diarrhea after receiving tetracyclines (especially with oral administration).

In ruminants, high oral doses can alter ruminal microbiota depression and cause ruminoreticular stasis. Rapid IV injection of undiluted propylene glycol-based products can cause intravascular hemolysis with resultant hemoglobinuria. Propylene glycol-based products have also caused cardiodepressant effects when administered to calves. When administered IM, local reactions, yellow staining, and necrosis may be seen at the injection site.

Tetracycline therapy (especially long-term) may result in overgrowth of non-susceptible bacteria or fungi (superinfections).

Tetracyclines have also been associated with photosensitivity reactions and, rarely, hepatotoxicity, formation of anti-nuclear antibodies, or blood dyscrasias. Risk for hepatotoxicity may be increased with pre-existing renal or hepatic impairment.

Reproductive/Nursing Safety

Animal studies indicate that tetracyclines cross the placenta, are found in fetal tissues, and can have toxic effects on the developing fetus. Because tetracyclines can delay fetal skeletal development and discolor deciduous teeth, they should only be used in the last half of pregnancy when the benefits outweigh the fetal risks. Oxytetracycline and tetracycline are considered more likely to cause these abnormalities than either doxycycline or minocycline. Evidence of embryotoxicity has also been noted in animals when given tetracycline during early pregnancy.[5]

Tetracycline had no effect on fertility when administered in the diet to male and female rats at a daily intake of 25 times the human dose. Tetracyclines are excreted in milk but because much of the drug will be bound to calcium in milk, it is unlikely to be of significant risk to nursing animals. Short-term use of tetracycline is considered compatible with breastfeeding.[6]

Overdose/Acute Toxicity

Tetracyclines are generally well tolerated after acute overdoses. Dogs given more than 400 mg/kg/day orally or 100 mg/kg/day IM of oxytetracycline did not demonstrate any toxicity. Oral overdoses would most likely be associated with GI disturbances (vomiting, anorexia, and/or diarrhea). Should the patient develop severe emesis or diarrhea, fluids and electrolytes should be monitored and replaced if necessary. Chronic overdoses may lead to drug accumulation and nephrotoxicity.

Rapid IV injection of tetracyclines has induced transient collapse and cardiac arrhythmias in several species, presumably due to chelation with intravascular calcium ions. Overdose quantities of drug could exacerbate this effect if given too rapidly IV. If the drug must be given rapidly IV (in less than 5 minutes), some clinicians recommend pretreating the animal with IV calcium gluconate. Rapid IV injection of undiluted propylene glycol-based products can cause intravascular hemolysis with resultant hemoglobinuria.

High oral doses given to ruminants can alter ruminal microbiota and cause ruminoreticular stasis.

For patients that have experienced or are suspected to have experienced an overdose, consultation with a 24-hour poison consultation center specializing in providing veterinary-specific information is recommended. For general information related to overdose and toxin exposures, as well as contact information for poison control centers, refer to ***Appendix.***

Drug Interactions

The following drug interactions have either been reported or are theoretical in humans or animals receiving tetracyclines and may be of significance in veterinary patients. Unless otherwise noted, use together is not necessarily contraindicated, but weigh the potential risks and perform additional monitoring when appropriate.

- **Atovaquone**: Tetracyclines have caused decreased atovaquone concentrations.
- **Beta-Lactam or Aminoglycoside Antibiotics**: Bacteriostatic drugs, like the tetracyclines, have been historically thought to interfere with bactericidal activity of the penicillins, cephalosporins, and aminoglycosides but the clinical significance of this interaction is unknown.
- **Digoxin**: Tetracyclines have increased the bioavailability of digoxin in a small percentage of human patients and caused digoxin toxicity. These effects may persist for months after discontinuation of the tetracycline.
- **Divalent or Trivalent Cations** (eg, oral antacids, saline cathartics or other GI products containing aluminum, calcium, iron, magnesium, zinc, or bismuth cations): When orally administered, tetracyclines can chelate divalent or trivalent cations that can decrease the absorption of the tetracycline or the other drug if it contains these cations; it is recommended that all oral tetracyclines be given at least 1 to 2 hours before or after the cation-containing products.
- **Methoxyflurane**: Fatal nephrotoxicity has occurred in humans when used with tetracycline.
- **Neuromuscular Blocking Agents**: Tetracyclines may potentiate neuromuscular blockade.
- **Sucralfate**: Sucralfate may impair the oral absorption of tetracycline; separate dosing by at least 2 hours to minimize this effect.
- **Warfarin**: Tetracyclines may depress plasma prothrombin activity and patients on anticoagulant therapy may need dosage adjustment.

Laboratory Considerations

- Tetracyclines (not minocycline) may cause falsely elevated values of urine catecholamines when using fluorometric methods of determination.
- Tetracyclines can reportedly cause false positive urine glucose results if using the cupric sulfate method of determination (Benedict's reagent, *Clinitest*®), but this may be the result of ascorbic acid that is found in some parenteral formulations of tetracyclines. Tetracyclines have also reportedly caused false negative results in determining urine glucose when using the glucose oxidase method (*Clinistix*®, *Tes-Tape*®).

Dosages

DOGS:

Adjunctive treatment of sterile inflammatory or autoimmune diseases (extra-label): Tetracycline is typically used in combination with niacinamide. Recommended dosages are empirical and vary.

- Dogs 10 kg (22 lb) or less: tetracycline 250 mg/dog (NOT mg/kg) PO 3 times daily in combination with niacinamide 250 mg/dog (NOT mg/kg) PO 3 times daily[7]
- Dogs more than 10 kg (22 lb): tetracycline 500 mg/dog (NOT mg/kg) PO 3 times daily in combination with niacinamide 500 mg/dog (NOT mg/kg) PO 3 times daily[7]

NOTES:

1. If efficacious, may reduce niacinamide dose to twice-daily administration and then taper further over time when possible.
2. Tetracycline may be replaced with doxycycline 5 – 10 mg/kg PO every 12 hours OR minocycline 5 – 10 mg/kg PO every 12 hours.[8]
3. Some clinicians have used 15 kg (33.1 lb) as the weight cutoff (ie, dogs 15 kg [33.1 lb] or less receive 250 mg/dog [NOT mg/kg]; dogs more than 15 kg [33.1 lb] receive 500 mg/dog [NOT mg/kg]).[9] Other clinicians have suggested niacinamide 45 mg/kg PO every 8 hours in combination with tetracycline 45 mg/kg PO every 8 hours.[10]

Susceptible infections (extra-label): 22 mg/kg PO every 8 hours for 14 to 28 days

CATS:

Susceptible infections (extra-label): 15 – 22 mg/kg PO every 8 hours for 14 to 28 days

FERRETS:

Susceptible infections (extra-label): 25 mg/kg PO 2 to 3 times daily[11]

RABBITS, RODENTS, SMALL MAMMALS:

a) **Rabbits**: 50 – 100 mg/kg PO every 8 to 12 hours[12]
b) **Chinchillas**: 50 mg/kg PO every 8 to 12 hours[13]
c) **Chinchillas, Guinea Pigs, Rats**: 20 mg/kg PO every 12 hours. **Mice**: 20 mg/kg PO every 12 hours or 50 – 60 mg/L of drinking water, **Hamsters**: 30 mg/kg PO every 6 hours or 400 mg/L of drinking water. **Gerbils**: 20 mg/kg PO or IM once a day.[14]

CATTLE:

Susceptible infections in calves (label dosage; FDA-approved): 22 mg/kg/day PO in drinking water for up to 5 days.[15] Prepare fresh solution once or twice daily.

Digital dermatitis in cow (extra-label): 2 – 25 g applied topically to affected foot as a paste or powder, with or without bandaging[16,17]

SHEEP:

Susceptible infections (extra-label): using previously available FDA-approved product, 11 mg/kg PO twice daily for up to 5 days[18]

SWINE:

Susceptible infections (label dosage; FDA-approved): 22 mg/kg/day PO in drinking water for 3 to 5 days.[15] Prepare fresh solution once or twice daily.

POULTRY:

Susceptible infections (label dosage; FDA-approved): 200 to 800 mg/gallon drinking water for 7 to 14 days[15]

BIRDS:

Chlamydiosis; mild respiratory disease (especially flock treatment) (extra-label):

a) Using tetracycline soluble powder containing 324 g tetracycline/pound, mix ¼ teaspoon of soluble powder per gallon of drinking water. Used as an adjunct for psittacosis with other tetracycline forms. Will not reach therapeutic concentrations by itself. Prepare fresh solution twice daily, as potency is rapidly lost.[19]

b) Using tetracycline soluble powder containing 324 g tetracycline/pound, mix ¼ teaspoon of soluble powder per gallon of drinking water and administer for 5 to 10 days. Prepare fresh solution 2 to 3 times daily, as potency is rapidly lost. For converting regimen to pelleted feeds, administer oral suspension by gavage at 200 – 250 mg/kg once or twice daily until feeds are accepted; this is not an adequate therapy for long-term treatment of chlamydiosis (psittacosis).[20]

Monitoring

- Adverse effects
- Clinical efficacy
- Long-term use or in susceptible patients: periodic renal, hepatic, thyroid, and hematologic evaluations

Client Information

- This medicine is best given without food. Avoid giving this medicine orally within 1 to 2 hours of milk or other dairy products.
- If gastrointestinal upset occurs, giving with a small amount of food may help, but this may also reduce the amount of drug absorbed.

Chemistry/Synonyms

An antibiotic obtained from *Streptomyces aureofaciens* or derived semisynthetically from oxytetracycline, tetracycline HCl occurs as a moderately hygroscopic, yellow, crystalline powder. Approximately 100 mg/mL is soluble in water and 10 mg/mL soluble in alcohol.

Tetracycline base has a solubility of ≈0.4 mg per mL of water and 20 mg per mL of alcohol. Commercially available tetracycline HCl for IM injection also contains magnesium chloride, procaine HCl, and ascorbic acid.

Tetracycline may also be known as tetracyclini hydrochloridum; many trade names are available.

Storage/Stability

Unless otherwise instructed by the manufacturer, tetracycline oral tablets and capsules should be stored in tight, light-resistant containers at room temperature (15°C-30°C [59°F-86°F]).

Compatibility/Compounding Considerations

No specific information noted.

Dosage Forms/Regulatory Status

VETERINARY-LABELED PRODUCTS:

Tetracycline HCl Soluble Powder (as a water additive): 324 g/lb in 5 lb containers; FDA-approved for use in swine, cattle, and poultry. (OTC at time of writing). Not to be used in pre-ruminating calves or calves to be processed for veal. Not for use in turkeys or chickens producing eggs for human consumption. Withdrawal times: swine, 4 days; calves, 5 days; chicken, 4 days. For topical applications, a milk withdrawal time of 24 hours is recommended[21]; however, it has been suggested that a more conservative 36-hour withdrawal may be needed.[22]

HUMAN-LABELED PRODUCTS:

Tetracycline HCl Capsules: 250 mg and 500 mg; generic; (Rx)

References

For the complete list of references, see **wiley.com/go/budde/plumb**

Theophylline

(thee-***off***-i-lin)

Phosphodiesterase Inhibitor Bronchodilator

Prescriber Highlights

- ► Bronchodilator with mild diuretic activity used as adjunctive therapy in dogs with cough and in cats with asthma.
- ► Narrow therapeutic index in humans, but dogs appear to be less susceptible to toxic effects at higher plasma concentrations
- ► Doses should be calculated using lean body weight in obese animals.
- ► Many drug interactions are possible; fluoroquinolones (eg, enrofloxacin) can increase theophylline concentrations substantially.
- ► Availability can be an issue; check with a reputable compounding pharmacy for availability.

Uses/Indications

Theophyllines (ie, aminophylline, theophylline) are used primarily for their bronchodilatory effects, especially in dogs with cough and cats with asthma. Theophylline may also be considered when managing sick sinus syndrome and other bradycardias.[1] In coughing dogs with heart disease and evidence of concurrent tracheal instability or chronic small airway disease, clinical improvement may be seen with a bronchodilator such as theophylline. Theophylline has also been used as a bronchodilator in horses; however, some do not recommend its use in this species due to its narrow therapeutic index.[2]

Pharmacology/Actions

Theophylline competitively inhibits phosphodiesterase (PDE) III (and PDE IV to a lesser extent), thereby increasing amounts of cyclic AMP (cAMP) that then increase the release of endogenous epinephrine. The elevated concentrations of cAMP may also inhibit the release of histamine and slow reacting substance of anaphylaxis (SRS-A). The myocardial and neuromuscular transmission effects of theophylline may be a result of translocating intracellular ionized calcium. Adenosine antagonism may contribute to CNS stimulant effects.

Theophylline directly relaxes smooth muscles in the bronchi and pulmonary vasculature; smooth muscle relaxant effects also occur in the uterus, biliary, and GI tracts. In addition, theophylline may induce diuresis, vasodilate arterioles and veins, increase gastric acid secretion and corticosteroid activity, improve mucociliary clearance, and inhibit mast cell release. Theophylline has weak chronotropic and inotropic action, improves diaphragm contractility, stimulates the CNS, and can cause respiratory stimulation (centrally mediated). Theophylline also has anti-inflammatory effects, including diminished activity of inflammatory and immune cells, especially eosinophils, within the airways.[3,4]

Pharmacokinetics

Oral absorption of theophylline from commercial extended-release formulations is variable.[5] Bioavailability of compounded modified-release theophylline products was ≈96% in dogs, and peak concentrations were reached 7.1 to 8.9 hours after administration.[6,7] Theophylline is distributed throughout extracellular fluids and body tissues. In dogs, only ≈10% is bound to plasma proteins at therapeutic serum concentrations.[8] The volume of distribution of theophylline in dogs has been reported to be 0.5 to 0.8 L/kg.[9] After IV administration of aminophylline (=7.88 mg/kg theophylline) to greyhounds, mean theophylline volume of distribution (steady-state) was 0.72 L/kg, mean clearance was 0.935 mL/minute/kg, and elimination half-life was ≈9 hours.[10] Clearance was 1.2 mL/minute/kg in puppies 1 week of age, and increased with age to peak at 7.1 mL/minute/kg in puppies 16 weeks of age.[11] It has been shown that herbal medicines, such as fenugreek and garden cress, can alter theophylline pharmacokinetics in beagles.[12] Elimination half-life was 8.7 to 10.5 hours following administration of compounded modified-release theophylline products.[6,7]

In cats, bioavailability was 96% (with aminophylline)[13] and ≈80% with extended-release formulations.[14] The volume of distribution in cats was reported to be 0.46 L/kg, and protein binding was 12%.[13] Elimination half-life was ≈8 hours[13] but was prolonged to ≈20 hours when the drug was administered in the evening (8 to 9 PM).[15] Transdermal administration of theophylline (15 mg/kg/day in either PLO or *Lipoderm*®) produced a therapeutic theophylline concentration in 2 of 7 cats in each formulation, and only 7 of the 56 total measurements were within the therapeutic range.[16]

In horses, oral bioavailability of immediate-release and extended-release formulations were 87% and 97%, respectively.[17] Protein binding was ≈13% to 23%[18]; volume of distribution was 0.85 to 1.6 L/kg[17-19]; and elimination half-life was 12 to 17 hours.[18,19] Pharmacokinetic values in donkeys were found to be similar to those of horses.[20]

In ruminating calves, oral bioavailability was 93%, volume of distribution was 0.8 L/kg, and elimination half-life was 6.4 hours.[21] In adult camels, protein binding was ≈33%, volume of distribution was ≈0.8 L/kg, and elimination half-life was ≈11 hours.[22] Oral bioavailability in goats and camels was 90%.[23] In goats, volume of distribution was 1.4 L/kg and elimination half-life was ≈2 hours.[23]

Because of the low volume of distribution and theophylline's low lipid solubility, obese patients should be dosed on a lean body weight basis. Theophylline is metabolized primarily in the liver (in humans) to 3-methylxanthine, which has weak bronchodilator activity. Renal clearance contributes only ≈10% to the overall plasma clearance of theophylline. In humans, there are wide interpatient variations in serum half-lives and resultant serum concentrations. It could be expected that similar variability exists in veterinary patients, particularly those with concurrent illnesses. Note that the pharmacokinetics of long-acting theophylline products vary with the modified (ie, extended) release mechanism, and duration of effect may vary between 8 to 24 hours in humans.

Contraindications/Precautions/Warnings

Theophylline is contraindicated in patients that are hypersensitive to xanthines (eg, aminophylline, theobromine, caffeine). Use in dogs with a history of epileptiform seizures is contraindicated.[24]

Theophylline should be administered with caution in patients with severe cardiac disease, gastric ulcers, hyperthyroidism, renal or hepatic disease, severe hypoxia, or hypertension. Theophylline clearance is decreased by ≈50% in patients with hepatic disease or CHF, and a 50% reduction in dosage has been suggested for patients in hepatic failure.[25] Clearance is reduced to a lesser extent by hypothyroidism, fever, and sepsis. Because it may cause or worsen pre-existing arrhythmias, caution and enhanced monitoring are advised in patients with cardiac tachyarrhythmias that receive theophylline. Neonatal and geriatric patients may have decreased clearances of theophylline and be more sensitive to its toxic effects.

In humans, exposure to secondhand smoke may increase theophylline clearance; whether the same occurs in animals is unknown.

Adverse Effects

Theophylline can produce CNS stimulation and GI irritation after administration by any route. Most adverse effects are related to the serum concentration of the drug and may be indicative of toxic blood concentrations; dogs appear to tolerate concentrations that may be toxic to humans.

Dogs and cats can exhibit clinical signs of nausea and vomiting, insomnia, increased gastric acid secretion, diarrhea, polyphagia, polydipsia, polyuria, dyspnea, tremors, agitation, nervousness, restlessness, and increased activity. In dogs, tachycardia was noted at a dose of 40 mg/kg twice daily with corresponding plasma theophylline concentration greater than 30 µg/mL.[26]

Adverse effects in horses are generally dose related and may include nervousness, excitability (with auditory, tactile, or visual stimulation), tremors, diaphoresis, tachycardia, and ataxia.[27]

Administration of theophylline with high-fat foods (eg, cheese, peanut butter) may increase the rate of absorption of some extended-release products, increasing the risk for adverse effects and toxic concentrations.

Reproductive/Nursing Safety

Theophylline has been shown to reduce uterine contractions. Theophylline crosses the placenta and is distributed into milk (70% of serum concentrations). In humans, theophylline is considered compatible with nursing.[28] Because safety has not been established in animals, this drug should only be used when the maternal benefits outweigh the potential risks to offspring.

Overdose/Acute Toxicity

In humans, clinical signs of toxicity (see ***Adverse Effects***) are usually associated with serum drug concentrations greater than 20 µg/mL and become more severe as the serum concentration exceeds that value. Tachycardia, arrhythmia, and CNS effects (eg, seizures, hyperthermia) are considered the most life-threatening aspects of toxicity. Hypokalemia and acid-base disturbances may also occur. Dogs and cats appear to tolerate serum concentrations greater than 20 µg/mL. Common clinical signs associated with overdose may include tachycardia.

Treatment of theophylline toxicity is supportive. GI decontamination with activated charcoal, which blocks theophylline absorption, can be considered and is more effective in reducing theophylline exposure than inducing emesis. Patients with seizures should have an adequate airway maintained and be treated with an IV benzodiazepine (eg, diazepam, midazolam) as indicated. Patients should be continuously monitored for cardiac arrhythmias and tachycardia. Hydration status and electrolytes should be monitored and corrected as necessary. Hyperthermia may be treated with phenothiazines[29] and tachycardia treated with propranolol if either condition is considered life-threatening. Theophylline is removed by hemodialysis, which may be an option in cases in which activated charcoal cannot be administered.

For patients that have experienced or are suspected to have experienced an overdose, consultation with a 24-hour poison consultation center specializing in providing veterinary-specific information is recommended. For general information related to overdose and toxin exposures, as well as contact information for poison control centers, refer to ***Appendix***.

Drug Interactions

The following drug interactions have either been reported or are theoretical in humans or animals receiving aminophylline or theophylline and may be of significance in veterinary patients. Unless otherwise noted, use together is not necessarily contraindicated, but weigh the potential risks and perform additional monitoring when appropriate.

- KETAMINE: Theophylline with ketamine can cause an increased incidence of seizures and cardiac arrhythmias.
- SYMPATHOMIMETICS (eg, **beta agonists** [eg, **albuterol**], **ephedrine, isoproterenol, phenylpropanolamine**): Toxic synergism (eg, CNS stimulation, arrhythmias) can occur if theophylline is used concurrently with sympathomimetics (especially ephedrine) or possibly isoproterenol. Concurrent use with beta-sympathomimetics is contraindicated.[24]

The following drugs can **decrease** theophylline concentrations:

- ALBENDAZOLE
- BARBITURATES (eg, **phenobarbital**): Can induce CYP enzymes and increase theophylline metabolism in dogs (not cats)
- BETA-2-ADRENERGIC RECEPTOR AGONISTS (eg, **albuterol**)
- CHARCOAL
- HERBAL AGENTS (eg, **fenugreek, garden cress**)[12]
- ISONIAZID: May increase or decrease concentrations
- ISOPROTERENOL
- KETOCONAZOLE
- LOOP DIURETICS (eg, **furosemide**): May increase or decrease concentrations
- PHENOBARBITAL
- PHOSPHATE BINDERS (eg, **aluminum hydroxide, calcium carbonate**): Can form an insoluble complex in the GI tract and inhibit drug absorption; separate administration by 2 hours
- RIFAMPIN
- SUCRALFATE: Can form insoluble complex in the GI tract and inhibit drug absorption; separate administration by 2 hours

The following drugs can **increase** theophylline concentrations:

- ALLOPURINOL
- BETA-ADRENERGIC RECEPTOR ANTAGONISTS, NONSELECTIVE (eg, **propranolol**): May also antagonize effects of theophylline
- CALCIUM CHANNEL BLOCKERS (eg, **diltiazem, verapamil**)
- CHLORAMPHENICOL: Consider reducing the dose of theophylline by 30% to 50% or extending the dosing interval
- CIMETIDINE
- CORTICOSTEROIDS (eg, **dexamethasone, prednis[ol]one**)
- ESTROGEN
- FLUCONAZOLE
- FLUOROQUINOLONES (eg, **ciprofloxacin, enrofloxacin, marbofloxacin**): Enrofloxacin reduced theophylline clearance by ≈50% in healthy beagles.[30] A similar effect was noted with oflaxacin.[31] Consider reducing the dose of theophylline by 30% to 50% or extending the administration interval. Monitor for toxicity and efficacy. Marbofloxacin reduces clearance of theophylline in dogs but not with clinical significance; however, in animals with renal impairment, marbofloxacin may interfere with theophylline metabolism in a clinically relevant manner.[32]
- INTERFERON ALFA
- MACROLIDES (eg, **clarithromycin, erythromycin**)
- METHOTREXATE
- MEXILETINE
- SELECTIVE SEROTONIN REUPTAKE INHIBITORS (SSRIs; eg, **fluoxetine**)
- THIABENDAZOLE
- THYROID HORMONES (in hypothyroid patients)

Theophylline may **decrease** the effects of the following drugs:

- BENZODIAZEPINES (eg, **diazepam, midazolam**)
- MACROLIDES (eg, **azithromycin, erythromycin**)
- PANCURONIUM
- PROPOFOL[33]

Laboratory Considerations

Theophylline can cause falsely elevated values of **serum uric acid** if measured by the Bittner or colorimetric methods. Values are not affected if using the uricase method.

Immunoassays are specific for theophylline. If using a spectrophotometric method of assay, theophylline serum concentrations can be falsely elevated by **furosemide, phenylbutazone, probenecid, theobromine, caffeine, sulfathiazole, chocolate**, or **acetaminophen**. **Cefazolin** may interfere with HPLC assays. The Schack and Wexler method of determining theophylline concentrations may be interfered with by large doses of **thiamine**.

Dosages

NOTES:

1. Theophyllines have a relatively low therapeutic index. Determine doses carefully; doses should be calculated using lean body weight in obese animals.
2. Extended-release oral dosage forms are generally used, but bioavailability of currently marketed human products can be variable in veterinary species; attentive monitoring for adverse effects and efficacy is recommended. Contact a pharmacist for the current availability of products. See ***Compatibility/Compounding***.
3. Dosage conversions between aminophylline and theophylline can be performed using the information found in ***Chemistry/Synonyms***.

DOGS:

Bronchodilator for small airway collapse/disease (extra-label):

a) Extended-release tablets: 10 mg/kg PO every 12 hours initially is recommended; titrate dosage to balance efficacy and tolerability. Dosages of 5 – 20 mg/kg PO every 12 to 24 hours can be used. Availability of commercial extended-release tablets may be problematic. Compounded modified-release theophylline products showed pharmacokinetic properties similar to previously available extended-release theophylline tablets.[6,34]

b) Immediate-release tablets: 9 mg/kg PO every 8 hours has been recommended.[35]

Bradyarrhythmias (eg, sick sinus syndrome, AV block) (extra-label): Using extended-release tablets, 10 mg/kg PO every 12 hours for sick sinus syndrome, as medical management may improve the clinical situation by reducing the impact of bradycardia episodes.[36] In one study, 54% of dogs with sinus node dysfunction had their clinical signs controlled with pharmacologic treatment; however, definitive treatment with recurrent episodes requires the placement of a pacemaker. In one case report in a German shepherd dog with syncope secondary to transient atrioventricular block with dilated cardiomyopathy and atrial fibrillation, an initial dose of 20 mg/kg once daily was used, but the dose was decreased to 10 mg/kg/day due to adverse GI effects; no syncope occurred after the dose reduction, and GI effects improved.[37]

CATS:

Bronchodilator (extra-label):

a) Extended-release tablets: 15 – 25 mg/kg (practically one 100 mg extended-release tablet/capsule) PO once daily in the evening has been suggested.[14] Some cats may only require dosing every other day.

b) Immediate-release tablets: 4.25 mg/kg PO every 12 hours. From a pharmacokinetic study using aminophylline[13,38]

HORSES:

Severe equine asthma (extra label): Loading dose of 12 mg/kg PO, followed by maintenance doses of 5 mg/kg PO every 12 hours

Monitoring

- Therapeutic efficacy and clinical signs of toxicity (eg, excitement, tremors, tachycardia, vomiting)
- Consider measuring serum theophylline concentrations for patients not responding to therapy or that have clinical signs of toxicity. Contact the laboratory for specific instructions on sample collection and handling as well as recommended therapeutic ranges. Therapeutic serum concentrations of theophylline in humans are ≈10 µg/mL. Dogs likely can tolerate higher peak con-

centrations. It is reported that sustained-release products peak 4 to 6 hours after administration in dogs and 8 to 12 hours after administration in cats, but variable bioavailability occurs.[25] Commercial immediate-release products generally peak 1.5 to 2 hours after administration.

Client Information

- This medicine can be given with or without food but giving with some food may prevent stomach upset or vomiting.
- Try to give the medicine in the same manner (ie, with or without food) and at the same time each day.
- Do not crush or allow animals to chew extended-release products.
- Report signs of agitation or excitement to your veterinarian.
- Keep out of reach of children and animals; overdose can be serious.

Chemistry/Synonyms

Theophylline is a naturally occurring xanthine derivative. Aminophylline differs from theophylline only by the addition of ethylenediamine to its structure and may have different amounts of molecules of water of hydration. 100 mg of hydrous aminophylline contains ≈79 mg of anhydrous theophylline; 100 mg of anhydrous aminophylline contains ≈86 mg anhydrous theophylline. Conversely, 100 mg of anhydrous theophylline is equal to 116 mg of anhydrous aminophylline and 127 mg of hydrous aminophylline.

Theophylline occurs as a bitter, odorless, white crystalline powder and has a melting point between 270°C and 274°C (518°F-525°F). It is sparingly soluble in alcohol and only slightly soluble in water at a pH of 7, but solubility increases with increasing pH.

Theophylline may also be known as anhydrous theophylline, teofillina, or theophyllinum; many trade names are available.

Storage/Stability

Theophylline oral dosage forms should be stored in tight containers at room temperature (15°C-30°C [59°F-86°F]). Avoid excessive heat.

Compatibility/Compounding Considerations

Compatibility is dependent on factors such as pH, concentration, temperature, and diluent used; specialized references or a hospital pharmacist can be consulted for more specific information.

Theophylline for injection is reportedly **compatible** when mixed with chlorpromazine, fluconazole, furosemide, lidocaine, methylprednisolone sodium succinate, and verapamil.

Theophylline for injection is reportedly **incompatible** (or data conflict) with ascorbic acid injection, ceftazidime, ceftriaxone, and phenytoin.

Modified-release products from some veterinary compounding pharmacies and from a 503B outsourcing facility have been validated for use in dogs.[6,7,34] Transdermal gel formulations prepared with pluronic lecithin organogel (PLO) or *Lipoderm*® applied once daily to the inner pinna of a cat's ears did not achieve therapeutic theophylline concentration.[16]

Dosage Forms/Regulatory Status

VETERINARY-LABELED PRODUCTS: NONE

The Association of Racing Commissioners International (ARCI) has designated this drug as a class 3 substance. Use of this drug may not be allowed in certain animal competitions. Check rules and regulations before entering in a competition while this medication is being administered. Contact local racing authorities for further guidance. See ***Appendix*** for further information.

HUMAN-LABELED PRODUCTS:

Theophylline Extended-Release Capsules and Tablets: 100 mg, 200 mg, 300 mg, 400 mg, 450 mg, and 600 mg (**NOTE**: Different products have different claimed release rates that may or may not correspond to actual times seen in veterinary patients.); *Theo-24*®, *Theochron*®, generic; (Rx). Availability of commercial extended-release products in strengths that are suitable for veterinary patients has been problematic. Check with a reputable compounding pharmacy for availability.

Theophylline Elixir: 80 mg/15 mL (26.7 mg/5 mL); *Elixophyllin*®; generic; (Rx)

References

For the complete list of references, see **wiley.com/go/budde/plumb**

Thiamine

Vitamin B_1

(***thye***-a-min)

Nutritional; B Vitamin

Prescriber Highlights

- ▶ Used for treatment or prevention of thiamine deficiency
- ▶ Adverse effects include tenderness or muscle soreness after IM injection, as well as hypersensitivity and anaphylactic reactions (rare).

Uses/Indications

Thiamine is indicated in the treatment or prevention of thiamine deficiency that may be secondary to either a lack of thiamine in the diet or the presence of thiamine-destroying compounds in the diet (eg, bracken fern, raw fish, sulfites,[1] amprolium, thiaminase-producing bacteria in ruminants).[2] Clinical signs of thiamine deficiency can manifest as GI (eg, anorexia, salivation), neuromuscular/CNS (eg, ataxia, cervical ventriflexion, seizures, loss of reflexes), ocular (eg, nystagmus, anisocoria, blindness), or cardiac (eg, brady- or tachyarrhythmias, cardiac hypertrophy) effects. Cats are more susceptible to thiamine deficiency than dogs, as their daily requirements are 3 times higher.[3] Evaluation of many cat foods, including canned and dry food as well as home-prepared diets, has shown suboptimal concentrations of thiamine.[4-7]

Thiamine may be supplemented in camelids and other species when long-term amprolium is used.[8]

Thiamine has also been used in the adjunctive treatment of lead poisoning and ethylene glycol toxicity to facilitate the conversion of glyoxylate to nontoxic metabolites.[9]

In animal models (eg, dogs, mice) and humans, thiamine has been used as adjunctive therapy for septic shock.[10,11]

Pharmacology/Actions

Thiamine combines with adenosine triphosphate (ATP) to form thiamine diphosphate/thiamine pyrophosphate that is used for carbohydrate metabolism without affecting blood glucose concentrations.

Absence of thiamine results in decreased transketolase activity in red blood cells and increased pyruvic acid blood concentrations. Without thiamine triphosphate, pyruvic acid is not converted into acetyl-CoA and diminished NADH results, with anaerobic glycolysis producing lactic acid. Lactic acid production is further increased secondary to pyruvic acid conversion. Lactic acidosis may occur.

Pharmacokinetics

Thiamine is absorbed from the GI tract and is rapidly metabolized by the liver. In humans, thiamine is distributed to all tissues with the highest concentrations in the liver, brain, kidney, and heart. The majority of the drug is eliminated as metabolites via the kidney.

Contraindications/Precautions/Warnings

Thiamine injection is contraindicated in animals that are hypersensitive to it or to any component of it. Anaphylactic reactions to parenteral thiamine have occurred after IM and IV administration.[9]

Adverse Effects

Hypersensitivity reactions have occurred following injection. Rarely, a vasovagal anaphylactic response (eg, cardiac arrest or severe bradycardia, cardiac arrhythmias, apnea, hypotension, collapse, seizure, or protracted neuromuscular weakness) has been observed in a small number of cats when thiaminewas administered SC. Some tenderness or muscle soreness may result after SC or IM injection. Thiamine can be diluted with sterile 0.9% sodium chloride to reduce the discomfort associated with SC administration.[3]

Reproductive/Nursing Safety

Thiamine administration to pregnant women has not been shown to cause fetal abnormalities; however, the possibility cannot be ruled out.[9] It is not known whether this drug is excreted in milk, but thiamine is considered compatible with breastfeeding in humans.[12]

Because safety has not been established in animals, this drug should only be used when the maternal benefits outweigh the potential risks to offspring.

Overdose/Acute Toxicity

Large overdoses of thiamine in laboratory animals have been associated with neuromuscular or ganglionic blockade, but the clinical significance is unknown. Transient cardiovascular depression[13] and respiratory depression may also occur with massive parenteral doses. Generally, no treatment should be required with most overdoses as excess drug will be excreted in the urine.

For patients that have experienced or are suspected to have experienced an overdose, consultation with a 24-hour poison consultation center specializing in providing veterinary-specific information is recommended. For general information related to overdose and toxin exposures, as well as contact information for poison control centers, refer to ***Appendix.***

Drug Interactions

- None noted

Laboratory Considerations

- Thiamine may cause false positive **serum uric acid** results when using the phosphotungstate method of determination or urobilinogen urine spot tests using Ehrlich reagent.
- The Schack and Wexler method of determining **theophylline concentrations** may be interfered with by large doses of thiamine.

Dosages

NOTE: Some references discourage the use of the IV route of administration due to risk for adverse hemodynamic effects[3,13,14]; however, these adverse effects are associated with dosages that are much higher than commonly recommended. Adverse cardiovascular effects have not been reported with orally administered thiamine.[14]

DOGS/CATS:

Thiamine deficiency (extra-label): The ideal dose of thiamine is unknown and dosage recommendations vary widely; however, thiamine has a relatively large margin for safety. One dosage recommendation for cats is 50 – 100 mg/cat (NOT mg/kg) parenterally (eg, SC, IM, slow IV) every 12 to 24 hours for 3 to 5 days, followed by PO administration for an additional 2 to 4 weeks.[3,13,14] Until further research determines optimal dosing recommendations, this recommendation for cats could also be used in dogs.[1,3,13,15]

Ethylene glycol toxicosis (extra-label): 50 mg/animal (NOT mg/kg) slow IV ever 6 hours[16]

Adjunctive treatment of refeeding syndrome after critical illness (extra-label): 10 – 100 mg/animal (NOT mg/kg) SC daily during the refeeding period[17]

HORSES:

Thiamine deficiency (extra-label): 0.5 – 5 mg/kg IV, IM, or PO[18]; 100 – 1000 mg/horse (NOT mg/kg) IM, SC, or IV (depending on formulation)[19]

Adjunctive treatment of perinatal asphyxia syndrome (eg, hypoxic ischemic encephalopathy) in foals (extra-label): 1 g/foal (NOT g/kg) in 1 L of fluids IV once a day[20]

Part of a parenteral nutrition (PN) formula (extra-label): B complex vitamins (thiamine 12.5 mg/mL; niacinamide 12.5 mg/mL; pyridoxine 5 mg/mL; d-panthenol 5 mg/mL; riboflavin 2 mg/mL; cyanocobalamin 5 mg/mL) should be supplied at a rate of 1 – 2 mL/45 kg (99 lb) daily, diluted in fluids or PN. Vitamin C should be supplied at a rate of 20 mg/kg/day enterally whenever possible.[21]

CATTLE:

Thiamine deficiency (polioencephalomalacia): 10 mg/kg IV or IM every 6 hours for 1 to 3 days, then daily. Prognosis is fair if the animals are still standing with some improvement within 24 hours; if still standing after a week, prognosis is good for a complete recovery.[22]

SHEEP & GOATS:

Thiamine deficiency (polioencephalomalacia) (extra-label): 10 mg/kg IV initially, then 10 mg/kg IV, IM, or SC every 6 hours for the first day. Dosing intervals may be tapered depending on the response to treatment; regaining appetite is a positive indicator.[23]

NEW WORLD CAMELIDS:

Prophylaxis when animals treated with amprolium for *Eimeria macusaniensis* for more than 5 days (extra-label): 10 mg/kg SC once a day after the fifth day of amprolium[8]

SWINE:

Thiamine deficiency (extra-label): 5 – 100 mg IM, SC, or IV (depending on formulation)[19]

Monitoring

- Clinical efficacy

Client Information

- A reason for thiamine deficiency (eg, diet, plants, raw fish) should be found with changes made to prevent recurrence.

Chemistry/Synonyms

A water-soluble B vitamin, thiamine HCl occurs as bitter-tasting, white, small hygroscopic crystals, or crystalline powder that has a characteristic yeast-like odor. Thiamine HCl is freely soluble in water, slightly soluble in alcohol, and has pK_as of 4.8 and 9.0. The commercially available injection has a pH of 2.5 to 4.5.

Thiamine HCl may also be known as aneurine hydrochloride, thiamin hydrochloride, thiamine chloride, thiamini hydrochloridum, thiaminii chloridum, vitamin B_1; many trade names available.

Storage/Stability

Thiamine HCl for injection should be protected from light and stored at temperatures less than 40°C (104°F) and preferably between 15°C and 30°C (59°F-86°F); avoid freezing.

Thiamine HCl is unstable in alkaline or neutral solutions or with oxidizing or reducing agents. It is most stable at a pH of 2.

Compatibility/Compounding Considerations

Compatibility is dependent upon factors such as pH, concentration, temperature, and diluent used; consult specialized references or a hospital pharmacist for more specific information.

Thiamine HCl is reportedly physically **compatible** with all commonly used IV replacement fluids.

Do **not** mix thiamine with alkaline drugs or alkalinizing agents (barbiturates, citrates, carbonates, acetates, copper ions) or oxidizing/reducing agents (eg, sulfites).

Dosage Forms/Regulatory Status

VETERINARY-LABELED PRODUCTS:

Thiamine HCl for Injection: 500 mg/mL; generic; (Rx). Labeled for use in dogs, cats, and horses.

Thiamine HCl as a supplement: Numerous oral vitamin/mineral/nutritional supplement products in tablet, gel, oral drench, chewable, and powder formulations; (OTC). Labeled for use in multiple species.

Thiamine monohydrate supplement: A component in numerous vitamin/mineral formulations; *DERM-TABS®*; (OTC). Labeled for use in dogs. Calf colostrum replacer and supplement; (OTC). Labeled for use in calves. Pelleted formulation; *Compose® 2X*; (OTC). Labeled for use in horses.

Thiamine mononitrate: Included as an ingredient in numerous oral vitamin/mineral/nutritional supplement/milk replacer products in tablet, gel, oral drench, and milk replacer powder formulations; (OTC). Labeled for use in multiple species. Also available as a type B or type C medicated feed drug that may contain neomycin and oxytetracycline; *Super Guard Plus®*; (VFD). Also available as *Calf Solutions® Balansure®* medicated with *CLARIFLY®* larvicide. (VFD) Labeled for use in calves for treatment of coccidiosis and contains an ionophore and fly control.

HUMAN-LABELED PRODUCTS:

Thiamine Tablets: 50 mg, 100 mg, 250 mg, and 500 mg; generic; (OTC)

Thiamine Capsules: 50 mg; generic; (OTC)

Thiamine HCl Injection: 100 mg/mL in 1 mL and 2 mL multi-dose vials; generic; (Rx)

References

For the complete list of references, see **wiley.com/go/budde/plumb**

Thiopental

(thye-oh-***pen***-tal) *Pentothal®*

Ultra-Short-Acting Thiobarbiturate

Prescriber Highlights

- Used for anesthesia induction or anesthesia for very short procedures. Not available in the US or Canada.
- Absolute contraindications: absence of suitable veins for IV administration, history of hypersensitivity reactions to barbiturates, status asthmaticus. Relative contraindications: severe cardiovascular disease or pre-existing ventricular arrhythmias, shock, increased intracranial pressure, myasthenia gravis, asthma, and conditions where hypnotic effects may be prolonged (eg, severe hepatic disease, myxedema, severe anemia, excessive premedication). Greyhounds (and other sighthounds) metabolize thiobarbiturates much more slowly than other breeds; consider using methohexital instead. Horses: pre-existing leukopenia; thiopental alone may cause excessive ataxia and excitement.
- Avoid: Extravasation, intracarotid or intra-arterial injections. Too rapid IV administration can cause significant vascular dilatation and hypoglycemia.
- Adverse Effects: Dogs: Ventricular bigeminy. Cats: Apnea after injection, mild arterial hypotension. Horses: Excitement and severe ataxia (if used alone); transient leukopenias, hyperglycemia, apnea, moderate tachycardia, mild respiratory acidosis
- Severe CNS toxicity and tissue damage have occurred in horses receiving intracarotid injections of thiobarbiturates.
- DEA Schedule IV (C-IV) controlled substance

Uses/Indications

Because of its rapid action and short duration, in young, healthy animals, thiopental has been used as an induction agent (rapid IV bolus) for general anesthesia with other anesthetics or as the sole anesthetic agent for very short procedures. In sick or debilitated animals, thiopental may be used in a more cautious manner (IV, slowly to effect). Once widely used, thiopental is no longer available in many markets, including in the US and Canada.

Pharmacology/Actions

Because of their high lipid solubility, thiobarbiturates (also known as ultra short-acting barbiturates) rapidly enter the CNS and produce profound hypnosis and anesthesia. They act directly on the CNS neurons in a manner similar to that of the inhibitory transmitter GABA.

Pharmacokinetics

Following IV injection of therapeutic doses, hypnosis and anesthesia occur within 1 minute and usually within 15 to 30 seconds. The drug rapidly enters the CNS and then redistributes to muscle and adipose tissue in the body. The short duration of action (10 to 30 minutes) after IV dosing of thiopental is not due to rapid metabolism, but rather to this redistribution out of the CNS and into muscle and fat stores. Greyhounds and other sighthounds may exhibit longer recovery times than other breeds. This may be due to these breeds' low body fat concentrations and differences in the metabolic handling of the thiobarbiturates. Although anesthesia is short, recovery periods may require several hours. Prolonged recovery can also be noticed in horses[1] and bovine youngstock[2] when compared to ketamine.

Thiopental is metabolized by the hepatic microsomal system, and several metabolites have been isolated. The elimination half-life in dogs has been reported as being ≈7 hours and in sheep as 3 to 4 hours. Little of the drug is excreted unchanged in the urine (0.3% in humans), so dose adjustments are not necessary for patients with chronic renal failure.

Thiopental is highly protein-bound (75%).

Contraindications/Precautions/Warnings

The following are considered **absolute contraindications** to the use of thiopental: absence of suitable veins for IV administration, history of hypersensitivity reactions to the barbiturates, and status asthmaticus. **Relative contraindications** include severe cardiovascular disease or pre-existing ventricular arrhythmias, shock, hypotension, hypovolemia, increased intracranial pressure, myasthenia gravis, asthma, and conditions where hypnotic effects may be prolonged (eg, severe hepatic disease, myxedema, severe anemia, excessive premedication). The intracranial pressure (ICP) might increase due to respiratory depression and hypoventilation with a consequent increase in CO_2. If the patient is ventilated properly, thiopental decreases both ICP and cerebral metabolic oxygen consumption rate ($CMRO_2$), resulting in a neuroprotective effect. The decrease in mean arterial pressure (MAP) causes a decrease in cerebral blood flow (CBF), but the decrease in $CMRO_2$ helps maintain the ratio of CBF and $CMRO_2$ unchanged. Although MAP decreases, the cerebral perfusion pressure (CPP) remains unchanged due to the decrease in ICP (CPP = MAP – ICP). These relative contraindications do not preclude the use of thiopental, but dose adjustments and specific management of the patient must be considered, and the drug must be given cautiously.

Patients with renal dysfunction, acidemia, or hypoproteinemia may show increased sensitivity to thiopental.

Because greyhounds (and other sighthounds) metabolize thiobarbiturates much more slowly than methohexital, many clinicians recommend using methohexital instead. In horses, thiopental should not be used if the patient has pre-existing leukopenia. Some clinicians feel that thiopental should not be used alone in the horse as it may cause excessive ataxia and excitement. In young cattle, it is recommended that thiopental be avoided due to slower metabolism and long recovery times.

Concentrations of less than 2% in sterile water should not be used as they may cause hemolysis. Extravasation and intra-arterial injections should be avoided because of the high alkalinity of the solution. Severe CNS toxicity and tissue damage have occurred in horses receiving intracarotid injections of thiobarbiturates.

Adverse Effects

In dogs, thiopental has an arrhythmogenic incidence of ≈40%. Ventricular bigeminy is the most common arrhythmia seen; it is usually transient and generally responds to additional oxygen. Administration of catecholamines, xylazine, halothane, and methoxyflurane may exacerbate the arrhythmogenic effects of the thiobarbiturates, while lidocaine may inhibit it. Cardiac output may also be reduced but is probably only clinically significant in patients experiencing heart failure. Dose-related apnea and hypotension may be noted.

Cats are susceptible to developing apnea after injection and may develop mild arterial hypotension.

Horses can exhibit clinical signs of excitement and severe ataxia during the recovery period if the drug is used alone. Horses can develop transient leukopenia and hyperglycemia after administration. A period of apnea, moderate tachycardia, and mild respiratory acidosis may also develop after dosing.

Too rapid IV administration can cause significant vascular dilatation and hypoglycemia. Repeated administration of thiopental is not advised as recovery time can become significantly prolonged. Parasympathetic adverse effects (eg, salivation, bradycardia) can be managed with the use of anticholinergic agents (atropine, glycopyrrolate).

Prolonged recoveries may occur when repeated dosages of thiopental are administered.

The high pH of thiopental (10 to 11) can cause significant tissue irritation and necrosis if administered perivascularly; administration through an IV catheter is advised.

Reproductive/Nursing Safety

Thiopental readily crosses the placental barrier and should be used with caution during pregnancy.

Small amounts of thiopental may appear in milk following administration of large doses but are unlikely to be of clinical significance in nursing animals.

Because safety has not been established in animals, this drug should only be used when the maternal benefits outweigh the potential risks to offspring.

Overdose/Acute Toxicity

Treatment of thiobarbiturate overdosage consists of supporting respirations (eg, O_2, mechanical ventilation) and giving cardiovascular support; do not use catecholamines (eg, epinephrine).

For patients that have experienced or are suspected of having experienced an overdose, consultation with a 24-hour poison consultation center specializing in providing veterinary-specific information is recommended. For general information related to overdose and toxin exposures, as well as contact information for poison control centers, refer to ***Appendix***.

Drug Interactions

The following drug interactions have either been reported or are theoretical in humans or animals receiving thiopental and may be of significance in veterinary patients. Unless otherwise noted, use together is not necessarily contraindicated, but weigh the potential risks and perform additional monitoring when appropriate.

- **Clonidine**: IV clonidine prior to induction may reduce thiopental dosage requirements by up to 37%.[3]
- **CNS Depressants, Other** (eg, **methocarbamol**): May enhance respiratory and CNS depressant effects
- **Diazoxide**: Potential for hypotension
- **Epinephrine, Norepinephrine**: The ventricular fibrillatory effects of epinephrine and norepinephrine may be potentiated when used with thiobarbiturates and halothane.
- **Ketoprofen**: Anesthesia recovery time was prolonged[4]
- **Metoclopramide**: Given prior to induction may reduce thiopental dosage requirements
- **Midazolam**: May potentiate hypnotic effects
- **Opioids** (eg, **buprenorphine, fentanyl, morphine, tramadol**): Given prior to induction may reduce thiopental dosage requirements
- **Phenothiazines** (eg, **acepromazine**): May potentiate thiopental effects; hypotension possible

Dosages

NOTE: Atropine sulfate (or glycopyrrolate) is often administered prior to thiobarbiturate anesthesia to prevent parasympathetic adverse effects; however, some clinicians question whether routine administration of anticholinergic agents is necessary. Thiobarbiturates are administered strictly to effect; listed dosages are guidelines only.

DOGS/CATS:

Labeled dose (No longer marketed in the US): 13.2 – 26.4 mg/kg IV depending on the duration of anesthesia required[5]

Extra-label doses:

a) Usually dosed at 12 – 15 mg/kg, with ⅓ of the drug administered rapidly and any additional amount administered to effect. Repeated doses will accumulate, resulting in prolonged recoveries; residual effects may last several hours.[6]

b) Dogs: 15 – 17 mg/kg IV; Cats: 9 – 11 mg/kg IV[7]

RABBITS, RODENTS, SMALL MAMMALS:

Chemical restraint (extra-label): **Mice**: 50 mg/kg IP; **Rats**: 40 mg/kg IP; **Hamsters/Gerbils**: 30 – 40 mg/kg IP; **Guinea pigs**: 15 – 30 mg/kg IV; **Rabbits**: 15 – 30 mg/kg IV[8]

CATTLE:

General Anesthesia in premedicated cattle (extra-label): Cattle: 8.1 – 9.9 mg/kg IV; calves: 4.5 mg/kg IV[7]

HORSES:

General Anesthesia in premedicated horses (extra-label): 5.9 – 12.9 mg/kg IV.[7] A dose of thiopental 4 mg/kg IV, after premedication with medetomidine and midazolam, achieved induction and recovery quality comparable to ketamine 2.5 mg/kg IV; however, the recovery was longer when thiopental was used.[1]

SWINE:

General Anesthesia (extra-label): 5 – 11 mg/kg IV[7]

SHEEP:

General Anesthesia (extra-label): 9 – 14 mg/kg IV[7]

Monitoring

- Level of hypnosis/anesthesia
- Respiratory status; cardiac status (eg, heart rate and rhythm and blood pressure)

Client Information

This drug should only be used by professionals familiar with its effects, and in a setting where adequate respiratory support can be performed.

Chemistry/Synonyms

Thiopental, a thiobarbiturate, occurs as a bitter-tasting, white to off-white, crystalline powder or a yellow-white hygroscopic powder. It is soluble in water (1 g in 1.5 mL) and alcohol. Thiopental has a pK_a of

7.6 and is a weak organic acid. Thiopental solutions are very alkaline (pH greater than 10).

Thiopental sodium may also be known as thiopentone sodium, natrium isopentylaethylthiobarbituricum, penthiobarbital sodique, thiomebumalnatrium cum natrii carbonate, thiopentalum natricum, thiopentobarbitalum solubile, tiopentol sodico, *Anesthal®*, *Bensulf®*, *Farmotal®*, *Hipnopento®*, *Inductal®*, *Intraval®*, *Nesdonal®*, *Pensodital®*, *Pentothal®*, *Sandothal®*, *Sodipental®*, *Thionembutal®*, *Thiopentax®*, *Tiobarbital®*, or *Trapanal®*.

Storage/Stability

When stored in the dry form, thiopental sodium is stable indefinitely. Thiopental should be diluted with only sterile water for injection, 0.9% sodium chloride or 5% dextrose. Do not use concentrations of less than 2% in sterile water as they may cause hemolysis. After reconstitution, solutions are stable for 3 days at room temperature and 7 days if refrigerated; however, as no preservative is present, consider using it within 24 hours after reconstitution. After 48 hours, there are reports of the solution attacking the glass bottle in which it is stored. Thiopental may also adsorb to plastic IV tubing and bags. Do not administer any solution that has a visible precipitate.

Compatibility/Compounding Considerations

Compatibility is dependent upon factors, such as pH, concentration, temperature, and diluent used; consult specialized references or a hospital pharmacist for more specific information.

Preparation of Solution for Administration: Use only sterile water for injection, 0.9% sodium chloride, or 5% dextrose to dilute. A 5 g vial diluted with 100 mL will yield a 5% solution, and diluted with 200 mL will yield a 2.5% solution. Discard reconstituted solutions after 24 hours.

The following agents have been reported to be physically **compatible** when mixed with thiopental: aminophylline, chloramphenicol sodium succinate, hyaluronidase, hydrocortisone sodium succinate, neostigmine methylsulfate, oxytocin, pentobarbital sodium, phenobarbital sodium, potassium chloride, propofol (1:1 mixture), scopolamine HBr, sodium iodide, and tubocurarine chloride (recommendations **conflict** with regard to tubocurarine; some clinicians recommend not mixing with thiopental).

The following agents have been reported to be physically **incompatible** when mixed with thiopental: lactated Ringer's solution, amikacin sulfate, atropine sulfate, chlorpromazine, codeine phosphate, dimenhydrinate, diphenhydramine, ephedrine sulfate, glycopyrrolate, hydromorphone, insulin (regular), meperidine, morphine sulfate, norepinephrine bitartrate, penicillin G potassium, prochlorperazine edisylate, promazine HCl, promethazine HCl, succinylcholine chloride, and tetracycline HCl.

Dosage Forms/Regulatory Status

VETERINARY-LABELED PRODUCTS:

None presently marketed in the United States

The Association of Racing Commissioners International (ARCI) has designated this drug as a class 2 substance. Use of this drug may not be allowed in certain animal competitions. Check rules and regulations before entering a competition while this medication is being administered. Contact local racing authorities for further guidance. See ***Appendix*** for more information.

HUMAN-LABELED PRODUCTS:

Thiopental remains unavailable in the United States market.

References

For the complete list of references, see **wiley.com/go/budde/plumb**

Thyrotropin Alfa

(thye-roe-***troe***-pin) Thyroid-Stimulating Hormone, TSH Hormone

Prescriber Highlights

- ▶ Used for thyroid-stimulating hormone (TSH) test of thyroid function
- ▶ Contraindications include adrenocortical insufficiency, hyperthyroidism, coronary thrombosis, hypersensitivity to bovine thyrotropin. Cannot be used to evaluate thyroid function in patients receiving levothyroxine.
- ▶ Adverse effects include hypersensitivity (especially with repeated injections).
- ▶ Expense (human product) may be an issue.

Uses/Indications

The labeled indication for the formerly available bovine-source veterinary product *Dermathycin®* was *for the treatment of acanthosis nigricans and for temporary supportive therapy in hypothyroidism in dogs*. However, TSH is used more commonly as a diagnostic agent in the TSH stimulation test to diagnose primary hypothyroidism in many species. It can also be used for the diagnosis of congenital hypothyroidism. Commercially available TSH is supplied as a recombinant human product (rhTSH). While rhTSH enhances radioactive iodine uptake in hyperthyroid cats,[1] inconsistent results were noted when used to evaluate radioactive iodine uptake in dogs with thyroid tumors.[2]

Pharmacology/Actions

Thyrotropin increases iodine uptake by the thyroid gland and increases the production and secretion of thyroid hormones and thyroglobulin. With prolonged use, hyperplasia of thyroid cells may occur.

Pharmacokinetics

No specific information was located; exogenously administered TSH apparently exerts maximal increases in circulating T_4 ≈4 to 8 hours after IM or IV administration. In humans, peak TSH concentrations occur at ≈10 hours after administration and the elimination half-life is ≈25 hours.

Contraindications/Precautions/Warnings

A previous veterinary drug manufacturer (Coopers) listed adrenocortical insufficiency and hyperthyroidism as contraindications to TSH use for treatment purposes in dogs. In humans, TSH is contraindicated in patients with coronary thrombosis, untreated Addison's disease, or hypersensitivity to bovine thyrotropin.

Levothyroxine supplementation can cause thyroid atrophy and should be discontinued before thyroid testing with TSH. After discontinuing levothyroxine, a washout period of 6 to 8 weeks before performing the TSH stimulation test has been proposed.[3]

Adverse Effects

Because the commercially available product is derived from human sources, hypersensitivity reactions are possible in patients sensitive to human proteins, particularly with repeated use. To date, no reports of anaphylaxis in animals receiving rhTSH have been reported. Nausea, vomiting, diarrhea, and fatigue have been reported in humans.

Reproductive/Nursing Safety

It is not known whether the drug is excreted in milk, but it is unlikely to be clinically significant when used for diagnostic purposes.

Because safety has not been established in animals, this drug should only be used when the maternal benefits outweigh the potential risks to offspring.

Overdose/Acute Toxicity

Chronic administration at high dosages can produce clinical signs of hyperthyroidism. Massive overdoses can cause clinical signs resembling thyroid storm. Refer to the levothyroxine monograph for more information on treatment.

For patients that have experienced or are suspected of having experienced an overdose, consultation with a 24-hour poison consultation center specializing in providing veterinary-specific information is recommended. For general information related to overdose and toxin exposures, as well as contact information for poison control centers, refer to ***Appendix.***

Drug Interactions

No specific drug interactions were reported, but see the information regarding levothyroxine (see ***Contraindications/Precautions/Warnings*** section). Concurrent use of levothyroxine while using thyrotropin alfa for provocative thyroid testing may skew test results.

Laboratory Considerations

- Prior or concurrent levothyroxine supplementation may skew results of TSH stimulation testing (see ***Contraindications/Precautions/Warnings*** section).

Dosages

DOGS:

TSH stimulation test (extra-label):

a) From two studies where dogs received either 75 µg/dog or 150 µg/dog (NOT µg/kg) IV of the human recombinant product. Blood samples were taken before and 6 hours after rhTSH administration for determination of total serum thyroxine (T_4) concentration. The authors concluded that the TSH-stimulation test with rhTSH is a valuable diagnostic tool to assess thyroid function in selected dogs in which a diagnosis of hypothyroidism cannot be based on basal T_4 and canine TSH concentrations alone. Using the higher dose of rhTSH resulted in a higher discriminatory power with regard to differentiating between primary hypothyroidism and non-thyroidal disease and the authors recommend the higher dose (150 µg/dog [NOT µg/kg]) of rhTSH for performing a TSH stimulation test in a diseased animal or an animal on medication, especially if testing cannot be delayed.[4,5]

b) Using rhTSH: 75 – 150 µg/dog (NOT µg/kg) IV. The higher dose of TSH is recommended in dogs with concurrent disease and those receiving medication that might suppress thyroid function. Measure serum total T_4 at 0 hours (presample) and 6 hours postdosing. Hypothyroidism is confirmed by a pre- and post-total T_4 concentration below the reference range for basal total T_4 concentration (less than 1.5 µg/dL). Euthyroidism is confirmed by a post total T_4 concentration greater than 2.5 µg/dL and at least 1.5 times the basal T_4 concentration.[6]

CATS:

TSH stimulation test (extra-label):

a) 25 µg/cat (NOT µg/kg) IV. Draw pre- and postdosing total T_4 levels. Can be useful for differentiating feline iatrogenic hypothyroidism from non-thyroidal illness.[3]

b) Using rhTSH: 25 µg/cat (NOT µg/kg) IV. Measure serum total T_4 at 0 hours (presample) and 6 hours postdosing.[7]

BIRDS:

TSH stimulation test (extra-label): 20 - 200 µg/kg IM. Draw T_4 sample at baseline (predose) and 4 to 6 hours after dose.[8]

FERRETS:

TSH stimulation test (extra-label): 100 µg/ferret (NOT µg/kg) IM. Postlevel (T_4) drawn at 4 hours. Authors concluded that the results suggested that rhTSH can be used for TSH testing in ferrets when administered IM. Based on the results, a euthyroid ferret should have an increase of ≈30% in plasma T_4 concentration 4 hours after rhTSH injection.[9]

SMALL MAMMALS:

TSH stimulation test (guinea pigs) (extra-label): 100 µg/guinea pig (NOT µg/kg) IM. Postlevel (T_4) drawn at 3 to 4 hours. Authors concluded that the results suggested that rhTSH can be used for TSH testing in guinea pigs when administered IM. Based on the results, authors suggest that the thyroxine concentration in a euthyroid guinea pig should at least double 3 to 4 hours after rhTSH injection.[10]

Chemistry/Synonyms

Commercially available thyrotropin (human; rhTSH) is now available only as a lyophilized powder for reconstitution obtained via DNA recombinant technology. Thyrotropin is a highly purified preparation of thyroid-stimulating hormone (TSH). Thyrotropin is a glycoprotein and has a molecular weight of ≈28,000 – 30,000. Thyrotropin is measured in International Units (IU), which is abbreviated as units in this reference. 7.5 µg of thyrotropin are ≈equivalent to 0.037 units. The formerly available veterinary product was obtained from bovine anterior pituitary glands.

Thyrotropin may also be known as thyroid-stimulating hormone, thyrotrophic hormone, thyrotrophin thyrotropin, TSH, *Thyrogen*®, or *Tirogen*®.

Storage/Stability

Thyrotropin alfa (non-reconstituted) should be stored between 2°C and 8°C (36°F-46°F). If necessary, the reconstituted solution can be stored up to 24 hours at 2°C to 8°C (36-46°F); avoid microbial contamination. However, it is reportedly stable if kept refrigerated (2°C-8°C [36°F-46°F]).) up to 4 weeks and up to 12 weeks if frozen (-20°C [-4°F). Protect from light.

Compatibility/Compounding Considerations

Compatibility is dependent on factors such as pH, concentration, temperature, and diluent used; specialized references or a hospital pharmacist should be consulted for more specific information.

After reconstitution visually inspect each vial for particulate matter or discoloration before use. Do not use any vial exhibiting particulate matter or discoloration. Do not use after the expiration date on the vial.

Dosage Forms/Regulatory Status

VETERINARY-LABELED PRODUCTS: NONE

HUMAN-LABELED PRODUCTS:

Recombinant (human) Thyrotropin (Thyroid-Stimulating Hormone) Powder for Injection, Lyophilized: 1.1 mg per vial; *Thyrogen*®; (Rx)

References

For the complete list of references, see **wiley.com/go/budde/plumb**

Thyrotropin-Releasing Hormone (TRH)

(thye-roe-***troe***-pin ree-***lee***-seen ***hor***-mohn)
Hormone

Prescriber Highlights

- Most commonly used for diagnosing pituitary pars intermedia dysfunction (PPID) in horses. Can also be used for some thyroid-related tests.
- Adverse effects in horses include transient muscle trembling, yawning, lip smacking, flehmen, and coughing.
- In the United States, must be compounded

Uses/Indications

Thyrotropin-releasing hormone (TRH; protirelin) is most commonly used in veterinary medicine as a diagnostic agent (TRH stimulation test) for diagnosing pituitary pars intermedia dysfunction (PPID) in horses. While safe and fast, when measuring cortisol as the marker, false-positive results are relatively common. Combining this test with a dexamethasone suppression test can improve diagnostic test sensitivity and specificity, but increases testing times and sampling requirements.[1] Measuring plasma corticotropin (ACTH) instead of cortisol after TRH now appears to offer the highest diagnostic sensitivity compared with other tests for PPID and may allow for earlier detection.[2] Because of seasonal variations in ACTH levels, the TRH stimulation test should be performed during winter or spring.[3-6]

In dogs, the TRH test can potentially be used to differentiate primary from secondary hypothyroidism. It is not a reliable test to diagnose primary hypothyroidism.

TRH or its analogues may improve physical function after acute intervertebral disk herniation.

Pharmacology/Actions

Thyrotropin-releasing hormone directly stimulates thyrotropin secretion by the pituitary gland, thereby indirectly stimulating synthesis and secretion of thyroid hormones.

In horses, thyrotropin-releasing hormone (TRH) can stimulate the equine pars intermedia and appears to directly stimulate equine melanotropes. In healthy horses, plasma alpha-melanocyte-stimulating hormones can be increased more than 400% after TRH. Normal horses will have slight increases in ACTH after TRH administration, subclinical PPID horses have a moderate increase in ACTH, while clinically ill PPID horses have dramatic increases in ACTH after TRH. Response to TRH is greater in autumn months than at other times of the year.

Pharmacokinetics

No specific information for veterinary species was noted. Onset of action after IV administration appears to be within minutes. In humans, buccal administration yielded statistically significant increases in thyrotropin concentrations above baseline at 30 and 60 minutes, although at 30 minutes both the thyrotrophic effect and adverse effects were less in some subjects. Deamidase, peptidase, and imidopeptidase enzymes in the CNS and serum metabolize TRH to active and inactive metabolites. Elimination half-life is ≈5 minutes.

Contraindications/Precautions/Warnings

Contraindicated in patients that are hypersensitive to it. Use with caution in patients with seizure disorders as IV administration has rarely caused seizures in humans.

Adverse Effects

Hypersalivation, vomiting and restlessness were noted in healthy dogs.[7] In horses, IV administration of TRH can cause transient muscle trembling, yawning, lip-smacking, flehmen, and coughing.

In humans, TRH given by rapid IV injection or intranasally can cause nausea, a desire to urinate, flushing, dizziness, and a strange taste. Intranasal administration has rarely caused bronchospasm. IV administration can cause transient increases in pulse rate, and changes in blood pressure; convulsions have rarely occurred.

Reproductive/Nursing Safety

It is not known whether TRH is excreted in milk, but it is unlikely to be clinically significant when used for diagnostic purposes.

Because safety has not been established in animals, this drug should only be used when the maternal benefits outweigh the potential risks to offspring.

Overdose/Acute Toxicity

No specific information was located; determine doses and drug volumes carefully.

For patients that have experienced or are suspected to have experienced an overdose, consultation with a 24-hour poison consultation center specializing in providing veterinary-specific information is recommended. For general information related to overdose and toxin exposures, as well as contact information for poison control centers, refer to ***Appendix***.

Drug Interactions

The following drug interactions have either been reported or are theoretical in humans or animals receiving TRH and may be of significance in veterinary patients. Unless otherwise noted, use together is not necessarily contraindicated, but weigh the potential risks and perform additional monitoring when appropriate.

- **Corticosteroids** (eg, **dexamethasone**): At high doses, may cause decreased thyrotropin response to TRH. Dexamethasone suppression test may be performed concurrently with TRH testing in horses.[8,9]
- **Cyproheptadine**: May cause decreased thyrotropin response to TRH
- **Dopamine Blocking Drugs** (eg, **domperidone, metoclopramide**): May cause increased thyrotropin response to TRH
- **Gonadorelin and Gonadorelin Analogues**: May cause increased thyrotropin response to TRH
- **Salicylates**: May cause decreased thyrotropin response to TRH
- **Thyroid Hormones** (eg, **levothyroxine**): May decrease thyrotropin response to TRH

Laboratory Considerations

- Contact your laboratory for specific sampling guidelines and shipping requirements.

Dosages

DOGS:

Assess pituitary and thyroid gland function:

a. **Differentiate primary from secondary hypothyroidism** (extra-label): Collect a pre-TRH blood sample; administer 0.2 mg/dog (NOT mg/kg) IV of TRH; collect a 4-hour post-TRH blood sample. Measure pre- and post-TRH serum T_4 concentrations. **NOTE**: For measurement of thyrotropin (TSH) collect blood samples pre- and 30 minutes post-TRH administration.[10]

b. **Differentiate primary hypothyroidism from nonthyroidal illness** (extra-label): Collect a pre-TRH blood sample; administer 0.01 mg/kg IV of TRH; collect a 30- minute post-TRH blood sample. Measure pre- and post-TRH serum TSH concentrations. TSH will be elevated in dogs without thyroidal illness.[7,11]

CATS:

Assess thyroid gland function for hyperthyroidism (extra-label): Collect a pre-TRH blood sample; administer 0.1 mg/kg IV of TRH; collect a 4-hour post-TRH blood sample. Measure pre- and post-TRH serum T_4 concentrations. Hyperthyroid cats have little to no post-TRH elevation in T_4.[12]

HORSES:

Diagnosis of pituitary pars intermedia dysfunction (PPID) using the TRH stimulation test (extra-label):

Using plasma ACTH as the marker:

Protocol 1: The most accurate results are obtained when diagnostic testing is performed winter or spring. Contact your diagnostic laboratory for specific sample requirements. Collect baseline (usually plasma) sample for ACTH analysis. Inject TRH 1 mg IV. Collect plasma sample at 10 and/or 30 minutes following TRH. A 10-minute and/or a 30-minute post-TRH ACTH level of 110 nanograms/L and 65 nanograms/L, respectively,[5,13,14] are the current diagnostic cut-offs, but these may vary depending on the laboratory used.[2,3,15]

Protocol 2: An alternative testing procedure is as above, but TRH 0.5 mg IV is used for ponies and the post-TRH sample is drawn at 30 minutes. At Auburn University Endocrine Diagnostic Laboratory: ACTH concentrations at T = 0, 10, and 30 minutes should all be <35 picograms/mL, with even lower concentrations expected between December and June. Note: Can also be used to simultaneously rule out hypothyroidism by collecting samples for T_3 and T_4 at 0, 2, and 4 hours. Normal horse: A doubling of T_4 after 4 hours and ≈tripling of T_3 after 2 hours is expected. A normal horse will have a small increase in ACTH concentration after 30 minutes (refer to seasonal reference ranges). PPID horse: T_3 and T_4 will increase the same as a normal horse, and the ACTH at T = 0 will be elevated, and at 30 minutes ACTH will be markedly elevated. Hypothyroid horse: No marked increase in T_3 or T_4. (Resting T_3 and T_4 concentrations are not very useful.)[16]

Combined dexamethasone suppression/TRH stimulation test using plasma cortisol as the marker: Collect plasma between 8 AM and 10 AM. Administer dexamethasone 0.04 mg/kg IM. Three hours later administer TRH 1 mg IV. Collect plasma 30 minutes after TRH was given and again 24 hours after the dexamethasone dose (21 hours post-TRH). Compared to baseline, a plasma cortisol greater than 1 µg/dL at 24 hours post-dexamethasone sample or a greater than or equal to 66% increase for the 3-hour post-TRH sample suggests PPID. **NOTE**: Some diagnostic laboratories prefer to use serum for measurement of cortisol levels. The effect of season on the combined test has not been assessed but would likely result in similar incidence of false-positive results as each of the component tests do.[9,17]

Chemistry/Synonyms

TRH (protirelin) is a synthetic tri-peptide with the same sequence of amino acids as the natural hypothalamic neuro-hormone. It occurs as a white or yellowish-white hygroscopic powder that is very soluble in water and freely soluble in methyl alcohol.

Thyrotropin-releasing hormone may also be known as Abbott-38579, TRH, thyrotrophin-releasing hormone, lopremone, protirelin, thyroliberin, thyrotropin-releasing factor (TRF), *Antepan*®, or *Relefact*®.

Storage/Stability

TRH (protirelin) powder should be stored at 2°C to 8°C (36°C-46°C) and protected from light and moisture. If using a compounded preparation, store as labeled.

Compatibility/Compounding Considerations

No specific information noted

Dosage Forms/Regulatory Status

VETERINARY-LABELED PRODUCTS: NONE

HUMAN-LABELED PRODUCTS:

There are no commercially available products marketed in the United States at present, but TRH may be available from compounding pharmacies.

References

For the complete list of references, see **wiley.com/go/budde/plumb**

Tiamulin

(tye-***am***-myoo-lin) *Denagard*®

Diterpine Pleuromutilin Antibiotic

Prescriber Highlights

- ▶ Antibiotic approved for use in swine; may be used extra-label in chickens and turkeys
- ▶ Contraindications include in animals with access to feeds containing polyether ionophores (eg, monensin, lasalocid, narasin, or salinomycin) and in swine over 113.4 kg (250 lb).
- ▶ Adverse effects are unlikely.
- ▶ Variable withdrawal times depending on dosage.

Uses/Indications

Tiamulin is FDA-approved for use in swine to treat pneumonia caused by susceptible strains of *Actinobacillus pleuropneumoniae* and swine dysentery caused by *Brachyspira hyodysenteriae*. Tiamulin has demonstrated activity against *Brachyspira hampsonii*.[1] In the UK, tiamulin is approved for use in turkeys and chickens for the reduction in the severity of disease caused by mycoplasmas; in pigs for dysentery, colitis, and pneumonia; and in rabbits for enterocolitis.[2]

The World Health Organization (WHO) has designated tiamulin as an Important antimicrobial for human medicine.[3] The Office International des Epizooties (OIE) Antimicrobial Classification has designated tiamulin as a Veterinary Highly Important antimicrobial.[4]

Pharmacology/Actions

Tiamulin is a pleuromutilin antibiotic that is usually bacteriostatic but can be bactericidal in high concentrations against susceptible organisms. The drug acts by binding to the 50S ribosomal subunit, thereby inhibiting bacterial protein synthesis; it has good intracellular penetration.

Tiamulin has good activity against many gram-positive cocci, including most staphylococci and streptococci (not group D streptococci). It also has good activity against *Mycoplasma* spp and spirochetes. With the exceptions of *Haemophilus* spp, most isolates of *Lawsonia intracellularis*, and some *Escherichia coli* and *Klebsiella* spp strains, tiamulin activity is quite poor against gram-negative organisms. Tiamulin does not have apparent efficacy against *Histomonas meleagridis*.

Pharmacokinetics

Tiamulin is well absorbed orally by swine. Approximately 85% of a dose is absorbed and peak levels occur between 2 to 4 hours after a single oral dose. Tiamulin is apparently well distributed, with the highest levels found in the lungs.

Tiamulin is extensively metabolized to over 20 metabolites, with some of the metabolites having antibacterial activity. Approximately 30% of these metabolites are excreted in the urine with the remainder excreted in the feces.

Contraindications/Precautions/Warnings

Tiamulin should not be administered to animals that have access to feeds containing polyether ionophores (eg, monensin, lasalocid, narasin, salinomycin), as adverse reactions may occur. Do not use tiamulin in swine over 113.4 kg (250 lb).

Tiamulin inhalation has been reported to result in QT prolongation and ventricular tachyarrhythmia in humans; wear appropriate protective equipment when handling.[5]

Reproductive/Nursing Safety

Teratogenicity studies done in rodents demonstrated no teratogenic effects at doses up to 300 mg/kg. The manufacturer has concluded that the drug is not tumorigenic, carcinogenic, teratogenic, or mutagenic.

Adverse Effects

Adverse effects occurring with this drug at usual doses are considered unlikely. Rarely, redness of the skin, primarily over the ham and underline, has been observed in swine. If this occurs, it is recommended to discontinue the medication, provide clean drinking water, and hose down the housing area or move affected animals to clean pens.

Overdose/Acute Toxicity

Oral overdoses in swine may cause transient salivation, vomiting, and CNS depression (calming effect). Discontinue drug and treat symptomatically and supportively if necessary.

For patients that have experienced or are suspected to have experienced an overdose, consultation with a 24-hour poison consultation center specializing in providing veterinary-specific information is recommended. For general information related to overdose and toxin exposures, as well as contact information for poison control centers, refer to ***Appendix.***

Drug Interactions

The following drug interactions have either been reported or are theoretical in humans or animals receiving tiamulin and may be of significance in veterinary patients. Unless otherwise noted, use together is not necessarily contraindicated, but weigh the potential risks and perform additional monitoring when appropriate.

- **Polyether Ionophores** (eg, **monensin, lasalocid, narasin, salinomycin**): Tiamulin should not be administered to animals that have access to feeds containing polyether ionophores, as adverse reactions may occur.
- **Lincosamides, Macrolides** (eg, **clindamycin, lincomycin, erythromycin, tylosin**): Although not confirmed with this drug, concomitant use with other antibiotics that bind to the 50S ribosome could lead to decreased efficacy secondary to competition at the site of action.

Dosages

SWINE:

Swine dysentery (label dosage; FDA-approved): 7.7 mg/kg PO daily in drinking water for 5 days. See package directions for dilution instructions.[6]

Swine pneumonia (label dosage; FDA-approved): 23.1 mg/kg PO daily in drinking water for 5 days. See package directions for dilution instructions.[6]

Medicated premix: See the label for the product.

POULTRY:

***Mycoplasma* spp disease in chicken and turkey** (extra-label): 25 mg/kg bodyweight administered in drinking water as 0.025% solution for 3 – 5 days (chicken) or for 5 days (turkey)[2]

Monitoring

- Clinical efficacy

Client Information

- Prepare fresh medicated water daily.
- Avoid contact with skin or mucous membranes as irritation may occur.

Chemistry/Synonyms

A semisynthetic diterpene-class antibiotic derived from pleuromulin, tiamulin is available commercially for oral use as the hydrogen fumarate salt. It occurs as white to yellow, crystalline powder with a faint but characteristic odor. Approximately 60 mg of the drug are soluble in 1 mL of water.

Tiamulin may also be known as 81723-hfu, SQ-14055, SQ-22947 (tiamulin fumarate), or *Denagard®*.

Storage/Stability

Protect from moisture; store in a dry place at controlled room temperature (59°F-77°F [15°C-25°C]). In unopened packets, the powder is stable up to 5 years. Fresh solutions should be prepared daily when using clinically.

Compatibility/Compounding Considerations

No specific information is noted.

Dosage Forms/Regulatory Status

VETERINARY APPROVED PRODUCTS:

Tiamulin Medicated Premix: 10 g/1 lb in 35 lb bags; *Denagard® 10*; (OTC). FDA-approved for use in swine not weighing over 113.4 kg (250 lb). Slaughter withdrawal period at the 35 g/ton use is 2 days; at the 200 g/ton dose it is 7 days.

Tiamulin Solution as tiamulin hydrogen fumarate in an aqueous base; *Triamulox® Liquid Concentrate* (12.3% solution in 32 oz bottles); *Denagard® Liquid Concentrate* (12.5% solution in 1000 mL and 5000 mL bottles; (OTC). FDA-approved for use in swine not weighing over 113.4 kg (250 lb). Slaughter withdrawal: treatment at 3.5 mg/lb = 3 days; at 10.5 mg/lb = 7 days. The UK label lists slaughter withdrawal of 2 days for chicken and 5 days for turkey; there is no withdrawal time for eggs laid by chickens.

Tiamulin solution for injection: 162 mg/mL; *Vetmulin®*; (Not available in the United States). For treatment and prevention of dysentery in swine in individuals with known exposure; not for herd-level treatment. Withdrawal time is 21 days.[7]

There is also a chlortetracycline/tiamulin premix approved by the FDA.

HUMAN APPROVED PRODUCTS: NONE

References

For the complete list of references, see **wiley.com/go/budde/plumb**

Tigilanol Tiglate

(tih-*gil*-an-ol tig-late) *Stelfonta®*
Antineoplastic

Prescriber Highlights

- FDA-approved for intratumoral injection for treatment of dogs with nonmetastatic cutaneous mast cell tumors (MCTs) anywhere on the body and nonmetastatic subcutaneous MCTs at or distal to the elbow or the hock
- Destruction of the tumor produces a wound at the treatment site that typically heals within ≈6 weeks.
- Tigilanol tiglate **must** be used concomitantly with a corticosteroid (eg, prednis(ol)one), an H_1-receptor antagonist (eg, diphenhydramine), and an H_2-receptor antagonist (eg, famotidine) to minimize severe systemic reactions caused by mast cell degranulation.
- Has been used in an extra-label manner to treat skin tumors in horses; concomitant medications and dosages for horses differ from those used in dogs
- Contraindicated for treatment of subcutaneous MCT above the elbow or the hock, of MCT volume exceeding 10 cm³, and in dogs with metastatic disease. Total dose must not exceed 5 mL/dog and 0.25 mL/kg.
- Do not administer into the tumor margin, beyond the tumor periphery, or by any route other than directly in the tumor.
- Use with extreme caution in MCTs that are ulcerated; use cautiously with mucocutaneous MCTs and in animals with conditions associated with impaired wound healing.
- Adverse effects include extensive wound formation, tissue sloughing, and cellulitis that occurs at, and may extend from, the tumor site. Injection site reactions (eg, pain, swelling, erythema, bruising) are common. In dogs, lameness in the treated limb and GI effects (eg, hyporexia/anorexia, vomiting, diarrhea) may also occur.
- Handle this drug with extreme caution, as accidental self-injection or needlestick injury may result in severe wound formation. Wear appropriate personal protective equipment when preparing or administering this drug. Those who are pregnant or planning to become pregnant should not handle this drug.
- Provide the manufacturer's client information sheet to owners before the drug is administered.

Uses/Indications

In dogs with a tumor volume less than 10 cm³, tigilanol tiglate is administered via intratumoral injection to treat nonmetastatic cutaneous mast cell tumor (MCTs) located anywhere on the body or nonmetastatic **subcutaneous** MCTs at or distal to the elbow or the hock. Intratumoral tigilanol tiglate administration destroys the tumor over ≈1 week, and the resulting wound typically heals within ≈6 weeks. In a field study, 75% of treated dogs achieved complete response in the target tumor 28 days after receiving 1 injection.[1] In dogs with an incomplete response, a second injection 1 month later resulted in a cumulative complete response rate of ≈87%. Efficacy proved higher in tumors of lower cytologic grade when compared with tumors of higher grade (ie, 72% vs 38%).[1] At 12 weeks after treatment, a complete response was maintained in 93% of dogs.[1] In a separate evaluation, 89% of evaluable dogs remained tumor free at the treatment site 12 months after treatment,[2] and most cases of recurrence were noted within 12 weeks after treatment.

Tigilanol tiglate **must** be used in combination with a corticosteroid and antihistamines (see ***Contraindications/Precautions/Warnings*** and ***Dosages***).[3]

Tigilanol tiglate was successfully used intratumorally in 2 horses to treat local disease (fibroblastic sarcoid, periocular squamous cell carcinoma); tumor response followed a pattern similar to that observed in dogs.[4]

Pharmacology/Actions

Tigilanol tiglate disrupts mitochondrial function, resulting in oncolysis.[3,5,6] This effect is immediate, short-lived, and limited to the area of injection. In addition, the drug preferentially activates beta II (alpha-, beta I-, and gamma-isoforms of protein kinase C [PKC] are also activated[3,7]), producing an acute (2 to 4 days) inflammatory response in and around the tumor that restricts tumor blood supply, as well as recruiting and activating the cellular immune response (ie, neutrophils and macrophages). Activating PKC also increases tumor vascular permeability that leads to destruction of the tumor vasculature.[3,5,6] Tumor destruction and necrosis are typically seen 4 to 7 days after administration.[3,5,6]

Tigilanol tiglate does not prevent MCT development in dogs.[5,6]

Pharmacokinetics

The pharmacokinetics of tigilanol tiglate have been described in dogs receiving intratumoral administration.[3,5,6] A relatively small amount of the drug is absorbed into systemic circulation. Peak plasma concentration (C_{max}) ranged from 0.356 to 13.8 ng/mL (mean 5.9 ng/mL), and elimination half-life was 2.85 to 36.87 hours. Tigilanol tiglate exposure (C_{max} and AUC_{last}) demonstrated no relationship with tumor location or total tigilanol tiglate dose.[3] The systemic exposure of tigilanol tiglate following intratumoral injection is not sufficient to treat MCT at other sites or to treat metastatic disease.[6]

Although tigilanol tiglate treatment is not administered by the IV route, following 0.025 – 0.075 mg/kg IV infusion in dogs, tigilanol tiglate C_{max} was 11 – 57 ng/mL,[8] and half-life was 0.54 hours.[5,6,8]

Contraindications/Precautions/Warnings

Tigilanol tiglate is contraindicated in patients hypersensitive to it or to propylene glycol, which is present in the commercial formulation. Do not inject tigilanol tiglate in MCTs with volume greater than 10 cm³, or in the margins of a surgically resected MCT[5,6]; SC injection in locations above the elbow or hock may result in severe systemic reactions due to mast cell degranulation and must be avoided.[3] Use tigilanol tiglate with extreme caution in MCTs that are ulcerated or have broken skin, as drug leakage from the site could lead to an underdose and unintentional drug exposure[5,6]; consider applying a bandage to the treated area. Use tigilanol tiglate with caution in MCTs located in mucocutaneous regions (eg, conjunctiva, lip margins, vulva, prepuce, anus) and at the extremities (eg, tail, paws)[5,6] and in patients with conditions associated with impaired wound healing (eg, uncontrolled diabetes mellitus, hyperadrenocorticism).[3] In completely subcutaneous MCTs, an incision may be needed to allow drainage of necrotic tissue.[5,6] Safe use of tigilanol tiglate in dogs younger than 3.5 years old was not evaluated during United States approval studies,[3] but European Union authorization provides for use in dogs 12 months of age and older.[5]

When treating MCT in dogs, an anti-inflammatory dose of a corticosteroid **must** be started 2 days prior to tigilanol tiglate injection. Both H_1- and H_2-receptor antagonists (eg, diphenhydramine, famotidine) **must** be started the day of tigilanol tiglate injection. See ***Dosages***. These concomitant treatments **must** continue for an additional 7 days after tigilanol tiglate administration (ie, 10 total days of corticosteroid and 8 total days of both antihistamines). Failure to administer these treatments for the full duration has resulted in death due to mast cell degranulation.[3]

Tigilanol tiglate does not treat metastatic disease, as it is only effective at the injection site.[5,6] Tumor necrosis and wound formation are expected outcomes of tigilanol tiglate administration and occur ≈ 4 to 7 days after injection. The size (ie, surface area) of the resulting wound is increased with larger tumor volume, enlarged regional lymph nodes, and higher cytologic tumor grade.[9] Fully healed wounds were noted at 4, 6, and 12 weeks after administration in ≈58%, ≈75%, and ≈97% of dogs, respectively.[3,6,9] NOTE: Histologic tumor grading after tigilanol tiglate treatment is unlikely to be accurate following necrosis of the tumor. Cytologic grading prior to treatment is recommended.[3]

Tigilanol tiglate is a skin and eye irritant.[10] Wear appropriate personal protective equipment (eg, gloves, gown, eye protection) when preparing and administering tigilanol tiglate. Accidental human self-injection of tigilanol tiglate may cause severe wound formation. Do not recap needles. In case of accidental self-injection, the manufacturer advises that the area be rinsed with water and to immediately seek medical attention; give the package insert to the attending physician.[3]

Sedation of the patient may be necessary to reduce the risk for needlestick injury. A Luer-lock syringe must be used to administer tigilanol tiglate. If leakage occurs following removal of syringe, rinse injection site with saline to wash tigilanol tiglate from skin surface.

As there is little information available regarding the teratogenic potential of tigilanol tiglate, the manufacturer recommends those who are pregnant or planning to become pregnant avoid preparing or administering the drug.

Tigilanol tiglate is intended only for intratumoral administration. Severe systemic reactions may result from inadvertent IV injection.

Tigilanol tiglate dosage is based on tumor volume. Consider using calipers to measure tumor dimensions[8] and instituting practices such as redundant drug dosage, volume checking, and special alert labels.

Do not confuse *Stelfonta*® with *Stelazine*® or *Stelara*®—or tigilanol with tigecycline, timolol, or *Tigan*®.

Adverse Effects

Swelling and bruising at the injection site, which may occur as soon as 2 hours after administration, on the day of treatment occurs in over 90% of treated dogs, whereas pain and heat are noted in ≈50% to 70% of dogs ≈24 hours after injection. Treatment site exudate occurs ≈7 days after injection and may be serous, serosanguinous, sanguineous, seropurulent, or purulent. Wound size following administration is frequently, but not always, proportional to the tumor size.[6]

The most frequently reported adverse effects following tigilanol tiglate injection include (in decreasing order)[3]: injection site pain (52%), lameness in the treated limb (25%), vomiting (21%), diarrhea (21%), hypoalbuminemia (18%), anorexia/hyporexia (12%), regional lymph node enlargement (11%), tachycardia (10%), weight loss (10%), dermatitis (8%), injection site infection (7%), tachypnea (6%), lethargy (5%), and pyrexia (3%). Tachypnea and lethargy were transient in a pilot field study.[8] Most adverse effects occurred in the first 7 days after injection.[3]

Anemia, neutrophilia, hypoalbuminemia, leukocytosis, monocytosis, and elevated creatine kinase have been documented following intratumoral injection.[3,6]

Reproductive/Nursing Safety

Safe use of tigilanol tiglate in pregnant, breeding, or lactating dogs has not been evaluated.[3,6]

Overdose/Acute Toxicity

Tigilanol tiglate administered IV (**NOTE**: not labeled route of administration) across a range of doses resulted in retching and vomiting during or immediately following the infusion, salivation, tremors, swaying gait, tachypnea, and lateral recumbency.[3,5,6] These effects were dose-related and considered serious but self-limiting and typically resolved 1 to 4 hours postinfusion. Tachycardia was observed with 0.075 mg/kg IV infusion,[3] and seizures and death occurred following 0.225 mg/kg IV infusion.[5,6] Infusion site reactions, including wound formation, were noted.[3]

There is no known antidote for toxic tigilanol tiglate exposure; treat clinical signs with supportive therapy.

For patients that have experienced or are suspected to have experienced an overdose, it is strongly encouraged to consult with the drug manufacturer, or if unavailable, contact one of the 24-hour poison consultation centers that specialize in providing information specific for veterinary patients. For general information related to overdose and toxin exposures, as well as contact information for poison control centers, refer to ***Appendix***.

Drug Interactions

Antibiotics, sedatives, and analgesics, including opioids, have been coprescribed for dogs receiving tigilanol tiglate.[3,6] The following drug interactions have either been reported or are theoretical in humans or animals receiving tigilanol tiglate and may be of significance in veterinary patients. Unless otherwise noted, use together is not necessarily contraindicated, but weigh the potential risks and perform additional monitoring when appropriate.

- **Antineoplastic Agents** (eg, **toceranib, vinblastine**): Use of other antineoplastic agents 2 months prior to tigilanol tiglate was prohibited in field studies.[8] Use together cautiously, if at all.
- **Immunosuppressive Agents** (eg, **cyclosporine, lokivetmab, oclacitinib**): Use of immunosuppressive agents 14 days prior to tigilanol tiglate was prohibited in field studies. Use together cautiously.[8]
- **NSAIDs** (eg, **carprofen, deracoxib, firocoxib, meloxicam**): In dogs being treated for MCT, a corticosteroid must be administered concomitantly with tigilanol tiglate; therefore, NSAIDs may need to be avoided during periods of corticosteroid use. Use of NSAIDs 7 days prior to tigilanol tiglate administration was prohibited in field studies.[8]

Laboratory Considerations

Histologic tumor grading after tigilanol tiglate treatment is unlikely to be accurate due to tumor necrosis; cytologic grading prior to treatment should be considered.[3]

Dosages

DOGS:

Nonmetastatic cutaneous MCT anywhere on the body or nonmetastatic subcutaneous MCT at or distal to the elbow or hock (label dosage; FDA-approved): 0.5 mL/cm^3 of tumor volume injected into (not under) a single MCT[3] with maximum tumor volume of 10 cm^3

Concomitant medications

An anti-inflammatory dose of a corticosteroid ***must*** be started 2 days prior to tigilanol tiglate injection, and histamine H_1- and H_2-receptor antagonists ***must*** be started on the day of tigilanol tiglate injection (see ***Contraindications/Precautions/Warnings***). The manufacturer's protocol uses the following dosages:

- Prednis(ol)one 0.5 mg/kg PO twice daily for 7 days (2 full days before treatment, the day of treatment, and for 4 days after treatment), decreased to 0.5 mg/kg PO once daily for 3 additional days (10 days total)
- Diphenhydramine 2 mg/kg PO twice daily, beginning the morning of the day of treatment and for 7 additional days (8 days total)
- Famotidine 0.5 mg/kg PO twice daily beginning the morning of the day of treatment and for 7 additional days (8 days total)

Calculating the dose to be administered

1. Tumor volume is calculated as 0.5 × [length (cm) × width (cm) × height (cm)]; it is highly recommended to use calipers to obtain tumor measurements.[8]

2. Number of mL of tigilanol tiglate to administer = 0.5 mL × tumor volume.
3. Confirm that tigilanol tiglate dose does not exceed 0.25 mL/kg.
4. The minimum dose is 0.1 mL, and the maximum dose is 5 mL, regardless of body weight, tumor volume, or number of tumors. **NOTE**: In a small dose-finding study, using dosages less than what is listed on the label demonstrated lower efficacy and a higher rate of adverse effects.[11]

Administration

1. Shaving the tumor slightly beyond the margins is recommended, unless doing so requires excessive manipulation of the tumor or causes the dog stress.[11]
2. Consult the product label for administration technique. A Luer-lock syringe ***must*** be used with a 23-gauge needle to inject tigilanol tiglate into the tumor with a dispersed (ie, fanning) pattern such that the tumor is fully perfused. Do not inject in a blood vessel or tumor margins, beyond tumor periphery, or deep into the tumor. Avoid manipulation of the tumor prior to injection to minimize the risk for mast cell degranulation.
3. Sedation of the patient may be necessary to decrease risk of accidental self-injection.

Dogs with an incomplete response may be given a second dose 30 days after the first injection. The corticosteroid and antihistamines described above are also required for the second treatment. Tigilanol tiglate dose for the second treatment must be based on the tumor volume calculated at the time of the second treatment.

Nonresectable, nonmetastatic cutaneous MCT or nonmetastatic subcutaneous MCT at or distal to the elbow or hock (extra-label): 0.5 mL/cm^3 of tumor volume, following the calculations, limits, cautions, and techniques presented in the FDA-approved labeled-dosage protocol above, with the following exceptions: maximum tumor volume is 8 cm^3, maximum dosage is 4 mL/dog (not to exceed 0.15 mg/kg), and, if needed, a second dose may be repeated 28 days after the first dose. The tumor must be accessible for intratumoral injection. More than 1 MCT may be treated per dog provided the preceding limits are not exceeded.[5,6]

HORSES:

Treatment of equine sarcoid or squamous cell carcinoma (extra-label): 0.35 mg/cm^3 (not mL/ cm^3) of tumor volume injected with a Luer-lock syringe using a dispersed pattern to fully perfuse the lesion.[4] Minimum dose of 0.05 – 0.1 mg/horse and maximum dose of 0.2 – 2 mg/horse; dose may vary based on lesion location. Standing sedation and local or regional anesthesia may be used. Surgical excision of the sarcoid pedicle was performed to measure and treat the tumor base.

Concomitant medication

- Immediately following tigilanol tiglate injection, administer flunixin 1.1 mg/kg IV.
- After tigilanol tiglate treatment, administer phenylbutazone 4.4 mg/kg PO twice daily for 3 days, followed by 2.2 mg/kg PO twice daily for the next 7 days if required.
- For ocular mucocutaneous and peri-orbital lesions, a subpalpebral lavage system must be placed at the time of treatment to administer an ophthalmic NSAID (eg, ketorolac, 0.1 mL every 6 hours) *and* atropine 1% (0.1 mL every 6 hours); a UV-protecting head veil is required.

Monitoring

- Clinical efficacy
- Signs of systemic mast cell degranulation for up to 7 days after treatment may include vomiting, diarrhea, anorexia/hyporexia, lethargy, urticaria, hypotension, altered breathing, and edema or bruising at or away from the MCT treatment site
- CBC, general chemistry, albumin, creatine kinase

Client Information

- Your veterinarian will provide an information sheet prior to administration of this drug.
- Tigilanol tiglate will be administered by your veterinarian. Sedation of your dog may be required to allow safe administration of the drug.
- At least 3 other medications are used with tigilanol tiglate. It is absolutely essential that these medications are administered exactly as prescribed, as death has occurred when these medications were not used, or were used improperly (eg, not giving the full 8- or 10-day treatment).
- Tigilanol tiglate destroys the mast cell tumor. In doing so, a wound will form where the drug was administered within a week of administration. This is a normal and expected part of treatment.
- Reactions (eg, swelling, redness, heat, pain) at the treatment site may begin as soon as 2 hours after injection and may last up to 1 week or longer. These reactions may be painful; talk to your veterinarian if you think your dog may need pain relievers.
- As the tumor breaks down, the skin at the injection site may darken or break open. A pocket, or wound, with a red and healthy-appearing border will develop at the site and progressively heal over several weeks. In some cases, the size of the wound may exceed the size of the original tumor. Antibiotics may be required if an infection develops in or around the wound.
- The wound is typically left uncovered. Discharge from the treatment site can be cleaned with warm water when necessary. Wear disposable gloves while cleaning. Use of preventive measures (eg, Elizabethan collar, bandage) may be needed if your dog is excessively grooming (licking) the treatment site. Other pets should be prevented from grooming the treatment site.
- Wound healing typically occurs 4 to 6 weeks after injection but may take longer in some dogs.
- Drinking water should be made accessible to treated dogs.
- Contact your veterinarian if your dog stops eating, develops lameness, has repeated vomiting or diarrhea, has difficulty breathing, or shows signs of severe pain, or if the treatment site appears to be increasing in size, is irritated, or has extensive swelling, redness, or bruising.
- Thoroughly wash any human skin that comes in contact with the treatment site, wound discharge, or materials contaminated with wound discharge (eg, bedding). Wash soiled items separately from other laundry.
- If there are multiple animals in the house, they may need to be separated to prevent grooming or trauma to the treated site.

Chemistry/Synonyms

Tigilanol tiglate is a phorbol ester with a molecular weight of 563. The commercial product is a clear colorless solution that also contains propylene glycol (40% v/v). Tigilanol tiglate is an epoxytigliane isolated from the seed of *Fontainea picrosperma*, a tree native to Australia.[7]

Tigilanol tiglate may also be known as EBC-46, phorbol triacetate, tigliane, TT, or *Stelfonta*®.

Storage/Stability

Tigilanol tiglate injection must be stored refrigerated at 2°C to 8°C (36°F-46°F). Do not freeze. Store in the manufacturer's carton to protect from light. Discard unused portion in accordance with routine medical waste.

Compatibility/Compounding Considerations

None noted

Dosage Forms/Regulatory Status

VETERINARY-LABELED PRODUCTS:

Tigilanol Tiglate Injection: 1 mg/mL solution in 2 mL single-use vials; *Stelfonta*®, (Rx). NADA# 141-541

HUMAN-LABELED PRODUCTS: NONE

References

For the complete list of references, see **wiley.com/go/budde/plumb**

Tildipirosin

(til-di-***pir***-oh-sin) *Zuprevo*®

Macrolide Antibiotic

Prescriber Highlights

- Injectable macrolide antibiotic used as a single SC dose in beef and nonlactating dairy cattle
- Used as a single IM dose in swine (not approved in the United States)
- Precautions: do not use the cattle product in swine; do not administer IV; do not use in chickens or turkeys.
- Do not use in automatically powered syringes. In case of human injection, contact a physician immediately. Use precautions when handling any tildipirosin product.
- Pain and swelling at the injection site are the most common adverse effects.

Uses/Indications

Tildipirosin is an injectable macrolide antibiotic that is approved by the FDA for the treatment of bovine respiratory disease (BRD) associated with *Mannheimia haemolytica, Pasteurella multocida,* and *Histophilus somni* in beef and nonlactating dairy cattle and for the control of respiratory disease in beef and nonlactating dairy cattle at high risk for developing BRD associated with *Mannheimia haemolytica, Pasteurella multocida,* and *Histophilus somni.* A study in heifers comparing metaphylactic antimicrobial administration of tildipirosin, tulathromycin, or placebo administered 10 days before experimental inoculation with *Mannheimia haemolytica* concluded that tildipirosin-treated animals had less pulmonary damage and fewer clinical signs of illness when compared to the other groups.[1]

In the EU, tildipirosin is also approved for the treatment of swine respiratory disease (SRD) associated with *Actinobacillus pleuropneumoniae, Pasteurella multocida, Bordetella bronchiseptica,* and *Haemophilus parasuis* sensitive to tildipirosin.

The World Health Organization (WHO) has designated tildipirosin as a Critically Important, Highest Priority antimicrobial for human medicine.[2] The Office International des Epizooties (OIE) Antimicrobial Classification has designated tildipirosin as a Veterinary Critically Important antimicrobial.[3]

Pharmacology/Actions

Similar to other macrolides, the antimicrobial activity of tildipirosin is due to its binding to the ribosomal 50S subunit of bacterial cells and inhibiting bacterial protein synthesis. Tildipirosin is generally classified as a time-dependent antibiotic, although it may be concentration-dependent (AUC/MIC ratio) against some isolates of *Mannheimia haemolytica* and *Pasteurella multocida.*

Significant increases in MIC of *P multocida* and *M haemolytica* to tildipirosin can be conveyed by the presence of the *erm*(42) gene.[4]

Macrolides inhibit the secretion of proinflammatory cytokines, phospholipase activity, and the release of leukotrienes and have anti-inflammatory effects on bovine macrophages and neutrophils.[5]

Pharmacokinetics

In cattle, after a single 4 mg/kg SC injection, bioavailability was 78%, and peak plasma concentrations of 0.7 to 0.8 µg/mL occurred within 1 hour of dosing. Concentrations of tildipirosin in lung and bronchial fluid far exceed those in plasma. Lung:plasma ratios range from 28 times at 4 hours to 214 times at 240 hours. Bronchial fluid:plasma ratios are 5 times at 4 hours; up to 72 times at 240 hours. The elimination half-life was ≈9 days in plasma and 10 to 11 days in lung and bronchial fluid.[6,7] Because of the extensive partitioning of macrolides into tissues and because of their multi-fold greater concentrations in bronchial fluid relative to that observed in the blood, plasma drug concentrations underestimate concentrations at the site of action.

A research publication suggests that upon administration to beef cattle and pigs at the recommended dose, colonic tildipirosin activity remains at subinhibitory concentrations far below the MICs against bovine and porcine foodborne pathogens and commensal bacteria.[8]

In pigs, after 4 mg/kg IM, peak plasma concentrations occurred within 23 minutes. Only ≈30% is bound to porcine plasma proteins. The mean terminal half-life was ≈4.4 days. Concentrations in the lung peaked about 1 day after dosing, and the lung half-life was ≈7 days.[9,10]

Contraindications/Precautions/Warnings

Tildipirosin is contraindicated in animals hypersensitive to it or other macrolide antibiotics. Tildipirosin is **NOT** for use in chickens or turkeys, and the 18% product must **NOT** be used in swine. Tildipirosin must **NOT** be given IV.

Cross-resistance can occur with other macrolides, and use with other macrolides or lincosamides is not advised. SC injection in cattle may result in local tissue reactions that can persist beyond the slaughter withdrawal period and may result in trim loss of edible tissue at slaughter.

Care must be taken to avoid accidental injection in humans, as toxicology studies in laboratory animals (including dogs) showed cardiovascular effects after IM administration. Do not use automatically powered syringes that do not have an additional protection system. In case of human injection, seek medical advice immediately and show the package insert or label to the physician. Avoid direct contact with skin and eyes. If accidental eye exposure occurs, rinse eyes with clean water. If accidental skin exposure occurs, wash the skin immediately with soap and water. Wash hands after use. Tildipirosin may cause sensitization by skin contact.

Adverse Effects

In cattle, pain and swelling at injection sites are the most commonly reported adverse effects, with pain on palpation persisting for 1 day in most treated cattle. Swelling can last at the injection site for up to 21 days posttreatment, and tissue lesions have been noted at 35 days postinjection.[7,11] Swelling and inflammation, which may be severe, may be seen at the injection site after administration. SC injection may result in local tissue reactions, which persist beyond the slaughter withdrawal period. This may result in trim loss of edible tissue at slaughter.

In pigs, swelling at the injection site after IM injection can persist for up to 3 days but is not painful upon palpation. Injection site reactions resolved completely within 21 days of injection.[10] Shock-like reactions with fatal outcomes can occur rarely.[10]

Reproductive/Nursing Safety

The safety of the veterinary medicinal product has not been established during pregnancy and lactation; however, no evidence for any selective developmental or reproductive effects was noted in any of the laboratory studies.

The product is not labeled for use in lactating dairy cattle.

Because safety has not been established in animals, this drug should only be used when the maternal benefits outweigh the potential risks to offspring.

Overdose/Acute Toxicity

Limited information is available. In cattle, dosages up to 5 times recommended caused little demonstrable effects other than localized tissue reactions.[7]

Some piglets that were given 3 times (12 mg/kg) and 5 times (20 mg/kg) the normal doses IM developed muscle tremors, weakness, or showed subdued activity. One animal developed a shock-like syndrome after 20 mg/kg and was euthanized. Mortality was seen at dosages of 25 mg/kg or greater.[10]

Dogs given IM doses of 20 mg/kg caused a slight but significant decrease in blood pressure.[11,12]

For patients that have experienced or are suspected of having experienced an overdose, consultation with a 24-hour poison consultation center specializing in providing veterinary-specific information is recommended. For general information related to overdose and toxin exposures, as well as contact information for poison control centers, refer to ***Appendix.***

Drug Interactions

No specific drug interactions were noted, although the EU label states: *There is cross resistance with other macrolides. Do not administer with antimicrobials with a similar mode of action such as other macrolides or lincosamides.*[13]

Laboratory Considerations

None were noted.

Dosages

CATTLE:

Treatment of bovine respiratory disease (BRD) associated with *Mannheimia haemolytica, Pasteurella multocida,* and *Histophilus somni* in beef and nonlactating dairy cattle and for the control of respiratory disease in beef and nonlactating dairy cattle at high risk for developing BRD associated with *Mannheimia haemolytica, Pasteurella multocida,* and *Histophilus somni* (label dose, FDA-approved): 4 mg/kg SC as a single dose in the neck. Do not inject more than 10 mL per injection site.[7]

SWINE:

Treatment of swine respiratory disease (SRD) associated with *Actinobacillus pleuropneumoniae, Pasteurella multocida, Bordetella bronchiseptica,* and *Haemophilus parasuis* sensitive to tildipirosin (extra-label): **NOTE**: The 18% cattle product must not be used in swine; the swine product (EU) is 40 mg/mL (4%). Administer 4 mg/kg IM once only. The injection volume should not exceed 5 mL per injection site. Start treatment in the early stages of the disease and re-evaluate within 48 hours; if clinical signs persist or increase, antibiotic treatment should be changed.[10]

Monitoring

Clinical efficacy. The product information for the UK products states: *In cattle, evaluate the response to treatment within 2 to 3 days after injection. If clinical signs of respiratory disease persist or increase, treatment should be changed to using another antibiotic.*[13] In pigs, it is recommended to evaluate the response to treatment within 48 hours after injection. If clinical signs of respiratory disease persist, increase, or if relapse occurs, treatment should be changed to using another antibiotic.[10]

Client Information

- Understand and follow use restrictions and withdrawal times for food animals.
- Humans with a known drug allergy to macrolide antibiotics (eg, erythromycin, clarithromycin) should avoid contact with the medication.
- Do not use automatically powered syringes that do not have an additional protection system. In case of accidental self-injection, seek medical advice immediately and show the package leaflet or label to the physician. In case of skin or eye exposure, wash/flush with clean water.

Chemistry/Synonyms

Tildipirosin (CAS Registry: 328898-40-4; ATCvet code: QJ01FA96) is a 16-membered semisynthetic macrolide antimicrobial agent.

The injectable solution is a clear, yellowish solution. Excipients in the injectable solution include citric acid monohydrate, propylene glycol, and water for injection.

Tildipirosin may also be known as 20, 23-di-piperidynyl-mycaminosyl-tylonolide, or PMT. The trade name is *Zuprevo®*.

Storage/Stability

Store the injectable solution at temperatures at or below 30°C (86°F). Do not freeze. The EU label states not to store above 25°C (77°F). The maximum storage time after the first puncture is 28 days at or below 25°C (77°F). Do not puncture 50 mL and 100 mL vial stoppers more than 8 times or the 250 mL vial stopper more than 16 times.

Compatibility/Compounding Considerations

No specific information was noted. The EU label states: *In the absence of compatibility studies, this veterinary medicinal product must not be mixed with other veterinary medicinal products.*

Dosage Forms/Regulatory Status

VETERINARY-LABELED PRODUCTS:

Tildipirosin Injection: 180 mg/mL (18%) in 50 mL, 100 mL, and 250 mL multidose vials; *Zuprevo®*; (Rx). FDA-approved (NADA# 141-334) for use in cattle. Not for use in female dairy cattle 20 months of age or older or in pre-ruminating calves. Do not use in calves to be processed for veal. Withdrawal time is 21 days. (Withdrawal time in EU label is 47 days.)

Tildipirosin 40 mg/mL injection for use in swine is available in EU (not available in the US).

HUMAN-LABELED PRODUCTS: NONE

References

For the complete list of references, see **wiley.com/go/budde/plumb**

Tiletamine/Zolazepam

(tye-***let***-a-meen/zoe-***laze***-a-pam) *Telazol®*

Injectable Anesthetic/Tranquilizer

Prescriber Highlights

- Combination similar to ketamine/diazepam but with a longer duration of effect
- Contraindications include pancreatic disease, New Zealand white rabbits, severe cardiac or pulmonary disease, or during pregnancy.
- Use with caution in patients that have renal disease and in large exotic cats.
- Apply ophthalmic lubricant after administration
- Dosages may need to be reduced in geriatric or debilitated animals, or in animals with renal dysfunction.
- Adverse effects include respiratory depression, pain after IM injection, athetoid movements, tachycardia (especially dogs), emesis during emergence, excessive salivation and bronchial/tracheal secretions, transient apnea, vocalization, erratic and/or prolonged recovery, involuntary muscular twitching, hypertonia, cyanosis, cardiac arrest, pulmonary edema, muscle rigidity, and either hypertension or hypotension.
- Monitor body temperature (may cause hypothermia)
- DEA Schedule III (C-III) controlled substance

Uses/Indications

In dogs, tiletamine/zolazepam is labeled for induction of anesthesia and for restraint and minor procedures of short duration (≈30 minutes) that require mild to moderate analgesia. Tiletamine/zolazepam is also labeled for restraint or anesthesia combined with muscle relaxation in cats. Although tiletamine/zolazepam is not FDA-approved for other species, it has been used in many domestic, exotic, and wild species. A potential disadvantage of this product is that it is a fixed-ratio combination and the pharmacokinetics of each drug can vary significantly among species.

Pharmacology/Actions

Tiletamine is a dissociative anesthetic and zolazepam is a benzodiazepine. The pharmacology of this drug combination is similar to that of ketamine combined with diazepam or midazolam.

In cats, tiletamine can briefly (≈1 minute) decrease blood pressure after IV injections, but this parameter increases above baseline after this brief period.[1] In dogs, a persistent tachycardia is followed by decreased blood pressure, although cardiac output typically remains unchanged. It can cause apneustic breathing (like ketamine); however, normal minute ventilation and pCO_2 is maintained.[2,3] In dogs, induction with tiletamine IV had no clinical effects on intraocular pressure.[4] The same outcomes were noted when this drug was administered IM and intranasal in cats.[5]

Pharmacokinetics

In dogs, the onset of action following IM injection averages 7.5 minutes. The mean duration of surgical anesthesia is ≈27 minutes, with recovery times averaging ≈4 hours. The duration of the tiletamine effect is longer than that of zolazepam, so there is a shorter duration of tranquilization and muscle relaxation than there is anesthesia. Less than 4% of the drugs are reported to be excreted unchanged in the urine in dogs. Reported elimination half-life for tiletamine is 1.25 to 2.5 hours, and 1.5 hours for zolazepam.

In cats, the onset of action is reported to be within 5 to 12 minutes after IM injection. Duration of anesthesia is dose dependent, but is usually≈21 to 60 minutes at peak effect, which is reported to be ≈3 times the duration of ketamine anesthesia. The duration of effect of the zolazepam component is longer than that of the tiletamine, so there is a greater degree of tranquilization than anesthesia during the recovery period. The recovery times vary in length from ≈1 to 5.5 hours. Reported elimination half-life for tiletamine is 2.5 hours and 4.5 hours for zolazepam. These differences in half-life result in less predictable anesthetic effects when multiple doses are administered.

In xylazine-sedated horses, tiletamine/zolazepam 1.5 mg/kg IV (over 15 seconds) produced the following pharmacokinetic data (means reported): For tiletamine and zolazepam: clearance, 96 mL/minute/kg and 6.7 mL/minute/kg; volume of distribution, 0.79 L/kg and 0.76 L/kg; terminal half-life, 29 minutes and 235 minutes. Tiletamine is cleared much more rapidly than zolazepam. At this dose, recumbency lasted for 30 to 43 minutes, and the mean time to standing was 39 minutes. The authors judged recoveries to be excellent.

In pigs, higher concentrations of zolazepam were observed in pig plasma and it was cleared more slowly compared with tiletamine. Apparent clearance was 11 L/hour (zolazepam) versus 134 L/hour (tiletamine); and half-life was 2.76 hours (zolazepam) versus 1.97 hours (tiletamine). Three metabolites of zolazepam and 1 metabolite of tiletamine were identified in pig urine, plasma, and microsomal incubations.[6]

Contraindications/Precautions/Warnings

Tiletamine/zolazepam should only be used in situations in which sufficient monitoring and patient-support capabilities (eg, intubation, ventilation) are available. Tiletamine/zolazepam is contraindicated in animals with pancreatic disease and severe cardiac or pulmonary disease. Animals with renal insufficiency may have prolonged duration of anesthetic action or recovery times.

Because tiletamine/zolazepam may cause hypothermia, susceptible animals (eg, small body surface area, low ambient temperatures) should be monitored carefully and a supplemental heat source should be provided if needed. Like ketamine, tiletamine/zolazepam does not abolish pinnal, palpebral, pedal, laryngeal, and pharyngeal reflexes, and its use (alone) may not be adequate if surgery is to be performed on these areas.

It has been reported that this drug is contraindicated in New Zealand white rabbits due to renal toxicity.[7] Other breeds seem to be unaffected.

Tiletamine/zolazepam is often avoided for use in large, exotic cats, as it reportedly can cause seizures, prolonged recovery, permanent neurologic abnormalities, or death. Although several clinicians have suggested that tiletamine/zolazepam is contraindicated in tigers (*Panthera tigris*), an evaluation of the literature suggests that although adverse effects can occur, tiletamine/zolazepam is not contraindicated.[8] A study found no major differences in pharmacokinetics between tigers and leopards (*Panthera pardus*).[9] A study evaluating the effects of tiletamine/zolazepam in combination with detomidine (TZD) in 9 tigers found it to be effective in immobilizing captive healthy tigers and no neurologic and/or important adverse reactions were noted; however, hypertension and ataxia may be seen during recovery.[10]

Animals' eyes remain open after receiving tiletamine/zolazepam; they should be protected from injury and an ophthalmic lubricant should be applied to prevent excessive drying of the cornea. When dissociative anesthetic agents (ie, ketamine, tiletamine) are used, animals maintain the swallowing reflex, making intubation challenging, especially in cats. The use of sedatives before the administration of tiletamine/zolazepam may improve the outcome. Topical lidocaine (on the arytenoid cartilages) or rocuronium IV (with ventilatory support)[11] has been used in cats to facilitate tracheal intubation.

The effects of tiletamine (eg, anesthesia with concurrent athetosis, muscle rigidity, convulsions) typically outlast the duration of zolazepam effects in dogs, which may cause agitated recoveries. See ***Adverse Effects***.

Dosages may need to be reduced in geriatric or debilitated animals or animals with renal dysfunction.

Adverse Effects

Respiratory depression is a possibility, especially when higher doses are administered. Apnea may occur; observe animal carefully. Pain after IM injection (especially in cats) has been noted, which may be a result of the low pH of the solution. Athetoid movements (eg, constant succession of slow, writhing, involuntary movements of flexion, extension, pronation) may occur; do not give additional tiletamine/zolazepam in an attempt to diminish these actions. Large doses given SC or IM (vs small doses given IV) may result in longer, rougher recoveries. Recoveries in dogs can be rougher than those usually seen in cats.

In dogs, tachycardia may be a common effect and last for 30 minutes. Insufficient anesthesia after recommended doses has been reported in dogs.

Tiletamine/zolazepam has been implicated in causing nephrosis in lagomorphs and prolonged recovery, neurologic signs, and death in large cats (specifically in tigers).

Other adverse effects include emesis during emergence, excessive salivation and bronchial/tracheal secretions (if atropine not administered beforehand), transient apnea, vocalization, erratic and/or prolonged recovery, involuntary muscular twitching, hypertonia, cyanosis, cardiac arrest, pulmonary edema, muscle rigidity, seizure activity, and either hypertension or hypotension.[12] Atropine 0.04 mg/kg IV, IM, or SC can be used concurrently to control hypersalivation.

Reproductive/Nursing Safety

Tiletamine/zolazepam crosses the placenta and may cause respiratory depression in newborns; use for cesarean sections is contraindicated.[12] The teratogenic potential of the drug is unknown, and it is not recommended for use during any stage of pregnancy or during lactation.

Overdose/Acute Toxicity

The manufacturer claims a 2 times margin of safety in dogs, and a 4.5 times margin of safety in cats. Lethal doses can occur at ≈5 to 10 times the labeled IM doses. A preliminary study in dogs suggests that doxapram 5.5 mg/kg will enhance respirations and arousal after tiletamine/zolazepam.[13] In massive overdoses, it is suggested that mechanically assisted ventilation be performed if necessary and other clinical signs treated supportively. Use of flumazenil to reverse zolazepam is not commonly done, as its use will exacerbate the effects of tiletamine, which cannot be reversed.

High doses of tiletamine have caused acute tubular necrosis in New Zealand white rabbits.[14,15]

Drug Interactions

Little specific information is available presently on drug interactions with this product. The following drug interactions either have been reported or are theoretical in animals receiving tiletamine/zolazepam and may be of significance. Unless otherwise noted, use together is not necessarily contraindicated, but weigh the potential risks and perform additional monitoring when appropriate.

- **ANESTHETICS, INHALATIONAL** (eg, **isoflurane, sevoflurane**): Dose may need to be reduced when used concomitantly with tiletamine/zolazepam.
- **BARBITURATES** (eg, **phenobarbital**): Dose may need to be reduced when used concomitantly with tiletamine/zolazepam.
- **CHLORAMPHENICOL**: In cats, anesthesia is prolonged an average of ≈30 minutes by chloramphenicol; however, in dogs, chloramphenicol apparently has no effect on recovery times.
- **PHENOTHIAZINES** (eg, **acepromazine**): Can cause increased respiratory and cardiac depression

The following are interactions for the related compounds ketamine and midazolam and could apply to tiletamine/zolazepam:

Ketamine:

- **NEUROMUSCULAR BLOCKERS** (eg, **succinylcholine, tubocurarine**): May cause enhanced or prolonged respiratory depression
- **THYROID HORMONES**: Combination has induced hypertension and tachycardia in humans; beta-blockers (eg, **propranolol**) may be of benefit in treating these effects.

Midazolam:

- **ANESTHETICS, INHALATIONAL** (eg, **isoflurane, sevoflurane**): Midazolam may decrease the dosages required.
- **AZOLE ANTIFUNGALS** (eg, **fluconazole, itraconazole, ketoconazole**): May increase midazolam concentrations
- **CALCIUM CHANNEL BLOCKERS** (eg, **diltiazem, verapamil**): May increase midazolam concentrations
- **CIMETIDINE**: May increase midazolam concentrations
- **CNS DEPRESSANTS, OTHER**: May increase the risk for respiratory depression
- **MACROLIDES** (eg, **clarithromycin, erythromycin**): May increase midazolam concentrations
- **OPIOIDS**: May increase the hypnotic effects of midazolam; hypotension has been reported when used with meperidine.
- **PHENOBARBITAL**: May decrease peak concentrations and AUC of midazolam
- **RIFAMPIN**: May decrease peak concentrations and AUC of midazolam

Dosages

NOTE: Listed dosages are for the combined amounts of tiletamine/zolazepam.

DOGS:

NOTE: The label dosages for dogs is considered to be greater than is necessary for most indications. The label indications and dosages are provided below but the use of lower, extra-label dosages should be considered.

Restraint for diagnostic purposes (label dosage; FDA-approved): 6.6 – 9.9 mg/kg IM[12]

Minor procedures of short duration (label dosage; FDA-approved): 9.9 – 13.2 mg/kg IM.[12] If supplemental doses are necessary, give doses less than the initial dose; total dose should not exceed 26.4 mg/kg.

Induction of anesthesia (label dosage; FDA-approved): 2.2 – 4.4 mg/kg IV slowly over 30 to 45 seconds.[12] Additional drug may be given if the depth of anesthesia is not sufficient 60 seconds after administration; total dose of 4.4 mg/kg IV should not be exceeded. Maintain anesthesia with an inhalant anesthetic.[12]

Anesthetic induction (extra-label): 3 – 4.5 mg/kg IV followed by isoflurane anesthesia[16]

Aggressive (difficult to handle) dogs (extra-label): 1 – 2 mg/kg IM. Use only if there is insufficient sedation from a combination of opioid, higher dose medetomidine, and midazolam.[17] Anecdotally, 5 mg/kg IM in combination with an opioid (eg, morphine, hydromorphone)

CATS:

NOTE: The label dosages for cats is considered to be greater than is necessary for most situations. The label indications and dosages are provided below but the use of lower, extra-label dosages should be considered.

Procedures such as dentistry, abscess treatment, foreign body removal (label dosage; FDA-approved): 9.7 – 11.9 mg/kg IM [12]

Minor procedures of short duration that require mild to moderate levels of analgesia (eg, lacerations, castration) (label dosage; FDA-approved): 10.6 – 12.5 mg/kg IM[12]

Ovariohysterectomy and onychectomy (label dosage; FDA-approved): 14.3 – 15.8 mg/kg IM.[12] If supplemental doses are necessary, give doses in increments that are less than the initial dose; total dose should not exceed 72 mg/kg.

Procedures that require relief of mild pain (extra-label): 2 – 5 mg/kg IV or 5 – 10 mg/kg IM. The tiletamine/zolazepam vial can be reconstituted with butorphanol 2.5 mg (using 10 mg/mL solution) and dexmedetomidine 2.5 mL (using 0.5 mg/mL solution) and given IM.[18]

Procedures that require relief of moderate to severe pain (extra-label): Tiletamine/zolazepam 3 mg/kg IM in combination with methadone 0.2 mg/kg and given IM provided superior sedation and similar recovery when compared to acepromazine-methadone combination.[19]

Sedation of healthy cats prior to blood donation (extra-label): 5 mg/kg IM[20]

Oral transmucosal (OTM) administration (extra-label): 10 – 15 mg/kg OTM effectively restrained healthy cats under experimental conditions.[21]

Restraint of aggressive cats: Anecdotally, 3 – 5 mg/kg IM in combination with an opioid (eg, hydromorphone) results in profound sedation.

HORSES:

Anesthesia (extra-label): Xylazine 1.1 mg/kg IV, 5 minutes prior to tiletamine/zolazepam 1.65 – 2.2 mg/kg IV. Recumbency lasted 30 to 43 minutes, and mean time to stand was 39 minutes. Both induction and recovery quality were subjectively evaluated as excellent.[22,23]

Immobilization (extra-label): Tiletamine/zolazepam 2.4 mg/kg IM in combination with detomidine 0.04 mg/kg IM. Time to sternal recumbency was 76 minutes, and time to standing was 118 minutes.[24]

RUMINANTS:

Chemical restraint (extra-label):

Combining tiletamine/zolazepam with ketamine and xylazine (TKX-Ru) for capturing intractable ruminant patients and large exotic hoof stock: Reconstitute a 500 mg vial of tiletamine/zolazepam with ketamine 250 mg (2.5 mL) and large animal xylazine 100 mg (1 mL), yielding a final volume of 4 mL. Use 1.25 – 1.5 mL/110 to 115 kg (242.5 lb to 253.5 lb) body weight for smaller-sized ruminant patients, and 1 mL/110 to 115 kg (242.5 lb to 253.5 lb) body weight for large-sized ruminant patients. Typically administered via a dart gun or pole syringe. Patients generally become compliant and recumbent in 5 to 10 minutes.[25]

Combining tiletamine/zolazepam with ketamine and detomidine (TZDK) in free-range cattle: Prepare solution of tiletamine/zolazepam 52.6 mg/mL in combination with detomidine 4.2 mg/mL and ketamine 52.6 mg/mL. Administer 1 mL/100 kg (220.5 lb) body weight (body weight estimated visually) IM[26,27]

Sheep undergoing surgical procedures (extra-label):

a) 8 – 12 mg/kg IV[28]

b) 12 mg/kg IM yields surgical anesthesia lasting 30 minutes[28]

NEW WORLD CAMELIDS:

Sedative/analgesic with xylazine (extra-label): Tiletamine/zolazepam 2 mg/kg in combination with xylazine 0.2 or 0.4 mg/kg IM provided antinociceptive effects for ≈30 to 50 minutes.[29] Transient hypoxemia can be seen with xylazine administration; however, this is not clinically relevant in healthy llamas. Tiletamine/zolazepam alone was deemed suitable only for immobilization for non-painful procedures.

Sedative/analgesic with dexmedetomidine (extra-label): In adult male alpacas, tiletamine/zolazepam 2 mg/kg IM in combination with dexmedetomidine 0.01 – 0.02 mg/kg IM significantly increased the duration of lateral recumbency, time to standing, and response to painful stimuli compared with tiletamine/zolazepam alone.[30]

SWINE:

Sedative/analgesic in combination with ketamine and xylazine (extra-label): Reconstitute a 500 mg vial of tiletamine/zolazepam with ketamine 250 mg (2.5 mL) and large animal xylazine 250 mg (2.5 mL), yielding a final volume of 5 mL and a concentration of 50 mg/mL of each drug. For sedation: 0.01 mL/kg IM; for surgical anesthesia: 0.02 mL/kg IM. **WARNING**: Anecdotally, this combination has been associated with deaths after recovery.[31]

Sedative/analgesic in companion pigs (extra-label): For procedures of short duration (15 to 30 minutes), 2 mg/kg IM; procedures of longer duration (30 to 60 minutes): 3 – 4 mg/kg IM[32]

Anesthesia/sedation (extra-label):

a) A variety of protocols have been used in pigs. The use of tiletamine/zolazepam alone is not recommended due to insufficient CNS depression and analgesia, rough recovery, paddling, vocalization, and hypersalivation. Can be used in combination with ketamine and xylazine. Combine ketamine 250 mg (2.5 mL of 100 mg/mL) with xylazine 250 mg (2.5 mL of 100 mg/mL) to a vial of tiletamine/zolazepam. Use 1 mL per 35 to 75 kg IM, depending on sedation required. Use one-half of these doses when administering to pot-bellied pigs.[33]

b) Short-term anesthesia in domestic pigs: Tiletamine/zolazepam 8 mg/kg IM with methadone 0.2 mg/kg IM in neck muscles provided adequate anesthesia for minor procedures lasting ≈30 minutes but was associated with poor recovery.[34]

c) A study compared induction and anesthesia of tiletamine/zolazepam/ketamine/xylazine (4.4/2.2/2.2 mg/kg), tiletamine/zolazepam/xylazine (4.4/2.2 mg/kg), tiletamine/zolazepam/xylazine (4.4/4.4 mg/kg), and ketamine/xylazine (2.2/2.2 mg/kg). All combinations were administered IM. Both tiletamine/zolazepam/xylazine combinations were deemed to be superior.[35]

d) In miniature pigs, tiletamine/zolazepam 3.5 mg/kg IM has been combined with xylazine 1.32 mg/kg IM and tramadol 1.8 mg/kg IM to increase depth and duration of anesthesia.[36] This combination can be antagonized with atipamezole, flumazenil, and naloxone.[37]

FERRETS:

Sedative/analgesic (extra-label): Tiletamine/zolazepam 22 mg/kg IM.[38] Tiletamine/zolazepam 1.5 mg/kg in combination with xylazine 1.5 mg/kg IM; may reverse xylazine with yohimbine 0.05 mg/kg IM. Tiletamine/zolazepam 1.5 mg/kg with xylazine 1.5 mg/kg and butorphanol 0.2 mg/kg IM; may reverse xylazine with yohimbine 0.05 mg/kg IM.[39]

SMALL MAMMALS:

Chemical restraint in small rodents (extra-label): 6 – 10 mg/kg IM is adequate prior to inhalation anesthesia. Advantages over ketamine include better muscle relaxation, small volume of injection, rapid induction time, and a wide margin of safety. Disadvantages of this drug combination are increased respiratory secretions, variability in recovery times, and short shelf-life after reconstitution.[40] Not recommended for New Zealand white rabbits.[41]

REPTILES:

NOTE: Significant interspecies and interpatient differences in effectiveness can be seen.

a) **Large snakes**: 3 mg/kg IM to facilitate handling and anesthesia. Administer 30 to 45 minutes prior to handling. Sedation may persist for up to 48 hours. May also be used in crocodilians at 4 – 8 mg/kg[42]

b) 3 – 10 mg/kg IM. Lizards and snakes can generally be treated with lower end of dosage range and chelonians may require high end. If sedation is inadequate, may give incrementally up to the maximum dose. Monitor closely for apnea and ventilate if required[43]

c) At lower doses of 4 – 10 mg/kg, sedation may be sufficient for some procedures (eg, venipuncture, gastric lavage, intubation for inhalation anesthesia). At higher doses of 15 – 40 mg/kg, recovery may be greatly prolonged. Starting dose: 7 – 15 mg/kg[44]

d) Best used for sedation and tranquilization or to facilitate intubation, especially in large boas, crocodilians, and venomous species. Author starts with a dose of 5 mg/kg IM and repeats if needed. Higher doses of 6 mg/kg are associated with very long recovery times, especially in chelonians (72 hours).[45]

e) **Anesthetic induction of chelonians** (extra-label): Aquatic or box turtles, 5 mg/kg IM, SC; tortoises, 10 – 20 mg/kg IM in brachial muscle; intubation is usually possible 20 minutes after administration.[46]

Monitoring

- Depth of anesthesia and degree of analgesia
- Ventilation (eg, $ETCO_2$), pulse oximetry (PaO_2), cardiovascular status (eg, heart rate and rhythm, blood pressure)
- Monitor eyes to prevent drying out or injury
- Body temperature

Client Information

Tiletamine/zolazepam should only be administered by authorized veterinary professionals that are familiar with its use. Some manufacturers state that women who are pregnant, or are suspected to be pregnant, should not handle the product.

Chemistry/Synonyms

Tiletamine is an injectable anesthetic agent chemically related to ketamine. Zolazepam is a diazepinone minor tranquilizer. The pH of the injectable product (after reconstitution) is 2.2 to 2.8.

Tiletamine HCl may also be known as CI-634, CL-399, or CN-54521-2; zolazepam HCl may also be known as CI-716.

Tiletamine/zolazepam may also be known as *Telazol®*, *Tilzolan®*, *Tzed®*, or *Zoletil®*.

Storage/Stability

Tiletamine/zolazepam is a schedule III (C-III) controlled substance that should be stored in an area that is substantially constructed and securely locked. Follow applicable local, state, and federal rules regarding disposal of unused or wasted controlled drugs.

Store unreconstituted vials at controlled room temperature (20°C-25°C [68°F-77°F]). After reconstitution with sterile water for injection, solutions may be stored for 7 days at room temperature and 56 days if refrigerated. Use only clear solutions; color may vary from colorless to light amber.

Compatibility/Compounding Considerations

Reconstitute with 5 mL sterile water.

Dosage Forms/Regulatory Status

VETERINARY-LABELED PRODUCTS:

Tiletamine/zolazepam has been designated as a Class 2 substance by the Association of Racing Commissioners International (ARCI). Use of this drug may not be allowed in certain animal competitions. Check rules and regulations before entering in a competition while this medication is being administered. Contact local racing authorities for further guidance. See ***Appendix***.

Tiletamine HCl (equivalent to 250 mg free base) and Zolazepam HCl (equivalent to 250 mg free base) as lyophilized powder/vial in 5 mL vials. When 5 mL of sterile diluent (sterile water) is added, a concentration of 50 mg/mL of each drug (100 mg/mL combined) is produced; *Telazol®*, generic; (Rx, C-III). FDA-approved for use in cats and dogs. NADA# 106-111

No guidelines for milk or meat withdrawal intervals are available.[47]

HUMAN-LABELED PRODUCTS: NONE

References

For the complete list of references, see **wiley.com/go/budde/plumb**

Tilmicosin

(til-mi-***coe***-sin) *Micotil®, Pulmotil®*

Macrolide Antibiotic

Prescriber Highlights

- ► Injectable macrolide antibiotic used in cattle, sheep, and sometimes rabbits; oral concentrate used in swine
- ► **Fatal to cattle and sheep when the injection is administered IV**; give by the SC route only. **May be fatal if injected** by any route in swine, horses, or goats. Severe reactions reported in camelids
- ► **Accidental injection can be fatal in humans.** Do not use in automatically powered syringes. In case of human injection, contact a physician immediately. Use precautions when handling any tilmicosin product.
- ► Adverse effects include SC injection site edema, lameness, and decreased food and water intake; accidental IM injection may cause a local tissue reaction, resulting in trim loss.

Uses/Indications

Tilmicosin injection is indicated for the treatment of bovine respiratory disease (BRD) associated with *Mannheimia haemolytica*, *Pasteurella multocida*, and *Histophilus somni*, for the treatment of ovine respiratory disease associated with *M haemolytica*, and for the treatment of swine respiratory disease (SRD) associated with *Mannheimia haemolytica*. It is also indicated for the control of respiratory disease in cattle at high risk for developing BRD associated with *Mannheimia haemolytica*. For oral use (in drinking water), tilmicosin is indicated for the control of swine respiratory disease associated with *Pasteurella multocida* and *Haemophilus parasuis* in groups of swine in buildings where a respiratory disease outbreak is diagnosed. It is also used for the control of SRD associated with *Mycoplasma hyopneumoniae* in the presence of porcine reproductive and respiratory syndrome virus (PRRSV) in groups of swine in buildings where a respiratory disease outbreak is diagnosed.

In other countries, tilmicosin injection is indicated for use in cattle for the treatment of interdigital necrobacillosis and in sheep for the treatment of foot rot or acute ovine mastitis,[1] and the oral concentrate is added to drinking water for the treatment and metaphylaxis of respiratory disease[2] in chickens and turkeys.

The World Health Organization (WHO) has designated tilmicosin as a Critically Important, Highest Priority antimicrobial for human medicine.[3] The Office International des Epizooties (OIE) Antimicrobial Classification has designated tilmicosin as a Veterinary Critically Important antimicrobial.[4]

Pharmacology/Actions

Like other macrolides, tilmicosin has activity primarily against gram-positive bacteria, although some gram-negative bacteria are affected, and the drug reportedly has some activity against mycoplasma. Preliminary studies have shown that 95% of studied isolates of *Pasteurella multocida* are sensitive. Bacterial isolates susceptible to tilmicosin at concentrations of less than or equal to 8 µg/mL are reported as susceptible to tilmicosin. The MIC_{90} value reported for *M. haemolytica* and *P. multocida* in cattle with BRD is 32 µg/mL. Oral tilmicosin does not have activity against *Cryptosporidium* spp in goats.[5]

Pharmacokinetics

Tilmicosin apparently concentrates in lung tissue. A single SC injection of *Micotil®* 10 mg/kg of body weight dose in cattle resulted in peak tilmicosin concentrations within 1 hour and detectable concentrations (0.07 µg/mL) in serum beyond 3 days. At 3 days postinjection, the lung:serum ratio is ≈60:1. MIC_{95} concentrations

(3.12 µg/mL) for *P. haemolytica* persist for a minimum of 3 days after a single injection.

Contraindications/Precautions/Warnings

Injections in humans can be fatal; exercise extreme caution when handling injectable products. Do not use in automatically powered syringes. Never carry a syringe of tilmicosin with a needle attached.[1] Keep needles capped until ready to use; only attach the needle to fill the syringe or administer injection; keep syringe and needle separate at all other times. Ensure animals are properly restrained before attempting to administer. Do not work alone when using tilmicosin injectable.[1] In case of accidental injection, seek medical attention immediately. Emergency treatment includes applying ice to the injection site and contacting a physician immediately. Elanco emergency medical telephone numbers are 1-800-722-0987 or 1-800-428-4441.

Avoid contact with eyes.

Do not inject by any route in swine, goats, nonhuman primates, or horses as fatalities may result. Do not administer IV to sheep or cattle, as deaths of cattle have been observed with a single IV dose of 5 mg/kg. There have been anecdotal reports of severe reactions in some camelids.

When using oral concentrate in drinking water, do not use rusty containers for medicated water as product integrity may be affected.[2] Oral concentrate must be diluted before administration. Do not allow horses or other equines access to water containing tilmicosin.

Adverse Effects

In cattle: injection site swelling and inflammation, lameness, collapse, anaphylaxis/anaphylactoid reactions, decreased food and water consumption, and death.

In sheep: dyspnea and death. Injection lesions are described as being generally more severe and occurred at higher frequency rates in the animals treated with higher doses of tilmicosin. If administered IM, a local tissue reaction may occur, resulting in the trim loss. Edema may be noted at the site of SC injection.

In swine: decreased water consumption has been observed in healthy pigs receiving tilmicosin via drinking water.

In rabbits receiving SC tilmicosin, local swelling and necrosis at the injection site, as well as weakness, pallor, tachypnea, and sudden death have been observed.[6]

Reproductive/Nursing Safety

Safe use in pregnant or lactating animals or animals to be used for breeding purposes has not been demonstrated.

Because safety has not been established in animals, this drug should only be used when the maternal benefits outweigh the potential risks to offspring.

Overdose/Acute Toxicity

The cardiovascular system is apparently the target of toxicity in animals. The primary cardiac effects are increased heart rate (tachycardia) and decreased contractility (negative inotropy). In cattle, doses up to 50 mg/kg IM did not cause death, but 150 mg/kg SC did cause fatalities, as well as 5 mg/kg IV. Doses as low as 10 mg/kg in swine caused increased respiration, emesis, and seizures; 20 mg/kg IM caused deaths in most animals tested. In monkeys, 10 mg/kg administered once caused no signs of toxicity, but 20 mg/kg caused vomiting; 30 mg/kg caused death.

In cases of human injection, contact a physician immediately. The manufacturer has emergency telephone numbers to assist in dealing with exposure: 1-800-722-0987 or 1-800-428-4441.

For patients that have experienced or are suspected of having experienced an overdose, consultation with a 24-hour poison consultation center specializing in providing veterinary-specific information is recommended. For general information related to overdose and toxin exposures, as well as contact information for poison control centers, refer to ***Appendix.***

Drug Interactions

In swine, **epinephrine** increased the mortality associated with tilmicosin. No other specific information was noted; refer to the ***Erythromycin*** monograph for possible interactions.

Dosages

CATTLE:

Treatment of BRD associated with *Mannheimia haemolytica, Pasteurella multocida,* and *Histophilus somni* or control of respiratory disease in cattle at high risk for developing BRD associated with *Mannheimia haemolytica* (FDA-approved): 10 – 20 mg/kg SC as a single dose. Injection under the skin in the neck is suggested. If not accessible, inject under the skin behind the shoulders and over the ribs. Do not inject more than 10 mL per injection site. If no improvement is noted within 48 hours, the diagnosis should be re-evaluated.[7]

SHEEP:

Treatment of ovine respiratory disease associated with *Mannheimia haemolytica* (FDA-approved): In sheep greater than 15 kg (33 lb), 10 mg/kg SC as a single dose. Injection under the skin in the neck is suggested. If not accessible, inject under the skin behind the shoulders and over the ribs. Do not inject more than 10 mL per injection site. If no improvement is noted within 48 hours, the diagnosis should be re-evaluated.[7]

SWINE:

Control of SRD associated with *Pasteruella multocida* and *Haemophilus parasuis* in groups of swine in buildings where a respiratory disease outbreak is diagnosed (FDA-approved): Using oral concentrate, administer it in drinking water at a concentration of 200 mg tilmicosin per liter of drinking water for 5 consecutive days. Replace the water every 24 hours. One 960 mL bottle is sufficient to medicate 1200 L (320 gallons) of drinking water for pigs. When using water medicating pump with a 1:128 inclusion rate, add 1 bottle (960 mL) of *Pulmotil AC®* per 2.5 gallons of stock solution.[2]

SMALL MAMMALS:

Rabbits:

Pasteurellosis[6] (extra-label):

a) 25 mg/kg SC once[8]; repeat in 3 days if necessary
b) 5 mg/kg SC on day 0; if no reaction, give 10 mg/kg SC on days 7 and 14

Monitoring

- Efficacy
- Signs of water refusal or dehydration (medicated drinking water[2])
- Cardiovascular status following SC injection

Client Information

- If clients are administering the drug, warn them about the potential toxicity to humans, swine, and horses in case of accidental injection.
- Carefully instruct in proper injection techniques.
- Avoid contact with eyes.

Chemistry/Synonyms

Tilmicosin phosphate, a semisynthetic macrolide antibiotic, is commercially available in a 300 mg/mL (of tilmicosin base) injection with 25% propylene glycol.

Tilmicosin may also be known as EL-870, LY-177370, *Micotil®*, or *Pulmotil®*.

Storage/Stability

Store the injection at or below room temperature 30°C (86°F). Avoid exposure to direct sunlight. The UK label states to discard 28 days after the first puncture.

Store the oral liquid at or below 30°C (86°F). Protect from direct sunlight. The UK label states to use within 3 months of opening. Discard medicated water after 24 hours. Discard medicated milk replacer after 6 hours. Do not freeze; protect from frost.[2]

Compatibility/Compounding Considerations

Compatibility is dependent on factors such as pH, concentration, temperature, and diluent used; specialized references or a hospital pharmacist should be consulted for more specific information.

No specific information was noted.

Dosage Forms/Regulatory Status

VETERINARY-LABELED PRODUCTS:

Tilmicosin for Subcutaneous Injection: 300 mg/mL in 250 mL multidose vials; *Micotil® 300 Injection*; (Rx). FDA-approved (NADA# 140-929) for use in cattle and sheep. Not FDA-approved for use in female dairy cattle 20 months or older. Do not use in lactating ewes if milk is to be used for human consumption. Do not use in veal calves. Slaughter withdrawal (at labeled doses) is 42 days.

Tilmicosin Phosphate 250 mg/mL Aqueous Concentrate for oral use in drinking water in 960 mL bottles; *Pulmotil® AC, Tilmovet® AC*; (Rx). FDA-approved (NADA# 141-361) for use in swine. Slaughter withdrawal is 7 days.

Tilmicosin medicated article is available for incorporation into the feed of swine, beef and nonlactating dairy cattle.

HUMAN-LABELED PRODUCTS: NONE

References

For the complete list of references, see **wiley.com/go/budde/plumb**

Tiludronate

Tiludronic Acid

(til-yoo-***droe***-nate) *Tildren®*

Bisphosphonate; Bone Resorption Inhibitor

Prescriber Highlights

- Used as an IV treatment for navicular syndrome in horses
- Must be given slowly and evenly as an IV infusion over 90 minutes
- Contraindications include horses that are hypersensitive to tiludronate or mannitol and horses with a history of renal impairment.
- Use with caution in horses with conditions that cause mineral or electrolyte imbalance (eg, HYPP, hypocalcemia) and conditions that may be exacerbated by hypocalcemia (eg, cardiac disease).
- Adverse effects include signs of colic, muscle tremor (hypocalcemia), fatigue/lassitude, sweating, injection site effects, salivation, and tail hypertonia.

Uses/Indications

Tiludronate (tiludronic acid) is indicated for the control of clinical signs associated with navicular syndrome in horses.[1] It may be beneficial in managing lameness isolated to the navicular bone and distal tarsal osteoarthritis by decreasing bone resorption and inflammation.[2,3] Treatment earlier in the course of the disease apparently results in greater efficacy.

Tiludronate appeared to inhibit the radiographic progression of osteoarthritis after traumatic injury of the fetlock joint but was associated with increased markers of cartilage damage.[4]

Pharmacology/Actions

Tiludronate, like other bisphosphonates, inhibits osteoclastic bone resorption by inhibiting osteoclast function after binding to bone hydroxyapatite, thereby helping to regulate bone remodeling.

Pharmacokinetics

After IV injection in horses, the drug is rapidly distributed to the bone. Binding is greater to cancellous bone than cortical bone. Plasma protein binding is reported to be ≈85%, and the elimination half-life is ≈4 hours. Repeated daily doses do not result in accumulation in plasma. Tiludronate undergoes minimal metabolism. The unbound drug is eliminated unchanged in the urine. Approximately 25% to 50% of a single IV dose is eliminated in the urine over 96 hours. Quantifiable concentrations of tiludronate in the bone can be detected up to 1 year postdose,[1] and in the plasma for up to 3 years.[5]

Contraindications/Precautions/Warnings

Tiludronate is contraindicated in horses with known hypersensitivity to tiludronate disodium or to mannitol. It should not be used in horses with impaired renal function or a history of renal disease, as conditions causing renal impairment may increase plasma bisphosphonate concentrations, resulting in an increased risk for adverse reactions. Horses should be well hydrated prior to administration because of the potential nephrotoxic effects.[1]

Safe use has not been evaluated in horses less than 4 years of age. Bisphosphonates affect bone turnover and therefore may affect bone growth.[1] Increased bone fragility has been observed after high doses or a long duration of use.

Tiludronate can affect plasma concentrations of certain minerals and electrolytes, including calcium, magnesium, and potassium, immediately after treatment and can last up to several hours. Use caution when administering tiludronate to horses with conditions affecting mineral or electrolyte homeostasis (eg, hyperkalemic periodic paralysis (HYPP), hypocalcemia) and conditions which may be exacerbated by hypocalcemia (eg, cardiac disease).

Adverse Effects

Adverse effects reported in horses are most commonly seen during the infusion period or within 4 hours of beginning the infusion. Adverse effects include signs of abdominal pain or colic (eg, pawing, evidence of pawing, getting up and down, pacing, restlessness, rolling, trying to roll, looking at or biting at the side, stretching out/straining, kicking at belly/walls, and shifting weight), muscle tremors/fasciculation, fatigue/lassitude, and sweating. Colic signs occur in ≈30% to 45% of horses and generally resolve without treatment.[1] If these signs persist, conventional colic treatments (NOT including NSAIDs) are recommended. Muscle tremors may be treated with IV calcium if required. Horses with HYPP appear to be at increased risk for adverse effects.[1]

Adverse reactions occurring between 4 and 24 hours posttreatment include increased frequency of urination with or without increased drinking, reduced appetite, sore or stiff neck, fever, and uncomplicated colic.

Up to 9% of patients develop local reactions at the injection site (eg, phlebitis), particularly after the fourth injection. Other adverse effects reported include polydipsia/polyuria, decreased feed intake, recumbency, salivation, and tail hypertonia.

Tiludronate has caused acute renal failure.[6] Assess renal function and hydration status prior to administration.

The drug may be safely administered to horses within 24 to 36 hours after bone scintigraphy.[7]

Reproductive/Nursing Safety

Bisphosphonates should not be used in pregnant or lactating mares or mares intended for breeding.[1] Bisphosphonates have been shown to cause fetal developmental abnormalities in laboratory animals. The uptake of bisphosphonates into fetal bone may be greater than into maternal bone, creating a possible risk for skeletal or other abnormalities in the fetus.

Many drugs, including bisphosphonates, may be excreted in milk and may be absorbed by nursing animals.

Studies performed in male and female rats at tiludronate doses as high as 75 mg/kg/day demonstrated no effects on fertility. Studies in pregnant rabbits given 2 to 5 times the human-recommended dosages showed no skeletal abnormalities. Pregnant mice given 7 times the human-recommended dosages showed some adverse effects (eg, decreased litter size, malformed paws in 6 fetuses from 1 litter). Rat studies have shown decreased litter sizes[8] but no teratogenic effects.

Overdose/Acute Toxicity

Limited information is available. The manufacturer reports that dosing horses 3 times at monthly intervals caused an increased frequency of adverse effects, particularly signs of colic and muscle tremor. A dose-dependent increase in the frequency and severity of hypocalcemia and hyperphosphatemia was noted.

For patients that have experienced or are suspected of having experienced an overdose, consultation with a 24-hour poison consultation center specializing in providing veterinary-specific information is recommended. For general information related to overdose and toxin exposures, as well as contact information for poison control centers, refer to ***Appendix***.

Drug Interactions

The following drug interactions have either been reported or are theoretical in humans or animals receiving tiludronate and may be of significance in veterinary patients. Unless otherwise noted, use together is not necessarily contraindicated, but weigh the potential risks and perform additional monitoring when appropriate.

- **Aminoglycosides** (eg, **amikacin, gentamicin**): Concurrent use may increase the risk for nephrotoxicity and hypocalcemia.
- **Amphotericin B**: Concurrent use with nephrotoxic drugs may increase the risk for nephrotoxicity.
- **Nonsteroidal Anti-Inflammatory Drugs** (NSAIDs; eg, **flunixin**): The product label warns that NSAIDs should not be used concurrently with tiludronate. Concurrent use may increase the risk for renal toxicity and acute renal failure. Acute renal failure has been reported in horses concurrently administered NSAIDs and tiludronate within a 48-hour period. Additionally, horses concurrently administered both drugs in field studies demonstrated statistically significant increases in serum BUN and creatinine concentrations but were not always associated with clinical signs of renal dysfunction. Appropriate washout periods should be observed, and BUN and creatinine should be monitored. If treatment for discomfort is required after tiludronate administration, a non-NSAID treatment should be used.
- **Tetracyclines** (eg, **oxytetracycline**): May increase the risk for hypocalcemia

Laboratory Considerations

No specific concerns were noted.

Dosages

HORSES:

Control of clinical signs associated with navicular syndrome (label dose; FDA-approved): A single dose of 1 mg/kg as an IV infusion in 1000 mL of 0.9% sodium chloride. Administer slowly and evenly over 90 minutes (to minimize adverse reactions) through a suitable IV catheter inserted into a jugular vein and connected to the infusion bag using sterile infusion tubing.[1] Maximum effect may not occur until 2 months posttreatment. Infusion of the labeled dose diluted in 5000 mL of 0.9% sodium chloride solution appears to be a common practice.

Control of clinical signs associated with navicular syndrome (extra-label): Ten bolus doses of 0.1 mg/kg IV every 24 hours for 10 consecutive days.[9] Used in horses particularly sensitive to adverse effects of tiludronate

Monitoring

- Clinical efficacy
- Serum calcium
- BUN and serum creatinine prior to administration of NSAIDs following dosing
- Adverse effects (particularly within the first 4 hours after dosing)

Client Information

- A veterinary professional should administer this medication.
- Observe the animal for up to 4 hours postadministration for signs of hypocalcemia (eg, muscle tremors) or colic. Monitor food and water intake, urinary frequency, and body temperature for a few days after administration.
- Allow the horse to lie down, as this is an expected behavior after the infusion is complete.
- Consult with your veterinarian prior to giving anti-inflammatory medications (NSAIDs) following tiludronate administration.

Chemistry/Synonyms

Tiludronate disodium is a non-nitrogen-containing bisphosphonate that occurs as a white powder with a molecular weight of 380.6. Commercially available products contain the disodium salt of tiludronic acid. 120 mg of tiludronate disodium is equivalent to 100 mg of tiludronic acid.

Tiludronate disodium or tiludronic acid may also be known as ME-3737, SR-41319, acidum tiludronicum, *Tildren*®, or *Skelid*®.

Storage/Stability

Store unreconstituted powder at controlled room temperature 20°C to 25°C (68°F-77°F). After preparation, either administer the infusion within 2 hours of preparation or store it for up to 24 hours under refrigeration at 2°C to 8°C (36°F-46°F) and protect it from light.

Compatibility/Compounding Considerations

Do **not** reconstitute or mix this product with calcium-containing solutions or other solutions containing divalent cations, such as lactated Ringer's solution, as it may form complexes with these ions.

Preparation of the reconstituted solution (20 mg/mL): Use strict aseptic technique. Remove 25 mL of solution from a 1-liter bag of sterile 0.9% sodium chloride and add to a vial of *Tildren*®. Shake gently until the powder is completely dissolved. This reconstituted solution contains 20 mg of tiludronate disodium per mL. After reconstitution, further dilution is required before administration.

Preparation of the solution for infusion: Using strict aseptic technique, withdraw the appropriate volume of the reconstituted solution based on the horse's body weight. Inject that volume back into the 1-liter bag of sterile 0.9% sodium chloride. Horses greater than 550 kg (1210 lb) will require a second vial of reconstituted solution. Invert the infusion bag several times to mix the solution before infusion. Label the infusion bag to ensure proper use.

After preparation, the infusion should be administered either within 2 hours of preparation, or it can be stored for up to 24 hours under refrigeration at 2°C to 8°C (36°F-46°F) and protected from light.

Administer for infusion through a suitable IV catheter inserted into a jugular vein and connected to the infusion bag using sterile infusion tubing.

Dosage Forms/Regulatory Status

VETERINARY-LABELED PRODUCTS:

Tiludronic Acid: 500 mg (as tiludronate disodium) lyophilized powder for reconstitution per vial; *Tildren*®; (Rx). FDA-approved for horses. NADA #141-420

HUMAN-LABELED PRODUCTS: NONE

References

For the complete list of references, see **wiley.com/go/budde/plumb**

Tinidazole

(tye-***ni***-dah-zole) *Tindamax*®

Nitroimidazole Antiprotozoal/Antibiotic

Prescriber Highlights

- Drug similar to metronidazole, but does not appear to have significant advantages over metronidazole or ronidazole
- Used primarily as an alternative treatment for giardiasis. Potentially useful for treating anaerobic infections (especially in the mouth), trichomoniasis, amebiasis, and balantidiasis.
- Little experience in veterinary medicine. Most likely adverse effects are GI-related; like other nitroimidazole agents, neurotoxicity is possible.

Uses/Indications

Little information is presently available on the use of tinidazole in veterinary species. Because of its antiprotozoal effects, it has been used as an alternative for treating giardiasis in small animals. Tinidazole could have efficacy against amebiasis, trichomoniasis, or balantidiasis, but documentation of efficacy is not available. Tinidazole potentially could be useful for treating anaerobic infections in small animals, particularly those associated with dental infections.[1] Tinidazole has a longer duration of action than metronidazole in dogs and cats.

In a small study done in cats experimentally infected with *Tritrichomonas foetus*, tinidazole 30 mg/kg PO once daily for 14 days decreased fecal shedding of *T foetus* but failed to eradicate the infection from 2 of 4 cats.[2] However, results from a pilot study indicated that tinidazole 30 mg/kg, formulated in a gastro-resistant capsule coated with guar gum, PO once daily for 14 days resolved *T foetus* infections and improved the clinical condition in 5 FIV-positive cats and was also effective against concomitant *Giardia duodenalis* infection in the 4 affected cats.[3]

In humans, oral tinidazole is FDA-approved for treating extraintestinal and intestinal amebiasis (ie, *Entamoeba histolytica*), giardiasis (ie, *Giardia duodenalis* and *G lamblia*), and trichomoniasis (ie, *Trichomonas vaginalis*).

The World Health Organization (WHO) has designated tinidazole as an Important antimicrobial for human medicine.[4]

Pharmacology/Actions

Tinidazole is a 5-nitroimidazole similar to metronidazole. It is bactericidal against susceptible bacteria. Its exact mechanism of action is not completely understood, but it is taken up by anaerobic organisms where it is reduced to an unidentified polar compound. It is believed that this compound is responsible for the drug's antimicrobial activity by disrupting DNA and nucleic acid synthesis in the bacteria.

Tinidazole has activity against many obligate anaerobes and *Helicobacter pylori*. It has excellent activity against *Porphyromonas* spp found in canine gingiva.[1]

Tinidazole is also trichomonacidal and amebicidal.[5] Its mechanism of action for its antiprotozoal activity is not well understood. It has therapeutic activity against *Entamoeba histolytica*, *Trichomonas* spp, and *Giardia* spp.

Pharmacokinetics

In dogs and cats,[6] tinidazole is practically completely absorbed after oral administration. Apparent volumes of distribution are 0.66 L/kg in dogs and 0.54 L/kg in cats. Dogs clear the drug about twice as fast as cats; elimination half-lives are ≈4.4 hours in dogs and 8.4 hours in cats.

In horses,[7] tinidazole is practically completely absorbed after oral administration. Apparent volume of distribution is 0.66 L/kg and elimination half-life is ≈5.2 hours.

Contraindications/Precautions/Warnings

Tinidazole is contraindicated in patients documented to be hypersensitive to it or other 5-nitroimidazoles (eg, metronidazole). In humans, tinidazole is contraindicated in the first trimester of pregnancy.

Tinidazole is metabolized by the liver; use with caution in patients with hepatic dysfunction. Tinidazole should be used with caution in patients with blood dyscrasias.

As other 5-nitroimidazoles (eg, metronidazole, ronidazole) have been associated with neurotoxic signs in dogs and cats and seizures have been reported rarely with tinidazole use in humans, use with caution in animals susceptible to seizures.

The human labeling for tinidazole carries a black box warning stating: *Carcinogenicity has been seen in mice and rats treated chronically with another agent in the nitroimidazole class (eg, metronidazole). Although such data has not been reported for tinidazole, avoid unnecessary use of tinidazole. Reserve its use for the conditions for which it is indicated.*

Adverse Effects

The adverse effect profiles for dogs, cats, or horses are not well described since clinical use of this medication has been limited. GI effects including vomiting, inappetence, and diarrhea are most likely. Giving the medication with food may help alleviate these effects. Other 5-nitroimidazoles (eg, metronidazole, ronidazole) have been associated with neurotoxic signs in dogs and cats.

Although metronidazole has been shown to significantly decrease food intake in chinchillas, equivalent doses of tinidazole did not affect food intake.[8]

In humans, tinidazole reportedly has fewer side effects than metronidazole.[9] GI effects (eg, dysgeusia, nausea, decreased appetite) are the most commonly reported adverse effects. Rare adverse effects in humans include seizures, transient myelosuppression, and hypersensitivity reactions.[5]

Reproductive/Nursing Safety

In studies performed on male rats, tinidazole decreased fertility and caused testicular histopathology.

Tinidazole crosses the placenta. While studies in mice and rats have not demonstrated significant fetal effects, because of its mutagenic potential, it is stated that it should <u>not be used in women during the first trimester</u> of pregnancy. If considering use of this product in a pregnant animal, weigh the potential benefits of treatment versus the risks.

Tinidazole is distributed into maternal milk at levels approximating those found in serum. It is suggested that milk replacer be used if tinidazole is necessary for treating a nursing dam.

Overdose/Acute Toxicity

Limited information is available. In studies done in rats and mice, the oral LD_{50} was greater than 3.6 g/kg for mice and greater than 2 g/kg for rats. Treatment of acute overdoses of tinidazole is symptomatic and supportive. Gastric lavage or induction of emesis may be helpful. Hemodialysis can remove ≈43% of the amount in the body (human) in a 6-hour session.

For patients that have experienced or are suspected of having experienced an overdose, consultation with a 24-hour poison consultation center specializing in providing veterinary-specific information is recommended. For general information related to overdose and toxin exposures, as well as contact information for poison control centers, refer to ***Appendix.***

Drug Interactions

The following drug interactions have either been reported or are theoretical in humans or animals receiving metronidazole (a related compound) and may be of significance in veterinary patients. Unless otherwise noted, use together is not necessarily contraindicated, but weigh the potential risks and perform additional monitoring when appropriate.

- **Busulfan**: Tinidazole may increase the serum concentration of busulfan.
- **Cholestyramine**: May decrease metronidazole absorption; interaction may apply to tinidazole
- **Cimetidine**: May decrease the metabolism of tinidazole and increase the likelihood of dose-related side effects occurring
- **Cisapride**: Tinidazole may increase the serum concentration of cisapride; contraindicated in humans.
- **Cyclosporine, Tacrolimus** (systemic): Tinidazole may increase the serum concentration of cyclosporine or tacrolimus.
- **Ethanol**: May induce a disulfiram-like (nausea, vomiting, cramps) reaction
- **Fluorouracil** (systemic): Tinidazole may increase the serum concentration of fluorouracil and increase the risk of toxicity.
- **Ketoconazole**: May decrease the metabolism of tinidazole and increase the likelihood of dose-related side effects occurring
- **Oxytetracycline**: Reportedly, may antagonize the therapeutic effects of metronidazole; interaction may apply to tinidazole
- **Phenobarbital**: May increase the metabolism of tinidazole, thereby decreasing blood concentration
- **Rifampin**: May increase the metabolism of tinidazole, thereby decreasing blood concentration
- **Warfarin**: Metronidazole (and potentially tinidazole) may prolong the prothrombin time (PT) in patients taking warfarin or other coumarin anticoagulants. Avoid concurrent use if possible; otherwise, intensify monitoring.

Laboratory Considerations

- **AST, ALT, LDH, Triglycerides, Hexokinase glucose**: Tinidazole, like metronidazole, may interfere with enzymatic coupling of the assay to oxidation-reduction of nicotinamide adenine. Falsely low values, including zero, may result.

Dosages

DOGS:

Giardiasis (extra-label): 44 mg/kg PO every 24 hours for 6 days. Potentially useful for treating trichomoniasis, amebiasis, and balantidiasis, but efficacy data are lacking for animals.[10] Another source lists the same dosage but treats for 3 days.[11]

CATS:

Giardiasis (extra-label): 30 mg/kg PO once daily for 7 to 10 days.[12] Another source lists the same dosage but treats for 3 days.[11]

Tritrichomonas foetus (extra-label): 30 mg/kg PO once daily for 14 days decreased detection of *T foetus* in 50% of experimentally infected cats

Monitoring

- Clinical efficacy in treating the infection

Client Information

- Give this medication with food.
- Animals should not have access to alcohol when receiving this medication.
- If gastrointestinal signs (eg, vomiting, lack of appetite, diarrhea) are severe or persist, contact your veterinarian.
- Contact your veterinarian immediately if animal shows signs of behavior changes, eyes moving back and forth (nystagmus), convulsions, or if it has difficulty walking, climbing stairs; these could be signs that drug toxicity is occurring.

Chemistry/Synonyms

Tinidazole occurs as an almost white or pale-yellow crystalline powder. It is practically insoluble in water, soluble in acetone, and sparingly soluble in methyl alcohol.

Tinidazole may also be known as CP-12574 or tinidazolum or tinidatsoli. International trade names include: *Estovyn-T*®, *Fasigyn*®, *Tindamax*®, *Tiniba*®, *Tiniameb*®, or *Tinidazol*®.

Storage/Stability

Store tinidazole tablets at controlled room temperature (20°C-25°C [68°F-77°F]) protected from light.

Compatibility/Compounding Considerations

The manufacturer label states an oral suspension can be made by pulverizing four 500 mg oral tablets with a mortar and pestle. Add ≈10 mL of cherry syrup to the powder and mix until smooth. Transfer the suspension to a graduated amber container. Use several small rinses of cherry syrup to transfer any remaining drug in the mortar to the final suspension for a final volume of 30 mL (67 mg/mL). This suspension is stable for 7 days at room temperature. When this suspension is used, it should be shaken well before each administration.[13]

Tinidazole reportedly is very bitter tasting. If using compounded products, consider using capsules or having a flavored suspension prepared.

Dosage Forms/Regulatory Status

VETERINARY-LABELED PRODUCTS: NONE

As tinidazole is a nitroimidazole, its use is prohibited in animals to be used for food.

HUMAN-LABELED PRODUCTS:

Tinidazole Tablets (scored): 250 mg and 500 mg; *Tindamax*®, generic; (Rx)

References

For the complete list of references, see **wiley.com/go/budde/plumb**

Tiopronin

(tye-oh-***proe***-nin) *Thiola*®

Antiurolithic (Cystine)

Prescriber Highlights

- Used in combination with dietary therapy, high fluid intake, and urinary alkalinization for prevention and dissolution of cystine urolithiasis in dogs
- Avoid use in cats.
- Use with caution in animals with agranulocytosis, aplastic anemia, thrombocytopenia or other significant hematologic abnormality, impaired renal or hepatic function, or sensitivity to either tiopronin or penicillamine.
- Adverse effects include Coombs-positive regenerative spherocyte anemia, aggressive behavior, proteinuria, thrombocytopenia, elevations in liver enzymes, dermatologic effects, and myopathy.
- Cost and availability may be problematic.

Uses/Indications

Tiopronin may be added to the treatment regimen for the prevention and dissolution of cystine urolithiasis in dogs when dietary therapy (ie, low-protein, low-sodium diet), high fluid intake, and urine alkalinization are not completely effective.[1-5]

Pharmacology/Actions

Tiopronin is a chelator that is considered an antiurolithic agent. It undergoes thiol-disulfide exchange with cystine (cysteine-cysteine disulfide) to form tiopronin-cystine disulfide. This complex is more water-soluble and readily excreted thereby preventing cystine calculi from forming. Its effects on cystine reduction are dose-related and typically begin within the first day of treatment. Given the relatively rapid elimination of drug, twice daily dosing is recommended.

Pharmacokinetics

Tiopronin has a rapid onset of action, and in humans, up to 48% of a dose is found in the urine within 4 hours of dosing.[6] Tiopronin has a relatively short duration of action, and its effect in humans disappears in ≈10 hours. Elimination is primarily via renal routes.

Contraindications/Precautions/Warnings

Tiopronin is contraindicated in patients that are hypersensitive to it or in those patients with obstructive urolithiasis. Tiopronin's risks vs benefits should be considered before using in patients with agranulocytosis, aplastic anemia, thrombocytopenia, or other significant hematologic abnormalities. Use with caution in patients with impaired renal or hepatic function or sensitivity to penicillamine. In humans, it is recommended to start tiopronin at a lower dose in patients with history of severe toxicity to penicillamine.

Avoid use of tiopronin in cats as they reportedly do not tolerate the drug well and dissolution of cystine uroliths has not been successful.[7]

Adverse Effects

There is limited information available on the adverse effect profile of tiopronin in dogs. In a retrospective study evaluating tiopronin treatment for cystinuria, ≈13% of treated dogs experienced adverse events including proteinuria, thrombocytopenia, anemia, increased liver enzymes and bile acids, lethargy, dermatologic effects (small pustules of the skin, dry crusty nose), aggression, sulfur odor of the urine, or myopathy (noted as staggering and difficulty chewing).[3] Adverse effects manifested between 1 month and 36 months (mean of 7.8 months) of therapy and resolved with discontinuation of therapy. Tiopronin has been associated with Coombs-positive regenerative spherocyte anemia in dogs. If this effect occurs, the drug should be discontinued and appropriate treatment started as needed (eg, corticosteroids, blood component therapy).

If adverse reactions occur, stop treatment for 4 weeks. Check blood and urine analysis every 1 to 2 weeks until remission of signs. When the adverse reactions disappear, start tiopronin again, gradually increasing the dose from 10 – 15 mg/kg every 12 hours. If the adverse reactions reappear despite a lowered dose, tiopronin treatment has to be abandoned.[3]

In cats, GI signs, liver disease, and anemia have been reported.[7]

In humans, common adverse effects include dermatologic effects (ecchymosis, itching, rashes, mouth ulcers, jaundice) and GI distress. Less frequently reported adverse effects include allergic reactions (specifically adenopathy), arthralgias, dyspnea, fever, hematologic abnormalities, edema, and nephrotic syndrome.[6]

Reproductive/Nursing Safety

There is limited information on the reproductive safety of tiopronin. No adverse developmental outcomes were noted in rats given up to 4 times the recommended human dose.[8] Skeletal defects, cleft palates and increased resorptions were noted when rats were given 10 times the human dose of penicillamine and, therefore, may also be of concern with tiopronin. In humans, tiopronin is contraindicated during pregnancy except in severe cases of cystinuria in which the potential benefits outweigh possible hazards.

Because tiopronin may be excreted in milk, it is not recommended for use in nursing animals.

Because safety has not been established in animals, this drug should only be used when the maternal benefits outweigh the potential risks to offspring.

Overdose/Acute Toxicity

There is little information available. It is suggested to contact an animal poison control center for further information in the event of an overdose situation.

For patients that have experienced or are suspected to have experienced an overdose, consultation with a 24-hour poison consultation center specializing in providing veterinary-specific information is recommended. For general information related to overdose and toxin exposures, as well as contact information for poison control centers, refer to ***Appendix.***

Drug Interactions

Potentially, use of tiopronin with **other drugs causing nephrotoxicity, hepatotoxicity, or myelosuppression** could cause additive toxic effects. Clinical significance is not clear.

Dosages

DOGS:

Prevention and dissolution of cystine urinary calculi (extra-label):

a) **Prevention of uroliths**: 15 mg/kg PO every 12 hours. Increase water intake and urine diuresis. Alkalinize urine (pH 6.5 to 7.0) using potassium citrate. In cases with low cystine excretion and low urolith recurrence rate, tiopronin dose may be individually decreased (less than 30 mg/kg) or stopped.[2-4]

b) **Dissolution of uroliths**: Approximately 20 mg/kg PO every 12 hours. Reevaluation of uroliths with ultrasound or radiography every 4th week. After urolith dissolution, give preventive dose of tiopronin. If urolith dissolution is not achieved after 2 to 3 months, surgery is recommended.[2-4]

Monitoring

- Re-examination is recommended 1, 3, 6, and 12 months after starting treatment, and if well controlled, every 6 to 12 months thereafter.
- Physical examination
- Ultrasonography/radiography of the urinary tract
- Urinalyses with sediment using first morning urine samples
- CBC with platelet count
- Liver enzymes (ALP, ALT)

Client Information

- Clients should be counseled on the importance of adequate compliance with this medicine to maximize efficacy and detailed on the clinical signs to watch for regarding adverse effects.
- Give this medicine at the same time each day, at least one hour before or two hours after meals.

Chemistry/Synonyms

A sulfhydryl compound related to penicillamine, tiopronin has a molecular weight of 163.2. It occurs as a white crystalline powder that is freely soluble in water.

Tiopronin may also be known as SF 522, N-(2-Mercaptopropionyl)-glycine (MPG), 2-MPG, thiopronine, *Acadione®*, *Captimer®*, *Epatiol®*, *Mucolysin®*, *Mucosyt®*, *Sutilan®*, *Thiola®*, *Thiosol®*, or *Tioglis®*.

Storage/Stability

Store tablets in tight containers at room temperature 25°C (77°F) with excursions permitted to 15°C -30°C (59°F -86°F).

Compatibility/Compounding Considerations

No specific information noted

Dosage Forms/Regulatory Status

VETERINARY-LABELED PRODUCTS: NONE

HUMAN-LABELED PRODUCTS:

Tiopronin Tablets: 100 mg; *Thiola®*; (Rx)

Tiopronin Delayed Release Tablets: 100 mg, 300 mg; *Thiola EC*®; (Rx)

References

For the complete list of references, see **wiley.com/go/budde/plumb**

Tobramycin, Systemic

(toe-bra-***mye***-sin) *Nebcin*®

Aminoglycoside Antibiotic

See also ***Tobramycin Ophthalmic***

Prescriber Highlights

- Parenteral aminoglycoside antibiotic that is active against a variety of bacteria, predominantly gram-negative aerobic bacilli
- Because of potential adverse effects, systemic use is usually reserved for serious infections; may be less nephrotoxic than gentamicin.
- Adverse effects may include nephrotoxicity, ototoxicity, and neuromuscular blockade.
- Cats may be more sensitive to toxic effects.
- Risk factors for nephrotoxicity include pre-existing renal disease, age (both neonatal and geriatric), fever, sepsis, and dehydration.

Uses/Indications

Tobramycin can be useful clinically to treat serious gram-negative infections in most species. It is often used in settings where gentamicin-resistant bacteria are a clinical problem or when amikacin is unavailable. The inherent toxicity of the aminoglycosides limits their systemic use to serious infections when there is either a documented lack of susceptibility to other less potentially toxic antibiotics or when the clinical situation dictates the immediate treatment of a presumed gram-negative infection before culture and susceptibility results are reported.

Whether tobramycin is less nephrotoxic than either gentamicin or amikacin when used clinically is somewhat controversial, but in controlled laboratory animal studies, it was less nephrotoxic.

The World Health Organization (WHO) has designated tobramycin as a Critically Important, Highest Priority antimicrobial for human medicine.[1] The Office International des Epizooties (OIE) Antimicrobial Classification has designated tobramycin as a Veterinary Critically Important antimicrobial.[2]

Pharmacology/Actions

Tobramycin, like the other aminoglycoside antibiotics, acts on susceptible bacteria, presumably by irreversibly binding to the 30S ribosomal subunit, thereby inhibiting protein synthesis. It is considered a bactericidal concentration-dependent antibiotic.

Tobramycin's spectrum of activity includes coverage against many aerobic gram-negative and some aerobic gram-positive bacteria, including most species of *Escherichia coli*, *Klebsiella* spp, *Proteus* spp, *Pseudomonas* spp, *Salmonella* spp, *Enterobacter* spp, *Serratia* spp, *Shigella* spp, *Mycoplasma* spp, and *Staphylococcus* spp. Tobramycin has more activity against *Pseudomonas* spp isolates than gentamicin.

The antimicrobial activity of the aminoglycosides is enhanced in an alkaline environment, but pus or cellular debris can reduce efficacy.

The aminoglycoside antibiotics are inactive against fungi, viruses, and most anaerobic bacteria.

Pharmacokinetics

Tobramycin, like the other aminoglycosides, is not appreciably absorbed after oral or intrauterine administration, but it is absorbed from topical administration (not skin or urinary bladder) when used in irrigations during surgical procedures. Patients receiving oral aminoglycosides with hemorrhagic or necrotic enteritis may absorb appreciable quantities of the drug. SC injection results in slightly delayed peak levels and more variability than after IM injection. Bioavailability from IM or SC injection is greater than 90%.

The pharmacokinetics of tobramycin in horses have been reported.[3-5] In a study where horses were given 4 mg/kg IV,[5] the following approximate values were reported (**NOTE**: First value is a calculated value from a microbiologic assay, and the second is from an HPLC assay): volume of distribution (steady-state) (Vd), 0.24 to 0.55 L/kg; clearance (Cl), 101 to 130 mL/kg/hour; and elimination half-life ($t_{1/2}$), 2.5 to 4 hours. Another study where horses were administered 4 mg/kg IV, IM, or IV with concurrent IA[3] reported the following (means) after IV administration: Vd, 0.18 L/kg; Cl, 1.18 mL/kg/minute; and $t_{1/2}$, 4.6 hours. IM mean bioavailability was 81%, but there was wide variability (±44%). Concurrent IA administration did appear to alter IV pharmacokinetics.

A 2008 review article of pharmacokinetic studies of aminoglycosides in various mammals showed the following mean values for tobramycin: dogs: $t_{1/2}$, 56 minutes; Vd, 4.1 L/kg; Cl, 53.7 mL/kg/minute; cats: $t_{1/2}$, 1.5 hours; Vd, 0.8 L/kg; and Cl, 6.3 mL/kg/minute.[6]

After absorption, aminoglycosides are distributed primarily in the extracellular fluid. They are found in ascitic, pleural, pericardial, peritoneal, synovial, and abscess fluids and high levels are found in sputum, bronchial secretions, and bile. Aminoglycosides (other than streptomycin) are minimally protein-bound (less than 20%) to plasma proteins. Aminoglycosides do not readily cross the blood–brain barrier or penetrate ocular tissue. CSF levels are unpredictable and range from 0% to 50% of those found in the serum. Therapeutic levels are found in bone, heart, gallbladder, and lung tissues after parenteral dosing. Aminoglycosides tend to accumulate in certain tissues, such as the inner ear and kidneys, which may help explain their toxicity.

Elimination of aminoglycosides after parenteral administration occurs almost entirely by glomerular filtration. Patients with decreased renal function can have significantly prolonged half-lives. In humans with normal renal function, elimination rates can be highly variable with the aminoglycoside antibiotics.

Contraindications/Precautions/Warnings

Aminoglycosides are contraindicated in patients that are hypersensitive to them. Because these drugs are often the only effective agents in severe gram-negative infections, there are no other absolute contraindications to their use; however, they should be used with extreme caution in patients with pre-existing renal disease, with concomitant monitoring and dosage interval adjustments made. Other risk factors for the development of toxicity include age (both neonatal and geriatric patients), fever, sepsis, and dehydration.

Because aminoglycosides can cause irreversible ototoxicity, they should be used with caution in working dogs (eg, seeing-eye dogs, herding, police dogs, and dogs for the hearing impaired). Topical preparations for the treatment of otitis externa should only be used when an intact tympanic membrane is present.

Aminoglycosides should be used with caution in patients with neuromuscular disorders (eg, myasthenia gravis) because of their neuromuscular blocking activity.

Aminoglycosides are generally considered contraindicated in rabbits and hares, as they adversely affect the GI flora balance in these animals.

Adverse Effects

The aminoglycosides possess nephrotoxic and ototoxic effects. The nephrotoxic (tubular necrosis) mechanisms of these drugs are not completely understood but are likely related to accumulation in the renal convoluted tubules, interfering with phospholipid metabolism in the lysosomes of proximal renal tubular cells, resulting in leakage of proteolytic enzymes into the cytoplasm. Nephrotoxicity normally manifests by azotemia and decreases in urine specific gravity and creatinine clearance. Proteinuria and cells or casts may also be seen in the urine. Nephrotoxicity is usually reversible once the drug is discontinued. Although tobramycin may be less nephrotoxic than the other aminoglycosides, the potential for nephrotoxicity remains, and equal caution and monitoring are required.

Ototoxicity (eighth cranial nerve toxicity) from aminoglycosides can manifest with either auditory and/or vestibular clinical signs and may be irreversible.[7] Vestibular clinical signs are more frequent with streptomycin, gentamicin, or tobramycin. Auditory clinical signs are more frequent with amikacin, neomycin, or kanamycin, but any manifestation can occur with any of the drugs. Cats are apparently sensitive to the vestibular effects of aminoglycosides.

The aminoglycosides can also cause neuromuscular blockade, facial edema, pain or inflammation at the injection site, peripheral neuropathy, and hypersensitivity reactions. Rarely GI clinical signs, hematologic, and hepatic effects have been reported.

Reproductive/Nursing Safety

Aminoglycosides cross the placenta, and fetal concentrations range from 15% to 50% of those found in maternal serum. Tobramycin can concentrate in fetal kidneys and, although rare, cause eighth cranial nerve toxicity or nephrotoxicity in fetuses. Total irreversible deafness has been reported in some human babies whose mothers received tobramycin during pregnancy. Because the drug should only be used in serious infections, the benefits of therapy may exceed the potential risks.

Tobramycin is excreted in breast milk, but because of poor oral absorption, it is unlikely to have systemic effects on the infant. However, it could alter gut flora.

Because safety has not been established in animals, this drug should only be used when the maternal benefits outweigh the potential risks to offspring.

Overdose/Acute Toxicity

If an inadvertent overdose is administered, hemodialysis is very effective in reducing serum levels of the drug. Peritoneal dialysis will also reduce serum levels but is much less efficacious.

For patients that have experienced or are suspected of having experienced an overdose, consultation with a 24-hour poison consultation center specializing in providing veterinary-specific information is recommended. For general information related to overdose and toxin exposures, as well as contact information for poison control centers, refer to ***Appendix.***

Drug Interactions

The following drug interactions have either been reported or are theoretical in humans or animals receiving tobramycin and may be of significance in veterinary patients. Unless otherwise noted, use together is not necessarily contraindicated, but weigh the potential risks and perform additional monitoring when appropriate.

- **Anesthetics, General** (eg, **alfaxalone, isoflurane, ketamine, propofol**): Concurrent use could potentiate neuromuscular blockade.
- **Beta-Lactam Antibiotics** (eg, **penicillins, cephalosporins**): May have synergistic effects against some bacteria; some potential for inactivation of aminoglycosides in vitro (do not mix together) and in vivo (patients in renal failure). Cephalosporins could cause additive nephrotoxicity when used with aminoglycosides, but this interaction has only been well documented with cephaloridine and cephalothin (both no longer marketed).
- **Diuretics, Loop** (eg, **furosemide, torsemide**): Concurrent use may increase the risk for nephrotoxicity and/or ototoxicity.
- **Diuretics, Osmotic** (eg, **mannitol**): Concurrent use may increase the nephrotoxic or ototoxic potential of aminoglycosides.
- **Nephrotoxic Drugs, Other** (eg, **amphotericin B, cisplatin, cyclosporine, polymyxin B, vancomycin**): Increased risk for nephrotoxicity
- **Neuromuscular Blocking Agents** (eg, **atracurium**): Concurrent use could potentiate neuromuscular blockade.
- **Nonsteroidal anti-inflammatory drugs** (**NSAIDs**; eg, **carprofen, meloxicam, robenacoxib**): May increase tobramycin concentration

Laboratory Considerations

- Tobramycin serum concentrations may be falsely decreased if the patient is also receiving some **beta-lactam antibiotics** and the serum is stored prior to analysis. It is recommended that if the assay is delayed, samples be frozen and, if possible, drawn at times when the beta-lactam antibiotic is at a trough level.

Dosages

NOTE: There is significant interpatient variability with aminoglycoside pharmacokinetic parameters. To ensure therapeutic levels and minimize the risks for toxicity, consider monitoring serum levels. See ***Monitoring***.

DOGS & CATS:

Susceptible infections (extra-label): Dogs: 9 – 14 mg/kg IV, IM, or SC once daily. Cats: 5 – 8 mg/kg IV, IM, or SC once daily

HORSES:

Susceptible infections (extra-label): 4 mg/kg IV once daily. IM administration will somewhat reduce peak concentration and corresponding efficacy against some Enterobacteriaceae.[3]

LLAMAS:

Susceptible infections (extra-label): 4 mg/kg IV once a day[8]

BIRDS:

Susceptible infections (extra-label):

a) 5 mg/kg IM every 12 hours[9]

b) 2.5 – 5 mg/kg/day; must be given parenterally[10]

REPTILES:

Susceptible infections (extra-label): 2.5 mg/kg once daily IM[11]

Monitoring

- Efficacy (cultures, clinical signs associated with infection)
- Gross monitoring of vestibular or auditory toxicity is recommended.
- Tobramycin serum concentration, if possible (see below)
- Nephrotoxicity (see below)

The following recommendations are from the International Renal Interest Society (IRIS) to prevent aminoglycoside-induced acute kidney injury (AKI; in dogs and cats).

Prior to aminoglycoside treatment*:

- Carefully consider the potential risk factors: dehydration, concomitant treatment with furosemide, use of other nephrotoxic drugs, arterial hypotension, hypokalemia, previous history of AKI, pre-existing chronic kidney disease (CKD). When such factors are identified, alternatives to aminoglycoside treatment should be considered.
- Perform urinalysis: measure urine specific gravity, examine for glycosuria, proteinuria (UPC), and abnormal sediment. If abnormalities are detected, investigate carefully to determine the underlying cause before deciding whether to prescribe aminoglycosides.
- Blood tests: determine blood creatinine concentration. Consider avoiding the use of aminoglycosides if the blood creatinine concentration is at the borderline between stage I and stage II or al-

ready in stage II. In borderline cases, further investigations might be considered to evaluate renal risk.
- Imaging: abdominal radiograph and/or ultrasonographic examination
- Measurement of arterial blood pressure: high-risk hypertension: systolic BP greater than 180 mm Hg is indicative of renal damage and risk.

**This list was adapted from IRIS. Preventing Aminoglycoside-induced AKI. http://www.iris-kidney.com/education/education/prevention.html.*

During the treatment*:
- Assess the hydration status of the patient (body weight, total plasma protein concentration, and hematocrit) once weekly.
- If therapeutic drug monitoring is available, ensure the plasma tobramycin concentration has decreased to below 1 mg/L (1 µg/mL) before the next dose is administered.
- Carefully re-assess the pretreatment urine and blood variables indicated above
- Repeat these assessments every 3 to 4 days to detect any change. If there is any doubt of renal damage, perform the GGT:creatinine ratio in the urine (when available in the laboratory); an increase is an early indicator of nephrotoxicity.
- Continue monitoring for 1 week after discontinuing the treatment, as AKI may occur later as aminoglycosides accumulate inside proximal tubular cells and persist for long periods after dosing.
- The risk for nephrotoxicity increases with the duration of the treatment, as aminoglycoside nephrotoxicity is cumulative.
- If findings suggest the development of AKI (urine: the presence of renal casts in the sediment, glycosuria, low specific gravity; blood: azotemia): Immediately stop aminoglycoside therapy. Hospitalize the patient and monitor urine production. Nonoliguric AKI generally occurs and is reversible. Oliguric AKI has a poor prognosis. Start adequate IV fluid therapy. Monitor BUN, creatinine, and electrolytes (hypokalemia is frequent in nonoliguric AKI and should be corrected)
- If AKI is worsening, consider renal substitutive therapy (hemodialysis). After apparent recovery from aminoglycoside-induced AKI, some dogs may remain renally impaired.

**This list was adapted from IRIS. Preventing Aminoglycoside-induced AKI. http://www.iris-kidney.com/education/education/prevention.html.*

Client Information
- Tobramycin must be injected if it is used for treating serious infections. It does not work if it is given by mouth.
- This medicine can damage the nerves, hearing, and kidneys. Monitor your animal for symptoms such as vomiting, not eating, lethargy, and difficulty walking.
- Cats may be more likely to have damage to their hearing.
- Give this medicine once daily either in the vein (by your veterinarian) or under the skin (subcutaneous).
- This medicine can be used topically (in the eye, ear, on the skin) for certain infections.
- While your animal is taking this medication, it is important to return to your veterinarian for blood and urine tests. Do not miss these important follow-up visits.

Chemistry/Synonyms
Tobramycin, an aminoglycoside derived from *Streptomyces tenebrarius*, occurs as a white to off-white, hygroscopic powder that is freely soluble in water and very slightly soluble in alcohol. The sulfate salt is formed during the manufacturing process. The commercial injection is a clear, colorless solution, and the pH is adjusted to 6 to 8 with sulfuric acid and/or sodium hydroxide.

Tobramycin sulfate may also be known as tobramycin sulphate, *Nebcin®*, *Nebcine®*, *Tobra®*, or *TOBI®*.

Storage/Stability
Store tobramycin sulfate for injection at room temperature (15°C to 30°C [59°F-86°F]); avoid freezing and temperatures above 40°C (104°F). Do not use the product if discolored. After reconstitution, keep the solution in a refrigerator and use it within 96 hours. If kept at room temperature, use the solution within 24 hours.

Compatibility/Compounding Considerations
Compatibility is dependent on factors such as pH, concentration, temperature, and diluent used; specialized references or a hospital pharmacist should be consulted for more specific information.

Although the manufacturers state that tobramycin should not be mixed with other drugs, it is reportedly physically **compatible** and stable in most commonly used IV solutions (**NOT compatible** with dextrose and alcohol solutions, *Polysal®*, *Polysal® M*, or *Isolyte® E, M,* or *P*) and **compatible** with the following drugs: aztreonam, bleomycin sulfate, calcium gluconate, cefoxitin sodium, ciprofloxacin lactate, clindamycin phosphate (not in syringes), metronidazole (with or without sodium bicarbonate), ranitidine HCl, and verapamil HCl.

The following drugs or solutions are reportedly physically **incompatible** or only **compatible** in specific situations with tobramycin: furosemide and heparin sodium. Compatibility is dependent upon factors such as pH, concentration, temperature, and diluent used; consult specialized references or a hospital pharmacist for more specific information.

In vitro inactivation of aminoglycoside antibiotics by beta-lactam antibiotics is well documented; see the information in the ***Drug Interactions*** and ***Laboratory Consideration*** sections.

Dosage Forms/Regulatory Status
VETERINARY-LABELED PRODUCTS: NONE

HUMAN-LABELED PRODUCTS:

Tobramycin Sulfate Solution for Injection: 10 mg/mL in 2 mL vials, and 40 mg/mL in 2 mL, 30 mL, and 50 mL vials; generic; (Rx)

Tobramycin Sulfate Powder for Injection: 1.2 g (40 mg/mL after reconstitution), preservative-free in 30 mL bulk package vial; generic; (Rx)

Also available in ophthalmic preparations as well as products (solution, powder [capsule]) for inhalation.

References
For the complete list of references, see **wiley.com/go/budde/plumb**

Toceranib
(toe-***ser***-a-nib) *Palladia®*

Tyrosine Kinase Inhibitor Antineoplastic

Prescriber Highlights
- ► FDA-approved for grades II or III canine mast cell tumors (MCTs) in dogs
- ► Discontinue toceranib therapy at least 3 days prior to, and 2 weeks following, surgery.
- ► Most common adverse effects are diarrhea, decreased/loss of appetite, lameness, weight loss, and hematochezia.
- ► Adverse effects can be serious and require treatment delay or dose reduction.
- ► Monitoring is essential.
- ► Toceranib should be handled as a hazardous drug; personal protective equipment (PPE) should be used accordingly.

Uses/Indications

Toceranib is indicated for the treatment of Patnaik grade II or III, recurrent, cutaneous mast cell tumors (MCTs) with or without regional lymph node involvement in dogs.

Toceranib may prove useful for treating a variety of tumors in dogs, including heart-base tumors,[1] sarcomas, carcinomas, melanomas, multidrug-resistant lymphoma,[2] and multiple myeloma. Toceranib has been investigated in combination with radiation therapy[3] and in combination with other targeted therapies such as calcitriol,[4] carboplatin,[5,6] low-dose continuous (metronomic) cyclophosphamide alone[7] or with piroxicam,[8] doxorubicin,[9] lomustine,[10-12] piroxicam,[13] prednisone, and vinblastine.[14-16]

Preliminary data suggest that toceranib is tolerated in cats at a similar dose range and schedule as that recommended for dogs.[17-22] Early evidence of biological activity against feline MCTs,[17,22] pancreatic carcinoma,[23,24] and oral squamous cell carcinoma[20] has been demonstrated.

Pharmacology/Actions

Toceranib is a small molecule tyrosine kinase inhibitor (TKI) that selectively inhibits the tyrosine kinase activity of several split receptor tyrosine kinases (RTKs), including vascular endothelial growth factor receptor-2 (VEGFR2), platelet-derived growth factor receptor-beta (PDGFR-beta), and KIT (stem cell growth factor receptor), among others. These kinases are believed to be involved in growth, pathologic angiogenesis, and metastatic processes of certain tumors. Toceranib competitively inhibits ATP binding in target RTKs, preventing receptor phosphorylation and subsequent downstream signal transduction. Toceranib can induce cell cycle arrest and apoptosis in canine tumor cell lines expressing activating mutations in KIT. As canine mast cell tumors (MCTs) universally express KIT and a subset possess activating mutations, toceranib administration can be associated with objective antitumor activity in a large minority of dogs with MCTs. Aberrant KIT localization and/or activation mutation may influence treatment response, although conflicting data exist.[3,25,26] Toceranib's activity against VEGFR2 and PDGFR-beta has the potential to exert antiangiogenic effects in multiple tumor types. Additional information suggests that toceranib administration may be associated with a reduction in immunosuppressive regulatory T cells in the peripheral blood.[7]

Pharmacokinetics

The oral bioavailability of toceranib phosphate in dogs is ≈77%. The presence of food does not significantly impact absorption. Binding to canine plasma proteins is ≈94%, and the volume of distribution is very large (ie, greater than 20 L/kg). The terminal elimination half-life is 31 hours after oral administration. Although the metabolic fate of toceranib has not been completely determined, it appears that the drug is metabolized via cytochrome P450 and/or flavin monooxygenase to an N-oxide metabolite in the liver.[27,28]

A study evaluating toceranib peak plasma concentrations after administration of lower oral dosages (2.5 – 2.75 mg/kg PO every other day) resulted in an average 6- to 8-hour postdose plasma concentration ranging from 100 – 120 ng/mL.[29] These were significantly above the 40 ng/mL concentration that is associated with inhibition of KIT phosphorylation, and the adverse event profile was substantially reduced from the one associated with the label dosage of 3.25 mg/kg every other day.

Contraindications/Precautions/Warnings

Toceranib use has not been evaluated in dogs less than 24 months of age or weighing less than 5 kg (11 lb). Because toceranib can cause vascular dysfunction leading to edema and thromboembolism (including pulmonary emboli) and may impair wound healing, it is recommended that toceranib be discontinued at least 3 days prior to, and 2 weeks following, surgery.

When toceranib is used for the treatment of bulky mast cell tumors (MCTs), significant mast cell degranulation may occur with resultant adverse effects; systemic mastocytosis should be ruled out prior to starting toceranib.[30]

Toceranib can cause clinical signs similar to those seen with aggressive MCTs. When these occur, the drug should be stopped and the patient re-evaluated. When signs resolve, treatment may be re-instituted at a lower dose or reduced frequency. The package insert has specific monitoring requirements with dose adjustment or therapy pause guidelines when certain adverse effects (eg, severe diarrhea, GI bleeding) occur or when laboratory monitoring indicates toxicity. See ***Monitoring***.

Toceranib in combination with lomustine and prednisolone in dogs with advanced MCTs caused severe adverse effects in all 10 enrolled dogs, including grade 3 and 4 neutropenia (n = 9), GI toxicity (n = 5), and hepatotoxicity and pancreatitis (n = 1 each), requiring temporary discontinuation of therapy in 9 dogs, and 4 dogs died or were euthanized due to treatment-related adverse effects.[12]

Toceranib should be handled as a hazardous drug; personal protective equipment (PPE) should be used accordingly to minimize the risk for exposure.[6] Refer to the Occupational Safety and Health Association (OSHA) website for more information.

Adverse Effects

The most common adverse effects observed with toceranib in dogs include diarrhea, decreased/loss of appetite, lameness, weight loss, and hematochezia. Severe diarrhea or GI bleeding requires immediate treatment and necessitates dose interruption or reduction (see ***Monitoring***). Other potential adverse effects include vomiting, anemia, thrombocytopenia, lethargy, azotemia, hyperphosphatemia, increased ALT, muscle cramping/pain, neutropenia, hypoalbuminemia, thromboembolic disease, vasculitis, pancreatitis, nasal depigmentation, change in coat or skin color, epistaxis, seizures, and pruritus. Increased systolic blood pressure (SBP) has been noted in dogs receiving toceranib, with an average increase of 11 to 16 mm Hg, and 37% to 45% of dogs developing SBP greater than 160 mm Hg.[31,32] Proteinuria occurred in 20% to 25% of dogs.[31,33] Over a 90-day study period, laboratory assessments of thyroid function remained with the laboratory reference interval but trended toward reduced thyroid dysfunction.[34] Case reports describe nephrotic syndrome developed in a dog after 328 days of toceranib treatment for a mast cell tumor,[35] as well as secondary lymphoma in another dog after 3 months of toceranib treatment for a GI stromal tumor.[36]

One source[37] suggests starting certain drugs 4 to 7 days prior to staring toceranib to reduce the likelihood of toxicity. These drugs include antacids (eg, famotidine, omeprazole), H_1 blockers (eg, diphenhydramine), prednisone (to reduce tumor inflammation and possibly decrease mast cell tumor mediators' effects), and sucralfate (if dog has a positive stool hemoccult). Additionally, in dogs that experience hyporexia or vomiting after therapy has begun, administration of metoclopramide, ondansetron, or maropitant may be effective. Loperamide can be given on toceranib dosing days to help prevent or lessen diarrhea; other clinicians have found metronidazole useful. Another study reported that continuation of prednisone after treatment was begun, but only given on days when toceranib is not given, was well tolerated.[3]

In cats that have received toceranib, reported adverse effects include GI toxicity, myelosuppression, azotemia, hepatopathy, and alopecia.[17-21]

Reproductive/Nursing Safety

Toceranib is a likely teratogen and should not be used in pregnant females. It is labeled as contraindicated in breeding, pregnant, or lactating bitches. For sexually intact patients, verify pregnancy status prior to administration.

Because reproductive/nursing safety has not been established in animals, this drug should only be used when the maternal benefits outweigh the potential risks to offspring.

Overdose/Acute Toxicity

No acute toxicity data are available, but toceranib has a narrow margin of safety. For patients that have experienced or are suspected to have experienced an overdose, consultation with a 24-hour poison control center specializing in providing veterinary-specific information is recommended. For general information related to overdose and toxin exposures, as well as contact information for poison control centers, refer to ***Appendix.***

Drug Interactions

The following drug interactions either have been reported or are theoretical in animals receiving toceranib and may be of significance in veterinary patients. Unless otherwise noted, use together is not necessarily contraindicated, but weigh the potential risks and perform additional monitoring when appropriate.

- **Calcitriol**: An in vitro study found that calcitriol had synergistic effects with toceranib against canine C2 mastocytoma cells. The authors concluded that calcitriol combination therapies might have significant clinical utility in the treatment of canine mast cell tumors (MCTs) but refinement of the calcitriol-dosing regimen must be carried out.[4]
- **Nonsteroidal Anti-Inflammatory Drugs (NSAIDs; eg, carprofen, meloxicam)**: The package insert states to use NSAIDs with caution in conjunction with toceranib due to an increased risk for GI ulceration or perforation. Although NSAIDs (eg, **piroxicam**) are sometimes used with toceranib as part of metronomic drug protocols,[13] it is recommended that they not be given on the same day as toceranib as GI toxicity can be exacerbated.[37]
- **CYP3A4 Inhibitors** (eg, **clarithromycin, fluconazole, grapefruit juice, itraconazole, ketoconazole, verapamil**): May increase toceranib concentrations. This interaction with toceranib has not been documented in dogs to date and presently is speculative; however, use caution.
- **Other Cytotoxic Antineoplastic Agents** (eg, **doxorubicin, lomustine, vinblastine**): Potentiation of myelosuppression (neutropenia) with toceranib co-administration, necessitating reductions in dosage and/or frequency of administration of the cytotoxic agent, has been reported.[9-11,14] Use in combination with caution.

Laboratory Considerations

- None noted

Dosages

NOTE: There is a significant amount of ongoing research evaluating toceranib for use with other drugs, other species, and for extra-label indications and since chemotherapy indications, treatment protocols, monitoring and safety guidelines often change, the following dosages should be used only as a general guide. Consultation with a veterinary oncologist and referral to current veterinary oncology references[38-42] are strongly recommended.

DOGS:

NOTE: The label dosage for dogs is considered by most clinicians to be greater than is necessary and is associated with more adverse effects. The label indications are provided below, but the use of lower, extra-label dosages is strongly recommended.

Patnaik grade II or III, recurrent, cutaneous mast cell tumors (MCTs) with or without regional lymph node involvement (label dosage; FDA-approved): Initial dose 3.25 mg/kg PO every other day (every 48 hours).[30] Dose reductions of 0.5 mg/kg (to a minimum dose of 2.2 mg/kg) every other day and dose interruptions (cessation of treatment) for up to 2 weeks may be utilized, if needed, to manage adverse reactions. May be administered with or without food. Do not split tablets.

Chemotherapeutic agent (extra-label): Clinical experience with toceranib in dogs suggests that 2.4 – 2.75 mg/kg every other day is better tolerated than the label dosage, resulting in less toxicity, better owner compliance, and fewer drug holidays.[29] Some dogs do not tolerate this dosing regimen even at the 2.4 mg/kg dose rate. Medical oncologists have found that a Monday/Wednesday/Friday schedule of dosing may be better tolerated by some dogs. This may be particularly useful when toceranib is combined with other drugs such as NSAIDs. When a dog cannot tolerate the Monday/Wednesday/Friday schedule, every-third-day dosing may be attempted, but this is not ideal and may result in subtherapeutic drug exposure.[37]

CATS:

Chemotherapeutic agent (extra-label): A target dosage of 3.25 mg/kg every other day or Monday/Wednesday/Friday appears to be tolerated. Practically, each dose equates to 10 mg/cat (NOT mg/kg), which results in doses ranging from 2 to 4 mg/kg for the average 2.5 to 5 kg (5.5 to 11 lb) cat and is tolerated by the majority of cats and is recommended by some clinicians.[22]

Monitoring

- Baseline and periodic CBC, hematocrit, and serum albumin, creatinine, and phosphate. The manufacturer recommends weekly (approximately) veterinary assessment for the first 6 weeks of therapy and approximately every 6 weeks thereafter. The package insert states:

  Temporarily discontinue drug if anemia, azotemia, hypoalbuminemia, and hyperphosphatemia occur simultaneously. Resume treatment at a dose reduction of 0.5 mg/kg after 1 to 2 weeks when values have improved and albumin is >2.5 g/dL. Temporary treatment interruptions may be needed if any one of these occurs alone: hematocrit <26%, creatinine ≥2 mg/dL, or albumin <1.5 g/dL. Then resume treatment at a dose reduction of 0.5 mg/kg once the hematocrit is >30%, the creatinine is <2.0 mg/dL, and the albumin is >2.5 g/dL. Temporarily discontinue the use of toceranib if neutrophil count is ≤1000/mL. Resume treatment after 1 to 2 weeks at a dose reduction of 0.5 mg/kg, when neutrophil count has returned to >1000/mL. Further dose reductions may be needed if severe neutropenia recurs.[30]
- Other laboratory tests that have been suggested for monitoring (every 6 to 8 weeks) include urinalysis, full chemistry panel, thyroid function, and urine protein:creatinine ratio.
- Adverse effects (diarrhea): If 4 or more watery stools/day or diarrhea persists for 2 days, stop drug and institute supportive care until formed stools recur. When dosing is resumed, decrease dose by 0.5 mg/kg.
- Adverse effects (eg, GI bleeding): If fresh blood in stool or melena for more than 2 days, or frank hemorrhage or blood clots in stool are noted, stop drug and institute supportive care until resolution of all clinical signs of blood in stool, then decrease dose by 0.5 mg/kg.
- Blood pressure (every 6 to 8 weeks)[31]
- Tumor size

Client Information

- Always provide Client Information Sheet with prescription. In addition, it is highly recommended to verbally reiterate some of the key points found on the client information sheet.
- This medication may be given with or without food; do not split or crush tablets.
- Toceranib is a chemotherapy (anticancer) drug. The drug can be

hazardous to other animals and people that come in contact with it. On the day your animal gets the drug and then for a few days afterward, all bodily waste (eg, urine, feces, litter), blood, or vomit should only be handled while wearing disposable gloves. Seal the waste in a plastic bag, then place both the bag and gloves in with the regular trash.

- Do not wash any items soiled with stool, urine, or vomit from your dog with regular laundry.
- Store toceranib out of the reach of children or pets.

Chemistry/Synonyms

Toceranib phosphate is an idolinone with a molecular weight of 494.46. Toceranib may also be known as PHA-291639, SU-11654, UNII-59L7Y0530C, toceranibum, or tocéranib.

Storage/Stability

Toceranib phosphate tablets should be stored at controlled room temperature 20°C-25°C (68°F-77°F).

Compatibility/Compounding Considerations

No specific information was noted.

Dosage Forms/Regulatory Status

VETERINARY-LABELED PRODUCTS:

Toceranib Phosphate Oral Tablets: 10 mg, 15 mg, and 50 mg; *Palladia*®; (Rx) NADA # 141-295

HUMAN-LABELED PRODUCTS: NONE

References

For the complete list of references, see **wiley.com/go/budde/plumb**

Tolazoline

(toe-***laz***-oh-leen) *Tolazine*®

Alpha-Adrenergic Antagonist

Prescriber Highlights

- Alpha-adrenergic antagonist used primarily in horses and other large animals as a reversal agent for xylazine or other alpha-2 agonists
- Reversal effects may be partial and transitory.
- Contraindications in horses include stress, debilitation, cardiac disease, sympathetic blockage, hypovolemia, shock, hypersensitivity, or coronary artery or cerebrovascular disease.
- Use caution or avoid use in foals.
- Adverse effects in horses include transient tachycardia, peripheral vasodilation presenting as sweating and injected mucous membranes, hyperalgesia of the lips (eg, licking, flipping of lips), piloerection, clear lacrimal and nasal discharge, muscle fasciculations, and apprehensiveness.
- Ruminants and camelids may be more susceptible to the adverse effects of tolazoline, especially when given IV or at high doses.
- Availability may be an issue; may be obtained from compounding pharmacies.

Uses/Indications

Tolazoline is FDA-approved and indicated for the reversal of sedative and analgesic effects associated with xylazine in horses. Tolazoline antagonizes the effects of detomidine more completely, hastens recovery, and lasts longer than atipamezole[1]; however, effects can be transient, and sedative effects may reoccur.[2,3]

Tolazoline has also been used for reversing the effects of xylazine and other alpha-2 agonists (eg, dexmedetomidine, detomidine, medetomidine) in horses and in a variety of other species, but fewer safety and efficacy data are available.

Pharmacology/Actions

By directly relaxing vascular smooth muscle, tolazoline has peripheral vasodilating effects and decreases total peripheral resistance. Tolazoline also is a competitive alpha-1- and alpha-2-adrenergic blocking agent, helping explain its mechanism for reversing the effects of xylazine. It may stimulate GI secretions and motility via parasympathomimetic or histamine type-2 agonist effects.

Tolazoline is rapid-acting (usually within 5 minutes of IV administration) but may not fully reverse effects on sedation or heart rate and rhythm. It has a short duration of action; repeat doses may be required.

In horses that received detomidine 0.04 mg/kg sublingually (SL), then tolazoline 4 mg/kg IV 1 hour later, tolazoline's effect on detomidine-induced changes in the chin-to-ground distance was minimal, and detomidine-induced changes in heart rate and rhythm only persisted for 15 to 20 minutes.[2]

After tolazoline doses of 4 mg/kg IV in horses, average heart rate decreased beginning 2 minutes postinjection, with heart rate nadir at 45 minutes. No apparent effect on chin-to-ground distance was noted. PCV significantly increased in all horses throughout the times sampled with the maximal change at 15 minutes. Serum glucose concentrations increased significantly in all horses at the first time point measured through 1.5 hours postinjection.[4]

Pharmacokinetics

After a single tolazoline 4 mg/kg IV injection in 6 horses, tolazoline had a mean volume of distribution (steady-state) of 1.68 L/kg, clearance of 0.757 L/hour/kg, and elimination half-life of 2.08 hours.[4] In a subsequent study, after horses (n = 9) were first given detomidine 0.04 mg/kg SL, then tolazoline 4 mg/kg IV 1 hour later; mean tolazoline pharmacokinetic values included volume of distribution (steady-state) of 1.9 L/kg, clearance of 11.2 mL/minute/kg, and elimination half-life of 3.51 hours.[2] An older preapproval study done in ponies reported the elimination half-life of ≈1 hour.[5]

Animal studies have demonstrated that tolazoline concentrates in the liver and kidneys.

Contraindications/Precautions/Warnings

The manufacturer does not recommend use in horses exhibiting signs of stress, debilitation, cardiac disease, sympathetic blockage, hypovolemia, or shock. Safe use for foals has not been established, and some clinicians believe it should not be used in foals, as adverse reactions and fatalities have been reported.

Tolazoline should be considered contraindicated in patients known to be hypersensitive to it or with coronary artery or cerebrovascular disease. Humans that have any of the conditions listed above should use extra caution when handling the agent.

Adverse Effects

In horses, adverse effects that may occur include transient tachycardia; peripheral vasodilatation presenting as sweating and injected mucous membranes of the gingiva and conjunctiva; hyperalgesia of the lips (eg, licking, flipping of lips); piloerection; clear lacrimal and nasal discharge; muscle fasciculations; and apprehensiveness. Adverse effects should diminish with time, and generally disappear within 2 hours of dosing. The potential for adverse effects increases if tolazoline is given at higher than recommended dosages or if xylazine has not been previously administered.

Ruminants and camelids appear to be more sensitive to tolazoline's effects than horses. In cattle, 1.5 mg/kg IV can cause coughing, increased frequency of defecation, and mild increases in breathing effort. At higher doses (2 – 10 mg/kg IV), bright red conjunctival mucous membranes, coughing, nasal discharge, salivation, labored breathing, CNS depression, signs of abdominal pain, straining, head pressing, restlessness, and severe diarrhea can be observed. Rapid IV injection has been reported to cause significant cardiac stimulation, tachycardia, increased cardiac output, vasodilation, and GI distress.

Reproductive/Nursing Safety

Safety during pregnancy in breeding or lactating animals has not been established. It is unknown if the drug crosses the placenta or enters maternal milk.

Overdose/Acute Toxicity

In horses given tolazoline alone (no previous xylazine), 5 times the recommended doses resulted in GI hypermotility, with resultant flatulence and defecation or attempt to defecate. Some horses exhibited mild colic and transient diarrhea. Intraventricular conduction may be slowed when horses are overdosed, with a prolongation of the QRS-complex noted. Ventricular arrhythmias may occur, resulting in death with higher overdoses (5 times the recommended doses). In humans, ephedrine (**NOT** epinephrine or norepinephrine) has been recommended to treat serious tolazoline-induced hypotension.

A llama that received 4.3 mg/kg IV and again 45 minutes later (≈5 times overdose) developed signs of anxiety, hyperesthesia, profuse salivation, GI tract hypermotility, diarrhea, convulsions, hypotension, and tachypnea. Treatment, including IV diazepam, phenylephrine, IV fluids, and oxygen, was successful.[6]

Tolazoline 8 mg/kg IV has reportedly caused a fatality in a sheep.

Apnea, fasciculations, and muscle tensing were observed in mule deer that received dosages of 6.1 – 8.4 mg/kg IV; however, no adverse effects were observed in black-tailed deer that received an average dosage of 8.1 mg/kg IV.[7]

For patients that have experienced or are suspected of having experienced an overdose, consultation with a 24-hour poison consultation center specializing in providing veterinary-specific information is recommended. For general information related to overdose and toxin exposures, as well as contact information for poison control centers, refer to ***Appendix.***

Drug Interactions

The following drug interactions have either been reported or are theoretical in humans or animals receiving tolazoline and may be of significance in veterinary patients. Unless otherwise noted, use together is not necessarily contraindicated, but weigh the potential risks and perform additional monitoring when appropriate.

- **Dopamine**: Concurrent use may cause severe hypotension.
- **Epinephrine, Norepinephrine**: If large doses of tolazoline are given with either norepinephrine or epinephrine, a paradoxical drop in blood pressure can occur, followed by a precipitous increase in blood pressure.
- **Ethanol**: Accumulation of acetaldehyde can occur if tolazoline and alcohol are given simultaneously.

Dosages

DOGS/CATS:

Reversal of xylazine effects (extra-label): 2 – 4 mg/kg slow IV (administration rate should approximate 1 mL/second).[8] **WARNING**: If reversal is warranted, the high concentration (100 mg/mL) of the veterinary drug may make accurate dosing difficult. Tolazoline is not FDA-approved for use in dogs or cats, and the United States manufacturer does not recommend its use.

EQUINE:

Horses: Reversal of xylazine effects (label dosage; FDA-approved): 4 mg/kg slow IV; administration rate should approximate 1 mL/second. [9]

Horses: Reversal of xylazine effects (extra-label): 0.5 – 2 mg/kg IM (preferred) or slow IV; if administering IV, dividing the dose into multiple smaller doses has been suggested.[10]

Horses: Reversal of low-dose alpha-agonist effects after dental procedures (extra-label): Following sedation with 1.1 – 2.2 mg/kg IM xylazine, reverse with tolazoline 0.04 mg/kg slow IV; may repeat 0.02 mg/kg slow IV 20 to 30 minutes later if needed.[11]

Donkeys: Reversal of detomidine (extra-label): Tolazoline 4 mg/kg IV, given 15 minutes after detomidine 0.04 mg/kg IV, reduced the degree and duration of sedation, ataxia, and analgesia.[12]

RUMINANTS (CATTLE, SHEEP, GOATS):

NOTE: Not FDA-approved for use in cattle, sheep, goats, or other food animals

Reversal of alpha-2 agonists (extra-label): 0.5 – 1.5 mg/kg IV. Other clinicians have suggested that IV administration of tolazoline should be avoided, except in emergency situations, to prevent adverse effects such as cardiac asystole.[13,14]

CAMELIDS:

Reversal of alpha-2 agonists (extra-label):

a) Preferred reversal agent for xylazine is tolazoline 1 – 2 mg/kg IM or SC.[15-17]. IV administration (especially the labeled dose—4 mg/kg) should be avoided as adverse effects have occurred.[6]
b) 0.5 – 1.5 mg/kg IV. Today, these lower doses are now recommended for use in all ruminants, including camelids. Other clinicians have suggested that IV administration of tolazoline should be avoided, except in emergency situations, to prevent adverse effects such as cardiac asystole.[13]

SWINE:

Reversal of alpha-2 agonists (extra-label): 2 – 4 mg/kg IV or 2 mg/kg IM[18,19]

DEER:

NOTE: Not FDA-approved for use in food animals

Reversal of xylazine (extra-label):

a) 2 – 4 mg/kg slow IV; titrate to effect[8]
b) 2 – 4 mg/kg IV, or 50% of dose given IV, 50% given IM[7,20,21]

BIRDS:

Reversal of alpha-2-adrenergic agonists (eg, xylazine, detomidine) (extra-label): 15 mg/kg IV[22]

Monitoring

- Efficacy (ie, reversal of xylazine effects)
- Adverse effects (eg, tachycardia, sweating, mucous membrane injection, lip licking, ocular and nasal discharge, fasciculations, and restlessness)

Client Information

- Because of the risks associated with the use of xylazine and reversal by tolazoline, only veterinary professionals should administer and monitor these drugs.

Chemistry/Synonyms

Tolazoline HCl is an alpha-adrenergic blocking agent that is structurally related to phentolamine. It occurs as a white to off-white, crystalline powder possessing a bitter taste and a slight aromatic odor. Tolazoline is freely soluble in ethanol or water. The commercially available (human) injection has a pH between 3 and 4.

Tolazoline HCl may also be known as benzazoline hydrochloride, phenylmethylimidazoline, tolazolinium chloratum, *Priscol®*, *Priscoline®*, *Tolazine®*, or *Vaso-Dilatan®*.

Storage/Stability

Store commercially available injection products between 15°C and 30°C (59°F and 86°F) and protected from light. Color change or crystallization may occur with refrigeration.

Compatibility/Compounding Considerations

Compatibility is dependent on factors such as pH, concentration, temperature, and diluent used; specialized references or a hospital pharmacist should be consulted for more specific information.

The drug is reportedly physically **compatible** with the commonly used IV solutions.

Dosage Forms/Regulatory Status

VETERINARY-LABELED PRODUCTS:

Tolazoline HCl Injection: 100 mg/mL in 100 mL multi-dose vials; *Tolazine*®; (Rx). FDA-approved for use in horses; not to be used in foodproducing animals. Cattle slaughter withdrawal: 8 days; mild discard 2 days. Deer slaughter withdrawal = 30 days. While this product is still listed in FDA's Green Book of approved animal drugs, it may no longer be commercially available in the US. [11]

The Association of Racing Commissioners International (ARCI) has designated this drug as a class 3 substance. Use of this drug may not be allowed in certain animal competitions. Check rules and regulations before entering a competition while this medication is being administered. Contact local racing authorities for further guidance. See ***Appendix*** for more information.

HUMAN-LABELED PRODUCTS: NONE

References

For the complete list of references, see **wiley.com/go/budde/plumb**

Tolfenamic Acid

(tole-fen-*a*-mik) *Tolfedine*®

Nonsteroidal Anti-inflammatory Agent (NSAID)

Prescriber Highlights

- ► Oral and injectable NSAID approved in various countries for dogs, cats, cattle, and swine. No approved products in the United States
- ► Relatively safe for short-term use.
- ► Contraindicated in patients with active GI bleeding or ulceration and those that are hypersensitive to it or other drugs in its class
- ► Use caution in patients with renal or hepatic insufficiency and those that are dehydrated, hypovolemic, or hypotensive.
- ► Not recommended prior to surgery due to its effects on platelet function

Uses/Indications

Tolfenamic acid is an anti-inflammatory, antipyretic, and analgesic agent approved in other countries for use in dogs, cats, cattle, and swine.

Tolfenamic acid may be useful for the treatment of acute or chronic pain and/or inflammation in dogs and acute pain/inflammation in cats.

In some countries, tolfenamic acid is approved for the treatment of pneumonia and acute mastitis in cattle and metritis mastitis agalactia in swine.[1]

Pharmacology/Actions

Tolfenamic acid exhibits pharmacologic actions similar to those of aspirin. It is a potent inhibitor of cyclooxygenase, thereby inhibiting the release of prostaglandins. It also has direct inhibition of prostaglandin receptors. Tolfenamic acid has significant antithromboxane activity and is not recommended for use presurgically because of its effects on platelet function.

Pharmacokinetics

Tolfenamic acid is absorbed after oral administration. In dogs, peak concentrations occur from 2 to 4 hours after dosing. Enterohepatic recirculation is increased if given with food. This effect can increase the bioavailability but also creates more variability in bioavailability than when given to fasted dogs. The volume of distribution in dogs is reported to be 1.2 L/kg, and it has an elimination half-life of ≈6.5 hours. The duration of the anti-inflammatory effect is 24 to 36 hours. Dogs with experimentally induced renal failure had significantly increased clearances of the drug, presumably via increasing hepatic metabolism or enterohepatic recycling of tolfenamic acid.[2]

Contraindications/Precautions/Warnings

Tolfenamic acid is contraindicated in animals hypersensitive to it or to other drugs in its class (eg, meclofenamic acid). Like other NSAIDs, it should not be used in animals with active GI bleeding or ulceration. Use with caution in patients with decreased renal or hepatic function. Avoid use in dehydrated, hypovolemic, or hypotensive animals.[3]

Use in animals under 6 weeks of age is not recommended.[3]

Adverse Effects

Tolfenamic acid is relatively safe when given as recommended in dogs and cats. Vomiting and diarrhea have been reported after oral use. Experimental studies did not demonstrate significant renal or GI toxicity until doses were more than 10 times labeled. Potentially, long-term use could cause renal failure, especially in cats. However, 1 small (n = 7) study, where healthy cats received 4 mg/kg PO once daily for 14 days, did not find significant changes in renal scintigraphy or biochemical profiles when compared to baseline.[4]

Because of its anti-thromboxane activity and resultant effects on platelet function, tolfenamic acid is not recommended for use presurgically.

Reproductive/Nursing Safety

No specific information was located; like other NSAIDs, tolfenamic acid should be used with caution in pregnancy.

Because safety has not been established in animals, this drug should only be used when the maternal benefits outweigh the potential risks to offspring.

Overdose/Acute Toxicity

No specific information was located. It is suggested that if an acute overdose occurs, treatment follows standard overdose procedures (empty gut following oral ingestion). Supportive treatment should be instituted as necessary, and diazepam IV used to help control seizures. Monitor for GI bleeding. Because tolfenamic acid may cause renal effects, monitor electrolyte and fluid balance carefully and manage renal failure using established guidelines.

For patients that have experienced or are suspected of having experienced an overdose, consultation with a 24-hour poison consultation center specializing in providing veterinary-specific information is recommended. For general information related to overdose and toxin exposures, as well as contact information for poison control centers, refer to ***Appendix.***

Drug Interactions

The following drug interactions have either been reported or are theoretical in humans or animals receiving tolfenamic acid or other NSAIDs and may be of significance in veterinary patients. Unless otherwise noted, use together is not necessarily contraindicated, but weigh the potential risks and perform additional monitoring when appropriate.

- **Aspirin**: May increase the risk for GI toxicity (eg, ulceration, bleeding, vomiting, diarrhea)
- **Corticosteroids**: As concomitant corticosteroid therapy may increase the occurrence of gastric ulceration, avoid the use of these drugs when also using tolfenamic acid.
- **Digoxin**: NSAIDs may increase serum levels.
- **Fluconazole**: Administration has increased plasma levels of celecoxib in humans and potentially could also affect tolfenamic acid levels in dogs.

- **Furosemide**: NSAIDs may reduce saluretic and diuretic effects; may increase the risk for nephrotoxicity.
- **Methotrexate**: Serious toxicity has occurred when NSAIDs have been used concomitantly with methotrexate; use together with extreme caution.
- **Nephrotoxic Drugs** (eg, **aminoglycosides, amphotericin B**): May enhance the risk for nephrotoxicity
- **NSAIDs, Other** (eg, **meloxicam, flunixin**): May increase the risk for GI toxicity (eg, ulceration, bleeding, vomiting, diarrhea)
- **Warfarin**: Closely monitor patients also receiving drugs that are highly bound to plasma proteins (eg, **warfarin**), as tolfenamic acid and its active metabolite are 98% to 99% protein-bound in the dog and may displace warfarin from plasma proteins.

Dosages

DOGS:

NSAID (extra-label):

a) Acute pain: 4 mg/kg once daily SC, IM, or PO for 3 to 5 days. Chronic pain: 4 mg/kg, PO once daily for 3 to 5 consecutive days per week. The injectable is suggested for the first dose only.[5]

b) Injectable: 4 mg/kg SC once; if necessary, can repeat 4 mg/kg SC once 24 hours after initial injection. Oral: 4 mg/kg PO once daily for 3 days; oral treatment may be repeated once a week (ie, 3 days of medication followed by 4 days without medication). Oral and injectable treatments may be combined (ie, give initial injection of 4 mg/kg once SC followed 24 hours later by 4 mg/kg PO once daily for 3 days).[6,7]

CATS:

Acute pain (extra-label): 4 mg/kg once daily SC, IM, or PO for 3 to 5 days. The injectable is suggested for the first dose only.[5]

Anti-inflammatory; Adjunctive treatment of upper respiratory disease in association with antimicrobial therapy (injectable) or for treatment of febrile syndromes (oral); (extra-label): 4 mg/kg SC or PO (with food) once a day for 3 to 5 days. Injectable is labeled as a single injection or can be repeated 1 time.[6,8]

CATTLE:

NOTE: Other countries may have different withdrawal requirements; refer to the product label. This drug is not approved in the US, and its administration would not be legal unless a veterinarian could provide justification for its use.[9]

Pneumonia (extra-label): 2 mg/kg by IM injection high in the neck.[7] Treatment may be repeated once only after 48 hours. Another course of treatment should not be administered within 28 days. **DO NOT** inject cattle other than into muscle tissues high on the side of the neck. Meat withdrawal = 10 days (IM); Milk withdrawal = 12 hours

Acute mastitis (extra-label): 4 mg/kg as a single IV injection.[7] Meat withdrawal = 4 days (IV); Milk withdrawal = 12 hours

SWINE:

NOTE: Other countries may have different withdrawal requirements; refer to the product label. This drug is not approved in the United States, and its administration would not be legal unless a veterinarian could provide justification for its use.[9]

Metritis-mastitis-agalactia (extra-label): 2 mg/kg IM into the rump once.[7] Another course of treatment should not be administered within 21 days. Meat withdrawal = 6 days.[8] (Label Information; *Tolfejec*®—Troy Labs, Australia)

Monitoring

- Clinical efficacy
- Adverse effects

Client Information

- The weekly dosing regimen (3 to 5 consecutive days per week for dogs) is important to follow to minimize the risks for side effects. Do not give longer to cats than your veterinarian prescribes.
- Should give oral medicine with food.
- Vomiting and diarrhea have been reported as side effects in dogs and cats.
- Report any changes in appetite, water consumption, or GI distress to your veterinarian.

Chemistry/Synonyms

Tolfenamic acid, a nonsteroidal anti-inflammatory agent in the anthranilic acid (fenamate) category, is related chemically to meclofenamic acid.

Tolfenamic acid may also be known as acidum tolfenamicum, *Bifenac*®, *Clotam*®, *Clotan*®, *Fenamic*®, *Flocur*®, *Gantil*®, *Migea*®, *Polmonin*®, *Purfalox*®, *Rociclyn*®, *Tolfamic*®, *Tolfedine*®, *Tolfejec*®, or *Turbaund*®.

Storage/Stability

Unless otherwise labeled, store tolfenamic acid products at room temperature. Protect from light. Refer to the injectable product label for discard dating following the first vial puncture.

Compatibility/Compounding Considerations

No specific information was noted.

Dosage Forms/Regulatory Status

VETERINARY-LABELED PRODUCTS:

None in the United States; in New Zealand, Australia, UK, and/or Europe: Tolfenamic Acid Tablets: 6 mg, 20 mg, and 60 mg; Tolfenamic Acid Oral Suspension: 20 mg/mL; and Tolfenamic Acid Injection: 40 mg/mL are available.

HUMAN-LABELED PRODUCTS: NONE

References

For the complete list of references, see **wiley.com/go/budde/plumb**

Toltrazuril

(tole-***traz***-yoo-ril) *Baycox*®

Antiprotozoal/Anticoccidial

Prescriber Highlights

- Approved in some countries for treating coccidial infections in calves, lambs, piglets, and poultry
- Not commercially available in the United States; must be legally imported or compounded by a reputable pharmacy
- May be considered as an alternative for treating coccidiosis in companion animals (eg, dogs, cats, and rabbits) and the oocyst shedding stage of toxoplasmosis in cats
- Adverse effect profile not well described, but appears relatively safe

Uses/Indications

Toltrazuril is an antiprotozoal agent that is approved in some countries to treat *Isospora suis* in piglets and coccidiosis in lambs (*Eimeria crandalis* and *Eimeria ovinoidalis*) and calves (*Eimeria bovis* or *Eimeria zuernii*). The drug also may be considered as an alternative treatment for coccidiosis in dogs, cats, camelids, birds, rabbits, mice, and reptiles.

Toltrazuril has activity against parasites of the genus *Hepatozoon* spp, but other drugs (eg, imidocarb, primaquine, doxycycline) are generally used. Toltrazuril can induce initial excellent clinical responses in dogs with American canine hepatozoonosis (ACH) but cannot completely eliminate the parasites, and remission is transient in most dogs.[1] A combination of toltrazuril and emodepside (*Procox*®) with clindamycin reduced infectivity but did not completely clear the organism.[2] Toltrazuril has been used for treating the oocyst shedding stage of toxoplasmosis in cats.

Although toltrazuril has been used to treat equine protozoal myeloencephalitis (EPM) caused by *Sarcocystis neurona*, the use of FDA-approved products (eg, ponazuril, pyrimethamine/sulfadiazine) is preferred.

Toltrazuril failed to eradicate *Neospora caninum* in congenitally infected lambs.[3]

Pharmacology/Actions

Toltrazuril is the parent compound to ponazuril (toltrazuril sulfone). Its mechanism of action is not well understood, but it appears to inhibit protozoal enzyme systems and cell division and damages intracellular structures. Light and electron microscope studies show that toltrazuril is active against all intracellular stages of coccidia, including schizonts and micro- and macrogamonts.[4] It interferes with the division of the protozoal nucleus and the activity of the mitochondria, and damages the wall-forming bodies in the microgametes. Toltrazuril produces severe vacuolization of the protozoal endoplasmic reticulum in all intracellular development stages.

Toltrazuril has activity against *Hepatozoon* spp, *Isospora* spp, *Sarcocystis* spp, *Toxoplasma* spp, and all intracellular stages of *Coccidia* spp.

Pharmacokinetics

Toltrazuril is slowly absorbed after oral administration. The highest concentrations are found in the liver; it is rapidly metabolized into the sulfone derivative (ponazuril). Plasma half-lives are 72 hours in calves, 170 hours in lambs, and 51 hours in piglets. There is little enterohepatic recirculation. It is primarily excreted in the feces.

In rabbits, the pharmacokinetics of toltrazuril were compared using a compounded toltrazuril formulation to improve solubility (prepared by solid dispersion technology using DMSO, PEG 400, and PEG 6000 as a carrier for drinking water) with a commercially available (in China) 0.5% premix product. With the compounded preparation, peak plasma levels were ≈3 times greater, and AUC was ≈2 times greater. The authors concluded that using toltrazuril prepared with solid dispersion technology could provide better anticoccidial activity via the attainment of higher blood concentrations.[5]

Contraindications/Precautions/Warnings

Toltrazuril should not be used in patients that have had prior hypersensitivity reactions to it or other triazinone (triazine) antiprotozoals (eg, ponazuril, diclazuril).

The principal metabolite of toltrazuril (toltrazuril sulfone, ponazuril) reportedly persists in the environment, and undiluted manure from treated animals can contaminate groundwater. There appears to be little risk for significant environmental contamination when toltrazuril is used in dogs, cats, or other companion animals (eg, pet birds, reptiles).

Do not confuse toltrazuril with toltrazuril sulfone (ponazuril) as the dosages differ.

Adverse Effects

Toltrazuril appears to be well tolerated in birds. An adverse effect profile in mammals is not well described. Potentially, GI signs could occur. Some horses receiving the related drug ponazuril developed blisters on their nose and mouth, and others developed a rash or hives during field trials.[6]

Reproductive/Nursing Safety

No reproductive or nursing safety information was located; weigh the potential risks versus benefits of use during pregnancy or lactation.

Because safety has not been established in animals, this drug should only be used when the maternal benefits outweigh the potential risks to offspring.

Overdose/Acute Toxicity

Doses up to 5 times the label recommendations in calves, lambs, and piglets resulted in no adverse hematologic or pathologic effects.[4] Doses of up to 10 times the label recommendations in horses were tolerated without significant adverse effects. Five times overdoses in poultry have been tolerated without clinical signs noted. Decreased water intake has been seen if overdoses are greater than 5 times.

For patients that have experienced or are suspected of having experienced an overdose, consultation with a 24-hour poison consultation center specializing in providing veterinary-specific information is recommended. For general information related to overdose and toxin exposures, as well as contact information for poison control centers, refer to ***Appendix.***

Drug Interactions

- None were reported.

Laboratory Considerations

- No issues were noted.

Dosages

DOGS:

Coccidiosis (extra-label): 10 – 30 mg/kg PO once daily for 1 to 3 days[7,8]

CATS:

Enteroepithelial cycle (oocyst shedding) of toxoplasmosis (extra-label): 5 – 10 mg/kg PO once daily for 2 days[9]

Coccidiosis (extra-label): 20 – 30 mg/kg PO once.[10] Repeating the dose in 10 days improves efficacy.

CATTLE:

Prevention of clinical signs of coccidiosis and reduction of coccidia shedding in calves on farms with a confirmed history of coccidiosis caused by *Eimeria bovis* or *Eimeria zuernii* (extra-label): 15 mg/kg PO once for each animal.[11] For the treatment of a group of animals of the same breed and same or similar age, the dosing should be done according to the heaviest animal of this group. To obtain maximum benefit, animals should be treated before the expected onset of clinical signs (ie, in the prepatent period). Not for calves weighing greater than 80 kg (176 lb) or in fattening units such as veal or beef calves. Not for dairy animals

SHEEP:

Prevention of clinical signs of coccidiosis and reduction of coccidian shedding in lambs on farms with a confirmed history of coccidiosis caused by *Eimeria crandallis* and *Eimeria ovinoidalis* (extra-label): 20 mg/kg PO as a single dose.[4] To obtain maximum benefit, sheep should be treated in the prepatent period before the expected onset of clinical signs. The prepatent period of *E ovinoidalis* is 12 to 15 days, and the prepatent period of *E crandalis* is 15 to 20 days. If animals are to be treated collectively rather than individually, they should be grouped according to their body weight and dosed accordingly. In order to maximize effectiveness, it is important to time therapy according to individual farm management and the lifecycle of the organism involved. Not for use in dairy sheep

CAMELIDS:

Coccidiosis caused by *Eimeria* spp (extra-label): 5 – 20 mg/kg PO once daily for up to 3 days. The higher doses and longer courses are for the treatment of individuals; the lower doses may be used for control.[12]

SWINE:

Preclinical coccidiosis due to *Isospora suis* in neonatal piglets

(extra-label): 20 mg/kg body weight PO once at 3 to 4 days of age.[4] Weigh 3 representative litters at 3 days of age to determine an average piglet weight. Not for use in suckling or barbecue pigs

BIRDS:

Coccidiosis in chickens and turkey (extra-label): 7 mg/kg per day orally in drinking water for 2 consecutive days.[13] Consult product label for instruction on preparing and administering medication via drinking water systems. Do not use in laying birds producing eggs for human consumption

Coccidiosis in raptors (extra-label): 7 mg/kg PO once daily for 2 to 3 days[14]

SMALL MAMMALS:

Coccidiosis (extra-label):

a) **Rabbits**: In the study, a single oral dose of toltrazuril 2.5 mg/kg or 5 mg/kg PO reduced oocyte counts by 98.1% and 99.6%, respectively.[15] The authors concluded that there appeared to be no advantage to using the higher dose and 2.5 mg/kg PO once recommended.

b) **Mice**: Toltrazuril 0.5% 10 – 20 mg/kg PO given for 3 days, pause for 5 days, and then repeat once more[16]

c) **Guinea pigs**: Coccidiosis, 2.5 – 5 mg/kg PO twice, 5 days apart[17]

REPTILES:

Parasitism in bearded dragons (extra-label): 5 – 15 mg/kg PO once daily for 3 days[18]

Coccidiosis in tortoises (extra-label): 15 – 20 mg/kg PO every 48 hours for 3 months reduced mortality.[19]

Monitoring

- Clinical efficacy: fecal egg count reduction testing before and up to 10 to 14 days after treatment

Client Information

- Used to treat certain types of protozoal infections found in your animal's feces. Not currently available in the United States but may be legally imported by your veterinarian.
- This medicine may be given with food or on an empty stomach. If your animal vomits or acts sick after getting it on an empty stomach, give it with food or a small treat to see if this helps. If vomiting continues, contact your veterinarian.
- Avoid direct contact with the medication. Wear disposable gloves and wash hands after giving medication.
- This medicine appears to be well tolerated by all animals.
- Manure from treated animals contains residual medication that can negatively affect groundwater and the growth of certain crops. Manure from treated animals must be diluted with 3 times the amount of manure from untreated animals before being spread onto land.

Chemistry/Synonyms

Related to other antiprotozoals, such as ponazuril, toltrazuril is a triazinone (triazine) antiprotozoal (anticoccidial) agent. The commercially available (in Europe) 2.5% oral solution is an alkaline, clear, colorless to yellow-brown solution that also contains triethanolamine 30 mg/mL and polyethylene glycol 80.7 mg/mL. Toltrazuril has a molecular weight of 425.4.

Toltrazuril may also be known as Bay-Vi-9142, toltrazurilo, toltrazurilum, and *Baycox®*, *Cevauril®*, *Chanox® Multi*, *Tolracol®*, *Zorabel®*.

Storage/Stability

Store the 2.5% solution at temperatures at 25°C (77°F) or below. Store oral 5% suspensions at temperatures at 30°C (86°F) or below.

Dilutions in drinking water more concentrated than 1:250 (4 mL of the 2.5% solution to 1 L of water) may precipitate. After dilution, the resulting solution is stable for 24 hours. It is recommended to discard medicated drinking water not consumed after 24 hours.

Compatibility/Compounding Considerations

Do not mix toltrazuril solution for drinking water with other medications.[11,13]

Dosage Forms/Regulatory Status

VETERINARY-LABELED PRODUCTS:

None in the United States; in some countries, toltrazuril 2.5% (25 mg/mL) solution for dilution in drinking water and/or 5% (50 mg/mL) oral suspension are available. Refer to the specific product label for withdrawal times or other restrictions for use.

A combination oral suspension for dogs and cats containing toltrazuril and emodepside (*Procox®*) is also available in some markets. A combination injection product (*Forceris®*) containing toltrazuril and iron (as gleptoferrin) for use in piglets also may be available.

HUMAN-LABELED PRODUCTS: NONE

References

For the complete list of references, see **wiley.com/go/budde/plumb**

Topiramate

(toe-***pie***-rah-mate) *Topamax®*

Anticonvulsant

Prescriber Highlights

- May be useful for refractory seizure disorders in dogs, particularly for partial seizure activity; may be of benefit in treating cats, but little information is available.
- Very short half-life in dogs (2 to 4 hours), but therapeutic activity may persist secondary to high affinity for receptors in the brain.
- Adverse effects may include GI distress, sedation, ataxia, inappetence, and irritability in dogs; in cats, sedation and inappetence have been noted.
- Expense may be an issue, but generic products are now available.
- The National Institute for Occupational Safety and Health (NIOSH) classifies topiramate as a hazardous drug; use appropriate precautions when handling.

Uses/Indications

Topiramate may be useful for treating refractory seizures in dogs, particularly partial seizure activity. It may also be of benefit in treating cats, but little information is available. A case report of a cat with feline idiopathic ulcerative dermatitis treated with topiramate has been published.[1]

Pharmacology/Actions

Although the exact mechanism for its antiseizure action is unknown, topiramate possesses three properties that may play a role in its activity: Topiramate blocks, in a time-dependent manner, action potentials elicited repetitively by a sustained depolarization of neurons; it increases the frequency that GABA activates $GABA_A$ receptors; and it antagonizes the kainite/AMPA receptors without affecting the NMDA receptor subtype. Topiramate's actions are concentration-dependent; effects can first be seen at 1 micromole and maximize at 200 micromoles. Topiramate is a weak inhibitor of carbonic anhydrase isoenzymes CA-II and CA-IV; it is believed that this effect does not contribute significantly to its antiepileptic actions but may influence the drug's adverse effect profile.

Pharmacokinetics

In dogs, topiramate is rapidly absorbed after oral administration, but absolute bioavailability varies between 30 and 60%. Half-life ranges from 2 to 4 hours after multiple doses.[2] Comparatively, the half-life in humans is ≈21 hours in adults, but shorter in children.[3] In humans, the drug is not extensively metabolized and is ≈70% is excreted unchanged in the urine.

No information on sustained-release topiramate product (eg, 24-hour topiramate sprinkles) pharmacokinetics in dogs or cats was located.

Contraindications/Precautions/Warnings

Topiramate is contraindicated in patients hypersensitive to it.[3] In humans, topiramate should be used with caution in patients with impaired hepatic or renal function.

The National Institute for Occupational Safety and Health (NIOSH) classifies topiramate as a hazardous drug; personal protective equipment (PPE) should be used accordingly to minimize the risk for exposure.[4]

Adverse Effects

Because this drug has not commonly been used in veterinary patients, an accurate adverse effect profile is not well described. In dogs, the most prevalent adverse effects reported include GI distress, sedation, ataxia, inappetence, weight loss and irritability; signs often subsided or lessened in severity over time.[5] In cats, sedation and inappetence have been noted.[1] A case of renal tubular acidosis in a cat has been reported, which resolved with discontinuation of topiramate and supportive care.[6]

In humans, the most likely adverse effects include somnolence, dizziness, nervousness, confusion, and ataxia. Rarely, acute myopia with secondary angle closure glaucoma has been reported. Incidence of kidney stones is ≈2 to 4 times higher in patients taking topiramate than in the general population. Topiramate can cause a hyperchloremic metabolic acidosis and reduce citrate excretion in the urine, thus increasing urine pH, leading to calcium phosphate renal calculi.

Reproductive/Nursing Safety

Teratogenic effects were noted in mice and rats given topiramate at dosages equivalent to those used in humans.[3] Topiramate enters maternal milk; use with caution in nursing patients.

Overdose/Acute Toxicity

Overdoses in humans have caused convulsions, drowsiness/lethargy, slurred speech, blurred and double vision, impaired mentation, stupor, ataxia, metabolic acidosis, hypotension, agitation, and abdominal pain.[3]

Clinical signs reported in dogs and cats with a topiramate overdose include lethargy, ataxia, and vomiting (cats).

Treatment consists of GI decontamination if the ingestion was recent, and supportive therapy. Hemodialysis enhances the elimination of topiramate from the body.

For patients that have experienced or are suspected of having experienced an overdose, consultation with a 24-hour poison consultation center specializing in providing veterinary-specific information is recommended. For general information related to overdose and toxin exposures, as well as contact information for poison control centers, refer to ***Appendix***.

Drug Interactions

The following drug interactions have either been reported or are theoretical in humans or animals receiving topiramate and may be of significance in veterinary patients. Unless otherwise noted, use together is not necessarily contraindicated, but weigh the potential risks and perform additional monitoring when appropriate.

- **Amitriptyline**: Topiramate may increase amitriptyline concentration.
- **Carbonic Anhydrase Inhibitors** (eg, **acetazolamide, dichlorphenamide**): Concurrent use may increase the risk for renal calculus formation.
- **CNS Depressant Drugs, Other** (eg, **acepromazine, cannabidiol, gabapentin, trazodone**): Other CNS depressant drugs may exacerbate the CNS adverse effects of topiramate.
- **Furosemide**: Concurrent use may increase the risk for hypokalemia.
- **Hydrochlorothiazide**: Concurrent use may result in increased topiramate exposure and increase the risk for hypokalemia.
- **Methenamine**: Topiramate may alter urine pH and decrease the efficacy of methenamine
- **Opioids** (eg, **buprenorphine, hydrocodone, tramadol**): May exacerbate the CNS adverse effects of topiramate
- **Phenobarbital**: Concurrent use may decrease topiramate serum concentration.
- **Posaconazole**: Concurrent use may result in increased topiramate plasma concentration and topiramate toxicity.

Laboratory Considerations

- No specific laboratory interactions or considerations were noted.

Dosages

DOGS:

Add-on drug (to phenobarbital or bromides) for refractory epilepsy (extra-label): No controlled clinical studies were noted that support clinical use or any dosage. Initially, 2 mg/kg PO twice daily for 2 weeks, then increase to 5 mg/kg PO twice daily and continue for ≈2 months. If seizure frequency is not reduced by at least 50% (compared with prior to topiramate) and no adverse effects occurred, increase dose to 10 mg/kg PO twice daily. Reassess again after ≈2 months and if the prior criteria were met, increase dose to 10 mg/kg PO 3 times daily. Dogs that were responders received dosages within the range of 5 – 10 mg/kg PO twice daily.[5]

CATS:

Refractory epilepsy (extra-label): No controlled clinical studies were noted that support clinical use or any dosage. Anecdotally, 12.5 – 25 mg/cat (≈2.4 – 5 mg/kg) PO twice daily has been noted. To reduce adverse effects, dose is usually started low and increased as tolerated. Inappetence can be dose-limiting.

Feline idiopathic ulcerative dermatitis (extra-label): 5 mg/kg PO twice daily. From a case report, remission occurred within 4 weeks and control was maintained for 30 months. Two attempts to withdraw topiramate led to relapse within 24 hours.[1]

Monitoring

- Efficacy
- Adverse effects
- Plasma concentrations of topiramate are usually not monitored in humans, but therapeutic levels are thought to range from 2 to 25 mg/L.

Client Information

- Give this medicine as directed by your veterinarian. Do not skip doses. Try to give the medicine at the same time each day.
- This medicine may be given with or without food. If your animal vomits or acts sick after getting it on an empty stomach, give the medicine with food or small treat to see if this helps. If vomiting continues, contact your veterinarian.
- Do not suddenly stop giving this medicine to your animal or seizures may occur again.
- It is recommended to maintain a seizure diary to help determine how well this medicine is working.
- Possible side effects may include gastrointestinal distress (nausea, vomiting, loss of appetite) or sedation (sleepiness, lack of energy). Report these or any other unexpected changes to your veterinarian right away.

- This medication is considered to be a hazardous drug as defined by the National Institute for Occupational Safety and Health (NIOSH). Talk with your veterinarian or pharmacist about the use of personal protective equipment when handling this medicine.

Chemistry/Synonyms

A sulfamate-substituted derivative of D-fructose antiepileptic, topiramate occurs as a white crystalline powder with a bitter taste. Its solubility in water is 9.8 mg/mL; it is freely soluble in alcohol.

Topiramate may also be known as McN-4853, RWJ-17021, *Epitomax®*, *Topamac®*, *Topamax®*, or *Topimax®*.

Storage/Stability

Topiramate tablets should be stored in tight containers at room temperature (15°C-30°C [59°F-86°F]); protect from moisture. Topiramate sprinkle capsules should be stored in tight containers at temperatures below 25°C (76°F); protect from moisture.

Compatibility/Compounding Considerations

No specific information noted

Dosage Forms/Regulatory Status

VETERINARY-LABELED PRODUCTS: NONE

The Association of Racing Commissioners International (ARCI) has designated this drug as a class 2 substance. Use of this drug may not be allowed in certain animal competitions. Check rules and regulations before entering in a competition while this medication is being administered. Contact local racing authorities for further guidance. See ***Appendix*** for more information.

HUMAN-LABELED PRODUCTS:

Topiramate Oral Tablets and Caplets: 25 mg, 50 mg, 100 mg, and 200 mg; *Topamax®*, *Topiragen®*, generic; (Rx)

Topiramate Sprinkle Capsules: 15 mg and 25 mg; *Topamax® Sprinkle*, generic; (Rx)

Topiramate Sprinkle Capsules Extended-Release (24-hr for humans): 25 mg, 50 mg, 100 mg, 150 mg, and 200 mg; *Qudexy XR®*, *Trokendi® XR*, generic; (Rx)

Topiramate Oral Solution: 25 mg/mL in 473 mL bottle; *Eprontia®*; (Rx)

References

For the complete list of references, see **wiley.com/go/budde/plumb**

Torsemide

(***tor***-se-myde) *Demadex®*

Loop Diuretic

Prescriber Highlights

- Used as adjunctive treatment of CHF in dogs and cats, especially in cases that have stopped responding to furosemide
- ≈10 to 20 times more potent than furosemide with longer diuretic action
- Contraindicated in patients with anuria, hypersensitivity, dehydration, or serious electrolyte depletion
- Adverse effects include GI (vomiting, diarrhea, anorexia) and renal effects (polyuria, increased renal values, renal insufficiency or failure).

Uses/Indications

Torsemide is a loop diuretic similar to furosemide but is ≈10 to 20 times more potent, and its diuretic effects can persist for a longer period (≈12 hours). Therefore, the starting dose should be 5% to 10% of the required furosemide dose, and dosing frequency may be reduced.[1] It may be a useful adjunctive treatment for congestive heart failure (CHF) in dogs and cats, particularly in patients that have become refractory to furosemide.

The parenteral form of torsemide has been discontinued in the US, so use is limited to oral therapy.[2]

In dogs, torsemide is an option for dogs with myxomatous mitral valve disease (MMVD) in stages C and D of heart failure, which are no longer responsive to furosemide.[3] A study in dogs with MMVD that compared oral furosemide vs oral torsemide (dosed at 10% of the furosemide dose divided into twice-daily doses) concluded that torsemide is equivalent to furosemide at controlling clinical signs of CHF and is likely to achieve greater diuresis vs furosemide.[4] Two larger-scale studies have also found that torsemide given every 24 hours is noninferior to furosemide for MMVD dogs with CHF.[5,6] In dogs with first-time CHF related to MMVD that were naïve to diuretics, torsemide was noninferior to furosemide for reducing pulmonary edema and clinical cough scores without worsening of dyspnea or exercise intolerance.[6] Torsemide was associated with a 64% reduction in risk for cardiac death, euthanasia due to worsening CHF, or study withdrawal due to worsening CHF. However, adverse effects were more frequent in dogs receiving torsemide. Another study in dogs with CHF related to MMVD found torsemide to be noninferior to furosemide based on clinical improvement or stabilization of CHF.[5] Additionally, torsemide was associated with a 2-fold reduction in risk for reaching the composite cardiac endpoint (spontaneous cardiac death, euthanasia for HF, or CHF class worsening) within the first 12 weeks of treatment compared to furosemide.[5]

A small retrospective study found that torsemide was tolerated in cats with spontaneous CHF as first-line and second-line treatments.[7]

One pharmacokinetic study in horses concluded that torsemide might be a reasonable alternative to furosemide because of good absorption after oral administration, reasonable half-life, and sustained diuretic effect.[8]

Pharmacology/Actions

Torsemide, like furosemide, inhibits sodium and chloride reabsorption in the ascending loop of Henle via interference with the chloride-binding site of the 1Na+, 1K+, 2Cl- cotransport system.

Torsemide increases renal excretion of water, sodium, potassium, chloride, calcium, magnesium, hydrogen, ammonium, and bicarbonate. Torsemide is able to suppress almost total water reabsorption in dogs.[1] In healthy dogs, diuretic resistance developed after 14 days of furosemide but not torsemide.[9]

In dogs, excretion of potassium is affected much less than sodium (20:1); this is ≈2 times the ratio of Na:K excreted than with furosemide. The diuretic activity begins within 1 hour of dosing, peaks at ≈2 hours, and persists for ≈12 hours. In dogs, torsemide appears to have differing effects on aldosterone than furosemide. When compared to furosemide, torsemide increases plasma aldosterone levels and inhibits the amount of receptor-bound aldosterone; however, additional research must be performed to determine the clinical significance of these effects.

In cats, torsemide's effects on potassium excretion appear to be similar to that of furosemide. Peak diuresis occurs ≈4 hours postdose and persists for 12 hours.[10]

Pharmacokinetics

Limited information is available. Oral bioavailability has been reported to be between 80% and 100% in dogs and cats. Plasma protein binding in dogs is greater than 98%. ≈60% of the dose is excreted unchanged in the urine.[11] Elimination half-life in dogs is ≈10 hours and is ≈13 hours in cats.[1,12]

In horses, 1 study found that torsemide was orally absorbed and reached plasma concentrations similar to those reported in dogs, rabbits, rats, and humans. A single dose of 6 mg/kg PO resulted in a maximum plasma concentration of 10.14 µg/mL ≈3 hours after dosing and a half-life of 9.2 hours.[8]

In humans, torsemide has high oral bioavailability; patients may be switched between IV and PO forms with no change in dose. Bioavailability in dogs has been reported at 80% to 100%. It is extensively bound to plasma proteins in humans (greater than 99%). The major metabolite in humans is the carboxylic acid derivative, which is biologically inactive.

Contraindications/Precautions/Warnings

Torsemide should not be used in patients with known hypersensitivity to it or other sulfonylureas. Caution in patients with other sulfonamide hypersensitivities; cross-reactivity between antibiotic sulfonamides and non-antibiotic sulfonamides is theoretically possible.[13] Torsemide should not be used with other loop diuretics, in dehydrated or hypovolemic patients, or in anuric patients.[11]

Use torsemide cautiously in patients with significant hepatic dysfunction, hyperuricemia (may increase serum uric acid), or diabetes mellitus (may increase serum glucose). Torsemide can cause excessive diuresis that could potentially cause symptomatic dehydration, decreased blood volume and hypotension, and worsening renal function. Acute renal failure is possible; concomitant use of nephrotoxic drugs increases this risk. Symptomatic electrolyte abnormalities are possible. Use of torsemide at higher than recommended doses, in patients with severe renal impairment, or patients with hyponatremia may increase the risk for ototoxicity.[14]

Adverse Effects

Adverse effect profiles for dogs and cats have not been fully established because of the limited use of this drug in veterinary medicine. In clinical studies, the most common adverse effects seen were GI effects (vomiting, diarrhea, anorexia) and renal effects (polyuria, increased renal values, renal insufficiency or failure).[5,6] One study in healthy dogs given torsemide daily for 26 weeks reported dose-dependent adverse effects, including dryness of oral mucosa, decreased food intake, increased water intake, electrolyte imbalances, increased urine pH, decreased urine specific gravity, and increased serum aldosterone concentrations.[15] In healthy dogs, diuretic resistance developed after 14 days of furosemide but not torsemide, and both drugs were associated with increased BUN and plasma creatinine concentrations when compared with values before treatment.[9]

Torsemide can induce fluid and electrolyte abnormalities. Patients should be monitored for hydration status and electrolyte imbalances (especially potassium, calcium, magnesium, and sodium). Prerenal azotemia may result if moderate to severe dehydration occurs. Hyponatremia is probably the greatest concern, but hypocalcemia, hypokalemia, and hypomagnesemia may all occur. Animals with normal food and water intake are much less likely to develop water and electrolyte imbalances than those that do not.

Other potential adverse effects include hematologic effects (eg, anemia, leukopenia), weakness, and restlessness. Torsemide, unlike furosemide, apparently only rarely causes significant ototoxic effects in humans; high doses in laboratory animals have induced ototoxicity.

Reproductive/Nursing Safety

No effects on fertility were noted when female and male rats were administered up to 25 mg/kg/day.

No adverse teratogenic effects were seen when pregnant rats and rabbits were administered up to 15 times (human dose) and 5 times (human dose), respectively. Larger doses increased fetal resorptions, decreased average body weight, and delayed fetal ossification.

It is unknown if torsemide enters milk, but furosemide is distributed in milk. Clinical significance for nursing offspring is unknown.

Because safety has not been established in animals, this drug should only be used when the maternal benefits outweigh the potential risks to offspring.

Overdose/Acute Toxicity

In dogs, the oral LD_{50} is greater than 2 g/kg. Fluid and electrolyte imbalance is the most likely risk associated with an overdose. Consider GI decontamination for very large or quantity unknown ingestions. Acute overdoses should generally be managed by observation with fluid, electrolyte, and acid-base monitoring; supportive treatment should be initiated if required.

For patients that have experienced or are suspected of having experienced an overdose, consultation with a 24-hour poison consultation center specializing in providing veterinary-specific information is recommended. For general information related to overdose and toxin exposures, as well as contact information for poison control centers, refer to ***Appendix.***

Drug Interactions

The following drug interactions have either been reported or are theoretical in humans or animals receiving torsemide and may be of significance in veterinary patients. Unless otherwise noted, use together is not necessarily contraindicated, but weigh the potential risks and perform additional monitoring when appropriate.

- ANGIOTENSIN-CONVERTING ENZYME INHIBITORS (ACEIs; eg, **enalapril, benazepril**): Slightly increased risk for hypotension, particularly in patients that are volume or sodium depleted secondary to diuretics
- AMINOGLYCOSIDES (eg, **gentamicin, amikacin**): Other diuretics have been associated with increasing the ototoxic or nephrotoxic risks of aminoglycosides. It is unknown if torsemide can also have these effects and, if so, what the clinical significance may be.
- AMPHOTERICIN B: Loop diuretics may increase the risk for nephrotoxicity development.
- CHOLESTYRAMINE: Concomitant administration may decrease torsemide absorption; administer separately.
- CISPLATIN: Concomitant use may increase the risk for worsening renal function or renal failure.
- CORTICOSTEROIDS (eg, **dexamethasone, predniso(lo)ne**): Increased risk of hypokalemia
- DIGOXIN: Can increase the area under the curve of torsemide by 50% but is unlikely to be of significance clinically; torsemide-induced hypokalemia may increase the potential for digoxin toxicity.
- IOHEXOL: Increased risk for nephrotoxicity
- NONSTEROIDAL ANTI-INFLAMMATORY DRUGS (NSAIDs; eg, **carprofen, flunixin**): NSAIDs may reduce the natriuretic effects of torsemide. Concomitant use with NSAIDs may increase the risk for worsening renal function or renal failure.
- PROBENECID: Can reduce the diuretic efficacy of torsemide.
- SALICYLATES (eg, **aspirin**): Torsemide can reduce the excretion of salicylates.

Laboratory Considerations

Torsemide can affect **serum electrolytes, glucose, uric acid,** and **BUN** concentrations.

Dosages

DOGS/CATS:

Diuretic for adjunctive treatment of heart failure (extra-label): Initial dose 0.1 – 0.3 mg/kg PO every 24 hours.[3,5-7] Torsemide dosages are ≈5% to 10% of furosemide doses, as torsemide is ≈10 to 20 times more potent than furosemide; if switching from furosemide, torsemide dose should be started at 5% to 10% of the total daily furosemide dose.

HORSES:

Diuretic for fluid overload (extra-label): Based on a pharmacokinetic study, 0.5 – 1 mg/kg PO every 12 hours appears to be a reasonable starting dose.[8]

Monitoring

- Serum electrolytes, BUN, creatinine, glucose (if diabetic)
- Hydration status
- Blood pressure, if indicated
- Clinical signs of edema, patient weight, if indicated

Client Information

- While taking this medicine, your animal will drink and urinate more often than usual. Be sure your animal always has access to freshwater. You may give this medicine with or without food.
- While your animal is taking this medicine, your veterinarian will need to monitor your animal closely. Do not miss these important follow-up visits.
- Contact your veterinarian immediately if you notice excessive thirst, weakness, collapse (passing out), head tilt, lack of urination, or a racing heartbeat.

Chemistry/Synonyms

Torsemide is a lipophilic anilinopyridine sulfonylurea loop diuretic that occurs as white to off-white, crystalline powder. It is practically insoluble in water and slightly soluble in alcohol.

Torsemide may also be known as torasemide, AC-3525, AC 4464, BM-02.015, JDL-464, and *Demadex*®. International trade names include *Isemid*®, *Torem*®, and *Unat*®.

Storage/Stability

Store torsemide tablets below 40°C (104°F); preferably between 15°C and 30°C (59°F and 86°F).

Compatibility/Compounding Considerations

No specific information was noted.

Dosage Forms/Regulatory Status

VETERINARY-LABELED PRODUCTS: NONE IN THE US.

The Association of Racing Commissioners International (ARCI) has designated this drug as a class 3 substance. Use of this drug may not be allowed in certain animal competitions. Check rules and regulations before entering a competition while this medication is being administered. Contact local racing authorities for further guidance. See ***Appendix*** for more information.

HUMAN-LABELED PRODUCTS:

Torsemide Oral Tablets: 5 mg, 10 mg, 20 mg, and 100 mg; *Demadex*®, generic; (Rx)

Torsemide Injection: 10 mg/mL; generic; (Rx). **NOTE**: This product has been discontinued.

References

For the complete list of references, see **wiley.com/go/budde/plumb**

Tramadol

(***tram***-ah-doll) *Ultram*®

Opioid Agonist

Prescriber Highlights

- ► Synthetic mu-receptor partial opioid agonist that also inhibits the reuptake of serotonin and norepinephrine
- ► Appears useful as an analgesic in cats, but studies in dogs provide conflicting evidence of analgesia; may take up to 2 weeks for full analgesic activity in chronic pain states
- ► It is contraindicated in patients hypersensitive to it and other opioids, and in those with GI obstruction. Use with caution in patients with a history of seizures or patients receiving other CNS or respiratory depressants.
- ► Appears well tolerated in dogs; sedation is the most likely adverse effect.
- ► Several potential clinically significant drug interactions exist; avoid use with selective serotonin reuptake inhibitors (SSRIs; eg, fluoxetine) or monoamine oxidase inhibitors (MAOIs; eg, selegiline).
- ► DEA Schedule IV (C-IV) controlled substance

Uses/Indications

Tramadol is used for adjunct treatment of postoperative or chronic pain in many species. It is most useful when used in combination with NSAIDs or other analgesic drugs (eg, amantadine, gabapentin, alpha-2 agonists).[1] Tramadol use as an analgesic was widely adopted in veterinary medicine in part based on its low cost and previous status as a noncontrolled drug; however, evidence of efficacy is conflicting and studies demonstrating tramadol's efficacy as a sole analgesic[2-5] are outweighed by studies that cite its limitations.[1,6-11] A meta-analysis that reviewed the efficacy of tramadol for postoperative pain management in dogs found that tramadol likely results in a decreased need for rescue analgesia compared to no treatment or placebo, but the certainty of the evidence was determined to be low.[12] Studies of tramadol in dogs with osteoarthritis did not show benefits compared to placebo.[10,13] Anecdotally, tramadol has also been used as an anti-tussive agent; however, evidence of efficacy is lacking.

Tramadol's efficacy as an analgesic in cats is more robust.[14-19]

In horses, tramadol administered as an epidural may also be useful as an analgesic, but no appropriate commercial dosage forms are available in the United States; however, studies evaluating the antinociceptive effects in horses after IV administration have found that IV tramadol is not an effective analgesic in horses when used alone.[20,21] Some studies have shown benefits when used in combination therapy.[21,22] In donkeys, tramadol used with lidocaine as an epidural has a shorter onset and longer duration of action than when lidocaine is used alone.[23]

Tramadol administered systemically in sheep, camels, and camelids has noticeable adverse effects and a lack of efficacy and should not be used in those species.[24-28]

Pharmacology/Actions

Tramadol is a centrally acting partial opioid agonist with primarily mu-receptor activity. It also weakly inhibits the reuptake of serotonin and norepinephrine. Analgesic activity is due to the parent compound and its active metabolite, M1 (O-desmethyltramadol [ODT]). When compared with tramadol in laboratory animal studies, M1 was 20 times more potent in binding to mu receptors and was 6 times more potent as an analgesic.

Naloxone only partially antagonizes the analgesic effects of tramadol; other partial antagonists include yohimbine and ondansetron.

Pharmacokinetics

Bioavailability is ≈65% after oral administration of immediate-release tablets in dogs, but there is significant interpatient variability. Rectal bioavailability is ≈10%. The volume of distribution (V_D), total body clearance, and half-life are 3.8 L/kg, 55 mL/kg/minute, and 1.7 hours, respectively.[29] Tramadol is extensively metabolized via several pathways to at least 20 metabolites. The active M1 metabolite is formed by cytochrome P450 2D15 (CYP2D15) but is a minor metabolite in dogs.[30,31] M1 has a half-life of ≈2 hours after oral tramadol administration.[29] Dogs appear to produce substantial quantities of the inactive metabolite M2 via CYP2B11. M1 and M2 are further metabolized to M5 (N,O-didesmethyltramadol) via CYP2C21 and 2D15.[30,32] Pharmacokinetics of tramadol have been reported for young and middle-aged dogs. After IV administration at 4 mg/kg, the V_D, elimination half-life, and total body clearance were 4.77 ± 1.07 L/kg, 1.91 ± 0.26 hours, and 29.9 ± 7.3 mL/kg/minute, respectively, in young dogs and 4.73 ± 1.43 L/kg, 2.39 ± 0.97 hours, and 23.7 ± 5.4 mL/kg/minute, respectively, in middle-aged dogs. Excretion was significantly prolonged in older animals.[33] In greyhounds, tramadol's half-life is slightly shorter (ie, 1.1 hours).[34]

After intranasal administration in dogs, tramadol was rapidly absorbed into the systemic circulation, becoming detectable after 5 minutes and reaching maximum concentrations ≈40 minutes after administration. Bioavailability was determined to range from 3.3% to 20.6%. In general, plasma concentrations were low and variable. Tramadol half-life was ≈1 hour. M1 was largely undetectable. Plasma concentrations were low, and because they did not correlate with analgesic effect it was hypothesized that tramadol bypassed systemic circulation and traveled directly to the CNS.

A study of 8 cats that received the immediate-release oral tablet showed high interpatient variability in absorption (2 cats had inadequate data and could not be analyzed). The main metabolite produced in cats is the active M1 metabolite. The elimination half-life for the parent compound was ≈2.25 to 3.5 hours and was 4.5 hours for the M1 metabolite.[35] Another study in 6 cats demonstrated the following approximate values: 60% oral bioavailability, 2 L/kg volume of distribution at steady state (V_{SS}), 12 mL/kg/minute clearance, and 3.2 hours terminal half-life. The terminal half-life of M1 after oral administration was ≈4.8 hours. After transdermal application of a compounded tramadol gel, a dose of ≈2.8 mg/kg resulted in undetectable or very low plasma concentrations.[36]

In adult horses, tramadol had relatively poor oral absorption (≈3% to 10%)[37,38] and an elimination half-life of ≈1.5 to 2.5 hours after IV or IM administration and up to 10 hours when given orally.[37–41] The M1 active metabolite half-life was ≈4 hours. Oral doses of 10 mg/kg yielded concentrations of tramadol and M1 that are believed to be therapeutic, whereas lower doses (3 to 6 mg/kg) were inconsistent and transient.[41–44] M2 appears to be the main metabolite produced by horses, with very low and variable M1 concentrations.[37,45] In donkeys given single IV doses of 2 mg/kg, the half-life of the parent compound was ≈1 hour, and the halflife of the M1 metabolite was ≈8.5 hours.[46]

Tramadol has different pharmacokinetics in neonatal and weaned foals. After oral administration, higher bioavailability (53% vs 20%), shorter time to peak concentration (1 hour vs 1.25 hours), and peak levels occurred with neonatal (2 weeks of age) vs weaned (4 months of age) foals. The elimination half-life did not significantly differ (≈2 hours). The active metabolite (M1) remained above the reported therapeutic concentration for humans for 3 hours in neonatal foals and 8 hours in weaned foals.[47] In another study, the elimination half-life was ≈1.5 hours in foals up to 6 weeks of age.[48]

In llamas administered 2 mg/kg IV, tramadol and M1 pharmacokinetics values (approximate means) were: V_{SS}, 4 L/kg and 26.5 L/kg; clearance, 1.7 L/kg/hour and 2.03 L/kg/hour; half-life, 2.1 hours and 10.4 hours. IM (2 mg/kg) bioavailability was high.[49] Data in camels were similar to those in llamas.[24] In alpacas, oral bioavailability was poor (6% to 19%).[28] After IV administration (3.4 to 4.4 mg/kg), V_D was 5.50 ± 2.66 L/kg, total body clearance was ≈4.6 L/kg/hour, and half-life was ≈0.9 hours. The M1 metabolite was not detected.

The elimination half-life of tramadol in sheep receiving IV tramadol (4 and 6 mg/kg) was 0.6 hours and 1.2 hours for M1.[27] Bioavailability in goats given tramadol at 2 mg/kg IV and PO was 37%, and the half-life was ≈1 hour (IV) and 2.7 hours (PO). The M1 half-life was 2.9 hours after IV administration but was undetectable after oral administration.[50]

In red-tailed hawks given an oral dose of 11 mg/kg, plasma levels of tramadol reached or exceeded concentrations associated with analgesia in humans for at least 4 hours after administration. The elimination half-lives were 1.3 hours (tramadol) and 1.9 hours (M1).[51] Single IV doses given to Hispaniolan Amazon parrots resulted in half-lives of 1.54 hours (tramadol) and 2.55 hours (M2). Oral bioavailability was ≈24%.[52]

Contraindications/Precautions/Warnings

Tramadol is contraindicated in patients that are hypersensitive to it or other opioids. The combination product containing acetaminophen is contraindicated in cats. In humans, the drug is contraindicated in patients with GI obstruction or paralytic ileus and in children younger than 12 or undergoing tonsillectomy or adenoidectomy.

Caution should be used when tramadol is given in conjunction with other drugs that can cause CNS or respiratory depression. Because tramadol has caused seizures in humans, it should be used with caution in animals with pre-existing seizure disorders, at increased risk for seizures (eg, head trauma, CNS infections), or receiving other drugs that may reduce the seizure threshold. Similar to other opioidlike compounds, tramadol should be used with caution in geriatric or severely debilitated animals and in those with severe asthma. Animals with impaired renal or hepatic function may need dosage adjustments.

Although the risk for physical dependence is less than that of several other opioids, it has been reported in humans. The drug should be withdrawn gradually in animals that receive it chronically. Humans can potentially abuse tramadol, and significant diversion of the drug reportedly occurs. Clinicians should be alert to pet owners seeking tramadol.

Extended-release tablets, which are not currently recommended or used in veterinary patients, should not be broken, crushed, or chewed because toxicity could occur.

Care should be taken not to confuse traMADol with traZODone.

Adverse Effects

Tramadol appears to be well tolerated in dogs and appears to have fewer adverse effects than methadone or morphine.[53] Tramadol has the potential to cause a variety of adverse effects associated with its pharmacologic actions, including CNS effects (eg, excessive sedation, agitation, anxiety, tremor, dizziness) or GI effects (inappetence, vomiting, constipation, diarrhea).

Limited information is available on the adverse effects in cats. Vomiting, sedation, mydriasis, dysphoria or euphoria, and constipation have been reported. In a study, neurologic effects (eg, mydriasis, dysphoria) were seen in 25% of cats, and the drug was observed to be unpalatable to cats.[54] Unpalatability may lead to dose avoidance.

In horses, tramadol 5 mg/kg IV caused excitement[20]; ataxia and muscle spasms were more frequently seen in donkeys after 4 mg/kg IV administration.[46]

In humans receiving tramadol, ≈10% develop pruritus. Injectable tramadol may cause respiratory and cardiac depression.

Reproductive/Nursing Safety

Laboratory animals have experienced embryotoxicity and fetotoxicity at doses administered 0.6 to 3.6 times the maximum daily human dose. Chronic tramadol administration in pregnant patients may result in opioid withdrawal in the offspring. Tramadol was embryotoxic and fetotoxic in laboratory animals when given at dosages 3 to 15 times the recommendation.

Humans receiving long-term opioid therapy have experienced hypogonadism, resulting in an impairment of reproductive functions.

Tramadol and its active M1 metabolite enter maternal milk. This drug is not recommended for use while nursing.

Overdose/Acute Toxicity

Acute oral overdoses can cause signs of CNS depression or serotonin syndrome. Clinical signs associated with an overdose in dogs include sedation/lethargy, vomiting, tachycardia, vocalizing, ataxia, agitation, or tremor. In cats, mydriasis, hypersalivation, lethargy, ataxia, tachycardia, and vomiting have been reported. Signs of serotonin syndrome due to overdose (80 mg/kg PO) have been described in a cat.[55]

Treatment is primarily supportive (eg, maintaining respiration, treating seizures with benzodiazepines or barbiturates). Naloxone may NOT be useful in tramadol overdoses, as it may only partially reverse some of the effects of the drug and may increase the risk for seizures. Naloxone did not decrease the drug's lethality in tramadol overdoses given to mice. Cyproheptadine and phenothiazines can be used to treat stimulatory signs. Tramadol and the M1 metabolite are not removed by dialysis.[56]

For patients that have experienced or are suspected of having experienced an overdose, it is strongly encouraged to consult with a 24hour poison consultation center that specializes in providing information specific for veterinary patients. For general information related to overdose and toxin exposures, as well as contact information for poison control centers, refer to ***Appendix***.

Drug Interactions

Tramadol is metabolized by CYP2B, CYP2D, and CYP3A enzyme families. The following drug interactions have either been reported or are theoretical in humans or animals receiving tramadol and may be of significance in veterinary patients. Unless otherwise noted, use together is not necessarily contraindicated, but weigh the potential risks and perform additional monitoring when appropriate.

- **Amantadine**: Concomitant use with tramadol may increase the risk for seizures because tramadol at high doses has caused seizures in humans[56], and amantadine can lower the seizure threshold[57]; however, an increased risk for seizures with this drug combination appears unlikely in a clinical setting at recommended dosages. Monitor for sedation or other neurologic adverse effects if using this combination.
- **Amiodarone**: May increase tramadol concentrations and decrease M1 (active metabolite) concentrations
- **Anticholinergic Agents** (eg, **atropine, glycopyrrolate**): Concurrent use may increase the risk for anticholinergic effects (eg, constipation, urinary retention).
- **Antidepressants, Miscellaneous** (eg, **mirtazapine, trazodone**): Increased risk for serotonin syndrome
- **Antihistamines** (eg, **diphenhydramine, hydroxyzine, promethazine**): Increased risk for CNS depression
- **Azole Antifungals** (eg, **fluconazole, ketoconazole**): Fluconazole inhibits tramadol metabolism to the inactive M2 metabolite without inhibiting the formation of the active M1 metabolite. In dogs that were receiving fluconazole and that were given tramadol, tramadol and M1 concentrations increased by 31-fold and 39-fold, respectively.[58] Ketoconazole may increase tramadol exposure and risk for toxicity.[59]
- **Benzodiazepines** (eg, **alprazolam, diazepam**): Increased risk for respiratory depression
- **Cimetidine**: May increase tramadol exposure and risk for toxicity[59]
- **CNS Depressants, Miscellaneous** (eg, **dexmedetomidine, gabapentin, levetiracetam, methocarbamol**): Increased risk for CNS depression
- **Cyproheptadine**: May decrease efficacy of tramadol
- **Digoxin**: In humans, tramadol has been rarely linked to digoxin toxicity.
- **Erythromycin**: May increase tramadol exposure and risk for toxicity
- **Iohexol**: Concurrent use may increase the risk for seizures.
- **Ketamine**: Increased risk for CNS and respiratory depression
- **Metoclopramide**: Increased risk for seizures
- **Mitotane**: May reduce tramadol levels and efficacy
- **Monoamine Oxidase Inhibitors** (MAOIs; eg, **amitraz, selegiline**): Potential for serotonin syndrome; MAOI use within the past 14 days or use together should be avoided.
- **Ondansetron**: In humans, use together may reduce the effectiveness of both drugs.
- **Opioid Analgesics** (eg, **buprenorphine, butorphanol, methadone**): May increase the risk for seizures, serotonin syndrome, and CNS and respiratory depression; methadone may inhibit tramadol metabolism.
- **Phenobarbital**: Increased risk for CNS depression. Tramadol may lower the seizure threshold. Phenobarbital may decrease tramadol levels.
- **Quinidine**: May increase tramadol concentrations and decrease M1 (active metabolite) concentrations
- **Rifampin**: May reduce tramadol levels and efficacy
- **S-Adenosyl Methionine (SAMe)**: Theoretically, concurrent use of SAMe with tramadol could cause additive serotonergic effects.
- **Sevoflurane**: Pretreatment with tramadol reduced minimum alveolar concentration (MAC) values by 22% to 30% in dogs[60,61] and 40% in cats.[62]
- **Selective-Serotonin Reuptake Inhibitors** (SSRIs; eg, **fluoxetine, paroxetine, sertraline**): Can inhibit the metabolism of tramadol to its active metabolites, thereby decreasing its efficacy and increasing the risk for toxicity (serotonin syndrome, seizures)
- **Terbinafine**: May increase tramadol levels and reduce the formation of M1 metabolite due to CYP2D6 inhibition. In humans, this effect may persist for weeks after discontinuing terbinafine.
- **Tricyclic Antidepressants** (eg, **amitriptyline, clomipramine**): Increased risk for seizures and serotonin syndrome; amitriptyline may inhibit tramadol metabolism.
- **Yohimbine**: May antagonize (partial) the pharmacologic effects of tramadol
- **Warfarin**: In humans, increased prothrombin time in patients taking tramadol has been reported (relatively rare).

Laboratory Considerations

- No specific laboratory interactions or considerations were noted.

Dosages

DOGS:

Analgesic (extra-label): 4 – 10 mg/kg PO every 8 hours; pharmacokinetic data suggest administration every 6 hours may be necessary. Tramadol's efficacy as a single agent appears questionable. The long-term efficacy of tramadol may decrease with time.[10]

CATS:

Analgesic (extra-label): Most recommendations for administration in cats are 1 – 2 mg/kg PO every 12 hours. There is no clear dosage for tramadol in cats based on prospective studies. Some clinicians suggest that some cats may only need to be dosed every 24 hours; others suggest doses up to 4 mg/kg. Tramadol has an unpleasant taste, and avoidance may be an issue. Neurologic and opioid adverse effects can be seen, particularly in geriatric cats at doses greater than 2 mg/kg.[17]

HORSES:

Analgesic (extra-label):

a) Based on pharmacokinetic studies and treated patients: 10 mg/kg PO every 12 hours[41–44]

b) **Chronic laminitis pain**:

i. 5 – 10 mg/kg PO every 12 hours,[42,63] although the 5 mg/kg dose did not reliably produce analgesia.[42]

ii. Tramadol 5 mg/kg PO twice daily for 7 days—with ketamine 0.6 mg/kg/hour IV CRI over 6 hours each day for the first 3 days of treatment.[63]

BIRDS:

Analgesic (extra-label):

a) **Red-tailed hawks**: From a pharmacokinetic study, authors concluded that an oral dose of 15 mg/kg PO every 12 hours would be a reasonable starting point; additional pharmacodynamic and repeat dose pharmacokinetic studies are needed.[51]

b) **Hispaniolan Amazon parrots**: From pharmacokinetic and antinociceptive studies, 30 mg/kg PO every 6 to 8 hours may provide clinical analgesia. Further studies are needed to fully evaluate the analgesic effects of tramadol in psittacines.[52,64,65]

SMALL MAMMALS:

Analgesic (extra-label):

a) **Sugar gliders**: 2 – 6 mg/kg PO every 12 hours[66]

b) **Chinchillas, guinea pigs, rodents**: 5 – 10 mg/kg PO every 12 hours[67]

c) **Companion pigs**: 4 – 6 mg/kg PO every 12 hours[68]

REPTILES:

Analgesic (extra-label):

a) **Red-eared slider turtles**: 5 – 10 mg/kg PO[69]

b) **Reptiles/chelonians**: 5 – 10 mg/kg PO every 48 to 72 hours. Good analgesic efficacy with relatively long duration when administered PO in chelonians; less respiratory depression than other opioids[70]

Monitoring

- Clinical efficacy
- Adverse effects

Client Information

- Contact your veterinarian if you suspect your animal's pain is not controlled.
- This medicine may be given with or without food. Putting the medicine in a small amount of canned food may hide its bitter taste. If your animal vomits or acts sick after receiving this drug on an empty stomach, give the medicine with food or a small treat. If vomiting continues, contact your veterinarian.
- This medicine may cause changes in alertness or behavior. Use it with caution in working or service dogs.
- The combination product with acetaminophen (*Ultracet*®) should NOT be used in cats.
- Tramadol is a controlled substance in the United States. It is against the law to give away or sell this medication and to use it without a prescription.

Chemistry/Synonyms

Tramadol HCl, a mu-receptor opioid agonist, occurs as a white crystalline powder that is freely soluble in water or alcohol and very slightly soluble in acetone. Tramadol is not derived from opium, nor is it a semisynthetic opioid, but it is entirely synthetically produced.

Tramadol HCl may also be known as CG-315, CG-315E, tramadoli hydrochloridum, or U-26225A; many trade names are available.

Storage/Stability

Unless otherwise labeled, store tramadol tablets at a controlled room temperature of 20°C to 25°C (68°F-77°F); excursions are permitted between 15°C and 30°C (59°F-86°F). Dispense in tight, light-resistant containers. Tramadol is a controlled substance and should be stored in an area that is substantially constructed and securely locked, in accordance with US Drug Enforcement Administration regulations.

Compatibility/Compounding Considerations

Tramadol suspensions, 5 mg/mL[71] and 10 mg/mL,[72] made by crushing tramadol tablets and suspending in appropriate vehicles, have demonstrated potency and stability for up to 90 days when refrigerated or stored at room temperature.

Dosage Forms/Regulatory Status

VETERINARY-LABELED PRODUCTS: NONE

The Association of Racing Commissioners International (ARCI) has designated this drug as a class 2 substance. Use of this drug may not be allowed in certain animal competitions. Check rules and regulations before entering in a competition while this medication is being administered. Contact local racing authorities for further guidance. See ***Appendix*** for more information.

HUMAN-LABELED PRODUCTS:

Tramadol HCl Oral Tablets (film-coated): 50 mg; *Ultram*®, generic; (Rx); (C-IV)

Tramadol HCl Extended-Release Tablets and Capsule: 100 mg, 200 mg, and 300 mg; *Ultram ER*®, *Ryzolt*®, generic [tablets], *ConZip*® [capsules]; (Rx); (C-IV). **NOTE**: Dogs apparently do not absorb these products as well as humans and potentially could overdose if they chew on the tablets or capsules.

Tramadol HCl Oral Solution: 5 mg/mL; *Qdolo*®; (Rx); (C-IV)

Tramadol is also available in a fixed-dose combination of tramadol HCl 37.5 mg and acetaminophen 325 mg tablets. United States trade name is *Ultracet*®; (Rx); (C-IV). **WARNING**: This combination product should **not** be used in cats.

In several countries outside the United States, tramadol injection is available commercially.

References

For the complete list of references, see **wiley.com/go/budde/plumb**

Tranexamic Acid

(tran-ex-***am***-ik ***as***-id) *Cyklokapron*®, *Lysteda*®

Fibrinolysis Inhibitor

Prescriber Highlights

- ► Used to prevent or reduce bleeding in dogs and cats
- ► Contraindications include hypersensitivity and in patients with a history of, risk for, or active thromboembolic disease.
- ► Causes dose-dependent vomiting; may be useful as an emetic
- ► Thromboembolic events and visual disturbances have occurred in humans.
- ► Inadvertent intrathecal administration is rapidly fatal.

Uses/Indications

Tranexamic acid is used to prevent and reduce postoperative bleeding and to stop traumatic bleeding in dogs and cats. It may be effective in controlling hyperfibrinolysis associated with *Angiostrongylus vasorum* infection.[1] It has also been used as an emetic in dogs.[2]

Pharmacology/Actions

Tranexamic acid reduces bleeding by inhibiting the breakdown of fibrin. It reversibly binds to lysine binding sites on plasminogen to prevent the binding of plasminogen to fibrin and thus prevents the formation of plasmin. Inhibiting plasmin-mediated fibrin dissolution stabilizes the blood clot matrix. In horses, tranexamic acid is ≈10 times more potent in vitro than aminocaproic acid; in dogs, it is ≈4 times more potent.[3,4] The minimum plasma concentration of tranexamic acid required to completely inhibit experimentally induced hyperfibrinolysis is ≈145 µg/mL in dogs[3] and ≈6 µg/mL in horses.[4]

Tranexamic acid is emetogenic in dogs, causing dose-dependent vomiting within 2 to 3 minutes of administration. Dogs vomited only once or twice, and the emetogenic effect persisted for 4 to 5 minutes.[2] In a larger cohort of dogs, vomiting occurred in 85% of dogs receiving tranexamic acid. The median time to onset of vomiting was ≈2 minutes, median duration of emesis was ≈2.5 minutes, and median of 2 episodes of emesis.[5] Emetogenic effects of tranexamic acid may be mediated by NK1 receptors.[2] It can antagonize GABA and glycine receptors, and these actions may contribute to its proconvulsive effect.[6]

Pharmacokinetics

No veterinary pharmacokinetic information was located.

In humans, tranexamic acid is ≈45% bioavailable after oral administration, with peak concentrations occurring at 3 hours.[7] Absorption appears unaffected by food. It is widely distributed with a volume of distribution of ≈0.4 L/kg. It passes into aqueous humor, breast milk, and crosses the placenta. It does not bind to plasma proteins. Tranexamic acid is not appreciably metabolized and is excreted unchanged in the urine with a terminal elimination half-life of ≈2 hours after IV administration[8] and ≈11 hours after oral administration.[8]

Contraindications/Precautions/Warnings

Tranexamic acid is contraindicated in patients that are hypersensitive to it and in patients with a history of, risk for, or active thromboembolic disease. In humans, it is contraindicated in patients with subarachnoid hemorrhage as cerebral edema has occurred.[7,8] Patients with renal impairment require dosage reduction.

In humans, inadvertent intrathecal administration has resulted in seizures and cardiac arrhythmias.[8] Thrombosis and thromboembolism have been reported with IV administration. Tranexamic acid should be discontinued if ocular or vision disturbances occur. Patients treated for upper urinary tract bleeding have developed ureteral obstruction caused by clot formation.

Adverse Effects

Vomiting can occur immediately or within minutes of IV administration, is dose dependent, and more likely with rapid IV bolus administration.[2,9] Administration of maropitant IV 10 minutes before treatment with tranexamic acid has been shown to prevent emesis.[10] Tonic-clonic seizures have been reported in dogs.[11,12]

In humans, nausea, vomiting, and diarrhea are dose related; musculoskeletal pain, thrombosis, and visual changes, including ocular or retinal occlusion, have been reported.[7,8] Hypotension can occur when administered IV too rapidly. Anaphylactic reactions have been reported, and convulsions have been reported during surgery.

Reproductive/Nursing Safety

Tranexamic acid crosses the placenta and reaches concentrations approximating those found in maternal blood.[7,8] No impairment of fertility or evidence of fetal harm was observed in studies with laboratory animals, including doses up to 4 times the maximum human oral dose; however, safe use of tranexamic acid during pregnancy has not been established.

Tranexamic acid is distributed into milk; use with caution in lactating patients or consider milk replacer.

Because safety has not been established in animals, this drug should only be used when the maternal benefits outweigh the potential risks to offspring.

Overdose/Acute Toxicity

GI distress, hypotension, myoclonus, and thromboembolic events may occur. Retinal changes, including degeneration, have occurred in dogs, cats, and rats that received 3 to 40 times the human dose for 6 days to 1 year.[7,8] GI decontamination should not be necessary but can be considered in patients that did not vomit. Provide supportive and symptomatic treatment.

Inadvertent intrathecal administration can be rapidly fatal; contact an animal poison control center immediately.

For patients that have experienced or are suspected to have experienced an overdose, consultation with a 24-hour poison consultation center specializing in providing veterinary-specific information is recommended. For general information related to overdose and toxin exposures, as well as contact information for poison control centers, refer to ***Appendix***.

Drug Interactions

The following drug interactions have either been reported or are theoretical in humans or animals receiving tranexamic acid and may be of significance in veterinary patients. Unless otherwise noted, use together is not necessarily contraindicated, but weigh the potential risks and perform additional monitoring when appropriate.

- **Chlorpromazine**: May increase risk for bleeding
- **Estrogens**: Increased risk for thrombotic events with combined use
- **Thrombolytics** (eg, **alteplase**): Concomitant use may reduce efficacy of both agents.

Laboratory Considerations

- None noted

Dosages

DOGS:

Adjunctive treatment of bleeding (extra-label): 10 mg/kg IV over 2 minutes, followed by 10 mg/kg/hour IV CRI for 3 hours[9]

Control of hyperfibrinolysis associated with *Angiostrongylus vasorum* infection (extra-label): 10 – 20 mg/kg IV over 15 to 20 minutes; repeat 6 to 8 hours later based on thromboelastography (TEG) testing[1]

Induce emesis (extra-label): In one study, 50 mg/kg IV bolus induced vomiting in all dogs (n = 10) without adverse effects; lower doses (20 – 40 mg/kg IV) were not uniformly effective to induce emesis.[2]

CATS:

Control of bleeding during surgical carcinoma and sarcoma removal (extra-label): 15 mg/kg IV bolus given during anesthetic induction reduced surgical blood loss and shortened the activated clotting time (ACT) without altering prothrombin time (PT) or activated prothrombin time (aPTT).[13]

Monitoring

- Thromboelastography (TEG analysis)
- Baseline and periodic CBC and platelets as indicated by clinical condition

- Vision changes or deficits

Client Information

- Humans have rarely experienced changes in vision or vision loss with this drug. It is unclear if this occurs in veterinary patients. Contact your veterinarian if you are concerned that your animal is developing vision problems.

Chemistry/Synonyms

Tranexamic acid is a synthetic lysine derivative that occurs as a white, crystalline powder. It is freely soluble in water and practically insoluble in alcohol. The solution for injection has a pH of 6.5 to 8.

Tranexamic acid is also known as CL-65336, acidum tranexamicum, *Cyklokapron®*, *Hexakapron®*, and *Lysteda®*.

Storage/Stability

Tranexamic acid tablets and injection should be stored at room temperature (20°C-25°C [68°F-77°F]), with excursions permitted between 15°C-30°C (59°F-86°F).

Compatibility/Compounding Considerations

Compatibility is dependent on factors such as pH, concentration, temperature, and diluent used; specialized references or a hospital pharmacist should be consulted for more specific information.

According to the manufacturer, tranexamic acid injection is **compatible** with most solutions for infusion, including saline or balanced electrolyte solutions, carbohydrate solutions, amino acid solutions, and Dextran solutions; heparin may be added to tranexamic acid injection. Tranexamic acid injection should **NOT** be mixed with blood and is **incompatible** with penicillins (eg, penicillin G, ampicillin, piperacillin).

Dosage Forms/Regulatory Status

VETERINARY-LABELED PRODUCTS: NONE

The Association of Racing Commissioners International (ARCI) has designated this drug as a class 4 substance. Use of this drug may not be allowed in certain animal competitions. Check rules and regulations before entering in a competition while this medication is being administered. Contact local racing authorities for further guidance. See ***Appendix*** for more information.

HUMAN-LABELED PRODUCTS:

Tranexamic Acid for Injection: 100 mg/mL in 10 mL ampules and single-dose vials; *Cyklokapron®*, generic; (Rx)

Tranexamic Acid Tablets: 650 mg; *Lysteda®*, generic; (Rx)

References

For the complete list of references, see **wiley.com/go/budde/plumb**

Trazodone

(***traz***-oh-done) *Desyrel®*

Serotonin (5-HT$_{2A}$) Antagonist/Reuptake Inhibitor

Prescriber Highlights

- Antidepressant used for adjunctive treatment of behavior disorders (particularly those that are anxiety- or phobia-related) and to facilitate postoperative confinement in dogs; also used for transport- and examination-related anxiety in cats
- Commonly used as an anxiolytic prior to veterinary appointments in dogs and cats
- Efficacy in facilitating postoperative confinement in dogs has been described, although there may be a large placebo effect.
- Well tolerated after oral administration. IV use of compounded formulations in dogs and horses has resulted in aggression and excitation.

Uses/Indications

Trazodone may be useful in treating behavior disorders in small animals, particularly when it is used as an adjunctive treatment in patients that do not adequately respond to conventional therapies.[1] Trazodone appears to be effective in providing short-term relief of anxiety during hospitalization and postoperative confinement after orthopedic surgery[2,3]; however, a placebo-controlled study found no difference between postoperative dogs given trazodone and those given a placebo to facilitate calmness and ease of confinement.[4]

Trazodone is commonly used as an anxiolytic prior to veterinary appointments[5]; it is also used to reduce anxiety in high-stress situations (eg, shelter housing).[6]

A recent study showed that when trazodone was administered before induction of general anesthesia in healthy dogs undergoing orthopedic surgery, the hemodynamic and propofol-sparing effects of trazodone were comparable to those of acepromazine.[7] The use of trazodone premedication also demonstrated an isoflurane minimum alveolar concentration (MAC)-sparing effect in dogs.[8]

Trazodone has been used anecdotally to decrease the hyperesthetic effects associated with strychnine toxicity.

Pilot studies in cats suggest trazodone is an effective sedative[9,10] or anxiolytic and may improve tractability during veterinary examinations.[11] Systolic blood pressure was significantly decreased in healthy cats undergoing an echocardiogram, with no altered echocardiographic results.[10]

Trazodone use in horses undergoing stall rest and exhibiting adverse behaviors resulted in significant calming in 17 out of 18 horses.[12]

In humans, trazodone is used for treating depression, aggressive behavior, alcohol or cocaine withdrawal, panic disorder, migraines, and insomnia.

Pharmacology/Actions

Trazodone is classified as a 5-HT$_{2A}$ and 5-HT$_{2C}$ antagonist/reuptake inhibitor (SARI) that primarily potentiates serotonin activity in the CNS. In laboratory animals, trazodone is shown to selectively inhibit serotonin uptake by brain synaptosomes and potentiate behavior changes induced by the serotonin precursor 5-hydroxytryptophan. Trazodone can antagonize alpha-1 adrenergic receptors and reduce blood pressure. Because trazodone can antagonize 5-HT$_2$ receptors and cause their downregulation, it can augment the efficacy of selective serotonin reuptake inhibitors (SSRIs).[13] It has fewer anticholinergic effects as compared with tricyclic antidepressants and is among the antidepressants with the lowest seizure risk.

Pharmacokinetics

In dogs, administration of 8 mg/kg IV resulted in a mean volume of distribution of 2.53 L/kg, a mean elimination half-life of 169 minutes, and a mean plasma total body clearance of 11.15 mL/minute per kg.[14] Administration of 8 mg/kg PO resulted in bioavailability of 85% and an elimination half-life of 166 minutes; peak plasma concentrations occurred at 445 minutes (mean), but there was wide intersubject variation (± 271 minutes).

In horses, the oral bioavailability of trazodone powder (4 mg/kg mixed into moistened feed) was 63%.[15] Peak concentrations of trazodone and its active metabolite (ie, m-chlorophenylpiperazine [m-CPP]) were reached within 1.7 to 2.5 hours and 0.5 to 1.8 hours, respectively, following 7.5 or 10 mg/kg.[12,15] Active metabolite accounted for ≈1% to 4% of total drug exposure.[12] The terminal half-life of trazodone was 7 to 8 hours; the m-CPP half-life was more variable (ie, 4 to 7 hours)[12,15] and concentration-dependent.[12] Half-life was prolonged in 2 horses, and the authors suggested genetic polymorphism of cytochrome P450 enzymes as a possible explanation.[15]

In humans, the oral bioavailability of trazodone (tablets) is ≈65%; the presence of food increases absorption (ie, area under the curve

[AUC] is increased) but decreases C_{max} (ie, peak plasma concentration) and delays T_{max} (ie, time of peak concentration).[16] Peak plasma concentrations occur ≈1 hour after a dose when trazodone is given on an empty stomach and after ≈2 hours when given with food. Trazodone is ≈90% to 95% bound to plasma proteins. The volume of distribution ranges from 0.47 to 0.84 L/kg. Metabolization is extensive and occurs primarily in the liver. m-CPP is also an active metabolite in humans and is formed via oxidative cleavage by CYP3A4 and further metabolized to inactive compounds via CYP2D6. Excretion is mostly (ie, 70% to 75%) via renal mechanisms, with only a small amount (ie, 0.13%) excreted unchanged in the urine. ≈21% of a dose is excreted in feces. The elimination half-life of the parent compound is ≈7 hours.

Contraindications/Precautions/Warnings

Trazodone is contraindicated in patients that are hypersensitive to it or in those receiving, or that have recently used, monoamine oxidase inhibitors (MAOIs; see ***Drug Interactions***). Trazodone should be used with caution in patients with severe cardiac disease or hepatic or renal impairment. Trazodone may dilate the pupils, which could trigger an acute crisis in patients with angle-closure glaucoma.

Do not confuse traZODone with traMADol.

Adverse Effects

Trazodone appears to be well tolerated in most patients. In dogs, the most common adverse effects are GI disturbances (eg, nausea, vomiting, diarrhea, or colitis), ataxia, and sedation.[1,3,14] Tachycardia, increased anxiety, behavior disinhibition, and aggression have also been reported. Trazodone appears to exert qualitatively different and less pronounced cardiac conduction effects in dogs than do tricyclic antidepressants. Transient priapism in a dog has also been reported.[7]

In pharmacokinetic studies in horses, excitation, tremors, and ataxia were observed after trazodone 1.5 mg/kg was given IV (over 1 minute)[15]; and sedation occurred following oral administration of 4 mg/kg[15]; and oversedation, muscle fasciculations, and transient arrhythmias occurred after oral administration of 7.5 or 10 mg/kg.[12,15]

Trazodone alone is unlikely to cause serotonin syndrome at clinically used dosages, but it is possible when trazodone is used with other serotonergic drugs. The most common clinical signs observed with serotonin syndrome in dogs include (in descending order) vomiting, diarrhea, seizures, hyperthermia, hyperesthesia, depression, mydriasis, vocalization, death, blindness, hypersalivation, dyspnea, ataxia/paresis, disorientation, hyperreflexia, and coma.[17]

In humans, the most common adverse effects include lethargy or somnolence, blurred vision, confusion, dizziness, dry mouth, orthostatic hypotension, sweating, and hyponatremia. QT prolongation can occur but is much less common in humans treated with trazodone than those treated with tricyclic antidepressants. Priapism has been reported rarely in men taking trazodone.

Reproductive/Nursing Safety

Trazodone appears to be relatively safe to use during pregnancy. At very high doses (ie, 15 to 50 times the recommended dose) in rats and rabbits, some increase in fetal death/resorption rates and congenital abnormalities were noted.[16]

Trazodone is excreted into human milk at very low concentrations.[16]

Because safety has not been established in animals, this drug should only be used when the maternal benefits outweigh the potential risks to offspring.

Overdose/Acute Toxicity

No specific information was located regarding trazodone overdoses in veterinary patients. Clinical signs associated with an overdose in dogs and cats commonly include sedation or lethargy, ataxia, and vomiting. In humans, the incidence of serious toxicity from trazodone overdose (alone) was low as compared with tricyclic antidepressant overdoses; however, in the event of a substantial overdose of trazodone, it is recommended to contact an animal poison control center for further guidance.

For patients that have experienced or are suspected to have experienced an overdose, consultation with a 24-hour poison control center specializing in providing veterinary-specific information is recommended. For general information related to overdose and toxin exposures, as well as contact information for poison control centers, refer to ***Appendix.***

Drug Interactions

The following drug interactions have either been reported or are theoretical in humans or animals receiving trazodone and may be of significance in veterinary patients. Unless otherwise noted, use together is not necessarily contraindicated, but the potential risks must be weighed and additional monitoring performed when appropriate.

- **Aspirin**: Increased risk for GI bleeding; monitoring is needed
- **Azole Antifungals** (eg, **ketoconazole, fluconazole**): May increase trazodone blood concentrations; concurrent use is contraindicated in humans.
- **Cisapride**: Increased risk for QT prolongation. Concurrent use is contraindicated in humans, but the incidence of QT prolongation in dogs and cats is unknown.
- **CNS Depressants** (eg, **alpha-2 agonists** [eg, **dexmedetomidine**], **benzodiazepines, opioids**): Use with trazodone may cause additive CNS depressant effects.
- **Digoxin**: Trazodone may increase digoxin concentrations.
- **Diuretics** (eg, **furosemide**): May increase risk for hyponatremia
- **Fluoroquinolones** (eg, **ciprofloxacin**): Increased risk for QT prolongation
- **Hypotensive Drugs** (eg, **amlodipine, enalapril, telmisartan**): Trazodone may increase reductions in blood pressure and cause hypotension.
- **Isoflurane**: Premedication with trazodone (8 mg/kg) 2 hours prior to induction resulted in a mean MAC reduction of 17%.[8]
- **Linezolid**: Increased risk for serotonin syndrome; concomitant use is contraindicated in humans.
- **Macrolide Antibiotics**: (eg, **erythromycin, clarithromycin**): May increase trazodone blood concentrations
- **Methylene blue**: Increased risk for serotonin syndrome; concomitant use is contraindicated in humans.
- **Mirtazapine**: Increased risk for CNS depression, serotonin syndrome, and/or QT prolongation
- **Monoamine Oxidase Inhibitors** (**MAOIs**; eg, **amitraz, selegiline**): Increased risk for serotonin syndrome; concurrent use is contraindicated in humans.
- **Metoclopramide**: Increased risk for serotonin syndrome
- **Ondansetron**: Increased risk for QT prolongation
- **Phenothiazines** (eg, **acepromazine**): May increase trazodone blood concentrations; can cause additive CNS effects
- **Selective Serotonin Reuptake Inhibitors** (**SSRIs**; eg, **fluoxetine**): Increased risk for serotonin syndrome. Trazodone is commonly used together with SSRIs, but patients should be observed for signs associated with serotonin syndrome (see ***Adverse Effects***). Fluoxetine may also inhibit the metabolization of trazodone.
- **Tramadol**: Increased risk for serotonin syndrome
- **Tricyclic Antidepressants** (eg, **amitriptyline, clomipramine**): Increased risk for serotonin syndrome

Laboratory Considerations

- None noted

Dosages

DOGS:

Adjunctive treatment of anxiety-related disorders (extra-label):

a) From a retrospective study of 56 dogs: The initial dose was ≈2.5 – 5 mg/kg PO every 12 to 24 hours for 3 days to allow dogs to become tolerant to the drug and avoid potential GI adverse effects.[1] The average final dose was ≈7.5 mg/kg/day PO, regardless of the dog's size. Wide interpatient dose variability existed, with oral doses ranging ≈2 – 19.5 mg/kg/day. The maximum individual dose was 300 mg. All dogs had an individually tailored behavior management program, and trazodone was added to other behavior-modifying drugs.

Body weight	Initial dose (total; NOT mg/kg) range	Target dose (total; NOT mg/kg)range
<10 kg (22 lb)	≤25 mg every 8-24 hours	≤50 mg every 8-24 hours
≥10-20 kg (22-44 lb)	50 mg every 12-24 hours	100 mg every 8-24 hours
≥20-40 kg (44-88 lb)	100 mg every 12-24 hours	200 mg every 8-24 hours
>40 kg (88 lb)	100 mg every 12-24 hours	200 – 300 mg every 8-24 hours

b) 2 – 10 mg/kg PO up to every 8 hours is recommended for daily modification of anxiety when the dog is at home in a low-stress situation and when sedation is undesired

c) Trazodone can be given as needed in addition to daily (or routine) use of another/different serotonergic agent (eg, clomipramine, fluoxetine). It is given ≈1 hour prior to the onset of anxiety, with a typical starting dose between 2 and 5 mg/kg and adjusting upward as necessary to get control (maximum dose, 14 mg/kg/day).[18] Because of the wide interpatient variability in metabolism of trazodone, test doses are recommended (when possible) to determine the time to onset of antianxiety effect before implementing its use for an expected/known anxiety-producing event.

Anxiolytic prior to veterinary visits (extra-label):

a) **As a single agent administered at least 90 minutes prior to travel**: 5 – 7.5 mg/kg PO[5] as needed up to 19.5 mg/kg PO daily[1] in aggressive dogs or those with high fear/anxiety/stress. 9 – 12 mg/kg PO also has been used.[19] The maximum recommendation is 300 mg/dose.[20] **NOTE**: Sedation may occur at the high end of the dose, which may be acceptable and preferred with high-anxiety situations (eg, transportation, hospitalization). In dogs with high fear/anxiety/stress or aggression, the same dose should also be administered the night before travel.

b) **In combination with gabapentin**: Trazodone 5 mg/kg PO in combination with gabapentin 10 mg/kg PO administered 2 hours prior to veterinary visits[21]

c) **As an adjunct to the Chill Protocol** (anecdotal):

i. <u>Replace</u> gabapentin with trazodone 5 – 10 mg/kg PO and administer the evening before the hospital visit and the morning of the hospital visit at least 2 hours prior to travel. Administer melatonin (small dogs, 0.5 – 1 mg PO; medium dogs, 1 – 3 mg PO; large dogs, 5 mg PO) with the morning dose of trazodone; administer acepromazine 0.025 – 0.05 mg/kg OTM 30 minutes before travel.

ii. Trazodone may be <u>added</u> to the Chill Protocol for dogs that do not experience adequate sedation or anxiolysis with the original Chill Protocol: Trazodone 5 – 10 mg/kg PO along with gabapentin 10 – 20 mg/kg PO administered the evening before the hospital visit and the morning of the hospital visit at least 2 hours prior to travel. Administer melatonin (small dogs, 0.5 – 1 mg PO; medium dogs, 1 – 3 mg PO; large dogs, 5 mg PO) with the morning dose of trazodone and gabapentin; administer acepromazine 0.025 to 0.05 mg/kg OTM 30 minutes before travel.

Anxiolytic for postsurgical confinement and stress during hospitalization (extra-label):

a) **As a single agent during hospitalization**: 4 mg/kg PO every 12 hours. Doses can be increased to 10 – 12 mg/kg, or the frequency of administration can be increased to every 8 hours when needed for desired calming and anxiolytic effects. The amount given did not exceed 300 mg/dose or 600 mg/24 hours.[20]

b) **In combination with tramadol**: Trazodone ≈3.5 mg/kg PO every 12 hours in combination with tramadol 4 – 6 mg/kg PO every 8 to 12 hours for the first 3 postoperative days (see ***Drug Interactions***), then tramadol discontinued, and trazodone increased to ≈7 mg/kg PO every 12 hours for at least 4 weeks.[3] A separate pharmacokinetic and hemodynamic study concluded that trazodone might be most useful in patients after surgery following complete recovery from anesthesia. In this study, trazodone doses of 8 mg/kg PO were well tolerated, but because of substantial variability in time to maximum plasma concentrations, individualized approaches to dose intervals may be necessary. At the authors' institution, trazodone treatment is instituted 12 to 24 hours after surgery for anxious patients, and clinicians often prescribe trazodone for a treatment duration of weeks to months for surgical patients to facilitate cage rest and activity restriction, particularly following orthopedic procedures. Further studies are warranted.[14]

CATS:

Anxiolytic prior to veterinary visits (extra-label):

a) **As a single agent administered at least 90 minutes prior to travel**: In a placebo-controlled study of 10 client-owned cats with a history of signs of anxiety during transport and/or veterinary examination, trazodone 50 mg/cat (NOT mg/kg) PO (equals 10.9 mg/kg based on average body weight [range, 7.7 – 15.2 mg/kg]) was given 60 to 90 minutes prior to a veterinary visit. No cat in the trazodone group displayed any signs of transportation- or examination-related anxiety, and stress scores and ease of examination were significantly better in cats treated with trazodone as compared with those receiving a placebo. Vocalization was common in both groups prior to transportation to the clinic and became less intense after trazodone administration.[11] A higher trazodone dose (100 mg/cat [NOT mg/kg] PO, ≈20 – 33 mg/kg) given to purpose-bred cats caused sedation and decreased activity level 2 hours after administration but did not improve behavioral response to physical examination.[9]

b) **In combination with gabapentin**: Trazodone 5 mg/kg PO in combination with gabapentin 10 mg/kg PO administered 2 hours prior to veterinary visits[21]

HORSES:

Facilitation of stall rest and treatment of abnormal behaviors (extra-label): 2.5 mg/kg PO once daily to 10 mg/kg PO twice daily depending on clinical reponse.[22] Duration of treatment lasted from 1 to 70 days.

Monitoring

- Clinical efficacy and adverse effects

Client Information

- Trazodone is used in dogs to treat anxiety-related conditions, including thunderstorms or firework phobias. The use of a combination of trazodone with other medications is common to help reduce anxiety.
- This medicine is also used when activity restriction (eg, cage rest) is needed after surgery.
- Trazodone may be given with food or on an empty stomach. If the animal vomits or acts sick after receiving trazodone on an empty stomach, give the medicine with a small amount of food or a small treat. It is important to contact your veterinarian if vomiting continues.
- Full calming effect may take up to 2 weeks of routine use, especially when trazodone is used alone.
- The most common side effects are sleepiness and decreased activity. Call your veterinarian if you observe shivering, dilated pupils, or agitation.
- Caution is advised when giving trazodone to working/service dogs, as they may be unable to perform their duties while on this medication.
- With chronic use, withdrawal signs may occur if the daily dose is not gradually reduced. Do not discontinue this medicine without first speaking with your veterinarian.

Chemistry/Synonyms

Trazodone is a triazolopyridine antidepressant agent. It occurs as an odorless, white to off-white crystalline powder and is sparingly soluble in water, alcohol, or chloroform. Trazodone tablets contain trazodone hydrochloride.

Trazodone may also be known as AF-1161, trazodona, trazodon, or sleepeasy. A common trade name is *Desyrel*®.

Storage/Stability

Store trazodone between 20°C and 25°C (68°F-77°F); excursions at 15°C to 30°C (59°F-86°F). Keep the medication in an airtight container and protect it from light.

Compatibility/Compounding Considerations

No specific information was noted.

Dosage Forms/Regulatory Status

VETERINARY-LABELED PRODUCTS: NONE

The Association of Racing Commissioners International (ARCI) has designated this drug as a class 2 substance. Use of this drug may not be allowed in certain animal competitions. Check rules and regulations before entering a competition while this medication is being administered. Contact local racing authorities for further guidance. See ***Appendix*** for more information.

HUMAN-LABELED PRODUCTS:

Trazodone Oral Tablets: 50 mg, 100 mg, 150 mg, and 300 mg; generic; (Rx)

References

For the complete list of references, see **wiley.com/go/budde/plumb**

Triamcinolone

Triamcinolone Acetonide

(trye-am-***sin***-oh-lone) *Vetalog*®

Glucocorticoid

Prescriber Highlights

- ► Oral, parenteral, topical, and inhaled glucocorticoid that is 4 to 10 times (some say up to 40 times) more potent than hydrocortisone; no appreciable mineralocorticoid activity. Commonly used for intra-articular injection (especially in horses)
- ► Contraindications include systemic fungal infections, viral infections, animals with arrested tuberculosis, peptic ulcer, corneal ulcer, or hyperadrenocorticism.
- ► Use cautiously in the presence of diabetes, osteoporosis, predisposition to thrombophlebitis, hypertension, CHF, renal insufficiency, and active tuberculosis.
- ► If using systemically, the goal is to use as little as possible for as short a time as possible.
- ► Primary adverse effects with sustained use are cushingoid in nature (eg, polyuria, polydipsia, polyphagia, muscle wasting, osteoporosis).
- ► Many potential drug and laboratory interactions

Uses/Indications

Labeled indications include the treatment of inflammation and related disorders in dogs, cats, and horses; and management and treatment of acute arthritis, and allergic and dermatologic disorders in dogs and cats.[1,2]

Although glucocorticoids have been used to treat many conditions in humans and animals, triamcinolone has 4 primary uses with accompanying dosage ranges: 1) replacement or supplementation (eg, relative adrenal insufficiency associated with septic shock) for glucocorticoid deficiency secondary to hypoadrenocorticism; 2) anti-inflammatory agent; 3) immunosuppression, and 4) antineoplastic agent. High-dose use is not supported for hemorrhagic or hypovolemic shock, head trauma, spinal cord trauma[3], or sepsis. In general, when administering glucocorticoids, the following principles should be followed:

- A specific diagnosis is needed before glucocorticoids are administered as they can mask disease.
- A course of treatment should be determined prior to treatment.
- A therapeutic endpoint should be determined prior to treatment.
- The least potent glucocorticoid should be used at the lowest dose for a minimal amount of time.
- It is important to understand when glucocorticoid use is inappropriate (eg, acute infection, diabetes).[4]

See ***Glucocorticoid Agents, General Information.***

In working dogs with naturally occurring hip osteoarthritis, intra-articular (IA) injection of triamcinolone with hyaluronic acid into the hip joint reduced pain scores for up to 5 months.[5]

In horses, combining triamcinolone with a local anesthetic (eg, mepivacaine) has been shown to not alter the potency or duration of action of triamcinolone IA injections and may be useful to both confirm the joint causing lameness and to reduce synovitis.[6] In healthy horses, IA triamcinolone acetonide diffused directly from the distal interphalangeal joint with or without hyaluronic acid and may prove to be useful in treating navicular syndrome, but further studies are needed.[7] However, more lame horses receiving IA triamcinolone injection achieved clinical success 3 weeks after treatment than horses receiving the IA combination of triamcinolone and hyaluronate.[8] Triamcinolone given IM improves lung function in horses with severe equine asthma for up to 28 days.[9]

Intralesional injection of triamcinolone into esophageal[10,11] and rectal[12] strictures has been done in dogs and cats prior to dilation in an attempt to prolong the time needed between dilation procedures; more studies are needed to make specific recommendations for this use.[11]

Pharmacology/Actions

Triamcinolone acetonide is considered an intermediate-acting (metabolic activity of 24 to 48 hours when given orally) glucocorticoid that is ≈4 to 10 times more potent than hydrocortisone. Triamcinolone has negligible mineralocorticoid effects. When injected IM, duration of activity may persist for 4 to 6 (and sometimes up to 8) weeks. A study in cats with allergic pruritus found triamcinolone to be ≈7 times more potent than methylprednisolone.[13]

Intra-articular injection can reduce articular protein, inflammatory cell infiltration, intimal hyperplasia, and subintimal fibrosis, and increase synovial levels of hyaluronan and glycosaminoglycan.

Glucocorticoids have effects on virtually every cell type and system in mammals. For more information, refer to ***Glucocorticoid Agents, General Information***.

Pharmacokinetics

Like other corticosteroids, plasma concentrations are not a good indicator of biologic activity. A pharmacokinetic study to establish appropriate withdrawal times in thoroughbred horses after IM or intra-articular (IA) injection found: a plasma terminal elimination half-life of 11.4 (± 6.53) days for IM and 0.78 (±1) days for IA administration. Concentrations were below the limit of detection after IM injection by days 52 (plasma) and 60 (urine), and after IA injection by day 7 (plasma) and day 8 (urine). Triamcinolone acetonide was also undetectable in any of the joints sampled following IM administration and remained above the limit of quantitation for 21 days following IA administration.[14]

IA administration to horses results in systemic effects, including suppression of cortisol for up to 4 days following administration,[15] and improvement of lung function in horses with severe asthma.[9]

Contraindications/Precautions/Warnings

Triamcinolone is contraindicated in patients that are hypersensitive to it. Systemic use of glucocorticoids is generally considered contraindicated in viral or systemic fungal infections (unless used for replacement therapy in hypoadrenocorticism), in animals with tuberculosis, chronic nephritis, or hyperadrenocorticism when administered IM in patients with idiopathic thrombocytopenia. Sustained-release injectable glucocorticoid use is considered contraindicated for chronic corticosteroid treatment of systemic diseases.

Relative contraindications include the presence of diabetes mellitus, osteoporosis, or CHF. Corticosteroids should not be used to alleviate inflammation or pain caused by infections. Corticosteroids may mask signs of infection (eg, fever).

Patients that have received corticosteroids chronically should be tapered off slowly as endogenous ACTH and corticosteroid function may return slowly. If the animal undergoes a stressful event (eg, surgery, trauma, illness) during the tapering process or until normal adrenal and pituitary function resume, additional glucocorticoids should be administered.

Aseptic preparation of the injection site should precede all intra-articular (IA) injections. Inadvertent administration into adjacent soft tissue is the most common reason for inadequate response after IA injection.[1] IA injections given to horses with undiagnosed asthma may mask clinical signs related to asthma and delay diagnosis.[9]

Triamcinolone induced rapid death of mesenchymal stem cells (MSC) in an in vitro cell culture,[16] and the authors concluded that concomitant use of corticosteroids is likely to have a detrimental effect on cell viability during MSC treatment.

Adverse Effects

Adverse effects are generally associated with long-term administration of these drugs, especially if the drugs are administered at high doses or not on an alternate-day regimen. Effects typically manifest as clinical signs of hyperadrenocorticism. Glucocorticoids can delay growth when administered to young, growing animals. A list of potential effects is outlined in ***Glucocorticoid Agents, General Information***.

In dogs, polyuria (PU), polydipsia (PD), and polyphagia (PP) may occur during short-term burst therapy and on days when the drug is administered during alternate-day maintenance therapy. Other adverse effects in dogs receiving triamcinolone chronically can include dull/dry coat, weight gain, panting, vomiting, diarrhea, increased liver enzymes, GI ulceration (especially with high parenteral or oral dosages), hypercoagulability, hyperlipidemia, activation or worsening of diabetes mellitus, muscle wasting, and/or behavior changes (eg, depression, lethargy, aggression). Discontinuation of the drug may be necessary; changing to an alternate steroid may also alleviate adverse effects. Adverse effects associated with anti-inflammatory treatment are relatively uncommon, with the exception of PU, PD, and PP. Adverse effects associated with immunosuppressive dosages are more common and potentially more severe.

Glucocorticoids appear to have a greater hyperglycemic effect in cats than other species. Occasionally, PU, PD, and PP with weight gain, diarrhea, and/or depression will be present. Long-term, high-dose treatment can lead to cushingoid effects.

In horses, the potential for dexamethasone or triamcinolone playing a contributory role in the development of laminitis has been a traditional concern; however, a large, retrospective observational cohort study of horses found that intrasynovial triamcinolone administration did not increase the risk of laminitis.[17] Also there is no evidence that intra-articular corticosteroids cause harm to subchondral bone or promote catastrophic injury.[18] Another review article on this subject states:

Although the association of laminitis with elevated serum cortisol in pituitary pars intermedia dysfunction suggests that chronic exposure to glucocorticoids may be part of laminitis pathogenesis, review of published reports and databases suggests that glucocorticoid-induced laminitis is a relatively rare occurrence. . . . Generally, local glucocorticoid administration presents little risk as does systemic treatment of recurrent airway obstruction without concurrent disease. Caution should be used however in horses that are overweight and/or insulin resistant, or have had a recent bout of acute laminitis of alimentary or endotoxic origin.[19]

Reproductive/Nursing Safety

Endogenous glucocorticoids are likely necessary for normal fetal development. They may be required for adequate surfactant production and development of myelin, retinal tissue, the pancreas, and mammary tissue.

Glucocorticoids administered to pregnant dogs have resulted in congenital abnormalities, including deformed forelegs, phocomelia, and anasarca. Additionally, cleft palate has been reported in dogs, rabbits, and rodents. Systemic glucocorticoids administered to animals may induce the first stage of parturition when used during the last trimester of pregnancy and may precipitate premature parturition followed by dystocia, fetal death, retained placenta, and metritis.

Corticosteroids appear in milk and could suppress growth, interfere with endogenous corticosteroid production, or cause other unwanted effects in the nursing offspring. Use with caution in nursing dams.

Overdose/Acute Toxicity

Glucocorticoids, when given short term, are unlikely to cause harmful effects, even in massive doses. If clinical signs occur, use supportive treatment if required.

For patients that have experienced or are suspected to have experienced an overdose, consultation with a 24-hour poison consultation center specializing in providing veterinary-specific information is recommended. For general information related to overdose and toxin exposures, as well as contact information for poison control centers, refer to ***Appendix.***

Drug Interactions

The following drug interactions have either been reported or are theoretical in humans or animals receiving triamcinolone systemically and may be of significance in veterinary patients. Unless otherwise noted, use together is not necessarily contraindicated, but weigh the potential risks and perform additional monitoring when appropriate.

- **Amphotericin B**: When administered concomitantly with glucocorticoids, may cause hypokalemia
- **Anesthetics, Local** (eg, **epidural injections**): Combination with glucocorticoids in epidurals has caused serious CNS injuries and death.
- **Anticholinesterase Agents** (eg, **pyridostigmine, neostigmine**): In patients with myasthenia gravis, concomitant glucocorticoid and anticholinesterase agent administration may lead to profound muscle weakness. If possible, discontinue anticholinesterase medication at least 24 hours prior to corticosteroid administration.
- **Azole Antifungals** (eg, **itraconazole, ketoconazole**): May decrease the metabolism of glucocorticoids and increase triamcinolone blood concentrations; ketoconazole may induce adrenal insufficiency when glucocorticoids are withdrawn by inhibiting adrenal corticosteroid synthesis.
- **Cyclophosphamide**: Glucocorticoids may also inhibit the hepatic metabolism of cyclophosphamide; dosage adjustments may be required.
- **Cyclosporine**: Concomitant administration of glucocorticoids and cyclosporine may increase the blood concentrations of each, by mutually inhibiting the hepatic metabolism of each other; the clinical significance of this interaction is not clear.
- **Digoxin**: Secondary to hypokalemia, increased risk for arrhythmias
- **Diuretics, Potassium-Depleting** (eg, **furosemide, thiazides**): Administered concomitantly with glucocorticoids may cause hypokalemia
- **Ephedrine**: May increase metabolism of glucocorticoids
- **Estrogens** (eg, **DES, estriol**): The effects of triamcinolone, and possibly other glucocorticoids, may be potentiated by concomitant administration with estrogens.
- **Insulin**: Insulin requirements may increase in patients receiving glucocorticoids.
- **Isoniazid**: Triamcinolone may decrease isoniazid concentrations.
- **Macrolide Antibiotics** (eg, **clarithromycin, erythromycin**): May increase triamcinolone concentrations
- **Mitotane**: May alter the metabolism of steroids; higher than usual doses of steroids may be necessary to treat mitotane-induced adrenal insufficiency
- **Nonsteroidal Anti-Inflammatory Drugs** (eg, **carprofen, flunixin, meloxicam, phenylbutazone**): Administration of ulcerogenic drugs with glucocorticoids may increase the risk for GI ulceration.
- **Opioids** (eg, **morphine**): Combination with glucocorticoids in epidurals has caused serious CNS injuries and death.
- **Phenobarbital**: May increase the metabolism of glucocorticoids and decrease triamcinolone blood concentrations
- **Rifampin**: May increase the metabolism of glucocorticoids and decrease triamcinolone blood concentration
- **Salicylates** (eg, **aspirin, bismuth subsalicylate**): Glucocorticoids may reduce salicylate blood concentrations.
- **Vaccines, Modified Live**: Patients receiving corticosteroids at immunosuppressive dosages should generally not receive live attenuated-virus vaccines as virus replication may be augmented; a diminished immune response may occur after vaccine, toxoid, or bacterin administration in patients receiving glucocorticoids.
- **Warfarin**: Triamcinolone may affect clotting times; monitor.

Laboratory Considerations

- Glucocorticoids may increase **serum cholesterol**.
- Glucocorticoids may increase **serum and urine glucose** concentrations.
- Glucocorticoids may decrease **serum potassium**.
- Glucocorticoids can suppress the release of thyroid stimulating hormone (TSH) and reduce T_3 and T_4 values. Thyroid gland atrophy has been reported after chronic glucocorticoid administration. Uptake of I^{131} by the thyroid may be decreased by glucocorticoids.
- Reactions to **skin tests** may be suppressed by glucocorticoids.
- False negative results of the **nitroblue tetrazolium** test for systemic bacterial infections may be induced by glucocorticoids.
- Glucocorticoids may cause **neutrophilia** within 4 to 8 hours after dosing with return to baseline within 24 to 48 hours after drug discontinuation.
- Glucocorticoids can cause **lymphopenia**, which can persist for weeks after drug discontinuation in dogs.

Dosages

NOTE: When used systemically (PO, IM, or SC), initial doses of triamcinolone acetonide can be given at dosages that are ≈7 to 8 times lower than the prednis(ol)one dosage. For example: If the dosage of prednisone for the indication to be treated is 1 mg/kg PO, a corresponding dosage of triamcinolone acetonide would be ≈0.125 mg/kg PO. Triamcinolone has negligible mineralocorticoid effects, and its biologic activity may persist for 36 to 48 hours. If given on a daily basis, treatment for longer than 1 to 2 weeks will suppress the HPA axis and recovery will take longer than 1 week. Therefore, if triamcinolone is used for longer than a few days, when discontinuing, dosage should be tapered off using alternate-day, then every-third-day therapy.

DOGS/CATS:

Glucocorticoid effects (label dosage; FDA-approved):

a. **Using tablets**: 0.11 mg/kg PO initially once daily, may increase to 0.22 mg/kg PO once daily if initial response is unsatisfactory. As soon as possible, but not later than 2 weeks, reduce dosage gradually to 0.028 – 0.055 mg/kg/day.[20]
b. **Injectable product**: 0.11 – 0.22 mg/kg IM or SC for inflammatory or allergic disorders, and 0.22 mg/kg IM or SC for dermatologic disorders.[1] Effects generally persist for 7 to 15 days; if clinical signs recur, may repeat or institute oral therapy.
c. **Intralesional injection**: 1.2 – 1.8 mg/lesion (total dose; NOT mg/kg) is divided in several injections around the lesion at 0.5 to 2.5 cm intervals; administer well into the cutis.[1] When injecting, do not exceed 0.6 mg at any one site or a total dose of 6 mg when treating multiple lesions. May repeat after 3 or 4 days if indicated.
d. **Intra-articular (IA) and intrasynovial injection**: Dose for IA or intrasynovial administration is dependent on the size of the joint to be treated and on the severity of clinical signs. A single injection of 1 – 3 mg/dog (NOT mg/kg) IA.[1] After 3 to 4 days, dose may be repeated, depending on the severity of clinical signs and the clinical response. If initial results are inadequate or too transient, dose may be increased, but the recommended dose should not be exceeded. Routine aseptic preparation of

the area should be made prior to all IA injections. A thorough understanding of the pertinent anatomic relationships is essential. The inadvertent administration of the corticosteroid into the soft tissues surrounding a joint is not harmful but is the most common cause of failure to achieve the desired local results.

Anti-inflammatory agent (extra-label):

a) **Induction**: 0.05 – 0.22 mg/kg PO once daily. Maintenance: 0.05 – 0.1 mg/kg (or lower if possible) PO every 48 to 72 hours. Taper dose slowly if discontinuing.
b) **Adjunctive treatment of pruritus in allergic cats**: Initial induction dosage was 0.5 mg/cat (NOT mg/kg) PO once daily for cats weighing less than or equal to 5 kg (11 lb), and 0.75 mg/cat (NOT mg/kg) PO once daily for cats more than 5 kg (11 lb). Cats that did not achieve remission by day 7 had their once-daily induction dose doubled for the next 7 days. Mean dosage required for induction of remission was 0.18 mg/kg (range 0.09 – 0.26 mg/kg) PO once daily; 94% of treated cats achieved remission by the end of the second week. Dosages used to achieve remission were then given every other day and tapered (from 100% to 25% of induction dose in 25% increments) to the lowest every other day dosage that maintained remission. Mean alternate-day dosages were 0.08 mg/kg.[13]
c) **Canine hip osteoarthritis**: 0.2 mg/kg IA into the affected hip joint(s).[21] Alternatively, 20 mg/joint (NOT mg/kg) IA.[5] For both dosing options, administer IA triamcinolone injection in combination with 1 to 2 mL of hyaluronic acid IA.

Immunosuppressive agent (extra-label):

a) **Autoimmune skin diseases**: Induction: 0.4 – 0.6 mg/kg PO once daily. Maintenance: 0.1 – 0.2 mg/kg PO every 48 to 72 hours[22]
b) **Feline pemphigus foliaceus**: Induction: 0.6 – 2 mg/kg PO once daily. Maintenance: 0.6 – 1 mg/kg PO every 2 to 7 days. Cats receiving triamcinolone had significantly fewer adverse effects than cats receiving prednisolone and chlorambucil.[23]

Intralesional injection (extra-label):

a) **Preventing re-stricture after esophageal dilation**:
   i. Using an endoscopically directed needle, triamcinolone 2 – 10 mg (total dose; NOT mg/kg) is divided and injected submucosally into each of 4 quadrants (≈0.5 – 2.5 mg/quadrant), placed circumferentially around the stricture site *before* the balloon dilation procedure.[24–26]
   ii. Dilute triamcinolone 40 mg (total dose; NOT mg/kg) 1:1 with 0.9% sodium chloride and divide solution to inject submucosally into 4 quadrants (≈10 mg/quadrant), placed circumferentially around the stricture site *before* the balloon dilation procedure.[10]
b) **Preventing re-stricture after rectal dilation in dogs**: 5 – 10 mg (total dose; NOT mg/kg) divided and injected submucosally into 4 quadrants, placed circumferentially around the stricture site *before* the balloon dilation procedure[27]
c) **Preventing re-stricture after rectal dilation in cats**: 0.8 mg (total dose; NOT mg/kg) was injected submucosally into each of 4 quadrants, placed circumferentially around the stricture site *before* the balloon dilation procedure[12]
d) **Mast cell tumors**: 1 – 2 mg triamcinolone per cm of tumor length based on the longest tumor dimension. Treatment interval varied from weekly doses (20%), one-time doses (40%), or clinician's discretion (40%).[28]
e) **Ciliary body ablation for chronic glaucoma in dogs**: Triamcinolone 1 – 2 mg (total dose; NOT mg/kg) in combination with gentamicin 30 – 50 mg (total dose; NOT mg/kg) administered intravitreally[29]

HORSES:

Inflammation and related disorders (label dosage; FDA-approved):

a) **Oral**: 0.011 – 0.022 mg/kg PO twice daily[30]
b) **Injection**: 0.022 – 0.044 mg/kg IM or SC; usual dose, 12 – 20 mg/horse (NOT mg/kg)[1]
c) **Intra-articularly or intrasynovially**: 6 – 18 mg/joint (NOT mg/kg) IA, depending on the joint size and severity of inflammation. Do not exceed 18 mg/dose. May repeat after 3 or 4 days if indicated.[1]

Noninfectious synovitis or/and osteoarthritis (extra-label): 12 mg/horse (NOT mg/kg) as a single IA injection[8]

Severe equine asthma exacerbation (extra-label): 40 mg/horse (NOT mg/kg) IM improved lung function for 28 days[9]

Equine recurrent uveitis (extra-label): 5 mg/eye (NOT mg/kg) injected into the suprachoroidal space for horses that have responded poorly to other treatments[31]

Monitoring

Monitoring of glucocorticoid therapy is dependent on its reason for use, dosage, agent used (amount of mineralocorticoid activity), dosing schedule (daily vs alternate-day therapy), route of administration, duration of therapy, and the animal's age and condition. The following list may not be appropriate or complete for all animals; use clinical assessment and judgment should adverse effects be noted:

- Weight, appetite, signs of fluid retention
- Serum and/or urine electrolytes
- Total plasma proteins and albumin
- Blood glucose
- Urine culture
- Growth and development in young animals

Client Information

- Give oral products with food.
- The goal of treatment is to find the lowest dose possible and use it for the shortest period of time. Follow your veterinarian's instructions on how to give this medicine.
- Many side effects are possible, especially when used long term or when given in higher doses. The most common side effects are increased appetite, thirst, and need to urinate.
- In dogs, stomach or intestinal ulcers, perforation, or bleeding can occur while taking this medicine. Contact your veterinarian right away if your animal stops eating or if you notice a high fever, black tarry stools, or bloody vomit (will look like coffee grounds).
- Do not stop treatment abruptly without your veterinarian's guidance, as serious side effects could occur.
- Be sure to tell your veterinarian what other medication (including vitamins, supplements, or herbal therapies) you give your animal.

Chemistry/Synonyms

Triamcinolone acetonide, a synthetic glucocorticoid, occurs as a slightly odorous, white to cream-colored, crystalline powder with a melting point between 290°C and 294°C (554°F-561°F). It is practically insoluble in water, very soluble in dehydrated alcohol and slightly soluble in alcohol.

The commercially available sterile suspensions have a pH range of 5 to 7.5.

Triamcinolone acetonide may also be known as triamcinoloni acetonidum; many trade names are available.

Storage/Stability

Triamcinolone acetonide products should be stored at room temperature (15°C-30°C [59°F-86°F]). The injection should be stored upright inside the manufacturer's carton, protected from light and freezing.

Compatibility/Compounding Considerations

No specific information was noted.

Dosage Forms/Regulatory Status

VETERINARY-LABELED PRODUCTS:

The Association of Racing Commissioners International (ARCI) has designated this drug as a class 4 substance. See ***Appendix*** for more information. Use of this drug may not be allowed in certain animal competitions. Check rules and regulations before entering in a competition while this medication is being administered. Contact local racing authorities for further guidance.

Triamcinolone Acetonide Tablets: 0.5 mg and 1.5 mg; *Vetalog®*, generic; (Rx). FDA-approved for use in dogs and cats

Triamcinolone Acetonide Suspension for Injection: 2 mg/mL in 25 mL and 100 mL vials; 6 mg/mL in 3 mL, 5 mL and 25 mL vials; *Vetalog® Parenteral*; (Rx). FDA-approved for use in dogs, cats, and horses not intended for food

Triamcinolone Acetonide Oral Powder: 15 g of powder contains 10 mg of triamcinolone acetonide; *Vetalog®* Oral Powder; (Rx). FDA-approved for use in horses. Product is listed in the FDA Green Book but does not appear to be commercially available.

Triamcinolone is available as a topical spray, and in combination with other agents as a topical cream or ointment.

HUMAN-LABELED PRODUCTS:

Triamcinolone Acetonide Injection: 10 mg/mL and 40 mg/mL suspension in 1 mL, 5 mL, and 10 mL vials; *Kenalog®-10* and *-40*; (Rx)

Many topical preparations are available, alone and in combination with other agents. Oral mucosal paste and inhaled products are also FDA-approved. All are Rx.

References

For the complete list of references, see **wiley.com/go/budde/plumb**

Triamterene

(trye-***am***-te-reen) *Dyrenium®*

Potassium-Sparing Diuretic

Prescriber Highlights

- May be considered as an alternative to spironolactone for adjunctive treatment of CHF in dogs
- Rarely used in veterinary medicine; limited clinical experience in dogs and cats
- Contraindications include anuria, severe or progressive renal disease, severe hepatic disease, hypersensitivity to triamterene, or pre-existing hyperkalemia. Triamterene should not be used with other potassium-sparing agents (spironolactone, amiloride) or potassium supplements.
- Most common adverse effect is hyperkalemia; monitoring serum potassium is required.

Uses/Indications

Triamterene is a potassium-sparing diuretic that may be considered as an alternative to spironolactone for the adjunctive treatment of congestive heart failure in dogs; however, there is little experience associated with its use in dogs or cats and it is rarely recommended.

Pharmacology/Actions

By exerting a direct effect on the distal renal tubule, triamterene inhibits the reabsorption of sodium in exchange for hydrogen and potassium ions. It is a relatively weak diuretic since only ≈2% to 3% of filtered sodium is resorbed in the terminal portion of the distal tubule. Unlike spironolactone, it does not competitively inhibit aldosterone. Triamterene increases renal excretion of sodium, calcium, magnesium, and bicarbonate; urine pH may be slightly increased. Serum concentrations of potassium and chloride may be increased. When used alone, triamterene has little effect on blood pressure. Triamterene can reduce GFR slightly, probably by affecting renal blood flow; this effect is reversible when the medication is discontinued.

Pharmacokinetics

Pharmacokinetic data for dogs or cats were not located. In humans, triamterene is rapidly absorbed after oral administration and oral bioavailability is ≈85%. Onset of diuresis occurs in 2 to 4 hours, peaks at ≈6 hours and diuresis can persist up to 12 to 16 hours post-dose. Triamterene is metabolized in the liver to 6-p-hydroxytriamterine and its sulfate conjugate. These metabolites are eliminated in the bile/feces and urine; elimination half-life is ≈2 hours.

Contraindications/Precautions/Warnings

Triamterene is contraindicated for human patients (and presumably dogs and cats) with anuria, severe or progressive renal disease, severe hepatic disease, hypersensitivity to triamterene, pre-existing hyperkalemia, or history of triamterene-induced hyperkalemia. Concurrent therapy with another potassium-sparing agent (spironolactone, amiloride) or potassium supplementation is also contraindicated.

In humans, hyperkalemia from potassium-sparing agents such as triamterene is more likely in patients with renal impairment and diabetes, and in elderly or severely ill patients.[1]

Adverse Effects

Because triamterene has been infrequently used in veterinary medicine, an accurate adverse effect profile for small animal species is not known. Hyperkalemia is possible and monitoring of electrolytes and renal function are necessary. In humans, hyperkalemia rarely occurs in patients with normal urine output and potassium intake.

Less common adverse effects reported in humans include headache, dizziness, GI effects (eg, nausea, vomiting, diarrhea), azotemia, hyponatremia, and an increased sensitivity to sunlight. Rarely, hypersensitivity reactions have occurred in human patients taking triamterene.[1] Other rare adverse effects include triamterene-nephrolithiasis, liver enzyme abnormalities, agranulocytosis, nephrotoxicity, thrombocytopenia, or megaloblastosis.

Reproductive/Nursing Safety

Studies to determine triamterene's effects on fertility in human have not been performed; however, studies in pregnant rats given triamterene at 6 to 20 times the human dose did not show adverse effects to the fetuses.[1] Triamterene crosses the placental barrier.

Triamterene is distributed into milk. Although unlikely to pose much risk to nursing animals, safety during nursing cannot be assured.

Because safety has not been established in animals, this drug should only be used when the maternal benefits outweigh the potential risks to offspring.

Overdose/Acute Toxicity

The oral LD_{50} for triamterene in mice is 380 mg/kg.[1] Fluid and electrolyte imbalance is the most likely risk associated with an overdose. GI effects or hypotension are also possible. Consider GI decontamination protocols for very large or quantity unknown ingestions. Acute overdoses should generally be managed by observation and supportive treatment with fluid diuresis as well as electrolyte (especially serum potassium) and acid-base monitoring.

For patients that have experienced or are suspected to have experienced an overdose, consultation with a 24-hour poison consultation center specializing in providing veterinary-specific information is recommended. For general information related to overdose and toxin exposures, as well as contact information for poison control centers, refer to ***Appendix***.

Drug Interactions

The following drug interactions have either been reported or are theoretical in humans or animals receiving triamterene and may be of significance in veterinary patients. Unless otherwise noted, use together is not necessarily contraindicated, but weigh the potential risks and perform additional monitoring when appropriate.

- Angiotensin Converting Enzyme Inhibitors (ACEIs; eg, **enalapril, benazepril**): Increased risk for hyperkalemia
- Antidiabetic Agents (eg, **insulin, oral hypoglycemic agents** [eg, **glipizide**]): Triamterene may increase blood glucose levels.
- Antihypertensive Agents: Possible potentiation of hypotensive effects
- Diuretics, Potassium-sparing (eg, **spironolactone, amiloride**): Increase risk for hyperkalemia; use of these drugs with triamterene in humans is contraindicated.
- Lithium: Triamterene may reduce lithium clearance.
- Nonsteroidal Anti-Inflammatory Drugs (NSAIDs): Triamterene with NSAIDs (especially indomethacin) may increase the risks of nephrotoxicity.
- Potassium Supplements or High Potassium Foods: Increased risk for hyperkalemia

Laboratory Considerations

- **Quinidine**: Triamterene may interfere with fluorescent assay of quinidine.

Dosages

DOGS:

Adjunctive treatment of heart failure (extra-label): Anecdotally, 1 – 2 mg/kg PO twice daily or 2 – 4 mg/kg PO daily. Limited published evidence to support use or any dosage; if a potassium-sparing diuretic is used, spironolactone is usually preferred.

Monitoring

- Baseline and periodic serum electrolytes (especially potassium), BUN, creatinine
- Hydration status; patient body weight
- Blood pressure, if indicated
- Signs of edema

Client Information

- Give this medication with food to help prevent stomach upset.
- Your animal's urine may develop a bluish hue while it is taking this medicine. This color change is normal and will go away when the medication is stopped.
- Because this medication has not been used very much in dogs or cats, report any unusual side effects to your veterinarian.

Chemistry/Synonyms

Triamterene is structurally related to folic acid and occurs as a yellow, odorless, crystalline powder. It is practically insoluble in water and very slightly soluble in alcohol. At 50°C, it is slightly soluble in water. In acidified solutions, triamterene gives off a blue fluorescence.

Triamterene may also be known as NSC-77625, KF-8542, FI-6143, triamteren, trimaterenum, triamtereen, or *Dyrenium*®. International trade names include *Dytac*® and *Triteren*®. There are many trade names for combination products with hydrochlorothiazide.

Storage/Stability

Triamterene capsules should be stored between 15-30°C (59-86°F) in tight, light-resistant containers.

Compatibility/Compounding Considerations

No specific information noted

Dosage Forms/Regulatory Status

VETERINARY-LABELED PRODUCTS: NONE

The Association of Racing Commissioners International (ARCI) has designated this drug as a class 4 substance. Use of this drug may not be allowed in certain animal competitions. Check rules and regulations before entering in a competition while this medication is being administered. Contact local racing authorities for further guidance. See ***Appendix***.

HUMAN-LABELED PRODUCTS:

Triamterene Capsules: 50 mg and 100 mg; *Dyrenium*®; (Rx)

In humans, triamterene is often prescribed as a fixed-dose combination with hydrochlorothiazide; many preparations are available.

References

For the complete list of references, see **wiley.com/go/budde/plumb**

Trientine

(***trye***-en-teen) *Syprine*®

Chelating Agent

Prescriber Highlights

- ► Oral copper chelating agent for copper hepatopathy. Limited veterinary experience with this drug
- ► Give on an empty stomach, 1 to 2 hours prior to meals
- ► Likely fewer adverse effects than penicillamine, but acute kidney injury possible
- ► More expensive than penicillamine; not readily available commercially and may need to be compounded into smaller dosages

Uses/Indications

Trientine may be useful for the treatment of copper-associated hepatopathy in dogs,[1] particularly when dogs cannot tolerate the adverse effects (eg, vomiting) associated with penicillamine.

In humans, trientine is indicated for patients with Wilson disease who cannot tolerate penicillamine.

Pharmacology/Actions

Trientine is an effective chelator of copper and increases its elimination via urinary excretion. It apparently has a greater affinity for copper in plasma than penicillamine, but penicillamine has a greater affinity for tissue copper.

Pharmacokinetics

No animal data were located. In humans, trientine is poorly absorbed and then extensively metabolized, primarily by acetylation. The drug and metabolites are excreted in the urine, with an elimination half-life of ≈2 to 4 hours.

Contraindications/Precautions/Warnings

Trientine is contraindicated in patients that are hypersensitive to it. Patients receiving trientine should be closely monitored for evidence of iron deficiency anemia.

In case of skin contact, promptly wash the area with water as contact dermatitis is possible. Capsules should not be opened or chewed.[2]

Adverse Effects

Adverse effects of trientine in dogs treated for copper hepatotoxicity are minimal, but the veterinary experience is limited. Acute kidney injury has been reported, particularly when used in dogs with high liver copper levels and at higher doses.

In humans, nausea may occur, especially at the beginning of therapy.[3] Dystonias, muscle spasms, myasthenia gravis, and iron deficiency anemia have been noted after long-term use. Paradoxical neurologic deterioration has been reported.[4–6]

Reproductive/Nursing Safety

Trientine is a potential teratogen. It was teratogenic in rats that were given doses similar to those for humans.[2]

It is not known whether this drug is excreted in breast milk. Exercise caution when administering to nursing patients.

Because safety has not been established in animals, this drug should only be used when the maternal benefits outweigh the potential risks to offspring.

Overdose/Acute Toxicity

Little information is available; a case of a human ingesting 30 g of trientine without significant morbidity has been reported.

For patients that have experienced or are suspected of having experienced an overdose, consultation with a 24-hour poison consultation center specializing in providing veterinary-specific information is recommended. For general information related to overdose and toxin exposures, as well as contact information for poison control centers, refer to ***Appendix.***

Drug Interactions

The following drug interactions have either been reported or are theoretical in humans or animals receiving trientine and may be of significance in veterinary patients. Unless otherwise noted, use together is not necessarily contraindicated, but weigh the potential risks and perform additional monitoring when appropriate.

- **IRON**: Iron and trientine inhibit the absorption of one another; if iron therapy is needed, give doses at least 2 hours apart from one another.
- **ZINC**: Because trientine may also chelate zinc or other minerals, avoid concomitant therapy (most do not recommend using zinc for copper reduction until copper chelation therapy with penicillamine or trientine is completed) or separate dosages by at least 2 hours.

Dosages

DOGS:

Chelator for copper hepatotoxicity (extra-label): 5 – 7.5 mg/kg PO twice daily.[1] Administer 1 to 2 hours prior to meals. Doses up to 10 – 15 mg/kg PO twice daily have been suggested.[7]

Monitoring

- Periodic liver biopsies for quantitative hepatic copper levels and response to therapy
- Free and total serum copper
- Baseline and periodic renal and hepatic function tests
- Iron status, anemia

Client Information

- It is best to give this medicine 1 to 2 hours before feeding or giving other medications. If your dog vomits after getting it, contact your veterinarian to see if giving it with a small amount of food is okay.
- Trientine may cause skin reactions. Administer as whole capsules. Wash any area that may come in contact with capsule contents.

Chemistry/Synonyms

Trientine HCl, an oral copper chelator, occurs as a white to pale-yellow crystalline powder. It is hygroscopic, freely soluble in water, and slightly soluble in alcohol.

Trientine HCl may also be known as MK-0681, TJA-250, 2,2,2-tetramine, TETA, trien hydrochloride, triethylenetetramine dihydrochloride, trientine hydrochloride, *Metalite*®, or *Syprine*®.

Storage/Stability

Store trientine capsules in the refrigerator at 2°C to 8°C (36°F-46°F) in tightly closed containers.

Compatibility/Compounding Considerations

Trientine may need to be compounded into smaller capsules to give appropriate doses to dogs.

One sources states: *Modification of 2,2,2-tetramine (trientine) to 2,3,2-tetramine increases potency as a copper-chelating agent. Use of 2,3,2-tetramine in affected Bedlington terriers reduced liver copper concentrations significantly after 200 days of treatment at a dose of 15 mg/kg body weight. This drug is not commercially available, but can be obtained from chemical supply companies in the form of N,N'-bis(2-aminoethyl)-1,3-propanediamine and prepared as a salt for oral administration.*[8]

Dosage Forms/Regulatory Status

VETERINARY-LABELED PRODUCTS: NONE

HUMAN-LABELED PRODUCTS:

Trientine HCl Oral Capsules: 250 mg; *Syprine*®, generic; (Rx)

References

For the complete list of references, see **wiley.com/go/budde/plumb**

Trilostane

(***try***-low-stane) *Vetoryl*®

Adrenal Steroid Synthesis Inhibitor

Prescriber Highlights

- ► Reduces the synthesis of cortisol, aldosterone, and adrenal androgens via competitive inhibition of 3-beta hydroxysteroid dehydrogenase
- ► May be useful in dogs for the treatment of pituitary-dependent hyperadrenocorticism (PDH), hyperadrenocorticism caused by adrenocortical tumors when surgery is not an option, and alopecia X; in cats for the treatment of feline PDH; and in horses for the treatment of pituitary pars intermedia dysfunction (PPID)
- ► Treatment goals often include resolution of clinical signs and avoiding oversuppression of the adrenal axis. For safe administration, appropriate rechecks with laboratory testing are required. Ideally, for each individual patient, the timing of trilostane administration and ACTH stimulation testing should remain consistent when monitoring therapy.
- ► A lower, twice-daily regimen appears to be effective and associated with fewer significant adverse effects.
- ► Potential adverse effects in dogs include lethargy, inappetence, vomiting, electrolyte abnormalities, and diarrhea; iatrogenic hypoadrenocorticism and death have been reported.
- ► Give with food for improved bioavailability.
- ► Use of licensed product is recommended; use compounded products with caution.
- ► Do not handle trilostane if pregnant or trying to conceive.

Uses/Indications

Trilostane is approved for the treatment of pituitary-dependent hyperadrenocorticism (PDH) and for the treatment of hyperadrenocorticism (HAC) associated with adrenocortical tumors (AT) in dogs when surgery is not an option. Doses lower than the label-recommended amounts given twice daily appear to be as effective and better tolerated than the labeled dose.[1,2] Trilostane may also be useful in the treatment of alopecia X.[3-5]

Trilostane appears to be a viable, well-tolerated medical treatment option in cats with HAC.[6-8] Trilostane may be useful for the treatment of pituitary pars intermedia dysfunction (PPID) in horses.[9]

Pharmacology/Actions

Trilostane is a competitive inhibitor of 3-beta hydroxysteroid dehydrogenase and reduces synthesis of cortisol, aldosterone, and adrenal androgens. Inhibition is reversible and apparently dose dependent.

In dogs with PDH, cortisol concentrations decreased markedly

2 to 4 hours after trilostane administration. From baseline, significant increases occurred in endogenous adrenocorticotropic hormone (ACTH) concentrations between hours 3 and 12, significant increases in aldosterone concentrations occurred between hours 16 and 20 (not clinically significant), and significant increases in renin activity occurred between hours 6 and 20. Potassium concentrations decreased significantly between hours 0.5 and 2 but were not of clinical significance.[10] Another study in dogs with PDH assessed the effects of mitotane and trilostane on aldosterone secretory reserve and whether the aldosterone concentration correlates with serum electrolyte concentrations. Aldosterone concentrations in the mitotane- and trilostane-treated dogs at 30- and 60-minutes post-ACTH were significantly lower than in clinically healthy dogs, and treated dogs had a greater decrease in aldosterone secretory reserve at 30 minutes than at 60 minutes. No correlation between aldosterone and serum electrolyte concentrations was observed.[11]

Pharmacokinetics

In dogs, orally administered trilostane is rapidly but erratically absorbed, with peak concentrations occurring between 1.5 and 2 hours postadministration. Absorption is enhanced when given with food. Trilostane is metabolized in the liver to several metabolites, including ketotrilostane, which is active. An ex vivo study in canine adrenal glands found that ketotrilostane was 4.9 times and 2.4 times more potent than trilostane in inhibiting cortisol and corticosterone secretion, respectively.[12]

Contraindications/Precautions/Warnings

Trilostane is contraindicated in animals hypersensitive to it. The manufacturer cautions to not use the drug in patients with primary hepatic disease or renal insufficiency. In field studies, treated patients had a statistically significant decrease in RBC parameters (ie, hematocrit, hemoglobin, RBC count) as compared with pretreatment values; however, the posttreatment values remained within the normal range. Although this effect is not commonly reported, monitoring CBC in dogs with underlying anemia should be considered.

Hypoadrenocorticism can develop at any dose and at any time during therapy and does not appear to be dose dependent,[13,14] and although adrenal suppression caused by trilostane is reversible in most cases, adrenal necrosis and death have rarely occurred in dogs.[2,14] **Owners should be warned about this life-threatening complication**, counseled on the clinical signs of an Addisonian crisis, and, if there is any suspicion of an Addisonian crisis, instructed to discontinue trilostane therapy, administer glucocorticoids, and seek veterinary care immediately. Owners should always be provided a small supply of predniso(lo)ne or dexamethasone tablets when trilostane is prescribed in order to initiate emergency treatment for a possible Addisonian crisis. Dexamethasone is the preferred corticosteroid for treatment, as it will not interfere with the ACTH stimulation test. If prednisone or prednisolone are used, an ACTH stimulation test cannot be accurately performed for at least 24 hours after administration because of cross-reactivity of these drugs in cortisol assays.

When used to control clinical signs of HAC in dogs with adrenal tumors, trilostane does not shrink tumors, and adrenal glands may increase in size during treatment. Treatment with trilostane may not reduce the risk for HAC-induced pancreatitis.[15] HAC may mask signs of osteoarthritis or atopic dermatitis, and signs of these conditions may emerge during trilostane treatment as endogenous cortisol concentration decreases.

During periods of stress (eg, boarding, surgery), animals treated with trilostane may require short-term exogenous corticosteroid (see ***Dexamethasone, Prednisolone/Prednisone***) supplementation.

Do not handle trilostane if pregnant or trying to conceive.[16] Trilostane has been associated with teratogenic effects and early pregnancy loss in laboratory animals.

Adverse Effects

Trilostane appears to be relatively well tolerated in dogs, but dogs can develop lethargy, mild electrolyte abnormalities (eg, hyponatremia, hyperkalemia), vomiting, diarrhea, and inappetence during the first few days of therapy secondary to steroid withdrawal.[17] These effects are usually mild and self-limiting; however, signs cannot be attributed to drug intolerance alone and could be indicative of hypoadrenocorticism.

In cats with HAC, adverse effects associated with trilostane therapy have included lethargy, anorexia, and dulled mentation.

No adverse effects were noted in a study of trilostane given to 20 horses with equine PPID.[18]

Reproductive/Nursing Safety

Trilostane is contraindicated during pregnancy. The drug can significantly reduce the synthesis of progesterone in vivo and is associated with teratogenic effects and early pregnancy loss in laboratory animals.[16] Safe use has not been evaluated in male dogs intended for breeding.

Because safety has not been established in lactating animals, this drug should only be used when the maternal benefits outweigh the potential fetal risks.

Overdose/Acute Toxicity

Death occurred in 50% of healthy beagles administered 20.1 to 33.5 mg/kg PO twice daily for 90 days.[16] If clinical signs of hypoadrenocorticism are present, treatment with corticosteroids, mineralocorticoids, and IV fluids may be required; blood pressure, hydration status, and electrolyte balance should be monitored. Because the drug's effects are relatively short, monitoring of patients without complications should only be required for a few days after ingestion.

For patients that have experienced or are suspected to have experienced an overdose, consultation with a 24-hour poison consultation center specializing in providing veterinary-specific information is recommended. For general information related to overdose and toxin exposures, as well as contact information for poison control centers, refer to ***Appendix***.

Drug Interactions

The following drug interactions have either been reported or are theoretical in humans or animals receiving trilostane and may be of significance in veterinary patients. Unless otherwise noted, use together is not necessarily contraindicated, but weigh the potential risks and perform additional monitoring when appropriate.

- **ANGIOTENSIN-CONVERTING ENZYME INHIBITORS (ACEIs**; eg, **benazepril, enalapril**): May increase risk for hyperkalemia
- **KETOCONAZOLE**: May potentiate the effects of trilostane and lead to hypoadrenocorticism
- **MITOTANE**: May potentiate the effects of trilostane and lead to hypoadrenocorticism. Wait at least 1 month after discontinuing mitotane before initiating trilostane.
- **POTASSIUM-SPARING DIURETICS** (eg, **spironolactone**): May increase risk for hyperkalemia
- **POTASSIUM SUPPLEMENTS; HIGH POTASSIUM FOODS**: May increase risk for hyperkalemia

Laboratory Considerations

- None

Dosages

CAUTION: Hypoadrenocorticism can develop at any dose and at any time during therapy and does not appear to be dose dependent. Animals should always be sent home with glucocorticoid supplementation in the event of an Addisonian crisis. See ***Contraindications/Precautions/Warnings***.

DOGS:

CAUTION: The label dosage for dogs is considered by most clinicians to be greater than is necessary for most patients. The label dosage is provided below; however, the use of lower, extra-label dosages (listed below label dosage) is recommended.

Hyperadrenocorticism (HAC) (label dosage; FDA-approved): Starting dose is 2.2 – 6.7 mg/kg (based on body weight and capsule size) PO once daily with food; after giving this dose for ≈10 to 14 days, re-examination is required and a 4- to 6-hour post-administration ACTH stimulation test and serum biochemical test (eg, electrolytes, renal and hepatic function) should be performed. If physical examination results are acceptable, adjust the dose according to post-ACTH serum cortisol based on Table 1 in the package insert.[16] Individual dose adjustments and close monitoring are essential. Re-examine and conduct an ACTH stimulation test 10 to 14 days after <u>every</u> dose alteration. Care must be taken during dose increases to monitor the dog's clinical signs and serum electrolyte concentrations. Once-daily administration is recommended; however, if clinical signs are not controlled for the full day, twice-daily dosing may be needed. To switch from a once-daily dosing regimen to a twice-daily dose, divide the total daily dose into 2 portions given 12 hours apart; it is not necessary for the doses to be equal. If applicable, the larger dose should be administered in the morning and the smaller dose in the evening.[16] **NOTE**: Extra-label use of twice daily doses permits use of a lower total daily trilostane dosage that appears equally effective and better tolerated.[19] See extra-label dosages below.

Hyperadrenocorticism (HAC) (extra-label):

Twice-daily administration:

a) In dogs weighing less than 5 kg: ≈0.5 – 1 mg/kg (0.78 ± 0.26 mg/kg) PO every 12 hours for 4 weeks, and then was adjusted based on clinical signs and ACTH stimulation testing.[1] No dogs required more than the manufacturer's lowest recommended starting dose of 3 mg/kg per day to control disease.[2] Slow adjustment of the treatment protocol to achieve clinical improvement may be needed on a case-by-case basis. There is some evidence that as body weight increases, especially in dogs weighing more than 30 kg (66 lb), the amount of trilostane (mg/kg/dose as well as mg/kg/day dosage) required to control clinical signs decreases.[5]

b) 0.21 – 1.1 mg/kg PO every 12 hours (mean, 0.86 mg/kg every 12 hours). Slow adjustment of the treatment protocol to achieve clinical improvement may be needed on a case-by-case basis. Most (≈75%) of the dogs in the study did not need more than 3 mg/kg per day to control disease throughout the 1-year follow-up. Author concluded that the results of the present study indicated that trilostane is both potent and effective in dogs at doses less than those recommended by the manufacturer and that a lower dose administered twice daily should be considered as it minimizes the incidence and severity of adverse effects and trilostane's effects have been shown to last less than 12 hours.[2]

c) Average initial dose of 0.78 – 3.1 mg/kg PO every 12 hours; average final dose of 1.43 – 3.75 mg/kg PO every 12 hours. It is recommended to start at a dosage of 0.5 – 1 mg/kg PO every 12 hours, with a maximum initial <u>*daily*</u> dose of 30 mg/dog (NOT mg/kg) for dogs weighing more than 30 kg (66 lb).[20]

Once-daily administration:

a) ≈2 mg/kg (based on body weight and available capsule sizes) PO once daily with food. Titrate dose slowly according to individual response, using lowest dose necessary to control clinical signs. If signs of HAC are not adequately controlled, increase dose by 50% and split into 2 evenly divided doses. Doses of 10 mg/kg per day or higher may be required in a small number of dogs.[15]

b) Average initial dose of 2.9 – 6.4 mg/kg PO every 24 hours; average final dose of 2.8 – 19 mg/kg PO every 24 hours[20]

Alopecia X (extra-label):

a) 3 – 3.6 mg/kg PO twice daily for 4 to 6 months. From a case series ($n = 3$)[3]; no adverse effects were reported.

b) In dogs weighing less than 10 kg (22 lb), average trilostane dose was 10.85 mg/kg PO per day given either once daily or divided and given twice daily for 4 to 8 weeks.[4]

c) A study in Pomeranians reported 1 mg/kg PO given twice daily to be a positive therapeutic option.[21]

CATS:

Hyperadrenocorticism (extra-label): Average dosages were 4.3 mg/kg PO once daily or 3.3 mg/kg PO twice daily; dosages ranged from 10 – 30 mg/cat (NOT mg/kg) PO every 12 to 24 hours to 12 mg/kg PO every 12 hours.[6-8,22]

HORSES:

Equine pituitary pars intermedia dysfunction (PPID; formerly known as equine Cushing's syndrome) (extra-label): 0.4 – 1 mg/kg (total dose of 120 – 240 mg/horse [NOT mg/kg]) PO once daily.[18] **NOTE**: Trilostane may be beneficial to those horses with PPID associated with adrenal gland hyperplasia and hypercortisolemia but has no effect on the excessive production of other pituitary-derived hormones.[23]

SMALL MAMMALS:

Hyperadrenocorticism in guinea pigs (extra-label): 2 – 6 mg/kg PO every 24 hours[24,25]

Monitoring

- Clinical effects. Clinical signs may correlate poorly with cortisol concentrations or ACTH stimulation test results.[26] Asking caregivers to keep a daily diary of their animal's clinical signs can help ascertain clinical control over time and help to make informed decisions about trilostane dosage adjustments.
- Adverse effects. Addisonian crisis is a life-threatening adverse effect of trilostane therapy. Monitor patients closely during therapy for this potential complication. Dispense oral dexamethasone at the time of discharge for owners to administer in case of an Addisonian crisis.
- Baseline and periodic (at 30 days, 90 days, and then every 3 months) history and physical examination[16]
- Baseline and periodic (at 30 days, 90 days, and then every 3 months) CBC and serum chemistry profiles with particular attention paid to electrolytes and renal and liver parameters[16]
- Urinalysis and (possibly) urine cortisol:creatinine ratio (UCCR). Of note, no advantage has been demonstrated in a UCCR evaluation on each re-evaluation, but measurement of urine specific gravity, glucose, and protein or checking for evidence of infection (ie, urine culture) may be helpful in assessing dogs treated long-term with trilostane.[2]
- ACTH stimulation testing is imperative to ensure safe continuation of trilostane therapy. Familiarity with and understanding of testing methods are necessary to ensure consistency of results and safe continuation of therapy. Ideally, for each individual patient, the timing of trilostane administration and ACTH stimulation testing should remain consistent when monitoring therapy. Different strategies include:
  - For long-term monitoring once an optimum dose has been reached, an ACTH stimulation test 4 to 6 hours after trilostane administration should be perfomed.[16] Results from 2 studies suggest the optimal time point for an ACTH stimulation test is

2 to 4 hours after trilostane administration.[10,27] A post-ACTH stimulation test that results in a cortisol of less than 1.45 µg/dL (less than 40 nmol/L), with or without electrolyte abnormalities, may precede the development of clinical signs of hypoadrenocorticism.[16] Good control is indicated by favorable clinical signs as well as post-ACTH serum cortisol of 1.45 – 9.1 µg/dL (40 to 250 nmol/L). If the ACTH stimulation test result is less than 1.45 µg/dL (less than 40 nmol/L) and/or if electrolyte imbalances characteristic of hypoadrenocorticism (eg, hyperkalemia, hyponatremia) are found, trilostane should be temporarily discontinued until recurrence of clinical signs consistent with hyperadrenocorticism and ACTH stimulation test results return to normal (1.45 – 9.1 µg/dL or 40 –250 nmol/L). Trilostane may then be re-introduced at a lower dose. One study concluded that a baseline cortisol concentration collected 4 to 6 hours after trilostane administration in dogs with hyperadrenocorticism provided clinically useful information about control of adrenal gland function,[28] but another study concluded baseline cortisol, endogenous ACTH, and the cortisol/ACTH ratio could not replace the ACTH stimulation test for monitoring trilostane therapy.[29]

- A second ACTH stimulation test performed 9 to 12 hours post-trilostane administration and ≈6 hours after the first ACTH stimulation test may provide additional therapy guidance in dogs that are clinically well-regulated and have cortisol less than 2 µg/dL before and after the first ACTH stimulation test.[30]
- Cortisol concentration measured pre-trilostane and 3-hours post-trilostane administration also may be a useful monitoring method,[31] although inconsistencies were noted in pre-trilostane cortisol measurements obtained 1 hour apart.[32]
- In dogs showing no signs of hypoadrenocorticism, cortisol concentrations in the normal range, measured by pre-trilostane cortisol concentration, could provide necessary information for management of the case. If the pre-trilostane cortisol concentration is low, additional cortisol testing (such as ACTH stimulation testing) should be performed to ensure safe continuation of therapy. Alternatively, if the pre-trilostane cortisol concentration is low in dogs showing no signs of hypoadrenocorticism, the trilostane dose could be decreased.[32]

Client Information

- Give this medicine exactly as prescribed by your veterinarian. Do not stop or give more of the drug unless you first talk to your veterinarian.
- Discontinue trilostane and contact your veterinarian immediately if any vomiting, diarrhea, lethargy, poor/reduced appetite, weakness, or collapse are observed.
- Give each dose with food, unless otherwise directed by your veterinarian. If directed to administer this medicine once daily, give it in the morning.
- If a dose is missed, give the dose at the next scheduled dose administration time.
- Wash your hands after handling this medicine. Do not empty capsule contents or do not attempt to divide the capsules. Do not handle the capsules if you are pregnant or trying to conceive.
- Report any side effects to your veterinarian.
- Keep this medicine out of reach of children and animals.
- Trilostane helps manage your animal's condition but is not a cure. Improvements in your animal's condition occur gradually and may be difficult to see on a daily basis.

Chemistry/Synonyms

Trilostane, a synthetic steroid analogue, has a molecular weight of 329.4 and its chemical name is 4-alpha, 5-alpha-epoxy-17-beta-hydroxy-3-oxoandrostane-2-alpha-carbonitrile. It is relatively insoluble in water.

Trilostane may also be known as WIN 24540, trilostaani, *Vetoryl®*, *Desopan®*, *Modrastane®*, or *Modrenal®*.

Storage/Stability

Commercially available trilostane capsules should be stored at room temperature (25°C [77°F]), with excursions between 15°C to 30°C (59°F-86°F) permitted.

Compatibility/Compounding Considerations

An evaluation of compounded trilostane capsules obtained from 8 compounding pharmacies found that 38% of compounded batches were outside the acceptance criteria for content (content ranged from 39% to 152% of stated label), and 20% did not meet the established criteria for dissolution. Reformulation of the licensed trilostane product into a novel capsule size by a trained pharmacist did not affect dissolution characteristics and the target dose was achieved. The authors concluded, *On the basis of these findings, compounded trilostane products should be used with caution as they may jeopardize the management of dogs with hyperadrenocorticism and potentially impact patient safety.*[33]

Trilostane 5 mg/mL oral suspension in cod liver oil (prepared using *Vetoryl®* capsules) retained potency within 90% to 105% of labeled value for 60 days when stored in amber glass vials at room temperature. Potency fell below 90% of the labeled value when stored in amber plastic bottles at room temperature.[34]

Dosage Forms/Regulatory Status

VETERINARY-LABELED PRODUCTS:

Trilostane Oral Capsules: 5 mg, 10 mg, 30 mg, 60 mg, and 120 mg packaged in aluminum foil blister cards of 10 capsules; *Vetoryl®*; (Rx). NADA 141-291

HUMAN-LABELED PRODUCTS:

Modrastane® was withdrawn from the United States market in 1994.

References

For the complete list of references, see **wiley.com/go/budde/plumb**

Trimeprazine/Prednisolone

(trye-***mep***-ra-zeen/pred-***niss***-oh-lone) *Temaril-P®*
Phenothiazine Antihistamine, Corticosteroid
See also ***Prednisolone/Prednisone***

Prescriber Highlights

- Indicated for relief of pruritus and as an antitussive in dogs
- Goal of therapy should be to use the lowest dose possible for the least amount of time to treat and control patient's condition.
- Relatively contraindicated in animals with systemic fungal infection, hypovolemia, shock, tetanus, or strychnine intoxication
- Caution is advised in animals with hepatic dysfunction, cardiac disease, active bacterial or viral infections, peptic ulcer, corneal ulcer, hyperadrenocorticism (Cushing syndrome), diabetes, osteoporosis, predisposition to thrombophlebitis, hypertension, congestive heart failure, renal insufficiency, or general debilitation and in very young animals.
- Primary adverse effects include sedation, significant hypotension, cardiac rate abnormalities, hypo- or hyperthermia, and hyperadrenocorticism with sustained use.
- Many potential drug and laboratory interactions

Uses/Indications

Trimeprazine/prednisolone is indicated for treatment of pruritic and inflammatory conditions (especially if induced by allergic conditions such as atopic dermatitis) or as an antitussive.[1] There is anecdotal evidence that treatment with trimeprazine/prednisolone combinations require less prednisolone to control pruritus.[2,3]

Pharmacology/Actions

Trimeprazine has antihistaminic, sedative, antitussive, and antipruritic qualities. The veterinary FDA-approved product contains prednisolone in its formulation, providing additional antipruritic and anti-inflammatory effects.

See ***Glucocorticoid Agents, General Information***.

Pharmacokinetics

The pharmacokinetics of trimeprazine have apparently not been studied in animals. In humans, peak concentration occurs 3.5 to 4.5 hours after oral administration in adults and 1 to 2 hours in children. Protein binding is 90%. Half-life is ≈5 hours in adults and ≈7 hours in children.[4,5]

See ***Glucocorticoid Agents, General Information***.

Contraindications/Precautions/Warnings

Like other phenothiazines, trimeprazine is contraindicated in patients with a known hypersensitivity to it or other phenothiazines. It should not be used for patients in comatose states due to large amounts of CNS depressants or for tetanus or strychnine intoxication due to its effects on the extrapyramidal system. It is relatively contraindicated in patients with hypovolemia, dehydration, or shock, and should be used cautiously in animals with CNS depression, hepatic dysfunction, cardiac disease, or general debilitation.

Systemic use of glucocorticoids is generally contraindicated in animals with systemic fungal infections (with some exceptions such as when used for replacement therapy in animals with hypoadrenocorticism or to help reduce severe inflammation), corneal ulceration, or hypersensitivity to the drug. Use with caution in animals with concomitant renal disease, as they may be at increased risk for GI adverse effects. Animals, particularly cats, at risk for diabetes mellitus or with concurrent cardiovascular disease should not receive glucocorticoids or should receive them with caution because of the potent hyperglycemic effect of these agents. In humans, long-term glucocorticoids may increase intraocular pressure and increase the risk for cataracts and osteoporosis.

Systemic glucocorticoids suppress adrenal function. The drug should be tapered off slowly in animals receiving it chronically, as endogenous ACTH and corticosteroid function may return slowly. Additional glucocorticoids should be administered to animals undergoing a stressor (eg, surgery, trauma, illness) during the tapering process or until normal adrenal and pituitary functions resume.

Adverse Effects

For trimeprazine, possible adverse effects include sedation, depression, hypothermia, hypotension, and extrapyramidal reactions (eg, rigidity, tremors, weakness, restlessness).

For the product containing corticosteroids, additional adverse effects include elevated liver enzymes, weight loss, muscle wasting, polyuria/polydipsia, vomiting, and diarrhea. Iatrogenic hyperadrenocorticism may develop. Worsening of diabetes mellitus, GI ulceration and immunosuppression are possible, particularly at higher dosages.

Additional adverse effects of the combination product include sodium retention and potassium loss, negative nitrogen balance, suppressed adrenocortical function, delayed wound healing, osteoporosis, possible increased susceptibility to and/or exacerbation of bacterial infection, sedation, protruding nictitating membrane, and blood dyscrasias.[1] In addition, intensification and prolongation of the action of sedatives, analgesics, or anesthetics, as well as potentiation of organophosphate toxicity and procaine activity, may be noted.

Reproductive/Nursing Safety

Corticosteroids can induce the first stages of parturition if administered during the last trimester of pregnancy.[1] Small amounts of both trimeprazine and prednisolone are excreted into human milk; use with caution in nursing animals or consider milk replacer. Because safety has not been established in animals, this drug should only be used when the maternal benefits outweigh the potential risks to offspring.

Overdose/Acute Toxicity

The most likely effects of an overdose include sedation and ataxia. Gut decontamination and supportive treatment should be used. It is especially advised to contact a veterinary poison center for treatment of seizures and/or hypotension that are nonresponsive to crystalloid fluid therapy.

For patients that have experienced or are suspected to have experienced an overdose, consultation with a 24-hour poison consultation center specializing in providing veterinary-specific information is recommended. For general information related to overdose and toxin exposures, as well as contact information for poison control centers, refer to ***Appendix***.

Drug Interactions

The following drug interactions have either been reported or are theoretical in humans or animals receiving promethazine (a related phenothiazine antihistamine) or prednisolone and may be of significance in veterinary patients. Unless otherwise noted, use together is not necessarily contraindicated, but weigh the potential risks and perform additional monitoring when appropriate.

- AMPHOTERICIN B: May cause hypokalemia when administered concomitantly with glucocorticoids
- ANTACIDS, ALUMINUM-, CALCIUM-, OR MAGNESIUM-CONTAINING: May cause reduced GI absorption of oral phenothiazines
- ANTICHOLINESTERASE AGENTS (eg, **neostigmine, pyridostigmine**): In animals with myasthenia gravis, concomitant glucocorticoid use with these agents may lead to profound muscle weakness. If possible, discontinue anticholinesterase medication

at least 24 hours prior to corticosteroid administration.

- **Antidiarrheal Mixtures** (eg, **bismuth subsalicylate mixtures, kaolin/pectin**): May cause reduced GI absorption of oral phenothiazines
- **Cholestyramine**: May reduce prednisolone absorption
- **Cisapride**: Increased risk for cardiac arrhythmia when used with phenothiazines
- **CNS Depressant Agents** (eg, **anesthetics, methocarbamol**): May cause additive CNS depression if used with phenothiazines
- **Cyclophosphamide**: Glucocorticoids may inhibit the hepatic metabolism of cyclophosphamide; dosage adjustments may be required.
- **Cyclosporine**: Concomitant administration with glucocorticoids may increase blood concentrations of each by mutually inhibiting the hepatic metabolism of each other; the clinical significance of this interaction is not clear.
- **Digoxin**: Secondary to hypokalemia, increased risk for arrhythmia
- **Diuretics, Potassium-Depleting** (eg, **furosemide, thiazides**): May cause hypokalemia when administered concomitantly with glucocorticoids
- **Ephedrine**: May increase metabolism of glucocorticoids
- **Epinephrine**: Contraindicated in the treatment of acute hypotension produced by phenothiazine-derivative tranquilizers, as further depression of blood pressure can occur
- **Estrogens**: The effects of hydrocortisone, and possibly other glucocorticoids, may be potentiated by concomitant administration with estrogens.
- **Fluoroquinolones** (eg, enrofloxacin, marbofloxacin, pradofloxacin): Concurrent use may increase the risk for tendinitis and tendon rupture.
- **Insulin**: Insulin requirements may increase in patients receiving glucocorticoids.
- **Ketoconazole**: May decrease metabolism of glucocorticoids
- **Macrolide Antibiotics** (eg, clarithromycin, erythromycin): May decrease glucocorticoid metabolism
- **Metoclopramide**: Phenothiazines may potentiate the extrapyramidal effects of metoclopramide.
- **Mitotane**: May alter the metabolism of steroids; higher-than-usual doses of steroids may be necessary to treat mitotane-induced adrenal insufficiency.
- **Mycophenolate**: Prednisolone increased the in vitro unbound (active) fraction of mycophenolic acid in dogs.6
- **Nonsteroidal Anti-Inflammatory Drugs** (NSAIDs; eg, carprofen, meloxicam): Administration of other ulcerogenic drugs with glucocorticoids may increase the risk for gastric ulcers.
- **Organophosphate Agents**: Phenothiazines should not be given within 1 month of deworming with these agents, as their effects may be potentiated.
- **Opioids** (eg, buprenorphine, morphine, tramadol): May cause additive CNS depression
- **Paraquat**: Toxicity of the herbicide paraquat may be increased by prochlorperazine.
- **Phenobarbital**: May increase the metabolism of glucocorticoids. Additive sedation may occur with phenobarbital.
- **Procaine**: Activity may be enhanced by phenothiazines.
- **Propranolol**: Increased concentrations of both drugs are possible.
- **Rifampin**: May increase the metabolism of glucocorticoids
- **Salicylates** (eg, aspirin, bismuth subsalicylate): Glucocorticoids may reduce salicylate blood concentrations.
- **Selective Serotonin Reuptake Inhibitors** (**SSRIs**; eg, fluoxetine, paroxetine): May increase phenothiazine plasma concentrations
- **Vaccines**: Animals receiving corticosteroids at immunosuppressive doses should generally not receive live attenuated virus vaccines, as virus replication may be augmented. A diminished immune response may occur after vaccine, toxoid, or bacterin administration in animals receiving glucocorticoids.

Laboratory Considerations

- Glucocorticoids may increase serum **cholesterol** and **alkaline phosphatase** concentrations.
- Glucocorticoids may increase **urine glucose** concentrations
- Glucocorticoids may decrease **serum potassium.**
- Glucocorticoids can suppress the release of **thyroid stimulating hormone (TSH)** and reduce T_3 and T_4 values. Thyroid gland atrophy has been reported after chronic glucocorticoid administration. Uptake of I^{131} by the thyroid may be decreased by glucocorticoids.
- Phenothiazine metabolites may darken the urine and cause false positive results for **amylase, urobilinogen, uroporphyrins, porphobilinogens,** and **5-hydroxyindolacetic acid.**
- Reactions to **allergen tests** may be suppressed by glucocorticoids and/or trimeprazine. The actual effect of trimeprazine with prednisolone on allergen-specific intradermal tests (IDT) and allergen-specific IgE serological (ASIS) tests has not been reported.[7] A 2- to 4-week withdrawal time prior to IDT or ASIS is recommended.[7,8]
- False negative results of the **nitroblue tetrazolium test for systemic bacterial infections** may be induced by glucocorticoids.

Dosages

DOGS:

Antipruritic and antitussive therapy (label dosage; FDA-approved): Dosed according to body weight: up to 4.5 kg (10 lb) = ½ tablet PO twice daily; 4.9 to 9 kg (11 to 20 lb) = 1 tablet PO twice daily; 9.5 to 18.1 kg (21 to 40 lb) = 2 tablets PO twice daily; over 18.1 kg (40 lb) = 3 tablets PO twice daily. After 4 days, reduce dose to ½ of initial dose or to an amount just sufficient to maintain remission of clinical signs; adjust as necessary.[1]

Adjunctive treatment of chronic pruritus (extra-label): 1 tablet/5 kg (11 lb) PO every 12 hours for 4 to 7 days, then 1 tablet/5 kg (11 lb) PO once daily for 4 to 7 days, and finally, 1 tablet/5 kg (11 lb) PO every other day. This schedule may be changed according to each animal's needs; however, the goal for long-term glucocorticoid therapy is to give the lowest dose possible to maintain control while administering the dose every other day or less frequently if possible. However, because antihistamines should be administered daily for optimal effect, this complicates the use of this fixed dose combination product.[8]

CATS:

Pruritus (extra-label): Anecdotally, trimeprazine 5 mg/prednisolone 2 mg has been used at 1 tablet/cat (NOT mg/kg) PO twice daily.

Monitoring

- Efficacy
- Degree of sedation and anticholinergic effects
- Adverse effects associated with corticosteroids
- Baseline and periodic (eg, every 6 to 12 months) CBC, serum chemistry profile, urinalysis, and urine culture (especially for geriatric animals) when used long-term[8]

Client Information

- Give this medicine as directed by your veterinarian. This medicine is a combination of an antihistamine and a cortisone-like steroid used to reduce itching. It may also be used to treat cough.

- This medicine can cause drowsiness, muscle tremors, and rigidity (stiffness), increased thirst, appetite, and amount of urine produced. It is important to not limit your animal's access to water to avoid these signs. Instead, make sure your animal has plenty of opportunities to eliminate outside to avoid accidents.
- Long-term use of this medicine can cause changes in the hair coat, thin skin, poor wound healing, potbellied appearance, muscle wasting, and increased chances for infection.
- This medicine is meant to be given for the shortest amount of time and at the lowest dose necessary to control your animal's signs.
- Contact your veterinarian if any of the side effects are worrisome.

Chemistry/Synonyms

Trimeprazine tartrate, a phenothiazine antihistamine related to promethazine, occurs as an odorless, white to off-white crystalline powder. It deteriorates on exposure to light and air. Approximately 0.5 gram is soluble in 1 mL water, and 0.05 gram is soluble in 1 mL of alcohol. Trimeprazine tartrate may also be known as alimemazine tartrate, *Panectyl®*, *Temaril®*, or *Vanectyl®*.

Prednisolone occurs as an odorless, white to practically white crystalline powder that is very slightly soluble in water and slightly soluble in alcohol. Prednisolone is also known as deltahydrocortisone or metacortandralone.

Storage/Stability

Store trimeprazine/prednisolone products in a cool, dry place at room temperature not above 25°C (77°F).

Compatibility/Compounding Considerations

No specific information noted

Dosage Forms/Regulatory Status

VETERINARY-LABELED PRODUCTS:

No single-agent trimeprazine products are FDA-approved for veterinary medicine.

Trimeprazine 5 mg with Prednisolone 2 mg Tablets; *Temaril-P® Tablets*; (Rx). FDA-approved for use in dogs. NADA# 012-437

The Association of Racing Commissioners International (ARCI) has designated this drug as a class 4 substance. See ***Appendix*** for more information. Use of this drug may not be allowed in certain animal competitions. Check rules and regulations before entering in a competition while this medication is being administered. Contact local racing authorities for further guidance.

HUMAN-LABELED PRODUCTS: NONE

References

For the complete list of references, see **wiley.com/go/budde/plumb**

Tripelennamine

(tri-pel-***ehn***-a-meen) *Re-Covr®*

Antihistamine

Prescriber Highlights

- ▶ Injectable antihistamine FDA-approved for use in horses and cattle
- ▶ IV administration is contraindicated in horses
- ▶ Adverse effects include CNS stimulation (if given IV to horses), sedation, depression, ataxia, and GI effects.

Uses/Indications

Tripelennamine is a first-generation antihistamine that is FDA-approved for use in horses and cattle for treating conditions in which antihistaminic therapy may be expected to alleviate some signs of disease.[1] It has been used as a CNS stimulant in downer cows when administered slowly IV.

Pharmacology/Actions

Tripelennamine is a first-generation antihistamine that competitively inhibits histamine at H_1 receptor sites. It does not inactivate or prevent the release of histamine but can prevent histamine's action on the cell. Besides their antihistaminic activity, these agents also have varying degrees of anticholinergic and CNS activity (sedation). Tripelennamine is considered to have moderate sedative activity and minimal anticholinergic activity when compared with other first-generation antihistamines.

Pharmacokinetics

The pharmacokinetics of tripelennamine have apparently not been thoroughly studied in domestic animals or humans. One study performed on horses and camels showed that after IV administration, similar pharmacokinetic profiles were obtained for both species.[2] Terminal elimination half-lives were around 2-plus hours; volumes of distribution steady-state were ≈1.5 to 3 L/kg; protein binding was 80%, and total body clearance was ≈1 L/hour/kg.

Contraindications/Precautions/Warnings

Tripelennamine is contraindicated in patients that are hypersensitive to it. IV administration is contraindicated in horses (see ***Adverse Effects***).

Do not use tripelennamine in beef calves less than 2 months, dairy calves, or veal calves; it should not be used in horses intended for human consumption.

In humans, contraindications to tripelennamine included narrow-angle glaucoma bladder neck obstruction, pyloroduodenal obstruction, and asthma.

Adverse Effects

Adverse effects include CNS depression, ataxia, and GI disturbances. CNS stimulation (eg, hyperexcitability, nervousness, muscle tremors) lasting up to 20 minutes has been noted in horses after administration of label-recommended dosages.

Reproductive/Nursing Safety

No information was located. Because safety has not been established in animals, this drug should only be used when the maternal benefits outweigh the potential fetal risks.

Overdose/Acute Toxicity

Overdoses of tripelennamine reportedly can cause CNS excitation, seizures, and ataxia. Treat the patient supportively if clinical signs are severe.

For patients that have experienced or are suspected to have experienced an overdose, consultation with a 24-hour poison consultation center specializing in providing veterinary-specific information is recommended. For general information related to overdose and toxin exposures, as well as contact information for poison control centers, refer to ***Appendix***.

Drug Interactions

The following drug interactions have either been reported or are theoretical in humans or animals receiving tripelennamine and may be of significance in veterinary patients. Unless otherwise noted, use together is not necessarily contraindicated, but weigh the potential risks and perform additional monitoring when appropriate.

- CNS Depressants (eg, **detomidine, methocarbamol**): Increased sedation can occur if tripelennamine is combined with other CNS depressant drugs.
- Heparin: Antihistamines may partially counteract the anticoagulation effects of heparin or warfarin.
- Monoamine Oxidase Inhibitors (MAOIs; eg, **amitraz,**

linezolid, selegiline): Concomitant use is considered contraindicated in humans; veterinary significance is unknown.

- **Warfarin**: Antihistamines may partially counteract the anticoagulation effects of heparin or warfarin.

Laboratory Considerations

- Antihistamines can decrease the wheal and flare response to **antigen skin testing**. In dogs, the recommended optimal withdrawal time of antihistamines prior to intradermal allergy testing is 7 days (the minimum recommended withdrawal time is 2 days).[3]

Dosages

NOTE: It is recommended to warm the solution to near body temperature before injecting; give IM injections into large muscle groups of the hind legs or cervical area.

HORSES:

Antihistamine (label dosage; FDA-approved): 1.1 mg/kg IM every 6 to 12 hours as needed.[1] **NOTE**: Do **NOT** administer IV to horses.

CATTLE:

Antihistamine (label dosage; FDA-approved): 1.1 mg/kg IV or IM every 6 to 12 hours as needed. Administer IV if more immediate effect is needed.

Monitoring

- Clinical efficacy
- Adverse effects

Chemistry/Synonyms

Tripelennamine HCl, an ethylenediamine-derivative antihistamine, occurs as a white, crystalline powder that will slowly darken upon exposure to light. It has a melting range of 188°C to 192°C (370°F-378°F) and pK_as of 3.9 and 9. One gram is soluble in 1 mL of water or 6 mL of alcohol.

Tripelennamine HCl may also be known as tripelennaminium chloride, *Pyribenzamine*®, or *Re-Covr*®.

Storage/Stability

Store the injection at room temperature (20°C-25°C [68°F-77°F]), with excursions permitted between 15°C to 30°C (59°F-86°F). Protect this product from light and avoid freezing or excessive heat. The vial should be punctured a maximum of 30 times.[1]

Compatibility/Compounding Considerations

No specific information was noted.

Dosage Forms/Regulatory Status

VETERINARY-LABELED PRODUCTS:

Tripelennamine HCl for Injection: 20 mg/mL in 100 mL, 250 mL, and 500 mL multiple-dose vials; *Re-Covr*®; (Rx). FDA-approved for use in cattle and horses. Not for use in horses to be used for food purposes. Not for use in beef calves less than 2 months, dairy calves, or veal calves. Meat withdrawal is 4 days; milk withdrawal is 24 hours.

The Association of Racing Commissioners International (ARCI) has designated this drug as a class 3 substance. Use of this drug may not be allowed in certain animal competitions. Check rules and regulations before entering a competition while this medication is being administered. Contact local racing authorities for further guidance. See ***Appendix***.

HUMAN-LABELED PRODUCTS: NONE

References

For the complete list of references, see **wiley.com/go/budde/plumb**

Tulathromycin

(too-***la***-throe-***mye***-sin) *Draxxin*®

Injectable Macrolide Antibiotic

Prescriber Highlights

- ▶ Labeled for cattle and swine
- ▶ Single-dose treatment; long tissue half-lives
- ▶ Different withdrawal times in cattle based upon formulation of product used
- ▶ Not for lactating dairy cattle or veal calves
- ▶ Local injection site reactions most likely adverse effect

Uses/Indications

In beef and non-lactating dairy cattle, tulathromycin (100 mg/mL formulation) is indicated for the treatment of bovine respiratory disease (BRD) associated with *Mannheimia haemolytica, Pasteurella multocida, Histophilus somni* (*Haemophilus somnus*), and *Mycoplasma bovis*; and for the control of respiratory disease in cattle at high risk of developing BRD, associated with *Mannheimia haemolytica, Pasteurella multocida, Histophilus somni* (*Haemophilus somnus*), and *Mycoplasma bovis*. It is also FDA-approved for the treatment of bovine foot rot (interdigital necrobacillosis) associated with *Fusobacterium necrophorum* and *Porphyromonas levii* and for the treatment of infectious bovine keratoconjunctivitis (IBK) associated with *Moraxella bovis*.[1] In suckling calves, dairy calves and veal calves, tulathromycin (both 100 mg/mL and 25 mg/mL formulations) is indicated for the treatment of BRD associated with *M haemolytica, P multocida, H somni*, and *M bovis*.[1,2]

Tulathromycin (both 100 mg/mL and 25 mg/mL formulations) is indicated for the treatment of swine respiratory disease (SRD) associated with *Actinobacillus pleuropneumoniae, Pasteurella multocida, Bordetella bronchiseptica, Haemophilus parasuis,* and *Mycoplasma hyopneumoniae;* and for the control of SRD associated with *Actinobacillus pleuropneumoniae, Pasteurella multocida*, and *Mycoplasma hyopneumoniae* in groups of pigs where SRD has been diagnosed.[1,2]

Tulathromycin may be effective in treating various infections in commercial bison, white-tailed deer, small ruminants, and rabbits.

The World Health Organization has designated tulathromycin as a Critically Important, Highest Priority antimicrobial for human medicine.[3] The Office International des Epizooties (OIE) has designated tulathromycin as a Veterinary Critically Important Antimicrobial (VCIA) Agent in bovine and swine species.[4]

Pharmacology/Actions

Although tulathromycin is a macrolide antibiotic, it is structurally unique in that it has three amine groups (tribasic), while erythromycin and azithromycin have one (monobasic) and two (dibasic) groups, respectively. The tribasic group of compounds are called triamilide macrolides.

As with other macrolides, tulathromycin is effective against a range of gram-positive bacteria, with enhanced activity against gram negatives. It is believed that tulathromycin's tribasic structure allows it to better penetrate gram-negative bacteria and its low affinity for bacterial efflux pumps may allow the drug to remain and accumulate within bacteria.

The mechanism of action of tulathromycin is similar to other macrolides. It inhibits protein synthesis by penetrating the cell wall and binding to the 50S ribosomal subunits in susceptible bacteria. It is considered a bacteriostatic antibiotic although there is the potential for time-dependent bactericidal action, particularly with high concentrations. The drug possesses bactericidal activity particularly for *Mannheimia haemolytica* and *Pasteurella multocida*. A postantibiotic effect can be produced; the duration is both drug and pathogen dependent.

Tulathromycin's efficacy is enhanced by its ability to accumulate and persist in pulmonary epithelial lining fluid, macrophages and neutrophils. The drug shows notable accumulation and long persistence in lung tissue. Neither time-dependent nor concentration-dependent models may accurately predict or describe the drug's efficacy. The efficacy of some modern macrolides (eg, azithromycin) may be more predictive by assessing the total drug exposure to the pathogen; the AUC:MIC ratio may be helpful.

Tulathromycin reportedly possesses immunomodulatory effects in leukocytes in vitro and anti-inflammatory effects in pigs in experimental models of *A pleuropneumoniae* infection and nonmicrobial-induced pulmonary inflammation. This suggests that in addition to its antimicrobial properties, tulathromycin may dampen severe proinflammatory responses and drive resolution of inflammation in pigs with microbial pulmonary infections.[5] The accumulation of macrolides in anti-inflammatory cells is widely recognized.[6]

Bacterial isolates susceptible to tulathromycin at concentrations of 16 µg/mL or less are reported as susceptible to tulathromycin. The MIC_{90} values reported for *M haemolytica* and *P multocida* in cattle with BRD are 2 µg/mL and 1 µg/mL, respectively. To date, resistance development to tulathromycin has not been a major problem; however, greater resistance against tulathromycin in *M haemolytica* isolates has been identified from 2013 to 2017 when compared to isolates from 2008 to 2012.[7]

Pharmacokinetics

In feeder calves given 2.5 mg/kg SC (in the neck), tulathromycin is rapidly and nearly completely absorbed (bioavailability greater than 90%). Peak plasma concentrations generally occur within 15 minutes after dosing. Volume of distribution is very large (≈11 L/kg) and total systemic clearance is ≈170 mL/hour/kg. This extensive volume of distribution is largely responsible for the long elimination half-life of this compound. In plasma, elimination half-life is ≈2.75 days, but in lung tissue it is ≈8.75 days. Tulathromycin is eliminated from the body primarily unchanged via biliary excretion with half of the dose being eliminated in the feces. Effective concentrations of tulathromycin against pathogens commonly associated with BRD are maintained for up to 10 days after administration to cattle.[8]

In a pharmacokinetic study of 6 healthy adult horses following IM administration of tulathromycin at 2.5 mg/kg, half-life was 54.8 hours, bioavailability was 99.4%, and time to peak concentration was 0.75 hours. After IV administration of the same dose, half-life was 59.8 hours and volume of distribution was 16.8 L/kg.[9] Tulathromycin reaches high concentrations in the pulmonary epithelial lining fluid (PELF) and bronchoalveolar lavage cells (BALC) in horses after both IM and IV administration of 2.5 mg/kg.

Following IM administration to feeder pigs at a dosage of 2.5 mg/kg, tulathromycin is readily and rapidly absorbed (bioavailability 88%) with peak levels occurring in ≈15 minutes. Tulathromycin rapidly distributes into body tissues, and the volume of distribution is 13 to15 L/kg. Plasma half-life is ≈60 to 90 hours, but lung tissue half-life is ≈5.9 days. Tulathromycin is eliminated from the body primarily unchanged via the feces and urine. In pigs, two-thirds of the dose is eliminated in the feces.

Results from a manuscript detailing the administration of a single injection of tulathromycin 2.5 mg/kg SC in deer reports similarity in maximal serum concentrations between deer and cattle and high lung concentrations in deer, suggesting the recommended cattle dosage is effective in deer. Tissue concentrations persisted for 56 days suggesting a need for longer withdrawal times in deer than cattle.[10]

The pharmacokinetics of tulathromycin in sheep appear to be similar enough to those in goats and cattle to recommend similar dosing (2.5 mg/kg SC), assuming that the target pathogens have similar inhibitory concentrations.[11]

Contraindications/Precautions/Warnings

Tulathromycin is contraindicated in animals with a prior hypersensitivity reaction to the drug.

Adverse Effects

At labeled dosages, adverse effects appear to be minimal in cattle and swine. At therapeutic doses, transient hypersalivation, head shaking, and pawing at the ground have been reported. One feeder calf in a field study developed transient dyspnea. Injection site reactions are most commonly reported and there have been some reports of anorexia in cattle to the FDA's Adverse Drug Reporting database. Subcutaneous or intramuscular injection can cause a transient local tissue reaction that may result in trim loss at slaughter.

In foals, self-limiting diarrhea, elevated temperature, and swelling at the injection site have been reported. In horses, significant injection site reactions and systemic reactions (sweating, pawing, lateral recumbency) have been documented following IM and SC injections.[9]

All goats used in a pharmacokinetic study developed injection site reactions.[12]

Reproductive/Nursing Safety

The effects of tulathromycin on reproductive performance, pregnancy and lactation have not been determined.[1,2]

Because safety has not been established in animals, this drug should only be used when the maternal benefits outweigh the potential risks to offspring.

Overdose/Acute Toxicity

In cattle (feeder calves), single SC doses of up to 25 mg/kg caused transient indications of pain at the injection site, including head shaking and pawing at the ground. Injection site swelling, discoloration of the subcutaneous tissues at the injection site and corresponding histopathologic changes were seen in animals in all dosage groups.

The SC administration of 12.5 to 15 mg/kg (5 to 6 times the labeled dosage) of tulathromycin to feeder calves caused no clinical signs of cardiovascular toxicity and no macroscopic tissue lesions. Minimal to mild myocardial degeneration was reported in 1 of 6 calves given a single dose of 12.5 mg/kg and 2 of 6 calves given 15 mg/kg.

In swine, single IM doses of up to 25 mg/kg caused transient indications of pain at the injection site, restlessness, and excessive vocalization. Tremors occurred briefly in one animal receiving 7.5 mg/kg BW.

No systemic treatment for single overdoses should be necessary; localized treatment at the injection site (eg, ice pack) to reduce swelling and pain as well as FDA-approved analgesic medications can be considered.

For patients that have experienced or are suspected to have experienced an overdose, consultation with a 24-hour poison control center specializing in providing veterinary-specific information is recommended. For general information related to overdose and toxin exposures, as well as contact information for poison control centers, refer to ***Appendix.***

Drug Interactions

- No drug interactions are noted in the product labels, and none could be found in other references for tulathromycin.

Laboratory Considerations

- None noted

Dosages

CATTLE:

Susceptible infections, labeled indications (label dosage; FDA-approved):

a) **Using 100 mg/mL product**: 2.5 mg/kg (1.1 mL/100 lb) SC as a single dose in the neck.[1] Do not inject more than 10 mL per injection site.

b) **Using 25 mg/mL product**: 2.5 mg/kg (1 mL/22 lb) SC as a single dose in the neck.[2] Do not inject more than 11.5 mL per injection site.

SWINE:

Susceptible infections, labeled indications (label dosage; FDA-approved):

a) **Using 100 mg/mL product**: 2.5 mg/kg (0.25 mL/22 lb) IM as a single dose in the neck.[1] Do not inject more than 2.5 mL per injection site.

b) **Using 25 mg/mL product**: 2.5 mg/kg (1 mL/22 lb) IM as a single dose in the neck.[2] Do not inject more than 4 mL per injection site.

GOATS:

Pneumonia associated with *Mannheimia haemolytica, Pasteurella multocida,* and *Mycoplasma* spp. (extra-label): 2.5 mg/kg SC; repeat in 7 days if necessary.[12,13] Dosage is based on pharmacokinetic studies in meat and dairy goats. After a single dose, a 34-day meat withdrawal interval and a 45-day milk withdrawal time are recommended.[12–14]

DEER:

Susceptible infections (extra-label): Authors report using the cattle dose at 2.5 mg/kg SC once with the need to have a longer withdrawal time compared to cattle.[10]

Monitoring

- Clinical efficacy

Client Information

- Follow dosing guidelines exactly. Withdrawal times in cattle differ between products.
- Not for female dairy cattle 20 months or older or in poultry
- Cattle are dosed subcutaneously in the neck. Swine are dosed intramuscularly in the neck.

Chemistry/Synonyms

Tulathromycin is a semi-synthetic macrolide antibiotic of the subclass triamilide. It occurs as white to off-white crystalline powder that is readily soluble in water at pH less than 8. At a pH of 7.4 (physiological pH), tulathromycin (a weak base) is ≈50 times more soluble in hydrophilic than hydrophobic media.

The commercially available injections contain tulathromycin as the free base in an equilibrated mixture of the two isomeric forms of tulathromycin in a 9:1 ratio. The injectable vehicle consists of 50% propylene glycol, monothioglycerol (5 mg/mL); citric and hydrochloric acids are added to adjust pH, and it has a relatively low viscosity.

Tulathromycin may also be known as tulathromycine, tulathromycinum, CP-472295 (component A), CP-547272 (component B), or *Draxxin*®.

Storage/Stability

Tulathromycin injection should be stored at or below 25°C (77°F); some products allow for excursions up to 40°C (104°F). The number of times a vial may be punctured varies by vial size and by manufacturer, as does the length of time the vial may be used after first puncture; consult product labels for specific information.

Compatibility/Compounding Considerations

No specific information noted

Dosage Forms/Regulatory Status

VETERINARY-LABELED PRODUCTS:

Tulathromycin Injection: 100 mg/mL in 50 mL, 100 mL, 250 mL, and 500 mL vials; *Draxxin*®, generic; (Rx). FDA-approved for use in beef and non-lactating cattle, and suckling calves, including dairy and veal calves, and swine. Cattle intended for human consumption must not be slaughtered within 18 days from the last treatment, and the swine withdrawal is 5 days. Do not use in female dairy cattle 20 months of age or older. NADA# 141-244

Tulathromycin Injection: 25 mg/mL in 50 mL, 100 mL, and 250 mL vials; *Draxxin® 25*; (Rx). FDA-approved for use in suckling calves, dairy calves, veal calves and swine. Not for use in ruminating cattle. When used as labeled; swine withdrawal = 5 days and calves = 22 days. NADA# 141-349

Tulathromycin and Ketoprofen Injection: Tulathromycin 100 mg/mL and Ketoprofen 120 mg/mL in 50 mL, 100 mL, 250 mL, and 500 mL vials; *Draxxin® KP*; (Rx). FDA approved for use in beef steers, beef heifers, beef calves 2 months of age and older, beef bulls, dairy bulls, and replacement dairy heifers. Not for use in reproducing animals over one year of age, or in dairy or veal calves less than 2 months of age. When used as labeled, withdrawal time is 18 days. NADA# 141-543

HUMAN-LABELED PRODUCTS: NONE

References

For the complete list of references, see **wiley.com/go/budde/plumb**

Tylosin

(**tye**-loe-sin) *Tylan*®

Macrolide Antibiotic

Prescriber Highlights

- ► Approved for use in cattle, swine, poultry, and honey bees; can be used in dogs and cats with diarrhea
- ► Contraindications include animals with a hypersensitivity to it or other macrolide antibiotics, and in horses and possibly other hindgut fermenters.
- ► Adverse effects include pain and local reactions after IM injection and GI upset (eg, anorexia, diarrhea) after PO administration; may cause severe diarrhea if administered orally to ruminants. Swine can experience edema of rectal mucosa and mild anal protrusion with pruritus, erythema, and diarrhea.
- ► Use in food animals (including honey bees) requires a prescription (soluble powder) or a veterinary feed directive (medicated feed).

Uses/Indications

Oral tylosin is commonly recommended for the adjunctive treatment of acute and chronic diarrhea in dogs, cats, and some small mammals. There is good evidence supporting the use of tylosin in the treatment of chronic diarrhea in dogs.[1–3]

Although oral tylosin has been anecdotally used in dogs to treat tear staining caused by chronic epiphora, supporting evidence for this use is weak, and there are concerns about the use of antimicrobials for nonantimicrobial indications.[4] Tylosin has demonstrated efficacy in the treatment of canine superficial and deep pyoderma caused by *Staphylococcus intermedius*.[5–8] Although tylosin is not commonly used as first-line therapy for treatment of pyoderma, it may be useful in cases for which resistance occurs.

In beef and nonlactating dairy cattle, tylosin is indicated for the treatment of bovine respiratory complex, foot rot, calf diphtheria, and metritis. In swine, it is indicated for the treatment of arthritis, pneumonia, erysipelas, and dysentery or enteropathies. Tylosin is also used clinically (extra-label) in cattle and swine for the treatment of infections caused by susceptible organisms; however, other approved antibiotics are generally preferred for systemic therapy.

The World Health Organization (WHO) has designated macrolides as Critically Important, Highest Priority antimicrobials for human medicine.[9] The Office International des Epizooties (OIE) has designated macrolides as Veterinary Critically Important Antimicrobial (VCIA) Agents in veterinary species.[10]

Pharmacology/Actions

Tylosin, a bacteriostatic antibiotic, is thought to have the same mechanism of action as erythromycin (ie, binds to 50S ribosome and inhibits protein synthesis) and exhibits a similar spectrum of activity. Tylosin has activity primarily against gram-positive bacteria, including streptococci and staphylococci (eg, *Staphylococcus pseudintermedius*).[7] There is some activity against gram-negative bacteria, but it is limited. Tylosin has some activity against *Campylobacter* spp but is not a recommended first-line agent for that bacteria. Good activity against *Mycoplasma* spp is present.[11] Over 50% of *Enterococcus faecalis* canine isolates from healthy dogs were resistant to tylosin in a study.[12] Tylosin may increase concentrations of enterococci in the jejunum, resulting in probiotic effects (ie, improved microbiota and clinical signs).[13,14] Tylosin may also have direct anti-inflammatory effects[15] and immunomodulatory effects on cell-mediated immunity.

Pharmacokinetics

In mammals, tylosin tartrate is well absorbed from the GI tract, primarily from the intestine. The phosphate salt is not as well absorbed after oral administration. Bioavailability after IM injection is ≈70% to 95%.[16,17] Peak concentration is reached in 1.5 to 2 hours in cows and swine[17-20] and ≈3 to 4 hours in sheep and goats.[16,21] Similar to erythromycin, tylosin is well distributed in the body after systemic absorption, with the exception of penetration into the CSF. The volume of distribution of tylosin is reportedly 1.7 L/kg in small animals and 1 – 2.3 L/kg in cattle.[18,22] In lactating dairy cattle, the milk to plasma ratio is ≈5.[18,20]

Tylosin is eliminated in the urine and bile, apparently as unchanged drug. The elimination half-life of tylosin is reportedly 54 minutes in dogs,[23] 139 minutes in newborn calves, 64 minutes in calves 2 months of age or older, and 80 to 97 minutes in cows.[18,24] The elimination half-life is ≈4.5 hours in swine, sheep, and goats.[16,17]

In chickens, oral bioavailability of tylosin tartrate is 27%. Peak concentration of 0.44 µg/mL is reached ≈1.3 hours after oral administration. Elimination half-life is 1.34 hours.[25]

Contraindications/Precautions/Warnings

Tylosin is contraindicated in patients that are hypersensitive to it or other macrolide antibiotics (eg, erythromycin). Tylosin is contraindicated in horses, as severe and sometimes fatal diarrhea may result; the drug should be used with extreme caution, if at all, in other hindgut fermenters (eg, rabbits).

Adverse reactions, including shock and death, may result from overdose in baby pigs.[26,27] Do not attempt injection into pigs weighing less than 11.4 kg (25 lb) with the 200 mg/mL formulation; in these pigs it is recommended to use the 50 mg/mL injection with a syringe that can accurately measure 0.1 mL.

Adverse Effects

The most likely adverse effects are pain and local reactions at IM injection sites and mild GI upset (eg, anorexia, diarrhea). Tylosin may induce severe diarrhea if administered orally to ruminants or by any route to horses. In swine, reported adverse effects include edema of rectal mucosa and mild anal protrusion with pruritus, erythema, and diarrhea.

Reproductive/Nursing Safety

Safety of tylosin in pregnant animals has not been established, but other macrolides are considered safe for use during pregnancy. Tylosin is excreted into milk at concentration up to 5 times higher than is found in serum.[18] Because safety has not been established in animals, this drug should only be used when the maternal benefits outweigh the potential risks to offspring.

Overdose/Acute Toxicity

Tylosin is relatively safe in most overdose situations. LD_{50} in pigs is greater than 5 g/kg PO and ≈1 g/kg IM. Dogs have been reported to tolerate oral doses of 800 mg/kg. Long-term (ie, 2-year) oral administration of up to 400 mg/kg produced no organ toxicity in dogs. Shock and death have been reported in piglets overdosed with tylosin.

For patients that have experienced or are suspected to have experienced an overdose, consultation with a 24-hour poison consultation center that specializes in providing veterinary-specific information is recommended. For general information related to overdose and toxin exposures, as well as contact information for poison control centers, refer to ***Appendix.***

Drug Interactions

The following drug interactions have either been reported or are theoretical in humans or animals receiving tylosin and may be of significance in veterinary patients. Unless otherwise noted, use together is not necessarily contraindicated, but weigh the potential risks and perform additional monitoring when appropriate. Refer to ***Erythromycin*** for more information on potential interactions.

- **Bentonite**: Simultaneous administration of tylosin (in drinking water or feed) and bentonite (mixed in feed as a mycotoxin binder) should be avoided, as there is significant reduction in tylosin plasma levels and area under the curve (AUC) in chickens.[28]
- **Digoxin**: May increase digoxin blood concentrations with resultant toxicity

Laboratory Considerations

- Macrolide antibiotics may cause falsely elevated **ALT** (SGPT) and **AST** (SGOT) values when using colorimetric assays.
- Fluorometric determinations of **urinary catecholamines** can be altered by concomitant macrolide administration.

Dosages

DOGS/CATS:

NOTES:

1. Using volumetric containers (eg, teaspoons) to measure tylosin soluble powders is not necessarily accurate; however, 1 level teaspoon (5 mL) of powder contains ≈2.5 – 2.7 g of tylosin, and ⅛ level teaspoon contains ≈325 mg of tylosin.
2. Powder is unpalatable.

Antibiotic-responsive diarrhea and adjunctive treatment of inflammatory bowel disease (IBD) in dogs; (extra-label): 20 – 25 mg/kg PO once daily has been studied,[1-3] while 20 mg/kg PO every 8 to 12 hours has also been suggested.[29] Duration is poorly defined; 7 days has been used in some studies, but 4 to 6 weeks has been recommended.[30] Diarrhea often reappears within weeks after discontinuation (some dogs with tylosin-responsive diarrhea remain clinically normal while treatment continues). A lower dose of 5 – 15 mg/kg PO once daily has been effective in dogs that have relapsed.[1-3]

Adjunctive treatment of colitis (extra-label): 10 – 15 mg/kg PO every 8 hours for 14 to 28 days, then maintain with 5 mg/kg PO every 24 hours[31]

Campylobacteriosis (extra-label): 11 mg/kg PO every 8 hours[32]

***Clostridium perfringens*-associated diarrhea** (extra-label): Although there is little objective information on when and how to provide treatment, tylosin 10 – 20 mg/kg PO every 12 to 24 hours has been recommended.[32]

***Cryptosporidium* spp-associated diarrhea in cats** (extra-label):

10 – 15 mg/kg PO every 12 hours will sometimes resolve diarrhea. Tylosin can be a GI irritant; if a positive response has been noted in the first 7 days of therapy, and if there is no toxicity, continue treatment for 1 week after clinical resolution of diarrhea. Some cats with *Cryptosporidium* spp infection (with or without *Giardia* spp coinfection) require several weeks of treatment prior to resolution of diarrhea.[33]

Canine pyoderma (extra-label): 10 – 20 mg/kg PO every 12 hours; continue treatment for 7 days after resolution of active lesion.[6,8]

CATTLE:

Susceptible infections in beef and nonlactating dairy cattle (label dosage; FDA-approved): 17.6 mg/kg IM once daily. Continue treatment for 24 hours after clinical signs have resolved, not to exceed 5 days. Do not inject more than 10 mL per site. Use the 50 mg/mL formulation in calves weighing less than 91 kg (200 lb).[26]

SWINE:

Susceptible infections (label dosage; FDA-approved):

a) **Injection**: 8.8 mg/kg IM twice daily. Continue treatment for 24 hours after clinical signs have resolved, not to exceed 3 days.[26] Do not inject more than 5 mL per site. Use the 50 mg/mL formulation for piglets weighing less than 11.3 kg (25 lb).[27]

b) **In drinking water**: 250 mg tylosin soluble powder is added per gallon of sole source drinking water for 3 to 10 days; subsequent treatment with tylosin medicated feed may be necessary.[11]

POULTRY:

Chickens (label dosage; FDA-approved):

a) **Necrotic enteritis**: 851 – 1419 mg/gallon of sole source drinking water for 5 days[11]

b) **Chronic respiratory disease**: 2000 mg/gallon of sole source drinking water for 3 days; treatment duration of 1 to 5 days may be considered based on severity of infection.[11]

Turkeys (label dosage; FDA-approved): 2000 mg/gallon of sole source drinking water for 3 days; treatment duration of 2 to 5 days may be considered based on severity of infection.[11]

Reduction in severity of effects of infectious sinusitis associated with *Mycoplasma gallisepticum*: 2000 mg/gallon of sole source drinking water for 3 days; treatment duration of 2 to 5 days may be considered based on severity of infection.[11]

FERRETS:

Susceptible enteric infections (extra-label): 10 mg/kg PO once to twice daily[34]

RABBITS, RODENTS, SMALL MAMMALS:

NOTE: Use with caution in hindgut fermenters.

Rabbits: 10 mg/kg SC or IM every 12 to 24 hours[35]

Gerbils, Hamsters, Rats: 10 mg/kg SC once a day[36]

HONEY BEES:

Control of American foulbrood (label dosage; FDA-approved): 200 mg tylosin mixed in 20 g confectioners/powdered sugar and dusted over the top bars of the brood chamber once weekly for 3 weeks. Apply early in the spring or fall before the main honey flow begins.[11]

Monitoring

- Clinical efficacy
- Adverse effects, including signs of enterocolitis in hindgut fermenters

Client Information

- This medicine is most commonly used in dogs and cats to treat diarrhea and inflammation of intestines; it may also be used to treat respiratory infections in birds (including chickens) and reptiles.
- Do not give this medicine to horses or ponies.
- Oral doses may be given with or without food. Give this medicine with food if stomach upset or vomiting occurs.
- The powder has an extremely bitter taste. The animal may be more likely to accept the medication if the powder is placed in an empty gelatin capsule.
- Tylosin is usually well tolerated when it is given orally to small animals (ie, dogs and cats). Contact your veterinarian if your animal experiences side effects.
- When tylosin is given in drinking water, prepare a fresh solution every 3 days. First mix the appropriate amount of tylosin powder with 1 gallon of drinking water, then further dilute it according to the product label.

Chemistry/Synonyms

Tylosin, a macrolide antibiotic composite structurally related to erythromycin, is produced from *Streptomyces fradiae* and may contain tylosin B, C, and D in addition to the main component. It occurs as an almost white to buff-colored powder with a pK_a of 7.1. It is slightly soluble in water and soluble in alcohol. Tylosin is considered to be highly lipid soluble. The tartrate salt is soluble in water. The injectable form of the drug (as the base) is in a 50% propylene glycol solution.

Tylosin may also be known as desmycosin, tilosina, tylosiini, tylosinum, tylozin, tylozyna, or *Tylan*®.

Storage/Stability

Unless otherwise instructed by the manufacturer, injectable tylosin should be stored in well-closed containers at 25°C (77°F). Tylosin, like erythromycin, is unstable in acidic (pH less than 4) media.

Compatibility/Compounding Considerations

Because converting volume measurements into weights is not very accurate for powders, it is recommended to weigh powders when using them for pharmaceutical purposes. However, if this is not possible, 1 level teaspoon (5 mL) of commercially available tylosin tartrate (*Tylan*® *Soluble*) contains ≈2.5 to 2.7 g of tylosin; ⅛ level teaspoon contains ≈325 mg of tylosin.

Tylosin tartrate powder added to food can be unpalatable for dogs or cats. Placing the proper dose in a gelatin capsule may be more preferable than mixing it into food. Another suggestion for dogs or cats that absolutely will not eat food with tylosin in it is to melt ≈¼ teaspoon of butter, pour into mini ice tray compartments, add the appropriate dose of tylosin powder, mix well, and freeze. (**NOTE**: Stability information for this procedure has not been performed.) Alternatively, the medication can be compounded. See ***Appendix*** for finding a quality assured pharmacy.

It is not recommended to mix tylosin for injection with other drugs, as precipitation of tylosin may result.[26,27]

Dosage Forms/Regulatory Status

VETERINARY-LABELED PRODUCTS:

A prescription or veterinary feed directive is required to treat any food animals (including honey bees) with tylosin.

Tylosin Injection: 50 mg/mL and 200 mg/mL; *Tylan*®, generic; (OTC). FDA approved for use in nonlactating dairy cattle, beef cattle, and swine. Slaughter withdrawal (at labeled doses): cattle = 21 days; swine = 14 days. Not for use in calves intended to be processed for veal, preruminating calves, or female dairy cattle 20 months of age or older (including dry cows).

Tylosin Tartrate Powder: (≈2.5 – 2.7 g/level teaspoon) in 100 g bottles; *Tylan*® *Soluble, generic*; (Rx). FDA-approved for use in turkeys (not layers), chickens (not layers), swine, and honey bees. Slaughter withdrawal swine = 2 days; chickens = 1 day; turkeys = 5 days. Complete honey bee treatments at least 4 weeks prior to the main honey flow.

There are many FDA-approved tylosin phosphate products available via veterinary feed directive for use in beef cattle, swine, and honey bees. Many of these products have other active ingredients included in their formulations.

HUMAN-LABELED PRODUCTS: NONE

References

For the complete list of references, see **wiley.com/go/budde/plumb**

Ursodiol

Ursodeoxycholic acid (UDCA)

(ur-soe-***dye***-ole) *Actigall®, URSO®*

Choleretic; Bile Acid; Hepatoprotectant

Prescriber Highlights

- Bile acid that may be useful for adjunctive treatment of hepatobiliary disease in dogs and cats, particularly cholestatic disorders; may also be effective in treating biliary sludge (microlithiasis)
- Contraindicated in the presence of extrahepatic bile duct obstruction or vanishing bile duct syndrome; do not use in rabbits and other hindgut fermenters because of bacterial metabolism to the hepatotoxic bile acid, lithocholic acid.
- Appears to be well tolerated in dogs and cats; should be given with food

Uses/Indications

In small animal species, ursodiol may be useful as adjunctive therapy for the medical management of acute and chronic cholestatic hepatobiliary disorders by ameliorating the progression of inflammatory and degenerative changes associated with these conditions[1-7]; it may also aid in the resolution of biliary sludge accumulation (ie, microlithiasis).[8,9] Ursodiol can also be used as part of the medical management of gallbladder mucoceles by protecting against hepatobiliary epithelial damage that occurs with this condition; however, there is no evidence that ursodiol aids in the medical dissolution of mature gallbladder mucoceles and surgical correction is indicated in many patients.[10,11]

Although ursodiol is approved to dissolve cholesterol choleliths in humans,[12] it will not dissolve choleliths in small animal species as they are commonly composed of calcium carbonate (dogs) or calcium bilirubinate (cats), not cholesterol.

Pharmacology/Actions

Ursodiol is a noncytotoxic bile acid that has several pharmacologic actions.[13-15] After oral administration, ursodiol decreases intestinal absorption of cholesterol and suppresses hepatic synthesis and secretion of cholesterol, and ultimately reduces cholesterol saturation in the bile. In veterinary medicine, ursodiol is used for its choleretic (increased bile flow) properties. It increases the expression of membrane transport proteins on the canalicular membrane of hepatocytes that are responsible for the movement of bile acids from hepatocytes to the bile canaliculi. Secretion of ursodiol into the bile ducts stimulates the flow of bicarbonate-rich bile and promotes the elimination of toxic bile acids. A process known as cholehepatic shunting allows for the recirculation of ursodiol from the cholangiocytes back to the hepatocytes.

Ursodiol has antioxidant, anti-inflammatory, and some mild immunomodulatory effects. It promotes hepatobiliary cytoprotection by replacing the more toxic hydrophobic bile acids (eg, lithocholic acid, deoxycholic acid), which accumulate in the bile acid pool with cholestatic liver disease. Additionally, it is antiapoptotic through its ability to stimulate cell survival pathways; ursodiol also acts as a molecular chaperone and protects against endoplasmic reticulum-mediated hepatobiliary cellular stress caused by toxic bile acids.

Pharmacokinetics

Ursodiol is well absorbed from the small intestine after oral administration. In humans, up to 90% of the dose is absorbed from the small intestine into the portal circulation. Absorption is improved in the presence of food.[12] Once it reaches the liver, it is extracted from the portal circulation, conjugated with either taurine or glycine in hepatocytes, then secreted into bile. Ursodiol concentrates in the gallbladder, and the concentration in bile plateaus at ≈30% to 50% of total bile acid after ≈3 weeks. After biliary secretion into the duodenum, the majority of conjugated ursodiol is extracted by the apical bile acid transporter in the ileum, deposited into the portal circulation, and transported back to the liver. A small portion of conjugated ursodiol in the intestinal tract may be deconjugated by bacterial enzymes and either be absorbed there or pass to the colon where it may be eliminated or converted to other bile acids (including the potentially hepatotoxic bile acid, lithocholic acid), which also are eliminated in the feces. In most species, with the exception of hindgut fermenters, the amount of this hepatotoxic bile acid generated is minimal and inconsequential.

The very small quantities of unconjugated ursodiol that enter the systemic circulation are bound (70%) to plasma proteins, and less than 1% is excreted in the urine. Ursodiol has been detected in the serum of dogs and cats following oral administration.[3,16]

Contraindications/Precautions/Warnings

Ursodiol is contraindicated in rabbits and other hindgut fermenters as it is converted into the hepatotoxic bile acid, lithocholic acid.[17] It is also contraindicated in patients hypersensitive to it or other bile acid products and in patients with complete extrahepatic bile duct obstruction. Ursodiol should also be used cautiously in dogs and cats with histologically confirmed hepatic ductopenic disorders (eg, cholangitis, cholangiohepatitis) as it may lead to progressive biliary damage. The benefits of using ursodiol should be weighed against its risks in patients with complications associated with choleliths (eg, biliary obstruction, biliary fistulas, cholecystitis, pancreatitis, cholangitis). Ursodiol does not dissolve radiopaque, calcified cholesterol, or radiolucent bile pigment choleliths.[12]

Adverse Effects

Ursodiol appears to be well tolerated in dogs and cats.[16,18-20] A study in 20 healthy dogs given ursodiol 10 to 15 mg/kg PO daily showed no changes in hepatic ultrasound, serum liver enzymes, total bilirubin, cholesterol, or triglyceride concentrations after 6 to 8 weeks of administration.[20] An additional study in 12 healthy dogs at the same dose showed no changes in serum bile acids testing and hepatic histopathology after 7 days of therapy.[19] Two studies in normal cats given ursodiol showed no changes in CBC, biochemical panel, urinalysis, ultrasound, or hepatic histopathology, but a significant decrease in serum cholesterol was noted.[16,18] See ***Laboratory Monitoring***.

In humans taking ursodiol, elevated liver enzymes, diarrhea, abdominal pain, and other GI effects have rarely been noted.[12] Although hepatotoxicity has not been associated with ursodiol therapy in humans, there are some patients with an inability to sulfate lithocholic acid (a naturally occurring bile acid and also a metabolite of ursodiol). These patients are at risk for increased concentrations of lithocholic acid as bile acid sulfation is a mechanism for bile acid detoxification. The clinical significance of this information for dogs and cats is unclear.

Reproductive/Nursing Safety

No evidence of impaired fertility or fetal harm was found in pregnant rabbits or rats given ursodiol 7 times or 22 times, respectively, the maximum human labeled dose.[12] It does not cross the placenta and has been safely used in the treatment of intrahepatic cholestasis of pregnancy in women.[21]

It is not known whether ursodiol is excreted in breast milk. Because minimal drug is systemically absorbed, clinical effects on nursing animals are unlikely.

Overdose/Acute Toxicity

Overdoses of ursodiol would most likely cause diarrhea, although salivation and vomiting have been noted in dogs. Treatment, if required, could include supportive therapy, oral administration of an aluminum-containing antacid (eg, aluminum hydroxide suspension), or gastric emptying (if large overdose) with concurrent administration of activated charcoal or cholestyramine suspension.

For patients that have experienced or are suspected of having experienced an overdose, consultation with a 24-hour poison consultation center specializing in providing veterinary-specific information is recommended. For general information related to overdose and toxin exposures, as well as contact information for poison control centers, refer to ***Appendix***.

Drug Interactions

The following drug interactions have either been reported or are theoretical in humans or animals receiving ursodiol and may be of significance in veterinary patients. Unless otherwise noted, use together is not necessarily contraindicated, but weigh the potential risks and perform additional monitoring when appropriate.

- ALUMINUM-CONTAINING ANTACIDS: May bind to ursodiol, thereby reducing its efficacy
- CHOLESTYRAMINE: May bind to ursodiol, thereby reducing its efficacy
- CYCLOSPORINE: May increase cyclosporine serum concentrations
- ESTROGENS: May increase hepatic cholesterol secretion and counteract ursodiol effects in humans; significance in veterinary patients is unknown.
- FENOFIBRATE: Fibrates increase cholesterol formation and may counteract ursodiol effects in humans; significance in veterinary patients is unknown.
- GEMFIBROZIL: Fibrates increase cholesterol formation and may counteract ursodiol effects in humans; significance in veterinary patients is unknown.
- TAURINE: Although not documented, concern has been raised that chronic administration of ursodiol in cats may lead to taurine deficiency.

Laboratory Considerations

- Ursodiol may falsely elevate total **serum bile acid test** results, although the magnitude of this change may not be clinically relevant.[16,19,20] It is recommended to stop ursodiol for a minimum of 2 to 3 days before performing total serum bile acid testing.

Dosages

DOGS:

Medical treatment of biliary sludge (microlithiasis) and adjunctive treatment of acute and chronic nonobstructive cholestatic disorders or chronic hepatitis (extra-label): 10 – 15 mg/kg PO with food once daily day or divided twice daily[22]

CATS:

Adjunctive treatment of nonobstructive acute and chronic cholestatic disorders (extra-label): 10 – 15 mg/kg PO with food once daily day or divided twice daily[6]

Lymphocytic cholangitis: 15 mg/kg PO with food daily produced morphologic and immunohistochemical improvements, although prednisolone reduced inflammation to a greater extent and promoted longer survival.[1,2]

BIRDS:

Adjunctive treatment of liver disease (extra-label): 10 – 15 mg/kg PO once daily[23]

Monitoring

- Periodic abdominal ultrasonography based on the clinical presentation of the underlying condition being treated (eg, biliary sludge)
- Baseline and periodic (eg, every 3 to 6 months) serum liver chemistry panel (eg, ALT, ALP, GGT, total bilirubin)

Client Information

- Ursodiol is used to help animals with liver, pancreas, and/or gallbladder problems.
- This medicine works best when given with food. It also has a bitter taste that can often be masked when the medicine is given with food.
- Ursodiol is usually well-tolerated by dogs and cats. Diarrhea is the most common side effect. Contact your veterinarian if you have any concerns about your animal's condition.
- Do not give this medicine to rabbits, guinea pigs, rodents, or horses.

Chemistry/Synonyms

Ursodiol, also known as ursodeoxycholic acid, is a naturally occurring bile acid. It occurs as a white or almost white, bitter-tasting crystalline powder that is practically insoluble in water and freely soluble in alcohol.

Ursodiol may also be known as acidum ursodeoxycholicum, UDCA, or ursodesoxycholic acid; many trade names are available, including *Actigall®*.

Storage/Stability

Unless otherwise specified by the manufacturer, store ursodiol at room temperature (20°C to 25°C [68°F-77°F]) in tight containers. Half tablets maintain acceptable quality for up to 28 days when stored in the bottle at room temperature. Because of the bitter taste, store the segments separately from whole tablets.

Compatibility/Compounding Considerations

Ursodiol 50 mg/mL oral suspension can be compounded from commercially available tablets. Triturate 20 ursodiol 250 mg tablets with 50 mL of *Ora-Plus®* and qs ad to 100 mL with *Ora-Sweet®*. The resulting suspension retains 90% potency for 90 days when stored at both 5°C (41°F) or 25°C (77°F). Compounded preparations of ursodiol should be protected from light and shaken well before use.[24]

Dosage Forms/Regulatory Status

VETERINARY-LABELED PRODUCTS: NONE

HUMAN-LABELED PRODUCTS:

Ursodiol Oral Capsules: 300 mg; *Actigall®*, generic; (Rx)

Ursodiol Oral Tablets: 250 mg and 500 mg; *URSO®-250* and *-Forte*, generic; (Rx)

References

For the complete list of references, see **wiley.com/go/budde/plumb**

Valacyclovir

(*val*-ay-*sye*-kloe-veer) *Valtrex®*
Antiviral

Prescriber Highlights

- ► Potentially useful for treating equine herpes viral infection; however, definitive proof is lacking
- ► Prodrug of acyclovir with improved oral absorption
- ► Should not be used in cats due to lack of efficacy and profound toxicity (ie, nephrotoxicity, hepatotoxicity, myelosuppression)
- ► Use with caution and consider dose reduction in patients with renal insufficiency.
- ► Patients must be adequately hydrated during treatment.
- ► Appears to be well tolerated in horses, but experience is limited

Uses/Indications

Valacyclovir may be effective for treating equine herpesvirus 1 (EHV-1) infection, although evidence to support this use is limited. In horses experimentally exposed to EHV-1, valacyclovir was effective in reducing viral replication as measured by decreased viral load in blood, nasal secretions, and bronchoalveolar fluid; however, viral load in the CSF did not differ from placebo.[1] Clinical signs improved when valacyclovir was given prior to EHV-1 exposure as well when given up to 2 days after viral challenge. In ponies experimentally infected with EHV-1 that received valacyclovir 1 hour prior to inoculation, the drug reduced respiratory signs, but not other clinical signs.[2] These findings resemble the experience in humans, where treatment is more likely to be successful when initiated early (ie, with the earliest symptom or sign of disease).

Valacyclovir treatment was reported in a retrospective study of 7 naturally occurring cases of EHV-1.[3] Another report of 31 horses treated with valacyclovir also found a strong decrease of EHV-1 viral load in nasal secretions and blood in all treated horses.[4] Successful valacyclovir use was reported in 2 stallions during an outbreak of equine coital exanthema[5] and in a single case of equine multinodular pulmonary fibrosis[6]; however, valacyclovir failed to reduce viral load in 6 horses diagnosed with equine multinodular pulmonary fibrosis, and 5 horses were euthanized due to progression of clinical signs.[7]

Valacyclovir did not suppress FHV-1 replication in cats.[8]

In humans, valacyclovir is used for treatment, suppression, and/or prevention of herpes and varicella viral infections, and, at high doses, for prevention of cytomegalovirus infections in immunocompromised patients.

Pharmacology/Actions

As a prodrug, valacyclovir is rapidly and almost completely hydrolyzed to the nucleoside analogue acyclovir and L-valine. Viral-specific thymidine kinase then converts acyclovir to acyclovir monophosphate, which is further phosphorylated to the active acyclovir triphosphate. Acyclovir triphosphate is incorporated into the viral DNA to cause viral DNA chain termination and thereby inhibits viral DNA synthesis and replication. Variations in acyclovir sensitivity and resistance are likely mediated by differing sensitivity, or outright deficiency of, viral thymidine kinase.[9,10]

The primary goal of antiherpetic therapy is to decrease viral replication until the immune system mounts an appropriate response and controls active infection.[9]

In humans, valacyclovir has antiviral activity against herpes labialis, herpes simplex, herpes zoster, varicella zoster, and cytomegalovirus. Resistance of herpes simplex and varicella zoster to acyclovir has been reported in humans and can result from changes in thymidine kinase or DNA polymerase.[11]

Pharmacokinetics

In horses, oral absorption of valacyclovir is 8-fold greater than acyclovir,[12] with bioavailability reported as 26%[12] and up to 50% when the drug is administered after intragastric lavage.[13] The effect of food on oral absorption is uncertain. The pharmacokinetic profile of valacyclovir at 20 mg/kg PO was nearly identical to acyclovir at 10 mg/kg administered as an IV infusion over 1 hour.[12] Peak serum concentration was reached ≈50 minutes after administration.[12,13] Volume of distribution was 9.8 L/kg,[12] but penetration into the CSF was minimal.[10] Protein binding was low at 10% to 20%.[12] Elimination half-life of unbound acyclovir was 8.8 hours.[12] Following administration of valacyclovir 40 mg/kg PO every 8 hours (mixed in applesauce), acyclovir serum concentration remained above 3 µg/mL (the EC_{50}[12]) for 60% of the dosing interval,[10] and concentrations from nasal swabs were 50% to 100% of serum concentration.[2] Serum acyclovir concentration (mean peak concentration, 1.5 µg/mL on day 4) was lower than expected in 6 horses with EHV-5 that received valacyclovir 30 mg/kg PO every 8 hours for 48 hours, then 20 mg/kg every 12 hours for 8 additional days.[7]

After a single dose of valacyclovir 40 mg/kg was given orally in eastern box turtles, peak concentration of 1.9 µg/mL was reached 13 hours after dosing, and half-life was 15.2 hours. In this species, valacyclovir 40 mg/kg PO every 24 hours is predicted to maintain concentrations above 0.45 µg/mL.[14]

In humans, valacyclovir is rapidly absorbed, with peak concentrations reached after 1.5 hours. Bioavailability is ≈55% and is not affected by food. Conversion to acyclovir occurs with first-pass hepatic and intestinal metabolism. Acyclovir is widely distributed into most tissues, and protein binding is ≈15%. Acyclovir undergoes minimal hepatic metabolism and is excreted equally via the kidneys (47%) and in the feces (46%). Elimination half-life is ≈3 hours but increases to 14 hours in patients with end-stage renal disease. Hepatic impairment does not alter acyclovir pharmacokinetics.

Contraindications/Precautions/Warnings

Valacyclovir should not be used in patients that are hypersensitive to valacyclovir or acyclovir.[11] Valacyclovir should not be used in cats, as it has caused significant toxicity (eg, severe myelosuppression, coagulative necrosis of the renal tubular epithelium, centrilobular atrophy and hepatic necrosis) in this species.[8]

Valacyclovir should be used with caution in patients with renal insufficiency, and in those that are geriatric (with or without diminished renal function), dehydrated, or receiving nephrotoxic drugs, as use under these conditions has resulted in acute kidney injury in humans[11]; dosage modification may be considered in patients with significant renal impairment. Maintaining hydration in patients receiving valacyclovir is critical, as the drug may precipitate in—and cause damage to—the renal tubules.[11]

Do not confuse valACYclovir with valGANciclovir or VANcomycin.

Adverse Effects

Valacyclovir appeared to be well tolerated in horses enrolled in pharmacokinetic or experimental studies.

In cats infected with feline herpesvirus 1 (FHV-1), lethargy, dehydration, and significant decreases in WBC and neutrophil counts were noted 6 to 9 days after initiation of valacyclovir at 60 mg/kg PO every 6 hours; histologic changes included bone marrow suppression, coagulative necrosis in the renal tubules, centrilobular atrophy, and hepatic necrosis.[8] The drug did not suppress FHV-1 replication.

In humans, GI distress (eg, nausea, vomiting, abdominal pain), CNS depression, agitation, confusion, seizures, encephalopathy, and ophthalmologic, hematologic, and dermatologic conditions have also been reported.[11] CNS adverse reactions are more common in geriatric patients; however, they have also been reported in adults and pediatric patients with or without reduced renal function. Increased liver enzymes and crystal formation in renal tubules has also occurred.

Reproductive/Nursing Safety

Valacyclovir is rapidly metabolized to acyclovir, which is found in amniotic fluid and crosses the placenta. No evidence of embryo-fetal toxicity or teratogenicity has been observed in animal studies.[11]

Although valacyclovir is not detected in milk, low levels of the metabolite acyclovir are present in breast milk of women taking valacyclovir. This drug should be used with caution in lactating patients.[11]

Because safety has not been established in animals, this drug should only be used when the maternal benefits outweigh the potential fetal risks.

Overdose/Acute Toxicity

Vomiting and diarrhea are the predominant signs of acyclovir toxicity; acute kidney injury is theoretically possible with higher doses. Acute oral overdose is unlikely to cause significant toxicity. Crystalluria and elevated renal values occurred after administration of acyclovir at 188.7 mg/kg in a dog.

GI decontamination can be considered with ingestions of valacyclovir at 150 mg/kg or higher if done within 60 to 90 minutes of ingestion. Below 150 mg/kg, GI signs (eg, vomiting, diarrhea) will likely predominate. Nephrotoxicity, hepatotoxicity, and myelosuppression occurred in cats receiving 240 mg/kg/day.[8] Acyclovir is removed via hemodialysis.

For patients that have experienced or are suspected to have experienced an overdose, consultation with a 24-hour poison consultation center specializing in providing veterinary-specific information is recommended. For general information related to overdose and toxin exposures, as well as contact information for poison control centers, refer to ***Appendix.***

Drug Interactions

The following drug interactions have either been reported or are theoretical in humans or animals receiving valacyclovir and may be of significance in veterinary patients; unless otherwise noted, use together is not necessarily contraindicated, but the potential risks should be weighed and additional monitoring should be performed when appropriate:

- CIMETIDINE: Concurrent use in humans increases acyclovir area under the curve (AUC) by 32%, but this effect is considered to be clinically insignificant
- MEPERIDINE: Concurrent use may increase risk for CNS stimulation and excitation.
- MYCOPHENOLATE: Concurrent valacyclovir and mycophenolate may increase serum concentration of each.
- NEPHROTOXIC MEDICATIONS (eg, aminoglycosides, amphotericin B, cyclosporine, and ifosfamide): Concomitant administration of valacyclovir with nephrotoxic medications may increase the potential for nephrotoxicity.[11] Renal function should be monitored.
- PROBENECID: Concurrent use in humans increases acyclovir AUC by 49%, but this effect is considered clinically insignificant.
- THEOPHYLLINE, AMINOPHYLLINE: May increase serum concentration of theophylline or theophylline derivatives
- VACCINES FOR VIRAL ENCEPHALOMYELITIS INFECTIONS (EG, EEE, VEE, WEE, WEST NILE VIRUS): Concurrent valacyclovir may diminish vaccine effectiveness.
- ZIDOVUDINE: Concurrent use may increase risk for CNS depression.

Laboratory Considerations

- No specific laboratory interactions or considerations have been noted.

Dosages

HORSES:

Prevention or reduction of clinical signs in horses infected with equine herpesvirus 1 (EHV-1) (extra-label): 27 – 30 mg/kg PO every 8 hours for 6 doses, followed by 18 – 20 mg/kg PO every 12 hours for 1 to 2 weeks[1,3,10]

Equine coital exanthema (ECE) caused by equine herpesvirus 3 (EHV-3) (extra-label): 27 mg/kg PO every 8 hours for 6 doses, followed by 18 mg/kg PO every 12 hours for 10 or 11 days was believed to prevent lesions from expanding; stallions returned to mating 7 to 9 days after discontinuation of the drug.[5]

Monitoring

- Viral load in blood and nasal secretions via quantitative PCR[15]
- Clinical efficacy
- Adverse effects
- Baseline and periodic serum renal chemistries (eg, serum BUN and creatinine) and urinalysis
- Hydration status

Client Information

- This medicine can be given with or without food. If GI upset (eg, diarrhea, lack of an appetite) occurs, give the medicine with a small amount of food. Contact your veterinarian if the problem continues.
- Be sure your animal has access to fresh drinking water at all times.

Chemistry/Synonyms

Valacyclovir is the L-valine ester of acyclovir. Commercial dosage forms contain valacyclovir hydrochloride, which occurs as a white to off-white powder with aqueous solubility of 174 mg/mL at 25°C (77°F). 1 mg valacyclovir is equal to 1.11 mg valacyclovir HCl.

Valacyclovir may also be known as 256U87; *Valtrex®*, *Shilova®*, *Vaclovir®*, and *Valvir®* are examples of the many trade names available in different countries.

Storage/Stability

Valacyclovir tablets should be stored at a controlled room temperature of 15°C to 25°C (59°F-77°F) in a tightly closed container out of reach of children and animals.

Compatibility/Compounding Considerations.

A 50 mg/mL oral suspension may be made with caplets, *ORA-Plus®*, and either *ORA-Sweet®* or *ORA-Sweet® SF* (similar suspending vehicles may be used). Crush ten 500 mg tablets in a mortar and reduce to a fine powder. Sequentially add four 5 mL portions of *ORA-Plus®* (20 mL total) and mix to a uniform paste; transfer to an amber glass bottle calibrated to 100 mL, rinse mortar with 10 mL of *ORA-Plus®* 3 times, then add quantity of syrup (*ORA-Sweet®* or *ORA-Sweet® SF*) sufficient to make 100 mL. Label "shake well" and "refrigerate." Stable for 28 days refrigerated between 2°C to 8°C (36°F-46°F).[16] If a less concentrated suspension is desired, use five 500 mg tablets to make 25 mg/mL and follow previously described process for 100 mL total volume.[13]

Dosage Forms/Regulatory Status

VETERINARY-LABELED PRODUCTS: NONE

HUMAN-LABELED PRODUCTS:

Valacyclovir Oral Tablets: 500 mg and 1000 mg; *Valtrex®*, generic; (Rx). Some presentations may be scored.

References

For the complete list of references, see **wiley.com/go/budde/plumb**

Vancomycin

(van-koe-***mye***-sin) *Vancocin®*

Glycopeptide Antibiotic

Prescriber Highlights

- IV antibiotic reserved for life-threatening, multidrug-resistant staphylococcal or enterococcal infections. It may also be used PO to treat *Clostridioides difficile* diarrhea.
- When used systemically, must be given IV; severe pain and tissue injury occur with SC or IM injection.
- Oral vancomycin is not absorbed systemically and is only useful for treating intraluminal enteric infections.
- Nephrotoxic drug with limited understanding of optimal dosing regimens
- If decreased renal function, decrease dosage and/or frequency
- Use in veterinary medicine is controversial because of the drug's importance in human medicine. Veterinary infectious disease specialists should be consulted prior to treatment. Use should be reserved for infections with confirmed susceptibility and for infections that are resistant to first- and second-tier options.

Uses/Indications

Because vancomycin is used for severe multidrug-resistant infections in humans, its use in veterinary medicine should be reserved for confirmed infections where culture and susceptibility testing demonstrates resistance to all other options (usually methicillin-resistant *Staphylococcus* spp [eg, MRSA, MRSP] or multidrug-resistant *Enterococcus* spp) and when the infection is considered treatable and consultation with an infectious disease expert has concluded that vancomycin is a viable and reasonable treatment.[1-3] Empirical use should be discouraged. Oral vancomycin may be useful for oral treatment of *Clostridioides difficile* enteric infections, although treatment of this infection is rarely required and other treatment options (ie, metronidazole) are available for instances when treatment is indicated.

Vancomycin may also be useful for local therapy, such as through implantation of antimicrobial-impregnated substances (eg, PMMA beads, gels),[4,5] intra-articular injection, and regional limb perfusion. Uses that do not result in appreciable systemic or enteric concentrations are not associated with the same concerns of emergence of resistance in the patient's microbiome.

The World Health Organization (WHO) has designated vancomycin as a Critically Important, Highest Priority antimicrobial for human medicine.[6]

Pharmacology/Actions

Vancomycin inhibits cell wall synthesis and bacterial cell membrane permeability. It also affects bacterial RNA synthesis. It is only effective against gram-positive bacteria, including many strains of streptococci, staphylococci, and enterococci. Vancomycin is generally a bactericidal, time-dependent antibiotic, but is bacteriostatic against enterococci. Vancomycin also has activity against *Clostridioides (Clostridium) difficile*, *Rhodococcus equi*, *Listeria monocytogenes*, *Corynebacterium* spp, and *Actinomyces* spp. Vancomycin and aminoglycosides can have synergistic action against susceptible bacteria. Pus and cellular debris may bind to vancomycin and reduce its efficacy.

Resistance to vancomycin by certain strains of enterococci and staphylococci is an increasing concern in human medicine and potentially in veterinary patients. The global prevalence of vancomycin-resistant enterococci (VRE) in companion animals has been estimated to be 14.6%,[7] although regional variability exists.[8,9]

Pharmacokinetics

When given orally, vancomycin is not appreciably absorbed. A single dose study in dogs showed a bioavailability of 0.27% to 1.66% after oral administration.[10] After IV administration, vancomycin is widely distributed. Therapeutic concentrations can be found in pleural, ascitic, pericardial, and synovial fluids. At usual serum concentrations, it does not readily distribute into the CSF.

In humans, the elimination half-life of vancomycin in patients with normal renal function is ≈4 to 6 hours.[2] Prolonged dosing can allow the drug to accumulate. The drug is eliminated primarily via glomerular filtration; small amounts are excreted into the bile.

Contraindications/Precautions/Warnings

Vancomycin is an important antibiotic for treating multidrug-resistant infections in humans. It should not be used in veterinary patients when other antibiotics can be used to successfully treat the infection. Some clinicians believe that the drug should never be used in veterinary patients and its use in animals is banned in some countries. Nephrotoxicity is a concern.

IV vancomycin can be fatal in rabbits.

Patients with decreased renal function that require vancomycin should have doses reduced or dosing interval extended. Serum peak and trough concentrations should be monitored.

Adverse Effects

When given parenterally, nephrotoxicity and ototoxicity are the most serious potential adverse effects of vancomycin. In humans, the incidence of nephrotoxicity is relatively high in some patient populations[11]; however, it is usually reversible. In humans, dermatologic reactions and hypersensitivity can occur[2]; it is unknown if these effects are issues for veterinary patients. Reversible neutropenia has been reported in humans, particularly when the dose is high and prolonged.

Do not administer vancomycin IV rapidly or as a bolus; thrombophlebitis, severe hypotension, and cardiac arrest (rare) have been reported.[2] Vancomycin must be given over at least 30 minutes as a dilute solution. Do not give vancomycin IM, SC, or IP. Severe tissue damage and pain may occur.

Oral therapy may cause adverse GI effects (eg, nausea, inappetence, vomiting, diarrhea).

Reproductive/Nursing Safety

Because vancomycin should only be used for serious infections, the potential benefits of therapy will probably outweigh the risks in most circumstances.

Vancomycin is excreted into milk.[2] Because the drug is not appreciably absorbed through the GI tract, it is unlikely to pose significant harm to nursing animals, although diarrhea could occur.

Overdose/Acute Toxicity

IV overdoses of vancomycin may cause an increased risk for adverse effects, particularly ototoxicity and nephrotoxicity. Supportive care is advised. Hemodialysis does not appear to remove the drug in significant amounts.

For patients that have experienced or are suspected to have experienced an overdose, consultation with a 24-hour poison consultation center specializing in providing veterinary-specific information is recommended. For general information related to overdose and toxin exposures, as well as contact information for poison control centers, refer to ***Appendix.***

Drug Interactions

The following drug interactions have either been reported or are theoretical in humans or animals receiving vancomycin and may be of significance in veterinary patients. Unless otherwise noted, use together is not necessarily contraindicated, but weigh the potential risks and perform additional monitoring when appropriate.

- **Aminoglycosides**: Vancomycin may increase the risk for aminoglycoside-related ototoxicity or nephrotoxicity. Because this combination of drugs may be medically required (there is evidence of synergy against staphylococci and enterococci), enhanced monitoring is suggested.
- **Anesthetic Agents**: In children, vancomycin used with anesthetic agents has caused erythema and a histamine-like flushing.
- **Nephrotoxic Drugs, Other** (eg, **amphotericin B, cisplatin**): Use with caution with other nephrotoxic drugs.

Laboratory Considerations

- No specific concerns were noted.

Dosages

DOGS/CATS:

Susceptible gram-positive, systemic, life-threatening infections (extra-label):

a) 15 mg/kg IV over 30 to 60 minutes every 6 to 8 hours[12]

b) 3.5 mg/kg IV and follow with 1.5 mg/kg/hour IV CRI[13]

Oral treatment of documented *Clostridioides difficile* infection unresponsive to metronidazole (extra-label): 10 – 20 mg/kg PO every 6 hours for 5 to 7 days. **NOTE**: Oral vancomycin is not appreciably systemically absorbed and is only effective for susceptible enteric infections.

HORSES:

Susceptible gram-positive, systemic, life-threatening infections (extra-label): Average dosage was 7.5 mg/kg IV over 30 minutes every 8 hours from a retrospective study in 15 horses. The authors recommend that the use of vancomycin in horses be limited to cases in which culture and susceptibility results clearly indicate that this agent is likely to be effective and in which there is no reasonable alternative.[14]

Susceptible gram-positive, systemic, life-threatening infections; IV regional limb perfusion (IVRLP) or intraosseous regional limb perfusion (IORLP); (extra-label): Vancomycin 300 mg diluted in 60 mL 0.9% sodium chloride and infused IV (using an IV pump) or IO (administered manually) over 30 minutes. IVRLP or IORLP administration maintained their targeted trough drug concentration in synovial fluid. The authors concluded that IVRLP and IOPLP were safe and may be clinically useful in horses. IVRLP may be better for distal interphalangeal (DIP) joints and IORLP for metacarpophalangeal (MTCP) joints. Mean vancomycin concentration in the MTCP joint was 4 µg/mL for 24 hours after IORLP. [5,15,16]

Monitoring

When used parenterally:

- Baseline and periodic serum renal chemistry profile
- Monitoring trough drug concentrations is sometimes used in human medicine, mainly in patients with decreased renal function, advanced age, or other complicating factors. The target is to achieve a trough vancomycin concentration between 10 – 15 µg/mL, with 15 – 20 µg/mL recommended for serious MRSA infections.[17,18] The low end, or slightly lower, may be appropriate if an aminoglycoside is being used concurrently. There is little indication for routine peak drug concentration monitoring. Whether the same concentrations apply to veterinary patients is unknown but if drug monitoring is performed, human targets are reasonable to apply to animals.
- Baseline and periodic CBC with prolonged therapy

Client Information

- This medicine is most commonly given in the vein, by your veterinarian, while your animal is hospitalized.
- Oral vancomycin may be used for outpatient treatment. Be sure to give this medicine as directed by your veterinarian. It may be given with a small amount of food.
- Your veterinarian will need to monitor your animal closely while it is taking this medicine. Do not miss these important follow-up visits.

Chemistry/Synonyms

A glycopeptide antibiotic, vancomycin HCl occurs as an odorless, tan to brown free-flowing powder. It is freely soluble in water. A 5% aqueous solution has a pH of 2.5 to 4.5.

Vancomycin may also be known as vanco, vancomycini, or *Vancocin®*; there are many registered international trade names available.

Storage/Stability

Vancomycin should be stored at room temperature in tight containers that are protected from light. Once reconstituted (see administration instructions in the product label or in ***Dosages***), the injectable or oral solutions are stable for 14 days if refrigerated. If diluted further with 5% dextrose or 0.9% sodium chloride for parenteral administration, solutions are stable for 24 hours at room temperature and 2 months if refrigerated. Vancomycin solution in 5% dextrose should be stored at or below -20°C (-4°F); once thawed they are stable at room temperature for 72 hours, or 30 days if refrigerated. Do not refreeze thawed solutions.

Compatibility/Compounding Considerations

Compatibility is dependent on factors such as pH, concentration, temperature, and diluent used; consult specialized references or a hospital pharmacist for more specific information.

Vancomycin is **compatible** with 5% dextrose, 0.9% sodium chloride, and lactated Ringer's injection. To prepare a parenteral solution using vancomycin 500 mg or 1 g powder for injection: Reconstitute the 500 mg for injection vial by adding 10 mL of sterile water for injection; add 20 mL if using the 1 g vial. Before administering to patient, further dilute reconstituted solutions with (at least 100 mL for 500 mg; 200 mL for 1 g vial) a compatible diluent (eg, 5% dextrose, lactated Ringer's, 0.9% sodium chloride). Frozen containers of vancomycin solution in 5% dextrose should be thawed at room temperature (25°C[77°F]) or under refrigeration (5°C[41°F]); do not force thaw with hot water bath or by microwave.

Vancomycin injection is reportedly **Y-site compatible** with the following drugs: atropine sulfate, calcium salts, ciprofloxacin, clindamycin phosphate, dexamethasone sodium phosphate, diphenhydramine hydrochloride, famotidine, gentamicin, ketamine hydrochloride, metoclopramide, midazolam, ondansetron, potassium chloride, sodium bicarbonate, and tobramycin.

Vancomycin injection is reportedly **incompatible** with ampicillin, amphotericin B, cefazolin, ceftazidime, diazepam, furosemide, hydrocortisone sodium succinate, pantoprazole, and propofol.

Dosage Forms/Regulatory Status

VETERINARY-LABELED PRODUCTS: NONE

HUMAN-LABELED PRODUCTS:

Vancomycin HCl Powder for Injection (IV) Solution: 500 mg, 750 mg, 1 g, 5 g, and 10 g vials; (some preservative free); generic; (Rx)

Vancomycin for IV Injection in dextrose (frozen): 500 mg/100 mL, 750 mg/150 mL, 1 g/200 mL, 1.25 g/250 mL, 1.5 g/300 mL, and 2 g/400 mL; generic; (Rx)

Vancomycin HCl Oral Capsules: 125 mg and 250 mg; *Vancocin®*, generic; (Rx). **NOTE**: Not for systemic infections; not appreciably absorbed

Vancomycin Oral Solution: 25 mg/mL in 150 mL and 300 mL bottles, and 50 mg/mL in 80 mL, 150 mL and 300 mL bottles; *First-Vancomycin®-25, -50*; (Rx). **NOTE**: Not for systemic infections; not appreciably absorbed

References

For the complete list of references, see **wiley.com/go/budde/plumb**

Vasopressin

(vay-soe-***press***-in) *Vasostrict®*

Hormone; Pressor Agent

Prescriber Highlights

- ► Used primarily as a diagnostic agent and for the adjunctive treatment of shock syndromes and cardiopulmonary resuscitation
- ► Contraindications include chronic nephritis until nitrogen retention is resolved to reasonable levels, and in patients that are hypersensitive to it. Use with caution in patients that have vascular disease, seizure disorders, heart failure, or asthma.
- ► Adverse effects include nausea, GI pain/cramping, local irritation at the injection site (including sterile abscesses), extravasation injuries, skin reactions, abdominal pain, hematuria, and, rarely, a hypersensitivity (urticarial) reaction.
- ► Overdoses can lead to exacerbation of adverse effects, and possibly water intoxication.
- ► Cost of the drug may be an issue.

Uses/Indications

Vasopressin is used as a diagnostic agent (after a modified water deprivation test) and for the adjunctive treatment of shock syndromes and cardiopulmonary resuscitation in small animal species. Vasopressin has some potential advantages over epinephrine for treatment of ventricular asystole or pulseless electrical activity. Vasopressin can act as a vasoconstricting agent even when acidosis is present, and it may cause less vasoconstriction of the coronary and renal vasculature, thereby increasing myocardial perfusion and reducing myocardial oxygen consumption. Additionally, it does not have the arrhythmogenic or chronotropic effects that are associated with epinephrine.

Vasopressin has been documented to increase blood pressure in dogs with systemic inflammatory response syndrome (SIRS) and sepsis-induced hypotension. A case report in 5 dogs with dopamine-resistant SIRS or sepsis-induced hypotension found, in all cases, that the mean arterial blood pressure increased within 15 minutes of adding vasopressin to the treatment regimen.[1] Vasopressin is a common second-line agent (after norepinephrine) for the treatment of vasodilatory hypotension in both dogs and cats.[2]

In human medicine, vasopressin has been used to treat acute GI hemorrhage and stimulate GI peristalsis. Vasopressin CRI is also being used for the treatment of hypotensive septic patients that are unresponsive to conventional vasopressor. Prior to radiographic procedures, it has been used in humans to dispel interfering gas shadows or help concentrate contrast media.[3,4]

Pharmacology/Actions

Vasopressin or antidiuretic hormone (ADH) acts through at least 5 different receptors (3 subtypes: V1, V2, V3; the oxytocin receptor; and the purinergic P2 receptor) to maintain serum osmolality. Via V2 receptors, vasopressin promotes the renal reabsorption of solutefree water in the distal convoluted tubules and collecting duct. ADH increases cyclic adenosine monophosphate (cAMP) at the tubule, which increases water permeability at the luminal surface, resulting in increased urine osmolality and decreased urine flow. Without vasopressin, urine flow can be increased up to 90% greater than normal.

At doses above those necessary for antidiuretic activity, vasopressin V1 receptor stimulation and blockade of K+ -sensitive ATP channels can cause smooth muscle contraction. Capillaries and small arterioles are most affected, with resultant decreased blood flow to several systems. Hepatic flow may actually be increased, however.

Vasopressin can cause contraction of the smooth muscle of the bladder and gall bladder and increase intestinal peristalsis, particularly of the colon. Vasopressin may decrease gastric secretions and increase GI sphincter pressure; gastric acid concentration remains unchanged.

Vasopressin possesses minimal oxytocic effects, but at large doses, it may stimulate uterine contraction. Vasopressin V3 receptor stimulation causes the release of corticotropin, growth hormone, and follicle-stimulating hormone (FSH).

Pharmacokinetics

Vasopressin is destroyed in the GI tract prior to being absorbed and therefore must be administered either intranasally or parenterally. After IM or SC administration in dogs, aqueous vasopressin has an antidiuretic activity for 2 to 8 hours. Vasopressin is distributed throughout the extracellular fluid. The hormone apparently is not bound to plasma proteins. Vasopressin is rapidly destroyed in the liver and kidneys. The plasma half-life has been reported to be only 10 to 20 minutes in humans.

Contraindications/Precautions/Warnings

In humans, vasopressin is contraindicated in patients that are hypersensitive to it, as well as in patients with chronic nephritis until nitrogen retention is resolved to reasonable levels.

Because of its effects on other systems, particularly at high doses, vasopressin should be used with caution in patients with vascular disease, seizure disorders, heart failure, or asthma.

In humans, IV or IO vasopressin is considered a high alert medication (medications that require special safeguards to reduce the risk for errors). Consider instituting practices such as redundant drug dosage and volume checking with special alert labels.

Adverse Effects

Vasopressin adverse effects include local irritation at the injection site (extravasation necrosis possible), bronchoconstriction, arrhythmias, skin reactions, platelet aggregation, hyperbilirubinemia, nausea, abdominal pain and cramping, hematuria, and, rarely, a hypersensitivity (urticarial) reaction.[5]

Reproductive/Nursing Safety

Although the drug has minimal effects on uterine contractions at usual doses, it should be used with caution in pregnant animals.

Information on vasopressin levels in maternal milk was not located. Because vasopressin is not orally absorbed, adverse effects on nursing animals would not be expected. Because safety has not been established in animals, this drug should only be used when the maternal benefits outweigh the potential risks to offspring.

Overdose/Acute Toxicity

Acute overdoses would likely exacerbate the adverse effects listed above. Heart rate and rhythm as well as blood pressure should be monitored. Early clinical signs of overdose-induced water intoxication can include listlessness or depression. More severe intoxication clinical signs can include coma, seizures, and eventually death. Treatment for mild intoxication is stopping vasopressin therapy and restricting water access until it has resolved. Severe intoxication may require the use of osmotic diuretics (eg, mannitol, urea, dextrose) with or without furosemide.

For patients that have experienced or are suspected of having experienced an overdose, consultation with a 24-hour poison consultation center specializing in providing veterinary-specific information is recommended. For general information related to overdose and

toxin exposures, as well as contact information for poison control centers, refer to ***Appendix***.

Drug Interactions

The following drug interactions have either been reported or are theoretical in humans or animals receiving vasopressin and may be of significance in veterinary patients. Unless otherwise noted, use together is not necessarily contraindicated, but weigh the potential risks and perform additional monitoring when appropriate.

ISOFLURANE: In horses undergoing isoflurane anesthesia, IV administration of vasopressin raised blood pressure and caused mucous membrane ischemia within 1 minute, cardiac arrest within 5 to 10 minutes of administration in 8 of 10 horses.[6]

The following drugs may **inhibit** the antidiuretic activity of vasopressin:

- **ETHANOL**
- **EPINEPHRINE** (large doses)
- **HEPARIN**
- **NOREPINEPHRINE** (large doses)

The following drugs may **potentiate** the antidiuretic effects of vasopressin:

- **CYCLOPHOSPHAMIDE**
- **ENALAPRIL**
- **FLUDROCORTISONE**
- **FUROSEMIDE**
- **TRICYCLIC ANTIDEPRESSANTS** (eg, **amitriptyline, clomipramine**)
- **VINCRISTINE**

Dosages

NOTES:

1. Do not confuse dosages listed as units/kg/minute; units/kg per hour, milliunits/kg/minute.
2. Prior to IV administration, vasopressin should be diluted in 0.9% sodium chloride or 5% dextrose solutions to a final concentration of 0.1 – 1 unit/mL.[5]

DOGS/CATS:

Diagnostic agent for diabetes insipidus in conjunction with a modified water deprivation test (extra-label): A clear understanding of the limitations and risks for this test is required for patient safety during the test and to achieve an accurate diagnosis. Prior to administration, it is recommended to consult with a veterinary internal medicine specialist or refer to a current small animal endocrinology text for specific information about the protocol, precautions, endpoints, and contraindications for this type of testing.

a) 0.2 – 0.4 units/kg (maximum total dose of 5 units/animal [NOT units/kg]) IM[7]
b) **Dogs**: 2 – 3 units/dog (NOT units/kg) SC[8]
c) **Cats**: 0.55 units/kg SC [8]

Adjunctive treatment during cardiopulmonary resuscitation (extra-label):

a) 0.8 units/kg IV or IO as a substitute for or in combination with epinephrine every 3 to 5 minutes may be considered. Vasopressin is administered after every other basic life support cycle. If IV or IO access is not possible, intratracheal (IT) administration can be considered. Dilute in sterile saline or sterile water and administer via a catheter longer than the endotracheal tube. If giving IT, the dosage has not been fully determined, but 1.2 units/kg IT is currently recommended.[9]
b) With pulseless electrical activity or ventricular asystole, vasopressin may be beneficial for myocardial and cerebral blood flow: 0.2 – 0.8 units/kg, IV once[8]
c) In dogs, 0.4 – 0.8 units/kg IV, followed by 1 – 4 milliunits/kg per *MINUTE* IV CRI[10]

Adjunctive treatment of hypotension associated shock (extra-label):

a) **Adjunctive post-CPR treatment**: 0.5 – 5 milliunits/kg/*MINUTE* (0.03 – 0.3 units/kg/*HOUR*) IV CRI [9,10]
b) **Patients with vasodilatory shock unresponsive to fluid resuscitation and catecholamine (dobutamine, dopamine, norepinephrine) administration**: 0.01 – 0.04 units/*MINUTE* (NOT units/kg/*MINUTE*) IV. (**NOTE**: This dose is not dependent on patient weight.) DO NOT exceed 0.04 units/*MINUTE* (NOT units/kg/*MINUTE*), as there is a risk for myocardial ischemia. DO NOT use in patients with cardiogenic shock.[10,11]
c) **Adjunctive treatment of dogs with septic shock or severe systemic inflammatory response syndrome** (extra-label): The goal is to raise the diastolic pressure to 70 to 90 mm Hg, which is usually associated with a mean pressure of 110 to 140 mm Hg and a systolic of 140 to 180 mm Hg. If norepinephrine between 0.5 – 1 µg/kg/*MINUTE* IV CRI does not maintain the goal, consider adding vasopressin 1 – 4 milliunits/kg/*MINUTE* IV CRI. Infusion is started at the low end of the range and titrated upwards in response to need. Supplementation with low doses of vasopressin can restore catecholamine and hemodynamic response.[12]
d) **Hypotension that persists in dogs despite volume resuscitation** (extralabel): 0.5 – 5 milliunits/kg/*MINUTE* (0.03 – 0.3 units/kg/*HOUR*) IV CRI. Although arterial blood pressure may improve, it should be used cautiously, as excessive vasoconstriction (particularly to the splanchnic and renal circulation, thereby causing GI and renal ischemia) may occur. In the dog, splanchnic vasoconstriction may exacerbate the sepsis by promoting the loss of the gut barrier function and then bacterial translocation to the bloodstream.[13]

HORSES:

Refractory hypotension in critically ill neonatal foals (extra-label): 0.1 – 2.5 milliunits/kg/*MINUTE* IV CRI.[14] From the retrospective study, vasopressin dosages were titrated to the minimum infusion rate needed to achieve a mean arterial pressure (MAP) greater than 65 mm Hg. All foals also received dobutamine and other supportive treatment. Vasopressin use was associated with a significant increase in MAP and urinary output, and a significant decrease in heart rate.

Monitoring

- Blood pressure; heart rate and rhythm
- Hydration, body weight; fluid and electrolyte status
- Urine output, specific gravity, and/or osmolality
- Water consumption

Chemistry/Synonyms

Vasopressin, a hypothalamic hormone stored in the posterior pituitary, is a 9-amino acid polypeptide with a disulfide bond. In most mammals (including dogs and humans), the natural hormone is arginine vasopressin, while in swine, the arginine is replaced with lysine. Lysine vasopressin has only about ½ the antidiuretic activity of arginine vasopressin. Previously available vasopressin products were a combination of arginine or lysine vasopressin derived from natural sources or synthetically prepared, while the currently available product is synthetic arginine vasopressin. The products are standardized by their pressor activity in rats (USP posterior pituitary [pressor] units); their antidiuretic activity can be variable. Commercially available vasopressin has little, if any, oxytocic activity at usual doses.

Vasopressin occurs as a white to off-white amorphous powder. Vasopressin injection is a clear, colorless or practically colorless liquid with a faint, characteristic odor. Vasopressin is soluble in water.

Vasopressin may also be known as ADH, antidiuretic hormone, 8-arginine vasopressin, beta-hypophamine, *Neo-Lidocaton*®, *Pitressin*®, or *Pressyn*®.

Storage/Stability

Store vasopressin (aqueous) injection at controlled cold temperatures, 2°C to 8°C (36°F-46°F), but it may be stored at room temperature for up to 12 months or until the manufacturer's expiry date; avoid freezing. After first use, refrigerate the multiple-dose vial and discard it after 30 days. Discard the solutions diluted for IV infusion and kept at room temperature 18 hours after mixing or 24 hours if refrigerated.

Compatibility/Compounding Considerations

Compatibility is dependent upon factors such as pH, concentration, temperature, and diluent used; consult specialized references or a hospital pharmacist for more specific information.

Vasopressin is **Y-site compatible** with aminocaproic acid, amiodarone, buprenorphine, butorphanol, calcium gluconate/chloride, cefazolin, ciprofloxacin, dexamethasone sodium phosphate, diltiazem, dobutamine, dopamine, epinephrine, famotidine, fentanyl citrate, gentamicin, heparin, hydroxyethyl starch 130/0.4 in sodium chloride, imipenem/cilastatin, lidocaine, magnesium sulfate, mannitol, meropenem, metoclopramide, metronidazole, midazolam, morphine sulfate, nitroglycerin, norepinephrine, pantoprazole, phenylephrine, piperacillin/tazobactam, procainamide, sodium bicarbonate, and voriconazole. It is **incompatible** with ampicillin, diazepam, furosemide, insulin (regular), and phenytoin.

If the aqueous injection is to be administered as an IV or intra-arterial infusion, it should be diluted in either 5% dextrose or 0.9% sodium chloride. For infusion use in humans, it is usually diluted to a concentration of 0.1 to 1 unit/mL.

Dosage Forms/Regulatory Status

VETERINARY-LABELED PRODUCTS: NONE

HUMAN-LABELED PRODUCTS:

Vasopressin Injection: 20 pressor units/mL in 1 mL and 10 mL vials; *Vasostrict*®; (Rx)

Vasopressin Tannate Sterile Suspension in oil is no longer commercially available.

References

For the complete list of references, see **wiley.com/go/budde/plumb**

Vecuronium

(vek-yew-***roe***-nee-um) *Norcuron*®

Nondepolarizing Neuromuscular Blocker

Prescriber Highlights

- ► Used primarily in dogs and cats as an adjunct to general anesthesia to produce muscle relaxation during surgical procedures or mechanical ventilation and facilitate endotracheal intubation
- ► Use with caution in animals with severe renal dysfunction, myasthenia gravis, or hepatic or biliary disease.
- ► Not for use as a single agent; no analgesic or sedative actions
- ► High alert drug; ensure appropriate respiratory support, reversal agents, and error-reducing safeguards are in place to minimize risk of patient harm.

Uses/Indications

Vecuronium is indicated as an adjunct to general anesthesia to produce muscle relaxation during surgical procedures or mechanical ventilation and facilitate endotracheal intubation. In dogs it has been used during general anesthesia to decrease respiratory motion and allow for controlled respiratory cycles during radiation therapy of heart base tumors.[1] Vecuronium causes very minimal cardiac effects and generally does not cause the release of histamine. It has been used topically to cause mydriasis in birds to facilitate fundoscopic exam.[2]

Pharmacology/Actions

Vecuronium is a nondepolarizing neuromuscular blocking agent and acts by competitively binding at cholinergic receptor sites on the motor end-plate resulting in paralysis of striated muscles. Vecuronium, when compared to pancuronium (on a weight basis), has been described as being equipotent to up to 3 times more potent.

The potency of vecuronium as a neuromuscular blocker appears to be lower in horses than other species and some horses appear to be relatively resistant to its effect.[3,4]

Pharmacokinetics

The onset of neuromuscular blockade after IV injection is dose-dependent. Dogs given 50 µg/kg IV (also receiving halothane anesthesia) experienced complete paralysis.[5] Duration of effect is ≈20-30 minutes when given as a bolus. Vecuronium has a shorter duration of action than pancuronium (≈⅓ to ½ as long), but similar to that of atracurium.

In cats, after injection of vecuronium 0.6 mg/kg IV, the steady state volume of distribution was 0.23 L/kg, half-life was 31 minutes, and clearance was 11 mL/minute/kg. Vecuronium or its metabolites were recovered in the bile (40%), urine (15%), and liver (15%).[6]

Vecuronium is partially metabolized; it and its metabolites are excreted into the bile and urine. Prolonged recovery times may result in patients with significant renal or hepatic disease.

In humans, vecuronium is up to 80% bound to plasma proteins.[7] The half-life ranges from 65 to 75 minutes. Patients with hepatic function impairment or cirrhosis exhibited prolonged plasma half-lives and almost double the recovery time compared to patients with normal function.

Contraindications/Precautions/Warnings

Vecuronium is contraindicated in patients hypersensitive to it. Lower doses may be necessary in patients with hepatic or biliary disease. In patients with myasthenia gravis, neuromuscular blocking agents (NMBA) should be administered with caution using doses much lower than typical (15%-20% of recommended dose) and with continuous monitoring of neuromuscular transmission.[8]

Vecuronium should only be used in patients that are adequately anesthetized as it has no analgesic or sedative/anesthetic actions. Respiratory support (eg, intubation, mechanical ventilation), neuromuscular blocker reversal agents, and staff experienced in the use of of these agents must be readily available. Inadvertent administration of neuromuscular blocking agents to patients for which they were not intended may cause significant harm, including death. Neuromuscular blocking agents should be sequestered from other medications, and with access limited to those familiar with their use.[9] Prominent placement of warning labels (eg, "paralyzing agent- causes respiratory arrest," "causes respiratory paralysis; patient must be ventilated") on storage containers is highly recommended.

Vecuronium's duration of action is shorter in dogs with diabetes mellitus.[10]

In horses, vecuronium should be used with caution due to possible failure to produce complete paralysis and its prolonged action in this species.[3,11]

Adverse Effects

Other than the effects associated with pharmacologic neuromuscular blockade, vecuronium appears to be well tolerated in the limited number of animals studied.

Reproductive/Nursing Safety

It is unknown whether vecuronium causes fetal harm or if the drug is excreted into maternal milk. Because safety has not been established in animals, this drug should only be used when the maternal benefits outweigh the potential risks to offspring.

Overdose/Acute Toxicity

The LD_{50} reported for mice and rats following IV administration was 0.051 and 0.2 mg/kg, respectively. Overdoses with neuromuscular blocking agents may result in prolonged neuromuscular blockade. The primary treatment is maintenance of the patient's airway, mechanical ventilation and oxygenation, and adequate sedation until recovery function is assured. Only after evidence of recovery is seen should administration of an anticholinesterase drug with an anticholinergic agent be considered. Blood pressure, heart rate, ventilation and oxygenation (end tidal CO_2, SpO_2, and blood gas analysis) should be monitored during an overdose with any necessary supportive treatment performed.

Reversal of blockade might be accomplished by administering an anticholinesterase agent (eg, neostigmine) with an anticholinergic agent (eg, atropine, glycopyrrolate). See ***Neostigmine***. A case report of the anticholinesterase edrophonium (not currently commercially available) failing to reverse prolonged vecuronium-induced neuromuscular blockade in a dog has been published.[12] Vecuronium can be reversed by the drug sugammadex, a binding agent that is specific for vecuronium and rocuronium.[13]

For patients that have experienced or are suspected of having experienced an overdose, consultation with a 24-hour poison consultation center specializing in providing veterinary-specific information is recommended. For general information related to overdose and toxin exposures, as well as contact information for poison control centers, refer to ***Appendix***.

Drug Interactions

The following drug interactions have either been reported or are theoretical in humans or animals receiving vecuronium and may be of significance in veterinary patients. Unless otherwise noted, use together is not necessarily contraindicated, but weigh the potential risks and perform additional monitoring when appropriate.

- MEDETOMIDINE: May shorten the duration of vecuronium effect[14]
- NON-DEPOLARIZING MUSCLE RELAXANT DRUGS, OTHER: May have a synergistic effect if used with vecuronium
- SUCCINYLCHOLINE: May speed the onset of action and enhance the neuromuscular blocking actions of vecuronium; do not give vecuronium until succinylcholine effects have subsided.

The following agents may enhance or prolong the neuromuscular blocking activity of vecuronium:

- AMINOGLYCOSIDE ANTIBIOTICS (eg, gentamicin)
- ANESTHETICS, GENERAL (eg, isoflurane)
- ANTIARRHYTHMIC AGENTS (eg, procainamide, quinidine)
- BACITRACIN, POLYMYXIN B (systemic): Consider therapy modification.
- CALCIUM CHANNEL BLOCKERS (eg, amlodipine, diltiazem)
- CYCLOSPORINE (systemic)
- LINCOSAMIDE ANTIBIOTICS (eg, clindamycin)
- MAGNESIUM SALTS, SYSTEMIC
- TETRACYCLINE DERIVATIVES (eg, doxycycline, minocycline)
- VANCOMYCIN

Laboratory Considerations

- None noted

Dosages

DOGS:

Neuromuscular relaxation/blockade (extra-label):

a) 100 µg/kg (0.1 mg/kg) IV[15-17]; additional doses of 0.05 mg/kg IV can be administered if prolonged blockade is required.[15] Initial doses of up to 200 µg/kg (0.2 mg/kg) IV have also been used to prolong blockade; however, this higher dose will prolong the recovery period.[15]

b) From a study done in female beagles: 25 µg/kg (0.025 mg/kg) IV over 5 seconds. This dose of vecuronium was chosen after pilot studies and was expected to produce partial block without causing apnea. In 9 of the 10 dogs, vecuronium at this dose produced a twitch reduction of greater than 80%. Significant residual neuromuscular block could be measured at the hind limb with acceleromyography when ventilation spontaneously returned.[18] In another study, complete paralysis was induced at dosages of 50 µg/kg (0.05 mg/kg), suggesting that under inhalational anesthesia, the ED_{90} of vecuronium in dogs is likely much lower than the previously reported 90 µg/kg (0.09 mg/kg).[5] The authors concluded that monitoring spontaneous ventilation, including end-tidal CO_2, expired tidal volume, peak inspiratory flow or minute ventilation, cannot be used as a surrogate for objective neuromuscular monitoring, and this practice may increase the risk of postoperative residual paralysis.

c) **If using CRI propofol-fentanyl anesthesia**: vecuronium 0.2 mg/kg/*HOUR* IV CRI for maintenance[19]

d) **If using isoflurane or sevoflurane with fentanyl IV CRI anesthesia**: vecuronium 0.1 mg/kg/*HOUR* IV CRI for maintenance[20]

CATS:

Neuromuscular relaxation/blockade (extra-label): 20 – 40 µg/kg (0.02 – 0.04 mg/kg) IV[21-23]

Monitoring

- Degree of neuromuscular blockade; the manufacturer recommends use of a peripheral nerve stimulator to determine drug response, the need for additional doses, and to evaluate recovery.
- Cardiac rate and blood pressure

Client Information

- This drug should only be used by professionals familiar with using neuromuscular blocking agents in a supervised setting with adequate ventilatory support.

Chemistry/Synonyms

Structurally similar to pancuronium, vecuronium bromide is a synthetic, nondepolarizing neuromuscular blocking agent. It contains the steroid (androstane) nucleus but is devoid of steroid activity. It occurs as white to off-white or slightly pink crystals or crystalline powder. In aqueous solution, it has a pK_a of 8.97, and the commercial injection has a pH of 4 after reconstitution. 9 mg are soluble in 1 mL of water; 23 mg are soluble in 1 mL of alcohol.

Vecuronium bromide may also be known as Org-NC-45, *Curlem®*, *Norcuron®*, *Rivecrum®*, *Vecural®*, or *Vecuron®*.

Storage/Stability

The commercially available powder for injection should be stored at controlled room temperature (20°C-25°C [68°F-77°F]) and protected from light. After reconstitution with sterile water for injection, vecuronium bromide is stable for 24 hours at 2°C to 8°C (36°F-46°F).[5] As it contains no preservative, unused portions should be discarded after reconstitution.

Compatibility/Compounding Considerations

Compatibility is dependent on factors such as pH, concentration,

temperature, and diluent used; specialized references or a hospital pharmacist should be consulted for more specific information.

Compatible with 0.9% sodium chloride, 5% dextrose in water, 5% dextrose in 0.9% sodium chloride, and lactated Ringer's for dilution.

It should not be mixed in the same IV bag or syringe, or given through the same needle with alkaline drugs (eg, barbiturates) or solutions (eg, sodium bicarbonate) as precipitation may occur.

Dosage Forms/Regulatory Status

VETERINARY-LABELED PRODUCTS: NONE

The Association of Racing Commissioners International (ARCI) has designated this drug as a class 2 substance. Use of this drug may not be allowed in certain animal competitions. Check rules and regulations before entering a competition while this medication is being administered. Contact local racing authorities for further guidance. See ***Appendix*** for more information.

HUMAN-LABELED PRODUCTS:

Vecuronium Bromide Powder for Injection: 10 mg and 20 mg in 10 mL and 20 mL vials; generic; (Rx)

Vecuronium Bromide Solution for Injection: 1 mg/mL in 10 mL prefilled syringes or 100 mL vials; generic; (Rx)

References

For the complete list of references, see **wiley.com/go/budde/plumb**

Verapamil

(ver-***ap***-a-mill) *Calan®, Verelan®*

Calcium Channel Blocker

Prescriber Highlights

- Used for supraventricular tachycardias in dogs and cats
- Contraindications include cardiogenic shock or severe CHF (unless secondary to a supraventricular tachycardia), hypotension, sick sinus syndrome, second- or third-degree AV block, digoxin intoxication, or hypersensitivity to verapamil. IV administration is contraindicated within a few hours of IV beta-blocker administration.
- Use with caution in patients with heart failure, hypertrophic cardiomyopathy, hepatic impairment, or renal impairment. Use cautiously in patients with atrial fibrillation and Wolff-Parkinson-White (WPW) syndrome.
- Verapamil is a P-glycoprotein substrate and should be used with caution in dogs with the *MDR1* gene mutation (also known as *ABCB1*-1delta).
- Adverse effects include hypotension, bradycardia, tachycardia, exacerbation of CHF, peripheral edema, AV block, pulmonary edema, nausea, constipation, dizziness, headache, or fatigue.
- Many possible drug interactions

Uses/Indications

In dogs and cats, verapamil may be useful for the treatment of supraventricular tachycardias and, possibly, treatment of atrial flutter or fibrillation. If systolic dysfunction is present, calcium channel blockers are often drugs of choice for atrial or AV nodal tachycardia. When oral therapy is indicated, most clinicians prefer using diltiazem instead of verapamil.

Pharmacology/Actions

Verapamil is a slow-channel calcium (L-type) blocking agent and a phenylalkylamine that is classified as a class IV antiarrhythmic drug. Verapamil exerts its actions by binding the L-type calcium channels and blocking the transmembrane influx of extracellular calcium ions across membranes of vascular smooth muscle cells and myocardial cells. The result of this blocking is inhibition of the contractile mechanisms of vascular, which causes systemic and coronary vasodilation, and inhibition of the contractile mechanisms of cardiac smooth muscle. Verapamil has inhibitory effects on the cardiac conduction system, and these effects produce its antiarrhythmic properties.

Electrophysiologic effects include an increased effective refractory period of the AV node, decreased automaticity, and substantially decreased AV node conduction. On ECG, heart rate and RR intervals can be increased or decreased; PR and AH intervals are increased. Verapamil has negative effects on myocardial contractility, and it decreases peripheral vascular resistance.

Verapamil is a P-glycoprotein inhibitor, which could increase toxicity risk for other substrate drugs but also could be used for therapeutic advantage (eg, overcoming P-glycoprotein-mediated multidrug resistance by blocking efflux of some chemotherapy drugs).

Pharmacokinetics

In dogs, 90% of an oral dose is absorbed, but because of a high first-pass effect, bioavailability is only 10% to 23%. The volume of distribution has been reported to be ≈4.5 L/kg in dogs. Serum half-lives of 1.8 hours and 2.5 hours have been reported in dogs, which appears to be significantly faster than in humans. Biotransformation occurs in the liver, and like humans, several metabolites are formed, including some that have activity. Elimination occurs primarily via the bile/feces in dogs.

No pharmacokinetic information was located for cats.

In humans, ≈90% of a dose of verapamil is rapidly absorbed after oral administration, but because of a high first-pass effect, only ≈20% to 30% is available to the systemic circulation. Patients with significant hepatic dysfunction may have considerably higher percentages of the drug systemically bioavailable. Food will decrease the rate and extent of absorption of the sustained-release tablets, but less so with the conventional tablets. Verapamil's volume of distribution is between 4.5 and 7 L/kg; ≈90% of the drug in the serum is bound to human plasma proteins. Verapamil crosses the placenta, and milk concentrations may approach those in the plasma.

Verapamil is metabolized in the liver to at least 12 separate metabolites, with norverapamil being the most predominant. The majority of the amounts of these metabolites are excreted into the urine. Only 3% to 4% is excreted unchanged in the urine. In humans, the half-life of the drug is 2 to 8 hours after a single IV dose, but it can increase after 1 to 2 days of oral therapy (presumably due to a saturable process of the hepatic enzymes).

Contraindications/Precautions/Warnings

Verapamil is contraindicated in patients with cardiogenic shock or severe CHF (unless secondary to a supraventricular tachycardia amenable to verapamil therapy), hypotension (less than 90 mm Hg systolic), sick sinus syndrome, second- or third-degree AV block, digoxin intoxication, or hypersensitivity to verapamil.

IV verapamil is contraindicated within a few hours of IV beta-adrenergic blocking agents (eg, propranolol), as they both can depress myocardial contractility and AV node conduction. The use of this combination in patients with wide complex ventricular tachycardia (QRS greater than 0.11 seconds) can cause rapid hemodynamic deterioration and ventricular fibrillation.

Verapamil should be used with caution in patients with heart failure, hypertrophic cardiomyopathy, and hepatic or renal impairment. Toxicity may be potentiated in patients with hepatic dysfunction. It should be used cautiously in patients with atrial fibrillation that have Wolff-Parkinson-White (WPW) syndrome, as fatal arrhythmias may result; this is considered a contraindication in humans.[1]

Verapamil should be used with caution in diabetic animals because it may increase blood glucose in dogs.[2,3]

Verapamil is a P-glycoprotein inhibitor, which could increase the risk for toxicity in animals with the *MDR1* gene mutation (also known as *ABCB1*-1delta) that are concurrently receiving P-glycoprotein substrates.

Adverse Effects

Possible adverse effects include hypotension, bradycardia, tachycardia, exacerbation of CHF, peripheral edema, AV block, pulmonary edema, nausea, constipation, dizziness, or fatigue.

Reproductive/Nursing Safety

Verapamil crosses the placenta and can be detected in umbilical vein blood at delivery. Oral verapamil in rats with doses 1.5 to 6 times the human dose was embryocidal and retarded fetal growth and development, likely due to reduced weight gains in dams.[1]

Verapamil is excreted in milk.[1] Consider discontinuing nursing if the dam requires verapamil therapy.

Because safety has not been established in animals, this drug should only be used when the maternal benefits outweigh the potential risks to offspring.

Overdose/Acute Toxicity

Clinical signs of overdose are extensions of verapamil's adverse effect profile, and may include lethargy, bradycardia, hypotension, QT interval prolongation, hyperglycemia, junctional rhythms, and second- or third-degree AV block.[4] Sinus tachycardia is also possible, presumably due to carotid sinus reflex stimulation. Other clinical signs that may be noted include GI upset, vomiting, hypothermia, CNS depression, noncardiogenic pulmonary edema, hypokalemia, metabolic acidosis, and increased lactate production. Rarely CNS stimulation (eg, seizures, agitation, ataxia, tremors) occurs.

If overdose is secondary to recent oral ingestion (less than 2 hours) and the patient is asymptomatic, GI decontamination (eg, emesis, activated charcoal ± sorbitol) should be considered. Treatment is generally supportive in nature; vigorously monitor cardiac and respiratory functions. IV calcium salts have been suggested to treat the negative inotropic clinical signs but may not adequately treat clinical signs of heart block. See ***Calcium, IV (-Borogluconate, -Chloride, -Gluconate)***. The use of fluids and pressor agents (eg, dopamine, norepinephrine) may be utilized to treat hypotensive clinical signs. The AV block and/or bradycardia can be treated with isoproterenol, norepinephrine, atropine, or cardiac pacing. Patients that develop a rapid ventricular rate after verapamil because of antegrade conduction in flutter/fibrillation with Wolff-Parkinson-White (WPW) syndrome have been treated with direct current (DC) cardioversion, lidocaine, or procainamide. Other therapies may include glucagon, insulin/glucose, and IV lipid emulsion.[4,5]

Because of the potential for severe toxic effects and the potentially complicated management of calcium channel blocker overdoses, consultation with a 24-hour poison consultation center specializing in providing veterinary-specific information is recommended. For general information related to overdose and toxin exposures, as well as contact information for poison control centers, refer to ***Appendix***.

Drug Interactions

The following drug interactions have either been reported or are theoretical in humans or animals receiving verapamil and may be of significance in veterinary patients. Unless otherwise noted, use together is not necessarily contraindicated, but weigh the potential risks and perform additional monitoring when appropriate.

- **Angiotensin-Converting Enzyme Inhibitors (ACEIs; eg, benazepril, enalapril)**: May cause additive hypotensive effects
- **Alpha-Adrenergic Receptor Antagonists (eg, prazosin)**: May cause additive hypotensive effects
- **Beta-Adrenergic Receptor Antagonists (eg, propranolol)**: May cause additive negative cardiac inotrope and chronotrope effects
- **Bupivacaine/Mepivacaine**: Concurrent use may increase the risk for heart block.
- **Buspirone**: Concurrent use may result in an increased risk for enhanced buspirone effects.
- **Calcium**: Concurrent use may result in reversal of hypotensive effects.
- **Clonidine**: Concurrent use may result in an increased incidence of sinus bradycardia.
- **Clopidogrel**: Concurrent use may result in decreased antiplatelet effect and increased risk for thrombotic events.
- **Cyclosporine**: Verapamil may increase levels and risk for toxicity.
- **Dantrolene**: Cardiovascular collapse is reported in animals when used with verapamil.
- **Digoxin**: Verapamil may increase the blood levels of digoxin; monitoring of digoxin levels is recommended.
- **Diuretics**: May cause additive hypotensive effects
- **Doxorubicin**: Verapamil may increase concentrations.
- **Erythromycin, Clarithromycin**: May increase verapamil levels
- **Fluconazole**: Concurrent use may result in increased verapamil exposure and risk for toxicity.
- **Fentanyl**: Concurrent use may result in increased risk for fentanyl toxicity.
- **Hydrocodone**: Concurrent use may increase hydrocodone exposure and risk for increased or prolonged opioid effects.
- **Ivermectin**: In rabbits, concurrent use increased ivermectin plasma concentration and AUC, and prolonged elimination half-life.[6] In vitro studies using canine cells demonstrate verapamil inhibits P-glycoprotein transport of ivermectin.[7,8]
- **Ketoconazole**: Concurrent use may result in increased ketoconazole and verapamil exposure.
- **Midazolam**: Concurrent use may result in increased/prolonged sedation.
- **Morphine**: Concurrent use may increase morphine exposure.
- **Neuromuscular Blockers (eg, atracurium)**: Neuromuscular blocking effects of nondepolarizing muscle relaxants may be enhanced by verapamil.
- **P-Glycoprotein Substrates, Other (eg, butorphanol, loperamide, vincristine)**: Because verapamil is a P-glycoprotein inhibitor, combination could increase the risk for toxicity for animals with the MDR1 gene mutation (also known as *ABCB1*-1delta) that are concurrently receiving P-glycoprotein substrates.
- **Phenobarbital**: May reduce verapamil concentrations
- **Quinidine**: Additive alpha-adrenergic blocking activity; increased hypotensive effect; verapamil can block quinidine's AV conductive effects and increase quinidine levels.
- **Rifampin**: May reduce verapamil levels
- **Theophylline, Aminophylline**: Verapamil may increase serum levels of theophylline and lead to toxicity.
- **Vincristine**: Calcium channel blockers may increase intracellular vincristine by inhibiting the drug's outflow from the cell.

Laboratory Considerations

- Verapamil may elevate blood glucose in dogs and confuse **blood glucose** determinations.

Dosages

DOGS:

Supraventricular tachycardia (extra-label): Initially, 0.05 mg/kg IV given over 1 to 2 minutes while continuously monitoring ECG. If not effective, may repeat dose every 5 to 10 minutes until a total dose of 0.15 mg/kg has been administered. If effective, control may last only for 30 minutes (or less). For longer control, a

2 – 10 μg/kg/minute IV CRI can be administered.[9,10]

CATS:

Supraventricular tachycardia (extra-label): Initially, 0.025 mg/kg IV given over 1 to 2 minutes while continuously monitoring ECG. If not effective, may repeat every 5 to 10 minutes until a total dose of 0.15 mg/kg has been administered. If effective, control may last only for 30 minutes (or less). For longer control, a 2 – 10 μg/kg per minute IV CRI can be administered.[11]

HORSES:

Controlling ventricular rate in atrial fibrillation (extra-label): 0.025 – 0.05 mg/kg IV every 30 minutes, not to exceed a total dose of 0.2 mg/kg[12]

SMALL MAMMALS:

a) **Hamsters**: 0.25 – 0.5 mg/hamster (NOT mg/kg) SC[13]
b) **Rabbits**: 8 – 16 mg/kg PO daily in combination with 0.5 – 2 mg/kg SC once daily[13,14]

Monitoring

- Heart rate and rhythm; blood pressure
- Clinical signs of toxicity (see ***Adverse Effects***)
- Blood pressure, particularly during acute IV therapy

Client Information

- This medicine is used in dogs and cats to treat heart rhythm problems.
- This medicine is not commonly used in animals, so side effects are not well known. Possible side effects include swelling of the limbs, too fast or too slow heartbeats, gastrointestinal effects (eg, vomiting, constipation), and drowsiness/tiredness/lack of energy. Contact your veterinarian if you have any concerns about your animal.
- It is very important that your animal receives each dose. If you miss a dose, give it when you remember, but it if it close to the time for the next dose, skip the dose you missed and give it at the next scheduled time. After that, return to the regular dosing schedule.
- Your veterinarian will need to monitor your animal while it is taking this medicine. Do not miss these important follow-up visits.

Chemistry/Synonyms

Verapamil HCl is a calcium channel blocking agent that occurs as a bitter-tasting, nearly white, crystalline powder. It is soluble in water, and the injectable product has a pH of 4 to 6.5.

Verapamil HCl tablets should be stored at room temperature (15°C-30°C [59°F-86°F]); the injectable product should be stored at room temperature (15°C-30°C [59°F-86°F]) and protected from light and freezing.

Verapamil may also be known as CP-16533-1, D-365, iproveratril hydrochloride, or verapamili hydrochloridum; many trade names are available.

Compatibility/Compounding Considerations

Compatibility is dependent on factors such as pH, concentration, temperature, and diluent used; specialized references or a hospital pharmacist should be consulted for more specific information.

Verapamil HCl for injection is physically **compatible** when mixed with all commonly used IV solutions. However, a crystalline precipitate may form if verapamil is added to an infusion line with 0.45% sodium chloride with sodium bicarbonate running. Verapamil is reported to be physically **compatible** with the following drugs: amikacin sulfate, aminophylline, ampicillin sodium, ascorbic acid, atropine sulfate, calcium chloride/gluconate, cefazolin sodium, cefotaxime sodium, cefoxitin sodium, chloramphenicol sodium succinate, cimetidine HCl, clindamycin phosphate, dexamethasone sodium phosphate, diazepam, digoxin, dobutamine HCl (slight discoloration due to dobutamine oxidation), dopamine HCl, epinephrine HCl, furosemide, gentamicin sulfate, heparin sodium, hydrocortisone sodium phosphate, hydromorphone HCl, insulin, isoproterenol, lidocaine HCl, magnesium sulfate, mannitol, meperidine HCl, methylprednisolone sodium succinate, metoclopramide HCl, morphine sulfate, multivitamin infusion, nitroglycerin, norepinephrine bitartrate, oxytocin, pancuronium Br, penicillin G potassium/sodium, pentobarbital sodium, phenobarbital sodium, phentolamine mesylate, phenytoin sodium, potassium chloride/phosphate, procainamide HCl, propranolol HCl, protamine sulfate, quinidine gluconate, sodium bicarbonate, sodium nitroprusside, tobramycin sulfate, vasopressin, and vitamin B complex with C.

The following drugs have been reported to be physically **incompatible** with verapamil: albumin injection, amphotericin B, hydralazine HCl, and trimethoprim/sulfamethoxazole.

Dosage Forms/Regulatory Status

VETERINARY-LABELED PRODUCTS: NONE

The Association of Racing Commissioners International (ARCI) has designated this drug as a class 4 substance. Use of this drug may not be allowed in certain animal competitions. Check rules and regulations before entering a competition while this medication is being administered. Contact local racing authorities for further guidance. See ***Appendix*** for more information.

HUMAN-LABELED PRODUCTS:

Verapamil HCl Tablets: 40 mg, 80 mg, and 120 mg; *Calan*®, generic; (Rx)

Verapamil HCl Sustained-Release Tablets: 120 mg, 180 mg, and 240 mg; *Calan® SR*, generic; (Rx); Tablets may be split in ½ without altering sustainedrelease characteristics.

Verapamil HCl Extended-Release Capsules: 100 mg, 120 mg, 180 mg, 200 mg, 240 mg, 300 mg, and 360 mg; *Verelan*®, *Verelan® PM*, generic; (Rx). Capsules may be opened, and contents sprinkled on soft food, but capsule contents should not be crushed or chewed.

Verapamil HCl for Injection: 2.5 mg/mL in 2 mL and 4 mL vials, ampules, and syringes; generic; (Rx)

References

For the complete list of references, see **wiley.com/go/budde/plumb**

Verdinexor

(ver-dih-***nex***-or) *Laverdia®-CA1*
Antineoplastic

Prescriber Highlights

- Conditionally approved oral treatment for dogs with lymphoma and must therefore only be used as labeled
- Must be administered immediately after feeding a small meal
- Contraindications include dogs with a hypersensitivity to the drug, or those that are pregnant, nursing, or intended for breeding. Dogs weighing less than 9 kg (19.8 lb) may not be accurately dosed or undergo dose adjustments.
- Adverse effects include anorexia, vomiting, diarrhea, weight loss, lethargy, polydipsia, polyuria, elevated liver enzymes, and thrombocytopenia.
- Disposable chemotherapy-resistant gloves should be used when handling verdinexor and the treated dog's bodily fluids and waste. Disposable chemotherapy-resistant gloves should also be worn when handling the dog's toys and food and water bowl. This medicine can affect male and female fertility. Women who are pregnant, may become pregnant, or breast-feeding should not handle the drug.
- Include the Client Information Sheet (CIS) when dispensing the drug. The CIS states that unused tablets are to be returned to the veterinarian for disposal.

Uses/Indications

Verdinexor is conditionally approved (pending a full demonstration of effectiveness) by the FDA for the treatment of lymphoma in dogs. In a field study, a complete response (CR) or partial response (PR) occurred in 20 of 58 dogs with T-cell or B-cell lymphoma (34.5%, CR = 1, PR = 19).[1] In dogs with lymphoma the median time to tumor progression (TTP) was 29.5 days (range, 7 to 244 days),[2] but TTP was 43 days in naïve lymphoma patients compared to 24 days for relapsed patients.[3] Clinical benefit (ie, CR, PR, or stable disease) was also demonstrated in 64% of dogs with non-Hodgkin lymphoma in a separate study.[4] In both studies,[3,4] concurrent corticosteroid use was allowable but was not part of the designed study protocol.

As a conditionally approved drug, it is a violation of US federal law to use this product other than as directed on the label.

Pharmacology/Actions

Verdinexor is a selective inhibitor of nuclear export (SINE) that reversibly inhibits chromosome region maintenance 1 (CRM1, also known as exportin-1 [XPO1]). CRM1 is an export protein responsible for transporting macromolecules, including RNA, tumor suppressor proteins (TSP; eg, p53, RB1), and growth regulatory proteins (GRP; eg, p21) from the cell nucleus into the cytoplasm.[5–7] Inhibition of CRM1 by verdinexor prevents the export of TSP and GRP, and the resulting restoration of TRP and GRP within the nucleus renders the cell susceptible to apoptosis.[4,8] As CRM1 is overexpressed and/or mutated in cancer patients,[7–9] verdinexor exerts its activity preferentially in cancer cells or in cells with genomic damage.[10,11] In addition to lymphomas, verdinexor has demonstrated biologic activity against cell lines for canine mammary carcinoma,[12] mast cell tumor,[4] melanoma,[9] osteosarcoma,[4] and transitional cell carcinoma.[12]

As a class, SINEs block thrombopoietin signaling and reversible thrombocytopenia is a common adverse effect.[13]

Verdinexor has demonstrated antiviral activity,[14,15] including against eastern and western equine encephalitis.[16]

Pharmacokinetics

The oral bioavailability of verdinexor in recently fed dogs is 3-fold to 5-fold greater than in fasted dogs.[1] In healthy and recently fed dogs receiving a single oral verdinexor dose, the time to peak plasma concentration is ≈1 to 4 hours after administration, and plasma half-life was ≈2 to 6 hours.[1] In dogs with lymphoma, at steady-state the mean peak verdinexor concentration of 278 ng/mL occurred ≈5 hours after administration, mean AUC was 1971 ng·t/mL, and half-life was ≈5 hours.[3] Verdinexor is thought to be metabolized by glutathione conjugation.[2]

Contraindications/Precautions/Warnings

Verdinexor is contraindicated in patients hypersensitive to it. Do not use the drug in dogs that are pregnant, lactating, or intended for breeding.[2]

Dogs weighing less than 9 kg (19.8 lb) may not be accurately dosed or undergo dose adjustments.[2] Dogs weighing 9 to 9.6 kg (19.8-21.1 lb) cannot undergo dosage increase from 1.25 mg/kg to 1.5 mg/kg. Verdinexor has not been evaluated in dogs younger than 7 months of age; with diabetes mellitus, cardiovascular, hepatic or renal disease; with concurrent serious infections or malignancy; or with clinically relevant hypercalcemia.

Oral absorption is dramatically increased when verdinexor is administered with food.[1] Because anorexia may be a dose-limiting adverse effect,[4] appetite stimulants appropriate for dogs and low-dose corticosteroids may be needed to maintain the dog's appetite during the course of therapy.[3,4]

Verdinexor has a narrow margin of safety. See ***Overdose/Acute Toxicity***.

Verdinexor is an antineoplastic agent, and disposable chemotherapy-resistant gloves are to be used when handling. Pregnant women, women who may become pregnant, and nursing women should not handle or administer verdinexor, or come in contact with the treated dog's waste or bodily fluids.

Adverse Effects

Adverse effects are dose-related.[4] All dogs in a field study of dogs with lymphoma experienced at least one adverse effect.[2] Common adverse effects included anorexia (45% to 74%), vomiting (26% to 59%), diarrhea (12% to 52%), weight loss (31% to 48%), and lethargy (17% to 41%).[1,3] Polydipsia (33%) and polyuria (31%) have also been observed,[1] although concurrent corticosteroid use was common. Other adverse effects seen in more than or equal to 10% of dogs in the field trial included fever, weakness, generalized pain, and cough/dyspnea. Hematological toxicity reported in a field study included thrombocytopenia (31%), lymphopenia (29%), neutrophilia (26%), anemia (22%), leukopenia (21%), and neutropenia (16%).[1] In the dogs with thrombocytopenia, 2 experienced bruising and 1 had epistaxis.[2]

Changes in serum chemistry values included elevated liver enzymes including ALP (48%), ALT (36%), and AST (10%); increased BUN (26%); hypercalcemia (17%); hypochloremia (14%); hyperphosphatemia (12%); and hypoproteinemia (10%). Prolonged partial thromboplastin time has also been noted.[1] A protein-losing nephropathy was reported in one dog.[23]

Hematuria, UTI, low urine specific gravity, and proteinuria were abnormalities noted on urinalysis.[2]

Reproductive/Nursing Safety

Verdinexor is contraindicated in dogs that are pregnant, lactating, or intended for breeding. The drug is embryotoxic and teratogenic in rats.[2] Reduced male and female fertility has been documented in animal studies and in humans.

Overdose/Acute Toxicity

In dogs given 1 – 1.75 mg/kg orally 3 times per week, in addition to the drug's typical adverse effects, other clinical signs included thin body condition, excessive shedding, loss of skin elasticity, lacrimation, slight depression, and slight decrease of forelimb strength.[2] Reduced lymphocytes, eosinophils, and monocytes were observed as was increased fibrinogen, albumin, and BUN.

For patients that have experienced or are suspected to have experienced an overdose, it is strongly encouraged to consult with one of the 24-hour poison consultation centers that specialize in providing information specific for veterinary patients. For general information related to overdose and toxin exposures, as well as contact information for poison control centers, refer to ***Appendix.***

Drug Interactions

The effects of concurrent drugs on verdinexor metabolism have not been studied. The product label states that verdinexor was administered concomitantly with other drugs such as corticosteroids (eg, predniso(lo)ne), proton pump inhibitors (eg, omeprazole), histamine H_2 receptor antagonists (eg, famotidine), antibiotics, antiemetics (eg, ondansetron), GI motility modifiers (eg, loperamide, metoclopramide), and opioids (eg, morphine).[1]

- **Chemotherapy, Other**: Safe and effective use of verdinexor with other chemotherapeutic agents has not been evaluated.[2]
- **Vaccines**: Verdinexor may diminish the response to vaccines.

The product label cautions that concurrent administration of verdinexor with drugs that undergo glutathione conjugation (eg, acetaminophen) should be minimized. Possible substrates of glutathione S-transferase include:

- **Acetaminophen** (metabolite)
- **Anthracyclines** (eg, **doxorubicin, mitoxantrone**)
- **Busulfan**
- **Cisplatin**
- **Cyclophosphamide**
- **Spinosad**
- **Thiotepa**

Laboratory Considerations

None noted

Dosages

DOGS:

Lymphoma (label dosage; conditionally approved by FDA): 1.25 mg/kg PO immediately after feeding twice per week with at least 72 hours between doses (eg, Monday and Thursday, or Tuesday and Friday)

- If tolerated after 2 weeks, increase dosage to 1.5 mg/kg PO twice per week with at least 72 hours between doses.
- To manage adverse effects, dosage may be reduced by increments of 0.25 mg/kg; dosage interruptions may also be considered. Minimum dosage is 1 mg/kg PO twice per week with at least 72 hours between doses.
- See product label for dosing tables with the necessary combinations of tablet strengths for 1 mg/kg, 1.25 mg/kg, and 1.5 mg/kg dosages.[2]

Monitoring

- Although the exact schedule for recheck appointments and blood work testing has not been determined, the phase II study performed rechecks weekly during the first 28 days, then every other week.[3]
- Baseline and periodic physical examinations and blood work (eg, CBC, serum chemistry [including liver enzymes, albumin, total protein]) are recommended as needed based on the patient's response to therapy (especially after starting therapy or increasing the dose) and occurrence of any adverse effects.
- Baseline and periodic (as clinically indicated) urinalysis, urine culture, and urine protein:creatinine (UPC) ratio
- Appetite, food intake, body weight
- Tumor dimensions, response to therapy

Client Information

- Verdinexor is an antineoplastic (anticancer) medicine. This medicine can be hazardous to other animals and people that come in contact with it. On the day of verdinexor treatment, and for 3 days afterward:
    - Chemotherapy-resistant gloves are to be worn (check with your veterinarian to ensure you have the appropriate gloves):
        - when handling or administering verdinexor (this is particularly important with broken tablets, or if your dog spits out verdinexor tablet(s))
        - to prevent contact with your dog's feces, urine, saliva, and vomit
        - when handling your dog's food and water dishes or toys
    - Clean wastes or bodily fluids using disposable absorptive materials (eg, paper towels) and discard in a securely sealed plastic bag.
    - Wash any items that come in contact with your dog's feces, urine, saliva, or vomit separately from normal household laundry.
- Children, as well as women who are nursing, pregnant, or attempting to become pregnant, should not handle verdinexor tablets, or the dog's waste or bodily fluids (saliva, vomit, urine). This medicine can also affect male fertility.
- Do not eat, drink, or smoke while handling this medicine.
- Do not store this medicine near food, in or near a food preparation area, or with medications intended for use in humans.
- Wash skin with soap and water in case of accidental contact with verdinexor tablets, or with your dog's feces, urine, saliva, or vomit within 3 days after verdinexor administration.
- With accidental eye exposure, rinse eyes with a large amount of tap water for 10 minutes while holding back the eyelid. Remove contact lenses. Seek medical advice immediately and show package insert or label to the physician.
- Seek medical attention in case of accidental human ingestion of verdinexor, or with significant exposure to your dog's feces, urine, vomit, or saliva on the day of treatment or for 3 days afterward.
- Do not crush or split tablets. Administer your dog's dose promptly after the tablets are removed from the bottle.
- Administer immediately after feeding. Ensure your dog consumes the entire dose. Placing tablets in your dog's food bowl is not recommended.
- There must be at least 72 hours separating each verdinexor dose. If you miss a dose, do not make up the dose, but give the next regularly scheduled dose.
- The most frequent side effects include reduced or loss of appetite, weight loss, vomiting, diarrhea, low energy level (weakness). Contact your veterinarian if you notice your dog refusing to eat for longer than 1 day, has repeated vomiting or diarrhea, has a low energy level, or any other changes that concern you.
- Overdoses can be very serious; administer each dose exactly as prescribed.
- Keep verdinexor tablets out of reach of children and animals.
- Your veterinarian will need to perform examinations and blood work on your dog while it is taking this medicine. Do not miss these important follow-up visits.
- Do not throw unused verdinexor tablet in the trash. Unused verdinexor tablets should be returned to your veterinarian for disposal.

Chemistry/Synonyms

Verdinexor occurs as a crystalline solid. It is soluble in DMSO and sparingly soluble in ethanol.[17] It has an oil:water partition coefficient of 4.1.[18]

Verdinexor may also be known as KPT-335 or *Laverdia®-CA1*.

Storage/Stability

Store verdinexor tablets at room temperature between 20°C to 25°C (68°F-77°F). Store out of reach of children and pets. Do not store verdinexor tablets near other drugs, food, or in a food preparation area.

Compatibility/Compounding Considerations

No information available

Dosage Forms/Regulatory Status

VETERINARY-LABELED PRODUCTS:

Verdinexor Coated Tablets: 2.5 mg, 10 mg, and 50 mg in 50-count bottles; *Laverdia®-CA1*, (Rx). Conditional Approval Application Number 141-526. Extra-label use of conditionally approved drugs is not permitted by FDA.

HUMAN-LABELED PRODUCTS: NONE

References

For the complete list of references, see **wiley.com/go/budde/plumb**

Vinblastine

(vin-***blas***-teen) *Velban®*

Antineoplastic

Prescriber Highlights

- ▶ Vinca alkaloid antineoplastic used for a variety of tumors in dogs and cats
- ▶ Contraindications include pre-existing leukopenia or granulocytopenia (unless a result of the disease being treated) or active bacterial infection; reduce dose if hepatic insufficiency. Use it with caution in herding breeds (eg, collies) that may have the *MDR1* mutation (also known as *ABCB1*-1delta).
- ▶ Adverse effects include nausea/vomiting (less than with vincristine), myelosuppression (more so than with vincristine); it may also cause constipation, alopecia, stomatitis, ileus, inappropriate ADH secretion, jaw and muscle pain, and loss of deep tendon reflexes.
- ▶ Cats can develop neurotoxicity, causing constipation or paralytic ileus and aggravating hyporexia; cats can also develop reversible axon swelling and paranodal demyelination.
- ▶ Extravasation can cause significant tissue irritation and cellulitis.
- ▶ Many drug interactions
- ▶ Hazardous drug; use appropriate precautions and wear gloves and protective clothing when preparing or administering. Potential teratogen

Uses/Indications

Vinblastine may be used in the treatment of lymphomas, carcinomas, and mast cell tumors in small animal species. It may be more effective than vincristine in the treatment of canine mast cell tumors.

The combination of vinblastine and toceranib for the treatment of canine mast cell tumors was evaluated in a phase I trial. Although an objective response rate of 71% was noted, vinblastine dosing required a 50% reduction due to dose-limiting toxicity when compared to single-agent use. The use of this combination is not supported based on current drug combination paradigms.[1]

A prospective clinical trial in cats ($n = 40$) to compare vincristine and vinblastine response rates, outcomes, and toxicity in a COP-based protocol for lymphoma found that both arms had similar response rates, progression-free survival (PFS) times, and lymphoma-specific survival (LSS) times, but vincristine-treated cats had a higher incidence of GI adverse effects.[2]

Vinblastine has been evaluated in a retrospective analysis for response in relapsed canine lymphoma. The approximate response rate was 25% and was short in duration, with a median of 29.5 days.[3]

A prospective clinical trial in dogs ($n = 28$) using vinblastine to treat bladder transitional cell carcinoma found that 36% had a partial response, 50% had stable disease, and 14% had disease progression. The majority of dogs (27 of 28) did not have clinically relevant adverse effects, but 61% required dosage reduction (from the initial 3 mg/m² IV every 2 weeks) due to neutropenia. The authors concluded vinblastine could be considered another treatment option.[2] Another study found that, when used in combination with piroxicam in dogs with urethral carcinoma, piroxicam enhanced the activity of vinblastine and extended the progression-free survival. However, overall survival was significantly longer in dogs receiving vinblastine monotherapy.[4] There was no added survival benefit found when combining vinblastine with toceranib.[5]

Pharmacology/Actions

Vinblastine binds to microtubular proteins (tubulin) in the mitotic spindle, thereby preventing cell division during metaphase. It also interferes with amino acid metabolism by inhibiting glutamic acid utilization and preventing purine synthesis, citric acid cycle, and urea formation.

Pharmacokinetics

After IV administration, vinblastine is rapidly distributed to tissues. In humans, ≈75% is bound to tissue proteins, and the drug does not appreciably enter the CNS. Vinblastine is extensively metabolized by the liver and is primarily excreted in the bile/feces; lesser amounts are eliminated in the urine. CYP3A12 is the major cytochrome P450 isoform responsible for the metabolism of vinblastine in dogs.[6]

Contraindications/Precautions/Warnings

Vinblastine is contraindicated in patients with pre-existing leukopenia or granulocytopenia (unless a result of the disease being treated) or active bacterial infection. Doses of vinblastine should be reduced in patients with hepatic disease. In humans, a 50% reduction in dose is recommended when transaminases are 2 to 3 times the upper limit of normal.[7]

Because vinblastine is potentially neurotoxic as well as a substrate of P-glycoprotein, it should be used with caution in herding breeds (eg, collies) that may have *MDR1* mutation (also known as *ABCB1*-1delta) causing nonfunctional proteins. Myelosuppression and GI toxicity (anorexia, vomiting, diarrhea) are more likely to occur at standard dosages in dogs with the *MDR1* mutation. To reduce the likelihood of severe toxicity in these dogs (mutant/normal or mutant/mutant), the Veterinary Clinical Pharmacology Laboratory at Washington State University recommends reducing the dose by 25% to 30% and carefully monitoring these patients.[8]

Vinblastine is for IV use only and may be fatal if given by other routes.[9]

Do not confuse vinBLAStine with vinCRIStine; consider using "tall man lettering" when writing orders.

The National Institute for Occupational Safety and Health (NIOSH) classifies vinblastine as a hazardous drug[10]; wash hands after handling and use personal protective equipment (PPE) accordingly to minimize the risk for exposure.

Adverse Effects

Vinblastine can cause GI toxicity, including nausea and vomiting, which generally lasts less than 24 hours. Vinblastine is reported to cause less GI toxicity than vincristine.[2] It can be myelosuppressive at usual dosages (nadir at 4 to 9 days after treatment; recovery at 7 to 14 days). Vinblastine is considered more myelosuppressive than vincristine. Neutropenia is generally the doselimiting toxicity in dogs and humans.[9,11] At high doses, vinblastine may cause peripheral neurotoxic effects similar to those seen with vincristine. Additionally, vinblastine may cause constipation, alopecia, stomatitis, ileus, inappropriate ADH secretion, jaw and muscle pain, and loss of deep tendon reflexes.

Cats can develop neurotoxicity that can be associated with constipation or paralytic ileus, thereby aggravating anorexia. They may develop reversible axon swelling and paranodal demyelination.

Other adverse effects in humans include hypertension, ototoxicity, and acute shortness of breath or severe bronchospasm.[9]

Vinblastine is considered a vesicant, and extravasation may cause significant tissue irritation and cellulitis. If clinical signs of extravasation are noted, discontinue infusion immediately at that site and apply moderate heat to the area to help disperse the drug. Injections of hyaluronidase have also been suggested to help diffuse the drug. Ice is not recommended for vinca alkaloid extravasation as it has been shown to significantly increase skin ulceration.[12] Topical dimethyl sulfoxide (DMSO) has also been recommended by some to treat the area involved.

Reproductive/Nursing Safety

Little is known about the effects of vinblastine on developing fetuses, but it is believed that the drug possesses some teratogenic and embryotoxic properties. It may also cause aspermia in males.

It is not known whether vinblastine is excreted in milk, but because of the potential for serious adverse reactions in nursing offspring, the use of milk replacer is recommended if the dam requires vinblastine.

Because safety has not been established in animals, this drug should only be used when the maternal benefits outweigh the potential risks to offspring.

Overdose/Acute Toxicity

The LD_{50} in mice and rats following IV administration is 15 mg/mL and 2 mg/mL, respectively. In dogs, the lethal dose for vinblastine has been reported as 0.2 mg/kg. In addition to the exacerbations of the expected adverse effects, neurotoxicities similar to those associated with vincristine may also be noted.

In a cat that received 4 times the recommended IV dose, the following clinical signs were noted: within hours depression and inability to jump; Days 1 to 11 anorexia; Days 2 to 6 neutropenia with a fever on Day 4; Days 2 to 10 thrombocytopenia and anemia; Days 4 to 10 vomiting and diarrhea, and on Days 3 to 10 syndrome of inappropriate ADH (SIADH). Aggressive therapeutic interventions supporting the patient resulted in recovery.[13]

In humans, cardiovascular and hematologic monitoring is performed after an overdose. Treatment can include anticonvulsants and the prevention of ileus. Additionally, an attempt is made to prevent the effects associated with the syndrome of inappropriate antidiuretic hormone (SIADH) with fluid restriction and loop diuretics to maintain serum osmolality.

For patients that have experienced or are suspected of having experienced an overdose, consultation with a 24-hour poison consultation center specializing in providing veterinary-specific information is recommended. For general information related to overdose and toxin exposures, as well as contact information for poison control centers, refer to ***Appendix.***

Drug Interactions

The following drug interactions have either been reported or are theoretical in humans or animals receiving vinblastine and may be of significance in veterinary patients. Unless otherwise noted, use together is not necessarily contraindicated, but weigh the potential risks and perform additional monitoring when appropriate.

- **Ototoxic Drugs** (eg, cisplatin, carboplatin): May cause additive risk for ototoxicity
- **Immunosuppressive Drugs** (eg, azathioprine, cyclophosphamide, corticosteroids): Use with other immunosuppressant drugs may increase the risk for infection.
- **Macrolide Antibiotics** (except azithromycin): Macrolide antibiotics may increase the serum concentration of vinblastine; consider therapy modification.
- **Myelosuppressive Agents** (eg, antineoplastics, immunosuppressants, iron chelators): Concurrent use with other bone marrow depressant medications may result in additive myelosuppression; avoid combination when possible.
- **Vaccines** (live and inactivated): Vinblastine may diminish vaccine efficacy and enhance adverse effects of vaccines.

Caution is advised if using other drugs that can inhibit **P-glycoprotein,** particularly in those dogs at risk for *MDR1* genetic mutation (eg, collies, Australian shepherds, shelties, long-haired whippets, "white feet" breeds), unless tested homozygous normal for the gene locus. Drugs and drug classes involved include:

- **Amiodarone**
- **Azole Antifungals** (eg, **ketoconazole, itraconazole**)
- **Carvedilol**
- **Cyclosporine**
- **Diltiazem**
- **Erythromycin; Clarithromycin**
- **Quinidine**
- **Spironolactone**
- **Tamoxifen**
- **Verapamil**

Laboratory Considerations

- Vinblastine may significantly increase both blood and urine concentrations of **uric acid** (potentially significant for Dalmatians).

Dosages

NOTE: Because of the potential toxicity of this drug to patients, veterinary personnel, and clients, and since chemotherapy indications, treatment protocols, and monitoring and safety guidelines often change, the following dosages should be used only as a general guide. Consultation with a veterinary oncologist and referral to current veterinary oncology references[14-18] are strongly recommended.

DOGS/CATS:

Antineoplastic agent (extra-label): Depending on the protocol and the disease treated, vinblastine doses are usually 1.5 – 3 mg/m^2 (NOT mg/kg) IV every 1 to 2 weeks, often in combination with other chemotherapy drugs (eg, cyclophosphamide and prednisolone in dogs).[19,20] One small observational study found that for mast cell tumors in dogs, a higher dose of 3 mg/m^2 (NOT mg/kg) resulted in a lower rate of recurrence than a lower 2 mg/m^2 (NOT mg/kg) dose.[21]

Monitoring

- Efficacy
- Baseline and periodic complete blood counts with platelets
- Baseline and periodic liver enzymes prior to therapy and repeated as necessary

Client Information

- Vinblastine is a chemotherapy (anticancer) medicine. The medicine can be hazardous to other animals and people that come in contact with it. On the day your animal gets the medicine and then for a few days afterward, handle all bodily waste (urine, feces, litter), blood, or vomit only while wearing chemotherapy-resistant gloves. Seal the waste in a plastic bag and then place both the bag and gloves in with the regular trash. Those who are pregnant, attempting to conceive, or nursing should not clean up the animal's waste.

- Do not wash any items soiled with waste, vomit, or saliva from your dog with other laundry. Take precautions in handling the dog's toys, food bowl, and water bowl; wash separately from other items.
- Your veterinarian will need to perform regular monitoring, including blood tests and/or radiographs, to be sure this drug is not causing toxic effects to your animal. Do not miss these important follow up visits.
- Observe your dog for lack of appetite, vomiting, or diarrhea. If these signs are severe, or if you notice difficulty breathing or signs of infection, contact your veterinarian immediately.
- Bone marrow suppression can occur. The greatest effects on bone marrow usually occur within a week after treatment. Your veterinarian will do blood tests to watch for this, but if you see bleeding, bruising, fever (indicating an infection), or if your animal becomes tired easily, contact your veterinarian right away. Do not miss important follow-up visits with your veterinarian.
- Cats can develop nerve toxicity from vinblastine, resulting in severe constipation and loss of appetite.

Chemistry/Synonyms

Vinblastine sulfate, a vinca alkaloid, is isolated from the plant *Catharanthus roseus* (*vinca rosea Linn*) and occurs as a white or slightly yellow hygroscopic, amorphous, or crystalline powder that is freely soluble in water. The commercially available injection has a pH of 3 to 5.5.

Vinblastine may also be known as 29060-LE, NSC-49842, sulfato de vimblastina, vinblastini sulfas, vincaleukoblastine sulphate, VBL, *Alkaban®*, *Blastovin®*, *Cellblastin®*, *Cytoblastin®*, *Ifabla®*, *Lemblastine®*, *Periblastine®*, *Serovin®*, *Solblastin®*, *Velban®*, *Velbe®*, *Velsar®*, or *Xintoprost®*.

Storage/Stability

Store intact vials between 2°C to 8°C (36°F-46°F) and protect them from light. Dispose of any unused product or waste materials in accordance with proper procedures for cytotoxic drugs.

Compatibility/Compounding Considerations

Compatibility is dependent upon factors such as pH, concentration, temperature, and diluent used; consult specialized references or a hospital pharmacist for more specific information.

Vinblastine sulfate is reportedly **compatible** with 0.9% sodium chloride, lactated Ringer's, or 5% dextrose in water for dilution. It is also reportedly physically **compatible** with the following IV solutions and drugs: 5% dextrose with bleomycin sulfate and **compatible in syringes or at Y-sites** with bleomycin sulfate, cisplatin, cyclophosphamide, droperidol, fluorouracil, leucovorin calcium, methotrexate sodium, metoclopramide HCl, mitomycin, and vincristine sulfate.

Vinblastine sulfate **compatibility information conflicts** or is dependent on diluent or concentration factors with doxorubicin HCl and heparin sodium (in syringes).

Vinblastine sulfate is reportedly physically **incompatible** with furosemide and cefepime.

Dosage Forms/Regulatory Status

VETERINARY-LABELED PRODUCTS: NONE

HUMAN-LABELED PRODUCTS:

Vinblastine Sulfate Injection: 1 mg/mL in 10 mL and 25 mL vials; generic; (Rx)

Vinblastine Powder for Injection: 10 mg in vials; *Velban®*, generic; (Rx)

References

For the complete list of references, see **wiley.com/go/budde/plumb**

Vincristine

(vin-***kris***-teen) *Oncovin®, Vincasar PFS*

Antineoplastic

Prescriber Highlights

- ▶ Vinca alkaloid antineoplastic used for a variety of tumors (primarily lymphoid, hematopoietic neoplasms, and hemangiosarcoma) in dogs and cats
- ▶ Used for the treatment of immune-mediated thrombocytopenia and induces thrombocytosis when given at low doses
- ▶ Contraindications include patients with pre-existing leukopenia or granulocytopenia (unless as a result of the disease being treated) or active bacterial infection; reduce dose if hepatic disease is present.
- ▶ Use with caution in dogs that may have the *MDR1* genetic mutation.
- ▶ Less myelosuppressive than vinblastine but may cause more peripheral neurotoxic effects; neuropathic clinical signs can include proprioceptive deficits, spinal hyporeflexia, or paralytic ileus with resulting constipation.
- ▶ Cats can develop neurotoxicity causing constipation or paralytic ileus, aggravating anorexia; vinblastine may be substituted.
- ▶ Potentially teratogenic and embryotoxic. The National Institute for Occupational Safety and Health (NIOSH) classifies vincristine as a hazardous drug; use appropriate precautions when handling. Advise clients to use caution when handling animal waste.
- ▶ For IV use *only*. Vesicant, avoid extravasation

Uses/Indications

Vincristine is used as an antineoplastic primarily in combination drug protocols in the treatment of lymphoid hematopoietic neoplasms (CHOP) and hemangiosarcoma (VAC) in dogs and cats. In dogs, the drug may be used as a single agent in the therapy of transmissible venereal neoplasms.

A prospective clinical trial in cats ($n = 40$) to compare vincristine and vinblastine response rates, outcomes, and toxicities in a COP-based protocol for lymphoma, found that both arms had similar response rates, progression-free survival (PFS) times, and lymphoma-specific survival (LSS) times, but vincristine-treated cats had a higher incidence of GI adverse effects.[1] As a result, vinblastine is most commonly substituted for vincristine in cats.

Because vincristine can induce thrombocytosis (at low doses) and has some immunosuppressant activity, it may also be employed in the treatment of immune-mediated thrombocytopenia (ITP). A prospective, randomized study in dogs ($n = 20$) comparing the effect of hIVIG versus vincristine on platelet recovery in dogs with ITP found no significant differences in groups in platelet recovery time, hospitalization time, or survival at discharge or 6 months or 1 year after entry into the study. The authors concluded that because of lower cost and ease of administration, vincristine should be considered for first-line adjunctive treatment for the acute management of canine ITP.[2]

Pharmacology/Actions

By binding to beta-tubulin, vincristine blocks microtubule formation and prevents mitotic spindle formation; arresting cell division is thus arrested in metaphase. It also interferes with amino acid metabolism by inhibiting glutamic acid utilization and preventing purine synthesis, citric acid cycle, and urea formation. Tumor resistance to one vinca alkaloid does not imply resistance to another.

Vincristine can induce thrombocytosis (mechanism unknown) and has some immunosuppressant activity.

Pharmacokinetics

After IV administration, vincristine is rapidly distributed to tissues. In humans, ≈75% is bound to tissue proteins, and the drug does not appreciably enter the CNS. Vincristine is extensively metabolized by the liver and primarily excreted in the bile and/or feces; lesser amounts are eliminated in the urine. In dogs, the pharmacokinetics are reportedly biphasic with a volume of distribution of 0.66 L/kg and elimination half-life of ≈48 minutes.[3] Vincristine residue was detected in urine for 3 days after administration to dogs.[4]

Contraindications/Precautions/Warnings

Vincristine is contraindicated in patients with pre-existing leukopenia or granulocytopenia (unless as a result of the disease being treated) or active bacterial infection and should be used with caution in patients with hepatic diseases, biliary obstruction (hepatic, posthepatic), leukopenia, infection, or pre-existing neuromuscular disease.

Doses of vincristine should be reduced in patients with hepatic disease and/or biliary obstruction (hepatic, posthepatic). Complete avoidance or an empirical 50% reduction in dose should be considered if serum bilirubin concentrations are greater than 2 mg/dL.

Because vincristine is a substrate of P-glycoprotein, it should be used with caution in dogs (eg, Australian shepherds, collies) that may have the *MDR1* genetic mutation.[5] Bone marrow suppression (eg, decreased blood cell counts, particularly neutrophils) and GI toxicity (eg, anorexia, vomiting, diarrhea) are more likely to occur at normal doses in dogs with either the homozygous (mutant/mutant) or heterozygous (normal/mutant) *MDR1* mutation. To reduce the likelihood of severe toxicity in these dogs (mutant/normal or mutant/mutant), the Veterinary Clinical Pharmacology Laboratory at Washington State University recommends reducing the dose by 25% to 30% and carefully monitoring these patients.[5]

Border collies, unrelated to their *MDR1* status, appear to be more susceptible to developing vincristine-associated myelosuppression.[6]

Do not confuse vinBLAStine with vinCRIStine; writing part of the drug's name using tall man lettering on prescriptions/orders may reduce the risk of errors.

In humans, it is recommended to use 0.9% sodium chloride to dilute vincristine into a flexible sterile container to prevent inadvertent administration by any route other than IV. IV administration should be done over 5 to 10 minutes.

The National Institute for Occupational Safety and Health (NIOSH) classifies vincristine as a hazardous drug; personal protective equipment (PPE) should be used accordingly to minimize the risk for exposure.[7]

Adverse Effects

Although structurally related to and having a similar mechanism of action as vinblastine, vincristine has a different adverse effect profile. Vincristine is much less myelosuppressive (causing mild leukopenia) at usual doses but may cause more peripheral neurotoxicity. Neuropathic clinical signs may include proprioceptive deficits, spinal hyporeflexia, or paralytic ileus with resulting constipation. In humans, vincristine commonly causes mild sensory impairment and peripheral paresthesias. These additional neurotoxic effects may also occur in animals; additional caution should be exercised in patients with a predisposing neuropathic disorder (ie, degenerative myelopathy). Cats can develop neurotoxicity associated with constipation or paralytic ileus, thereby aggravating anorexia[8]; they may also develop reversible axon swelling and paranodal demyelination.[9]

In addition, in small animals, vincristine may cause vomiting, diarrhea, anorexia, impaired platelet aggregation, increased liver enzyme activity, inappropriate ADH secretion, jaw pain, alopecia, stomatitis, or seizures. Compared with other chemotherapy treatments, GI effects are considered frequent but mild.[10] Many dogs receiving chemotherapy will have minor hair coat changes (eg, shagginess, loss of luster). Breeds with continuously growing hair coats (eg, poodles, terriers, Afghan hounds, old English sheepdogs) are more likely to experience significant alopecia.

A case report of a cat developing pulmonary edema attributed to vincristine administration has been published.[11]

In dogs, vincristine can cause erythrocyte dysplasia, although this effect is deemed clinically insignificant.[12]

Vincristine is a vesicant, and extravasation may cause localized tissue irritation and cellulitis. Administer IV following a single, clean venipuncture attempt through an IV catheter (indwelling or butterfly). If clinical signs of extravasation are noted, discontinue infusion immediately at that site and apply moderate, dry heat to the area to help disperse the drug and promote vascular absorption. Injections of hyaluronidase have also been suggested to help diffuse the drug.

Reproductive/Nursing Safety

For sexually intact patients, verify pregnancy status prior to administration. Vincristine is teratogenic and embryotoxic (including malformations; embryo resorption and death) when given at recommended dosages in laboratory animals.[13] It may also cause aspermia in males.

It is not known whether this drug is excreted in milk. Because of the potential for serious adverse effects in nursing offspring, the use of milk replacer is recommended if the dam requires vincristine.

Overdose/Acute Toxicity

Following IV administration, the LD_{50} in mice and rats is 3 mg/kg and 1 mg/kg, respectively.

In dogs, the maximum tolerated vincristine dose is reported to be 0.06 mg/kg every 7 days for 6 weeks. Animals receiving this dose showed signs of mild anemia, leukopenia, increased liver enzyme activity, and neuronal shrinkage in the peripheral nervous system and CNS. Megaesophagus and hemorrhagic diarrhea occurred in 1 dog following accidental overdose.[14]

If the overdose is acute (≈6 hours), plasmapheresis may be considered.[15] Other treatment considerations include activated charcoal and cholestyramine (which sequesters intestinal secretion of many acidic drugs and increases their rate of elimination). For subsequent GI signs, a metoclopramide CRI and use of other prokinetic agents (eg, cisapride, erythromycin) may be useful to prevent severe ileus. For severe myelosuppression, filgrastim (G-CSF) may be started prophylactically along with broad-spectrum antibiotics.

In humans, multiple products have been used to reduce neurotoxicity, including rescue with folinic acid (leucovorin) 18 mg every 3 hours 16 times and pyridoxine 50 mg IV or PO every 8 hours[16]; glutamic acid (glutamine) 500 mg PO 3 times daily for 1 month was reported to decrease vincristine neurotoxicity with no additional adverse effects.[17]

In cats, the lethal dose of vincristine is reportedly 0.1 mg/kg. Cats receiving toxic doses showed weight loss, seizures, leukopenia, and general debilitation. A cat receiving vincristine 5 mg/m^2 (NOT mg/kg; 10 times the recommended dose) died 72 hours following the overdose despite intensive treatment with calcium folinate.[14]

In humans, cardiovascular and hematologic monitoring are performed after an overdose. Treatment can include anticonvulsants and prevention of ileus. In addition, an attempt should be made to prevent the effects associated with syndrome of inappropriate antidiuretic hormone (SIADH) by using fluid restriction and loop diuretics to maintain serum osmolality.

For patients that have experienced or are suspected to have experienced an overdose, consultation with a 24-hour poison consultation center specializing in providing veterinary-specific information

is recommended. For general information related to overdose and toxin exposures, as well as contact information for poison control centers, refer to ***Appendix***.

Drug Interactions

The following drug interactions have either been reported or are theoretical in humans or animals receiving vincristine and may be of significance in veterinary patients. Unless otherwise noted, use together is not necessarily contraindicated, but weigh the potential risks and perform additional monitoring when appropriate.

- ASPARAGINASE: Additive neurotoxicity and myelosuppression may occur; effects are less common when asparaginase is administered after vincristine or when doses are separated by 24 hours.
- CHOLESTYRAMINE: Pretreatment with cholestyramine blocks enterohepatic vincristine reuptake and enhances vincristine fecal excretion in dogs. No data are available regarding its use for treatment of vincristine overdose.
- IMMUNOSUPPRESSIVE DRUGS (eg, **azathioprine, corticosteroids, cyclophosphamide**): Use with other immunosuppressant drugs may increase the risk for infection.
- MITOMYCIN: In humans who have previously or simultaneously received mitomycin-C with vinca alkaloids, severe bronchospasm has occurred.
- MYELOSUPPRESSIVE AGENTS (eg, **antineoplastics, iron chelators**): Concurrent use with other bone marrow depressant medications may result in additive myelosuppression; avoid combination when possible.
- VACCINES (live and inactivated): Vincristine may diminish vaccine efficacy and enhance adverse effects of vaccines.

Caution is advised if using vincristine with drugs that can inhibit P-glycoprotein, which may increase intracellular vincristine concentration, particularly in those dogs at risk for *MDR1* genetic mutation (eg, collies, Australian shepherds, Shetland sheepdogs, long-haired whippets, "white feet" breeds), unless they are negative (normal/normal) for the mutation. Drugs and drug classes involved include:

- AMIODARONE
- AZOLE ANTIFUNGALS (eg, **itraconazole, ketoconazole**)
- CARVEDILOL
- CYCLOSPORINE
- DILTIAZEM
- MACROLIDE ANTIBIOTICS (eg, **erythromycin, clarithromycin** but NOT **azithromycin**)
- QUINIDINE
- SPIRONOLACTONE
- TAMOXIFEN
- VERAPAMIL

Laboratory Considerations

- Vincristine may significantly increase both blood and urine concentrations of **uric acid**.

Dosages

NOTES:

1. Because of the potential toxicity of this drug to patients, veterinary staff, and pet owners, and because chemotherapy indications, treatment protocols, monitoring, and safety guidelines often change, the following dosages should be used only as a general guide. Consultation with a veterinary oncologist and referral to current veterinary oncology references[18-22] are strongly recommended.
2. Do NOT confuse mg/kg with mg/m² dosages.

DOGS:

Neoplastic diseases (extra-label): Usually used in combination protocols with other drugs; consultation with a veterinary oncologist is encouraged before use; see **NOTES**. Vincristine is usually administered at 0.5 – 0.75 mg/m² (NOT mg/kg) IV every 1 to 2 weeks.

Transmissible venereal tumor (extra-label)

a) Vincristine is used as sole therapy, usually at 0.5 mg/m² (NOT mg/kg; maximum dose 1 mg) IV once weekly for 4 to 6 weeks.
b) Vincristine 0.025 mg/kg IV weekly. Can be used in combination with intratumoral interferon alpha-2α.[23]
c) Vincristine 0.025 mg/kg IV every other week, alternating with L-asparaginase 5000 units/m² (NOT mg/kg) SC every other week for an 8-week treatment period that includes a total of 4 doses of each drug[24]

Adjunctive treatment of immune-mediated thrombocytopenia (extra-label): In a study, dogs received vincristine 0.02 mg/kg IV bolus once. Dogs also received glucocorticoids (usually prednisone 1.5 – 2 mg/kg PO every 12 hours) and doxycycline until results of serologic testing were negative for tick-borne disease. In dogs that did not have an increase in platelet count 7 days after treatment, azathioprine 2 mg/kg PO once daily was added. **NOTE**: At this dose of vincristine, clinically significant myelosuppression has not been described.[2]

CATS:

Neoplastic diseases (extra-label): Consultation with a veterinary oncologist is encouraged before use; see **NOTES**. Vincristine is usually administered at 0.5 – 0.75 mg/m² (NOT mg/kg) IV every 1 to 3 weeks. Intraperitoneal (IP) vincristine administration was considered a safe and effective alternative route of administration.[25]

HORSES:

Neoplastic diseases (extra-label): Consultation with a veterinary oncologist is encouraged before use; see **NOTES**. Usual dosages are 0.5 mg/m² (NOT mg/kg; usually 2.5 – 3 mg total dose per horse) IV weekly.

Adjunctive therapy for generalized lymphoma as part of the CAP protocol (extra-label): The following are starting dosages; total doses can be increased by 20% to 30% without the expectation of complications. Cytarabine (cytosine arabinoside) at an average dose of 1 – 1.2 g (total dose) SC or IM once every 1 to 2 weeks; cyclophosphamide 1 g (total dose) IV every 2 weeks (alternating with cytarabine); and prednisolone 1 mg/kg PO every other day. Vincristine 2.5 mg (total dose) IV is added on the weeks when cytarabine is administered if there is no response.

- With remission, the starting doses are maintained for 2 to 3 months, then the horse is switched to a maintenance protocol. The first cycle of maintenance therapy increases the treatment interval for each drug by 1 week (except prednisolone, which is kept at the same frequency but with a reducing dose). If the horse is still in remission 2 to 3 months after the first cycle, the second cycle is started by adding an additional week to the treatment intervals of each drug.[26]

FERRETS

Neoplastic disease (extra-label): 0.12 mg/kg IV once weekly for 3 weeks, then every 3 weeks as part of a modified COP protocol[27]

Monitoring

- Verify pregnancy status prior to administration.
- Physical and neurologic examinations
- Baseline and periodic (prior to each treatment) CBC, and serum liver profile
- Adverse effects: development of peripheral motor and/or sensory deficits, fever, constipation, icterus

Client Information

- Vincristine is a chemotherapy (anticancer) drug. The drug can be hazardous to other animals and humans that come into contact with it. On the day your animal receives the drug and then for a minimum of 3 days afterward, all bodily waste (eg, urine, feces), litter, blood, and vomit should only be handled while wearing disposable gloves. Seal the waste in a plastic bag, then place both the bag and gloves in the regular trash. Those who are pregnant, attempting to conceive, or nursing should not clean up the animal's waste.
- In the interest of safety to other animals and humans, do not take your dog to a dog park or allow your animal to urinate and defecate in public places until your veterinarian tells you that it is okay to do so.
- Bone marrow suppression can occur. The greatest effects on bone marrow usually occur within a few weeks after treatment. Your veterinarian will need to do blood tests to watch for this problem. Do not miss these important follow up visits.
- Your veterinarian will need to do periodic examinations and blood tests on your animal after it receives this medication. Do not miss these important follow-up visits.
- Your animal should not receive vaccines containing live (or modified live) viruses while receiving this medication.
- Contact your veterinarian right away if you see bleeding, bruising, or fever (indicating an infection) or if your animal becomes tired easily.
- Contact your veterinarian right away if you notice pain, redness, or swelling in the area where the injection was given.
- Vincristine can cause serious neurologic toxicity that can result in weakness, severe constipation, and loss of appetite.
- Your animal should not participate in animal competitions while on this drug. Exposure to other animals may put your animal at serious risk of infections during chemotherapy treatment. Talk with your veterinarian about when itis safe to return to these events.

Chemistry/Synonyms

Vincristine sulfate, commonly referred to as a vinca alkaloid, is isolated from the plant *Catharanthus roseus* (*Vinca rosea Linn*) and occurs as a white or slightly yellow, hygroscopic, amorphous, or crystalline powder that is freely soluble in water and slightly soluble in alcohol. The commercially available injection has a pH of 3 to 5.5. Vincristine sulfate has pK_as of 5 and 7.4.

Vincristine sulfate may also be known as leurocristine sulfate, VCR, LCR compound 37231, leurocristine sulphate, NSC-67574, 22-oxovincaleukoblastine sulphate, sulfato de vincristina, vincristini sulfas, and *Oncovin*®; many other trade names are available.

Storage/Stability

Intact vials should be stored upright between 2°C to 8°C (36°F-46°F) and protected from light. Diluted solutions are stable for 7 days at refrigerated temperatures or 2 days at room temperature.

Compatibility/Compounding Considerations

Compatible with normal saline or dextrose 5% in water for dilution. Vincristine sulfate is reportedly physically **compatible** with bleomycin sulfate, cytarabine, fluorouracil, and methotrexate sodium and in syringes or at Y-sites with bleomycin sulfate, cisplatin, cyclophosphamide, doxorubicin HCl, droperidol, fluorouracil, heparin sodium, leucovorin calcium, methotrexate sodium, metoclopramide HCl, mitomycin, and vinblastine sulfate.

Vincristine sulfate is reportedly physically **incompatible** with furosemide.

Compatibility is dependent on factors such as pH, concentration, temperature, and diluent used; consult specialized references or a hospital pharmacist for more specific information.

Dosage Forms/Regulatory Status

VETERINARY-LABELED PRODUCTS: NONE

HUMAN-LABELED PRODUCTS:

Vincristine Sulfate Injection: 1 mg/mL in 1 mL, 2 mL, and 5 mL vials; *Vincasar® PFS*, generic; (Rx)

References

For the complete list of references, see **wiley.com/go/budde/plumb**

Vinorelbine

(vin-***or***-el-been) *Navelbine*®

Antineoplastic

Prescriber Highlights

- ▶ A semisynthetic vinca alkaloid antineoplastic used to treat a variety of tumors in dogs and cats
- ▶ Contraindications include pre-existing anemia, thrombocytopenia, or granulocytopenia (unless a result of the disease being treated) or active bacterial infection; reduce dose for patients with hepatic dysfunction.
- ▶ Adverse effects in dogs include gastroenterocolitis (eg, nausea, vomiting, diarrhea), myelosuppression; peripheral neuropathy appears less likely than with other vinca alkaloids.
- ▶ Extravasation injury is possible; ensure the IV catheter is well placed and freely flowing.
- ▶ Adverse effects in cats include anemia, neutropenia, weight loss, and/or vomiting.
- ▶ Wear gloves and protective clothing when preparing and administering. Vinorelbine is a hazardous drug as defined by the National Institute for Occupational Safety and Health (NIOSH). Potentially teratogenic

Uses/Indications

Vinorelbine is an antineoplastic drug that has been studied in dogs for the treatment of hemangiosarcoma,[1] locally aggressive or metastatic cutaneous mast cell tumors,[2] bronchoalveolar carcinoma,[3] primary pulmonary carcinoma[4] histiocytic sarcoma,[4] and with piroxicam for urinary bladder carcinoma.[5]

Vinorelbine use in cats appears to be limited; there is 1 phase I study in cats with a variety of tumor types published.[6]

In humans, vinorelbine is indicated for the treatment of non-small cell lung cancers (first-line, locally advanced, or metastatic) and is also used in the treatment of breast cancer; carcinomas of the esophagus and cervix; head, neck, and salivary gland cancer; Hodgkin's lymphoma; mesothelioma; ovarian cancer; and small cell lung cancer.

Pharmacology/Actions

Vinca alkaloids bind tubulin in the mitotic spindle, which prevents microtubule formation, interferes with axonal neurotransmitter movement, and causes microtubule depolymerization, thereby preventing cell division during metaphase. Vinorelbine also interferes with amino acid metabolism by inhibiting glutamic acid utilization and preventing purine synthesis, citric acid cycle, and urea formation.

Pharmacokinetics

In dogs receiving vinorelbine IV, a rapid distribution phase was noted. Protein binding was 90%, and the terminal half-life was 34.5 hours.[7]

In humans, ≈85% of circulating vinorelbine is bound to cellular components (≈75% to platelets and other cells, ≈10% to plasma proteins). Vinorelbine is rapidly distributed to tissues, although the drug does not appreciably enter the CNS. It reaches 300-fold greater concentration in lung tissue than in plasma.

Vinorelbine is extensively metabolized in the liver by CYP3A, and at least 2 active metabolites are formed. The drug is primarily excreted in the bile and/or feces (≈45%), with lesser amounts (11% to 18%) of the unchanged drug eliminated in the urine. Terminal halflife is ≈40 hours.

Contraindications/Precautions/Warnings

Vinorelbine is contraindicated in patients with pre-existing leukopenia or granulocytopenia, thrombocytopenia, or active bacterial infections.[8] Severe myelosuppression resulting in serious infection, septic shock, and death can occur. Doses should be delayed or reduced for patients with decreased neutrophil counts. In humans, a dose reduction of 50% is suggested if neutrophil count is 1000 cells/mm^3 to 1499 cells/mm^3, and delaying treatment is advised if neutrophil count is less than 1000 cells/mm^3. Previous fever, sepsis, or delayed treatments warrant a 25% dose reduction.

Doses of vinorelbine should be reduced in patients with hepatic disease. In humans, a 50% dose reduction is recommended if serum bilirubin levels are greater than 2 mg/dL, and a 75% dose reduction is recommended for bilirubin greater than 3 mg/dL.[8] Vinorelbine use should be avoided in patients receiving radiation therapy in fields that include the liver.

Other vinca alkaloids (ie, vinblastine, vincristine) are substrates of P-glycoprotein and should be used with caution in herding breeds (eg, collies) that may have the the *MDR1* mutation (also known as *ABCB1*-1delta) causing nonfunctional proteins, as adverse effects may be more likely. However, vinorelbine does not appear to be a significant substrate for P-glycoprotein, and it is, therefore, unclear whether testing for the *MDR1* mutation (also known as *ABCB1*-1delta) prior to initiating vinorelbine therapy is warranted.[9]

Intrathecal administration of vinca alkaloids must be avoided, as this route of administration may result in ascending paralysis and death.

In humans, vinorelbine can cause severe and fatal paralytic ileus, constipation, intestinal obstruction, necrosis, and perforation.[8] Pulmonary toxicity, including severe bronchospasm, interstitial pneumonitis, and acute respiratory distress syndrome, can also occur.

The National Institute for Occupational Safety and Health (NIOSH) classifies vinorelbine as a hazardous drug; personal protective equipment (PPE) should be used accordingly to minimize the risk for exposure.[10]

Adverse Effects

In 16% to 46% of dogs, vinorelbine can cause gastroenterocolitis (nausea/vomiting and diarrhea),[2-5] which generally lasts less than 24 hours; it is not considered highly emetogenic.

Myelosuppression was noted in 32% to 54% of dogs[2-5] and can occur at usual dosages. Granulocyte nadir is at 7 to 10 days after treatment; recovery is 7 to 14 days later. Myelosuppression may be cumulative.[3,4] Thrombocytopenia (grade 1 or 2) occurred in 7% of dogs in 1 retrospective study.[4] Vinorelbine is considered more myelosuppressive than vincristine.

Hepatic cirrhosis was noted in 1 dog[3] and nonspecific abdominal pain with elevated liver enzymes occurred in another dog,[4] although it was unclear whether those effects were directly attributable to vinorelbine. Vinorelbine may cause peripheral neurotoxic effects (eg, jaw and muscle pain, peripheral neuropathy, loss of deep tendon reflexes). One case of bilateral hind limb ataxia in a dog has been noted.[4]

In a phase I study in 19 cats, the following adverse effects were noted: anemia (32%), neutropenia (21%), weight loss (16%), persistent vomiting (11%), thrombocytopenia (5.2%), and grade 4 acute renal injury (5.2%).[6]

Administration site reactions (eg, phlebitis, erythema) occur more commonly with rapid IV injection or when administered into peripheral veins. Vinorelbine is considered a vesicant, and extravasation can cause significant tissue irritation, cellulitis, and necrosis. If clinical signs of extravasation are noted, discontinue infusion immediately and attempt to aspirate the drug back. Apply moderate heat to the area to help disperse the drug. Injections of hyaluronidase (150 units/mL, 1 to 6 mL through IV site; or 0.2 mL SC or intradermally in 5 sites [1 mL total] at the leading edge of extravasated drug) may help diffuse the drug. Ice is not recommended for vinca alkaloid extravasation as it can significantly worsen skin ulceration.[11] Topical dimethyl sulfoxide (DMSO) can be considered to treat the area involved. Never administer vinorelbine via SC or IM routes.

Reproductive/Nursing Safety

Vinorelbine possesses teratogenic and embryotoxic properties and should only be used in pregnant patients if the potential benefits to the dam outweigh the risk to the developing fetus. Placental transfer in rats was less than 1%.[7] Vinorelbine may also cause aspermia in males.

Concentrations of vinorelbine in rat mammary glands exceeded that of plasma concentration.[7] It is not known whether vinorelbine is excreted in milk, but because of the potential for serious adverse reactions in nursing offspring, the use of milk replacer is recommended if the dam requires vinorelbine.

For sexually intact patients, verify pregnancy status prior to administration.

Because safety has not been established in animals, this drug should only be used when the maternal benefits outweigh the potential risks to offspring.

Overdose/Acute Toxicity

In humans, death has occurred after a 5-fold overdose. In addition to the exacerbations of the expected adverse effects (eg, ileus, myleosuppression), neurotoxicity similar to those associated with vincristine (eg, loss of reflexes, paresthesias) may also be noted.

In humans, treatment is supportive and can include anti-infectives, hematopoietic drugs, and/or blood transfusions. Additionally, an attempt is made to prevent the effects associated with the syndrome of inappropriate antidiuretic hormone (SIADH) with fluid restriction and close monitoring of fluid and electrolyte status.

For patients that have experienced or are suspected of having experienced an overdose, consultation with a 24-hour poison consultation center specializing in providing veterinary-specific information is recommended. For general information related to overdose and toxin exposures, as well as contact information for poison control centers, refer to ***Appendix.***

Drug Interactions

Vinorelbine is a CYP3A substrate. The following drug interactions have either been reported or are theoretical in humans or animals receiving vinorelbine and may be of significance in veterinary patients. Unless otherwise noted, use together is not necessarily contraindicated, but weigh the potential risks and perform additional monitoring when appropriate.

- **AMPHOTERICIN B**: May increase the risk for nephrotoxicity, bronchospasm, and hypotension by an undetermined mechanism
- **ANTIDIURETIC HORMONE** (eg, **desmopressin, vasopressin**): May increase the risk for water intoxication and/or hyponatremia
- **AZOLE ANTIFUNGALS** (eg, **itraconazole, ketoconazole, voriconazole**): May increase serum concentration of vinorelbine; consider reducing the vinorelbine dose.
- **CYP3A INHIBITORS** (eg, **amiodarone, fluvoxamine, grapefruit juice**): Concurrent use may increase vinorelbine concentration and risk for toxicity.
- **HEPARINS** (eg, **dalteparin, enoxaparin, heparin**): Concurrent use may increase the risk for bleeding.

- Immunosuppressive Drugs (eg, **azathioprine, cyclophosphamide, corticosteroids**): Use with other immunosuppressant drugs may increase the risk for infection.
- Macrolide Antibiotics (except **azithromycin**): Macrolide antibiotics may increase the serum concentration of vinorelbine; consider reducing the vinorelbine dose.
- Myelosuppressive Agents (eg, **antineoplastics, immunosuppressants, iron chelators**): Concurrent use with other myelosuppressive medications may result in additive myelosuppression; avoid combination when possible.
- Neuropathy-inducing Drugs (eg, **carboplatin, dapsone, isoniazid, metronidazole, nitrofurantoin**): Concurrent use may increase the risk for peripheral neuropathy.
- Ototoxic Drugs (eg, **aminoglycosides, cisplatin, carboplatin**): May cause additive risk for ototoxicity
- Vaccines (live and inactivated): Vinorelbine may diminish vaccine efficacy and enhance adverse effects of vaccines.

Laboratory Considerations

- Vinorelbine may significantly increase both blood and urine concentrations of **uric acid** (potentially significant for Dalmatians).

Dosages

NOTE: Because of the potential toxicity of this drug to patients, veterinary personnel, and clients, and because chemotherapy indications, treatment protocols, and monitoring and safety guidelines often change, the following dosages should be used only as a general guide. Consultation with a veterinary oncologist and referral to current veterinary oncology references[12-16] are strongly recommended.

DOGS:

Neoplastic disease (extra-label): Initial dosage is usually 15 mg/m^2 (NOT mg/kg) IV into a freely flowing IV catheter over 6 to 10 minutes as a solution diluted to a concentration of 1 – 3 mg/mL; flush IV line after administration. The frequency of administration is typically every 1 to 2 weeks. Dosage escalation to 16 – 18 mg/m^2 (NOT mg/kg) IV can be considered based on tolerability. Dosage may be decreased by 10% to 20% if myelosuppression occurs.[2-5]

CATS:

Neoplastic disease (extra-label): Recommended starting dose is 11.5 mg/m^2 (NOT mg/kg) administered as a 1.5 mg/mL solution IV over 5 minutes every 7 days for up to 4 treatments; continuation with doses every 2 weeks may be considered. Dosage may be decreased by 10% to 25% if myelosuppression occurs.[6]

Monitoring

- Efficacy
- Baseline and periodic (ie, prior to each dose) CBC with platelet count
- Baseline and periodic liver enzymes

Client Information

- Vinorelbine is a chemotherapy (anticancer) medicine. The medicine can be hazardous to other animals and people that come in contact with it. On the day your animal gets the drug and then for a few days afterward, handle all bodily waste (urine, feces, litter), blood, or vomit only while wearing chemotherapy-resistant gloves. Seal the waste in a plastic bag, then place both the bag and gloves in the regular trash.
- Those who are pregnant, attempting to conceive, or nursing should not clean up the animal's waste.
- Do not wash any items soiled with waste, vomit, or saliva from your dog with other laundry. Take precautions in handling the dog's toys, food bowl, and water bowl; wash separately from other items.
- Your veterinarian will need to perform regular monitoring, including blood tests and/or radiographs, to be sure this drug is not causing toxic effects to your animal. Do not miss these important follow up visits.
- Observe your dog for lack of appetite, vomiting, or diarrhea. If these signs are severe, or if you notice difficulty breathing or signs of infection, contact your veterinarian immediately.
- Bone-marrow suppression can occur. The greatest effects on bone marrow usually occur within a week after treatment. Your veterinarian will do blood tests to watch for this, but if you see bleeding, bruising, fever, or other signs of an infection or if your animal becomes tired easily, contact your veterinarian right away.

Chemistry/Synonyms

Vinorelbine is a semisynthetic vinca alkaloid derived from the plant *Catharanthus roseus*. Pharmaceutical formulations contain vinorelbine tartrate; 1 mg of vinorelbine is equivalent to 1.385 mg of vinorelbine tartrate. Vinorelbine tartrate occurs as a white, yellow, or light-brown, hygroscopic, amorphous powder that is freely soluble in water. The commercially available injection has a pH of 3.3 to 3.8.

Vinorelbine may also be known as 5'-nor-anhydrovinblastine and *Bagovir*®, *Vinelbine*®, or *Navelbine*®.

Storage/Stability

Store intact vials between 2°C and 8°C (36°F-46°F) and protect them from light. The commercially available injection is packaged under inert gas. Diluted solutions at concentrations between 0.5 mg/mL and 2 mg/mL are stable for up to 24 hours at 5°C to 30°C (41°F-86°F).[17] Dispose of any unused product or waste materials in accordance with proper procedures for cytotoxic drugs.

Compatibility/Compounding Considerations

Compatibility is dependent upon factors such as pH, concentration, temperature, and diluent used; consult specialized references or a hospital pharmacist for more specific information.

Compatible with lactated Ringer's, Ringer's, 0.45% and 0.9% sodium chloride, and 5% dextrose in water or 0.45% sodium chloride.

Vinorelbine is reportedly **syringe** or **Y-site compatible** with amiodarone, bleomycin sulfate, butorphanol, calcium salts, carboplatin, ceftazidime, ciprofloxacin, cyclophosphamide, dexamethasone sodium phosphate, dexmedetomidine, doxorubicin, famotidine, fentanyl, fluconazole, hydromorphone, leucovorin calcium, lidocaine hydrochloride, meropenem, metoclopramide HCl, midazolam, naloxone, pamidronate, potassium salts, and zoledronic acid.

Vinorelbine sulfate **compatibility information conflicts** with heparin sodium (in syringes).

Vinorelbine sulfate is reportedly physically **incompatible** with ampicillin sodium, amphotericin B (all forms), cefazolin, ceftriaxone, diazepam, furosemide, nitroprusside sodium, pantoprazole, phenobarbital, piperacillin-tazobactam, and sodium bicarbonate.

Dosage Forms/Regulatory Status

VETERINARY-LABELED PRODUCTS: NONE

HUMAN-LABELED PRODUCTS:

Vinorelbine Sulfate Injection: 10 mg/mL in 1 mL and 5 mL vials; generic; (Rx)

References

For the complete list of references, see **wiley.com/go/budde/plumb**

Vitamin A

Vitamin (Retinoid)

Prescriber Highlights

- ► Potentially useful for adjunctive treatment of some types of dermatoses in dogs. Evidence is weak to support its use, but it is usually tolerated well.
- ► Give with food; may require 1 to 2 months before efficacy can be noted
- ► Must be given IM or SC; do not administer parenteral doses by the IV route.
- ► Keratoconjunctivitis or increased liver enzymes possible

Uses/Indications

In dogs, although evidence supporting the use of vitamin A is weak, exogenously administered (nondietary) vitamin A may be useful for treating vitamin A–responsive dermatosis in cocker spaniels (and other breeds), sebaceous adenitis, primary idiopathic seborrhea and other primary keratinization disorders, follicular disorders (eg, color dilution alopecia), and keratoacanthoma. It also can be used to treat hypovitaminosis A in other species, including chelonians and birds.

One retrospective study (n = 24) using oral vitamin A (mean dosage was 1037 units/kg/day) for a minimum of 1 month to treat sebaceous adenitis has been published.[1] All but 2 dogs also received other treatments, including systemic antibiotics, systemic antifungal medications, fatty acid supplementation, or various topical treatments. At follow-up, ≈½ of the owners were satisfied with the overall appearance of their dogs, reporting at least 25% improvement in clinical signs, but almost ⅓ of owners reported no improvement. The authors concluded that no correlations could be made between vitamin A dosage and response to treatment; prognoses could not be made based on clinical and histopathologic findings.

Pharmacology/Actions

Vitamin A (and its derivatives) is necessary for growth, bone and dental development, vision, reproduction, cortisol synthesis, immunity, and the integrity of mucosal and epithelial surfaces. Vitamin A is a cofactor in various biochemical reactions, including mucopolysaccharide synthesis, cholesterol synthesis, and hydroxysteroid metabolism. Retinol combines with opsin to form rhodopsin in rod cells (responsible for motion detection and night vision) and iodopsin in cone cells (responsible for light and color vision). All retinoids have some antiproliferative, anti-inflammatory, and immunomodulatory effects.

Pharmacokinetics

Orally administered vitamin A (except retinoic acid) must be converted to retinol by pancreatic and mucosal hydrolases before it is absorbed in the small intestine and re-esterified in mucosal cells. Absorption may be reduced with impaired hepatic or pancreatic function. These retinyl esters (primarily retinyl palmitate) enter the systemic circulation via the lymphatics after they are bound by chylomicrons and are then cleared from the circulation and stored by the liver. Retinoic acid is directly absorbed unchanged and then transported into systemic circulation via albumin. It is metabolized by glucuronidation pathways.

Contraindications/Precautions/Warnings

Exogenously administered vitamin A is contraindicated in patients that are known to be hypersensitive to it or in patients with hypervitaminosis A. Vitamin A dosages in excess of the recommended daily requirements are contraindicated during pregnancy. Anaphylactic shock and death have occurred in humans after IV administration.

To avoid hypervitaminosis A, consider all sources of vitamin A (eg, dietary, other supplements, topicals) when prescribing vitamin A.

Adverse Effects

Dogs appear to tolerate oral vitamin A well. Potential adverse effects in dogs can include GI effects, erythema, pruritus, and behavioral changes. Long-term oversupplementation can cause hypervitaminosis A, which is exhibited by localized or generalized papules (firm center), poor coat quality, alopecia, scaling, excessive bleeding, liver disease, and, rarely, keratoconjunctivitis sicca. Adverse effects generally resolve after drug discontinuation.

Cats appear to be susceptible to chronic vitamin A toxicity. A case report of hypervitaminosis A in a cat that was fed raw liver and developed hepatic fibrosis and stellate cell lipidosis has been published.[2]

Reproductive/Nursing Safety

Exogenously administered vitamin A is contraindicated in pregnancy.

Safety to nursing offspring is not known, but vitamin A requirements in dams increase while nursing.

Because safety has not been established in animals, this drug should only be used when the maternal benefits outweigh the potential risks to offspring.

Overdose/Acute Toxicity

Data on acute toxicity from oral vitamin A in dogs or cats were not located. Oral LD_{50} in rats is 2000 mg/kg.[3]

In humans, acute toxic effects can include GI effects (eg, nausea, vomiting), drowsiness, headache, and vertigo. In adults, blurred vision has been reported, and in infants, bulging fontanelles. Toxic (1 time) doses reported are 350,000 units per dose for infants and children less than 6 years old, and greater than 2,000,000 units per dose for adults, or ≈25,000 units/kg. Long-term overdosing appears to hold the greater risk for dogs (and cats); refer to the ***Adverse Effects*** section for more information. Treatment consists of discontinuation of vitamin A and supportive therapy.

For patients that have experienced or are suspected of having experienced an overdose, consultation with a 24-hour poison consultation center specializing in providing veterinary-specific information is recommended. For general information related to overdose and toxin exposures, as well as contact information for poison control centers, refer to ***Appendix.***

Drug Interactions

The following drug interactions have either been reported or are theoretical in humans or animals receiving vitamin A and may be of significance in veterinary patients. Unless otherwise noted, use together is not necessarily contraindicated, but weigh the potential risks and perform additional monitoring when appropriate.

- **Cholestyramine**: May reduce vitamin A absorption; separate dosages by at least 2 hours if using concomitantly
- **Clopidogrel**: High doses of vitamin A may increase the risk for bleeding.
- **Heparin**: High doses of vitamin A may increase the risk for bleeding.
- **Isotretinoin** (eg, other **retinoids**): Increased risk for vitamin A toxicity
- **Mineral Oil**: May reduce the amount of vitamin A absorbed from the gut. Separate dosages by at least 2 hours if using concomitantly.
- **Neomycin**: May reduce vitamin A absorption
- **Tetracyclines** (eg, **doxycycline, minocycline**): Concurrent use may increase the risk for pseudotumor cerebri (benign intracranial hypertension).
- **Warfarin**: High doses of vitamin A may increase the risk for bleeding.

Laboratory Considerations

- Vitamin A may falsely elevate **bilirubin** when determined by Ehrlich's reagent.

Dosages

NOTE: Dosages are not well defined, and little evidence exists to support any dosing regimen.

DOGS:

Adjunctive treatment of canine sebaceous adenitis (extra-label): Initially, 8000 – 10,000 units/dog (NOT units/kg) PO twice a day; can increase to 20,000 – 30,000 units/dog (NOT units/kg) PO twice a day.[4] From a retrospective study (n = 24): doses varied from 380 – 2667 units/kg/day PO (mean dosage was 1037 units/kg per day for a minimum of 1 month).[1]

Vitamin A-responsive dermatosis, primary idiopathic seborrhea, follicular disorders, keratoacanthoma (extra-label): 625 – 800 units/kg PO once a day or 10,000 – 50,000 units/dog (NOT units/kg) PO once a day with a fatty meal. It may take 4 to 8 weeks before any improvement can be seen.[5]

REPTILES:

Adjunctive treatment of hypovitaminosis A in chelonians (extra-label): In addition to adding carrots and cod liver oil to the diet, vitamin A injection at 2000 units/kg IM can be given.[6]

Hypovitaminosis A in geckos (extra-label): 0.01 mL of vitamin A+D for injection (containing 500,000 units/mL vitamin A) SC; repeat in 14 days[7]

Monitoring

- Efficacy
- Schirmer tear test (STT) if using it long term. Recommendation for frequency for rechecking STT varies; every 3 weeks to every 6 to 12 months have been suggested.
- Liver enzymes if using it long term; baseline and every 6 to 12 months
- Other adverse effects as they arise

Client Information

- Give this medicine with food (meals), preferably food that is high in fat.
- This medicine may be taken 1 to 2 months before it causes any improvement in condition.
- Do not give more of this medicine than your veterinarian prescribes. Vitamin A can be toxic, especially if high doses are given for a long time.
- Watch for dry eyes.

Chemistry/Synonyms

Vitamin A may consist of retinol, or its esters formed from edible fatty acids, principally acetic and palmitic acids. In liquid form, vitamin A is a light yellow to red oil that may solidify upon refrigeration. In solid form, it takes on the appearance of any diluent that has been added. Vitamin A can be practically odorless, or it may have a mild fishy odor (but no rancid odor or taste). It is unstable in air and light. In liquid form, vitamin A is insoluble in water or glycerol and soluble in dehydrated alcohol or vegetable oils. In solid form, vitamin A may be dispersible in water.

Sources of vitamin A can be via retinols or provitamins. Retinols include retinol, retinal, and retinoic acid and are found in foods such as milk, meat, or eggs. Provitamins are plant-derived and include alpha-, beta- and gamma-carotene, which are converted to vitamin A in the body. Food processing, such as freezing, may reduce the amount of vitamin A in foods.

Formerly, vitamin A recommended daily allowances (RDA; for humans) were expressed in units, but now units has been replaced by retinol activity equivalents (RAE), where 1 RAE = retinol 1 µg, beta-carotene (from supplements) 0.2 µg, beta-carotene (from food) 12 µg, alpha-carotene 24 µg, or beta-cryptoxanthin 24 µg. (Note that pharmacologic doses continue to be expressed in units.)

Vitamin A may also be known as axerophthol, oleovitamin A, retinol, or retinyl palmitate.

Storage/Stability

Store oral products in tight, light-resistant containers away from heat. Store the injection between 2°C and 8°C (36°F and 46°F); do not freeze. Protect products from air and light.

Compatibility/Compounding Considerations

No specific information was noted.

Dosage Forms/Regulatory Status

VETERINARY-LABELED PRODUCTS:

Vitamin A for injection can be found in combination with the other fat-soluble vitamins (vitamin D and/or E) labeled for use in newborn or adult cattle, sheep, and swine; FDA approval status is uncertain (OTC).

HUMAN-LABELED PRODUCTS:

Vitamin A Oral Capsules: 7500 units, 8000 units, 10,000 units, and 25,000 units; generic; (OTC)

Vitamin A Palmitate (Retinyl Palmitate) for IM Injection: 50,000 units/mL (15 mg retinol/mL); *Aquasol-A*®; (Rx). **NOTE**: IV administration is contraindicated.

References

For the complete list of references, see **wiley.com/go/budde/plumb**

Vitamin E ± Selenium

Alpha-tocopherol

(***vye***-ta-min-***ee;*** se-***lee***-nee-um)

Nutritional; Vitamin

Prescriber Highlights

- Vitamin E (alone) has been used for various skin-related conditions (immune-mediated, ischemic dermatopathies); as an adjunctive treatment for hepatopathies and feline pansteatitis; and vitamin E deficiency states caused by dietary deficiency, pancreatitis, or genetics.
- Vitamin E with selenium is used for the treatment or prophylaxis of selenium-tocopherol deficiency (STD) syndromes in ewes and lambs (white muscle disease); sows, weanling and baby pigs (hepatic necrosis, mulberry heart disease, white muscle disease); calves and breeding cows (white muscle disease); and horses (myositis associated with STD).
- Contraindications: vitamin E/selenium products should only be used in the species for which they are FDA-approved.
- Adverse effects include anaphylactoid reactions; IM injections may cause transient muscle soreness. Selenium overdoses can cause depression, ataxia, dyspnea, blindness, diarrhea, muscle weakness, and a garlic odor on the breath. Selenium overdoses can be extremely toxic.

Uses/Indications

Vitamin E may be useful as adjunctive treatment of discoid lupus erythematosus, symmetrical lupoid onychodystrophy,[1] pemphigus complex, and demodicosis in dogs. A review article on canine ischemic dermatopathies states: *The mainstay for pharmacologic management of ischemic dermatopathies is pentoxifylline in combination with vitamin E.*[2]

Vitamin E may also be of benefit in the adjunctive treatment of hepatic fibrosis or adjunctive therapy of copper-associated hepatopathy in dogs and pansteatitis in cats. There is some evidence that vitamin E and silymarin have synergistic effects on hepatocytes and a study in dogs found evidence that silymarin and vitamin E provided some efficacy in preventing gentamicin-induced nephrotoxicity.[3] However, with respect to using vitamin E for canine liver disease, an article reviewing the evidence states: ...*vitamin E supplements have been recommended for dermatologic and hepatobiliary diseases (cholestatic and necro-inflammatory hepatopathies) in which antioxidant activity may be of benefit. However, no scientific data support their use for any of these indications.* The results of one study showed a potential clinical benefit of oral vitamin E as adjunctive treatment of canine atopic dermatitis.[4]

Supplemental vitamin E appears useful for treating retinal pigment epithelial dystrophy (RPED) with neuroaxonal degeneration in English cocker spaniels (and presumably other breeds).[5]

A double-blinded and randomized pilot study (n = 8 in treatment group) in a canine experimental osteoarthritis model found some evidence that dogs treated with vitamin E (≈400 units/dog [NOT units/kg] PO per day) showed a reduction in inflammation joint markers and histological expression, as well as a trend to improving signs of pain.[6]

Some dogs and cats with dilated cardiomyopathy have low vitamin E concentrations, but it is unknown if vitamin E supplementation has any clinical effect. Vitamin E supplementation in cats with chronic kidney disease did not improve anemia or measures of oxidative stress.[7]

Depending on the product and target species, vitamin E/selenium is indicated for the treatment or prophylaxis of selenium-tocopherol deficiency (STD) syndromes in ewes and lambs (white muscle disease); sows, weanling and baby pigs (hepatic necrosis, mulberry heart disease, white muscle disease); calves and breeding cows (white muscle disease); and horses (myositis associated with STD). A small, noncontrolled study indicated that vitamin E/selenium may be useful as adjunct therapy to a miticide (ivermectin) for treating canine sarcoptic mange.[8]

Pharmacology/Actions

Both vitamin E and selenium are involved with cellular metabolism of sulfur. Vitamin E has antioxidant and anti-inflammatory properties and with selenium, protects against red blood cell hemolysis and prevents the action of peroxidase on unsaturated bonds in cell membranes.

Pharmacokinetics

After absorption, vitamin E is transported in the circulatory system via beta-lipoproteins. Water-soluble (water-dispersible) oral forms appear to be more bioavailable. Impaired hepatic or pancreatic function may reduce absorption. Vitamin E is distributed to all tissues and stored in adipose tissue. Vitamin E is only marginally transported across the placenta. Vitamin E is metabolized in the liver via glucuronidation and excreted primarily into the bile. Absorption of vitamin E may be impaired in patients with severe cholestatic liver disease or in animals with fat malabsorption syndromes.

Pharmacokinetic parameters for selenium were not located.

Contraindications/Precautions/Warnings

Vitamin E (alone) should be used with caution in patients with coagulation disorders.

Vitamin E/selenium products should only be used in the species for which they are FDA-approved. Because selenium can be extremely toxic, the indiscriminate use of these products can be dangerous. Give slowly when administering IV to horses.

Adverse Effects

Oral administration of vitamin E appears to be well-tolerated, with a wide margin of safety. Anaphylactoid reactions have been reported. IM injections may be associated with transient muscle soreness. Other adverse effects are generally associated with overdoses of selenium (see ***Overdose/Acute Toxicity***).

Reproductive/Nursing Safety

Because safety has not been established in all animal species, this supplement should only be used when the maternal benefits outweigh the potential risks to offspring.

Overdose/Acute Toxicity

Large overdoses of vitamin E can cause coagulopathies.

Selenium is toxic in overdose quantities but has a fairly wide safety margin. Cattle have tolerated chronic doses of 0.6 mg/kg/day with no adverse effects (approximate therapeutic dose is 0.06 mg/kg). Clinical signs of selenium toxicity include depression, ataxia, dyspnea, blindness, diarrhea, muscle weakness, and a garlic odor on the breath. Horses suffering from selenium toxicity may become blind, paralyzed, slough their hooves, and lose hair from the tail and mane. Dogs may exhibit signs of anorexia, vomiting, and diarrhea at high doses.

For patients that have experienced or are suspected to have experienced an overdose, consultation with a 24-hour poison consultation center specializing in providing veterinary-specific information is recommended. For general information related to overdose and toxin exposures, as well as contact information for poison control centers, refer to ***Appendix***.

Drug Interactions

The following drug interactions have either been reported or are theoretical in humans or animals receiving vitamin E/selenium and may be of significance in veterinary patients. Unless otherwise noted, use together is not necessarily contraindicated, but weigh the potential risks and perform additional monitoring when appropriate.

- **ANTICOAGULANT AGENTS** (eg, **heparins, rivaroxaban, warfarin**): Risk for bleeding may be increased.
- **ANTIPLATELET AGENTS** (eg, **aspirin, clopidogrel**): Risk for bleeding may be increased.
- **CHOLESTYRAMINE**: May reduce the absorption of orally administered vitamin E
- **IRON**: Large doses of vitamin E may delay the hematologic response to iron therapy in patients with iron deficiency anemia.
- **MINERAL OIL**: May reduce the absorption of orally administered vitamin E
- **NONSTEROIDAL ANTI-INFLAMMATORY DRUGS** (eg, **carprofen, flunixin, meloxicam, phenylbutazone**): Risk for bleeding may be increased.
- **VITAMIN A**: Absorption, utilization, and storage may be enhanced by vitamin E.

Laboratory Considerations

- None noted

Dosages

The following dosages are for vitamin E as a single agent; for dosages of vitamin E/selenium veterinary-labeled products see ***Dosage Forms/Regulatory Status***. Do not confuse dosages of units/animal with units/kg.

DOGS:

Ischemic dermatopathies (extra-label): 200 units/small-sized dog (NOT units/kg); 400 units/medium-sized dog (NOT units/kg); 600 units/large-sized dog (NOT units/kg) PO every 12 hours. The ideal oral dosage of vitamin E for maximum cutaneous protection has not been elucidated, but it has a wide margin of safety for oral supplementation. Used in combination with pentoxifylline 15 mg/kg PO every 8 hours to 30 mg/kg PO every 12 hours.[2]

Atopic dermatitis (extra-label): 8.1 units/kg PO once daily improved clinical sign scores in dogs with atopic dermatitis.[4]

Adjunctive treatment of immune-mediated skin diseases (eg, discoid lupus erythematosus, canine demodicosis, or derma-

tomyositis) (extra-label): Anecdotally, 200 – 800 units/dog (NOT units/kg) PO twice daily.

Adjunctive treatment of hepatopathies or as an antioxidant hepatoprotective (extra-label): Anecdotally, 50 – 400 units/dog (NOT units/kg) PO once daily. Some recommend water-soluble (water-dispersible) dosage forms as oral bioavailability may be higher.[9]

Tocopherol deficiency associated with exocrine pancreatic disease (extra-label): 100 – 400 units/dog (NOT units/kg) PO once daily for 1 month then every 1 to 2 weeks as needed.[10]

Retinal pigment epithelial dystrophy (RPED) (extra-label): 600 – 900 units/dog (NOT units/kg) PO twice daily.[5]

CATS:

Pansteatitis (extra-label): 10 – 15 units/kg PO once daily. **NOTE**: One study in 4 cats with pansteatitis showed good clinical response in 3 cats (one was lost to follow-up) after treatment with oral vitamin E 50 mg/kg once a day, in combination with prednisolone (2 mg/kg/day for 1 week and then every other day for an additional 1 to 2 weeks) and dietary changes.[11]

HORSES:

Vitamin E deficiency (extra-label): Natural-source water-dispersible forms of vitamin E (*Elevate W.S.*®) 10 units/kg PO (assume per day—*Plumb*) are 5 to 6 times more bioavailable than synthetic vitamin E acetate, and a 5000 units/horse (NOT units/kg) (*assume per day—Plumb*) more than doubles serum vitamin E levels within 12 hours. Foals should receive 5 – 6.6 units/kg/day PO using a liquid formulation. Before implementing supplementation, it is important to measure serum alpha-tocopherol concentrations to determine if there is an underlying deficiency and to monitor the efficacy of supplementation.[12-14] **NOTE**: Donkeys may have a lower selenium requirement than horses.[15]

Equine metabolic syndrome (extra-label): 1000 units/horse (NOT units/kg) PO daily added to diet[16]

Adjunctive treatment of neurologic disease (extra-label): There are many recommendations for using high levels of vitamin E supplementation for horses with neurologic disease, ranging from 1,500 – 23,000 units/500 kg (1102 lb) horse daily. The use of vitamin E for these conditions is empirically based on a belief that it could be neuroprotective in disorders not related to a deficiency of vitamin E. There appears to be no scientific evidence that supplementation with doses of vitamin E above the 2007 National Research Council (NRC) recommended dose will have a therapeutic effect in horses other than those associated with a vitamin E deficiency. Many of these dosage recommendations exceed the NRC upper safety recommendation of 20 units/kg (10,000 units/500 kg horse). Furthermore, many of these studies were performed before the development of natural forms of vitamin E in horses and these amounts might be excessive if natural vitamin E is used therapeutically.[17]

Monitoring

- Clinical efficacy
- Blood selenium concentrations (when using the combination product). Normal values for selenium have been reported as: more than 1.14 µmol/L in calves, more than 0.63 µmol/L in cattle, more than 1.26 µmol/L in sheep, and more than 0.6 µmol/L in pigs. Values indicating deficiency are: less than 0.40 µmol/L in cattle, less than 0.60 µmol/L in sheep, and less than 0.20 µmol/L in pigs. Intermediate values may result in suboptimal production.
- Optionally, glutathione peroxidase activity may be monitored.

Client Information

- Vitamin E is used to treat some skin, liver, and eye conditions and is safe when given as directed.
- Large overdoses can cause bleeding. Contact your veterinarian if your animal develops bleeding from the gums, low energy level, or blood in the urine or feces.
- If using the vitamin E and selenium injection, do not give more than your veterinarian recommends; selenium can be toxic if too much is given.

Chemistry/Synonyms

Vitamin E is a lipid-soluble vitamin that can be found in either liquid or solid forms. The liquid forms occur as clear, yellow to brownish red, viscous oils that are insoluble in water, soluble in alcohol, and miscible with vegetable oils. Solid forms occur as white to tan-white granular powders that disperse in water to form cloudy suspensions. Vitamin E may also be known as alpha tocopherol. In 2000, one unit of vitamin E was redefined to equal the biologic activity of 1 mg all racemic-alpha-tocopheryl acetate, or 0.91 mg (910 µg) all racemic-alpha-tocopheryl. Potencies expressed in International units or USP units are no longer current.

Selenium in commercially available veterinary injections is found as sodium selenite. Each mg of sodium selenite contains ≈460 µg (46%) of selenium.

Storage/Stability

Vitamin E/selenium for injection should be stored at temperatures less than 25°C (77°F); protect from freezing.

Compatibility/Compounding Considerations

No specific information noted.

Dosage Forms/Regulatory Status

VETERINARY-LABELED PRODUCTS:

Vitamin E Oral Liquid

Many products may be labeled for use in animals and as they are considered supplements and not drugs, they are not necessarily FDA-approved animal drugs. Some products with horse indications and dosages are: *Elevate*® *W.S* 500 units/mL and *Elevate*® *Maintenance Powder 1000 units/7 grams*; (OTC).

Vitamin E (Alone) Injection

Vitamin E Injection: 300 units/mL in 250 mL vials; *Emulsivit*® *E-300*; (Rx). For SC or IM administration.

Vitamin E Injection: 500 units/mL in 250 mL vials; *Vital E*®*-500*; (OTC). For SC or IM administration.

Vitamin E/Selenium Oral

Equ-SeE®: Each teaspoon (5 cc) contains ≈1 mg selenium and 220 units vitamin E; (OTC).

Other top dress equine products containing vitamin E and selenium include *Elevate*® *SE* (1500 units vitamin E plus 1 mg selenium per 7 grams); (OTC)

Vitamin E/Selenium Injection

Mu-Se®: Each mL contains: selenium 5 mg (as sodium selenite); vitamin E 68 units; 100 mL vial for injection. FDA-approved for use in weanling calves, nonlactating dairy cattle, and breeding beef cattle. (Rx) Slaughter withdrawal (at label dosages) = 30 days. Dose: For weanling calves: 1 mL/ 90.9 kg (200 lb) body weight IM or SC. For breeding beef cows: 1 mL/90.9 kg (200 lb) body weight during middle third of pregnancy and 30 days before calving IM or SC.

Bo-Se®: Each mL contains selenium 1 mg (as sodium selenite) and vitamin E 68 units; 100 mL vial for injection. FDA-approved for use in calves, swine, and sheep. (Rx) Slaughter withdrawal (at label dosages) = 30 days (calves); 14 days (lambs, ewes, sows, and pigs). Dose: Calves: 2.5 – 3.75 mL/45.5 kg (100 lb) body weight (depending on severity of condition and geographical area) IM or SC. Lambs (2 weeks of age or older): 1 mL/18.2 kg (40 lb) body weight IM or SC (1 mL minimum). Ewes: 2.5 mL/45.5 kg (100 lb) body weight IM or SC. Sows and weanling pigs: 1mL/18.2 kg (40 lb) body weight IM or SC (1 mL minimum). Do not use on newborn pigs.

E-Se®: Each mL contains selenium 2.5 mg (as sodium selenite) and vitamin E 68 units in 100 mL vials. FDA-approved for use in horses. (Rx) Equine dose: 1 mL/45.5 kg (100 lb) body weight slow IV or deep IM (in 2 or more sites; gluteal or cervical muscles). May be repeated at 5- to 10- day intervals.

Vitamin E for injection is also available in combination with vitamins A and D. Vitamin E may also a component of feed additives, milk replacers and topical products.

HUMAN-LABELED PRODUCTS:

Vitamin E Tablets: 100 units, 200 units, 400 units, generic; (OTC)

Vitamin E Capsules: 200 units, 400 units, and 1000 units; *Vita-Plus E®, Alph E®, Vita-Plus E®*, generic; (OTC)

Vitamin E Drops: 15 units/0.3 mL in 12 mL and 30 mL; *Aquasol E®*; (OTC)

Vitamin E Liquid: 400 units/15 mL in 30 and 60 mL; *Nutr-E-Sol®*; (OTC)

Topicals are available. There are no FDA-approved vitamin E/selenium products for humans, but there are many products that contain either vitamin E (alone or in combination with other vitamins ± minerals) or selenium (as an injection alone or in combination with other trace elements) available.

References

For the complete list of references, see **wiley.com/go/budde/plumb**

Voriconazole

(vor-ih-***koh***-nah-zohl) *Vfend®*

Second-Generation Triazole Antifungal

See also ***Voriconazole Ophthalmic***

Prescriber Highlights

- Broad-spectrum oral/parenteral triazole antifungal
- Cats appear to be susceptible to adverse effects. Until further pharmacokinetic and safety studies can be done, it should only be used in cats as a last resort.
- Like other compounds in this class, there are many potential drug interactions.
- The National Institute for Occupational Safety and Health (NIOSH) classifies voriconazole as a hazardous drug; use appropriate precautions when handling.

Uses/Indications

Voriconazole may be useful to treat a variety of fungal infections in veterinary patients, particularly against *Blastomyces* spp, *Cryptococcus* spp, *Coccidioides* spp,[1,2] and *Aspergillus* spp. It has high oral bioavailability in a variety of species and can cross into the CNS. There is limited clinical experience using voriconazole in veterinary patients. Because of adverse effects in cats, it is generally only recommended as a last resort. There is considerable interest in using voriconazole for treating aspergillosis in pet birds, as their relatively small size may make the drug more affordable; additional research must be performed before dosing regimens are available.

The drug may be used for horses with fungal keratomycosis.[3-5] See also ***Voriconazole Ophthalmic***.

Pharmacology/Actions

Voriconazole is a synthetic derivative of fluconazole, which has broad-spectrum antifungal activity against a variety of organisms, including *Candida* spp, *Aspergillus* spp, *Trichosporon* spp, *Histoplasma* spp, *Cryptococcus* spp, *Blastomyces* spp, and *Fusarium* spp. Like the other azole/triazole antifungals, it inhibits a fungal cytochrome P450-dependent demethylation enzyme that produces ergosterol in the cell membrane. The resultant intracellular accumulation of methylated sterols weakens the cellular membranes of susceptible fungi, increasing membrane permeability, allowing leakage of cellular contents, and impairing uptake of purine and pyrimidine precursors.

Unlike fluconazole, voriconazole also inhibits 24-methylene dehydrolanosterol demethylation in molds such as *Aspergillus* spp, giving it more activity against these fungi.

Pharmacokinetics

In dogs, voriconazole is rapidly and essentially completely absorbed after oral administration. Absorption is decreased when voriconazole is given with food but is not affected by drugs that raise gastric pH. Peak concentrations occur ≈3 hours after oral dosing. Voriconazole is only moderately (51%) bound to canine plasma proteins and the volume of distribution is ≈1.3 L/kg. Concentrations attained in CSF, aqueous humor, and synovial fluid are 43% to 53% that of plasma.[6] It is metabolized in the liver to a variety of metabolites with the N-oxide metabolite being the primary circulating metabolite. This metabolite has only weak antifungal activity (less than 100 times as active as the parent). The elimination pharmacokinetics of voriconazole in dogs is very complex. Both dose-dependent nonlinear elimination and auto-induced metabolism after multiple dosages are seen, complicating any dosage regimen; dosages may need to be increased over time. Autoinduction of metabolism apparently does not occur in humans, rabbits, or guinea pigs. Terminal half-life in one study was 3.3 hours.[6]

In fasted cats receiving single oral doses of 4 – 6 mg/kg, peak concentrations of 2.2 to 2.5 µg/mL occurred within 1.5 hours after administration. Volume of distribution was 1.7 to 2.1 L/kg. All 4 cats that received tablet formulations had trough voriconazole concentrations above 1 µg/mL for at least 72 hours after administration. Oral administration of a loading dose of 25 mg/cat (NOT mg/kg) followed by 12.5 mg/cat (NOT mg/kg) every other day caused voriconazole accumulation over the 2-week study period. Terminal half-life averaged 43 hours.[7]

In horses, voriconazole is well absorbed after oral administration with peak concentrations at ≈1 to 3 hours postdose. Voriconazole has low protein binding (31%); volume of distribution is ≈1.35 to 1.6 L/kg. The drug is distributed into the CSF, tears, and synovial fluid. Elimination half-life is ≈13 hours after oral dosing. Mean half-life in tear film is ≈25 hours. It is not known if voriconazole self-induces hepatic metabolism after multiple doses in a horse.[5,8,9]

After single oral doses to alpacas, voriconazole had a low bioavailability (≈24%), but IV doses of 4 mg/kg yielded plasma concentrations above 0.1 µg/mL for at least 24 hours. Elimination half-life was ≈8 hours.[10]

In Hispaniolan Amazon parrots, oral voriconazole had a short half-life (≈1 hour). The authors concluded that the drug could be safely administered to this species at a dose of 18 mg/kg PO every 8 hours for 11 days, but that further studies were necessary to determine safety and efficacy of long-term treatment.[11]

Contraindications/Precautions/Warnings

Voriconazole is contraindicated in patients that are hypersensitive to it or other azole antifungals, although evidence is lacking regarding cross-reactivity between voriconazole and other azole antifungal agents.

Voriconazole should be used with extreme caution in cats, as they appear to be prone to serious adverse effects. It should be given with caution to patients with hepatic dysfunction or proarrhythmic conditions. Electrolytes (eg, potassium, magnesium, calcium) should be corrected before starting voriconazole therapy. Infusion reactions are uncommon, but infusion should be stopped immediately if there is development of flushing, fever, sweating, tachycardia, dyspnea, nausea, or pruritis.

The voriconazole IV product contains 3200 mg of sulfobutyl ether beta-cyclodextrin sodium (SBECD) per vial; this compound can accumulate in patients with decreased renal function.

The National Institute for Occupational Safety and Health (NIOSH) classifies voriconazole as a hazardous drug; personal protective equipment (PPE) should be used accordingly to minimize the risk for exposure.[12]

Adverse Effects

Accurate adverse effect profiles are unknown for veterinary species. Liver enlargement and up to a 2- to 3-fold increase in cytochrome P450 hepatic microsomal enzyme concentrations were noted in dogs orally dosed for 30 days. This may significantly impact the metabolism of other drugs that are hepatically metabolized (see ***Drug Interactions***). Mild to moderate adverse GI effects have been noted in dogs receiving oral voriconazole.[6] A dog treated with an IV infusion of voriconazole developed significant pyrexia and tachypnea after the infusion.[13] In dogs, high serum voriconazole concentration was associated with a reversible neurotoxicosis and increased liver enzymes.[14]

Cats appear to be susceptible to developing adverse effects from voriconazole. Two cats initially treated with 10 mg/kg PO once daily developed significant adverse reactions, including azotemia, inappetence, lethargy, and weight loss.[15] One developed a presumed cutaneous drug reaction, which resolved when voriconazole was discontinued, and the other cat developed ataxia and hind limb paresis. In another published case report, 3 cats receiving voriconazole at doses of 10 – 13 mg/kg PO once daily developed neurologic signs that included ataxia in all subjects, 2 of the 3 cats developed paraplegia, and 2 of the 3 cats had ophthalmic signs (eg, mydriasis, decreased or absent pupillary light responses, reduced menace response).[16] One cat developed an arrhythmia and in another, hypokalemia was noted. In a pharmacokinetic study, severe miosis and ptyalism were noted in cats receiving voriconazole tablets and suspension; ptyalism caused by voriconazole suspension prevented drug absorption in one cat.[7]

In humans, commonly encountered adverse effects include visual disturbances (eg, blurring, spots, wavy lines) usually within 30 minutes of dosing or if higher drug concentrations are attained, and rashes (usually mild to moderate in severity). Less frequent adverse effects include GI effects (eg, nausea, vomiting, diarrhea), hepatotoxicity (eg, jaundice, abnormal liver function tests), hypertension/hypotension, tachycardia, peripheral edema, hypokalemia, and hypomagnesemia. Rarely, eye hemorrhage, exfoliative dermal reactions, anemia, leukopenia, thrombocytopenia, pancytopenia, QT prolongation, torsade de pointes, and nephrotoxicity have been reported. Hallucinations have also been reported.[17]

Reproductive/Nursing Safety

Voriconazole was teratogenic in rats at low doses (10 mg/kg) and embryotoxic in rabbits at higher doses (100 mg/kg).[18] In humans, voriconazole has a high risk for major birth defects and miscarriage. It is unknown if voriconazole enters milk. Because safety has not been established in animals, this drug should only be used when the maternal benefits outweigh the potential risks to offspring.

Overdose/Acute Toxicity

The minimum lethal dose in rats and mice was 300 mg/kg (4 to 7 times maintenance dose). Toxic effects included increased salivation, mydriasis, ataxia, depression, dyspnea, and seizures. Accidental single overdoses of up to 5 times the recommended dose in human pediatric patients caused only brief photophobia. No antidote is known for voriconazole overdoses. GI decontamination should be considered for large oral overdoses, followed by close observation and supportive treatment if required. Hemodialysis may assist in the removal of voriconazole and the sulfobutyl ether beta-cyclodextrin sodium (SBECD) vehicle.

For patients that have experienced or are suspected to have experienced an overdose, consultation with a 24-hour poison consultation center specializing in providing veterinary-specific information is recommended. For general information related to overdose and toxin exposures, as well as contact information for poison control centers, refer to ***Appendix.***

Drug Interactions

There are many potential drug interactions involving voriconazole. Voriconazole is a substrate of CYP450 2C and inhibitor of CYP450 3A isoenzymes. The following partial listing includes reported or theoretical interactions in humans receiving voriconazole that may also be of significance in veterinary patients. Because, in dogs, voriconazole induces hepatic microsomal enzymes (in humans it does not), additional interactions and further clarification may be reported, as clinical use increases in veterinary patients. Unless otherwise noted, use together is not necessarily contraindicated, but weigh the potential risks and perform additional monitoring when appropriate.

- **Amiodarone**: Potential for serious cardiac arrhythmias such as torsade de pointes; concurrent use is contraindicated in humans
- **Benzodiazepines** (eg, **alprazolam, midazolam**): Voriconazole may increase benzodiazepine concentrations.
- **Bromocriptine**: Voriconazole may increase serum concentrations of bromocriptine.
- **Buspirone**: Voriconazole may increase serum concentrations of buspirone.
- **Calcium Channel Blockers** (eg, **amlodipine, diltiazem, verapamil**): Voriconazole may increase serum concentrations; dosage adjustment may be required.
- **Cisapride**: Voriconazole may increase serum concentrations of cisapride and increase risk for serious cardiac arrhythmias; use is contraindicated.
- **Corticosteroids** (eg, **prednisolone**): Potentially increased AUC for prednisolone
- **Cyclosporine**: Increased cyclosporine concentrations; 50% reduction in cyclosporine dose recommended
- **Doxorubicin**: Voriconazole may increase serum concentrations of doxorubicin; concurrent use is contraindication in humans.
- **Fentanyl, Alfentanil**: Voriconazole may increase plasma concentrations; monitor for toxicity and adjust dosage if necessary.
- **Glipizide, Glyburide**: Voriconazole may increase serum concentrations of these drugs and increase risk for hypoglycemia.
- **Methadone**: Voriconazole may increase plasma concentrations of R-methadone; monitor for methadone toxicity and adjust dosage if necessary.
- **Phenobarbital**: May decrease voriconazole concentrations resulting in therapeutic failure; use together is contraindicated.
- **Procainamide**: Potential for serious cardiac arrhythmias such as torsade de pointes
- **Proton Pump Inhibitors** (**PPIs**; eg, **omeprazole**): Voriconazole may increase omeprazole (and potentially other PPIs) concentrations.
- **Quinidine**: Potential for serious cardiac arrhythmias such as torsade de pointes; concurrent use is contraindicated in humans.
- **Rifampin**: Decreased voriconazole concentrations; use together contraindicated

- **Sildenafil**: Voriconazole may increase plasma concentrations; monitor for toxicity and adjust dosage if necessary.
- **Sotalol**: Potential for serious cardiac arrhythmias such as torsade de pointes
- **Vinca Alkaloids** (eg, **vinblastine, vincristine**): Possible increased Vinca alkaloid concentrations; monitor for toxicity.
- **Warfarin**: Voriconazole may potentiate warfarin's effects.

Laboratory Considerations

- No specific concerns were noted; see ***Monitoring*** for additional information.

Dosages

DOGS:

NOTE: In dogs, voriconazole may induce its own metabolism (see ***Pharmacokinetics***); dosages may need to be increased over time.

Coccidioidomycosis (extra-label): 4 mg/kg PO every 12 hours[1]

Systemic aspergillosis (extra-label): 4 – 5 mg/kg PO every 12 hours[19]

Sinonasal aspergillosis postsurgical debridement of fungal plaques (extra-label): From a case series ($n = 3$), 2.5 – 3.3 mg/kg PO every 12 hours[14]

CATS:

Aspergillosis (extra-label): From a pharmacokinetic study, a loading dose of 25 mg/cat (NOT mg/kg) PO, followed by 12.5 mg/cat (NOT mg/kg) every 72 hours.[7] **NOTE**: Case reports have documented significant toxicity at 10 mg/kg PO daily.[15,16]

HORSES:

Susceptible, systemic fungal infections (extra-label): Based on pharmacokinetic studies, 3 – 4 mg/kg PO once daily or 3 mg/kg PO twice daily should be sufficient to treat aspergillosis, but higher doses (4 – 5 mg/kg PO once daily) are probably necessary to treat infections with *Fusarium* spp.[8,9,20]

Guttural pouch mycosis (extra-label): 3 mg/kg PO every 12 hours; used in combination with topical 1% enilconazole[21]

Keratomycosis (extra-label): Based on a pharmacokinetic study, 4 mg/kg PO once daily is expected to achieve voriconazole concentration in tear fluid at the AUC:MIC ratio associated with treatment efficacy against *Aspergillus* spp.[5]

BIRDS:

Susceptible, systemic fungal infections (extra-label): Based on a pharmacokinetic study in Hispaniolan Amazon parrots, the authors concluded that the drug could be safely administered to this species at a dose of 18 mg/kg PO every 8 hours for 11 days, but that further studies were necessary to determine safety and efficacy of long-term treatment. [11]

Avian aspergillosis: 12.5 mg/kg PO twice daily for 60 to 90 days or by nebulization as a 1 mg/mL solution for 60 minutes once daily.[22] In a pharmacokinetic study involving racing pigeons, a suggested dosage is 10 mg/kg PO twice daily or 20 mg/kg PO once daily.[23]

REPTILES:

Susceptible, systemic fungal infections (extra-label):

a) **Red-eared sliders**: Based on pharmacokinetic study, 5 mg/kg SC[24]

b) **Chrysosporium anamorph of *Nannizziopsis vriesii* (CANV) in bearded dragons**: 10 mg/kg PO every 24 hours for 4 to 9 weeks[24]

Monitoring

- Efficacy
- Adverse effects
- Baseline and periodic serum liver chemistry panel and electrolytes
- Voriconazole plasma concentration (target range 1 to 4 µg/mL)[25]

Client Information

- Give this medicine to your animal at least 1 hour before or 1 hour after feeding.
- Report any possible side effects to your veterinarian immediately, including itching/rash; yellowing of the whites of the eyes, gums, or skin; reduced appetite; difficulty walking; vision problems.
- This medication is considered to be a hazardous drug as defined by the National Institute for Occupational Safety and Health (NIOSH). Talk with your veterinarian or pharmacist about the use of personal protective equipment when handling this medicine especially if you are pregnant or trying to conceive.

Chemistry/Synonyms

A triazole antifungal, voriconazole occurs as a white to light-colored powder with a molecular weight of 349.3. Aqueous solubility is 0.7 mg/mL.

Voriconazole may also be known as UK-109496, voriconazol, voraconazolum, or *Vfend*®.

Storage/Stability

Voriconazole tablets should be stored at 15°C to 30°C (59°F-86°F).

The unreconstituted powder for oral suspension should be stored in the refrigerator (2°C-8°C [36°F-46°F]). Once reconstituted, it should be stored in tightly closed containers at room temperature (15°C-30°C [59°F-86°F]); do not refrigerate or freeze. After reconstitution, the suspension is stable for 14 days. The suspension should be shaken well for 10 seconds prior to each administered dose.

The powder for injection should be stored at room temperature (15°C-30°C [59°F-86°F). After reconstituting with 19 mL of sterile water for injection, the manufacturer recommends using immediately; however, chemical and physical stability remain for up to 24 hours if stored in the refrigerator (2°C-8°C [36°F-46°F]). Discard solution if it is not clear or if particles are visible.

Compatibility/Compounding Considerations

Compatibility is dependent on factors such as pH, concentration, temperature, and diluent used; specialized references or a hospital pharmacist should be consulted for more specific information.

The injectable solution must be further diluted to a concentration of 5 mg/mL or less for administration over 1 to 2 hours. Suitable diluents for IV infusion include (partial list): 0.9% sodium chloride, lactated Ringer's solution, 5% dextrose in lactated Ringer's solution, and 5% dextrose. Voriconazole is **not compatible** with simultaneous infusion with blood products or concentrated electrolyte solutions.

Voriconazole tablets can be crushed and made into a 2.5 mg/mL oral suspension by mixing a crushed 200 mg tablet with 20 mL water, then adding 60 mL *OraPlus*®. Thoroughly mix the suspension (eg, shaken, vortex mixed) until no particles are visible. Suspension should also be shaken for ≈30 to 60 seconds prior to each use. The suspension will remain stable for 14 days if kept under refrigeration.[11,26] A voriconazole 40 mg/mL suspension can also be compounded using 200 mg tablets and a vehicle comprised of a commercial suspending agent and either water (3:1 v/v) or sweetening (1:1 v/v) agents. To prepare, thoroughly mix a crushed 200 mg tablet with 5 mL of vehicle. The resultant suspension is stable for up to 30 days at room temperature or refrigerated.[27]

Dosage Forms/Regulatory Status

VETERINARY-LABELED PRODUCTS: NONE

HUMAN-LABELED PRODUCTS:

Voriconazole Tablets: 50 mg and 200 mg; *Vfend*®, generic; (Rx)

Voriconazole Powder for Oral Suspension: 45 g (40 mg/mL after reconstitution) in 75 mL bottles; *Vfend*®, generic; (Rx)

Voriconazole Powder for Injection, Lyophilized: 200 mg in single-use vials; *Vfend I.V.*®, generic; (Rx). Also contains sulfobutyl ether beta-cyclodextrin sodium (SBECD, a solubilizing agent) 3200 mg/vial. See ***Contraindications/Precautions/Warnings.***

References

For the complete list of references, see **wiley.com/go/budde/plumb**

Warfarin

(***war***-far-in) *Coumadin*®

Anticoagulant

Prescriber Highlights

- ► Coumarin derivative anticoagulant uncommonly used for long-term thromboprophylaxis, primarily in dogs. Requires careful monitoring and dosage adjustment
- ► Use in cats is not recommended.
- ► Full anticoagulant effect requires several days to be achieved; may need additional anticoagulant (eg, heparin) during this time.
- ► Contraindications include pre-existent hemorrhage; pregnancy; patients undergoing or contemplating eye or CNS surgery, major regional lumbar block anesthesia, or surgery of large, open surfaces; active bleeding from the GI, respiratory, or GU tract; aneurysm; acute nephritis; cerebrovascular hemorrhage; blood dyscrasias; uncontrolled or malignant hypertension; hepatic insufficiency; pericardial effusion; and visceral carcinomas.
- ► Adverse effects include dose-related hemorrhage; death is possible.
- ► Many potentially significant drug interactions
- ► Teratogenic. The National Institute for Occupational Safety and Health (NIOSH) classifies warfarin as a hazardous drug; use appropriate precautions when handling.

Uses/Indications

In veterinary medicine, warfarin has been used for the oral, long-term treatment (or prevention of recurrence) of thrombotic conditions, primarily in dogs. Use of warfarin in veterinary species is controversial due to unproven benefit in reducing mortality, increased expense associated with monitoring, and potential for serious effects (bleeding); many clinicians do not recommend its use.[1]

Pharmacology/Actions

Warfarin inhibits vitamin K epoxide reductase (VKORC1), which interferes with the action of vitamin K_1 in the synthesis of the coagulation factors II, VII, IX, and X, as well as the anticoagulant proteins C and S. Warfarin acts indirectly as an anticoagulant (it has no direct anticoagulant effect) to prevent the extension of an existing thrombus and reduce formation of new clots. Sufficient amounts of vitamin K_1 can override this effect. Depletion of existing clotting factors occurs gradually over the first several days of treatment, and additional anticoagulant therapy (eg, heparin) may be required. Warfarin is administered as a racemic mixture of S (+) and R (-) warfarin. The S (+) enantiomer is a significantly more potent vitamin K antagonist than the R (-) enantiomer in species studied.

Pharmacokinetics

Warfarin is rapidly and completely absorbed in humans after oral administration. In cats, warfarin is also rapidly absorbed after oral administration.

After absorption, warfarin is ≈99% bound to plasma proteins in humans. Only free (unbound) warfarin is active. It is reported that there are wide species variations with regard to protein binding; in cats, greater than 96% of the drug is protein bound, and horses have a higher free (unbound) fraction of the drug than do sheep, swine, or rats. Although other coumarin and indanedione anticoagulants are distributed in human milk, warfarin does not enter milk.

Warfarin is principally metabolized in the liver to inactive metabolites that are excreted in urine and bile (and then reabsorbed and excreted in the urine). The plasma half-life of warfarin may be several hours to several days depending on the patient (and possibly species). In cats, the terminal half-life of the S enantiomer is ≈23 to 28 hours and the terminal half-life of R enantiomer is ≈11 to 18 hours.

Contraindications/Precautions/Warnings

Warfarin is contraindicated in patients with pre-existent hemorrhagic tendencies or diseases, as well as patients undergoing or contemplating eye or CNS surgery, major regional lumbar block anesthesia, or surgery of large, open surfaces. It should not be used in patients with active bleeding from the GI, respiratory, or GU tract. Other contraindications include aneurysm, acute nephritis, cerebrovascular hemorrhage, blood dyscrasias, uncontrolled or malignant hypertension, hepatic insufficiency, pericardial effusion, pregnancy, and visceral carcinomas. Warfarin should not be used in patients with heparin-induced thrombocytopenia until platelet counts have stabilized. Anticoagulated patients have experienced hematomas after spinal or epidural anesthesia. Clients must be willing to comply with the frequency and expense of routine monitoring.

Use warfarin with extreme caution in cats. Most clinicians no longer recommend use of warfarin in cats due to an increased mortality rate and a high rate of significant adverse events, including fatal hemorrhage.[1]

Excessive anticoagulation can be managed by withholding one to several doses, with or without administration of vitamin K and/or blood products, with a subsequent dose reduction. Presurgical management may require withholding warfarin for up to several days prior to surgery and use of alternative anticoagulants (eg, heparin), although warfarin may continue uninterrupted if the surgical bleeding risk is low.

The National Institute for Occupational Safety and Health (NIOSH) classifies warfarin as a hazardous drug[2]; personal protective equipment (PPE) should be used accordingly to minimize the risk for exposure.

Adverse Effects

The principal adverse effect of warfarin use is dose-related hemorrhage, which may manifest with clinical signs of anemia, thrombocytopenia, weakness, hematomas and ecchymoses, epistaxis, hematemesis, hematuria, melena, hematochezia, hemarthrosis, hemothorax, intracranial and/or pericardial hemorrhage, and death. In humans, skin necrosis, calciphylaxis, and cholesterol microemboli have been reported.

Reproductive/Nursing Safety

Warfarin is embryotoxic, can cause congenital malformations, and is considered contraindicated during pregnancy. If anticoagulant therapy is required during pregnancy, most clinicians recommend using unfractionated or low-molecular weight heparin.

Based on limited published data, warfarin has not been detected in the breast milk of humans treated and is generally considered safe to use in nursing patients, but the nursing infant should be monitored for bruising or bleeding.

Overdose/Acute Toxicity

Acute overdoses of warfarin may result in life-threatening hemorrhage. In dogs and cats, single doses of 5 – 50 mg/kg have been associated with toxicity. It must be remembered that a lag time of 2 to 5 days may occur before signs of toxicity occur, and animals must be monitored and treated accordingly. Cumulative toxic doses of warfarin have been reported as 1 – 5 mg/kg for 5 to 15 days in dogs and 1 mg/kg for 7 days in cats. Common clinical signs associated with overdose may include anorexia, hematuria, lethargy, and vomiting.

If overdose is detected early, prevent absorption from the gut using standard protocols. If clinical signs are noted, they should be treated with blood products and vitamin K_1 (phytonadione). Refer to ***Phytonadione (Vitamin K_1)*** monograph for more information.

For patients that have experienced or are suspected of having experienced an overdose, it is strongly encouraged to consult with one of the 24-hour poison consultation centers that specialize in providing information specific for veterinary patients. For general information related to overdose and toxin exposures, as well as contact information for poison control centers, refer to ***Appendix***.

Drug Interactions

Drug interactions with warfarin are perhaps the most important in human medicine. Warfarin is metabolized principally by CYP2C9, but also by many other CYP enzymes. The following drug interactions have either been reported or are theoretical in humans or animals receiving warfarin and may be of significance in veterinary patients. Unless otherwise noted, use together is not necessarily contraindicated, but weigh the potential risks and perform additional monitoring when appropriate.

A multitude of drugs have been documented or theorized to interact with warfarin. The following drugs or drug classes may **increase the anticoagulant response** of warfarin (not necessarily a complete list):

- Acetaminophen
- Allopurinol
- Amiodarone
- Anabolic Steroids (eg, **boldenone**)
- Azole Antifungals (eg, **fluconazole, itraconazole, voriconazole**)
- Cephalosporins (eg, **cefazolin, cefpodoxime, cephalexin**)
- Chloramphenicol
- Cisapride
- Clopidogrel
- Danazol
- Fatty Acids, Omega-3
- Fluoroquinolones (eg, **enrofloxacin**)
- Glucosamine
- Heparins (unfractionated and low molecular weight heparins)
- Lactulose
- Macrolide Antibiotics (eg, **azithromycin, clarithromycin, erythromycin**)
- Metronidazole
- Mirtazapine
- Neomycin
- Nonsteroidal Anti-Inflammatory Drugs (NSAIDs; eg, **carprofen, meloxicam, phenylbutazone**)
- Penicillins (eg, **amoxicillin, dicloxacillin, penicillin G, piperacillin**)
- Pentoxifylline
- Proton Pump Inhibitors (PPIs; eg, **omeprazole, pantoprazole**)
- Quinidine
- Salicylates (eg, **aspirin**[3])
- Selective Serotonin Reuptake Inhibitors (SSRIs; eg, **fluoxetine, sertraline**)
- Sulfonamides (including combinations with ormetoprim and trimethoprim)
- Thyroid Medications
- Tramadol
- Vitamin E

The following drugs or drug classes may **decrease the anticoagulant response** of warfarin (not necessarily a complete list):

- Barbiturates (eg, **phenobarbital**)
- Corticosteroids (eg, **dexamethasone**)
- Cyclosporine: Additionally, warfarin may reduce cyclosporine efficacy.
- Estrogens
- Griseofulvin
- Mercaptopurine
- Rifampin
- Phenobarbital
- Spironolactone
- Sucralfate
- Vitamin K

Should concurrent use of any of the above drugs with warfarin be necessary, enhanced monitoring is required.

Laboratory Considerations

- Warfarin may cause falsely decreased **theophylline values** if using the Schack and Waxler ultraviolet method of assay.

Dosages

NOTE: Warfarin is not recommended as an anticoagulant due to an inconsistent anticoagulant effect, the need for close monitoring, and the risk for significant adverse effects including death due to hemorrhage.[1]

DOGS:

Anticoagulant (extra-label):

a) Initial dose of 0.05 – 0.2 mg/kg PO once daily, with dosage adjusted (see ***Monitoring***) to achieve an INR of 2 to 3. The 2 most important principles in adjusting the warfarin dose were to make adjustments to the total weekly dose rather than the total daily dose, and to keep the dose adjustments small (10% to 15% of the total weekly dose).[4-7]

b) Initial (loading) dose of 0.2 mg/kg PO once daily for 2 days, followed by 0.1 mg/kg PO once daily has been suggested.[8]

HORSES:

Anticoagulant (extra-label): Rarely recommended. Anecdotally, for adjunctive treatment of laminitis, 0.0198 mg/kg PO once daily; monitor prothrombin time until prolonged 2 to 4 seconds beyond baseline.[9]

Monitoring

NOTE: The frequency of monitoring is controversial, and dependent on several factors including dose, the patient's condition, and concomitant problems.

- Although prothrombin times (PT) or international normalized ratio (INR; not validated for veterinary patients[1]) are most commonly used to monitor warfarin, proteins induced by vitamin K antagonists (PIVKA) have been suggested as being more sensitive. Prothrombin times during treatment with warfarin are usually recommended to be 1.5 to 2 times normal and INRs to be between 2 and 3.[5,6,10,11] A retrospective study in dogs used INR to adjust dosage. In that study, some dogs required weekly or biweekly dose adjustments based on the INR value for the first 2 to 4 weeks. Based on concurrent disease processes or concomitant drug therapy, it is recommended that dogs have an INR value checked at least every 3 months with chronic treatment.[4]
- Platelet counts and packed cell volume (PCV) should be done periodically.
- Monitor for bleeding, including feces and urine
- Clinical efficacy

Client Information

- Other medications and foods can interact with warfarin and can either increase the risk for bleeding or reduce warfarin's anticoagulant effects. Talk with your veterinarian before changing diets or starting a new medicine (including those sold over the counter and supplements) or stopping medications that your animal is currently taking.
- Do not allow your animal to be in situations where it could be injured or cut, as serious bleeding may occur. If abnormal bleeding is seen, contact your veterinarian immediately.
- To assure the dose is correct, routine blood tests will be needed. Do not miss these important follow-up visits.
- If a dose is missed, it should be taken as soon as possible on the same day. Do not double up doses the next day.

Chemistry/Synonyms

A coumarin derivative, warfarin sodium occurs as a slightly bitter tasting, odorless, white, amorphous or crystalline powder that discolors in light. It is very soluble in water and freely soluble in alcohol. The commercially available products contain a racemic mixture of the two optical isomers.

Warfarin sodium may also be known as sodium warfarin, warfarinum natricum, *Coumadin®, Jantoven®, or Panwarfin®*; there are many other trade names internationally.

Storage/Stability

Warfarin sodium tablets should be stored in tight, light-resistant containers at room temperature 20°C to 25°C (68°F-77°F).

Compatibility/Compounding Considerations

Compatibility is dependent on factors such as pH, concentration, temperature, and diluent used; specialized references or a hospital pharmacist should be consulted for more specific information.

Dosage Forms/Regulatory Status

VETERINARY-LABELED PRODUCTS: NONE

The Association of Racing Commissioners International (ARCI) has designated this drug as a class 5 substance. Use of this drug may not be allowed in certain animal competitions. Check rules and regulations before entering in a competition while this medication is being administered. Contact local racing authorities for further guidance. See ***Appendix*** for more information.

HUMAN-LABELED PRODUCTS:

Warfarin Sodium Oral Tablets (scored): 1 mg, 2 mg, 2.5 mg, 3 mg, 4 mg, 5 mg, 6 mg, 7.5 mg, and 10 mg; *Coumadin®, Jantoven®*, generic; (Rx)

References

For the complete list of references, see **wiley.com/go/budde/plumb**

Xylazine

(***zye***-la-zeen) *Rompun®, AnaSed®*

Alpha-2-Adrenergic Agonist

Prescriber Highlights

- Used as a sedative and analgesic agent in a variety of species; used as an emetic in cats
- Contraindicated in animals receiving epinephrine or having active ventricular arrhythmias. Do **not** give to animals that are exhausted, dehydrated, or with urinary tract obstruction. Avoid intra-arterial injection as it may cause severe seizures and collapse.
- Use with extreme caution in patients that have pre-existing cardiac dysfunction, hypotension or shock, respiratory dysfunction, severe hepatic or renal insufficiency, pre-existing seizure disorders, or if severely debilitated. Xylazine should generally not be used in the last trimester of pregnancy, particularly in cattle. Horses may kick after a stimulatory event (usually auditory); use caution.
- Use xylazine with caution in patients treated for intestinal impactions and in horses during the vasoconstrictive development phase of laminitis.
- Adverse effects in dogs include muscle tremors, bradycardia with partial atrioventricular (AV) block, reduced respiratory rate, movement in response to sharp auditory stimuli, emesis, and bloat from aerophagia, which may require decompression.
- Adverse effects in cats include emesis, muscle tremors, bradycardia with partial AV block, reduced respiratory rate, movement in response to sharp auditory stimuli, increased urination.
- Adverse effects in horses include muscle tremors, bradycardia with partial AV block, reduced respiratory rate, movement in response to sharp auditory stimuli, sweating, increased intracranial pressure, decreased GI motility, and decreased mucociliary clearance.
- Adverse effects in cattle include salivation, ruminal atony, bloating, regurgitation, hypothermia, diarrhea, bradycardia, premature parturition, and ataxia.
- Yohimbine, tolazoline, and atipamezole may be used alone or in combination to reverse effects or speed recovery times.
- Dosages between species can be very different; be certain of product concentration when preparing doses, especially if treating ruminants.

Uses/Indications

Xylazine is FDA-approved for use in dogs, cats, horses, deer, and elk to produce a state of sedation with a shorter period of analgesia and as a preanesthetic agent before local anesthesia. It is also approved as a preanesthetic agent before general anesthesia in dogs, cats, and horses. In horses, xylazine is often used in combination with other agents (eg, opioids, ketamine, guaifenesin) to induce anesthesia or perioperative sedation and analgesia.[1]

Xylazine use in small animal species is somewhat controversial. It is usually reserved for healthy animals because it can cause arrhythmias, reduce cardiac output, and increase the risk for general anesthesia-related death. Newer alpha-2 agonists (eg, dexmedetomidine) are preferred over xylazine, as they have fewer adverse effects in dogs and cats.

In cats, xylazine causes emesis and can be used to induce vomiting after toxin ingestion or drug overdoses.[2-4]

Pharmacology/Actions

Xylazine, a potent alpha-2-adrenergic agonist, is classified as a sedative/analgesic agent with muscle relaxant properties. Xylazine possesses several of the same pharmacologic actions as morphine. However, it does not cause CNS excitation in cats, horses, or cattle but causes sedation and CNS depression. In horses, the visceral analgesia produced has been demonstrated to be superior to that produced by meperidine, butorphanol, or pentazocine.[5]

Xylazine can also have alpha-1 agonist activity and is less selective for alpha-2 receptors than detomidine, romifidine, or dexmedetomidine. The alpha-2: alpha-1 receptor selectivity of xylazine is 160:1 (detomidine = 260:1, romifidine = 340:1, medetomidine and dexmedetomidine = 1620:1).

Emesis is often seen in cats and occasionally in dogs receiving xylazine. Although it is thought to be centrally mediated, neither dopaminergic blockers (eg, phenothiazines) nor alpha-blockers (eg, yohimbine, tolazoline) block the emetic effect. Xylazine does not cause emesis in cattle, sheep, or goats. Xylazine depresses thermoregulatory mechanisms and either hypo- or hyperthermia is a possibility, depending on ambient air temperatures.

Effects on the cardiopulmonary system include an initial increase in peripheral vascular resistance with increased blood pressure followed by a longer period of lowered blood pressures (below baseline). An initial reflex bradycardia may occur in response to alpha-1-mediated vasoconstriction and can be seen with some animals developing a second-degree atrioventricular (AV) block or other arrhythmias. An overall decrease in cardiac output of up to 30% may be seen. Xylazine, with or without concurrent halothane, has been demonstrated to enhance the arrhythmogenic effects of epinephrine in dogs.

Xylazine's effects on respiratory function are usually clinically insignificant; however, at high doses, xylazine can cause respiratory depression with decreased tidal volumes and respiratory rates and an overall decreased minute volume. Xylazine causes skeletal muscle relaxation through inhibition of centrally mediated pathways, which may result in dyspnea in brachycephalic dogs and horses with upper airway disease.

Xylazine can increase blood glucose secondary to decreased pancreatic secretion of insulin. In nondiabetic animals, there appears to be little clinical significance associated with this effect, although an osmotic diuresis may result from transient hyperglycemia, and polyuria may occur due to decreased production of vasopressin (antidiuretic hormone [ADH]).

In dogs, clinical doses decrease tear production in a dose-related manner[6] but do not affect intraocular pressure and pupil size.[7]

In horses, signs of sedation include a lowering of the head with relaxed facial muscles and drooping of the lower lip. The retractor muscle is relaxed in male horses, but unlike with acepromazine, there are no reports of permanent penile paralysis. Although the animal may appear to be thoroughly sedated, auditory stimuli may provoke arousal with kicking and avoidance responses.

Differences are seen with regard to the sensitivity of species to xylazine. Domestic ruminants are extremely sensitive to xylazine when compared with dogs, cats, or horses, and they generally require ≈10% of the dose that is required for horses to exhibit the same effect. Pigs are less sensitive and require higher doses (≈20 times compared with the ruminant's dose). Xylazine, in combination with ketamine or tiletamine/zolazepam, is commonly used in swine for chemical restraint.

Pharmacokinetics

Absorption is rapid following IM injection, but the bioavailability is incomplete and variable. Bioavailability ranges of 40% to 48% in horses, 17% to 73% in sheep, and 52% to 90% in dogs have been reported after IM administration.

In dogs and cats, the onset of action following an IM or SC dose is ≈10 to 15 minutes and 3 to 5 minutes following an IV dose. The analgesic effects may persist for only 15 to 30 minutes, but the sedative actions may last for 1 to 2 hours, depending on the dose given. The serum half-life of xylazine in dogs has been reported as averaging 30 minutes. Complete recovery after dosing may take 2 to 4 hours in dogs and cats.

In horses, the onset of action following IV administration occurs within 1 to 2 minutes, with a maximum effect observed 3 to 10 minutes after injection. The duration of effect is dose dependent but may last for ≈1.5 hours. After a single dose of xylazine, the serum half-life is ≈50 minutes in a horse. Recovery times generally take from 2 to 3 hours. Intraosseous xylazine administration resulted in no significant differences in pharmacokinetic parameters or physiologic response as compared to IV administration.[8] Intra-articular administration resulted in systemic drug absorption (bioavailability = 58%) and occurrence of systemic effects.[9]

Contraindications/Precautions/Warnings

Do not give xylazine to animals that are dehydrated, debilitated, or with urinary tract obstruction. Xylazine is contraindicated in animals receiving epinephrine or having active ventricular arrhythmias. It should be used with extreme caution in animals with pre-existing cardiac dysfunction, hypotension or shock, respiratory dysfunction, severe hepatic or renal insufficiency, or pre-existing seizure disorders.

Do not confuse IV and IM dosages. Avoid intracarotid injection as it may cause severe seizures and collapse. Be certain of product concentration when drawing up into the syringe, especially if treating ruminants, as ruminants are extremely sensitive to the sedative effects of alpha-2 agonists.

Large animal species, including horses, may become ataxic following dosing, and caution should be observed. Use with caution in horses after xylazine administration, as they have been known to kick after a stimulatory event (usually auditory) even when horses to be appear sedated. The addition of opioids (eg, butorphanol) may help temper this effect. Because xylazine may inhibit GI motility, use it with caution in patients treated for intestinal impactions. Use cautiously in horses during the development of the vasoconstrictive phase of laminitis, as xylazine has been shown to reduce digital flow of blood for about 8 hours after administration.

Adverse Effects

Emesis is generally seen within 3 to 5 minutes after xylazine administration in cats and occasionally in dogs. To prevent aspiration, do not induce further anesthesia until this time has lapsed. Other adverse effects noted in dogs and cats after xylazine administration include muscle tremors, bradycardia with second-degree atrioventricular (AV) block, reduced respiratory rate, movement in response to sharp auditory stimuli, and increased urination.

Xylazine can reduce tear production and cause diuresis in dogs and cats.[6,10]

Adverse effects for horses include muscle tremors, bradycardia with second-degree AV block, reduced respiratory rate, movement in response to sharp auditory stimuli, and sweating (rarely profuse).[11] Additionally, horses receiving xylazine may develop transient hypertension, increased urine production, decreased gastric emptying, decreased motility of duodenum, jejunum and pelvic flexure, increased intrauterine pressure/contractions, and reduced mucociliary clearance rates. Ataxia occurs in a dose-dependent fashion.[12]

In cattle, adverse reactions associated with xylazine include salivation, ruminal atony, bloating and regurgitation, hypothermia, diarrhea, and bradycardia.

Reproductive/Nursing Safety

Limited information was located on the safety of xylazine in pregnancy. No reports of teratogenicity in animals were located.

Xylazine can have an oxytocin-like effect on the uterus of pregnant cattle and may induce premature parturition. Because it may induce premature parturition, it should generally not be used in the last trimester of pregnancy, particularly in cattle. For horses, one review concludes "...alpha-2 agonists are safe in pregnant animals, but close monitoring is advised."[13] Reduced fetal survival rates have been noted when xylazine is used as a premedication for cesarean deliveries.[14]

Xylazine does not appear to be excreted in detectable quantities in cows' milk.

Because safety has not been established in animals, this drug should only be used when the maternal benefits outweigh the potential risks to offspring.

Overdose/Acute Toxicity

In the event of an accidental overdose, emesis, cardiac arrhythmias, hypotension, and profound CNS and respiratory depression may occur. Seizures have also been reported after overdoses. There has been much interest in using alpha-blocking agents as antidotes or reversal agents to xylazine. Yohimbine, atipamezole, and tolazoline have been suggested to be used alone and in combination to reverse the effects of xylazine or speed recovery times. See ***Yohimbine, Tolazoline,*** and ***Atipamezole*** for more information.

For patients that have experienced or are suspected to have experienced an overdose, consultation with a 24-hour poison consultation center specializing in providing veterinary-specific information is recommended. For general information related to overdose and toxin exposures, as well as contact information for poison control centers, refer to ***Appendix.***

Drug Interactions

The following drug interactions have either been reported or are theoretical in humans or animals receiving xylazine and may be of significance in veterinary patients. Unless otherwise noted, use together is not necessarily contraindicated, but weigh the potential risks and perform additional monitoring when appropriate.

- ACEPROMAZINE: Concurrent use of acepromazine with xylazine is generally considered safe; however, there is potential for additive hypotensive effects after the first hypertensive phase of xylazine. Manufacturers warn against using xylazine in conjunction with tranquilizers. Thus, this combination should be used cautiously in animals susceptible to hemodynamic complications.
- ANESTHETIC AGENTS (eg, **alfaxalone, isoflurane, ketamine, propofol**): May cause additive CNS depression if used with xylazine. Dosages of these agents may need to be reduced.
- ANTICHOLINERGIC AGENTS (eg, **atropine, butylscopolamine, glycopyrrolate**): Use of anticholinergic agents with alpha-2 agonists may significantly increase arterial blood pressure, heart rate, and the incidence of arrhythmia.[15,16] Clinical use of atropine or glycopyrrolate to prevent or treat bradycardia caused by alpha-2 agonists is controversial and use together is discouraged; this may be particularly important when using higher doses of the alpha-2 agonist.
- ANTIEMETIC AGENTS (eg, **maropitant, metoclopramide, ondansetron**): Antiemetics may decrease the emetogenic effects of xylazine.
- ATIPAMEZOLE: Used clinically to reverse to effects of xylazine
- BENZODIAZEPINES (eg, **diazepam, midazolam**): May cause additive CNS depression if used with xylazine. Dosages of these agents may need to be reduced.
- CHLORAMPHENICOL: Prolonged sedation and GI stasis possible[17]
- CNS DEPRESSANT AGENTS, OTHER (eg, **barbiturates, methocarbamol, trazodone**): May cause additive CNS depression if used with xylazine. Dosages of these agents may need to be reduced.
- EPINEPHRINE: The use of epinephrine with xylazine, with or without the concurrent use of halothane, may induce ventricular arrhythmias.
- OPIOIDS (eg, **buprenorphine, morphine, tramadol**): May cause additive CNS depression if used with xylazine. Dosages of these agents may need to be reduced
- RESERPINE: A case of a horse developing colic-like clinical signs after reserpine and xylazine has been reported. Until more is known about this potential interaction, the use of these 2 agents together should be avoided.
- YOHIMBINE: May reverse the effects of medetomidine; however, atipamezole is preferred for clinical use to reverse the drug's effects because atipamezole is more selective for the alpha receptors and is unlikely to cause hypotension, which is common following administration of yohimbine.

Laboratory/Diagnostic Interactions

- In horses, xylazine infusion caused overestimation of lithium dilution method for cardiac output (LiDCO) measurements.[18]
- The use of xylazine before abdominal radiography can make test interpretation difficult in animals that develop gaseous distention of the stomach or bloat.

Dosages

NOTE: A reversal agent should always be on hand; reversal of sedative effects also reverses analgesic effects.

DOGS:

NOTE: Most clinicians prefer using newer alpha-2 agonists (eg, dexmedetomidine) that have a greater selectivity for the alpha-2 adrenergic receptor.

Sedation accompanied by a short period of analgesia; pre-anesthetic agent (label dosage; FDA-approved): 1.1 mg/kg IV OR 1.1 – 2.2 mg/kg IM or SC.[19] NOTE: The label dosage for dogs is considered by most clinicians to be greater than is necessary for most indications. The labeled indications are provided below, but the use of lower, extra-label dosages should be considered.

Preanesthetic agent (extra-label): 0.2 – 1 mg/kg IV, IM, or SC[20]

Analgesic adjunct (extra-label): 0.05 – 0.5 mg/kg IV, IM, or SC

CATS:

NOTE: Except for its use as an emetic, most clinicians prefer using newer alpha-2 agonists (eg, dexmedetomidine) that have greater selectivity for the alpha-2 adrenergic receptor.

Sedation accompanied by a short period of analgesia; pre-anesthetic agent (label dosage; FDA-approved): 1.1 mg/kg IV OR 2.2 mg/kg IM or SC.[11] NOTE: The label dosage for cats is considered by most clinicians to be greater than is necessary for most indications. The labeled indications are provided below, but the use of lower extra-label dosages should be considered.

Emetic (extra-label): 0.4 – 1.1 mg/kg IM or SC; will not work with toxicants that target the CRTZ. After emesis, effects can be reversed with yohimbine 0.1 mg/kg IV, tolazoline 0.5 – 1 mg/kg IV, or atipamezole 0.05 0.2 mg/kg IM can be considered. Tolazoline may be superior to yohimbine to reverse the emetic effects of xylazine in the cat.[3,21,22]

Preanesthetic agent (extra-label dose): 0.2 – 1 mg/kg IV, IM, or SC[20]

Analgesic adjunct (extra-label): 0.05 – 0.5 mg/kg IV, IM, or SC

Anxiolytic agent (extra-label): 0.05 – 0.2 mg/kg IV or IM[23]

HORSES:

Sedation accompanied by a short period of analgesia; pre-anesthetic agent (label dosage; FDA-approved): 1.1 mg/kg IV;

2.2 mg/kg IM.[24] Allow the animal to rest quietly until full effect is reached.

NOTE: FDA-approved dosages usually produce sedation lasting 1 to 2 hours and analgesia lasting for 15 to 30 minutes.

NOTE: More information for extra-label protocols for the use of xylazine as part of drug combinations for injectable sedation, anesthesia/analgesia protocols can be found in other references.[25] The following are some examples of published recommended dosages and protocols:

a) **Standing sedation and analgesia** (extra-label): Full dose is 1 mg/kg IV; for intraoperative use, IV dose is usually lower than the full dose, or an IV CRI can be used. CRI dosages reported range from 0.5 – 1 mg/kg/hour IV.[26] Epidural dosages range from 0.17 – 0.25 mg/kg.[13] Alternately, 0.5 – 1.1 mg/kg IV (onset of peak action in 2 to 5 minutes; duration ≈30 minutes); 1 – 2 mg/kg IM (onset of peak action in 15 minutes; duration ≈30 minutes). For prolonged procedures: 0.5 mg/kg IV, followed by a CRI of 0.65 mg/kg/hour.[27]
b) **Field anesthesia**: (extra-label): Sedate with xylazine 1 mg/kg IV OR 2 mg/kg IM given 5 to 10 minutes (longer for IM route) before induction of anesthesia with ketamine 2 mg/kg IV. The horse must be adequately sedated (chin to the metacarpals) before giving the ketamine (ketamine can cause muscle rigidity).[28]
c) **Part of induction protocols** (extra-label):
<u>Normal healthy patients</u>: 0.44 – 0.66 mg/kg IV. Wait for sedation and muscle relaxation to occur (≈5 minutes) before induction of general anesthesia. Higher doses (up to 2 mg/kg IV) may be needed depending on the horse's level of excitation.
<u>Compromised patients</u>: Use a very modest dose of xylazine 0.22 – 0.44 mg/kg IV, depending on status and demeanor, to minimize its cardiovascular effects in compromised patients. Slow administration of guaifenesin (5% solution) can be used to gradually create the desired level of sedation, followed by a more rapid administration of guaifenesin and ketamine.[29]
d) **IV anesthesia (greater than 30 minutes) using "GKX" or "triple-drip"** (extra-label): Guaifenesin (50 mg/mL), ketamine (1 – 2 mg/mL; 2 mg/mL concentration used for more painful or noxious procedures), and xylazine (0.5 mg/mL). Most practitioners prefer to induce with xylazine/ketamine or xylazine/diazepam/ketamine, and then use GKX for maintenance. Typically, the CRI runs at 1.5 – 2.2 mL/kg/hour IV, depending on the procedure, patient response, and ketamine concentration.
e) **Recovery after inhalant anesthesia** (extra-label): 0.2 – 0.5 mg/kg IV can be administered after inhalant anesthesia to improve recovery.[30,31]
f) **Supplementation of general anesthesia** (extra-label): Xylazine 0.5 – 1 mg/kg/hour IV CRI has been used with ketamine and isoflurane anesthesia.[26,32,33]
g) **Low-dose sedation to facilitate lameness evaluations** (extra-label): 0.3 mg/kg (route not stated, assume IV- *Plumb*) did not mask lameness (measured with body-mounted inertial sensors) or cause ataxia, despite all horses receiving xylazine showing subjective signs of sedation within 5 minutes of administration and reduced chin-to-ground measurement at a 20-minute observation point.[34]

CATTLE:

CAUTION: Cattle are extremely sensitive to xylazine's effects; be certain of dose and dosage form. <u>Use only the 20 mg/mL solution</u> for this species.

NOTE: Xylazine is approved for use in cattle in several countries; withdrawal times vary depending on labeling in each country. In the United States, xylazine is not FDA-approved for use in cattle. Xylazine withdrawal intervals vary based on the dose and route of administration. Withdrawal intervals may be lengthened if xylazine sedation is reversed with tolazoline or yohimbine. Consult FARAD for further information.

Chemical restraint and injectable anesthesia (extra-label): The reader is encouraged to refer to the in-depth review by Abrahamsen[35] where detailed discussions on the use of alpha-2 agonists alone and in combination with other anesthetic adjuncts (eg, ketamine stun) for both standing and recumbent procedures can be found. Examples:

a) **Analgesia and restraint for standing procedures in cattle** (extra-label): Butorphanol 0.01 – 0.025 mg/kg in combination with xylazine 0.02 – 0.05 mg/kg and ketamine 0.04 – 0.1 mg/kg and administered IM or SC, depending on dose route and patient demeanor. The higher end of these dosages is likely to result in the animal becoming recumbent.[35] For a 450 kg (992.1 lb) animal, total doses (NOT mg/kg) of butorphanol 5 mg, xylazine 10 mg, and ketamine 20 mg would constitute the low end of the dosing range. Up to an hour of cooperation was accomplished using this protocol, but more fractious patients may require increased doses. For animals weighing more than 450 kg (992.1 lb), it is suggested to give no more than butorphanol 10 mg (total dose, NOT mg/kg) or xylazine 20 mg (total dose, NOT mg/kg) for the initial dose.[36]
b) **Standing sedation** (extra-label): The following xylazine dosages would be expected to produce standing sedation with a low incidence of recumbency for facilitating short diagnostic or therapeutic procedures. Patients will generally tolerate mildly uncomfortable stimuli, but these dosages should not be counted on to provide significant analgesia. Duration of effect generally lasts about 30 to 40 minutes. **NOTE**: IM administration of doses intended to be given IV reduces the chance for recumbency.[35]

Patient type	IV (mg/kg)	IM (mg/kg)
Quiet dairy breeds	0.0075 – 0.01	0.015 – 0.02
Tractable cattle	0.01 – 0.02	0.02 – 0.04
Anxious cattle	0.02 – 0.03	0.04 – 0.06
Extremely anxious or unruly cattle	0.025 – 0.05	0.05 – 0.1

Sedation/analgesia: 0.1 – 0.3 mg/kg IM; 0.05 – 0.15 mg/kg IV; 0.05 – 0.07 mg/kg epidurally. When xylazine is used IV/IM, analgesia can be short-lived (½ hour).[37]

DEER/ELK:

Sedative/analgesic (label dosage; FDA-approved): **NOTE**: FDA-approved dosages usually produce sedation lasting 1 to 2 hours and analgesia lasting for 15 to 30 minutes.

a) **Fallow deer**: 4.4 – 8.8 mg/kg IM
b) **Mule, sika, or white-tailed deer**: 2.2 – 4.4 mg/kg IM
c) **Elk**: 0.55 – 1.1 mg/kg IM[24]

Sedative/analgesic (extra-label): For chemical immobilization, reconstitute 1 vial of tiletamine/zolazepam using xylazine 400 mg/4 mL; administer 1 mL/45.5 kg (1 mL/100 lb).[38]

SHEEP & GOATS:

NOTE: Use xylazine with extreme caution in these species due to the risk for acute pulmonary edema and hypoxemia, low pulse oximetry readings, and subsequent cyanosis.[39–41] <u>Use only the 20 mg/mL solution</u>. Consult FARAD for xylazine meat and milk withdrawal intervals, which vary based on dose and route of administration. More information using xylazine as part of drug combinations for injectable sedation, anesthesia/analgesia protocols can be found in other references.[35,42,43]

Light, standing sedation (extra-label): 0.01 mg/kg IV for light standing sedation to 0.2 mg/kg IM for recumbency of an hour's duration. Goats are a bit more sensitive than sheep. Dosage ranges of 0.05 – 0.1 mg/kg IV (goats) and 0.1 – 0.4 mg/kg IV (sheep) have also been recommended. When beginning to use these drugs, it is advisable to start with a conservative dose until one develops a feel for the level of sedation provided.[44,45]

CAMELIDS:

Procedural pain (eg, castrations) when recumbency (up to 30 minutes) is desired (extra-label): Alpacas: Xylazine 0.46 mg/kg in combination with butorphanol 0.046 mg/kg and ketamine 4.6 mg/kg and administered IM. Llamas: Xylazine 0.37 mg/kg in combination with butorphanol 0.037 mg/kg and ketamine 3.7 mg/kg and administered IM. May administer 50% of the original dose of xylazine and ketamine during anesthesia to prolong the effect up to 15 minutes. Expect 20 minutes of surgical time; the patient should stand 45 to 60 minutes after injection.[46]

Standing sedation and restraint (extra-label): Xylazine 0.1 mg/kg in combination with ketamine 0.2 mg/kg and *either* morphine 0.1 mg/kg OR butorphanol 0.05 mg/kg and administered IM. This combination provides ≈15 minutes of standing restraint. An additional dose of ketamine 0.01 mg/kg IM will extend the duration for another 5 to 10 minutes.[47]

Sedative/analgesic with tiletamine/zolazepam (extra-label): Xylazine 0.2 or 0.4 mg/kg in combination with tiletamine/zolazepam 2 mg/kg and administered IM produces significant antinociception. Transient hypoxemia was associated with xylazine administration, which is not considered clinically important in healthy llamas.[48] Adding morphine to the combination of xylazine and tiletamine/zolazepam resulted in a longer duration of analgesia.[49]

Sedative/analgesic (extra-label): 0.2 mg/kg IV OR 0.3 mg/kg IM or SC may provide profound sedation for 10 to 20 minutes and an additional 10 to 20 minutes of mild sedation, but overall effects are often unpredictable.[47]

SWINE:

NOTE: Xylazine dosages in swine are higher than those used in other species.

Sedative/analgesic (extra-label):

a) Xylazine 1 – 2.5 mg/kg IM in combination with ketamine 10 – 12 mg/kg IM[50,51] or xylazine 2 mg/kg IM in combination with ketamine 20 mg/kg IM and midazolam 0.25 mg/kg IM[51,52]
b) 0.5 – 4 mg/kg IM, alone or in combination with ketamine[53,54]

Induction of general anesthesia (extra-label): Xylazine 1 – 2 mg/kg in combination with tiletamine/zolazepam 4 – 6 mg/kg IM[51]

Maintenance of anesthesia (extra-label): Triple drip (ie, guaifenesin/ketamine/xylazine [GKX]) -- To 500 or 1000 mL of guaifenesin (50 mg/mL), add xylazine 1 mg (NOT mg/kg) plus ketamine 1 – 2 mg (NOT mg/kg) per mL of guaifenesin. Run solution at 2.2 mL/kg/hour IV CRI for up to 2 hours.[51]

BIRDS:

Sedative/analgesic (extra-label):

a) 1 – 4 mg/kg IM; provides sedation for ketamine anesthesia. Xylazine has been used at dosages of up to 10 mg/kg in small psittacines.[55,56]
b) Xylazine 2 – 6 mg/kg in combination with ketamine 10 – 30 mg/kg and administered IM; birds weighing less than 250 g require a higher dose (on a mg/kg basis) than birds weighing greater than 250 g.[57]

FERRETS:

Sedative/analgesic (extra-label):

a) 0.5 – 2 mg/kg IM or SC. Usually combined with atropine 0.05 mg/kg OR glycopyrrolate 0.01 mg/kg and administered IM
b) Xylazine 2 mg/kg in combination with butorphanol 0.2 mg/kg and administered IM[58,59]
c) Xylazine 1.5 mg/kg in combination with tiletamine/zolazepam 1.5 mg/kg +/- butorphanol 0.2 mg/kg and administered IM

RABBITS, RODENTS, SMALL MAMMALS:

Sedative/analgesic (extra-label)[60]:

a) **Rabbits**:
   i. Xylazine 5 mg/kg in combination with ketamine 35 mg/kg and administered IM; surgical anesthesia for 20 to 30 minutes, good relaxation, sleep time is 60 to 120 minutes, some effects reversible with atipamezole
   ii. Xylazine 5 mg/kg in combination with ketamine 25 mg/kg and butorphanol 0.1 mg/kg and administered IM; surgical anesthesia for 60 to 90 minutes, good relaxation, sleep time is 120 to 180 minutes
   iii. Xylazine 5 mg/kg in combination with ketamine 25 mg/kg and acepromazine 1 mg/kg and administered IM; surgical anesthesia for 45 to 75 minutes, good relaxation, sleep time is 100 to 150 minutes
b) **Gerbils**: Xylazine 2 mg/kg in combination with ketamine 50 mg/kg and administered IP
c) **Guinea pigs**: Xylazine 5 mg/kg in combination with ketamine 40 mg/kg and administered IP
d) **Hamsters**: Xylazine 10 mg/kg in combination with ketamine 200 mg/kg and administered IP
e) **Mice**: Xylazine 10 mg/kg in combination with ketamine 80 mg/kg and administered IP
f) **Rats**: Xylazine 10 mg/kg in combination with ketamine 75 mg/kg and administered IP

Monitoring

- Level of sedation and analgesia
- Heart rate and rhythm, blood pressure, respiratory depth and rate, $ETCO_2$, pulse oximetry (SpO_2), and body temperature should be considered in all patients, and mandatory in higher risk patients.
- Hydration status

Client Information

- Xylazine should only be used by individuals familiar with its use.

Chemistry/Synonyms

Xylazine HCl is an alpha-2-adrenergic agonist that is structurally related to clonidine. It occurs as a colorless, white or almost white crystalline powder that is freely soluble in water. The pH of the commercially prepared injections is ≈5.5. Dosages and bottle concentrations are expressed in terms of the base.

Xylazine HCl may also be known as Bay-Va-1470, *Rompun*®, *AnaSed*®, *Chanazine*®, *Nerfasin*®, *Sedazine*®, *Tranquived*®, *X-Ject E*®, *Xylamax*®, or *Xylamed*®.

Storage/Stability

Do not store above 30°C (86°F). Some manufacturers state to store at 20°C to 25°C (68°F-77°F) and permit excursions up to 40°C (104°F).

Compatibility/Compounding Considerations

Compatibility is dependent on factors such as pH, concentration, temperature, and diluent used; specialized references or a hospital pharmacist should be consulted for more specific information.

Xylazine is reportedly physically **compatible** in the same syringe with several compounds, including acepromazine, buprenorphine, butorphanol, chloral hydrate, and meperidine. Anecdotally, xylazine is physically **compatible** when combined in the same vial with ketamine and/or tiletamine/zolazepam, and in IV solution with guaifenesin and ketamine (ie, "triple drip"). However, the stability and potency of these combinations have not been studied and cannot be recommended.

A study evaluated the stability, sterility, pH, particulate formation, and efficacy of compounded ketamine, acepromazine, and xylazine (KAX) in laboratory rodents. The results supported the finding that the drugs are stable and effective for at least 180 days after mixing if stored at room temperature in the dark. Compounded ketamine/xylazine combinations at concentrations intended for laboratory rodents demonstrated 3 months' stability at any temperature when diluted in saline.[61] Undiluted ketamine/xylazine was stable for 3 months only if refrigerated. The ketamine/acepromazine/xylazine combination was only stable for 1 month if refrigerated, and the unrefrigerated combination was not stable at any temperature.[62]

Dosage Forms/Regulatory Status

VETERINARY-LABELED PRODUCTS:

The Association of Racing Commissioners International (ARCI) has designated this drug as a class 3 substance. The use of this drug may not be allowed in certain animal competitions. Check rules and regulations before entering a competition while this medication is being administered. Contact local racing authorities for further guidance. See ***Appendix*** for more information.

Xylazine Injection: 20 mg/mL in 20 mL vials or 100 mg/mL in 50 mL vials: *Rompun*®, *AnaSed*®, generic; (Rx). FDA-approved for use (depending on strength and product) in dogs, cats, horses, deer, and elk. Do not use in horses intended for human consumption or in *Cervidae* less than 15 days before or during hunting season.

Xylazine is not FDA-approved for use in cattle in the United States; however, in Canada, at label dosages, it reportedly has been assigned withdrawal times of 3 days for meat and 48 hours for milk. Consult FARAD for meat and milk withdrawal intervals, which vary based on dose and route of administration.

HUMAN-LABELED PRODUCTS: NONE

References

For the complete list of references, see **wiley.com/go/budde/plumb**

Yohimbine

(yo-***him***-been) *Yobine*®, *Antagonil*®

Alpha-2-Adrenergic Antagonist

Prescriber Highlights

- Used to reverse xylazine, other alpha-2 agonists, and, potentially, amitraz; may be used prophylactically before amitraz dips
- Use with caution in patients that have renal disease or seizure disorders.
- Reversal effects may diminish before the agonist's effects dissipate.
- Adverse effects include transient apprehension or CNS excitement, muscle tremors, salivation, hypertension, increased cardiac and respiratory rates, and hyperemic mucous membranes; more likely in small animal species and horses.
- Many potential drug interactions

Uses/Indications

Yohimbine is indicated to reverse the effects of xylazine in dogs, but it is used clinically to reverse the effects of other alpha-2 agonists and in several other species as well.

Yohimbine may be efficacious in reversing some of the toxic effects associated with other agents (eg, amitraz) and can be used prophylactically before amitraz dips.

Pharmacology/Actions

Yohimbine is an alpha-2-adrenergic antagonist that can competitively antagonize the effects of xylazine and other alpha-2-adrenergic agonists. Alone, yohimbine increases heart rate and can decrease blood pressure (at high doses),[1] causes CNS stimulation and antidiuresis, and has hyperinsulinemic effects. A study in cats found that yohimbine could antagonize xylazine- and medetomidine-induced diuresis in healthy cats.[2] It can increase borborygmi and GI sounds in horses[3] and act as an antiemetic in cats.[4]

A study in horses that received detomidine 0.03 mg/kg IV followed 15 minutes later by yohimbine 0.2 mg/kg IV found that yohimbine rapidly reversed the sedative effects of detomidine, effectively returned heart rate and the percent of atrioventricular conduction disturbances to pre-detomidine values, and effectively reduced detomidine-induced hyperglycemia.[5] Another study in horses after they received sublingual detomidine showed the effects of yohimbine 0.075 mg/kg IV on detomidine-induced changes in the chin-to-ground distance were minimal, and that the effects on detomidine-induced changes in heart rate and rhythm only persisted for 15 to 20 minutes.[6]

By blocking central alpha-2 receptors, yohimbine enhances sympathetic outflow (norepinephrine). Peripheral alpha-2 receptors are also found in the cardiovascular system, genitourinary system, GI tract, platelets, and adipose tissue.

Pharmacokinetics

A study (using 2 compartmental analyses) where yohimbine 0.12 mg/kg IV was administered to horses found a large volume of distribution (mean, 3.2 L/kg), a low clearance (mean, 13.6 mL/kg per minute), and a long elimination half-life (4.4 hours).[7] A separate study from the same group, using IV doses of 0.1, 0.2, and 0.4 mg/kg IV, reported similar results.[8] The main metabolite, hydroxy-yohimbine, can be detected in urine samples for as long as 96 hours post-administration.[7]

A study reported the pharmacokinetics of yohimbine in steers and dogs.[9] The apparent volume of distribution (steady-state) was ≈5 L/kg in steers and 4.5 L/kg in dogs. The total body clearance was ≈70 mL/minute/kg in steers and 30 mL/minute/kg in dogs. The half-life of the drug was ≈0.5 to 1 hour in steers and 1.5 to 2 hours in dogs.

Yohimbine is believed to penetrate the CNS quite readily. When it is used to reverse the effects of xylazine, the onset of action generally occurs within 3 minutes.

The metabolic fate of the drug is not fully understood, but in humans, 90% of the drug is metabolized in the liver primarily by hydroxylation. In horses, at least 2 metabolites were detected in a pharmacokinetic study, both of which appeared to be hydroxylated metabolites.[8] Whether any metabolites have activity is not known, but in humans, there have been reports that the major metabolite, 11-hydroxy yohimbine, may have pharmacologic activity.

Contraindications/Precautions/Warnings

Yohimbine is contraindicated in patients that are hypersensitive to it. In humans, yohimbine is contraindicated in patients with renal disease.

Yohimbine should be used cautiously in patients with seizure disorders. When used to reverse the effects of xylazine, normal pain perception may result. The alpha-2-adrenergic antagonist effects of yohimbine may diminish before the effects of the agonist dissipate.

Prolonged withdrawal periods for horses in athletic events may be necessary.

Adverse Effects

Yohimbine may cause transient apprehension or CNS excitement, muscle tremors, hypertension, tachycardia,[10] salivation, increased respiratory rates, and hyperemic mucous membranes. Adverse effects appear to be more probable in small animal species and horses.

An in vitro study found that yohimbine inhibited collagen-induced aggregation of bovine and equine platelets.[11] Clinical significance is not known.

Reproductive/Nursing Safety

Safe use of yohimbine in pregnant animals or animals intended for breeding has not been established. No information on safety during lactation was located.

Because safety has not been established in animals, this drug should only be used when the maternal benefits outweigh the potential risks to offspring.

Overdose/Acute Toxicity

Dogs receiving 0.55 mg/kg (5 times the recommended dose) exhibited transient clinical signs of seizures and muscle tremors.

Yohimbine is commonly found in combination with other stimulants in over-the-counter medications. The most common signs are hyperactivity, tachycardia, anxiety, diarrhea, hind limb weakness, hyperthermia, injected sclera, and vocalization.

For patients that have experienced or are suspected of having experienced an overdose, consultation with a 24-hour poison consultation center specializing in providing veterinary-specific information is recommended. For general information related to overdose and toxin exposures, as well as contact information for poison control centers, refer to ***Appendix.***

Drug Interactions

Little information is available; use yohimbine with caution with **other alpha-2-adrenergic antagonists** or **other drugs that can cause CNS stimulation**.

- **ANTIHYPERTENSIVES** (eg, **angiotensin-converting enzyme inhibitors [ACEIs], calcium channel blockers** [eg, **amlodipine**], **hydralazine**): Reduced effectiveness of antihypertensive medications has been noted.
- **DETOMIDINE**: In horses, a study found that giving yohimbine after prior administration of detomidine caused yohimbine clearance and volume of distribution to decrease with resultant increases in yohimbine peak plasma levels. The authors concluded that this increases the potential for untoward effects and warrants further study into the physiologic effects of this combination of drugs.[12]
- **RESERPINE**: Concurrent administration of high doses (1 mg/kg IV of each drug) was uniformly fatal to dogs.[1]
- **TRICYCLIC ANTIDEPRESSANTS** (eg, **amitriptyline, clomipramine**): In humans, yohimbine is not recommended for use with antidepressants or other mood-altering agents; hypertension has been reported with tricyclic antidepressants.

Dosages

DOGS:

Xylazine reversal (label dosage; FDA-approved): 0.11 mg/kg IV slowly[13]

Reversal or prevention of amitraz toxicity (extra-label): If atipamezole is unavailable, yohimbine 0.1 mg/kg IV or 0.25 mg/kg IM[14,15]; some clinicians recommend using yohimbine in combination with atipamezole 50 μg/kg IM.[14,16]

CATS:

Reversal of xylazine-containing anesthetic combinations (extra-label): 0.5 mg/kg IV at the end of the procedure[17]

HORSES:

Alpha-2-adrenergic agonist reversal (extra-label): The less specific alpha-2 agonists—xylazine, detomidine, and romifidine—are typically reversed using yohimbine 0.05 – 0.2 mg/kg administered IM or slowly IV.[18] A study where yohimbine was given at 0.2 mg/kg IV 15 minutes after IV detomidine found that it effectively reversed detomidine-induced sedation, bradycardia, atrioventricular heart block, and hyperglycemia.[19]

CATTLE:

Alpha-2-adrenergic agonist (xylazine) reversal (extra-label): 0.1 – 0.125 mg/kg IM. Consider IV administration in an emergency situation. If ketamine or tiletamine/zolazepam have been used, allow 30 to 45 minutes before reversing xylazine (nonemergency situation) to avoid rough recovery.[20-22]

LLAMAS:

Xylazine reversal (extra-label): 0.125 – 0.25 mg/kg IV or IM[23,24]

SWINE:

Reversal of dexmedetomidine combination with butorphanol and midazolam (extra-label): 0.3 mg/kg IM[25]

Reversal of xylazine, ketamine, tiletamine/zolazepam anesthesia in sows (extra-label): 0.1 mg/kg IM[26,27]

BIRDS:

Reversal agent for alpha-2-adrenergic agonists (eg, xylazine): 0.1 mg/kg IV[28]

RABBITS, RODENTS, SMALL MAMMALS:

Reversing the effects of xylazine and to partially antagonize the effects of ketamine and acepromazine (extra-label):

a) **Rabbits:** 0.2 mg/kg IV as needed[29]

b) **Mice/Rats:** 0.2 mg/kg IP as needed[29]

Monitoring

- CNS status (arousal level)
- Cardiac rate; rhythm (if indicated), blood pressure (if indicated and practical)
- Respiratory rate

Client Information

- This agent should only be used by veterinary professionals.

Chemistry/Synonyms

Yohimbine HCl, a Rauwolfia or indolealkylamine alkaloid, has a molecular weight of 390.9. It is chemically related to reserpine.

Yohimbine may also be known as aphrodine hydrochloride, chlorhydrate de quebrachine, corynine hydrochloride, *Aphrodyne®*, *Dayto Himbin®*, *Pluriviron mono®*, *Prowess Plain®*, *Urobine®*, *Virigen®*, *Yobine®*, *Yocon®*, *Yocoral®*, *Yohimex®*, *Yohydrol*, *Yomax®*, or *Zumba®*.

Storage/Stability

Store yohimbine injection at room temperature (15°C-30°C [59°F-86°F]) and protected from light and heat.

Compatibility/Compounding Considerations

No specific information was noted.

Dosage Forms/Regulatory Status

VETERINARY-LABELED PRODUCTS:

The Association of Racing Commissioners International (ARCI) has designated this drug as a class 2 substance. Use of this drug may not be allowed in certain animal competitions. Check rules and regulations before entering a competition while this medication is being administered. Contact local racing authorities for further guidance. See ***Appendix*** for more information.

Yohimbine Sterile Solution for Injection: 2 mg/mL in 20 mL vials; *Yobine®*; (Rx). FDA-approved for use in dogs. NADA# 140-866.

The United States product label states yohimbine is not for use in food-producing animals.

HUMAN-LABELED PRODUCTS:
No FDA-approved products were located; 2 mg, 5.4 mg, and 6 mg tablets are available in Canada (Rx) but unlikely to be of veterinary benefit.

References
For the complete list of references, see **wiley.com/go/budde/plumb**

Zidovudine

(zid-o-***vew***-den) *Retrovir®*
Antiretroviral

Prescriber Highlights
- ▶ Antiretroviral agent that may be useful for adjunctive treatment of FeLV or FIV in cats
- ▶ Use with caution in patients with renal, hepatic, or bone marrow dysfunction.
- ▶ Nonregenerative anemia is the most common adverse effect in cats.
- ▶ The National Institute for Occupational Safety and Health (NIOSH) classifies zidovudine as a hazardous drug; use appropriate precautions when handling.

Uses/Indications

In veterinary medicine, zidovudine may be useful for treating feline immunodeficiency virus (FIV) or feline leukemia virus (FeLV). Although zidovudine can reduce the viral load in infected cats and improve clinical signs, it may not alter the natural course of the disease to a great extent.

A double-blind placebo-controlled trial assessed the efficacy of human interferon-alpha2a 100,000 IU/kg SC every 24 hours, zidovudine 5 mg/kg PO every 12 hours, and a combination of both drugs in cats infected naturally with FeLV. This study reported that although there was a trend for improved clinical status in treated cats, they were unable to demonstrate measurable statistically significant efficacy of either drug alone or together when given for 6 weeks.[1]

As drug resistance can be seen, one source recommends that zidovudine treatment is likely best reserved for those situations where symptomatic/supportive measures are not working.[2] Drug resistance can be seen as early as 6 months after starting treatment.[3]

Pharmacology/Actions

Zidovudine is considered an antiretroviral agent. Although its exact mechanism of action is not fully understood, zidovudine is converted in vivo to an active metabolite (triphosphate) that interferes with viral RNA-directed DNA polymerase (reverse transcriptase). This causes a virustatic effect in retroviruses.

Zidovudine has some activity against gram-negative bacteria and can be cytotoxic as well.

Pharmacokinetics

Zidovudine is well absorbed after oral administration. In cats, oral bioavailability is ≈95%. When zidovudine is administered with food, peak concentrations may be decreased, but the total area under the curve may not be affected; peak concentrations occur ≈1 hour post-dosing in cats. The drug is widely distributed, including into the CSF. It is only marginally bound to plasma proteins. Zidovudine is rapidly metabolized and excreted in the urine. Half-life in cats is ≈1.5 hours.[4]

Contraindications/Precautions/Warnings

Zidovudine is contraindicated in patients that have developed life-threatening hypersensitivity reactions to it in the past.[5]

Use zidovudine with caution in patients with bone marrow, renal, or hepatic dysfunction. The European Advisory Board on Cat Diseases (ABCD) guidelines on prevention and management of feline immunodeficiency advise against the use of zidovudine in cats with myelosuppression. Dosage adjustment may be necessary for cats with renal or hepatic dysfunction.

In humans, hematologic toxicity, including neutropenia and severe anemia, has been associated with zidovudine use.[5] Symptomatic myopathy has also occurred with prolonged use. Lactic acidosis and severe hepatomegaly with steatosis have been reported with nucleoside analogues. In humans, rapid infusions or bolus injections should be avoided, and zidovudine should not be given IM.

The National Institute for Occupational Safety and Health (NIOSH) classifies zidovudine as a hazardous drug[6]; personal protective equipment (PPE) should be used accordingly to minimize the risk for exposure

Adverse Effects

In cats, reductions in RBCs, PCV, and hemoglobin are the most common adverse effects reported. Anemia may be nonregenerative and is most commonly seen with the higher end of the dose range (10 – 15 mg/kg). If hematocrit drops below 20%, treatment should be discontinued, and anemia then usually resolves within a few days.[3] Diarrhea and weakness have also been reported.

In a controlled trial with a total of 22 cats receiving zidovudine, no notable adverse effects were detected.[1]

Although there are many adverse effects reported in humans, granulocytopenia and GI effects, especially nausea, vomiting, and anorexia, appear to be the most likely to occur.[5] The frequency and severity of adverse effects in humans are greater in patients with more advanced infection at the time of treatment initiation.

Reproductive/Nursing Safety

Zidovudine given to rats in doses up to 7 times the usual adult (human) doses had no effect on conception rates. Fetal toxicity occurred in rats receiving up to 450 mg/kg/day and in rabbits given 500 mg/kg/day.

Zidovudine is excreted in milk. Clinical significance is not clear for nursing offspring. Because safety has not been established in animals, this drug should only be used when the maternal benefits outweigh the potential risks to offspring.

Overdose/Acute Toxicity

Human adults and children have survived oral overdoses of up to 50 g without permanent sequelae.[5] Vomiting and transient hematologic effects are the most consistent adverse effects reported with overdoses.

For patients that have experienced or are suspected of having experienced an overdose, consultation with a 24-hour poison consultation center specializing in providing veterinary-specific information is recommended. For general information related to overdose and toxin exposures, as well as contact information for poison control centers, refer to ***Appendix.***

Drug Interactions

The following drug interactions have either been reported or are theoretical in humans or animals receiving zidovudine and may be of significance in veterinary patients. Unless otherwise noted, use together is not necessarily contraindicated, but weigh the potential risks and perform additional monitoring when appropriate.

- **Antifungals, Azole** (eg, **fluconazole, ketoconazole**): May increase zidovudine serum concentration
- **Atovaquone**: May increase zidovudine serum concentration
- **Doxorubicin**: May antagonize each other's effects; avoid use together.
- **Interferon Alfa**: Increased risk for hematologic and hepatic toxicity

- **Methadone**: May increase serum concentration of zidovudine
- **Myelotoxic/Cytotoxic drugs** (eg, chloramphenicol, doxorubicin, flucytosine, vincristine, vinblastine): Administered with zidovudine may increase the risk for hematologic toxicity
- **Probenecid**: May increase zidovudine serum concentration
- **Rifampin**: May decrease serum concentration (AUC) of zidovudine

Laboratory Considerations

- None were noted.

Dosages

CATS:

Adjunctive therapy of feline leukemia virus (FeLV) and feline immunodeficiency virus (FIV) (extra-label): 5 – 10 mg/kg PO or SC every 12 hours.[3,7,8] The higher dose should be used carefully as adverse effects (eg, nonregenerative anemia) can develop. When using the injectable formulation SC, the product should be diluted (see ***Compatibility/Compounding Considerations***) prior to administration to avoid local irritation[3]; dilution to 4 mg/mL is advised.[5]

Monitoring

- Baseline and weekly CBC for the first month during treatment, then monthly if stable[3]
- CD4/CD8 rates, if possible
- Clinical efficacy

Client Information

- For this medication to work properly, give it exactly as your veterinarian has prescribed.
- Side effects can include anemia, diarrhea, and weakness. If your cat seems overly tired or has no energy, contact your veterinarian right away.
- Your veterinarian will need to monitor you cat while it is taking this medicine. Do not miss these important follow-up visits.

Chemistry/Synonyms

Zidovudine, a thymidine analogue, is synthetically produced and occurs as a white to beige-colored, odorless, crystalline solid. ≈20 mg is soluble in 1 mL of water.

Zidovudine may also be known as ZDV, azidodeoxythymidine, 3'-azido-2',3'-dideoxythymidine, azidothymidine, AZT, BW-A509U, BW-509U, compound-S, zidovudinum, and *Retrovir*®; many other trade names are available.

Storage/Stability

Store zidovudine oral tablets, capsules, and solution at room temperature 15°C to 25°C (59°F-77°F). Protect from heat, light, and moisture.

Store zidovudine injection at room temperature (20-25°C [68-77°F]) and protect from light. Once diluted, it is stable for 24 hours at room temperature or 48 hours if refrigerated at 2°C to 8°C (36°F-46°F).

Compatibility/Compounding Considerations

Compatibility is dependent upon factors such as pH, concentration, temperature, and diluent used; consult specialized references or a hospital pharmacist for more specific information.

Zidovudine for injection is **compatible** with 5% dextrose, 0.9% sodium chloride, 5% dextrose with 0.45% sodium chloride, lactated Ringer's, and 5% dextrose with lactated Ringer's solutions.[9] It is reported as **Y-site compatible** with amikacin, clindamycin phosphate, dexamethasone sodium phosphate, dexmedetomidine, dobutamine, fluconazole, gentamicin sulfate, heparin sodium, hydromorphone, metoclopramide, metronidazole, ondansetron, pantoprazole, potassium chloride, trimethoprim/sulfamethoxazole, and voriconazole.

Dosage Forms/Regulatory Status

VETERINARY-LABELED PRODUCTS: NONE

HUMAN-LABELED PRODUCTS:

Zidovudine Oral Tablets: 300 mg; *Retrovir*®, generic; (Rx)

Zidovudine Oral Capsules: 100 mg; *Retrovir*®, generic; (Rx)

Zidovudine Oral Syrup: 50 mg/5 mL (10 mg/mL) in 240 mL; *Retrovir*®, generic; (Rx)

Zidovudine Injection Solution: 10 mg/mL in 20 mL single-use vials; *Retrovir*®; (Rx)

References

For the complete list of references, see **wiley.com/go/budde/plumb**

Zinc (Systemic)

(zeenk)

Nutritional; Trace Element

See also ***Zinc Gluconate (Neutralized), Topical***

Prescriber Highlights

- ► Metal nutritional agent that may be used for zinc deficiency, to reduce copper toxicity in susceptible dog breeds (eg, Bedlington terriers, West Highland white terriers) with hepatic copper toxicosis, and treat hepatic fibrosis in dogs
- ► Contraindications include animals taking penicillamine and those that are hypersensitive to it.
- ► Use caution or avoid use in animals that may have copper deficiency or elevated zinc concentration; consider obtaining copper and zinc serum concentrations before treating.
- ► Adverse effects related to large doses of zinc supplementation may include GI disturbances or hematologic abnormalities (usually hemolysis), particularly if a coexistent copper deficiency exists.
- ► Zinc overdoses (eg, United States pennies minted after 1982) can be serious.

Uses/Indications

Zinc sulfate is used systemically as a nutritional supplement in a variety of species. Oral zinc acetate has been shown to reduce copper toxicity in dog breeds that are susceptible to hepatic copper toxicosis (eg, Bedlington terriers, West Highland white terriers). Zinc therapy may also be of benefit in the treatment of hepatic fibrosis and zinc-responsive dermatosis. In dogs and cats, zinc has been used for adjunctive therapy for superficial necrolytic dermatitis (metabolic epidermal necrosis; hepatocutaneous syndrome).

Pharmacology/Actions

Zinc is a necessary nutritional supplement; it is required by over 200 metalloenzymes for proper function. Enzyme systems that require zinc include DNA polymerase, ALP, alcohol dehydrogenase, carbonic anhydrase, and RNA polymerase. Zinc is also necessary to maintain the structural integrity of cell membranes and nucleic acids. Zinc catalyzes essential biochemical reactions, such as activation of substrates of carbonic anhydrase in erythrocytes. Zinc-dependent physiological processes include sexual maturation and reproduction, cell growth and division, vision, night vision, wound healing, immune response, and taste acuity. In dogs with hepatitis, zinc induces the intestinal copper-binding protein metallothionein, resulting in antifibrotic and hepatoprotective properties.[1]

When administered orally, large doses of zinc can inhibit the intestinal absorption of copper and inhibit the reabsorption of secreted copper (eg, from bile or feces).

Pharmacokinetics

About 20% to 30% of dietary zinc is absorbed, principally from the duodenum and ileum. Bioavailability is dependent on the food in which it is present. Phytates can chelate zinc and form insoluble complexes in an alkaline pH; high concentrations of dietary calcium or phosphorus may also impair absorption. Food may have a similar effect on the bioavailability of zinc supplements. Zinc is stored mostly in red and white blood cells but is also found in the muscle, skin, bone, retina, pancreas, liver, kidney, and prostate gland. Serum zinc is bound to albumin and amino acids. Elimination is primarily via the feces, but some zinc is also excreted by the kidneys and in sweat. Zinc found in feces may be reabsorbed in the colon.

Contraindications/Precautions/Warnings

Zinc supplementation should be avoided or used cautiously in patients with copper deficiency.

Zinc sulfate injection is NOT for direct IV infusion and it is only intended for use in parenteral nutrition solutions. Solutions with an osmolarity of 900 mOsm/L or greater must be infused through a central catheter. Zinc sulfate injection contains aluminum; prolonged administration may lead to aluminum toxicity, particularly in animals with renal insufficiency.

Do not confuse dosages or concentrations of zinc salts with those of elemental zinc.

Adverse Effects

Large doses of zinc may cause GI disturbances; zinc acetate or methionine may be less irritating to the GI than other salts and mixing the contents of the capsule with a small amount of tuna or hamburger may also minimize vomiting. Hematologic abnormalities (usually hemolysis) may occur with large doses or serum concentrations greater than 1000 µg/dL (1 mg/dL), particularly if a coexistent copper deficiency exists.

Reproductive/Nursing Safety

Zinc requirements increase during pregnancy. Although zinc deficiency during pregnancy has been associated with adverse perinatal outcomes, other studies report no such occurrences. In humans, since zinc deficiency is very rare, the routine use of zinc supplementation during pregnancy is not recommended. No evidence of impaired fertility or fetal harm was noted in laboratory animals receiving up to 6 times the recommended human dose.

Zinc is excreted in breast milk; use it with caution in lactating animals.

Overdose/Acute Toxicity

Signs associated with overdoses of zinc in mammals include hemolytic anemia, neutropenia, hypotension, acute pancreatitis, jaundice, vomiting, and pulmonary edema. The most common clinical signs associated with a zinc overdose in dogs and cats include vomiting, diarrhea, polydipsia, and lethargy.

Zinc toxicosis in dogs ingesting topical zinc oxide includes vomiting, diarrhea, and hemolytic anemia.[2]

Zinc intoxication in birds is relatively common, but clinical signs of intoxication in birds are varied and nonspecific. They include lethargy, anorexia, regurgitation, polyuria, polydipsia, hematuria, hematochezia, pallor, dark or bright green diarrhea, foul-smelling feces, paresis, seizures, and sudden death.[3] Treatment involves removing the source of zinc, chelation therapy (edetate calcium disodium, penicillamine,[4] or succimer), and supportive care.

For patients that have experienced or are suspected of having experienced an overdose, consultation with a 24-hour poison consultation center specializing in providing veterinary-specific information is recommended. For general information related to overdose and toxin exposures, as well as contact information for poison control centers, refer to ***Appendix***.

Drug Interactions

The following drug interactions have either been reported or are theoretical in humans or animals receiving zinc and may be of significance in veterinary patients. Unless otherwise noted, use together is not necessarily contraindicated, but weigh the potential risks and perform additional monitoring when appropriate.

- **Calcium Supplements, Oral**: May potentially inhibit oral zinc absorption
- **Copper**: Large doses of zinc can inhibit copper absorption in the intestine; if this interaction is not desired, separate copper and zinc supplements by at least 2 hours.
- **Fluoroquinolones** (eg, enrofloxacin, ciprofloxacin): Zinc salts may reduce the oral absorption of some fluoroquinolones.
- **Iron Supplements, Oral**: May potentially inhibit oral zinc absorption; zinc salts may reduce the oral absorption of iron.
- **Penicillamine**: May potentially inhibit oral zinc absorption; zinc salts may reduce the oral absorption of penicillamine; the combination is considered contraindicated in dogs with hepatopathy.
- **Tetracyclines**: Zinc salts may chelate oral tetracyclines and reduce their absorption; tetracyclines may reduce zinc absorption; separate doses by at least 2 hours.
- **Ursodiol**: May potentially inhibit oral zinc absorption; the clinical significance is not clear.

Dosages

NOTE: Zinc products may be labeled with concentrations expressed as salt OR as elemental zinc. Assume the labeled concentration per tablet or capsule is elemental zinc unless the labeled ingredients and concentrations state otherwise. Dosages below are for elemental zinc unless otherwise noted.

DOGS:

Adjunctive treatment and prophylaxis of primary copper hepatopathy (extra-label): 8 – 10 mg/kg elemental zinc PO every 12 hours. Separate dose from meals by 1 to 2 hours. Monitor concentrations every 2 to 3 months and adjust the dose as necessary.[5]

Hepatic fibrosis (extra-label): Empirical dosage is 15 mg/kg of elemental zinc per day (or 200 mg elemental zinc per medium-sized dog per day, tapered to 50 – 100 mg/dog (NOT mg/kg) PO per day based on serum zinc concentrations). Zinc should ideally be given on an empty stomach (1 hour before or after a meal); mix with tuna oil if nausea is noted.[1,6]

Prevention of copper accumulation associated with chronic hepatitis (extra-label): 100 mg elemental zinc/dog (NOT mg/kg) PO daily for 3 to 6 months, then reduce to 50 mg elemental zinc/dog (NOT mg/kg) PO per day.

Adjunctive therapy for superficial necrolytic dermatitis or zinc-responsive dermatosis (extra-label): 2 – 3 mg/kg PO once a day of elemental zinc with food either once daily or divided every 12 hours.[7,8] Doses may need to be adjusted based on response to therapy. The addition of low-dose glucocorticoid therapy may benefit cases that do not respond solely to zinc supplementation. In syndrome I patients (fed balanced diets) that do not respond to oral zinc supplementation and low-dose glucocorticoid therapy, slow IV or IM injections with sterile zinc sulfate solutions at 10 – 15 mg/kg weekly (maximum of 600 mg/month) for at least 1 month have been recommended. Syndrome I patients require lifelong therapy. Syndrome II patients (fed diets low in zinc or high in phytates [cereal grains, soy-based or corn-based diets] or with high concentrations of minerals [calcium, iron, or copper] that may bind dietary zinc) can have zinc supplementation discontinued after the diet has been corrected and clinical signs resolve.[8]

CATS:

Adjunctive therapy of severe hepatic lipidosis (extra-label): 7 – 10 mg/kg PO once daily, in B-complex mixture if possible[9]

Primary copper hepatopathy (extra-label): 2 – 4 mg/kg elemental zinc PO every 12 to 24 hours

Superficial necrolytic dermatitis (extra-label): Dosages are not well described; doses used in dogs could possibly be extrapolated for cats.[8]

Monitoring

- Hepatic diseases:
- Plasma zinc concentration: The goal is above 200 µg/dL but less than 800 µg/dL.[10]
- Copper quantification when possible; serum ALT serially when copper quantification is not feasible.
- There is a poor correlation between serum zinc concentrations and zinc-deficient states in dogs, and zinc concentrations may have more value in the detection of potentially toxic intake or corroboration of a clinical diagnosis of toxicity or deficiency.[11]
- Periodically measure CBC to monitor for hemolytic anemia.[12]

Client Information

- Although it is best to give oral zinc on an empty stomach, if vomiting occurs, mix it with hamburger or tuna fish to decrease this side effect.
- Do not give more than prescribed; zinc can be very toxic (especially in dogs).
- While your animal is taking this medication, it is important to return to your veterinarian for blood tests. Do not miss these important follow-up visits.

Chemistry/Synonyms

Zinc acetate occurs as white crystals or granules. It has a faint acetous odor and effloresces slightly. One gram is soluble in 2.5 mL of water or 30 mL of alcohol. Zinc acetate contains 30% elemental zinc (100 mg zinc acetate = 30 mg elemental zinc).

Zinc sulfate occurs as a colorless granular powder, small needles, or transparent prisms. It is odorless but has an astringent metallic taste. 1.67 g are soluble in 1 mL of water. Zinc sulfate is insoluble in alcohol and contains 23% zinc by weight (100 mg zinc sulfate = 23 mg elemental zinc).

Zinc gluconate occurs as a white or practically white powder or granules. It is soluble in water and very slightly soluble in alcohol. Zinc gluconate contains 14.3% zinc (100 mg zinc gluconate = 14.3 mg elemental zinc).

Zinc methionine contains 18% to 21% elemental zinc. For every 5 mg of zinc methionine, there is ≈1 mg of elemental zinc.

Zinc acetate may also be known as E650 or zinci acetas dihydricus.

Zinc sulfate may also be known as zinc sulphate, zinci sulfas, or zincum sulfuricum; many trade names are available.

Storage/Stability

Store zinc acetate crystals in tight containers. Unless otherwise recommended by the manufacturer, store zinc sulfate products in tight containers at room temperature of 15°C to 30°C (59°F-86°F).

Compatibility/Compounding Considerations

If using bulk chemical powder: Zinc acetate contains 30% elemental zinc; zinc gluconate contains 14.3% elemental zinc; zinc sulfate contains 23% elemental zinc; zinc methionine contains 18% to 21% elemental zinc. One milligram of elemental zinc is provided by the following: 2.8 mg zinc acetate, 2.09 mg zinc chloride, 7.14 mg zinc gluconate, and 4.4 mg zinc sulfate. Zinc for injection is intended only as an additive to parenteral nutrition; do not administer the undiluted drug.

Dosage Forms/Regulatory Status

VETERINARY-LABELED PRODUCTS:

None as single-ingredient products for systemic use located; several vitamin/mineral supplements contain zinc, however. *NutriVed Chewable Zinpro®* Tablets contain 15 mg elemental zinc and 30 mg methionine; (OTC).

HUMAN-LABELED PRODUCTS:

Zinc Acetate is available from chemical supply houses.

Zinc Capsules: 25 mg and 50 mg elemental zinc (as zinc acetate or zinc sulfate), *Galzin®*, generic; (Rx/OTC)

Zinc Injection: 1 mg/mL (as 2.46 mg sulfate) in 5 mL and 10 mL vials; 5 mg/mL (as 21.95 mg sulfate) in 5 mL vials; 1 mg/mL (as 2.09 mg chloride) in 10 mL vials; and 3 mg/mL (as 7.41 mg sulfate) in 10 mL vials; generic; (Rx)

Zinc Tablets: 10 mg, 15 mg, 25 mg, 30 mg, and 50 mg elemental zinc (usually as zinc gluconate or zinc sulfate); generic; (OTC)

Zinc is also available in topical dermatologic and ophthalmic preparations.

References

For the complete list of references, see **wiley.com/go/budde/plumb**

Zoledronate

Zoledronic Acid

(***zoe***-le-***dron***-ik ***as***-id) *Zometa®, Reclast®*

Bisphosphonate

Prescriber Highlights

- ▶ Used IV for treating hypercalcemia of malignancy and for adjuvant analgesic treatment of malignant osteolytic bone pain most commonly associated with osteosarcoma
- ▶ Administer as an infusion in saline or dextrose over no less than 15 minutes (shorter than required for pamidronate administration).
- ▶ Appears well tolerated in veterinary patients with comorbidities including hypercalcemia but may cause electrolyte abnormalities and renal toxicity
- ▶ Check renal function prior to administration.
- ▶ The National Institute for Occupational Safety and Health (NIOSH) classifies zoledronic acid as a hazardous drug; use appropriate precautions when handling.

Uses/Indications

Zoledronate may be useful as an adjunctive analgesic for treating osteolytic bone pain associated with primary and metastatic skeletal malignancies including osteosarcoma in dogs and hypercalcemia associated with malignancy.[1-6] The drug had a chondroprotective effect in dogs with experimentally induced osteoarthritis.[7]

Zoledronate appears to slow tumor growth and reduce pathologic bone turnover in cats with oral squamous cell carcinoma.[8]

Horses with bone fragility disorder treated with zoledronate demonstrated both clinical and scintigraphic improvement.[9]

Pharmacology/Actions

Bisphosphonates, at therapeutic concentrations, inhibit bone resorption and do not inhibit bone mineralization via binding to hydroxyapatite crystals. Bisphosphonates impede osteoclast activity and induce osteoclast apoptosis, an effect that may be seen with monotherapy[10] or in combination with chemotherapy.[11,12] Zoledronate's primary target is the osteoclast enzyme farnesyl pyrophosphate synthase. Urinary calcium and phosphorus excretion is increased, and hypocalcemia, hypophosphatemia, and hypermagnesemia may result. Markers of bone turnover are reduced in healthy dogs as well as dogs with experimentally induced disease.[13,14] Zoledronate has ≈100 times greater relative antiresorptive potency as compared with pamidronate.[15]

Bisphosphonates in vitro have direct cytotoxic or cytostatic effects on human and canine osteosarcoma cell lines.[16] Additionally, zoledronate demonstrates bone-preserving activities at the primary tumor in a mouse model of canine osteosarcoma.[17] Zoledronate may also have antiangiogenic effects and inhibit cell migration in certain cancers.[8]

Pharmacokinetics

Zoledronate was administered by 15-minute IV infusion to 4 healthy dogs; the volume of distribution was ≈0.3 L/kg, and half-life was 2.2 hours.[18]

In 8 healthy horses receiving 0.057 mg/kg of an experimental zoledronic acid formulation administered by 30-minute IV infusion, the volume of distribution was 1.5 L/kg, and the elimination half-life was 2.2 hours.[19]

In humans, after IV infusion, ≈50% to 75% is incorporated into bone; the balance is largely excreted unchanged in the urine. It is not metabolized and does not alter the metabolism of other drugs. It has a terminal elimination half-life of ≈146 hours. Total drug exposure (area under the curve) is increased with increasing renal impairment. The shorter half-life reported in animals presumably reflects a shorter sampling period.

Contraindications/Precautions/Warnings

Zoledronic acid is contraindicated in patients with hypersensitivity to it and in patients with hypocalcemia or severe renal impairment.[20] Dosage adjustments are not necessary in patients with mild to moderate renal impairment. Zoledronic acid may cause renal injury and should be used with caution in patients that are receiving nephrotoxic drugs or that have moderate renal impairment, electrolyte imbalances, or disorders affecting mineral metabolism. Patients should be adequately hydrated prior to receiving zoledronic acid.

The National Institute for Occupational Safety and Health (NIOSH) classifies zoledronic acid as group 3 (*non-antineoplastic agents that primarily have adverse reproductive effects*).[21]

Do not confuse the trade name *ZOMeta®* (zolendronate) with *ZIMeta®* (dipyrone).

Adverse Effects

Zoledronate administered by 15-minute IV infusions appears to be well tolerated in veterinary patients.[22] One retrospective study reported adverse effects in dogs that included azotemia, vomiting, and diarrhea; however, concurrent medications could not be ruled out as the cause of these effects.[22] Acute kidney injury has also been reported in dogs but this effect appears infrequent and mild to moderate in severity.[23] Hypocalcemia has been noted, and osteonecrosis of the jaw has been reported.[24] Irritation may occur if extravasated.[5]

In humans, nausea, musculoskeletal pain, osteonecrosis of the jaw, atypical fractures, anemia, iritis/uveitis, hypotension, hypermagnesemia, hypophosphatemia, hypocalcemia, hypocalcemia-related cardiac or neurologic adverse effects, thrombocytopenia, and agranulocytosis have been reported.[20] Postinfusion pyrexia, fatigue, myalgia, and arthralgia commonly occur, and analgesic or antipyretic medication may be used to limit these effects. Infusion site reactions (eg, redness, swelling) occur infrequently. Adverse effects can occur days to months after administration.

Reproductive/Nursing Safety

In pregnant rats, administration of zoledronate during gestation at doses greater than 2.4 times the recommended human systemic exposure amount resulted in pre- and postimplantation losses and fetal skeletal, visceral, and external malformations; maternal mortality also increased.[20]

It is unknown if zoledronic acid is excreted in milk.[20] As neonatal exposure could have effects persisting for weeks to months, use with extreme caution in lactating animals; consider milk replacer.

Because safety has not been established in animals, this drug should only be used when the maternal benefits outweigh the potential risks to offspring.

Overdose/Acute Toxicity

Clinically significant hypocalcemia, hypophosphatemia, and hypomagnesemia may occur and should be corrected. Severe hypocalcemia has caused tetany and has been associated with atrial fibrillation. In humans, the risk for renal toxicity increases with 5-minute IV infusion times and doses of 8 mg.

For patients that have experienced or are suspected to have experienced an overdose, consultation with a 24-hour poison consultation center specializing in providing veterinary-specific information is recommended. For general information related to overdose and toxin exposures, as well as contact information for poison control centers, refer to ***Appendix.***

Drug Interactions

The following drug interactions have either been reported or are theoretical in humans or animals receiving zoledronate and may be of significance in veterinary patients. Unless otherwise noted, use together is not necessarily contraindicated, but weigh the potential risks and perform additional monitoring when appropriate.

- **AMINOGLYCOSIDES**: May enhance hypocalcemic effects of zoledronate; monitor.
- **CORTICOSTEROIDS** (eg, **dexamethasone, fludrocortisone, prednis(ol)one**): Zoledronate must be used carefully (with monitoring) when used in conjunction with other drugs that can affect calcium.
- **LOOP DIURETICS** (eg, **furosemide**): Loop diuretics promote calcium excretion and may result in additive effects on calcium concentrations.
- **NEPHROTOXIC DRUGS** (eg, **aminoglycosides, amphotericin B, cisplatin**): Use with caution; potential for increased risk for nephrotoxicity
- **NONSTEROIDAL ANTI-INFLAMMATORY DRUGS** (**NSAIDs**; eg, **carprofen, flunixin, meloxicam**): Use with caution; potential for increased risk for nephrotoxicity
- **THIAZIDE DIURETICS** (eg, **hydrochlorothiazide**): Thiazide diuretics promote calcium retention and may impair the hypocalcemic effects of zoledronate.

Laboratory Considerations

- None noted

Dosages

NOTE: See ***Compatibility/Compounding Considerations*** prior to administration.

DOGS:

Adjunctive treatment of hypercalcemia of malignancy (extra-label): 4 mg/dog (NOT mg/kg) IV infusion over 15 minutes.[25] Administration of doses ranging from 0.1 – 0.32 mg/kg have been reported.[5,22]

Palliative treatment of bone pain associated with osteosarcoma (extra-label): 0.1 mg/kg IV infusion over 15 minutes on the second of 2 days of ionizing radiation and repeated every 4 weeks[26]

CATS:

Adjunctive treatment of bone-invasive oral squamous cell carcinoma (extra-label): 0.2 mg/kg IV infusion over 15 minutes every 28 days[8]

HORSES:

Bone fragility disorder (extra-label): 0.075 mg/kg IV infusion over 30 minutes. Zoledronic acid solution was compounded immediately before administration using pharmaceutical grade zoledronate, citric acid, and mannitol solution.[9]

Monitoring

- Baseline and periodic serum renal chemistry panel and electrolytes (eg, calcium [total, ionized], phosphorous, potassium, magnesium) and hydration status should be monitored before starting each dose and especially for patients with pre-existing azotemia or for those receiving concurrent nephrotoxic drugs.
- Baseline and periodic CBC
- Baseline and periodic markers of bone turnover (eg, bone-specific ALP, urine N-telopeptide)[1]
- Baseline and periodic urinalysis

Client Information

- Your pet may have an elevated temperature or loss of appetite after receiving this medicine. Some animals may also experience muscle, bone, or joint pain for several days after treatment. Contact your veterinarian if you think your pet is in pain.
- This medicine must be given in your veterinarian's clinic. It cannot be administered at home.
- Your veterinarian will need to monitor your pet while it is being treated with this medicine. Do not miss these important follow-up visits.
- This medication is considered to be a hazardous drug as defined by the National Institute for Occupational Safety and Health (NIOSH). Talk with your veterinarian or pharmacist about the use of personal protective equipment when handling your animals waste (eg, urine, feces, vomit).

Chemistry/Synonyms

Zoledronic acid is an imidazole bisphosphonate acid analogue of pyrophosphate that occurs as a white crystalline powder. It is sparingly soluble in water, and practically insoluble in organic solvents.

Zoledronic acid is also known as zoledronate, CGP-42446, zoledronsyra, *Reclast*®, *Aclasta*®, and *Zometa*®.

Storage/Stability

Store zoledronate at room temperature 25°C (77°F); excursions to 15°C to 30°C (59°F-86°F) are permitted.

Zoledronic acid concentrate (0.8 mg/mL) that has been diluted for infusion should be stored refrigerated at 2°C to 8°C (36°F-46°F). The total time between dilution and completion of administration must not exceed 24 hours.

Compatibility/Compounding Considerations

Compatibility is dependent on factors such as pH, concentration, temperature, and diluent used; specialized references or a hospital pharmacist should be consulted for more specific information.

Do **not** mix zoledronate with any IV fluid containing divalent cations (eg, calcium and magnesium containing fluids such as lactated Ringer's solution [LRS], *Plasmalyte*®, Ringer's). It is recommended to use a 0.9% sodium chloride or 5% dextrose IV solution and a dedicated IV line. Refrigerated solutions should equilibrate to room temperature before administration.

Zoledronate is reportedly **Y-site compatible** with the following drugs (partial list): aminocaproic acid, ampicillin/sulbactam, azithromycin, buprenorphine, butorphanol tartrate, carboplatin, cefazolin, cefotaxime, ceftazidime, cisplatin, clindamycin, cyclophosphamide, cytarabine, dacarbazine, dexamethasone sodium phosphate, dexmedetomidine, dexrazoxane, diphenhydramine, dopamine, dobutamine, doxorubicin HCl (also liposome form), doxycycline, erythromycin lactobionate, famotidine, fentanyl citrate, fluconazole, fluorouracil, gemcitabine, heparin, hydromorphone, hydroxyzine, imipenem-cilastatin, lidocaine HCl, mannitol, metoclopramide, methylprednisolone sodium succinate, midazolam, mitoxantrone, morphine, ondansetron, pantoprazole, piperacillin-tazobactam, potassium chloride, ranitidine, vinblastine, and vincristine.

Zoledronate is reportedly **incompatible** with dantrolene, diazepam, and phenytoin sodium.

Dosage Forms/Regulatory Status

VETERINARY-LABELED PRODUCTS: NONE

HUMAN-LABELED PRODUCTS:

Zoledronic Acid Injection: 4 mg in 5 mL (0.8 mg/mL) concentrated solution in single-dose vials and 4 mg and 5 mg in 100 mL ready-to-use IV solution; *Reclast*®, *Zometa*®, generic; (Rx).

References

For the complete list of references, see **wiley.com/go/budde/plumb**

Zonisamide

(zoh-***niss***-a-mide) *Zonegran*®

Anticonvulsant

Prescriber Highlights

- May be useful as an add-on drug for refractory epilepsy. May also be considered for initial treatment as monotherapy in dogs
- Half-life of 15 hours in dogs allows for twice-daily administration, and half-life of 33 hours in cats allows for once-daily administration.
- Increase in dose may be needed when used in conjunction with phenobarbital.
- Common adverse effects include sedation, ataxia, and inappetence. Rarely, hepatopathy, urinary calculi, and metabolic and acute tubular acidosis have been reported.
- Known teratogen in dogs
- The National Institute for Occupational Safety and Health (NIOSH) classifies zonisamide as a hazardous drug; use appropriate precautions when handling.

Uses/Indications

In dogs, zonisamide has demonstrated effectiveness as monotherapy[1-3] and as an add-on drug for the treatment of refractory epilepsy.[4] Open-label studies in dogs with zonisamide used as monotherapy or as an add-on drug reported 58% to 81% response rates.[1,3,4] Based on the limited available evidence, zonisamide is recommended as monotherapy or as add-on treatment for canine epilepsy.[5]

Limited use in cats has occurred with anecdotal success in controlling seizures.[6]

Pharmacology/Actions

Although the exact mechanism of action for zonisamide is not known, it is postulated to produce antiseizure activity at sodium and T-type calcium channels, reducing transient inward currents and thereby stabilizing neuronal membranes and suppressing neuronal hypersynchronization.[7,8] Zonisamide may potentiate serotoninergic and dopaminergic neurotransmission but does not appear to potentiate gamma-aminobutyric acid (GABA). It has carbonic anhydrase inhibitory activity and can scavenge for free radicals in the brain.

Zonisamide reduced the number of paroxysmal electroencephalogram (EEG) discharges in cats with familial spontaneous epilepsy.[9]

Pharmacokinetics

In dogs, zonisamide is well absorbed (oral bioavailability ≈68%), with a volume of distribution of ≈0.8 L/kg and an average protein binding of 40%.[10,11] Plasma T_{max} after a single oral dose was reported to be 0.44 hours, and C_{max} was observed to be 14.4 µg/mL; C_{max} after repeated administration over 8 weeks was 58 µg/mL.[10,12,13] Concentrations of zonisamide are known to be higher in whole blood and RBCs as compared with plasma, so terminal half-life between RBC and plasma varies considerably. Oral plasma terminal half-life after repeated administration for 8 weeks was ≈23 hours,[10] but RBC half-life was reported at ≈37 hours; plasma half-life following a single oral dose was found to be 17.2 hours. Plasma clearance after a single oral dose was reported to be ≈32 mL/hour/kg. Most of the drug is excreted via the kidneys into the urine but ≈20% is metabolized, primarily in the liver. Unlike in humans, zonisamide exhibits linear pharmacokinetics (dose to plasma trough concentrations) in dogs at doses between 5 – 30 mg/kg PO twice daily.[11,14] Zonisamide administered rectally (10 – 30 mg/kg) failed to reach therapeutic concentration.[15,16]

In cats, zonisamide has an onset of action of ≈4 hours and a half-life of ≈33 hours; steady state is likely reached within 7 days.[17,18]

In Hispaniolan parrots, 20 mg/kg PO every 12 hours resulted in plasma concentrations within the known therapeutic range. Elimination half-life was ≈10 hours.[19]

Human metabolism of zonisamide includes acetylation and glucuronidation of an intermediate metabolite.[20] Approximately ⅔ of a dose is eliminated renally as unchanged drug and metabolites.

Contraindications/Precautions/Warnings

In humans, zonisamide is contraindicated in patients that are hypersensitive to it or any sulfonamide drug.[21] Use zonisamide with caution in patients with significant renal impairment; dosage reduction may be required. Although it is unlikely that a sulfa hypersensitivity reaction can be elicited, use caution in animals with keratoconjunctivitis sicca or other previous sulfonamide-related adverse effects.

The National Institute for Occupational Safety and Health (NIOSH) classifies zonisamide as a hazardous drug (nonantineoplastic agent representing an occupational hazard to healthcare workers); personal protective equipment (PPE) should be used accordingly to minimize the risk for exposure.[22] See ***Controlling Occupational Exposure to Hazardous Drugs*** for more information.

Adverse Effects

A systematic review and meta-analysis of adverse effects of antiepileptic drugs in dogs showed a weak level of evidence for zonisamide safety profile when used as monotherapy and adjunctive therapy.[23] The most common type I adverse effects (ie, dose dependent, predictable) were sedation followed by ataxia, vomiting, and decreased serum ALP activity; less common effects included increased serum ALT and glutamate dehydrogenase (GLDH) activity, aggression, anorexia, emaciation, and decreased T_4 and serum albumin.[23] When zonisamide was used as monotherapy, increased serum ALT and GLDH activity was not reported; however, in a recent review on incidence of hepatopathies in dogs on oral zonisamide, less than 1% of dogs experienced acute, potentially life-threatening hepatopathy associated with oral zonisamide therapy within the first 3 weeks of therapy.[24] Subclinical abnormalities in ALT and ALP activity were also noted in less than 10% of dogs during long-term therapy; clinical signs of liver disease were not observed.

Type II adverse effects (ie, idiosyncratic, nondose dependent, unpredictable) were idiosyncratic hepatotoxicity and mixed acid-base disorder.[23] A reduction in total T_4 was observed in one study, while free T_4 decreased slightly but remained within the reference range.[10] There are case reports of dogs developing zonisamide-associated apparent acute idiopathic hepatic necrosis,[25,26] pseudolymphoma,[27] urinary calculi,[25] hepatopathy,[28] acute tubular acidosis,[29] febrile neutropenia,[30] erythema multiforme,[31,32] and abnormal behavior (eg, sudden aggression, insomnia, restlessness, constant attention-seeking behavior).[33]

In a combined pharmacokinetic and toxicity study in cats, 50% of the cats receiving zonisamide 20 mg/kg per day developed adverse effects including inappetence, diarrhea, vomiting, ataxia, and somnolence; however, weight loss did not occur.[18] Zonisamide-related hypersensitivity syndrome in a cat has been reported.[34] Anorexia necessitated drug discontinuation in a cat.[35] Although a systematic review found that the majority of cats receiving zonisamide did not have adverse effects in reported studies, the efficacy and safety profile of zonisamide in cats was considered weak.[36]

Zonisamide is a sulfonamide-containing compound, but it does **not** contain the arylamine group known for causing a reactive intermediate, which may become a hapten for immunogenicity, ultimately leading to a sulfa allergy. Cross-reactivity between zonisamide and sulfa antibiotics has been demonstrated in vitro but has not been confirmed to be cross-reactive in humans. Based on currently available information, zonisamide is unlikely to cause keratoconjunctivitis sicca or other sulfonamide-related adverse effects in dogs or cats.

In a pharmacokinetic study of 10 birds, zonisamide did not alter appetite, body weight, or hematologic or serum chemistry panel values.[19]

In humans, the most common adverse effects include anorexia, nausea, dizziness, somnolence, agitation, and headache.[21] Rarely, serious dermatologic reactions (eg, Stevens-Johnson syndrome, toxic epidermal necrolysis [TEN]), blood dyscrasias, oligohidrosis, and hyperthermia have been reported in humans. Nephrolithiasis occurs in 4% of humans. Anorexia and weight loss in humans have also been noted.

Reproductive/Nursing Safety

Zonisamide is teratogenic in dogs, mice, and rats.[21] Zonisamide 10 or 30 mg/kg/day (approximate therapeutic doses in dogs) administered to pregnant dogs resulted in ventricular septal defects, cardiomegaly, and various valvular and arterial anomalies at the higher dose.[14] A plasma zonisamide concentration of 25 µg/mL was the threshold level for malformation. Owners of pregnant dogs should be made aware of and accept the significant risks associated with the use of this drug.

Zonisamide enters maternal milk at levels of 40% to 80% that of maternal plasma concentration. Use zonisamide with caution in nursing animals.[37] Because safety has not been established in animals, this drug should only be used when the maternal benefits outweigh the potential risks to offspring.

Overdose/Acute Toxicity

The LD_{50} of zonisamide in dogs is reportedly 1 g/kg. Human patients have survived zonisamide overdoses of ≈7.5 g (total dose) without complications.[38] In humans, overdoses may cause coma, bradycardia, hypotension, and respiratory depression.[21] Clinical signs associated with toxicity in dogs include sedation/lethargy, anxiety, ataxia, and/or vomiting. In cats, toxicity effects (eg, anorexia, vomiting, diarrhea, lethargy, ataxia) were noted in 50% of cats in a study.[18]

Treatment recommendations include GI decontamination, if ingestion was recent, and supportive therapy. Supportive care may be required for several days because of the drug's long half-life.

For patients that have experienced or are suspected to have experienced an overdose, it is strongly encouraged that a 24-hour poison consultation center that specializes in providing information specific for veterinary patients be consulted. For general information related to overdose and toxin exposures, as well as contact information for poison control centers, refer to ***Appendix.***

Drug Interactions

In humans, zonisamide is a substrate of CYP3A4.[21] It did not alter P-glycoprotein efflux in an experimental model.[39,40] The following drug interactions have either been reported or are theoretical in humans or animals receiving zonisamide and may be of significance in veterinary patients. Unless otherwise noted, use together is not necessarily contraindicated, but weigh the potential risks and perform additional monitoring when appropriate.

- **CYP3A Inducers** (eg, **dexamethasone, rifampin**): May shorten the half-life of zonisamide and require dose adjustment[8]
- **Carbonic Anhydrase Inhibitors (CAIs;** eg, **acetazolamide)**: Concurrent use with CAIs may increase the risk for metabolic acidosis and kidney stone formation.[41]
- **Phenobarbital**: In dogs, phenobarbital may increase the clearance of zonisamide and decrease the peak concentrations, half-life, and area under the curve (AUC) of zonisamide[12,13,42,43]; this effect persisted up to 10 weeks after phenobarbital discontinuation.[13] Zonisamide dose may need to be increased by up to 50%.[12] In dogs, if zonisamide will be given in conjunction with phenobarbital, it is recommend that zonisamide be given at the high end of the dose range[44-47]; however, one source recommends reducing the phenobarbital dose by 25%.[48]

Laboratory Considerations

- Zonisamide may decrease total T_4 levels.[10]

Dosages

DOGS:

Seizure control (extra-label):

a) For dogs _not_ already receiving phenobarbital, begin with 5 mg/kg PO every 12 hours.[1,4,5,49]

b) For dogs already receiving phenobarbital, begin with 7 – 10 mg/kg PO every 12 hours.[5,49] See ***Monitoring***.

CATS:

Monotherapy for seizure control (extra-label): 2.5 – 5 mg/kg PO every 12 hours[9]

Adjunctive seizure control for cats refractory to phenobarbital (extra-label): Anecdotally, 5 mg/kg PO every 12 to 24 hours.[17,35] From a case series, 6 – 17 mg/kg PO once daily.[6] Because of its long half-life in cats, doses of 5 – 10 mg/kg PO once daily are likely to be appropriate.

Monitoring

- Anticonvulsant efficacy
- Adverse effects (eg, inappetence, vomiting)
- Therapeutic drug monitoring may be useful in veterinary patients when seizures are not controlled. Therapeutic concentrations for zonisamide are thought to be 10 – 40 µg/mL.[1,4,5] One recommendation is to monitor trough levels (ie, within 1 hour prior to next scheduled dose) 1 to 2 weeks after initiating therapy or after dose changes and whenever seizure frequency changes.[5] Consider measuring peak zonisamide concentrations (ie, within 3 to 4 hours postdosing) for patients taking phenobarbital concurrently and that have poor seizure control. Samples obtained from whole blood yield higher zonisamide concentration than samples from plasma.[11] Consult with the veterinary diagnostic laboratory measuring drug concentrations to ensure appropriate samples are collected and to gain guidance on dosage adjustments.
- Baseline and periodic (eg, after 1 month of therapy, then every 3 to 6 months if no problems) CBC and serum chemistry panel[5,7] for hepatic enzyme activity (eg, ALT, ALP), BUN, electrolytes (especially bicarbonate), and venous blood–gas analysis.

Client Information

- This medicine may be given with or without food. If your animal vomits or acts sick after getting it on an empty stomach, give the medicine with food or a small treat.
- Do not stop giving this medicine to your animal without discussing with your veterinarian first, as it may cause seizures to occur.
- Keep a seizure diary to help determine how well this medicine is working.
- Contact your veterinarian immediately if your animal stops eating, has a lack of appetite, becomes overly tired or develops a yellowish tint to the eyes, skin, or gums (jaundice).
- This medicine is considered to be hazardous as defined by the National Institute for Occupational Safety and Health because it may affect the reproductive ability of men or women actively trying to conceive, women who are pregnant or may become pregnant, and women who are breastfeeding. It is recommended that you wear gloves when administering this medication to your animal and wash your hands thoroughly afterwards. If you have questions about this medication's hazards, contact your veterinarian or pharmacist.

Chemistry/Synonyms

Zonisamide, a sulfonamide unrelated to other antiseizure drugs, occurs as a white powder with a pK_a of 10.2. It is moderately soluble in water (0.8 mg/mL).

Zonisamide may also be known as AD-810, CI-912, PD-110843, *Excegran*®, or *Zonegran*®.

Storage/Stability

Zonisamide capsules should be stored at 25°C (76°F); excursions are permitted between 15°C to 30°C (59°F-86°F). Store in a dry place and protect from light.

Compatibility/Compounding Considerations

The preparation and stability of extemporaneously compounded (from 100 mg capsules) zonisamide 10 mg/mL suspensions in simple syrup or methylcellulose (0.5%) have been published.[50] The simple-syrup suspension was stable for at least 28 days when stored at room temperature or under refrigeration and the methylcellulose (0.5%) suspension was stable for 28 days when stored under refrigeration and for 7 days when stored at room temperature.

Dosage Forms/Regulatory Status

VETERINARY-LABELED PRODUCTS: NONE

HUMAN-LABELED PRODUCTS:

Zonisamide Capsules: 25 mg, 50 mg, and 100 mg; *Zonegran*®, generic; (Rx)

References

For the complete list of references, see **wiley.com/go/budde/plumb**

Ophthalmic Agents, Topical

ALISON CLODE, DVM, DACVO
Port City Veterinary Referral Hospital
InTown Veterinary Group
Portsmouth, New Hampshire

The following section lists the majority of veterinary-labeled ophthalmic topical products and some of the more commonly used human-labeled products in veterinary medicine; written by Alison Clode, DVM, DACVO, based on previous work by Gigi Davidson, DICVP, and Michael Davidson, DVM, DACVO. Section editor: James A. Budde, PharmD, DICVP. Drugs are listed in alphabetical order.

For additional information, an excellent review on veterinary ophthalmic pharmacology and therapeutics can be found in the following textbooks: *Slatter's Fundamentals of Veterinary Ophthalmology*, 6th Edition. Maggs DJ, Miller PE, and Ofri R, Eds. Saunders, 2017 and *Veterinary Ophthalmology*, 5th Edition; Gelatt KN, Gilger BC, Kern TJ, Eds. Wiley-Blackwell, 2013.

Routes of Administration for Ophthalmic Drugs

The route of administration selected to deliver therapy for an ocular condition is critical to successful therapy. The following table lists advantages and disadvantages of each route of administration for ocular medications. **NOTE:** Unless otherwise indicated, **small animals** (dogs and cats) receive 1 drop of solutions per administration, or ¼ – ½ inch of ointments per administration; **horses** receive 1 – 2 drops (administered directly to the eye) or 0.1 mL (administered via subpalpebral lavage (SPL) catheter or squirted directly into the eye) of solutions, or ¼ – ½ inch of ointments per administration.

Route	Target tissues	Dosage forms	Advantages	Disadvantages	Comments
Topical	Conjunctiva, cornea, anterior uvea, lids	**Solutions, suspensions**	▪ General ease of administration ▪ Minimal interference with vision ▪ Low incidence of contact dermatitis ▪ Minimal toxicity to interior of eye in presence of penetrating wound	▪ Imprecise dosing ▪ Potential for contamination ▪ Short contact time with eye ▪ Requires more frequent application than ointment ▪ Diluted by tearing ▪ Systemic absorption ▪ Difficult to administer to horses without SPL catheter placement	▪ Doses greater than 1 drop rarely indicated in small animals (maximum tear capacity is 10 – 20 μ Ls, volume of a drop is 25 – 50 μLs) ▪ Allow 5 minutes between drops ▪ Instill in order of least viscous to most, solutions prior to suspensions, and aqueous base prior to oil base ▪ Owners should be counseled to avoid contact of applicator tip with eye.
		Ointments	▪ Longer contact time ▪ Less frequent administration than drops ▪ Protect cornea from drying ▪ Not diluted by tearing	▪ Contribute to volume of ocular discharge ▪ Temporarily blur vision ▪ More difficult to administer ▪ Contact dermatitis ▪ Should not be applied to penetrating corneal wounds as vehicles cause granulomatous uveitis ▪ Difficult to determine exact dose ▪ Metal tubes may fatigue and split before all medication is used.	▪ Owners should be counseled to avoid contact of application tube with eye. ▪ Observe patient for brief period after application due to temporarily blurred vision ▪ Instill solutions and suspensions prior to ointments
Subconjunctival injection	Cornea, anterior uvea	**Sterile solutions and suspensions**	▪ High local concentrations with smaller total dose minimizes systemic effects ▪ Circumvents poor patient compliance with topical administration	▪ Uncertain drug disposition following administration ▪ May create scar tissue ▪ Drug cannot be removed once applied. ▪ Drug vehicle residues may persist. ▪ Inadvertent globe perforation	▪ Indicated for poorly compliant owners and/or uncooperative patients ▪ Indicated for drugs with poor corneal penetration
Intracameral injection	Anterior segment	**Sterile, non-preserved solutions and suspensions**	▪ Allows very high local drug concentrations	▪ Risk for infection ▪ Risk for hemorrhage, retinal detachment, cataract formation, and retinal degeneration ▪ Risk for intraocular toxicity	▪ Indicated to dissolve fibrin and blood clots in the anterior chamber (eg, tPA) ▪ Indicated for intraocular surgery (local anesthetics, viscoelastic substances) ▪ With caution, indicated for severe intraocular infections

Route	Target tissues	Dosage forms	Advantages	Disadvantages	Comments
Intravitreal injection	Posterior segment	**Sterile, non-preserved solutions and suspensions**	▪ Allows very high local drug concentrations	▪ Risk for infection ▪ Risk for hemorrhage, retinal detachment, cataract formation, and retinal degeneration ▪ Risk for intraocular toxicity	▪ Indicated to manage end-stage glaucoma (gentamicin/steroid) ▪ With caution, indicated for severe intraocular infections ▪ With caution, indicated for intractable uveitis
Retrobulbar and peribulbar injection	Posterior segment, optic nerve	**Sterile solutions and suspensions**	▪ Allows very high local drug concentrations	▪ Risk for infection ▪ Risk for globe perforation, optic nerve trauma, retrobulbar hemorrhage	▪ Indicated prior to enucleation (local anesthetics) ▪ Indicated for intraocular surgery when neuromuscular blockade is not possible
Systemic drugs (oral, SC, IM, IV)	Lids, posterior segment, optic nerve, anterior uvea (occasionally)	**Tablets, capsules, sterile solutions and suspensions**	▪ Allows drug penetration to areas topical therapy will not reach	▪ Systemic effects, including toxicities, occur ▪ Limited penetration into the cornea	▪ See specific monographs for use of systemic agents.

Principles of Compounding Ophthalmic Products

GIGI DAVIDSON, BSPharm, DICVP

Physiochemical Considerations for Compounding Ophthalmic Preparations

The availability of suitable commercially available products for every veterinary ophthalmic indication is highly unlikely. Many agents used in veterinary ophthalmology are no longer or were never commercially available. Examples of agents that are commonly used by veterinarians but are not currently commercially available include acetylcysteine, amphotericin B, chloramphenicol, cidofovir, tacrolimus, and voriconazole ophthalmic solutions and/or ointments. Even if commercially available, products may be of inappropriate concentration to achieve a therapeutic effect in a given patient (eg, cyclosporine) or may have agents and excipients that may have adverse effects in animal patients (eg, polymyxin B in cats). In other cases, no product is commercially available and must be compounded from other nonophthalmic drugs or from bulk chemicals (eg, acetylcysteine ophthalmic solution and disodium edetate ophthalmic solution). For these reasons, pharmacists are frequently called upon to compound products to be used in the animal eye. These products may be administered topically in the form of solutions, suspensions, or ointments or administered by periocular or intraocular injection, by drug-implanted collagen shields, or by drug-impregnated disposable contact lens delivery systems. The quality and sterility of these products are critical, and preparations for injection into the eye must meet endotoxin limits. To ensure adequate stability, uniformity, and sterility, both the American Society of Health-Systems Pharmacists and the United States Pharmacopoeia (USP) Convention have published standards (eg, USP General Chapter <797> *Pharmaceutical Compounding—Sterile Preparations*) for pharmacy-prepared ophthalmic products. These standards address the following areas of concern.

Validation of Formulation

Before compounding any preparation for ophthalmic use, the pharmacist should obtain documentation that substantiates the stability, safety, and benefit of the requested formulation. Pharmacists may call the manufacturer of the drug, refer to primary literature, call regional eye centers, or call professional compounding organizations to obtain such information. If no such documentation is available, the pharmacist must employ professional judgment in determining a suitable formulation for ophthalmic administration and then apply the most conservative beyond-use dates established in USP <797>. Factors to consider when making this judgment include sterility, tonicity, endotoxin burden, pH and buffering, the toxicity of the drug, need for preservatives, solubility, stability in the chosen vehicle, particle size in suspensions, viscosity, packaging, and any precautions necessary to keep drug residues from occurring in any food-producing animals.

Documentation

A readily retrievable document (electronic or written), known as a Master Formulation Record, must be maintained for each ophthalmic preparation compounded. This Master Formulation Record must indicate the name of the preparation, the dosage form, the specifications and source of each ingredient used, the weights and measures of each ingredient used, the equipment required, a complete description of each step in the compounding process with a special notation of aseptic techniques to be utilized and which method of sterilization is employed, beyond-use dating, storage requirements, specific packaging requirements, sample label and auxiliary labeling, quality control testing that must be performed (eg, pH, sterility, endotoxin testing for injections), and references for the formula. The expected visual appearance of the final preparation must also be described in the Master Formulation Record. Compounding Records for each compound prepared must also be made (electronic or written) and must include the date of compounding, lot or batch number assigned, the quantity of each ingredient used to prepare the compound, the manufacturer, lot number, and expiration date of each ingredient used, results of any quality testing, a sign-off provision for compounder and checker, the amount compounded, and the projected beyond-use date for the compounded preparation.

Sterility

Ophthalmic dosage forms must be compounded in aseptic conditions. Sterile compounding standards must be consulted in the United States Pharmacopeia General Chapter <797>. Sterility is the most important consideration for ophthalmic products. Contaminated ophthalmic products can result in eye infections leading to blindness or even loss of the eye, especially if pathogens, such as Pseudomonas, are present. Eye infections from contamination can also lead to systemic infections requiring hospitalization and may even result in death. All ophthalmics should be compounded in a primary engineering control (PEC; eg, laminar flow hood or compounding aseptic isolator) that maintains an ISO 5 level of air quality. PECs must be certified at least annually for acceptable performance and maintenance of expected environmental quality. The compounding pharmacist must also be appropriately garbed as described in USP <797> and must use impeccable aseptic technique when handling products intended for use in the eye. All products must be rendered sterile after formulation in the laminar flow hood and maintain sterility throughout their labeled beyond-use date.

Sterilization of the final preparation for ophthalmic solutions is most easily achieved through filtration through vehicle-compatible 0.2 μm sterilizing filters, which also remove particulate matter. Note that this method is not suitable for ophthalmic suspensions or ointments. Ophthalmic suspensions and ointments must be sterilized by other means (such as autoclaving, dry heat, or irradiation) to avoid filtering out active drugs. Preservatives may also be added to prevent bacterial growth, especially if the container is intended for multiple uses. FDA has established maximum potency per unit dose thresholds for preservative agents in FDA-approved ophthalmic products, which can be found at https://www.accessdata.fda.gov/scripts/cder/iig/index.cfm. USP <797>, places limits on beyond-use dates for nonpreserved aqueous ophthalmic preparations. The preservative selected must be compatible with the active drug and excipients as well as nontoxic to the eye or to the patient.

Clarity

Drugs prepared as ophthalmic solutions should meet requirements for particle size and quantity as standardized in USP <789> *Particulate Matter in Ophthalmic Solutions*. Drugs prepared as ophthalmic suspensions cannot be filtered but must be of a particle size that does not irritate or scratch the cornea, typically less than 25 μm. A general rule of thumb is that particles that can be felt when rubbing a drop of the preparation between the thumb and forefinger are too large to be used in the eye. The use of an ointment mill is highly recommended to decrease the particle size for ophthalmic ointments.

Tonicity

Ophthalmic products do not need to be isotonic if the contact time with the cornea is only a few minutes. The eye can tolerate a range of 200 to 600 mOsm/L for short periods of time. Some ophthalmic preparations are intentionally hypertonic in order to reduce corneal edema. For ointments, irrigations, and products that will remain in contact with the eye longer than a few minutes, isotonic products should be used. Hypotonic agents may cause corneal edema, and hypertonic agents may dehydrate the cornea and cause pain. Tear fluid and normal saline have identical osmotic pressures, making 0.9% sodium chloride an excellent vehicle for ophthalmic products. For products that are hypotonic, sodium chloride equivalencies can be used to determine how much sodium chloride is necessary to render the product isotonic. An extensive list of sodium chloride equivalents for drugs has been published.[1]

Buffering and pH

Ophthalmic preparations are generally buffered in a range from 4.5 to 11.5. Buffering is necessary to provide maximal stability of the drug or for the comfort and safety of the patient. Alkaloids, such as atropine and pilocarpine, are usually buffered. If the activity and stability of the drug are not pH-dependent, and the pH of the product is not irritating, then buffers may be omitted from the formulation. Commonly used buffers for ophthalmic preparations include Palitzsch buffer, boric acid buffer, boric acid/sodium borate buffer, sodium acetate/boric acid buffer, Sorensen's modified phosphate buffer, Atkins and Pantin buffer solution, Feldman buffer, and Gilford ophthalmic buffer. Formulations for these solutions and ratios required to achieve the desired pH have been published.[2]

Viscosity Enhancers

Because tears and blinking reflexes reduce the total amount of drug available for penetration, an increase in residence time in the eye will increase drug absorption. Increasing the viscosity of the drug is the most common way to prolong contact time. Methylcellulose derivatives (eg, carboxymethylcellulose, hydroxyethylcellulose, and hydroxypropylmethylcellulose) are the most commonly used agents. Polyvinyl alcohol and polyvinylpyrrolidone have also been used. The FDA has established maximum potency per unit dose thresholds for carboxymethylcellulose and for viscosity agents in FDA-approved ophthalmic products, which can be found at https://www.accessdata.fda.gov/scripts/cder/iig/index.cfm.

Quality Control

Finished preparations should be thoroughly inspected visually for clarity and uniformity of suspension. The pH of the final preparation should always be checked, and the value should be recorded on the master formula record for that batch. Most compounded preparations should have a pH of 5 to 7 unless otherwise indicated for stability or penetration of ocular tissue. Sterility testing and endotoxin testing should be performed where required.

Packaging

Ophthalmic preparations should be packaged in sterile dropper bottles (glass or plastic), or individual doses can be placed in sterile syringes with sterile tip caps. Ointments should be packaged in sterile ointment tubes and heat-sealed. Preparations that are sensitive to light and moisture should be packaged in tight, light-resistant containers.

Beyond-Use Dating

Beyond-use dates must be assigned according to the limits specified in the most current official USP Chapter <797>. Limits are assigned based on the risk for contamination according to the method of preparation, use of nonsterile ingredients, and presence or absence of preservatives.

Considerations for the Use of Ophthalmics in Veterinary Patients

Veterinary patients experience many of the same ophthalmic diseases and conditions as humans, and treatments are often based on human therapy. Animals, however, have a variety of species-related characteristics that might cause human-designed therapies to fail or be toxic. Behavioral characteristics, such as grooming, may significantly reduce the contact time of ophthalmic agents with the eye and increase systemic exposure through ingestion. Anatomical differences, such as size and tear capacity volume, must be considered when formulating ophthalmic therapies. Ease of administration must also be considered. Horses and other large animals may simply elevate their eyes out of a caregiver's reach if ophthalmic treatments are objectionable. Specialized delivery devices have been created to treat these patients. Subcutaneous palpebral lavage systems are tunneled under the skin over the animal's brow into the upper eyelid and allow for the passage of medication through long catheters that are easily reachable by caregivers. Food-producing animals require special consideration, as systemic absorption of ophthalmic agents in animals could result in violative drug residues in food intended for human consumption. Finally, the use of active pharmaceutical ingredient powders (ie, bulk drug substances) to prepare compounds for animals is allowed only under the regulatory discretion provided by CVM FDA's Guidance for Industry #256.

References

For the complete list of references, see **wiley.com/go/budde/plumb**

General Principles of Ocular Penetration

GIGI DAVIDSON, BSPharm, DICVP

Corneal penetration

Drugs must generally be administered topically to treat corneal and intraocular conditions. Although the eye would appear to be an easy target for topical administration, the eye has several anatomical barriers to prevent penetration by foreign substances. Instantaneous tear production, strong blinking reflexes, and alternating layers of lipophilic and hydrophilic tissue all work in conjunction to prevent the entry of foreign substances. The clear tissue known as the cornea covers the visible outer surface of the eye between the lids. The cornea must be clear to allow for vision, and nature has accomplished this by omitting blood vessels in the cornea. Because of this lack of vascular tissue, systemically administered drugs rarely penetrate the cornea. Additionally, the cornea is composed of several layers of lipophilic (outer layers) and hydrophilic (inner layer) tissue. For a topically administered drug to fully penetrate the cornea, the drug must be able to exist in ready equilibrium between both ionized and nonionized forms in order to cross these layers (eg, chloramphenicol, atropine, and pilocarpine). Most antibiotics are water-soluble and will not penetrate the lipophilic outer layer of the cornea unless ulcers are present. Small molecular weight (less than 350) and high local concentration of drugs will increase penetration, however, even if the drugs are ionized and hydrophilic. Thus, topical administration is ideal as it allows for very high local concentrations of the drug on the cornea. For a topically administered drug to reach the anterior chamber and bind to intraocular structures (eg, ciliary body, iris, aqueous humor) to exert a clinical effect, the drug must pass through the cornea. Drugs may also reach the anterior chamber to some extent by passive absorption through the conjunctiva.

Key points for corneal penetration of drugs:

- Lipophilic
- Equilibrium between ionized and nonionized forms
- Small molecular weight (less than 350)
- High local concentrations

Intravitreal Penetration

Topically administered drugs reach the vitreous only in very small concentrations. To treat severe conditions of the anterior chamber (uveitis) as well as intravitreal conditions, drugs may be administered by periocular or intraocular injection. The periocular routes include subconjunctival injection and sub-Tenon's membrane injection, while the intraocular routes are intracameral injection (directly into the aqueous humor) or intravitreal injection (directly into the vitreous humor). Periocular injections can be administered under sedation and topical anesthesia. Intraocular injections are usually only performed while the patient is very heavily sedated or under general anesthesia. Both periocular and intraocular routes bypass the outermost chemical and physical ocular defenses and allow for a better concentration of drugs in the vitreous. The volume of administration for these routes is relatively small: periocular injections should not exceed 0.5 to 1 mL in small animals and 2 mL in large animals, and intraocular injections should not exceed 0.1 mL in small animals and 0.25 mL in large animals because of the risk for increased intraocular pressure. Drugs injected into the eye should be free of preservatives and buffers and must be sterile and meet endotoxin limits for injections.

Route of Therapy for Given Ocular Target

Target tissue	Routes of administration
Eyelids	Topical, systemic
Corneal surface	Topical
Anterior segment	Topical if good penetration or mild disease Systemic if poor penetration or severe disease
Posterior segment	Systemic or intraocular injection (rarely)

Questions to Ponder Prior to Compounding Ophthalmic Products

- Where is the target of therapy? (eyelids, corneal surface, cornea, anterior segment, posterior segment)
- What is the character of the drug?
    - Lipophilic? Hydrophilic?
    - What is the molecular weight?
    - What is the inherent toxicity of the drug to the eye (gentamicin)? To the caregiver (chloramphenicol)? To the patient (polymyxin B in cats)?
    - Are there data to support what concentration is necessary for corneal penetration?
    - Is the drug soluble in a vehicle that is not toxic to the eye?
    - If not soluble, will the particle size of the suspension or the ointment scratch the corneal or conjunctiva?
    - What is the pH of the final product? Is this in an acceptable range to avoid irritation (4.5 to 11.5)?
    - What is the tonicity of the final product? Hypertonic? Hypotonic? How long will the product be in contact with the cornea if not isotonic?
    - Will the viscosity need to be enhanced to prolong contact with the eye? Which agent is compatible?
    - What is the duration of therapy? Will the product require preservation if used long-term and/or multiple times? Which preservative is compatible?

Topical Ophthalmic Agents Listed by Class/Indication

NOTE: Some agents are listed in more than one category.

Analgesics (see also **NSAIDs and Anesthetics, Ocular)**
Morphine
Nalbuphine

Anesthetics, Ocular
Benoxinate
Lidocaine
Proparacaine
Tetracaine

Antibacterials, Single-Agent
Amikacin
Azithromycin
Besifloxacin
Chloramphenicol
Ciprofloxacin
Erythromycin
Gatifloxacin
Gentamicin
Levofloxacin
Moxifloxacin
Ofloxacin
Povidone Iodine
Silver Sulfadiazine
Sulfacetamide
Tobramycin
Vancomycin

Antibiotic Combinations
Bacitracin/Polymyxin B
Neomycin/Polymyxin B/Bacitracin
Neomycin/Polymyxin B/Gramicidin
Oxytetracycline/Polymyxin B

Antibiotic Corticosteroid Combinations
Gentamicin/Prednisolone
Neomycin/Polymyxin B with Dexamethasone
Neomycin/Polymyxin B with Hydrocortisone
Neomycin/Polymyxin B/Bacitracin with Hydrocortisone
Sulfacetamide/Prednisolone
Tobramycin/Dexamethasone
Tobramycin/Loteprednol etabonate

Anticollagenase Agents
Acetylcysteine
Edetate Disodium

Antifungals
Amphotericin B
Itraconazole
Miconazole
Natamycin
Silver Sulfadiazine
Voriconazole

Antihistamines (see also **Mast Cell Inhibitors)**
Alcaftadine
Azelastine
Bepotastine
Cromolyn
Epinastine
Ketotifen
Lodoxamide
Nedocromil sodium
Olapatadine

Antineoplastics
Fluorouracil
Mitomycin

Antiseptics
Povidone Iodine
Silver Sulfadiazine

Antivirals
Acyclovir
Cidofovir
Ganciclovir
Idoxuridine
Trifluridine

Chelating Agents
Edetate Disodium

Corticosteroids, Single-Agent
Dexamethasone
Difluprednate
Fluorometholone
Hydrocortisone
Loteprednol
Prednisolone

Decongestants
Phenylephrine

Diagnostics
Fluorescein Sodium
Lissamine Green
Phenylephrine
Rose Bengal

Fibrinolytics
Alteplase (Tissue Plasminogen Activator [tPA])

Glaucoma, Ocular Hypertension Agents

Alpha-Adrenergic Agonists
Apraclonidine
Brimonidine

Beta-Blockers
Betaxolol
Carteolol
Levobunolol
Timolol

Carbonic Anhydrase Inhibitors
Brinzolamide
Dorzolamide

Miotics, Cholinesterase Inhibitors
Demecarium

Miotics, Direct-Acting
Pilocarpine

Prostaglandin Analogues
Bimatoprost
Latanaprost
Tafluprost
Travoprost

Fixed-Dose Combinations
Brimonidine/Timolol
Brinzolamide/Brimonidine
Dorzolamide/Timolol

Hyperosmotic Agents
Sodium Chloride, Hypertonic

Immunologics
Cyclosporine
Pimecrolimus
Tacrolimus

Irrigating Solutions

Mast Cell Stabilizers
Cromolyn
Nedocromil

Mydriatics and Cycloplegic

Mydriatics
Atropine
Cyclopentolate
Phenylephrine (mydriatic)
Tropicamide

Mydriatic Combinations
Cyclopentolate/Phenylephrine
Hydroxyamphetamine/Tropicamide

Nonsteroidal Anti-Inflammatory Drugs (NSAIDs)
Bromfenac
Diclofenac
Flurbiprofen
Ketorolac
Nepafenac

Ocular Lubricants

Surgical Adjuncts
Fluorouracil (5-FU)
Mitomycin

Acetylcysteine Ophthalmic

(a-***see***-tuhl-***sis***-teen)

Anticollagenase Agent

Prescriber Highlights

- ► Mucolytic agent with antioxidant and anti-inflammatory effects; used to stop digestion of the cornea by collagenases and proteases
- ► Used to improve tear film stability
- ► Foul odor is usual and does not affect drug activity

Uses/Indications

Acetylcysteine is used topically to prevent corneal melting caused by proteinases and collagenases that are present when bacterial and/or fungal infection of ulcers occurs. Acetylcysteine at concentrations greater than 0.5% reduces such enzymatic activity in vitro.[1,2] Additionally, acetylcysteine is beneficial in stabilizing the tear film in quantitative and qualitative tear film deficiency disorders.[3]

Pharmacology/Actions

Acetylcysteine inhibits collagenase activity by reducing disulfide bonds and chelating the cofactors zinc and calcium. Additionally, acetylcysteine inhibits matrix metalloproteinase-9 (MMP-9) production by corneal epithelial cells.[4] Although MMPs play a role in initial corneal wound healing, down-regulation is necessary to prevent corneal digestion and allow corneal wound healing.

Contraindications/Precautions/Warnings

Acetylcysteine is contraindicated in patients that have a history of hypersensitivity to it or any component of the formulation.

Acetylcysteine exposure to the pulmonary tree may result in severe bronchospasm, so this medicine should be used with caution in asthmatic patients.

Adverse Effects

Adverse effects reported in humans or animals include irritation, redness, and tearing of the eyes. If inhaled, acetylcysteine can rarely cause bronchoconstriction and tracheal irritation. Concentrations of acetylcysteine greater than 10% are irritating to the eye.

Acetylcysteine may decrease corneal epithelial migration.[4]

Dosages

Corneal ulcers (extra-label): 1 drop to the affected eye(s) every 1 to 2 hours for the first 24 hours, followed by 3 to 4 times daily until clinical improvement occurs

Dry eye (extra-label): 1 drop to the affected eye(s) every 12 to 24 hours as long as clinical improvement is present

Monitoring

- Clinical efficacy as demonstrated by control of corneal melting and subsequent corneal wound healing, or signs of improved tear film quantity and quality

Client Information

- Use this medication as directed by your veterinarian.
- Wait 5 to 10 minutes after applying this medication before applying any other medications to the eye(s).
- Foul, rotten-egg odor is normal with this drug and does not affect how well it works.
- Store solutions in the refrigerator. Do not freeze.
- Do not use this medication if the color changes, if it becomes cloudy, or if there are particles in the solution.

Storage/Stability

Store this product in the refrigerator (2°C-8°C [35.6°F-46.4°F]) away from moisture and sunlight; do not freeze. Compounded 5% or 10% solutions of acetylcysteine are reported as stable for 60 days in the refrigerator, protected from light.[5]

Compatibility/Compounding Considerations

Acetylcysteine ophthalmic preparations should not be mixed directly with any other ophthalmic medications.

Dosage Forms/Regulatory Status

VETERINARY-LABELED PRODUCTS: NONE

HUMAN-LABELED PRODUCTS: NONE

Acetylcysteine ophthalmic solution (1% to 5%) must be compounded by a qualified compounding pharmacist.

References

For the complete list of references, see **wiley.com/go/budde/plumb**

Acyclovir Ophthalmic

(a-***sye***-klo-veer)

Antiviral

For systemic use of acyclovir, refer to ***Acyclovir***

Prescriber Highlights

- ► Used as an ophthalmic ointment in cats to treat feline herpesvirus-1 (FHV-1) with variable reported efficacy
- ► Requires frequent administration (ie, 5 to 6 times daily)
- ► This medication should NOT be used systemically in cats because of myelotoxicity, poor bioavailability, and poor efficacy against FHV-1.
- ► In the United States, acyclovir is not commercially available as an ophthalmic preparation; it must be compounded.

Uses/Indications

Acyclovir has been used topically as an ophthalmic ointment in cats with feline herpesvirus-1 (FHV-1), although inferior in vitro efficacy against herpesvirus-1 (FHV-1) and requirements for frequent administration limit its clinical usefulness.[1-4]

Pharmacology/Actions

Acyclovir is an acyclic nucleoside analogue that inhibits viral replication through the inhibition of feline herpesvirus-1 (FHV-1) DNA polymerase. In the first of 3 activation steps, acyclovir is selectively phosphorylated by viral thymidine kinase, with the 2 subsequent steps performed by host cell enzymes. Poor efficacy against FHV-1 is due to poor selectivity of viral thymidine kinase for FHV-1.

Contraindications/Precautions/Warnings

Acyclovir is contraindicated in patients that have a history of hypersensitivity to it or drugs like it (valacyclovir) or to any component of the formulation. Systemic use of acyclovir is contraindicated in cats as it could lead to leukopenia, acute anemia, and nephrotoxicity.[5]

Adverse Effects

When acyclovir is used systemically, adverse effects reported in humans or animals include bone marrow suppression, nephrotoxicity, and hepatotoxicity. When acyclovir is applied topically to the eyes, mild stinging and blepharitis may occur after application.

Dosages

Feline herpesvirus-1 (extra-label): ¼ – ½ inch strip to the affected eye(s) 5 times daily[4]; decreased frequency of administration is associated with decreased clinical effect.

Monitoring

- Resolution of clinical signs associated with corneal ulceration, corneal vascularization, conjunctivitis
- Baseline and periodic CBC and serum renal chemistries with prolonged topical therapy

Client Information

- This medicine must be given 5 times daily to be effective.
- Store acyclovir according to package instructions. Discard this medicine if the color changes or if it becomes cloudy.
- Do not allow cats to lick this medicine when grooming.

Storage/Stability

Because this compound must be compounded (in the United States), storage recommendations can vary; follow storage requirements listed on the packaging.

Compatibility/Compounding Considerations

Acyclovir ophthalmic preparations should not be mixed directly with any other ophthalmic medications.

Dosage Forms/Regulatory Status

VETERINARY-LABELED PRODUCTS: NONE

HUMAN-LABELED PRODUCTS: NONE

Acyclovir is not approved in an ophthalmic dosage form, but sterile ophthalmic ointment may be compounded by qualified compounding pharmacists.

References

For the complete list of references, see **wiley.com/go/budde/plumb**

Alcaftadine Ophthalmic

(al-***kaf***-ta-deen) *Lastacaft®*

Antihistamine

Prescriber Highlights

- ► H1 receptor antagonist and mast cell stabilizer
- ► Indicated for allergic conjunctivitis
- ► May cause ocular burning, stinging, and irritation

Uses/Indications

Alcaftadine may be used in animals to alleviate the clinical signs of allergic conjunctivitis. No reports of clinical efficacy or tolerability in animals have been published.

Pharmacology/Actions

Alcaftadine is a histamine-1 (H_1) receptor antagonist and mast cell stabilizer. Inhibition of histamine receptor activation decreases the early-phase response in allergic conjunctivitis. Mast cell stabilization controls the late-phase allergic response in the conjunctiva by inhibiting the release of cytokines and lipid mediators. In humans, itching is prevented within 3 minutes after administration and this effect lasts up to 24 hours.[1]

Contraindications/Precautions/Warnings

Alcaftadine is contraindicated in patients that have a history of hypersensitivity to it or any component of the formulation.

Adverse Effects

Adverse effects reported in humans include irritation, burning and stinging on application, redness, and pruritus. Evaluation of adverse effects has not been performed in animals. Discontinue use if pruritus worsens. Alcaftadine has demonstrated less cytotoxicity in corneal epithelial cell cultures compared with other topical antiallergic medications.[2]

Dosages

Allergic conjunctivitis (extra-label): 1 drop to the affected eye(s) once daily

Monitoring

- Clinical efficacy: resolution of ocular pruritus

Client Information

- Use this medication as directed by your veterinarian.
- Use proper administration techniques to avoid contamination of the solution. Keep the dropper bottle tightly closed when the medication is not in use.
- Wait for 5 minutes after applying this medication before applying any other medications to the eye.
- Store this medication at room temperature away from moisture and sunlight. Do not freeze.
- Do not use this medication if the color changes, becomes cloudy, or if there are particles in the solution.

Storage/Stability

Store this product at controlled room temperature (15°C-25°C [59°F-77°F]) away from moisture and sunlight.

Compatibility/Compounding Considerations

Alcaftadine ophthalmic preparations should not be mixed directly with any other ophthalmic medications.

Dosage Forms/Regulatory Status

VETERINARY-LABELED PRODUCTS: NONE

HUMAN-LABELED PRODUCTS:

Alcaftadine 0.25% Ophthalmic Solution (containing alcaftadine 0.25%; benzalkonium chloride 0.005%; edetate disodium; sodium phosphate, monobasic; purified water; NaCl; NaOH and/or HCl to adjust pH to 7, with osmolality of 290 mOsm/kg); 3 mL in sterile ophthalmic dropper bottle; *Lastacaft®*; (Rx)

References

For the complete list of references, see **wiley.com/go/budde/plumb**

Alteplase Ophthalmic
Tissue Plasminogen Activator (tPA)

(***ahl***-teh-plays) *Activase®*

Fibrinolytic

Prescriber Highlights

- ► Used via intracameral (anterior chamber) injection to lyse intraocular fibrinohemorrhagic clots
- ► Does not lead to fibrinolysis when administered topically
- ► Toxic to the corneal endothelium in intracameral doses greater than 50 µg
- ► Not approved for intraocular injection; must be prepared from the injectable form intended for intracatheter administration

Uses/Indications

Alteplase ophthalmic is most commonly injected intracamerally to lyse intraocular fibrin and blood clots. Intraocular fibrin clots, which form as a result of intraocular inflammation and/or bleeding, can induce synechiae formation and obstruct aqueous humor flow and drainage, thus predisposing affected eyes to the development of glaucoma. Intracameral injection of alteplase in humans following cataract surgery dissolves fibrin clots and reduces posterior synechiae without resulting in re-bleeding.[1]

Immediate postoperative intracameral injection of alteplase in dogs undergoing cataract surgery does not significantly impact postoperative development of anterior chamber fibrin or postoperative ocular hypertension.[2] Topical application of alteplase does not lyse intraocular clots.[3] In dogs and cats, intracameral injection of alteplase 25 µg results in fibrinolysis without corneal toxicity, whereas alteplase doses of 50 µg lead to corneal endothelial toxicity.[3,4]

Pharmacology/Actions

Alteplase (tissue plasminogen activator) is an enzyme (serine protease) that binds to fibrin in clots, which converts the plasminogen component of the clot to plasmin, thus inducing local fibrinolysis.

Contraindications/Precautions/Warnings

Tissue plasminogen activator is contraindicated in patients that have a history of hypersensitivity to it or any component of the formulation. The most frequent adverse reaction associated with thrombolytics in approved indications is bleeding. Caution should be exercised with patients that have thrombocytopenia, other hemostatic defects (including those secondary to severe hepatic or renal disease), or any condition for which bleeding constitutes a significant hazard.[5] Intracameral doses of 50 µg have resulted in toxicity to the corneal epithelium in dogs and cats.[3,4]

Adverse Effects

Adverse effects reported in humans or animals include increased risk for bleeding following administration. Corneal toxicity is likely with intracameral alteplase doses of 50 µg but does not occur with doses of 25 µg.[3,4]

Dosages

Intraocular fibrinolysis (extra-label): Intracameral injection of 0.1 mL of a 0.25 mg/mL sterile solution (25 µg total dose)

Monitoring

- Clinical efficacy
- Resolution of the intraocular clot, which generally occurs within 24 to 48 hours.[6] Observe the patient for signs of re-bleeding.

Client Information

- This medication is not administered outside of veterinary clinics.

Storage/Stability

Refer to individual packaging for storage information; generally, this product is kept under refrigeration (2°C-8°C [36°F-46°F]). Protect the lyophilized material during extended storage from excessive exposure to light. After reconstitution, the drug may be stored between 2°C and 30°C (36°F-86°F) and used within 8 hours. Discard any unused solution after administration is complete. Alteplase contains no preservatives. Store aliquots of reconstituted and further diluted solutions in an ultralow (-80°C [-112°F]) freezer for 45 days unless extended stability and sterility testing has been conducted. Do not re-freeze aliquots once thawed. Discard this product if the color changes, if it becomes cloudy, or if there are particles in the solution.

Compatibility/Compounding Considerations

Alteplase ophthalmic preparations should not be mixed directly (in vitro) with any other ophthalmic medications. It is not available as an ophthalmic injection. For intraocular injection, *Cathflo Activase®* is further diluted with normal saline to a final concentration of 0.25 mg/mL.

Dosage Forms/Regulatory Status

VETERINARY-LABELED PRODUCTS: NONE

HUMAN-LABELED PRODUCTS: NONE

Alteplase is not approved for ophthalmic use.

Cathflo Activase® is available (containing alteplase 2.2 mg [which includes a 10% overfill], L-arginine 77 mg, polysorbate-80 0.2 mg, and phosphoric acid for pH adjustment. Each reconstituted vial will deliver 1 mg/mL of alteplase at a pH of ≈7.3). For intraocular injection, this solution is further diluted with normal saline to a final concentration of 0.25 mg/mL.

Activase® is available as 50 and 100 mg lyophilized powder vials with diluent (sterile water for injection) included.

References

For the complete list of references, see **wiley.com/go/budde/plumb**

Amikacin Ophthalmic

(am-uh-***kay***-sin)

Aminoglycoside Antibiotic

For systemic use, see ***Amikacin***

Prescriber Highlights

- ► Topical ophthalmic aminoglycoside antibiotic used for susceptible ocular bacterial infections that are resistant to other aminoglycoside antibiotics
- ► Amikacin is not commercially available as an ophthalmic preparation in the United States; it must be compounded.
- ► Cats may be more subject to toxic effects of amikacin than other species.

Uses/Indications

Although an amikacin ophthalmic formulation is not commercially available, it can be compounded for use in ophthalmic infections caused by susceptible strains of *Pseudomonas* spp, *Escherichia coli*, *Proteus* spp, *Klebsiella* spp, and other gram-negative bacteria.[1] Amikacin has activity against penicillinase and nonpenicillinase-producing species of *Staphylococcus* spp, but low activity against other gram-positive organisms. Amikacin is less toxic to the posterior segment compared with other aminoglycoside antibiotics and the injectable dosage form is sometimes used as an intravitreal injection to treat bacterial endophthalmitis.

The World Health Organization (WHO) has designated amikacin as a Critically Important, High Priority antimicrobial for human medicine.[2] The Office International des Epizooties (OIE) has designated amikacin as a Veterinary Critically Important Antimicrobial (VCIA) Agent in equine species.[3]

Pharmacology/Actions

Amikacin sulfate, an aminoglycoside, is actively transported into the bacterial cell. It binds to a specific receptor protein on the 30S subunit of bacterial ribosomes. It consequently interferes with an initiation complex between mRNA (messenger RNA) and the 30S subunit, inhibiting protein synthesis by inducing misreading of the mRNA. Aminoglycosides are bactericidal, whereas most other antibiotics that interfere with protein synthesis are bacteriostatic. Although topical administration does not produce substantial aqueous humor concentrations, subconjunctival injections of amikacin solutions may achieve therapeutic concentrations in the cornea and the aqueous humor.[4]

Contraindications/Precautions/Warnings

Amikacin is contraindicated in patients that have a history of hypersensitivity to it or any component of the formulation.

Adverse Effects

When amikacin is used systemically, it can cause nephrotoxicity and neurotoxicity (ototoxicity and vestibular toxicity). Cats are more susceptible to the toxic effects of amikacin, and it is recommended that all patients receiving topical amikacin be monitored for systemic toxicity. Although uncommon, topical aminoglycoside preparations have been reported to cause local reactions such as lid itching, swelling, and conjunctival erythema in humans.

Dosages

Susceptible ocular infections (extra-label): Apply 1 drop to the affected eye(s) every 1 to 2 hours for the first 24 hours, followed by every 4 to 6 hours, pending clinical improvement

Monitoring

- Clinical efficacy: cytology and culture to evaluate for the presence of bacteria. Clinical resolution of signs of ocular surface infection
- Adverse effects (eg, signs of vestibular or auditory toxicity or nephrotoxicity)
- Urinalysis with sediment to check for casts in the urine, which may be an early indicator for nephrotoxicity

Client Information

- Give this medicine as directed by your veterinarian.
- Use proper administration techniques to avoid contamination of the medication. Keep the cap tightly closed when this medicine is not in use.
- Wait for 5 minutes after applying this medicine before applying any other medications to the eye.
- Store this medicine according to the directions on the product label, protected from light. Do not freeze.
- Do not use this medicine if the color changes, if it becomes cloudy, or if there are visible particles in the solution.

Storage/Stability

Store product as directed on the product label, protected from light.

Compatibility/Compounding Considerations

Amikacin sulfate ophthalmic solution should not be mixed directly with any other ophthalmic medications.

Dosage Forms/Regulatory Status

VETERINARY-LABELED PRODUCTS: NONE

HUMAN-LABELED PRODUCTS: NONE

Amikacin is not approved in an ophthalmic dosage form, but sterile solutions of amikacin 1% to 5% may be compounded by qualified compounding pharmacists.

References

For the complete list of references, see **wiley.com/go/budde/plumb**

Amphotericin B Ophthalmic

(am-foe-***ter***-i-sin ***bee***)

Polyene Antifungal

Prescriber Highlights

- ▶ Antifungal agent used to treat ocular surface fungal infections
- ▶ Not commercially available in an ophthalmic dosage form
- ▶ Solutions made from the formulation for IV injection may be used topically or injected subconjunctivally.

Uses/Indications

Amphotericin B is used primarily in horses to treat fungal keratitis. It is effective against yeast and dimorphic fungal organisms, including *Histoplasma* spp, *Coccidioides* spp, *Candida albicans*, *Blastomyces* spp, *Cryptococcus* spp, *Sporothrix* spp, and *Mucor* spp, with variable activity against filamentous organisms (more efficacy for *Aspergillus* spp than *Fusarium* spp).

Amphotericin B has demonstrated in vitro ability to reduce biofilm formation by *Candida* spp, thus decreasing virulence.[1] Topical administration is minimally effective. There is evidence supporting the beneficial effect of subconjunctival and intrastromal injections in humans.[2,3]

Pharmacology/Actions

Amphotericin B acts by binding fungal sterols in cell membranes, resulting in leakage of intracellular constituents. Amphotericin B is usually fungistatic but can be fungicidal in higher concentrations.

Contraindications/Precautions/Warnings

Amphotericin B is contraindicated in patients that have a history of hypersensitivity to it or any component of the formulation.

Adverse Effects

Adverse effects reported in humans or animals include mild burning, stinging, irritation, or redness. Topical application may be toxic to the corneal epithelium,[4] whereas subconjunctival injection of nonliposomal forms may induce ocular irritation.[5]

Dosages

Topical administration (extra-label; 0.15% to 0.5% solution): 1 – 2 drops in the affected eye(s), or 0.1 mL in the subpalpebral lavage (SPL) catheter, every 2 to 6 hours, depending upon severity of infection

Subconjunctival injection (extra-label): Inject 0.3 mL of a 0.5 mg/mL solution under the bulbar conjunctiva every 48 to 96 hours.[2]

Monitoring

- Clinical efficacy and evaluation for clinical signs suggestive of continued infection
- Corneal scraping to determine the resolution of fungal infection

Client Information

- Give this medication to your animal as directed by your veterinarian.
- Use proper administration techniques to avoid contamination of the medication. Keep the cap tightly closed when the medication is not in use.
- Wait for 5 minutes after applying this medication before applying any other medications to the eye.
- Store this medication in a refrigerator protected from light.
- Discard this medication if the color changes, if it becomes cloudy, or if there are particles in the solution.

Storage/Stability

Store the product in the refrigerator (2°C-8°C [35.6°F-46.4°F]) away from moisture and sunlight; do not freeze.

Compatibility/Compounding Considerations

Amphotericin B should not be mixed with salt-containing solutions and should not be mixed directly (in vitro) with any other drugs. Amphotericin B is not available as an ophthalmic preparation but may be prepared as a topical solution (0.15% to 0.5% in dextrose 5% or sterile water) or as a subconjunctival injection (0.5 mg/mL in sterile water). Historically, only the nonliposomal injection was recommended for compounding topical solutions; however, studies demonstrate that topical liposomal amphotericin B ophthalmic solutions are equally effective and less irritating.[6] Although stability is concentration-dependent, most solutions are chemically stable for 7 days in the refrigerator protected from light. Additionally, recent evidence suggests that ophthalmic solutions prepared from liposomal amphotericin B retain chemical potency for up to 6 months.[7]

Dosage Forms/Regulatory Status

VETERINARY-LABELED PRODUCTS:

None are available, but amphotericin B may be compounded by reconstituting the injection as a 0.15% to 0.5% solution and used as an ophthalmic solution. See ***Compatibility/Compounding Considerations***.

HUMAN-LABELED PRODUCTS: NONE

References

For the complete list of references, see **wiley.com/go/budde/plumb**

Apraclonidine Ophthalmic

(a-pra-***cloe***-ni-deen) *Iopidine®*

Alpha-Adrenergic Anti-Glaucoma Agent

Prescriber Highlights

- ► Used to manage glaucoma
- ► Uncommonly used in veterinary species
- ► Do not use in cats, as bradycardia and vomiting may occur.
- ► Results in dry nose and mouth, headaches, cardiac arrhythmias, and fatigue in humans
- ► Tachyphylaxis may occur with long-term use.

Uses/Indications

Apraclonidine ophthalmic may be used as a short-term adjunct for patients that are maximally treated with other anti-glaucoma agents but still require additional lowering of intraocular pressure (IOP). Although reports of the use of apraclonidine in veterinary patients are sparse, one report documented control of IOP for ≈8 months in a dog in conjunction with dorzolamide/timolol ophthalmic medications.[1]

Pharmacology/Actions

Apraclonidine is a relatively selective alpha-2-adrenergic agonist. Activation of presynaptic alpha-2 receptors leads to inhibition of norepinephrine release, and activation of postsynaptic alpha-2 receptors on the nonpigmented ciliary body epithelial cells leads to decreased intracellular cyclic adenosine monophosphate (cAMP), both of which decrease aqueous humor production and intraocular pressure (IOP). Additionally, aqueous humor outflow may be increased by a direct effect on uveoscleral outflow, as well as structural alterations to conventional outflow tract that decrease resistance to outflow. Tachyphylaxis (loss of effect) may occur over time, usually in less than 1 month in humans.

Contraindications/Precautions/Warnings

Apraclonidine is contraindicated in patients that have a history of hypersensitivity to it or any component of the formulation.

Apraclonidine should not be used in patients that are receiving clonidine or monoamine oxidase inhibitors (MAOIs). Do not use apraclonidine in cats, as it can cause bradycardia, hypersalivation, diarrhea, and vomiting.[2] Apraclonidine should be used with caution, if at all, in animals with hepatic or renal insufficiency.

Adverse Effects

Adverse effects reported in humans or animals include conjunctival blanching, eyelid elevation, and mydriasis. Dogs may experience vomiting and diarrhea.[3] Rarely, ophthalmic use of apraclonidine may cause dry mouth, dry eye, tachycardia, hypertension, and tachypnea.

Dosages

Glaucoma (extra-label): 1 drop to the affected eye(s) every 8 to 12 hours

Monitoring

- Clinical efficacy
- Intraocular pressure (IOP)

Client Information

- Use this medication as directed by your veterinarian.
- Use proper administration techniques to avoid contamination of the medication. Keep the cap tightly closed when the medication is not in use.
- Wait for 5 minutes after applying this medication before applying any other medications to the eye.
- Store this medication as directed on the product label away from moisture and sunlight. Do not freeze.
- Do not use this medication if the color changes, if it becomes cloudy, or if there are particles in the solution.

Storage/Stability

Store product in the refrigerator or at controlled room temperature (2°C-25°C [36°F-77°F]) away from moisture and sunlight; do not freeze.

Compatibility/Compounding Considerations

Apraclonidine ophthalmic preparations should not be mixed directly with any other ophthalmic medications.

Dosage Forms/Regulatory Status

VETERINARY-LABELED PRODUCTS: NONE

HUMAN-LABELED PRODUCTS:

Apraclonidine 0.5% Ophthalmic Solution (containing benzalkonium chloride 0.01%, NaCl, sodium acetate, NaOH and/or HCl [pH 4.4 to 7.8], and purified water) in 5 mL and 10 mL sterile ophthalmic dropper bottles; *Iopidine®*; (Rx)

Apraclonidine 1% Ophthalmic Solution (containing benzalkonium chloride 0.01%, NaCl, sodium acetate, NaOH and/or HCl [pH 4.4 to 7.8], and purified water), 0.1 mL in plastic ophthalmic dispensers, packaged 2 per pouch enclosed in foil overwrap; *Iopidine®*; (Rx)

References

For the complete list of references, see **wiley.com/go/budde/plumb**

Atropine Ophthalmic

(***ah***-troe-peen) *Isopto Atropine®*

Mydriatic/Cycloplegic

For systemic use, refer to ***Atropine***

Prescriber Highlights

- ► Used therapeutically to dilate the pupil, paralyze the ciliary body, and stabilize the blood–aqueous barrier in animals with anterior uveitis
- ► Used to perform cycloplegic refraction; not intended to induce mydriasis for diagnostic evaluation of the posterior segment as mydriasis will persist for days to weeks
- ► Use with caution in affected and unaffected eyes of animals diagnosed with primary glaucoma.

Uses/Indications

Atropine ophthalmic is primarily used to reverse miosis and treat ciliary body spasm associated with anterior uveitis. It stabilizes the blood–aqueous barrier and lessens the occurrence of pupillary adhesions by minimizing intraocular exudation of proteins and cells caused by uveal inflammation.

Pharmacology/Actions

Atropine is a nonselective muscarinic receptor antagonist, leading to parasympatholytic activity. In the eye, anticholinergic activity produces mydriasis and cycloplegia by blocking stimulation of the iris sphincter muscle and the ciliary body accommodative muscle. It induces mydriasis in ≈1 hour, and the effects may persist up to 120 hours in dogs, 144 hours in cats, and days to weeks in horses.[1]

Contraindications/Precautions/Warnings

Atropine ophthalmic is contraindicated in patients that have a history of hypersensitivity to it or any component of the formulation. Atropine ophthalmic should also not be used in patients with primary glaucoma or in dogs that are predisposed to developing glaucoma, as elevation in intraocular pressure (IOP) may result.[2] Atropine ophthalmic may induce colic in horses secondary to systemic absorption, but this is rare.[3] Avoid using the ointment formulation on penetrating corneal wounds because of the potential for intraocular damage associated with exposure of the ointment's inactive ingredients to the intraocular environment.

Adverse Effects

Adverse effects reported in animals include sensitivity to bright light or sunlight and burning and irritation upon application. Cats and dogs may experience transiently decreased tear production; thus, concurrent administration of topical tear replacers is appropriate. Hypersalivation, which may occur because of drainage of the bitter-tasting solution into the nasopharynx, can be avoided by use of ointment formulations. Atropine ophthalmic causes tachycardia in healthy dogs.[4]

Dosages

Mydriasis and cycloplegia (extra-label): Initially, 1 drop or a ¼ – ½ inch strip to the affected eye(s) 2 to 3 times daily and then once daily or every other day afterward to achieve mydriasis

Monitoring

- Clinical efficacy: confirm continued mydriasis and degree of patient comfort

Client Information

- Wash your hands prior to and after applying this medicine to your animal's eye(s) to prevent human exposure and unintended exposure of your animal's eye.
- Excessive drooling may occur (especially in cats).
- Use proper administration techniques to avoid contamination of the medication. Do not touch the dropper (or ointment) tip or allow it to touch your animal's eye or any other surface to prevent contamination.
- Keep the cap tightly closed when this medicine is not in use.
- This medicine may cause your animal's tear production to decrease. Your veterinarian may also recommend the use of an over-the-counter (OTC) tear replacement solution or ointment for your animal's eye(s) to alleviate this problem.
- Wait for 5 to 10 minutes after applying atropine before applying any other medications to the eye.

Storage/Stability

Store at controlled room temperature (20°C-25°C [68°F-77°F]) away from moisture and sunlight; do not freeze.

Compatibility/Compounding Considerations

Atropine sulfate ophthalmic preparations should not be mixed directly with any other ophthalmic medications.

Dosage Forms/Regulatory Status

VETERINARY-LABELED PRODUCTS: NONE

HUMAN-LABELED PRODUCTS: NONE

Atropine Sulfate 1% Ophthalmic Ointment USP (containing atropine sulfate 10 mg; white petrolatum; mineral oil; lanolin oil; purified water) in 3.5 g ophthalmic tubes; generic; (Rx)

Atropine Sulfate 1% Ophthalmic Solution, USP (containing atropine sulfate 20 mg; benzalkonium chloride 0.01%, dibasic sodium phosphate; edetate disodium; hypromellose (2910); monobasic sodium phosphate; NaOH and/or HCl to adjust pH to 3.5 to 6; water for injection), 2 mL, 5 mL, and 15 mL in sterile ophthalmic dropper bottles; *Isopto Atropine*®, generic; (Rx)

References

For the complete list of references, see **wiley.com/go/budde/plumb**

Azelastine Ophthalmic

(a-za-***las***-teen)

Antihistamine

Prescriber Highlights

- ▶ Used for the treatment of allergic conjunctivitis
- ▶ Rapid onset of action (3 minutes) and long duration of action (8 hours) in humans

Uses/Indications

Azelastine is used to relieve pruritus caused by allergic conjunctivitis. No studies describing the efficacy and safety of azelastine after topical administration have been performed in veterinary patients.

Pharmacology/Actions

Azelastine is an H_1- and H_2-receptor antagonist, which also inhibits the release of histamine from mast cells and the production of leukotrienes involved in the allergic response.[1] Azelastine has a rapid onset of action (3 minutes) and a long duration of antipruritic action (8 hours) in humans.

Contraindications/Precautions/Warnings

Azelastine is contraindicated in patients that have a history of hypersensitivity to it or any component of the formulation.

Adverse Effects

Adverse effects reported in humans include transient burning or stinging upon instillation in the eye (greater than experienced with other ophthalmic solutions, possibly related to the moderate pH of 5 to 6.5) and a bitter taste. Asthma, conjunctivitis, dyspnea, eye pain, fatigue, influenza-like symptoms, pharyngitis, pruritus, rhinitis, and temporary blurring are other reported adverse effects (some of these effects were indistinguishable from the disease being treated).[2]

Dosages

Allergic conjunctivitis (extra-label): 1 drop to the affected eye(s) 2 times daily

Monitoring

- Clinical efficacy. Resolution of pruritus and conjunctivitis

Client Information

- Use this medicine as directed by your veterinarian.
- Use proper administration techniques to avoid contamination of the medication. Keep the cap tightly closed when not in use.
- Wait for 5 minutes after applying this medication before applying any other medications to the eye.
- Store this medicine in the refrigerator or at room temperature away from moisture and sunlight. Do not freeze.
- Do not use if the color changes, becomes cloudy, or if there are particles in the solution.

Storage/Stability

Store upright between 2°C and 25°C (36°F-77°F) away from moisture and sunlight.

Compatibility/Compounding Considerations

Azelastine ophthalmic preparations should not be mixed directly (in vitro) with any other ophthalmic medications.

Dosage Forms/Regulatory Status

VETERINARY-LABELED PRODUCTS: NONE

HUMAN-LABELED PRODUCTS:

Azelastine HCl 0.05% Ophthalmic Solution (containing 0.5 mg azelastine hydrochloride; disodium edetate dehydrate; hypromellose; sorbitol solution; NaOH; water for injection; benzalkonium chloride

0.125 mg; pH of ≈5 to 6.5; osmolarity of ≈271 – 312 mOsm/kg), 6 mL in a sterile ophthalmic dropper bottle; generic; (Rx)

References

For the complete list of references, see **wiley.com/go/budde/plumb**

Azithromycin Ophthalmic

(uh-***zith***-roe-***mye***-sin) *Azasite®*

Macrolide Antibiotic

For systemic use, refer to ***Azithromycin***

Prescriber Highlights

- ▶ Used to treat ocular surface bacterial infections
- ▶ May cause reversible phospholipid accumulation in the cornea
- ▶ Prolonged use of antibiotic preparations may result in overgrowth of nonsusceptible organisms, including fungi.

Uses/Indications

Azithromycin ophthalmic solution is used to treat susceptible strains of *Haemophilus* spp, *Streptococcus* spp, and *Staphylococcus* spp. In vitro efficacy against some *Chlamydia* spp and *Mycoplasma* spp has also been reported.[1] Reports of clinical efficacy and/or toxicity/tolerability of azithromycin ophthalmic in animals are not available.

The World Health Organization (WHO) has designated azithromycin as a Critically Important, Highest Priority antimicrobial for human medicine.[2]

Pharmacology/Actions

Azithromycin is a bacteriostatic macrolide antibiotic that binds to the 50S ribosomal subunit of susceptible microorganisms and interferes with microbial protein synthesis.

Contraindications/Precautions/Warnings

Azithromycin ophthalmic solution is contraindicated in patients that have a history of hypersensitivity to it or any component of the formulation. Azithromycin ophthalmic solution is indicated for topical ophthalmic use only; it should not be administered systemically, injected subconjunctivally, or introduced directly into the anterior chamber of the eye.[1]

Adverse Effects

Adverse effects reported in humans include burning, stinging, and irritation on application. Systemic azithromycin has also caused phospholipidosis (intracellular phospholipid accumulation) in dogs, mice, and rats, and cytoplasmic microvacuolation of the cornea was observed in rabbits following ocular administration, which resolved when the medication was discontinued.[1]

Dosages

Bacterial conjunctivitis (extra-label): 1 drop to the affected eye(s) 2 times daily the first 2 days, followed by once daily for 5 days

Monitoring

- Clinical efficacy: resolution of bacterial conjunctivitis

Client Information

- Give this medicine exactly as your veterinarian has prescribed.
- Wash your hands before applying this medicine to your animal's eye(s).
- Be sure you understand how to give this medicine to your animal to avoid contamination of the medicine, which could worsen the eye condition.
- Wait for 5 minutes after applying this medicine before applying any other medicines to the eye.
- Keep the cap on the medicine tightly closed when it is not in use.
- Store this medicine in the refrigerator. After opening, the medicine can be stored at room temperature. Discard the medicine 14 days after opening or if if the color of the solution changes, if it becomes cloudy, or if there are particles.

Storage/Stability

Store this product in the refrigerator (2°C-8°C [36°F-46°F]) away from moisture and sunlight; do not freeze. Discard this product 14 days after opening.

Compatibility/Compounding Considerations

Azithromycin ophthalmic preparations should not be mixed directly with any other ophthalmic medications.

Dosage Forms/Regulatory Status

VETERINARY-LABELED PRODUCTS: NONE

HUMAN-LABELED PRODUCTS:

Azithromycin 1% Ophthalmic Solution (containing azithromycin 10 mg [1%]; mannitol; citric acid; sodium chloride; poloxamer 407; polycarbophil; edetate disodium; water for injection; NaOH to adjust pH), 2.5 mL in a sterile ophthalmic dropper bottle; *Azasite®*; (Rx)

References

For the complete list of references, see **wiley.com/go/budde/plumb**

Benoxinate Ophthalmic
Oxybuprocaine Ophthalmic

(bin-***ak***-sin-ate) *Altafluor®, Fluress®, Flurox®*

Topical Ocular Anesthetic

Prescriber Highlights

- ▶ Rapid-acting topical anesthetic used for ocular diagnostic procedures
- ▶ Should never be prescribed for therapeutic administration
- ▶ Only available in combinations with the vital dye fluorescein sodium
- ▶ Chronic use results in tear film instability and corneal epithelial and stromal damage, which may progress to vision loss.
- ▶ Less burning, stinging, and chemosis than tetracaine

Uses/Indications

Like other topical anesthetic agents, benoxinate is indicated for use in ophthalmic diagnostic procedures, including measurement of intraocular pressure (tonometry), ocular ultrasonography, gonioscopy, and corneal and conjunctival sampling for cytology and culture. Benoxinate is also indicated for therapeutic procedures in the hospital, including removing foreign bodies and sutures from the cornea, eyelid and conjunctival surgery, corneal grafting procedures, and cataract extraction. It is only available in ophthalmic solutions combined with the vital dye fluorescein. In dogs, benoxinate causes fewer adverse reactions (burning, stinging, and chemosis) than tetracaine.[1,2] Benoxinate has demonstrated comparable corneal anesthesia to that achieved by topical proparacaine in normal horses and donkeys.[3]

Pharmacology/Actions

Benoxinate induces local anesthesia by inhibiting neuronal depolarization, thus preventing the generation of an action potential. The action occurs due to the binding of the local anesthetic molecule to the intracellular portion of the voltage-gated sodium channel within the neuron, thus inhibiting the intracellular movement of sodium. Variations in the structure of different local anesthetics influence their relative potencies; however, all local anesthetics have decreased efficacy in the acidic environment of inflammation, whereas alkaline environments improve intracellular penetration, thus increasing efficacy. The duration of action is dose- and species-dependent, with a total duration of corneal anesthesia following a single drop of 55 minutes in dogs and 45 minutes in cats.[1,2]

Contraindications/Precautions/Warnings

Benoxinate is contraindicated in patients that have a history of hypersensitivity to it or any component of the formulation. It should never be prescribed as an ocular analgesic as prolonged use of a topical ocular anesthetic will produce significant corneal epithelial and stromal disease, as well as tear film instability, and may result in loss of vision.[4]

Adverse Effects

Benoxinate is usually well-tolerated, but local irritation (conjunctival redness, lacrimation, or squinting) may occur several hours after administration. These signs occur less frequently with benoxinate than with tetracaine.[3] Although patients that are sensitive to other local anesthetics may be less likely to react to benoxinate, local or systemic sensitivity may still occur and rarely manifest as a pseudoallergic (anaphylactoid) reaction mimicking an IgE-mediated vasodilatory event. Cardiovascular, respiratory, and CNS depressant effects that may result from local anesthetics are extremely rare with appropriate use of topical local anesthetics. However, care should be exercised when administering to small veterinary patients (ie, puppies, kittens, "pocket pets") or those with pathways that may increase absorption (ie, amphibians). Its use as a therapeutic analgesic leads to superficial punctate keratitis, which may advance to diffuse necrotizing keratitis, severe infiltrative keratitis, persistent epithelial defects, or damage to Descemet's membrane.[4]

Dosages

Ophthalmic procedures requiring local anesthesia (extra-label): 1 – 2 drops to the target eye(s) prior to examination or performing procedure. May repeat adding 1 drop every 5 to 10 minutes for 2 to 3 additional times. With further applications, the duration of corneal anesthesia can be extended to 55 minutes in dogs. Additional doses should be avoided in small patients (ie, puppies, kittens, "pocket pets").

Monitoring

- Onset of action as indicated by awake patient, permitting diagnostic procedures to be performed
- Onset of action as indicated by a reduction in anesthetic requirements when administered pre- and intra-operatively
- Damage to corneal epithelium indicated by a positive fluorescein stain test

Client Information

- Animal owners must not administer benoxinate in the home. It is reserved for diagnostic procedures at veterinary clinics.

Storage/Stability

Store the product in the refrigerator (2°C-8°C [36°F-46°F]). Once opened, the medication can be stored at room temperature for up to 1 month.[5] Keep this product away from moisture and sunlight; do not freeze.

Discard this medication if the color of the solution changes, if it becomes cloudy, or if it develops particles.

Compatibility/Compounding Considerations

Benoxinate ophthalmic preparations should not be mixed directly (in vitro) with any other ophthalmic medications.

Dosage Forms/Regulatory Status

VETERINARY-LABELED PRODUCTS: NONE

HUMAN-LABELED PRODUCTS:

Benoxinate HCl 0.4% and Fluorescein Sodium 0.25% (containing fluorescein sodium 2.5 mg; benoxinate hydrochloride 4 mg; boric acid; povidone; purified water; HCl to adjust pH to 4.3 to 5.3; chlorobutanol 1%); 5 mL in sterile ophthalmic dropper bottles; *Altaflu-or*®, *Fluress*®, *Flurox*®; (Rx). No benoxinate ophthalmic products have been approved by the US FDA.

References

For the complete list of references, see **wiley.com/go/budde/plumb**

Bepotastine Ophthalmic

(be-po-***tas***-teen) *Bepreve*®

Antihistamine

Prescriber Highlights

- ► H_1 receptor antagonist used in the management of allergic conjunctivitis

Uses/Indications

Bepotastine is used to relieve pruritus caused by allergic conjunctivitis. The efficacy and safety of topical bepotastine has not been evaluated in veterinary species.

Pharmacology/Actions

Bepotastine is a direct histamine-1 (H_1) antagonist and mast cell stabilizer, with inhibitory effects on other inflammatory mediators, such as leukotrienes and eosinophils. The onset of action (control of itching) in humans is 15 minutes following instillation, with a duration of effect up to 8 hours.[1]

Contraindications/Precautions/Warnings

Bepotastine is contraindicated in patients that have a history of hypersensitivity to it or any component of the formulation. Use it with caution in pregnant or nursing patients.[2]

Adverse Effects

Adverse effects reported in humans include transient burning or stinging upon instillation in the eye, nasal irritation, and a bad taste in the mouth.[1]

Dosages

Allergic conjunctivitis (extra-label): 1 drop to the affected eye(s) 2 times daily

Monitoring

- Clinical efficacy: resolution of pruritus and conjunctivitis

Client Information

- Use this medicine as directed by your veterinarian.
- Use proper administration techniques to avoid contamination of the medication. Keep the cap tightly closed when the medication is not in use.
- Wait for 5 minutes after applying this medication before applying any other medications to the eye.
- Store at room temperature away from moisture and sunlight. Do not freeze.
- Do not use this medicine if the color changes, if it becomes cloudy, or if there are particles in the solution.

Storage/Stability

Store at controlled room temperature (15°C-25°C [59°F-77°F]) away from moisture and sunlight; do not freeze.

Compatibility/Compounding Considerations

Bepotastine ophthalmic preparations should not be mixed directly (in vitro) with any other ophthalmic medications.

Dosage Forms/Regulatory Status

VETERINARY-LABELED PRODUCTS: NONE

HUMAN-LABELED PRODUCTS:

Bepotastine Besilate 1.5% Ophthalmic solution (containing bepotastine besilate 15 mg; benzalkonium chloride 0.005%; monobasic sodium phosphate dehydrate; NaCl; NaOH to adjust pH to 6.8; water for injection, USP, with an osmolality of 290 mOsm/kg), 5 mL and 10 mL in sterile ophthalmic dropper bottles; *Bepreve®*; generic (Rx)

References

For the complete list of references, see **wiley.com/go/budde/plumb**

Besifloxacin Ophthalmic

(be-si-***flocks***-a sin) *Besivance®*

Fourth-Generation Fluoroquinolone Antibiotic

Prescriber Highlights

- ► Available in ophthalmic formulation only
- ► Used to treat bacterial conjunctivitis or keratitis
- ► Physically incompatible with many drugs; therefore, should not be directly mixed with other ophthalmic medications
- ► As with other topical antibiotics, prolonged use may result in overgrowth of nonsusceptible organisms.

Uses/Indications

Besifloxacin ophthalmic is used to treat bacterial conjunctivitis and keratitis. It is generally effective against gram-negative, gram-positive, and anaerobic organisms, particularly *Staphylococcus* spp, *Streptococcus* spp, *Haemophilus* spp, and *Pseudomonas aeruginosa*.

Pharmacology/Actions

Besifloxacin is a fourth-generation fluoroquinolone antibiotic that acts, via inhibition of both topoisomerase II (DNA gyrase) and topoisomerase IV, to impair bacterial DNA synthesis. Inhibition of both enzymes decreases the development of resistance to this class of fluoroquinolones in general, and organisms have demonstrated even lower resistance to besifloxacin due to this balanced inhibition.[1] Besifloxacin achieves superior aqueous humor concentrations in normal dogs relative to gatifloxacin and moxifloxacin (other fourth-generation fluoroquinolones)[2]; however, other studies have demonstrated effective ocular surface concentrations of besifloxacin following topical administration, with lesser aqueous humor concentrations.[1] The currently available formulation of besifloxacin is formulated with a mucoadhesive polymer that increases contact time with the ocular surface, which is favorable for concentration-dependent fluoroquinolone antibiotics.[1,3]

Contraindications/Precautions/Warnings

Besifloxacin is contraindicated in patients with a history of hypersensitivity to besifloxacin, other fluoroquinolones, or any component of the formulation. For topical ophthalmic use only, not for injection subconjunctivally or into the anterior chamber of the eye.[3] Fluoroquinolone-induced retinal toxicity in domestic cats has not been demonstrated with this product.

Adverse Effects

Adverse effects reported in humans or animals include blurred vision, tearing, eye pain, conjunctival redness, itching, and a bad taste in the mouth. Temporary punctate keratitis, which resolves with discontinuation of medication, has also been reported rarely in humans.[4]

Dosages

Conjunctivitis (extra-label): 1 drop to the affected eye(s) 3 times daily

Keratitis (extra-label): 1 drop to the affected eye every 2 to 8 hours

Monitoring

- Clinical efficacy. Corneal cytology with culture and susceptibility testing to evaluate for the persistence of bacteria, and evaluation for clinical signs suggestive of continued infection

Client Information

- Give this medicine to your animal as directed by your veterinarian. Be sure you understand how to safely give to your animal.
- Invert the bottle and shake once before use. Do not give your animal this medicine if the color changes, if it becomes cloudy, or if particles are seen in the solution.
- Crystals may develop on the surface of the eye during treatment but will not cause harm.
- Do not mix this medicine with other eye medications.
- If you are giving your animal other eye medications, wait 5 minutes after applying this medicine before applying any other medications to the eye.
- Do not freeze this medicine. Store this medicine at room temperature, away from light and moisture.

Storage/Stability

Store this product at controlled room temperature 20°C to 25°C (68°F-77°F) away from moisture and sunlight; do not freeze.

Compatibility/Compounding Considerations

Fluoroquinolone antibiotics interact with many other drugs, including those containing cations (eg, iron, aluminum, magnesium, calcium). Besifloxacin should not be mixed with any other drugs.

Dosage Forms/Regulatory Status

VETERINARY-LABELED PRODUCTS: NONE

HUMAN-LABELED PRODUCTS:

Besifloxacin 0.6% (6 mg/mL) Ophthalmic Suspension (containing besifloxacin 0.6%; benzalkonium chloride 0.01%; polycarbophil; mannitol; poloxamer 407; NaCl; edetate disodium dehydrate; NaOH; water for injection, with an osmolality of ≈290 mOsm/kg), 5 mL in a sterile ophthalmic dropper bottle; *Besivance®*; (Rx)

References

For the complete list of references, see **wiley.com/go/budde/plumb**

Betaxolol Ophthalmic

(be-***tax***-uh-lol) *Betoptic®, Betoptic S®*

Beta-1-Selective Beta-Adrenergic Blocker

Prescriber Highlights

- ► Beta-blocker that decreases intraocular pressure (IOP) as a treatment for glaucoma
- ► More effective reduction in IOP using 0.5% solution relative to 0.25% solutions in veterinary patients; however, increased risk for adverse effects exists when using the higher concentration
- ► Delays onset of glaucoma in the normal eye of dogs with unilateral glaucoma
- ► Use with caution in asthmatic patients because of the potential to induce bronchospasm.

Uses/Indications

Betaxolol is a beta-1-selective beta-blocker used to reduce intraocular pressure (IOP) in primary glaucoma and as prophylaxis to prevent glaucoma in the normal eye of animals with unilateral glaucoma.[1] In combination with tafluprost, betaxolol leads to a greater reduction of IOP in normal dogs compared to timolol.[2]

Pharmacology/Actions

Betaxolol works through the blockade of the beta-receptors in the ciliary body epithelium to reduce intraocular pressure (IOP) by decreasing aqueous humor production. Several mechanisms have been postulated for this effect, including beta-blockade, particularly beta-2 receptors, reducing norepinephrine-induced tonic sympathetic stimulation, leading to decreased activation of cAMP in the ciliary body; inhibition of Na+K+ATPase activity; or vasoactive mechanisms on the iris and ciliary body. Betaxolol also inhibits glutamine-induced increases in intracellular calcium and sodium, thereby providing a potential protective effect against ischemic insult to the retina.[3] Because of betaxolol's beta-1-selective activity, its hypotensive effect may be less than that of nonselective beta-blockers, as beta-2 blockade is of greater importance to aqueous humor production.

Contraindications/Precautions/Warnings

Betaxolol is contraindicated in patients that have a history of hypersensitivity to it or any component of the formulation. Betaxolol should be used carefully in patients with heart block, bradycardia, heart failure, asthma, chronic bronchitis, or other cardiopulmonary conditions, although systemic cardiopulmonary adverse effects are not likely with ocular use of betaxolol. Beta-blockers should be used with caution in patients with diabetes mellitus, as these drugs may mask signs of acute hypoglycemia. Beta-blockers should be used with caution in patients with hyperthyroidism, as these drugs may mask indications of this condition. Abrupt discontinuation of beta blockers should be avoided.

Adverse Effects

Adverse effects reported in humans or animals include transient burning, stinging, and irritation upon application to the eye, as well as keratitis, anisocoria, and photophobia. Bradycardia, heart block, congestive heart failure, pulmonary distress, insomnia, dizziness, headaches, lethargy, and depression have been reported in humans. Other topically applied beta-blockers produce significant reductions in heart rate in healthy cats.[4]

Dosages

Glaucoma (extra-label): 1 drop to the affected eye(s) twice daily

Monitoring

- Clinical efficacy
- Monitor intraocular pressure (IOP)
- Observe asthmatic and diabetic patients for respiratory difficulty or acute hypoglycemia, respectively.

Client Information

- Use this medication as directed by your veterinarian.
- Suspension formulations must be shaken well before using.
- Use proper administration techniques to avoid contamination of the medication. Keep the cap tightly closed when the medication is not in use.
- Wait for 5 minutes after applying this medication before applying any other medications to the eye.
- Store this medication in the refrigerator or at room temperature away from moisture and sunlight. Do not freeze.
- Do not use this medication if the color changes, if it becomes cloudy, or if there are particles in the solution.

Storage/Stability

Store this product in the refrigerator (2°C-8°C [36°F-46°F]) or at controlled room temperature (20°C-25°C [68°F-77°F]) away from moisture and sunlight; do not freeze.

Compatibility/Compounding Considerations

Betaxolol ophthalmic preparations should not be mixed directly with any other ophthalmic medications.

Dosage Forms/Regulatory Status

VETERINARY-LABELED PRODUCTS: NONE

HUMAN-LABELED PRODUCTS:

Betaxolol HCl 0.5% Ophthalmic Solution (containing 5.6 mg betaxolol HCl equivalent to 5 mg betaxolol; benzalkonium chloride 0.01%; edetate disodium; NaCl, HCl, and/or NaOH to adjust pH; purified water) in 2.5 mL, 5 mL, 10 mL, and 15 mL sterile ophthalmic dropper bottles; *Betoptic*®, generic; (Rx)

Betaxolol HCl 0.25% ophthalmic solution (containing betaxolol HCl 2.8 mg equivalent to 2.5 mg betaxolol; benzalkonium chloride 0.01%; mannitol; poly (styrene-divinyl benzene); edetate disodium; NaOH and/or HCl to adjust pH; purified water) in sterile 10 mL and 15 mL ophthalmic dropper bottles; *Betoptic*®*-S*; (Rx)

References

For the complete list of references, see **wiley.com/go/budde/plumb**

Bimatoprost Ophthalmic

(bi-***mat***-oh-prost) *Lumigan*®*, Latisse*®*, Durysta*®

Prostaglandin Analogue Anti-Glaucoma Agent

Prescriber Highlights

- Used to decrease intraocular pressure (IOP) in patients with primary glaucoma or ocular hypertension
- Not effective for feline glaucoma, and unlikely to be effective for equine glaucoma
- Do not use if intraocular inflammation is present, as the drug may worsen the inflammation or lead to pupillary block glaucoma
- Twice-daily dosing results in less fluctuation of IOP.
- Lower concentration of benzalkonium chloride than latanoprost or travoprost; therefore, bimatoprost causes less ocular discomfort on administration
- May increase brown pigment, resulting in discoloration of light-colored irises and increased eyelash growth

Uses/Indications

Bimatoprost is used to lower intraocular pressure (IOP) in the management of glaucoma in dogs. It is indicated as a treatment for primary glaucoma; however, secondary glaucomas (caused by uveitis, lens luxation, or intraocular tumor) are not appropriately treated with bimatoprost. Due to differences in intraocular receptors, bimatoprost is ineffective in lowering the IOP in cats, although it does produce miosis.[1,2] Although once-daily administration is indicated in humans, twice-daily administration has been demonstrated to more consistently lower IOP in dogs.[3] Significant miosis also occurs following administration.[3] An intracameral sustained-release bimatoprost implant has demonstrated increased IOP-lowering efficacy in comparison with topical administration of varied concentrations of bimatoprost in normotensive dogs.[4]

Pharmacology/Actions

Bimatoprost, a prostaglandin analogue, is a synthetic structural analogue of prostaglandin derived from a fatty acid precursor, anandamide. It selectively mimics the effects of naturally occurring prostamides. Bimatoprost is believed to lower intraocular pressure (IOP) by increasing the outflow of aqueous humor through both the trabecular meshwork and uveoscleral routes.[5] In humans, the onset of action is in 4 hours, with a total duration of 8 to 12 hours.

Contraindications/Precautions/Warnings

Bimatoprost is contraindicated in patients that have a history of hypersensitivity to it or any component of the formulation. Bimatoprost should be used with caution in the presence of anterior uveitis and secondary glaucoma, particularly in cases already exhibiting significant miosis, as this treatment may exacerbate miosis, promote synechiae formation, and worsen glaucoma. Bimatoprost should also be used with caution in dogs with primary anterior lens luxation, as the miosis that results may trap the lens and/or vitreous within the pupillary aperture, thus creating pupillary block glaucoma. Bimatoprost is not contraindicated in dogs with secondary posterior lens luxation, as the miosis may (favorably) trap the lens in the posterior segment.

Adverse Effects

Adverse effects reported in humans or animals include stinging, burning, erythema (conjunctival hyperemia), and irritation on administration. Macular edema has been reported in humans using bimatoprost. Bimatoprost may cause increased eyelash growth, may worsen intraocular inflammation through prostaglandin-mediated mechanism, and/or cause darkening of the iris through direct stimulation of iris melanocytes.

Dosages

Glaucoma (extra-label):

a. Solution: Initially, 1 drop to the affected eye(s) once daily in the evening; increase to twice daily as glaucoma progresses. Twice-daily administration of bimatoprost may be more effective in dogs.
b. Sustained-release implant: Intracameral injection of the sustained-release implant is performed using the associated ophthalmic drug delivery system. Repeat implantation should not be performed in an eye that has received a prior implant.

Monitoring

- Clinical efficacy measured through sustained reduction of intraocular pressure (IOP)

Client Information

- Use this medication as directed by your veterinarian.
- Use proper administration techniques to avoid contamination of the medication. Keep the cap tightly closed when the medication is not in use.
- Wait for 5 minutes after applying this medication before applying any other medications to the eye.
- Store this medication in the refrigerator or at room temperature away from moisture and sunlight. Do not freeze.
- Do not use this medication if the color changes, if it becomes cloudy, or if there are particles in the solution.

Storage/Stability

Store solution in the refrigerator or at controlled room temperature (2°C-25°C [36°F-77°F]) away from moisture and sunlight; do not freeze.

Store implant in the refrigerator (2°C-8°C [36°F-46°F]).

Compatibility/Compounding Considerations

Bimatoprost ophthalmic preparations should not be mixed directly with any other ophthalmic medications.

Dosage Forms/Regulatory Status

VETERINARY-LABELED PRODUCTS: NONE

HUMAN-LABELED PRODUCTS:

Bimatoprost 0.01% Ophthalmic Solution (containing bimatoprost 0.1 mg/mL; benzalkonium chloride 0.02%; NaCl; sodium phosphate, dibasic; citric acid; purified water; NaOH and/or HCl to adjust pH to 6.8 to 7.8, with an osmolality of 290 mOsm/kg) in sterile 2.5 mL, 5 mL, and 7.5 mL ophthalmic dropper bottles; *Lumigan®*, generic; (Rx)

Bimatoprost 0.03% Ophthalmic Solution (containing bimatoprost 0.3 mg; benzalkonium chloride 0.005%; NaCl; sodium phosphate, dibasic; citric acid; purified water; NaOH and/or HCl to adjust pH to 6.8 to 7.8, with an osmolality of 290 mOsm/kg) in sterile 2.5 mL, 5 mL, and 7.5 mL ophthalmic dropper bottles; *Latisse®*, generic; (Rx). **NOTE:** *Latisse®* is approved for topical use only for inducing eyelash growth and should not be used in the eye.

Bimatoprost 10 µg Ophthalmic Implant (containing 10 µg bimatoprost in a single-use applicator that is packaged in a sealed foil pouch containing desiccant, NDC 0023-9652-01); *Durysta®* (Rx)

References

For the complete list of references, see **wiley.com/go/budde/plumb**

Brimonidine Ophthalmic

(bri-***moe***-ni-deen) *Alphagan P®, Combigan®, Qoliana®, Simbrinza®*

Alpha-Adrenergic Agonist; Anti-Glaucoma Agent

Prescriber Highlights

- Used to decrease intraocular pressure (IOP) in patients with glaucoma
- Produces less severe adverse effects than apraclonidine, but it is not a first-line anti-glaucoma agent in veterinary species
- Greenish-yellow color of the solution is a characteristic and not a sign of degradation or contamination

Uses/Indications

Brimonidine may be used to treat elevated intraocular pressure (IOP) in patients with glaucoma or ocular hypertension. Its use in glaucomatous beagles 2 to 3 times daily has demonstrated no consistent clinical effect.[1] Administration of brimonidine to normotensive horses, with or without timolol, has not shown any clinically significant effect.[2]

Pharmacology/Actions

Brimonidine is a relatively selective alpha-2-adrenergic agonist. Activation of presynaptic alpha-2 receptors inhibits norepinephrine release, and activation of postsynaptic alpha-2 receptors on the nonpigmented ciliary body epithelial cells decreases intracellular cAMP, both of which result in decreased aqueous humor production and decreased intraocular pressure (IOP). Additionally, aqueous humor outflow may be increased by a direct effect on uveoscleral outflow, as well as structural alterations to the conventional outflow tract that decrease resistance to outflow.

Contraindications/Precautions/Warnings

Brimonidine is contraindicated in patients that have a history of hypersensitivity to it or any component of the formulation. Brimonidine should be used cautiously, if at all, in patients with vascular insufficiency syndromes (eg, laminitis, cerebral, or coronary vascular insufficiency). Concomitant use of monoamine oxidase inhibitors (MAOIs; eg, amitraz, selegiline) may potentiate the risk for systemic hypotension. Instruct pet owners to keep it out of reach of household animals, as ingestion of brimonidine ophthalmic solution has caused serious cardiovascular toxicities.[3] Overdoses of brimonidine can be treated with atipamezole, yohimbine, and other alpha-2 antagonists. Caution should be exercised if brimonidine is used in conjunction with beta-blockers (ophthalmic and systemic), antihypertensives, and/or cardiac glycosides. When brimonidine is used in humans, the clinical effect diminishes over time and requires careful monitoring.

Adverse Effects

Adverse effects reported in humans or animals are numerous and include (but are not limited to) oral dryness, allergic conjunctivitis, conjunctival hyperemia, ocular pruritus, burning, stinging, foreign body sensation, irritation, eyelid and conjunctival edema, dizziness, muscular pain, and hypertension. Use of brimonidine in dogs is associated with miosis and bradycardia.[4] Administration of brimonidine in cats consistently results in vomiting, which may be ameliorated by premedication with oral maripotant.[5] Brimonidine in cats also produces dose-dependent sedation, bradycardia, and hypotension.[6]

Dosages

Glaucoma (extra-label): 1 drop to the affected eye(s) 2 to 3 times daily

Monitoring

- Clinical efficacy measured through continued control of intraocular pressure (IOP)
- Baseline and periodic heart rate and blood pressure, particularly in dogs and cats

Client Information

- Use this medicine as directed by your veterinarian.
- Keep this medicine out of reach of household animals and children, as ingestion of brimonidine ophthalmic solution can cause serious heart problems.
- Use proper administration techniques to avoid contamination of the medication. Keep the cap tightly closed when the medication is not in use.
- Wait for 5 minutes after applying this medication before applying any other medications to the eye.
- Store this medication at room temperature away from moisture and sunlight. Do not freeze.
- Do not use this medication if the color changes, if it becomes cloudy, or if there are particles in the solution.

Storage/Stability

Store at controlled room temperature (20°C-25°C [68°F-77°F]) away from moisture and sunlight; do not freeze.

Compatibility/Compounding Considerations

Brimonidine ophthalmic preparations should not be mixed directly with any other ophthalmic medications.

Dosage Forms/Regulatory Status

VETERINARY-LABELED PRODUCTS: NONE

HUMAN-LABELED PRODUCTS:

Brimonidine Tartrate 0.1% Ophthalmic Solution (containing brimonidine tartrate 0.1%; boric acid; calcium chloride; magnesium chloride; potassium chloride; purified water; *PURITE®* 0.005% as preservative; sodium borate; sodium carboxymethylcellulose; NaCl; HCl and/or NaOH to adjust pH to 7.7), 5 mL, 10 mL, or 15 mL in sterile ophthalmic dropper bottles; *Alphagan-P®*; (Rx)

Brimonidine Tartrate 0.15% Ophthalmic Solution (containing brimonidine tartrate 0.15%; boric acid; calcium chloride; magnesium chloride; potassium chloride; purified water; *PURITE®* 0.005% as preservative; sodium borate; sodium carboxymethylcellulose; NaCl; HCl and/or NaOH to adjust pH to 7.7), 5 mL, 10 mL, or 15 mL in sterile ophthalmic dropper bottles; *Alphagan-P®*; (Rx)

Brimonidine Tartrate 0.15% Ophthalmic Solution (containing brimonidine tartrate 1.5 mg/mL; *POLYQUAD®* (polyquaternium-1) 0.01 mg/mL; povidone; boric acid; sodium borate; calcium chloride; magnesium chloride; potassium chloride; mannitol; sodium chloride; purified water; HCl and/or NaOH to adjust pH), 5 mL, 10 mL, or 15 mL in sterile ophthalmic dropper bottles; *Qoliana®*; (Rx)

Brimonidine Tartrate 0.2% Ophthalmic Solution (containing brimonidine tartrate 0.2%; benzalkonium chloride 0.005%; polyvinyl alcohol; NaCl; citric acid; purified water; HCl and/or NaOH to adjust pH to 5.6 to 6.6, with an osmolality of 280 – 330 mOsm/kg) in a 5 mL, 10 mL, and 15 mL dropper bottle; generic; (Rx)

HUMAN-LABELED COMBINATION PRODUCTS:

Brimonidine Tartrate 0.2% and Timolol Maleate 0.5% Ophthalmic Solution (containing brimonidine tartrate 0.2%; timolol 0.5%; benzalkonium chloride 0.005%; purified water; sodium phosphate, dibasic; sodium phosphate, monobasic; HCl and/or NaOH to adjust pH to 6.5 to 7.3, with an osmolality of 280 – 330 mOsm/kg), 5 mL, 10 mL, or 15 mL in sterile ophthalmic dropper bottles; *Combigan®*, generic; (Rx)

Brimonidine Tartrate 0.2% and Brinzolamide 1% Ophthalmic Suspension (containing brinzolamide 10 mg; brimonidine tartrate 2 mg, equivalent to 1.32 mg free base; benzalkonium chloride 0.03 mg; propylene glycol; carbomer 974P; boric acid; mannitol; NaCl; tyloxapol; purified water; HCl and/or NaOH to adjust pH), 8 mL in sterile ophthalmic dropper bottle; *Simbrinza®*; (Rx)

References

For the complete list of references, see **wiley.com/go/budde/plumb**

Brinzolamide Ophthalmic

(bryn-***zoe***-la-mide) *Azopt®, Simbrinza®*

Carbonic Anhydrase Inhibitor Anti-Glaucoma Agent

Prescriber Highlights

- ► Decreases intraocular pressure (IOP) by reducing the production of aqueous humor
- ► May be better tolerated than dorzolamide because of less acidic pH
- ► Sulfonamide derivative; caregivers with sulfa allergies should avoid direct contact with the medicine.

Uses/Indications

Brinzolamide is used to decrease intraocular pressure (IOP) in glaucoma and ocular hypertension. It may be used in cases of primary glaucoma or secondary glaucoma (caused by uveitis, lens luxation, or intraocular tumors) in dogs, cats, and horses. Brinzolamide effectively lowers the IOP in normal horses but does not decrease the IOP in normal cats.[1,2] Efficacy of prophylactic brinzolamide administration for preventing manifestation of primary glaucoma in unaffected eyes of dogs with contralateral primary glaucoma has not been demonstrated.[3]

Pharmacology/Actions

Carbonic anhydrase (CA) is an enzyme found in many body tissues, including the eye. CA inhibitors reduce the formation of hydrogen and bicarbonate ions from carbon dioxide and water by noncompetitive, reversible inhibition of the enzyme CA, thereby reducing the availability of these ions for active transport into secretions. In humans, CA exists as a number of isoenzymes, with CA-II being the most relevant to glaucoma management. Inhibition of CA in the ciliary processes of the eye decreases aqueous humor secretion, presumably by slowing the formation of bicarbonate ions with subsequent reduction in sodium and fluid transport, which results in a reduction in intraocular pressure (IOP).[4] Brinzolamide is more lipophilic than dorzolamide, resulting in increased intraocular concentrations following topical administration.[5]

Contraindications/Precautions/Warnings

Brinzolamide is contraindicated in patients that have a history of hypersensitivity to it or any component of the formulation or drugs like it, such as sulfonamides. Caregivers with sulfonamide allergies should use caution when applying brinzolamide.

Adverse Effects

Adverse effects reported in humans or animals include stinging, burning, and irritation upon application. Corneal edema may occur in patients with low corneal endothelial cell counts. Humans experience headaches and a bitter taste in the mouth after brinzolamide administration. It is possible that animals experience these adverse effects. Carbonic anhydrase (CA) inhibitors, including brinzolamide, have been implicated in the development of significant ulcerative and nonulcerative keratitis following long-term administration.[6]

Dosages

Glaucoma (extra-label): 1 drop to the affected eye(s) 2 to 3 times daily

Monitoring

- Clinical efficacy
- Confirm maintenance of intraocular pressure (IOP) within the normal range for the species being treated
- Monitor for corneal edema

Client Information

- Use this medication as directed by your veterinarian.
- Shake this medication well before using.
- Use proper administration techniques to avoid contamination of the medication. Keep the cap tightly closed when the medication is not in use.
- Wait for 5 minutes after applying this medication before applying any other medications to the eye.
- Store in the refrigerator or at room temperature away from moisture and sunlight. Do not freeze.
- Do not use this medication if the color changes.

Storage/Stability

Store this product in the refrigerator or at controlled room temperature (4°C-30°C [39°F-86°F]) away from moisture and sunlight; do not freeze.

Compatibility/Compounding Considerations

Brinzolamide ophthalmic preparations should not be mixed directly with any other ophthalmic medications.

Dosage Forms/Regulatory Status

VETERINARY-LABELED PRODUCTS: NONE

HUMAN-LABELED PRODUCTS:

Brinzolamide 1% Ophthalmic Suspension (containing brinzolamide 10 mg; benzalkonium chloride 0.01%; mannitol; carbomer 974P; tyloxapol; edetate disodium; NaCl; purified water; HCl and/or NaOH to adjust pH to 7.5; osmolality of 300 mOsm/kg), 10 mL or 15 mL in sterile ophthalmic dropper bottles; *Azopt®*; (Rx)

HUMAN-LABELED COMBINATION PRODUCTS:

Brinzolamide 1% and Brimonidine Tartrate 0.2% Ophthalmic Suspension (containing brinzolamide 10 mg; brimonidine tartrate 2 mg, equivalent to 1.32 mg as brimonidine free base; benzalkonium chloride 0.03 mg; propylene glycol; carbomer 974P; boric acid; mannitol; sodium chloride; tyloxapol; purified water; HCl and/or NaOH to adjust pH), 8 mL in sterile 10 mL ophthalmic dropper bottle; *Simbrinza®*; (Rx)

References

For the complete list of references, see **wiley.com/go/budde/plumb**

Bromfenac Ophthalmic

(***brome***-fen-ak) *Bromsite®, Prolensa®*

Nonsteroidal Anti-Inflammatory Drug (NSAID)

Prescriber Highlights

- Used to control anterior segment inflammation
- Longer duration of action than diclofenac
- May delay ocular wound healing and increase risk for intraocular bleeding

Uses/Indications

Bromfenac is indicated for controlling anterior segment inflammation (eg, conjunctivitis, keratitis, anterior uveitis) and for providing analgesia following surgical removal of cataracts. In a prospective study evaluating inflammation, postoperative ocular hypertension, and posterior capsular opacification (PCO) in dogs following cataract surgery, the effectiveness of prednisolone acetate was compared with artificial lens implants that were impregnated with celecoxib (NSAID) or topically applied bromfenac. Over the long-term follow-up period of 56 weeks, bromfenac was comparable to prednisolone acetate in controlling inflammation and did not lead to an increased incidence of ocular hypertension, and it effectively managed PCO.[1] In contrast, bromfenac was associated with an increased incidence of elevated intraocular pressure (IOP) relative to flurbiprofen in dogs 6 weeks following surgical cataract removal.[2]

Pharmacology/Actions

Bromfenac is an NSAID that blocks prostaglandin synthesis by inhibiting cyclooxygenase 1 and 2. Prostaglandins mediate many adverse effects that occur because of intraocular inflammation, including disruption of the blood-aqueous humor barrier, vasodilation, increased vascular permeability, leukocytosis, and increased intraocular pressure (IOP).[3] Blocking prostaglandin production, therefore, minimizes the adverse short- and long-term effects of intraocular inflammation.

Contraindications/Precautions/Warnings

Bromfenac is contraindicated in patients that have a history of hypersensitivity to it or any component of the formulation. The potential for cross-sensitivity to acetylsalicylic acid, phenylacetic acid derivatives, and other NSAIDs exists. Topical NSAIDs may result in corneal epithelial breakdown and corneal thinning, erosion, or ulceration.[3] Topical NSAIDs may slow or delay corneal wound healing. As topical corticosteroids are also known to slow or delay healing, concomitant use of topical NSAIDs and topical steroids may increase the potential for healing problems. Because of interference with thrombocyte aggregation, ophthalmic NSAIDs may cause increased bleeding of ocular tissues (including hyphema) in conjunction with ocular surgery. It is recommended that bromfenac ophthalmic solution be used with caution in patients with known bleeding tendencies or those receiving other medications that may prolong bleeding times.[3]

Adverse Effects

Adverse effects associated with bromfenac that have been reported in humans or animals include burning, stinging, and irritation upon application; conjunctival hyperemia; risk for ocular bleeding; and delayed corneal wound healing.

Dosages

Anterior segment inflammation (extra-label): 1 drop to the affected eye(s) every 8 hours initially, then reduced to lowest effective dose

Postoperative ocular analgesia (extra-label): 1 drop to the affected eye(s) every 6 to 8 hours as needed to control pain

Monitoring

- Clinical efficacy through evidence of efficacious analgesia and control of intraocular inflammation

Client Information

- Use this medication as directed by your veterinarian.
- Use proper administration techniques to avoid contamination of the medication. Keep the cap tightly closed when the medicine is not in use.
- Wait for 5 minutes after applying this medication before applying any other medications to the eye.
- Store this medication at room temperature away from moisture and sunlight; do not freeze.
- Do not use this medication if the color changes, if it becomes cloudy, or if there are particles in the solution.

- Discard compounded gels by the discard date indicated by the compounding pharmacist.

Storage/Stability

Store this product at controlled room temperature (15°C-25°C [59°F-77°F]) away from moisture and sunlight; do not freeze.

Compatibility/Compounding Considerations

Bromfenac ophthalmic preparations should not be mixed directly with any other ophthalmic medications.

Dosage Forms/Regulatory Status

VETERINARY-LABELED PRODUCTS: NONE

HUMAN-LABELED PRODUCTS:

Bromfenac 0.09% Ophthalmic Solution (containing bromfenac sodium sesquihydrate 0.1035% equivalent to 0.09% bromfenac-free acid; benzalkonium chloride 0.05 mg/mL; boric acid; polysorbate 80; povidone; sodium borate; sodium sulfite anhydrous; NaOH to adjust pH; water for injection), in sterile 2.5 mL and 5 mL ophthalmic dropper bottle; generic; (Rx)

Bromfenac 0.07% Ophthalmic Solution (containing bromfenac sodium hydrate 0.805 mg; benzalkonium chloride 0.005%; boric acid; edetate disodium; povidone; sodium borate; sodium sulfite; tyloxapol; NaOH to adjust pH; water for injection), in sterile 1.6 mL or 3 mL ophthalmic dropper bottle; *Prolensa*®; (Rx)

Bromfenac 0.075% Ophthalmic Solution (containing bromfenac sodium sesquihydrate 0.81 mg equivalent to bromfenac-free acid 0.76 mg; boric acid; sodium borate; citric acid; sodium citrate; poloxamer 407; polycarbophil; NaCl; edetate disodium; water for injection; NaOH to adjust pH; benzalkonium chloride 0.05 mg/0.005%), in sterile 5 mL ophthalmic dropper bottle; *Bromsite*®; (Rx)

References

For the complete list of references, see **wiley.com/go/budde/plumb**

Carteolol Ophthalmic

(kar-***tay***-uh-lol)

Nonselective Beta-Blocker

Prescriber Highlights

- ► Nonselective (beta-1 and beta-2) beta-blocker that decreases aqueous humor production to decrease intraocular pressure (IOP) as a treatment for glaucoma
- ► May delay onset of glaucoma in the normal eye of dogs with unilateral glaucoma
- ► Use with caution in asthmatic patients due to the potential to induce bronchospasm

Uses/Indications

Carteolol may be used to reduce intraocular pressure (IOP) in primary glaucoma and as prophylaxis to prevent glaucoma in the normal eye of animals with unilateral glaucoma. The evaluation of its efficacy in animals has not been performed.

Pharmacology/Actions

Carteolol is a nonselective beta-adrenergic blocking agent with associated intrinsic sympathomimetic activity and without significant membrane-stabilizing activity.[1] Blockade of ciliary body beta-receptors (particularly beta-2-receptors) reduces intraocular pressure (IOP) by decreasing aqueous humor production. Several mechanisms of action have been postulated for this effect, including beta-blockade (particularly beta-2-receptors) reducing norepinephrine-induced tonic sympathetic stimulation, which then leads to decreased activation of cAMP in the ciliary body; inhibition of Na+K+ATPase activity; or vasoactive mechanisms on the iris and ciliary body. Topically administered beta-blockers also inhibit glutamine-induced increases in intracellular calcium and sodium, thereby providing a potential protective effect against ischemic insult to the retina.[2]

Contraindications/Precautions/Warnings

Carteolol is contraindicated in patients that have a history of hypersensitivity to it or any component of the formulation. Carteolol should be used carefully in patients with heart block, bradycardia, heart failure, asthma, chronic bronchitis, or other cardiopulmonary conditions, although systemic cardiopulmonary adverse effects are not likely with ocular use of carteolol.

Beta-blockers should be used with caution in patients with diabetes mellitus, as these drugs may mask signs of acute hypoglycemia. Beta-blockers should also be used with caution in patients with hyperthyroidism, as these drugs may mask indications of this condition. Abrupt discontinuation of beta-blockers should be avoided.

Adverse Effects

Adverse effects reported in humans or animals include transient burning, stinging, and irritation upon application to the eye. Although not specifically evaluated, it is possible that carteolol could lead to reduction in heart rate following topical administration in veterinary species.[3]

Dosages

Glaucoma (extra-label): 1 drop to the affected eye(s) 2 times daily

Monitoring

- Clinical efficacy
- Monitor intraocular pressure (IOP)
- Observe asthmatic and diabetic patients for respiratory difficulty or acute hypoglycemia, respectively

Client Information

- Use this medication as directed by your veterinarian.
- Use proper administration techniques to avoid contamination of the medication. Keep the cap tightly closed when the medication is not in use.
- Wait for 5 minutes after applying this medication before applying any other medications to the eye.
- Store this medication at room temperature away from moisture and sunlight. Do not freeze.
- Do not use this medication if the color changes, if it becomes cloudy, or if there are particles in the solution.

Storage/Stability

Store this product at controlled room temperature (15°C-25°C [59°F-77°F]) away from moisture and sunlight; do not freeze.

Compatibility/Compounding Considerations

Carteolol ophthalmic preparations should not be mixed directly with any other ophthalmic medications.

Dosage Forms/Regulatory Status

VETERINARY-LABELED PRODUCTS: NONE

HUMAN-LABELED PRODUCTS:

Carteolol HCl 1% Ophthalmic Solution (containing carteolol HCl 10 mg; benzalkonium chloride 0.05 mg; NaCl; monobasic and dibasic sodium phosphate; NaOH and/or HCl to adjust pH to 6 to 8; purified water), in a 5 mL, 10 mL, and 15 mL dropper bottle; generic; (Rx)

References

For the complete list of references, see **wiley.com/go/budde/plumb**

Chloramphenicol Ophthalmic

(klor-am-***fen***-uh-kol)

Broad-Spectrum Antibiotic

For systemic use, refer to ***Chloramphenicol***

Prescriber Highlights

- ► Used to provide antibacterial coverage in the presence of corneal ulcerations or therapeutic antibacterial coverage for susceptible ocular surface infections, particularly feline *Mycoplasma* spp or *Chlamydia* spp infections
- ► Chloramphenicol has caused acute toxicity and death in humans; instruct caregiver to wear gloves and avoid contact with this drug.
- ► Chloramphenicol ophthalmic preparations are no longer commercially available but may be compounded by a qualified compounding pharmacist.
- ► The National Institute for Occupational Safety and Health (NIOSH) classifies chloramphenicol as a hazardous drug; use appropriate precautions when handling.

Uses/Indications

Chloramphenicol is used for the treatment of surface ocular infections involving the conjunctiva and/or cornea caused by chloramphenicol-susceptible organisms.[1]

The World Health Organization (WHO) has designated chloramphenicol as a Highly Important antimicrobial for human medicine.[2] The Office International des Epizooties (OIE) has designated amphenicol as a Veterinary Critically Important Antimicrobial (VCIA) Agent in veterinary species.[3]

Pharmacology/Actions

Chloramphenicol is a broad-spectrum, bacteriostatic antibiotic that inhibits protein synthesis by interfering with the transfer of activated amino acids from soluble RNA to ribosomes, thus preventing protein elongation. It generally has good activity against gram-positive, gram-negative, and intracellular organisms, common to the ocular surface; the activity against *Pseudomonas* spp is consistently poor. Development of resistance to chloramphenicol is uncommon for *Staphylococcus* spp and *Streptococcus* spp.[4-7]

Chloramphenicol is found in measurable amounts in the aqueous humor following topical application to the eye.

Contraindications/Precautions/Warnings

Chloramphenicol is contraindicated in patients that have a history of hypersensitivity to it or any component of the formulation.

Chloramphenicol may induce dose-dependent bone marrow suppression or idiosyncratic aplastic anemia, both of which have a low risk of occurring following topical ophthalmic administration.[8,9] Caregivers should be instructed to wear gloves and wash hands after handling this drug. Chloramphenicol is banned for use in food-producing animals.

The National Institute for Occupational Safety and Health (NIOSH) classifies chloramphenicol as a hazardous drug; personal protective equipment (PPE) should be used accordingly to minimize the risk for exposure.

Adverse Effects

Adverse effects reported in animals include occasional burning or stinging on application. Bone marrow suppression and blood dyscrasias have been reported following the use of systemic chloramphenicol.

Dosages

Bacterial conjunctivitis (extra-label): ¼ – ½ inch strip or 1 drop in the affected eye(s) every 6 to 8 hours

Monitoring

- Cytology and culture to evaluate for the presence of bacteria
- Clinical resolution of signs related to ocular surface infection
- Baseline and periodic CBC to monitor for bone marrow suppression

Client Information

- Humans should avoid direct contact with this medicine. Wear gloves during administration and wash hands after handling this medicine.
- Use proper administration techniques to avoid contamination of the medication. Do not touch the dropper (or ointment) tip or allow it to touch your animal's eye or any other surface to prevent contamination.
- Keep cap tightly closed when not in use.
- Wait 5 minutes after applying this medication before applying any other medications to the eye.
- Do not use if the color changes, becomes cloudy, or if there are particles in the solution.
- This medication is considered to be a hazardous drug as defined by the National Institute for Occupational Safety and Health (NIOSH). Talk with your veterinarian or pharmacist about the use of personal protective equipment when handling this medicine.

Storage/Stability

Store at controlled room temperature (20°C-25°C [68°F-77°F]) away from moisture and sunlight; do not freeze.

Compatibility/Compounding Considerations

Chloramphenicol should not be mixed directly (in vitro) with any other drugs.

Dosage Forms/Regulatory Status

VETERINARY-LABELED PRODUCTS: NONE

HUMAN-LABELED PRODUCTS: NONE

Chloramphenicol was formerly available as a 0.5% ophthalmic solution or a 1% ointment but is no longer commercially available. A qualified compounding pharmacist may prepare it if needed.

References

For the complete list of references, see **wiley.com/go/budde/plumb**

Cidofovir Ophthalmic

(sye-***doe***-fo-veer)

Antiviral

Prescriber Highlights

- ► Used as an ophthalmic antiviral agent in cats with feline herpesvirus-1 (FHV-1)
- ► Less frequent administration and shorter treatment duration when compared to other ophthalmic antiviral agents
- ► Cidofovir has caused hypospermia and birth defects in humans and should not be used in animals intended for breeding.
- ► Not commercially available in an ophthalmic dosage form but can be compounded as a 0.5% ophthalmic solution
- ► The National Institute for Occupational Safety and Health (NIOSH) classifies cidofovir as a hazardous drug; use appropriate precautions when handling.

Uses/Indications

Cidofovir is compounded into a 0.5% ophthalmic solution for the topical treatment of feline herpesvirus-1 (FHV-1) keratitis in cats. In vitro efficacy of cidofovir against FHV-1 is consistently high.[1,2]

Because cidofovir is effective when administered twice daily for 10 days,[3] it has a significant therapeutic advantage over other antiviral ophthalmic agents (eg, trifluridine, vidarabine, and idoxuridine) which must be administered 4 to 6 times daily for 2 to 3 weeks.

Cidofovir decreases viral shedding in dogs experimentally infected with ocular canine herpesvirus-1 infections; however, it causes local irritation and toxicity.[3] Although the efficacy of cidofovir has not been evaluated in horses for treatment of keratitis associated with equine herpesvirus-2, it has demonstrated mild in vitro efficacy versus other equine alpha-herpesviruses.

Pharmacology/Actions

Cidofovir suppresses viral replication by inhibiting the synthesis of viral DNA. Cidofovir diphosphate, the active intracellular metabolite, demonstrates much greater selectivity for viral, rather than human, DNA. Because cidofovir is incorporated into the growing DNA chain, it reduces the rate of viral DNA synthesis, thereby having a virustatic effect.

Contraindications/Precautions/Warnings

Cidofovir is contraindicated in patients that have a history of hypersensitivity to it or any component of the formulation. Do not use cidofovir in animals intended for breeding, as cidofovir has been shown to cause hypospermia and is mutagenic and teratogenic in humans. Following IV administration, cidofovir has caused death by irreversible nephrotoxicity[4]; do not use in animals with pre-existing renal impairment or concurrently with nephrotoxic drugs. Direct intraocular injection is contraindicated.[4]

The National Institute for Occupational Safety and Health (NIOSH) classifies cidofovir as a hazardous drug; personal protective equipment (PPE) should be used accordingly to minimize the risk for exposure.

Adverse Effects

Adverse effects reported in humans or animals following topical administration include burning or stinging on application and nasolacrimal occlusion in rabbits and humans following prolonged (weeks) treatment. Severe adverse effects reported in humans following IV administration include nephrotoxicity (after even a single IV dose), neutropenia, metabolic acidosis, and uveitis/ocular hypotony. Although these reactions reported with IV administration have not been reported following ocular administration, nephrotoxicity is theoretically possible. Topical ocular administration of cidofovir to dogs has led to signs of irritation (eg, conjunctival pigmentation, blepharitis).[3]

Dosages

Feline herpesvirus-1 keratitis (extra-label): 1 drop to the affected eye(s) 2 times daily for 10 days[5]

Canine herpesvirus-1 ocular infections (extra-label): 1 drop to the affected eye(s) twice daily for 14 days[3]

Monitoring

- Clinical resolution of signs related to herpesvirus ocular infections (eg, corneal ulceration, corneal vascularization, conjunctivitis)
- Consider baseline and periodic renal chemistry panels

Client Information

- Humans should avoid direct contact with this drug. Wear gloves during administration and wash hands after each treatment is done.
- Use proper administration techniques to avoid contamination of the medication. Do not touch the dropper (or ointment) tip or allow it to touch your animal's eye or any other surface to prevent contamination.
- Keep cap tightly closed when this medicine is not in use.
- Wait 5 minutes after applying this medicine before applying any other medications to the eye.
- Do not use if the color changes or becomes cloudy or if there are particles in the solution.
- This medication is considered to be a hazardous drug as defined by the National Institute for Occupational Safety and Health (NIOSH). Talk with your veterinarian or pharmacist about the use of personal protective equipment when handling this medicine.

Storage/Stability

Store in the refrigerator (2°C-8°C [35.6°F-46.4°F]) away from moisture and sunlight; do not freeze.

The reported chemical stability of this solution is 180 days when stored in glass at 4°C (39.2°F), -20°C (-4°F), and -80°C (-112°F).[6] Storage times should be determined by the results of individual extended stability and sterility testing or compendial standards.

Compatibility/Compounding Considerations

Cidofovir should not be mixed directly (in vitro) with any other drugs.

Dosage Forms/Regulatory Status

VETERINARY-LABELED PRODUCTS: NONE

HUMAN-LABELED PRODUCTS: NONE

Cidofovir is not approved for use as an ophthalmic dosage form, but a cidofovir 0.5% ophthalmic solution can be prepared by a qualified compounding pharmacist.

References

For the complete list of references, see **wiley.com/go/budde/plumb**

Ciprofloxacin Ophthalmic

(sip-roe-***flox***-a sin) *Ciloxan®*

Fluoroquinolone Antibiotic

For systemic use, refer to ***Ciprofloxacin***

Prescriber Highlights

- ► Used to treat bacterial conjunctivitis or keratitis
- ► Physically incompatible with many drugs; therefore, should not be directly mixed with other ophthalmic medications
- ► Crystalline drug precipitates may be noted in the superficial portion of corneal defects during use.

Uses/Indications

In veterinary patients, ciprofloxacin ophthalmic may be used for the treatment of bacterial conjunctivitis or keratitis caused by susceptible strains of *Staphylococcus* spp, *Streptococcus* spp, *Pseudomonas aeruginosa*, *Chlamydia* spp, and *Haemophilus* spp.[1]

The World Health Organization (WHO) has designated ciprofloxacin as a Critically Important, Highest Priority antimicrobial in human medicine.[2]

Pharmacology/Actions

Ciprofloxacin is a bactericidal and concentration-dependent antibiotic, with susceptible bacteria cell death occurring within 20 to 30 minutes of exposure. Ciprofloxacin has demonstrated a significant postantibiotic effect in both gram-negative and gram-positive bacteria and is active in both the stationary and growth phases of bacterial replication. Its mechanism of action is not thoroughly understood, but it is believed to act by inhibiting bacterial DNA-gyrase (a type-II topoisomerase), thereby preventing DNA supercoiling and DNA synthesis.

Although ciprofloxacin is considered to have greater efficacy against gram-negative organisms as compared with gram-positive, studies involving ocular isolates obtained from dogs and horses with bacterial keratitis indicate good efficacy with minimal resistance against *Streptococcus* spp, *Staphylococcus* spp, and *Pseudomonas aeruginosa*.[3–6] However, more recent reports involving isolates from humans with ocular infections indicate lower susceptibility of *Staphylococcus* spp to ciprofloxacin.

Contraindications/Precautions/Warnings

Ciprofloxacin is contraindicated in patients that have a history of hypersensitivity to it, other fluoroquinolones, or any component of the formulation. Ophthalmic preparations are for topical ophthalmic use only. They are not for injection subconjunctivally or into the anterior chamber of the eye. Fluoroquinolone-induced retinal toxicity in domestic cats has not been demonstrated with a topical formulation of ciprofloxacin.

Adverse Effects

Adverse effects reported in humans or animals include blurred vision, tearing, eye pain, redness, itching, and a bad taste in the mouth.[7] Crystalline drug precipitates may be observed in the superficial portion of corneal defects during use; however, this effect did not adversely affect clinical and visual outcomes in human clinical studies.[7] The arthropathy that occurs in immature animals associated with oral administration of quinolones has not been noted following topical ophthalmic administration.

Dosages

Conjunctivitis (extra-label): 1 drop or ¼ – ½ inch strip to the affected eye(s) every 2 to 8 hours

Keratitis (extra-label): 1 drop or ¼ – ½ inch strip to the affected eye every 2 to 8 hours

Monitoring

- Corneal cytology and culture to evaluate for the persistence of bacteria
- Evaluation for clinical signs suggestive of persistent infection

Client Information

- Use this medication as directed by your veterinarian.
- Use proper administration techniques to avoid contamination of the medication. Do not touch the dropper tip or allow it to touch your animal's eye or any other surface to prevent contamination.
- Wait 5 minutes after applying this medicine before applying any other medicine to your animal's eye(s).
- Crystals may appear on the surface of your animal's eye during treatment. This change is not harmful and will go away once treatment is complete.
- Keep cap tightly closed when not in use. Store this medication in the refrigerator or at room temperature away from moisture and sunlight. Do not freeze.
- Do not use this medication if the color changes, becomes cloudy, or if there are particles in the solution.

Storage/Stability

Store this product in the refrigerator (2°C-8°C [35.6°F-46.4°F]) or at controlled room temperature (20°C-25°C [68°F-77°F]) away from moisture and sunlight; do not freeze.

Compatibility/Compounding Considerations

Fluoroquinolone antibiotics interact with many other drugs, including those containing cations (eg, iron, aluminum, magnesium, or calcium). Ciprofloxacin should not be mixed directly (in vitro) with any other drugs.

Dosage Forms/Regulatory Status

VETERINARY-LABELED PRODUCTS: NONE

HUMAN-LABELED PRODUCTS:

Ciprofloxacin 0.3% Ophthalmic Solution (containing ciprofloxacin HCl 3.5 mg equivalent to 3 mg base; benzalkonium chloride 0.006%; sodium acetate; acetic acid; mannitol; edetate disodium; HCl and/or NaOH may be used to adjust pH to 4.5; purified water; osmolality is 300 mOsm/kg), 2.5 mL, 5 mL, or 10 mL in sterile ophthalmic dropper bottles; *Ciloxan*®, generic; (Rx)

Ciprofloxacin 0.3% Ophthalmic Ointment (containing ciprofloxacin HCl 3.33 mg equivalent to 3 mg base; mineral oil; white petrolatum), in 3.5 g sterile ophthalmic ointment tubes; *Ciloxan*®; (Rx)

References

For the complete list of references, see **wiley.com/go/budde/plumb**

Cromolyn Ophthalmic

(***kroh***-mah-lin)

Mast Cell Stabilizer

Prescriber Highlights

- Used for seasonal allergic conjunctivitis or atopic conjunctivitis
- Administer 2 to 6 times daily
- Mild transient stinging and burning may occur upon application

Uses/Indications

Mast cell-stabilizing ophthalmic agents are used to control the clinical signs of allergic and atopic conjunctivitis. Response to therapy (eg, decreased itching, tearing, redness, and discharge) is usually evident within a few days, but longer treatment for up to 6 weeks may be required. Once improvement has been established, therapy should be continued for as long as needed to sustain improvement.[1] If required, corticosteroids may be used concomitantly with cromolyn ophthalmic solution. Efficacy of cromolyn as treatment for conjunctivitis in veterinary species has not been established.

Pharmacology/Actions

Cromolyn inhibits the degranulation of sensitized mast cells and blocks the release of histamine and slow-releasing substance of anaphylaxis from mast cells following antigen recognition. Cromolyn does not have intrinsic vasoconstrictor, antihistaminic, cyclooxygenase inhibition, or other anti-inflammatory properties. Cromolyn is poorly absorbed when applied topically.

Contraindications/Precautions/Warnings

Cromolyn is contraindicated in patients that have a history of hypersensitivity to cromolyn or any component of the formulation.

Adverse Effects

Adverse effects reported in humans or animals include a transient mild stinging and burning upon application.

Dosages

Allergic conjunctivitis (extra-label): 1 drop to each eye 2 to 6 times daily

Monitoring

- Clinical efficacy: resolution of clinical signs associated with allergic conjunctivitis

Client Information

- Use proper administration techniques to avoid contamination of the medication. Keep the cap tightly closed when the medicine is not in use.

- Wait for 5 minutes after applying this medicine before applying any other medicines to the eye.
- Store this medicine at room temperature away from moisture and sunlight. Do not freeze.
- Do not use the medicine if the color changes, if it becomes cloudy, or if there are particles in the solution.

Storage/Stability

Store this product at room temperature (15°C-30°C [59°F-86°F]) away from moisture and sunlight; do not freeze.

Compatibility/Compounding Considerations

Cromolyn ophthalmic preparations should not be mixed directly with any other ophthalmic medications.

Dosage Forms/Regulatory Status

VETERINARY-LABELED PRODUCTS: NONE

HUMAN-LABELED PRODUCTS:

Cromolyn Sodium 4% Ophthalmic Solution (containing cromolyn sodium 40 mg; benzalkonium chloride 0.01%; edetate disodium 0.1%; purified water; HCl and/or NaOH to adjust pH to 4 to 7), 10 mL in sterile ophthalmic dropper bottle; generic; (Rx)

References

For the complete list of references, see **wiley.com/go/budde/plumb**

Cyclopentolate Ophthalmic

(sye-kloe-***pen***-toe-late) *Cyclogyl® Cyclomydril®, Akpentolate®, Pentolair®*

Anticholinergic Cycloplegic/Mydriatic Agent

Prescriber Highlights

- Primarily used as a diagnostic agent to facilitate mydriasis and cycloplegia
- Rapid and intense onset of mydriasis and cycloplegia in 15 to 60 minutes; heavily pigmented irises may require an increased frequency of administration or stronger concentrations. May increase intraocular pressure (IOP); therefore, use cautiously in patients with glaucoma
- Higher concentrations (*at least 1%*) cause stinging on application.
- Available as a combination product with phenylephrine (*Cyclomydril®*) to facilitate mydriasis with less cycloplegia

Uses/Indications

Cyclopentolate is primarily used to induce rapid mydriasis and cycloplegia to enable funduscopic examination and cycloplegic refraction to be performed. It is also available as a combination with phenylephrine to accomplish greater mydriasis with lesser cycloplegia.

Pharmacology/Actions

Cyclopentolate blocks the responses of the sphincter muscle of the iris and the accommodative muscle of the ciliary body to cholinergic stimulation, resulting in pupillary dilation (mydriasis) and paralysis of accommodation (cycloplegia).[1] Cyclopentolate acts rapidly, producing maximal dilation in less than 1 hour in dogs[2] and cats,[3] and within 12 hours in horses,[4,5] with a total duration of mydriasis from 2 to 4 days. Complete recovery of accommodation usually takes 6 to 24 hours. Heavily pigmented irises may require an increased frequency of administration or stronger concentrations than lightly pigmented irises.[1] When cyclopentolate is combined with phenylephrine (an adrenergic drug), synergistic mydriasis occurs, with less accompanying cycloplegia due to the lower concentration of cyclopentolate in the combination product.

Contraindications/Precautions/Warnings

Cyclopentolate is contraindicated in patients that have a history of hypersensitivity to it or any component of the formulation. Although a single drop of cyclopentolate did not elevate intraocular pressure (IOP) in normal dogs,[2] cyclopentolate may cause an increase in IOP and therefore should be used cautiously in patients with glaucoma. Administration to normal cats[3] and horses[4] has been associated with increased IOP in studies; however, another study documented no effect on IOP in normal horses.[5] Reduction in STT has been reported in cats.[3]

Adverse Effects

Adverse effects reported in humans or animals include burning and stinging on application.[1] Increased intraocular pressure (IOP), photophobia, blurred vision, irritation, hyperemia, conjunctivitis, blepharoconjunctivitis, punctate keratitis, and synechiae have also been reported.[1] Burning and stinging are usually associated with higher concentrations (*at least 1%*). CNS and cardiovascular disturbances are often noted in human pediatric patients and may occur when used in smaller animals.

Dosages

Mydriasis and cycloplegia (extra-label): 1 drop to the desired eye(s) followed by a second drop 5 minutes later if necessary. **NOTE**: Use of a single drop may avoid adverse systemic effects in smaller animals. Administer this medicine 40 to 50 minutes prior to a diagnostic procedure to ensure full effects.

Monitoring

- Clinical efficacy: desired mydriasis and cycloplegia achieved; full recovery in 24 hours

Client Information

- This medicine is rarely used at home.
- This medicine may make your animal sensitive to light for ≈24 hours after administration. Keep your animal out of bright sunlight until pupils return to normal size.
- Wash your hands after use to prevent accidental contact with eyes (causes pupil dilation).
- Use proper administration techniques to avoid contamination of the medication. Keep the cap tightly closed when the medicine is not in use.
- Wait for 5 minutes after applying this medicine before applying any other medicines to the eye.
- Store this medicine at room temperature away from moisture and sunlight. Do not freeze.
- Do not use this medicine if the color changes, if it becomes cloudy, or if there are particles in the solution.

Storage/Stability

Store this product at controlled room temperature (20°C-25°C [68°F-77°F]) away from moisture and sunlight; do not freeze.

Compatibility/Compounding Considerations

Cyclopentolate ophthalmic preparations should not be mixed directly with any other ophthalmic medications.

Dosage Forms/Regulatory Status

VETERINARY-LABELED PRODUCTS: NONE

HUMAN-LABELED PRODUCTS:

Cyclopentolate HCl Ophthalmic Solution 0.5% (containing cyclopentolate HCl 0.5%; benzalkonium chloride 0.01%; boric acid; edetate disodium; sodium carbonate and/or HCl to adjust pH to between 3 and 5.5; purified water), 15 mL in sterile ophthalmic dropper bottles; *Cyclogyl®*, generic; (Rx)

Cyclopentolate HCl Ophthalmic Solution 1% (containing cyclopentolate HCl 1%; benzalkonium chloride 0.01%; boric acid; edetate disodium; sodium carbonate and/or HCl to adjust pH to between 3 and 5.5; purified water), 2 mL, 5 mL, or 15 mL in sterile ophthalmic dropper bottles; *Cyclogyl®*, *Pentolair®*, *Akpentolate®*; (Rx)

Cyclopentolate HCl Ophthalmic Solution 2% (containing cyclopentolate HCl 2%; benzalkonium chloride 0.01%; boric acid; edetate disodium; sodium carbonate and/or HCl to adjust pH to between 3 and 5.5; purified water), 2 mL, 5 mL, or 15 mL in sterile ophthalmic dropper bottles; *Cyclogyl®*; (Rx)

Human-Labeled Combination Products:

Cyclopentolate HCl 0.2% and Phenylephrine HCl 1% Ophthalmic Solution (containing cyclopentolate HCl 0.2%; phenylephrine HCl 1%; benzalkonium chloride 0.01%; edetate disodium; boric acid; HCl and/or sodium carbonate to adjust pH; purified water), 2 mL or 5 mL in sterile ophthalmic dropper bottles; *Cyclomydril®*; (Rx)

References

For the complete list of references, see **wiley.com/go/budde/plumb**

Cyclosporine Ophthalmic

(**sye**-klo-**spore**-in) *Cequa®, Ciclosporin, Cyclosporin A, Optimmune®, Restasis®*

Immunosuppressive Agent

See also ***Cyclosporine (Systemic)***

Prescriber Highlights

- ► Approved as an ophthalmic ointment for the treatment of keratoconjunctivitis sicca (KCS) in dogs and for other ocular surface inflammatory diseases in other species
- ► Poor intraocular penetration requires alternate routes of administration to manage intraocular inflammatory diseases
- ► Animals that do not respond to the approved (0.2%) ophthalmic ointment may benefit from higher concentrations (1% to 2%) of cyclosporine ophthalmic solution, which must be compounded.
- ► Weeks of therapy may be required to cause an increase of tear production; however, discontinuation of therapy can quickly (within days) result in loss of normal tear production.
- ► The National Institute for Occupational Safety and Health (NIOSH) classifies cyclosporine as a hazardous drug; use appropriate precautions when handling.

Uses/Indications

Topical ophthalmic cyclosporine is approved for the treatment of keratoconjunctivitis (KCS) in dogs; it may also be used to treat other ocular surface inflammatory conditions, such as chronic superficial keratitis (CSK; pannus), immune-mediated keratitis (IMMK), eosinophilic keratitis, pigmentary keratitis, and postoperative keratitis in dogs and other species.[1,2] Topical cyclosporine 1.5% has demonstrated efficacy for the management of eosinophilic keratitis in cats.[3] Sustained-released cyclosporine implants have been developed for suprachoroidal and episcleral implantation; the former is for the treatment of equine recurrent uveitis (ERU), and the latter for IMMK in horses and KCS in dogs.[4-9]

Pharmacology/Actions

Cyclosporine, a calcineurin inhibitor, is an immunosuppressive agent that focuses on cell-mediated immune responses, with some humoral immunosuppressive action. Cyclosporine binds to T-cell cyclophilin and blocks calcineurin-mediated T-cell activation. T-helper lymphocytes are the primary target, but T-suppressor cells are also affected. Cyclosporine can also inhibit cytokine production and release (including IL-2 and interferon-gamma in dogs[10-12] and IL-3, IL-4, and tissue necrosis factor-alpha in humans), thereby affecting the function of eosinophils, mast cells, granulocytes, and macrophages.

The immunosuppressive effects make cyclosporine useful when it is administered locally in animals with ocular diseases that are suspected to be immune-mediated, such as keratoconjunctivitis (KCS) and chronic superficial keratitis (CSK). Cyclosporine increases lymphocyte apoptosis and decreases corneal epithelial apoptosis in dogs with KCS,[13] thus protecting the ocular surface. However, other mechanisms likely improve tear production, as tear production is increased by topical administration of cyclosporin in dogs without KCS. For this reason, cyclosporine is thought to have direct stimulatory effects on the lacrimal gland, possibly by altering neurotransmitter release.[14] After initiation of cyclosporine therapy, effective tear production takes several weeks; however, cessation of therapy results in the return of clinical signs in a matter of days.[1] Clinical improvement in cases of KCS is not necessarily dependent on an increase in aqueous tear production as measured by the Schirmer tear test (STT) because other components of the tear film that are not assessed by the STT may also improve with topical cyclosporine administration.[15]

Because of the frequent need for the chronic daily administration of topical cyclosporine, the sustained-release cyclosporine devices are surgically placed in the episcleral space in horses with immune-mediated keratitis (IMMK). The duration of drug release is ≈18 months.[4] Due to limited penetration to the intraocular environment, the sustained release cyclosporine disc devices are surgically implanted suprachoroidally in horses with equine recurrent uveitis (ERU). The duration of drug release is ≈2 to 3 years.[7]

Contraindications/Precautions/Warnings

Cyclosporine is contraindicated in patients that have a history of hypersensitivity to it or any component of the formulation. Use in the presence of ocular viral or fungal infections should be undertaken with caution. Cyclosporine is available as an ophthalmic solution for humans (0.05% to 0.09%); however, these formulations are not effective in controlling keratoconjunctivitis (KCS) in dogs. More concentrated solutions of cyclosporine ophthalmic (1% to 2%) may be prepared (compounded) by qualified compounding pharmacists. It is not recommended to administer cyclosporine ophthalmic ointment or solutions compounded in oil via subpalpebral lavage catheter because of the likely irreversible obstruction of the catheter, necessitating replacement.

The National Institute for Occupational Safety and Health (NIOSH) classifies cyclosporine as a hazardous drug; personal protective equipment (PPE) should be used accordingly to minimize the risk for exposure.

Adverse Effects

Adverse effects reported in humans or animals include local irritation, periocular erythema, lid spasm, rubbing of the eye, alopecia, and epiphora. Many adverse effects are believed to be induced by the vehicle preparation used in compounded formulations rather than by cyclosporine itself. In dogs with herpesvirus keratitis, the administration of topical ophthalmic cyclosporine has not been shown to induce recrudescence of clinical signs.

Dosages

Keratoconjunctivitis sicca and chronic superficial keratitis in dogs (label dosage; FDA-approved): ¼ inch strip to the affected eye(s) every 12 hours[17]

Inflammatory ocular surface diseases (extra-label):

a. Ointment: ¼ – ½ inch strip to the affected eye(s) every 12 hours
b. Cyclosporine solutions (1% to 2%): 1 drop to the affected eye(s) every 12 hours

Immune-mediated keratitis (extra-label): Surgical implantation of a sustained-release device created for episcleral implantation should be performed by a board-certified veterinary ophthalmologist. The implant contains cyclosporine for continued release over ≈12 to 18 months.

Equine recurrent uveitis (ERU) (extra-label): Surgical implantation of a sustained-release device created for suprachoroidal implantation should be performed by a board-certified veterinary ophthalmologist. The implant contains cyclosporine for continued release over ≈2 to 3 years.

Monitoring

- Clinical effect for keratoconjunctivitis (KCS). Evaluate Schirmer tear test, as well as a reduction in mucoid ocular discharge and conjunctival hyperemia.
- Clinical effect for ocular surface inflammatory conditions (topical administration; episcleral device). Evaluate for lack of progression (and possibly regression) of chronic inflammatory changes, such as corneal pigmentation, vascularization, and fibrosis.
- Clinical effect for equine recurrent uveitis (ERU; suprachoroidal device): Evaluate markers of intraocular inflammation (eg, flare, hypopyon, ocular hypotony, miosis, vitreal debris) and frequency of recurrence.

Client Information

- Make sure you understand how to give this medication to your animal. Keep the cap tightly closed when the medicine is not in use.
- Wait for 5 to 10 minutes after applying this medicine before applying any other medicines to the eye.
- Store cyclosporine ointment in the refrigerator or at room temperature away from moisture and sunlight. Handle and squeeze the tube gently so the metal will not crack and leak.
- Store cyclosporine solutions at room temperature (do not refrigerate or freeze).
- Do not use this medicine if the color of the solution changes, if it becomes cloudy, or if there are particles in the solution.
- This medication is considered to be a hazardous drug as defined by the National Institute for Occupational Safety and Health (NIOSH). Talk with your veterinarian or pharmacist about the use of personal protective equipment when handling this medicine.

Storage/Stability

Store the commercially available ophthalmic ointment in the refrigerator (2°C-8°C [35.6°F-46.4°F]) or at controlled room temperature (20°C-25°C [68°F-77°F]) away from moisture and sunlight. Do not refrigerate or freeze compounded cyclosporine solutions.

The long-term stability of a 1% solution in corn oil determined by USP is 180 days. Storage times should be determined by the results of individual extended stability and sterility testing or compendial standards.

Compatibility/Compounding Considerations

Cyclosporine should not be mixed directly (in vitro) with any other drugs.

Do not administer cyclosporine ophthalmic ointment or solutions compounded in oil in a subpalpebral lavage catheter, because of the likely irreversible obstruction of the catheter.

Dosage Forms/Regulatory Status

VETERINARY-LABELED PRODUCTS:

Cyclosporine 0.2% Ophthalmic Ointment (containing cyclosporine 2 mg/g, USP; petrolatum, USP; corn oil, NF; petrolatum and lanolin alcohol), in a 3.5 g ophthalmic ointment tube; *Optimmune*®; (Rx). Approved for use in dogs.

Cyclosporine 1% to 2% Ophthalmic Solutions in fixed oils may be compounded by qualified compounding pharmacists.

HUMAN-LABELED PRODUCTS:

Cyclosporine 0.05% Ophthalmic Emulsion (containing cyclosporine 0.05%; glycerin; castor oil; polysorbate 80; carbomer copolymer type A; purified water; NaOH to adjust pH), 30 or 60 sterile, single-use LDPE vials (0.4 mL each), or 5.5 mL sterile multi-dose ophthalmic dropper; *Restasis*®; (Rx). **NOTE:** This solution is not effective in controlling keratoconjunctivitis (KCS) in dogs.

Cyclosporine 0.09% Ophthalmic Solution (containing cyclosporine 0.09%; polyoxyl 40 hydrogenated castor oil; octoxynol-40; sodium phosphate, monobasic, dihydrate; sodium phosphate, dibasic, anhydrous; sodium chloride; povidone K90; hydrochloric acid; sodium hydroxide; water), in 6 pouches with 10 single-use vials (0.25 mL each) per pouch; *Cequa*®; (Rx). **NOTE:** This solution is not effective in controlling KCS in dogs.

References

For the complete list of references, see **wiley.com/go/budde/plumb**

Demecarium Ophthalmic

(deh-meh-***kar***-ee-um)

Anticholinesterase Ocular Antihypertensive

Prescriber Highlights

- ► Used primarily for preventive management of glaucoma in the unaffected eye of canine patients diagnosed with primary glaucoma in the fellow eye
- ► Product must be compounded as it is no longer commercially available.
- ► Used 1 to 2 times daily

Uses/Indications

Demecarium ophthalmic is used for preventive management of glaucoma in the contralateral eye of canine patients diagnosed with primary glaucoma in the fellow eye.[1,2] Demecarium's therapeutic efficacy for managing active glaucoma is minimal relative to other commercially available medications.

Pharmacology/Actions

Demecarium is an anticholinesterase that prolongs the effect of acetylcholine by inactivating the cholinesterases that break down acetylcholine, which has been released at the neuroeffector junction of parasympathetic postganglionic nerves. Demecarium inactivates both pseudocholinesterase and acetylcholinesterase. It causes constriction of the iris sphincter muscle (miosis) and the ciliary body muscle. These actions facilitate the outflow of aqueous humor, leading to a reduction in intraocular pressure (IOP). Demecarium is an organophosphate and may cause severe and even fatal dose-related toxicity associated with a decrease in systemic acetylcholinesterase levels, especially in cats.[3] See ***Adverse Effects.***

Contraindications/Precautions/Warnings

Demecarium is contraindicated in patients that have a history of hypersensitivity to it or any component of the formulation. Demecarium is contraindicated in pregnant animals; caregivers that are pregnant or intend to become pregnant should be warned to avoid contact with this medication.

Adverse Effects

Adverse effects reported in humans or animals include stinging, burning, and ocular irritation. Demecarium can cause severe and even fatal dose-related systemic toxicity, especially in cats.[3] Signs of systemic toxicity include vomiting, anorexia, diarrhea, lethargy, and weakness. Short-term (8 days) induction of aqueous humor flare occurs following the administration of demecarium in normal dogs.[4]

Dosages

Prophylaxis of glaucoma in the normal eye (extra-label): 1 drop to the nonglaucomatous eye 1 to 2 times daily

Monitoring

- Clinical efficacy; maintenance of normal intraocular pressure (IOP) in the contralateral eye of dogs with unilateral glaucoma
- Monitor for signs of systemic toxicity (vomiting, anorexia, diarrhea, lethargy, and weakness)

Client Information

- Use this medicine as directed by your veterinarian.
- Use proper administration techniques to avoid contamination of the medicine. Keep the cap tightly closed when the medicine is not in use.
- Wait for 5 minutes after applying this medicine before applying any other medicines to the eye.
- Store this product as directed on the product labeling, away from moisture and sunlight. Do not freeze.
- Do not use this medicine if the color changes, if it becomes cloudy, or if there are particles in the solution.

Storage/Stability

Store this product as directed on the product labeling away from moisture and sunlight; do not freeze.

Compatibility/Compounding Considerations

Demecarium ophthalmic preparations should not be mixed directly with any other ophthalmic medications.

Dosage Forms/Regulatory Status

VETERINARY-LABELED PRODUCTS: NONE

HUMAN-LABELED PRODUCTS: NONE

Demecarium bromide is no longer commercially available but may be prepared (compounded) as a 0.125% or 0.25% ophthalmic solution by qualified compounding pharmacists.

References

For the complete list of references, see **wiley.com/go/budde/plumb**

Dexamethasone Ophthalmic

(decks-uh-***meth***-uh-sown) *Maxidex®, Dexasporin®, Maxitrol®, Tobradex®*

Corticosteroid

For systemic use, refer to ***Dexamethasone***

Prescriber Highlights

- Topical corticosteroid used to treat ocular surface and intraocular inflammatory conditions
- May be combined with antibiotics (eg, neomycin, polymyxin B)
- Contraindications include a hypersensitivity to dexamethasone; an existing or suspected bacterial, viral, or fungal ocular infection; and in the presence of a corneal abrasion or ulceration.

Uses/Indications

Dexamethasone ophthalmic can be used to treat inflammation following ocular injury or cataract surgery or to treat generalized inflammatory conditions of the anterior segment (eg, conjunctivitis, keratitis, anterior uveitis). Evaluation of relative efficacy of dexamethasone ophthalmic in veterinary patients has not been performed.

Dexamethasone is available in many combinations with antimicrobial agents for topical ophthalmic use.

Pharmacology/Actions

Corticosteroids have broad immunomodulatory and anti-inflammatory actions, which are mediated via direct effects on gene expression, as well as by nongenomic effects on cell membranes and receptors. Ultimately, corticosteroids decrease pro-inflammatory gene transcription, production of pro-inflammatory prostaglandins and leukotrienes, B- and T-cell number and function, cell-mediated immunity, and humoral immunity.[1] Specific mechanisms involved in controlling ocular inflammatory conditions are not definitively known. Dexamethasone is a potent base steroid (relative glucocorticoid potency of 30 versus 4 for prednisolone and 1 for hydrocortisone). Greater intraocular penetration, and therefore potential clinical efficacy in cases of anterior uveitis, is achieved with dexamethasone alcohol formulations relative to sodium phosphate formulations; however, intraocular penetration of dexamethasone alcohol and sodium phosphate preparations is less than that of prednisolone acetate suspensions.

Following the topical administration of dexamethasone sodium phosphate, measurable concentrations of dexamethasone are present in the anterior segment of normal cat and dog eyes.[2,3]

Contraindications/Precautions/Warnings

Dexamethasone is contraindicated in patients that have a history of hypersensitivity to it or any component of the formulation. Due to inhibition of epithelial wound healing and potentiation of infection, dexamethasone ophthalmic is also contraindicated when corneal ulceration is suspected or present or in the presence of corneal infection (bacterial, fungal, or viral).[4] Topical administration of glucocorticoids may produce systemic effects. For more, refer to ***Glucocorticoid Agents, General Information***. Use dexamethasone ophthalmic with caution in patients with endocrine diseases (eg, diabetes mellitus, acromegaly), infectious diseases, chronic kidney disease, congestive heart failure, systemic hypertension, or gastric ulceration. When use of dexamethasone ophthalmic is necessary to treat a patient with these conditions, the minimal effective dose should be administered for the shortest possible time.

Adverse Effects

Adverse effects reported in humans include development of cataracts (via altered glucose or lenticular metabolic effects), increased intraocular pressure (IOP; via activation of glucocorticoid receptors in the trabecular meshwork), infection (via immunosuppression), decreased wound healing (via increased collagenolytic activity), mydriasis, and calcific keratopathy. In some animals, IOP may increase with chronic use; however, most reports suggest the change is reversible when the treatment is discontinued.[5,6] Cats with glaucoma have demonstrated a potentially clinically significant increase in IOP with administration of topical dexamethasone.[7] Systemic effects with topical ophthalmic administration are rare but include hepatopathy, suppression of endogenous glucocorticoid production, and focal alopecia. Concurrent use of systemic steroids increases the risk for these adverse effects.

Dosages

Conjunctivitis, keratitis, anterior uveitis (extra-label): 1 drop or ¼ inch strip to the affected eye(s) as frequently as every 2 hours until clinical improvement occurs, then gradually (over days to weeks) decrease the frequency of administration, provided clinical improvement is maintained.

Post-cataract removal (extra-label): 1 drop to the affected eye(s) every 8 to 12 hours

Monitoring

- Clinical efficacy
- Resolution or development of signs of inflammation
- Intraocular pressure (IOP; especially in cats) and ocular surface

integrity (eg, fluorescein stain) as needed based on clinical presentation
- Blood or urine glucose changes based on development of clinical signs (eg, polyuria, polydipsia) in diabetic animals

Client Information
- This medicine can be given for various lengths of time. Be sure you understand how often and for how long your animal should be given this medicine.
- Shake suspensions well before using.
- Use proper administration techniques to avoid contamination of the medication. Keep the cap tightly closed when the medicine is not in use.
- Wait 5 minutes after applying this medication before applying any other medications to the eye.
- Contact your veterinarian as soon as possible if your animal's eye condition worsens or does not improve while using this medicine.
- Your veterinarian will need to monitor your animal's eye condition while taking this medicine. Do not miss these important follow-up visits.
- Store this medicine as directed on the product label. Do not freeze.
- Do not use this medicine if the color changes, becomes cloudy, or if there are visible particles in the solution.

Storage/Stability
Storage recommendations can vary; follow storage requirements listed on packaging. Most commonly, this product is recommended to be stored at controlled room temperature 68°F to 77°F [20°C-25°C]) away from moisture and sunlight; do not freeze.

Compatibility/Compounding Considerations
Dexamethasone ophthalmic solutions should not be mixed directly with any other ophthalmic medications.

Dosage Forms/Regulatory Status

VETERINARY-LABELED PRODUCTS: NONE

HUMAN-LABELED PRODUCTS:

Dexamethasone Sodium Phosphate 0.1% Ophthalmic Suspension (containing dexamethasone 0.1%; benzalkonium chloride 0.01%; hypromellose 0.5%; NaCl; dibasic sodium phosphate; polysorbate 80; edetate disodium; citric acid and/or NaOH to adjust pH; purified water), 5 mL or 15 mL in sterile ophthalmic dropper bottle; *Maxidex*®; generic; (Rx)

Dexamethasone Sodium Phosphate 0.1% Ophthalmic Solution (containing dexamethasone 0.1%; benzalkonium chloride 0.01%; hypromellose 0.5%; NaCl; dibasic sodium phosphate; polysorbate 80; edetate disodium; citric acid and/or NaOH to adjust pH; purified water), 5 mL or 15 mL sterile ophthalmic dropper bottle; generic; (Rx)

HUMAN-LABELED COMBINATION PRODUCTS:

Neomycin and Polymyxin B Sulfates and Dexamethasone Ophthalmic Suspension (containing neomycin sulfate equivalent to neomycin 3.5 mg, polymyxin B sulfate 10,000 units, dexamethasone 0.1%, benzalkonium chloride 0.004%, hypromellose 2910 0.5%, sodium chloride, polysorbate 20, HCl and/or NaOH to adjust pH, purified water), in a 5 mL sterile ophthalmic dropper bottle; *Maxitrol*®, *Dexasporin*®; (Rx)

Neomycin and Polymyxin B Sulfates and Dexamethasone Ophthalmic ointment (containing neomycin sulfate equivalent to neomycin 3.5 mg, polymyxin B sulfate 10,000 units, dexamethasone 0.1%, methylparaben 0.05%, propylparaben 0.01%, white petrolatum, anhydrous liquid lanolin), in a sterile 3.5 g tube; *Maxitrol*®, generic; (Rx)

Tobramycin and Dexamethasone Ophthalmic Ointment (containing tobramycin 0.3%, dexamethasone 0.1%, chlorobutanol 0.5% , mineral oil, white petrolatum), in a sterile 3.5 g tube; *Tobradex*®; (Rx)

Tobramycin and Dexamethasone Ophthalmic Suspension (containing tobramycin 0.3%, dexamethasone 0.1%, benzalkonium chloride 0.01%, tyloxapol, edetate disodium, NaCl, hydroxyethyl cellulose, sodium sulfate, sulfuric acid and/or NaOH to adjust pH, purified water), in a sterile 2.5 mL ophthalmic dropper; *Tobradex*®, generic; (Rx)

Tobramycin and Dexamethasone Ophthalmic Suspension (containing tobramycin 0.3%, dexamethasone 0.05%, xanthan gum, tyloxapol, disodium edetate, NaCl, propylene glycol, sodium sulfate, benzalkonium chloride 0.01%, NaOH and/or HCl to adjust pH, purified water), in a sterile 5 mL ophthalmic dropper; *Tobradex*®; (Rx)

References
For the complete list of references, see **wiley.com/go/budde/plumb**

Diclofenac Ophthalmic

(dye-***kloe***-fen-ak) *Voltaren*®

Nonsteroidal Anti-inflammatory Drug (NSAID)

*For topical cream, refer to **Diclofenac, Topical***

Prescriber Highlights
- ► Used to control anterior segment inflammation
- ► May delay ocular wound healing and increase risk for intraocular bleeding
- ► Sulfite preservatives in diclofenac may trigger asthma attacks in susceptible patients.

Uses/Indications
Diclofenac ophthalmic is indicated for controlling anterior segment inflammation (eg, conjunctivitis, keratitis, anterior uveitis), inducing mydriasis during cataract-removal surgery, and for providing analgesia following surgical removal of cataracts. In dogs and cats, diclofenac significantly reduces clinical signs associated with experimentally induced intraocular inflammation[1,2]; however, it has not demonstrated reliable reduction in corneal sensitivity in normal dogs.[3,4]

Pharmacology/Actions
Diclofenac is an NSAID that blocks prostaglandin synthesis by inhibiting cyclooxygenase 1 and 2. Prostaglandins mediate many of the adverse effects of intraocular inflammation, including disruption of the blood-aqueous barrier, vasodilation, increased vascular permeability, leukocytosis, and increased intraocular pressure (IOP). Blocking prostaglandin production therefore minimizes the adverse short- and long-term effects of intraocular inflammation. Prostaglandins also appear to play a role in the miotic response produced during ocular surgery by constricting the iris sphincter independently of cholinergic mechanisms. Thus, diclofenac inhibits miosis induced during cataract surgery.[4]

Contraindications/Precautions/Warnings
Diclofenac is contraindicated in patients that have a history of hypersensitivity to it or any component of the formulation. The potential for cross-sensitivity to acetylsalicylic acid, phenylacetic acid derivatives, and other NSAIDs exists.[5] Topical NSAIDs may result in corneal epithelial breakdown and corneal thinning, erosion, or ulceration, which could cause delayed corneal wound healing; concurrent use of topical NSAIDs and topical corticosteroids may further delay healing and increase the potential for development of adverse effects.[5] Due to interference with thrombocyte aggregation, ophthalmic NSAIDs may cause increased bleeding of ocular tissues (eg, hyphema) in conjunction with ocular surgery. It is recommended

that diclofenac ophthalmic solution be used with caution in patients with known bleeding tendencies (eg, severe liver disease) or in those receiving anticoagulant medications (eg, heparins, rivaroxaban), which may prolong bleeding time.[5]

Adverse Effects

Adverse effects reported in humans or animals include transient ocular burning or stinging on administration.[5] Superficial punctate keratitis has been reported with long-term use. NSAIDs may also cause direct cellular damage, causing delayed healing and/or deterioration of existing corneal wounds. Although unlikely, systemic adverse effects may occur with the use of topical NSAIDs, including increased risk for gastric ulceration, decreased platelet aggregation, worsening of asthma and cardiac disease, and renal toxicity. Concurrent use of systemic NSAIDs and corticosteroids increases the risk for systemic adverse effects. The increased bleeding tendency of ocular tissues in conjunction with ocular surgery has also been reported. A comparison of the anti-inflammatory effects of topically administered diclofenac and prednisolone acetate in dogs with cataracts and well-regulated diabetes did not detect differences in measured parameters indicative of diabetes control (eg, fructosamine, body weight), although the authors concluded more research is warranted.[6] Although diclofenac administration was not associated with an elevation in intraocular pressure (IOP) in dogs with normal eyes,[7] it did result in increased IOP in dogs with experimentally induced uveitis.[8]

Dosages

Postoperative cataract surgery (extra-label): 1 drop to the affected eye(s) every 6 hours throughout the first 2 weeks of the postoperative period

Anterior segment inflammation (extra-label): 1 drop to the affected eye(s) every 6 to 12 hours

Monitoring

- Clinical efficacy (eg, decreased or absent anterior segment inflammation)
- Adverse effects (eg, delayed wound healing)

Client Information

- Use this medicine as directed by your veterinarian.
- Do not use this medicine if the color changes, if the solution becomes cloudy, or if there are particles in the solution.
- Diclofenac ophthalmic may cause burning or stinging on administration. It may also increase the risk for bleeding and may slow down healing in the eye.
- Use proper administration techniques to avoid contamination of the medication. Keep the cap tightly closed on the medicine when it is not in use.
- Wait for 5 minutes after applying this medicine before applying any other medications to the eye.
- Store this medicine at room temperature away from moisture and sunlight. Do not freeze.
- Your veterinarian will need to monitor your animal while it is taking this medicine. Do not miss these important follow-up visits.

Storage/Stability

Store this product at controlled room temperature (68°F to 77°F [20°C-25°C]) away from moisture and sunlight; do not freeze.

Compatibility/Compounding Considerations

Diclofenac ophthalmic solutions should not be mixed directly with any other ophthalmic medications.

Dosage Forms/Regulatory Status

VETERINARY-LABELED PRODUCTS: NONE

HUMAN-LABELED PRODUCTS:

Diclofenac Sodium 0.1% Ophthalmic Solution (containing 1 mg diclofenac sodium; polyoxyl 35 castor oil; boric acid; tromethamine; sorbic acid (2 mg/mL); edetate disodium (1 mg/mL); purified water), in a 5 mL ophthalmic dropper bottle; *Voltaren*®, generic; (Rx)

References

For the complete list of references, see **wiley.com/go/budde/plumb**

Difluprednate Ophthalmic

(dye-floo-***pred***-nate) *Durezol*®

Corticosteroid

Prescriber Highlights

- Used for treatment of anterior segment inflammatory conditions
- Exerts clinical effect equal to that of prednisolone acetate
- Do not use in patients with an existing or suspected bacterial, viral, or fungal ocular infection or in the presence of corneal ulceration

Uses/Indications

Difluprednate ophthalmic can be used to treat inflammation following ocular injury or cataract surgery or to treat generalized inflammatory conditions of the anterior segment (eg, conjunctivitis, keratitis, anterior uveitis). It has been shown to exert comparable efficacy to prednisolone acetate in humans[1] and in dogs with experimentally induced anterior chamber inflammation.[2]

Pharmacology/Actions

Corticosteroids have broad immunomodulatory and anti-inflammatory actions, which are mediated via direct effects on gene expression, as well as by nongenomic effects on cell membranes and receptors. Ultimately, corticosteroids decrease proinflammatory gene transcription, production of proinflammatory prostaglandins and leukotrienes, B- and T-cell number and function, cell-mediated immunity, and humoral immunity.[3] Specific mechanisms involved in regulating ocular inflammation are not known.

Contraindications/Precautions/Warnings

Difluprednate is contraindicated in patients that have a history of hypersensitivity to it or any component of the formulation. Due to inhibition of epithelial wound healing and potentiation of infection, difluprednate ophthalmic is contraindicated when corneal ulceration is suspected or present or in the presence of corneal infection (bacterial, fungal, or viral),[4] infectious diseases, chronic renal failure, congestive heart failure, systemic hypertension, or gastric ulceration. When use of difluprednate is necessary in these conditions, the minimal effective dose should be administered for the shortest possible time.

Adverse Effects

Adverse effects reported in humans include development of cataracts (via altered glucose or lenticular metabolic effects), increased intraocular pressure (IOP; via activation of glucocorticoid receptors in the trabecular meshwork), infection (via immunosuppression), decreased wound healing (via increased collagenolytic activity), mydriasis, and calcific keratopathy. Increased IOP may occur in some animals with long-term use of difluprednate; however, most reports suggest the change is reversible.[5,6] Systemic effects are rare but include hepatopathy, suppression of endogenous glucocorticoid production, and focal alopecia. Concurrent use of systemic steroids increases the risk for these adverse effects.

Dosages

Conjunctivitis (extra-label): 1 drop in affected eye(s) every 4 to 8 hours, then gradually decrease the dose over days to weeks, provided clinical improvement is maintained

Keratitis (extra-label): 1 drop in affected eye(s) every 4 to 8 hours, then gradually decrease the dose over days to weeks, provided clinical improvement is maintained

Anterior uveitis (extra-label): 1 drop in affected eye(s) 4 times daily for 14 days, then gradually decrease the dose over days to weeks, provided clinical improvement is maintained

Post-cataract removal (extra-label): 1 drop in the surgical eye 4 times daily, beginning 24 hours after surgery and continuing 2 weeks postoperative, then decrease to 2 times daily for 1 week, then continue to taper dosage based on clinical response

Monitoring

- Clinical efficacy
- Resolution or development of signs of inflammation
- Intraocular pressure (IOP; especially in cats) and ocular surface integrity (eg, fluorescein stain) as needed based on clinical presentation
- Blood or urine glucose changes based on development of clinical signs (eg, polyuria, polydipsia) in diabetic animals

Client Information

- This medicine can be given for various lengths of time. Be sure you understand how often and for how long your animal should be given this medicine.
- Use proper administration techniques to avoid contamination of the medication. Keep the cap tightly closed when the medicine is not in use.
- Wait 5 minutes after applying this medication before applying any other medications to the eye.
- Contact your veterinarian as soon as possible if your animal's eye condition worsens or does not improve while using this medicine.
- Your veterinarian will need to monitor your animal's eye condition while taking this medicine. Do not miss these important follow-up visits.
- Store this medicine as directed on the product label. Do not freeze.
- Do not use this medicine if the color changes, if it becomes cloudy, or if there are visible particles in the solution.

Storage/Stability

Store this product at controlled room temperature (20°C-25°C [68°F-77°F]) away from moisture and sunlight; do not freeze.

Compatibility/Compounding Considerations

Difluprednate ophthalmic preparations should not be mixed directly with any other ophthalmic medications.

Dosage Forms/Regulatory Status

VETERINARY-LABELED PRODUCTS: NONE

HUMAN-LABELED PRODUCTS:

Difluprednate 0.05% Ophthalmic Emulsion (containing difluprednate 0.05%; sorbic acid 0.1%; boric acid; castor oil; glycerin; polysorbate 80; water for injection; sodium acetate; sodium EDTA; NaOH to adjust the pH to 5.2 to 5.8, with tonicity of 304 – 411 mOsm/kg), in 5 mL ophthalmic dropper bottle; *Durezol*®; (Rx)

References

For the complete list of references, see **wiley.com/go/budde/plumb**

Dorzolamide Ophthalmic

(dor-***zoe***-la-mide) *Trusopt*®, *Cosopt*®, *Cosopt*® *PF*

Carbonic Anhydrase Inhibitor Anti-Glaucoma Agent

Prescriber Highlights

- ▶ Decreases intraocular pressure (IOP) by reducing the production of aqueous humor
- ▶ Three-times-daily dosing recommended over twice-daily dosing
- ▶ More stinging on application compared with brinzolamide, due to more acidic pH of dorzolamide
- ▶ Sulfonamide derivative; caregivers with sulfa allergies should avoid direct contact with the medicine.
- ▶ Available as a single agent or in combination with timolol maleate

Uses/Indications

Dorzolamide ophthalmic (alone or in combination with timolol) is used to decrease intraocular pressure (IOP) in patients with glaucoma and ocular hypertension. In dogs with and without glaucoma, dorzolamide leads to a significant IOP reduction, which is more consistent when it is dosed 3 times daily versus 2 times daily.[1,2] When dorzolamide ophthalmic is administered in combination with a beta blocker, the IOP-lowering effects are additive.[3,4] Reduced IOP also occurs in normal cats and horses,[5] and similar to dogs, improved efficacy may result when dorzolamide is administered in combination with timolol in horses.[6,7] Efficacy of prophylactic dorzolamide administration for preventing manifestation of primary glaucoma in unaffected eyes of dogs with contralateral primary glaucoma has not been demonstrated.[8]

Pharmacology/Actions

Carbonic anhydrase (CA) is an enzyme found in many body tissues, including the eye. CA inhibitors reduce the formation of hydrogen and bicarbonate ions from carbon dioxide and water by noncompetitive, reversible inhibition of the enzyme CA, thereby reducing the availability of these ions for active transport into secretions.[9] In humans, CA exists as multiple isoenzymes, with CA-II being the most relevant to glaucoma management. Inhibition of CA in the ciliary processes of the eye decreases aqueous humor secretion, presumably by slowing the formation of bicarbonate ions with subsequent reduction in sodium and fluid transport, which results in a decrease in intraocular pressure (IOP).[9] Dorzolamide equilibrates between acidic and basic forms, allowing for both lipid and water solubility and greater corneal and scleral penetration.

Contraindications/Precautions/Warnings

Dorzolamide is contraindicated in patients that have a history of hypersensitivity to it or sulfonamides or any component of the formulation.

Adverse Effects

Adverse effects reported in humans or animals include burning and stinging upon application (due to low pH), superficial punctate keratitis, local hypersensitivity reactions, and corneal edema. Systemic adverse effects are not usually observed with the topical application; however, renal tubular acidosis and hypokalemia have been reported in a cat due to topical carbonic anhydrase inhibitor (CAI) administration.[10] CAIs, including dorzolamide, have been implicated in the development of significant ulcerative and nonulcerative keratitis following long-term administration.[11]

Dosages

Glaucoma (extra-label): 1 drop in the affected eye(s) or 0.1 mL in the subpalpebral lavage (SPL) catheter every 8 to 12 hours

Monitoring

- Clinical efficacy
- Confirm maintenance of intraocular pressure (IOP) within the normal range for the species being treated
- Monitor for corneal edema

Client Information

- Use this medication as directed by your veterinarian.
- Use proper administration techniques to avoid contamination of the medicine. Keep the cap tightly closed when the medicine is not in use.
- Wait for 5 minutes after applying this medication before applying any other medications to the eye.
- Store at room temperature away from moisture and sunlight. Do not freeze.
- Do not use this medication if the color changes.

Storage/Stability

Store this product at controlled room temperature (20°C-25°C [68°F-77°F]) away from moisture and sunlight.

Compatibility/Compounding Considerations

Dorzolamide ophthalmic preparations should not be mixed directly with any other ophthalmic medications.

Dosage Forms/Regulatory Status

VETERINARY-LABELED PRODUCTS: NONE

HUMAN-LABELED PRODUCTS:

Dorzolamide HCl 2% Ophthalmic Solution (containing dorzolamide HCl 22.3 mg equivalent to 20 mg dorzolamide; benzalkonium chloride 0.0075%; hydroxyethyl cellulose; mannitol; sodium citrate dehydrate; NaOH to adjust pH; water for injection), in 5 mL and 10 mL ophthalmic dropper bottles; *Trusopt*®, generic; (Rx)

HUMAN-LABELED COMBINATION PRODUCTS:

Dorzolamide HCl 2% and Timolol maleate 0.5% Ophthalmic Solution (containing dorzolamide HCl equivalent to 20 mg dorzolamide; timolol maleate 6.8 mg equivalent to 5 mg timolol; benzalkonium chloride 0.0075%; sodium citrate; hydroxyethyl cellulose; NaOH; mannitol; water for injection, with a pH of 5.65 and an osmolality of 242 – 323 mOsm/kg), in sterile 10 mL ophthalmic dispenser bottles. *Cosopt*®, generic; (Rx)

Dorzolamide HCl 2% and Timolol maleate 0.5% Ophthalmic Solution, preservative-free (containing 22.3 mg dorzolamide HCl equivalent to 20 mg dorzolamide; 6.8 mg timolol maleate equivalent to 5 mg timolol; hydroxyethyl cellulose; mannitol; sodium citrate; NaOH to adjust pH; water for injection), in 15 sterile single-use containers, 0.2 mL per container; *Cosopt® PF*; (Rx)

References

For the complete list of references, see **wiley.com/go/budde/plumb**

Edetate Disodium Ophthalmic

Sodium EDTA

(ed-uh-***tayt*** dye-***so***-dee-um)

Chelating Agent

Prescriber Highlights

- Used for dissolution of corneal calcium deposits
- Also used to decrease corneal digestion due to collagenase activity in infected ulcers
- Do not mix with calcium-containing drugs
- No longer commercially available; must be compounded

Uses/Indications

Edetate disodium is used topically to remove calcific corneal deposits that occur in the superficial cornea, which may cause pain or impair vision. Corneal calcium deposits may form in association with chronic keratitis, chronic uveitis, or hypercalcemia. These deposits may be dissolved from the conjunctiva, corneal epithelium, and anterior stroma following EDTA administration. Calcium deposits in the deep stroma are not affected, as edetate disodium is lipid-insoluble and does not penetrate the corneal epithelium. Topical administration of EDTA also decreases collagenase activity in infected corneal ulcers, thus helping to control corneal melting.[1,2] Edetate disodium has been used as an emergency treatment to decontaminate the eye after injury by zinc chloride, and for emergency management and follow-up treatment of calcium hydroxide burns in the eye.

Pharmacology/Actions

Edetate disodium forms a soluble complex with calcium ions and other divalent and trivalent metals, which leads to the dissolution of calcium deposits from the ocular surface. As calcium (and other) ions serve as cofactors for enzymes responsible for collagenolysis, binding the ions makes them unavailable to the enzymes, thus decreasing enzymatic activity.[1]

Contraindications/Precautions/Warnings

Edetate disodium ophthalmic should not be used in patients that are hypersensitive to it or any component of the formulation.

Adverse Effects

Adverse effects reported in humans or animals include swelling of the stroma (usually following application of concentrations greater than 1%), stinging on application, and swelling of the eyelids. Toxic effects have been demonstrated in vitro to corneal epithelial cells.[3]

Dosages

Calcium chelation for corneal deposits and/or collagenolysis (extra-label): 1 drop of the solution (0.35% to 1.85%, but most commonly 1%) to the affected eye(s) initially 4 to 6 times daily and then 3 to 4 times daily as indicated

Zinc chloride injury (extra-label): Topical, to the cornea, as a 1.7% (0.046 M) solution as irrigation for 15 minutes; more likely to be effective if started within 2 minutes of exposure

Monitoring

- Clinical efficacy
- Monitor mineral deposits in the cornea
- Monitor corneal digestion (melting)

Client Information

- Use this medicine as directed by your veterinarian.
- Use proper administration techniques to avoid contamination of the medication. Keep the cap tightly closed when the medicine is not in use.
- Wait 5 minutes after applying this medication before applying any other medications to the eye.
- Store this medicine as directed on the product label. Do not freeze.
- Do not use this product if the color changes, if it becomes cloudy, or if there are particles in the solution.
- Discard this product by the date indicated on the label.

Storage/Stability

Store this product as directed on the product labeling; do not freeze.

Compatibility/Compounding Considerations

Edetate disodium ophthalmic preparations should not be mixed directly with any other ophthalmic medications, especially those containing calcium.

Dosage Forms/Regulatory Status

VETERINARY-LABELED PRODUCTS: NONE

HUMAN-LABELED PRODUCTS: NONE

Edetate disodium ophthalmic solution must be prepared (compounded) by a qualified compounding pharmacist. It is usually prepared as a 1% solution in an artificial tear solution not containing calcium.

References

For the complete list of references, see **wiley.com/go/budde/plumb**

Epinastine Ophthalmic

(ep-i-***nas***-teen) *Elestat®*

Antihistamine

Prescriber Highlights

- ► H_1-selective antihistamine with H_2-blocking and mast cell stabilizing activity
- ► Used to relieve signs of allergic conjunctivitis (particularly pruritus)
- ► Duration of action allows for twice-daily dosing

Uses/Indications

Epinastine is used to treat and prevent pruritus associated with allergic conjunctivitis.

Pharmacology/Actions

Epinastine is a topically active, direct histamine-1 (H_1) receptor antagonist and an inhibitor of histamine release from the mast cell. Epinastine is selective for the H_1 receptor and has an affinity for the histamine-2 (H_2) receptor. Epinastine also possesses an affinity for the alpha-1, alpha-2, and 5-HT_2 receptors.[1] No evaluation of its use as a topical ophthalmic agent has been performed in veterinary species.

Contraindications/Precautions/Warnings

Epinastine is contraindicated in patients that have a history of hypersensitivity to it or any component of the formulation.

Adverse Effects

Adverse effects reported in humans include burning sensation in the eye, folliculitis, hyperemia, pruritus, and epiphora.[1] The most frequently reported nonocular adverse reactions include cold symptoms and upper respiratory infections, headache, rhinitis, sinusitis, increased cough, and pharyngitis. Some of these adverse effects may be related to the underlying disease being treated.

Dosages

Allergic conjunctivitis (extra-label): 1 drop in the affected eye(s) every 12 hours

Monitoring

- Clinical efficacy: resolution of signs related to allergic conjunctivitis (eg, pruritus, tearing, squinting)

Client Information

- Use this medicine as directed by your veterinarian.
- Use proper administration techniques to avoid contamination of the medicine. Keep the cap tightly closed when the medicine is not in use.
- Wait for 5 minutes after applying this medication before applying any other medications to the eye.
- Store this medication at room temperature away from moisture and sunlight. Do not freeze.
- Do not use this medicine if the color changes, if it becomes cloudy, or if there are particles in solution.

Storage/Stability

Store at controlled room temperature (20°C-25°C [68°F-77°F]) away from moisture and sunlight; do not freeze.

Compatibility/Compounding Considerations

Epinastine ophthalmic preparations should not be mixed directly with any other ophthalmic medications.

Dosage Forms/Regulatory Status

VETERINARY-LABELED PRODUCTS: NONE

HUMAN-LABELED PRODUCTS:

Epinastine HCl 0.05% Ophthalmic Solution (containing epinastine 0.05%; benzalkonium chloride 0.01%; edetate disodium; purified water; NaCl; sodium phosphate, monobasic; NaOH and/or HCl to adjust pH to 7; osmolality range of 250 – 310 mOsm/kg), in a 5 mL sterile ophthalmic dropper bottle; *Elestat®*, generic; (Rx)

References

For the complete list of references, see **wiley.com/go/budde/plumb**

Erythromycin Ophthalmic

(eh-***rith***-rowe-***mye***-sin)

Macrolide Antibiotic

For systemic use, refer to ***Erythromycin***

Prescriber Highlights

- ► Used to treat susceptible ocular surface infections (eg, *Mycoplasma* spp and *Chlamydia* spp in cats)
- ► Only available as an ophthalmic ointment
- ► Used up to 6 times daily
- ► Use with caution in pocket pets that may ingest the drug via grooming.

Uses/Indications

Erythromycin ophthalmic ointment is used for the treatment of superficial ocular infections involving the conjunctiva and/or cornea caused by organisms that are susceptible to erythromycin. See ***Pharmacology/Actions***. Administration of topical erythromycin to normal cat eyes did not induce significant changes in normal ocular surface microflora.[1]

The World Health Organization (WHO) has designated erythromycin as a Critically Important, Highest Priority antimicrobial for human medicine.[2] The Office International des Epizooties (OIE) has designated macrolides as Veterinary Critically Important Antimicrobial (VCIA) Agents in avian, bovine, caprine, equine, lagomorphs, ovine, and swine species.[3]

Pharmacology/Actions

Erythromycin inhibits protein synthesis by binding the 50S subunit of the bacterial ribosome, thus inhibiting the formation of peptide bonds between amino acids by a variety of specific mechanisms. Erythromycin is usually active against *Streptococcus* spp, *Staphylococcus* spp, *Mycoplasma* spp, and *Chlamydia* spp.[4]

Erythromycin is considered ineffective against *Pseudomonas aeruginosa*.[5]

Contraindications/Precautions/Warnings

Erythromycin is contraindicated in patients that have a history of hypersensitivity to it or any component of the formulation. Topical macrolides should be used carefully, if at all, in pocket pets (eg, hamsters, chinchillas) and rabbits, as these animals may ingest macrolides while grooming, which increases the potential for GI adverse effects.

Adverse Effects

Adverse effects reported in humans or animals include mild **ocular** stinging, burning, irritation, and redness. Pocket pets ingesting macrolides may suffer from acute and potentially fatal diarrhea.

Dosages

Susceptible ocular infections (extra-label): ¼ – ½ inch strip in the affected eye(s) up to 6 times daily depending on the severity of infection

Monitoring

- Corneal cytology and culture to evaluate for the presence of bacteria
- Clinical efficacy: improvement and resolution of clinical signs associated with bacterial infection
- GI clinical signs; discontinue administration if diarrhea occurs following use on pocket pets.

Client Information

- Use this medicine as directed by your veterinarian
- Do not give this medicine to pocket pets (eg, hamsters, chinchillas) or rabbits without frequent examinations by your veterinarian.
- To prevent contamination, do not touch the dropper tip or allow it to touch your animal's eye or any other surface. Keep the cap tightly closed on the medication when it is not in use.
- If you are administering more than 1 eye medication to your animal, wait 5 minutes between each medication before giving the next. Use eye drops before eye ointments to allow the drops to absorb into the eye.
- Your veterinarian will need to monitor your animal while it is receiving this medicine. Do not miss these important follow-up visits.
- Store this medicine at room temperature; do not freeze. Do not use the medicine if the color or consistency changes.

Storage/Stability

Store erythromycin ophthalmic formulations at controlled room temperature (20°C-25°C [68°F-77°F]); do not freeze.

Compatibility/Compounding Considerations

Erythromycin should not be mixed directly (in vitro) with any other drugs. Erythromycin is not available as an ophthalmic solution.

Dosage Forms/Regulatory Status

VETERINARY-LABELED PRODUCTS: NONE

HUMAN-LABELED PRODUCTS:

Erythromycin 0.5% Ophthalmic Ointment (containing erythromycin 5 mg/g in a sterile ophthalmic base of mineral oil and white petrolatum), in a 3.5 g ointment tube; generic; (Rx)

References

For the complete list of references, see **wiley.com/go/budde/plumb**

Fluorescein Stain Ophthalmic

(***flur***-e-seen)

Ocular Diagnostic Agent

Prescriber Highlights

- Used clinically to delineate full-thickness loss of corneal epithelium (corneal ulcer), to evaluate tear film breakup time, and to determine patency of nasolacrimal outflow system (Jones test)
- Yellow-green dye binds to corneal stroma but not to the corneal epithelium or Descemet membrane
- Available in combination with topical anesthetic (oxybuprocaine) to minimize discomfort on application and to facilitate additional diagnostic tests
- IV injection of its approved formulations is used diagnostically during fluorescein angiography.
- Fluorescein should **not** be used during intraocular surgery.

Uses/Indications

Topical application of fluorescein solutions to the ocular surface enables identification of corneal ulcers, evaluation of tear film breakup time (an indicator of tear film quality), and determination of patency of the nasolacrimal system (Jones test). Manufactured solutions of fluorescein, with or without topical anesthetics, are available for use, whereas dilution of individually wrapped fluorescein strips with eyewash is an alternative method that also decreases the risk for contamination between patients. Visualization of fluorescein retention by the cornea or conjunctiva, with either white or cobalt blue light, indicates epithelial loss (ulceration). The rapid appearance of breaks in fluorescein within the tear film suggests tear film quality disturbances. The appearance of fluorescein at the nostril following application to the ocular surface indicates functional patency of the nasolacrimal duct system (positive Jones test). IV injection of fluorescein solutions is used to evaluate blood flow patterns within the eye in the diagnostic procedure fluorescein angiography.

Pharmacology/Actions

Fluorescein is a water-soluble dye that is not retained by normal cornea because it does not pass through the hydrophobic epithelium. If the epithelium is absent, fluorescein penetrates the hydrophilic corneal stroma and stains it bright yellow-green. The green color is best visualized utilizing blue light from a cobalt filter attached to a penlight transilluminator, or a Wood's lamp. It may also be visible with ambient white light. Defects in the corneal stroma that extend to the deepest layer (Descemet membrane) will not retain fluorescein in the deepest aspect, as Descemet membrane is hydrophobic. In fluorescein angiography, vessels in the active areas of inflammation and neovascularization demonstrate leakage of fluorescein associated with increased vascular permeability. Fluorescein fluoresces in light with a wavelength between 485 and 500 nm, with maximal emission between 520 and 530 nm.

Contraindications/Precautions/Warnings

Fluorescein is contraindicated in patients that have a history of hypersensitivity to it or any component of the formulation. Fluorescein should not be used during intraocular surgery.

Adverse Effects

Adverse effects reported in humans or animals following the application of the strips include local hypersensitivity reactions and transient discomfort. Temporary staining of the skin and fur may result after use. Adverse effects following IV administration can be severe and include nausea, vomiting, GI distress, headache, syncope, hypotension, and signs of hypersensitivity. In humans, cardiac arrest, basilar artery ischemia, severe shock, convulsions, thrombophlebitis at the injection site, and, in rare cases, death have been reported. Extravasation of the solution at the injection site causes intense pain at the site and dull aching pain in the injected limb.[1]

Dosages

Determination of corneal injury: Wet fluorescein strip with 1 to 2 drops of normal saline solution. Apply moistened tip to conjunctiva or fornix. Allow patient to blink several times after application. Wait 60 seconds, rinse with sterile irrigating solution, and examine with the use of a light source; a cobalt filter may be attached to the light surface for better visualization. Defects in the corneal epithelium illuminate the stroma bright green. In deep corneal lesions, the lesion's center may fail to take up the stain and appears black, indicating that a descemetocele is present.

Tear film breakup time: Wet fluorescein strip with 1 to 2 drops of normal saline solution. Apply moistened tip to conjunctiva or fornix. Allow patient to blink once, and then hold lids open and monitor tear film for breaks, which appear as dark lines within the green.

Normal values are greater than 20 seconds in dogs, with shorter times indicating qualitative tear film deficiency.

Nasolacrimal outflow patency (Jones test): Wet fluorescein strip with 1 to 2 drops of normal saline solution. Apply moistened tip to conjunctiva or fornix. It is recommended that the patient's nose be tipped downward to facilitate drainage of fluorescein-laden tears through the nasolacrimal system, at which point fluorescein will be visible at the nares; a cobalt filter may be attached to a light surface for better visualization. Normal times are 2 to 5 minutes in dogs and up to 10 minutes in cats.

Fluorescein angiography: Rapid IV injection (≈1 mL/second) of 2 to 5 mL of fluorescein 100 mg/mL in the antecubital vein is followed by ocular vasculature visualization, using a cobalt filter light source and appropriate magnification. Time to filling and pattern of filling of vasculature within the anterior and posterior segments are noted and correlated with normal versus disease states. (This procedure is performed by board-certified veterinary ophthalmologists.)

Monitoring

- Diagnostic product; no monitoring is required

Client Information

- Do not use fluorescein strips at home.

Storage/Stability

Store this product at controlled room temperature (20°C-25°C [68°F-77°F]) away from moisture and sunlight; do not freeze.

Compatibility/Compounding Considerations

Fluorescein ophthalmic preparations should not be mixed directly with any other ophthalmic medications.

Dosage Forms/Regulatory Status

VETERINARY-LABELED PRODUCTS: NONE

HUMAN-LABELED PRODUCTS:

Although IV fluorescein solutions have been approved by the US FDA, no topical ophthalmic fluorescein products have been approved.

Fluorescein Sodium 10% Injection (containing fluorescein 100 mg/mL and sterile water for injection; NaOH and/or HCl to adjust pH), in 5 mL single-use glass vials; *Fluorescite*®; (Rx)

Fluorescein Sodium 10% Injection (containing fluorescein 100 mg/mL and sterile water for injection; NaOH and/or HCl to adjust pH), in 5 mL single-dose glass vials; *AK-FLUOR 10%*®; (Rx)

Fluorescein Sodium 25% Injection (containing fluorescein 250 mg/mL and sterile water for injection; NaOH and/or HCl to adjust pH), in 2 mL single-dose glass vials; *AK-FLUOR 25%*; (Rx)

Fluorescein Sodium Ophthalmic Strips USP 1 mg per strip; individually wrapped strips in cartons of 50, 100, or 300; *Dry Eye Test*®, *Ful-Glo*®, *Bioglo*®, *Glostrips*®; (Rx)

COMBINATION PRODUCTS APPROVED FOR USE IN HUMANS:

Fluorescein Sodium and Benoxinate Hydrochloride Ophthalmic Solution 0.25%/0.4% (containing fluorescein sodium 2.5 mg; benoxinate hydrochloride 4 mg; povidone; hydrochloric acid; boric acid; sodium hydroxide; water for injection; hydrochloric acid and/or sodium hydroxide to adjust pH to 4.3 to 5.3), in sterile 5 mL ophthalmic dropper bottle; *Altafluor Benox*®, generic; (Rx)

Fluorescein Sodium and Benoxinate Hydrochloride Ophthalmic Solution 0.25%/0.4% (containing fluorescein sodium 2.5 mg; benoxinate hydrochloride 4 mg; chlorobutanol 10 mg; boric acid; povidone; sodium hydroxide and/or hydrochloric acid may be added to adjust pH to 4.3 to 5.3; purified water), in sterile 5 mL ophthalmic dropper bottle; *Fluress*®, generic; (Rx)

References

For the complete list of references, see **wiley.com/go/budde/plumb**

Fluorometholone Ophthalmic

(flew-roe-***meth***-oh-lone) *Flarex*®, *FML*®, *FML Forte*®

Corticosteroid

Prescriber Highlights

- ▶ Used to treat anterior segment inflammatory conditions
- ▶ Contraindications include the presence of corneal ulceration and existing or suspected bacterial, viral, or fungal ocular infection.
- ▶ Use with caution in avian species, as systemic adrenal suppression may result.
- ▶ Shake suspension well before using.

Uses/Indications

Fluorometholone ophthalmic can be used to treat inflammation following ocular injury or cataract surgery or to treat generalized inflammatory conditions of the anterior segment (eg, conjunctivitis, keratitis, anterior uveitis). Evaluation of relative efficacy of fluorometholone ophthalmic in veterinary patients has not been performed.

Pharmacology/Actions

Corticosteroids have broad immunomodulatory and anti-inflammatory actions, mediated via direct effects on gene expression, as well as by nongenomic effects on cell membranes and receptors. Ultimately, corticosteroids decrease pro-inflammatory gene transcription, production of pro-inflammatory prostaglandins and leukotrienes, B- and T-cell number and function, cell-mediated immunity, and humoral immunity.[1] The specific mechanisms involved in regulating ocular inflammation are not known. Fluorometholone alcohol preparations are most effective for ocular surface inflammation, rather than intraocular inflammation, due to comparatively poor transcorneal penetration relative to the acetate preparations.

Contraindications/Precautions/Warnings

Fluorometholone is contraindicated in patients that have a history of hypersensitivity to it or any component of the formulation. Ocular corticosteroids should not be used in animals with bacterial, fungal, or viral ocular infections, or if corneal ulceration is present, as they may potentiate infection and decrease epithelial wound healing.

Adverse Effects

Adverse effects reported in humans include development of cataracts (via altered glucose or lenticular metabolic effects), increased intraocular pressure (IOP; via activation of glucocorticoid receptors in the trabecular meshwork), infection (via immunosuppression), decreased wound healing (via increased collagenolytic activity), mydriasis, and calcific keratopathy. Some animals may develop increased IOP with chronic use; however, most reports suggest the change is reversible.[2,3] Additionally, fluorometholone is associated with less risk of IOP elevation compared with other topical corticosteroids. Systemic effects are rare but include hepatopathy, suppression of endogenous glucocorticoid production, and focal alopecia. Concurrent use of systemic steroids increases the risk for these adverse effects.

Dosages

Conjunctivitis (extra-label): 1 drop or ¼ inch strip in the affected eye(s) as frequently as every 4 hours until clinical improvement occurs, then gradually (over days to weeks) decrease the dosage, provided clinical improvement is maintained

Keratitis (extra-label): 1 drop or ¼ inch strip in the affected eye(s) as frequently as every 4 hours until clinical improvement occurs, then gradually (over days to weeks) decrease the dosage, provided clinical improvement is maintained

Anterior uveitis (extra-label): 1 drop or ¼ inch strip in the affected eye(s) as frequently as every 4 hours until clinical improvement occurs, then gradually (over days to weeks) decrease the dosage, provided clinical improvement is maintained

Monitoring

- Clinical efficacy through resolution of signs of inflammation
- Monitor intraocular pressure (IOP) and ocular surface integrity
- Blood or urine glucose changes based on development of clinical signs (eg, polyuria, polydipsia) in diabetic animals

Client Information

- Use this medicine as directed by your veterinarian.
- It is important to shake the suspension well before giving this medicine to your animal.
- Use proper administration techniques to avoid contamination of the medication. Keep the cap tightly closed when the medicine is not in use.
- Wait for 5 to 10 minutes after applying this medicine before applying any other medicines to the eye.
- Store this medicine in the refrigerator or at room temperature away from moisture and sunlight. Do not freeze.
- Do not use this medicine if the color changes or if there are particles in the suspension.

Storage/Stability

Store this product in the refrigerator or at controlled room temperature (2°C-25°C [36°F-77°F]) away from moisture and sunlight; do not freeze.

Compatibility/Compounding Considerations

Fluorometholone ophthalmic preparations should not be mixed directly with any other ophthalmic medications.

Dosage Forms/Regulatory Status

VETERINARY-LABELED PRODUCTS: NONE

HUMAN-LABELED PRODUCTS:

Fluorometholone 0.1% Ophthalmic Suspension (containing fluorometholone 1 mg/mL; benzalkonium chloride 0.01%; sodium chloride; monobasic sodium phosphate; edetate disodium; hydroxyethyl cellulose; tyloxapol; HCl and/or NaOH to adjust pH; purified water), 5 mL or 10 mL in sterile ophthalmic dropper bottles; *FML®*, *Flarex®*; (Rx)

Fluorometholone 0.25% Ophthalmic Suspension (containing fluorometholone 2.5 mg/mL; benzalkonium chloride 0.005%; edetate disodium; polysorbate 80; polyvinyl alcohol 1.4%; purified water; NaCl; sodium phosphate, dibasic; sodium phosphate, monobasic; NaOH to adjust the pH from 6.2 to 7.5), 5 mL or 10 mL in sterile ophthalmic dropper bottles; *FML Forte®*; (Rx)

Fluorometholone 0.1% Ophthalmic Ointment (containing fluorometholone 1 mg/mL; phenylmercuric acetate (0.0008%); mineral oil; petrolatum (and) lanolin alcohol; white petrolatum), in 3.5 g ophthalmic ointment tubes; *FML®*; (Rx)

References

For the complete list of references, see **wiley.com/go/budde/plumb**

Fluorouracil Ophthalmic

(flewr-oh-***your***-uh-sil)

Antineoplastic Agent

*For systemic use, see **Fluorouracil***

Prescriber Highlights

- ► Antifibrotic agent used adjunctively in periocular surgeries (most commonly in glaucoma implant procedures)
- ► Antineoplastic used for susceptible cutaneous tumors
- ► **Do NOT use in cats** or in patients with myelosuppression or serious infections.
- ► Adverse effects include dose-dependent myelosuppression, GI toxicity, and neurotoxicity.
- ► Known teratogen
- ► The National Institute for Occupational Safety and Health (NIOSH) classifies fluorouracil as a hazardous drug; use appropriate precautions when handling.

Uses/Indications

Fluorouracil ophthalmic is used as an adjunct in ocular surgeries, particularly in those that treat glaucoma through placement of drainage shunts or alteration of the natural aqueous humor outflow tracts, because of fluorouracil's ability to reduce fibroblastic proliferation and prevent subsequent scarring.[1] Fluorouracil ophthalmic is also used to treat ocular surface neoplastic conditions, such as squamous cell carcinoma and sarcoids.

Pharmacology/Actions

Fluorouracil is a pyrimidine analogue that is converted through intracellular mechanisms into multiple active metabolites which interfere with DNA and RNA synthesis, inhibit cell growth, and promote cell death.[2]

Contraindications/Precautions/Warnings

Fluorouracil is contraindicated in patients that are hypersensitive to it or any component of the formulation. <u>Fluorouracil is absolutely contraindicated in cats by any route of administration</u>, including ophthalmic administration, as cats develop a severe, potentially fatal neurotoxicity when they are exposed to fluorouracil by any route. Do not use fluorouracil in patients that are pregnant or in those that are myelosuppressed or have concurrent serious infections. Although systemic adverse effects are less likely after topical application of fluorouracil in other species, they can occur.

The National Institute for Occupational Safety and Health (NIOSH) classifies fluorouracil as a hazardous drug; personal protective equipment (PPE) should be used accordingly to minimize the risk for exposure.

Adverse Effects

Although less likely after topical administration, adverse effects reported in humans or animals include myelosuppression, GI toxicity (eg, diarrhea, GI ulceration, sloughing, stomatitis), and neurotoxicity (seizures). The most frequent adverse reactions with ophthalmic fluorouracil administration occur locally and are often related to an extension of the pharmacological activity of the drug.[3] These effects include burning, crusting, allergic contact dermatitis, erosions, erythema, hyperpigmentation, irritation, pain, periorbital alopecia, photosensitivity, pruritus, scarring, rash, soreness, and ulceration.

Dosages

NOTE: Multiple protocols exist for use during surgical procedures for correction of glaucoma; these protocols vary with the type of procedure and other patient parameters. As these procedures should be performed by board-certified veterinary ophthalmologists, the protocols are not detailed here.

Ocular surface neoplasia (extra-label): Fluorouracil 1% ophthalmic solution (compounded), 1 drop in affected eye(s) 4 times daily for 1 week; may be repeated in regular cycles.[4,5] Use of a *topical* 1% fluorouracil ointment applied 4 times daily also has been described.[6,7]

Monitoring

- Clinical efficacy
- Maintenance of patency of the glaucoma implant, which leads to control of intraocular pressure
- Cell or tissue samples for evaluation to confirm remission of neoplasia

Client Information

- This is a chemotherapy (anticancer) drug. The drug and its byproducts can be hazardous to other animals and humans. Pregnant women and sick or immunocompromised individuals should avoid contact.
- Wear protective gloves and a mask when administering this medicine. After administration, seal these gloves, mask, and other waste products in a plastic bag, and then place in the regular trash. Wash your hands immediately after each application.
- Loss of hair around the eyes may occur after use.
- Wait for 5 to 10 minutes after applying this medicine before applying any other medicines to the eye.
- Store this medicine according to instructions on the bottle or prescription label.
- Do not use this medicine if the color changes, if it becomes cloudy, or if there are particles in the solutions.

Storage/Stability

Store this product as directed on the product label.

Compatibility/Compounding Considerations

Fluorouracil ophthalmic preparations should not be mixed directly with any other ophthalmic medications. Fluorouracil ophthalmic preparations are not commercially available but may be prepared by qualified compounding pharmacists by utilizing the 50 mg/mL injectable solution. Fluorouracil 1% ophthalmic solution prepared this way is reported to be stable for 3 weeks.[8]

Dosage Forms/Regulatory Status

VETERINARY-LABELED PRODUCTS: NONE

HUMAN-LABELED PRODUCTS:

Fluorouracil ophthalmic formulations must be prepared (compounded) by a qualified compounding pharmacist. See ***Compounding: How to Find a Quality Assured Pharmacy.***

References

For the complete list of references, see **wiley.com/go/budde/plumb**

Flurbiprofen Ophthalmic

(flur-bi-***proe***-fin) *Ocufen®*

Nonsteroidal Anti-inflammatory Drug (NSAID)

Prescriber Highlights

- ▶ Used to control anterior segment inflammation
- ▶ May cause transient increases in intraocular pressure (IOP)
- ▶ May delay ocular wound healing and increase risk for intraocular bleeding

Uses/Indications

Flurbiprofen ophthalmic is indicated for controlling anterior segment inflammation (eg, conjunctivitis, keratitis, anterior uveitis), inducing mydriasis during cataract-removal surgery, and for providing analgesia following surgical removal of cataracts. In dogs, flurbiprofen significantly reduced clinical signs associated with experimentally induced intraocular inflammation,[1] whereas it demonstrated poor efficacy in cats.[2] Flurbiprofen did not decrease corneal sensitivity in normal dogs, suggesting its use as an ophthalmic analgesic may be limited[3]; however, analgesic effects may improve in the presence of ocular pain.

Pharmacology/Actions

Flurbiprofen is an NSAID that blocks prostaglandin synthesis by inhibiting cyclooxygenase 1 and 2. Prostaglandins mediate many of the adverse effects of intraocular inflammation, including disruption of the blood–aqueous barrier, vasodilation, increased vascular permeability, leukocytosis, and increased intraocular pressure (IOP). Blocking prostaglandin production therefore minimizes the adverse short- and long-term effects of intraocular inflammation. Prostaglandins also appear to play a role in the miotic response produced during ocular surgery by constricting the iris sphincter independently of cholinergic mechanisms. Thus, flurbiprofen inhibits miosis induced during cataract surgery.[4]

Contraindications/Precautions/Warnings

Flurbiprofen is contraindicated in patients that have a history of hypersensitivity to it or any component of the formulation. The potential for cross-sensitivity to acetylsalicylic acid, phenylacetic acid derivatives, and other NSAIDs exists.[4] Topical NSAIDs may result in corneal epithelial breakdown and corneal thinning, erosion, or ulceration, which could cause delayed corneal wound healing; concurrent use of topical NSAIDs and topical corticosteroids may further delay healing and increase the potential for development of adverse effects.[4] Due to interference with thrombocyte aggregation, ophthalmic NSAIDs may cause increased bleeding of ocular tissues (eg, hyphema) in conjunction with ocular surgery. It is recommended that flurbiprofen ophthalmic solution be used with caution in patients with known bleeding tendencies (eg, severe liver disease) or in those receiving anticoagulant medications (eg, heparins, rivaroxaban), which may prolong bleeding time.[4]

Adverse Effects

Adverse effects reported in humans or animals include transient ocular burning or stinging on administration.[4] Additional adverse reactions reported with the use of flurbiprofen ophthalmic include fibrosis, miosis, and mydriasis. NSAIDs may also cause direct cellular damage, causing delayed healing and/or deterioration of existing corneal wounds. Although unlikely, systemic adverse effects may occur with the use of topical NSAIDs, including increased risk for gastric ulceration, decreased platelet aggregation, worsening of asthma and cardiac disease, and renal toxicity. Concurrent use of systemic NSAIDs and corticosteroids increases the risk for systemic adverse effects. The increased bleeding tendency of ocular tissues in conjunction with ocular surgery has also been reported. Flurbiprofen has been documented to elevate intraocular pressure (IOP) in dogs,[5,6] and decrease the IOP-lowering effect of latanoprost in normal canine eyes6 and canine eyes following surgical cataract removal.[7] Flurbiprofen increased corneal sensitivity when it was administered to normal canine eyes; therefore, it is suspected to be associated with an ocular irritant effect.[8]

Dosages

Preoperative for cataract surgery (extra-label): 1 drop every 30 minutes for 4 applications beginning 2 hours prior to surgery

Anterior segment inflammation (extra-label): 1 drop in affected eye(s) every 8 hours; frequency may be reduced to once daily after resolution of initial inflammation

Monitoring

- Clinical efficacy (eg, decreased or absent anterior segment inflammation)
- Adverse effects (eg, delayed wound healing)

Client Information

- Use this medicine as directed by your veterinarian.
- Do not use this medicine if the color changes, if it becomes cloudy, or if there are particles in the solution.
- Flurbiprofen ophthalmic may cause burning or stinging on administration. It may also increase the risk for bleeding and may slow down healing in the eye.
- Use proper administration techniques to avoid contamination of the medication. Keep the cap tightly closed on the medicine when it is not in use.
- Wait for 5 minutes after applying this medicine is before applying any other medications to the eye.
- Store this medicine at room temperature away from moisture and sunlight. Do not freeze.
- Your veterinarian will need to monitor your animal while it is taking this medicine. Do not miss these important follow-up visits.

Storage/Stability

Store as directed on package labeling (15°C-25°C [59°F-77°F]) away from moisture and sunlight; do not freeze.

Compatibility/Compounding Considerations

Flurbiprofen ophthalmic solutions should not be mixed directly with any other drugs.

Dosage Forms/Regulatory Status

VETERINARY-LABELED PRODUCTS: NONE

HUMAN-LABELED PRODUCTS:

Flurbiprofen sodium 0.03% Ophthalmic Solution (containing flurbiprofen 0.3 mg/mL; thimerosal 0.005%; citric acid; edetate disodium; polyvinyl alcohol 1.4%; potassium chloride; purified water; NaCl; sodium citrate; HCl and/or NaOH to adjust pH to 6 to 7; osmolality of 260 – 330 mOsm/kg), in 2.5 mL ophthalmic dropper bottles; *Ocufen*®, generic; (Rx)

References

For the complete list of references, see **wiley.com/go/budde/plumb**

Ganciclovir Ophthalmic

(gan-***sye***-kloe-veer) *Zirgan*®

Antiviral Agent

Prescriber Highlights

- ▶ Used as an ophthalmic antiviral in cats with feline herpesvirus-1 (FHV-1) and dogs with canine herpesvirus-1 (CHV-1)
- ▶ May cause myelosuppression and nephrotoxicity in cats if ingested
- ▶ In vitro efficacy versus FHV-1 is 2 to 10 times greater than similar antivirals.

Uses/Indications

In veterinary patients, ganciclovir may be used to treat feline herpesvirus-1 (FHV-1)-induced ocular surface disease in cats. In vitro efficacy of ganciclovir versus FHV-1 has been demonstrated at various concentrations1 and is 2 times greater than cidofovir and penciclovir and 10 times greater than acyclovir.[2,3] When ganciclovir was administered to cats with healthy eyes 3 times daily, no signs of ocular irritation developed.[1]

Evaluation of ganciclovir in experimentally induced canine herpesvirus-1 infections (CHV-1) indicated good efficacy without signs of ocular toxicity.[4] In vitro evaluation of ganciclovir suggests efficacy against equine alpha-herpesviruses[5,6] ; however, evaluation of ganciclovir's use in vivo has not been performed.

Pharmacology/Actions

Ganciclovir is a guanosine derivative that, upon phosphorylation, inhibits DNA replication of herpes simplex viruses (HSV). Ganciclovir is transformed by viral and cellular thymidine kinases (TK) to ganciclovir triphosphate, which works as an antiviral agent by competitive inhibition of viral DNA-polymerase and prevents DNA elongation.

Contraindications/Precautions/Warnings

Ganciclovir is contraindicated in patients that have a history of hypersensitivity to it or any component of the formulation.

Myelosuppression and nephrotoxicity may occur in cats after systemic treatment. Ganciclovir has been shown to be embryotoxic in rabbits and mice and teratogenic in rabbits following IV administration.[7] Because safety has not been established in animals, this drug should only be used when the maternal benefits outweigh the potential risks to offspring. Do not allow cats to ingest the topical formulation; an e-collar may be required to avoid unintentional ingestion during grooming.

Adverse Effects

Adverse effects reported in humans or animals include blurred vision, eye irritation, punctate keratitis, chemosis, and conjunctival hyperemia and discharge.[1,7] Myelosuppression and nephrotoxicity are possible in cats after ingestion by grooming.

Dosages

Herpes keratitis (extra-label): 1 drop in affected eye(s) up to 5 times daily until the corneal ulcer has healed, then 3 times daily for 7 days

Monitoring

- Clinical efficacy: resolution of clinical signs associated with herpes keratitis (eg, corneal ulceration, corneal vascularization, conjunctivitis)
- Baseline and periodic CBC and chemistry panel for cats to detect myelosuppression and nephrotoxicity

Client Information

- Wipe the cat's face after applying. Do not let cats lick this medication, as it can be toxic when ingested.
- Use proper administration techniques to avoid contamination of the medication. Keep the cap tightly closed when the medication is not in use.
- Wait for 5 minutes after applying this medication before applying any other medications to the eye.
- Store this product at room temperature away from moisture and sunlight. Do not freeze.
- Do not use this medication if the color changes, if it becomes cloudy, or if there are particles in the gel.

Storage/Stability

Store this product at controlled room temperature (20°C-25°C [68°F-77°F]) away from moisture and sunlight.

Compatibility/Compounding Considerations

Ganciclovir should not be mixed directly (in vitro) with any other drugs.

Dosage Forms/Regulatory Status

VETERINARY-LABELED PRODUCTS: NONE

HUMAN-LABELED PRODUCTS:

Ganciclovir 0.15% Ophthalmic Gel (containing ganciclovir 1.5 mg/mL; carbopol; water for injection; NaOH (to adjust the pH to 7.4); mannitol; benzalkonium chloride 0.075 mg), in a 5 g ophthalmic gel tube; *Zirgan*®; (Rx)

References

For the complete list of references, see **wiley.com/go/budde/plumb**

Gatifloxacin Ophthalmic

(gat-i-**flocks**-a sin) *Zymaxid®, Zymar®*

Fourth-Generation Fluoroquinolone Antibiotic

Prescriber Highlights

- ► Fluoroquinolone antimicrobial available in ophthalmic formulation only; used to treat bacterial conjunctivitis or keratitis
- ► Appropriately used as a therapeutic antibiotic in cases with known ocular surface infection; not appropriate for prophylactic use
- ► Physically incompatible with many drugs; therefore, it should not be directly mixed with other ophthalmic medications
- ► Crystalline drug precipitates may be noted in the superficial portion of corneal defects during use.

Uses/Indications

Gatifloxacin ophthalmic may be useful for treating bacterial conjunctivitis or keratitis caused by susceptible strains of *Staphylococcus* spp, *Streptococcus* spp, *Pseudomonas aeruginosa*, *Chlamydophila* spp, and *Haemophilus* spp. Gatifloxacin has demonstrated good in vitro activity versus *Pseudomonas* spp organisms cultured from dogs with ulcerative keratitis,[1] particularly in relation to the second-generation fluoroquinolone ciprofloxacin.[2] In comparison to moxifloxacin and besifloxacin, gatifloxacin demonstrated lower corneal and aqueous humor concentrations when administered to dogs with normal eyes.[3] Gatifloxacin should be used to treat, rather than prevent, bacterial ocular infections.

Pharmacology/Actions

Gatifloxacin is a fluoroquinolone antibiotic that acts via inhibition of both topoisomerase II (DNA gyrase) and topoisomerase IV to impair bacterial DNA synthesis. Inhibition of these 2 enzymes decreases the development of resistance to this class of fluoroquinolones. In comparison with besifloxacin, gatifloxacin is reported to have slightly greater in vitro efficacy versus gram-negative organisms, with slightly lesser in vitro efficacy versus gram-positive organisms.[4]

Contraindications/Precautions/Warnings

Gatifloxacin is contraindicated in patients that have a history of hypersensitivity to it, other fluoroquinolones, or any component of the formulation. This drug should only be used as a topical ophthalmic. Do not inject gatifloxacin subconjunctivally or into the anterior chamber of the eye. Fluoroquinolone-induced retinal toxicity in domestic cats has not been demonstrated with this product.

Adverse Effects

Adverse effects reported in humans or animals include blurred vision, tearing, eye pain, redness, itching, and a bad taste in the mouth. Crystalline drug precipitates may be noted in the superficial portion of corneal defects during use.

Dosages

Conjunctivitis (extra-label): 1 drop in affected eye(s) every 2 to 8 hours

Keratitis (extra-label): 1 drop in the affected eye every 2 to 8 hours

Monitoring

- Clinical efficacy. Corneal cytology and culture to evaluate for persistence of bacteria, and evaluation for clinical signs suggestive of continued infection

Client Information

- Use this medicine as directed by your veterinarian.
- Use proper administration techniques to avoid contamination of the medication. Keep the cap tightly closed when the medicine is not in use.
- Crystals may appear on the ocular surface after initiation of treatment.
- This medicine may precipitate when mixed with other ophthalmic medicines. Therefore, when giving this medicine to your horse through a subpalpebral lavage catheter, it is important to flush the catheter well with air between medications.
- Wait 5 minutes after applying this medicine before applying any other medicines to the eye.
- Store this medicine at room temperature away from moisture and sunlight. Do not freeze.

Storage/Stability

Store this product at controlled room temperature (20°C-25°C [68°F-77°F]) away from moisture and sunlight; do not freeze.

Compatibility/Compounding Considerations

Gatifloxacin ophthalmic preparations should not be mixed directly with any other ophthalmic medications and is considered physically incompatible with many drugs.

Dosage Forms/Regulatory Status

VETERINARY-LABELED PRODUCTS: NONE

HUMAN-LABELED PRODUCTS:

Gatifloxacin 0.3% Ophthalmic Solution (containing gatifloxacin 3 mg/mL; benzalkonium chloride 0.005%; edetate disodium; purified water and NaCl; HCl and/or NaOH to adjust pH to ≈6; osmolality of 260 to 330 mOsm/kg) in 5 mL ophthalmic dropper bottles; *Zymar®*, generic; (Rx)

Gatifloxacin 0.5% Ophthalmic Solution (containing gatifloxacin 5 mg/mL; benzalkonium chloride 0.005%; edetate disodium; purified water and NaCl; HCl and/or NaOH to adjust pH to ≈6; osmolality of 260 to 330 mOsm/kg), 2.5 mL in a sterile ophthalmic dropper bottle; *Zymaxid®*, generic; (Rx)

References

For the complete list of references, see **wiley.com/go/budde/plumb**

Gentamicin Ophthalmic

(**jen**-ta-mye-sin **sul**-fate) *Genoptic®, Gentocin®, Gentak®*

Aminoglycoside Antibiotic

*For systemic use, see **Gentamicin***

Prescriber Highlights

- ► Topical ophthalmic aminoglycoside antibiotic used as a treatment for susceptible ocular surface bacterial infections
- ► Do not use if a full-thickness corneal wound is present, as gentamicin is toxic to the eye's interior.
- ► Fortified solutions of gentamicin sulfate up to 13.6 mg/mL may be compounded for use in susceptible infections of equine bacterial keratitis.

Uses/Indications

Gentamicin ophthalmic is primarily used for patients with ocular infections caused by gram-negative aerobes, such as *Pseudomonas aeruginosa*.[1,2] Gentamicin does not demonstrate consistent efficacy against versus *Staphylococcus* spp or *Streptococcus* spp isolates.[1,3] As the spectrum of gentamicin is weighted toward gram-negative organisms, and as it is more toxic to the corneal epithelium, gentamicin should not be considered a first-line prophylactic antibiotic in veterinary ophthalmology.[4,5]

In horses with end-stage glaucoma, intravitreal injection of gentamicin at higher doses is used to chemically ablate the ciliary body, thus reducing the production of aqueous humor and lowering intraocular pressure (IOP)[6]; lower doses may be used to manage equine recurrent uveitis (ERU).[7,8] See ***Gentamicin***.

The World Health Organization (WHO) has designated gentamicin as a Critically Important, High Priority antimicrobial for human medicine.[9] The Office International des Epizooties (OIE) has designated gentamicin as a Veterinary Critically Important Antimicrobial (VCIA) Agent in equine species.[10]

Pharmacology/Actions

Gentamicin sulfate, an aminoglycoside, is actively transported into the bacterial cell. It binds to a specific receptor protein on the 30S subunit of bacterial ribosomes. It consequently interferes with an initiation complex between mRNA (messenger RNA) and the 30S subunit, inhibiting protein synthesis by inducing misreading of the mRNA. Aminoglycosides are bactericidal, whereas most other antibiotics that interfere with protein synthesis are bacteriostatic.

Contraindications/Precautions/Warnings

Gentamicin is contraindicated in patients that have a history of hypersensitivity to it or any component of the formulation. Gentamicin should not be used if a full-thickness corneal wound is present, as gentamicin is toxic to the eye's interior.

Adverse Effects

Adverse effects reported in humans or animals include ocular burning and irritation upon drug instillation, nonspecific conjunctivitis, conjunctival epithelial defects, and conjunctival hyperemia. Other adverse reactions that have rarely been reported include allergic reactions, thrombocytopenic purpura, and hallucinations (humans).[11] In dogs and cats, although causation has not been proven, intravitreal gentamicin injections for ciliary body ablation may be linked to the development of intraocular tumors.[12,13] In horses, cataract formation and diffuse retinal degeneration have been reported following the intravitreal injection of low-dosage gentamicin for equine recurrent uveitis (ERU) management.[8]

When gentamicin is used systemically, it can cause nephrotoxicity and neurotoxicity (ototoxicity and vestibular toxicity). Cats are more susceptible to the toxic effects of gentamicin, and it is recommended that all patients receiving topical gentamicin be monitored for systemic toxicity.

Dosages

Susceptible ocular infections (extra-label): 1 drop of the solution or ¼ – ½ inch strip in the affected eye(s) 4 to 6 times daily. The frequency may be increased to every 30 to 60 minutes for a few hours if needed.

Monitoring

- Clinical efficacy: cytology and culture to evaluate for presence of bacteria; clinical resolution of signs of ocular surface infection and or recurrent inflammation
- Intraocular pressure (IOP) when used as adjunctive treatment for equine glaucoma or recurrent uveitis
- Urinalysis with sediment to check for casts in the urine, which may be an early indicator for renal toxicity

Client Information

- Give this medicine as directed by your veterinarian.
- Use proper administration techniques to avoid contamination of the medication. Keep cap tightly closed when not in use.
- Wait 5 minutes after applying this medication before applying any other medications to the eye.
- Store this medicine according to the directions on the product label, protected from light. Do not freeze.
- Do not use this medicine if the color changes, if it becomes cloudy, or if there are particles in the solution.

Storage/Stability

Store this product as directed on the product label, protected from light; do not freeze.

Compatibility/Compounding Considerations

Gentamicin sulfate should not be mixed directly (in vitro) with any other drugs.

Dosage Forms/Regulatory Status

VETERINARY-LABELED PRODUCTS:

Gentamicin Sulfate 0.3% Ophthalmic solution (containing gentamicin sulfate equivalent to 3 mg gentamicin base; disodium phosphate; monosodium phosphate; NaCl; benzalkonium chloride; aqueous solution with pH 6.8 to 7.3), in sterile 5 mL dropper bottle; generic; (Rx)

VETERINARY-LABELED COMBINATION PRODUCTS:

Gentamicin Sulfate 0.3% and Betamethasone Ophthalmic solution (containing gentamicin sulfate equivalent to 3 mg gentamicin base; 1 mg betamethasone acetate equivalent to 0.89 mg betamethasone alcohol; polyoxyol 40 stearate; polyethoxy 35 castor oil; edetate disodium; 0.1 mg benzalkonium chloride as a preservative; water for injection), supplied in a sterile 5 mL dropper bottle; *Gentocin® Durafilm®*; (Rx)

HUMAN-LABELED PRODUCTS:

Gentamicin 0.3% Ophthalmic Solution (containing gentamicin sulfate equivalent to 3 mg/mL gentamicin base; benzalkonium chloride; edetate disodium; polyvinyl alcohol 1.4%; purified water; NaCl; sodium phosphate, dibasic; HCl and/or NaOH to adjust the pH in an aqueous, buffered solution with a pH of 6.5 to 7.5), in 5 mL ophthalmic dropper bottles; *Genoptic®*, *Gentak®*; (Rx)

Gentamicin 0.3% Ophthalmic Ointment (containing gentamicin sulfate equivalent to 3 mg/mL of gentamicin in a base of white petrolatum and mineral oil, with methylparaben and propylparaben as preservatives), in a 3.5 g ophthalmic ointment tube; generic; (Rx)

HUMAN-LABELED COMBINATION PRODUCTS:

Gentamicin and Prednisolone Acetate Ophthalmic Ointment 0.3%/0.6% (containing gentamicin sulfate equivalent to 0.3% gentamicin base; prednisolone acetate 0.6%; chlorobutanol (chloral derivative) 0.5%; mineral oil; petrolatum (and) lanolin alcohol; purified water; white petrolatum), in a sterile 3.5 g ophthalmic tube; *Pred-G®*; (Rx)

Gentamicin and Prednisolone Acetate Ophthalmic Suspension 0.3%/1% (containing gentamicin sulfate equivalent to 0.3% gentamicin base; prednisolone acetate (microfine suspension) 1%; benzalkonium chloride 0.005%; edetate disodium; hypromellose; polyvinyl alcohol 1.4%; polysorbate 80; purified water; sodium chloride; sodium citrate dehydrate; NaOH and/or HCl to adjust pH (5.4 to 6.6), in a sterile 5 mL ophthalmic dropper bottle; *Pred-G®*; (Rx)

References

For the complete list of references, see **wiley.com/go/budde/plumb**

Hydrocortisone Ophthalmic

(hye-droe-***kor***-ti-zone)

Corticosteroid Anti-inflammatory Agent

Prescriber Highlights

- Ophthalmic corticosteroid used to treat ocular surface inflammation
- Only commercially available formulation is in combination with neomycin/polymyxin B +/-bacitracin
- NOT effective for deep corneal or intraocular inflammation (uveitis)
- Contraindications include a hypersensitivity to dexamethasone; an existing or suspected bacterial, viral, or fungal ocular infection; and in the presence of a corneal abrasion or ulceration.
- Use with caution in avian species due to risk for systemic corticosteroid effects.

Uses/Indications

Hydrocortisone is used in combination with topical antibiotics (eg, neomycin, polymyxin, ± bacitracin) for inflammatory conjunctivitis.

Pharmacology/Actions

Hydrocortisone is a naturally occurring corticosteroid that is produced by the adrenal glands. Corticosteroids have broad immunomodulatory and anti-inflammatory actions, which are mediated via direct effects on gene expression, as well as by non-genomic effects on cell membranes and receptors. Ultimately, corticosteroids decrease pro-inflammatory gene transcription, production of pro-inflammatory prostaglandins and leukotrienes, B- and T-cell number and function, cell-mediated immunity, and humoral immunity.[1] Specific mechanisms involved in controlling ocular inflammatory conditions are not definitively known. Hydrocortisone has a relative glucocorticoid potency of 1 (versus 4 for prednisolone and 30 for dexamethasone and betamethasone), which correlates with weak clinical efficacy.

Hydrocortisone is a weak base steroid with poor intraocular penetration; therefore, it is ineffective for treating intraocular inflammation (uveitis).

Contraindications/Precautions/Warnings

Hydrocortisone is contraindicated in patients that have a history of hypersensitivity to it or any component of the formulation. Due to inhibition of epithelial wound healing and potentiation of infection, hydrocortisone ophthalmic is also contraindicated when corneal ulceration is suspected or present, or in the presence of corneal infection (bacterial, fungal, or viral).[2,3] Topical administration of glucocorticoids may produce systemic effects. For more information, refer to ***Glucocorticoid Agents, General Information***. Use hydrocortisone ophthalmic with caution in patients with endocrine diseases (eg, diabetes mellitus, acromegaly), infectious diseases, chronic kidney disease, congestive heart failure, systemic hypertension, or gastric ulceration. When use of hydrocortisone ophthalmic is necessary to treat a patient with these conditions, the minimal effective dose should be administered for the shortest possible time. Ophthalmic steroids should be used with extreme caution in avian species due to increased risk for systemic adverse effects.

Adverse Effects

Adverse effects reported in humans or animals include burning, stinging, and irritation upon application to the eye.[3] Systemic absorption may result in suppression of the hypothalamus-pituitary-adrenal axis. The use of corticosteroids may result in posterior subcapsular cataract formation, glaucoma, and secondary ocular infections due to bacteria, fungi, or viruses.[4] With the chronic use of hydrocortisone, intraocular pressure (IOP) may increase in some animals; however, most reports suggest the change is reversible.[5–7]

Dosages

Inflammatory conjunctivitis (extra-label): ¼ – ½ inch strip in the affected eye(s) up to 4 times daily

Monitoring

- Clinical efficacy
- Resolution of signs of inflammation
- Intraocular pressure (IOP; especially in cats) and ocular surface integrity (eg, fluorescein stain)
- Blood or urine glucose changes based on clinical signs (eg, polyuria, polydipsia) in diabetic animals

Client Information

- Available only as an ointment form, in combination with antibiotics.
- Use proper administration techniques to avoid contamination of the medication. Keep the cap tightly closed when the medication is not in use.
- Wait for 5 minutes after applying this medication before applying any other medications to the eye.
- Store this medicine as directed on the product label. Do not freeze.
- Discard this medicine if the color change occurs.

Storage/Stability

Store at controlled room temperature (68°F-77°F [20°C-25°C]), away from moisture and sunlight.

Compatibility/Compounding Considerations

Hydrocortisone ophthalmic should not be mixed directly (in vitro) with any other drugs. Instruct caregivers to wait for 5 minutes after applying this medication before applying any other medications to the eye.

Dosage Forms/Regulatory Status

VETERINARY-LABELED PRODUCTS:

No ophthalmic products containing only hydrocortisone are available; available commercially in combination with antimicrobial agents.

Neomycin/Bacitracin/Polymyxin/Hydrocortisone Ophthalmic Ointment (containing neomycin sulfate equivalent to 3.5 mg neomycin base, polymyxin B sulfate equivalent to 10,000 polymyxin B units, bacitracin zinc equivalent to 400 bacitracin units, hydrocortisone 10 mg/g, and white petrolatum), in a 3.5 g ophthalmic ointment tube; *Vetropolycin HC*®, (Rx)

HUMAN-LABELED PRODUCTS:

Neomycin/Bacitracin/Polymyxin/Hydrocortisone Ophthalmic Ointment (containing neomycin sulfate equivalent to 3.5 mg neomycin base, polymyxin B sulfate equivalent to 10,000 polymyxin B units, bacitracin zinc equivalent to 400 bacitracin units, hydrocortisone 10 mg/g, and white petrolatum), in a 3.5 g ophthalmic ointment tube; generic, (Rx)

Neomycin/Polymyxin/Hydrocortisone Ophthalmic Ointment (containing neomycin sulfate equivalent to 3.5 mg neomycin base, polymyxin B sulfate equivalent to 10,000 polymyxin B units, hydrocortisone 10 mg/g, and white petrolatum), in a 3.5 g ophthalmic ointment tube; generic, (Rx)

References

For the complete list of references, see **wiley.com/go/budde/plumb**

Idoxuridine Ophthalmic

(eye-docks-***yoor***-uh-deen)

Antiviral (Nucleoside Analogue)

Prescriber Highlights

- ► Topical antiviral agent used in cats with feline herpesvirus-1 (FHV-1)
- ► Must be used 4 to 5 times daily
- ► In vitro efficacy is less than trifluridine and comparable to or greater than other antivirals.
- ► No longer commercially available; must be compounded as an ointment, solution, or suspension

Uses/Indications

Idoxuridine is used topically in cats to treat conjunctivitis and keratitis associated with feline herpesvirus-1 (FHV-1) infections. Idoxuridine has also demonstrated efficacy in the treatment of canine herpesvirus-1 (CHV-1) keratitis.[1] Although relative efficacy versus other antiviral agents is not known and direct causation of clinical effect is difficult to determine, idoxuridine was associated with improvement in keratoconjunctivitis caused by equine herpesvirus-2 (EHV-2) in foals.[2]

Pharmacology/Actions

Idoxuridine is chemically similar to thymidine, and its substitution into viral DNA causes misreading of the viral genetic code, thereby inhibiting viral replication. Because idoxuridine is a nonspecific inhibitor of DNA synthesis, it affects any cellular function requiring thymidine and is not suitable for systemic use. Even with topical therapy, corneal toxicity can occur. Idoxuridine is virustatic. Idoxuridine's in vitro efficacy is less than trifluridine, comparable to ganciclovir, greater than cidofovir, and much greater than acyclovir.[3,4]

Contraindications/Precautions/Warnings

Idoxuridine is contraindicated in patients that have a history of hypersensitivity to it or any component of the formulation.

Adverse Effects

Adverse effects reported in humans or animals include acute ocular irritation, including burning, corneal stippling, vascularization, and clouding. Following prolonged use of idoxuridine, ocular irritation characterized by follicular conjunctivitis, blepharitis with punctal swelling, bulbar conjunctival hyperemia, and corneal epithelial staining has also been reported. Treatment with idoxuridine should be discontinued if adverse effects occur.

Dosages

Keratitis caused by feline herpesvirus-1 (FHV-1), canine herpesvirus-1 (CHV-1), or equine herpesvirus-2 (EHV-2) (extra label): 1 drop in affected eye(s) every 2 to 3 hours for 48 hours, then 4 to 5 times daily for a week beyond the resolution of clinical signs

Monitoring

- Resolution of clinical signs of herpetic keratitis (eg, corneal ulceration, corneal vascularization, conjunctivitis)

Client Information

- Give this medicine to your animal as directed by your veterinarian.
- Use proper administration techniques to avoid contamination of the medication. Keep the cap tightly closed when the medication is not in use.
- Wait for 5 minutes after applying this medication before applying any other medications to the eye.
- Store this medication as directed on the product label. Do not freeze and protect from light.
- Do not use this medication if the color changes, if it becomes cloudy, or if there are particles in solutions.

Storage/Stability

Because this compound must be compounded (in the United States), storage recommendations can vary; follow storage requirements listed on the packaging. Do not freeze.

Compatibility/Compounding Considerations

Idoxuridine should not be mixed directly (in vitro) with any other drugs.

Dosage Forms/Regulatory Status

VETERINARY-LABELED PRODUCTS: NONE

HUMAN-LABELED PRODUCTS: NONE

No ophthalmic dosage form of idoxuridine is approved for use; however, Idoxuridine may be compounded as a 0.1% to 0.5% solution, suspension, and/or ointment by a qualified compounding pharmacist.

References

For the complete list of references, see **wiley.com/go/budde/plumb**

Irrigating Solutions, Ophthalmic

BSS®, Collyrium®

Ocular Irrigant

Prescriber Highlights

- ► Available for either intraocular or extraocular use
- ► Extraocular (eyewashes) products should NOT be used intraocularly.

Uses/Indications

Extraocular eyewash preparations are used to irrigate the nasolacrimal duct system, remove debris from the eye, and remove the excess stain after diagnostic staining (eg, fluorescein) of the cornea.

Intraocular irrigation solutions are used during intraocular surgery (eg, cataract removal, vitreal surgery) to maintain the shape of the anterior chamber, cool phacoemulsification handpieces, and lavage emulsified lens and surgical byproducts from the eye.

Pharmacology/Actions

OTC extraocular eyewash preparations are sterile isotonic solutions that contain preservatives and are intended to be used for general external ophthalmic use only.

Intraocular sterile irrigating solutions are sterile, preservative-free, physiologically balanced salt solutions that mimic the composition of the aqueous humor in terms of physiologic pH, osmolality, and ion composition; they contain electrolytes required for normal cellular metabolic functions. Some intraocular irrigating solutions also contain glutathione, which is responsible for stabilizing endothelial cell junctions and intraocular pumping functions.

Contraindications/Precautions/Warnings

Extraocular eyewash preparations are contraindicated for intraocular use, as preservative components are toxic to the corneal endothelium. They are also contraindicated if the patient is hypersensitive to any component of the formulation. Adding drugs or other fluids to intraocular irrigating solutions may damage intraocular tissue.

In humans with diabetic mellitus who are undergoing vitrectomy, caution is recommended with the use of intraocular irrigating solutions, as intraoperative lens changes have been noted in some patients; the same recommendation may apply to diabetic animals. Caution should be used in diabetic animals undergoing vitrectomy for other causes (eg, trauma, neoplasia, endophthalmitis).

Adverse Effects

Intraocular irrigation solutions have caused corneal clouding and edema in some patients due to endothelial damage. In humans, lens changes have been noted in some diabetic patients who are undergoing vitrectomy. A study evaluating cooled versus room temperature irrigating solutions demonstrated no significant adverse effects between the 2 temperatures.[1]

Dosages

Extraocular eyewash (extra-label): Flush affected eye(s) as needed; control rate of flow by exerting pressure on the bottle.

Intraocular use during surgery (extra-label): Use a sterile, preservative-free balanced salt solution (NOT an OTC eyewash) according to the established practices for each surgical procedure.

Monitoring

- When intraocular solutions are used, monitor for development or worsening of corneal clouding or edema or opacification of the lens.
- In diabetic patients, monitor for lens changes post-vitrectomy.

Client Information

- If you are using an over-the-counter eyewash solution, use proper administration techniques to avoid eye injury or contamination of the product. Keep the cap tightly closed when the medication is not in use.

- Wait 5 minutes after using the eyewash before applying any medications to the eye.
- Store this product at room temperature away from moisture and sunlight. Do not freeze.
- Discard this product if the color changes or the solution becomes cloudy.

Storage/Stability

Store OTC eyewash products as labeled, usually at controlled room temperature away from moisture and sunlight; do not freeze.

Store solutions for intraocular use at 8°C to 30°C (46°F-86°F); avoid excessive heat, and do not freeze. Discard solution after 6 hours. Store *BSS Plus®* solutions at 2°C to 25°C (36°F-77°F); do not freeze. Discard prepared solution after 6 hours. Do not use unfinished solutions on a different patient.

Compatibility/Compounding Considerations

It is not recommended to add any other solutions or drugs to intraocular or extraocular irrigating solutions; however, extra-label additives in some protocols have included heparin, epinephrine, antibiotics, or local anesthetics.

For reconstituting *BSS Plus®* solutions: Reconstitute solution just prior to use in surgery. Follow the same strict aseptic reconstitution procedures used for IV solution additives. Remove the blue flip-off seal from the part 1 (480 mL) bottle. Remove the blue flip-off seal from the part 2 (20 mL) vial. Clean and disinfect the rubber stoppers on both containers by using sterile alcohol wipes. Transfer the contents of the part 2 vial to the part 1 bottle using the vacuum transfer device (provided). An alternative method of solution transfer may be accomplished by using a syringe to remove precisely 20 mL of the part 2 solution and transfer to the part 1 container through the outer target area of the rubber stopper. **NOTE:** An excess volume of the part 2 solution is provided in each vial; discard unused solution. Gently agitate the contents to mix the solutions. Place a sterile cap on the bottle if the solution is not going to be used immediately. Remove the tear-off portion of the label. Record the time and date of reconstitution and the patient's name on the bottle label.

Dosage Forms/Regulatory Status

VETERINARY-LABELED PRODUCTS:

Several products are marketed as eye washes or rinses for animal patients, including *Clear Eyes®*, *Conquer Hy-Optic®*, *Nutri-Vet® Dog Eye Rinse*, and *Vetericyn® Plus Eye Wash*. Ingredients vary significantly, and some are labeled only as tear stain removers. None of these products appear to be FDA-approved, and they should NOT be used for intraocular procedures.

HUMAN-LABELED PRODUCTS:

Irrigating Solutions, Intraocular

Balanced Salt Solution Irrigating Solution in 15 mL, 18 mL, 30 mL, 250 mL, or 500 mL; preservative-free containing 0.64% NaCl, 0.075% KCl, 0.03% magnesium chloride, 0.048% calcium chloride, 0.39% sodium acetate, 0.17% sodium citrate, and NaOH or HCl; *BSS®*, generic; (Rx)

Balanced Salt Solution Plus; in 2 parts in 10 mL (part 1) and 240 mL (part 2) in a 250 mL bottle; preservative-free containing 0.0154% calcium chloride, 0.714% sodium chloride, 0.038% potassium chloride, 0.02% magnesium chloride, 0.42% sodium phosphate, 0.2% sodium bicarbonate, 0.092% dextrose, 0.0184% glutathione disulfide; *BSS Plus®*; (Rx)

References

For the complete list of references, see **wiley.com/go/budde/plumb**

Itraconazole Ophthalmic

(it-ruh-***kon***-uh-zohl) *Sporanox®*

Azole Antifungal Agent

Prescriber Highlights

- ► Used as a treatment for ocular surface fungal infections
- ► Not commercially available as an ophthalmic preparation; must be compounded
- ► Compounded forms contain 10% to 30% DMSO, which may be irritating when administered.
- ► Warn caregivers to wear nitrile gloves when applying this medication to protect them from DMSO exposure.

Uses/Indications

Itraconazole ophthalmic preparations are primarily used to treat fungal keratitis in horses[1,2]; however, they have successfully been used in dogs with fungal keratitis.[3]

Pharmacology/Actions

Itraconazole interacts with 14 alpha-sterol demethylase, a cytochrome P-450 enzyme involved in the conversion of lanosterol to ergosterol. Ergosterol is an essential component of the fungal cell membrane, and preventing its synthesis may increase cellular permeability and cause leakage of cellular contents. Other possible effects of itraconazole include inhibition of endogenous respiration, purine uptake and yeast to mycelial transformation, and impairment of triglyceride and phospholipid biosynthesis. Targeted oxidative enzymes of fungal species, rather than mammalian cells, increase efficacy and decrease host toxicity. Itraconazole is usually effective against *Aspergillus* spp, with variable efficacy versus *Candida* spp and consistently lower efficacy against *Fusarium* spp.[1,2] Identification of fungal species prior to treatment is critical to the success of treatment.[4]

Contraindications/Precautions/Warnings

Itraconazole is contraindicated in patients that have a history of hypersensitivity to it or any component of the formulation. Compounded itraconazole 1% in DMSO 30% may cause irritation to the cornea. A solution of DMSO 1% is commonly used as a control for corneal irritation in ophthalmic drug studies.[5]

Adverse Effects

Adverse effects reported in humans or animals include stinging and irritation from the DMSO component. Although systemic absorption of topically applied ointments is unlikely, systemic exposure to itraconazole has resulted in hepatotoxicity and hearing loss in humans. Compared with miconazole and natamycin, itraconazole demonstrates lower toxic effects on corneal epithelial cells in vitro.[6]

Dosages

Fungal keratitis (extra-label): 1 – 2 drops, ½ inch strip, or 0.1 mL in the subpalpebral lavage (SPL) catheter to the affected eye(s) every 2 to 3 hours initially, followed by tapering of frequency based on clinical response

Monitoring

- Clinical efficacy: corneal scrapings with cytology and cultures to determine the clearing of fungal organisms
- Resolution of clinical signs of infection
- Toxicity: monitor for ocular irritation (eg, corneal edema, chemosis, blepharospasm) from DMSO

Client Information

- Use this medicine as directed by your veterinarian.
- A garlic-like odor is normal (from the DMSO solvent).
- Wear nitrile gloves when applying to prevent absorption of DMSO solvent found in the medicine.

- Use proper administration techniques to avoid contamination of the medicine. Keep the cap tightly closed when the medicine is not in use.
- Wait 5 minutes after applying this medicine before applying any other medicines to the eye.
- Store as directed on package labeling away from moisture and sunlight Do not freeze. Discard if the color or consistency changes.

Storage/Stability

Store this product as directed on the label from the compounding pharmacy. Keep this product away from moisture and sunlight; do not freeze.

Compatibility/Compounding Considerations

Itraconazole ophthalmic preparations should not be mixed directly with any other ophthalmic medications. Itraconazole ophthalmic preparations are not commercially available, but a compounded preparation containing 30% DMSO has been described.[7,8]

Dosage Forms/Regulatory Status

VETERINARY-LABELED PRODUCTS: NONE

HUMAN-LABELED PRODUCTS: NONE

Itraconazole ophthalmic products are not commercially available and must be prepared (compounded) by a qualified compounding pharmacist. Itraconazole has been compounded into a 1% ophthalmic ointment in a base containing 10% to 30% DMSO or into a 1% ophthalmic solution containing 30% DMSO.

References

For the complete list of references, see **wiley.com/go/budde/plumb**

Ketorolac Ophthalmic

(kee-***toe***-role-ak) *Acular®, Acular LS®, Acuvail®*

Nonsteroidal Anti-inflammatory Drug (NSAID)

Prescriber Highlights

- ► Used to control anterior segment inflammation, particularly in association with seasonal allergic conjunctivitis
- ► May cause transient increases in intraocular pressure (IOP)
- ► May delay ocular wound healing and increase risk for intraocular bleeding

Uses/Indications

Ketorolac ophthalmic is indicated for controlling anterior segment inflammation (eg, conjunctivitis, keratitis, anterior uveitis), inducing mydriasis during cataract-removal surgery, and for providing analgesia following surgical removal of cataracts. In diabetic patients, ketorolac may be useful to avoid the systemic effects of topically applied corticosteroids. Ketorolac is also indicated to alleviate the signs of allergic conjunctivitis. Ketorolac did not decrease corneal sensitivity in the eyes of normal dogs,[1] suggesting that its use as an ophthalmic analgesic may be limited; however, analgesic effects might improve in the presence of ocular pain.

Pharmacology/Actions

Ketorolac is an NSAID that blocks prostaglandin synthesis by inhibiting cyclooxygenase 1 and 2. Prostaglandins mediate many of the adverse effects of intraocular inflammation, including disruption of the blood-aqueous humor barrier, vasodilation, increased vascular permeability, leukocytosis, and increased intraocular pressure. Blocking prostaglandin production, therefore, minimizes the adverse short- and long-term effects of intraocular inflammation. Prostaglandins also appear to play a role in the miotic response produced during ocular surgery by constricting the iris sphincter independently of cholinergic mechanisms.

Contraindications/Precautions/Warnings

Ketorolac is contraindicated in patients that have a history of hypersensitivity to it or any component of the formulation. The potential for cross-sensitivity to acetylsalicylic acid, phenylacetic acid derivatives, and other NSAIDs exists.[2] In humans that have either a known hypersensitivity to aspirin or NSAIDs or a past medical history of asthma, there have been reports of bronchospasm or exacerbation of asthma associated with the use of ketorolac tromethamine ophthalmic solution. Therefore, caution should be used when treating individuals that have previously exhibited sensitivities to these drugs. Topical NSAIDs may result in corneal epithelial breakdown, delayed corneal wound healing, and corneal thinning, erosion, or ulceration. As such, ketorolac ophthalmic should be used with caution in patients with complicated or repeated ocular surgeries, corneal denervation, corneal epithelial defects, diabetes mellitus, and corneal surface diseases (eg, KCS).[2] As topical corticosteroids are also known delay healing, concomitant use with topical NSAIDs may increase the potential for delayed or impaired healing. Due to interference with thrombocyte aggregation, ophthalmic NSAIDs may cause increased bleeding of ocular tissues (eg, hyphema) in conjunction with ocular surgery. It is recommended that ketorolac ophthalmic solution be used with caution in patients with known bleeding tendencies (eg, severe liver disease) or in those receiving anticoagulant medications (eg, heparins, rivaroxaban), which may prolong bleeding time.[1]

Adverse Effects

Adverse effects reported in humans or animals include transient stinging and burning on instillation, corneal edema, iritis, ocular inflammation, ocular irritation, superficial keratitis, and superficial ocular infections.[1] Ocular bleeding may occur because of interference with thrombocyte aggregation. Other adverse effects that have rarely occurred in humans include corneal infiltrates, corneal ulcers, eye dryness, headaches, and visual disturbance (blurry vision).

Although unlikely, systemic adverse effects may occur with the use of topical NSAIDs, including increased risk for gastric ulceration, decreased platelet aggregation, worsening of asthma and cardiac disease, and renal toxicity. Concurrent use of systemic NSAIDs and corticosteroids increases the risk for systemic adverse effects.

Dosages

Allergic conjunctivitis: 1 drop to the affected eye(s) 2 to 4 times daily

Anterior segment inflammation (extra-label): 1 drop to the affected eye(s) 2 to 4 times daily

Postoperative analgesia: 1 drop to the surgical eye 2 to 4 times daily, beginning one day prior to surgery and continuing for 2 weeks postoperative

Monitoring

- Clinical efficacy (eg, decreased or absent anterior segment inflammation)
- Adverse effects (eg, delayed wound healing)

Client Information

- Use this medicine as directed by your veterinarian.
- Do not use this medicine if the color changes, if it becomes cloudy, or if there are particles in solutions.
- Ketorolac ophthalmic may cause burning or stinging on administration. It may also increase the risk for bleeding and may slow down healing in the eye.
- Use proper administration techniques to avoid contamination of the medication. Keep the cap tightly closed when the medication is not in use.

- Wait 5 minutes after applying this medication before applying any other medications to the eye.
- Store this medicine in the refrigerator or at room temperature away from moisture and sunlight. Do not freeze.
- Your veterinarian will need to monitor your animal while it is taking this medicine. Do not miss these important follow-up visits.

Storage/Stability

Store as directed on package labeling (15°C-25°C [59°F-77°F]) away from moisture and sunlight; do not freeze.

Compatibility/Compounding Considerations

Ketorolac should not be mixed directly with any other drugs. Ketorolac is not available as an ophthalmic ointment.

Dosage Forms/Regulatory Status

VETERINARY-LABELED PRODUCTS: NONE

HUMAN-LABELED PRODUCTS:

Ketorolac Tromethamine 0.5% Ophthalmic Solution (containing ketorolac tromethamine 5 mg/mL; benzalkonium chloride 0.01%; edetate disodium 0.1%; octoxynol 40; purified water; NaCl; HCl and/or NaOH to adjust the pH to 7.4 and osmolality of 290 mOsm/kg), in a 5 mL ophthalmic dropper bottle; *Acular*®, generic; (Rx)

Ketorolac Tromethamine 0.4% Ophthalmic Solution (containing ketorolac tromethamine 0.4%; benzalkonium chloride 0.006%; edetate disodium 0.015%; octoxynol 40; purified water; NaOH; HCl and/or NaOH to adjust pH to ≈7.4), 5 mL in a 10 mL sterile ophthalmic dropper bottle; *Acular LS*®, generic; (Rx)

Ketorolac Tromethamine 0.45% Ophthalmic Solution (containing ketorolac tromethamine 0.45%; carboxymethylcellulose; NaCl; sodium citrate dehydrate; purified water; NaOH and/or HCl to adjust pH), in 30 single-use vials of 0.4 mL each; *Acuvail*®; (Rx)

References

For the complete list of references, see **wiley.com/go/budde/plumb**

Ketotifen Ophthalmic

(kee-toe-***tye***-fin) *Alaway*®, *Zaditor*®

Antihistamine Agent

Prescriber Highlights

- ▶ Relatively selective H_1 blocker used to treat allergic conjunctivitis
- ▶ Use up to 2 times daily

Uses/Indications

In veterinary patients, ketotifen is used to provide temporary relief of the clinical signs associated with allergic conjunctivitis.

Pharmacology/Actions

Ketotifen is a relatively selective, noncompetitive histamine antagonist (H_1 receptor) and mast cell stabilizer. Ketotifen inhibits the release of mediators (eg, histamine, leukotrienes C4 and D4 [SRS-A], platelet-activating factor) from mast cells, during hypersensitivity reactions; ketotifen also decreases chemotaxis and activation of eosinophils. Evaluation of the effectiveness of the topical ocular application of ketotifen in veterinary species has not been performed.

Contraindications/Precautions/Warnings

Ketotifen is contraindicated in patients that have a history of hypersensitivity to it or any component of the formulation.

Adverse Effects

Adverse effects reported in humans include conjunctival injection, rhinitis, ocular allergic reactions, burning or stinging of the eye, conjunctivitis, eye discharge, dry eye, eye pain, eyelid disorder, itching eye, keratitis, lacrimation disorder, mydriasis, photophobia, rash, and pharyngitis.

Dosages

Allergic conjunctivitis (extra-label): 1 drop in the affected eye(s) twice daily

Monitoring

- Clinical efficacy
- Resolution or relief of signs of allergic conjunctivitis (pruritus, tearing, squinting, erythema)

Client Information

- Use proper administration techniques to avoid contamination of the medication. Keep the cap tightly closed when the medication is not in use.
- Wait for 5 to 10 minutes after applying this medication before applying any other medications to the eye.
- Store this medication in the refrigerator or at room temperature away from moisture and sunlight; do not freeze. Do not use this medication if the color changes, if it becomes cloudy, or if there are particles in solutions.

Storage/Stability

Store this medication in the refrigerator or at controlled room temperature away from moisture and sunlight; do not freeze.

Compatibility/Compounding Considerations

Ketotifen should not be mixed directly (in vitro) with any other drugs. Ketotifen is not available as an ophthalmic ointment.

Dosage Forms/Regulatory Status

VETERINARY-LABELED PRODUCTS: NONE

HUMAN-LABELED PRODUCTS:

Ketotifen Fumarate 0.025% Ophthalmic Solution (containing: ketotifen fumarate equivalent to 0.25 mg ketotifen per milliliter; benzalkonium chloride 0.01%; glycerol; NaOH/HCl to adjust pH to 4.4 to 5.8; water for injection; with an osmolality of 210 to 300 mOsm/kg), in a 5 mL ophthalmic dropper bottle; *Alaway*®, *Zaditor*®, generic; (OTC)

Ketotifen Fumarate 0.035% Ophthalmic Solution (containing: ketotifen fumarate equivalent to 0.25 mg ketotifen per milliliter; benzalkonium chloride 0.01%; glycerol; NaOH/ HCl to adjust pH to 4.4 to 5.8; water for injection; with an osmolality of 210 – 300 mOsm/kg), in a 5 mL ophthalmic dropper bottle; *Alaway*®, generic; (OTC)

Latanoprost Ophthalmic

(la-***ta***-noe-prost) *Rocklatan*®, *Vyzulta*®, *Xalatan*®, *Xelpros*®

Prostaglandin Analogue

Prescriber Highlights

- ▶ Used to decrease intraocular pressure (IOP) in patients with primary glaucoma or ocular hypertension
- ▶ Not effective for most cases of feline or equine glaucoma
- ▶ Do not use if IOP inflammation is present, as it may worsen inflammation or lead to pupillary block glaucoma.
- ▶ Twice-daily dosing results in less fluctuation of IOP.
- ▶ Preservatives may cause ocular irritation.

Uses/Indications

In dogs, latanoprost is used to reduce intraocular pressure (IOP) to manage primary glaucoma. Up to 60% reduction in IOP can be achieved with either once-daily[1] or twice-daily administration in dogs, with twice-daily administration resulting in lower and less variable IOP.[2] When it is administered in combination with a topical NSAID to normotensive canine eyes, latanoprost's ocular hypotensive effects are lessened,[3] whereas administration with a topical corticosteroid to normotensive canine eyes does not adversely impact the ocular hypotensive effects.[4]

Latanoprost is generally not indicated for use in cats with glaucoma, as it does not lower IOP in normal feline eyes,[1] and glaucoma in cats is frequently secondary to uveitis (latanoprost is contraindicated in the presence of uveitis). Although encountered uncommonly in clinical practice, primary congenital glaucoma in cats may be effectively managed with latanoprost, with an IOP reduction of up to 60% initially and efficacy decreasing over 3 weeks of treatment.[5]

Use in horses is generally not indicated due to relatively poor IOP-lowering effect and an association with a high incidence of adverse effects (eg, ocular discomfort)[6]; however, concurrent administration of topical latanoprost and diclofenac to normal equine eyes has demonstrated IOP reduction and reduced signs of discomfort.[7]

Pharmacology/Actions

Prostaglandin analogues are chemically modified versions of prostaglandin F2-alpha, an endogenous inflammatory molecule that mediates ocular hypotensive effects by increasing outflow of aqueous humor through both the trabecular meshwork and uveoscleral outflow routes. In addition to reducing intraocular pressure (IOP), latanoprost leads to miosis.

Contraindications/Precautions/Warnings

Latanoprost is contraindicated in patients that have a history of hypersensitivity to it or any component of the formulation. Latanoprost should be used with caution in the presence of anterior uveitis and secondary glaucoma, particularly in cases already exhibiting significant miosis, as this treatment may exacerbate miosis, promote synechiae formation, and worsen glaucoma. Latanoprost should also be used with caution in dogs with primary anterior lens luxation, as the miosis that results may trap the lens and/or vitreous within the pupillary aperture, thus creating pupillary block glaucoma. Latanoprost is not contraindicated in dogs with secondary posterior lens luxation, as the miosis may (favorably) trap the lens in the posterior segment.

Adverse Effects

Adverse effects reported in humans or animals include blurred vision, burning and stinging, conjunctival hyperemia, foreign body sensation, itching, increased pigmentation of the iris, and punctate epithelial keratopathy. Latanoprost may worsen intraocular inflammation. Latanoprost may cause darkening of the iris through direct stimulation of iris melanocytes, and it may also cause eyelash changes (eg, increased length, thickness, pigmentation, and the number of lashes) and eyelid skin darkening. Macular edema, including cystoid macular edema, has been reported after the use of latanoprost in humans. Horses develop conjunctival hyperemia, epiphora, and blepharospasm with latanoprost's administration.[8]

Dosages

Glaucoma (extra-label): 1 drop in the affected eye(s) once to twice daily

Monitoring

- Confirm maintenance of intraocular pressure (IOP) within the normal range for the species being treated

Client Information

- Use this medicine as indicated by your veterinarian.
- Use proper administration techniques to avoid contamination of the medicine. Keep the cap tightly closed when the medicine is not in use.
- Wait 5 minutes after applying this medicine before applying any other medicines to the eye.
- Store unopened bottle(s) under refrigeration. Do not freeze. Once a bottle is opened for use, it may be stored at room temperature (up to 25°C [77°F]), protected from light, for up to for 6 weeks.
- Do not use this medicine if the color changes, if it becomes cloudy, or if there are particles in solutions.

Storage/Stability

Protect this product from light. Store unopened bottle(s) under refrigeration at 2°C to 8°C (36°F-46°F)[9]; do not freeze. During shipment to the owner, the bottle may be maintained at temperatures up to 40°C (104°F) for a period not exceeding 8 days. Once a bottle is opened for use, it may be stored at room temperature up to 25°C (77°F) for 6 weeks.

Compatibility/Compounding Considerations

Latanoprost ophthalmic preparations should not be mixed directly with any other ophthalmic medications.

Dosage Forms/Regulatory Status

VETERINARY-LABELED PRODUCTS: NONE

HUMAN-LABELED PRODUCTS:

Latanoprost 0.005% Ophthalmic Solution (containing 50 µg of latanoprost per milliliter; benzalkonium chloride 0.02%; NaCl; sodium dihydrogen phosphate monohydrate; disodium hydrogen phosphate anhydrous; water for injection, with a pH of ≈6.7 and an osmolality of ≈267 mOsm/kg), in 2.5 mL ophthalmic dropper bottles; *Xalatan*®, generic; (Rx)

Latanoprost 0.005% Ophthalmic Solution (containing 50 µg of latanoprost; potassium sorbate 4.7 mg; castor oil; sodium borate; boric acid; propylene glycol; edetate disodium; polyoxyl 15 hydroxystearate; sodium hydroxide; hydrochloric acid; water for injection), in 2.5 mL ophthalmic dropper bottles; *Xelpros*® (Rx)

HUMAN-LABELED COMBINATION PRODUCTS:

Netardusil 0.02% and latanoprost 0.005% Ophthalmic Solution (containing netarsudil 0.285 mg; latanoprost 0.050 mg; benzalkonium chloride 0.20 mg; mannitol; boric acid; sodium hydroxide to adjust pH; water for injection), in 2.5 mL ophthalmic dropper bottles; *Rocklatan*® (Rx)

References

For the complete list of references, see **wiley.com/go/budde/plumb**.

Levobunolol Ophthalmic

(lee-voe-***byoon***-uh-lol) *Akbeta®, Betagan®*

Nonselective Beta-Adrenergic Blocker

Prescriber Highlights

- Decreases aqueous humor production to lower intraocular pressure (IOP) as a treatment for glaucoma
- May delay onset of glaucoma in the normal eye of dogs with unilateral glaucoma
- Use with caution in asthmatic patients due to the potential to induce bronchospasm.

Uses/Indications

Levobunolol is used to reduce intraocular pressure (IOP) in primary glaucoma and as prophylaxis to prevent glaucoma in the normal eye of animals with unilateral glaucoma. In dogs, the magnitude of reduction in IOP is less with levobunolol alone as compared with the combination of levobunolol and dorzolamide,[1] and timolol and dorzolamide.[2]

Pharmacology/Actions

Levobunolol is a nonselective beta-adrenergic blocking agent with associated intrinsic sympathomimetic activity but without significant membrane-stabilizing activity; the significance of which is not fully understood in ophthalmic use. Blockade of ciliary body beta receptors, particularly beta-2 receptors, reduces intraocular pressure (IOP) by decreasing aqueous humor production. The exact mechanism of the ocular hypotensive effect of beta-blockers is not clear. Several mechanisms have been postulated for this effect, including beta-blockade of norepinephrine-induced tonic sympathetic stimulation, leading to decreased activation of cAMP in the ciliary body, inhibition of Na+K+ATPase activity, or vasoactive mechanisms on the iris and ciliary body. Topically administered beta-blockers also inhibit glutamine-induced increases in intracellular calcium and sodium, thereby providing a potential protective effect against ischemic insult to the retina.[3]

Contraindications/Precautions/Warnings

Levobunolol is contraindicated in patients that have a history of hypersensitivity to it or any component of the formulation. Levobunolol should be used cautiously, if at all, in patients with heart block, bradycardia, heart failure, asthma, chronic bronchitis, or other cardiopulmonary conditions.[1]

Adverse Effects

Adverse effects reported in humans or animals include transient burning, stinging, and irritation upon application to the eye. Topically applied levobunolol led to a significant reduction in heart rate in healthy dogs, thus supporting its limited use in dogs with cardiopulmonary conditions.

Dosages

Glaucoma (extra-label): 1 drop in the affected eye(s) twice daily

Monitoring

- Clinical efficacy
- Confirm maintenance of intraocular pressure (IOP) within the normal range for the species being treated
- Observe asthmatic and diabetic patients for respiratory difficulty or acute hypoglycemia, respectively.
- Heart rate

Client Information

- Use this medicine as directed by your veterinarian.
- Use proper administration techniques to avoid contamination of the medicine. Keep the cap tightly closed when the medicine is not in use.
- Wait for 5 to 10 minutes after applying this medicine before applying any other medicines to the eye.
- Store this medicine at room temperature away from moisture and sunlight. Do not freeze.
- Do not use this medicine if the color changes, if it becomes cloudy, or if there are particles in solutions.

Storage/Stability

Store this product at controlled room temperature (15°C-25°C [59°F-77°F]) away from moisture and sunlight; do not freeze.

Compatibility/Compounding Considerations

Levobunolol ophthalmic preparations should not be mixed directly with any other ophthalmic medications.

Dosage Forms/Regulatory Status

VETERINARY-LABELED PRODUCTS: NONE

HUMAN-LABELED PRODUCTS:

Levobunolol 0.25% Ophthalmic Solution (containing levobunolol HCl 0.5%; benzalkonium chloride 0.004%; polyvinyl alcohol 1.4%; edetate disodium; sodium metabisulfite; sodium phosphate, dibasic; potassium phosphate, monobasic; NaCl; HCl or NaOH to adjust the pH; purified water), in 5, 10, and 15 mL ophthalmic dropper bottles; *Akbeta®*, *Betagan®*; (Rx)

Levobunolol 0.5% Ophthalmic Solution (containing benzalkonium chloride 0.004%; polyvinyl alcohol 1.4%; edetate disodium; sodium metabisulfite; sodium phosphate, dibasic; potassium phosphate, monobasic; NaCl; HCl or NaOH to adjust the pH; purified water), in 5, 10, and 15 mL ophthalmic dropper bottles; *Akbeta®*, *Betagan®*, generic; (Rx)

References

For the complete list of references, see **wiley.com/go/budde/plumb**

Levofloxacin Ophthalmic

(lev-oh-***flocks***-a sin)

Third-Generation Fluoroquinolone Antibiotic

Prescriber Highlights

- ► Used to treat confirmed bacterial conjunctivitis or keratitis based on culture and susceptibility; prophylactic use is not recommended.
- ► Physically incompatible with many drugs; therefore, it should not be directly mixed with other ophthalmic medications.
- ► Crystalline drug precipitates may be noted in the superficial portion of corneal defects when levofloxacin is used on the eye.

Uses/Indications

Levofloxacin ophthalmic may be used to treat bacterial conjunctivitis or keratitis caused by susceptible strains of *Staphylococcus* spp, *Streptococcus* spp, *Pseudomonas aeruginosa*, *Chlamydophila* spp, and *Haemophilus* spp.[1] Levofloxacin is effective against other gram-positive and gram-negative organisms; however, its potency is not considered significantly greater than that of second-generation fluoroquinolones (eg, ciprofloxacin), particularly versus *Staphylococcus* spp.[1,2] The increased clinical efficacy of levofloxacin may be afforded by increased penetration to ocular tissues.[3]

The World Health Organization (WHO) has designated levofloxacin as a Critically Important, Highest Priority antimicrobial in human medicine.[2]

Pharmacology/Actions

Levofloxacin is a third-generation fluoroquinolone antibiotic that acts via the inhibition of bacterial topoisomerase II (DNA gyrase), leading to impaired DNA replication and repair.

Contraindications/Precautions/Warnings

Levofloxacin should not be used prophylactically and is contraindicated in patients that have a history of hypersensitivity to it, other fluoroquinolones, or any component of the formulation. It should only be used as a topical ophthalmic. It should not be injected subconjunctivally or into the anterior chamber of the eye. Fluoroquinolone-induced retinal toxicity in domestic cats has not been demonstrated with this product.

Adverse Effects

Adverse effects reported in humans or animals include blurred vision, tearing, eye pain, redness, itching, and a bad taste in the mouth. Crystalline drug precipitates may be noted in the superficial portion of corneal defects when levofloxacin is used.[4]

Dosages

Conjunctivitis (extra-label): 1 drop in affected eye(s) every 2 to 8 hours

Keratitis (extra-label): 1 drop in affected eye(s) every 2 to 8 hours, or 0.1 mL in the subpalpebral lavage (SPL) catheter every 2 to 8 hours. May precipitate when mixed with other ophthalmic medications; therefore, it is important to flush SPL catheter well with air between medications.

Monitoring

- Corneal cytology and culture to evaluate for the presence of bacteria
- Clinical efficacy: improvement and resolution of clinical signs associated with bacterial infection
- If blepharospasm, uveitis, worsening of ulceration, or no improvement in infection occur within 7 days, reassess microbial susceptibility.

Client Information

- Use this medication as directed by your veterinarian.
- Crystals may appear on the surface of the eye during treatment with levofloxacin ophthalmic.
- Do not mix this medicine with other eye medications.
- Wait 5 minutes after applying this medicine before applying any other medications to the eye.
- Use proper administration techniques to avoid contamination of the medication. Keep the cap tightly closed when the medication is not in use.
- Your veterinarian will need to monitor your animal while it is receiving this medicine. Do not miss these important follow-up visits.
- Store this medication in the refrigerator or at room temperature. Do not freeze.
- Do not use this medication if the color changes, if it becomes cloudy, or if there are particles in the solutions.

Storage/Stability

Store this product in the at controlled room temperature (15°C-25°C [59°F-77°F]) away from moisture and sunlight; do not freeze.

Compatibility/Compounding Considerations

Fluoroquinolone antibiotics interact with many other drugs, including those containing cations (eg, iron, aluminum, magnesium, calcium). Levofloxacin should not be mixed directly (in vitro) with any other drugs. Levofloxacin is not available as an ophthalmic ointment.

Dosage Forms/Regulatory Status

VETERINARY-LABELED PRODUCTS: NONE

HUMAN-LABELED PRODUCTS:

Levofloxacin 0.5% ophthalmic solution (containing levofloxacin 5 mg/mL, benzalkonium chloride 0.005%, NaCl, and water. May also contain HCl and/or NaOH to adjust pH to 6.5 with an osmolality of ≈300 mOsm/kg), in a 5 mL ophthalmic dropper bottle; generic; (Rx)

References

For the complete list of references, see **wiley.com/go/budde/plumb**

Lidocaine Ophthalmic

(***lye***-doe-kane)

Topical Ocular Anesthetic

For other uses of lidocaine, see ***Lidocaine, Systemic; Lidocaine, Local Anesthetic; Lidocaine, Topical***

Prescriber Highlights

- ► Injectable local anesthetic that may be used for analgesia for ocular diagnostic and therapeutic procedures
- ► Should never be prescribed for at-home administration
- ► Dose- and species-dependent duration, with maximal effect generally between 1 and 5 minutes in dogs, cats, and horses

Uses/Indications

Lidocaine is a local anesthetic available as an injectable solution or an ophthalmic topical gel that can be administered topically to facilitate ophthalmic diagnostic and therapeutic procedures, including measurement of intraocular pressure (tonometry), corneal and conjunctival sampling for cytology and culture, ocular ultrasonography, and gonioscopy. Lidocaine is indicated as an adjunctive anesthetic for performing therapeutic procedures in the hospital, including removal of foreign bodies and sutures from the cornea, eyelid and conjunctival surgeries, corneal grafting procedures, and cataract extraction. Lidocaine demonstrates maximal effect generally between 1 and 5 minutes, lasting around 20 to 25 minutes in dogs[1,2] and ≈45 to 55 minutes in horses.[3-5] The degree of anesthesia in normal canine eyes was comparable to that of topically applied bupivacaine and ropivacaine.[6] Due to the likelihood of developing ocular surface toxicities with prolonged or repeated use, it should never be prescribed for use as an ocular analgesic.

Pharmacology/Actions

Lidocaine induces local anesthesia by inhibiting neuronal depolarization, thus preventing the generation of an action potential. This action occurs due to the binding of the local anesthetic molecule to the intracellular portion of the voltage-gated sodium channel within the neuron, thus inhibiting the intracellular movement of sodium. Variations in the structure of different local anesthetics influence their relative potencies. All local anesthetics have increased efficacy in alkaline environments due to improved intracellular penetration; efficacy is decreased in the acidic environment of inflammation.

Contraindications/Precautions/Warnings

Lidocaine is contraindicated in patients with a history of hypersensitivity to it or any component of the formulation. Prolonged use of a topical ocular anesthetic will likely produce significant corneal epithelial and stromal disease, as well as tear film instability, and may result in loss of vision.[7]

Adverse Effects

Instillation of lidocaine may result in local irritation (eg, blepharospasm, conjunctival hyperemia) several hours after administration. Patients sensitive to other local anesthetics may be less likely to react to proparacaine; however, local or systemic sensitivity may still occur and manifest as a pseudo-allergic (anaphylactoid) reaction mimicking an IgE-mediated vasodilatory event. Cardiovascular, respiratory, and CNS depressant effects that may result from other local anesthetics are extremely rare with the appropriate use of topical anesthetics. Care should be exercised, however, when administering to small veterinary patients (ie, puppies, kittens, "pocket pets", amphibians) that may be more susceptible to the effects of systemically absorbed drug. Use as a therapeutic analgesic leads to superficial punctate keratitis, which may progress to diffuse necrotizing keratitis, severe infiltrative keratitis, persistent epithelial defects, or damage to Descemet's membrane. Application of the topical ophthalmic and nonophthalmic gels in normal dog[1,2] and horse[3] eyes induced conjunctival hyperemia and punctate epithelial damage.

Dosages

Ophthalmic procedures requiring local anesthesia in small animal species (extra-label): 1 – 2 drops in the target eye(s) prior to examination or procedure. May repeat 1 drop every 5 to 10 minutes for 2 to 3 additional times. **Additional doses should be avoided in small patients (puppies, kittens, "pocket pets", amphibians).**

Ophthalmic procedures requiring local anesthesia in horses (extra-label): Using an ophthalmic topical gel, 0.2 mL in the target eye(s) prior to examination or procedure.[3,5,8] Onset of analgesia is within 1 to 5 minutes and duration is ≈45 to 55 minutes.

Monitoring

- Clinical effect. The onset of action indicated by an awake patient that is permitting diagnostic procedures to be performed and by a reduction in anesthetic requirements when administered preoperatively

Client Information

- Animal owners must **not** administer lidocaine in the home. Its use is limited to diagnostic procedures performed in the veterinary clinical setting.

Storage/Stability

Store at controlled room temperature 15°C to 25°C (59°F-77°F) and protected from sunlight; do not freeze. Discard single-use containers after use.

Compatibility/Compounding Considerations

Lidocaine should not be mixed directly with any other ophthalmic drugs.

Dosage Forms/Regulatory Status

VETERINARY-LABELED PRODUCTS: NONE

HUMAN-LABELED PRODUCTS:

Lidocaine HCl 3.5% ophthalmic gel (containing 35 mg lidocaine HCl per mL; hypromellose; NaCl; purified water; HCl, and/or NaOH to adjust pH), in 1 mL tubes and 5 mL in a 10 mL round plastic dropper bottle; *Akten*® (Rx)

References

For the complete list of references, see **wiley.com/go/budde/plumb**

Lissamine Green Ophthalmic

(***lis***-ah-meen) *Green Glo*®

Ocular Diagnostic Agent

Prescriber Highlights

- Vital dye that demonstrates corneal and conjunctival epithelial cell damage, as well as deficiency in ocular surface mucins
- Less stinging on administration than is associated with rose bengal
- Requires broader interpretive experience than fluorescein staining
- Unapproved drug with periodic market shortages

Uses/Indications

Lissamine green is used as a diagnostic agent when superficial corneal or conjunctival epithelial damage is suspected. Lissamine green does not sting on application like rose bengal, but interpretation of the results requires broader evaluative experience than that for rose bengal and fluorescein. A grading scale that implements slit-lamp biomicroscopy to evaluate the regions of uptake is used in humans, and lissamine green has recently been demonstrated to be an effective adjunctive diagnostic test for the evaluation of qualitative and quantitative tear film deficiencies in dogs.[1,2]

Pharmacology/Actions

Lissamine green stains the cornea and conjunctiva blue upon instillation, resulting in speckling of the cornea and conjunctiva if ulcerations or dry patches from muco-deficient or damaged epithelial cells are present.

Contraindications/Precautions/Warnings

Lissamine green is contraindicated in patients that have a history of hypersensitivity to it or any component of the formulation. Lissamine green has demonstrated antimicrobial activity against gram-positive and gram-negative organisms; thus, samples for bacterial culture should be collected before administration of lissamine green.[3]

Adverse Effects

Adverse effects of lissamine green reported in humans or animals include stinging on instillation.

Dosages

Detection of corneal change: Wet the surface of the lissamine green strip with 1 to 2 drops of normal saline solution. Apply moistened tip to the conjunctiva or fornix as required. Allow the patient to blink several times after application to disperse the dye across the surface of the eye. Wait 60 seconds, then read with a white light source. Blue speckling will be evident for areas of the damaged or muco-deficient cornea.

Monitoring

- Lissamine green ophthalmic is a diagnostic agent. Monitoring is not required.

Client Information

- Lissamine green is not used at home by animal caregivers.

Storage/Stability

Store this product in a well-ventilated place protected from moisture and light; do not freeze.[4]

Compatibility/Compounding Considerations

Lissamine green ophthalmic preparations should not be mixed directly with any other ophthalmic medications.

Dosage Forms/Regulatory Status

VETERINARY-LABELED PRODUCTS: NONE

HUMAN-LABELED PRODUCTS:

Lissamine Green 1.5 mg Strips (containing 1.5 mg of lissamine green per strip), in individually wrapped strips in containers of 100 strips; *Green Glo*®; (Rx). There are no FDA-approved forms of lissamine green strips.

References

For the complete list of references, see **wiley.com/go/budde/plumb**

Lodoxamide Ophthalmic

(loe-***doks***-a-mide) *Alomide*®

Mast Cell Stabilizer

Prescriber Highlights

- Topical mast cell stabilizer used to treat seasonal conjunctivitis

Uses/Indications

Lodoxamide may be used to treat allergic conjunctivitis. No studies describing the efficacy and safety of lodoxamide after topical administration have been performed in veterinary patients.

Pharmacology/Actions

Lodoxamide is a mast cell stabilizer with efficacy in treatment of type I hypersensitivity reactions (IgE-mediated). Mast cell inhibition decreases vascular permeability, thus diminishing the signs associated with conjunctivitis. It does not possess vasoconstrictor, antihistaminic, cyclooxygenase inhibition, or other anti-inflammatory activity.

Contraindications/Precautions/Warnings

Lodoxamide is contraindicated in patients that have a history of hypersensitivity to it or any component of the formulation.[1]

Adverse Effects

Adverse effects reported in humans include transient burning, stinging, or discomfort on instillation.[1] Additional adverse effects that were infrequently reported include ocular itching, blurred vision, dry eye, tearing, discharge, hyperemic, crystalline deposits, foreign body sensation, corneal erosion/ulcer, lid/lash scales, eye pain, ocular edema/swelling, ocular warming sensation, ocular fatigue, chemosis, anterior chamber cells, keratopathy/keratitis, blepharitis, allergy, stick sensation, and epitheliopathy. Nonocular adverse events that were infrequently reported include headache, heat sensation, dizziness, somnolence, nausea, stomach discomfort, sneezing, dry nose, and rash.

Dosages

Conjunctivitis (extra-label): 1 drop in the affected eye(s) 4 times daily for up to 3 months

Monitoring

- Clinical efficacy: resolution of conjunctival redness, itching, and discomfort

Client Information

- Use this medicine as directed by your veterinarian.
- Use proper administration techniques to avoid contamination of the medicine. Keep the cap tightly closed when the medicine is not in use.
- Wait for 5 minutes after applying this medicine before applying any other medicines to the eye.
- Store at room temperature away from moisture and sunlight. Do not freeze.
- Do not use this medicine if the color changes or if there are particles in the solution.

Storage/Stability

Store this product at controlled room temperature (20°C-25°C [68°F-77°F]) away from moisture and sunlight.

Compatibility/Compounding Considerations

Lodoxamide ophthalmic preparations should not be mixed directly with any other ophthalmic medications.

Dosage Forms/Regulatory Status

VETERINARY-LABELED PRODUCTS: NONE

HUMAN-LABELED PRODUCTS:

Lodoxamide Tromethamine Ophthalmic Solution 0.1% (containing lodoxamide tromethamine 1.78 mg, equivalent to 1 mg lodoxamide; benzalkonium chloride 0.007%; mannitol; hypromellose 2910; sodium citrate; tyloxapol; citric acid; edetate disodium; NaOH and/or HCl to adjust pH; purified water), in sterile 10 mL ophthalmic dropper bottle; *Alomide*®; (Rx)

References

For the complete list of references, see **wiley.com/go/budde/plumb**

Loteprednol Ophthalmic

(lote-uh-***pred***-nole) *Lotemax*®, *Alrex*®, *Zylet*®, *Eysuvis*®, *Inveltys*®

Corticosteroid Anti-Inflammatory Agent

Prescriber Highlights

- ▶ A topical corticosteroid used to treat ocular surface and anterior segment inflammatory conditions
- ▶ Do not use in bacterial, fungal, or viral keratitis or if corneal abrasion or ulceration are suspected.
- ▶ Use with caution in avian species due to risk for systemic corticosteroid effects.

Uses/Indications

Loteprednol ophthalmic is used to treat inflammatory conditions of the palpebral and bulbar conjunctiva, cornea, and anterior segment of the globe (eg, blepharitis, conjunctivitis, keratitis, anterior uveitis). In humans with dry eye syndrome, loteprednol has demonstrated benefit in the initial management of the condition before initiation or in conjunction with topically administered cyclosporine.[1,2] No studies describing the efficacy and safety of loteprednol after topical administration have been performed in veterinary patients.

Pharmacology/Actions

Corticosteroids have broad immunomodulatory and anti-inflammatory actions, which are mediated via direct effects on gene expression, as well as by nongenomic effects on cell membranes and receptors. Ultimately, corticosteroids decrease pro-inflammatory gene transcription, production of pro-inflammatory prostaglandins and leukotrienes, B- and T-cell number and function, cell-mediated immunity, and humoral immunity.[3] The specific mechanisms involved in regulating ocular inflammation are not known. Loteprednol is a "soft" steroid (a metabolically labile moiety that undergoes hydrolysis to its active form within the cornea, thus allowing local anti-inflammatory effects to predominate relative to harmful adverse effects).

Contraindications/Precautions/Warnings

Loteprednol is contraindicated in patients that have a history of hypersensitivity to it or any component of the formulation. Topical corticosteroids are contraindicated in known or suspected corneal ulceration or corneal infection (eg, bacterial, fungal, or viral). Use loteprednol with caution in patients with diabetes mellitus or other endocrine diseases, infectious diseases, chronic renal failure, congestive heart failure, systemic hypertension, or gastric ulceration. When use of loteprednol is necessary in these conditions, the minimal effective dose should be administered for the shortest possible time.

Adverse Effects

Adverse effects reported in humans include development of cataracts (via altered glucose or lenticular metabolic effects), increased intraocular pressure (IOP; via activation of glucocorticoid receptors in the trabecular meshwork), infection (via immunosuppression), decreased wound healing (via increased collagenolytic activity), mydriasis, and calcific keratopathy. Increased IOP and development of cataracts are minimized with loteprednol relative to other topically administered corticosteroids.[4-6] Systemic effects are rare but include hepatopathy, suppression of endogenous glucocorticoid production, and focal alopecia. Concurrent use of systemic steroids increases the risk for these adverse effects.

Dosages

Conjunctivitis (extra-label): 1 drop or ¼ inch strip in the affected eye(s) every 4 to 8 hours, then gradually decrease the dosage, provided clinical improvement is maintained

Keratitis (extra-label): 1 drop or ¼ inch strip in the affected eye(s) every 4 to 8 hours, then gradually decrease the dosage, provided clinical improvement is maintained

Keratoconjunctivitis sicca (extra-label): 1 drop in the affected eye(s) 4 times daily for 2 weeks

Anterior uveitis (extra-label): 1 drop or ¼ inch strip in the affected eye(s) every 4 to 8 hours, then gradually decrease the dosage, provided clinical improvement is maintained

Perioperative cataract removal (extra-label): 1 drop in the surgical eye(s) 4 times daily, beginning 24 hours after surgery, continuing for 2 weeks

Monitoring

- Clinical efficacy: resolution of inflammation
- Monitor intraocular pressure (IOP) and observe for signs of infection or delayed wound healing
- Monitor for blood and/or urine glucose changes in diabetic animals

Client Information

- Use this medicine as directed by your veterinarian.
- Shake suspensions well before using.
- Use proper administration techniques to avoid contamination of the medicine.
- Keep the cap tightly closed when the medicine is not in use.
- Wait for 5 minutes after applying this medicine before applying any other medicines to the eye.

- Store this medicine at room temperature away from moisture and sunlight. Do not freeze.
- Do not use this medicine if the color changes or if there are particles in the solutions.

Storage/Stability

Store this product at room temperature (15°C-25°C [59°F-77°F]) away from moisture and sunlight.

Compatibility/Compounding Considerations

Loteprednol ophthalmic preparations should not be mixed directly with any other ophthalmic medications.

Dosage Forms/Regulatory Status

VETERINARY-LABELED PRODUCTS: NONE

HUMAN-LABELED PRODUCTS:

Loteprednol Etabonate 0.2% Ophthalmic Suspension (containing loteprednol etabonate 2 mg, edetate disodium, glycerin, povidone, purified water, tyloxapol, HCl and/or NaOH may be added to adjust the pH, and benzalkonium chloride 0.10%, as an isotonic suspension of 250 – 310 mOsm/kg), in 10 mL sterile ophthalmic dropper bottle; *Alrex*®; (Rx)

Loteprednol Etabonate 0.25% Ophthalmic Suspension (containing loteprednol etabonate 2.5 mg, glycerin, sodium citrate dihydrate, sodium chloride, poloxamer 407, edetate disodium dihydrate, citric acid, water for injection, and benzalkonium chloride 0.01%), in 10 mL sterile ophthalmic dropper bottle; *Eysuvis*®; (Rx)

Loteprednol Etabonate 0.38% Ophthalmic Gel (containing loteprednol etabonate 3.8 mg, boric acid, edetate disodium dihydrate, glycerin, hypromellose, poloxamer, polycarbophil, propylene glycol, sodium chloride, water for injection, sodium hydroxide to adjust pH, and benzalkonium chloride 0.003%), in 10 mL ophthalmic dropper bottle; *Lotemax SM*®; (Rx)

Loteprednol Etabonate 0.5% Ophthalmic Gel (containing loteprednol etabonate 5 mg, boric acid, edetate disodium dehydrate, glycerin, polycarbophil, propylene glycol, NaCl, tyloxapol, water for injection, NaOH to adjust pH to 6 to 7, and benzalkonium chloride 0.003%), in sterile 5 g ophthalmic tube; *Lotemax*®; (Rx)

Loteprednol Etabonate Ophthalmic Ointment 0.5% (containing loteprednol etabonate 5 mg, white petrolatum, and mineral oil), in a sterile 3.5 g ophthalmic tube; *Lotemax*®; (Rx)

Loteprednol Etabonate 0.5% Ophthalmic Suspension (containing loteprednol etabonate 5 mg, edetate disodium, glycerin, povidone, purified water, tyloxapol, HCl and/or NaOH to adjust the pH, and benzalkonium chloride 0.01%, as an isotonic suspension of 250 – 310 mOsm/kg), in 5 mL, 10 mL, and 15 mL ophthalmic dropper bottles; *Lotemax*®, generic; (Rx)

Loteprednol Etabonate 1% Ophthalmic Suspension (containing loteprednol etabonate 10 mg, glycerin, sodium citrate dihydrate, poloxamer 407, sodium chloride, edetate disodium dihydrate, citric acid, water for injection, and benzalkonium chloride 0.01%), in 2.8 mL sterile ophthalmic dropper bottle; *Inveltys*®; (Rx)

Loteprednol Etabonate 0.5% and Tobramycin 0.3% Ophthalmic Suspension (containing loteprednol etabonate 5 mg, tobramycin 3 mg, edetate disodium, glycerin, povidone, purified water, tyloxapol, sulfuric acid and/or NaOH to adjust the pH, and benzalkonium chloride, as an isotonic suspension of 260 – 320 mOsmol/kg), in sterile 5 mL and 10 mL ophthalmic dropper bottles; *Zylet*®; (Rx)

References

For the complete list of references, see **wiley.com/go/budde/plumb**

Miconazole Ophthalmic

(mye-***kon***-uh-zohl)

Azole Antifungal Agent

Prescriber Highlights

- ▶ Used to treat ocular surface fungal infections
- ▶ Not commercially available as an ophthalmic preparation; must be compounded
- ▶ Penetrates the cornea more efficiently than natamycin

Uses/Indications

Miconazole ophthalmic solution is primarily used to treat fungal keratitis in horses; however, it has been successfully used to treat keratomycosis in a dog.[1] Miconazole has a broad antifungal spectrum against most fungi and yeasts of veterinary interest. Sensitive organisms include *Blastomyces dermatitidis*, *Paracoccidioides brasiliensis*, *Histoplasma capsulatum*, *Candida* spp, *Coccidioides immitis*, *Cryptococcus neoformans*, and *Aspergillus fumigatus*. Some *Aspergillus* spp and *Fusarium* spp are only marginally sensitive.

Pharmacology/Actions

Miconazole interacts with 14-alpha-sterol demethylase, a cytochrome P-450 enzyme involved in the conversion of lanosterol to ergosterol. Ergosterol is an essential component of the fungal cell membrane; preventing its synthesis increases cellular permeability and causes leakage of cellular contents. Other **antifungal** effects of miconazole include inhibition of endogenous respiration, purine uptake, the transformation of yeasts to mycelial forms, and impairment of triglyceride and phospholipid biosynthesis.

Miconazole has a wide antifungal spectrum against most fungi and yeasts of veterinary interest; however, susceptibility of isolates of normal ocular surface microflora and isolates from horses with fungal keratitis indicates variable efficacy. Thus, culture and susceptibility testing should be performed in horses with cytologically confirmed or suspected fungal keratitis.[1-5]

Contraindications/Precautions/Warnings

Miconazole is contraindicated in patients that have a history of hypersensitivity to it or any component of the formulation.

Adverse Effects

Adverse effects reported in humans or animals include transient burning or stinging on application. Miconazole may cause local irritation if it is injected subconjunctivally. Although systemic absorption of topically applied solutions is unlikely, systemic exposure to miconazole has resulted in hepatotoxicity and hearing loss in humans. Miconazole had more cytotoxic effects on cultured corneal epithelial cells than itraconazole, but miconazole had less cytotoxic effects than natamycin.[6]

Dosages

Equine fungal keratitis (extra-label): 1 – 2 drops to the affected eye(s) or 0.1 mL in the subpalpebral lavage (SPL) catheter every 2 to 3 hours initially, then taper the frequency based on clinical response

Monitoring

- Clinical efficacy: improvement and resolution of clinical signs associated with the fungal infection
- Corneal scrapings with cytology and cultures to determine the clearing of fungal organisms

Client Information

- Use this medication as directed by your veterinarian.
- Use proper administration techniques to avoid contamination of the medication. Keep the cap tightly closed when the medication is not in use.

- Wait 5 minutes after applying this medication before applying any other medications to the eye.
- Your veterinarian will need to monitor your animal while it is receiving this medicine. Do not miss these important follow-up visits.
- Store this medication as directed on the product label. Do not freeze.
- Do not use this medication if the color changes, if it becomes cloudy, or if there are particles in solutions.

Storage/Stability

Store this product in the refrigerator (2°C-8°C [36°F-46°F]) or at controlled room temperature (20°C- 25°C [68°F-77°F]); check individual labels for details, as recommendations vary by product. Do not freeze. Keep product away from moisture and sunlight.

Compatibility/Compounding Considerations

Miconazole should not be mixed directly (in vitro) with any other drugs.

Dosage Forms/Regulatory Status

VETERINARY-LABELED PRODUCTS: NONE

HUMAN-LABELED PRODUCTS: NONE

Miconazole has been compounded into a 1% ophthalmic solution that mimics the formerly commercially available *Monistat IV®*. Miconazole topical creams and ointments for dermatological use should **NOT** be used in the eye.

References

For the complete list of references, see **wiley.com/go/budde/plumb**

Mitomycin Ophthalmic

(***mye***-toe-***mye***-sin) *Mitosol®, Mitomycin C*

Cytotoxic Agent

Prescriber Highlights

- ► Antifibrotic agent used adjunctively in periocular surgeries (most commonly used in glaucoma implant procedures)
- ► Antineoplastic agent used for susceptible periocular and ocular surface tumors
- ► Product is normally blue in color.
- ► May cause periocular alopecia following treatment
- ► The National Institute for Occupational Safety and Health (NIOSH) classifies mitomycin as a hazardous drug; use appropriate precautions when handling.

Uses/Indications

Because of its ability to reduce fibroblastic proliferation and prevent subsequent scarring, mitomycin is used adjunctively in ocular surgeries, particularly to treat glaucoma by placement of drainage shunts or alternation of the natural aqueous humor outflow tracts; however, efficacy is unknown.[1-3] Mitomycin is also used as an adjunct to surgical removal for treatment of cutaneous and ocular surface neoplastic conditions (eg, squamous cell carcinoma, hemangiosarcoma) to prevent recurrence.[4-8]

Pharmacology/Actions

Mitomycin binds DNA, which leads to cross-linking of DNA and subsequent inhibition of DNA synthesis and function. Evidence suggests that at high concentrations of the drug, cellular RNA and protein synthesis are also suppressed.

Contraindications/Precautions/Warnings

Mitomycin is contraindicated in patients that have a history of hypersensitivity to it or any component of the formulation. Mitomycin is contraindicated in patients with thrombocytopenia, coagulation disorder, or an increase in bleeding tendency due to other causes. Pregnant women or women attempting to become pregnant should avoid contact with this drug.

The National Institute for Occupational Safety and Health (NIOSH) classifies mitomycin as a hazardous drug; personal protective equipment (PPE) should be used accordingly to minimize the risk for exposure. Refer to the Occupational Safety and Health Association (OSHA) website for more information.

Adverse Effects

Adverse effects reported in humans or animals include burning and stinging on application, corneal irritation, and edema formation.[4] Periocular alopecia has been reported in horses after topical application.[5] Topical administration in the presence of corneal epithelial defects has been associated with stromal ulceration and bullous keratopathy.[5] The systemic use of mitomycin has been associated with myelosuppression, particularly thrombocytopenia and leukopenia, nephrotoxicity, and pulmonary toxicity, although these effects are unlikely with topical therapy.

Dosages

Equine periocular squamous cell carcinoma (extra-label): ½ inch strip of a 0.04% ointment to the affected site 3 times daily for 21 days in a cycle of 7 days of drug application, followed by a 7-day drug vacation.[5,6] If using a subpalpebral lavage (SPL) system, instill 0.1 mL of a 0.04% solution 3 times daily for 21 days in a cycle of 7 days of drug application, followed by a 7-day drug vacation; maintain catheter patency by flushing the line with air after each dose.

Adjunctive antifibrotic agent for glaucoma implant surgery (extra-label): A single, 5-minute intraoperative application of 0.5 mg/mL solution at the filtration site following surgical placement of the shunt.[1] **NOTE:** Multiple protocols exist for use during surgical procedures for correcting glaucoma, varying with the type of procedure and other patient parameters. As these procedures should be performed by board-certified veterinary ophthalmologists, the protocols are not detailed here.

Monitoring

- Clinical efficacy depending on indication:
  - Maintenance of patency of the glaucoma implant, leading to control of intraocular pressure (IOP)
  - Cell or tissue samples for evaluation to confirm remission of neoplasia

Client Information

- This medicine is a chemotherapy drug. Pregnant women and sick or immunocompromised individuals should avoid contact with this medicine.
- Personal protective equipment (eg, gloves, mask) should be worn when giving this medicine to your animal. Dispose of any waste in a doubled plastic bag, then place the bag in a secure disposal location that children and animals cannot access.
- Use proper administration techniques to avoid contamination of the medicine. Keep the cap tightly closed when the medicine is not in use.
- Wait for 5 minutes after applying this medicine before applying any other medicines to the eye.
- Store this medicine in the refrigerator. Do not freeze.
- Do not use this medicine if the color changes (it is normally blue), if it becomes cloudy, or if there are particles in the solution.
- This medication is considered to be a hazardous drug as defined by the National Institute for Occupational Safety and Health (NIOSH). Talk with your veterinarian or pharmacist about the use of personal protective equipment when handling this medicine.

Storage/Stability

Store this product in the refrigerator (2°C-8°C [36°F-46°F]), away from moisture and sunlight. Store compounded products as stated on product label.

Compatibility/Compounding Considerations

Mitomycin ophthalmic preparations should not be mixed directly with any other ophthalmic medications. Mitomycin ophthalmic solution is not commercially available, but mitomycin lyophilized powder for injection can be compounded into appropriate ophthalmic solutions as follows:

- If using the 5 mg vial, reconstitute vial with 12.5 mL sterile 0.9% sodium chloride injection to make a 0.4 mg/mL (0.04%) solution.
- If using the 20 mg vial, reconstitute with 50 mL sterile 0.9% sodium chloride injection to make a 0.4 mg/mL (0.04%) solution.

NOTE: Commercially available mitomycin 20 mg vials may not contain 50 mL volume. Use caution when reconstituting, and when volume restrictions require, aseptically transfer contents into a 50 mL empty sterile vial.

Mitomycin ophthalmic ointments are not commercially available but may be prepared by qualified compounding pharmacists.

Dosage Forms/Regulatory Status

VETERINARY-LABELED PRODUCTS: NONE

HUMAN-LABELED PRODUCTS:

Mitomycin ophthalmic topical solution for multi-use is not commercially available, but mitomycin lyophilized powder for injection (5 mg or 20 mg vial) can be compounded into a suitable ophthalmic. A commercially available kit for mitomycin ophthalmic topical (single use) as an adjunct to ab externo glaucoma surgery is available; *Mitosol®*, generic; (Rx).

References

For the complete list of references, see **wiley.com/go/budde/plumb**

Morphine Ophthalmic

(***mor***-feen)

Opioid

Prescriber Highlights

- ► Opioid analgesic that may be beneficial in the treatment of ocular pain
- ► Must be compounded by a qualified compounding pharmacist, as no ophthalmic dosage forms are commercially available
- ► Do not use in animals receiving naloxone, nalbuphine, or nalorphine, as these drugs have opioid antagonist properties.
- ► DEA Schedule II (C-II) controlled substance

Uses/Indications

Morphine ophthalmic solution may be used to manage ocular pain. Dogs with experimentally induced corneal ulcers that received morphine solution 3 times daily experienced a reduction in signs of ocular pain without prolonged healing times[1]; however, in a clinical trial of dogs and cats with naturally occurring corneal ulcers, a single drop of morphine solution did not improve clinical signs of pain.[2] Combined topical administration and subconjunctival injection did not appear to provide ocular pain relief (as evaluated by changes in blepharospasm, conjunctival hyperemia, blinking rates, tearing) in dogs following phacoemulsification surgery.[3] Topical morphine did not affect corneal sensitivity when it was administered to normal equine eyes.[4,5]

Pharmacology/Actions

Morphine is primarily an opioid mu receptor agonist that interacts with mu binding sites located in the brain, as well as within the spinal cord and on peripheral sensory nerves. They are present in the cornea in smaller numbers than delta receptors in the canine cornea.[1] The analgesic effects on the cornea can be variable. It is possible that receptor specificity and localization, frequency of administration, and location of pain stimulus relative to drug penetration all impact clinical efficacy. Topical ocular morphine administration to eyes of normal horses results in measurable intraocular and systemic morphine concentrations, without local or systemic adverse effects.[4]

Contraindications/Precautions/Warnings

Morphine ophthalmic is contraindicated in patients with a history of hypersensitivity to it or any component of the formulation. Adverse effects may occur following concomitant use with monoamine oxidase inhibitors (eg, amitraz, linezolid, selegiline) or within 14 days of such treatment. Because of potential systemic absorption, morphine ophthalmic should be used with caution in patients with respiratory insufficiency or depression; severe CNS depression; bronchoconstrictive disorders (eg, asthma); heart failure secondary to pulmonary hypertension; arrhythmias; increased intracranial or cerebrospinal pressure (eg, head injury, brain tumor); or seizures.

Adverse Effects

Adverse effects reported in humans or animals include stinging and burning on application. Although systemic adverse effects are unlikely with topical administration, they could occur. See ***Morphine***.

Dosages

Corneal ulcers: 1 drop of a morphine 1% solution in the affected eye(s) every 8 hours

Monitoring

- Clinical efficacy: control of signs of ocular discomfort (eg, blepharospasm, conjunctival hyperemia, tearing)

Client Information

- Use this medicine as directed by your veterinarian.
- This medicine is a controlled substance and may not be refilled without a new prescription.
- Use proper administration techniques to avoid contamination of the medicine. Keep the cap tightly closed when the medicine is not in use.
- Wait for 5 minutes after applying this medicine before applying any other medicines to the eye.
- Store this medicine as directed on package label. Keep product away from moisture and sunlight. Do not freeze.
- Do not use this medicine if the color changes, if it becomes cloudy, or if there are particles in the solution.

Storage/Stability

Store this product as directed on the package labeling away from moisture and sunlight; do not freeze.

Compatibility/Compounding Considerations

Morphine ophthalmic preparations should not be mixed directly with any other ophthalmic medications.

Dosage Forms/Regulatory Status

VETERINARY-LABELED PRODUCTS: NONE

HUMAN-LABELED PRODUCTS: NONE

Morphine sulfate ophthalmic solution is not commercially available; it must be compounded. Preservative-free morphine sulfate injection may be aseptically diluted with sterile 0.9% sodium chloride injection to achieve a 1% (10 mg/mL) aseptic ophthalmic solution.

References

For the complete list of references, see **wiley.com/go/budde/plumb**

Moxifloxacin Ophthalmic

(mox-ih-***flox***-uh-sin) *Vigamox®, Moxeza®*

Fourth-Generation Fluoroquinolone Antimicrobial

Prescriber Highlights

- ▶ Used to treat confirmed bacterial conjunctivitis or keratitis based on culture and susceptibility; prophylactic use is not recommended
- ▶ Physically incompatible with many drugs; therefore, it should not be directly mixed with other ophthalmic medications
- ▶ Crystalline drug precipitates may be noted in the superficial portion of corneal defects when moxifloxacin is used on the eye.

Uses/Indications

Moxifloxacin ophthalmic may be used to treat bacterial conjunctivitis or keratitis caused by susceptible strains of *Staphylococcus* spp, *Streptococcus* spp, *Pseudomonas aeruginosa*, *Chlamydophila* spp, and *Haemophilus* spp. Moxifloxacin is effective against other gram-positive and gram-negative organisms. *Pseudomonas aeruginosa* isolates from dogs with bacterial keratitis showed slightly greater resistance in vitro to moxifloxacin than to other fluoroquinolones,[1] whereas *Staphylococcus pseudintermedius* isolates from dogs with bacterial keratitis demonstrated lower rates of resistance in vitro to moxifloxacin than to other fluoroquinolones.[2] Penetration of topical ophthalmic moxifloxacin into the tears, cornea, and aqueous humor of horses with normal eyes was significantly greater than with the second-generation fluoroquinolone ciprofloxacin.[3,4]

The World Health Organization (WHO) has designated moxifloxacin as a Critically Important, Highest Priority antimicrobial in human medicine.[2]

Pharmacology/Actions

Moxifloxacin is a fourth-generation fluoroquinolone antibiotic that acts via inhibition of bacterial topoisomerase II (DNA gyrase) and topoisomerase IV, leading to impaired DNA replication and repair. The inhibition of both enzymes decreases the rates of resistance as compared to earlier generations of fluoroquinolones.

Contraindications/Precautions/Warnings

Moxifloxacin is contraindicated in patients that have a history of hypersensitivity to moxifloxacin, to other fluoroquinolones, or to any of the components of this medication. This medication should only be used as a topical ophthalmic; it should not be injected subconjunctivally or into the anterior chamber of the eye. Moxifloxacin should not be used prophylactically. Fluoroquinolone-induced retinal toxicity in domestic cats has not been demonstrated with this product.

Adverse Effects

Adverse effects reported in humans or animals include blurred vision, tearing, eye pain, redness, itching, and a bad taste in the mouth. Crystalline drug precipitates may be noted in the superficial portion of corneal defects when moxifloxacin is used.

Dosages

Conjunctivitis (extra-label): 1 drop in the affected eye(s) every 2 to 8 hours

Keratitis (extra-label): 1 drop in the affected eye(s), or 0.1 mL in the subpalpebral lavage (SPL) catheter, every 2 to 8 hours. May precipitate when mixed with other ophthalmic medications; therefore, it is important to flush SPL catheter well with air between medications

Monitoring

- Corneal cytology and culture to evaluate for the persistence of bacteria
- Clinical efficacy: improvement and resolution of clinical signs associated with bacterial infection
- If blepharospasm, uveitis, worsening of ulceration, or no improvement in infection occur within 7 days, reassess microbial susceptibility.

Client Information

- Use this medication as directed by your veterinarian.
- Crystals may appear on the surface of the eye during treatment with moxifloxacin ophthalmic.
- Do not mix this medicine with other eye medications.
- Wait 5 minutes after applying this medication before applying any other medications to the eye.
- Use proper administration techniques to avoid contamination of the medication. Keep the cap tightly closed when the medication is not in use.
- Your veterinarian will need to monitor your animal while it is receiving this medicine. Do not miss these important follow-up visits.
- Store this medication in the refrigerator or at room temperature away from moisture and sunlight. Do not freeze.
- Do not use this medication if the color changes, if it becomes cloudy, or if there are particles in solutions.
- Dispose of unused medication in regular trash; do not put it into the sewer system.

Storage/Stability

Store this product in the refrigerator (2°C-8°C [36°F-46°F]) or at controlled room temperature (20°C-25°C [68°F-77°F]); check individual labels for details as recommendations vary by product. Do not freeze. Keep product away from moisture and sunlight.

Compatibility/Compounding Considerations

Fluoroquinolone antibiotics interact with many other drugs, including those containing cations (eg, iron, aluminum, magnesium, or calcium). Moxifloxacin should not be mixed directly (in vitro) with any other drugs.

Dosage Forms/Regulatory Status

VETERINARY-LABELED PRODUCTS: NONE

HUMAN-LABELED PRODUCTS:

Moxifloxacin 0.5% Ophthalmic Solution (containing moxifloxacin HCl 5.45 mg, boric acid, NaCl, purified water, and HCl and/or NaOH to adjust pH), 3 mL in sterile ophthalmic dropper bottle; *Vigamox®*, generic; (Rx)

Moxifloxacin 0.5% Ophthalmic Solution (containing NaCl, xanthan gum, boric acid, sorbitol, tyloxapol, purified water, and HCl and/or NaOH to adjust pH), 3 mL in sterile ophthalmic dropper bottle; *Moxeza®*; (Rx)

References

For the complete list of references, see **wiley.com/go/budde/plumb**

Nalbuphine Ophthalmic

(***nal***-byoo-feen) *Nubain®*

Opioid Agonist/Antagonist Analgesic Agent

Prescriber Highlights

- ▶ Used to provide ocular analgesia in patients
- ▶ Do not use in combination with other opioid ocular analgesics (eg, morphine sulfate).

Uses/Indications

Nalbuphine may be compounded as an ophthalmic preparation to provide ocular surface analgesia. In dogs, nalbuphine 1% administered 3 times daily after the creation of a corneal epithelial wound was not effective as an analgesic,[1] whereas nalbuphine 0.8% administered 3 times daily following phacoemulsification reduced corneal sensitivity and signs of ocular discomfort.[2] Corneal sensitivity was not decreased in normal horses following a single administration of 1.2% nalbuphine.[3] Additionally, 1.2% nalbuphine did not decrease corneal sensation in rabbits.[4]

Pharmacology/Actions

Nalbuphine is a synthetic opioid agonist/antagonist analgesic of the phenanthrene series. Nalbuphine's analgesic potency is essentially equivalent to that of morphine on a milligram basis. The opioid antagonist activity of nalbuphine is one-fourth as potent as nalorphine and 10 times as potent as pentazocine. Nalbuphine, by itself, has potent opioid antagonist activity at doses equal to or lower than its analgesic dose. When nalbuphine is administered following or concurrently with mu-agonist opioid analgesics (eg, morphine, oxymorphone, fentanyl), it may partially reverse or block opioid-induced respiratory depression from the mu-agonist analgesic.[5]

Contraindications/Precautions/Warnings

Nalbuphine is contraindicated in patients that have a history of hypersensitivity to it or any component of the formulation. Nalbuphine is a partial opioid antagonist and should not be used in patients receiving other opioid agents as analgesia may be reversed by nalbuphine. When nalbuphine is used systemically, it has potential to depress respiratory and cardiac systems; however, these effects are unlikely when the drug is used topically.

Adverse Effects

Adverse effects reported in humans or animals include burning, stinging, and irritation on application. Systemic adverse effects, although unlikely following topical use, include respiratory and cardiovascular depression, somnolence, and ataxia.

Dosages

Corneal analgesia (extra-label): 1 drop in the affected eye(s) every 8 hours

Monitoring

- Clinical efficacy as demonstrated by adequate ocular analgesia

Client Information

- Use this medicine as directed by your veterinarian.
- Use proper administration techniques to avoid contamination of the medicine. Keep the cap tightly closed when the medicine is not in use.
- Wear gloves when administering the medicine to avoid inadvertent contact with it.
- Wait 5 minutes after applying this medicine before applying any other medicines to the eye.
- Store this medicine as directed on the package labeling, away from moisture and sunlight. Do not freeze.
- Do not use this medicine if the color changes, if it becomes cloudy, or if there are particles in the solutions.

Storage/Stability

Because this medication must be compounded, storage recommendations can vary; follow storage requirements listed on the packaging, away from moisture and sunlight. Do not freeze.

Compatibility/Compounding Considerations

Nalbuphine ophthalmic preparations should not be mixed directly with any other ophthalmic medications. Nalbuphine is not commercially available and must be compounded by a qualified compounding pharmacist.

Dosage Forms/Regulatory Status

VETERINARY-LABELED PRODUCTS: NONE

HUMAN-LABELED PRODUCTS: NONE

Nalbuphine is not commercially available as an ophthalmic preparation but may be compounded by qualified compounding pharmacists into 0.8% to 1.2% ophthalmic solution.

References

For the complete list of references, see **wiley.com/go/budde/plumb**

Natamycin Ophthalmic

(nat-uh-***mye***-sin) *Natacyn®*

Polyene Antifungal

Prescriber Highlights

- ▶ Commercially available ophthalmic suspension used to treat fungal keratitis, primarily associated with *Fusarium* spp
- ▶ Poorly soluble and does not efficiently penetrate corneal epithelium following topical administration
- ▶ Well tolerated following topical administration
- ▶ Natamycin suspensions may block subpalpebral lavage (SPL) catheters; therefore, ensure catheter patency by flushing the line with air after each dose.
- ▶ Expensive

Uses/Indications

Natamycin is primarily used to treat equine fungal keratitis caused by *Fusarium* spp. As natamycin is not as effective for deep stromal lesions, efficacy may be enhanced by creation of superficial ulceration (ie, therapeutic penetrating keratoplasty) to increase transcorneal penetration.[1]

Pharmacology/Actions

Natamycin is a tetraene polyene antibiotic derived from *Streptomyces natalensis*. It possesses in vitro activity against various yeasts and filamentous fungi, including *Candida* spp, *Aspergillus* spp, *Cephalosporium* spp, *Fusarium* spp, and *Penicillium* spp; culture and susceptibility testing is recommended to ensure appropriate therapy.[2–4] The mechanism of action appears to be through binding to the sterol moiety of the fungal cell membrane, thus altering membrane permeability and allowing leakage of essential fungal intracellular constituents. Although the activity against fungi is dose-related, natamycin is predominantly fungicidal.

Contraindications/Precautions/Warnings

Natamycin is contraindicated in patients that have a history of hypersensitivity to it or any component of the formulation.[5]

Adverse Effects

Adverse effects reported in humans or animals include corneal opacity, eye discomfort, eye edema, eye hyperemia, foreign body sensation, paresthesia, and tearing.[5] Allergic reactions, dyspnea, and chest pain have been reported in humans that were administered natamycin.

Dosages

Equine fungal keratitis (extra-label): 0.1 mL to the affected eye(s) every 2 to 6 hours, depending upon the severity of infection (can be used more frequently initially). If administering via subpalpebral lavage (SPL) catheter, maintain catheter patency by flushing the line with air after each dose.

Monitoring

- Corneal scrapings with cytology and culture and susceptibility testing to determine the clearance of fungal organisms
- Resolution of clinical signs of infection

Client Information

- Give this medicine to your animal as directed by your veterinarian.
- Use proper administration techniques to avoid contamination of the medication. Keep the cap tightly closed when the medication is not in use.

- Shake the medication well before using.
- Wait 5 minutes after applying this medication before applying any other medications to the eye.
- Store this medication at room temperature away from moisture and sunlight; do not freeze.
- Avoid exposure to light and excessive heat.
- Do not use this medication if the color changes.

Storage/Stability

Store this medication at 2°C to 24°C (36°F-75°F) away from moisture and sunlight (dispensed in a brown bottle to minimize exposure to light); do not freeze.[5]

Compatibility/Compounding Considerations

Natamycin should not be mixed directly (in vitro) with any other drugs.

Dosage Forms/Regulatory Status

VETERINARY-LABELED PRODUCTS: NONE

HUMAN-LABELED PRODUCTS:

Natamycin 5% Ophthalmic Suspension (containing natamycin 50 mg/mL, benzalkonium chloride 0.02%, NaOH and/or HCl to adjust the pH to 5 to 7.5, and purified water), in a 15 mL amber glass dropper bottle; *Natacyn*®; (Rx)

References

For the complete list of references, see **wiley.com/go/budde/plumb**

Nedocromil Ophthalmic

(ne-doe-***krow***-mill) *Alocril*®

Mast Cell Stabilizing Ophthalmic Agent

Prescriber Highlights

- ► Topical mast cell stabilizer used to treat allergic conjunctivitis

Uses/Indications

Nedocromil may be used for the treatment of ocular itching associated with allergic conjunctivitis. The efficacy of nedocromil in animals following topical ocular administration has not been evaluated.

Pharmacology/Actions

Nedocromil is a mast cell stabilizer and inhibits histamine release from mast cells. Decreased chemotaxis and decreased activation of eosinophils (anti-inflammatory effects) have also been demonstrated following administration of nedocromil.[1]

Contraindications/Precautions/Warnings

Nedocromil is contraindicated in patients that have a history of hypersensitivity to it or any component of the formulation.

Adverse Effects

Adverse effects reported in humans include ocular burning, irritation and stinging, unpleasant taste, and nasal congestion. Approximately 40% of humans report headaches and a bad taste in their mouths after use.[2] Other less common adverse effects associated with nedocromil administration include asthma, conjunctivitis, eye redness, photophobia, and rhinitis.

Dosages

Allergic conjunctivitis (extra-label): 1 drop in the affected eye(s) twice daily. Treatment should be continued throughout exposure (ie, until exposure to the offending allergen is terminated), even when clinical signs are absent.

Monitoring

- Clinical efficacy: resolution of signs of allergic conjunctivitis

Client Information

- Use this medicine as directed by your veterinarian.
- Use proper administration techniques to avoid contamination of the medicine. Keep the cap tightly closed when the medicine is not in use.
- Wait for 5 minutes after applying this medicine before applying any other medicines to the eye.
- Store this medicine in the refrigerator or at room temperature away from moisture and sunlight. Do not freeze.
- Do not use this medicine if the color changes, if it becomes cloudy, or if there are particles in the solution.

Storage/Stability

Store this product in the refrigerator (2°C-8°C [35.6°F-46.4°F]) or at controlled room temperature (20°C-25°C [68°F-77°F])[2] away from moisture and sunlight; do not freeze.

Compatibility/Compounding Considerations

Nedocromil ophthalmic preparations should not be mixed directly with any other ophthalmic medications.

Dosage Forms/Regulatory Status

VETERINARY-LABELED PRODUCTS: NONE

HUMAN-LABELED PRODUCTS:

Nedocromil 2% Ophthalmic Solution (containing nedocromil 20 mg/mL; benzalkonium chloride 0.01%; edetate disodium 0.05%; purified water; NaCl 0.5%, buffered to a pH of 4 to 5.54 with an osmolality range of 270 – 330 mOsm/kg), in a 5 mL ophthalmic dropper bottle; *Alocril*®, generic; (Rx)

References

For the complete list of references, see **wiley.com/go/budde/plumb**

Nepafenac Ophthalmic

(ne-***paf***-en-ak) *Nevanac*®, *Ilevro*®

Nonsteroidal Anti-Inflammatory Drug (NSAID)

Prescriber Highlights

- ► Used to control anterior segment inflammation, particularly in association with surgical removal of cataracts
- ► Prodrug to amfenac, which is bioavailable to the posterior segment
- ► May increase risk for intraocular bleeding, inhibit corneal wound healing, and promote corneal melting

Uses/Indications

Nepafenac is used to decrease inflammation following cataract surgery. It may also be used to control other anterior segment inflammatory conditions (eg, conjunctivitis, keratitis, anterior uveitis).[1] Studies evaluating efficacy in veterinary patients have not been performed.

Pharmacology/Actions

Nepafenac is an NSAID and analgesic prodrug. After topical ocular dosing, nepafenac penetrates the cornea, where it is converted by ocular tissue hydrolases to amfenac, which inhibits the action of prostaglandin H synthase (cyclooxygenase), an enzyme required for prostaglandin production. Prostaglandins mediate many of the adverse effects of intraocular inflammation, including disruption of the blood-aqueous humor barrier, vasodilation, increased vascular permeability, leukocytosis, and alterations in intraocular pressure (IOP). Blocking prostaglandin production, therefore, minimizes the adverse short- and long-term effects of intraocular inflammation.

Contraindications/Precautions/Warnings

Nepafenac is contraindicated in patients that have a history of hypersensitivity to it or any component of the formulation or other NSAIDs. Caution should be employed when using nepafenac in patients that have previously exhibited sensitivity to other NSAID drugs, as there is potential for cross-sensitivity. Nepafenac has been associated with increased bleeding of ocular tissues (including hyphema) in conjunction with ocular surgery due to interference with platelet aggregation. All topical NSAIDs may slow or delay epithelial wound healing. Concomitant use with topical steroidal agents may increase the potential for delayed healing. Nepafenac should be used cautiously in patients receiving systemic anticoagulants (eg, aspirin, clopidogrel, warfarin, and heparin), as concomitant use may increase the risk for intraocular bleeding. Use of topical NSAIDs may result in keratitis due to epithelial breakdown, corneal thinning, corneal erosion, corneal ulceration, or corneal perforation. It should be discontinued immediately in patients exhibiting evidence of corneal epithelial breakdown.

Postmarketing experience with topical NSAIDs suggests that use more than 24 hours before surgery or beyond 14 days after surgery may increase patient risk for the occurrence of corneal adverse effects.[2]

Adverse Effects

Adverse effects reported in humans or animals include capsular opacity, decreased visual acuity, foreign body sensation, increased intraocular pressure (IOP), and sticky sensation.[2] Other ocular adverse effects include conjunctival edema, corneal edema, dry eye, lid margin crusting, ocular discomfort, ocular hyperemia, ocular pain, ocular pruritus, photophobia, tearing, and vitreous detachment. Some of these effects may be the consequence of the cataract surgical procedure.[3] Nonocular adverse effects reported by humans include headache, hypertension, nausea, vomiting, and sinusitis.[2] Increased bleeding time, delayed corneal wound healing, keratitis, and corneal weakening have also been reported.

Although unlikely, systemic adverse effects may occur with the use of topical NSAIDs, including increased risk for gastric ulceration, decreased platelet aggregation, worsening of asthma and cardiac disease, and renal toxicity. Concurrent use of systemic NSAIDs and corticosteroids increases the risk for systemic adverse effects.

Dosages

Perioperative for cataract surgery (extra-label): 1 drop in the affected eye(s) 1 to 3 times daily for up to 2 weeks following cataract surgery

Anterior segment inflammation (extra-label): 1 drop in the affected eye(s) every 8 hours

Monitoring

- Clinical efficacy: decreased or absent inflammation. Monitor for delayed wound healing

Client Information

- Use this medicine as directed by your veterinarian.
- Shake this medicine well before using.
- Use proper administration techniques to avoid contamination of the medication. Keep the cap tightly closed when the medication is not in use.
- Wait for 5 minutes after applying this medication before applying any other medications to the eye.
- Store in the refrigerator or at room temperature away from moisture and sunlight. Do not freeze.
- Do not use this medicine if the color changes.

Storage/Stability

Store in the refrigerator (2°C-8°C [35.6°F-46.4°F]) or controlled room temperature (20°C-25°C [68°F-77°F])[2] away from moisture and sunlight; do not freeze.

Compatibility/Compounding Considerations

Nepafenac ophthalmic preparations should not be mixed directly with any other ophthalmic medications.

Dosage Forms/Regulatory Status

VETERINARY-LABELED PRODUCTS: NONE

HUMAN-LABELED PRODUCTS:

Nepafenac 0.1% Ophthalmic Solution (containing nepafenac 1 mg/mL; mannitol; carbomer 974P; NaCl; tyloxapol; edetate disodium; benzalkonium chloride 0.005%; NaOH and/or HCl to adjust pH to 7.4; purified water, USP, with an osmolality of 305 mOsm/kg), 3 mL in a sterile 4 mL ophthalmic dropper bottle; *Nevanac*®; (Rx)

Nepafenac 0.3% Ophthalmic Suspension (containing nepafenac 0.3%; boric acid, propylene glycol; carbomer 974P; NaCl; guar gum; carboxymethylcellulose sodium; edetate disodium; benzalkonium chloride 0.005%; NaOH and/or HCl to adjust pH; purified water, USP), 1.7 mL in a sterile 4 mL ophthalmic dropper bottle, or 3 mL in a sterile 4 mL ophthalmic dropper bottle; *Ilevro*®; (Rx)

References

For the complete list of references, see **wiley.com/go/budde/plumb**

Ocular Lubricants

Tear Replacement and Ocular Lubricating Agents

Prescriber Highlights

- Used in the temporary enhancement of the quality and quantity of precorneal tear film
- Hyaluronate/hyaluronic acid-containing preparations may exert a beneficial effect on corneal ulcer healing.
- Most artificial tears and ocular lubricants are labeled for humans and are available OTC.
- Preservative-free solutions are less likely to cause stinging or corneal damage with long-term use.
- Petroleum-based ocular products should not be used in procedures where combustion may occur (eg, electrocautery, laser) or when contact with the intraocular environment is possible (eg, penetrating corneal wound).
- Basic components of an artificial tear/ocular lubricant include demulcent (soothing agent), emollient (a fat-based agent that softens and protects tissues), inactive ingredients (impact viscosity, tonicity, and pH), and preservatives (to prevent bacterial growth).

Uses/Indications

Artificial tear solutions and ocular lubricants are used when there is a decrease in tear production, an increase in tear loss through evaporation, and a decrease in the tear film's break up time, such as in the presence of qualitative and quantitative keratoconjunctivitis sicca (KCS)[1], buphthalmos (enlarged globe that adversely affects the ability to blink), or lagophthalmos (inability to blink due to the conformational or functional abnormality of the eyelid). Ocular lubricants are also beneficial during sedation and anesthesia to prevent corneal desiccation[2] and as a vehicle for compounding water-soluble medications for ocular application. Although the evidence is variable, preparations containing hyaluronic acid/sodium hyaluronate may accelerate the healing of corneal ulcers.[3,4]

Pharmacology/Actions

Improving the quality (eg, viscosity, osmolarity, retention time) of the precorneal tear film results in improvement in comfort for patients with tear film deficiencies, as well as reduction in ocular surface inflammation and damage. Preparations include a demulcent that acts as a soothing and anti-inflammatory agent, an emollient to protect tissues and prevent drying, inactive ingredients to stabilize the preparation for ocular administration, and preservatives to prevent contamination.[5]

Demulcents may include polyethylene glycol (PEG), propylene glycol (PG), glycerin, cellulose derivatives, hydroxymethylcellulose (HMC), hydroxypropylcellulose (HPC), hydroxypropylmethylcellulose (HPMC), and polyvinyl alcohol (PVA). Although each demulcent varies slightly in a specific function, broadly, they are all responsible for increasing viscosity of the preparation, decreasing viscosity and osmolarity of the tear film, protecting mucous membranes, relieving inflammation, and improving the stability of the tear film.[6]

Emollients may include lanolin, mineral oil, petrolatum, paraffin, and wax. Although each emollient varies slightly in a specific function, broadly, they are all responsible for lubrication and soothing, stabilizing the lipid layer of the tear film, and sealing in moisture.[6]

Inactive ingredients may include sorbitol, hyaluronic acid (HA), sodium hyaluronate, L-carnitine and erythritol, hydroxypropyl guar, polyacrylic acid, tyloxapol, and tromethamine. Although each inactive ingredient varies slightly in a specific function, they are responsible for lowering the osmolarity of the tear film, stabilizing the viscosity of the tear film, prolonging contact time of active ingredients, promoting appropriate corneal epithelial metabolism, and maintaining hydration.[6]

Preservatives may include benzalkonium chloride, polyquad, sodium perborate, stabilized oxychloro complex, edetate disodium, and chlorobutanol. Although each preservative varies in a specific function, broadly, they are responsible for decreasing bacterial contamination of the preparation, increasing drug penetration, and increasing shelf life.[6] Some preservatives (eg, benzalkonium chloride) are known ocular irritants and cause destabilization of the tear film, which is beneficial in some conditions to allow for improved penetration of active ingredients. Although this action may be beneficial for some ocular conditions (eg, glaucoma), the resulting epithelial cell damage can be harmful in ocular surface diseases (eg, corneal ulceration). Thus, preservatives have been developed that are stable in solution but degrade upon contact to minimize ocular surface damage.

The combination of demulcent and emollient, as well as other inactive ingredients and preservatives, decreases friction on the ocular surface and increases tear retention and tear film moisture while minimally impacting ocular clarity.

Contraindications/Precautions/Warnings

Artificial tear solutions are contraindicated in patients that have a history of hypersensitivity to any component of the formulation. Interactions between topical ocular lubricants and other ocular preparations may occur, leading to alterations in viscosity of the lubricant, decreased efficacy in stabilizing the precorneal tear film, precipitate formation, or patient irritation or discomfort.

Adverse Effects

Adverse effects reported in animals include eye pain, burning or stinging on instillation, and redness. Preservative-free solutions may decrease these adverse effects. Blurred vision is commonly reported in humans after the application of ocular ointments; thus, many OTC preparations are formulated as solutions with varied demulcent and emollient proportions. Sticky eyelashes and increased sensitivity to light are commonly reported by humans using solutions containing hydroxypropyl cellulose.

Dosages

Tear replacement (extra-label): 1 drop or a ¼ – ½ inch strip to the affected eye(s) every 2 to 3 hours or as often as possible

Ocular lubrication during anesthetic procedures (extra-label): ½ – 1 inch strip to each eye every 90 minutes. Do not use in procedures where the combustion of petroleum-based ocular lubricants or contact of the lubricant with the intraocular environment may occur.

Monitoring

- Clinical efficacy
- Monitor corneal surface for signs of damage, as chronic use of preserved solutions may cause corneal damage.

Client Information

- Place these drops in your animal's eye(s) as often as possible during the day. Administer longer-acting ointments at bedtime.
- If you notice any increase in squinting, eye discharge, or ocular redness, discontinue use and contact your veterinarian.
- Use proper administration techniques to avoid contamination of the medication. To prevent contamination, do not touch the dropper tip (or ointment) or allow it to touch your animal's eye or any other surface.
- Keep the cap tightly closed when the medicine is not in use.
- If applying multiple medications to your animal's eye(s), apply lubricating medications last, at least 5 minutes following administration of other eye medications.
- Store this medicine at room temperature away from moisture and sunlight. Do not freeze.
- Do not use this medicine if the color changes, if the solution becomes cloudy, or if there are particles in the solution.

Storage/Stability

Store at controlled room temperature (20°C-25°C [68°F-77°F]) away from moisture and sunlight.

Compatibility/Compounding Considerations

Artificial tears and ocular lubricants are often used as vehicles when compounding topical ocular medications. Check to ensure compatibility of all ingredients and preservatives before compounding.

Dosage Forms/Regulatory Status

VETERINARY-LABELED PRODUCTS:

None are FDA-approved.

Hyaluronic Acid-Containing Products

Active ingredients (formulation)	Label status; size(s)	Trade names/additional information
water for injection; sodium chloride; 0.25% viscoadaptive hyaluronan; glycerin; sodium phosphate; potassium sorbate; EDTA	OTC; 10 mL in a sterile ophthalmic dropper bottle	*I-Drop® Vet Plus Lubricant* **NOTE**: There is also a 0.3% gel, *I-Drop® Vet Gel.*
sterile water; sorbitol; carbomer; sodium hydroxide; disodium EDTA; cetrimide	OTC; 0.7 oz tube	*OptixCare® Eye Lube*
sterile water; sorbitol; carbomer; hyaluron; sodium hydroxide; disodium EDTA; cetrimide	OTC; 0.7 oz tube	*OptixCare® Eye Lube Plus*
water; 0.4% Hyasent-S (modified, cross-linked HA); sodium chloride; disodium; phosphate; potassium chloride; potassium phosphate	Rx; 10 mL in a sterile ophthalmic dropper bottle	*Remend® Eye Lubricating Drops* **NOTE**: There is also a 0.75% gel that is marketed as a corneal repair gel for superficial corneal ulcers: *Remend®* Corneal Repair Gel.

HUMAN-LABELED PRODUCTS:

There are many products marketed, and this list is not comprehensive:

Polyvinyl Alcohol-Containing Products

Active ingredients (formulation)	Label status; size(s)	Trade names/additional information
polyvinyl alcohol 1%; polyethylene glycol 400 1%; benzalkonium chloride 0.1 mg/mL; dextrose; edetate disodium; purified water; HCl and/or NaOH to adjust pH	OTC; 15 mL in a sterile ophthalmic dropper bottle	*HypoTears®*
polyvinyl alcohol 0.5%; povidone 0.6%; benzalkonium chloride; dextrose; edetate disodium; potassium chloride; purified water; sodium bicarbonate; sodium chloride; sodium citrate; sodium phosphate (mono- and dibasic)	OTC; 15 mL in a sterile ophthalmic dropper bottle	*Murine Tears®*

Polyvinylpyrrolidone-Containing Products

Active ingredients (formulation)	Label status; size(s)	Trade names/additional information
polyvinyl pyrrolidone 2%; polyvinyl alcohol 2.7%; boric acid; disodium edetate dihydrate; ethanol; glycerin; lecithin; polixetonium; polysorbate-80; potassium chloride; purified water; sodium chloride	OTC; 15 mL in a sterile ophthalmic dropper bottle	*Freshkote®*

Carboxymethylcellulose-Containing Products

Active ingredients (formulation)	Label status; size(s)	Trade names/additional information
sodium carboxymethylcellulose 1%; borate buffers; calcium chloride; magnesium chloride; potassium chloride; purified water; sodium bicarbonate; NaCl; sodium phosphate	OTC; 0.6 mL single-use vials	*TheraTears® Liquid Gel*
sodium carboxymethylcellulose 0.25%; borate buffers; calcium chloride; *Dequest®*; potassium chloride; purified water; sodium bicarbonate; sodium borate; sodium chloride; magnesium chloride; sodium perborate; sodium phosphate; trehalose	OTC; 15 mL in a sterile ophthalmic dropper bottle	*TheraTears® Lubricant Eye Drops*

Hydroxypropyl Methylcellulose-Containing Products

Active ingredients (formulation)	Label status; size(s)	Trade names/additional information
dextran 70 0.1%; hydroxypropyl methylcellulose 2910 0.3%; calcium chloride; magnesium chloride; potassium chloride; purified water; sodium bicarbonate; NaCl; zinc chloride; HCl and/or NaOH and/or carbon dioxide to adjust pH	OTC; 0.4 mL single-use containers in cartons of 28	*Bion Tears®*
dextran 70 0.1%; glycerin 0.2%; hypromellose 0.3%; boric acid; calcium chloride; glycine; HCl and/or NaOH to adjust pH; magnesium chloride; POLYQUAD (polyquaternium-1) 0.002% preservative; polysorbate 80; potassium chloride; purified water; sodium chloride; zinc chloride	OTC; 15 mL in a sterile ophthalmic dropper bottle	*Genteal® Moderate Lubricating Liquid* **NOTE**: Many other *Genteal®* formulations exist.
glycerin 0.2%; hydroxypropyl methylcellulose 0.2%; polyethylene glycol 400 1%; ascorbic acid; benzalkonium chloride; boric acid; dextrose; disodium phosphate; glycine; magnesium chloride; potassium chloride; purified water; sodium borate; sodium chloride; sodium citrate; sodium lactate	OTC; in a sterile 15 mL or 30 mL ophthalmic dropper bottle	*Visine Tears® Dry Eye Relief* **NOTE**: Many other *Visine®* formulations exist.

Hydroxypropyl Guar-Containing Products

Active ingredients (formulation)	Label status; size(s)	Trade names/additional information
hydroxypropyl methylcellulose 0.3%; carbopol 980; phosphonic acid; purified water; sodium perborate; sorbitol	OTC; 10 g in sterile ophthalmic dropper bottles	*Systane® Lubricant Eye Gel* **NOTE**: Many other *Systane®* formulations exist.

Polyethylene Glycol/Hyaluronate-Containing Products

Active ingredients (formulation)	Label status; size(s)	Trade names/additional information
polyethylene glycol 400 0.25%; boric acid; calcium chloride; magnesium chloride; potassium chloride; purified water; sodium borate; sodium chloride; sodium chlorite (*Ocupure*® brand); sodium hyaluronate	OTC; 15 mL in a sterile ophthalmic dropper bottle	*Blink*® *Gel Tears* NOTE: Many other *Blink*® formulations exist.

Petroleum-Based Products

Active ingredients (formulation)	Label status; size(s)	Trade names/additional information
mineral oil 15%; white petrolatum 85%	OTC; 3.5 g ophthalmic ointment tube	*Genteal*® *Night-Time Ointment*
light mineral oil 1%; mineral oil 4.5%	OTC; 15 mL ophthalmic dropper bottle	*Soothe XP*®
mineral oil 20%; white petrolatum 80%	OTC; 3.5 g ophthalmic ointment tube	*Tears Again*®

References

For the complete list of references, see **wiley.com/go/budde/plumb**

Ofloxacin Ophthalmic

(o-***flocks***-uh-sin) *Ocuflox*®

Second-Generation Fluoroquinolone Antimicrobial

Prescriber Highlights

- Used to treat bacterial conjunctivitis or keratitis
- Physically incompatible with many drugs; therefore, it should not be directly mixed with other ophthalmic medications.
- Crystalline drug precipitates may be noted in the superficial portion of corneal defects during use.

Uses/Indications

Ofloxacin ophthalmic may be used for the treatment of bacterial conjunctivitis or keratitis caused by susceptible strains of *Staphylococcus* spp, *Streptococcus* spp, *Pseudomonas aeruginosa*, *Chlamydophila* spp, and *Haemophilus* spp.[1] Ofloxacin achieves greater aqueous humor concentrations than ciprofloxacin following topical administration to dogs.[2] In the UK, horses with bacterial keratitis did not demonstrate increased resistance to ofloxacin.[3]

The World Health Organization (WHO) has designated fluoroquinolones as a Critically Important, Highest Priority antimicrobial in human medicine.[4]

Pharmacology/Actions

Ofloxacin is a bactericidal and concentration-dependent fluoroquinolone antibiotic that is believed to act by inhibiting bacterial DNA-gyrase (a type-II topoisomerase), thereby preventing DNA supercoiling and DNA synthesis. The activity of ofloxacin is greater against gram-negative organisms than gram-positive organisms. *Staphylococcus* spp demonstrates lower susceptibility to second-generation fluoroquinolones than most other gram-positive agents.[1]

Contraindications/Precautions/Warnings

Ofloxacin is contraindicated in patients that have a history of hypersensitivity to ofloxacin, to other fluoroquinolones, or to any of the components of this medication. Ofloxacin should only be used as a topical ophthalmic. Do not inject ofloxacin subconjunctivally or into the anterior chamber of the eye. Fluoroquinolone-induced retinal toxicity in domestic cats has not been demonstrated with this product.

Adverse Effects

Adverse effects reported in humans or animals include blurred vision, tearing, eye pain, redness, and itching.[5] Crystalline drug precipitates may be noted in the superficial portion of corneal defects during use. The arthropathy that occurs in immature animals associated with oral administration of quinolones has not been noted following topical ophthalmic administration.[5] Alterations in ocular surface microflora, with the increased population of resistant organisms, have been documented in dogs during 6 weeks of topical ofloxacin therapy following cataract surgery.[6]

Dosages

Conjunctivitis (extra-label): 1 drop in the affected eye(s) every 2 to 8 hours

Keratitis (extra-label): 1 drop in the affected eye(s), or 0.1 mL in the subpalpebral lavage (SPL) catheter, every 2 to 8 hours. It may precipitate when mixed with other ophthalmic medications; therefore, it is important to flush the SPL catheter well with air between medications.

Monitoring

- Corneal cytology and culture to evaluate for the persistence of bacteria
- Evaluation for clinical signs suggestive of continued infection

Client Information

- Use this medication as directed by your veterinarian.
- Use proper administration techniques to avoid contamination of the medication. Do not touch the dropper tip or allow it to touch your animal's eye or any other surface to prevent contamination.
- Crystals may appear on the ocular surface after initiation of treatment with ofloxacin.
- Wait 5 minutes after applying this medication before applying any other medications to the eye.
- Keep the cap tightly closed when the medication is not in use. Store this medication in the refrigerator or at room temperature away from moisture and sunlight. Do not freeze.
- Do not use this medication if the color changes, if it becomes cloudy, or if there are particles in the solution.

Storage/Stability

Store this medication in the refrigerator (2°C-8°C [35.6°F-46.4°F]) or at controlled room temperature (20°C-25°C [68°F-77°F]) away from moisture and sunlight; do not freeze.[5]

Compatibility/Compounding Considerations

Fluoroquinolone antibiotics interact with many other drugs, including those containing cations (eg, iron, aluminum, magnesium, or calcium). Ofloxacin should not be mixed directly (in vitro) with any other drugs.

Dosage Forms/Regulatory Status

VETERINARY-LABELED PRODUCTS: NONE

HUMAN-LABELED PRODUCTS:

Ofloxacin 0.3% Ophthalmic Solution (containing ofloxacin 3 mg/mL; benzalkonium chloride 0.005%; NaCl; HCl and/or NaOH to adjust pH to a range of 6 to 6.8; purified water; with an osmolality of 300 mOsm/kg), in a 5 mL and 10 mL ophthalmic dropper bottle; *Ocuflox*®, generic; (Rx)

References

For the complete list of references, see **wiley.com/go/budde/plumb**

Olopatadine Ophthalmic

(o-la-***pat***-a-deen) *Pataday*®, *Patanol*®, *Pazeo*®

H_1 and H_2 Receptor Antagonist Antihistamine Agent

Prescriber Highlights

- Used to relieve pruritus caused by allergic conjunctivitis
- Longer duration of action allows once- to twice-daily dosing

Uses/Indications

Olopatadine ophthalmic is used to relieve pruritus caused by allergic conjunctivitis. Evaluation of olopatadine's clinical efficacy in veterinary species has not been performed.

Pharmacology/Actions

Olopatadine is a selective, noncompetitive H_1 and H_2 receptor antagonist and a mast cell stabilizer. It is also an inhibitor of proinflammatory mediators such as leukotrienes and thromboxane.[1]

Contraindications/Precautions/Warnings

Olopatadine is contraindicated in patients that have a history of hypersensitivity to it or any component of the formulation.

Adverse Effects

Adverse effects reported in humans include transient burning or stinging on instillation in the eye, although instillation was more comfortable compared with other ophthalmic antihistamines.[1]

Dosages

Allergic conjunctivitis (extra-label): 1 drop in the affected eye(s) once daily (*Pataday*®, *Pazeo*®) or twice daily (*Pataday*®, *Patanol*®)

Monitoring

- Clinical efficacy: resolution of pruritus and conjunctivitis

Client Information

- Use this medicine as directed by your veterinarian.
- Use proper administration techniques to avoid contamination of the medication. Keep the cap tightly closed when the medicine is not in use.
- Wait 5 minutes after applying this medicine before applying any other medicines to the eye.
- Store this medicine in refrigerator or at room temperature away from moisture and sunlight. Do not freeze.
- Do not use this medicine if the color changes, if it becomes cloudy, or if there are particles in the solutions.

Storage/Stability

Store this product in the refrigerator (2°C-8°C [35.6°F-46.4°F]) or at controlled room temperature (20°C-25°C [68°F-77°F]) away from moisture and sunlight; do not freeze.

Compatibility/Compounding Considerations

Olopatadine ophthalmic preparations should not be mixed directly with any other ophthalmic medications.

Dosage Forms/Regulatory Status

VETERINARY-LABELED PRODUCTS: NONE

HUMAN-LABELED PRODUCTS:

Olopatadine 0.1% Ophthalmic Solution (containing 1.11 mg olopatadine HCl equivalent to 1 mg olopatadine per mL; povidone; dibasic sodium phosphate; NaCl; edentate disodium; benzalkonium chloride 0.01%; HCl/NaOH to adjust pH to ≈7; purified water, with an osmolality of ≈300 mOsm/kg), in 2.5 mL ophthalmic dropper bottles; *Pataday*®, *Patanol*®; generic; (Rx)

Olopatadine 0.2% Ophthalmic Solution (containing 2.22 mg olopatadine HCl equivalent to 2 mg olopatadine per mL; povidone; dibasic sodium phosphate; NaCl; edentate disodium; benzalkonium chloride 0.01%; HCl/NaOH to adjust pH to ≈7; purified water, with an osmolality of ≈300 mOsm/kg), in 2.5 mL ophthalmic dropper bottles; *Pataday*®; generic; (Rx)

Olopatadine 0.7% Ophthalmic Solution (containing 7.76 mg olopatadine HCl equivalent to 7 mg olopatadine per mL; povidone; hydroxypropyl-gamma-cyclodextrin; polyethylene glycol 400; hydroxypropyl methylcellulose; boric acid; mannitol; benzalkonium chloride 0.015%; HCl/NaOH to adjust pH; purified water), in 2.5 mL ophthalmic dropper bottles; *Pataday*®, *Pazeo*®; generic; (Rx)

References

For the complete list of references, see **wiley.com/go/budde/plumb**

Oxytetracycline/Polymyxin B Ophthalmic

(ocks-ih-***tet***-rih-sye-kleen/pol-lee-***mix***-in) *Terramycin*®

Combination Antibiotic

For information related to systemic use, see ***Oxytetracycline*** *and* ***Polymyxin B***

Prescriber Highlights

- Used to treat superficial ocular bacterial infections in dogs, cats, horses, cattle, and sheep
- Frequently effective for treating *Chlamydia* spp and *Mycoplasma* spp conjunctivitis in cats
- *Chlamydia* spp infections should be treated for 3 to 4 weeks beyond resolution of clinical signs to disrupt *Chlamydia* spp reproductive cycle.
- Some cats experience local irritation or more severe anaphylactic reactions that necessitate discontinuation of treatment.
- Used to decrease keratomalacia induced by matrix metalloproteinases in response to corneal infections
- May accelerate corneal epithelial wound healing in dogs

Uses/Indications

Oxytetracycline/Polymyxin B is used to prevent or treat superficial ocular infections involving the conjunctiva and/or cornea caused by gram-positive, gram-negative, and intracellular bacteria. It is commonly used to treat known or suspected *Chlamydia* spp and *Mycoplasma* conjunctivitis in cats.

Following a single dose of topical oxytetracycline/polymyxin B administered to normal canine eyes, tear film concentrations surpass MICs for common ocular pathogens.[1] Topical tetracyclines have variable effects on the rate of corneal epithelial wound healing in dogs without bacterial ocular surface infections.[2,3] Topical tetracyclines are useful in decreasing keratomalacia occurring due to bacterial infections of corneal ulcers[4]; however, the twice-daily dosing advised by the manufacturer may not be sufficient to achieve sustained collagenolytic activity within the tear film of normal canine eyes.[1]

Pharmacology/Actions

The reversible binding of tetracyclines to the 30S ribosomal subunits of susceptible organisms inhibits the binding of the tRNA and its associated amino acid to the mRNA-ribosome complex, which disrupts protein synthesis. Tetracyclines demonstrate good activity against *Rickettsia* spp, *Borrelia* spp, *Chlamydia* spp, *Mycoplasma* spp, *Moraxella* spp, and *Brucella* spp, with variable activity against *Staphylococcus* spp and *Streptococcus* spp. Tetracyclines are not effective against *Pseudomonas* spp.

The increased healing rate of uninfected corneal ulcers in dogs treated with topical tetracyclines is thought to be due to upregulation of transforming growth factor-beta.[2] Oxytetracycline is also a potent inhibitor of matrix metalloproteinase-9 and a moderate inhibitor of matrix metalloproteinase-2. The reduction of keratomalacia occurring in infected corneal ulcers is due to inhibition of matrix metalloproteinases (MMP), which is induced by tetracyclines binding calcium and zinc (cofactors necessary for MMP activity).[5]

Polymyxin B sulfate, one of a group of related antibiotics derived from *Bacillus polymyxa*, is rapidly bactericidal. This action is exclusively effective against gram-negative organisms, particularly *Pseudomonas aeruginosa*.[6] Polymyxin B sulfate interacts with the lipopolysaccharide of the cytoplasmic outer membrane of gram-negative bacteria, altering membrane permeability and causing cell death; it does not need to enter the cell. Polymyxin B sulfate has a bactericidal action against almost all gram-negative bacilli except the Proteus group. It is ineffective against gram-positive bacteria, gram-negative cocci, or obligate anaerobes. It lacks activity against viral, fungal, or parasitic pathogens. Pus and cellular debris reduce effectiveness.

Contraindications/Precautions/Warnings

Oxytetracycline and polymyxin are contraindicated in patients that have a history of hypersensitivity to either drug, drugs in the same class, or any component of the formulation.

Adverse Effects

Adverse effects reported in humans or animals are rare. Oxytetracycline with polymyxin B sulfate is well tolerated by the epithelial membranes and other tissues of the eye. Allergic or inflammatory reactions due to individual hypersensitivity are rare; however, some cats may have an anaphylactic reaction to the polymyxin B component.[6,7]

Dosages

Conjunctivitis, keratitis (label dosage; FDA approved): ¼ inch strip in the affected eye(s) 2 to 4 times daily[6]

Monitoring

- Clinical efficacy
- Resolution of conjunctivitis or keratitis

Client Information

- Use this medication as directed by your veterinarian.
- Use proper administration techniques to avoid contamination of the medication. Do not touch the dropper tip or allow it to touch your animal's eye or any other surface to prevent contamination.
- Wait 5 minutes after applying this medicine before applying any other medicine to your animal's eye(s).
- Crystals may appear on the surface of your animal's eye during treatment. This change is not harmful and will go away once treatment is complete.
- Keep the cap tightly closed when the medication is not in use. Store this medication at room temperature away from moisture and sunlight. Do not freeze.
- Do not use this medication if the color changes.

Storage/Stability

Store at controlled room temperature (20°C-25°C [68°F-77°F]), with excursions between 15°C to 30°C (59°F-86°F), away from moisture and sunlight; do not freeze.

Compatibility/Compounding Considerations

Oxytetracycline should not be mixed directly (in vitro) with any other drugs.

Dosage Forms/Regulatory Status

VETERINARY-LABELED PRODUCTS:

Oxytetracycline HCl and Polymyxin B Ophthalmic Ointment (containing oxytetracycline 5 mg/g; polymyxin B sulfate 10,000 units/g; white petrolatum; liquid petrolatum), in 3.5 g ointment tubes; *Terramycin*®; (Rx)

HUMAN-LABELED PRODUCTS: NONE

References

For the complete list of references, see **wiley.com/go/budde/plumb**

Phenylephrine Ophthalmic

(fen-il-*ef*-rin) *Cyclomydril*®

Alpha Agonist Vasoconstrictor

For systemic use, refer to ***Phenylephrine***

Prescriber Highlights

- ► Direct-acting sympathomimetic agent (alpha-1 agonist)
- ► Used to augment mydriasis, most commonly during intraocular surgical procedures and to limit bleeding during minor ocular surface procedures
- ► Not an effective mydriatic in cats or horses when used alone but may increase mydriatic effect when combined with atropine
- ► Used to differentiate second- from third-order Horner syndrome
- ► Local discomfort may occur after application.
- ► Cardiovascular adverse effects are more likely in small dogs and cats and following use of 10% concentrations.

Uses/Indications

Phenylephrine is most commonly used to induce mydriasis prior to phacoemulsification for cataract removal. It is also used prior to minor ocular surface procedures (eg, conjunctival biopsy) to limit bleeding. Phenylephrine is also used to distinguish second- from third-order lesions in Horner syndrome because of the phenomenon of denervation hypersensitivity. In dogs, maximal pupillary dilation occurs in 55 minutes[1]; however, phenylephrine alone does not lead to mydriasis in cats[2] and horses.[3]

Pharmacology/Actions

Phenylephrine is a direct alpha-1-adrenergic receptor agonist with potent local vasoconstrictor effects. Mydriatic effects are variable and are achieved through direct stimulation of the radial iris dilator muscle.

Contraindications/Precautions/Warnings

Phenylephrine is contraindicated in patients that have a history of hypersensitivity to it or any component of the formulation. Phenylephrine should be used cautiously in patients with thyrotoxicosis or hypertension, as adverse cardiovascular effects may occur.

Adverse Effects

Adverse effects reported in humans or animals include eye pain and stinging on instillation, temporary blurred vision and photophobia, and conjunctival sensitization. Cardiovascular effects following topical administration have been reported in dogs[3] and cats[4] due to systemic absorption, which may result in adverse cardiovascular effects (eg, marked increase in blood pressure, syncope, myocardial infarction, bradycardia, and ventricular and supraventricular arrhythmias) that could require therapeutic intervention.[4-6] The systemic effects can be severe and may require intervention. The effects of phenylephrine will be increased when it is administered after topical local anesthetic agents because of epithelial damage induced by topical local anesthetic agents. In normal dogs, phenylephrine leads to a statistically (but not necessarily clinically) significant increase in intraocular pressure (IOP) following topical administration.[1]

Dosages

Diagnosis of Horner syndrome (extra-label): 1 drop of phenylephrine 0.25% solution in each eye. Patients suffering from third-order Horner syndrome will experience mydriasis from this low concentration, whereas healthy patients will not. If there is no response in 20 to 30 minutes, apply 1 drop of a 2.5% solution to each eye. If mydriasis occurs, second-order Horner syndrome is likely.

Preoperative cataract removal (extra-label): 1 drop of phenylephrine 2.5% or 10% in the affected eye(s) as a single dose or every 15 minutes for 2 hours. Severe cardiovascular adverse effects are more likely with small dogs and cats and following use of the 10% solution, thus caution should be exercised both with the concentration and the frequency of administration. Effects are augmented when it is administered following topical anesthetic agents.

Monitoring

- Clinical efficacy
- Monitor degree of pupillary dilation
- Monitor bleeding after minor ocular surface surgical procedures
- Monitor heart rate and blood pressure

Client Information

- This medicine is rarely (if ever) indicated for administration to animals at home.
- Use proper administration techniques to avoid contamination of the medicine. Keep the cap tightly closed when the medicine is not in use.
- Wait 5 minutes after applying this medicine before applying any other medicines to the eye.
- Store this medicine as directed on package labeling away from moisture and sunlight; do not freeze.
- Do not use this medicine if the color changes, if it becomes cloudy, or if there are particles in the solution.

Storage/Stability

Store this product as directed on package labeling either in the refrigerator (2°C-8°C [35.6°F-46.4°F]) for 10% concentration or at controlled room temperature (20°C-25°C [68°F-77°F]) for 2.5% concentration; do not freeze.

Compatibility/Compounding Considerations

Phenylephrine ophthalmic preparations should not be mixed directly with any other ophthalmic medications.

Dosage Forms/Regulatory Status

VETERINARY-LABELED PRODUCTS: NONE

HUMAN-LABELED PRODUCTS:

Phenylephrine HCl 2.5% Ophthalmic Solution (containing phenylephrine hydrochloride 25 mg (2.5%); sodium phosphate monobasic; sodium phosphate dibasic; boric acid; water for injection; hydrochloric acid and/or sodium hydroxide (to adjust pH); benzalkonium chloride), in a sterile 15 mL ophthalmic dropper bottle; generic; (Rx)

Phenylephrine HCl 10% Ophthalmic Solution (containing phenylephrine hydrochloride 100 mg (10%); sodium phosphate monobasic; sodium phosphate dibasic; boric acid; water for injection; hydrochloric acid and/or sodium hydroxide (to adjust pH); benzalkonium chloride), in a sterile 10 mL ophthalmic dropper bottle; generic; (Rx)

Phenylephrine HCL 1% and Cyclopentolate HCl 0.2% Ophthalmic Solution (containing cyclopentolate hydrochloride 0.2%; phenylephrine hydrochloride 1%; benzalkonium chloride 0.01%; edetate disodium; boric acid; hydrochloric acid and/or sodium carbonate (to adjust pH); purified water), in sterile 5 mL ophthalmic dropper bottle; *Cyclomydril*®; (Rx)

References

For the complete list of references, see **wiley.com/go/budde/plumb**

Pilocarpine Ophthalmic

(***pye***-loe-***kar***-peen) *Isopto Carpine*®

Cholinergic Miotic Agent

Prescriber Highlights

- Primarily used to treat neurogenic keratoconjunctivitis sicca (KCS). It may also be used to treat primary glaucoma in dogs but has largely been replaced by other treatments.
- Contraindicated in cases of secondary glaucoma (eg, caused by uveitis or lens luxation) because of the risk for pupillary block
- Ophthalmic solution may be administered to the affected eye or be given orally on food as a treatment for neurogenic KCS.
- Monitor for ocular and systemic toxicity.

Uses/Indications

The primary use of pilocarpine in veterinary patients is for the treatment of neurogenic keratoconjunctivitis sicca (KCS), which is caused by interrupted neurologic signaling to the otherwise normal lacrimal glands. In dogs with coinciding xeromycteria (dryness of the nasal mucous membranes), pilocarpine also increases nasal secretions. Oral administration and topical ocular administration, alone or in combination, increases tear production in dogs.[1-3] Pilocarpine, administered topically to the eye, may also be used to diagnose parasympathetic denervation of the iris sphincter caused by lesions of or trauma to the oculomotor nerve (cranial nerve III). Pilocarpine may also be used topically to treat primary glaucoma in dogs,[4] but it has largely been replaced by beta-blockers, carbonic anhydrase inhibitors, and prostaglandin agents. Pilocarpine does not reduce intraocular pressure (IOP) in horses and is therefore not used to treat equine glaucoma.[5]

Pharmacology/Actions

Pilocarpine mimics acetylcholine and acts as a direct-acting cholinergic agonist at the neuromuscular junctions. In the eye, this cholinergic stimulation leads to lacrimal secretion, and can therefore be used to treat neurogenic keratoconjunctivitis sicca (KCS; ie, lacrimal gland tissue is normal, but innervation is interrupted). Cholinergic stimulation also leads to ciliary body muscle contraction, which places posteriorly directed tension on the base of the iris to mechanically pull open the iridocorneal angle, increasing aqueous humor outflow in dogs with elevated intraocular pressure (IOP).

Contraindications/Precautions/Warnings

Pilocarpine is contraindicated in patients that have a history of hypersensitivity to it or any component of the formulation. Avoid its use in dogs with glaucoma secondary to uveitis or lens luxation, as the induction of miosis may lead to blockage of aqueous humor flow through the pupil, thus worsening glaucoma (pupillary block glaucoma).

Adverse Effects

Adverse effects reported in humans or animals include significant irritation (due to the low pH) upon application, which may result in inflammation of the uveal tract.[1,6] Local irritation has been reported in dogs within the first 2 days of treatment, but it appears to improve and cause minimal problems thereafter.[7] Long-term use may result in irreversible miosis due to dilator muscle atrophy and sphincter muscle fibrosis. Systemic absorption of pilocarpine, which occurs when the medication is administered orally, may result in vomiting, diarrhea, increased salivation, increased urination, bronchiolar spasm, and pulmonary edema.

Dosages

Diagnosis of ocular parasympathetic denervation (oculomotor nerve [cranial nerve III]) lesions (extra-label): 1 drop of diluted pilocarpine (0.1-0.2%) solution in the affected eye(s)[8]

Neurogenic keratoconjunctivitis sicca (KCS; extra-label): 1 drop of pilocarpine 0.25% solution in the affected eye(s) 4 times daily, alone or in combination with 2 drops/9.1 kg (20 lb) of a pilocarpine 2% solution in food to be consumed orally twice daily.[9] The dose is increased weekly until signs of toxicity occur or until clinical signs are controlled. If signs of toxicity develop, the dose must be decreased.

Primary glaucoma (extra-label): 1 drop of pilocarpine 1% or 2% solution in the affected eye(s) 3 times daily. **NOTE**: Topical pilocarpine is not recommended for first-line or chronic therapy.

Monitoring

- Clinical efficacy (neurogenic keratoconjunctivitis sicca [KCS]): improved tear production as assessed by Schirmer tear test, patient comfort, and decreased ocular redness and irritation
- Clinical efficacy (primary glaucoma): decrease in/control of intraocular pressure (IOP)
- Observe for signs of systemic toxicosis, including vomiting, diarrhea, increased salivation, increased urination, bronchiolar spasm (coughing), and pulmonary edema, which may occur with both oral and topical administration.
- Monitor for signs of ocular irritation (eg, redness, squinting, cloudiness) when the drug is administered topically.

Client Information

- Give this medication as directed by your veterinarian.
- Observe your animal for signs of toxicity, including vomiting, diarrhea, increased salivation, increased urination, and coughing. Contact your veterinarian if any of these signs occur.
- Use proper administration techniques to avoid contamination of the medication. Keep the cap tightly closed when the medication is not in use.
- Wait 5 minutes after applying this medication before applying any other medications to the eye.
- Store this medicine at room temperature away from moisture and sunlight. Do not freeze.
- Do not use this medicine if the color changes, if it becomes cloudy, or if there are particles in the solutions.

Storage/Stability

Store this medication at controlled room temperature (15°C-25°C [59°F-77°F]) away from moisture and sunlight; do not freeze.

Compatibility/Compounding Considerations

Pilocarpine should not be mixed directly (in vitro) with any other drugs.

Dosage Forms/Regulatory Status

VETERINARY-LABELED PRODUCTS: NONE

HUMAN-LABELED PRODUCTS:

Pilocarpine HCl 1%, 2%, or 4% Ophthalmic Solution (containing pilocarpine 10 mg/mL, 20 mg/mL, or 40 mg/mL, respectively; benzalkonium chloride 0.01%; monobasic sodium phosphate; hypromellose; edetate disodium; dibasic sodium phosphate, purified water; NaOH and/or HCl may be added to adjust pH to 3.5 to 5.5), in a 15 mL ophthalmic dropper bottle; *Isopto Carpine®*, generic; (Rx).

References

For the complete list of references, see **wiley.com/go/budde/plumb**

Pimecrolimus Ophthalmic

(pi-mek-***kroe***-li-mus)

T-cell Immunosuppressive Lacromimetic Agent

Prescriber Highlights

- ► Used to treat dogs with keratoconjunctivitis sicca (KCS), chronic superficial keratitis (CSK), and other immune-mediated ocular surface inflammatory conditions
- ► Useful for cyclosporine-resistant cases of KCS
- ► Not commercially available, must be compounded. *Elidel®* topical (skin) pimecrolimus ointment should NOT be used in the eye.
- ► Advise caregivers to wear gloves when handling pimecrolimus.

Uses/Indications

Pimecrolimus is used to stimulate tear production in dogs with keratoconjunctivitis sicca (KCS) that do not respond to topical cyclosporine. Pimecrolimus 1% administered 3 times daily to patients with KCS and chronic superficial keratitis (CSK) produced favorable improvement in clinical signs.[1] A prospective study in dogs comparing pimecrolimus 1% with cyclosporine 0.2% over an 8-week period found significantly greater improvement in clinical signs that were treated with pimecrolimus rather than cyclosporine.[2] Topical ophthalmic pimecrolimus has not been evaluated in cats or horses.

Pharmacology/Actions

Pimecrolimus is a calcineurin inhibitor (like cyclosporine) that reversibly inhibits T-cell proliferation and prevents the release of pro-inflammatory cytokines. Pimecrolimus binds to intracellular macrophilin, forming a complex that subsequently binds to and inhibits calcineurin. In blocking calcineurin, translocation of the cytoplasmic component of the nuclear factor of activated T cells to the nucleus is prevented. This prevention of translocation impairs transcription of the genes encoding IL-2 and other cytokines, thereby suppressing T-cell proliferation and normal immune function.

Contraindications/Precautions/Warnings

Pimecrolimus is contraindicated in patients that have a history of hypersensitivity to it or any component of the formulation. Caregivers should be advised to avoid contact with pimecrolimus, as skin contact with pimecrolimus has been associated with the development of cancer in humans.

Adverse Effects

Adverse effects to ocular use of pimecrolimus are rare but include orbital alopecia, which may be related to oil vehicles used to compound pimecrolimus solutions.

Dosages

Keratoconjunctivitis sicca (KCS) (extra-label): 1 drop of a pimecrolimus 1% solution in affected eye(s) 2 to 3 times daily

Chronic superficial keratitis (CSK) (extra-label): 1 drop of a pimecrolimus 1% solution in affected eye(s) 2 to 3 times daily

Monitoring

- Baseline and periodic Schirmer tear test, as well as reduction in mucoid ocular discharge and conjunctival hyperemia. Evaluate for lack of progression (and possibly regression) of chronic inflammatory changes, such as corneal pigmentation, vascularization, and fibrosis

Client Information

- Use this medicine as directed by your veterinarian.
- This is a lifelong medicine and must be given daily. Missed doses may cause return of keratoconjunctivitis sicca (KCS) or chronic superficial keratitis (CSK).
- Wear gloves when handling pimecrolimus. Use proper administration techniques to avoid contamination of the medicine. Keep the cap tightly closed when the medicine is not in use.
- Wait 5 minutes after applying this medicine before applying any other medicines to the eye.
- Store this medicine as directed on the package labeling away from moisture and sunlight; do not freeze.
- Do not use this medicine if the color changes, if it becomes cloudy, or if particles are seen in solutions.

Storage/Stability

Store this product as directed on the package labeling away from moisture and sunlight.

Compatibility/Compounding Considerations

Pimecrolimus ophthalmic preparations should not be mixed directly with any other ophthalmic medications.

Dosage Forms/Regulatory Status

VETERINARY-LABELED PRODUCTS: NONE

HUMAN-LABELED PRODUCTS: NONE

Pimecrolimus ophthalmic preparations are not commercially available but have been prepared (compounded) by qualified compounding pharmacists in 1% solutions in oil vehicles including olive oil, corn oil, and medium-chain triglyceride oil.

References

For the complete list of references, see **wiley.com/go/budde/plumb**

Povidone-Iodine Ophthalmic

(***poe***-veh-done ***eye***-oh-dyne) *Betadine®*

Ocular Disinfectant

Prescriber Highlights

- ► Primarily used as a component of preoperative periocular surface preparation
- ► An inexpensive alternative to traditional antifungal, antibacterial, or antiviral ophthalmic agents
- ► May be used to debride nonvital corneal epithelium from indolent ulcers
- ► Solutions greater than 1% must be thoroughly lavaged from the eye within 5 minutes of administration to avoid corneal toxicity.
- ► Topical administration causes discomfort.

Uses/Indications

Povidone-iodine ophthalmic solutions (1% to 5%) are used as a component of periocular surface preparation for all surgical procedures. Additionally, they may be used to chemically debride loose epithelium associated with superficial chronic corneal epithelial defects (SCCED; also called indolent ulcer), or as treatment for bacterial, fungal, and viral infections of the ocular surface. Contrary to what may be expected, lower concentrations (less than 1%) of povidone-iodine demonstrate greater bactericidal activity than higher (10%) concentrations.[1] Povidone-iodine 1.25% led to comparable clinical improvement relative to topical neomycin/polymyxin B/gramicidin and ciprofloxacin in human patients with bacterial keratitis caused by various organisms.[2]

Pharmacology/Actions

Povidone-iodine is an iodophor that damages bacterial cell walls and organelle membranes through interactions with fatty acid double bonds. Additionally, povidone-iodine induces oxidative damage to amino acids and nucleotides. These actions lead to formation of pores in membranes, producing bactericidal and virucidal, and, potentially, fungicidal and sporicidal activity, depending on organism and contact time.

Contraindications/Precautions/Warnings

Povidone-iodine is contraindicated in patients with a history of hypersensitivity to it or any component of the formulation.

Adverse Effects

Adverse effects reported in humans or animals include local burning and stinging on application, as well as chemosis and conjunctival hyperemia; however, concentrations less than 1% are better tolerated than more concentrated preparations. Some patients may experience a local hypersensitivity reaction. Solutions of 0.25% to 10% demonstrate varying degrees of toxicity to ocular surface cells in vitro.[3]

Dosages

Periocular preoperative preparation (extra-label): Saturate sterile swabs or ocular gauze with povidone-iodine solution and apply to surgical area as disinfectant component of presurgical preparation; irrigate the ocular surface with sterile saline solution, leaving it in contact with the surgical area for 2 minutes. Residual solution should be removed via irrigation with sterile saline solution.

Fungal, bacterial, or herpesvirus keratitis (extra-label): 1 drop of a 5% solution to the affected eye(s) once every 24 hours. Treated eye(s) must be thoroughly lavaged with sterile saline solution not more than 5 minutes after administration to avoid corneal damage.

Debridement of nonvital epithelium in superficial chronic corneal epithelial defects (SCCED) ulcers (extra-label): 1 – 2 drops of a 5% solution to the affected eye(s) once. Irrigate thoroughly with sterile saline solution to remove all povidone-iodine not more than 5 minutes after application to avoid damage to the healthy corneal epithelium.

Monitoring

- Clinical efficacy

Client Information

- Use this medicine as recommended by your veterinarian.
- Rinse the animal's eyes thoroughly with sterile eyewash solution within 5 minutes of application.
- Use proper administration techniques to avoid contamination of the medicine. Keep the cap tightly closed when the medicine is not in use.
- Store at room temperature away from moisture and sunlight. Do not freeze.
- Do not use this medicine if the color changes, if it becomes cloudy, or if particles are seen in the solution.

Storage/Stability

Store at controlled room temperature (20°C-25°C [68°F-77°F]) away from moisture and sunlight; do not freeze.

Compatibility/Compounding Considerations

Povidone-iodine preparations should not be mixed directly with any other medications. Sterile povidone-iodine ophthalmic preparation is available as a 5% solution intended for application to the eyes, but solutions of 0.5% to 1% may be prepared by diluting this solution with sterile normal saline. Nonsterile povidone-iodine solutions should not be administered to the eye.

Dosage Forms/Regulatory Status

VETERINARY-LABELED PRODUCTS: NONE

HUMAN-LABELED PRODUCTS:

Povidone-Iodine 5% Ophthalmic Prep (containing povidone-iodine 5%, with 0.5% available iodine; purified water; citric acid; glycerin; nonoxynol-9; NaCl; NaOH; and dibasic sodium phosphate) in a sterile 30 mL bottle; *Betadine Sterile Ophthalmic Prep*®; (Rx)

References

For the complete list of references, see **wiley.com/go/budde/plumb**

Prednisolone Ophthalmic

(pred-***niss***-oh-lone) *Pred Forte*®, *Omnipred*®, *Blephamide*®, *Pred G*®

Corticosteroid

For systemic use, refer to ***Prednisolone/Prednisone***

Prescriber Highlights

- ► Topical corticosteroid used to treat ocular surface and intraocular inflammatory conditions
- ► Superior penetration into the anterior segment compared with other topical corticosteroids, particularly in acetate formulation (versus phosphate)
- ► Use cautiously in small diabetic patients to avoid blood glucose dysregulation.
- ► Contraindications include a hypersensitivity to prednis(ol)one; an existing or suspected bacterial, viral, or fungal ocular infection; and the presence of a corneal abrasion or ulceration.

Uses/Indications

Prednisolone ophthalmic is used to treat inflammatory conditions of the palpebral and bulbar conjunctiva, the cornea, and the anterior segment of the globe (eg, blepharitis, conjunctivitis, keratitis, anterior uveitis). Greater intraocular penetration (and therefore potential clinical efficacy) is achieved with acetate formulations relative to phosphate. Administration of prednisolone acetate to the eyes of cats reduced experimentally induced uveitis more significantly than dexamethasone, flurbiprofen, and diclofenac.[1]

Prednisolone is available in combination with antimicrobial agents for topical ophthalmic use.

Pharmacology/Actions

Corticosteroids have broad immunomodulatory and anti-inflammatory actions, which are mediated via direct effects on gene expression, as well as by nongenomic effects on cell membranes and receptors. Ultimately, corticosteroids decrease pro-inflammatory gene transcription, production of pro-inflammatory prostaglandins and leukotrienes, B- and T-cell number and function, cell-mediated immunity, and humoral immunity.[2] Specific mechanisms involved in controlling ocular inflammatory conditions are not known. Prednisolone has a relative glucocorticoid potency of 4 (versus 1 for hydrocortisone and 25 for dexamethasone); however, its superior intraocular penetration when in the acetate formulation leads to increased clinical efficacy relative to dexamethasone ophthalmic formulations.

Contraindications/Precautions/Warnings

Prednisolone is contraindicated in patients with a history of hypersensitivity to it or any component of the formulation. Due to inhibition of epithelial wound healing and potentiation of infection, prednisolone ophthalmic is contraindicated when corneal ulceration is suspected or present or in the presence of corneal infection (bacterial, fungal, or viral),[3] infectious diseases, chronic renal failure, congestive heart failure, systemic hypertension, or gastric ulceration. When use of prednisolone is necessary in these conditions, the minimal effective dose should be administered for the shortest possible time.

Adverse Effects

Adverse effects reported in humans include development of cataracts (via altered glucose or lenticular metabolic effects), increased intraocular pressure (IOP; via activation of glucocorticoid receptors in the trabecular meshwork), infection (via immunosuppression), decreased wound healing (via increased collagenolytic activity), mydriasis, and calcific keratopathy. Increased IOP may occur in some animals with long-term use of prednisolone; however, most reports suggest the change is reversible.[4,5] Systemic effects are rare but include hepatopathy, suppression of endogenous glucocorticoid production, and focal alopecia. Concurrent use of systemic steroids increases risk for these adverse effects.

Dosages

Conjunctivitis (extra-label): 1 drop or ¼ inch strip in the affected eye(s) every 6 hours until clinical improvement occurs, then gradually decrease, provided clinical improvement is maintained

Keratitis (extra-label): 1 drop or ¼ inch strip in the affected eye(s) every 6 hours until clinical improvement occurs, then gradually decrease, provided clinical improvement is maintained

Anterior uveitis (extra-label): 1 drop or ¼ inch strip in the affected eye(s) every 6 hours until clinical improvement occurs, then gradually decrease, provided clinical improvement is maintained

Post-cataract removal (extra-label): 1 drop in the affected eye(s) every 6 hours

Monitoring

- Clinical efficacy
- Resolution or development of signs of inflammation
- Intraocular pressure (IOP; especially in cats) and ocular surface integrity (eg, fluorescein stain) as needed based on clinical presentation
- Blood or urine glucose changes based on development of clinical signs (eg, polyuria, polydipsia) in diabetic animals

Client Information

- This medicine can be given for various lengths of time. Be sure you understand how often and for how long your animal should be given this medicine.
- Shake suspensions well before using.
- Use proper administration techniques to avoid contamination of the medication. Keep the cap tightly closed when the medicine is not in use.
- Wait 5 minutes after applying this medication before applying any other medications to the eye.
- Contact your veterinarian as soon as possible if your animal's eye condition worsens or does not improve while using this medicine.
- Your veterinarian will need to monitor your animal's eye condition while taking this medicine. Do not miss these important follow-up visits.
- Store this medicine as directed on the product label. Do not freeze.
- Do not use this medicine if the color changes, if it becomes cloudy, or if there are visible particles in the solution.

Storage/Stability

Storage recommendations can vary; follow storage requirements listed on packaging. Most commonly, this product is recommended to be stored at controlled room temperature (20°C-25°C [68°F-77°F]) away from moisture and sunlight; do not freeze.

Compatibility/Compounding Considerations

Prednisolone ophthalmic preparations should not be mixed directly with any other ophthalmic medications.

Dosage Forms/Regulatory Status

VETERINARY-LABELED PRODUCTS: NONE

HUMAN-LABELED PRODUCTS:

Prednisolone Acetate 0.12% Ophthalmic Suspension (containing prednisolone acetate [microfine suspension] 0.12%, benzalkonium chloride, boric acid, edetate disodium, hypromellose, polysorbate 80, purified water, sodium bisulfite, sodium chloride, and sodium citrate) in 10 mL sterile ophthalmic dropper bottle; *Pred Mild*®; (Rx)

Prednisolone Acetate 1% Ophthalmic Suspension (containing prednisolone acetate [microfine suspension] 1%; benzalkonium chloride; boric acid; edetate disodium; hypromellose; polysorbate 80; purified water; sodium bisulfite; NaCl; and sodium citrate, with a pH of 5 to 6) in 5 mL and 10 mL ophthalmic dropper bottles; *Pred Forte* 1%, *Omnipred*® generic; (Rx)

Prednisolone Sodium Phosphate 1% Ophthalmic Solution (containing prednisolone sodium phosphate 10 mg/mL [equivalent to 9.1 mg/mL prednisolone phosphate] in a buffered isotonic solution; hypromellose; monobasic and dibasic sodium phosphate; NaCl, edetate disodium and purified water; NaOH and/or HCl may be added to adjust the pH to 6.2 to 8.2) in 5 mL and 10 mL ophthalmic dropper bottles; generic; (Rx)

HUMAN-LABELED COMBINATION PRODUCTS:

Gentamicin and Prednisolone Acetate Ophthalmic Ointment 0.3%/0.6% (containing gentamicin sulfate equivalent to 0.3% gentamicin base, prednisolone acetate 0.6%, chlorobutanol [chloral derivative] 0.5%, mineral oil, petrolatum [and] lanolin alcohol, purified water, and white petrolatum) in a sterile 3.5 g ophthalmic tube; *Pred-G*®; (Rx)

Gentamicin and Prednisolone Acetate Ophthalmic Suspension 0.3%/1% (containing gentamicin sulfate equivalent to 0.3% gentamicin base, prednisolone acetate [microfine suspension] 1%, benzalkonium chloride 0.005%, edetate disodium, hypromellose, polyvinyl alcohol 1.4%, polysorbate 80, purified water, sodium chloride, sodium citrate dehydrate, NaOH and/or HCl to adjust pH [5.4 to 6.6]) in a sterile 5 mL ophthalmic dropper bottle; *Pred-G*®; (Rx)

Sulfacetamide Sodium and Prednisolone Acetate Ophthalmic Ointment (10%/0.2%) (containing sulfacetamide sodium 10%, prednisolone acetate 0.2%, phenylmercuric acetate 0.0008%, white petrolatum, mineral oil, and petrolatum and lanolin alcohol) in a sterile 3.5 g ophthalmic tube; *Blephamide S.O.P.*®; (Rx)

Sulfacetamide Sodium and Prednisolone Acetate Ophthalmic Suspension (10%/0.2%) (containing sulfacetamide sodium 10%, prednisolone acetate 0.2%, benzalkonium chloride 0.004%, edetate disodium, polysorbate 80, polyvinyl alcohol 1.4%, potassium phosphate monobasic, purified water, sodium phosphate dibasic, sodium thiosulfate, and HCl and/or NaOH to adjust the pH [6.6 to 7.2]); *Blephamide*®; (Rx)

References

For the complete list of references, see **wiley.com/go/budde/plumb**

Proparacaine Ophthalmic

(proe-***pare***-a-kane) *Alcaine*®, *Flucaine*®

Topical Ocular Anesthetic

Prescriber Highlights

- Rapid-acting topical anesthetic used for ocular diagnostic procedures
- Should never be prescribed for therapeutic administration
- Dose- and species-dependent duration, with maximal effect generally between 5 and 15 minutes in dogs, cats, and horses
- Long-term use results in tear film instability and globe-threatening corneal epithelial and stromal damage.
- Some products must be stored in the refrigerator; consult product label.

Uses/Indications

Proparacaine is indicated for use in ophthalmic diagnostic procedures, including measurement of intraocular pressure (tonometry), corneal and conjunctival sampling for cytology and culture, ocular ultrasonography, and gonioscopy. Proparacaine is indicated as an adjunctive anesthetic for performing therapeutic procedures in the hospital, including removal of foreign bodies and sutures from the cornea; eyelid and conjunctival surgeries; corneal grafting procedures; and cataract extraction. Proparacaine has dose- and species-dependent duration of action, with maximal effect between ≈5 and 15 minutes in dogs, cats, and horses, and duration of effect lasting around 30 minutes.[1-5] The degree of maximal effect of proparacaine is less than that of viscous tetracaine in dogs.[2] Favorably, administration of topical proparacaine has not been associated with decreased positive bacterial or fungal cultures in dogs, cats, or horses.[6,7] Because of the likelihood of developing ocular surface toxicities with prolonged or repeated use, proparacaine should never be prescribed for use as an ocular analgesic.

Pharmacology/Actions

Proparacaine induces local anesthesia by inhibiting neuronal depolarization, which prevents generation of an action potential. This action occurs due to binding of the local anesthetic molecule to the intracellular portion of the voltage-gated sodium channel within the neuron, thus inhibiting intracellular movement of sodium. Variations in the structure of different local anesthetics influence their relative potencies. All local anesthetics have increased efficacy in alkaline environments due to improved intracellular penetration; efficacy of local anesthetics is decreased in acidic environments, such as when there is inflammation.

Contraindications/Precautions/Warnings

Proparacaine is contraindicated in patients with a history of hypersensitivity to it or any component of the formulation. Prolonged use of a topical ocular anesthetic will likely produce significant corneal epithelial and stromal disease, as well as tear film instability, and may result in loss of vision.[8]

Adverse Effects

Instillation of proparacaine may result in local irritation several hours after administration. Although patients that are sensitive to other local anesthetics may be less likely to react to proparacaine, local or systemic sensitivity may manifest as a pseudo-allergic (anaphylactoid) reaction mimicking an IgE-mediated vasodilatory event. Cardiovascular, respiratory, and CNS depressant effects that may result from other local anesthetics are extremely rare with appropriate use of topical anesthetics. Care should be exercised, however, when proparacaine is administered to small veterinary patients (ie, puppies, kittens, "pocket pets"), or those more susceptible to systemic absorption (ie, amphibians). Use of proparacaine as a therapeutic analgesic leads to superficial punctate keratitis, which may progress to diffuse necrotizing keratitis, severe infiltrative keratitis, persistent epithelial defects, or damage to the Descemet membrane.

Dosages

Ophthalmic procedures requiring local anesthesia (extra-label): 1 – 2 drops in the target eye(s) prior to examination or procedure. May repeat 1 drop every 5 to 10 minutes 2 to 3 additional times. With additional applications, the duration of corneal anesthesia can be extended to 55 minutes in dogs. Additional doses should be avoided in small patients (ie, puppies, kittens, "pocket pets").

Monitoring

- Clinical effect: Onset of action is indicated by awake patient permitting diagnostic procedures to be performed, and by a reduction in anesthetic requirements when administered preoperatively.

Client Information

- Proparacaine is **not** administered by pet owners in the home. It is reserved for diagnostic procedures in the veterinary practice.

Storage/Stability

Store this product in a refrigerator or at controlled room temperature (depending on the product label) away from moisture and sunlight; do not freeze.[9]

Discard this product if the solution changes color, if it becomes cloudy, or if it develops particles.

Compatibility/Compounding Considerations

Proparacaine should not be mixed directly (in vitro) with any other drugs.

Dosage Forms/Regulatory Status

VETERINARY-LABELED PRODUCTS: NONE

HUMAN-LABELED PRODUCTS:

Proparacaine HCl 0.5% ophthalmic solution (containing 5 mg/mL proparacaine; benzalkonium chloride 0.01%; glycerin; HCl and/or NaOH to adjust pH; purified water) in 15 mL ophthalmic dropper bottles; *Alcaine®*, generic; (Rx)

Proparacaine HCl 0.5% with Fluorescein Sodium Ophthalmic Solution (containing proparacaine 5 mg/mL; fluorescein sodium 2.5 mg/mL; povidone; boric acid; water for injection; NaOH and/or HCl to adjust pH; methylparaben), 5 mL, in sterile plastic or glass ophthalmic dropper bottles; *Flucaine®*, generic; (Rx)

References

For the complete list of references, see **wiley.com/go/budde/plumb**

Rose Bengal Stain, Ophthalmic

(rose ***ben***-gall) *Glostrips®*

Ocular Diagnostic Agent

Prescriber Highlights

- ► Vital dye that demonstrates corneal and conjunctival epithelial cell damage, as well as deficiency in ocular surface mucins
- ► Full-thickness loss of corneal epithelium is not necessary to cause rose bengal uptake by epithelial cells (in contrast to fluorescein).
- ► Very toxic to cornea; irrigate eye(s) well after use
- ► Stings upon application

Uses/Indications

Rose bengal stain is used to detect epithelial cell damage prior to full-thickness epithelial cell loss (ulceration), as most commonly occurs with viral infections. Rose bengal staining may also be used as an adjunctive diagnostic procedure for nonulcerative epithelial and subepithelial keratomycosis in horses.[1] Rose bengal uptake also occurs in patients with qualitative (mucin) tear deficiency syndromes. Rose bengal stain has recently been demonstrated to be an effective adjunctive diagnostic test for evaluation of quantitative tear film deficiencies in dogs.[2]

Pharmacology/Actions

Rose bengal stains both the nuclei and cell walls of dead or degenerated epithelial cells of the cornea and conjunctiva. In contrast to fluorescein stain, rose bengal does not require full-thickness loss of corneal epithelium to indicate damage to the cornea. Rose bengal uptake is decreased in cells that are covered appropriately by mucin, a component of the tear film.

Contraindications/Precautions/Warnings

Rose bengal is contraindicated in patients with a history of hypersensitivity to it or any component of the formulation. Topical anesthetic agents may be indicated to prevent stinging on application. Rose bengal is very toxic to the cornea, and treated eye(s) should be thoroughly irrigated after exposure. Rose bengal is virucidal and may confound results of diagnostic tests for viral keratitis; therefore, culture samples should be obtained prior to application of the stain.

Adverse Effects

Adverse effects reported in humans or animals include burning and stinging upon application.

Dosages

Detection of corneal and conjunctival cell damage (extra-label; NOT FDA-approved): Wet the surface of the rose bengal strip with 1 – 2 drops of normal saline solution. Apply moistened tip of strip or instill 1 drop of rose bengal 1% solution to conjunctival fornix. Examine the eye with white light or with a red-free absorption filter. Degenerated or dead epithelial cells will appear red in color. Flush eye(s) after exposure.

Monitoring

- Evaluate corneas for signs of toxicity (eg, ulceration)

Client Information

- Rose bengal strips should not be used by pet owners at home.

Storage/Stability

Store this product in the refrigerator or at controlled room temperature (below 30°C) away from moisture and sunlight as directed on packaging or by compounding pharmacist; do not freeze. Unpreserved solutions of rose bengal carry a high risk of contamination with bacteria. Store this product as directed and observe all assigned beyond-use dates.

Compatibility/Compounding Considerations

Rose bengal ophthalmic preparations should not be mixed directly with any other ophthalmic medications. Rose bengal solution is no longer commercially available but may be compounded as a 1% solution either with or without preservatives; however, preservation systems are strongly recommended to prevent microbial and fungal contamination.[3]

Dosage Forms/Regulatory Status

VETERINARY-LABELED PRODUCTS: NONE

HUMAN-LABELED PRODUCTS:

Rose Bengal 0.13% Strips (containing rose bengal 1.3 mg/strip) as individually wrapped strips in containers of 100 sterile strips; *Glostrips®*, generic; (Rx). No FDA-approved dosage forms of rose bengal are currently available.

Rose bengal may be prepared (compounded) by qualified compounding pharmacists into a 1% sterile solution in sterile water for injection.

References

For the complete list of references, see **wiley.com/go/budde/plumb**

Silver Sulfadiazine (SSD) Ophthalmic

(***sil***-ver sul-fa-***dye***-ahy-zeen) *Silvadene®, SSD®, Thermazene®*

Broad-Spectrum Antibacterial; Antifungal Agent

Prescriber Highlights

- ► Antibacterial and antifungal dermatologic topical cream used as treatment for fungal keratitis in horses
- ► Long-term use may result in discoloration of the sclera due to argyrism.
- ► Do not use this medication in subpalpebral lavage (SPL) catheters, as occlusion will result.
- ► Best dispensed in 1 mL sterile tuberculin syringes with sterile tip caps for administration to the ocular surface
- ► Warn caregivers with sulfonamide allergies to avoid contact with this medication.

Uses/Indications
Silver sulfadiazine is used as a broad-spectrum antibacterial and antifungal ophthalmic agent. It is used most commonly as a less expensive alternative to conventional therapy for fungal keratitis in horses. Silver sulfadiazine was found to be superior to natamycin in sensitivity testing for fungal isolates in horses with fungal keratitis.[1]

Pharmacology/Actions
A specific mechanism of action has not been determined for silver sulfadiazine's antibacterial and antifungal activity; however, its effectiveness may be from either synergistic interactions between the silver and sulfadiazine components, or actions of each component individually. Silver is a biocide that binds to a broad range of targets, thus exerting a variety of effects, such as enzyme inhibition, protein denaturation, or membrane leakage, depending upon the target bound. Sulfadiazine interferes with microbial folic acid synthesis via competitive inhibition of bacterial dihydropteroate synthetase.

Contraindications/Precautions/Warnings
Silver sulfadiazine is contraindicated in patients that have a history of hypersensitivity to it or any component of the formulation. It should not be administered through subpalpebral lavage (SPL) catheters as occlusion will result. The package labeling of the topical cream clearly states that it is **NOT** for use in the eye. As such, it is recommended to obtain informed consent from owners before prescribing.

Adverse Effects
Adverse effects reported in humans or animals include argyrism (bluish discoloration of the skin and sclera due to silver accumulation), pain, burning, and itching. Although rare, systemic effects that may occur in association with the sulfonamide component include transient leukopenia, skin rashes and inflammation, blood dyscrasias, GI reactions, hepatitis, and toxic nephrosis.

Dosages
NOTE: All dosages are extra-label, and the package insert of the topical cream clearly states that it is **NOT** for use in the eye. As such, it is recommended to obtain informed consent from owners before prescribing.

Bacterial or fungal keratitis: ¼ – ½ inch strip or 0.1 – 0.2 mL in the conjunctival sac of the affected eye(s) every 1 to 2 hours initially, then tapered to every 4 hours and then per clinical response. Avoid long-term use.

Monitoring
- Clinical efficacy: resolution of keratitis as evidenced by cytology and cultures
- Sclera: discontinue use if sclera becomes blue or gray in color (argyrism)

Client Information
- Use this medicine as directed by your veterinarian.
- Do not use this medicine in subpalpebral lavage (SPL) catheters.
- Use proper administration techniques to avoid contamination of the medication. Keep the cap tightly closed when the medicine is not in use.
- Wait 5 minutes after applying this medicine before applying any other medicines to the eye.
- Store this product at room temperature away from moisture and sunlight. Do not freeze.
- Do not use this medicine if the color changes.

Storage/Stability
Store this product at controlled room temperature (20°C-25°C [68°F-77°F]) away from moisture and sunlight; do not freeze.

Compatibility/Compounding Considerations
Silver sulfadiazine should not be mixed directly with any other ophthalmic medications.

Dosage Forms/Regulatory Status
VETERINARY-LABELED PRODUCTS: NONE

HUMAN-LABELED PRODUCTS: NONE

Silver sulfadiazine is **NOT** approved for ophthalmic use. The package insert of all brands of silver sulfadiazine topical creams warns against use in the eye. As such, it is recommended to obtain informed consent from owners before prescribing. It is available as a topical cream, silver sulfadiazine 10 mg/g in a water miscible base in 20 g, 50 g, 400 g, and 1000 g containers. It is optimally dispensed in sterile, single-use tuberculin syringes tipped with a sterile tip cap (needle removed) for administration in the conjunctival sac.

References
For the complete list of references, see **wiley.com/go/budde/plumb**

Sodium Chloride (Hypertonic) Ophthalmic

(soe-dee-um ***klor***-ide [hye-per-ton-ik]) *Muro 128®, Altachlore®, Sochlor®*

Hyperosmotic Agent

Prescriber Highlights
- Used for temporary reduction of corneal edema
- Ointment forms have longer contact time and are preferred relative to solution forms.
- Available without prescription
- Compromise of the corneal surface (eg, corneal ulcer) may diminish the benefits of hypertonic sodium chloride due to loss of a functional epithelial barrier.

Uses/Indications
Hypertonic sodium chloride ophthalmic is used for the temporary reduction of corneal edema and associated bullous keratopathy, superficial corneal erosions, and chronic corneal edema that develop due to endothelial dysfunction induced by a variety of causes. Reduction of edema is short-lived; however, the reduction may be sufficient to favorably impact corneal clarity. Topical administration of 5% sodium chloride ophthalmic ointment to normal canine corneas resulted in decreased corneal thickness.[1] Although topical hypertonic saline has been administered to dogs with spontaneous chronic corneal epithelial defects (SCCEDs) undergoing various debridement techniques,[2] use of 5% sodium chloride ophthalmic did not significantly change the rate of corneal healing, and even prolonged healing time in some cases.[3]

Pharmacology/Actions
Tear film and aqueous humor are continuously absorbed by the hydrophilic corneal stroma; fluid balance is controlled by a normally functioning corneal epithelium and endothelium. When this balance is disrupted because of endothelial dysfunction, fluid accumulates in the corneal stroma and migrates to the surface of the cornea, causing opacification, bullae formation, ulceration, and visual impairment. The use of topical hypertonic saline may reduce the fluid accumulation in the corneal stroma.

Contraindications/Precautions/Warnings
Hypertonic sodium chloride is contraindicated in patients with a history of hypersensitivity to any component of the formulation. It may have lesser efficacy in the presence of corneal ulceration, as intact corneal epithelium is required to create the concentration gradient by which fluid is drawn from the bullae. Application of hypertonic sodium chloride may further increase discomfort associated with ulcerative keratitis.

Adverse Effects

Adverse effects reported in humans or animals include temporary burning and stinging upon application. Short-term application of hypertonic sodium chloride to normal canine eyes did not induce signs of toxicity.[1]

Dosages

Corneal Edema (extra-label): 1 – 2 drops or a ¼ – ½ inch strip in the affected eye(s) every 3 to 4 hours

Monitoring

- Clinical efficacy
- Observe for resolution of corneal edema. Treatment should be discontinued if discomfort or corneal ulceration develop.

Client Information

- Use this medication as directed by your veterinarian.
- This medication is available without a prescription. Only use products recommended by your veterinarian.
- Use proper administration techniques to avoid contamination of the medication. Keep the cap tightly closed when the medication is not in use.
- Wait 5 to 10 minutes after applying this medication before applying any other medications to the eye.
- Store this medication as directed on the product label. Do not freeze.
- Do not use this medication if the color changes, if it becomes cloudy, or if there are visible particles in the solution.

Storage/Stability

Store at controlled room temperature (20°C-25°C [68°F-77°F]) away from moisture and sunlight; do not freeze. Discard this medication if the color changes, if it becomes cloudy, or if particles are observed in the solution.

Compatibility/Compounding Considerations

Hypertonic sodium chloride should not be mixed directly (in vitro) with any other drugs to avoid dilution of the active ingredient.

Dosage Forms/Regulatory Status

VETERINARY-LABELED PRODUCTS: NONE

HUMAN-LABELED PRODUCTS:

Sodium Chloride 5% Ophthalmic Ointment (containing sodium chloride 50 mg/mL, lanolin oil, mineral oil, water for injection and white petrolatum) in a 3.5 g ophthalmic ointment tube; *Muro 128®*, *Altachlore®*, *Sochlor®*; (OTC)

Sodium Chloride 2% or 5% Ophthalmic Solution (containing sodium chloride 20 mg/mL or 50 mg/mL, methylparaben 0.023%, propylparaben 0.01% boric acid, hypromellose, propylene glycol, purified water, sodium borate, NaOH and/or HCl to adjust pH) in a 15 mL ophthalmic dropper bottle; *Muro 128®*, *Altachlore®*, *Sochlor®*; (OTC)

References

For the complete list of references, see **wiley.com/go/budde/plumb**

Sulfacetamide Ophthalmic

(sul-fa-***seet***-uh-mide) *Bleph-10®, Blephamide®*

Sulfonamide Antimicrobial Agent

Prescriber Highlights

- Topical antimicrobial used to treat ocular surface bacterial infections
- Warn caregivers with sulfonamide allergies to avoid contact with this medication.
- Some sulfacetamide ophthalmic products are combined with prednisolone; do not use these formulations in patients with bacterial, viral, or fungal keratitis.

Uses/Indications

Sulfacetamide is used to treat conjunctivitis and other superficial ocular infections due to susceptible microorganisms. Sulfacetamide is considered active against *Escherichia coli*, *Staphylococcus aureus*, *Streptococcus pneumoniae* and *Streptococcus viridans*, *Haemophilus*, *Klebsiella*, and *Enterobacter*. Sulfacetamide has no activity when it is applied topically for *Neisseria* spp, *Serratia marcescens*, or *Pseudomonas aeruginosa*. A significant percentage of staphylococcal isolates are completely resistant to sulfa drugs. Sulfacetamide is also found in combination products with prednisolone (eg, *Blephamide®*).

Pharmacology/Actions

All sulfonamides are bacteriostatic agents with a similar spectrum of activity. Sulfonamides inhibit bacterial synthesis of dihydrofolic acid via competitive inhibition of dihydropteroate synthetase. Resistant strains have altered dihydropteroate synthetase with reduced affinity for sulfonamides or produce increased quantities of aminobenzoic acid.[1]

Contraindications/Precautions/Warnings

Sulfacetamide is contraindicated in patients that have a history of hypersensitivity to it or any component of the formulation. Sulfacetamide may induce serious allergic reactions and blood dyscrasias, but this is rare following topical ophthalmic administration.[1] Patients with corneal infections due to bacterial, viral, or fungal organisms should not receive corticosteroid-containing sulfacetamide products.

Adverse Effects

Adverse effects reported in humans or animals following ocular administration include local irritation, stinging, and burning.[1] Although rare, systemic effects that may occur in association with the sulfonamide component include transient leukopenia, skin rashes and inflammation, toxic epidermal necrolysis, blood dyscrasias, GI reactions, fulminant hepatic necrosis, and toxic nephrosis.

In dogs, systemic sulfonamides are known to cause keratoconjunctivitis sicca (KCS) due to a direct toxicity to the lacrimal acinar cells; however, there have been no reports of topical sulfacetamide causing KCS. This toxic effect to the lacrimal acinar cells is caused by the nitrogen-containing pyridine and pyrimidine rings in sulfonamides and is dose-related. The estimated incidence of KCS is 15% to 25% in dogs treated with sulfonamides and may be latent in onset.[2] Dogs exhibiting blepharospasm or excess mucus ocular discharge should be evaluated for KCS. This condition may be reversible if sulfonamide use is discontinued in time. See ***Monitoring***.

Dosages

Susceptible bacterial conjunctivitis and ocular infections (extra-label): 1 drop or ¼ – ½ inch strip on the affected eye(s) every 2 to 3 hours initially and then tapered according to clinical response. Duration of therapy is usually 7 to 10 days.

Monitoring

- Clinical efficacy: resolution of bacterial conjunctivitis as evidenced by cytology and cultures
- Baseline and periodic Schirmer tear testing, especially in predisposed breeds. Dogs should be observed for signs of developing KCS (eg, mucus ocular discharge, blepharospasm).

Client Information

- Use this medicine as directed by your veterinarian.
- Caregivers with sulfa allergies should avoid contact with this medicine.
- Observe dogs for signs of dry eye (eg, squinting, excessive mucus eye discharge, redness of the whites of the eyes) and consult your veterinarian if this occurs.
- Use proper administration techniques to avoid contamination of

the medicine. Keep the cap tightly closed when the medicine is not in use.

- Wait 5 minutes after applying this medicine before applying any other medicines to the eye.
- Store this medicine at room temperature away from moisture and sunlight. Do not freeze.
- Do not use this medicine if it becomes cloudy, or if particles are seen in the solutions. Sulfacetamide solutions will darken over time. The medicine should be thrown away if this occurs.

Storage/Stability

Store this product at controlled room temperature (20°C-25°C [68°F-77°F]) away from moisture and sunlight; do not freeze.

Compatibility/Compounding Considerations

Sulfacetamide ophthalmic preparations should not be mixed directly with any other ophthalmic medications.

Dosage Forms/Regulatory Status

VETERINARY-LABELED PRODUCTS: NONE

HUMAN-LABELED PRODUCTS:

Sulfacetamide Sodium 10% Ophthalmic Solution (containing sulfacetamide sodium 10%; benzalkonium chloride 0.005%; edetate disodium; polysorbate 80; polyvinyl alcohol 1.4%; purified water; sodium phosphate dibasic; sodium phosphate monobasic; sodium thiosulfate; and HCl and/or NaOH to adjust pH to 6.8 to 7.5), 5 mL in sterile 10 mL ophthalmic dropper bottles; *Bleph-10®*, generic; (Rx)

Sulfacetamide Sodium 10% Ophthalmic Ointment (containing sulfacetamide sodium USP 100 mg; white petrolatum; mineral oil) in 3.5 g tubes; generic; (Rx)

HUMAN-LABELED COMBINATION PRODUCTS:

Sulfacetamide Sodium 10% and Prednisolone Acetate 0.2% Ophthalmic Suspension (containing sulfacetamide sodium 10%; prednisolone acetate 0.2%; benzalkonium chloride 0.004%; edetate disodium; polysorbate 80; polyvinyl alcohol 1.4%; potassium phosphate monobasic; purified water; sodium phosphate dibasic; sodium thiosulfate; and HCl and/or NaOH to adjust the pH to 6.6. to 7.2), 5 mL in 10 mL bottle, and 10 mL in 15 mL bottle; *Blephamide®*; (Rx)

Sulfacetamide Sodium 10% and Prednisolone Sodium Phosphate 0.23% Ophthalmic Suspension (containing sulfacetamide sodium 100 mg; prednisolone sodium phosphate 2.5 mg, equivalent to prednisolone phosphate 2.3 mg; poloxamer 407; boric acid; edetate disodium; purified water; NaOH and/or HCl to adjust pH to 6.5 to 7.5) in 5 mL and 10 mL; generic; (Rx)

Sulfacetamide Sodium 10% and Prednisolone Acetate 0.2% Ophthalmic Ointment (containing sulfacetamide sodium 10%, prednisolone acetate 0.2%, phenylmercuric acetate 0.0008%, white petrolatum, mineral oil, petrolatum (and) lanolin alcohol) in sterile 3.5 g ophthalmic tube; *Blephamide®*; (Rx)

References

For the complete list of references, see **wiley.com/go/budde/plumb**

Tacrolimus Ophthalmic

(ta-***kroe***-li-mus)

T-cell Inhibitor Immunosuppressive Agent

Prescriber Highlights

- ► Used to treat dogs with keratoconjunctivitis sicca (KCS), chronic superficial keratitis (CSK), and other immune-mediated ocular surface inflammatory conditions
- ► Useful for cyclosporine-resistant cases of KCS
- ► It is not commercially available; it must be compounded (*Protopic®* topical dermal tacrolimus ointment should **NOT** be used in the eye).
- ► The National Institute for Occupational Safety and Health (NIOSH) classifies tacrolimus as a hazardous drug; use appropriate precautions when handling.

Uses/Indications

Tacrolimus is used to stimulate tear production in dogs with quantitative and qualitative keratoconjunctivitis sicca (KCS). Tacrolimus 0.03% has been demonstrated to be equally efficacious as cyclosporine 2% for canine KCS.1 Concentrations of 0.01% to 0.03% have been reported to be successful in controlling canine KCS.[1-4] Tacrolimus can also manage other ocular surface inflammatory conditions, such as chronic superficial keratitis (CSK). Tacrolimus topical ophthalmic use has not been evaluated in cats or horses.

Pharmacology/Actions

Tacrolimus is a macrolide antibiotic that has a T-cell suppressant activity similar to that of cyclosporine, but the potency is ≈100 times that of cyclosporine. Reversible T-cell suppression results from inhibition of calcineurin by tacrolimus. Within T cells, the binding of tacrolimus with the intracellular protein (FK-506) forms a complex that subsequently binds to and inhibits intracellular calcineurin. Inhibition of calcineurin prevents transcription of pro-inflammatory cytokines and T-cell signal transduction, resulting in immunosuppressive effects.

Contraindications/Precautions/Warnings

Tacrolimus is contraindicated in patients that have a history of hypersensitivity to it or any component of the formulation. The degree of systemic absorption from ophthalmic preparations is not known; use with caution in small-sized animals.

The National Institute for Occupational Safety and Health (NIOSH) classifies tacrolimus as a hazardous drug; personal protective equipment (PPE) should be used accordingly to minimize the risk for exposure.

Adverse Effects

Adverse effects associated with the ocular use of tacrolimus are rare but include orbital alopecia, which may be related to oil vehicles used to compound tacrolimus solutions.

Dosages

Keratoconjunctivitis sicca (KCS) (extra-label): 1 drop in each eye 2 times daily

Chronic superficial keratitis (CSK) (extra-label): 1 drop in each eye 2 times daily

Monitoring

- Clinical efficacy: baseline and periodic Schirmer tear test, reduction in mucoid ocular discharge and conjunctival hyperemia, and lack of progression (and possibly regression) of chronic inflammatory changes, such as corneal pigmentation, vascularization, and fibrosis

Client Information

- Use this medicine as directed by your veterinarian.

- This is a lifelong medication and must be given daily to be effective. Missed doses may cause rapid (within days) return of keratoconjunctivitis sicca (KCS).
- Use proper administration techniques to avoid contamination of the medicine. Keep the cap tightly closed when the medicine is not in use.
- Wait for 5 minutes after applying this medication before applying other medications to the eye.
- Store this medicine as directed on the package labeling away from moisture and sunlight. Do not freeze.
- Do not use this medicine if the color changes, if it becomes cloudy, or if there are particles in the solutions.
- This medication is considered to be a hazardous drug as defined by the National Institute for Occupational Safety and Health (NIOSH). Talk with your veterinarian or pharmacist about the use of personal protective equipment when handling this medicine.

Storage/Stability

Store this product as directed on the package labeling away from moisture and sunlight; do not freeze.

Compatibility/Compounding Considerations

Tacrolimus ophthalmic preparations should not be mixed directly with any other ophthalmic medications.

It is not commercially available and must be prepared (compounded) by a qualified compounding pharmacist.

Dosage Forms/Regulatory Status

VETERINARY-LABELED PRODUCTS: NONE

HUMAN-LABELED PRODUCTS: NONE

Tacrolimus ophthalmic preparations are not commercially available but may be compounded by qualified compounding pharmacists in concentrations varying from 0.01% to 0.03% in oil vehicles including olive oil, corn oil, and medium-chain triglyceride oil.

References

For the complete list of references, see **wiley.com/go/budde/plumb**

Tafluprost Ophthalmic

(***ta***-floo-prost) *Zioptan®*

Prostaglandin Analogue

Prescriber Highlights

- ► Used as a treatment for primary glaucoma in dogs
- ► Unlikely to be effective for feline or equine glaucoma
- ► Twice-daily dosing of tafluprost may result in less fluctuation of intraocular pressure (IOP).
- ► Preservative-free and may be better tolerated than preservative-containing prostaglandin analogues
- ► May worsen intraocular inflammation through prostaglandin-mediated mechanisms

Uses/Indications

Tafluprost is indicated to reduce intraocular pressure (IOP) in canine glaucoma. It has not been evaluated as a treatment for feline or equine glaucoma; however, other prostaglandin analogues are minimally effective in those species.

Pharmacology/Actions

Prostaglandin analogues are chemically modified versions of prostaglandin F2-alpha. Prostaglandin F2-alpha, an endogenous inflammatory mediator, mediates ocular hypotensive effects, presumably by increasing the outflow of aqueous humor through the trabecular meshwork and uveoscleral routes. In addition to lowering intraocular pressure (IOP), tafluprost induces miosis by activating prostaglandin receptors. In normal canine eyes, tafluprost significantly decreased IOP and induced miosis following a single administration.[1] When combined with betaxolol or timolol, a single administration of tafluprost to normal canine eyes produced a greater IOP reduction than tafluprost alone.[2]

Contraindications/Precautions/Warnings

Tafluprost is contraindicated in patients that have a history of hypersensitivity to it or any component of the formulation. Tafluprost should be used with caution in the presence of anterior uveitis and secondary glaucoma, particularly in cases already exhibiting significant miosis, as this treatment may exacerbate miosis, promote synechiae formation, and worsen glaucoma. Also, in dogs with primary anterior lens luxation, tafluprost should be used with caution, as the resulting miosis may trap the lens and/or vitreous within the pupillary aperture, thus creating pupillary block glaucoma. Tafluprost is not contraindicated in dogs with secondary posterior lens luxation, as the miosis may (favorably) trap the lens in the posterior segment.

Adverse Effects

Adverse effects associated with tafluprost reported in humans or animals include blurred vision, burning and stinging, conjunctival hyperemia, foreign body sensation, itching, increased pigmentation of the iris, and punctate epithelial keratopathy. Tafluprost may cause darkening of the iris through direct stimulation of iris melanocytes, and it may cause increased eyelash growth. Tafluprost may worsen intraocular inflammation. Macular edema, including cystoid macular edema, has also been reported after the use of tafluprost in humans.

Dosages

Glaucoma (extra-label): 1 drop in the affected eye(s) 1 to 2 times daily

Monitoring

- Clinical efficacy: maintenance of normal intraocular pressure (IOP)

Client Information

- Use this medicine as directed by your veterinarian.
- Use proper administration techniques to avoid contamination of the medicine. Keep the cap tightly closed when the medicine is not in use.
- Wait 5 minutes after applying this medicine before applying any other medicines to the eye.
- The solution from one individual unit is to be used immediately in one or both eyes. Because sterility cannot be maintained after the individual unit is opened, the remaining contents should be discarded immediately after administration.
- Store this medicine in the original pouch in the refrigerator. After opening the pouch, the unopened single-use containers may be stored in the opened foil pouch for up to 28 days at room temperature. Protect this medicine from light and moisture. Discard any unused containers 28 days after first opening the pouch.
- Do not use this medicine if the color changes, if it becomes cloudy, or if there are particles in the solutions.

Storage/Stability

Store this product in the original pouch in the refrigerator (2°C-8°C [36°F-46°F]). After opening the pouch, the unopened single-use containers may be stored in the opened foil pouch for up to 28 days at room temperature (20°C-25°C [68°F-77°F]). Protect this product from light and moisture. Discard any unused containers 28 days after first opening the pouch.

Compatibility/Compounding Considerations

Tafluprost ophthalmic preparations should not be mixed directly with any other ophthalmic medications.

Dosage Forms/Regulatory Status

VETERINARY-LABELED PRODUCTS: NONE

HUMAN-LABELED PRODUCTS:

Tafluprost 0.0015% Ophthalmic Solution (containing tafluprost 0.015 mg/mL; glycerol; sodium dihydrogen phosphate dihydrate; disodium edetate; polysorbate 80; water for injection; HCl and/or NaOH to adjust pH to 5.5 to 6.75 and an osmolality of 260 – 300 mOsm/kg), in 0.3 mL single-use containers in boxes of 30 or 90 pouches; *Zioptan*®, generic; (Rx)

References

For the complete list of references, see **wiley.com/go/budde/plumb**

Tetracaine Ophthalmic

(***teh***-trah-kane) *Altacaine*®, *Tetravisc*®

Topical Ocular Anesthetic

Prescriber Highlights

- Rapid-acting topical anesthetic for ocular diagnostic procedures; it should not be prescribed for therapeutic administration, as it will cause ocular surface toxicity
- Anesthetic duration of the solution is 20 to 30 minutes; viscous forms have a longer duration of action.
- Comparable efficacy to oxybuprocaine, as evaluated in dogs; increased efficacy relative to proparacaine, as evaluated in horses
- Increased ocular surface irritation as compared with proparacaine and oxybuprocaine
- Long-term use results in tear film instability and corneal epithelial and stromal damage, and it may progress to vision loss.

Uses/Indications

Tetracaine is indicated for use in ophthalmic diagnostic procedures, including measurement of intraocular pressure (tonometry), corneal and conjunctival sampling for cytology and culture, ocular ultrasonography, and gonioscopy. Tetracaine is indicated as an adjunctive anesthetic for therapeutic procedures in the hospital, including removal of foreign bodies and sutures from the cornea; eyelid and conjunctival surgeries; corneal grafting procedures; and cataract extraction. In veterinary patients, tetracaine may produce a more rapid and deeper plane of local anesthesia relative to proparacaine.[1] A single application of 1% solution in dogs induces anesthesia for a duration of 30 minutes,[2] whereas viscous tetracaine has a significantly longer duration of action than proparacaine solution and lidocaine gel.[3] With a single application of 0.5% in horses, the anesthesia is 20 to 30 minutes long; additional applications of 1% solution prolongs anesthesia up to 1 hour.[4] A formulation of viscous tetracaine decreases corneal sensitivity and has a longer duration of action (1 hour) in horses compared with proparacaine or nonviscous tetracaine.[1]

Because of the likelihood of developing ocular surface toxicities with prolonged, repeated use, tetracaine should never be prescribed for use as an ocular analgesic. See ***Adverse Effects***.

Pharmacology/Actions

Tetracaine induces local anesthesia by inhibiting neuronal depolarization, which prevents the generation of an action potential. This action occurs due to the binding of tetracaine to the intracellular portion of the voltage-gated sodium channel within the neuron, thus inhibiting the intracellular movement of sodium. Variations in the structure of different local anesthetics influence their relative potencies; however, all local anesthetics have increased efficacy in alkaline environments due to improved intracellular penetration (efficacy is decreased in the acidic environment of inflammation).

Contraindications/Precautions/Warnings

Tetracaine is contraindicated in patients that have a history of hypersensitivity to it or any component of the formulation. Prolonged use of a topical ocular anesthetic leads to significant corneal epithelial and stromal disease, as well as tear film instability, and may result in loss of vision.[5]

Adverse Effects

Upon initial administration, instillation of tetracaine in the eye, at recommended concentration and dosage, may produce mild irritation, conjunctival redness, lacrimation, or squinting; however, some local irritation may occur several hours after the instillation, and this irritation may be greater than that seen with proparacaine.[2] Tetracaine appears safe for use in patients that are sensitive to other local anesthetics, but local or systemic sensitivity occasionally occurs and rarely may manifest as a pseudo-allergic (anaphylactoid) reaction mimicking an IgE-mediated vasodilatory event. Cardiovascular, respiratory, and CNS depressant effects that may result from other local anesthetics are rare with the appropriate use of topical anesthetics. Care should be exercised when administering tetracaine to small patients (ie, puppies, kittens, "pocket pets") or animals known to have increased absorption of the drug (ie, amphibians). The use of tetracaine as a therapeutic analgesic leads to superficial punctate keratitis, which may progress to diffuse necrotizing keratitis, severe infiltrative keratitis, persistent epithelial defects, or damage to the Descemet membrane. In horses, reduction in the tear film breakup time has been reported, which is indicative of decreased stability of the precorneal tear film.[6]

Dosages

Ophthalmic procedures requiring local anesthesia (extra-label): 1 – 2 drops in the target eye(s) before examination or procedure. May repeat 1 drop every 5 to 10 minutes for 2 to 3 additional times. With a single application of tetracaine 0.5% in horses, the duration of anesthesia is 20 to 30 minutes; additional applications, application of 1% solution, or application of viscous formulation may prolong anesthesia for as long as 1 hour in horses. Additional doses should be avoided in small patients (ie, puppies, kittens, and "pocket pets").

Monitoring

- Clinical effect. The onset of action is indicated by awake patients permitting diagnostic procedures to be performed and by a reduction in anesthetic requirements when tetracaine is administered preoperatively.

Client Information

- This medicine is only given in the veterinary clinic for use on your animal's eye to allow for examination.

Storage/Stability

Storage recommendations can vary; follow storage requirements listed on packaging. Most commonly, this product is recommended to be stored at controlled room temperature (20°C-25°C [68°F-77°F]) away from moisture and sunlight; do not freeze. Discard the medication if the solution changes color, if it becomes cloudy, or if it develops particles.

Compatibility/Compounding Considerations

Tetracaine ophthalmic preparations should not be mixed directly with any other ophthalmic medications.

Dosage Forms/Regulatory Status

VETERINARY-LABELED PRODUCTS: NONE

HUMAN-LABELED PRODUCTS:

Tetracaine HCl 0.5% Viscous Ophthalmic Solution (containing tetracaine HCl 0.5%; benzalkonium chloride; boric acid; edetate disodium; hypromellose; potassium chloride; sodium borate; NaCl; water for injection) in 0.6 mL single unit dose plastic containers and 5 mL ophthalmic dropper bottles; *Tetravisc*®; (Rx) (not US FDA-approved)

Tetracaine HCl 0.5% Ophthalmic Solution (containing tetracaine HCl 5 mg; boric acid; potassium chloride; edetate disodium; purified water; NaOH and/or HCl to adjust pH to 3.7 to 6; chlorobutanol 0.4%) in 15 mL ophthalmic dropper bottles; generic; (Rx)

References

For the complete list of references, see **wiley.com/go/budde/plumb**

Timolol Ophthalmic

(**tim**-oh-lol) *Timoptic*®, *Betimol*®, *Istalol*®, *Combigan*®, *Cosopt*®
Nonselective Beta-Blocker

Prescriber Highlights

- Beta-blocker that decreases aqueous humor production to decrease intraocular pressure (IOP) in patients with glaucoma
- Although less effective than 0.5% concentrations, 0.25% concentrations of timolol are associated with fewer systemic adverse effects.
- Delays onset of glaucoma in the normal eye of dogs with unilateral glaucoma
- Use with caution in asthmatic patients due to the potential to induce bronchospasm.

Uses/Indications

Timolol is used to reduce intraocular pressure (IOP) in primary glaucoma and to prevent glaucoma in the normal eye of animals with unilateral glaucoma. The 0.25% concentration has minimal ocular hypotensive effects in animals and the 0.5% concentration is preferentially employed; however, the potential for systemic adverse effects is greater with the 0.5% solution.[1,2] The maximal IOP-lowering effect is ≈20% to 25% in normotensive dogs[3,4] and horses,[5] and 10% in cats.[6] Gel-forming 0.5% solutions of timolol (meant to increase ocular surface residence time by utilizing the interaction of xanthum gum with tears) reduce IOP by a mean of 5.3 mm Hg in dogs.[7] However, IOP reduction in glaucomatous cats is less consistent.[8] Reduction of IOP following the administration of timolol 0.5% in combination with dorzolamide 2% twice daily in normal eyes of horses is variable but has been reported to be as high as 17%.[5,9,10] Although timolol may also be combined with alpha-adrenergic agonists (eg, brimonidine) to potentiate ocular hypotensive effects through the increased outflow of aqueous humor and decreased aqueous humor production, the adverse effects of brimonidine decrease its utility in small animal patients. This combination does not produce a clinically significant IOP reduction in normal horses.[11]

Pharmacology/Actions

Timolol is a nonselective beta-adrenergic receptor blocking agent with intrinsic sympathomimetic activity, but it lacks membrane-stabilizing activity. Blockade of ciliary body beta-receptors, particularly beta-2 receptors, reduces intraocular pressure (IOP) by decreasing aqueous humor production. The exact mechanism of the ocular hypotensive effect of beta-blockers has not been definitively demonstrated; however, several mechanisms have been postulated for this effect including beta blockade of norepinephrine-induced tonic sympathetic stimulation, leading to decreased cAMP activation in the ciliary body, inhibition of Na+K+ATPase activity, or vasoactive activity on the iris and ciliary body. Topically administered beta-blockers also inhibit glutamine-induced increases in intracellular calcium and sodium thereby providing a potential protective effect against ischemic insult to the retina.[12]

Contraindications/Precautions/Warnings

Timolol is contraindicated in patients that have a history of hypersensitivity to it or any component of the formulation. Timolol should be used cautiously, if at all, in patients with atrioventricular block, bradycardia, heart failure, asthma, chronic bronchitis, or other cardiopulmonary conditions. Use this product cautiously in diabetic patients, as timolol can mask clinical signs associated with hypoglycemia.

Adverse Effects

Adverse effects reported in humans or animals include transient burning, stinging, and irritation upon application to the eye. In dogs, cats, and horses, the administration of timolol may cause slight miosis. It may trigger attacks in cats with asthma. Timolol produces significant reductions in heart rate in healthy cats, thus supporting its limited use in patients with known cardiopulmonary disease.[1]

Dosages

Glaucoma or prophylaxis in the normal eye of unilateral glaucoma (extra-label): 1 drop in the affected eye(s) twice daily

Monitoring

- Clinical efficacy
- Intraocular pressure (IOP) and disease progression
- Respiratory rate in asthmatic patients; blood glucose in diabetic patients; heart rate and resting respiratory rate in cardiac patients (especially cats)

Client Information

- Use this medicine as directed by your veterinarian.
- This medication may delay the onset of glaucoma in the normal eye of dogs with glaucoma in their other eye.
- Wait 5 minutes after applying this medication before applying any other medications to the eye.
- Tell your veterinarian about any conditions or diseases your animal may have now or has had in the past, especially asthma or diabetes.
- Use proper administration techniques to avoid contamination of the medication. Do not touch the dropper (or ointment) tip or allow it to touch your animal's eye or any other surface to prevent contamination.
- Keep the cap tightly closed when the medication is not in use.
- Do not use this medicine if the color changes, if it becomes cloudy, or if there are particles in solutions.
- Your veterinarian will need to monitor your animal's eye condition while taking this medicine. Do not miss these important follow-up visits.

Storage/Stability

Store this medication at controlled room temperature (15°C-25°C [59°F-77°F]) away from moisture and sunlight; do not freeze. Discard this medication if the solution color change, if it becomes cloudy, or if there are particles in the solution.

Compatibility/Compounding Considerations

Timolol maleate ophthalmic preparations should not be mixed directly with any other ophthalmic medications.

Dosage Forms/Regulatory Status

VETERINARY-LABELED PRODUCTS: NONE

HUMAN-LABELED PRODUCTS:

Timolol 0.25% Ophthalmic Solution (containing 2.56 mg timolol hemihydrate equivalent to 2.5 mg timolol; monosodium and disodium phosphate dehydrate to adjust pH; water for injection; benzalkonium chloride 0.01%), in 5 mL, 10 mL, and 15 mL sterile ophthalmic dropper bottles; *Betimol*®; (Rx)

Timolol 0.5% Ophthalmic Solution (containing 5.12 mg timolol hemihydrate equivalent to 5 mg timolol; monosodium and disodium phosphate dehydrate to adjust pH; water for injection; benzalkonium chloride 0.01%), in 5 mL, 10 mL, and 15 mL sterile ophthalmic dropper bottles; *Betimol*®, *Istalol*®; (Rx)

Timolol 0.25% Ophthalmic Solution (containing 3.4 mg timolol maleate equivalent to 2.5 mg timolol; monobasic and dibasic sodium phosphate; NaOH to adjust pH; purified water; benzalkonium chloride 0.01%), in sterile 5 mL and 10 mL ophthalmic dropper bottles; *Timoptic*®, generic; (Rx)

Timolol 0.5% Ophthalmic Solution (containing 6.8 mg timolol maleate equivalent to 5 mg timolol; monobasic and dibasic sodium phosphate; NaOH to adjust pH; purified water; benzalkonium chloride 0.01%), in sterile 5 mL and 10 mL ophthalmic dropper bottles; *Timoptic*®, generic; (Rx).

Timolol 0.25% Gel-Forming Solution (containing 3.4 mg of timolol maleate equivalent to 2.5 mg timolol; gellan gum; tromethamine; mannitol; water for injection; benzododecinium bromide 0.012%), in sterile 5 mL ophthalmic dropper bottles; *Timoptic-XE*®, generic; (Rx)

Timolol 0.5% Gel-Forming Solution (containing 6.8 mg of timolol maleate equivalent to 5 mg timolol; gellan gum; tromethamine; mannitol; water for injection; benzododecinium bromide 0.012%), in sterile 5 mL ophthalmic dropper bottles; *Timoptic-XE*®, generic; (Rx)

HUMAN-LABELED COMBINATION PRODUCTS:

Timolol 0.5% and Dorzolamide 2% Ophthalmic Solution (containing 20 mg/mL dorzolamide (22.26 mg of dorzolamide HCl) and 5 mg/mL timolol (6.83 mg timolol maleate); benzalkonium chloride 0.0075%; sodium citrate; hydroxyethyl cellulose; NaOH; mannitol; water for injection, with a pH of ≈5.65 and an osmolarity of 242 – 323 mOsm/kg), in 10 mL ophthalmic dropper bottles; *Cosopt*®; (Rx)

Timolol 0.5% and Dorzolamide 2% Ophthalmic Solution (containing 20 mg/mL dorzolamide (22.3 mg of dorzolamide HCl) and 5 mg/mL timolol (6.8 mg timolol maleate); hydroxyethyl cellulose; mannitol; sodium citrate; NaOH (to adjust pH); water for injection), supplied in a foil pouch containing 15 low-density polyethylene 0.2 mL single-use containers; *Cosopt PF*®; (Rx)

Brimonidine Tartrate 0.2% and Timolol Maleate 0.5% Ophthalmic Solution (containing brimonidine tartrate 0.2%; timolol maleate 0.5%; benzalkonium chloride 0.005%; citric acid; polyvinyl alcohol; NaCl; sodium citrate; purified water; HCl and/or NaOH added to adjust pH to 5.6 to 6.6, with an osmolality of 280 – 330 mOsm/kg), in a 10 mL dropper bottle; *Combigan*®, generic; (Rx)

References

For the complete list of references, see **wiley.com/go/budde/plumb**

Tobramycin Ophthalmic

(tobe-ra-***mye***-sin) *Tobrex*®, *AkTob*®, *Tobradex*®, *Tobradex ST*®, *Zylet*®

Aminoglycoside Antimicrobial Agent

For systemic use, see ***Tobramycin***

Prescriber Highlights

- Used as a treatment for susceptible bacterial infections of the ocular surface
- Do not confuse pure tobramycin ophthalmic preparations with preparations containing glucocorticoids.
- Fortified solutions of tobramycin greater than 13.5 mg/mL may be compounded for use in susceptible infections where commercially available products are not concentrated enough to achieve inhibitory concentrations.

Uses/Indications

Tobramycin ophthalmic is primarily used to treat ocular surface infections caused by *Pseudomonas aeruginosa*; however, susceptibility of *Pseudomonas* spp isolates may be decreasing.[1] Preparations of tobramycin in combination with a glucocorticoid are used primarily in the management of inflammatory conditions of the conjunctiva that are associated with or at risk for developing a superficial bacterial infection[2]; it may also be used postoperatively following ocular surface or intraocular surgical procedures.

The World Health Organization (WHO) has designated tobramycin as a Critically Important, High Priority antimicrobial for human medicine.[3] The Office International des Epizooties (OIE) has designated tobramycin as a Veterinary Critically Important Antimicrobial (VCIA) Agent in equine species.[4]

Pharmacology/Actions

Tobramycin is actively transported into bacteria and binds to a specific aminoglycoside receptor on the 30S subunit of bacterial ribosomes and interferes with an initiation complex between mRNA and the 30S subunit to inhibit protein synthesis. Aminoglycosides are bactericidal, whereas most other antibiotics that interfere with protein synthesis are bacteriostatic. Tobramycin's spectrum of activity includes coverage against many aerobic gram-negative bacteria, including most species of *Escherichia coli*, *Klebsiella* spp, *Proteus* spp, *Pseudomonas* spp, *Salmonella* spp, *Enterobacter* spp, *Serratia* spp, and *Shigella* spp. Efficacy against *Staphylococcus* spp is limited, and efficacy against *Streptococcus* spp is negligible.[5,6]

The antimicrobial activity of the aminoglycosides is enhanced in an alkaline environment; the acidic nature of pus or cellular debris can reduce efficacy.

The aminoglycoside antibiotics are inactive against fungi, viruses, and anaerobic bacteria.

Contraindications/Precautions/Warnings

Tobramycin is contraindicated in patients that have a history of hypersensitivity to it or any component of the formulation. Cross sensitivity of tobramycin with other aminoglycosides has been known to occur.[7]

Commercially available tobramycin solutions and ointments may not achieve inhibitory concentrations in the eye and may be either compounded in fortified concentrations (greater than or equal to 13.5 mg/mL) or injected subconjunctivally.[8,9]

Adverse Effects

Adverse effects associated with tobramycin reported in humans or animals include ocular burning and irritation upon drug instillation, nonspecific conjunctivitis, conjunctival epithelial defects, and conjunctival hyperemia.

When tobramycin is used systemically, it can cause nephrotoxicity and neurotoxicity (ototoxicity and vestibular toxicity).[7] Because cats are more susceptible to these toxic effects of aminoglycosides, it is recommended that all cats receiving topical tobramycin be monitored for systemic toxicity.

Dosages

Susceptible ocular surface infections (extra-label): 1 drop or ¼ – ½ inch strip in the affected eye(s) 4 to 6 times daily. The frequency may be increased to every 30 to 60 minutes for treating significant infections.

Management of inflammatory conditions of the conjunctiva associated with or at risk for developing a superficial bacterial infection | Postoperative ocular surface or intraocular procedures (extra-label): Using a tobramycin/glucocorticoid combination preparation, 1 drop or ¼ – ½ inch strip in the affected eye(s) 3 to 4 times daily. The frequency is decreased following control of ocular surface inflammation, with a corresponding reduced risk for infection.

Monitoring

- Clinical efficacy: corneal cytology with culture and susceptibility testing to evaluate for the persistence of bacteria. Evaluate clinical signs suggestive of continued infection.
- Baseline and periodic urinalysis with sediment evaluation to check for casts, which may be an early indicator for renal toxicity

Client Information

- Use this medicine as directed by your veterinarian.
- Use proper administration techniques to avoid contamination of the medicine. Keep the cap tightly closed when the medicine is not in use.
- Wait 5 minutes after applying this medicine before applying any other medicines to the eye.
- Store this medicine in the refrigerator or at room temperature away from moisture and sunlight. Do not freeze.
- Do not use this medicine if the color changes, if becomes cloudy, or if there are particles in the solution.

Storage/Stability

Store this product in the refrigerator or at controlled room temperature (2°C-25°C [46°F-77°F]) as directed in product labeling, away from moisture and sunlight; do not freeze.

Compatibility/Compounding Considerations

Tobramycin ophthalmic preparations should not be mixed directly with any other ophthalmic medications. Tobramycin may be compounded into a fortified ophthalmic solution in concentrations of greater than or equal to 13.5 mg/mL by aseptically adding tobramycin injection in appropriate amounts to commercially available tobramycin ophthalmic solution.[8]

Dosage Forms/Regulatory Status

VETERINARY-LABELED PRODUCTS: NONE

HUMAN-LABELED PRODUCTS:

Tobramycin 0.3% Ophthalmic Solution; *Tobrex*®; *Aktob*®; generic; (Rx)

Tobramycin 0.3% Ophthalmic Ointment; *Tobrex*®; (Rx)

HUMAN-LABELED COMBINATION PRODUCTS:

Tobramycin and Dexamethasone Ophthalmic Ointment (containing tobramycin 0.3% (3 mg), dexamethasone 0.1% (1 mg), chlorobutanol 0.5% (5 mg), mineral oil, white petrolatum), in a sterile 3.5 g tube; *Tobradex*®; (Rx)

Tobramycin and Dexamethasone Ophthalmic Suspension (containing tobramycin 0.3% (3 mg), dexamethasone 0.1% (1 mg), benzalkonium chloride 0.01%, tyloxapol, edetate disodium, NaCl, hydroxyethyl cellulose, sodium sulfate, sulfuric acid and/or NaOH to adjust pH, purified water), in a sterile 2.5 mL ophthalmic dropper; *Tobradex*®, generic; (Rx)

Tobramycin and Dexamethasone Ophthalmic Suspension (containing tobramycin 0.3% (3 mg), dexamethasone 0.05% (0.5 mg), xanthan gum, tyloxapol, disodium edetate, NaCl, propylene glycol, sodium sulfate, benzalkonium chloride 0.01%, NaOH and/or HCl to adjust pH, purified water), in a sterile 5 mL ophthalmic dropper; *Tobradex ST*®; (Rx)

Tobramycin 0.3% and Loteprednol 0.5% Ophthalmic Suspension in 5 mL and 10 mL; *Zylet*®; (Rx)

References

For the complete list of references, see **wiley.com/go/budde/plumb**

Travoprost Ophthalmic

(***trav***-oh-prost) *Travatan Z*®

Prostaglandin Analogue

Prescriber Highlights

- ► Used to decrease intraocular pressure (IOP) in dogs with primary glaucoma or ocular hypertension
- ► Based on receptor differences, it is not effective in feline glaucoma and unlikely to be effective in equine glaucoma.
- ► Do not use it if intraocular inflammation is present, as it may worsen inflammation or lead to pupillary block glaucoma.
- ► Twice-daily dosing of travoprost results in less fluctuation of IOP.
- ► Preservative systems may cause ocular irritation and discomfort.

Uses/Indications

Travoprost is used in dogs to reduce intraocular pressure (IOP) to manage primary glaucoma. It has not been evaluated for efficacy in either cats or horses. In normotensive canine eyes, once-daily administration of travoprost reduced IOP comparably to latanoprost. It also resulted in miosis and conjunctival hyperemia.[1] In glaucomatous canine eyes, once- and twice daily administration of travoprost 0.004% significantly reduced IOP,[2] whereas concentrations above 0.0001% were necessary to mediate ocular hypotension and miosis in a dose-response study.[3]

Pharmacology/Actions

Prostaglandin analogues are chemically modified versions of prostaglandin F2-alpha, an endogenous inflammatory mediator that mediates ocular hypotensive effects by increasing outflow of aqueous humor through both the trabecular meshwork and uveoscleral routes. In addition to reducing intraocular pressure (IOP), travoprost leads to miosis.

Contraindications/Precautions/Warnings

Travoprost is contraindicated in patients that have a history of hypersensitivity to it or any component of the formulation. Travoprost should be used with caution in the presence of anterior uveitis and secondary glaucoma, particularly in cases already exhibiting significant miosis, as this treatment may exacerbate miosis, promote synechiae formation, and worsen glaucoma. In addition, in dogs with primary anterior lens luxation, travoprost should be used with caution, as the resulting miosis may trap the lens and/or vitreous within the pupillary aperture, thus creating pupillary block glaucoma. Travoprost is not contraindicated in dogs with secondary posterior lens luxation, as the miosis may (favorably) trap the lens in the posterior segment.

Adverse Effects

Adverse effects associated with travoprost reported in humans or animals include blurred vision, burning and stinging, conjunctival hyperemia, foreign body sensation, itching, increased pigmentation of the iris, increased eyelash growth, and punctate epithelial keratopathy. Travoprost may cause darkening of the iris through direct stimulation of iris melanocytes, and it may worsen intraocular inflammation. Macular edema, including cystoid macular edema, has been reported after the use of travoprost in humans.

Dosages

Glaucoma (extra-label): 1 drop in the affected eye(s) once to twice daily

Monitoring

- Clinical efficacy: sustained reduction of intraocular pressure (IOP)

Client Information

- Use this medicine as directed by your veterinarian.
- Use proper administration techniques to avoid contamination of the medicine. Keep the cap tightly closed when the medicine is not in use.
- Wait 5 minutes after applying this medicine before applying any other medicines to the eye.
- Store this medicine in the refrigerator or at room temperature. Do not freeze.
- Do not use this medicine if the color changes, if it becomes cloudy, or if there are particles in the solution.

Storage/Stability

Store this product in the in the refrigerator or at room temperature (2°C-25°C [36°F-77°F]) away from moisture and sunlight; do not freeze.

Compatibility/Compounding Considerations

Travoprost preparations should not be mixed directly with any other medications.

Dosage Forms/Regulatory Status

VETERINARY-LABELED PRODUCTS: NONE

HUMAN-LABELED PRODUCTS:

Travoprost 0.004% Ophthalmic Solution (containing travoprost 0.04 mg; benzalkonium chloride 0.015%; polyoxyl 40 hydrogenated castor oil; tromethamine; boric acid; mannitol; edetate disodium; NaOH and/or HCl to adjust pH; water for injection), in sterile 2.5 mL and 5 mL ophthalmic dropper bottles; generic; (Rx)

Travoprost 0.004% Ophthalmic Solution (containing travoprost 0.04 mg; polyoxyl 40 hydrogenated castor oil; sofzia® [boric acid, propylene glycol; sorbitol; zinc chloride]; NaOH and/or HCl to adjust pH; purified water), in a sterile 2.5 mL ophthalmic dropper bottle; *Travatan Z*®; (Rx)

References

For the complete list of references, see **wiley.com/go/budde/plumb**

Trifluridine Ophthalmic

Trifluorothymidine (TFT)

(try-***floor***-ih-deen) *Viroptic*®

Antiviral (Nucleoside Analogue)

Prescriber Highlights

- ► Topical antiviral agent used in cats with feline herpesvirus-1 (FHV-1)
- ► Effective as treatment of dogs with experimentally induced canine herpesvirus-1 (CHV-1) infection
- ► Must be used 4 to 5 times daily
- ► In vitro efficacy of trifluridine is greater than that of acyclovir and idoxuridine.
- ► May cause more irritation and pain upon administration as compared with other topical antiviral agents
- ► Trifluridine is a corneal toxin and should not be used for more than 3 weeks at a time.
- ► The National Institute for Occupational Safety and Health (NIOSH) classifies trifluridine ophthalmic as a hazardous drug; use appropriate precautions when handling.

Uses/Indications

Trifluridine is used for topical treatment of feline herpesvirus-1 (FHV-1) keratitis. It may also be used for canine herpesvirus-1 (CHV-1) keratitis.[1,2] Evaluation of trifluridine's efficacy for equine herpesvirus-2 (EHV-2) keratitis has not been performed.

Pharmacology/Actions

Trifluridine interferes with DNA synthesis; however, its antiviral mechanism of action is not completely known. It is believed that trifluridine incorporates into viral DNA, as well as reversibly inhibits thymidylate synthetase, an essential enzyme in DNA synthesis. Trifluridine's in vitro efficacy is consistently greater than that of acyclovir and idoxuridine.[3,4] Trifluridine is virustatic.

Contraindications/Precautions/Warnings

Trifluridine is contraindicated in patients that have a history of hypersensitivity to it or any component of the formulation.

The National Institute for Occupational Safety and Health (NIOSH) classifies trifluridine ophthalmic as a hazardous drug; personal protective equipment (PPE) should be used accordingly to minimize the risk for exposure.

Adverse Effects

Adverse effects reported in humans or animals include acute ocular irritation, including burning, corneal stippling, vascularization, and clouding. The irritation associated with administration of trifluridine may be more intense than the inflammation caused by FHV-1. Following prolonged use of trifluridine, ocular irritation characterized by follicular conjunctivitis, blepharitis with punctal swelling, bulbar conjunctival hyperemia, and corneal epithelial staining have also been reported. In any of these cases, the drug should be discontinued.

Dosages

Keratitis caused by feline herpesvirus-1 (FHV-1) or canine herpesvirus-1 (CHV-1) (extra-label): 1 drop in the affected eye(s) every 2 to 3 hours for 48 hours and then 4 to 5 times daily for a week beyond the resolution of clinical signs. Trifluridine is a corneal toxin and should not be used for greater than 3 weeks at a time.

Monitoring

- Clinical efficacy: resolution of clinical signs (eg, corneal ulceration, corneal vascularization, conjunctivitis)

Client Information

- Give this medicine to your animal as directed by your veterinarian.
- Do not use this medication for more than 3 consecutive weeks.
- Trifluridine may cause stinging upon administration.
- Use proper administration techniques to avoid contamination of the medication. Keep the cap tightly closed when the medication is not in use.
- Wait for 5 minutes after applying this medication before applying any other medications to the eye.
- Store this medication in the refrigerator away from moisture and sunlight. Do not freeze.
- Do not use this medication if the color changes, if it becomes cloudy, or if there are particles in the solutions.
- This medication is considered to be a hazardous drug as defined by the National Institute for Occupational Safety and Health (NIOSH). Talk with your veterinarian or pharmacist about the use of personal protective equipment when handling this medicine.

Storage/Stability

Store in the refrigerator (2°C-8°C [36°F-46°F]) away from moisture and sunlight; do not freeze.

Compatibility/Compounding Considerations

Trifluridine should not be mixed directly with any other ophthalmic medications. Trifluridine is not available as an ophthalmic ointment.

Dosage Forms/Regulatory Status

VETERINARY-LABELED PRODUCTS: NONE

HUMAN-LABELED PRODUCTS:

Trifluridine aqueous 1% Ophthalmic Solution (containing trifluridine 10 mg in an aqueous solution with glacial acetic acid and sodium acetate (buffers); NaCl; thimerosal 0.001%), in a 7.5 mL ophthalmic dropper bottle; *Viroptic*®; generic; (Rx)

References

For the complete list of references, see **wiley.com/go/budde/plumb**

Triple Antibiotic Ophthalmic

(Neomycin/Polymyxin B/Bacitracin; Neomycin/Polymyxin B/Gramicidin)

Double Antibiotic Ophthalmic

(Bacitracin/Polymyxin B)

Broad-Spectrum Antimicrobial Combination Agent

Prescriber Highlights

- First choice for prophylactic antimicrobial coverage in dogs and horses with ocular surface inflammatory conditions, including ulcerative keratitis
- First choice for therapeutic antimicrobial coverage in dogs and horses with ulcerative keratitis until culture and sensitivity results are available
- Available as an ointment (neomycin/polymyxin B/bacitracin; polymyxin B/bacitracin) or solution (neomycin/polymyxin B/gramicidin)
- Some animals, particularly cats, may be hypersensitive to neomycin or polymyxin components in ointments.
- Do not confuse hydrocortisone-containing triple antibiotic ophthalmic ointment with those that lack corticosteroids.
- Prolonged use of antibiotic preparations may result in overgrowth of nonsusceptible organisms, including fungi.

Uses/Indications

Triple antibiotic ophthalmic products are used for topical treatment of superficial infections of the external eye and its adnexa caused by susceptible bacteria. Triple antibiotic ophthalmic is often used as prophylactic antimicrobial treatment prior to and following ophthalmic surgery. Triple antibiotic ophthalmic is also used for antimicrobial prophylaxis of corneal injuries and wounds. Triple antibiotic ophthalmic ointments may also contain a corticosteroid; thus, it is important to ensure that the appropriate formulation is selected. Specifically, corticosteroid-containing preparations should not be administered in patients with ulcerative keratitis. Triple antibiotic ophthalmic solutions substitute gramicidin for bacitracin. Double antibiotic ophthalmic preparations do not contain neomycin.

Pharmacology/Actions

Neomycin sulfate, an aminoglycoside, is actively transported into the bacterial cell and binds a specific receptor protein on the 30S subunit of bacterial ribosomes. It consequently interferes with the initiation complex between messenger RNA (mRNA) and the 30S subunit, inhibiting protein synthesis by inducing misreading of the mRNA. Aminoglycosides are bactericidal, whereas most other antibiotics that interfere with protein synthesis are bacteriostatic. Aminoglycosides are used primarily in infections involving aerobic, gram-negative bacteria, such as *Pseudomonas* spp, *Acinetobacter* spp, and *Enterobacter* spp. Infections caused by gram-positive bacteria, such as *Staphylococcus* spp and *Streptococcus* spp, are significantly less susceptible to neomycin.[1-4] Aminoglycosides are mostly ineffective against anaerobic bacteria, fungi, and viruses.

Polymyxin B increases the permeability of the bacterial cell membrane by interacting with the phospholipid components of the membrane for a variety of gram-negative organisms, with lesser efficacy versus gram-positive organisms such as *Streptococcus* spp.[1-4] It is bactericidal.

Bacitracin, a polypeptide antibiotic, inhibits bacterial cell wall synthesis by preventing transfer of mucopeptides into the growing cell wall. It has bactericidal activity in vitro against a variety of gram-positive organisms and a few gram-negative organisms. In practice however, topical bacitracin is most useful for gram-positive bacillus infections. Importantly, bacitracin is effective against beta-hemolytic *Streptococcus equi* ocular infections, whereas efficacy against *Pseudomonas aeruginosa* is negligible.[2-4] Bacitracin poorly penetrates the cornea and therefore is of limited value in deep corneal or intraocular infections.

In combination, neomycin sulfate, polymyxin B sulfate, and bacitracin zinc are considered active against *Staphylococcus aureus*; streptococci, including *Streptococcus pneumoniae*; *Escherichia coli*; *Haemophilus influenzae*; *Klebsiella* spp; *Enterobacter* spp; *Neisseria* spp; and *Pseudomonas aeruginosa*.

Gramicidin has activity against gram-positive organisms (not gram-positive bacilli) and some gram-negative organisms. Its mechanism of action is to bacterial cell wall permeability to inorganic cations.

Contraindications/Precautions/Warnings

Triple antibiotic combinations are contraindicated in patients that have a history of hypersensitivity to any component of the formulation. Some cats are hypersensitive to the neomycin or polymyxin component of triple antibiotic ointments.[5] This hypersensitivity has not been associated with steroid-containing triple antibiotic products. Although there is concern that prolonged use of antibiotic preparations may result in overgrowth of nonsusceptible organisms, including fungi, minimal impact on the ocular surface microbiome of dogs or horses was noted after 7 days of administration to normal eyes.[6,7]

Adverse Effects

Adverse effects reported in humans or animals include irritation and swelling upon instillation. Ophthalmic antibiotics, especially those containing neomycin sulfate and polymyxin B, may cause cutaneous sensitization and anaphylaxis, particularly in cats.[5] Clinical signs associated with sensitization to topical antibiotics can include itching, reddening, and edema of the conjunctiva and eyelid but may progress to anaphylaxis. Clinical signs usually subside quickly on withdrawing the medication, and death has been rarely reported.[8]

Dosages

Ulcerative conjunctivitis or keratitis: 1 drop of solution or ¼ inch strip of ointment in the affected eye(s) 3 to 4 times daily until resolution of ulceration and infection or until microbial susceptibilities necessitate a change to another antimicrobial agent

Nonulcerative conjunctivitis or keratitis: 1 drop of solution or ¼ inch strip of ointment in the affected eye(s) 3 to 4 times daily until resolution of infection and inflammation

Monitoring

- Clinical efficacy. Resolution of conjunctivitis or keratitis as evidenced by cytology, cultures, or remission of clinical signs

Client Information

- Use this medication as directed by your veterinarian.
- Cats may have a severe allergic reaction to one of the components of this medication. Contact your veterinarian immediately if your cat has difficulty breathing or has facial swelling after receiving this medication.
- Use proper administration techniques to avoid contamination of the medication. Do not touch the dropper/ointment tip or allow it to touch animal's eye or any other surface to prevent contamination.

- Wait for 5 to 10 minutes after applying any other medicine to your animal's eye.
- Keep the cap tightly closed when the medication is not in use. Store this medicine at room temperature away from moisture and sunlight. Do not freeze.
- Do not use this medicine if the color changes or becomes cloudy.

Storage/Stability

Store at controlled room temperature (20°C-25°C [68°F-77°F]) away from moisture and sunlight; do not freeze.

Compatibility/Compounding Considerations

Triple antibiotic ophthalmic preparations should not be mixed directly with any other ophthalmic medications.

Dosage Forms/Regulatory Status

VETERINARY-LABELED PRODUCTS:

Neomycin/Polymyxin B/Bacitracin Ophthalmic Ointment (containing neomycin sulfate equivalent to 3.5 mg neomycin base, polymyxin B sulfate equivalent to 10,000 polymyxin B units, bacitracin zinc equivalent to 400 bacitracin units, and white petrolatum and mineral oil, q.s.), in a 3.5 g ophthalmic ointment tube; *Vetropolycin®*; (Rx)

Neomycin/Polymyxin B/Bacitracin with Hydrocortisone Ophthalmic Ointment; each gram contains bacitracin zinc USP 400 units, neomycin sulfate 0.5% (equivalent to 3.5 mg neomycin base), polymyxin B sulfate USP 10,000 units, and hydrocortisone acetate USP 1% in a base of white petrolatum and mineral oil; *Vetropolycin HC®*; (Rx)

HUMAN-LABELED PRODUCTS:

Neomycin/Polymyxin B/Bacitracin Ointment (containing neomycin sulfate equivalent to 3.5 mg neomycin base, polymyxin B sulfate equivalent to 5,000 or 10,000 polymyxin B units, bacitracin zinc equivalent to 400 bacitracin units, and white petrolatum, q.s.), in a 3.5 g ophthalmic ointment tube; *Neosporin®*, *Lumi-Sporyn®*, generic; (Rx)

Neomycin/Polymyxin B/Gramicidin Ophthalmic Solution (containing polymyxin B equivalent to 1.75 mg polymyxin B base, polymyxin B sulfate equivalent to 10,000 polymyxin B units, gramicidin 0.025 mg/mL, alcohol 0.5%, thimerosal 0.001%, propylene glycol, polyoxyethylene polyoxypropylene compound, NaCl, and water for injection), in a 10 mL ophthalmic dropper bottle; *Neosporin®*, generic; (Rx)

Bacitracin and Polymyxin B Sulfate Ophthalmic Ointment (containing polymyxin B sulfate equivalent to 10,000 polymyxin B units, bacitracin zinc equivalent to 500 bacitracin units, and white petrolatum, q.s.), *AK-Poly-Bac®*, generic; (Rx)

HUMAN-LABELED COMBINATION PRODUCTS:

Neomycin and Polymyxin B Sulfates and Dexamethasone Ophthalmic Suspension (containing neomycin sulfate equivalent to neomycin 3.5 mg, polymyxin B sulfate 10,000 units, dexamethasone 0.1%, benzalkonium chloride 0.004%, hypromellose 2910 0.5%, sodium chloride, polysorbate 20, HCl and/or NaOH to adjust pH, and purified water), in a 5 mL sterile ophthalmic dropper bottle; *Maxitrol®*, *Dexasporin®*; (Rx)

Neomycin and Polymyxin B Sulfates and Dexamethasone Ophthalmic ointment (containing neomycin sulfate equivalent to neomycin 3.5 mg, polymyxin B sulfate 10,000 units, dexamethasone 0.1%, methylparaben 0.05%, propylparaben 0.01%, white petrolatum, and anhydrous liquid lanolin), in a sterile 3.5 g tube; *Maxitrol®*, generic; (Rx)

References

For the complete list of references, see **wiley.com/go/budde/plumb**

Tropicamide Ophthalmic

(troe-***pik***-uh-myde) *Mydriacyl®, Paremyd®, Tropicacyl®*

Anticholinergic Mydriatic; Cycloplegic Agent

Prescriber Highlights

- ▶ Mydriatic agent with mild cycloplegic action
- ▶ Used to produce short-term dilation for funduscopic examination or to prevent synechiae formation following cataract surgery
- ▶ More rapid onset and shorter duration of mydriasis compared with atropine
- ▶ Poor cycloplegic ability compared with atropine, resulting in minimal control of ciliary body muscle spasm
- ▶ Good corneal penetration due to lack of ionization at physiological pH
- ▶ May increase intraocular pressure (IOP); use with caution in patients with glaucoma

Uses/Indications

Tropicamide is used to produce rapid- and short-acting mydriasis for funduscopic evaluation. Tropicamide has also been used to break down synechiae in uveitis and to prevent synechiae formation following cataract surgery. It is not as effective as atropine in inducing cycloplegia and is consequently a poor choice for controlling ocular pain caused by ciliary spasm. Tropicamide has been demonstrated to overcome the miosis induced by topical ophthalmic latanoprost[1] and parenteral butorphanol[2] administration in dogs with normal eyes, without leading to elevated intraocular pressure, and thus can be used to facilitate posterior segment examination.

Pharmacology/Actions

Tropicamide causes anticholinergic effects by blocking the muscarinic receptors of the sphincter muscle of the iris and the ciliary body muscle, which produces pupillary dilation (mydriasis) and, to a lesser degree, paralysis of accommodation (cycloplegia). Tropicamide induces mydriasis in about 15 to 30 minutes, and the pupil returns to normal in 6 to 12 hours.

Contraindications/Precautions/Warnings

Tropicamide is contraindicated in patients that have a history of hypersensitivity to it or any component of the formulation. It should not be used in patients with primary glaucoma as it can induce increases in intraocular pressure (IOP).[3]

Adverse Effects

Adverse effects reported in humans include sensitivity to bright light, burning and irritation upon application, and superficial punctate keratitis. Dry mouth, tachycardia, headache, nausea, vomiting, pallor, psychotic reactions, CNS disturbances, muscle rigidity, behavioral disturbance, and vasomotor and cardiorespiratory collapse have also been reported. Hypersalivation has been reported in cats and dogs due to bitter taste. Tear production may be decreased for several hours after application of tropicamide ophthalmic in cats and horses,[4,5] and intraocular pressure (IOP) may increase in cats and dogs.[3,6]

Dosages

Mydriasis (extra-label): 1 to 2 drops repeated in 5 minutes in the eye to be examined to achieve pupillary dilation[7]

Mydriasis post-cataract removal surgery (extra-label): 1 to 2 drops into the affected eye(s) once to twice daily postoperatively to facilitate pupil mobility

Monitoring

- Clinical efficacy
- Confirm continued pupillary dilation
- Intraocular pressure (IOP)

Client Information

- Use this medicine as directed by your veterinarian.
- Use proper administration techniques to avoid contamination of the medication. Do not touch the dropper (or ointment) tip or allow it to touch your animal's eye or any other surface to prevent contamination.
- Dogs and cats may drool excessively after administration of this medication due to the bitter taste.
- Wash your hands after application to prevent accidentally getting the medicine into your eyes, which can cause pupil dilation.
- Wait 5 minutes after applying this medication before applying any other medications to the eye.
- Keep the cap tightly closed when the medication is not in use. Store this medicine at room temperature away from moisture and sunlight; do not freeze.
- Do not use this medicine if the color changes, if it becomes cloudy, or if there are particles in solutions.
- Your veterinarian will need to monitor your animal's eye condition while taking this medicine. Do not miss these important follow-up visits.

Storage/Stability

Store at controlled room temperature (20°C-25°C [68°F-77°F]) away from moisture and sunlight; do not freeze.

Compatibility/Compounding Considerations

Tropicamide should not be mixed directly with any other ophthalmic medications.

Dosage Forms/Regulatory Status

VETERINARY-LABELED PRODUCTS: NONE

HUMAN-LABELED PRODUCTS: NONE

Tropicamide 0.5% Ophthalmic Solution, USP (containing tropicamide 5 mg/mL; benzalkonium chloride 0.01%; NaCl; edetate disodium; purified water; HCl and/or NaOH to adjust pH to 4 to 5.8), in 3 mL and 15 mL dropper bottles; *Tropicacyl*®, generic; (Rx)

Tropicamide 1% Ophthalmic Solution, USP (containing tropicamide 10 mg/mL; benzalkonium chloride 0.01%; NaCl; edetate disodium; purified water; HCl and/or NaOH to adjust pH to 4 to 5.8), in 3 mL and 15 mL dropper bottles; *Mydriacyl*®, generic; (Rx)

HUMAN-LABELED COMBINATION PRODUCTS:

Hydroxyamphetamine hydrobromide 1% and Tropicamide 0.25% Ophthalmic Solution (containing hydroxyamphetamine 1%; tropicamide 0.25%; benzalkonium chloride 0.005%; edetate disodium 0.015%; NaCl; HCl and/or NaOH to adjust pH to 4.2 to 5.8; purified water), in sterile 15 mL ophthalmic dropper bottle; *Paremyd*®; (Rx)

References

For the complete list of references, see **wiley.com/go/budde/plumb**

Vancomycin Ophthalmic

(***van***-kohe-***mye***-sin)

Glycopeptide Antimicrobial Agent

For systemic use, refer to ***Vancomycin***

Prescriber Highlights

- ▶ Topical use reserved for treatment of ocular surface and intraocular infections caused by methicillin-resistant gram-positive organisms
- ▶ Not effective against gram-negative bacteria
- ▶ Not approved in an ophthalmic dosage form in the United States, although ocular dosage forms are approved in other countries

Uses/Indications

Vancomycin can be used for treating ocular surface infections caused by methicillin-resistant microorganisms, such as methicillin-resistant *Staphylococcus aureus* (MRSA) or *Staphylococcus pseudintermedius* (MRSP). Vancomycin compounded into 0.3% to 1% ophthalmic ointment has been shown to be effective in treating methicillin-resistant *Staphylococcus aureus* keratitis in a dog,[1] rabbits,[2] and humans; however, it has also been demonstrated that vancomycin is not necessary for all MRSA ocular infections, as chloramphenicol, rifampicin, and tetracyclines, among others, show varied in vitro efficacy.[3,4] Vancomycin can also be administered intravitreally for severe cases of methicillin-resistant endophthalmitis. Intracameral injection of vancomycin nanoparticles has also demonstrated good prophylactic activity against MRSA in rabbits with minimal adverse effects.[5]

The World Health Organization (WHO) has designated vancomycin as a Critically Important, Highest Priority antimicrobial for human medicine.[6]

Pharmacology/Actions

The bactericidal action of vancomycin results from inhibition of cell wall biosynthesis, which is induced by binding of the antibiotic to cell wall precursor molecules. Vancomycin is not active in vitro against gram-negative bacteria (due to different mechanisms for cell wall formation), mycobacteria, or fungi.

Contraindications/Precautions/Warnings

Vancomycin is contraindicated in patients that have a history of hypersensitivity to it or any component of the formulation.

Adverse Effects

Adverse effects reported in humans or animals include burning or stinging on application, ocular discharge, regional pruritus, and conjunctival hyperemia. Nephrotoxicity, ototoxicity, dermal toxicities, vasculitis, and severe gram-negative colitis have been associated with systemic use of vancomycin; however, these adverse effects are not likely to occur following ophthalmic use.

Dosages

Methicillin-resistant bacterial conjunctivitis or keratitis (extra-label): 1 drop of solution or ¼ inch strip of ointment applied to the affected eye(s) 4 to 5 times daily

Monitoring

- Clinical efficacy: corneal cytology and culture to evaluate for bacteria. Evaluate clinical signs suggestive of progressive infection.

Client Information

- Use this medicine as directed by your veterinarian.
- Use proper administration techniques to avoid contamination of the medicine. Keep the cap tightly closed when the medicine is not in use.
- Wait for 5 to 10 minutes after applying this medicine before applying any other medications to the eye.
- Store this product as directed on the package labeling away from moisture and sunlight. Do not freeze.
- Do not use this medicine if the color changes, if it becomes cloudy, or if there are particles in the solutions.

Storage/Stability

Store this product as directed on package labeling away from moisture and sunlight; do not freeze.

Compatibility/Compounding Considerations

Vancomycin preparations should not be mixed directly with any other medications.

Dosage Forms/Regulatory Status

VETERINARY-LABELED PRODUCTS: NONE

HUMAN-LABELED PRODUCTS: NONE

Vancomycin ophthalmic preparations are not commercially available in the United States, but vancomycin ointments and ophthalmic solutions (0.3% to 1%) have been prepared (compounded) by qualified compounding pharmacists.

References

For the complete list of references, see **wiley.com/go/budde/plumb**

Voriconazole Ophthalmic

(vohr-uh-***kon***-uh-zohl) *VFend*®

Azole Antifungal Agent

Prescriber Highlights

- ► Used as a treatment for ocular surface fungal infections
- ► Although this medication is not commercially available as an ophthalmic preparation, the commercially available IV form may be administered topically to the eye.
- ► Penetrates cornea efficiently and achieves effective concentrations in the aqueous humor
- ► Considerably more effective against filamentous fungal organisms than polyene or other azole antifungal agents
- ► The National Institute for Occupational Safety and Health (NIOSH) classifies voriconazole ophthalmic as a hazardous drug; use appropriate precautions when handling.

Uses/Indications

Ocular administration of voriconazole is primarily used to treat fungal keratitis, most commonly in horses but also in other species.[1,2] Voriconazole 1% solution for IV injection, prepared according to the package instructions, achieves effective antifungal concentrations in the aqueous humor while causing minimal to no irritation when it is administered to normal eyes of horses.[3] The same or higher concentrations have been associated with treatment success following intracorneal and subconjunctival injection in horses.[4-6] Voriconazole was associated with successful control of keratomycosis due to both filamentous and yeast organisms in dogs[2,7,8] and filamentous organisms in a cat.[1,9] Intravitreal administration is used in humans as treatment for fungal endophthalmitis.[10]

Pharmacology/Actions

Voriconazole interacts with 14-alpha-sterol demethylase, a cytochrome P-450 enzyme involved in the conversion of lanosterol to ergosterol. Ergosterol is an essential component of the fungal cell membrane and preventing its synthesis may increase cellular permeability and cause leakage of cellular contents. Other possible effects of voriconazole include inhibition of endogenous respiration, purine uptake and the transformation of yeasts to mycelial forms, and impairment of triglyceride and phospholipid biosynthesis. Because voriconazole specifically targets oxidative enzymes of fungal species, it has higher efficacy and lower host toxicity. Voriconazole has a broad antifungal spectrum against most fungi and yeasts of veterinary interest. Sensitive organisms include *Aspergillus* spp, *Candida* spp, *Fusarium* spp, and *Aspergillus* spp.[11-13]

Contraindications/Precautions/Warnings

Voriconazole is contraindicated in patients that have a history of hypersensitivity to it or any component of the formulation.

The National Institute for Occupational Safety and Health (NIOSH) classifies voriconazole ophthalmic as a hazardous drug; personal protective equipment (PPE) should be used accordingly to minimize the risk for exposure.

Adverse Effects

Adverse effects reported in humans or animals include transient burning or stinging on application. Although not reported following topical administration, neurologic signs have resulted in cats following oral administration of voriconazole.[14]

Dosages

Fungal keratitis (extra-label): 1 drop to the affected eye(s) or 0.1 mL in the subpalpebral lavage (SPL) catheter, every 2 to 3 hours initially, followed by tapering of frequency based on clinical response. Voriconazole may be administered through a SPL catheter; however, its use with constant-rate infusion pumps in conjunction with a SPL catheter is not advised due to crystallization of voriconazole within the unit.[4]

Monitoring

- Clinical efficacy: corneal scrapings with cytology and cultures to determine to clear fungal organisms; resolution of clinical signs of infection

Client Information

- Use this medication up to 10 to 12 times daily initially, with a reduction in frequency occurring as the infection resolves.
- Use proper administration techniques to avoid contamination of the medication. Keep the cap tightly closed when the medication is not in use.
- Wait 5 minutes after applying this medication before applying any other medications to the eye.
- Store this medication in the refrigerator; do not freeze.
- Do not use this medication if the color changes, if it becomes cloudy, or if there are particles in the solutions.
- This medication is considered to be a hazardous drug as defined by the National Institute for Occupational Safety and Health (NIOSH). Talk with your veterinarian or pharmacist about the use of personal protective equipment when handling this medicine.

Storage/Stability

Store this medication in the refrigerator (2°C-8°C [35.6°F-46.4°F]); do not freeze. Reconstituted solutions (see ***Compatibilty/Compounding Considerations***) are stable for 14 days (in the absence of sterility testing) when refrigerated.[15]

Compatibility/Compounding Considerations

Voriconazole ophthalmic preparations should not be mixed directly with any other ophthalmic medications. Voriconazole is not approved in an ophthalmic dosage form. A 1% ophthalmic solution can be created by aseptically reconstituting the powder in a 200 mg vial for injection with 19 mL of sterile water for injection or normal saline, according to the package instructions.[16]

Dosage Forms/Regulatory Status

VETERINARY-LABELED PRODUCTS: NONE

HUMAN-LABELED PRODUCTS: NONE

Voriconazole is available as a 200 mg lyophilized powder (*VFend*®, generic) for reconstitution to a 1% solution following the addition of 19 mL water for injection. This reconstituted solution can be safely used for topical ophthalmic administration. Voriconazole may be compounded to a 1% ointment by a qualified, licensed compounding pharmacist.

References

For the complete list of references, see **wiley.com/go/budde/plumb**

Dermatologic Agents, Topical

SANDRA KOCH, DVM, MS, DACVD
University of Minnesota, St. Paul, MN

The following section lists many of the active ingredients and examples of corresponding preparations used topically for their local action in veterinary medicine. The list includes both veterinary-labeled products and some useful human-labeled dermatologic products. In the marketplace, the drug sponsor, availability, and formulation of these products tend to change rapidly, so this listing should be used as a basic guide; always refer to the specific product label. Active ingredients are listed by therapeutic class. Products that are applied topically but are absorbed systemically and used primarily for their systemic effects are found in the systemic monograph section.

Portions of this section are adapted from Koch SN, Torres SMF, Plumb, DC. *Canine and Feline Dermatology Drug Handbook*. John Wiley & Sons, 2012. This reference provides additional detail on these and other compounds and products.

Anti-Inflammatory/Anti-Pruritic Agents, Topical

Corticosteroid Agents, Topical

NOTE: There are at least 20 chemical entities (plus a variety of salts) used in humans for topical corticosteroid therapy. The following section includes many veterinary topical products and some human products that may be of use in veterinary medicine. See also ***Otic Agents*** for more products.

Betamethasone, Topical

(bet-ah-***meth***-ah-zone)

For systemic use, refer to ***Betamethasone****.*

For otic use, refer to ***Corticosteroid/Antimicrobial Agents, Otic****.*

Indications/Actions

Betamethasone is considered a high-potency topical corticosteroid. It may be beneficial for adjunctive treatment of localized pruritic or inflammatory conditions. Because risks associated with betamethasone (eg, HPA axis suppression, systemic corticosteroid effects, skin atrophy) are higher than with hydrocortisone, betamethasone products are generally reserved for severe localized pruritic conditions or conditions for which hydrocortisone is not efficacious. Most veterinary-labeled topical betamethasone products also contain gentamicin, and labeled indications are for treating infected superficial lesions caused by bacteria sensitive to gentamicin. Additional otic products that contain an antimicrobial (eg, gentamicin) and an antifungal (eg, clotrimazole) are available. See ***Corticosteroid/Antimicrobial Agents, Otic***. These products can be used extra-label for treating localized mixed bacterial and yeast infections when potent anti-inflammatory activity is also desired. Topical dosage forms containing betamethasone as a sole ingredient are only available in products labeled for humans.

Glucocorticoids are nonspecific anti-inflammatory agents. They likely act by inducing phospholipase A2 inhibitory proteins (lipocortins) in cells, thereby reducing the formation, activity, and release of endogenous inflammatory mediators (eg, histamine, prostaglandins, kinins). Glucocorticoids also mitigate DNA synthesis via an antimitotic effect on epidermal cells. Topically applied corticosteroids also inhibit the migration of leukocytes and macrophages to the area, thereby reducing erythema, pruritus, and edema.

Ointments are the most potent vehicle, as they are the most occlusive, whereas creams tend to be less potent than ointments of the same medication/strength, followed by lotions and gels.[1]

Suggested Dosages/Uses

Betamethasone formulations are best suited for focal (eg, pedal) or multifocal lesions for relatively short durations (ie, less than 2 months). See ***Precautions/Adverse Effects***. Initially, topical glucocorticoids are used sparingly 1 to 4 times per day, and then the frequency is tapered when control is achieved. Long-term, frequent use can cause HPA axis suppression; risk can be reduced by treating for only as long as necessary on as small an area as possible. Refer to the individual product label for specific dosing recommendations.

Precautions/Adverse Effects

Several veterinary topical products list pregnancy as a contraindication. Systemic glucocorticoids can be teratogenic or induce parturition during the third trimester of pregnancy in animals. If considering use during pregnancy, weigh the respective risks with treating versus the potential benefits. Owners should wash their hands after application or wear gloves when applying. Avoid contact with eyes. Do not allow the animal to lick or chew at affected sites for at least 20 to 30 minutes after application. Occlusive dressings increase glucocorticoid penetration and can increase the risk for systemic side effects.

- Reactions to allergen **intradermal skin tests** may be suppressed by glucocorticoids.[2,3] A 2-week (14-day) withdrawal time before intradermal skin testing is recommended for dogs and cats[4,5]; no withdrawal time is required before serum IgE testing to identify sensitizing allergens in cats.[5]

Use care when treating large areas or when using on small-sized patients. Higher potency, increased concentration, or long duration of use increases risks for HPA axis suppression, immune suppression, systemic glucocorticoid effects (eg, PU/PD, polyphagia, vomiting, diarrhea), and complications caused by skin atrophy (eg, skin fragility, alopecia, localized pyoderma, comedones, weakened barrier function). Betamethasone may delay wound healing, primarily if used longer than 7 days. Vomiting and diarrhea have been reported after ingestion of topical products containing betamethasone. Local skin reactions (eg, burning, itching, redness) are possible but uncommon.

Veterinary-Labeled Products

NOTE: There are no veterinary-labeled topical products in the United States that contain betamethasone as a single active ingredient.

Active ingredients (formulation)	Species	Label status; size(s)	Trade names/additional information
Gentamicin 0.57 mg/mL, betamethasone valerate 0.284 mg/mL (spray) Other ingredients: propylene glycol, isopropyl alcohol, parabens	Labeled for dogs	Rx; depending on the product: 60 mL, 72 mL, 120 mL, and 240 mL	*Gentocin*®; *GentaCalm*®; *GentaSpray*®; *Betagen*®; *Gentamicin*®; *Gentaved*®; *GentaSoothe*®; *GenOne*®; *Relifor*®

Human-Labeled Products

NOTE: This is a partial listing. Do not confuse products containing *augmented* betamethasone dipropionate (eg, *Diprolene*®) with betamethasone dipropionate. Augmented betamethasone dipropionate is more potent than betamethasone dipropionate. For more information on human-labeled betamethasone products, refer to a comprehensive human drug reference or contact a pharmacist.

Active ingredients (formulation)	Label status; size(s)	Trade names/additional information
Betamethasone dipropionate 0.05% (ointment)	Rx; 15 g, 45 g	generic
Betamethasone dipropionate 0.05% (cream)	Rx; 15 g, 45 g	generic
Betamethasone dipropionate 0.05% (lotion)	Rx; 60 mL	generic
Betamethasone valerate 0.1% (ointment)	Rx; 30 g, 45 g	generic
Betamethasone valerate 0.1% (cream)	Rx; 15 g	generic
Betamethasone valerate 0.1% (lotion)	Rx; 60 mL	generic
Betamethasone valerate 0.12% (foam)	Rx; 300 g	*Luxiq*®; generic
Clotrimazole 1%, betamethasone dipropionate 0.05% (lotion)	Rx; 30 mL	generic
Clotrimazole 1%, betamethasone dipropionate 0.05% (cream)	Rx; 15 g, 45 g	*Lotrisone*®

References

For the complete list of references, see **wiley.com/go/budde/plumb**

Hydrocortisone, Topical

(hye-droe-***kor***-ti-zone)

Indications/Actions

Hydrocortisone is a topical corticosteroid that may be useful for adjunctive treatment of localized pruritic and/or inflammatory conditions. Due to its low potency, hydrocortisone is a reasonable first choice for larger focal areas or for small-sized patients. Some products contain additional ingredients (eg, Burow's solution [aluminum acetate], pramoxine) that may have additional antipruritic effects.

Topical glucocorticoids are nonspecific anti-inflammatory agents. They are thought to act by inducing phospholipase A_2 inhibitory proteins (lipocortins) in cells, thereby reducing the formation, activity, and release of endogenous inflammatory mediators (eg, histamine, prostaglandins, kinins). Glucocorticoids also reduce DNA synthesis via an antimitotic effect on epidermal cells. Topically applied glucocorticoids also inhibit the migration of leukocytes and macrophages to the area, reducing erythema, pruritus, and edema.

Suggested Dosages/Uses

Hydrocortisone formulations are best suited for focal (eg, pedal) or multifocal lesions for relatively short durations (ie, less than 2 months; see ***Precautions/Adverse Effects***).

Initially, topical glucocorticoid creams and ointments are applied 1 to 4 times daily, and then the frequency is tapered after control is achieved. In contrast to some more potent topical corticosteroids, hydrocortisone can be applied more frequently and over a greater surface area, with less risk for local or systemic adverse effects; however, long-term frequent use can still cause HPA axis suppression. Risk can be reduced by treating patients for only as long as necessary on the smallest area possible.

Shampoos containing hydrocortisone are generally used from once a week up to once a day. They typically should remain in contact with the skin for at least 10 minutes before rinsing.

Precautions/Adverse Effects

Several veterinary topical products list pregnancy as a contraindication. Owners should wash their hands after application or wear gloves when applying. Avoid contact with eyes. Do not allow the animal to lick or chew at affected sites for at least 20 to 30 minutes after application. Occlusive dressings increase glucocorticoid penetration and can increase the risk for systemic adverse effects. The risks associated with hydrocortisone are significantly less when compared with higher potency corticosteroids (eg, betamethasone).

Local skin reactions are possible but uncommon. Atrophy associated with skin fragility, superficial follicular cysts (milia), and comedones may be seen with long-term frequent use, but these conditions occur more commonly when using more potent topical corticosteroids (eg, betamethasone). Although systemic absorption is rare with hydrocortisone, long-term use may lead to HPA axis suppression. Accidental ingestion may cause GI signs such as nausea, vomiting, or diarrhea.[1]

Reactions to allergen intradermal skin tests may be suppressed by glucocorticoids.[2,3] A 2-week (14-day) withdrawal time before intradermal skin testing is recommended for dogs and cats[4,5]; no withdrawal time is required before serum IgE testing to identify sensitizing allergens in cats.[5]

Veterinary-Labeled Products

Refer to the individual product labeling for specific dosing recommendations and inactive ingredients.

Active ingredients (formulation)	Species	Label status; size(s)	Trade names/additional information
Hydrocortisone 0.5% (lotion)	Labeled for dogs	OTC; 4 oz	*Dogswell®*
Hydrocortisone 1% (lotion)	Labeled for dogs, cats, and horses	OTC; 8 oz	*Vetergen Hydrocortisone; AtopiCream HC*
Hydrocortisone 0.5% (cream)	Labeled for dogs and cats	OTC; 1 oz	*Zymox®*
Hydrocortisone 1% (cream)	Labeled for dogs and cats	OTC; 1 oz	*Zymox®*
Hydrocortisone 0.5% (spray)	Labeled for dogs	OTC; 5 oz	*Hartz®*
Hydrocortisone 1% (spray)	Labeled for dogs and cats	OTC; 2 oz	*Zymox®*
Hydrocortisone 1%, chlorhexidine 4%, (spray)	Labeled for dogs, cats, and horses	OTC; 8 oz	*TrizCHLOR® 4HC*
Hydrocortisone 1%, pramoxine 1% (spray)	Labeled for dogs and cats	OTC; 4 oz, 8 oz	*Comfort HC®; Vetraseb®* HC
Hydrocortisone 1%, acetic acid 1%, boric acid 2%, ketoconazole 0.15% (spray)	Labeled for dogs, cats, and horses	OTC; 8 oz	*MalAcetic® ULTRA*
Hydrocortisone 1%, Burow's solution 2% (solution)	Labeled for dogs and/or cats	OTC or Rx; 1 oz, 2 oz, and 16 oz bottle	*Cort/Astrin®; Corti-Derm®; Bur-O-Cort 2:1®; Hydro-B 1020®; Hydro-Plus®*
Hydrocortisone 0.5%, chlorhexidine 2%, ketoconazole 1% (salve)	Labeled for dogs, cats, and horses	OTC; 4 oz	*EquiShield® CK HC*
Hydrocortisone 1%, chlorhexidine 4% (shampoo)	Labeled for dogs, cats, and/or horses	OTC; 8 oz, 16 oz	*TrizCHLOR 4HC; Chlorhexidine 4% HC*
Hydrocortisone 1%, chlorhexidine 2%, ketoconazole 1% (shampoo)	Labeled for dogs, cats, and horses	OTC; 12 oz	*EquiShield® CK HC*
Hydrocortisone 1%, acetic acid 1%, boric acid 2%, ketoconazole 0.15% (shampoo)	Labeled for dogs and cats	OTC; 8 oz	*MalAcetic® ULTRA*
Hydrocortisone 1%, acetic acid 1%, boric acid 1% (wipes)	Labeled for dogs and cats	OTC; 25 count jar	*MalAcetic® HC*

Human-Labeled Products

NOTE: Partial listing; there are many branded products available with hydrocortisone. For more information on human-labeled hydrocortisone products, refer to a comprehensive human drug reference (eg, *Facts and Comparisons*) or contact a pharmacist.

Active ingredients (formulation)	Label status; size(s)	Trade names/additional information
Hydrocortisone 0.5%, hydrocortisone 1% (ointment)	OTC/Rx; 25 g, 28 g, 28.35 g, 28.4 g, 30 g, 56 g, 110 g, 430 g, and 454 g	Status determined by labeling
Hydrocortisone 2.5% (ointment)	Rx; 20 g, 28.35 g, 435.6 g, and 454 g	
Hydrocortisone 0.5%, hydrocortisone 1% (cream)	OTC/Rx; 1 g, 1.5 g packets, 14 g, 14.2 g, 15 g, 20 g, 26 g, 28 g, 28.3 g, 28.35 g, 28.4 g, 30 g, 42 g, 56 g, 120 g, and 454 g	Status determined by labeling
Hydrocortisone 2.5% (cream)	Rx; 15 g, 20 g, 28 g, 28.35 g, 30 g, and 454 g	
Hydrocortisone 1% (lotion)	OTC/Rx; 30 mL, 59 mL, 60 mL, 88.7 mL, 99 mL, 113 mL, 114 mL, 118 mL, and 120 mL	Status determined by labeling
Hydrocortisone 2%, hydrocortisone 2.5% (lotion)	Rx; 29.6 mL (2% only), 59 mL and 118 mL (2.5% only)	*Ala Scalp®; Scalacort®;* generic
Hydrocortisone 1% (gel)	OTC; 28 g, 30 g, 42.53 g, and 56 g	
Hydrocortisone 2.5% (gel)	Rx; 43 g	
Hydrocortisone 10% (gel compounding kit)	Rx; 60 g jar	*First-Hydrocortisone®*
Hydrocortisone 1%, hydrocortisone 2.5% (solution)	OTC/Rx; 30 mL, 44 mL, 59 mL, and 120 mL	
Hydrocortisone 1% (foam)	OTC; 88.7 mL	*Itch-X®*
Hydrocortisone 1% (applicator)	OTC; 36 mL	*Cortizone-10 Easy Relief®*

References

For the complete list of references, see **wiley.com/go/budde/plumb**

Isoflupredone Combinations, Topical

(eye-soe-***floo***-preh-dohn)

Indications/Actions

Isoflupredone is a high-potency topical corticosteroid. In combination with neomycin and tetracaine, isoflupredone is indicated in dogs as a dressing for minor cuts and abrasions, as a postsurgical therapy, and for treating anal gland infections and moist dermatitis.[1] It is indicated in cats and horses as a dressing for minor cuts and abrasions and as postsurgical therapy.[1,2]

Because risks associated with isoflupredone (eg, HPA axis suppression, systemic corticosteroid effects, skin atrophy) are higher than with hydrocortisone, these products are generally reserved for severe localized pruritic conditions or for conditions when hydrocortisone is not efficacious.

Corticosteroids are nonspecific anti-inflammatory agents. They are thought to act by inducing phospholipase A2 inhibitory proteins (lipocortins) in cells, thereby reducing the formation, activity, and release of endogenous inflammatory mediators (eg, histamine, prostaglandins, kinins). Corticosteroids also mitigate DNA synthesis via an anti-mitotic effect on epidermal cells. Topically applied corticosteroids also inhibit the migration of leukocytes and macrophages to the area, reducing erythema, pruritus, and edema.

Suggested Dosages/Uses

Clean the affected area prior to application of isoflupredone. Apply a small amount of ointment or powder 1 to 3 times daily as needed and continue based on clinical response.[1,2]

Precautions/Adverse Effects

Topical corticosteroids are often considered contraindicated in patients that are pregnant or have tuberculosis of the skin. Systemic corticosteroids can be teratogenic or induce parturition during the third trimester of pregnancy in animals. If isoflupredone is being considered for use during pregnancy, weigh the risks for treating versus the potential benefits.

Residual activity may affect intradermal or allergy serum tests; it is recommended to discontinue use of isoflupredone 2 weeks before allergy testing.[3] Isoflupredone may delay wound healing, particularly when used longer than 7 days.

Isoflupredone products may be harmful if swallowed; prevent treated animals from licking or chewing at affected sites for at least 20 to 30 minutes after application. Powdered formulations may cause allergy or asthma symptoms if inhaled.[2]

Wear gloves or wash hands after application. Avoid contact with eyes.

Use isoflupredone cautiously on large treatment areas and on small-sized patients. Treat the smallest area possible for the minimum duration. The prolonged use of corticosteroid products increases the risk for HPA axis suppression, systemic corticosteroid effects (eg, polydipsia, polyuria, iatrogenic hyperadrenocorticism, skin atrophy). Local skin reactions (eg, burning, itching, redness) or hypersensitivity reactions are possible.

Veterinary-Labeled Products

Active ingredients (formulation)	Species	Label status; size(s)	Trade names/additional information
Isoflupredone acetate 0.1%, neomycin sulfate 0.5%, tetracaine HCl 0.5% (ointment)	Labeled for dogs, cats, and horses	Rx; 10 g tube	*Neo-Predef® with Tetracaine; Tritop®*
Isoflupredone acetate 0.1%, neomycin sulfate 0.5%, tetracaine HCl 0.5% (powder)	Labeled for dogs, cats, and horses	Rx; 15 g insufflator bottle	*Neo-Predef® with Tetracaine* Store in a dry place. Do not allow the tip of the bottle to contact moisture.

Human-Labeled Products

None

References

For the complete list of references, see **wiley.com/go/budde/plumb**

Mometasone, Topical

(moe-***met***-a-zone)

For otic use, see ***Corticosteroid/Antimicrobial Agents, Otic.***

Indications

Mometasone is a high-potency topical corticosteroid. It may be beneficial for adjunctive treatment of pruritic and inflammatory conditions. Mometasone products are generally reserved for severe pruritic conditions or for hydrocortisone treatment failures, as the risks associated with mometasone (eg, HPA axis suppression, skin atrophy) are higher than with hydrocortisone.

Mometasone is found in several veterinary-labeled otic suspensions in combination with antibiotics and antifungals. These otic combination products have been used topically extra-label for yeast and bacterial skin infections when a potent anti-inflammatory effect is needed but should only be used when there is evidence of bacterial or yeast infections.

Corticosteroids are non-specific anti-inflammatory agents. They are thought to induce phospholipase A2 inhibitory proteins (lipocortins) in cells, thereby reducing the formation, activity, and release of endogenous inflammatory mediators (eg, histamine, prostaglandins, kinins). Corticosteroids also reduce DNA synthesis via an anti-mitotic effect on epidermal cells. Topically applied corticosteroids also inhibit the migration of leukocytes and macrophages to the area, reducing erythema, pruritus, and edema.

Suggested Dosages/Uses

Mometasone should be applied sparingly, initially 1 to 2 times daily then less frequent as clinical signs improve. Mometasone formulations are best suited for focal (eg, pedal) or multifocal lesions that require relatively short treatment durations (ie, less than 2 months). Frequency of application and duration of treatment should be based on the severity of clinical signs. For veterinary-labeled products, refer to the specific product label for additional usage information.

Precautions/Adverse Effects

Safe use of mometasone during pregnancy is not established; it should only be used when the benefits outweigh the risks. Use cautiously on large treatment areas or in small-sized patients due to risk for systemic absorption. Treat only for as long as necessary on as small of an area as possible to reduce the risk for toxicities such as HPA axis suppression, systemic corticosteroid effects (eg, polydipsia, polyuria, iatrogenic Cushing's, adverse GI effects), and cutaneous atrophy associated with skin fragility. Other potential adverse effects that occur with increases in product concentrations and prolonged duration of use include alopecia, localized pyoderma, superficial follicular cysts (milia), and comedones. Local skin reactions (eg, burning, pruritus, erythema) are possible but unlikely. Mometasone may delay wound healing, particularly if used longer than 7 days. Do not let treated animals lick or chew at affected areas for at least 20 to 30 minutes after application; ingestion may result in GI upset. Occlusive dressings increase steroid penetration and can increase the risk for systemic adverse effects.

Reactions to allergen intradermal skin tests may be suppressed by glucocorticoids. A 2-week (14-day) withdrawal time before intradermal skin testing is recommended for dogs and cats[1]; no withdrawal time is required before serum IgE testing to identify sensitizing allergens in cats.[2]

Wash hands after handling or wear gloves during application. Avoid contact with eyes.

Veterinary-Labeled Products

Active ingredients (formulation)	Species	Label status; size(s)	Trade names/additional information
Mometasone 1 mg/g, gentamicin 3 mg/g, clotrimazole 10 mg/g (suspension)	Labeled for otic use in dogs	Rx; 7.5 g, 15 g, 30 g, and 215 g tubes	*Mometamax®; Malmetazone®; Mometavet®; Maxi-Otic®; MotaZol®* Topical use is extra-label.
Mometasone 1 mg/g, orbifloxacin 10 mg/g, posaconazole 1 mg/g (suspension)	Labeled for otic use in dogs	Rx; 7.5 g, 15 g, and 30 g tubes	*Posatex®* Topical use is extra-label.

Human-Labeled Products

NOTES:

1. Mometasone furoate is the salt generally used in pharmaceutical products.
2. Many commercial products exist. Below is a representative list of available products. For more information on human-labeled mometasone products, refer to a comprehensive human drug reference or contact a pharmacist.

Active ingredients (formulation)	Label status; size(s)	Trade names/additional information
Mometasone furoate 0.1% (cream)	Rx; 15 g and 45 g	generic
Mometasone furoate 0.1% (ointment)	Rx; 15 g and 45 g	generic
Mometasone furoate 0.1% (lotion)	Rx; 30 mL and 60 mL	*Elocon®*; generic
Mometasone furoate 0.1% (solution)	Rx; 30 mL and 60 mL	generic
Mometasone furoate 50 µg/100 mg (nasal spray)	OTC; 10 mL and 17 mL bottle	*Nasonex®* Extra-label when used topically

References

For the complete list of references, see **wiley.com/go/budde/plumb**

Triamcinolone, Topical

(trye-am-***sin***-oh-lone)

For systemic use, see ***Triamcinolone.***

For otic use, see ***Corticosteroid/Antimicrobial Agents, Otic.***

Indications/Actions

Triamcinolone is generally considered a medium potency corticosteroid at concentrations less than 0.5%. It may be beneficial for adjunctive treatment of pruritic or inflammatory conditions. Triamcinolone products are typically reserved for severe pruritic conditions or for conditions when hydrocortisone is not efficacious, as the risk for HPA axis suppression and skin atrophy are higher than with hydrocortisone.

Triamcinolone can be found as a sole agent in some veterinary creams or sprays, although most of these contain an antibiotic and/or antifungal agent. These products can be used for treating localized mixed bacterial and yeast infections when potent anti-inflammatory activity is also desired. Additional otic products that contain an antibiotic and an antifungal are available. See ***Corticosteroid/Antimicrobial Agents, Otic***.

Corticosteroids are non-specific anti-inflammatory agents. They are thought to induce phospholipase A2 inhibitory proteins (lipocortins) in cells, thereby reducing the formation, activity, and release of endogenous inflammatory mediators (eg, histamine, prostaglandins, kinins). Corticosteroids also mitigate DNA synthesis via an anti-mitotic effect on epidermal cells. Topically applied corticosteroids also inhibit the migration of leukocytes and macrophages to the area, reducing erythema, pruritus, and edema.

Suggested Dosages/Uses

Topical triamcinolone is best suited for focal (eg, pedal) or multifocal lesions for relatively short durations (ie, less than 2 months). Triamcinolone ointment should be applied sparingly, initially 1 to 4 times daily and then tapered when control is achieved. Triamcinolone spray is labeled for use twice daily for 7 days, then once daily for 7 days, then every other day for 14 days. For veterinary products, refer to the specific product label for dosing recommendations.

Precautions/Adverse Effects

Systemic corticosteroids can be teratogenic or induce parturition during the third trimester of pregnancy in animals. If considering use during pregnancy, weigh the risks of treating versus potential benefits. Wear gloves when applying and wash hands after application. Spray should be applied in a well-ventilated area. Avoid contact with eyes. Do not allow animals to lick or chew at affected sites for at least 20 to 30 minutes after application; oral ingestion may result in GI upset.

Reactions to allergen intradermal skin tests may be suppressed by glucocorticoids. A 2-week (14-day) withdrawal time before intradermal skin testing is recommended for dogs and cats[1]; no withdrawal time is required before serum IgE testing to identify sensitizing allergens in cats.[2]

Long-term, frequent use can cause HPA axis suppression. Treat for only as long as necessary on as small of an area as possible using the lowest effective concentration to reduce the risk for HPA axis suppression, cutaneous effects (eg, skin atrophy, skin fragility, alopecia, localized pyoderma, comedones), and other systemic corticosteroid effects (eg, polydipsia, polyuria, iatrogenic Cushing's, GI effects). Use with caution when treating small-sized patients or large areas. Triamcinolone may delay wound healing, mainly if used longer than 7 days. Local skin reactions (eg, burning, itching, redness) are also possible.

Veterinary-Labeled Products

Active ingredients (formulation)	Species	Label status; size(s)	Trade names/additional information
Triamcinolone acetonide 0.015% (spray)	Labeled for dogs	Rx; 8 oz, 16 oz bottle	*Genesis*®
Triamcinolone acetonide 0.1% (cream)	Labeled for dogs	Rx; 7.5 g, 15 g	*Medalone*®; *Vetalog*® Although these products are still listed in the FDA Green Book of approved animal drugs, they may no longer be commercially available.
Triamcinolone acetonide 1 mg/g, neomycin 2.5 mg/g, thiostrepton 2500 units/g, nystatin 100,000 units/g (cream)	Labeled for dogs and cats	Rx; 7.5 g, 15 g tube	*Animax*®; *Derma-Vet*®; *Panalog*® Although these products are still listed in the FDA Green Book of approved animal drugs, they may no longer be commercially available.
Triamcinolone acetonide 1 mg/mL, neomycin 2.5 mg/mL, thiostrepton 2500 units/mL, nystatin 100,000 units/mL, (ointment)	Labeled for dogs and cats	Rx; 7.5 mL, 15 mL, 30 mL, and 240 mL	*Animax*®; *Derma-Vet*®; *Dermalog*®; *Dermalone*®; *EnteDerm*®; *Quadritop*®; *Quadruple*®; *Resortin*®; *VetaDerm Tetrafect*®

Human-Labeled Products

NOTE: For more information on human-labeled triamcinolone products, refer to a comprehensive human drug reference or contact a pharmacist.

Active ingredients (formulation)	Label status; size(s)	Trade names/additional information
Triamcinolone acetonide 0.025% (ointment)	Rx; 15 g, 80 g, 454 g	generic
Triamcinolone acetonide 0.05% (ointment)	Rx; 430 g	*Trianex*®; generic
Triamcinolone acetonide 0.1% (ointment)	Rx; 15 g, 80 g, 454 g	generic
Triamcinolone acetonide 0.5% (ointment)	Rx; 15 g	generic
Triamcinolone acetonide 0.025% (cream)	Rx; 15 g, 85.2 g, 454 g	*Triderm*®; generic
Triamcinolone acetonide 0.1% (cream)	Rx; 28.4 g, 85.2 g	*Triderm*®; generic
Triamcinolone acetonide 0.5% (cream)	Rx; 15 g, 454 g	*Triderm*®; generic
Triamcinolone acetonide 0.025% (lotion)	Rx; 60 mL	generic
Triamcinolone acetonide 0.1% (lotion)	Rx; 60 mL	generic
Triamcinolone acetonide 0.147 mg/g (spray)	Rx; 63 g, 100 g	*Kenalog*®; generic 10.3% alcohol
Triamcinolone acetonide 0.1%, nystatin 100,000 units/g (cream)	Rx; 15 g, 30 g, 60 g	generic
Triamcinolone acetonide 0.1%, nystatin 100,000 units/g (ointment)	Rx; 15 g, 30 g, 60 g	generic

References

For the complete list of references, see **wiley.com/go/budde/plumb**

Non-Corticosteroid Agents, Topical

Aluminum Acetate Solution, Topical
Burow's Solution

(ah-***loo***-mi-num ***ass***-ih-tate)

Astringent

For otic use, see ***Corticosteroid Agents, Otic.***

Indications/Actions

Aluminum acetate solution (Burow's solution, modified Burow's solution) is an astringent antipruritic agent that can be used for adjunctive treatment of minor skin irritations, such as insect bites and localized inflamed and exudative skin conditions (eg, acute moist dermatitis, fold dermatitis [intertrigo], contact dermatitis). This solution can also be used to reduce inflammation associated with otitis externa (see ***Corticosteroid Agents, Otic***). In addition to astringent and antipruritic actions, aluminum acetate solution also has acidifying effects and it is mildly antiseptic. The exact mechanisms of action for each of these effects is not fully understood; it was shown to have an antibacterial effect against Staphylococcus aureus and Pseudomonas aeruginosa through alterations and damage to the cell wall and bacteriolysis.[1]

Suggested Dosages/Uses

Topical use of aluminum acetate as a single agent is usually via a wet compress, dressing, or soak. Application for 15 to 30 minutes is generally recommended, and the affected area is air-dried between applications. Use can be as often as necessary, but every 4 to 6 hours is often employed. As aluminum acetate solution products come in various dosage forms (powder or tablets for dissolving, liquid), refer to package directions for proper dilutions; dilutions of 1:40, 1:20, or 1:10 are commonly used. Various generic products exist. **NOTE**: The commercially prepared, veterinary-labeled products that also contain hydrocortisone may be directly applied without dilution. See ***Hydrocortisone, Topical***.

Precautions/Adverse Effects

Do not cover application site with plastic or occlusive dressing to try to prevent product evaporation. Use cool or warm[2] water for dissolving powder/tablets. Avoid contact with eyes. Pet owners should wash their hands after application. Aluminum acetate solution may cause dry skin or skin irritation in some patients. For products containing hydrocortisone, prolonged use should be avoided or limited to 1 to 2 weeks at a time to prevent potential skin atrophy and systemic absorption. A minimum of a 2-week withdrawal period is recommended for these products before intradermal or allergy serum testing. See ***Hydrocortisone, Topical***.

Veterinary-Labeled Products

Active ingredients (formulation)	Label status; size(s)	Trade names/additional information
Aluminum acetate 2%, hydrocortisone 1% (solution) Other ingredients: water, propylene glycol	OTC; 1 oz, 2 oz, 16 oz	*Cort/Astrin®; Corti-Derm®; Hydro-B 1020*

Human-Labeled Products

NOTE: In some products, aluminum acetate solution may be listed as aluminum sulfate and calcium acetate combined in water.

Active ingredients (formulation)	Label status; size(s)	Trade names/additional information
Aluminum sulfate tetradecahydrate, 1347 mg; calcium acetate monohydrate, 952 mg (powder)	OTC; packets of various concentrations (12/box)	*Domeboro®* Dilute as directed. When combined with water, the active ingredient (aluminum acetate) is formed.
Aluminum acetate 0.5% (gel)	OTC; 3 oz	*Domeboro®*
Aluminum acetate 0.2% (gel) Other ingredients: dehydroacetic acid, ethylhexylglycerin, glycine, hexylene glycol, malic acid	OTC; 2 oz	*TriCalm®*

References

For the complete list of references, see **wiley.com/go/budde/plumb**

Camphor/Menthol/Phenol, Topical

(***kam***-for; ***men***-thol; ***fee***-nol)

Indications/Actions

When used in low concentrations, camphor/menthol/phenol products can be used as counterirritants; they may be added to proprietary or compounded products, primarily as antipruritics. Camphor and phenol may also have some antiseptic properties. Camphor and menthol act by stimulating and desensitizing nociceptors.[1] Camphor produces a warming sensation, whereas menthol produces a cooling effect.[2]

Precautions/Adverse Effects

These compounds may cause local irritation and should not be used around or in the eyes. Products containing phenol should NOT be used on cats.

Veterinary-Labeled Products

NOTE: There are also several over-the-counter (OTC) products containing menthol, phenol, or camphor; these products are not listed below and are used primarily on equine patients for overexertion, soreness, or stiffness. These include a variety of liniments (eg, white liniment, Choate's liniment) or gels (eg, *Cool Gel*®, *Ice-O-Gel*®, *Shin-O-Gel*®).

Active ingredients (formulation)	Species	Label status; size(s)	Trade names/additional information
Menthol 7.5 mg/mL, oil of camphor 7.5 mg/mL, oil of eucalyptus 7.5 mg/mL, oil of pine 7.5 mg/mL, oil of thyme 2.8 mg/mL, Peru balsam 1.5 mg/mL, phenol 7.5 mg/mL, biebrich scarlet red 100 ppm (spray)	Labeled for superficial cuts, wounds, and burns for horses and mules	OTC; 500 mL	Many trade names Shake well

References

For the complete list of references, see **wiley.com/go/budde/plumb**

Colloidal Oatmeal, Topical

(ko-***loyd***-al ***ote***-meel)

Indications/Actions

Colloidal oatmeal is made from oat grains (*Avena sativa*) and is used topically as an anti-inflammatory, antipruritic, and emollient agent. It ameliorates and provides soothing effects in pruritic, inflamed, and dry and/or scaly skin disorders, such as atopic dermatitis and irritant skin reactions. Although colloidal oatmeal's mechanism of action is not completely understood, avenanthramides, one of its antioxidant phenolic compounds, have been shown to exert anti-inflammatory effects in the skin by inhibiting activities of pro-inflammatory cytokines in human epidermal keratinocytes.[1] Avenanthramides were also shown to inhibit histamine release, prostaglandin biosynthesis, and cleavage of arachidonic acid from phospholipids in keratinocytes. In animal models, avenanthramides also reduced scratching and inflammatory cytokines implicated in pruritus; the antipruritic effect appears to increase as the oatmeal concentration increases. Colloidal oatmeal also forms a hydrophilic film that retains and replenishes moisture in the stratum corneum, and it also helps to normalize the skin's pH. Moreover, colloidal oatmeal was found to improve the epidermal skin barrier by inducing and upregulating the expression of important skin barrier markers in human equivalent keratinocytes.

Suggested Dosages/Uses

Spray formulations can be used 2 to 3 times per day or as needed for itching or pain. Shampoo or conditioner is usually used once a day to once a week. Shampoo should be in contact with the skin for at least 5 to 10 minutes and then rinsed well. Refer to each product's label for further details.

Precautions/Adverse Effects

Colloidal oatmeal has been known to be very safe. In humans, there are some reports of contact dermatitis associated with its use; however, most data indicate a low potential for oatmeal-containing products to cause irritation or allergic sensitization. Some animals might develop sensitivity (eg, pruritus, erythema) to some of these topical agents, in which case the product should be discontinued. Because colloidal oatmeal has a potential antihistamine effect, a minimum of a 2-week withdrawal period is recommended before intradermal testing.

Veterinary-Labeled Products

NOTE: Products listed are representative of those containing only colloidal oatmeal as the principal active ingredient.

Active ingredients (formulation)	Species	Label status; size(s)	Trade names/additional information
Colloidal oatmeal (leave-on spray) Other ingredients: ceramides, safflower oil	Labeled for dogs, cats, and horses	OTC; 8 oz, 12 oz, and 1 gallon	*Dermallay*®

Active ingredients (formulation)	Species	Label status; size(s)	Trade names/additional information
Colloidal oatmeal 1% (cream rinse) Other ingredients: lactic acid, propylene glycol	Labeled for dogs, cats, and horses	OTC; 8 oz, 16 oz, and 1 gallon	*Epi-Soothe®*
Colloidal oatmeal (conditioner); other ingredients vary	Labeled for dogs and cats	OTC; 16 oz, 17 oz, 1 gallon	*Aloe & Oatmeal Skin and Coat; Aloe & Oatmeal®*
Colloidal oatmeal (shampoo); other ingredients vary	Labeled for dogs and cats; some products labeled for horses	OTC; 4 oz, 8 oz, 12 oz, 16 oz, 17 oz, 1 gallon	*Aloe & Oatmeal®; Dermallay®*(soap free); *Epi-Soothe®; Vet Solutions Aloe & Oatmeal®; Simply Pure®; Aloe and Oatmeal* (soap and alcohol-free); *Aloe Oatmeal* (soap-free)

Human-Labeled Products

NOTE: There are several human products available containing colloidal oatmeal, including creams, lotions, and products, to be added to the bath. Common trade names include *Aveeno®*, *Geri Silk®*, and *Actibath®*.

References

For the complete list of references, see **wiley.com/go/budde/plumb**

Diphenhydramine, Topical

(dye-fen-***hye***-dra-meen) *Benadryl®*

For systemic use, see ***Diphenhydramine.***

Indications/Actions

Diphenhydramine is a first-generation antihistamine that has some local anesthetic activity. This activity is probably its primary antipruritic mechanism of action. Diphenhydramine may be absorbed in small amounts transdermally but is unlikely to cause systemic adverse effects with typical use.

Suggested Dosages/Uses

Topical creams, ointments, gels, lotions, or sprays are usually applied 1 to 3 times a day as needed. The shampoos and conditioners are generally used once a week to once a day after bathing, respectively. Shampoos should remain in contact with the skin for at least 10 minutes before being rinsed. Check product label for specific instructions.

Precautions/Adverse Effects

Avoid contact with eyes or mucous membranes. Do not apply to blistered or oozing areas of the skin. Fatalities have rarely been reported in children after excessive exposure (ie, application to a large percentage of body surface area with open sores); veterinary significance is uncertain. Pet owners should wash their hands after application or wear gloves when applying.

Prolonged use could potentially cause local irritation and/or hypersensitization. Residual activity may affect intradermal or allergy serum tests. It has been suggested to stop using this product 2 weeks before allergy intradermal testing.

Veterinary-Labeled Products

Active ingredients (formulation)	Species	Label status; size(s)	Trade names/additional information
Diphenhydramine 1%, pramoxine 1%, (conditioner spray)	Labeled for dogs and cats	OTC; 8 oz	*Benasoothe®* Other ingredients: ceramides, phytosphingosine, safflower oil, *Aloe barbadensis*, glycerin, lanolin cholesterol, glycerin, lanolin

Human-Labeled Products

Active ingredients (formulation)	Label status; size(s)	Trade names/additional information
Diphenhydramine 2% (spray), diphenhydramine 2% (gel), diphenhydramine 1% (cream), diphenhydramine 2% (cream), diphenhydramine 2% (ointment), diphenhydramine 2% (stick), diphenhydramine 12.5 mg (strip)	OTC; various sizes available	*Benadryl®; Banophen®; CareOne®; Allergy Relief®* Other ingredients may include calamine, zinc oxide, acetate, pyrilamine, tripelennamine, menthol, camphor.

Fatty Acids (Omega), Topical

For systemic use, see ***Fatty Acids, Omega-3***

Indications/Actions

Essential fatty acids are polyunsaturated fatty acids that are not synthesized by the body and must be obtained from external sources. The 2 main types of essential fatty acids are omega-3 and omega-6 fatty acids. Essential fatty acids are indicated primarily for pruritic and inflammatory conditions (eg, atopic dermatitis, sebaceous adenitis) and keratinization disorders (eg, seborrhea). They may also be used to improve coat quality and dry skin. Some products may contain other active ingredients and natural oils, and therefore, may have additional indications.

The exact mechanism of action of essential fatty acids is not well understood; however, essential fatty acids affect the arachidonic acid concentrations in plasma lipids and platelet membranes. They decrease the production of inflammatory prostaglandins in the body, thereby reducing inflammation and pruritus. Essential fatty acids may also play a role in restoring the skin barrier.

Suggested Uses/Dosages

Sprays, wipes, and mousses are typically applied up to 2 to 3 times daily as needed. Spot-on treatments vary from weekly to every 2 weeks. Shampoos and crème rinses can be applied daily to weekly. Shampoos should generally be left in contact with the skin for 5 to 10 minutes before rinsing.

Precautions/Adverse Effects

No specific precautions or adverse effects are described for topical essential fatty acids; however, sensitivity reactions are possible. If signs such as pruritus or erythema occur, discontinue use.

Veterinary-Labeled Products

Below is a representative sample of the products available. **NOTE:** Refer to specific product labels for details on inactive ingredients and instructions for use.

Active ingredients (formulation)	Species	Label status; size(s)	Trade names/additional information
Essential fatty acids from safflower oil (shampoo)	Labeled for dogs and cats; some products labeled for horses	OTC; 4 oz, 12 oz, 16 oz, 1 gallon	*HyLyt®; DermaLyte®; EFA Essential Fatty Acid®* Soap-free
Essential fatty acids from safflower oil with oatmeal (shampoo)	Labeled for dogs, cats, and horses	OTC; 12 oz, 1 gallon	*DermAllay®* Soap-free
Essential fatty acids from safflower oil (creme rinse)	Labeled for dogs and cats; some products labeled for horses	OTC; 8 oz, 1 gallon	*HyLyt®*; generic
Essential fatty acids from hemp seed oil (spot-on)	Labeled for dogs, cats, horses, and small mammals	OTC; boxes of 4 pipettes in the following sizes: Dogs: Under 10 kg (22 lb): 0.6 mL 10 - 20.5 kg (22-45 lb): 1.2 mL 20.5 - 40.9 kg (45-90 lb): 2.4 mL Cats: 0.4 mL Small mammals: 0.6 mL Horses: 30 mL bottles	*Essential 6®* Directions: Initially, 1 dose weekly for 2 months, then 1 dose every 2 weeks for maintenance. Do not bathe within 2 days before and 2 days after application. Brush application site 24 hours after applying to remove product residue.
Essential fatty acids from hemp seed oil and tamanu oil (spot-on)	Labeled for dogs	OTC; boxes of 4 pipettes in the following sizes: **Dogs:** under 10 kg (22 lb): 0.6 mL Dogs 10 - 20.4 kg (22-45 lb): 1.2 mL 20.4 - 40.8 kg (45-90 lb): 2.4 mL	*PYOspot®* Directions: 1 pipette weekly Do not bathe during 2 days before and 2 days after application. Brush application site 24 hours after applying to remove product residue.
Essential fatty acids from hemp seed oil (mousse)	Labeled for dogs, cats, and small mammals	OTC; 150 mL	*Essential 6®* Soap-free and rinse-free. Shake before use.

Active ingredients (formulation)	Species	Label status; size(s)	Trade names/additional information
Essential fatty acids from soybean oil (balm)	Labeled for dogs	OTC; 1.67 oz jar	*BIO BALM®* Occlusive and water-resistant
Essential fatty acids from hemp seed oil (wipes)	Labeled for dogs and cats	OTC; pack of 20 wipes	*PYOClean®* Soap-free and alcohol-free
Essential fatty acids from safflower oil (spray)	Labeled for dogs, cats, and horses	OTC; 8 oz, 12 oz, and 1 gallon	*Dermallay®* Soap-free, oatmeal spray conditioner

Human-Labeled Products

NOTE: Several human over-the-counter products are available in the United States but may contain additional ingredients and generally are not used in dogs and cats.

Lidocaine/Lidocaine Combinations, Topical

(***lye***-doe-kane)

For systemic use of lidocaine, please refer to ***Lidocaine (Intravenous; Systemic)****. For local anesthetic use, please refer to* ***Lidocaine, Local Anesthetic****.*

Indications/Actions

Lidocaine is used topically as a dermal anesthetic or antipruritic. It is included in several products used for acute moist dermatitis, pruritic lesions, and painful skin conditions. When combined with prilocaine, it may provide dermal anesthesia before painful or invasive procedures such as catheter placements.

Lidocaine exerts its anesthetic properties by altering sodium ion permeability across the cell membrane, thereby inhibiting conduction from sensory nerves.

Suggested Dosages/Uses

Lidocaine can be applied in a thin layer every 3 to 4 hours as needed. For veterinary-labeled products, refer to the specific product label for details on use.

Precautions/Adverse Effects

Although topical lidocaine may be absorbed systemically, systemic toxicity is unlikely. Applying to a significant percentage of body area, using for prolonged times, using high concentrations, applying to irritated or broken skin, or covering the application site may increase the risk for systemic absorption and subsequent toxicity. Use with caution in patients receiving Class-I antiarrhythmics such as systemic lidocaine or mexiletine. Patches can cause serious adverse effects if chewed.[1]

Possible adverse effects include hypersensitivity reactions or skin irritation such as burning or tenderness. Products containing prilocaine may be more likely to cause methemoglobinemia or systemic toxicity; however, these effects occur rarely.[2] Some products may also contain antiseptics, such as chlorhexidine and povidone-iodine.

Wear gloves when applying and wash hands after handling. Avoid contact with eyes. Do not use in ears unless the product is explicitly labeled for otic use.

Veterinary-Labeled Products

Active ingredients (formulation)	Species	Label status; size(s)	Trade names/additional information
Lidocaine 2.4% (spray)	Labeled for dogs and horses	OTC; 2 oz	*Silver L®; BioCalm®*
Lidocaine 2.4%, benzalkonium chloride 0.1% (spray)	Labeled for dogs	OTC; 4 oz	*Allercaine® with Bittran® II*
Lidocaine 2.46%, benzalkonium chloride 0.2% (spray)	Labeled for dogs, cats, and horses	OTC; 4 oz	*Hexa-Caine®*
Lidocaine 0.5%, chlorhexidine 0.2% (solution)	Labeled for dogs, cats, and horses	OTC; 4 oz	*Dermachlor Flush Plus®* These products may no longer be commercially available.
Lidocaine 2%, povidone-iodine 2% (solution)	Labeled for dogs, cats, and horses	OTC; 16 oz	*Barrier® II*

Human-Labeled Products

NOTE: Many commercial products exist. Below is a representative list of available products.

Active ingredients (formulation)	Label status; size(s)	Trade names/additional information
Lidocaine 2% (cream)	OTC; various	*Xolido®*

Active ingredients (formulation)	Label status; size(s)	Trade names/additional information
Lidocaine 4% (cream)	OTC; various	*Anecream*®; *Bengay*®; *Aspercreme*®; *LC-4*; *LMX-4*
Lidocaine 5% (cream)	OTC; various	*Anecream*® *5*; *LC-5*; generic
Lidocaine 3% (lotion)	Rx; 4 oz, 6 oz	*Lidosorb*®; generic
Lidocaine 5% (ointment)	Rx; 30 g, 35.44 g, or 50 g tube, 50 g, 150 g, or 250 g jar	*Xylocaine*®; generic
Lidocaine 1.8% (patch)	Rx; box of 30 patches	*ZTlido*®
Lidocaine 4% (patch)	OTC; various	*Aspercreme*®; generic
Lidocaine 5% (patch)	Rx; box of 30 patches	*Dermalid*®; *Lidoderm*®; generic
Lidocaine 0.5% (spray)	OTC; various	*Burnamycin*®; generic
Lidocaine 4% (spray)	OTC; various	*Aspercreme*®; generic
Lidocaine 2% (gel/jelly)	Rx; 6 mL or 11 mL prefilled syringes; 5 mL, 10 mL, or 20 mL *Uro-Jet*® syringes; 5 mL or 30 mL tube	*Xylocaine*®; generic
Lidocaine 4% (gel/jelly)	OTC; various	*Alocane*®; *Topicaine*®; generic
Lidocaine 5% (gel/jelly)	OTC; various	*Topicaine*®; generic
Lidocaine 2.5%, prilocaine 2.5% (cream)	Rx; 5 g, 15 g, and 30 g	*EMLA*®; generic

References

For the complete list of references, see **wiley.com/go/budde/plumb**

Phytosphingosine, Topical

(fye-tos-***fin***-goh-seen)

Indications/Actions

Phytosphingosine products are indicated for localized and generalized inflammatory conditions of the skin associated with pruritus and dryness, including allergic diseases such as atopic dermatitis. Some products are also indicated for use as a liquid wound dressing for localized inflammation and after surgery (could be sprayed on sutures). Some products are marketed for seborrheic conditions. There is some evidence supporting the role of phytosphingosine on skin barrier restoration in dogs.[1]

Phytosphingosine acts as a ceramide precursor, and it is a salient molecule in the natural defense mechanism of the skin. Ceramides comprise 40% to 50% of the main lipids responsible for maintaining the cohesion of the stratum corneum. Therefore, ceramides are essential for restoring the skin lipid barrier, controlling local flora, and maintaining the correct moisture balance. Phytosphingosine is also anti-inflammatory; it has anti-IL-1 activity, impairing the production of PGE2, and it inhibits kinase protein C.

Suggested Dosages/Uses

Phytosphingosine spray should be applied every 3 days for 2 to 3 weeks.[2] Gel should be applied once daily as needed for itching relief.[3] Mousse should be applied to dry hair and should be used every 3 days for 2 to 3 weeks.[4] Shampoo should be used 2 to 3 times weekly for 1 to 2 weeks.[5] Leave the shampoo in contact with the skin for at least 5 to 10 minutes before rinsing well. Shake products well before use. Refer to specific product label for details on use.

Precautions/Adverse Effects

Discontinue use if skin redness or irritation occurs. Avoid contact with the eyes.

Veterinary-Labeled Products

NOTE: *Be aware when selecting products that different combinations of active ingredients may be marketed under similar trade names. For products containing other active ingredients, including* ***Chlorhexidine, Topical*** *and* ***Pramoxine, Topical****, please refer to their respective monographs.*

Active ingredients (formulation)	Species	Label status; size(s)	Trade names/additional information
Phytosphingosine salicyloyl 0.2% (gel)	Labeled for dogs and cats	OTC; 2 oz	*Douxo*® *Calm*
Phytosphingosine salicyloyl 0.05% (micro-emulsion spray)	Labeled for dogs and cats	OTC; 6.8 oz	*Douxo*® *Calm*
Phytosphingosine salicyloyl 0.05%, chlorhexidine gluconate 3% (micro-emulsion spray)	Labeled for dogs and cats	OTC; 6.8 oz	*Douxo*® *Chlorhexidine*
Phytosphingosine hydrochloride 0.2% (mousse)	Labeled for dogs and cats	OTC; 8 oz	*SkinGuard*® *Balance*
Phytosphingosine salicyloyl 0.05%, chlorhexidine gluconate 3%, climbazole 0.5% (mousse)	Labeled for dogs and cats	OTC; 6.8 oz	*SkinGuard*® *Restore*

Active ingredients (formulation)	Species	Label status; size(s)	Trade names/additional information
Phytosphingosine salicyloyl 0.05%, pramoxine hydrochloride 1% (mousse)	Labeled for dogs and cats	OTC; 6.8 oz	*SkinGuard® Relieve*
Phytosphingosine salicyloyl 0.05%, chlorhexidine gluconate 3%, climbazole 0.5% (pads)	Labeled for dogs and cats	OTC; 30 pads	*SkinGuard® Restore*
Phytosphingosine hydrochloride 0.1% (shampoo)	Labeled for dogs and cats	OTC; 8 oz	*SkinGuard® Balance*
Phytosphingosine hydrochloride 0.05%, benzoyl peroxide 3%, salicylic acid 2%, sodium thiosulfate 2% (shampoo)	Labeled for dogs and cats	OTC; 8 oz	*SkinGuard® Clear*
Phytosphingosine salicyloyl 0.05%, chlorhexidine gluconate 3%, climbazole 0.5% (shampoo)	Labeled for dogs and cats	OTC; 8 oz	*SkinGuard® Restore*
Phytosphingosine salicyloyl 0.05%, pramoxine hydrochloride 1% (shampoo)	Labeled for dogs and cats	OTC; 8 oz	*SkinGuard® Relieve*

Human-Labeled Products

NOTE: There are several over-the-counter human cosmetic products containing phytosphingosine in the United States. These products mainly target lipid barrier restoration and are generally not used in dogs and cats.

References

For the complete list of references, see **wiley.com/go/budde/plumb**

Pramoxine, Topical

(pra-***moks***-een)

Indications/Actions

Pramoxine is a topical anesthetic that is often combined with other topical medications to temporarily reduce pain and itching.

Pramoxine affects peripheral nerves and has been shown to antagonize histamine-mediated pruritus; however, the mechanism of action is unknown. Pramoxine is not structurally related to procaine-type anesthetics. Peak local anesthetic effects occur within 3 to 5 minutes of application.

Suggested Dosages/Uses

Pramoxine sprays are typically labeled for daily use as needed. Shampoos are typically labeled for use up to 2 to 3 times weekly and may be used as often as once daily. Allow shampoo to remain in contact with the skin for at least 5 to 10 minutes before rinsing well. Mousse products are labeled for use every 3 days and should be applied to dry hair, massaged in, and left to air dry. Rinses may be applied daily to once weekly, separately or after baths. Ointment is labeled for use every other day. Labeled doses may differ based on active ingredient combinations; refer to specific product labels for detailed use instructions.

Precautions/Adverse Effects

Avoid contact with eyes; pramoxine is too irritating for ophthalmic use. Wear gloves when applying or wash hands after application. Adverse effects are uncommon; however, localized dermatitis is possible. Discontinue use if redness, irritation, swelling, or pain occurs or increases with use.

Pramoxine shows an antagonizing impact on histamine-mediated pruritus. Therefore, at least a 2-week withdrawal period before intradermal testing is recommended.

Veterinary-Labeled Products

Active ingredients (formulation)	Species	Label status; size(s)	Trade names/additional information
Pramoxine HCl 1% (spray)	Labeled for dogs and cats; some products also labeled for horses	OTC; 8 oz, 12 oz	*Comfort; Micro-Pearls Advantage Dermal-Soothe®; Pramox-1®; Relief®*
Pramoxine HCl 0.5%, hydrocortisone 1% (spray)	Labeled for dogs and cats; some products labeled for horses	OTC; 4 oz, 8 oz	*Dermabliss®*
Pramoxine HCl 1%, hydrocortisone 1% (spray)	Labeled for dogs and cats; some products also labeled for horses	OTC; 4 oz, 8 oz	*Comfort HC; EquiShield® IR; Pramoxine HC; Suffusion® HC; VetraSeb® HC*
Pramoxine HCl 1%, phytosphingosine salicyloyl 0.05% (spray)	Labeled for dogs and cats	OTC; 8 oz	*VetraSeb® P; Suffusion® P +PS*
Pramoxine HCl 1%, diphenhydramine HCl 1% (spray)	Labeled for dogs and cats	OTC; 8 oz	*Benasoothe®*

Active ingredients (formulation)	Species	Label status; size(s)	Trade names/additional information
Pramoxine HCl 1% (shampoo)	Labeled for dogs and cats; some products also labeled for horses	OTC; 8 oz, 12 oz, 16 oz, 1 gallon	*BioCalm®; CeraSoothe®; Comfort Shampoo; Dermabliss®; Micro-Pearls Advantage Dermal-Soothe®; Pramox-1®; Relief®; Suffusion® P; VetraSeb® CeraDerm® P*
Pramoxine HCl 1%, diphenhydramine HCl 1% (shampoo)	Labeled for dogs and cats	OTC; 12 oz	*Benasoothe®*
Pramoxine HCl 1%, hydrocortisone 1% (shampoo)	Labeled for dogs, cats, and horses	OTC; 12 oz	*EquiShield® IR*
Pramoxine HCl 1%, phytosphingosine salicyloyl 0.05% (shampoo)	Labeled for dogs and cats; some products also labeled for horses	OTC; 8 oz, 16 oz	*Phyto P; Suffusion® P +PS; VetraSeb® P*
Pramoxine HCl 1% (rinse)	Labeled for dogs and cats; some products also labeled for horses	OTC; 12 oz, 16 oz, 1 gallon	*Comfort; Micro-Pearls Advantage Dermal-Soothe®; Pramox*
Pramoxine HCl 1%, phytosphingosine salicyloyl 0.05% (rinse)	Labeled for dogs, cats, and horses	OTC; 8 oz	*Phyto P*
Pramoxine HCl 1% (mousse)	Labeled for dogs and cats; some products also labeled for horses	OTC; 6.8 oz	*CeraSoothe®; Suffusion® P; VetraSeb® CeraDerm® P;*
Pramoxine HCl 1%, phytosphingosine salicyloyl 0.05% (mousse)	Labeled for dogs and cats	OTC; 6.8 oz	*Phyto P; Suffusion® P +PS; VetraSeb® P*
Pramoxine HCl 1% (ointment)	Labeled for dogs and cats	OTC; 15 g	*Deter-X®*

Human-Labeled Products

NOTE: Partial listing; there are many branded combination products available that also contain pramoxine. For more information on human-labeled products, refer to a comprehensive human drug reference (eg, *Facts and Comparisons*) or contact a pharmacist.

Active ingredients (formulation)	Label status; size(s)	Trade names/additional information
Pramoxine 1% (lotion)	OTC; 7.5 oz, 8 oz	*Sarna Sensitive®*, generic
Pramoxine 1% (spray)	OTC; 2 oz	*Itch-X®*; generic
Pramoxine 1% (gel)	OTC; 35.4 g	*Itch-X®*
Pramoxine HCl 1% (wipes)	OTC; 30 count	generic

Zinc Gluconate (Neutralized), Topical

*For otic use, see **Cleaning/Drying Otic Agents**.*

Indications/Actions

Zinc gluconate can be used as a sole agent for mild pruritus or as an adjunct treatment for moderate to severe pruritic conditions, mild bacterial infections, or dry skin. It can also be used for minor skin irritations, such as insect bite reactions, acute moist dermatitis, acral lick dermatitis, fold dermatitis (intertrigo), feline acne, and postsurgical wounds.

The exact mechanism of action of topical zinc is unknown. Zinc plays a role in extracellular matrix remodeling, wound healing, connective tissue repair, inflammation, and cell proliferation. Zinc also has antiseptic and astringent properties.

Suggested Dosages/Uses

Zinc gluconate may be applied to affected areas as needed up to twice daily to relieve itching and soothe the skin. For veterinary products, refer to specific product label for details on use. Do not let animals lick or chew at affected areas for at least 20 to 30 minutes after application.

Precautions/Adverse Effects

Avoid contact with eyes and mucous membranes.

Veterinary-Labeled Products

Active ingredients (formulation)	Species	Label status; size(s)	Trade names/additional information
Zinc gluconate (spray)	Labeled for dogs, cats, horses, and some exotic pets	OTC; 2 oz, 4 oz	*Maxi/Guard® Zn7 Derm*
Zinc gluconate (gel)	Labeled for dogs, cats, horses, and some exotic pets	OTC; 1 oz, 2 oz	*Maxi/Guard® Zn7 Derm*

Human-Labeled Products

There are a variety of human-labeled OTC zinc gluconate products, some in combination with other active ingredients.

Antimicrobial Agents, Topical

Antibacterial Agents, Topical

See also:
Sulfur, Precipitated, Topical (Keratolytic Agents)

Bacitracin, Topical

(bass-ih-***trase***-in)

Antibiotic

For ophthalmic use, see ***Triple Antibiotic Ophthalmic****.*

Indications/Actions

Bacitracin is used topically to treat and prevent infection after dermal lacerations, scrapes, minor burns, and surgical procedures. Bacitracin acts by inhibiting cell wall synthesis of susceptible bacteria by preventing the formation of peptidoglycan chains. It is either bactericidal or bacteriostatic, depending on drug concentration and bacterial susceptibility. Bacitracin is primarily active against gram-positive bacteria, but *Staphylococcus* spp are becoming increasingly resistant; therefore, bacitracin ideally should be used only after confirmation of bacterial skin infections in dogs and cats. Bacitracin activity is not impaired by blood, pus, necrotic tissue, or large inocula.

Suggested Dosages/Uses

Bacitracin may be applied up to 3 times daily and be covered by a suitable dressing. Administration of bacitracin is usually not recommended to continue for more than 1 week.

Precautions/Adverse Effects

Bacitracin topical ointment should not be used in or around the eyes, for the treatment of ulcerated lesions, chronic canine dermatoses, or in patients that are known to be hypersensitive to it. There have been reports of cats developing fatal anaphylactic reactions after administration of triple-antibiotic ophthalmic ointment containing bacitracin.[1] Bacitracin is also well documented as causing allergic contact dermatitis after topical administration in humans with the potential for anaphylaxis.[2] Deep puncture wounds, animal bites, or deep cutaneous infections may require systemic antibiotic therapy. Although topical administration generally results in negligible systemic levels, if bacitracin is used over large areas of the body or on serious burns or puncture wounds, measurable absorption and potential toxicity may occur. Do not let animal lick or chew at affected areas for at least 20 to 30 minutes after application. Pet owners should wash their hands after application.

Veterinary-Labeled Products

None

Human-Labeled Products

Bacitracin ointment is available alone as 500 units/g in various tube sizes. There are many OTC human products available with various combinations of antibiotics. Some products may also contain pramoxine hydrochloride for soothing and pain relief.

Active ingredients (formulation)	Label status; size(s)	Trade names/additional information
Bacitracin zinc 500 units/g (ointment) Other ingredients (depending on the manufacturer): white petrolatum, mineral oil	OTC; 14 g, 14.2 g, 28 g, 28.4 g, and 120 g tubes; 454 g jar	generic
Bacitracin zinc 500 units/g, polymyxin B sulfate 10,000 units/g (ointment)	OTC; 28.3g tube	*Polysporin*®
Bacitracin zinc 400 units/g, neomycin 3.5 mg/g, polymyxin B sulfate 5000 units/g (ointment)	OTC; 14.2g, 28.3g tube	*Neosporin*®; generic

References

For the complete list of references, see **wiley.com/go/budde/plumb**

Benzoyl Peroxide, Topical

(ben-***zoyl*** per-***oks***-ide)

Antibacterial

Indications/Actions

Benzoyl peroxide products are available as gels, shampoos, or cream rinses for topical use. Shampoos are generally used for oily dermatoses (eg, seborrhea oleosa), superficial and deep pyodermas, and furunculosis. Benzoyl peroxide shampoos can also be used as adjunctive therapy for generalized demodicosis and schnauzer comedo syndrome. Gels may be useful for treating localized superficial and deep pyodermas, chin acne, fold pyodermas, and localized lesions caused by *Demodex* spp.

Benzoyl peroxide is an antibacterial agent with comedolytic ("follicular flushing"), keratolytic,[1] and antiseborrheic actions. It also has some mild antipruritic activity and wound healing effects. Benzoyl peroxide is lipophilic and penetrates into the stratum corneum, where it is converted to benzoic acid. The antibacterial activity of benzoyl peroxide is due to free radical formation that oxidizes bacterial proteins.[2]

Suggested Dosages/Uses

Gels are commonly administered once to twice daily; shampoos may be used anywhere from once daily to once weekly. Shampoos should remain in contact with the skin for 5 to 10 minutes before rinsing well. For veterinary products, refer to the product label for details on use.

Precautions/Adverse Effects

Avoid contact with the eyes or mucous membranes. Benzoyl peroxide will bleach colored fabrics, jewelry, clothing, or carpets and might bleach the animal's haircoat. Owners should be advised to keep treated animals away from fabrics during treatment. Do not let the animal lick or chew at treated areas for a few minutes after application.

In some animals, benzoyl peroxide can be drying or irritating. Adverse effects can include erythema, pruritus, or pain at the treated site, particularly when higher concentrations (greater than 5%) are used. Reducing the frequency of use, applying emollients after bathing, or using shampoos with moisturizing microvesicles may alleviate or prevent these effects. Benzoyl peroxide causes photosensitivity in humans.[3] Limit sun exposure for dogs with light or thin coats. **NOTE:** Benzoyl peroxide shampoos do not lather well.

Veterinary-Labeled Products

CREAM RINSE

Active ingredients (formulation)	Species	Label status; size(s)	Trade names/additional information
Benzoyl peroxide 2.5%	Labeled for dogs and cats	OTC; 12 oz	generic

GEL

Active ingredients (formulation)	Species	Label status; size(s)	Trade names/additional information
Benzoyl peroxide 5% Other ingredients: propylene glycol, docusate sodium, DMDM hydantoin	Labeled for dogs and cats	OTC; 30 g bottle	*Micro BP*

SHAMPOOS

Active ingredients (formulation)	Species	Label status; size(s)	Trade names/additional information
Benzoyl peroxide 2.5% Other ingredients: *Novasome*® microvesicles	Labeled for dogs and cats	OTC; 12 oz, 1 gallon	*Micro-Pearls Advantage Benzoyl-Plus*®
Benzoyl peroxide 2.5%	Labeled for dogs and cats	OTC; 12 oz, 1 gallon	generic
Benzoyl peroxide 2.5% Other ingredients: glycolic acid 1%	Labeled for dogs and cats	OTC; 8 oz	*GlycoBenz*®
Benzoyl peroxide 2.5%, salicylic acid 1%, sulfur 1% (shampoo)	Labeled for dogs and cats	OTC; 12 oz	*Sulfur Benz*®
Benzoyl peroxide 2.5%, sulfur 2%	Labeled for dogs and cats	OTC; 16 oz	generic
Benzoyl peroxide 3%	Labeled for dogs and cats	OTC; 16 oz, 1 gallon	*BPO-3*®
Benzoyl peroxide 3%, salicylic acid 2%, sulfur 2%	Labeled for dogs and cats	OTC; 8 oz, 12 oz, and 16 oz	*Oxibenz-3*®; *Peroxiderm*®; generic

Human-Labeled Products

There are many human products available that contain benzoyl peroxide (2.5% to 10%); however, with the possible exception of the 5% gel products, the veterinary formulations would be more suitable for dogs or cats. Benzoyl peroxide 5% gel can be labeled as either Rx or OTC, depending on the product, and are available as generics or with the following trade names: *Benzac*®, *Desquam-X*®, or *PanOxyl*®.

References

For the complete list of references, see **wiley.com/go/budde/plumb**

Clindamycin, Topical

(klin-da-***mye***-sin) *Cleocin*®, *ClinzGard*®

For systemic use, see ***Clindamycin.***

Indications/Actions

Topical clindamycin may be used for treating feline acne or other localized skin infections caused by bacteria susceptible to it. It has been recommended by some veterinary dermatologists that topical clindamycin only be used when other topical antibiotics, such as gentamicin, have failed. Ideally, treatment should be based on culture and susceptibility results. Clindamycin is a lincosamide antibiotic and inhibits bacterial protein synthesis by binding to the 50S ribosomal subunit. Its primary activity is against anaerobic and gram-positive aerobic bacteria. For more information on clindamycin pharmacology, see ***Clindamycin***.

Suggested Dosages/Uses

When used for feline acne, topical clindamycin is generally applied in a thin film once to twice daily. *ClinzGard®* is used as a single dose application in bite and puncture wounds, surgical incisions, and anal sacs after cleaning and debridement (when applicable).

Precautions/Adverse Effects

In patients with a history of hypersensitivity to clindamycin or lincomycin, topical clindamycin should not be used. Avoid contact with eyes. Clients should wash their hands after application or wear gloves when applying. Contact reactions (pain, burning, erythema, itching, drying, peeling) are possible. Clindamycin lotions and gels may cause less burning than topical solutions or foams. Because clindamycin can be absorbed through the skin, systemic adverse effects are possible. Although clindamycin-related diarrhea and colitis are rare in animals, severe diarrhea, bloody diarrhea, and severe colitis have been reported in humans with topical use.

Veterinary-Labeled Products

Active ingredients (formulation)	Species	Label status; size(s)	Trade names/additional information
Clindamycin hydrochloride 1% (gel)	Labeled for dogs and cats	Rx; sterile 1 or 2 mL single-dose syringes (box with 4 units)	*ClinzGard®* Indicated for anal sac disease, tissue abscesses, bites, puncture wounds, and surgical incisions. Single-dose with a sustained release over 7 to 10 days. Must be applied to clean and debrided (if necessary) surfaces

Human-Labeled Products

Active ingredients (formulation)	Label status; size(s)	Trade names/additional information
Clindamycin phosphate 1% (lotion)	Rx; 60 mL	*Clindamax®*; *Cleocin T®*; generic
Clindamycin phosphate 1% (gel)	Rx; 30 g, 60 g, 40 mL, and 75 mL	*Clindagel®*; *Clindamax®*; *Cleocin T®*; generic
Clindamycin phosphate 1% (solution)	Rx; 30 mL, 60 mL	*Cleocin T®*; generic
Clindamycin phosphate 1% (aerosol foam) Other ingredients: cetyl alcohol, ethanol 58%, stearyl alcohol, propylene glycol	Rx; 50 g, 100 g	*Evoclin®* Dispense into cap or onto a cool surface, then use fingertips to apply small amounts. Dispensing directly onto hands or affected area(s) will cause the foam to melt on contact. If the foam seems runny or warm, run canister under cold water.
Clindamycin phosphate 1% (pledgets) Other ingredients: isopropyl alcohol, propylene glycol	Rx; 60 per box/jar	*Cleocin T®*; *Clindacin®*; *Clindacin®-P*; *Clindets®*; generic

Gentamicin, Topical

(jen-ta-***mye***-sin)

*For systemic use, see **Gentamicin**.*
*For otic use, see **Corticosteroid/Antimicrobial Agents, Otic**.*

Indications/Actions

Topical gentamicin can be useful for treating both primary and secondary superficial bacterial skin infections caused by susceptible bacteria. Some products indicate prophylactic use after lacerations, abrasions, or after minor surgery; however, dermatologists recommend using topical gentamicin only to treat confirmed bacterial skin infections, as resistance may occur. Therefore, the use of gentamicin solely for the treatment of yeast and/or inflammation without evidence of bacterial infection should also be avoided. In small animal medicine, topical gentamicin is frequently used in combination with a corticosteroid (typically betamethasone or mometasone) to treat superficial lesions, including "hot spots" (acute moist dermatitis and pruritic lesions).

Some products containing betamethasone or mometasone and clotrimazole are labeled for otic use but can also be used extra-label for bacterial and yeast skin infections that are sensitive to gentamicin and clotrimazole when an anti-inflammatory effect is also desired. Formulations containing a corticosteroid are best suited for focal (eg, pedal) or multifocal lesions for relatively short durations (ie, less than 2 months). Initially, topical gentamicin/corticosteroid products are used 1 to 4 times daily until control is achieved, and then the frequency is tapered. Sole ingredient gentamicin sulfate topical forms are available with human labeling.

Gentamicin is an aminoglycoside antibiotic. It binds to the bacterial 30S ribosomal unit and inhibits protein synthesis. It has minimal activity against *Streptococcus* spp, variable activity against *Staphylococcus* spp, and good activity against gram-negative bacteria, including

Klebsiella spp, *Escherichia coli*, and some strains of *Pseudomonas* spp. Gentamicin-resistant strains of *Pseudomonas* spp are an ongoing issue.

Suggested Dosages/Uses

Topical gentamicin creams, ointments, or suspensions are generally applied to affected areas up to 4 times daily. Topical gentamicin/corticosteroid sprays are labeled for use 1 to 4 times daily for up to 7 days. Creams are typically used for infections associated with greasy skin, whereas ointments are typically used for infections associated with dry skin.

Precautions/Adverse Effects

Topical gentamicin may be systemically absorbed if it is used on ulcerated, burned, or denuded skin. Creams are more likely to be absorbed than are ointments; however, systemic toxicity is unlikely to occur unless gentamicin is applied to a significant percentage of body surface area or is used for prolonged times. Do not let the animal lick or chew at treated areas for at least 20 to 30 minutes after application.

Products that contain corticosteroids can cause HPA axis suppression with long-term or frequent use, cutaneous atrophy that can be associated with skin fragility, superficial follicular cysts (milia), reduced or lack of hair regrowth, and comedones. Risk can be reduced by only treating for as long as necessary on the smallest area possible. Mometasone is considered a "soft steroid", delivering its potent anti-inflammatory effect close to its site of action while reducing the degree of systemic exposure and thus limiting the associated systemic and local adverse effects. Nevertheless, care should be taken to avoid excessive or prolonged use. Residual activity may affect intradermal or serum allergy tests, and it has been suggested to discontinue use of corticosteroid-containing products 2 weeks before allergy testing.[1]

Avoid contact with eyes. Clients should wash their hands after application or wear gloves when applying.

Veterinary-Labeled Products

Refer to the individual product labeling for specific dosing recommendations and inactive ingredients.

NOTE: There are no topical gentamicin-only labeled veterinary products in the United States.

Active ingredients (formulation)	Species	Label status; size(s)	Trade names/additional information
Gentamicin 3 mg/g, clotrimazole 10 mg/g, mometasone 1 mg/g (suspension)	Approved for otic use in dogs	Rx; 7.5 g, 15 g, 30 g, and 215 g tubes	*Mometamax®; Mometavet®* Extra-label when used topically in dogs and cats
Gentamicin 3 mg/mL, betamethasone 1 mg/mL (solution)	Approved for otic use in dogs and cats	Rx; 7.5 mL, 15 mL, 240 mL	*Vet Beta-gen®* Extra-label when used topically
Gentamicin 0.57 mg/mL, betamethasone 0.284 mg/mL (spray)	Approved for use in dogs	Rx; 15 g, 30 g, 60 mL, 72 mL, 120 mL, and 240 mL	*Betagen®; Gentacalm®; GentaSoothe®; GentaSpray®; Genta Ved®; Gentocin®*
Gentamicin 3 mg/g, clotrimazole 10 mg/g, betamethasone 1 mg/g (ointment)	Approved for otic use in dogs	Rx; 7.5 g, 10 g, 15 g, 20 g, 25 g, 30 g, and 210 g bottles or tubes	*MalOtic®; Otomax®; Tri-Otic®; Vetromax®* Extra-label when used topically in dogs and cats

Human-Labeled Products

Active ingredients (formulation)	Label status; size(s)	Trade names/additional information
Gentamicin 0.1% (cream and ointment)	Rx; 15g, 30 g tubes	generic

References

For the complete list of references, see **wiley.com/go/budde/plumb**

Honey, Topical

Topical Antibacterial Agent *HoneyCure®, Medihoney®*

Indications/Actions

Honey is a natural product that is generally made from flower nectar by honey bees. Honey is composed of over 200 biologically active compounds, including sugars, proteins, vitamins, minerals, phenols, and plant- and bee-derived enzymes. Medical-grade honey is honey that has been filtered to a higher level than food-grade honey and has been sterilized to kill, remove, or inactivate bacteria, fungi, protozoa, and spores. Medical-grade Manuka honey is commonly used for medicinal purposes and is produced by honey bees foraging only from flowers of the Manuka tree (*Leptospermum scoparium*) from Australia and New Zealand. Other monofloral (eg, honeydew, Scottish Heather) or regionally derived (eg, Saudi, Italian, Portugese) honeys have also been studied for potential medicinal purposes. Medical-grade honey can be used as an alternative or adjunctive therapy for many dermatologic conditions (eg, traumatic wounds, burn wounds) in animals.

Honey is considered to be an effective broad-spectrum topical antibacterial agent, and unlike traditional antibiotics, resistance to its killing effects has not been reported.[1] Honey's antimicrobial properties have been attributed to its osmotic action and low pH (3.4 to 6.1) as well as to the presence of hydrogen peroxide. Additionally, Manuka honey also has nonperoxide bacteriostatic properties due to the presence of methylglyoxal (MGO), which may inhibit bacterial protein synthesis.[1-3] In vitro studies have shown honey to have potent antimicrobial effects against important skin microbes, including *Staphylococcus aureus, Staphylococcus pseudintermedius, Acinetobacter baumannii, and Escherichia coli,* in addition to antibiotic-resistant strains of bacteria such as methicillin-resistant *Staphylococcus aureus* (MRSA) and *Pseudomonas aeruginosa.*[3-8] It has also been demonstrated to be effective against fungal organisms such as *Malassezia pachydermatis and Candida albicans* and viruses.[7,9]

Suggested Dosages/Uses

NOTE: Ensure that enough honey is in full contact with the wound bed and that honey dressings extend to cover any areas of inflammation surrounding the wound. If a nonadherent dressing is used between the honey dressing and the wound bed, it must be sufficiently porous to allow the honey to diffuse through.

Honey gels, ointments, or creams: Clean and dry wound. Apply product directly to the affected skin, beyond wound edges, as a thin layer once daily or more often according to the severity of the treated wounds or lesions. Cover with bandage if needed.

Honey dressings: Commercially available honey-impregnated dressings facilitate the application of honey to wounds, especially those that need to be maintained in place or protected longer. Alternatively, honey dressings may be prepared in the clinic by applying medical-grade honey to a clean, dry dressing (eg, sterile gauze pad, adhesive bandage); apply the dressing to the skin, then apply a suitable secondary dressing, such as a semi-occlusive dressing, to prevent leakage of honey. Replace the dressing when drainage from the wound saturates the dressing. Change the dressings frequently enough to prevent the honey from being washed away or excessively diluted by wound exudate. The frequency of dressing change will vary but the typical interval is every 2 to 3 days. As the wound heals, the dressing changes will likely be less frequent. When using honey to debride hard eschar, softening the eschar by soaking with saline will allow better penetration of the honey. Owners may be instructed on how to replace the dressings so that it can be done at home.

Precautions/Adverse Effects

Honey is safe when applied to healthy skin and wounds. Although it is safe if ingested, if applying honey without a bandage, do not let the animal lick or chew affected areas for at least 20 to 30 minutes to prevent removing the honey from the treated area(s). An Elizabethan collar may be helpful. Do not use honey to control heavy bleeding, in third-degree burns, and in patients with known sensitivity to honey. Honey may crystalize, making it difficult to use. If crystalized, gently warm the honey, mix it well, and allow it to cool before use. Honey applied directly to the skin (instead of the bandage) may be "messy" (eg, ooze or leak from or around application site).

Veterinary-Labeled Products

Many different brands of medical-grade honey or medical-grade Manuka honey exist. Listed below are representative examples of products available. Refer to specific product labels for further details.

Active ingredients	Label status/sizes	Trade names; other information
Manuka honey	OTC; labeled for use on dogs; 1 oz and 2 oz tubes; 2 oz, 4 oz, 16 oz, 32 oz jars	*HoneyCure®*
Manuka honey 10%, *MicroSilver BG®* 0.1% (spray gel)	OTC; labeled for use on all animals; 8 oz bottle	*Silver Honey® Hot Spot and Wound Repair; Silver Honey® Rapid Wound Repair*
Manuka honey 11%, *MicroSilver BG®* 0.2% (ointment)	OTC; labeled for use on all animals; 2 oz tube	*Silver Honey® Hot Spot and Wound Repair; Silver Honey® Rapid Wound Repair*
Manuka honey 40% (gel)	OTC; labeled for use on large and small animals; 1.75 oz tube	*L-Mesitran®*
Untreated raw honey (cream)	OTC; labeled for use on horses; 190 mL jar	*HoneyHeel®*

Human-Labeled Products

Many different brands of medical-grade honey or medical-grade Manuka honey exist. Listed below are representative examples of products available. Refer to specific product label for further details.

Active ingredients	Label status/sizes	Trade names; other information
Manuka honey 30% (cream)	OTC; 0.5 oz tube	*First Honey®*
Manuka honey 63% impregnated hydrogel colloidal sheet (nonadhesive dressing)	OTC; 2.4" x 2.4" and 8" x 12" sheets of 1/pack, 10/pack	*MediHoney® HCS*
Manuka honey 80% (gel)	OTC; 1.5 oz tube	*MediHoney®*
Manuka honey 100% (adhesive dressing)	OTC; 1" x 3.25" adhesive dressings of 12/box, 3" x 4" adhesive dressings of 6/box	*FirstHoney®*
Manuka honey 100% (gel)	OTC; 0.5 oz and 1.5 tubes. Single-use, 10/box or individual tube	*TheraHoney®*

Active ingredients	Label status/sizes	Trade names; other information
Manuka honey 100% (hydrocolloid paste)	OTC; 0.5 oz, 1.5 oz, and 3.5 oz tubes. 1/pack, 4/pack, 10/pack, 12/pack	*MediHoney®*
Manuka honey 100% (ointment)	OTC; 0.5 oz tube	*First Honey®*
Manuka honey 100% (impregnated in calcium alginate pads)	OTC; single-use sheets: 2" x 2", 4" x 5", and ¾" x 12" sheets of 1/pack, 5/pack, 10/pack, and 100/case	*MediHoney® Calcium Alginate Dressing* Calcium alginate provides wound fluid absorption capabilities.
Manuka honey 100% (impregnated in sheets [nonadhesive dressing])	OTC; single-use sheets; can be cut to fit within the wound edges. 2" x 2", 4" x 5" sheets of 10/box; rope: 1" x 12"; 4" x 4" flexible foams of 10/box	*TheraHoney®; TheraHoney® HD; TheraHoney® Foam Flex*

References

For the complete list of references, see **wiley.com/go/budde/plumb**

Mupirocin, Topical

Pseudomonic Acid A

(myoo-***pye***-roe-sin)

Indications/Actions

Mupirocin is FDA-approved for the treatment of bacterial skin infections in dogs caused by susceptible strains of *Staphylococcus aureus* or *Staphylococcus pseudintermedius,* including beta-lactamase producing and methicillin-resistant strains. Mupirocin can be used to treat superficial pyoderma, fold pyoderma, interdigital cysts, draining tracts, acne, and pressure point pyodermas. It may also be used in other species for conditions such as feline acne or equine pyoderma.

Mupirocin also has activity against other gram-positive pathogens, including strains of *Corynebacterium* spp, *Clostridium* spp, *Proteus* spp, and *Actinomyces* spp., Although it has activity against some gram-negative bacteria, it is not used clinically for gram-negative infections. *Pseudomonas* spp is particularly resistant to mupirocin. Mupirocin has anecdotally been reported to have some effect against Malassezia spp in dogs and cats.

Mupirocin is an antibiotic isolated from the bacterium *Pseudomonas fluorescens.* It is unique in that it belongs to the monocarboxylic acid class and is structurally related to other commercially available antibiotics. Pseudomonic acid A represents 90% to 95% of the mixture and is the main compound of mupirocin. It acts by inhibiting bacterial protein synthesis by binding and inhibiting bacterial isoleucyl transfer-RNA synthetase. It is bacteriostatic at low concentrations or bactericidal at high concentrations. While bacterial resistance is rare in animals, resistant strains of *Staphylococcus* spp have been identified. Resistance transference is thought to be plasmid-mediated and thought to occur more frequently when mupirocin is used on large areas of the skin for prolonged durations. Therefore, mupirocin may be best suited for short-term treatment on small, localized areas. Cross-resistance with other antimicrobials has not been identified. Because this antibiotic is a salient treatment used in humans with resistant infections, its use should be limited to select or resistant cases in veterinary patients.

Mupirocin is not significantly absorbed through the skin into the systemic circulation but does penetrate well into granulomatous and deep pyoderma lesions. It is not suitable for application to burns.

Suggested Dosages/Uses

After cleansing the lesion, mupirocin should be applied to completely cover the affected area. It is labeled for twice daily application on dogs. It requires 10 minutes of contact time to be active. The maximum duration of treatment is 30 days.[1]

In cats with chin acne, once- to twice-daily applications have been shown to be effective for treating secondary infections.[2]

Precautions/Adverse Effects

Mupirocin is contraindicated in patients with a history of hypersensitive reactions to it or other ointments containing polyethylene glycol. Use veterinary labeled products with caution on extensive deep lesions due to risk for nephrotoxicity from absorption of large quantities of polyethylene glycol.[1] Do not let animals lick or chew treated areas for at least 20 to 30 minutes after application. Avoid contact with eyes; not for ophthalmic use.

Mupirocin is typically well tolerated. Contact reactions such as pain, erythema, and itching are possible. Overgrowth of non-susceptible organisms (superinfection) is also possible with prolonged use.

Veterinary-Labeled Products

Active ingredients (formulation)	Species	Label status; size(s)	Trade names/additional information
Mupirocin 2% (ointment)	Labeled for use on dogs	Rx; 15 g, 22 g	*Muricin®*; generic

Human-Labeled Products

Active ingredients (formulation)	Label status; size(s)	Trade names/additional information
Mupirocin 2% (ointment)	Rx; 1 g, 15 g, 22 g, and 30 g	*Bactroban®; Centany®*; generic
Mupirocin 2% (cream)	Rx; 15 g, 30 g	*Bactroban®*; generic

References

For the complete list of references, see **wiley.com/go/budde/plumb**

Nitrofurazone, Topical

(nye-troe-***fur***-ah-zone) *Furazone®*

Indications/Actions

Nitrofurazone is FDA-approved for prevention or treatment of surface bacterial infections of wounds, burns, and cutaneous ulcers in dogs and horses; some products are also approved for cats.[1] It is a synthetic nitrofuran with a broad-antibacterial spectrum. Nitrofurazone is bactericidal against many bacteria involved in surface infections, including gram-positive (eg, *Staphylococcus aureus*, *Streptococcus* spp) and gram-negative (eg, *Escherichia coli*) bacteria; however, evidence supporting clinical efficacy is unavailable. Nitrofurazone has also anecdotally been used for the adjunctive treatment of myiasis.

The mechanism of action of nitrofurazone is thought to be associated with inhibiting bacterial enzymes that primarily degrade glucose and pyruvate.

Suggested Dosages/Uses

Nitrofurazone ointment should be applied directly to the affected area with a spatula or placed on gauze that is then applied to the lesion.[1] Dressing may be changed several times a day or left in place for longer periods of time, but the ointment should remain in contact with the lesion for at least 24 hours. Nitrofurazone powder should be applied to the affected areas daily to several times per day.[2] Refer to specific product labels for details on use.

Precautions/Adverse Effects

Nitrofurazone has been shown to cause mammary tumors when fed in high doses to rats and ovarian tumors in mice. **Federal law prohibits the use of nitrofurazone products in or on food animals, including horses intended to be used for food**. Wear gloves and wash hands after applying.

Ointments may contain polyethylene glycols. If used on large areas of denuded skin, significant amounts of polyethylene glycol could be absorbed, which can cause nephrotoxicity.[3] Avoid contact with eyes and mucous membranes. Do not allow animals to lick or chew treated areas for at least 30 minutes. Avoid exposing products to sunlight, strong fluorescent lighting, excessive heat, or alkaline materials.

Topical nitrofurazone is typically well tolerated. Hypersensitivity reactions and skin reactions, including pain, erythema, and itching, are possible but uncommon. Discontinue use of this product if redness, irritation, or swelling persists or increases. Overgrowth of nonsusceptible organisms (superinfection) is also possible with the prolonged use of nitrofurazone.

Veterinary-Labeled Products

Active ingredients (formulation)	Species	Label status; size(s)	Trade names/additional information
Nitrofurazone 0.2% (ointment)	Labeled for dogs, cats, and horses	OTC; 1 lb jars	*Fura-Septin®; NFZ® Wound Dressing;* generic
Nitrofurazone 0.2% (ointment)	Labeled for horses	OTC; 1 lb jars	*Fura-Zone®*
Nitrofurazone 0.2% (powder)	Labeled for dogs, cats, and horses	OTC; 45 g	*NFZ® Puffer;* generic Shake or rotate to loosen powder. Restricted drug in California

Human-Labeled Products

None. Nitrofurazone products are no longer available for humans in the United States.

References

For the complete list of references, see **wiley.com/go/budde/plumb**

Silver Sulfadiazine, Topical

(***sil***-ver sul-fa-***dye***-ah-zeen)

Indications/Actions

Silver sulfadiazine (SSD) is used in veterinary medicine to treat localized bacterial skin infections, particularly those caused by *Pseudomonas* spp. In humans, topical SSD is labeled for prophylaxis and treatment of second- and third-degree burns.

SSD has extensive antimicrobial activity. It is bactericidal against many gram-positive and gram-negative bacteria and is also effective against yeasts. SSD disrupts microbial cell membranes and cell walls; this differs from the antibacterial actions of silver nitrate or sodium sulfadiazine. It can enhance epithelization but can impair granulation.

Suggested Dosages/Uses

For burns, silver sulfadiazine (SSD) is applied once to twice daily at a thickness of ≈1/16th of an inch (1 to 2 mm). Dressings may be applied over the cream. For localized bacterial infections, once- to twice-daily application is recommended. Apply to affected area(s) and massage the cream into the skin.

Precautions/Adverse Effects

Use with caution in patients that are hypersensitive to sulfonamides, as they may also react to silver sulfadiazine (SSD). Patients with significant hepatic or renal dysfunction have increased risk for drug accumulation, particularly when used over large areas. Because SSD can impair granulation, avoid use in non-granulated wounds. Avoid contact with eyes. Wear gloves or wash hands after applying. Do not let animals lick or chew at affected areas for at least 20 to 30 minutes after application.

Adverse effects of systemic sulfonamides are possible, such as blood dyscrasias and keratoconjunctivitis sicca (KCS). Use over large areas or use for extended durations can increase the risk for systemic adverse effects. Refer to ***Sulfa-/Trimethoprim*** for more information. In humans, transient leukopenia has been reported with SSD treatment. However, leukocyte normalization occurs even with continuation of therapy. Other uncommon adverse effects in humans include skin necrosis, erythema multiforme, skin discoloration, rashes, and interstitial nephritis.

Veterinary-Labeled Products

There are no topical SSD products labeled for veterinary patients. An otic preparation (*Baytril® Otic*) contains silver sulfadiazine (SSD). See ***Antibacterials, Otic*** for more information.

Active ingredients (formulation)	Species	Label status; size(s)	Trade names/additional information
Silver sulfadiazine 1%, enrofloxacin 0.5% (emulsion)	Labeled for otic use in dogs	Rx; 15 mL, 30 mL	*Baytril®* Extra-label when used topically

Human-Labeled Products

Active ingredients (formulation)	Label status; size(s)	Trade names/additional information
Silver sulfadiazine 1% (cream)	Rx; 20 g, 25 g, 50 g, 85 g, 400 g, and 1000 g	*Silvadene®; SSD®; Thermazene®*

Antifungal Agents, Topical

Clotrimazole, Topical

(kloe-***trye***-ma-zole) *Lotrimin®*

For otic products containing clotrimazole, see ***Corticosteroid/Antimicrobial Agents, Otic.***

Indications/Actions

Topical clotrimazole has activity against dermatophytes and yeasts; it may be useful for localized lesions associated with *Malassezia* spp. There is limited information regarding its efficacy for the treatment of dermatophytosis in cats and dogs. Most veterinary clotrimazole products also contain gentamicin and a glucocorticoid and are labeled for otic use; these products may be used in an extra-label manner for bacterial and yeast skin infections with concurrent inflamed, pruritic skin.

Intranasal instillation of clotrimazole via sinus trephination or direct frontal sinuscopy may also be used for the treatment of sinonasal aspergillosis in dogs, with or without systemic antifungal therapy.[1-3]

Clotrimazole is an imidazole antifungal that inhibits the biosynthesis of ergosterol, a component of fungal cell membranes, leading to increased membrane permeability and probable disruption of membrane enzyme systems.

Suggested Dosages/Uses

If sprays are prescribed, twice-daily applications are usually recommended. Ointments are generally applied to affected areas up to 4 times daily. For veterinary products, refer to the product label for details on individual use.

Precautions/Adverse Effects

Avoid contact with eyes and mucous membranes. Clients should wash their hands after application or wear gloves when applying. Skin irritation is possible but unlikely to occur with products containing only clotrimazole. Avoid contact with eyes. Do not allow the animal to lick or chew at affected sites for at least 20 to 30 minutes after application.

Cribriform plate damage has historically been suggested as a contraindication for topical antifungal treatment for sinonasal aspergillosis; however, small retrospective reviews of dogs with cribriform plate lysis cases found no neurologic adverse effects following infusion of clotrimazole 1% into the frontal sinuses.[4,5]

Products containing clotrimazole in combination with a glucocorticoid (eg, betamethasone):
Several veterinary topical products list pregnancy as a contraindication. Systemic glucocorticoids can be teratogenic or induce parturition during the third trimester of pregnancy in animals. If considering use during pregnancy, weigh the respective risks with treating versus potential benefits. Clients should wash their hands after application or wear gloves when applying. Avoid contact with eyes. Do not allow the animal to lick or chew at affected sites for at least 20 to 30 minutes after application. Residual activity from glucocorticoids may affect intradermal or serum allergy tests; it has been suggested to stop use 2 weeks prior to allergy testing.

Use care when treating large areas or when using on smaller patients. Risks can be reduced by treating for only as long as necessary on as small an area as possible. When higher concentrations of glucocorticoids are used or with longer durations of therapy (ie, longer than 7 days), there is an increased risk for HPA axis suppression, systemic glucocorticoid effects (eg, polydipsia, polyuria, polyphagia), skin changes (eg, atrophy, skin fragility, alopecia, localized pyoderma, comedones), and delayed wound healing. Vomiting and diarrhea have been reported with the use of products containing betamethasone. Local skin reactions (burning, itching, redness) are possible but unlikely to occur.

Veterinary-Labeled Products

Active ingredients (formulation)	Species	Label status; size(s)	Trade names/additional information
Clotrimazole 1% (ointment) Other ingredients: bentonite, jojoba oil, magnesium oxide, peppermint oil, silver oxide, tea tree oil, white wax, zinc oxide	Not specified	OTC, not FDA approved; 100 g	*Aardora®*
Clotrimazole 1% (solution)	Labeled for dogs and cats	OTC, not FDA approved or Rx; 30 mL	*ClotrimaTop®*
Clotrimazole 1% (spray or dropper) Other ingredients: propylene glycol, SD alcohol 40, benzoyl alcohol, chloroxylenol	Labeled for dogs and cats	OTC, not FDA approved; 1 oz dropper, 2 oz spray	*Clotrimazole Antifungal®*

Human-Labeled Products

Active ingredients (formulation)	Label status; size(s)	Trade names/additional information
Clotrimazole 1% (solution)	OTC/Rx (status determined by labeling); depending on the product: 10 mL, 30 mL	generic
Clotrimazole 1% (cream)	OTC/Rx (status determined by labeling); depending on the product: 10 mL, 30 mL	*Lotrimin AF®; Desenex®*

References

For the complete list of references, see **wiley.com/go/budde/plumb**

Enilconazole, Topical

(ee-nil-***kon***-a-zole) *Imaverol®*

Indications/Actions

Although no dosage forms are currently commercially available for topical use in the United States, compounded enilconazole is used topically for treating dermatophytosis in small animals and horses. In other countries, a commercially available topical rinse is available for canine, equine, and bovine species. The use of topical enilconazole on cats with dermatophytosis is somewhat controversial as no products are labeled for feline use; however, there are reports of successful use of enilconazole as a sole therapy or in combination with oral itraconazole for cats with dermatophytosis.

Intranasal instillation of enilconazole after plaque debridement has also been shown useful in treating nasal aspergillosis in small animal species.[1]

A poultry environmental disinfectant product (*Clinafarm EC®*) is available in the United States and has been used extra-label to treat dermatophytosis; however, as this product is regulated by the EPA, it is illegal to use it in a manner inconsistent with its labeling.

Enilconazole, like other azoles, inhibits the biosynthesis of ergosterol, an essential component of fungal cell membranes, leading to increased membrane permeability and allowing leakage of intracellular components.

Suggested Dosages/Uses

The commercial product should be diluted by adding 1 part of concentrated solution to 50 parts warm water, which yields a 2 mg/mL emulsion. Remove crusts with a hard brush that has been soaked in the diluted emulsion. It is highly recommended that the animal be sprayed entirely at the first treatment to reach subclinical lesions as well.

Dogs: Clip longhaired dogs prior to treatment, and wash with the diluted emulsion 4 times at 3 to 4 day intervals.[2] During application, the hair should be brushed thoroughly in the opposite direction of hair growth to make sure that the skin is thoroughly wet. Alternatively, dogs may be dipped in a bath of the diluted emulsion.[3]

Horses: The lesions and surrounding skin are to be washed with the diluted emulsion 4 times at 3 to 4 day intervals.[2]

Cattle: Wash with diluted emulsion or apply with a sprayer or high-pressure cleaning unit 3 to 4 times at 3-day intervals.[3]

Dispose of all unused diluted solutions. Refer to the product label for details on use.

Precautions/Adverse Effects

Avoid contact with eyes. Clients should wear gloves and eye protection when applying.

When enilconazole is used topically in cats, hypersalivation, vomiting, anorexia, weight loss, muscle weakness, and a slight increase in serum ALT levels have been reported.

Veterinary-Labeled Products

Active ingredients (formulation)	Species	Label status; size(s)	Trade names/additional information
Enilconazole 10% (concentrate)	Labeled for dogs and horses; also labeled for cattle in some countries	50 mL, 100 mL, 1 L	*Imaverol®; Austrazole®* Not available in the United States. Refer to specific product labels for withdrawal periods.

Human-Labeled Products

None

References

For the complete list of references, see **wiley.com/go/budde/plumb**

Ketoconazole, Topical

(kee-toe-***kah***-na-zole) *Nizoral®, KetoChlor®*

*For systemic use, see **Ketoconazole.***

*For otic use, see **Corticosteroid/Antimicrobial Agents, Otic.***

Indications/Actions

Topical ketoconazole has activity against dermatophytes and yeasts, and ketoconazole shampoos can be an effective treatment for *Malassezia* spp dermatitis and dermatophytosis; however, topical ketoconazole shampoos are generally ineffective or minimally effective when used alone for dermatophytosis. Patients with severe, generalized infections may require additional systemic therapy.

Ketoconazole, like other azoles, inhibits the biosynthesis of ergosterol, an essential component of fungal cell membranes, leading to increased membrane permeability and allowing leakage of intracellular components.

Suggested Dosages/Uses

Sprays and wipes should be applied 1 to 2 times daily. Shampoos and conditioners can be used daily to weekly. Shampoo should typically be left in contact with the skin for at least 10 minutes prior to rinsing; see specific product label for details.

Precautions/Adverse Effects

Avoid contact with eyes; skin irritation is possible. Clients should wash their hands after application or wear gloves when applying. Do not allow animals to chew or lick application site for at least 20 to 30 minutes after application.

Veterinary-Labeled Products

Active ingredients (formulation)	Species	Label status; size(s)	Trade names/additional information
Ketoconazole 1%, chlorhexidine 2%, TrisEDTA (spray)	Labeled for dogs and cats	OTC; 8 oz	*Mal-A-Ket® Plus*
Ketoconazole 1%, chlorhexidine 2%, phytosphingosine 0.02% (spray)	Labeled for dogs and cats	OTC; 8 oz	*Vetraseb®* CK
Ketoconazole 0.3%, chloroxylenol 0.3% (spray)	Labeled for dogs, cats, and horses	OTC; 4 oz, 8 oz	*Pharmaseb®*
Ketoconazole 0.15%, hydrocortisone 1%, acetic acid 1%, boric acid 2% (spray)	Labeled for dogs, cats, and horses	OTC; 8 oz	*MalAcetic® ULTRA*
Ketoconazole 0.15%, hydrocortisone 1%, acetic acid 1%, boric acid 2% (shampoo)	Labeled for dogs, cats, and horses	OTC; 8 oz	*MalAcetic® ULTRA*
Ketoconazole 1%, chlorhexidine 2%, acetic acid 2% (shampoo)	Labeled for dogs, cats, and horses	OTC; 8 oz, 1 gallon	*Mal-A-Ket®*
Ketoconazole 1%, chlorhexidine 2% (shampoo)	Labeled for dogs and cats; some products also labeled for horses	OTC; 8 oz, 16 oz, and 1 gallon	*KetoHex®; Ceraven CHX+KET; VetraSeb® CeraDerm® CK*
Ketoconazole 1%, chloroxylenol 2% (shampoo)	Labeled for dogs, cats, and horses	OTC; 8 oz, 16 oz, and 1 gallon	*Pharmaseb®*
Ketoconazole 1%, chlorhexidine 2.3% (shampoo)	Labeled for dog and cats	OTC; 8 oz, 16 oz	*KetoChlor®*
Ketoconazole 1%, chlorhexidine 2%, phytosphingosine 0.05% (shampoo)	Labeled for dogs, cats, and horses	OTC; 8 oz, 16 oz	*Phyto CHX+KET®; Ketoseb +PS®*
Ketoconazole 1%, chlorhexidine 2%, glycolic acid 1% (shampoo)	Labeled for dogs, cats, and horses	OTC; 8 oz	*GlyChlorK®*
Ketoconazole 17 mg, chlorhexidine 20 mg, phytosphingosine 0.4 mg (wipes)	Labeled for dogs and cats	OTC; 50 count jar	*Ketoseb +PS*
Ketoconazole 1%, chlorhexidine 2% (wipes)	Labeled for dogs, cats, and horses	OTC; 50 count jar	*KetoHex®; VetraSeb®; CeraDerm® CK*
Ketoconazole 1%, chlorhexidine 2%, acetic acid 2% (wipes)	Labeled for dogs and cats	OTC; 50 count jar	*Mal-A-Ket®*
Ketoconazole 0.3%, chloroxylenol 0.3% (wipes)	Labeled for dogs, cats, and horses	OTC; 50 count	*Pharmaseb®*

Active ingredients (formulation)	Species	Label status; size(s)	Trade names/additional information
Ketoconazole 1%, chloroxylenol 2% (mousse)	Labeled for dogs, cats, and horses	OTC; 7 oz	*Pharmaseb®*
Ketoconazole 1%, chlorhexidine 2% (mousse)	Labeled for dogs and cats; some products also labeled for horses	OTC; 6.8 oz	Ceraven CHX+KET; *VetraSeb®*; *CeraDerm®* CK
Ketoconazole 1%, chlorhexidine 2%, phytosphingosine 0.05% (mousse)	Labeled for dogs and cats	OTC; 6.8 oz	*Ketoseb+PS*
Ketoconazole 0.1%, TrisEDTA (flush)	Labeled for dogs, cats, and horses	OTC; 4 oz, 12 oz	*T8 Keto®*
Ketoconazole 0.15%, chlorhexidine 0.15%, TrisEDTA (flush)	Labeled for dogs and cats	OTC; 4 oz, 12 oz	*Mal-A-Ket® Plus*
Ketoconazole 0.3%, chloroxylenol 0.3% (flush)	Labeled for dogs, cats, and horses	OTC; 4 oz, 8 oz	*Pharmaseb®*
Ketoconazole 0.15%, TrisEDTA (flush)	Labeled for dogs, cats, and horses	OTC; 4 oz, 12 oz	*TrizUltra® + Keto*
Ketoconazole 0.2%, chlorhexidine 0.2% (flush)	Labeled for dogs, cats, and horses	OTC; 4 oz	*KetoHex®*
Ketoconazole 0.1%, phytosphingosine 0.01% (flush)	Labeled for dogs and cats	OTC; 4 oz, 16 oz	*VetraSeb® CeraDerm® Tris*
Ketoconazole 0.2%, chlorhexidine 0.2%, phytosphingosine 0.02% (flush)	Labeled for dogs and cats	OTC; 4 oz, 16 oz	*Ketoseb+PS®*

Human-Labeled Products

Active ingredients (formulation)	Label status; size(s)	Trade names/additional information
Ketoconazole 1% (shampoo)	OTC; 4 oz, 7 oz	*Nizoral A-D®*
Ketoconazole 2% (shampoo)	Rx; 4 oz	*Nizoral®*; generic
Ketoconazole 2% (cream)	Rx; 15 g, 30 g, 60 g	*Nizoral®*; generic
Ketoconazole 2% (foam)	Rx; 50 g, 100 g	*Extina®*; *Ketodan®*; generic
Ketoconazole 2% (gel)	Rx; 45 g	*Xolegel®*

Lime Sulfur, Topical

(*lyme sul*-fur)

Indications/Actions

Lime sulfur is used as a generalized topical treatment for dermatophytosis. It is considered one of the most effective agents against *Microsporum canis.* In addition, it is efficacious for treatment of demodicosis in cats.[1] Lime sulfur can also be useful as an adjunctive treatment of *Malassezia* spp dermatitis, cheyletiellosis, chiggers, sarcoptic and notoedric mange, fur mites, lice, canine demodicosis, and sarcoptic mange, in addition to chorioptic mange in horses.

Lime sulfur has antibacterial and antifungal properties secondary to the formation of pentathionic acid and hydrogen sulfide after application. Lime sulfur may also have keratolytic, keratoplastic, antiparasitic, and antipruritic effects.

Suggested Dosages/Uses

Concentrated dips should be shaken well prior to use and must be diluted. Typically, 4 oz of concentrate should be diluted in 1 gallon of water, mixed well, and carefully applied to affected areas.[2] For chronic or resistant cases, 8 oz of concentrate may be diluted per gallon of water. Treatment may be repeated every 5 to 7 days. See specific product label for detailed dilution and application instructions. Do not rinse or blow-dry animals after application. Do not allow animals to ingest lime sulfur; apply a protective collar until dry if necessary to prevent ingestion.

When used for dermatophytosis, twice-weekly treatments have been recommended if tolerated.[3] Continue treatment until 2 consecutive negative cultures at weekly intervals are obtained.

For confirmed cases of feline surface demodicosis, applications are recommended every 5 to 7 days for a total of 6 treatments. For surface demodicosis treatment trials, 3 applications should be performed; if a significant improvement in clinical signs is noted, 3 more applications should be performed to complete treatment. If no significant improvement is seen after 3 applications, demodicosis should be ruled out and other diagnoses should be considered.

Precautions/Adverse Effects

Use caution when handling lime sulfur as adverse effects may occur after accidental dermal exposure, oral ingestion, or inhalation. Wear gloves and wash hands after handling. Avoid contact with eyes and mucous membranes; safety glasses are recommended.[2] Lime sulfur can stain porous surfaces such as concrete and porcelain and can permanently discolor jewelry. Lime sulfur should only be used in a well-ventilated area, or a respirator should be worn during application.

Lime sulfur is safe to use on pregnant and nursing animals and kittens/puppies over 2 to 3 weeks of age.

Lime sulfur may cause skin irritation or drying. Lime sulfur can temporarily stain light-colored fur and can rarely cause hair loss on the pinnae in cats. The odor of lime sulfur may persist on treated animals after application but is generally tolerable after drying. Oral ingestion can rarely cause nausea and oral ulcers, particularly in cats; an Elizabethan collar can help prevent ingestion from licking and grooming. Systemic toxicosis secondary to dermal exposure of lime sulfur has been reported after improper dilution of the concentrate.[4] Therefore, detailed dilution instructions are important for owners when recommending this therapy.

Veterinary-Labeled Products

Active ingredients (formulation)	Species	Label status; size(s)	Trade names/additional information
Lime sulfur 97.8% (dip)	Labeled for dogs, puppies, kittens, and cats; some products also labeled for horses	OTC; 4 oz, 16 oz, 1 gallon	*LimePlus*®; generic Shake well and dilute before use.

Human-Labeled Products

None

References

For the complete list of references, see **wiley.com/go/budde/plumb**

Miconazole, Topical

(mye-***kah***-nah-zole)

For ophthalmic use, see ***Miconazole Ophthalmic***

For otic use, see ***Antifungal Agents, Otic*** *and* ***Corticosteroid/Antimicrobial Agents, Otic***

Indications/Actions

Topical miconazole is used for the treatment of *Malassezia* spp dermatitis and infections caused by *Microsporum canis, Microsporum gypseum, and Trichophyton mentagrophytes.*[1] Lotions, sprays, and creams are generally used for localized lesions; patients with severe, generalized infections may require systemic antifungal therapy. Topical miconazole products are typically only minimally effective for dermatophytosis when used as a single agent; adjunctive systemic treatment is commonly required.

Miconazole is an imidazole antifungal with activity against dermatophytes and yeast. Its actions are a result of altering the permeability of fungal cellular membranes and interfering with peroxisomal and mitochondrial enzymes, leading to intracellular necrosis. Miconazole products are fungicidal with repeated application. Miconazole has been shown to be active against a series of gram-positive bacteria and to help repair the skin barrier function and mitigate some inflammatory cell reactions.[2]

Suggested Dosages/Uses

Sprays, creams, lotions, or wipes should be applied 1 to 2 times daily. Shampoos and conditioners may be used daily to weekly. Typically, shampoo should be left in contact with the skin for at least 10 minutes prior to rinsing. For veterinary products, refer to the specific product label for details on use.

Precautions/Adverse Effects

Avoid contact with eyes. Wash hands thoroughly after application to prevent the spread of fungal infections.[1] Do not allow treated animals to lick or chew at affected areas for at least 20 to 30 minutes after application.

Skin irritation is uncommon but possible. Wipes and sprays that contain alcohol may be severely irritating to inflamed, eroded, or ulcerated skin.

Veterinary-Labeled Products

NOTE: Miconazole nitrate is the salt generally used in pharmaceutical products. Some products express concentration as base, others express concentrations of the salt.

Active ingredients (formulation)	Species	Label status; size(s)	Trade names/additional information
Miconazole 1% (spray)	Labeled for dogs and cats	Rx; 60 mL, 120 mL, 240 mL	*MicaVed*®; *Micazole*®; *Priconazole*®; *Conzol*®
Miconazole nitrate 2% (spray)	Labeled for dogs, cats, and horses	OTC; 4 oz, 16 oz	generic
Miconazole nitrate 2%, chlorhexidine 2% (spray)	Labeled for dogs, cats, and horses	Rx; 8 oz	*Malaseb*®
Miconazole nitrate 2%, chlorhexidine 2%, TrisEDTA (spray)	Labeled for dogs, cats, and horses	OTC; 8 oz, 12 oz, 32 oz	*MiconaHex+Triz*®
Miconazole nitrate 0.2%, chlorhexidine 0.2% (flush)	Labeled for dogs, cats, and horses	Rx; 4 oz, 12 oz	*Malaseb*®
Miconazole 0.1% (flush)	Labeled for dogs and cats	OTC; 4 oz, 16 oz	*BioTris*®

Active ingredients (formulation)	Species	Label status; size(s)	Trade names/additional information
Miconazole 1% (lotion)	Labeled for dogs and cats	Rx; 30 mL, 60 mL	*Conzol®; Priconazole®; MicaVed®; Miconosol®; Micazole®*
Miconazole nitrate 2%, chlorhexidine 2%, TrisEDTA (wipes)	Labeled for dogs, cats, and horses	OTC; 50 count jar	*MiconaHex+Triz®*
Miconazole nitrate 15.1 mg/mL, gentamicin sulfate 1.5 mg/mL, hydrocortisone aceponate 1.11 mg/mL (suspension)	Labeled for otic use in dogs	Rx; 10 mL	*Easotic®* Topical use is extra-label.
Miconazole nitrate 23 mg/mL, polymyxin B sulfate 0.5293 mg/mL, prednisolone acetate 5 mg/mL (suspension)	Labeled for otic use in dogs	Rx; 15 mL, 30 mL	*Surolan®* Topical use is extra-label.
Miconazole nitrate 2%, chlorhexidine 2% (shampoo)	Labeled for dogs, cats, and horses	Rx; 8 oz, 16 oz	*Malaseb®*
Miconazole nitrate 2%, chlorhexidine 2%, TrisEDTA (shampoo)	Labeled for dogs, cats, and horses	OTC; 8 oz, 16 oz, 1 gallon	*MiconaHex+Triz®*
Miconazole nitrate 2%, chloroxylenol 1%, salicylic acid 2% (shampoo)	Labeled for dogs, cats, and horses	OTC; 8 oz, 12 oz, 1 gallon	*Sebozole®*
Miconazole 2% (shampoo)	Labeled for dogs and cats	OTC; 12 oz	generic
Miconazole nitrate 2%, colloidal oatmeal 2% (shampoo)	Labeled for dogs, cats, puppies, and kittens	OTC; 12 oz, 1 gallon	generic
Miconazole nitrate 2%, chlorhexidine 2% (shampoo)	Labeled for dogs and cats	OTC; 8 oz, 12 oz, 16 oz, 1 gallon	*BioHex®; Micoseb®*
Miconazole nitrate 2%, chlorhexidine 2%, TrisEDTA (mousse)	Labeled for dogs, cats, and horses	OTC; 7.1 oz	*MiconaHex+Triz®*

Human-Labeled Products

In addition to the products listed below, there are 2% topical vaginal creams, vaginal suppositories, 2% powders, and spray powders available. Most human-labeled products are OTC.

Active ingredients (formulation)	Label status; size(s)	Trade names/additional information
Miconazole 2% (ointment)	OTC; depending on the product: 4 g, 30 g, 57 g, 56.7 g, 113 g, and 142 g packages	generic
Miconazole 2% (aerosol spray or powder)	OTC; 30 g, 43 g, 85 g, 90 g, 113 g, and 133 g cans	generic
Miconazole 2% (cream)	OTC; many sizes available	generic

References

For the complete list of references, see **wiley.com/go/budde/plumb**

Nystatin/Nystatin Combinations, Topical

(nye-***sta***-tin)

For systemic use, see ***Nystatin.***

Indications/Actions

Nystatin is typically used in combination with antibiotics and glucocorticoids in small animal medicine; it is generally not used as a single agent due to limited dosage forms and alternative antifungal agents. Combination products containing neomycin, thiostrepton, and triamcinolone are FDA-approved in dogs and cats for treatment of inflammatory dermatologic disorders, particularly associated with bacterial or *Candida albicans* infections.[1] Use for topical yeast infections without a bacterial component should be avoided to prevent antibiotic resistance.

Nystatin is active against many yeasts and yeast-like fungi, such as *Malassezia spp* and *Candida* spp. Nystatin binds to sterols in fungal cell membranes, thereby increasing membrane permeability and allowing leakage of intracellular components. Nystatin does not have activity against bacteria and is ineffective against other fungi.

Suggested Dosages/Uses

Although nystatin is rarely used as a single topical agent, human products can be used if needed. In humans, creams are preferred to ointments in intertriginous areas; topical powders are used for moist lesions.

After cleaning affected areas, nystatin combination products should be applied sparingly in a thin film. Frequency of application is based on severity of infection and may range from once daily to once weekly for mild infections and up to 2 to 3 times daily for severe infections.[1] Frequency can be decreased as infection improves. Products that contain triamcinolone are best suited for focal (eg, pedal) or multifocal lesions that require relatively short treatment durations (eg, less than 2 months).

Precautions/Adverse Effects

Avoid empiric use of combination products or use in the absence of concurrent bacterial infection to help prevent bacterial resistance.

Avoid contact with eyes. Wear gloves or wash hands after application. Do not let the animal lick or chew at the treated area(s) for at least 20 to 30 minutes after application.

Topical nystatin is considered nontoxic and is generally well-tolerated, although hypersensitivity reactions are possible.[2] Potential adverse effects reported in humans include burning, itching, rash, and eczema.[3] The combination veterinary products are usually well-tolerated when used on the skin; however, neomycin can cause localized sensitivity, and glucocorticoids can potentially cause cutaneous atrophy or HPA-axis suppression.[1] At least a 2-week withdrawal period is recommended prior to intradermal or allergy serum testing for products containing corticosteroids, such as triamcinolone.[4]

Veterinary-Labeled Products

Active ingredients (formulation)	Species	Label status; size(s)	Trade names/additional information
Nystatin 100,000 units/g, neomycin sulfate 2.5 mg/g, thiostrepton 2500 units/g, triamcinolone acetate 1 mg/g (cream)	Labeled for dogs and cats	Rx; 7.5 g, 15 g	*Animax®*
Nystatin 100,000 units/g, neomycin sulfate 2.5 mg/g, thiostrepton 2500 units/g, triamcinolone acetonide 1 mg/g (ointment)	Labeled for dogs and cats	Rx; 7.5 mL, 15 mL, 30 mL, and 240 mL	*Animax®*; *Quadritop®*; *Derma-Vet®*; *Dermalog®*; *Dermalone®*; *EnteDerm®*

Human-Labeled Products

Active ingredients (formulation)	Label status; size(s)	Trade names/additional information
Nystatin 100,000 units/g (powder)	Rx; 15 g, 30 g, and 60 g	*Nyamyc®*; *Nystop®*; generic
Nystatin 100,000 units/g (ointment)	Rx; 15 g, 30 g	generic
Nystatin 100,000 units/g (cream)	Rx; 15 g, 30 g	generic
Nystatin 100,000 units/g, triamcinolone acetate 1mg/g (ointment)	Rx; 15 g, 30 g, and 60 g	generic
Nystatin 100,000 units/g, triamcinolone acetate 1 mg/g (cream)	Rx; 15 g, 30 g, and 60 g	generic

References

For the complete list of references, see **wiley.com/go/budde/plumb**

Selenium Sulfide, Topical

(si-***leen***-ee-um ***sul***-fide)

Indications/Actions

Selenium sulfide may be useful in dogs for treating seborrheic disorders (mainly for seborrhea oleosa) and for the adjunctive treatment of *Malassezia* dermatitis, particularly in dogs exhibiting signs of waxy, greasy, or scaly (seborrheic) dermatitis.

Selenium sulfide possesses antifungal and sporicidal activity, keratolytic, keratoplastic, and degreasing properties. It alters epidermal turnover in cells of the epidermis and follicular epithelium and interferes with hydrogen bond formation of keratin, thereby reducing corneocyte production. The antifungal mechanism of action of selenium sulfide is not well understood.

Suggested Dosages/Uses

Selenium sulfide shampooing frequency is patient dependent. In general, medicated shampoos should remain in contact with the skin for 10 minutes. Alternatively, allow 3 to 5 minutes of contact time, rinse thoroughly, and then repeat the procedure. Thoroughly rinse off the shampoo to prevent skin irritation and excessive drying.

Precautions/Adverse Effects

Selenium sulfide products should not be used on cats. Avoid contact with eyes and mucous membranes. Selenium sulfide can damage or discolor jewelry. Clients should wear gloves when using these products.

Selenium sulfide can be irritating, especially to the scrotal area. It can also cause excessive drying and hair-coat staining or discoloration. Do not use these products on broken or inflamed skin. After discontinuation, rebound seborrhea can occur and can be more severe than pretreatment presentation.

GI effects such as nausea, vomiting, or diarrhea may occur if selenium sulfide is ingested orally. Neurologic signs are possible if large quantities are ingested. In case of substantial oral ingestion, consultation with a 24-hour poison consultation center specializing in providing veterinary-specific information is recommended. For general information related to overdose and toxin exposures, as well as contact information for poison control centers, refer to ***Appendix***.

Veterinary-Labeled Products

There are no veterinary labeled products containing selenium sulfide currently available in the United States; products may be available in other countries.

Human-Labeled Products

Active ingredients (formulation)	Label status; size(s)	Trade names/additional information
Selenium sulfide 1% (shampoo)	OTC; 11 oz	*Selsun Blue®*, generic
Selenium sulfide 2.25% (shampoo)	Rx; 6 oz	generic
Selenium sulfide 2.3% (shampoo)	Rx; 6 oz	generic
Selenium sulfide 2.5% (lotion)	Rx; 4 oz	generic
Selenium sulfide 2.25% (foam)	Rx; 2.5 oz	*Tersi®* Marketing status uncertain

Terbinafine, Topical

(ter-***bin***-a-feen)

For systemic use, see ***Terbinafine.***

For otic use, see ***Corticosteroid/Antimicrobial Agents, Otic.***

Indications/Actions

Terbinafine is an allylamine antifungal agent that may be useful for localized lesions associated with *Malassezia* infections. In an in vitro study, topical 1% terbinafine was shown to have good efficacy as adjuvant focal therapy against *Microsporum canis* with good residual activity.[1]

Terbinafine inhibits the biosynthesis of ergosterol by inhibiting the fungal squalene epoxidase enzyme. The resultant depletion of ergosterol within the fungal cell membrane and the intracellular accumulation of squalene are believed to be responsible for the fungicidal effect of terbinafine. It is fungicidal against dermatophytes but may only be fungistatic against yeast organisms.

Suggested Dosages/Uses

Topical terbinafine may be applied to skin areas affected with *Malassezia* once to twice a day. Based on in vitro data, less frequent application (ie, once daily to every other day) may be sufficient for adjuvant therapy of *M canis* skin infections due to the demonstrated residual activity of terbinafine.[1]

Precautions/Adverse Effects

Avoid contact with eyes and mucous membranes. Wash hands after application. Do not allow animals to lick or chew at the treated area(s) for at least 30 minutes after application.

Local irritation is possible, including burning, pruritis, or rash.

Veterinary-Labeled Products

None labeled for use on skin.

Human-Labeled Products

Active ingredients (formulation)	Label status; size(s)	Trade names/additional information
Terbinafine hydrochloride 1% (cream)	OTC; 12 g, 15 g, 24 g, 30 g, 42 g	*Lamisil AT®*; generic
Terbinafine hydrochloride 1% (spray)	OTC; 125 mL	*Lamisil AT®*

References

For the complete list of references, see **wiley.com/go/budde/plumb**

Antiseptic Agents, Topical

Acetic Acid/Boric Acid, Topical

(ah-***see***-tik ***ass***-id; ***bor***-ik ***assi***-id)

For otic products, refer to ***Antiseptic Agents, Otic***

Indications/Actions

Acetic and boric acids are indicated for the topical treatment of skin infections caused by bacteria, including *Staphylococcus* spp,[1] *Pseudomonas* spp,[2,3] and yeast, such as *Malassezia* spp. They are also indicated for fold dermatitis, acute moist dermatitis, pododermatitis, and seborrhea oleosa.

Acetic and boric acids are potent antibacterial and antifungal agents with a rapid killing effect. They also possess ceruminolytic, keratolytic, keratoplastic, and astringent properties.

Some products also contain other antimicrobials, such as chlorhexidine and ketoconazole, or anti-inflammatory agents, such as hydrocortisone for anti-pruritic effects.

Suggested Uses/Dosages

Sprays and wipes may be applied up to 2 to 3 times a day. Shampoos and conditioners can be used daily to weekly, during or after routine bathing. Leave shampoos in contact with the skin for at least 10 minutes prior to rinsing. Refer to the product label for specific instructions.

Acetic acid and boric acid topical products have concentrations ranging from 1% to 2% for each acid. One study found that acetic acid and boric acid concentrations as low as 0.5% have bactericidal effects against *Staphylococcus pseudintermedius* in vitro.[1]

Precautions/Adverse Effects

Skin redness and irritation may occur. Do not let the animal lick or chew at affected areas for at least 20 to 30 minutes after application. For products that also contain hydrocortisone, caution should be used to avoid excessive or frequent use due to its potential cutaneous and systemic adverse effects.

Veterinary-Labeled Products

SHAMPOOS

Acetic acid 2%, boric acid 2%	Labeled for dogs, cats, and horses	OTC; 12 oz, 16 oz, and 1 gallon	*MalAcetic®*
Ketoconazole 0.15%, hydrocortisone 1%, acetic acid 1%, boric acid 2% Other ingredients: ceramide complex	Labeled for dogs, cats, and horses	OTC; 8 oz	*MalAcetic® ULTRA*
Ketoconazole 1%, acetic acid 2%, chlorhexidine 2%	Labeled for dogs, cats, and horses	OTC; 8 oz and 1 gallon	*Mal-A-Ket®*
Ketoconazole 1%, acetic acid 2%, chlorhexidine 2%		OTC; 12 oz	*HexaChlor-K®*

SPRAYS

Active ingredients (formulation)	Species	Label status; size(s)	Trade names/additional information
Acetic acid 2%, boric acid 2%	Labeled for dogs, cats, and horses	OTC; 8 oz, 16 oz	*MalAcetic®*
Ketoconazole 0.15%, hydrocortisone 1%, acetic acid 1%, boric acid 2% Other ingredients: ceramide complex	Labeled for dogs, cats, and horses	OTC; 8 oz	*MalAcetic® ULTRA*
Ketoconazole 1% acetic acid 2%, chlorhexidine 2%	Labeled for dogs and cats	OTC; 8 oz	*HexaChlor-K®*

WIPES

Active ingredients (formulation)	Species	Label status; size(s)	Trade names/additional information
Acetic acid 2%, boric acid 2%	Labeled for dogs and cats	OTC; 25 count, 100 count jar	*MalAcetic®*
Ketoconazole 1%, acetic acid 2%, chlorhexidine 2%	Labeled for dogs and cats	OTC; 50 count jar	*HexaChlor-K®*; *Mal-A-Ket®*
Hydrocortisone 1%, acetic acid 1%, boric acid 1%; other ingredients: ceramide complex	Labeled for dogs and cats	OTC; 25 count jar	*MalAcetic® HC*

Human-Labeled Products

There are several OTC human products available containing acetic acid or boric acid (alone or containing other ingredients). For more information on human-labeled acetic acid or boric acid products, refer to a comprehensive human drug reference or contact a pharmacist.

References

For the complete list of references, see **wiley.com/go/budde/plumb**

Chlorhexidine, Topical

(klor-***heks***-ih-deen) *Nolvasan®*

Indications/Actions

Chlorhexidine is a synthetic phenol-related bisbiguanide that exists as acetate, gluconate, and hydrochloride salts. It is a topical antiseptic that has activity against many bacteria and fungi. It appears to have greater efficacy for bacterial infections, particularly *Staphylococcus* spp, than for yeast or dermatophyte infections. Chlorhexidine prevents the outgrowth of bacterial spores but does not prevent germination and is not sporicidal. It can be bacteriostatic or bactericidal depending on concentration.[1] Chlorhexidine is a membrane-active agent that acts by damaging bacterial cytoplasmic membranes. Antifungal activity can be obtained with chlorhexidine concentrations of 2% or higher.

Because chlorhexidine causes less drying and is usually less irritating than benzoyl peroxide, it is sometimes used in patients that cannot tolerate benzoyl peroxide. However, it does not have the keratolytic, comedolytic, or degreasing effects of benzoyl peroxide. Chlorhexidine possesses some residual effects and can remain active on the skin after rinsing.

In one study comparing in vitro efficacy of shampoos, chlorhexidine was shown to be the most effective biocide against *Pseudomonas* spp, methicillin-susceptible and methicillin-resistant *Staphylococcus* spp, and *Malassezia* spp.[2] Another controlled clinical study showed that bathing twice weekly with a 4% chlorhexidine-based shampoo for 4 weeks was as effective as systemic therapy with amoxicillin/clavulanic acid for the treatment of canine superficial pyoderma associated with susceptible and methicillin-resistant *Staphylococcus pseudintermedius*.

Another study found chlorhexidine 2% solution with alcohol had similar efficacy as povidone-iodine 7.5% in reducing total skin bacteria load and preventing surgical site infections in dogs.[3]

Chlorhexidine products may also contain other ingredients, such as antifungals (eg, ketoconazole, miconazole, climbazole), which provide superior antifungal activity as compared with chlorhexidine alone, salicylic acid, phytosphingosine, and hydrocortisone.

Suggested Dosages/Uses

For wound irrigation or foot soaking, diluting the chlorhexidine solution with water to 0.05% to 0.1% is recommended. Sprays, mousses, and wipes/pads are typically applied 1 to 2 times daily. Shampoos and conditioners are typically used daily to weekly. Shampoos should be left in contact with the skin for at least 10 minutes prior to rinsing. For veterinary products, refer to the product label for details and specific instructions.

A nosocomial outbreak of chlorhexidine-resistant *Serratia marcescens* has been linked to improper disinfectant procedures in one veterinary hospital.[4]

Precautions/Adverse Effects

Keep chlorhexidine products away from the eyes. Chlorhexidine is safely used on cats, although irritation and corneal ulcers have been reported. Chlorhexidine may impair wound healing; it is not recommended for long-term use, particularly on granulating lesions.

Hypersensitivity and local skin irritant reactions are possible. Clients should wash their hands after application or wear gloves when applying. The likelihood of irritation increases with increased concentrations. Do not let the animal lick or chew treated areas for at least 20 to 30 minutes after application. Advise clients that blue chlorhexidine solutions can stain furniture, carpets, and the animal.

Veterinary-Labeled Products

Several teat dip and udder wash products, a lubricant, and oral rinses are also available. Several trade names are used for chlorhexidine products, including *Nolvasan®*, *Chlorhexiderm®*, *Dermachlor®*, *Chlorasan®*, *Chloradine®*, *Privasan®*, and *Chlorhex®*.

OINTMENTS

Active ingredients (formulation)	Species	Label status; size(s)	Trade names/additional information
Chlorhexidine 1%		OTC; 7 oz, 16 oz	*Chlorhex®; Nolvasan®*
Chlorhexidine 2%	Labeled for dogs, cats, and horses	OTC; 7 oz, 16 oz	
Chlorhexidine 4%	Labeled for dogs, cats, and horses	OTC; 1 lb	*Vetasan®*

SPRAYS

Active ingredients (formulation)	Species	Label status; size(s)	Trade names/additional information
Chlorhexidine (various concentrations)	Labeled for dogs, cats, and horses	OTC; various sizes	Some products contain aloe.
Chlorhexidine 4%, TrizEDTA	Labeled for dogs, cats, and horses	OTC; 8 oz, 16 oz	*TrizChlor 4®*
Hydrocortisone 1%, chlorhexidine 4%, TrizEDTA	Labeled for dogs, cats, and horses	OTC; 8 oz	*TrizChlor 4HC®* Avoid excessive or prolonged use due to product's steroid content.
Ketoconazole 1%, chlorhexidine 2%, TrizEDTA	Labeled for dogs and cats	OTC; 8 oz	*Mal-A-Ket® Plus*
Miconazole 2%, chlorhexidine 2%, TrizEDTA Other ingredients: ceramide complex	Labeled for dogs, cats, and horses	OTC; 8 oz, 16 oz, and 32 oz	*MiconaHex®*
Ketoconazole 1%, chlorhexidine 2%, phytosphingosine 0.02% Other ingredients: aloe barbadenis, lactic acid	Labeled for dogs and cats	OTC; 8 oz	*VetraSeb CK*
Chlorhexidine 3%, phytosphingosine 0.05%	Labeled for dogs and cats	OTC; 6.8 oz	*DOUXO®*
Chlorhexidine 4% Other ingredients: isopropyl alcohol 4%	Labeled for dogs and cats	OTC; 8 oz	*Chlorhex®*

SHAMPOOS

Active ingredients (formulation)	Species	Label status; size(s)	Trade names/additional information
Chlorhexidine 4%	Labeled for dogs, cats, and horses	OTC; 8 oz, 12 oz, 16 oz, 1 gallon	*ChlorhexiDerm®; Chlorhex®; Max Chlorhexidine®*
Chlorhexidine 4%, TrizEDTA	Labeled for dogs, cats, and horses	OTC; 8 oz, 1 gallon	*TrizCHLOR®*
Hydrocortisone 1%, chlorhexidine 4%, TrizEDTA	Labeled for dogs, cats, and horses	OTC; 8 oz	*TrizCHLOR®4HC* Avoid excessive or prolonged use due to its steroid content.
Chlorhexidine 4% Other ingredients: ceramide III, microsilver	Labeled for dogs and cats	OTC; 8 oz, 16 oz, and 1 gallon	*Hexaderm®* Soap-free
Chlorhexidine 2%		OTC; 8 oz, 16 oz, and 1 gallon	
Chlorhexidine 3%, ophytrium 0.5%	Labeled for dogs and cats	OTC; 200 mL, 500 mL	*DOUXO S3® PYO*
Ketoconazole 1%, chlorhexidine 2%, phytosphingosine salicyloyl 0.05%	Labeled for dogs and cats	OTC; 6.8 oz	*Vetraseb CK®*
Ketoconazole 1%, hydrocortisone 1%, chlorhexidine 2% Other ingredients: vitamin-rich emollients	Labeled for dogs, cats, and horses	OTC; 16 oz	*EquiShield®*
Ketoconazole 1%, acetic acid 2%, chlorhexidine 2%	Labeled for dogs, cats, and horses	OTC; 8 oz, 1 gallon	*Mal-A-Ket®*
Miconazole 2%, chlorhexidine 2%, TrizEDTA Other ingredients: ceramide complex	Labeled for dogs, cats, and horses	OTC; 8 oz, 16 oz, and 1 gallon	*MiconaHex®*
Ketoconazole 1%, chlorhexidine 2% Other ingredients: gylcerin, isopropyl alcohol	Labeled for dogs and cats	OTC; 8 oz, 16 oz, and 1 gallon	*KetoHex®*
Ketoconazole 1%, chlorhexidine 2.3% Other ingredients: alkyl polyglucoside (polysaccharide); chitosanide; D-mannose, D-galactose, L-rhamnose (monosaccharides); *Spherulite®* microcapsules	Labeled for dogs and cats	OTC; 8 oz, 16 oz, and 1 gallon	*KetoChlor®*
Miconazole nitrate 2%, chlorhexidine 2%	Labeled for dogs, cats, and horses	OTC; 8 oz, 12 oz, 16 oz, and 0.5 gallon	*Malaseb®*
Miconazole nitrate 2%, chlorhexidine 2% Other ingredients: ceramide III, microsilver	Labeled for dogs and cats	OTC; 8 oz, 16 oz, and 1 gallon	*BioHex®* Soap-free

SOLUTIONS, FLUSHES, AND SCRUBS

Active ingredients (formulation)	Species	Label status; size(s)	Trade names/additional information
Chlorhexidine 2% (solution)	May be labeled for use on dogs, horses, cattle, and swine	OTC; 16 oz, 1 gallon	
Chlorhexidine 20% (solution)		OTC	*Chlorhexidine®* For 1%: Dilute 6 oz into 1 gallon of water or shampoo. For 2%: Dilute 12 oz into 1 gallon of water or shampoo.
Chlorhexidine (flush)		OTC; 4 oz, 12 oz	
Chlorhexidine 0.2% (flush) Other ingredients: glycerin, isopropyl alcohol	Labeled for dogs and cats	OTC; 4 oz	*Chlorhexis®*
Chlorhexidine 0.15%, TrizEDTA (flush)	Labeled for dogs and cats	OTC; 4 oz	*TrizChlor®*
Ketoconazole 0.15%, chlorhexidine 0.15%, TrizEDTA (flush)	Labeled for dogs and cats	OTC; 4 oz, 12 oz	*Mal-A-Ket®* A multi-cleanse flush to aid in the treatment of bacterial and fungal (dermatophytosis and *Malassezia* spp) infections
Chlorhexidine 0.2%, lidocaine 0.5% (flush) Other ingredients: benzoic acid, glycerin, malic acid, propylene glycol, salicylic acid		OTC; 4 oz	*Dermachlor®*
Miconazole 2%, chlorhexidine 2% (flush)	Labeled for dogs, cats, and horses	OTC; 4 oz, 12 oz	*Malaseb®*
Chlorhexidine 2% (flush)		OTC; 4 oz, 8 oz, and 16 oz	
Ketoconazole 1%, chlorhexidine 2%, phytosphingosine 0.02% (flush)	Labeled for dogs and cats	OTC; 4 oz, 16 oz	*Ketoseb®*
Ketoconazole 1%, chlorhexidine 2%, phytosphingosine salicyloyl 0.05% (flush)	Labeled for dogs and cats	OTC; 6.8 oz	*Vetraseb CK®*
Chlorhexidine 2%, chlorhexidine 4% (scrub)		OTC; 1 gallon	

WIPES

Active ingredients (formulation)	Species	Label status; size(s)	Trade names/additional information
Chlorhexidine 3%, ophytrium 0.5%	Labeled for dogs and cats	OTC; 30 count jar	*DOUXO S3® PYO* Alcohol-free
Ketoconazole 17 mg, chlorhexidine 20 mg, phytosphingosine 0.4 mg	Labeled for dogs and cats (*Ketoseb+PS®*) and horses (*PhytoVet CK®*)	OTC; 50 count jar	*Ketoseb+PS®; PhytoVet CK®*
Ketoconazole 1%, chlorhexidine 2%, phytosphingosine salicyloyl 0.04% Other ingredients: glycerin, lactic acid, propylene glycol	Labeled for dogs and cats	OTC; 60 count jar	*Vetraseb CK®*
Ketoconazole 17 mg, chlorhexidine 20 mg	Labeled for dogs, cats, and horses	OTC; 50 count jar	*KetoHex®*

Ketoconazole 1%, acetic acid 2%, chlorhexidine 2%	Labeled for dogs and cats	OTC; 50 count jar	*Mal-A-Ket®*
Miconazole 2%, chlorhexidine 2%, TrizEDTA Other ingredients: ceramide complex	Labeled for dogs, cats, and horses	OTC; 50 count jar	*MiconaHex®*
Chlorhexidine 4%, TrizEDTA	Labeled for dogs and cats	OTC; 50 count jar	*TrizChlor®*
Climbazole, chlorhexidine 2% Other ingredients: ceramide III, microsilver	Labeled for dogs and cats	OTC; 50 count jar	*BioHex®*

MOUSSES

Active ingredients (formulation)	Species	Label status; size(s)	Trade names/additional information
Chlorhexidine 3%, ophytrium 0.5%	Labeled for dogs and cats	OTC; 5 oz	*DOUXO S3® PYO* Water-based. Leave-on. To be used between bathing or when bathing is not practical
Miconazole 2%, chlorhexidine 2%	Labeled for dogs and cats	OTC; 6.8 oz	*Ketoseb®* Water-based. Leave-on. To be used between bathing or when bathing is not practical
Chlorhexidine 4%, TrizEDTA	Labeled for dogs, cats, and horses	OTC; 7.1 oz	*TrizChlor 4®*
Miconazole 2%, chlorhexidine 2%, TrizEDTA Other ingredients: ceramide complex	Labeled for dogs, cats, and horses	OTC; 7.1 oz	*Miconahex+Triz®*
Climbazole 0.5%, ceramides III 0.05%, chlorhexidine 3%, microsilver 1%	Labeled for dogs and cats	OTC; 6.8 oz	*BioHex®* Leave-on. To be used between bathing or when bathing is not practical

ORAL RINSES

Active ingredients (formulation)	Species	Label status; size(s)	Trade names/additional information
Chlorhexidine 0.12%	Labeled for dogs and cats	OTC; 8 oz	*Dentahex®* For daily use after each meal. Avoid touching tip of bottle to gums.
Chlorhexidine 0.13%	Labeled for dogs and cats	OTC; 8 oz	*Clenz-a-dent®* Orange flavored

Human-Labeled Products

There are several topical skin cleansers available in the 2% to 4% range. Trade names include *Hibiclens®*, *Hibistat®*, *Betasept®*, *Exidine®*, *Dyna-Hex®*, and *BactoShield®*.

References

For the complete list of references, see **wiley.com/go/budde/plumb**

Chloroxylenol, Topical

PCMX

(kloro-**zye**-len-ol)

For otic use, see ***Cleaning/Drying Agents, Otic*** *and* ***Antiseptic Agents, Otic.***

Indications/Actions

Chloroxylenol is an antiseptic with demonstrated efficacy against gram-negative and gram-positive bacteria, in addition to a wide variety of fungal organisms, and against RNA and DNA viruses. It is slower acting than other antiseptic agents[1] and has minimal residual effects.[2] It can be used in presurgical preparation of the skin; in cleaning wounds; and in the treatment of bacterial, fungal, and yeast skin infections. An in vitro study comparing the efficacy of antimicrobial shampoos showed that a shampoo containing chloroxylenol 2% was not effective against *Pseudomonas* spp and methicillin-susceptible and methicillin-resistant *Staphylococcus* spp; however, it was effective against *Malassezia* spp.[3] Another in vitro study found that chloroxylenol was inferior to chlorhexidine against MRSA biofilms.[4]

Chloroxylenol, also known as PCMX, is a chlorinated phenolic antiseptic. Its antibacterial action is thought to be due to the disruption of bacterial membranes.

Suggested Uses/Dosages

Shampoos should be left in contact with the skin for at least 10 minutes prior to rinsing. Refer to product label for details on individual use. Sprays and wipes/pads can be applied 1 to 3 times daily according to the patient's needs. Do not let the animal lick or chew at treated areas for at least 20 to 30 minutes after application.

Precautions/Adverse Effects

Chloroxylenol may cause skin irritation.

Veterinary-Labeled Products

This list represents only products where chloroxylenol is one of the main active ingredients.

Active ingredients (formulation)	Species	Label status; size(s)	Trade names/additional information
Chloroxylenol 2% (scrub) Other ingredients: deionized water, hydroxyethylcellulose, polysorbate-20, polyquaternium-7, propylene glycol, sodium laureth sulfate, sodium lauryl sulfate		OTC; 16 oz, 1 gallon	Used for surgical scrub and preoperative skin preparation. Do not dilute.
Chloroxylenol 2%, salicylic acid 2%, sodium thiosulfate 2% (shampoo) Other ingredients: citric acid, propylene glycol	Labeled for dogs and cats	OTC; 16 oz, 1 gallon	Has antiseborrheic effect
Miconazole nitrate 2%, chloroxylenol 1% (shampoo) Other ingredients: propylene glycol, salicylic acid	Labeled for dogs, cats, and horses	OTC; 8 oz, 16 oz, and 1 gallon	*Sebozole®* Has antibacterial, antifungal, and antiseborrheic activity. Shake well.
Ketoconazole 1%, chloroxylenol 2% (shampoo)	Labeled for dogs, cats, and horses	OTC; 8 oz, 16 oz, and 1 gallon	*Pharmaseb®*
Ketoconazole 0.3%, chloroxylenol 0.3% (wipes)	Labeled for dogs, cats, and horses	OTC; 60 count	*Pharmaseb®* Water-based
Ketoconazole 0.3%, chloroxylenol 0.3% (flush) Other ingredients: benzyl alcohol, propylene glycol	Labeled for dogs, cats, and horses	OTC; 4 oz, 8 oz	*Pharmaseb®* Water-based. Can be used as a cleansing agent for the skin and ears
Ketoconazole 0.33%, chloroxylenol 0.33% (flush) Other ingredients: benzyl alcohol, propylene glycol, sodium borate decahydrate	Labeled for dogs, cats, and horses	OTC; 8 oz	*Ketomax®* Contains sodium borate decahydrate to obtain pH of 8.5
Ketoconazole 0.3%, chloroxylenol 0.3% (spray) Other ingredients: benzyl alcohol, propylene glycol	Labeled for dogs, cats, and horses	OTC; 4 oz, 8 oz	*Pharmaseb®* Water-based

Human-Labeled Products

There are several topical products available containing chloroxylenol that are usually combined with other ingredients, such as hydrocortisone, menthol, pramoxine, and benzocaine. They are presented in different forms (creams, ointments, lotions, and shampoos) but are not commonly used in dogs and cats. Trade names include *Aurinol®*, *Calamycin®*, *Cortamox®*, *Cortane-B®*, *Dermacoat®*, and *Foille®*.

References

For the complete list of references, see **wiley.com/go/budde/plumb**

Enzymes, Topical (Lactoperoxidase, Lysozyme, Lactoferrin)

*For otic use, see **Cleaning/Drying Agents, Otic.***

Indications/Actions

Lactoperoxidase, lysozyme, and lactoferrin are topical enzymes that work synergistically when combined and are reported to be effective against bacterial, fungal, and viral microorganisms. They are listed by the manufacturer to be effective against *Staphylococcus* spp, *Pseudomonas* spp, *Malassezia* spp, *Candida albicans*, and *Microsporum* spp. Lactoperoxidase combined with hydrogen peroxide, thiocyanate, and/or iodide produces hypothiocyanite or hypoiodite ions that are bactericidal by oxidizing components of bacterial cell walls. Hypoiodite also is fungicidal. Lactoferrin acts as a bacteriostatic agent against many bacteria by depriving them of iron.

They can be used alone but are often used in combination with hydrocortisone for mild itching or as an adjunctive treatment for more severe itching, such as atopic dermatitis.

Suggested Uses/Dosages

Sprays and creams are labeled for use 1 to 2 times a day. Shampoos and conditioners should be used daily to weekly. Shampoo should be in contact with the skin for 3 to 5 minutes prior to rinsing well. Products are labeled as worry-free if licked, but animals should be prevented from licking or chewing treated areas for at least 20 to 30 minutes after application if possible. Refer to product label for details on individual product use.

Precautions/Adverse Effects

Overall, these products appear to be safe. There are no reported adverse effects, but skin irritation is possible. Caution should be used to avoid excessive or long-term use of products containing glucocorticoids due to potential adverse effects such as cutaneous atrophy and systemic absorption.

Veterinary-Labeled Products

Refer to each product label for details on use, inactive ingredients, and any precautions.

Active ingredients (formulation)	Species	Label status; size(s)	Trade names/additional information
Lactoferrin, lactoperoxidase, lysozyme (spray)	Labeled for all pets of all ages	OTC; 2 oz	*Zymox®*
Lactoferrin, lactoperoxidase, lysozyme, hydrocortisone 0.5% (spray)	Labeled for all pets of all ages	OTC; 2 oz	*Zymox®*
Lactoferrin, lactoperoxidase, lysozyme, hydrocortisone 1% (spray)	Labeled for all pets of all ages	OTC; 2 oz	*Zymox®*
Lactoferrin, lactoperoxidase, lysozyme (cream)	Labeled for companion animals	OTC; 1 oz	*Zymox®*
Lactoferrin, lactoperoxidase, lysozyme, hydrocortisone 0.5% (cream)	Labeled for companion animals	OTC; 1 oz	*Zymox®*
Lactoferrin, lactoperoxidase, lysozyme, hydrocortisone 1% (cream)	Labeled for companion animals	OTC; 1 oz	*Zymox®*
Lactoferrin, lactoperoxidase, lysozyme (shampoo)	Labeled for all pets of all ages	OTC; 12 oz, 1 gallon	*Zymox®*
Lactoferrin, lactoperoxidase, lysozyme (leave-on conditioner)	Labeled for all pets of all ages	OTC; 12 oz, 1 gallon	*Zymox®*
Lactoferrin, lactoperoxidase, lysozyme (shampoo)	Labeled for horses	OTC; 12 oz, 1 gallon	*Zymox® Equine Defense*
Lactoferrin, lactoperoxidase, lysozyme (conditioner)	Labeled for horses	OTC; 12 oz, 1 gallon	*Zymox® Equine Defense*
Lactoferrin, lactoperoxidase, lysozyme (spray)	Labeled for horses	OTC; 8 oz	*Zymox® Equine Defense*
Lactoferrin, lactoperoxidase, lysozyme (cream)	Labeled for horses	OTC; 2.5 oz	*Zymox® Equine Defense*

Human-Labeled Products

None

Hypochlorous Acid, Topical

(hye-poe-***klor***-us ***ass***-id)

For ophthalmic use, see ***Irrigating Solutions, Ophthalmic.***

For otic use, see ***Antiseptic Agents, Otic*** *and* ***Cleaning/Drying Agents, Otic.***

Indications/Actions

Topical hypochlorous acid is used for the management of wounds, abscesses, cuts, abrasions, skin irritations, ulcers, postsurgical incision sites, burns, wound odors, and to accelerate healing. It may be used for the prevention or treatment of bacterial skin infections, including methicillin-resistant *Staphylococcus* spp and *Pseudomonas* spp; however, one small, controlled study investigating the efficacy of hypochlorous acid 0.011% applied to the skin twice daily for 4 weeks for the treatment of canine superficial pyoderma showed no statistically significant difference as compared with placebo. Hypochlorous acid also has antifungal and antiviral properties and is reported to reduce inflammation, pain, and itching.

Hypochlorous acid products act rapidly against gram-positive and gram-negative bacteria and fungal/yeast organisms. Some products contain oxychlorine (bleach-like) compounds; many products have a neutral pH.

The mechanism of action of hypochlorous acid is to disrupt the cellular membrane of single-cell organisms. Because the mechanism of action is primarily chemical in nature, resistance appears unlikely.

Suggested Dosages/Uses

Clip hair if necessary and apply to affected areas up to 3 times daily; may be used with dressing applications on wounds or in combination with a cleanser. These products are generally safe to use around the eyes, nose, and mouth, and no rinsing is typically required; refer to specific product labels for details on use.

Precautions/Adverse Effects

No precautions or adverse effects have been reported. Hypochlorous acid products are generally non-toxic and safe if licked or ingested. Although they do not sting or irritate the skin, the treated area may redden secondary to increased blood flow. Clients should be warned about possible bleaching/staining of carpets, clothing, and jewelry.

Veterinary-Labeled Products

Below is a representative sample of the products available.

Active ingredients (formulation)	Species	Label status; size(s)	Trade names/additional information
Hypochlorous acid 0.009% (liquid)	Labeled for cats	OTC; 2 oz	*Vetericyn Plus® Feline Facial Therapy*
Hypochlorous acid 0.012% (spray)	Labeled for all animals	OTC; 3 oz, 4 oz, 8 oz, and 16 oz	*Vetericyn Plus® Reptile Wound and Skin Care; Vetericyn Plus® Poultry Care; Vetericyn Plus® All Animal Wound and Skin Care; Vetericyn Plus® Equine Wound and Skin Care*
Hypochlorous acid 0.012% (spray gel)	Labeled for all animals	OTC; 4 oz, 8 oz, and 16 oz	*Vetericyn Plus® Hydrogel; Vetericyn Plus® Feline Hydrogel*
Hypochlorous acid 0.015% (spray)	Labeled for all animals	OTC; 16 oz	*Vetericyn® Pink Eye Spray*

Human-Labeled Products

Active ingredients (formulation)	Label status; size(s)	Trade names/additional information
Hypochlorous acid 0.008%, sodium hypochlorite 0.002% (spray/gel/solution)	Depending on the labeling: OTC/Rx; 1.5 oz to 990 mL	*Microcyn®*
Hypochlorous acid 0.00025%, sodium hypochlorite 0.0036% (spray)	OTC; 2 oz	*Myclyns®* pH: 6.2 to 7.8.

Povidone Iodine, Topical

(***poe***-vi-done ***eye***-oh-dine) *Betadine®*

Indications/Actions

Povidone iodine is used as a topical first-aid agent and a presurgical skin antiseptic. It may be used for superficial pyoderma and *Malassezia* spp dermatitis; however, it is infrequently used in small animal dermatology due to its drying, irritating, and staining effects.

Povidone iodine, an iodophor antiseptic, is rapidly bactericidal at low concentrations against both gram-positive and gram-negative bacteria. It is also fungicidal and sporicidal as a 1% aqueous solution. Povidone acts by slowly releasing iodine to tissues. It has prolonged activity (4-6 hours) but is not as long acting as chlorhexidine. Povidone iodine also has mild degreasing and debriding activity.

Suggested Dosages/Uses

Thoroughly wet affected area(s) to ensure complete coverage. For veterinary products, refer to the specific product label for details on use.

Precautions/Adverse Effects

Povidone may be drying and irritating to skin and can be extremely irritating to the scrotal skin and external ears. Use with emollients may alleviate the drying effects. It may also stain skin, hair, and fabrics. Avoid contact with eyes.

Wear gloves or wash hands after application. Use with caution on deep or puncture wounds or on serious burns. Systemic absorption can result in renal and thyroid dysfunction.

Veterinary-Labeled Products

NOTES:

1. The following products are only representative and not meant to be all-inclusive. There are many available povidone iodine products, including hoof dressings, teat dips, boluses (to prepare a solution), and udder washes. Povidone iodine products are also available in combination with lidocaine and as a combination of povidone and potassium iodine.
2. 10% povidone iodine yields 1% titratable iodine; labels may be confusing. Povidone iodine may also be listed as polyvinylpyrrolidone iodine. Products below are listed as povidone iodine.

Active ingredients (formulation)	Label status; size(s)	Trade names/additional information
Povidone iodine 5% (shampoo)	OTC; Depending on the manufacturer: 8 oz, 16 oz, 32 oz, 1 gallon	*Aloedine*®, generic
Povidone iodine 5% (spray)	OTC; 16 oz	generic
Povidone iodine 7.5% (scrub)	OTC; 32 oz, 1 gallon	*Vetadine*®; *Pivodine*®; *Povidine*®; *Poviderm*®
Povidone iodine 10% (gel)	OTC; 20 oz	*Biozide*®
Povidone iodine 10% (solution)	OTC; 32 oz, 1 gallon	*Poviderm*®; *Prodine*®; *Vetadine*®

Human-Labeled Products

NOTE: There are a large number of povidone iodine products available. In addition to those listed, vaginal gels, swabs, sponges, and foaming skin cleansers are also available.

Active ingredients (formulation)	Label status; size(s)	Trade names/additional information
Povidone iodine 5% (powder spray)	OTC; 2 oz	*Betadine*®
Povidone iodine 5% (spray)	OTC; 3 oz	*Betadine*®
Povidone iodine 7.5% (scrub)	OTC; 4 oz, 16 oz, 32 oz, 1 gallon	*Betadine*®; generic
Povidone iodine 10% (ointment)	OTC; 1 g (packet), 28.4 g	generic
Povidone iodine 10% (solution)	OTC; 0.5 oz, 4 oz, 8 oz, 16 oz, 32 oz, 1 gallon	*Betadine*®; generic

Antiparasitic Agents, Topical

For topical agents that are administered topically but absorbed systemically through the skin to treat ecto- and endoparasites (eg, ***Eprinomectin, Fluralaner, Ivermectin, Moxidectin, Selamectin),*** refer to the respective monographs in the systemic section.

Amitraz Collar, Topical

(a-mi-***traz***) *Preventic*®

Indications/Actions

A water-resistant amitraz collar is available for dogs 12 weeks of age and older that is labeled to kill and detach ticks for up to 3 months[1]; the collar does not control fleas. It starts working within 24 hours of placement. **Do NOT apply the amitraz collar to cats or rabbits as it will cause toxicity.**

Topical amitraz dip was FDA-approved for the treatment of generalized demodicosis in dogs; however, this product is no longer marketed. It was also used to treat canine sarcoptic mange, cheyletiellosis, and feline surface (*Demodex gatoi)* or follicular demodicosis (*Demodex cati*), and as a general insecticidal/miticidal agent in several other species.

Amitraz is thought to act through agonism of octopamine receptors in ectoparasites. Octopamine receptors are considered the invertebrate equivalent to adrenergic receptors in vertebrates. The overstimulation of octopamine receptors leads to overexcitation, paralysis, and death.[2,3]

Suggested Dosages/Uses

DOGS:

Kill and detach ticks (label dosage; EPA-approved): Apply collar based on dog's body weight. Dogs up to 27.3 kg (60 lb): 18-inch adjustable collar; dogs over 27.3 kg (60 lb): 25-inch adjustable collar. The collar must be worn tightly enough to make contact with the skin. Replace collar every 90 days.

Precautions/Adverse Effects/Drug Interactions

Do not reuse the collar or container; wrap it in a newspaper and throw it in the trash. Do not use the collar on puppies under 12 weeks of age.

Amitraz can be toxic to cats and rabbits and should not be used in these species.

Amitraz collars may cause toxicity if swallowed (by either animals or humans). Treatment should consist of emesis, retrieval of the collar using endoscopy if possible, and administration of activated charcoal and a cathartic to remove any remaining collar fragments. Yohimbine 0.11 – 0.2 mg/kg IV (start with low dosage) may be of benefit to treat adverse effects associated with the overdose. Because yohimbine has a short half-life, it may need to be repeated, particularly if the animal has ingested an amitraz-containing collar that could has not been retrieved from the GI tract. See ***Yohimbine***. Atipamezole has also been used to treat amitraz toxicity; see ***Atipamezole.*** For patients that have experienced or are suspected to have experienced an overdose, consultation with a 24-hour poison consultation center specializing in providing veterinary-specific information is recommended. For general information related to overdose and toxin exposures, as well as contact information for poison control centers, refer to ***Appendix.***

Veterinary-Labeled Products

Active ingredients (formulation)	Species	Label status; size(s)	Trade names/additional information
Amitraz 9% (collar)	Labeled only for dogs 12 weeks of age and older	OTC (EPA); 18 inches (for dogs less than 27.2 kg [60 lb]), 25 inches (for dogs more than 27.2 kg [60 lb])	*Preventic*® Adjustable (cut off excess). Effective for 3 months

Human-Labeled Products

None

References

For the complete list of references, see **wiley.com/go/budde/plumb**

Crotamiton, Topical

(***kroe***-ta-mye-ton)

Indications/Actions

Crotamiton is a topical miticide/scabicide used primarily for adjunctive treatment (with ivermectin) of mite infections (eg, *Knemidocoptes* spp) in birds. Crotamiton has both miticidal and antipruritic actions. Its miticidal mechanism of action is unknown; however, its antipruritic effect is reported to be due to its inhibition of the transient receptor potential vanilloid 4 (TRPV4) channel that is expressed on the skin peripheral neurons and keratinocytes.[1]

Suggested Dosages/Uses

Once- to twice-daily application is usually recommended. Shake well before use.

Precautions/Adverse Effects

Do not apply around the eyes or mouth. Little is known of the compound's safety profile. Irritation or hypersensitivity reactions are possible; do not use on patients with a known hypersensitivity to it.[2] Discontinue if irritation or sensitization develops. Do not apply to acutely inflamed skin or raw, weeping skin.

Prevent grooming or preening after application, as oral ingestion can cause irritation of the buccal, esophageal, and gastric mucosa; nausea; vomiting; and abdominal pain.

Adverse effects in humans include dermatitis, pruritis, and rash.[2]

For patients that have experienced or are suspected to have experienced an overdose, consultation with a 24-hour poison consultation center specializing in providing veterinary-specific information is recommended. For general information related to overdose and toxin exposures, as well as contact information for poison control centers. See ***Appendix***.

Veterinary-Labeled Products

None

Human-Labeled Topical Products

Active ingredients (formulation)	Label status; size(s)	Trade names/additional information
Crotamiton 10% (lotion) Other ingredients: cetyl alcohol, emollient base	Rx; 60 g, 227 g, 454 g	*Crotan*®, *Eurax*®

References

For the complete list of references, see **wiley.com/go/budde/plumb**

Deltamethrin/Deltamethrin Combination Products, Topical

(del-ta-***meeth***-rin)

Indications/Actions

In the United States, deltamethrin-impregnated collars are labeled for killing fleas (ie, *Ctenocephalides* spp) and ticks[1] (ie, *Amblyomma americanum, Rhipicephalus sanguineus, Dermacentor variabilis, Ixodes scapularis, I pacificus*) and repelling mosquitoes on dogs for up to 6 months.[2] Treatment with deltamethrin has been shown to be an effective strategy to reduce the incidence of leishmaniasis by repelling and killing mosquitos and phlebotomine sandflies, which are important vectors.[3] The mosquito repellent activity may also help reduce the incidence of heartworm infection[4]; further research is needed.

Deltamethrin is a synthetic pyrethroid insecticide and acts by disrupting the sodium channel conduction in arthropod nerve cell membranes, resulting in paralysis and death. Some collars are combined with pyriproxyfen, an insect growth regulator.

Suggested Dosages/Uses

Collars should be worn continuously and be replaced every 6 months.[1,2] Maximum effect may not occur until 2 to 3 weeks after collar placement; therefore, it is recommended to apply the collar before the start of flea/tick season.[5] Wipe the collar with a damp paper towel prior to application to remove dust. The collar is placed so that 2 to 3 fingers can easily fit between the collar and neck. The collar does not need to be removed for bathing or swimming. Follow specific product label for use instructions.

Precautions/Adverse Effects

Do not use deltamethrin on cats. Collars containing deltamethrin should not be used on dogs younger than 12 weeks.[1,2] Collars may cause irritation if placed too tightly. Skin reactions (erythema, localized dermatitis, pruritis) and hair loss at the application site are possible.[6] In extremely rare cases, neurologic signs such as tremor or lethargy have been reported.[6] Use with caution in debilitated, pregnant, nursing, geriatric, or medicated animals.[1,2]

If a collar is ingested, uncoordinated movements, tremor, drooling, vomiting, or rigidity are possible. Treatment is supportive, and clinical signs usually subside within 48 hours.[6] For patients that have experienced or are suspected to have experienced an overdose, consultation with a 24-hour poison consultation center specializing in providing veterinary-specific information is recommended. For general information related to overdose and toxin exposures, as well as contact information for poison control centers, refer to ***Appendix***.

Avoid contact with eyes, skin, or clothing. Wash hands after handling. Mammalian exposure to deltamethrin is classified as safe; however, deltamethrin is highly toxic to aquatic animals (especially fish) and should be used very carefully around water sources.

Veterinary-Labeled Products

Active ingredients (formulation)	Species	Label status; size(s)	Trade names/additional information
Deltamethrin 4% (collar)	Labeled for dogs 12 weeks of age or older **Do NOT use on cats.**	OTC (EPA)	*Activyl®; Adams®; PetArmor®; Proact®; Sentry®; Zodiac®* Adjustable (one size fits all). Water-resistant
Deltamethrin 4% (collar)	Labeled for dogs 12 weeks of age or older **Do NOT use on cats.**	OTC (EPA)	*Protect®; Salvo®; Sentry®* Available for small, medium, and large dogs. Water-resistant
Deltamethrin 4%, pyriproxyfen 1% (collar)	Labeled for dogs 12 weeks of age or older **Do NOT use on cats.**	OTC (EPA)	*PetArmor®* One size fits all. Waterproof

Human-Labeled Products

None

References

For the complete list of references, see **wiley.com/go/budde/plumb**

Dinotefuran/Pyriproxyfen Combinations, Topical

(die-noh-te-***fyoor***-an, pye-ri-***proks***-i-fen)

Indications/Actions

Dinotefuran/pyriproxyfen combinations are used in dogs and cats for the treatment and control of external parasites. The combination of dinotefuran and pyriproxyfen controls adult fleas and all immature flea stages, including eggs, larvae, and pupae. Some canine combination products also contain permethrin, which broadens the spectrum to also repel and kill ticks, mosquitos, lice, mites (excluding mange), biting flies, and sand flies. Some feline combination products contain fipronil, providing rapid speed of kill and added protection against ticks and chewing lice.

Dinotefuran is a nitroguanidine, neonicotinoid insecticide with a structure similar to acetylcholine. It permanently binds to the same insect receptor sites as acetylcholine and activates the nerve impulse at the synapse, which cause stimulation that results in tremors, incoordination, and insect death. Dinotefuran does not bind to mammalian acetylcholine receptor sites.

Pyriproxyfen is a second-generation insect growth regulator that mimics insect juvenile growth hormone, halting development during metamorphosis and larval development. It also concentrates in female flea ovaries, which causes nonviable eggs to be produced. When dinotefuran is combined with an adulticide (eg, permethrin, fipronil), all stages of the parasite are killed, and re-infestation is less likely. It is more resistant to UV light than is methoprene.

Suggested Dosages/Uses

Dinotefuran/pyriproxyfen combination products are recommended once monthly for dogs and cats. Refer to the package labeling for specific dosages and application instructions.

Apparently, bathing or swimming does not interfere with efficacy of canine products; however, the authors do not recommend bathing the pet until 2 days after application. Cats should be completely dry before the *Catego®* product is applied and they should remain dry for 24 hours after application.[1]

Precautions/Adverse Effects

The dog product containing permethrin (*Vectra 3D®*) **must not be used on cats or on dogs that cohabitate with cats.** The manufacturer recommends not using *Vectra 3D®* or *Vectra®* on debilitated, aged, medicated, pregnant, or nursing animals or on animals known to be sensitive to pesticide products. Mild transitory skin erythema may occur at the application site. Avoid eye and oral contact since dinotefuran can cause substantial but temporary eye irritation. *Vectra 3D®* was reported to be associated with the development of pemphigus foliaceus-like disease occurring at the site of application and at distant sites in 3 dogs.[1]

Veterinary-Labeled Products

Active ingredients (formulation)	Species	Label status; size(s)	Trade names/additional information
Dinotefuran 22%, pyriproxyfen 3% (spot-on solution)	Labeled for dogs and puppies 8 weeks of age or older	OTC (EPA) 1.1 - 4.5 kg (2.5-10 lb): 1.3 mL/dose 5 - 9 kg (11-20 lb): 2 mL/dose 9.5 - 25 kg (21-55 lb): 4 mL/dose 25 - 45.4 kg (56-100 lb): 6 mL/dose	*Vectra®*
Dinotefuran 22%, pyriproxyfen 3% (spot-on solution)	Labeled for cats and kittens 8 weeks of age or older	OTC (EPA) 0.9 - 4.1 kg (2-9 lb): 0.8 mL/dose 4.1 kg (9 lb) or over: 1.2 mL/dose	*Vectra®*
Dinotefuran 22%, pyriproxyfen 3%, fipronil 8.92% (spot-on solution)	Labeled for cats and kittens 8 weeks of age or older	OTC (EPA) All cats weighing over 0.7 kg (1.5 lb): 0.5 mL/dose	*Catego®*
Dinotefuran 4.95%, pyriproxyfen 0.44%, permethrin 36.08% (spot-on solution)	Labeled ***only*** for dogs and puppies 8 weeks of age or older	OTC (EPA) 2.3 - 4.5 kg (5-10 lb): 0.8 mL/dose 5 - 9 kg (11-20 lb): 1.6 mL/dose 9.5 - 25 kg (21-55 lb): 3.6 mL/dose 25.4 - 43.1 kg (56-95 lb): 4.7 mL/dose Over 43.1 kg (95 lb): 8 mL/dose	*Vectra 3D®* **Must NOT be used on cats. In households where a dog cohabitates with cats, keep cat separated from treated dog for 24 hours.**

Human-Labeled Products

None

References

For the complete list of references, see **wiley.com/go/budde/plumb**

Fipronil/Fipronil Combinations, Topical

(**fip**-roe-nil) *Frontline®*

See also ***Permethrin/Permethrin Combinations, Topical; Pyriproxyfen/Pyriproxyfen Combinations, Topical***

Indications/Actions

In the United States, fipronil is indicated for the treatment of fleas, ticks, and chewing lice infestations in dogs and cats. It has also been used successfully for *Trombicula autumnalis* (chigger) infestation, sarcoptic mange, cheyletiellosis, and otoacariasis.

Fipronil is a phenylpyrazole antiparasitic agent that interferes with the passage of chloride ions in GABA-regulated chloride channels in invertebrates, thereby disrupting CNS activity and causing death of the parasite. Fipronil collects in the oils of the skin and hair follicles and continues to be released over a period of time, which results in a long residual activity. When topically applied, the drug spreads over the body in ≈24 hours via translocation.

When fipronil is combined with the insect growth regulator (S)-methoprene, flea eggs and flea larvae are also killed. (S)-methoprene mimics flea juvenile growth hormone, which halts development during metamorphosis and larval development. It also concentrates in female flea ovaries, causing nonviable eggs to be produced. Additional combination products with permethrin, etofenprox, cyphenothrin, and pyriproxyfen (synthetic pyrethroids) or amitraz are available.

Suggested Dosages/Uses

Spot-on solutions are generally applied in one or more spots on the back of the neck or between the shoulder blades. The hair should be parted so the solution can be applied directly to the skin.

When applying spray, use one gloved hand to ruffle the coat while spraying sides, back, legs, abdomen, shoulders, and neck. To apply this product to the head and eye area, spray a gloved hand and gently rub into the coat. Alternatively, a towel soaked with fipronil may be used to treat the face. Apply this product until coat is thoroughly wet.[1]

Fleas, ticks, or chewing lice: Monthly treatments are generally recommended when fipronil is used for treatment and prevention of fleas, ticks, or chewing lice. See product labels for specific directions on administration and recommendations on bathing and swimming after administration. In some cases, for better efficacy, the interval between applications needs to be shortened to every 14 days.

Trombicula autumnalis **infestation:** Monthly application of fipronil *spray* (0.25%) has been successful in dogs. Apply the *spray* to the entire body, thoroughly wetting the coat, with particular emphasis on the areas typically affected (eg, feet, ears, face, perineum, and tail). Monthly applications should be administered throughout the trombiculid season at the dose of 3 – 6 mL/kg. In some cases, application every 14 days may be required. Fipronil seemed to have a shorter duration of effect in cats, with reinfestation seen after 7 to 10 days.[2]

Sarcoptic mange: Fipronil *spray* (0.25%) is recommended for confirmed cases using 2 protocols:

a) Apply once weekly for 4 weeks[3]
b) Apply every 2 to 3 weeks for 3 treatments[4]

Dosages ranging from 3 mL/kg to 39 mL/kg were used in these reports. Thoroughly wet the coat, paying special attention to the areas typically affected by the disease (eg, ears, face, ventrum, and extremities). A decrease in pruritus may be noticed as early as 7 days after the first application. Fipronil use is not recommended in treatment trials (ie, high clinical suspicion of mite infestation but mites not found on skin scrapings) because of anecdotal reports of treatment failures with this product.

Cheyletiellosis: Fipronil *spray* (0.25%) has been successfully used at a dose of 3 mL/kg to ensure complete and thorough body coverage, along with environmental permethrin treatment. Repeat fipronil treatment after 30 days.[5] Fipronil use is only recommended for confirmed cases and is not recommended in treatment trials (ie, high clinical suspicion of mite infestation but mites not found on skin scrapings) because of anecdotal reports of treatment failures.

Otoacariasis: Instill 1 drop of fipronil solution inside each ear canal and apply the rest of the dosing tube between the shoulder blades.[6] Fipronil needs to be applied in the ear canals to be effective. Resolution of clinical signs can be seen as early as 7 days posttreatment. Additional applications may be needed.

Precautions/Adverse Effects

Do not use fipronil on puppies or kittens less than 8 weeks of age. Fipronil compounds are reported to be contraindicated in rabbits, as toxicity deaths have occurred with the spray. Do not apply fipronil to or spray in or near the eyes. Temporary irritation may occur at the site of administration. Hypersensitivity has rarely been reported; animals that have demonstrated hypersensitivity reactions to fipronil should not be retreated. Use fipronil with caution on debilitated, elderly, or medicated patients.

Dispose of containers properly to avoid contamination of food or water sources. Avoid human contact with skin, eyes, or clothing. Wash well with soap and water if skin contact occurs. Wear gloves when applying fipronil and wash hands thoroughly after handling. Use sprays only in a well-ventilated area. Avoid contact with treated animals until coat is dry.

Most products are labeled as remaining effective after bathing, water immersion, or exposure to sunlight; however, avoid shampooing within 48 hours of application. Spotted areas may appear wet or oily for up to 24 hours after application.

Veterinary-Labeled Products

NOTE: This is not an all-inclusive list but is representative of the types of products available.

Active ingredients (formulation)	Species	Label status; size(s)	Trade names/additional information
Fipronil 0.29% (spray)	Labeled for use on dogs, cats, puppies, and kittens 8 weeks of age or older	OTC (EPA); 8.5 oz, 17 oz	*Frontline®*
Fipronil 0.29%, (S)-methoprene 0.27% (spray)	Labeled for use on dogs, cats, puppies, or kittens 8 weeks of age or older	OTC (EPA); 8 oz, 16 oz	*Martin's FLEE® Plus*
Fipronil 9.7% (spot-on solution)	Labeled for use on dogs, cats, puppies, and kittens 8 weeks of age or older	OTC (EPA); various formulations and packages depending on each product	*Hartz® First Defense®; Pronyl OTC®; Sentry Fiproguard®; Spectra Sure®* The indication may differ among these products.
Fipronil 9.7% (spot-on solution)	Labeled for use on cats and kittens 8 weeks of age or older and over 0.7 kg (1.5 lb)	OTC (EPA); single-dose applicators 0.5 mL in packages of 3 and 6	*Adams Fortress®; Hartz® First Defense®; Sentry Fiproguard®*
Fipronil 9.8%, (S)-methoprene 11.8% (spot-on solution)	Labeled for use on cats or kittens 8 weeks of age or older and over 0.7 kg (1.5 lb)	OTC (EPA); single-dose applicators 0.5 mL in packages of 3 and 6	*Frontline®* Plus; *Martin's FLEE® Plus;* PetAction® *Plus; PetArmor® Plus; Pronyl OTC Plus®; Sentry Fibroguard®; Spectra Sure® Plus*
Fipronil 9.8%, (S)-methoprene 8.8% (spot-on solution)	Labeled for dogs and puppies 8 weeks of age or older **Do NOT use on cats.**	OTC (EPA); single-dose applicators in packages of 3 and 6: up to 10 kg (22 lb): 0.67 mL; 10.4 - 20 kg (23-44 lb): 1.34 mL; 20.4 - 39.9 kg (45-88 lb): 2.68 mL; 40.4 - 59.9 kg (89-132 lb): 4.02 mL	*EctoAdvance® Plus; Frontline® Plus; PetAction® Plus, PetArmor® Plus; Pronyl OTC® Plus; Spectra Sure® Plus*

Active ingredients (formulation)	Species	Label status; size(s)	Trade names/additional information
Fipronil 9.8%, etofenprox 15% (spot-on solution)	Labeled for all cats over 12 weeks of age	OTC (EPA); single-dose applicators 0.5 mL in packages of 3	*Martin's FLEE® Prefurred*
Fipronil 9.8%, cyphenothren 5.2%, (S)-methoprene 8.8% (spot-on solution)	Labeled for use on dogs 12 weeks of age or older and at least 1.8 kg (4 lb)	OTC (EPA); single-dose applicators in packages of 3	*Frontline® Trita®*
Fipronil 9.8%, etofenprox 15%, (S)-methoprene 11.8% (spot-on solution)	Labeled for use on cats or kittens 12 weeks of age or older	OTC (EPA); single-dose applicators 0.5 mL in packages of 3	*Frontline® Tritak*
Fipronil 9.8%, pyriproxyfen 0.25%, (S)-methoprene 11.8% (spot-on solution)	Labeled for cats and kittens 8 weeks of age or older and less than or equal to 0.7 kg (1.5 lb)	OTC (EPA); single-dose applicators 0.5 mL in packages of 3 and 6	*Frontline® Gold*
Fipronil 9.58%, pyriproxyfen 11.65% (spot-on solution)	Labeled for cats and kittens 8 weeks of age or older and less than or equal to 0.7 kg (1.5 lb)	OTC (EPA); single-dose applicators 0.5 mL in packages of 3	*Effipro®*
Fipronil 9.78%, pyriproxyfen 2.94% (spot-on solution)	Labeled for dogs and puppies 8 weeks of age or older **Do NOT use on cats.**	OTC (EPA); single-dose applicators in packages of 3: 2.3 - 10.4 kg (5-22.9 lb): 0.67 mL; 10.4 - 20 kg (23-44.9 lb): 1.34 mL; 20.4 - 40.3 kg (45-88.9 lb): 2.68 mL; 40.4 - 59.9 kg (89-132 lb): 4.02 mL	*Effipro®*
Fipronil 9.8%, cyphenothrin 5.2% (spot-on solution)	Labeled for dogs and puppies 12 weeks of age or older **Do NOT use on cats.**	OTC (EPA); single-dose applicators in packages of 3: up to 10 kg (22 lb): 0.67 mL; 10.4 - 20 kg (23-44 lb): 1.34 mL; 20.4 - 39.9 kg (45-88 lb): 2.68 mL; 40.4 - 59.9 kg (89-132 lb): 4.02 mL	*Martin's Prefurred® Plus; Parastar® Plus*
Fipronil 9.8%, cyphenothrin 5.2%, (S)-methoprene 8.8% (spot-on solution)	Labeled for use on dogs 12 weeks of age or older and at least 1.8 kg (4 lb) **Do NOT use on cats.**	OTC (EPA); single-dose applicators in packages of 3: up to 10 kg (22 lb): 0.67 mL; 10.4 - 20 kg (23-44 lb): 1.34 mL; 20.4 - 40.3 kg (45-88 lb): 2.68 mL; 40.4 - 59.9 kg (89-132 lb): 4.02 mL	*Frontline® Tritak*
Fipronil 6.01%, permethrin 44.88% (spot-on solution)	Labeled for dogs and puppies at least 8 weeks of age **Do NOT use on cats.**	OTC (EPA); single-dose applicators in packages of 3: 2.3 - 5 kg (5-10.9 lb): 0.5 mL; 5 - 10.4 kg (11-22.9 lb): 1 mL; 20.4 - 40.3 kg (45-88.9 lb): 4 mL; 40.4 - 59.9 kg (89-132 lb): 6 mL	*Effitix®*
Fipronil 6%, permethrin 44.8%, pyriproxyfen 1.8% (spot-on solution)	Labeled for dogs and puppies at least 8 weeks of age **Do NOT use on cats.**	OTC (EPA); single-dose applicators in packages of 3: 2.3 - 5 kg (5-10.9 lb): 0.5 mL; 5 - 10.4 kg (11-22.9 lb): 1 mL; 20.4 - 40.3 kg (45-88.9 lb): 4 mL; 40.4 - 59.9 kg (89-132 lb): 6 mL	*Effitix® Plus; Frontline® Shield*
Fipronil 8.92%, dinotefuran 22%, pyriproxyfen 3% (spot-on solution)	Labeled for cats and kittens over 0.7 kg (1.5 lb) and over 8 weeks of age	OTC (EPA); packages of 3 and 6	*Catego®*
Fipronil 9.8%, (S)-methoprene 8.8%; Amitraz 22.1% (spot-on solution)	Labeled for dogs and puppies 8 weeks of age or older and at least 2.3 kg (5 lb) body weight **Do NOT use on cats.**	OTC (EPA); 1.7 mL, 2.14 mL, 4.28 mL, and 6.42 mL per applicator	*Certifect®*

Human-Labeled Products

None

References

For the complete list of references, see **wiley.com/go/budde/plumb**

Imidacloprid/Imidacloprid Combinations, Topical

(eye-mi-da-***kloe***-prid) *Advantage®*, Seresto®

For systemic use, see ***Imidacloprid, Systemic and Moxidectin/Moxidectin Combination Products***

Indications/Actions

Imidacloprid topical solution is indicated for the prevention and treatment of flea infestations in cats and flea and lice infestations in dogs. Imidacloprid is effective against both adult fleas and flea larvae.[1] The combination of imidacloprid and pyriproxyfen is indicated for the prevention and treatment of all flea stages in dogs and cats and lice infestations in dogs. The combination of imidacloprid, pyriproxyfen, and permethrin is indicated in dogs only for the prevention and treatment of fleas, ticks, mosquitoes, biting flies, and lice.

The combination of imidacloprid and flumethrin impregnated into a slow-release collar is indicated for the prevention and treatment of ticks, fleas, and lice in dogs and prevention and treatment of ticks and fleas in cats. It has also been shown to prevent babesiosis[2] and leishmaniosis[3] in dogs and is indicated for the prevention of leishmaniosis in some countries.

Imidacloprid's mechanism of action as an insecticide is to act on nicotinic acetylcholine receptors on the postsynaptic membrane, causing CNS impairment and death of the ectoparasite. Certain insect species are more sensitive to these agents than are mammalian receptors. This is a different mechanism of action than other insecticidal agents (organophosphates, pyrethrins, carbamates, insect growth regulators [IGRs], and insect development inhibitors [IDIs]). Imidacloprid is reported to be nonteratogenic, nonhypersensitizing, nonmutagenic, nonallergenic, noncarcinogenic, and nonphotosensitizing. When applied topically, imidocloprid is not absorbed into the bloodstream or internal organs. Permethrin and flumethrin, found in some imidacloprid products, are neurotoxins that slow the movement of sodium ions through sodium channels in neuron membranes of the ectoparasite. Pyriproxyfen may also be found in some imidacloprid products; it mimics insect juvenile growth hormone, halting development during metamorphosis and larval development. It also concentrates in female flea ovaries, causing non-viable eggs to be produced.

Suggested Dosages/Uses

Refer to the package information for product-specific application instructions. Imidacloprid products are generally administered once monthly; however, extra-label dosages, such as once weekly or every other week, have been used. Although swimming, bathing, and rain do not significantly affect the duration of action, animals that have been shampooed repeatedly may require additional treatment(s) before the next monthly dosing interval, not to exceed once weekly administration.

Precautions/Adverse Effects

When used as directed, imidacloprid topical solutions are usually well tolerated and adverse effects are minimal. Dermal irritation has been reported at the site of application.

Imidacloprid and pyriproxyfen combinations are contraindicated in puppies younger than 7 weeks, dogs weighing less than 3 lbs, and kittens younger than 7 or 8 weeks (depending on product). Use with caution in debilitated, older, pregnant, or nursing animals.

Combination products that contain permethrin must not be used on cats. They should be used with caution in households with cats, particularly if cats are in close contact with or will groom treated dogs.

Avoid contact with the eyes and mouth; oral contact may cause excessive salivation. If eye contact occurs in humans or animals, flush well with an ophthalmic irrigation solution or water. Wearing gloves is not required during administration but is recommended to avoid contact with human skin. Wash hands with soap and water after handling. Keep out of reach of children. Store products away from food sources to avoid the possibility of contamination. Carefully dispose of products in the trash.

Most toxicities are seen following oral dosing of topical products. In cats, clinical signs may include hypersalivation, vomiting, lethargy, and hiding; oral ulcers have also been rarely reported in cats. In dogs, reported clinical signs include vomiting, hypersalivation, and trembling.

Veterinary-Labeled Products

Active ingredients (formulation)	Species	Label status; size(s)	Trade names/additional information
Imidacloprid 9.1% (spot-on solution)	Dogs and puppies 7 weeks of age and older; cats and kittens 8 weeks of age and older	OTC (EPA); packages of 4 or 6 applicators: Cats 4.1 kg (9 lb) and under: 0.4 mL Cats over 4.1 kg (9 lb): 0.8 mL Dogs under 4.5 kg (10 lb): 0.4 mL Dogs 5 - 9.1 kg (11-20 lb): 1 mL Dogs 9.5 - 25 kg (21-55 lb): 2.5 mL Dogs over 25 kg (55 lb): 4 mL	*Advantage®* (product no longer available in the United States)
Imidacloprid 10%, flumethrin 4.5%, (collar)	Dogs and puppies 7 weeks of age and older; cats and kittens 10 weeks of age and older	OTC (EPA); available in 3 collar sizes: Cat: 15 inches Small dog (up to 8.2 kg [18 lb]): 15 inches Large dog (over 8.2 kg [18 lb]): 27.5 inches	*Seresto®*

Active ingredients (formulation)	Species	Label status; size(s)	Trade names/additional information
Imidacloprid 9.1%, pyriproxyfen 0.46% (spot-on solution)	Dogs and puppies 7 weeks of age and older; cats and kittens 8 weeks of age and older	OTC (EPA); packages of 4 or 6 applicators: Cats 0.9 - 2.3 kg (2-5 lb): 0.23 mL Cats 2.3 - 4.1 kg (5-9 lb): 0.4 mL Cats over 4.1 kg (9 lb): 0.8 mL Dogs 1.4 - 4.5 kg (3-10 lb): 0.4 mL Dogs 5 - 9.1 kg (11-20 lb): 1 mL Dogs 9.5 - 25 kg (21-55 lb): 2.5 mL Dogs over 25 kg (55 lb): 4 mL	*Advantage® II; Adventure Plus®*
Imidacloprid 9.1%, pyriproxyfen 0.46% (spot-on solution)	Cats and kittens at least 7 weeks of age	OTC (EPA); packages of 4 applicators: 2.3 - 4.1 kg (5-9 lb): 0.4mL (red) Over 4.1 kg (9 lb): 0.8 mL (purple)	*Provecta® II*
Imidacloprid 7.12%, permethrin 35.6%, pyriproxyfen 0.36% (spot-on solution)	Dogs and puppies over 7 weeks of age **Do NOT use on cats.**	OTC (EPA); packages of 4 applicators for use on dogs ONLY: 1.8 - 4.5 kg (4-10 lb): 0.48 mL 5 - 9.1 kg (11-20 lb): 1.2 mL 9.5 - 25 kg (21-55 lb): 3 mL Over 25 kg (55 lb): 4.8 mL	*Activate® II*
Imidacloprid 8.8%, permethrin 44%, pyriproxyfen 0.44% (spot-on solution)	Dogs and puppies 7 weeks of age **Do NOT use on cats.**	OTC (EPA); packages of 4 or 6 applicators for use on dogs ONLY: 1.8 - 4.5 kg (4-10 lb): 0.4 mL 5 - 9.1 kg (11-20 lb): 1 mL 9.5 - 25 kg (21-55 lb): 2.5 mL Over 25 kg (55 lb): 4 mL	*K9 Advantix® II; Provecta® Advanced*

Human-Labeled Products

None

References

For the complete list of references, see **wiley.com/go/budde/plumb**

Isopropyl Myristate, Topical

(eye-so-***proe***-pil ***meer***-is-tate) *Resultix®*

Indications/Actions

Isopropyl myristate is a noninsecticidal product labeled for the removal and killing of attached and crawling ticks on dogs and cats. It acts by dissolving the outer wax layer covering the hard shell (cuticle) of the tick, resulting in uncontrollable water loss and death. Ticks generally die and fall off within 3 hours.

Suggested Dosages/Uses

Spray tick until it is covered with solution, ≈2 sprays. Tick should be dead within 3 hours and will either fall off the animal or will be immobile when it is removed. If the tick has not fallen off after 3 hours, carefully remove it with gloves or tweezers. Dispose of the tick by placing it in a sealable plastic bag. Wash hands after handling product, and after any accidental exposure to ticks.

Isopropyl myristate can be used as often as needed.[1]

Precautions/Adverse Effects

Do not use near the eyes or on irritated skin. Discontinue use if skin irritation or skin infection develops.

Isopropyl myristate is toxic to invertebrates and fish.[1] Never dispose of product down any drain; do not discharge into lakes, streams, ponds, estuaries, oceans, or other waters where aquatic invertebrates or fish may be found.

Veterinary-Labeled Products

Active ingredients (formulation)	Species	Label status; size(s)	Trade names/additional information
Isopropyl myristate 50% (spray)	Labeled for dogs and cats	OTC (EPA); 20 mL	*Resultix®*

Human-Labeled Products

None

References

For the complete list of references, see **wiley.com/go/budde/plumb**

Methoprene/Methoprene Combinations, Topical

(meth-oh-***preen***)

Indications/Actions

Methoprene is an insect growth regulator that prevents the maturation of flea and mosquito eggs and larva. Methoprene mimics insect juvenile growth hormone, halting development during metamorphosis and larval development. It also concentrates in female flea ovaries, resulting in the production of nonviable eggs.

Methoprene is typically combined with an adulticide to kill all stages of the parasites and prevent reinfestation. Fipronil and pyrethroids (eg, cyphenothrin, etofenprox, permethrin) are commonly used in combination with methoprene. These agents also provide coverage against additional parasites; see specific product labels for details on parasite activity.

Suggested Dosages/Uses

For use and dosage recommendations, refer to the specific product insert.

Precautions/Adverse Effects

Methoprene is commonly found in products containing **pyrethroids that are toxic to cats**, especially small kittens. **Only use products on cats that are specifically labeled for use on cats.** Use pyrethroid-containing products cautiously on dogs that cohabitate with cats.

Hypersensitivity reactions and skin irritation are possible with methoprene-containing products. Avoid eyes and mucous membranes during application. When used as a single agent, methoprene has low toxicity in mammals.

Additional precautions and adverse effects vary based on other active ingredients; refer to specific product insert.

Methoprene products should be protected from light as methoprene is broken down by UV light.

Veterinary-Labeled Products

NOTES:

1. Methoprene is available in a variety of combinations. Use caution selecting products labeled for different species as different combinations of active ingredients may be marketed under the same trade name.
2. There is an extensive number of products marketed, including collars, topical sprays, foggers, and spot-on solutions; the following products are only representative.

Active ingredients (formulation)	Species	Label status; size(s)	Trade names/additional information
Methoprene 2.9% (spot-on solution)	Labeled for cats and kittens 12 weeks of age and older	OTC (EPA); single-dose 1 mL applicators in packages of 3	*Hartz® UltraGuard® OneSpot®*
Methoprene 3%, permethrin 45% (spot-on solution)	Labeled for dogs 6 months of age and older **Do NOT use on cats.**	OTC (EPA); single-dose applicators per weight in packages of 4	*Zodiac® Spot On® for Dogs*
Methoprene 3.6%, etofenprox 40% (spot-on solution)	Labeled for kittens 12 weeks of age and older	OTC (EPA); single-dose 1.8 mL applicators in packages of 3 for cats 2.3 kg (5 lb) and over	*Hartz® UltraGuard Plus® for Cats; Hartz® UltraGuard Pro® for Cats*
Methoprene 4.05%, etofenprox 46%	Labeled for cats and kittens 12 weeks of age and older	OTC (EPA); single-dose applicators per weight in packages of 3	*Adams® Plus for Cats*
Methoprene 8.8%, fipronil 9.8% (spot-on solution)	Labeled for dogs or puppies 8 weeks of age and older	OTC (EPA); single-dose applicators per weight in packages of 3 and 6	*Frontline® Plus for Dogs; Onguard® Plus for Dogs; PetArmor® Plus for Dogs; Sentry® Fiproguard Plus for Dogs*
Methoprene 8.8%, fipronil 9.8%, cyphenothrin 5.2% (spot-on solution)	Labeled for use on dogs 12 weeks of age and older **Do NOT use on cats.**	OTC (EPA); single-dose applicators per weight in packages of 3	*Frontline® Tritak® for Dogs*
Methoprene 11.8%, fipronil 9.8% (spot-on solution)	Labeled for use on cats or kittens 8 weeks of age and older	OTC (EPA); single-dose applicators of 0.5 mL in packages of 3 and 6	*Frontline® Plus for Cats; Onguard® Plus for Cats; PetArmor® Plus for Cats; Sentry® Fiproguard Plus for Cats*
Methoprene 11.8%, fipronil 9.8%, etofenprox 15% (spot-on solution)	Labeled for use on cats or kittens 12 weeks of age or older	OTC (EPA); single-dose applicators of 0.5 mL in packages of 3	*Frontline® Tritak® for Cats*

Active ingredients (formulation)	Species	Label status; size(s)	Trade names/additional information
Methoprene 8.8%, fipronil 9.8%, pyriproxyfen 0.25% (spot-on solution)	Labeled for dogs and puppies 8 weeks of age and older	OTC (EPA); single-dose applicators of 0.5 mL in packages of 3 and 6 per weight	*Frontline® Gold for Dogs*
Methoprene 11.8%, fipronil 9.8%, pyriproxyfen 0.25% (spot-on solution)	Labeled for cats and kittens 8 weeks of age and older	OTC (EPA); single-dose applicators of 0.5 mL in packages of 3 and 6 for cats 0.7 kg (1.5 lb) or greater	*Frontline® Gold for Cats*
Methoprene 0.27%, piperonyl butoxide 0.37%, pyrethrins 0.2% (spray)	Labeled for use on dogs, cats, puppies, kittens, horses, and ponies **NOT for puppies or kittens less than 12 weeks old**	OTC (EPA); 16 oz, 24 oz, 1 gallon	*Vet-Kem Ovitrol Plus®; Bio-Spot®*
Methoprene 0.27%, fipronil 0.29% (spray)	Labeled for use on cats or kittens 8 weeks of age or older	OTC (EPA); 6.5 oz (aerosol spray), 8 oz (trigger spray)	*Martin's FLEE®*
Methoprene 1.1%, piperonyl butoxide 1.05%, pyrethrins 0.15% (shampoo)	**NOT for puppies or kittens less than 12 weeks old**	OTC (EPA); 12 oz	*Vet-Kem®*
Methoprene 1.02%, tetrachlorvinphos 14.55% (collar)	Labeled for dogs and cats	OTC (EPA); sizing based on neck circumference and varies based on manufacturer	*Hartz® UltraGuard Plus®; Hartz® UltraGuard Pro®; PetArmor® for Cats; Adams® Plus*
Methoprene 1.02%, deltamethrin 4% (collar)	Labeled for dogs 12 weeks and older	OTC (EPA); one size, fits dogs with necks up to 26"	*Hartz® InControl®; Hartz® UltraGuard ProMAX*

Human-Labeled Products

None

Permethrin/Permethrin Combinations, Topical

(per-***meth***-rin)

Indications/Actions

Permethrin is a synthetic pyrethroid insecticide that acts as an adulticide and miticide. It has knockdown activity against fleas, ticks, lice, and some mites, including *Cheyletiella* spp and *Sarcoptes scabiei*. Permethrin also has repellant activity against flies, gnats, and mosquitoes.

In dogs, permethrin is primarily used to prevent fleas and ticks. In large animal and food animal species, it is primarily used for flies, lice, mites, mosquitoes, ticks, and keds.

Permethrin acts by disrupting the sodium channel current in arthropod nerve cell membranes, resulting in paralysis and death.

Suggested Dosages/Uses

Permethrin products can typically be applied every 2 weeks or every 4 weeks; refer to specific product label for details on use.

Precautions/Adverse Effects

Permethrin and other synthetic pyrethroids are toxic to cats, especially small kittens. Do not use permethrin-containing products on cats and avoid use on dogs that cohabitate with cats.

Permethrin may cause hypersensitivity reactions. Do not use permethrin near the eyes or mucous membranes. Adverse effects are uncommon but can include pruritus or mild skin irritation at the application site.

Wear gloves and wash hands after application. In case of skin contact, wash off with water.

Permethrin is extremely toxic to aquatic organisms and bees. Apply and dispose of products with caution as not to contaminate the environment.

Veterinary-Labeled Products

NOTES:

1. This is not an inclusive list; there are an extensive number of products marketed, including shampoos, pour-ons, sprays, foggers, and dusts. Use caution selecting products, as different combinations of active ingredients may be marketed under the same trade name.
2. **Permethrin products must NOT be used on cats** and should not be used on dogs that cohabitate with cats.

Active ingredients (formulation)	Species	Label status; size(s)	Trade names/additional information
Permethrin 45% (spot-on solution)	Labeled for horses over 3 months of age	OTC (EPA); single-dose applicators in packages of 3 or 6	*Equi-Spot®*

Active ingredients (formulation)	Species	Label status; size(s)	Trade names/additional information
Permethrin 50% (spot-on solution)	Labeled for horses over 3 months of age	OTC (EPA); single-dose applicators in packages of 3 or 6	*Pro-Force®50*
Permethrin 45%, pyriproxyfen 1.9% (spot-on solution)	Labeled for dogs over 3 months of age	OTC (EPA); single-dose applicators in packages of 3: 6.8 kg (15 lb) and under: 1 mL 6.8 - 15 kg (15-33 lb): 1.5 mL 15 -30 kg (33-66 lb): 3 mL 30 kg (66 lb) and over: 4.5 mL	*Sentry®*
Permethrin 45%, pyriproxyfen 5% (spot-on solution)	Labeled for dogs older than 3 months of age	OTC (EPA); single-dose applicators in packages of 4: 2.3 - 6.8 kg (5-15 lb): 1 mL 7.3 - 15 kg (16-33 lb): 1.5 mL 15.4 - 30 kg (34-66 lb): 3 mL Over 30 kg (66 lb): 4.5 mL	*ShieldTec Plus®*
Permethrin 44%, imidacloprid 8.8%, pyriproxyfen 0.44% (spot-on solution)	Labeled for dogs 7 weeks of age and older	OTC (EPA); in packages of 2, 4, or 6: 1.8 - 4.5 kg (4-10 lb): 0.4 mL 5 - 9.1 kg (11-20 lb): 1 mL 9.5 - 25 kg (21-55 lb): 2.5 mL Over 25 kg (55 lb): 4 mL	*K9 Advantix® II*
Permethrin 35.6%, imidacloprid 7.12%, pyriproxyfen 0.36% (spot-on solution)	Labeled for dogs 7 weeks of age and older	OTC (EPA); in packages of 4: 1.8 - 4.5 kg (4-10 lb): 0.48 mL 5 - 9.1 kg (11-20 lb): 1.2 mL 9.5 - 25 kg (21-55 lb): 3 mL Over 25 kg (55 lb): 4.8 mL	*Activate® II*
Permethrin 36.08%, dinotefuran 4.95%, pyriproxyfen 0.44% (spot-on solution)	Labeled for dogs 7 weeks of age and older	OTC (EPA); in packages of 3 or 6: 2.3 - 4.5 kg (5-10 lb): 0.8 mL 5 - 9.1 kg (11-20 lb): 1.6 mL 9.5 - 25 kg (21-55 lb): 3.6 mL 25.4 -4 3.1 kg (56-95 lb): 4.7 mL Over 43.1 kg (95 lb): 8 mL	*Vectra 3D®*
Permethrin 45%, methoprene 3% (spot-on solution)	Labeled for dogs 6 months of age and older	OTC (EPA); in packages of 4: 3.2 6.8 kg (7-15 lb): 0.65 mL 7.3 - 13.6 kg (16-30 lb): 1 mL 14.1 - 27.2 kg (31-60 lb): 2 mL Over 27.2 kg (60 lb): 3 mL	*Zodiac®*
Permethrin 0.1%, 2-[1 methyl-2-(4-phenoxyphenoxy) ethoxy] pyridine 0.125%, N-octyl bicycloheptene dicarboximide 0.479%, pyrethrins 0.112% (spray)	Labeled for dogs over 6 months of age	OTC (EPA); 8 oz bottle	*Veterinary Formula Clinical Care®*
Permethrin 0.1%, piperonyl butoxide 0.5%, pyrethrins 0.05% (spray)	Labeled for dogs over 3 months of age	OTC (EPA); 32 oz bottle	*Flea Halt®*

Human-Labeled Products

Active ingredients (formulation)	Label status; size(s)	Trade names/additional information
Permethrin 1% (creme rinse)	OTC; 59 mL	*Nix®*; generic Labeled for treatment of head lice in humans
Permethrin 5% (cream)	Rx; 60 g	*Acticin®*; *Elimite®*; generic Labeled for treatment of scabies in humans

Pyrethrin/Pyrethrin Combinations, Topical

(pye-***ree***-thrin)

For otic use, see ***Antiparasitic Agents, Otic.***

Indications/Actions

Pyrethrins are natural insecticides derived from the pyrethrum flower that have knockdown activity against fleas, lice, ticks, and *Cheyletiella* spp. In small animal medicine, pyrethrins are used primarily to treat fleas and ticks on dogs and cats. In large animal and food animal medicine, there are many products available for pour-on, dusting, and spray use.

The natural pyrethrins are made up of 6 compounds. They act by disrupting the sodium channel current in arthropod nerve cell membranes, resulting in paralysis and death. Pyrethrins are often found in combination with insect growth regulators, such as methoprene or pyriproxyfen, or with synergistic agents such as piperonyl butoxide. Insect growth regulators add activity against egg and larval growth stages. Piperonyl butoxide inhibits insect metabolic enzymes (P450 system), which prevents the breakdown of primary insecticides and allows for a lower dose to be used.

Suggested Dosages/Uses

For dosage recommendations, refer to the specific product label.

Precautions/Adverse Effects

Pyrethrins are generally considered to be some of the safest insecticidal products. Avoid contact with the eyes and mucous membranes. Do not apply over wounds or irritated skin. Wear gloves when applying or wash hands after handling.

Cats are more susceptible to pyrethrin toxicity than other species. **Only use products on cats that are specifically labeled for cats.** Use pyrethrin products with caution in dogs that cohabitate with cats, and do not allow cats to groom application areas before dry. Avoid applying to hypothermic patients or applying when ambient temperatures are low. Pyrethrin products are toxic to fish and aquatic animals; do not allow products to enter drains or other water sources during application or disposal.

Adverse effects are uncommon but may include pruritus or mild skin irritation at the application site. Hypersensitivity reactions can also occur.

Veterinary-Labeled Products

There are a wide variety of available products, including shampoos, pour-ons, sprays, dusts, and ointments. The following is not an all-inclusive list.

Active ingredients (formulation)	Species	Label status; size(s)	Trade names/additional information
Pyrethrins 0.2%, piperonyl butoxide 0.37%, (S)-methoprene 0.27% (spray) Other ingredients: N-octyl bicycloheptene dicarboximide 0.62%	Labeled for use on dogs, cats over 3 pounds and 12 weeks of age; horses; and ponies.	OTC (EPA); 16 oz, 1 gallon	*Vet-Kem Ovitrol Plus®*
Pyrethrins 0.05%, permethrin 0.1%, piperonyl butoxide 0.5% (spray)	Labeled for dogs older than 3 months of age. **Do NOT use on cats or on dogs that cohabit with a cat.**	OTC (EPA); 8 oz, 32 oz, 40 oz	*Flea Halt®*
Pyrethrins 0.18%, 2-[1-Methyl-2-(4-phenoxyphenoxy) ethoxy] pyridine 0.125%, N-octyl bicycloheptene dicarboximide 0.957% (spray)	Labeled for dogs over 6 months of age or cats over 7 months of age	OTC (EPA); 8 oz, 15 oz	*Advantage®*
Pyrethrins 0.18%, N-octyl bicycloheptene dicarboximide 0.479%, piperonyl butoxide 0.3% (spray)	Labeled for dogs and puppies over 6 months of age	OTC (EPA); 8 oz, 15 oz	*Advantage®*
Pyrethrins 0.05%, piperonyl butoxide 0.5% (shampoo)	Labeled for dogs and cats over 12 weeks of age	OTC (EPA); 12 oz	*Zodiac®*
Pyrethrins 0.15%, piperonyl butoxide 1.88%, (S)-methoprene 0.1% (shampoo)	Labeled for dogs and cats over 12 weeks of age	OTC (EPA); 12 oz	*Adams® Plus*
Pyrethrins 0.15%, piperonyl butoxide 1.88%, (S)-methoprene 0.1% (shampoo)	Labeled for dogs and cats over 12 weeks of age	OTC (EPA); 12 oz	*Vet-Kem® Ovitrol Plus*
Pyrethrins 0.15%, N-oxyl bicycloheptene dicarboximide 0.5%, piperonyl butoxide 0.3% (shampoo)	Labeled for dogs and cats over 12 weeks of age	OTC; 12 oz, 1 gallon	*Davis®*
Pyrethrins 0.15%, N-octyl bicycloheptene dicarboxamide 0.479%, piperonyl butoxide 0.3% (shampoo)	Labeled for dogs, cats, ferrets, and horses over 12 weeks of age	OTC (EPA); 16 oz, 1 gallon	*Veterinary Formula®*

Active ingredients (formulation)	Species	Label status; size(s)	Trade names/additional information
Pyrethrins 0.97%, di-n-propyl isocinchomerate 1.94%, N-octyl bicycloheptene dicarboxamide 5.7%, piperonyl butoxide 3.74% (dip)	Labeled for dogs and cats over 12 weeks of age	OTC (EPA); 4 oz	*Adams Plus®*
Pyrethrins 0.3%, piperonyl butoxide 3% (dip)	Labeled for dogs and cats over 12 weeks of age	OTC (EPA); 8 oz, 1 gallon	*Bio-Groom®*

Human-Labeled Products

Active ingredients (formulation)	Label status; size(s)	Trade names/additional information
Pyrethrins 0.33%, piperonyl butoxide 4% (shampoo)	OTC; 2 oz, 4 oz, 8 oz	*Rid®*; generic Indicated for treatment of lice in humans

Pyriproxyfen/Pyriproxyfen Combinations, Topical

(pye-ri-***proks***-i-fen)

See also ***Deltamethrin, Dinotefuran/Pyriproxyfen Combinations, Fipronil/Fipronil Combinations, Imidacloprid/Imidacloprid Combinations, Methoprene/Methoprene Combinations, Permethrin/Permethrin Combinations,*** *and* ***Pyrethrin/Pyrethrin Combinations***

Indications/Actions

Pyriproxyfen is a second-generation insect growth regulator and is added to topical and environmental products to extend the insecticidal spectrum to include eggs and larva.

Pyriproxyfen mimics insect juvenile growth hormone, halting development during metamorphosis and larval development. It also concentrates in female flea ovaries, causing non-viable eggs to be produced. Pyriproxyfen is combined with adulticides such as permethrin or fipronil to kill all stages of targeted parasites, making re-infestation less likely.

Suggested Dosages/Uses

For dosage recommendations, refer to the specific product label.

Precautions/Adverse Effects

Pyriproxyfen can be found in products that contain **permethrin, which is toxic to cats**, particularly small kittens. **Only use products containing pyrethroids that are specifically labeled for use on cats**. Pyriproxyfen has low toxicity in mammals, but skin irritation and hypersensitivity reactions are possible.

Wear gloves when applying products containing insecticides and wash hands after handling. Pyriproxyfen is more resistant to UV light than is methoprene.

Veterinary-Labeled Products

NOTE: This is not an all-inclusive list but is representative of the types of products available.

Active ingredients (formulation)	Species	Label status; size(s)	Trade names/additional information
Pyriproxyfen 0.46%, imidacloprid 9.1% (spot-on solution)	Labeled for dogs and puppies 7 weeks of age and older; cats and kittens 8 weeks of age and older	OTC (EPA); packages of 3, 4 or 6 applicators: Cats 0.9 - 2.3 kg (2-5 lb): 0.23 mL Cats 2.3 - 4.1 kg (5-9 lb): 0.4 mL Cats over 4.1 kg (9 lb): 0.8 mL Dogs 1.4 - 4.5 kg (3-10 lb): 0.4 mL Dogs 5 - 9.1 kg (11-20 lb): 1 mL Dogs 9.5 - 25 kg (21-55 lb): 2.5 mL Dogs over 25 kg (55 lb): 4 mL	*Advantage®II; Adventure Plus®; Cross Block® II; Pet Armor Advanced® II*
Pyriproxyfen 0.46%, imidacloprid 9.1% (spot-on solution)	Labeled for cats and kittens 7 weeks of age and older	OTC (EPA); packages of 4 applicators: 2.3 - 4.1 kg (5-9 lb): 0.4 mL (red) Over 4.1 kg (9 lb): 0.8 mL (purple)	*Provecta® II*
Pyriproxyfen 0.44%, imidacloprid 8.8%, permethrin 44% (spot-on solution)	Labeled for dogs and puppies 7 weeks of age and older **Do NOT use on cats or on dogs that cohabitate with a cat.**	OTC (EPA); packages of 4 or 6 applicators for use on dogs ONLY: 1.8 - 4.5 kg (4-10 lb): 0.4 mL 5 - 9.1 kg (11-20 lb): 1 mL 9.5 -25 kg (21-55 lb): 2.5 mL Over 25 kg (55 lb): 4 mL	*K9 Advantix® II; Provecta® Advanced*

Active ingredients (formulation)	Species	Label status; size(s)	Trade names/additional information
Pyriproxyfen 0.36%, imidacloprid 7.12%, permethrin 35.6% (spot-on solution)	Dogs and puppies over 7 weeks of age **Do NOT use on cats or on dogs that cohabitate with a cat.**	OTC (EPA); packages of 4 applicators for use on dogs ONLY: 1.8 - 4.5 kg (4-10 lb): 0.48 mL 5 - 9.1 kg (11-20 lb): 1.2 mL 9.5 - 25 kg (21-55 lb): 3 mL Over 25 kg (55 lb): 4.8 mL	*Activate®II*
Pyriproxyfen 0.44%, dinotefuran 4.95%, permethrin 36.08% (spot-on solution)	Labeled for dogs over 7 weeks of age **Do NOT use on cats or on dogs that cohabitate with a cat.**	OTC (EPA); in packages of 3 or 6: 2.3 – 4.5 kg (5-10 lb): 0.8 mL 5 - 9.1 kg (11-20 lb): 1.6 mL 9.5 -25 kg (21-55 lb): 3.6 mL 56 to 95 lb: 4.7 mL Over 95 lb: 8 mL	*Vectra 3D®*
Pyriproxyfen 1.9%, permethrin 45%, (spot-on solution)	Labeled for dogs over 3 months of age **Do NOT use on cats or on dogs that cohabitate with a cat.**	OTC (EPA); single-dose applicators in packages of 3: 6.8 kg (15 lb) and under: 1 mL 6.8 - 15 kg (15-33 lb): 1.5 mL 15 - 29.9 kg (33-66 lb): 3 mL 29.9 kg (66 lb) and over: 4.5 mL	*Sentry®*
Pyriproxyfen 5%, permethrin 45% (spot-on solution)	Labeled for dogs over 3 months of age **Do NOT use on cats or on dogs that cohabitate with a cat.**	OTC (EPA); single-dose applicators in packages of 4: 2.3 - 6.8 kg (5-15 lb): 1 mL 7.3 - 15 kg (16-33 lb): 1.5 mL 15.4 - 29.9 kg (34-66 lb): 3 mL Over (29.9 kg) 66 lb: 4.5 mL	*ShieldTec Plus®*
Pyriproxyfen 3%, dinotefuran 22%, fipronil 8.92% (spot-on solution)	Labeled for cats and kittens over 8 weeks of age	OTC (EPA); available in packages of 3 or 6 applicators for cats over 0.7 kg (1.5 lb)	*Catego®*
Pyriproxyfen 2%, cyphenothrin 40%, (spot-on solution)	Labeled for use on dogs more than 12 weeks of age **Do NOT use on cats or on dogs that cohabitate with a cat.**	OTC (EPA); available in packages of 3 applicators: 4.1 - 9.1 kg (9 - 20 lb), 9.5 - 17.7 kg (21 - 39 lb), 18.1 - 27.2 kg (40 - 60 lb), and at least 27.7 kg (61 lb)	*TriForce®*

Human-Labeled Products

None

Spinetoram, Topical

(***spin***-et-oh-ram)

Indications/Actions

Spinetoram is an insecticide used for the prevention and treatment of flea infestations in cats.

Spinetoram is a semi-synthetic, second-generation derivative of the natural insecticide spinosad. It acts on both GABA and nicotinic acetylcholine receptors in the CNS of insects, leading to CNS hyperexcitation, followed by paralysis and death. Spinetoram begins to act within 30 minutes after application.[1]

Suggested Dosages/Uses

To treat and prevent flea infestations, spinetoram should be applied once monthly to the skin at the base of the head. For detailed application instructions, refer to the specific product label.

Precautions/Adverse Effects

Spinetoram should not be used on kittens less than 8 weeks of age. Do not allow cats to ingest product. Only a single dose should be applied at one time, regardless of the weight of the cat (ie, large cats do not require additional doses). Use spinetoram with caution on debilitated, aged, pregnant, or nursing animals, or any animal known to be sensitive to pesticides. Avoid contact with the eyes or mouth. Spinetoram should not be used in dogs, as they are more sensitive to the toxic effects of spinetoram than mice, rats, or cats.[2]

The primary adverse effects are application site reactions, including hair loss, hair changes (eg, greasing, clumping, matting), redness, inflammation, and itching. Other reported adverse effects include inactivity, vomiting, and inappetence.[3] Do not allow cats to groom after application in order to prevent ingestion. Application at the base of the head, rather than the shoulder blades, decreases the risk for direct ingestion.

Spinetoram has been shown to produce reproductive adverse effects in female rats including treatment-related depletion of primordial ovarian follicles, growing ovarian follicles, dystocia and other parturition abnormalities, late resorptions or retained fetuses, and increased postimplantation loss. However, no adverse effects were observed on the offspring at dose levels that produced parental toxicity. The developmental toxicity and reproduction studies indicated no evidence of increased susceptibility of the offspring with pre- and/or postnatal exposures.[2]

Veterinary-Labeled Products

Active ingredients (formulation)	Species	Label status; size(s)	Trade names/additional information
Spinetoram 11.2% (spot-on solution)	Labeled for cats and kittens 8 weeks of age and older	OTC (EPA); in packs of 1, 3, or 6: Cats and kittens over 0.82 kg (1.8 lb): 0.77 mL	*Cheristin*®

Human-Labeled Products

None

References

For the complete list of references, see **wiley.com/go/budde/plumb**

Antiseborrheic Agents, Topical

Refer to:
Benzoyl Peroxide, Topical (Antimicrobial Agents, Topical; Antibacterial Agents)
Coal Tar/Coal Tar Combinations, Topical (Keratolytic Agents)
Fatty Acids (Omega), Topical (Antipruritic/Anti-Inflammatory Agents, Topical; Non-Corticosteroid Agents)
Phytosphingosine, Topical (Antipruritic/Anti-Inflammatory Agents, Topical; Non-Corticosteroid Agents)
Salicylic Acid, Topical (Keratolytic Agents)
Selenium Sulfide, Topical (Antimicrobial Agents, Topical; Antifungal Agents)
Sulfur, Precipitated, Topical (Keratolytic Agents)

Immunomodulator Agents, Topical

Imiquimod, Topical

(ih-***mi***-kwih-mod) *Aldara*®, *Zyclara*®

Indications/Actions

Imiquimod is an immune response modifier that may be useful in the treatment of a variety of topical conditions in animals. In dogs and cats, it may be beneficial in treating actinic keratosis, squamous cell carcinoma, pigmented epidermal plaques, cutaneous viral papillomatosis, localized solar dermatitis, and solar carcinoma in situ. It may also be useful for feline herpesvirus dermatitis, feline Bowen's disease, and canine melanocytomas. Many of these indications are based on anecdotal evidence, as there are very few studies published for veterinary use. In horses, imiquimod has been anecdotally used for treating equine sarcoids, aural plaques, and epitrichial sweat gland ductal carcinoma. In humans, it is labeled as a treatment for genital or perianal warts, superficial basal cell carcinomas, and actinic keratoses of the face and scalp.

Imiquimod is an imidazoquinoline compound that binds to toll-like receptor 7 and stimulates the immune system to release various cytokines, including interferon-alpha and interleukin-12. These locally generated cytokines induce a Th1 immune response with the generation of cytotoxic effectors. Imiquimod itself does not have in vitro activity against wart viruses but stimulates monocytes and macrophages to release cytokines that induce regression in viral protein production.

Suggested Dosages/Uses

Use of imiquimod in animals is limited and further studies are needed. Doses and treatment regimens vary depending on the disease treated and tolerance to the drug. Doses range from applying a thin film once daily to applying every other week. Exudate and crusts should be gently cleaned prior to application of imiquimod. Treatment duration and frequency may be adjusted depending on patient response and adverse reactions.

Precautions/Adverse Effects

Wear gloves when applying imiquimod. Avoid exposing the eyes and mucous membranes to imiquimod; however, dogs with oral mucosal papilloma and horses with corneal squamous cell carcinomas have been treated without significant problems. Although systemic absorption is unlikely, do not allow treated animals to lick or groom the application site.

Local skin reactions are common and expected with imiquimod therapy, including erythema, burning, tenderness, pain, irritation, oozing/exudate, and erosion. Treatment duration and frequency may require adjustment depending on irritant reactions. Depigmentation and hair loss may occur at application sites as posttreatment sequelae.

Increased liver enzymes, neutropenia, partial anorexia, and vomiting were reported in cats in one small study, possibly associated with ingestion postcutaneous application.[1] Consider a baseline hepatic profile with periodic monitoring. Do not cover application site with occlusive dressings. It is thought that imiquimod may increase risk for sunburn; avoid exposing application site to sunlight.

Veterinary-Labeled Products

None

Human-Labeled Products

Active ingredients (formulation)	Label status; size(s)	Trade names/additional information
Imiquimod 2.5% (cream)	Rx; 7.5 g pump bottle, single-use 250 mg packets in boxes of 28	*Zyclara®*
Imiquimod 3.75% (cream)	Rx; 7.5 g pump bottle	*Zyclara®*; generic
Imiquimod 5% (cream)	Rx; single-use 250 mg packets in boxes of 12 or 24	*Aldara®*; generic

References

For the complete list of references, see **wiley.com/go/budde/plumb**

Pimecrolimus, Topical

(pim-e-***kroe***-li-mus)

Indications/Actions

Topical pimecrolimus may be beneficial for the adjunctive treatment of atopic dermatitis, discoid lupus erythematosus, pemphigus erythematosus or foliaceous, pinnal vascular disease or other cutaneous vasculopathies, alopecia areata, vitiligo, perianal fistulas (concurrent therapy or as maintenance treatment after cyclosporine therapy), and for feline proliferative and necrotizing otitis externa. Unlike topical corticosteroids, pimecrolimus does not have atrophogenic or metabolic effects associated with long-term use or large treatment areas.

Pimecrolimus is a calcineurin inhibitor that acts similarly to cyclosporine and tacrolimus. It inhibits T-lymphocyte activation primarily by inhibiting the phosphatase activity of calcineurin. It also inhibits the release of inflammatory cytokines and mediators from mast cells and basophils. The mechanism of pimecrolimus may not be identical to tacrolimus, as pimecrolimus did not impair the primary immune response (as did tacrolimus) in mice after a contact sensitizer was applied. Both drugs did impair the secondary response, however. Any clinical significance associated with this difference is not yet clear.

Suggested Dosages/Uses

There is limited experience with pimecrolimus in veterinary patients. It is typically recommended to use twice daily until signs are controlled, then decrease to the least frequent application that controls clinical signs.

Precautions/Adverse Effects

Although a causal relationship has not been established, skin malignancy and lymphoma have rarely been reported in humans using topical pimecrolimus. Therefore, long-term use is not recommended in humans, and pimecrolimus application should be limited to only the affected area(s). The long-term adverse effects of topical pimecrolimus in veterinary patients are currently unknown. Close monitoring is recommended for patients using this medication on a continuous maintenance basis. When long-term treatment is required, the ultimate goal should be to achieve the lowest possible dose that controls clinical signs. Pimecrolimus should not be used in patients that are receiving systemic immunosuppressant therapy or are otherwise immunocompromised.

Wear gloves or use an applicator (eg, cotton swab) when applying the cream and wash hands after handling. Do not allow animals to lick or chew at the treated area(s) for at least 20 to 30 minutes after application to avoid ingestion and allow the medication to work.

Although topical pimecrolimus appears well tolerated in dogs, localized irritation and pruritus have been reported in both humans and dogs. Pimecrolimus has been anecdotally reported to be less irritating than tacrolimus in dogs; however, it may also be less effective. Pimecrolimus may be cost prohibitive.

Veterinary-Labeled Products

None

Human-Labeled Products

Active ingredients (formulation)	Label status; size(s)	Trade names/additional information
Pimecrolimus 1% (cream)	Rx; 30 g, 60 g, and 100 g	*Elidel®*; generic

Tacrolimus, Topical

(ta-***kroe***-li-mus)

Indications/Actions

Tacrolimus ointment may be beneficial in veterinary patients as a sole or adjunctive treatment of atopic dermatitis, discoid lupus erythematosus, pemphigus erythematosus or foliaceous, pinnal vascular disease, alopecia areata, vitiligo, dermal arteritis of the nasal philtrum, perianal fistulas (adjunctive or maintenance treatment after cyclosporin therapy), sterile canine panniculitis, and feline proliferative and necrotizing otitis externa. Unlike topical corticosteroids, tacrolimus does not have atrophogenic or metabolic effects associated with long-term use or large treatment areas.

Tacrolimus is a calcineurin inhibitor that inhibits T-lymphocyte activation. It also inhibits the release of inflammatory cytokines and mediators from mast cells and basophils.

Suggested Dosages/Uses

There is limited experience with topical tacrolimus in veterinary patients. Twice-daily application is typically recommended until signs are controlled. Application can then be reduced to the minimum frequency needed to control clinical signs.

Precautions/Adverse Effects

Although a causal relationship has not been established, skin malignancy and lymphoma have rarely been reported in humans using topical tacrolimus. Therefore, long-term use is not recommended in humans, and tacrolimus application should be limited to only the affected area(s). The long-term adverse effects of topical tacrolimus in veterinary patients are currently unknown, and thus close monitoring is recommended for patients using this medication on a continuous maintenance basis. When long-term treatment is required, the ultimate goal should be to achieve the lowest possible dose that controls clinical signs. Tacrolimus should not be used in patients that are receiving systemic immunosuppressant therapy or are otherwise immunocompromised. Do not use this ointment on premalignant or malignant skin conditions.

Wear gloves or use an applicator (eg, cotton swab) when applying the ointment and wash hands after handling. Do not allow animals to lick or chew at the treated area(s) for at least 20 to 30 minutes after application to avoid ingestion and allow the medication to work.

The commercially available ointment should not be used as (or compounded into) an ophthalmic preparation for treating KCS in dogs, as it contains propylene carbonate, a known ocular toxin.

Although topical tacrolimus appears well tolerated in dogs, localized irritation and pruritus have been reported in both humans and dogs. Pimecrolimus has been anecdotally reported as less irritating than tacrolimus in dogs; however, it may also be less effective. The cost of topical tacrolimus may be prohibitive.

The National Institute for Occupational Safety and Health (NIOSH) classifies tacrolimus as a hazardous drug; personal protective equipment (PPE) should be used accordingly to minimize the risk for exposure.

Veterinary-Labeled Products

None

Human-Labeled Products

Active ingredients (formulation)	Label status; size(s)	Trade names/additional information
Tacrolimus 0.03% (ointment)	Rx; 30 g, 60 g, and 100 g	*Protopic®*; generic
Tacrolimus 0.1% (ointment)	Rx; 30 g, 60 g, and 100 g	*Protopic®*; generic

Keratolytic Agents, Topical

See also:
Benzoyl Peroxide, Topical (Antimicrobial Agents, Topical; Antibacterial Agents)
Phytosphingosine, Topical (Antipruritic/Anti-Inflammatory Agents, Topical; Non-Corticosteroid Agents)
Selenium Sulfide, Topical (Antimicrobial Agents, Topical; Antifungal Agents)

Coal Tar/Coal Tar Combinations, Topical

(kole tar)

Indications/Actions

The use of coal tar containing shampoos in veterinary medicine is somewhat controversial, particularly since almost all veterinary-labeled products have been withdrawn from the market. However, coal tar shampoos have been used for many years to treat greasy dermatoses (seborrhea oleosa) in dogs.

Coal tar possesses keratoplastic, keratolytic, vasoconstrictive, antipruritic, and degreasing actions. Coal tar's mechanism of keratoplastic (keratoregulating) action is probably secondary to decreasing mitosis and DNA synthesis of basal epidermal cells.[1]

Suggested Dosages/Uses

The frequency of shampooing will vary according to the patient's needs. When using a medicated shampoo, allow 10 minutes of contact time. Another acceptable regimen is to allow the shampoo to act for 3 to 5 minutes, rinse it thoroughly, then repeat the procedure. Refer to specific product labels for directions, as contact time recommendations may vary. Completely rinse to prevent skin irritation and/or excessive drying.

Precautions/Adverse Effects

The carcinogenic risks associated with coal tar products are debated. At present, most (including the FDA) believe that coal tar products with concentrations of 5% or less are safe for human use. However, should they be used on animals, clients should wear gloves when applying and wash off any product that contacts their skin. Carcinogenic risk assessment for dogs using coal tar products was not located. **Coal tar products should not be used on cats**, patients that have prior sensitivity reactions to tar products, or patients that have dry scaling dermatoses.

Be careful comparing coal tar concentrations on labels. Coal tar solution contains ≈20% coal tar extract or refined tar. For example, a 10% coal tar solution contains ≈2% coal tar (refined).

Photosensitization, skin drying, and skin irritation are possible with coal tar therapy. Adverse effects are more likely with coal tar concentrations greater than 3%. Residual odor is often bothersome to clients. Tar may stain fabrics or haircoats and discolor jewelry.

Veterinary-Labeled Products

Active ingredients (formulation)	Species	Label status; size(s)	Trade names/additional information
Coal tar solution 3%, chloroxylenol 0.6%, salicylic acid 2%, sulfur 2% (shampoo)	Labeled for dogs **Do NOT use on cats.**	OTC; 8 oz	*Imrex®*

Active ingredients (formulation)	Species	Label status; size(s)	Trade names/additional information
Coal tar solution 2%, sulfur 2% (shampoo) Other ingredients: allantoin, aloe vera extract, citric acid, sodium laureth sulfate	Labeled for dogs **Do NOT use on cats.**	OTC; 4 oz, 8 oz, and 12 oz	*Sulfodene®*
Coal tar solution 5% (equivalent to 1% refined coal tar) (shampoo)	Labeled for dogs **Do NOT use on cats.**	OTC; 12 oz, 1 gallon	*Nova Pearls®* Slow-release power moisturizers encapsulated in *Novasome®* microcarriers
Coal tar solution 2%, menthol 1%, salicylic acid 3% (shampoo)	Labeled for dogs **Do NOT use on cats.**	OTC; 16 oz, 1 gallon	*Pharmasal-T®*
Coal tar solution 1%, salicylic acid 0.22%, sulfur 2% (shampoo) Other ingredients: aloe vera, menthol, zinc oxide	Labeled for dogs **Do NOT use on cats.**	OTC; 12 oz, 1 gallon	

Human-Labeled Products

Several products labeled for human use and containing coal tar—including ointments, lotions, and creams—are available in concentrations ranging from 0.5% to 5% coal tar (not coal tar extract).

Active ingredients (formulation)	Label status; size(s)	Trade names/additional information
Coal tar 0.5% (shampoo)	OTC; 120 mL, 177 mL, 240 mL, 355 mL, and 480 mL	*DHS Tar®; Polytar®; Tera-Gel®*
Coal tar 1% (shampoo)	OTC; 180 mL, 473 mL	*Ionil T®; PC-Tar®; Zetar®*
Coal tar 2% (shampoo)	OTC; 132 mL, 255 mL, and 480 mL	*Neutrogena® T/Gel Original®*
Coal tar 3% (shampoo)	OTC; 120 mL, 240 mL	*MG 217 Medicated Tar®*

References

For the complete list of references, see **wiley.com/go/budde/plumb**

Salicylic Acid, Topical

(sal-i-***sil***-ic ***ass***-id)

Indications/Actions

Salicylic acid is used to treat seborrheic disorders with mild to moderate scaling and mild waxy or keratinous debris, including seborrhea sicca and oleosa. Salicylic acid is often combined with sulfur or benzoyl peroxide. In higher concentrations, salicylic acid can be used to remove localized excessive tissues associated with hyperkeratotic disorders, such as calluses and idiopathic thickening of the planum nasale and footpads. Salicylic acid is also used in some wound cleansers.

Salicylic acid has mild antipruritic, antibacterial (bacteriostatic), keratoplastic, and keratolytic actions. Lower concentrations are primarily keratoplastic, and higher concentrations are keratolytic. Salicylic acid lowers skin pH, increases corneocyte hydration, and dissolves the intercellular binder between corneocytes. Salicylic acid and sulfur are thought to be synergistic in their keratolytic actions.

Suggested Dosages/Uses

Salicylic acid shampoos are typically labeled for use 2 to 3 times weekly; however, the frequency will vary according to the patient's needs. Allow medicated shampoos to remain in contact with the skin for 5 to 10 minutes before rinsing well. Alternatively, allow for 3 to 5 minutes of contact time, rinse thoroughly, then repeat the procedure. Ensure shampoo is rinsed completely to prevent skin irritation and excessive drying. Refer to specific product labels for complete directions.

Precautions/Adverse Effects

Salicylic acid products that are combined with coal tar must not be used on cats.

Avoid contact with eyes and mucous membranes. Do not allow animals to lick during bathing in order to avoid ingestion. Avoid using on broken skin unless product is specifically labeled for wounds. Wash hands after application, as skin irritation is possible. Salicylic acid products may bleach colored fabrics.

Possible adverse effects include burning, itching, pain, erythema, and swelling at the application site, particularly when used in concentrations greater than 2%. A rebound seborrheic effect can occur.

Veterinary-Labeled Products

Active ingredients (formulation)	Species	Label status; size(s)	Trade names/additional information
Salicylic acid 6.6% (gel)	Labeled for dogs, cats, and horses	OTC; 1 oz	*Solva-Ker®*
Salicylic acid 1.6%, benzocaine 1.5% (ointment)	Labeled for dogs	OTC; 2 oz	*Sulfodene® 3-Way Ointment*

Active ingredients (formulation)	Species	Label status; size(s)	Trade names/additional information
Salicylic acid, benzoic acid, malic acid (cream)	Labeled for dogs and cats	OTC; 1 oz, 14 oz	*Derma-Clens®*
Salicylic acid 2% (shampoo)	Labeled for dogs and cats; some products also labeled for horses	OTC; 8 oz, 16 oz	*BioSeb®; CeraSoothe® SA; KeraSeb®, Ceraven SA®*
Salicylic acid 1%, benzoyl peroxide 2.5% (shampoo)	Labeled for dogs, cats, and horses	OTC; 12 oz, 1 gallon	*DermaBenSs®*
Salicylic acid 2%, benzoyl peroxide 3% (shampoo)	Labeled for dogs, cats, and horses	OTC; 12 oz, 1 gallon	*EZ-Derm®*
Salicylic acid 2%, chloroxylenol 2%, sodium thiosulfate 2% (shampoo)	Labeled for dogs, cats, and horses	OTC; 16 oz, 1 gallon	*Universal Medicated Shampoo*
Salicylic acid 2%, sulfur 2% (shampoo)	Labeled for dogs and cats	OTC; 4 oz, 8 oz, 16 oz	*Exfolux®*
Salicylic acid 2%, selenium sulfide 1%, sulfur 2% (shampoo)	Labeled for dogs, cats, and horses	OTC; 16 oz	*Siccaderm®*
Salicylic acid 2%, benzoyl peroxide 3%, sulfur 2% (shampoo)	Labeled for dogs and cats	OTC; 12 oz	*Pet MD®*
Salicylic acid 0.22%, sulfur 2%, coal tar solution 1%, zinc oxide 0.22% (shampoo)	Labeled for dogs **Do NOT use on cats.**	OTC; 12 oz, 1 gallon	*Sulfur & Tar®*
Salicylic acid 1%, benzoyl peroxide 2.5% (shampoo)	Labeled for dogs and cats	OTC; 12 oz	*Peroxiderm®*
Salicylic acid 1% (mousse)	Labeled for dogs and cats	OTC; 6.8 oz	*CeraSoothe® SA*
Salicylic acid 2% (mousse)	Labeled for dogs, cats, and horses	OTC; 6.8 oz	*BioSeb®*

Human-Labeled Products

NOTE: In addition to the prescription products listed, there are a wide variety of human-labeled topical salicylic acid products in a range of concentrations available OTC, including creams, ointments, transdermal patches, liquids, and gels. These products are typically labeled for wart removal or treatment of acne. There are also a wide variety of OTC skin cleansers and shampoos containing salicylic acid, often in combination with sulfur, coal tar, or menthol. For more information on these products, refer to a comprehensive human drug reference or contact a pharmacist.

Active Ingredients (formulation)	Label status; size(s)	Trade names/additional information
Salicylic acid 3% (ointment)	Rx; 30 g	*Bensal HP®; Keralyt®*; generic
Salicylic acid 6% (cream)	Rx; 16 oz	*Salex®*
Salicylic acid 6% (lotion)	Rx; 8 oz	*Salex®*
Salicylic acid 6% (foam)	Rx; 7.1 oz	*Salvax®*
Salicylic acid 6% (gel)	Rx; 40 g, 100 g	*Keralyt®*; generic

Sulfur, Precipitated, Topical

(***sul***-fer)

Indications/Actions

Sulfur-containing shampoos are often used to treat patients with seborrheic disorders exhibiting mild to moderate scaling, with mild waxiness and keratinous debris. Sulfur is often found in combination with salicylic acid.

Sulfur has keratoplastic and keratolytic actions. Lower concentrations of sulfur are primarily keratoplastic secondary to assisting the conversion of cysteine to cystine, which is thought to be an important factor in the maturation of corneocytes. Like salicylic acid, the keratolytic effects of sulfur increase with concentration. Salicylic acid and sulfur are believed to be synergistic in their keratolytic actions. Sulfur also has mild degreasing effects and can be mildly antipruritic. Sulfur has antibacterial, antifungal, and antiparasitic effects secondary to sulfur conversion to hydrogen sulfide and pentathionic acid by bacteria and keratocytes.

Suggested Dosages/Uses

Sulfur shampoo label directions range from once daily to once weekly; the frequency of use will vary depending on the patient. Allow medicated shampoos to remain in contact with the skin for 5 to 10 minutes before rinsing well. Alternatively, allow for 3 to 5 minutes of contact time, rinse thoroughly, then repeat the procedure. Ensure shampoo is rinsed completely to prevent skin irritation and excessive drying. Refer to the specific product label for complete instructions.

Precautions/Adverse Effects

Avoid contact with eyes, mucous membranes, and open cuts or sores. Wear gloves when applying and wash hands after application. Residual odor can be bothersome, and sulfur may stain fabrics and hair.

Sulfur can be irritating or drying and can cause pruritus. A rebound seborrheic effect can occur with sulfur-containing products.

Veterinary-Labeled Products

Active ingredients (formulation)	Species	Label status; size(s)	Trade names/additional information
Sulfur 2% (shampoo)	Labeled for dogs **Do NOT use on cats.**	OTC; 12 oz	*Sulfodene*®
Sodium thiosulfate 2%, chloroxylenol 2%, salicylic acid 2% (shampoo)	Labeled for dogs, cats, and horses	OTC; 16 oz, 1 gallon	*Universal Medicated Shampoo*® Sodium thiosulfate serves as source of soluble sulfur.
Sulfur 2%, salicylic acid 2%, selenium sulfide 1% (shampoo)	Labeled for dogs, cats, and horses	OTC; 16 oz	*Siccaderm*®
Sulfur 1%, benzoyl peroxide 2.5%, salicylic acid 1% (shampoo)	Labeled for dogs and cats	OTC; 12 oz, 1 gallon	*Sulfur Benz*®
Sulfur 2%, coal tar solution 1%, salicylic acid 0.22%, zinc oxide 0.22% (shampoo)	Labeled for dogs **Do NOT use on cats.**	OTC; 12 oz, 1 gallon	*Sulfur & Tar*®
Sulfur 2%, salicylic acid 2% (shampoo)	Labeled for dogs and cats	OTC; 4 oz, 8 oz, 16 oz	*Exfolux*®

Human-Labeled Products

NOTE: There are several topical products containing sulfur labeled for human use, including creams, lotions, shampoos, and soaps that are typically labeled for acne or dandruff. For more information on these products, refer to a comprehensive human drug reference or contact a pharmacist.

Retinoid Agents, Topical

Tretinoin, Topical

All-Trans Retinoic Acid; Vitamin A Acid

(***tret***-in-oyn)

Indications/Actions

Topical tretinoin has been used anecdotally for treating localized follicular or hyperkeratotic disorders, such as idiopathic nasal and footpad hyperkeratosis, Schnauzer comedo syndrome, callous pyodermas, and chin acne.

The exact mechanism of action of tretinoin is not well understood, but it stimulates cellular mitotic activity, increases cell turnover, and decreases the cohesiveness of follicular epithelial cells. Similar to other retinoids, tretinoin is derived from vitamin A. It **may have anti-inflammatory and immunomodulatory effects by stimulating cytotoxic T-cells and natural killer cells, inhibiting polymorphonuclear cells and suppressing lymphocyte proliferation. Retinoids also have antineoplastic effects by maintaining epithelial cell differentiation and inhibiting tumor cell proliferation.**

Suggested Dosages/Uses

In small animal species, topical tretinoin is often used initially at a concentration of 0.05% and is applied once daily. Treatment is continued until clinical signs are controlled or until treatment is no longer tolerated. Once clinical signs are controlled, tretinoin frequency is then reduced to only as needed. In animals that are unable to tolerate therapy, a lower concentration of 0.025% to 0.01% may be tried to minimize adverse effects.

Precautions/Adverse Effects

Avoid excessive sun exposure during treatment with tretinoin. Avoid contact with eyes, nostrils, inner ears, and mouth. Wear gloves when applying and wash hands after handling. **Do not use this product in pregnant or nursing animals. Do not let animals lick or chew at the treated area(s) for at least 20 to 30 minutes after application. Some gel products contain soluble fish proteins and should be used with caution in patients with fish allergies.**

Adverse effects can include hypersensitivity reactions and local irritation (eg, erythema, dryness, peeling, pruritus).

The National Institute for Occupational Safety and Health (NIOSH) classifies tretinoin as a hazardous drug; personal protective equipment (PPE) should be used accordingly to minimize the risk for exposure.

Veterinary-Labeled Products

None

Human-Labeled Products

Active ingredients (formulation)	Label status; size(s)	Trade names/additional information
Tretinoin 0.02% (cream)	Rx; 20 g, 40 g, 44 g, 60 g	*Renova*®
Tretinoin 0.025% (cream)	Rx; 20 g, 45 g	*Avita*®; *Retin-A*®; generic
Tretinoin 0.05% (cream)	Rx; 20 g, 40 g	*Refissa*®; *Retin-A*®; generic
Tretinoin 0.1% (cream)	Rx; 20 g	*Retin-A*®; generic
Tretinoin 0.01% (gel)	Rx; 15 g, 45 g	*Retin-A*®; generic
Tretinoin 0.025% (gel)	Rx; 15 g, 20 g, 45 g	*Avita*®; *Retin-A*®; generic
Tretinoin 0.05% (gel)	Rx; 45 g	*Atralin*®; generic
Tretinoin 0.04% (gel microspheres)	Rx; 20 g, 45 g, 50 g	*Retin-A Micro*®; generic
Tretinoin 0.06% (gel microspheres)	Rx; 50 g	*Retin-A Micro*®
Tretinoin 0.08% (gel microspheres)	Rx; 50 g	*Retin-A Micro*®
Tretinoin 0.1% (gel microspheres)	Rx; 20 g, 45 g, 50 g	*Retin-A Micro*®; generic
Tretinoin 0.05% (lotion)	Rx; 20 g, 45 g, 50 g	*Altreno*®

Otic Agents, Topical

Although this is not a complete list, the following examples are representative of the types of topical otic preparations that are available to veterinarians. Included are both veterinary-labeled and human-labeled products that may be of use in veterinary medicine. Portions of this section are adapted from Koch SN, Torres SMF, Plumb, DC. *Canine and Feline Dermatology Drug Handbook.* John Wiley & Sons, 2012. This reference provides additional detail on these and other compounds and products.

Antibacterial Agents, Otic

See also ***Corticosteroid/Antimicrobial Agents, Otic***

Indications/Actions

Antibacterial ear preparations are commonly used to treat infections caused by various bacteria, such as *Staphylococcus* spp or *Pseudomonas* spp. Ear cytology should be performed to confirm a bacterial infection prior to prescription of topical antibiotics, mainly to prevent antibiotic overuse and bacterial resistance. In long-term cases and when rods are seen on cytology, culture and susceptibility may be recommended to identify multidrug-resistant organisms, such as *Pseudomonas* spp. Very few otic products that contain solely an antibiotic are commercially available to treat bacterial otitis; therefore, ophthalmic products, compounded products, or injectable products applied topically into the ear canals are sometimes used to treat these infections, mainly when steroids and antifungals are not needed. Listed below are the commercial products containing an antibiotic agent exclusively.

Suggested Dosages/Uses

These products should be used 2 to 3 times daily in adequate amounts to coat the entire ear canal. When using acidifying ear cleansers with an aminoglycoside- or fluoroquinolone-containing agent, it is recommended to use these products about 1 hour apart since low pH can decrease the activity of aminoglycosides and fluoroquinolones. Advise the client to discontinue the medication and contact the veterinarian if the animal's ears become redder or more inflamed at any time during treatment.

Patients should be rechecked before discontinuing treatment, and treatment must be continued until 1 week after negative cytology is obtained.

Precautions/Adverse Effects

There is little information available regarding ototoxicity from topical antibiotics use in dogs and cats; therefore, caution should be used when prescribing various topical otic medications in patients with ruptured tympanic membranes due to potential ototoxicity. Ototoxicity has been reported with aminoglycosides in dogs and cats, and cats may be more sensitive to their potential ototoxicity; however, this concern may be overstated. One study showed no vestibulotoxic or ototoxic effects from 21 days of otic gentamicin applied every 12 hours to ears with ruptured tympanic membranes. Another study showed that instillation of aqueous solutions of tris-EDTA combined with marbofloxacin or gentamicin into the middle ear of dogs with otitis media either did not change or improved the brainstem auditory-evoked responses (BAER); however, tobramycin solution impaired the BAER. Based on this study, the concern for ototoxicity is higher with tobramycin compared with marbofloxacin and gentamicin.[1]

Veterinary- and Human-Labeled Products

Refer to each product's label for inactive ingredients and precautions or contraindications.

Active ingredients (formulation)	Species	Label status; size(s)	Trade names/additional information
Enrofloxacin 0.5%, silver sulfadiazine (SSD) 1%	Labeled for dogs	Rx; 15 mL, 30 mL	*Baytril®*
Gentamicin sulfate 0.3% (solution, ointment)	Labeled for dogs and cats	Rx; 5 mL (solution), 3.5 g (ointment)	*Gentocin®* Extra-label use in the ears. Many human ophthalmic products are also available.
Oxytetracycline hydrochloride 5 mg/g, polymixin B 10,000 units/g (ointment)	Labeled for dogs, cats, and horses	3.5 g tube	*Terramycin®* Extra-label use in the ears
Ciprofloxacin hydrochloride 0.3% (solution, ointment)	Human-labeled product	Rx; 5 mL, 10 mL (solution), 3.5 g (ointment)	*Ciloxan®*; generic Extra-label use in the ears
Ciprofloxacin hydrochloride 0.2% (solution)	Human-labeled product	Rx; 0.25 mL single use	*Cetraxal®*; generic
Ofloxacin 0.3% (solution)	Human-labeled product	Rx; 5 mL, 10 mL	*Floxin®*; generic
Tobramycin 0.3% (solution, ointment)	Human-labeled product	Rx; 5 mL	*Tobrex®*; generic Extra-label use in the ears

References

For the complete list of references, see **wiley.com/go/budde/plumb**

Antibiotic-Potentiating Agents, Otic

Tromethamine-ethylenediaminetetraacetic acid (tris-EDTA) has antimicrobial and antibiotic potentiating activity. Cell surfaces of gram-negative bacteria are damaged when exposed to EDTA. Tromethamine (tris) enhances the effects of EDTA, and the tris-EDTA combination is bacteriostatic.[1] Exposure to tris-EDTA results in increased permeability to extracellular solutes and leakage of intracellular solutes. Cell surfaces of gram-positive bacteria are more resistant to tris-EDTA than gram-negative bacteria.[2] Tris-EDTA has also shown synergistic effects with various antibiotics, such as aminoglycosides and fluoroquinolones in vitro.[1–4] Tris-EDTA also has antibiofilm activity through inhibition of bacterial adhesion.[5]

Tris-EDTA is non-ototoxic and safe to use in the middle ear. Tris-EDTA–containing products are most effective when applied 15 to 30 minutes before the topical antibiotic. Products containing tris-EDTA are available as a sole ingredient or combined with chlorhexidine or ketoconazole. When recommending ear flushing as part of the treatment regimen, it is important to demonstrate the cleaning technique in the examination room and advise the client to discontinue application and contact the veterinarian if the ears become redder or more inflamed at any time during the course of cleaning. The frequency of cleaning varies according to the needs of the individual patient. ***Refer to each product's label for inactive ingredients and precautions or contraindications.***

Active ingredients (formulation)	Species	Label status; size(s)	Trade names/additional information
Tris-EDTA (flush)	Labeled for dogs, cats, and horses	4 oz, 16 oz	*TrizEDTA®*
Tris-EDTA (crystals flush)	Labeled for dogs and cats	4 oz, 16 oz	*TrizEDTA crystals®*
Tris-EDTA, chlorhexidine 0.15% (flush)	Labeled for dogs and cats	4 oz	*TrizCHLOR®*
Tris-EDTA, ketoconazole 0.15% (flush)	Labeled for dogs, cats, and horses	4 oz, 12 oz	*TrizULTRA + Keto®*
Tris-EDTA, chlorhexidine 0.15%, ketoconazole 0.15% (flush)	Labeled for dogs and cats	4 oz, 12 oz	*Mal-A-Ket Plus TrizEDTA®*

References

For the complete list of references, see **wiley.com/go/budde/plumb**

Antifungal Agents, Otic

See also ***Corticosteroid/Antimicrobial Agents, Otic***

Indications/Actions

Antifungal ear preparations are usually used to treat otitis caused by *Malassezia* spp and rarely other otic fungal diseases, such as aspergillosis and candidiasis. Most commercially available products also contain an antibiotic and/or a glucocorticoid. Therefore, ear cytology should be performed to confirm a fungal/yeast infection prior to prescription of topical antifungals, particularly if an antimicrobial and antibiotic combination is being considered.

Topical azole antifungals, such as miconazole and clotrimazole, have been shown to possess in vitro activity against *Staphylococcus* spp. Listed in the ***Veterinary-Labeled Products*** section are exclusively the products without antibiotic or glucocorticoid agents. These products are not labeled as otic medications but have commonly been used in veterinary patients.

Suggested Dosages/Uses

Most products are labeled to be used 1 to 2 times daily in adequate amounts to coat the patient's entire ear canal.

Precautions/Adverse Effects

Advise owners to discontinue the medication and contact their veterinarian if their animal's ears become redder or more inflamed at any time during treatment. There is little information available regarding ototoxicity from topical antifungal use in dogs and cats; therefore, caution should be used when prescribing various topical otic medications in animals with ruptured tympanic membranes. In one study in dogs, administration of clotrimazole (15 g tube [2% cream] mixed 50:50 with sterile water) did not change the BAER score, and vestibular signs were not reported.[1] No other safety studies in dogs or cats with otic antifungals are available. Patients should be rechecked before discontinuing treatment, and treatment should be continued until 1 week after negative cytology is obtained.

Refer to each product's label for inactive ingredients and precautions or contraindications. Some inactive ingredients, including alcohol or alcohol-based solvents such as propylene glycol, can be irritating and cause inflammation, particularly in sensitive, eroded, or ulcerated ears, and these ingredients should be avoided in ears with ruptured tympanum.

Veterinary-Labeled Products

Active ingredients (formulation)	Species	Label status; size(s)	Trade names/additional information
Clotrimazole 1% (solution)	Labeled for dogs and cats	Rx; 10 mL, 30 mL, and 60 mL	*ClotrimaTop®; Clotrimazole®*
Miconazole nitrate 1.15% (equivalent to 1% miconazole base by weight) (lotion)	Labeled for dogs and cats	Rx; 60 mL, 120 mL	*Conzol®; MicaVed®; Miconosol®*

References

For the complete list of references, see **wiley.com/go/budde/plumb**

Antiparasitic Agents, Otic

NOTE: This monograph includes only preparations labeled to be applied directly into the ear canals for the treatment of otoacariosis; however, parasiticides with systemic or more generalized effect are preferred because *Otodectes cynotis* mites are known to also live outside ear canals and can re-infest the ears. See also ***Afoxolaner; Fipronil/Fipronil Combinations, Topical; Fluralaner; Sarolaner; Selamectin***. Refer to specific product labels for complete instructions regarding use, inactive ingredients, precautions, and contraindications.

Active ingredients (formulation)	Species	Label status; size(s)	Trade names/additional information
Piperonyl butoxide 0.5%, pyrethrins 0.05%	Labeled for dogs and cats 12 weeks of age or older	OTC; 3 mL, 9 mL, 0.5 oz, 1 oz	*Adams®; Happy Jack Mitex®; Hartz UltraGuard®* Clean ears. Apply daily for 7 to 10 days. Repeat in 2 weeks if necessary
Piperonyl butoxide 0.6%, pyrethrins 0.06%	For use on dogs and cats 12 weeks of age or older	OTC; 1 oz, 3 oz, 4 oz	*No-Bite®; PetArmor; Sentry HC EARMITE free®; Sergeant's Vetscription MITEaway®* Clean ears. Apply twice daily until ticks/mites are eliminated
Piperonyl butoxide 1%, pyrethrins 0.15%	Labeled for dogs; some products labeled for cats and horses NOT for use on puppies or kittens under 12 weeks old OR for use on horses/foals intended for slaughter	OTC; 4 oz, 6 oz	*Ear-Rite®* (dogs); *Ear Mite®* (dogs, cats, horses) Clean ears. Apply daily for 7 to 10 days. Do not repeat treatment for 3 to 5 days if used as a repellent. Horses are treated daily for 2 to 3 days, then every 3 to 5 days as needed for controlling ectoparasites (eg, ticks, gnats).
Piperonyl butoxide 1.05%, pyrethrins 0.1%	For use on dogs 12 weeks of age or older	OTC; 0.75 oz	*Ear Mite Remedy* Clean ears. Apply once. If needed, repeat every other day until the infestation is resolved.

Active ingredients (formulation)	Species	Label status; size(s)	Trade names/additional information
Piperonyl butoxide 1.5%, pyrethrins 0.15%	Species depends on product No products available for use on dogs, cats, or rabbits under 12 weeks of age	OTC; 0.5 oz, 1 oz	*Ear-Rite*® (cats and kittens); *Eradimite*® (dogs and cats); *Otomite*® *Plus* (dogs, cats, puppies, kittens) Clean ear. Apply as a single dose. May repeat every 2 days until the condition has cleared up or repeat in 7 days depending on product directions. As a preventative treatment, apply every 15 days
Piperonyl butoxide 1%, pyrethrins 0.15% (lotion)	For use on dogs and cats at least 12 weeks old	OTC; 6 oz	*Performer*® Clean ears. Apply for 7 to 10 days
Piperonyl butoxide 1.5%, pyrethrins 0.15% (lotion)	For use on dogs and cats over 12 weeks of age	OTC; 12 mL, 22 mL	*Mita-Clear*® Clean ear; instill enough to wet ear canal and massage. Do not reapply for 7 days
Milbemycin oxime 0.1% (solution)	For use on cats or kittens 4 weeks of age or older	Rx; box of 10 pouches of 2 tubes of 0.25 mL each	*MilbeMite*® Clean ear. Apply entire contents of tube in the external ear canal; one tube per ear. Repeat in 30 days, if recommended by the veterinarian Safe use in cats used for breeding purposes, pregnant, or lactating has not been evaluated.
Ivermectin 0.01% (suspension)	For use in cats and kittens 4 weeks of age or older	Rx; box of 12 foil pouches of 2 ampules of 0.5mL each	*Acarexx*® Apply 0.5 mL in each ear. Repeat 1 time if necessary based on ear mite life cycle and response to treatment
Neomycin sulfate 0.25%, thiabendazole 4%, dexamethasone 0.1%	Labeled for otoacariasis and bacterial and fungal otitis in dogs and cats for a maximum of 1 week duration	OTC; 7.5 mL, 15 mL	*Tresaderm*® Clean ears. Apply twice daily until the infestation is resolved

Antiseptic Cleaning Agents, Otic

See also ***Cleaning/Drying Agents, Otic***

Indications/Actions

Topical antiseptic ear flushes include acetic acid, salicylic acid, boric acid, chlorhexidine, ketoconazole, miconazole, hypochlorous acid, and microsilver-containing products. These products are typically used as adjunctive therapy for ear infections (eg, bacterial and/or yeast) but can also be used as sole treatment in mild, first-time infections and for maintenance in some cases. Acetic and boric acids work as an acidifying, drying, and antimicrobial agent. Chlorhexidine has activity against gram-positive and gram-negative bacteria and fungi. Chloroxylenol is mostly active against bacteria. Ketoconazole and miconazole are fungistatic antifungals, although miconazole has been shown to be fungicidal against *Candida* spp. Hypochlorous acid is a broad-spectrum antimicrobial with rapid activity against gram-positive and gram-negative bacteria and fungal/yeast organisms. Its mode of action against micro-organisms mimics that of neutrophils in the body. The main route of attack against microorganisms is disruption of the cellular membrane. Microsilver has both antibiofilm and antibacterial properties, generating silver ions that kill gram-positive and gram-negative bacteria, such as *Pseudomonas aeruginosa*, *Staphylococcus* spp, *Streptococcus* spp, including multidrug-resistant organisms, in addition to *Malassezia* spp.

Suggested Dosages/Uses

When recommending ear flushing as part of the treatment regimen, it is important to demonstrate the cleaning technique in the examination room and advise the client to discontinue application and contact the veterinarian if the ears become redder or more inflamed at any time during the course of cleaning.

The frequency of cleaning varies according to the needs of the individual patient. Some of these products may also be used as antiseptics for the skin. Refer to each product label for inactive ingredients, details on use, and any precautions.

Precautions/Adverse Effects

There is little information regarding the ototoxicity of ear cleaners in dogs and cats. Agents that are believed to be safe in dogs and cats for ear flushing in the presence of ruptured tympanic membrane include sterile water, sterile saline, tris-EDTA, and possibly chlorhexidine at a concentration of less than 0.05%. More concentrated chlorhexidine-containing products should be used cautiously in ear canals with ruptured tympanic membranes because of the potential for ototoxicity, particularly in cats.

Alcohol-containing products should be avoided if the status of the tympanic membrane cannot be determined or if it is ruptured. Avoid products containing alcohol for eroded, ulcerative, and/or painful and sensitive ears as that alcohol can be irritant.

Veterinary-Labeled Products

Active ingredients (formulation)	Species	Label status; size(s)	Trade names/additional information
Acetic acid 2%, boric acid 2% (cleanser)	Labeled for dogs and cats	OTC; 4 oz, 8 oz, and 16 oz	*MalAcetic®* Other ingredients: water, glycerin, polysorbate 20, fragrance, sodium hydroxide
Acetic acid 2% (solution)	Labeled for dogs and cats	OTC; 4 oz, 16 oz	*OtoCetic®* Other ingredients: water, witch hazel, benzyl alcohol, polysorbate 80, DMDM hydantoin (as preservative), fragrance
Acetic acid 1%, ketoconazole 0.15%, hydrocortisone 1% (cleanser)	Labeled for dogs, cats, and horses	OTC; 2 oz, 8 oz	*MalAcetic® Ultra* Other ingredients: ceramide complex
Acetic acid 1%, boric acid 2%, hydrocortisone 1%, ketoconazole 0.15% (flush)	Labeled for dogs and cats	OTC; 8 oz	*Oticetic®* Other ingredients: propylene glycol, ceramides, glycerin, polysorbate, triethanolamine, fragrance
Chlorhexidine 0.15%, ketoconazole 0.15%, tris-EDTA (flush)	Labeled for dogs and cats	OTC; 4 oz, 12 oz	*Mal-A-Ket Plus TrizEDTA®* Other ingredients: decolorized aloe vera, glycerine, glycolic acid, methylisothiazolinone, nonoxynol-9, tris-EDTA, water
Chloroxylenol 0.2%, ketoconazole 0.2% (flush)	Labeled for dogs, cats, and horses	OTC; 4 oz, 8oz	*Pharmaseb®*
Chloroxylenol 0.33%, ketoconazole 0.33% (flush)	Labeled for dogs, cats, and horses	OTC; 8 oz	*Ketomax®* Other ingredients: benzyl alcohol, fragrance, propylene glycol, purified water, sodium borate decahydrate
Hypochlorous acid (HOCl) 0.009% (rinse)	Safe for use on all animals	OTC; 3 oz	*Vetericyn Plus® Antimicrobial Ear Rinse* Other ingredients: electrolyzed water (H_2O), sodium chloride (NaCl), sodium hypochlorite (NaOCl)
Ketoconazole 0.1% (flush)	Labeled for dogs and cats	OTC; 12 oz	*Curaseb®* Other ingredients: purified water, SDA-40, nonoxynol-9, benzyl alcohol, disodium EDTA, tromethamine technical grade, fragrance
Ketoconazole 0.1%, phytosphingosine HCl 0.01% (flush)	Labeled for dogs and cats	OTC; 4 oz, 16 oz	*VetraSeb® TRIS* Other ingredients: water, SDA 40B 190 proof, nonoxynol-9, tromethamine, disodium EDTA, methylisothiazolinone
Miconazole 0.1% (flush)	Labeled for dogs and cats	OTC; 4 oz, 16 oz	*BioTris®* Other ingredients: disodium EDTA, methylchloroisothiazolinone, methylisothiazolinone, N-octadecanoylphytosphingosine (ceramide Ill), PEG-40 hydrogenated castor oil, propylene glycol, purified water, tromethamine (Tris USP)
Microsilver 0.5%. climbazole 0.5% (concentrate)	Labeled for dogs and cats	OTC; 6 mL	*UltraOtic® Concentrate* Other ingredients: avicel RC-591, benzyl alcohol, glycerin, N-octadecanoylphytosphingosine (ceramide Ill), phenoxyethanol, polysorbate 80, purified water, sodium benzoate, titanium dioxide, triton x100/OP10, xanthan gum

Active ingredients (formulation)	Species	Label status; size(s)	Trade names/additional information
Microsilver 0.2%, lactic acid 1% (rinse)	Labeled for dogs and cats	OTC; 4 oz	*UltraOtic®* Antiseptic/antibiofilm activity. May be used prior to *UltraOtic® Concentrate* for additional benefit Other ingredients: carboxymethyl cellulose, fragrance, glycerin, magnesium aluminum silicate, methylchloroisothiazolinone, methylisothiazolinone, octoxynol-10, purified water
Salicylic acid 0.15%, ketoconazole 0.1% (ear rinse)	Labeled for dogs and cats	OTC; 4 oz	*PetArmor® Medicated Ear Rinse* Other ingredients: glycerin, potassium sorbate, propyelene glycol, purified water, sodium benzoate

Cerumenolytic Agents, Otic

Indications/Actions

Cerumenolytic agents soften hardened cerumen and make it easier to remove. Cerumenolytic agents can be classified as water-based agents, oil-based agents, or agents that are neither water nor oil based. Docusate sodium (DSS) and triethanolamine polypeptide oleate are water-based agents that act as surfactants to emulsify and disperse cerumen. Oil-based agents, such as propylene glycol, squalane, and various oils, soften and loosen cerumen without disintegrating it.[1] Squalane is the most potent of these agents. Some agents are neither water nor oil based, such as carbamide peroxide (urea-hydrogen peroxide) and glycerin. Carbamide peroxide is a foaming agent that releases oxygen to help break up debris. Glycerin acts by softening and loosening cerumen, similar to oil-based agents.

Docusate sodium, calcium sulfosuccinate (docusate calcium), and carbamide peroxide are considered potent cerumenolytic agents. Squalane and triethanolamine polypeptide oleate are less potent agents. Propylene glycol, glycerin, and oils are considered very mild cerumenolytic agents.

Evidence in humans suggests that no cerumenolytic agent is superior to any other, but any type of cerumenolytic agent tends to be superior to no treatment.[2]

Suggested Dosages/Use

These agents work best when they are applied 10 to 15 minutes prior to cleaning an area with an astringent or drying cleaner. Demonstrate proper cleaning technique in the examination room if cerumenolytic products will be administered at home by an owner. Advise owners to discontinue product application and contact their veterinarian if their animals' ears become redder or more inflamed at any time during the course of cleaning.

Precautions/Adverse Effects

Cerumenolytic agents should not be used with ruptured tympanic membranes (especially in cats) because of the potential for ototoxicity, with the exception of squalane.[3] If cerumenolytic agents are needed during in-hospital ear-flushing procedures, use of these products should be followed by multiple flushes with warm sterile isotonic saline. Alcohol-containing products should be avoided if the status of the tympanic membrane cannot be determined, or if the tympanic membrane is ruptured. Avoid products containing alcohol for eroded, ulcerative, and/or painful and sensitive ears, as the alcohol can be an irritant. The frequency of cleaning varies according to the needs of the individual animal. Some of these products may also be used as antiseptics for the skin. Refer to each product label for details on use and any precautions.

Veterinary-Labeled Products

Active ingredients (formulation)	Species	Label status; size(s)	Trade names/additional information
Squalane 25% in isopropyl myristate and light mineral oil	Labeled for dogs and cats	OTC; 4 oz	*Cerumene®*
Phytosphingosine 0.2% in alcohol, water, and propylene glycol	Labeled for dogs and cats	OTC; 4.2 oz, 8.4 oz	*Douxo® Micellar*
Carbamide peroxide 6.5%, glycerin base	Labeled for dogs and cats	OTC; 4 oz	*Earoxide®*
Propylene glycol, salicylic acid, glycerin	Labeled for dogs and cats	OTC; 8 oz, 12 oz	*EpiKlean®*
Squalane 22%, isopropyl myristate, white mineral oil	Labeled for dogs and cats	OTC; 4 oz	*KlearOtic®*
Methylchloroisothiazolinone, methylisothiazolinone, micellar solution (cetrimonium bromide, disodium EDTA, PEG-6 caprylic/capric glycerides, polysorbate 80, water), N-octadecanoyl-phytosphingosine (ceramide III)	Labeled for dogs and cats	OTC; 8 oz	*Milytic®*

Active ingredients (formulation)	Species	Label status; size(s)	Trade names/additional information
Calendula, capryloyl glycine (*Lipacide*® C8G), glycerin, isopropyl alcohol, labrasol, lemon synthetic perfume, polysorbate 80, transcutol V, tromethamine, undecylenoyl glycine (*Lipacide*® UG), water	Labeled for dogs and cats	OTC; 4 oz	*pH•notix*®
Phytosphingosine hydrochloride 0.01%, salicylic acid 0.15%	Labeled for dogs and cats	OTC; 8 oz	*SkinGuard*® *Cleanse*
Denatured alcohol 10%, lactic acid 1.76%, propylene glycol, docusate sodium, salicylic acid	Labeled for dogs and cats	OTC; 4 oz, 8 oz, and 16 oz	*Vet Solutions*®

References

For the complete list of references, see **wiley.com/go/budde/plumb**

Cleaning/Drying Agents, Otic

Indications/Actions

Cleaning and drying agents are typically used after debris or exudate has been removed from the ear canals with a cerumenolytic agent; however, they may also be used as a sole ear cleanser. The primary ingredients are astringents, such as isopropyl alcohol or aluminum acetate, and acids, such as boric acid or salicylic acid. Some cleaning and drying agents may have antimicrobial effects, and some may also be used as antiseptics for the skin.

Suggested Dosages/Use

The frequency of cleaning varies according to the needs of the individual patient. Cleaning and drying ear solutions can be used on a maintenance regimen to help prevent ear infections and after bathing or swimming to keep the external ear canals dry. It is important to demonstrate the cleaning technique in the examination room.

Precautions/Adverse Effects

Advise the client to discontinue the application and contact the veterinarian if the ears become redder or more inflamed at any time during the course of cleaning.

There is little information regarding the ototoxicity of ear cleaners in dogs and cats. Agents that are believed to be safe in dogs and cats for ear flushing in the presence of ruptured tympanic membrane include sterile water, sterile saline, tris-EDTA, and possibly chlorhexidine at a concentration of less than 0.05%. Propylene glycol- and alcohol-containing products should be avoided if the status of the tympanic membrane cannot be determined or if it is ruptured. Avoid products containing alcohol for eroded, ulcerative, and/or painful and sensitive ears as that alcohol can be irritant.

Veterinary-Labeled Products

Refer to each product label for specific details on use, inactive ingredients, and any precautions.

There is an overwhelming number of these products marketed, and the following are representative; they do not appear to be FDA-approved products. Many products also contain cerumenolytic ingredients. See also ***Cerumenolytic Otic Agents***.

Active ingredients (formulation)	Species	Label status; size(s)	Trade names/additional information
Isopropyl alcohol, glycerin (lotion)	Labeled for dogs and cats	OTC; 4 oz, 6 oz, 8 oz, 12 oz, 32 oz, 1 gallon	*ADL*® *Ear Flushing Drying Lotion*
Dioctyl sodium sulfosuccinate, glycerin, lactic acid, salicylic acid, SD alcohol (solution)	Labeled for dogs and cats	OTC; 4 oz, 8 oz, 1 gallon	*Aloe vera otic cleanser (formerly AloeClens*®*); Aurocin*®*; Clean Ear*® *with Aloe Vera; Conquer*® *Hy-Otic*
Lactic acid 1.76%, salicylic acid 0.1%, SD alcohol 10% (solution)	Labeled for dogs and cats	OTC; 4 oz, 8 oz, 16 oz, and 1 gallon	*Ear Cleansing Solution*
Acetic acid, boric acid, ethanol (flush)	Labeled for dogs and cats	OTC; 12 oz, 1 gallon	*EarMed*® *Boracetic*®
Ethanol (solution)	Labeled for dogs and cats	OTC; 12 oz, 1 gallon	*EarMed*® *Cleansing Solution and Wash*
Ethanol (wipes)	Labeled for dogs and cats	OTC; 40 wipes 5 x 6, 50 wipes 5 x 8.5, and 160 wipes 6 x 7	*EarMed*®
Propylene glycol 3%, salicylic acid 0.05%, SD alcohol (cleanser)	Labeled for dogs and cats	OTC; 8 oz, 12 oz, 32 oz	*EpiKlean*®
Dioctyl sodium sulfosuccinate, chloroxylenol 0.1%, EDTA 0.5%, salicylic acid 0.2% (solution)	Labeled for dogs and cats	OTC; 4 oz, 8 oz	*Epi-Otic*® *Advanced*
Eucalyptus oil, malic acid, salicylic acid (solution)	Labeled for dogs and cats	OTC; 4 oz, 16 oz	*Eucalyptus Oil (formerly Euclens*®*)*

Active ingredients (formulation)	Species	Label status; size(s)	Trade names/additional information
Acetic acid 2%, boric acid 2% (cleanser)	Labeled for dogs and cats	OTC; 4 oz, 8 oz, and 16 oz	*MalAcetic®*
Acetic acid 1%, hydrocortisone 1%, ketoconazole 0.15% (cleanser)	Labeled for dogs, cats, and horses	OTC; 2 oz, 8 oz	*MalAcetic ULTRA®*
Boric acid, zinc gluconate (liquid)	Recommended for dogs, cats, and exotics	OTC; 2 oz, 4 oz	*Maxi/Guard® zn 4.5*
Isopropyl alcohol (solution)	Labeled for dogs and cats	OTC; 4 oz, 16 oz	*Nolvasan®*
Malic acid, salicylic acid (solution)	Labeled for dogs and cats	OTC; 4 oz	*Oti-Clens®*
Dioctyl sodium sulfosuccinate, lactic acid, propylene glycol, salicylic acid, SD alcohol (solution)	Labeled for dogs and cats	OTC; 8 oz	*Otiderm®*
Boric acid 2%, glycolic acid 2% (solution)	Labeled for dogs and cats	OTC; 16 oz	*Otiderm® Advanced*
Glycerin, dioctyl sodium sulfosuccinate, lactic acid, salicylic acid (solution)	Labeled for dogs and cats	OTC; 8 oz	*OtiRinse®*
Acetic acid, alcohol (cleanser)	Labeled for dogs and cats	OTC; 4 oz	*Sulfodene®*
Chloroxylenol, SD alcohol (gel)	Labeled for dogs	OTC; 4 oz	*Swimmer's Ear Astringent*
Glycerin, lactic acid 1%, microsilver 0.2% (rinse)	Labeled for dogs and cats	OTC; 4 oz	*UltraOtic®*
Hypochlorous acid (HOCI) 0.009% (rinse)	Safe for all animals	OTC; 3 oz	*Vetericyn Plus®*
Glycerin, lactic acid 2.7%, salicylic acid 0.15%, sodium dioctyl sulfosuccinate, SD alcohol (solution)	Labeled for dogs and cats	OTC; 8 oz, 16 oz	*VetOtic®*
Coco-glucoside, glucose oxidase, glycerin, lactoferrin, lactoperoxidase, lysozyme, zinc gluconate (cleanser)	Labeled for dogs and cats	OTC; 4 oz, 1 gallon	*Zymox®* Ear Cleanser

Corticosteroid Agents, Otic

See also ***Corticosteroid/Antimicrobial Agents, Otic***

Indications/Actions

Corticosteroid-containing ear medications are used in cases of acute or chronic otitis with the goal of reducing inflammation, edema, tissue hyperplasia, pain, and pruritus. In addition, they are helpful in decreasing secretions from sebaceous and apocrine glands, thereby reducing the buildup of debris in ear canals. Otic solutions that contain glucocorticoids without an antibiotic can be used as maintenance therapy, if needed, in cases of allergic otitis.

Suggested Dosages/Uses

The frequency of applications should be according to the patients' needs, usually 1 to 4 times daily.

Precautions/Adverse Effects

When using corticosteroid preparations as maintenance therapy, use the least potent glucocorticoid at the lowest possible frequency to balance efficacy and prevent undesirable adverse effects, including skin atrophy, alopecia, and adrenocortical suppression effects from systemic absorption. Some glucocorticoids, such as dexamethasone and fluocinolone, are believed to be safe for use in the middle ear; however, the combination of fluocinolone and dimethyl sulfoxide (DMSO; *Synotic®*) may not be safe for administration in the ear if the tympanic membrane is ruptured as DMSO may cause ototoxicity.[1]

Veterinary-Labeled Products

Refer to each product's label for inactive ingredients and precautions or contraindications. Some inactive ingredients, including alcohol or alcohol-based solvents such as propylene glycol, can be irritating and cause inflammation, particularly in sensitive, eroded, or ulcerated ears, and should be avoided in ears with ruptured tympanum.

Active ingredients (formulation)	Species	Label status; size(s)	Trade names/additional information
Fluocinolone 0.01%, DMSO 60% (solution)	Labeled for dogs	Rx; 8 mL, 60 mL	*Synotic®*

Active ingredients (formulation)	Species	Label status; size(s)	Trade names/additional information
Hydrocortisone 0.5% (solution)	Labeled for dogs and cats	OTC; 1.25 oz	*Zymox®*
Hydrocortisone 1% (solution)	Labeled for dogs and cats	OTC; 1.25 oz	*Zymox®*, *Zymox® Plus*
Hydrocortisone 1%, Burow's solution 2% (solution)	Labeled for dogs	OTC; 1 oz, 16 oz	*Cort/Astrin®*

Human-Labeled Products

Active ingredients (formulation)	Species	Label status; size(s)	Trade names/additional information
Fluocinolone acetonide 0.01% (oil)	Labeled for humans	Rx; 20 mL	*DermOtic®*; generic

References

For the complete list of references, see **wiley.com/go/budde/plumb**

Corticosteroid/Antimicrobial Agents, Otic

See also **Corticosteroid Agents, Otic**

Indications/Actions

Most otic antimicrobial preparations for veterinary use that are commercially available combine an antifungal, an antibiotic, and a glucocorticoid agent. These medications should be used when anti-inflammatory and/or anti-pruritic effects are needed in the presence of concurrent bacteria and yeast infections. Ear cytology should be performed to confirm an infection prior to prescription of ear medications containing antimicrobials, particularly antibiotics, to help prevent antibiotic overuse and bacterial resistance. In chronic cases or when rods are seen on cytology, culture and susceptibility may be recommended to identify multidrug-resistant organisms, such as *Pseudomonas* spp. If only bacteria or yeast are present, more targeted otic antimicrobials, with or without glucocorticoids, may be considered.

Suggested Dosages/Uses

Most of these products should be used 2 to 3 times daily in adequate amounts to coat the entire ear canal. Refer to each product's label for detailed usage instructions. Patients should be rechecked before discontinuing treatment, and treatment must be continued until 1 week after negative cytology is obtained.

Precautions/Adverse Effects

Advise the client to discontinue the medication and contact the veterinarian if the ears become redder or more inflamed at any time during treatment and to avoid contact with the animal's mouth and eyes.

Use with caution when prescribing various topical otic medications in patients with ruptured tympanic membranes due to potential ototoxicity. Cats may be more sensitive to irritation and ototoxicity from topical otic agents.[1] Use of aminoglycosides in the presence of a ruptured tympanic membrane is controversial. One study showed no vestibulotoxic or ototoxic effects from 21 days of otic gentamicin applied every 12 hours to ears with ruptured tympanic membranes. Another study measured brainstem auditory-evoked responses (BAER) and found that although tobramycin significantly impaired hearing, gentamicin did not[2]; however, ototoxicity from topical aminoglycoside administration has been shown in many chinchilla and guinea pig studies.[3–6] In dogs, administration of clotrimazole 2% cream mixed 50:50 with sterile water did not change the BAER score, and vestibular signs were not reported. Some glucocorticoids, such as dexamethasone and fluocinolone, are believed to be safe for use in the middle ear. One dog developed pemphigus vulgaris after 1 week of otic polymyxin B application.[7]

Veterinarians and owners must use caution when handling these medications to prevent potential accidental human exposure, especially direct skin and eye contact. *Claro®* and *Osurnia®* contain specific warnings regarding ocular injuries in humans, including corneal ulcers.[8,9] Eye protection is recommended during administration, and dogs should be restrained to minimize postapplication head shaking.

Veterinary- and Human-Labeled Products

Refer to each product's label for inactive ingredients and precautions or contraindications. Some inactive ingredients, including alcohol or alcohol-based solvents, such as propylene glycol, can be irritating and cause inflammation, particularly in sensitive, eroded, or ulcerated ears, and should be avoided in ears with ruptured tympanum.

Active ingredients (formulation)	Species	Label status; size(s)	Trade names/additional information
Florfenicol 16.6 mg/mL, terbinafine 14.8 mg/mL, mometasone furoate 2.2 mg/mL (solution)	Labeled for dogs	Rx; 1 mL single-dose dropperette	*Claro®* 1 tube per ear; 30-day duration of effect. Shake before use. To be administered in the clinic.
Gentamicin sulfate 0.3%, clotrimazole 1%, betamethasone valerate 0.1% (ointment)	Labeled for dogs	Rx; 7.5 g, 10 g, 15 g, 25 g, 30 g, and 215 g	*Gentizol®*, *MalOtic®*, *Otibiotic®*, *Otomax®*

Active ingredients (formulation)	Species	Label status; size(s)	Trade names/additional information
Gentamicin sulfate 1.5 mg/mL, miconazole nitrate 17.4 mg/mL, hydrocortisone aceponate 1.11 mg/mL, (suspension)	Labeled for dogs	Rx; 10 mL (10 doses)	*Easotic®* Oily suspension; shake well before use. Labeled for once-daily dosage for 5 days. Prime pump before first use.
Gentamicin sulfate 3 mg/mL, betamethasone valerate 1 mg/mL (solution)	Labeled for dogs and cats	Rx; 7.5 mL, 15 mL, and 240 mL	*GenOne®, GentaOtic®, GentaVed®, Vet Beta-Gen®*
Ketoconazole 0.15%, hydrocortisone 1% (thermally activated gel)	Labeled for dogs and cats	OTC; 2 oz	*KC-Oto Pack®*
Gentamicin 3 mg/g, clotrimazole 10 mg/g, mometasone 1 mg/g (suspension)	Labeled for dogs	Rx; 7.5 g, 15 g, 30 g, and 215 g	*LoZatom®, Malmetazone®, Maxi-Otic®, Mometamax®, Mometavet®, MotaZol®* Once-daily dosing. Shake well before use.
Neomycin sulfate 0.25%, thiostrepton 2500 units/mL, nystatin 100,000 units/mL, triamcinolone acetonide 0.1% (ointment)	Labeled for dogs and cats	Rx; 7.5 mL, 15 mL, 30 mL, and 240 mL	*Animax®, Dermalone®, Derma-Vet®, EnteDerm®, Quadritop®*
Florfenicol 10 mg/mL, terbinafine 10 mg/mL, betamethasone acetate 1 mg/mL (gel)	Labeled for dogs	Rx; single-dose 1 mL tube	*Osurnia®* 1 tube per ear; repeat in 7 days. To be administered in the clinic. Do not clean ear canal for 45 days after initial treatment.
Orbifloxacin 10 mg/g, posaconazole 1 mg/g, mometasone furoate 1 mg/g (suspension)	Labeled for dogs	Rx; 7.5 g, 15 g, and 30 g	*Posatex®* Once-daily dosing. Shake well before use.
Polymyxin B 0.5293 mg/mL, miconazole 23 mg/mL, prednisolone acetate 5 mg/mL (suspension)	Labeled for dogs	Rx; 15 mL, 30 mL	*Surolan®* Shake well before use.
Neomycin 3.2 mg/mL, thiabendazole 40 mg/mL, dexamethasone 1 mg/mL (solution)	Labeled for dogs and cats	Rx; 7.5 mL, 15 mL	*Tresaderm®*
Neomycin sulfate 0.5%, isoflupredone acetate 0.1%, tetracaine hydrochloride 0.5% (ointment)	Labeled for dogs, cats, and horses	Rx; 10 g	*Tritop®*

Human-Labeled Products

Active ingredients (formulation)	Species	Label status; size(s)	Trade names/additional information
Ciprofloxacin 0.3%, dexamethasone 0.1% (suspension)	Human-labeled product	Rx; 7.5 mL	*Ciprodex®* Shake before use.
Ciprofloxacin 0.2%, hydrocortisone 1% (suspension)	Human-labeled product	Rx; 10 mL	*Cipro® HC* Shake well before use.
Colistin 3 mg/mL, neomycin 3.3 mg/mL, thonzonium bromide 0.5 mg/mL, hydrocortisone 10 mg/mL (suspension)	Human-labeled product	Rx; 10 mL	*Coly-Mycin S®, Cortisporin-TC®* Shake well before use.
Neomycin 3.5 mg/mL, polymyxin B 10,000 units/mL, hydrocortisone 10 mg/mL (solution)	Human-labeled product	Rx; 7.5 mL and 10 mL	generic
Tobramycin 0.3%, dexamethasone 0.05% (suspension)	Human-labeled product	Rx; 2.5 mL and 5 mL	*TobraDex® ST* Extra-label use in the ear.
Tobramycin 0.3%, dexamethasone 0.1% (suspension)	Human-labeled product	Rx; 2.5 mL, 5 mL, and 10 mL	*TobraDex®* Extra-label use in the ear.

References

For the complete list of references, see **wiley.com/go/budde/plumb**

Appendix

Veterinarian's Guide to Writing Prescriptions

A growing number of pet owners opt to have prescriptions filled at community or online pharmacies to obtain medications for their animals. In accordance with this trend, at least 40 states require veterinarians to provide pet owners with written prescriptions upon request.[1] Additionally, these pharmacies may be needed to fill prescriptions for medications that are compounded or not stocked in the veterinarians' clinic. Legally, animal prescriptions are treated the same as human prescriptions and must meet the same requirements in order to be filled. The following best practices will assist veterinarians to write legally compliant prescriptions while also minimizing the risk for medication errors and reduce potential harm to animal patients.

Prescription Requirements

Prescriptions are legal documents, and the information required on prescriptions, veterinary or otherwise, varies by state. Check with your state's Pharmacy and Veterinary boards to ensure all legal requirements are met.

LEGAL PRESCRIPTION REQUIREMENTS

- Patient name and species
- Pet owner's name and address
- Date prescription was written
  - Do not postdate; however, it may be acceptable to write "Do not fill until ___" to prevent early filling.
- Drug Information
  - Drug name
  - Strength
  - Dosage form (eg, tablet, capsule, suspension)
  - Quantity
  - Instructions for use ("sig"): dose, route, and frequency of administration
- Number of refills. The use of "PRN" generally authorizes refills for 1 year from written date.
- DEA # for controlled substance prescriptions
- Prescriber's name, address, and phone number
- Prescriber signature
- Withdrawal time (if applicable)

HELPFUL ITEMS THAT MAY NOT BE LEGALLY REQUIRED

Think of the pharmacist as the last safety check before the medication reaches the patient. The more information provided on the prescription, the more the safety of patients and their owners can be assured.

- Client phone number
- Patient's breed
- Patient's current body weight
- Indication for use
- Duration of use
- Patient date of birth
- Usage (ie, companion versus food/fiber animal)

Controlled Substances

Controlled substances are drugs that have the potential for abuse or dependence and are classified into 5 schedules according to their medical use, as well as relative abuse potential and dependence liability. Controlled substances are regulated both by individual states as well as by the Federal government. In order to prescribe controlled substances, practitioners must be authorized in the jurisdiction where they are licensed to practice and also be registered with the Drug Enforcement Agency (DEA). As controlled substance requirements vary between states, consult your state's controlled substance act to ensure compliance.

- **All controlled substances prescriptions must include the prescriber's DEA registration number.**
- **Schedule II (C-II) prescriptions** (eg, hydrocodone combinations)
  - Must be a physical (written or printed) prescription with original, manual signature (cannot be called in or faxed). Note that electronic prescribing of C-II prescriptions is permitted by DEA, but current veterinary practice management systems often do not meet DEA requirements.
  - Refills are not permitted – a new prescription must be generated each time
  - States may specify a time limit (eg, 30 or 60 days) within which C-II prescriptions must be filled; unfilled prescriptions become void after this time limit has passed.
  - Quantity limits (eg, 30-day maximum supply) may be mandated by the state
- **Schedule III-IV (CIII-IV) prescriptions** (eg, benzodiazepines, phenobarbital, tramadol)
  - Fax and verbal (ie, telephone) transmission is allowed
  - For chronic medications, a new prescription is required every 6 months
  - Refills are permitted, up to a maximum of 5 refills in 6 months
  - Quantity limits (eg, 90-day maximum supply) may be mandated by the state

Best Practices for Prescription Writing

- Manually written prescriptions should be in blue or black ink.
- Write the quantity to be dispensed both numerically and alphabetically for clarity and to avoid potential diversion (eg, #30 [thirty] tablets).
- When a patient requires a specific brand or manufacturer of a product (eg, *Novolin® N*), write the prescription for the required product name or manufacturer, and notate on the prescription for the pharmacist to "dispense as written."
- Do not pre-sign blank prescriptions.
- Prescribers are not obligated to provide their DEA number for noncontrolled prescriptions and may instead provide a state-issued license number.
  - The National Provider Identifier (NPI) is used for human insurance billing purposes and as such is not intended to be held by veterinarians.

Medication Errors and Patient Safety

The human health care system has given considerable attention to reducing medical errors, including those involving medications. Although prescription abbreviations are used throughout many references and are generally well recognized, they increase the potential for errors to occur. The Institute for Safe Medication Practices (ISMP) and the Joint Commission on Accreditation of Healthcare Organizations (JCAHO) focus on medication safety and have identified certain abbreviations and dose expressions that should be avoided due to the documented increased risk for medication errors. When writing a prescription, writing out the directions in plain English and avoiding the use of error-prone abbreviations help to ensure patient safety.

Style to avoid	Example	Potential problem	Use instead
Naked decimals	.5 mg	Read as 5 mg (10x overdose)	0.5 mg
Trailing zeros	5.0 mg	Read as 50 mg (10x overdose)	5 mg
Examples of error-prone abbreviations (not a complete list)	SID*	Read as BID, QID, 5/day	Write out "daily" or "every 24 hours"
	QD, q.d., q1d	Read as QID	Write out "daily" or "every 24 hours"
	QOD, EOD	Read as QD or other frequency	Write out "every other day" or "every 48 hours"
	QID	Read as QD or other frequency	Write out "four times daily" or "every 6 hours"
	IU or u	Read as "IV" or 10; read as 0	Write out "units"
	ng	Read as mg	Write out "nanogram"
	Gr	Read as "gram" instead of "grain"	Write out "grain" or use metric system (eg, mg equivalent)
	AD, AS, AU	Read as "OD", "OS", or "OU"	Write out "right ear", "left ear", or "both ears"
	hs, qhs	Read as "half strength"	Write out "at bedtime"
	SQ, sq, or sub q	Read as "SL" or "5 every"	SUBQ or write out "subcutaneously"
Drug name shorthand	MgSO4	Read as morphine sulfate	Write out magnesium sulfate
	Bute	Read as butorphanol	Write out "phenylbutazone"

*SID is an abbreviation that is virtually unknown to health professionals outside of veterinary medicine, and most pharmacists do not recognize it. SID should be eliminated from usage and replaced with "daily" or "once daily." The additional time taken to write out "once daily" could prevent a potentially serious, avoidable error.

Commonly Used Abbreviations

Listed below are some commonly used abbreviations; however, the use of any abbreviation can increase the potential for errors to occur.

Abbreviation	Meaning
ac	before meals
amp	ampule
c̄ , c	with
cap	capsule
disp	dispense
g or gm	gram
gtt(s)	drop(s)
h, hr	hour
IA	intra-articular
ID	Intradermal
IM	intramuscular
IO	intraosseous
IP	intraperitoneal
IV	intravenous
kg	kilogram
lb	pound
m^2	meter squared
mg	milligram

Abbreviation	Meaning
mL	milliliter (ensure L is capitalized)
OD	right eye
OS	left eye
OU	both eyes
pc	after meals
PO	by mouth
prn	as needed
q	every
q4h	every 4 hours
qs; qs ad	quantity sufficient; quantity sufficient to make
Sig	directions to patient
SL	sublingual
stat	immediately
susp	suspension
tab	tablet
Tbsp, T	tablespoon (15 mL)
tsp, t	teaspoon (5 mL)
UD, ut dict	as directed

References

For the complete list of references, see **wiley.com/go/budde/plumb**

Pharmacist's Quick Guide to Veterinary Prescriptions: A Whole Different Animal

Dogs are not furry versions of people, and cats are not small dogs

Veterinarians may prescribe approved animal and human drugs in an extra-label (off-label) manner for therapeutic purposes to their patients as long as there is no threat to public health and certain other criteria are met, including a valid veterinarian–client–patient relationship (VCPR). Because often there are significant differences in the use of medications in animals versus humans, pharmacists must understand that information applicable to human patients may not be valid for veterinary patients. The following points are essential to consider.

Pharmacokinetics/Pharmacodynamics

The pharmacokinetics/pharmacodynamics can differ significantly for many drugs used in veterinary versus human patients. Some key species-specific examples follow.

DOGS

Dogs have nearly 30% more blood/kg than humans do, which can affect drug concentrations in the blood.

Dogs have a faster glomerular filtration rate, so renal elimination of drugs may be more rapid.

CATS

Cats are deficient or limited in several metabolic pathways, including hepatic glucuronidation, hydroxylation, and demethylation.

As compared to humans, animals—especially cats—may use different hepatic CYP isoenzymes to metabolize drugs.

For example, cats may not adequately convert prednisone to prednisolone.

OF NOTE

Doses and dose frequency can differ radically between humans and animals.

Thyroid supplementation: Levothyroxine doses for hypothyroid dogs can be 10 times (or more) the doses used in hypothyroid humans and may be given twice daily (q12h).

Seizure control: Doses for seizure medications can be much higher than those prescribed for human patients.

Antibiotics: Some antibiotic doses are very large (eg, ciprofloxacin dose for dogs) as compared to doses needed for human patients.

Different breeds of a species may have varying pharmacokinetics for a given drug.

Toxicities/Adverse Effects

Compounds that are considered relatively nontoxic for human patients can cause serious toxicity or adverse effects in veterinary patients. Key examples follow.

DOGS

Over-the-counter (OTC) NSAIDs (eg, aspirin, ibuprofen, naproxen): Relatively low doses can cause serious GI bleeding and/or renal toxicity.

Xylitol (common sweetener, sugar alcohol) can cause life-threatening hypoglycemia and acute hepatic failure in dogs.

Phenobarbital can cause hepatotoxicity in dogs.

CATS

Acetaminophen in cats: As little as 10 mg/kg can cause fatal methemoglobinemia.[1]

Cats can develop serious renal toxicity from the use of NSAIDs.

Dry-pilling doxycycline in cats can cause esophageal erosions and strictures.

Permethrin-containing products are toxic to cats.

OF NOTE

Be wary of pet owners' requests to give food with their pet's oral medications (to increase patient acceptance) without seeking a veterinarian's guidance. Many common foods (eg, chocolate, grapes/raisins) can be toxic to animals.

Understanding the Prescription

Veterinarians use different terminology and abbreviations than physicians and often prescribe drugs differently than pharmacists are accustomed to seeing.

OF NOTE

Pet owners may be referred to as "clients." The pet is the patient.

Veterinarians are taught to use the abbreviation SID (derived from the Latin *semel in die*, meaning once a day) in dosing instructions. Do not confuse this abbreviation with other abbreviations.

Veterinarians will rarely prescribe oral liquids as per 5 mL. Example: Amoxicillin 250 mg/5 mL suspension may be prescribed as 50 mg/mL.

KEY INFORMATION

A few key reminders may help pharmacists avoid medication errors and ensure animal health in partnership with the veterinarian and animal's owner.

KEY REMINDERS

What applies to human patients may not be relevant or valid for veterinary patients.

Refer to a trusted veterinary drug reference or contact the prescribing veterinarian if there are any questions or concerns about a prescription as written.

Do not assume that take-home information intended for human patients, including patient information sheets, is appropriate for animal patients.

Some drugs are used exclusively in animal patients (eg, enrofloxacin).

Veterinary-only drugs may interact with human-labeled drugs being concurrently administered extra-label.

All insulin products require a prescription when used in animals.

OTC drugs labeled for humans (eg, diphenhydramine) require a veterinary prescription to be used in animals, as veterinary use of these drugs is extra-label.

KEY DO NOTS

Do not substitute drug products (especially insulins) or dose forms without first contacting the veterinarian. 10% of veterinarians responding to recent polls indicated that some patients had been harmed when outside pharmacies made unauthorized substitutions.[2]

Do not recommend use of human OTC products or supplements in animal patients without seeking guidance from the animal's veterinarian, as some OTC products may contain combinations of drugs that could be toxic to animals (eg, phenylephrine).

Do not ask veterinarians for their NPI number—it is illegal for veterinarians to have one. A DEA number is not an appropriate substitution.

FOR MORE INFORMATION:

Use of prescription drugs in veterinary medicine. American Veterinary Medical Association: avma.org/resources-tools/avma-policies/use-prescription-drugs-veterinary-medicine.

Veterinary Pharmacy Education (Resolution No: 110-5-14). National Association of Boards of Pharmacy: nabp.pharmacy/news/news-releases/veterinary-pharmacy-education-resolution-110-5-14/. Passed May 30, 2014. NABP 110th Annual Meeting, Phoenix, AZ.

References

For the complete list of references, see **wiley.com/go/budde/plumb**

Important Contact Information

Poison Control Centers

In the US:

There are many regional poison centers that may be of assistance with animal poisonings; refer to your local poison control center for more information. The following are known 24-hour poison control centers in the US that specialize in providing information specific for veterinary patients.

- **Arizona Poison and Drug Information Center:**
  - 800-222-1222
  - expertise with management of snake bite envenomation
  - azpoison.com
- **ASPCA Animal Poison Control Center:**
  - 888-426-4435
  - consultation fee applies
  - aspca.org/pet-care/animal-poison-control
- **Pet Poison Helpline:**
  - 855-764-7661
  - consultation fee applies
  - petpoisonhelpline.com

In the UK:

- **Veterinary Poisons Information Center**:
  - +44 20 7305 5055 (for veterinarians)
  - +44 12 0250 9000 (pet owners)
  - subscription service
  - vpisglobal.com

In Australia:

- **Australian Animal Poisons Centre:**
  - +61 1300 869 738
  - animalpoisons.com.au

Governmental Veterinary Drug-Related Websites

In the US:

- **Center for Disease Control and Prevention, National Institute for Occupational Safety and Health (NIOSH):**
  - Useful document: List of Hazardous Drugs (cdc.gov/niosh/docs/2016-161/default.html)
  - cdc.gov/niosh/index.htm
- **Drug Enforcement Administration (DEA):**
  - 800-882-9539 (toll-free number for registration information)
  - deadiversion.usdoj.gov
- **Food and Drug Administration Center for Veterinary Medicine (FDA-CVM):**
  - General questions: email askCVM@fda.hhs.gov
  - Report an adverse event for a pharmaceutical:
    - For FDA-approved or indexed products, contact the drug company directly to report the adverse drug event.
    - Alternatively, file a report by downloading and completing the 1932a electronic form from fda.gov/animal-veterinary/report-problem/how-report-animal-drug-and-device-side-effects-and-product-problems#report See *How Do I Report A Problem (Adverse Events for Animal Drugs and Devices)?*
  - Call 888-332-8387 (888-FDA-VETS)
  - Emergency: 866-300-4374 or 301-796-8240
  - For after hours, call and leave a recorded message
  - Importation of veterinary products: The burden of importation appears to rest upon the exporter in completing necessary Customs and Border Patrol (CBP) documents that will allow the drugs to clear US Customs upon entry into the United States. It is important to note that drug shipments may still be seized by US Customs and returned to the exporter despite efforts to provide necessary documentation.
    - For more information: fda.gov/media/71776/download
    - Questions regarding importation of unapproved animal drugs should be emailed to the FDA Center for Veterinary Medicine, Office of Surveillance and Compliance, Division of Compliance at CVMImportRequests@fda.hhs.gov.
- **Food Animal Residue Avoidance & Depletion Program (FARAD):**
  - 1-888-USFARAD (1-888-873-2723)
  - farad.org
- **US Department of Agriculture (USDA) Animal and Plant Health Inspection Service (APHIS):**
  - Report an adverse event for an immunobiological agent (eg, vaccines, bacterins) or diagnostic kits:
    - For USDA-approved products, contact the manufacturer directly to report the adverse event.
    - Alternatively, call the USDA at 800-752-6255 or file a report by downloading and completing the USDA Adverse Event Reporting form from www.aphis.usda.gov/aphis/ourfocus/animalhealth/veterinary-biologics/adverse-event-reporting/CT_Vb_adverse_event
- **US Environmental Protection Agency (EPA):**
  - Most of the products used topically for the control of ectoparasites and insects on animals are regulated by the Environmental Protection Agency (EPA) under the *Federal Insecticide Fungicide and Rodenticide Act.* The National Pesticide Information Center (NPIC) is a collaboration between Oregon State University and the EPA.
  - Report an adverse event related to topical pesticides:
    - For EPA-approved products, contact the manufacturer directly to report the adverse event.
    - Alternatively, call NPIC at 800-858-7378 or report the adverse on the NPIC web portal located at npic.orst.edu/vet

In Australia:

- Australian Pesticides and Veterinary Medicines Authority (APVMA Website):
  - apvma.gov.au

In Canada:

- Health Canada website with many veterinary links:
  - canada.ca/en/health-canada.html

In New Zealand:

- New Zealand Food Safety Authority Ag Compounds and Vet Medicines:
  - www.mpi.govt.nz/agriculture/agricultural-compounds-vet-medicines

In the UK:

- Veterinary Medicines Directorate:
  - www.gov.uk/government/organisations/veterinary-medicines-directorate
- Centre for Agriculture and Bioscience International (CABI):
  - maintains a listing of global and country/region specific websites and databases pertaining to veterinary drug products
  - cabi.org/ahpc/more-resources/drug-databases

Drug Shortage Websites

- The Food and Drug Administration (FDA) maintains a drug shortage website:
  - email notification service is available
  - fda.gov/drugs/drug-safety-and-availability/drug-shortages
  - download the app for Android and iOS: FDA Drug Shortages
- The American Society of Health-System Pharmacists (ASHP) has a website for drug shortages related to human drugs:
  - ashp.org/drug-shortages/current-shortages

Drug Store Toxins in Small Animal Species

Products or compounds may be found in retail settings, pharmacies, or in human drugs that may be potentially toxic to dogs, cats, or other pets. Below is a partial list only. This list is not meant to be inclusive of all potentially toxic items. In addition, there are many human prescription drugs with significant toxic potential for small animal species; refer to the respective systemic monograph section. If the drug is not listed, consult with an animal poison control center for more information. The following known 24-hour poison control centers specialize in providing information specific for veterinary patients. Consultation fees apply.

- **ASPCA Animal Poison Control Center:** 888-426-4435; aspca.org/pet-care/animal-poison-control
- **Pet Poison Helpline (US):** 855-764-7661; petpoisonhelpline.com
- **Veterinary Poisons Information Service (UK):** 0207 305 5055; vpisglobal.com (membership required)
- **Australian Animal Poisons Centre (AU/NZ):** 1300 869 738 (AU) or 0800 869 738 (NZ); animalpoisons.com.au

Over-the-Counter (OTC) Medications

- **5-Hydroxytryptophan** (5-HTP, *Griffonia* seed extract): Human dietary supplement; serotonin precursor. Toxic to dogs and cats, as it induces serotonin syndrome. Clinical signs include sedation at low doses. High doses cause agitation, tremors, seizures, hyperthermia, GI upset, ataxia, abdominal pain, hyperesthesia, and transient blindness. The minimum oral toxic dose for dogs is 24 mg/kg; the minimum oral lethal dose for dogs is 128 mg/kg.[1]
- **Acetaminophen** (eg, *Tylenol*®; also known as APAP, paracetamol): Human analgesic and antipyretic. Contraindicated in cats at any dose and not recommended for ferrets. In cats, this medication can cause methemoglobinemia, hepatic necrosis, and death. Clinical signs include shock, brown mucous membranes, respiratory distress, cyanosis, lethargy, depression, coma, and edema of the face and paws. In dogs, hepatotoxicity and methemoglobinemia can also occur; doses above 100 mg/kg are considered toxic. Clinical signs include anorexia, nausea, vomiting, lethargy, abdominal pain, icterus, hepatic encephalopathy, and coma.[2]
- **Alpha lipoic acid** (thioctic acid, ALA): Dietary supplement used to manage diabetes mellitus. Dose-dependent toxicity in dogs and cats; cats are more sensitive. Clinical signs develop in 30 minutes to several hours, with acute hypoglycemia as the primary concern. Other clinical signs include hypersalivation, vomiting, ataxia, tremors, and seizures. Anecdotal therapeutic dose in cats is 1 – 5 mg/kg daily; the minimum toxic dose is 13 mg/kg. ALA is considered 10 times more toxic to cats than dogs.[3] In dogs, the experimental maximum tolerated dose is 126 mg/kg,[4] but suspicious deaths have been reported at 100 mg/kg.
- **Aspirin** (ASA): NSAID and antiplatelet agent. Toxicity is dose dependent—see the ***Aspirin*** monograph for more information. This medication is used therapeutically in dogs and cats but at very different doses. Cats are very sensitive to salicylates, which have half-lives of 38 to 45 hours at 25 mg/kg in this species. Severe intoxication occurs at more than 80 mg/kg in cats and 100 to 500 mg/kg in dogs. Clinical signs include vomiting, GI ulceration, hematemesis, melena, Heinz body anemia (cats), metabolic acidosis, hyperthermia, and renal and liver damage.
- **Caffeine** (eg, *No-Doze*®, also found in analgesics, coffee, energy drinks, gels and gums, foods such as chocolate): Toxic to dogs and cats. Clinical signs include vomiting, diarrhea, polyuria, polydipsia, hyperactivity, ataxia, tachycardia, tachypnea, hypertension, weakness, cardiac arrhythmias, tremors, seizures, and coma. Death can result from cardiac arrhythmia or respiratory failure. Clinical signs begin at 15 mg/kg. The oral LD_{50} in dogs is 140 mg/kg and 80 – 150 mg/kg in cats.[5]
- **Dextromethorphan** (eg, *Delsym*®, *Robitussin-DM*®): Human cough suppressant—see the ***Dextromethorphan*** monograph for more information. Toxicity is dose dependent. Dextromethorphan has been used anecdotally in dogs at 2 mg/kg PO twice daily to treat cough and repetitive behavioral disorders. Clinical signs of toxicity include agitation, hallucination, nervousness, mydriasis, shaking, facial edema (dogs), vomiting, and diarrhea. Some clinical signs may be similar to serotonin syndrome, such as tremors, seizures, hyperesthesia, hyperthermia, hypersalivation, and death.[5]
- **Ibuprofen** (eg, *Advil*®, *Motrin*®): Human NSAID. Toxic to dogs, cats, and ferrets; not recommended for veterinary use. GI ulceration may occur, as evidenced by hematemesis, diarrhea, melena, weakness, pale mucous membranes, abdominal pain, lethargy, and inappetence. With larger ingestions, acute renal failure, liver failure, and neurologic signs such as tremors or seizures can develop. In ferrets, toxicity affects GI, renal, and central nervous systems.[6]
- **Imidazolines** (eg, oxymetazoline [*Afrin*®], tetrahydrozoline [*Visine*®], naphazoline, tolazoline): Toxic to all pets. Not recommended for veterinary use. Poisoning occurs most commonly after pets chew open product vials. Clinical signs of intoxication may include vomiting, bradycardia, cardiac arrhythmias, poor capillary refill time, hypotension or hypertension, panting, depression, weakness, nervousness, hyperactivity, or shaking. These signs appear within 30 minutes to 4 hours postexposure. In general, imidazoline decongestant exposure may affect the GI, cardiopulmonary, and nervous systems. Veterinary alpha-2-adrenergic antagonists such as atipamezole (*Antisedan*®) or yohimbine may be antidotal.
- **Iron** (Fe): Found in OTC iron supplements (see the ***Ferrous Sulfate*** monograph), multivitamins, prenatal vitamins, fertilizers, pesticides, single-use hand warmers or heating pads such as *ThermaCare*®, and oxygen absorber sachets in food packaging (eg, beef jerky). Toxicity in dogs has been observed at doses greater than 20 mg/kg of elemental iron. Clinical signs include vomiting, bloody diarrhea, lethargy, abdominal pain, and GI ulcerations. More severe signs such as metabolic acidosis, shock, hypotension, hypovolemia, tachycardia, coagulation deficits, hepatic necrosis,

tremors, seizures, and coma can occur. The amount of elemental iron ingested should be determined to assess toxicity. Oxygen absorbers used in food packaging are commonly mistaken for silica gel packets, which are nontoxic.[7]

- **Naproxen** (eg, *Aleve*®): Human NSAID. Highly toxic to dogs, cats, and ferrets. This medication is not recommended for veterinary use in small animal species. In dogs, doses of 5 mg/kg may result in GI irritation or ulceration, and doses greater than 10 – 20 mg/kg may result in acute renal failure. Stomach ulcers, bloody vomiting, diarrhea, melena, weakness, pale gums, abdominal pain, lethargy, and inappetence may occur.
- **Permethrin:** Topical insecticide. Toxic to cats in concentrated formulas (typically greater than 5% to 7%). OTC lice treatment products typically contain 1% permethrin or pyrethrins/piperonyl butoxide and are not usually of concern. Cats are highly sensitive to pyrethrins and pyrethroids; application of concentrated products could be fatal. The most common clinical signs observed are nervous system effects such as hyperesthesia, generalized tremors, muscle fasciculation, hyperthermia, and seizures. Clinical signs can develop within hours or may be delayed up to 72 hours and generally last 2 to 3 days.[8]
- **Phenazopyridine** (eg, *Pyridium*®; PAP): Human urinary analgesic. This medication is not recommended for veterinary use, as it is metabolized to acetaminophen. Cyanosis, methemoglobinemia, rhabdomyolysis, and hepatotoxicity are possible.[9]
- **Phenylephrine** (eg, *Sudafed-PE*®): Human oral decongestant. May be toxic to dogs and cats at high doses. Ingestion can result in hyperactivity, agitation, vomiting, mydriasis, tachycardia, hypertension, hyperthermia, cyanosis, arrhythmias, tremors, and seizures. Pet owners purchasing antihistamines for their pets may unwittingly select a combination product that also contains decongestants like phenylephrine.[5]
- **Pseudoephedrine** (eg, *Sudafed*®): Human oral decongestant with sympathomimetic properties. Pseudoephedrine can be highly toxic to dogs and cats. In dogs, 5 – 6 mg/kg results in moderate to severe clinical signs, with death possible at 10 –12 mg/kg. Ingestion can result in hyperactivity, agitation, vomiting, mydriasis, tachycardia, hypertension, hyperthermia, cyanosis, arrhythmias, tremors, and seizures. Pet owners purchasing antihistamines for their pets may unwittingly select a combination product that also contains decongestants such as pseudoephedrine. See the ***Pseudoephedrine*** monograph for additional information.[5]
- **Vitamin D** (ergocalciferol [D_2], cholecalciferol [D_3]): Found in rodenticides, as a single-agent vitamin, and in multivitamin products. Ingestion of cholecalciferol-rodenticides and single-agent vitamins carries a greater risk for toxicosis than ingestion of multivitamins. Intoxication results from hypercalcemia and hyperphosphatemia followed by metastatic mineralization, typically presenting as acute renal failure. Clinical signs are observed within the first 48 hours of overdose and can include vomiting, lethargy, muscle weakness, bloody diarrhea, depression, polyuria, and polydipsia. With high doses, death from acute renal failure can result.[10]

Medicinal Oils, Solvents, or Excipients

- **Benzyl alcohol**: Preservative. Commonly found in injectable drug products. Cats may be very susceptible to toxic effects. Clinical signs include ataxia, hyperesthesia, muscle fasciculation, depression, coma, respiratory failure, and death.[11]
- **Peppermint oil** (menthol): Toxic to cats. Ingested peppermint oil may cause GI upset, CNS depression, and hepatotoxicity. Inhalation may cause aspiration pneumonia.
- **Propylene glycol**: Commonly found in automotive antifreeze as an alternative to ethylene glycol (also known as pet-safe antifreeze, RV antifreeze), as well as hair dyes, disinfectants, paints, and varnishes; occasionally used in injectable drug products. The canine oral LD_{50} is 9 mL/kg of undiluted propylene glycol. Initial clinical signs can include depression, weakness, ataxia, polyuria, and polydipsia. Lactic acidosis occurs later. Heinz body anemia occurs in cats with chronic ingestion. Hypotension, cardiovascular collapse, and seizures can occur.[12]
- **Tea tree oil** (melaleuca oil): Topical antibacterial agent. Toxicosis is common following exposure to 100% oil (oral or dermal exposure). As little as 7 drops of oil have caused poisoning in pets. Cats are more susceptible to toxicosis than dogs. Clinical signs observed include ataxia, hypothermia, dehydration, muscle tremors, and coma. Tea tree oil may be hepatotoxic to cats.[13] Toxicosis in birds has also been reported.[14]
- **Xylitol**: Natural sweetener with a low glycemic index. Commonly found in many sugar-free foods (eg, peanut butter) and chewing gum, breath mints, nicotine gum, baked goods, oral care products, nasal sprays, chewable vitamins, and some prescription medications, including gabapentin oral liquid, and some oral dispersing tablet (ODT) formulations. It can be toxic to dogs; clinical signs may be delayed up to 12 hours after ingestion and include hypoglycemia, lethargy, vomiting, ataxia, and collapse, and seizures can occur. Acute liver failure is possible. Dogs ingesting greater than 0.1 g/kg of xylitol are considered at risk for developing hypoglycemia; doses greater than 0.5 g/kg may be hepatotoxic. Decontamination is suggested for dogs with exposure greater than 50 mg/kg.[15]

Foods

- ***Allium*-containing foods** (eg, garlic, onion, leeks, chives): May be toxic to dogs and cats. Oral consumption can lead to toxicosis. Clinical signs result from hemolytic anemia and often include depression, hemoglobinuria, icterus, tachypnea, tachycardia, weakness, and exercise intolerance. Inappetence, abdominal pain, and diarrhea may also occur. Development of clinical signs is delayed; they may not be observed until several days after ingestion.[16]
- **Bread/Yeast dough:** Dough containing yeast continues to rise after ingestion, releasing gas that may result in bloating and torsion.[17] Ethanol also can be produced, resulting in ethanol toxicosis. Clinical signs include vomiting, ataxia, lethargy, blindness, abdominal distension, and coma.
- **Chocolate**: Toxic to dogs and cats. Chocolate contains methylxanthines, including caffeine, although the primary toxic component is theobromine, which varies in concentration between brands and types of chocolate products. Clinical signs occur 6 to 12 hours after ingestion. Dogs that ingest 20 mg/kg of methylxanthine content generally display mild GI signs, but cardiotoxic and neurotoxic effects may be seen after ingestion of 40 to 50 mg/kg and more than 60 mg/kg, respectively. Initial signs include polydipsia, vomiting, diarrhea, and restlessness, followed by hyperactivity, polyuria, ataxia, tremors, and seizures. Other effects include tachycardia, premature ventricular contractions, tachypnea, cyanosis, hypertension, hyperthermia, and coma. Pancreatitis can occur 24 to 72 hours after ingestion, due to the high-fat content in chocolate. Death can result from cardiac arrhythmias or respiratory failure. Dogs can easily ingest a toxic dose of chocolate.[18]
- **Grapes, raisins, currants, tamarinds**: These foods are toxic to dogs, as they contain tartaric acid, which dogs are highly sensitive to.[19] Clinical signs can appear within hours and include vomiting, diarrhea, lethargy, and polydipsia. Acute kidney injury may develop within 24 hours to several days after exposure. A toxic dose can be difficult to clinically ascertain, as fruits contain varying amounts of tartaric acid. As such, all exposures are concerning.
- **Macadamia nuts:** Toxic to dogs. Common clinical signs of mac-

adamia nut ingestion include weakness, depression, vomiting, ataxia, tremors, joint pain, lameness, hind limb weakness, hyperthermia, recumbency, and abdominal pain. Clinical signs are typically seen at doses greater than 2 g/kg. Clinical signs have been reported at doses as low as 0.7 mg/kg.[20]

- **Xylitol:** See ***Medicinal Oils, Solvents, or Excipients***

Household Products/Solvents

- **Acids** (eg, drain/toilet bowl cleaners, hair wave neutralizers, metal cleaners, rust removers, vinegar): Tissue damage is related to pH and concentration. Products with a pH of 2 to 4 can cause mild to moderate tissue irritation. Products with a pH less than 2 are corrosive; some examples include acetic acid (concentrations more than 50%), aluminum sulfate (concentrations more than 20%), hydrochloric acid (concentrations more than 10%), and sulfuric acid (concentrations more than 10%). Clinical signs include oral/dermal/GI ulcerations, dysphagia, vomiting, hematemesis, abdominal pain, stridor, and coughing. Induction of emesis is not recommended.[5]
- **Alkalis/Bases** (eg, drain cleaners, dry cell batteries, hair relaxers, lye, nonchlorine bleach, oven cleaners): Tissue damage is related to pH and concentration. Products with a pH of 10 to 11 can cause mild tissue irritation. Products with a pH of 11 to 12 may cause corrosive tissue injury; examples include sodium hypochlorite (concentrations more than 10%), sodium carbonate (concentrations more than 15%), sodium hydroxide (concentrations more than 2%), and sodium silicate (concentrations more than 20%). Clinical signs include ulcerations, dysphagia, vomiting, hematemesis, abdominal pain, stridor, and coughing. Induction of emesis is not recommended.[5]
- **Rodenticides, anticoagulants**: Toxic to all mammals and birds; dogs are more sensitive than cats. Active ingredients (eg, brodifacoum, bromadiolone, chlorophacinone, difethialone, diphacinone, warfarin) antagonize vitamin K epoxidase. Clinical signs typically develop 3 to 5 days after ingestion. Most common clinical signs following ingestion can include dyspnea, coughing, lethargy, exercise intolerance, and hemoptysis. Nonspecific signs can include lethargy, anorexia, or lameness. Signs of bleeding can occur such as hematuria, hematemesis, melena, hyphema, and epistaxis. Vitamin K_1 (phytonadione) is the antidote for these toxicities. See the ***Phytonadione Vitamin K_1*** monograph for more information. **NOTE:** As of April 2015, retail stores in the United States are no longer allowed to carry rodenticide products that contain brodifacoum, bromadiolone, or difethialone for residential use.
- **Rodenticides, bromethalin**: Toxic to all species; however, cats are more sensitive than dogs. Intoxication is due to cerebral edema (white matter vacuolization). No antidote is available, although IV lipid emulsion may be effective to reverse the clinical signs associated with bromethalin.[21-23] The minimum lethal dose in dogs is 2.5 mg/kg active ingredient, and in cats it is 0.3 mg/kg. Dogs may exhibit ataxia, weakness, paralysis, tremors, seizures, and coma. Cats are more prone to paralytic signs.[24]
- **DEET** (eg, *Off*®; N,N-diethyl-meta-toluamide): Found in insect repellants. Neurologic signs (eg, tremors, hyperexcitation, ataxia, and seizures), skin irritation, hypersalivation, and vomiting can result. Up to 13% of DEET is absorbed through the skin in dogs.
- **Ethanol** (alcohol, *Purell*® and other hand sanitizers): Ingesting large amounts of ethanol may cause hypoglycemia, hypothermia, and hypotension. Clinical signs include weakness, lethargy, vomiting, collapse, hypothermia, weak respirations, and coma. The minimum oral lethal dose in dogs is 5.55 g/kg. See the ***Ethanol*** monograph for additional information.
- **Ethylene glycol** (found in automotive antifreeze): The minimum lethal dose of undiluted ethylene glycol antifreeze is 4.2 to 6.6 mL/kg in dogs and 1.5 mL/kg in cats. Toxicity typically occurs in 3 stages. The first stage occurs within 30 minutes to 12 hours and clinical signs include nausea, vomiting, polyuria, polydipsia, ataxia, and metabolic acidosis. The second stage occurs 12 to 24 hours after ingestion, and is characterized by dehydration, tachypnea, and tachycardia. The third stage occurs 12 to 24 hours after ingestion in cats and 36 to 72 hours in dogs. Clinical signs include renal failure, anorexia, depression, lethargy, oral ulcers, hypersalivation, coma, and seizures. Products such as wall paint and printer ink that contain less than 5% ethylene glycol rarely cause problems. See the ***Fomepizole*** and ***Ethanol*** monographs for additional information.[25]
- **Ice melts containing calcium chloride:** Exposure may cause severe skin and GI tract irritation, and electrolyte imbalance. Clinical signs associated with exposure include salivation, depression, disorientation, polydipsia, diarrhea, vomiting, and anorexia.[26]
- **Metaldehyde** (found in some snail/slug baits): Concentrations of active ingredient range from 3.25% to 4%, which are toxic to pets. Clinical signs are similar in dogs and cats and may appear minutes to hours after ingestion. Typical signs include anxiety, tachycardia, nystagmus, mydriasis, hyperpnea, panting, hypersalivation, and ataxia. Vomiting, diarrhea, tremors, hyperesthesia, continuous seizures, metabolic acidosis, rigidity, opisthotonos, and severe hyperthermia may also be seen. Delayed signs that may develop are depression, coma, and liver failure. Death from respiratory failure can occur within a few hours of exposure.[27]
- **Methanol** (organic solvent found in windshield washer fluid, paint thinners, household cleaning products): Toxic to dogs and cats. The canine oral LD_{50} of undiluted methanol is 5 to 11.25 mL/kg. Clinical signs in dogs and cats are similar to ethanol intoxication and include ataxia, depression, lethargy, sedation, hypothermia, and metabolic acidosis. It does not cause blindness in dogs and cats as it does in humans.[5]
- **Mothballs** (naphthalene or paradichlorobenzene [PDB]): Toxic to all species via ingestion, inhalation, or dermal contact. Ingestion may cause severe GI upset, neurologic stimulation followed by depression (PDB), hemolytic anemia (naphthalene), and liver and kidney damage. Dogs that ingested 1.5 g/kg of naphthalene mothballs developed hemolytic anemia. PDB is ≈50% less toxic than naphthalene. Mothballs typically weigh 2.7 g to 4 g each.[28]
- **Polyurethane glues** (eg, *Gorilla*®, *Elmer's*® *ProBond*®): Expanding adhesive glues that contain isocyanates. Although not poisonous, the glue expands significantly once ingested to create a firm, foam-like foreign body that can cause gastric or esophageal obstructions.[28] Clinical signs can be seen 15 minutes to 20 hours after ingestion and include vomiting, abdominal distension, stomach pain, inappetence, and lethargy. Surgical removal is almost always necessary. Inducing emesis is not often recommended.

Miscellaneous Items

- **Glow-in-the-dark jewelry and toys** (liquid-filled plastic necklaces, earrings, plastic wands, safety sticks): Mildly toxic to dogs and cats. These products contain dibutyl phthalate, a chemical that has a bitter taste and is capable of causing immediate eye, skin, and mucous membrane irritation. Most commonly, cats are exposed after piercing jewelry with their teeth. Significant but self-limiting hypersalivation results but is of little toxicologic concern.
- **Lily plants** (*Lilium* spp, *Hemerocallis* spp): Highly toxic to cats. *Lilium* spp (eg, Easter lily, stargazer lily, tiger lily, Asiatic hybrids) are frequently sold as cut flowers in retail settings, as they are inexpensive, fragrant, and long lasting. *Hemerocallis* spp (day lilies) are more often sold in pots for outdoor planting. Small ingestions of leaves, petals, pollen, or vase water can cause kidney injury in cats within 1 to 2 days. If untreated, the prognosis is grave.

- **Liquid potpourri** (simmer pot potpourri): Cats are more susceptible to toxicosis than dogs. Products may contain cationic detergents and essential oils. Ingestion of cationic detergents can result in ulceration or severe inflammation of the mouth and upper GI tract. Essential oils are absorbed across the skin and mucous membranes and result in tissue irritation, GI upset, CNS depression, and dermal hypersensitivity. Inducing emesis is not recommended.[29]
- **Lithium-ion disc batteries:** Ingestion can be toxic to dogs and cats. Tissue necrosis is caused by electric current flow in the GI tract. The greatest concern is for esophageal necrosis followed by perforation, potential aortic fistula, and fatal hemorrhage. Clinical signs include ulceration of the gums, teeth discoloration, hypersalivation, food/water refusal, abdominal pain, shock and pallor, and abdominal distension.[5]
- **Pennies from the United States**: Pennies minted after 1982 are toxic to dogs and cats due to high (97%) zinc content. Ingestion can cause acute GI distress and oxidative damage to red blood cells that results in hemolytic anemia. Additionally, damage to the kidneys, liver, GI tract, pancreas, and red blood cells can occur.[30]

References

For the complete list of references, see **wiley.com/go/budde/plumb**

Overdose and Toxin Exposure Decontamination Guidelines

Contacting a poison control center to manage overdose and toxin exposures is strongly encouraged. The following known 24-hour poison control centers specialize in providing information specific for veterinary patients:

- **ASPCA Animal Poison Control Center**: 888-426-4435; aspca.org/pet-care/animal-poison-control
- **Pet Poison Helpline (US):** 855-764-7661; petpoisonhelpline.com
- **Veterinary Poisons Information Service (UK):** 0207 305 5055; vpisglobal.com
- **Australian Animal Poisons Centre:** 1300 869 738 (AU) or 0800 869 738 (NZ); animalpoisons.com.au

All patients should be stabilized prior to attempts at decontamination to prevent or limit systemic absorption of toxicants. The choice of decontamination method(s) to be administered is guided by the species being treated and the circumstances related to the exposure (eg, duration since exposure, drug or toxin properties). When a patient has ingested a potentially toxic dose of a substance, the clinician has many options for GI decontamination including, but not limited to, dilution, induction of emesis, gastric lavage, the use of adsorbents or cathartics, and administration of enemas. In many cases, the best treatment plan will include more than one of these methods.

Dilution using a small amount of milk or water is recommended in cases where irritant or corrosive materials have been ingested. A dose of 2 – 6 mL/kg is suggested (ie, ≈1 to 2 teaspoons/cat [NOT teaspoons/kg]).[1,2] Administration of the diluent in small volumes is important because giving excessive amounts may lead to emesis and cause the esophagus to be re-exposed to the damaging material.[3] Fruits and vegetables with high water content can be fed to accomplish dilution in some patients, especially birds and reptiles. Dilution methods should not be used for patients with an increased risk for aspiration (eg, actively seizing, obtunded).[3] Dilution with milk, yogurt, or cottage cheese may be useful for patients with oral irritation after ingesting oxalate-containing plants (eg, *Philodendron* spp).[4]

Emetics are often most effective when administered within 2 to 3 hours postingestion.[3] Induction of emesis beyond 3 hours may still be effective for some ingested substances, such as those that coalesce to form a bezoar in the stomach (eg, chewable medications, chocolate[5]) or those that delay gastric emptying. In general, administration of an emetic will empty ≈40% to 60% of the stomach contents when emesis is induced within an hour of toxin ingestion[2,6,7]; however, the amount of vomitus produced will diminish as time passes.[7] If the patient has not recently eaten, emetic efficacy (ie, productive emesis) may be increased by feeding a small meal prior to administration.

Emetics can be administered to dogs, cats, potbelly pigs, and ferrets; however, they should not be administered to horses, ruminants, birds, rabbits, or rodents. Horses and rodents are physically unable to vomit, and induction of emesis may put them at risk for gastric rupture.

Emesis may not be warranted for patients that have already vomited. Patients that are exhibiting clinical signs such as coma, seizures, or recumbency should not be given an emetic. Additionally, if the patient has ingested a CNS stimulant and is already agitated, the additional stimulation of vomiting could lead to seizures.[3] Do not induce emesis (ie, emesis is **contraindicated**) in patients that have ingested corrosive agents (eg, alkalis, acids) because the lining of the esophagus may become ulcerated when the product is swallowed. Re-exposure of the esophageal lining to the corrosive agent during emesis will increase the risk for esophageal ulceration, perforation, and scarring.[6] Emesis is also not recommended after petroleum distillate ingestion due to the risk for aspiration.

Caution is advised when inducing emesis in patients with underlying conditions (eg, severe cardiac disease, seizures) that may impact the patient's ability to safely vomit; carefully consider the risk versus benefit to induing emesis in these patients.

Apomorphine, Dexmedetomidine, Hydrogen Peroxide 3%, Hydromorphone, Ropinirole, and ***Xylazine*** are emetics that are commonly used in veterinary medicine. Emesis was successful in 95% of dogs that received ropinirole[8] and in over 90% of dogs that received either apomorphine or hydrogen peroxide[9]; however, hydrogen peroxide has fallen out of favor due to its associated adverse effects (eg, protracted emesis, esophageal irritation/injury) and should only be used when no other option is available (eg, patient is too far away from veterinary care). Apomorphine is ineffective as an emetic in cats; dexmedetomidine and hydromorphone are a preferred emetics in this species.[10,11]

Historically, other agents such as table salt, dishwashing liquid, syrup of ipecac, and powdered mustard have been used to induce vomiting; however, they are no longer recommended due to the increased risk for adverse effects.[3,6]

Gastric lavage may be considered for patients when emesis is contraindicated, not possible, or has been unsuccessful (eg, presence of bezoars in the stomach); however, it should also not be used to remove caustic materials or volatile hydrocarbons for the same reasons emesis is contraindicated in such cases.[3] The efficacy of gastric lavage is limited by the substance ingested and the diameter of the stomach tube that can be passed. Lavage is not a routinely chosen decontamination method, as it is unlikely to be as effective as emesis[6] and is associated with significant potential risks (eg, aspiration, general anesthesia).[3]

General anesthesia with endotracheal intubation is required to perform gastric lavage to minimize the risk for aspiration. Rodents with cheek pouches should have these spaces gently emptied with a finger or swab prior to the lavage. Risks associated with gastric lavage include damage to or perforation of the esophagus and/or stomach, electrolyte abnormalities (eg, hypo-/hypernatremia depending on lavage solution used), hypothermia, and unintentional placement of the stomach tube into the trachea with subsequent instillation of fluid into the patient's lungs.[3]

Adsorbents bind to chemicals/toxicants in the GI tract to prevent further systemic absorption of a toxicant; they may be used as a single agent or in addition to administration of an emetic or performing gastric lavage. Activated charcoal (AC) is the most commonly used adsorbent. See also ***Charcoal, Activated*** for more information. Many AC products also contain sorbitol, a cathartic to aid in the elimination of the toxicant. See ***Cathartics*** below. When administering these products, it is important to note which product is being administered to avoid adverse effects caused by overuse of the cathartic.

AC is composed of large porous particles that have a large binding surface area to trap organic compounds within the GI tract, including any orally administered medications given concurrently at the time of decontamination. Over-the-counter charcoal tablets and capsules labeled to control flatulence and bloating are not recommended, as the amount of charcoal is often low, and the binding area is much smaller when compared to the AC products specifically intended for GI decontamination.[12]

Repeated doses of AC can be considered in some instances where toxicants are known to undergo enterohepatic recirculation. Examples of toxicants known to undergo this type of recycling include bromethalin, cholecalciferol, ivermectin, and some NSAIDs. If medications are excreted in the bile, AC can be beneficial regardless of the route the medication was administered.

AC does not bind to all compounds equally. Efficiency of adsorption increases with the molecular size of the toxin, and poorly water-soluble organic substances are better adsorbed than small, polar, water-soluble organic compounds. Chemicals that are not effectively bound include ethanol, methanol, fertilizer, fluoride, petroleum distillates, heavy metals, iodides, nitrates, nitrites, sodium chloride, and chlorate. Animals that have ingested caustic substances should not receive AC, as AC is unlikely to bind these products. Additionally, AC may compound the mucosal surface irritation caused by the caustic substance and complicate the identification of oral and esophageal burns.[12]

Animals with no clinical signs may freely consume the charcoal suspension if administered via syringe. A small amount of food may be added to enhance palatability.[4] In animals exhibiting clinical signs, administration of activated charcoal suspensions may be done via a nasogastric tube, as it may be better accepted (especially in cats) and offer a greater margin of safety. Always ensure adequate airway protection, as AC administration carries a risk for aspiration, which carries a poor prognosis.

Cholestyramine may also be used to treat toxicoses of enterohepatically recirculated agents[13] (eg, cholecalciferol,[14,15] amiodarone, digoxin, NSAIDs,[16] vincristine).[17] Cholestyramine is an anion exchange resin that binds with bile acids in the intestine to prevent their reabsorption; toxins that require binding to bile acids for reabsorption (eg, cholecalciferol, piroxicam, indomethacin) will be excreted in the feces. See ***Cholestyramine*** for more information.

Cathartics promote elimination of substances, including the therapeutically administered AC, from the GI tract. When used in combination with AC, the cathartic is given immediately following or mixed with the charcoal.

Cathartics are contraindicated when corrosive substances were ingested or if the animal is dehydrated or hypotensive or has ileus, diarrhea, intestinal obstruction or perforation, history of recent abdominal trauma, or significant electrolyte imbalance.[7] Saline cathartics should also not be used in birds or reptiles and in patients with renal insufficiency.

Osmotic cathartics cause free water to enter the GI tract; the resulting increase of the lumen volume stimulates GI motility and expulsion of the feces. ***Sorbitol*** and ***Saline Cathartics*** are most commonly used for decontamination procedures and may be combined with AC in commercially prepared products.

Other cathartics are classified as bulk and lubricant cathartics. The most commonly used bulk cathartic is ***Psyllium***; in dogs and cats, unspiced canned pumpkin or squash also can be fed. In birds and reptiles, diluted peanut butter, fruit, or vegetables can also be used as bulking agents. Timothy hay can be used in rabbits. Historically, mineral oil was the most commonly used lubricant cathartic, especially in horses; however, mineral oil is no longer recommended in dogs and cats due to the aspiration risk and limited efficacy. Because all cathartics alter the water balance in the GI tract, hydration needs to be maintained.

Enemas using warm water may be indicated when elimination of toxicants (eg, extended-release or controlled-release drugs) from the lower GI tract is desired.[6,18] Commercially prepared phosphate enema solutions should be avoided due to the risk for electrolyte and acid-base disturbances.[6]

References

For the complete list of references, see **wiley.com/go/budde/plumb**

Multidrug Sensitivity (*MDR1* Mutation) in Dogs and Cats

KATRINA L. MEALEY, DVM, PHD, DACVIM, DACVCP
College of Veterinary Medicine, Washington State University

Editor's Note: The following information is adapted, with permission, from Washington State University, College of Veterinary Medicine Program in Individualized Medicine (PrIMe) website: prime.vetmed.wsu.edu/.

Introduction

P-glycoprotein, encoded by the multidrug sensitivity gene (*MDR1* gene, also known as *ABCB1* gene), is a drug transport pump that plays an important role in limiting drug distribution to the brain, as well as pumping many drugs into the bile for excretion from the body. Both canine-specific and feline-specific mutations in the respective *MDR1* genes have been identified such that affected animals have either no P-glycoprotein function, in the case of homozygous animals, or decreased P-glycoprotein function, in the case of heterozygous animals.[1,2] Affected dogs and cats have a decreased ability to limit brain distribution of P-glycoprotein substrate drugs and biliary excretion of those same drugs, which may lead to serious toxicity.

Distribution of Canine and Feline Breeds Affected by the *MDR1* Gene Mutation

Dogs: The canine *MDR1* mutation (also known as *ABCB1*-1delta) is most commonly found in the dog breeds listed in the table below; however, it is important to note that the mutation can occur in any breed, and clinicians should not rely solely on breed predispositions. Genetic testing is the only definitive way to know which dogs are affected.

Breed	Allele frequency (approximate)
Australian shepherd	50%
Australian shepherd, mini	50%
Border collie	Less than 5%
Chinook	25%

Breed	Allele frequency (approximate)
Collie	70%
English shepherd	15%
German shepherd	10%
Herding breed cross	10%
Long-haired whippet	50%
McNab	30%
Mixed breed	5%
Old English sheepdog	5%
Shetland sheepdog	15%
Silken windhound	30%

Cats: Current data do not suggest a breed predilection for the feline *MDR1* mutation.

Problem Drugs

P-glycoprotein function can be reduced by drugs that are P-glycoprotein substrates (eg, ketoconazole) and not solely by the *MDR1* mutation itself.[3]

The following drugs have been documented to cause problems in dogs and cats with the *MDR1* mutation. These are general recommendations and are intended to be a starting point; clinical conditions (eg, *MDR1* genotype, health status) and concurrently administered drugs or supplements must be factored in when deciding how to proceed with the use of these drugs in a particular patient. It is recommended to consult a veterinary clinical pharmacologist for details related to a specific patient.

- **Acepromazine**: In dogs with the MDR1 mutation, acepromazine tends to cause more profound and prolonged sedation.4 It is recommended to reduce the dose by 25% in dogs heterozygous for the MDR1 mutation (mutant/normal) and by 30% to 50% in dogs homozygous for the MDR1 mutation (mutant/mutant).
- **Apomorphine**: Apomorphine can cause CNS depression in dogs homozygous for the *MDR1* mutation at standard doses.[5]
- **Butorphanol**: Anecdotally, butorphanol tends to cause more profound and prolonged sedation in dogs with the *MDR1* mutation. It is recommended to reduce the dose by 25% in dogs heterozygous for the *MDR1* mutation (mutant/normal) and by 30% to 50% in dogs homozygous for the *MDR1* mutation (mutant/mutant).
- **Cyclosporine**: Excessive immunosuppression (T-cell suppression) occurred in a dog heterozygous for the *MDR1* mutation (mutant/normal) receiving a relatively low (6.6 mg/kg/day) cyclosporine dose.[6]
- **Doxorubicin**: Dogs with the *MDR1* mutation are more sensitive to adverse effects to these antineoplastic drugs. Myelosuppression (eg, decreased blood cell counts, particularly neutrophils) and GI toxicity (eg, anorexia, vomiting, diarrhea) are more likely to occur at normal doses in dogs with the *MDR1* mutation.[7-10] To reduce the likelihood of severe toxicity in these dogs, *MDR1* mutant/normal dogs should have their initial dose reduced by 25%, whereas *MDR1* mutant/mutant dogs should have their initial dose reduced by 50%; subsequent doses can be increased by 10% if the initial dose is well tolerated. It has been suggested that these dosage reductions may reduce clinical efficacy,[9] but there are no clinical data to support this. These patients should be closely monitored for adverse effects.
- **Emodepside**: Use of emodepside in dogs and cats with the *MDR1* mutation has resulted in neurologic toxicity.[1,11]
- **Eprinomectin**: Eprinomectin used at label dosages in cats with the *MDR1* mutation has resulted in neurologic toxicity.[12]
- **Grapiprant**: Self-limited vomiting occurred in one collie dog homozygous for the *MDR1* mutation. It is recommended to reduce the dose by 25% in dogs heterozygous for the *MDR1* mutation (mutant/normal) and by 30% to 50% in dogs homozygous for the *MDR1* mutation (mutant/mutant).[13]
- **Ivermectin**: Although the dose of ivermectin used to prevent heartworm infection (6 μg/kg) is safe in dogs with the mutation, higher doses, such as those used for treating mange (300 – 600 μg/kg), will cause neurologic toxicity in dogs that are homozygous for the *MDR1* mutation (mutant/mutant) and can cause less severe neurologic toxicity in dogs that are heterozygous for the mutation (mutant/normal).[1,2,14]
- **Loperamide**: At doses used to treat diarrhea, this drug will cause neurologic toxicity in dogs with the *MDR1* mutation. This drug should be avoided in all dogs with the *MDR1* mutation.[15,16]
- **Maropitant**: Maropitant has been noted to cause mild to moderate CNS depression in dogs with the *MDR1* mutation.[17]
- **Milbemycin**: Like ivermectin, milbemycin is safe in dogs with the mutation when it is used for heartworm prevention at the labeled dosages; however, higher doses have been documented to cause neurologic toxicity in dogs with the *MDR1* mutation.[18]
- **Moxidectin**: Similar to ivermectin, moxidectin is safe for use in dogs and cats with the mutation when it is used for heartworm prevention at the labeled dosages. Higher doses (generally 10 to 20 times higher than the heartworm prevention dose) and oral ingestion of topical products have been documented to cause neurologic toxicity in dogs with the *MDR1* mutation.
- **Selamectin**: Like ivermectin, selamectin is safe in dogs and cats with the mutation when it is used for heartworm prevention at the labeled dosages; however, higher doses and oral ingestion of topical products have been documented to cause neurologic toxicity in pets with the *MDR1* mutation.[1,19,20]
- **Vinca alkaloids** (eg, **vinblastine, vincristine, vinorelbine**): Dogs with the *MDR1* mutation are more sensitive to adverse effects to these antineoplastic drugs.[7,8] Myelosuppression (eg, decreased blood cell counts, particularly neutrophils) and GI toxicity (eg, anorexia, vomiting, diarrhea) are more likely to occur at normal doses in dogs with the *MDR1* mutation.[7-10] To reduce the likelihood of severe toxicity in these dogs, *MDR1* mutant/normal dogs should have their initial dose reduced by 25%, whereas *MDR1* mutant/mutant dogs should have their initial dose reduced by 50%; subsequent doses can be increased by 10% if the initial dose was well tolerated. It has been suggested that these dosage reductions may reduce clinical efficacy,[9] but there are no clinical data to support this. These patients should be closely monitored for adverse effects.

The following drugs have been reported to be pumped by P-glycoprotein in humans, but there are currently no data stating whether they are canine or feline P-glycoprotein substrates and should be used with caution until more data are available.

- Domperidone
- Etoposide
- Ondansetron

There are many additional drugs that are P-glycoprotein substrates in humans and data continue to emerge regarding their effects in dogs and cats with the *MDR1* mutation.

Testing

Only genetic diagnostic testing can identify animals with normal

P-glycoprotein function (*MDR1* normal/normal), heterozygote animals (*MDR1* mutant/normal), or homozygote mutant animals (*MDR1* mutant/mutant). Washington State University College of Veterinary Medicine offers *MDR1* genotyping for dogs and cats as well as counseling for dosing patients tested through Washington State University: https://prime.vetmed.wsu.edu/

Further Reading:

Mealey KL, Fidel J. P-glycoprotein mediated drug interactions in animals and humans with cancer. *Journal of Veterinary Internal Medicine.* 2015;29(1):1-6.

Mealey KL. Adverse drug reactions in veterinary patients associated with drug transporters. *Vet Clin North Am Small Anim Pract.* 2013;43(5):1067-1078.

References

For the complete list of references, see **wiley.com/go/budde/plumb**

How to Find a Quality-Assured Compounding Pharmacy

GIGI DAVIDSON, RPH, DICVP, FSVHP (HONORARY), FACVP

VetPharm Consulting and College of Veterinary Medicine, North Carolina State University

Compounded medications are often required in veterinary medicine to provide for the specialized needs of a patient that cannot be met with commercially available dosage forms. However, choosing a "quality" compounding pharmacy among the many available can be challenging. The following guidelines can help the clinician narrow their choices to best provide for their patients. —Donald Plumb, PharmD

1. When choosing a compounding pharmacy, look for the designation "ACHC Accredited Compounding Pharmacy" (www.achc.org).

Accreditation by the Accreditation Commission for Healthcare (ACHC, formerly Pharmacy Compounding Accreditation Board or ACHC) means the pharmacy has independent, external validation that it meets nationally accepted quality assurance, quality control, and quality improvement standards. ACHC's national standards are based on the consensus of industry experts on those elements that should exist in a pharmacy that adheres to high-quality standards. While all pharmacies must be licensed, ACHC accredited pharmacies have gone the "extra mile" to assure quality.

Only when a pharmacy has met ACHC's rigorous standards is accreditation issued. In order to demonstrate compliance with ACHC standards and earn ACHC accreditation, pharmacies voluntarily participate in an off-site and on-site evaluation process that includes:

- Verification by ACHC that the pharmacy is not on probation for issues related to compounding quality, public safety, or controlled substances.
- Verification that the pharmacy is properly licensed in each state in which it does business.
- An extensive on-site evaluation by an ACHC surveyor, all of whom are compounding pharmacists trained in evaluating compliance with ACHC's quality standards. For example, this evaluation includes:
  - An assessment of the pharmacy's system for assuring and maintaining compliance with all of the United States Pharmacopeia (USP) Standards for Compounding. (eg, Chapters <795>, <797>, and <800>.)
  - An assessment of the pharmacy's system for assuring and maintaining staff competency.
  - A review of facilities and equipment.
  - Review of records and procedures required to prepare quality compounded medications.
  - Verification that the pharmacy uses ingredients manufactured in FDA-registered facilities.
  - Review of the pharmacy's program for the quality testing of compounded preparations.

2. In addition to accreditation by ACHC or other compounding accreditation organizations (eg, NABP or the Joint Commission), inquire about specialized training and expertise in compounding dosage forms for delivery to veterinary patients.

- Many active and inactive ingredients (eg, sweeteners, flavors, preservatives, solvents, vehicles, dyes) used to compound preparations for humans can be toxic in nonhuman species. It is critical that pharmacists preparing compounds for animals are aware of these toxicities.
- Specialized administration devices (eg, subpalpebral lavage catheters, tom cat catheters for rectal administration of antiepileptic medications, and enteral feeding tubes) are also used in veterinary patients. Qualified compounding pharmacists preparing medications for administration through these devices must be aware of compound components and qualities (eg, viscosity, causticity, absorbency) that could obstruct or otherwise damage these administration devices.
- Quality veterinary compounding pharmacies maintain a variety of species-specific and species-appropriate flavoring agents and can customize compounded therapies to individual veterinary patients as indicated.

3. Request evidence for assigned beyond-use dates (expiration dates for compounded preparations).

Chemical and physical stability, as well as sterility storage times for compounded preparations, should be supported by scientific evidence or national quality standards, such as the United States Pharmacopeia (USP) Chapters <795> (nonsterile compounds) and <797> (sterile compounds). USP beyond use dating limits for compounds can be found in the current official versions of those General Chapters at www.usp.org and also in USP's Compounding Compendium on USP's website. If a pharmacy assigns longer beyond-use dates (BUDs) than the limits stated in the current official versions of those chapters, a request should be made to the compounding pharmacy to provide supporting scientific evidence.

Glucocorticoid Agents, General Information

Glucocorticoid Comparison Table

Drug	Equivalent anti-inflammatory dose (mg)	Relative anti-inflammatory potency	Relative mineral-corticoid activity	Plasma half-life dogs (minutes) [humans]	Duration of action after oral/IV	Ester form: solubility/release durations (IM)
Hydrocortisone (Cortisol)	20	1	1-2	52-57 [90]	Less than 12 hours (8-12 hours)	Sodium succinate: very/minutes
Betamethasone	0.6	25	0	* [300+]	More than 36 hours (36-54 hours)	Sodium succinate or phosphate: very/minutes
Dexamethasone	0.75	30	0	119-136 [200-300+]	More than 36 hours (36-54 hours)	Sodium succinate or sodium phosphate: very/minutes Phenylpropionate or isonicotinate: moderate/days to weeks
Flumethasone	1.5	15-30	*	*	*	Very/minutes
Isoflupredone	*	17	*	*	*	Acetate: duration of action up to 48 hours
Methylprednisolone	4	5	0	91 [200]	12-36 hours	Sodium succinate: very/minutes Acetate: moderate/days to weeks
Prednisolone	5	4	1	69-197 [112-212]	12-36 hours	Sodium succinate: very/minutes Acetate: moderate/days to weeks
Prednisone	5	4	1	*[60]		*
Triamcinolone	4	5	0	[200+]	24-48 hours	Acetonide: poorly/weeks

*Data not available

Uses/Indications

Although glucocorticoids have been used to treat many conditions in humans and animals, dexamethasone has 5 primary uses with accompanying dosage ranges: 1) as a diagnostic agent to test for hyperadrenocorticism, 2) as a replacement or supplementation (eg, relative adrenal insufficiency associated with septic shock) for glucocorticoid deficiency secondary to hypoadrenocorticism, 3) as an anti-inflammatory agent, 4) for immunosuppression, and 5) as an antineoplastic agent.[1,2]

Glucocorticoids are used in the treatment of endocrine conditions (eg, adrenal insufficiency), autoimmune and immune-mediated diseases (eg, rheumatoid arthritis, systemic lupus, masticatory myositis[3]), severe allergic conditions, anaphylaxis, envenomation, respiratory diseases (eg, asthma), dermatologic diseases (eg, pemphigus, allergic dermatoses), hematologic disorders (eg, thrombocytopenia, autoimmune hemolytic anemia), neoplasias, nervous system disorders (eg, increased CSF pressure), GI diseases (eg, ulcerative colitis exacerbations, inflammatory bowel disease), renal diseases (eg, nephrotic syndrome), and induction of fetal maturation. Some glucocorticoids are used topically on the eye and skin or are injected intra-articularly or intralesionally. This list is not exhaustive. High-dose glucocorticoid use in the treatment of hemorrhagic or hypovolemic shock, head trauma, spinal cord trauma, and/or sepsis is not supported.[4]

In general, when administering glucocorticoids, the following principles should be followed:

- A specific diagnosis is needed before glucocorticoids are administered, as they can mask disease.
- A course of treatment should be determined prior to treatment.
- A therapeutic endpoint should be determined prior to treatment.
- The least potent glucocorticoid should be used at the lowest dose for the shortest amount of time.
- It is important to understand when glucocorticoid use is inappropriate (eg, acute infection, diabetes).[5]

Pharmacology/Actions

Glucocorticoids have effects on virtually every cell type and system in mammals. An overview of the effects of these agents follows:

- **Cardiovascular system**: Glucocorticoids can reduce capillary permeability and enhance vasoconstriction, and a clinically insignificant positive inotropic effect can occur after glucocorticoid administration.
- **Cells**: Glucocorticoids inhibit fibroblast proliferation, macrophage response to migration inhibiting factor, sensitization of lymphocytes and the cellular response to mediators of inflammation; they can also stabilize lysosomal membranes.
- **CNS/autonomic nervous system**: Glucocorticoids can lower seizure threshold, alter mood and behavior, diminish the response to pyrogens, stimulate appetite, and maintain alpha rhythm. Glucocorticoids are necessary for normal adrenergic receptor sensitivity.
- **Endocrine system**: When an animal is not stressed, glucocorticoids suppress the release of corticotropin (adrenocorticotropic hormone [ACTH]) from the anterior pituitary, which reduces or prevents the release of endogenous corticosteroids. Stress factors (eg, renal disease, liver disease, diabetes) may occasionally nullify the suppressing aspects of exogenously administered steroids. The release of thyroid-stimulating hormone (TSH), follicle-stimulating hormone (FSH), prolactin, and luteinizing hormone may be reduced when glucocorticoids are administered at pharmacological doses. Conversion of thyroxine (T4) to triiodothyronine (T3) may be reduced by glucocorticoids, and plasma levels of parathyroid hormone may be increased. Glucocorticoids may inhibit osteoblast function. Vasopressin (antidiuretic hormone [ADH]) activity is reduced at the renal tubules, and diuresis may occur. Glucocorticoids inhibit insulin binding to insulin receptors and the post-receptor effects of insulin.
- **Fluid and electrolytes balance**: Glucocorticoids can increase renal potassium and calcium excretion, sodium and chloride reabsorption, and extracellular fluid volume. Hypokalemia and/or hypocalcemia rarely occur. Diuresis may develop following glucocorticoid administration.
- **GI tract and hepatic system**: Glucocorticoids increase the secretion of gastric acid, pepsin, and trypsin. Glucocorticoids alter the structure of mucin and decrease mucosal cell proliferation. Iron salts and calcium absorption are decreased while fat absorption is increased. Hepatic changes can include increased fat and glycogen deposits within hepatocytes, increased serum levels of ALT, and gamma-glutamyl transpeptidase (GGT). Significant increases can be seen in serum ALP levels. Glucocorticoids can cause minor increases in bromosulfophthalein (BSP) retention time.
- **Hematopoietic system**: Glucocorticoids can increase the number of circulating platelets, neutrophils, and red blood cells, but platelet aggregation is inhibited. Decreased amounts of lymphocytes (peripheral), monocytes, and eosinophils can be seen, as glucocorticoids can sequester these cells in the lungs and spleen and can decrease the release from bone marrow; removal of old red blood cells becomes diminished. Glucocorticoids can cause involution of lymphoid tissue.
- **Immune system** (also see Cells and Hematopoietic system): Glucocorticoids can decrease circulating levels of T lymphocytes; inhibit lymphokines; inhibit neutrophil, macrophage, and monocyte migration; reduce production of interferon; inhibit phagocytosis, chemotaxis, and antigen processing; and diminish intracellular killing. Specific acquired immunity is affected less than nonspecific immune responses. Glucocorticoids can also antagonize the complement cascade and mask the clinical signs of infection. Mast cells are decreased in number and histamine synthesis is suppressed. Many of these effects only occur at high doses and different species have different responses.
- **Metabolic effects**: Glucocorticoids stimulate gluconeogenesis. Lipogenesis is enhanced in certain areas of the body (eg, abdomen) and adipose tissue can be redistributed away from the extremities to the trunk. Fatty acids are mobilized from tissues, and their oxidation is increased. Plasma levels of triglycerides, cholesterol, and glycerol are increased. Protein is mobilized from most areas of the body (except the liver).
- **Musculoskeletal**: Glucocorticoids may cause muscular weakness, atrophy, and osteoporosis. Bone growth can be inhibited via growth hormone and somatomedin inhibition, increased calcium excretion, and inhibition of vitamin D activation. Resorption of bone can be enhanced. Fibrocartilage growth is also inhibited.
- **Ophthalmic**: Prolonged glucocorticoid use (both systemic or topically to the eye) can cause increased intraocular pressure and glaucoma, cataracts, and exophthalmos.
- **Skin**: Thinning of dermal tissue and skin atrophy can be seen with chronic glucocorticoid therapy. Hair follicles can become distended, and alopecia may occur.

Contraindications/Precautions/Warnings

Systemic use of glucocorticoids is generally considered contraindicated in systemic fungal infections (unless used for replacement therapy for treatment of hypoadrenocorticism), when administered IM in patients with idiopathic thrombocytopenia, and in patients that are hypersensitive to a particular glucocorticoid. Concurrent use of sustained-release injectable glucocorticoids is contraindicated for chronic corticosteroid therapy of systemic diseases. Corticosteroid use may be contraindicated in horses predisposed to laminitis or exhibiting endocrinopathies.

Patients that have received systemic glucocorticoids for more than 2 weeks should be slowly tapered off the drug to allow return of endogenous ACTH and corticosteroid function. If the animal undergoes a stressful event (eg, surgery, trauma, illness) during the tapering process and/or until normal adrenal and pituitary function resume, additional glucocorticoids should be administered.

Adverse Effects

Adverse effects are associated with long-term administration of these drugs, especially if the drugs are administered at high doses or not on an alternate-day regimen. Effects typically manifest as clinical signs of hyperadrenocorticism. Glucocorticoids can delay growth when administered to young, growing animals. See ***Pharmacology***.

In dogs, polyuria (PU), polydipsia (PD), and polyphagia (PP) may occur during short-term burst therapy and on days when the drug is administered during alternate-day maintenance therapy. Adverse effects in dogs can include dull/dry coat, weight gain, panting, vomiting, diarrhea, elevated liver enzymes (ALP more than ALT), vacuolar hepatopathy, GI ulceration/perforation (especially with high parenteral or oral doses), hypercoagulability, hyperlipidemia, activation or worsening of diabetes mellitus, muscle wasting, and behavior changes (eg, depression, lethargy, aggression).[6] Glucocorticoids have been known to delay growth in young animals. Discontinuation of the drug may be necessary; changing to an alternative glucocorticoid may also alleviate adverse effects. Adverse effects associated with anti-inflammatory therapy are relatively uncommon, with the exception of PU, PD, and PP. Adverse effects (eg, secondary infections) associated with immunosuppressive doses are more common and potentially more severe.

Cats generally require higher dosages than dogs for clinical effect, but typically develop fewer adverse effects. Glucocorticoids appear to have a greater hyperglycemic effect in cats than in other species. Occasionally, PU, PD, PP with weight gain, diarrhea, or depression can be seen. Long-term, high-dose therapy can lead to Cushingoid effects.

Administration of dexamethasone or triamcinolone may play a role in the development of laminitis in horses, **but this is thought to only occur rarely. In a study of healthy adult horses, hyperglycemia**

and hyperinsulinemia returned to baseline values within 2 to 3 days of discontinuing dexamethasone, but recovery of insulin secretion was delayed by ≈2 weeks.[7]

Reproductive/Nursing Safety

Glucocorticoids are necessary for normal fetal development. They may be required for adequate surfactant production, myelin, retinal, pancreatic, and mammary development. Excessive doses early in pregnancy may lead to teratogenic effects. In horses and ruminants, exogenous steroid administration may induce parturition when administered in the latter stages of pregnancy.

Glucocorticoids are present in human breast milk.[8] High doses or prolonged administration to dams may potentially inhibit the growth of nursing newborns. In humans, several studies suggest that amounts excreted in human breast milk are negligible with prednisone or prednisolone doses of 20 mg/day or less, or methylprednisolone doses of less than or equal to 8 mg/day. Large doses for short periods of time may not harm the infant. Waiting 3 to 4 hours after administration before allowing offspring to nurse and using prednisolone rather than prednisone may result in a lower corticosteroid exposure for the offspring.

Overdosage/Acute Toxicity

When given short-term, glucocorticoids are unlikely to cause harmful effects, even in massive doses. One incidence of a dog developing acute CNS effects after accidental ingestion of glucocorticoids has been reported. Should clinical signs occur, supportive treatment should be implemented if necessary.

For patients that have experienced or are suspected to have experienced an overdose, consultation with a 24-hour poison consultation center specializing in providing veterinary-specific information is recommended. For general information related to overdose and toxin exposures, as well as contact information for poison control centers, refer to ***Appendix***.

Drug Interactions

The following drug interactions have either been reported or are theoretical in humans or animals receiving glucocorticoids and may be of significance in veterinary patients. Unless otherwise noted, use together is not necessarily contraindicated, but the potential risks should be weighed, and additional monitoring performed when appropriate.

- **AMPHOTERICIN B**: When administered concomitantly with glucocorticoids, may cause hypokalemia
- **ANTICHOLINESTERASE AGENTS** (eg, **neostigmine, pyridostigmine**): In patients with myasthenia gravis, concomitant glucocorticoid with these agents may lead to profound muscle weakness. If possible, discontinue anticholinesterase medication at least 24 hours prior to corticosteroid administration.
- **ASPIRIN (SALICYLATES)**: Glucocorticoids may reduce salicylate blood levels.
- **CYCLOPHOSPHAMIDE**: Glucocorticoids may inhibit the hepatic metabolism of cyclophosphamide; dosage adjustments may be required.
- **CYCLOSPORINE**: Concomitant administration may increase the blood levels of each, by mutually inhibiting the hepatic metabolism of each other; clinical significance of this interaction is not clear.
- **DIGOXIN**: Secondary to hypokalemia, increased risk for arrhythmias
- **DIURETICS, POTASSIUM-DEPLETING** (eg, **furosemide, thiazides**): When administered concomitantly with glucocorticoids, may cause hypokalemia
- **EPHEDRINE:** May increase metabolism
- **ESTROGENS**: The effects of hydrocortisone, and possibly other glucocorticoids, may be potentiated by concomitant administration with estrogens.
- **INSULIN**: Requirements may increase in patients receiving glucocorticoids.
- **KETOCONAZOLE**: May decrease metabolism
- **MITOTANE**: May alter the metabolism of glucocorticoids; higher than usual doses of glucocorticoids may be necessary to treat mitotane-induced adrenal insufficiency.
- **NONSTEROIDAL ANTI-INFLAMMATORY DRUGS** (**NSAIDs**; eg, **carprofen, meloxicam**): Administration of other ulcerogenic drugs with glucocorticoids may increase ulceration risk.
- **PHENOBARBITAL**: May increase the metabolism of glucocorticoids
- **RIFAMPIN**: May increase the metabolism of glucocorticoids
- **VACCINES**: Patients receiving corticosteroids at immunosuppressive dosages should generally not receive live attenuated-virus vaccines, as virus replication may be augmented; a diminished immune response may occur after vaccine, toxoid, or bacterin administration in patients receiving glucocorticoids.

Laboratory Considerations

- Glucocorticoids may increase serum **cholesterol** and **urine glucose** levels.
- Glucocorticoids may decrease serum **potassium.**
- Glucocorticoids may induce **ALP activity** in dogs.
- Certain glucocorticoids (eg, prednisone, prednisolone, hydrocortisone) will interfere with **cortisol assays** (**ACTH stimulation testing**). **NOTE:** Dexamethasone does not interfere.
- Glucocorticoids can suppress the release of thyroid-stimulating hormone (TSH) and reduce T_3 and T_4 values. Thyroid gland atrophy has been reported after chronic glucocorticoid administration. Uptake of I^{131} by the thyroid may be decreased by glucocorticoids.
- Reactions to allergen **intradermal skin tests** may be suppressed by glucocorticoids.[9,10] A 2-week (14-day) withdrawal time before intradermal skin testing is recommended for dogs and cats[11,12]; no withdrawal time is required before serum IgE testing to identify sensitizing allergens in cats.[12]
- False negative results of the **nitroblue tetrazolium test for systemic bacterial infections** may be induced by glucocorticoids.

Monitoring

Monitoring of glucocorticoid therapy is dependent on its reason for use, dosage, agent used (amount of mineralocorticoid activity), dosage schedule (daily versus alternate day therapy), duration of therapy, and the animal's age and condition. The following list may not be appropriate or complete for all animals; use clinical assessment and judgment should adverse effects be noted:

- Weight, appetite, and/or signs of fluid retention
- Serum and/or urine electrolytes
- Total plasma proteins and albumin
- Blood glucose
- Urine culture
- Growth and development in young animals
- ACTH stimulation test to rule out iatrogenic hyperadrenocorticism

Client Information

- Clients should carefully follow the dosage instructions and should not discontinue the drug abruptly without consulting with veterinarian beforehand.
- Clients should be briefed on the potential adverse effects that can be seen with these drugs and instructed to contact the veterinarian should these effects progress or become severe.

References

For the complete list of references, see **wiley.com/go/budde/plumb**

Insulin, General Information

Insulin preparations are used for the treatment of diabetic ketoacidosis (DKA) and uncomplicated diabetes mellitus and as adjunctive therapy in treating hyperkalemia. Veterinary use of insulin has primarily been in dogs and cats, and there are 2 insulin products with FDA approval for use in these species: lente (*vetsulin*®) and recombinant human protamine zinc (*ProZinc*®) insulin. Insulin administration has also been reported for use in other species including, but not limited to, horses, cattle, camelids, birds, ferrets, and guinea pigs. (Information on the individual species and insulins with their exact application can be found in the relevant monographs.)

Goals of insulin therapy in diabetic patients include resolution of clinical signs associated with diabetes mellitus and minimizing the risk for complications such as hypoglycemia or ketosis. Often, hypoglycemia occurring secondary to insulin treatment can be more life-threatening than the hyperglycemia being treated. Diabetic dogs are typically permanently insulin-dependent (similar to a type 1 diabetes in humans) with an inability to produce insulin and require lifelong exogenous insulin. However, diabetic cats tend to develop an early insulin resistance (more consistent with type 2 diabetes in humans), which results in a combination of impaired insulin action (ie, resistance, beta cell dysfunction/failure) and culminates in insulin dependence. Achieving diabetic remission in cats should be considered as a possible treatment goal in newly diagnosed diabetic cats.[1] Increasing the chances for successful remission in cats is often accomplished by instituting more rigorous diabetic management interventions to achieve glycemic control as early as possible after the initial diagnosis.

Treatment of diabetes mellitus is complex. In sick diabetic patients (ie, those with DKA), insulin is only one component of therapy and treatment may require fluid and electrolyte replacement, management of acid/base disturbances, dietary adjustments, and antimicrobial therapy. These patients are typically stabilized with short-acting insulins before transitioning to long-acting insulin therapy; however, in cats, the use of a long-acting insulin (ie, glargine) has been found to be an effective and safe alternative treatment for the management of DKA.[2] Adequate monitoring is mandatory for all patients.

When treating uncomplicated diabetic patients, insulin choice is generally based on efficacy and duration of action in the species being treated. Recommended first-choice insulin products are porcine lente, recombinant human protamine zinc insulin (rPZI), or NPH insulin in dogs and protamine zinc insulin (rPZI) or glargine insulin in cats.[3]

Uses/Indications

Rapid or short-acting insulin:

Rapid or short-acting insulin is commonly used for stabilization of the sick diabetic patient, and as adjunctive therapy for the treatment of hyperkalemia. It is administered by IM and SC injection or by IV infusion. IV insulin administration is recommended in patients with poor tissue perfusion, in shock or cardiovascular collapse, or in those that require adjunct therapy for hyperkalemia.

Regular insulin (or R insulin) is the most commonly used short-acting insulin for diabetic emergencies. If regular insulin is not available or is cost prohibitive, other short-acting insulin preparations include insulin lispro or aspart. All short-acting insulin preparations are human products in U100 (100 units insulin/mL) concentration; higher concentrations may be available for some products, but their use has not been studied in veterinary species.

Regular insulin (*Humulin*® *R*, *Novolin*® *R*)
Lispro insulin (*HumaLOG*®, *Admelog*®, or *Lyumjev*®)
Aspart insulin (*NovoLog*®, *Fiasp*®)

Intermediate-acting insulin:

Intermediate-acting insulin preparations can be used for initial and long-term management of diabetes, especially in dogs.

Porcine lente insulin (*vetsulin*®) is a U40 (40 units insulin/mL) insulin and is FDA-approved for use in dogs and cats.

Recombinant human neutral protamine hagedorn (NPH) insulin (*Humulin*® *N*, or *Novolin*® *N*) is a U100 insulin approved for use in humans. *Novolin*® *N* and *Humulin*® *N* are essentially interchangeable; however, veterinary endocrinologists often recommend using only one brand after therapy is initiated. This insulin is not recommended for use in cats due to its short duration of action in this species.[3]

Long-acting insulin:

Although these insulins are categorized as long-acting, twice-daily therapy is often required. Long-acting insulin preparations can be considered when intermediate-acting insulin preparations are too short in duration of action. Long-acting insulin preparations are often used as first-line insulin choices in diabetic cats.

Glargine insulin is available in U100 concentration (*Lantus*®, *Basaglar*®, *Rezvoglar*®, *Semglee*®); a U300 (300 units insulin/mL) concentration (*Toujeo*®) is available. Glargine insulin also can be considered as an alternative to regular insulin CRI for the management of DKA.[4]

Protamine zinc insulin (*ProZinc*®) is a U40 insulin and is FDA-approved for use in dogs and cats.

Detemir insulin (*Levemir*®) is a U100 insulin. Use this product cautiously in dogs, as they exhibit a strong hypoglycemic response to detemir.

Degludec insulin (*Tresiba*®) is a U100 insulin that is ultra-long-acting in humans. There are insufficient data and experience in veterinary clinical patients to make a dosing recommendation for this insulin type at this time.

Pharmacology/Actions

Insulin is a hormone secreted by beta cells in the pancreatic islets of Langerhans. Eliciting multiple biologic responses, insulin initiates its actions by binding to cell-surface receptors, which are present in varying numbers in virtually all mammalian cells. This binding results in a cascade of intracellular events that can be studied in detail by consulting a physiology text.

Insulin is the primary hormone responsible for controlling the uptake, utilization, and storage of cellular nutrients. Insulin primarily affects liver, muscle, and adipose tissues but also exerts potent regulatory effects on other cell types. Insulin stimulates carbohydrate metabolism in cardiac, skeletal, and adipose tissue by facilitating glucose uptake into the cells. Other tissues, such as brain, nerve, intestinal, liver, and kidney tubules, do not require insulin for glucose transport. Insulin is involved in hepatic conversion of glucose to glycogen (for storage), and the hypothalamus requires insulin for glucose entry into the satiety center.

Insulin secretion is a tightly regulated process designed to provide stable concentrations of glucose in blood during fasting and feeding. This regulation is achieved by the coordinated interplay of nutrients, GI and pancreatic hormones, and autonomic neurotransmitters. The primary stimulus for secretion of endogenous insulin is glucose. Insulin also has direct effects on fat and protein metabolism. The hormone stimulates lipogenesis, increases protein synthesis, and inhibits lipolysis and free fatty acid release from adipose tissues. Insulin promotes an intracellular shift of potassium and magnesium. Exogenous insulin elicits all the pharmacologic responses usually produced by endogenous insulin.

Contraindications/Precautions/Warnings

There are no alternatives for insulin used for diabetic indications;

thus, there are no absolute contraindications to its use except during episodes of hypoglycemia. The likelihood that significant amounts of insulin antibodies will form is directly related to how divergent the administered insulin molecule is from the species being treated. Porcine insulin is identical to canine insulin and is considered the insulin source of choice for diabetic dogs. Cats have been shown to develop anti-insulin antibodies when given human, beef, and beef/pork insulins[5]; dogs have developed anti-insulin antibodies when given beef and pork insulins.[6] The presence of insulin antibodies may increase, decrease, or have no effect on glycemic control.[5,7] Anti-insulin antibodies should be investigated only after other etiologies for poor control (eg, expired insulin, concurrent disease, medication interference) are ruled out. In dogs with significant (ie, greater than 40%) anti-insulin antibodies and poor glycemic control, consider switching to a porcine or recombinant human insulin source or an insulin preparation devoid of protamine. It is unknown if veterinary patients produce antibodies to insulin analogues (eg, glargine, detemir).

Patients presented with severe ketoacidosis, anorexia, lethargy, and/or vomiting should be treated with short-acting insulin (eg, regular) and appropriate supportive therapy until their condition is stabilized. Alternatively, glargine administration was determined to be an effective and safe alternative to the standard regular insulin IV CRI protocol for the management of diabetic ketoacidosis (DKA) in cats.[4]

For obese patients, dose calculations should be based on the individual patient's ideal body weight to avoid inadvertent insulin overdose.

Long-term repeated SC/IM injections of insulin at the same site may cause lipodystrophic reactions, which could interfere with insulin absorption.

Insulin syringes are designed for use with a specific strength of insulin, with the needle covers color-coded according to strength (U40 syringes have a red top, whereas U100 syringes have an orange top). When dosing from a vial, caution must be used to ensure the correct syringes are being used for the insulin strength (eg, U40 syringes for U40 insulin) and that they are not mismatched (eg, U40 syringes for U100 insulin). U40 syringes contain 0.5 mL and have 20 unit marks. One unit mark in a U40 syringe will contain 1 unit of U40 insulin. U100 syringes are available in 0.3 mL, 0.5 mL, and 1 mL size. One unit mark in a U100 syringe will contain 1 unit of U100 insulin. Some brands of 0.3 mL syringes include half unit markings.

Tuberculin (TB) syringes can also be used but are not generally recommended because the potential for dose calculation confusion is substantial.

Using syringe sizes that do not match the insulin type is not recommended due to the increased risk for (potentially catastrophic) dosing errors; however, if the appropriate syringe is not available, conversions can be carefully calculated. Always double-check the conversion before administering to the patient. **NOTE**: Inadvertently using a U40 syringe for U100 insulin will result in a 2.5 times overdose of insulin; similarly, using U100 syringes with U40 insulin will result in a 2.5 times underdose of insulin.

- **If using U100 syringes to measure U40 insulin doses:**
  - Determine the required dose of U40 insulin.
  - Multiply the required units of U40 insulin by 2.5. Example: If the required U40 insulin dose is 10 units, then 10 units × 2.5 = 25 units of U40 insulin when using U100 syringes to administer.
- **If using TB syringes to measure U40 insulin doses:**
  - Determine the required dose of U40 insulin.
  - Multiply the required units of U40 insulin × 0.025. Example: If the required U40 insulin dose is 10 units, then 10 units × 0.025 = 0.25 mL of U40 insulin when using TB syringes to administer.
- **Be sure to double-check all calculations before administering to patient.**

When using pen devices, ensure the needles being used are designed specifically for the product being given.

When writing prescriptions, do not abbreviate units as "U," as it has been shown to increase the rate of transcription and dosage errors. In human medicine, insulin is considered a "high alert" medication (ie, medication that requires special safeguards to reduce the risk for errors). Consider instituting practices such as redundant drug dosage and volume checking, and special alert labels.

Adverse Effects

Adverse effects of insulin therapy may include hypoglycemia (see ***Overdose/Acute Toxicity***), hypokalemia, hypophosphatemia (diabetic ketoacidosis [DKA] only), and injection site reactions to the "foreign" proteins. In cases of hypoglycemia caused by excessive insulin, rebound hyperglycemia may follow (ie, Somogyi effect) due to release of counter-regulatory hormones in response to hypoglycemia or rapid rates of glucose decline following insulin administration. It is important to recognize this phenomenon when making insulin adjustments to avoid complications caused by inadvertent increases in insulin doses when in fact the dose needs to be decreased.

Reproductive/Nursing Safety

The safe use of veterinary-labeled insulins (ie, *vetsulin*®, *ProZinc*®) in breeding or pregnant animals has not been studied. Refer to specific insulin monographs for further information.

In humans, insulin is considered a treatment of choice for gestational diabetes[8]; insulin is compatible with nursing.

Overdose/Acute Toxicity

Insulin overdose leads to hypoglycemia. Signs may include weakness, shaking, head tilt, lethargy, ataxia, seizures, blindness, unusual behavior, and coma. Other signs may include restlessness, hunger, and muscle fasciculations. Electrolyte disturbances, including hypokalemia, may occur. Prolonged hypoglycemia can result in permanent brain damage or death.

Mild hypoglycemia can be treated by offering the animal its usual food. More serious signs (eg, seizures) should be treated with oral dextrose solutions (eg, *Karo*® syrup) applied to the buccal mucosa or by IV injections of 50% dextrose solutions (small amounts: usually 2 – 15 mL [0.5 – 1 mL/kg], diluted and slowly administered[9]; see ***Dextrose 50% injection***). For in-clinic management, glucagon may also be considered on an as-needed basis for an insulin overdose. See ***Glucagon*** for more information. If the animal is seizing, fingers should not be placed in the animal's mouth. Once the animal's hypoglycemia is alleviated (response usually occurs within 1 to 2 minutes), the animal should be closely monitored (both by physical observation and serial blood glucose concentrations) to prevent a recurrence of hypoglycemia (especially with the slower-absorbed/longer-acting products) and to prevent hyperglycemia from developing. Future insulin dosages or feeding habits should be evaluated or adjusted based on consultation with the clinician to prevent further occurrences of hypoglycemia.

For patients that have experienced or are suspected to have experienced an overdose, consultation with a 24-hour poison consultation center specializing in providing veterinary-specific information is recommended. For general information related to overdose and toxin exposures, as well as contact information for poison control centers, refer to ***Appendix.***

Drug Interactions

The following drug interactions have either been reported or are theoretical in humans or animals receiving insulin and may be of importance in veterinary patients. Unless otherwise noted, use together is not necessarily contraindicated, but weigh the potential risks and perform additional monitoring when appropriate.

- **Beta-Adrenergic Antagonists** (eg, **atenolol, propranolol**): Can have variable effects on glycemic control and can mask the signs associated with hypoglycemia
- **Clonidine**: Can mask the signs associated with hypoglycemia
- **Digoxin**: Because insulin can reduce serum potassium concentrations, patients receiving concomitant digoxin therapy—particularly patients receiving concurrent diuretic therapy—should be closely monitored.
- **Diuretics** (eg, **furosemide, hydrochlorothiazide**): Insulin shifts extracellular potassium into the intracellular space; serum potassium concentration should be closely monitored in patients receiving concomitant diuretic therapy. Diuretics may also *decrease* the hypoglycemic activity of insulin (ie, increase insulin requirements).
- **Reserpine**: Can mask the signs associated with hypoglycemia

The following drugs or drug classes may potentiate the hypoglycemic activity of insulin (ie, decrease insulin requirements):

- **Alcohol**
- **Anabolic Steroids** (eg, **boldenone, stanozolol, testosterone**)
- **Angiotensin II Receptor Blockers** (ARBs; eg, **telmisartan**)
- **Angiotensin-Converting Enzyme Inhibitors** (ACEIs; eg, **benazepril, enalapril**)
- **Disopyramide**
- **Fenofibrate**
- **Fluoroquinolones** (eg, **ciprofloxacin, enrofloxacin**)
- **Fluoxetine**
- **Hypoglycemic Agents, Oral** (eg, **acarbose, glipizide, metformin**)
- **Monoamine Oxidase Inhibitors** (MAOIs; eg, **amitraz, linezolid, selegiline**)
- **Pentoxifylline**
- **Salicylates** (eg, **aspirin, bismuth subsalicylate**)
- **Somatostatin Derivatives** (eg, **octreotide**)
- **Sulfonamides** (eg, **sulfadimethoxine, sulfamethoxazole**)

The following drugs or drug classes may decrease the hypoglycemic activity of insulin (ie, increase insulin requirements):

- **Alpha-2-Adrenergic Agonists** (eg, **dexmedetomidine, medetomidine, xylazine): May cause hyperglycemia and temporarily interfere with glycemic control**
- **Beta-Adrenergic Agonists** (eg, **albuterol, terbutaline**)
- **Corticosteroids** (eg, **dexamethasone, prednis(ol)one**)
- **Danazol**
- **Diazoxide**
- **Estrogens** (eg, **diethylstilbestrol** [**DES**], **estriol**)
- **Isoniazid**
- **Niacin**
- **Phenothiazines** (eg, **acepromazine, chlorpromazine**)
- **Progestins** (eg, **megestrol**)
- **Thyroid Hormones**: Can elevate blood glucose concentrations in diabetic patients when thyroid hormone therapy is first initiated

Monitoring

Diabetic patients should be closely monitored, especially during the first month of insulin therapy. Each patient requires an individualized treatment plan, frequent reassessment, and adjustments of the plan based on the response of the patient. It is encouraged to review a veterinary endocrinology reference text or consult with a veterinary emergency and critical care and/or endocrinology specialist for further information related to regulating diabetic patients and insulin adjustments. The overarching goal when monitoring diabetic patients is control of clinical signs related to hyperglycemia (eg, polyuria, polydipsia) while avoiding hypoglycemia.[3] Interpret all monitoring strategies based on clinical signs. Results from the monitoring options below may conflict in regards to achieving good glycemic and clinical control.

- Patient status and control of clinical signs: body weight, appetite, fluid intake, urine output
- Glucose (blood or interstitial). Experience with continuous interstitial glucose monitoring in dogs and cats indicates that these devices are easy to apply, user friendly, and provide useful information surrounding glycemic control while the patient is in the clinic or home environment.[10-14] A blood glucose curve should be considered at the following times[3]:
  a) At the discretion of the supervising veterinarian, after the first dose of a new insulin type, blood glucose can be checked regularly after administration. The goal for monitoring following the first dose of insulin would be solely to identify hypoglycemia. The insulin dose should NOT be increased based on the first-day blood glucose evaluation. If blood glucose falls below 150 mg/dL during the glucose curve, frequency of monitoring should increase to hourly until the blood glucose is greater than 150 mg/dL.[3] Although the insulin dose should never be increased on the first day of therapy, the dose should be decreased by 10% to 50% in dogs and 0.5 units in cats if blood glucose is less than 150 mg/dL at any time during the day.[3] Repeat glucose curves on subsequent days (and decrease insulin dose if necessary) until nadir is greater than 150 mg/dL.
  b) 7 to 14 days after starting insulin or an insulin dose change
  c) At least every 3 months, even in animals with well-controlled diabetes
  d) Any time clinical signs recur in an animal with previously well-controlled diabetes
  e) When hypoglycemia is suspected. **NOTE**: For patients that have experienced or are suspected to have experienced repeated or unexplained hypoglycemia, it is strongly encouraged to consult with a veterinary emergency and critical care and/or endocrinology specialist or reference text that specializes in providing information specific for treatment of hypoglycemia.
- Urine glucose monitoring is typically only helpful for documenting prolonged hypoglycemia (eg, persistently negative urine glucose testing when monitoring for diabetic remission in cats). As most diabetic patients spend time above the renal threshold for urinary glucose spillage, even patients with well-controlled diabetes may be intermittently glucosuric throughout the day.
- Fructosamine or glycosylated hemoglobin can be measured if available and warranted.
- Additional monitoring for patients with diabetic ketoacidosis (DKA)[15]:
  - Glucose measurement every 1 to 2 hours initially; adjust insulin therapy and begin dextrose infusion when blood glucose decreases below 250 mg/dL (14 mmol/L). See ***Dosages*** section of specific insulin type being administered.
  - Hydration status, respiration, pulse every 2 to 4 hours
  - Serum electrolytes (eg, magnesium, phosphorous, potassium), plasma ketones, and total venous CO_2 concentrations every 4 to 8 hours
  - Urine output, glycosuria urine ketones every 4 to 8 hours
  - Body weight, packed cell volume, temperature, and blood pressure every 6 to 8 hours
  - Additional monitoring as applicable to address concurrent disease

Client Information

- **NOTES for veterinarian**:
  1. Correct injection techniques should be taught and practiced with the client before the animal's discharge.

2. Emphasis should be placed on matching the appropriate syringe and insulin concentration (eg, do not interchange U40 insulin and syringes with U100 insulin and syringes) and correct needles with pens/devices.
3. Both veterinary-approved insulins have owner information sheets, client-friendly handouts, and websites to provide client support on administration and use of insulin.

- For this medication to work safely, give the insulin exactly as your veterinarian has prescribed. Your veterinarian will teach you correct injection techniques before your animal is discharged. Only use the syringes provided by your veterinarian.
- Always double-check the dose in the syringe before you inject your animal. Overdoses may be fatal.
- Do not give this medicine if your animal is not eating.
- The insulin bottle should be visually inspected prior to use. Some insulins will be clear and colorless, whereas others may appear as a uniform milky suspension. There should never be clumps or unexpected particles. Your veterinarian will show you what the vial contents should look like.
- Some insulins require gentle rolling or shaking of the vial prior to withdrawing a dose.
- Unused insulin is stored in the refrigerator. After the vial or pen/device is first used, the insulin will need to be either kept at room temperature or refrigerated depending on the type of insulin. After measuring the dose from a refrigerated insulin into a syringe, allow the contents to come to room temperature before injection.
- The injection site should be frequently changed, with the main sites being the back of the neck, side of the animal, or shoulder area.
- Place the used needles and syringes in a sharps disposal container immediately after use, making sure you do not attempt to disconnect the needle from the syringe or recap the needle. Your veterinarian or pharmacist will help you obtain these containers. Do not reuse needles or syringes.
- Signs of low blood sugar (*hypoglycemia*) include weakness, depression, lack of energy, sluggishness, staggering gait (ie, stumbling) when walking, behavior changes, muscle twitching, seizures (convulsions), or coma. **If your animal is unconscious or having a seizure, this is a medical emergency.** Take your animal to the veterinarian immediately. **If your animal is conscious and able to swallow**, rub ≈1 tablespoon of corn syrup (*Karo*®) or honey on your animal's gums until it is alert enough to eat. Feed the usual meal and contact your veterinarian for recommendations. Some animals may not show any obvious physical signs of low blood sugar. If your animal is not acting normally, contact your veterinarian to make sure your animal's blood sugar concentrations are in a safe range.
- Contact your veterinarian at your earliest convenience if you notice excessive thirst, increased frequency of urination, or increased appetite in your animal, as these signs may indicate the insulin dose needs to be adjusted.
- Keep insulin products out of temperature extremes. When traveling, insulin should not be left in carry-on luggage that will pass through airport surveillance equipment. Generally, insulin stability is not affected by a single pass-through surveillance equipment; however, longer than normal exposure or repeated passes through surveillance equipment may alter insulin potency.
- Do not stop giving this medication to your animal unless instructed to do so by your veterinarian.
- Your veterinarian will need to closely monitor your animal during treatment. Do not miss these important follow-up visits.
- **Keep insulin out of the reach of children. Avoid contact with eyes. In case of contact, immediately flush eyes with running water for at least 15 minutes. Accidental injection may cause hypoglycemia. In case of accidental injection, seek medical attention immediately.**

Chemistry/Synonyms

The endocrine component of the pancreas is organized as discrete islets (islets of Langerhans) that contain 4 cell types, each of which produces a different hormone. Insulin is produced in the beta cells, which comprise 60% to 80% of the islet. Insulin is a protein consisting of 2 chains, designated A and B, with 21 and 30 amino acids, respectively, that are connected by 2 disulfide bonds. Human insulin has a molecular weight of 5808.

The amino acid composition of insulin has been determined in various animal species. The insulin of dogs and pigs is identical in structure. Dogs, horses, cattle, sheep, and goats differ only in positions 8, 9, and 10 of the A chain. Porcine insulin differs from human insulin by 1 amino acid (alanine instead of threonine at the carboxy terminal of the B chain [ie, in position B 30]), and bovine insulin differs by 2 additional alterations in the A chain (threonine and isoleucine in positions A8 and A10 are replaced by alanine and valine, respectively). Of the domestic species, feline insulin is most similar to bovine insulin, differing by only 1 amino acid (at position 18 of the A chain). Human insulin differs from rabbit insulin by a single amino acid. There is a single insulin gene and a single protein product in most mammalian species (multiple insulins appear to occur frequently among fish). Recombinant DNA technology is used to manufacture most insulins, in which the insertion of the insulin gene into the DNA of nonpathogenic bacteria or yeast allows the organisms to produce the insulin protein.

For therapeutic purposes, doses and concentrations of insulin are expressed in units. This is sometimes abbreviated as "U," but this practice is discouraged to reduce the chance for transcription and dosing errors. One unit of insulin is equal to the amount required to reduce the concentration of blood glucose in a fasting rabbit to 45 mg/dL. All commercial preparations of human-labeled insulin currently manufactured in the United States are supplied in solution or suspension at a concentration of 100 units/mL, which is ≈3.6 mg/mL of insulin (one notable exception is detemir, which contains 14.2 mg/mL of insulin). Likewise, one unit of insulin equals ≈35 µg of insulin, and 1 mg insulin is ≈28.8 units.[16]

All human and purified pork insulin products have a neutral pH of ≈7 to 7.8, except for insulin glargine, which has an acidic pH of ≈4.

Storage/Stability

All insulin manufacturers state that unopened insulin products should be stored in the refrigerator and protected from temperature extremes and direct sunlight. Freezing (less than 2°C [36°F]) may alter the protein structure and decrease potency. Particle aggregation and crystal damage may not be visible to the naked eye. Higher temperature extremes (greater than 30°C [86°F]) and direct exposure to sunlight may produce insulin transformation products and fibril formation. Manufacturers allow room-temperature storage of most in-use vials, but recommendations for duration of use and storage vary by manufacturer and product.

Although manufacturers recommend discarding opened bottles of insulin after 4 to 6 weeks (or expiration date, whichever comes first), studies support that insulin potency and stability is maintained for longer durations.[17,18] Veterinary internal medicine specialists indicate that the vial may be used for 3 to 6 months after opening and possibly beyond the listed expiration date as long as it is handled carefully, stored in the refrigerator, and the solution does not develop discoloration, flocculent precipitates, or changes in consistency. If a lack of diabetes regulation is noted when using the product beyond the expiration date (3 to 6 months after starting therapy), it may be prudent to replace with new insulin prior to adjusting insulin therapy.[3]

Compatibility/Compounding Considerations

Compatibility is dependent on factors such as pH, concentration, temperature, and diluent used; consult a pharmacist or specialized references for more specific information.

Diluting insulin: Not all insulin solutions can or should be diluted. Refer to specific insulin monographs for detailed information.

Dosage Forms

Insulin preparations are available for injection from a vial or as an insulin pen. For some pet owners, insulin pens may provide more accuracy with dosing, especially when administering low or half doses of insulin. See specific insulin monographs for details related to available dosage forms.

For humans, insulins are FDA-licensed (approved) biological products. Some insulin types have biosimilar or interchangeable biosimilar products available. Please refer to the FDA's Purple Book for more information about FDA-approved biologics, including biosimilar and interchangeable products.

References

For the complete list of references, see **wiley.com/go/budde/plumb**

Opioids, General Information

Receptors for opioid analgesics are found in high concentrations in the limbic system, spinal cord, thalamus, hypothalamus, striatum, and midbrain. They are also found in tissues, such as the GI tract, urinary tract, and in other smooth muscles.

Opioid receptors are further broken down into 3 main subgroups:

1. *Mu (MOP)* receptors are found primarily in the pain-regulating areas of the brain. They are responsible for analgesia but also many of the associated adverse effects, including euphoria, respiratory depression, sedation, physical dependence, miosis, decreased GI motility, nausea, vomiting, and hypothermic actions of opioids.
2. *Kappa (KOP)* receptors are located primarily in the deep layers of the cerebral cortex and spinal cord. They are thought to contribute to analgesia, nociception, diuresis, sedation, and miosis.
3. *Delta (DOP)* receptors are located in the limbic areas of the CNS, such as the neocortex and amygdala. They are thought to contribute to analgesia, decreased GI motility, and inhibition of dopamine release.

The nociceptin orphanin peptide receptor [NOP, also known as orphan receptor L1, ORL1]) has a structure that is very similar to the other opioid receptors; however, it does not respond in a classic fashion to opioid antagonists, and its classification as an opioid receptor remains controversial. Previously, several other opioid receptor subtypes (including sigma and epsilon) were proposed but have been reclassified as nonopioid receptors as they have little to no affinity for opioids and morphine-like compounds.[1-4]

All opioids in clinical practice act primarily at the MOP receptor with varying degrees of activity on the KOP and DOP receptors. Opioids can be classified according to origin: naturally occurring (eg, morphine, codeine), semisynthetic (eg, oxycodone, buprenorphine), and synthetic (eg, methadone, fentanyl). Additionally, they can be classified according to their effect on the receptors: agonist (eg, morphine, fentanyl), partial agonist (eg, buprenorphine), and antagonist (eg, naloxone, naltrexone).

The primary pharmacologic effects of opioids include analgesia, antitussive activity, respiratory depression, sedation, emesis, physical dependence, and intestinal effects (constipation, defecation).

Secondary pharmacologic effects include:

- CNS: Euphoria, excitement
- Cardiovascular: Bradycardia, peripheral vasodilation, decreased peripheral resistance, and baroreceptor inhibition, which may result in orthostatic hypotension and syncope
- Urinary: Diuresis, increased bladder sphincter tone can induce urinary retention

Various species may exhibit paradoxical effects from these agents. For example, in contrast to the expected effects of sedation and constipation after morphine administration, horses, cattle, swine, and cats may develop excitement while dogs may defecate. Dogs and humans may develop miosis, while other species (especially cats) may develop mydriasis. For more information, see the individual monographs for each agent.

References

For the complete list of references, see **wiley.com/go/budde/plumb**

Penicillins, General Information

Uses/Indications

Penicillins are beta-lactam antimicrobials that are used for a wide range of infections in various species. FDA-approved indications/species, as well as non-FDA-approved uses, are listed in the ***Uses/Indications*** and ***Dosages*** section for each drug.

Pharmacology/Actions

Penicillins are beta-lactam antimicrobials that disrupt bacterial cell wall synthesis by binding penicillin-binding proteins (PBPs) within the bacterial cell wall, which inhibits peptidoglycan synthesis. This results in a defective barrier and an osmotically unstable spheroplast. The number and type of PBPs vary between different bacteria, as do the different affinities for various beta-lactams. This helps explain the differences in spectrums of activity the drugs have, which are not explained by the influence of beta-lactamases. Penicillins are time-dependent antimicrobials, usually bactericidal, and like other beta-lactam antibiotics, they are generally considered more effective against actively growing bacteria. The penicillins have no activity against rickettsia, mycobacteria, *Mycoplasma* spp, fungi and viruses. There are several classes of penicillins with various spectrums of activity.

Natural penicillins: penicillin G and V

In general, the natural penicillins are susceptible to the effects of beta-lactamases and are unable to penetrate the cell membrane of gram-negative bacteria. Therefore, their spectrum of activity is mainly aerobic gram-positive cocci, including streptococci and non–penicillinase-producing staphylococci. They also have activity against some aerobic and anaerobic gram-positive bacilli, such as *Bacillus anthracis*, *Clostridium* spp, *Fusobacterium* spp, and *Actinomyces* spp. In addition, they have activity against some nonpenicillinase-producing gram-negative aerobic cocci and against most spirochetes. The natural penicillins are inactive against most aerobic and anaerobic gram-negative bacilli. The natural penicillins are available as sodium, potassium, procaine, or benzathine salt forms. Procaine and benzathine salts slow absorption, leading to a longer duration of action. However, the slow absorption of benzathine penicillin G can result in inadequate penicillin concentration.

Penicillinase-resistant penicillins: nafcillin, cloxacillin, dicloxacillin, oxacillin

The penicillinase-resistant penicillins have a narrower spectrum of activity than the natural penicillins but are resistant to degradation by penicillinases. Their antimicrobial efficacy is aimed directly against penicillinase-producing strains of gram-positive cocci, particularly staphylococcal species. Their spectrum of activity is mainly methicillin-susceptible staphylococci and streptococci; they are inactive against methicillinresistant staphylococci and extended-spectrum beta-lactamase-producing Enterobacteriaceae. In general, this class is more hepatically excreted than other classes of penicillins and is less likely to require dose adjustments for patients with renal insufficiency.

Aminopenicillins: ampicillin, amoxicillin

The aminopenicillins (sometimes referred to as broad-spectrum or ampicillin penicillins) have increased activity against many strains of gram-negative aerobes, including *Escherichia coli*, *Klebsiella* spp, *Proteus mirabilis,* and *Haemophilus* spp. Like the natural penicillins, they are susceptible to inactivation by beta-lactamases. They also have some activity against many anaerobic bacteria, including clostridial organisms. They are inactive against *Pseudomonas aeruginosa*, *Serratia* spp, indole-positive *Proteus* spp (*Proteus vulgaris*), *Citrobacter* spp, and *Acinetobacter* spp.

Extended-spectrum penicillins (anti-pseudomonal penicillins): piperacillin

The extended-spectrum penicillins have increased activity against gram-negative aerobes and are sometimes called anti-pseudomonal penicillins. These agents have similar spectrums of activity as the aminopenicillins but with additional activity against several gramnegative organisms of the family Enterobacteriaceae, as well as many strains of *Pseudomonas aeruginosa*. Like the aminopenicillins, these agents are susceptible to inactivation by beta-lactamases. The primary agent in this class (ie, piperacillin) is only available as a piperacillin/tazobactam combination.

Potentiated penicillins: amoxicillin/clavulanic acid, ampicillin/sulbactam, piperacillin/tazobactam

In order to reduce the inactivation of penicillins by beta-lactamases, beta-lactamase inhibitors, such as clavulanic acid, sulbactam, and tazobactam, have been developed to inactivate these enzymes. These compounds have little to no inherent antimicrobial activity but can inactivate beta-lactamases, rendering beta-lactamase-producing bacteria susceptible to the penicillin component of the combination. This is an effective approach against many resistant bacteria, particularly staphylococci and Enterobacteriaceae. The effect of these betalactamase inhibitors depends on the type of beta-lactamase that is being produced. Extended-spectrum beta-lactamases (ESBLs), an increasing problem in human and veterinary medicine, are variably susceptible to beta-lactamase inhibitors.

Resistance mechanisms:

In addition to the production of beta-lactamases, other resistance mechanisms against penicillins exist. Some bacteria, such as *Staphylococcus aureus* (MRSA), *Enterococcus* spp, and *Streptococcus pneumonia,* have PBP mutations or alterations that have decreased affinity for penicillins.[1] Resistance may also occur through decreased entry through membrane porins or removal of the drug via efflux pumps.

Pharmacokinetics (General)

The oral absorption characteristics of the penicillins are dependent upon their class. Penicillin G is the only available oral penicillin that is substantially affected by gastric pH and can be completely inactivated at a pH of less than 2. The other orally available penicillins are resistant to acid degradation. Effects of food vary between the penicillins. Of the orally administered penicillins, penicillin V and amoxicillin tend to have the greatest bioavailability in their respective classes.

Penicillins are generally distributed widely throughout the body. Most drugs attain therapeutic concentrations in the kidneys, liver, heart, skin, lungs, intestines, bile, bone, and peritoneal, pleural, and synovial fluids. Penetration into the CSF and eye only occur with inflammation and may not reach therapeutic concentrations. Penetration into the prostate is poor.[2] Penicillins are bound in varying degrees to plasma proteins and cross the placenta.

Most penicillins are rapidly excreted largely unchanged by the kidneys into the urine via glomerular filtration and tubular secretion and, therefore, achieve high concentrations in the urine. Probenecid can prolong half-lives and increase serum concentrations by blocking the tubular secretion of penicillins. Except for the penicillinase-resistant penicillins, hepatic inactivation and biliary secretion are minor routes of excretion.

Contraindications/Precautions/Warnings

Penicillins are contraindicated in patients with a history of hypersensitivity to them. Because there may be cross-reactivity, use penicillins cautiously in patients that are documented hypersensitive to other beta-lactam antibiotics (eg, cephalosporins, cephamycins, carbapenems).

Do not administer systemic antibiotics orally in patients with septicemia, shock, or other grave illnesses, as absorption of the medication from the GI tract may be significantly delayed or diminished. Parenteral (preferably IV) routes should be used for these cases. Certain species (eg, snakes, birds, turtles, guinea pigs, and chinchillas) are reportedly sensitive to procaine penicillin G.

Do not use oral penicillins in hindgut fermenting species, such as horses and rabbits, as they can cause a fatal GI disease.

High doses of penicillin G sodium or potassium, particularly in small animals with a pre-existing electrolyte abnormality, renal disease, or congestive heart failure, may cause electrolyte imbalances, including hypokalemia. Other injectable penicillins, such as ampicillin, have significant quantities of sodium per gram and may cause electrolyte imbalances when used in large dosages in susceptible patients.

Adverse Effects

Penicillins are typically well tolerated. When given orally, penicillins may cause GI effects (eg, anorexia, vomiting, diarrhea). Because the penicillins may also alter gut flora, antibiotic-associated diarrhea can occur.

Hypersensitivity reactions, unrelated to dose, can occur with these agents and manifest as rashes, fever, eosinophilia, neutropenia, agranulocytosis, thrombocytopenia, leukopenia, anemias, lymphadenopathy, or anaphylaxis. In humans, it is estimated that up to 15% of patients hypersensitive to cephalosporins will also be hypersensitive to penicillins.[3] The incidence of cross-reactivity in veterinary patients is unknown.

Neurotoxicity (eg, ataxia in dogs) has been associated with very high doses or prolonged use. Although the penicillins are not considered hepatotoxic, elevated liver enzymes have been reported. Other effects reported in dogs include tachypnea, dyspnea, edema, and tachycardia.

Some penicillins (ticarcillin, piperacillin, and nafcillin) have been implicated in causing bleeding problems in humans. These drugs are infrequently used systemically in veterinary species, so the ramifications of this effect are unclear.

Reproductive/Nursing Safety

Penicillins have been shown to cross the placenta. Safe use during pregnancy has not been firmly established, but no teratogenic reports have been documented either.

Penicillins are excreted in maternal milk in low concentrations; use potentially could cause diarrhea, candidiasis, or allergic response in the nursing offspring.

Because safety has not been established in animals, this drug should only be used when the maternal benefits outweigh the potential risks to offspring.

Overdose/Acute Toxicity

Acute oral penicillin overdoses are most likely to cause GI distress, but other effects are possible (see ***Adverse Effects***). In humans, very high dosages of parenteral penicillins, especially in patients with renal disease, have induced CNS effects.

For patients that have experienced or are suspected of having experienced an overdose, consultation with a 24-hour poison consultation center specializing in providing veterinary-specific information is recommended. For general information related to overdose and toxin exposures, as well as contact information for poison control centers, refer to ***Appendix.***

Drug Interactions

The following drug interactions have either been reported or are theoretical in humans or animals receiving penicillins and may be of significance in veterinary patients. Unless otherwise noted, use together is not necessarily contraindicated, but weigh the potential risks and perform additional monitoring when appropriate.

- **AMINOGLYCOSIDES**: In vitro studies have demonstrated that penicillins can have synergistic or additive activity against certain bacteria when used with aminoglycosides or cephalosporins. Penicillins and aminoglycosides should not be administered in the same syringe because of the potential for inactivation.
- **BACTERIOSTATIC ANTIBIOTICS** (eg, **chloramphenicol, erythromycin, tetracyclines**): Use with penicillins is generally not recommended, particularly in acute infections where the organism is rapidly proliferating as penicillins tend to perform better on actively growing bacteria.
- **PROBENECID**: Competitively blocks the tubular secretion of most penicillins, thereby increasing serum levels and serum half-lives

Laboratory Considerations

- Penicillins may cause false-positive **urine glucose** determinations when using cupric-sulfate solution (Benedict's solution, *Clinitest*®). Tests utilizing glucose oxidase (*Tes-Tape*®, *Clinistix*®) are not affected by penicillin.
- In humans, clavulanic acid and high dosages of piperacillin have caused a false-positive direct **Coombs test**.
- Penicillins may cause false-positive **urine protein** determinations and falsely elevated **urine, serum,** or **CSF protein** in a variety of testing methods.

Monitoring

- Clinical signs of efficacy
- Culture and susceptibility as indicated for clinical condition being treated
- CBC and electrolytes may be indicated in some cases.
- Adverse effects including hypersensitivity reactions and GI disturbances (ie, vomiting, diarrhea, inappetence)
- Serum levels and therapeutic drug monitoring are not routinely done with these agents.

Client Information

- Gastrointestinal side effects are most common.
- Compliance with the therapeutic regimen should be stressed. It is important to complete the full course of therapy, even after clinical signs improve.

References

For the complete list of references, see **wiley.com/go/budde/plumb**

Antimicrobials in Human and Veterinary Medicine: A Global Classification

ERICA EARNHARDT WASSACK, PHARMD, DICVP, FSVHP, FACVP

College of Veterinary Medicine, Mississippi State University

Antimicrobial agents used in human and veterinary medicine are drugs used to kill or inhibit the growth of microorganisms such as bacteria and fungi. These drugs are essential for human and animal health and welfare. Human and veterinary antimicrobial use has created a global health concern regarding antimicrobial resistance.[1,2]

The World Health Organization (WHO), in collaboration with the Food and Agriculture Organization of the United Nations (FAO) and the World Organization for Animal Health (OIE), addressed the public health consequences of using antimicrobial agents in food producing animals and concluded that:

1. Antimicrobial resistance was a global public and animal health concern that has been impacted by the use of antimicrobial agents in all sectors.
2. Evidence existed of human health consequences as a product of nonhuman use of antimicrobials resulting in resistant microorganisms.
3. The volume and pattern of nonhuman antimicrobial use have affected the human exposure to resistant bacteria.
4. The consequences of antimicrobial resistance were severe in pathogens resistant to antimicrobials critically important in humans.

As a result, WHO appointed an expert committee to develop a list of antimicrobial agents considered critically important in human medicine [Critically Important Antimicrobials for Human Medicine[1]]. WHO also recommended that OIE develop a list of critically important antimicrobial agents in veterinary medicine [OIE List of Antimicrobial Agents of Veterinary Importance[2]]. These lists should be used to ensure that all antimicrobials, especially critically important antimicrobials, are used prudently in both human and veterinary medicine to minimize the risk for antimicrobial resistance.

Additionally, antimicrobials listed as critically important (eg, fluoroquinolones, third- and fourth-generation cephalosporins, and colistin) in the WHO and OIE veterinary guidelines should be used with the following antimicrobial stewardship recommendations:

- Antimicrobials are not to be used as preventive treatment applied via feed or water in the absence of clinical signs in animal(s) to be treated.
- Antimicrobials are not to be used as a first-line treatment unless justified. When antimicrobials are used as second-line treatment, their use should ideally be based on results of bacteriological tests.
- Extra-label use should be limited and reserved for instances where no alternatives are available.
- Antimicrobials should be phased out for use as growth promotors.

WHO Critically Important Antimicrobials for Human Medicine

The WHO list of Critically Important Antimicrobials for Human Medicine is a reference to help public health authorities as well as practitioners formulate and prioritize risk assessment and management strategies to preserve antimicrobial effectiveness and minimize risk for transmission of resistance to the human population.[1] The list takes into account pathogens likely to transfer from animals, food products, or the environment to humans.

The ranking of antimicrobial agents helps identify which veterinary antimicrobials pose a higher risk to humans.

As stated in the Critically Important Antimicrobials for Human Medicine document,[1] categorization of medically important antimicrobial classes is determined by two criteria:

Criterion 1: Antimicrobial class is the sole, or one of limited available therapies, to treat serious bacterial infections in humans.

Criterion 2: Antimicrobial class is used to treat infections in humans caused by either:

1. Bacteria that may be transmitted to humans from nonhuman sources, or
2. Bacteria that may acquire resistance genes from nonhuman sources.

Based on the above criteria, antimicrobial agents are placed into three categories:

- **Critically Important**: Antimicrobial class meets *both* criterion 1 and criterion 2
- **Highly Important**: Antimicrobial class meets *either* criterion 1 or criterion 2
- **Important**: Antimicrobial class does not meet *either* criterion

Antimicrobial agents within the Critically Important category are further prioritized to determine which agents need the most resources allocated to provide risk management strategies. Antimicrobial classes in this group that also meet all three of the following criteria are considered the Critically Important, *Highest* Priority; those that meet only one or two of these additional criteria are considered Critically Important, *High* Priority.

1. Antimicrobial class used to treat a large number or proportion of humans being treated for serious infections for which there are limited antimicrobial choices available.
2. Antimicrobial class has high frequency of use for any indication in human medicine, or high proportion of use for serious infection in healthcare settings; use in these situations may increase microbial resistance.
3. Antimicrobial class used to treat infections in people with existing evidence that animal sources transmit *resistant bacteria* (eg, nontyphoidal *Salmonella* spp and *Campylobacter* spp) or *resistance genes* (eg, *Escherichia coli* and *Enterococcus* spp).

OIE Antimicrobial Agents of Veterinary Importance

The development of the OIE List of Antimicrobial Agents of Veterinary Importance took into consideration any antimicrobial agent authorized for use in veterinary medicine according to the criteria of quality, safety, and efficacy defined by the *Terrestrial Animal Health Code*.[2] Therefore, all antimicrobial agents used in food-producing animals (avian, bee, bovine, caprine, camel, equine, rabbit, ovine, fish, swine) were divided into three categories: critically important, highly important, and important. **NOTE**: The OIE list of antimicrobials was compiled for antimicrobial importance in *food-producing* animals only and differs from the WHO classification listed above.

The criteria to define veterinary important antimicrobial agents took into account the vast number of species treated in veterinary medicine.

Categorization of important antimicrobial classes used in veterinary medicine is determined by two criteria.

Criterion 1: Majority (greater than 50%) of OIE Member Country contributions response to questionnaire identified the importance of antimicrobial class.

Criterion 2: Compounds within the antimicrobial class were identified as essential against specific infections and sufficient therapeutic alternatives were lacking.

Categorization of antimicrobials of veterinary importance is similar to the WHO guidelines:

Veterinary Critically Important Antimicrobial Agents (VCIA): Antimicrobial class meets *both* criterion 1 and criterion 2

Veterinary Highly Important Antimicrobial Agents (VHIA): Antimicrobial class meets *either* criterion 1 or criterion 2

Veterinary Important Antimicrobial Agents (VIA): Antimicrobial class meets *neither* criterion 1 nor criterion 2

Summary of the Current WHO and OIE Antimicrobial Classifications

WHO Abbreviations

CI-Highest: Critically Important, Highest Priority
CI-High: Critically Important, High Priority
Highly: Highly Important
Important: Important
NC: Not classified

OIE Abbreviations

VCIA: Veterinary Critically Important Antimicrobial Agents
VHIA: Veterinary Highly Important Antimicrobial Agents
VIA: Veterinary Important Antimicrobial Agents
NC: Not classified

*Veterinary-approved drug only

Antimicrobial class	Example of antimicrobials(s)	WHO	OIE
Amdinopenicillins	Mecillinam, Pivmecillinam	Highly	VCIA
Aminocoumarin	Novobiocin	NC	VIA
Aminocyclitols	Spectinomycin	Important	VCIA
Aminoglycosides	Amikacin, Arbekacin, Apramycin*, Bekanamycin, Dibekacin, Dihydrostreptomycin, Framycetin, Gentamicin, Isepamicin, Kanamycin, Neomycin, Netilmicin, Ribostamycin, Streptomycin, Tobramycin	CI-High	VCIA
Amphenicols	Chloramphenicol, Florfenicol*, Thiamphenicol	Highly	VCIA
Ansamycins	Rifabutin, Rifampicin, Rifaximin, Rifapentine, Rifamycin	CI-High	VHIA
Arsenical	Nitarsone, Roxarsone	NC	VIA
Bicyclomycin	Bicozamycin	NC	VIA
Carbapenems and other penems	Biapenem, Doripenem, Ertapenem, Faropenem, Imipenem, Meropenem, Panipenem	CI-High	NC
Cephalosporins, first generation	Cefacetrile, Cefadroxil, Cefaloridine, Cefalexin, Cefalonium*, Cefalotin, Cefaparin, Cefatrizine, Cefazedone, Cefazolin, Cefradine, Cefroxadine, Ceftezole	Highly	VHIA

Antimicrobial class	Example of antimicrobials(s)	WHO	OIE
Cephalosporins, second generation	Cefaclor, Cefamandole, Cefbuperazone, Cefmetazole, Cefminox, Cefonicid, Ceforanide, Cefotetan, Cefotiam, Cefoxitin, Cefprozil, Cefuroxime	Highly	VHIA
Cephalosporins, third generation	Cefcapene, Cefdinir, Cefditoren, Cefetamet, Cefixime, Cefmenoxime, Cefodizime, Cefoperazone, Cefoperazone/Sulbactam, Cefotaxime, Cefpiramide, Cefpodoxime, Cefovecin*, Cefsulodin, Ceftazidime, Ceftazidime/Avibactam, Ceftibuten, Ceftiofur*, Ceftizoxime, Ceftriaxone, Ceftriazone/sulbactam, Latamoxef, Tazobactam	CI-Highest	VCIA
Cephalosporins, fourth generation	Cefepime, Cefoselis, Cefozopran, Cefpirome, Cefquinome*	CI-Highest	VCIA
Cephalosporins, fifth generation	Ceftaroline fosamil, Ceftobiprole, Ceftolozane	CI-Highest	NC
Cephamycins	Flomoxef, Loracarbef	Highly	NC
Cyclic polypeptides	Bacitracin, Enramycin, Gramicidin	Important	VHIA
Drugs used solely to treat tuberculosis and mycobacterial diseases	Bedaquiline, Calcium aminosalicylate, Capreomycin, Cycloserine, Delamanid, Ethambutol, Ethionamide, Isoniazid, Morinamide, Para-aminosalicylic acid, Protionamide, Pyrazinamide, Sodium aminosalicylate, Terizidone, Tiocarlide	CI-High	NC
Fluoroquinolones	Besifoxacin, Cinoxacin, Ciprofloxacin, Danofloxacin*, Delafloxacin, Difloxacin*, Enoxacin, Enrofloxacin*, Fleroxacin, Garenoxacin, Gatifloxacin, Gemifloxacin, Grepafloxacin, Bafloxacin*, Levofloxacin, Lomefloxacin, Marbofloxacin*, Moxifloxacin, Nadifloxacin, Norfloxacin, Ofloxacin, Orbifloxacin*, Pazufloxacin, Pefloxacin, Pipemidic acid, Piromidic acid, Pradofloxacin*, Prulifloxacin, Rosoxacin, Rufloxacin, Sitafloxacin, Sparfloxacin, Temafloxacin	CI-Highest	VCIA
Fusidic acid	Fusidic acid	NC	VIA
Glycopeptides and lipoglycopeptides	Avoparcin*, Dalbavancin, Oritavancin, Teicoplanin, Telavancin, Vancomycin	CI-Highest	NC
Glycylcyclines	Tigecycline	CI-High	NC
Ionophores	Lasalocid, Maduramycin, Monensin, Narasin, Salinomycin, Semduramicin	NC	VHIA
Lincosamides	Clindamycin, Lincomycin, Pirlimycin*	Highly	VHIA
Lipopeptides	Daptomycin	CI-High	NC
Macrolides and ketolides	Azithromycin, Cethromycin, Clarithromycin, Dirithromycin, Erythromycin, Fidaxomicin, Flurithromycin, Gamithromycin*, Josamycin, Kitasamycin*, Midecamycin, Miocamycin, Oleandomycin, Ramoplanin, Rokitamycin, Roxithromycin, Solithromycin, Spiramycin, Telithromycin, Tildipirosin*, Tilmicosin*, Troleandomycin, Tulathromycin*, Tylosin*, Tylvalosin*	CI-Highest	VCIA
Monobactams	Aztreonam, Carumonam	CI-High	NC
Nitrofurantoins	Furaltadone*, Furazolidone, Nifurtoinol, Nitrofural, Nitrofurantoin	Important	NC
Nitroimidazoles	Metronidazole, Ornidazole, Tinidazole	Important	NC
Orthosomycins	Avilamycin	NC	VIA
Oxazolidinones	Cadazolid, Linezolid, Radezolid, Tedizolid	CI-High	NC
Penicillins (anti-staphylococcal)	Cloxacillin, Dicloxacillin, Flucloxacillin, Oxacillin, Nafcillin	Highly	VCIA
Penicillins (natural, aminopenicillins, antipseudomonal)	Amoxicillin, Amoxicillin/Clavulanate, Ampicillin, Ampicillin/Sulbactam, Aspoxicillin*, Azidocillin, Azlocillin, Bacampicillin, Carbenicillin, Carindacillin, Clometocillin, Epicillin, Hetacillin, Metampicillin, Meticillin, Mezlocillin, Panamecillin, Penethamate hydriodide*, Penicillin G (benzylpenicillin), Penicillin V (phenoxymethylpenicillin), Pheneticillin, Piperacillin, Piperacillin/Tazobactam, Pivampicillin, Propicillin, Sulbenicillin, Sultamicillin, Talampicillin, Temocillin, Ticarcillin, Ticarcillin/Clavulanate	CI-High	VCIA
Phosphoglycolipids	Bambermycin (Lavomycin)	NC	NC
Phosphonic acid	Fosfomycin	CI-High	VHIA
Pleuromutilins	Retapamulin, Tiamulin*, Valnemulin*	Important	VHIA

Antimicrobial class	Example of antimicrobials(s)	WHO	OIE
Polymyxins	Colistin, Polymyxin B	CI-Highest	VHIA
Pseudomonic acids	Mupirocin	Highly	NC
Quinolones, first generation	Flumequine, Miloxacin, Nalidixic acid, Oxolinic acid	CI-Highest	VHIA
Quinoxalines	Carbadox, Olaquindox	NC	VIA
Riminofenazines	Clofazimine	Highly	NC
Steroid antibacterials	Fusidic acid	Highly	VIA
Streptogramins	Quinupristin/Dalfopristin, Pristinamycin, Virginiamycin*	Highly	VIA
Sulfonamides, dihydrofolate reductase inhibitors, and combinations	Brodimoprim, Formosulfathiazole*, Iclaprim, Phthalylsulfathiazole*, Pyrimethamine, Sulfadiazine, Sulfadimethoxine, Sulfadimidine, Sulfafurazole, Sulfaisodimidine, Sulfalene, Sulfamazone, Sulfamerazine, Sulamethizole, Sulfamethoxazole, Sulfamethoxypyridazine, Sulfametomidine, Sulfametoxydiazine, Sulfametrole, Sulfamoxole, Sulfanilamide, Sulfaperin, Sulfaphenazole, Sulfapyridine, Sulfathiazole, Sulfathiourea, Tetroxoprim, Trimethoprim	Highly	VCIA
Sulfones	Aldesulfone, Dapsone	Highly	NC
Tetracyclines	Chlortetracycline, Clomocycline, Demeclocycline, Doxycycline, Lymecycline, Metacycline, Minocycline, Omadacycline, Oxytetracycline, Penimepicycline, Rolitetracycline, Tetracycline	Highly	VCIA
Thiostrepton	Nosiheptide	NC	VIA

Further Reading:

Prestinaci F, Pezzotti P, Pantosti A. Antimicrobial resistance: a global multifaceted phenomenon. *Pathog Glob Health.* 2015;109(7):309–318.

Weese JS, Giguère S, Guardabassi L, et al. ACVIM consensus statement on therapeutic antimicrobial use in animals and antimicrobial resistance. *J Vet Intern Med.* 2015;29(2):487-98.

References

For the complete list of references, see **wiley.com/go/budde/plumb**

ARCI UCGFS Classifications

The Association of Racing Commissioners International (ARCI), Inc. is a not-for-profit corporation that *exists to assist in the coordination of the collective efforts of its members who are responsible for ensuring compliance with government laws and regulations designed to protect the general public and racing industry participants, including the equine and canine athletes.*

The organization's website has the most current information on the *Uniform Classification Guidelines for Foreign Substances (UCGFS) and Recommended Penalties Model Rule.* It can be accessed at: https://www.arci.com/wp-content/uploads/2020/12/Uniform-Classification-Guidelines-Version-14.4.pdf

Extra-Label Drug Use

JAMES A. BUDDE, PHARMD, FSVHP, DICVP

VetMedux

The following information is adapted from the FDA website: https://www.fda.gov/AnimalVeterinary/GuidanceComplianceEnforcement/ActsRulesRegulations/ucm085377.htm

The Animal Medicinal Drug Use Clarification Act of 1994 (AMDUCA) permits veterinarians to prescribe extra-label use of certain approved new animal drugs and approved human drugs for animals under certain conditions. *Extra-label use* refers to the use of an approved drug in a manner that is not in accordance with the approved label directions. This includes, but is not limited to, use in species not listed in the labeling, use for indications (disease or other conditions) not listed in the labeling, use at dosage levels, frequencies, or routes of administration other than those stated in the labeling, and deviation from the labeled withdrawal time based on these different uses. Under AMDUCA and its implementing regulations published at Title 21, Code of Federal Regulations, Part 530 (21 CFR 530), any extra-label use of an approved new animal or human drug must be by or on the lawful order of a veterinarian within the context of a veterinarian-client-patient relationship (VCPR).

There are additional specific conditions that must be met for extra-label use of approved animal and approved human drugs in food-producing animals. The following conditions appear in 21 CFR 530.20:

- There is no approved animal drug that is labeled for such use and that contains the same active ingredient in the required dosage form and concentration, except where a veterinarian finds, within the context of a valid VCPR, that the approved animal drug is clinically ineffective for its intended use.
- Before prescribing or dispensing an approved animal drug or approved human drug for extra-label use in food animals, the veterinarian must:
  1. make a careful diagnosis and evaluation of the conditions for which the drug is to be used;
  2. establish a substantially extended withdrawal period prior to marketing of milk, meat, eggs, or other edible products supported by appropriate scientific information, if applicable;
  3. institute procedures to assure that the identity of the treated animal or animals is carefully maintained; and
  4. take appropriate measures to assure that assigned time frames for withdrawal are met and no illegal drug residues occur in any food-producing animal subjected to extra-label treatment.

The following additional conditions must be met for a permitted extra-label use, in food-producing animals, of an approved human drug, or of an animal drug approved only for use in animals not intended for human consumption:

- Such use must be accomplished in accordance with an appropriate medical rationale.
- If scientific information on the human food safety aspect of the use of the drug in food-producing animals is not available, the veterinarian must take appropriate measures to assure that the animal and its food products will not enter the human food supply.
- Extra-label use of an approved human drug in a food-producing animal is not permitted if an animal drug approved for use in food-producing animals can be used in an extra-label manner for the particular use.

Any drug prescribed and dispensed for extra-label use by a veterinarian or dispensed by a pharmacist on the order of a veterinarian must bear or be accompanied by labeling information adequate to assure the safe and proper use of the drug.(21 CFR 530.12) At a minimum, such information shall include the following:

- the name and address of the prescribing veterinarian. If the drug is dispensed by a pharmacy on the order of a veterinarian, the labeling shall include the name of the prescribing veterinarian and the name and address of the dispensing pharmacy, and may include the address of the prescribing veterinarian
- the established name of the drug (active ingredient), or, if formulated from more than one active ingredient, the established name of each ingredient
- any directions for use specified by the veterinarian (including class/species or identification of the animal(s) being treated; dosage, frequency, and route of administration; and the duration of therapy)
- any cautionary statements
- the veterinarian's specified withdrawal, withholding, or discard time(s) for meat, milk, eggs, or any food which might be derived from the treated animal(s).

AMDUCA provides specific conditions under which extra-label use from compounding of approved animal drugs or approved human drugs is permitted. The compounding must be in compliance with all relevant provisions of 21 CFR 530. The extra-label drug use regulation does not permit animal drug compounding from active pharmaceutical ingredients (bulk drugs). FDA/CVM issued the final compounding drug guidance for veterinarians and pharmacists in 2022. For more information, consult guidance document #256 Compounding Animal Drugs from Bulk Drug Substances; CVM GFI #256 - Compounding Animal Drugs from Bulk Drug Substances | FDA

Under the AMDUCA provisions, FDA has the right to prohibit extra-label uses of certain drugs in animals.

FDA may prohibit the extra-label use of an approved animal drug or approved human drug or class of drugs in food-producing animals if FDA determines that:

- An acceptable analytical method needs to be established and such method has not been established or cannot be established.
- The extra-label use of the drug or class of drugs presents a risk to the public health.
- A prohibition may be a general ban on the extra-label use of the drug or class of drugs or may be limited to a specific species, indication, dosage form, route of administration, or combination of factors. FDA may prohibit the extra-label use of an animal or human drug in nonfood-producing animals if FDA determines that such extra-label use presents a risk to the public health.

The following drugs, families of drugs, and substances are prohibited for extra-label animal and human drug uses in food-producing animals (21CFR 530.41 Drugs prohibited for extra-label use in animals)**:**

- Chloramphenicol
- Clenbuterol
- Diethylstilbestrol (DES)
- Dimetridazole
- Ipronidazole
- Other nitroimidazoles
- Furazolidone
- Nitrofurazone
- Sulfonamide drugs in lactating dairy cattle (except approved use of sulfadimethoxine, sulfabromomethazine, and sulfaethoxypyridazine)
- Fluoroquinolones
- Glycopeptides
- Phenylbutazone in female dairy cattle 20 months of age or older
- Cephalosporins (not including cephapirin) in cattle, swine, chickens, or turkeys:
  (i) for disease prevention purposes;
  (ii) at unapproved doses, frequencies, durations, or routes of administration; or
  (iii) if the drug is not approved for that species and production class.

The following drugs, or classes of drugs, that are approved for treating or preventing influenza A, are prohibited from extra-label use in chickens, turkeys, and ducks:

- Adamantanes
- Neuraminidase inhibitors

To clarify extra-label use of cephalosporins, a cephalosporin may be used for an extra-label indication to treat cattle, swine, chickens, or turkeys provided the cephalosporin product being administered is approved for use in that species for another indication, and the dosage used adheres to the labeled dose, route of administration, frequency and duration of use for that species. The following examples of extra-label drug use are prohibited:

- Use of cefpodoxime tablets in a pig because cefpodoxime is not labeled for use in that species
- Administration of ceftiour sodium (*Naxcel*®) 5 mg/kg SC in a cow, because only the labeled dose of 1.1 – 2.2 mg/kg may be used
- Administration of ceftiour sodium (*Naxcel*®) to healthy cattle prior to shipment to prevent shipping fever, as cephalosporins may not be used for disease prevention
- Administration of ceftiofur crystalline free acid (*Excede*®) to cattle intramuscularly because it is only labeled for subcutaneous use
- administration of ceftiofur crystalline free acid (*Excede*®) to cattle subcutaneously but at a site other than the posterior aspect of the ear, because it is only labeled to be administered in the posterior aspect of the ear

Veterinary Feed Directive

JAMES A. BUDDE, PHARMD, DICVP
VetMedux

Per the Federal Register, *In 1996, Congress enacted the Animal Drug Availability Act (ADAA) to facilitate the approval and marketing of new animal drugs and medicated feeds. In passing the ADAA, Congress created a new regulatory category for certain animal drugs used in or on animal food (animal feed) called veterinary feed directive drugs (or VFD drugs).*[1] Per the FDA, *This category was created to provide veterinary supervision without invoking state pharmacy laws for prescription drugs that were unworkable for the distribution of medicated feed.*[2] VFD drugs are not prescription drugs. In 2015, the Food and Drug Administration (FDA) amended the new animal drug regulations to implement the VFD drugs section of the ADAA, with full implementation beginning in December 2016. The VFD requirements apply to all VFD drugs for use in major or minor species.

The FDA approves drugs that require veterinary supervision and oversight for their use. These drugs are classified into 2 separate regulatory categories. When the drug being approved is not for use in or on animal feed, the drug is approved as a prescription drug. When the drug being approved is for use in or on animal feed (a medicated feed), the FDA approves these drugs as a VFD drug.

Per the FDA: *A veterinary feed directive (VFD) is a written (nonverbal) statement issued by a licensed veterinarian in the course of the veterinarian's professional practice that authorizes the use of a VFD drug or combination VFD drug in or on an animal feed. This written statement authorizes the client (the owner of the animal or animals or other caretaker) to obtain and use animal feed bearing or containing a VFD drug or combination VFD drug to treat the client's animals only in accordance with the conditions for use approved, conditionally approved, or indexed by the FDA. A VFD is also referred to as a VFD order.*[2]

To issue a VFD, a veterinarian must meet all the following requirements*:

- Be licensed to practice veterinary medicine
- Be operating in the course of the veterinarian's professional practice and in compliance with all applicable veterinary licensing and practice requirements
- Write VFD orders in the context of a valid client–patient relationship
- Issue a VFD compliant with the conditions for use approved, conditionally approved, or indexed for the VFD drug or combination VFD drug (ie, **Extra-label use of VFD is NOT permitted.**)
- Prepare and sign a written VFD providing all required information
- Enter additional discretionary information to more specifically identify the animals to be treated/fed the VFD feed (See ***Optional information on the VFD*** below for more information)
- Include required information when a VFD drug is authorized for use in a drug combination that includes more than 1 VFD drug
- Restrict or allow the use of the VFD drug in combination with 1 or more OTC drug(s)
- Provide the feed distributor with a copy of the VFD via hardcopy, facsimile (fax), or other electronic means
- Provide the client with a copy of the VFD
- Retain the original VFD in its original form (electronic or hardcopy) for 2 years
- Provide VFD orders for inspection and copying by FDA on request.

**This list was adapted from US FDA. Veterinary Feed Directive Requirements for Veterinarians. https://www.fda.gov/animal-veterinary/development-approval-process/veterinary-feed-directive-requirements-veterinarians.*

Use of medicated feed is authorized by a VFD, not by a prescription (Rx). A lawful VFD must be complete. The following information is required on a lawful VFD*:

- Veterinarian's name, address, and telephone number
- Client's name, business or home address, and telephone number
- Premises at which the animals specified in the VFD are located
- Date of VFD issuance
- Expiration date of the VFD (the expiration date specifies the last day the VFD feed can be fed)
- Name of the VFD drug(s) (**NOTE**: By default, the VFD feed manufacturer may use an approved substitute, but the VFD may specify that a substitution is not allowed)
- Species and production class of animals to be fed the VFD feed
- Approximate number of animals to be fed the VFD feed by the expiration date of the VFD
- Indication for which the VFD is issued
- Level of VFD drug in the feed and duration of use (Duration of use determines the length of time [established as part of the approval, conditional approval, or index listing process] that the animal feed containing the VFD drug is allowed to be fed to the animals.)
- Withdrawal time, special instructions, and cautionary statements necessary for use of the drug in conformance with the approval
- Number of reorders (refills) authorized, if permitted by the drug approval, conditional approval, or index listing (refills may not be authorized if a drug approval is silent on refills)
- Statement: *Use of feed containing this veterinary feed directive (VFD) drug in a manner other than as directed on the labeling (extra-label use), is not permitted.*[1]
- An affirmation of intent for combination VFD drugs as described in 21 CFR 558.6(b)(6)
- Veterinarian's electronic or written signature

**This list was adapted from US FDA. Veterinary Feed Directive Requirements for Veterinarians. https://www.fda.gov/animal-veterinary/development-approval-process/veterinary-feed-directive-requirements-veterinarians.*

Optional information on the VFD*:

- A more specific description of the location of the animals (eg, by site, pen, barn, stall, tank, or other descriptor the veterinarian deems appropriate)
- Approximate age range of the animals
- Approximate weight range of the animals
- Any other information the veterinarian deems appropriate to identify the animals at issue

**This list was adapted from US FDA. Veterinary Feed Directive Requirements for Veterinarians. https://www.fda.gov/animal-veterinary/development-approval-process/veterinary-feed-directive-requirements-veterinarians.*

The following definitions may be useful*:

- VFD drug: a drug intended for use in or on animal feed, which is limited to use under the professional supervision of a licensed veterinarian.
- Combination VFD drug: an approved combination of new animal drugs intended for use in or on animal feed under the professional supervision of a licensed veterinarian, and at least 1 of the new animal drugs in the combination is a VFD drug.
- Category I drugs: drugs that do not require a withdrawal period at the lowest use level in each species for which they are approved.
- Category II drugs: drugs that require a withdrawal period at the lowest use level for at least 1 species for which they are approved or are regulated on a "no-residue" basis or with a zero tolerance because of a carcinogenic concern, regardless of whether a withdrawal period is required.
- Type A medicated articles are the most concentrated form of the new animal drug and are used in the manufacture of another Type A medicated article, or a Type B or C medicated feed. (**NOTE**: To reduce the potential to create unsafe drug residues, the manufacturing of medicated feeds with Category II Type A medicated articles is restricted to licensed feed mills.)
- Type B medicated feed is intended solely for the manufacture of other Type B or Type C medicated feeds and contains a substantial quantity of nutrients with the new animal drug.
- Type C medicated feed is intended as the complete feed for the an-

imal, or may be added on top of a usual ration, or may be offered as a supplement with other animal feed. A Type C medicated feed has the lowest concentration of the new animal drug.

This list was adapted from US FDA. Veterinary Feed Directive Requirements for Veterinarians. https://www.fda.gov/animal-veterinary/development-approval-process/veterinary-feed-directive-requirements-veterinarians

FDA resources:
Guidance for Industry (GFI) documents:

- #120, Small Entity Compliance Guide: Veterinary Feed Directive Regulation Questions and Answers, last updated March 2019.
- #209, The Judicious Use of Medically Important Antimicrobial Drugs in Food-Producing Animals, published April 2012.
- #213, New Animal Drugs and New Animal Drug Combination Products Administered in or on Medicated Feed or Drinking Water of Food-Producing Animals: Recommendations for Drug Sponsors for Voluntarily Aligning Product Use Conditions with GFI #209, published December 2013.
- #233, Veterinary Feed Directive Common Format Questions and Answers, published September 2016.

Websites:
US FDA. Veterinary Feed Directive (VFD). www.fda.gov/animal-veterinary/development-approval-process/veterinary-feed-directive-vfd
US FDA. FACT SHEET: Veterinary Feed Directive Final Rule and Next Steps. www.fda.gov/animal-veterinary/development-approval-process/fact-sheet-veterinary-feed-directive-final-rule-and-next-steps
US FDA. Veterinary Feed Directive Requirements for Veterinarians. www.fda.gov/animal-veterinary/development-approval-process/veterinary-feed-directive-requirements-veterinarians
National Archives. Code of Federal Regulations. ecfr.gov/current/title-21/chapter-I/subchapter-E/part-558

References
For the complete list of references, see **wiley.com/go/budde/plumb**

Conversion Tables for Weight in Kilograms to Body Surface Area (m^2)

The following tables are derived from the equation:

DOGS
Approximate body surface area in m^2 =
10.1 (body weight in grams)$^{2/3}$ ÷ 10,000

Weight in kg	m^2
0.5	0.06
1	0.1
2	0.15
3	0.2
4	0.25
5	0.29
6	0.33
7	0.36
8	0.4

Weight in kg	m^2
9	0.43
10	0.46
11	0.49
12	0.52
13	0.55
14	0.58
15	0.6
16	0.63
17	0.66

Weight in kg	m^2
18	0.69
19	0.71
20	0.74
21	0.76
22	0.78
23	0.81
24	0.83
25	0.85
26	0.88
27	0.9
28	0.92
29	0.94
30	0.96
32	1.01
34	1.05

Weight in kg	m^2
36	1.09
38	1.13
40	1.17
42	1.21
44	1.25
46	1.28
50	1.36
54	1.44
58	1.51
62	1.58
66	1.65
70	1.72
74	1.78
80	1.88

CATS
Approximate body surface area in m^2 =
10 (body weight in grams)$^{2/3}$ ÷ 10,000

Weight in kg	m^2
2	0.159
2.5	0.184
3	0.208
3.5	0.231
4	0.252
4.5	0.273
5	0.292
5.5	0.311
6	0.33
6.5	0.348
7	0.366
7.5	0.383
8	0.4
8.5	0.416
9	0.432
9.5	0.449
10	0.464

Conversion of Conventional Chemistry Units to SI Units

The Système Internationale d'Unites (SI), or the International System of Units, was recommended for use in the health professions by the World Health Assembly in 1977. It is slowly being adopted in the United States and many journals now require its use. The following is an abbreviated table of conversion values for some of the more commonly encountered tests that may now be reported in SI units.

Chemistry analyte	Conventional unit	Conversion factor	SI unit
Albumin	g/dL	x 10	= g/L
Ammonia	µg/dL	x 0.5872	= µmol/L
Bilirubin	mg/dL	x 17.10	= µmol/L
Calcium	mg/dL	x 0.2495	= mmol/L
Cholesterol	mg/dL	x 0.0259	= mmol/L
CO_2 pressure, pCO_2	mm Hg	x 0.1333	= kPa
Creatinine	mg/dL	x 88.4	= µmol/L
Glucose	mg/dL	x 0.0555	= mmol/L
Lactate	mg/dL	x 0.1110	= mmol/L
Magnesium	mg/dL	x 0.4114	= mmol/L
O_2 pressure, pO_2	mm Hg	x 0.1333	= kPa
Phosphorus	mg/dL	x 0.3229	= mmol/L
Protein	g/dL	x 10	= g/L
Urea nitrogen	mg/dL	x 0.3570	= mmol/L
Amylase	IU/L	x 1	= units/L
AST (SGOT)	IU/L	x 1	= units/L
ALT (SGPT)	IU/L	x 1	= units/L
Lipase	IU/L	x 1	= units/L
ALP	IU/L	x 1	= units/L
SDH (Sorbitol)	IU/L	x 1	= units/L
Bicarbonate	mEq/L	x 1	= mmol/L
Chloride	mEq/L	x 1	= mmol/L
Potassium	mEq/L	x 1	= mmol/L
Sodium	mEq/L	x 1	= mmol/L
CO_2 (total)	mEq/L	x 1	= mmol/L

Conversion: Weights; Temperature; Liquids

WEIGHTS:

1 ounce (oz) = 28.4 grams
1 pound (lb) = 0.454 kilogram = 454 grams = 16 ounces (oz)
1 kilogram (kg) = 2.2 pounds = 1000 grams
1 gram (g) = 1000 milligrams = 15.43 grains

1 milligram (mg) = 1000 micrograms (µg or mcg)
1 microgram (mcg or µg) = 1000 nanograms (ng)
1 grain (gr) = 64.8 mg (often rounded to 60 mg or 65 mg)

TEMPERATURES:

°F = (°C + 1.8) + 32
°C = (°F – 32) ´ 0.56

LIQUIDS:

1 gallon (gal) = 4 quarts = 8 pints = 128 fluid ounces = 3.785 liters = 3785 mL
1 quart (qt) = 2 pints = 32 fluid ounces = 946 mL
1 pint = 2 cups = 16 fluid ounces = 473 mL
1 cup = 8 fluid ounces = 237 mL = 16 tablespoons
1 fluid ounce = 30 mL
1 tablespoon = 15 mL = 3 teaspoons
1 teaspoon = 5 mL
4 liters = 1.06 gallons
1 liter (L) = 1000 mL = 10 deciliters
1 deciliter (dL) = 100 mL
1 milliliter (mL) = 1 cubic centimeter (cc) = 1000 microliters (µL; mcL)

Milliequivalents and Molecular Weights

The term milliequivalent (mEq) is typically used to express the quantities of electrolytes administered to patients. A mEq is 1/1000 of an equivalent (Eq). For pharmaceutical purposes, an equivalent may be thought of as equal to the equivalent weight of a given substance. In practical terms, an equivalent is the molecular weight of the substance divided by the valence or the radical. Examples:

How many milligrams equal 1 mEq of potassium chloride (KCl)?

Equivalent weight = molecular weight ÷ valence
[Molecular weight of KCl = 74.5 (K^+ = **39.1** + Cl^-= **35.4**) grams; Valence = 1 (K^+; Cl)]
Equivalent weight = 74.5 ÷ 1 = 74.5 grams ÷ 1000 = 0.0745 grams
Milliequivalent weight of KCl = 0.0745 grams × 1000 mg/1 gram = 74.5 mg = 1 mEq KCl

How many milligrams equal 1 mEq of anhydrous calcium chloride ($CaCl_2$)?

Equivalent weight = molecular weight ÷ valence
[Molecular weight of anhydrous $CaCl_2$ = 111 (Ca^{2+} = **40** + Cl^-= 35.4 × 2 = **71**) grams; Valence = 2 (Ca^{2+}; 2-Cl^-)]
Equivalent weight = 111 ÷ 2 = 55.5 grams ÷ 1000 = 0.0555 grams
Milliequivalent weight of anhydrous $CaCl_2$ = 0.0555 grams × 1000 mg/1 gram = 55.5 mg = 1 mEq anhydrous $CaCl_2$

Listed below are some commonly used electrolytes with their molecular weights and valences in parentheses:

Electrolyte	Molecular weight (valence)
Sodium chloride	58.44 (1)
Sodium bicarbonate	84 (1)
Sodium acetate, anhydrous	82 (1)
Sodium acetate, trihydrate	136 (1)
Sodium lactate	112 (1)
Potassium chloride	74.55 (1)
Potassium gluconate	234.25 (1)
Calcium gluconate	430.4 (2)
Calcium lactate, anhydrous	218.22 (2)
Calcium chloride, anhydrous	111 (2)
Calcium chloride, dihydrate	147 (2)

Electrolyte	Molecular weight (valence)
Magnesium sulfate, heptahydrate	246.5 (2)
Magnesium sulfate, anhydrous	120.4 (2)
Magnesium chloride, anhydrous	95.21 (2)
Magnesium chloride, hexahydrate	203.3 (2)

Solubility Definitions

The following definitions are used throughout the book in the chemistry section for each agent:

Descriptive term	Parts of solvent for 1 part of solute
Very soluble	Less than 1
Freely soluble	From 1 to 10
Soluble	From 10 to 30
Sparingly soluble	From 30 to 100
Slightly soluble	From 100 to 1000
Very slightly soluble	From 1000 to 10,000
Practically insoluble or insoluble	More than 10,000

Parenteral Fluids

(Not a complete listing; includes both human- and veterinary-approved products)

Sodium chloride solutions	Sodium (mEq/L)	Chloride (mEq/L)	Osmolality (mOsm/L)	Volumes available (mL)
Sodium chloride 0.45% (half-normal saline)	77	77	155	3, 5, 500, 1000
Sodium chloride 0.9% (normal saline)	154	154	308	1, 2, 2.5, 3, 4, 5, 10, 20, 25, 30, 50, 100, 130, 150, 250, 500, 1000
Sodium chloride 3%	513	513	1027	500
Sodium chloride 5%	855	855	1710	500
Sodium chloride 7.2%	1232	1232	2464	1000
Sodium chloride 7.5%	1283	1283	2567	1000

Dextrose solutions	Dextrose (g/L)	Calories (kCal/L)	Osmolality (mOsm/L)	Volumes available (mL)
Dextrose 2.5%	25	85	126	250, 500, 1000
Dextrose 5%	50	170	253	10, 25, 50, 100, 130, 150, 250, 400, 500, 1000
Dextrose 10%	100	340	505	250, 500, 1000
Dextrose 20%	200	680	1010	500, 1000
Dextrose 25%	250	850	1330	in 10 mL syringes
Dextrose 30%	300	1020	1515	500, 1000
Dextrose 38.5%	385	1310	1945	1000
Dextrose 40%	400	1360	2020	500, 1000
Dextrose 50%	500	1700	2525	50, 250, 500, 1000
Dextrose 60%	600	2040	3030	500, 1000
Dextrose 70%	700	2380	3535	250, 500, 1000

Dextrose/Saline solutions	Sodium (mEq/L)	Chloride (mEq/L)	Dextrose (g/L)	Calories (kCal/L)	Osmolality (mOsm/L)	Volumes available (mL)
Dextrose 2.5% and 0.45% sodium chloride	77	77	25	85	280	250, 500, 1000
Dextrose 5% and 0.11% sodium chloride	19	19	50	170	290	500, 1000
Dextrose 5% and 0.2% sodium chloride	34	34	50	170	320	250, 500, 1000
Dextrose 5% and 0.33% sodium chloride	56	56	50	170	365	250, 500, 1000
Dextrose 5% and 0.45% sodium chloride	77	77	50	170	405	250, 500, 1000
Dextrose 5% and 0.9% sodium chloride	154	154	100	170	560	250, 500, 1000
Dextrose 10% and 0.45% sodium chloride	77	77	100	340	660	1000
Dextrose 10% and 0.9% sodium chloride	154	154	100	340	815	500, 1000

Electrolyte solutions	Sodium (mEq/L)	Potassium (mEq/L)	Calcium	Magnesium (mEq/L)	Chloride (mEq/L)	Gluconate (mEq/L)	Lactate (mEq/L)	Acetate (mEq/L)	Osmolarity (mOsm/L)	Volumes available (mL)
Ringer's injection	147	4	4.5	–	156	–	–	–	310	250, 500, 1000
Lactated Ringer's solution	130	4	2.7	–	109	–	28	–	273	250, 500, 1000, 5000
Plasma-Lyte® 148	140	5	–	3	98	23	–	27	294	500, 1000
Plasma-Lyte® *A*; *Normosol*®*-R* pH 7.4	140	5	–	3	98	23	–	27	294	500, 1000, 5000
Isolyte® *S pH* 7.4	141	5	–	3	98	23	–	27	295	500, 1000
Hartmann's solution	131	5	4	–	111	–	29	–	278	1000, 5000

Dextrose/ electrolyte solutions	Dextrose (g/L)	Calories (kCal/L)	Sodium (mEq/L)	Potassium (mEq/L)	Calcium (mEq/L)	Magnesium (mEq/L)	Creatinine (mEq/L)	Gluconate (mEq/L)	Lactate (mEq/L)	Acetate (mEq/L)	Osmolarity (mOsm/L)	Volumes available (mL)
Half-strength lactated Ringer's and dextrose 2.5%	25	89	65.5	2	1.4	–	54	–	14	–	263	250, 500, 1000
Lactated Ringer's and dextrose 5%	50	179	130	4	2.7	–	109	–	28	–	527	250, 500, 1000
Normosol®*-M* and dextrose 5%	50	170	40	13	–	3	40	–	–	16	363	500, 1000
Normosol®*-R* and dextrose 5%	50	185	140	5	–	3	98	23	–	27	547	1000
Ringer's and dextrose 5%	50	170	140	4	4.5	–	156	–	–	–	562	500, 1000

Normal Vital Signs

Species	Temperature °C (°F)*	Resting heart rate/minute	Resting respiratory rate/minute
Dog, young	37.5-39.2 (99.5-102.5)	110-120	15-30
Dog, adult medium breed	37.5-39.2 (99.5-102.5)	–	–
Dog, adult large breed	37.5-39.2 (99.5-102.5)	60-90	15-30
Cat, young	37.8-39.5 (100-102.5)	130-140	20-30
Cat, senior	37.8-39.5 (100-102.5)	100-120	20-30
Cattle, up to 1 year old	38.6-39.4 (101.5-103.5)	100-120	15-40
Cattle, over 1 year old	37.8-39.2 (100-102.5)	55-80	10-30
Chicken	40.5-43 (105-109.4)	250-300	–
Chinchilla	37-38 (98.6-100.4)	100-150	–
Ferret	37.8-39.2 (100-102.5)	200-400	33-36
Gerbil	38.2 (100.8)	260-600	85-160
Goat	38.5-40.2 (101.3-104.5)	70-120	10-30
Guinea pig	–	200-300	–
Hamster	37.6 (99.7)	300-600	38-110
Hedgehog, African	35.5-37 (95.7-98.6)	180-280	25-50
Horse, foal	37.5-39.3 (99.5-102.7)	64-128	10-14
Horse, 3 to 24 months	37.5-39.3 (99.5-102.7)	40-80	10-14
Horse, adult	37.2-38.5 (99-101.3)	28-40	10-14
Mouse	37.1 (98.8)	450-750	90-210
Rat	37.7 (99.9)	250-400	71-146
Rabbit	38.5-39.3 (100.4-105)	150-350	50-60
Sheep	38.5-40 (101.3-104)	66-115	10-30
Swine, piglet	38.9-40 (102-104)	100-130	24-36
Swine, adult	37.8-38.9 (100-102)	60-90	8-18
Sugar glider	36.3 (97.3)	200-300	16-40

***Temperature (Rectal):** Temperatures will normally fluctuate over the course of the day. The following things may increase body temperature: time of day (evening), food intake, muscular activity, approaching estrus, during gestation, and high external temperatures. The following conditions may decrease body temperature: intake of large quantities of cool fluids, time of day (morning), and low atmospheric temperature. Small-breed dogs tend to have higher normal temperatures than large-breed dogs.

Reference Laboratory Ranges

NOTE: The following reference ranges are as a general reference only. For clinical use, refer to the designated normal values published by the specific laboratory used. Values were originally published by **Marshfield Clinic Laboratories, Veterinary Diagnostic Service**.

Ferret values were adapted from ***Biology and Diseases of the Ferret,* 3rd Edition**. Fox, JG and Marini, RP, Eds; Wiley-Blackwell, 2014.

Rabbit values were adapted from ***Animal Models in Toxicology*, 3rd Edition**. Gad, SC, Ed; CRC Press, 2013.

Rat hematology values were adapted from ***Schalm's Veterinary Hematology*, 3rd Edition**. Weiss, DJ and Wardrop, KJ, Eds; Wiley-Blackwell, 2010.

Chemistry: Companion/Small Animal Species

Values were originally published by Marshfield Clinic Laboratories, Veterinary Diagnostic Service.

Test	Units	Canine	Feline	Ferret	Rat	Rabbit
Albumin	gm/dL	2.6-4	2.3-3.9	3.5-4.2	3.2-3.7	3.5-5.5
Alkaline phosphatase (ALP)	units/L	13-289	8 -115	9-84	232-632	40-140
Alanine aminotransferase (ALT)	units/L	14-151	23-145	78-149	59-166	15-50
Amylase	units/L	268-1653	627-1572	**	545-847	**
Anion gap	–	17-28	17-32	**	24-39	**
Aspartate aminotransferase (AST)	units/L	18-86	14-68	28-120	90-345	15-45
Beta-hydroxybutyrate	mg/dL	0.2-0.8	0.3-1.9	**	2.2-5.1	**
Bicarbonate	mmol/L	16-31	11-21	20-28	18-27	**
Bile acids, fasting	μmol/L	0-12	0-5	**	NA	**
Bile acids, postprandial (or nonfasting)	μmol/L	5-25	5-15	**	2.2-5.1	**
Bilirubin – Direct	mg/dL	0-0.2	0-0.2	**	0-0	**
Bilirubin – Total	mg/dL	0.1-0.5	0 -0.4	0-0.1	0-0.1	0.1-0.5
Blood urea nitrogen (BUN)	mg/dL	8-30	13-36	11-25	13-19	11-25
Calcium	mg/dL	8.7-12	8.1-11.8	8.7-9.4	9.5-13.9	12.5-15.5
Chloride	mmol/L	100-121	114-130	118-126	98 104	96-106
Cholesterol	mg/dL	98-300	81-275	119-201	50-92	30-100
Creatine kinase (CK)	units/L	50-554	52-462	–	113-692	**
Creatinine	mg/dL	0.4-2	0.5-2.5	0.4-0.9	0.3-0.5	0.9-1.7
Fructosamine	μmol/L	180-330	164-356	**	139-176	**
Gamma glutamyl transferase (GGT)	units/L	3-19	0-2	1-8	0-0	0-10
Globulin	g/dL	2.2-4.1	2.8-5.4	**	2.6-3.5	**
Glucose	mg/dL	74-145	65-155	107-138	70-308	100-190
Haptoglobin	mg/mL	1-5	0.5-3.8	**	0.9-2.1	**
Insulin	μunits/mL	5-65	NA	4.9-34.8	NA	**
Iron	μg/dL	46-214	43-226	**	184-497	**
Lactate	mmol/L	0.99-4.77	0.83-4.95	–	1.60-17.29	**
Lactate dehydrogenase (LDH)	units/L	19-162	35-325	241-752	364-1706	**
Lipase	units/L	109 -750	15-246	**	14-41	**
Magnesium	mg/dL	1.6-2.3	1.7-2.6	**	3.8-5.5	**
Phosphorus	mg/dL	2.5-7.9	2.7-7.3	5.2-7.6	5.6-16.8	2-9
Potassium	mmol/L	3.4-5.6	3.4-5.4	4.3-5.3	3.8-5.6	3.5-6
Sorbitol dehydrogenase (SDH)	units/L	0.7-20	1.8-22.1	**	27.3-118.5	**
Thyroid-stimulating hormone (TSH)	ng/mL	0.03-0.32	NA	NA	NA	NA
Sodium	mmol/L	141-159	151-164	146-160	146-151	133-150
Symmetric dimethylarginine (SDMA)	μg/dL	0-14	0-14	**	**	**
Total T_4 (tT_4)	μg/dL	0.4-3.7	0.6-3.6	0.7-8.3	0.6-3.9	**
Total protein (TP)	g/dL	5-8.3	5.7-8.6	6.2-7.1	5.8-7.1	5.2-7.5
Triglycerides	mg/dL	36-240	24-169	10-32	101-369	30-180
Uric acid	ng/dL	0.2-0.7	0-0.4	0.8-3.1	3.7-9.1	**

**No normal range established in this laboratory

Hematology: Companion/Small Animal Species

Values were originally published by Marshfield Clinic Laboratories, Veterinary Diagnostic Service.

Test	Units	Canine	Feline	Ferret	Rat	Rabbit
Red blood cell (RBC) count	x $10^6/\mu L$	4.48-8.53	5.80-11	7.30-12.18	5-7.20	7-9
Hemoglobin	g/dL	10.5-20.1	8.6-16	12-17.4	10.5-15	13.7-16.8
Hematocrit	%	33-58.7	28-47	36-61	32-45	37.9-49.9
Mean corpuscular volume (MCV)	fL	63-78.3	37.7-50	42.6-51	55-70	49.9-58.3
Mean corpuscular hemoglobin (MCH)	pg/cell	21-27	12.3-17.2	13.7-16	19-23	17.8-29
Mean corpuscular hemoglobin concentration (MCHC)	g/dL	30.8-35.9	31.1-36	30.3-34.9	30-35	33.2-37.9
Red cell distribution width (RDW)	%	11.9-18.1	17-24	7.3-12.2	**	10.5-14.9
Platelet count	x $10^3/\mu L$	140-540	160-660	297-910	300-750	680-1280
White blood cell (WBC) count	x $10^3/\mu L$	4-18.2	3.7-20.5	4.4-19.1	4-13	1.1-7.5
Segmented neutrophil absolute #	x $10^3/\mu L$	2.5-15.7	1.3-15.7	1.3-3.7	1-6	0.2-1.5
Band neutrophil absolute #	x $10^3/\mu L$	0-0.20	0-0.5	0-0.10	0-0.10	0-0.10
Lymphocyte absolute #	x $10^3/\mu L$	0.3-3.9	1-7.9	1.5-6.7	2-9	0.8-5.7
Monocyte absolute #	x $10^3/\mu L$	0-1.4	0-1	0.1-0.8	0-0.5	0-0.2
Eosinophil absolute #	x $10^3/\mu L$	0-1.3	0.10-2	0.1-0.9	0-0.4	0-0.2
Basophil absolute #	x $10^3/\mu L$	0-0.1	0-0.1	0-0.1	0-1	0-0.3

**No normal range established in this laboratory

Chemistry: Equine, Food, and Fiber Animal Species

Values were originally published by Marshfield Clinic Laboratories, Veterinary Diagnostic Service.

Test	Units	Alpaca	Bovine	Camelid (Llama)	Caprine	Equine	Ovine	Porcine
Albumin	g/dL	2.7-4.4	3.1-4.3	1.9-4.9	2.3-3.4	2.4-3.7	2.8-3.7	3.2-4.2
Alkaline phosphatase (ALP)	units/L	17-232	12-154	15-115	18-220	96-385	47-681	61-147
Alanine aminotransfer-ase (ALT)	units/L	5-21	10-33	5-18	11-28	5-13	11-26	30-53
Amylase	units/L	561-1211	11-21	**	10-73	1-5	5-40	744- 2330
Anion gap	—	11-22	10-25	**	12-20	10-24	14-21	13-30
Aspartate aminotrans-ferase (AST)	units/L	73-282	48-204	98-256	60-118	204-390	52-122	17-63
Beta-hydroxybutyrate	mg/dL	0.4-0.9	1.9-14.8	0.3-1.2	2.3-4.9	1.2-4.4	0.6-5.4	0.2-1.2
Bicarbonate	mmol/L	20-32	22-29	13-38	23-3 2	21-33	21-32	18-32
Bile acids, fasting	µmol/L	NA	NA	**	NA	NA	NA	NA
Bile acids, postprandial (or nonfasting)	µmol/L	11-82	1.9-14.8	**	5-69	1.2-4.4	3-86	1-31
Bilirubin – Direct	mg/dL	0-0	0-0.2	**	0-0.7	0-0.4	0-0	0-0.2
Bilirubin – Total	mg/dL	0-0.1	0-0.2	0.1-0.2	0-0.1	0.2-2.2	0-0.1	0-0.1
Blood urea nitrogen (BUN)	mg/dL	13-30	8-22	8-34	7-22	9-27	13-28	10-24
Calcium	mg/dL	8.5-10.1	7.9-10.5	7.8-10.7	8.2-10.3	10.2-13.4	9.4-11	10.1-11.8
Chloride	mmol/L	107-116	100-109	106-129	101-109	92-107	100-112	91-109
Cholesterol	mg/dL	15-63	112-331	16-57	52-120	59-125	31-85	41-89
Creatine kinase (CK)	units/L	31-232	50-271	**	98-267	131-548	47-273	136-1609
Creatinine	mg/dL	0.8-2	0.3-0.8	0.4-3.1	0.4-0.9	0.4-1.9	0.5-0.9	0.8-1.7
Fructosamine	µmol/L	222-386	186-243	**	187-273	227-347	182-278	217-299

Test	Units	Alpaca	Bovine	Camelid (Llama)	Caprine	Equine	Ovine	Porcine
Gamma glutamyl transferase (GGT)	units/L	12-29	4-41	9-41	31-58	6-32	26-75	34-82
Globulin	g/dL	1.4-5.5	2-4	0.8 -4.5	3.5-5.3	2.3-5.3	2.5-4.5	5.3-6.4
Glucose	mg/dL	93-137	44-75	61-173	40-76	54-118	45-85	44-91
Haptoglobin	mg/mL	0.3 -1.6	0.1-1.7	**	0-4.9	0.9-5	0.1-1.8	0-1.8
Insulin	µunits/mL	NA	NA	**	NA	0.5-10	NA	NA
Iron	µg/dL	53-206	97-261	—	13-215	98-213	90-310	109-222
Lactate	mmol/L	0.31-5.06	0.38 -1.83	**	0.67-4.43	0.60-7.97	8.18-15.14	1.43-5.52
Lactate dehydrogenase (LDH)	units/L	171-445	744 -1592	**	172-441	244-802	280-597	328-782
Lipase	units/L	2-130	1-10	**	11-42	10-32	10-38	2-12
Magnesium	mg/dL	1.8-2.5	1.8-2.9	**	2.1-3.2	1.5-2.4	1.9-2.7	1.9-3.1
Phosphorus	mg/dL	2.8-9	4.1-8.3	1.5-8.9	3.8-9.6	1.4-5.9	4.5-9.2	6-9.3
Potassium	mmol/L	4-5.8	3.7-5.6	3.7-5.8	4.4-6.5	3.2-5.5	4.1-5.9	4.5-7.6
Sorbitol dehydrogenase (SDH)	u/L	1.5-16	6.6-37.8	**	19.7-71.9	3.3-15.5	10.2-54.3	4.7-18.8
Thyroid-stimulating hormone (TSH)	ng/mL	NA	NA	NA	NA	NA	NA	NA
Sodium	mmol/L	145-153	135-145	145-166	139-147	130-140	139- 150	128-151
Total T_4 (tT_4)	µg/dL	5.5-12	1.5-5.3	5.5-12	4.1-8.9	0.5-3.1	4-9.6	2.4-7.1
Total protein (TP)	g/dL	4.8-8.7	5.6-7.8	3.3-8.8	6.3-8.2	5.2-8.2	5.7-7.7	5.8-8.1
Triglycerides	mg/dL	11-55	4-26	6-41	11-66	10-61	10-32	34-165
Uric acid	mg/dL	0-0.1	0.5-1.6	**	0-0.2	0.1- 0.6	0-0.2	0-02

**No normal range established in this laboratory

Hematology: Equine, Food, and Fiber Animal Species

Values were originally published by Marshfield Clinic Laboratories, Veterinary Diagnostic Service.

Test	Units	Alpaca	Bovine	Camelid (Llama)	Caprine	Equine	Ovine	Porcine
Red blood cell (RBC) count	x 10^6/µL	8.6-15.9	5-10	9.33-17.06	12.2-20	5.63-12.09	9.9-14.5	6.4-8
Hemoglobin	g/dL	8.6-16.5	8-15	10.6-17.3	7-12	9.8-17.1	10.2-14.3	12.9-15.9
Hematocrit	%	21.1-41.8	24-46	25.8-45.6	19.2-33	27-47.5	32.3-47.4	38.3 – 47.8
Mean corpuscular volume (MCV)	fL	21.6-29.9	40-60	23.3-31	13.2-19.7	33.5-55.8	28.6-36.7	55.1-65.1
Mean corpuscular hemoglobin (MCH)	pg/cell	8.6-11.7	11-17	9.2-12.1	5.1-6.7	12.2-19.3	8.9-11.2	18.2-22
Mean corpuscular hemoglobin concentration (MCHC)	g/dL	38.1-41.1	30-36	36.3-41.9	33.1-40	32.4-37.4	29.3-32.3	31.4-35.1
Red cell distribution width (RDW)	%	18.8-31.4	14-31	20.3-29.6	24.9-41.2	20.6-29	19.9-26.4	14.2-17.7
Platelet count	x 10^3/µL	269-912	230-690	185-1007	300-600	95-385	78-1309	157-618
White blood cell (WBC) count	x 10^3/µL	4.7-28.6	4-12	5.9-18.9	9.5-30.5	4.1-14.3	3.7-11.7	10.9-21.8
Segmented neutrophil absolute #	x 10^3/µL	1.3-12	0.6-4	2.6-13.1	4.2-17.5	1.7-10.4	0.8-3.6	3.2-13.1
Band neutrophil absolute #	x 10^3/µL	0-0.1	0-0.1	0-0.05	0-0.1	0-0.1	0-0.1	0-0.1
Lymphocyte absolute #	x 10^3/µL	0.6-11	2.5-7.5	0.73-6.90	1.6-9.6	0.6-6.7	0.8-7.4	3.3-11.5

Test	Units	Alpaca	Bovine	Camelid (Llama)	Caprine	Equine	Ovine	Porcine
Monocyte absolute #	x $10^3/\mu L$	0-4.7	0-0.8	0-0.61	0.1-1.5	0-0.9	0-0.4	0-1.9
Eosinophil absolute #	x $10^3/\mu L$	0.3-6.4	0-2.4	0-4.32	0-3.5	0-0.5	0-1.10	0-1.5
Basophil absolute #	x $10^3/\mu L$	0-3.6	0-0.2	0-0.27	0-0.6	0-0.2	0-0.4	0-0.2

Coagulation: Bovine, Canine, Equine, Feline

Values were originally published by Marshfield Clinic Laboratories, Veterinary Diagnostic Service.

Test	Units	Canine	Feline	Equine	Bovine
Antithrombin (AT)	%	75-108	87-143	10-1000	10-1000
Activated partial thromboplastin time (APTT)	seconds	9.1-15.6	9.9-23.4	33-55	21.3-35.8
Fibrinogen, quantitative	mg/dL	200-400	50-300	100-400	300-700
Fibrinogen, semi-quantitative	mg/dL	100-500	50-300	100-400	300-700
Prothrombin time (PT)	seconds	5.4-8.8	7.2-12.5	9.1-12.6	16.8-20.7

Urinalysis: Canine, Feline

Values were originally published by Marshfield Clinic Laboratories, Veterinary Diagnostic Service.

Test	Units	Canine	Feline
Specific gravity	–	1.001-1.070	1.001-1.080
pH	–	5.5-7.5	5.5-7.5
Volume	mL/kg/day	24-41	22-30
Osmolality	mOsmol/kg $H_2 0$	500-1200 50 minutes; 2400 maximum	50 minutes; 3000 maximum
Sediment: RBCs/hpf	cells/hpf	0-5	0-5
Sediment: WBCs/hpf	cells/hpf	0-5	0-5
Sediment: casts/hpf	cells/hpf	0	0
Glucose	mg/dL	0	0
Ketones	mg/dL	0	0
Bilirubin	mg/dL	0–trace	0
Calcium	mEq/L	2-10	**
Creatinine	mg/dL	100-300	110-280
Chloride	mEq/L	0-400	**
Magnesium	mg/kg/24 hours	1.7-3	3
Phosphorus	mEq/L	50-180	**
Potassium	mEq/L	20-120	**
Sodium	mEq/L	20-165	**
Urea nitrogen	mg/kg/24 hours	140-2302	374-1872

**No normal range established in this laboratory

Cerebral Spinal Fluid: Canine, Feline

Values were originally published by Marshfield Clinic Laboratories, Veterinary Diagnostic Service.

Test	Units	Canine	Feline
Pressure	mm H_20	Less than 170	Less than 100
Specific gravity	–	1.005-1.007	1.005-1.007
Lymphocytes/µL	–	Less than 5	Less than 5
Pandy test	–	Negative–trace	Negative
Protein	mg/dL	Less than 25	Less than 25
Creatine kinase (CK)	units/L	9-28	**
Potassium	mEq/L	3.5-6	**
Chloride	mEq/L	96-106	**
Triglycerides	mg/dL	30-180	**
Gamma glutamyl transferase (GGT)	units/L	0-10	**

**No normal range established in this laboratory

Estrus and Gestation Periods: Dogs and Cats

	Dog	Cat
Appearance of first estrus at the age of:	7-9 months	4-12 months
Estrous cycle in animals not served:	Mean = 7 months Range = every 5-8 months	Every 4-30 days (14-19 day model) if constant photoperiod
Duration of estrus period:	7-42 days (proestrus plus estrus)	2-19 days
First occurrences after parturition:	Pregnancy does not alter interval	7-9 days
Gestation period	Mean = 63 days; Range 58-71 days	Mean = 63 days; Range 58-70 days
Number of young	8-12 large breeds 6-10 medium breeds 2-4 small breeds	4-6
Suckling period	3-6 weeks	3-6 weeks

Systemic Drugs Sorted by Therapeutic Class or Major Indication

This appendix lists systemic drugs or combination drug products by their therapeutic class or major indication. Classifications are based on the American Society of Health-System Pharmacists (ASHP) drug classification system. As some drugs have multiple indications, there may not be a specific dosage listed for a specific indication for every species. As such, the following species codes are used in parentheses after the drug name to indicate for which species a dosage is presented:

A = Avian
B = Bovine, Cattle
C = Cat, Feline
D = Dog, Canine
Fer = Ferret
Fi = Fish
H = Horse, Equine
Hb = Honey Bees
L = Llama, Alpacas, New World Camelids, Camels
Po = Pocket Pets, Rabbits, Small Mammals
R = Reptiles/Amphibians
Ru = Ruminants
Sh = Sheep/Goats; Ovine/Caprine; Small Ruminants
Sw = Swine, Pigs
Z = Wildlife/Zoo Animals

Antihistamines

Cetirizine (D, C, H)
Chlorpheniramine (D, C, H, A, Fer)
Clemastine (D, C)
Cyproheptadine (D, C, H)
Diphenhydramine (D, C, H, B, A, Fer, Po)
Doxepin (D, C, H, A)
Fexofenadine (D, C)
Hydroxyzine (D, C, H, A, Fer, Po)
Loratadine (D, C)
Meclizine (D, C, Po)
Promethazine (D, C, H)
Pyrilamine (H)
Trimeprazine/Prednisolone (D, C)
Tripelennamine (H, B)

Central Nervous System Drugs

(including anti-inflammatories, analgesics, muscle relaxants)

CNS/Respiratory Stimulants

Caffeine (D, H)
Doxapram (D, C, H, B, Sw, A, Fer, Po, R)

Analgesics, Nonsteroidal Anti-Inflammatory Drugs (NSAIDs)

Aspirin (D, C, H, B, Fer, Po)
Carprofen (D, C, H, B, Sh, A, Fer, Po, R)
Deracoxib (D)
Diclofenac, Topical (H)
Dimethyl Sulfoxide (DMSO) (D, H)
Dipyrone (D, C, H)
Etodolac (D, H)
Firocoxib (D, H)
Flunixin (B, H, Sh, Sw, Fer, Po)
Grapiprant (D)
Ketoprofen (D, C, H, B, Sh, Sw, A, Fer, Po)
Ketorolac (D, Po)
Mavacoxib (D)
Meloxicam (D, C, H, B, Sh, L, Sw, A, Fer, Po, R)
Phenylbutazone (D, H, Ru)
Piroxicam (D, C, H, Po)
Robenacoxib (D, C)
Tolfenamic Acid (D, C, B, Sw)

Analgesics, Opioid Agonists

Alfentanil (D, C)
Codeine (D, C, Po)
Fentanyl Injection (D, C, H, Sh, Fer, Po)
Fentanyl Transdermal Patch (D, C, H, Sh, L, Sw, A, Po)
Hydrocodone Combinations (D)
Hydromorphone (D, C, H, Fer, Po, R)
Meperidine (D, C, H, B, Fer, Po)
Methadone (D, C, H, Sh)
Morphine (D, C, H, Sh, L, Po)
Oxymorphone (D, C, H, Sh, A, Fer, Po)
Remifentanil (D, C, H)
Sufentanil (D, C)
Tramadol (D, C, H, B, A, Po, R)

Analgesics, Opioid Agonist/Antagonists

Buprenorphine (D, C, H, Sh, Sw, Fer, Po)
Butorphanol (D, C, H, B, Sh, L, A, Fer, Po)
Nalbuphine (D, C, B, Po)

Analgesics, Other

Acetaminophen (D, H, Po)
Amantadine (D, C)
Clonidine (D, C, B)
Frunevetmab (C)
Gabapentin (D, C, A)
Ketamine (D, C, H, B, Ru, L, Sw, A, Fer, Po, R)
Lidocaine (Intravenous; Systemic) (D, C, H, Sh, Po)
Medetomidine/Vatinoxan (D)
Pregabalin (D, C, H)

Antipyretics

Acetaminophen (D, H)
Aspirin (D, C)
Dipyrone (H)
Flunixin (B, Sw)
Ketoprofen (B, Sh, Sw)

Behavior-Modifying Agents

Alprazolam (D, C, H)
Amitriptyline (D, C, A)
Buspirone (D, C)
Clomipramine (D, C, A)
Clonazepam (D, C)
Clorazepate (D, C)
Diazepam (D, H, Sh, A)
Doxepin (D, C, H, A)
Fluoxetine (D, C, H)
Fluvoxamine (D, C)
Gabapentin (D, C)
Imepitoin (D, C)
Imipramine (D)
L-Theanine (D, C)
Lorazepam (D, C)
Methylphenidate (D)
Oxazepam (D, C)
Paroxetine (D, C, A)
Pheromones (D, C, H)
Pregabalin (C)
Sertraline (D, C)
Trazodone (D, C, H)

Cannabinoids

Cannabidiol (CBD) (D)

Tranquilizers/Sedatives

Acepromazine (D, C, H, B, Sh, Sw, Fer, Po)
Alfaxalone (D, C, B, Po)
Alprazolam (D, C, H)
Chlorpromazine (D, C, B, Sh, Sw)
Detomidine (D, C, H, B, Sh, L, A)
Dexmedetomidine (D, C, H, Po)
Diazepam (D, C, H, Sh, L, A, Fer, Po)
Ketamine (D, C, H, B, Ru, L, Sw, A, Fer, Po, R)
Lorazepam (D, C)
Medetomidine (D, C, H, B, Sh, L, A, Fer, Po, R)
Medetomidine/Vatinoxan (D)
Midazolam (D, C, H, Ru, A, Po)
Pentobarbital (H)
Reserpine (H)
Romifidine (D, C, H, B)
Tiletamine/Zolazepam (D, C, H, Ru, L, Sw, Fer, Po, R)
Xylazine (D, C, H, B, Sh, L, Sw, A, Fer, Po, Z)

Anesthetic Agents, Barbiturates

Pentobarbital (D, C, H, Po)
Thiopental (D, C, H, B, Sh, Sw, Po)

Anesthetic Agents, Inhalants

Desflurane (D, C, H, L, Po)
Isoflurane (D, C, H, Sh, A, Fer, Po, R)
Sevoflurane (D, C, H, Sh, L, A, Po, R)

Anesthetic Agents, Local

Bupivacaine (D, C, H, B, Sh, Po, R)
Bupivacaine Liposomal (D, C)
Lidocaine, Local Anesthetic (D, C, H, B, Sh, L, Po, R)

Mepivacaine (D, C, H, B, Sh, Sw)
Ropivacaine (D, C, H, B, Sh, Sw)

Anesthetic Agents, Miscellaneous
Alfaxalone (D, C, H, B, Sh, Fer, Po)
Alfentanil (D, C)
Etomidate (D, C, Fer, Po)
Fentanyl Injection (D, C, H, Sh, Fer, Po)
Ketamine (D, C, H, B, Ru, L, Sw, A, Fer, Po, R)
Propofol (D, C, H, Sh, L, Po, R)
Remifentanil (D, C, H)
Sufentanil (D, C)
Tiletamine/Zolazepam (D, C, H, Ru, L, Sw, Fer, Po, R)

Reversal Agents
Atipamezole (D, C, H, B, Sh, L, A, Po, R)
Flumazenil (D, C, H, A, R)
Naloxone (D, C, H, Po, R)
Naltrexone (D, C)
Neostigmine (D, C, H)
Tolazoline (D, C, H, Ru, L, Sw, A, Z)
Yohimbine (D, C, H, B, L, Sw, A, Po)

Anticonvulsants
Bromides (D)
Clonazepam (D, C)
Clorazepate (D, C)
Diazepam (D, H)
Felbamate (D)
Gabapentin (D, C, A)
Imepitoin (D, C)
Levetiracetam (D, C, H)
Lorazepam (D, C)
Phenobarbital (D, C, H, Fer)
Pregabalin (D, C, H)
Topiramate (D, C)
Zonisamide (D, C)

Neuromuscular Blockers
Atracurium (D, C, H, Sh, L, Po)
Rocuronium (D, C, H)
Succinylcholine (D, C, H, Ru, R)
Vecuronium (D, C)

Muscle Relaxants, Skeletal
Dantrolene (D, H)
Diazepam (D)
Guaifenesin, Intravenous (H, Sh, L)
Methocarbamol (D, C, H)

Euthanasia Agents
Euthanasia Agents with Pentobarbital (D, C, Large Animals)
Potassium (-Acetate, -Chloride, -Gluconate) (H, Ru)

Cardiovascular Agents
Inotropic Agents
Digoxin (D, C, Fer)
Dobutamine (D, C, H, A)
Pimobendan (D, C)

Antiarrhythmic Drugs
Amiodarone (D, H)
Digoxin (D, C, H, B)
Diltiazem (D, C, H, Fer, Po)
Lidocaine (Intravenous; Systemic) (D, C, H, Po)
Mexiletine (D, C)
Procainamide (D, C, H)
Quinidine (D, H) Verapamil (D, C, H, Po)
See also, Beta-Blockers

Anticholinergics (Parasympatholytics)
Atropine (D, C, H, B, Sh, L, Sw, A, Fer, Po, R)
Butylscopolamine (H)
Glycopyrrolate (D, C, H, Ru, Fer, Po, R)
Hyoscyamine (D)

Angiotensin Converting Enzyme Inhibitors (ACEIs)
Benazepril (D, C, H)
Enalapril (D, C, A, Fer)
Imidapril (D)
Lisinopril (D, C)
Ramipril (D, C)

Calcium Channel Blocking Agents
Amlodipine (D, C, A)
Diltiazem (D, C, H, Fer, Po)
Verapamil (D, C, H, Po)

Vasodilating Agents
Hydralazine (D, C, H)
Isoxsuprine (H, A)
Nitroglycerin, Transdermal (D, C, Fer)
Nitroprusside (D, C)
Pimobendan (D, C)
Sildenafil (D, C)
Tadalafil (D)

Agents Used to Treat Hypotension and Shock
Dobutamine (D, C, H, A)
Dopamine (D, C)
Ephedrine (D, C, H)
Epinephrine (D, C, H, Ru, Sw, A, Po, R)
Isoproterenol (D, C)
Norepinephrine (D, C, H, Sh, L)
Phenylephrine (D, C, H, Sh)
Vasopressin (D, C, H)

Alpha-Adrenergic Blocking Agents
Phenoxybenzamine (D, C, H)
Prazosin (D, C)

Beta-Adrenergic Blocking Agents
Atenolol (D, C, Fer)
Carvedilol (D)
Esmolol (D, C)
Metoprolol (D, C)
Propranolol (D, C, H, Fer)
Sotalol (D, C, H)

Angiotensin Receptor Blockers (ARBs)
Irbesartan (D, C)
Losartan (D)
Telmisartan (D, C)

Antihypertensive Agents, Miscellaneous
Fenoldopam (D, C, H)
Nitroprusside (D, C)

Other Cardiovascular Agents
Carnitine (D, C)
Taurine (D, C)

Respiratory Drugs
Sympathomimetics
Albuterol (D, C, H, B)
Clenbuterol (H, B)
Ephedrine (D, C, H)
Epinephrine (D, C, H, Ru, Sw)
Isoproterenol (D, C)
Pseudoephedrine (C)
Terbutaline (C, A, R)

Xanthines
Aminophylline (D, C, H, B)
Caffeine (D, H)
Theophylline (D, C)

Antitussives
Butorphanol (D)
Codeine (D)
Diphenoxylate/Atropine (D)
Hydrocodone Combinations (D)

Mucolytics
Acetylcysteine (D, C, H)

Other Respiratory Agents
Ciclesonide (H)
Cromolyn (H)
Fluticasone (D, C, H)
Ipratropium (H, Po)
Montelukast (C)

Renal and Urinary Tract Agents
Diuretics, Carbonic Anhydrase Inhibitors
Acetazolamide (D, C, H)
Dichlorphenamide (D, C)
Methazolamide (D, C)

Diuretics, Thiazides
Chlorothiazide (D, C)
Hydrochlorothiazide (D, C, H, A)

Diuretics, Loop
Furosemide (D, C, H, B, A, Fer, Po, R, Fi)
Torsemide (D, C)

Diuretics, Potassium Sparing
Spironolactone (D, C)
Triamterene (D)

Diuretics, Osmotic
Glycerin, Oral (D, C)
Mannitol (D, C, H, B, Sh, Sw, Fer, Po)

Agents for Urinary Incontinence or Retention
Bethanechol (D, C, H)
Dantrolene (D, C, Po)
Diazepam (D)
Diethylstilbestrol (DES) (D)
Ephedrine (D)
Estriol (D)
Imipramine (D, C)
Oxybutynin (D, C)
Phenoxybenzamine (D, C, H)
Phenylpropanolamine (D, C)
Prazosin (D, C)
Pseudoephedrine (D)
Tamsulosin (D, C)

Urinary Alkalinizers
Citrate, Potassium (D, C)
Sodium Bicarbonate (D, C, H, Ru, A)

Urinary Acidifiers
Ammonium Chloride (D, C, H, Sh)
Methionine (D, C, Sh)

Agents for Urolithiasis
Allopurinol (D, A, R)
Ammonium Chloride (D, C, H, Sh)
Citrate, Potassium (D, C)
Methionine (D, C, Sh)
Tiopronin (D)

Renal/Urinary Agents, Miscellaneous
Amitriptyline (D, C, A)
Colchicine (D, A)
Probenecid (R)

Gastrointestinal (GI) Agents

Antiemetic Agents
Acepromazine (D, C)
Chlorpromazine (D, C)
Dimenhydrinate (D, C)
Diphenhydramine (D, C)
Dolasetron (D, C)
Granisetron (D, C)
Maropitant (D, C)
Meclizine (D, C, Po)
Metoclopramide (D, C)
Mirtazapine (D, C)
Ondansetron (D, C)
Prochlorperazine (D, C)
Promethazine (D, C)

Antacids, Oral
Aluminum Hydroxide (D, C, H, B, Po, R)
Calcium Acetate (D, C)
Calcium, Oral (-Carbonate, -Gluconate, -Lactate) (D, C)
Magnesium Hydroxide (D, C, B, Sh)
Sodium Bicarbonate (D, C, H, Ru, A)

Histamine-2 Antagonists
Cimetidine (D, C, H, Fer, Po)
Famotidine (D, C, H, B, Fer, Po)
Nizatidine (D, C)
Ranitidine (D, C, H, Fer, Po)

Gastromucosal Protectants
Sucralfate (D, C, H, A, Fer, R)

Prostaglandin E Analogues
Misoprostol (D, C, H, B, Sh)

Proton Pump Inhibitors
Esomeprazole (D, C, H)
Omeprazole (D, C, H, Sw, Fer)
Pantoprazole (D, C, H, L)

Appetite Stimulants
Capromorelin (D, C)
Cyproheptadine (D, C)
Mirtazapine (D, C)
Oxazepam (C)

GI Antispasmodics-Anticholinergics
Hyoscyamine (D)
Butylscopolamine (H)
Propantheline (D, C, H)

GI Stimulants/Prokinetic
Cisapride (D, C, H, Po)
Erythromycin (D, C, H, B)
Lidocaine (Intravenous; Systemic) (H)
Metoclopramide (D, C, H, Po)
Neostigmine (H, B, Sh, Sw)
Nizatidine (D, C)
Ranitidine (D, C, Po)

Digestive Enzymes
Pancrelipase (D, C, A, Po)

Laxatives
Bisacodyl (D, C)
Docusate (D, C, H, Sh)
Lactulose (D, C, A, R)
Magnesium Hydroxide (D, C, B, Sh)
Mineral Oil (D, C, H, B, Sh, Sw, A, Po)
Polyethylene Glycol 3350 (PEG 3350) (D, C)
Psyllium (D, C, H)
Saline Cathartics (D, C, H, Ru)
Sorbitol (D, C, H)

Antidiarrheals
Bismuth Subsalicylate (D, C, H, B, Sw, Fer)
Cholestyramine (D, Po)
Clonidine (D, C)
Crofelemer (D)
Diphenoxylate/Atropine (D, C)
Kaolin/Pectin (D, C, H, B, Sh, Sw, A, Fer, Po)
Loperamide (D, C, Po)

Emetics
Apomorphine (D, Fer)
Hydrogen Peroxide 3% (D, Sw, Fer)
Hydromorphone (D, C)
Ropinirole (D)
Xylazine (C)
Tranexamic Acid (D)

GI Drugs, Miscellaneous
Bismuth Subsalicylate (D, C, H, B, Sw, Fer)
Budesonide (D, C)
Colchicine (D, A)
Olsalazine (D)
Phenobarbital (D)
S-Adenosyl Methionine ± Silybin (D, C)
Sulfasalazine (D, C, H, Fer)
Ursodiol (D, C, H, A)

Hormones/Endocrine/ Reproductive Agents

Sex Hormones, Estrogens
Diethylstilbestrol (DES) (D)
Estradiol (H)
Estriol (D)

Sex Hormones, Progestins
Altrenogest (D, H, Sw)
Medroxyprogesterone (D, C, H)
Megestrol (D, C)

Sex Hormones, Androgens
Testosterone (D, B)

Anabolic Steroids
Stanozolol (D, C, H, A, Fer, Po, R)

Posterior Pituitary Hormones
Desmopressin (D, C, H, A)
Vasopressin (D, C, H)

Oxytocics
Oxytocin (D, C, H, B, Sh, L, Sw, A, Po, R)

Adrenal Cortical Steroids
Corticotropin (ACTH) (D, H, A)
Cortisone (D)
Cosyntropin (D, C, H)

Mineralocorticoids
Desoxycorticosterone Pivalate (DOCP) (D, C)
Fludrocortisone (D, C, Fer)

Glucocorticoids
Betamethasone (D, H)
Budesonide (D, C, H)
Ciclesonide (H)
Dexamethasone (D, C, H, B, Sw, Po)
Flumethasone (D, C, H)
Fluticasone (D, C, H)
Hydrocortisone (D, C)
Isoflupredone (H, B, Sw)
Methylprednisolone (D, C, H)

Prednisolone/Prednisone (D, C, H, B, L, A, Po, R)
Triamcinolone (D, C, H)

Adrenal Steroid Inhibitors

Metyrapone (C)
Mitotane (D, Fer)
Selegiline (D)
Trilostane (D, C, H, Po)

Antidiabetic Agents

Acarbose (D, C)
Exenatide (C)
Glipizide (C)
Glyburide (C)
Insulin, Aspart (D, C, B)
Insulin, Detemir (D, C)
Insulin, Glargine (D, C, H, Fer, Po)
Insulin, Lente (D, C)
Insulin, Lispro (D, C)
Insulin, NPH (D, H, L, A, Fer, Po)
Insulin, Protamine Zinc (PZI) (D, C, H, B, L)
Insulin, Regular (Crystalline Zinc) (D, C, H, L, A)
Metformin (C, H)

Glucose Elevating Agents

Diazoxide (D, Fer, Po)
Glucagon (D, C, B, Fer)
Octreotide (D, H, Fer)

Thyroid Hormones

Levothyroxine (D, C, H, A, R)
Liothyronine (D, C)
Thyrotropin (TSH) (D, C, A, Fer, Po)

Antithyroid Drugs

Carbimazole (C)
Methimazole (C, Po)

Prostaglandins

Cloprostenol (D, C, H, B, Sh, L, Sw)
Dinoprost (D, C, H, B, Sh, Sw)

Endocrine/Reproductive Drugs, Miscellaneous

Aglepristone (D, C, Sh, Po)
Bromocriptine (D, C, H)
Cabergoline (D, C, A)
Calcitriol (D, C)
Chorionic Gonadotropin (HCG) (D, C, H, B, Sh, Sw, A, Fi)
Clenbuterol (H, B)
Cyproheptadine (H)
Deslorelin (D, H, Fer)
Finasteride (D, Fer)
Gonadorelin (D, C, B)
Imipramine (H)
Leuprolide (A, Fer, Po)
Melatonin (D, C, H, Sh, Fer, Z)
Metergoline (D, C)
Misoprostol (D, C, H, B, Sh)
Osaterone (D)
Pergolide (H)
Somatotropin (D, B)
Terbutaline (D, C)
Thyrotropin (TSH) (D, C, H, A, Fe, Po)
Thyrotropin-Releasing Hormone (TRH) (D, C, H)

Anti-infective Drugs

Antiparasitics, Ectoparasiticides

Afoxolaner (D, C, Sw, A)
Doramectin (D, C, H, B, L, Sw, Po)
Eprinomectin (C, H, B, Sh, L)
Fluralaner (D, C, Po)
Imidacloprid, Systemic (D)
Ivermectin (D, C, H, B, Sh, L, Sw, A, Fer, Po, R, Z)
Ivermectin/Clorsulon (B)
Lotilaner (D, C)
Lufenuron (D, C, Po)
Milbemycin Oxime (D, C)
Moxidectin (D, C, H, B, Sh, L, Fer)
Nitenpyram (D, C, R)
Sarolaner (D, C)
Selamectin (D, C, Fer, Po)
Selamectin/Sarolaner (C)
Spinosad (D, C)

Antiparasitics, Endoparasiticides

Albendazole (B, Sh, L, Po)
Allopurinol (D, C, A, R)
Amprolium (D, C, B, Sh, L, Sw, A, Fer, Po)
Atovaquone (D, C)
Decoquinate (D, B, Sh, L, A)
Diclazuril (D, C, H, B, Sh, A, Po)
Diminazene (D, H, B, Sh, Po)
Doramectin (D, C, H, B, L, Sw, Po)
Emodepside/Praziquantel (D, C, R)
Eprinomectin (C, H, B, Sh, L)
Eprinomectin/Praziquantel (C)
Epsiprantel (D, C)
Febantel (D, C)
Fenbendazole (D, C, H, B, Sh, L, Sw, A, Fer, Po, R, Z)
Furazolidone (C)
Imidocarb (D, C, H, B)
Ivermectin (D, C, H, B, Sh, L, Sw, A, Fer, Po, R, Z)
Ivermectin/Clorsulon (B)
Levamisole (D, H, B, Sh, Sw, R)
Meglumine Antimoniate (D)
Melarsomine (D)
Metronidazole (D, C, A, Po, R)
Milbemycin Oxime (D, C)
Miltefosine (D, Fer)
Morantel (B, Sh)
Moxidectin (D, C, H, B, Sh, L, Fer)
Nitazoxanide (D, C, H)
Oxfendazole (H, B, Sh, Sw)
Oxibendazole (H, Po)
Paromomycin (D, C, Sh, L, R)
Piperazine (D, C, Sw, A, Po, R)
Ponazuril (D, C, H, Sh, L, A, Po, R)
Praziquantel/Praziquantel Combination Products (D, C, H, Sh, L, A, Po, R)
Primaquine (C)
Pyrantel (D, C, H, L, A, Po)
Pyrimethamine (D, C, H, A)
Pyrimethamine/Sulfadiazine (H)
Quinacrine (D, C, R)
Ronidazole (D, C)
Selamectin (D, C, Fer, Po)
Selamectin/Sarolaner (C)
Sodium Stibogluconate (D)
Sulfadiazine (H)
Sulfamethoxazole (D, C, Fer, A, Po, R)
Sulfadimethoxine (D, C, B, L, Fer, Po, R)
Tinidazole (D, C)
Toltrazuril (D, C, B, Sh, L, Sw, A, Po, R)

Antibiotics, Aminoglycosides, and Aminocyclitols

Amikacin (D, C, H, L, A, Fer, Po, R, Fi)
Apramycin (B, Sw, A, Po)
Gentamicin (D, C, H, Sw, A, Fer, Po, R)
Neomycin (D, C, B, Sh, Sw, A, Fer)
Spectinomycin (Sw, A, Po)
Tobramycin (D, C, H, L, A, R)

Antibiotics, Carbapenems

Ertapenem (D, C)
Imipenem/Cilastatin (D, C, H)
Meropenem (D, C, H)

Antibiotics, Cephalosporins

Cefaclor (D, C)
Cefadroxil (D, C, Fer)
Cefazolin (D, C, H, R)
Cefepime (D, C, H)
Cefixime (D, C)
Cefotaxime (D, C, H, A, R)
Cefotetan (D, C)
Cefovecin (D, C)
Cefoxitin (D, C, H)
Cefpodoxime (D, C, H)
Cefquinome (H, B)
Ceftazidime (D, C, H, R)
Ceftiofur Crystalline Free Acid (H, B, Sh, Sw, Po)
Ceftiofur HCl (B, Sw)
Ceftiofur Sodium (D, C, H, B, Sh, Sw, A, R)
Ceftriaxone (D, C, H)
Cefuroxime (D, C, Sh)
Cephalexin (D, C, A, Fer, Po, R)
Cephapirin (B)

Antibiotics, Macrolides

Azithromycin (D, C, H, B, A, Po)
Clarithromycin (D, C, H, Fer)
Erythromycin (D, C, H, B, A, Fer)
Gamithromycin (H, B, Sh, Sw)
Tildipirosin (B, Sw)
Tilmicosin (B, Sh, Sw, Po)
Tulathromycin (B, Sh, Sw, Z)
Tylosin (D, C, B, Sw, A, Fer, Po, Hb)

Antibiotics, Penicillins
Amoxicillin (D, C, B, A, Fer, Po, R)
Amoxicillin/Clavulanate (D, C, A, Fer)
Ampicillin (D, C, H, B, Fer, Po, R)
Ampicillin/Sulbactam (D, C)
Cloxacillin (B)
Dicloxacillin (D, C)
Oxacillin (D, C, H)
Penicillin G (D, C, H, B, Ru, Sw, A, Fer, Po)
Penicillin V (D, C)
Piperacillin/Tazobactam (D, C, A, R)

Antibiotics, Tetracyclines
Chlortetracycline (C, A, Po)
Doxycycline (D, C, H, A, Po, R)
Minocycline (D, C, H)
Oxytetracycline (D, C, H, B, Sh, Sw, A, R, Z)
Tetracycline (D, C, B, Sh, Sw, A, Fer, Po)

Antibiotics, Lincosamides
Clindamycin (D, C, A, Fer, R)
Lincomycin (D, C, Sw, A, Fer)
Pirlimycin (B)

Antibiotics, Quinolones
Ciprofloxacin (D, C, H, A, Fer, Po)
Danofloxacin (B, R)
Enrofloxacin (D, C, H, B, L, Sw, A, Fer, Po, R)
Marbofloxacin (D, C, A, Po, R)
Orbifloxacin (D, C, H, A, Po)
Pradofloxacin (D, C, A)

Antibiotics, Sulfonamides
Sulfa-/Trimethoprim (D, C, H, A, Fer, Po, R)
Sulfadiazine/Pyrimethamine (H)
Sulfadimethoxine (D, C, H, B, L, Fer, Po, R)
Sulfadimethoxine/Ormetoprim (D)

Antibiotics, Antibacterials, Miscellaneous
Chloramphenicol (D, C, H, A, Fer, Po, R)
Clofazimine (D, C, A)
Dapsone (D, H)
Ethambutol (D, C, A)
Florfenicol (B, Sh, L, Sw)
Fosfomycin (D)
Isoniazid (INH) (D, C, B, Ru)
Linezolid (D, C)
Methenamine (D, C)
Metronidazole (D, C, H, A, Fer, Po, R)
Nitrofurantoin (D, C, H)
Novobiocin (B)
Polymyxin B (C, H, Sh)
Rifampin (D, C, H)
Rifaximin (D)
Ronidazole (D, C)
Tiamulin (Sw, A)
Tinidazole (D, C)
Vancomycin (D, C, H)

Antifungal Agents
Amphotericin B (D, C, H, L, A, Po, R)
Caspofungin (D, C)
Fluconazole (D, C, H, A, Po, R)
Flucytosine (D, C)
Griseofulvin (D, H, Po)
Iodide (Potassium-, Sodium-) (D, C, H, B, Sh)
Itraconazole (D, C, H, A, Po, R)
Ketoconazole (D, C, H, A, Po, R)
Nystatin (D, C, H, A, R)
Posaconazole (D, C)
Terbinafine (D, C, A, Po, R)
Voriconazole (D, C, H, A, R)

Antiviral Agents
Acyclovir (D, H, A)
Amantadine (D, C)
Famciclovir (C)
Interferon Alfa, Human Recombinant (D, C)
Interferon Omega, Feline Origin (D, C)
Lysine (C)
Oseltamivir (D, H)
Valacyclovir (H)
Zidovudine (C)

Blood Modifying Agents

Anticoagulants/Antithrombotics
Aspirin (D, C, H, Po)
Clopidogrel (D, C, H)
Cobalamin (Po)
Dalteparin (D, C, H)
Enoxaparin (D, C, H)
Heparin (D, C, H)
Rivaroxaban (D, C)
Warfarin (D, H)

Erythropoietic Agents
Cobalamin | Vitamin B_{12} (D, C, H, B, Sw, Po)
Darbepoetin Alfa (D, C)
Epoetin Alfa (D, C, Fer, Po)
Ferrous Sulfate (D, C)
Folic Acid | Vitamin B_9 (D, C, H, Po)
Iron Dextran (D, C, Sw, A, Fer)
Leucovorin (D, C H)

Blood Modifying Agents, Miscellaneous
Aminocaproic Acid (D, H)
Fenofibrate (D)
Filgrastim (D, C, H, L)
Gemfibrozil (D, C)
Hemoglobin Glutamer-200 (Bovine) (D, C)
Pentoxifylline (D, C, H)
Tranexamic Acid (D, C)
Vitamin K_1 | Phytonadione (D, C, H, B, Sh, Sw, A, Po)

Fluid and Electrolyte Modifiers

Albumin, Human (D, C)
Aluminum Hydroxide (D, C, Po, R)
Calcitonin (D, R)
Calcitriol (D, C)
Calcium Acetate (D, C)
Calcium, Oral (-Carbonate, -Gluconate, -Lactate) (D, C)
Calcium, IV (-Borogluconate, -Chloride, -Gluconate) (D, C, H, B, Sh, Sw, A, R)
Dextran 70 (D, C, B)
Dextrose 50% Injection (D, C, H, B, Sh, Sw)
Ergocalciferol (D, C)
Hydroxyethyl Starch (HES) Colloids (D, C, H, L, A)
Hypertonic Saline (7% – 7.5%) (D, C, H, B, A)
Lanthanum (D, C)
Magnesium Hydroxide (D, C, B, Sh)
Magnesium, IV (D, C, H, B, Sh, Sw)
Phosphate, (Potassium-, Sodium-) IV (D, C)
Potassium (-Acetate, -Chloride, -Gluconate) (D, C, H, Ru)
Sevelamer (D, C)

Antineoplastics

Antineoplastics, Alkylating Agents
Carboplatin (D, C)
Chlorambucil (D, C, H, Fer)
Cisplatin (D, H)
Cyclophosphamide (D, C, H, Fer, Po)
Dacarbazine (DTIC) (D)
Ifosfamide (D, C)
Lomustine (D, C)
Mechlorethamine (D, C)
Melphalan (D, C)
Procarbazine (D, C)

Antineoplastics, Antimetabolites
Cytarabine (D, C, H)
Fluorouracil (D, H)
Methotrexate (D, C, H)
Rabacfosadine (D)

Antineoplastics, Antibiotics
Bleomycin (D, C)
Dactinomycin (D, C)
Doxorubicin (D, C, H, Fer)
Epirubicin (D, C)
Streptozocin (D)

Antineoplastics, Mitotic Inhibitors
Vinblastine (D, C)
Vincristine (D, C, H, Fer)
Vinorelbine (D, C)

Antineoplastics, Miscellaneous
Asparaginase (D, C)
Gemcitabine (D, C)
Hydroxyurea (D, C)

Interferon Alfa, Human Recombinant (D)
Mitoxantrone (D, C)
Mitotane (D)
Piroxicam (D, C, H)
Tigilanol Tiglate (D, H)
Toceranib (D, C)
Verdinexor (D)

Immunomodulators

Immunosuppressive Drugs

Azathioprine (D, H, Fer)
Cyclosporine (D, C)
Dexamethasone (D, C, H, B, Sw, Po)
Flumethasone (D, C, H)
Hydroxychloroquine (D)
Immune Globulin, Intravenous (IVIG) (D)
Leflunomide (D, C)
Methotrexate (D, C, H)
Methylprednisolone (D, C, H)
Mycophenolate (D, C)
Niacinamide (D)
Oclacitinib (D, C)
Prednisolone/Prednisone (D, C, H, B, L, A, Po, R)
Triamcinolone (D, C, H)

Gold Compounds

Auranofin (D, C)

Immunostimulants

Mycobacterial Cell Wall Fraction Immunomodulator (D, H, B)
Parapox Ovis Virus Immunomodulator (H)
Propionibacterium acnes Injection (D, C, H)
Staphylococcal Phage Lysate (D)

Antidotes/Antivenoms/Reversal Agents

Acetylcysteine (D, C)
Antivenom, Black Widow Spider (D, C)
Antivenom, Crotalidae (D, C, H)
Antivenom, North American Coral Snake (D, C, H)
Atipamezole (D, C, H, B, Sh, L, A, Po, R)
Atropine (D, C, H, B, Sh, L, Sw, A, Fer, Po, R)
Charcoal, Activated (D, C, H, Ru, Fer)
Cobalamin (D)
Deferoxamine (D, C, H)
Dexrazoxane (D)
Dimercaprol (BAL) (D, C, H, Ru)
Domperidone (D, H)
Edetate Calcium Disodium (CaEDTA) (D, C, H, Food Animals, L, A, Po)
Ethanol (D, C, H)
Flumazenil (D, C, H, A, R)
Glycopyrrolate (D, C, H)
Fomepizole (D, C)
Leucovorin (D, C, H)
Lipid Emulsion, Intravenous (ILE) (D, C, H, Sh, Po, R)
Methylene Blue (D, C, H, Ru)
Molybdates (D, Food Animals, Sh)
Naloxone (D, C, H, Po, R)
Penicillamine (D, C, Ru, A)
Phenobarbital (B)
Physostigmine (D, H, B)
Polymyxin B (C, H, Sh)
Pralidoxime (2-PAM) (D, C, H, Ru, L, A)
Pyridoxine (Vitamin B_6) (D, C)
S-Adenosyl Methionine (SAMe) ± Silybin (D, C)
Sodium Thiosulfate (D, C, H, Ru)
Succimer (D, C, H, A)
Trientine (D)
Vitamin K_1 | Phytonadione (D, C, H, B, Sh, Sw, A, Po)
Zinc, Systemic (D, C)

Bone/Joint Agents

Alendronate (D, C)
Allopurinol (A, R)
Clodronate (H)
Glucosamine/Chondroitin (D, C, H)
Hyaluronate (D, H)
Pamidronate (D, C, H)
Pentosan Polysulfate (D, C, H)
Polysulfated Glycosaminoglycan (D, C, H, Po)
Tiludronate (H)
Zoledronic Acid (D, C, H)

Dermatologic Agents (Systemic)

Amitriptyline (D, C, A)
Interferon Omega, Feline Origin (D, C)
Isotretinoin (D, C)
Lokivetmab (Canine Atopic Dermatitis Immunotherapeutic, CADI) (D)
Pentoxifylline (D, C, H)
Terbutaline (H)
Topiramate (C)

Vitamins and Minerals/Nutrients

Ascorbic Acid | Vitamin C (D, C, H, B, Po)
Calcitriol (D, C)
Calcium, IV (-Borogluconate, -Chloride, -Gluconate) (D, C, H, B, Sh, Sw, A, R)
Calcium, Oral (-Carbonate, -Gluconate, -Lactate) (D, C)
Carnitine (D, C)
Cobalamin (D, C, H, B, Sh, Sw, Po)
Ergocalciferol | Vitamin D_2 (D, C)
Fatty Acids, Omega-3 (D, C, H)
Ferrous Sulfate (D, C)
Folic Acid | Vitamin B_9 (D, C, H, Po)
Iron Dextran (D, C, Sw, A, Fer)
Leucovorin (D, C H)
Lipid Emulsion, Intravenous (ILE) (small, large animal species)
Lysine (C)
Magnesium, IV (D, C, H, B, Sh, Sw)
Medium Chain Triglycerides (MCT Oil) (D)
Melatonin (D, C, H, Sh, Fer, Z)
Methionine (D, C, Sh)
Niacinamide (D)
Phosphate, (Potassium-, Sodium-) IV (D, C)
Potassium (-Acetate, -Chloride, -Gluconate) (D, C, H, Ru)
Pyridoxine | Vitamin B_6 (D, C)
Taurine (D, C)
Thiamine | Vitamin B_1 (D, C, H, B, Sh, L, Sw)
Vitamin A (D, R)
Vitamin E ± Selenium (D, C, H)
Vitamin K_1 | Phytonadione (D, C, H, B, Sh, Sw, A, Po)
Zinc, Systemic (D, C)

Cholinergic Muscle Stimulants

Edrophonium (D, C, H)
Pyridostigmine (D, C, Fer)

Systemic Acidifiers

Acetazolamide (D, C, H)
Acetic Acid (H, B, Ru)

Systemic Alkalinizers

Citrate, Potassium (D, C)
Sodium Bicarbonate (D, C, H, Ru, A)

Unclassified

Iohexol (D, C, H, A, Po, R)

Index

Note: For clarity, ® or ™ have been removed.